RC952
CWT 100

HAZ
GERIATRIC ...NE
AND GERONTOLOGY

HAZZARD'S GERIATRIC MEDICINE AND GERONTOLOGY

Sixth Edition

EDITORS

JEFFREY B. HALTER, MD
Professor of Internal Medicine
Chief, Division of Geriatric Medicine
Director, Geriatrics Center and Institute of Gerontology
University of Michigan
Ann Arbor, Michigan

JOSEPH G. OUSLANDER, MD
Professor and Associate Dean for Geriatric Programs
Charles E. Schmidt College of Biomedical Science
Professor (Courtesy), Christine E. Lynn College of Nursing
Florida Atlantic University
Professor of Medicine (Voluntary)
Division of Gerontology and Geriatric Medicine
University of Miami Miller School of Medicine
Boca Raton, Florida

MARY E. TINETTI, MD
Gladys Phillips Crofoot Professor of Medicine, Epidemiology, and Public Health
Director, Program on Aging
Yale University School of Medicine
New Haven, Connecticut

STEPHANIE STUDENSKI, MD, MPH
Professor, Department of Medicine (Geriatrics)
University of Pittsburgh
Staff Physician, VA Pittsburgh GRECC
Pittsburgh, Pennsylvania

KEVIN P. HIGH, MD, MS
Professor of Medicine, Sections on Infectious Diseases,
Hematology/Oncology and Molecular Medicine
Chief, Section on Infectious Diseases
Wake Forest University Health Sciences
Winston-Salem, North Carolina

SANJAY ASTHANA, MD
Duncan G. and Lottie H. Ballantine Chair in Geriatrics
Professor and Head, Section of Geriatrics & Gerontology
University of Wisconsin School of Medicine and Public Health
Director, Geriatric Research, Education and Clinical Center (GRECC)
William S. Middleton Memorial Veterans Hospital
Associate Director, Wisconsin Alzheimer's Institute
Madison, Wisconsin

EDITOR EMERITUS AND SENIOR ADVISOR

WILLIAM R. HAZZARD, MD
Professor of Medicine
University of Washington
Director, Geriatrics and Extended Care
VA Puget Sound Health Care System
Seattle, Washington

SENIOR EDITORIAL ASSISTANT

NANCY F. WOOLARD
Wake Forest University Health Sciences
Winston-Salem, North Carolina

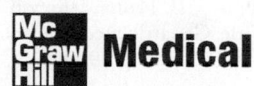

New York   Chicago   San Francisco   Lisbon   London   Madrid   Mexico City
Milan   New Delhi   San Juan   Seoul   Singapore   Sydney   Toronto

The McGraw·Hill Companies

6 7 8 9 10 QVS/QVS 17 16 15 14

ISBN 978-0-07-148872-3
MHID 0-07-148872-3

This book was set in Adobe Garamond by Aptara®, Inc.
The editors were Jim Shanahan and Karen G. Edmonson.
The production supervisor was Phil Galea.
Project management was provided by Samir Roy, Aptara, Inc.
The designer was Janice Bielawa; the cover designer was Maria Scharf.
This book is printed on acid-free paper.

Library of Congress Cataloging-in-Publication Data

Hazzard's geriatric medicine and gerontology. – 6th ed. / editors, Jeffrey B. Halter . . . [et al.].
    p. ; cm.
  Rev. ed. of: Principles of geriatric medicine and gerontology / editors, William R. Hazzard . . .
[et al.]. 5th ed. c2003.
  Includes bibliographical references and index.
  ISBN-13: 978-0-07-148872-3 (alk. paper)
  ISBN-10: 0-07-148872-3 (alk. paper)
  1. Geriatrics. 2. Gerontology.   I. Hazzard, William R., 1936-   II. Halter, Jeffrey B.
III. Principles of geriatric medicine and gerontology.   IV. Title: Geriatric medicine and gerontology.
  [DNLM: 1. Geriatrics. 2. Health Services for the Aged. WT 100 H431g 2009]
  RC952.P752 2009
  618.97–dc22

                                                     2008049545

Contents

Part I
PRINCIPLES OF GERONTOLOGY

Part II
PRINCIPLES OF GERIATRICS

SECTION A   Assessment

SECTION B   Organization of Care

Color Plate appears between pages 772 and 773.

Contributors

INTERNATIONAL ADVISORY BOARD

Spain   Dr. Francisco Javier Ortiz Alonso
Associate Professor in Health Sciences
Departamento de Medicina
Universidad Complutense de Madrid
Chief Geriatric Section
Hospital General Universitario Gregorio
    Maranon
Madrid, Spain

Switzerland   Dr. Jean-Pierre Michel
Professor of Medicine
Chair of Rehabilitation and Geriatrics
University of Geneva Medical School
Geneva University Hospitals - Geriatric
    Department
Geneva, Switzerland

Sweden   Professor Bengt Winblad, MD, PhD
Professor of Geriatric Medicine and Chief
    Physician
Karolinska Institute
Neurotec
Karolinska University Hospital
Stockholm, Sweden

United Kingdom   Professor Gary Ford
Professor of Pharmacology of Old Age
Director Clinical Research Centre
University of Newcastle upon Tyne
Newcastle upon Tyne, United Kingdom

CHAPTER AUTHORS

Numbers in brackets refer to the chapters written or co-written by the contributor

Azhar Afaq, MD
Fellow, Department of Endocrinology
University of Oklahoma Health Sciences Center
Oklahoma City, Oklahoma [80]

Steven M. Albert, PhD, MSPH
Professor of Behavioral & Community Health Sciences
Graduate School of Public Health
University of Pittsburgh
Pittsburgh, Pennsylvania [7]

Neil B. Alexander, MD
Professor of Internal Medicine
Division of Geriatric Medicine
Director, Mobility Research Center
Research Professor, Institute of Gerontology
University of Michigan
Director, VA Ann Arbor Health Care System GRECC
Ann Arbor, Michigan [113]

Sonia Ancoli-Israel, PhD
Professor of Psychiatry
University of California, San Diego
Director, Sleep Disorders Clinic
VA San Diego Health System
San Diego, California [55]

Danielle L. Anderson, MD
Postdoctoral Fellow, Section of Geriatric Psychiatry and
Neuropsychiatry
Johns Hopkins University
Baltimore, Maryland [71]

Julia A.M. Anderson, MBChB, BSc, MD, FRCP(Edin),
    FRCPath
Associate Professor, Consultant Hematologist
Department of Clinical and Laboratory Hematology
Royal Infirmary of Edinburgh
Edinburgh, United Kingdom [106]

Derek C. Angus, MD, MPH
Professor and Chair, Department of Critical Care Medicine
University of Pittsburgh School of Medicine
Pittsburgh, Pennsylvania

James A. Ashton-Miller, PhD
Albert Schultz Collegiate Research Professor of
    Mechanical Engineering
College of Engineering,
    Research Professor, Institute of Gerontology
University of Michigan
Ann Arbor, Michigan [113]

Sanjay Asthana, MD, FRCP(C)
Duncan G. and Lottie H. Ballantine Chair in Geriatrics
Professor and Head, Section of Geriatrics & Gerontology
University of Wisconsin School of Medicine and Public Health
Director, GRECC
William S. Middleton Memorial Veterans Hospital
Associate Director, Wisconsin Alzheimer's Institute
Madison, Wisconsin [65]

James L. Bailey, MD
Professor of Medicine, Renal Division
Emory University School of Medicine
Atlanta, Georgia [86]

Rajbir Bakshi, MD
Assistant Professor of Psychiatry
University of Texas Southwestern Medical Center
Dallas, Texas [72]

Courtney Barancin, MD
Instructor in Medicine
Division of Gastroenterology and Hepatology
University of Wisconsin
Madison, Wisconsin [90]

Steven Barczi, MD
Associate Professor of Medicine
Director, Geriatric Medicine Fellowship
University of Wisconsin Medical School
Associate Director—Clinical
William S. Middleton Memorial Veterans Hospital GRECC
Madison, Wisconsin [41]

Barbara Bates-Jensen, RN, PhD
Associate Adjunct Professor of Medicine
Division of Geriatrics
Anna & Harry Borun Center for Gerontological Research
David Geffen School of Medicine at UCLA
Reseda, California [58]

Susan M. Bell, MBBS, BSc
Clinical Fellow, Division of Cardiovascular Medicine
Vanderbilt University Medical Center
Nashville, Tennessee [75]

Mark Benson, MD
Fellow, Division of Gastroenterology and Heptology
Department of Medicine
University of Wisconsin
Madison, Wisconsin [90]

Roberto Bernabei, MD
Professor of Internal Medicine
Universita Cattolica del Sacro Cuore
Dipartimento di Scienze Gerontologiche-Geriatriche e Fisiatriche
Roma, Italy [6]

Cheryl D. Bernstein, MD
Assistant Professor of Anesthesiology
UPMC Pain Medicine
University of Pittsburgh
Pittsburgh, Pennsylvania [123]

Richard W. Besdine, MD, FACP, AGSF
Professor of Medicine
Division of Geriatric Medicine
Center for Gerontology and Health Care Research
Brown Medical School
Providence, Rhode Island [56]

John D. Birkmeyer, MD
George D. Zuidema Professor of Surgery
Chair, Surgical Outcomes Research
University of Michigan
Ann Arbor, Michigan [37]

Marc R. Blackman, MD
Veteran's Affairs Medical Center
Washington, DC [25]

Caroline Blaum, MD
Associate Professor of Internal Medicine
Division of Geriatric Medicine
University of Michigan
Research Scientist, VA Ann Arbor Healthcare System GRECC
Ann Arbor, Michigan [17]

Daniel G. Blazer, MD, PhD
Professor of Psychiatry
Duke University Medical Center
Durham, North Carolina [70]

Jacob B. Blumenthal, MD
Assistant Professor of Medicine
Division of Gerontology and Geriatric Medicine
University of Maryland School of Medicine
Veteran Affairs Maryland Health Care System
Baltimore, Maryland [110]

Maureen Bolon, MD, MS
Assistant Professor of Medicine
Division of Infectious Diseases
Northwestern University Feinberg School of Medicine
Chicago, Illinois [125]

Chad E. Boult, MD, MPH, MBA
Professor of Health Policy and Management
Director, Lipitz Center for Integrated Health Care
Johns Hopkins School of Public Health
Baltimore, Maryland [15]

Jennifer S. Brach, PhD, PT, GCS
Assistant Professor of Physical Therapy
University of Pittsburgh
Pittsburgh, Pennsylvania [115]

Lawrence R. Brawley, PhD
Canada Research Chair in Physical Activity in Health
 Promotion and Disease Prevention
University of Saskatchewan
Saskatoon, Saskatchewan, Canada [28]

Cynthia J. Brown, MD, MSPH
Assistant Professor of Medicine
Division of Gerontology and Geriatric Medicine
University of Alabama-Birmingham
Birmingham, Alabama [29]

Kenneth Brummel-Smith, MD
Charlotte Edwards Maguire Professor and Chair
Department of Geriatrics
Florida State University
College of Medicine
Tallahassee, Florida [23]

Ferdinand Buonanno, MD
Assistant Professor of Neurology
Harvard Medical School
Massachusetts General Hospital
Stroke Service
Boston, Massachusetts [64]

Cynthia M. Carlsson, MD, MS
Assistant Professor of Medicine
Section on Geriatrics and Gerontology
University of Wisconsin School of Medicine and Public Health
William S. Middleton Memorial Veterans Hospital GRECC
Madison, Wisconsin [65]

Bruce A. Carnes, PhD
Professor, Donald W. Reynolds Department of Geriatric Medicine
University of Oklahoma Health Sciences Center
Oklahoma City, Oklahoma [119]

Iain G. Carpenter, MD
Professor, Centre for Health Services Studies
University of Kent
Canterbury, Kent, United Kingdom [6]

Annette M. Chang, MD
Assistant Professor of Internal Medicine
Division of Metabolism, Endocrinology & Diabetes
University of Michigan Health System
VA Ann Arbor Healthcare System
Ann Arbor, Michigan [109]

Julie E. Chang, MD
Assistant Professor of Medicine
Section on Hematology/Oncology
University of Wisconsin School of Medicine and Public Health
Madison, Wisconsin [99]

Susan L. Charette, MD
Geriatric Medicine
University of California, Los Angeles Health System
Los Angeles, California [30]

Gurkamal S. Chatta, MD
Associate Professor of Medicine
Division of Hematology-Oncology
UPMC Cancer Institute
University of Pittsburgh Medical Center
Chief, Hematology-Oncology
VA Pittsburgh Health Care System
Pittsburgh, Pennsylvania [101]

Paulo H.M. Chaves, MD, PhD
Assistant Professor of Medicine
Division of General Internal Medicine
Core Faculty, Center on Aging and Health
Johns Hopkins University
Baltimore, Maryland [102]

Susan Cheng, MD
Fellow, Cardiovascular Medicine, Brigham and Women's
    Hospital
Department of Medicine
Divisions of Gerontology and Geriatric Medicine and
    Cardiovascular Medicine
Harvard Medical School
Boston, Massachusetts [75]

Brenna Cholerton, MD
Clinical Assistant Professor of Psychiatry and Behavioral
    Sciences
University of Washington School of Medicine
VA Puget Sound Health Care System GRECC
Seattle, Washington [62]

Colleen Christmas, MD
Assistant Professor of Medicine
Division of Geriatric Medicine
Johns Hopkins University School of Medicine
Baltimore, Maryland [118]

Audrey Chun, MD
Assistant Professor, Brookdale Department of
    Geriatrics and Adult Development
Director, Martha Stewart Center for Living
Mt. Sinai School of Medicine
New York, New York [31]

Harvey Jay Cohen, MD
Walter Kempner Professor and Chair, Department of Medicine
Director, Center for the Study of Aging and Human
    Development
Duke University Medical Center
Durham, North Carolina [94]

Mairav Cohen-Zion, PhD
Assistant Research Scientist, Department of Psychiatry
University of California, San Diego
San Diego, California [55]

Eric A. Coleman, MD, MPH
Professor of Medicine
Division of Health Care Policy and Research
University of Colorado Health Sciences Center
Aurora, Colorado [16]

Leo M. Cooney, Jr. MD
Humana Foundation Professor of Medicine
Chief, Section of Geriatric Medicine
Yale University School of Medicine
Yale–New Haven Hospital
New Haven, Connecticut [121]

Suzanne Craft, PhD
Professor of Psychiatry and Behavioral Sciences
University of Washington School of Medicine
VA Puget Sound Health Care System
Seattle, Washington [62]

Timothy J. Daaleman, DO, MPH
Associate Professor of Family Medicine
Research Fellow, Program on Aging, Disability &
    Long-Term Care
Cecil G. Sheps Center for Health Services Research
University of North Carolina at Chapel Hill
Chapel Hill, North Carolina [33]

Osvaldo DelBono, MD, PhD
Professor of Internal Medicine
Section on Gerontology and Geriatric Medicine
Wake Forest University School of Medicine
Winston-Salem, North Carolina [112]

Mary Catherine Dennis, MSW
Doctoral Candidate, Joint Program in Social Work
    and Social Science
School of Social Work
University of Michigan
Ann Arbor, Michigan [27]

Nikhila Deo, BS, MEng
University of Wisconsin School of Medicine and Public Health
Madison, Wisconsin [77]

Margaret A. Drickamer, MD
Associate Professor of Medicine
Section of Geriatric Medicine
Yale University School of Medicine
New Haven, Connecticut [13]

Catherine E. DuBeau, MD
Professor of Medicine
Section of Geriatrics
Director, Geriatric Continence Clinic
University of Chicago
Chicago, Illinois [50]

Ruth E. Dunkle, PhD
Wilbur J. Cohen Collegiate Professor of Social Work
School of Social Work
University of Michigan
Ann Arbor, Michigan [27]

Gustavo Duque, MD, MPH
Associate Professor of Medicine
Head of the Discipline of Geriatric Medicine
Director of the Aging Bone Research Program at Nepean
    Clinical School
University of Sidney
Sidney, Australia [117]

Niloo M. Edwards, MD
Professor and Chairman, Division of Cardiothoracic Surgery
University of Wisconsin School of Medicine and Public Health
Madison, Wisconsin [77]

Paul L. Enright, MD
Professor of Medicine
College of Public Health
University of Arizona
Tucson, Arizona [82]

Peter C. Enzinger, MD
Instructor in Medicine
Harvard Medical School
Boston, Massachusetts [98]

William B. Ershler, MD
Deputy Clinical Director
National Institute on Aging
Baltimore, Maryland [104]

Stanley Fahn, MD
Professor of Neurology
Neurological Institute
Columbia University Medical Center
New York, New York [66]

Michael A. Fearing, PhD
Research Fellow, Aging Brain Center
Institute for Aging Research
Harvard Medical School
Boston, Massachusetts [53]

Bruce A. Ferrell, MD
Professor of Clinical Medicine
Division of Geriatrics
UCLA David Geffen School of Medicine
Los Angeles, California [30]

Luigi Ferrucci, MD, PhD
Director, Baltimore Longitudinal Study of Aging
National Institute on Aging
Baltimore, Maryland [5] [52]

Emily Finlayson, MD, MS
Assistant Professor of Surgery
Division of Colon & Rectal Surgery
University of Michigan
Ann Arbor, Michigan [37]

Ellen Flaherty, PhD, APRN, BC
Vice President for Quality Improvement
Village Care of New York
New York, New York [26]

Scott A. Flanders, MD
Associate Professor of Medicine
University of Michigan
Ann Arbor, Michigan [17]

Gary A. Ford, MB, BCh
Professor of Pharmacology of Old Age
Director, Clinical Research Centre
School of Clinical & Laboratory Sciences
University of Newcastle upon Tyne
Newcastle upon Tyne, United Kingdom [8]

Christina E. Forsyth, HSc
Rotman Research Institute at Baycrest
Toronto, Ontario, Canada [63]

Marilisa Franceschi, MD
Research Fellow Istitudo di Ricovero e Cura a
    Carattere Scientifico (IRCCS)
Casa Sollievo della Sofferenza Hospital
San Giovanni Rotondo, Italy [91]

Linda P. Fried, MD, MPH
Dean and DeLamar Professor of Public Health
Professor of Epidemiology and Medicine
Senior Vice President, Columbia University Medical Center
New York, New York [52]

Brant E. Fries, PhD
Professor of Health Management and Policy
School of Public Health
Research Professor, Institute of Gerontology
University of Michigan
Chief, Health System Research
VA Ann Arbor Healthcare System GRECC
Ann Arbor, Michigan [6]

Terry Fulmer, PhD, RN, FAAN
Dean of the College of Nursing and the Erline
    Perkins McGriff Professor
New York University
New York, New York [26]

James Galvin, MD, MPH
Associate Professor of Neurology, Psychiatry and Neurobiology
Director, Memory Diagnostic Center
Hope Center for Neurological Disorders
Washington University School of Medicine
St. Louis, Missouri [12]

Giovanni Gambassi, MD
Associate Professor, Centro Medicina dell'Invecchiamento
Universita Cattolica del Sacro Cuore
Rome, Italy [6]

Andrew W. Gardner, PhD
CMRI Hobbs-Rechnagel Professor
General Clinical Research Center
University of Oklahoma Health Sciences Center
Oklahoma City, Oklahoma [80]

Lowell W. Gerson, PhD
Professor Emeritus of Epidemiology
Department of Community Health Sciences
Northeastern Ohio Universities College of Medicine
Senior Scientist, Emergency Medicine Research Center
Bonita Springs, Florida [18]

Shahyar M. Gharacholou, MD
Fellow, Divisions of Geriatrics and Cardiology
Duke University Medical Center
Durham, North Carolina [76]

Sudeep S. Gill, MD, MSc, FRCPC
Assistant Professor of Medicine
Queens University, St. Mary's of the Lake Hospital
Kingston, Ontario, Canada [24]

Jeffrey Ginsberg, MD
Professor of Medicine
Division of Hematology and Thromboembolism
McMaster University
Hamilton, Ontario, Canada [105]

Cary E. Gleason, PhD
Senior Scientist, Department of Medicine
Section of Geriatrics and Gerontology
University of Wisconsin School of Medicine and Public Health
William S. Middleton Memorial Veterans Hospital GRECC
Madison, Wisconsin [65]

Ronald M. Glick, MD
Assistant Professor of Psychiatry and Physical Medicine and
    Rehabilitation
Medical Director, Center for Integrative Medicine
University of Pittsburgh Medical Center
Pittsburgh, Pennsylvania [25]

Andrew P. Goldberg, MD
Professor of Medicine, Division of Gerontology
University of Maryland School of Medicine
Director, GRECC, Baltimore VA Maryland Health Care System
Baltimore, Maryland [110]

Ramaswamy Govidan, MD
Associate Professor of Medicine, Division of Oncology
Washington University School of Medicine
St. Louis, Missouri [97]

Len Gray, MB, BS, MMed, PhD, FRACP
Professor of Geriatric Medicine
Department of Medicine
University of Queensland
Princess Alexandra Hospital
Woolloongabba, Australia [6]

David A. Greenwald, MD
Associate Professor of Clinical Medicine
Division of Gastroenterology
Montefiore Medical Center
Bronx, New York

Tomas Griebling, MD
Associate Professor and Vice Chair of Urology
Assistant Scientist, Center on Aging
University of Kansas School of Medicine
Kansas City, Kansas [48]

Professor Beatrix Grubeck-Loebenstein
Director, Institute for Biomedical Aging Research
Austrian Academy of Sciences, Immunology Division
Innsbruck, Austria [3]

David A. Gruenewald, MD
Associate Professor of Medicine
University of Washington School of Medicine
VA Puget Sound Health Care System
Seattle, Washington [107]

Jack M. Guralnik, MD, PhD
Senior Investigator
Chief, Epidemiology and Demography Section
National Institute on Aging
Bethesda, Maryland [5]

Jerry H. Gurwitz, MD
Executive Director, Myers Primary Care Institute
University of Massachusetts
Worcester, Massachusetts [24]

Karen E. Hall, MD, PhD
Associate Professor of Internal Medicine
Division of Geriatric Medicine
University of Michigan Health System
Research Scientist, GRECC
Ann Arbor VAMC
Ann Arbor, Michigan [89]

Jeffrey B. Halter, MD
Professor of Internal Medicine
Chief, Division of Geriatric Medicine
Director, Geriatrics Center and Institute of Gerontology
University of Michigan
Ann Arbor, Michigan [109]

Joseph T. Hanlon, PharmD, MS
Professor of Medicine, Division of Geriatrics
Research Health Scientist
University of Pittsburgh
Pittsburgh, Pennsylvania [25]

Danielle Harari, MB, BS
Consultant Physician & Clinical Lead in Elderly Medicine
Honorary Senior Lectuere (KCL)
Department of Ageing and Health
St. Thomas' Hospital
London, England [93]

Tamara B. Harris, MD, MS
Senior Investigator and Chief, Geriatrics Epidemiology Section
Laboratory of Epidemiology, Demography, and Biometry
Intramural Research Program
National Institute on Aging
Bethesda, Maryland [39]

Rowan H. Robins Harwood, MSc, MD
Professor, Community Health Sciences
Nottingham City Hospital
Nottingham, United Kingdom [6]

Sima R. Hassani, DO
Clinical Instructor in Medicine
David Geffen School of Medicine at UCLA
Kaiser Permanente Medical Center
Woodland Hills, California [108]

Jennifer Hayashi, MD
Assistant Professor of Medicine
Johns Hopkins University School of Medicine
Baltimore, Maryland [22]

William R. Hazzard, MD
Professor of Medicine
University of Washington
Director, Geriatrics and Extended Care
VA Puget Sound Health Care System
Seattle, Washington [9][45]

Arthur E. Helfand, DPM
Professor Emeritus and Retired Chair
Department of Community Health, Aging & Health Policy
Temple University School of Podiatric Medicine
Narbeth, Pennsylvania [122]

Jean Claude Henrard, MD
Professor, Centre de Gerontologie
Hospital Sainte Perine
Paris, France [6]

Jerome M. Hershman, MD, MACP
Distinguished Professor of Medicine
David Geffen School of Medicine at UCLA
VA Greater Los Angeles Healthcare System
Los Angeles, California [108]

Kevin P. High, MD, MS, FACP
Professor of Medicine, Sections on Infectious Diseases,
Hematology/Oncology and Molecular Medicine
Chief, Section on Infectious Diseases
Wake Forest University Health Sciences
Winston-Salem, North Carolina [124]

Sarah N. Hilmer, PhD, FRACP
Senior Lecturer in Medicine
Department of Clinical Pharmacology and Aged Care
University of Sydney, Royal North Shore Hospital
St. Leonards, New South Wales, Australia [8]

Jacqueline Hind, MS, CCC-LP, BRS-S
Outreach Program Manager
University of Wisconsin School of Medicine and Public Health
William S. Middleton Memorial VA Hospital
Madison, Wisconsin [41]

John Hirdes, PhD
Professor of Health Studies and Gerontology
University of Waterloo
Waterloo, Ontario, Canada [6]

Mustafa M. Husain, MD
Professor of Psychiatry and Internal Medicine
Chief, Division of Geriatric Psychiatry
University of Texas Southwestern Medical Center
Dallas, Texas [72]

Kathryn Hyer, PhD, MPP
Associate Professor, School of Aging Studies
Florida Policy Exchange Center on Aging
University of South Florida
Tampa, Florida [26]

Naoki Ikegami, MD
Professor and Chair of Health Policy and Management
Keio University School of Medicine
Shinjuku-ku, Tokyo, Japan [6]

Sharon K. Inouye, MD, MPH
Professor of Medicine
Harvard Medical School
Beth Israel Deaconess Medical Center
Institute for Aging Research
Roslindale, Massachusetts [53]

Nadine A. Jackson, MD, MPH
Clinical Fellow, Medical Oncology
Dana-Farber Cancer Institute
Boston, Massachusetts [98]

Arshad Jahangir, MD
Associate Professor of Medicine
Mayo Clinic
Scottsdale, Arizona [79]

Brian D. James, M Bioethics
Center on Aging and Health
Johns Hopkins Bloomberg School of Public Health
Baltimore, Maryland [34]

Larry E. Johnson, MD, PhD
Associate Professor of Geriatrics & Family and Preventive
  Medicine
University of Arkansas for Medical Sciences
Central Arkansas Veteran's Healthcare System
North Little Rock VA Hospital
North Little Rock, Arkansas [38]

Sterling C. Johnson, PhD
Associate Professor of Medicine
University of Wisconsin School of Medicine and Public Health
William S. Middleton Memorial Veterans Hospital
Madison, Wisconsin [68]

Theodore M. Johnson, II, MD, MPH
Associate Professor of Medicine
Emory University
Manager, Geriatrics and Extended Care Service Line
Atlanta VA Medical Center
Decatur, Georgia [59]

Timothy M. Johnson, MD
Lewis and Lillian Becker Professor of Dermatology
University of Michigan
Ann Arbor, Michigan [100]

Palmi V. Jonsson, MD, FACP
Professor and Chief of Geriatrics
Landspitali University Hospital
University of Iceland School of Medicine
Reykjavik, Iceland [6]

Yvette L. Ju, DO
Intramural Research Program
National Institute on Aging
Bethesda, Maryland [116]

Mary E. Jung, MSc
University of Saskatchewan
Saskatoon, Saskatchewan, Canada [28]

Amy C. Justice, MD, PhD
Associate Professor of Medicine
Yale University School of Medicine
Chief, Section of General Medicine
West Haven VA Healthcare System
West Haven, Connecticut [128]

Marshall B. Kapp, JD, MPH, FCLM
Garwin Distinguished Professor of Law & Medicine
Co-Director, Center for Health Law & Policy
Southern Illinois University School of Law
Carbondale, Illinois [32]

Jason H.T. Karlawish, MD
Professor of Medicine
Ralston-Penn Center
University of Pennsylvania
Philadelphia, Pennsylvania [34]

Leslie I. Katzel, MD, PhD
Associate Professor of Medicine
Division of Gerontology and Geriatric Medicine
University of Maryland School of Medicine
Associate Director, Clinical
Veteran Affairs Maryland Health Care System GRECC
Baltimore, Maryland [110]

Clive Kearon, MB, MRCP (I), FRCP (C), PhD
Professor of Medicine
McMaster University
Head, Clinical Thrombosis Service
Henderson General Hospital
Hamilton, Ontario, Canada [105]

Rose Anne Kenny, MD, FRCPI, FRCP
Professor, Geriatric Medicine/Consultant
Medical Gerontology
Trinity Centre, St. James Hospital
Trinity College Dublin, College Green
Dublin, Ireland [57]

Gretchen G. Kimmick, MD, MS
Associate Professor of Medicine
Division of Medical Oncology
Duke University Medical Center
Durham, North Carolina [95]

Mary B. King, MD
Assistant Professor of Clinical Medicine
University of Connecticut School of Medicine
Hartford Hospital Geriatric Program
Hartford, Connecticut [54]

Thomas B.L. Kirkwood, PhD
Professor of Medicine and Institute Director
Institute for Aging and Health
Newcastle University
Newcastle upon Tyne, United Kingdom [2]

J. Philip Kistler, MD
Professor of Neurology
Harvard Medical School
Director, Stroke Service
Massachusetts General Hospital
Boston, Massachusetts [64]

Dalane W. Kitzman, MD
Professor of Internal Medicine
Sections on Cardiology and Gerontology and Geriatric Medicine
Wake Forest University Health Sciences
Winston-Salem, North Carolina [74]

Heidi D. Klepin, MD
Assistant Professor of Internal Medicine
Section on Hematology and Oncology
Wake Forest University Health Sciences
Winston-Salem, North Carolina [103]

Wendy M. Kohrt, PhD
Professor of Medicine, Division of Geriatrics
University of Colorado Denver
Aurora, Colorado [114]

George A. Kuchel, MD, FRCP
Professor of Medicine
Travelers Chair in Geriatrics and Gerontology
Director, UConn Center on Aging
Chief, Division of Geriatric Medicine
University of Connecticut Health Center
Farmington, Connecticut [51]

Mark S. Lachs, MD, MPH
Professor of Medicine
Co-Director, Division of Geriatric Medicine and Gerontology
Weill Medical College of Cornell University
New York, New York [60]

James M. Lai, MD
Postdoctoral Fellow, Section of Geriatrics
Yale University School of Medicine
New Haven, Connecticut [13]

Agnes Y.Y. Lee, MD, MSc, FRCPC
Associate Professor of Medicine
Division of Hematology and Thromboembolism
Medical Director, Thrombosis Program
McMaster University
Hamilton, Ontario, Canada [106]

Bruce Leff, MD
Associate Professor of Medicine
Johns Hopkins University School of Medicine
Baltimore, Maryland [22]

Ilo E. Leppik, MD
Professor of Neurology
University of Minnesota School of Medicine
MINCEP Epilepsy Care
Minneapolis, Minnesota [69]

Stacy Tessler Lindau, MD, MAPP
Assistant Professor
Departments of Obstetrics and Gynecology and
  Medicine-Geriatrics
Chicago Core on Biomeasures in Population Based
  Health and Aging Research
University of Chicago
Chicago, Illinois [47]

Shari M. Ling, MD
Staff Clinician, Clinical Research Branch
Translational Research and Medical Services Section
National Institute on Aging
Baltimore, Maryland [116]

David A. Lipschitz, MD, PhD
Longevity Center-St Vincent Senior Health
Little Rock, Arkansas [101]

XiaoKe Liu, MD
Heart Center for Excellence
Kalamazoo, Michigan [79]

Noelle K. LoConte, MD
Assistant Professor of Medicine
Section of Hematology/Oncology
University of Wisconsin School of Medicine and Public Health
Madison, Wisconsin [99]

Mark B. Loeb, MD
Professor of Pathology and Molecular Medicine and of Clinical
  Epidemiology and Biostatistics
McMaster University
Hamilton, Ontario, Canada [130]

Richard F. Loeser, Jr., MD
The Dorothy Rhyne Kimbrell and Willard Duke Kimbrell
  Professor of Arthritis and Rheumatology
Chief, Section on Molecular Medicine
Wake Forest University Health Sciences
Winston-Salem, North Carolina [112]

Dan L. Longo, MD
Scientific Director
National Institute on Aging
Baltimore, Maryland [104]

Michael Lucey, MD
Professor of Medicine
Head, Section of Gastroenterology and Hepatology
University of Wisconsin School of Medicine and Public Health
Madison, Wisconsin [90]

Mathew W. Ludgate, MB, ChB
Lecturer, Department of Dermatology
University of Michigan
Ann Arbor, Michigan [100]

Kenneth W. Lyles, MD
Professor of Medicine
Vice-Chair for Clinical Research
Duke University Medical Center
VA Medical Center
Durham, North Carolina [111]

William L. Lyons, MD
Assistant Professor of Internal Medicine
Section of Geriatrics and Gerontology
University of Nebraska Medical Center
Omaha, Nebraska [16]

Jay Magaziner, PhD, MSHyg
Professor and Director, Division of Gerontology
Department of Epidemiology and Preventive Medicine
University of Maryland School of Medicine
Baltimore, Maryland [118]

Preeti N. Malani, MD
Assistant Professor of Internal Medicine
Divisions of Geriatric Medicine and Infectious Diseases
University of Michigan Health System
Veterans Affairs Ann Arbor Healthcare System
Ann Arbor, Michigan [35]

Leon S. Maratchi, MD
Gastroenterology Consultants, P.A. – Hollywood
Hollywood, Florida

Edward R. Marcantonio, MD, SM
Associate Professor of Medicine
Harvard Medical School
Director of Research, Division of General Medicine and
    Primary Care
Beth Israel Deaconess Medical Center
Brookline, Massachusetts [20][53]

Thomas J. Marrie, MD
Professor of Medicine
Dean, Faculty of Medicine and Dentistry
University of Alberta
Edmonton, Alberta, Canada [126]

Alvin M. Matsumoto, MD
Professor of Medicine
University of Washington School of Medicine
Associate Director, GRECC
VA Puget Sound Health Care System
Seattle, Washington [107]

Mark P. Mattson, PhD
Gerontology Research Center
National Institute on Aging
Baltimore, Maryland [61]

Shawn M. McClintock, PhD
Postdoctoral Fellow, Department of Psychiatry
University of Texas Southwestern Medical Center
Dallas, Texas [72]

Eric B. Milbrandt, MD, MPH, FCCP
Assistant Professor, CRISMA Laboratory
Department of Critical Care Medicine
University of Pittsburgh School of Medicine
Pittsburgh, Pennsylvania [19]

Myron Miller, MD
Professor of Medicine
Johns Hopkins University School of Medicine
Baltimore, Maryland [88]

Bruce Miller, MD
Professor of Neurology
Director, UCSF Alzheimer's Disease Research Center
University of California, San Francisco
San Francisco, California [67]

Karen L. Miller, MD
Associate Professor of Obstetrics and Gynecology
University of Utah
Salt Lake City, Utah [48]

Ram R. Miller, MD, CM
Assistant Professor
Epidemiology and Preventive Medicine
University of Maryland School of Medicine
Baltimore, Maryland [118]

Richard A. Miller, PhD
Professor of Pathology
Associate Director, Geriatric Center
University of Michigan
Investigator, VA Ann Arbor, GRECC
Ann Arbor, Michigan [1]

Daniel Morgensztern, MD
Assistant Professor of Medicine
Section on Medical Oncology
Washington University School of Medicine
St. Louis, Missouri [97]

John N. Morris, PhD
Co-Director, Hebrew Senior Life Institute for Aging Research
The Alfred A. and Gilda Slifka Chair in Social Gerontological
    Research
Harvard Medical School
Boston, Massachusetts [6]

R. Sean Morrison, MD
Director, National Palliative Care Research Center
Hermann Merkin Professor of Palliative Care
Professor of Geriatrics and Medicine
Brookdale Department of Geriatrics and Adult Development
Mt. Sinai School of Medicine
New York, New York [31]

Suzanne B. Murray, MD
Assistant Professor of Psychiatry and Behavioral Sciences
University of Washington School of Medicine
Seattle, Washington [73]

Hyman B. Muss, MD
Professor of Medicine
University of Vermont and Vermont Cancer Center
Burlington, Vermont [95]

Yuri R. Nakasato, MD, MBA
Assistant Professor of Rheumatology and Geriatrics
Department of Rheumatology
University of North Dakota
MeritCare Health Systems
Fargo, North Dakota [119]

Aman Nanda, MD
Assistant Professor of Medicine
Division of Geriatrics
Rhode Island Hospital
Brown Medical School
Providence, Rhode Island [56]

Anne B. Newman, MD, MPH
Professor of Epidemiology and Medicine
Director, Center for Aging and Population Health
University of Pittsburgh
Pittsburgh, Pennsylvania [83]

Lindsay E. Nicolle, MD
Professor of Medicine and Medical Microbiology
University of Manitoba
Winnipeg, Manitoba, Canada [127]

Martin O'Donnell, MB, PhD, MRCPI
Associate Professor of Medicine
McMaster University
Hamilton General Hospital
Hamilton, Ontario, Canada [105]

Graziano Onder, MD, PhD
Assistant Professor, Centro Mefdicina dell'Invecchiamento
Universita Cattolica del Sacro Cuore
Rome, Italy [6]

Mark B. Orringer, MD
John Alexander Distinguished Professor of Thoracic Surgery
Head, Department of Thoracic Surgery
University of Michigan
Ann Arbor, Michigan [35]

Joseph G. Ouslander, MD
Professor and Associate Dean for Geriatric Programs
Charles E. Schmidt College of Biomedical Science
Professor (Courtesy), Christine E. Lynn College of Nursing
Florida Atlantic University
Professor of Medicine (Voluntary)
Division of Gerontology and Geriatric Medicine
University of Miami Miller School of Medicine
Boca Raton, Florida [59]

Miguel A. Paniagua, MD
Assistant Professor of Clinical Medicine
Division of Gerontology and Geriatric Medicine
University of Miami Miller School of Medicine
Miami VA Medical Center
Miami, Florida [9]

Marcella Pascualy, MD
Associate Professor of Psychiatry
Director, Geriatric Psychiatry Fellowship
University of Washington
VA Puget Sound Health Care System
Seattle, Washington [73]

Sanjeevkumar R. Patel, MD, MS
Assistant Professor of Internal Medicine
University of Michigan
Ann Arbor, Michigan [85]

Claire Peel, PhD, PT, FAPTA
Associate Provost for Faculty Development/Affairs
University of Alabama-Birmingham
Birmingham, Alabama [29]

Xiaomei Pei, PhD
Professor, Department of Sociology
Tsinghua University
Beijing, China [6]

Michael C. Perry, MD, MS, FACP
Professor and Director
Division of Hematology and Medical Oncology
University of Missouri/Ellis Fischel Cancer Center
Columbia, Missouri [97]

Elaine Peskind, MD
Professor of Psychiatry
University of Washington School of Medicine
VA Puget Sound Health Care System
Seattle, Washington [73]

Eric Petrie, MD
Associate Professor of Psychiatry
Division of Psychiatric Neurosciences
University of Washington School of Medicine
VA Puget Sound Health Care System
Seattle, Washington [73]

Eric D. Peterson, MD, MPH
Professor of Medicine
Division of Cardiology
Associate Vice Chair for Quality
Director of CV Research
Associate Director, Duke Clinical Research Institute
Duke University Medical Center
Durham, North Carolina [76]

Elizabeth A. Phelan, MD
Assistant Professor of Medicine
Division of Geriatrics and Gerontology
Harborview Medical Center
University of Washington School of Medicine
Seattle, Washington [9]

Kenneth J. Pienta, MD
Professor of Internal Medicine and Urology
University of Michigan
Ann Arbor, Michigan [96]

Alberto Pilotto, MD
Director, Department of Medical Sciences
Head, Geriatrics Unit & Gerontology-Geriatric Laboratory
    Research
Istitudo di Ricovero e Cura a
    Carattere Scientifico (IRCCS)
Casa Sollievo della Sofferenza Hospital
San Giovanni Rotondo, Italy [91]

Paula M. Podrazik, MD
Associate Professor of Medicine
Section of Geriatrics
University of Chicago
Chicago, Illinois [17]

Bruce G. Pollock, MD, PhD
Professor of Psychiatry
The Rotman Research Institute
Baycrest Center for Geriatric Care
Toronto, Ontario, Canada [63]

Bayard L. Powell, MD
Professor of Internal Medicine
Chief, Section on Hematology and Oncology
Wake Forest University Health Sciences
Winston-Salem, North Carolina [103]

Luigi Puglielli, MD, PhD
Assistant Professor of Medicine
Section of Geriatrics and Gerontology
University of Wisconsin School of Medicine and Public
    Health
William S. Middleton Memorial Veterans Hospital
    GRECC
Madison, Wisconsin [65]

Kip E. Queenan, MD
Assistant Professor of Psychiatry
University of Texas Southwestern Medical Center
Dallas, Texas [72]

Peter V. Rabins, MD
Professor of Psychiatry
Division of Geriatric Psychiatry and Neuropsychiatry
Johns Hopkins University
Baltimore, Maryland [71]

Annette Hylen Ranhoff, MD, PhD
Professor, Ullevaal University Hospital
Diakonhjemmet Hospital
Medical Department
Oslo, Norway [6]

Arati V. Rao, MD
Assistant Professor of Medicine
Divisions of Medical Oncology and Geriatrics
Duke University Medical Center
Durham VA Medical Center
Durham, North Carolina [94]

Keith L. Rapp, MD, CMD
CEO, Geriatric Associates of America, PA
Webster, Texas [21]

Mary Pat Rapp, PhD, RN, GNP-BC
Assistant Professor of Nursing
University of Texas School of Nursing
Houston, Texas [21]

Mark Reger, PhD
Research Neuropsychologist
Department of Psychology
Madigan Army Medical Center
Tacoma, Washington [62]

W. Jack Rejeski, PhD
Professor of Health and Exercise Science
Wake Forest University
Winston-Salem, North Carolina [28]

David B. Reuben, MD
Professor of Medicine
Chief, Geriatric Medicine & Gerontology
David Geffen School of Medicine at UCLA
Los Angeles, California [11]

Justin C. Rice, MD
Iowa Clinic
West Des Moines, Iowa [90]

Michael W. Rich, MD
Professor of Medicine
Washington University School of Medicine
Director, Cardiac Rapid Evaluation Unit
Barnes-Jewish Hospital
St. Louis, Missouri [78]

Ian H. Robbins, MD, PhD
Professor of Medicine and Neurology
Medical Oncology Section
University of Wisconsin School of Medicine and Public Health
Madison, Wisconsin [99]

JoAnne Robbins, PhD
Professor of Medicine, Radiology, Nutritional
 Sciences, and Biomedical Engineering
University of Wisconsin School of Medicine and Public Health
Associate Director of Research/GRECC
William S. Middleton Memorial VA Hospital
Madison, Wisconsin [41]

Paula Rochon, MD, MPH
Professor, Department of Medicine
Senior Scientist, Institute for Clinical Evaluative Sciences
Assistant Director, Kunin-Lunenfeld Applied Research
 Unit – Baycrest Centre
University of Toronto
Toronto, Ontario, Canada [24]

G. Alec Rooke, MD, PhD
Professor of Anesthesiology
Visiting Professor of Anesthesia, Critical Care and Pain Medicine
Beth Israel Deaconess Medical Center
Boston, Massachusetts [36]

Caterina Rosano, MD, MPH
Assistant Professor of Epidemiology
Graduate School of Public Health
Center for Aging and Population Health
University of Pittsburgh
Pittsburgh, Pennsylvania [115]

Sonja Rosen, MD
Assistant Clinical Professor of Medicine
Division of Geriatric Medicine
UCLA School of Medicine
Santa Monica, California [11]

Mary H. Samuels, MD
Professor of Medicine
Division of Endocrinology, Diabetes and Clinical Nutrition
Program Director, Clinical and Translational Research Center
Oregon Health & Science University
Portland, Oregon [108]

Jeff M. Sands, MD
Juha P. Kokko Professor of Medicine and Physiology
Director, Renal Division
Associate Dean for Clinical and Translational Research
Emory University
Atlanta, Georgia[86]

Jochen Schacht, MD
Professor of Biological Chemistry
Director, Kresge Hearing Research Institute
Department of Otorhinolaryngology
University of Michigan
Ann Arbor, Michigan [44]

Lynn E. Schlanger, MD
Assistant Professor of Medicine
Renal Division
Emory University School of Medicine
Atlanta, Georgia[86]

Kenneth E. Schmader, MD
Professor of Medicine
Chief, Division of Geriatrics
Duke University Medical Center
Director, Durham VA Medical Center GRECC
Durham, North Carolina [129]

Richard Schulz, PhD
Professor of Psychiatry, Epidemiology, Sociology, Psychology,
 Community Health, and Health and Rehabilitation Sciences
Director, University Center for Social and Urban Research
Associate Director, Institute on Aging
University of Pittsburgh
Pittsburgh, Pennsylvania [7]

Robert S. Schwartz, MD
Goodstein Professor of Medicine
Division Head, Geriatric Medicine
University of Colorado Health Sciences Center
Aurora, Colorado [114]

Todd P. Semla, MS, PharmD
VA Pharmacy Benefits Management Service
Hines, Illinois [63]

Su-Hua Sha, MD
Research Investigator
Kresge Hearing Research Institute
Director, Molecular Otology and Signal Transduction Laboratory
University of Michigan
Ann Arbor, Michigan [44]

Win-Kuang Shen, MD
Professor of Medicine
Mayo Clinic
Rochester, Minnesota [79]

Jonathan A. Ship, DMD*
Professor, Department of Oral Medicine
New York University College of Dentistry
Director, Bluestone Center for Clinical Research
New York, New York [42]

Jeffrey H. Silverstein, MD
Professor of Anesthesiology
Associate Dean for Research
Mt. Sinai School of Medicine
New York, New York [36]

Don D. Sin, MD, MPH
Canadian Research Chair in Chronic Obstructive Lung Disease
Associate Professor of Medicine
University of British Columbia
James Hogg iCAPTURE Centre for Cardiovascular and
 Pulmonary Research, St. Paul's Hospital
Vancouver, British Columbia, Canada [83]

*deceased

Aneesh Bhim Singhal, MD
Assistant Professor of Neurology
Harvard Medical School
Assistant Neurologist
J. Philip Kistler MGH Stroke Research Center
Massachusetts General Hospital
Boston, Massachusetts [64]

Eric Edward Smith, MD, MPH
Assistant Professor of Neurology
Harvard Medical School
Assistant Neurologist
J. Philip Kistler MGH Stroke Research Center
Massachusetts General Hospital
Boston, Massachusetts [64]

John D. Sorkin, MD, PhD
Associate Professor of Medicine, Gerontology
Chief, Biostatistics and Informatics
University of Maryland School of Medicine
Baltimore VA Medical Center
Baltimore, Maryland [80][110]

MaryFran R. Sowers, MS, PhD
Professor of Epidemiology
John G. Searle Professor of Public Health
Director, Center for Integrated Approaches to Complex Diseases
University of Michigan
Ann Arbor, Michigan [46]

Knight Steel, MD
Professor, Hackensack University Medical Center
Hackensack, New Jersey [6]

Sharon E. Strauss, MD
Associate Professor of Medicine
University of Calgary and University of Toronto
Foothills Medical Centre
Calgary, Alberta, Canada [10]

Stephanie Studenski, MD, MPH
Professor, Department of Medicine (Geriatrics)
University of Pittsburgh
Staff Physician, VA Pittsburgh GRECC
Pittsburgh, Pennsylvania [115]

Dennis H. Sullivan, MD
Professor of Medicine and Geriatrics
Vice Chairman, Donald W. Reynolds Department of Geriatrics
University of Arkansas for Medical Sciences
Director, VA Little Rock GRECC
Little Rock, Arkansas [38]

Mark A. Supiano, MD
Professor and Chief, Division of Geriatrics
University of Utah School of Medicine
University of Utah Center on Aging
Director, VA Salt Lake City GRECC
Salt Lake City, Utah [81]

George E. Taffet, MD
Associate Professor of Medicine
Chief, Section on Geriatrics
Section on Cardiovascular Sciences
Baylor College of Medicine
Houston, Texas [74]

Andra E. Talaska, BS
Research Associate
Department of Biological Chemistry
University of Michigan
Ann Arbor, Michigan [44]

Joyce Lisa Tenover, MD, PhD
Professor of Medicine
Division of Geriatrics Medicine and Gerontology
Wesley Woods Center of Emory University
Emory University School of Medicine
Atlanta, Georgia [49]

Victor J. Thannickal, MD
Associate Professor of Medicine
Division of Pulmonary and Critical Care Medicine
University of Michigan Health System
Ann Arbor, Michigan [84]

Mary E. Tinetti, MD
Gladys Phillips Crofoot Professor of Medicine,
    Epidemiology, and Public Health
Director, Program on Aging
Yale University School of Medicine
New Haven, Connecticut [10]

Jennifer Tjia, MD, MSCE
Assistant Professor of Medicine
Division of Geriatric Medicine
University of Massachusetts Medical School
Worcester, Massachusetts [24]

Galen B. Toews, M.D.
Professor of Internal Medicine
Chief, Division of Pulmonary and Critical Care Medicine
University of Michigan Health System
Ann Arbor, Michigan [84]

Bruce R. Troen, MD
Associate Professor of Medicine
University of Miami Leonard M. Miller School of Medicine
Miami VA Medical Center
Miami, Florida [117]

Jack I. Twersky, MD
Associate Clinical Professor of Medicine
Duke University Medical School
Durham VA Medical Center
Durham, North Carolina [129]

Mark L. Unruh, MD, MS
Assistant Professor of Medicine
Renal-Electrolyte Division
University of Pittsburgh School of Medicine
Pittsburgh, Pennsylvania [87]

Peter V. Vaitkevicius, MD
Associate Professor of Medicine
Chief, Department of Cardiology
Wayne State University School of Medicine
John D. Dingell VA Medical Center
Detroit, Michigan [35]

Victor Valcour, MD
Adjunct Clinical Assistant Professor of Geriatrics in Neurology
Memory and Aging Center
University of California, San Francisco
San Francisco, California [67]

Jeffrey I. Wallace, MD, MPH
Associate Professor of Medicine
Division of Gerontology and Geriatric Medicine
University of Colorado Health Sciences Center
Aurora, Colorado [40]

Jeremy D. Walston, MD
Associate Professor of Medicine
Division of Geriatric Medicine and Gerontology
Johns Hopkins University
Baltimore, Maryland [4][52]

Louise C. Walter, MD
Associate Professor of Medicine
University of California, San Francisco
Staff Physician, San Francisco VA Medical Center
San Francisco, California [14]

Lucy Y. Wang, MD
Senior Fellow, Department of Psychiatry and Behavioral Sciences
University of Washington School of Medicine
VA Puget Sound Health Care System
Seattle, Washington [10]

Timothy S. Wang, MD
Associate Professor of Dermatology
University of Michigan
Ann Arbor, Michigan [73][100]

Gale R. Watson, MEd, CLVT
National Director, Blind Rehabilitation Service
RS-OPS, Veterans Health Central Office
Washington, DC [43]

Stephen G. Weber, MD, MS
Assistant Professor of Medicine
Section of Infectious Diseases
University of Chicago
Chicago, Illinois [125]

Birgit Weinberger
Institute for Biomedical Aging Research
Immunology Division
Austrian Academy of Sciences
Innsbruck, Austria [3]

Debra K. Weiner, MD
Associate Professor of Medicine, Psychiatry and Anesthesiology (Geriatrics)
University of Pittsburgh Medical Center Pain Medicine Program
University of Pittsburgh
Pittsburgh, Pennsylvania [123]

Daniela Weiskopf
Institute for Biomedical Aging Research
Immunology Division
Austrian Academy of Sciences
Innsbruck, Austria [3]

Chad Whelan, MD
Associate Professor of Medicine
University of Chicago
Chicago, Illinois [17]

Jocelyn Wiggins, BM, BCh, MRCP
Assistant Professor of Internal Medicine
Division of Geriatric Medicine
University of Michigan
Ann Arbor, Michigan [85]

Scott T. Wilber, MD, FACEP
Associate Professor of Emergency Medicine
Northeastern Ohio Universities College of Medicine
Director, Emergency Medicine Research Center
Summa Health System
Akron, Ohio [18]

Aaron Van Wright III, MD
Associate Clinical Professor
Department of Psychiatry
University of Texas Southwestern Medical Center
Dallas, Texas [72]

Sachin Yende, MD, MS
Assistant Professor of Critical Care Medicine
University of Pittsburgh School of Medicine
Pittsburgh, Pennsylvania [83]

Raymond Yung, MB, ChB
Associate Professor of Internal Medicine
Divisions of Geriatric Medicine and Rheumatology
University of Michigan
Associate Director, Research
VA Ann Arbor GRECC
Ann Arbor, Michigan [120]

Mark Yurkofsky, MD, CMD
Chief of Extended Care, Palliative Medicine and Intensive
  Home-based Programs
Harvard Vanguard Medical Associates Medical Director
The Boston Center for Rehabilitative and Subacute Care
Instructor of Medicine
Harvard Medical School
Boston, Massachusetts [20]

Susan J. Zieman, MD, PhD
Assistant Professor of Medicine
Divisions of Cardiology and Geriatric Medicine
John Hopkins University School of Medicine
Baltimore, Maryland [75]

Foreword

Publication of the 6th edition marks an important milestone in the evolution of this work-in-progress—passing the baton from the last of the original editors to a new (albeit thoroughly seasoned) group from the next generation of geriatricians and gerontologists, expanded now to 6 under the senior leadership of Jeffrey Halter, who bring the latest and the best in this growing field to students and practitioners of our discipline on behalf of the aging patients we serve.

This orderly succession gives me an enormous sense of pride and confidence that the progressive maturation of this textbook over the first 5 editions will continue unabated for the foreseeable future. From the outset this has been buttressed by the unflagging commitment to our field demonstrated by McGraw-Hill since this project was but a gleam in the eye of Derek Jeffers, senior publisher's editor for *Harrison's Principles of Internal Medicine*. In the late 1970s he conceived it as an important and timely initiative on behalf of our new field to bring students and practitioners up to modern standards in caring for the already burgeoning numbers of elderly patients. He first enlisted the collaboration of Edwin L. Bierman, who had recently added Gerontology to his title as head of the Division of Metabolism in the Department of Medicine at the University of Washington, to develop a new textbook for our field to serve as a companion to *Harrison's* and the first such American contribution in this discipline. Ed, mentor from metabolism fellowship days at the University of Washington, turned in rapid order first to his long-time friend and colleague, Reubin Andres, clinical director of the Gerontology Research Center (GRC) of the National Institute on Aging in Baltimore, to serve as senior editor and soon thereafter to me, as a junior member of his division, to join in a tripartite effort to launch the first edition of the *Principles of Geriatric Medicine and Gerontology*. This came to fruition over the next 5 years, during which I moved to Baltimore to join the Department of Medicine at Johns Hopkins as vice-chairman and to develop a new Geriatric program based principally at the East Baltimore (now Hopkins Bayview) campus that was the site of the GRC. And with the steady support of Jeffers and the editorial assistance of Ellen Hazzard, in 1985 the first edition was published, receiving favorable reviews and an enthusiastic reception from members of our still fledgling field.

Encouraged by this promising beginning, the accelerating pace of progress in aging research, and the recognition of Geriatrics as a legitimate, scientifically-based medical discipline (and by the thousands of practitioners and fellows who were certified through the first examination developed as a joint effort by the American Board of Internal Medicine and the American Board of Family Practice in 1988), we proceeded to assemble the 2nd edition as an expanded volume, notably through the contributions of a of fourth editor for the neural sciences (John Blass), and a section devoted to the Geriatric Syndromes, which was published in 1990. With its solid reputation established, the 3rd edition (with Nancy Woolard as editorial assistant) followed in 1994, with additional editors in Jeffrey Halter (another endocrinologist turned geriatrician) and Walter H. Ettinger, Jr. (a rheumatologist but also the first fellowship-trained geriatrician on the panel), and the first turnover on the editorial board in the retirement of Andres from the panel. The 4th edition was published in 1999 with Joseph Ouslander, another trained geriatrician, succeeding Ed Bierman following his death in 1995. Subsequently, as Ettinger left the board, he was succeeded by Mary Tinetti, another card-carrying geriatrician, and the 5th edition was published in 2003. A token of appreciation given to all contributors to the 5th edition visually summarized this history of the *Principles of Geriatric Medicine and Gerontology*: a photograph on a mouse pad of the first five volumes standing between the book-ends that exemplify the enduring philosophy of editions of this textbook: our enduring commitment to aging, both "successful" and "usual"(Figure 1), portraying a striving runner on one end symbolizing the price and rewards of a robust old age while on the other end the discouraged, frail old person to whom much of our professional effort is devoted with heart, mind, and soul.

Now with the publication of the 6th edition in 2009 the editorial succession is complete as the last members of the early boards leave with the retirement of John Blass and my "promotion" to emeritus status, Jeffrey Halter assumes the reins of leadership, and three vigorous new members join to expand and broaden the effort: Sanjay Asthana, a geriatrician with primary professional expertise in the neural sciences (notably Alzheimer's Disease and related disorders); Kevin High, an infectious disease subspecialist with broad interests and ties in subspecialty internal medicine and

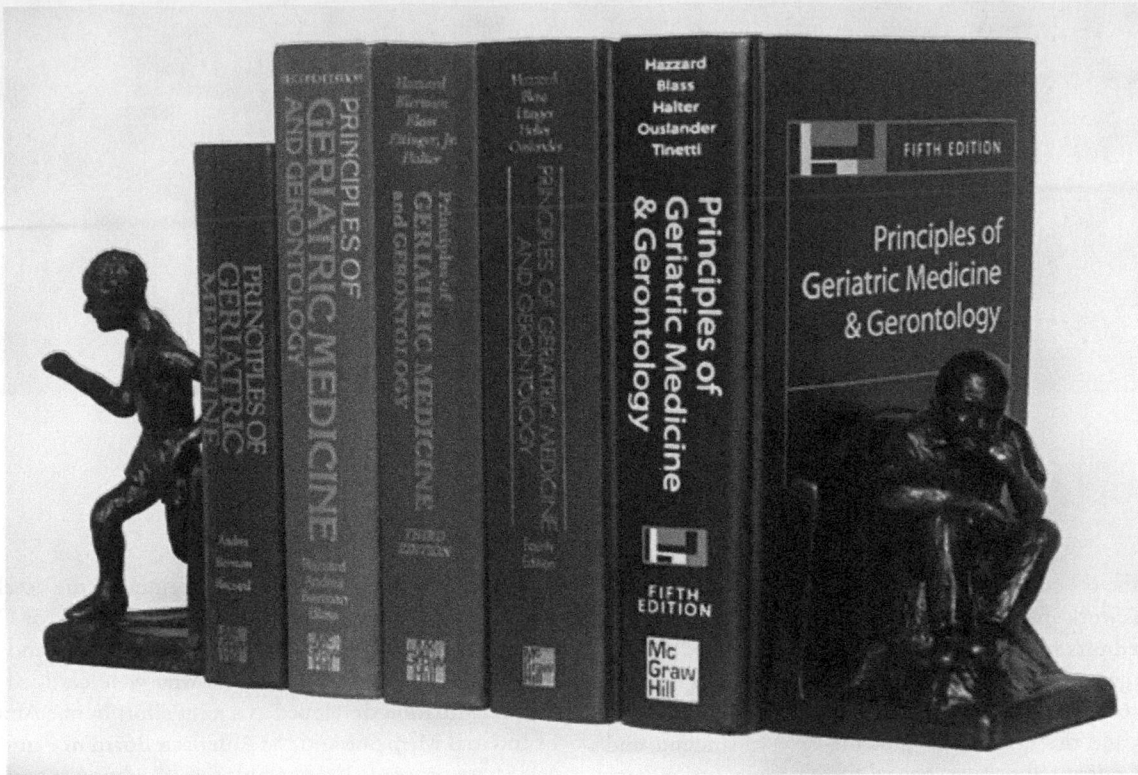

FIGURE 1.

geriatrics; and Stephanie Studenski, a geriatrician and rheumatologist/rehabilitation specialist.

I am proud to remain associated with this tradition of excellence and I am entirely confident that the solid principles upon which this textbook were founded will assuredly remain undiminished with the strong support of James Shanahan at McGraw-Hill and the leadership of the board of editors of the 6th edition:

- To publish a timely, comprehensive, state-of-the-art textbook as an icon and practical, day-to-day tool of our discipline that is anchored in science, evidence-based medicine, and the balanced, patient-centered practice of our specialty.

- To focus our information and our chapters upon the learning needs of those who will lead our field as it continues to evolve and its scientific underpinnings become evermore secure and comprehensive: most clearly the fellows in training who will become the future practitioners, researchers, and educators in this rapidly advancing field and whose contributions will be leveraged maximally among the broad array of students and practitioners whom they instruct and with whom they collaborate.

- To hold our aging and elderly patients squarely in the center of our vision for the future of our field, for they are and always will be the raison d'etre of our discipline.

William R. Hazzard
2009

Preface

On behalf of the Editors, it is an honor and privilege to provide this Preface to *Hazzard's Geriatric Medicine and Gerontology*, 6th Edition. In an accompanying Foreword for the 6th edition, Bill Hazzard provides a brief history of this textbook, which has become a mainstay of the rapidly developing field of geriatric medicine. Adding to the already rich history of this book, first published in 1985, the 6th edition emerges renewed and vibrant. It is particularly special that it is the first edition of this textbook to carry the name of its founding editor Bill Hazzard in its title. What we and our publisher McGraw-Hill have done is to simply formalize the reality of the imprint that Bill Hazzard has made, as the textbook has been known informally as Hazzard's Textbook already for many years.

The 6th edition is substantially different from its predecessors, reflecting the substantial growth and increasing sophistication of geriatrics as a defined medical discipline. The main sections of this edition have been reorganized to make the sections more functionally aligned. Vitality and continued rejuvenation has been enhanced through the addition of 9 new chapters: Inflammation and Aging, International Gerontology, General Principles of Pharmacology, Transitions (of care), Emergency Room Care, Rural Aging, Social Work, Psychoactive Drug Therapy, and Appropriate Antibiotic Use. Furthermore, we have recruited new authors for over 40% of the chapters. As Bill Hazzard has outlined in his Foreword, three new editors have played a critical role in the renewal of this textbook: Sanjay Asthana. Kevin High and Stephanie Studenski. They have joined me (my 4th edition), Joe Ouslander (his 3rd edition) and Mary Tinetti (her 2nd edition) to make a vital new editorial team. Fortunately for all of us, Bill Hazzard has stayed actively involved as Editor Emeritus and Senior Advisor.

The 6th edition acknowledges and recognizes the worldwide growth of the field of geriatric medicine in several ways. A distinguished International Advisory Board has been created; the previously mentioned, new chapter on International Gerontology summarizes a number of important issues around the world; and we are very pleased that 11 of the chapters in the 6th edition have been written by authors who are in countries outside of the United States. Overall, our authors are a large and diverse group including many geriatricians but also a substantial number of other specialists, who come from a range of medical and surgical disciplines. In addition multiple health professions and disciplines are represented among the authors. Two of the textbook's editors are women, and nearly 30% of the lead authors of chapters, as well as many other co-authors, are women.

A major step forward is the online version of the 6th edition. One of the original goals of working with McGraw-Hill as the publisher of this textbook, as described in Bill Hazzard's Foreword, was to provide a link with *Harrison's Principles of Internal Medicine*. While there have been a number of parallels with Harrison's over previous editions, the link becomes substantial with the online version of *Hazzard's Geriatric Medicine and Gerontology*, 6th Edition. Both Harrison's Online and Hazzard's are part of McGraw-Hill's Access Medicine, a comprehensive online resource for medical students, residents, clinicians, and researchers. In addition to Harrison's Online and Hazzard's, Access Medicine includes the ability to quickly search across more than 50 titles from McGraw-Hill's Clinical and Lange Libraries. There are a number of important implications of our textbook becoming a part of McGraw-Hill's Access Medicine. First, it adds a living presence to the textbook as additional material can be added as needed as online updates. We anticipate that such updates will be available for many chapters of the textbook on a regular basis. We are especially pleased that students of the health professions, both undergraduate and postgraduate, will have full access to our textbook through the online version if they are at an institution that subscribes to Access Medicine. Finally, our authors are no longer encumbered by page limits for the published text. Additional complementary material and illustrations, as well as educational materials, can now be made available through the online edition.

Thus just as our population is inexorably aging, and medicine is faced with an ever growing number of older patients with multiple and complex problems, we have been able to bring together the best minds and leaders in the field to provide authoritative guidance, including a highly diverse and breadth of thinking that has not previously existed in our textbook of geriatric medicine. We hope to reach a broader audience through the availability of the electronic version of the textbook and to keep it a living and growing document that encompasses the rapid stream of new information which is helping us to provide an evidence base for more effective care for our elderly population.

Putting together a textbook of this magnitude requires enormous effort by many people. Again on behalf of the editors, I wish to particularly thank the many chapter authors who have contributed to the book. Their dedication and commitment is exemplified by Jonathan Ship, whose untimely death in 2008 is a major loss to the field of geriatric dentistry. Jonathan wrote the Oral Cavity chapter for the last three editions. Because it has become a classic, I asked Jonathan if he would be willing to revise and update the chapter for the 6th edition. We both knew that he had a terminal diagnosis and would not likely live to see the final publication. However, I was not surprised when Jonathan immediately accepted the invitation to revise his chapter, which he did with his usual vigorous and thorough effort. A little bit of Jonathan thus lives on in the 6th edition.

The editors also greatly appreciate the strong and effective working relationship that we have with McGraw-Hill. This relationship is made possible by the outstanding efforts of James Shanahan and colleagues who have ensured the progress of the publication and the important next steps in the textbook's evolution. We especially appreciate the efforts of Nancy Woolard from Wake Forest University School of Medicine, who has served as a senior editorial assistant for four previous additions. Her role has been critical to provide a strong link to our past history and as the final common pathway for assembly of the 6th edition. We also wish to acknowledge the staff that provided support for editorial efforts from our academic offices. These include Jane Harlow and Beverly Williams at the University of Michigan, Jane Mallory at Yale University, Lori Hasse at the University of Wisconsin, Sheila Rutledge at Wake Forest University, and Susan Ratliff at Emory University.

Jeffrey B. Halter
2009

PRINCIPLES OF GERONTOLOGY

Biology of Aging and Longevity

Richard A. Miller

Aging is the process that converts young adults, most of them healthy and in no need of assistance from physicians, into older adults whose deteriorating physiological fitness leads to progressively increasing risks of illness and death. The effects of aging are so familiar to health professionals and aging adults that it is viewed by both parties as something immutable, taken for granted, an arena in which diseases and their treatments take place, but not itself subject to intervention or modulation. The major discovery in biogerontology, gradually emerging from decades of work in animal model systems, is that this old-fashioned viewpoint is wrong, and that the aging process can be delayed or decelerated in mammals, built very much like human beings, by simple manipulations of nutritional signals and genetic circuits similar to those already well-documented in people. It is now absolutely routine to extend lifespan, in rats and mice, by about 40%, i.e., about 10 times the increase in active life expectancy that would ensue from a complete elimination of all neoplastic illnesses, or all heart attacks, in a human population. It thus seems plausible that a more detailed understanding of the factors that determine aging and the processes by which aging increases the risk of such a wide range of lethal and nonlethal illnesses and disabilities could, in the foreseeable future, have a profound impact on preventive medicine.

Aging is a mystery, in the same sense that infectious disease was once a mystery, and consciousness still is: an area of investigation in which well-informed researchers cannot really be confident that they have selected a line of investigation bound to be productive. Until recently, most published papers in biogerontology journals consisted of descriptions of the ways in which young mice, rats, or people differed from older ones, originally in terms of anatomy and physiology, as indicated by levels of enzymes or hormones, and more recently by exhaustive catalogs of protein and mRNA levels. This descriptive era is gradually being superseded by one focused on specific molecular hypotheses about the key factors that regulate aging. The foundation of this modern approach to the biology of aging was the development of genetic models and nutritional manipulations which could delay aging, and the exploitation of this leverage to

test molecular ideas about the basis for the retardation of the aging process.

WHAT IS AGING?

This question—what is aging?—is posed not as an invitation to semantic quibbling, but to initiate reexamination of facts so familiar that they are seldom examined. A case history of an individual who has mild arthritis, some loss of hearing acuity, some evidence of incipient cataract, loss of muscle mass and strength, a progressive decline in capacity for aerobic exercise, troubles with learning and remembering, and an increased vulnerability to infectious illness would lead any physician to assume that the individual described is a man or woman of 60 or more years of age. But the list of signs and symptoms refers with equal accuracy to a 20-year-old horse, or a 10-year-old dog, or a 2-year-old mouse. The specific list of deficits and impairments shifts a bit from person to person, and from species to species, but it is extremely rare to find an 80-year-old person, or 3-year-old mouse, or 14-year-old dog that has avoided all of these age-associated problems. The aging process is synchronized, in that it is common to see all of these difficulties in older people, horses, dogs, and mice, but rare to encounter any of them in young adults just past puberty. This synchrony, though entirely familiar to schoolchildren, physicians, and scientists alike, is the central challenge in biological gerontology: how is it that such a process affects so many cells, tissues, organs and systems at a rate that varies, even among mammals, over a 100-fold range from the shortest lived shrews to the longest lived whales? Structural features of shrews, mice, dogs, and people are remarkably similar at scales from the arrangement of DNA and histones in the nucleus, to the architecture of the kidney, heart, and thymus, to the role of the central nervous system (CNS) and endocrine systems in regulating responses to heat and cold, hunger and thirst, infection, and predators. Why, then, in molecular terms, will the eye, kidney, immune system, brain, and joints of a mouse last only 2 to 3 years under optimal conditions, while the same cells and organs and systems persevere for 50 or more years in people, and longer still in some species of whales?

The definition proposed at the beginning of this chapter—aging as a process for turning young adults into distinctly less healthy old ones—is straightforward enough to appear simple-minded, but in practice draws some prominent distinctions. In this view, aging is not a disease: Diseases are certainly among the most salient consequences of aging, but aging produces many changes not classified as diseases, and many diseases also affect young people. Similarly, lifespan and mortality risks are influenced by many factors besides aging. Thus, evidence that a gene or diet or public health measure has altered life expectancy, upwards or downwards, does not imply that the effects have been achieved by an effect on aging. In the context of the whole organism definition of aging used in this chapter, it is hard to interpret the meaning of changes that occur as individual cells "age" in tissue culture. While cell culture studies can provide valuable information of great relevance to ideas about aging, the two processes are likely to be fundamentally different.

From a biological standpoint, a critical distinction is the difference between aging and development. Development creates a healthy young adult from a fertilized egg, and is strongly molded by natural selection. Genetic mutations that impair development, creating a slower falcon, a near-sighted chipmunk, or a chimpanzee uninterested in social cues, are rapidly weeded from the gene pool. But the force of natural selection diminishes dramatically at ages that are seldom reached. Mice, for example, typically live only 6 months or so in the wild, before they succumb to predation, starvation, or other natural hazard. There is strong selective pressure against mutations that cause cataracts in the first few months of mouse life, but little or no pressure against genotypes that postpone cataract formation for 2 years. Mice protected, in a laboratory setting, against predation, starvation, and other risks typically do develop cataracts in their second or third year. In wolves, however, a genotype that delayed cataracts for only 2 years would be a disaster; natural selection favors wolf genes that preserve lens transparency for a decade or more. A similar process, working on our ancestors in environments where survival to 15 was common, but survival to 55 distinctly uncommon, has filled our own genome with alleles that postpone cancer, osteoarthritis, coronary disease, Alzheimer's, presbycusis, cataracts, sarcopenia, immune senescence, and many other familiar maladies, for about 50 to 60 years. Thus, although aging and development seem, superficially, to be similar processes in that both lead to changes in form and function, they are different in a fundamental and critical way: Development is molded directly by the forces of Darwinian selection and the changes of aging are the consequence of the failure of these selective processes to preserve function at ages seldom reached by individuals in any given species.

Aging as a Coordinated, Malleable Process

The definition of aging as a process that turns young adults into old ones conflicts with a view of aging as instead a collection of processes, some that lead to arterial disease, some that affect endocrine function, some that impair cognition or cause neoplastic transformation, etc. Because each of these ailments is itself the outcome of a complex interaction among many factors, including genes, diet, accidents, viruses, toxins, antibiotics, and physicians, and because each of these diseases, and many others, seems an inextricable part of

aging, it has seemed implausible to regard aging as less complex than its (apparent) constituents. Considering aging as a process, rather than a collection of complex processes, has thus seemed to be an oversimplification.

However, two lines of evidence support the merits of the view of aging as a unitary process, with its own (still ill-defined) physiological and molecular basis, which underlies and tends to synchronize the multiple changes seen in older individuals. The first of these discoveries was caloric restriction: The observation that rodents allowed to eat only 60% of the amount of food they would voluntarily consume would live 40% longer than controls permitted free access to food. This observation, first made by McCay in the 1930s, has now been repeated in more than a dozen species in scores of laboratories, and ongoing studies in rhesus monkeys have now produced preliminary, but highly suggestive, evidence that similar benefits may accrue in our own order of mammals. The key point is not merely that lifespan is extended, but that nearly all of the consequences of aging are coordinately delayed. Caloric restriction delays changes in cells that proliferate continuously (such as gut epithelial cells), cells that can be triggered to proliferate when called upon (such as lymphocytes), and those that never proliferate (such as most neurons), as well as on tissues that are extracellular or acellular (such as lens tissue and extracellular collagen fibrils). It delays aspects of aging characterized by excess proliferation, such as neoplasias, and those characterized by failure to proliferate (such as immune senescence). It delays or decelerates age change at the tissue level (such as degradation of articular cartilage) and those involving complex interplay among multiple cells and tissues (such as loss of cognitive function and endocrine control circuits). Because caloric restriction alters, in parallel, so vast an array of age-associated changes, it seems inescapable that these many changes, distinct as they are, must be in some measure timed, i.e., synchronized by a mechanism altered by caloric intake.

A second, more recent, set of experiments leads to the same inference. In 1996, Bartke and his colleagues showed that Ames dwarf mice, in which a developmental defect in the pituitary impairs production of growth hormone (GH), thyrotropin, and prolactin, had an increase of more than 40% in both mean and maximal lifespan compared to littermates with the normal allele at the same locus. Since then studies of this mutant, and the closely similar Snell dwarf, have documented delay in kidney pathology, arthritis, cancer, immune senescence, collagen cross-linking, cataracts, and cognitive decline, making a strong case that these genetic changes in endocrine levels do indeed modulate the aging process as a whole, with consequent delay in a very wide range of age-synchronized pathology. Since 1996, mouse researchers have documented increased lifespan in at least nine other mutations, of which five others, like the Ames and Snell mutations, lead to lower levels of or responses to GH and/or its mediator insulin-like growth factor I (IGF-I).

These observations, on calorically restricted (CR) rodents and now also in mutant mice, justify a sea change in thinking about aging and its relationship to disease. The new framework includes two key tenets: (1) the aging process, despite the complexity of its many effects, can usefully be considered as a single, coordinating mechanism and (2) the rate at which aging progresses can be decelerated in mammals as well as in other taxa. From this perspective, a fundamental challenge to biogerontologists is to develop and test models of how age-dependent changes are themselves coregulated, during middle age, to produce old people or old mice or old worms. Studies of the aged, as opposed to studies of aging, are relevant to this challenge only insofar as they are exploited to generate or test ideas about coregulation and synchrony, rather than ideas about disease-specific pathogenesis. The key resource for meeting the challenge is not comparisons between young and old donors, but rather comparisons between young or middle-aged adults who are known to be aging at different rates. Fortunately, the same experiments that have documented the malleability of aging rate have done so by producing sets of animals that do indeed age at normal or slower-than-normal paces. With luck, future studies may produce at least tentative answers to the two key questions in biogerontology: How does aging produce the signs and symptoms of aging and what controls the rate of this process in mammals?

Key Themes from Studies of Invertebrate Models

Four main ideas have emerged, in the period 1990–2008, from studies of genetically convenient invertebrate models, the nematode worm *Caenorhabditis elegans* and the fruit fly *Drosophila melanogaster*. (1) Single gene mutations—lots of them—can extend lifespan in worms and flies (and mice). Most mutations discovered so far are "loss of function," in which eliminating or crippling the gene product leads to slower aging and lifespan extension. (2) The genes whose elimination slows aging are typically those used by the normal animal to notice and respond to environmental poverty; they are selected, by evolution, to permit the animal to take on alternate forms or functions to deal with the relative absence of nutritional conditions optimal for rapid growth and reproduction. Many of these genes are familiar to physicians and biological scientists: they encode insulin, insulin-like growth factors, possibly thyroid hormones, and other regulators of fuel usage and metabolic fluxes, as well as the intracellular proteins that change cell properties in response to these hormones. (3) The mutations that extend lifespan in worms and flies (and perhaps in mice) render the animals more resistant to lethal injury, such as that resulting from heavy metals, ultraviolet irradiation, heat, oxidizing agents, and chemicals that damage DNA. It thus seems plausible that augmentations of stress resistance are the mechanism by which these mutant genes slow aging. (4) This three-way association, connecting aging to stress to signals about nutrition, has very deep evolutionary roots and can be noted (albeit with species-specific nuances) in yeast, flies, worms, and mice. The suggestion here is that the pathways tying nutrition to stress to aging rate evolved extremely early in the eukaryotic lineage, in an ancestor predating the branch points between yeast, flies, worms, and vertebrates. The key implication is that investigations into the cell biology of these linked processes in conveniently short-lived organisms may provide valuable insights into aging and disease in humans.

Molecular Leads for Further Study

Studies of the invertebrate model systems have also called attention to a range of intracellular pathways that influence longevity, perhaps through regulation of resistance to a variety of forms of lethal and metabolic stress. Components of these pathways are now under scrutiny to see if they also affect aging and disease in rodents. Many of the antiaging mutations in worms, for example, act by increasing the actions of a DNA-binding factor called Daf-16, whose targets include genes that modulate resistance to oxidative damage, DNA repair, and other modes of cellular defense. The mammalian equivalent to Daf-16, a member of the FoxO group of transcription factors,

has already been implicated in control of cell death in human and rodent cells, and studies of the role of FoxO family members in aging are under way. A second family of proteins, the sirtuins, was initially implicated in lifespan regulation in studies of the budding yeast *Saccharomyces cerevisiae*, but then shown also to be able to increase lifespan in nematode worms. There is some evidence that members of the sirtuin family may contribute to the improved health and longevity of mice on a calorie-restricted diet, and interest in these proteins has been spurred by observations that median lifespan of mice on a diet high in saturated fat can be increased significantly by resveratrol, whose many biochemical effects include stimulation of sirtuin activity. Work with invertebrates has also brought new attention to the possible role of TOR, the "target of rapamycin," in control of lifespan and responses to dietary interventions. TOR plays a major role, conserved throughout the evolutionary tree, in regulating protein translation rates in response to both external cellular stress and the available supply of amino acids. TOR inhibition by rapamycin is a mainstay of clinical immunosuppressive therapy after organ transplantation, and TOR inhibitors also show promise as antineoplastic agents. Other molecular circuits, including those triggered by the p66 (shc) protein, the tumor-suppressor p53, and the stress-responsive kinase JNK, were initially discovered through work with rodents and now are also being examined in the context of invertebrate models for aging. Each of these biochemical pathways has powerful and still only partially defined links to hormonal signals, neoplastic transformation, stem cell homeostasis, and the balance between cell growth and cell death, so their elucidation is likely to provide both rationale and direction for translational work aimed at slowing the aging process and retarding age-related disease and dysfunction.

Delayed Aging in Mice and Rats

Caloric Restriction

Mice or rats fed approximately 30% or 40% less food than they would ordinarily consume typically live up to 40% longer than freely fed animals. These CR animals stay healthy and active, with good physical, sensory, and cognitive function, at ages at which most of the controls have already died. The intervention extends lifespan if initiated at very young ages (e.g., at weaning), or when started early in adulthood (e.g., at 6 months, in a species where puberty occurs at 2 months and median survival is about 28 months). Whether CR diets extend lifespan when initiated in animals already older than half the median lifespan is controversial, with some early studies suggesting little or no response, and some more recent experiments leading to a positive result. Lifespan can be extended using CR diets of widely varying composition, and there is strong evidence that total caloric intake, rather than proportions of specific fuel sources (carbohydrates, fats, proteins), is responsible for the beneficial effects. CR diets do not, except in the first few months after their imposition, alter metabolic rate or oxygen consumption per gram of lean body mass because CR rodents lose weight, or if adolescent fail to gain weight, so that lean body mass matches calorie supply once equilibrium is established. Although CR rodents are less obese than control animals, it seems unlikely that the effect of CR diets on aging is caused entirely by avoidance of obesity, in part because CR diets extend lifespan in mice genetically engineered to lack leptin (ob/ob mice). When placed on a CR diet, ob/ob mice are both longer lived and more obese than normal mice with normal caloric intake. There is some evidence that CR diets can delay at least some aspects of aging, for example, changes in immune function, in nonobese rhesus monkeys, but definitive evidence, based on lifespan data, is not yet available.

Mice and rats on CR diets show delay or deceleration in a very wide range of age-dependent processes, including neoplastic and nonneoplastic diseases, changes in structure and function of nearly all tissues and organs evaluated, endocrine and neural control circuits, and ability to adapt to metabolic, infectious, and cardiovascular challenges. Mouse stocks that have been engineered for vulnerability to specific lethal diseases, such as models of lupus or early neoplasia, also tend to live longer when placed on a CR diet. Intensive study of CR rodents in the past 20 years has suggested many ideas about the mechanism of its effects, including ideas about altered levels and responses to glucocorticoids and/or insulin, increases in stress-resistance pathways including resistance to oxidative injury, diminished inflammatory responses, changes in stem cell self-renewal, and many others, each plausible, none of them at this point more than plausible. Further work on the early and midterm effects of CR diets is among the most attractive avenues for testing basic ideas about aging in mammals.

Methionine-Restricted Diets

Rats fed a diet containing much reduced levels of the essential amino acid methionine were shown, in 1993, to live 40% longer than rats, on a standard diet, and more recent work has shown a similar, though smaller, effect on mice. These animals are not calorically restricted—they eat more calories, per gram of lean body mass, than control rats, and rats pair-fed normal food at levels that match the total caloric intake of a methionine-restricted (MR) rat show a much smaller degree of lifespan extension. MR diets could, in principle, affect aging by causing changes in protein translation or rate of protein turnover, by changes in DNA methylation (which depends upon metabolites of methionine), by alterations in levels or distribution of the antioxidant glutathione (also a metabolite of methionine), by changes in hormone levels (MR mice show low levels of insulin, glucose, and insulin-like growth factor 1, IGF-I), or by induction, through hormesis, of augmented stress response pathways at the cellular level. Some of these ideas could be tested using diets that restrict levels of other amino acids, and there is older, fragmentary evidence that such diets, too, may induce lifespan extension in rodents. MR is thus the second confirmed method for extending lifespan in mammals and comparisons of similarities and differences between CR and MR rodents are likely to prove highly informative.

Single-Gene Mutations That Extend Mouse Lifespan

The initial reports in the 1980s and 1990s that mutations of single genes in worms, and then in flies, could produce dramatic increases in lifespan were the strongest support, along with the CR data, for viewing aging as a unitary process that could be decelerated. The report in 1996 by Bartke and his colleagues that the lifespan of mice could be extended more than 40% by mutation of a gene required for pituitary development opened the door to new genetic models for study of aging in mammals. This Ames dwarf gene (Prop1) leads to an endocrine syndrome featuring low levels of growth hormone (GH), IGF-I, thyrotropins and the thyroxines, and prolactin. The observation that longevity in mice could be improved by reduction

of hormones in the insulin/IGF family, i.e., the same family of signals implicated in lifespan extension in worms and (later) flies, provided a key foundation for exploiting comparative cell biology in biogerontology research. Subsequent work then showed that similar degrees of lifespan extension could be seen in Snell dwarf mice, whose endocrine defects are very similar to those of Ames dwarfs, and also in mice that lack the GH receptor (GHR-KO mice) (Figure 1-1). This last observation, together with documented lifespan extension in mice lacking GH-releasing hormone receptor (GHRHR) and in mice with diminished expression of the IGF-I receptor (IGF1R heterozygotes), suggested strongly that a common factor, i.e., low production of or response to IGF-I, is a major cause of lifespan extension in all five models, although it is certainly possible that other factors, such as altered insulin sensitivity, thyroid tonicity, adipokine levels, etc., may contribute to antiaging effects in some of these mouse models. Male and female mice are affected by each of these mutations except that the effect of the IGF1R mutation seems stronger in females than in males. Mice in which tissue levels of IGF-I are reduced by genetic manipulation of a protease that controls local concentrations of IGF-I binding proteins are also long-lived, again consistent with models in which abnormally low IGF-I levels cause lifespan extension in mice. Studies of Snell and Ames dwarf mice have shown that the exceptional longevity of these mice is accompanied by a delay or deceleration of age-dependent changes in T lymphocytes, skin collagen, renal pathology, lens opacity, cognitive function, and neoplastic progression; taken with the lifespan data, these observations suggest strongly that these mutations, like the CR diet, act to slow the aging process itself.

In addition to the six mutations that lead to lower levels of IGF-I signals, there are now five other mutations that have been shown, in each case in a single unreplicated report, to extend lifespan in mice. Table 1-1 presents a summary of these 11 published mutations that extend maximal lifespan in mice. Transgenic overexpression of urokinase-type plasminogen activator in the brain has been reported to produce a significant extension of lifespan, perhaps by suppression of appetite with consequent mimicry of a CR diet. Mice in which the insulin receptor has been inactivated specifically in adipose tissue show an 18% lifespan increase, consistent with the idea that altered insulin sensitivity or adipokine levels might play a role in aging rate in this species. Transgenic mice overexpressing the klotho protein, a cofactor for fibroblast growth factor (FGF) signals whose absence leads to early death by elevation of vitamin D levels, have been reported to live 19% to 31% longer than controls, perhaps reflecting the ability of klotho to block insulin or IGF-I signals. A mutation that inactivates the 66 kDa splice variant of the Shc protein, involved in the pathway to programmed cell death after exposure to hydrogen peroxide or ultraviolet light, also extends longevity (by about 28%), as does transgenic overexpression, in mitochondria, of catalase, an enzyme involved in detoxification of hydrogen peroxide (a 20% lifespan increase). These last two reports, if confirmed in other laboratories, may give new insights into the connections linking aging and late-life diseases to agents that damage DNA or induce oxidative injury at intracellular sites.

More work is needed to determine to what extent these mutations influence common pathways, to see whether they do or do not influence aging through the same mechanism. It is possible, for example, that some of these mutations diminish risk of cancer, a common cause of death in many inbred mouse strains, without effect on any other age-dependent trait, while others may modulate the effects of aging on multiple organ systems, thus diminishing mortality risk

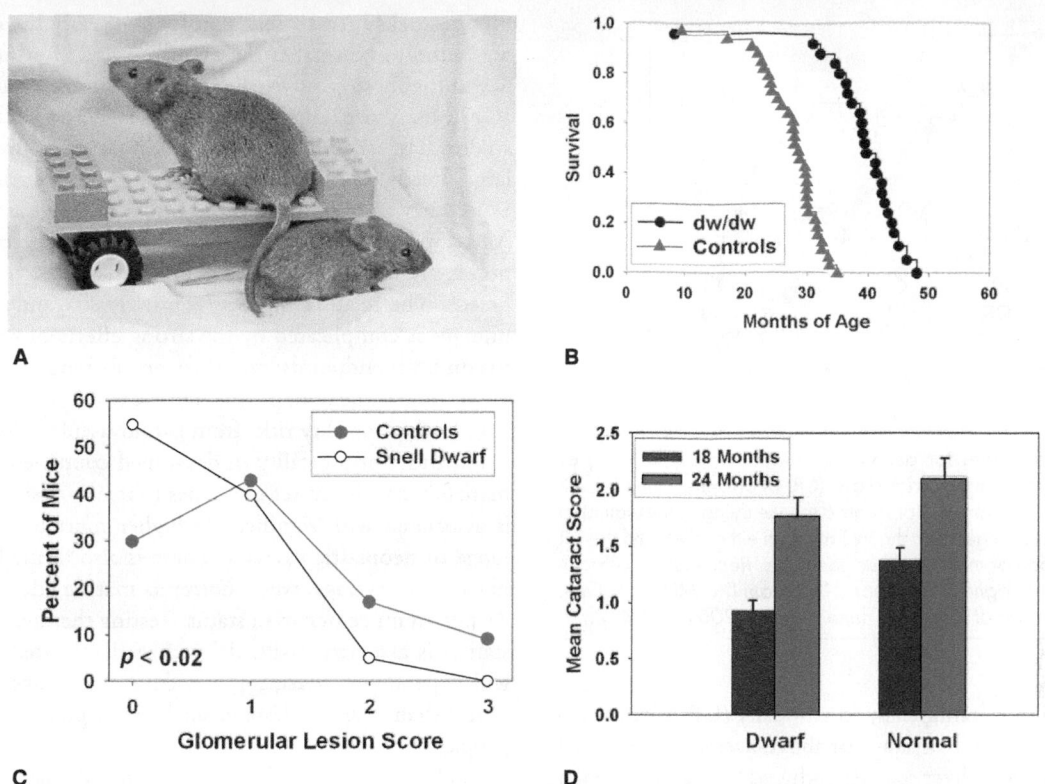

FIGURE 1-1. (A) A young adult Snell dwarf mouse, with a littermate control (on the vehicle). (B) Survival curves for Snell dwarf (dw/dw) mice and littermate controls. (C) Glomerular basement pathology scores, at terminal necropsy, for Snell dwarf ($N = 40$) and control ($N = 46$) mice. Higher scores indicate a greater degree of kidney pathology. Despite living 40% longer, a higher percent of Snell dwarfs had 0 scores at necropsy and a smaller percent had scores of 2 or 3. (D) Cataract scores determined by slit lamp examination in Snell dwarf and littermate control mice at 18 and 24 months of age. $p < 0.001$ for the difference between dwarfs and controls at each age. (B) *Data from Flurkey K, Papaconstantinou J, Miller RA, Harrison DE. Lifespan extension and delayed immune and collagen aging in mutant mice with defects in growth hormone production. Proc Natl Acad Sci U S A. 2001;98(12):6736–6741.* (C and D) *Data from Vergara M, Smith-Wheelock M, Harper JM, Sigler R, Miller RA. Hormone-treated Snell dwarf mice regain fertility but remain long-lived and disease resistant. J Gerontol Biol Sci. 2004;59:1244–1250.*

from both neoplastic and nonneoplastic diseases. There are hints, for example, that CR diets and the Ames dwarf gene may affect longevity by different mechanisms. As shown in Figure 1-2, caloric restriction extends lifespan in normal as well as in dwarf mice, and the Ames mutation extends lifespan on both CR and control diets, showing

that the effects are at least partly additive. The survival curves in Figure 1-2 also suggest that the Ames dwarf mutation may be affecting the age at which deaths begin to occur ("delay" of aging), and that the CR diet may affect, instead, the rate at which deaths occur once mortality risks become detectable ("deceleration" of aging). Dwarf

TABLE 1-1

Mouse Mutants That Improve Longevity

MUTATION	EFFECT ON LIFESPAN (%)	COMMENT
Ames dwarf (df), Prop1	50	Low GH, IGF-I, thyrotropin, thyroxine, prolactin
Snell dwarf (dw), Pit	42	Low GH, IGF-I, thyrotropin, thyroxine, prolactin
GHRHR (lit, little)	23	Low GH, IGF-I Survival increase on low-fat diet only
GHR-KO	42	Low IGF-I
IGF-I receptor	26	Heterozygous mice; significant only in females only
Pregnancy-associated plasma protein A, PAPP-A	38	Protease for IGF-I binding proteins
Klotho transgenic	19–31	Impairs insulin and IGF-I signals
Insulin receptor; FIRKO	18	Receptor diminished in adipose cells only
Shc-66	28	Lower apoptosis after UV, H_2O_2
Urokinase-type plasminogen activator, uPA	18	Transgenic, expressed in brain; may suppress appetite.
Catalase transgenic, MCAT	19	Overexpression in mitochondria only

FIRKO, fat-specific insulin receptor knockout; GH, growth hormone; GHRHR, growth hormone–releasing hormone receptor; GHR-KO, growth hormone receptor knockout; IGF-I, insulin-like growth factor I; MCAT, mitochondria-specific catalase transgenic; PAPP-A, pregnancy-associated plasma protein A; UV = ultraviolet; Pit-1, POU domain, class 1, transcription factor 1; Prop-1, prophet of Pit-1; Shc-66, 66 kDa splicing isoform of Src homology 2 domain containing transforming protein 1.

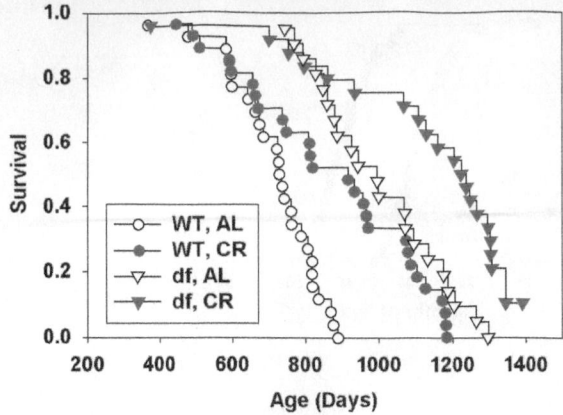

FIGURE 1-2. Survival curves for genetically normal (wild-type [WT]) or Ames dwarf (df) mice on caloric-restricted diet (CR) or on unrestricted ad libitum (AL) food intake. Each symbol represents a mouse dying at the indicated age. The dwarf mice live longer than the WT mice on either diet, and the CR diet extends the life span of mice of either genotype. *Reproduced with permission from Bartke A, Wright JC, Mattison JA, Ingram DK, Miller RA, Roth, GS. Extending the lifespan of long-lived mice. Nature. 2001;414:412.*

and CR mice also differ dramatically in adiposity (CR mice are extremely lean; dwarf mice have average or above-average proportions of fat), and in resistance to liver toxicity induced by acetaminophen poisoning. Analysis of the mechanisms by which each of the mutations shown in Table 1-1 affects lifespan and age-dependent traits will help to sort out questions about whether initial mortality rate and mortality rate doubling time are under separate physiological control.

As Table 1-1 suggests, the evidence from mice indicates that diminution of IGF-I levels, either in early life, adult life, or perhaps both, can create mice that are long-lived compared to controls. The association has also been noted using experimental designs in which individual mice are tested for IGF-I levels as young adults: those mice with the lowest IGF-I levels were found to live significantly longer than those with higher IGF-I concentrations. Similarly,

mouse stocks bred by selection for slow early life growth trajectory are found to be smaller than controls and also longer-lived. There is also highly suggestive evidence for a similar relationship between IGF-I, body size, and lifespan in dogs and horses. For dogs, several studies have shown greater longevity in small-size breeds than in large breeds, and a strong relationship between body size and life expectancy among mixed-breed (mongrel) dogs as well (Figure 1-3). Anecdotal and limited published data suggest that pony breeds of horses are also substantially longer lived than horses of full-sized breeds. The relationship between body size and life expectancy in humans is complicated by the strong effects of socioeconomic status on both endpoints: wealthier people tend to be both taller and longer-lived than poor people. On the whole, tall stature is associated with lower mortality risks from cardiovascular diseases, which are a major cause of mortality in developed countries. In contrast, a remarkably consistent set of studies (Table 1-2) show that tall stature is associated with significantly higher mortality risk from a wide range of neoplastic diseases. There is also limited data that centenarians, on average, were shorter as mature adults than those who do not attain centenarian status. Testing the idea that short midlife stature is associated with delayed or decelerated aging in humans will depend on measuring a wide range of age-dependent traits, rather than merely lifespan, on large populations of middle-aged people.

Stress Resistance and Aging

Mutations that extend lifespan in invertebrates typically render the animals resistant to multiple forms of lethal injury, whether the threat comes from oxidative agents, heat, heavy metals, or irradiation. Indeed, this stress resistance seems likely to represent the mechanism by which these mutations delay the aging process. Thus presumably much of the cellular and extracellular pathology that produces dysfunction and increases mortality risk in older animals is held in abeyance by the same, poorly defined, defenses that permit nematodes and flies to survive when exposed to external stress in an experimental setting. Genetic dissection of the relevant pathways has

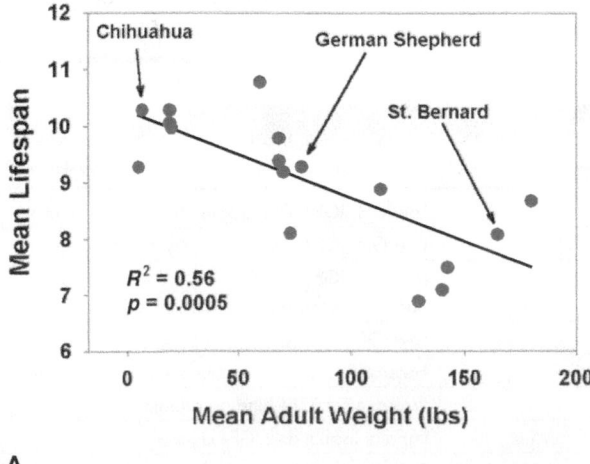

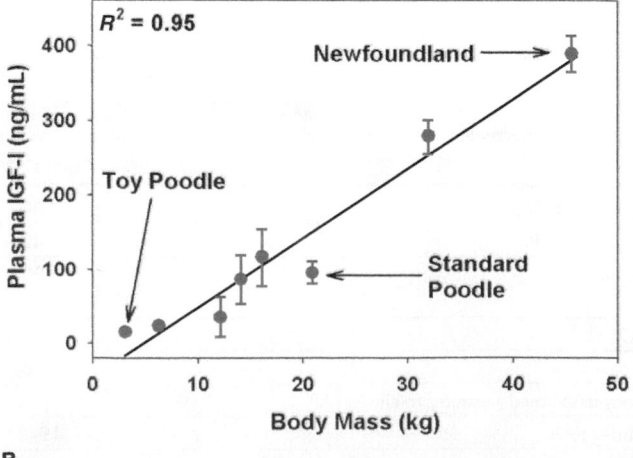

A

B

FIGURE 1-3. Longevity, size, and insulin-like growth factor I (IGF-I) levels among breeds of purebred dogs. Left panel shows mean breed lifespan as a function of mean breed weight for each of 16 breeds of dogs; three breeds are indicated by arrows. *Data from Li Y, Deeb B, Pendergrass W, Wolf N. Cellular proliferative capacity and life span in small and large dogs. J Gerontol A Biol Sci Med Sci. 1996;51(6):B403–B408.* Right panel shows mean plasma IGF-I levels as a function of body mass in eight breeds of purebred dogs. *For details and citations see Miller and Austad. Growth and aging: why do big dogs die young? In: Masoro EJ, Austad, SN, eds. Handbook of the Biology of Aging. 6th ed., New York, New York: Academic Press; 2006.*

TABLE 1-2

Population-Based Association Between Short-Stature and Lower Mortality Risk for Multiple Neoplastic Diseases

TEST POPULATION	TALL PEOPLE DO BETTER	SHORT PEOPLE DO BETTER
15,000 Scots	All-cause stroke Coronary disease	Colorectal, prostate, hematopoietic cancers
12,000 NHANES (United States); men		Cancers; 40–60% effect; adjusted for race, smoking, income
NHANES women		Breast and colorectal cancer
22,000 U.S. male physicians		Cancer; adjusted for age, BMI, exercise, smoking
570,000 Norwegian women		Breast cancer
400,000 American women		Breast cancer, postmenopause
1.1 million Norwegians		Esophageal cancer
England and Wales (by county)	All-cause mortality Ischemic heart disease	Breast, prostate, ovarian cancer

NHANES, National Health and Examination Survey.
For reference citations, see Miller RA, Austad, SN. Growth and aging: why do big dogs die young? In: Masoro EJ, Austad SN, eds. Handbook of the Biology of Aging. 6th ed. New York, New York: Academic Press; 2006:512–533.

shown, surprisingly, that in normal, nonmutant worms, the levels of stress resistance, and thus resistance to aging, are actively diminished by specific DNA-binding transcription factors. These factors, whose human homologs are members of the FoxO family, are retained by evolutionary pressures because they provide reproductive advantages in the natural environment, in which animals must be able to quickly take advantage of transient access to nutrients. Genetic inactivation of these FoxO pathways in the laboratory produces mutant animals that are not ideally suited for natural conditions, but which are resistant to many kinds of stress and which age more slowly than normal. Studies of gene expression patterns in the long-lived mutant worms have shown that the FoxO proteins can trigger transcription of over 100 genes that together protect against many different forms of cellular damage. The list includes enzymes that destroy free radicals, heat shock proteins, and other chaperones that guard against misfolded proteins, proteins that protect against infection, and chelating agents that bind toxic metal ions, among others.

The connection between induction of these stress-resistance pathways and late-life diseases has been shown by two sets of informative experiments. In the first, genetically identical worms were exposed to a brief, nonlethal heat stress, and physically separated into those that showed a strong response of chaperone proteins and those that did not. Worms with the most robust response to transient stress were found to be longer lived than those with lower stress responses. A second approach involved worms bearing genetic variants that cause aggregation of proteins and neurodegeneration (Huntington's disease) in people; neurological dysfunction in these worms can be delayed, and in some cases prevented entirely, by augmentation of the FoxO-dependent stress-resistance pathways. Similarly, age-dependent increases in susceptibility to stress-induced cardiac arrhythmias in *Drosophila* can be significantly postponed by activation of FoxO-dependent protective pathways.

Studies of the relationship of stress resistance to aging in mammals are underway, but suggestive data have begun to emerge. Both CR diets and at least some of the long-lived endocrine mutant stocks show elevated levels of enzymes with antioxidant action, heavy metal chelators, and intracellular chaperone proteins, as well as have lower levels of oxidative damage to DNA, proteins, and lipids. Cells grown, in tissue culture, from long-lived Snell and Ames dwarf mutant mice, or from mice lacking GH receptor, are resistant to lethal injury caused by cadmium, peroxide, heat, a DNA alkylating agent (MMS), ultraviolet light, and paraquat (which induces mitochondrial damage by free radical generation). Mice prepared by CR or MR diets are resistant to liver damage induced by the oxidative hepatotoxin acetaminophen, and long-lived mutant mice are somewhat more resistant to death induced by paraquat injection. Stress resistance also seems to play a role in evolution of long-lived species in that cells from long-lived rodents and other mammals are resistant in culture to several forms of oxidative and nonoxidative damage. This work provides initial support for models that attribute variations in aging rate to differences in stress resistance pathways, but many questions remain unanswered at this early stage. Figure 1-4 shows representative results for resistance to stress in long-lived mutant worms and cells from long-lived mutant mice, as well as data on resistance of CR and MR mice to an oxidative hepatotoxin. Figure 1-5 presents data from two studies showing stress resistance in culture of cells from longer-lived mammalian species.

Genetic Approaches to Analysis of Aging in Humans

Attempts to find genetic variations that influence aging in humans have been plagued with practical and conceptual problems in addition to the obvious difficulty that selection of mating partners is not amenable to experimental control. For one thing, heritability calculations show that only about 15% to 20% of the variation in lifespan among humans can be attributed to genetic factors. Furthermore, an unknown but potentially large fraction of this genetic variation probably reflects genetic variants that influence susceptibility to diseases of childhood, infectious agents, and specific common illnesses of old age. For example, genetic variants that cause Huntington's disease or type 1 diabetes or which triple the normal risk of myocardial infarction by the age of 50 years would all contribute to the measured heritability of lifespan, but do so by altering mortality risks from a specific form of illness rather than by alteration of aging with its effects on multiple late-life traits. Thus genetic variants that mold lifespan by effects on aging per se, if they exist at all, are likely to influence only a small fraction of variation (perhaps 5%) in how long people live.

Formal analyses of the genetics of human aging have so far relied mostly on candidate gene approaches, in which the investigator

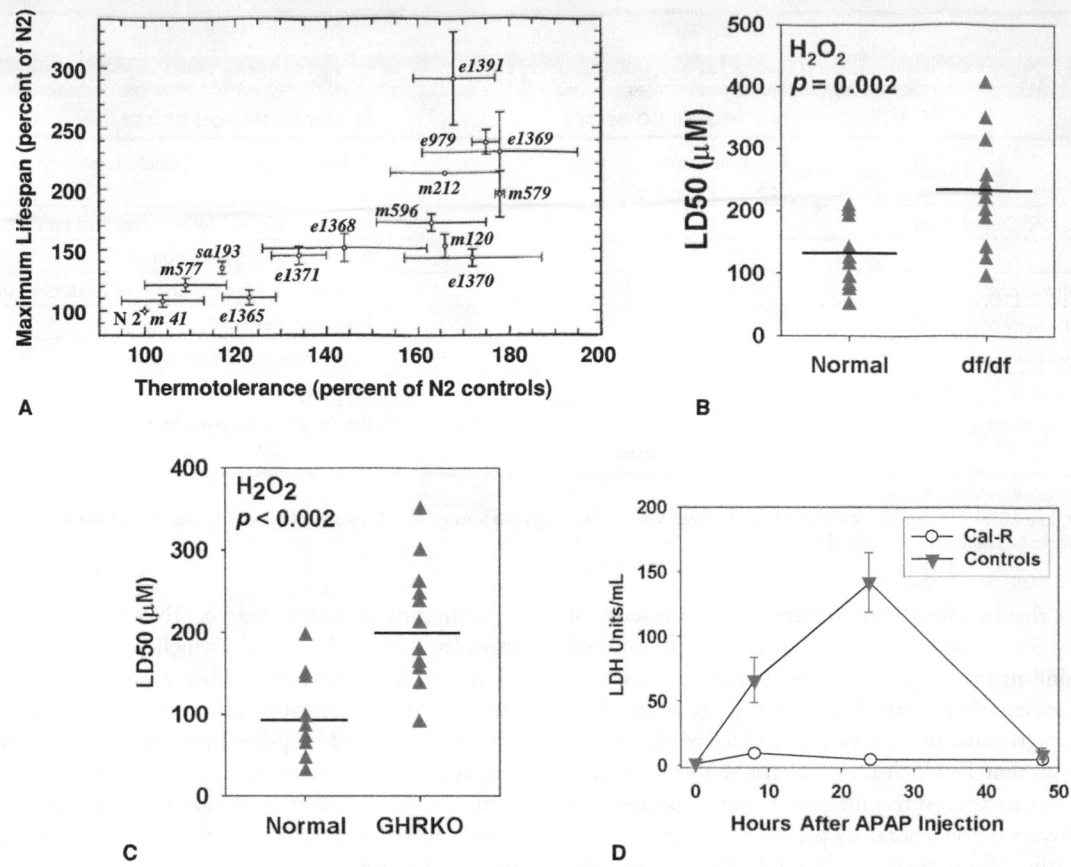

FIGURE 1-4. Association of stress resistance to longevity. (A) Resistance to heat shock (thermotolerance) is higher in mutant worms that have extended longevity. Each point is the mean for one mutant strain. (B) Resistance of skin-derived fibroblasts to lethal hydrogen peroxide concentrations is higher in cells from Ames dwarf (df/df) mice compared to controls. Each symbol shows an individual mouse. (C) Hydrogen peroxide (H_2O_2) resistance of skin-derived fibroblasts from long-lived growth hormone receptor knock out (GHRKO) mice. LD50 is the amount of peroxide that kills 50% of the cells. (D) Resistance of calorie-restricted (Cal-R) mice to liver injury induced by injection of acetaminophen (APAP); serum LDH levels indicate the level of damage to hepatocytes at varying intervals after a single injection (unpublished data of Chang and Miller). (A) *Reproduced with permission from Gems D, Sutton AJ, Sundermeyer ML, et al. Two pleiotropic classes of daf-2 mutation affect larval arrest, adult behavior, reproduction and longevity in Caenorhabditis elegans. Genetics. 1998;150:129–155. (B and C) Reproduced with permission from Salmon AB, Murakami S, Bartke A, Kopchick J, Yasumura K, Miller RA. Fibroblast cell lines from young adult mice of long-lived mutant strains are resistant to multiple forms of stress. Am J Physiol Endocrinol Metab. 2005;289(1):E23–E29.*

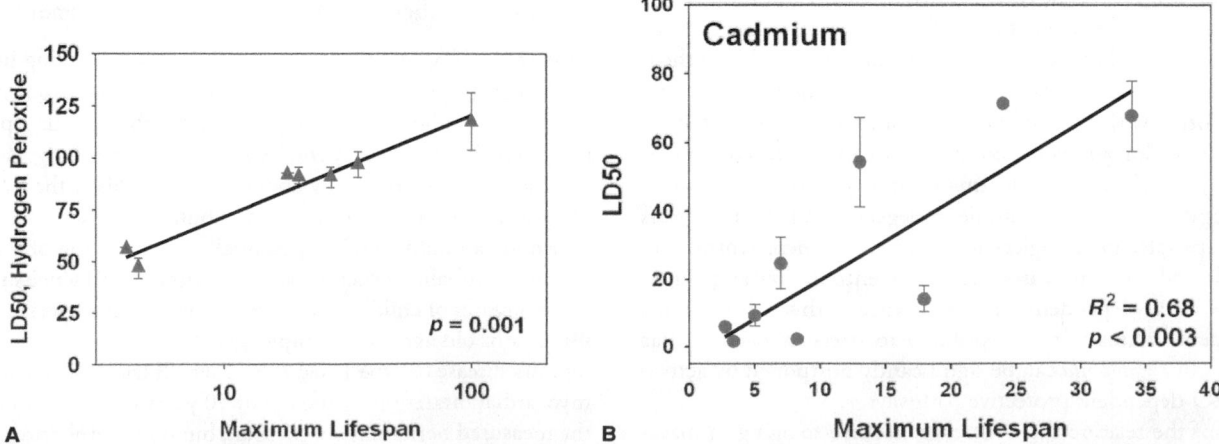

FIGURE 1-5. Stress resistance in fibroblasts from animals of long-lived species. Left panel: Resistance of cultured skin fibroblasts to hydrogen peroxide as a function of species maximum lifespan in years. Species, from left to right, are hamster, rat, rabbit, sheep, pig, cow, and human. *Reproduced with permission from Kapahi P, Boulton ME, Kirkwood TB. Positive correlation between mammalian life span and cellular resistance to stress. Free Radic Biol Med. 1999;26(5–6):495–500.* Right panel: Resistance of cultured skin fibroblasts to cadmium as a function of species maximum lifespan in years. Species, left to right, are laboratory mouse, wild-caught mouse, rat, red squirrel, white-footed mouse, deer mouse, fox squirrel, porcupine, beaver, and little brown bat. LD50 is the amount of hydrogen peroxide or cadmium that kills 50% of the cells. *Reproduced with permission from Harper JM, Salmon AB, Leiser SF, Galecki AT, Miller RA. Skin-derived fibroblasts from long-lived species are resistant to some, but not all, lethal stresses and to the mitochondrial inhibitor rotenone. Aging Cell. 2007;6:1–13.*

evaluates long-lived and control populations for variations at one or a small number of genetic loci, selected on theoretical grounds as most likely to be involved in aging or disease processes. The alternate approach, whole genome screening of large populations for association of longevity to hundreds of thousands of genetic variants, is also beginning to produce initial results at an accelerating pace. Although most of the published studies, and those in progress, focus on nuclear genes, there are tantalizing suggestions from studies of large families that a surprisingly high proportion of inherited effects on lifespan may come through the maternal line alone, suggesting that variations in mitochondrial gene sequences (which are inherited almost entirely from mothers to both sons and daughters) may also influence life expectancy in humans.

A major problem with all these approaches, from the perspective of biological gerontology, is the lack of a defensible phenotype: a measure of aging better than lifespan. There are now several dozen reports of candidate loci at which particular alleles are overrepresented among centenarians or near-centenarians, and advocates of this strategy hope that among this collection are some loci that control aging rate. But skeptics note that alleles that increase risk of cardiac disease, or Alzheimer's disease, or stroke, or various common forms of cancer, or severe osteoporosis are likely to have contributed to disease and death before the age of 90 or 100 years, and thus to have been eliminated or greatly reduced among the very old. Thus it should be assumed that a collection of genetic loci whose frequency discriminates very old people from others of the same birth cohort will include many genes with influence over common forms of lethal illnesses rather than genes that modulate aging per se. This problem is not one that can be solved by technological innovation or larger numbers of tested subjects; it requires development of a phenotype that provides more information about health in old age than merely a record of the age at death. For example, a genetic allele that identified, among 70-year-old people, those most likely to have excellent eyesight and hearing, no history of cancer, angina, diabetes, or arthritis, above-average responses to vaccination, and retention of baseline levels of cognition and muscle strength would be a much stronger candidate for an authentic "antiaging" gene than one that predicted survival to the age of 100 years.

Models of Accelerated Aging

There are a small number of rare, inherited, diseases, of which Werner's syndrome and Hutchinson-Gilford syndrome are the most celebrated, that have been mooted as possible examples of "accelerated" aging. Some of the physical features and symptoms of these diseases do resemble, at least superficially, some of the changes that typically affect older people, including in particular changes in skin and connective tissues. Hutchinson-Gilford syndrome, sometimes called "progeria," is now known to be caused by mutations in the gene for Lamin A, a component of the nuclear membrane. Werner's syndrome patients usually have mutations in an enzyme ("WRN") that has activity as a DNA helicase (unwinding coiled DNA) and as an endonuclease. Patients with Hutchinson-Gilford syndrome typically survive to their early teens, and Werner's syndrome patients frequently survive to their mid-forties, about 10 years after the age of typical diagnosis.

However, it is highly debatable whether either of these diseases provides strong clues about the molecular or cellular basis for age-related changes in normal individuals. Werner's patients do resemble elderly people in some ways: they frequently suffer from cataracts and premature graying of the hair, and by their early thirties often develop osteoporosis, diabetes, and atherosclerosis. On the other hand, many features of normal aging are not seen in Werner's patients and many features of Werner's syndrome are not seen in normal old individuals. Werner's syndrome patients, for example, do not show signs of Alzheimer's disease or other amyloidoses, hypertension, or immune failure. Mesenchymal tumors, which are rare in normal people, are about 100-fold more frequent in Werner's patients, but the epithelial and hematopoietic tumors characteristic of normal aging are not seen in Werner's syndrome patients. Furthermore, Werner's patients exhibit many features that are not seen in normal aging, including subcutaneous calcifications, altered fat distribution, vocal changes, flat feet, malleolar ulcerations, high levels of urinary hyaluronic acid, and a number of other idiosyncrasies not seen commonly in elderly individuals. Mice with mutations in the WRN gene live a normal lifespan and do not show signs of premature senescence. It seems possible that investigation of the pathogenesis of Werner's syndrome may provide key clues to the mechanisms of age-related diseases. But it seems at least equally plausible that the WRN mutation, perhaps through alteration of cells responsible for connective tissue maintenance, induces multiorgan failure through processes quite distinct from the changes that impair some of the same organs in normal aging.

AGING, CELLULAR SENESCENCE, TELOMERES, AND CANCER

The famous observation of Hayflick that human diploid fibroblasts cease to grow in culture after a limited number of population doublings sparked a line of experimentation that continues to yield important insights into the molecular control of cell growth, differentiation, and neoplastic transformation. Human fibroblasts placed in tissue culture will continue to divide until approximately 50 cell doublings have occurred, after which the remaining cells can survive indefinitely in a healthy but nondividing state. In the 1970s and 1980s, this "clonal senescence" model seemed to be an attractive approach to study the genetics and cell biology of aging. It is now clear that growth cessation of continuously passaged human fibroblasts is caused principally by the progressive loss of telomeric DNA at the ends of each chromosome at each mitosis. The chemistry of DNA replication requires that duplication of the end of each DNA molecule be conducted by a specialized enzyme complex called telomerase, and telomeres will therefore become shorter at each cell division except in cells, like most tumor cells, that express telomerase. The very short telomeres that eventually develop in proliferating cells then trigger, through steps not yet fully defined, expression of new genes that block further mitotic cycles but do not lead to cell death.

The challenge of showing that this in vitro system can deliver important clues about the biology of aging, that is, about the process that converts healthy young adults into old people, has remained a serious hurdle. The most obvious possibility is that some of the diseases and disabilities of the elderly population might represent a loss, with age, in proliferative capacities of one or more cell types. But there are many reasons to be skeptical of analogies between growth cessation of cells in continuous culture and the complex network of reinforcing failures that lead to aging of intact organisms. For one thing, aging clearly leads to dysfunction of many cell types that do not divide at all, like neurons and skeletal muscle myocytes, and to dysfunction of extracellular structures like teeth, cartilage, and lens, and it is difficult to see how clonal senescence can affect these processes. Telomere erosion has been postulated to contribute to dysfunction of memory T cells in elderly subjects; but it is hard on this ground to explain the equally poor function, in the same subjects, of naïve memory T cells, whose telomeres are similar in old age to those of memory cells found in young adults. In addition, there are many cell types, such as intestinal crypt stem cells and hematopoietic progenitor cells, that can divide many thousands of times over the course of a lifespan, but which nonetheless show age-related functional decline. In addition, telomere-dependent replicative failure cannot be responsible for the effects of aging in mice or rats, or indeed in the many other species known to have longer telomeres and shorter lives than humans. If 70 years of human lifespan are just sufficient to produce perceptible shortening of the 6 to 10 kilobases of human telomeres, it is hard to see how the 2 to 3 years of rodent lifespan could have much impact on the 20 to 100 kilobases of telomeric deoxyribonucleic acid (DNA) with which rats and mice are endowed. Furthermore, genetic manipulations have produced lines of mice whose telomeres are indeed at the same, short length seen in proliferating cell types in elderly humans. While these mice show specific abnormalities (skin ulceration, infertility, frequently lethal gastrointestinal lesions, and increased frequencies of certain forms of neoplasia), they do not resemble normal aged mice in most respects.

The possibility that clonal senescence might contribute to some of the signs of aging thus faces some serious obstacles, but perhaps not insuperable ones. There is evidence that the cellular changes ("cell senescence") induced in human cells by overshort telomeres might be triggered, in human and nonhuman cells, as a response to other forms of DNA damage, and it is thus possible that senescent cells could accumulate, with advancing age, through different mechanisms in long-lived and short-lived species. Early work based on histological assays suggested that senescent cells were rare (less than 0.1%), even in biopsies from very old donors, although new methods for detecting other aspects of the senescent phenotype have led to upward revisions of this estimate. It remains a challenge, however, to develop and test models to explain how properties of tissues, organs, and multiorgan systems (like the brain and endocrine circuits) might be altered by the presence of a small admixture of nondividing senescent cells. Senescent cells in vitro express a suite of secreted enzymes and cytokines that are not produced by dividing fibroblasts and it is possible that these may contribute to aging at the tissue or organ level.

Telomere-dependent clonal senescence does seem to play a critical role in the protection of humans from many forms of late-life cancer. The key finding was the observation that telomerase is turned on, and telomere diminution prevented or reversed, in approximately 90% of clinically significant human neoplasias. It thus seems likely that short telomeres and stringently repressed telomerase gene expression evolved during the course of human evolution to protect us against fatal neoplasias that would otherwise arise early in life. Because most cancers are clonal, and each clinically significant tumor represents the outcome of several stages of selection for rare cellular variants for independence from growth control, resistance to immune defenses, and barriers to metastasis, evolution of large-bodied species, with a much higher number of potential target cells for neoplas-

tic transformation should require development of strong antitumor defenses not needed in smaller creatures. The average human has approximately 3000 times as many cells as a mouse; if each had the same annual likelihood of neoplastic transformation as a mouse cell, the annual cancer incidence in humans would be 3000 times higher than in mice. In fact, however, humans usually avoid neoplasia over a lifetime that is 30 times longer than the mouse's lifespan; evolution has developed strategies that reduce per cell transformation rate by a factor of about 90 000 in evolving humans from shorter-lived, smaller progenitor species. These defenses may well include telomere-based clonal senescence responses, as well as improvements in repair of somatic mutations and reduction of intracellular levels of DNA-modifying agents. There is no reason to believe, however, that evolved defenses against cancer in humans could not be further improved: similar considerations show that whale cells, for example, are about 10 000-fold more resistant than human cells to neoplastic transformation.

Recent work on stem cell biology has suggested a key role for a specific protein, p16/INK4a, as a mediator of the balance between anticancer and antiaging mechanisms. INK4a is induced as part of the process by which cellular senescence halts cell proliferation. An increase in levels of INK4a in many tissues of aging mice, but particularly in stem cells, has suggested that senescent stem cells may indeed accumulate as a consequence of normal aging and may represent an evolved mechanism to prevent early life neoplasia. New evidence suggests that INK4a may lead, in parallel, to diminished stem cell function in the aging bone marrow, brain, and pancreas. Mice engineered to have lower levels of INK4a have now been shown to retain stem cell activities at ages at which these cells perform poorly in normal animals, even though the same mice are somewhat more cancer-prone than normal controls. Interventions that prevent age-related induction of INK4a might be an attractive approach to diminishing many forms of late-life illness in parallel if the intervention did not simultaneously increase cancer risk.

AGING RESEARCH AND PREVENTIVE MEDICINE

The central rationale for biological gerontology is the hope that discoveries in this field will lead to innovations in preventive medicine: an authentic antiaging drug that produced the same demographic changes seen in rodents on CR or MR diets would yield about 10-fold greater improvement in mean life expectancy than would the complete elimination of cancers or of myocardial infarctions (Figure 1-6). A detailed understanding of the molecular pathways that lead to coordinated stress resistance in cells of dwarf mice, or of the adjustments that render CR rats resistant to autoimmune, neoplastic, and degenerative diseases, or of the evolutionary changes that permit large animals to survive cancer-free and cataract-free for many decades should in principle suggest avenues to preventive medical care that could dramatically postpone disability and lethal illnesses. Empirical testing of drugs that are thought likely to slow the aging process in mice has already documented two compounds that can extend median lifespan significantly, either in mice consuming a high-fat diet (resveratrol) or in mice consuming a normal diet (nordihydroguiaretic acid); data on extension of maximum lifespan extension from these or other agents are likely to emerge in the next few years.

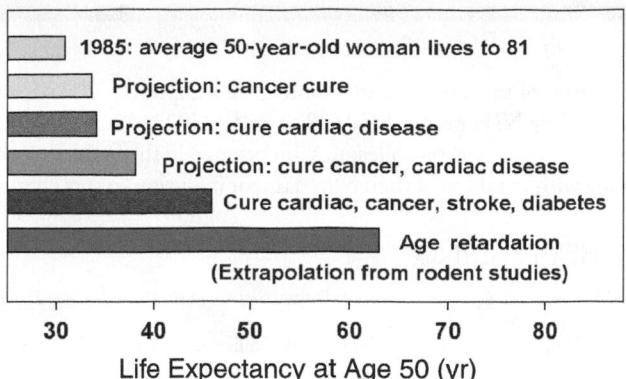

FIGURE 1-6. Theoretical remaining life expectancy of a 50-yr-old white woman in the United States under a variety of demographic assumptions. The top bar shows remaining life expectancy with disease-specific mortality rates that prevailed in 1985. The four middle bars show projected life expectancy under the assumption that mortality risks for the indicated diseases were in fact zero. *Data from Olshansky SJ et al. Science 1990;250:634.* The bottom line shows projected longevity if it were possible to retard human aging to the same degree that is obtained in the typical study of caloric restriction in rats or mice. *Figure reprinted with permission from Miller RA. Extending life: scientific prospects and political obstacles. Milbank Quart 2002;80:155–174.*

But the pathway connecting discovery in this area of basic science to intervention is strewn with obstacles, some scientific, but others political, economic, and legal. Even if research in mice or rats were to demonstrate a dramatic effect of a specific agent on the aging process, producing (for example) a 40% increase in mean and maximal lifespan, showing that the agent was able to safely extend human lifespan would require vast resources and treatment of young or middle-aged adult subjects for many decades. Pharmaceutical firms have little commercial incentive for embarking on expensive tests that might (or might not) demonstrate safety and efficacy of an agent many decades in the future, and governmental agencies, already strained by limited resources and competition among medical researchers with alternate priorities, are also unlikely to be able to support such an ambitious long-term undertaking. Indeed, the laws that govern testing of candidate drugs in the United States permit investigative studies only of agents proposed to treat or prevent a specific disease and explicitly exclude aging from consideration as a "disease" for the purposes of this classification. Nor are many scientists eager to devote their careers to an experiment whose conclusions are unlikely to emerge around the time of their own planned retirement. A hypothetical agent that is active in those already old could, in principle, be tested with a relative short follow-up, i.e., over a period of 5 to 10 years. However, there is at present no empirical evidence, or theoretical basis, for assuming that interventions that retard the aging process could be effective in older subjects in which this process has already led to major disruptions in cellular and tissue functions.

Introduction of authentic antiaging compounds into the practice of health care is thus likely to involve relatively unconventional pathways. The public has shown an unbridled appetite for consumption of compounds and mixtures, labeled as "nutritional supplements," which are exempt from laws that govern prescription and nonprescription drugs, and are purported to oppose the effects of aging. Thus far, there is no evidence that any of the agents so touted, in-cluding melatonin, dehydroepiandrosterone (DHEA), homeopathic remedies, and many others, can retard, delay, or reverse aging in humans or animal models. However, it seems possible that agents that did prove, in animal studies, to have the ability to delay or decelerate aging might make their way into human use, or into clinical trials. The high value placed by many dog and cat owners on the health of their pets may lead to sponsorship of trials of antiaging medications in these carnivores, whose lifespan is intermediate between rodents and humans; such trials might lead to further evidence of health and efficacy of the agents tested in a large mammal model. If a promising agent can be shown through typical short-term clinical tests to be useful for the treatment or prevention of a specific disease, Food and Drug Administration (FDA) approval for administration of the agent might then lead to further study of disease prevention and enhanced survival.

ANTIAGING RESEARCH: SOCIAL OBSTACLES AND ETHICAL CONCERNS

Serious research into the basic biology of aging, and proposed translational research to turn gerontological discoveries into antiaging medicines have long been hobbled by pessimism, specifically the assumption that aging is immutable, and by stigma, arising from claims made for allegedly effective antiaging potions promoted unscrupulously for commercial gain. For these reasons, many political and scientific leaders have been understandably shy of lending support for research efforts whose goal is to develop antiaging interventions for human use. Journalists, who are often aware of promising discoveries in biological gerontology, are nonetheless often drawn ineluctably toward promotion of extreme claims, which, while entertaining, go well beyond scientific evidence and thus further impair the credibility of the antiaging research enterprise. Although several decades of evidence has now clearly refuted the common assumption that the aging process is too complex or too stable to be altered, the attitudes and expectations of opinion leaders and the lay public greatly undermine and complicate efforts to attract support for this research agenda.

A related concern is often posed as a question of ethics: if the goal of antiaging research is to help keep people alive and healthy for several decades beyond their current "natural" lifespan, would not realization of this goal greatly complicate efforts to solve the current set of Malthusian dilemmas? In a world where resource depletion, food shortages, and environmental degradation already consign billions to great suffering, would not methods that delay aging and death lead to unacceptable exacerbations of these and related problems? Arguments along these lines are often influenced by the unstated assumption that old people are typically ill, unhappy, and unproductive, and a desire to avoid creating a society in which an ever-increasing proportion of the population has the problems that can afflict people at the very end of life.

This concern that development of antiaging medicines would be unethical is widespread, but easy to refute. Most of modern medical research is designed to help prevent or treat diseases with a high risk of mortality and thus to increase the likelihood that patients will enjoy additional years or decades of good health. Efforts to develop vaccines for influenza, or to eradicate residual tumor burden by adjuvant chemotherapy, or to correct arrhythmias, or the symptoms of diabetes or gall stones are all designed to allow patients to remain healthy and active as long as possible. These research efforts are appropriately considered ethical and indeed heroic, even though patients so treated are quite likely to encounter additional illnesses, often associated with suffering, at later ages. A similar motivation and justification underlies translational research in biological gerontology. Clearly, there is no pressing need for agents that merely prolong life in people who are in the final stages of a dementing illness or nearing death in great pain, and developing drugs that extend lifespan without improvements in health would not be an attractive goal. Fortunately, each of the dietary and genetic manipulations shown in rodent models to extend longevity does so by an increase in the length of healthy lifespan; postponement of death goes hand in hand (and is almost certainly caused by) postponement of a very wide range of diseases and forms of disabilities. A society in which many people remain active and productive at ages of 80–100 years or so would indeed require economic adjustments and alterations of assumptions about retirement ages and family structure, just as adjustments of this kind have been required as societies have experienced reductions in infant and childhood mortality that greatly increase the proportion of newborns that reach the ages of 20 to 50 years. Such adjustments are not trivial, but such fears have not raised concerns about the ethical merit of insulin therapy, vaccination programs, smoking cessation clinics, or adjuvant chemotherapy, and from this perspective it is hard to understand why success in antiaging research should be considered pernicious.

There is, however, a serious ethical concern about antiaging interventions that deserves more attention than it has received. There is some basis for believing that agents that decelerate aging, either by alteration of IGF-I signals or through the still undiscovered mechanisms used by CR and MR diets, might be more effective if imposed early in life, perhaps as early as the childhood years. In such a case, decisions about use of such preventive treatments might have to be made by parents on behalf of their young children. If such agents had side effects, such as postponement of puberty, or permanent short stature, would parents be acting ethically to impose these side effects on their children in order to provide them with additional decades of excellent health in adult life? Conversely, would parents be acting ethically to deny their children additional decades of healthy life just to allow them to grow to what is now considered "normal" height? Questions of this kind are harder to answer than concerns about whether postponement of late-life illnesses is or is not desirable on its own merits.

ACKNOWLEDGMENTS

Preparation of this chapter, and some of the unpublished data, was supported by NIH grants AG024824 and AG023122. I appreciate the willingness of several colleagues, mentioned in the figure legends, to share with me some of their own data for inclusion in this chapter.

FURTHER READING

Austad SN. *Why We Age: What Science Is Discovering About the Body's Journey Through Life*. Chichester: Wiley; 1999.

Bartke A, Wright JC, Mattison JA, Ingram DK, Miller RA, Roth GS. Extending the lifespan of long-lived mice. *Nature*. 2001;414:412.

Chen D, Guarente L. SIR2: a potential target for calorie restriction mimetics. *Trends Mol Med*. 2007;13:64–71.

Flurkey K, Papaconstantinou J, Miller RA, Harrison DE. Lifespan extension and delayed immune and collagen aging in mutant mice with defects in growth hormone production. *Proc Natl Acad Sci USA*. 2001;98(12):6736–6741.

Gems D, Sutton AJ, Sundermeyer ML, et al. Two pleiotropic classes of daf-2 mutation affect larval arrest, adult behavior, reproduction and longevity in *Caenorhabditis elegans*. *Genetics*. 1998;150:129–155.

Harper JM, Salmon AB, Leiser SF, Galecki AT, Miller RA. Skin-derived fibroblasts from long-lived species are resistant to some, but not all, lethal stresses and to the mitochondrial inhibitor rotenone. *Aging Cell* 2007;6:1–13.

InfoAging Web site. http://websites. afar.org [Accessed August 1, 2008]

Kapahi P, Boulton ME, Kirkwood TB. Positive correlation between mammalian life span and cellular resistance to stress. *Free Radic Biol Med*. 1999;26(5–6):495–500.

Kirkwood T. *Time of Our Lives: The Science of Human Aging*. Chichester: Oxford University Press; 2000.

Li Y, Deeb B, Pendergrass W, Wolf N. Cellular proliferative capacity and life span in small and large dogs. *J Gerontol A Biol Sci Med Sci*. 1996;51(6):B403–B408.

Miller RA. Extending life: scientific prospects and political obstacles. *Milbank Quart*. 2002;80:155–174.

Miller RA. Kleemeier Award Lecture: are there genes for aging? *J Gerontol Biol Sci*. 1999;54A:B297–B307.

Morimoto RI. Stress, aging, and neurodegenerative disease. *N Engl J Med*. 2006;355: 2254–2255.

Olshansky SJ, Hayflick L, Perls TT. Anti-aging medicine: the hype and the reality. *J Gerontol Ser A Biol Sci Med Sci*. 2004;59:B513–B514.

Olshansky SJ, Perry D, Miller RA, Butler RN. In pursuit of the longevity dividend: what should we be doing to prepare for the unprecedented aging of humanity? *Scientist*. March 2006:28–36.

Salmon AB, Murakami S, Bartke A, Kopchick J, Yasumura K, Miller RA. Fibroblast cell lines from young adult mice of long-lived mutant strains are resistant to multiple forms of stress. *Am J Physiol Endocrinol Metab* 2005;289(1):E23–E29.

Science of Aging Knowledge Environment. http://sageke.sciencemag.org/ [Accessed August 1, 2008]

Tatar M, Bartke A, Antebi A. The endocrine regulation of aging by insulin-like signals. *Science*. 2003;299:1346–1351.

Vergara M, Smith-Wheelock M, Harper JM, Sigler R, Miller RA. Hormone-treated Snell dwarf mice regain fertility but remain long-lived and disease resistant. *J Gerontol Biol Sci*. 2004;59:1244–1250.

Weindruch R, Sohal RS. 1997. Caloric intake and aging. *N Engl J Med*. 1997;337: 986–994.

Genetics of Age-Dependent Human Disease

Thomas B. L. Kirkwood

THE BIOLOGICAL NATURE OF INTRINSIC AGING

Understanding the biology of intrinsic aging is important for geriatricians because of the insights it provides into: (i) why and how the body becomes progressively more vulnerable to disability and disease as we grow older; (ii) how we might intervene in the underlying mechanisms; and (iii) what is the exact nature of the relationship between "normal" aging and age-related diseases. Although there is significant variability in how aging affects individuals, certain underlying processes appear to follow a common course. Furthermore, humans share some features of aging with a wide range of other animal species. Thus, even though much of the research on intrinsic aging is done using simple animal models such as the roundworm *Caenorhabditis elegans* or the fruitfly *Drosophila melanogaster*, it appears that common regulatory pathways are at least partially conserved across the spectrum that includes mammals, and in particular humans. This is especially the case for fundamental mechanisms that protect cells against shared threats such as damage to DNA arising from endogenous stressors like reactive oxygen species (ROS), which are essential molecular by-products of the body's dependence on oxygen to provide energy.

Why Aging Occurs

One of the central questions in the biology of aging is the nature of the genetic contribution to longevity. How do genes act on the aging process, and how does an individual's genetic endowment contribute to their longevity?

Aging and longevity are clearly influenced by genes. Firstly, the life spans of human monozygotic twin pairs are more similar than life spans of dizygotic twins. Secondly, there are differences in life span between different genetically inbred strains of any given laboratory animal, such as the mouse. Thirdly, studies of simple organisms like fruit flies, nematode worms, and yeast have identified gene muta-

tions that affect duration of life. However, although genes influence longevity, genes appear to account for only about 25% of the variance in human life span.

The nature of the genetic contribution to the aging process has received much attention, both from the perspective of evolutionary theory and through experimentation. The evolutionary angle is valuable because it can tell us a great deal about the kinds of genes that are likely to underlie the aging process. A commonly held belief is that aging evolved as an evolutionary necessity—for instance, to remove older individuals who might otherwise consume resources needed by the young. However, there is little support for the idea that aging does actually fulfill such a role. In nature, the vast majority of animals die young, long before they could become obstructive to the interests of the next generation. Out of a population of newborn wild mice, for example, nine out of 10 of them will be dead before 10 months even though half of the same animals reared in captivity would still be alive at 2 years. Thus, aging in mice is seen only in protected environments, and until relatively recently the same would have been true for human populations. It is only in the last 200 years that human life expectancy, even in the most advantaged countries, exceeded 40 years.

Since it is rare that an animal survives long enough to show any sign of aging, a genetically programmed means to limit population size and avoid overcrowding, if it exists, is not often brought into play. Furthermore, the idea that aging could be beneficial needs to be set against the fact that even if an animal did reach older age, the adverse effects of intrinsic senescence on fertility and risk of dying are far from beneficial as far as the individual is concerned. The idea of programmed aging rests on the notion that organisms should weaken and die altruistically, for the "good of the species." While there may be instances where natural selection has produced apparently altruistic outcomes, evolutionary biologists have carefully delineated the rather special circumstances required for this kind of selection force to work. Aging does not fit these requirements. The argument against programmed aging can be summarized by observing that if such a program did exist, what would prevent a mutation occurring that abrogated the program and allowed the mutant to survive indefinitely? The fact that such mutants are never observed is empirical support that backs up the other objections.

The evidence from nature is that instead of being programmed to die, organisms are genetically programmed to survive. However, in spite of a formidable array of survival mechanisms, most species appear not to be programmed well enough to last indefinitely. A key to understanding why this should be so, and what governs how long a survival period there should be, comes from studying survival patterns in wild populations. If 90% of wild mice are dead by the 10 months, any investment in programming for survival much beyond this point can benefit at most 10% of the population. This immediately suggests that there will be little evolutionary advantage in programming long-term survival capacity into a mouse. The argument is further strengthened by the observation that nearly all of the survival mechanisms required by the mouse to combat intrinsic deterioration (DNA damage, protein oxidation, etc.) require metabolic resources. Metabolic resources are scarce, as is evidenced by the fact that the major cause of mortality for wild mice is cold, due to insufficient energy to maintain body temperature. From a Darwinian point of view, the mouse will benefit more from investing any spare resource into thermogenesis or reproduction than into better DNA repair capacity than its need for longevity.

This concept, with its explicit focus on evolution of optimal levels of cell maintenance, is termed the "disposable soma" theory. In essence, the investments in durability and maintenance of somatic (nonreproductive) tissues are predicted to be sufficient to keep the body in good repair through the normal expectation of life in the wild environment, with some measure of reserve capacity. Thus, it makes sense that mice (with 90% mortality by 10 months) have intrinsic life spans of around 3 years, while humans (who probably experienced something like 90% mortality by the age of 50 years in our ancestral environment) have intrinsic life spans limited to about 100 years. The distinction between somatic and reproductive tissues is important because the reproductive cell lineage, or germ line, must be maintained at a level that preserves viability across the generations, whereas the soma needs only to support the survival of a single generation.

This concept helps to explain why species differ in their intrinsic life spans. It is noteworthy, for example, that species of birds and bats tend to have greater longevity than flightless species. The reason is thought to be that flight is a very successful way of reducing an animal's mortality risk, since it is possible to escape many predators and to forage over a greater range, thereby lessening the risk of starvation caused by a local food shortage. If risk is reduced, the statistical chance of living a bit longer is increased, and so it becomes worthwhile to invest in a higher level of somatic maintenance and repair. Studies comparing the biochemistry of cellular repair among long- and short-lived species bear this prediction out. Cells from long-lived organisms exhibit greater capacity to repair molecular damage and withstand biochemical stresses than cells from short-lived species.

The disposable soma theory provides a bridge between understanding not only why aging occurs but also how aging is caused in molecular and cellular terms. It thus extends earlier considerations by Medawar, who suggested that because organisms die young there is little force of selection to oppose the accumulation within the genome of mutations with late-acting deleterious effects, and

by Williams, who suggested that genes with beneficial effects would be favored by selection even if these genes had adverse effects at later ages. This is known as the theory of "antagonistic pleiotropy," the term pleiotropy meaning that the same gene can have different effects in different circumstances.

The current synthesis of evolutionary ideas about why aging occurs can thus be summarized in four points:

1. There are no specific genes for aging.
2. Genes of particular importance for aging and longevity are those governing durability and maintenance of the soma.
3. There may exist other genetically determined trade-offs between benefits to young organisms and their viability at older ages.
4. There may exist a variety of gene mutations with late deleterious effects that contribute to the senescent phenotype.

Given these points, it is clear that multiple genes contribute to the aging phenotype. A cornerstone of the current research agenda is to identify these genes and discover which are the most important.

Mechanisms of Aging

Aging appears to be driven by the progressive accumulation through life of a variety of random molecular defects that build up within cells and tissues. These defects start to arise very early in life, probably *in utero*, but in the early years, both the fraction of affected cells and the average burden of damage per affected cell are low. However, over time the faults increase, resulting eventually in age-related functional impairment of tissues and organs (Figure 2-1). This concept makes clear the life-course nature of the underlying mechanisms. Aging is a continuous process, starting early and developing gradually, instead of being a distinct phase that begins in middle to late life.

Since there are multiple kinds of molecular and cellular damage, and a corresponding variety of mechanisms to protect against and repair them, aging is a highly complex process involving multiple mechanisms at different levels. This multiplicity of candidate mechanisms can easily become confusing, particularly since those researching a specific mechanism have a tendency to suggest that their preferred choice is *the* mechanism that drives aging. It will be

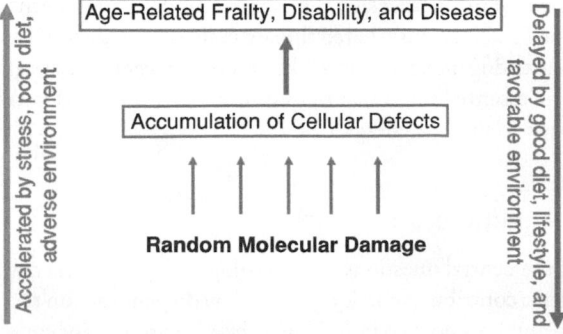

FIGURE 2-1. The aging process is driven by a lifelong accumulation of molecular damage, resulting in gradual increase in the fraction of cells carrying defects. After sufficient time has passed, the increasing levels of these defects interfere with both the performance and functional reserves of tissues and organs, resulting in age-related frailty, disability, and disease. Stress, adverse environment, and poor nutrition can increase the rate at which molecular damage arises. Intrinsic maintenance mechanisms, such as DNA repair and antioxidants, can slow the rate of accumulation.

apparent from the previous section that, in fact, it is highly unlikely that any single mechanism can tell the whole story. We will consider the prominent hypothesized mechanisms below. For each mechanism, there is evidence supporting the hypothesis that it is indeed an agent of senescence. However, the extent of the contribution to senescence is generally too small for the mechanism to be a sufficient explanation of age-related degeneration. The clear inference is that aging is multicausal and that the various mechanisms all play their part and are likely to interact synergistically. For example, a build-up of mitochondrial DNA mutations will lead to a decline in the cell's energy production, and this will reduce the capacity to carry out energy-dependent protein clearance. In recent years, novel methods based on computer modeling of interactions and synergism between different aging mechanisms have begun to build a better integrated picture of how cells break down with age and there is growing experimental evidence that interactions between multiple mechanisms are important.

Oxidative Damage

An important theme linking several different kinds of damage is the action of ROS (also known as free radicals), which are produced as by-products of the body's essential use of oxygen to produce cellular energy. Of particular significance are the contributions of ROS-induced damage to cellular DNA through (i) damage to the chromosomal DNA of the cell nucleus, resulting in impaired gene function, (ii) damage to telomeres—the protective DNA structures that appear to "cap" the ends of chromosomes (analogous to the plastic tips of shoelaces), and (iii) damage to the DNA that exists within the cell's energy-generating organelles, the mitochondria, resulting in impaired energy production.

DNA Damage and Repair

Damage to DNA is particularly likely to play a role in the lifelong accumulation of molecular damage within cells, since damage to DNA can readily result in permanent alteration of the cell's DNA sequence. Cells are subject to mutation all the time, both through errors that may become fixed when cells divide and as a result of ROS-induced damage, which can occur at any time. Numerous studies have reported age-related increases in somatic mutation and other forms of DNA damage, suggesting that an important determinant of the rate of aging at the cell and molecular level is the capacity for DNA repair.

A key player in the immediate cellular response to DNA damage is the enzyme poly(ADP-ribose) polymerase-1 (PARP-1). There is a strong, positive correlation of PARP-1 activity with the life span of the species: cells from long-lived species having higher levels of PARP-1 activity than cells from short-lived species. Similarly, human centenarians, who have often maintained remarkably good general health, appear to have a greater poly(ADP-ribosyl)ation capacity than the general population.

Telomeres

In many human somatic tissues, a decline in cellular division capacity with age appears to be linked to the fact that the telomeres, which protect the ends of chromosomes, get progressively shorter as cells divide. This is due to the absence of the enzyme telomerase, which

in humans is normally expressed only in germ cells (in testis and ovary) and in certain adult stem cells. Some studies have suggested that in dividing somatic cells, telomeres act as an intrinsic "division counter," perhaps to protect us against runaway cell division as happens in cancer but causing aging as the price for this protection. Erosion of telomere length below a critical length appears to trigger activation of cell cycle "checkpoints," especially the p53/p21/pRb system, resulting in permanent arrest of the cell's capacity for further division.

The loss of telomeric DNA is often attributed mainly to the so-called "end-replication" problem—the inability of the normal DNA copying machinery to copyright to the very end of the strand in the absence of telomerase. However, biochemical stress has an even bigger effect on the rate of telomere loss. Telomere shortening is greatly accelerated (or slowed) in cells with increased (or reduced) levels of stress. The clinical relevance of understanding telomere maintenance and its interaction with biochemical stress is considerable. A growing body of evidence suggests that telomere length is linked with aging and mortality. Not only do telomeres shorten with normal aging in several tissues (e.g., lymphocytes, vascular endothelial cells, kidney, liver), but also their reduction is more marked in certain disease states. For example, there appears to be a 100-fold higher incidence of vascular dementia in people with prematurely short telomeres. Furthermore, the psychological stress associated with provision of long-term care for those with chronic illness has also been associated with premature shortening of telomeres, presumably through biochemical sequelae to the chronic activation of stress hormones. Short telomeres may therefore serve as a general indicator of previous exposure to stress and as a prognostic indicator for disease conditions in which stress plays a causative role.

Mitochondria

An important connection between oxidative stress and aging is suggested by the accumulation of mitochondrial DNA (mtDNA) deletions and point mutations with age. Mitochondria are intracellular organelles, each carrying its own small DNA genome, which are responsible for generating cellular energy. As a by-product of energy generation, mitochondria are also the major source of ROS within the cell, and they are therefore both responsible for, and a major target of, oxidative stress. Any age-related increase in the fraction of damaged mitochondria is likely to contribute to a progressive decline in the cell and tissue capacity for energy production. Age-related increases in frequency of cytochrome c oxidase (COX)-deficient cells have been reported in human muscle and brain, associated with increased frequency of mutated mtDNA.

Initial evidence for age-related accumulation of mtDNA mutations came mainly from tissues such as brain and muscle where cell division in the adult, if it occurs at all, is rare. This led to the idea that accumulation of mtDNA mutation was driven mainly by the dynamics of mitochondrial multiplication and turnover within nondividing cells. However, there is now strong evidence of age-dependent accumulation of mtDNA mutations in human gut epithelium, which has the highest cell division rate of any tissue in the body. Thus, it appears that accumulation of defects in mitochondria may be a widespread phenomenon. This is also supported by the discovery that mitochondrial dysfunction may be an important driver of the contribution to cellular senescence that is made by the shortening of telomeres, confirming the synergism and interaction between different molecular mechanisms of aging.

Proteins

In addition to damage affecting cellular DNA, damage to protein molecules occurs to a considerable extent, and accumulation of faulty proteins contributes to important age-related disorders such as cataract, Parkinson's disease, and Alzheimer's disease. In some ways, the accumulation of defective proteins is harder to explain than the accumulation of DNA damage, since individual protein molecules are subject to a continual cycle of synthesis and breakdown. Thus, damaged individual protein molecules should be cleared as soon as that molecule is degraded. However, there is evidence that the protein degradation mechanisms themselves deteriorate in function with aging. This is thought to occur because these mechanisms eventually become overwhelmed by a build-up of defective protein molecules that are resistant to breakdown, for example, because they form aggregates large enough to withstand the normal removal systems. It is the build-up of such aggregates that is commonly linked with cell and tissue pathology.

THE RELATIONSHIP BETWEEN NORMAL AGING AND DISEASE

The relationship between normal aging and age-related disease has long been controversial. At stake is the question of whether the term "normal aging" should be reserved for individuals in whom identifiable pathology is absent, whereas specific age-related diseases, such as Alzheimer's disease, are seen as distinct entities. However, this concept gives rise to a conundrum. As a cohort ages, the fraction that can be said to be aging "normally" declines to a very low level. Whether the word "normal" can usefully be applied to such an atypical subset is debatable.

In a clinical context, it often makes sense to try and draw a distinction between normal aging and disease, since this may have implications for treatment. However, if the aim is to understand the *mechanisms* responsible for age-related conditions, such a distinction can obscure what is really going on, since the boundary between aging and disease pathogenesis may be somewhat arbitrary. For the vast majority of chronic, degenerative conditions, such as dementia, osteoporosis, and osteoarthritis, age is the biggest single risk factor predisposing to the disease in question. What is it about aging that renders the older cell or tissue more vulnerable to pathology?

Aging involves the progressive accumulation of cellular and molecular lesions, and the same is generally true of the age-associated diseases. Thus, there is considerable potential for overlap between the causative pathways leading to normal aging and age-related diseases. In the case of osteoporosis, for example, progressive bone loss from the late twenties onwards is the norm. Whether an individual reaches a critically low bone density, making him or her highly susceptible to fracture, is governed by how much bone mass they had to start with and by their individual rate of bone loss. The process that leads eventually to osteoporosis is thus entirely "normal," but what distinguishes whether or not this process results in an overtly pathological outcome is a range of moderating factors. In the case of Alzheimer's disease, most people above the age of 70 years have extensive cortical amyloid plaques and neurofibrillary tangles (the

Multistage Progression of Age-Related Disease

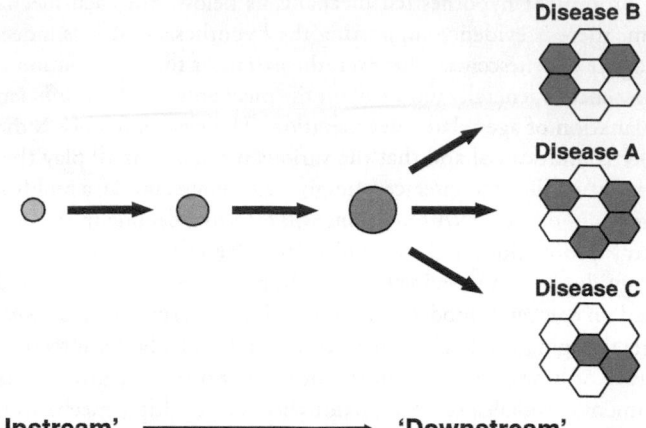

FIGURE 2-2. Multistage progression of age-dependent diseases. The intrinsic aging process, as well as most age-dependent diseases, are driven by the gradual accumulation of molecular and cellular faults. Although individual age-dependent diseases may be defined by particular "end-stage" cellular pathology, common upstream processes, such as DNA damage or oxidative damage to proteins, are shared between many age-related diseases and intrinsic aging. Intervention in these upstream processes has the potential, therefore, to be effective against multiple age-related diseases.

so-called hallmarks of classic Alzheimer's disease) even though they may show no evidence of major cognitive decline. In this instance, what determines whether or not the diagnosis of Alzheimer's disease is called for may be not so much the presence of lesions as which specific targets are affected.

As the upstream mechanisms giving rise to age-related diseases often involve the kind of damage that is thought to contribute to intrinsic aging, similar damaging processes may contribute to the pathogenesis of multiple disorders, even though the final nature of the end-stage lesions may be different (Figure 2-2). For example, oxidative stress may be a factor in protein aggregation in neurodegenerative diseases, in cell defects contributing to atherogenesis in cardiovascular diseases, and in impaired function of osteoblasts in osteoporosis. If this concept is correct, future interventions that target underlying processes of normal aging may postpone multiple age-related diseases.

The role played by basic cell maintenance systems both in securing longevity and in protecting against a spectrum of age-associated conditions is nicely illustrated by the human CDKN2a locus, which intriguingly codes for two different proteins via different open reading frames. One of these proteins is $p16^{INK4a}$, a cyclin-dependent protein kinase inhibitor; the other is ARF, a potent regulator of p53. The level of $p16^{INK4a}$ is associated with cellular aging in skin, pancreatic islets, and hematopoietic and neuronal stem cells, and $p16^{INK4a}$, together with ARF, is involved in regulating cell senescence and tumor suppression. At the population level, polymorphism at the CDKN2a locus is associated with risk for type 2 diabetes and with the preservation of physical function at older age. It seems likely that further study of the gene and its protein products will reveal important interconnections with aging and age-related diseases.

Through increased understanding of how fundamental maintenance systems are involved in protection against both aging and disease, it can be expected that future interventions will be found that can target underlying processes of normal aging, with the benefit of postponing multiple age-related diseases.

GENETIC AND NONGENETIC EFFECTS ON AGING

The disposable soma theory predicts that at the heart of the evolutionary explanation is the principle that organisms have been acted upon by natural selection to optimize the utilization of metabolic resources (energy) between competing physiological demands, such as growth, maintenance, and reproduction. Consistent with this prediction, it is striking that insulin signaling pathways appear to have effects on aging that may be strongly conserved across the species range. Insulin signaling regulates responses to varying nutrient levels. Allied to the role of insulin signaling pathways is the discovery that a class of proteins called sirtuins appears to be centrally involved in fine-tuning metabolic resources in response to variations in food supply. As described in Chapter 1, restricted intake of calories in laboratory rodents simultaneously suppresses reproduction and upregulates a range of maintenance mechanisms, resulting in an extension of life span and the simultaneous postponement of age-related diseases. Although dietary restriction may not have an effect of similar magnitude in humans, it will be surprising if there are no metabolic consequences of varying food supply.

One of the clearest examples of how metabolic signaling affects aging and longevity comes from a study on genes of the insulin/insulin-like growth factor 1 (IGF-1) signaling pathway in *C. elegans*. When threatened with overcrowding, which the larval worm detects by the increasing concentration of a pheromone, its development is diverted from the normal succession of larval molts into a long-lived, dispersal form called the "dauer" larva. Dauers show increased resistance to stress and can survive very much longer than the normal form, reverting to complete their development should more favorable conditions be detected. An insulin/IGF-1-receptor gene, *daf-2*, heads the gene regulatory pathway that controls the switch into the dauer form, and mutations in *daf-2* produce animals that develop into adults with substantially increased life spans. In common with other members of the evolutionarily conserved insulin/IGF-1 signaling pathway, *daf-2* also regulates lipid metabolism and reproduction. The *daf-2* gene product exerts its effects by influencing "downstream" gene expression, in particular via the actions of another gene belonging to the dauer-formation gene family, *daf-16*, which it inhibits.

Gene expression profiling has identified more than 300 genes that appear to have their expression levels altered by *daf-16* regulation. This large number suggests that, as predicted by the evolutionary theory, many genes are involved in determining longevity. The genes modulated by *daf-16* can be grouped into several broad categories. The first category includes a variety of stress-response genes, including genes for antioxidant enzymes. A second group of genes encode antimicrobial proteins, which are important for survival in this organism because its death is commonly caused by proliferation of bacteria in the gut. A miscellaneous third group included genes involved in protein turnover, which is an important cellular maintenance system.

The picture that emerges from both evolutionary theory and the empirical evidence is that the genetic control of longevity is mediated through a large array of mechanisms specifying individual maintenance and repair systems (Figure 2-3). Acting above these may exist a hierarchy of genes that serve to sense the quality of the

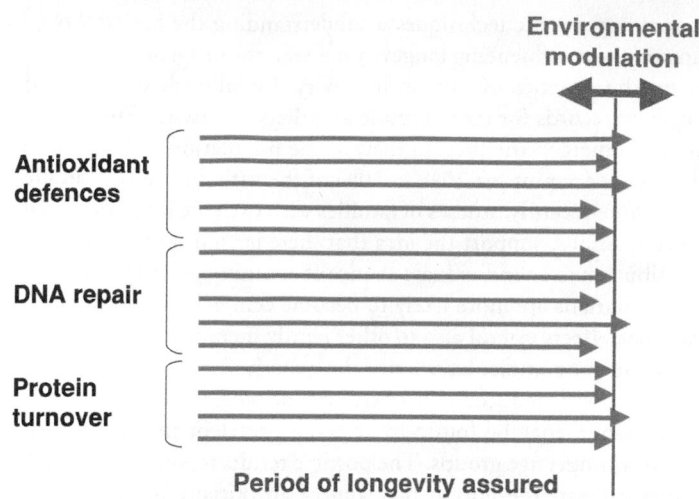

FIGURE 2-3. Gene regulation of longevity is effected through the genetic specification of many individual pathways for maintenance and repair of somatic cells and tissues. Among these pathways are those for antioxidant defense, DNA repair, and protein turnover. Natural selection is thought to have tuned these mechanisms to provide similar periods of "longevity assured" before the lesions resulting from the imperfect nature of the maintenance and repair processes give rise to age-dependent frailty, disability, and disease. In some organisms, there appears to have evolved a capacity to respond to changes in the environment, e.g., the availability of food, to fine-tune the overall settings of maintenance and repair processes so as to optimize the investments in maintenance and repair to suit different circumstances. One such example is the effect of dietary restriction in small animals, which results in suspension of reproduction and a coordinated increase in maintenance and repair, which in turn postpones both intrinsic aging and age-dependent diseases. The extent to which such capacity for environmental modulation exists in humans is as yet unclear, but it is likely to be less than in small animals for which reproduction constitutes a much greater fraction of the organism's energy budget.

environment, e.g., the abundance of food, and adjust metabolism accordingly. The discoveries that have been made during the current expansion of research on genetic and nongenetic factors affecting aging in nonhuman animal models are now beginning to be extended to human health and disease. Broad similarities are expected to exist, although in view of the different ecological circumstances affecting humans, as compared to a small animal like a nematode worm, the existence and nature of the higher-level, environment-sensing genetic pathways cannot be assumed to be identical.

GENETICS OF HUMAN LONGEVITY AND THE IMPLICATIONS FOR AGE-DEPENDENT DISEASE

While genetics is unlikely to have played any important part in the near doubling of human life expectancy over the last two centuries, the emergence of large numbers of people attaining great age has revealed information about the genetic contribution to human longevity that was unavailable previously. Population genetics explains how much of the variation in a trait—in this case, longevity—is due to innate differences in gene endowment and how much is due to the environment. When few individuals survived to the limit of the biological potential, the genetic contribution was masked by the large contribution to variance that arose from the environment and also, of course, from luck. During the last two decades, the possibility of applying genetic techniques to understanding the heritability of innate factors influencing longevity has seen the burgeoning of studies on the genetics of human longevity. Initially, these examined longevity records for monozygotic and dizygotic twins. From these analyses emerged the finding that, in the population at large, gene differences account for 20% to 30% of the variation in human life span. More recently, studies of families with extreme longevity, such as centenarians, support the idea that there is an important genetic contribution to an individual's chance of attaining great age. Siblings of centenarians are more likely to become centenarians themselves, and these effects extend also to other family members. A number of candidate-gene studies have tested the hypothesis that specific alleles associated with reduced risk of disease, or with improved somatic maintenance, may be found to be more prevalent in centenarians than in younger age groups. The positive results reported from such studies support the notion that, out of an initially heterogeneous cohort, those with a genetic endowment predisposing to somatic durability and freedom from disease will become increasingly numerous, as a fraction of the surviving members, while the cohort grows ever older.

The advent of rapid genome analysis techniques has made possible the scanning of the entire human genome for genetic markers that are associated with longevity in kin groups, without requiring any prior hypothesis as to the nature of the genes associated with these markers. Several current studies are exploiting these techniques using, for example, DNA from surviving nonagenarian siblings to search for markers that might confer familial predisposition for healthy aging. The rationale for these studies is that while, for an individual, surviving to great age might be a matter of chance, the fact that two or more individuals from the same family have done so makes it more likely that something in their shared genetic endowment is responsible.

Early results from genetic studies on human longevity are now emerging. In line with the evidence from nonhuman animal models, there is some indication that long-lived humans have decreased levels of IGF-1, consistent with the hypothesis that insulin/IGF-1 response is associated with longevity. Further studies on gene polymorphisms linked to the insulin/IGF-1-signaling pathways are likely to reveal this association in further detail. Similarly, there is growing interest in the possibility that polymorphisms in members of the sirtuin gene family (proteins that influence the activity of essential factors regulating the general patterns of gene expression), already shown to be important in connection with longevity-associated metabolism in yeast and animal models, may have connections with life span regulation in humans.

Among the factors that directly affect cellular maintenance, predicted by evolutionary theory to be central to regulating aging and longevity, there is growing evidence that genes regulating fundamental DNA repair processes are linked to life span. The human progeroid condition Werner's syndrome is caused by mutation in the *WRN* gene, which codes for an enzyme that has multiple roles in DNA maintenance and repair, while Hutchinson-Gilford syndrome (a more extreme form of progeria) is associated with mutation in the *LMNA* gene coding for a component of the external envelope of the cell nucleus.

Other gene associations with aging are being discovered among genes that regulate the cellular response to damage. When a cell detects that it has suffered damage, particularly to its DNA, it may activate a pathway that leads to programmed cell death (apoptosis) or another pathway that leads to permanent cell cycle arrest. Which of these routes is taken depends in large part on the risk, posed by the damage, of potentially initiating a tumor. If the cell is a stem cell, it is more likely to undergo apoptosis. Teleologically this appears to make sense, since the cancer transformation risk of preserving a cell that belongs to a highly proliferative tissue compartment is greater, and so it is logical for the cell to be deleted and replaced. On the other hand, if the cell belongs to a more general category, such as a fibroblast, it is less likely that apoptosis will be triggered and the cell instead is subjected to permanent arrest, or senescence. Various genes influence the likelihood of adopting one or another of these alternatives. Furthermore, experimental modulation of these genes or naturally occurring polymorphisms have been found to influence the outcome. For example, if the function of the tumor suppressor p53 is genetically enhanced, apoptosis is more likely, and this is found to be associated with a reduced lifetime risk of cancer. However, this protection comes at a cost, since in mouse models, at least, the process of intrinsic aging, caused by age-dependent tissue loss of cellularity, is accelerated by genetic enhancement of p53 activity. Life span is reduced and various age-dependent pathological changes occur earlier.

In terms of the genetics of specific age-dependent diseases, there is likely to be considerable overlap between the underlying pathways contributing to intrinsic aging generally and to the lesions associated with individual diseases. It is striking that even in the cases where gene polymorphisms have been linked to particular diseases, such as Alzheimer's, the dominant risk factor in sporadic cases, i.e., those not associated with strongly familial, early-onset presentation, is age rather than genotype. Thus, in pursuing the genetics of these kinds of age-dependent conditions, the research question is more likely to be answered if it is formulated in terms of addressing how specific genes affect the underlying pathogenesis of intrinsic aging, rather than driving a pathway that is mechanistically distinct.

MALLEABILITY OF THE HUMAN AGING PROCESS

One of the striking features of the increase in human life expectancy in recent decades is that, contrary to demographic forecasts of the major national and international agencies, life span has continued to increase steadily. This was initially surprising because it was thought that there was a fixed ceiling on human life expectancy imposed by the intrinsic, programmed nature of the aging process itself. By this logic, once death rates in the early and middle years had been pushed down to the low levels seen in most developed countries, there would be little opportunity for life expectancy to climb further.

The failure of the limited life span paradigm can, however, be understood within the framework for the intrinsic biology of aging outlined previously. If there is no intrinsic genetic program for aging, then the mechanisms that drive the aging process—accumulation of molecular and cellular damage—are amenable to environmental modulation. Aging is the result of a gradual but progressive accumulation of *damage* to cells, tissues, and organs. However, the process is not entirely passive, since the rate of accumulation is strongly resisted by maintenance and repair processes, which are controlled by *genes*. Furthermore, both the incidence of damage and the regulation of these genes may be influenced by extrinsic factors. This picture readily accommodates the roles of at least five major elements contributing to the individuality of the human aging process: genes, nutrition, lifestyle (e.g., exercise), environment, and chance.

The recognition of this interplay of factors is likely to be crucial for integrating biological, clinical, and social gerontology. For example, environment is often defined by social factors such as housing, transport, and income. Poor environments may adversely affect an individual's opportunities for healthy aging in terms of nutrition, lifestyle, etc. In particular, a poor environment can reinforce a tendency for the older person to suffer social isolation, which in turn can exacerbate psychological and physical deterioration. On the positive side, the understanding that we now have of the biological science of human aging supports the idea that the aging process is much more malleable than has hitherto been recognized. It is likely that the continuing increase in human life expectancy reflects the increasingly favorable conditions of life in most developed countries. This opens the way to a range of interventions that may further improve health in old age and extend quality of life. Conversely, the threat exists that with rising levels of obesity and declining levels of physical activity, the future may see the increase in longevity slow down or even reverse.

FURTHER READING

Burkle A, Beneke S, Brabeck C, et al. Poly(ADP-ribose) polymerase-1, DNA repair and mammalian longevity. *Exp Gerontol.* 2002;37:1203–1205.

Christensen K, Johnson TE, Vaupel JW. The quest for genetic determinants of human longevity: challenges and insights. *Nat Rev Genet.* 2006;7:436–448.

Collado M, Blasco MA, Serrano M. Cellular senescence in cancer and aging. *Cell.* 2007;130:223–233.

Cournil A, Kirkwood TBL. If you would live long, choose your parents well. *Trends Genet.* 2001;17:233–235.

Esiri MM, Matthews F, Brayne C, et al. Pathological correlates of late-onset dementia in a multicentre, community-based population in England and Wales. *Lancet.* 2001;357:169–175.

Finch CE, Tanzi R. The genetics of aging. *Science.* 1997;278:407–411.

Gems D, Partridge L. Insulin/IGF signalling and aging: seeing the bigger picture. *Curr Opin Genet Dev.* 2001:11;287–292.

Kapahi P, Boulton ME, Kirkwood TBL. Positive correlation between mammalian life span and cellular resistance to stress. *Free Radic Biol Med.* 1999:26;495–500.

Kenyon C, Chang J, Gensch E, Rudner A, Tabtiang R. A *C. elegans* mutant that lives twice as long as wild-type. *Nature.* 1993:366;461–464.

Kim S, Kaminker P, Campisi J. Telomeres, aging and cancer: in search of a happy ending. *Oncogene.* 2002;21:503–511.

Kirkwood TBL. The origins of human aging. *Phil Trans R Soc Lond B.* 1997;352: 1765–1772.

Kirkwood TBL. *Time of Our Lives: the Science of Human Ageing.* New York, New York: Oxford University Press; 1999.

Kirkwood TBL. Understanding the odd science of aging. *Cell.* 2005;120:437–447.

Larsen PL, Albert P, Riddle DL. Genes that regulate both development and longevity in *Caenorhabditis elegans. Genetics* 1995:139;1567–1583.

Medawar PB. *An Unsolved Problem of Biology.* London: Lewis; 1952.

Melzer D, Frayling TM, Murray A, et al. A common variant of the p16^{INK4a} genetic region is associated with physical function in older people. *Mech Ageing Dev.* 2007;128:370–377.

Murphy CT, McCarroll SA, Bargmann CI, et al. Genes that act downstream of DAF-16 to influence the lifespan of *Caenorhabditis elegans. Nature* 2003;424: 277–284.

Perls T, Kohler IV, Andersen S, et al. Survival of parents and siblings of supercentenarians. *J Gerontol A Biol Sci Med Sci.* 2007;62:1028–1034.

Taylor RW, Barron MJ, Borthwick GM, et al. Mitochondrial DNA mutations in human colonic crypt stem cells. *J Clin Invest* 2003;112:1351–1360.

von Zglinicki T. Oxidative stress shortens telomeres. *Trends Biochem Sci.* 2002;27:339–344.

von Zglinicki T, Serra V, Lorenz M, et al. Short telomeres in patients with vascular dementia: an indicator of low antioxidative capacity and a possible prognostic factor? *Lab Invest.* 2000;80:1739–1747.

Williams GC. Pleiotropy, natural selection and the evolution of senescence. *Evolution.* 1957;11:398–411.

Immunology and Aging

Birgit Weinberger ■ *Daniela Weiskopf* ■ *Beatrix Grubeck-Loebenstein*

GENERAL ASPECTS OF IMMUNOSENESCENCE

The immune system undergoes profound age-related changes, collectively termed immunosenescence. This process affects various cell types including hematopoietic stem cells (HSCs), lymphoid progenitor cells in the bone marrow and in the thymus, the thymus itself, mature lymphocytes in peripheral blood and secondary lymphatic organs and also elements of the innate immune system. These immunological changes contribute to elevated susceptibility to infectious diseases, to more severe symptoms, prolonged duration and poorer prognosis of infections and to decreased protective effects of vaccinations. Reactivation of Varicella-Zoster virus leading to herpes zoster is observed by far more frequently in elderly compared to young adults. Infections with influenza virus are associated with more severe symptoms in elderly patients and with an increased risk for secondary complications. Additionally, risks for many other infections are increased in elderly people. As the elderly population is particularly susceptible to infection and vulnerable in case of disease, vaccination is of special importance. Unfortunately, the efficacy of various vaccines, e.g., influenza, hepatitis A and hepatitis B, is lower in elderly people. New strategies are needed to improve vaccination and to develop vaccines that specifically target and stimulate the aged immune system.

EFFECT OF AGING ON DIFFERENT CELL TYPES

Hematopoietic Stem Cells and Lymphoid Progenitor Cells

Hematopoiesis

All circulating blood cells of an adult individual including immature lymphocytes are generated in the bone marrow. Both liver and spleen can also be recruited as sites for haematopoiesis in case of increased need for newly generated blood cells or if the bone marrow is injured. All blood cells originate from a common stem cell (HSC) and become committed to develop along particular lineages. The first step of differentiation leads to the separation of myeloid and lymphoid progenitors. Myeloid progenitors further differentiate to become erythrocytes, platelets, basophils, eosinophils, neutrophils, monocytes, macrophages, mast cells, or dendritic cells (DC). Lymphoid progenitors give rise to B lymphocytes, T lymphocytes, and natural killer (NK) cells (Figure 3-1A). Maturation of B cells, which includes rearrangement and expression of immunoglobulin genes as well as selection for cells with functional immunoglobulins and against self-reactive B cells, takes place in the bone marrow. Mature B cells then enter the circulation and lymphoid organs where they encounter their specific antigens. T lymphocytes leave the bone marrow in an immature state and migrate to the thymus where maturation with somatic recombination and expression of the T cell receptor (TCR) genes occur. Additionally, positive selection for functional TCRs and negative selection against self-reactive T cells take place in the thymus. Like B cells, mature T cells finally migrate to lymphoid organs and are also found in the blood stream (Figure 3-1B) (Color Plate 1).

Age-Related Changes of Hematopoiesis

The overall amount of hematopoietic tissue in the bone marrow is decreased with age. Changes of the hematopoietic microenvironment and alterations of hormone production disturb self-renewal and lineage commitment of HSCs. HSCs themselves are also affected by aging as indicated, e.g., by shortening of telomeres. In combination, these two effects may lead to fewer and less functional HSCs with increasing age. Interestingly, the lymphoid lineage is far more compromised by age-related changes than the myeloid lineage. Fewer pro-B cells are generated in aging and fewer of these cells transit through the next differentiation steps. As a consequence, the

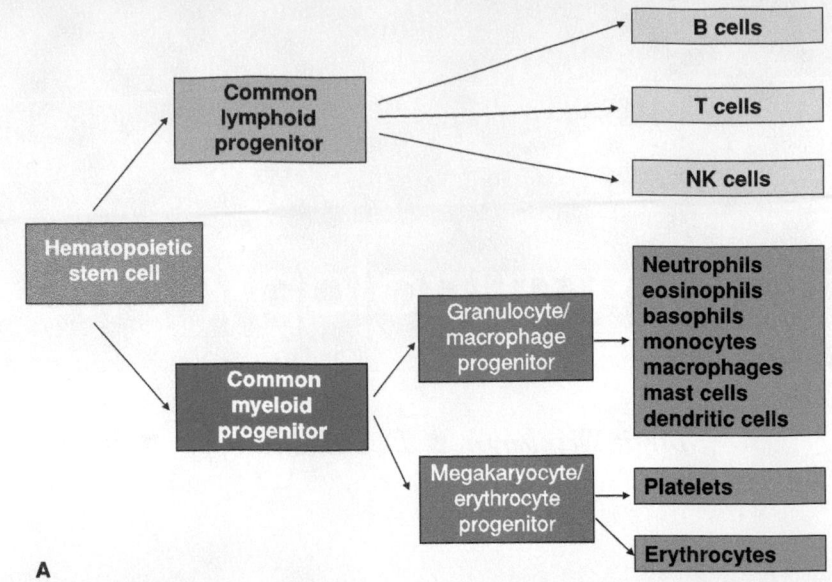

A

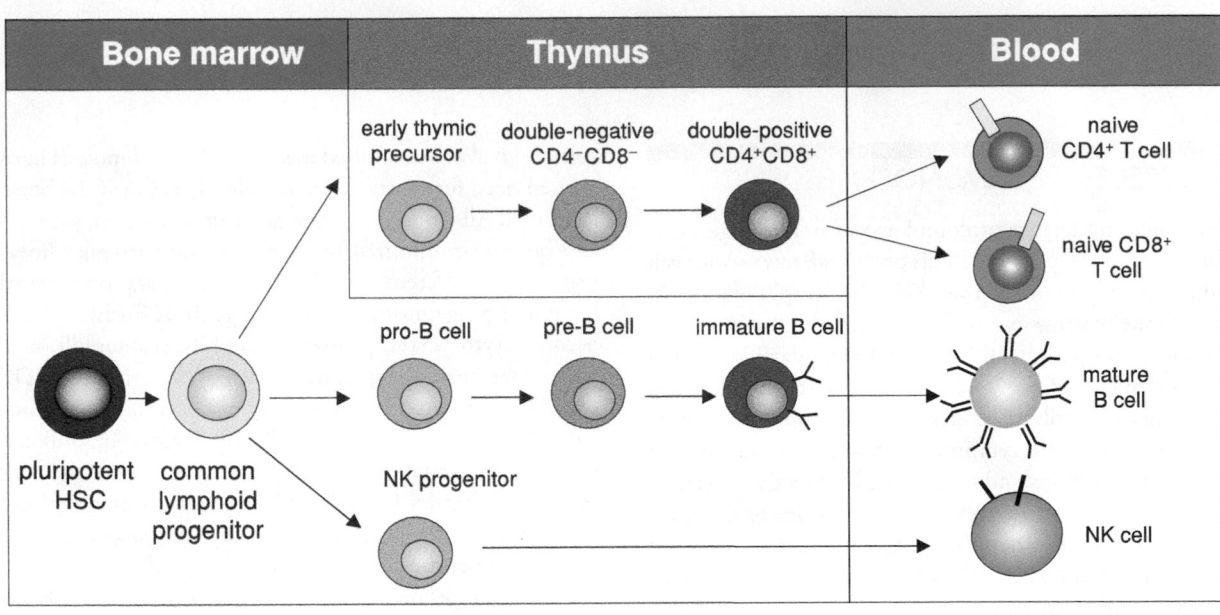

B

FIGURE 3-1. Hematopoiesis and maturation of lymphoid cells. (A) Schematic representation of hematopoiesis. Hematopoietic stem cells differentiate into lymphoid and myeloid progenitors that give rise to the different cell types found in peripheral blood. (B) Maturation of lymphoid cells. Maturation of T cells takes place in the thymus, whereas B cells and NK cells undergo maturation in the bone marrow. All mature lymphocytes migrate into the periphery and can be found in blood.

number of mature B cells leaving the bone marrow is lower. T cell precursors seem to be less affected by aging. However, due in part to dramatic alterations in the thymus, where the maturation of T cells takes place, the T cell compartment undergoes substantial changes with age.

Involution of the Thymus

Maturation of T cells takes place in the thymus, a bilobed organ situated in the upper anterior thorax, just above the heart. It is divided into multiple lobules that consist of an outer cortex that is densely populated with thymocytes and an inner medulla that is sparsely populated with thymocytes. Other cell types found in the thymus

are nonlymphoid epithelial cells, macrophages, and lymphoid DC. They provide important stimuli (e.g., cytokines and physical interaction via major histocompatibility complex (MHC) molecules) for the development of mature T lymphocytes. Immature T cells enter the thymus where they proliferate and differentiate into mature T lymphocytes. During this differentiation, the T cells migrate from the outer cortex to the medulla from where they exit the thymus and spread to the periphery. The very complex maturation process includes proliferation, recombination of the TCR genes to assure diversity of the T cell repertoire, negative selection, and extensive apoptosis of self-reactive or nonreactive T cells and positive selection of expedient T cells, which recognize foreign antigens presented by MHC complexes. The T cells that exit from the thymus are called

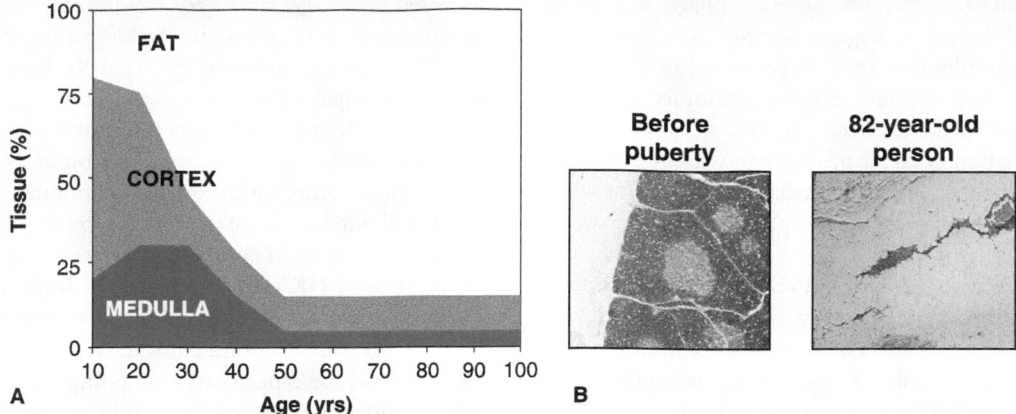

FIGURE 3-2. Thymic involution and loss of functional thymic tissue. (A) With increasing age, functional thymic tissues (medulla and cortex) are replaced by fat. Depicted are percentages of thymic tissues and fat tissue against donor age. (B) Histological pictures of human thymic tissue derived from a child or an 82-yr-old person stained with hematoxylin. In the pediatric thymus areas of cortex (outer darker staining) and medulla (inner lighter staining) tissue are prominent. Thymic tissue from elderly individuals shows dramatic reduction of functional tissue and invasion of adipose tissue. Magnification = 120×. Reprinted from George AJT, Ritter MA. Thymic involution with ageing: obsolescence or good housekeeping? Immunol. Today. 1996;17;267. With permission from Elsevier.

naïve as they have never had contact with their specific antigen. Naïve T cells make up the reservoir of cells that is needed to respond to neoantigens that are encountered throughout life.

One of the hallmarks of immunosenescence is the involution of the thymus, which is characterized by a reduction in the overall size of the organ and by a replacement of the functional cortex and medulla tissue by fat. These changes start early in life and are almost complete by the age of 40 to 50 years. Figure 3-2 illustrates the redistribution of tissues in the thymus with increasing age and depicts histological changes. Involution of the thymus could be caused by both defects in the T cell precursor cells and changes of the thymic stromal cells. This working model postulates that these changes could occur simultaneously in each compartment or one could precede the other. In either case, age-associated degeneration of the one compartment negatively influences the other, leading to progressive loss of thymic function. As a consequence, the number of thymocytes and of naïve T cells exiting the thymus is dramatically decreased with age. The missing output of newly generated naïve T cells leads to crucial changes in the T cell repertoire and the composition of the T cell compartment. However, the overall role of thymus involution in age-related changes of peripheral immune cells remains to be determined.

Innate Immune System

Components and Functions of the Innate Immune System

The innate immune system is the first line of defense against infection. It consists of cellular and biochemical defense mechanisms that respond to infectious agents by recognizing common structures shared by pathogens. It is not able to distinguish between fine differences of antigens. The innate immune system reacts faster than the adaptive immune system. However, due to a lack of memory mechanisms, the innate immune system is not able to "remember" antigens. There are therefore no differences between primary and subsequent responses to the same pathogen. The major components of innate immunity are physical barriers (epithelia), phagocytic cells

(neutrophils, macrophages, DCs), NK cells, the complement system, and a variety of cytokines that regulate and coordinate innate immune responses (Table 3-1). Toll-like receptors (TLR) are highly conserved receptors that are expressed on different cell types of the innate immune system and recognize distinct classes of pathogens. To date, over 20 mammalian TLR have been identified recognizing, for example, lipopolysaccharide (LPS), other bacterial proteoglycans, or unmethylated CpG nucleotides found in bacteria or viruses. Each TLR seems to be crucial in the responses to distinct classes of infectious pathogens. Binding of microbial components to the TLR leads to activation of innate immune cells and induces production of cytokines.

TABLE 3-1

Components and Functions of the Innate Immune System	
COMPONENT	**FUNCTION**
Epithelial barriers	Prevention of microbial entry
Complement	Opsonization of microbes, killing of microbes, activation of leukocytes
Mannose-binding lectin	Opsonization of microbes, activation of complement
Cytokines	Inflammation, activation of phagocytes, stimulation of IFN-γ production
Dendritic cells	Antigen uptake in peripheral sites, antigen presentation in lymph nodes
Neutrophils	Phagocytosis, killing of pathogens
Eosinophils	Killing of antibody-coated parasites
Mast cells and basophils	Release of granules containing histamine and active agents, induction of inflammation and tissue responses
Macrophages	Phagocytosis, killing of pathogens, cytokine release, antigen presentation
Natural killer cells	Release of lytic granules, killing of infected cells and tumor cells

The main function of neutrophils and macrophages is to recognize, internalize, and destroy pathogens. Macrophages also process foreign proteins to peptides that are then presented to T lymphocytes. This link between innate and adaptive immunity will be described in more detail in the next section. DC are of crucial importance for the initiation of an adaptive immune response to new antigens. They are found under the epithelia of many organs where they capture antigens, process them, and present them to naïve T cells after migrating to lymph nodes.

NK cells are able to directly kill target cells by releasing perforin and granzymes. Perforin creates pores in the target cells through which granzymes enter the cells. These enzymes activate caspases and induce apoptosis of the cell. NK cell function is regulated by a balance of activating and inhibiting receptors. Activation is induced by molecules that are expressed on infected or otherwise stressed host cells. NK cells are thus able to identify, for example, virus-infected cells. MHC class I molecules, which are present on all host cells, act as inhibitory signals and prevent killing of healthy cells by NK cells. As a variety of viruses induce down-regulation of MHC class I in order to avoid recognition by the adaptive immune response, the lack of MHC expression indicates viral infection and is also used by NK cells to identify these cells.

Additionally, cells of the innate immune system produce cytokines that cause inflammation, induce the release of inflammatory plasma proteins, and activate innate and adaptive immune cells, which are recruited to the site of infection (see Chapter 4).

Age-Related Changes of the Innate Immune System (Table 3-2)

While most humoral components of the innate immune system such as the complement system are not affected by the aging process, age-related changes of innate immune cells occur, leading to alterations in cell function and in the production of cytokines and chemokines. The overall number of neutrophils remains constant, but there are characteristic age-related functional changes. Both their phagocytic capacity as well as their efficiency of killing internalized microbes is decreased in old age. This leads to an overall reduction of bactericidal activity. A decreased ability to kill pathogens has also been observed in aged macrophages. Additionally, their antigen-presenting function is impaired due to a decreased expression of MHC class II molecules, leading to defects in the activation of CD4$^+$ T cells. Alterations in the expression and function of TLRs also add to age-related impairments within the innate immune system.

NK cell numbers increase with age, but their cytotoxic potential and the production of cytokines decrease on a per cell basis. Proliferation of aged NK cells in response to stimulatory cytokines like IL-2 is reduced. How DC are affected by age is still not fully understood. In aged mice and humans, the number of DC in the skin is decreased and the capacity of DC to migrate to lymph nodes after antigen contact is impaired. Little is known about age-related functional changes of human DC. Animal models suggest that antigen presentation is decreased in old age; however, so far this has not been confirmed in humans. DC differentiated in vitro from monocytes derived from aged humans are indistinguishable from their young counterparts.

Subclinical inflammatory processes gradually increase with age in a variety of species (see Chapter 4). Elevated plasma concentrations of interleukin-6 (IL-6), IL-1β, and tumor necrosis factor-alpha (TNF-α) have been described in elderly populations and were postulated as predictive markers of functional disability and mortality. This progressive proinflammatory state in elderly persons has been referred to as "inflamm-aging." Such chronic inflammatory processes may support the development and progression of age-related diseases, such as osteoporosis, neurodegeneration, and atherosclerosis. At first sight, "inflamm-aging" seems to contradict the functional defects observed in innate immune cells. However, it is believed that chronic subclinical inflammation is caused by chronic stimulation of the innate immune system by products of degradation processes and/or by the partial inability of the aged immune system to eliminate certain pathogens. This could lead to chronic, yet inefficient innate immune responses.

Genetic factors, like polymorphisms in genes encoding for cytokines like IFN-γ, IL-6, and IL-10 can also influence the severity of inflammatory responses in old age. Chemokines, which direct the movement of circulating lymphocytes to sites of injury of infection, play a crucial role in initiating adaptive immune responses and in directing movement of immune cells through the body. Approximately 50 human chemokines have been described. Alterations in serum concentrations of some of them have been reported in elderly people. However, for most of the proteins studied, conflicting results have been obtained. Some reports show increased concentrations of the proinflammatory, IFN-γ inducible chemokines MIG (CXCL9) and IP-10 (CXCL10). Elevated levels of MCP-1 (CCL2), which also acts proinflammatory by regulating T cell and monocyte recruitment toward sites of inflammation, have been described in elderly people; however, other studies were not able to confirm these findings.

Adaptive Immune System

Components and Principal Functions of the Adaptive Immune System

The adaptive immune system consists of lymphocytes, namely, T and B cells, and antibodies, which are produced by B cells. Both

TABLE 3-2

Age-Related Changes of Innate Immune Cells		
	AGE-RELATED DECREASE	**AGE-RELATED INCREASE**
Neutrophils	Phagocytic capacity Oxidative burst Bactericidal activity	Membrane viscosity
Macrophages	Phagocytic capacity Oxidative burst MHC class II expression	

NK cells	Cytotoxicity
	Production of
	  proinflammatory
	  cytokines and
	  chemokines
	Proliferative response to IL-2
		Number of cells

Cytokines and chemokines		Serum concentration of IL-6, IL-1β, TNF-α Serum concentration of MIG (CXCL9) and IP-10 (CXCL10)

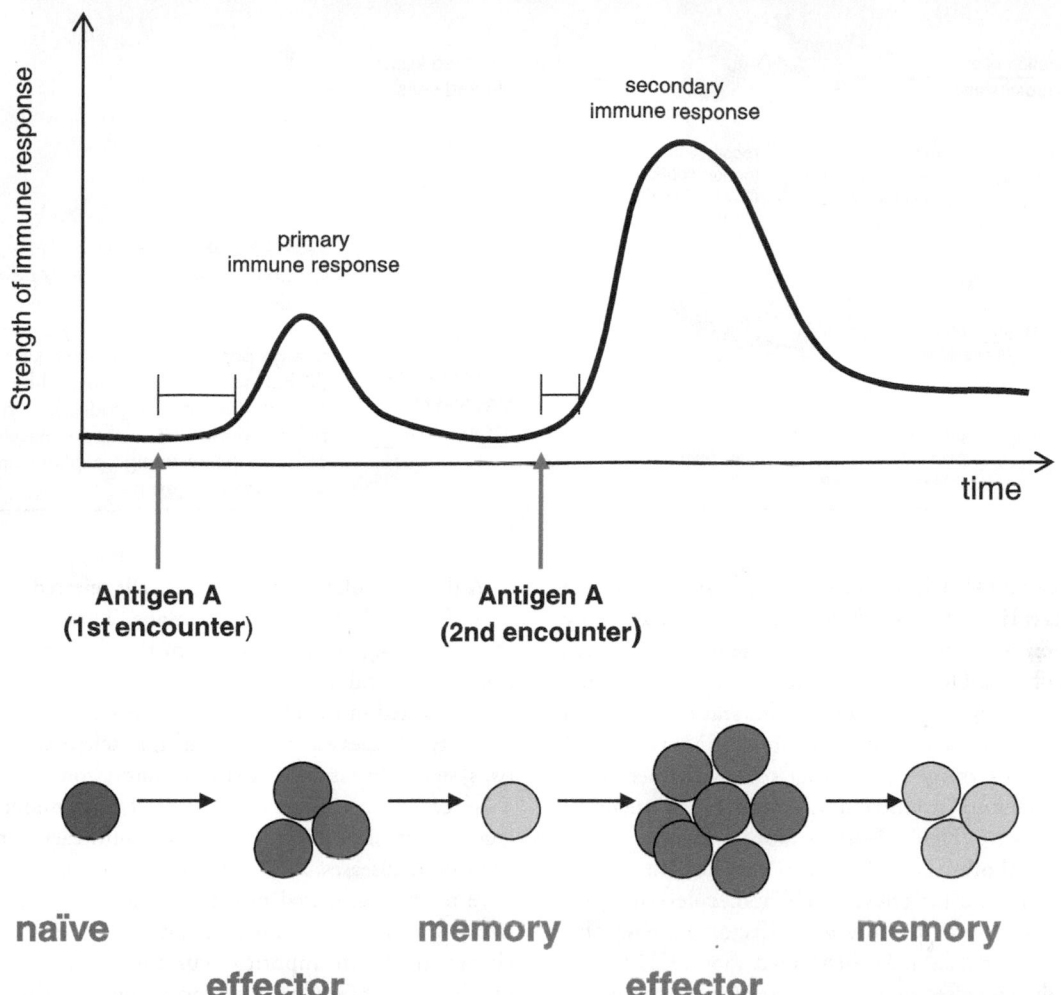

FIGURE 3-3. Primary and secondary immune response. The upper panel shows a schematic depiction of the strength of the immune response as measured, e.g. by antibody titers or numbers of effector T cells. The secondary immune response after repeated encounter with the same antigen is faster and more pronounced compared to the primary immune response. After repeated stimulation with the same antigen immune responses are sustained at a higher level. The lower panel depicts the expansion and differentiation of lymphocytes in the course of primary and secondary immune responses. Naïve cells differentiate into effector cells after encountering their antigen. Most effector cells are eliminated by apoptosis after clearance of the pathogens. Few cells remain in the body as long-lived memory cells and are able to quickly and efficiently differentiate into effector cells in case of a second contact with the same antigen. After clearance of the pathogens, most effector cells are again eliminated; however, more long-lived memory cells are generated.

B and T lymphocytes can be divided into naïve, memory, and effector cells with regard to their differentiation status. Lymphocytes that have not yet encountered their specific antigen are called naïve. Upon contact with their antigen, these cells proliferate and differentiate into memory and effector lymphocytes. This antigen-triggered response increases in magnitude and effectiveness with each encounter of a particular infectious agent (Figure 3-3) (Color Plate 2). After the first encounter with the antigen, it takes several days for the adaptive immune response to fully respond and activate effector cells. Once the pathogen is cleared, most of the activated effector cells are eliminated. However, long-lived memory cells remain in the body and ensure that the response to a second contact with the same antigen is faster and more pronounced compared to the primary response. Both T and B lymphocytes recognize their antigens via highly diverse surface molecules called T cell receptor (TCR) or B cell receptor (BCR), respectively. The diversity of these molecules is due to extensive somatic recombination of the genes encoding the TCR or BCR during the maturation of lymphocytes. The total

number of specificities of the lymphocytes in an individual, called the immunological repertoire, is estimated to be 10^7 to 10^9.

T Lymphocytes

T cells can be divided into CD4$^+$ and CD8$^+$ T cells. CD4$^+$ T cells are called T-helper cells and are required for stimulation of B cells and activation of macrophages. CD8$^+$ T cells or cytotoxic T lymphocytes (CTL) directly interact with virally infected and tumor cells and kill these target cells. T cells are not able to directly recognize foreign antigens. Their highly diverse T cell receptors interact with molecules of the MHC that are associated with peptides derived from antigenic proteins. MHC class I molecules are present in all nucleated cells. All proteins that are synthesized within a cell are processed into peptides and presented via MHC class I on the surface of the cells. CD8$^+$ T cells interact with the MHC–peptide complexes and distinguish between self and nonself peptides. Cells presenting foreign peptides, e.g. viral components on infected cells, are targeted for

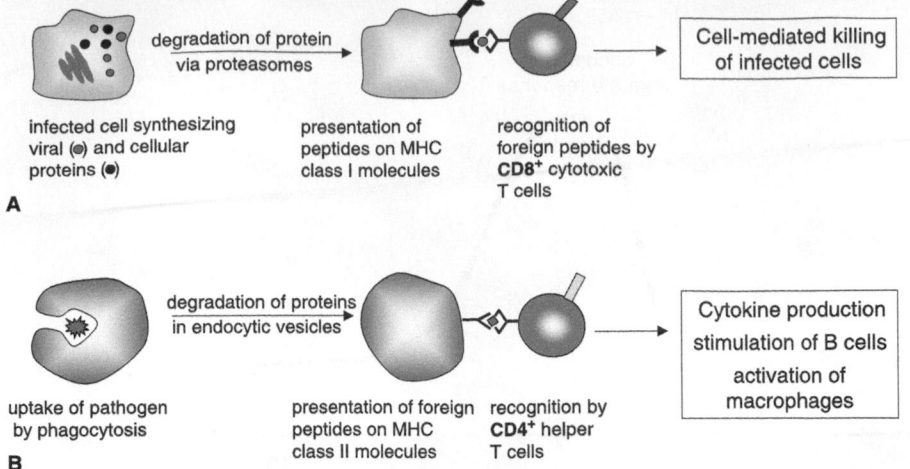

A

infected cell synthesizing viral (●) and cellular proteins (●) → degradation of protein via proteasomes → presentation of peptides on MHC class I molecules → recognition of foreign peptides by **CD8+** cytotoxic T cells → Cell-mediated killing of infected cells

B

uptake of pathogen by phagocytosis → degradation of proteins in endocytic vesicles → presentation of foreign peptides on MHC class II molecules → recognition by **CD4+** helper T cells → Cytokine production stimulation of B cells activation of macrophages

FIGURE 3-4. Processing and presentation of antigens via MHC class I or class II. (A) Synthesized proteins are degraded via proteasomes and presented on MHC class I molecules. CD8+ cytotoxic T cells recognize foreign peptides and mediate killing of infected cells. (B) Pathogens are internalized by antigen presenting cells; proteins are degraded in endocytic vesicles and presented on MHC class II molecules. CD4+ helper T cells recognize foreign peptides and stimulate B cells and macrophages.

killing (Figure 3-4A). CD4+ T-helper cells recognize peptides in the context of MHC class II molecules. These proteins are present only on specialized antigen-presenting cells of the innate immune system (monocytes, macrophages, DC) and on B cells. Antigen-presenting cells recognize foreign antigens, internalize them, and process them into peptides, which are presented in the context of MHC class II molecules. Interaction of antigen-presenting cells with specific T-helper cells induces cytokine production in T cells and stimulates B cells to produce antibodies (Figure 3-4B) (Color Plate 3).

When naïve T cells (both CD4+ and CD8+) make contact with cells presenting their specific antigen via MHC molecules, they proliferate and differentiate into memory and effector T cells. This process is called clonal expansion. As mentioned above, CD8+ and CD4+ T cells exert distinct effector functions. As described above for NK cells, effector CD8+ T cells also release perforin and granzymes to induce apoptosis in infected or tumor cells. CD4+ effector cells stimulate phagocytes of the innate immune system. NK cells induce cytokine production in T cells to enhance immune responses and are required for efficient antibody production by B cells (Figure 3-5A) (Color Plate 4). On the basis of their cytokine profile and effector functions, T_{H1} and T_{H2} subpopulations have been characterized within the T-helper cells. Both subsets differentiate from the same precursors, namely naïve CD4+ T cells. The T_{H1} differentiation pathway is mainly triggered by the cytokine IL-12, which is produced by innate immune cells in response to microbes that infect or activate macrophages and DC. T_{H1} cells produce proinflammatory cytokines, such as IFN-γ and TNF-α. These cytokines stimulate the microbicidal activity of phagocytes and the production of opsonizing and complement-fixing IgG antibodies. Microbes can then be efficiently phagocytozed and eliminated by phagocytes.

T_{H2} responses mainly occur in response to helminths and allergens, which cause chronic T cell stimulation, often in the absence of macrophage activation or pronounced innate immune responses. T_{H2} differentiation is induced by IL-4, which is produced mainly by the T_{H2} cells themselves. T_{H2} cells produce IL-4, IL-5, IL-10, and IL-13, stimulate B cells, and antagonize the phagocyte-stimulating effect of IFN-γ. As both differentiation pathways are self-enhancing, immune responses are often polarized in either the one or the other direction. However, T cells with a T_{H0} phenotype, which are able to produce T_{H1} and T_{H2} cytokines, have also been described.

A third population of T helper cells referred to as T_{H17} cells has been described in mice and humans. These cells are generated in response to signals different from the ones needed for the induction of T_{H1} and T_{H2} responses and secrete IL-17. T_{H17} cells have been detected in the blood and tissues from patients suffering from a variety of diseases such as multiple sclerosis, rheumatoid arthritis, systemic lupus erythematosus, and Crohn's disease. The role of T_{H17} cells in host defense is not yet fully understood, but many studies suggest that they may trigger autoreactive responses and autoimmune diseases. Additionally, the so-called "regulatory" T cells have recently attracted much attention. Several subtypes of regulatory T cells, which downregulate immune responses, have been characterized. An important current research focus in the field is on CD4+ TREGs ("naturally occurring" regulatory T cells). These cells express high levels of the α-chain of the IL-2 receptor CD25 and of the transcription factor forkhead box P3 (FOXP3). Autoimmune diseases, chronic infections, and cancer have been linked to quantitative and/or qualitative defects of TREGs.

For in vitro analysis and isolation, different cells of the immune system can be characterized and identified by expression of particular surface proteins. These markers are used to distinguish between different cell types and cell subsets especially in the T cell compartment. Table 3-3 summarizes frequently used surface markers and gives an overview about their expression on different cell types.

Age-Related Changes in the T Cell Compartment

The size of the mature T cell pool remains stable over the lifetime of an individual. However, the proportionate representation of different T cell subsets, namely, of naïve, memory, and effector cells, undergoes substantial changes with increasing age (Figure 3-5A). Figure 3-6 (Color Plate 5) illustrates the phenotype and functional properties of naïve, memory, and effector T cells.

Aging leads to a decrease of naïve T cells, while memory and effector cells accumulate (Figure 3-7A). Generally, the changes are more pronounced in the CD8+ than in the CD4+ compartment. A relatively diverse naïve CD4+ T cell compartment is maintained for decades despite decreasing thymic output. However, after the age of 70 years, a dramatic decline of diversity occurs, resulting in a severely contracted repertoire. Similar changes within the CD8+

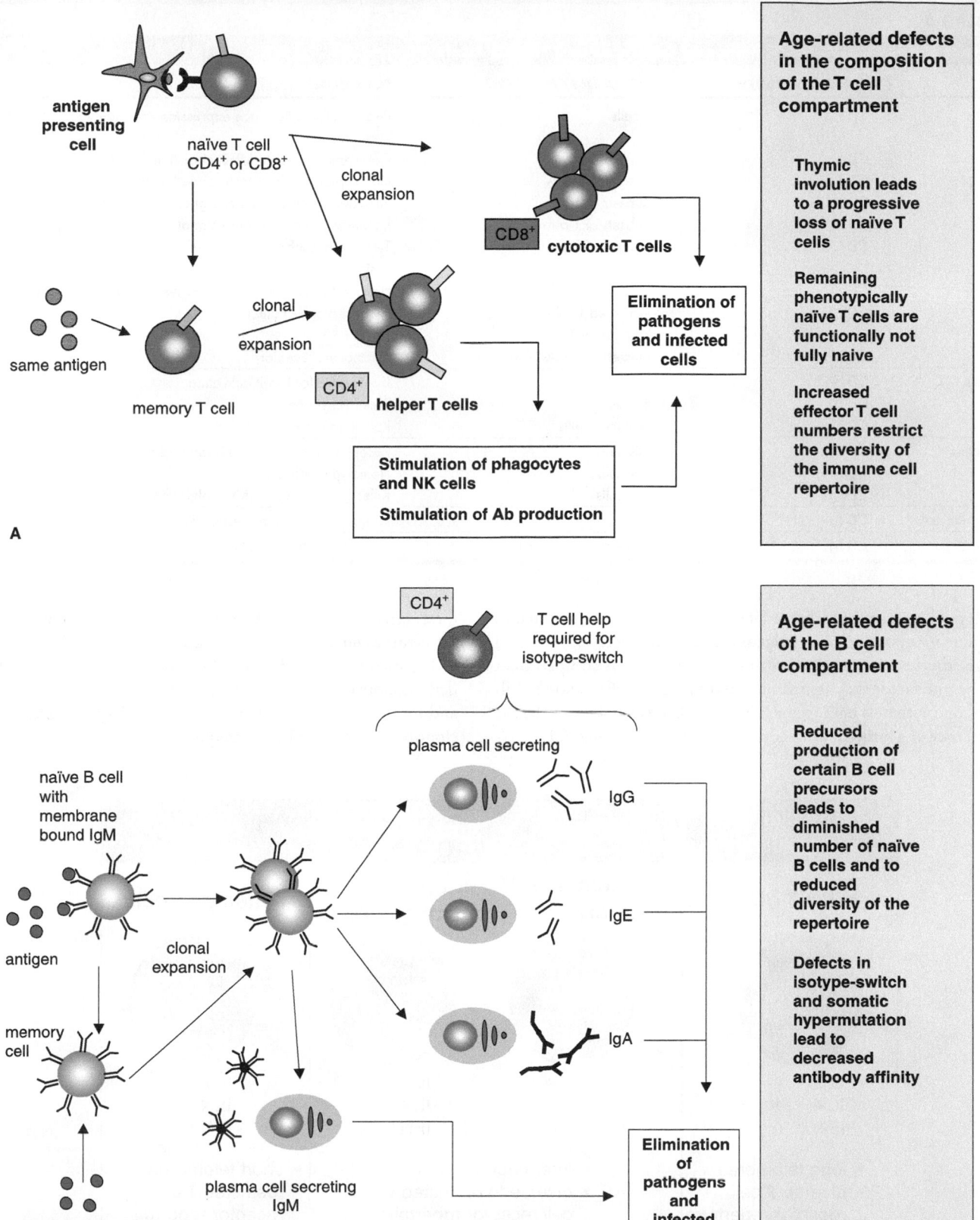

FIGURE 3-5. Schematic representation of adaptive immune responses and age-related changes. (A) Antigen presenting cells present foreign peptides to naïve T cells, which expand and differentiate into memory and effector T cells. CD8+ cytotoxic T cells directly eliminate infected cells. CD4+ helper T cells stimulate phagocytes and NK cells and are crucial for the induction of antibody production. Thus they indirectly contribute to elimination of pathogens and infected cells. (B) Antigens bind to the membrane-bound antibodies on naïve B cells which expand and differentiate into memory and effector B cells, which are called plasma cells and secrete antibodies. Contact with T helper cells and stimulation by cytokines leads to recombination events in the genes encoding for heavy chains of antibodies. Depending on the stimulus IgG, IgE or IgA antibodies are generated and secreted in order to eliminate pathogens.

TABLE 3-3

Surface Markers Used for Definition of Cell Types and T Cell Subsets

	SURFACE MARKER	CELLULAR EXPRESSION	FUNCTION
T cells	CD3	T cells	Required for cell-surface expression and signal transduction of the T cell receptor
	CD4	T helper cells	Coreceptor, binds to MHC class II molecule
	CD8	Cytotoxic T cells	Coreceptor, binds to MHC class I molecule
	CD27	Subsets of T cells	Receptor for costimulatory signal
	CD28	Subsets of T cells	Receptor for costimulatory signal
	CD45RA	Subsets of T cells	Tyrosine phosphatase, involved in antigen-receptor mediated signaling
	CD62L	Subsets of T cells	Homing to peripheral lymph nodes, adhesion to endothelial cells
	CD25	Activated T cells Regulatory T cells	IL-2 receptor α-chain
	CCR7	Subsets of T cells	Chemokine receptor
B cells	CD19	B cells	Coreceptor for B cell activation
	CD20	B cells	B cell activation
	CD22	Mature B cells	Regulation of B cell activation
NK cells	CD16	NK cells	Receptor for Fc part of IgG antibodies
	CD56	NK cells	Homotypic adhesion
	CD158	NK cells	Killer Ig-like receptor (KIR), inhibition or activation of NK cells
Dendritic cells	CD1a	DC	Nonpeptide antigen presentation
Monocytes	CD14	Myelomonocytic cells	Lipopolysaccharide (LPS) receptor

T cell pool occur even earlier in life. As naïve T cells are required to adequately respond to new antigens that have not been encountered before, the loss of diversity within the naïve T cell compartment may be one factor that contributes to diminution of the host's ability to cope with new pathogens. Effector cells are characterized by the occurrence of a limited number of large, expanded clones. CD8+ effector cells frequently exhibit specificity for persistent viruses, mainly for cytomegalovirus (CMV) but also for Epstein–Barr virus (EBV) or hepatitis C virus (HCV). CMV-specific CD8+ T cells from elderly donors exhibit a terminally differentiated effector phenotype and occur as few largely expanded clones. Expanded CD4+ T cell clonotypes appear to be less frequent.

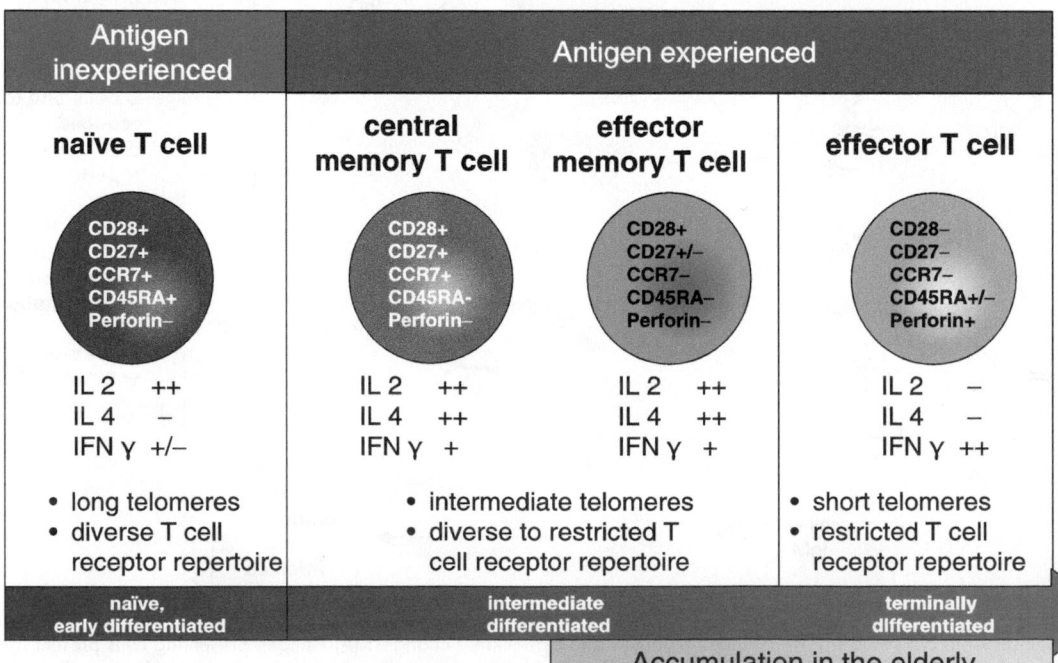

FIGURE 3-6. Characteristics of different T cell subsets upon differentiation. Antigen inexperienced (naïve) and antigen experienced (memory and effector) T cells are shown with respect to their surface marker expression, telomere length, and T cell receptor repertoire. Central memory and effector memory T cells can be distinguished within the memory compartment. Effector memory and effector T cells accumulate in the elderly.

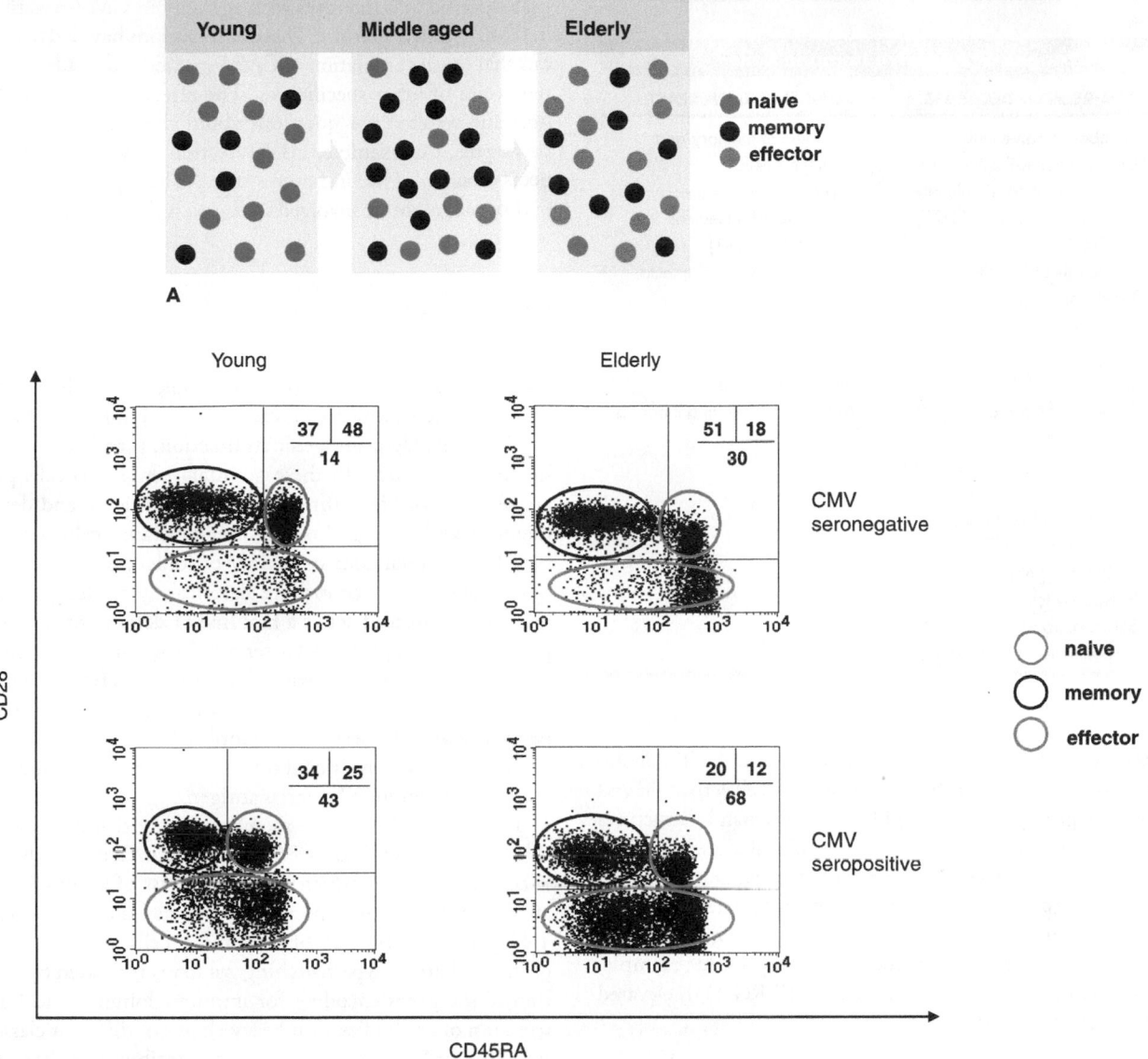

FIGURE 3-7. Age-related changes of the composition of the T cell compartment and influence of latent CMV-infection. (A) Schematic representation of changes in the quantitative distribution of naïve (blue), memory (black), and effector (gray) T cells in peripheral blood. (B) Representative FACS data are shown for young and old CMV-negative and CMV-positive donors. Naïve, memory, and effector CD8$^+$ T cells are defined by expression of CD45RA and CD28 and are highlighted in blue, black, or gray respectively. Percentages of the individual subsets are depicted in the upper right corner. With increasing age the percentage of naïve cells decreases, whereas effector T cells accumulate. CMV-seropositivity significantly enhances these changes. *Reprinted with modifications from Almanzar G, et al. Long-term cytomegalovirus infection leads to significant changes in the composition of the CD8+ T cell repertoire, which may be the basis for an imbalance in the cytokine production profile in elderly persons J Virol. 2005;79:3675. With permission from the American Society for Microbiology.*

Age-related changes in the composition of the T cell pool are accompanied by alterations in the cytokine production profile. Cytokines are crucial for communication processes among immune cells and for the regulation of immunological responses. Murine studies suggest an age-related shift from a T_{H1}-like to a T_{H2}-like response with decreased levels of IL-2 and IFN-γ and an increase in the production of IL-4, IL-6, and IL-10. This shift, however, could not be confirmed in humans, in whom a polarization toward type 1 responses has been shown. This discrepancy may reflect different response patterns in different species, but also differences in experimental protocols.

The influence of aging on T_{H17} cells and their potential role in immunosenescence has not yet been analyzed. A possible role for regulatory T cells (TREGs) in aging has been discussed, but so far no consensus has been reached about if and how this specific T cell type changes with aging.

Age-Related Changes of T Cells on the Single Cell Level (Table 3-4)

Age-related defects also occur at the single cell level. Both signaling deficiencies and changes of immunological synapses that are formed upon interaction of T cells with antigen presenting cells contribute to the altered activation potential of some aged T cells. Hyporesponsiveness to antigenic challenge has been especially observed in CD4$^+$ T cells. This may be due to cell-type-specific changes in the

TABLE 3-4

Age-Related Changes of Adaptive Immune Cells

	AGE-RELATED DECREASE	AGE-RELATED INCREASE
T cells	Number of naïve cells Diversity of the T cell repertoire Expression of co-stimulatory molecules (CD28, CD27, CD40L) Proliferative capacity T cell signaling Activation potential of naïve cells	Numbers of memory and effector cells Expression of senescence-associated molecules (CD57, KLRG-1) Expanded clones of effector cells
B cells	Generation of B cell precursors Diversity of the B cell repertoire Size and number of germinal centers Expression of costimulatory molecules (CD27, CD40) Antibody affinity Isotype switch Serum antibody response to specific foreign antigens	Number of B1 cells Autoreactive serum antibodies

plasma membrane. Lipid raft formation is essential for T cell signalling and may play a role in the regulation of T cell activation and other immunological processes. Lipid rafts are dynamic structures of the plasma membrane where signaling molecules are organized and recruited/excluded in a time-dependent manner. Due to an age-dependent increase of the cholesterol content of plasma membranes, the dynamics of lipid rafts are altered in aged cells. The expression of molecules that are prototypic markers for NK cells, for example, CD57 and killer cell lectin-like receptor G 1 (KLRG-1), is elevated on effector T cells from elderly persons.

Factors That Accelerate Age-Related Changes in the T Cell Pool

Aging is not only a risk factor for infection, but pathogens themselves may contribute to immunosenescence, as repeated exposure to antigens directly shapes the T cell compartment in the aging individual. CMV, a herpes virus that infects the majority of the adult population and establishes lifelong latency in the host, is one example that has been studied in the context of immunosenescence. Infection with CMV induces characteristic changes in the CD4$^+$ as well as in the CD8$^+$ compartment. The age-related decrease of naïve T cells and the accumulation of terminally differentiated effector T cells are enhanced in persons infected with CMV compared to CMV-seronegative elderly persons (Figure 3-7B). Longitudinal studies of individuals above the age of 86 years with a follow-up of up to 8 years found that 2-year mortality could be predicted using the so-called "immune risk phenotype" (IRP) defined by immunological parameters like a low CD8$^+$/CD4$^+$ ratio and a poor response of T cells after stimulation with mitogens. The IRP was also associated with CMV seropositivity.

Chronic infection with CMV appears to affect the capacity of the immune system to respond to other pathogens. For example, the immune response to EBV is also impaired, as the number of EBV-specific cells increases with age only in CMV-negative but not in CMV-positive persons. These observations have led to the hypothesis that the accumulation of CMV-specific cells leads to a shrunken repertoire of other specificities. The effects of CMV on the aging immune system raise questions about the role of other persistent pathogens. For example, HIV infection may accelerate certain aspects of aging of the immune system. Thus, persistent or recurrent pathogens might be involved in the complex process of immunosenescence.

B Lymphocytes

Generally, B cells can be divided into three subsets: follicular (B2), marginal zone (MZ), and B1 B cells. Follicular B cells originate from primary follicles, which are areas within the lymph nodes where naïve B cells reside. Upon antigenic stimulation, germinal centers develop in the lymph node. In these germinal centers, B cells proliferate, are selected for high-affinity binding to antigen, and develop into memory B cells and antibody-producing plasma cells. The peripheral blood B cell pool consists mainly of follicular B cells. In contrast, MZ B cells do not contribute significantly to the germinal center reaction but instead act as a first line of defense against pathogens, particularly encapsulated bacteria, which enter the blood stream. The subset of B cells known as B1 cells differs from the majority of B cells. Generally only 5% to 10% of the total B cell pool in the periphery and the secondary lymphoid organs are B1 cells. They express a relatively restricted repertoire of immunoglobulins mainly recognizing common bacterial antigens.

Resting B cells express membrane-bound immunoglobulin M (IgM), also referred to as BCR. Upon contact with their antigen, B cells secrete IgM, which is the first class of antibodies produced after stimulation. In response to cytokines and direct contact with T helper cells, a fraction of activated B cells undergoes the process of heavy chain isotype switching, which is mediated by recombination of the genes encoding for immunoglobulins and leads to the secretion of antibodies with heavy chains of different classes such as IgG, IgA, or IgE (Figure 3-5B). These antibody classes perform distinct effector functions. IgG antibodies block the entry of pathogens into cells and mediate phagocytosis by macrophages. These antibodies are needed for effective defense against most viral and bacterial pathogens. IgA antibodies are mainly produced by B cells in mucosal tissues, as these antibodies are most efficiently transported into mucosal secretions where they eliminate microbes entering through the epithelia. IgE antibodies are generated in response to helminths and also mediate allergic reactions. In a further step of maturation, somatic recombination occurs in the variable region of the genes encoding for immunoglobulins in order to generate antibodies with higher affinity. Long-lived memory B cells and plasma cells reside in the body for up to several decades and ensure efficient "recall" responses in the case of subsequent encounter of the same pathogen.

Age-Related Changes of the B Cell Compartment

Primary antibody responses in aged humans are often weaker, antibody levels drop faster, and the antibodies bind their antigen with lower affinity compared to young adults. These responses have been studied in detail in the context of vaccination and it has been concluded that the protective effect of vaccinations against *Streptococcus pneumoniae*, influenza, hepatitis B, and tetanus is decreased with age.

Additionally, aging is also associated with an increased prevalence of autoantibodies. These antibodies are in the majority of cases present in low concentrations and are frequently directed against cellular components such as nuclei or mitochondria. They rarely contribute to autoimmune diseases, which classically occur earlier in life.

The impact of aging on peripheral B cells is complex and involves a variety of changes of single cells as well as of the repertoire. The number of B2 cells is reduced in elderly people. In contrast, there are more B1 cells, which means that fewer of the classical, antibody-producing B cells that are essential for defense against pathogens are present. Some of the changes observed in the B cell compartment seem to parallel the ones observed in the T cell pool. Thus the number of naïve B cells decreases in some elderly people while memory cells accumulate, leading to clonal expansions of certain B cell specificities. These expansions may limit the diversity of the repertoire.

As mentioned above, isotype switching is required to produce high-affinity IgG antibodies that eliminate pathogens. Defects in isotype switching lead to the accumulation of B cells producing IgM and a concomitant lack of IgG-secreting cells. IgM antibodies have a lower affinity to antigens. Age-related defects in somatic mutation also lead to a reduced affinity of antibodies from aged individuals (Table 3-4).

Age-Related Defects in Interactions Between T and B Cells

As interactions with T cells are essential for B cell activation and antibody production, it is difficult to attribute defects in the humoral immune response exclusively to intrinsic alterations of B cells. Low-level and transient production of specific antibodies in elderly persons is frequently due to a combination of age-related defects in the generation and maturation of B cells and dysregulated or defective T cell help.

Aged CD4$^+$ T cells produce less IL-2 and as a consequence express less CD40L, which is a crucial molecule in the interaction of B and T cells. Less efficient T cell help leads to a reduced antigen-specific B cell expansion and differentiation as well as to decreased IgG production and germinal center formation. T helper cells also play a crucial role in isotype switching and the affinity maturation of antibodies. A defective T helper function thus contributes to diminished high-affinity B cell responses in old age. In fact, in mouse models, there is little evidence of intrinsic age-dependent defects in B cell function. Rather, age-related loss of B cell function is a result of poor T cell stimulation.

Cutaneous Immune System

The specialized immune system that is found in the skin is called the cutaneous immune system and consists of lymphocytes and antigen-presenting cells. The epidermis is composed of keratinocytes, melanocytes, Langerhans cells (LC), and intraepidermal T cells. Keratinocytes and melanocytes play no role for the adaptive immune response; however, keratinocytes are capable of producing cytokines that contribute to innate immune responses and local inflammation. Langerhans cells are immature DC and are specialized for capturing antigens that enter the body through the skin. After contact with the antigen, they mature, migrate into the dermis, and via lymphatic vessels to the lymph nodes, where they act as antigen-presenting cells and stimulate T cells. Only a small fraction of the skin-associated lymphocytes reside in the epidermis, and most of them are CD8$^+$ T cells. The majority of cutaneous T cells (both CD4$^+$ and CD8$^+$) are found in the dermis. Most of these T cells show an activated or memory phenotype. However, it is unclear whether these cells permanently populate the skin compartment or are circulating between blood, lymphatic vessels, and tissues. Macrophages are also present in the dermis.

Age-associated changes of T cells and macrophages as described above also affect these cell types in the skin and contribute to the impaired immunological properties of aged skin. Langerhans cells, which are found exclusively in the epidermis, also undergo age-related alterations. The number of Langerhans cells decreases with age. Morphological changes like reduced formation of dendrites have been observed in LC from aged individuals. In animal models, the capability of LC to trap antigen, present it to T cells, and stimulate T cell proliferation decreases with age. However, these functional defects have not been confirmed in humans. Migration of LC from the epidermis to local lymph nodes is essential for antigen presentation and activation of adaptive immune responses. Migration of LC following administration of TNF-α is impaired with aging. However IL-1β-induced mobilization of LC seems to be intact in aged individuals.

Keratinocytes produce a variety of pro- and anti-inflammatory cytokines like interleukins, interferons, growth factors, and chemokines upon stimulation by UV light, allergens, or infectious agents. Only a few cytokines have been analyzed in the context of skin aging. As an example, keratinocytes of elderly persons produce less IL-1 and more of the antagonist of the IL-1 receptor, reducing the overall IL-1 activity. Therefore local inflammation and activation of innate immune responses could be reduced at the site of infection.

In addition to age-related changes of ubiquitous immune cells and of skin-specific immunologically active cells like keratinocytes and Langerhans cells, morphological and structural changes of the aged skin contribute to the increased incidence of skin infections in elderly people.

Mucosal Immune System

The mucosal surfaces of the gastrointestinal and respiratory tracts are colonized by lymphocytes and antigen-presenting cells that initiate immune responses against ingested or inhaled antigens. However, little is known about age-related changes of the immune function of the respiratory mucosa. More is known about aging effects on the gastrointestinal tract. Lymphocytes are found within the epithelial layer as well as in the lamina propria and in organized structures called Peyer's patches with distinct cell populations at the different sites. Like lymph nodes and lymphoid follicles in the spleen, the Peyer's patches contain B cell-rich areas, which contain germinal centers that are essential for initiation of immune responses. The gastrointestinal tract is permanently colonized by the gut flora. The mucosal immune system on the one hand establishes tolerance to the indigenous microflora and to food proteins and on the other hand fights pathogens by the production of IgA antibodies and the activation of T cells. Total IgA levels are unchanged or even elevated in elderly people, whereas the response to specific antigens as measured by specific IgA is lower in aged animals. Aged mice also exhibit decreased susceptibility to oral tolerance induction. The precise cellular and molecular regulatory mechanisms in the induction of mucosal tolerance and immunity and their alterations in aging are currently not fully understood. However, it seems reasonable to argue that increased susceptibility to infectious agents that enter the body through mucosal surfaces is at least partly due to age-related defects in mucosal immunity.

CLINICAL IMPLICATIONS OF IMMUNOSENESCENCE

Infectious Diseases

A thorough review of "Infections in Older Adults" can be found in Chapter 124, and individual chapters throughout this textbook. The high rate of infection-related hospitalization in elderly people is not only due to increased incidence of infection but also because of more severe symptoms and underlying comorbidity. Most common infections have a poorer prognosis in elderly patients, partially due to decreased immune function. In addition, underlying diseases that cause tissue damage and age-related changes (e.g. of the epithelium) facilitate infection. Fever is generally less common in elderly patients. Less than 50% of frail, very elderly patients with infection will develop temperatures high enough to be considered fever.

Immunosenescence and Cancer

The immune system plays a crucial role in controlling cancer and protecting the individual. As immune function declines with age, it seems reasonable to hypothesize that immunosenescence might be involved in the dramatic age-related increase of many cancers (see Chapter 94). However, despite provocative findings described below, the relevance of immunosenescence to tumor development and immune evasion remains controversial.

Enhanced inflammatory responses may contribute to tumor development in the elderly people. Genetic polymorphisms, resulting in distinct expression levels of cytokines like IL-6 and IL-10, could theoretically affect tumor incidence and progression. Additionally, the limited pool of naïve T cells and the impaired processing and presentation of antigens might contribute to a decreased recognition of emerging tumor antigens and to the increased incidence of tumors with aging. Some evidence suggests that at least some of the mechanisms that are used by tumor cells to escape immune surveillance are more effective in elderly people. Tumors often express fas ligand (FasL), which interacts with its receptor (FasR) on the surface of lymphocytes and induces apoptosis in the T cells that attack the tumor. As the expression of FasR is elevated on aged cells, T cells infiltrating the tumor might be killed more effectively in elderly people, allowing tumor growth. Several tumors release immunosuppressive cytokines to suppress antitumor immune responses. This immunosuppressive strategy of the tumor could be more effective in the already proinflammatory milieu of the aged immune system. Other factors involved in cancer-induced immunosuppression are prostaglandins that are produced by tumor cells. Aged lymphocytes may be more sensitive to prostaglandins, which inhibit activation of antitumor lymphocytes.

Thus, a variety of links may connect immunosenescence, tumor incidence, and tumor growth. However, more research is required to elucidate the interplay of immunosenescence, age-related changes of other body systems, environmental influences, and stochastic events in tumorigenesis.

IMMUNOLOGICAL INTERVENTIONS

Vaccines

Vaccination is the most cost-effective measure to prevent infection-related disease. More than 25 different infectious diseases can be prevented by vaccination. Large-scale vaccination programs have led to the eradication of smallpox and to a dramatic reduction of diseases like poliomyelitis, diphtheria, tetanus, measles, mumps, and many more. However, vaccination efficacy is generally lower in the elderly population, and this particularly vulnerable cohort may not be fully protected following immunization. For some vaccines such as tetanus, diphtheria, and pertussis, vaccination induces lower concentrations of antibodies in the elderly people. Additionally, antibody titers decline more rapidly in aged individuals compared to young adults. The quality and specific type of antibody may also be important in determining the effectiveness of vaccination in an elderly patient.

Recommendations for Vaccination

Several vaccinations are specifically recommended for elderly people in various developed countries. Vaccination against influenza is recommended for everybody above the age of 60 or 65 years as influenza is associated with a high risk of severe disease and death in this age group. Due to the occurrence of various viral subtypes and a high rate of mutation, the influenza vaccine is matched with circulating strains every year. Thus, annual vaccination with the new vaccine is required to obtain protection. Vaccination rates have increased since the 1990s, but depending on the region they still only range from 30% to 60% of the elderly population. Although influenza vaccination efficacy decreases with advancing age, hospitalization and death due to influenza are reduced by vaccination (see Chapter 130 for additional details on influenza vaccine and other preventive measures).

Another vaccine that is generally recommended for elderly individuals is the 23-valent polysaccharide vaccine directed against *Streptococcus pneumonia*. Case–control studies suggest that the incidence of invasive pneumococcal disease is reduced by 65% in vaccinated elderly people. However, protection of high-risk groups with underlying comorbidities is lower. Vaccine efficacy with regard to pneumonia is generally low. The poor efficacy of the vaccine for preventing pneumonia and the associated apathy of patients and providers accounts for some of the relatively low vaccination coverage in elderly populations (see Chapter 126 for additional information on preventing pneumonia and pneumoccocal vaccination).

Reactivation of Varizella-Zoster virus, which manifests as herpes zoster, occurs in old age, in part because the immune response established after primary infection weakens with time. However, individuals who frequently come in contact with the virus, e.g. via children with varicella, have a reduced risk of herpes zoster. Vaccination to prevent herpes zoster has now been approved in the United States and in Europe for use in elderly people. The attenuated live vaccine contains a higher dose of the same virus strain that is also used for vaccination of infants. The vaccination is recommended for individuals over the age of 60 years. Incidence of herpes zoster and postherpetic neuralgia is reduced by approximately 50% and 67%, respectively. Currently, the maximum follow-up of the first large clinical trials is 3 years, which means that it is not yet clear how long the protective effect will last and whether booster vaccinations will be necessary (see Chapter 129 for details on herpes zoster and its prevention).

As the number of elderly individuals vaccinated against yellow fever has increased in recent years, it has become apparent that this age group might be at a higher risk of developing severe adverse effects. It has been postulated that the aged immune system might be failing to control the attenuated vaccine virus, leading to systemic infection.

Improving Vaccination Efficacy

It is now apparent that specific vaccination strategies and vaccines are needed for elderly people. Most vaccines currently used aim to induce serum antibodies. For efficient induction of antibody production, B cells need to be stimulated by $CD4^+$ T helper cells. Thus, vaccines specifically targeting enhanced $CD4^+$ T cell responses might also be successful in increasing antibody production. This strategy could lead to more efficient vaccines that are able to raise protective antibody levels in the elderly people. However, conjugation of polysaccharides to protein (e.g., pneumococcal and meningococcal polysaccharide conjugate vaccines) that significantly enhances $CD4^+$ T cell responses and vaccine efficacy in very young children has not markedly improved responses in older adults. The reasons for this remain uncertain. Possible explanations could be the nature of the protein conjugate, prior immunity, or age-related defects of the innate immune system.

For various pathogens like influenza, tuberculosis, hepatitis B, and herpes zoster, $CD8^+$ cytotoxic T cells play a key role in the control of infection as they eliminate infected cells and prevent further spread of the infection. Vaccinations against these pathogens could be designed to induce not only specific antibodies but also long-lasting $CD8^+$ T cell memory.

Several approaches are currently being investigated in order to improve vaccination efficacy for elderly people. Attenuated live vaccines are highly immunogenic and induce strong T and B cell responses. However, as observed for vaccination against yellow fever, live vaccines in old age might be associated with an increased risk of side effects. The use of live-attenuated vaccines early in life and/or during young adulthood followed by booster vaccination with inactivated vaccines in old age could be one possible strategy to overcome this problem. It has been shown, for example, that previous vaccination with polio live vaccine enhances the effect of booster with the inactivated vaccine later in life.

In order to increase immunogenicity of inactivated vaccines, they can be supplemented with adjuvants, which facilitate an effective immune response. Different classes of adjuvants improve processing and presentation of the antigen, stimulate components of the innate immune response, or provide the appropriate cytokine environment to elicit T and B cell responses. However, very few adjuvants are currently approved for use in humans. Many vaccines are supplemented with aluminum salts, which enhance antibody production but have little effect on cellular immunity. MF59® is an oil-in-water emulsion that is used as an adjuvant in influenza vaccines. The adju-

vanted vaccine seems to be more efficient in elderly people, leading to higher rates of seroconversion compared to conventional vaccines. Numerous adjuvants are currently being tested in animal studies or in early clinical trials. Of particular interest are immunomodulatory adjuvants that might overcome the specific deficits of the aging immune system.

The effect of booster vaccinations is dependent on the time since the last vaccination and particularly on the antibody titer before booster. It is therefore of crucial importance to increase public awareness that regular booster vaccinations during adulthood are essential to maintain the ability to respond to recall antigens in old age. Shortened intervals of booster vaccinations for individuals above 60 years might also be a possible strategy to ensure protective antibody levels.

Unfortunately, it is necessary to emphasize that vaccination coverage remains suboptimal in elderly populations. Only 60% of elderly people are vaccinated against influenza or pneumococcal infection despite clear efficacy of these vaccines. Regular boosters and increased vaccination coverage could be efficient short-term tools to increase protection of the vulnerable aged population.

Caloric Restriction

For several decades, experiments have been performed in different model organisms in which caloric intake was reduced. When supplemented with vitamins and essential elements to avoid malnutrition, caloric restriction of ~30% increases life span of invertebrates (*Coenorhabditis elegans, Drosophila melanogaster*), rodents (mice, rats, hamsters), and other vertebrates (birds, zebra fish) significantly (see Chapter 1). Various mechanisms have been postulated to be responsible for this effect, including the delay of immunosenescence. Generally, dietary restriction is particularly effective when applied long-term and before the onset of aging. Trials conducted with non-human primates (*Macacus rhesus*) in which CR was applied for 10 to 17 years have confirmed physiological and immunological effects that were observed in dietary-restricted smaller animals. CR prevented the loss of naïve T cells and preserved the diversity of the T cell repertoire. Additionally, T cell function was improved and less inflammatory cytokines were produced by memory T cells. Primate studies are still ongoing and aim to eventually elucidate the influence of caloric restriction on life span.

Additional Measures to Improve Immune Function

In order to overcome age-related defects of the immune system, several interesting approaches to delay or even reverse immunosenescence are being investigated using animal models. As described above, involution of the thymus and the resulting loss of newly generated naïve T cells may contribute to the deterioration of immune function with age. For this reason, thymic regeneration might reduce immunosenescence. Some experiments with mice have shown that it is possible to partially restore thymopoiesis and to stimulate regrowth of the thymus to a certain extent. However, other studies have been less compelling and full rejuvenation of the thymus and regeneration to its previous size has not yet been achieved.

Another driving force for age-related changes of the immune system is chronic stimulation by immunodominant pathogens that favor the accumulation of highly differentiated T cell clones, replacing naïve and functional memory T cells. It has been suggested that a reduction of antigenic stimulation by eradication of chronic subclinical infections as they are found in the oral cavity, the gastrointestinal tract, and the urinary tract could improve the immune status in old age. As described above latent infection with CMV may accelerate immunosenescence and accumulation of senescent effector T cells. Whether early life vaccination to prevent CMV infection could affect CMV-associated immunological changes in old age has not been tested.

Alternatively, the highly differentiated, clonally expanded T cells that result from chronic antigenic stimulation could be depleted in order to give room for more "useful" T cells. However, it would be essential to remove only dysfunctional T cells without interfering with functionally intact, less differentiated T cells. It has also been proposed to isolate T cells early in adulthood and to store them in vitro until a person needs "fresh" T cells in old age. With this approach, it would theoretically be possible to manipulate the cells before reperfusion, for example, by expanding selected T cell subpopulations or T cells of certain specificities that promise the greatest benefit for the recipient.

CONCLUSION

One major challenge of the future will be to prolong healthy life in which quality of life is maintained. Overcoming the detrimental effects of immunosenescence may be one important step in achieving this goal. Infectious diseases harbor a substantial risk for illness, loss of independence, disabilities, and death for elderly people. Whereas vaccinations constitute an effective measure to prevent infection, age-related defects of the immune system impede protection following vaccination of older adults. New vaccines and vaccination strategies that specifically target the aged immune system may help ensure protection of the vulnerable elderly population. Deeper insight into and an even better understanding of the immunological changes that occur with age will without doubt help to delay or even reverse the deleterious effects of immune dysfunction in the elderly people.

FURTHER READING

Allman D, Miller JP. B cell development and receptor diversity during aging. *Curr Opin Immunol.* 2005;17:463.

Artz AS, Ershler WB, Longo DL. Pneumococcal vaccination and revaccination of older adults. *Clin Microbiol Rev.* 2003;16:308.

Bader MS, McKinsey DS. Viral infections in the elderly. The challenges of managing herpes zoster, influenza, and RSV. *Postgrad Med.* 2005;118:45.

Cambier J. Immunosenescence: a problem of lymphopoiesis, homeostasis, microenvironment, and signaling. *Immunol Rev.* 2005;205:5–6.

Chen J. Senescence and functional failure in hematopoietic stem cells. *Exp Hematol.* 2004;32:1025.

Cunningham-Rundles S. The effect of aging on mucosal host defense. *J Nutr Health Aging* 2004;8:20.

Dejaco C, Duftner C, Schirmer M. Are regulatory T-cells linked with aging? *Exp Gerontol.* 2006;41:339.

Gardner EM, Murasko DM. Age-related changes in Type 1 and Type 2 cytokine production in humans. *Biogerontology.* 2002;3:271.

Gavazzi G, Krause KH. Ageing and infection. *Lancet Infect Dis.* 2002;2:659.

Gomez CR, Boehmer ED, Kovacs EJ. The aging innate immune system. *Curr Opin Immunol.* 2005;17:457.

Goodwin K, Viboud C, Simonsen L. Antibody response to influenza vaccination in the elderly: a quantitative review. *Vaccine.* 2006;24:1159.

Gravekamp C. Cancer vaccines in old age. *Exp Gerontol.* 2007;42:441.

Kovaiou RD, Herndler-Brandstetter D, Grubeck-Loebenstein B. Age-related changes in immunity: implications for vaccination in the elderly. *Expert Rev Mol Med.* 2007;9:1.

Linton PJ, Dorshkind K. Age-related changes in lymphocyte development and function. *Nat Immunol.* 2004;5:133.

Messaoudi I, Warner J, Fischer M, et al. Delay of T cell senescence by caloric restriction in aged long-lived nonhuman primates. *Proc Natl Acad Sci USA.* 2006; 103:19448.

Pawelec G, Akbar A, Caruso C, et al. Human immunosenescence: is it infectious? *Immunol Rev.* 2005;205:257.

Plackett TP, Boehmer ED, Faunce DE, et al. Aging and innate immune cells. *J Leukoc Biol.* 2004;76:291.

Provinciali M, Smorlesi A. Immunoprevention and immunotherapy of cancer in ageing. *Cancer Immunol Immunother.* 2005;54:93.

Salvioli S, Capri M, Valensin S, et al. Inflamm-aging, cytokines and aging: state of the art, new hypotheses on the role of mitochondria and new perspectives from systems biology. *Curr Pharm Des.* 2006;12:3161.

Shurin GV, Yurkovetsky ZR, Chatta GS, et al. Dynamic alteration of soluble serum biomarkers in healthy aging. *Cytokine.* 2007;39:123.

Shurin MR, Shurin GV, Chatta GS. Aging and the dendritic cell system: implications for cancer. *Crit Rev Oncol Hematol.* 2007;64:90.

Taub DD, Longo DL. Insights into thymic aging and regeneration. *Immunol Rev.* 2005;205:72.

Weinberger B, Herndler-Brandstetter D, Schwanninger G, et al. Biology of immune responses to vaccines in elderly persons. *Clin Inf Dis.* 2008;46:1078.

Wilson NJ, Boniface K, Chan JR, et al. Development, cytokine profile and function of human interleukin 17-producing helper T cells. *Nat Immunol.* 2007;8:950.

Inflammation and Aging

Jeremy D. Walston

In recent years, multiple studies of older adults have identified strong relationships between serum markers of inflammation and frailty, worsening chronic disease, disability, and mortality. Although these studies are not proof that the chronic activation of inflammatory pathways causes these adverse health care outcomes, recent biological evidence supports that chronic exposure to inflammatory mediators leads to alterations in multiple physiological systems. These in turn contribute to the older adult's vulnerability to adverse health outcomes. Because the activation of inflammatory pathways appear to be so intricately linked to many aging systems, some investigators have propagated use of the term "inflammaging" as a summary of the physiological and molecular changes consistent with the aging process that are known to be associated with chronic activation of inflammatory pathways. Other investigators now utilize "chronic inflammation" as a descriptor for the ongoing activation of the innate immune system that has been observed in some older individuals. The rising use of these terms in aging research and in clinical practice signifies the emerging importance of inflammation as an important contribution, adverse health outcomes in older adults. The study of the clinical utility of relevant inflammatory biomarkers, the understanding of the specific age-related mechanisms that activate and sustain chronic inflammation in older adults, and exploration of the impact that inflammatory mediators and pathway activation have on specific physiological systems and on the overall vulnerability observed in older adults are certain to impact both research and clinical agendas for older adults in the coming years. Given this crucial focus and the importance of understanding this emerging area of investigation for those who care for older adults, and the high likelihood that both investigators and clinicians will likely encounter this important and evolving area of aging research in the coming years, this chapter will (1) describe evolving definitions of inflammation used in the context of aging research and clinical practice, (2) provide a review of the robust relationships between activation of inflammatory pathways and adverse health outcomes previously identified in older adults, (3) describe the pertinent areas of the molecular biol-

ogy of inflammation necessary to understand how and why older adults are more vulnerable to inflammatory pathway activation, (4) characterize the relationships between inflammatory pathway activation, multisystem decline, and the biological vulnerability observed in older adults, and (5) highlight the current and potential future clinical relevance of inflammation in older adults.

INFLAMMATION IN THE CONTEXT OF AGING AND ADVERSE HEALTH OUTCOMES

Inflammation, often referred to as the activation of the innate immune system, is a complex and important physiological response to external threats. In general, it is a critical housekeeping function that acts to fight acute infections and repair wounds through common biological pathways that in turn activate hormonal, thrombotic, and cytokine pathways (Figure 4-1). These pathways function throughout the life span to attenuate or eliminate countless infections and injuries from becoming life-threatening events. This inflammatory signaling is in general a self-limiting process that ends when the infection or injury is resolved and the local and systemic inflammatory pathways return to a state of inactivation. Common clinical examples that lead to the activation of inflammatory pathways and that are attenuated by inflammatory processes at any age include responses to localized superficial injuries such as skin lacerations, localized infections such as urinary tract infections or small abscesses, systemic bacterial infections, and major trauma such as bone fractures or organ injury. In the most superficial processes, inflammation is localized and does not usually result in a measurable systemic response. However, in major infections or injuries, systemic activation of inflammatory pathways result in measurable elevations in circulating inflammatory cytokines and other acute-phase reactant proteins, cortisol, and sympathetic nervous system activation.

In most cases, these small or large innate immune system responses are largely self-limited by negative feedback mechanisms

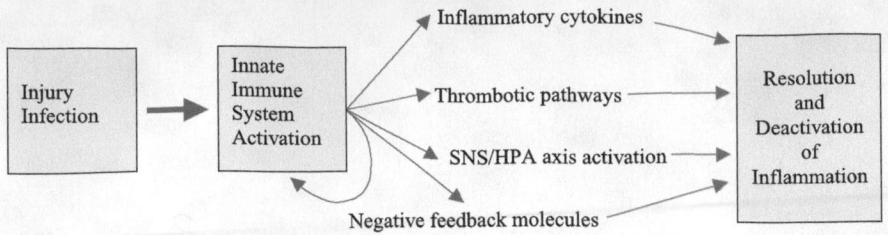

FIGURE 4-1. Normal inflammatory response to injury or infection, with activation of multiple physiological pathways and ultimately resolution of response.

and by the resolution of initial injury or infection (Figure 4-1). However, recent evidence from population studies of older adults suggests that many older individuals who have no obvious injury or infection have ongoing activation of inflammatory processes even when multiple acute and chronic conditions are accounted for. The inflammatory measurements of total white blood cells, neutrophils, and inflammatory cytokines, even after adjustment for disease states, are usually highly correlated with each other. These studies also provide important evidence of a link between inflammatory pathway activation and adverse health outcomes as detailed below.

Part of the evidence that the chronic activation of inflammatory pathways in older adults may be pathological comes from dozens of well-performed association studies that have identified significant inverse relationships between the common adverse health outcomes of disability, frailty, and mortality and elevated serum interleukin-6 (IL-6) and/or C-reactive protein (CRP). A study by Ferrucci et al. demonstrated a 76% increased risk of developing mobility disability over 4 years in previously nondisabled participants of the Established Populations for Epidemiologic Studies of the Elderly who were in the highest tertile of IL-6 compared to those in the lowest tertile. This study identified a serum IL-6 level of 2.5 pg/mL as an important threshold point beyond which the risk for developing disability rises exponentially. In the Cardiovascular Health Study, investigators identified an odds ratio for being frail of 2.80 in those older adults with a CRP level above 5.77 μg/mL even after excluding those participants with cardiovascular disease and diabetes. In a later study, Puts et al. identified an odds ratio of 1.69 for incident frailty in older adults with a CRP level between 3 and 10 mg/mL. Other investigators have identified strong inverse relationships between inflammatory mediators and mortality in older adults. In the study of osteoporotic fractures, Tice et al. identified an eightfold risk for cardiovascular mortality over 6 years in those with CRP levels above 3.0 mg/mL. Harris et al. identified an 1.9-fold increased relative risk for death over 4.6 years in those participants in the Iowa 65+ Rural Health Study with IL-6 levels greater than 3.19 pg/mL compared to those with low IL-6 levels. Similarly, CRP levels over 2.78 mg/mL also predicted a relative risk for death of 1.6 over the same period of time. Importantly, combining IL-6 and CRP in the analysis increased the sensitivity of identifying those at increased risk of all-cause mortality by identifying a 2.6-fold risk of dying over the same period if both inflammatory markers were elevated compared to the group with neither elevated. Interestingly, many of these studies either excluded participants with severe or chronic disease states known to activate inflammatory pathways, or at least adjusted for them in statistical models, suggesting that this elevation is not purely a result of chronic disease. Although it is not possible to conclude that the activation of inflammatory pathways is causal in these adverse health outcomes for these mostly cross-sectional association studies, their consistency suggests an important connection between chronic inflammatory pathway activation and adverse health outcomes. Further support for the importance of the connection between inflammation and adverse clinical outcomes has come from the many clinical and basic biological studies that have helped to better elucidate the mechanisms by which inflammatory pathways and adverse health outcomes are connected as described below.

MOLECULAR BIOLOGY OF INFLAMMATION

Clues to etiology logically extend from recently developed knowledge about age-related physiological and molecular changes and from improved understanding of the signal transduction pathways that activate or deactivate the inflammatory process. Although triggers for inflammation may vary, the key gateway molecular signal transduction system centers around the nuclear transcription factor nuclear factor kappa B (NFκB) (Figure 4-2). NFκB, when activated by specific stress or inflammatory signals, facilitates the expression of multiple inflammatory mediators and in general leads to a cascade

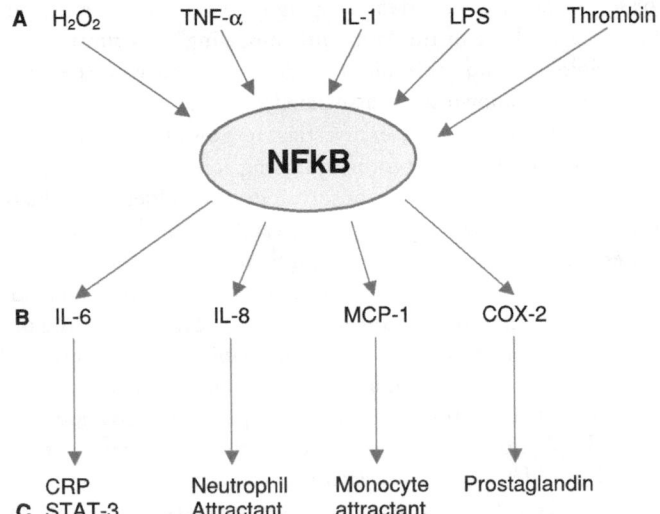

FIGURE 4-2. Schematic of the inflammatory gateway nuclear transcription factor NFκB (center circle), along with inflammatory triggers (row A), and inflammatory outflow (rows B and C). Row A shows specific inflammatory stimuli that lead to NFκB activation via specific cell receptors and specific signal transduction pathways (not shown). Activated subunits of NFκB (center circle) in turn leads to the expression of proteins that provide negative feedback for inflammation (not shown) or that propagate inflammatory message (row B) and influence the activation of other pathways (row C) that influence inflammatory response, thrombosis, and the expression of other proteins.

of molecular messages that in sum represents an inflammation (Figure 4-2, row B). Embedded in this response are connections to other important signals that provide negative feedback necessary to attenuate inflammatory responses, and to other signals that provide connections toward or away from apoptosis. Because of the complexity of this signal transduction pathway, a detailed discussion of this biology is well beyond the scope of this chapter. However, because this biology will likely be relevant to the future clinical care of older adults, it is important to understand how and why these pathways may be chronically active in some older adults, and how their downstream effects contribute to many of the pathophysiological changes and even symptoms that older adults experience. Understanding these molecular pathways also helps to facilitate the understanding of the biology that makes older adults more vulnerable to a host of diseases and adverse outcomes, and may provide some future specificity as investigators begin to target these pathways in pharmaceutical interventions for older adults.

Inflammatory Signal

A set of cell surface receptors (Figure 4-2A) act through cell signal transduction pathways to activate NFκB. This links the message of "stress" to the cell nucleus, where inflammatory mediators are in turn generated (Figure 4-2, row B). One of the more important triggers of NFκB-induced inflammatory pathway activators include the tumor necrosis factor alpha (TNF-α). TNF-α is secreted very early in the inflammatory process, usually from immune system cells in response to infections. TNF-α, originally discovered as a serum factor related to cancer, is also secreted in high amounts from the connective tissue surrounding malignancies, and from adipocytes. It has several subtypes of specific cell surface receptors that act to transmit the message of inflammation, which in turn activates NFκB and leads to the expression of a host of inflammatory mediators as described below. Interleukin-1 (IL-1) is most often secreted in response to infections and injury, and activates and amplifies inflammatory signaling through its own cell surface receptor. In addition, IL-1 has recently been identified as a major cytokine that is secreted from senescent cells, providing support that may play an important role in late life activation of inflammatory pathways.[7] In addition to these early inflammatory cytokine signals, the bacterial surface antigen lipopolysaccharide (LPS) and some viral particles bind to a family of cell surface toll-like receptors (TLR), which in turn set off a separate signal transduction pathway that in turn amplifies NFκB-related inflammatory signaling. This pathway to inflammatory activation is certainly crucial for the protection of the organism against acute infections, and likely also helps in organized defense against chronic infections. Recent evidence suggests that thrombin, a clotting component, may also activate inflammatory pathways through its own receptor. This provides a link between injury and inflammation. Finally, and potentially very important for aging-related activation of inflammatory systems, the free radicals superoxide and hydrogen peroxide activate inflammatory pathways via signal transduction pathways that facilitate NFκB-mediated inflammatory gene production (Figure 4-2, row A). In sum, all of these specific activating molecules, cell surface receptors, and signal transduction pathways, no matter what the ultimate triggering mechanisms is, transmit the message of stress to the nucleus of the cell, where NFκB-related activity induces the expression of inflammatory mediators that act to either amplify the inflammatory message or exert nega-

tive feedback that brakes inflammatory signaling as described below (Figure 4-2).

Inflammatory Message

The molecules that are generated by inflammatory signaling give specificity to the inflammatory message that in sum activates inflammatory pathways or leads to an attenuation of that signal (Figure 4-2, rows B and C). The complexity of these pathways and the limited understanding of what drives inflammatory specificity limits the following discussion to a general overview relevant to previously published aging studies. The molecules that are most known for being elevated in older adults that make up the most easily measurable systemic inflammatory response include IL-6 and CRP. IL-6 is a pleiotropic cytokine that in combination with cell-bound and circulating IL-6 receptor plays a crucial role in both inflammatory and anti-inflammatory balancing in acute inflammation. Chronic IL-6 production also leads to the expression of CRP, a commonly measured inflammatory mediator that likely functions at the interface between inflammation and thrombosis and is therefore an increasingly important marker of cardiovascular disease risk. Both of these NFκB pathway-induced molecules have been repeatedly shown to associate with adverse outcomes in older adults. Other potent inflammatory mediators produced by NFκB activation include (1) cyclooxygenase 2 (COX 2), best known for its role in joint inflammation and its key role in prostaglandin production, (2) interleukin-8 (IL-8), a potent neutrophil attractant factor, and (3) monocyte chemoattractant protein 1 (MCP-1), a protein that amplifies monocyte inflammatory response. Each of these factors, and multiple others known to be stimulated by NFκB-related activation, serve to amplify inflammatory signaling both locally and systemically, and provide some specificity in response.

In addition to these inflammation-specific functions, NFκB signaling also leads to the expression of proteins that provide negative feedback to NFκB. NFκB-related signal transduction also plays an important role at the interface between inflammatory signaling, apoptosis, and the development of cellular senescence. Although the details of these pathways are beyond the scope of this chapter, more detailed understanding of the balance between inflammation, apoptosis, and cell senescence may help elucidate many of the important questions underlying late life declines in multiple physiological systems.

WHY ARE OLDER ADULTS MORE LIKELY TO HAVE HIGHER LEVELS OF INFLAMMATORY CYTOKINES?

Several NFκB pathway triggering mechanisms intrinsic to the aging process lead to the production of inflammatory mediators including: (1) increased numbers of dysfunctional, cytokine secreting senescent cells, (2) increases in TNF-α- and IL-6-producing adipocytes related to increased body fat in older adults, (3) age-related increases in free radicals of oxygen, which are known to directly trigger NFκB activity and lead to the increased generation of inflammatory mediators, and (4) age-related declines in levels of hormones known to attenuate NFκB activity. In addition, multiple chronic disease states can contribute to increased serum levels of inflammatory cytokines and variation in inflammation-related genes that are unmarked in the face of disease states of increased cytokine levels. These reasons are

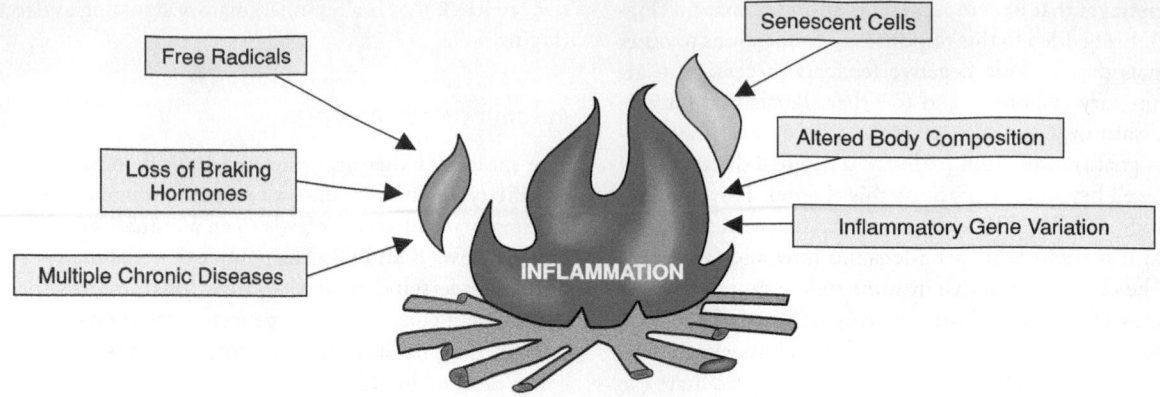

Feeding the Fire of Inflammation in Older Adults

FIGURE 4-3. Feeding the fire of inflammation: Multiple age-related molecular and physical alterations account for the increased propensity toward higher levels of inflammatory pathway activation in older adults.

likely additive, and at least are hypothesized to activate a fire of inflammation (Figure 4-3).

With increasing age and increasing numbers of cell cycle passage, many cell types take on senescent characteristics that include inability to undergo apoptosis or reproduction, altered gene expression that results in altered cell function (or dysfunction), and increased tendency to secrete inflammatory cytokines. These senescent characteristics have been observed in multiple cell types, including endothelial cells, adipocytes, fibroblasts, and immune system cells. Next, body composition changes associated with aging are also likely to contribute to increased cytokine production, especially related to the increase in the less metabolically active adipocytes that often take the place of more metabolically active muscle or fibrous tissue. These fat cells are much more likely to secrete both TNF-α and IL-6, both of which amplify inflammatory signaling. Levels of free radicals of oxygen also tend to increase with increasing age, which is due to both age-related declines in enzymes that suppress free radical production and increased production. These free radical molecules such as hydrogen peroxide and superoxide are potent stimulators of the NFκB signal transduction cascade, leading to production of inflammatory mediators. These factors can either activate inflammation, which makes it more likely that older adults will have chronically increased levels of circulating inflammatory mediators such as IL-6. Finally, age-related declines of dehydroepandrosterone-sulfate (DHEA-S), testosterone, and estrogen also likely play an important role in the activation of inflammation. DHEA-S works in part by blocking NFκB activation, while the sex steroid normally binds gene transcription sites for inflammatory cytokines such as IL-6. This braking action gradually declines as these hormones subside late in life.

In addition to these purely age-related changes that result in chronic activation of inflammatory pathways, many chronic disease states common in older adults are known to activate inflammatory pathways. These chronic diseases include those with known inflammatory components such as active rheumatoid arthritis, polymyalgia rheumatica, and most types of cancer. Many chronic disease states not traditionally thought to be inflammatory diseases, including renal failure, congestive heart failure, and atherosclerotic vascular disease trigger the production of inflammatory mediators such as IL-6 and TNF-alpha. These disease states, along with the aging-related

alterations in cell type and oxidative stress, are likely an important trigger for the elevated levels of inflammatory mediators detectable in the serum of many older adults. These mediators, especially if they include IL-1 or TNF-α, act to further ramp up inflammatory system activation and lead to the more chronic production of the more stable molecules IL-6 and CRP, two molecules that have most often been associated with adverse health outcomes and disease states in older adults. These age- and disease-related triggers of inflammation help to explain the increasing late-life inflammatory burden, and increase the vulnerability in late life to inflammatory changes. Finally, variation in genes that code for inflammatory mediators have been shown to be increasingly relevant late in life. This appears to be in part related to chronic and acute disease states that trigger inflammatory mediators, which in turn worsen disease states. For example, at least two studies show that older men with myocardial infarction (MI) and IL-6 gene promoter variant were much more likely to die of MI-related complications than those without the promoter variant.

CHRONIC INFLAMMATION CONTRIBUTES DIRECTLY TO PATHOPHYSIOLOGICAL CHANGES IN OLDER ADULTS

Although multiple studies now demonstrate strong associations between the activation of inflammatory pathways, chronic disease states, and adverse health care outcomes, there is no one clear mechanism that connects inflammation to the vulnerability to decline frequently observed in older adults with chronic activation of inflammatory pathways. Recent evidence from multiple molecular biological studies suggest that many of the inflammatory mediators found to be associated with adverse health outcomes actually contribute directly to the decline in multiple physiological systems. Furthermore, there is increasing evidence that chronically activated inflammatory pathways actually contribute to the development and exacerbation of other disease states, hence further contributing to the vulnerability to adverse health outcomes of disability, frailty, and mortality.

Evidence for inflammatory activation playing a role in multiple system decline in late life comes from both from association studies in populations of older adults and from molecular studies. For example, one of the most critical physiological systems for preserving function and well being in older adults is skeletal muscle. Declines in skeletal muscle strength, an important contributor to disability and frailty, is strongly associated with elevated inflammatory markers. In a recent manuscript by Schaap et al., older Dutch participants in a longitudinal study of aging were found to have a two- to threefold increased risk of losing 40% of their grip strength over 3 years if their IL-6 level was greater than 5 pg/mL and their CRP was greater than 6 mg/mL. Cesari et al. demonstrated a significant decline in strength over 3 years in older participants in those InCHIANTI participants with the highest levels of IL-6, CRP, and IL-1 receptor antagonist (IL-1RA). IL-1 RA production is stimulated by IL-6 and it is utilized as a surrogate measure for the strongly proinflammatory cytokine IL-1. For molecular evidence, consider a study of IL-6$^{-/-}$ mice injected with IL-6, where marked gastrocnemius muscle atrophy and protein degradation by cathepsin L and B was demonstrated. Other molecular studies directly link NFκB activation to the down-regulation of MyoD, a critical factor in skeletal muscle differentiation and repair.

Chronic exposure to inflammatory mediators also influences other critical physiological systems, which in turn influences late-life vulnerability. One in vivo study performed in young rhesus monkeys helps to illustrate multisystemic influence of the inflammatory cytokines. These monkeys were injected with low doses of human recombinant the IL-6 for 30 days. During this period, those injected lost 10% lean body mass, developed depression, mild anemia, osteopenia, and increased levels of CRP. Many other studies focused on individual systems have also demonstrated direct effects of inflammatory mediators on systems that impact late-life vulnerability. For example, osteoclastogenesis, which is an important component of osteoporosis, is directly upregulated by IL-6 neurologic damage in Alzheimer's disease and other neurodegenerative conditions have been directly linked to both Cox-2 and IL-6 expression. TNF-α has been demonstrated to alter iron absorption and utilization in red blood cells, which in turn decreases red blood cell production. In immune system cells, chronic IL-6 signaling activates the STAT 3 pathway and the expression of antiapoptotic factors such as BCL-2 that in turn lead to the accumulation of inflammation-reinforcing T-cells. Chronic IL-6 expression also stimulates the anorexic proteins including leptin, neuropeptide Y, melanocortin, and orexin that suppress hunger. These studies and many others provide substantial evidence that NFκB pathway activation and its downstream products can induce profound tissue changes and can facilitate the pathogenesis of many common disease states.

CHRONIC INFLAMMATION CONTRIBUTES TO CHRONIC DISEASE IN OLDER ADULTS

While it is increasingly clear that elevated serum levels of inflammatory mediators strongly associate with many disease states and adverse health outcomes common in older adults, clues as to causality or even directionality of the activation of inflammatory pathways have not been identified in these mainly cross-sectional studies. However, recent evidence supports that inflammatory mediators per se, even if they are generated by chronic disease states, go on to have a potent biological impact on the exacerbation of chronic diseases and con-

tribute to the development of new disease states. For example, recent laboratory evidence demonstrates that NFκB-related inflammatory mediators contributes directly to malignancy promotion. Furthermore, other studies suggest that inflammation is an integral part of the development of both vascular lesions that lead to chronic blockages in blood vessels, and to the acute process that results in infarctions through activation of thrombotic pathways. These studies and many others provide substantial evidence that inflammatory mediators can induce pathophysiologic change in multiple physiologic systems, and can and do contribute to multiple disease states and distal outcomes of frailty, disability, and mortality in older adults.

POTENTIAL CLINICAL UTILITY OF INFLAMMATORY MARKERS AND ANTI-INFLAMMATORY INTERVENTIONS

As more and more studies are published that document the increased risk for adverse health outcomes associated with the elevation in serum-based inflammatory mediators, increased interest has developed to utilize these markers as part of clinical practice. Despite the fact that mild IL-6 and CRP elevations are associated with adverse health outcomes, no studies have demonstrated the clinical utility of such measurements. This is in part because there is no known way to prove that lowering inflammatory activation will attenuate inflammation in older adults, especially when it is not related to a specific inflammatory condition. As measurement of individual inflammatory mediators become easier and cheaper, as more specificity is assigned to these markers, and as specific, targeted, and safe interventions targeting inflammatory pathways are developed, serum inflammatory markers may well evolve into a more useful clinical tool that can help identify the most vulnerable older adults and guide therapeutic or preventive interventions.

To date, anti-inflammatory medications, including aspirin (ASA) and nonsteroidal anti-inflammatory drugs (NSAIDs), have mostly been used as over-the-counter pain medications. ASA has certainly been shown to reduce the incidence of clotting-related conditions, and is therefore frequently used in older adults as a safe and effective medication. However, it has not yet been demonstrated to have an impact on function or frailty or other nonspecific adverse health outcome frequently measured in older adults. Epidemiological studies of NSAIDs in relationship to cognition have shown mixed evidence related to long-term impact on slowing cognitive decline. However, there is little doubt that these agents are important components of shorter-term pain management for geriatric conditions such as osteoarthritis.

Over the past several years, many other more specific anti-inflammatory medications have been utilized to treat other geriatric conditions such as anorexia and weight loss, usually in a specific disease state rather than aging or frailty per se. For example, pentoxifylline, an agent that blocks TNF-α RNA transcription, was tested in a group of cancer patients and in human immunodeficiency virus (HIV) patients. There was no evidence that it provided a clear weight gain or appetite benefit, and there was a suggestion that the agent may increase the risk for infection. Thalidomide, a drug that degrades TNF-α RNA and hence blocks inflammatory signal propagation, has shown more promise in clinical trials of

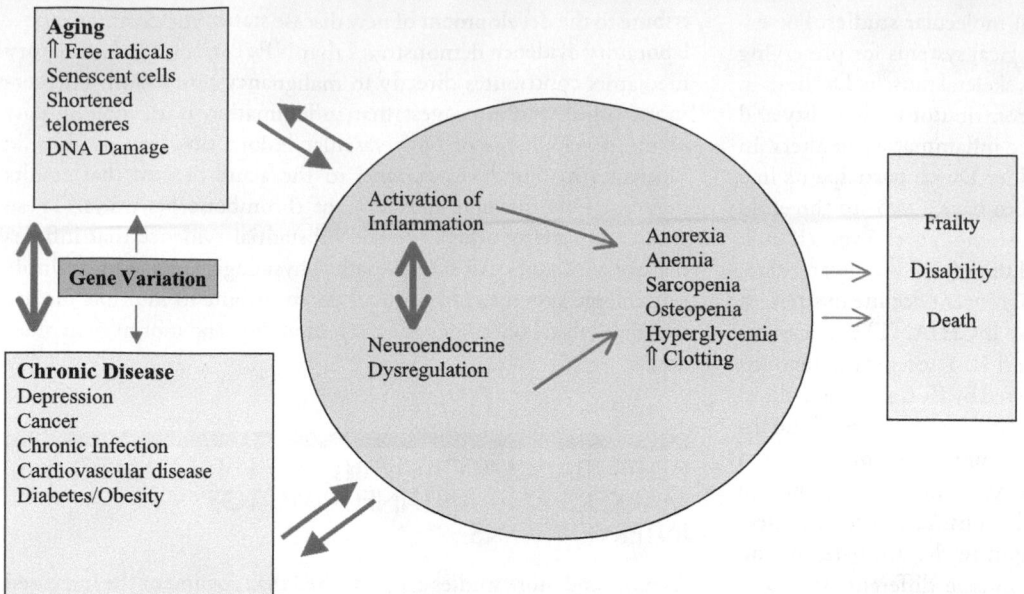

FIGURE 4-4. Integrated model representing connections between aging, gene variation, and chronic disease and the activation of inflammation and neuroendocrine changes, which ultimately alters physiologic systems and adverse health outcomes in older adults. The left and in the middle of the figure represent a platform of altered biology from which age-related vulnerability to adverse health outcomes evolve.

patients with pancreatic cancer. In clinical trials, it appears to be well tolerated and may influence weight gain in HIV and in pancreatic cancer, despite the fact that it offered no survival advantage. Megestrol, a hormonal agent known to block IL-6 transcription, has also been shown to be beneficial in HIV and cancer-related cachexia. It has been tolerated with minimal side effects, and is probably safe but not clearly effective at stimulating appetite in most geriatric populations.

As more and more disease specific and cytokine specific blocking agents are developed in the coming years, extreme caution must be taken in any future use in older populations given the increased risk and vulnerability to life-threatening infections or sepsis that is inherent in agents that target key components of the inflammatory cascade such as TNF-α or IL-6. Future studies of agents or activities that modulate or attenuate inflammation rather than block the inflammation, or perhaps agents that treat the underlying cause of the chronic activation of inflammation may be safer and more effective than agents that block these pathways.

SUMMARY: DOES CHRONIC INFLAMMATION CONTRIBUTE TO AN ALTERED BIOLOGICAL PLATFORM FOR LATE-LIFE VULNERABILITY?

This chapter has presented an overview of studies that connect elevated levels of inflammatory mediators with a range of adverse health outcomes, and an overview of the biological reasons that older adults are more likely to develop chronic inflammation than younger adults. In addition, emerging evidence that inflammatory mediators themselves directly impact multiple physiological systems and acute and chronic disease states has been reviewed. Developed with this background in mind, Figure 4-4 shows inflammatory triggers, pathophysiologic change related to inflammation, and related adverse health outcomes in one comprehensive overview model. The underlying molecular changes, the disease states, and the altered physiology on the left side of the figure represents a platform from which the increased vulnerability to adverse health outcomes

observed in older adults with increased levels of inflammatory mediators can develop (Figure 4-4). Future studies of this vulnerability would benefit from a better understanding of the interface between molecular change and disease development, and how interventions may attenuate inflammation without adverse outcomes.

FURTHER READING

Bermudez EA, Rifai N, Buring J, Manson JE, Ridker PM. Interrelationships among circulating interleukin-6, C-reactive protein, and traditional cardiovascular risk factors in women. *Arterioscler Thromb Vasc Biol.* 2002;22(10):1668–1673.

Binkley NC, Sun WH, Checovich MM, Roecker EB, Kimmel DB, Ershler WB. Effects of recombinant human interleukin-6 administration on bone in rhesus monkeys. *Lymphokine Cytokine Res.* 1994;13(4):221–226.

Campisi J. Senescent cells, tumor suppression, and organismal aging: good citizens, bad neighbors. *Cell.* 2005;120(4):513–522.

Cohen HJ, Harris T, Pieper CF. Coagulation and activation of inflammatory pathways in the development of functional decline and mortality in the elderly. *Am J Med.* 2003;114(3):180–187.

Ershler WB, Keller ET. Age-associated increased interleukin-6 gene expression, late-life diseases, and frailty. *Annu Rev Med.* 2000;51:245–270.

Ferrucci L, Harris TB, Guralnik JM, et al. Serum IL-6 level and the development of disability in older persons [see comments]. *J Am Geriatr Soc.* 1999;47(6):639–646.

Franceschi C, Capri M, Monti D, et al. Inflammaging and anti-inflammaging: a systemic perspective on aging and longevity emerged from studies in humans. *Mech Ageing Dev.* 2007;128(1):92–105.

Iwasaki Y, Asai M, Yoshida M, Nigawara T, Kambayashi M, Nakashima N. Dehydroepiandrosterone-sulfate inhibits nuclear factor-kappaB-dependent transcription in hepatocytes, possibly through antioxidant effect. *J Clin Endocrinol Metab.* 2004;89(7):3449–3454.

Krtolica A, Campisi J. Cancer and aging: a model for the cancer promoting effects of the aging stroma. *Int J Biochem Cell Biol.* 2002;34(11):1401–1414.

Kurihara N, Bertolini D, Suda T, Akiyama Y, Roodman GD. IL-6 stimulates osteoclast-like multinucleated cell formation in long term human marrow cultures by inducing IL-1 release. *J Immunol.* 1990;144(11):4226–4230.

Leng S, Xue QL, Huang Y, et al. Total and differential white blood cell counts and their associations with circulating interleukin-6 levels in community-dwelling older women. *J Gerontol A Biol Sci Med Sci.* 2005;60(2):195–199.

Lukiw WJ, Bazan NG. Strong nuclear factor-kappaB-DNA binding parallels cyclooxygenase-2 gene transcription in aging and in sporadic Alzheimer's disease superior temporal lobe neocortex. *J Neurosci Res.* 1998;53(5):583–592.

Maggio M, Guralnik JM, Longo DL, Ferrucci L. Interleukin-6 in aging and chronic disease: a magnificent pathway. *J Gerontol A Biol Sci Med Sci.* 2006;61(6):575–584.

Pedersen M, Bruunsgaard H, Weis N, et al. Circulating levels of TNF-alpha and IL-6-relation to truncal fat mass and muscle mass in healthy elderly individuals and in patients with type-2 diabetes. *Mech Ageing Dev* 2003;124(4):495–502.

Pikarsky E, Porat RM, Stein I et al. NF-kappaB functions as a tumour promoter in inflammation-associated cancer. *Nature.* 2004;431(7007):461–466.

Puts MT, Visser M, Twisk JW, Deeg DJ, Lips P. Endocrine and inflammatory markers as predictors of frailty. *Clin Endocrinol. (Oxf)* 2005;63(4):403–411.

Thomas DR. The relationship between functional status and inflammatory disease in older adults. *J Gerontol A Biol Sci Med Sci.* 2003;58(11):995–998.

Ting AY, Endy D. Signal transduction. Decoding NF-kappaB signaling. *Science.* 2002 November 8;298(5596):1189–1190.

Walston J, McBurnie MA, Newman A, et al. Frailty and activation of the inflammation and coagulation systems with and without clinical morbidities: Results from the Cardiovascular Health Study. *Arch Intern Med.* 2002;162:2333–2341.

Yeh SS, Schuster MW. Geriatric cachexia: the role of cytokines. *Am J Clin Nutr.* 1999;70(2):183–197.

Demography and Epidemiology

Jack M. Guralnik ■ *Luigi Ferrucci*

INTRODUCTION

Over the past century, there have been truly remarkable changes in the numbers and characteristics of older persons throughout the world. The growth of the older population has resulted from a general increase in the overall population size but has been particularly affected by major declines in several of the leading causes of mortality. The increased survival of older persons has also been accompanied by declining birth rates; so the proportion of the population aged 65 years and older has increased dramatically and will continue to increase for the next 50 years. These demographic transformations have an effect on society that reverberates well beyond the increased medical care needs associated with an older population.

As more people live to advanced old age, it is important to gain a greater understanding of more than just the individual diseases that affect them. It is critical to appreciate the global picture of older persons who may have multiple chronic conditions, decrements in functional abilities, and social and psychological problems that may have an impact on many facets of their health and quality of life. In contrast to the previous stereotype, older people become more heterogeneous, not more alike, as they age, and understanding this process is a key challenge of geriatric medicine. Adding to the clinical perspective on single patients or small samples of patients, geriatric epidemiology has provided a useful tool with which to approach these challenges by studying representative populations of older persons. Going beyond the demographic focus of counting and projecting the number of older people in the population, epidemiology has made additional contributions to our understanding of the health status and functional trajectory of the older population. Since the 1980s, epidemiologic researchers either have utilized previously initiated cohort studies that include persons who have aged during the study or have begun new cohorts focusing on older people. These epidemiologic studies have assessed the distribution and determinants of specific diseases and have evaluated issues of relevance to an aging population, such as quality of life, geriatric

syndromes, comorbidity, functional status, and end-of-life issues. Many of the chapters in this book refer to epidemiologic research on specific diseases and conditions. This chapter focuses on the more general or "geriatric" outcomes, particularly disability, that have also been the subject of much epidemiologic investigation.

The chapter begins by documenting the rapid growth and impressive increases in the number of older persons in the United States and other countries. It then examines improvements in survival and life expectancy. Selected demographic characteristics are then considered, including living situation and labor force participation across many developed countries.

The second section, on mortality, depicts current causes of death in the older population in the United States and considers the change in death rates with increasing age. Data on overall and disease-specific changes in mortality rates from 1950 through 2004 show the dramatic changes in these rates. The third section addresses chronic disease in the older population by using data from national surveys on self-reporting of chronic conditions, ambulatory medical visits, and hospital discharges. Data are then presented for two conditions, cancer and dementia, as examples of conditions where the use of only mortality data would provide an incomplete picture. The fourth section presents epidemiologic data on disability in older persons. This section describes the prevalence of disability, its causes and consequences, individual transitions in functional status, population changes in disability prevalence, and measurement issues. Finally, the chapter provides a description of important behavioral risk factors for chronic disease, injury, and disability and the prevalence rates of these risk factors in the older population.

DEMOGRAPHICS

Aging of the Population in the United States

One-hundred-fifty years of aging in America are summarized in Table 5-1, beginning with 1900 and including projections till 2050.

TABLE 5-1

Actual and Projected Growth of the Older U.S. Population, 1900–2050 (Millions)

	TOTAL POPULATION (ALL AGES)	≥65 YEARS		≥85 YEARS	
		Number	% of Total	Number	% of ≥65
1900	76.1	3.1	4.1	0.1	3.2
1950	152.3	12.3	8.2	0.6	4.9
2000	276.1	34.9	12.6	4.4	12.6
2050	403.7	82.0	20.3	19.4	23.7

Source: Population Division, U.S. Census Bureau, Washington, DC, 20233.

This table demonstrates how the older population has grown, as well as how the oldest segment of the older population has grown even more rapidly. In 1900, only 4.1% of the 76 million persons in the United States were aged 65 years and older, and among those in this age group only 3.2% were aged 85 years and older. By 1950, more than 8% of the total population was aged 65 years and older, and by 2000, this percentage had increased to 12.6%. The U.S. Census Bureau creates several alternative mortality scenarios when developing population projections, and according to their middle mortality assumption, there will be 82 million persons aged 65 years and older in the United States in 2050. If mortality declines faster than projected under this assumption, the number of older people will be even higher. In 2050, one in five Americans will be aged 65 years or older. The growth of the 85 years and older population, termed by some the oldest old, will be even more dramatic. By 2050, when the current baby boom generation will be in this age group, it is projected that over 19 million persons, representing nearly a quarter of all persons aged 65 years and older, will be 85 years and older. There will be more than four times as many people in the 85 years and older age group as there are now, and almost 200 times as many as there were in 1900. Thus, the number of older people is rising dramatically; the proportion of the total population aged 65 years and older is increasing; and the older population itself is getting older, with increasing proportions in the 85 years and older subgroup.

Aging of the Population and Life Expectancy Around the World

Population aging is taking place throughout the world. Figure 5-1 presents data on the current and projected percentage of the population aged 65 years and older for six regions of the world. Change in the proportion of a population that is elderly depends on changes both in the survival of older persons and in the birthrate. Improved survival at older ages and a low birthrate have resulted in European countries having the oldest populations in the world. In fact, the Population Research Bureau estimates that of the world's 25 countries with the oldest populations (not including small island countries), 24 are in Europe. Italy and Germany are estimated to have the oldest populations in Europe and the second and third oldest in the world at approximately 19% each. Sometime around 2004, Japan surpassed Italy to become the oldest major country in the world, with 20% of its population being 65 years or older. Japan remains the only major country not in Europe on the list of the oldest 25 populations. Considering countries of all sizes, the tiny country of Monaco surpasses Japan to become the country with the highest proportion of the population aged 65 years and older, at approximately 22%. Europe will continue to have the oldest populations in the world in the twenty-first century, with almost one in four Europeans projected to be aged 65 years or older by 2030. The current percentage aged 65 years and older in Latin America, the Caribbean, Asia, the Near East, and North Africa is low, ranging from about 4% to 6%. However, growth of the older population will be rapid in these countries, and it is projected that in 2030, the proportion of the population in this age range will double. Sub-Saharan Africa has few older persons, and it is expected that the percentage of older people in the general population will not grow substantially in the future.

Populations have aged at different speeds and during different time periods throughout the world. Figure 5-2 shows the number of years it took, or is projected to take, for specific countries to

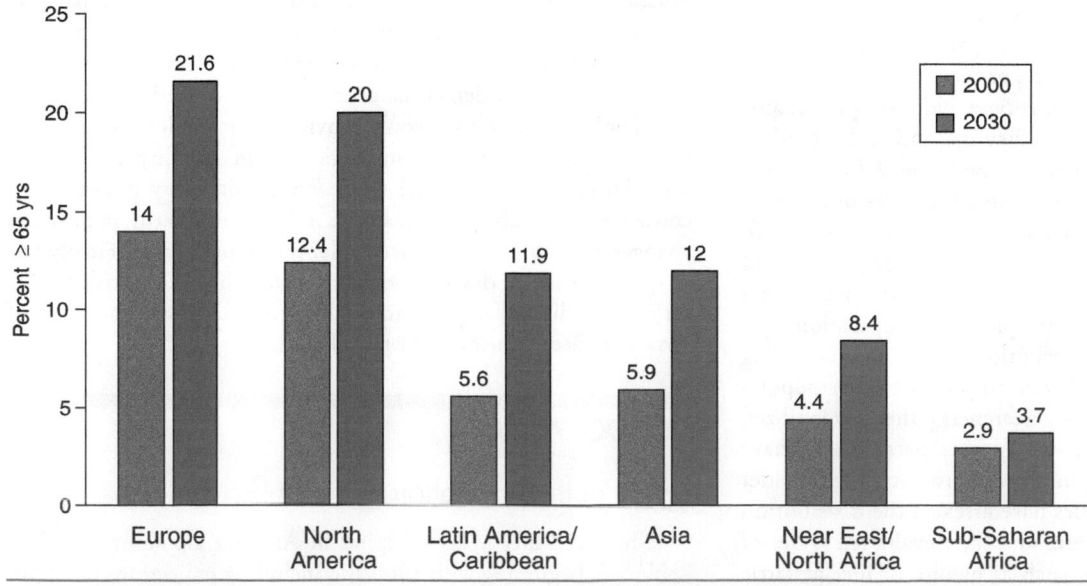

FIGURE 5-1. Percent of population age 65 yrs and older, 2000 and projected for 2030. U.S. Census Bureau, 2004, "Life Tables," International Data Base, at http://www.census.gov/ipc/www/idbnew.html Accessed on February 21, 2007.

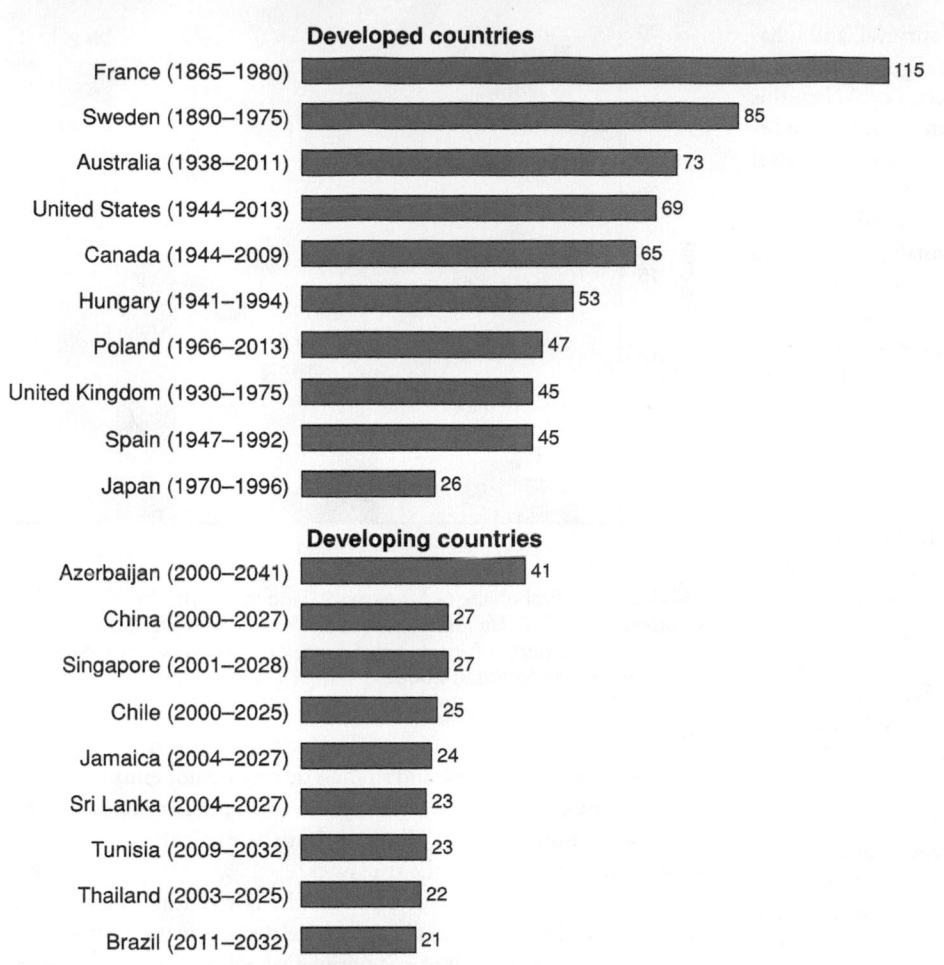

Developed countries

Country	Years
France (1865–1980)	115
Sweden (1890–1975)	85
Australia (1938–2011)	73
United States (1944–2013)	69
Canada (1944–2009)	65
Hungary (1941–1994)	53
Poland (1966–2013)	47
United Kingdom (1930–1975)	45
Spain (1947–1992)	45
Japan (1970–1996)	26

Developing countries

Country	Years
Azerbaijan (2000–2041)	41
China (2000–2027)	27
Singapore (2001–2028)	27
Chile (2000–2025)	25
Jamaica (2004–2027)	24
Sri Lanka (2004–2027)	23
Tunisia (2009–2032)	23
Thailand (2003–2025)	22
Brazil (2011–2032)	21
Colombia (2017–2037)	20

FIGURE 5-2. Speed of aging: number of years and time period in which percent of population aged 65 and over doubled or will double from 7% to 14%. *Reprinted with permission from Kinsella K, Velkoff VA. An Aging World: 2001. U.S. Census Bureau, Series P95/01–1. Washington, DC: US Government Printing Office; 2001.*

progress from having 7% of the population aged 65 years and older to having 14% of the population in this age range. The United States is expected to reach 14% in 2013 and will have taken 69 years to make the transition. Sweden and the United Kingdom reached the 14% level in 1975, with Sweden taking 85 years to go from 7% to 14% and the United Kingdom taking about half that time. Japan has already reached the 14% mark and took only 26 years to do so.

A particularly clear message about the speed of aging in developing countries is presented in Figure 5-2. Although the developing countries shown will generally not reach the 14% mark until the third decade of this century, they will have spent less than 27 years making the transition. The rapid aging of these countries will certainly have a large societal impact, with less ability to adapt than in countries that have aged more slowly.

Life Expectancy at Different Ages

Better survival at all ages has had a major impact on the size and age distribution of the older population. Figure 5-3 depicts survival curves for the total U.S. population over the course of the twentieth century and into the twenty-first century. In 1900, there was substantial mortality in infancy and early childhood, with the survival curve in midlife being somewhat steeper than at the end of the twentieth century. By 1950, a large proportion of early-life mortality had

been removed, although survival in this age range was still improving by the end of the century. By 1990, a large proportion of persons were living to age 60 years, and only at age 70 years did the survival curve start to fall rapidly. The survival curve continued to shift to the right through 2003. The change observed in the shape of survival

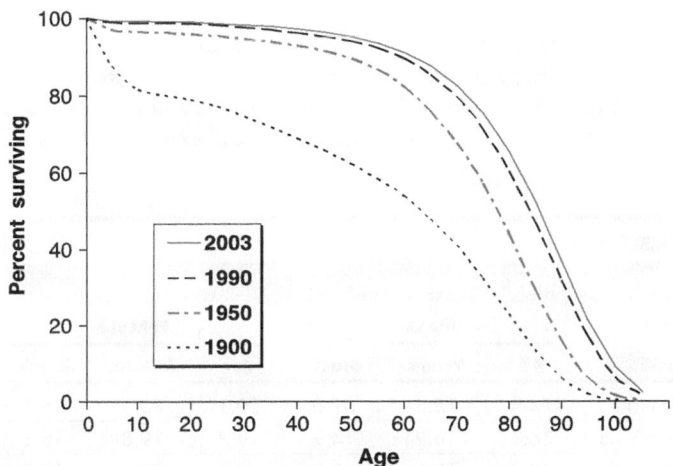

FIGURE 5-3. Survival curves for U.S. population. *Arias E. United States Life Tables, 2003. National Vital Statistics Reports, vol. 54, no. 14. Hyattsville, MD: National Center for Health Statistics; 2006.*

curves has been termed the rectangularization of survival, and it has been proposed that at some point in time full rectangularization will be reached, with no further increases in life expectancy. When this will occur is not yet clear, but the U.S. Census Bureau and Social Security Administration are projecting continued increases in survival for at least the next 50 years.

Life expectancy at age x is defined as the average number of years remaining to be lived by a member of a survivorship group who is exactly age x. Most life expectancy estimates use current life tables, meaning that they use the age-specific mortality experience of the current population. With this approach, life expectancy at birth gives an estimate of the average length of life of a cohort of children who are born now and then experience today's age-specific mortality rates as they proceed through life. This is an artificial construct, but it provides a way to represent the overall mortality experience of a current population and allows us to compare this experience across countries and over time. If mortality rates continue to decline, as is expected, the average child born today will live considerably longer than the estimate shown on a current life table. Given these caveats, it is nonetheless useful to examine changes in life expectancy over the last century and life expectancy at specific ages. Life expectancy at birth was only 47.3 years in 1900 and rose to 68.2 years by 1950, affected to a large extent by improvements in infant and child mortality. Life expectancy continued to rise through the second half of the twentieth century, driven mainly by increases in survival in middle and old age. Table 5-2 shows life expectancy at birth and at ages 65, 75, and 85 years for the year 2003. At every age, females have a higher life expectancy than males, with the differential at birth being 5.3 years. The gender differential for blacks (7.1 years) is greater than for whites (5.2 years). Blacks have a lower life expectancy than whites through age 75 years and then have a higher life expectancy at age 85 years. The observations of importance to geriatric medicine in these estimates are that the average 75-year-old man will live about 10 more years and the average 75-year-old woman will live more than 12 additional years. At age 85, the average person can still expect to live another 6 to 7 years.

The estimates shown in Table 5-2 do not include Hispanics. Although the National Center for Health Statistics does publish data on Hispanic mortality rates, these data come with warnings of problems associated with their accuracy. The denominator for Hispanic rates comes from the U.S. Census, where Hispanic ethnicity is self-reported. At the time of death, Hispanic ethnicity is reported by the person completing the death certificate, and there is likely a large amount of underreporting. It is also known that a not insignificant number of Hispanic persons return to their native countries to spend

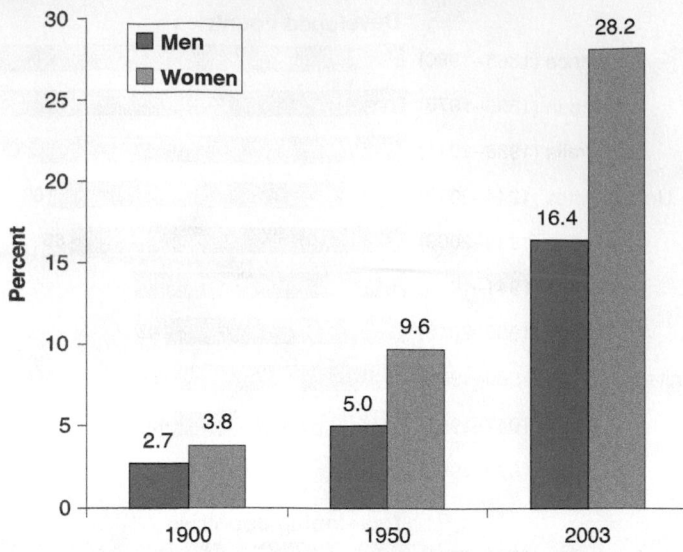

FIGURE 5-4. Probability of 50-year-old living to 90 yrs, 1900 to 2003. *Computed from U.S. life tables in Arias E. United States Life Tables, 2003. National Vital Statistics Reports, vol. 54, no. 14. Hyattsville, MD: National Center for Health Statistics; 2006.*

the last years of their lives, and so their deaths are not enumerated as deaths in the United States. Thus, there is substantial underascertainment of the numerator for Hispanic death rate calculations, leading to an underestimation of the true rates.

The improvements in survival over the last century are relevant to the field of geriatric medicine, as the decline in mortality rates throughout life has resulted in a population with a large proportion of individuals who will survive to advanced old age. This point is made compellingly by the data shown in Figure 5-4. This figure was generated using data from 1900, 1950, and 2003 life tables and illustrates the proportion of 50-year-old men and women who can expect to live to age 90 years or older. Only about 3% of 50-year-olds could expect to live to this age in 1900. By 1950, this proportion had hardly risen at all in men but had gone up to nearly 10% in women. The large decreases in old-age mortality in the second half of the century led to large changes by 2003, when over 16% of 50-year-old men and more than 28% of 50-year-old women could expect to reach the age of 90 years or older. All these estimates are derived from current life tables; so if mortality continues to decline, these percentages will be even higher in the current cohort of 50-year-olds. The consequence of these changes is that an unprecedented proportion of the current middle-aged population will live to very old age.

Extreme Longevity

There has always been a fascination with extreme longevity, but the demographics of very long life have been formally studied only in recent years. Examples of persons who lived to 100 years are mentioned at the time of the Imperial Rome and, although these reports cannot be directly validated, there is no reason to believe that a few rare individuals might not have reached extreme longevity. However, as the percentage of centenarians has risen, especially in the last century, centenarians are no longer rare and virtually all geriatricians have dealt with a centenarian patient. Studying centenarians

TABLE 5-2

Life Expectancy in 2003 (Years)						
	MALE			**FEMALE**		
AGE	**All**	**White**	**Black**	**All**	**White**	**Black**
At birth	74.8	75.3	69.0	80.1	80.5	76.1
At 65 yrs	16.8	16.9	14.9	19.8	19.8	18.5
At 75 yrs	10.5	10.5	9.8	12.6	12.6	12.4
At 85 yrs	6.0	5.9	6.4	7.2	7.1	7.8

Source: Arias, E. United States Life Tables, 2003. National Vital Statistics Reports, Vol. 54, No. 14. Hyattsville, MD: National Center for Health Statistics; 2006.

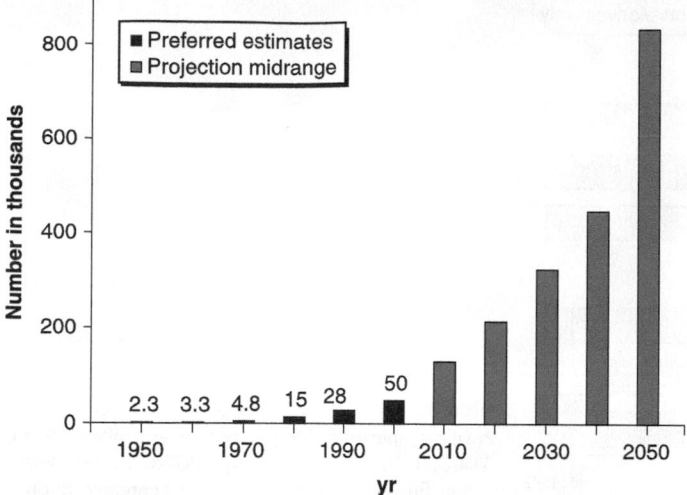

FIGURE 5-5. Number (thousands) of centenarians in the United States using preferred estimates (1950–2000) and midrange projections (2010–2050). Projected numbers adapted from Day JC. Population Projections of the United States by Age, Sex, Race, and Hispanic Origin: 1995–2050, U.S. Bureau of the Census, Current Population Reports, P25–1130. Washington, DC: U.S. Government Printing Office; 1996. Preferred estimates for 1950–2000 acquired from He W, Sungupta M, Velkoff VA, DeBarros KA. U.S. Census Bureau, Current Population Reports, P23-209, 65+ in the United States, 2005. Washington, DC: U.S. Government Printing Office; 2005.

provides a magnified view of the aging process, but the study of long-lived individuals can also provide results that are important in geriatric practice. In fact, little is known about the factors that predict decline in health status, disability, and mortality in individuals in their nineties.

Previous claims for the world record for longevity were often unsubstantiated, and pockets of the world where claims were made for general high longevity usually turned out to be no different than other parts of the world. However, recent data from places like Sardinia, Italy, have identified areas of increased longevity that have been meticulously validated. There is currently no solid explanation about why centenarians are concentrated in these geographical areas.

Better age documentation has made it possible to be more confident about the numbers of centenarians and changes in these numbers. It has been estimated that the number of centenarians in western Europe has doubled every decade since 1950, and estimates for the United States also show a doubling between 1980 and 1990 and again from 1990 to 2000, when the total number of centenarians rose from 28,000 to more that 50,000 (Figure 5-5). In 2005, the United States had 55,000 centenarians, more than any other country in the world and about 12% of the estimated living world centenarians. In comparison, the population of the United States represents only 4.6% of the world population. However, future increases will be spectacular. It has been estimated that between 2000 and 2050, the number of centenarians will increase more than 16-fold, with a projected 850,000 centenarians in the United States in 2050.

In 1990, 78% of U.S. centenarians were non-Hispanic whites. However, since then, the Hispanic and black population have expanded much faster than the white population. Thus, centenarians in the future are expected to be much more ethnically diverse. In all reported series, with the single exception of Sardinia, there are fewer male than female centenarians. However, men reaching this age are

considerably less likely to have significant mental and cognitive disability than women.

Although family and twin studies suggest a strong genetic predisposition to extreme longevity and candidate genes have been described, the full mechanism is not understood. The secret is probably a combination of favorable genetic background and environmental factors that exert their influence in critical periods over the life span. In fact, many centenarians report that they were completely independent in self-care activities of daily living and free of disabling condition up to their late nineties. In addition, a sizable proportion of centenarian "escapers" are totally independent and free of major medical condition. Super-centenarians, individuals 110 years old or older, appeared around 200 years ago and their number is currently estimated at about 300 to 400. However, age has been validated in less than 100 of these people. In spite of many claims, only two persons have been clearly documented to have lived to 120 years.

Demographic Characteristics of the Aging Population

Further demographic characteristics relevant to the social environment in which older persons find themselves living are shown in Figures 5-6 and 5-7. In Figure 5-6, the elderly ratio, defined as the number of persons aged 65 years and older divided by the number of persons aged 20 to 64 years, multiplied by 100, is shown for the total population and racial and ethnic subgroups in 2000 and projected to 2050. With the faster growth of the older population and the less rapid increase in the younger population, this ratio will rise dramatically in the future. Currently there are about 21 older people for every 100 persons aged 20 to 64 years. By 2050, there will be 38 older people for every 100 persons in the younger age group, the group who will be called on to care for older parents and grandparents and whose Social Security payments will be used to provide for retirees. Now and in the future, the elderly ratio is highest in whites. Blacks currently have a higher ratio than Hispanics, but by 2050 there will be about 26 elderly blacks, Hispanics, and persons of other races for every 100 people aged 20 to 64 years.

Living situation is determined by health, financial factors, and widowhood and varies considerably by gender and age, as seen in Figure 5-7. Among community-living persons in the United States, women are much more likely to live alone, with almost 60% of

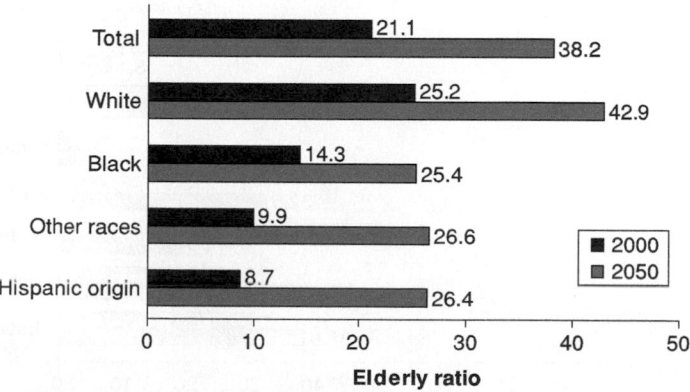

FIGURE 5-6. Elderly ratio: number of persons aged 65 yrs and older divided by number of persons aged 20 to 64, times 100. *He W, Sungupta M, Velkoff VA, DeBarros KA. U.S. Census Bureau, Current Population Reports, P23-209, 65+ in the United States, 2005. Washington, DC: U.S. Government Printing Office; 2005.*

Alone
With spouse
With other relatives
With nonrelatives only
Women
65 to 74 yrs
75 to 84 yrs
85 years and over
Men
65 to 74 yrs
75 to 84 yrs
85 years and over
0
20
40
60
80
100
Percent

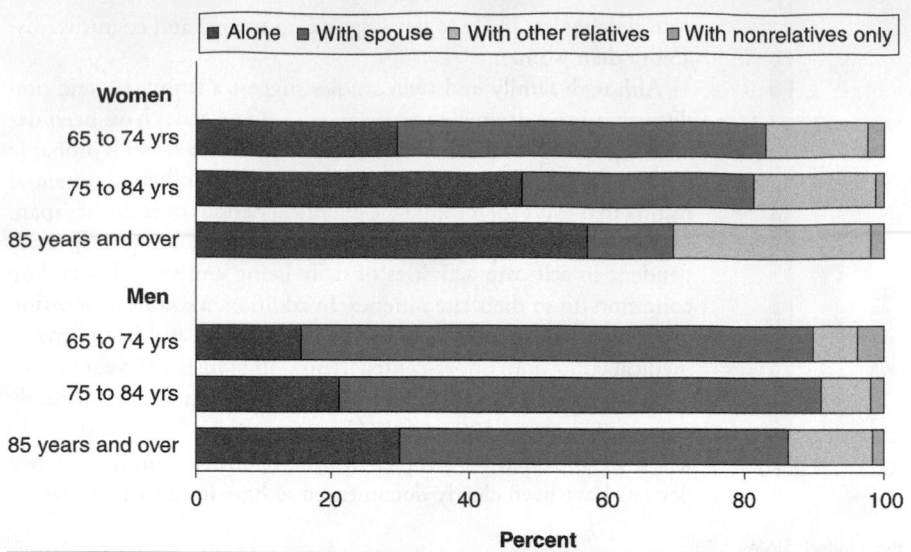

FIGURE 5-7. Living arrangements of community-dwelling persons 65 yrs and over United States, 2003. U.S. Census Bureau, 2003a, Current Population Survey, Annual Social and Economic Supplement, detailed tables.

women aged 85 years and older living alone. A large proportion of men live with their spouses. Women are more likely to outlive their husbands not only because they live longer but also because they tend to marry older men. Modest percentages of older persons live with other relatives, and a very small proportion live with nonrelatives.

Employment

In recent years, the percentage of older people who work and the average age of retirement have fallen throughout the developed countries. In Figure 5-8, the percentage of persons working is shown for the early 1970s and the late 1990s for the 60 to 64-year age group,

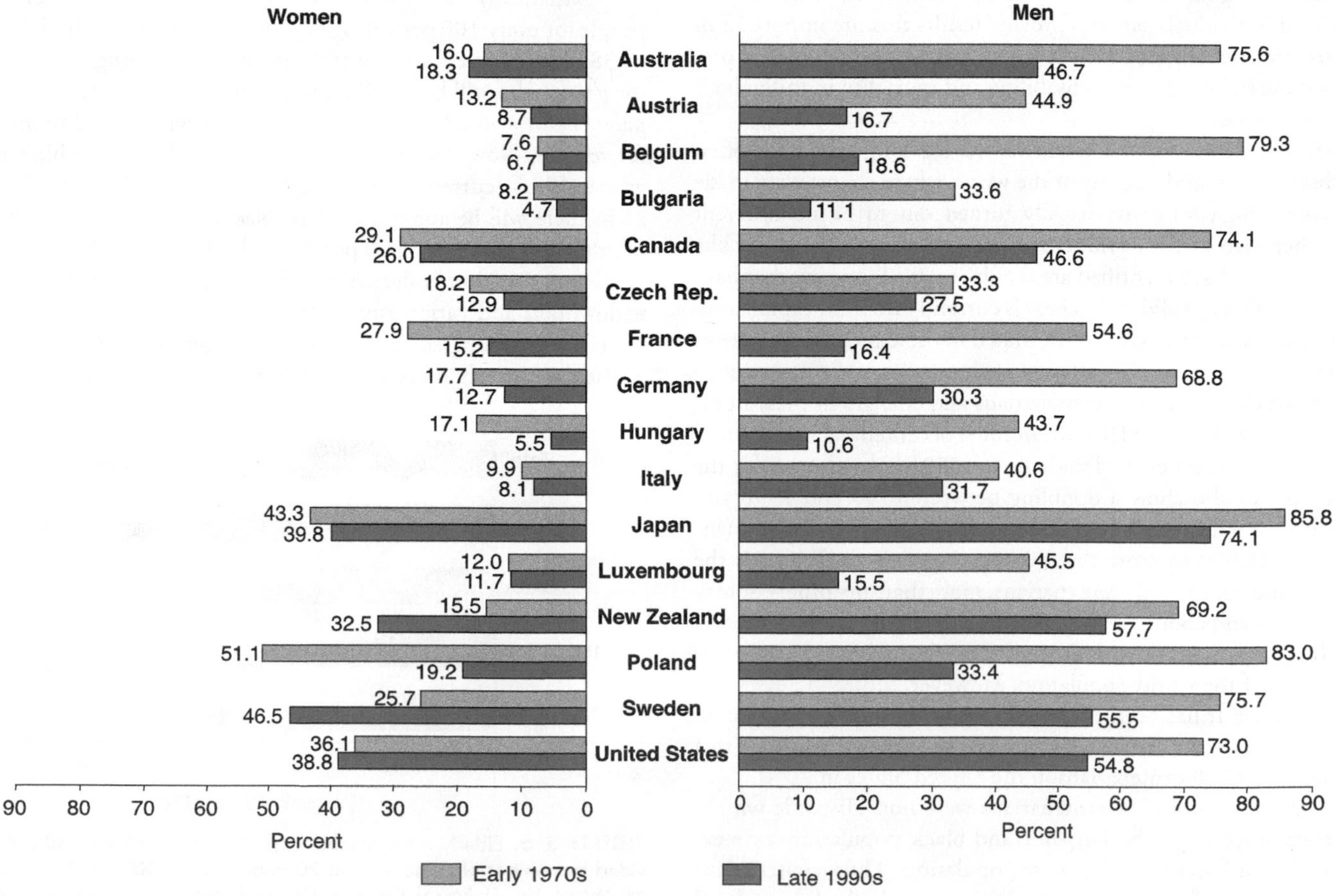

Women
Men
Australia 16.0 18.3 75.6 46.7
Austria 13.2 8.7 44.9 16.7
Belgium 7.6 6.7 79.3 18.6
Bulgaria 8.2 4.7 33.6 11.1
Canada 29.1 26.0 74.1 46.6
Czech Rep. 18.2 12.9 33.3 27.5
France 27.9 15.2 54.6 16.4
Germany 17.7 12.7 68.8 30.3
Hungary 17.1 5.5 43.7 10.6
Italy 9.9 8.1 40.6 31.7
Japan 43.3 39.8 85.8 74.1
Luxembourg 12.0 11.7 45.5 15.5
New Zealand 15.5 32.5 69.2 57.7
Poland 51.1 19.2 83.0 33.4
Sweden 25.7 46.5 75.7 55.5
United States 36.1 38.8 73.0 54.8
90 80 70 60 50 40 30 20 10 0
0 10 20 30 40 50 60 70 80 90
Percent
Percent
Early 1970s
Late 1990s

FIGURE 5-8. Labor force participation rates for men and women aged 60–64 yrs in developed countries, early 1970s and late 1990s. *Reprinted with permission from Kinsella K, Velkoff VA. An Aging World: 2001. U.S. Census Bureau, Series P95/01-1. Washington, DC: US Government Printing Office; 2001.*

TABLE 5-3

Leading Causes of Death Among Persons at Least 65 Yrs Old in 2004

CAUSE OF DEATH	NUMBER OF DEATHS	DEATH RATE (PER 100,000 POPULATION)	% OF ALL DEATHS IN PERSONS ≥65 YRS
Heart disease	533,302	1536.5	30.4
Malignant neoplasms	385,847	1111.6	22.0
Cerebrovascular disease	130,538	376.1	7.4
Chronic lower respiratory disease	105,197	303.1	6.0
Alzheimer's disease	65,313	188.2	3.7
Diabetes mellitus	53,956	155.5	3.1
Influenza and pneumonia	52,760	152.0	3.0
Nephritis, nephrotic syndrome, and nephrosis	35,105	101.1	2.0
All other accidents	27,939	80.5	1.6
Septicemia	25,644	73.9	1.5
Motor vehicle accidents	7081	20.4	0.4
All other causes (residual)	332,987	959.4	19.0
Total	1755,669	5058	100.0

Source: Miniño AM, Heron M, Murphy SL, Kochanek KD. Deaths: Final data for 2004. Health E-Stats. Hyattsville, MD: National Center for Health Statistics; 2006.

the group that was traditionally preretirement. Overall, women work less than men, but in a few countries, including the United States, the percentage of women working rose during this time. In many countries, there have been extremely large declines in the percentage of men in this age group who work. For example, the percentage of men 60 to 64 years old who were employed declined over this 25-year period from 76% to 47% in Australia, from 79% to 19% in Belgium, from 55% to 16% in France, and from 69% to 30% in Germany. An increase in societal wealth has been the main driving force for decreased workforce participation, but other factors include obsolescence of the skills of older workers, pressure for older workers to leave their jobs to make room for younger workers in countries with high unemployment, and the growth of financial incentives for early retirement. The percentage of persons in the 65 years and older age group who work has also declined. For example, in the United States, the percentage of men in this age group who work dropped from 24.8% in the early 1970s to 16.9% in the late 1990s. The corresponding percentages for men in Germany were 16% and 4.5%, in France 10.7% and 2.3%, and in Japan 54.5% and 35.5%. With earlier retirement and longer life expectancy, the number of years people live after retirement has increased greatly. The Organization for Economic Cooperation and Development (OECD) has estimated that in 1960 men in developed countries could expect to spend 46 years in the labor force and a little more than 1 year in retirement. By 1995, years in the labor force had decreased to 37, whereas years in retirement had increased to 12.

MORTALITY

Leading Causes of Death

The increasingly greater life expectancy of the population has been driven in part by reduced mortality at older ages. It is instructive to review the U.S. vital statistics data on causes of death in the older population, changes in these rates with increasing age, and trends in overall and disease-specific mortality over time. Table 5-3 lists the leading causes of death in the population age 65 years and older in 2004. It employs the ICD-10 classification system, which was first used for national data in 1999. As in younger individuals, heart disease is by far the most common cause of death, followed by cancer. The five leading causes of death—heart disease, cancer, stroke, chronic lower respiratory tract disease, and Alzheimer's disease account for 69.5% of all deaths. Alzheimer's disease, which in the past was rarely assigned as the underlying cause of death and was not on the list of leading causes of death, was the seventh leading cause of death in older persons in 2000 and in 2003 rose to the fifth leading cause of death, responsible for 3.7% of deaths. This is still likely a gross underestimation. The contribution of Alzheimer's disease in the future will probably grow substantially. It is well recognized that assigning a single underlying cause of death is fraught with problems when an individual dies in advanced old age and has multiple chronic conditions. What is surprising is that despite this difficulty the distribution of causes of death in the United States remains quite stable from year to year.

Age-specific mortality rates for selected leading causes of death are depicted in Figure 5-9. On this logarithmic scale, a straight-line increase indicates an exponential increase in mortality rate with age. An exponential increase is present for all causes of death and parallel increases are seen for heart disease, cerebrovascular disease, and pneumonia and influenza. The exponential rise with age for Alzheimer's disease mortality is substantially steeper. The mortality rates for cancer and lower respiratory tract disease do not maintain as steep a rise with increasing age, perhaps because the people who contribute in large part to these categories are smokers, who die at younger ages and are less represented in the oldest segment of the population. Diabetes mortality rates also do not show an exponential increase with advancing age, again because diabetic patients may die disproportionately at younger ages. The one condition in this figure for which the mortality rate slope becomes steeper with advancing age is accidents. Although motor vehicle accidents are an issue of real concern in older persons, it is important to note, as shown in Table 5-3, that there are four times as many deaths from other types of accidents, primarily falls, as from motor vehicle accidents.

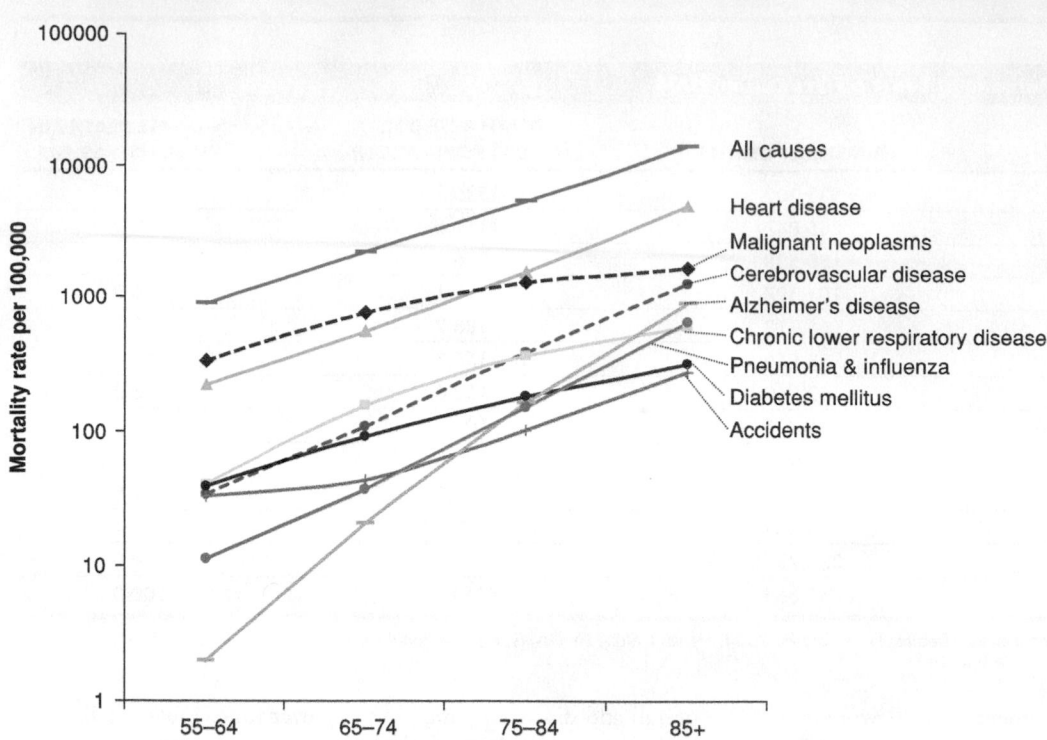

FIGURE 5-9. Age-specific death rates for leading cause of death in the older population, United States, 2004. Centers for Disease Control and Prevention, National Center for Health Statistics, National Vital Statistics System; Vital statistics of the United States, 2004 annual mortality file.

Mortality Rates

The graph of the exponential rise in mortality with increasing age, which has been described for many species, has been termed the Gompertz curve. It has been difficult to evaluate whether the exponential increase is maintained to the very end of life, as the numbers of extremely old individuals available for study have traditionally been quite small. Recently, larger populations of very old humans and other species have been evaluated to examine whether the Gompertz curve continues to describe mortality rates at advanced old age. Figure 5-10 shows death rates for humans and fruit flies at the extremes of old age, and in both these examples the Gompertz function, which is represented as a straight line in the human example, is not consistent with the data. The conclusion from these studies and from studies on a variety of other species is that the force of mortality declines somewhat in individuals who survive to very old age, although the causes of this phenomenon remain unclear.

The first half of the twentieth century saw large declines in mortality in infants and children, but in the second half of the century, there were unprecedented declines in mortality in the older segment of the population. In the total population, mortality rates between 1950 and 2004 fell by 41.9% in males and 45.1% in females (Figure 5-11). What was notable during the latter half of the century was that this magnitude of decline was also seen in men and women in the 65- to 74-year-old and 75- to 84-year-old age groups. Even for people 85 years and older, there was a mortality rate decline that exceeded 30%.

Mortality change over this time period is further explored in Table 5-4, which lists 1950 and 2004 death rates and percentage changes in these rates for heart disease, stroke, and cancer, diseases that account for 60% of deaths in older adults. For the total population, heart disease mortality declined more than 60%, and stroke mortality dropped more than 70%, a truly remarkable decline in

these diseases that reflects major advances in both prevention and treatment as well as a secular trend that is not fully understood. For both these diseases, the declines in the 65- to 74-year-old and 75- to 85-year old age groups generally exceeded the percentage decline seen for the total population. In persons aged 85 years and older, heart disease mortality declined by more than 45%, with stroke mortality dropping by more than 60% in men and more than 55% in women, impressive declines in this very old segment of the population. Unfortunately, the declines in mortality seen for heart disease and stroke were not seen for cancer. In women, the overall population

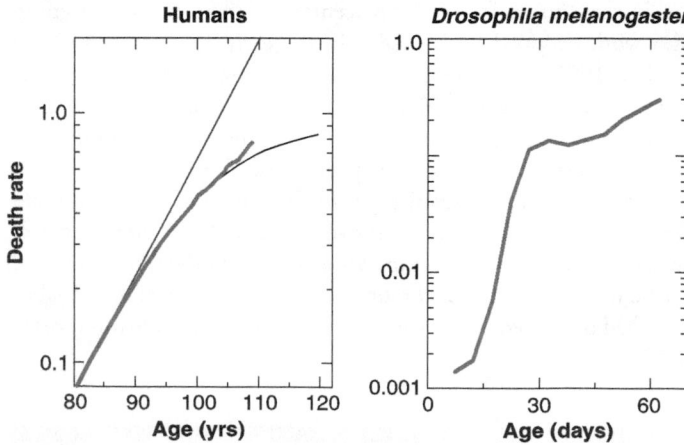

FIGURE 5-10. Death rates at advanced old age in women and from age 0–60 days for a genetically homogeneous line of *Drosophila melanogaster*. Human estimates come from data aggregated from 14 countries for which data were available over the period from 1950 to 1990 for ages 80–109, and to 1997 for ages 110 and over. Data on *Drosophila* are from 6333 flies reared under usual laboratory conditions. *Reprinted with permission from Vaupel JW, Carey JR, et al. Biodemographic trajectories of longevity. Science. 1998;280:855.*

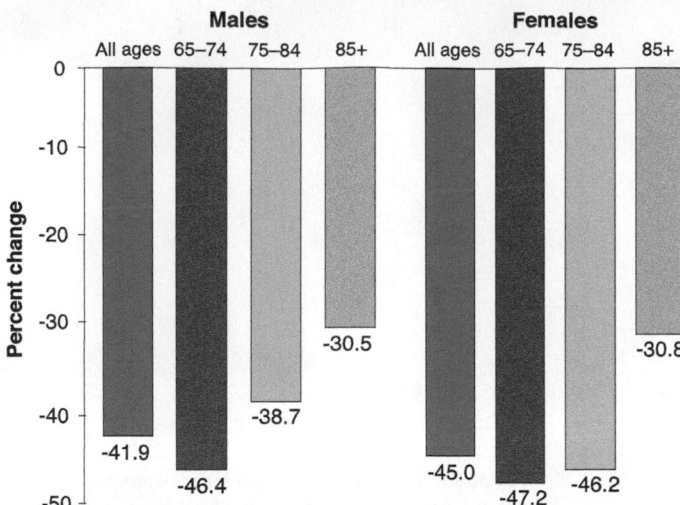

FIGURE 5-11. Percent change in mortality rates, United States, 1950–2004, for all ages (age-adjusted using yr 2000 standard population) and for older age groups. Calculated from data in National Center for Health Statistics. *Health, United States, 2006 with Chartbook on Trends in the Health of Americans.* Hyattsville, MD: National Center for Health Statistics; 2006.

showed a modest decline in cancer mortality, but the older population had a slight rise in rates. Cancer mortality rates rose in older men, with increases of 25% in men 75 to 84 years and 40% in men 85 years and older. Heavy cigarette smoking in the cohort of men who were in the older age groups at the end of the last century was probably a major contributing factor to this increase in cancer rates. Figure 5-12 depicts change in mortality from cancers of the lung, trachea, and bronchus over the past half century. Mortality in men was much higher than in women and rose very steeply in men 75 to 84 years and 85 years and older until the early 1990s, when it leveled off. Cancer mortality rose less steeply in men 65 to 74 years, leveled off in the late 1980s and is now showing a downturn. Mortality from cancer of the lung, trachea, and bronchus in older women rose slowly after 1960, with a slightly steeper rise in those 75 to 84 years beginning in the 1980s.

Mortality from acquired immunodeficiency syndrome (AIDS) has had a small but not insubstantial impact on older persons compared to the younger population. Figure 5-13 shows trends in age groups beginning at age 45 years. The steep rise and then fall in AIDS mortality in the 45 to 54 years age group is reflected in similar but increasingly less pronounced patterns in each succeeding age group.

DISEASE STATUS

Prevalence of Common Diseases

Although there is much useful information to be gained by observing the diseases responsible for mortality, a full picture of disease status in the older population cannot be obtained by looking only at diseases that cause death. A number of ascertainment approaches that work well to characterize morbidity in the general population are used here to give an overview of important diseases prevalent in

TABLE 5-4

Age-Adjusted* and Age-Specific Mortality, U.S., During 1950 and 2004 and the Percent Change

		1950	2004	CHANGE
Diseases of the Heart				
Males				
	All ages	697.0	267.9	–61.6
	65–74	2292.3	723.8	–68.4
	75–84	4825.0	1893.6	–60.8
	85+	9659.8	5239.3	–45.8
Females				
	All ages	484.7	177.3	–63.4
	65–74	1419.3	388.6	–72.6
	75–84	3872.0	1245.6	–67.8
	85+	8796.1	4741.5	–46.1
Cerebrovascular Disease				
Males				
	All ages	186.4	50.4	–73.0
	65–74	589.6	121.1	–79.5
	75–84	1543.6	402.9	–73.9
	85+	3048.6	1118.1	–63.3
Females				
	All ages	175.8	48.9	–72.2
	65–74	522.1	96.6	–81.5
	75–84	1462.2	374.9	–74.4
	85+	2949.4	1303.4	–55.8
Malignant Neoplasms				
Males				
	All ages	208.1	227.7	9.4
	65–74	791.5	907.6	14.7
	75–84	1332.6	1662.1	24.7
	85+	1668.3	2349.5	40.8
Females				
	All ages	182.3	157.4	–13.7
	65–74	612.3	627.1	2.4
	75–84	1007.7	1023.5	1.6
	85+	1299.7	1340.1	3.1

*Data for "all ages" is age-adjusted by using the U.S. 2000 standard population.
Source: National Center for Health Statistics. Health, United States, 2006 with Chartbook on Trends in the Health of Americans. Hyattsville, MD: National Center for Health Statistics; 2006.

older persons. This overview is not meant to provide a comprehensive epidemiology of all medical conditions that often develop with aging but to show data that allow for a comparison of rates across the major conditions.

When a medical history is obtained, a clinician begins to construct a profile of disease status from self-reporting by the patient. In extending this approach to surveys of large, representative samples of older persons, it has been found that self-reporting works quite well for most diseases. Table 5-5 lists the most commonly reported chronic conditions among people aged 65 years and older in the United States. The most commonly reported condition is hypertension, reported by nearly half of older persons. Nearly one-quarter of men and 17% of women reported coronary heart disease and stroke history is reported by over 8% of older persons. Arthritis and chronic joint symptoms were reported by a large proportion of older persons and they, like many of the conditions on the list, have a large impact on overall health and quality of life but do not appear on the list of the most common conditions causing death. There

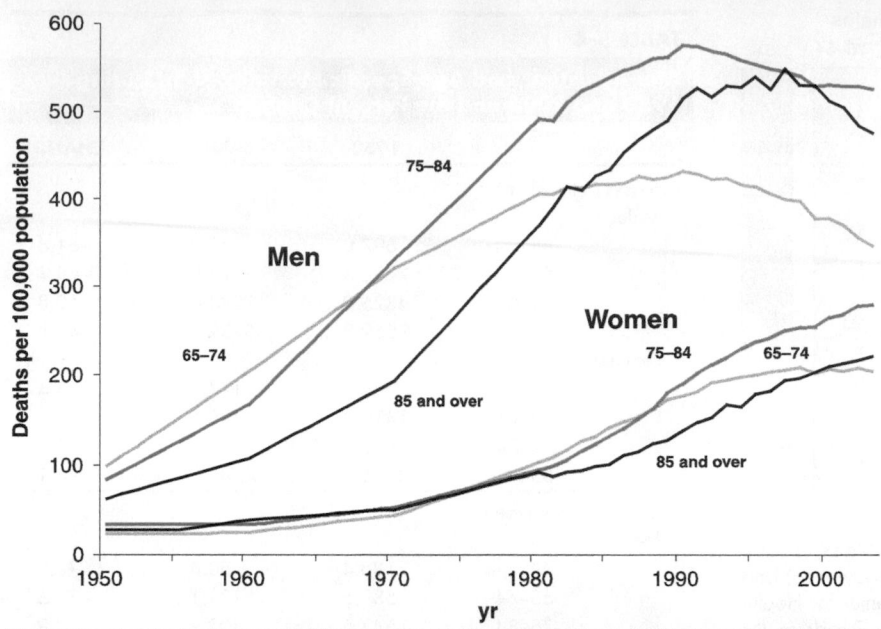

FIGURE 5-12. Mortality rate for malignant neoplasms of the trachea, bronchus, and lung by age, sex, and year: United States, 1950–2004. Miniño AM, Heron M, Murphy SL, Kochanek KD. Deaths: Final data for 2004. *Health E-Stats*. Hyattsville, MD: National Center for Health Statistics; 2006.

are some differences in the prevalence rates of chronic conditions according to race and ethnicity. For example, in persons aged 70 years and older, diabetes is more common in non-Hispanic black and Hispanic persons than in non-Hispanic whites. Non-Hispanic blacks have 1.5 times as much hypertension as non-Hispanic whites. Non-Hispanic white men report more heart disease than Hispanic whites or non-Hispanic blacks, whereas non-Hispanic black women report more stroke than non-Hispanic whites or Hispanics.

Co-occurrence of Multiple Chronic Conditions

An important aspect of disease status that distinguishes the older population from the younger population is the high rate of the cooccurrence of multiple chronic conditions, termed comorbidity or multiple morbidity. Because the risk of developing most diseases increases progressively with age, the increased prevalence and severity of comorbidity is not surprising. However, several lines of research

suggest that the observed prevalence of comorbidity is higher than the prevalence expected based on the rates of individual diseases, implying a clustering of diseases in certain individuals. The concept of comorbidity is a useful one in considering the burden of disease in older people. However, the operationalization of a definition for comorbidity depends on the number of conditions being ascertained and the intensity of the diagnostic effort to identify prevalent diseases. The longer the list of conditions and the harder one works to find prevalent diseases, the greater the prevalence of comorbidity. In a national survey that used self-reporting of nine common conditions, comorbidity was present in almost 50% of persons aged 60 years and older. Among those aged 80 years and older, 70% of women and 53% of men had comorbidity. Although comorbidity is a characteristic of older patients that is dealt with regularly by clinicians, there has been a limited amount of research on the classification of specific patterns of comorbidity and on the impact of comorbidity. In particular, certain combinations of conditions seem to occur at a higher

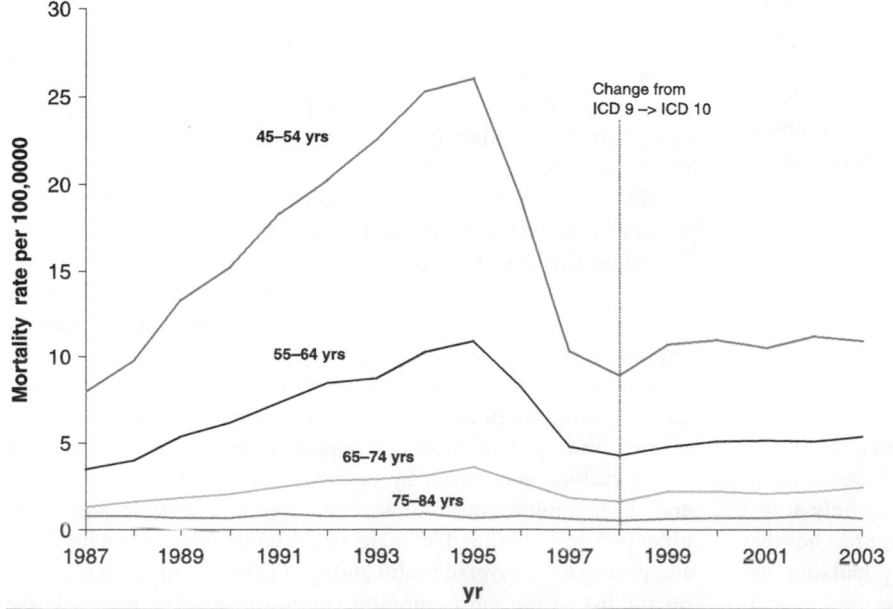

FIGURE 5-13. Mortality rate for HIV/AIDS by age and year in the United States, 1987–2003. Miniño AM, Heron M, Murphy SL, Kochanek KD. Deaths: Final data for 2004. *Health E-Stats*. Hyattsville, MD: National Center for Health Statistics; 2006.

TABLE 5-5

Most Commonly Reported Chronic Conditions Per 100 Persons 65+ Yrs in 2005

CONDITION	MALE	FEMALE
Hypertension	44.6	51.1
Arthritis diagnosis	40.4	51.4
Chronic joint symptoms	39.7	47.7
Coronary heart disease	24.3	16.5
Cancer (any type)	23.2	17.5
Vision impairment	14.9	18.7
Diabetes	16.9	14.7
Sinusitis	11.5	16.0
Ulcers	13.1	10.4
Hearing impairment	14.8	8.4
Stroke	8.9	8.2
Emphysema	6.3	4.1
Chronic bronchitis	4.5	6.3
Kidney disorders	4.1	3.9
Liver disease	1.4	1.4

Source: Centers for Disease Control and Prevention, National Center for Health Statistics, National Health Interview Survey, sample adult questionnaire. Trends in Health and Aging. http://www.cdc.gov/nchs/agingact.htm. Accessed February 21, 2007.

rate than would be expected by chance alone, and certain pairs of conditions may have a synergistic effect on functional loss.

Health Care Utilization

Physician and Ambulatory Visits

Data on physician visits and hospitalizations can also provide insight into the disease status of older people. Table 5-6 shows data on medical visits and hospitalizations in 2004 for the full age spectrum.

With increasing age, the number of physician visits increases steadily, and persons aged 75 years and older make, on average, over seven visits per person per year. The proportion of each age group's visits that are for acute problems and for chronic problems are shown separately, and there is a clear trend in both, with acute problems decreasing steadily with increasing age and chronic problems rising with age and accounting for almost 60% of office visits in persons aged 75 years and older. The percentage of office visits at which four or more drugs are prescribed or continued also rises steeply with age, and one-quarter of ambulatory visits in persons aged 75 years and older involve patients taking this many drugs. Finally, the table lists overall rates of hospital discharge, which go up dramatically with increasing age. For every 1000 persons aged 65 to 74 years there are 259 hospital discharges in a year, and for every 1000 persons aged 75 years and older there are 427 hospital discharges in a year.

Table 5-7 demonstrates data from the National Ambulatory Medical Care Survey on the reasons for ambulatory visits to physicians' offices, hospital outpatient departments and emergency departments in 2001–2002. The three most common reasons for these visits were essential hypertension, diabetes, and arthropathies and related disorders. However, these three conditions accounted for less than 20% of ambulatory visits, with a wide range of problems accounting for the remainder. For all listed reasons, the visit rate per 100 persons is slightly higher in persons 75 years and older compared to the 65 to 74 years age group. Overall, the older group had 828 visits per 100 persons and the younger group 690 visits per 100 persons.

Causes of Hospitalization

The actual causes of hospitalization in persons aged 65 years and older are represented in Table 5-8, which uses data from the National Hospital Discharge Survey. Heart disease is the most important cause of hospitalization by far, with congestive heart failure a slightly more common cause of hospitalization than other manifestations of heart disease. Other diseases that are frequent causes of death in older adults (pneumonia, stroke and cancer) are also common reasons for

TABLE 5-6

Ambulatory Medical Visits, Reasons for the Visit* and Drug Prescription According To Age Group, and Hospital Discharges By Age Group, U.S., 2004

AGE GROUP	AVERAGE NUMBER OF VISITS PER PERSON PER YR†	PERCENT VISITS FOR ACUTE PROBLEMS	PERCENT VISITS FOR CHRONIC PROBLEMS (ROUTINE OR FLARE-UP)	PERCENT OF VISITS WITH 4+ DRUGS PRESCRIBED OR CONTINUED (1999)	NUMBER OF HOSPITAL DISCHARGES PER 1000 POPULATION
<15	2.4	51.7	18.5	5.3	42.3
15–24	1.7	40.5	24.9	3.0	74.2
25–44	2.4	36.2	33.4	5.6	86.6
45–64	3.8	30.8	47.6	15.0	117.8
65–74	6.2	24.6	56.3	21.6	259.2
75+	7.3	26.2	58.0	24.6	427.0

*Table does not account for pre- or postsurgery/injury follow-up, nonillness care, or unknown reason for visit.
†Per person estimates utilizing 2000 census numbers.
Sources: Hing E, Cherry DK, Woodwell DA. National Ambulatory Medical Care Survey: 2004 summary. Advance data from vital and health statistics; no 374. Hyattsville, MD: National Center for Health Statistics; 2006.
Cherry DK, Burt CW, Woodwell DA. National Ambulatory Medical Care Survey: 1999 summary. Advance data from vital and health statistics; no. 322. Hyattsville, Maryland: National Center for Health Statistics; 2001.
Lolak LJ, DeFrances CJ, Hall MJ. National Hospital Discharge Survey: 2004 Annual Summary with Detailed Diagnosis and Procedure Data. National Center for Health Statistics. Vital Health Stat. 2006;13(151).

TABLE 5-7

Top Reasons for Ambulatory Medical Visits to Physician Offices, Hospital Outpatient Departments, and Emergency Departments in the United States, 2001–02

	65–74 YEARS OF AGE			75+ YEARS OF AGE		
	Number of Visits (in thousands)	Percent	Number of Visits per 100 Persons	Number of Visits (in thousands)	Percent	Number of Visits per 100 Persons
Essential hypertension	10,587	8.5	58.6	10,617	8.1	67.3
Diabetes mellitus	7448	6.0	41.3	6935	5.3	43.9
Arthropathies and related disorders	5336	4.3	29.6	5586	4.3	35.4
Malignant neoplasms	4577	3.7	25.4	5552	4.2	35.2
Ischemic heart disease	4246	3.4	23.5	5171	4.0	32.8
Heart disease, excluding ischemic	3698	3.0	20.5	4518	3.5	28.6
Spinal disorders	3544	2.8	19.6	4021	3.1	25.5
Cataract	3522	2.8	19.5	3430	2.6	21.7
Rheumatisms, excluding back	3070	2.5	17.0	3220	2.5	20.4
Disorders of lipid metabolism	2463	2.0	13.6	2185	1.7	13.8
Injury	11,342	9.1	62.8	13,258	10.1	84.0
All other	64,819	52.0	421.8	66,134	50.6	419.1
All visits	124,652	100.0	690	130,627	100.0	828

Source: Schappert SM, Burt CW. Ambulatory care visits to physician offices, hospital outpatient departments, and emergency departments: United States, 2001–2002. National Center for Health Statistics. Vital Health Stat. 2006;13(159).

hospitalization, but so are diseases not as strongly associated with mortality, including fractures, osteoarthritis, chronic bronchitis, and psychosis. The presence of septicemia and volume depletion on this list of the leading causes of hospitalization reflects the fact that a portion of the older population is frail and at high risk for these kinds of illnesses.

TABLE 5-8

The Ten Leading Causes of Hospitalization in Persons Aged 65 and Older, First Listed Diagnosis. United States, 2004

	DISCHARGE RATE PER 10,000 POPULATION
1. Heart disease	767.9
Acute myocardial infarction	126.6
Coronary atherosclerosis	158.6
Cardiac dysrhythmias	145.0
Congestive heart failure	225.0
2. Pneumonia	220.4
3. Cerebrovascular disease	175.6
4. Malignant neoplasms	172.2
5. Fractures, all sites	147.0
Fractures, neck, of femur	79.6
6. Osteoarthrosis and allied disorders	117.7
7. Chronic bronchitis	88.9
8. Septicemia	78.5
9. Volume depletion	67.6
10. Psychoses	60.7

Source: Lolak LJ, DeFrances CJ, Hall MJ. National Hospital Discharge Survey: 2004 Annual Summary with Detailed Diagnosis and Procedure Data. National Center for Health Statistics. Vital Health Stat. 2006:13(151).

Cancer

Cancer mortality rates do not always reflect the incidence rates of newly diagnosed cancers. The latter data are available from the Surveillance, Epidemiology, and End Results (SEER) survey of the National Cancer Institute and other cancer registries. Figure 5-14 depicts the age-specific incidence of the most common cancers that affect men and women. The highest incidence rates in men are seen for prostate, lung, colon and rectum, and bladder cancers, and in women for breast, colon and rectum, lung, and uterine cancers. The incidence of most of these cancers rises steadily with increasing age, but several, including prostate, breast, and lung cancers, begin to drop in incidence at the oldest ages.

Dementia

Dementia is a condition of aging for which prevalence and incidence rates cannot be validly obtained from either national survey data or registries. Because of the complexities of diagnosing dementia, data on the occurrence of the condition must rely on well-designed epidemiologic studies in local geographic areas. A network of dementia studies in Europe used comparable diagnostic techniques, which allowed for the aggregation of data on both prevalence and incidence (Figure 5-15). These pooled results show that both incidence and prevalence increase with age, with a steep rise in prevalence after age 80 years, when the prevalence in women becomes somewhat higher than in men. The incidence data show a clear rise in women to age 90 years and older, but some leveling off in men after age 85 years. The incidence rates are about 15% to 30% of the prevalence rates. In a condition such as dementia, which cannot be cured, this relationship between incidence and prevalence indicates that mortality

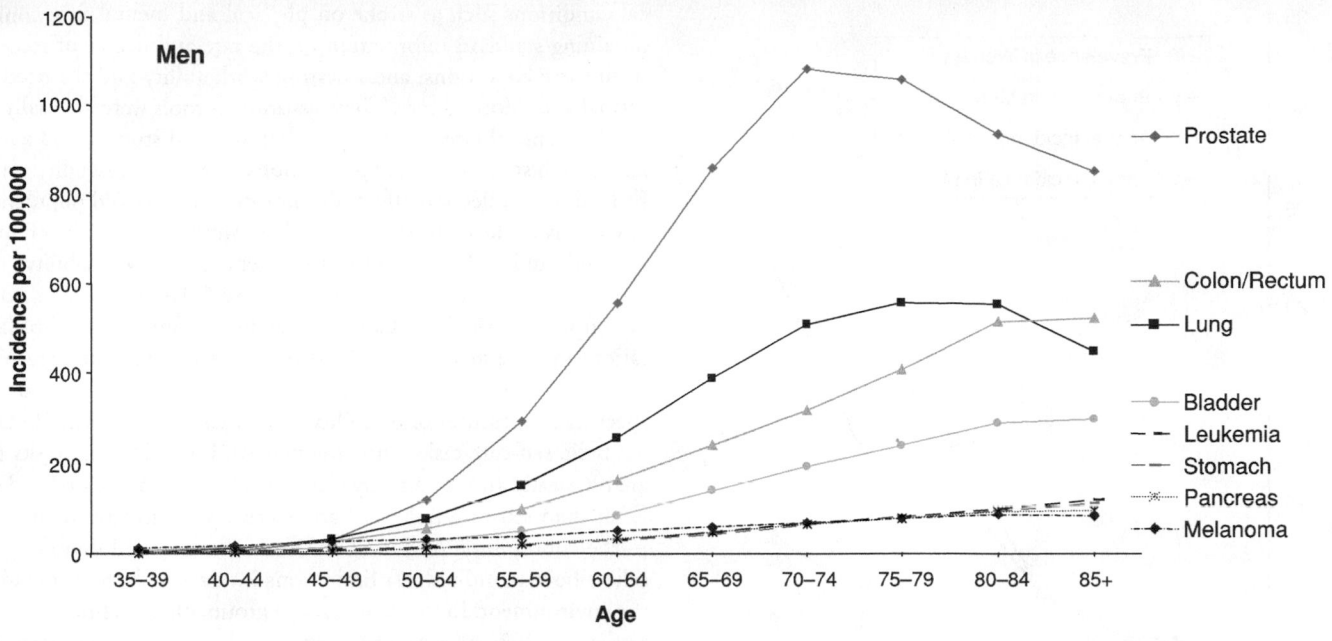

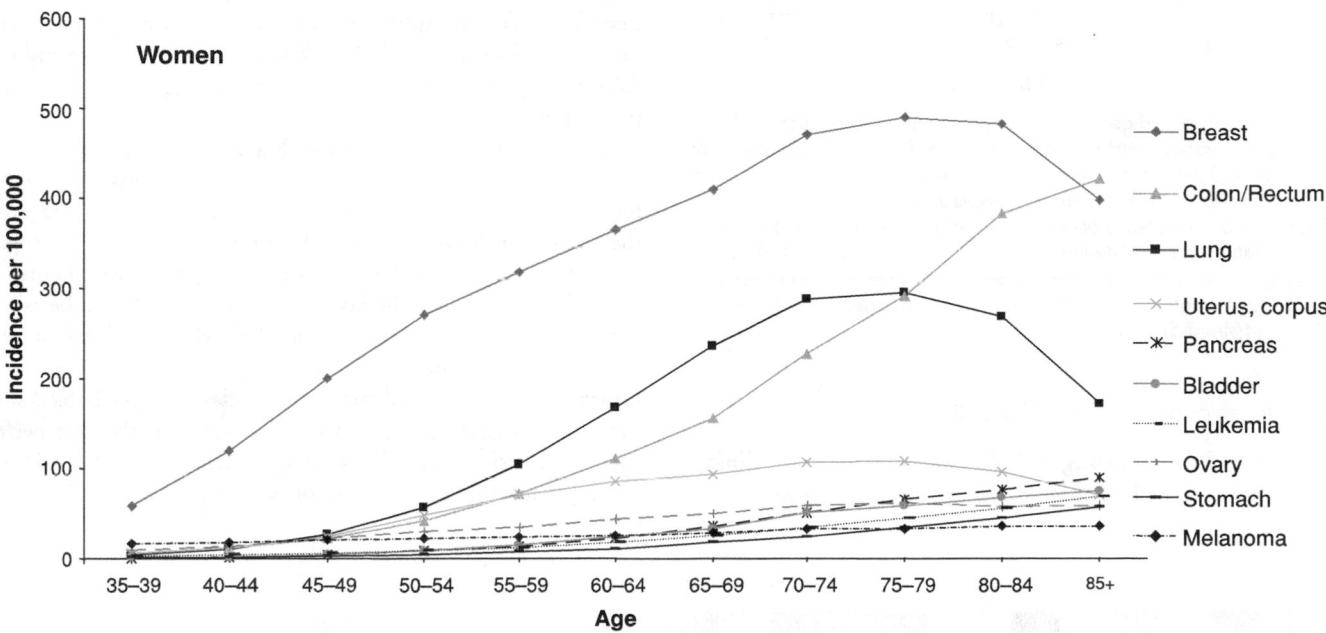

FIGURE 5-14. Incidence rates of specific cancers in men (top panel) and women (bottom panel) by age. SEER Cancer Statistics Review 1973–1998. Surveillance, Epidemiology and End Results Program, National Cancer Institute. http://seer.cancer.gov/csr/1973_1998/ Accessed on March 7, 2007.

occurs about 3 to 5 years after diagnosis. An even larger collection of studies on dementia incidence from around the world supported an exponential increase in dementia with age and demonstrated that rates tend to be lower in East Asia than in Europe and the United States.

DISABILITY

A hallmark of geriatrics is emphasis on the functional ability of older patients, and this subject is discussed from a clinical point of view in several chapters in this book. This approach recognizes that although individual diseases are important and that our system of modern medicine is oriented toward the diagnosis and treatment of specific diseases, the consequences of single and multiple diseases can be understood best by evaluating the functional status of the patient. A large body of epidemiologic work undertaken over the past two decades has treated disability as a condition that can be studied in much the same way as if it were a well-defined chronic disease by using epidemiologic tools to assess prevalence, incidence, and a wide range of risk factors. This work has led to a greater understanding of the occurrence, determinants, and consequences of disability in the older population and has provided insights into strategies for the prevention of disability.

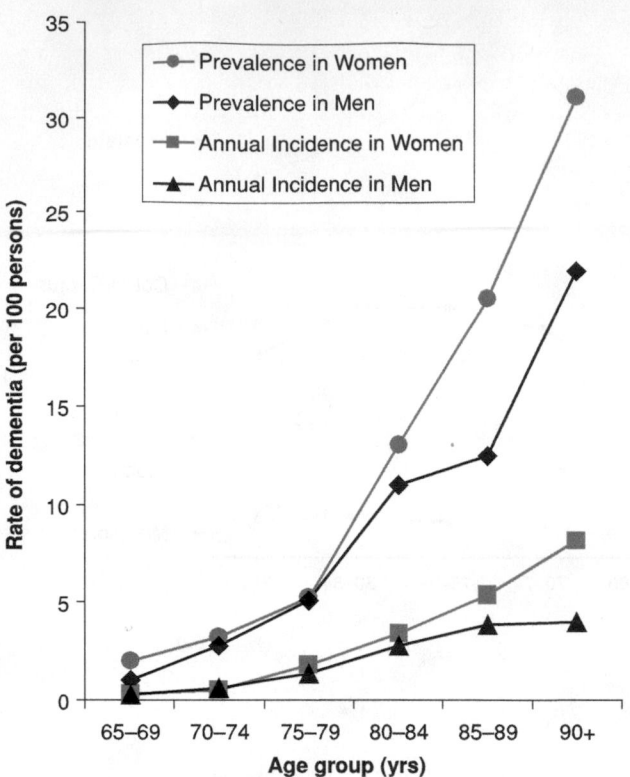

FIGURE 5-15. Age- and gender-specific prevalence and annual incidence of dementia in persons aged 65 and older. Data from pooled analyses of 11 studies carried out in eight European countries (prevalence) and in eight studies in seven countries (incidence). *Adapted with permission from Lobo A, Launer LJ, et al. Prevalence of dementia and major subtypes in Europe: A collaborative study of population-based cohorts. Neurology. 2000;54(suppl 5):S4. Fratiglioni L, Launer LJ, et al. Incidence of dementia and major subtypes in Europe: A collaborative study of population-based cohorts. Neurology. 2000;54(suppl 5):S10.*

Measures of Function and Disability

Measures of disability were originally developed for use in the clinical setting and were aimed at quantifying the impact of severe medi-

cal conditions such as stroke on physical and mental functioning, obtaining standard information on the rate and degree of recovery from these conditions, and assessing work ability and the need for formal and informal care. These assessment tools were gradually applied in clinical research and population-based studies, and almost all research studies in older populations now assess disability status. Federal data collection efforts did not include very old populations as recently as the early 1980's, but these surveys now have no upper age limit and include various instruments to assess disability. This type of assessment is illustrated in Figure 5-16, which is based on data from the Medicare Current Beneficiary Survey. Physical limitations include such basic tasks as standing, reaching, and grasping. These tasks represent the building blocks of functioning but are not specifically measures of disability. Activities of daily living (ADLs) are basic self-care tasks. Instrumental ADL (IADLs) are tasks that are physically and cognitively somewhat more complicated and difficult than self-care tasks and are necessary for independent living in the community. ADL and IADL are measures of disability and reflect how an individual's limitations interact with the demands of the environment. In the youngest age group, physical limitations are present in 40% of men and women and there is a low prevalence difficulty with ADLs. With increasing age, the prevalence of ADL disability increases rapidly and the proportion of persons with no limitations decreases to under 10% in persons 85 years and older. Additionally, the prevalence of disability is higher in women compared to men of the same age.

Disability has been assessed with a wide variety of instruments, and even when instruments contain the same items, they may differ in how they assess specific aspects of performing the task or the severity of limitation in performing the task. For example, it is always debatable whether it is better to ask people whether they actually perform a specific task or whether they should be asked to judge whether they could perform the task even if they have not done it for long time. The former approach gives more concrete information, but respondents could be classified as disabled simply because they have chosen not to do a task that they are perfectly capable of performing. The latter approach allows for classification of people regardless of whether or not they have actually done the

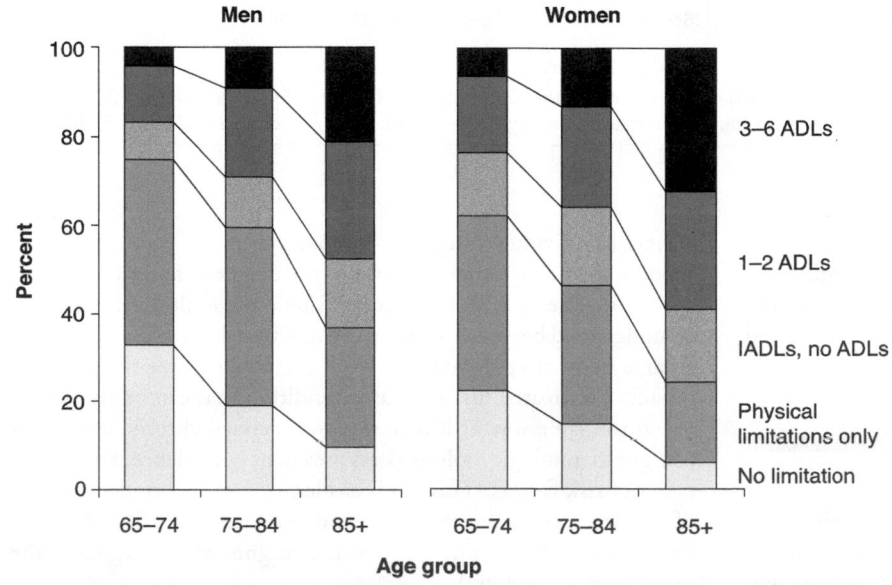

FIGURE 5-16. Physical limitations and disability according to age and sex, U.S., 2004. Physical limitations are defined as any difficulty doing one or more of the following: stooping, lifting, reaching, grasping, and walking 1/4 mile. Instrumental activities of daily living (IADLs) are defined as any difficulty doing one or more of the following: using the telephone, doing light housework, doing heavy housework, preparing meals, shopping, and managing money. Activities of daily living (ADLs) are defined as any difficulty doing one or more of the following: bathing or showering, dressing, eating, getting in or out of bed or chair, walking across a room, and using the toilet. Functional limitations of Medicare beneficiaries by age, residence, sex, race, and ethnicity from the Medicare Current Beneficiary Survey, 1992–2004. (MAHSE04) National Center for Health Statistics, Trends in Health and Aging. http://www.cdc.gov/nchs/agingact.htm. Accessed on February 21, 2007.

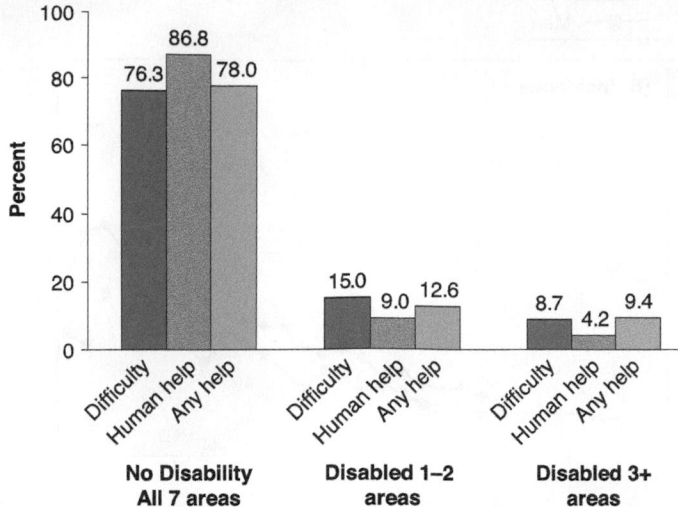

FIGURE 5-17. Disability estimates using three different measurements methods. *Reprinted with permission from Jette AM. How measurement techniques influence estimates of disability in older populations. Soc Sci Med. 1994;38:937.*

task recently but is limited because respondents who have not done the task are required to speculate as to their ability. For this and other issues in disability assessment, there is no single best way to perform an assessment, and there is therefore no single instrument that is ideal. The lack of standardization that results from the use of different instruments makes it difficult to compare rates of disability across studies. The differences in prevalence rates that different methods of assessment yield are demonstrated in the methodologic study of ADL disability shown in Figure 5-17. Disability classified as

having any difficulty or being unable to perform a task had a higher prevalence than disability classified as requiring human assistance or being unable to perform. Disability classified as requiring human help or help from an assistive device had a higher prevalence rate than disability requiring human help only and was similar in prevalence to the classification using difficulty. This study found that for individual ADLs the assessments that relied on difficulty produced estimates of disability 1.2 to 5 times greater than assessments that used human assistance as the criterion for disability. Thus, in evaluating research that reports on disability rates, it is critical to examine the way questions are asked and how responses are used to determine the presence of disability.

Disability as an Indicator of Health Status and Prognosis

Disability status has been demonstrated in epidemiologic studies to be one of the most potent of all health status indicators in predicting adverse outcomes. This is probably because disability measures are able to capture the impact of the presence and severity of multiple pathologies, including physical, cognitive, and psychological conditions, as well as the potential synergistic effects of these conditions on overall health status. The powerful prognostic power of disability presence is illustrated in Figure 5-18, which considers a hierarchy of disability statuses that are defined as independent in ADLs, independent but reporting some difficulty with ADLs, and dependent on personal assistance for ADLs. For these three groups, there were different cumulative probabilities over a 4-year follow-up period of the two outcomes shown here—admission to a nursing home and mortality. These results support the discussion in the previous paragraph that different disability criteria can identify population subgroups with different prognoses. They also support the validity of disability

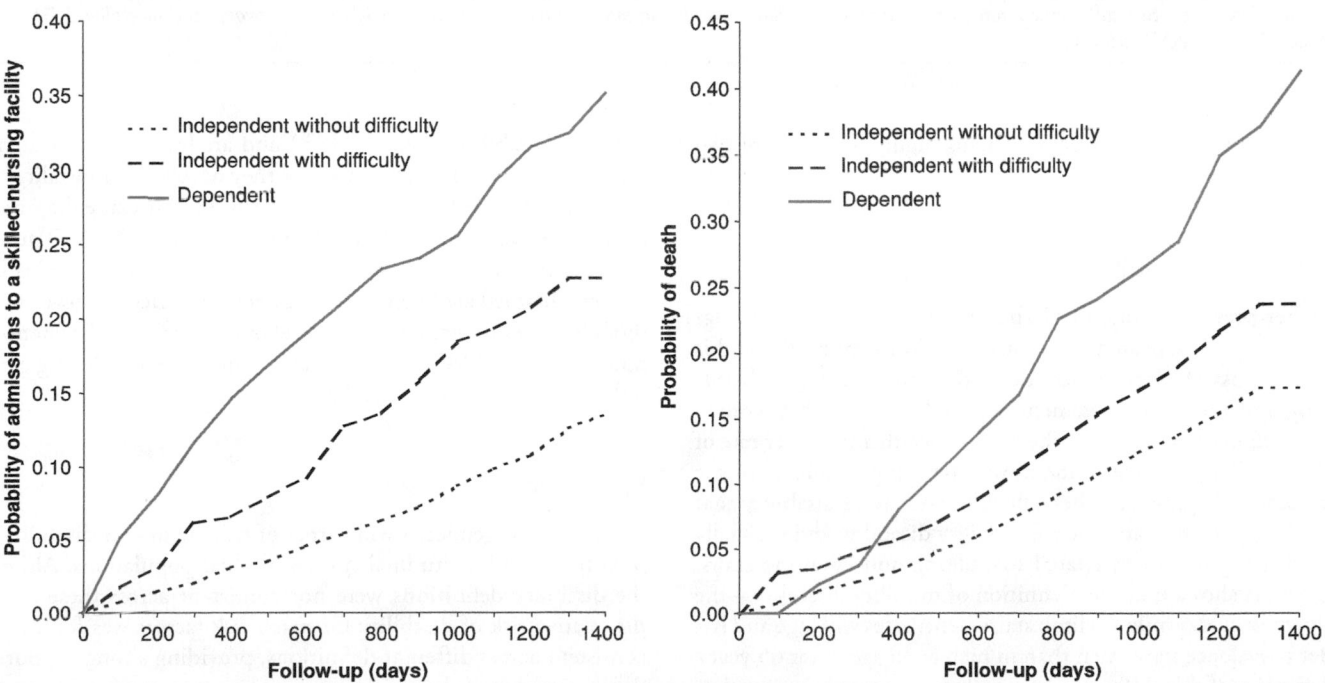

FIGURE 5-18. Cumulative probability of admission to a skilled-nursing facility (left) and death (right) for three basic activities of daily living groups. *Reprinted with permission from Gill TM, Robison JT, et al. Difficulty and dependence: Two components of the disability continuum among community-living older persons. Ann Intern Med. 1998;128:96.*

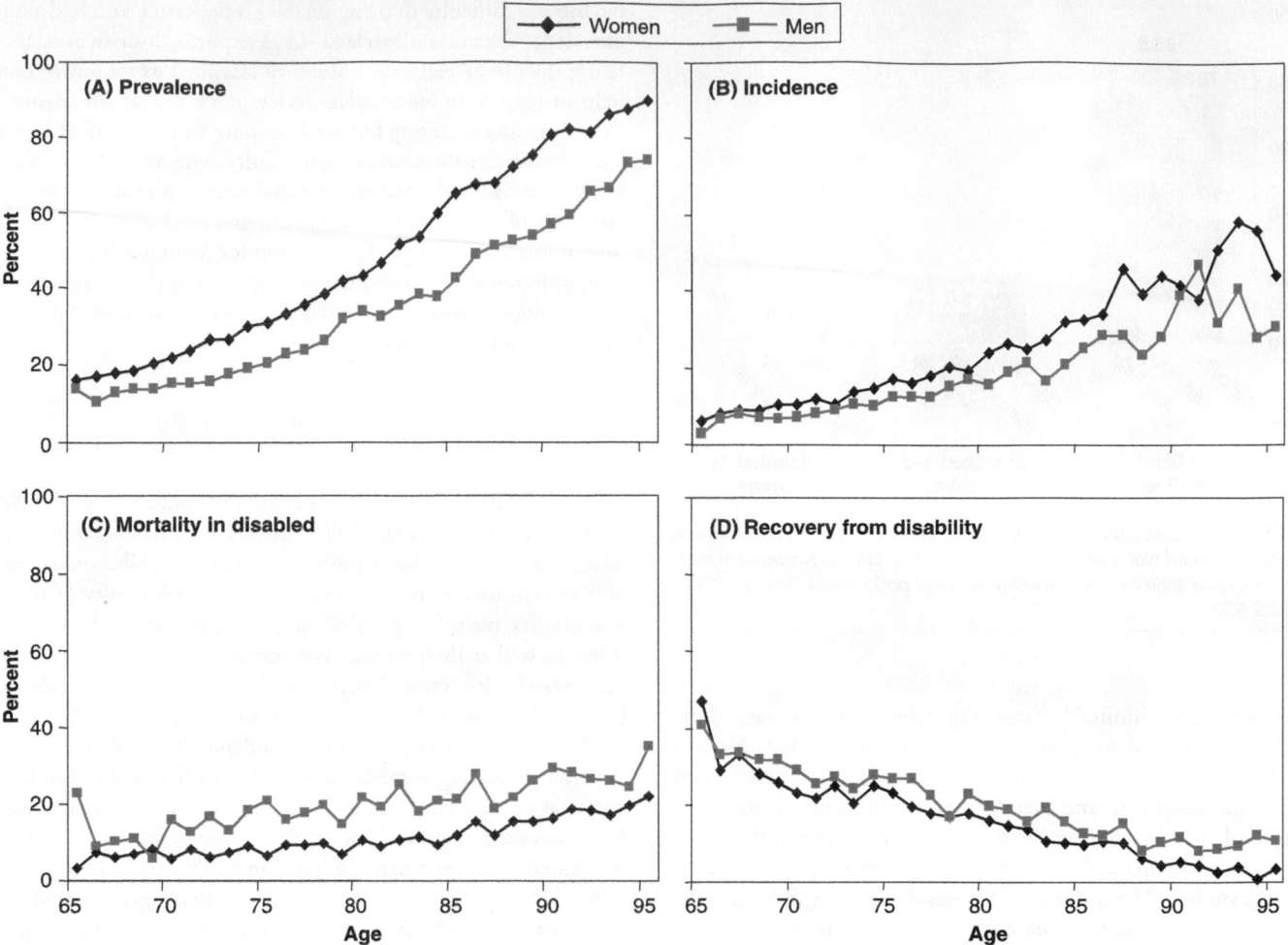

FIGURE 5-19. Women's and men's prevalence of mobility disability (a), 1-year incidence among nondisabled persons (b), and 1-year mortality (c) and recovery (d) among disabled persons, by age. Established Populations for the Epidemiologic Study of the Elderly. *Reprinted with permission from Leveille SG, Penninx BW, et al. Sex differences in the prevalence of mobility disability in old age: the dynamics of incidence, recovery, and mortality. J Gerontol B Psychol Sci Soc Sci. 2000:55:S41.*

measurement, with level of disability being highly predictive of two important outcomes.

Prevalence of Disability

The higher prevalence rate of disability in women, shown in Figure 5-16, has been repeatedly demonstrated in many studies and is consistent across a variety of measures and in studies using both self-reporting and objective assessments. Indeed, the fact that women live longer than men in spite of their worse health and higher rate of disability at all ages is one of the most interesting paradoxes in the epidemiology of aging. Another valuable measure of disability that has received increasing attention is mobility disability and is usually evaluated using questions related to walking and climbing stairs. Figure 5-19A shows that one definition of mobility disability—the inability to walk 0.5 mile or climb stairs—increases with age and has a higher prevalence in women than in men at all ages after 65 years. The dynamics of this difference in prevalence are highly instructive. Prevalence is a snapshot at a single point in time and is a function of the flow into and out of the condition being assessed. In the case of mobility disability, women have a higher incidence (new occur-

rence) of disability (Figure 5-19B) and are less likely to exit from the disabled state than men because they have lower mortality than men when they are disabled (Figure 5-19C) and because they are less likely to recover from disability than men (Figure 5-19D). Thus, the prevention of disability and better treatment of women who have become disabled are likely to have a beneficial effect in lowering the disability rates of women to the level of those of men. Reduction in mortality in disabled men would also contribute to reducing gender differences in disability prevalence.

Risk Factors for Disability

In addition to gender, a wide array of risk factors for disability has been found in longitudinal studies in older populations. Although the disability definitions were not consistent across these studies, the relative risk of disability for many risk factors was found to be consistent across different definitions, providing strong support for the importance of these risk factors. The most commonly and consistently reported risk factors for disability are listed in Table 5-9, which comes from a review of 78 community-based longitudinal studies that assessed factors related to decline in functional status

TABLE 5-9

Risk Factors for Functional Status Decline

Behavioral Risk Factors and Individual Characteristics
    Low physical activity
    Smoking
    High and low body mass index, weight loss
    Heavy and no alcohol consumption
    Increased age
    Lower socioeconomic status (income, education)
    High medication use
    Poor self-rated health
    Reduced social contacts

Chronic Conditions
    Cardiovascular disease
        Hypertension
        Coronary heart disease
        Myocardial infarction
        Angina pectoris
        Congestive heart failure
        Stroke
        Intermittent claudication
    Osteoarthritis
    Hip fracture
    Diabetes
    Chronic obstructive pulmonary disease
    Cancer
    Visual impairment
    Depression
    Cognitive impairment

Comorbidity

Source: Stuck et al., Soc Sci Med. 1999;48:445–469.

in older persons. Risk factors are divided into behavioral and individual characteristics, and specific chronic conditions. There is a great deal of interdependence among these risk factors. Behavioral risk factors such as physical inactivity and smoking can promote the development of a variety of diseases, which can then go on to cause disability. It is becoming evident that these behavioral risk factors may also have direct effects of their own. For example, physical inactivity may be a risk factor for the onset of specific diseases, and it also may have a direct negative impact on muscle, bone, and the central and peripheral nervous systems. These changes can move an individual closer to the physiologic and functional threshold beyond which functioning is impaired to the point that disability occurs. Figure 5-20 shows the relative contributions of specific conditions to disability according to age group. These data were obtained by asking persons who reported a limitation in their activities (work limitation or need for assistance in ADLs or IADLs) to specify the health condition that they thought was responsible for that limitation. Arthritis and heart or other circulatory diseases were by far the most commonly reported conditions contributing to physical limitations but it is notable that sensory limitations are also reported to make large contributions. Dementia is reported by proxies to be a substantial contributor to activity limitations in those age 85 years and older.

The role that cognitive impairment plays in physical disability has been generally underappreciated in epidemiologic studies. For clinicians attending to severely disabled persons in nursing homes,

however, it is evident that dementia itself prevents these individuals from being independent. Figure 5-21, based on data from population-based studies in Tuscany, Italy, shows estimates of the numbers of men and women with ADL disability in 1999 according to age. It also separates these people into those with and without dementia. There is an overall increase in the number of disabled persons through the mid-eighties in men and through the late eighties in women, with a drop-off in the numbers after that because of the decline in the total number of persons in the population at these advanced ages. The obvious gap in these otherwise smooth curves is a result of the low birthrate during and just after World War I, which translated into a smaller population 80 years later. In both men and women, most ADL disability before age 75 years is not associated with dementia. From age 75 to 90 years, about half of ADL disability is accompanied by dementia, and after age 90 years, the majority of persons with ADL disability have dementia. It should be noted that these data do not prove that dementia is what caused the disability in these individuals. Serious physical impairments and diseases co-occur with dementia, and it may not be possible to always understand just what the cause of disability is. Nevertheless, it is impressive that such a large proportion of disabled persons have dementia, and it is clear that cognitive functioning must be considered when developing interventions to prevent or treat disability.

Recovery from Disability

Longitudinal epidemiologic studies have revealed much about the dynamics of disability onset and progression. It has been found that, contrary to previous belief, a substantial proportion of individuals who are disabled report improvement on subsequent assessments. In effect, disability is a product of the disease or diseases from which an individual suffers, sedentary lifestyle or disuse, and physiologic declines that may be the result of aging or pathologic processes that are not specific diseases but result from factors such as inflammation or endocrine changes. As these predisposing conditions change, they have an impact on the initiation of disability and on changes in the status of already established disability. Figure 5-22 shows data on recovery from a study that assessed community-dwelling persons age 70 years and over on a monthly basis. Results are shown for the percent with disability who recovered for 2 or more months and 6 or more months according to the pattern of disability they initially reported. For persons with any disability, recovery rates were high and long-term recovery was also quite common. Recovery rates were also high in persons who had disability reported for 2 or more consecutive months (persistent disability) and 3 or more consecutive months (chronic disability). Other studies have observed high rates of improvement in disability status over intervals ranging from 1 to 3 years. These studies are conservative in their estimates of recovery because they are missing transient improvement due to the long time interval between assessments. Observed improvement in function could result from inaccurate self-reporting of disability over time (unreliability of instrument), a true change in disability status, or both. There is some evidence that both these explanations play a role, but there is consistent evidence that there is a certain amount of real improvement in disability. Both community-based studies and studies on persons hospitalized after an acute event have evaluated factors that predict recovery from disability. Age less than 85 years, good cognitive function, remaining physically mobile, absence of

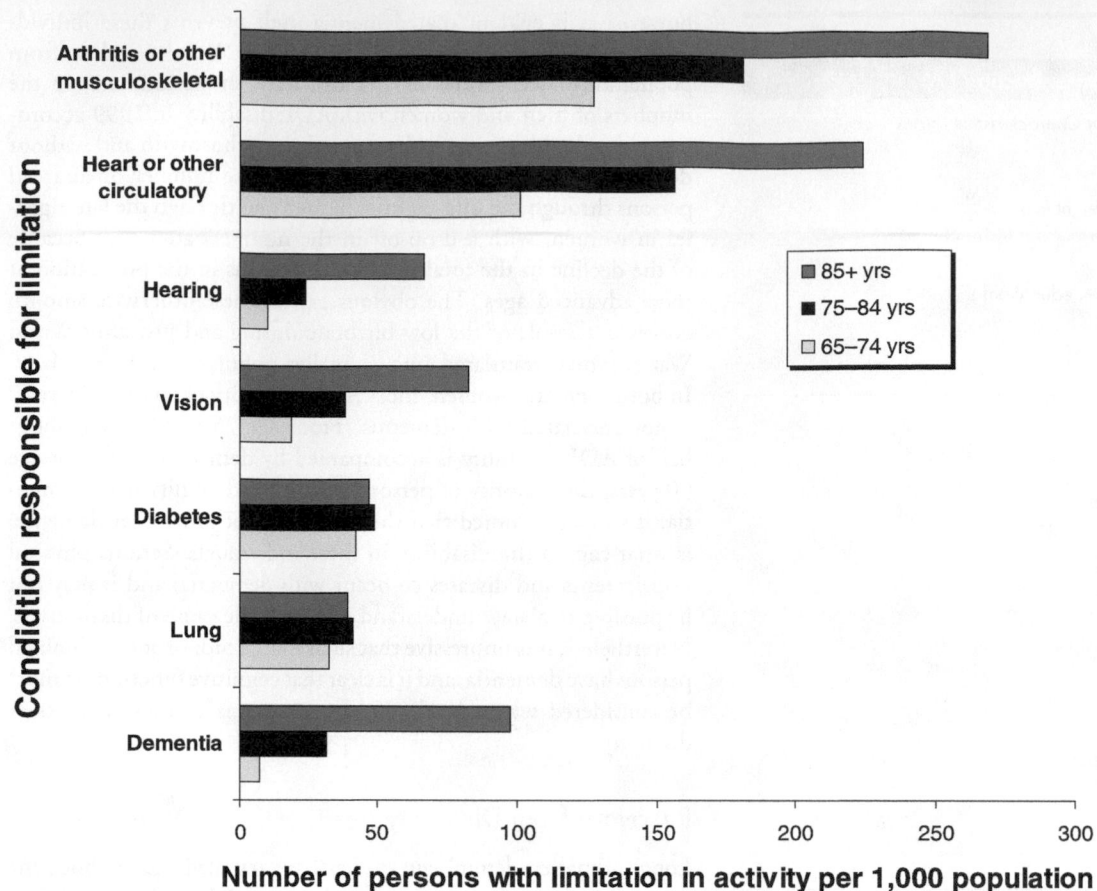

FIGURE 5-20. Reported chronic conditions responsible for self-reported activity limitation by age group: NHIS, 2003–2004. Activity limitation defined as work limitations or need for assistance with ADLs (eating, bathing, dressing, and getting around inside the home) or IADLs (household chores, doing necessary business, and shopping or running errands). If any limitations are identified, the respondent is asked to specify the health condition(s) causing the limitation(s) and indicate how long he or she has had each specified condition. U.S. Census Bureau 2004, National Health Interview Survey, 1997–2000, Prevalence of selected chronic conditions by age, sex, race, and Hispanic origin: United States, Data Warehouse on Trends in Health and Aging, NHICO1c, National Center for Health http://www.cdc.gov/nchs/agingact.htm. Statistics. Accessed on February 21, 2007.

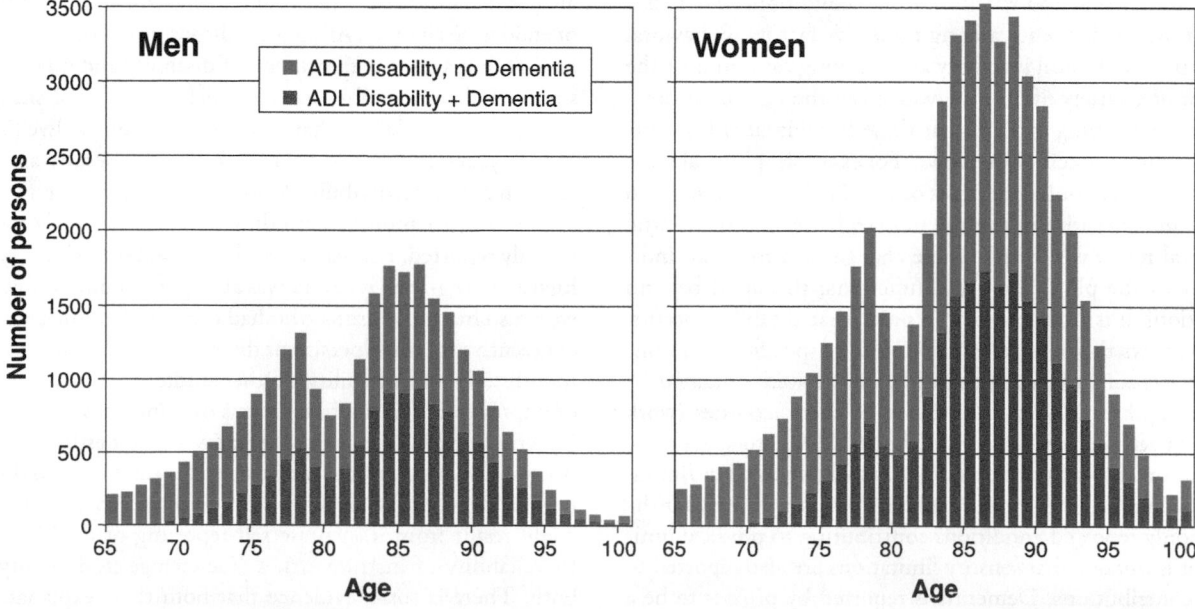

FIGURE 5-21. Estimated number of men and women with activities of daily living disability (need for help of another person) with and without an additional diagnosis of dementia according to age, Tuscany, Italy, 1999. The figure was obtained by applying estimates from three large population-based epidemiologic studies in the Tuscany population, the Italian Longitudinal Study on Aging, JCARE Dicomano, and InCHIANTI. The original analyses and population estimates are from Istituto Nazionale di Statistica: National Statistical Institute of Italy, 1999. Internet address www.istat.it. Accessed February 21, 2007.

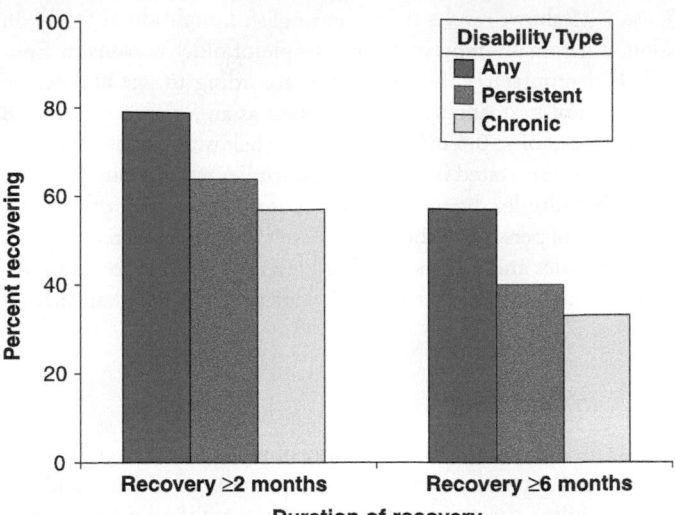

FIGURE 5-22. Percent recovering function after 2 months and after 6 months according to disability type. Any disability is defined at monthly visits as any new need for help or inability to perform one or more of the following ADLs: bathing, dressing, walking, and transferring. "Persistent" disability is defined as a new disability that was present for at least two consecutive months. "Chronic" disability is defined as a new disability that was present for at least 3 consecutive months. *Adapted from Hardy SE, Gill TM. Recovery from disability among community-dwelling older persons. JAMA. 2004;291:1596–1602.*

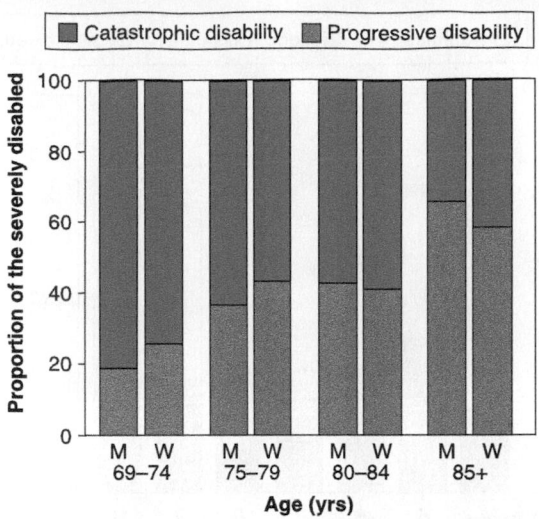

FIGURE 5-23. Proportion of population needing help with three or more activities of daily living (ADL) who have catastrophic disability (no ADL disability in preceding year) and progressive disability (need for help with one or two ADL in previous year), by age and gender. *Reprinted with permission from Ferrucci L, et al. Progressive versus catastrophic disability: a longitudinal view of the disablement process. J Gerontol A Biol Sci Med Sci. 1996;51:M123.*

depression, and good social support have all been associated with a greater probability of recovery.

Types of Disability Progression

In understanding the dynamics of disability progression, it is useful to consider the pace at which disability develops. The terms "progressive disability" and "catastrophic disability" have been used, indicating a slow downhill course and a very rapid decline, respectively. Progressive disability results from one or more ongoing chronic conditions and causes disability over months or years, whereas catastrophic disability can occur in moments as a result of a stroke or a hip fracture. The prevalence of both progressive and catastrophic severe ADL disability, defined as needing help with three or more ADLs, increases with increasing age, although progressive disability rises faster than catastrophic disability. Among older persons with severe ADL disability, the proportion that has catastrophic ADL disability is much higher at younger ages, and the proportion that has progressive ADL disability is much higher at the oldest ages (Figure 5-23). A similar age pattern has been found for onset of severe mobility disability (inability to walk across a room), where it has been demonstrated that progressive disability is much more common in people who have three or more chronic conditions.

The dynamics of disability can also be approached by studying the pathologic changes that precede its onset. Different theoretical pathways have been proposed to describe the changes that occur as a person proceeds from disease to disability. The theoretical pathway that has received substantial empirical support in aging research is that proposed by Nagi and endorsed by the Institute of Medicine. In this pathway, two intermediate steps, impairment and functional limitation, follow disease and lead to disability (see Verbrugge and Jette, 1994). Impairment describes the dysfunction and structural abnormalities in specific body systems that result from pathology.

Functional limitation describes restrictions in basic physical and mental actions that result from impairments. Functional limitations are the basic building blocks of functioning, and the interaction of these components of functioning with the environmental demands faced by an individual determines whether that person is disabled (see Guralnik and Ferrucci, 2003). Conventional study of the consequences of disease describes the physiologic organ impairments that result from specific conditions. More recent work in aging has gone on to describe further steps in the pathway. The impacts of impairments such as poor balance, muscle weakness, and visual deficits on functional limitations and disability have been demonstrated. Furthermore, the relationship between functional limitations, such as reduced gait speed, and subsequent disability also supports the pathway.

Physical Performance Measures

Objective measures of physical performance have received increasing attention as assessments that can measure functioning in a standardized manner in both research and clinical settings. These measures can be used to represent impairments, functional limitations, or actual disability, but most are indicators of functional limitations. The standardized Short Physical Performance Battery (SPPB) was administered to a large number of participants in the Established Populations for the Epidemiologic Study of the Elderly (EPESE). This battery, which included gait speed, time required to rise from a chair and sit down five times, and hierarchic measures of balance, was used to create a summary score of lower extremity performance that ranged from 0 to 12 (see Guralnik et al., 1995). This measure has been found to predict mortality, the need for nursing home admission, and health care utilization in the overall older population. Furthermore, in a population that had no disability at the time the performance battery was administered, the score was found to be highly predictive of who developed ADL and mobility disability 1 and 4 years later (Figure 5-24). These findings have been replicated in other

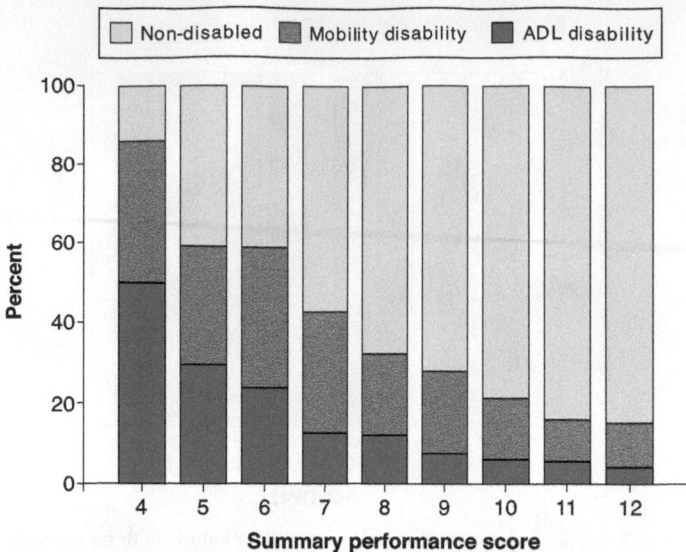

FIGURE 5-24. Disability status at four years according to baseline summary performance score in persons age 71 and older with no disability at baseline. *Reprinted with permission from Guralnik JM, Ferrucci L, et al. Lower extremity function in persons over the age of 70 yrs as a predictor of subsequent disability. N Engl J Med. 1995;332:556.*

populations and with other, similar performance measures and indicate that there is a state of preclinical disability, expressed as impairments and functional limitations, that indicates a high risk of proceeding to full-blown disability. This finding also provides a way of identifying high-risk older persons for whom preventive interventions may be highly effective.

Objective performance measures also provide a means of comparing functional status over time or across countries or cultures, where disability measures may lose comparability because of environmental differences or differential access to assistive devices.

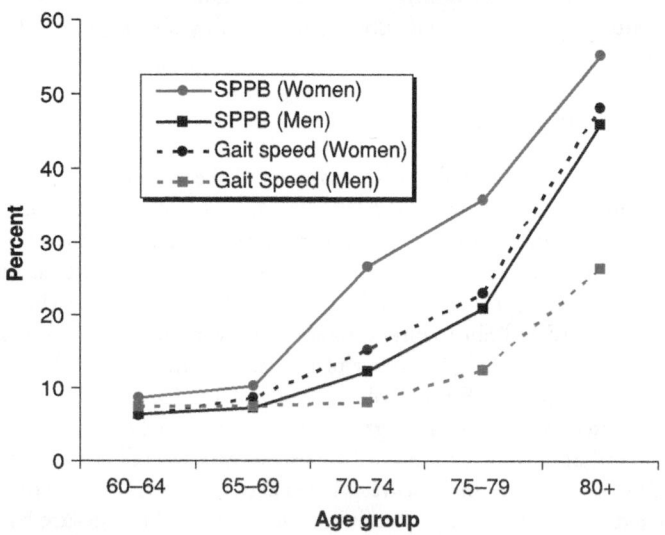

FIGURE 5-25. Percent of men and women with Short Physical Performance Battery score ≤ 8 and gait speed ≤ 0.5 m/s: England, 2002–2003. Institute for Fiscal Studies. Retirement, health, and relationships of the older population in England. The 2004 English Longitudinal Study of Aging (Wave 2). Tunbridge Well: Petersons, 2006. http://www.ifs.org.uk/elsa/report_wave2.php Accessed on February 21, 2007.

Figure 5-25 shows results from the English Longitudinal Study on Aging, a nationally representative sample of older persons in England. It demonstrates the prevalence according to age and sex of poor physical performance, documented as an SPPB score of ≤ 8 and gait speed of < 0.5 m/s. Performance below these cut-off points has been demonstrated in longitudinal studies to be strongly associated with multiple adverse outcomes. Poor performance affects only about 10% of persons in their sixties but the prevalence rises rapidly in the seventies and attains very high levels in persons above age 80 years. Women have higher rates of poor performance than men at all ages.

Trends in Disability

Because disability status is a good way of representing overall health status in older persons with complex patterns of disease, and because disability also has direct implications for the long-term care

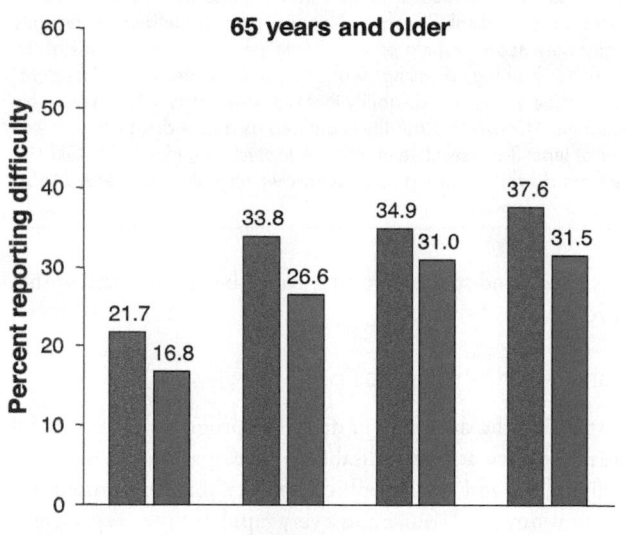

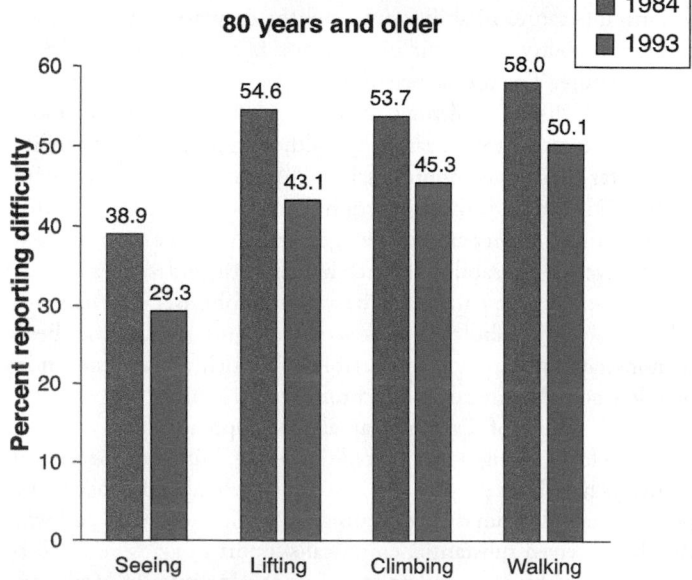

FIGURE 5-26. Prevalence of functional limitations, United States, 1984 and 1993. *Data from Freedman VA, Martin LG. Understanding trends in functional limitations among older Americans. Am J Public Health. 1998; 88:1457.*

needs of an older person, there has been much interest in evaluating disability trends over time. Although a number of national surveys now assess disability, uniform disability assessment done over time has been available only since the mid-1980s in just a few studies with nationally representative samples. Although these studies use different assessment instruments, a convincing decline in age- and gender-specific rates of disability was observed from the mid-1980s through the 1990s. The National Long Term Care Survey has similar assessments of ADL and IADL disability available from 1982 through 2005, and recent findings indicate that the decline in disability observed for the first 12 years of the study continued and actually accelerated from 1994 through 2005 (see Manton et al., 2006). In another study that utilized reports of functional limitations, including lifting and carrying 10 lb, climbing stairs, walking 1/4 mile, and seeing words in a newspaper, changes in prevalence were evaluated between 1984 and 1993. Declines were seen in the inability to perform all four of these tasks in the 65 years and older population and as well as the 80 years and older population (Figure 5-26). The functional limitations evaluated in this study, which assess more basic tasks than disability, are an excellent way to follow trends over time because they are influenced less by changing roles that can affect disability assessment (more men cooking in more recent surveys and more women managing money). The observed declines in disability and functional limitations can be attributed to a number of factors. Educational status is strongly associated with disability, and it has been estimated that anywhere from 25% to 75% of the observed functional declines are related to a higher educational level in more recent cohorts. Other factors proposed as

explanations for the decline in disability include reductions in the prevalence of several chronic diseases, changes in nutrition and public health at the time when these cohorts were young, and improved health promotion and medical therapy.

The interplay among time of disability onset, duration of disability, and time of death determines the number of years that older individuals live in the disability-free state, termed active life expectancy, and the number of years spent in the disabled state. Life table approaches have been used to calculate active and disabled life expectancy, utilizing data from population-based longitudinal studies on transitions from the nondisabled state to disability and death and from the disabled state to nondisability and death. Using this approach may provide insight into the mechanisms and risk factors that affect the quality of aging and suggest potential targets for intervention. In Figure 5-27, an example is shown using data from the EPESE study on the impact of race and educational status on total, active, and disabled life expectancy. This demonstrates that low education (less than 12 years) is associated with shorter total life expectancy and shorter active life expectancy in both black and white women and men but that, comparing persons with the same educational status, there are only small differences between blacks and whites. Alternative methods have been developed to estimate active life expectancy that utilize mortality data and prevalence of disability, which is easier to obtain in a national survey than 1-year transition probabilities. As more data become available to estimate both active and disabled life expectancy, we will gain more insight into the prospects for a compression of morbidity, which is the reduction in disabled life expectancy that results from compressing

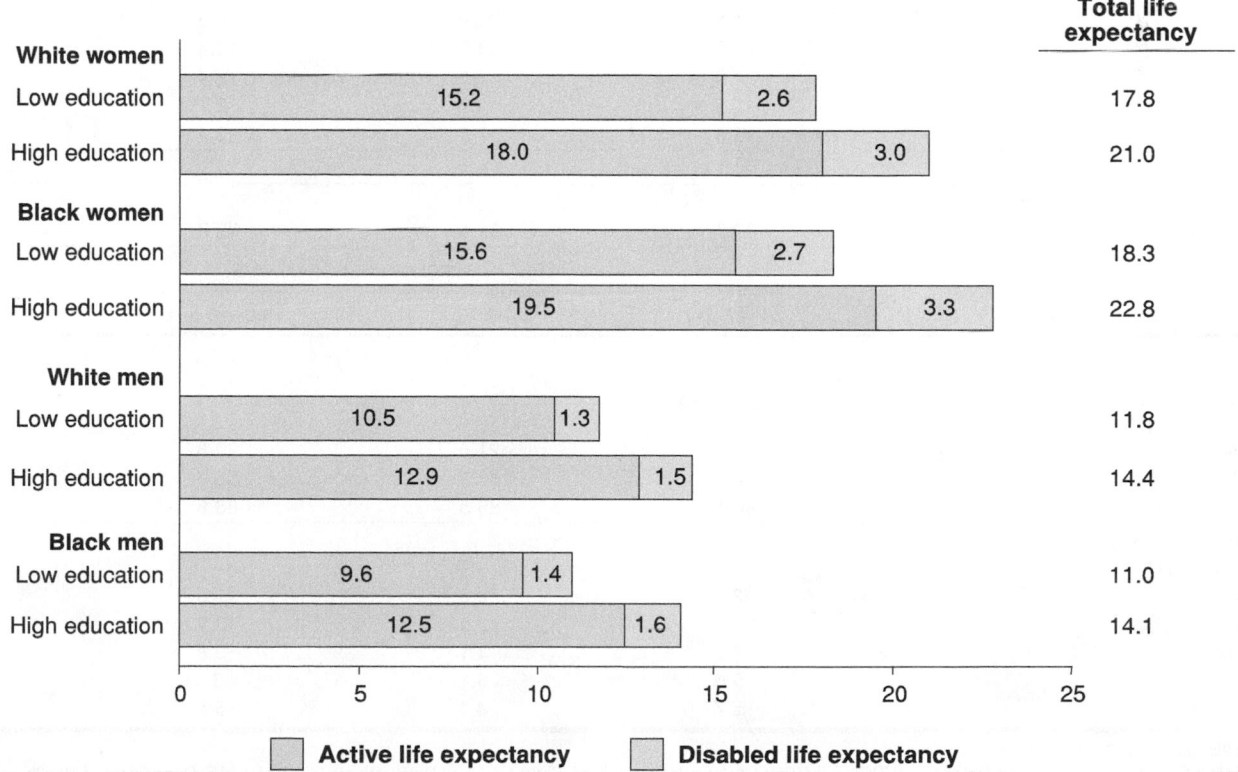

FIGURE 5-27. Total life expectancy, active (nondisabled) life expectancy, and disabled life expectancy at age 65 yrs according to gender, race, and educational status. Lower education defined as less than 12 yrs of school, and higher education as 12 or more years of school. *Data from Guralnik JM, Land KC, et al. Educational status and active life expectancy in older blacks and whites. N Engl J Med. 1993;329:110.*

TABLE 5-10

Behavioral Risk Factors in Middle-Aged and Older Persons, United States, 2004–2005

	PERCENT OF AGE GROUP			
	35–44 (yr)	45–54 (yr)	55–64 (yr)	65+ (yr)
Alcoholic beverages				
≥ One drink within the past 30 days	60.9	58.3	53.0	39.3
Men >2/day Women >1/day	5.1	4.7	4.2	2.9
5+ at one time	16.1	11.9	7.9	3.0
Cholesterol check				
Past 5 yrs	72.1	82.9	90.2	92.9
Never	21.7	11.6	6.5	4.9
BMI				
Overweight (25.0–29.9)	37.7	39.2	41.7	40.0
Obese (≥30.0)	25.3	27.0	29.3	20.3
Physical activities				
30+ moderate (5×) or 20+ vigor (3×)	49.7	51.5	55.3	61.0
20+ vigorous (3×)	29.9	56.6	21.1	14.1
Past month	78.6	76.9	73.4	65.9
Fruits and vegetables				
5 or more times per day	20.1	22.4	24.8	31.0
Dental visit in last year	72.4	74.4	72.5	66.1
Smoking status				
Everyday	17.7	17.2	14.6	6.6
Some days	5.4	5.0	3.8	2.2
Former	18.7	26.1	36.1	41.6
Never	57.9	49.8	46.1	48.8
Immunization				
Flu in past year	—	—	—	65.5
Pneumonia ever	—	—	—	65.7
Use of seatbelts*				
Always	69.5	70.9	70.3	74.4
Nearly always	13.9	14.2	13.4	12.1
Sometimes	7.5	7.5	7.4	5.3
Seldom	3.5	3.2	3.1	2.5
Never	3.8	3.5	3.5	3.2
Smoke detector in home*	97.1	96.1	94.9	93.5
Among persons with smoke detectors				
Smoke detector tested, past year*	82.7	81.6	82.7	82.7

	PERCENT OF AGE GROUP			
	40–49 (yr)	50–59 (yr)	60–64 (yr)	65+ (yr)
PSA test				
Within past 2 yrs	24.9	57.5	70.6	74.8
Colorectal screening				
Stool tested	—	21.6	29.8	30.4
Sigmoidoscopy or colonoscopy	—	42.3	55.7	63.2
Mammogram, ever*	80.1	88.5	88.8	84.3
Among women who had a mammogram				
Last mammogram*				
Past year	58	70.8	71.5	65.4
1–2 yrs	22.6	15.2	13.9	18.2
2–3 yrs	7.3	4.1	3.8	5.2
3–5 yrs	5.6	3.8	3	3.8
5+ yrs ago	5.7	4.5	5.5	7.2

*Most recent BRFSS data 1997.

Source: Centers for Disease Control and Prevention (CDC). Behavioral Risk Factor Surveillance System Survey Data. Atlanta, Georgia: U.S. Department of Health and Human Services, Centers for Disease Control and Prevention; 2005. http://apps.nccd.cdc.gov/brfss/index.asp

chronic disease and disability into a smaller number of years between disease and/or disability onset and mortality (see Fries, 1980).

Aging of Individuals with Life-Long Disabilities

In addition to the large number of persons who will develop disabilities in old age, there is a smaller cohort of persons with lifelong disabilities who will enter old age with these disabilities. Persons with developmental disabilities represent a heterogeneous population with varying abilities, and their disabilities may result from a variety of conditions such as cerebral palsy, mental retardation, learning disorders, autism, and epilepsy. It is estimated that in 2000, there were over 600,000 people in the United States with mental retardation and other developmental disabilities. Their numbers will double to 1.2 million by 2030 when all of the post–World War II "baby boom" generation will be in their sixties. Life expectancy of many persons with mental retardation and developmental disabilities has risen dramatically and many people with these disorders will live into advanced old age. Down's syndrome is an exception to this, however, with signs of accelerated aging and development of Alzheimer's disease at early ages. A further consideration related to the growing number of older persons with developmental disabilities is the continuation of their care when their own parents reach old age. Nearly two-thirds of persons with developmental disabilities live with their families and in one-quarter of these households the primary caregiver is 60 years or older. Over the next 30 years, there will be a considerable increase in the number of families where parents more than 80 years old are caring for an older child with a developmental disability.

BEHAVIORAL RISK FACTORS (see Chapter 28)

An important role for epidemiology is to elucidate risk factors for disease, injury, and disability. Many risk factors have been shown to have a large impact in older persons. Although certain risk factors that are potent predictors of major diseases in middle age may have less or no impact at old age, most behavioral risk factors continue to be important throughout old age (see Chapter 28). Cigarette smoking, for example, continues to predict mortality even in smokers who have survived past age 65 years, and stopping smoking even in old age is associated with better outcomes. The Centers for Disease Control and Prevention perform national surveys on a wide range of behavioral risk factors and include the older population in these assessments. Table 5-10 demonstrates the prevalence of risk factors

and protective factors across four age groups, from 35 to 44 years through 65 years and older. For almost all these health practices, older persons have similar or somewhat better rates than younger individuals.

These results are compatible with findings that adherence to physicians' recommendations and medication schedules is better in older than in younger persons. Thus, this is a population that faces increasing risk of disease and disability with increasing age but one that cares about its health, has a positive risk factor profile, and is willing to comply with interventions to prevent or improve adverse health outcomes. Applying what has been learned in epidemiologic studies on older populations so that effective prevention and treatment strategies will be available to older persons is a continuing challenge for the field.

ACKNOWLEDGMENT

This chapter was supported by the Intramural Research Program, National Institute on Aging, NIH.

FURTHER READING

Ettinger WH, Maradee AD, Neuhaus JM, et al. Long-term physical functioning in persons with knee osteoarthritis from NHANES I: Effects of comorbid medical conditions. *J Clin Epidemiol.* 1994;47:809.

Ferrucci L, Guralnik JM, Pahor M, et al. Hospital diagnoses, Medicare charges, and nursing home admissions in the year when older persons become severely disabled. *JAMA* 1997;277:728.

Fried LP, Guralnik JM. Disability in older adults: Evidence regarding significance, etiology, and risk. *J Am Geriatr Soc.* 1997;45:92.

Fries JF: Aging, natural death, and the compression of morbidity. *N Engl J Med.* 1980;303:130.

Gill TM, Robison JT, Tinetti ME. Predictors of recovery in activities of daily living among disabled older persons living in the community. *J Gen Intern Med.* 1997;12:757.

Guralnik JM. Assessing the impact of comorbidity in the older population. *Ann Epidemiol.* 1996;6:376.

Guralnik JM, Fried LP, Salive ME. Disability as a public health outcome in the aging population. *Ann Rev Public Health.* 1996;17:25.

Guralnik JM, Ferrucci L. Assessing the building blocks of function: Utilizing measures of functional limitation. *Am J Prev Med.* 2003;25:112.

Kramarow E, Lentzner H, Rooks R, et al. *Health and Aging Chartbook, Health, United States, 1999.* Hyattsville, MD; National Center for Health Statistics, 1999. http://www.cdc.gov/nchs/data/hus/hus99.pdf.

Manton KG, Gu X, Lamb VL. Change in chronic disability from 1982 to 2004/2005 as measured by long-term changes in function and health in the U.S. elderly population. *Proc Natl Acad Sci.* 2006;103:18374.

Stuck AE, Walthert JM, Nikolaus T, et al. Risk factors for functional status decline in community-living elderly people: a systematic literature review. *Soc Sci Med.* 1999;48:445.

Verbrugge LM, Jette AM. The disablement process. *Soc Sci Med.* 1994;38:1.

International Gerontology

Roberto Bernabei ■ Len Gray ■ John Hirdes ■ Xiaomei Pei ■ Jean Claude Henrard ■ Palmi V. Jonsson ■ Graziano Onder ■ Giovanni Gambassi ■ Naoki Ikegami ■ Annette Hylen Ranhoff ■ Iain G. Carpenter ■ Rowan H. Harwood ■ Brant E. Fries ■ John N. Morris ■ Knight Steel

IMPLICATIONS OF GLOBAL POPULATION AGING FOR HEALTH AND HEALTH CARE

Overview

Population aging is a pervasive, unprecedented global phenomenon. The trend is expected to continue into the twenty-first century. The older population is itself aging; the fastest growing age group is the oldest-old, those aged 80 years or older.

The chapter begins by highlighting the consequences and implications of the global aging of the population. In the economic area, population aging will have an impact on economic growth, savings, investments, and consumption, labor markets, pensions, and taxation. Also, this phenomenon will have a direct bearing on the intergenerational and intragenerational equity and solidarity that are the foundations of our societies. In the social sphere, population aging will affect health and health care, family composition and living arrangements, housing, and migration. Some of the inadequacies of health professional education and health care delivery systems in meeting the chronic health care needs of aging populations around the world are discussed.

The second section of the chapter describes how health care systems around the world are preparing to deal with patients with multiple chronic, degenerative diseases. Information is provided about developed countries in four continents including Canada and United States for North America; Iceland, Norway, United Kingdom, France, and Italy for Europe; Japan for Asia; and Australia for Oceania. The current situation in China is discussed as an example of the preparedness of the more densely populated developing countries and those with the fastest growing economies. For each country, the following information is presented: the principal char-acteristics of the health care system; the organizational approaches and the services available for older adults; and positive aspects, weaknesses, and specific peculiarities. Each nation's description ends with a description of what would happen in a hypothetical example of an 87-year-old widow hoping to return home after suffering a stroke with motor and speech deficits.

The third section of the chapter illustrates the difficulty in addressing these epidemiological changes without a global, standard way of assessing the needs of older individuals. The chapter describes the development of a minimum data set of information that can be applied, independent of nationality, language, and culture, to any health care setting. Data are presented to suggest that this global assessment is one strategy for capturing the essential aspects, variables, and solutions that make a local or a national health care system work more efficiently by responding to the needs of their older clients. Also, the chapter summarizes the results of the real-world application of such instruments by governmental mandate in the Canadian province of Ontario and in health services research conducted in Europe.

Finally, the chapter discusses the evidence that the unprecedented demographic changes, which had their origins in the nineteenth and twentieth centuries, are continuing well into the twenty-first century. The number of older persons has tripled over the last 50 years but it will more than triple again over the next 50 years. In contrast with the slow process of population aging experienced by the more developed countries, the aging process in most of the less developed countries is taking place in a much shorter period of time, and is occurring on larger population bases. Such rapid growth will require far-reaching economic and social adjustments in most countries. Effective and efficient health care for the chronic health problems facing this growing population of older adults will be a daunting challenge for all countries.

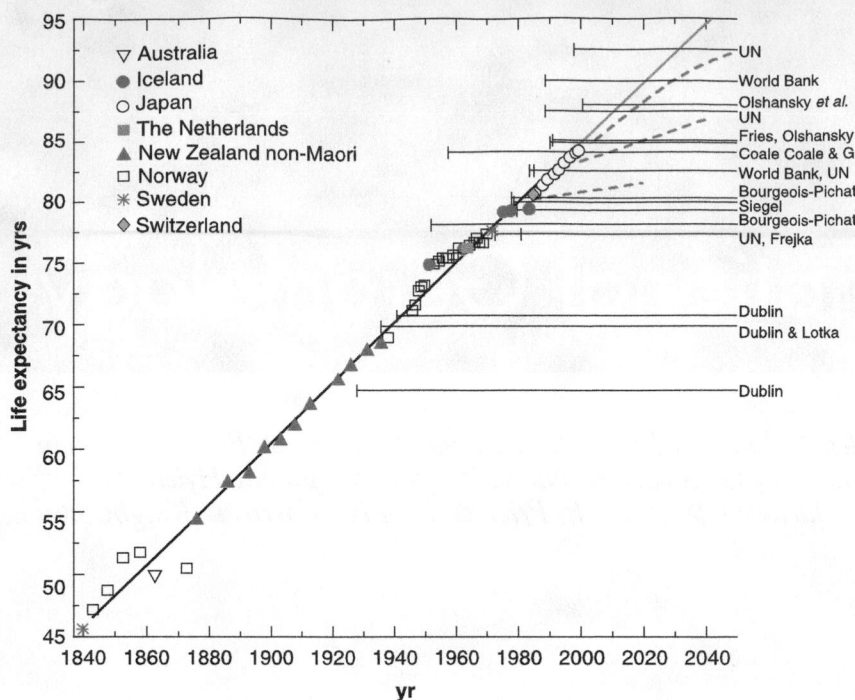

FIGURE 6-1. Increase in female life expectancy (in years) observed in selected countries since 1840 (solid lines) and extrapolated to 2040 (dashed lines). The horizontal black lines show asserted ceilings on life expectancy, with a short vertical line indicating the year of publication. *(Reprinted with permission from Oeppen J and Vaupel JW. Science 2002;296:1029–1031.)*

Demography of the Aging Global Population (see also Chapter 5)

Notwithstanding some heterogeneity, life expectancy is increasing across the globe. In most industrialized countries, this increase in life expectancy has mostly occurred over the last century. However, in the most recent decades, its pace has progressed at an unprecedented speed, reaching estimates far beyond those predicted by most international organizations such as the United Nations. The increase in life expectancy, seen in many countries throughout the world, does not seem to be levelling off (Figure 6-1).

The increase of life expectancy has resulted in increased proportion of individuals reaching the eight and ninth decade of life.

Individuals 80 years+ are consistently found to be the fastest growing segment of the population. Similarly, there is an unprecedented and increasing appearance of centenarians and supercentenarians (Figure 6-2).

The disproportionate life advantage favoring women over men has created a progressive feminization of the older population. Among individuals 85 years+, there are, on average, 55 men for every 100 women.

The increase in life expectancy has been paralleled—especially in the western world—by declining fertility rates. In most countries, the fertility rate is much below the mortality rate and below what it is considered the minimum for population replacement and conservation. The concomitance of an increased life expectancy with a

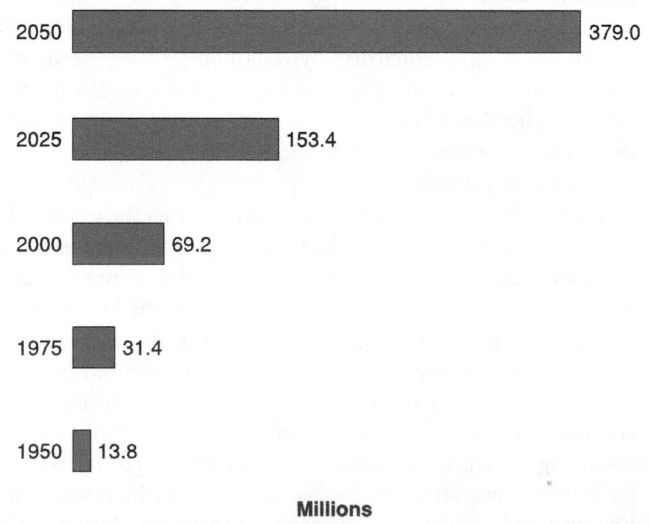

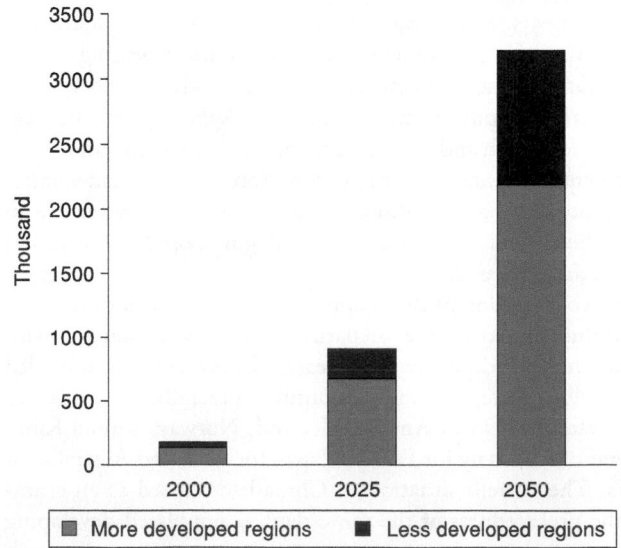

FIGURE 6-2. Population aged 80 yrs or older (in millions) in the period 1950 to 2050 (left panel); Distribution of world centenarians by development regions (2000–2050) (right panel). *(Reprinted with permission from World Population Aging 1950–2050, United Nations.)*

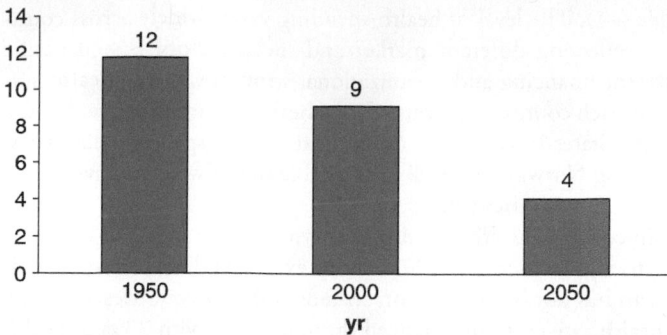

FIGURE 6-3. Potential support ratio: world, 1950–2050. *(Reprinted with permission from World Population Aging 1950–2050, United Nations.)*

reduced fertility rate has produced profound effects on the labor market, the financial resources, and other societal factors. One example is the potential support ratio, i.e., the number of persons aged 15 to 64 years per one older person aged 65 years and over. Between 1950 and 2000, the potential support ratio fell from 12 to 9 people per each person 65 years or older. By midcentury, the potential support ratio is projected to fall to 4 working-age persons for each person 65 years or older. Potential support ratios have important implications for social security schemes, particularly traditional systems in which current workers pay for the benefits of current retirees (Figure 6-3).

Effect of Population Aging on Health and Health Care

Epidemiological evidence shows that as age increases, there is a progressive, exponential increase in the occurrence of most chronic, degenerative, and progressive diseases, including cardiovascular disease, cancer, chronic obstructive pulmonary disease, dementia, and other degenerative conditions. Furthermore, there is an increase in the cooccurrence of these diseases, resulting in comorbidity.

Health care systems around the world have been modeled around the ideology of the disease model. Diagnosis and treatment is focused on eliminating or ameliorating the underlying pathology; health outcomes are determined by the disease. Also, functional impairment and quality of life are assumed to be improved by treating the "causative" disease. The disease model has resulted in the creation of health systems centered on acute care hospitals and disease-based specialists. This model has informed the way we have developed and accrued knowledge. For example, evidence-based medicine (EBM) has been promoted as the best approach to improving health and health care. The randomized, controlled trials on which EBM recommendations are based typically provide evidence of modest reductions in the relative risk of the disease-specific outcomes that are associated with the use of various interventions such as medications. Older patients and patients with multiple health conditions and therapies have been excluded from many evidence-generating randomized, controlled trials. Arguments have been made for extrapolating the evidence from such trials to subpopulations of elderly patients, but the generalizability of the results to these patients remains unknown.

Consequently, physicians and health personnel are facing a "new" type of patient who presents with an array of concomitant clinical conditions. These combinations of conditions result in varying degrees of functional deficits, cognitive deterioration, nutritional problems, and geriatric syndromes (delirium, falls, incontinence), often in the face of inadequate social support and financial resources.

This "new" complex, older patient presents a degree of complexity not previously considered by the traditional understanding of medicine and its role. The traditionally envisioned health care system, whether operating under universal coverage or private mechanisms, is challenged by this complex patient.

The response to the challenge of the complex older patient has been heterogeneous around over the world; differences in resource availability and economical and cultural issues have resulted in different organizations of health care systems. In addition, the methodological approaches adopted by systems to evaluate the needs of such complex patients have been highly variable and not standardized. In particular, the organization of services to care for geriatric patients, including geriatric assessment and management, remains highly variable. This variation is seen among nurses, physicians, therapists, nursing homes, home care services, and health systems.

To display this intercountry variability, each country's section will end with the description of likely sequences of events in a clinical case scenario. The clinical scenario is an 87-year-old widow who was independent in activities of daily living, cognitively intact, and living in her own house albeit with few social supports prior to suffering a stroke with resultant motor, speech, and swallowing deficits. Despite these deficits and lack of supports, she strongly wishes to return home. The types of treatments and services offered to her in each country will be presented.

INTERNATIONAL COMPARISONS

In order to illustrate the way countries in the most developed world have prepared to cope with population aging we have selected nine countries in four continents with large percentages of persons older than age 65, including Canada and the United States for North America, Iceland, Norway, United Kingdom, France, and Italy for Europe, Japan for Asia, and Australia for Oceania (Figure 6-4).

These countries have among the highest life expectancy at birth, well over 80 years for all but the United States and United Kingdom. The percentage of the population in that is aged 65 years and older ranges from 11% in Iceland to approximately 20% in Italy and Japan (Table 6-1). In the next 50 years, the percentage of older adults will

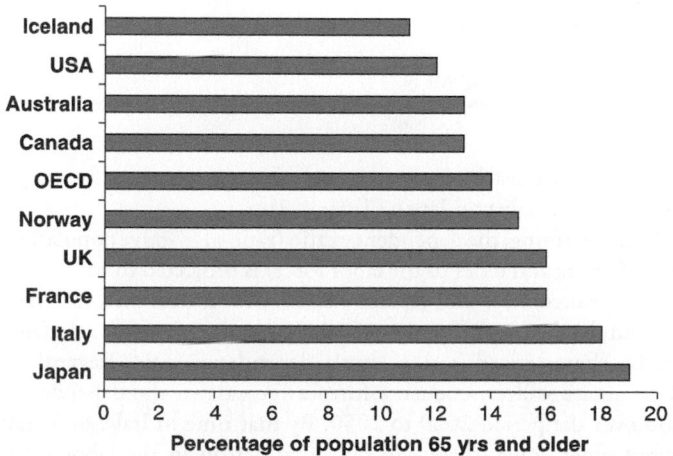

FIGURE 6-4. Percentage of population 65 yrs and older in nine Organization for Economic Cooperation and Development (OECD) countries compared with the mean OECD in the year 2005. *(Adapted from OECD Factbook 2007: Economic, Environmental and Social Statistics.)*

TABLE 6-1

Total Population, Percentage of Population At Least 65 Yrs Old, and Percentage of Gross Domestic Product Spend on Health Expenditures Across 10 Countries

America—United States
- Population—301.7 million
- Proportion 65+—11.9%
- Health expenditures—15.3% of GDP

America—Canada
- Population—32.6 million
- Proportion 65+—13.3%
- Health expenditures—10.2% of GDP

Europe—Iceland
- Population—293.000
- Proportion 65+—11.6%
- Health expenditures—10.2% of GDP

Europe—Norway
- Population—4.7 million
- Proportion 65+—14.7%
- Health expenditures—9.2% of GDP

Europe—United Kingdom
- Population—59.8 million
- Proportion 65+—16.1
- Health expenditures—8.3% of GDP

Europe—France
- Population—60.2 million
- Proportion 65+—16.6%
- Health expenditures—10.5% of GDP

Europe – Italy
- Population—58.5 million
- Proportion 65+—19.7%
- Health expenditures—8.4% of GDP

Asia – Japan
- Population—127.8 million
- Proportion 65+—20.2%
- Health expenditures—8.0% of GDP

Oceania—Australia
- Population—20.1 million
- Proportion 65+—13.1%
- Health expenditures—9.2% of GDP

Developing Countries—China
- Population—1306.3 million
- Proportion 65+—7.7%
- Health expenditures—5.6% of GDP

almost double in each country, estimated to reach over a third of the population in Italy and Japan (Table 6-2).

More alarming, the dependency ratio (ratio of inactive population aged 65 years and older to the labor force) is projected to be close to 50% in France, Italy, and Japan by 2020. This means that, for every older adult, there will be only two persons in the labor force. Iceland will be characterized by the lowest dependency ratio. Regardless, all countries will experience a further increase in the dependency ratio over the period 2020 to 2050. By that time in Italy, for every retired older adult, there will only one person in the labor force (Figure 6-5).

In most nine Organization for Economic Cooperation and Development (OECD) countries, expenditures on health are a large and growing share of both public and private expenditures (see

Table 6-1). The level of health spending varies widely across countries, reflecting different market and social factors as well as the different financing and organizational structures of the health system in each country. In terms of total health spending per capita, the United States is well ahead of the next highest spending countries, including Norway, and well over double the unweighted average of all OECD countries (Figure 6-6).

Since 1990, health spending has grown faster than gross domestic product in every OECD country except Finland, although this growth has not been constant. In most OECD countries, the bulk of health care costs are financed through taxes, with 73% of health spending, on average, being publicly funded in 2004.

The strategy and the organizational approach to deal with complex patients with multiple chronic conditions differ substantially across countries. In part, these differences are historical, cultural, demographic, and financial, and societal. For each country, we present key characteristics of the health care system, and organizational approaches and services available for older adults.

America: United States

Type of Health Care System

At the time this chapter is being written, the United States does not have universal health care. In the year 2007, as many as 50 000 000 Americans are uninsured. Nonetheless almost the entire older population is covered for some health care services under a federal insurance program known as Medicare (see Chapter 15).

Overall Organization and Services Available for Older Adults (see Chapter 15)

To be eligible to receive benefits, either the individual or the person's spouse must have worked for 10 years or more in a Medicare-covered capacity and be at least 65 years of age and a citizen or a legal resident of the country. Under most circumstances, enrolment in the program is automatic at age 65 years. Medicare Part A pays for most acute hospital level care services and many postacute care inpatient services for a limited period of time as well as some skilled home care and hospice services. For individuals who meet economic criteria, nonskilled home care services are provided by the states, using either Medicaid or state funds; their availability differs dramatically across the states.

Unlike Part A, the older person must request and pay for Medicare Part B insurance. This is the major payer for most physician services as well as ambulatory care. In 2007, it cost the individual about $100 per month, the exact amount being determined by the age at which the individual signs up for the plan.

Medicare Part D is an elective insurance plan that pays for pharmaceuticals. The individual desiring this insurance program usually must choose from among a large number of plans offered by different insurance companies, each of which may cost a different amount and have a somewhat different formulary.

Long-term care is not covered under Medicare. Multiple plans are offered by the insurance industry, each of which may differ with respect to the cost, waiting period for eligibility, and duration of coverage. Medicaid provides for long-term institutional care and many other health care services for the indigent population. However, the eligibility requirements and the exact services available vary from

TABLE 6-2

Population Aged 65 Yrs and older, Percentage of the Total Population 2000–2050							
COUNTRY	2000	2005	2010	2020	2030	2040	2050
OECD	13.0	13.8	14.7	17.8	21.3	23.9	25.5
United States	12.4	12.4	13.0	16.3	19.6	20.4	20.6
Canada	12.6	13.1	14.1	18.2	23.1	25.0	26.3
Iceland	11.6	11.7	12.4	15.5	19.2	20.9	21.5
Norway	15.2	14.7	15.1	18.0	20.6	22.9	23.2
UK	15.8	16.0	16.7	19.5	22.5	24.7	27.9
France	16.1	16.4	16.7	20.3	23.4	25.6	26.2
Italy	18.3	19.6	20.6	23.3	27.3	32.3	33.7
Japan	17.4	20.0	23.1	29.2	31.8	36.5	39.6
Australia	12.4	13.1	14.3	18.3	22.2	24.5	25.7

OECD, Organization for Economic Cooperation and Development.

state to state as Medicaid is a joint federal and state program of insurance.

The number of residential nursing home beds varies by state from a low of 21 beds per 1000 people older than 65 years to a high of 80 beds. The median is 49 beds. There are now more long-term care beds than there are acute care beds in the country. The percent of people aged 65 years and older with long-term care needs who do and do not reside in institutions and the proportion of the older Americans who reside in institutions are displayed in Figure 6-7.

An entirely separate health care system is provided by the Veterans Administration for military veterans who have limited assets. It has its own hospitals and ambulatory settings and employs its own physicians. Many of these facilities are attached to a varying degree to academic institutions.

There have been some important developments in the availability of physician services for older adults in the last 20 years. In 1988, geriatric medicine was recognized as an area of "Added Competence"

by both the American Board of Internal Medicine and the American Board of Family Medicine. Training programs in geriatric medicine for graduates of these two primary boards were designed and approved by the national accrediting body, the Accrediting Council for Graduate Medical Education. Similarly, geriatric psychiatry programs were established. In 2006, the American Board of Internal Medicine "upgraded" the field by making geriatric medicine a full specialty equivalent to, for example, cardiology and gastroenterology.

Nonetheless in the United States, geriatric medicine has recruited few physicians to its ranks with perhaps as few as 200 physicians entering the specialty annually. Likely, in no small part, this is a consequence of the marked difference in reimbursement for different types of services. For example, a comprehensive assessment of an older person is reimbursed at a far lesser amount than most any procedure that lasts a half an hour or more.

In the United States, most medical students have a limited geriatric experience, perhaps in part because of the inability of medical

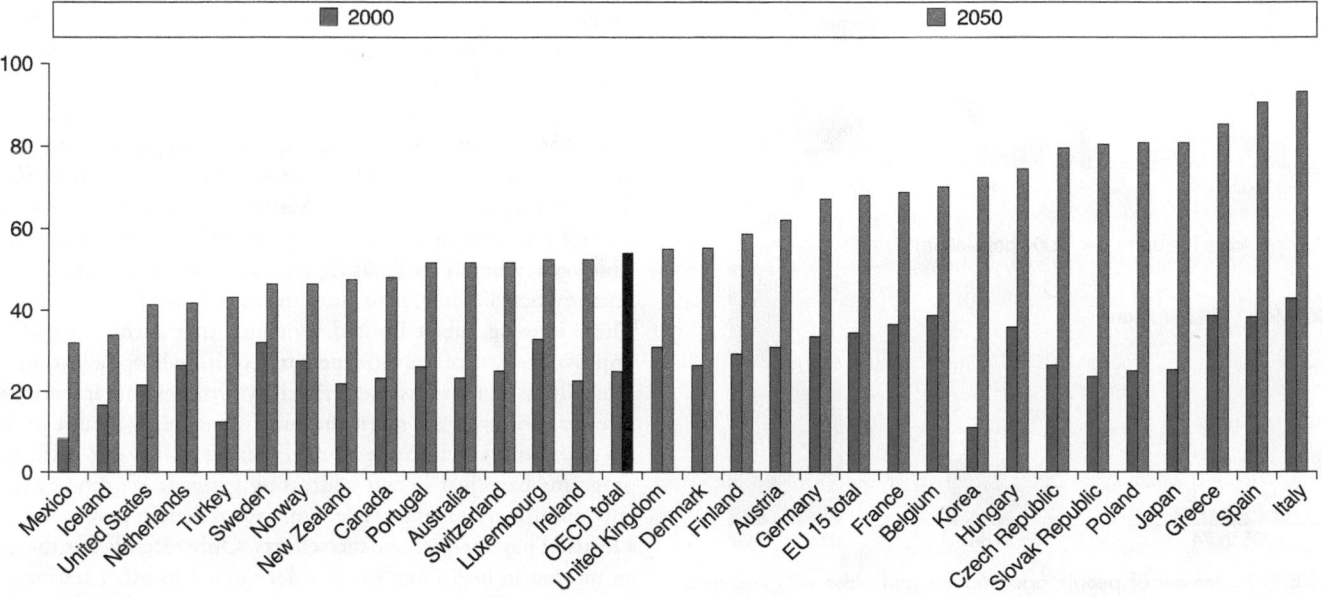

FIGURE 6-5. Ratio (percentage) of the retired population aged 65 yrs and older to the labor force, 2000–2050. *(Adapted from OECD Factbook 2007: Economic, Environmental and Social Statistics.)*

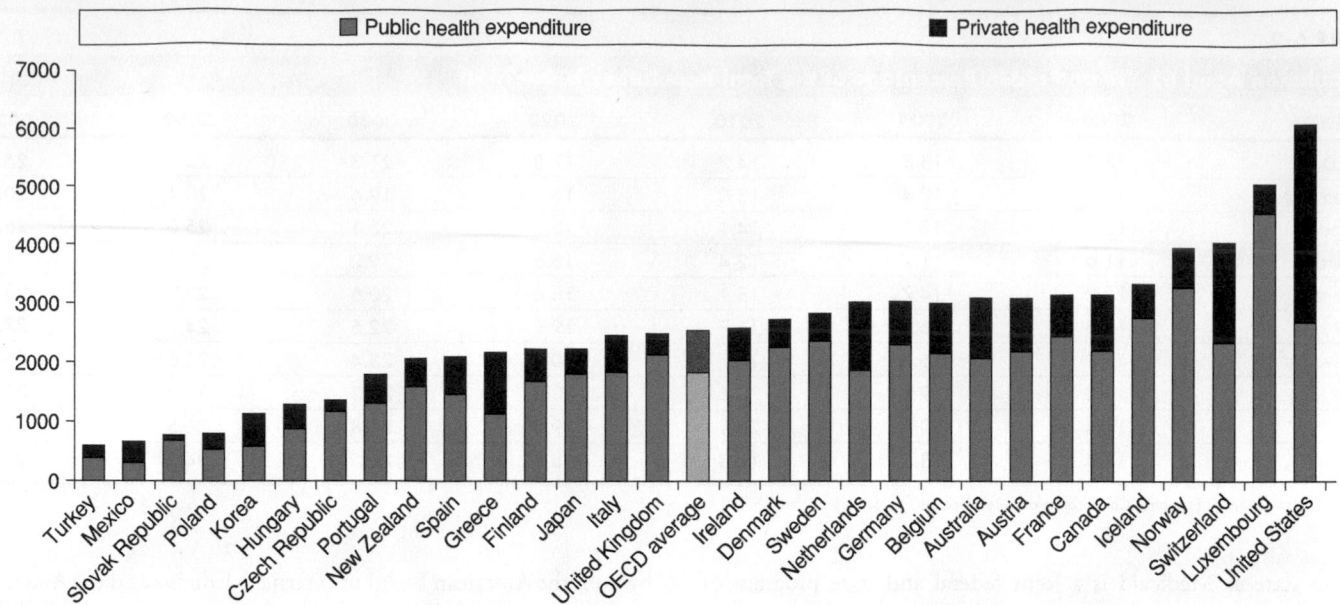

FIGURE 6-6. Public and private expenditure on health (U.S. dollars per capita, 2004 or latest available year.) *(Adapted from OECD Factbook 2007: Economic, Environmental and Social Statistics.)*

schools to be able to recruit sufficient numbers of faculty. In addition, elders usually have a multiplicity of chronic conditions whereas the traditional emphasis in the medical curriculum has been on acute medical issues in a hospital setting, and more recently but still to a lesser extent, on ambulatory medicine. Most medical students have little or no exposure to such concepts as functional status or to such sites of care as the home or the nursing home. Modest efforts are underway to encourage specialists who care for large numbers of elders, such as gynaecologists and urologists, to have exposure to geriatrics.

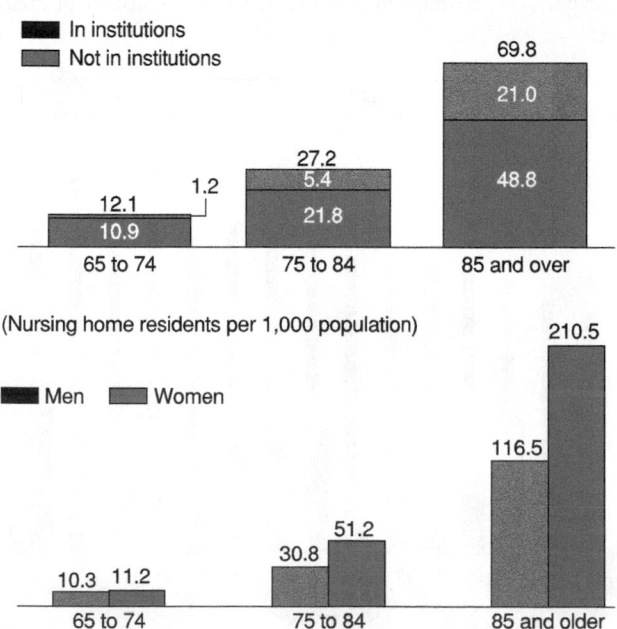

FIGURE 6-7. Percent of people aged 65 yrs and older with long-term care needs by age and place of residence: 1995 (upper panel); Nursing home residents among people aged 65 yrs and older by age and sex (lower panel). *(Reprinted with permission from US Census Bureau, Current Population Reports: 65+ in the United States.)*

The perception remains that the care of elders is not viewed as glamorously by either the public or the health profession as most other medical specialties. As elders tend to have multiple chronic conditions, multiple consultations may be viewed as necessary with the geriatrician serving in a lesser role, merely orchestrating the visits to specialists.

Peculiarities

The extraordinary cost of the health care system in the United States, as compared to other developed nations, has become increasingly visible to American industry, which traditionally has funded the health care insurance programs for its workers, to the American people, and to the politicians. Yet large numbers of citizens remain uninsured; the aging population is likely to need more care, increasing the per capita costs in the years ahead (Figure 6-8).

As a consequence of escalating costs, the health care system in the United States is changing. For example, under a pay-for-performance program, the Center for Medicare and Medicaid Services (CMS), the federal agency that oversees Medicare and Medicaid, has begun to offer financial incentives to improve the quality of medical care. This agency began by focusing attention on conditions such as an acute myocardial infarction and pneumonia in the hospital setting. There is some, albeit limited, evidence that such a program will improve the care of the older person requiring hospitalization for an acute illness. Symptoms and geriatric syndromes, rather than discrete diseases, however, are often the most concerning health problems for older adults in many settings (Figure 6-9). Pay-for-performance programs have just begun addressing geriatric syndromes such as falls and urinary incontinence. Functional deficits have not yet been a focus of pay-for-performance efforts. Only recently has there been an interest in beginning to consider quality in other settings, such as ambulatory care and postacute, nursing home care. CMS has at its disposal a wide variety of quality indictors that could be applied to persons in postacute and nursing home settings. Yet, long-term care and home care remain the stepchildren within the health care

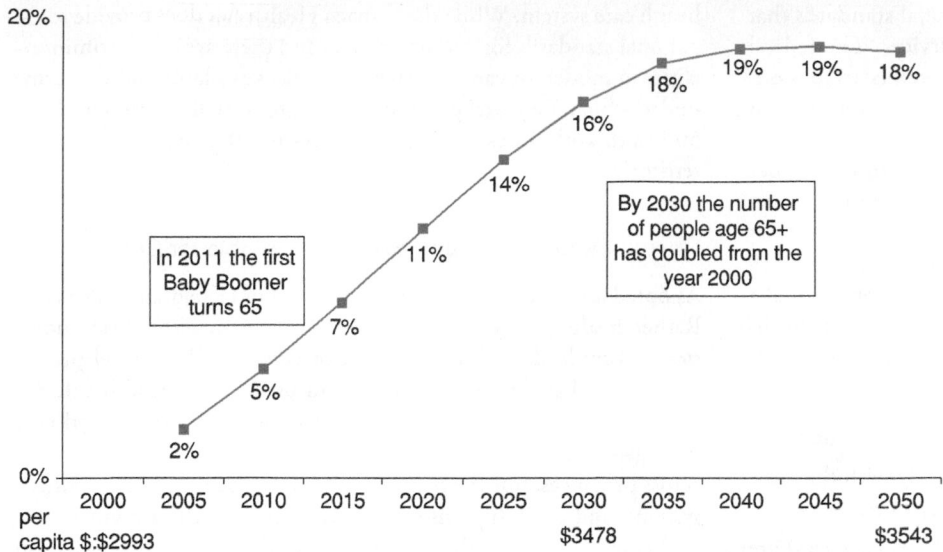

FIGURE 6-8. Cumulative percent change in health care per capita costs due to aging in the United States: 2000–2050. *(Martini EM, et al. Health Services Res. 2007;42:201–218.)*

system. Because Medicare does not pay for long-term care needs, it is not clear how this might change.

Difficulties and Solutions for a Typical Geriatric Patient

What type of treatment and services would likely be offered to an 87-year-old widow who was independent in activities of daily living (ADL) functioning, cognitively intact, and living in her own house but with few social supports who suffers a stroke with motor deficits and speech and swallowing troubles?

An 87-year-old widow who was living at home independently and presented to an Emergency Department with signs of an acute stroke would be evaluated immediately.

If seen within three hours of the onset of the symptoms she would undergo a computed tomography scan of her brain and likely a magnetic resonance imaging scan to determine if the stroke was due to a thrombosis or a bleed. If there was a thrombosis and if the elder did not have a contraindication, she might be treated with a drug intravenously with an eye to dissolving the thrombosis although few people get to the Emergency Department in time and few older persons are offered this treatment. She would have appropriate studies to rule out marked carotid artery stenosis as well as a myocardial infarction and a cardiac arrhythmia.

If no immediate intervention was indicated, she would be managed at an acute level of care for about 3 or 4 days. If she had a hemiplegia, she would be evaluated by a physical therapist, and possibly, an occupational therapist. She might also be evaluated for speech deficits and aphasia and likely would undergo a swallowing evaluation.

Most such individuals would then be transferred to an acute rehabilitation facility or perhaps to a subacute level of care for rehabilitation. If the individual was transferred to a subacute facility, she would first have had to spend three days (i.e., midnights) at an acute level of care before Medicare would pay for the service. If she were transferred directly to rehabilitation facility, this duration of acute care would not be necessary.

If the woman wished to return home and had no informal support, it would be necessary to determine her functional status. If it was felt that she could manage at home independently, then some home care services, such as nursing and physical therapy, and perhaps a home health aide, would be available for a limited period of time. However no long-term support services, such as assistance with bathing, shopping, or house cleaning, would be available unless the individual paid for them herself or was indigent and eligible for Medicaid. There are charitable organizations in some locations, but not all, that might offer to provide a very limited degree of support. But in all likelihood, these could not be counted on when arranging for discharge from a facility.

If she could not manage reasonably independently at home, it would be necessary for her to go to a long-stay nursing facility or, if she had a significant measure of functional ability, to an assisted living facility. Both would be quite expensive and only the former would be paid for by Medicaid if she had insufficient assets of her own.

America: Canada

Type of Health Care System

Health care in Canada is a joint federal–provincial responsibility. It is delivered and managed at the provincial–territorial level, with the majority of funding provided by provinces. The federal government transfers funds to the provinces and territories to pay for a portion of

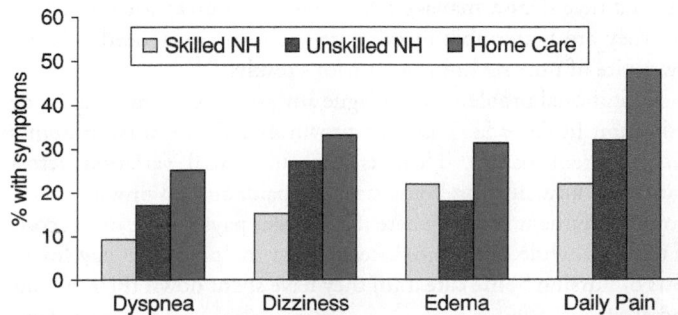

FIGURE 6-9. Persons in Home care and Nursing home care are compared on four types of symptoms. Data were collected with InterRAI-LTCF and InterRAI-HC instruments, which have these common identical assessment items.

public expenditures in health care, and sets national standards that govern the delivery of hospital and physician services. The federal government is also responsible for health protection related to product safety and pharmaceuticals, and it provides funding for research and health promotion at the national level.

Hospital and physician services have been publicly funded under a "single-payer" system in Canada since the 1957 Hospital Insurance and Diagnostic Services Act and the 1966 Medical Care Act established a shared approach to payment between the two layers of government. The Canada Health Act (CHA) of 1984 represented a major development in defining health care in Canada, by establishing five principles that would govern the delivery of services:

1. Public administration—provincial health care insurance must be operated and administered publicly on a not-for-profit basis.

2. Universality—all citizens must be covered equally with the same benefits and entitlements, irrespective of ability to pay.

3. Accessibility—no financial or other barriers (e.g., user fees) are permitted to ensure equity of access among citizens.

4. Portability—provides funding for Canadians visiting or moving to other parts of the country or travelling outside of Canada.

5. Comprehensiveness—ensures full coverage for "medically necessary services" provided by physicians or in hospitals (including dental surgery).

Following a protracted debate between federal and provincial governments, the Romanow Commission on the Future of Health Care in Canada was assembled to address issues such as the share of federal contributions to health expenditures and the scope of the Canada Health Act. The commission made numerous recommendations, but two that had the potential for a direct impact on the older persons were (1) expansion of the Canada Health Act to include home care and (2) addition of "accountability" to the Canada Health Act as a new principle governing health care in Canada. Ultimately, both recommendations were only partially implemented. Although almost every province provides substantial public funding for home care, there was tremendous resistance to its inclusion under the Canada Health Act. Following a meeting of the Prime Minister and provincial premiers, an agreement was reached that additional federal funds would flow to the provinces to expand existing home care services in targeted areas (mental health, postacute care, rehabilitation, and palliative care) without bringing it under the Canada Health Act. The Canadian Health Quality Council was established as a vehicle to improving accountability in health care, but it has not achieved full participation by all provinces and the Canada Health Act was not modified to include "accountability" as a new principle. Many provinces have launched their own accountability initiatives over the last 5 years, but there is no national consensus on what should be done to ensure quality, appropriateness, and cost-effectiveness of health care.

Another major development in the Canadian health care system has been the move toward regional management of health services. Provincial governments have played a diminishing role in the actual delivery of health care, with most organizational decision-making and resource allocation made at the local levels. The role of provincial ministries of health has changed to a stewardship function instead of direct management and oversight. While this model may mean that health care is delivered and managed in a way that is tailored to needs at the local level, it is increasingly difficult to speak of a "Canadian"

health care system. While the Canada Health Act does provide some national standards for certain services and there are many commonalities in models of care, the specific services available and the terms under which they are provided vary substantially between about 50 health authorities managing services in 10 provinces and three territories.

Overall Organization and Services Available for Older Adults

As noted above, there is no singular model of Canadian health care. Rather, health policy and service delivery in Canada are best understood as multiple variants on a set of common, high-level principles. With that caveat in mind, it can be said that health care for older adults in Canada involves several common services and care settings—home care, nursing homes, and hospitals are the constants across provinces, but the precise function of these services, payment systems, and eligibility criteria vary from province to province.

There is no exact estimate of the size of the home care population in Canada, in part because there are widely divergent definitions of home care. If one considers services such as nursing, personal support, home health aides, and rehabilitation, it would be reasonable to estimate that between 11% and 15% of older adults receive home care services. However, this value will generally be much higher if one expands the definition to include services such as transportation, meals on wheels, and other community supports offered by social service agencies.

A distinctive feature of home care in many provinces is the use of the case management approach to assessing needs, allocating resources, and managing community based services for frail older adults. For example, in Ontario, Community Care Access Centres (CCACs) use case managers to complete an assessment of long-stay home care clients (using the Resident Assessment Instrument for Home Care, the RAI-HC). Case managers use the assessment information to prioritize clients for access to community- and facility-based services and to establish a care plan based on the clinical findings of the assessment. They then contract with home care companies (both for-profit and not-for-profit) to provide the services needed by the client. Typical services include nursing for wound care and intravenous management, personal support for bathing and homemaking, and physical or occupational therapy; social work, speech language pathology, nutrition, and mental health services are only provided infrequently. A common concern in Ontario, however, is that caps on home care expenditures may limit the capacity of case managers to allocate services that would fully address clients' needs. In contrast, preliminary evidence from the Province of Manitoba suggests that if case managers have more resources for home care and they are better able to calibrate them to client needs, then a lower rate of nursing home admissions results.

Definitional problems also plague any estimates of nursing home utilization in Canada. Different provinces refer to nursing homes with different names. There is also substantial variation across Canada in how nursing home stays are paid. Several provinces employ a copayment system where the resident pays a share of the costs of the stay, while other provinces require the person to pay for all costs of nursing home care until they have spent down their income and assets.

An important change underway in Canada is the introduction of assisted living as a lower cost alternative to nursing home care for a population with lighter care needs. However, in some provinces, the movement toward assisted living appears to be driven by an interest in replacing regulated nursing home care with unregulated care.

As in other countries, acute hospitals in some Canadian provinces have employed a DRG-like system to manage hospital resources. Over the last two decades, this has resulted in dramatic reductions in average length of stay. However, in some provinces, a major concern has arisen with respect to alternative level of care (ALC) patients—those who no longer have acute care needs and are now in the hospital awaiting placement in a less intensive care setting. Frail older adults make up the vast majority of ALC; the size of this population has grown with the ongoing pressures to reduce hospital length of stay and the limited availability of long-term care beds or supportive housing options. This is further complicated by current case-mix systems for nursing homes that are not responsive to clinical complexity, resulting in a financial disincentive for these homes to accept heavy care residents.

Mental health services for older adults are provided in a variety of ways. In the community, home care services often exclude persons with severe mental illness. Instead, these individuals receive support from community mental health agencies that may or may not work in concert with home care. In addition, community mental health agencies often provide consultation services to nursing homes to assist them in meeting the needs of residents with complex psychiatric issues or high levels of behavior disturbance. However, it is not uncommon for nursing homes to discharge residents with frequent and severe behavior disturbance to inpatient geriatric psychiatry units because they do not have the expertise or resources to cope with these residents. Hence, there is a growing awareness in Canada of the need to find more cost-effective methods to respond to the mental health needs of nursing home residents.

Pecularities

About 80% of the population lives in urban settings, mainly in the southern regions of the country near the U.S. border. However, the rest of the population lives in rural settings, sometimes covering vast geographic areas that make it difficult to offer home care programs or nearby primary care services. About one-third (12.2 million) of the population of Canada lives in the province of Ontario. Toronto (the capital city of the province) has 2.5 million residents living in a 630 km^2 area with a population density of 3972 persons/ km^2. In contrast, the 10 000 residents of Yukon Territory who live outside its capital city (Whitehorse) in the northwest region of Canada are dispersed over a 474 000 km^2 area with a density of 0.1 persons per km^2.

A further consideration is that many residents of remote regions of the country are aboriginal peoples with unique cultural needs and health concerns. Persons with an aboriginal identity comprise 0.5% of the population of the city of Toronto and 1.7% of the Ontario population; however, they represent 15.9% and 36.8% of the population of Whitehorse and rural Yukon, respectively. Health care for aboriginal people on reserves is the responsibility of federal government, and off-reserve care is typically provided for by the provincial government. For most health indicators, persons of aboriginal origin are at disadvantage compared with general population. Although life expectancy has been improving, the gap between aboriginal and nonaboriginal people is 7.4 and 5.2 years for males and females, respectively. Morbidity rates are also notably higher in the aboriginal population for conditions like diabetes, heart disease, and tuberculosis.

Difficulties/Solutions for a Typical Geriatric Patient

What type of treatment and services would likely be offered to an 87-year-old widow who was independent in ADL functioning, cognitively intact, and living in her own house but with few social supports who suffers a stroke with motor deficits and speech and swallowing troubles?

An 87-year-old widow with an acute stroke and few comorbidities would typically receive care in a general medical ward of acute hospital ward. According to a 1999 study, only 4% of Ontario acute hospitals have a dedicated stroke unit. Rehabilitation in the postacute phase may be provided in a rehabilitation hospital or unit, or in a complex continuing care hospital (Ontario only). Depending on the patient's functional ability, medical condition, and access to informal support (in this case probably children), she may be transferred home with home care. Rehabilitation may be provided by the home care program or by community-based clinics. The home care program will also offer personal care, homemaking services, and nursing, if needed. If the patient's medical needs exceed the ability of family members to provide adequate support, then she may be placed in a long-term care home or an assisted living setting depending on the severity of impairment.

Europe: Iceland

Type of Health Care System

Iceland's health care system is nationalized, though there are private sector providers. On the purchaser side of the system, two structures fund services: (1) the National Institute of Social Security, which is financed through the central government's budget and through employers' and employees' contributions and (2) the central government's annual appropriation, financed through general taxation, which directly allocates financial resources to hospitals and primary care services. The rich and the less well-off use the same system, contributing copayments of 25% to 30% of the cost (with a limit on maximum expenditure). However, the copayments of older adults amount only to one-third of what actively working citizens pay; no copayments are required for hospitalization or rehabilitation or home nursing care for older adults.

Care of older adults has two components: health care and social services. Health care is organized regionally, through primary health care centers, and is paid for by the state, funded through the central government's budget. Social services are also organized regionally (albeit differently than health care) and are paid for by county councils, which are funded by local governments. Social services include assistance with home care and daycare. Geriatric hospital care, which has developed rapidly during the last 20 years, is financed by the state.

Nursing home placement costs the older person up to US$2000 per month (if their pensions are generous enough) and Iceland's national health insurance both pays the balance of about US$5000 per month (2006) and covers whatever portion of the cost is not covered by a resident's pension. Older adults do not have to spend down assets other than their pension fund to pay for their care.

The aim of the health care system is that every citizen should have one primary care provider, located at a primary health care center. However, the primary care providers do not have a gate-keeping function and all citizens can access ambulatory care specialists of their choice, although with slightly higher copayment than if a person was to seek primary care services. Hospital care has become increasingly specialized with the merging of hospitals, particularly in the Reykjavík area. Similarly, geriatric hospital care has been strengthened with consolidation of services at the University Hospital in Reykjavík. There are now 16 geriatricians and seven junior physician positions covering a population of 180 000. The geriatricians have all been trained abroad, in the United States, United Kingdom, and Sweden. The junior positions are both part of an internship year and residencies in internal and family medicine. The Department of Geriatrics is sectioned into acute geriatrics, consultation service, falls clinic, rehabilitation and respite care (four units), memory clinic and dementia units, palliative care unit, day hospital, and general outpatient unit. Geriatricians participate in nursing home care delivery along with family practitioners.

Overall Organization and Services Available for the Elderly

Until 25 years ago, the development of elderly care in Iceland was haphazard. In 1982, Iceland passed laws dealing specifically with issues relating to older adults, which were revised in 1989 and again in 1999. The law's underlying principle is that the autonomy of older adults shall be respected. Elderly persons have a legal entitlement to required services and the state must meet their needs in a way that is relevant and economically feasible. Elderly persons must be supported in their homes for as long as possible and have access to a nursing home when the need arises. A dedicated tax of about US$40 per person per year facilitates the development of care for older adults.

The laws mandated that a Nursing Home Preadmission Assessment (NHPA) be performed on anyone applying for nursing home placement to confirm and grade the need for long-term care. A multidisciplinary team performs the NHPA; the team consists of a physician, a nurse, a social worker, a representative of the municipality, and a representative of the Association of Elderly Citizens (this last team member participates only in planning decisions, not in the clinical assessment). The assessment is standard in form and content. It remains valid for up to 18 months, though it is supposed to be revised if the applicant's condition or situation changes during this time. The NPHA system generates national and regional waiting lists for the 3700 beds currently available. Although "homemade," this system opened the eyes of policymakers to the value of objective assessment and data gathering, and the NHPA had definite consequences on the further development of nursing home care in Iceland.

The content and quality of nursing home care were almost completely unknown in the early 1990s. Costs were considerable and the financing of nursing home care was variable. This began to change with implementation of the International Resident Assessment Instrument (InterRAI) system for nursing home care. Now all nursing home care is being financed based on case-mix or resource utilization groups derived from the assessment data. Other spin-off effects, which are being developed, include the monitoring of quality of care and the generation of clinical guidelines for identified problematic areas, working from a database accumulated through use of the standardized assessment instrument.

Nationwide, 13% of Iceland's elderly reside in nursing homes, although the figure is lower (9.7%) in Reykjavik. The average length of stay is slightly more than 3.5 years. About half of all nursing home residents in Iceland have dementia, but that figure rises to 80% in skilled nursing homes.

Other aspects of elderly care, however, remain as incompletely understood as nursing home care was. Health care policy allows older persons to stay at home as long as possible and supports them in doing so, but the needs of those in home care are not well-defined. There had long been interest in studying other forms of elderly care when such opportunities would arise, and so in 1997, when the InterRAI instrument for home care became available, such a study was performed. Collecting data at four community health centers in Reykjavik quickly raised questions about the quality of home care services. For example, older persons living in their own homes seem to have more untreated physical symptoms than similar residents of nursing homes. This may be due to the fact that there is less teamwork in the home care setting. The typical home care recipient may go for long periods of time without seeing a physician. That so many elderly persons are lonely and never get out of doors leads to question the wisdom of the policy of having people stay at home as long as possible. Regardless, the home care system should attend more carefully to issues of loneliness, depression, and mobility out of doors, perhaps by organizing elderly volunteers who could support their less-healthy peers and bring in the family practitioner in closer cooperation with home nurses. Home visits by family practitioners are all but extinct, except in emergencies, when it is just the on-call family practitioner who attends to the person and the primary care provider of that person is rarely involved.

Progress is also being made toward the eventual implementation of the other instruments in the InterRAI family. Thus in the year 2007, the InterRAI instruments for home care, mental health, and postacute care are being implemented. An acute care instrument is under study and thus Iceland may realize a seamless systematic and coordinated system of information on elderly care that brings information from one setting to the next electronically.

Peculiarities

Iceland's response to the need for elder care has been both empirical and somewhat chaotic. The philosophy of elder care is in many ways clear, but the system lacks comprehensive administration and is therefore fragmented (as is the health care system in general). The system's major drawbacks include:

1. Health care and social services within communities are not coordinated, in part because they are funded by different sources.

2. Nursing homes have autonomy regarding the admission of new residents and are not officially obliged either to accept first those persons on the waiting list who are in greatest need or those persons in hospitals who are waiting for nursing home beds. In areas where the need for nursing home beds exceeds the supply, some nursing homes admit applicants still living in the community before those persons in greater need who are waiting in hospitals.

3. Because of limited availability, primary health and home care services are insufficient to care adequately for elderly people living at home. This factor, combined with nursing homes' selection process, leads to the "bed blocking" of elderly persons in hospitals—an inefficient use of resources.

4. The quality of care received by Iceland's elderly persons is largely unknown.

Difficulties/Solutions for a Typical Geriatric Patient

What type of treatment and services would likely be offered to an 87-year-old widow who was independent in ADL functioning, cognitively intact, and living in her own house but with few social supports who suffers a stroke with motor deficits and speech and swallowing troubles?

An 87-year-old woman with acute stroke would most likely be admitted first to an inpatient neurology service, particularly if she is without cognitive problems and with limited comorbidities. If she had preexisting cognitive problems or several comorbid conditions, she would more likely be admitted to acute geriatrics.

If the woman was admitted to neurology, she would be transferred in a few days to either rehabilitation or postacute geriatric care. Occupational therapists could help reconfigure her apartment, if that would make it possible for her to return home. Physical therapists could go to her home to provide maintenance therapy; respite care could be organized. She could get meals-on-wheels, help with cleaning of the house, and home nursing care up to two times a day. Each professional would still make only very short visits. It is conceivable that she could go to a daycare center a few times of the week. The issue would be how she would feel being mostly alone. She would in any case get rehabilitation commensurate with her potential for recovery. With great determination, this person could possibly go home, but the situation would be precarious and with even minor additional insults or problems, it is likely that she would be admitted again to the hospital, where she might block a bed for months while awaiting nursing home placement. That would also be the case if she was not motivated to go home, in spite of her being cognitively intact.

Europe: Norway

Type of Health Care System

Norway has a national health service with universal coverage for medical care in hospitals, medications for chronic diseases, and also coverage for consultations with general practitioners (GPs), outpatient services, and physiotherapy when the yearly costs for the patients are over a certain limit (approximately €200). Home care services are partly covered by the municipalities, but patients have to pay a minimal fee. In some municipalities, the caring services are given by private organizations as a supplement to public care services. Long-term care in nursing home is covered for the first 3 months. For longer stays, the patient has to pay 85% of their income.

Overall Organization and Services Available for Older Persons

Generally, the health and caring services for elderly persons are viewed as satisfactory although services generally lack resources. The present government has declared the care of elderly persons a national priority.

Hospital Services In a National Survey in medical departments (1998), 35% of the patients were 75+ years and 11% had geriatric syndromes such as falls, cognitive impairment, and incontinence. Later figures show that 40% to 45% of patients in medical departments are 75+ years old.

Geriatric medicine is a subspecialty of internal medicine and most of the 70 practicing geriatricians are working in hospitals. The Universities in Oslo, Bergen, Trondheim, and Tromsoe have faculties of medicine, and all of them have geriatric medicine on their curriculum and university hospitals with geriatric departments. Most general hospitals have geriatric specialist services organized as geriatric departments in the larger hospitals (more than 4 to 500 beds) and geriatric sections in medical departments in middle sized hospitals (<200 beds). Some smaller hospitals have a geriatrician and geriatric outpatient services, but usually no dedicated beds for geriatric patients. Geriatric outpatient clinics in the hospitals are responsible for assessment of cognitive impairment and dementia, falls, urinary incontinence, and functional impairment. They have an interdisciplinary approach with specially trained nurses, physiotherapists, and occupational therapists.

Elderly units have been the preferred way to organize acute hospital care for the elderly. All stroke patients, independent of age, are recommended to be treated in acute stroke units, where internists or neurologists, and rarely geriatricians, are usually responsible. Despite these recommendations, there are still several hospitals where the acute geriatric patients are treated without geriatric expertise. In some places, the patients are transferred to a geriatric unit for rehabilitation after acute care, but many geriatric patients in the hospitals do not get access to geriatric specialist services at all.

Community Services Community care is the cornerstone in the care for elderly persons. All inhabitants have their own GP, responsible for the continuation and coordination of medical care.

Overall, 20% of elderly persons are receiving home care services, 5% are living in sheltered housing with care services, and 6% are living in nursing homes. Among persons 80+ years old, 10% are living in sheltered homes, and 14% in nursing homes. The municipalities also provide daycare centers for persons with dementia and physiotherapists and occupational therapists for assessment and rehabilitation.

Home-nursing and home-help services meet nursing needs and need for assistance in ADL and instrumental activities of daily living (IADL) and are received by more than half of persons 80+ years old. As in many other countries, the demands for services are higher than the supply. To allocate services to best meet the needs, many municipalities are using an "order and supply" model. Applications for home-care services (by letter, telephone, or personal contact) can be given from patients, proxies, and GPs to a public office in the municipality. The decision is detailed to type and objective of service and for how much time, and should give the patient a guarantee. The model is criticized for not being flexible and adaptable to the highly variable needs of frail elderly person.

During the last 20 years, retirement homes have been closed and sheltered housing with care services have been developed. They are suitable for elderly persons without major medical problems or great need for nursing care.

In some cities, it is possible to choose between public services and private agencies with the same coverage of the costs. Families with the necessary economic resources tend to organize private services as a supplement to the public services. Some nursing homes are run by private organizations, but with public financing.

Nursing homes are also part of community care. GPs or nursing home physicians are responsible for the medical services, rarely geriatricians. A survey of medical care in nursing homes in 2004 showed that doctors' hours per patient were low and the quality often insufficient. Nursing homes have three main functions; long-term care, respite care, and rehabilitation. Some nursing homes have special units for dementia care. The average age of the patients is 83 years and 70% to 80% suffer from dementia.

Peculiarities

Norway has the highest incidence of hip fractures worldwide. To organize a better care for these numerous patients, orthogeriatric units with comprehensive geriatric assessment and an interdisciplinary approach have been organized in some hospitals. The evidence of benefit from organizing such units is still sparse, but the practical experience is good.

Difficulties/Solutions for a Typical Geriatric Patient

What type of treatment and services would likely be offered to an 87-year-old widow who was independent in ADL functioning, cognitively intact, and living in her own house but with few social supports who suffers a stroke with motor deficits and speech and swallowing troubles?

An 87-year-old patient with a stroke should be treated in an acute stroke unit. If this happens, she will receive excellent care. However, often the stroke unit is full in which case she will be admitted to another medical ward where interdisciplinary care is lacking. At discharge, if she still has residual hemiparesis, she will get home care services and home rehabilitation. A nurse will come three times a day to give help with personal care and medication. During the first week, it is possible that four different nurses and nursing aids will visit. Every time the patient will have to tell her story and how she wants things to be done. Always the nurse is too busy to give more than basic nursing, and she never has the time to sit down for a chat. A home helper will come once per month to clean the flat. Our patient would receive home rehabilitation by a physiotherapist who will visit twice per week.

Europe: United Kingdom

Type of Health Care System

Organization and access to health care for older people is (in principle) no different from that available to the rest of the population. The predominant health care models are:

- a comprehensive National Health Service (NHS), funded from taxation and (mainly) free at the point of delivery and
- a system strongly based on primary care, both as provider of first-line medical management, and as gatekeeper to secondary care.

Since the foundation of the NHS in 1948, there have been frequent major reorganizations, as often as every 2 years. We have therefore seen repeated, and largely politically driven, changes of service. Currently health care is commissioned by Primary Care Trusts, in which GPs have a major leadership role. Commissioning is on the basis of a diagnosis-related group (DRG) model and a national tariff with funding allocated to commissioners by central government. Having been largely based on historical patterns of resource allocation, and central government direction on priorities (for example, various access targets, and the use of expensive drugs), funding is in-creasingly on a weighted capitation system to allow for regional variations in population and health profiles. At least five types of health care provider can be identified, including GPs, hospitals, newer NHS models, private providers, and local government.

Overall Organization and Services for Elderly Persons

General Medical Practices

These practices are mostly partnerships (with 1 to 12 medical partners), being self-employed contractors to the NHS, operating from locality-based premises. More recently, some practitioners are directly employed by the NHS. Practices employ their own nursing, counseling, and other staff. They undertake routine medical care for acute and chronic illnesses, including most immunization, vascular prevention, and screening of those older than 75-year-olds (once, but no longer, mandatory). The GPs are responsible for long-term prescribing and medication review. They provide the primary medical care for all care home residents. GPs under take a 3-year training programme, 2 years of which is spent in hospital specialities, but only some GPs will have training experience in geriatric medicine.

Hospitals

These are relatively large, and provide secondary and tertiary care for populations of about 200 000 to 600 000 persons. Emergency admissions are via GPs, or open-access emergency departments. Geriatric medicine is a well-established specialty, second in size only to anaesthesia. Geriatric training involves 5 years of higher specialist training following 3 years of junior hospital posts. Most geriatricians also practice general internal medicine, in particular for unselected medical emergency admissions. Some subspecialization occurs, including falls, movement disorders, continence, orthopedic, and old-age psychiatric liaison. All-age stroke medicine has emerged as a separate subspecialty, with the majority of stroke physicians being geriatricians (not neurologists). The majority of older persons will not be admitted to hospital under a geriatrician, however, and a lively debate continues about how to define the most appropriate specialist for a given patient. A variety of models exist (needs based, age-related, integrated with internal medicine). Geriatricians operate in multidisciplinary teams including nurses and various therapists. Some have duties outside hospital (community geriatricians) including care home and intermediate care support.

Acute medical emergencies are usually admitted to a single admissions ward under the care of a general physician, pending triage to specialty-based wards (including specialist acute geriatric medicine). Most older people will be discharged home from these wards, but postacute rehabilitation facilities (sometimes away from the main hospital site) are common.

Elective surgical patients will usually be "preassessed" and admitted on the day of operation. Those suffering complications or requiring prolonged rehabilitation will often be referred to geriatricians. In recent years, the UK government has made a major effort to reduce waiting times for elective surgery, which are rarely more than 3 to 6 months now, mostly benefiting older people.

Old-age psychiatry is also well established, but usually provided by separate psychiatric NHS organizations, with variable levels of integration with geriatric medicine. Over recent decades, they have concentrated on community-based services and have few in-patient beds. Older people with dementia who suffer a crisis are more likely to be admitted under physicians or geriatricians.

There is virtually no remaining hospital-based long-term care.

Newer Models of NHS Provision These models include a telephone consultation and triage service (NHS Direct), and nurse-led, open-access minor illness facilities (walk-in centres). Two notable developments have been intermediate care and community case management. Both aim to minimize acute hospital admission rates (increasing at 5% to 10% per year over recent decades) and reduce length of stay. Several intermediate care models exist, the most successful being home rehabilitation, sometimes supporting early hospital discharge. The other main model is rehabilitation provided in care homes, with medical oversight by GPs. Community case management, for older people with complex medical needs, provided by senior nurses, provides a surveillance and coordination function, with the aim of preventing escalation of medical crises.

Private Providers Traditional private provision (up to about 2000) accounted for 5% of total UK healthcare expenditure, mainly for elective surgery. For some procedures, such as joint replacement or cataract surgery, private sector providers undertook up to 30% of operations, encouraged by long NHS waiting times.

Since the 1980s, private providers have supplied the majority of care home places, divided between residential homes (board, lodging, and personal care) and nursing homes. Such care is classified as "social care" rather than "health care," and as such attracts user charges, albeit abated or subsidized depending on income. Private agencies also supply most home personal and domestic care.

Recently, the government has promoted a mixed-economy of provision with the introduction of commercial providers for NHS-funded outpatient clinic and elective surgical procedures, in part to increase capacity and reduce waiting times. Most dentistry and optometry is privately provided.

Local Government Authorities Local authorities are commissioners of "social care," but this includes domestic and personal home care (provided either directly or through private agencies), including meals at home, and daycare, and funding for care home placements, including respite care. Intermediate care schemes are mostly joint initiatives between primary health care and local authorities. Some home-based social care schemes are very intensive and sophisticated, such as specialist intensive home support for people with dementia. Local authorities employ social workers, some of whom are hospital-based, and are responsible for arranging home care and care home placements. However, resources are limited, and response times are often slow, causing prolonged hospital stays. For patients assessed as responsible for funding their own care, delays in finding care home places (usually the responsibility of their relatives) are common, however, there is wide regional variation.

Peculiarities

Peculiarities include the development of intermediate care rehabilitation schemes to reduce avoidable disability postacute illness intended to extend provision of multidisciplinary rehabilitation. However, usually there is no provision for specialist geriatrician input, medical care being the responsibility of GPs. Implementation has been widespread. Not all models have a strong evidence base to support their effectiveness, and their success in practice has been mixed. For example, some supported hospital early discharge schemes have worked very well. On the other hand, services are often reluctant to accept patients with cognitive impairment. Moreover the service has a strict 6-week timeframe, and concentrates more on restorative rehabilitation than the adaptive model that is more appropriate to chronic or progressive disabilities.

Community case management by specialist nurses intends to provide preemptive care to people living in their own homes at high risk of hospital admission in a crisis. The model of care is still evolving, in particular the means of selecting those to target, and also the extent to which links have been made with specialist geriatrician support (the main medical responsibility being with GPs). Case loads are about 50 per nurse. The service is popular, but evaluations of effectiveness have been equivocal.

The large number of geriatricians, long tradition of rehabilitation, relatively low level of reliance on care homes, emphasis on primary and out-of-hospital care, and the artificial division between "health" and "social" care, are all also peculiar features of United Kingdom.

Difficulties/Solutions for a Typical Geriatric Patient

What type of treatment and services would likely be offered to an 87-year-old widow who was independent in ADL functioning, cognitively intact, and living in her own house but with few social supports who suffers a stroke with motor deficits and speech and swallowing troubles?

UK policy is that elderly people should return to, and be maintained in, their own homes for as long as possible, although, in practice, patients or relatives may not agree with this. Requests for care home placements are rarely challenged (although the patient may be responsible for funding). Moreover, very intensive (and therefore expensive) home-based social care packages may not always be available. There has long been a rehabilitation culture, but there are also strong pressures to reduce hospital length of stay, and intermediate care rehabilitation often shuns more difficult cases (risking overreliance on potentially inappropriate care home discharges).

An 87-year-old with acute stroke, residual disabilities and social problems, and the will to return home, would almost certainly be able to return home. The policy is for her to be admitted under a specialist stroke service, although in some places, she may be admitted under a general geriatric service. Most stroke services provide comprehensive acute and rehabilitation care and are staffed by geriatricians, so the pattern of care would be very similar. Initial care would be multidisciplinary, with early medical, nursing, physiotherapy, and occupational therapy (and, if necessary, speech and language for communication or swallowing problems, and dietetics). Best practice would include early contact and information gathering from relatives, prior caregivers, and GP. Adherence to these guidelines is variable. However, the general standard of care for elderly people (typically those aged older than 75 years) in acute hospitals varies from hospital to hospital, with some having suboptimal staffing levels, and high rates of hospital-acquired infections compared with care for younger people. After medical stabilization, and when it had become clear that more prolonged rehabilitation would be required (probably after 1 to 2 weeks), she would be moved to a rehabilitation ward, either on the same hospital site or elsewhere. Depending on the local facilities available, she may move on to an intermediate care rehabilitation scheme. For someone living alone, typically this would be toward the end of rehabilitation, when specialized physiotherapy was no longer required, but when independent toileting was achieved. This would often be supported by a social care package providing up to four visits a day, for personal care, domestic tasks, shopping, and meals. Additional follow-up facilities might include hospital-based day hospitals, although many of these have lost their rehabilitation role to home-based intermediate care, and some have closed. Common difficulties will include timely access to the most appropriate admissions ward, delay in transfer to a rehabilitation ward, poor staffing of these wards, and delays in instituting social care (or care home if that is what she chose).

Europe: France

Type of Health Care System

The health care system provides universal care for all legal residents, choice of providers, free health programs for the poor and disabled, and significant cost reimbursement. The national health care system combines elements of public and private sectors, and Social Security consists of several public organizations, distinct from the state government, with separate budgets that refunds to patients the cost of care in both private and public facilities. It generally refunds patients 70% of most health care costs and 100% in case of costly or long-term ailments. Supplemental coverage may be bought from private insurers, most of them nonprofit, and from mutual insurers. Until recently, social security coverage was restricted to those who contributed to social security (generally, workers or retirees), excluding some poor segments of the population; only in recent years, has the government put into place universal health coverage.

Overall Organization and Services Available for Elderly Persons

Older persons seeking ambulatory care can elect to consult the general medical practitioner they have chosen. In the case of an emergency, patients are referred to the emergency department of a nearby local public hospital. When hospital care is required, the person has the freedom to choose the hospital. About 80% of beds are in public or nonprofit hospitals with physicians paid for by the government. The patient pays a daily flat rate (15 euros in 2006). The remaining 20% of beds are for-profit clinics with fee-for-service physicians paid entirely by patients. About 25% of beds are in rehabilitation wards and primarily used by older persons.

Since the mid-1980s, responsibility for organizing residential and home care has been decentralized at the level of the 100 local councils, assisted by the municipalities. There are various kinds of long-term care institutions for the elderly. Long-term care hospitals with full-time physicians are specifically intended for older persons who have lost their physical independence, regardless of the cause. In addition, there are nursing homes for dependent elderly people, public or nonprofit retirement homes, and private commercial residences with services. All these may have a part-time physician, but his or her responsibilities are not clear as residents usually have their own private physician. All together, in 2003, there were 51.2 long-term care beds per 1000 people aged 65 years and older.

Sheltered housing, providing a studio apartment with kitchen and bath room for one or two elderly persons has been progressively adapted to the needs of increasingly old occupants, with the installation of new technical equipment and the provision of some forms of care beside community services. Therefore such facilities may be considered as part of long-term care; they represent an additional 15.3 beds per 1000 aged 65 years and older.

Since the 1960s, the government has laid down a living-at-home policy that claims to be universal. Services implementation, however, has not achieved intended levels. The family still plays a major role in supporting and caring for older people. A national survey on impairment, disability, and handicap conducted in the year 2000 showed that family help represented more than 75% of all assistance.

Home-help services and home nursing services have been designed specifically for older people. The former have been in existence for 50 years. The latter were created in 1981 and have been developing slowly. A nurse coordinates and organises the various interventions by either registered or auxiliary nurses. The services most frequently carried out include help with activities of daily living, mobility, and the prevention of pressure sores. Since 1992, in order to facilitate employment, new home help services have been designed for domestic help and assistance to handicapped persons.

In 2002, an autonomy allowance was created, specifically for dependent elderly persons living at home or in an institution. Responsibility for this allowance has been given to the local councils although eligibility and the amount of allowance are related to disability assessment by a medicosocial team using a national scale. This team proposes a personalized care program of required interventions and appliances for those living at home. The person's copayment (15% on average, but up to 90%) is related to the person's income.

Public authorities have laid down a medicosocial policy for elderly persons that claims to be universal, but they have not provided the means for its development, especially for home care. Such development has been hindered by the seemingly impossible task of integrating policies from health sector and the scarcity of funds. The result today is that a distinction has been made between systems of care for handicapped adults and for dependent older people. Both are fragmented and usually characterized by numerous dysfunctions and inadequate responses to the complex care needs of these vulnerable populations. In the care sector for older persons, there are important geographical inequalities in accessibility to care. The lack of domiciliary care results in an overconsumption of acute hospital care. Moreover, there are inequalities in terms of quality of care due to differences in caregivers' qualification and the copayment amount relates to the status of care giver rather than the needs of the recipient.

The main issues at the present time are paying for long-term care insurance, integrating health and social care; increasing quantity and quality of care in both the residential and domiciliary settings; and increasing empowerment of older person in the determining their needs and how care will be provided.

Paying For Long-Term Care Less than 10% of the health care expenditure is used for long-term care provided to older persons. In contrast, three times more resources are provided for the long-term care of handicapped young adults.

There is currently a debate about creating long-term care insurance for handicapped persons, independent of their age. This should merge the different sources of financing in a national scheme, which includes long-term health and social care. The local responsibility for its implementation is still under discussion.

Integrating Health and Social Care Fragmentation of responsibilities for financing, organizing, and providing health and social long-term care, and poor coordination with acute care are particularly marked. The existing care system does not match the complex needs of older people with numerous, simultaneous, chronic, and disabling conditions. Integration of care may lead to more rational care processes, and would allow a more elaborate and flexible combination of interventions. It also may correct the insufficiencies in the supportive network and the housing condition of vulnerable older persons. During the last 20 years, demonstration projects have been undertaken to overcome the fragmentation of services and to reach a more coordinated care package for elderly persons. Newly promoted organizational models of care include improving case management programs within a multidisciplinary team, performing initial geriatric assessment and follow-up, linking primary health and social care givers together with geriatric team.

Increasing Quantity and Quality of Services Home care suffers from the lack of staff and of sufficient economic resources. Those obtained from the autonomy allowance are usually not sufficient to meet the needs of the most severely disabled. Therefore, those who can afford it will employ several unskilled persons. Persons unable to afford extra help will usually end up being admitted to an institution. Increasing the number of professional caregivers and giving them better training to improve their professional skill are priorities, which are regularly recognized but not fully implemented.

Increasing Empowerment of Older Persons On the whole, the wishes of the oldest old are not well represented. Rather, professionals and managers speak or decide for elderly persons. But some local programs now aim to take into account the users' viewpoint and the needs expressed by the oldest old persons in the definition of their needs and care.

Peculiarities

Several measures have been taken to help informal caregivers of disabled older adults. Respite care enables the older person living at home with family to be institutionalized periodically or to attend daycare several days a week. This allows a period of relief for a spouse or relatives who normally care for elderly persons. Financial measures, such as a tax relief, have been taken to encourage and maintain the ability of families to provide care.

Difficulties/Solutions for a Typical Geriatric Patient

What type of treatment and services would likely be offered to an 87-year-old widow who was independent in ADL functioning, cognitively intact, and living in her own house but with few social supports who suffers a stroke with motor deficits and speech and swallowing troubles?

In the best case scenario, a patient with a stroke will be admitted to a stroke unit and then discharged to a rehabilitation unit. Most often an elderly patient sustaining a stroke with moderate to severe disability would be admitted to an acute hospital. After a period of medical treatment (from 10 to 20 days), she will be transferred to a rehabilitation service, provided there is some prospect of returning to the community. Rehabilitation will be offered for up to 3 months, provided that functional gains continue and the prospect of returning home remains. At discharge, a home visit would be conducted and autonomy allowance may be provided. This allowance will provide a social life auxiliary to assist the elderly patient for personal care and domestic tasks. The amount of the allowance will be determined by the patient's disability level and a copayment percentage for which she will be responsible will depend on her income (up to 80%). Rehabilitation would be provided for several weeks or months, as required, by an independent physiotherapist paid on a fee-for-service basis. Severely disabled patients, particularly those without a coresident carer, will often be referred directly for permanent residential care in long-term care hospital or nursing home.

Europe: Italy

Type of Health Care System

Since 1978, Italy has a National Health Service, the Servizio Sanitario Nazionale (SSN), based on the principle of universal entitlement, with the central government providing free and equal access to preventive and medical care and to rehabilitation services to all residents. Citizens have a basically unlimited coverage, although they are asked to contribute minimal fees. These fees apply mainly to drug prescriptions (with the exception of so-called life-saving medications), laboratory tests, diagnostic investigations, and Emergency Room visits. Pressured by the economical outlook, the government has recently completed an unprecedented reform. Italy is adopting a semifederal organization of health care delivery. Each of the 20 regions, into which the country is divided, has now the responsibility to autonomously organize the services they feel appropriate based on the population needs. A national budget for health is set by the government each year (approximately 1000 euros per citizen) and then divided among the regions. In turn, the regions are required to allocate the necessary financial resources to each of nearly 300 local health agencies based on standard health-related indicators.

Overall Organization and Services Available for Elderly Persons

In the early-mid 1990s, Italy accounted for the lowest number of residential beds for elderly persons among western countries: 25 beds per 1000 people older than 65 years, while no other country had fewer than 60 beds. The numbers of elderly persons cared at home were even lower, less than 1% among those older than 65 years old, with a few exceptions in some northern regions.

The low number of nursing home beds and the shortage of home care services were due both to family structure and to the use of acute care hospitals. Italians have a family structure that—either because of choice or lack of availability—traditionally takes responsibility for the care of elderly persons, even when they become disabled. In southern Italy, this tradition is central to a culture that views care of elderly persons a natural responsibility of the family.

The other cause appears to be the use of acute hospital beds, which numbered 7 per 1000 inhabitants in the early 1990s, although there were marked differences between northern and southern regions. People relied upon acute care hospitals to solve a wide range of problems related to the assistance of elderly persons. As a result, the length of stay in internal medicine wards averaged 18 days in 1992, mostly because of delayed discharge. In 1993, a reform dramatically changed the approach to frail elderly patients needing long-term care; hospital reimbursement shifted from a fee-for-service to a prospective system based on the DRGs.

The aging of the population, with the rising number of older "clients" of the health agencies and the new prospective payment

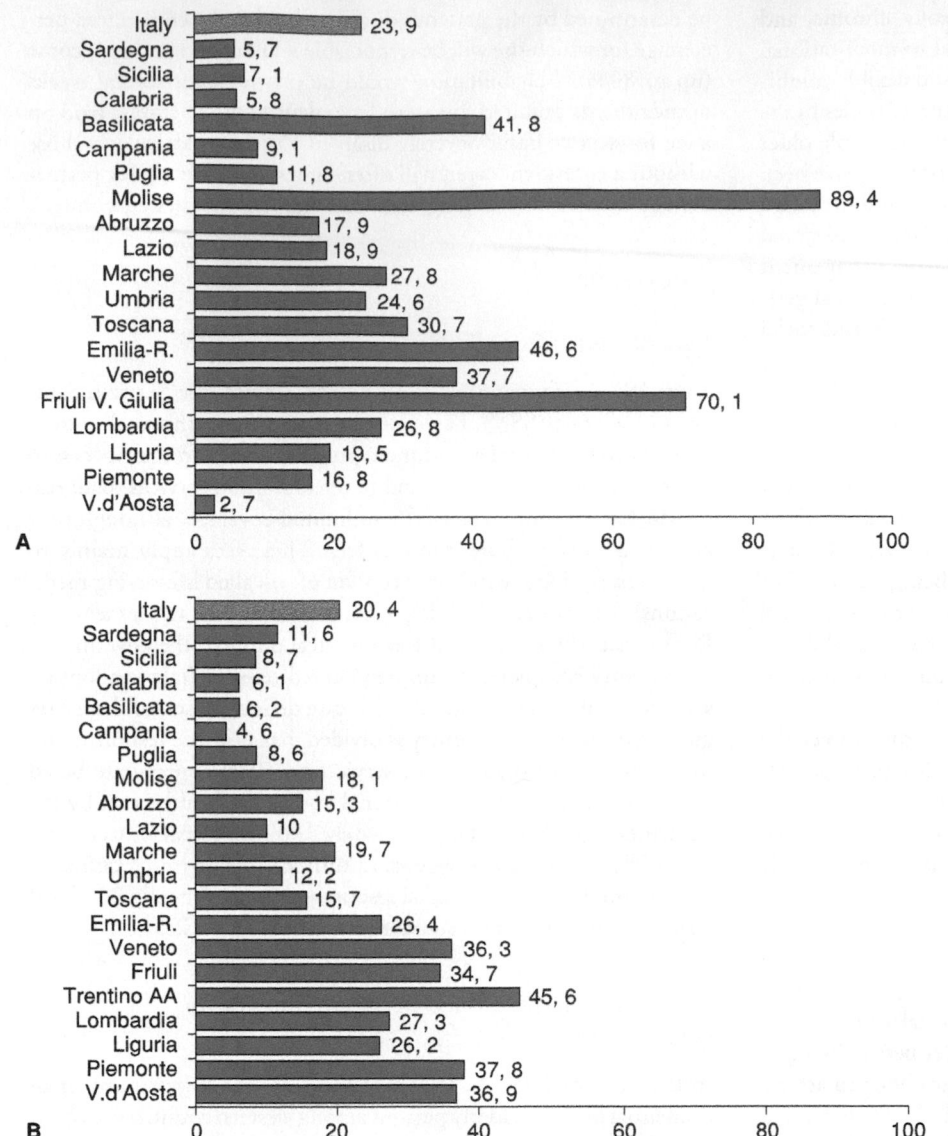

FIGURE 6-10. Number of persons 65 yrs or older/1000 in home care (panel A) and in long-term care (panel B) in 20 Italian regions in 2003. Data on home care are from CENSIS (www.censis.it) and data on long-term care are from ISTAT (www.istat.it). Datum on one region was not available for home care.

system, all led to redesign of the long-term care system and to the shift of resources from acute care hospitals to community services. Regional health authorities assign available resources based on central government's directives, local, and political needs. As a consequence, the availability of long-term care and home care services is highly different among the 20 Italian regions, which further widen already existing inequalities (Figure 6-10).

To guide and to coordinate the work of local health agencies, the Italian parliament promulgated a document in 1992 about frail elderly people needing continuing care. The "Progetto Obiettivo Salute dell'Anziano" (POSA), was not a law, but simply a series of suggestions and recommendations to health agencies.

The POSA identified the integration between health and social services as the key to satisfying the needs of these patients, delivering individualized and, at the same time, comprehensive care services. The POSA determined that the community-based geriatric evaluation unit (GEU) was the appropriate approach and that the GEU should include registered nurses, social workers, physiotherapists, and patient's GPs, and be coordinated by a geriatrician. Integrated home care (Assistenza Domiciliare Integrata [ADI]) and skilled nurs-

ing facility (Residenza Sanitaria Assistenziale [RSA]) were identified as the two major services.

Difficulties soon became evident. Health and social programs have been implemented irregularly in varying forms, mostly in northern regions and in rare, spotted areas of central Italy. In addition, community services are usually limited to social needs and the shift of health resources from hospital to community is not underway. Overall, the implementation of the POSA guidelines has been slow. Presently, 2% of persons aged 65 years or older are receiving home care and 2.4% are in a nursing home.

Peculiarities

Italy has traditionally emphasized family care giving, particularly by female members. Elderly persons in need of long-term care often prefer to live at home, rather than in an institution. This choice is rooted in cultural and religious values. It also depends on the very limited availability of long-term care beds on the one hand, and on the fact that more than 80% of elderly Italians own the house where they live, on the other hand.

In recent decades, triggered by societal forces, Italian women have been increasingly entering the labor market, limiting the time they can spend home caring for their loved ones. As a result, the need for in-home caregivers has quickly increased; this void has been filled by foreign-born caregivers (the *badanti*), paid either by elderly persons or by their families.

The high number of foreign-born caregivers is considered to be a panacea for the nationwide shortage of aides and services in general. Currently, there is an estimated 800 000 *badanti* and they cost Italian families about €8 billion each year. However, these caregivers are not licensed, they work outside the oversight of regulatory bodies, and nurture the "gray economy."

The Difficulties/Solutions for a Typical Geriatric Patient

What type of treatment and services would likely be offered to an 87-year-old widow who was independent in ADL functioning, cognitively intact, and living in her own house but with few social supports who suffers a stroke with motor deficits and speech and swallowing troubles?

Difficulties for a typical frail elderly person, having suffered a stroke but wishing to stay at home, are related to the limited availability of home care services. Only 2% of older adults in Italy receive home care services. Home care services are completely free, but given the paucity of resources, only young adults with cancer and/or disability or very frail and/or severely disabled older adults can be entitled to them. Therefore, older adults who are not admitted to home care and wishing to stay at home, the great majority, rely almost entirely (both socially and economically) on their families or on their own resources. Either members of the family, or more commonly, foreign caregivers (paid by the patient or by their family) care for the older adult at home.

Rehabilitation services provided by the National Health Service (and therefore free of charge) are also very limited, and preferentially reserved for young adults or healthy older adults without severe comorbidities. Private rehabilitation services are also available and easy to access if the patient or their family pay for it.

In cases in which she and her family cannot afford the social and economical costs needed to stay at home, long-term care may be the most reasonable solution. Long-term care is also paid for by the National Health Service, with a minimal copayment. However, due to the limited availability of beds, admission to long-term care may require a long wait (up to 6 months). Less than 3% of older adults aged 65 years or older in Italy are in long-term care.

Asia: Japan

Type of Health Care System

Since 1961, there has been universal coverage by a form of social insurance. Virtually all residents are compulsorily covered either by a health plan provided by the employer, or by the municipality where they reside if self-employed or retired. There is no choice of plans and all provide the same benefits including medications, dental care, and preventive services. The copayment is usually set at 10% for those 70 years and older. Copayment reaches 30% for those with incomes above the average worker. This affects about 10% of elderly persons. If copayment exceeds US $300 per month, then the rate for any additional payment is reduced to 1%. Although providers are reimbursed on a fee-for-service basis, service fees and drug prices are set and have been tightly controlled by the government. The percentage of the gross domestic product spent on health care is 8.0% and ranks 17th among the OECD countries. There is no gate-keeping, so patients may directly access virtually any provider in Japan. The delivery system is dominated by the private sector except for the high-tech medical centers that receive subsidies for their capital expenditures. Waiting lists are not a problem in acute care but are in long-term care (LTC) facilities. LTC is provided by the public LTC insurance, which was implemented in the year 2000.

Overall Organization and Services Available for Elderly Persons

Health care is highly accessible. A national survey showed that 11.5% of the population aged 65 years or older visited a health facility as outpatients on the day surveyed; the average interval between two visits was 9.6 days. Japan is unique among developed countries because most of the institutional LTC continues to be provided by hospitals. Almost 4% of the elderly population is currently hospitalized. This heavy reliance on hospitals was an unintended effect of making health care free for elders 70 years and older in 1973. Until that time, copayment rate was 50%. The fact that hospitals are reimbursed on an open-ended fee-for-service basis by health insurance combined with the fact that the majority of small- to medium-size hospitals are owned by doctors who could exercise their professional discretion on admission, led to rapid increment in the number of elderly inpatients. From the family's point of view, hospital care has the advantage that costs are covered by insurance and that it is socially acceptable. The establishment in 1986 of a new type of intermediate care facility, the Health Facilities for Elders (HFE), led to a decline in the proportion of older adults staying in acute care hospital, but to an increment in the absolute number of elderly inpatients.

Developments in social services generally lagged behind health care because they were financed entirely by taxes and limited by the budget. However, services began to improve after the government embarked on a 10-year plan to increase funding of local governments for developing LTC services in 1989 (referred to as the "Gold Plan"). By completion in 1999, the goal of increasing the number of full-time equivalent home-helpers from the 1990 level of 38 945 to 170 000 and the number of adult daycare centres from 1615 to 17 000 were met. However, access to services continued to be controlled by the local government welfare department, to be means-tested and to offer no choice of providers by the individual. Although restrictions based on income and availability of family support had officially been removed, the institutional culture of the social welfare agencies and budget limitations led to priority given to indigent elders living alone or with spouse.

These structural problems led to the implementation of the public LTC insurance that provides defined benefits as a universal entitlement for all elders 65 years and older who meet the eligibility criteria. For those 40 to 64 years old, benefits are limited to those having disabilities as a result of designated age-related diseases, such as stroke or Alzheimer's disease. Health and social LTC services have become integrated and coordinated by a care manager. Home-helpers for personal care (ADL support) and domestic tasks (IADL support), bathing service, loan of devices like wheelchairs, home reconstruction (putting in ramps and hand-bars etc.), and nursing homes were transferred from social services to the LTC insurance. Some hospital

LTC beds, all HFE beds, most visiting nurse and visiting rehabilitation services, and "medical management" (supervision of care by doctors) were transferred from health insurance to the LTC insurance. Adult daycare and temporary "respite" stays in institutional settings, which had been available from both sectors, were transferred but not unified and continued to maintain different staffing requirements. Doctors' services continue to be paid in the same way as before by health insurance. There are no cash benefits for family carers, partly because they were opposed by groups who claimed that their provision would further increase the social pressure to provide care for in-laws.

Eligibility is determined by the process shown in Figure 6-11: (1) completing a 79-item form on physical and mental status by a local government employee (usually a public health nurse) or individual under contract, (2) putting the results into a computer, which groups the individual into the seven levels of eligibility or ineligibility according to the algorithm, and (3) review by a local expert committee. This committee changes the level calculated by the computer, usually to a more severe level, based on the information in the forms written by the assessor and the attending physician. Income levels and the amount of informal care available are not taken into consideration. After eligibility has been determined, the individual can go to a certified care management agency of her choice for community care and be covered for LTC services up to the amount set for each level (from 49,700 Yen [US $200] to 358,300 Yen [US $3000] per month), or ask to be admitted to any LTC facility. There is a 10% copayment, with a ceiling for those with low incomes.

The LTC insurance is managed by the municipalities and financed by a combination of social insurance premiums and taxes. A method was devised to make the municipalities fiscally responsible for their LTC insurance programmes, while taking into account the differences in their income and demographic structure. The premiums of individuals aged 65 years and older reflect the LTC insurance expenditure levels of their municipality and are of six levels according to the individual's income. These premiums finance approximately one-sixth of the total expenditures. About twice this amount, one-third, is financed by premiums from those aged 40 to 64 years that are collected at the national level and redistributed to the municipalities, after adjusting for their income level and age distribution. The remaining half is financed by national and local taxes. Thus, although elderly persons who reside in municipalities using more services pay higher premiums (the maximum difference being threefold), their contributions compose only one-sixth of the total costs.

The implementation of the LTC insurance has led to dramatic increases in the number of elderly persons receiving services. The percentage of persons aged 65 years and older certified as being eligible increased from 10% in 2000 to 16% in 2005. In absolute terms, the number certified nearly doubled to 4.3 million in 2005, with the increase greater for the lighter eligibility levels and community care. Waiting lists for community care services have disappeared. Thus, the objectives were more than met, but expenditures increased more than projected. Instead of increasing from 4.3 trillion Yen in 2000 to 5.5 trillion Yen in 2005, expenditures increased to 6.8 trillion Yen (1.4% of GDP). In order to contain costs, service fees were cut in 2003 and 2006, partial payment of "hotel costs" was introduced in 2005, and benefits limited to preventive services (mainly light exercise in day care centres) for the two lightest eligibility levels in 2006. In addition, the 130,000 LTCI hospital beds will be phased out and converted to either a HFE or care home by the year 2012.

Peculiarities

The Japanese system is unique in that little reliance is placed on geriatricians or social workers. Geriatrics is not officially recognized as a specialty and only about one-quarter of the medical schools have such a department. Nor is general practice or family medicine recognized as a specialty. Although clinic-based physicians do not have access to hospital facilities and their patients are, for most part, primary care, they are usually trained in and have worked as specialists in hospitals before going into private practice. Consequently, social aspects of care tend to be neglected. Professionalism has also been lacking in social work, which was one reason why eligibility levels came to be determined by a computer program. Care managers were hastily created for the LTC insurance by allowing anyone who had worked for more than 5 years in a health or social care field to sit for the multiple-choice examination and, having passed, to participate in a 72-hour training program in order to obtain the license. By the year 2006, 370 000 individuals have cleared the examination and training, but there is little monitoring of their quality. No patient databases exist for quality monitoring purpose.

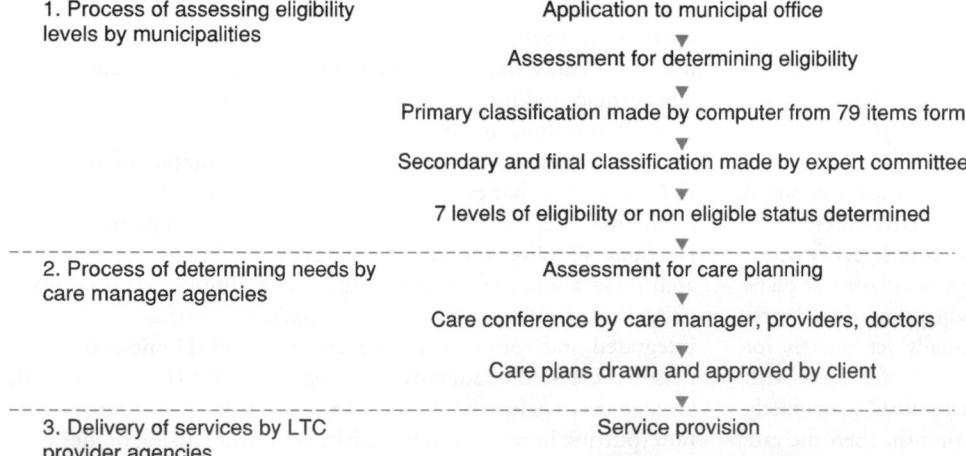

1. Process of assessing eligibility levels by municipalities

Application to municipal office
▼
Assessment for determining eligibility
▼
Primary classification made by computer from 79 items form
▼
Secondary and final classification made by expert committee
▼
7 levels of eligibility or non eligible status determined

2. Process of determining needs by care manager agencies

Assessment for care planning
▼
Care conference by care manager, providers, doctors
▼
Care plans drawn and approved by client

3. Delivery of services by LTC provider agencies

Service provision

FIGURE 6-11. Flow chart for receiving LTC services in Japan.

Difficulties/Solutions for a Typical Geriatric Patient

What type of treatment and services would likely be offered to an 87-year-old widow who was independent in ADL functioning, cognitively intact, and living in her own house but with few social supports who suffers a stroke with motor deficits and speech and swallowing troubles?

Under the best case scenario, the patient would be admitted to an acute stroke unit and then discharged to a rehabilitation unit, where the LTC insurance care manager would come and work with the hospital staff to draw the care plan: a weekly schedule for care workers to provide her with IADL and ADL support, and for visits by a nurse and a physiotherapist. If needed, ramps would be placed in her apartment before discharge. Her attending physician would visit her on a monthly basis to provide medical supervision and feedback the information to the care manager.

Under a more likely scenario, the patient would be admitted to the nearest hospital where the treatment and rehabilitation may not be up to standard. She would then be transferred to any LTC facility that has an empty bed. She would probably stay in the facility and may come to prefer it to her own home because of the security it provides and the lower costs. Her monthly out-of-pocket expenditures, assuming she has an average income, would be about US $200 in the case of the former, and about US $700 in the case of the latter.

Oceania: Australia

Type of Health Care System

The organization of the health care system in Australia is a complex blend of administrative and service provider arrangements. General community-based medical practice is provided largely by independent "private" practitioners. However, the fees are heavily subsidized by the national government through the "Medicare" scheme. Personal contributions by older and less well-off citizens are minimized. The scheme also subsidizes medical costs in private hospitals and the provision of pharmaceuticals (through the Pharmaceutical Benefits Scheme in the community and private hospital settings).

Hospital care is provided by public and private hospitals. Around 60% of admissions and 70% of bed days are provided in the public sector. Public hospitals are administered by state governments (there are nine states and territories, which comprise Australia), and are jointly funded by the national and state governments. Public hospital care is provided free of charge, regardless of financial status.

Citizens access private hospitals through the support of private health insurance which approximately 43% of the population elects to purchase from independent health insurance agencies. Persons holding private health insurance, however, can elect to use public hospitals and, when doing so, may elect to be admitted either as a "public" or "private" patient. In the latter instance, they may have some choice of their treating physician and access to slightly better physical facilities.

GPs act as "gate-keepers" to specialists, including geriatricians. Medicare subsidizes only specialist consultations that are referred by GPs.

Overall, the Australian government funds around two-thirds (68%) of total health expenditure. The remainder is sourced either directly from individuals at the point of service or indirectly through private health insurance. Hospital services account for 35% of all recurrent health expenditure.

In spite of the level of complexity, the overall impression of the Australian health care system is one of good accessibility and equity. By international standards, Australians enjoy good health status. Life expectancy at birth has risen significantly in recent decades to be among the highest in the world. Life expectancy at age 65 years is second only to Japan for males and third to Japan and France for females.

Overall Organization and Services Available for Elderly Persons

Specific services for elderly persons exhibit a similar level of complexity of administrative and service arrangements to those of the general health system. Long-term residential care is fully administered by the national government, whereas home care is a complex array of programs, some jointly administered by state and national governments and others administered by one or the other.

Long-term care is provided by a mixture of government, for-profit and not-for-profit organizations. Funding is provided on the basis of a locally developed dependency based system. User contributions are based on assets and means testing, and are netted off against the government funding. This results in the levels of funding available for care being approximately the same regardless of the resident's ability to pay.

The level of provision of services is governed in a variety of ways. Long-term residential care is tightly controlled by the national government according to a planning formula, which stipulates the ratio of beds to aged population (70+ years) at a state and regional level. Since this strategy was introduced in 1986, there has been increasing equity of provision across the nation. Certain aspects of community care are similarly regulated. So-called "packaged care" is made available on a places-per-aged population basis. These programs (entitled community-aged care packages) attract a subsidy-linked loosely to the equivalent cost to government of low level residential care. The other major community care program (the Home and Community Care program) provides a wide array of services but generally at a lower level of intensity than the packages referred to above. In both programs, the user contribution is modest, making home care highly affordable. Access can be limited, however, because service demand often exceeds supply.

Over the past 20 years, the national government policy has promoted a shift away from institutional to community care, although the level of provision of the former remains comparable to other developed nations. Government investment in community care is expanding considerably in real terms.

Eligibility for residential care is controlled through a national Aged Care Assessment Program, which comprises regionally based multidisciplinary teams of nurses, allied health personnel, and usually geriatricians. These services typically present themselves as services to individuals and families, offering advice and short-term case management in addition to their gate-keeping role for residential care and packaged community care.

Postacute community service provision is more complex with varying levels and types of services being provided across jurisdictions. In 2006, a national "transition care" program was established to provide short-term therapy and personal care services following hospital admission.

Specialist hospital-based geriatric services vary widely in availability across jurisdictions. They are state funded, but in some states, the establishment of such services is unplanned and often left to the discretion of individual hospitals. In other states, real attempts to plan services are made. Regardless, the majority of large hospitals operate some form of inpatient geriatric service. Predominantly these operate a "postacute" service model, accepting patients from acute hospital wards. Postacute care is rarely provided in long-term care institutions.

Inpatient rehabilitation services are widely available, although the lack of any planning framework results in some areas of poor availability. Rehabilitation is generally provided in the public hospitals but rehabilitation units also are common in the private sector. Many rehabilitation wards admit a mix of older and younger patients. Some hospital geriatric units provide a blend of acute and postacute geriatric assessment and rehabilitation services. Respite care is provided mainly in long-term care institutions.

Geriatric medicine is a rapidly expanding specialty, with geriatricians representing the second largest group after cardiology within specialist internal medicine. Geriatric practice is predominantly hospital-based, although many are linked to community assessment teams, ambulatory clinics, and day hospitals. Specialist geriatricians undergo training under the auspices of the Royal Australasian College of Physicians, the program comprising general or "basic" training followed by 3 years of "advanced" training within the specialty. Medical services for residents of long-term care facilities are provided by GPs.

Difficulties/Solutions for a Typical Geriatric Patient

What type of treatment and services would likely be offered to an 87-year-old widow who was independent in ADL functioning, cognitively intact, and living in her own house but with few social supports who suffers a stroke with motor deficits and speech and swallowing troubles?

An elderly patient sustaining a stroke with moderate to severe impairments would almost always be admitted to an acute hospital. After a period of medical treatment, around 10 to 20 days, transfer to a rehabilitation service would be typical, provided there was some prospect of returning to the community. Severely disabled patients, particularly those without a coresident carer, will often be referred directly for permanent residential care. Rehabilitation is offered for up to several months, provided functional gains continue and the prospect of returning home remains. A home visit would be conducted, with aids and appliances provided as needed. At discharge, a blend of in-home and centre-based rehabilitation would be offered, for at least 3 months if required. Subsequently, daycare, personal care assistance, and general home-maker services typically would be available.

Developing Countries: China

China is an excellent example of the future prospects for countries of the third and fourth world. In China, fertility rate dropped from 5.8 to 2.4 in just 10 years, from 1970 and 1980, and life expectancy increased almost 30 years, from 35 to 64 years, between 1950 and 1980. Thus, the transition, which took around 150 years in more developed countries, took 50 years in less developed countries, and only 10 to 20 years in China. Today, China's average is equal to that of the world in terms of the proportion of people aged 60+ years (10%) (Figure 6-12). However, by 2050, this proportion is expected to rise to 30%; in absolute numbers, this is an increase from 130 to 430 million people.

If current demographic rates in China are similar to those of developed countries, its economy and social welfare institutions are more similar to less developed countries. China plans to quadruple

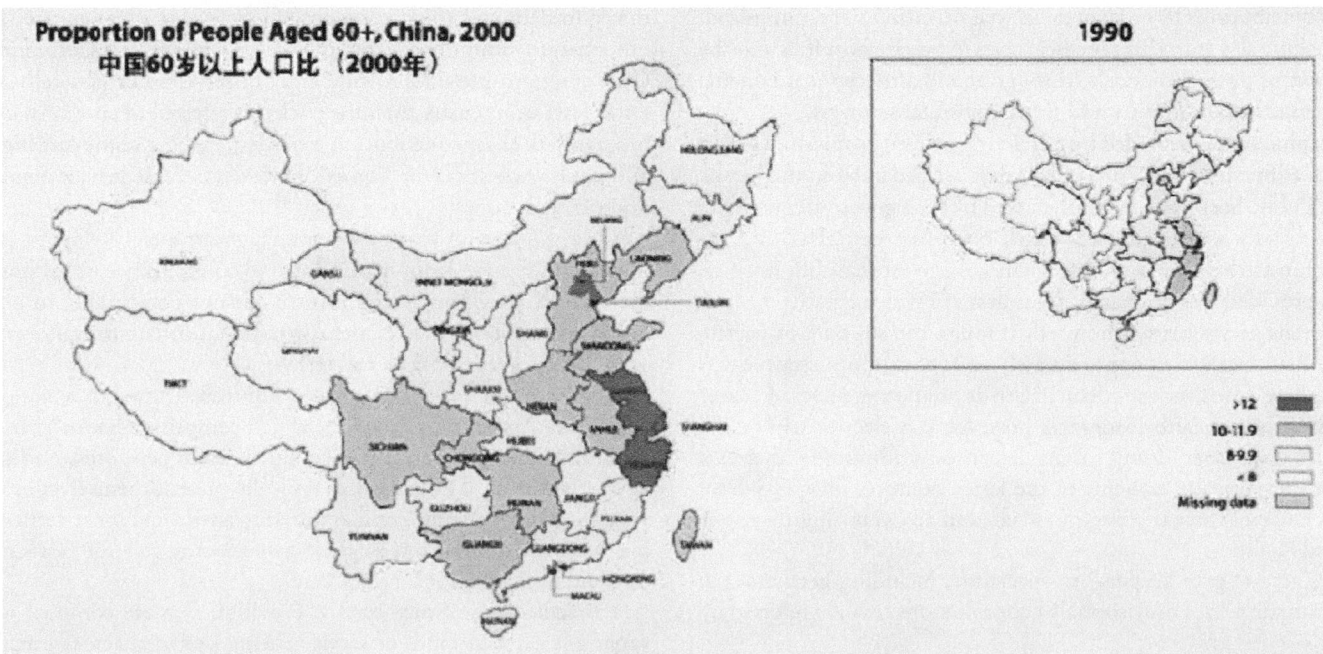

FIGURE 6-12. Proportion of people aged 60 yrs+ in China, by regions, 1990–2000. *(Reprinted with permission from Population ageing in China—facts and figures, UNPFA 2006.)*

its GDP per capita by 2020 but if the projections are correct, China will become old before it gets rich.

Type of Health Care System

The health care system in China is funded by a combination of state, social insurance, and private payments. In general, costs of primary health care are covered only in part by the state. Employees of the industrialized sectors are covered in part by the social medical insurance, financed by contributions by both the employee and the employer, and subsidized by the state. Farmers, who account for 60% of the total population, are covered in part by a cooperative medical insurance subsidized by the government at both the state and local levels. These insurances cover both medical and drug costs up to 50% to 100%, depending on the types of care received and sectors in which the care receiver is employed or was employed before retirement. As a result of the rising health care costs and limited coverage of the existing social medical insurance, health care cost increasingly becomes a burden to the majority of aged persons.

Overall Organization and Services Available for Elderly Persons

Care for elderly persons in China is administratively divided into two categories—medical services and residential care—which are supervised, respectively, by the Ministry of Health and the Ministry of Civil Affairs. Hospital care is the most frequently sought by aged persons. China's medical system was not originally designed to meet the chronic illnesses of elderly persons and there is a lack of well-trained professionals such as geriatricians and geriatric nurses. Although general hospitals in large cities currently tend to have geriatric wards to meet the needs of a rapidly growing aged population, physicians are usually not systematically trained as geriatricians. Indeed, few medical schools currently provide such training. Nevertheless, the annual hospitalization rate for those aged 65 years is around 8%. A somewhat good opinion about the quality of services in general hospitals and a lack of other options make the elderly population rely on acute care when they have to deal with health issues.

To reduce overuse of acute care resources and provide more appropriate care to aged persons, the Chinese government has made substantial effort over the last decade to develop community medical services. By 2004, 14 153 community health centers were operating in the urban areas. To attract elderly people away from large hospitals, most of the costs of community health care were reimbursed from social insurance. As a result, access to primary health care, which is one of the major concerns of aged community dwellers, has been improved.

Along with the declining overuse of acute care by aged patients, there has been a growth of a variety of services targeting the older population in the community, including rehabilitation and nursing care. An elderly patient being discharged from the hospital could receive home care, which would be delivered by health care workers from community health centers. Community health services are still at their early stage of development, and only present in urban areas, nevertheless, they provide elderly persons with a new alternative to family care.

The narrow coverage of the existing insurance programs, which only cover approximately 60% of elderly persons living in urban areas and less than 10% of those in rural areas, is a serious barrier for elderly persons needing access to health care. A considerable proportion of the urban elderly population and the majority of the rural elderly population have to rely totally on themselves and their family to pay for medical services. The sources of financial support for older adults in China by age are shown in Figure 6-13.

Another problem of the health care system in China is the lack of coordination between medical care and social care in terms of service organization and finance. When an elderly patient is discharged from hospital, it is likely that they will find it difficult to locate appropriate intermediate care between hospital and home. Long-term care facilities are confined to providing residential services under the regulations of the local bureaus of civil affairs. Very few facilities have qualified nursing staff to provide professional nursing care. For those who benefit from the social medical insurance, expenses related to long-term care are not covered by the program. There is currently no long-term care insurance, though the need for such insurance is growing rapidly.

In the country, there is a long tradition of family members caring for their elders at home. However, recent demographic changes have resulted in older persons living longer and have led to a decline in the availability of care by their families. By the year of 2001, the number of long-term care institutions reached 39 338. There were 893 000 persons, less than 1% of the aged population, residing in

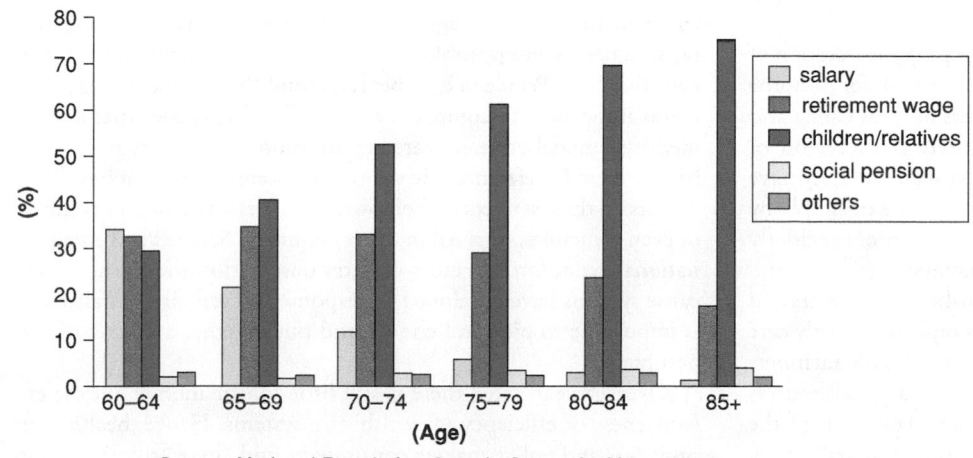

Source: National Population Sample Survey in China, 2004

FIGURE 6-13. Primary financial sources for the elderly by age in China in 2004. *(Reprinted with permission from Population ageing in China—facts and figures, UNPFA 2006.)*

these facilities. Long-term care institutions for elderly persons can be categorized by sources of funding as follows: (1) municipal institutions where funding for investment and operation directly comes from the local bureaus of civil affairs as public expenditures on social welfare and these institutions are owned by the city governments; (2) institutions funded by state enterprises in the urban areas or by township government in the rural areas and these institutions are owned by collectives; and (3) institutions funded and owned by private investors.

Three types of elderly persons become residents in the long-term care institutions: those who have no income and family, those who either themselves or their direct family members made publicly recognized contributions to the state, and all others who need care. For the first two types of elderly residents, the institutional services are paid for by the government agencies of civil affairs. For the last category, services are charged to the care receivers and their families. By the year of 2001, less than 25% of residents in urban facilities and about 6% of those in rural facilities were paying for services out-of-pocket.

Institutional long-term care for elderly persons is still underdeveloped, with currently insufficient capacity to meet the demand. Various empirical surveys have reported the significant proportions of elderly persons who need nursing care and assistance in daily life. On the other hand, the average occupancy rate of the existing facilities is only around 70%. Lack of funding for services, shortage of professional trained providers, and inadequacy in regulations to control the quality of care in these facilities are currently the major concerns about the development of elderly care services in China.

Peculiarities

Due to the cultural tradition of family care for the elderly and the scarcity of institutional long-term care resources, the overwhelming majority of the aged remain at their own homes when they are in need of care. However, the high rate of women's labor force participation and the reduction in the nation's birth rate has seriously challenged this tradition. With 78% of women aged 16 to 55 years employed outside the home, there has been a serious shortage of formal caregivers. In addition, since 1970s, China has implemented a family planning policy, which has dramatically reduced the average number of children per family. An unexpected consequence of such a policy is that more and more people grow old in an "empty nest."

To meet the need of elderly persons while keeping the tradition of family care, families in urban areas have started to look for in-home caregivers. As there is an oversupply of labourers in rural China and many migrate to urban areas seeking a job, there is a reservoir of potential in-home caregivers, most of whom are women. They have been introduced by commercial home service agencies or simply by friends to the families seeking care. They take daily care of the elderly persons and are paid by the client or family members.

There is no statistics about the number of in-home caregivers and the cost borne by the families, though it is now typical of elderly care in urban China. The practice of family care by nonfamily members is well accepted by the state as a way to absorb the surplus labourers from the rural areas and is sustained by the affordable cost of the services. As caregivers only have limited education and skills, they can only bargain for a wage much lower than the average income of urban residents. On the other hand, there is a lack of training, license, and supervision over the care provided.

Difficulties/Solutions for a Typical Geriatric Patient

What type of treatment and services would likely be offered to an 87-year-old widow who was independent in ADL functioning, cognitively intact, and living in her own house but with few social supports who suffers a stroke with motor deficits and speech and swallowing troubles?

A typical frail older woman discharged from the hospital after a stroke is most likely to go home directly as a result of difficulties in access to rehabilitation or nursing care. The number of rehabilitation facilities is limited and there is a lack of public funding to support the use of health care services other than hospital services. Once back home, she would have the problem of finding someone who could provide care to meet her health and daily living needs. She may find that her children are not always available even if she lives together with one of them unless this son or daughter is retired. She may also find that she cannot afford to seek long-term care without the financial support from her children, since few facilities are public funded and means-testing is required to be admitted to those facilities. Even if she could afford to fund her long-term care through private sources, she would soon find that most facilities are not prepared for people with comorbidities or hemiparesis.

In addition, she would have limited options to cope with the difficulties of resource scarcity and service inadequacy. She could hire an in-home caregiver to help when the family members are not available, an option that would be more affordable than institutional long-term care. Community services such as home beds or day care have been organized in recent years with the support of some local governments. Whether the elderly person in need could receive these services would depend on the availability of the services in the community where she resides. As these services are only available in large cities such as Beijing or Shanghai at present, only a small segment of elderly persons actually benefit from them.

NEED FOR STANDARD ASSESSMENT OF HEALTH NEEDS AND SERVICES ACROSS COUNTRIES

Health care systems in different countries worldwide have elected to confront the same demographic changes with a heterogeneous array of schemes and possible solutions. In the introduction to Home Care for Older People in Europe, Raymond Ilsley noted in 1991 that it was impossible to compare systems of different countries and to identify a model of health care organization and delivery that could be considered a reference. He wrote: "We were surprised at how little experts on these services in their own countries knew about practices, or even principles, pursued in other countries. Services had emerged nationally, not through cross-country observation and learning. Because systems have developed in response to local circumstances, it is impossible to pick and choose and put together a mosaic of the best bits."

Over 15 years later, there is still little information about the effectiveness or efficiency of health care systems. Hence, health care providers and policy makers continue to find "local" solutions, but these remain limited and nonreproducible experiences. In the field of geriatric medicine and health services organization for older people, there is no evidence on which to base efficient models of care. Currently, few data are available on health care organization; comparisons across different approaches in terms of patient outcomes and resources utilization have rarely been performed. A major obstacle to a systematic approach to evidence-based practice has been the use of different, noncomparable, assessment instruments, protocols, and procedures.

Comprehensive assessment (CGA) is considered the "technology" of geriatrics and its application is thought to result in a better quality of care by providing information on comorbidities, syndromes, socioeconomic problems, and functional and cognitive deficits. CGA facilitates development of specific and sensible care plans for individual patients. CGA typically is performed with variable measures and scales according to individual geriatrician's knowledge and access, limiting the ability to measure cross-population health and functional status. Health services are even less well studied. Thus, what constitutes best practices in terms of geriatric services remains largely unknown.

Standardized assessments that consider systematically several relevant areas appropriate to specific settings can provide evidence of health and health service needs across settings and locations. One such suite of comprehensive assessments has been developed by an international group of researchers gathered in a not-for-profit corporation, InterRAI.

InterRAI

InterRAI is a crossnational collaboration of geriatricians, researchers, and policy-makers, primarily experts in long-term care issues, dedicated to developing assessment systems. Its members come from 26 nations (Figure 6-14). InterRAI, since 1990, has worked to design second generation assessment systems characterized by comprehensiveness and health care setting specificity. Also, following their implementation, InterRAI has used the experiences of one nation to inform others, and to develop innovative research approaches using the data generated by these assessments. In 2006, InterRAI released a "suite," covering all of the major health care sectors devoted to elder care, thus creating the third generation of instruments. In particular, there are assessment systems that address the following populations: frail elderly persons in the community, home care, assisted living, nursing homes, postacute care, palliative care, acute care, and inpatient and community-based mental health.

These instruments use the same major items in common, facilitating clinical communication both between different caregiving professionals and across acute, postacute and long-term care settings. Thus, they can enhance multidisciplinary care planning and continuity of care, and provide the most effective use of information technology (Figures 6-15 and 6-16). These standardized instruments offer the opportunity to doctors, nurses, families, advocates, administrators, and public payers to track changes in the older adults' status across settings and over time. Each of these instruments has been developed to be rooted in care planning through a triggering system that enables the identification of the person's problems, but also to provide quality measures, case-mix systems, and eligibility screeners. Pre- versus postimplementation comparisons have suggested an impact on the quality of care being delivered. After the implementation of the Resident Assessment Instrument for nursing home patients (now called InterRAI-LTCF) for example, evidence of advanced directives increased by 60%, the use of restraints dropped by 40% particularly among cognitively intact residents, the use of indwelling catheter dropped significantly, while there was a dramatic increase in the use of preventive skin programs. The prevalence of pressure ulcers, dehydration, and poor nutrition declined. Finally, in the postimplementation phase, the hospitalization rate declined by 25% with no increase in mortality.

The instruments have also been adopted by 11 states in the United States, primarily for their home- and community-based (waiver) programs, where compatibility with the nursing home system has been crucial. When systematically collected in large databases, data from these standardized assessment instruments can help identify both individual and organizational level predictors of patients' outcomes and to evaluate the overall system of care.

InterRAI systems have been adopted nationwide in Iceland, Finland, and Estonia (both home care and nursing home); Switzerland and Hong Kong (home care), Japan (one of three recommended home care systems), and a major trial of the new suite is scheduled for a pilot in China, to name a few.

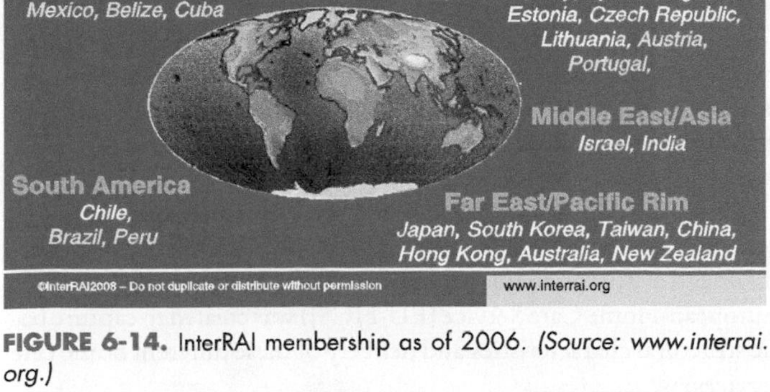

Experiences with InterRAI

Ontario's Experience Canada is the nation most advanced in adopting InterRAI instruments. It has designated three of the InterRAI instruments as national standards (home care, nursing home care, mental health) and is testing others in several communities (Figure 6-17). The province of Ontario, Canada, has made several steps forward in establishing an integrated health information system based on the InterRAI instruments. Complex continuing care hospitals/units were mandated in 1996 to use the Resident Assessment Instrument (now InterRAI-LTCF). By 2002, the RAI-Home Care (now InterRAI-HC) was mandated for all home care clients expected to be on service for 60 days or more. Case managers in single point entry agencies known as Community Care Access Centers (CCACs) now use the RAI-HC to assess needs and to contract services for home care clients. In 2005, the RAI-Mental Health (InterRAI-MH) was mandated for use in all adult in-patient beds in psychiatric hospitals/units, including acute, long stay, forensic, and

FIGURE 6-14. InterRAI membership as of 2006. *(Source: www.interrai. org.)*

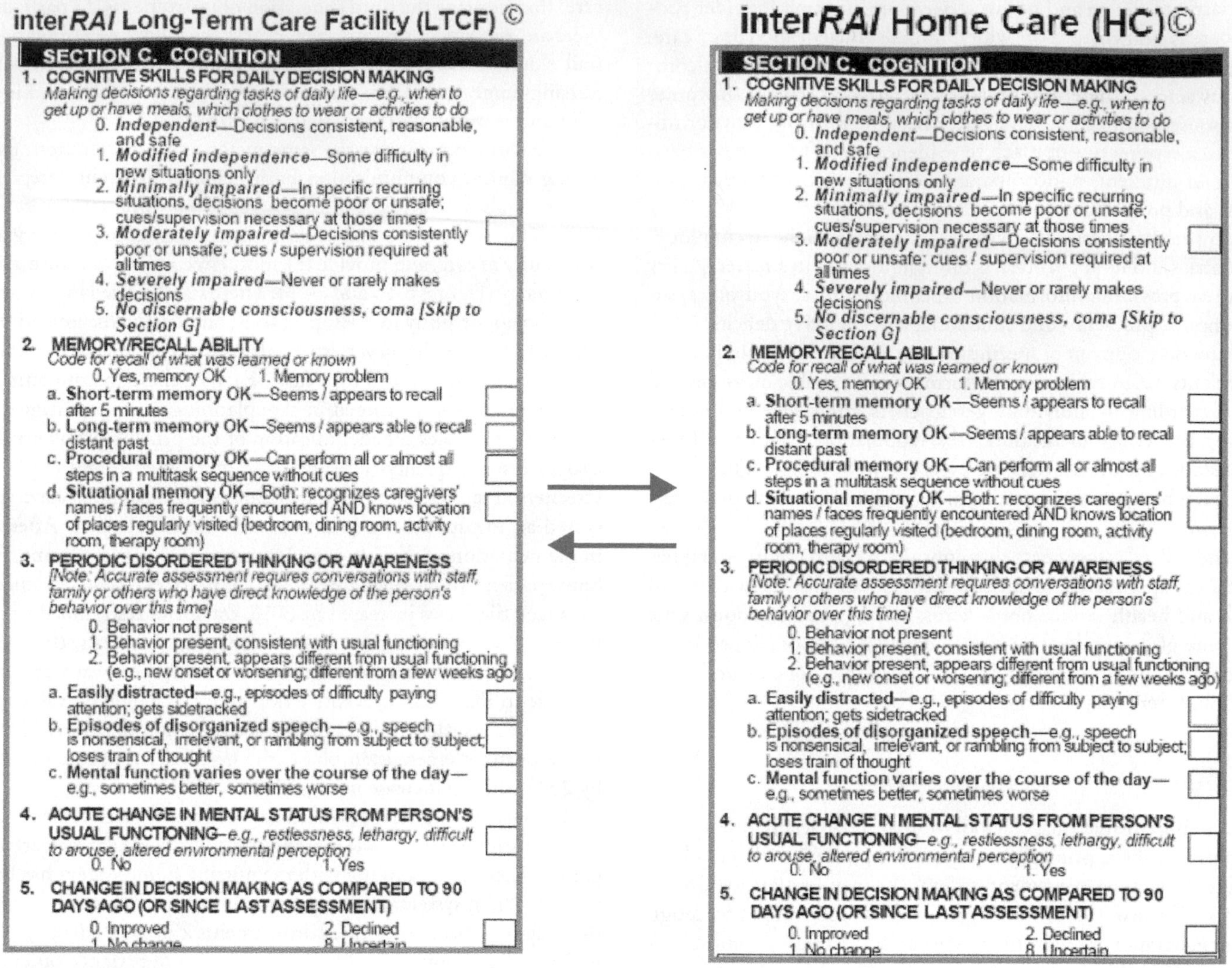

inter*RAI* Long-Term Care Facility (LTCF) ©

SECTION C. COGNITION

1. COGNITIVE SKILLS FOR DAILY DECISION MAKING
Making decisions regarding tasks of daily life—e.g., when to get up or have meals, which clothes to wear or activities to do
- 0. *Independent*—Decisions consistent, reasonable, and safe
- 1. *Modified independence*—Some difficulty in new situations only
- 2. *Minimally impaired*—In specific recurring situations, decisions become poor or unsafe; cues/supervision necessary at those times
- 3. *Moderately impaired*—Decisions consistently poor or unsafe; cues / supervision required at all times
- 4. *Severely impaired*—Never or rarely makes decisions
- 5. *No discernable consciousness, coma [Skip to Section G]*

2. MEMORY/RECALL ABILITY
Code for recall of what was learned or known
   0. Yes, memory OK   1. Memory problem
- a. **Short-term memory OK**—Seems / appears to recall after 5 minutes
- b. **Long-term memory OK**—Seems / appears able to recall distant past
- c. **Procedural memory OK**—Can perform all or almost all steps in a multitask sequence without cues
- d. **Situational memory OK**—Both: recognizes caregivers' names / faces frequently encountered AND knows location of places regularly visited (bedroom, dining room, activity room, therapy room)

3. PERIODIC DISORDERED THINKING OR AWARENESS
[Note: Accurate assessment requires conversations with staff, family or others who have direct knowledge of the person's behavior over this time]
- 0. Behavior not present
- 1. Behavior present, consistent with usual functioning
- 2. Behavior present, appears different from usual functioning (e.g., new onset or worsening; different from a few weeks ago)
- a. **Easily distracted**—e.g., episodes of difficulty paying attention; gets sidetracked
- b. **Episodes of disorganized speech**—e.g., speech is nonsensical, irrelevant, or rambling from subject to subject; loses train of thought
- c. **Mental function varies over the course of the day**—e.g., sometimes better, sometimes worse

4. ACUTE CHANGE IN MENTAL STATUS FROM PERSON'S USUAL FUNCTIONING—*e.g., restlessness, lethargy, difficult to arouse, altered environmental perception*
   0. No   1. Yes

5. CHANGE IN DECISION MAKING AS COMPARED TO 90 DAYS AGO (OR SINCE LAST ASSESSMENT)
   0. Improved   2. Declined
   1. No change   8. Uncertain

inter*RAI* Home Care (HC)©

SECTION C. COGNITION

1. COGNITIVE SKILLS FOR DAILY DECISION MAKING
Making decisions regarding tasks of daily life—e.g., when to get up or have meals, which clothes to wear or activities to do
- 0. *Independent*—Decisions consistent, reasonable, and safe
- 1. *Modified independence*—Some difficulty in new situations only
- 2. *Minimally impaired*—In specific recurring situations, decisions become poor or unsafe; cues/supervision necessary at those times
- 3. *Moderately impaired*—Decisions consistently poor or unsafe; cues / supervision required at all times
- 4. *Severely impaired*—Never or rarely makes decisions
- 5. *No discernable consciousness, coma [Skip to Section G]*

2. MEMORY/RECALL ABILITY
Code for recall of what was learned or known
   0. Yes, memory OK   1. Memory problem
- a. **Short-term memory OK**—Seems / appears to recall after 5 minutes
- b. **Long-term memory OK**—Seems / appears able to recall distant past
- c. **Procedural memory OK**—Can perform all or almost all steps in a multitask sequence without cues
- d. **Situational memory OK**—Both: recognizes caregivers' names / faces frequently encountered AND knows location of places regularly visited (bedroom, dining room, activity room, therapy room)

3. PERIODIC DISORDERED THINKING OR AWARENESS
[Note: Accurate assessment requires conversations with staff, family or others who have direct knowledge of the person's behavior over this time]
- 0. Behavior not present
- 1. Behavior present, consistent with usual functioning
- 2. Behavior present, appears different from usual functioning (e.g., new onset or worsening; different from a few weeks ago)
- a. **Easily distracted**—e.g., episodes of difficulty paying attention; gets sidetracked
- b. **Episodes of disorganized speech**—e.g., speech is nonsensical, irrelevant, or rambling from subject to subject; loses train of thought
- c. **Mental function varies over the course of the day**—e.g., sometimes better, sometimes worse

4. ACUTE CHANGE IN MENTAL STATUS FROM PERSON'S USUAL FUNCTIONING—*e.g., restlessness, lethargy, difficult to arouse, altered environmental perception*
   0. No   1. Yes

5. CHANGE IN DECISION MAKING AS COMPARED TO 90 DAYS AGO (OR SINCE LAST ASSESSMENT)
   0. Improved   2. Declined
   1. No change   8. Uncertain

FIGURE 6-15. Concordance across InterRAI instruments: assessment of cognitive function in InterRAI-LTCF and InterRAI-HC. *(Source: www.interrai.org.)*

geriatric psychiatry. Implementation of the Resident Assessment Instrument is currently underway for all long-term care facilities in the province, including for-profit and not-for-profit homes. Implementation of the InterRAI Contact Assessment (InterRAI CA) began in 2006, and it currently is used to determine (1) the need for comprehensive assessment with the RAI-HC; (2) urgency for initiation of services such as nursing or personal support, and (3) need for a referral for rehabilitation. The InterRAI CA will also be used as the basic assessment for short-stay home care clients with relatively uncomplicated care needs.

The use of InterRAI assessment instruments for each of these sectors has brought Ontario closer than many jurisdictions to the possibility of an integrated health information system, linking the major providers of health services to frail elderly people. The Canadian Institute for Health Information has established three national reporting systems to provide comparative reports on continuing care, home care, and mental health (see, for example, report on facility-based continuing care).

Many factors have contributed to the progress that Ontario has made to date, including strong leadership at all levels of the health care system; effective collaboration between key stakeholders; a clear commitment to standardization based on psychometrically sound

data and the establishment of an infrastructure to capture, compile, and report on the gathered data.

European Union Experience The "Aged in Home Care" (ADHOC) study (funded with a large grant from the European Union) was aimed at analyzing and comparing different models of home care for older persons in 11 European countries: the Czech Republic, Denmark, England, Finland, France, Germany, Iceland, Italy, the Netherlands, Norway, and Sweden. In each country, distinct municipalities providing formal home care services that were considered representative of the nation's urban areas were selected. The cities chosen were Amsterdam (the Netherlands), Copenhagen (Denmark), Helsinki (Finland), Oslo (Norway), Prague (Czech Republic), Reykjavik (Iceland), Stockholm (Sweden), Amiens (France), Ashford and Maidstone (UK), Monza (Italy), and Nuremberg and Bayreuth (Germany) (Figure 6-18).

Thousands of home care clients were assessed three times in one year in the 11 cities with the InterRAI Home Care instrument and a structured questionnaire on services' characteristics (the European-Home Care Service [EU-HCS]) was created to capture basic structural characteristics and delivery of these different home care services.

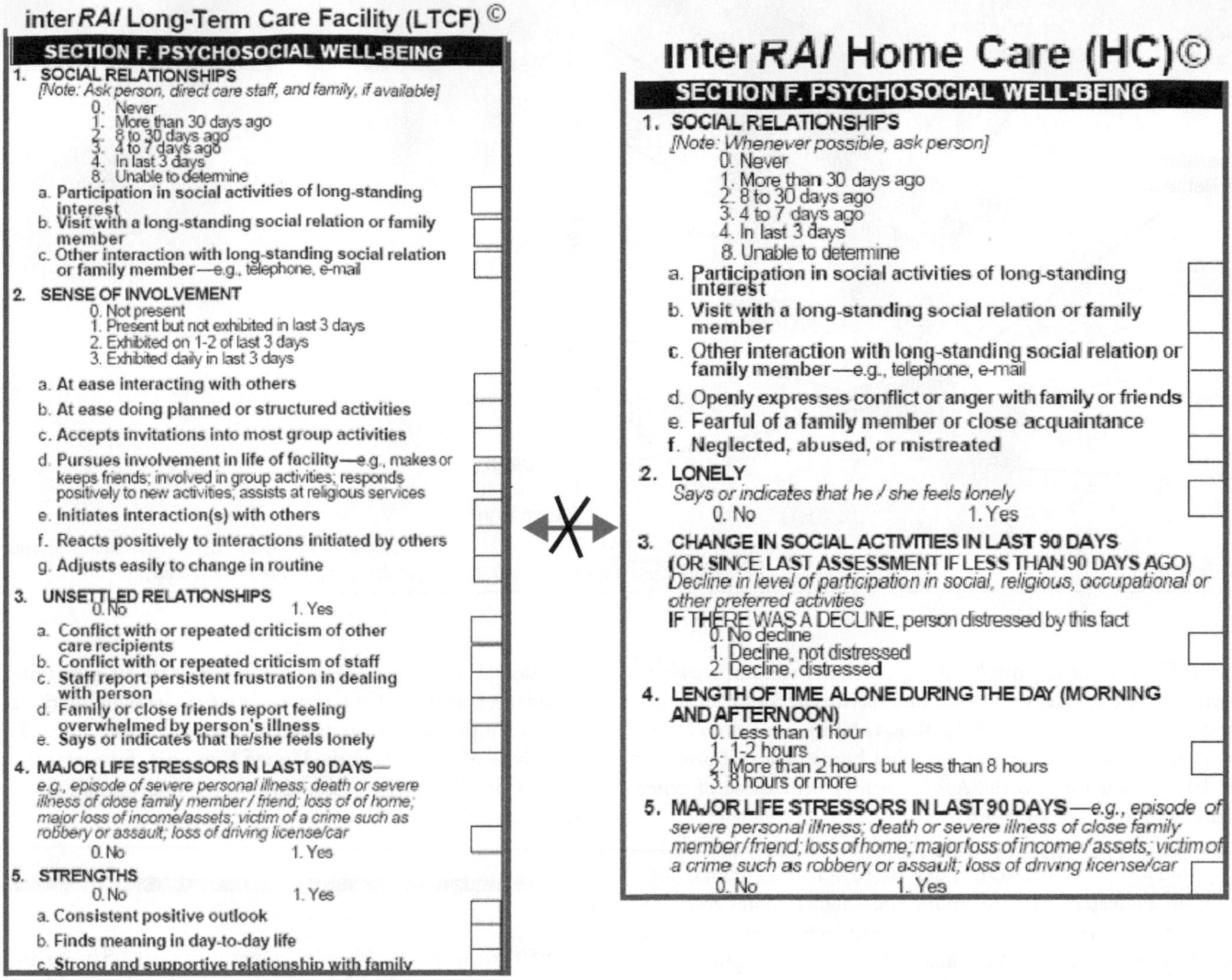

interRAI Long-Term Care Facility (LTCF) ©

SECTION F. PSYCHOSOCIAL WELL-BEING

1. SOCIAL RELATIONSHIPS
[Note: Ask person, direct care staff, and family, if available]
0. Never
1. More than 30 days ago
2. 8 to 30 days ago
3. 4 to 7 days ago
4. In last 3 days
8. Unable to determine

a. Participation in social activities of long-standing interest
b. Visit with a long-standing social relation or family member
c. Other interaction with long-standing social relation or family member—e.g., telephone, e-mail

2. SENSE OF INVOLVEMENT
0. Not present
1. Present but not exhibited in last 3 days
2. Exhibited on 1-2 of last 3 days
3. Exhibited daily in last 3 days

a. At ease interacting with others
b. At ease doing planned or structured activities
c. Accepts invitations into most group activities
d. Pursues involvement in life of facility—e.g., makes or keeps friends; involved in group activities; responds positively to new activities; assists at religious services
e. Initiates interaction(s) with others
f. Reacts positively to interactions initiated by others
g. Adjusts easily to change in routine

3. UNSETTLED RELATIONSHIPS
0. No   1. Yes

a. Conflict with or repeated criticism of other care recipients
b. Conflict with or repeated criticism of staff
c. Staff report persistent frustration in dealing with person
d. Family or close friends report feeling overwhelmed by person's illness
e. Says or indicates that he/she feels lonely

4. MAJOR LIFE STRESSORS IN LAST 90 DAYS—
e.g., episode of severe personal illness; death or severe illness of close family member / friend; loss of of home; major loss of income/assets; victim of a crime such as robbery or assault; loss of driving license/car
0. No   1. Yes

5. STRENGTHS
0. No   1. Yes

a. Consistent positive outlook
b. Finds meaning in day-to-day life
c. Strong and supportive relationship with family

interRAI Home Care (HC) ©

SECTION F. PSYCHOSOCIAL WELL-BEING

1. SOCIAL RELATIONSHIPS
[Note: Whenever possible, ask person]
0. Never
1. More than 30 days ago
2. 8 to 30 days ago
3. 4 to 7 days ago
4. In last 3 days
8. Unable to determine

a. Participation in social activities of long-standing interest
b. Visit with a long-standing social relation or family member
c. Other interaction with long-standing social relation or family member—e.g., telephone, e-mail
d. Openly expresses conflict or anger with family or friends
e. Fearful of a family member or close acquaintance
f. Neglected, abused, or mistreated

2. LONELY
Says or indicates that he / she feels lonely
0. No   1. Yes

3. CHANGE IN SOCIAL ACTIVITIES IN LAST 90 DAYS (OR SINCE LAST ASSESSMENT IF LESS THAN 90 DAYS AGO)
Decline in level of participation in social, religious, occupational or other preferred activities
IF THERE WAS A DECLINE, person distressed by this fact
0. No decline
1. Decline, not distressed
2. Decline, distressed

4. LENGTH OF TIME ALONE DURING THE DAY (MORNING AND AFTERNOON)
0. Less than 1 hour
1. 1-2 hours
2. More than 2 hours but less than 8 hours
3. 8 hours or more

5. MAJOR LIFE STRESSORS IN LAST 90 DAYS—*e.g., episode of severe personal illness; death or severe illness of close family member/friend; loss of home; major loss of income / assets; victim of a crime such as robbery or assault; loss of driving license/car*
0. No   1. Yes

FIGURE 6-16. Distinctions across InterRAI instruments: assessment of psychosocial well-being in InterRAI-LTCF and InterRAI-HC. *(Source: www.interrai.org.)*

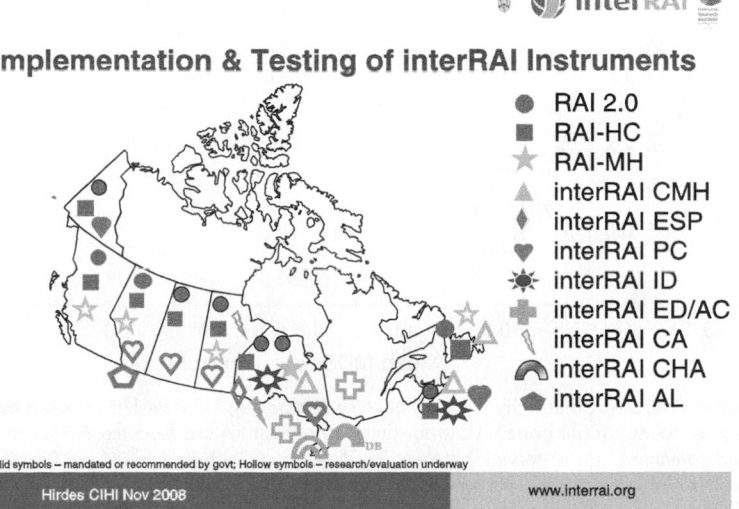

Implementation & Testing of interRAI Instruments

● RAI 2.0
■ RAI-HC
★ RAI-MH
▲ interRAI CMH
♦ interRAI ESP
♥ interRAI PC
☀ interRAI ID
✚ interRAI ED/AC
  interRAI CA
⌒ interRAI CHA
⬟ interRAI AL

Solid symbols – mandated or recommended by govt; Hollow symbols – research/evaluation underway

Hirdes CIHI Nov 2008   www.interrai.org

FIGURE 6-17. Implementation and testing of InterRAI instruments in Canada. *(Source: www.interrai.org.)*

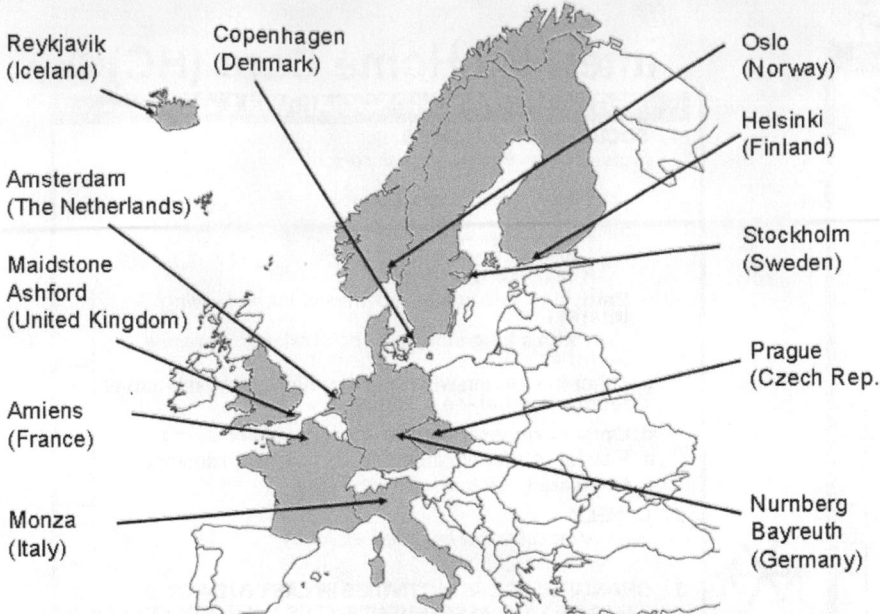

Reykjavik
(Iceland)

Copenhagen
(Denmark)

Oslo
(Norway)

Helsinki
(Finland)

Amsterdam
(The Netherlands)

Stockholm
(Sweden)

Maidstone
Ashford
(United Kingdom)

Amiens
(France)

Prague
(Czech Rep.)

Monza
(Italy)

Nurnberg
Bayreuth
(Germany)

FIGURE 6-18. Geographic distribution of countries participating in the AdHoc Study.

The AdHoc study also offered the opportunity to compare characteristics of care recipients in home care services in countries across Europe. For example, Figure 6-19 shows the functional and cognitive characteristics of patients receiving home care in European countries (participating to the AdHoc study) with those of other countries adopting the same instrument.

Functional status was measured by the seven-point ADL hierarchy and three-point IADL index based on meal preparation, medication management, and phone use (higher scores meaning more severe impairment). Cognitive status was measured using the seven-point Cognitive Performance Scale (CPS) (higher scores meaning more severe impairment). As shown in Figure 6-19, home care patients living in northern Europe present lower rate of functional and cognitive impairment compared to those living in south-

ern Europe (France and Italy), where home care recipients are very dependent. Patients in United States present a level of functional and cognitive impairment that resemble home care recipients in France and Italy much more than the United Kingdom, for example. Conversely, Canada presents a situation that is undistinguishable from that of United Kingdom.

CONCLUSION

In 1950, there were 205 million persons aged 65 years or over throughout the world. Fifty years later, the number had increased threefold to 606 million. By the year 2050, the number of older persons in the world will exceed the number of persons aged 5 years

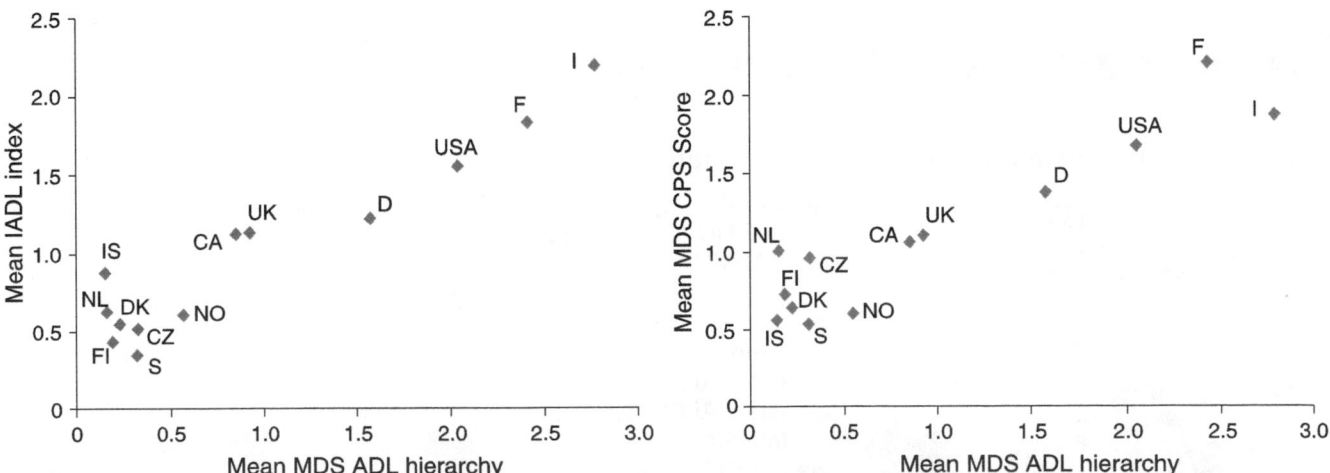

FIGURE 6-19. Relationship between mean MDS HC IADL index and mean MDS ADL hierarchy score by country (left panel); Relationship between mean MDS cognitive performance scale (CPS) and mean MDS ADL hierarchy by country (right panel). Data for European countries are from the AdHoc study. Data for United States are from Michigan MI Choice Waiver (home- and community-based services) in year 2005. CZ = Czech Republic, D = Germany, DK = Denmark, F = France, FI = Finland, I = Italy, IS = Iceland, NL = The Netherlands, NO = Norway, S = Sweden, UK = United Kingdom. *Data from Canada are from Ontario Community Care Access Services in year 2006.*

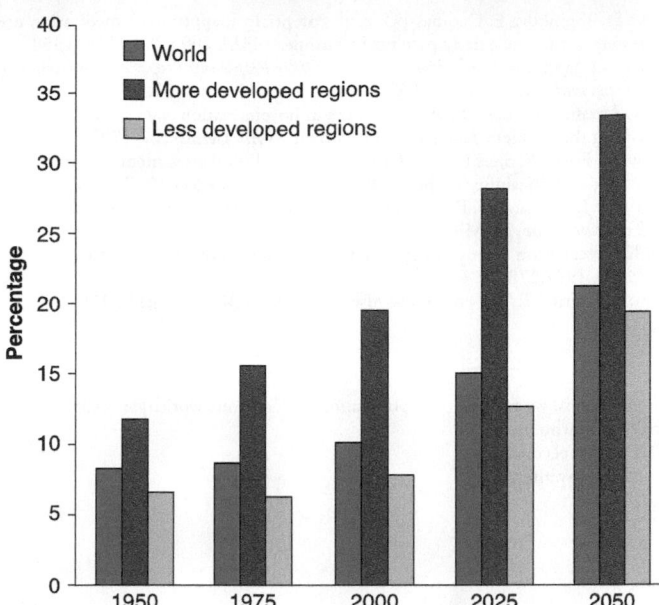

FIGURE 6-20. Proportion of population aged 60 yrs or older: world and development regions, 1950–2050. *(Reprinted with permission from World Population Aging 1950–2050, United Nations.)*

higher than the proportions in the less developed regions well into the twenty-first century (Figure 6-20).

In contrast with the slow process of population aging experienced in the past by most countries in the more developed regions, the aging process in most of the less developed countries is taking place in a much shorter period of time, and it is occurring on relatively larger population bases. As a result, the number of older people is increasingly larger in the less developed countries. Over the last century, the number of older adults increased globally by an average of 8 million persons every year. Of this increase, 66% occurred in the less developed countries. Over the next half century, this trend will intensify. In the more developed countries, the number of older adults will increase by about 70%, from 231 million in 2000 to 395 million in 2050. In contrast, in the less developed countries, the population aging will more than quadruple from 374 million to 1.6 billion. By 2050, nearly four-fifths of the world's older population will be living in the less developed countries (Figure 6-21).

This chapter has highlighted that even the richest countries in the world found themselves totally unprepared to confront the demographic changes. There is an extreme heterogeneity of the organization that each country has given to their respective health care services, and a substantial fragmentation into an array of services of unproven efficacy and efficiency. If this experience does not inform the policy decisions of the countries where most of the older adults will live in the future, it is highly foreseeable that there will be tremendous challenges for government and private spending in health care and, more generally, for economic growth and welfare.

One possible solution is to develop a more integrated and interdisciplinary care models of elderly services. The transition to this model will require a major reorganization of health care from education through delivery systems. Standardized assessment instruments that allow a cross-talk among different health care services

or less for the first time in history to reach nearly 2 billion. The older population is growing faster than the total population in practically all regions of the world, and the difference in growth rates is increasing.

However, the more developed countries are in general in a more advanced stage of the demographic transition. The proportions of older persons in those countries, therefore, will remain significantly

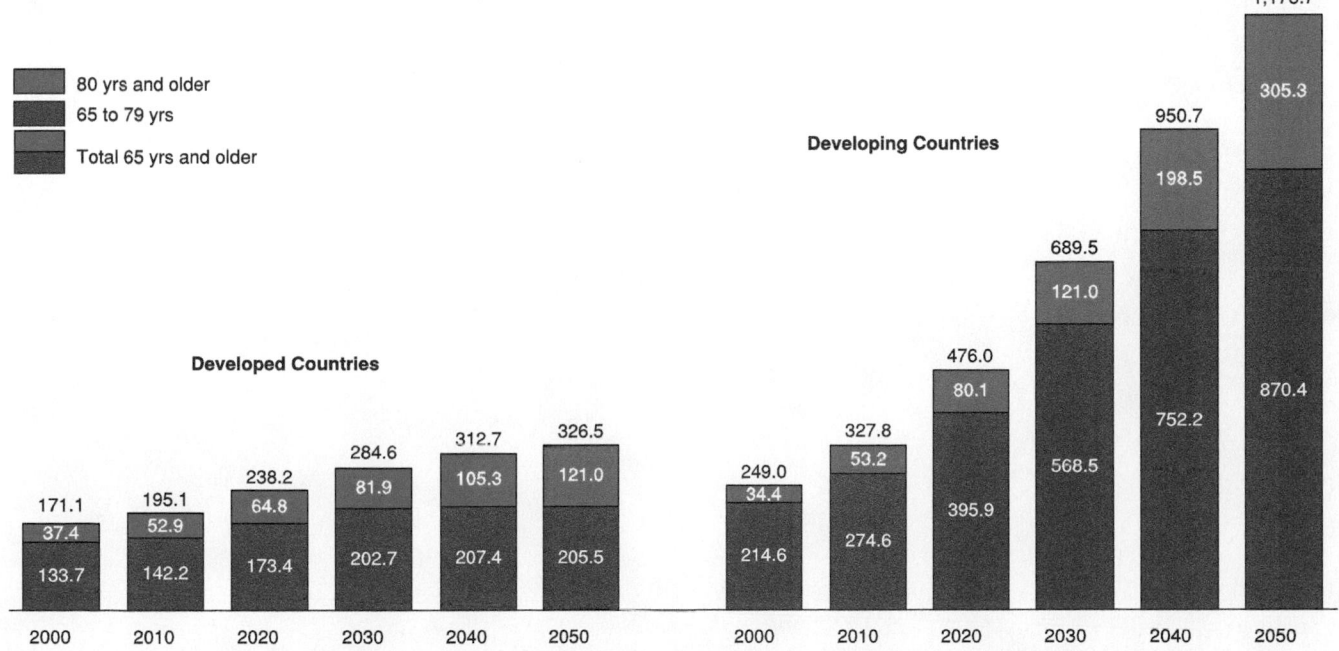

FIGURE 6-21. Population (in millions) aged 65 yrs and older for developed and developing countries by age: 2000–2050. *(Reprinted with permission from U.S. Census Bureau, Current Population Reports: 65+ in the United States.)*

can faciltate this transition to interdisciplinary care models, determine appropriate services based on need, and evaluate effectiveness and efficiency of specific services. Experiences in every country should inform practice and policy in other countries. Aging is a global issue.

FURTHER READING

Bernabei R, Gambassi G, Lapane K, et al. Management of pain in elderly patients with cancer. *JAMA*. 1998;279:1877.

Bernabei R, Gambassi G, Lapane K, et al. Characteristics of the SAGE database: a new resource for research on outcomes in long-term care. *J Gerontol A Biol Med Sci*. 1999;54:M25–33.

Carpenter I, Challis D, Hirdes J, et al., eds. *Care of Older People: a Comparison of Systems in North America, Europe and Japan*. London: Farrand Press; 1999.

Carpenter I, Gambassi G, Topinkova E, et al. Community care in Europe. The Aged in Home Care project (AdHOC). *Aging Clin Exp Res*. 2004;16:259.

Fialova D, Topinkova E, Gambassi G, et al. Potentially inappropriate medication use among home care elderly patients in Europe. *JAMA*. 2005;293:1348–1358.

Illsley R. In: Jamieson A, ed. *Home Care for Older People in Europe: A Comparison of Policies and Practices*. Oxford: Oxford University Press; 1991.

Mor V, Intrator O, Fries BE, et al. Changes in hospitalization associated with introducing the Resident Assessment Instrument. *J Am Geriatr Soc*. 1997;45:1002.

Morris JN, Fries BE, Steel K, et al. Comprehensive clinical assessment in community setting—Applicability of the MDS-HC. *J Am Geriatr Soc*. 1997;45:1017.

Rubenstein L, Wieland D, Bernabei R. In: Kurtis, ed. *Geriatric Assessment Technology: The State of the Art*. Milan; 1995.

Steel K. Research on ageing: an agenda for all nations individually and collectively. *JAMA*. 1997;278:1374.

Tinetti ME, Fried T. The end of the disease era. *Am J Med*. 2004;116:179.

Web Sites—General

United Nations, www.un.org/esa/population/publications/worldageing19502050/.

WHO, www.who.int.

OECD, www.oecd.org.

InterRAI, www.interrai.org.

Psychosocial Aspects of Aging

Richard Schulz ■ *Steven M. Albert*

Understanding the role of psychosocial factors in late life requires a high-altitude view of human development to identify the basic biological and social forces that fundamentally shape the development of the person and the ways in which they respond to life challenges. These forces are typically viewed as constraints and can be briefly summarized in four propositions.

1. Biological development follows a sequential pattern. Although there is considerable interindividual variability in biological development, the overall biological resources across the life span resemble an inverted U-function. During childhood and adolescence, cognitive and physical abilities increase and provide the basis for the development of complex motor and cognitive skills. Physical development plateaus during early adulthood and then later declines. In old age, declines in both physical and cognitive functioning are evident.

2. Societies impose age-graded sociostructural constraints on development. Life span psychologists and life course sociologists emphasize that all societies can be characterized as having age-graded systems, which constrain and provide a scaffold for life course patterns. These patterns provide predictability and structure at both individual and societal levels. A prototypical case is childbearing in women, which is shaped by both social institutions and biological constraints.

3. Life is finite. Whatever is to be achieved or experienced in life has to be done in a limited period of time, typically less than 80 years. At any given point in an individual's life, the anticipated amount of time left to live may shape behavior and affect in important ways.

4. Genetic endowment is a limiting factor on the biological and behavioral functioning of the individual. Although the potential behavioral repertoire of humans is vast, the capacity to achieve extraordinary levels of functioning in a given domain is often constrained by the genetic makeup of the individual.

This view of development emphasizes that accumulated resilience or adaptive capacity of individuals will vary as function of the individual's location in the life course. For example, the biological and physical reserves of an individual will generally be greater for persons in young adulthood than for persons in old age. Conversely, behavioral resources and psychological reserves may be greater at older ages because of accumulated life experiences, acquisition of skills, and increased knowledge. In addition, a given stressor will likely activate different psychological and behavioral processes in varying intensities as a function of the individual's location in the life course. Finally, because of fundamental changes in age-related biological functioning, the type and intensity of biological pathways activated by stressful encounters as well as the manifestation of overt disease will vary substantially as a function of the individual's location in the life course.

PSYCHOSOCIAL FACTORS, HEALTH, AND QUALITY OF LIFE

The number of topics that could legitimately be included in a discussion of psychosocial aspects of aging is vast. Work, retirement, migration, sexuality, stress, widowhood, emotionality, mental health, social support, and friendship are just a few of the domains that might be discussed within a psychosocial framework, and many of these topics are covered in other chapters of this book. The focus here is on psychosocial factors linked to health and quality of life. A broad conceptual framework identifying key psychosocial factors is presented in Figure 7-1. At the far left, the model identifies a broad array of *sociodemographic characteristics*, which directly and indirectly shape individual development, quality of life, and health throughout the life course. For example, many of the health disparities in our society have been linked to socioeconomic status, race, and gender. *Environmental and social resources and constraints* include multiple indicators known to affect health outcomes, including

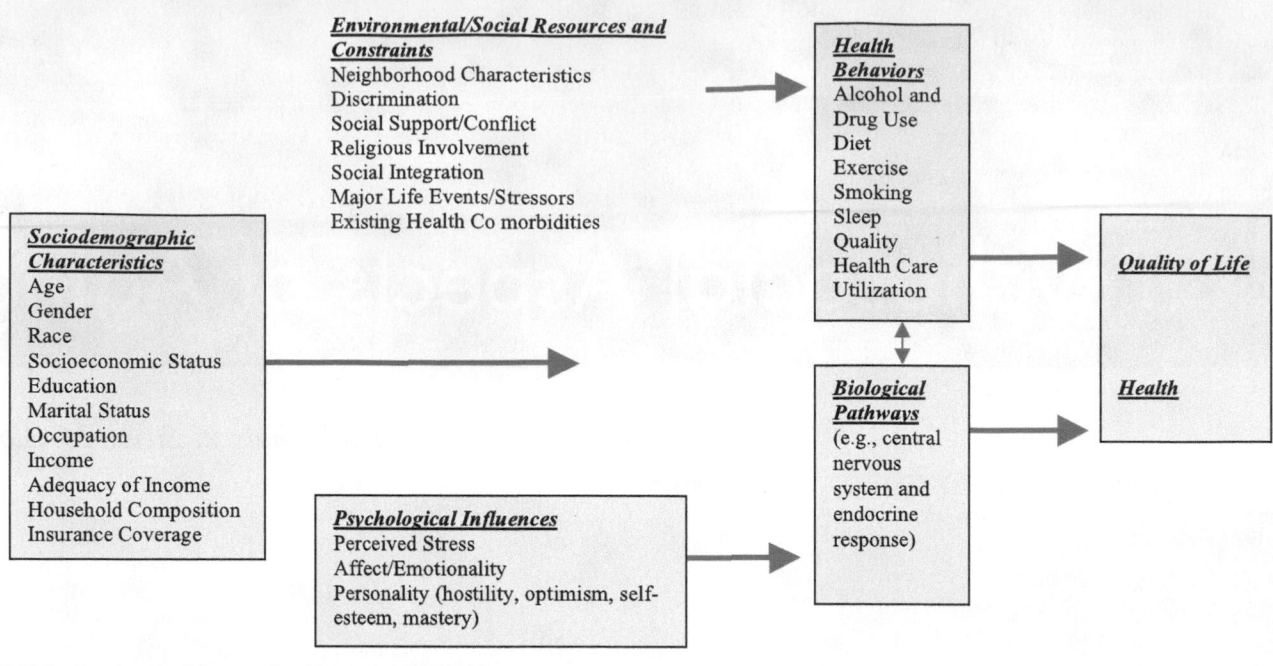

FIGURE 7-1. Psychosocial factors, health, and quality of life.

physical and social characteristics of the environment people live in. Discrimination, negative life events, and existing comorbidities can be major sources of constraint, while religious involvement and social support are often important protective resources (Figure 7-1).

Psychological influences include both positive and negative factors, including optimism, self-esteem, mastery, and control. Negative affect, such as depressive symptoms and perceived stress, affect health through their impact on behaviors and through biological pathways. The effects of psychological and social/environmental factors on health are often mediated through *health behaviors* and through *biological pathways* such as the central nervous system and endocrine response. Although there is still considerable debate regarding the causal links between these groups of variables, there is strong consensus that they are important contributors to health and quality of life. A detailed review of all of the variables identified within this model is beyond the scope of this chapter and would be redundant with other chapters in this volume. Thus, the goal here is to highlight core psychosocial factors and mechanisms linked to health and well-being. Specifically, the discussion that follows focuses on four psychosocial domains—social relationships, stress, personality and affect, and quality of life—that are critical to understanding aging and health.

SOCIAL RELATIONSHIPS

Maintaining social relationships is critical to promoting psychological and physical well-being in late life. Involvement in satisfying social relationships has been linked to decreased risk of cardiovascular disease, functional decline, and mortality. Social interactions and companionship also contribute to emotional well-being, life satisfaction, and happiness. Although the impact of social relationships on well-being is predominantly positive, there are circumstances when social relationships can be detrimental to the older individual. Thus, there is interest in determining which aspects of social relationships

are beneficial (and which are not) as well as the specific mechanisms by which they contribute to positive or negative health outcomes.

Three aspects of social relationships are typically identified: (1) *structural support*, often referred to as social integration or social connectedness, focuses on the quantity and types of social ties an individual has, (2) *social support* refers to the tangible or intangible benefits that people receive through social ties, and (3) *negative support* refers to the detrimental effects of social relationships.

Structural support is typically measured by counting the number and types (e.g., spouse, partner, friend, church member) of individuals in one's social network as well as the frequency of contact between members of the network. Numerous studies have shown that older individuals with more network ties are less likely to develop cognitive and physical disability, after controlling for baseline health and functional status characteristics. Other studies have shown slower rates of decline in functioning as well as longer survival among individuals with larger social networks and more frequent contact with network members. Put another way, low levels of social integration (i.e., social isolation) are a major risk factor for mortality, independent of traditional biomedical and other behavioral risk factors. The mechanisms responsible for the beneficial health effects of social integration have not been definitively established. Candidate mechanisms include improved health behaviors resulting from the positive influence of friends and relatives, reduced exposure to external stressors, a stronger sense of coherence and self-esteem, and improved biological resilience.

Social support typically identifies perceived support and received support, including four different types of support provided. Perceived support is the perception that support is available if needed, and received support refers to support that has actually been provided. The four types of support are as follows: (1) instrumental support, which refers to tangible goods and services such as financial assistance, help with self-care tasks; (2) informational support, which is defined as the provision of advice, information on how to solve problems, or guidance; (3) emotional support, which includes the provision of love, caring, and other positive feelings; and (4) appraisal support, which includes feedback given to help individuals evaluate themselves or a particular situation they may be struggling with. Although distinctions among the last three types of support are sometimes difficult to make in practice, they are useful in helping to understand what types of support are more or less beneficial under what circumstances. For example, emotional support has been shown to be particularly beneficial to promoting psychological well-being and cognitive and physical functioning. A number of mechanisms have been proposed to explain the beneficial effects of support including provision of needed material resources and services (instrumental support), reduction of the perceived severity of life stressors (appraisal support), or improvement of coping skills (informational or emotional support).

On the whole, the benefits of social relationships far outweigh their occasional *detrimental effects*. Nevertheless, interactions with network members are not always positive and may include criticism, neglect, demands, and other insensitive behaviors that negatively affect health and well-being. At the extreme, close network members may abuse their elderly relative with threats, economic exploitation, or physical harm. Close friends and relatives may also provide support that is well-intentioned but backfires, resulting in worse, rather than better, health outcomes. For example, receiving help with self-care tasks has been linked to disability onset and progression among originally high functioning older adults. Network members who are overprotective and provide too much support may foster dependency in older adults, leading to reduced physical activity and accelerated physical decline. Overprotection may also erode an older adult's confidence in being able to care for oneself, threaten feelings of autonomy, independence, and overall well-being.

Despite the potential for detrimental effects of social relationships, satisfaction with social relationships tends to be high in late life, even though social networks become somewhat smaller, and interactions with network members become less frequent. One reason is that older adults manage their social relationships to maximize positive support and companionship, and minimize relationships that are conflictual and difficult.

STRESS AND DISTRESS

Stress is the nonspecific result of a demand upon the body. It is a common pathway for a variety of physical, cognitive, and emotional challenges. The stressed person will experience adverse physiologic effects (primarily in the pituitary–adrenal axis and immune system) but also clinically appreciable effects on decision-making, problem-solving, vigilance, social inference, and perceptual and motor skills. In this case, stress, a normal feature of an individual's interaction with the environment, becomes distress, prolonged stress that overwhelms physiologic and psychologic regulatory mechanisms. Some research suggests that prolonged stress may even affect the rate of aging, as measured by telomeric shortening over successive cell replication cycles.

In older people, stress from health limitations and consequent social losses becomes more common. The rising prevalence of chronic disease and disability, increased awareness of cognitive or physical limitation, loss of valued social roles, and reduction in social networks through widowhood and loss of friendships all act as stressors that increase the risk of negative mental and physical states. The adverse effects of stress are lower for those who have strong social support systems and greater personal resources, but repeated losses in multiple domains may ultimately lead to the sense that one has lost control generally. Yet a robust finding from a variety of research settings is that older adults are able to maintain a sense of control even in quite challenging health circumstances. The elderly patient unable to leave home or nursing home floor may station herself in a strategic position to retain a view of activity and encourage social interaction. The elderly patient unable to ambulate in his home may sit in a chair by the window that affords the clearest view of what is happening outside the home. In these ways, older people with poor health and threats to autonomy or control may yet retain some command over features of their living space.

STRESSFUL LIFE EVENTS

Stressful life events have been linked to poor mental and physical health in individuals of all ages. Researchers interested in the relationship between stress and health have generally pursued two strategies to assess life stressors. Major life events such as illness and death of a loved one can be assessed using checklists or interviews to gauge their frequency and intensity. Alternatively, the ordinary hassles of day-to-day living (e.g., cooking, housework, work load, meeting deadlines, home repair, etc.) can be measured with structured self-report or interviewer-administered instruments. Older individuals, when compared to younger persons, experience fewer life events overall, although they experience more loss events, particularly those associated with declining health and loss of friends and loved ones. Younger individuals report more hassles in domains such as finances, work, home maintenance, personal life, and family and friends, whereas older men and women report more hassles in domains reflecting social issues, home maintenance, and health. Overall, for both younger and older individuals, daily hassles are more potent determinants of physical and psychological well-being than major life stressors. Older individuals demonstrate remarkable ability to successfully adapt to major life stressors such as the loss of a loved one. One important exception to this general observation occurs when older individuals are exposed to unrelenting chronic stressors such as having to care for a spouse with Alzheimer's disease. Under such circumstances, the chronicity, intensity, and variety of stressors impinging on the caregiver can exact a high price in terms of physical and psychiatric morbidity.

However, there is considerable variability in individual response to major life stressors. The concept of resilience, defined as the ability to recover from or benefit from adversity, has been introduced to account for this variability. Individuals able to overcome adversity are thought to have high levels of resilience, a combination of internal personality traits such as hardiness, high self-efficacy, mastery, and optimism, along with a strong external support system. Although intuitively engaging, the empirical and clinical utility of the concept of resilience remains open to debate.

BIOLOGICAL CONSEQUENCES OF STRESS

An important advance in recent decades is our increased understanding of the biological pathways through which psychosocial factors modulate changes in health. The field of psychoneuroimmunology focuses on linkages between psychosocial factors and nervous, neuroendocrine, and immune processes, which in turn have been linked to health. Much of this research has focused on stress, particularly chronic stress, and associated negative affective states such as depression, anxiety, and anger, as disruptors of these biological regulatory systems. Stress may influence immunity either through direct innervation of the central nervous system and immune system or directly through neuroendocrine immune pathways. Behavioral responses to stress may also affect immunity. For example, individuals experiencing stress may smoke more, drink more alcohol, eat poorly, and sleep less, all of which may influence immune response.

Because increasing age is associated with significant alterations in the functioning of many physiological systems, including endocrine and immune systems, old age has become a fertile ground for examining the relation between stress, biological mediators, and disease. For example, family caregiving is a chronic stressor with the ability to disrupt immune and neuroendocrine function. Compared to non-caregiver older adults, older caregivers have higher antibody titers for latent viruses, poor immune control over latent viral infections, reduced responsiveness of natural killer (NK) cells to cytokine signals, slower healing of wounds, poorer antibody responses to vaccination, and higher basal cortisol levels. Physical health effects of caregiving include greater risk of infectious disease, hypertensive changes in blood pressure, increased prevalence of cardiovascular disease, and mortality. Taken together, these findings suggest a strong link between stress, biological mediators, and illness; however, few studies have demonstrated the progression from stress to biological mediators to disease in the same individuals in the same study.

PERSONALITY, AFFECT, AND HEALTH

Personality is defined as the characteristics and attributes, and their associated behavioral patterns, which differentiate one person from another. Sometimes referred to as traits, dispositional tendencies, or fundamental human qualities, personality has long been of interest with respect to how it develops and may change across the life span. The five-factor model (FFM) of personality has been influential among gerontologists and claims that personality can be defined by five traits—openness to experience, conscientiousness, extraversion, agreeableness, and neuroticism—that remain relatively fixed until well into old age. Other important traits include mastery or control, the belief that important outcomes in life are under one's own control, as well as traits such as optimism and hostility. Despite the relative stability over time of key traits, personality traits may continue to change during midlife and beyond in response to specific goals, opportunities, and constraints. For example, functional declines in late life may erode one's sense of mastery, extraversion, or optimism about the future.

An important emerging area of research is focused on the link between two distinct dispositional attributes and health. Enduring negative affective styles such as anger, depression, and anxiety appear to be linked to greater morbidity and mortality, and conversely positive affect is linked to lower morbidity and decreased symptoms and pain. Positive affect is also associated with increased longevity among community-dwelling elderly. For example, one study coded autobiographical writing samples collected from a group of nuns when they were in their early twenties for positive emotion words and sentences. The greater the positive affect expressed in their writing, the greater the probability of being alive 60 years later (adjusting for age and education).

Multiple mechanisms might account for the relation between dispositional affect and morbidity and mortality, including health practices such as diet, exercise, and sleep quality, biological processes such as cardiovascular reactivity, as well as the stress hormones (such as epinephrine, norepinephrine, and cortisol). Positive affect has been associated with health-relevant hormones, including increases in oxytocin, growth hormone, and endogenous opioids. Inasmuch as individuals with positive affect are typically more pleasant to be around, they may also accrue health benefits through more positive social interactions and more attentive and higher quality health care from health care providers.

An important unresolved question is whether positive and negative affect are opposite sides of the same coin or two independent factors. If positive and negative affect are simple opposites, then being high on one necessarily means being low on the other, making it difficult to know whether salutary health effects are due to the presence of positive or the absence of negative affect. However, if individuals can simultaneously experience high levels of positive and negative affect, the two constructs might be independent and each uniquely contribute to health outcomes.

PSYCHOSOCIAL ASPECTS OF QUALITY OF LIFE AND VALUATION OF LIFE

Quality of life (QOL) includes two overlapping domains. Health-related quality of life specifies elements of daily function and well-being that change as a result of disease or therapeutic intervention. A satisfactory QOL measure in this sense allows researchers to rank different health conditions (and treatments) according to their impact on domains of health, such as mobility, independence in bathing and dressing, sensory acuity, mood, and absence of pain. The more negative the impact in these areas, the greater the quality of life impact of the health condition. Environment-based quality of life, by contrast, is not a health impact measure but rather registers the effect of personal resources or environmental factors on daily experience. Environment-related QOL domains include features of the natural and built environment (such as economic resources, housing, air and water quality, community stability, access to the arts and entertainment), as well as personal resources (such as the capacity to form friendships, appreciate nature, or find satisfaction in spiritual or religious life).

Maintaining the distinction between the two types of QOL is important. Health-related quality of life domains—patient reports of functional status, discomfort, pain, energy levels, social engagement—will track more closely with clinical measures of disease than environmental indicators. Recognizing this distinction eliminates much of the confusion about the "idiosyncrasy" of QOL ratings. However, the two types of QOL are also related in important ways. An impoverished environment (e.g., poor air quality, noise, lack of social stimulation) may affect health-related QOL. By the same token, health limitations may require environmental changes, such as reliance on assistive devices or personal assistance care, which affect environmental sources of QOL. The older adult with cognitive impairment faces threats to both dimensions of QOL: Dementia directly affects function and well-being and also forces environmental changes that may further reduce opportunities for quality in daily life.

A good test of whether a domain falls within the category of health-related QOL is whether this domain changes with successful medical treatment or change in care environment. Sample domains of this type, recorded in the Sickness Impact Profile (SIP), include ambulation, mobility, body care and movement, communication, alertness behavior, emotional behavior, social interaction, sleep and rest, eating, work, home management, and recreation. The Medical Outcomes Study (MOS SF36) identified a related set of eight domains: health perception, pain, physical function, social function, mental health, role limitation from physical causes, role limitation from mental health causes, and vitality. Others, such as the Health Utilities Index (HUI), stress still different domains, in this case a "within the skin" approach that restricts QOL to domains that are closely connected to clinical conditions.

QOL can be assessed as the difference between a population norm and mean value for patient samples, or more directly as a "utility" rating, that is, a numeric rating of how preferred (and thus how much better) one health state is relative to another. One common way to derive utilities for health states is to ask how many years of life people would be willing to give up to live without a health condition or disability.

The psychological analogue to quality of life is valuation of life. M. Powell Lawton raised this issue directly by examining psychological factors involved in people's reports of willingness to live in impaired states of health or with poor quality of life. Valuation of life (VOL) is "the extent to which the person is attached to his or her present life, for reasons related to a sense not only of enjoyment and absence of distress, but also hope, futurity, purpose, meaningfulness, persistence, and self-efficacy." VOL can be measured by reports of hope, the sense that life has meaning, and continued commitment to personal projects, that is, goal-driven activity. Valuation of life is an independent correlate of the wish to live even when we adjust for many factors associated with the wish to live, such as health state, cognitive capacity, mental health, perceived quality of life, and personal mastery. Valuation of life is a significant independent correlate of the wish to live under a great range of severe health limitations, including states of mobility impairment and severe pain, but not in the case of dementia or nursing home residence. It may be that perceived meaningfulness and purpose in life do not lead to the wish to live at any cost.

However it is measured, health-related QOL declines with age. This is a central, inescapable consequence of the increased prevalence of chronic disease with greater age and the effects of senescent changes in many physiologic domains. Older people adjust their daily lives to accommodate these decrements, and adjustment strategies may reduce the effects of such decrements on health-related QOL. Still, cross-sectional studies show strong declines in health-related QOL with increasing age. Valuation of life may not show so clear a pattern, but there is limited data on VOL over the life course. Investigations in this area will be important to help clarify decision-making at the end of life. A key issue is whether the wish for a shorter life is an expression of discouragement based on depression, or whether it is an expression of discouragement based on a judgment that life no longer has intrinsic value because impaired health does not allow meaning, purpose, or desired personal projects.

In contrast to health-related QOL, environment-related QOL may remain high throughout life and may even improve with greater age. With retirement, for example, older people have greater leisure time; and with children gone, houses paid for, and successful invest-ments, they may have greater disposable income as well. As a result, older people have increased opportunities to develop interests and create satisfying environments. These freedoms and opportunities counterbalance declines in health-related QOL and may be responsible for the great resiliency older people show in the face of declining health.

CONCLUSION

This chapter has described how psychosocial factors are critical contributors to the health and quality of life of older individuals. The chapter has focused on those factors that appear to be most promising in terms of explaining variability in health outcomes using a broad conceptual model that shows how psychosocial factors sequentially contribute to behaviors and biological processes linked to illness and quality of life. Although there is still much work to be done, one of the significant advances of the last decade is research showing how psychosocial factors get under the skin to affect the physiology and functioning of the organism. Continued advances in mind–body science along these lines will further enhance understating of the relationships between biology and psychology and will provide new opportunities for intervention.

A second theme of this chapter is the remarkable resilience of older individuals. Despite significant declines in multiple functional domains in late life, most older individuals adapt well to the challenges they face and maintain a high quality of life. This strength reflects finely tuned adaptive mechanisms that maximize the ability to cope with major life challenges.

A third and final theme is the importance of viewing aging in a life course context. No one is born old, and to be old means that one has accumulated experience, knowledge, social relationships, as well as physiological vulnerabilities. Understanding old age requires that we pay close attention to these factors in order to unravel the complexities of how life experiences contribute to functioning and development in late life.

FURTHER READING

Albert SM, Castillo-Castenada C, Sano M, et al. Quality of life in patients with Alzheimer's disease as reported by patient proxies. *J Am Geriatrics Soc.* 1996;44:1342–1347.

Albert SM, Logsdon RG, eds. *Assessing Quality of Life in Alzheimer's Disease.* New York, New York: Springer; 2000.

Aldwin CM, Park CL, Spiro AS. III, eds. *Handbook of Health Psychology and Aging.* New York, New York: Guilford Press; 2007.

Carstensen LL, Mikels JA, Mather M. Aging and the intersection of cognition, motivation and emotion. In: Birren J, Schaie, KW, eds. *Handbook of the Psychology of Aging,* 6th ed. San Diego, CA: Academic Press; 2006.

Cohen S. Social relationships and health. *Am Psychol.* 2004;59:676–684.

Cohen S, Pressman SD. Positive affect and health. *Curr Dir Psychol Sci.* 2006;15(3): 122–125.

Diener E, Seligman MEP. Beyond money: toward an economy of well being. *Psychol Sci Public Interest.* 2004;5:1–31.

Epel E, Burke HM, Adler N, Wolkowitz O, Sidney S, Seeman T. Socio-economic status and the anbolic/catabolic neuroendocrine balance. *Ann Behav Med.* 2006;31:50–80.

Jaeschke R, Singer J, Guyatt GH. Measurement of health status: ascertaining the minimal clinically important difference. *Control Clin Trial.* 1989;10: 407–415.

Lawton MP. A multidimensional view of quality of life in frail elders. In: Birren JE, ed. *The Concept and Measurement of Quality of Life in the Frail Elderly.* San Diego, CA: Academic Press; 1991.

Lawton MP, DeVoe MR, Parmelee P. Relationship of events and affect in the daily life of an elderly population. *Psychol Aging.* 1995;10(3):469–477.

Lawton MP, Kleban MH, Dean J. Affect and age: cross-sectional comparisons of structure and prevalence. *Psychol Aging.* 1993;8(2):165–175.

Lawton MP, Moss M, Hoffman C, Grant R, Ten Have T, Kleban MH. Health, valuation of life, and the wish to live. *Gerontologist.* 1999;39:406–416.

Lawton MP, Moss MS, Winter L, Hoffman C. Motivation in later life: personal projects and well-being. *Psychol Aging.* 2002;17(4):539–547.

Levine C, ed. *Family Caregivers on the Job: Moving Beyond ADLs and IADLs.* New York, New York: United Hospital Fund; 2004.

Penninx BW, van Tilburg T, Kriegsman DM, Deeg DJ, van Eijk JT. Effects of social support and personal coping resources on mortality in older age: the Longitudinal Aging Study Amsterdam. *Am J Epidemiol.* 1997;146(6):510–519.

Schulz R, Drayer RA, Rollman BL. Depression as a risk factor for non-suicide mortality in the elderly. *Biol Psychiatr.* 2002;52(3):205–225.

Schulz R, Heckhausen J. A life-span model of successful aging. *Am Psychol.* 1996;51:702–714.

Vitaliano PP, Zhang J, Scanlan JM. Is caregiving hazardous to one's physical health?: a meta-analysis. *Psychol Bull.* 2003;129(6):946–972.

Ware JF, Stewart AL. *Measuring Function and Well-Being.* Cambridge, MA: Harvard University Press; 1992.

General Principles of Pharmacology

Sarah N. Hilmer ■ *Gary A. Ford*

INTRODUCTION

The use of drug therapy in elderly individuals has increased substantially in recent years driven by increased numbers of older adults, the results of clinical trials including older adults, and a less nihilistic approach to therapy in this age group. As a consequence, the majority of drug therapy is prescribed to older adults. An understanding of the principles of pharmacology and appropriate application to the individual older person is necessary for all those who develop, regulate, and prescribe and monitor drug therapies in older adults. A further challenge is the need to optimally individualise drug therapy in older adults who constitute a very heterogeneous group ranging from healthy, fit community dwelling individuals taking no regular medication to frail institutionalized individuals with multiple comorbidities and polypharmacy.

When prescribing for older patients, it is important to consider pharmacokinetic and pharmacodynamic changes observed in normal aging, the likely effects of the individual's genetics and intercurrent disease, as well as evidence for therapeutic efficacy, and safety and the patient's total exposure to medications. In this chapter, we begin by describing the changes in pharmacokinetics and pharmacodynamics associated with aging and frailty. We then discuss adverse drug reactions and relevant issues in drug development, regulation, and pharmacoeconomics.

PHARMACOKINETICS

Pharmacokinetic processes determine the relationship between drug input (dose, dosage form, frequency, route of administration) and the concentration of drug achieved over time. The major components of pharmacokinetics are bioavailability, distribution, and clearance. While changes in many of these parameters have been described with aging, the most consistent and marked change in pharmacokinetics in older adults is the increase in interindividual variability.

Bioavailability

Bioavailability (F) is the proportion of drug reaching the systemic circulation after administration. Bioavailability depends on the route of administration, the chemical properties of the drug, the absorption of the drug, and the amount of drug that is cleared (first pass loss) before reaching the systemic circulation. Bioavailability of drugs administered by the intravascular route is 100% by definition, and is not affected by aging. Factors that influence bioavailability of medications for common extravascular routes of administration, and any known changes that occur with aging, are shown in Table 8-1. Bioavailability is the ratio of the area under the concentration–time curve (AUC) when the drug is given extravascularly to that when it is given intravenously (Figure 8-1). Bioavailability (F) is expressed as a fraction or percentage:

$$\text{Bioavailability } (F) = \frac{\text{AUC}_{\text{ev}}}{\text{AUC}_{\text{iv}}}.$$

The bioavailability of a drug given extravascularly can vary with age. As shown in Figure 8-1, with aging, absorption is often slower so the maximal plasma concentration is reached later (longer T_{max}) and is lower (lower C_{max}). However, the extent of absorption is usually complete in older adults so the area under the curve (bioavailability) is not affected. Drugs that require an acidic environment for absorption, such as ketoconazole, ampicillin, and iron, may have a reduced extent of absorption in the 5% to 10% of older adults with age-related hypochlorhydria secondary to atrophic gastritis, and in those taking medications that raise gastric pH such as H2-antagonists and proton pump inhibitors. In the case of oral administration where the medication undergoes first pass metabolism, which is often decreased in older adults, the area under the curve (bioavailability) may be increased.

TABLE 8-1

Factors Associated with Bioavailability of Drugs Administered Through Common Extravascular Routes and Description of Age-Related Changes

ROUTE	PROPERTIES OF DRUG	ABSORPTION Description	ABSORPTION Age-Related Changes	FIRST PASS CLEARANCE Description	FIRST PASS CLEARANCE Age-Related Changes
Oral	Particle size formulation Lipid solubility Ionization	Gut lumen decomposition Passive absorption Active transport (e.g., iron, vitamin B-12) Gut wall P-glycoprotein transports drugs back into lumen	Gastric pH may be less acidic, altering ionisation Complete but slower – Increased by longer gastrointestinal transit time and possible increase in permeability of epithelium – Decreased by reduced perfusion Probably decreased Not known	Gut wall CYP450 metabolism Hepatic metabolism	Not known Reduced 30–50%
Sublingual	Particle size Lipid solubility Potency	Rapid into blood vessels at base of tongue	Not known ?Reduced perfusion	Nil	
Rectal (local and systemic action)	Lipid solubility Ionisation	Varies with rectal contents	Not known ?Reduced perfusion	Nil	
Subcutaneous Injection	Particle size (small particles absorbed by capillaries, large particles absorbed by lymphatics) Protein complex pH Use of vasoconstrictors	Slow	Not known ?Reduced perfusion ?Changes to lymphatics	Nil ?Proteolysis of protein drugs in lymph nodes	
Intramuscular Injection	Lipid solubility Particle size (small particles absorbed by capillaries, large particles absorbed by lymphatics)	Slow (faster than subcutaneous due to better perfusion)	Not known ?Reduced perfusion ?Changes to lymphatics	Nil ?Proteolysis of protein drugs in lymph nodes	
Percutaneous	Lipid solubility	Slow Heat dependent	Not known ?Reduced perfusion	Nil	
Intranasal (local and systemic)	Lipid solubility	Variable	Not known ?Reduced perfusion	Nil	
Inhaled (local and systemic)	Particle size – Powders – Aerosol solutions inhaler (type and how used) Gases: gas partition coefficient (blood)	Minimal systemic absorption	Not known ?Effects of reduced alveolar area, low-grade inflammation, ventilation/perfusion mismatch, decreased diffusion and transport across alveolar capillary membrane	Lung metabolism and clearance	Not known
Ophthalmic (topical)	Formulation: drops, suspensions, ointments	Minimal (drainage through nasolacrimal canal)	Not known	Nil	

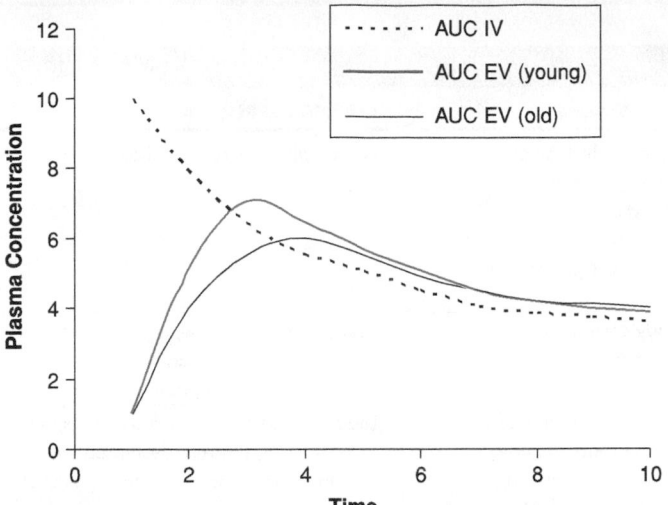

FIGURE 8-1. Theoretical plasma concentration–time curves for the same drug given intravascularly (IV) and extravascularly (EV). The bioavailability is the ratio of the area under the curve (AUC) for the EV route to the AUC for the IV route. The intravascular AUC is not affected by age. With aging, the extravascular curve shows delayed and lower maximal plasma concentration and AUC may be increased for drugs that undergo first pass hepatic metabolism.

Bioavailability defines the dose adjustment between intravascular and extravascular drug administration. Lower bioavailability drugs require higher doses when given extravascularly than intravascularly. Reduced first pass hepatic metabolism in older adults results in a lower dose requirement for oral active drugs that undergo hepatic clearance. Examples of prodrugs, which are administered as inactive compounds that must be metabolized into the active drug, include codeine, propranolol, enalopril, perindopril, and simvastatin. In older adults, there may be a higher dose requirement for prodrugs to obtain the same AUC for the active drug (metabolite) as in a young person.

The effects of aging on bioavailability of modified release oral formulations are not known. Modified release oral formulations tend be released for absorption lower in the gastrointestinal tract. In young adults, cytochrome P450 3A4 (CYP 3A4) has the highest content in the duodenum, followed by the jejunum, ileum, and colon. Drugs released lower in the gastrointestinal tract undergo less gut wall metabolism, increasing their bioavailability. Expression of CYP 3A4 in the gut wall has not been studied in aging. The activity of the transporter, P-glycoprotein (P-gp), which pumps drugs from the enterocytes back into the gut lumen, has its highest concentration in the ileum, followed by the colon, jejunum, and duodenum. Therefore, modified release formulations, released lower in the gastrointestinal tract, may undergo less P-gp efflux back into the gut lumen, increasing their absorption. There is no change in expression of P-gp in intestinal microsomes in aged rats; it is not known how intestinal wall transporter activity varies with age in humans. The combination of modified release medications, the possibility of less gut wall metabolism lower in the gastrointestinal tract and slower transit time with aging may increase drug bioavailability in older adults, although the different formulations of modified release medications may be differentially affected by age. Some formulations rely on pH to dissolve an external coat and may be affected by higher gastrointestinal pH in some older adults. Others have a

constant drug delivery rate independent of pH or gastrointestinal motility and may be less affected by changes of aging.

Distribution

Volume of distribution (V_d) is the apparent volume that the drug distributes into to achieve the plasma concentration (C_p). V_d is not a real anatomical volume. V_d may exceed the total real volume of the human body when there is significant binding to tissues. V_d is expressed by the equation:

$$V_d = \frac{\text{Amount of drug in body}}{C_p}.$$

The amount of drug in the body is known immediately after a known dose of the drug has been given intravenously, before it can be eliminated. Therefore, V_d can be calculated in humans from the dose given intravenously and the C_p immediately after administration.

The volume of distribution of a drug depends on plasma protein binding, lipid to water partition coefficient, tissue binding properties, and transporters. The main determinant of volume of distribution is the ratio of the strength of binding to plasma proteins to the strength of binding in tissues. Drugs that are bound more strongly to plasma proteins have a smaller V_d, and those that are bound more strongly to tissues have a larger V_d. Some examples include heparin and warfarin, which are highly plasma protein bound, and have V_d of 5 and 8 L, respectively, similar to blood volume. Digoxin is water-soluble but highly bound to muscle, with a V_d of 15 L. Imipramine is lipid soluble and has a V_d of 2100 L, which is far greater than the 42 L real volume of a 70 kg human. Alendronate adheres strongly to the bone surface, and has a V_d of 2580 L. The major determinants of V_d and how they are affected by normal aging are shown in Table 8-2.

The immediate volume of distribution is blood volume. Then the drug is distributed from the blood into various tissues at a rate that depends on the perfusion of the tissue, the ease with which the drug can pass through lipid membranes of cells and any active transport. Membrane permeability and passive transport may increase with age and malnutrition. The effects of aging on active transport is not well documented in humans, and in rats, varies between tissues, with an increase in P-glycoprotein expression and activity in the liver and lymphocytes, but not in the intestine or endothelium, with aging. With aging, the volume of distribution of verapamil (a substrate of P-glycoprotein) in the brain increases, consistent with dysfunction of the blood–brain barrier. Tissue perfusion may decrease with aging, which may slow distribution, particularly to less highly perfused tissues such as muscle and fat. The rate of distribution to or from the site of action of a drug may determine the onset or offset of drug effects.

The volume of distribution determines the loading dose of a drug. The loading dose is the dose required to achieve the desired C_p as soon as possible, and is calculated with the equation:

$$\text{Loading dose} = \text{Desired } C_p \times V_p$$

There may be small changes in loading dose in older adults due to the changes in V_d described above. For example, the volume of distribution of digoxin decreases from approximately 7 to 6 L/kg with aging, probably due to reduced muscle mass and reduced binding of digoxin to muscle. Therefore, loading dose should decrease by approximately 15%.

TABLE 8-2

Factors That Determine Volume of Distribution: Effects of Aging

FACTOR	EFFECT ON V_d	AGE-RELATED CHANGES	CLINICAL APPLICATION
Plasma protein binding	Highly protein bound drugs are generally less able to cross membranes and have smaller Vd	Decreased albumin which binds acidic drugs, e.g., warfarin, NSAIDs, phenytoin. Increased α1-acid glycoprotein which binds basic drugs, e.g., verapamil, propranolol.	Not usually clinically significant.
Tissue binding properties	Drugs which are tightly bound to tissues have large Vd	Changes in body composition (sarcopenia, increased adiposity) may affect Vd.	Drugs bound to muscle, e.g., digoxin, have decreased Vd with aging. Therefore decreased loading dose required.
Lipid: water coefficient	Lipid soluble drugs can pass through lipid membranes of cells more easily and have higher Vd than water soluble drugs	Relative increase in proportion of body fat and decrease in body water (muscle mass). Therefore, higher Vd for lipid soluble drugs and lower Vd for water soluble drugs with aging.	Loading dose of water soluble drugs, e.g., gentamicin, digoxin, decreased with aging to avoid toxicity from high initial Cp.
Transporters	Passive facilitated diffusion (move drug in same direction as concentration gradient). Active transport (use ATP to move drug against concentration gradient).	Unknown.	Drug interactions may occur at level of transporters. Passive transporters include the Organic Anion Transport Proteins (OAT-P) for benzyl penicillin, digoxin, and pravastatin. Active transporters include MDR1 (P-gp) for many cationic or neutral drugs, e.g., digoxin, macrolide antibiotics, verapamil.

Clearance

Clearance is the rate of elimination of a drug from the body. Clearance, CL, from each organ of elimination can be defined by the equation:

$$CL = Q \times E,$$

where Q is the flow rate to the organ and E is the extraction ratio. Total body clearance is the sum of the drug clearances by each organ, and can be expressed as

$$CL_{total} = CL_{hepatic} + CL_{renal} + CL_{other}.$$

Clinically, the clearance affects the maintenance dose of medications.

Hepatic Drug Clearance

Removal of a drug by the liver depends on portal and arterial hepatic blood flow and elimination by metabolism and/or secretion into the bile. The processes involved in hepatic clearance are shown in Figure 8-2 and changes in normal aging are shown in Table 8-3. Hepatic clearance of highly extracted substrates is determined mostly by hepatic blood flow and is known as flow-limited metabolism. This is consistently reduced in older adults. Hepatic clearance of poorly extracted substrates is described as capacity-limited metabolism because the intrinsic clearance (metabolising capacity) is the rate-limiting step and is less affected by old age. Protein binding may also affect the clearance of poorly extracted substrates. The effects of normal aging on flow-limited and capacity-limited hepatic clearance are shown in Figure 8-3.

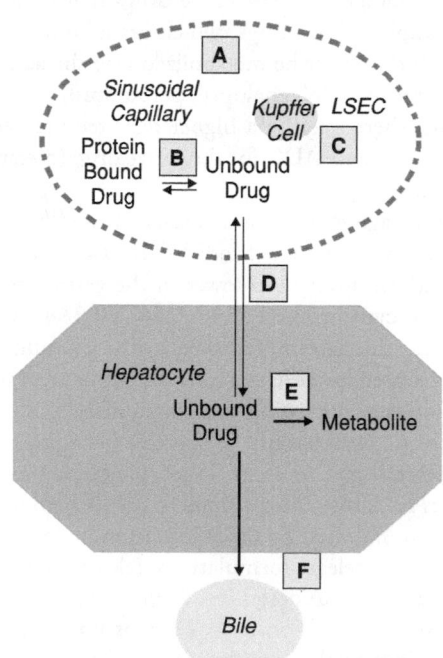

FIGURE 8-2. The processes involved in hepatic clearance. A, blood flow; B, protein binding; C, scavenger cells (Kupffer and Liver sinusoidal endothelial cells, LSECs); D, transfer across the LSECs and the hepatocyte apical membrane; E, metabolism; F, transport into bile ductule. *Adapted from Tozer TN, Rowland M. Introduction to Pharmacokinetics and Pharmacodynamics: The Quantitative Basis of Drug Therapy. Lippincott Williams and Wilkins; 2006, Fig 5–17.*

TABLE 8-3

Changes in Hepatic Clearance with Aging

PROCESS OF HEPATIC CLEARANCE	DESCRIPTION	AGE-RELATED CHANGES	CLINICAL APPLICATION
Hepatic blood flow	Portal venous flow (~80%) and hepatic arterial flow (~20%)	Decreases by 30–50%	Reduced clearance by 30–50% of high extraction ratio drugs, e.g., morphine and verapamil. Less impact on low extraction ratio drugs, e.g., carbamazepine, warfarin, diazepam.
Protein binding	Only free drug is cleared. Protein binding affected by disease and competition from other drugs.	Decreased albumin: acidic drugs have higher fraction unbound and increased hepatic clearance. Increased α1-acid glycoprotein: basic drugs have lower fraction unbound and decreased hepatic clearance.	Only significant for drugs that are highly protein bound (>90%) with low hepatic extraction ratios, e.g., warfarin, phenytoin, diazepam.
Scavenger cells	Kupffer cells scavenge large protein drugs. Liver sinusoidal endothelial cells (LSECs) may scavenge smaller particles.	Possible reduction in scavenger function (in animal studies).	Not known. May reduce hepatic clearance.
Transfer into hepatocyte	Transfer across the LSECs and the hepatocyte apical membrane by passive or active transport.	Structural changes in LSECs and the space of Disse may reduce transfer. Changes in hepatocyte membrane transport not known.	Not known. May reduce hepatic clearance.
Metabolism	Biotransformation to more hydrophilic metabolites that may be equally, less or more active than parent drug	Reduced phase I metabolism in vivo in normal aging by 30–50%. Phase II metabolism appears to be maintained in healthy aging, reduced in frail aged.	Probably preserved clearance of drugs that undergo capacity-limited phase II metabolism in healthy aging, e.g., temazepam, salicylic acid.
Transfer into bile ductule	Active transport into bile canaliculi. Bile enters small intestine and drug or metabolite reabsorbed (enterohepatic cycle) or excreted in faeces.	Unknown. In aged rodents, increased biliary P-glycoprotein expression and function.	Unknown.

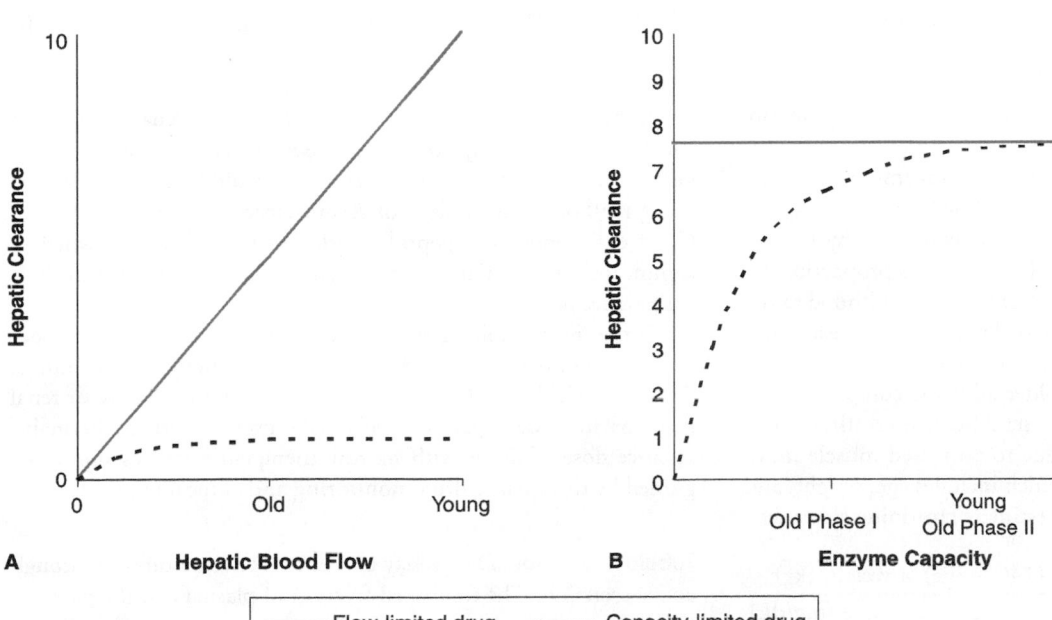

FIGURE 8-3. The effects of normal aging on hepatic drug clearance. With aging, hepatic blood flow is reduced by approximately 50%, which is associated with a 50% reduction in clearance of flow-limited drugs, but has little effect on clearance of capacity-limited drugs (A). In normal aging, phase I metabolism is reduced, which reduces hepatic clearance of capacity-limited drugs metabolized by these enzymes, while phase II metabolism is probably preserved, although it may be reduced in frailty. Changes in enzyme capacity do not affect the clearance of flow-limited drugs (B).

Flow-limited drug   - - - - Capacity-limited drug

TABLE 8-4

Changes in Renal Drug Clearance with Aging

PROCESS OF RENAL CLEARANCE	EFFECTS OF AGE	CLINICAL APPLICATION	EXAMPLE
Glomerular filtration	Decreased GFR, extent unclear, ~10–40%	Estimates used to adjust maintenance doses of drugs for renal impairment	Gentamicin clearance correlates with Cockcroft-Gault estimates of creatinine clearance.
Tubular secretion (active)	Decreased	Reduction in renal clearance may be greater than reduction in GFR.	Ratio of procainamide clearance to creatinine clearance decreases with aging.
		With polypharmacy, increase risk of drug-drug interactions through competition for transporters.	Digoxin excreted by passive glomerular filtration and active tubular secretion. Serum digoxin levels increase with number of concurrent P-gp inhibitors, e.g., verapamil, erythromycin, amiodarone, spironolactone, atorvastatin.
Tubular reabsorption (passive)	Unknown	If impaired, would reduce the effect of reduced glomerular filtration on clearance.	Changes in clearance of lithium, which, like sodium, is freely filtered at glomerulus and 80% reabsorbed in the proximal tubule, consistent with changes in GFR with aging.

Normal aging is only one of many factors that may influence hepatic clearance. For example, the hepatic clearance of flow-limited drugs may be decreased by diseases that reduce hepatic blood flow, such as heart failure, while hepatic clearance of capacity-limited drugs may be altered by other drugs that induce or block hepatic enzymes or by genetic polymorphisms.

Renal Clearance

The majority of drug elimination occurs through the kidneys. In the kidneys, drugs and their metabolites may undergo glomerular filtration, tubular secretion, and tubular reabsorption. These processes are summarized, with descriptions of any known age-related changes and relevant examples in Table 8-4.

Glomerular Filtration At the glomerulus, drugs and their metabolites are passively filtered from the afferent arterioles through the glomerular membrane to produce an ultrafiltrate of plasma within the capsular space of the glomerulus. Plasma proteins and cells are too large to cross the glomerular membrane so only free drug enters the capsular space of the glomerulus. The glomerular filtration rate (GFR) is the total volume of glomerular filtrate produced per unit time by all nephrons, and is approximately 120 mL/min in a young, healthy person (~10% of total renal blood flow). In normal aging, recent estimates suggest that GFR is moderately reduced by 15% to 40%. Effective renal plasma flow (ERPF) decreases proportionally more than GFR, by ~10% per decade from young adulthood to the age of 80 years. Older adults have increased renal vascular resistance, with impaired relaxation in response to vasodilators.

Estimation of renal function in older adults is complicated by confounders. Serum creatinine is not useful because creatinine production is reduced in older adults, due to decreased muscle mass. The Cockcroft-Gault equation [6], which includes age, weight, and serum creatinine, is used clinically to estimate creatinine clearance:

$$\text{Creatinine clearance (mL/min)} = \frac{(140 - \text{age}) \times \text{weight (kg)}}{72 \times \text{serum creatinine (mg/dL)}}$$
$$\times \ 0.85 \ \text{for females.}$$

Most dosing guidelines use the Cockcroft-Gault equation to adjust doses of renally excreted drugs with narrow therapeutic indices, such as gentamicin and low-molecular weight heparin, for renal function. However, the Cockcroft-Gault equation was derived from observational data from males receiving routine medical care for a range of illnesses, and may underestimate renal function in normal aging. Much of the age-related decline in renal function may be related to disease, particularly hypertension, atherosclerosis, and heart failure, rather than normal aging.

Recently, an equation to estimate the GFR, the modification of diet in renal disease (MDRD) equation, has been introduced to clinical practice. This equation has not been validated for extremes of age or dose adjustment. Unadjusted for body surface area, in the presence of the reduced height and weight observed in normal aging, the MDRD is likely to overestimate renal clearance in older adults. A study of elderly patients in long-term care demonstrated that only one-third of patients were classified in the same stage of renal impairment by both methods, with average MDRD estimates 20 mL/min/1.73 m² higher than those determined using Cockcroft-Gault, suggesting that the methods are not interchangeable for determining drug dose. Further validation studies are required to determine the best method for clinically determining renal impairment for the purposes of adjusting drug doses. Recently, it has been suggested that renal function in older adults could be better estimated using methods independent of serum creatinine, such as Cystatin C, an endogenous polypeptide marker of renal function, which is significantly elevated in older adults. The role of this marker in clinical practice is under investigation.

Currently available methods to estimate renal function in older adults are not reliable, particularly in frail or acutely ill older adults. While the Cockcroft-Gault equation can give an estimate of renal function for dose adjustment of renally excreted drugs, the maintenance dose of drugs with narrow therapeutic indices should be guided by therapeutic drug monitoring and clinical response.

Tubular Secretion Drugs may also enter the renal tubules through active secretion. The unfiltered fraction of plasma and the particles too large to enter the glomerular filtrate pass through the efferent arterioles to the vessels supplying the renal tubules. The majority of tubular secretion occurs in the proximal convoluted tubule and relies on active transport by specific pumps for anions and cations. Drugs bound to proteins or cells can undergo tubular secretion, but not glomerular filtration. These pumps are saturable and drugs may compete for transport into the renal tubule. There is a reduction in tubular secretion with aging to a similar and possibly greater extent than GFR.

Tubular Reabsorption Drugs that have been filtered at the glomerulus or secreted in the proximal convoluted tubule may be passively reabsorbed down the concentration gradient from the tubular fluid in the proximal and distal tubules. Reabsorption occurs for lipid-soluble drugs that are not ionized, and therefore may be influenced by the pH of the tubular fluid. Reabsorption is inversely related to urine flow rate. Changes in tubular reabsorption with aging are not well described. Proximal tubule functions are generally preserved in healthy aging, with near normal production of erythropoietin and normal sodium reabsorption in the proximal tubules. However, overall tubular function is decreased in the elderly, with impaired ability to concentrate or dilute urine maximally.

Nonhepatic, Nonrenal Clearance

Drug metabolism through cytochrome P450 and via conjugation can occur at many sites outside the liver. The effect of intestinal cytochrome P450 on bioavailability has been discussed in the section on bioavailability and in Table 8-1. Proteases and peptidases are found throughout the body and metabolise polypeptide drugs such as insulin, erythropoietin, and interferon. Circulating esterases also play a role in drug metabolism, including acetyl cholinesterase and carbonic anhydrase. Age-related changes in clearance outside the liver and kidney are not known.

Half-Life

Half-life ($t_{1/2}$) is the time taken to halve the amount of drug in the body (or the plasma concentration of the drug). Half-life depends on volume of distribution (V_d) and clearance (CL), and is calculated using the following equation:

$$t_{1/2} = \frac{0.693 \times V_d}{CL}.$$

The constant, 0.693, is the natural logarithm of 0.5.

A decrease in clearance, which is seen commonly with aging, results in an increase in half-life. An increase in volume of distribution, which occurs with lipid-soluble drugs with aging, would also result in an increase in half-life. Higher volume of distribution indicates that the drug is more concentrated in the tissues than the blood. Hepatic and renal clearance act on drug in the blood, so a smaller proportion of drug is eliminated with a larger volume of distribution. The theoretical effects of aging on half-life are shown in Figure 8-4.

The half-life determines the time course of drug accumulation and elimination, and the choice of dose interval. When a drug is started, plasma concentration reaches >90% of steady state after approximately four half-lives. When a drug that was at steady state is stopped, plasma concentration reaches <10% of steady state after approximately four half-lives. Dose interval is usually similar to half-life to maintain steady state.

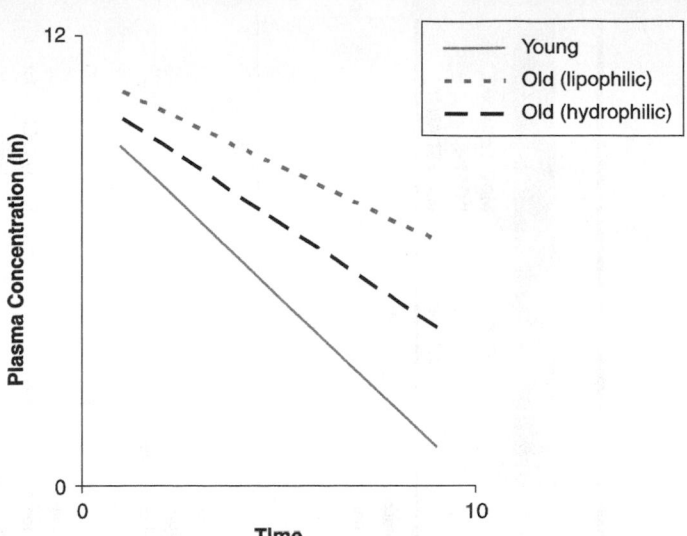

FIGURE 8-4. The theoretical effects of aging on half-life. The decrease in clearance with aging prolongs half-life. For lipid-soluble drugs, the increase in volume of distribution prolongs half-life further. For water-soluble drugs, the decrease in volume of distribution reduces half-life, but in most cases, the size of the effect of aging on volume of distribution is smaller than the effect on clearance, resulting in an overall increase in half-life compared to young subjects.

Changes in half-life with age will affect how long the drug takes to accumulate, to be eliminated, and the dosing interval of the drug. The increase in half-life that is observed for many drugs with aging means that it will take longer for drugs to reach steady state, longer to be eliminated after they are ceased, and dosing intervals may need to be increased.

Summary of Pharmacokinetic Changes with Aging

An increase in interindividual variability is the main change in pharmacokinetics with aging. Of the pharmacokinetic changes seen in normal aging, reduced hepatic and renal clearance are generally the most significant, and these affect maintenance dose and dosing interval. The changes in volume of distribution are smaller, and affect the half-life of drugs (to a lesser extent than the changes in clearance do) and the loading dose. The main changes in bioavailability with aging result from reduced first pass metabolism, with increased bioavailability of drugs that undergo significant first pass hepatic metabolism and decreased activation of prodrugs. Some important examples of age-related changes in pharmacokinetics and pharmacodynamics are shown in Table 8-5.

PHARMACODYNAMICS

Pharmacodynamics describes the effects of drugs on tissues and organs often described as "what the drug does to the body." Although the responses to a given weight-adjusted drug dose may be found to be altered in older healthy volunteers and patients, pharmacokinetic changes may account for most of the changes seen. Even when correcting for alterations in plasma drug concentrations, other modulatory neurohumoral influences may account for the altered response rather than any primary age-related sensitivity in cellular response of the relevant drug receptor.

TABLE 8-5

Changes in Pharmacokinetics and Pharmacodynamics with Aging and Suggested Dose Adjustments for Older Patients

THERAPEUTIC CLASS	MEDICATION	PHARMACOKINETICS			CHANGES IN NORMAL AGING				LOADING DOSE ADJUSTMENT	MAINTENANCE DOSE ADJUSTMENT
		Protein binding % (L, <50; M, 50–90; H, >90)	Volume of distribution L/kg (L, low, ≤0.55; M, 0.55–1.0; H, high, >1.0)	Route of elimination	Volume of distribution	Clearance	Half Life	Pharmacodynamics		
Antimicrobial	Erythromycin	M	M	Hepatic (CYP3A+ P-gp)	↔	↓	↑	No change in action of medications on microbes.	↔	↓
	Gentamicin	L	L	Renal	↔	↓, ↔	↑, ↔		↔	↓ By CrCl
	Metronidazole	L	M	Hepatic (CYP + gluc)	Slight ↓	?↓, ↔	?, ↔	Adaptive immune response ↓ with aging.	?, ↔	?, ↔, ↓
	Penicillin	M	L	Renal (tubular secretion)	?	?	?		?, ↔	?, ↓by CrCl, ↔ for efficacy
	Trimethoprim	L	H	Renal (acetylation)	↔	↓	↑		?, ↔	↓
	Vancomycin	L	L	Renal	?	↓	↑		↔	↓by CrCl
Cardiovascular	Amiodarone	H	H	Hepatic (CYP 2C, 3A)	?	↔	↔	? ↑ Sensitivity to therapeutic and toxic effects	→	→
	Digoxin	L	L	Renal	→	→	↑	? ↑ Sensitivity	→	↓by CrCl
	Furosemide	H	L	Hepatic, Renal	?↓, ↔	→	↑	Delayed response to diuretics due to reduced renal clearance.	?, ↔	→
	Metoprolol	L	H	Hepatic (CYP2D6)	?	↑, ↔	↑, ↔	↓responsiveness of beta receptors. Highly variable.	↔, →	↔
	Dihydropyridone Calcium Channel Antagonists	H	M	Hepatic (CYP3A)	↔	→	↑	Direct vasodilation intact. ↓reflex sympathetic stimulation.	↔	↓, ↔

Non-dihydropyridine Calcium Channel Antagonists	M (diltiazem); H (verapamil)	H	Hepatic (CYP3A)	↔	↔, ↓	↔, ↑	↑sensitivity sinoatrial node and ↓sensitivity atrio-ventricular node to conduction delay.	↓	↓	↓
ACE inhibitors	Varies between individual drugs	Varies between individual drugs	Renal > Hepatic (many are inactive prodrugs with active metabolites)	↔	↓	↑	↔	↓	↓	↓
Angiotensin II Receptor blockers	H	Varies between individual drugs	Hepatic (some inactive prodrugs with active metabolites)	↔	↔, ↓	↔, ↑	?	↔	↔	↔
Atorvastatin	H	H	Biliary; Hepatic (CYP3A4)	↓	↓	↑	?	?		? ↔, ↓
Antithrombotics										
Aspirin	M-H (decreases with increasing concentration)	L (increases with increasing concentration)	Hepatic, gut wall and plasma esterases	?	?, ↓ amount of plasma aspirin esterase in frailty	?	?	?, ↔	?, ↔	
Clopidogrel	H	L	Hepatic (CYP1A)	?	?	?	↔			
Warfarin	H	L	Hepatic (CYP3A4, 1A2, 2C9)	↔	↓, ↔	↑, ↔	↑	↔	↔	↓
Central nervous system acting drugs										
Phenytoin	H	M	Hepatic (CYP2C)	?	↔	↔	↑sensitivity to therapeutic effects and cardiotoxicity.	↔		↓

(continued)

TABLE 8-5

Changes in Pharmacokinetics and Pharmacodynamics with Aging and Suggested Dose Adjustments for Older Patients *(Continued)*

THERAPEUTIC CLASS	MEDICATION		PHARMACOKINETICS	CHANGES IN NORMAL AGING				LOADING DOSE ADJUSTMENT	MAINTENANCE DOSE ADJUSTMENT
	Amitryptiline	H	Hepatic (CYP3A4, 2C9, 2D6)	↑	↔	↑	↑ sensitivity to anticholinergic adverse effects	↓	↓
	Sertraline	H	Hepatic (CYP2D6)	?	↓	↑	Associated with hyponatremia and ↑ falls risk.	↓	↓
	Venlafaxine	L	Hepatic (CYP2D6)	↔	↓	↔	↑sensitivity to adverse effects.	↓	↓ + by CrCl
	Lithium	L	Renal	?, ↔	↓	↑	↑sensitivity to adverse effects, especially neurotoxicity.	↓	↓
	Diazepam	H	Hepatic	↑	↓	↑	↓EC$_{50}$ for sedation. ↑ risk of falls.	↓	↓
	Zolpidem	M	Hepatic	?	↓	↑	↑sensitivity to adverse effects.	↓	↓
	Haloperidol	H	Hepatic (CYP2D6)	?, ↑	↓	↑	↑sensitivity to adverse effects.	↓	↓
	Levodopa	-	Hepatic	↓	↔	↔	?	↓	↓
Gastrointestinal	Omeprazole	H	Hepatic (CYP2C, 3A)	↓	↓	↓	?	↔	↓, ↔
Endocrine	Estrogen	H	Hepatic (CYP3A4)	↓	↔, ↓	↑	? ↑sensitivity to adverse effects.	↓	↓
	Testosterone	H	Hepatic (CYP2)	?, ↓	↔, ↓	?, ↑	?	↓	↓

Drug								
Levothyroxine	H	H	?	Hepatic	?	?Decreased degradation of thyroxine	?↑ sensitivity to adverse effects	↑
								↓
Metformin	L	L	→	Renal	→	→	?	→
Glipizide	H	L	↔	Hepatic, renal	↔	↔	?↑risk factors for hypogly-caemia in	?, ↔
Rosiglitazone	H	L	↔	Hepatic	↔	↔		↔
Insulin	L	L	?	Hepatic, Renal	?	?	?	?, ↓ by CrCl
Alendronate	M	L	↔	Renal	↔	↔	? older adults	↔, ↓by CrCl
Analgesics								
Paracetamol (acetaminophen)	L	M	↔	Hepatic	↔	↓ (further ↓ in frailty)	?	↔, ?↓
Diclofenac	H	L	?	Hepatic	?	↔	?↑ sensitivity to adverse effects	?↓, ↔
Morphine	L	H	↔	Hepatic, Renal	↔	↔	?↑ sensitivity to therapeutic and toxic effects	?↔, ↓by CrCl

Most drug actions are mediated through interaction of part of the drug molecule with macromolecular components of the organism referred to as receptors. The majority of drug receptors are proteins involved in the regulation of hormones, neurotransmitters, enzymes, or transport processes. Other cellular components can also be drug targets such as nucleic acids in cancer chemotherapy. Many drug receptors are acted upon by and are highly selective for endogenous hormones or neurotransmitters. Drugs are usually either agonists at such receptors, causing activation of the receptor similar to that produced by the endogenous substance or antagonists, blocking the actions of the endogenous neurotransmitter or hormone. Most drug–receptor interactions involve reversible binding but sometimes if there is covalent binding, the interaction may be irreversible. Drug development seeks to identify target receptors that if activated or inhibited are likely to produce beneficial therapeutic effects, a process referred to as target identification. Target validation is the process where therapeutic efficacy is then demonstrated in preclinical and clinical development. In the last 20 years, a multitude of receptors have been identified through molecular cloning of expressed proteins but the biochemical, physiological, and clinical significance of most of these remains unknown. Receptor expression in cells may be modified by disease, aging, and the effect of drugs or endogenous agonists or antagonists.

The way drugs interact in reversible manner with receptors is described using a number of methods through drug receptor theory, with the maximum effect model (E_{max}) being one of the simplest most commonly used. This model assumes that the receptor when occupied by the drug forms a drug–receptor (DR) complex, which produces an effect and that the effect is proportional to the fraction of occupied receptors. The association and disassociation constants of the DR complex are referred to as k_1 and k_2 in the model and the KD (k_2/k_1) describes the equilibrium dissociation constant for the drug–receptor complex:

$$\text{Drug}\,(D) + \text{receptor}\,(R) \underset{k_2}{\overset{k_1}{\rightleftharpoons}} DR \rightarrow \text{effect}.$$

When the treatment effect is expressed against the drug or agonist concentration, a rectangular hyperbolic relationship is seen. Usually drug or agonist concentration is expressed in log terms and a sigmoidal relationship is seen, which can be described by three parameters:; EC_{50}, the concentration of drug at which 50% maximum drug effect occurs; E_{max}, the maximum drug effect, and n the slope of the curve (Figure 8-5). Understanding the dose–response curve is of critical importance in early development of a drug. A low EC_{50} identifies a selective agonist, which is preferred for drugs in development as at higher concentrations all drugs become less selective and act on other receptors and proteins. A high E_{max} identifies a drug with full agonist actions at the receptor. The steepness of the drug–receptor interaction informs the likely rate of change in response as drug concentration is increased. Depending on the individual variability in responsiveness, very steep or shallow slopes may be problematic in producing drugs for easy use in clinical practice. A key issue in drug development and in the treatment of older adults is that the EC_{50} and E_{max} often differ substantially between individuals. Large interindividual variability in response to a drug is not necessarily a problem for a drug with a high therapeutic index, i.e., a large difference between concentrations that produce efficacy and those that produce toxicity. With such drugs, a dose that produces a high concentration that produces near maximal effect in most subjects can be chosen for clinical use. Some antibiotics fall into this

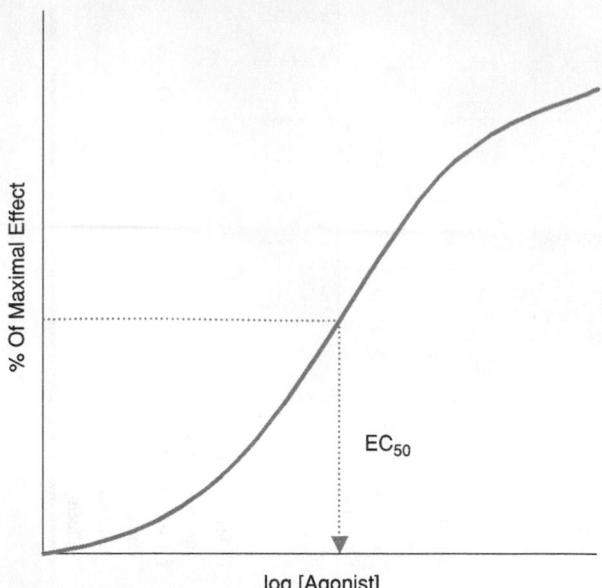

FIGURE 8-5. Sigmoid E_{max} dose–response curve showing the relationship between drug concentration in logarithmic units and the effect. The effect is proportional to the number of receptors occupied. E_{max} defines the maximal effect of the drug, EC_{50} the concentration at which half maximal effect occurs and n the steepness of the slope or response curve.

category. Where there is less margin between a therapeutic and toxic effect, referred to as a low therapeutic index, large interindividual variation make simple dosing regimens problematic as a dose that produces partial efficacy in one patient may produce drug toxicity in another.

Mechanisms of Aging Pharmacodynamic Changes

The underlying mechanisms of age-associated changes in drug responsiveness are not well understood. The β-adrenoceptor signal transduction system has been studied in some detail. This system is relatively well-characterized and aging changes in β-adrenergic responsiveness are well described. The β-adrenoceptor consists of a membrane-bound seven-loop protein with a receptor recognition site on the cell surface that binds to agonists or antagonists (Figure 8-6). The receptor is coupled to a stimulatory G protein. The G protein has three subunits (α, β, and γ) and exists in an active or inactive state. When the receptor binds to an agonist, the G protein undergoes a conformation change, which results in GTP binding to the α-subunit to form an α-GTP complex that activates adenylyl cyclase the catalytic component of the receptor, which converts ATP to cAMP. Increased intracellular cAMP activates protein kinases, which phosphorylate specific substrate proteins that lead to cellular responses such as the opening of ion channels or smooth muscle relaxation.

Main Pharmacodynamic Changes with Aging

Pharmacodynamic changes with aging are less well-characterized or understood than pharmacokinetic changes. The cardiovascular and central nervous systems are the two organs where the major aging changes have been described.

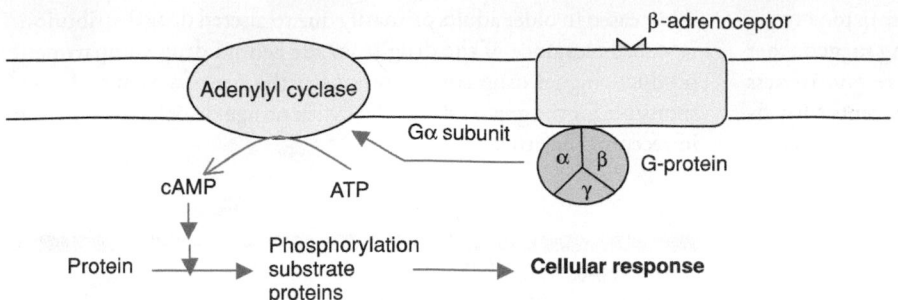

FIGURE 8-6. The β-adrenoceptor adenylyl cyclase complex and signal transduction system. The β-adrenoceptor binds with an agonist drug to undergo conformational change, resulting in the α-subunit of an associated stimulatory G protein binding to GTP. The α-GTP complex activates the catalytic moiety of adenylyl cyclise, resulting in conversion of ATP to cAMP, which activates protein kinases that phosphorylate substrate cellular proteins leading to cellular responses.

Cardiovascular System

The β-adrenergic system has been extensively studied. Aging is associated with a reduction in cardiac and vascular β-adrenergic responsiveness. The heart rate increase in response to intravenous bolus doses of the nonselective β-adrenoceptor agonist is reduced in older adults. Reduced β-adrenoceptor sensitivity has been observed in a number of animal species. Reduced cAMP second messenger response to β-adrenoceptor agonists has also been seen in in vitro studies of isolated human right atrial appendages. The reduced cardiac chronotropic responsiveness of older adults to isoproterenol is only partially due to reduced β-adrenoceptor sensitivity and is an example of the often complex multiple mechanisms underlying altered responsiveness of older adults to drugs. The increased heart rate response to isoproterenol is contributed to by increased efferent cardiac sympathetic activity and reduced parasympathetic activity produced by baroreceptor response to the fall in blood pressure secondary to peripheral vasodilatation mediated by activation of vascular β_2-adrenoceptors. The large age-associated difference in cardiac chronotropic responsiveness disappears when this response is blocked using autonomic blockade with atropine and clonidine. This result can be explained by the well-described reduction in baroreflex sensitivity that occurs with aging.

Older subjects are less sensitive to the hypotensive effect of β-adrenoceptor antagonists. Recent meta-analyses have suggested that β-adrenoceptor antagonists are less effective as initial therapy in the treatment of hypertension in older adults. However, there is little

convincing evidence that this is due to alterations in the affinity of the β-adrenoceptor for antagonists.

The acute blood pressure response to calcium-channel-blockers is more marked in older adults compared to younger adults. This result again can be explained by the reduced baroreflex activation that occurs with aging, rather than any alteration in effects on calcium channels in the peripheral vasculature.

The effect of age on vascular responsiveness has also been extensively studied. The availability of tools such as brachial artery infusion forearm blood flow and hand vein techniques have facilitated detailed study of the vascular system. The age-associated decline in β-adrenergic responsiveness has been demonstrated in both arteries and veins. While impaired β-adrenergic venodilator responses to infused isoproterenol are seen with age, α-adrenergic vasoconstrictor responses to α-adrenergic agonist phenylephrine are preserved (Figure 8-7). The maximal venodilator responsiveness to isoproterenol is reduced while sensitivity to isoproterenol as measured by the group E_{C50} is unchanged. This response was shown to be specific and not a generalized reduced impaired response to vasodilation because responses to some vasodilators including nitroglycerin, an NO donor, and bradykinin are preserved in older adults. An age-associated reduction in responsiveness to histamine, which acts through vascular H_2 receptors, is also found in dorsal hand veins. Both β-adrenergic and histamine venodilator responses are mediated through activation of adenylyl cyclase. In contrast, responses to prostaglandin E_2, which also acts by binding to membrane-bound receptors coupled to adenylyl cyclise are preserved. Prostaglandin

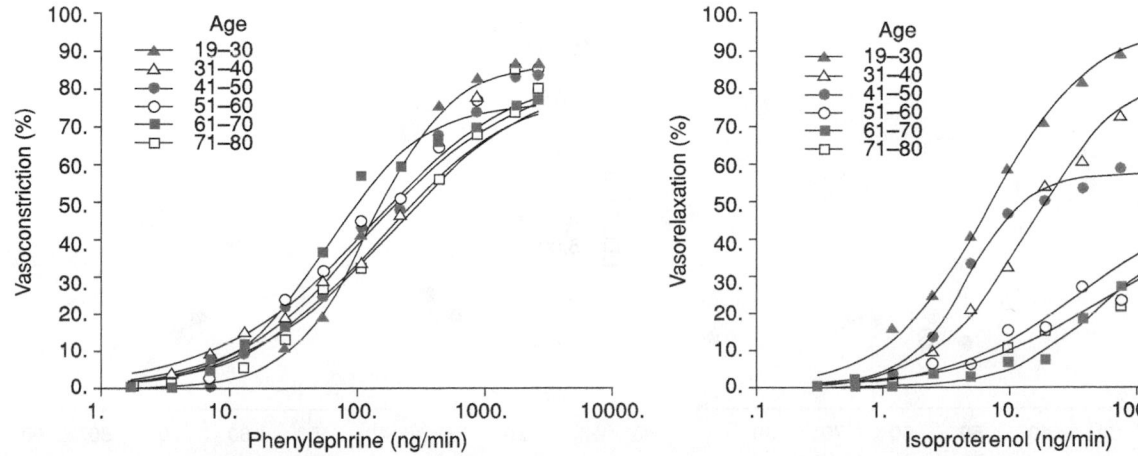

FIGURE 8-7. Human hand vein responsiveness to α_1- and β-adrenergic agonists. Vasoconstrictor effects to the α_1-adrenoceptor agonist phenylephrine and β-adrenoceptor agonist isoproterenol are shown in six healthy volunteer age groups. Age groups (yrs): ▲ 19–30; △ 31–40; ● 41–50; ○ 51–60; ■ 61–70; □ 71–80. (Reproduced from Pan HYM, Hoffman BB, Pershe RA, Blaschke TF. Decline in β-adrenergic receptor mediated vascular relaxation with aging in man. J Pharmacol Exp Ther. 1986;239:802–807.).

E_2 acts through membrane-bound prostanoid receptors to activate adenylyl cyclase and increase cAMP levels. This finding suggests that the reduction in vascular β-adrenergic and histamine responsiveness with aging is due to reduced affinity of the β-adrenoceptor for β-agonists or reduced coupling of the agonist occupied β-adrenoceptor to adenylyl cyclase.

Central Nervous System

Centrally acting drugs are frequently prescribed to older adults. Older adults are more sensitive to the sedative and respiratory depressant effects of benzodiazepines, for example, requiring lower doses of diazepam to produce adequate sedation for endoscopic procedures.

Older individuals experience more cognitive adverse effects with benzodiazepines than young individuals; older individuals with cognitive impairment are particularly vulnerable to these effects. Many studies have demonstrated that benzodiazepines are associated with falls in older adults. Benzodiazepines and other hypnotic drugs increase postural sway, which may at least partially explain this association. Benzodiazepines have also been reported to produce drops in systolic blood pressure. The increased sensitivity of older adults to benzodiazepines is due to three factors. Drug clearance is reduced; there is increased distribution of benzodiazepines to the older person's brain due to changes in lean body mass; and, finally, in animal models, there is increased pharmacodynamic sensitivity of the brain to any given concentration of benzodiazepine. Benzodiazepines bind to a central type benzodiazepine receptor and enhance affinity of the $GABA_A$ receptor to GABA, the main inhibitory neurotransmitter.

Older adults have increased sensitivity to narcotic and anesthetic agents. Brain sensitivity to the opiates fentanyl and alfentanil, measured using changes in electroencephalographic (EEG) frequency spectra, is increased in healthy older adults (Figure 8-8). Pharmacokinetics do not differ with age; animal studies suggest that the increased sensitivity may be due to altered expression of opiate receptors. Sensitivity to the anesthetic induction doses of thiopentone

is increased in older adults primarily due to altered drug distribution. Reduced clearance of the drug from the central drug compartment produces higher drug concentrations at the site of action and is responsible for the greater drug effect with no age-associated alteration in receptor sensitivity.

PHARMACOGENETICS AND PHARMACOGENOMICS

Genetic variation is one of many sources of variability in drug response and may affect any aspect of pharmacology. It is estimated that genetic factors account for between 20% and 95% of variability in drug disposition and drug effects, depending on the individual drug. Inherited sequence variants in genes encoding drug-metabolizing enzymes, drug transporters, or drug targets generally remain stable throughout a person's lifetime. However, gene expression may vary with age and with environmental factors.

Pharmacogenetics is the study of the effects of a drug in relation to a single or defined set of genes. Pharmacogenomics is the study of the effect of a drug in relation to the functions and interactions of all the genes in the genome. Most drug effects are determined by several gene products that modify pharmacokinetics and pharmacodynamics. The aging process itself and the diseases of aging have a variety of complex polygenic causes. Survival to extreme old age may be partly due to genetic variations that affect basic mechanisms of aging, which result in decreased susceptibility to age-associated diseases. Identification of these genetic variations may lead to the discovery of drug targets to enable longevity.

Drug responsiveness in older adults is influenced by genetic factors. Cytochrome P450 2D6 (CYP2D6), which metabolizes many psychoactive, cardiovascular, and analgesic medications, is polymorphic due to autosomal recessive inheritance of CYP2D6-inactivating alleles. Populations can be divided into poor, intermediate, and ultrarapid metabolizers. Age does not appear to affect the population prevalence of genotypes or genetically determined differences between poor, intermediate, and ultrarapid metabolizer phenotypes for

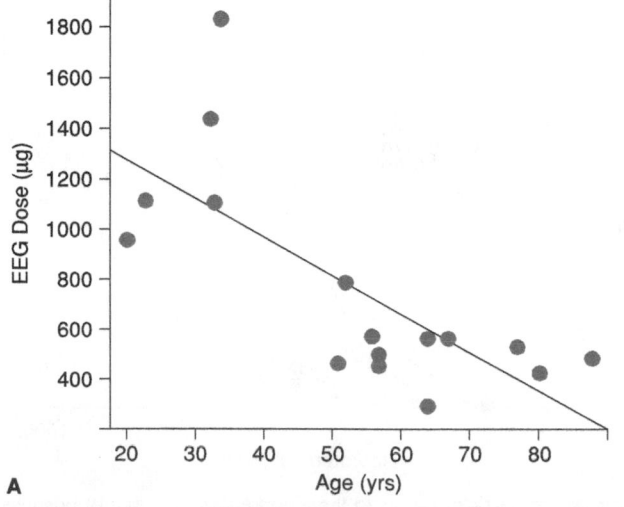

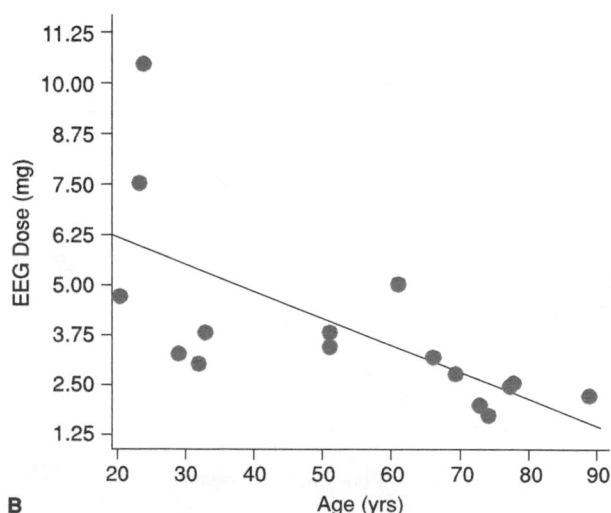

FIGURE 8-8. Sensitivity of health subjects to the anesthetic agents (a) fentanyl and (b) alfentanil. The drug dose that produces half the maximal change IC_{50} in EEG frequency measure is shown with a significant reduction in IC_{50} with increasing age. *(Reproduced from Scott JC, Stanski DR. Decreased fentanyl and alfentanil dose requirements with age. A simultaneous pharmacokinetic and pharmacodynamic evaluation. J Pharmacol Exp Ther. 1987;240:159–166.)*

CYP2D6. The response to a medication may be altered by polymorphisms in genes that are not responsible for its pharmacokinetics or its direct target. For example, variant alleles for sodium or potassium transporters may predispose to drug-induced long-QT syndrome.

Response to warfarin, an oral anticoagulant increasingly used by older adults, is partly determined by genetic factors that influence both pharmacokinetics and pharmacodynamics. The more active S-enantiomer of warfarin is predominantly metabolized by cytochrome P450 2C9 (CYP2C9). The CYP2C9*2 and CYP2C9*3 variants are associated with decreased metabolic efficiency, reduced S-warfarin clearance, and decreased warfarin dose requirements, with an increased risk of over anticoagulation, particularly during initiation of warfarin. Warfarin inhibits synthesis of vitamin-K dependent clotting factors by inhibiting vitamin K epoxide reductase complex 1 (VCORC1). Genetic variability in VCORC1 may account for more variation in warfarin maintenance dose requirements than variability in CYP2C9. Age, weight, smoking, exposure to CYP2C9 inducers and inhibitors, INR, and polymorphisms in warfarin metabolizing and drug target genes are all independently associated with warfarin dose, and together explain approximately 50% of the variability in maintenance dose requirements.

Pharmacogenetics currently plays a limited role in individualizing drug therapy. Consideration of pharmacogenetics to guide prescribing is recommended in Food and Drug Administration (FDA) labeling in limited situations to reduce risk of serious adverse drug reactions. Recommendations include considering the roles of CYP2C9 and VKORC1 in warfarin dosing, genotyping, or phenotyping thiopurine S-methyltransferase (TPMT) to guide dosing and reduce myelosuppression from azathioprine and 6-mercaptopurine and genotyping UGT1A1 to guide dosing and reduce neutropenia from irinotecan.

ADVERSE DRUG REACTIONS

Adverse drug reactions (see also Chapter 24) occur more frequently and are often more severe in older adults compared with younger adults. This increased risk is related to increased comorbidity, altered pharmacokinetics and pharmacodynamics, and polypharmacy. Randomized controlled studies of efficacy do not necessarily provide useful data on safety, particularly in older patients. Pharmacovigilance studies play a major role in this population, particularly those studies that investigate functional impairment as an important adverse drug event.

Adverse drug reactions account for 5% to 10% of hospital admissions among older adults and are the fourth to sixth largest cause of death in hospitalized patients in the United States. The increased risk of adverse drug reactions in older adults occurs with prescribed, over-the-counter, and complementary and alternative medicines. Reports of serious adverse drug events to the FDA are significantly more common in adults aged 65 years and over, controlling for population and medication exposure. The increased risk of adverse drug reactions in older adults has been attributed to increased comorbidity, altered pharmacokinetics and pharmacodynamics, and perhaps most importantly, polypharmacy.

Adverse drug reactions are classified as either Type A, which are related to the pharmacological actions of the drug, dose-related, and predictable, or Type B, which are usually unrelated to the pharmacological actions of the drug and are unpredictable. Type A adverse drug reactions include dose-related drug toxicity, drug side effects, and drug interactions. Type B adverse reactions include idiosyncratic and immunologic reactions. Most adverse drug reactions causing admission of older adults to hospital are classified as Type A reactions and hence are predictable and potentially preventable. Some type B reactions may also be more common and more severe in older adults.

The majority of type A adverse reactions in older adults are due to pharmacokinetic factors. However, altered pharmacodynamics also contribute to the increased incidence of adverse drug reactions with aging. For example drug-induced aplastic anemia is more frequent in older adults because of increased sensitivity of bone marrow cell lines. Extrapyramidal adverse drug reactions to centrally acting drugs occur more frequently in older adults and are differ in nature than in younger adults. Younger subjects experience acute dystonic reactions with metoclopramide and prochlorperazine, whereas dystonic reactions are very unusual in older adults but Parkinsonism and tardive dyskinesia are frequently seen. The age-associated reduction in basal ganglia dopaminergic neurones explains the increased incidence of drug-induced Parkinsonism with aging.

The increased risk of adverse drug events in older adults is often not detected in randomized controlled trials. Older adults, and particularly old frail adults with multiple comorbidites, may be specifically excluded from the trials. The majority of randomized controlled trials may be powered to look at efficacy rather than safety. Meta-analyses may be required to detect significant differences in adverse drug events. For example, a recent meta-analysis of randomized controlled trials in patients with symptomatic left ventricular dysfunction, comparing the combination of angiotensin II receptor blockers plus angiotensin converting enzyme (ACE) inhibitors against control treatment that included ACE inhibitors, found that combination treatment was associated with higher risks of medication discontinuation for adverse drug events, worsening renal function, hyperkalaemia, and symptomatic hypotension. These rates may be even higher outside the randomized controlled trial environment, where patients are less well monitored, have more comorbidities, and may be exposed to more polypharmacy with medications such as nonsteroidal anti-inflammatory drugs (NSAIDs) that contribute to renal impairment and hyperkalemia.

Observational pharmacovigilance studies have been used to detect adverse events in these populations. For example, the Randomized Aldactone Evaluation Study (RALES) demonstrated that spironolactone, in addition to ACE inhibitors, significantly improves outcomes in patients with severe heart failure, and only 2% of study patients treated with spironolactone developed hyperkalemia. In contrast, analysis of Canadian linked prescription-claims and hospital-admission data sets for more than 1.3 million adults aged 66 years or older found that among patients treated with ACE inhibitors who had recently been hospitalized for heart failure, the spironolactone-prescription rate increased fourfold after the publication of RALES (34 to 149 per 1000 patients), as did the rate of hospitalization for hyperkalaemia (from 2.4 to 11.0 per 1000 patients, $P < 0.001$) and the associated mortality (from 0.3 per 1000 to 2.0 per 1000 patients, $P < 0.001$), without significant decreases in the rates of readmission for heart failure or death from all causes.

Randomized controlled trials are seldom designed to detect increases in falls, functional impairment, and cognitive impairment, among the most important and common adverse drug events in older adults. There is an association between falls and the types and numbers of medications used. Exposure to any psychotropic medication, regardless of class, is associated with an almost twofold increased risk of falls in older adults. Newer psychotropic medications, such as selective serotonin reuptake inhibitors and atypical antipsychotics have been associated with similar falls risks in older adults compared to the older psychotropics. A randomized placebo-controlled trial of withdrawal of psychotropic medications in older subjects found a 76% reduction in falls over 44 weeks. There is a strong statistical association between polypharmacy and increased falls risk. This association may be explained by increased risk of prescription of specific classes of drugs that increase the risk of falls, such as sedatives, antipsychotics, and cardiovascular medications, with polypharmacy. However, some of the hazards attributed to polypharmacy may be related to the underlying comorbidities for which the medications are prescribed rather than to drug effects.

Drugs frequently play a major or contributory role in confusional states in older adults. Medications have been reported to be the cause of around one-quarter of cases of inpatient delirium. The drug classes most strongly associated with cognitive impairment and delirium are psychotropic and anticholinergic medications. The impairments in physical and cognitive functions associated with psychotropic and anticholinergic medications can be viewed as type A dose-dependent adverse drug reactions. Recent efforts have been made to quantify cumulative psychotropic and/or anticholinergic medication exposure and estimate the effects of this exposure on physical and cognitive functions in older adults, using tools such as the Drug Burden Index.

FRAILTY AND PHARMACOLOGY

Frailty is a poorly defined but increasingly studied condition characterized by high susceptibility to disease, impending decline in physical function and high risk of death. The most widely used definition of frailty includes measures of mobility (walk time), strength (grip strength), nutrition (weight loss), endurance (exhaustion), and physical activity. Interpretation of studies is limited by inconsistent definitions of frailty, small study size, and the increase in interindividual heterogeneity observed in the frail elderly. A key feature of frailty is loss of lean muscle mass, sarcopenia. Frailty is likely to have a major influence on pharmacokinetics, pharmacodynamics, and the therapeutic ratio of medications.

Pharmacokinetics and Frailty

Comparison of pharmacokinetics in frail older adults, nonfrail older adults, and young adults is limited to very few studies, most with small numbers of subjects. It appears that bioavailability is not significantly affected by frailty. Volume of distribution is likely to be affected by the increasing sarcopenia and relative adiposity seen in frailty. Hydrophilic drugs would have smaller and lipophilic drugs larger, volumes of distribution in frail older adults than in nonfrail older adults. Changes in hepatic clearance with frailty are varied. It appears that there is no change in phase I hepatic metabolism with frailty. Erythromycin clearance, a measure of CYP3A4 and P-glycoprotein function, is not significantly different in frail and nonfrail older adults. Phase II metabolism is probably maintained in healthy aging but reduced in frailty. Paracetamol and metoclopramide clearance per unit volume of liver, which rely on conjugation, are maintained in fit older adults but significantly reduced in frail adults. Renal clearance has not been well-described in this pop-

ulation, and there is currently no evidence of a further reduction in renal clearance in frailty. Some routes of nonhepatic, nonrenal clearance may be reduced in frailty. Plasma aspirin esterase is maintained in fit, but reduced in frail, older adults.

Pharmacodynamics and Frailty

There is little information on specific changes in pharmacodynamics in frail older adults. One study found that frail older adults reported more severe and prolonged sedation after intravenous metoclopramide than nonfrail older adults, independent of pharmacokinetic differences. Frailty predicts mortality in older adults with severe coronary artery disease, but it is not clear whether this is related to changes in pharmacologic response. There is some evidence that frailty is associated with a procoagulant state and chronic inflammation, and it is possible that such changes could affect pharmacodynamics, particularly those of anticoagulant and immune-modulating therapies. It is likely that frail older adults will respond differently to drug therapy in view of their reduced physiologic reserve and impaired adaptive responses.

Adverse Drug Events and Frailty

Frailty is associated with many risk factors for adverse drug events (Table 8-6). However, difficulties with the definition of frailty have limited formal assessment of the association between frailty and adverse events. One study found that one-third of frail elderly persons experience adverse drug reactions after discharge from hospital. For every dollar spent on drugs in nursing facilities, $1.33 in health care resources is consumed in the treatment of drug-related problems. Frail older adults do not tolerate some medications as well as nonfrail older adults. A study of antidepressants in depressed nursing home residents found that one in eight discontinued sertraline and one-third discontinued venlafaxine due to serious adverse events. These rates are at least four times higher than those observed in a

TABLE 8-6

Factors That May Increase the Risk of Adverse Drug Events in Frail Older Persons	
RISK FACTOR FOR ADVERSE DRUG EVENTS	**ASSOCIATION WITH FRAILTY**
Pharmacokinetics	Sarcopenia and reduced body weight alter volume of distribution
	Impaired phase II hepatic metabolism reduces clearance
	Wide heterogeneity therefore difficult to predict
Pharmacodynamics	Less physiologic reserve
	Wide heterogeneity so difficult to predict response
Medication Management	
Polypharmacy	Increased number of comorbidities
Compliance	Increased prevalence of cognitive and sensory impairment
Hospital admissions	Frequent admissions due to increased susceptibility to disease

study of treatment of major depression with comparable medications in geriatric outpatients aged over 65 years.

There are likely to be significant changes in pharmacokinetics and pharmacodynamics in frail older adults. Greater understanding of the physiology of frailty and further development of valid tools to recognize frailty in clinical practice are required to allow the study of pharmacologic changes in frail older adults. Understanding such changes will inform therapeutic decisions for frail older adults.

DRUG DEVELOPMENT AND REGULATION

In the last 50 years, all developed countries have introduced a process of evaluating new drug therapies before they are marketed to ensure safety and efficacy in the target group of patients to be treated. Drug regulation is undertaken by the FDA in the United States and by the European Medicines Evaluation Agency (EMEA) in Europe. For a drug to be approved, substantial preclinical and clinical data are required. There is an expectation that clinical studies should include the relevant population that will be treated including older adults (see also Chapter 24).

Phase I Studies

Clinical drug studies are categorized into four phases (I–IV). Following preclinical model studies to determine toxicity and likely pharmacokinetics in humans, phase I studies are undertaken in healthy volunteers to define tolerability, identify any major toxicity, and establish the drug's pharmacokinetics. Typically, phase I studies are performed in 12 to 20 male subjects with progressive dose escalation with close physiological monitoring and collection of plasma and urine to determine pharmacokinetics. Female subjects are usually excluded from phase 1 studies because of their childbearing potential and the potential risk of teratogenicity. Healthy older subjects are not usually studied in phase I studies in part because younger subjects are likely to be more resilient to any unanticipated toxicity. For some drug therapies where significant toxicity is anticipated, healthy volunteers are not used and studies to define pharmacokinetics and tolerability are undertaken in the relevant patient group for which it is considered ethically appropriate. For example, initial studies of cytotoxic drugs are usually undertaken in cancer patients with end-stage disease who have received all standard therapy.

There are clear examples in which different responses to drug therapy are seen between young and older subjects (see "Pharmacodynamics" section earlier). Studies in healthy older subjects may provide valuable insight into altered responsiveness or toxicity to inform the design and selected doses for phase II and III studies, which include older patients. For example, the majority of N-Methyl-D-Aspartate (NMDA) antagonists developed for acute stroke never achieved plasma concentrations associated with neuroprotection in phase II studies because of agitation, hallucinations, and confusion, which were particularly problematic in older patients with acute stroke.

Phase I studies had an excellent safety record until the recent incident with TNG 1412, a stimulatory monoclonal antibody being developed to treat rheumatoid arthritis, which led to near-fatal cytokine storm in six healthy volunteers studied in the UK. This has led to closer scrutiny by regulatory bodies of studies using newer biologic agents and the clinical environment in which such studies are conducted.

Phase II Studies

Phase II studies are usually placebo-controlled studies with a range of doses thought to produce a therapeutic response without major safety problems in a small group of patients with the target disease. The main aim of phase II studies is to demonstrate "proof of concept" rather than establishing a clinically useful response in a broad range of patients. For example, studies of a reperfusion drug for myocardial infarction or stroke would be designed to determine the extent to which the agent increases reperfusion as measured by angiography of the occluded blood vessel and monitor bleeding rates but not to necessarily demonstrate an improvement in mortality or disability. Prediction of the optimal dose to take forward in phase II studies is recognized to be challenging and maybe further complicated by dose-related differences in efficacy and toxicity between young and old patients. Bayesian adaptive dose design approaches in study design have been used to modify the allocation of doses informed by the response of previously randomized patients and end a study when there is clear evidence of the presence or absence of a predefined response. Phase II studies have proved very problematic for a number of disease areas in older adults particularly central nervous system (CNS) conditions such as acute stroke, pain, and neurodegenerative diseases.

Phase III Studies

Phase III studies are the key for establishing that a therapy has a benefit relevant to patient outcomes. In most therapy areas, the primary outcome in phase III trials is a clinically relevant disease-specific one that is able to demonstrate a clear benefit to patients in either survival or function and quality of life. In studies of acute stroke treatments, survival without disability is used. In studies of secondary prevention therapy for cardiovascular disease, a combined outcome of cardiovascular death, stroke, or myocardial infarction has been used.

Well-designed phase III trials should include patients who are representative of the population that will be treated if the drug is approved. Until recent years, Phase III trial protocols commonly had upper age limits. For example, many acute stroke studies (ECASS 1 and ECASS 2) had an upper age limit of 80 years and the large Heart Protection Study, which demonstrated the benefits of statins in patients at increased cardiovascular risk had an upper age limit of 75 years. Such age limits appear to have been introduced because of fears that a greater risk of adverse events in older adults might make the trial more likely to fail to achieve a positive outcome. There may be investigators with the view that preventing disease recurrence in older adults was not a worthwhile aim. Even when trials do not have an upper age limit, older adults often are excluded from enrolment in studies because of other protocol exclusion criteria such as comorbidities or concomitant drug therapy. The failure to include older adults in clinical trials leads to problems once the drug is approved. Sometimes the license will have an upper age limit such as alteplase for ischaemic stroke in Europe. Clinicians may be reluctant to treat older adults because of the lack of trial data in this group. Perhaps most importantly, we do not learn the benefits and harms of this age group, who then are given the medication without this knowledge.

International Guidelines on Drug Development now strongly recommend the inclusion of older adults in phase III trials, emphasizing the importance to seek patients 75 years and older and not excluding unnecessarily patients with concomitant illness. The older the population that is likely to use the drug after marketing the more important it is to include very elderly patients. A minimum of 100 patients is recommended to detect clinically important differences. For diseases such as Alzheimer's disease, it is expected that older patients will constitute the majority of the trial database. Pharmacokinetic studies in older adults and patients with renal impairment are recommended to detect age-associated pharmacokinetic differences.

Phase IV Studies

Phase IV trials are generally observational studies in large cohorts of patients following licensing and marketing. Well-conducted phase IV trials are larger than phase III trials and include the broad population of patients treated. They are important in detecting rare adverse drug events and in confirming the safety of therapy observed in clinical trials. They may also offer valuable information on drug effects in very elderly patients if these were not included in clinical trials.

PHARMACOEPIDEMIOLOGY

Pharmacoepidemiology uses the science of clinical epidemiology to measure patterns of medication use and outcomes in large populations. Pharmacoepidemiology allows assessment of the safety and efficacy of medications in large populations, which are often more diverse than the participants in randomized trials, over long periods of time.

Advantages of Pharmacoepidemiologic Studies

The advantages of pharmacoepidemiology over randomized controlled trials include (1) detection of adverse events that are too rare or too delayed to be detected in randomized trials; (2) assessment of efficacy over longer periods in a broader population; (3) correlation of medication use with outcomes that may not have been assessed in randomized trials; (4) assessment of safety and efficacy of medications beyond the stringent monitoring of a randomized trial.

Pharmacoepidemiology is a particularly useful tool to assess medications in older adults. Older adults are often excluded from randomized trials, either on the basis of age alone, or because of comorbidities, comedications, or functional impairment. Observational pharmacoepidemiologic studies can assess patterns of medication use, safety, and efficacy in frail individuals. It is particularly important to understand safety and efficacy over many years when deciding whether to continue or cease medications in older adults who have often been taking their medicines for decades. Many randomized trials only assess disease and mortality outcomes, and pharmacoepidemiologic studies can correlate medication exposure with functional and quality of life measures that may be more relevant to older adults. Pharmacoepidemiology assesses the effects of medications in the presence of medication management issues that occur in real clinical settings, e.g., limited adherence and monitoring.

Limitations of Pharmacoepidemiologic Studies

Pharmacoepidemiologic studies are limited by confounding and bias. Interpretation of studies is limited by variable prescribing patterns, variable comorbidities, confounding by indication, severity and prognosis, and controlling for the time dependency of drug use. Studies that rely on large epidemiologic data bases often contain very limited clinical information. There are several emerging approaches to manage confounders, including restricting study populations to more homogeneous groups, creating a propensity score to predict the probability of receiving a drug based on baseline covariates, and examining within-patient variability of drug exposure using crossover designs. Pharmacoepidemiology is likely to do much to inform prescribing for frail older adults.

PHARMACOECONOMICS

Pharmacoeconomics is the scientific subdiscipline of health economics that compares the value of one drug or drug therapy to another evaluating the cost, expressed in monetary terms, and effects, usually expressed in efficacy or quality of life of a drug. Pharmacoeconomic data can be used to guide optimal healthcare resource allocation. One important consideration in a pharmacoeconomic evaluation is to decide the perspective from which the analysis should be conducted, which may be institutional or societal.

Pharmacoeconomic studies compare two or more alternative courses of action in terms of their financial costs and benefits, usually a generic quality-of-life measure. The underlying aim is to achieve most health benefits across a specified patient population within available resources. The area has expanded in recent years because of the increasing problem of resource limitations in medical care and increasing numbers of often costly drug therapies coming to market. There are a number of different pharmacoeconomic approaches that can be used. Cost minimization analysis assumes or is based on data indicating clinical outcomes are equivalent and that the less costly intervention should be utilized. Cost effectiveness analysis examines outcomes measured in natural units such as life years, i.e. survival. Cost utility analysis examines outcomes measured in quality adjusted life years. Finally cost–benefit analysis examines costs and outcomes using only financial measures. Usually the results of clinical trials and costs of care are used to construct a lifetime model, which determines the cost difference between two treatment strategies and difference in health utility gain.

Cost effectiveness analysis has been used extensively in the United Kingdom by National Institute for Clinical Effectiveness (NICE), which has applied an approximate threshold of around £20,000 to £30,000 per quality adjusted life year gained in deciding whether to recommend therapies should be used in the publicly funded National Health Service. In the United States, managed care funds consider cost-effectiveness when deciding on the availability of drug therapy. There are some concerns that the cost-effectiveness approach may be prejudicial to older adults because their survival time is less than younger patients. However, for most preventative interventions, such as the treatment of cardiovascular risk factors or osteoporosis the greater absolute risk of experiencing an outcome event such as stroke, myocardial infarction, or fracture indicates intervention in older adults is more cost-effective, assuming a life expectancy at least as long as the time required to benefit. Thus consideration of cost effectiveness can facilitate health care systems appropriately directing resources to the treatment of older adults.

CONCLUSION

Knowledge of the age-related changes in pharmacokinetics and pharmacodynamics is important for researchers evaluating treatments in older adults and for clinicians treating older patients. Because of the increased risk of adverse drug effects in older adults, optimal prescribing is particularly critical in older patients. Making appropriate decision about drug therapy in the older individual requires careful consideration of the aims of treatment in the individual, risks of treatment from the drug, drugs–disease, and drug–drug interactions and careful review of the effect of treatment once initiated. This remains one of the major challenges of delivering high-quality geriatric care but when successfully delivered highly rewarding for both the physician and the older patient.

FURTHER READING

Campbell AJ, Robertson MC, Gardner MM, et al. Psychotropic medication withdrawal and a home-based exercise program to prevent falls: a randomized, controlled trial. *J Am Geriatr Soc.* 1999;47(7):850–853.

Gill J, Malyuk R, Djurdjev O, et al. Use of GFR equations to adjust drug doses in an elderly multi-ethnic group a cautionary tale. *Nephrol Dial Transplant.* 2007;22(10):2894–2899.

Hanlon JT, Pieper CF, Hajjar ER, et al. Incidence and predictors of all and preventable adverse drug reactions in frail elderly persons after hospital stay. *J Gerontol A Biol Sci Med Sci.* 2006;61(5):511–515.

Higashi MK, Veenstra DL, Kondo LM, et al. Association between CYP2C9 genetic variants and anticoagulation-related outcomes during warfarin therapy. *JAMA.* 2002;287(13):1690–1698.

Hilmer SN, Mager DE, Simonsick EM, et al. A drug burden index to define the functional burden of medications in older people. *Arch Intern Med.* 2007;167(8):781–787.

Lazarou J, Pomeranz BH, Corey PN. Incidence of adverse drug reactions in hospitalized patients: a meta-analysis of prospective studies. *JAMA.* 1998;279(15):1200–1205.

Le Couteur DG, Fraser, R, Hilmer S, et al. The hepatic sinusoid in aging and cirrhosis: effects on hepatic substrate disposition and drug clearance. *Clin Pharmacokinet.* 2005;44(2):187–200.

Leipzig RM, Cumming RG, Tinetti ME. Drugs and falls in older people: a systematic review and meta-analysis: I. Psychotropic drugs. *J Am Geriatr Soc.* 1999;47(1):30–39.

McLean AJ, Le Couteur DG. Aging biology and geriatric clinical pharmacology. *Pharmacol Rev.* 2004;56(2):163–184.

Moore AR, O'Keeffe ST. Drug-induced cognitive impairment in the elderly. *Drugs Aging.* 1999;15(1):15–28.

Moore TJ, Cohen MR, Furberg CD. Serious adverse drug events reported to the Food and Drug Administration, 1998–2005. *Arch Intern Med.* 2007;167(16):1752–1759.

Oslin DW, Ten Have TR, Streim JE, et al. Probing the safety of medications in the frail elderly: evidence from a randomized clinical trial of sertraline and venlafaxine in depressed nursing home residents. *J Clin Psychiatr.* 2003;64(8):875–882.

Routledge PA, O'Mahony MS, Woodhouse KW. Adverse drug reactions in elderly patients. *Br J Clin Pharmacol.* 2004;57(2):121–126.

Schwartz JB. Erythromycin breath test results in elderly, very elderly, and frail elderly persons. *Clin Pharmacol Ther.* 2006;79(5):440–448.

Toornvliet R, van Berckel BN, Luurtsema G, et al. Effect of age on functional P-glycoprotein in the blood-brain barrier measured by use of (R)-[(11)C]verapamil and positron emission tomography. *Clin Pharmacol Ther.* 2006;79(6):540–548.

Wilke RA, Lin DW, Roden DM, et al. Identifying genetic risk factors for serious adverse drug reactions: current progress and challenges. *Nat Rev Drug Discov.* 2007;6(11):904–916.

Yamada H, Dahl ML, Lannfelt L, et al. CYP2D6 and CYP2C19 genotypes in an elderly Swedish population. *Eur J Clin Pharmacol.* 1998;54(6):479–481.

Preventive Gerontology: Strategies for Optimizing Health Across the Life Span

Elizabeth A. Phelan ■ *Miguel A. Paniagua* ■ *William R. Hazzard*

INTRODUCTION

In developed societies, the success of disease prevention strategies over the last century, coupled with more effective treatments for many diseases, has resulted in a decline in mortality due to acute disease. However, this has been associated with a rise in chronic illness and attendant morbidity in the form of chronic disability in old age. The sheer magnitude of the elderly population of the near future will place critical demands on existing health care delivery systems. Continued independent functioning of the elderly population has therefore emerged as a major challenge to public health. The ability to perform activities of daily living is essential for ensuring independent living. Thus, preventive gerontology—the study of individual and population health strategies across the life span aimed at maximizing both the quality and quantity of human longevity—must now aim not just to retard chronic disease but also to prevent functional decline.

Aging is a lifelong process in which early- and mid-life events and behaviors can have an important influence on the health and functioning of individuals as they age. Development of chronic disease, functional decline, and loss of independence are not inevitable consequences of aging. Health and function in late life can be seen to a great degree as under one's own personal control. Disability is associated with chronic conditions that are potentially preventable, and changes in behavior and lifestyle will reduce risk factors that lead to many chronic conditions. This is true throughout life, and has been shown to apply even for persons of advanced age.

What should the primary care provider advise his/her young adult and middle-aged patients about how to maintain optimal health and function into their later years? Health promotion efforts at the level of the individual should ideally be established early in life and maintained throughout life. Chronic disease, an avoidable outcome intermediate in the pathway to functional decline or death (Figure 9-1), is unlikely to have a single cause but rather, to be the result of the interactions of multiple factors. Efforts to prevent such disease require a comprehensive approach that focuses primarily on behavioral modification.

Individuals who pursue a healthy lifestyle have a lower risk of developing a chronic disease. A healthy lifestyle can be conceptualized as one that involves avoidance of health-damaging behaviors along with the adoption of a proactive approach to one's health. This chapter will first examine those behaviors that should be avoided and then focus on those that should be adopted if one is to maximize the time spent in a state of independent functioning.

BEHAVIORS WITH ADVERSE HEALTH CONSEQUENCES

Achieving and maintaining health and function in advanced years can be aided by a commitment to a lifestyle that involves avoidance of smoking and other behaviors that adversely affect health. The Nurses Health Study found that middle-aged women who did not smoke, drank alcohol in moderate amounts, were not overweight, consumed a healthy diet, and exercised at least one-half hour daily had an 83% reduction in their risk of coronary events as compared with all the other women in the study. Each factor independently and significantly predicted risk, even after adjustment for age, family history, presence or absence of diagnosed hypertension, or diagnosed high cholesterol, and menopausal status. The online publication of Healthy People 2010, at http://www.healthypeople.gov/, contains links to reliable information about behavioral risk factors that lead to chronic disease and disability for individuals at every age (click on **Be a Healthy Person** link, and then click the **Online Health Checkups** link). Information on these topics can be found organized by age, race, ethnicity, and gender, and for parents, caregivers, and health professionals by clicking on the **Be a Healthy Person** link and then on **Health Information by Age**, **Gender**, **Race**. . . link.

The Task Force on Community Preventive Services, an independent, nonfederal, multidisciplinary group charged with reviewing

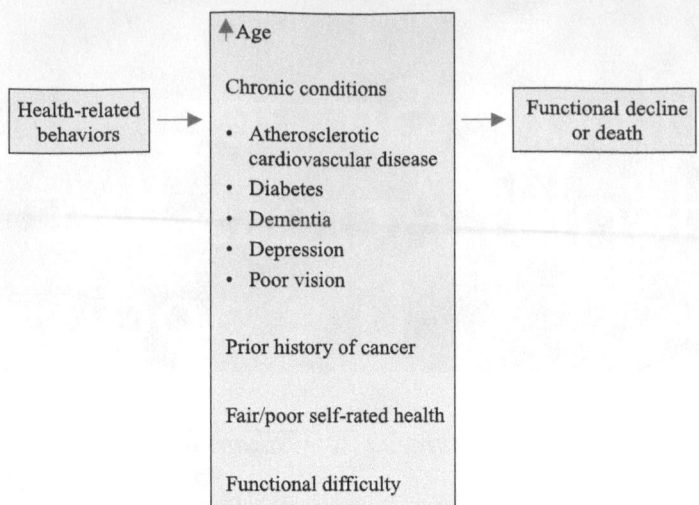

FIGURE 9-1. Conceptual model of how health behaviors impact the combined outcome of functional decline or death.

and assessing the quality of available evidence on the effectiveness and cost-effectiveness of essential community preventive health services, publishes reviews in an online document entitled, The Guide to Community Preventive Services. Topics coordinate with Healthy People 2010 objectives and address actual causes of death as described by McGinnis et al. in their 1993 JAMA article as well as prevalent risk behaviors. As topic reviews are completed, they are made available at http://www.thecommunityguide.org (click on a topic of interest under the heading, **Topics**).

Tobacco Use

Tobacco use is the largest single preventable cause of illness and premature deaths in the United States. Illnesses related to tobacco use (coronary artery disease (CAD), cancers of the lung, larynx, oral cavity, esophagus, pancreas, and urinary bladder, stroke, chronic obstructive pulmonary disease) account for one in every five deaths in the United States. Evidence from the National Health and Nutrition Examination Survey (NHANES) indicates that tobacco use predicts shorter survival time for middle-aged (45–54 years of age) and older (65–74 years of age) men. Although studies of prevalent cases have suggested that tobacco use either has no effect or is protective against Alzheimer's dementia, prospective data investigating incident cases found that, quite to the contrary, tobacco use is associated with an increased risk of dementia, including Alzheimer's dementia. Tobacco use can also multiply the risk associated with other carcinogenic agents: for example, heavy alcohol consumption, associated with esophageal cancer, carries an even greater risk when combined with cigarette smoking. Furthermore, the relative risk of developing lung cancer is at least additive among individuals who smoke and also have history of exposure to certain occupational agents such as arsenic, asbestos, chromium, nickel, and vinyl chloride.

It is increasingly evident that exposure to environmental tobacco smoke may also be a risk factor for lung cancer in lifelong nonsmokers. The adverse health effects of environmental tobacco smoke are far-reaching. In one case study, the attributable risk of death for second-hand smoke was similar to that of melanoma and motor vehicle collisions. A new report summarizing current evidence about second-hand smoke, entitled, The Health Consequences of Involuntary Exposure to Tobacco Smoke: A Report of the Surgeon General 2006, is available at http://www.ahrq.gov/path/tobacco.htm.

Tobacco dependence should be viewed as a chronic condition requiring ongoing assessment and repeated intervention. However, effective treatments are available that can lead to long-term, and in some cases, permanent abstinence. Studies have shown that individuals at any age can benefit from quitting the tobacco habit. Benefits include reduction in the risk of CAD, malignancy, stroke, and even hearing loss, along with improved pulmonary function, arterial circulation, and pulmonary perfusion.

Studies have found that only about 35% of adults are routinely asked about their tobacco habits or counseled to quit if they use tobacco. If providers do advise patients not to use tobacco, as many as 25% will quit or reduce the amount they use. Thus, providers should ask all patients at each clinic visit about tobacco use and advise all tobacco users about the importance of quitting, emphasizing factors that have been found to contribute most to successful attempts to quit: health concerns (symptoms); a desire to set an example for children; the expense of the habit; odor of breath, home, and clothing; and loss of taste for food. Providers should then assess a patient's willingness to attempt to quit. Patients who are unwilling to attempt to quit should be provided with a brief intervention designed to increase their motivation to quit. Patients who are willing to quit should be provided with treatments that have been identified as effective. First-line pharmacotherapies that have been shown to increase long-term smoking abstinence rates include bupropion and nicotine (gum, inhaler, nasal spray, or patch). Second-line therapies include clonidine and nortriptyline, the latter, a tricyclic antidepressant with anticholinergic activity, should be avoided unless there is a compelling contraindication to the other therapies. Additional information about these therapies, as well as descriptions of brief clinical interventions for patients willing and unwilling to make a quit attempt, can be found in the June 2000 guideline, "Treating tobacco use and dependence," available at http://www.ahrq.gov/clinic (click on **Clinical Practice Guidelines** link, then **Treating Tobacco Use and Dependence** box).

Substance Abuse

The harmful health effects of substance abuse are well documented. Studies have shown that individuals at any age can benefit from quitting these habits, and effective, brief interventions are available. Providers may consider participating in continuing education programs to hone screening and counseling skills.

Alcohol

Epidemiological studies support a survival benefit associated with moderate (up to two 8-ounce drinks per day) alcohol consumption, primarily through reduction of cardiovascular risk, including elevation of high-density lipoprotein (HDL) cholesterol. Additionally, both epidemiological and experimental studies suggest a protective effect against the development of cardiovascular disease with moderate consumption of red wine. The exact mechanism of the protective effect remains to be established, although it has been attributed to the properties of tannins or phenolic compounds, and to alcohol content, and moderate alcohol intake has been shown to be associated with less coronary atherosclerosis in a high-risk population. Weaker associations with moderate alcohol consumption include a protective effect against bone loss in older women, Alzheimer's disease, intermittent lower extremity claudication, ischemic stroke, and prevention of hearing loss.

However, consumption of alcohol beyond a moderate level can induce adverse effects on every organ system, including increased risk of hypertension; breast, colon, esophageal, liver, and head and neck cancer; cirrhosis; gastrointestinal bleeding; pancreatitis; cardiomyopathy; seizures; cerebellar degeneration; peripheral neuropathy; cognitive dysfunction; insomnia; depression; and suicide. Counseling about problem drinking following a few screening questions is a high-impact, cost-effective service (see "Priorities Among Effective Clinical Preventive Services: Results of a Systematic Review and Analysis" at http://www.prevent.org, under the "Tools and Resources" link). Screening can be accomplished by taking a careful history of alcohol use or by using a standardized screening questionnaire. All adults should be counseled on the health risks associated with excess alcohol consumption as well as the risk of injury (i.e., motor vehicle crashes or other equipment-related injury) after drinking alcohol. Nondependent heavy drinkers as well as those with alcoholism (a chronic illness involving a state of dependency) should be counseled about the benefits of decreasing alcohol intake. Brief counseling by primary care providers can result in a significant reduction in alcohol use. Dependent drinkers should be referred to formal alcohol treatment programs and considered for a trial of naltrexone, an opioid antagonist that reduces the pleasurable effects of alcohol and may reduce relapse to heavy drinking.

Illicit Drugs

The prevalence of injection drug use among older adults is unknown. Injection drug users typically initiate injection drug use during late adolescence (under age 21); however, a sizable subgroup begins injecting during early and late adulthood. Persons with a history of recreational drug use on only one or a few occasions are unlikely to self-identify; thus, clinicians should probe for such a pattern of usage.

Noninjection drug use (crack smokers, methamphetamine, intranasal heroin or cocaine, etc.) contributes to development of gastroduodenal ulcers, chest pain and myocardial infarction, and increased risk of death. As might be expected, higher levels of drug involvement also were associated with increased age-adjusted mortality. The United States Preventive Services Task Force (USPSTF) is currently updating its 1996 recommendations about screening for substance abuse.

Prescription Drug Misuse

Prescription drug misuse is poorly described in the medical literature but is a more prevalent problem than illicit drug use among older adults. Misuse of prescription medications may be related to insomnia, chronic pain, depression, and anxiety. The potential misuse of benzodiazepines is well recognized and has led to prescribing recommendations that suggest only short-term use and use only for intended indications. Amphetamine-like stimulants have abuse potential, but addiction to these drugs is seldom documented. Other medications that are often misused are sedative hypnotics, opioid analgesics, and barbiturates. Chronic use of such agents may lead to physical dependency and the development of withdrawal symptoms with attempts to discontinue use. Treatment may require detoxification followed by rehabilitation (see also Chapter 24).

Behaviors Increasing Risk of Injury

Head Trauma and Risk for Alzheimer's Disease

A number of case–control studies indicate that, in addition to maximizing one's years of education and minimizing exposure to neurotoxins, avoidance of significant head trauma (which resulted in loss of consciousness or seeking of medical attention) may lower the risk of eventual development of Alzheimer's disease. It therefore stands to reason that with implementation of cranioprotective measures during early life, such as wearing helmets during high-risk activities, and avoidance of high-risk behaviors that may put one at risk for head trauma, the risk of eventual cognitive decline may be reduced.

Ultraviolet Light and Risk for Skin Cancers and Cataracts

Increased risk of melanoma and nonmelanoma skin cancers as well as cataracts is associated with exposure to ultraviolet B (UV-B, or 280–320 nm) rays. More than five sunburns have been found to double the risk of melanoma, irrespective of the timing in life. Avoiding peak exposures, wearing protective clothing, avoiding artificial tanning devices (tanning lamps and beds) that emit UV radiation, and using sunscreen with a sun protection factor (SPF) of at least 30, indicating protection against UV-B, along with a star rating for Ultraviolet A (UV-A, or 320–400-nm rays) protection of 3 to 4 may reduce the risk of melanoma and other skin cancers. Wearing sunglasses that afford UV-B protection along with hats with brims can reduce the risk of cataracts by lowering eye exposure to UV-B light. Thus, patients should be advised to change behaviors that may increase the risk of skin cancer and cataracts. USPSTF, in its Guide to Clinical Preventive Services (available at http://www.ahrq.gov/clinic/prevenix.htm), concluded in 2001 that there is insufficient evidence to recommend for or against a periodic skin examination by clinicians; an update of this topic is in progress.

Prevention of Age-Related Macular Degeneration

Age-related macular degeneration (ARMD) is the leading cause of blindness in developed countries. The cause of ARMD is unknown; treatment is usually only partially effective, and thus prevention is an active area of investigation. Cigarette smoking appears to be a risk factor for the development and progression of ARMD; other risk factors appear to include hypertension, high cholesterol, high total fat intake, and obesity. The role of sunlight exposure is unclear. A high fish intake (more than four servings per week) may reduce the risk of ARMD. Observational studies examining the association between concentrations of antioxidant vitamins and ARMD development have yielded conflicting results. Published data from randomized controlled trials have thus far shown no clear benefit for vitamin E or beta carotene on the prevention of incident ARMD.

Excessive Noise and Risk for Hearing Loss

Noise-induced hearing loss ranks second only to presbycusis as a leading cause of sensorineural hearing loss, a well-described disability that is unarguably preventable. Such an insult can occur at any age and can affect one's life for years thereafter. Importantly, progression of cell death at the level of the cochlear cilia can be halted with avoidance of the offending recreational or occupational noise and using hearing protection, such as earplugs. Patients who have been exposed to excessive noise should be screened for hearing loss. When hearing loss is suspected, a thorough history, physical examination, and audiometry should be performed. If these examinations disclose evidence of hearing loss, referral for full audiologic evaluation is recommended.

Sleep Deprivation and Motor Vehicle Crash Fatalities

Impaired driving continues to be a considerable cause of morbidity and mortality in the United States. In 1998, alcohol was involved in 38% of all fatal motor vehicle collisions. Acute sleepiness, sleep deprivation, and nocturnal driving are other important risk factors for fatal motor vehicle accidents. Medical (i.e., obstructive sleep apnea, sedating medications) factors may contribute to daytime sleepiness, putting drivers at risk. Sleep deprivation can affect coordination, judgment, and reaction time and has been found to be involved in 16% to 60% of traffic accidents. Drivers' awareness of sleepiness while driving is not sufficient to prevent them from having an accident. Those who drive when sleepy need to be counseled to stop driving and rest before resuming driving.

Cell Phone Use While Driving and Motor Vehicle Crashes

A growing literature documents the hazards of cell phone use while driving. One study of nearly 500 drivers who had been involved in a motor vehicle crash, resulting in hospitalization showed that use of a cell phone (regardless of whether the phone was a hands-free type or not) up to 10 minutes prior to a crash was associated with an highly significant risk of crashing. Other studies have documented a dose–response relationship, wherein increasing frequency of cell phone use (not duration of use) is associated with a higher likelihood of an accident. Cell phone use may adversely affect driving via several mechanisms, including delaying response time, interfering with attention (e.g., failing to visually scan an intersection for traffic before proceeding through it), and impairing maintenance driving (e.g., staying within a lane).

Obesity

In adults, obesity is defined as a body mass index (BMI) of 30 kg/m^2 or more; overweight is a BMI of 25 to 29.9 kg/m^2 or more. Despite public health messages that focus on reducing fat intake and increasing energy expenditure, the prevalence of obesity in industrialized countries has reached epidemic proportions, with one in three being obese and another one in three being overweight.

Obesity is a major health hazard. There is strong evidence that obesity is associated with increased cardiovascular risk as well as a higher incidence of hypertension, hyperlipidemia, and type II diabetes mellitus (all associated with insulin resistance and "the metabolic syndrome"). Obesity is one of the factors associated with impaired mobility and other functional limitations, disabling conditions such as osteoarthritis; sleep apnea; gallbladder disease; nonalcoholic fatty liver disease; cancers of the breast, endometrium, and colon; and premature death. Moreover, those who are obese may suffer from social stigmatization, impaired social interaction, depression, and low self-esteem. Excess body weight or weight gain during middle age (especially early middle age, meaning age 25–50 years) contributes to the development of chronic conditions (cardiovascular disease, diabetes mellitus, hypertension, and osteoarthritis) in later years.

Because treatment and reversal of obesity is challenging, primary prevention is warranted. Efforts to maintain a healthy weight should start early in life and continue throughout adulthood, as this is likely to be more successful than efforts to lose substantial amounts of weight and maintain weight loss once obesity has developed. Data from NHANES I suggest that getting adequate rest may be important in obesity prevention. Sleeping less than 7 hours a night was shown to be a risk factor for subsequent obesity. This may be related to altered levels of leptin and ghrelin, two appetite-regulating hormones. Leptin is associated with appetite suppression and ghrelin is an appetite stimulant that is thought to play a role in long-term regulation of body weight. During sleep deprivation, leptin levels fall and ghrelin levels rise.

Adults who are trying to maintain a healthy weight after weight loss are advised to get even more physical activity than the 30 min/d (described below) that is currently recommended; the U.S. Department of Agriculture has recommended at least 60 min/d to manage weight. Weight management leading to a slow, steady weight loss is more beneficial that a pattern of weight cycling, which actually contributes to an elevated risk of mortality. The basal metabolic rate decreases with age, in parallel with a decline in lean body mass, and body fat increases proportionally. Thus, in order to most readily achieve normalization of body weight and body composition, an energy-sufficient (but not excessive) diet should be combined with a program of regular physical activity to permit maintenance of basal metabolic rate.

Obese individuals who are trying to lose a substantial amount of weight should seek the guidance of a health care provider prior to starting a weight-reduction program to ensure appropriate management of obesity as well as other health conditions. Current treatment of obesity involves combining either pharmacologic (e.g., orlistat, a gastrointestinal lipase inhibitor that restricts fat absorption, or sibutramine, a serotonin–norepinephrine reuptake inhibitor that enhances satiety and increases basal energy expenditure) or surgical treatments (e.g., gastric bypass, gastric banding) with dietary modification along with a physical activity program. Surgical intervention is limited to people with class II obesity (BMI $\geq$ 35 kg/m^2) and severe comorbidity or class III obesity (BMI $\geq$ 40 kg/m^2). A recent meta-analysis showed that dietary therapy (i.e., a very low calorie diet, less than 1100 kcal/d, or a low-calorie diet, with 1200–1500 kcal/d) provides <5 kg weight loss after 2 to 4 years, pharmacologic therapy provides 5 to 10 kg weight loss after 1 to 2 years, and surgical therapy provides 25 to 75 kg weight loss after 2 to 4 years. The same study showed that weight loss of $\geq$5% baseline weight improves lipids, blood pressure, and glycemic control but mainly among those with cardiovascular risk factors. However, the authors observed the majority of studies of weight loss have methodologic limitations (e.g., inadequate study duration, large proportions of subjects lost to follow-up, a lack of an appropriate usual care group) that limit the applicability of findings to obese persons in everyday clinical practice.

TAKING A PROACTIVE APPROACH TO PERSONAL HEALTH AND WELL-BEING

Achieving and maintaining health and function in advanced years—successful preventive gerontology—is rooted in a personal commitment to a lifestyle that promotes proper nutrition, physical fitness, social connections, and use of preventive health care. Whereas the advice and encouragement of the health care provider can facilitate preventive gerontology, it is the acceptance by the individual of primary responsibility in managing his or her health and behavior that is central to the concept.

Nutrition

A healthy diet can contribute to an increase in life expectancy and better health. Healthy diets have shown the potential to lower blood pressure and blood cholesterol. Optimal diets have also been associated with lower risk of chronic diseases, notably CAD, diabetes, obesity, and some forms of cancer. NHANES III data show potentially important decreases with age in median protein and zinc intakes as well as intakes of calcium, vitamin E, and other nutrients. Subclinical nutrient deficiencies can adversely affect health and physical functioning. Longitudinal studies have shown that caloric intake and macronutrient (fat, protein, and carbohydrate) intake decrease with age.

A diet with adequate calcium and vitamin D reduces the risk of osteoporosis, which is a major cause of fractures and concomitant disability and threatened independence, especially in postmenopausal women. Optimal serum levels of 25-hydroxy vitamin D [25(OH)D] (75–100 nmol/L) appear to not only have a salubrious effect on bone mineral density but may also reduce risk of colon cancer (via less cell proliferation and more cell differentiation), falls (via prevention of muscle weakness), and periodontal disease (independent of bone health). However, the currently recommended daily intakes of vitamin D (200 IU for younger adults, 600 IU for older adults) appear to be insufficient to achieve these optimal serum concentrations.

The traditional Mediterranean diet, dominated by consumption of olive oil, vegetables, nuts, and fruits, meets criteria for a healthy diet. Direct evidence in support of this diet has become available. For example, it has been associated with prevention of progression of cardiovascular disease and reversal of the metabolic syndrome. Such a diet appears to improve endothelial function, reduce serum markers of systemic vascular inflammation (C-reactive protein and the proinflammatory interleukins (IL) IL-6, IL-7, and IL-18), and decrease insulin resistance. A plausible mechanism by which this diet may reduce inflammation may lie in either the antioxidants or the fiber that are common elements in the different components of the diet. Either antioxidants or fiber may effect a reduction in the transient oxidative stress associated with macronutrient intake. The sixth edition of *Nutrition and Your Health: Dietary Guidelines for Americans*, available online at http://www.health.gov/dietaryguidelines/, can serve as a reference for providers in counseling adults about healthful eating patterns.

Physical Activity

Physical activity and physical fitness can help prevent or delay the onset of chronic illnesses such as CAD, type II diabetes, osteoporosis, and obesity; protect against the development of functional decline; improve mood; reduce stress; and, perhaps, increase life expectancy. Physical activities that improve endurance, strength, and flexibility will delay impairments in mobility and may preserve the ability to perform tasks of daily living. Regular, moderate-intensity physical activity increases muscle mass and oxidative capacity, improves immune function, increases antioxidant defense against oxygen free radicals, and reduces oxidative stress. The current recommendation that every American exercise at least 30 minutes on most, and preferably all days, derives from evidence that even moderate physical activity is associated with a substantial drop in all-cause mortality. The cumulative, lifetime activity pattern may be the most influential factor in terms of providing protection from most diseases, especially those with a long developmental period, as well as mediating secondary disease complications associated with CAD, diabetes, and hypertension. However, despite an enormous amount of information about the positive effects of exercise in preventing disease and increasing life expectancy, the majority of adults do not engage in regular, sufficient physical activity. For example, only 15% of the U.S. adult population met the 30 min/d goal in 1997, and 40% of adults engaged in no leisure-time physical activity. Women are less likely than men to report regular leisure time physical activity; the lowest levels typically are among women of Hispanic or African-American descent. Furthermore, aging appears to be associated with a rise in the prevalence of inactivity, especially among women, such that by age 75 years, one in three men and one in two women engage in *no* regular physical activity. Societal changes over the past 50 years, including increased dependence on cars for transportation, the advent of television and computers, and rise in number of desk jobs, have virtually engineered physical activity out of the daily routines of many Americans. Many mid-life and older adults are unaware of the benefits of physical activity. Thus, encouraging and prescribing physical activity for adults of all ages is imperative and can be viewed as a central tenet of preventive gerontology. Regular participation in activities of moderate intensity (such as brisk walking, climbing stairs, scrubbing floors, yard work), which increase caloric expenditure and maintain muscle strength, is recommended, as it is activity of moderate intensity that appears to allow health benefits to accrue. Current national guidelines suggest at least 30 minutes of moderate intensity exercise on 5 or more days per week (CDC) or vigorous intensity exercise (such as swimming laps, bicycling more than 10 miles per hour, jogging, or running) for 20 or more minutes on 3 or more days per week. The CDC, American College of Sports Medicine, and Surgeon General further state that daily physical activity requirements may be accumulated over the course of the day in short bouts of 10 to 15 minutes. Building activity into one's daily routine (e.g., taking the stairs rather than an elevator) is a practical and efficacious way to achieve a pattern of regular physical activity. Helpful, patient-centered information about how to become more active can be found at the CDC's Physical Activity for Everyone (http://www.cdc.gov/nccdphp/dnpa/physical/index.htm) and for overweight and obese adults, the Active at Any Size (http://www.healthfinder.gov/docs/doc11151.htm) Web sites.

Several psychological and environmental factors determine physical activity behavior throughout the life span. Self-efficacy, or confidence in one's ability to perform a particular behavior (in this case, regular exercise), is strongly associated with both adoption of and adherence to physical activity among adolescents, young adults, and older adults. Strategies suggested by Bandura to enhance self-efficacy, such as assessing readiness for exercise using a behavior change philosophy, using motivational interviewing techniques, weekly action planning and feedback, collaborative problem-solving, and addressing barriers to exercise may all enhance self-efficacy for exercise. These techniques can be learned and implemented by health care providers. Affective disorders such as depression and anxiety are inversely associated with physical activity participation at any age.

Thus, evaluation for the presence of these conditions and institution of treatment may be necessary before adoption of an exercise program can occur. Social influences on physical activity appear to be strong throughout the life span. Peer reinforcement is particularly important in youth, while social support from spouses and friends is correlated with vigorous activity in younger and older adult populations. Finally, environmental factors, particularly safety and accessibility, influence activity participation across the age span. These latter factors are increasingly becoming a focus of community intervention efforts.

Social Connections

Ongoing involvement in a social network permits social contact (integration), the provision of social support, and the opportunity for social influence, and is associated with positive health outcomes and self-assessed well-being. Through opportunities for social engagement, such as attending social functions, getting together with friends and family, and going to church, meaningful social roles are defined and reinforced, creating a sense of belonging and identity that is made possible by the network context. Measures of social integration or "connectedness" are powerful predictors of mortality likely because ties give meaning to an individual's life by enabling and obligating them to be fully involved in their community and thereby to feel attached to it.

In turn, there are several pathways most proximate to health by which social networks are thought to influence health: (1) a health behavioral pathway; (2) a psychological pathway; and (3) a physiologic pathway. Regarding the health behavioral pathway, social ties have been shown to influence the likelihood that certain behaviors will be adopted and that behavior will change (see also Chapter 28). Social influence refers to the way members of a social network obtain normative guidance about health-relevant behaviors (physical activity, smoking, etc.). For example, marriage and friendship ties have been shown in several studies to promote a healthier diet, more regular exercise, less smoking and drinking, and more cancer screening. Spouse pairs demonstrate a concordance in their level of exercise, smoking, and drinking. However, studies have also shown that family and friends carry the potential for encouraging detrimental health behaviors: for example, the presence of a smoker in one's social network has been associated with greater relapse in efforts to quit. Adherence and nonadherence to medical treatments have each been linked to the presence of more social ties. Thus, the evidence indicates that ties can serve as role models of appropriate or undesirable behavior. Evidence also suggests that social network size, or "connectedness," is inversely related to risk-related behaviors. Data from Alameda County show a gradient between increasing social disconnection and the prevalence of both health-damaging behaviors and mortality.

A second mechanism by which social networks influence health is via psychological pathways. Evidence suggests that ongoing participation in one's social network is essential for the maintenance of self-efficacy beliefs throughout life. For example, studies have observed the indirect influence of social support through enhanced self-efficacy in smoking cessation and exercise. In addition, it is generally accepted that social ties have a salutary effect on mental health and psychological well-being, regardless of whether an individual is under stress. Integration in a social network may also directly produce positive psychological states, such as a sense of self-worth,

purpose, and belonging. These positive states, in turn, may benefit mental health due to direct modulation of the neuroendocrine response to stress and may increase the likelihood of social support, protecting against psychological distress (depression and anxiety).

A third mechanism by which social networks influence health is via physiologic pathways. The basic premise is that human physiologic homeostasis is influenced by the social environment. Social relationships may influence health via alteration in immune response, by effects on the hypothalamic–pituitary–adrenal axis, or by cardiovascular reactivity. For example, a low number of contacts with acquaintances is associated with high resting plasma levels of epinephrine, and people with low social support have been found to have higher levels of urinary norepinephrine, regardless of their level of stress. Studies of medical students have shown that those who were lonely had lower levels of natural killer cell activity.

Cognitive Activity

Continuing cognitive activity has been shown to help maintain cognitive function. Crossword puzzle solving and reading are two examples of activities that can help maintain cognitive skills. Higher levels of education (and cognitive ability, for which education could be a marker) are associated with less age-related loss in cognitive function.

Napping

New evidence from the Greek European Prospective Investigation into Cancer and Nutrition Cohort, a population-based study involving Greek men and women, suggests that napping may have beneficial effects, particularly for men free of serious illness. Men and women taking midday naps of any duration or frequency had a 34% reduction in coronary mortality. Those who took an occasional nap had a 12% reduction in mortality, while those who napped on average at least 30 minutes, at least three times a week had a 37% reduction in mortality. In analyses stratified by gender, these effects appeared to be significant for men but not for women. The inverse association was significant among men who were currently working but nonsignificant among men who were not currently working (mainly retirees). The putative mechanism for this benefit, as described by the study authors, may be stress reduction.

Health Care

A primary purpose of health care in an aging society is to help each individual set and achieve personal health-related goals, i.e., goals that will enhance active life expectancy and quality of life. Adults should be instructed to seek medical attention early for bothersome symptoms. They should receive education about self-management of chronic conditions, including the importance of long-term adherence to medications (e.g., for treatment of hypertension or dyslipoproteinemia) prescribed to treat such conditions. Finally, they should be advised to participate fully in the periodic preventive screening and health care activities described below.

Blood Pressure Evaluations

A recent study supported by the National Heart, Lung, and Blood Institute indicates that middle-aged Americans face a 90% chance of developing high blood pressure at some time during the rest of their lives. All patients should be counseled that the development of high blood pressure is not an inevitability, and should be educated about the role of abstaining from smoking, following a healthy eating plan that includes low sodium, maintaining a healthy weight, being physically active, and consuming alcohol in moderation in the prevention of hypertension altogether.

The Framingham study showed that men aged 45 to 64 years with blood pressures above 160/95 have two to three times the CAD rate of those with pressures under 140/90. Among those with systolic pressures above 160, strokes are three times as frequent as among those with systolic pressures under 140. Thus, treating high blood pressure with lifestyle modification and medication will reduce the risk of CAD and stroke. There is also reasonably strong evidence that treatment of hypertension will decrease the risk of cognitive impairment.

Lipid Evaluations

Premature heart disease is unequivocally associated with elevated blood cholesterol levels. Data from the Framingham study indicate that for a 1% rise in cholesterol there is a 2% rise in CAD, while for a 1% rise in high-density lipoprotein (HDL) cholesterol, there is a 2% fall in risk of CAD. Strategies to increase HDL levels while lowering low-density lipoprotein (LDL) cholesterol to the total cholesterol: HDL cholesterol ratio of 3.5 or less are recommended. The USPSTF recommends that all adults (men beginning at age 35 years and women beginning at age 45 years) be screened routinely for lipid disorders to determine whether their cholesterol levels increase their risk for heart disease, and that providers treat abnormal lipids in people who are at increased risk for coronary heart disease. Screening should include total and high-density lipoprotein cholesterol. Providers should counsel all patients about lifestyle changes (reducing saturated fat in the diet, adequate intake of fruits and vegetables, exercising, and losing weight) that can improve their lipid levels. Individuals at highest risk may require medication to control their lipid abnormalities. Prediction tools can help guide treatment decisions; such tools provide a more accurate estimation of cardiovascular risk than does a count of the number of risk factors; see www.bmj.com/cgi/content/full/320/7236/709 for an example. An update of these (2001) recommendations is currently underway by the USPSTF.

The Adult Treatment Panel III (ATP III) National Cholesterol Education Program (NCEP) Update 2004: Implications of Recent Clinical Trials for the ATP III Guidelines (see http://www.nhlbi.nih.gov/guidelines/cholesterol/atp3upd04.htm) details current cholesterol treatment guidelines, including among others, the recommendations that (1) for very high-risk persons, an LDL-C goal of <70 mg/dL is a therapeutic option; (2) for high-risk persons with high triglycerides or low high-density lipoprotein cholesterol (HDL-C), the combination of a fibrate or nicotinic acid derivative with an LDL-C lowering drug should be considered. These recommendations need to be considered within the context of older adults' life expectancy, comorbidity, and preferences.

Glucose Monitoring

Diabetes is an important risk factor for CAD. Patients with diabetes tend to have more severe atherosclerosis, two to three times as many myocardial infarctions, and twice as many strokes as persons not having diabetes at the same age. This is especially germane for women, in whom diabetes appears to negate their relative (5 to 10 years) protection from CAD. In other words, a woman with diabetes is at equal risk of CAD at any given age as a man with diabetes. Current interventions for the prevention of type II diabetes mellitus are those targeted toward modifying risk factors such as reducing obesity and promoting physical activity. Awareness of risk factors for developing type II diabetes (i.e., strong family history of diabetes, age, obesity, physical inactivity, and having a personal history of gestational diabetes or being an offspring of a woman who had gestational diabetes) is important to permit screening, early detection, and treatment in high-risk populations.

Recent evidence suggests that weight reduction (via caloric restriction and increased physical activity) can reduce the risk of developing type II diabetes in overweight adults. This strategy appears to be more effective than pharmacological intervention (with metformin) in reducing insulin resistance (58% reduction in incidence of diabetes with lifestyle modification vs. 31% with metformin, each compared to placebo). Other lines of evidence (chiefly from clinical trials of statins that have included diabetics) underscore the importance and efficacy of CAD risk reduction in diabetics, in whom the risk of CAD events in the absence of clinical CAD is equivalent to that of persons not having diabetes with CAD. This has led to a more ambitious goal for LDL cholesterol reduction in patients with diabetes in the 2001 ATP III NCEP to 100 mg/dL or less, the same as in persons not having diabetes with CAD or other atherosclerotic vascular disease. The NCEP 2001 report can be viewed at http://www.nhlbi.nih.gov/guidelines/cholesterol/index.htm. These recommendations did not address older adults specifically and they need to be interpreted in the context of other comorbidities, life expectancy, likelihood of adverse consequences of preventive treatments, and preferences.

Cancer Screening

Cancers and cancer deaths can be prevented both by limiting exposure to known carcinogens and through early detection and treatment before a cancer has spread. Available screening procedures for colon and cervical cancer, if more widely applied to asymptomatic persons, would likely prevent many deaths from these diseases. For example, The Minnesota Colon Cancer Control Study showed that annual fecal occult-blood testing reduced mortality by 33%. The USPSTF, in its 2002 review, found insufficient evidence that newer screening technologies (e.g., computed tomographic colography) improve health outcomes. A large body of observational studies suggests that early detection through periodic Papanicolau (Pap) testing lowers mortality from cervical cancer by 20% to 60%. Most organizations recommend discontinuing Pap testing in older women who have multiple negative results and who have been tested regularly.

Mammographic screening for breast cancer remains controversial, given the risks (e.g., low sensitivity and specificity of mammography, false-positive results that generate additional testing and result in anxiety; overdiagnosis and unnecessary treatments) and costs associated with periodic (every 1–2 years beginning at the age of 40 years) screening. Debate continues over whether a survival benefit is derived from mass screening for breast cancer. Clinicians and women should discuss individual risk factors and personal preferences to determine when to have a first mammogram and how often to have them after that. Screening for early detection of prostate cancer also remains controversial, especially beyond age 70 years. The utility of screening for lung cancer remains an area of active investigation. In 2004, the USPSTF found poor evidence that any screening strategy (chest x-ray, sputum cytology, low-dose computerized tomography) for lung cancer results in decreased mortality. Studies are underway that should provide information about the effectiveness of more modern screening tests, including spiral computed tomography (CT). For more information, see http://www.cancer.gov/nlst (the National Lung Screening trial; results expected by 2009) and http://www.cancer.gov/prevention/plco/ (the Prostate, Lung, Colorectal, and Ovarian Cancer Screening Trial).

Depression Screening

Depression is a common and disabling condition. Those with a family history of depression, women, the unemployed, and those with chronic disease are at increased risk of depression. The USPSTF recommends screening adults for depression in clinical practices that have systems in place to ensure accurate diagnosis, effective treatment, and follow-up. This recommendation is comparable to those made by other groups, including the Canadian Task Force on Preventive Health Care (see http://www.ctfphc.org/).

Immunizations for Pneumococcal Pneumonia and Influenza

Both pneumococcal pneumonia and influenza can lead to hospitalization and disability. Vaccinations should be administered to any adult with a chronic condition regardless of age and universally for those over 65 years.

Aspirin for Primary Prevention of Myocardial Infarction

There is evidence that aspirin decreases the incidence of CAD in middle-aged and older adults who are at increased risk (i.e., a 5-year risk of 3% or more) but have never had a myocardial infarction or a cerebrovascular accident (CVA). Combined data from five clinical trials show that aspirin therapy lowers the risk of CAD by 28%. However, there is no reduction in the risk of CVA with aspirin; the risk of having a hemorrhagic CVA is actually slightly increased. There is also an increased risk of gastrointestinal bleeding with aspirin. Thus, the risk may outweigh the benefits for those who are at average or low risk for CAD. A risk calculator can be found at http://hin.nhlbi.nih.gov/atpiii/calculator.asp.

Low to Moderate Dose Aspirin for Reduction of All-Cause Mortality in Women

New data from the Nurses' Health Study suggest that use of low to moderate dose aspirin reduces mortality in women, especially for women who have cardiovascular risk factors or who are older. The benefit for cardiovascular mortality was evident within 5 years of use, while the benefit for cancer mortality required prolonged (10 years or more) use.

CONCLUSION

Adoption and maintenance of a healthy lifestyle should be emphasized from childhood through older adulthood. Sound health habits not only help people survive longer but postpone the onset of disability and compress functional loss into fewer years at the end of life. Among the most important self-care behaviors are those that involve adequate nutrition, avoidance of tobacco use, and regular physical activity. Healthy aging policy should emphasize modification of lifestyle risk factors across the life span and communities that support healthy eating and physical activity. As the population ages, the potential for strain on health care systems will increase, because the greatest use of health services has tended to occur during the last years of life. Thus, in the present health care environment, health promotion is an important focus for providers who care for individuals of any age.

FURTHER READING

Berkman LF, Kawachi I. *Social Epidemiology*. New York, New York: Oxford University Press; 2000.

Chan AT, Manson JE, Feskanich D, et al. Long-term aspirin use and mortality in women. *Arch Intern Med*. 2007;167:562–572.

Christen WG, Manson JE, Glynn RJ, et al. Beta carotene supplementation and age-related maculopathy in a randomized trial of US physicians. *Arch Ophthalmol*. 2007;125:333–339.

DiPietro L. Physical activity in aging: changes in patterns and their relationship to health and function. *J Gerontol A Biol Sci Med Sci*. 2001;56 Spec No 2:13–22.

Femia R, Natali A, L'Abbate A, et al. Coronary atherosclerosis and alcohol consumption: angiographic and mortality data. *Arterioscler Thromb Vasc Biol*. 2006;26:1607–1612.

Fleming MF, Barry KL, Manwell LB, et al. Brief physician advice for problem alcohol drinkers. A randomized controlled trial in community-based primary care practices. *JAMA*. 1997;277:1039–1045.

Gangwisch JE, Malaspina D, Boden-Albala B, et al. Inadequate sleep as a risk factor for obesity: analyses of the NHANES I. *Sleep*. 2005;28:1289–1296.

Knowler WC, Barrett-Connor E, Fowler SE, et al. Reduction in the incidence of type 2 diabetes with lifestyle intervention or metformin. *N Eng J Med*. 2002;346:393–403.

Maraldi C, Volpato S, Kritchevsky SB, et al. Impact of inflammation on the relationship among alcohol consumption, mortality, and cardiac events: the health, aging, and body composition study. *Arch Intern Med*. 2006;166:1490–1497.

McEvoy SP, Stevenson MR, McCartt AT, et al. Role of mobile phones in motor vehicle crashes resulting in hospital attendance: a case-crossover study. *Br Med J*. 2005;331:428.

Naska A, Oikonomou E, Trichopoulou A, et al. Siesta in healthy adults and coronary mortality in the general population. *Arch Intern Med*. 2007;167:296–301.

Olsen O, Gotzsche PC. Screening for breast cancer with mammography (Cochrane Review). Cochrane Database Syst Rev 4, 2001.

Popelka MM, Cruickshanks KJ, Wiley TL, et al. Moderate alcohol consumption and hearing loss: a protective effect. *J Am Geriatr Soc*. 2000;48:1273–1278.

Rollnick S, Mason P, Butler C. *Health Behavior Change: A Guide for Practitioners*. Philadelphia: Churchill Livingstone; 1999.

Taylor HR, Tikellis G, Robman LD, et al. Vitamin E supplementation and macular degeneration: randomised controlled trial. *Br Med J*. 2002;325:11.

Tyas SL, White LR, Petrovitch H, et al. Mid-life smoking and late-life dementia: the Honolulu-Asia Aging Study. *Neurobiol Aging*. 2003;24:589–596.

Venning, G. Recent developments in vitamin D deficiency and muscle weakness among elderly people. *Br Med J*. 2005;330:524–526.

Woodward A, Laugesen M. How many deaths are caused by second hand cigarette smoke? *Tob Control*. 2001;10:383–388.

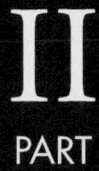

II
PART

PRINCIPLES OF GERIATRICS

Evaluation, Management, and Decision Making with the Older Patient

Sharon E. Strauss ■ *Mary E. Tinetti*

Clinical decision making, including diagnosis, treatment, and desired outcomes, differs between younger and older adult patients. The primary goal of medical care in younger adult patients usually is diagnosis of the disease causing the presenting symptoms, signs, and/or laboratory abnormalities. Treatment is targeted toward the pathophysiologic mechanisms deemed responsible for the disease. Relevant clinical outcomes are determined by the specific diseases and include cure if the disease is acute, and control or symptom modification if the disease is chronic.

The conventional disease-specific approach is not optimal in older patients for several reasons. First, age-related physiologic changes in most organ systems affect diagnostic test interpretation and response to treatments and may be difficult to differentiate from disease. In addition to age-related physiologic changes, the average 75-year-old suffers from 3.5 chronic diseases. With multiple coexisting chronic diseases, there is a less consistent relationship between pathology and disease or between disease and clinical manifestations. One disease may obscure or change the pathology, manifestations, or accuracy of laboratory evaluation of coexisting diseases. Treatment of one disease may increase the severity of another. With multiple coexisting diseases, it becomes difficult, and often impossible, to assess the severity or manifestations of individual diseases and to ascribe health and/or functional status to specific disease processes.

Second, many distressing symptoms or impairments among older persons, such as pain, dizziness, fatigue, sleep problems, sensory impairments, and gait disorders cannot be ascribed to a single disease; instead, they result from the accumulated effect of physical, psychological, social, environmental, and other factors. A clinical focus solely on diagnosing and treating discrete diseases may lead to expensive diagnostic testing with inconclusive results, to unnecessary, or even harmful, interventions, or, conversely, to ignoring potentially remediable symptoms. While clinicians may be reluctant to treat symptoms in younger and middle-aged patients without a specific diagnosis, treatment focused on improving symptoms in multiply ill and impaired older patients is often appropriate, because comfort and function are primary goals of health care in this population.

Third, diagnostic test characteristics may be altered by age and comorbidity, making selection and interpretation of tests more complicated than for younger patients. Furthermore, both the benefits and harms of treatment regimens may differ in the face of age-related physiologic changes and coexisting health conditions.

Fourth, older patients vary in the importance they place on potential health outcomes. When asked, older persons are able to prioritize among the often competing goals of increased survival, comfort, cognitive function, and physical function. Optimal clinical decision making in the care of older patients includes the articulation of patient preferences or goals of care; the identification of the diseases, impairments, and nondisease-specific factors affecting the attainment of these preferences and goals; and the selection of treatment options based on the modifiable impediments to individual patient goals. The multiplicity of impairments and diseases; the contribution of psychological, social, and environmental factors to health conditions; the enhanced likelihood of harm as well as benefit from many interventions; and the interindividual variability in patient preference all combine to make clinical decision making in the care of older persons very complex.

Fifth, clinical decision making is further complicated in older patients because other persons, including the spouse, adult children, other relatives, and significant others, are often actively involved, particularly when cognitive impairment is present. Involvement of family and friends is helpful and often crucial, since they may provide additional sources of information, facilitate adherence to treatment recommendations, and offer both emotional and instrumental support. Conflicts may arise, however, when goals of the patient and family differ. Striking a balance between patient confidentiality and family involvement, between independence and support, and between patient and family goals is a constant challenge. When based on an understanding of these factors, however, the clinical care of older persons is both effective and immensely gratifying.

PRESENTATION

At least three factors affect clinical presentation in older persons: underreporting of symptoms and impairments, changes in the patterns of presentation of individual illnesses, and an altered spectrum of health conditions. Contrary to a popular perception of older persons as complainers, they tend to underreport significant symptoms. One reason for underreporting is that both older persons and their clinicians often dismiss treatable symptoms and impairments as age-related changes for which nothing can be done. Denial, resulting from fear of economic, social, or functional consequences, is suggested as another reason for underreporting health conditions. Cognitive impairment and depressive symptoms may further limit the ability or desire of some older persons to report symptoms and health conditions. This tendency to underreport means that clinicians must actively inquire about symptoms and concerns.

Altered presentation is a second characteristic of illness in older persons. While both acute and chronic illnesses may, and often do, present with "classic" signs and symptoms, age-related changes and coexisting conditions may combine to obscure these classic presentations in older persons. Symptoms or signs of one condition may exacerbate or mask those of another condition, complicating clinical evaluation. For example, arthritis, if it limits physical activity, may mask the presence of severe cardiovascular disease. Manifestations of clinically important disease may be attenuated in older persons, particularly those who are frail. Chest pain may be absent in older persons presenting with myocardial infarction, as may shortness of breath in persons with congestive heart failure. Another common phenomenon is that symptoms in one organ system may reflect disease in another system. Pneumonia may present as confusion or anorexia; a urinary tract infection may present with behavioral or functional changes. A corollary of these altered presentations is that signs and symptoms are often nonspecific. That is, while suggesting that the older persons is experiencing an acute illness or an exacerbation of a chronic condition, the signs and symptoms may offer limited help in determining what the illness or condition might be. These altered presentations mean that the clinician must be particularly diligent in ascertaining all symptoms and signs. She must rely on combinations of findings from the history, physical examination, and ancillary testing to determine the diagnosis, or, as is often the case, to identify the treatable contributors to the illness or health condition.

Third, the spectrum of health conditions in older persons differs from younger patients. Important clinical entities include not only acute and chronic diseases but also geriatric syndromes as well as cognitive and physical disabilities. Geriatric syndromes are health conditions common in older persons that result from the accumulated effect of multiple predisposing factors and that may be precipitated by an acute insult. Examples described in other chapters include delirium, falls, and incontinence. Geriatric syndromes and disabilities are relevant because they may be the presenting manifestation of another underlying illness and because they are treatable causes of morbidity in their own right.

EVALUATION

Reason for Performing a Test or Evaluation

The process of establishing a diagnosis is complex for any patient. The goal may be to make a diagnosis in an ill patient, to generate a differential diagnosis for observed signs and symptoms, or to make an early diagnosis of presymptomatic disease among well individuals. Making diagnostic decisions is even more challenging in the older person because many have multiple conditions which can mask, mimic, or increase the symptoms of other diseases. Older persons may present atypically, and with nonspecific signs, symptoms and syndromes such as confusion or falls. Furthermore, contrary to the traditional clinical evaluation that is aimed at identifying the presence of discrete diseases, the aim of the clinical encounter in older patients maybe to identify the impairments, diseases, and other factors impeding the attainment of individual patient preferences and goals, as discussed below.

A clinical evaluation grounded in a clear understanding of these issues can be effective. These factors, however, dictate changes in the conventional clinical encounter in both the content and method of ascertainment for the history, the physical examination, and ancillary testing. It is important for clinicians to understand how to assess, interpret, and use the results of an evaluation.

Before deciding whether to pursue a diagnostic test, clinicians should take into account several issues related to the patient and to the characteristics of the test (Table 10-1). Clinicians should consider what they are going to do with the information obtained from the test and whether its consequences will help patients achieve their goals of care. For example, will the test be used to establish a diagnosis for which there is effective treatment? Is the patient willing to accept the treatment? Are there comorbid conditions or contraindications present that would preclude the patient from receiving the therapy? The diagnostic test is likely unnecessary if the patient is not interested in the therapy or if the therapy would result in significant risk of harm. The diagnostic test could also be done to assist with establishing a prognosis—but does the patient want this information? Will the diagnostic test lead to labeling, which can have

TABLE 10-1

Issues to Consider in Deciding Whether to Perform a Diagnostic Test and How to Interpret Results

- How will the results be used?
  - Establish a diagnosis
    - Is there a safe and effective treatment?
    - Do comorbid conditions preclude treatment or make it ineffective?
    - Will the patient accept the treatment?
  - Establish prognosis
    - Does patient want the information?
  - Monitor disease progression or response to therapy
- Definition and interpretation of normal (see Table 10-2)
- Is the test accurate in the patient for whom it is being considered?
- Can the test distinguish persons with and without the targeted condition?
- Do the potential consequences of the test justify its cost and inconvenience?
- Can the test be performed and interpreted in a competent fashion?

TABLE 10-2

Six Definitions of Normal

1. Gaussian: the mean ± 2 standard deviations—this definition assumes a normal distribution for all tests and results in all "abnormalities" having the same frequency.
2. Percentile: within the range, say, of 5–95%, has the same basic defect as the Gaussian definition.
3. Culturally desirable: when "normal" is that which is preferred by society, the role of medicine gets confused.
4. Risk factor: carrying no additional risk of disease; nicely labels the outliers, but does changing a risk factor necessarily change risk?
5. Diagnostic: range of results beyond which target disorders become highly probable.
6. Therapeutic: range of results beyond which treatment does more good than harm.

disastrous consequences? Diagnostic tests can also provide assistance in monitoring therapy once initiated. Finally, is the test being done for academic curiosity or simply because it is available?

The older population may have multiple target conditions but it may not be necessary or clinically useful to pursue all of these with diagnostic tests. An alternative strategy to consider in the elderly with multiple illnesses and symptoms is to focus on symptom modification.

Issues in Assessing and Interpreting Evaluation Results

Definition of Normal in Older Persons

If a diagnostic test is to be performed, then several issues in assessing and interpreting results need to be considered. Results of interview, examination, and ancillary tests typically are reported as "normal" or "abnormal." What is normal in the older person? There are at least six definitions of normal (Table 10-2) but this chapter will focus on the fifth definition, which refers to a range of results beyond which the target disorder becomes highly probable. The sixth definition is also worthy of consideration and includes the range of results beyond which treatment does more good than harm. This last definition is particularly important in the older population. Consider, for example, how the definition of normal blood pressure has changed over the past few decades as evidence accumulates that treatment of progressively less pronounced elevations in blood pressure does more good than harm.

Assessing Diagnostic Test Accuracy

Prior to performing a diagnostic test, clinicians should review and understand its accuracy in older patients with a spectrum of comorbidities. When attempting to determine the accuracy of a diagnostic test, three questions must be considered: (1) is the evidence about the accuracy of a diagnostic test valid? (2) Is there evidence that this test can accurately distinguish patients who do and do not have a specific disorder? and (3) How can this valid, accurate diagnostic test be applied to a specific patient? In assessing validity, the three key components to consider are: (1) independent, blind comparison with a reference standard of diagnosis (e.g., auscultation for a heart murmur

should occur independent of results of the echocardiogram; pathological interpretation of a biopsy should be done without knowledge of laboratory tests that precipitated the biopsy); (2) performance of the reference standard regardless of the diagnostic result (e.g., either performance of pulmonary angiography or long-term follow-up in the absence of anticoagulation therapy to determine negative test accuracy for suspected pulmonary embolism); and (3) evaluation of the diagnostic test in a spectrum of patients similar to those in whom it will be used in clinical practice. Methods for assessing validity using these components have been described in several excellent reviews. Of particular relevance is whether the diagnostic test was evaluated in older patients with a spectrum of comorbidities similar to those in whom you plan to apply the test.

Ability of Tests to Distinguish Patients Who Do and Do Not Have the Disease or Condition

Deciding whether a diagnostic test is important requires consideration of its ability to change the probability of disease prior to test completion (called the pretest probability of the target disorder) to a probability of the disease after test completion (called the posttest probability). Diagnostic tests that produce large changes from pretest to posttest probabilities are important and likely to be useful in clinical practice.

Consider, for example, a 76-year-old woman who is admitted to the hospital with community-acquired pneumonia. She responds nicely to appropriate antibiotics but her hemoglobin remains at 100g/L with a mean cell volume of 80. Her peripheral blood smear shows hypochromia. She is otherwise well and is on no incriminating medications. Her family physician found that her hemoglobin was 105 g/L 6 months prior to admission. She has never been investigated for anemia. A ferritin was ordered and the result is 60 mmoL/L. Does this patient have iron-deficiency anemia?

In a systematic review and meta-analysis of the accuracy of ferritin for diagnosing iron-deficiency anemia, displayed in Table 10-3, the prevalence of iron-deficiency anemia was 31%. The posttest probability, also known as the positive predictive value, of iron-deficiency anemia among patients with a serum ferritin <65 mmoL/L was 73%. Conversely, for a serum ferritin ≥65 mmoL/L, the posttest probability of iron-deficiency anemia is 5%, meaning that the probability of not having iron-deficiency anemia after a negative test result (serum ferritin ≥65 mmoL/L) is 95%, which is known as the negative predictive value. Thus, the probability of iron-deficiency anemia has shifted from 31% to either 73% or 5% depending on the test result.

But, what if the patient's pretest probability were greater than that of the population prevalence? A patient's pretest probability can be estimated from a variety of sources including clinical experience, regional or national prevalence statistics, practice databases, the study used for deciding test accuracy, and studies devoted specifically to determining pretest probabilities (or differential diagnosis). Clinicians might reasonably estimate this patient's pretest probability to be about 50%. The predictive value could be adjusted for this different pretest probability but it requires a lengthy equation. It is easier instead to calculate other measures of test accuracy such as likelihood ratios, which can be generated using sensitivity and specificity (Table 10-3). Using these two proportions, the patient's ferritin result would be about six (90%/15%) times as likely to be seen in someone

TABLE 10-3

Results of a Systematic Review of Serum Ferritin as a Diagnostic Test for Iron Deficiency Anemia

| | | TARGET DISORDER (IRON-DEFICIENCY ANEMIA) | | |
		Present	Absent	Total
Diagnostic test result (serum ferritin)	Positive (<65 mmol/L)	731	270	1001
		a	b	a + b
	Negative (≥65 mmol/L)	78	1500	1578
		c	d	c + d
Total		809	1770	2579
		a + c	b + d	a + b + c + d

Prevalence = $(a + c)/(a + b + c + d)$ = 809/2579 = 31%.
Positive predictive value = $a/(a + b)$ = 731/1001 = 73%.
Negative predictive value = $d/(c + d)$ = 1500/1578 = 95%.
Sensitivity = $a/(a + c)$ = 731/809 = 90%.
Specificity = $d/(b + d)$ = 1500/1770 = 85%.
Likelihood ratio (LR)+ = sensitivity/(1 – specificity) = 90%/15% = 6.
LR– = (1 – sensitivity)/specificity = 10%/85% = 0.12.
Study pretest odds = prevalence/(1 – prevalence) = 31%/69% = 0.45.
Posttest odds = pretest odds × likelihood ratio.
Posttest probability = posttest odds/(posttest odds + 1).
Modified with permission from Guyatt GH, Oxman AD, Ali M, et al. Laboratory diagnosis of iron-deficiency anemia: an overview. J Gen Intern Med. 1992;7:145–53.

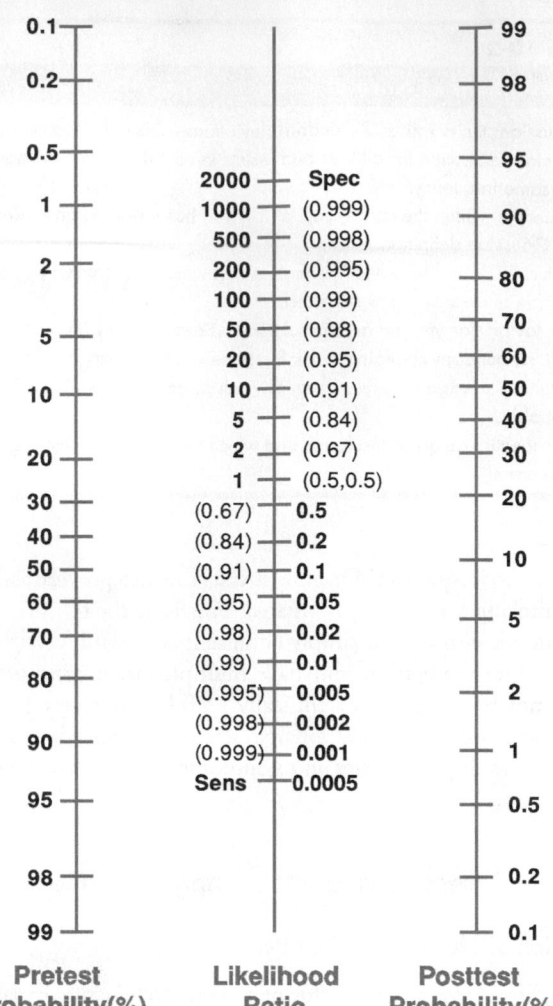

FIGURE 10-1. Nomogram developed by Fagan to calculate posttest probabilities. The left-hand column represents the pretest probability, the middle column represents the likelihood ratio, and the right-hand column shows the posttest probability. The posttest probability is obtained by anchoring a ruler at the pretest probability and shifting it until it lines up with the likelihood ratio for the observed test result.

with iron-deficiency anemia as compared to someone without the condition.

Likelihood ratios cannot be combined directly to pretest probabilities. Their use requires converting pretest probability to odds, multiplying the result by the likelihood ratio, and converting the consequent posttest odds into a posttest probability. An easier method is to use the nomogram developed by Fagan (Figure 10-1). For the serum ferritin example, following a positive test result, a pretest probability of 50% results in a posttest probability of 86%.

The likelihood ratio indicates how much a diagnostic test result will raise or lower the pretest probability of the target condition. A likelihood ratio of 1 means that the posttest probability is the same as the pretest probability. Likelihood ratios >1.0 increase the probability that the target disorder is present; and the higher the likelihood ratio, the greater is this increase. Conversely, likelihood ratios <1.0 decrease the probability of the target disorder.

Likelihood ratios are of particular use with multilevel tests, that is, when there is not a single, dichotomous "normal" or "abnormal" result. They also are useful when doing tests sequentially. For example, the posttest probability resulting from a first test becomes the pretest probability for a second, subsequent test. Expressing the accuracy of serum ferritin with level-specific likelihood ratios highlights how restricting a continuous result to just two levels can be misleading (Table 10-4). The likelihood ratio for a serum ferritin <15 mmoL/L is an impressive 52, which is sufficient to make a diagnosis of iron-deficiency anemia. Conversely, high levels of ferritin (>95 mmoL/L) are sufficient to rule out the diagnosis of iron deficiency. Returning to the clinical scenario, the patient had a pretest probability of 50% and a serum ferritin of 60 mmoL/L. This result generates a likelihood ratio of 1, which results in a posttest probability of 50%. This example highlights that the test, which was thought to be useful when considered as a two-level test, really is not been helpful in making a diagnosis.

TABLE 10-4

Results of Systematic Review of Serum Ferritin as a Diagnostic Test for Iron-Deficiency Anemia: Multilevel Results

| TEST RESULT | PRESENT | | ABSENT | | |
	No.	Prop.	No.	Prop.	LR
<15	474	0.59	20	0.01	51.85
15–34	175	0.22	79	0.04	4.85
35–64	82	0.10	171	0.11	1.05
65–94	30	0.04	168	0.09	0.39
≥95	48	0.06	1332	0.75	0.08

Modified with permission from Guyatt GH, Oxman AD, Ali M, et al. Laboratory diagnosis of iron-deficiency anemia: an overview. J Gen Intern Med. 1992;7: 145–53.

Deciding Whether a Diagnostic Test Should Be Performed in a Specific Patient

A test should not be performed unless its potential consequences justify its cost and it can be performed and interpreted in a competent, reproducible fashion. For example, there are many different D-dimer and B-type natriuretic peptide (BNP) assays—all with varying accuracy—resulting in a challenging interpretation for clinicians. Diagnostic tests often behave differently among different subsets of patients, generating higher likelihood ratios in later stages of florid disease and lower likelihood ratios in early, mild stages.

For any target disease, there are probabilities below which a clinician would dismiss a diagnosis and order no further tests to pursue that particular diagnosis. Similarly, there are probabilities above which a clinician would consider the diagnosis confirmed and would stop testing and initiate treatment. When the probability of the target disease lies between the test and treatment thresholds, further testing is considered. The treatment and test thresholds are a matter of judgment and they differ for different conditions depending on the risks of therapy (if risky, clinicians want to be more certain of the diagnosis) and the danger of the disease if left untreated (if the danger of missing the disease is high and effective therapy is available). The test-treatment threshold may not be crossed until several diagnostic tests are performed.

In older persons, there are additional issues to consider including the ability of the patient to complete the test and whether the test does more good than harm. A patient with significant gait impairment, for example, is not going to be able to complete an exercise stress test. And, it may not be appropriate to consider a particular diagnostic test in someone with multiple comorbidities and poor quality of life. For example, a diagnosis of dyslipidemia is not likely to be clinically relevant in someone with terminal cancer.

Establishing whether a test does more good than harm would theoretically require randomizing patients to a diagnostic strategy that includes the test under investigation or to one in which the test is not available and following patients in both groups forward in time to determine the frequency of patient-important outcomes. While such trials are rare, there are a few. Consider for example a recent Cochrane review of studies that evaluated the impact of screening for prostate cancer. Two randomized trials including more than 55 000 patients found no statistically significant difference in prostate cancer mortality between men randomized to prostate cancer screening and controls (RR: 1.01, 95% CI: 0.80–1.29). However, neither study assessed the effect of prostate cancer screening on quality of life, all-cause mortality, or cost effectiveness. Even in this trial, several relevant clinical questions remain unanswered. In the absence of studies that directly assess benefits and harms, we can look for studies assessing test accuracy. The value of an accurate test is then best determined by considering whether the target disorder is dangerous if left undiagnosed, the test has acceptable risks, and effective treatment exists. All three criteria are relevant, particularly in older patients with multiple health conditions and limited life expectancy. Otherwise it will often be the case that tests may be accurate and management may change as a result of their application, but their impact on important patient outcomes may be less certain.

These concerns in selecting, performing, and interpreting tests pertain to the clinical history, physical examination, laboratory testing, imaging, and other components of a clinical evaluation. In the next section, these and other issues relevant to the evaluation of the older patients are discussed. Illustrative examples are presented.

History/Interview

Setting and Source of Information

The clinical interview is an important element of the diagnostic process. It can be used to establish a diagnosis and monitor treatment and prognosis. The setting and sources of information may need to be adapted to the specific impairments of some older persons. Impairments in hearing, visual acuity, and cognition, each prevalent among older persons, mandate a quiet, well-lit, and unhurried setting—not easily obtained in today's health care environment—in order to obtain thorough and accurate information. Multiple encounters may be required to complete the history and to gather the necessary information. While the patient remains the key informant, the history often needs to be supplemented by information obtained from the family, friends, and other care providers, particularly if the older person has cognitive impairment.

Ascertainment of Goals and Preferences

Patient-centered care dictates that clinical decision making should occur within the context of individual preferences and goals. Ascertainment of these preferences, which are known to vary among older patients and among patients with multiple health conditions, should occur early and often. Older persons rarely volunteer their preferences. Active solicitation of priorities and preferences, therefore, needs to be an integral part of the patient and family interview. Much research attests to the difficulty that patients, especially older patients, have in choosing among a set of treatment options. Rather than having patients make specific treatment choices, which is difficult and often unreliable, encouraging patients to prioritize among different outcome domains allows them to express directly what is most important to them regarding their health care. The elicitation of priorities among general, often competing health outcome domains, including longevity, comfort/symptom relief, cognitive functioning, and physical functioning should drive all evaluation and management decisions. The articulation of specific, feasible goals within these domains then necessitates the identification of underlying diseases, impairments, health conditions, and other factors.

Components of the History and Interview

The altered, often attenuated, presentation of diseases, the coexistence of multiple processes and the underreporting of symptoms and conditions in older patients mandate a reordering of the importance of various components of the history. The chief complaint, the cornerstone of history-taking in younger patients, has decreased relevance in older persons. Indeed, overreliance on the chief complaint leads to the oft cited, though inaccurate, comment that older persons are "vague or poor historians." Older patients are not necessarily poor historians. Rather, they may be accurately reporting the often vague, nonspecific manner in which their illnesses present.

Review of Symptoms and Syndromes The review of systems takes on greater importance in older persons and is often the vehicle by which treatable health conditions are revealed. Complementary to the conventional review of systems, physicians should perform a review of syndromes, targeting modifiable multifactorial geriatric syndromes common in older persons including sleep problems, incontinence, pain, dizziness, falls, depressive symptoms, fatigue, anorexia, and weight loss. As noted earlier, these syndromes are both relevant targets of intervention themselves as well as clues to the existence of other acute and chronic illnesses. Difficulty, degree of dependence, and change in ability in both self-care or basic activities of daily living (ADL—eating, dressing, grooming, bathing, walking, and transferring) and instrumental activities of daily living (IADL—taking medication, handling finances, using transportation, preparing meals, housekeeping, communicating outside the home, and shopping) are integral components of the history in older persons constituting the inventory of functional status, as are frequency of participation in social and higher level physical activities. These functional activities often are the primary outcomes targeted in the treatment of older patients. Furthermore, changes in the frequency or difficulty in participating in these activities often herald the onset of a new, or worsening of an existing, illness.

Assessment of Mood, Affect, and Cognition The clinical history of older persons should also include assessments of cognitive function, affect, and mood (depressive symptoms), social supports, and economic and environmental factors because problems in these domains are prevalent in older persons, contribute to a wide range of health conditions, and are often modifiable. All patients should undergo quick screens of mood and affect, such as the two-question depressive screen (In the past month, have you been sad, blue, or down in the dumps? Have you lost interest in most things or been unable to enjoy them?) More formal, systematic assessments should be undertaken if there is any question of depression.

While the Mini Mental State Examination (MMSE) has good sensitivity (70%–92%) and specificity (77%–96%), shorter screening tests have been found to perform equally well. The Mini-Cog, for example, combines the three-item recall and the Clock Drawing Test (CDT). In a community-based study, the best performing scoring algorithm for the Mini-Cog was when the participant was judged to have dementia if either the three-item recall score was 0, or the three-item recall score was 1 to 2 and a CDT score was rated between 1 (mild) and 3 (severe). This scoring had a sensitivity of 99%, a specificity of 93%, a positive test likelihood ratio of 14.1, and a negative test likelihood ratio of 0.01. This scoring algorithm had a better sensitivity than the MMSE. The Mini-Cog has several advantages, which makes it a useful screening tool. It takes less than 5 minute to complete, is unaffected by language or education, and can be scored by untrained raters with minimal loss of accuracy. The high likelihood ratio of the best-performing algorithm reflected a population with a diagnosis of dementia and will be lower in populations with a low prevalence of dementia. A positive Mini-Cog should be followed by more comprehensive cognitive testing.

Physical Examination

The physical examination in older persons differs from younger persons in content and purpose. The purpose of the physical examination in younger persons is primarily to diagnose specific diseases. The physical examination in older persons, however, also serves to identify treatable impairments such as muscle weakness, gait instability, or sensory impairments, and to directly observe the performance of key functional tasks.

Functional Examination

While the technique of physical examination in an older person is often the same as in younger persons, direct observation and functional testing play particularly important roles in older persons. Observing the older patient as they walk down the hall, get on and off the examination table or in and out of bed, and arises from a chair and get dressed and undressed is a valuable and time-efficient way to ascertain relevant information concerning muscle strength, joint range of motion, and gait stability as well as difficulty with daily functional tasks. Similarly, buttoning and unbuttoning a shirt or blouse, taking shoes on and off, and writing a sentence are simple tests of fine-motor coordination, manual dexterity, and motor planning. Reading a prescription bottle or a magazine provides information on visual acuity. Observing a patient's ability to follow multiple-step commands such as during finger-to-nose testing provides valuable information on cognitive, as well as neurological, functioning. Information on nutritional status can be inferred from observations of the face (e.g., temporal wasting) and hands (e.g., interossei atrophy). Recent weight loss can be judged from clothing that is too large, especially at the collar and waist.

Interpreting Examination Findings

In interpreting physical examination findings, it is important to remember that the coexistence of multiple diseases and the occurrence of nondisease-specific physical impairments in older persons compromise the sensitivity and specificity and, consequently the predictive value of the physical examination in older persons. Abnormal findings may be linked to any of several diseases. Rales, for example, may result from any of congestive heart failure, interstitial fibrosis, or pneumonia, each common and often coexistent in older persons. A decreased neck range of motion may result from arthritis or be a secondary manifestation of voluntarily limiting neck turning because of dizziness caused by vestibular dysfunction. Conversely, the coexistence of multiple diseases may attenuate the physical findings of one or another disease process, such as when the sensitivity of the physical findings of congestive heart failure is compromised by the coexistence of chronic obstructive pulmonary disease.

Physical findings may also have important clinical and functional consequence, even when not linked to any specific disease. Peripheral neuropathy, manifested as decreased vibratory or position sense, for example, may be caused by any number of diseases, including diabetes mellitus, alcohol effect, or vitamin B-12 deficiency, or may occur in the absence of any clinically detectable disease process. Regardless of whether an underlying disease is causative, peripheral neuropathy is an important physical finding in its own right because it leads to gait unsteadiness and a predisposition to falling.

Selecting Components of the Physical Examination to Perform

While the content of the physical examination will be much the same for older, as for younger patients, given time constraints, high-yield, relevant, but not as yet traditional, examination items should substitute for low-yield items. Low-yield items are those that have low specificity in older persons or that do not provide useful information concerning diagnosis, prognosis, or treatment. Examples include the Weber and Rinne tests, undilated eye examinations, Papanicolaou (Pap) smear after age 65 years if previous results were normal, and routine testing of patellar reflexes because of the wide variation in "normal range." Conversely, high-yield items that should become part of the standard physical examination of older persons are defined as findings common in older persons that provide useful diagnostic or prognostic information or suggest the presence of a modifiable condition associated with morbidity. The functional tests described above are examples of high-yield items that should be part of the standard examination. Postural blood pressure, gait examination, inspection of ear canal for cerumen, hearing, visual acuity, and foot examination are other such examples.

Laboratory and Ancillary Tests

As for the physical examination, the coexistence of diseases and age-related changes may affect the sensitivity, specificity, predictive value, and interpretability of laboratory, imaging, and other ancillary tests. In addition, age-referenced normal values and ranges have been developed for some, albeit, not most laboratory tests.

In deciding whether to perform a laboratory, imaging, or other ancillary test, the clinician should consider the issues outlined in Table 10-1 and the principles described in this chapter. This decision process is illustrated for the example of noninvasive imaging for carotid stenosis, an area for which new technologies are constantly being developed. Consider for example, an 80-year-old patient who presents with a transient ischemic attack. A Carotid Doppler ultrasound is ordered and reveal >70% stenosis of the carotid artery on the affected side. Magnetic resonance angiography (MRA) is ordered and the patient's family wants to discuss whether to proceed with the test. Before the MRA is done, several issues should be considered in addition to ensuring that surgery is available and effective in your setting. Would the patient consider carotid endarterectomy? If the answer is no, further diagnostic testing is not warranted. Are there significant comorbidities or contraindications to the surgery? For example, if a patient has advanced dementia and poor functional status, the benefits of surgery would be questionable. If surgery might be contemplated, then it is appropriate to determine whether there are accurate and reliable tests for diagnosing carotid stenosis available in your setting.

A recent systematic review of the accuracy of noninvasive imaging tests compared with intra-arterial angiography for significant carotid stenosis in symptomatic patients can help with the last question noted above. Forty-one studies including 2541 patients were included in this review. The accuracy of the four imaging techniques for diagnosing significant carotid stenosis is provided in Table 10-5. For diagnosing 70% to 99% stenosis, the specificity was lowest for MRA and Doppler ultrasonography. Thus, MRA may result in inappropriate surgery in up to one in seven patients. This systematic review suggests that noninvasive testing cannot appropriately be used to recommend carotid endarterectomy. Patients should be made aware that they will likely require intra-arterial angiography, which does carry a small but real risk of complications. Unless the clinician considers patient outcome goals and risk preferences as well as the accuracy of the diagnostic tests, some patients will have surgery who do not need or desire it and some medically treated patients will have preventable strokes.

TABLE 10-5

Accuracy of Noninvasive Imaging Techniques for Diagnosing 70%–99% Carotid Stenosis Compared with Intra-Arterial Angiography

IMAGING TECHNIQUE	SENSITIVITY (95% CI)	SPECIFICITY (95% CI)	+LR	–LR
CEMRA	95% (88 to 97)	93% (89 to 96)	13	0.06
DUS	89% (85 to 92)	84% (77 to 89)	5.6	0.13
MRA	88% (82 to 92)	84% (76 to 97)	5.5	0.14
CTA	77% (68 to 84)	95% (91 to 97)	15	0.24

CEMRA, contrast-enhanced magnetic resonance angiography; DUS, Doppler ultrasonography; MRA, magnetic resonance angiography; CTA, computed tomographic angiography; LR, likelihood ratio.

Adapted with permission from Kelly A, Holloway RG. Noninvasive imaging techniques may be useful for diagnosing 70 to 99% carotid stenosis in symptomatic patients. ACP Journal Club 2006; Nov/Dec:77.

MANAGEMENT

Treatment decisions should be predicated on attaining feasible patient goals, particularly as treatment of one condition may worsen another and as many treatments adversely affect comfort and functioning. The increased chance of harm as well as benefit of most interventions in older persons dictates that a delineation and presentation of risks, benefits, and trade-offs should constitute an initial step in management. Furthermore, the coexistence of multiple conditions and the contribution of multiple factors to individual conditions require a prioritization of possible interventions to maximize adherence and benefit and minimize harm and burden.

Treatment focused on improving symptoms, rather than modifying disease, in multiply ill and impaired older patients is often appropriate, because comfort and function are primary goals of health care in this population. In contrast to a focus on disease management, which aims to reduce interindividual variability in treatment and monitoring, optimal management of older patients with multiple diseases, and variable health preferences and priorities is individualized.

Medication prescribing offers a particular challenge. There is an ever expanding list of medications available for treating chronic diseases and nondisease specific symptoms. Prescribing decisions need to be made within the context of patient preference and with an appreciation of total medication burden not solely the benefit and harm of each individual medication for an individual disease. The cost of medications is another significant medication-related issue in many older patients. Issues related to medication use in older patients are discussed in Chapter 24.

Because many health conditions in older persons result from the accumulated effect of psychological, social, and environmental, as well as purely medical, factors, a multicomponent, integrated treatment plan represents the most effective strategy. The use of nonpharmacologic interventions is one of the most effective ways to minimize medication use. For many health conditions, including diabetes mellitus, arthritis, congestive heart failure, depression, pain, and sleep disorders, treatment should include a combination of pharmacologic, rehabilitative, psychosocial, and environmental interventions. Exercise and physical activity are proven interventions for each of these conditions. Counseling and cognitive behavior therapies are important treatment components for depression, pain, and sleep disorders. Interdisciplinary teams, as discussed in Chapter 26 are essential to the successful implementation of these multicomponent interventions.

FURTHER READING

Boockvar KS, Lachs MS. Predictive value of nonspecific symptoms for acute illness in nursing home residents. *J Am Geriatr Soc.* 2003;51:1111–1115.

Boyd CM, Darer J, Boult C, et al. Clinical practice guidelines and quality of care for older patients with multiple comorbid diseases: implications for pay for performance. *JAMA.* 2005;294:716–724.

Fagan T. Nomogram for Bayes theorem. *N Eng J Med.* 1975;293:257.

Fried TR, Bradley EH, Towle VR, et al. Understanding the treatment preferences of seriously ill patients. *N Engl J Med.* 2002;346:1061–1066.

Ginsberg JS, Caco CC, Brill-Edwards PA, et al. Venous thrombosis in patients who have undergone major hip or knee surgery: detection with compression US and impedance plethysmography. *Radiology.* 1991;181:651–654.

Guyatt GH, Oxman AD, Ali M, et al. Laboratory diagnosis of iron-deficiency anemia: an overview. *J Gen Intern Med.* 1992;7:145–153.

Hirsch C. The Mini-cog had high sensitivity and specificity for diagnosing dementia in community-dwelling older adults. *ACP Journal Club* 2001;Sep/Oct:74.

Ilic D, O'Connor D, Green S, et al. Screening for prostate cancer. Cochrane Database of Systematic Reviews 2006, Issue 3. Art. No.: CD004720.

Kelly A, Holloway RG. Noninvasive imaging techniques may be useful for diagnosing 70 to 99% carotid stenosis in symptomatic patients. *ACP Journal Club* 2006;Nov/Dec:77.

Kim S, Goldstein D, Hasher L, et al. Framing effects in younger and older adults. *J Gerontol* 2005;60:P215–8.

Scanlan J, Borson S. The Mini-cog: receiver operating characteristics with expert and naïve raters. *Int J Geriatr Psych.* 2001;16:216–222.

Straus SE, Richardson WS, Glasziou P, et al. *Evidence Based Medicine: How to Practice and Teach It.* Edinburgh: Churchill Livingstone; 2005.

Tinetti ME, Bogardus ST Jr, Agostini JV. Potential pitfalls of disease-specific guidelines for patients with multiple conditions. *N Engl J Med.* 2004;351:2870–2874.

Tinetti ME, Fried T. The end of the disease era. *Am J Med.* 2004;116:179–185.

US Preventive Services Task Force. Guide to Clinical Preventive Services, 3rd Edition: Recommendations and systematic evidence reviews. Screening for dementia. AHRQ; 2000.

Wardlaw JM, Chappell FM, Best JJ, et al. Non-invasive imaging compared with intra-arterial angiography in the diagnosis of symptomatic carotid stenosis: a meta-analysis. *Lancet.* 2006;367:1503–1512.

Principles of Geriatric Assessment

David B. Reuben ■ *Sonja Rosen*

Geriatric assessment is a broad term used to describe the health evaluation of the older patient, which emphasizes components and outcomes different from that of the standard medical evaluation. This approach recognizes that the health status of older persons is dependent upon influences beyond the manifestations of their medical conditions. Among these are social, psychological and mental health, and environmental factors. Geriatric assessment also places high value upon functional status, both as a dimension to be evaluated and as an outcome to be improved or maintained.

Although in the strictest sense geriatric assessment is a diagnostic process, many use the term to include both evaluation and management. Moreover, geriatric assessment is sometimes used to refer to evaluation by the individual clinician and at other times is used to refer to a more interdisciplinary process, comprehensive geriatric assessment (CGA). The terminology is further clouded because the latter process has evolved since its inception with respect to sites where the assessment is provided, the participating health professionals, the nature of the assessment, and the amount of follow-up and management that is included. Accordingly, any discussion of geriatric assessment must be precise in its description of the process of interest.

This chapter is divided into four components: (1) geriatric assessment by the individual clinician, with an emphasis on the outpatient setting; (2) a strategic approach to geriatric assessment for the practicing clinician; (3) CGA and evidence for its effectiveness; and (4) lessons learned from geriatric assessment that have been applied to health care delivery of older persons.

GERIATRIC ASSESSMENT BY THE INDIVIDUAL CLINICIAN

Geriatric assessment (Figure 11-1) by the individual clinician extends beyond the traditional disease-oriented medical evaluation of older persons' health to include assessment of cognitive, affective, functional, social, economic, environmental, and spiritual status, as well as a discussion of patient preferences regarding advance directives. Assessment instruments can be used to guide these evaluations but do not substitute for clinical skills and judgment, including the skill of eliciting important items from the patient's history and physical examination. Information obtained from assessment instruments can direct the clinician's attention to issues that are particularly relevant to an individual patient. Systematic assessment of the multiple domains noted above ensures that the evaluation is comprehensive. Some clinicians may prefer to rely on less formal questions to probe into potential problems. Examples of potential open-ended questions are provided later in this chapter.

Geriatric assessment differs according to the setting where the patient is being evaluated. In the hospital setting, the initial assessment is usually directed at the acute medical problem that precipitated the hospitalization. As the patient begins to recover and plans are initiated for discharge, other components (e.g., social support, environment) assume increasing importance in the assessment. The inpatient setting can be problematic for geriatric assessment because of the rapidly changing status of several key dimensions. For example, a patient may temporarily become "dependent" on all measures of functional status when acutely ill and gradually improve prior to discharge. Because patients may overestimate their functional status based on their previous level of functioning, direct observational methods (e.g., by nurses or physical therapists) may provide a more accurate assessment. The patient's full potential to participate in rehabilitation may not be known until near the time of discharge.

Nursing home geriatric assessment requires that attention be directed to selected aspects of assessment such as nutritional status and self-care activities. Other components such as functional status at the instrumental activities of daily living level (e.g., shopping, meal preparation) are less relevant in this setting. Geriatric assessment conducted in the patient's home provides an opportunity for an entirely different type of assessment; environmental factors (e.g., home safety) and insights into functional status (e.g., cleanliness of

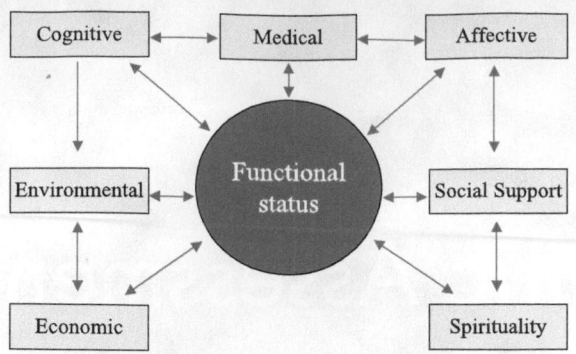

FIGURE 11-1. Interacting dimensions of geriatric assessment.

the home) can be directly assessed while other aspects of the traditional examination (e.g., the gynecologic examination) are much more difficult.

Because the primary site of most clinicians' practices is the office setting, assessment techniques are described primarily for this setting. When appropriate, differing, or particularly important information about assessment in other settings is added.

Components of the Geriatric Assessment

In addition to the standard medical history and physical examination, the clinician should systematically search for specific conditions that are common among older persons and that might have considerable impact on function. In the course of the traditional medical evaluation, these problems may go unnoticed because older patients fail to report them spontaneously. For example, they may not recognize that falling is a treatable medical problem. They may also be embarrassed to mention problems with maintaining urinary continence or with sexual function. Finally, they may believe that these symptoms, such as hearing loss, are normal aspects of aging that cannot be helped.

Visual Impairment

Visual impairment is a common and often under-reported problem in the older population. Each of the four major eye diseases (cataract,

age-related macular degeneration, diabetic retinopathy, and glaucoma) increases in prevalence with age. Moreover, presbyopia is virtually universal and the vast majority of older persons require eyeglasses. Visual impairment has been associated with increased risk of falls, functional and cognitive decline, immobility, and depression. The high rates of vision disorders and their associated sequalea, the brevity of the screening process, and the treatments available for visual impairment justify screening for visual impairment.

The standard method of screening for problems with visual acuity is the Snellen eye chart, which requires the patient to stand 20 ft from the chart and read letters, using corrective lenses. Patients fail the screen if they are unable to read all the letters on the 20/40 line with their eyeglasses (best corrected vision).

Several interviewer and self-administered instruments to detect functional problems caused by visual impairment have been developed, including the "Activities of Daily Vision Scale," VF-14, VFQ-25, and the Cataract Symptom Scale. These are primarily used in research settings, but may hold promise as screening instruments in the future.

Hearing Impairment

Hearing impairment is among the most common medical conditions reported by older persons, affecting approximately one-third of those 65 years of age or older. Hearing impairment is associated with reduced cognitive, emotional, social, and physical function in older persons and the use of amplification devices has led to improved functional status and quality of life of older persons.

Screening for hearing loss can be accomplished by several methods (Table 11-1). The most accurate of these is the Welch Allyn AudioScope 3 (Welch Allyn, Inc., Skaneateles Falls, NY), a handheld otoscope with a built-in audiometer. The AudioScope 3 can be set at several different levels of intensity, but should be set at 40 dB to evaluate hearing in older persons. A pretone at 60 dB is delivered and then four tones (500, 1000, 2000, and 4000 Hz) at 40 dB are delivered. Patients fail the screen if they are unable to hear either the 1000- or 2000-Hz frequency in both ears or both the 1000- and 2000-Hz frequencies in one ear, indicating the need for formal audiometric testing.

A simple alternative is to rely on patient's own subjective report of hearing loss. A self-reported hearing loss question involves asking

TABLE 11-1

Simple Tests of Hearing Loss		
QUESTION/TEST	**TIME TO ADMINISTER**	**COMMENTS**
Audioscope	1–2 minutes	Sensitivity 87–90%, specificity 70–90%
Single question: "Do you feel you have a hearing loss?"	<1 minute	Sensitivity 75–81%, specificity 64–70%
Whisper test	1 minute	Sensitivity 80–100%, specificity 82–89%
Hearing handicap	2 minutes	Sensitivity 48–63%, specificity 75–86% at cutpoint >8
Inventory for the elderly NHANES* battery Age >70 = 1 Male sex = 1 ≤12th grade education = 1 Previously saw doctor about trouble hearing =1 Without hearing aid, cannot hear whisper across the room = 1 Without hearing aid, cannot hear normal voice across the room = 2	<2 minutes	Sensitivity 80%, specificity 80% at cutpoint of >3

*National Health and Nutrition Examination Survey.

patients whether they feel they have hearing impairment. An affirmative answer is then considered to be a positive test for hearing loss, and patients should be referred to an audiologist.

Another alternative is the whispered voice test, which is administered by whispering three to six random words (numbers, words, or letters) at a set distance (6, 8, 12, or 24 inches) from the person's ear and then asking the patient to repeat the words. The examiner should be behind the person to prevent speech reading and the opposite ear should be covered or occluded during the examination. Patients fail the screen if they are unable to repeat half of the whispered words correctly.

Similar to vision screening, a self-administered test of emotional and social problems associated with impaired hearing, the Hearing Handicap Inventory for the Elderly—Screening Version (HHIE-S) was developed. Although this questionnaire is brief and easy to administer, its accuracy when compared to audiometry is less than the audiometer. Another screening instrument that uses sociodemographic information coupled with three simple questions (see Table 11-1) about hearing loss has high accuracy in identifying older persons with hearing loss.

Malnutrition/Weight Loss (See Also Chapter 38)

Malnutrition is a global term that encompasses many different nutritional problems that are associated with diverse health consequences. Both extremes of body weight place older people at risk for subsequent functional impairment, morbidity, and mortality. Among community-dwelling older persons, the most common nutritional disorder is obesity. In addition, a small percentage of community-dwelling older persons have energy or protein energy undernutrition, which places them at higher risk for death and functional decline. Protein energy undernutrition is defined by the presence of clinical (physical signs such as wasting, low body mass index) and biochemical (albumin or other protein) evidence of insufficient intake. Although the importance of low serum albumin and low cholesterol as prognostic factors for mortality in community-dwelling, hospitalized, and institutionalized older persons has been demonstrated, these tests may reflect inflammation rather than malnutrition.

Several methods of nutritional screening can be applied in office settings. On their initial visit, patients should be asked about weight loss within the previous 6 months. All patients should be weighed at every office visit. Height should also be measured on the initial visit to allow calculation of body mass index (weight in kg/[height in meters]^2). Several self-administered nutritional questionnaires are available, most notably the Nutrition Screening Initiative's 10-item checklist and the Mini-Nutritional Assessment (MNA). The use of the MNA can help detect risk of malnutrition while albumin and BMI are still in the normal range. Although the validity of these instruments has been questioned, they are being increasingly used in community-based screening programs.

In hospitalized older persons, malnutrition has been associated with higher mortality rates, delayed functional recovery, and higher rates of nursing home use. Therefore, energy and protein intake should be monitored closely in this setting. Intake can be measured through formal calorie counts. Laboratory monitoring may also be useful. Although serum albumin levels can drop acutely during inflammatory states, physiologic stress, and in response to trauma or surgical conditions, this protein has a long half-life (approximately 18 days). Accordingly, obtaining serum albumin level at the time of

hospital admission provides an idea of the patient's baseline nutritional status. Prealbumin, which has a much shorter half-life (approximately 2 days) may be a better means of monitoring response to nutritional treatment. Serum cholesterol may also be valuable in monitoring hospitalized patients as falling values have been associated with increased morbidity and mortality.

Urinary Incontinence

Urinary incontinence is common, especially among older women, and is underrecognized. Women may be embarrassed to raise the issue; they also may regard it as a normal aspect of aging. Urinary incontinence has been associated with depressive symptoms in older adults. Moreover, effective treatments are available for incontinence. As a result, screening for urinary incontinence has increasingly been recognized as an indicator of quality of care.

Asking two questions can screen for incontinence: (1) "In the last year, have you ever lost your urine and gotten wet?" and if so, (2) "Have you lost urine on at least six separate days?" In a research setting, those who answered positive to both questions had high rates (79% for women and 76% for men) of urinary incontinence as determined by a clinician's evaluation (see Chapter 59).

The 3IQ questionnaire is another interviewer-administered instrument that has been developed to distinguish between urinary stress and urge incontinence in primary care settings, (Table 11-2) and will need further validation in clinical settings.

TABLE 11-2

The Three Incontinence Questions (3IQ)

1. During the last 3 months, have you leaked urine (even a small amount?)
   Yes   No → Questionnaire completed

2. During the last 3 months, did you leak urine:
   (Check all that apply.)
   a. When you were performing some physical activity, such as coughing, sneezing, lifting, or exercise?
   b. When you had the urge or the feeling that you needed to empty your bladder, but you could not get to the toilet fast enough?
   c. Without physical activity and without a sense of urgency?

3. During the last 3 months, did you leak urine *most often*:
   (Check only one.)
   a. When you were performing some physical activity, such as coughing, sneezing, lifting, or exercise?
   b. When you had the urge or the feeling that you needed to empty your bladder, but you could not get to the toilet fast enough?
   c. Without physical activity and without a sense of urgency?
   d. About equally as often with physical activity as with a sense of urgency?

   Definitions of type of urinary incontinence are based on response to question 3:

Response to Question 3	Type of Incontinence
a. Most often with physical activity	Stress only or stress predominant
b. Most often with the urge to empty the bladder	Urge only or urge predominant
c. Without physical activity or sense of urgency cause	Other cause only or other predominant
d. About equally with physical activity and sense of urgency	Mixed

Balance and Gait Impairments and Falling

Over one-third of community-dwelling persons over age 65 years fall every year. Falls are independently associated with functional and mobility decline. Patients who have fallen or have a gait or balance problem are at higher risk of another fall. The risk of falling can be assessed by asking all older patients if they have fallen in the last year, and then performing a multifactorial falls assessment (Figure 11-2) by testing balance, gait, and lower extremity strength (see Chapter 54). Performing a multifactorial assessment on patients who screen positive for falls, and then treating their risk factors for

---

Reason for Visit: ☐ Fall *(Go to Q1)*
☐ Fear of falling ONLY *(Go to Q4)*

PATIENT LABEL

History:
→ *(Have patient lie down in preparation for orthostatic BP and P)*

1. When was last fall? ☐ Past 4 wks ☐ More than 4 wks

2. Circumstances of fall:	YES	NO
Loss of consciousness	☐	☐
Tripped/stumbled over something	☐	☐
Lightheadedness / palpitations	☐	☐
Unable to get up within 5 minutes	☐	☐
Needed assistance to get up	☐	☐

3. Orthostatics: *(Measure after 1 minute in specified position)*

Lying: BP: _____/_____ Pulse: _____

Standing: BP: _____/_____ Pulse: _____

4. Currently uses device for mobility?	YES	NO
Cane	☐	☐
Walker	☐	☐
Wheelchair	☐	☐
Other, *specify:* _____	☐	☐

5. Vision:		
Noticed recent vision change	☐	☐
Eye exam in past year	☐	☐

6. Visual acuity:

OS: 20/_____ OD: 20/_____ OU: 20/_____

7. Psychotropic medications *(specify)*:	YES	NO
Neuroleptics: _____	☐	☐
Antidepressants: _____	☐	☐
Benzodiazepines: _____	☐	☐

a) IF **YES** to benzodiazepines, dc'd? ☐ ☐ → Reason for continuation: _____

8. 2 or more drinks alcohol each day	YES ☐	NO ☐
9. Other conditions: _____	☐	☐

Examination:

1. 3-Item recall: ☐ **PASS** *(2-3 words)*
☐ **FAIL** *(0-1 word)* → Cognitive status: _____

2. Gait: ☐ **NORMAL** ☐ **ABNORMAL**

Abnormal if: -Hesitant start   -Heels do not clear toes of other foot
-Broad-based gait   -Heels do not clear floor
-Extended arms   -Path deviates

Timed-Up-and-Go:_____sec
(Normal ≤ 15 sec)

-Stand from chair NOT using arms,
-Walk 10 feet,
-Turn around,
-Walk back,
-Sit down

3. Balance:	YES	NO	If indicated:	YES	NO
Side-by-side, stable 10 sec	☐	☐	Can pick up penny off floor	☐	☐
Semi-tandem, stable 10 sec	☐	☐	Resistance to nudge	☐	☐
Full tandem, stable 10 sec	☐	☐			

4. Neuromuscular:	YES	NO		YES	NO
Quad strength: Can rise from chair w/o using arms	☐	☐	Rigidity *(e.g., cogwheeling)*	☐	☐
			Bradykinesia	☐	☐
If indicated, hip ROM and knee exam:			Tremor	☐	☐

Lab/Tests:
☐ EKG   ☐ Bone mineral density
☐ Holter   ☐ Other: _____

Impression:
☐ Strength problem   ☐ Parkinsonism
☐ Balance problem   ☐ Severe hip/knee OA
☐ Gait problem   ☐ Other: _____

Treatment:
☐ Exercises: ☐ Upper body ☐ Lower body
☐ Community exercise program
☐ Home safety checklist given
☐ Footwear discussion
☐ Community resource list given
☐ Falls education packet given
☐ Hip protectors
☐ Vitamin D 800 IU/day
☐ Ca carbonate 1200-1500 mg/day (Ca citrate if on PPI)

☐ Referral for PT
☐ Assistive device: _____ ☐ New ☐ Review
☐ Referral for home safety inspection/modifications
☐ Change in medication(s): _____
_____
☐ Referral for eye exam
☐ Cardiology consult
☐ Neurology consult
☐ Other: _____

FIGURE 11-2. Structured visit note to assess persons who have screened positive for falls. The information above dotted line is collected by office staff.

falling can reduce falls by 30% to 40%. Moreover, the assessment of these components may also help identify methods to improve the patient's function beyond reducing the risk of falling. Screening for falls and falls assessment, if the screen is positive, are recognized as indicators of quality of care.

Clinicians should ask their older persons specifically about falls and fear of falling, which should be included in the review of systems at the initial visit and at least annually. The use of a previsit questionnaire can also help elicit this information. The report of any fall should prompt subsequent questions by the clinician to determine the circumstances of the fall. Patients with recurrent falls or falls with any injury should receive a more detailed evaluation, including assessment of gait and balance, orthostatic blood pressure readings, vision testing, and reviewing medications that may contribute to the risk of falling (see Chapter 54).

Observing patients walking and performing balance maneuvers best assesses balance and gait disorders. Once the clinician is trained to assess gait, this evaluation can be performed while the patient is entering or leaving the examining room. Several simple tests of balance and mobility can also be performed quickly in the office setting, including the ability to maintain a side-by-side, semitandem, and full-tandem stance for 10 seconds; resistance to a nudge; and stability during a 360-degree turn (Table 11-3). Quadriceps strength can be briefly assessed by observing an older person arising from a hard armless chair without the use of his or her hands. The timed "up and go" test is a timed measure of the patients ability to rise arm chair, walk 3 m (10 ft), turn, walk back, and sit down again; those who take longer than 20 seconds to complete the test should receive further evaluation. Gait speed is also a helpful marker for recurrent falls. Patients who take more than 13 seconds to walk 10 m are more likely to have recurrent falls.

The Performance-Oriented Assessment of Mobility is a standardized battery that measures gait and balance; it has been widely used in research and in clinical settings, but may take too long to administer to be practical in most office settings as a screening test. The ability to stretch as measured by functional reach, a test of balance, can predict subsequent recurrent falls.

Polypharmacy (See Also Chapter 24)

Polypharmacy in older patients is associated with adverse drug reactions, reduced adherence, and inappropriate medication usage. Older persons often receive care from multiple providers and they may fill prescriptions at several pharmacies. Patients should be instructed, therefore, to bring in all current medications—both prescription and nonprescription medications—to each visit. Office personnel can check these against the medication list in the medical record and discrepancies can be brought to the clinician's attention at the time of the patient encounter. Several drug interaction programs are commercially available to check for potential drug–drug interactions. With the introduction of personal digital assistants and drug software programs, clinicians can easily assess the potential for drug–drug interactions at the time of prescribing any new medication. The use of four or more prescription and nonprescription medications should trigger a review and consideration of continued need for each medication given the increased risk of adverse drug effect with increasing number of medications.

Cognitive Assessment

Because the prevalence of Alzheimer's disease, other dementias, and cognitive impairment, rises considerably with advancing age, the yield of screening for cognitive impairment increases with age. The most commonly used screen is the Mini-Mental State Examination, a 30-item interviewer-administered assessment of several dimensions of cognitive function. However, it is too long for most practitioners to routinely incorporate as a screening test into their clinical practices. Several shorter screens (Table 11-4) have also been validated including recall of three items at 1 minute, the clock drawing test, and the Mini-Cog test, which combines three-item recall and clock drawing. The Time-and-Change test, which employs clock recognition and counting change, is another valid screening test. The clock drawing components of these tests evaluate executive function (which includes higher cognitive processing) and appear to be less influenced by educational level or culture than some other cognitive assessments. Although normal results on these tests vastly reduce the probability of dementia and abnormal results increase the likelihood that the patient has dementia, these tests are neither diagnostic for dementia nor do normal results exclude the possibility of this disorder. Patients who have abnormal findings on a cognitive screening test should receive more in-depth evaluation of memory, language, visual–spatial, and executive function.

Among hospitalized patients, mental status should be assessed at the time of hospital admission and then periodically because older persons are especially prone to develop delirium during the hospital stay. Abnormal findings on the mental status examination in hospitalized patients must be interpreted in the context of change from baseline and the clinical situation. The Confusion Assessment Method provides a guide to interpreting such changes (see Chapter 53).

Affective Assessment (See Also Chapter 70)

Although major depression is no more common among the elderly than the younger population, depression and other affective

---

TABLE 11-3

Simple Tests of Lower Extremities: Strength, Balance, Gait, and Fall Risk

QUESTION/TEST	TIME TO ADMINISTER	COMMENTS
Timed up and go	<1 minute	Sensitivity 88%, specificity 94% compared to geriatrician's evaluation using cutpoint >15 s
Gait speed over 10 m	< 30 s	>13 s predicts recurrent falls (Likelihood ratio: 2.0; 95% CI, 1.5–2.7)

Office-based maneuvers
  Observed gait
  Resistance to nudge
  Tandem/semitandem stand
  Rising from chair
  360° turn
	2–3 minutes	Some are part of performance-oriented assessment of mobility

Functional reach	2 minutes	Adjusted odds ratios for >2 falls within 6 mo
		  8.1 if unable to reach
		  4.0 if reach ≤6″
		  2.0 if reach ≥6″ but <10″

TABLE 11-4

Predictive Value of Brief Screening Questions for Cognitive Impairment

TEST	TEST RESULT	LIKELIHOOD RATIO
Orientation		
Day	Abnormal	6.3
	Normal	0.5
Month	Abnormal	16
	Normal	0.4
Year	Abnormal	37
	Normal	0.5
Forward digit-span	≤4 digits	7.1
	5 digits	2.0
	6 digits	0.8
	7 digits	0.1
Recall of 3 items	Recalls <2	3.1
	Recalls 2	0.5
	Recalls all 3	0.06
Clock drawing	Abnormal	24
	Almost normal	0.8
	Normal	0.2
Mini-Cog	Abnormal	14.1
	Normal	0.01
Time and Change	Abnormal	3.0
	Normal	0.2

Adapted with permission from Siu AL. Screening for dementia and investigating its causes. Ann Intern Med. 1991;115(2):122.

disorders are common and cause considerable morbidity. Depression in older adults may present atypically, and may be masked in patients with cognitive impairment or other neurologic diseases such as Parkinson's disease. A simple inquiry such as, "Do you often feel sad or depressed?" can be used as a screen. This single question, however, tends to be overly sensitive and may be better used in tandem with a second screen such as the Geriatric Depression Scale, which has 5-, 15-, and 30-item versions. A variety of other screens for depression are available and each has its advantages and disadvantages.

More recently, the Patient Health Questionnaire-9 (PHQ-9) has increasingly been used to detect and monitor depression symptoms. The PHQ-9 is a brief patient-administered depression scale, and provides a reliable and valid measure of depression severity. A score of >10 has a sensitivity of 88% and a specificity of 88% for major depression.

Assessment of Function

Measurement of functional status is an essential component of the assessment of older persons. The patient's ability to function can be viewed as a summary measure of the overall impact of health conditions in the context of his or her environment and social support system. Moreover, in older persons, the ability to function consistent with their personal lifestyle desires should be an important consideration in all-care planning. Therefore, changes in functional status should prompt further diagnostic evaluation and intervention. An early indicator of impending functional disability is self-perceived difficulty with performing functional tasks. Measurement of functional status is also valuable in monitoring response to treatment and may provide prognostic information that will help plan for long-term care.

Functional status can be assessed at three levels: basic activities of daily living (BADLs), instrumental or intermediate activities of daily living (IADLs), and advanced activities of daily living (AADLs). BADLs refer to self-care tasks such as bathing, dressing, toileting, continence, grooming, feeding, and transferring. Instrumental activities of daily living refer to the ability to maintain an independent household such as shopping for groceries, driving or using public transportation, using the telephone, meal preparation, housework, home repair, laundry, taking medications, and handling finances, whereas AADLs refer to the ability to fulfill societal, community, and family roles as well as participate in recreational or occupational tasks. These advanced activities vary considerably from individual to individual but may be valuable in monitoring functional status prior to the development of disability.

Scales that measure functional status at each of these levels have been developed and validated. Questions that ask about specific BADL and IADL functions have also been incorporated into a variety of more generic health-related quality-of-life instruments (e.g., the Medical Outcomes Study Short-Form 36 and its shorter version, the SF-12). Some AADLs (e.g., exercise and leisure time physical activity) can also be ascertained by using standardized instruments, but open-ended questions about how older persons spend their days might provide a better assessment of function in healthier older persons.

Over the past decade, there has been emerging interest in assessment of physical functioning by directly observing the performance of functional tasks. Instruments have been developed for use in ambulatory, nursing home, and hospital settings, and predictive validity has been demonstrated for many. To date, these instruments are rarely incorporated into clinical practice, but some demonstration projects are in place that are attempting to use performance-based instruments in practice, much like vital signs, to monitor patients. Some recent studies demonstrate that combining self-reported functional with performance-based measures can provide more refined prognostic information than either method alone.

Assessment of Social Support

The composition of the older patient's social support structure can be assessed by asking a few questions when obtaining the social history. The quality of these relationships should also be determined. For very frail older persons, the availability of assistance from family and friends is frequently the determining factor of whether a functionally dependent older person remains at home or is institutionalized. If dependency is noted during functional assessment, then the clinician should inquire as to who provides help for specific BADL and IADL functions and whether these persons are paid or voluntary help. Even in healthier older persons, it is often valuable to raise the question of who would be available to help if the patient becomes ill. Early identification of problems with social support may prompt planning to develop resources should the necessity arise.

Economic Assessment

Although some clinicians feel uncomfortable in assessing the economic status of their patients, insurance status is routinely collected by office staff. The patient's income can also be assessed and eligibility for state or local benefits (e.g., In Home Supportive Services through Medicaid) to provide services for the functionally impaired can be determined. For the frail and functionally impaired, physicians may need to begin discussions of planning to mobilize savings and other resources to provide personal attendant care.

Environmental Assessment

Environmental assessment encompasses two dimensions, the safety of the home environment and the adequacy of the patient's access to needed personal and medical services. Particularly among frail individuals and those with mobility and balance problems, the home environment should be assessed for safety. Although most physicians do not personally conduct environmental assessments, the National Safety Council has developed a home safety checklist that patients and their families can complete. For those receiving home health services, in-home safety inspections can be performed, including recommendations for installation of adaptive devices such as shower bars and raised toilet seats.

Older persons who begin to develop IADL dependencies should be evaluated for the geographic proximity of necessary services such as grocery shopping and banking, their need for use of such services, and their ability to use these services in their current living situations. Older drivers are at increased risk for motor vehicle accidents secondary to functional impairments, medications, and medical conditions. The Older Drivers Project, created by the American Medical Association (AMA) and the National Highway Traffic Safety Administration (NHTSA), have produced materials to help physicians approach this issue.

Spirituality

Spirituality, whether affiliated with a formal religious denomination or nonreligious intangible elements, has increasingly been recognized as an important influence on health. Recent data indicate that frequent attendance of religious services is associated with lower health care utilization and mortality rates. Formal instruments assessing spirituality have been developed but are not yet widely used in clinical practice. Simply asking older persons whether religion or spirituality is important to them may provide insights that may facilitate their care. Especially in hospital settings, involvement of pastoral care may be valuable in supporting the patient and in framing medical decisions in the context of the patient's personal belief system.

Advance Directives

Discussions of advance directives are important for all patients and should be initiated early on to discuss the patients' goals and preferences for care should they become unable to speak for themselves because of progressive cognitive impairment or acute illness. Physicians can assist patients by focusing on patients' overall goals of care, rather than specific detailed interventions, and incorporating these goals into the patients' current clinical situation. A particularly important time to discuss such preferences is prior to surgery because of the possibility of surgical complications or postoperative delirium, which may preclude discussions following the procedure. The durable power of attorney for health care, which asks the patient to designate a surrogate to make medical decisions if the patient loses decision-making capacity, is often less emotionally laden than specifying treatments that the patient may or may not want. Such discussions should be revisited any time there are significant changes in a patient's medical condition and a better understanding about prognosis becomes available. Patients often revise their thoughts about the benefits of treatment. Cultural differences regarding preferences for advance directives and end-of-life care should be recognized and respected.

A Strategic Approach to Geriatric Assessment

The practice of medicine in office settings is in a state of transition from a previous era of medicine when physicians practiced more like individual artisans to an approach in which physicians function as members of a health care team. Much of the germane information of the medical history can be obtained from old records, other professional or nonprofessional staff, or by self-report from patients or family members completing forms, rather than from direct physician interview. Although many physicians and patients lament such changes, this efficiency allows the physician to spend more time following up on issues raised by the available information, conducting the physical examination, discussing treatment, and providing health education.

One effort adopted by many clinical practices has been the use of previsit questionnaires that can be completed by the patient or proxy before the clinical encounter. These questionnaires typically gather information on past medical history, medications, preventive measures, and functional status, including information on who helps when the patient is functionally dependent. As a result, they can markedly reduce the time needed to conduct an initial assessment and can ensure a consistent level of comprehensiveness for every patient. By including validated screening instruments, they can also be used to case-find individuals with common geriatric syndromes. With the advance of technology and electronic health records, patients, families, or caregivers can complete such questionnaires electronically and the information obtained can be seamlessly integrated into the electronic health record.

A second method of streamlining the office visit is to delegate the administration of screening instruments for many of the important geriatric problems to trained office staff. Thus, the clinician may spend a short period of time reviewing the results of these screens and then decide which dimensions, if any, need greater evaluation. Several groups (Tables 11-5 and 11-6) have demonstrated the feasibility and yield of using office staff to administer case-finding and screening instruments that assess many of the dimensions described above. This approach can dramatically improve the practitioner's efficiency and increase the number of new and treatable problems detected in their older patients. However, using office-based staff to screen or case-find has cost implications. Office staff must be properly trained to administer these instruments, which can be quite time-consuming. One published method takes approximately 22 minutes to administer and another takes an estimated 10 minutes to administer. This time must be taken from other office tasks and the cost of screening may be considerable (see Table 11-6). Clinicians must also be able to effectively act on this information to improve clinical outcomes. Nevertheless, as physicians become increasingly pressured to increase their productivity, such methods may be the only way to feasibly ensure that older patients' diverse health needs are addressed comprehensively.

A third approach has been to integrate screening for geriatric conditions into the office workflow and then use structured clinical visit

TABLE 11-5

Multidimensional Screening Instruments

PROBLEM	SCREENING MEASURE	Positive Screen	SCREENING PACKAGE CHARACTERISTICS	
			Positive Predictive Value	Negative Predictive Value
Vision	Two parts: Ask: "Do you have difficulty driving, or watching television, or reading, or doing any of your daily actvites because of your eyesight?" If yes, then: Test each eye with Snellen chart while patient wears corrective lenses (if applicable).	Yes to question and inability to read greater than 20/40 on Snellen chart.	0.75	0.89
Hearing	Use audiometer set at 40 dB. Test hearing using 1000 and 2000 Hz	Inability to hear 1000 or 2000 Hz in both ears or either of these frequencies in one ear.	0.75	0.91
Leg mobility	Time the patient after asking: "Rise from the chair. Walk 20 feet briskly, turn, walk back to the chair and sit down."	Unable to complete task in 15 s.	0.91	0.92
Urinary incontinence	Two parts: Ask: "In the last year, have you ever lost your urine and gotten wet?" If yes, then ask: "Have you lost urine on at least 6 separate days?"	Yes to both questions.	0.86	0.96
Nutrition/weight loss	Two parts: Ask: "Have you lost 10 lbs over the past 6 months without trying to do so? Weigh the patient.	Yes to the question or weight <100 lb.	0.62	0.92
Memory	Three-item recall.	Unable to remember all three items after 1 minute.	0.60	0.92
Depression	Ask: "Do you often feel sad or depressed?"	Yes to the question.	0.71	0.90
Physical disability	Six questions: "... do strenuous activities such as fast walking or bicycling?" "... do heavy work around the house such as washing windows, walls, or floors?" "... go shopping for groceries or clothes?" "... get to places out of walking distance?" "... bathe, either a sponge bath, tub bath, or shower?" "... dress, such as putting on a shirt, buttoning and zipping, or putting on shoes?"	No to any of the questions.	0.88	0.77

Adapted with permission from Moore AA, Siu AL. Screening for common problems in ambulatory elderly: clinical confirmation of a screening instrument. Am J Med. 1996;100:438.

notes (example, Figure 11-2) to guide more detailed assessment and guide the clinician toward appropriate management steps. This approach has been demonstrated to improve the quality of care for falls and urinary incontinence. Portions of the structured visit note can be delegated to office staff, further increasing efficiency. Some practices have begun to incorporate this strategy into commercially available electronic health records. In this manner, the workflow of patient care can be redesigned, quality can be continuously monitored, and steps to improve quality can be implemented.

This approach to increasing efficiency can be applied to many geriatric conditions. Table 11-7 shows a strategy that optimizes the clinician's time by employing the most efficient methods to obtain assessment information. The initial step provides the clinician with basic information that can quickly be processed and followed with more extensive data gathering, when appropriate. Such a strategy begins with the previsit questionnaire and then is supplemented

by information obtained by office staff. These two data sources are reviewed by the clinician and additional information is obtained from the patient and family at the time of the visit.

COMPREHENSIVE GERIATRIC ASSESSMENT

CGA is based on the premise that a systematic evaluation of frail older persons by a team of health professionals may uncover treatable health problems and lead to better health outcomes. This evaluation typically includes four dimensions: physical health; functional status; psychological health, including cognitive and affective status; and socioenvironmental factors. Early randomized clinical trials provided convincing evidence that such programs conducted in hospital-based and rehabilitation units, which typically required several weeks of treatment, could lead to better survival rates, improved functional

TABLE 11-6

Multidimensional Case-Finding Instruments Used, with References and Average Performance Time			
PROBLEM	**INSTRUMENT (REFERENCE)**	**AVERAGE TIME TO PERFORM (MIN) (n = 37)**	**COST PER CASE RECEIVING A NEW DIAGNOSIS OR TREATMENT**
Cognitive impairment	Mini-Mental State Examination	9.2	$68
Depression	Geriatric Depression Scale	5.1	$17
Gait instability	Performance-Oriented Assessment of Mobility	2.5	$15
Malnutrition	Mid-arm circumference using gender-specific criteria	1.0	$15
Recent weight loss	Review of weights in chart	0.275	$8
Hearing impairment	Whisper test	0.55	<$1
Vision impairment	Hand-held Snellen chart	2.1	$10
Urinary incontinence	Specific question	0.275	<$1
Sexual problem	Questions regarding general function and specific problems	0.825	$14

Adapted with permission from Miller DK, Brunworth D, Brunworth DS, et al. Efficiency of geriatric case-finding in a private practitioner's office. J Am Geriatr Soc. 1995;43(5):533.

status, and more desirable placement (e.g., home rather than nursing home) following discharge from the hospital. Conceptually, CGA is a three-step process: (1) screening or targeting of appropriate patients, (2) assessment and development of recommendations, and (3) implementation of recommendations, including physician and patient adherence with recommendations. Each of these steps is essential if the process is to be successful at achieving health and functional benefits.

Within this broad conceptualization, CGA has been implemented using many different models in various health care settings (Table 11-8). Because of changes in length of hospital stays, an increasing number of CGA programs are relying on postdischarge and community-based assessment. Furthermore, most of the early programs focused on restorative or rehabilitative goals (tertiary pre-

vention), whereas many newer programs are aimed at primary and secondary prevention.

The purpose of the first step, targeting, is to distinguish elderly patients who are appropriate and will benefit from CGA, from those who are either too sick or are too well to benefit. To date, no easily administered targeting criteria have been demonstrated and validated to readily identify patients who are likely to benefit from CGA in different settings. Specific strategies used by CGA programs to identify older persons who are most appropriate for CGA have included chronological age, functional disability, physical illness, geriatric conditions, psychosocial conditions, and previous or predicted high health care utilization. All of these criteria have randomized clinical trial support for their effectiveness in identifying older persons likely to benefit from CGA. However, the definitions

TABLE 11-7

Strategy for Efficient Office-Based Assessment					
	METHOD AND DEPTH OF ASSESSMENT*				
Aspect Being Assessed	**Previsit Questionnaire**	**Office Staff Administered**	**Clinician Routine**	**Clinician As Needed**	**Referral† As Needed**
Past medical history	D		R		
Geriatric syndromes/health conditions					
Visual impairment	B	B	R		Ophthalmologist or optometrist
Hearing impairment	B	B (if needed)	R		Audiologist
Urinary incontinence	B	B	R	D	Geriatrician, urologist, or gynecologist
Malnutrition	D		R		Dietitian or social worker
Sexual dysfunction	B		R		Urologist or geriatrician
Polypharmacy	B		R		Pharmacist or geriatrician
Dental Problems	B		R		Dentist
Gait, balance, falls	B	B	B	D	Physical therapist
Affective problems	D		R	D	Psychiatrist
Cognitive problems		B	R	D	Geriatrician, psychiatrist, or neurologist
Functional disability	D		R	D	Physical or occupational therapist social worker
Environmental problems	D		R		Home health
Preventive services	D		R		

*B, brief screen (e.g., less than 2 min); D, detailed evaluation (usually 5 min or more); R, review of collected information.
†Examples of referrals to specific health professional or comprehensive geriatric assessment might be used.

TABLE 11-8

Spectrum of Comprehensive Geriatric Assessment like Interventions

	MOST INTENSIVE ⟵——————⟶ LEAST INTENSIVE		
Setting	CGA, GEM, and rehabilitation units	CGA consultation inpatient or outpatient	Community-based and in-home outreach programs
Targeting	Most restrictive		Least restrictive
Process	Large team, extensive evaluations		Screening and referral
Cost	Very expensive		Relatively inexpensive

CGA, comprehensive geriatric assessment; GEM, geriatric evaluation and management.

of these criteria and the interventions that have followed have varied from study to study.

Most CGA programs exclude patients who are unlikely to benefit because of terminal illness, severe dementia, complete functional dependence, and inevitable nursing home placement. Exclusionary criteria have also included identifying older persons who are "too healthy" to benefit.

The second step of CGA, the assessment process itself, continues to be highly variable across programs. The types of health care professionals included in the assessment team, the content of information collected, and the types and intensity of services provided have differed in studies of the effectiveness of CGA. In many settings, the CGA process relies on a core team consisting of a physician, nurse, and social worker and, when appropriate, draws upon an extended team of various combinations of physical and occupational therapists, nutritionists, pharmacists, psychiatrists, psychologists, dentists, audiologists, podiatrists, and opticians. Although these professionals are usually on staff in hospital settings and are available in the community, access to and reimbursement for these services have limited the effectiveness of the CGA process. Frequently, the composition of the team is determined by local expertise and availability of resources rather than programmatic needs. Increasingly, CGA programs are moving toward a "virtual team" concept in which members are included as needed, assessments are conducted at different locations on different days, and conferencing is completed via telephone or electronically.

Traditionally, the various components of the evaluation are completed by different members of the team. There is considerable variability in which professional conducts the assessments. For example, the medical assessment of older persons may be conducted by a physician, nurse practitioner, or physician's assistant. The core team may conduct only brief initial assessments or screens for some dimensions. These may be subsequently augmented with more in-depth evaluations by additional professionals. For example, a dietitian may be needed to assess dietary intake and provide recommendations; an audiologist may need to conduct a more extensive assessment of hearing loss and evaluate an older person for a hearing aid.

Components of Comprehensive Geriatric Assessment

The key elements of the process of care rendered by CGA teams can be divided into six steps: (1) data gathering; (2) discussion among the team; (3) development of a treatment plan; (4) implementation of the treatment plan; (5) monitoring response to the treatment plan; and (6) revising the treatment plan.

Data Gathering

In early studies of CGA, the data-gathering process simply identified the members of the team and mentioned that each conducted an evaluation. Such descriptions are problematic because of the variability of evaluations among health professionals. A formal training process can reduce this variability, but a popular approach is to standardize the assessment. Standardized assessments can either use instruments developed specifically for clinical purposes or assemble standard instruments that have previously been studied for validity and reliability. The advantage of the former is that teams can customize the information being gathered to best suit the clinical needs of the program. The advantage of the latter is that patients in the program can be compared to patients in other programs. Frequently, however, these instruments were developed for purposes other than to guide clinical decision-making and may provide information that is not very helpful in the care of patients.

Discussion among Team

Following initial data gathering, the team meets to discuss the patient's geriatric needs. Although any member of the team could theoretically lead the conference, the leadership is usually determined by local culture. Each conference typically begins with short discipline-specific presentations followed by interactive discussions among professionals. Sometimes additional information will need to be obtained before final recommendations can be made. The team then identifies problems that need action and might be responsive to treatment.

Development of the Treatment Plan

Based upon this discussion, the team develops an initial treatment plan and goals for the patient. Some CGA programs use protocols that are triggered by specific geriatric conditions whereas others rely on the experience and clinical judgment of the team. If the number of recommendations resulting from CGA is large, it is necessary to prioritize recommendations. CGA teams should advise primary care physicians and patients to focus on the major recommendations, those that are most likely to produce the desired outcomes. The urgency of recommendations must also be determined. Although some recommendations may need to be implemented immediately to confer short-term benefit such as stopping a medication that may be the cause of delirium, many more may be better implemented once the patient is stable.

At the time of the assessment, a plan for implementation of each recommendation must be developed. It needs to be determined who will assume responsibility for initiation and completion of the recommendation. Similarly, the team must establish a plan for monitoring the patient's progress as treatment is being delivered.

Implementation of the Treatment Plan

Because of the problem of poor adherence to CGA recommendations, the issue of implementation is particularly critical to the success of CGA consultation programs. Among inpatient CGA models, poor implementation rates may explain some negative trials of hospital consultation models of CGA. Failure to implement recommendations is usually attributable to three problems: (1) poor receptivity among primary care physicians whose patients have been assessed using consultative models; (2) inadequate resources to implement recommendations; and (3) poor continuity or follow-through on recommendations after hospital discharge. In ambulatory settings, patient adherence to recommendations emanating from CGA looms as an even larger obstacle to implementation. Patients may simply choose not to return to see the CGA team (in continuity of care models) or ignore recommendations in a consultative model.

A variety of options for implementation are available ranging from direct implementation of recommendations by the team to merely advising physicians and patients by a note in the chart or verbally. In consultative models of CGA in some ambulatory settings, patients have been provided with direct advice and instructions on how to approach their physicians to discuss CGA recommendations (patient empowerment). This method, coupled with direct communication to primary care physicians, has resulted in high implementation rates of CGA recommendations. Other approaches to improve adherence by primary care physicians have been by direct telephone contact, letters, faxes, and e-mail.

Monitoring

To ensure that recommendations are implemented and to follow a patient's progress through the treatment plan, patients must be monitored directly by the CGA team or by the primary care physician. If the team is to monitor the patient, key issues are how frequently and for how long this monitoring should occur. The more intensively and the longer patients are followed, the more resource-intensive the consultation becomes. In some models (described below), the CGA team may temporarily assume primary care for several months before returning the patient to the primary care physician for ongoing care.

Revising the Treatment Plan

By monitoring the patient, CGA teams can continually assess the patient's progress toward meeting the goals established by the team. If progress is not proceeding according to expectations, the team may need to reevaluate the patient and resume the team discussion. Treatment recommendations and implementation plans may need to be revised. Any modification will require additional monitoring. The frequency and extensiveness of reevaluations and additional discussions are important influences on the cost of CGA consultation.

Effectiveness of Comprehensive Geriatric Assessment

In virtually all studies of CGA, the process itself has resulted in improved detection and documentation of geriatric problems. However, such identification of problems has not always led to improved outcomes. Meta-analysis, a technique to pool the findings of individual trials to provide more precise estimates of effectiveness, has been used to evaluate five models of CGA (geriatric evaluation and management units, inpatient geriatrics consultation services, home assessment services, home assessment services for patients who had recently been discharged, and outpatient assessment services). The

first major CGA meta-analysis was published in 1993 and some components have been updated as new trials have been published.

Geriatric Evaluation and Management Units

Geriatric Evaluation and Management Units (GEMUs), which are often designed to be environmentally friendly to older persons, confer two advantages over consultation models. First, physicians staffing the unit generally assume primary care of the patient, thus facilitating the implementation of recommendations. Second, the availability and experience of a dedicated team of providers (e.g., nurses and therapists) increases the consistency and geriatric orientation of hospital and postacute care. The meta-analysis indicated that the hospital or rehabilitation unit model of CGA had the strongest and most consistent benefits on living at home and functional status. However, the geriatric evaluation and management unit may no longer confer the same benefits in the current American health care environment. A multisite randomized clinical trial within the U.S. Department of Veterans Affairs published in 2002 demonstrated little benefit of such units when compared to usual care, which may have improved considerably since the early 1980s. In addition, differences in health care delivery systems across various countries may help explain inconsistent results of more recent studies.

Inpatient Consultation

Both the 1993 meta-analysis and a subsequent large negative randomized clinical trial of inpatient geriatric assessment consultation have suggested little benefit from this model of CGA and it has largely been abandoned except in teaching settings.

Posthospital Discharge Assessment and Management

Similarly, posthospitalization CGA conducted in the home was ineffective in the meta-analysis in reducing mortality, functional decline, or readmission rates. Although a subsequent randomized clinical trial confirmed these negative findings, a nursing-led program of comprehensive discharge planning and home follow-up has been more effective. Key elements included use of targeting criteria to identify appropriate patients, a program of comprehensive discharge planning (including multidimensional assessment) and home follow-up with advanced practice nurses who visited the patients at least every other day during the hospitalization and at least twice during the 4 weeks following discharge. These visits were supplemented by telephone calls. In a randomized clinical trial, this intervention was associated with reduced hospital readmissions and costs.

Outpatient Consultation

The 1993 meta-analysis did not demonstrate any benefit from outpatient CGA consultation. A subsequent randomized clinical trial was also negative. More recently, a model that combines CGA with an adherence intervention has been developed and tested. This program provided outpatient CGA for community-dwelling older persons with functional disability, urinary incontinence, falls, or depressive symptoms. The assessment was then linked to an adherence intervention that was designed to empower the patient to take action and educate the physician. In a randomized clinical trial, this strategy was associated with less functional decline, less fatigue, and better social functioning and was cost-effective when compared with many commonly used treatments.

In-Home Assessment

Home assessment programs are a variation of CGA that focuses primarily on preventive rather than rehabilitative services and are aimed at patients at low rather than high risk of nursing home admission. A 2002 meta-analysis concluded that these programs were effective in reducing nursing home admissions only if they included at least five follow-up visits and in reducing functional decline only if they included multidimensional assessment. A beneficial effect on mortality was only found for younger patients (72.7–77.5 years).

Lessons Learned from Geriatric Assessment

Despite unresolved issues regarding the effectiveness of CGA, the principles of CGA have been incorporated into a number of programs that have been demonstrated to be effective. Several new models of outpatient care for older persons modify the basic structure of care delivery. These models adopt various components of CGA including targeting, assessment, and interventions.

Geriatric evaluation and continuity management is a direct outgrowth of CGA. These programs differ from CGA in that they become the source of ongoing primary care usually by interdisciplinary teams in geriatrics clinics. Randomized trials have indicated that this ongoing care has resulted in better perceived health, life satisfaction, affective health status, and quality of health and social care. One study demonstrated a significant benefit of GEM on instrumental activity of daily living functional status at 2 years. However, a large trial of GEM within the Department of Veterans Affairs demonstrated no effect on most outcomes. Another type of continuity GEM assumes primary care of older persons who are at high risk for high health care utilization for an average of 6 months and then returns patients to the care of their primary care physicians. When evaluated in a randomized clinical trial, this approach reduced the risk of functional decline and reduced the likelihood of depression at a modest cost ($1250 per person). Randomized trials of collaborative practice models using physicians, nurses, and case assistants, and physicians, nurses, and social workers for targeted patients have demonstrated reduced 2-year mortality and fewer hospitalizations, respectively.

Other new models that have yet to be evaluated in clinical trials also include core elements of CGA as part of the assessment and management functions of the care of older persons but may not include a CGA team as part of the process. Several of these bring CGA into primary care physicians' offices rather than creating a separate parallel delivery system or relying on primary care physicians' acceptance of CGA recommendations.

In addition, CGA has been adapted to specialty treatment of older persons including oncology, emergency department postdischarge management, inpatient orthopedic care, and the preoperative evaluation of elderly patients undergoing thoracic surgery. Elements of CGA have also been incorporated into disease management programs, including stroke and heart failure.

In summary, geriatric assessment continues to evolve as an integral component of the care of older persons. As assessment techniques become better standardized and validated, more efficient yet comprehensive approaches are possible. To date, implementation of such strategies has not occurred on a widespread basis. Cost, logistical, and training issues are still important barriers. However, as national initiatives to improve quality move forward, screening for geriatric conditions and appropriate assessment of patients who screen positive will gain more acceptance. Advances in technology and newer approaches to data collection have unleashed possibilities for incorporating geriatric assessment and management that could not have been imagined a decade ago. The research agenda still must include testing whether these more efficient strategies can lead to better health outcomes.

CGA has also changed considerably as medicine has become increasingly cost conscious. Though effective, the long-stay units can no longer be sustained and the emphasis must shift to extending the effective components and principles into less expensive settings and programs. Although several examples of such successful progeny have already been developed and tested, undoubtedly, additional generations of CGA-like interventions will be forthcoming.

FURTHER READING

Bagai A, Thavendiranathan P, Detsky AS. Does this patient have hearing impairment? *JAMA.* 2006;295(4):416–28.

Borson S, Scanlan J, Brush M, et al. The mini-cog: a cognitive 'vital signs' measure for dementia screening in multi-lingual elderly. *Int J Geriatr Psychiatry.* 2000;15(11):1021.

Brown JS, Bradley CS, Subak LL, et al. The sensitivity and specificity of a simple test to distinguish between urge and stress urinary incontinence. *Ann Intern Med.* 2006;144(10):715–723.

Cohen HJ, Feussner JR, Weinberger M, et al. A controlled trial of inpatient and outpatient geriatric evaluation and management. *N Engl J Med.* 2002;346(12):905.

Ellis G, Langhorne P. Comprehensive geriatric assessment for older hospital patients. *Br Med Bull.* 2005;71:45–59.

Ganz DA, Bao Y, Shekelle PG, et al. Will my patient fall? *JAMA.* 2007;297(1):77–86.

Guigoz Y. The Mini Nutritional Assessment (MNA ®) Review of the literature—What does it tell us? *J Nutr Health Aging.* 2006;10(6):466–487.

Inouye SK, van Dyck CH, Alessi CA, et al. Clarifying confusion: the confusion assessment method. A new method for detection of delirium. *Ann Intern Med.* 1990;113(12):941.

Kroenke K, Spitzer RL, Williams JBW. The PHQ-9. Validity of a brief depression severity measure. *J Gen Intern Med.* 2001;16(9):606–613.

Miller DK, Brunworth D, Brunworth DS, et al. Efficiency of geriatric case-finding in a private practitioner's office. *J Am Geriatr Soc.* 1995;43(5):533.

Moore AA, Siu AL. Screening for common problems in ambulatory elderly: clinical confirmation of a screening instrument. *Am J Med.* 1996;100:438.

Owen CG, Rudnicka AR, Smeeth L, et al. Is the NEI-VFQ-25 a useful tool in identifying visual impairment in an elderly population? *BMC Ophthalmol.* 2006;6:24.

Reuben DB, Greendale GA, Harrison GG. Nutrition screening in older persons. *J Am Geriatr Soc.* 1995;43(4):415.

Reuben DB, Roth C, Kamberg C, et al. Restructuring primary care practices to manage geriatric syndromes: the ACOVE-2 intervention. *J Am Geriatr Soc.* 2003;51(12):1787–1793.

Rubenstein LZ. Joseph T. Freeman award lecture: comprehensive geriatric assessment: from miracle to reality. *J Gerontol A Biol Sci Med Sci.* 2004;59(5):473–477.

Siu AL. Screening for dementia and investigating its causes. *Ann Intern Med.* 1991;115(2):122.

Stuck AE, Egger M, Hammer A, et al. Home visits to prevent nursing home admission and functional decline in elderly people: systematic review and meta-regression analysis. *JAMA.* 2002;287(8):1022–1028.

Stuck AE, Siu AL, Wieland,GD, et al. Comprehensive geriatric assessment: a meta-analysis of controlled trials. *J Lancet.* 1993;342:1032.

Tinetti ME. Performance-oriented assessment of mobility problems in elderly patients. *J Am Geriatr Soc.* 1986;34:119.

Tombaugh TN, McIntyre NJ. The Mini-Mental State Examination: a comprehensive review. *J Am Geriatr Soc.* 1992;40:922.

Mental Status and Neurological Examination in Older Adults

James E. Galvin

THE NEUROLOGY OF AGING

What Is Normal Neurological Aging?

The diagnosis of neurological disease in the older adult requires recognition not only of abnormal signs and symptoms but also an understanding of what changes are expected as part of the normal aging process. To distinguish neurological dysfunction related to disease from the neurological changes associated with normal aging, the clinician must conduct a comprehensive mental status and neurological examination. When establishing a neurological diagnosis, the clinical history (i.e., history of the present illness, past medical history, social habits, occupational experience, family illness, and disorders) assists the clinician in generating a differential diagnosis that can be further explored and refined by pertinent observations documented on the mental status and neurological examinations. The mental status assessment should evaluate cognition, emotion, and behavior. Because cognitive and affective disorders occur commonly in older adults, historical information should be obtained not only from the patient but a reliable informant such as the spouse, adult child, or caregiver. The neurological examination should be performed on all older adults regardless of the chief complaint as up to 60% of older patients have either a primary or secondary neurological sign or symptom. A complete mental status and neurological examination provides the necessary data to develop reasonable diagnostic hypotheses and drive the necessary laboratory, imaging, or specialized assessments to care for the patient.

Age-Related Changes in the Neurological Examination

Before discussion of the individual components of the examination, it would be useful to discuss changes that are expected as part of the aging process (Table 12-1). Normal age-related changes are due to progressive and irreversible changes associated with tissue senescence and the inability of nervous system to repair and regenerate secondary to the ravages of time. The frequency and qualitative characteristics of these changes vary from individual to individual but are present in many older adults.

Cognitive Changes

There continues to be a debate as the extent of cognitive changes associated with aging due largely to differences between cross-sectional and longitudinal study designs. When comparing older adults to young adults on similar cognitive tasks such as the Wechsler Adult Intelligence Scale, older adults generally score lower on both performance and verbal subtests. However, when differences in performance are considered in light of motor slowing and educational attainment, these changes are less apparent. Longitudinal evaluation of older adults has generally demonstrated little change in verbal intelligence with aging while performance is influenced significantly by motor and processing speed. Forgetfulness therefore is *not* part of normal aging. While it may take longer to process new information and retrieve well-learned information, new learning and memory formation occurs in older adults. This is one reason why delayed recall of word lists is effective in discriminating older adults with cognitive impairment from those without impairment.

Changes in Cranial Nerve Function

Visual and hearing changes are common in the older adult. Visual acuity declines because of a number of ophthalmologic (cataracts, glaucoma) and neurological (macular degeneration) causes. Pupillary size is typically smaller with age and pupils are less reactive to light and accommodation, forcing many older adults to use glasses for reading. There is also a restriction in eye movement in upward gaze. Also associated with aging is a decline in speech discrimination

TABLE 12-1

Neurological Changes Associated with Normal Aging

Psychomotor slowing
Decreased visual acuity
Smaller pupil size
Decreased ability to look upward
Decreased auditory acuity, especially for spoken language
Decreased muscle bulk
Mild motor slowing
Decreased vibratory sensation
Mild swaying on Romberg test
Mild lordosis and restriction of movement in neck and back
Depression of Achilles tendon reflex

due to presbycusis, a progressive elevation in the frequency threshold for hearing. There are also age-related degenerative changes in inner ear including loss of hair cells, atrophy of stria vascularis, and thickening of the basilar membrane.

Changes in Motor Function

There is a progressive decline in muscle bulk and strength associated with aging. Most of the muscle loss is found in the intrinsic muscles of the hands and feet, and around the shoulder. There is a weakening of the abdominal muscles, which may accentuate spinal lordosis and contribute to low back pain. Muscle loss is associated with denervation on electrophysiological studies and with type II atrophy on muscle biopsy. In addition to loss of strength and muscle bulk, changes in the speed and coordination of movement increases with advancing age. The changes may interfere with activities of daily living (dressing, putting away the dishes, getting out of a chair) and recreation activities (golfing, shuffleboard). On examination, these changes may manifest as mild bradykinesia and dysmetria on finger-nose-finger and heel-shin tests.

Changes in Sensory Function

By far the most common change will be the loss of vibration perception in the lower extremities and to a lesser extent position-sense may be affected as well. As vibration sensation becomes impaired in lower extremities, there is an ascending pattern, from toe to ankle and knee. Pain and temperature sensation is also diminished in the older adult, but in the absence of a pathological cause, usually does not elicit much symptomatology. The mild impairment in position sense often manifests as a mild swaying during the Romberg test.

Changes in Gait and Station

Changes in gait and station in old age may be attributed in part to decreased muscle strength, weakening of abdominal muscles, arthritis, and degenerative joint disease, diminished vibration and position sense, impairment in motor speed and coordination. These changes make it more difficult for older adults to tandem, heel, or toe walk for extended periods of time. Despite this, most older adults have adequate postural righting reflexes and are not likely to spontaneously fall (distinct from what is seen in Parkinson's disease).

Changes in Deep Tendon Reflexes

The most common age-associated change is the depression or loss of the Achilles tendon reflex. Other reflexes usually remain present but are diminished in response. An extensor plantar response (Babinski sign) is *not* a normal age-related change but instead is always associated with some underlying pathology in the upper motor neuron.

THE NEUROLOGICAL HISTORY

There is no substitution for a carefully elicited history detailing the onset, duration, quality, and location of symptoms. The history helps the clinician develop a differential diagnosis and focus on the neurological examination. The history will also guide the formulation of diagnostic evaluations and develop a treatment plan. In addition, a compassionate clinician will be able to build a trusting relationship with the patient that will enhance patient adherence to medical recommendations. As a general comment, to avoid bias, it is often useful to gather historical facts de novo and not read other records or review laboratory studies such as imaging before taking the history and performing the physical examination. In this section, we discuss two aspects of neurologic history taking—from the patient and, when available, from an informant.

Neurological History from the Patient

An accurate history requires that absolute attention is paid to detail, both verbal (what the patient is saying) and nonverbal (what the patient is doing). This is critical to match the chief complaint with the patient's body language. For example, someone complaining about severe low back pain but appears to be sitting comfortably in the chair may raise suspicion. Likewise, the older adult who offers no complaints but is noted to have a rest-tremor should prompt more detailed questioning. One of the most important attributes of a skilled clinician is the ability to be a good listener and to focus in on critical historical points. The most effective historians gather information by a combination of open-ended and structured questions. After asking the patient why they are in office and offer a chance to express concerns or worries in their own words, specific topics can be addressed by focused questioning.

Another important aspect of the history is to elicit qualitative and quantitative aspects of the chief complaint. It is not enough to elicit a history of a "headache" or "pain." What are the characteristics of the complaint, when did it start, what makes it better, what makes it worse? Has this happened before, and if so, did it present in the same fashion? Use simple scales to quantify the extent of the complaint by asking "On a scale of 1 to 10, with 10 being the worse (symptom)..." These qualities can help focus a differential diagnosis and helps to build trust with the patient.

Neurological History from an Informant

In many instances, gathering information from a third party will be invaluable in determining the onset, duration, and extent of the neurologic problem. In cases where there are problems with cognition or alertness, this may be the only reliable way to gather information. Again, using both open-ended and structured questions will often provide the clinician with important information about the chief complaint and assist in the development of a differential diagnosis.

MENTAL STATUS EXAMINATION

The elements of a comprehensive mental status examination include observational, cognitive, functional, and neuropsychiatric assessments. Although each of these elements is presented separately, they are interrelated and collectively characterize the neurobehavioral function of the patient. The initial contact with the patient affords the opportunity to assess whether a cognitive, attention, or language disorder is present. Questioning of an informant may bring to light changes in cognition, function, and behavior that the patient either is not aware of or denies.

Observational Assessment

Observation of a patient's level of arousal or alertness, appearance, emotion, behavior, movements, and speech provides insight into their mental status.

Level of Consciousness

An accurate assessment of a patient's mental status and neurologic function must first document the patient's alertness or level of arousal. Altered levels of consciousness can directly impact the patient's cognitive performance on mental status testing and influence the examiner's interpretation of the test results and maybe indicative of a medical or neurologic condition requiring immediate medical intervention (e.g., cardiopulmonary intervention, neurosurgical evaluation).

Abnormal patterns of arousal include hypoaroused or hyperaroused states. Decreasing levels of arousal include lethargy, obtundation, stupor, and coma. The lethargic patient is drowsy or fatigued and falls asleep if not stimulated; however while being interviewed, the patient will usually be able to attend to questioning. Obtundation refers to a state of moderately reduced alertness with diminished ability to consistently engage the environment. Even in the presence of the examiner, if not stimulated, the obtunded patient will drift off. The stuporous patient requires vigorous stimulation to be aroused. Responses are usually limited to simple "yes/no" responses or may consist of groans and grimaces. Coma, which represents the end of the continuum of hypoarousal states, is a state of unresponsiveness to the external environment. In the elderly, hypoarousal states can be associated with systemic infection, cardiac or pulmonary insufficiencies, meningoencephalitis, increased intracranial pressure, toxic-metabolic insults, traumatic brain injury, seizures, or cerebrovascular disease. Coma requires either bilateral hemispheric dysfunction or brainstem dysfunction. Another important consideration is the role of polypharmacy. Drug interactions are more common in the older adult and can significantly impair consciousness.

Hyperarousal states, on the other hand, are characterized by anxiety, autonomic hyperactivity (tachycardia, tachypnea, hyper-thermia), agitation or aggression, tremor, seizures, or exaggerated startle response. In the elderly, hyperarousal states are most often encountered in toxic-metabolic disorders including withdrawal from alcohol, opiates, or sedative-hypnotic agents. Other causes include tumors (both primary and metastatic), viral encephalitis (particularly herpes simplex), cerebrovascular, and hypoxemia. Some patients may experience fluctuating periods of both hypo- and hyperarousal.

Appearance

Assessment of a patient's physical appearance should acknowledge body size and type, apparent age, posture, facial expressions, eye contact, hygiene, dress, and general activity level. A disheveled appearance may indicate dementia, delirium, frontal lobe dysfunction, or schizophrenia. Wearing excessive makeup or flamboyant grooming or attire in an old individual should raise the suspicion of a manic episode or frontal lobe dysfunction. Patients with unilateral neglect may fail to dress, groom, or bathe one side of their body. Patients with Parkinson's disease may display a flexed posture, whereas patients with progressive supranuclear palsy have an extended, rigid posture. The overall appearance of an individual should also provide information regarding their general health status. The cachectic patient may harbor a systemic illness (e.g., cancer), or have anorexia or depression.

Emotional State and Affect

Affect describes the mental representation of external reality and the patient's internal feelings about external reality, while emotional state describes the objective display of emotion through facial grimaces, vocal tone, and body movements, and the subjective component of how the patient reports what he or she feels internally: "I feel sad, happy, apprehensive, cynical."

Depression is the most frequent mood disturbance in the older adult and occurs in a variety of neurologic disorders (Table 12-2). Euphoria or full-blown mania occurs less often than depression in the course of neurological illness. Euphoria is most common with

TABLE 12-2

Causes of Depression in the Older Adult
Idiopathic
Secondary to life situation (loss of spouse, child, friends)
Cerebrovascular accident
Hypothyroidism
Alzheimer's disease
Parkinson's disease
Frontotemporal dementia
Dementia with Lewy bodies
Head injury
Drug withdrawal
Drug intoxication (alcohol, barbiturates, sedative-hypnotics)
Medications (beta-blockers, reserpine, clonidine)
Multiple sclerosis
Epilepsy

TABLE 12-3

Common Movement Disorders and Signs

SIGN	DESCRIPTION	ETIOLOGY
Bradykinesia	Slowed initiation and sustained movements	Parkinson's disease, drug-induced, may be normal variant
Dyskinesia	Abnormal involuntary movements either slow or fast	Drug-induced, Huntington's disease, Parkinson's disease, idiopathic
Action or postural tremor	Fast frequency (10–15 Hz) associated with movement (action) or sustained posture (postural), may improve with small amount of alcohol	Benign, essential tremor, drug-induced
Rest tremor	Low-frequency (3–5 Hz) with pill rolling quality, may involve extremities or chin	Parkinson's disease, drug-induced
Intention tremor	High-frequency (10–15 Hz), worsening as approaching target	Cerebellar disease
Myoclonus	Lightning fast movements from brief muscle contractions	Stroke, sleep, Huntington's disease, epilepsy, Creutzfeldt-Jacob
Asterixis	Sudden loss of limb tone during sustained muscle contraction, sometime considered "negative" myoclonus	Hepatic, renal or pulmonary disease, drug-induced, encephalopathy, bacterial infection
Chorea	Brief, rapid, irregular contractions	Huntington's disease, Sydenham chorea, drug-induced
Ballismus	Large-amplitude, jerky movements with flinging of extremities	Subthalamic nucleus lesions
Tics	Sequenced coordinated movements or vocalizations that appear suddenly	Tourette's, drug-induced
Dystonia	Sustained muscle contraction with twisting or repetitive movements, may be painful	Idiopathic, infarcts, drug-induced
Athetosis	Slow, writhing movements predominantly proximal	Huntington's disease, infarcts
Akathisia	Internalized restlessness with urge to move	Drug-induced, encephalopathy, Parkinson's disease, Restless Legs Syndrome

frontal lobe dysfunction (trauma, frontotemporal degenerations, infections) and with secondary mania. Anxiety occurs in a variety of neuropsychiatric conditions including anxiety disorders, metabolic encephalopathies (e.g., hyperthyroidism, anoxia), toxic disorders (e.g., lidocaine toxicity), and degenerative diseases (e.g., Alzheimer's disease, Parkinson's disease). Objective and subjective emotional components may be incongruent in certain psychiatric disorders (e.g., schizophrenia and schizotypal personality disorder), and in neurologic conditions such as pseudobulbar palsy.

The range and intensity of the observable component of emotion should be noted. Constriction or flatness is observed in apathetic states; for example, in the context of negative symptoms of schizophrenia, severe melancholic depression, or in demented patients with apathy. Increased intensity, on the other hand, is seen in mood disorders such as bipolar illness, and in personality disorders such as borderline personality.

Lability is a disorder of emotional regulation. Patients with marked lability are irritable and shift rapidly among anger, depression, and euphoria. The emotional outbursts are usually short-lived. Labile mood is seen in mood disorders such as bipolar illness and in certain personality disorders such as borderline personality. It also may occur in frontotemporal dementia and pseudobulbar palsy.

Behavior

Behavioral observations can reveal important information regarding the mental status and neurological function of the patient. A variety of personality alterations can be encountered with focal brain lesions. Orbitofrontal dysfunction maybe characterized by impulsiveness or undue familiarity with the examiner, lack of judgment or lack of social anxiety, and antisocial behavior. Individuals with dorsolateral frontal lobe dysfunction may be inattentive and distractible. Apathy

(lack of motivation, energy, emotional reciprocity, social isolation) may be caused by medial frontal dysfunction. Dementias are associated with increased rigidity of though, egocentricity, diminished emotional responsiveness, and impaired emotional control.

Movement

Observation of patient's movements may provide evidence of parkinsonism, chorea, myoclonus, or tics (Table 12-3). Psychomotor retardation (i.e., slowed central processing and movement) may be indicative of vascular dementia, subcortical neurological disorders, parkinsonism, medial frontal syndromes, or depression. Psychomotor agitation may be indicative or a metabolic disorder, choreoathetosis, seizure disorder, mania, or anxiety.

Speech and Communication

Observation of spontaneous speech is the first step in formal language testing and can be assessed during history taking as well as in the course of the mental status examination. The examiner first observes spontaneity of speech as well as the timber, pitch, and modulation of voice. Mutism maybe encountered in several neurological conditions such as akinetic mutism, vegetative state, locked-in syndrome, catatonic unresponsiveness, or large left hemispheric lesions. Akinetic mutism is characterized by absent speech in the setting of alert-appearing immobility. The patient's eyes are open, and the individual may follow environmental events. The patient exhibits regular sleep–wake cycles but may be completely inert or display brief movements or postural adjustments spontaneously or in response to vigorous stimulation. Akinetic mutism may be seen with large frontal lobe injuries, bilateral cingulate gyrus damage, or midbrain pathology. Akinetic mutism should be distinguished from a vegetative state where the patient exhibits sleep–wake cycles with open eyes. A vegetative state can occur after severe brain injury. Locked-in syndrome occurs with bilateral pontine lesions, rendering the patient mute and paralyzed. Intellectual function, however, is not impaired and the patients can communicate by eye movements or eye blinks.

Spontaneous speech is characterized by its rate, rhythm, volume, response latency, and inflection. Accelerated speech may be encountered in mania, disinhibited orbitofrontal syndromes, or festinating parkinsonian conditions, whereas a reduced rate of speech output can occur as a component of psychomotor retardation. Response latencies may be prolonged or the patient may impulsively interrupt the examiner, anticipating the question. Perturbed speech prosody (loss of melody or inflection) can be encountered in brain disorders affecting the right hemisphere or the basal ganglia. Empty speech with hesitations or circumlocutions can be exhibited in patients with word-finding difficulties. Word-finding impairment may occur in aphasias, metabolic encephalopathies, physical exhaustion, sleep deprivation, anxiety, depression, or dorsolateral frontal lobe damage in the absence of an anomia.

Aphasia is characterized by impairment in oral and/or written communication. Deficits will vary depending on the location and extent of anatomic involvement. Aphasias are generally characterized as nonfluent or fluent (Table 12-4). Nonfluent aphasias are characterized by a paucity of speech, often with a hesitant quality. There is impairment in word searching and writing. The patient may appear frustrated or depressed because of awareness of the language deficit and the inability to communicate with family and health care providers. Fluent aphasias are characterized by empty speech. Word production is normal or maybe increased but there is a lack of comprehension about what words mean, often associated with impairment in reading ability. The patient often displays little insight to the language deficit and instead may become agitated because others are not following the conversation.

Cognitive Assessment

The assessment of cognitive function should be conducted methodically and should assess comprehensively the major domains of neuropsychological function (attention, memory, language, visuospatial skills, executive ability). The patient's age, handedness, educational level, and sociocultural background may all influence cognitive function and should be determined prior to initiating or interpreting the evaluation.

Attention

Two tests are useful in assessing attention: digit span forward and continuous performance tests. In the digit span forward test, the patient is asked to repeat increasingly long series of numbers (e.g. 1, 3–7, 4–6–3, 5–1–9–2, etc). The examiner says the numbers at a rate of one per second. A normal forward digit span is seven digits; fewer than five is abnormal. Concentration is evaluated by a continuous performance test. An example would be to say the months of the year in reverse order, starting with the last month of the year (December). Distractible patients tend to lose track and skip one or two months. Serial subtraction can also be used to test concentration but heavily dependent on educational attainment and mathematical abilities. Confusional states such as delirium are characterized by impaired attention.

Memory

Learning, recall, recognition, and memory for remote information are assessed in the course of mental status examination. Asking the patient to remember three words and then asking him or her to recall the words 3 minutes later can help assess learning, recall, and recognition. However, the shorter the list, the more easy it is to remember, particularly in high-functioning individuals. When told to remember items, patients will often remember the first two items heard (known as "primacy") and the last two items heard (known as "recency"), therefore longer lists of 10 words may be preferable. After a delay, recall of less than five words is considered abnormal. Patients having difficulty with recall may be given clues (e.g., the category of items to which the word belongs or a list of words containing the target) to distinguish between storage and retrieval deficits. Prompting and clues will not aid patients with storage deficits (e.g., amnesia); patients with intact storage but poor recall (e.g. retrieval-deficit syndrome) may be aided by clues. Amnestic deficits are thought to be causes by lesions in the hippocampal–thalamic circuit while retrieval deficits are likely due to lesions of frontal–basal ganglia circuitry.

Information is gathered on the patient's remote memory function while taking a history of the patient's illness, inquiring about the patient's life events (marriage, births of children, etc.), and asking about important historical events. An informant may also be helpful here to verify these events. The temporal profile of remote memory may be diagnostically important. Amnestic syndromes such as dementias usually feature normal, nonmemory cognitive functions, a period of retrograde amnesia following the onset of the disorder, variable periods of anterograde amnesia, and intact remote memory beyond the period of the retrograde amnesia. Psychogenic memory loss may include variable patterns of amnesia particularly in long-term events (e.g., not recall birth of children, not recall being married).

Language

Language assessment entails the evaluation of all aspects of communication including spontaneous speech, comprehension, repetition, naming, reading, and writing. Aphasic disturbances are characterized as fluent or nonfluent. Fluent aphasias are characterized by normal or excessive amounts of speech, preserved phrase length, intact speech melody, usually in combination with a paucity of information. Phonemic paraphasias (substitution of one phoneme for another); semantic paraphasias (the replacement of one word with another); or neologistic paraphasias (the construction of new words) may occur. Wernicke, transcortical sensory, conduction, and anomic aphasias are fluent aphasic syndromes.

Nonfluent aphasias feature reduced verbal output, short or one-word replies, agrammatism, poor speech initiation, reduced speech prosody, and dysarthria. There are few paraphasias. Broca, transcortical motor, global, and mixed transcortical aphasias are nonfluent aphasic disorders. Interestingly, nonfluent aphasic patients may have preserved abilities to curse fluently and sing well-learned songs (i.e., Happy Birthday) with few errors.

Primary progressive aphasia is a disorder seen in patients with asymmetric frontotemporal degeneration that involves dominant hemisphere. Progressive nonfluent aphasia involves primarily unilateral left frontal, left frontoparietal, or left frontotemporal degeneration and is characterized by agrammatism, paraphasias, and anomia. Bilateral temporal lobe atrophy and hypoperfusion with more

TABLE 12-4

Characteristics of Aphasias

FEATURE	BROCA APHASIA	WERNICKE APHASIA	CONDUCTION APHASIA	GLOBAL APHASIA	TRANSCORTICAL MOTOR	TRANSCORTICAL SENSORY	TRANSCORTICAL MIXED	PURE ANOMIA	THALAMIC
Anatomic localization	Inferior frontal (Broca's area)	Superior temporal (Wernicke's area)	Arcuate fasciculus	Middle cerebral artery distribution	Supplemental motor areas	Inferior parietal	Watershed areas	Angular/Supraminginal gyrus	Dorsomedial or ventral anterior nuclei
Fluency	Nonfluent	Fluent	Fluent	Nonfluent	Nonfluent	Fluent	Nonfluent	Fluent	Nonfluent
Repetition	Impaired	Impaired	Impaired	Impaired	Normal	Normal	Normal, may be only preserved language function	Normal	Normal
Rhythm of speech	Effortful with dysarthria	Quickened, long-winded, effusive	Normal	Severely impaired, mute	Slightly effortful	May appear normal	Effortful, slow	Normal	Effortful, slow
Content	Agrammatical, telegraphic	Mispronunciation and neologism (nonsense words)	Occasional use of wrong words	Abnormal	Agrammatical	Circumlocution, tangential	Variable impairment	Often normal, but uses descriptive language	Variable
Paraphasias	Common	Common	Common	Common	Variable	Variable	Variable	Common	Variable
Comprehension—Spoken	Good	Abnormal	Variable	Poor	Good	Abnormal	Abnormal	Normal	Abnormal
Comprehension—written	Worse than spoken	Better than spoken	May be normal	Poor	Good	Fair	Fair	Abnormal	Good
Writing	Impaired, with grammatical and spelling errors	Preserved, but inaccurate	Variable	Severely impaired	May be impaired	Preserved	Variable	Abnormal with spelling errors	Good
Naming	Poor	Poor	Fair	Poor	Poor	Good	Variable	Poor	Poor
Other findings	Hemiparesis, apraxia	Visual field deficits, hemisensory loss, apraxia	Mild hemiparesis, neglect	Hemiplegia, visual field deficits	Hemiparesis	Neglect, sensory loss	Variable with mild motor and sensory findings	Gerstmann syndrome (acalculia, agraphia, finger agnosia, left-right confusion)	Cognitive impairment, hemiataxia, hemiparesis, hemisensory loss

pronounced involvement of the left anterior temporal lobe may cause semantic dementia that is characterized by progressive loss of knowledge about objects, people, facts, and words, often accompanied by visual agnosia (inability to name or recognize objects presented visually).

Language comprehension is tested by asking the patient to follow increasingly complex linguistic constructions. The easiest commands are one-step orders such as "stand up" and "turn around," "open your mouth," and "stick out your tongue." Asking the patient to point to room objects or body parts is the next level of comprehension difficulty. Finally, more complex questions such as "If a lion is killed by a tiger, which animal is dead?" are asked. Impaired comprehension usually implies dysfunction of parietotemporal regions of the left hemisphere. Comprehension is abnormal in most fluent and global aphasic syndrome but may be preserved in nonfluent syndromes. In the elderly, it is important to establish that hearing is intact before testing comprehension. Failure to comprehend commands may reflect the inability to hear as opposed to impaired comprehension.

Repetition is assessed by asking the patient to repeat increasingly long phrases or sentences, generally beginning with simple phrases such as salutations ("Hello") and progress to more complex phrases ("Around the ragged rock, the rugged rascal ran"). Omissions and paraphasic substitutions may disrupt accurate repetition. Repetition is impaired in Wernicke, broca, conductive and global aphasia, but is generally preserved in transcortical aphasias.

Naming tests involve asking the patient to name objects, parts of objects, and colors. Errors include paraphasias, circumlocutory responses, and simply making no response. Aphasic patients may use descriptive terms rather than give the proper name. For example, a "watch" becomes "the thing you tell time with." Anomia occurs in aphasia, dementia, delirium, and can sometimes be seen as a consequence of head trauma. Adequate vision and object recognition must be ensured before errors are ascribed to naming deficits.

When assessing reading, the patient's ability to read aloud and to comprehend what is read must both be tested. Adequate vision must be ensured before failures are ascribed to an alexia. Most aphasias have concomitant alexias; however, the converse may not be true. In alexia with agraphia and alexia without agraphia, reading abnormalities may occur in the absence of other signs of aphasia.

Mechanical or aphasic abnormalities may cause agraphia. Micrographia is a characteristic aspect of parkinsonism in which the script becomes progressively smaller as the patient writes a sentence or extended series of numbers or letters, and mechanical agraphias occur in patients with limb paresis, limb apraxia, or movement disorders such as tremor and chorea. Aphasic agraphias accompany aphasic syndromes and errors similar to those noted in verbal output are present in written form. In Gerstmann syndrome (agraphia, acalculia, right–left disorientation, finger agnosia), alexia with agraphia, and disconnection agraphia (occurring with injury of the corpus callosum), agraphia occurs without aphasia. Agraphia also occurs in dementia and delirium.

Orientation

Orientation to time is tested by asking the patient to identify the correct day of the week, date, month, and year. Although some patients may make excuses (e.g., they are retired, they do not need to know, etc.), count only correct answers. This should be followed by asking the patient to guess the correct time of day without looking at a watch or clock. The patient should be within 1 hour of the correct time. Orientation to place is assessed by asking about city, county, state, and current location. If the patient is from out of town, major landmarks may be substituted for less well-known information such as county. Lastly, orientation to situation can be assessed by asking the patient why they are in the office today.

Abstraction

Similarities, differences, idioms, and proverb interpretation can all be used to assess abstracting capacity. These tests are heavily influenced by culture and educational attainment. Abstraction abnormalities are a nonspecific indicator of cerebral dysfunction. Patients with frontal lobe disorders have disproportionately severe abstracting disturbances.

Judgment and Problem Solving Abilities

Assessing judgment assists in exploring the patient's interpersonal and social insight. Judgment is impaired in many neurologic conditions. Damage to orbitofrontal subcortical circuit (e.g., in frontotemporal dementia, trauma, or focal syndromes) produces marked alterations in social judgment. Problem solving can be assessed by giving a scenario "If in a strange town, how would a person locate a friend they wished to see?" Correct answers might include use of phone book, the Internet, or city directory.

Visuospatial Skills

There are a number of visuospatial abilities including spatial attention, perception, construction, visuospatial problem solving, and visuospatial memory. Constructional tasks are most widely used to assess visuospatial ability. In the clock drawing test, the patient is asked to draw a clock and draw in the clock hands to indicate a specific time. The hands should be of different lengths. Watching the patient complete the clock is sometimes as informative as the finished product.

Patients with executive dysfunction may draw a clock face that is too small to contain the required numbers (poor planning), whereas patients with unilateral neglect will ignore half of the clock face.

Tests of copying involve having the patient reproduce figures such as a circle, intersecting circle and triangle, overlapping pentagons, cube, or more complex figures. Abnormalities include failures to reproduce the shapes accurately, perseveration on individual elements, drawing over the stimulus figure, or unilateral neglect. Drawing disturbances are common with many types of neurologic conditions including focal brain damage, degenerative disorders, and toxic and metabolic encephalopathies.

Calculation

In assessing calculation skills, patients are asked to add or multiply one or two digits mentally or to execute more demanding problems with pencil and paper. Calculation abilities are related to education and occupation. Acalculias may occur in association with a number of aphasic syndromes while visuospatial disorders lead to incorrect alignment of columns of numbers. Primary anarithmetias (inability to do math) are produced by damage to the posterior left hemisphere.

TABLE 12-5

The AD8, A Brief Informant Interview To Detect Dementia	YES, A CHANGE	NO, NO CHANGE	N/A, DON,T KNOW
Remember, "Yes, a change" indicates that there has been a change in the last several years caused by cognitive (thinking and memory) problems.			
1. Problems with judgment (e.g., problems making decisions, bad financial decisions, problems with thinking)			
2. Less interest in hobbies/activities			
3. Repeats the same things over and over (questions, stories, or statements)			
4. Trouble learning how to use a tool, appliance, or gadget (e.g., VCR, computer, microwave, remote control)			
5. Forgets correct month or year			
6. Trouble handling complicated financial affairs (e.g., balancing checkbook, income taxes, paying bills)			
7. Trouble remembering appointments			
8. Daily problems with thinking and/or memory			
TOTAL AD8 SCORE			

Executive Function

Executive function is assessed by asking the patient to perform tasks mediated by frontal–subcortical systems. Frontal–subcortical systems are complex neural circuits that include the dorsolateral prefrontal cortex, striatum, globus pallidus/substantia nigra, thalamic nuclei, and connecting white matter tracts. Patients with executive dysfunction manifest perseveration; motor programming abnormalities; reduced word list generation (left dorsolateral dysfunction); reduced nonverbal fluency (right dorsolateral dysfunction); poor set shifting; abnormal recall with intact recognition memory; loss of abstraction abilities; poor judgment; and impaired mental control. These abnormalities are common following head trauma, frontal lobe degenerations, frontal lobe neoplasms, multiple sclerosis, Huntington's disease and other basal ganglia disorders, subcortical infarctions, and in some brain infections such as syphilis.

Digit span backwards is a test of mental control and complex attention, as well as executive dysfunction. It entails saying increasingly long series of numbers and asking the patient to say them backwards (give 2–5-8, response should be 8–5-2). A normal digit span in reverse is five digits; fewer than three is abnormal.

Word List Generation

Word list generation is very useful and involves asking the patient to think of as many members of a specific category (most commonly animals) as possible within 1 minute. Normal individuals can name approximately 18 animals within 1 minute; less than 14 is considered abnormal. Word list generation deficits occur with anomia, frontal–subcortical systems dysfunction, and psychomotor retardation. It is a highly sensitive test but lacks specificity.

Informant Assessment

In many instances, asking questions of the informant will provide a wealth of information regarding the baseline abilities of the patient. There are several structured interviews that are short, easy to administer, and do not require specific training. Functional abilities and activities of daily living can be assessed with the Functional Activities Questionnaire, the Physical Self-Maintenance Scale, Instrumen-tal Activities of Daily Living Scale, or the Barthel Index. Baseline cognitive abilities can be assessed with brief informant interviews such as the AD8 (Table 12-5) or the IQCODE. The AD8 was developed in a research sample and validated in a clinic population and asks eight questions regarding change in the patient's memory, orientation, judgment and problem solving abilities, executive function, and interest level. Endorsement of two or more items suggests cognitive dysfunction and should trigger a more formal evaluation.

Neuropsychiatric Assessment

The neuropsychiatric interview of the patient includes the evaluation of thought form, thought content, and insight. The new onset of disturbances in any of these domains in the elderly is unusual in the absence of a brain disease. Their emergence should trigger the search for a neurologic or psychiatric condition.

Thought Form

Formal thought disorders such as tangentiality, circumstantiality, loose associations, illogicality, derailment, and thought blocking are much less common than disturbances of thought content as a manifestation of psychosis in neurologic diseases. Thought disorders have been observed in the psychoses accompanying epilepsy, Huntington's disease, and idiopathic basal ganglia calcification.

Perseveration and incoherence are disorders of the form of thought that are common in neuropsychiatric conditions. Perseveration refers to the inappropriate continuation of an act or thought after conclusion of its proper context. Intrusions are a special case of perseveration with late recurrences of words or thoughts from an earlier context. Perseverations and intrusions are seen in aphasias and dementing illnesses. Incoherence refers to the absence of logical association between words or ideas. It is observed in delirium, advanced dementias, and as part of the output of fluent aphasia.

Thought Content

Several types of disorders of thought content occur in neurologic diseases. Delusions are the most common manifestation of psychosis in neurologic disorders and are characterized by false beliefs based on incorrect inference about external reality. Common types of delusions encountered involve being followed or spied on, theft of personal property, spousal infidelity, or the presence of unwelcome strangers in one's home. Theme-specific delusions such as the Capgras syndrome (the belief that someone has been replaced by an identical-appearing impostor) may also be observed in neurologic illnesses. Delusions are common in a number of dementia etiologies including Alzheimer's disease and dementia with Lewy bodies, and may occur in vascular dementia, frontotemporal dementia, and Huntington's disease.

Hallucinations occur in many neurologic disorders. Hallucinations are sensory perceptions that occur without stimulation of the relevant sensory organ. Hallucinations and delusions occur together in psychosis; hallucinations are nondelusional when the patient recognizes the sensory experience to be unreal. Hallucinations may involve any sensory modality (visual, auditory, tactile, gustatory, olfactory) and maybe formed (e.g., people or things) or unformed (flashing lights or colors). Hallucinations occur with ocular and structural brain disorders as well as Charles Bonnet syndrome, epilepsy, narcolepsy, and migraine. Well-formed visual hallucinations (children, furry animals) are a prominent early sign in dementia with Lewy bodies. Less well-formed visual hallucinations occur in the moderate to severe stages of Alzheimer's disease. Gustatory or olfactory hallucinations are most common in seizure disorders, bipolar disorders, and schizophrenia, and with tumors located in the medial temporal lobe. Tactile hallucinations are most commonly associated with schizophrenia, affective disorders, or drug intoxication or withdrawal.

Insight

Patients with neuropsychiatric disease may display limited insight and be unaware of their medical conditions or limitations in function, thus assessment of a patient's insight into the severity of their illness can yield useful diagnostic information and assist in developing a therapeutic plan. For example, patients with Alzheimer's disease have impaired insight into their memory and cognitive difficulties, whereas patients with vascular dementia and dementia with Lewy bodies often exhibit more appropriate concern regarding their cognitive dysfunction. Lesions of the right parietal lobe are associated with unawareness, neglect, or denial of the abnormalities of the contralateral side.

Behavior and Personality

A variety of changes in personality and behavior have been described in neuropsychiatric disease in the older adult. Personality changes may include increased egocentricity and thought rigidity, impaired emotional control and diminished emotional responsiveness, loss of interest and apathy, and lack of concern for the feelings of others. No brief personality rating scales are available but in the proper setting the Neuroticism-Extroversion-Openness Five Factor Inventory (NEO-FFI) can be used to evaluate personality. Behavioral changes including irritability, depression, anxiety, hallucinations, delusions, and vegetative changes can be assessed with the Neuropsychiatric Inventory (NPI). There both long and short forms of the NPI available.

NEUROLOGICAL EXAMINATION

The neurologic examination includes assessment of cranial nerve function, strength, coordination, sensation, muscle stretch reflexes, pathologic/primitive reflexes, and neurovascular status. Examination of head and neck may provide additional important information.

Cranial Nerve Examination

Cranial Nerve I: Olfactory

In normal aging, loss of olfaction may be a nonspecific or clinically insignificant finding. Olfaction maybe impaired following head trauma, infection, zinc deficiency, Vitamin A deficiency, frontal lobe dysfunction, B-12 deficiency, and frontal lobe tumors (olfactory groove meniginoma). Olfaction is tested by asking the patient to identify a variety of odors. When testing, it is important to use simple and familiar odors (coffee beans, vanilla, or cinnamon). Complex scents such as perfumes and noxious agents (i.e. ammonia) should not be used. Ideally, the patient should close their eyes and each nostril should be tested separately.

Cranial Nerve II: Optic

Examination of the optic nerve includes visual inspection of the nerve head, testing of visual acuity, and mapping of the visual fields. In aging, visual acuity maybe impaired and can be due to a number of neurological and ophthalmologic causes. First, casual inspection of the corneal, sclera, and mucosal tissue should be carried out to evaluate structural abnormalities. Visual acuity can be evaluated with a Snellen visual chart or Rosenberg card held 14 inches from the eye. Screening should be done in a well-lit environment and to the patient's advantage allowing them to use their corrective lenses. If they do not have their glasses with them, refractive errors can be partly corrected by using a pinhole. Visual fields are tested at the bedside by confrontation. The examiner should face the patient, sitting or standing at a similar height and each eye should be tested independently. The patient is asked to look at the examiner's nose and the examiner's arms are extended laterally. The patient is asked to differentiate between one or two fingers. Each quandrant should be tested separately. After testing each eye individually, both eyes should be tested simultaneously for visual neglect. Monocular visual field deficits can be associated with glaucoma. Abrupt changes in visual fields or acuity should alert the clinician to potential vascular etiologies. Homonymous field deficits reflect disruption of the optic pathways posterior to the optic chiasm.

Pupillary examination should include evaluation of size and shape. Up to a 1 mm difference in size is generally considered normal. Pupillary responses are tested with a bright flashlight (not the ophthalmoscope). A normal pupil reacts to light by constricting; the contralateral pupil should also constrict. The pupils also constrict when shifting focus from a distant object to a near object (accommodation) and during convergence such as when patients are asked to look at their nose. Abnormalities of pupillary responses are associated with a number of neurologic disorders (Table 12-6). A review of medications is also important as a number of drugs can affect pupillary size. Mydriasis (pupillary diliation) can be caused

TABLE 12-6

Causes of Pupillary Changes in Older Adult

MIOSIS (PUPILLARY CONSTRICTION)	MYDRIASIS (PUPILLARY DILATATION)
Pontine lesion	Dorsal midbrain syndrome (Paranaud's)
Organophosphates	Amphetamines and sympathomimetics
Cholinergic agents	Anticholinergic agents
Opioids (except meperidine)	Meperidine
Pilocarpine-like agents	Atropine-like agents
Barbiturates	Cocaine
Phenothiazines	Phenothiazines
MAO inhibitors	Antihistamines
Phencyclidine (PCP)	Lysergic acid diethylamide (LSD)
Argyll-Robertson (syphilis)	Seizures/postictal state
Horner's syndrome (usually unilateral)	Thyrotoxicosis
Hypothermia	Hypermagnesemia
	Third nerve compression (usually unilateral)

SITE OF LESION	PUPIL SIZE	DIRECT RESPONSE	CONSENSUAL RESPONSE		ACCOMMODATION
			Ipsilateral	Contralateral	
Retina	Normal	Impaired	Impaired	Normal	Normal
Optic nerve	Normal	Lost	Lost	Normal	Normal
Optic chiasm	Normal	Normal	Normal	Normal	Normal
Optic tract	Normal	Normal	Normal	Normal	Normal
Optic radiation	Normal	Normal	Normal	Normal	Normal
Oculomotor nerve or nucleus	Dilated	Lost	Normal	Lost	Lost
Argyll-Robertson	Constricted	Lost	Normal	Lost	Normal
Sympathetic	Constricted	Normal	Normal	Normal	Normal

by atropine-like drugs, while miosis (pupillary constriction) can be caused by parasympathomimetic drugs.

A careful examination of the optic nerve should be performed in all patients. It is not always necessary to do a dilated examination, but the room should be darkened to increase pupillary size. The sharpness of optic disk margins, the ratio of optic cup to disk, venous pulsations, the caliber of blood vessels, and the presence of exudates, hemmorhages, emboli, and retinal pallor should be noted. Papilledema is characterized by blurring or elevation of the disk margins with the loss of normal venous pulsations and reflects raised intracranial pressure. As pressure increases, hemorrhages may be found adjacent to the disk. Glaucoma increases the size of the optic cup relative to the disk.

Cranial Nerves III, IV, and VI: Oculomotor, Trochlear, and Abducens

The oculomotor, trochlear, and abducens nerves mediate ocular motility, pupillary responses, and eyelid position. The trochlear nerve innervates the superior oblique muscle, the abducens nerve innervates the lateral rectus muscle, while the oculomotor nerve innervates the remainder of the extraocular muscles. The oculomotor nerve also innervated the levator muscles of the eyelid and carries parasympathetic nerves to the pupil. Testing each eye individually helps to identify ocular motility dysfunction. In aging, ocular motility may be reduced. Normal elderly can exhibit restricted convergence and limitation of conjugate upward gaze. Other nonspecific

concomitants of normal aging include the evolution of small sluggishly reactive pupils, loss of Bell phenomenon (upward eye deviation on eye closure), and the inability to dissociate ocular movements from head movements. The clinician should be concerned when an elderly patient exhibits new onset diplopia, pupillary asymmetry, nystagmus (Table 12-7), or extraocular movement disorders. Ptosis (drooping of the upper lid) can be caused by a number of disorders (Table 12-8). Isolated abducens palsies may be a sign of elevated intracranial pressure since the 6th nerve has the longest intracranial course.

Cranial Nerve V: Trigeminal

The trigeminal nerve is divided into three divisions: ophthalmic, maxillary, and mandibular. The first two divisions are pure sensory nerves mediating facial and corneal sensation. The third division carries both sensory fibers and innervates the muscles of mastication. The corneal reflex is mediated by the ophthalmic division and can be tested by lightly stimulating the cornea with a wisp of cotton. When the cornea on one side is stimulated, both eyes should close. Facial sensation is tested with a safety pin or cold handle of a tuning fork. Motor function is tested by asking the patient to bite down or open the jaw against resistance. Tumors of the middle fossa and in the cerebellopontine angle may compress the fifth cranial nerve and produce a cranial nerve syndrome with decreased corneal reflex and sensory loss on the ipsilateral face. Tic douleroux (trigeminal neuralgia) is a paraoxysmal pain disorder triggered by touching

TABLE 12-7

Types of Nystagmus and Ocular Oscillations		
MOVEMENT	**DESCRIPTION**	**LOCALIZATION**
Physiologic end stage	Fine, regular horizontal jerking at extremes of lateral gaze	No pathological significance
Jerk	Horizontal and rotary	Vestibular disorder
Vertical	Jerk movements in vertical plane	Posterior fossa disease, sedatives, anticonvulsants
Downbeating	Rhythmic, horizontal gaze still possible	Cervicomeduallary junction lesion
Upbeating	Rhythmic, horizontal gaze still possible	Lesion in pons, cerebellar vermis or medulla
Ocular bobbing	Arrhythmic, coarse movement with horizontal gaze palsy	Pontine lesion
Seesaw	Vertical dysconjugate movements with rotary component	Lesion by optic chiasm
Periodic alternating	Horizontal nystagmus with periodically alternating direction	Lower brainstem
Rebound	Horizontal jerk nystagmus transiently after sustained gaze to opposite side	Cerebellar pathways
Convergence-retraction	Eyes converge and move rhythmically back into the orbits on attempted upgaze	Periaqueductal gray (midbrain)
Ocular dysmetria	Overshoot or terminal oscillation of saccadic movements	Cerebellar pathways
Hypometric saccades	Slowed movements	Parkinson's disease, basal ganglia
Opsoclonus	Chaotic multidirectional conjugate saccades	Paraneoplastic syndrome (neuroblastoma, breast, lung)
Square-wave jerks	Small saccades interfering with visual fixation	Progressive supranuclear palsy
Ocular myoclonus	Rhythmic oscillations, usually vertical	Associated with palatal myoclonus, brainstem lesion

sensitive zones usually within the mandibular division. The cause may be idiopathic due to compressive lesions or demyelination at the root entry zone.

Cranial Nerve VII: Facial

The facial nerve supplies the facial musculature, lacrimal and salivary glands, and taste fibers of the anterior tongue. The motor function is tested by asking the patient to wrinkle their forehead, close their eyes, and smile. Unilateral weakness may cause a flattening of the nasolabial fold. If very weak, the patient may experience drooling. The eyelid is usually not severely affected with central lesions and the upper forehead is spared. In peripheral lesions such as Bell's palsy (Table 12-9), patients are unable close their eye or wrinkle their forehead. The facial nerve also innervates the stapedius muscle of the middle ear, which helps to modulate tympanic membrane vibration. This motor branch can be damaged during closed head trauma leading to hyperacusis, an increased perception of sound.

The sense of taste is not often tested, but can be done at the bedside using sugar, salt, or lemon juice. The patient is asked to stick their tongue out and a small amount of solution is placed on one side of the tongue. The patient is asked to describe the taste, and then allowed to drink some water before the next solution is applied.

Cranial Nerve VIII: Cochlear and Vestibular

Hearing and vestibular function are mediated by the eighth cranial nerve. Evaluation of hearing at the bedside is sometimes difficult. Use of a 512 Hz tuning fork can help discriminate conduction from sensorineural hearing loss. The Rinne test is done by placing a vibrating tuning fork on the mastoid process. As soon as the patient is unable to detect sound, the tuning fork is moved to a position near the external auditory canal. If the patient has normal hearing, air conduction should be better than bone conduction. If the patient has conduction deafness, the sound will not be heard because of pathology in the middle ear. In nerve deafness, air conduction is better than bone conduction but both will be reduced. The Weber test looks for

TABLE 12-8

Causes of Ptosis in the Older Adult
Congenital
Myopathic-causes
Myasthenia gravis
Oculopharyngeal muscular dystrophy
Myotonic dystrophy
Polymyositis
Hypothyroidism
Horner's syndrome
Vasculitis
Diabetes mellitus
Third nerve lesions (ptosis is rarely isolated finding)
Nuclear lesion in mesencephalon
Third nerve compression

TABLE 12-9

Causes of Bell's Palsy
Idiopathic
Pregnancy
Guillian-Barre syndrome
Lyme disease (may present as bifacial weakness)
Herpes Zoster (Ramsey-Hunt syndrome)
Neoplasms
Sarcoidosis
Head trauma
Acute intermittent porphyria
Lead poisoning
Brainstem infarction (rare)

TABLE 12-10

Differential Diagnosis of Tinnitus

TONAL TINNITUS	NONTONAL TINNITUS
Otitis media	Contraction of muscles in eustatian tube
Disorder of tympanic membrane	Contraction of stapedius muscle
Inner ear disorder (hair cells, organ of Corti)	Contraction of tensor tympani muscles
Cochlear nerve lesion	Palatal myoclonus
Acoustic Schwannoma	Carotid bruit
Meningioma	Arteriovenous malformations
Neurofibroma	Glomus jugulare tumor
Meniere's disease	
Head trauma	

lateralization. The tuning fork is placed in the middle of the skull and the patient asked to decide where they best hear the sound. In normal hearing, the sound is heard equally in both ears. In conduction deafness, vibrations are best heard in the abnormal ear. In nerve deafness, the sound is best appreciated in the normal ear. Decreased hearing for high-pitched sounds and lack of perception of background noise are common findings in normal aging and by themselves should not be considered a pathologic finding. Sensorineural deafness is characterized by loss of high-pitched sounds while conduction deafness is characterized by loss of low-pitched sounds. Tinnitus or ringing in the ears is a common symptom in adults. Tonal tinnitus is subjective and heard only by the patient. Nontonal tinnitus is more objective because in certain circumstances, the tinnitus can be heard by the examiner. The differential diagnosis of tinnitus is presented in Table 12-10.

Vestibular lesions produce nystagmus and vertigo. Vestibular nystagmus is horizontal or combined horizontal–rotatory and is typically accompanied by vertigo and nausea, whereas lesions disrupting vestibular connections in the central nervous system can produce nystagmus in any direction but are usually not associated with vertiginous or nauseous sensations. When characterizing nystagmus, only the fast component should be described. The complaint of dizziness in the elderly is not uncommon; however, the examiner must determine whether the dizzy patient is experiencing lightheadedness or true vertigo. If true vertigo is present, then the clinician should further discern whether it is peripheral (vestibular) or central (brainstem) in origin as well as associated features (Table 12-11). Causes of vertigo associated with vestibular disease include benign positional vertigo, Ménière's syndrome, and trauma.

Cranial Nerves IX and X: Glossopharyngeal and Vagus

The ninth and tenth cranial nerves control pharyngeal and laryngeal function, taste, and the gag reflex. Glossopharyngeal lesions cause asymmetric elevation of the palate and deviation of the uvula. Hoarseness, aphonia, and dysphagia occur with vagus nerve lesions. In normal aging, the gag reflex can be reduced and, when accompanied by a decrease in the cough reflex, can result in difficulty handling bronchial secretions. Glossopharyngeal neuralgia is a rare paroxysmal pain syndrome involving the posterior pharynx or tonsils usually triggered by excessively hot or cold foods or liquids.

Cranial Nerve XI: Accessory Nerve

The spinal accessory nerve innervates the upper half of the trapezius and the sternocleidomastoid muscle. In the normal elderly, frank weakness of the trapezius or sternocleidomastoid muscle is not a typical finding and, if present, should be investigated further. A delayed shrug may be an indication of a mild ipsilateral hemiparesis.

Cranial Nerve XII: Hypoglossal

The hypoglossal nerve innervates the tongue. Patients are asked to stick their tongue out; deviation to either side implies a lesion on the side of deviation. The tongue should also be examined for atrophy and spontaneous muscle contractions (fasciculation), suggesting upper motor neuron disease. Fasciculation is best detected on the lateral aspects of the tongue. Tongue weakness is also common in pseudobulbar palsy.

Motor System Examination

Muscle bulk, strength, tone, and coordination are assessed as part of the motor system examination.

Muscle Bulk

Muscle bulk is examined by visual inspection and palpation. Muscle wasting may occur with disuse; muscle, nerve, or spinal disease; and in generalized weight loss secondary to malnutrition, systemic illness, or advanced brain diseases. Mild muscular wasting without associated weakness can be encountered in normal aging most commonly involving the intrinsic hand and foot muscles, calf and shoulder girdle muscles.

Muscle Tone

Muscle tone maybe increased or decreased in neurologic disorders. Muscle tone is decreased in muscle and peripheral nerve disease, with cerebellar disorders, early in the course of many choreiform disorders, and acutely following an upper motor neuron lesion. Increased muscle tone is encountered in spasticity with pyramidal tract lesions and rigidity with extrapyramidal disorders. Cogwheel rigidity of Parkinson's disease is best palpated when manipulating the distal limbs, usually in a circular motion. "Gegenhalten" refers to the active resistance to movement encountered in advanced brain diseases.

Strength

Strength is graded as 0 (no evidence of muscle contraction), 1 (muscle contraction without movement of the limb), 2 (limb movement after gravity eliminated), 3 (limb movement against gravity), 4 (limb movement against partial resistance), or 5 (normal strength). Distal weakness is most indicative of peripheral neuropathies, whereas proximal weakness is more consistent with primary muscle disease. In aging, mild generalized weakness may occur; however, focal weakness is indicative of a neuropathologic process. Focal weakness often is subtle and maybe detected only with careful examination. Hemipareses occur with lesions of the pyramidal system. When testing strength, the examiner should attempt to isolate individual muscles (thumb abduction) rather than test whole groups (hand grip) to detect subtle signs of weakness. A pronator drift is seen with mild forms of weakness.

TABLE 12-11

Causes of Vertigo and Associated Findings

ANATOMIC LOCATIONS	CAUSES	OTOSCOPIC EXAMINATION	OTHER NEUROLOGICAL FINDINGS	TESTS OF EQUILIBRIUM	NYSTAGMUS	HEARING LOSS
Labyrinth	Benign postional, trauma, Meniere's, drug toxicity, viral infection	Usually negative	None	Ipsilateral past pointing, lateral pulsion to side of lesion	Horizontal or rotary to side opposite lesion, paroxysmal, positional	May be normal, sensorineural, or conduction deafness
Vestibular	Vestibular neuronopathy, herpes zoster	Zoster vesicles in auditory canal, tympanic membrane, and palate	7th and 8th cranial nerves	Ipsilateral past pointing, lateral pulsion to side of lesion	Positional	Sensorineural
Cerebellopontine angle tumor	Acoustic neuroma, menigioma, glioma, glomus jugulare	Normal	Ipsilateral 5th, 7th, 9th, and 10th cranial nerves, ataxia Increased intracranial pressure	Ataxia	Gaze-paretic, positional, coarser to side of lesion	Sensorineural
Brainstem and cerebellar lesions	Infarct, gliomas, encephalitis	Negative	Multiple cranial nerves, sensory or motor tract signs, ataxia, dysmetria	Ataxia	Horizontal and/or vertical, gaze-paretic	Normal
Cortical lesions	Infarct, glioma, trauma	Negative	Fluent aphasia, visual field cuts, hemimotor/sensory findings, seizures	Usually no change, mild ataxia	Usually absent	Normal

Abnormal Movements

During the interview and examination, the clinician should be observant for any movement that is not purposeful including tremor, chorea, dyskinesias, and ballismus. Tremor is usually described as action (associated with a movement) or rest (disappears with movement of affected extremities). "Essential" tremor is a usually benign hereditary condition associated with movement or sustained posture and may involve arms, legs, head, chin, or voice. Essential tremors often improve after drinking small amounts of alcohol.

Sensory Examination

Primary modalities, including light touch and temperature are tested to assess sensory function. Sensory examination is quite subjective and it is important to consider the consistency of responses and how sensory complaints relate to other signs and symptoms. Peripheral causes of sensory loss typically present bilaterally and are largely symmetric. Unilateral sensory loss occurs with lesions of primary sensory cortex or its projections.

Light Touch

Evaluation of light touch is not particularly helpful in discriminating pathology but is useful in defining the presence or loss of sensation. Lightly stroking the fingers or a wisp of cotton across the skin may help elicit dermatomal patterns of sensory loss for further evaluation.

Pain and Temperature

Pain and temperature sensation is carried by small unmyelinated fibers. Pain can be assessed with the use of a disposable safety pin while temperature can be assessed with the handle of the reflex hammer or tuning fork. The loss of pain sensation due to a metabolic or toxic peripheral neuropathy typically follows a stocking glove pattern, while lesions due to a radiculopathy follow a defined dermatome.

Vibration

Vibration is carried by large myelinated fibers and is assessed with a 128 Hz tuning fork. The tuning fork should be struck and placed on a bony prominence. Causes of pathologic decreased vibratory sensation include peripheral neuropathies, diabetes, tabes dorsalis, vitamin B-12 deficiency, and myelopathies.

Position

Proprioception is assessed by having the patient close their eyes and the examiner gently moves toes or fingers in the vertical plane. Skin proprioception can be assessed by lightly stroking the skin in an up or down fashion. The Romberg sign is performed to assess the intergrity of the dorsal columns. The patient is asked to stand with their feet together and eyes closed. The presence of a sway suggests a positive test. If the problem is due to a proprioceptive deficit, the patient is able to correct themselves with their eyes open. Position sense loss can be caused by peripheral neuropathies, diabetes, tabes dorsalis, vitamin B-12 deficiency, and myelopathies.

TABLE 12-12

Elements of Ataxia and Cerebellar Dysfunction

SIGN	DESCRIPTION
Dysmetria	Overshooting or undershooting a target
Dysdiadochokinesia	Impairment in rapid-alternating movements
Tremor	Coarse, rhythmic movement on action
Ataxic speech	Abnormal variability of volume, rate and phonation
Dysarthria	Slow and slurred speech
Gait Ataxia	Wide-based, unsteady

Cerebellar Examination

Cerebellar function and coordination maybe disrupted by many types of motor and sensory abnormalities. Tests of coordination include rapid alternating movements, fine finger movements, finger-to-nose movements, and heel-knee-shin maneuvers. During aging, there is an overall decrease in speed of coordinated movements that is of no pathologic consequence. However, gross abnormalities in cerebellar function are not anticipated and should be evaluated thoroughly (Table 12-12).

When unilateral cerebellar dysfunction is present, patient will overshoot target but may improve after a few trials. Dysdiadochokinesis occurs when the patient is asked to rapidly change hand or finger movements; difficulties in maintaining smooth movements are characteristic. Cerebellar lesions can also affect muscle tone causing hypotonia. Cerebellar tremors tend to be coarse and irregular, worsening in the terminal one-third of a movement.

Gait and Station

Gait and posture depend on motor, sensory, and cerebellar function. In normal aging, posture becomes more flexed, slowed, and may have a slightly unsteady quality. When assessing gait in the older adult, it is important to recognize gait abnormalities that may be secondary to joint pain and arthritic conditions. Gait is assessed by having the patient walk straight for at least 10 yards, making a turn and maneuvering in a tight corridor. It is important to note the presence of armswing and the distance of the stride. The patient should also be asked to tandem walk, walk on their toes and heels, and if possible walk up a few steps. Postural stability is assessed by asking the patient to stand with their shoulder-width apart. A forceful pull is given to their shoulders and the righting response is assessed. The clinician should be prepared to catch the patient. One step of retropulsion is considered normal. Table 12-13 lists common causes of gait disturbance in the elderly.

Muscle Stretch Reflexes

Decreased muscle stretch reflexes are found in muscle, peripheral nerve, and nerve root disorders, while increased reflexes occur with upper motor neuron lesions. Lateralized hyperactive reflexes in conjunction with spasticity and the Babinski sign are indicative of a contralateral lesion of the pyramidal system. In aging, deep tendon reflexes tend to become hypoactive. Ankle reflexes may be absent in normal aging, but knee reflexes persist. Reflexes are initially

TABLE 12-13

Gait Abnormalities in the Older Adult

GAIT	CAUSE	DESCRIPTION	ASSOCIATED SIGNS
Festinating	Parkinson's disease	Slow, shuffling picks up speed and may require wall or furniture to stop	Postural instability, rest tremor, bradykinesia, decreased arm swing, masked face, rigidity
Antalgic	Joint pain	Slow, gingerly pace	Facial grimaces
Spastic	Stroke	Stiff extremity, may require circumduction or scissor movements	Scuffing toe of affected leg across ground, weakness
Ataxic	Cerebellar disease	Wide-based	Dysmetria, dysdiadochokinesis
Sensory Ataxia	Peripheral neuropathy	Wide-based, high steps with foot slapping	Sensory loss, weakness
Apraxic	Normal pressure hydrocephalus	Feet appear "nailed" to floor, lower extremity bradykinesia	Dementia, urinary incontinence
Stooped	Lumbar stenosis	Forward flexion	Pain, lordosis, kyphoscoliosis
Myopathic	Proximal myopathy, myasthenia gravis	Uses arms to help push themselves up stairs or out of a chair (Gowers sign)	Muscle cramps, weakness, myoglobinuria
Astasia-Abasia	Psychosis, malingering	Wildly lurching, "hurky-jerky" movements, however patient does not fall	Signs of intoxication, delusions, hallucinations. Secondary gain.

hyperactive in cervical and lumbar spondylosis, however in advanced cases absent or diminished reflexes may be found as nerve roots become compromised.

Pathologic and Primitive Reflexes

The Babinski sign is dorsiflexion of the great toe with plantar stimulation. It is produced by upper motor neuron lesions. The grasp reflex (involuntary gripping of objects in or near the patient's hand) occurs in patients with advanced brain disease and with lesions restricted to the medial frontal lobes. The sucking reflex (sucking movements of the lips, tongue, and jaw elicited by stimulation of the lips) occurs in patients with frontal lobe and diffuse brain dysfunction.

The palmomental reflex (ipsilateral contraction of the mentalis muscle in response to stroking of the thenar eminence of the hand) can be seen in normal aged individuals and maybe regarded as pathologic when it is unilateral or when it does not fatigue with repeated palmar stimulation. The glabellar reflex (Myerson's sign) is elicited by tapping the patient between the eyes. After a few blinks, the patient should suppress further blinking. Patients with Parkinson's disease and other basal ganglia disorders will continue to blink.

Higher Cortical Function

Cortical sensory modalities, including two-point discrimination, graphesthesia, and stereognosis should be assessed. Two-point discrimination is best performed with calipers. Graphesthesia is performed with the patients eyes closed and numbers are traced onto the palm with the back of the reflex hammer. Stereognosis is also performed with the patients eyes closed. Common objects are placed into the patients' hand and they are allowed to move them about without using the other hand. Deficits imply dysfunction in the contralateral parietal lobe. Cortical sensory function should be assessed independently for each upper extremity. It is important to first assess primary sensory modalities. In the presence of prominent sensory loss, cortical sensory function cannot be assessed.

Neurovascular Assessment

Examination of vascular system, including auscultation for cranial and carotid bruits, palpation of peripheral pulses, and assessment of blood pressure (lying, sitting, and standing) complements the neurologic examination and should be performed on every patient.

CONCLUSION

A variety of neurologic disorders (e.g., stroke, Parkinson's disease, Alzheimer's disease) preferentially present in the older adult. A comprehensive mental status and neurologic examination should be performed in every patient to document changes in neurologic function (i.e., memory/cognition, behavior/personality, cranial nerves, motor function, and sensory perception) associated with pathologic conditions that affect the nervous system, and distinguish them from the functional changes associated with normal aging. Limited memory and cognitive function changes occur as one ages. Subtle changes in memory that do not interfere with normal functioning in society and that do not impair activities of daily living occur in normal aging. More significant declines in memory and cognitive function can be encountered in dementia (Table 12-14).

Altered cognitive function in the setting of a clear sensorium is consistent with dementia secondary to a neurodegenerative process or medical illness. Dementias (e.g., Alzheimer's disease, frontotemporal dementias, dementia with Lewy bodies) are characterized by a specific constellation of signs and symptoms. In Alzheimer's disease, the individual typically exhibits limited insight into their cognitive deficits that involve memory, language, and visuospatial skills. Patients with frontotemporal dementias present with a predominance of features consistent with frontal and/or temporal degeneration. These individuals exhibit early changes in behavior and personality, such as social inappropriateness, disinhibition, apathy, perseveration, and oral/dietary changes. Other accompanying features may include language/speech impairment, executive dysfunction, and preserved

TABLE 12-14

Differential Diagnosis of Dementia

Neurodegenerative disease
Alzheimer's disease
Dementia with Lewy bodies/Parkinson's disease
Frontotemporal dementia
Huntington's disease
Progressive supranuclear palsy
Corticobasal degeneration
Creutzfeldt-Jacob and other prion diseases
Wilson's disease
Neuronal ceroid lipofuscinosis

Vascular disease
Vascular dementia
Cerebral amyloid angiopathy
CADASIL
Vasculitis

Hydrocephalus

Demyelinating disorders
Multiple sclerosis
Leukodystrophies

Traumatic brain injury

Metabolic disorders
Hepatic encephalopathy
Hypothyroidism
Storage disorders
Electrolyte disorders (sodium, calcium)

Nutritional disorders
B-12 deficiency
Wernicke-Korsakoff syndrome (thiamine)

Mitochondrial disorders

Toxic disorders
Alcoholism
Drugs
Heavy metals

Neoplasia
Primary brain tumors (Meningiomas, Gliomas)
Metastatic disease
Paraneoplastic syndromes

Infection
HIV
Neurosyphillis
Progressive multifocal leukoencephalopathy
Subacute sclerosing panencephalitis
Whipple's disease

Epilepsy

posterior functions (e.g., visuospatial ability, calculations). In dementia with Lewy bodies, patients may exhibit fluctuating cognition, recurrent well-formed and detailed visual hallucinations, and extrapyramidal signs consistent with parkinsonism. Dementia can occur as a consequence of other neurological and medical illnesses such as cerebrovascular disease, vitamin B-12 deficiency, hypothyroidism, Parkinson's disease, and meningoencephalitis.

Delirium, on the other hand, causes alteration in sensorium and level of consciousness and is usually due to medications (Table 12-15), infection, head injury, or metabolic derangements. Associated features include disruption of sleep–wake cycle, intermittent drowsiness and agitation, restlessness, emotional lability, and frank psychosis (hallucination, illusions, delusions). Symptoms of delirium are often worse at night and occurs in up to 20% of hospitalized patients. The risk increases in the older adult the longer the hospital stay. Predisposing factors include advanced age, dementia, impaired physical or mental health, sensory deprivation (poor vision or hearing), and placement in intensive care units.

A functional decline in some aspects of cranial nerve function (e.g., vision, hearing, vestibular function, taste, and smell) can be anticipated in normal aging and should be distinguished from pathological conditions afflicting the nervous system. Similarly, older individuals experience decreased mobility as they age. Subtle changes in gait, posture, coordination, and strength are expected concomitants of aging. However, more profound changes that significantly alter mobility and/or present as focal weakness or impaired coordination should alert the clinician to the possibility of a neuropathologic disorder.

Alterations in sensory perception can be indicative of neuropsychiatric dysfunction. Subtle deficits in vibration and other primary sensory modalities may be encountered in normal aging. However,

TABLE 12-15

Medications Causing Delirium in the Older Adult

Alpha-methyl DOPA
Amantidine
Anticholinergics
Antihistamines
Antipsychotics
Atropine
Barbiturates
Benzodiazepines
Bromides
Chlordiazepoxide
Chloral hydrate
Cimetidine and other H2 blockers
Clonidine
Codeine and other opioids
Cocaine
Dextromethorophan
Digoxin
Dopamine agonists
Dopamine antagonists
Ethanol
Furosemide
Lithium
Levodopa
Nifedipine
Opioids
Phencyclindine (PCP)
Phenytoin
Prednisone and other steroids
Propanolol
Reserpine
Theophylline
Tricyclic antidepressants

marked deficits in sensory function are suggestive of neurologic disease and require further diagnostic testing.

In conclusion, neurologic findings of normal aging include subtle declines in cognitive function, mildly impaired motor function, and altered sensory perceptions. However, exaggerated impairments in cognitive, behavioral, motor, and sensory function suggest the onset of neurologic diseases that commonly afflict the older adult. A comprehensive mental status and neurologic examination is the foundation for identifying neuropathologic conditions that necessitate further laboratory and imaging investigation.

ACKNOWLEDGMENTS

This project was supported by a grants from the National Institute on Aging (P50 AG005681, P01 AG03991, P01 AG026276) and a generous gift from the Alan A and Edith L Wolff Charitable Trust.

REFERENCES

Adams RD, Victor M. *Principles of Neurology*, 5th ed. New York, New York: McGraw-Hill; 1993.

Aminoff MJ. *Neurology and General Medicine*, 2nd ed. New York, New York: Churchill-Livingstone; 1995.

Balsis S, Carpenter BD, Storandt M. Personality change preceded clinical diagnosis of dementia of the Alzheimer type. *J Gerontol B Psychol Sci Soc Sci.* 2005;60:98–101.

Blazer DG, Steffens DC, Busse EW. *Textbook of Geriatric Psychiatry*, 3rd ed. Washington DC: APA Publishing; 2004

Burns A, Lawlor B, Craig S. *Assessment Scales in Old Age Psychiatry.* London: Martin Dunitz; 1999.

Claussen CF. Subdividing tinnitus into bruits and endogenous, exogenous, and other forms. *Int Tinnitus J.* 2005;11:126–136.

Cummings JL. *The Neuropsychiatry of Alzheimer's Disease and Related Dementias.* London: Martin Dunitz; 2003.

Dronkers NF, Wilkins DP, Van Valin RD Jr, Redfern BB, Jaeger JJ. Lesion analysis of the brain areas involved in language comprehension. *Cognition.* 2004;92:145–177.

Galvin JE, Malcom H, Johnson DK, Morris JC. Personality traits distinguishing dementia with Lewy bodies from Alzheimer's disease. *Neurology.* 2007;68:1895–1901.

Galvin JE. Alzheimer's disease: understanding the challenges, improving the outcome. *Appl Neurol.* 2007;Suppl (Feb):3–13.

Galvin JE, Roe C, Coats M, et al. The AD8: a brief informant interview to detect dementia. *Neurology.* 2005;65:559–564.

Galvin JE, Powlishta KK, Wilkins K, et al. Predictors of preclinical Alzheimer's disease and dementia: a clinicopathologic study. *Arch Neurol.* 2005;62:758–765.

Galvin JE, Roe CM, Xiong C, Morris JC. The validity and reliability of the AD8 informant interview for dementia. *Neurology.* 2006;67:1942–1948.

Jones HR. *Netter's Neurology.* Teterboro, NJ: Icon Learning Systems; 2005.

Lord SR. Visual risk factors for falls in older people. *Age Ageing* 2006;35 Suppl 2:42–45.

Peters R. Ageing and the brain. *Postgrad Med J.* 2006;82:84–88.

Plum F, Posner JB. The Diagnosis of Stupor and Coma, 3rd ed. Philadelphia: FA Davis; 1982.

Rubin EH, Storandt M, Miller JP, et al. A prospective study of cognitive function and onset of dementia in cognitively healthy elders. *Arch Neurol.* 1998;55:395–401.

Tindall B. *Aids to Examination of the Peripheral Nervous System.* London: WB Saunders; 1986.

Assessment of Decisional Capacity and Competencies

Margaret A. Drickamer ■ *James M. Lai*

INTRODUCTION

The medical profession has been charged with the seemingly conflicting responsibilities of respecting patients' autonomy while protecting from harm those patients who are incapable of protecting themselves. Assessing a patient's capacity to make decisions is a role with which all clinicians should be familiar. Although certain situations may call for specialized assessment, generalists, internists, subspecialists, geriatricians, and advanced practice nurses, among other health professionals, should be sufficiently familiar with the principles and process to handle most situations. The purpose of this chapter is to explain some of the ethical underpinnings to this responsibility, to highlight the strengths and weaknesses of approaches to assessing decisional capacity, and to describe the types of situations in which the clinician may play a role.

Autonomy is defined as self-determination (see also Chapter 34). Respect for individual autonomy is understood to be an elemental principle of our society. Nonetheless, all of us face limitations on how much we can truly determine our fates. Limitations of resources and opportunity, societal and legal prohibitions, and the limits imposed by the rights of others not to have their autonomy infringed upon all limit one's self-determination. There are also limitations on who qualifies as an autonomous "self." The full right to self-determination is generally recognized to apply only to adults who are "of sound mind."

Paternalism is defined as limiting an individual's autonomy in order either to prevent that individual from doing harm to themselves or to prevent the person from missing a substantial benefit. The circumstances under which paternalism is acceptable are not defined by the action the individual may wish to undertake, or by the probable untoward consequences of an action, but rather by the individual's ability to make decisions. In other words, our wish to protect an individual from doing themselves harm does not justify paternalism; we cannot prevent an individual from doing things that may cause them harm (overeating, bungee jumping, etc.). We can only justify intervention if we judge that an individual lacks the capacity to make decisions. In such a case, we are responsible for protecting the person from the possible harm of an incapable decision.

The interplay between these concepts becomes apparent when the person is no longer felt to be "of sound mind." This chapter will focus on those individuals who have cognitive impairment or a clouded sensorium (fixed lesions, dementia, or delirium) and will not discuss the competence of individuals whose decisional capacity may be impaired by psychiatric illness. When patients are cognitively impaired, clinicians have an obligation to respect their rights, to protect their persons, and to consider the safety of the public. This often requires careful balancing of conflicting imperatives.

DEFINITION OF DECISIONAL CAPACITY

In the broadest sense of the word, for an individual to be competent, that individual must be well qualified to do whatever task they are doing. In the context in which we are talking, competence is viewed as a legal term. It refers to a judge's ruling as to whether an individual has been deemed capable of making their own decisions. An individual adjudicated to be incompetent must have a guardian appointed to make the decisions for the area (or areas) in which the person has been found to be incompetent. Although guidelines vary somewhat from state to state, it is generally accepted that a ruling of incompetence cannot be made solely on the basis of a medical diagnosis, age, level of education, or personal eccentricity. An adjudication of competence or incompetence is based on an assessment of the individual's decisional capacity and that individual's demonstrated ability or inability to carry out a plan. Therefore, the assessment of decisional capacity should include not just the patient's cognitive ability, but other factors that may be influencing their ability to decide. This would include emotional state, functional ability,

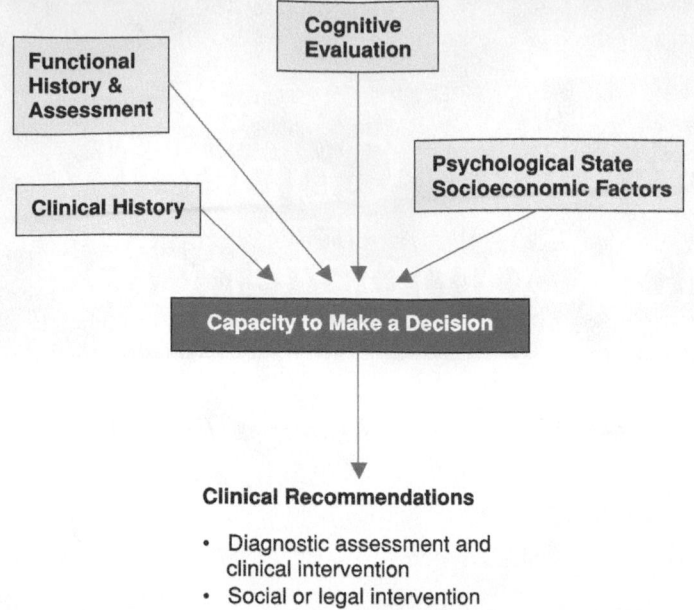

FIGURE 13-1. Components included in assessment of decisional capacity.

psychosocial situation (especially with regard to coercion), and financial and environmental limitations (Figure 13-1).

There are four necessary elements to making a capable decision; understanding, appreciation, reasoning, and expressing a choice (Table 13-1). First, the individual must be able to comprehend the information being considered sufficiently well to understand the important or relevant facts. That information must have been presented in a clear and concise manner with special attention taken to ensure that barriers such as hearing impairment, illiteracy, or language difference do not constitute the sole reasons that the person is unable to understand the information. Other issues, such as aphasia, delirium, or depression, may also interfere with the individual's ability to comprehend and retain information.

TABLE 13-1

Four Elements that Constitute Decision-Making Abilities

ABILITY	DESCRIPTION
Understanding	1. Comprehension of appropriately communicated information 2. Retention of information long enough to be able to recall it in discussion 3. Perception of the relationship between interventions and outcomes
Appreciation	1. Recognition of how the information relates to his or her own circumstances 2. Insight into the advantages and disadvantages of a proposed solution.
Reasoning	1. Manipulation of information to generate comparisons between different alternatives and their consequences 2. Justification of a rationale as a context for making these comparisons
Expressing a choice	Articulation of a clear choice with regard to a specific decision

Second, the individual must have the conceptual ability to appreciate the consequences of the decision that he or she is making. This includes both an appreciation of the risks and benefits of options and the ability to identify the consequences these risks and benefits will have on his or her life.

The individual must be able to reason, within their own frame of reference, why she or he is choosing a course of action. This is different than saying that a decision seems "reasonable" to the other parties involved, but rather it refers to the cognitive processing of values and beliefs in view of the information given. Judging the rationality of a decision can be tricky. Even if we feel—and even if most of society would feel—that an individual's decision is irrational, it does not give us grounds to negate the person's right to self-determination. Our society has a great respect for individuality and one's right to express that individuality in a wide variety of ways. Nonetheless, an individual's ability to give a plausible rationale for his or her decision is sometimes used as secondary evidence of decisional capacity. That is, demonstrating justification for one's choices (e.g. religious belief, personal value, etc.) provides another level of assurance that the patient's decision rests upon intact reasoning, rather than a set of delusional or incoherent beliefs that may often exist in the setting of cognitive impairment or psychiatric illness.

Finally, the person must be able to make a choice and communicate the decision. This is the lowest bar for decision-making capacity but one which may be impaired by specific damage in language or frontal lobe function as well as in severe global cognitive impairment.

One other consideration is sometimes used in judging an individual's decisional capacity: consistency of the person's decision. The inconsistency of an individual's decision with past decisions made by that person provides an important clue to possible underlying cognitive or psychiatric problems that deserve exploration. But, in itself, inconsistency does not negate the person's right to make decisions. Inconsistency of a specific decision over time may indicate that the individual has had difficulty with remembering or understanding the information provided and their cognitive abilities should also be explored.

LEGAL AND PRACTICAL ASPECTS IN DETERMINING DECISIONAL CAPACITY

In protecting an individual who is incapable of making decisions, one action that may need to be taken is applying to the local probate court asking that the individual be adjudicated to be incompetent and to have someone else appointed to make decisions. Although specifics of probate statutes vary among states, most follow a general pattern articulated in the Uniform Probate Code. Once an individual has been adjudicated incompetent, another person is appointed to represent his or her interests. This person is variably referred to as a guardian, conservator, or legal surrogate. We will use the term conservator. Although there are movements toward "limited conservatorship" that restrict the powers of the conservator to decision making in specific areas where a person has been shown to be incapable, there are two broad categories of conservatorship that are commonly used, those of finance and of person. Conservatorship of finance is a fairly self-evident term. Conservatorship of person grants a more global responsibility for assuring that the individual is kept safe and that decisions are made either as substituted judgment or on the basis of the individual's best interests (see Chapter 34). These decisions may involve, for example, medical care, where a person will live, what help the person will receive to maintain himself or herself. The person may retain the ability to make a will (testamentary competence), even when he or she has been adjudicated as incompetent of person and finance.

It should be emphasized that not all incapacitated individuals need to be conserved. There are no statistics available to say how many incapacitated individuals have informal care management by relatives and never require probate action. Personal experience would lead us to believe that most adults with cognitive deficits fall into this category. Probate adjudication of a conservator may not be needed if financial management has been allocated to a family member by a power of attorney prior to the individual becoming incapacitated, and if there is a general agreement among concerned and interested parties that decisions should be made either by a specific individual or group consensus. If the individual involved has granted someone a durable power of attorney for health affairs (see Chapter 34), there may not be a need for court action. Turning to a court will prove unnecessary even when interested parties disagree, provided they are willing to respect the individual's appointment of a surrogate decision maker.

Even when the court has been asked to take action, 75% to 85% of the time the court appoints a family member as conservator. The ability of an appointed conservator to act as an appropriate surrogate varies considerably. One advantage of having a court-appointed conservator is that the probate court has some oversight responsibilities for the management of the individual's affairs. Oversight by a judge may prove beneficial to individuals who might otherwise not be scrupulous about managing an incapacitated individual's funds. A judge who does not wish to choose a family member as conservator may appoint an individual from the community, an attorney, a social worker, or an agency to fill that role.

Although courts tend to see the ability to make decisions as an all-or-nothing phenomenon, a person's ability to make decisions falls on a continuum ranging from complete capability to incapacity. Furthermore, not only ability, but also circumstance, influences the need for intervention. For instance, a person's ability to capably manage financial affairs will be influenced by the size and complexity of the finances requiring management. If the need for complex medical decision making does not arise, then the ability of an individual to make those types of decisions is not questioned. If the individual is in a situation where others are managing household affairs and looking out for the person's needs, then the person's ability to care for self may not be examined. It is only when a problem arises that the individual's ability to make these types of decisions becomes an issue. Also, as mentioned above, even if the patient is incapable and others need to make decisions, this can often be handled without court participation.

Preventive legal measures, enacted in the course of patient care prior to episodes of incapacity, may negate the need to involve the court system. For example, a "springing" durable power of attorney may be drafted to designate a chosen person to have legal authority over financial matters at some time or event in the future when the patient is deemed unable to perform those actions. Other legal planning methods, such as designation of a conservator in advance of need or in vivo trusts, may also be useful mechanisms for securing appropriate surrogate decision makers for persons who may anticipate future incapacity.

PROCESS OF DETERMINING CAPACITY

The individual's inability to make decisions is determined in two different ways. Specific testing can measure cognitive dysfunction, and observing the person's decision-making process can demonstrate his or her inability to complete the decision-making task capably. In order to understand and apply both of these methods, one needs to understand the cognitive processes involved in decisional capacity. These processes can be understood both as discrete neuropsychiatric functions and as contributors to the holistic process of making decisions.

The brain functions that contribute to decision making are centered in the cortex and frontal lobes. Cortical (parietal and temporal lobe) functions involved in decision making include immediate memory and language. Immediate memory is defined as the ability to remember rehearsed or consolidated materials for 30 seconds to 30 minutes (e.g., first repeating three objects then recalling them in 5 min). Immediate memory is clearly important in the individual's ability to participate in a discussion around a specific decision. Cortical language abilities are those that affect comprehension and the ability to produce the intended words when expressing one's thoughts in both spoken and written communication. The ability to understand language is highly correlated with an individual's ability to comprehend the information needed to make a decision. Problems with expressive language ability from cortical lesions can lead to statements by the individual that misrepresent his or her thoughts (i.e., through misuse of words, word substitutions, or paraphrasic errors). The ability to understand and manipulate numbers may also be affected.

Frontal lobe functions involved in the process of making capable decisions include the abilities to concentrate, express oneself, use abstract reasoning, initiate actions, solve problems, monitor one's behavior, and use judgment. The frontal lobe is responsible for filtering out both internal and external stimuli that interfere with the individual's ability to concentrate and to understand instructions or explanations. Frontal lobe dysfunction can lead to inattention that interferes with the ability to complete necessary tasks appropriately. The intrusion of internal stimuli can lead to inappropriate and impulsive behaviors that can interfere with the individual's functioning and decision making.

Traditional Mental Status Tools

Tools commonly used for the assessment of cognition in patients, such as the Mini-Mental State Examination (MMSE) or the Executive Interview (EXIT), test specific cognitive functions (memory, language, praxis, concentration, etc.) or the integration of these functions into simple processes (three-step command, story telling). Looking at performance on individual items and extrapolating to predict how performance will affect the processes necessary for decision making may help the clinician to evaluate a patient. No single cut-off score on any of these tests will divide those capable of making a decision from those not capable. This is particularly true because different types of decisions require different skills. These tests also do not look at the patient's actual function. On the other hand, a score may signal a level of such diminished cognitive abilities that it is highly unlikely that persons with that score will be capable of making decisions. Looking at individual items on these tests and having knowledge of how the cognitive function tested may influence the individual's ability to make decisions is important. These tests may also serve as important triggers to further investigation of the individual's decisional capacity.

The MMSE is representative of tests for cortical function that have been shown to have some correlation with an individual's ability to make decisions. The MMSE tests skills, such as immediate memory, word finding, understanding simple verbal and written material, integrating that understanding into a simple action, and expressing basic ideas verbally or in writing, which may affect a person's ability to make decisions. MMSE scores of less than 10 have been shown to be diagnostic of a person so impaired that he or she is unable to make decisions.

Testing of frontal lobe or executive functioning is of great importance in assessing decisional capacity. The EXIT examination and clock drawing are the two measures most commonly used by clinicians. The EXIT 25 has been shown to have the best correlation with subjective measures of competency of any neuropsychological test. An overall score of 15 on the EXIT (higher being less capable) indicates very significant impairment. Again, recognizing errors on individual items and the correlative cognitive dysfunctions will be important in assessing less grossly impaired cases. Functions that may be most reflective of problems with decisional capacity include poor insight, impulsivity, poor self-monitoring, and impaired ability to plan and follow-through on the plan. Although individual items of these tests do not correlate directly with each of these functions, observing the individual as he or she does the test with these functions in mind can clarify areas of deficiency. For example, when the individual makes an obvious error, does he or she realize it and go back and correct the mistake? Is the person able to plan how to draw the face of a clock? If the person draws a clock face that is too small, does he or she notice this and correct it? Does the concrete stimulus of the numbers interfere with the abstraction of how the hands indicate time? Similar observations can be made while watching an individual take the EXIT examination. Does the person plan out how to approach a problem such as telling a story? Can the person correct errors in sequencing? Does the person let internal overlearned stimuli interfere with his or her ability to hear and repeat?

Test results can be deceptive: Individuals may have significant frontal lobe dysfunction, enough to impair their capacity for making decisions, and still score very well on the MMSE. There are more complex neuropsychological tests that can be done to test the same areas of function in more detail. These are not practical in the clinical setting, and the clinician should refer the patient to a neuropsychologist if there is any question of the nature or severity of neuropsychological deficits.

Tests of Decisional Capacity

There are tests that are specifically designed to assess an individual's capacity for making medical decisions. These tests may utilize hypothetical vignettes to demonstrate whether the individual is capable of the four elements of decision making, namely, understanding the vignette (usually written at a sixth-grade level), appreciation of the issues and the potential options involved in solving this issue, being able to reason with the material, and then being capable of verbalizing an opinion. An example of such a test is the Capacity to Consent to Treatment Instrument in which the individual must read a series of case vignettes and then consider two different treatment options.

The Hopkins Competency Assessment Test consists of a short essay that describes informed consent and durable power of attorney and a series of questions to assess the individual's comprehension of the material. The MacArthur Competence Assessment Tool-Treatment (MacCAT-T) is an example of a structured interview that allows the clinician to test the individual's ability to make a specific medical decision. The first two tests deal with theory or theoretical situations and have the advantage of being able to be used prior to the need for a decision. The MacCAT-T, however, focuses on an individual's ability to make a specific, real-time decision at the time of the testing.

CAPACITY TO MAKE SPECIFIC DECISIONS

It is not always possible to make a definitive and enduring diagnosis of decisional incapacity. This is because decisional incapacity is task-specific and may be time-limited. Although one may be adjudicated to be either incompetent or competent in the two broad legal categories of person and finance, the ability of an individual to make decisions or at least to participate in decisions needs to be thought of in much more flexible terms. We will discuss incapacity in matters of person (medical decisions and ability for self-care), finance, wills, advance directives, and research.

Medical Decisions

Because patients have the right to refuse medical interventions and they have the right to be informed before consenting to medical treatments, their ability to make these decisions has been widely discussed. The need to make a medical decision frequently prompts the first assessment of decisional capacity, often at a time when clinicians face pressure to make speedy judgments. For the patient facing these types of decisions, the neuropsychological functions of memory, language, and reasoning are the most crucial.

Although tests can help to measure the patient's ability to make medical decisions, observing the patient's ability to handle the information given is more valuable, and more important, than administering any test. Among tests, the EXIT examination has been shown to have the highest correlation (specificity and sensitivity) for testing medical decisional capacity when compared to expert assessment. Sometimes a formal structure or score is necessary, in which case the MacCAT-T provides a good framework from which to work. Here the interviewer is asked to stop and rate the individual's abilities in six steps of the process: (1) appreciation of the disorder, (2) understanding of the treatment and risks or discomforts, (3) appreciation of the treatment, (4) understanding of alternate treatments, (5) reasoning, and (6) expressing a choice.

Documentation of a formal score for any test is not necessary in most cases when a patient faces medical decisions. A thoughtful interview with the patient and a written description of the areas in which the patient is unable to function is usually sufficient for this purpose, although learning structured observation will enhance the clinician's ability to assess capacity.

Problems of Self-Care

Formal assessments of decision-making ability may be necessary when a patient demonstrates an inability to care for self or to accept the help needed to remain safe in his or her present environment.

Issues of cognitive impairment versus denial are difficult to sort through without formal testing. A person's tendency to be "eccentric" is not always easily distinguishable from dangerous behaviors stemming from increasing cognitive impairment and an inability to make decisions around self-care. Gross impairment of cortical functioning, especially short-term memory, can pose problems for day-to-day function. What is more evident is the impact of frontal lobe dysfunction. The inability to plan, initiate action, monitor one's behavior, and self-correct are essential to being able to care for oneself. A combination of findings on frontal lobe testing and demonstrated inability to care for oneself is often sufficient evidence for action, especially in combination with an inability to accept a level of care which would keep them safe. Alternatively, persons who demonstrate an inability to administer their own medications or safely prepare their own meals but who have accepted care, which will obviate these problems (e.g. home care, Meals-on-Wheels), may be regarded as having intact decision making with respect to solving these functional deficits.

There are as yet no clinical tools specifically designed to assist clinicians in assessing a person's ability to make a decisions related to self-care in the face of functional problems. A reasonable approach in this scenario, however, would involve a structured assessment where the patient must demonstrate an ability to: understand and appreciate a known functional problem; understand and appreciate the potential options to solving this problem, as well as the risks and benefits of those options; describe the consequences associated with these options; choose an option; and, then explain how this choice is superior to the other options not chosen. Similar to the MacCAT-T, this approach assesses decision-making ability with respect to the clinically relevant problem and measures decisional skills based on the legal standard.

Problems of Finances

There are times when an individual remains able to make medical decisions and decisions related to self-care but is no longer capable of managing the finances. When bills are going unpaid or gross mistakes are made in handling money, then someone else will need to take over financial management. Specific tests for measuring the ability to calculate, to understand a checkbook, to monitor bank accounts, or a more specific financial management assessment, such as the Financial Capacity Inventory, can be administered by an occupational therapist or a neuropsychologist, but usually a demonstrated problem with this area is sufficient to warrant supervision. If the individual has enough insight to understand the problem and a reliable person is available to help, granting that person a power of attorney for finances should suffice. If the incapacitated person is reluctant to relinquish control, or court monitoring is deemed advisable, then the family, the clinician, or other concerned party should seek a conservator of finance.

OTHER ISSUES OF DECISIONAL CAPACTIY AND CONSENT

Legal Documents

The ability to make a Last Will and Testament is felt to be retained even after the ability to handle finances and make decisions of person

have been lost. An individual's ability to remember what he or she is doing with the estate and to express some logic behind choices is usually sufficient evidence of capability. Despite the risk of exploitation of an impaired person, the courts are usually very liberal in allowing someone to change a will, even when the person has cognitive problems.

In contrast, the ability to grant someone Durable Power of Attorney for Health Affairs or to make a Living Will requires higher levels of cognitive function than does day-to-day decision making. Both of these areas deal with hypothetical situations that can often be hard even for cognitively intact individuals to fully understand and conceptualize. Scales such as the Hopkins Competency Assessment Test or the Capacity to Consent to Treatment Instrument may help to establish this ability, but these may not be practical for use in most clinical settings. At the very least, clinicians should question an individual's ability to fully understand the process if he or she has demonstrated problems with memory or language or has shown signs of frontal lobe dysfunction. The clinician must also recognize that even very cognitively impaired individuals may still be able to portray wishes and desires (see "Consent vs. Assent")

Temporary Loss of Decisional Capacity

Individuals may be transiently incapacitated for decision making or their ability to recover their cognition may not be known, such as when a patient is delirious or has suffered a recent stroke. In these situations, the clinician should seek an interim solution. An informal surrogate, the person granted durable power of attorney for health affairs, or a temporary conservator can make decisions while the clinician clarifies the prognosis for decisional capacity. The decisions needed during a time of uncertainty should fall on the side of aggressive protection of the individual's life or continued function until the person can make his or her wishes known or the permanence and extent of the impairment becomes clear.

Consent Versus Assent

Even when an individual is no longer able to give informed consent to a procedure or a change in living situation, he or she may still participate in the decision making process. Substituted judgment is the process that a surrogate (legal or otherwise) is supposed to apply as the basis on which a decision should be made. Substituted judgment enjoins one to take into account the patient's prior wishes and long-held beliefs as the basis for one's decision, "deciding as they would have decided" (see Chapter 34). Assent refers to the impaired individual's willingness to cooperate with a plan of care. It is, in essence, a way to take into consideration the individual's present desires when making a decision. Although it has been used primarily in the ethics and legal literature when looking at the role of adolescents in the process of medical decision making, the principles apply to impaired adults as well. In cognitively impaired adults, there is a continuum of incapacity, even amongst those who do not retain the full capacity to make decisions. An individual who is incapable of understanding the complexities of a situation or decision may retain high levels of understanding around specific aspects of the process and be able to express their opinions. Even very cognitively impaired patients can give indications of what brings them pleasure and what gives them pain. Clinicians and surrogates should consider this information in the decision-making process.

Clinicians trying to obtain consent for medical treatment or research protocols may wish to use a combination of surrogate consent and patient assent (shared decision making). This may be essential in some cases where the patient's ability to cooperate will be necessary in order to carry out the treatment or procedure. Even the courts are moving toward the recognition of the need for "limited conservatorship," which reflects that decisional capacity is not an all-or-nothing phenomenon. Decisional capacity is situation-dependent and can change with time.

Informed Consent in Research

An individual's ability to consent to participate in research is also difficult to judge. The understanding of the risks and benefits of being in a research study must be even greater than that for accepting or declining an established medical treatment. The risks and benefits are more theoretically based and therefore harder to make concrete to an individual who may be having difficulty with abstract thinking. This is an important time for dual decision making as outlined in the section above.

FURTHER READING

Grisso T, Appelbaum PS. *Assessing Competence to Consent to Treatment: A Guide for Physicians and Other Health Professionals.* New York, New York: Oxford University Press; 1998;6:124–125.

Grisso T, Appelbaum PS, Hill-Fotouhi C. The MacCAT-T: a clinical tool to assess patients' capacities to make treatment decisions. *Psychiatric Services* 1997;48:1415–1419.

Grisso T. *Evaluating Competencies: Forensic Assessments and Instruments.* New York, New York: Kluwer Academic/Plenum Publishers; 2003.

Holzer JC, Gansler DA, Moczynski NP, et al. Cognitive functions in the informed consent evaluation process: a pilot study. *J Am Acad Psychiatry Law.* 1997;25:531–540.

Janofsky JS, McCarthy RJ, Folstein MF. The Hopkins Competency Assessment Test: a brief method for evaluating patients' capacity to give informed consent. *Hospital and Community Psychiatry* 1992;43:132–136.

Kim SY, Karlawish JH, Caine ED, et al. Current state of research on decision-making competence of cognitively impaired elderly persons. *Am J Geriatr Psychiatry.* 2002;10:151–165.

Marson DC. Loss of competency in Alzheimer's disease: conceptual and psychometric approaches. *Int J Law Psychiatry.* 2001;24:267–283.

Royall DR, Mahurin RK, Gray KF. Bedside assessment of executive cognitive impairment: the executive interview. *J Am Geriatr Soc.* 1992;40:1221–1226.

Schindler BA, Ramchandani D, Matthews MK, et al. Competency and the frontal lobe: the impact of executive dysfunction on decisional capacity. *Psychosomatics.* 1995;36:400–4004.

Wendler D, Prasad K. Core safeguards for clinical research with adults who are unable to consent. *Ann Int Med.* 2001;135:514–523.

Principles of Screening in Older Adults

Louise C. Walter

This chapter focuses on the topic of screening, particularly the issues that need to be considered when making a decision to screen an older person for cancer. This decision highlights many of the special philosophical and practical challenges inherent in recommending preventive services to older persons. One obvious challenge to recommending cancer screening (and many other preventive services) to older adults is that few studies of preventive interventions have enrolled persons older than age 75 years. The absence of age-specific data requires clinicians to extrapolate data about the effectiveness of screening in younger persons and apply it to older persons. Furthermore, even if trials suggest that the effectiveness of screening is similar in younger and older populations, challenges remain about how to apply data from trials to an individual older person. Trials show the average effectiveness of an intervention, but they generally do not address individual patient characteristics, such as comorbid conditions or functional status, which may change the likelihood of receiving benefit or harm from screening. Given these challenges, the need to individualize screening decisions is especially important for older people, because individuals become increasingly unique in their particular combination of health, function, remaining life expectancy, and values with advancing age.

The important issues that need to be considered when making individualized screening decisions in elderly persons are not fully addressed by current guidelines. Although many screening guidelines that used to recommend upper age limits for stopping screening are now recommending screening an older person if the individual has a "reasonable life expectancy," current guidelines offer little guidance about how to estimate life expectancy or how patient preferences should factor into screening decisions. This chapter outlines a systematic framework for individualizing cancer screening decisions in older adults that includes consideration of an individual's life expectancy and the individual's preferences regarding the potential benefits and harms of screening (Figure 14-1).

Like many medical decisions, informed screening decisions are best made by using quantitative estimates of life expectancy and screening outcomes to anchor decisions, tempered by qualitative consideration of how an older person values the potential benefits and harms of screening. While potential benefits of screening include increased survival, this should be balanced against the potential harms of screening, which encompass adverse effects on survival, comfort, function, and psychological well-being emanating from all procedures that result from screening. For older patients who are bothered by the discomfort and risks of screening tests, the decrease in quality of life in the present may outweigh the small chance of future benefit.

GENERAL FRAMEWORK FOR MAKING INFORMED CANCER SCREENING DECISIONS

Estimate Life Expectancy

The first step in individualizing cancer screening recommendations is to estimate an older person's life expectancy, because life expectancy affects the likelihood of receiving benefit versus harm from screening. For example, finding an asymptomatic cancer in a person who will die of something else before the cancer would become symptomatic does not benefit the person and may cause considerable harm. The risk of such a scenario depends upon the life expectancy of the individual and the age-specific mortality rate of the particular cancer. With advancing age, the mortality rates of most cancers increase, yet overall life expectancy decreases. The need to weigh these two opposing factors when estimating the likelihood that a person will die of a screen-detectable cancer makes cancer screening decisions in older people complex.

In estimating life expectancy, it is useful to have a general idea of the distribution of life expectancies at various ages. For example, when estimating the life expectancy of an 80-year-old woman, it is useful to know that approximately 25% of 80-year-old women

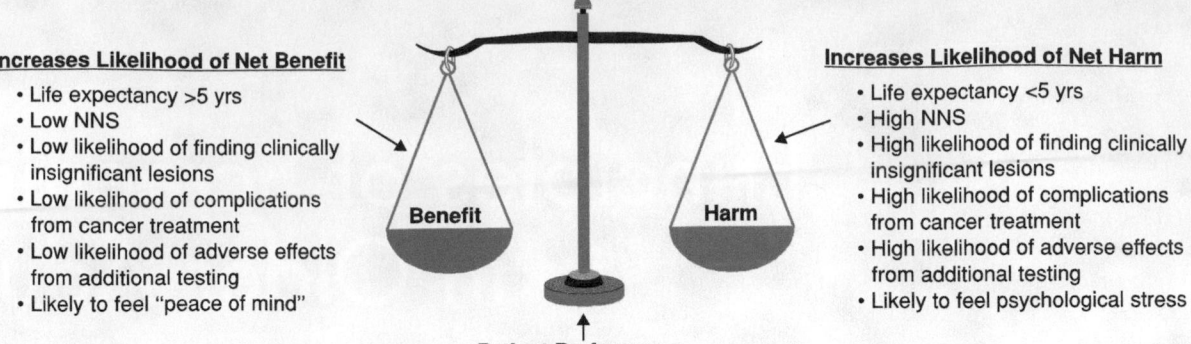

Increases Likelihood of Net Benefit

- Life expectancy >5 yrs
- Low NNS
- Low likelihood of finding clinically insignificant lesions
- Low likelihood of complications from cancer treatment
- Low likelihood of adverse effects from additional testing
- Likely to feel "peace of mind"

Benefit

Increases Likelihood of Net Harm

- Life expectancy <5 yrs
- High NNS
- High likelihood of finding clinically insignificant lesions
- High likelihood of complications from cancer treatment
- High likelihood of adverse effects from additional testing
- Likely to feel psychological stress

Harm

Patient Preferences

FIGURE 14-1. The benefits and harms that need to be weighed when making informed cancer screening decisions. Patient preferences act like a moveable fulcrum of a scale to shift the magnitude of the benefits or harms needed to tip the decision toward recommending the screening test (net benefit likely) or recommending against the screening test (net harm likely). NNS, number needed to screen to prevent one cancer-specific death.

will live more than 13 years, 50% will live at least 9 years, and 25% will live less than 5 years. Figure 14-2 presents the upper, middle, and lower quartiles of life expectancy for the U.S. population according to age and sex, and illustrates the substantial variability in life expectancy that exists at each age. Although it is impossible for clinicians to predict the exact life expectancy of an individual person, it is possible to make reasonable estimates of whether a person is likely to live substantially longer or shorter than an average person in his

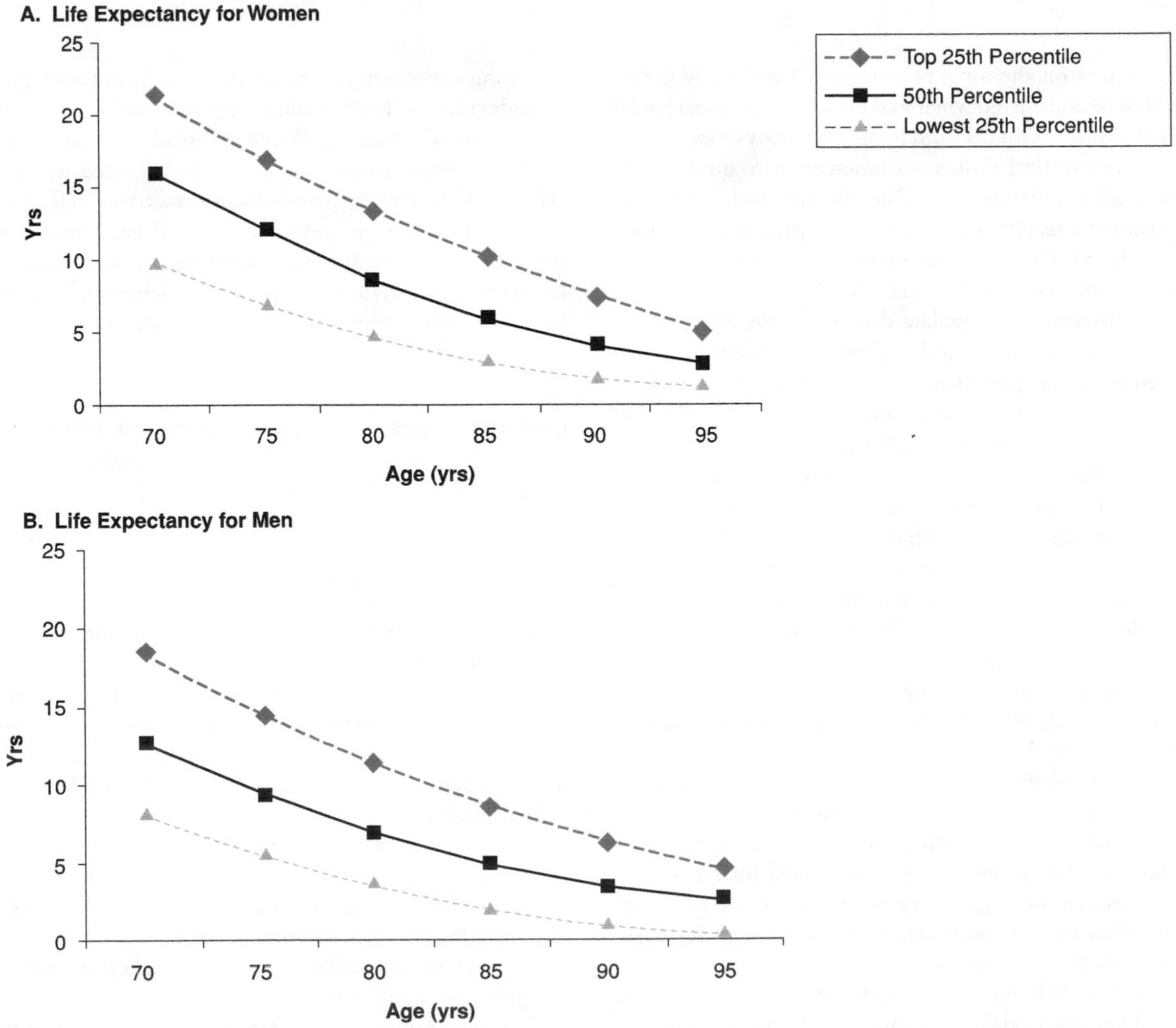

A. Life Expectancy for Women

(graph: Yrs vs Age (yrs), with legend)
- Top 25th Percentile
- 50th Percentile
- Lowest 25th Percentile

B. Life Expectancy for Men

(graph: Yrs vs Age (yrs))

FIGURE 14-2. Upper, middle, and lower quartiles of life expectancy for women and men at selected ages. Data from the Life Tables of the United States, 2001. *Adapted from Walter LC, Lewis CL, Barton MB. Screening for colorectal, breast, and cervical cancer in the elderly: a review of the evidence. Am J Med. 2005;118:1078.*

or her age cohort. Such estimates, while not perfect, would allow for better estimations of potential benefits and harms of screening than focusing on age alone.

There are many factors clinicians can use to estimate whether an older person is typical of someone at the middle of their age-sex cohort or is more like someone in the upper or lower quartiles. For example, the number and severity of comorbid conditions and functional impairments are much stronger predictors of mortality in older people than chronological age. Congestive heart failure, end-stage renal disease, oxygen-dependent chronic obstructive lung disease, severe dementia, or functional dependencies in several activities of daily living are examples of factors that would cause an elderly person to have a life expectancy substantially below the average for his or her age. The absence of significant comorbid conditions or presence of excellent functional status identifies older individuals who are likely to live longer than average.

Estimate Benefits of Cancer Screening

The next step is to consider the potential benefits of screening. The main benefit of cancer screening is the reduction in cancer mortality experienced by a few people whose early-stage disease is detected and treated, which otherwise would have been lethal during their remaining lifetime. While the impact of cancer screening on quality of life or functional decline has not been studied, there is good evidence that mammography, fecal occult blood testing (FOBT), and Papanicolaou (Pap) smears are effective in reducing cancer-specific mortality. However, the strength of the evidence that these tests are effective in older adults is limited by the small number of older patients included in screening trials. In addition, even screening tests likely to be effective in older populations may not provide survival benefit to individuals with short life expectancies, because the benefit from screening is not immediate. For example, in the randomized controlled trials of FOBT and mammography, the cancer-specific mortality curves between the screened and unscreened groups do not separate significantly until at least 5 years after the start of screening. This period is likely even longer for persons older than 70 years of age because some evidence suggests that the length of time that a screen-detectable cancer remains clinically asymptomatic increases with advancing age for both breast and colorectal cancer. This suggests that older persons who have life expectancies of less than 5 years will not derive survival benefit from cancer screening.

For patients with estimated life expectancies greater than 5 years, it is important to have a general idea of the potential benefit of screening tests in absolute terms. The absolute benefit of a screening test can be conveyed by the absolute risk reduction (the absolute difference in proportions of persons with a given outcome from two treatments or actions), or more effectively by calculating the number needed to screen (NNS), which is the reciprocal of the absolute risk reduction. Considering older persons at average risk for developing cancer, the approximate NNS to prevent one cancer-specific death is listed in Table 14-1 for screening tests that have been shown to be effective in reducing cancer-specific mortality. All the numbers in Table 14-1 assume a 5-year delay between the onset of screening and survival benefit. The numbers are presented according to age and life expectancy because life expectancy defines the potential number of years available for screening. For example, 240 very healthy 80-year-old women would have to be screened with mammography during their remaining lifetime to prevent one death from breast cancer. Table 14-1 emphasizes the importance of considering life expectancy when making cancer screening decisions, as illustrated by the example that an 85-year-old woman in the upper quartile of life expectancy is more likely to benefit from screening than a 75-year-old woman in the lowest quartile. The precision of the estimates of life expectancy, and, in turn, number needed to benefit, is greatly enhanced by considering comorbidity rather than chronological age alone.

Estimate Harms of Cancer Screening

The third step is to consider the potential harms of screening, as all screening tests pose direct and indirect harms. Harms that would be accepted to treat a symptomatic person with known disease are less acceptable when they are caused by screening tests, which benefit only a few individuals but expose all screened individuals to the harms. In addition, harms occur immediately, whereas it takes several years for a survival benefit to occur after cancer screening. Therefore, as the likelihood of benefit declines with decreasing life expectancy, the balance between harms and benefits from screening will shift in the direction of net harm.

Individuals who are found not to have cancer after work-up of an abnormal screening result (false-positive result) clearly have experienced harm from screening, as they were subjected to physical and psychological distress from additional testing and procedures that would not have been necessary had they not been screened. However, what is often forgotten is that in older persons some of the greatest harms from screening occur by finding and treating cancers that would never have become clinically significant. The risk of identifying an inconsequential cancer increases with decreasing life expectancy as well as with the increasing likelihood that screening will detect certain neoplasms that are unlikely to progress to symptoms in older persons, such as ductal carcinoma in situ (DCIS). Fewer than 25% of DCIS lesions progress to invasive cancer within 5 to 10 years, yet because of the inability to distinguish which lesions will progress, many older women with DCIS will undergo surgery. Women who have surgery for DCIS that would never have become symptomatic in their lifetime have suffered serious harm from screening.

In addition to physical harms, the psychological distress caused by cancer screening should be considered. Potential psychological harms range from the emotional pain of a diagnosis of cancer in persons whose lives were not extended by screening, through the alarm of false-positive results to the stress of undergoing the screening test itself. Many older persons may have cognitive, physical, or sensory problems that make screening tests and further work-up particularly difficult, painful, or frightening. Considering factors that increase the likelihood of harm is vital to making appropriate screening decisions.

Integrate Patient Values and Preferences

The final step is to assess how individuals value the potential harms and benefits of screening and to integrate their preferences into screening decisions. Because many cancer-screening decisions in older persons will not be answered solely by quantitative assessments of benefits and harms, talking to older persons about their values

TABLE 14-1

Number Needed to Screen Over Remaining Lifetime to Prevent One Cancer-Specific Death for Women and Men at Selected Ages and Life Expectancy Quartiles

	LIFE EXPECTANCY QUARTILE*														
	Age 70			Age 75			Age 80			Age 85			Age 90		
	Upper Quartile	Middle Quartile	Lower Quartile	Upper Quartile	Middle Quartile	Lower Quartile	Upper Quartile	Middle Quartile	Lower Quartile	Upper Quartile	Middle Quartile	Lower Quartile	Upper Quartile	Middle Quartile	Lower Quartile
Women															
Screening Test															
Mammography	142	242	642	176	330	1361	240	533	—	417	2131	—	1066	—	—
Pap smear	934	1521	4070	1177	2113	8342	1694	3764	—	2946	15056	—	7528	—	—
Fecal occult blood	178	340	1046	204	408	1805	262	581	—	455	2326	—	1163	—	—
Men															
Screening Test															
Fecal occult blood	177	380	1877	207	525	—	277	945	—	554	—	—	2008	—	—

*Life expectancy quartiles correspond to upper, middle, and lower quartiles as presented in Fig.14-2. Persons with life expectancies less than 5 yrs are unlikely to derive any survival benefit from cancer screening, which is denoted by "—."

Adapted from Walter LC, Covinsky KE. Cancer screening in elderly patients: A framework for individualized decision making. JAMA. 2001;285:2750.

and preferences is especially important. The value placed on different health outcomes will vary among older people, as will preferences for screening. For example, some women undergoing screening mammography value "peace of mind" after a negative screening result, whereas women with dementia likely receive no such comfort. In considering the benefits versus harm of screening, clinicians must elicit how individual persons value the trade-offs among longer survival, comfort, and functional status.

Clinicians should consider a person's usual approach to medical decision making to decide how to approach the discussion of screening. In some cases, clinicians will need to learn a person's values, apply them to the known benefits and harms of screening, and make a formal recommendation. For other people, the clinician will want to discuss the benefits and harms with the person and allow the person to apply his or her values to the outcomes and come to a decision together. For people with dementia, discussion about preferences should be held with an involved caregiver. However, it should be remembered that despite being unable to articulate consent, many persons with dementia can still effectively communicate refusal. Assent from a person with dementia is essential if invasive or potentially harmful testing or treatments are being considered (see Chapters 13 and 34). If a person with dementia is likely to be frightened or agitated by a screening test, the caregiver and clinician should forgo the test. Also, there should be a general discussion prior to screening about the possible procedures and treatments that may be required after an abnormal screening result. Persons who would not want further work-up or treatment of an abnormal result should not be screened.

APPLICATION OF SCREENING PRINCIPLES TO SPECIFIC CANCERS

Breast Cancer

Risk of Dying of Breast Cancer

For very healthy 75-year-old women who have life expectancies in the top twenty-fifth percentile, the lifetime risk of dying of breast cancer is approximately 2.8%. The risk of dying of breast cancer declines with decreasing life expectancy, such that unhealthy women older than age 75 years who have estimated life expectancies in the lowest twenty-fifth percentile for their age cohort have less than a 1% chance of dying of breast cancer.

Benefits of Breast Cancer Screening

Methods for screening for breast cancer are mammography and breast examination. Mammography has the strongest evidence for screening efficacy based on pooled evidence from randomized controlled trials showing an overall relative risk reduction in breast cancer-related mortality of 27% for women between the ages of 50 and 69 years. There is little information regarding the absolute benefits of screening mammography in women older than age 70 years, so data from trials in younger people must be extrapolated to older people (see Table 14-1). There are no data from randomized trials to indicate that clinical breast examination or breast self-examination,

without accompanying mammography, reduce mortality from breast cancer in any age group.

Harms of Breast Cancer Screening

On average, 1 in 15 elderly women sent for a screening mammogram will have a false-positive result and 1 in 1000 women will have DCIS detected, which would otherwise not have been found without screening. Most DCIS lesions are unlikely to have an effect on the life expectancy of older women, yet many will undergo surgery once DCIS has been found by screening. Frail older women are at increased risk for experiencing harms from screening. One study of frail community-living women found that 17% experienced burden from screening mammography as a result of work-up refusals, false-positive results, or identification of clinically insignificant lesions. Women with multiple comorbid conditions are also likely to experience adverse effects from surgery, radiation, and chemotherapy.

Recommendations

Most guidelines recommend mammography alone or supplemented by clinical breast examination (Table 14-2). There is no evidence of a specific age cut-off at which potential benefits of screening suddenly cease or potential harms suddenly become substantial for everyone, so most guidelines recommend continuing screening women over age 70 years, despite the lack of this age group in screening trials. Decisions to stop screening should be based on whether a woman has advanced age and comorbid conditions that limit her life expectancy. The author recommends against screening for breast cancer if a woman has an estimated life expectancy of less than 5 years. For women who have a life expectancy between 5 and 10 years, the decision to screen is a close call, and patient preferences should play a major role in the decision to screen. For healthy older women who have a life expectancy greater than 10 years, biennial screening mammography, regardless of age, is a reasonable recommendation based on the data available.

Colorectal Cancer

Risk of Dying of Colorectal Cancer

For very healthy 75-year-olds who have life expectancies in the top twenty-fifth percentile, the lifetime risk of dying of colorectal cancer is approximately 3.5% for men and 3.3% for women. The risk of dying of colorectal cancer declines with decreasing life expectancy, such that men and women older than age 70 years with life expectancies in the lowest twenty-fifth percentile for their age cohort have less than a 1% chance of dying of colorectal cancer.

Benefits of Colorectal Cancer Screening

Methods for screening for colorectal cancer include FOBT, flexible sigmoidoscopy, colonoscopy, and barium enema. Nonrehydrated FOBT has the strongest evidence for screening efficacy based on two randomized controlled trials, showing a relative risk reduction in colorectal cancer-related mortality of 15% to 18% for persons between the ages of 45 and 75 years. Table 14-1 lists estimates of absolute benefits of screening FOBT according to life expectancy. Case–control studies show that sigmoidoscopy provides protection

TABLE 14-2

Guideline Recommendations for Cancer Screening in Older Adults

Cancer Site	Test	Frequency	USPSTF Guideline	ACS Guideline	AGS Guideline
Colorectal	Fecal occult blood test or	Annual	Screen all adults ≥ 50 yr Discontinuing screening is reasonable in persons whose age and comorbid conditions limit life expectancy	Screen all adults ≥ 50 yr. Discontinuing screening is reasonable in persons with severe comorbidity that would preclude treatment	Screen all adults ≥ 50 yr Persons too frail to undergo colonoscopy and persons with short life expectancy (3–5 yr) should not be screened
	Sigmoidoscopy or	Every 5 yr			
	Colonoscopy or	Every 10 yr			
	Double-contrast Barium Enema	Every 5 yr			
Breast	Mammography with or without	Every 1–2 yr	Screen all women ≥ 40 yr Women with comorbid conditions that limit life expectancy are unlikely to benefit from screening	Screen all women ≥ 40 yr, continuing for as long as a woman is in good health and would be a candidate for treatment.	Screening should continue for older women who have a life expectancy ≥ 4 yr
	Clinical Breast Exam	Annually			
Cervical	Pap smear	Every 1–3 yr	Discontinue screening in women who have had a total hysterectomy and in women > 65 yr who are not at high risk for cervical cancer and have had adequate recent normal Pap smears	Immunocompetent women > 70 yr who have had ≥ 3 normal Pap smears in a row and no abnormal results within 10 yr may elect to stop. Screening may be stopped in women who have had a total hysterectomy and women with severe comorbid illness	It is acceptable to stop screening women > 70 yr who have had ≥ 2 normal Pap smears since age 60 and women who have a short life expectancy or would be unable to tolerate treatment

USPSTF, United States Preventive Services Task Force; ACS, American Cancer Society; AGS, American Geriatrics Society.
Adapted from Walter LC, Lewis CL, Barton MB. Screening for colorectal, breast, and cervical cancer in the elderly: a review of the evidence. Am J Med. 2005;118:1078..

from distal colorectal cancer that lasts up to 10 years. Case–control studies also suggest that colonoscopy has a long-lasting protective effect because persons who died of colorectal cancer were less likely to have had a colonoscopy in the prior 10 years (odds ratio = 0.43; 95% CI: 0.30–0.63). No randomized trials have examined the effectiveness of barium enema in reducing mortality from colorectal cancer, and studies of its accuracy are of poor methodological quality.

Harms of Colorectal Cancer Screening

Approximately 1 of 10 older adults who submit a screening non-rehydrated FOBT will have a false-positive result. Colonoscopy is the standard work-up following a positive FOBT and may have serious complications, such as perforation (1/1000), serious bleeding (3/1000), and cardiorespiratory events (5/1000). Complications may be higher if polypectomy is performed or if persons are in poor health. Discomfort from flexible sigmoidoscopy or colonoscopy may occur, and many older persons may experience substantial distress from the bowel preparation.

Recommendations

Most guidelines recommend annual screening FOBT and/or flexible sigmoidoscopy every 5 years or colonoscopy every 10 years for average-risk persons starting at age 50 years (see Table 14-2). There is no evidence available to determine which screening method is preferable or when screening should stop. Most guidelines do not recommend using upper age cut-offs to decide when to stop screening. Rather, most guidelines recommend that the decision to discontinue screening should be individualized, based on whether an older person has characteristics that considerably decrease the benefit-to-

risk ratio of screening (e.g., limited life expectancy or conditions that increase the risk of colonoscopy, such as cardiopulmonary disease or dementia). The author recommends against screening for colorectal cancer if a person has an estimated life expectancy of less than 5 years. For persons with life expectancies between 5 and 10 years, the decision to screen is a close call, and patient preferences should play a major role in the decision to screen. For healthy older people who have a life expectancy greater than 10 years, screening with FOBT and/or flexible sigmoidoscopy or colonoscopy, regardless of age, is a reasonable recommendation based on available data.

Cervical Cancer

Risk of Dying of Cervical Cancer

For very healthy 75-year-old women who have life expectancies in the top twenty-fifth percentile and who have not been previously screened for cervical cancer, the lifetime risk of dying of cervical cancer is approximately 0.2%. The risk of dying of cervical cancer declines with decreasing life expectancy and is extremely low for older women who have had normal screening examinations in the past.

Benefits of Cervical Cancer Screening

The principal method for screening for cervical cancer is through the use of cervical cytology. Since screening with Pap smears was initiated, population studies in the United States show a 20% to 60% decline in mortality rates from cervical cancer. Table 14-1 lists estimates of absolute benefits of screening Pap smears according to life expectancy. Decision models suggest that older women who have had repeated normal Pap smears during their reproductive years do not benefit from continued Pap testing beyond age 65 or 70 years. However, these models make variable recommendations about the number of normal Pap smears required prior to stopping screening.

Harms of Cervical Cancer Screening

For women older than age 70 years, the risk of a false-positive Pap smear result has not been studied, but for postmenopausal women with a normal Pap result in the previous 2 years, the positive predictive value of an abnormal cervical smear is less than 1%. Harms of false-positive results include needless patient concern and invasive procedures, such as colposcopy or biopsy. Discomfort and anxiety during Pap smears also occurs as does the identification and treatment of clinically unimportant cervical lesions.

Recommendations

Most guidelines recommend that Pap smears be performed in women over age 70 years who have not been regularly screened before. For these women, screening may stop after two normal Pap smears 1 year apart, although little data exist about benefits and harms of Pap smear screening in elderly women. For women who have been regularly screened, Pap smears may be performed less frequently (every 3 years) after three or more smears have been normal. Women with repeatedly normal Pap smears may stop screening at age 65 or 70 years, as can women at any age who have a life expectancy of less than 5 years or who no longer have a cervix (see Table 14-2).

Other Cancers

Although prostate-specific antigen (PSA) testing is frequently performed, no compelling evidence demonstrates that PSA testing reduces prostate cancer mortality at any age and the harms of screening are substantial, especially in older men. For example, the specificity of PSA decreases with advancing age, leading to higher rates of false-positive results requiring needle biopsies or cycles of repeat testing and anxiety. Even if prostate cancer is identified, modeling studies suggest that most cancers detected by screening men over age 70 years would never have produced symptoms during their lifetime. In addition, if prostate cancer identified by screening is treated, elderly men suffer more complications, including incontinence, impotence, and even death. Therefore, while controversy surrounds PSA screening in young, healthy populations, no organization currently recommends PSA screening in older men who have a life expectancy of less than 10 years. In addition, no organization currently recommends screening for lung, pancreatic, or ovarian cancer.

SCREENING FOR NONCANCEROUS DISEASES

Like cancer-screening decisions, decisions to screen older people for other types of diseases also need to be individualized by considering life expectancy, comparing potential benefits and harms, and understanding individual values and preferences. However, the role of life expectancy and individual preferences in other types of screening decisions may be different than that presented for cancer screening. The decision to recommend cancer screening to an older individual is highly dependent upon life expectancy because there is a substantial delay (generally more than 5 years) between when the screening test is performed and when benefit may occur. As a result, persons with limited life expectancies are very unlikely to derive survival benefit from cancer screening. However, the lag time between initiation of other screening tests and potential benefit often is much shorter than that for cancer screening. For example, the potential to benefit occurs quickly after initiating screening for depression or visual impairment, such that even persons with limited life expectancies may benefit from these screening tests. Similarly, individual preferences play less of a role when a preventive intervention has public health implications than when benefits and harms apply only to the individual being screened, as is the case for cancer screening. For example, prevention of contagious diseases by screening for tuberculosis is very important in nursing homes and should be universally recommended for patients and staff.

Survival is the benefit described for cancer screening as the effect on quality of life and function has not been studied. Many other screening tests in older people, however, are targeted at improving quality of life or at preventing functional decline, rather than improving survival. Much of the screening performed during a geriatric assessment, such as screening for incontinence or auditory impairment, for example, is aimed at improving quality of life rather than lengthening survival (see Chapter 11). Some types of screening have been associated with both improved survival and overall quality of life, such as screening older persons for hypertension. Several studies have shown that treatment of hypertension reduces the risk of stroke and cardiovascular events in older persons and may have a slight positive effect on cognitive and physical function and overall well-being.

In summary, the approach to making informed screening decisions is similar to that for many other medical decisions in which the potential risks and benefits are considered and patient preferences are understood. The emphasis should be on individualizing screening decisions by offering the best proven, least risky screening tests to those persons most likely to develop burdensome diseases. While the number of potential screening tests is large, prioritizing tests based on available evidence and estimations of life expectancy can help narrow the choices. For example, screening in older persons with limited life expectancies should prioritize quality of life outcomes and tests in which the lag time to benefit is short. By encouraging individualized decisions, screening may be more appropriately targeted to older persons for whom the potential benefits outweigh the potential harms.

FURTHER READING

American Geriatrics Society Ethics Committee: health screening decisions for older adults: position paper. *J Am Geriatr Soc.* 2003;51:270.

Barratt A, Irwig L, Glasziou P, et al. Users' guides to the medical literature, XVII: how to use guidelines and recommendations about screening. *JAMA.* 1999;281:2029.

Goldberg TH, Chavin SI. Preventive medicine and screening in older adults. *J Am Geriatr Soc.* 1997;45:344.

Gross CP, McAvay GJ, Krumholz HM, et al. The effect of age and chronic illness on life expectancy after a diagnosis of colorectal cancer: implications for screening. *Ann Intern Med.* 2006;145:646.

National Center for Health Statistics. Life Tables of the United States, 2001. Available at: http://www.cdc.gov/nchs/data/dvs/lt2001.pdf.

Raik BL, Miller FG, Fins JJ. Screening and cognitive impairment: ethics of forgoing mammography in older women. *J Am Geriatr Soc.* 2004;52:440.

Sawaya GF, Brown AD, Washington AE, et al. Current approaches to cervical cancer screening. *N Engl J Med.* 2001;344:1603.

Sox HC. Screening for disease in older people. *J Gen Intern Med.* 1998;13:424.

Takahashi PY, Okhravi HR, Lim LS, et al. Preventive health care in the elderly population: a guide for practicing physicians. *Mayo Clin Proc.* 2004;79:416.

U.S. Preventive Services Task Force: Recommendations for Adults: Cancer, in Guide to Clinical Preventive Services, 2005. http://www.ahrq.gov/clinic/pocketgd05.

Walter LC, Covinsky KE. Cancer screening in elderly patients: A framework for individualized decision making. *JAMA.* 2001;285:2750.

Walter LC, Eng C, Covinsky KE, et al. Screening mammography for frail older women: what are the burdens? *J Gen Intern Med.* 2001;16:779.

Walter LC, Lewis CL, Barton MB. Screening for colorectal, breast, and cervical cancer in the elderly: a review of the evidence. *Am J Med.* 2005;118:1078.

Welch HG. *Should I Be Tested for Cancer? Maybe Not and Here's Why.* Berkeley, CA: University of California Press; 2004.

Health Care System

Chad Boult

INTRODUCTION

This chapter describes and critiques the "system" that provides health care for older Americans. The system comprises many elements, including providers of health care, providers of supportive services, "alternative" healers, patients, families, insurers, regulators, and liaisons among these elements. The health care system is addressed primarily from the perspectives of health care professionals and their older patients, particularly patients with multiple chronic conditions and complex health care needs. Strategies for optimizing care within the system and examples of recent innovations designed to improve the system are described.

Strictly speaking, a system (from the Latin noun *systema*) is a set of procedures or structures that direct or coordinate the orderly flow of other processes. In the case of complex health care for chronically ill older Americans, however, the fragmentation, lack of coordination, and disorderly flow of information and interactions is not a true system of health care. Nevertheless, this chapter uses the term "health care system" to refer to the aggregate of the many elements involved in providing health care to older patients.

The chapter begins with brief introductory descriptions of individual elements of the current system, many of which are described in greater detail in the chapters that follow, e.g., care in hospitals, emergency departments, subacute facilities, rehabilitation units, and nursing homes; complementary and alternative care; and care during transitions between providers. The next section describes the present system's performance in addressing the multifaceted needs of chronically ill older patients, followed by a section on the roles of primary care clinicians in caring for this population. Later sections examine opportunities for creating a more effective, efficient, and patient-centered system and summarize some recent initiatives designed to improve the system's quality and outcomes.

THE ELEMENTS OF THE SYSTEM

The pluralistic U.S. health care system consists of five interacting elements: providers, patients and caregivers, insurers, liaisons, and regulators.

Providers

Providers include health care professionals, health care organizations, and supportive community services. Among health care professionals are primary care and specialty physicians, nurses, social workers, rehabilitative therapists, pharmacists, dentists, mental health professionals, health care aides, and complementary and alternative medicine (CAM) practitioners. In the past, primary care physicians (PCPs) managed their patients across settings of care, providing valuable continuity and advocacy as their patients moved through emergency departments, hospitals, and rehabilitation facilities. Today, increased specialization by site of care has constrained primary physicians mostly to providing ambulatory care. Hospitalists, emergency physicians, and skilled nursing facility specialists (SNFists) provide much of the care in institutions. Although such specialization may have improved some aspects of care within hospitals, emergency departments, and SNFs, it has also eroded continuity of care and contributed to the further fragmentation of an already fragmented system (see Chapter 16). Unfortunately, no one clinician may know the patient well.

The system's health care organizations include acute care hospitals, long-term care hospitals (LTCHs), emergency departments, rehabilitation units, home care agencies, house call practices, skilled nursing facilities (SNFs), hospice programs, long-term care facilities, personal care providers, and disease management companies. Some hospitals operate multidisciplinary Acute Care for Elders (ACE) units to meet the complex needs of older adults who become acutely ill or injured.

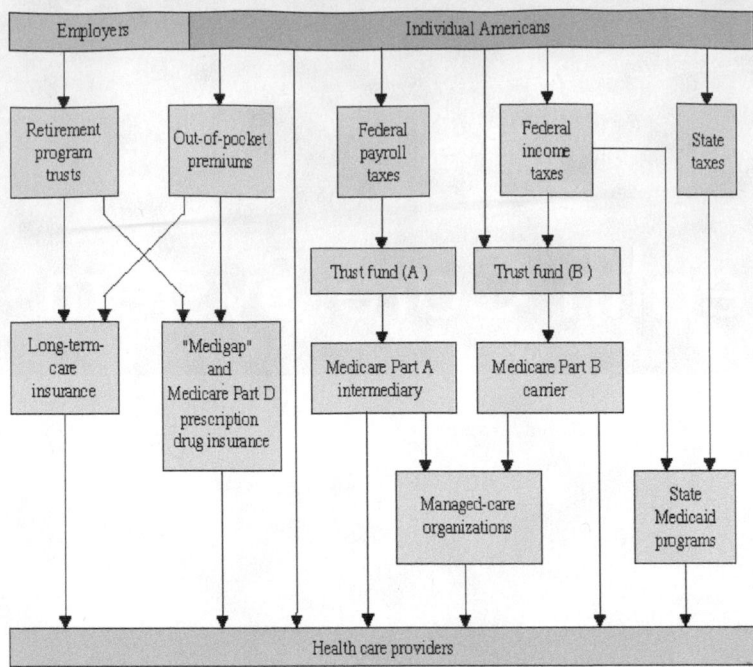

FIGURE 15-1. Flow of funds to providers of health care for older Americans.

A variety of organizations sponsor Programs of All-inclusive Care for the Elderly (PACE) that provide comprehensive community-based long-term care for older persons with significant disabilities. A few physician house call practices, often affiliated with medical schools, provide primary care at home to homebound patients. Although satisfying to patients and physicians, house call practices are challenged by low reimbursement.

Commercial disease management programs focusing on patients with congestive heart failure, diabetes, emphysema, or depression have proliferated in recent years as a new strategy for containing the high costs of these chronic illnesses. Disease managers, many of whom are nurses, follow standard protocols in communicating with patients by telephone to encourage them to see their physicians, use their medication appropriately, and adopt healthy behaviors. Most disease management programs work under contract with insurers; many use sophisticated health information technology (HIT) to remind patients to obtain appropriate preventive services and to track their use of health resources.

Community-based providers of supportive services include Area Agencies on Aging (AAA), Meals-on-Wheels, senior centers, transportation services, adult day care centers, condition-specific resources (e.g., the Alzheimer's Association), home modification programs, chore services, support groups, exercise programs, and congregate housing.

Patients and Caregivers

Most of the work of caring for chronic conditions is done (for better or for worse) by the patients who have the conditions and by their informal (i.e., unpaid) caregivers, such as family or friends. The degree to which patients are able adhere to medication regimens, healthy diets, physical activity programs, professional follow-up, and regular self-monitoring is a powerful determinant of the quality, cost, and clinical outcomes of their care. Out-of-pocket spending for health care by older patients and their families includes insurance premiums, deductibles, copayments, and the costs of products and services not covered by their health insurance, such as long-term care, eyeglasses, hearing aids, dental care, and medications. Such expenses can be significant. In 2000, older Americans' out-of-pocket spending for health care averaged 21.7% of their incomes. For low-income women in poor health, the figure was 51.6%.

Insurers

Both public and private organizations provide health insurance for older people. (Figure 15-1) Public health insurance programs include Medicare, Medicaid, the Veterans Health Administration, and Tricare (for military retirees). Private health insurance coverage for older Americans is provided by managed care organizations (MCOs), private indemnity insurers, and Medicare Part D providers.

Public Health Insurance

The Medicare program, which is administered by the federal Centers for Medicare and Medicaid Services (CMS), reimburses health care organizations and health care professionals for providing health care for Americans who are 65 years and older, disabled, or suffering from end-stage renal disease. As originally enacted, Medicare comprises two separate fee-for-service (FFS) plans (Part A and Part B), each of which pays predetermined amounts for specified health-related goods and services that are needed by its beneficiaries (Table 15-1). More than 80% of older Americans are covered by both plans.

Medicare Part A contracts with regional insurance companies ("intermediaries") to pay hospitals, nursing homes, home-care agencies, and hospice programs for the acute and subacute Medicare-covered services they provide. Older Americans (and their spouses) who have had Medicare taxes deducted from their paychecks for at least 10 years are entitled to coverage through Part A without paying premiums. Others may be able to purchase Part A coverage (for up to $423 per month, depending on how long Medicare taxes were deducted from their paychecks).

TABLE 15-1

Health Insurance Coverage for Older Americans

	FFS MEDICARE		SUPPLEMENTAL COVERAGE		MEDICARE HMO PLAN†
	Part A	**Part B**	**Medicaid***	**Medigap Policy**	
Covers the cost of:					
Hospitals	100%‡	—	$1024	$1024	100%
Postacute care in SNF	100%§	—	—	—	100%
Hospice	100%¶	—	—	—	—
Home care ("medically necessary")	100%	100%	—	—	100%
Durable medical equipment	80%**	80%**	20%	20%	100%
Diagnostic laboratory tests	—	100%	—	—	100%
Diagnostic imaging tests	—	80%	20%	20%	100%
Physicians, nurse practitioners	—	80%	20%	20%	100%
Outpatient PT, OT, ST	—	80%	20%	20%	100%
Outpatient services, supplies	—	80%	20%	20%	100%
Emergency care	—	80%	20%	20%	100%
Ambulance services	—	80%	20%	20%	100%
Preventive services	—	††	20%	20%	††,‡‡
Outpatient mental health care		50%	50%	50%	100%
Custodial care in nursing home	—	—	100%	—	—
Hearing, vision services	—	—	i	i	i
Outpatient medications	—	—	§§	§§	§§
Additional costs to patient:					
Deductibles	$1024¶¶	$135***	—	§§	§§
Monthly premiums	—	$96 to $238		§§	i§§

FFS, fee-for-service; HMO, health maintenance organization; OT, occupational therapy; PT, physical therapy; SNF, skilled nursing facility; ST, speech therapy.

*Under the Balanced Budget Act of 1997, state Medicaid programs were given the option whether or not to pay deductibles and co-insurance costs.

†Some Medicare Advantage plans require members to pay deductibles and co-payments.

‡For days 1–60 each benefit period, after the beneficiary or secondary insurer pays the deductible amount ($992).

¶For the first 20 days of SNF care following a hospital stay of at least 3 days.

§Patient makes co-payments of $5.00 per outpatient prescription and 5% of cost of respite care.

**When patient is receiving Medicare-covered home care.

††100% of allowed cost of fecal occult blood test, Pap smear interpretation, prostate-specific antigen test, blood tests for diabetes and cardiovascular disease, and influenza and pneumococcal vaccinations; 80% of allowed cost of mammograms and clinical examination of breast and pelvis (no deductible applies); after the annual Part B deductible has been paid, 80% of allowed cost of a general physical examination at age 65, glaucoma screening, sigmoidoscopy or colonoscopy or barium enema, digital examination of rectum (men), measurement of bone mass, hepatitis B vaccination, and diabetic education and equipment.

‡‡Some Medicare Advantage plans cover additional preventive services.

§§Benefits and costs vary widely among medigap insurance plans and state Medicaid plans.

¶¶Per benefit period (first 60 days following hospital admission).

***Annual.

Medicare Part B contracts with other regional insurance companies ("carriers") to pay physicians, nurse practitioners, social workers, psychologists, rehabilitation therapists, home-care agencies, ambulances, outpatient facilities, laboratory and imaging facilities, and suppliers of durable medical equipment for the Medicare-covered goods and services they provide. At age 65 years, people become eligible for Part B coverage if they are entitled to Part A coverage or if they are citizens or permanent residents of the United States. To obtain this coverage, eligible persons must enroll in Part B and pay monthly premiums ($96 to $238 in 2008), usually by agreeing to have them deducted from their monthly Social Security checks.

Physicians must choose whether to participate in the FFS Medicare program. For each Medicare-covered service provided, a participating physician submits a claim to the Part B carrier, accepts Medicare's fee for the service (80% of a preestablished "allowed" amount), and collects a 20% coinsurance payment from the patient or her secondary insurer. For services not covered by Medicare, the physician may bill the patient, if the patient agrees in advance in writing.

Physicians who choose to be "nonparticipants" in Medicare are permitted to bill patients directly for up to 15% more than 95% of Medicare's allowed amounts. Such patients pay their physicians

and then submit requests for partial reimbursement (i.e., for 80% of 95% of the allowed amounts) to the carrier. A few physicians choose to opt out of Medicare altogether; instead, they enter into "private contracts" with their older patients. Under these contracts, Medicare (and private "medigap" insurance plans) pay nothing, and patients pay physicians the full amount of the fees specified by the contracts.

Neither Part A nor Part B of the Medicare program covers periodic physical examinations, dental care, hearing aids, eyeglasses, orthopedic shoes, cosmetic surgery, care in foreign countries, or custodial long-term care at home or in nursing homes. Part B covers some preventive services (see Table 15-1). In 2008, beneficiaries paid out-of-pocket:

- Monthly payments for Part B ($96 to $238)
- Annual deductible for Part B ($135)
- The deductible for Part A ($1024 per benefit period, i.e., the first 60 days following a hospital admission)
- Coinsurance payments (usually 20%) for goods and services for which Medicare or other insurance pays a portion

- The full cost of those goods and services that are not covered by Medicare or other insurance.

CMS receives its mandates directly from Congress, with input from scientists and policymakers in the Congressional Budget Office. As such, CMS is subject to current Congressional law and, therefore, has limited authority to modify Medicare benefits or reimbursements beyond these provisions.

Medicaid is a joint federal-state health insurance program for some Americans—young and old—with low incomes and limited assets. With supervision and matching funds from CMS, each state operates its own unique Medicaid program that provides supplemental health insurance to low-income Medicare beneficiaries and primary health insurance to younger people of limited means. Most states' Medicaid programs pay the Part B premiums for Medicare beneficiaries who are also eligible for Medicaid ("dual eligibles"); some also pay their Medicare deductibles and coinsurance costs. The criteria for Medicaid eligibility and the additional benefits covered by Medicaid plans, such as eyeglasses, hearing aids, and dental services, vary considerably from state to state. Most important, Medicaid covers room and board in nursing homes for Medicaid-eligible, disabled people, many of whom have become eligible by liquidating their assets (i.e., by "spending down") to pay their medical and long-term care expenses. In many states, a limited number of disabled Medicaid recipients qualify (under "waiver" programs) for some long-term care services at home. Recently, several states have begun contracting with managed-care organizations to integrate Medicaid and Medicare benefits for "dual eligibles."

The Veteran's Health Administration (VHA) is a large, complex, integrated system that insures and provides comprehensive health care for "honorably discharged" military veterans. The VHA Medical Benefits Package covers preventive services, outpatient diagnostic and treatment services, inpatient medical and surgical care, medications (prescription and over-the-counter), and medical supplies. The VHA stratifies veterans into eight priority groups based on income, area of residence, and history of illness or injury during military service. The highest-priority patients, who are not required to make copayments, have service-connected health problems that are rated at least 50% disabling or that have caused them to be unemployable. Veterans receiving VHA benefits may simultaneously enroll in Medicare or Medicaid, giving them access to non-VA physicians and drugs that are not on the VA formulary. Unlike CMS, the VHA is authorized to bargain with pharmaceutical companies to limit the costs of prescription drugs through mass purchasing contracts.

The VHA underwent a major overhaul in the 1990s, driven by the aging of the veteran population, the growing burden of chronic health care needs, and Congressional concerns over poor quality and value of VHA services. The leadership of the VHA began to emphasize primary care, centralized goal-setting and resource management, standardized data reporting, information technology, and accountability for the quality of care. The VHA electronic health record system replaced paper charts throughout the network, making highly detailed patient records available at the point of clinical encounter. As a result of these changes, and of improvements in various quality indicators, the VHA is now considered by some to be a model of integrated health care.

Private Health Insurance

For older Americans who choose private health insurance, coverage is provided by MCOs, private indemnity insurers (e.g., "medigap" and long-term care insurance plans), and Medicare Part D providers. MCOs include Medicare health maintenance organizations (HMOs), which offer "Medicare Advantage" plans, as well as preferred provider organizations (PPOs) and point of service (POS) plans (Table 15-2).

Medicare Advantage

Medicare Advantage plans hold contracts with CMS specifying that, for each Medicare beneficiary they enroll, they will provide at least the standard Medicare benefits in return for risk-adjusted monthly "capitation" payments. In order to induce Medicare beneficiaries to switch from their traditional FFS Medicare coverage to a Medicare Advantage plan, some MCOs also cover additional benefits and charge low or no premiums, deductibles, and copayments. Medicare Advantage plans achieve cost savings by managing their enrollees' use of services within their networks of providers, with whom they negotiate price discounts in return for patient volume. As long as they provide at least the standard Medicare benefits to their enrollees, Medicare Advantage plans have considerable flexibility to test new models of care delivery without CMS's approval. Thus, some

TABLE 15-2

Advantages and Disadvantages of Four Types of Health Insurance		
TYPE OF INSURANCE	**PRIMARY ADVANTAGES**	**PRIMARY DISADVANTAGES**
FFS Medicare (Parts A, B and D)	Traditional Medicare benefits, choice of any provider that participates in the Medicare program, partial coverage for prescription medications	Cost of coinsurance, deductibles, noncovered goods and services (e.g., eyeglasses, hearing aids)
Medicaid	Coverage of coinsurance, deductibles, and some benefits* not covered by Medicare	Choice of providers restricted to a single network in some states
Medigap insurance	Coverage of coinsurance, deductibles, and some benefits† not covered by Medicare	Out-of-pocket monthly premiums range from $40 to $400, depending on the coverage provided by the policy purchased
Medicare Advantage plan	Traditional Medicare benefits plus coverage of additional goods and services†	Choice of providers restricted to a single network; potential for changes in premiums, copayments, deductibles, benefits, and providers at the discretion of the plan

FFS, fee-for-service; HMO, health maintenance organization.
*Benefits vary from state to state.
†Benefits vary from plan to plan.

Medicare Advantage plans may provide fertile ground for testing innovations in the health care system.

Each January, Medicare Advantage plans have the option of changing their premiums, benefits, and provider networks—or of discontinuing their plans in some or all of their service areas. Each November, beneficiaries covered by Medicare Part A and Part B have the option of joining any Medicare Advantage plan operating in their area; they cannot be denied enrollment because of health problems, except end-stage renal disease. Enrollees must continue to pay their monthly Medicare Part B premiums, and they must obtain their health care from the plan's provider network. They have the option of leaving the plan at any time and going back to the FFS Medicare program. Extensive information about all the options is available to consumers at each state's medical assistance office, at 1–800-MEDICARE (1–800-633–4227) or 1–877-486–2048 for hearing impaired TTY users, and at the Medicare Personal Plan Finder (www.medicare.gov/MPPF). In 2008, 20% of the Medicare population was enrolled in Medicare Advantage plans.

Supplemental Health Insurance

Private supplemental health insurance often covers health care costs that primary insurance, such as Medicare or VHA coverage, does not. Private insurance companies offer "medigap" plans of 12 types (A through L), classified according to the benefits they cover. A-level policies cover a person's Part A and Part B coinsurance costs, for example, 20% of Medicare's allowed fees for physicians' services and durable medical equipment. B-level plans cover Part A and Part B coinsurance, plus the Part A deductible ($1024 per benefit period). Each higher level of "medigap" policy provides additional benefits and costs more. J-level plans cover coinsurance, deductibles, care in foreign countries, and preventive services. Consumers can obtain "medigap" coverage with lower premiums by purchasing plans that require the insured to pay high deductibles (K- and L-level plans) or plans that cover the services of only selected physicians and hospitals ("Medicare SELECT" policies). Within 6 months of their initial enrollment in Medicare Part B, beneficiaries are entitled to purchase any "medigap" policy on the market at advertised prices. After this open enrollment period, "medigap" insurers can charge higher premiums or refuse to insure individual beneficiaries because of their past or present health problems.

Long-Term Health Insurance

The cost of long-term care in a nursing home averages more than $40,000 a year, and the cost of home care for disabled persons averages more than $6000 a year. Although more than a quarter of these long-term care costs are now paid directly out-of-pocket, fewer than 5% of Americans own long-term care insurance policies. Among older persons whose health qualifies them as eligible for long-term care insurance, only a small minority can afford to pay the premiums required for comprehensive long-term care policies, and less expensive policies may not provide adequate coverage for care at home or in a nursing home.

Medicare Part D

Medicare beneficiaries have the option of enrolling in one of many private Medicare Part D plans to obtain partial coverage for their prescription medications. Those who enroll pay annual premiums (about $300), deductibles ($285), and coinsurance (25% of the next $2295 of their medication costs). If their total medication costs exceed $2580, they then enter a coverage gap, or "doughnut hole," in which they pay 100% of the costs until their total out-of-pocket spending for drugs reaches $4050, after which their Part D plan pays 95% of any additional costs. Low-income beneficiaries may qualify for subsidized plans with lower premiums and cost-sharing requirements.

Regulators

Regulators are charged with the task of monitoring and improving the performance of specific elements of the system. For example, state medical and nursing boards regulate physicians and nurses; the Joint Commission on Accreditation of Healthcare Organizations (JCAHO) regulates hospitals and home care agencies; regional Quality Improvement Organizations (QIOs) assist providers in improving the quality of the care they deliver to Medicare beneficiaries; state insurance commissions regulate private health insurers; and state health departments regulate nursing homes. The roles of some of these regulatory groups are described in "Improving the Health Care System."

Care Management

Liaisons include care managers and case managers who coordinate the efforts of providers, patients, caregivers, and insurers to optimize the efficiency and the outcomes of patients' care. Care management services, usually provided by nurses or social workers, may be offered gratis to older persons for discrete episodes of illness by their insurance companies or for a fee indefinitely by private care management companies. Care management programs vary in their intensity of service, target population, focus (single disease or general), and intervention style (protocol-based, vs. individual discretion). Care managers' caseloads vary depending upon the intensity of involvement with each client.

PERFORMANCE OF THE SYSTEM

The United States leads the world in developing diagnostic and therapeutic technology, and almost all older Americans are covered by the Medicare program. As a result, the U.S. health care system provides most older Americans with unparalleled technical care for acute illnesses and injuries.

In caring for persons with chronic conditions requiring complex care, however, the system is less developed, less effective, and very inefficient. Figure 15-2 illustrates the "provider-centricity" of the present system. Patients and caregivers encounter many challenges when attempting to interact from the periphery with the multiple insurers and providers of the system.

As a result of deficiencies in all five elements of the health care system, care for older Americans with chronic conditions is marked by discontinuity, poor coordination, high costs, low quality, inaccessibility, and dissociation from patients' values and preferences. As the population of older Americans with chronic conditions grows rapidly in the decades ahead, the U.S. health care system, if not

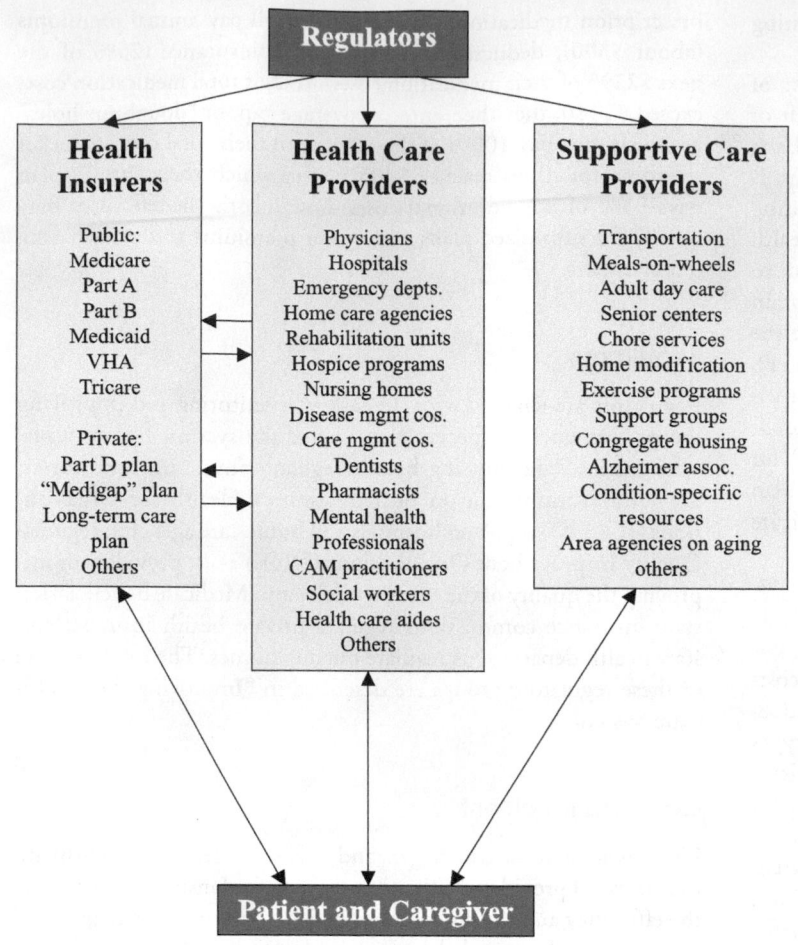

FIGURE 15-2. The present U.S. health care system.

transformed, will become increasingly inadequate and financially unsustainable.

At the root of the system's poor performance in chronic care has been the nation's unwillingness to make the substantial investments that would be required to transform all five elements of its health care system. Each element, therefore, continues to perform suboptimally.

- *Insurers.* By continuing to pay providers for each covered service they provide, insurance programs reward the provision of more (even duplicative) services, rather than the provision of higher quality or more effective services. By continuing to pay inadequately, if at all, for coordination of providers' efforts or for empowerment of patients or caregivers, insurers discourage providers from emphasizing these activities.

- *Regulators.* Because no regulatory agency evaluates coordination between providers, providers continue to operate as independent "silos." Because regulators' quality indicators focus on the completion of tests and the prescription of drugs, the quality of other processes that are essential to good chronic care, such as coordination, education, and empowerment, are not monitored, rewarded, or improved.

- *Providers.* Lacking potent financial and regulatory incentives to improve chronic care, many provider organizations do not expend significant resources to adopt networked HIT, to coordinate care across providers, or to encourage patients to manage their own chronic conditions. Physician groups, hospitals, and other organizations often function in isolation, providing care without

having complete information about the patient's condition or medical history, the services they have obtained in other settings, or the medications other clinicians have prescribed. Under the incentives of prospective payment, they often expedite patients' early transfer to other settings, further disrupting the continuity of care and increasing the probability of medical errors. Furthermore, most physicians are not well trained in the principles of high-quality chronic care, and they are not paid adequately for delivering such care.

- *Patients and caregivers.* Many older persons lack the knowledge, skills, and motivation to manage their chronic conditions proactively and to use providers appropriately. Instead, they have unhealthy life styles and rely on the health care system to take care of them when they get sick.

- *Liaisons.* Care management is a popular field for nurses and social workers, but limited investment has constrained the number of available positions. Little is known about which backgrounds, education, or activities of liaisons produce cost-effective health-related outcomes for their patients.

ROLE OF PRIMARY CARE CLINICIANS

Primary care clinicians, such as general internists, family physicians, geriatricians, and advanced practice nurses, play pivotal roles in the health care system's provision of chronic care. As chronically ill patients' primary point of contact with the system, these clinicians are well positioned to provide some essential chronic care services and to facilitate and coordinate others. In a sophisticated health care system, primary care clinicians, working individually or in teams, would provide chronically ill older patients with the following:

1. Comprehensive assessment of crucial health-related domains, such as medical, psychological, functional, cognitive, social, and nutritional status—and of values and advance directives

2. Preventive services, such as screening tests and evaluations, immunizations, and support for healthy lifestyles

3. Treatment of chronic conditions with prescriptions for medications, diets, behavior modification, and physical activity

4. Referrals to specialist physicians and community agencies

5. Coordination of care with all other providers

6. Education and encouragement for patients to manage their chronic conditions

7. Information and support for informal caregivers

8. Proactive monitoring of health status, medication effects, and adherence to plans

9. Oversight of transitions between sites of care, including reconciling different medication lists

Unfortunately, most primary care clinicians are unable to provide many of these services routinely. The majority of U.S. primary care providers operate in solo or small-group practices with only rudimentary HIT that does not support disease registries, the sharing of clinical information, identification of high-risk patients, evidence-based clinical decision-making, or prompts for preventive interventions like mammograms or influenza vaccinations.

Except for geriatricians, most American physicians have received little training in the principles of chronic disease management. Medicare and most supplemental insurers remunerate many of these services insufficiently (# 1 and 2) or not at all (# 4–9), and their payments for treating diseases (#3) are inadequate and shrinking each year in relation to inflation (Table 15-3). Many physicians compensate by focusing mostly on treating diseases (# 3), scheduling shorter and more frequent patient visits, and discontinuing the practice of caring for their patients through hospital, rehabilitation, and nursing home settings.

Steadily increasing administrative pressures on the primary care practice environment distracts clinicians from providing high-quality chronic care. Clinicians must master and monitor the ever-changing idiosyncrasies of Medicare's requirements for documenting clinical services and submitting bills, as well as attending to the other complex, unpaid responsibilities of operating an office practice. These pressures have produced several unintended consequences. Some primary care providers are limiting the number of Medicare beneficiaries their practices will accept. The number of young physicians choosing careers in family medicine has decreased by 50% in recent years; and the proportion of internal medicine residents choosing to become generalists has also decreased by half. The nation's workforce of board-certified geriatricians has been declining since 1998.

Care for individuals is increasingly provided by specialists who focus on single diseases. The average older patient is cared for by 3.5 different care providers. There is often little coordination among these providers, resulting in uncoordinated, fragmented care with increased potential for medical errors. The capacity of the U.S. health care system to provide sustainable chronic care, which is already minimal, is threatened further by these trends toward diminishing roles in the system for primary care providers.

IMPROVING THE HEALTH CARE SYSTEM

Chronic Care Model

Structural change does not come easily or quickly in the pluralistic U.S. health care system, but major structural changes will be

TABLE 15-3

Fee-for-Service Reimbursement by Medicare, Year 2008				
E&M SERVICE	E&M CODE	"ALLOWED" AMOUNT($)*	80%	CMS PAYMENT($)†
Comprehensive office visit, new patient	99205	180	× 0.80 =	144
Detailed office visit, established patient	99213	62	× 0.80 =	50
Detailed office visit (mental health problem), established patient	99213	62	× 0.50 =	31
Comprehensive office consult	99245	228	× 0.80 =	182
Comprehensive inpatient consultation‡	99255	198	× 0.80 =	158
Complex hospital admission	99223	176	× 0.80 =	141
Complex hospital follow-up visit	99233	93	× 0.80 =	74
Comprehensive nursing facility initial assessment	99305	109	× 0.80 =	87
Detailed nursing facility follow-up visit	99308	60	× 0.80 =	48
Comprehensive initial home visit	99345	197	× 0.80 =	158
Detailed follow-up home visit	99349	114	× 0.80 =	91
Home-health certification	G0181	108	× 0.80 =	86

E&M, evaluation and management; CMS, Centers for Medicare and Medicaid Services.

*For physicians who participate in Medicare; amounts vary by location (see http://www.cms.hhs.gov/physicians/mpfsapp/ for local rates and annual updates).

†For eligible services provided by nurse practitioners, payment is 85% of the amount shown.

‡Hospital or nursing facility consultation.

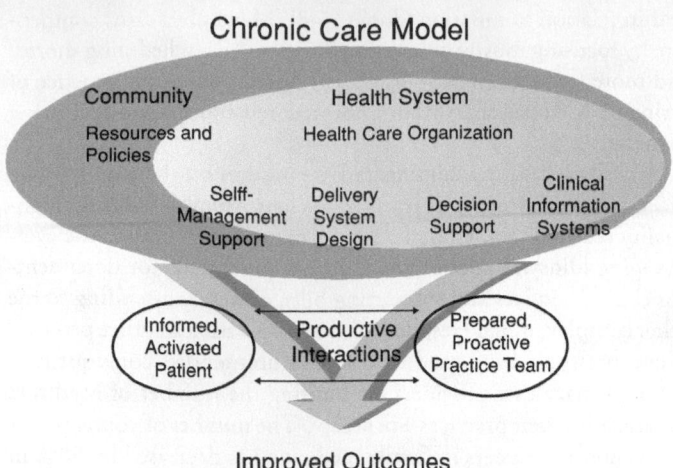

FIGURE 15-3. The chronic care model.

necessary to improve the quality of health care for chronically ill older Americans. The "Chronic Care Model" provides a guide to the changes in health care organizations, providers, patients, and caregivers that would improve chronic care in the U.S. health care system (Figure 15-3). The Chronic Care Model postulates that improved functional and clinical outcomes could be achieved through productive interactions between prepared, proactive practice teams and informed, activated patients and families. These enhanced interactions could result from changes in six areas of the health care system: (1) tighter links between health professionals and community resources; (2) enlightened, committed leadership of health care delivery organizations; (3) better patient self-management of chronic conditions; (4) evidence-based clinical decision-making by providers; (5) redesign of the delivery system; and (6) improved clinical information systems.

The changes called for by the Chronic Care Model could be invoked both from "top–down" decisions and actions by the U.S. Congress and other national organizations and from "bottom–up reform" by individual clinicians, academicians, patients, and family caregivers.

Top–Down Organizational Change

As shown in Figure 15-4, the top–down approach involves a panoply of organizations lobbying legislators to use the power of the U.S. Congress to influence the priorities and programs of the elements of the health care system over which it has direct control: CMS, the Veterans Health Administration, the Administration on Aging (AoA), and regulatory agencies. The actions of these elements, in turn, influence the actions of other elements of the system: providers, insurers, liaisons, patients, and caregivers.

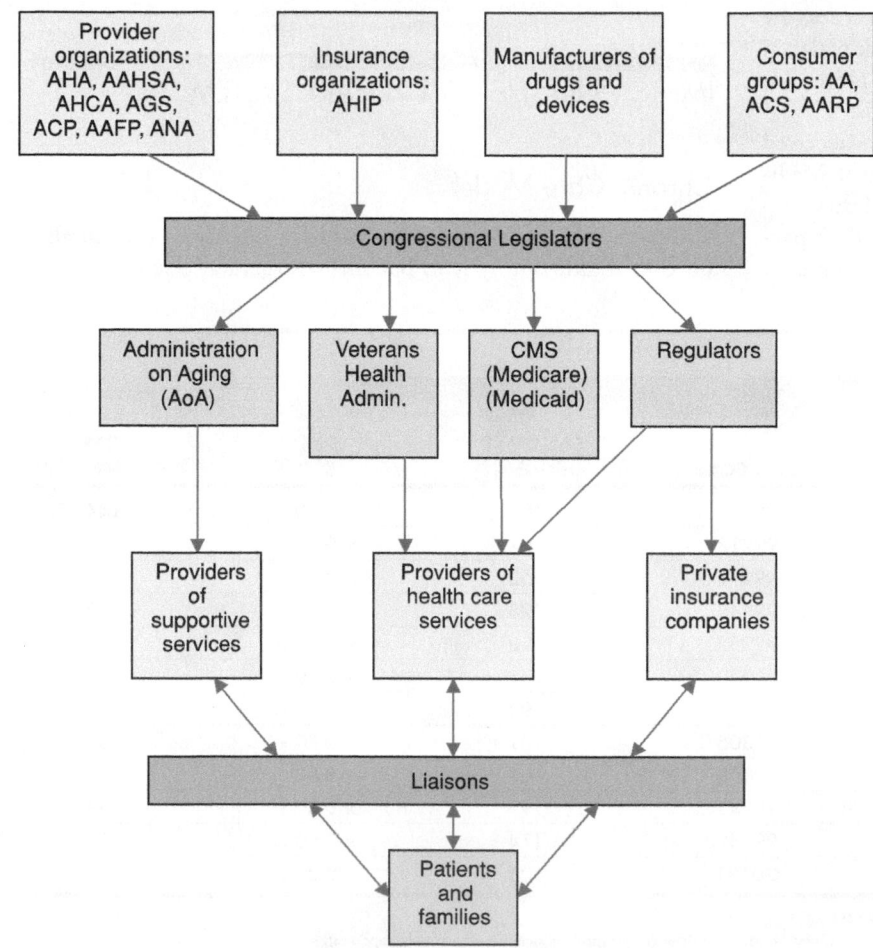

FIGURE 15-4. The top–down policy approach to improving the system. AHA, American Hospital Association; AAHSA, American Association of Homes and Services for the Aging; AHCA, American Health Care Association; AGS, American Geriatrics Society; ACP, American College of Physicians; AAFP, American Academy of Family Physicians; AHIP, America's Health Insurance Plans; AA, Alzheimer's Association; ACS, American Cancer Society.

Ultimately, the most profound improvements in the performance of the health care system will occur when national and state legislators commit to fundamental long-term reforms in large health care programs, such as Medicare, Medicaid, the Veterans Health Administration, and the Administration on Aging. Older patients and their family caregivers could accelerate such reform "from the top–down" by supporting consumer organizations and by voting preferentially for "pro-chronic care" political candidates and "from the bottom–up" by "shopping" for high-quality care, by asserting their care preferences to their providers, and by becoming informed, active "self-managers" of their own health conditions.

Bottom–Up Change

The bottom–up approach to improving the system also involves actions by clinicians, educators, researchers, provider organizations, and private insurers. Clinicians who are committed to high-quality chronic care could help propel improvements in its quality and cost-effectiveness by:

- Participating actively in medical education about the principles of chronic care, as both learners and teachers

- Advocating for access to HIT that would facilitate evidence-based medical decision-making, electronic sharing of clinical information among providers, identification of high-risk patients, maintenance of disease registries, and prompts for preventive and follow-up care

- Embracing novel chronic care practice designs, e.g., group visits and collaboration with patient liaisons and interdisciplinary teams

- Contributing to the relevant clinical, educational, and governmental programs of professional organizations such as local and state medical societies, the American Geriatrics Society, the American College of Physicians, the American Academy of Family Physicians, and other professional societies

- Providing expert testimony at governmental hearings about the obstacles to and opportunities for improving the quality and efficiency of health care for older Americans

Role of Academic Health Centers

Academic health professionals have additional opportunities to improve the health care system by conducting research and improving education in chronic care. Conducting and reporting the results of rigorous research on innovative approaches to chronic care is a crucial process for improving the health care system. Innovations that succeed in improving outcomes in research settings must then be translated into widespread clinical practice. For such diffusion to occur rapidly, innovations must be acceptable to insurers, providers, patients, families, and regulators—and they must be promoted to each of these elements for many years. Innovations are most likely to permeate the health care system if they rely on accessible technology and labor pools and provide immediate benefits to most of the elements of the system (i.e., cost savings for insurers, increased revenue or decreased net costs for providers, and improved quality of life for patients and families) without running afoul of existing regulations. Innovations which improve only clinical outcomes or

have unknown effects on costs are unlikely to be adopted widely by all the elements of the system.

Most U.S. physicians and nurses are under-trained to provide state-of-the-art comprehensive care for older patients with chronic conditions. Academicians have opportunities to improve chronic care education by leading curricular reform in their home institutions and by participating in national campaigns to remediate the curricula of

- Medical schools (e.g., through the Association of American Medical Colleges)

- Nursing schools (e.g., through the American Association of Colleges of Nursing)

- Residencies (e.g., through specialty certification boards, the Accreditation Council for Graduate Medical Education, and CMS, which funds most residency education)

- Programs of continuing education (e.g., through specialty recertification requirements and the Accreditation Council for Continuing Medical Education)

Some academicians and clinicians with advanced knowledge and skills in management have additional opportunities to assume leadership roles to help facilitate improvement in the quality of the education and chronic care provided by their organizations. Under the influence of top–down forces (e.g., changes in funding and regulation) and bottom–up initiatives (e.g., new research findings and a sharper focus on high-quality chronic care by clinicians, educators, patients and families), executives of provider and insurance organizations would be motivated to transform chronic care by implementing the Chronic Care Model. As chronic care becomes increasingly important to their business plans, these leaders will perceive greater incentives to invest in sophisticated HIT, innovative delivery models, health care professionals trained in chronic care, and ongoing programs for improving the quality and efficiency of chronic care.

RECENT QUALITY IMPROVEMENT INITIATIVES

Numerous initiatives intended to improve the quality of health care for older persons with chronic conditions have been launched during the past decade. Some have emanated (top–down) from Congressional policy mandates to CMS, while others have evolved (bottom–up) from clinical innovations by health care providers.

Policy-Driven Initiatives

To improve the quality of health care for Medicare beneficiaries during the past decade, CMS has implemented several mandatory systems for collecting, reporting, and acting on information about the quality of care provided by Medicare Advantage plans, nursing homes, home care agencies, hospitals, and physicians. Medicare Advantage plans must collect and report performance data, e.g., the Health Plan Employer Data and Information Set (HEDIS) and the Health Outcomes Survey (HOS). Plans must also operate Quality Improvement Systems for Managed Care (QISMC) to enhance beneficiaries' health status and functional independence. CMS also requires the ongoing collection and reporting of standardized quality data by nursing homes (i.e., the Minimum Data Set [MDS]), by home health agencies (i.e., the Older Americans Standardized Information System [OASIS]), and by hospitals (e.g., care for beneficiaries with heart attacks, heart failure, and pneumonia). These data are available at www.Medicare.gov.

The Medicare Modernization Act of 2003 (MMA 03) required CMS to implement

- the optional "Medicare Part D" program, which covers part of the cost of participating beneficiaries' prescription medications,

- a pilot test of eight large regional disease management programs (now called the "Medicare Health Support" programs) involving hundreds of thousands of beneficiaries with diabetes, heart disease, or emphysema, and

- several Medicare demonstration projects.

In response to this and previous legislation, CMS is now conducting dozens of demonstration projects designed to improve the quality and outcomes of care for beneficiaries with chronic conditions. In most of these demonstrations, CMS is paying supplemental capitated fees to provider or managed care contractors who are providing case management or disease management services to high-cost beneficiaries with chronic conditions, such as heart failure, diabetes mellitus, or other "special needs."

Many of the recently designed demonstrations are based on the principle of "pay for performance" (P4P) according to which CMS pays the capitation fees only to the extent that the contractor attains preestablished performance standards, e.g., performing specified diagnostic tests in certain percentages of the population, prescribing medications according to evidence-based practice guidelines, reducing Medicare's overall FFS payments, and receiving high satisfaction ratings by beneficiaries. Despite the intuitive appeal of linking payment to quality, little is known about the most effective ways to make this linkage. For example, which quality indicators should be included, what is the right amount of payment, should payment emphasize improved quality or high quality, and how much quality improvement and cost savings can be expected? The results of evaluations of many of the ongoing P4P demonstration and pilot programs are expected by the end of the decade.

In January of 2006, CMS launched an initiative designed to improve the quality of care that physicians provide to FFS Medicare beneficiaries: the Physician Voluntary Reporting Program (PVRP). Initially, participating physicians reported to CMS their adherence to a set of quality indicators in caring for their Medicare patients, e.g., ordering specific screening tests and prescribing proper medications. The next phase of implementation (called the Physician Quality Reporting Initiative [PQRI]) began in July of 2007. In this voluntary "pay for reporting" phase, participating physicians received a bonus of up to 1.5% of their FFS Medicare payments for reporting their adherence to dozens of predefined quality indicators for specified health conditions. Evaluations of the PVRP and the PQRI as well as plans for a subsequent P4P phase were incomplete when this chapter went to press.

In December 2006, Congress passed the Tax Relief and Health Care Act, which required CMS to conduct a national demonstration of a concept called the "Patient-Centered Medical Home" (Figure 15-5). In this model of care, Medicare beneficiaries select physician practices to function as medical homes. Medicare then pays the practice a supplemental capitation fee in return for the

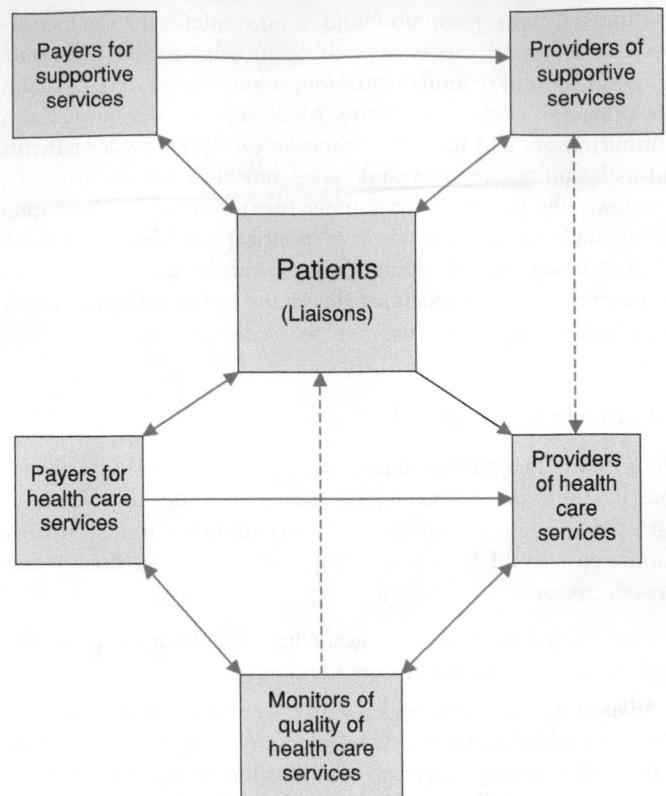

FIGURE 15-5. A patient-centered health care system.

practice team's provision of care coordination, patient education and empowerment, and communication with family caregivers. Additional details about this demonstration were not available when this chapter went to press.

Provider-Driven Initiatives

Several recent innovations with potential to improve the system's performance for chronically ill older patients have originated with health care providers. Some focus primarily on patients, caregivers, and/or liaisons, while several others are designed to improve providers' performance.

A "Chronic Disease Self-Management" (CDSM) program provides structured training and peer support that empowers older persons to assume an active role in managing their chronic conditions. In this program, groups of 10 to 15 older persons with chronic conditions meet weekly for six sessions with trained laypersons to learn self-management methods and to discuss the challenges they face. Participants learn to create and implement "action plans" for dealing with pain, functional deficits, physician visits, and health behaviors such as diet and physical activity. Randomized trials by Lorig et al. have demonstrated that CDSM participants have improved self-management skills, enhanced quality of life, and reductions in the use of health care services.

Other promising programs are centered on health care liaisons who facilitate older adults' transitions across health care settings. One model relies on the expertise of advance practice nurses to identify hospitalized older adults who are at risk for early readmission and to coordinate their care as they return home after discharge. These nurses collaborate with the patient, the caregiver(s), the primary care provider, and the patient's other providers to ensure that the gains made in the hospital are sustained in the postacute setting. As discussed in Chapter 16, this model of transitional care is effective in decreasing readmissions and reducing insurance expenditures.

Several initiatives have created interdisciplinary teams to strengthen the role of primary care in the health care system. In one initiative, a dyad consisting of a nurse practitioner and a primary care provider provides and coordinates care for residents of long-term care facilities. By evaluating and treating residents in their living environments, the nurse practitioner and primary care provider gain accurate insight into residents' functional status, which informs care plans that are tailored to their needs and available resources. The dyad works closely with the nursing home staff and administration to increase the probability that emerging health and behavioral problems are detected early and can be treated on site. Studies have demonstrated that this model leads to high resident satisfaction and significant cost savings, primarily through the early detection and management of acute problems, thus averting the need for transfers to emergency departments and hospitals.

Another innovation is the provision of primary care to groups of patients who have several chronic conditions. The primary goal of the group meeting is to facilitate self-management of chronic illness through targeted education, strategies to promote self-care, peer and professional support, and attention to the psychosocial challenges of living with chronic conditions. Group visits are designed to complement rather than replace the traditional one-on-one office visit. The visits are held monthly and typically last 90 minutes. Participants include the primary care provider and nursing staff, a pharmacist, and 8 to 12 older patients and their caregivers. Physical therapists, dietitians, and social workers participate on an ad hoc basis, leading discussions on topics relevant to their professional fields. The meetings begin with a brief socialization period to facilitate cohesion among the participants. A health care practitioner then gives a presentation on a health topic, such as medication management, nutrition, or advance directives. Following the presentation, the health care team provides primary health services to the patients, including immunizations, blood pressure assessment, and medication refills. The group then discusses the session's health topic and shares personal strategies for overcoming barriers to managing their condition and living with particular symptoms. The remaining time is devoted to brief one-on-one visits, if necessary, with the primary care provider or nurse. Group visits have been shown to decrease the use of hospital and emergency services and to improve patients' self-management, quality of life, and satisfaction with health care. Their effects on health status, however, have been less impressive. A recent two-year, randomized, controlled trial of group outpatient visits for chronically ill older adults by Scott et al. found no significant changes in functional or health outcomes.

Depression is common and costly among older persons. Although medications and counseling can control most depressive symptoms, few depressed older patients receive effective treatment. A recent innovation in primary care has shown promise for improving the care and the quality of life for such patients. In this approach, a depression care manager—a nurse or psychologist trained to deliver a structured, multisession model of psychotherapy—collaborates with the patient's primary care provider in providing education, pharmacotherapy, counseling, and care coordination for a year. A multi-center randomized controlled trial by Unutzer et al. showed that the likelihood of recovery from depression was 3.5 times greater for older patients who received such care, compared to those who received "usual" care. Efforts to disseminate this approach throughout the U.S. health care system are ongoing.

A similar collaborative modification of primary care has been designed and tested for older patients with Alzheimer's disease and their caregivers. In this approach, an advance practice nurse leads an interdisciplinary team that uses standard protocols in collaborating with the patient's caregiver and primary care provider to manage the psychological and behavioral symptoms of dementia. In a randomized controlled trial by Callahan et al., patients who received care under this model had significantly fewer behavioral and psychological symptoms of dementia after 18 months, and their caregivers reported significant improvements in distress and depression.

Low-income persons often have difficulty obtaining needed health-related services as they grow older. A recent innovation in health care is designed to meet these needs in collaboration with the patient's primary care provider. An interdisciplinary geriatrics team uses care protocols and an electronic medical record to help the primary care provider assess, manage care, and coordinate a wide range of community-based services. In a randomized controlled trial by Counsell et al., this approach improved low-income patients' mental health, vitality, and social functioning, while decreasing the use of emergency and hospital services by those at highest risk for hospitalization.

A comprehensive interdisciplinary model of primary care designed to improve the quality of life and efficiency of resource use among chronically ill older patients is known as "Guided Care." In this model, primary health care is infused with the operative principles of several proven innovations. A registered nurse who has completed a supplemental educational curriculum works in a practice with several primary care providers to provide comprehensive chronic care to 50 to 60 of their multimorbid older patients. Using an electronic health record, the Guided Care nurse collaborates with the patient's primary care provider in conducting eight clinical processes: assessing the patient and primary caregiver at home, creating an evidence-based care plan, promoting patient self-management, monitoring the patient's conditions monthly, coaching the patient to practice healthy behaviors, coordinating the patient's transitions between sites and providers of care, educating and supporting caregivers, and facilitating access to community resources. The effects of Guided Care are now being measured in a 5-year, multisite, cluster-randomized, controlled trial in the mid-Atlantic region of the United States. Early results include improved quality of care and reduced use and cost of health services.

CONCLUSION

The aging of the baby-boom generation, coupled with technology-driven increases in health care spending and a decline in the number of workers per Medicare beneficiary, will soon create serious financial challenges for the Medicare program. Similarly, increases in the number of older Americans with serious disabilities will soon surpass most states' ability to pay for their long-term care. To improve the performance of the health care system rapidly, the nation needs both prompt, profound reform of its health care policies and bold leadership by innovative health professionals.

FURTHER READING

Bodenheimer T. Primary care—will it survive? *N Engl J Med.* 2006;355(9):861–864.

Bodenheimer T, Wagner EH, Grumbach K. *JAMA.* 2002;288(14):1775–1779.

Boult C, Reider L, Frey K et al. Early effects of "Guided Care" on the quality of health care for multimorbid older persons: a cluster-randomized controlled trial. *J Gerontol A Biol Sci Med Sci.* 2008;63(3):321–327.

Callahan CM, Boustani MA, Unverzagt FW, et al. Effectiveness of collaborative care for older adults with Alzheimer's disease in primary care: a randomized controlled trial. *JAMA.* 2006;295(18):2148–2157.

Centers for Medicare and Medicaid Services, Department of Health and Human Services. *Medicare: Resident and New Physician Guided: Helping Health Professionals Navigate Medicare.* Rockville, MD: US Government Printing Office; 2007.

Coleman EA, Parry C, Chalmers S, et al. The care transitions intervention: results of a randomized controlled trial. *Arch Intern Med.* 2006;166(17):1822–1828.

Counsell SR, Callahan CM, Clark DO, et al. Geriatric care management for low-income seniors: a randomized controlled trial. *JAMA.* 2007;298(22):2623–2633.

Feder J, Komisar HL, Niefeld M. Long-term care in the United States: an overview. *Health Aff (Millwood).* 2000;19(3):40–56.

Institute of Medicine. *Crossing the Quality Chasm: A New Health System for the 21st Century.* Washington, DC: National Academy Press; 2001.

Health Care Financing Administration. 2007 Guided to Health Insurance for People with Medicare. Pub. No. HCFA 02110. Rockville, MD: US Government Printing Office; 2007. Available at www.Medicare.gov/publications/home.asp.

Health Care Financing Administration. Medicare and You. Pub. No. HCFA 10050. Rockville, MD: US Government Printing Office; 2007. Available at www.Medicare.gov/publications/home.asp.

The Henry J. Kaiser Family Foundation. Medicare at a glance fact sheet. February 2007.

Jha AK, Perlin JB, Kizer KW, et al. Effect of the transformation of the Veterans Affairs health care system on the quality of care. *N Engl J Med.* 2003;348(22):2218–2227.

Lorig KR, Ritter P, Stewart AL, et al. Chronic disease self-management program: 2-year health status and health care utilization outcomes. *Med Care.* 2001;39(11):1217–1223.

Maxwell S, Moon M, Segal M. Growth in Medicare and out-of-pocket spending: impact on vulnerable beneficiaries. The Urban Institute; January 2001.

Mays J, Brenner M, Neuman T, et al. Estimates of Medicare beneficiaries' out-of-pocket drug spending in 2006: modeling the impact of the MMA. Actuarial Research Corporation and the Henry J. Kaiser Family Foundation; November 2004.

Medicare. The Official U.S. Government Site for People with Medicare. www.Medicare.gov.

Naylor MD, Brooten DA, Campbell RL, et al. Transitional care of older adults hospitalized with heart failure: a randomized, controlled trial. *J Am Geriatr Soc.* 2004;52(5):675–684.

Oliver A. : The Veterans Health Administration: an American success story? *Milbank Q.* 2007;85(1):5–35.

Scott JC, Conner DA, Venohr I, et al. Effectiveness of a group outpatient visit model for chronically ill older health maintenance organization members: a 2-year randomized trial of the cooperative health care clinic. *J Am Geriatr Soc.* 2004;52(9):1463–1470.

Unutzer J, Katon W, Williams JW, Jr, et al. Improving primary care for depression in late life: the design of a multicenter randomized trial. *Med Care.* 2001;39(8):785–799.

Winter J, Balza R, Caro F, et al. Medicare prescription drug coverage: consumer information and preferences. *Proc Natl Acad Sci USA.* 2006;103(20):7929–7934.

Transitions

William L. Lyons ■ *Eric A. Coleman*

INTRODUCTION

In developed countries the care of complex older patients commonly entails their transfer from one health care setting to another and from one team of providers to another, as their medical and functional needs evolve. In theory, this allows an economical application of specialized resources to be applied at each stage. As an example (Figure 16-1), an elderly woman may be admitted to an acute hospital for diagnosis and initial management of community-acquired pneumonia. After stabilization and initiation of treatment, she is transferred to a skilled nursing facility (SNF) for rehabilitation, continued antibiotic treatment, and close monitoring by nursing. If she decompensates in some manner in the nursing facility (for example, by becoming acutely delirious), she may be transferred to an emergency department (ED) for urgent physician evaluation; rehospitalization may follow. After further diagnostic work and treatment, she returns to the nursing facility to complete her rehabilitative program before finally returning to her home in the community, where a visiting nursing agency assists family in her care. In this sequence her changing care needs prompted physical transfers and encounters with a succession of professionals—hospitalists and acute care nursing in the hospital; then a new provider, nursing, and rehabilitation staff at the SNF; then new providers and nursing in the ED; probably new hospitalists and nurses on her rehospitalization; and finally a new set of nurses, rehabilitation team, and outpatient provider when she returns home. To keep this patient from falling through the cracks, her various providers (and their organizations) must exercise considerable diligence and attention to detail. Active involvement from the patient and her family is necessary as well.

This chapter discusses transitional care, the actions taken to ensure coordination and continuity of health care as patients are transferred among various care settings. Good transitional care entails not just the physical transfer of a patient, but the orderly transfer of responsibility of care of the patient as well. The chapter is meant to

be of particular use for those clinicians (physicians, physician assistants, and nurse practitioners) charged with direct responsibility for managing care transitions.

For a number of reasons, the challenges of transitional care appear to be growing in the United States. Compared to the situation faced by physicians a century ago, our patients are much older, with longer problem (and medication) lists, and greater functional disability. Families may live in other cities and offer little ability or willingness to provide care at home. Health care venues have proliferated and become specialized. Typical care settings found in many large American cities are listed in Table 16-1. Providers themselves have also become more specialized, and in some instances (as with hospitalists, intensivists, SNFists, or emergency medicine physicians), their specialty is defined by the setting in which they practice. Changes in medical education are introducing new challenges as well, with resident work hour limits forcing more handoffs than existed before. Finally, coordination and continuity of care is made more difficult by the fact that the United States lacks a health care "system" per se.

Transitional care is at the confluence of two ascendant movements in modern health care—improved patient safety and patient-centered care. Poorly executed transitions place patients at risk of injury and other adverse events. Well-executed transitions intrinsically incorporate patients' individual goals, needs, and values. The quality of transitions also influences resource use, such as ED utilization and need for rehospitalization. For all these reasons (Table 16-2), a number of influential advisory, professional, and funding organizations have shown interest in the topic. The Institute of Medicine has called for greater integration of care delivery across health care settings. The Society of Hospital Medicine, the American Geriatrics Society, and the American Board of Internal Medicine all have urged greater professional commitment to transitional care. The Joint Commission on the Accreditation of Healthcare Organizations (JCAHCO) has adopted a patient tracer methodology, which allows surveyors to determine how a patient fares during a sequence of transitions. JCAHCO also has begun confirming that surveyed organizations

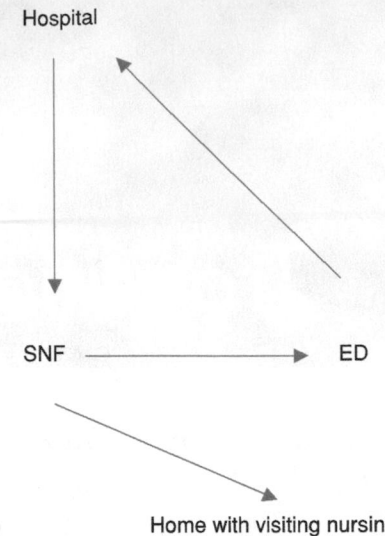

FIGURE 16-1. Common traffic pattern for older patients undergoing health care transitions. SNF, skilled nursing facility; ED, emergency department.

employ medication reconciliation (discussed below) and standardized approaches for patient handoffs.

Hospitals are required, as part of Medicare Conditions of Participation, to employ a discharge planning process for all patients, with policies and procedures in writing. Further, hospitals must identify

TABLE 16-1

Venues of Care Available in Typical Urban Centers	
DOMAIN	**CHARACTERISTICS**
Hospital	Medically and technologically intense. Minimal emphasis on longitudinal management of acute or chronic illness.
Postacute skilled nursing/subacute	Continuation of care begun in hospital. Less physician contact and diagnostic emphasis. Greater emphasis on skilled nursing and rehabilitation.
Long-term care	Nursing and supportive care for physically frail and cognitively impaired.
Assisted living	Wide spectrum of care, with scant regulation. Nursing and supportive care for physically frail and cognitively impaired, but residents less frail than in long-term care, and professional nursing staff may be minimal.
Acute rehabilitation	Intense inpatient provision (several hours daily by multiple disciplines) of rehabilitation therapy, typically for patients who have suffered acute orthopedic or neurologic injury.
Home care	Generally for "homebound" elders with "skilled needs". Care provided primarily by RN, PT, OT, ST, SW, aides.
Hospice	Inpatient (limited capacity) or home. Palliation of symptoms and maintenance of dignity for persons whose life expectancy is anticipated to be less than 6 months.

RN, registered nurse; PT, physical therapy; OT, occupational therapy; ST, speech therapy; SW, social work.

TABLE 16-2

Effects of Poorly Executed Transitions
• Adverse events in peridischarge period (e.g. medication discrepancies or errors)
• Recidivism to the emergency department or hospital
• Reduced patient, family, provider satisfaction
• Increased cost of care

all patients who are likely to suffer adverse health consequences after discharge in the absence of adequate discharge planning. Hospitals also are required to provide for the initial implementation of the discharge plan. Despite Medicare's evident interest in promoting high-quality transitional care, the program currently lacks vigorous monitoring and reimbursement incentives.

Beyond an appropriate alignment of "sticks and carrots," improvements in transitional care quality will require research advances, inculcation, and cultural change within health care organizations and professions, and discipline-specific training. In that spirit, this chapter is intended to provide didactic material for training health care providers who are responsible for managing the care transitions of elders with complex care needs. Much of the data presented and recommendations made apply to transfers from acute hospitals, but the key principles apply to transitions involving other health care settings as well.

TRANSITIONS TRAFFIC AND TRANSITIONS QUALITY

With increasing pressures to shorten hospital lengths of stay, it is becoming less common for an older patient to be cared for in the hospital until she feels well, at which time she is discharged home in the care of her family. National statistics from 2004 for Medicare patients discharged from acute hospitals show that about a quarter of them were transferred to another institution (such as a nursing home or rehabilitation facility), and an additional 14% were discharged to their home with the involvement of home health professionals. Recent work also confirms many providers' impressions that the period immediately following hospital discharge can be characterized by continued movement from place to place. A recent study of Medicare beneficiaries examined the 30-day period following hospital discharge, and found that 60% of patients made a single transfer, 18% made two transfers, 9% made three transfers, and 4% made four or more. These frequent transfers represent discontinuities in patients' care where vital information may be lost and care plans become fragmented.

The risk for hospital readmission is greatest in the period immediately after discharge. A study of patients with hip fracture discharged from New York City hospitals, for example, found that 32% were readmitted within a 6-month period, and over a third of these readmissions occurred within the first month after discharge. It is increasingly recognized that the "peridischarge" period is a dangerous time for patients. In one prospective cohort study of patients discharged home from the medical service of an academic medical center, 6% of patients had suffered preventable adverse events by about 3 weeks after discharge. An additional 6% experienced adverse events whose severity might have been reduced by improved quality of care. In another single-institution study of patients discharged from an academic medical service, researchers examined inpatient and outpatient records for evidence of three types of errors arising from discontinuity of care: (a) medication continuity errors, (b) test follow-up errors (in which test results were pending at the time of hospital discharge, but were not acknowledged in the outpatient chart), and (c) work-up errors (in which an outpatient test was recommended or scheduled by the inpatient team, but did not take place). About half of the patients' charts were found to contain at least one of these discontinuity errors, and those patients with work-up errors were over six times more likely to be rehospitalized than patients without these errors.

A major cause of the peridischarge hazard may be communication failures between hospital physicians and physicians who see patients soon after discharge. Historically, the same physician attended to the patient in hospital and in clinic, but the increased use of hospitalists and covering physicians creates opportunities for information discontinuities. In one study, only 3% of primary care doctors reported discussions with hospital physicians about discharge plans. In other studies, about half of discharge summaries are received by primary care physicians by 4 weeks of discharge; a quarter of summaries never reach the primary physician. And those summaries that are received commonly lack important information. Diagnostic test results are missing in 38%, consultant recommendations in 52%, discharge medications in 21%, and test results pending at discharge in 65%. There is a pressing need to improve the fidelity of information transfer from hospitals to primary care providers and other physicians and care providers.

Poor communication between hospital providers and patients (or families) probably contributes as well to peridischarge risk. Patients often report that they do not understand potential adverse effects of their discharge medications, when they may resume normal activities, which questions to ask and whom to address them to, and which warning signs to watch for. More globally, many patients express a lack confidence in their ability to make sure the care plan reflects their particular preferences, goals, and needs.

Metrics are needed to implement a quality improvement effort in transitional care. Coleman et al. developed the Care Transitions Measure (CTM), a patient-focused instrument that can be used to track performance changes over time. Two versions of the instrument, one with three items and another with 15, can be found at www.caretransitions.org. The CTM encompasses four domains of quality in transitional care (Table 16-3). The first domain is the fidelity of information transfer. Is accurate information transferred from sending clinicians to receiving clinicians in a reliable and timely manner? The second domain is patient and family preparation. Do they understand the purpose of the new care setting? If the patient is going home, do they understand the things they are responsible for managing in the care plan? The third domain is support for

TABLE 16-3

Four Domains of Quality in Transitional Care

1. Fidelity of information transfer
2. Preparation of patient, family, caregiver
3. Support for patient self-management
4. Patient empowerment to assert goals and preferences

With permission from Coleman EA, Smith JD, Frank JC, et al. Development and testing of a measure designed to assess the quality of care transitions. Int J Integr Care [online]. 2002;2 Jun 1. Available at: www.ijic.org

patient self-management. Does the patient know the warning signs and symptoms to watch for after discharge, and the purpose and adverse effects of the medications? Finally, the fourth domain is patient empowerment to assert individual goals and preferences. Does the patient feel the hospital staff took into account her particular goals when determining what her health care needs are, and where they could best be met after discharge? Lower CTM scores have been shown to predict reduced likelihood of ED use and rehospitalization in the postdischarge period. While developed for quality improvement efforts, all clinicians would benefit from considering the CTM items or Table 16-3 when contemplating individual patient transfers. The National Quality Forum has endorsed the CTM for use in public reporting.

PREDICTORS OF PROBLEMATIC TRANSITIONS

Experienced clinicians develop a sense for which patients are likely to experience difficulties after a transition to a new setting. In hospital jargon these patients are potential "bounce-backs" or candidates for early readmission. One statistical model that helps to identify such at-risk patients is provided in a study by Coleman et al. (Posthospital care transitions: patterns, complications, and risk identification. *Health Serv Res*, 2004;39(5):1449). A consensus of factors that help to identify patients at risk of hospital readmission is listed in Table 16-4. Several of the items are not surprising—older patients, those with more serious illnesses, those with need for activity-of-daily-living assistance but with marginal support, and those with a history of previous hospitalizations are all more likely to require rehospitalization soon after discharge. In addition to physical ailments, however, depression predicts readmission, as does a worse self-rating of patient health. Patients who have difficulty with treatment adherence (to medication regimens or follow-up appointments) are at risk as well. Finally, patients (or families) who have not received education around the time of discharge are more likely to suffer complicated transitions.

TABLE 16-4

Risk Factors for Complicated Care Transitions*

DEMOGRAPHICS	MEDICAL DIAGNOSES	PSYCHOSOCIAL	OTHER
Increased age	Heart disease	Medicare and Medicaid eligible	Prior hospital use
	Stroke history	Caregiver needed for ADL assistance	Worse self-rating of health
	Diabetes mellitus	Inadequate social support	Inadequate patient/family preparation
	Cancer	Depression	Instructions given without regard to health literacy or cognitive ability
	High Charlson comorbidity score		

*A complicated transition is one that transfers a patient to a higher-acuity care setting.

Knowledge of risk factors for problematic transitions is important for clinical leaders who are contemplating new programs and innovations in transitional care. Such programs may be time- and labor-intensive; administrative leaders or funding agencies will look for evidence of cost-effectiveness. A key strategy in creating a cost-effective program is to employ targeting criteria that help in identifying patients most in need of special help. Patients who lack such criteria (such as those shown in Table 16-4) are less likely to require costly interventions in order to avoid transitions-related mishaps.

INNOVATIONS IN TRANSITIONAL CARE

A number of interventions to improve care transitions have been studied; the majority involve discharge from the acute hospital. One systematic review of 54 randomized, controlled trials involving interventions designed to improve outcomes of discharge of elders from hospitals found that the location of the intervention appeared to be an important factor. The most successful interventions, in terms of reducing readmission risk, were those that took place in the patients' homes, or in both hospital and at home, but not exclusively in the acute setting. One such landmark trial, reported by Rich and coworkers, focused on the discharge of high-risk elders with congestive heart failure (CHF). This diagnosis is the leading cause of hospital admission for Medicare patients and is associated with frequent readmission. Rich's multifactorial intervention included intensive education about CHF provided by nurses; social work involvement for help with discharge planning and arrangement of care after discharge; review of the drug regimen by a geriatric cardiologist; dietary assessment and education by a dietician; high-intensity follow-up by the hospital's home care services; and additional home visits and telephone consultation as needed by the research team. Those patients in the intervention arm of this prospective, randomized, controlled trial demonstrated a lower risk of readmission, reduced cost of care, and greater quality-of-life scores.

A later study by Naylor and colleagues considered a broader range of diagnoses for hospitalized elders being discharged to the community. The study population in this prospective, randomized trial included elders with one of several medical or surgical diagnoses, and known to be at risk (using predetermined criteria) for poor discharge outcomes. The intervention made use of advanced practice nurses who assumed responsibility for transitional care from the time of admission to the hospital. These advance practice nurses followed their patients into the home following discharge, and substituted for visiting nurses during the first 4 weeks after patients left the hospital. As with the Rich study, the Naylor study found that the intervention reduced risk of readmission, as well as total cost of care.

Coleman and colleagues reported on the results of the Care Transitions Intervention, which introduced two conceptual innovations. First, this intervention was designed to encourage older patients (and their caregivers) to assert their own preferences, and to acquire self-management skills relating to transitions across care settings. Second, the intervention introduced the role of a "transition coach," who, although a nurse practitioner by training, did not function as a health care provider. Rather, she encouraged self-management and direct communication with primary care providers. The transition coach visited patients in the hospital and at home, and also made frequent follow-up telephone calls. Patients worked with the transition coach for about 28 days after their discharge to home.

Major areas of emphasis included medication self-management; use of a patient-centered record (maintained by the patient, and listing medical problems, medications, and other vital information); empowerment of the patient to schedule and complete follow-up visits with physicians; and patient's understanding of events that suggest that a health condition is worsening. Patients who received this program were significantly less likely to be readmitted to the hospital and the benefits were sustained for 5 months after the end of the 1-month intervention. More than simply managing posthospital care in a reactive manner, the Care Transitions Intervention imparted self-management skills that proved beneficial after the end of the program. Anticipated cost savings for 350 chronically ill adults extending from an initial hospitalization over 12 months is almost $296 000. Patients who received this program were also more likely to achieve self-identified personal goals around symptom management and functional recovery.

A number of hospitalist programs have set up postdischarge follow-up clinics in which patients are seen soon after discharge by the physician who provided care in the acute setting. The benefits of these programs have not yet been demonstrated in large, prospective trials. Nevertheless, a large cohort study using an administrative data base for hospitalized patients in Ontario, Canada, found that patients who followed up after discharge with their inpatient provider had a reduced combined rate of readmission and 30-day mortality.

Several pharmacist-led transitions interventions have been recently reported. One intervention involved simply a follow-up phone call placed by pharmacists to patients 2 days after discharge, during which patients were asked whether they had obtained their medicines and understood how to take them. Patients receiving the phone call returned to the ED less often than those who did not (10% vs. 24% at 30 days). Another randomized study examined the effect of pharmacists counseling patients at hospital discharge, and calling 3 to 5 days later. Patients receiving the intervention showed a lower rate of preventable adverse drug events 1 month after hospital discharge. The process of medication reconciliation (discussed below), conducted by pharmacists, was tested in a preintervention/postintervention study involving patients who resided at a nursing home, were hospitalized, and subsequently discharged back to the nursing facility. After the intervention began a pharmacist reconciled the nursing home and hospital medication lists, and reported discrepancies to patients' physicians. Compared to the preintervention group, the postintervention group showed significantly reduced odds of suffering discrepancy-related adverse drug events (odds ratio 0.11, $p = 0.05$).

Use of electronic methods to transfer patient information between various sites of care (e.g., hospitals, nursing facilities, EDs) is being piloted in a number of locations. Preliminary reports suggest these methods may improve outcomes, such as reducing the number of hospital readmissions. Although these approaches present challenges (nursing homes would need to master electronic interfaces and equipment and to use federally endorsed standards), they appear promising.

ROLES AND RESPONSIBILITIES

A crucial first step in making systematic improvements in transitional care is for the various parties in this activity—the team of

TABLE 16-5

Roles and Responsibilities in Transitional Care

Sending Team
- Ensures that patient is clinically stable for transfer
- Confirms the receiving venue can meet patient's medical, nursing, and rehabilitation needs
- Ensures that patient/caregiver understand purpose of transfer
- Communicates necessary information (e.g. via transfer summary) to receiving team in a timely manner
- Ensures recommendations from consulting physicians and other professionals (e.g., social work, occupational therapy, physical therapy, clinical pharmacy, psychology) are transmitted to receiving team
- Arranges and communicates timely follow-up appointments with appropriate health care professionals
- Is available for questions after transfer (and provides contact information)

Receiving Team
- Reviews transfer information and orders prior to or upon patient's arrival
- Identifies and clarifies discrepancies or questions (regarding patient's status, goals, care plan, etc.) directly with sending care team

Both Sending and Receiving Teams
- Begin planning for next transition at time of admission to own setting
- Elicit goals and preferences from patient/caregivers, and incorporates these into care plan
- Identify patient's system of social support
- Determine current and baseline level of function
- Use preferred mode of communication (phone, fax, e-mail, etc.) for professionals in other care settings.

Patient/Family/Caregiver
- Participates in decisions about transfer destination and purpose
- Knows whom to contact (and how) if questions arise during transfer
- Understands which medications to take, how to take them, why they have been prescribed, and potential side effects. Has a "system" for organizing and taking medications
- Is knowledgeable about their major health conditions, knows which symptoms to watch out for, and whom to call should they arise
- Asks questions of doctor or nurse before transfer from current location
- Understands follow-up arrangements with next provider or with primary provider

From Coleman EA. Aspen Transitional Care Conference proceedings.

clinicians sending a patient to a new setting, the receiving team, and the patient (and family)—to clearly understand their respective roles and responsibilities. As shown in Table 16-5, certain responsibilities belong to one party alone, but some are common or shared.

When the sending team plans to transfer a patient from a higher-acuity to a lower-acuity setting, it is incumbent on them to make a determination that the patient is clinically stable for the move. Predictors of instability for patients leaving a hospital include new incontinence, chest pain, dyspnea, or confusion; pronounced vital sign abnormalities, including fever and oxygen desaturation; poor oral intake; and wound infection. The sending team is also obliged to confirm that the new setting can meet the patient's needs for medical, nursing, and rehabilitative care. The sending team has several communication responsibilities. First, they must explain the purpose of the transfer and confirm that the patient (or caregiver) understands. Second, they must communicate essential information (described further below) to the receiving team and in a timely manner. This information includes recommendations made by consulting physicians and other health professionals of various disciplines. The sending team arranges follow-up appointments (e.g., with primary care providers, surgeons, consulting physicians), and notifies the patient, family, and receiving team. The sending team must provide contact information and be available for questions (from receiving team, patient, family) after transfer.

The receiving team has two general responsibilities in the transfer process. First, before or at the time of the patient's arrival, they must review the information and orders transmitted by the sending team. Second, after this review, and after their independent evaluation of the patient, they should identify any questions or discrepancies, and contact the sending team for assistance. An expected but missing beta-blocker on the medication list, for example, may represent an oversight or a deliberate decision.

A number of responsibilities are common to both the sending and receiving teams of clinicians. Both teams should begin planning for transfer of the patient at the time of admission to their own setting. Both elicit care goals and preferences (e.g., recovery of function, "comfort care") from patients and families, and incorporate these into the care plan at their own setting. Both must identify their patients' social support (family, friends, church group, etc.), and surrogate decision makers. Both must determine their patients' baseline and current functional abilities, including activities of daily living and mobility. And both should attempt to employ the mode of communication (phone, fax, e-mail) preferred by clinicians in other care settings.

The division of these responsibilities among various disciplines (medicine, nursing, pharmacy, for example) on a team at a given setting divide will depend on local custom and capabilities. An organization choosing to launch a quality improvement program in care transitions might begin by convening a meeting of leaders of various disciplines, clarifying responsibilities, and obtaining commitments to fill the roles listed in Table 16-5.

Patients and families have important responsibilities as well. They need to participate in discussions with clinicians about the destination and purpose of contemplated transfers. They should keep a record of whom to contact if questions come up during or after their transfer. They need a basic understanding of their medication regimen—which drugs are on the list and why, how to take them, what side effects to watch for—as well as a system (such as a pillbox) for organizing them. Similarly, they must have a good understanding of their major health conditions, including what symptoms constitute "red flags" that should be reported, and to whom. Patients and families should remember or write down questions they should pose to their doctor or nurse before transfer. Finally, they should note and understand the follow-up arrangements that have been made for the next provider, their primary provider, and consultants.

STRATEGIES FOR EXCELLING AT TRANSITIONAL CARE

Clinical teams or organizations endeavoring to provide outstanding transitional care first need consensus about the information that must be transmitted to the next care setting along with each patient. Table 16-6 offers a list of essential data elements in nine domains. Although it is not necessary or customary for clinicians to transmit each indicated piece of information, sending organizations should assign some member of the clinical team the responsibility for communicating each item.

Overall care goals refers to what the patient and family hope to accomplish at the new care setting. Examples of general goals include recovery from an acute illness, followed by return to the previous residence; custodial care for the remainder of the patient's life; or hospice care.

TABLE 16-6

Essential Information to be Passed to New Care Setting	
DOMAIN	**INFORMATION**
Overall care goals	E.g., recovery of previous function with return to community versus maintenance of comfort
Medical	Admitting medical problems and others complicating management Status of these problems and prognosis
Functional	Baseline and current basic and instrumental activities of daily living; mobility
Treatments	Comprehensive medication list Drug allergies, intolerances, adverse effects history Physical therapy, occupational therapy, speech therapy, psychology, etc.
Social background and support	Primary caregiver (name, relationship, contact information) Ability and willingness to provide ongoing care Community-level support Patient's previous residence
Communication and Culture	Language, literacy, health beliefs
Advance directives	Preferences (e.g., for CPR, ventilator support, artificial nutrition/hydration, dialysis) Power of attorney
Durable medical equipment	Current needs, vendor's name and contact information
Coverage/benefits/ insurance/suppliers	Provider network for SNFs, home health agencies, hospice, respite, durable medical equipment

CPR, cardiopulmonary resuscitation; SNF, skilled nursing facility.

Medical information comprises the bulk of a typical hospital discharge summary, with an enumeration of the patient's various diagnoses, how they were treated, and how the patient fared.

Functional information includes the patient's self-care abilities (basic and instrumental activities of daily living), mobility, need for assistance, and assistive devices.

Treatments include a listing of the scheduled and as-needed medications, history of drug-related ill effects, and recommended nonpharmacogic therapies to be provided at the new setting (rehabilitative, psychological, etc.).

Social background and support provides vital background information about the patient's family and/or caregivers, their willingness to provide assistance to the patient, the presence of additional help from the community (e.g., from church groups), and the patient's previous (and ultimate) residence.

Communication and culture refers to important aspects of how patients comprehend health-related information and make decisions about their care. If a patient's primary language is other than English, this formation needs to be passed along. Low levels of literacy, if known, also should be communicated so that the receiving team does not provide written materials without the necessary assistance. Health beliefs (for example, a fatalistic view about stroke risk in a patient with atrial fibrillation) and decision-making style (for example, all major decisions are discussed with adult children) should be documented as well.

Advance directives must accompany patients to new care venues. These may be as simple as the designation of a surrogate, such as a durable power of attorney for health care, or may be more involved, such as instructions regarding the use of life-supporting technologies or resuscitation attempts.

Patients frequently need specialized *durable medical equipment* at their new site of care. Examples might include wound vacuum devices for use in the nursing home or provision of a hospital bed at home. Although not typically spelled out in detail by physicians, this information (devices, vendors' names) should be provided by the responsible disciplines at the sending institution.

Physicians also are unlikely to provide the receiving team or institution with information about details of *insurance benefits and coverage*, home health agencies, or provider networks. This responsibility should be assumed by a defined member of the sending team.

A succinct yet informative transfer summary is an important component of good transitional care. We offer as an example Table 16-7, a hospital discharge summary for a representative 85-year-old woman admitted for pneumonia. Several features of this model summary are worth noting. First, the discharge diagnoses list not only the usual medical problems (pneumonia, diabetes, and so forth), but also cognitive diagnoses (dementia from Alzheimer's disease), behavioral problems ("sundowning"), affective disorders (depression), and functional problems (gait disorder with history of falls). The Hospital Course portion of the summary includes multiple, brief, problem-labeled paragraphs; this format has been shown to be preferred to a chronological recollection of the hospital stay. The discharge instructions include red flags to watch for (worsening dyspnea, fatigue, etc.), as well as where to call if these problems arise.

The discharge medications section of Table 16-7 contains information that will be essential for the receiving care team, and which too often is neglected in hospital discharge summaries. In addition to the dose, route, and frequency for each drug, an indication is provided. Tapering schedules or stop dates (for drugs like systemic

TABLE 16-7

Sample Hospital Discharge Summary

Patient name: Jane Q. Doe.

Medical record number: 12345678

Admission date: 1-2-07

Discharge date: 1-9-07

Attending physician: Ralph Green, M.D.

Referring physician: Susan Brown, M.D.

Resident physician: Sally White, M.D.

Discharge diagnoses:

Community-acquired pneumonia.

Dementia secondary to Alzheimer's disease.

Delirium, with episodic "sundowning"

Diabetes mellitus, type II

Depressive disorder

Hypertension

Multifactorial gait disorder with falls, due to Parkinson's disease and knee osteoarthritis

Procedures performed during hospitalization:

Right-sided thoracentesis performed by Dr. Steven Gray in Interventional Radiology

Hospital Course:

Mrs. Doe is an 85 yr-old woman who was admitted to the Medical Service on January 2nd for 3 days of worsening dyspnea, cough, confusion, and poor oral intake. Please see the dictated admission note from that date for additional information about her admitting physical examination and laboratory data.

1. Pneumonia. Her admitting chest film showed a right lower lobe infiltrate and right-sided pleural effusion. Blood cultures were sterile, but her admission white cell count was 15 000, and her oxygen saturation was 88% on room air. She was treated with IV ceftriaxone and azithromycin for 6 days before being switched to oral levofloxacin on the day before discharge. A modified barium swallow showed no evidence of aspiration. Thoracentesis showed her right-sided effusion to be exudative. Culture of the pleural fluid is no-growth. Oxygenation on the morning of discharge was 94% on room air.

2. Delirium. Mrs. Doe was oriented to her own name at admission, and showed episodes of verbal aggressiveness early during her stay. By hospital day five she had returned to baseline (oriented to self and place). Haloperidol was used as needed the first three days of her admission.

3. Diabetes. To reduce the risk of lactic acidosis, her outpatient drug, metformin, was held. She required minimal doses of sliding scale regular insulin to maintain glucose under 140. We will leave it to her outpatient physician whether to start an alternate oral diabetic agent.

4. Gait disorder (see below). Physical therapy evaluated Mrs. Doe for gait and balance training, and has recommended that she employ a wheeled walker. Physical therapy instructed her on its use. Prosthetics provided her with a walker at discharge.

5. Parkinson's disease. Her carbidopa/levodopa was continued without change in dose from the outpatient setting.

6. Knee osteoarthritis. We urged her to discontinue use of ibuprofen, and she agreed to try scheduled acetaminophen.

7. Hypertension. Hydrochlorothiazide was continued without change.

Discharge instructions: Mrs. Doe should resume her previous diet (prudent diabetic) and employ her new walker when ambulating. If she experiences worsening dyspnea, fatigue, confusion, or reduced oral intake, her daughter Kate agrees to call the Medical Clinic at 555–1234.

Discharge medications:

Drug	Dosing	Indications	Remarks
Levofloxacin	250 mg PO qd	Pneumonia	Last dose 1/15/07
Citalopram	40 mg PO qd	Depression	Unchanged from outpatient
HCTZ	12.5 mg PO qd	Hypertension	Unchanged from outpatient
Carbidopa/levodopa (25/100)	One tab PO qid	Parkinson's disease	Unchanged from outpatient
Acetaminophen	650 mg PO qid	Knee arthritis	New

Note that metformin and ibuprofen (previously in outpatient regimen) have been *stopped.*

Rehabilitation orders: The hospital team has deemed Mrs. Doe to be homebound. She will be seen in her home by visiting nursing, and we have asked for an in-home physical therapy assessment by the agency as well.

Follow-up appointments: With primary care physician Dr. Brown on 1/16/07 at 2 pm, and with neurologist Dr. Black on 2/1/07 at 10 am.

Pending laboratory studies: Await final cytology reading on pleural fluid specimen.

Family/caregiver/surrogate decision maker: Patient's daughter, Kate, lives with her and is her durable power of attorney for health care. Kate's cell phone is 555–0000.

Goals/Preferred Intensity of Care/Code Status: We reviewed Mrs. Doe's overall prognosis, in light of her moderate Alzheimer's disease, comorbidities, and functional status. Kate took part in the conversation as well. They still desire that Mrs. Doe be "full code" in the event of cardiopulmonary arrest, but they are very clear that she would not wish to receive artificial nutrition and hydration in the event of end-stage dementia.

Functional status at transfer: (see also Nursing documentation) Requires assistance with bathing and dressing; now employing wheeled walker to ambulate.

Dictated by: Sally White, M.D.

CC: Susan Brown, M.D.

TABLE 16-8

Information for the Preadmission Medication History

- Which medications taken at which times
- Identities of prescribing providers
- Identities of pharmacies dispensing medications
- Non-oral medications used (eye drops, suppositories, patches, inhalers, creams, etc.)
- Assessment of patient's (or caregiver's) understanding of drug indications
- OTCs and herbals/vitamins/supplements
- Allergies and adverse drug reactions history
- Assessment of adherence (e.g., number of doses missed per week)
- How patient (or caregiver) manages the regimen at home (e.g., use of pill box)

OTCs, over-the-counter medications.

TABLE 16-9

Items to Fax or E-mail to Primary Care Provider Upon Hospital Discharge

- Discharge diagnoses
- Discharge medications
- Results of major tests and procedures
- Tests still pending
- Follow-up arrangements, and ideal follow-up interval
- Contingency plans
  - What may go wrong, and what to do
  - Immediate follow-up needs at first posthospital visit

From Kripalani S, Jackson AT, Schnipper JL, et al. Promoting effective transitions of care at hospital discharge: a review of the literature. J Hosp Med 2007;2(5):314–323.

corticosteroids, antibiotics, or anticoagulants) are given as needed. Finally, the transfer medication list is *reconciled* with the regimen at entry to the facility. In the case of a hospital discharge, the discharge medication list would be compared to the patient's earlier outpatient list. Properly performed, medication reconciliation answers three questions: (a) Which of the patient's transfer medications are new, that is, were not taken until after the patient was admitted to the current venue? (b) Which of the patient's previous medications are to be stopped? (c) For those medications that have been continued from the earlier setting, which doses have changed?

A well-reconciled discharge medication regimen requires complete understanding of the preadmission regimen. Table 16-8 lists components of a thorough preadmission medication history. This includes not only information that is essential for the subsequent reconciliation (drugs, doses, use of over-the-counter remedies and herbals, etc.), but other beneficial items like identities of prescribing providers and pharmacies, assessment of the patient's understanding of the regimen, impression of adherence to the prescribed regimen, method of administration at home (pill boxes, etc.), history of adverse drug reactions, indication, and consideration of continued need.

Some additional important sections follow the discharge medications list in Table 16-7. Follow-up appointments, arranged before transfer, spell out which provider is to be seen and when. Pending laboratory studies highlight tests whose results are still outstanding. This situation occurs more frequently with short lengths of stay. The specification of caregiver/surrogate decision maker and of goals/preferred intensity of care in Table 16-7 illustrates how this information (called for in Table 16-6) might be spelled out in practice to good effect. Finally, information on functional status at transfer is typically provided in greater detail by documents prepared by nursing and rehabilitation disciplines, but deserves mention in a synthesized way by the physician as well.

Hospital discharge summaries ideally are available for review by the next care team or primary care clinician before their encounter with the discharged patient. Unfortunately, these summaries all too often fail to reach primary providers in a timely manner. To assure that these providers have access to vital information about their patients at the time of hospital discharge, we recommend that certain information (Table 16-9) be faxed or e-mailed by hospital providers. At the time of hospital discharge, a patient's primary provider should be apprised of the discharge diagnoses (with emphasis on the reason for the hospitalization), the complete list of discharge medications,

results of major tests, a listing of tests that have been done but whose results are still outstanding (biopsy results, for example), and follow-up arrangements (especially those involving the primary provider and visiting nursing). A couple of other items also deserve inclusion in this abbreviated summary and may require a bit of thought on the part of the transferring clinicians. First, given what is known about the patient in question, what problems might arise soon after discharge, related perhaps to potential disease exacerbations or family dynamics? What action might be taken if these problems occur? Second, which issues will require follow-up attention at the first postacute visit?

Up to this point, we have emphasized communications between sending and receiving clinicians involved in a transfer. Excellent transitional care requires that effective communication take place with the patient (or caregiver) as well. Table 16-10 lists informational items that must be communicated to the patient, as well as tips on performing this function. It is not necessary that all these items be communicated by a physician—some might better be discussed by nursing or pharmacy personnel—but leaders in the transferring organization should assure that lines of responsibility are clear. Because of variations in the health literacy of patients and their families, transfer instructions should be provided at about a 6th grade level.

Important new diagnoses (particularly those that precipitated an acute illness episode) should be shared with the patient around the time of discharge, if this has not occurred already. The discharge

TABLE 16-10

Communications with Patient/Caregiver at Time of Transfer

- Review important discharge diagnoses.
- Review the reconciled medication list.
- Review possible adverse effects of medications.
- Discuss necessary activity limitations (e.g., joint range-of-motion, showering).
- Share functional prognosis, if known.
- Review worrisome signs/symptoms or red flags, along with whom to contact.
- Discuss what to expect at any new site of care.
- Review new self-care tasks (e.g., wound care, fingerstick glucose testing).
- Review dates of follow-up.
- Minimize jargon.
- Provide written materials.
- Check for understanding (have patient repeat back what she has heard; have her demonstrate important self-care tasks).
- Finish with "What questions about your transfer can I answer?", and make time to answer these.

medication list should also be reviewed, including the indications for the drugs, the changes made from the regimen the patient had followed before, and potential adverse drug reactions. Important limitations in the patient's activity, such as physical exertion or bathing concerns, should be discussed. Patients and families should be apprised of functional prognoses: "I think you have a good chance of getting back to your previous ability to walk around your home after about four to six weeks of rehabilitation at the nursing facility." Signs or symptoms that may signal early trouble should be related, along with information on what the patient should do should they arise. Important follow-up appointments (with primary providers, surgeons, or specialists) should be made and communicated to patient and family.

If the patient is headed to a new care venue, such as a SNF, it is helpful to say a few words about what to expect there: "You will not be seeing your doctor or nurse practitioner at the rehabilitation center as often as you have in the hospital, particularly if things are progressing well. The emphasis there will be much more on rehabilitation. You and the therapy staff will be working hard to recover your ability to walk like before and take care of yourself." Important self-care tasks, such as wound care techniques or glucose self-monitoring, must be taught or reviewed prior to discharge. To confirm that patients and families are learning what they need to know, clinical personnel should check for understanding by having them repeat back what they have heard and by demonstrating the requisite self-care skills: "Just to be sure I have done a good job of teaching you how to change this dressing, let's have you try it now."

A great deal of information is transmitted by clinicians to patients and families around the time of transfer. Some communication routines may help to maximize the chances that this information is understood and remembered. First, information and instructions should be given in lay language: avoid jargon and Latin abbreviations. Second, written materials should be provided for later review and reference. Finally, at the completion of the discharge instructions, the patient and family should be asked, "What questions about your transfer can I answer?"

The Care Transitions Intervention, discussed earlier, was specifically designed to be low-intensity, low-cost, and brief in duration. One particular strategy was the encouragement of patient "ownership" over core elements of their medical history through the use of a portable personal health record. This record included medical diagnoses, current medications, allergies, and primary care providers. A second strategy was the employment of Transition Coaches. Several leading health care organizations, operating under different financial structures, have adopted the Care Transitions Intervention.

Clinician leaders (e.g., chiefs of medical staff) and managers of health care organizations may wish to employ well-established methods of quality improvement to foster better transitional care. One such method involves the collection of vital process data—such as the fraction of discharge summaries that include a reconciled medication list, the fraction of discharged patients who were given follow-up appointments, or patient satisfaction survey data—and the use of these data in Deming cycles (Plan-Do-Study-Act) designed to improve the studied measure. Another method is the use of regular "customer–supplier" exchanges. Regularly scheduled meetings between representatives of hospitals and postacute nursing homes, or between hospitalists and primary providers, allow for the identification of interface concerns, prioritization of improvement efforts, and the nurturing of improved communication and rapport.

SPECIAL CASES OF CARE TRANSITIONS

More than a quarter of nursing home residents are transferred each year at least once to an ED for urgent evaluation. These transfers are often perilous given their urgency, the difficulties of many nursing home residents in recalling and relating their history, and the problems of reaching families or surrogate decision makers. Conversely, when nursing home residents return, facility staff often report confusion about diagnostic findings or therapeutic recommendations from the ED. A recent study reported on the results of focus groups involving nursing home staff, ED personnel, and emergency medical services providers. Table 16-11 summarizes the authors' findings on recommended information exchange between health professionals working in the two care settings. ED personnel need to know the reason for transfer, as well as whom to contact at the nursing facility for additional information. The patient's physician (with contact information) should be identified. Important clinical information the ED will need includes the patient's past medical history, medications and drug allergies, baseline cognitive and physical function, latest vital signs, and recent laboratory and x-ray results. Advance directives and surrogate decision maker or family contact are vital as well. Finally, in the event that the ED is contemplating a return of the patient to the nursing facility with new orders, it will be important for ED providers to be made aware of the capabilities of the facility to provide technical or nursing-intensive care, such as intravenous medication administration. Nursing home leaders (medical directors or directors of nursing) may wish to create a blank form listing the items from Table 16-11, and assure that nurses who transfer patients for emergency evaluation complete the form and send along photocopies of related documents.

TABLE 16-11

Information Exchange Between Nursing Homes and Emergency Departments

Information from Nursing Home to Emergency Department
- Name and contact information for nursing home
- Physician's name and contact information
- Patient's demographics (name, age, birthdate)
- Reason for transfer to emergency department
- Past medical history
- Medications and allergies
- Baseline cognitive and physical function
- Advance directives ("code status", living will)
- Power of attorney or family contact
- Most recent vital signs
- Recent laboratory and radiologic results
- Nursing home capabilities (e.g., wound care, IV antibiotics)

Information from Emergency Department to Nursing Home Providers
- Working diagnosis from emergency department
- Treatment provided by the emergency department
- Emergency department vital signs
- Tests performed, with results
- Pending results, with plans for transmission to nursing home staff
- Recommendations for further treatment
- Legible copy of emergency department chart, including consultants' notes
- Contact information for any outpatient follow-up

From Terrell KM, Miller DK. Challenges in transitional care between nursing homes and emergency departments. J Am Med Dir Assoc. 2006;7:499.

Information needed by nursing home personnel when residents return from the ED includes the working diagnosis rendered by emergency personnel, vital signs from the ED, results of testing performed there, treatment provided in the ED, and recommendations for further treatment or follow-up. A legible copy of the chart from the ED is generally essential. Just as nursing facility leaders may implement a standardized transfer form for patients sent to the ED, leaders from emergency medicine and nursing may institute their own transfer-back-to-nursing-home form or checklist, and employ quality improvement methods to confirm that the needed information is reliably transmitted.

Another common transition involving older patients is the admission to the program of a home health nursing agency. As with transfers between nursing homes and EDs, it is helpful to employ a checklist (Table 16-12) of informational items that the home nursing agency will need. Much of this is "the usual"—provider name and contact information, patient name and demographics, medical history and problem list, medication list and drug allergies, functional status, advance directives, and names of surrogate decision makers. A few items are more peculiar to the home care setting. First, if the home health program services are to be covered by Medicare, it will be important to specify the skilled care needs and to state that the patient meets "homebound" criteria. Second, what are the goals of care that the nursing personnel should keep in mind? Articulating these will not only help to prioritize their work, but will indicate when discharge from their program is appropriate. Third, what are the clinical and psychosocial issues (e.g., laboratory values, functional improvements) that are to be reported?

A third common care transition involving elders is the handoff of the hospitalized patient from one physician to another, such as for night or weekend coverage. Solet and coworkers reviewed the literature on such handoffs (few high-quality studies exist), and evaluated the handoff process at the four hospitals staffed by one Midwestern internal medicine residency program. Based on their work, they make four overall recommendations. First, handoffs of hospitalized patients should generally be made face to face, to allow the doctor assuming care of the patients to ask questions, to practice read-back skills, and to register nonverbal information such as facial expression, tone of voice, and body language. Second, the format for information transfer should be highly standardized. Third, the skill of handing off the care of complex and potentially unstable patients to another provider needs to be explicitly taught. And fourth, handoff skills need to be practiced repetitively, as is done by professionals in other

high-risk occupations, such as air traffic handling. We believe these are reasonable recommendations, based on the information available to date, and we also endorse the authors' list of essential elements that should be passed on at the time of handoff. These elements include: patient identification, location, date of admission, a brief synopsis of the patient's admitting presentation, a list of currently active and pertinent past medical problems, medications and drug allergies, venous access (and how important it is that this be maintained), code status, key laboratory data, foreseeable problems with recommended contingency plans, and psychosocial concerns. Some or all of this information should be transmitted in written or electronic form (via computer or personal data assistant) as well as orally.

EDUCATING PROFESSIONALS IN CARE TRANSITIONS

Educational scholarship in the field of transitional care is at an embryonic stage. Reports of needs assessments have been few in number and have involved small sample sizes. One such assessment employed focus groups and surveys to determine the educational needs in geriatrics for medical students and internal medicine residents. Trainees perceived training gaps in four major areas; one of these was in transitional care (primarily involving discharge from the hospital). Another needs assessment performed at a single internal medicine residency of an academic medical center found that house staff received little instruction in, or role modeling of, good transitional care; that residents learned to create better discharge summaries primarily from experience; and that resident-generated discharge summaries demonstrated a need for improved format and information content.

Few reports are available describing transitional care educational interventions and their effects. Some medical schools are beginning to incorporate the topic into their curriculum using teaching methodologies such as lectures, video, group discussions, and interdisciplinary exercises. A number of residencies have also incorporated instruction on the subject, primarily on how to compose a proper hospital discharge summary. Educational techniques have included didactic instruction, individualized feedback to residents, and technologies that permit the incremental preparation of discharge summaries during a patient's hospital course.

Although we cannot (yet) cite studies to support our views, we believe that trainees will receive improved transitions education if a few approaches are adopted. First, attending physicians should be role models for excellence in this area. They should demonstrate mastery of the assessment and communication skills required to manage care transitions. Increased faculty development efforts at many centers will probably be required to assure that teaching faculty members master the needed skills. Second, attending physicians must evaluate their learners for transitional care performance, provide generous and specific feedback, and incorporate their assessments into learners' end-of-rotation formal evaluations. Third, transitional care topics should be incorporated into teaching conferences. One natural place to do so is the "M&M" (morbidity and mortality) conference. While usually a forum to discuss cases in which a patient suffered from a hard-to-diagnose malady, or in which some procedural misfortune ensued, the M&M conference presents an opportunity to dissect a systems breakdown, such as a fumbled patient handoff.

TABLE 16-12

Information Needed by Home Health Nursing for Patients Admitted to Their Care

- Name of physician overseeing care, with contact information and preferred mode of communication
- Patient name and demographics
- Medicare: Skilled care needs? Homebound?
- Past medical history, medications, allergies
- Cognitive and physical function
- Advance directives, surrogate decision makers
- Overall goals of care and preliminary care plan
- Issues to monitor and report

An indication that a training program has succeeded in incorporating transitional care into its curriculum is that its trainees give as much effort and thought to patient transfers as they do to admissions.

SUMMARY

A confluence of trends in American health care is pushing transitional care quality onto the agendas of professional leaders, certifying and regulatory bodies, third-party payers, and patient advocacy groups. Well-executed transitional care is patient-centered and improves patient safety. Given the aging of the population, the accretion of chronic medical and functional problems, the specialization of care venues, the pressure to reduce lengths of stay, and increasing disincentives for many clinicians to provide care across a continuum of settings, transitional care will only grow in prominence.

Research has shown that older patients and members of other vulnerable populations are most likely to suffer mishaps during handoffs of care. Nevertheless, we are learning which approaches and techniques seem to improve the odds of good outcomes. There is a growing consensus about what informational elements should be transmitted to patients, families, and the next team of providers. Empowering patients and their caregivers is vital. Employing professionals, such as transition coaches, whose role definition includes navigating patients through the health care system, has proven beneficial. And providing explicit, dedicated training in care transitions to physicians, physician assistants, nurse practitioners, nurses, and pharmacists is imperative.

Yet substantial improvement in the quality of American health care transitions will require a combination of approaches and strategies. First, the scientific foundation for the field is still being constructed, and important research questions abound. What are the best measures of transitional care quality? Which factors predict transitions mishaps? Which transitional care interventions are beneficial and cost-effective?

Second, a commitment to improve care transitions creates a demand for educating the professionals who plan and execute these transitions. Health professions educators will need to incorporate the topic into an already crowded curriculum. Particularly challenging is that the best method for teaching the subject may require a genuinely interdisciplinary approach.

Finally, a refined scientific database at the disposal of committed and energetic teachers may only yield improvement around the edges. Health care professionals, being human, still respond to the mix of incentives and disincentives they face. The fee-for-service model that dominates provider payment in the United States hinders efforts at providing coordinated care for patients. Whether substantial and widespread improvements in transitional care can occur in the United States without extensive modifications of the payment system is open to doubt.

FURTHER READING

Coleman EA. Falling through the cracks: challenges and opportunities for improving transitional care for persons with continuous complex care needs. *J Am Geriatr Soc.* 2003;51:549.

Coleman EA. Aspen Transitional Care Conference proceedings. http://www.uchsc.edu/hcpr/documents/AspenTransitionProceedings.pdf Accessed March 10, 2007.

Coleman EA and Boult C. The American Geriatrics Society Health Care Systems Committee: improving the quality of transitional care for persons with complex care needs. *J Am Geriatr Soc.* 2003;51:556.

Coleman EA and Fox PD. One patient, many places: managing health care transitions, Part I: introduction, accountability, information for patients in transition. *Ann. Long-Term Care.* 2004;12(9):25.

Coleman EA, Min SJ, Chomiak A, et al. Posthospital care transitions: patterns, complications, and risk identification. *Health Serv Res,* 2004;39(5):1449.

Coleman EA, Parry C, Chalmers S, et al. The Care Transitions Intervention: results of a randomized controlled trial. *Arch Intern Med.* 2006;166:1822.

Coleman EA, Smith JD, Frank JC, et al. Development and testing of a measure designed to assess the quality of care transitions. *Int J Integr Care* [online]. 2002;2 Jun 1. www.ijic.org

Drickamer MA, Levy B, Irwin KS, et al. Perceived needs for geriatric education by medical students, internal medicine residents, and faculty. *J Gen Intern Med.* 2006;21(12):1230.

Dudas V, Bookwalter T, Kerr KM, et al. The impact of follow-up telephone calls to patients after hospitalization. *Am J Med.* 2001;111(9B):26S.

Halasyamani L, Kripalani S, Coleman E, et al. Transition of care for hospitalized elderly patients—development of a discharge checklist for hospitalists. *J Hosp Med.* 2006;1:354.

Kind AJH, Smith MA, Frytak JR, et al. Bouncing back: patterns and predictors of complicated transitions 30 days after hospitalization for acute ischemic stroke. *J Am Geriatr Soc.* 2007;55:365.

Kripalani S, LeFevre F, Phillips CO, et al. Deficits in communication and information transfer between hospital-based and primary care physicians: implications for patient safety and continuity of care. *JAMA.* 2007;297:831.

Kripalani S, Jackson AT, Schnipper JL, et al. Promoting effective transitions of care at hospital discharge: a review of the literature. *J Hosp Med* 2007;2(5):314–323.

Moore C, Wisnivesky J, Williams S, et al. Medical errors related to discontinuity of care from an inpatient to an outpatient setting. *J Gen Intern Med.* 2003;18:646.

Naylor MD, Brooten D, Campbell R, et al. Comprehensive discharge planning and home follow-up of hospitalized elders: a randomized clinical trial. *JAMA.* 1999;281:613.

Rich MW, Beckham V, Wittenberg C, et al. A multidisciplinary intervention to prevent the readmission of elderly patients with congestive heart failure. *N Engl J Med.* 1995;333:1190.

Roy CL, Poon EG, Karson AS, et al. Patient safety concerns arising from test results that return after hospital discharge. *Ann Intern Med.* 2005;143(2):121.

Schnipper JL, Kirwin JL, Cotugno MC, et al. Role of pharmacist counseling in preventing adverse drug events after hospitalization. *Arch Intern Med.* 2006;166(5):565.

Solet DJ, Norvell JM, Rutan GH, et al. Lost in translation: challenges and opportunities in physician-to-physician communication during patient handoffs. *Acad Med.* 2005;80:1094.

Terrell KM and Miller DK. Challenges in transitional care between nursing homes and emergency departments. *J Am Med Dir Assoc.* 2006;7:499.

Terrell KM and Miller DK. Critical review of transitional care between nursing homes and emergency departments. *Ann. Long-Term Care Clinical Care Aging.* 2007;15(2):33.

Web Sites

www.caretransitions.org

www.hospitalmedicine.org (visit the "Resource Center")

Acute Hospital Care

Scott A. Flanders ■ *Paula M. Podrazik*
■ *Chad Whelan* ■ *Caroline Blaum*

The nearly 25% of adults 65 years and older who are hospitalized each year represents a higher proportion than for any other age group. Many of these older adults experience protracted or permanent functional decline and worsening health after their acute hospital stay. Although people 65 years and older comprise only about 12% of the U.S. population, they account for one-third of acute hospital admissions and about 46% of the national costs for acute hospital care.

National data show that older hospitalized patients have a more complex hospital course than younger hospitalized patients (Table 17-1). In 2003, the length of stay for patients 65 years and older was 1.7 days longer than for those under 65 years old, although the length of stay for the major discharge diagnoses has dropped since 1997. The mean total hospital costs were 46% higher for the 65 years and older group compared with the younger group. Hospital costs for older patients have increased over 25% since 1997. Although hospital deaths are decreasing, people 65 years and older have nearly five times the in-hospital mortality as younger hospitalized patients.

While many principles of acute hospital care are the same for all age groups, the elderly patient population is at increased risk of collecting comorbidities and accompanying medications, functional decline, cognitive impairment, and dwindling social supports. Therefore, there are several issues related to the hospital admission, hospital stay, and discharge that deserve specific attention when considering the care of the geriatric population. The care of hospitalized elders requires a systematic approach to the evaluation and management of commonly seen geriatric conditions and perhaps implementation of structural changes specifically designed to address the needs of this often medically complex and potentially vulnerable population.

HOSPITAL ADMISSION

Reasons for Admission for Geriatric Patients

The major diagnoses for which older adults are hospitalized are related to chronic diseases and respiratory conditions. The 15 most common conditions, accounting for 48% of the hospital admission diagnoses, are listed in Table 17-2. Also common and important to recognize, but less likely to be reported as the reason for admission, are conditions more likely to occur in older adults such as failure to thrive, falls, adverse drug effects, or change in mental status. In addition, older adults maybe admitted with an atypical presentation of another condition, such as when change in mental status is due to underlying fluid and electrolyte disorder or urinary tract infection (UTI). Often the reported diagnosis for a hospitalized older patient may not fully capture the underlying reasons that necessitated the admission and does not explain the hospital course and subsequent health status of the patient. While many of the 15 most frequent conditions reported as causes for hospitalizations among older adults represent acute exacerbations of chronic diseases, the reasons why a stable older adult with heart failure suddenly decompensates or a 90-year-old assisted living resident is admitted with a broken hip, often relate as much to the physical and/or social vulnerability of many older adults as to their complex health status.

In addition to the primary problems that led to the admission, the effect of comorbid chronic diseases must be considered. Over 60% of Medicare patients have two or more major chronic diseases and 24% have four or more. In 2004, people 65 years and older admitted to the hospital had an average of 2.3 comorbid conditions. Comorbid chronic diseases have several consequences for the hospitalized

TABLE 17-1

Characteristics of Hospitalizations Among Nonelderly and Elderly Populations, 2003

	YOUNGER THAN 65 YR	65 YR AND OLDER
Percentage of U.S. population	88%	12%
Percent of hospital stays	65.3%	34.7%
Mean length of stay (days)	4.0	5.7
Admitted through emergency department (%)	36.2%	57.4%
Died in hospital (%)	0.9%	4.7%

Source: AHRQ, Center for Delivery, Organization, and Markets, Healthcare Cost and Utilization project, Nationwide Inpatient Sample, 2003.

TABLE 17-2

Most Frequent Conditions Causing Hospitalizations among Older Patients, 2003

RANK	PRINCIPAL DIAGNOSIS	% OF ALL HOSPITALIZATIONS IN OLDER ADULTS
1	Heart failure	6.3
2	Pneumonia	5.8
3	Coronary atherosclerosis	5.1
4	Cardiac dysrhythmias	3.7
5	Acute myocardial infarction	3.4
6	Chronic obstructive pulmonary disease	3.1
7	Stroke	3.0
8	Osteoarthritis	2.8
9	Rehabilitation care, fitting prostheses, adjustment of devices	2.5
10	Fluid and electrolyte disorders	2.3
11	Chest pain	2.2
12	Urinary tract infection	2.1
13	Hip fracture	2.1
14	Complication of medical device, implant, or graft	2.0
15	Septicemia	1.9
Total admissions for top 15 conditions	6.4 million	48.3

Source: AHRQ, Center for Delivery, Organization, and Markets, Healthcare Cost and Utilization project, Nationwide Inpatient Sample, 2003.

elder and for the clinician. Multiple diseases often mean multiple outpatient physicians, complicating communication between inpatient and outpatient providers. Multiple diseases lead to the use of multiple medications. Multiple medications, even if indicated, can result in confusion about medications, difficulty with medication reconciliation and drug adherence, and adverse drug events (ADEs) including amplified side effects, drug–drug or drug–disease interactions, and errors in drug administration. A high burden of chronic disease can lead to self-care difficulties, patient and caregiver frustration and burnout, and physiological instability for the patient.

In older patients, especially those 75 years and older, common conditions such as vision or hearing impairment, mobility impairment and fall risk, poor nutrition, incontinence, depression, cognitive impairment, and functional impairment often occur in conjunction with the major chronic diseases that lead to hospital admissions. For example, 2004 data from the Health and Retirement Survey (HRS), a nationally representative health interview survey sponsored by the National Institute on Aging demonstrate that the geriatric conditions of falls and incontinence are common in older adults with heart failure, coronary heart diseases, and diabetes (Table 17-3).

Conditions commonly seen in older patients often labeled as "geriatric" conditions can contribute to the need for the acute ad-

mission, and substantially influence the hospital course and discharge plans. Cognitive impairment, one such geriatric condition, is a major risk for delirium. At admission, it may be impossible to distinguish between delirium and dementia or to determine a patient's baseline cognitive performance. Delirium is associated with longer

TABLE 17-3

Proportion of Respondents aged 65 yrs and Older with Index Disease or Condition Who Have Other Diseases/Conditions*

INDEX DISEASE OR CONDITIONS (% OF TOTAL SAMPLE)	WEIGHTED PERCENTAGES[2]						
	Coronary Disease	Heart Failure	Diabetes	Incontinence	Falls	≥1 Other Condition	≥2 Other Conditions
Coronary Disease (8.7%)		24.1% (20.9–27.6)	30.4% (27.2–33.8)	33.4% (29.3–37.9)	38.6% (35.1–42.3)	72.6% (68.9–76.0)	37.0% (32.9–41.3)
Heart Failure (4.8%)	43.8% (38.6–49.1)		36.5% (31.3–42.0)	36.7% (32.2–41.5)	43.0% (38.3–47.7)	82.2% (77.9–85.9)	49.7% (44.8–54.6)
Diabetes (19.4%)	13.6% (12.1–15.4)	9.0% (7.6–10.6)		28.2% (26.1–30.4)	28.8% (26.7–30.9)	52.4% (49.7–55.1)	20.5% (18.5–22.6)
Incontinence (25.0%)	11.6% (10.2–13.3)	7.0% (6.0–8.3)	21.9% (20.1–23.8)		36.6% (34.6–38.7)	55.0% (52.8–57.1)	16.7% (15.1–18.4)
Falls (23.2%)	14.5% (12.8–16.3)	8.9% (7.6–10.3)	24.0% (22.2–25.9)	39.4% (37.2–41.6)		60.4% (58.2–62.5)	19.9% (18.0–21.9)

*From the Health and Retirement Study, 2004 wave; n = 11 113.

†Weighted percentages are derived using the Health and Retirement Study (HRS) respondent population weights to adjust for the complex sampling design of the HRS survey. Row percentages are shown. For example, among older adults with reported coronary heart disease, 24.1% report heart failure and 38.6% report falls.

hospital length of stay, greater functional disability, and increased mortality following hospitalization. Several prospective studies have documented that hospital mortality is related to nutritional status, cognitive dysfunction, and functional disability. These factors independently predict mortality even when the comorbid diseases and diseases leading to hospitalization are considered.

Often physicians caring for an acutely ill, unstable or unsafe older adult who requires acute hospitalization are advised to identify or "screen" for frailty. There is as yet no universally accepted definition or measure of frailty. The term "frail" tends to be used to refer to an older adult who is physiologically or socially vulnerable. Recently, researchers have tried to develop empiric definitions of frailty, which, while promising, may not yet be clinically applicable. The idea of a vulnerable or at-risk elderly person may be clinically more helpful. The presence of comorbid conditions, functional decline, cognitive impairment, or inadequate or abusive social situations suggests vulnerability. Since functional decline and cognitive impairments increase with age, the advanced age of a patient (e.g., >75 years) may strongly factor into a clinician's decision to "screen" for risk of frailty and perform screens of memory, functional status, hearing, and sight, and take an in-depth social history during the hospitalization. These issues require attention from the admission process through discharge planning and postacute care transitions.

Geriatric conditions can be the reason for admission. Examples include falls or "failure to thrive," defined as poor nutrition and weight loss associated with diseases, dementia, functional disability, and sometimes inadequate caregiving. Assessment of comorbidities and geriatric conditions (e.g., falls, failure to thrive, dementia, urinary incontinence) upon admission and during the hospitalization with simple screening questions and physical evaluation will help the clinician operationalize the ideas of "vulnerable" and frail, and provide targets for therapy such as increased nutrition, physical therapy, glasses, and hearing aids. Social issues, such as inability to buy medications, inadequate caregiving and/or insufficient help at home, elder neglect and abuse, and elder self-neglect are unfortunately relatively common. They can be missed if they are not specifically considered and investigated.

Admission Screening

At the time of admission, much of the focus is on evaluation and management of a disease-specific, perhaps life-threatening illness. However, the admission also provides an opportune time to screen for issues of importance in the care of elderly patients, particularly issues likely to affect the course, treatment, and prognosis of the illness that precipitated the hospitalization. Important components of the admission screen are described.

Communication with Family and Primary Care Providers

While many patients can provide accurate descriptions of their home situations and presenting symptoms, every effort should be made to discuss these issues with family members who can often provide additional information about social issues that may have contributed to admission or who may describe symptoms or events that help clarify the admitting diagnosis. Older patients often present with complex symptoms and atypical presentations of disease requiring increased attention to the factors that led up to the admission. Similarly, the patient's primary outpatient provider of care should be contacted. It is increasingly common for patients to be cared for by inpatient physicians, such as hospitalists, who do not care for patients in the outpatient setting. This means many elderly patients are being "handed-off" at admission. Studies have shown that most primary care providers want to be contacted at admission. Primary providers can help clarify the acute problem and can provide a more complete medical history including other comorbid conditions, previous diagnostic testing, and response to previous treatments. Depending on the reason for admission and the hospital course, communication with the patient's specialist physicians may also be necessary.

Medication Reconciliation

Hospital admission is an important time for medication review. Clarification of the patient's medications, often prescribed by multiple physicians, and identification of potential adverse drug reactions (ADRs) are two important aspects of medication review. ADRs may lead to hospital admission and are more common as numbers of medications and comorbid illness increase. While age alone is not an independent predictor of ADRs, older patients are more likely to have multiple comorbid conditions and be on multiple medications. In addition, there are certain medications or classes of medications that have been identified by expert consensus panels as being at high risk for ADRs in elderly patients with relatively low clinical benefit and often a safer alternative medication exists. These high-risk medications should likewise be identified and discussed with the primary care physician. Careful attention should be paid to medications most likely to lead to ADRs including analgesics, sedatives, cardiovascular medications, and psychoactive drugs. Regulatory bodies, such as the Joint Commission for Accreditation of Healthcare Organizations (JCAHO), are requiring that all institutions have a process in place to reconcile, or review, medication lists for high-risk or unnecessary medications. This process needs to happen throughout the hospitalization, but is especially important at admission. Medication reconciliation is a time-consuming, but important process involving a rigorous review of each medication for appropriateness in conjunction with comorbidities and the other medications the patient is taking and requires discussion with the primary care physician and, often, specialty physicians at the point of discharge for continuity of care, best drug choices, and safety. Aspects of medication reconciliation can be aided by computerized physician order entry systems and clinical pharmacists.

Identify Frailty

While precise definitions of frailty are elusive, studies have shown that patients of advanced age (e.g., >80 years) or with functional impairments are the most vulnerable and should be considered "frail." At least one survey of a general medicine service in an urban medical center estimated 25% of elderly patients were frail or vulnerable, according to the Vulnerable Elderly Survey-13 tool that scores age, self-perceived health, and aspects of functional status to predict increased risk of morbidity and mortality. Frailty puts patients at risk for further functional and cognitive decline, delirium, prolonged hospitalization, increased costs, and mortality. Identification of frailty at admission should alert the hospital physician to the need to further evaluate for dementia and other geriatric conditions and can help frame discussions about prognosis. It also signals the need to start advanced discharge planning.

Functional Screen

Functional measures are stronger predictors of mortality and contribute more to prognosis in the hospitalized older patient than comorbid illness, disease severity, and diagnoses. Assessing activities of daily living (ADLs) and instrumental activities of daily living (IADLs) are well-known measures of functional impairment. The hospital physician should also be comfortable in performing routine assessments of mobility, such as the "Get Up and Go" test (see Chapter 115). Any documented mobility or ADL impairment should trigger physical therapy and/or occupational therapy assessments and should signal the need to institute early mobilization and early institution of discharge planning.

Dementia Screen

Screening for dementia is particularly important in the elderly patient who is losing weight, noncompliant with medications, admitted from a nursing home or readmitted to the hospital. Impaired judgment and insight can impact a patient's ability to make health decisions, discuss end-of-life issues, and live independently after discharge. It also identifies patients at risk for the development of delirium in the hospital and readmission after discharge. While diagnosis of dementia is based on DSM-IV criteria, two common screening tools, the Mini-Mental Status Examination (MMSE) and the Mini-Cog (see Chapters 11 and 12), can be used to quickly identify patients at high risk for dementia. Both tests have similar sensitivities, but the MMSE is the only one to have been validated in the hospital setting, while the Mini-Cog is faster to perform. Impairments on either test should result in active planning for cognitive stimulation during the hospitalization, comprehensive discharge planning instituted at the beginning of the hospital stay, and family/caregiver involvement.

HOSPITAL STAY

Hospitalization presents many hazards for older patients. While the outcome of hospitalization is dependent on the severity and type of acute illness and the patient's baseline vulnerability, elderly patients are at five times increased risk for iatrogenic complications during hospitalization. Older patients have an average 35% risk of functional decline during acute hospitalization. In addition, they are at increased risk for the development of delirium. After discharge, they are at increased risk for needing institutionalization and hospital readmission. While the hospital may be considered "unsafe" for vulnerable elderly patients, hospitalization is often necessary to treat acute illness. Thus, considerable attention must be given to creating a systematic approach to preventing and treating common hospital complications in the geriatric population. This topic has appropriately generated considerable attention recently among researchers, payors, regulatory bodies such as JCAHO and the federal government, as well as patients and their families.

Common Problems in Hospitalized Elderly Patients

Delirium

The incidence of delirium in hospitalized older patients is as high as 50% and is associated with increased mortality, hospital length of stay, and need for placement in long-term care. Because delirium in elderly patients can present atypically (such as the hypoactive form), it often goes unrecognized by physicians and nurses. Understanding risk factors, making the diagnosis, and instituting strategies for prevention of delirium are critical for the hospital physician.

In a study group of patients >70 years old, risk factors for delirium included severe illness, cognitive impairment (MMSE<24), and BUN / Cr ratio $\geq$ 18. Precipitating factors for delirium were use of restraints or a bladder catheter, $\geq$ 3 medications added, an iatrogenic event, and malnutrition (see Chapter 53). Patients at risk for delirium should have targeted strategies to prevent its development. Many institutions have put formal delirium prevention programs into place. These programs are designed to prevent cognitive impairment, sleep deprivation, immobility, dehydration, as well as vision and hearing impairment. The Hospital Elder Life Program (HELP) uses an orientation board and a program of cognitive stimulation to reduce the rate of confusion from 26% to 8%. Even in the absence of a formal program, the hospital physician should have the patient's family stay overnight if possible, remove unnecessary foley catheters, avoid restraints, eliminate unnecessary medications, order early mobilization and visual / hearing aids, and address dehydration. While attention to these issues by individual physicians is important, the case can also be made for a more systematic, interdisciplinary approach.

Over a 6-month period, a community hospital was able to demonstrate a 14% reduction in the rate of delirium and cost savings of over $600,000 for a 40-bed unit by implementing portions of the HELP program. The program showed sustained results including higher nursing and patient satisfaction. This program succeeded despite limited resources that required them to eliminate portions of the original HELP program.

Immobility and Falls

During an acute hospital stay, the older patient is at high-risk for falls. These inpatient falls are not only common, but carry significant risk of short- and long-term adverse effects for the frail elderly patient. Estimates for inpatient falls among all hospitalized patients range from two to seven falls per 1000 patient-days. However, not all hospitalized patients face the same risk. In a single urban academic center, rates for medical patients were significantly higher (6.2 falls/1000 patient days) as compared to surgical patients (2.18 falls/1000 patient days).

Inpatient falls are frequently associated with injury, with estimates of one-third to almost one-half of falls resulting in injuries. Most concerning is that an estimated 8% of falls result in moderate to severe injuries. These falls and injuries are associated with significant in-hospital adverse outcomes. Patients who suffer falls with injury have longer lengths of stay and higher costs than similar patients who do not suffer a fall. In addition to the in-hospital effects, a fall with injury may lead to serious long-term health outcomes as well. Falls among elderly patients with and without injuries are risk factors for increased use of health care resources in the future, functional decline, loss of independence, higher rates of discharge to extended care facilities, and even death.

While all elderly patients are at risk for falling, as the risk of falls increases with age, in hospitalized patients, there are multiple well-described risk factors that can better identify patients at the highest risk (Table 17-4). These risk factors include patient-specific baseline characteristics, patient-specific effects of the acute

TABLE 17-4

Risk Factors for Falling among Hospitalized Patients

Increasing age
History of falls
Dementia/delirium
Visual deficits
Dehydration
Frequent toileting/incontinence
Dizziness
Difficulty in balance, transfers, or walking
Polypharmacy
Use of sedatives/hypnotics
Lower extremity muscle weakness
High patient to nurse ratio

illness superimposed on baseline risk, and environmental factors. As may be expected, multiple risk factors increase the risk of falling for patients. In one study, elderly patients with four risk factors had a 10-fold increased risk of falling as compared to those with no risk factors. Although this study was conducted in community dwelling elderly persons, it is likely that this increase in fall risk with each additional risk factor is similar for hospitalized elderly patients as well.

Given the well-described risk factors for falls among hospitalized elderly patients, a tool for identifying those patients at highest risk would prove very useful. Several tools designed to screen for risk of falls have been developed and are easy to use. However, these currently available tools have been found to have significant limitations when evaluated outside of the initial population used for development of the instruments. The major limitation is that the tools often have very high sensitivities and low specificities so that they tend to identify a large percentage of patients as high-risk. Understanding this limitation of risk assessment tools is important as a high sensitivity/low specificity tool is a reasonable method of screening for at-risk patients. The Morse Fall Scale, consisting of questions addressing history of falls, presence of multiple diagnoses, use of ambulatory aids, presence of intravenous therapy or heparin lock, gait and transfer ability, and mental status and the St. Thomas's Risk Assessment Tool in Falling Elderly Inpatients (STRATIFY) instrument, consisting of five items that address risk factors for falling: history of falling, patient agitation, visual impairment affecting everyday function, need for frequent toileting, and transfer ability and mobility are two of the most commonly used falls screens in the acute hospital setting.

While all clinicians caring for elderly hospitalized patients should be aware of the risks and implications of falls, systematic interventions have proven most successful to date in lowering the risk of falls. These systematic interventions rely on identifying at-risk patients using baseline risk, preventing or minimizing the effects of the acute illness/injury on risk of falls, and affecting environmental changes that limit the falls as well as reducing the risk of injury from any falls that do occur. Reductions in total in-hospital falls have been reduced by as much as 19% with an even more dramatic 77% reduction in falls with injuries with reductions sustained for as long as 2 years. These interventions have utilized a multipronged approach and it is unclear as to what aspects of the programs are most effective. It is important to note that not all published reports have been able

to demonstrate this level of effectiveness. While additional work is required to better understand the components of an effective falls and injury prevention program, it is appropriate for hospitals and clinicians caring for elderly patients in the acute care setting to develop local programs modeled on successful programs and then to evaluate their programs locally.

Nutrition

Poor nutritional status is common among hospitalized elderly patients. Studies have estimated that up to 50% of all hospitalized older patients are nutritionally at risk and up to 25% meet criteria for malnourished. The causes of these nutritional deficiencies are usually multiple and are related to issues including chronic host issues, effects of the acute illness, and environmental factors prior to hospitalization. Among hospitalized older patients, poor nutritional status is associated with worse clinical outcomes than matched nutritionally intact patients. During the hospitalization, nutritionally at-risk patients are more likely to suffer from a hospital-acquired complication, particularly infection. Compared with patients with good nutritional status, poor nutritional status is associated with longer length of stay, higher readmission rates, increased likelihood of being discharged to an extended care facility, and higher mortality rates.

Given the prevalence and importance of poor nutritional status in the older hospitalized patient, strategies aimed at early identification and intervention should be instituted. Several screening tools have been developed included the Chandra scale, the Nutrition Screening Initiative, and the Mini Nutritional Assessment. The Mini Nutritional Assessment has been shown to be predictive for in-hospital mortality, longer length of stay, and greater likelihood to be discharged to a long-term care facility. None of these instruments should be used as diagnostic tools; they are reasonable to use as part of a system of nutritional screening that can be followed up by a more thorough assessment.

Interventions on at-risk patients can be effective at improving nutritional markers. These interventions include dietary counseling, oral supplementation, or enteral feeding in select populations. When possible, oral feeding is the optimal method for nutritional repletion and maintenance. While these interventions can improve nutritional markers, there is less clear evidence that they affect important clinical outcomes. Despite this lack of evidence in the hospitalized older patient, it is reasonable to provide these nutritional interventions given the positive effects seen on intermediate outcomes.

A difficult situation that often arises in the hospital setting is the question of whether to place a gastrostomy tube (or equivalent) for long-term nutritional support. These feeding tubes do have a role in patients who have reversible deficits in oral feeding ability (e.g., postesophageal surgery) and in patients who are cognitively intact but may have a long-term need for enteral feedings due to mechanical issues. However, often the decision in the acute hospital setting involves older patients who have underlying cognitive deficits, most often dementia, who are no longer able to maintain adequate oral nutrition even with oral supplements. It is important to recognize that this is a marker of end-stage dementia and that there is harm associated with placing feeding tubes in these patients with no benefit to cognitive or functional status and can negatively impact quality of life. This can be a difficult decision for family members to make and can be a trigger to begin or continue discussions about goals of care in these patients.

Preventing Nosocomial Infections

Infections are one of the most common adverse events in health care, affecting over 2 million people, contributing to over 90 000 deaths, and costing over $4.5 billion yearly in the United States. Up to 10% of patients admitted to acute care hospitals develop hospital-acquired infections; this rate is rising. The majority of hospital-acquired infections are due to UTIs, pneumonia, surgical site infections, and bloodstream infections. A full discussion of the management of all these infections is beyond the scope of this chapter, but older patients are disproportionately affected by UTIs, pneumonia, and increasingly, *Clostridium difficile* infections. Putting strategies in place to address these infections (and in particular, preventing them) and practicing good infection control is critical for inpatient physicians focused on the care of elderly patients.

Hospital-Acquired Urinary Tract Infections

UTI is the most common hospital acquired infection, accounting for up to 40% of all nosocomial infections. Hospitals acquired UTIs lead to bacteremia in up to 4% of patients, and carry a mortality rate between 15% and 30%. Females, older patients, and patients with severe underlying illness are at greatest risk. Urinary catheterization is a contributing factor in the majority of infections in hospitalized patients. The National Nosocomial Infection Surveillance (NNIS) System reports a median rate of catheter associated UTI per 1000 catheter days of 3.9. While classic UTIs present with dysuria, frequent urination, and urgency, these symptoms are less common in older patients, and are difficult to evaluate in the patient with a catheter in place or with cognitive impairment. In addition, asymptomatic bacteriuria in hospitalized patients is a common finding. Its significance in patients with a catheter remains unknown, and most experts recommend against treatment in the absence of symptoms. When symptomatic, most cases of UTI in the hospital are caused by *Escherichia coli*, Enterococcus, *Pseudomonas aeruginosa*, *Klebsiella pneumoniae*, and Candida species.

Most of the focus on preventing nosocomial UTIs is on mitigating the risk imposed by urinary catheters. Indwelling urinary catheter (IUC) use varies by hospital unit and patient type, but they are used in up to 25% of elderly hospitalized patients. In addition to contributing to infection risk, catheters are known to increase the risk of delirium and falls and have been referred to as a "one-point restraint." While systematic reviews have shown that some types of antimicrobial catheters (nitrofurazone or silver alloy coated) reduce rates of bacteriuria in hospitalized patients, most effort has been spent on trying to avoid catheters in the first place. Appropriate use of catheters includes patients unable to void, postanesthesia use, monitoring of urine output in patients unable to comply with collection, protection of an open wound in an incontinent patient, and use in palliative care. Unnecessary use is common; some reports have suggested that up to 30% of hospital physicians are unaware that their patients even have a catheter. One of the most important risk prevention strategies is avoiding unnecessary catheter use. In institutions with computerized order entry, clinical decision support, electronic reminders, and automatic stop orders have been effective at reducing the overall use and duration of use of urinary catheters. Paper reminders are also effective in institutions lacking computerized order entry. In male patients who require a urinary catheter (other than for urinary retention), recent work has shown that condom catheters in addition to being rated as more comfortable, reduce the composite risk of bacteriuria, symptomatic UTIs, and death. Of note, most of the benefit was in the reduction of asymptomatic bacteriuria. This protective effect of condom catheters maybe diminished in patients with dementia who frequently pull off their catheters. Each time the condom catheter is replaced, swabbing of the meatus is required which may increase the risk of bacteriuria and subsequent infection when it occurs repeatedly.

Hospital-Acquired Pneumonia

Hospital-acquired pneumonia, also referred to as nosocomial pneumonia, includes both ventilator-associated pneumonia and nonventilator-associated pneumonia that develops 48 or more hours after hospitalization. Almost all the data on hospital-acquired pneumonia comes from intensive care units (ICUs) and the study of ventilator-associated pneumonia. Extrapolation to the non-ICU population may not be appropriate. A third class of nosocomial pneumonia that is increasingly common and important for the geriatric population is health care-associated pneumonia. Patients at risk for health care-associated pneumonia include patients receiving home IV antibiotics, home nursing or home wound care, residence in a nursing home or long-term care facility, patients who have been hospitalized for ≥2 days in the past 90 days, and patients who have received dialysis or IV therapy at a hospital-based clinic in the past 30 days. Health care associated pneumonia develops in the community, but has a spectrum of causative organisms, and an approach to management that is similar to hospital-acquired pneumonia.

Pneumonia is the second most common nosocomial infection with an incidence of 5 to 10 cases per 1000 hospitalizations. The rates in patients with endotracheal tubes are up to 20 times higher. The mortality attributable to nosocomial pneumonia is debated, but maybe as high as 30%. An episode of nosocomial pneumonia clearly increases hospital length of stay and costs.

Nosocomial pneumonia results from microbial invasion of sterile lung parenchyma as a result of microaspiration of contaminated oropharyngeal or gastric secretions. A defect in host defenses, aspiration of a large inoculum of organisms, or aspiration of a particularly virulent organism may contribute to parenchymal infection. Risk factors for the development of nosocomial pneumonia that are commonly found in older patients are listed in Table 17-5. Understanding the risk factors is critical to implementing effective prevention strategies. Many prevention strategies for ventilator-associated pneumonia have been well-described elsewhere and are best directed at the ICU physicians and other ICU personnel. However, there are several important strategies to prevent nosocomial pneumonia that are important for physicians caring for hospitalized elders in the non-ICU setting.

One of the best ways to prevent pneumonia is to avoid intubation in patients with respiratory failure. Increasingly, the use of noninvasive ventilation has been effective in reducing the need for intubation. In selected patients with acute COPD or heart failure exacerbations, noninvasive ventilation reduced the need for intubation and was associated with less pneumonia, shorter hospital length of stay, and in some studies, lower mortality. Patients with facial trauma and altered mental status are generally not recommended for noninvasive ventilation due to increased risk of complications such as aspiration.

Keeping patients upright, or semirecumbent, has been shown to reduce rates of pneumonia. In one study, elevating the head of the

TABLE 17-5

Risk Factors for Nosocomial Pneumonia in Elderly Patients

Impaired host defenses/increased aspiration
  Endotracheal tubes
  Nasogastric tubes
  Enteral feeding tubes
  Supine positioning
  Impaired mental status
  Sedation
Large inoculum of organisms
  Bacterial colonization
  Gastric alkalinization (enteral feeds/H2-receptor blockers, proton pump
    inhibitors)
  Iatrogenic (forced hand ventilation)
  Sinusitis
  Malnutrition
  Contaminated respiratory equipment
Overgrowth of virulent organisms
  Prolonged antibiotic use
  Iatrogenic (inadequate hand washing)
  Central venous lines
  Comorbid illness
  Frequent hospitalizations
  Prolonged hospital stays

bed >45° reduced rates of ventilator-acquired pneumonia significantly. While little data exist for this practice outside the ICU, head of bed elevation is likely to reduce episodes of hospital-acquired pneumonia outside the ICU, especially in patients at risk for aspiration. Stress ulcer prophylaxis increases gastric pH and allows for colonization of the gastrointestinal tract by potentially pathogenic organisms. Studies have suggested that use of medications that raise gastric pH (primarily H2-antagonists) is associated with an increased risk of pneumonia. While these medications are necessary in some patients, they are likely overused and may contribute to episodes of hospital-acquired pneumonia. In general, the only patients shown to benefit from stress ulcer prophylaxis are those with shock, respiratory failure, and coagulopathy. Data on risks for the use of proton pump inhibitors (PPI) in hospitalized patients is limited. However, studies in the community setting link these agents to increased rates of community-acquired pneumonia suggesting similar mechanisms. In the hospitalized elder, every effort should be made to assure an appropriate indication exists for continued use of H2-antagonists or PPIs. Given the role of colonizing oropharyngeal bacteria, it would seem that improving oral hygiene could prevent nosocomial pneumonia. While no study has been performed in hospitalized patients, improved oral hygiene in nursing home residents—by the use of antiseptic mouthwash, brushing teeth after meals, and weekly plaque removal—has been linked to reduced rates of aspiration pneumonia. Improved oral hygiene in hospitalized elderly patients (mouthwash and brushing), is low cost, can involve the family in resource-constrained environments, and may prevent pneumonia.

Clostridium difficile

Clostridium difficile is the most common cause of health care–acquired diarrhea, occurring at a rate of 61 cases per 100 000 discharges in 2003. In the past few years, several outbreaks in hospitals and nursing homes have been described. These outbreaks have been associated with high morbidity and mortality. Concurrent with recent outbreaks are reports of poor response to therapy, and high rates of relapse. Many of the epidemic outbreaks that have been associated with highly morbid disease have been linked to a previously uncommon strain, B1/NAP1.

The biggest risk factors for infection include antibiotic use and hospitalization. Additional risk factors relevant to the care of a geriatric population include advanced age, severity of illness, use of proton pump inhibitors, and use of tube feeding. While clindamycin is classically associated with *C. difficile*, any antibiotic (including metronidazole and vancomycin used to treat the disease) can cause infection. Cephalosporins are widely used and commonly cause *C. difficile* infection. More recently, fluoroquinolone use has been associated with outbreaks of the B1/ NAP1 strain.

Prevention of *C. difficile* requires both infection control measures and antibiotic stewardship. Outbreaks have been successfully controlled by patient isolation in a single room, implementation of contact precautions (gown and gloves for anyone entering the room) and, because clostridia spores are not easily killed by alcohol-based hand rubs, liberal handwashing with soap and water for all persons entering and leaving the patient's room. The implementation of formal antibiotic rotation programs and restriction of particular antibiotics during outbreaks may also be required to combat *C. difficile*.

Infection Control

Prevention of hospital-acquired infections also includes careful attention to hand hygiene and preventing the spread of antimicrobial resistance. With careful hand washing before and after patient contact, the incidence of nosocomial infection is reduced. Existing data suggest that plain soap and water, antibacterial soaps (chlorhexidine based), and alcohol-based hand rinses have equivalent effect. The use of alcohol-based rinses in bedside dispensers may improve compliance with hand hygiene recommendations.

The numbers of organisms in U.S. hospitals displaying resistance and the mechanisms by which they develop resistance have both increased dramatically in recent years. Particular problem organisms include among the gram positives, methicillin-resistant *Staphylococcus aureus* (MRSA), and vancomycin-resistant enterococcus (VRE), and among the gram negatives, drug-resistant *Pseudomonas aeruginosa*, *Acinetobacter baumannii*, and extended spectrum beta-lactamase-producing Enterobacteriaceae. Infections with these organisms are associated with increased morbidity, mortality, and costs. Physicians should be familiar with their institution's resistance profile and understand when infection with these organisms is possible in order to give timely, appropriate antibiotic therapy. Delay in the initiation of adequate antibiotic therapy (i.e., antibiotics that are active against the organism that is ultimately isolated) has been associated with increased mortality in many types of infection.

Preventing the development and spread of these organisms is critical. The use and misuse of antibiotics has been associated with the development of resistance. Considerable attention has been given to antibiotic stewardship programs that focus on development of appropriate antibiotic formularies and treatment recommendations, restricted use of certain agents, and feedback to providers on prescribing practices. Many of these programs have been effective in controlling the emergence of resistance and in stopping outbreaks of highly resistant organisms. Prevention of the transmission of these organisms once they emerge is also critical. Preventing person-to-person spread has been most successful with gram-positive organisms. Contact precautions (i.e., gowns, gloves) and isolation of infected patients in private rooms are the usual strategies. Caution is warranted when caring for elderly patients who are placed in isolation. Studies have shown that patients in isolation are less likely to be examined by health care providers. This potentially places these patients at increased risk of a missed diagnosis. It can also mean less physical therapy, less contact with nursing and family, and the potential for development of delirium. Extra effort may be required to continue the best practices of geriatric care for elderly patients who are in contact isolation.

Venous Thromboembolism Prophylaxis

Prevention of venous thromboembolism (VTE), which includes deep venous thrombosis (DVT) and pulmonary embolism (PE), is an important consideration in hospitalized patients, leading to serious morbidity and mortality. Venous thromboembolism, while not uncommon in hospitalized medical patients, is often unrecognized. While there is no consensus on quantifying patient-specific risk factors, patients admitted with heart failure, severe respiratory disease, or malignancy, patients confined to bed, and older patients are considered to be at increased risk for VTE. Multiple studies, including several meta-analyses, have demonstrated the efficacy of pharmacologic prophylaxis against VTE in high-risk hospitalized patients. These studies have shown that both low molecular weight heparin (LMWH) and unfractionated heparin reduce the risk of both DVT and PE without a significant increased risk of major bleeding (minor bleeding episodes, including development of hematomas, maybe more common in patients receiving pharmacologic prophylaxis). Prophylaxis has not been associated with a mortality benefit and its cost-effectiveness has not been well studied. For patients at high risk of bleeding, the use of intermittent pneumatic leg compression is a reasonable substitute for heparin products.

The use of standard order sets and reminders built into computerized order entry systems facilitate routine use of VTE prophylaxis in high-risk patients. The effect of avoiding bedrest and encouraging frequent mobilization on reducing the occurrence of DVTs and PEs has not yet been studied.

Patient Safety

Hospitalized older adults are more likely than hospitalized younger adults to suffer iatrogenic complications of hospitalization because older adults have longer, more complex hospitalizations, and greater physiological vulnerability. Since the Institute of Medicine Report focusing on patient safety, some of these "iatrogenic" complications are now understood as patient safety problems. For example, infectious complications of catheters and devices are common among older patients, who often have urinary catheters, other lines, and devices. Thromboembolic events, nosocomial infections, falls, ADEs, and drug errors due to incorrect reconciliation of a complex medical regimen, all are more common in older hospitalized patients and are targets of patient safety improvement. National Patient Safety Goals, approved by the Joint Commission on the Accreditation of Health Care Organizations in 2008, address many risks faced by older adult hospital patients. The goals include reducing risk of health care-associated infections, reconciling medications accurately across the care continuum, reducing falls and fall risk, preventing pressure ulcers, and assessing risk of pressure ulcer development. Geriatricians and other physicians and providers caring for older hospitalized patients should be actively involved with planning and implementing patient safety interventions in the acute hospital setting.

Palliative Care

In contrast to the ideal vision of death in which most people see themselves dying at home with family, many Americans die in hospitals. As recently as 2001, it was estimated that nearly 50% of people who died did so in hospitals. In some cases death is unexpected, but in most cases it is not. Despite the fact that many people die in hospitals, we do not yet do a good job of delivering end-of-life care. Surveys of patients and families have shown that patients dying in hospitals believe they do not have enough contact with physicians, emotional support, information about what to expect of the dying process, and unfortunately, a substantial percentage report moderate or severe pain in the last 3 days of life. Delivering high-quality end-of-life care requires experience, as well as a substantial investment in time. Providers working in today's hospitals recognize these problems, yet struggle with increasingly complex patients, as well as demands for both increased quality and efficiency of care. As a result, many hospitals have developed formal palliative care programs to adequately address the needs of dying patients. Most palliative care programs focus on maximizing comfort and quality of life rather than delivering curative therapy. Formal palliative care programs focus on pain and symptom control, communication challenges, addressing spiritual needs, and facilitating care transitions. As of 2002, it was estimated that 26% of academic medical centers and 17% of all hospitals had hospital-based palliative care programs. While many hospitals use a variety of practitioners to staff their programs, geriatricians, hospitalists, and oncologists are well-represented in most programs. There now are formal palliative care fellowships and plans for board certification in this discipline. Any comprehensive approach to care of the hospitalized elder must address issues of end-of-life care. A full discussion of end-of-life care can be found in Chapter 31.

HOSPITAL DISCHARGE AND CARE TRANSITIONS (see also Chapter 16)

The transition of elderly patients from the inpatient to outpatient setting is fraught with risk. At discharge patients are routinely transitioned from the care of an inpatient physician to that of their primary care provider, one or more specialist physicians, or a health care provider at a nursing home or rehabilitation facility. This "handoff" creates the opportunity for information to be lost or miscommunicated, resulting in the potential for adverse clinical consequences. The Institute of Medicine (IOM) report, "To Err is Human," estimated that after discharge 49% of patients experience at least one medical error; 19% to 23% of patients suffer adverse events. These adverse events are associated with deficiencies in health literacy, patient education, communication among providers within and between systems, medical follow-up, and medication issues. The medication issues at discharge are well documented. Recent research has shown that 14% of patients experience one or more medication discrepancies after discharge, and that at 30 days, readmissions were twice as common in patients who had experienced a discrepancy.

Other studies have shown an ADE rate of 11% at 3 weeks after discharge. Patients who recalled having medication side-effects explained to them prior to discharge had fewer ADEs. While these transition problems are not unique to the geriatric population, older patients are disproportionately affected.

There is widespread agreement among health care professionals that improving safety during transitions of geriatric patients from the inpatient to outpatient setting is a health system priority. Unfortunately, there are no national standards outlining criteria for assessing the adequacy of discharge planning for older adults and there is no consensus on the best strategy to optimize the discharge process. A systematic review of the literature indicated little evidence for the effectiveness of discharge planning as a means of reducing length of stay, mortality, or costs.

The problems that occur at discharge highlight the need for systems-level solutions to track information and facilitate communication during this transition. Four key areas need to be addressed at discharge:

1. *Hospital physician–primary care (and specialist if indicated) provider communication:* While communication with a patient's primary physician is valuable at key points of the patient's hospitalization, it is critical at discharge. A phone call at discharge to the primary care provider is preferred, but timely communi-cation of a summary of the patient's course, medication changes, and required follow-up can be automated and sent by e-mail or fax. The Society of Hospital Medicine has developed a discharge checklist that can be used to identify elements to include in a discharge summary and information that needs to be communicated to the physician following the patient as an outpatient (Table 17-6).

2. *Medication reconciliation:* Reconciliation ensures that an accurate up-to-date list of medications is maintained and is consistent with the patient's plan of care. Regulatory agencies require that this occurs at discharge. A standardized approach needs to be developed by the inpatient team; the approach can include physician- or nurse-based reconciliation and education. The process can be automated or can involve the use of clinical pharmacists. Several studies have shown that involving clinical pharmacists in the medication reconciliation process at discharge leads to fewer ADEs after discharge and in some cases has reduced readmissions. Many of the more robust pharmacist-based programs also call patients after discharge to troubleshoot medication problems.

3. *Pending tests and labs:* Many patients are discharged with labs and test results pending. Studies have shown that physicians are often unaware of tests requiring review and follow-up after hospital discharge. While automated mechanisms to track pending

TABLE 17-6

A Hospital Checklist for the Ideal Discharge of the Elderly Patient

DATA ELEMENTS	Discharge Summary	PROCESS — Patient Instructions	PROCESS — Communication to Follow-Up Clinician on Day of Discharge
Presenting problem that precipitated hospitalization	x	x	x
Key findings and test results	x		x
Final primary and secondary diagnoses	x	x	x
Brief hospital course	x	x	x
Condition at discharge, including functional status and cognitive status if relevant	x—Functional status o—Cognitive status		
Discharge destination (and rationale if not obvious)	x		x
Discharge Medications:			
Written schedule	x	x	x
Include purpose and cautions for each	o	x	o
Comparison with pre-admission medications,			x
(e.g. new, changes in dose/frequency unchanged, medications that should no longer be taken)	x	x	
Follow-up appointments with name of provider, date, address, phone number, visit purpose, suggested management plan	x	x	x
All pending labs or tests, responsible person to whom results will be sent	x		x
Recommendation of and sub-specialty consultants	x		o
Documentation of patient education and understanding	x		o
Any anticipated problems and suggested interventions	x	x	x
24/7 call back number	x	x	
Identify referring and receiving providers	x	x	
Resuscitation status and any other pertinent end-of-life issues	o		

x, required element; O, optional element.

Reprinted with permission from Halasyamani L, Kripilani S, Coleman E, et al. Transition of care for hospitalized elderly patients-development of a discharge checklist for hospitalists. J Hosp Med. 2006;1:354–360.

results are the ideal, they remain uncommon. Checklists, creating extra layers of safety for important results (i.e., more than one care provider scheduled follow up appointment), and careful communication of what action should be taken based on the pending test result will help ensure important results do not fall through the cracks.

4. *Patient/family empowerment/discharge coaches:* Involving the patient or their family in the discharge process has been associated with improved outcomes and provides an extra layer of safety for follow-up of test results pending at discharge and communication of important events that occurred during the hospitalization. Studies have shown that encouraging patients to take a more active role in their care, and providing tools and guidance in the form of "transition coaches" can lower hospital costs and readmission rates for elderly patients. This patient-centered care is a useful strategy to improve care transitions.

MODELS OF HOSPITAL CARE AND THE ELDERLY PATIENT

The care of hospitalized elders is occurring within a dynamic hospital environment that is changing, in part to address financial and other challenges for providers but also to better meet the needs of the geriatric population, and the increasing demands to provide safer, higher quality, and more cost-effective care. In this section of the chapter, we address some of the changes in models of hospital care relevant for the healthcare provider focused on the high-quality care of hospitalized elders.

Hospitalist

Concurrent with the increased attention to the needs of hospitalized elders has been the emerging presence of hospitalists. The hospitalist physician, usually a general internist, focuses clinical activity almost exclusively on caring for hospitalized patients. Varied forces have driven the hospitalist movement, including improved efficiency of hospital care, physician ownership of inpatient quality and safety initiatives, and the dual clinical and financial challenges of managing patients in both the office and hospital. Teaching hospitals

also employ hospitalists to mitigate pressures resulting from resident work hour reductions. The rapid growth of the hospitalist field has been supported, in part, by direct financial support from physician group practices, hospitals, and academic medical centers.

There are currently 15,000 practicing hospitalists in the United States, with numbers expected to double by 2010 (Figure 17-1). The American Hospital Association (AHA) found that nearly 30% of U.S. hospitals had hospital medicine groups; the percentage exceeded 60% for hospitals with more than 200 beds. Similar penetration exists at academic medical centers (AMCs). Over half of teaching hospitals and 66% of major teaching hospitals (defined as a member of the Council of Teaching Hospitals and Health Systems) have developed hospital medicine groups. The hospitalist programs at these academic centers tend to be quite large, with an average of 17 hospitalists per program.

As hospital medicine programs have grown, so have the roles of hospitalists. The hospitalist's primary task has not changed since the formation of the field, namely, the day-to-day clinical care of complex medical patients, in both academic and nonacademic settings. However, in many institutions, they have expanded their scope of practice by establishing palliative care programs as well as quality improvement and patient safety programs all of particular applicability and potential benefit to the hospitalized elderly patient. In addition, hospitals have supported the creation of surgical comanagement programs that focus on both outpatient preoperative assessment and inpatient postoperative management. With the hospital setting as their "office," hospitalists are often in leading administrative roles within hospitals and academic medical centers.

Teaching hospitals need to support residency programs; this need has catalyzed hospitalist growth in those settings. Driven by the need for increased educational oversight and Medicare billing requirements, academic medical centers have increasingly turned to hospitalists to staff resident teaching services. More recently, in an effort to prevent adverse outcomes related to overly tired trainees, in July 2003, the Residency Review Committee (RRC) began enforcing rules that prevent residents from working more than 80 hours in 1 week or for more than 30 hours in a single shift. Faced with increasing bed occupancy, increasingly complex patient populations, and the perception that the floats, hand-offs, and patchwork coverage solutions were adversely affecting patient care, academic medical centers looked for other options. Many chose to decompress the

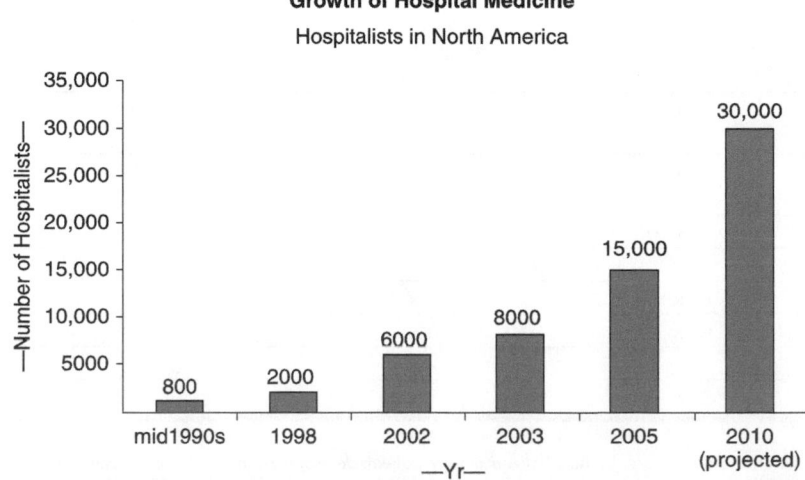

Growth of Hospital Medicine

Hospitalists in North America

FIGURE 17-1. Growth of hospital medicine. *Source*: Society of Hospital Medicine.

numbers of patients seen on resident services to nonresident services, which are now commonly staffed by hospitalists.

As the hospitalist model of care has spread, the field has changed the way clinical problems are approached and managed. New research questions have been raised regarding the clinical approach to hospitalized patients, implementation of best practices, care transitions, and how to improve patient safety, again with potentially significant benefit to the medically complex and/or potentially vulnerable elderly patient. Representative research topics currently being explored by hospitalist investigators include identifying biomarkers predictive of perioperative outcomes, evaluating methods to prevent health care-associated infection, examining the utility of a variety of care processes for common inpatient diagnoses like pneumonia, studying the intersection between resident education and inpatient safety, and exploring techniques to improve quality during transitions of patient care.

Hospitalists are both ideally suited and situated to play a central role in improving quality and safety of the care of hospitalized elders. As a site-defined specialty, hospitalists spend more time in the hospital than do many other physicians, allowing them to gain insight into the problems commonly encountered in geriatric care and some potential solutions. By working closely with hospital personnel and administration, hospitalists can take the lead in the development and refinements of interdisciplinary teams designed to enhance the quality and safety of inpatient geriatric care.

Acute Care of the Elderly Units

Acute Care of the Elderly (ACE) units were described and studied in community and academic settings in the mid-1990s. The ACE unit intervention consisted of environmental interventions (rugs, lighting, handrails), patient-centered care model that emphasized independence and rehabilitation from the beginning of the hospital stay, and a multidisciplinary care team consisting of nurses, physicians, therapists, social workers, and nutritionists and pharmacists providing coordinated care within a dedicated inpatient unit. Findings from the randomized controlled trial in 1995 found significantly improved functional status and decreased admission to nursing homes in patients randomized to the ACE unit interventions. Lengths of stay and hospital charges were similar in both groups. Recent retrospective studies have confirmed ACE unit benefits on function and quality of life, without increased hospital charges. Despite favorable results, ACE units are not widely disseminated in U.S. hospitals, largely due to the capital expenditures incurred in creation of such a unit, difficulty in recruiting the qualified specialist leaders, and future concerns with not having enough room for the rapidly expanding elderly patient population in such a space-defined unit. A review in 2003 surveyed hospitals associated with medical schools that had a geriatrics program and found that only 16 had ACE units. The number of community hospitals with ACE units is unknown. Some hospitals or academic medical centers have preferred to develop a virtual ACE team, rather than a dedicated ACE unit. The virtual ACE team is a multidisciplinary geriatrics consult team involving physician, nurse, social work, pharmacy and physical therapy that is designed to improve patients' hospital course and expedite discharge planning and transitional care. The virtual ACE team model provides the expertise and systems approach to the care of the elderly hospitalized population, particularly the vulnerable and medically complex outside the confines of a defined unit.

Stroke Units

Stroke units use a care delivery model analogous to ACE unit models. A stroke unit is a multidisciplinary team specifically dedicated to the care of the stroke patient. Physicians, nurses, and therapists are involved in a coordinated effort to support the care and rehabilitation of stroke patients. The stroke unit maybe a dedicated hospital unit, a mobile team than manages patient along with the primary inpatient team, or may function within a rehabilitation unit. Stroke units were reviewed in a Cochrane report in 2001, which analyzed results from 23 randomized and quasirandomized trials and concluded that there was evidence that stroke units improved function at discharge, rates of discharge to home, and stroke survival. There was some evidence that dedicated stroke units had better outcomes. Whether there are aspects of poststroke care that can be generalized and systematized to improve elderly patient health care outcomes outside such a unit needs further investigation.

FURTHER READING

Amador LF, Loera JA. Preventing postoperative falls in the older adult. *J Am Coll Surg.* 2007;204:447–453.

Boyd CM, Xue QL, Simpson CF, et al. Frailty, hospitalization, and progression of disability in a cohort of disabled older women. *Am J Med.* 2005;118:1225–1231.

Curriculum for the Hospitalized Aging Medical Patient (CHAMP). Available on the Portal of Online Geriatrics Education. http://www.pogoe.org. Supported by the Donald W. Reynolds Foundation.

Dentali F, Douketis JD, Gianni M, et al. Meta-analysis: anticoagulant prophylaxis to prevent symptomatic venous thromboembolism in hospitalized medical patients. *Ann Intern Med.* 2007;146:278–288.

Flanders SA, Collard HR, Saint S. Preventing nosocomial pneumonia. In: Lautenbach E, Woeltje K, eds. *The Society for Healthcare Epidemiology of America: Practical Handbook for Healthcare Epidemiologists.* Thorofare, NJ: Slack; 2004:69–78.

Flanders SA, Wachter RM. Hospitalists: the new model of inpatient medical care in the United States. *Eur J Intern Med.* 2003;14:65–70.

Forster AJ, Murff HJ, Peterson JF, et al. Adverse drug events occurring following hospital discharge. *J Gen Intern Med.* 2005;20:317–323.

Gasink LB, Lautenbach E. Prevention and treatment of healthcare-acquired infections. *Med Clin N Am.* 2008;92:295–313.

Gill TM, Allore HG, Holford TR, et al. Hospitalization, restricted activity, and the development of disability among older persons. *JAMA.* 2004;292:2115–2124.

Gillick MR. Rethinking the role of tube feeding in patients with advanced dementia. *N Eng J Med.* 2000;342:206–210.

Halasyamani L, Kripilani S, Coleman E, et al. Transition of care for hospitalized elderly patients- development of a discharge checklist for hospitalists. *J Hosp Med.* 2006;1:354–360.

Hitcho EB, Krauss MJ, Birge S, et al. Characteristics and circumstances of falls in a hospital setting: a prospective analysis. *J Gen Intern Med.* 2004;19:732–739.

Inouye SK, Bogardus ST, Baker DI, et al. The Hospital Elder Life Program: a model of care to prevent cognitive and functional decline in older hospitalized patients. *J Am Geriar Soc.* 2000;48:1697–1706.

Inouye SK, Charpentier PA. Precipitating factors for delirium in hospitalized elderly persons: predictive model and interrelationship with baseline vulnerability. *JAMA.* 1996;275:852–857.

Inouye SK, Peduzzi PN, Robinson JT, et al. Importance of functional measures in predicting mortality among older hospitalized patients. *JAMA.* 1998;279:1187–1193.

Inouye SK, van Dyck CH, Alessi CA, et al. Clarifying confusion: the confusion assessment method. A new method for detecting delirium. *Ann Intern Med.* 1990;113:941–948.

Kaboli PJ, Hoth AB, McClimon BJ, et al. Clinical pharmacists and inpatient medical care: a systematic review. *Arch Intern Med.* 2006;166:955–964.

Loo VG, Poirier L, Miller MA, et al. A predominantly clonal multi-institutional outbreak of *Clostridium difficile*-associated diarrhea with high morbidity and mortality. *N Engl J Med.* 2005;353:2442–2449.

Mathias S, Navak US, Isaacs B. Balance in elderly patients: the "get-up and go" test. *Arch Phsy Med Rehabil.* 1986;67:387–389.

Nagamine M., Jiang J, Merrill CT. Trends in elderly hospitalizations, 1997–2004. *Statistical Brief #14.* Rockville, MD: AHRQ; 2006.

National Nosocomial Infections Surveillance. National Nosocomial Infections Surveillance (NISS) System Report, data summary from January 1992 through June 2004, issued October 2004. *Am J Infect Control.* 2004;32:470–485.

National Patient Safety Goals: Facts about the 2008 National Patient Safety Goals. 2007. http://www.jointcommmission.org/PatientSafety.

Rubin FH, Williams JT, Lescisin DA, et al. Replicating the Hospital Elder Life Program in a community hospital and demonstrating effectiveness using quality improvement methodology. *J Am Geriatr Soc.* 2006;54:969–974.

Russo CA and Elixhauser A. Hospitalizations in the elderly. *Statistical Brief #6.* Rockville, MD; AHRQ; 2006.

Saint S, Flanders SA. Hospitalists in teaching hospitals: opportunities but not without danger. *J Gen Intern Med.* 2004;19:392–393.

Saint S, Kaufman SR, Rogers MA, et al. Condom versus indwelling urinary catheters: a randomized trial. *J Am Geriatr Soc.* 2006;54:1055–1061.

Saint S, Lipsky BA, Goold SD. Indwelling urinary catheters: a one-point restraint ? *Ann Intern Med.* 2002;137:125–127.

Saint S, Savel RH, Matthay MA. Enhancing the safety of critically ill patients by reducing urinary and central venous catheter-related infections. *Am J Respir Crit Care Med.* 2002;165:1475–1479.

Van Nes MC, Herrmann FR, Gold G, et al. Does the mini nutritional assessment predict hospitalization outcomes in older people. *Age Ageing.* 2001;30:221–226.

Emergency Department Care

Scott T. Wilber ■ *Lowell W. Gerson*

The emergency department (ED) plays a unique and essential role in the care of the older adult. The ED is open 24 hours a day, seven days a week, 365 days a year. It provides access to the millions of people who have no other entry point for health care. It gives care to people who have no established community provider and acts as the gatekeeper between the community and the hospital.

The prevailing model of care in EDs has been established for over 40 years but does not conform well to the needs of the older adult. Based on principles proposed in 1962 by the Committee on Trauma of the American College of Surgeons (ACS), EDs are designed for rapid evaluation and treatment of the emergent and urgent needs of acutely ill and injured patients. ED care differs from care delivered in other settings. Typically, there is no preexisting relationship between the patient and the physician. The process rewards speed, the timeframe is immediate, and the focus is on the patient's complaint. It is not friendly to the older patient with complex needs who require thorough assessment and evaluation and whose care process is slow-moving.

In the 1990s, the Society for Academic Emergency Medicine (SAEM) Geriatric Task Force proposed a model of emergency care for older patients (Table 18-1). The model appreciates differences in disorders and diagnoses by age, atypical presentation of disease, altered physiology of aging, the complexity of diagnosis, and management of older patients, and the need to consider other issues beyond the presenting complaint. The Geriatric Task Force recognized that symptoms may be nonspecific, comorbidities are common, and response to therapy is often difficult to predict. The Task Force proposed a biopsychosocial model of emergency care for older patients. The model has evolved over time and reflects the current thinking about basic principles for emergency care of the older patient.

The ED plays a crucial role in care for seniors. Older people use the ED at higher rates than other populations, present more often with urgent and emergent conditions, and are more frequently transported by ambulance. In addition, the ED is a major care provider for nursing home residents; one of four nursing home residents is transported to an ED yearly.

Emergency medicine has only recently identified the older population as a group with special needs, but interest in the area is growing exponentially. The first journal article to address the emergency care of elders was by published in 1967 and concerned emergency surgery. There were 39 other articles cited for the years 1966 to 1970. From 2001 to 2005, there were 1267 entries, which represents over a 30-fold increase. A major contributor to the growth of geriatric emergency room (ER) medicine was a seminal series of articles in the *Annals of Emergency Medicine*. The articles emerged from a project to evaluate the care of elders in United States EDs, funded by the John A. Hartford Foundation and carried out by the SAEM Geriatric Emergency Medicine Task Force. The task force reviewed the literature and conducted surveys of emergency physicians and residency program directors, reviewed ER records, and held focus groups. The task force found that the evidence base for ED care of the older adult was small and that the discipline had failed to plan ED care to meet the needs of elders. Given the expected growth of the aging population in coming decades and the high volume of ED use among them, there was concern that emergency medicine training programs have no organized content on care for older ED patients and that there have been no organized advocates within either emergency medicine or geriatrics to spearhead change in emergency health care for seniors.

It cannot be known whether the SAEM reports stimulated action to address these concerns, or whether change was inevitable. Without question, the reports brought ED care for the older adult to the attention of leaders within emergency medicine and geriatrics. Today, the SAEM and the American College of Emergency Physicians (ACEP) are represented on a Council of Medical Specialties hosted by the American Geriatrics Society. Moreover, both SAEM and ACEP have developed working groups who focus on older emergency patients. Today, emergency medicine training programs include geriatric content and the qualifying examinations include questions directed at care of older patients.

TABLE 18-1

Geriatric Emergency Care Model Developed by the SAEM Geriatrics Task Force

- The patient's presentation is frequently complex.
- Common diseases may present atypically.
- Comorbid conditions must be considered.
- Polypharmacy is common and may be a factor in presentation, diagnosis, and management.
- Cognitive impairment is possible and mental status should be evaluated.
- Standard values for diagnostic tests may not be applicable.
- With age comes decreased functional reserve and this must be anticipated.
- Social support systems are important in care of older patients and should be considered in planning for care.
- Knowledge of baseline functional status is essential in evaluating new complaints.
- Medical problems must be evaluated for psychosocial adjustment.
- The encounter is an opportunity to assess important conditions in the patient's personal life.

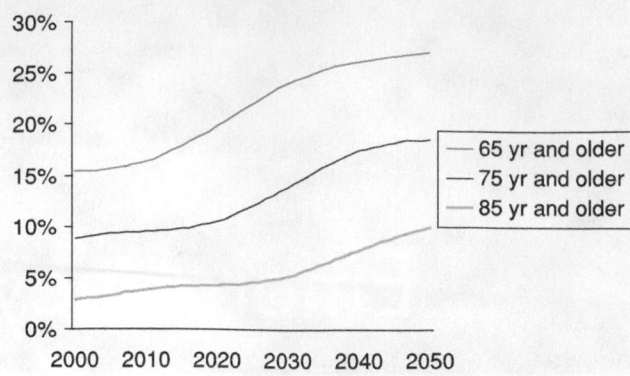

FIGURE 18-1. Projected change in ED visits by older patients.

EPIDEMIOLOGY

The aging of the U.S. population poses a challenge to health care delivery, as older patients consume a disproportionate share of health care resources. Emergency care is one area of heavy resource use by older patients. In 2004, approximately 14% of the 110 million ED visits were by patients aged 65 years and older. Compared to younger patients, older patients have higher levels of disease acuity and the probability of hospital admission from the ED is higher. In one study, 40% of older adults in the ED were admitted, compared to 10% of younger adults. Older adults were also more likely to be admitted to critical care units (4% vs. <1%), more likely to undergo laboratory and radiographic testing, and had longer ED lengths of stay.

Given the high rate of ED use by older adults and the projected growth of the older populations, ED use by older adults will increase further in the future (Figure 18-1). Assuming stable visit rates, the proportion of ED visits that are by older patients will increase to approximately 25% by the year 2030. In recent years, however, ED visit rates by older people have grown 26%, which is higher than any other segment of the population. Thus the combined effects of an aging population and increasing ED use rates could push the proportion of older adults in the ED even higher.

The presenting complaints of older patients differ from those of younger patients. The most common ED-presenting complaint for both older and younger patients is injury, though this complaint is even more common in younger patients (37%) than older patients (26%). Other common reasons for ED visits are shown in Figure 18–2 and include dyspnea, chest pain, and abdominal pain. The 10 chief complaints in Figure 18-2 comprise about two-thirds of all ED chief complaints for older patients.

PATHOPHYSIOLOGY AND PRESENTATIONS

In past years, the role of the emergency physician was primarily triage—determining which patients were ill and required further inpatient work-up and which were safe to be discharged. With the substantial increase in the quality and quantity of available diagnostic tests, this role has shifted. The primary role of the emergency

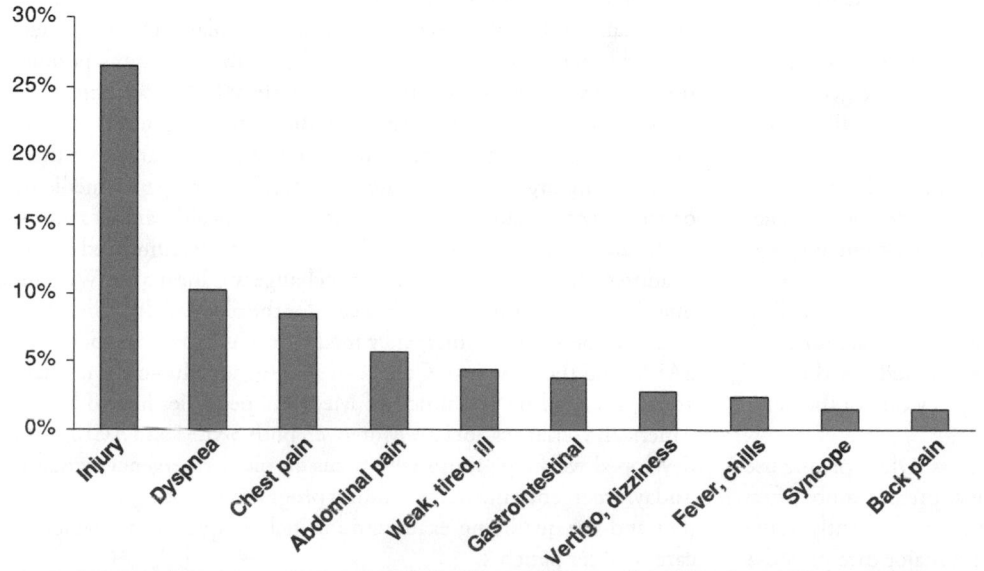

FIGURE 18-2. Common reasons for ED visits in older patients.

physician is now diagnosis. Most often, the correct diagnosis will be made in the ED. However, there are times when making the correct diagnosis is not possible and the focus is on ruling out serious disease. In many instances, emergency physicians also treat the disease they have diagnosed, though it is not uncommon for the patients to require treatment that exceeds the capability of the emergency physician. Given the high proportion of older patients who require hospital admission, the treatment of many older patients exceeds the care that can be provided in the ED.

ED use sometimes has negative connotations. Many physicians seem apologetic when referring a patient to the ED and an ED visit is sometimes even considered a type of adverse outcome in research. These negative connotations may be based on a faulty perception of the role of the ED in the care of older patients. Since the older patient has a higher probability of serious disease, the ED may provide the best place to accomplish diagnosis and treatment of potentially dangerous undifferentiated complaints with relative speed compared to traditional inpatient and outpatient settings.

Typical ED approaches to diagnosis may not work well with the older patient. Older patients may present with undifferentiated complaints that have a broad differential diagnosis encompassing numerous serious diseases. Common diseases may present atypically. Cognitive impairment may limit the ability to obtain an accurate history. Older patients may tend to minimize symptoms; attributing a symptom to a benign rather than a more serious condition. For example, an older ED patient may suggest that their chest pain is due to indigestion rather than heart attack or their abdominal pain is constipation rather than ischemic bowel. Typical presenting signs and symptoms may be absent, and diagnostic tests may be normal despite serious diseases. For these reasons, an extensive evaluation may be appropriate to sort out the complexities of the situation. While commonly considered a sign of poor judgment and derogatively described as "shotgunning," with the complex older patient, extensive evaluation may be the most thoughtful approach.

Acute cardiac ischemia may be especially difficult to diagnose in the older patient. In the younger-old (e.g., 65–85 years), the majority of patients have chest pain, although atypical presentations can occur. After age 85 years, atypical presentations of cardiac ischemia outnumber typical ones by a 2:1 margin. Common atypical presentations include altered mental status, abdominal pain, dyspnea, and arrhythmia. In fact, acute delirium or change in level of consciousness (stupor or coma) can sometimes be the single presenting symptom of what turns out to be acute cardiac ischemia. Conversely, altered mental status is only rarely due to acute cardiac ischemia; it is the cause of record in only 1% of patients who present to the ED with acute mental status changes.

Abdominal pain in the older adult also presents challenges in the ED. For example, among older patients with acute cholecystitis, most do not have epigastric or right upper quadrant pain, and 5% do not have any pain at all. Over half will be afebrile, and nearly half will have a normal white blood cell count. Only one in five older patients with appendicitis present classically, less than half have an elevated temperature, and a quarter have atypical tenderness on examination that is either diffuse or localized to an area other than the right lower quadrant. In contrast to younger patients with abdominal pain, lack of abnormal laboratory studies or a normal body temperature in an older patient would not help rule out the need for surgical intervention. The nonspecific presentation of serious abdominal disease in the older adults has led to increased reliance on the use of computed

tomography, which has a much higher sensitivity and specificity than the clinical examination in the evaluation of the older patient with abdominal pain.

EVALUATION

The Geriatric Emergency Care Model (Table 18-1) outlines an approach to older ED patients that differs from the approach to younger patients. In addition to assessing the chief complaint, the care model encourages routine assessment of cognitive and functional status.

Older patients who present to the ED may have cognitive impairment. This impairment may limit the reliability of the medical history and reduce their understanding of and compliance with discharge instructions. Cognitive impairment may be previously diagnosed or unrecognized. Delirium is an important cause of cognitive impairment in older ED patients. About 10% of older ED patients have delirium, but is recognized as delirium in only one-third of cases. The failure to diagnose delirium in ED patients can increase mortality two- to threefold. Screening instruments for cognitive impairment that are useful in other settings may be of limited use in the ED. The Mini-Mental Status Examination, for instance, takes up to 15 minutes to complete in ED patients and some tasks, such as writing, can be limited in patients with extremity injuries or IVs. These limitations make its use impractical for emergency physicians who must therefore use brief, sensitive tests to assess for cognitive dysfunction, leaving more in-depth assessment to primary care physicians and consultants. Examples of brief tests include the Orientation Memory Concentration Test, the Six-Item Screener, and the Clock Drawing Test.

Functional status and the potential for functional decline after discharge are critical but rarely addressed issues in the ED. Factors that contribute to post-ED functional decline are listed in Table 18-2. People with subacute or chronic illnesses often visit the ED at a point where the illness has developed a significant impact on function, especially the ability to transfer and walk. Injuries can produce functional impairment either from the injury itself or from the treatments such as splints and slings. Patients whose basic activities of daily living are affected by their illness or injury require further evaluation or admission to the hospital, even if the treatment of the illness or injury would not require hospitalization. In the ED of the authors, mobility is assessed in older patients with a "Get Up and Go" test (assessing the ability to transfer and ambulate) with or without a walker as appropriate. Those who are unable to adequately

---

TABLE 18-2

Factors Associated with Post-ED Functional Decline and Adverse Outcomes

- Cognitive impairment
- ADL/IADL impairment (walking, transferring, transportation)
- Requires assistance from caregivers or home nurses
- Recent (30-day) ED use
- Recent (3–6 month) hospitalization
- Multiple medications (>3–5 meds)
- Lives alone, no caregiver
- Visual problems
- ED nursing recommendation

complete the test should not be discharged home from the ED without intensive home support. If such support cannot be assured, it is essential to explore alternatives to discharge, such as hospitalization or admission to a skilled nursing facility.

MANAGEMENT

Medication

There are multiple aspects of geriatric pharmacotherapy that are important in the ED. Elders use more prescription and over-the-counter drugs than any other age group. They consume a third of all prescription medications and half of the over-the-counter preparations. Adverse drug events including drug–drug interactions and adverse drug reactions are thought to account for more that 10% of ED visits and a quarter of hospital admissions for older patients.

Many patients receive new prescriptions when they are discharged from the ED. New medications can precipitate problems, such as unanticipated interactions with ongoing medications. The emergency physician may be unaware of the potential interactions or may not have complete information about ongoing medications. Only about 40% of community-dwelling older ED patients can either correctly identify their prescription medications or provide a written list. A third of the lists that are brought to the ED are not accurate.

Inappropriate prescribing can occur in the ED. Using the Beers criteria to identify potentially inappropriate prescriptions, about 4% of ED prescriptions are considered inappropriate. The Beers criteria have not been validated for use in the ED setting and it is possible that short-term use of selected medications deemed inappropriate in the Beers criteria would be acceptable, so 4% may be an overestimate. Inappropriate prescribing is a correctable problem and system changes, like placing a pharmacist in the ED or using warnings as a part of computerized prescription order entry might help minimize these problems.

Processes and Environment

Older adults are generally satisfied with ED care but are able to identify many areas for improvement. The majority of older patients express satisfaction with the quality of medical care they receive in the ED. They say that their medical problems were handled well and that they had no problems as a result of their care. On the other hand, older adults can identify concerns about the ED process. ED process concerns include long waits, lack of communication with staff and feeling abandoned, difficulty in arranging transportation home when discharged, and the billing processes. Feelings of anxiety are common because patients come to the ED with a suspected serious or life-threatening condition and are frightened by the prospects of care. Anxiety can be reduced by ED personnel who can help by providing updates about the condition, the proposed ED care, and plans for care after ED discharge. The ED environment is another area of concern to both patients and providers. ED patients note that the ED is too cold, there are not enough blankets, the gurneys are uncomfortable, especially for prolonged periods, pillows are not available, and the ED is noisy with disconcerting sights and sounds. ED professionals add that floors can be slippery and in-

crease risk of falls. The physical design of the ED limits interaction with staff; signage is confusing and lighting is harsh. There is often no source of external light. The ED environment is obviously not elder-friendly.

There is a movement to modify EDs along the lines developed by Acute Care of the Elderly (ACE units) (see Chapter 17 on ACE units). Some leaders in geriatric emergency medicine are considering ways of "ACE-ifying" the ED. and some even have suggested the development of geriatric-specific EDs, similar to pediatric EDs. One hospital demonstration project has created an emergency care unit staffed by geriatricians. The concept of the "ACE-ified" ED is consistent with the Geriatric Emergency Care Model proposed by the SAEM Task Force.

Teamwork is crucial for optimum emergency care of older patients. EDs can provide access to team members who can help with elder care, such as geriatric nurse practitioners, social workers, pharmacists, and physical therapists. These team members are especially valuable for communication, coordination of care, and discharge planning. Nonprofessional or volunteer staff can help improve the patient's comfort by responding to requests for blankets, temperature control, and information.

Changes to the ED environment may also improve care to older patients. The hard gurneys used in EDs are helpful for patient transportation but can be painful for patients. Reclining chairs like those used for dialysis can reduce pain and increase satisfaction for older patients. Other potential changes include sound-proof curtains between beds, nonskid surfaces on floors, rails on walls, large print signage, and large-faced clocks. Since older patients can arrive at the ED without eyeglasses and hearing aids, the ED could have a standing supply of necessary items for sensory problems. A supply of magnifiers, reading glasses, and electronic sound amplifiers can promote communication and make the older patient feel more comfortable. The revolution in computerized medical records afforded by modern information technology (IT) holds great promise for improving the ED care of older patients. Reliable medical records could reduce the time needed to obtain the medical history. Medical errors might be reduced since important information would be automatically downloaded at ED registration. Important information to be accessed should include past medical history, current diseases, recent imaging and laboratory studies, last known medications, allergies, dates of recent admissions, social history, and baseline cognitive and functional status.

PREVENTION

Accessing Vulnerable Populations

As noted above, the ED provides a safety net for underserved, vulnerable patients who lack access to routine care in the community. For this reason, there has been an interest in using the ED to provide preventive care. In 2000, SAEM's Public Health Task Force published a systematic review of the preventive activities recommended by the U.S. Preventive Services Task Force (USPTF) to assess their potential for ED use. Seventeen topics were reviewed, of which two (falls prevention and pneumococcal vaccination) were specific to older patients. Pneumococcal vaccination programs were recommended and the task force reported that falls prevention programs showed promise and should be further evaluated.

ED-based pneumococcal vaccination programs have been evaluated. They do not affect patient's length of stay, and require only about 4 minutes of staff time. The SAEM Task Force did not consider influenza immunization for older ED patients as part of their review. However, studies have shown that offering influenza vaccine to older ED patients may be an effective approach to reducing influenza morbidity and mortality and also reduce ED crowding during the flu season.

Nearly 2 million people older than 65 years are treated in the ED for a fall each year. Falls prevention activities recommended by the USPTF include exercise (particularly training to improve balance), safety-related skills and behaviors, and environmental hazard reduction, monitoring and adjusting medications, visual acuity testing, hormone replacement therapy, screening for dementia and osteoporosis, and postfall assessment and intervention. Given time constraints and the difficulty in evaluating acutely ill patients, most of these activities are unlikely to be conducted in the ED. However, the ED can educate older patients about falls and provide information and referral to reduce their risk of falling again. The ED visit might be a unique "teachable moment" for patients who have come to the ED because of falls. Patients who have fallen or are increased risk for falls may also be referred for geriatric assessment or falls prevention evaluation. While these activities have been recommended, it should be emphasized that there are few tests of effectiveness of these promising activities.

Prevention of Post-ED Decline

Elder ED visitors are susceptible to suffering health declines following an ED visit. Between 20% and 50% of older persons experience a significant deterioration in function after an ED visit. The vulnerability to decline in functional status after an ED visit is most likely due to a combination of chronic health conditions, acute illness or injury, coexisting medical and psychiatric problems, lack of social support, and iatrogenic issues such as medication errors. Factors associated with post-ED functional decline are listed in Table 18-2.

Regardless of the reasons for the decline, the ED would be ideal for community surveillance for elders at risk for functional decline who could benefit from multidisciplinary, community-based care management programs. But results of studies in different countries and using different approaches have shown mixed results. One problem is that available ED-based screening instruments have a low specificity and thus find too many cases, resulting in a referral rate that overwhelms community services. Successful programs share three features: identifying patients most likely to benefit, clinical control of care, and long-term follow-up.

There are barriers to providing preventive care in the ED. Those who work in an ED have conflicting priorities and a different approach to patients compared to providers in geriatric inpatient or outpatient settings. While emergency physicians realize that older patients frequently have unique needs and complex clinical presentations, they are pressed by time and the need to prioritize to focus on the presenting complaint and the need to rule out emergent conditions. Linkages between ED and geriatric outpatient units may help reduce barriers to preventive care for older ED patients. These patients could be screened in the ED for suitability for a community program. Those who are suspected of being at high risk could be referred. This approach has been used with fall prevention programs and in the care management programs noted above.

While not always anticipated, the patients themselves may present barriers to referral to community agencies. Older ED patients are frequently unwilling to participate in community services. The authors attempted to link patients in their ED with a multidisciplinary Medicaid Waiver Program of the local Area Agency on Aging. The ED used the Agency's screening instrument to identify at risk patients who were being discharged home. While many patients screened positive, few were willing to have the home-based assessment. It is possible that EDs with onsite geriatric nurses, care managers, or social workers could perform more focused screening. They might also help educate ED patients to encourage participation in the community agency programs and be directly involved in scheduling appointments.

SPECIAL ISSUES

Emergency Medical Services

Emergency Medical Services (EMS) use for older patients ranges between 100 and 167 per 1000 older adults per year. This rate exceeds that for other age groups and has important implications for EMS operations. As with emergency medicine and other areas in general, the EMS community has been slow to modify equipment, training, and procedures to reflect the needs of older adult patients. EMS administrators, government officials, and public health leaders must plan for an increased volume of EMS patients.

In the United States, EMS is generally provided by local communities and overseen by the state. However, the National Highway Traffic Safety Administration (NHTSA) created standard curricula, which have been adopted by many states. There are several levels of training for EMS providers. In the National Standard Curriculum for lower level providers (First Responders and EMT-basic), there is a specific focus on children (who represent 4% of EMS patients), but no similar focus on older persons (who represent one-third of EMS patients). The curricula for higher level providers (EMT-intermediate or EMT-paramedic) do have a specific focus on geriatrics. The curriculum for EMT-paramedic training includes comprehensive sections on physiology across the life span and geriatrics. Overall, this dedicated geriatrics training represents about 1% of the 1000- to 1200-hour curriculum.

The American Geriatrics Society (AGS) and the National Council of State EMS Training Coordinators recognized the deficiency in geriatric training for EMTs and created a coalition of 13 national organizations, which developed a continuing education course, Geriatrics Education for EMS (GEMS). Future cooperation between the EMS community and geriatric professionals is essential to ensure that their training is appropriate and adequate.

EMS equipment and protocols must be adapted to the older patient. For instance, the standard approach to patients with potential neck injuries is to place them in a rigid cervical collar and a backboard with head immobilizing blocks. This approach may be difficult or impossible in older patients with kyphoscoliosis. Immobilization for prolonged periods can also lead to skin breakdown. An alternative is the use of long vacuum splints that can immobilize patients with kyphoscoliosis in a more comfortable position.

Providers of prehospital care have a rare opportunity among healthcare providers—the ability to assess patients in their homes during their acute illness. Programs have been developed to use EMTs to screen older adults for social issues including abuse and neglect and to assess the home environment. EMTs are trained to identify potential problems, refer at-risk patients to the appropriate agencies for assessment and link the patient to community services. Evaluations of such programs have found a benefit to individual patients.

Geriatricians and the ED

There are not enough geriatricians for the present population and prospects for reducing this shortfall seem unlikely. Other specialists must develop sufficient geriatric expertise to attend to the special needs of the older patient. There is increasing growth in the number of emergency physicians who identify with geriatric emergency medicine. Part of this growth is a result of the AGSs' initiative to increase geriatric expertise among surgical and related medical specialists. Emergency Medicine has been an active participant in this project from its outset. The project's initial efforts were directed at increasing the geriatric content of residency education and the improving the quantity and quality of research. This project, a collaboration between specialty societies developed a cadre of young leaders and improved the outlook for geriatric expertise in the surgical specialties, especially in emergency medicine.

Geriatricians can actively participate in increasing expertise among emergency physicians. They can contribute to the educational program for emergency physicians in training and in continuing education for board certified physicians. Geriatricians can participate in rounds and can give didactic material to those in training. The future of continuing education is likely to be in computer-based interactive educational modules. Geriatricians can participate in the development of these modules.

Geriatricians and advance practice nurses have been active and important consultants to emergency physicians. Emergency physicians appreciate the difficulty in diagnosis and management of older patients. A cooperative geriatric consulting service is of benefit to both the geriatrician and the emergency physician. Emergency physicians are responsive to service programs that will improve outcomes for their patients. Increasing interest in geriatric emergency care makes emergency physicians particularly amenable to programs that improve outcomes for older patients. Having a relationship of mutual respect further fosters willingness to cooperate. Geriatricians with an idea for a program that links the ED with a service, e.g., a fall prevention or geriatric assessment, will find an ally if they wish to develop that program. Similarly, geriatricians should accept overtures from emergency physicians with ideas.

The Emergency Department's Relationship with Long-Term Care

Nearly a quarter of nursing home residents are transported at least once each year to the ED. Compared to community dwelling older adults, nursing home residents tend to present to the ED with less information and are more likely to have a nonspecific chief complaint. Thus they are most likely to require special adaptation in ED care. Two-thirds of nursing home residents who present to the ED are cognitively impaired and cannot provide a clear medical history. Often, families are not immediately available or are unaware of recent changes in the patient's condition. For this reason, communication between the nursing home and ED is crucial. However, 10% of nursing home residents are transported to the ED without *any* written documentation and important patient information often is missing in the 90% who arrive with paperwork. If baseline cognitive and functional status is not reported, it is impossible to determine if changes have occurred. The ED is also often a poor communicator when older patients are discharged back to the nursing home. Nursing home personnel report that residents often return from the ED without notification, written documentation, or recommendations for care.

Nursing home to ED and ED to nursing home transfers are a frequent and important type of transition in care. Poor communication during these transitions increases the cost of care, leads to greater use of health care services, and jeopardizes the patient's safety. The interaction between nursing homes and EDs is one area where geriatricians, nursing home personnel, and emergency physicians can interact to improve the care of the older patient.

Alternatives to Hospitalization

The ED is a gatekeeper between the community and the hospital. The decision to admit a patient to the hospital or to discharge a patient is made in the ED. As noted above, this difficult decision must take into account medical, functional, and social issues. There are several potential alternatives to hospitalization following an ED evaluation. One is the "Hospital at Home" concept. "Hospital at Home" programs have been evaluated for a variety of medical conditions including pneumonia, congestive heart failure (CHF), cellulitis, and chronic obstructive pulmonary disease (COPD). These programs have demonstrated improved satisfaction, lower rates of depression, and lower rates of nursing home admissions, without a difference in functional status or mortality. Another alternative is direct ED admission to skilled nursing facilities. Currently, Medicare requires a three-day inpatient hospital stay to qualify for Medicare skilled nursing facility coverage. Thus a Medicare patient can only be covered for a direct admission from the ED to a nursing home if they have had a qualifying hospital stay in the prior 30 days. For patients with private insurance or who belong to a Medicare health maintenance organization (HMO), the requirement for prior hospitalization may not be applicable. The requirement for prior hospitalization was created decades ago, prior to the many changes in inpatient, ED, and skilled nursing facility care. A change in this rule might lead to improved transitions and more efficient use of health care.

Cooperation between emergency physicians, primary care physicians, and geriatricians is essential to create successful alternatives to hospitalization. Guidelines could help match care settings with appropriate subsets of acutely ill older adults and treatment protocols to ensure patient and caregiver satisfaction, cost-effectiveness, low mortality, and good functional outcomes.

Disaster Planning

Older people are at increased risk and have unique needs in natural and human-made disasters. However, they often are not recognized as a vulnerable group during disaster planning and response. Recent disasters demonstrate their vulnerability. In the 2004 Indian Ocean tsunami, there were more deaths in people older than 60 years than in any other age group. Nearly half of those who died in hurricane Katrina, were 75 years or older and 70% were older than 60 years. Even power outages can be a significant problem for elderly who need oxygen, nebulizers, or who depend on motorized wheelchairs or other electric devices.

Elders, especially those with disabilities or chronic medical conditions, do not have the functional reserve to respond to a disaster. Social isolation, impaired mobility, economic constraints, functional dependence, and the need for specialized medical treatments such as dialysis affect the ability of older persons to cope with disasters. Geriatric specialists can help those involved in disaster planning and response understand the unique needs of the older population.

Standard disaster shelters often are unable to accommodate elders who are not functionally independent. Special needs shelters can be created to help care for chronically ill or functionally impaired patients, though these shelters may require patients to be accompanied by a caregiver. Special needs patients often present to hospital EDs during a disaster, even without acute medical emergencies, because their needs cannot be met elsewhere. Unfortunately, they may spend considerable time in the ED or require hospitalization if no other location for care is identified. Since both EDs and hospitals may be functioning at or beyond capacity during a disaster, these limited resources are strained by the nonmedical demands of these special needs patients, and more appropriate settings are preferable for both the patient and the system.

CONCLUSIONS

The art and science of care for older ED patients is in its infancy. We only now are beginning to understand the complexities in caring for the growing number of older persons. The anticipated growth of older population makes it imperative that we increase the number of health care professionals with expertise in caring for older patients in the ED and that we develop systems of care that are elder friendly. This requires the cooperation of researchers, educators and clinicians to improve outcomes for our older patients.

FURTHER READING

Adams JG, Gerson LW. A new model for emergency care of geriatric patients. *Acad Emerg Med.* 2003;10:271–274.

Bibler DD Jr, Merendino KA. Nonpenetrating chest trauma in the geriatric patient. *Geriatrics.* 1967;22:119–126.

Caplan GA, Williams AJ, Daly B, et al. A randomized, controlled trial of comprehensive geriatric assessment and multidisciplinary intervention after discharge of elderly from the emergency department—the DEED II study. *J Am Geriatr Soc.* 2004 Sep;52(9):1417–1423.

Gerson LW, Schelble DT, Wilson JE. Using paramedics to identify at-risk elderly, *Ann Emerg Med.* 1992;21:688–691.

Hastings SN, Heflin MT. A systematic review of interventions to improve outcomes for elders discharged from the emergency department. *Acad Emerg Med.* 2005;12(10):978–986.

Meldon SW, Mion LC, Palmer RM, et al. A brief risk-stratification tool to predict repeat emergency department visits and hospitalizations in older patients discharged from the emergency department. *Acad Emerg Med.* 2003;Mar;10(3):224–232.

Mion LC, Palmer RM, Meldon SW, et al. Case finding and referral model for emergency department elders: a randomized clinical trial. *Ann Emerg Med.* 2003;Jan;41(1):57–68.

McCaig LF, Nawar EN. National hospital ambulatory medical care survey: 2004 emergency department summary. Advance data from vital and health statistics, no. 372, Hyattsville, MD: National Center for Health Statistics; 2006.

McCusker J, Bellavance F, Cardin S, et al. Detection of older people at increased risk of adverse health outcomes after an emergency visit: the ISAR screening tool. *J Am Geriatr Soc.* 1999;47:1229–1237.

Parker JS, Vukov LF, Wollan PC. Abdominal pain in the older: use of temperature and laboratory testing to screen for surgical disease. *Fam Med.* 1996;28:193–197.

Sanders AB. Care of the elderly in emergency departments: conclusions and recommendations. *Ann Emerg Med.* 1992;21:830–834.

Sanders AB, ed. *Emergency Care of Elder Persons.* St. Louis, CO: Beverly Cracom; 1996.

Wilber ST, Gerson LW. A research agenda for geriatric emergency medicine. *Acad Emerg Med.* 2003;10:251–260.

Wilber ST, Gerson LW, Terrell KT, et al. Geriatric emergency medicine and the 2006 IOM report on the future of emergency care. *Acad Emerg Med.* 2006;13:1345–1351.

Wilber ST. Geriatric emergency medicine. In: Solomon DH, LoCicero J, Roesnethal RA, eds. *New Frontiers in Geriatric Research. An Agenda for Surgical and Related Medical Specialties.* New York, New York: American Geriatrics Society; 2004: 53–83.

Critical Care

Eric B. Milbrandt ■ *Derek C. Angus*

One in five Americans dies in the intensive care unit (ICU) or shortly after an ICU stay. Regardless of the precise age threshold used to define "elderly," it is clear that a sizeable proportion of ICU patients are older adults. In the United States, those aged 65 years or older constitute nearly 50% of ICU admissions, a percentage which will grow considerably with the aging of the population. While the proportion of elderly ICU patients maybe higher in the United States than in other countries, most developed countries have seen substantial ICU use by patients older than age of 65 years. Importantly, most studies support that age alone is not an independent predictor of outcome in the ICU and that age should not be used as a criterion for determining which patients can "benefit" from intensive care. Rather, the key issue is the reversibility of the acute illness in the context of the overall health of the patient.

As a group, the elderly present with a unique set of challenges and opportunities for critical care providers. Many of these are well-defined and known, while others are poorly defined and relatively understudied. In this chapter, we briefly review some of the physiologic changes associated with aging and their implications for intensive care. We discuss some of the common admitting diagnoses and associated conditions seen in elderly patients and present data about outcomes of intensive care in the aged. We then explore interventions that may improve outcomes of intensive care, not only for patients, but for their loved ones as well.

AGE-RELATED CHANGES IN PHYSIOLOGY

Much has been written about the physiology of aging and the reader may refer to the Chapters in Part IV on organ systems for more detail for a thorough review of the topic. Rather than duplicate what has already been written, we focus on some of the key physiologic changes associated with aging and their implications for intensive care. These changes can be summarized as a gradual decline in organ function and physiologic reserve with an increased prevalence of chronic disease and vulnerability to disease.

The aging cardiovascular system can affect critical illness in two ways. The first is through increased prevalence of cardiovascular disease, which may be the primary reason for presenting to the ICU or a complicating factor when a patient with a noncardiovascular admitting diagnosis subsequently develops acute cardiovascular illness, such as cardiac ischemia. The second way cardiovascular disease can affect critical illness is through decreased cardiac reserve. Though this decrease may not be sufficient to alter daily activities in otherwise healthy subjects, the acute "stress test" of critical illness is often sufficient to make it manifest.

Maximal heart rate, ejection fraction, and cardiac output decrease with age, as does the responsiveness to sympathetic stimulation. The aging heart is therefore somewhat limited in its ability to increase cardiac output in response to stress, relying primarily on increased filling and stroke volume, rather than increased heart rate. This leads to greater preload dependency and amplifies the cardiac output compromising effects of hypovolemia. However, because of age-related stiffening of the ventricles, diastolic dysfunction also becomes common, increasing the risk of pulmonary edema with overly aggressive fluid resuscitation. Ventricular stiffening results in an increased reliance on "atrial kick" for diastolic filling and poor tolerance of atrial fibrillation. Taken together, these changes mandate careful attention to volume status and control of atrial arrhythmias.

Pulmonary function gradually declines with age due to changes in the lung and chest wall. Vital capacity, or the maximum amount of air that can be exhaled after a maximum inhalation, decreases, as does the speed with which it can be exhaled. Because of ventilation–perfusion mismatching and increased airway closure, the oxygen content of arterial blood decreases with a resultant widening the alveolar-to-arterial oxygen gradient. In other words, less of the oxygen that is delivered to the lung is taken up by the body. The sum of these changes leaves elderly subjects less able to respond to the increase respiratory requirements of critical illness even in the absence of overt respiratory pathology, such as chronic obstructive pulmonary disease.

There is a significant decline in renal function with aging, including decreased renal blood flow, glomerular filtration rate (GFR), and creatinine clearance (CrCl). Urine concentrating and diluting ability also decrease, leaving the elderly patient less prepared to deal with electrolyte and volume status changes. Elimination of renally excreted drugs decreases in parallel with GFR. Approximations of GFR, such as CrCl, should therefore be used to adjust the dosage of these medications. A variety of equations can be used to estimate CrCl, with the Cockcroft and Gault equation most commonly utilized:

$$CrCl = \text{creatinine clearance}$$
$$= \frac{[(140 - age) \times IBW \, (\times 0.85 \text{ for females})]}{(Scr \times 72)}$$

In this equation, Scr is serum creatinine and IBW the ideal body weight. For males, IBW = 50 kg + 2.3 kg for each inch over 5 feet; for females, IBW = 45.5 kg + 2.3 kg for each inch over 5 feet.

Age-related changes in hepatic metabolism are much more difficult to predict. Unlike renal function, there is no measure to assess hepatic metabolism. Put simply, hepatic elimination of drugs is either reduced or unaltered. Host factors, such as blood flow, concurrent drug use, nutritional status, gender, disease states, and genetic differences in enzymatic activity, result in considerable metabolic variability from patient to patient. In the setting of known hepatic insufficiency, such as cirrhosis, clinicians should either avoid or reduce the dosage of hepatically eliminated drugs. In such patients, clinicians should also be on the watch for coagulation abnormalities and hypoalbuminemia, the latter of which may require reduced dosing for drugs that are highly albumin bound.

Aging is associated with significant changes in immune function that may have important implications for elderly ICU patients. The term "immunosenescence" has been used to describe these changes, which include unresponsiveness, hyporesponsiveness, or aberrant responsiveness to tissue damage and/or infection. With advancing age, T and B lymphocyte compartments of the immune system deteriorate progressively while the respiratory burst of macrophages and neutrophils becomes impaired rendering them less able to destroy bacteria. This leaves the elderly less responsive to vaccinations and more prone to developing invasive bacterial infections, whether community- or hospital-acquired. Furthermore, aging brings an imbalance of pro- and anti-inflammatory cytokines, leading to either inadequate or overabundant response when the system is challenged. As such, older subjects may not be able to adequately activate the immune system or stop it once it is started. Whether these cytokine imbalances make the elderly ICU patient more likely to develop cytokine-mediated organ dysfunction in the setting of tissue damage or infection is not known, though it seems likely.

In addition to organ system changes, aging brings about a gradual decrease in lean body mass and total body water with an increase in body fat. These body composition changes lead to changes in volume of distribution for many drugs. Fat soluble drugs, such as the sedative propofol, may have an increased volume of distribution, with fatty tissues serving as a slowly clearing drug reservoir once the medication is stopped. Water-soluble drugs, on the other hand, may have a decreased volume of distribution, with a potential need for loading dose reductions. For an excellent review of pharmacokinetics in the elderly, the reader is referred to Mayersohn. Changes in body composition and physical activity also lead to a decrease in resting energy expenditure. Even so, risk of protein-calorie malnutrition increases, especially during acute illness, highlighting the importance of early nutritional support.

COMMON ADMITTING DIAGNOSES

Table 19-1 lists some of the more common ICU admitting diagnoses seen in the elderly, many of which represent exacerbations of chronic conditions or diseases to which the elderly are particularly vulnerable. Rather than focusing on management principles of each disease, which are well covered in just about any critical care text, we review two quintessential diseases of the elderly, community-acquired pneumonia (CAP) and severe sepsis.

Pneumonia is often called the old man's friend because, as pointed out by Sir William Osler more than 100 years ago, pneumonia is a frequent, nonpainful, lethal event in elderly patients. Since Osler's time, there have been considerable advances in the management of pneumonia, not the least of which is the discovery of antibiotics. Nevertheless, CAP remains common and is still one of the leading causes of hospital admission and death throughout the world. In an analysis of 150 000 elderly Medicare recipients hospitalized with CAP in the first quarter of 1997, Kaplan and colleagues found that almost half of all elderly patients admitted for CAP die in the subsequent year, with most deaths occurring after hospital discharge. One of three elderly patients who survived hospitalization for CAP died in the year following hospital discharge. Their data confirm Osler's notion and show that even today, with many preventive and therapeutic measures, there is a high risk of death in elderly patients discharged from the hospital after an episode of CAP. These data have important implications for patient prognostication, family counseling, and medical decision making, such as whether to continue life support and aggressive medical care. They also highlight the fact that hospital mortality is not an appropriate outcome measure for studies in elderly patients with CAP, since beneficial or detrimental aspects of interventions may not manifest within this time frame. Given the overall poor prognosis that CAP portends for the elderly, preventative measures, such as pneumococcal and influenza vaccination and smoking and alcohol cessation, will remain key.

TABLE 19-1

Common ICU Admitting Diagnoses in the Elderly

Acute respiratory failure due to	Kidney or urinary tract infection
• Pneumonia	Gastrointestinal hemorrhage
• Congestive heart failure	Nutritional and metabolic disorders
• Chronic obstructive pulmonary disease	• Uncontrolled diabetes mellitus
Cardiovascular conditions	Severe sepsis
• Myocardial infarction/unstable angina	Postoperative states
• Arrhythmias and conduction disorders	• Coronary artery bypass
Falls and fractures	• Cardiac catheterization/percutaneous intervention
Stroke or transient ischemic attacks	• Hip replacement or fracture repair
	• Major bowel procedures

Severe sepsis is a common, expensive, and frequently fatal condition, with as many deaths annually as those from acute myocardial infarction. It is especially common in the elderly and is likely to increase substantially as the U.S. population ages. Angus and colleagues examined the incidence, cost, and outcome of severe sepsis in the 1995 hospital discharge records from seven large states. The authors found that the incidence of severe sepsis increased >100-fold with age (0.2/1000 in children to 26.2/1000 in those >85 years old). The most commonly identified sites of infection were respiratory, genitourinary, abdominal, and wound/soft tissue. Mortality was 28.6%, or 215 000 deaths nationally, and also increased with age, from 10% in children to 38.4% in those >85 years old. Women had lower age-specific incidence and mortality, but the difference in mortality was explained by differences in underlying disease and site of infection. Average costs per case were $22 100, with annual total costs of $16.7 billion nationally. Incidence was projected to increase by 1.5% per annum.

The observation that sepsis is a disease of the elderly mandates consideration of the appropriateness of care, including determination of patient preferences. Data suggest that there are already differences in the aggressiveness of treatment in the very old, with lower length of stay, ICU use, and hospital costs in those aged >85 years. Yet, aggressive care is not necessarily futile in the elderly, and the majority of elderly septic patients survive to hospital discharge. Unfortunately, there are limited data on postdischarge survival or quality of life after sepsis in the elderly. Such information will be crucial in determining optimal healthcare policy as the U.S. population ages and the number of cases of sepsis increases.

ASSOCIATED CONDITIONS THAT MAY COMPLICATE ICU CARE

In addition to age-related changes in physiology, there are a number of associated conditions that may complicate the care and management of critically ill elderly patients (Table 19-2). Atypical presentations of common medical conditions, such as myocardial infarction and CAP, are common in the elderly, which may lead to delayed or incorrect diagnoses and which mandate broad initial differential diagnosis lists. Anemia may be preexisting or a consequence of critical illness. Current guidelines recommend restricting red blood cell transfusion to those patients with hemoglobin values of ≤ 7 g/dL, as long as active bleeding or ischemia is not present. Drug-resistant organisms are increasingly encountered, especially in nursing home residents or those who are frequently hospitalized. While it is important to avoid antibiotic overuse, careful attention to risk factors and local resistance patterns should guide antibiotic selection.

The proportion of elderly patients who are undernourished is high and undernutrition has serious health implications in the ICU, including immune dysfunction, poor wound healing, and increased mortality risk. Dysphagia, poor dentition, swallowing disorders, and constipation not only put patients at risk of aspiration, but may also significantly impair nutritional support measures. Polypharmacy is widespread, increasing the likelihood of drug interactions and life-threatening side-effects. Medication lists should therefore be "trimmed" regularly and reconciled with each care setting transition.

Pressure sores may be a reason for admission, such as when they are a source of infection, or a complication of care, especially if skin care is not meticulously addressed. Skin integrity can be further compromised by urinary or bowel incontinence, though collecting devices, such as urinary catheters, may exacerbate other conditions, such as delirium. Vision and hearing difficulties are frequent and efforts should be made to avoid sensory deprivation due to misplaced glasses or hearing aids. Alcoholism is present in around 10% of ICU patients and even more common is certain patient populations, such as those admitted for trauma. Early recognition of alcohol abuse and dependence is essential and should prompt consideration of several alcohol-specific diagnoses that have important prognostic and therapeutic implications, including alcohol withdrawal, cardiomyopathy, arrhythmias, and electrolyte disorders.

DEMENTIA AND DELIRIUM

Two associated conditions, dementia and delirium, require special consideration. There are currently 2.2 million Americans living with dementia. Projections suggest that this number will grow to greater than 10 million by 2040 due to the aging of the population and increasing life expectancy among those affected. Although there are no data to support it, there is a prevailing notion in the medical community that patients with dementia have worse outcomes from intensive care than those without dementia. This has led some to suggest that the use of critical care services be restricted for demented patients.

Challenging this notion is a study by Pisani and colleagues that examined short-term outcomes in medical ICU patients with ($n = 66$) or without dementia ($n = 329$). Despite the fact that patients with dementia were older, slightly sicker, and more likely to have a do-not-resuscitate/do-not-intubate order on admission, there were no differences in outcomes between demented and nondemented patients. In fact, ICU and hospital mortality rates were actually lower in patients with dementia, although these differences were not statistically significant. Not surprisingly, patients with dementia were more likely to have their code status changed to less aggressive care. Yet, overall aggressiveness of ICU care, as measured by the use of ICU interventions, was not different between groups. The authors concluded that presumptions of less favorable outcomes of critical care in patients with dementia should not drive treatment decisions in the ICU, with the possible exception of code status determinations.

The findings of Pisani and colleagues raise some interesting ethical challenges. Most critically, how does one elicit preferences for aggressive care from patients with dementia, given that they may or may not have clearly articulated their preferences before cognitive

TABLE 19-2

Associated Conditions that may Complicate Care of Elderly ICU Patients	
Atypical presentations of common medical conditions	Polypharmacy
Anemia	Pressure sores
Drug resistant organisms	Urinary or bowel incontinence
Malnutrition/undernutrition	Vision and hearing difficulties
Dysphagia/swallowing disorders	Alcoholism
Constipation	Dementia
Poor dentition	Delirium

impairment became too severe? Furthermore, with less than half of dementia cases being recognized by bedside physicians in the Pisani study, one can envision scenarios where decision-making ability is presumed, yet not present. How can we try to help this process along, and what is the role of the intensivist? A good place to start might be to engage in ICU exit interviews to help families think about what they would do the next time their loved one becomes ill. Better yet would be to get patients better oriented to their potential future and more involved in advanced decision making well before dementia has become too advanced and the window of opportunity has closed.

Delirium is a form of acute cognitive dysfunction that manifests as a fluctuating change in mental status, with inattention and altered level of consciousness. Delirium is very common in the ICU, occurring in as many as 80% of mechanically ventilated ICU patients. Many clinicians consider ICU delirium to be expected, iatrogenic, and without consequence. However, recent data associate delirium with increased duration of mechanical ventilation and ICU stay, worse 6-month mortality, and higher costs. Although there are clearly defined risk factors for delirium, there is little understanding of the underlying pathophysiology. The precise mechanisms are unknown and there are likely to be multiple mechanisms at work in any given patient (Table19-3). For an in-depth review of potential mechanisms, the reader is referred to Milbrandt and Angus.

Attending to modifiable risk factors is a central tenet of delirium prevention. Areas to consider include: avoiding polypharmacy; minimizing the use of anticholinergics and sedatives while appropriately treating pain; promoting good sleep hygiene by establishing a sleep–wake cycle and avoiding noise and light pollution; preventing sensory deprivation by ensuring use of glasses and hearing aides; and frequent orientation. In the hospital wards, Inouye and colleagues found an intervention that consisted of standardized protocols for the management of six risk factors for delirium (cognitive impairment, sleep deprivation, immobility, visual impairment, hearing impairment, and dehydration) significantly reduced the number and duration of delirium episodes in hospitalized older patients. To date, no such trial has been conducted in the ICU.

When nonpharmacologic measures fail to prevent or remedy ICU delirium, national guidelines recommend treatment with antipsychotics. Haloperidol has been used for many years to manage agitation in mechanically ventilated ICU patients, and it is the recommended drug for treatment of ICU delirium. Kalisvaart and colleagues compared the effect of haloperidol prophylaxis (1.5 mg/day preoperatively and up to 3 days postoperatively) with that of placebo in 430 elderly hip surgery patients at risk for delirium. Although there was no difference in the incidence of postoperative delirium between treatment and control groups, those in the haloperidol group had significantly reduced severity and duration of delirium (5.4 days vs. 11.8 days; $P < 0.001$). Haloperidol also appeared to reduce the length of hospital stay among those who developed delirium (17.1 days vs. 22.6 days; $P < 0.001$). In a retrospective cohort study that examined haloperidol use in 989 patients who were mechanically ventilated for longer than 48 hours, Milbrandt and colleagues found that patients treated with haloperidol had significantly lower hospital mortality than did those who never received the drug (20.5% vs. 36.1%; $P = 0.004$), an association that persisted after adjusting for potential confounders. Because of the observational nature of the study and the potential risks associated with haloperidol use, these findings require confirmation in a randomized, controlled trial before being applied to routine patient care. Anecdotally, the use of atypical antipsychotics, such as risperidone, olanzapine, or ziprasidone, is in vogue. However, they are no more effective than haloperidol for treating ICU delirium and, like haloperidol, these agents all have the potential to cause QT-interval prolongation and cardiac arrhythmias. Furthermore, the newer medications are 10- to 20-fold more expensive than generic haloperidol.

OUTCOMES OF INTENSIVE CARE

It is perhaps self-evident that ICU patients have high short-term mortality, the rate of which depends primarily on the admitting diagnosis, the severity of physiological derangement, and the underlying chronic health state of the patient, rather than age itself. For those that survive to hospital discharge, a traditional measure of therapeutic success, subsequent survival trajectories differ markedly from the general population. In other words, survivors of critical illness are at increased risk of mortality long after the acute illness has resolved. In diseases like severe sepsis, this effect may be seen as far out as a year after the illness.

The specialty of critical care has made significant advances in the care of severely ill patients. Mortality rates for many commonly encountered critical illnesses such as severe sepsis and acute respiratory distress syndrome (ARDS) have declined sharply over the past two decades. However, as greater numbers of patients survive intensive care, it is becoming increasingly evident that quality of life after critical illness is not always optimal.

Late nonmortal sequelae of critical illness include deficits in physical function, cognition, and mental health. The majority of studies that have examined post-ICU physical function have focused on survivors of ARDS, a population that tends to be younger than general ICU patient populations. For example, Herridge and colleagues found that 1 year after the illness, the majority of ARDS survivors reported persistent functional disability primarily due to

TABLE 19-3

Pathophysiological Mechanisms Thought to Underlie Delirium

Predisposing factors	*Iatrogenic and environmental*
• Age	• Sedatives and analgesics
• Preexisting cognitive deficits	• Sleep deprivation
• Multiple comorbidities	• Pain and anxiety
• Poor functional status	• Unfamiliar environment
• Vision and hearing impairment	• Physical restraints
• Drug or alcohol abuse	• Bladder catheterization
• Malnutrition	*Neurotransmitter abnormalities*
• HIV	• ↓ Acetylcholine
• Genetics (ApoE4)	• ↑ Dopamine, 5-HT, GABA, glutamate, NE
Metabolic derangements	*Occult diffuse brain injury due to*
• Dehydration, hyperosmolarity	• Local and systemic hypoxia
• ↑ Na+, Ca++	• Hypoperfusion and hypotension
• Uremia	• Hyperglycemia
• Liver failure	• Cytokine-mediated inflammation and microvascular thrombosis

HIV, human immunodeficiency virus; Apo, apolipoprotein; 5-HT, serotonin; GABA, γ-aminobutyric acid; NE, norepinephrine.

nonpulmonary conditions such as muscle weakness and fatigue. Though the distance walked in 6 minute improved over the 12 months after ICU discharge, at 1 year, it was still only two-thirds predicted. Less than half had returned to work. The absence of systemic corticosteroid treatment or ICU-acquired illnesses as well as the rapid resolution organ dysfunction was associated with better functional status during the 1-year follow-up. At 2 years, exercise limitation persisted while health-related quality of life remained below that of the normal population.

Studies that have specifically examined functional outcomes in elderly ICU survivors have been relatively small and methodologically limited, as reviewed by Hennessy and colleagues. An important underlying theme that emerges from such studies is that elderly ICU survivors, while clearly at risk of post-ICU physical disability, are more frequently satisfied with their post-ICU lives than younger survivors and report preservation of health-related quality of life. This apparent paradox is not unique to ICU-based studies and is well-described in health utility theory. Clinicians and family members, therefore, should not presume that elderly patients who are either premorbidly functionally limited or likely to suffer from post-ICU limitations would not want aggressive care during their acute illness. Ideally, such decisions should be made based on the patient's own expressed wishes. When this is not possible, decision makers should be careful not to discount too heavily the value, or utility, that a functionally impaired life might represent for the patient.

Evidence from a variety of cohort studies suggests that 25% to 78% of ICU survivors experience neurocognitive impairments. For instance, nearly half of ARDS survivors manifest neurocognitive sequelae 2 years after their illness, falling to below the sixth percentile of the normal distribution of cognitive function. Considering Terri Fried's observation that 89% of Americans would not wish to be kept alive if they had severe, irreversible neurologic damage, these findings are quite concerning. In general, difficulty with memory is the most frequently observed deficit, followed by executive function and attention deficits, as shown by Hopkins and colleagues. Impairments tend to improve during the first 6 to 12 months after hospital discharge, with little additional improvement after 1 year. Elderly subjects seem to be at greatest risk, especially in the setting of preexisting mild neurocognitive impairment or dementia. Furthermore, ICU-acquired cognitive insults may accelerate the trajectory of cognitive decline, leading to what some have called "ICU-accelerated dementia." Data regarding the potential mechanisms underlying ICU-acquired neurocognitive deficits are quite limited, though evidence suggests roles for hypoxemia, hypotension, hyperglycemia, delirium, sedatives, and analgesics.

Psychiatric symptoms and disorders, such as depression, anxiety, and posttraumatic stress disorder (PTSD), affect 15% to 35% of ICU survivors months or even years after their acute medical illness, as reviewed by Weinert. In one study of 154 survivors of >48 hours of mechanical ventilation, 32% suffered from depression (Center for Epidemiologic Studies Depression Scale (CES-D) score ≥ 16) 1 year after their illness. The results were nearly identical to those obtained at the initial 2-month follow-up, suggesting that the burden of depression for ICU survivors may not improve over time. Other studies in survivors of ARDS or other forms of respiratory failure have shown similarly high rates of depression symptoms.

It is not difficult to understand why the experience of critical illness might lead to symptoms of anxiety and PTSD. Similar to combat or natural disaster, there are a number of extreme psycho-logical stresses in the ICU, including fearing of losing one's life, being routinely subjected to painful procedures, sleep deprivation, drug-induced hallucinations, and a perceived loss of control. Of survivors of ARDS, 28% scored above the threshold value on the Posttraumatic Stress Syndrome Inventory (PTSS-10), which is highly suggestive of the diagnosis of PTSD. Studies of other ICU patient groups, such as survivors of septic shock and those undergoing cardiac surgery, show a similarly high risk of PTSD symptoms. In the ARDS study, those with recall of ICU events seemed to fair worse, suggesting that memories of ICU events were associated with psychologic distress. However, others have shown that the content of recalled ICU memories may be key, in that those with delusional memories and no factual recall appear to be at greater risk of post-ICU depression, anxiety, and PTSD.

Small randomized trials show that depression and posttraumatic stress symptoms can be reduced by interventions during or after critical illness. Kress and colleagues found that mechanically ventilated patients who had their sedation interrupted each day had a trend toward a lower incidence of PTSD (0% vs. 32%, $P = 0.06$) in addition to shorter duration of mechanical ventilation. Jones and colleagues demonstrated that a self-help rehabilitation manual was effective in aiding physical recovery and reducing depression in survivors of mechanical ventilation. In patients suffering from stroke, two studies have shown that prophylactic administration of antidepressants prevents the emergence of depressive symptoms, even when started several weeks after the stroke. Whether such a preventative approach would work in other ICU patient groups at high risk of depression remains to be seen. It is clear, however, that antidepressants can be helpful in established postillness depression, such as after acute coronary ischemia or stroke.

CAREGIVER OUTCOMES

More than 40 million Americans serve as informal caregivers to their ill loved ones, and often suffer physical, psychologic, and financial burden as a result. Most evidence for caregiver burden relates to the care of the chronically ill, but studies are beginning to show that informal caregivers of ICU survivors and family members of current ICU patients also have significant burden, including increased risk for depression and PTSD. For instance, in the longest longitudinal follow-up to date of the informal caregivers ($n = 169$) of critical illness survivors, Van Pelt and colleagues found an elevated and persistent risk of depression, disruption in lifestyle, and reduction in employment over a 12-month period after the onset of critical illness. One-third of caregivers were at risk of depression (CES-D ≥ 16) at 2 months. Although the proportion of caregivers at risk of depression decreased over time, this difference was not statistically significant. At 2 months, only 28.7% of caregivers were employed and 13.0% indicated that they had stopped working in order to provide care. Similar to depression risk, there was no statistically significant change in either employment status or lifestyle disruption over time.

Comparing caregivers of ICU survivors with other caregiver populations provides important insight into the negative impact of critical illness. The findings of Van Pelt and colleagues demonstrate lifestyle disruption and risk for depression that are much greater than that of the general population and similar to caregivers of Alzheimer's patients. Considering the tremendous caregiver burden that frequently results from caring for those with dementia, these findings underscore the severity of the downstream impairment that can occur after critical illness. This study strengthens growing evidence that the negative societal impact of critical illness goes beyond short-term mortality to include significant lifestyle disruption not only for ICU survivors but also their informal caregivers.

TOWARD IMPROVING OUTCOMES OF INTENSIVE CARE IN THE ELDERLY

There are a variety of interventions that improve outcomes in ICU patients regardless of patient age (Table 19-4). Adherence to these and other measures can be increased by the use of checklists, such as the ICU Quality Improvement Checklist developed by the Kansas Critical Care Collaborative (see http://www.kscritcare.org). In addition, there are a variety of interventions that are particularly well-suited to address specific conditions experienced more commonly in elderly ICU patients. Delirium prevention strategies, which were discussed above, have the potential to reduce medical complications, length of stay, and cost, yet remain largely untested in the ICU. The importance of avoiding polypharmacy to prevent dangerous drug interactions and side-effects cannot be overstated. Yet, a casual review of medication records in most ICUs reveals medication lists that are often much larger than is perhaps necessary.

Prolonged bed rest has well-known adverse physiologic effects, including cardiovascular deconditioning and skeletal muscle atrophy. In healthy volunteers, a mere 14 days of bed rest can produce a 1.7% decrease in lean body mass, with a 4.1% decrease in lean thigh mass. After 6 weeks of bed rest, 25% to 30% of quadriceps strength is lost. Although other factors, such as illness severity and exposure to corticosteroids, no doubt play a role in post-ICU physical disability, the contribution of bed rest should not be discounted. Because of the nature of critical illness and the modalities used to manage it, prolonged bed rest seems to be the rule in the ICU. Physical rehabilitation, which has the potential to restore lost function, is traditionally not started until after ICU discharge. One small study by Bailey and colleagues evaluated the feasibility and safety of early physical activity in 103 patients (mean age 62.5 years) with respiratory failure who required >4 days of mechanical ventilation.

"Early" was defined as the interval starting with initial physiologic stabilization and ending with ICU discharge. Activity events were sitting on the edge of the bed, sitting in a chair, and ambulating with or without assistance. Remarkably, nearly 70% of survivors were able to ambulate >100 ft before ICU discharge. Since the ability to ambulate is often an important determinant of a patient's ability to return to home, this finding is quite impressive. Participation in activity events was not limited by advanced age, comorbidities, or the presence of an endotracheal tube. Adverse events were infrequent, easily remedied, and did not result in complications that required additional therapy, extra cost, or longer length of stay.

Though many ICU admissions are unanticipated and emergent, a sizeable proportion is anticipated due to elective operative procedures. For these anticipated ICU admissions, preoperative assessment can identify previously undiagnosed or inadequately treated comorbidities. Subsequent medical optimization may reduce postoperative morbidity and mortality, as has been shown for cardiorespiratory optimization prior to major thoracic or abdominal surgeries. Patients undergoing nonthoracoabdominal procedures may also benefit from this approach. In a before and after study, Harari and colleagues found that preoperative comprehensive geriatric assessment incorporating prediction of adverse outcomes combined with targeted interventions reduced postoperative medical complications, such as pneumonia and delirium, and length of stay in elective orthopedic patients aged 65 years and over. There were also improvements in pressure sores, pain control, early mobilization, and inappropriate catheter use. Limiting the broad application of the results of this study are the significant amount of time and resources that comprised the intervention, including both pre- and posthospitalization clinic visits and in-home physical therapy as well as active in-hospital assessment by a geriatrician and nurse.

ICU follow-up clinics have been proposed as a means of identifying and addressing the myriad of potential late sequelae that elderly ICU survivors may face. While still uncommon in the United States, as many as 30% of ICUs providing care to high-level ICU patients in the United Kingdom offered outpatient follow-up their patients in 2006 as shown by Griffiths and colleagues. ICU follow-up clinics can be nurse- or doctor-led and are commonly run on multidisciplinary lines, with patients potentially benefiting from inputs that include physical therapy, dietetics, urology, ear, nose, and throat (ENT), psychology, and psychiatry. Where extended ICU follow-up exists, patients report great satisfaction with the service. A multicenter randomized control trial of the effectiveness of ICU follow-up clinics in improving longer-term outcomes of critical illness, the PRaCTICaL trial (ISRCTN24294750), is currently underway.

Family satisfaction is an important measure of the quality of ICU care. Yet, attention to objective measurement and improvement of family satisfaction is a relatively recent phenomena in the ICU. Clinician–family communication is possibly the most important factor driving family satisfaction. Other factors that may improve family satisfaction include allowing family members more time to speak during conferences, avoiding contradictions in provided clinical information, helping resolve conflicts among family members, and implementing flexible visitation policies.

Having a loved one die in the ICU is an extraordinarily stressful event. Studies of families of dying patients identify effective communication between caregivers and families and having support from caregivers throughout the decision-making process to be important

TABLE 19-4

Interventions to Improve Outcomes in ICU Patients Regardless of Age	
INTERVENTION	OUTCOME
Subcutaneous heparin	↓ Deep venous thrombosis
H2-blockers	↓ Gastric "stress" ulcers
Low tidal volume ventilation	↓ Ventilator-induced lung injury ↓ Mortality
Goal-directed sedation with daily sedation interruption	↓ Duration of mechanical ventilation
Spontaneous breathing trials	↓ Duration of mechanical ventilation
Attention to skin care	↓ Skin breakdown
Tight blood glucose control	↓ Mortality
Lower transfusion thresholds	↓ Mortality
Hand hygiene	↓ Hospital-acquired infections

to family members. Yet, communication and support are sometimes inadequate due to the many competing priorities in a busy ICU. Lautrette and colleagues evaluated the effect of a proactive communication strategy in family members of 126 patients dying in 22 ICUs in France. The intervention consisted of an end-of-life family conference conducted according to specific guidelines and that concluded with the provision of a brochure on bereavement. In the control group, interactions between the family and the ICU staff, including the end-of-life conference, occurred according to the usual practice at each center. The authors found that those in the intervention group had longer conferences and more time for family members to talk. Furthermore, intervention family members had decreased symptoms of anxiety, depression, and PTSD 90 days after the patient's death, suggesting that the intervention may lessen the burden of bereavement.

Palliative care is medical care focused on the relief of suffering and support for the best possible quality of life for patients and families facing life-threatening illness. Many clinicians consider intensive care and palliative care to be diametrically opposed. Yet, as pointed out by Ira Byock, each discipline's primary goal (extending life for critical care and comfort and quality of life for palliative care) represents an important secondary goal for the other. ICU care providers are beginning to realize the benefits of early and programmatic palliative care involvement for their sickest patients. Recent successful interventions have included processes for symptom (especially pain) assessment and management; mandatory family meetings; daily patient-specific goal setting; advance care planning; and addressing patient and family emotional and spiritual health. A recent special supplement of Critical Care Medicine introduced by Ira Byock discusses these interventions and other issues surrounding palliative care in the ICU in greater detail.

FURTHER READING

Angus DC, Barnato AE, Linde-Zwirble WT, et al. Use of intensive care at the end of life in the United States: an epidemiologic study. *Crit Care Med.* 2004;32(3):638–643.

Angus DC, Linde-Zwirble WT, Lidicker J, Clermont G, Carcillo J, Pinsky MR. Epidemiology of severe sepsis in the United States: analysis of incidence, outcome, and associated costs of care. *Crit Care Med.* 2001;29(7):1303–1310.

Bailey P, Thomasen GE, Spuhler VJ, et al. Early activity is feasible and safe in respiratory failure patients. *Crit Care Med.* 2006;35(1):139–145.

Byock I. Improving palliative care in intensive care units: identifying strategies and interventions that work. *Crit Care Med.* 2006;34(11 Suppl):S302-S305.

Fried TR, Bradley EH, Towle VR, Allore H. Understanding the treatment preferences of seriously ill patients. *N Engl J Med.* 2002;346(14):1061–1066.

Griffiths JA, Barber VS, Cuthbertson BH, Young JD. A national survey of intensive care follow-up clinics. *Anaesthesia.* 2006;61(10):950–955.

Harari D, Hopper A, Dhesi J, Babic-Illman G, Lockwood L, Martin F. Proactive care of older people undergoing surgery ('POPS'): designing, embedding, evaluating and funding a comprehensive geriatric assessment service for older elective surgical patients. *Age Ageing.* 2007;36(2):190–196.

Hennessy D, Juzwishin K, Yergens D, Noseworthy T, Doig C. Outcomes of elderly survivors of intensive care: a review of the literature. *Chest.* 2005;127(5):1764–1774.

Herridge MS, Cheung AM, Tansey CM, et al. One-year outcomes in survivors of the acute respiratory distress syndrome. *N Engl J Med.* 2003;348(8):683–693.

Hopkins RO, Jackson JC. Long-term neurocognitive function after critical illness. *Chest.* 2006;130(3):869–878.

Inouye SK, Bogardus ST, Jr., Charpentier PA, et al. A multicomponent intervention to prevent delirium in hospitalized older patients. *N Engl J Med.* 1999;340(9):669–676.

Jones C, Skirrow P, Griffiths RD, et al. Rehabilitation after critical illness: a randomized, controlled trial. *Crit Care Med.* 2003;31(10):2456–2461.

Kalisvaart KJ, de Jonghe JF, Bogaards MJ, et al. Haloperidol prophylaxis for elderly hip-surgery patients at risk for delirium: a randomized placebo-controlled study. *J Am Geriatr Soc.* 2005;53(10):1658–1666.

Kaplan V, Clermont G, Griffin MF, et al. Pneumonia: still the old man's friend? *Arch Intern Med.* 2003;163(3):317–323.

Kress JP, Gehlbach B, Lacy M, Pliskin N, Pohlman AS, Hall JB. The long-term psychological effects of daily sedative interruption on critically ill patients. *Am J Respir Crit Care Med.* 2003;168(12):1457–1461.

Lautrette A, Darmon M, Megarbane B, et al. A communication strategy and brochure for relatives of patients dying in the ICU. *N Engl J Med.* 2007;356(5):469–478.

Mayersohn M. Pharmacokinetics in the elderly. *Environ Health Perspect.* 1994;102 Suppl 11:119–124.

Milbrandt EB, Angus DC. Bench-to-bedside review: critical illness-associated cognitive dysfunction—mechanisms, markers, and emerging therapeutics. *Crit Care.* 2006;10(6):238.

Milbrandt EB, Kersten A, Kong L, et al. Haloperidol use in mechanically ventilated patients is associated with lower hospital mortality. *Crit Care Med.* 2005;33(1):226–229.

Pisani MA, Redlich CA, McNicoll L, Ely EW, Friedkin RJ, Inouye SK. Short-term outcomes in older intensive care unit patients with dementia. *Crit Care Med.* 2005;33(6):1371–1376.

Van Pelt DC, Milbrandt EB, Qin L, et al. Informal caregiver burden among survivors of prolonged mechanical ventilation. *Am J Respir Crit Care Med.* 2007;175(2):167–173.

Weinert C. Epidemiology and treatment of psychiatric conditions that develop after critical illness. *Curr Opin Crit Care.* 2005;11(4):376–380.

Subacute Care

Edward R. Marcantonio ■ *Mark Yurkofsky*

A recently aired radio advertisement states, "Nursing Homes: not just for the end of life anymore." While the number of elderly persons residing permanently in nursing homes has remained stable over the past several years, increasing numbers are admitted to nursing homes for short-term stays, usually for rehabilitation or continuing medical management after an acute hospitalization. Indeed, the past 15 years has seen the establishment of a whole new area of medicine, termed "subacute care," "postacute care," or "transitional care," along with units that specialize in this care. While subacute care can be delivered in both free-standing skilled nursing facilities (SNFs) and in hospital-based transitional care units, the former have come to dominate the industry over the past 5 years. Subacute care is an important component of the continuum of care for elderly persons, and care in this setting is frequently provided by geriatricians and geriatric nurse practitioners. In fact, subacute care is an important clinical niche of geriatric medicine.

This chapter discusses the fundamentals of subacute care from the perspective of clinicians delivering care in this setting. After defining subacute care and its providers, the chapter follows the timeline of subacute care, beginning at the hospital, to subacute admission, assessment, care planning, medical management, and discharge planning. The chapter also briefly touches upon the financial and medicolegal aspects of providing care in this setting and highlights aspects of medical management and decision making that may be unique in the subacute setting.

DEFINITION OF SUBACUTE CARE

There is some debate about the exact definition of subacute care. In fact, there is a great deal of variation in the settings, patients, and providers encompassed within subacute care. In this chapter, subacute care is defined as the management of discrete episodes of illness requiring medical management and/or functional rehabilitation within the SNF. The intensity of the medical management is generally less than that provided on a general medical/surgical unit in an acute care hospital, but greater than what can be provided in the traditional nursing home setting, or at home. The level of functional rehabilitation provided is less intense than in a specialized rehabilitation hospital, but greater than that provided at home. Usually, but not always, subacute care provides a continuation of a treatment plan initiated in the hospital. The frequency of medical encounters and the costs of care are also intermediate between the hospital and long-term care settings.

A major distinction between acute care and subacute care is a focus on function. This makes it an ideal setting for geriatricians. Acute care in hospitals is focused on diagnosis and targeted aggressive treatment of acute medical problems. Unfortunately, as a result of hospitalization, many elderly persons suffer nosocomial complications and functional decline that persist well after the acute problem is corrected. Innovative models have been developed to reduce the risk of delirium and functional decline in acute care hospitals; nonetheless, these problems remain rampant, particularly in frail individuals with underlying dementia or chronic medical illnesses. Add to this the continuing pressure to shorten length of stay, and many acutely hospitalized elderly persons are unable to return to their residences at discharge. Subacute care has filled the need for a place where these patients can receive ongoing medical and nursing care, in addition to skilled rehabilitation and discharge planning for eventual return to the community. Length of stay in subacute care varies widely, from less than 1 week up to 100 days (the Medicare limit), but the average is generally 1 to 3 weeks.

Subacute care plays a particularly important role in the managed care system for several reasons. First, the cost pressures engendered under managed care require treating patients in the least costly environment that meets their needs. Second, many managed care plans have per diem rates with acute care hospitals, leading to even more intense pressure for discharge than the traditional Medicare diagnosis-related group (DRG) system. Third, managed care plans are exempt from the "3-day" hospital rule (in traditional Medicare, patients must be hospitalized for at least 3 nights to qualify for a skilled nursing benefit), so that these patients can access their SNF benefit with a shorter hospital stay, or even be directly admitted from the community (often via the doctor's office or emergency department). For all of these reasons, managed care plans tend to admit sicker patients to SNFs for shorter lengths of stay, and managed care providers have been the leaders in developing expertise in subacute care. Foremost has been the establishment of teams of physicians and nurse practitioners who spend most or all of their professional lives delivering subacute care. These teams have developed protocols for facilitating hospital transfers, assessing patients, delivering sophisticated medical care, addressing acute medical problems, minimizing rehospitalizations, providing case management, and proactive discharge planning. Each of these is discussed in greater detail later in this chapter.

SUBACUTE CARE PATIENTS

Compared to the usual nursing home population, subacute patients tend to be younger (average age in seventies rather than late eighties), more acutely ill, but less likely to have dementia or major chronic functional limitations. Most patients admitted for subacute care come directly from hospitals and are expected to return to their homes after a specific, planned treatment course. However, a small but significant fraction of subacute patients (10% to 33%) never achieve discharge goals and "convert" to long-stay nursing home patients. Another significant fraction of patients become medically unstable in the subacute setting and need to be rehospitalized (up to 25%). A third group of patients present with advanced illness and receive end-of-life care and die in the subacute setting. These figures depend on the acuity of illness and underlying frailty of the population, as well as on the quality of care provided at the facilities. Except for the dying patients, maximizing return to the community, and minimizing rehospitalizations and long-term care placements are worthy goals of subacute care. Typical subacute diagnoses include hip fracture, other fractures (upper extremity or vertebral), stroke, cardiac and pulmonary conditions (including pneumonia), pressure and vascular ulcers, postoperative care, and deconditioning. Subacute patients may need intensive medical management, functional rehabilitation, or a combination of both. As noted above, some also receive formal hospice or hospice-like services in the subacute setting.

SUBACUTE CARE PHYSICIANS

Delivering effective care to the subacute population requires a much greater physician presence than traditional long-term care. Just as the term *hospitalist* denotes physicians working primarily in the hospital, *SNFist* and *subacutist* are terms occasionally used to describe clinicians practicing primarily in the subacute environment. Practicing as a long-term care and subacute care clinician requires a special set of skills. Physicians working in SNFs and subacute units are usually geriatricians or other clinicians with strong geriatric skills such as internists, osteopathic physicians, and family practitioners.

A number of clinical, administrative, and interpersonal skills are important for a physician to achieve success in the area of subacute care. To properly manage this challenging patient population, the

TABLE 20-1

Areas of Clinical Expertise in Subacute Care

Geriatric syndromes including delirium, dementia, and urinary incontinence
Postoperative orthopedic and surgical patients
Pressure ulcer prevention and management
Pain and symptom control in the dying patient
Non-ICU hospital conditions such as congestive heart failure and infections
Medication administration and dosing in an elderly population
Wound care
Geriatric rehabilitation

nursing facility clinician must have *clinical expertise* in managing conditions that are a blend of office, hospital, and geriatric practice (Table 20-1).

Leadership skills are highly desirable in the physicians practicing in this setting. The physician is the leader of the facility interdisciplinary team whose members include rehabilitation specialists, nurses, social service, and case management. The subacute setting is an environment that benefits greatly from a physician leading the geriatric care team.

Administrative skills are also important for the subacute care practitioner. Nursing facilities have a relatively simple administrative structure. The administrator and director of nursing are the primary salaried personnel that run the facility. There is a facility medical director as well. Attending physicians have the opportunity to work closely with these three individuals in a facility. Attending physicians, even if they are not the medical director, can make significant contributions to the quality of care of subacute patients (Table 20-2).

Interpersonal skills are the third key area for subacute care practitioners. The ability to form trusting collaborative relationships with patients and families quickly is critical to effective care in nursing facilities. Patients currently entering nursing facilities are often critically ill, are more dependent than previously, fear loss of independence, have caregivers under great stress, and often have financial and housing pressures. They may also be suspicious of nursing facilities and may not understand all of the medical issues. Table 20-3 summarizes the interpersonal skills needed in a subacute care provider in order to handle these issues.

ROLE OF ADVANCED PRACTICE CLINICIANS

Daily rounding by a clinician with round-the-clock phone availability is essential to providing effective subacute care. To provide

TABLE 20-2

Areas of Administrative Expertise in Subacute Care

Improving care transitions from hospital to subacute facility
Improving facility systems regarding ancillary supports (especially lab, x-ray, and pharmacy), training staff, documentation, and communication
Knowledge regarding OBRA* regulations
Working effectively within the constraints of the reimbursement system for nursing facilities under Medicare and managed care

*OBRA, Omnibus Budget Reconciliation Act of 1987.

TABLE 20-3

Interpersonal Skills Needed to Provide Effective Subacute Care
Understand and appreciate the nursing home culture
Be a skilled leader of the interdisciplinary team
Work well with families regarding discharge planning and end-of-life care
Teach staff within the facility
Interface effectively with hospital and outpatient clinicians
Be a good listener and a good communicator

this enhanced clinical coverage, physicians may collaborate with advanced practice clinicians (APCs) such as nurse practitioners and physician's assistants. APCs play a major role in providing care in many subacute units. States and facilities vary regarding the scope of practice for APCs. In some locales, nurse practitioners practice as independent clinicians, while in others, direct physician supervision is required. Many facilities require written guidelines that describe the scope of practice of the APC as well as the manner by which physician supervision will be provided.

The physician working in a subacute care setting may find tremendous benefit from working with an APC. Many APCs have specialized areas of expertise that complement the skills and knowledge of the physician. Table 20-4 lists the roles and duties an APC can assume in a subacute unit.

A physician practicing with an APC has the opportunity to form a team that can improve the quality of care provided and can improve job satisfaction for both providers. As in other teams, excellent communication, trust, availability, and support are essential.

The model of physician–APC collaboration in the subacute setting has many similarities to an inpatient hospital model. The APC may operate much like a first-year resident, managing day-to-day issues, identifying new issues, and requesting support from the physician when needed. By rounding together on a regular basis the MD–APC care team have the opportunity to assess patients together. Patients can be reassured seeing their care team together. There is no substitute for a bedside evaluation in assessing issues such as pain control, cognitive status, anxiety, and medical stability. APCs are able to participate in night and weekend on-call duties. It is essential that if an APC is taking "first call" that there always be a physician available for consultative support.

It is preferable to have a model of on-call coverage that uses clinicians who not only know the patient but also the capabilities of the facility. When it is not possible to have a clinician who is a direct caregiver providing on-call coverage, effective signouts are important. Key clinical information can be transmitted by direct

verbal communication or, with HIPAA appropriate safeguards to ensure patients confidentiality, by written summaries that can be faxed or e-mailed to the covering clinician.

SUBACUTE CARE REGULATIONS

Subacute care units are licensed and regulated under the same regulations as nursing homes. In 1987, a set of regulations regarding patient care in nursing facilities was enacted in the Omnibus Budget Reconciliation Act (OBRA). These regulations laid out a number of principles that were used to standardize care in nursing facilities. In 1995, the nursing home certification and enforcement regulations took effect. Unless nursing facilities were found to comply with the standards laid out in OBRA, they would not be allowed to participate in the Medicare and Medicaid programs. Table 20-5 summarizes key aspects of the OBRA regulations. These principles provide a framework for providing appropriate clinical care. Physicians must work collaboratively with nursing facility staff to maintain compliance with OBRA regulations. It is particularly challenging managing a high turnover, higher acuity population under these regulations. Excellent assessment skills, complete and accurate documentation, and a well-functioning interdisciplinary team are necessary to meet regulatory requirements, and are also the cornerstone of good subacute care.

DEFINING QUALITY IN SUBACUTE CARE

Quality in subacute care goes beyond traditional medical process and outcome measures emphasized in hospitals. Perhaps most important is the quality and availability of the nursing staff. Because of the stress of managing high-acuity patients in the nursing home setting, many subacute facilities are chronically understaffed, or experience high staff turnover, especially of licensed nurses and nursing aides. Significant use of "agency" personnel, with little knowledge of the facility or its patients, can have a major negative impact on quality. Additional issues that are of great importance in the subacute setting include the quality of the rehabilitation services for patients with medical conditions that are likely to improve, and palliative care services for patients whose clinical status is likely to deteriorate. Subacute facilities are also judged on their hotel services in addition to their medical services. Good food, pleasant ambience, television, and clean rooms are all part of the reasonable expectations of patients and their families. Subjective measures, such as patient and family satisfaction, and the facility's reputation in the community, can be good overall measures of quality.

TABLE 20-4

Roles of Advanced Practice Clinicians in Subacute Care
Specialized areas of expertise including management of dementia, pressure ulcers, wounds, gynecological issues, and congestive heart failure
Patient/family education regarding diabetes, home safety, medication administration, medication simplification
Training facility staff
Working out problems with nurses, nurses' aides, patient, and family

TABLE 20-5

Key Aspects of the OBRA* Regulations
The medical regimen must be comprehensive and part of an interdisciplinary care plan
A decline in the resident's physical, mental, and psychosocial well-being must be demonstrably unavoidable
Restraint use requires rigorous individual clinical assessment
The resident's drug regimen must be justifiable

*OBRA, Omnibus Budget Reconciliation Act of 1987.

ADMITTING A SUBACUTE PATIENT: THE HOSPITAL PERSPECTIVE

The vast majority of subacute patients are transferred from acute care hospitals. The providers at the hospitals have a critical role in ensuring the success of the subacute stay. Often, hospital providers operate with little knowledge of the facilities to which they are sending their patients. A brief communication between the hospital and subacute clinicians can help to answer questions about appropriateness, timing of transfer, specific treatments, and overall goals of care. Unfortunately, this type of communication is more the exception than the rule. In general, if the acute care hospital providers have any questions or concerns about transfer of a patient, it is best to ask before acting.

The first question to be asked is who should be sent to subacute care, and who should not? Subacute facilities vary widely in terms of their capabilities, so there is no general answer. Hospital physicians often make the naïve assumption that the nurses "screening" patients for facilities have intimate knowledge of them and can make appropriate referrals. Often, these screeners work for large corporations that may have several facilities in a large urban area. The screeners focus more on "filling beds," and leave it up to the clinicians to determine appropriateness. It is also important to note that once a patient is accepted by a facility, the actual transfer may not take place for 1 to 2 days. During that time period, the patient may change clinically so it is important to reassess for clinical appropriateness at the time of transfer.

A few rules of the thumb hold: in general, a patient requiring the intensive care unit (ICU) is *not* appropriate for subacute care. The rare exception is a stable ventilated patient who is being transferred from an ICU to a specialized pulmonary subacute facility. In addition to ICU care, few subacute facilities have sophisticated cardiac monitoring, and so patients with active cardiac issues such as unstable angina, poorly controlled congestive heart failure, or arrhythmias requiring continuous monitoring are rarely good candidates for subacute care.

Nursing care in subacute facilities is much less intensive than in acute care hospitals. While hospitals rarely have more than 7 patients per nurse, subacute units may have from 12 to 20 or more patients per nurse—in an 8-h shift, this averages to as little as 20 minutes per patient. Therefore, patients with hemodynamic instability, on multiple intravenous medications, or other situations requiring close nursing monitoring, maybe poor candidates for subacute care. It is therefore critical that an assessment is made to be sure that the needs of the patient can be met with the staffing available. In general, patients with a relatively straightforward treatment plan for acute illness that has shown evidence of improvement, combined with established treatment of chronic illnesses and functional rehabilitation needs, are the most ideal for this setting.

On the opposite end of the spectrum is a patient who will likely be able to go home within a few days. For these patients, an additional facility transfer is probably not worthwhile or necessary, and runs the risk of introducing further discontinuity. In general, subacute stays substantially shorter than 1 week should be avoided in favor of direct discharge to home.

Another issue is selecting the best facility for the patient. This is a complex issue that involves both clinical and psychosocial factors. Screeners and hospital case managers often need to be focused on getting a bed quickly rather than finding the best facility for the

patient. In addition, bed availability can at times be an issue. Facilities vary widely in their capabilities, and some have specialized programs in specific areas, such as orthopedics and stroke care. In general, knowledge of a proven track record of success handling a particular kind of patient is the best proof of the wisdom of transfer. In addition to these clinical issues, patients and family members may prefer a facility close to home, which can facilitate family visits and the like. These preferences should be honored if all else is equal. However, it should be explained to patients and family members that because only a short-term stay is anticipated, established medical care linkages and proven clinical excellence should outweigh geographic convenience to ensure the best possible outcome.

The optimal time for transfer can be defined as the point when the patient's needs can be met as well or better at the subacute facility as in the hospital. In practice, this is often hard to define, and discharge is often dictated by bed availability or "critical pathways" that predetermine length of stay. Ultimately, it is the physician's responsibility to determine whether the patient is clinically ready for transfer, and for ensuring adequate transfer of information with the patient for continued implementation of the plan of care. It is better to keep the patient for an extra day in the hospital than to risk a rapid readmission for medical instability or poorly coordinated transfer.

When the time for transfer comes, it is crucial that the appropriate information accompany the patient. Table 20-6 describes the key information required by the SNF. In addition, the physicians at the hospital should review the discharge summary and other key transfer documents to ensure that there are no discrepancies—if so, these should be remedied.

Developing better systems whereby receiving facilities and sending hospitals coordinate the transitions of care is crucial to improving patient care and optimizing outcomes. One approach can be

---

TABLE 20-6

Key Data Needed for Transfer to a Subacute Unit

A list of clinical problems
Complete medication list matched with the clinical diagnosis
Summary of hospital course
Code status/advance directives
Name of health care proxy/guardian
Wound-care instructions
Weight-bearing instructions
Recent significant laboratory test results
Key health care providers involved in care and how to contact them
Diet including consistency of food/liquids if swallowing is impaired
If on tube feeding, type of tube, rate/time of feeding, amount/time of water flushes
Recent focused physical exam findings
Goals for the subacute stay
Pending tests and how to follow up
Follow-up appointments
Clear anticoagulation orders with recent PT/INR results, INR goals
Indications for urinary catheter if present and when it can be removed
Last bowel movement
Family contacts with accurate names, phone numbers, and addresses
Type of intravenous access

INR, international normalized ratio, PT, prothrombin time.

achieved through sharing information via computer systems. Clearly, this is easiest for onsite transitional care units (which are becoming less common). However, even free-standing subacute facilities can have dial-up or hard-wired computer links with sending hospitals. Only certain members of the subacute staff (particularly the physicians, who may also be on staff at the sending hospital) receive access to key elements of the patient's record, as well as the ability to e-mail hospital providers.

Understanding the limitations of subacute care facilities can help hospital providers better manage the transfer of care. First, consider the timing of transfer. Unfortunately, most patients arrive for admission to SNFs between 4 and 7 P.M. However, staffing at most SNFs is best on the day (7 A.M. to 3 P.M.) shift. Therefore, hospitals should attempt to transfer the patient as early as possible during the day, preferably before noon. Before sending the patient, hospital providers should ensure that all patient needs, including nutritional, are met for the next several hours. Second, consider that most SNFs do not have onsite pharmacies and that it may take several hours for ordered medications to be delivered to the patient. Therefore, all medications, particularly pain medications that the patient will need over the next 4 to 6 hours, should be administered prior to transfer. Finally, SNFs may have difficulty inserting and maintaining intravenous access. Therefore, stable access should be ensured prior to transfer. If the patient will need more than 1 to 2 days of treatment, a more permanent "long-line" catheter is advisable.

One special case deserves mention: direct admissions from the community to subacute care. Because of Medicare's "3-day rule," direct admissions come only in managed care patients (who are exempt from this rule), or patients who have had a 3-day hospital admission in the previous 30 days. Direct admissions should be medically stable and should not require immediate diagnostic or therapeutic intervention. In these cases, it is crucial that appropriate information, including reason for admission, medical history, physical examination, medications, treatments, allergies, and the like, be transmitted from the emergency department or doctor's office. A direct dialog between the sending and receiving physician is often required. Only systems that can care for high-acuity subacute patients should consider direct admission.

ADMITTING A SUBACUTE PATIENT: THE FACILITY PERSPECTIVE

Those who work in a subacute environment need to understand the crucial role played by the first 24 hours postadmission. From a clinical outcome, patient satisfaction, and a risk management perspective, the first day and night in the facility is key. Case 1 illustrates some of the perils of the hospital–subacute transfer.

Case 1: Transition of Care Issues in the First 24 Hours

An 85-year-old male retired professor is admitted with a hip fracture, hypertension, and diabetes. Here are some common issues that arise that can impact outcomes in a subacute setting:

1. *Family communication:* The patient's daughter does not know if and when her father is going to the subacute facility and does not know how to get to the subacute facility.

2. *Timing of admission:* The patient is scheduled for a 2 P.M. arrival, but arrives at 6 P.M. because the hospital nurse had another sick patient and did not get the paperwork done. The patient left the hospital before dinner was served and arrived at the subacute facility after dinner was over.

3. *Avoidable complications:* His blood glucose was 40 mg/dL and he was lethargic by the time his dinner arrived.

4. *Missing information:*

   The weight-bearing status is not given on the hospital referral.

   The page 1 referral had a "titrate Coumadin to INR of 2.0" order but no dose and no INRs.

   The discharge summary did not arrive with the patient.

   The hospital was not aware that the patient took glaucoma drops and therefore these medications were not noted on the referral form.

5. *Facility issues:*

   Physical therapy had left by the time the patient arrived and nursing was not comfortable transferring the patient out of bed to the toilet.

   Diapers were placed on the patient irrespective of continence status.

   The room smelled because the patient was incontinent.

   Pain medicine was ordered but was not delivered until the next morning.

The daughter arrives, sees her father in diapers, in pain, more confused, and the nurses unsure about his medications, and wants to send the patient back to the hospital and says she is going to write a complaint letter to the Department of Public Health.

The issues that arise in Case 1 are not unusual. Patients arrive unexpectedly, sometimes with medical issues requiring prompt attention, and the information transmitted is inadequate and sometimes contradictory. Interagency referral forms maybe done at different times than discharge summaries and can contain conflicting information.

Nursing home clinicians often manage new SNF admissions telephonically for the first 24 hours. Accurate, complete nursing assessments are important to the SNF clinician who is attempting to manage a patient he or she has never met over the phone. Nurses who work on subacute units need to work effectively with their off-site physician colleagues. An important aspect of this collaboration is judgment as to when to page the physician/APC and what information to have available. Nurses need to perform an appropriate assessment of the patient based on the clinical situation. In addition, it is important to have information on medications being given, as well as recent laboratory results.

A comprehensive history and physical examination is required within 48 to 72 hours of subacute admission. It is best practice if this can be performed within the first 24 hours. In addition to understanding the medical problems identified at the hospital, key issues for the subacute clinician to consider when admitting a new patient include understanding the goals for the SNF stay, making sure medications are appropriately dosed, and assessing pain, bowel status, and cognition. If the patient has an indwelling bladder catheter, the reason it was placed and the ongoing need for it should be assessed.

In addition to the history and physical by the physician–APC team, the newly admitted subacute patient must have a number of assessments performed by many disciplines. The physician or APC, as leader of the interdisciplinary team, needs to be aware of key findings from these team members and integrate them into the initial

TABLE 20-7

Initial Assessment of the New Patients by Subacute Staff

Rehabilitation team	Screens by physical, occupational, therapy, and speech
Nursing	Skin, cognition, fall risk, pain, bowel/bladder, medication review and reconciliation
Dietary	Nutritional needs/diet
Kitchen	Food preferences
Social service	Psychosocial evaluation, end-of-life preferences
Case management	Discharge planning including equipment and home care
Administration	Valuables assessment

treatment plan. Table 20-7 provides examples of the assessments that need to be done and the disciplines that do them.

Patients not only have medical issues identified by the hospital, but may arrive with unidentified issues, such as fever, delirium, skin breakdown, constipation, pain, and urinary retention, which may require immediate attention. The subacute clinician has to organize this information and prioritize issues that need immediate attention.

Nursing facilities do not have onsite pharmacies. Delivery of medications can take several hours. To help with this issue, facilities have drug "emergency boxes" that contain dozens of frequently used medications including intravenous antibiotics and a small selection of opioids. Familiarity with the contents of these boxes is important for the subacute care provider to practice effectively. At times, short-term substitutions must be made until the exact medication can be delivered. In addition, like hospitals, facilities have formularies. Medications may need to be changed to meet formulary requirements.

PATIENT/FAMILY/STAFF INTERACTIONS

In addition to being astute and thorough when assessing a new patient, the subacute clinician must be skilled at establishing trusting relationships with the patient and key family members as soon as possible after admission. Any time a patient changes setting and new caregivers assume care, there are opportunities and dangers. The initial hours after admission are therefore an important window period in which the receiving clinicians can form a strong collaborative relationship with the patient and the family.

Family members provide important clinical and functional information that may otherwise be unavailable. Speaking with family members may help to identify areas of concern related to past care and can point to special issues on which to focus immediately on admission. The physician can establish themselves as a patient advocate and a problem solver. By establishing an early, strong family connection, the subacute clinician is better able to identify and ultimately meet the goals of care, and overcome barriers to discharge.

PHYSICIAN'S ROLE IN REHABILITATION

In the subacute setting, an interdisciplinary team meeting plays a crucial role in formulating and assessing the plan of care. At the team meeting, key issues of function, medical condition, cognition, mood, and interactions between family, patient, and staff can be shared. The interdisciplinary team needs to gather and communicate information regarding medical condition, treatment and prognosis, rehabilitation potential and level of function, psychosocial needs, financial options, and family/patient teaching needs. Most internists, primary care physicians, family practitioners, and general practitioners do not receive formal training in rehabilitation. Many physicians working in nursing facilities do not take an active role in assessing the patient's rehabilitation needs, goals, and progress. There is a vital role that a subacute physician can play in this regard that benefits the facility and the patients, as well as the patients' families.

The physician understands the pathophysiology of disease processes better than any other member of the interdisciplinary care team. Therefore, the physician has a critical role to play in leading the team in identifying realistic functional goals for patients, understanding, and explaining the impact of intercurrent medical illnesses on patient function, and communicating with patients, staff, and families regarding realistic goals and expected level of function. The physician does not need to know how best to identify weakness in a particular muscle group and what exercises to do to strengthen it, nor what the best assistive device will be for a patient. However, the physician does need to understand whether the goals of treatment outlined by the therapy team are realistic based on the patient's physical ability, cognitive capacity, as well as their home environment and supports.

How to get the patient walking again is often the major challenge to face nursing facility staff. Generally, physical and occupational therapists are able to provide 1 to 3 hours of therapy per day, 5 to 6 days per week, in the subacute setting. It is essential that other members of the care team provide an environment that encourages patients to get out of bed and ambulate when the therapists are not working with the patient. Nurses and aides need to be taught by the therapists how best to transfer the patient, to observe any weight-bearing precautions, and to learn which assistive devices need to be used. Often schedules need to be set up to get the patient washed, fed, dressed, and out of bed. Identifying what is not working well and brainstorming with other members of the care team to identify solutions is an important role for the physician. There are a number of roles that the physician maybe required to fill in the interdisciplinary team (Table 20-8).

Clear communication between all members of the interdisciplinary team is essential (see Chapter 26). The physician, nurse practitioner, and physician assistant play an important role in helping set realistic goals and making sure that each member of the care team is providing care that is geared towards achieving those goals. They also play a key role in communicating with family members.

Case 2 outlines the key role of physicians in communicating between providers and altering the plan of care to optimize patient outcomes.

Case 2: Importance of Communication in Subacute Care

A 78-year-old female with a left hip fracture repair and a history of mild dementia presents to the nursing facility for rehabilitation. The patient arrives with a non weight-bearing status on her left leg. The physician sees the patient and finds she has poor memory and impaired judgment. She lives with her frail but independent husband in a home with eight stairs separating the bedroom and kitchen. The physician orders occupational and physical therapy evaluations.

TABLE 20-8

Physician's Roles in the Interdisciplinary Team

Provide medical expertise on prognosis

Determine realistic, achievable functional goals

Determine whether medical improvement is likely, resulting in improved function, or whether medical status has plateaued or will deteriorate with stable or reduced function

Adjust treatment based on input from team members (pain/bowel/anxiety, etc.)

Gather input from specialists and share with team members

Participate in brainstorming to identify solutions

Guide discussions around ethical issues

Determine when skilled care is not beneficial or needed

Facilitate family communication

Determine when discharge to another setting is appropriate

Provide constructive feedback

Assess/improve teamwork between rehabilitation/nurses/nurses aides

On day 2 of the admission, the physician realizes that the patient's functional and cognitive deficits will likely prevent her from keeping weight off the operated leg. Furthermore, it is clear that very few 78-year-olds can ambulate safely on one leg using a walker or crutches. In such situations, the end result is often that until the weight-bearing restriction is removed, which generally takes 1 to 2 months, the patient will not be able to ambulate and will require a prolonged nursing home stay. This places the patient at high risk for needing permanent long-term care. The physician calls the operating surgeon and explains the dilemma. Upon further reflection, the surgeon states that the fracture was minimally displaced, the alignment was good, the repair was reasonably strong, and the patient is only 105 pounds and advances her to a weight-bearing as tolerated status. The treatment plan for this patient has now changed dramatically. Achieving independence with transfers now becomes a realistic possibility. She may be able to negotiate stairs. The plan is now for a 1- to 2-week stay with discharge to a home setting with community supports and the family paying for extra assistance.

Patients with advanced dementia may have great difficulty learning new strategies or compensatory techniques. The physician plays a vital role in identifying patients who can benefit from therapy. In addition to dementia, patients with delirium, depression, pain, or other medical illnesses may have difficulty participating in and benefiting from a rehabilitation program. The physician must identify and treat the depression, pain, or congestive heart failure that is limiting participation in and benefit from the rehabilitation program.

It is often appropriate and necessary to teach nursing facility staff such as nurses' aides how best to feed, transfer, and ambulate patients. The goal is to provide for the patient's safety while maximizing their autonomy. There is a tension at times between getting things done quickly by helping the patient and having the same task be done more slowly but with the patient doing all the work. The patient may take 20 minutes to get dressed, needing periodic verbal cues from the nurses' aide during the process. If the nurses' aide did more of the work the job might be done in 10 minutes. The patient may even prefer to have the aide do more of the work. However, a cornerstone of care for the elderly patient is to encourage as much independence as possible, and this is even more important in the subacute setting when the goal is to return home.

PHYSICIAN'S ROLE IN FAMILY MEETINGS

Family meetings are an invaluable means of sharing information, reviewing goals, making decisions, and identifying action steps. Family meetings should generally take place after there has been an interdisciplinary team meeting without the family present. Complex information needs to be presented in an organized manner that allows time for questions, discussion, and identifying action steps. Ideally, all this needs to be done in less than 45 minutes, so that staff can resume other duties and patients and family members are not overwhelmed. Family meetings can include the patient, key family members, the physician/nurse practitioner/physician's assistant; case manager; social service; the rehabilitation team, including physical, occupational, and speech therapy; nursing; and even aides. Formulating an agenda and goals for the meeting ahead of time helps identify who needs to be present. Table 20-9 summarizes common goals for family meetings.

A staff member such as the physician, case manager, or social worker should run the meeting. It is often very helpful for the senior clinician to provide a brief update regarding the medical issues and prognosis. Knowing what different team members are going to recommend is essential for family meetings to go well. Major differences in the treatment plan between team members should be addressed before the family meeting. For example, the therapist may find the confused patient with a resolving pneumonia is not participating in rehabilitation. However, the physician maybe able to explain that the confusion is likely related to a delirium and may improve quickly as the pneumonia responds to antibiotics. Without the physician present to provide this input, the facility caregivers and family members may not have an accurate picture regarding disease progression, clinical improvement, and overall prognosis. Providing a clear, realistic picture of function and medical prognosis is also a critical part of the discharge planning process.

Several conditions are especially common among subacute patients. Key aspects of these conditions relevant to subacute care are

TABLE 20-9

Goals of Family Meetings

Information gathering regarding:
    Previous function
    Caregiver supports
    Financial resources
    Home environment
    Goals of care

Decision making regarding:
    End-of-life care
    Rehabilitation goals that need to be attained
    Discharge site, e.g., home, long-term care, assisted living
    Setting a discharge date

Resolving areas of conflict:
    Between family members
    Between family and patient
    Regarding facility services

discussed below. Other chapters in this text discuss these conditions in more detail.

MEDICAL MANAGEMENT IN THE SUBACUTE SETTING

Pain Management

It is well recognized that pain, especially in the elderly person, is often unrecognized and undertreated. Effective pain relief is an essential aspect of subacute care. Table 20-10 outlines some of the negative consequences of untreated pain.

Recognizing and relieving pain are critical skills for the subacute clinician. It is beyond the scope of this chapter to review the broad area of pain relief. However, opioid use in the subacute setting merits special mention.

Opioids play an important role in pain control. Whether for postoperative pain or end-stage cancer, a sound knowledge of principles of pain control and an understanding of nursing facility regulations regarding opioid use is essential. Opioids can be delivered in several different forms. Familiarity with the different routes of administration for opioids is an important aspect of providing pain management. Table 20-11 summarizes routes of administration. Patients arriving from hospitals may have orders written for intravenous "push" opioids. Nurses in nursing facilities do not generally give opioids, or other medications, in this manner. The clinician in the nursing facility needs to reorder these medications in a form that is appropriate for the facility.

The regulatory issues in nursing facilities can, at times, complicate and impair the provision of good pain control. Unlike the hospital setting, nursing facilities regulations require a prescription for each opioid order. The physician must either fax a prescription to the pharmacy or call the pharmacy to obtain an emergency 72-hour supply of the medication. In nursing facilities, exact doses and parameters for "as needed" indications are required, for instance: "Percocet (5/325 mg) 1 tablet orally q4h prn for moderate hip pain (4 to 7 on pain scale) and 2 tablets orally q4h prn for severe hip pain (8 to 10 on pain scale)." Sliding scale dosing orders, such as "Morphine sulfate 1–4 mg subcutaneously Q 1–4 hours PRN," are not allowed.

TABLE 20-10

Impact of Pain in Subacute Patients
Decreased mobility
Incontinence
Constipation/impaction
Pressure ulcers
Delirium
Depression
Anxiety
Malnutrition
Pneumonia
Increased risk of needing long-term care
Family stress

TABLE 20-11

Routes of Opioid Administration
Oral tablets in both short- and long-acting form
Oral liquids
Sublingual liquids in concentrate form
Rectal suppositories
Transdermal patches
Subcutaneous injections
Subcutaneous infusions

Many patients may experience a roller coaster effect when given prn doses of short acting pain medications. The result is many hours of discomfort with just a few hours of pain relief. Familiarity with and use of sustained-release oral opioids is an essential aspect to being able to provide successful pain control in the nursing facility. It should also be noted that most extended release medications should not be crushed. If the patient is not able to swallow the tablet, then an alternate dosing route needs to be considered, such as a transdermal patch.

Finally, a standing bowel program needs to be ordered along with the opioids. Orders for "milk of magnesia prn" or routine stool softeners are inadequate for most patients on opioids. Table 20-12 summarizes key points regarding opioid use in subacute care.

Urinary Incontinence and Catheters

Many patients arriving at subacute facilities have indwelling catheters or were incontinent at the hospital. Urinary catheters are most commonly used to monitor urine output when patients are first admitted to the hospital. Most patients arriving with catheters from the hospital can have them removed immediately. From both an infection control and a nursing home regulatory perspective, urinary catheters should be used in very limited situations. The two main ones are in the setting of urinary retention when intermittent catheterization is not practical and in the case of severe skin wounds when healing would be impaired by urine from an incontinent patient. Before committing a patient to permanent catheterization for urinary retention, it is important to determine whether there is a reversible cause for the retention, such as stool impaction or a medication side effect. Anticholinergic medications are particularly likely to inhibit proper bladder emptying.

TABLE 20-12

Key Issues Regarding Opioid Use in Subacute Care
Be specific regarding dosing/frequency when ordering opioids
Know the contents of the facility's "emergency box"
Prompt faxing/phoning reduces delays in getting opioids
Order a bowel program with opioids
Evaluate whether a sustained release product is needed with prn "rescue" doses
For new admissions, consider developing a system where it is known what the medications (including opioids) will be before the patients arrives and preorder them so there will not be delays

TABLE 20-13

Assessing and Managing Incontinence
Treat a diaper as a red flag: ask why it is on and if not needed make sure it stays off
Do a rectal exam: stool impaction is commonly overlooked and is very treatable
Consider a bedside commode if the patient is slow transferring and ambulating
Make sure there is not a problem with delays answering call lights; if there are delays, involve the director of nursing in formulating a solution
Avoid anticholinergics, especially in men, as they may cause urinary retention or confusion
Get a good history from the patient/family regarding prehospitalization continence
Consider obtaining a postvoid residual volume to rule out urinary retention
Review medications and lab work for causes of incontinence

TABLE 20-14

Speech Therapist's Role in Aspiration Management
Screening new admissions for swallowing difficulties
Assessing swallowing capabilities
Recommending food and liquid consistency
Teaching the patient compensatory swallowing strategies, e.g., chin tuck
Deciding whether further diagnostic studies are needed, e.g., modified barium swallow
Training facility staff and family members proper techniques

fact that elderly patients entering nursing facilities often have poor dentition, ill-fitting, or missing dentures.

The role of the speech therapist in reducing aspiration risk includes items listed in Table 20-14. Table 20-15 summarizes the physician's role in helping to manage the patient with swallowing difficulties.

Falls

A significant challenge in managing patients in nursing facilities is the tension between safety and autonomy. Many patients in nursing facilities have cognitive impairment as well as a functional deficit that hinders transfers or ambulation. The physician plays a vital role in working with facility staff in identifying risk factors for falls and reducing those risks. Table 20-16 identifies some of the common causes of falls in a subacute setting.

If a patient does fall, a review of the above issues needs to be undertaken to determine why the fall occurred and to take corrective measures. The use of restraints, whether physical or chemical, to prevent activities or behaviors that increase the risk of falls needs to be carefully scrutinized. Physical restraints may result in injury or even death if improperly used or monitored. Chemical restraints (e.g., sedating psychotropic drugs) have significant morbidity associated with them as well. Finding ways to manage problematic behaviors to decrease the risk of falls or to keep patients safer is challenging (Table 20-17).

The attending physician or facility medical director maybe asked to review cases prior to admission where restraints could be required. Proper documentation in the medical record regarding fall evaluation and restraint use or nonuse is very important. Occasionally, physicians will need to speak with state surveyors investigating an injury related to a fall. Having a clear, well-documented plan on how to manage the patient who is at risk for falls can be very helpful in this situation in preventing citations or even monetary penalties for the facility.

The hospitalized patient with new incontinence often has an etiology that can be diagnosed and treated in the nursing facility without sophisticated studies. It is important to determine the prehospitalization continence status and the etiology for the incontinence. Infections, medications (diuretics), delirium, immobility, fecal impaction, urinary retention, and deconditioning are common causes of incontinence that are readily treated. Nurses' aides, nurses, and therapists are very important to the clinician as a source of information regarding continence. An interdisciplinary meeting is an excellent way in which to obtain information on continence and to develop a plan to manage it. Table 20-13 summarizes some ways of rapidly assessing and managing incontinence in the nursing facility (see also Chapter 59 on incontinence).

Swallowing Issues

An appropriate diet and feeding plan can be crucial in the subacute setting. Hospitals may not always supply detailed information on food and beverage consistencies for patients at the time of admission to the nursing facility. Patients with strokes, impaired cognition, and other neuromuscular disorders require special types of diets because of dysphagia. The subacute clinician should be familiar with these diets. Solid foods can be ground or pureed to facilitate swallowing. Liquids can be thickened to nectar or honey-thick consistencies to reduce aspiration risk. Contacting the sending hospital prior to feeding the patient may be necessary to determine the proper diet in a patient with dysphagia.

Speech therapists are important members of the rehabilitation team in nursing facilities. Speech therapists have a dual role. They work on communication techniques and strategies and also screen for and evaluate swallowing difficulties. Speech therapists can assess whether food consistencies are appropriate and whether other interventions are needed such as elevation of the head of the bed, tucking the chin, or turning the head with swallowing.

Swallowing difficulties can develop in the setting of an acute or a chronic illness. Delirium and dementia contribute to swallowing problems, especially if an acute medical illness develops. Stroke, neuromuscular illnesses, anatomical abnormalities, and infections also may cause dysphagia. Coupled with swallowing problems is the

TABLE 20-15

Physician's Role in Aspiration Management
Order appropriate food and fluid consistencies
Order aspiration precautions when appropriate
Coordinate the interdisciplinary team to ensure that the proper diet is provided at all times
Assess whether a feeding tube might be indicated
Identify reversible medical causes of dysphagia

TABLE 20-16

Causes of Falls in Subacute Settings
Medication-related postural hypotension
Medication-related confusion
Pain
Poorly fitting footwear
Inadequate lighting
Delays in answering call lights
Incontinence causing a slip and fall
Lack of familiarity with environment
Environmental hazards such as oxygen tubing, bedside trays that roll when leaned on
New stroke or fracture causing weakness in a limb(s)

TABLE 20-18

Conditions Placing Patients at High Risk for Skin Breakdown
End-stage diseases
Poor nutritional status
Cognitive impairment
Immobility from fracture or neurological deficit
Incontinence of urine and stool
Dehydration
Infections
Sensory Impairment
Pain

Pressure Ulcers

Clinicians practicing in nursing facilities must have a good understanding of preventing and managing pressure ulcers. Pressure ulcers can result in pain, immobility, catheter use, infections, malnutrition, prolonged SNF stays, and hospital admissions. While some pressure ulcers are avoidable, many others are unavoidable. Similar to falls, clinicians and facilities must realize that these ulcers are potential areas for litigation. Excellent documentation and a thorough knowledge of techniques for preventing and treating pressure ulcers are areas with which the subacute clinician must be familiar.

Nursing facilities do skin assessments as part of the admitting process, and again periodically during the stay. It is worthwhile to familiarize yourself with the screening tool used in your facility and to review it once it is completed on new admissions. High-risk patients can be identified in this manner. However, changes can occur in which a low-risk patient can quickly become high risk. For instance, a patient may develop diarrhea and weakness. The physician–APC team must recognize a new increased risk for skin breakdown. Table 20-18 identifies the patients at highest risk for skin breakdown.

By recognizing the at-risk patient population, steps can be implemented that can reduce the likelihood of skin breakdown (see Chapter 58). Even if pressure ulcers develop, demonstrating that preventive measures were in place and being monitored can protect the facility and the clinician from censure by local health departments and from litigation (Table 20-19).

Medication Issues

A growing awareness of the impact of medication-related morbidity has taken place in recent years (Table 20-20). The subacute practitioner needs to have a good understanding of the medication delivery and administration systems. As described above, very few nursing facilities have an in-house pharmacy. Medications are delivered after being called or faxed in to an outside pharmacy. It generally takes several hours to deliver medications.

Physicians in nursing facilities must be aware of medications that should be avoided or dose adjusted in older patients. Patients may arrive from hospitals on medications that have a high risk of side effects in this population. It is incumbent on the subacute clinician to carefully review each medicine for necessity, proper dosing, and potential interactions with other medication being administered. Adjusting doses for reduced creatinine clearance is another important aspect of medication management in the subacute setting.

Case 3 illustrates a useful example on medication ordering.

Case 3: Issues in How Medications Are Ordered

An 80-year-old woman with a history of hypertension, angina, and atrial fibrillation is on metoprolol 50 mg bid. The admitting

TABLE 20-17

Fall/Injury Reducing Interventions in Subacute Settings
Identifying the high risk patient
Using a bell instead of a call button—better for some demented patients
Physical/occupational therapy evaluation
Bed or chair alarm—although these often go off after the patient is on the ground
Implement a toileting schedule—this needs to work on all 21 shifts per week
Low beds or putting mattress on the floor
Placing a pad next to the bed
Hip protectors
Encourage time spent in group activities
Use half instead of full bed rails
Identify correlating events, e.g., postprandial hypotension

TABLE 20-19

General Measures That May Avoid or Minimize Pressure Ulcers
Pressure-reducing mattresses
Turning schedules
Optimizing nutrition
Vitamin supplements such as zinc and vitamin C
Maintaining hydration
Controlling moisture and soiling from incontinence
Avoiding prolonged sitting
Pressure-relieving devices on chairs
Managing other medical conditions
Using protective devices such as multipodous boots for heel protection

TABLE 20-20

Common Medication Issues in Nursing Facilities
Late doses
Missed doses
Giving medications to the wrong patient
Wrong dose administered
Patient refused medication and physician not informed
Mislabeled medication from pharmacy
Wrong dose of medication sent from pharmacy
Medications ordered that should be avoided in the elderly population (e.g., anticholinergics, long-acting benzodiazepenes)

TABLE 20-21

Strategy to Manage Persistent Delirium in Post-acute Care
Structured mental status assessment on admission with application of the Confusion Assessment Method to detect delirium.
If delirium detected, contact the physician/APC
Workup to identify and treat reversible causes and contributors to delirium.
Institute measure to prevent or manage common complications of delirium
Avoid physical and chemical restraints, and sedatives at night if possible
Create an environmental milieu conducive to recovery from delirium, including provision of appropriate sensory aids, orientating devices such as clocks, calendars, and an orientation board, consistency of staff (if possible), cognitive and physical rehabilitation.
Educate family members about delirium, and engage them to help reorient the patient

physician is asked by the nurse to provide parameters for the order so "metoprolol 50 mg bid, hold if blood pressure is under 100 systolic or pulse under 55" is written. Two days later, the patient is sent to the emergency department complaining of chest pain and is found to be in atrial fibrillation with a ventricular response of 140 bpm.

On review of the medial record, it is found that the patient had a blood pressure in the 90s and metoprolol was held for three doses. The initial parameters for the metoprolol were written to avoid hypotension or bradycardia. However, the medication was needed for rate control and angina treatment. As in most other aspects of nursing home care, excellent communication is the key to success. Modifying the original order to read "metoprolol 50 mg bid, hold *and call MD* if blood pressure under 100 systolic or pulse under 55" could have alerted the physician to the fact that multiple doses were being missed. The dose could be reduced or another medication used that could ultimately have avoided a hospitalization.

DEALING WITH COMPLICATIONS OF THE ACUTE HOSPITAL

Subacute providers must often treat complications of hospitalization. In fact, the necessity for postacute care maybe determined more by these complications than by the primary diagnosis itself. Both the principles of geriatrics and empiric research suggest that the most effective approach for dealing with these complications is to prevent them. Unfortunately, subacute providers are not in a preventive position and must effectively manage problems that develop in the hospital.

Foremost among hospital-acquired complications is delirium, or acute confusion, which affects up to one-third of hospitalized patients aged 70 years or older. While some delirious patients clear quickly in the hospital, others remain confused for weeks to months. Because patients with persistent confusion are usually unable to return home, a large percentage of these patients are discharged to subacute facilities. In subacute care, residual delirium may profoundly impact the medical or rehabilitation plan, so that these patients are at high risk of "bouncing back" to the acute hospital, or failing to meet their rehabilitation goals.

Patients with delirium must be identified promptly and evaluated to ensure that all medical problems or medications that perpetuate delirium are eliminated. Probably the most common error among subacute practitioners is to attribute symptoms of delirium to an underlying dementia, and therefore neglecting potential op-

portunities to restore a patient's cognitive and functional status. To combat this, a brief but structured mental status assessment should be performed on all new admissions to subacute care, with particular focus on identifying key symptoms of delirium as described in the Confusion Assessment Method. Once delirium is recognized, in addition to identifying and treating its causes, a comprehensive cognitive and functional rehabilitation program that recognizes and abates the effect of delirium should be put into place. While "failure to abate delirium" has been introduced as a Medicare quality measure for subacute care, knowledge about detection and management of delirium among subacute care providers remains scant, and delirium abatement programs are far from being implemented at most facilities. Key steps in the management of delirium in subacute care are described in Table 20-21.

Another major problem inherited from hospitals is deconditioning. Elderly patients at bed rest lose muscle strength (and bone mineral density) rapidly, so that after a prolonged hospitalization, many frail elderly patients are unable to walk, even though their primary disease process had nothing to do with ambulation (e.g., pneumonia). Cardiovascular deconditioning may lead to severe orthostatic hypotension that may take months to resolve. Prolonged muscle and cardiovascular reconditioning may be required to restore these patients to their preillness status.

Depression is also very common in elderly patients after acute hospitalization. The presence of significant depressive symptoms, even in the absence of clinical depression, exerts a powerful negative influence on functional recovery in the weeks to months following acute illness. Subacute patients should be evaluated for depression or depressive symptoms using both informal staff observations and a structured assessment tool such as the Geriatric Depression Scale. Those with evidence of depression should be referred for appropriate mental health consultation and/or initiated on antidepressant medication. Because antidepressant medication may take weeks to become effective, psychostimulants such as methylphenidate can be quite useful as a short-term "bridge" in severely depressed postacute patients.

Finally, a mundane but serious consequence of hospitalization is the loss of glasses, dentures, hearing aids, or other assistive devices that elderly persons need for communication, eating, and the like. Often, these are not brought in to the hospital; in this case, the family should be asked to bring these into the subacute facility as part of the patient's rehabilitative plan. If the devices are indeed lost, prompt replacement maybe required, often at financial hardship to the patient. An old pair or glasses or pocket amplifier hearing devices may serve as a temporary substitute while a permanent replacement is obtained.

ACUTE MEDICAL PROBLEMS IN SUBACUTE CARE

The subacute population comprises individuals unable to return home after a hospitalization. These are sick, frail, and medically complex patients, which places them at higher risk for the development of an acute medical problem. Estimates suggest that between 10% and 33% of the subacute population must be urgently transferred back to the hospital. However, the rate of "bounce backs" varies widely among facilities and practitioners. Keeping patients in the facility is a worthy goal and facilities need to be more proactive with medical management and advance directives to achieve this goal. However, some acutely ill patients clearly need to go back to the hospital. We briefly discuss some of the most common acute problems in subacute care, and some of the key issues in determining whether to transfer the patient back to the hospital.

Fever is perhaps the most common acute problem in this setting. The first step is to determine whether the patient is clinically and hemodynamically stable. If so, the ability to perform a prompt diagnostic work-up is a key issue in determining the need for transfer. In addition to the ubiquitously ordered urinalysis and culture, a targeted physical examination, chest x-ray, and blood tests should be part of a basic fever work-up. Results should be available in hours, not days. Once results return, intravenous therapy, either for antibiotics and/or fluids to treat concomitant dehydration, is often required, at least for a few days. When the facility can provide prompt and appropriate evaluation and treatment is often a major determinant as to whether the workup can be done on-site or requires transfer to the emergency department.

Shortness of breath is another common presenting acute problem in subacute care, with many possible etiologies. Prompt work-up will include examination of the lungs and heart, testing for oxygen saturation, and possible electrocardiogram or chest x-ray. Treatment may include oxygen, bronchodilator treatments, diuretics, and respiratory therapy. In addition to clinical severity, facility capabilities may determine whether the patient needs to be transferred.

Perhaps the most vexing issue in subacute care is acute mental status change, or incident delirium. This should be distinguished from prevalent or residual delirium that was present at the time of hospital transfer. Proactive measures, such as careful documentation of a baseline mental status examination, are a key to the proper management of this problem. If new acute mental status change is detected, prompt and thorough evaluation for adverse drug effects and acute medical problems by a physician or APC is required. Often, medical management is relatively straightforward and should be attempted in the nursing facility when possible. At times, the patient's behavior and inability to cooperate with the staff rather than the medical condition itself necessitates transfer. Use of chemical or physical restraints should be avoided, if possible.

ADVANCE DIRECTIVES AND END-OF-LIFE ISSUES

Every subacute patient should have advance directives discussed, including identifying a substitute decision maker and describing advance care wishes. The default is often to continue the advance directives from the hospital; however, these should be readdressed at the time of subacute admission. If not already in place, a health care proxy should be completed. Resuscitation status, transfer back to the hospital, and any limits to care, including use of artificial hydration or feeding, should be discussed with the patient and/or family and carefully documented in the medical record.

While most of this chapter has focused on patients whose goal is to return home and to premorbid functioning, subacute care is also being increasingly used as a place for the dying. In the past, hospitals would care for patients during the dying process, which may extend from a few days to weeks. Now, however, hospitals face intense pressure to discharge these patients as soon as the decision is made to no longer pursue aggressive medical care. Subacute care facilities have filled a niche for such patients who are unable to go home and can provide a comfortable, supportive environment for the dying patient and the patient's family.

Effectively managing the dying process in subacute care requires expertise and effort that may exceed the capability of facility staff. The staff may need help with pain control and symptom relief or have inadequate time to adequately provide emotional support for the patient and/or family. In this case, involvement of a hospice program in the subacute facility is advised. Depending on the acuity of the dying process, hospice may provide occasional consultation or constant onsite direct-care management. It is often most effective if hospice can have adequate time to develop relationships with the staff, patient, and family before the acute dying process. Learning to recognize the optimal time to involve hospice is an art that can be developed through experience managing these patients. Effectively integrating a formal hospice program into a subacute setting requires strong leadership and commitment, as well as intensive collaboration and education support between hospice and subacute facility staff.

DISCHARGE PLANNING IN SUBACUTE CARE

Discharge planning from the subacute setting needs to be individualized; however, a number of basic principles and concepts can be applied to all individuals. Discharge planning should begin on or before admission. Patients should be sent to a subacute facility with clear goals for the stay. Often these goals involve rehabilitation to improve mobility, working toward independence with activities of daily living (ADLs) and stabilizing ongoing medical problems. Identifying these goals is helpful in establishing a treatment plan that will reduce barriers to discharge.

A common problem faced by the subacute interdisciplinary team is whether the patient will be safe at home. Common issues are how well someone needs to walk or transfer to be allowed to go home. Autonomy must be balanced with safety. Enlisting extra home supports from family members, friends, and home care agencies, or getting a personal safety alarm, can increase the comfort level of the care team to attempt a discharge to a home setting.

Many people have input into when a patient should be discharged. While the physician has ultimate responsibility for the discharge order, therapists, social workers, insurers, and family members may play a major role in the discharge decision. The physician needs to be skilled at assessing the input received from team members in making this decision. Except in the case of the hospice-type patient, medical stability is a major criterion for discharge.

Independence in the ability to transfer, ambulate, perform ADLs, and take medications properly is not essential if proper supports are in place.

A home visit by the therapy team maybe helpful in assessing what additional goals need to be reached, what equipment needs to be obtained and whether discharge is feasible. Equipment such as walkers and wheelchairs require living spaces without excess clutter and adequate doorways. Stairs, railings, and bathrooms can be assessed as well. Home modifications such as ramps, grab bars, raised toilet seats, and railings may need to be installed prior to discharge.

There is an opportunity when discharging a patient to do a complete review of all medications and treatments. Ideally, this review should be performed by a physician or nurse practitioner because a facility registered nurse cannot make medication or treatment changes. Removing unnecessary prn medications, simplifying dosing schedules, writing out prescriptions, and educating on medication taking are just some of the issues that need to be addressed. The facility case manager needs to work with the physician–APC in deciding on the appropriate home care services and ordering them. Discharge is also a time to update the primary care physician on the patient's medical status and to make sure that appropriate follow-up appointments are in place.

Sometimes, despite the best efforts of subacute clinicians and facilities, a patient fails to recover sufficiently to return home and needs to be placed in long-term care. This may require discharge to a new nursing home, moving to a different unit within the same facility, or merely "decertification" of a bed. Regardless of the physical arrangement, this move has major financial ramifications because the cost of care must now be borne by the patient, Medicaid, or if this has been purchased, a long-term care insurance provider. At times, it is determined that the patient no longer has skilled medical or rehabilitative needs prior to the use of all possible "Medicare days." In this case, decertification is sometimes contentious and may require input from the medical director in addition to the attending physician. It is best to give the patient and family as much advance notice as possible of impending decertification, especially if transfer of facility is required.

RISK MANAGEMENT IN SUBACUTE CARE

Nursing facilities are, in many parts of the country, a growing venue for litigation. There are a number of areas of risk management in nursing facilities that are quite different from those of the ambulatory setting. Practitioners need to educate themselves about these areas of increased risk. As in any clinical situation, documentation is critical to demonstrate that appropriate care has been provided. When there is a lawsuit related to the care of a nursing home patient, the facility is often named as a defendant. The physician might also be named. Table 20-22 describes common causes of lawsuits against nursing facilities.

SUBACUTE FACILITY REIMBURSEMENT

Beginning in 1999, a dramatic change occurred regarding Medicare nursing home reimbursement, which has driven many individually owned and large national for-profit nursing home chains into bankruptcy. This change in reimbursement is called Prospective

TABLE 20-22

Common Causes of Litigation in Nursing Facilities
Falls
Pressure ulcers
Elopement
Restraints
Weight loss
Physical, emotional, or sexual abuse
Medication errors
Aspiration

Payment System (PPS). Under PPS, nursing facilities must categorize and group each patient into one of several dozen categories. These categories, or Resource Utilization Groups (RUGs), have different daily rates of reimbursement for the facility from Medicare. The medical, rehabilitation, and nursing needs of each patient must be properly and accurately identified in order to obtain the proper RUG classification. The RUG classification is determined by the Minimum Data Set (MDS). The MDS is an assessment tool used for all nursing home patients, including those receiving subacute care. The MDS assists the facility in developing a plan of care for the patient, and also identifies the appropriate RUG category.

The reimbursement that the facility receives from Medicare covers essentially all aspects of care, including rehabilitation, laboratory, x-ray, supplies, and pharmacy. Only by effectively managing these ancillary costs can facilities cover their costs. Achieving success under PPS requires excellent identification and documentation of patient needs and function, cost-effective use of x-ray, laboratory, and pharmacy services, including those services provided outside of the facility, such as ambulance, emergency room, and diagnostic services. Managed care contracts, for the most part, are similar to PPS in that the per diem rate covers rehabilitation, x-ray, laboratory, and pharmacy services. Medicaid and private payments are used primarily for long-term institutional care rather than for subacute care.

Subacute physicians and APCs are instrumental in helping nursing facilities succeed under PPS and managed care. The clinical expertise provided by these practitioners enables facilities to better evaluate the scope and severity of clinical conditions for each patient. Having enhanced clinical presence in the nursing facility can help to identify and treat new illnesses sooner, thereby implementing less-costly interventions and avoiding complications. For example, identifying and treating pneumonia before the patient becomes delirious, dehydrated, and septic is certainly better for the patient and can lead to a reduced need for intravenous therapies, emergency department visits, ambulance services, and hospitalization. The result is a better financial outcome for the facility, as well as a better clinical outcome for the patient.

REIMBURSEMENT FOR PHYSICIANS

A nursing home practice has some distinct advantages over an office practice. For instance, a nursing home practice can have lower overhead costs. A physician who only practices in SNFs does not have to pay rent on a large office with multiple examination rooms, needs less nursing and administrative staff, and does not have to pay for as much equipment and other office supplies.

Physician billing in nursing facilities is currently based on 10 codes organized into three categories. The first two categories are codes related to discharges and follow-up visits. The third category relates to the performance of a full history and physical examination on admission, or at a yearly physical. Nurse practitioners and physician's assistants can bill Medicare for the care they provide in nursing facilities. At present, the Medicare fee schedule is 85% of the physician payment for the same level of service code. Individual states and insurance carriers may not view coding similarly. It is suggested that physicians learn about coding guidelines in their specific geographic regions. The American Medical Directors Association is an excellent resource for obtaining up to date billing information (www.amda.com).

SUBACUTE CARE AS A SAFETY NET

Subacute care is an important setting to provide medical and rehabilitative services, as well as end-of-life and palliative care. The interdisciplinary approach upon which subacute care is based should benefit patients and society from both quality of care and cost perspectives. Hospitals are discharging increasingly complex patients just getting over a critical illness, often on new medications, and with functional decline. Many of these patients have conditions that are continuing to evolve in the days immediately post hospital discharge. By providing enhanced clinical support services, the subacute site serves as a safety net in the continuum of care for older persons. A large cadre of physicians and APCs with expertise in managing complex illnesses, as well as strong skills in geriatrics and palliative care, are needed to care for the growing numbers of patients who can benefit from subacute care.

FURTHER READING

Bergmann MA, Murphy KM, Kiely DK, Jones RN, Marcantonio ER. A model for management of delirious post-acute patients. *J Am Geriatr Soc.* 2005;53:1817–1825.

Burl JB, et al. Geriatric nurse practitioners in long-term care: demonstration of effectiveness in managed care. *J Am Geriatr Soc.* 1998;46:506.

Buxbaum RC. The evolution of subacute care. *Long Term Care Interface.* 2006;7:29–32.

Coleman EA, Min SJ, Chomiak A, Kramer AM. Posthospital care transitions: patterns, complications, and risk identification. *Health Serv Res.* 2004;39:1449–1465.

Cotterill PG, Gage BJ. Overview: Medicare post-acute care since the Balanced Budget Act of 1997. *Health Care Financ Rev.* 2002 Winter;24:1–6.

Creditor MC. Hazards of hospitalization of the elderly. *Ann Intern Med.* 1993;118:219.

Friedman M, et al. Post-acute and ongoing assessment of elders: where to begin? *2000 Post-Acute Outcomes Sourcebook.* New York, New York: Faulkner and Grey's Healthcare Information Center; 2000.

Hutt E, et al. Precipitants of emergency room visits and acute hospitalization in short-stay medicare nursing home residents. *J Am Geriatr Soc.* 2002;50:223.

Levenson SA. *Subacute and Transitional Care Handbook: Defining, Delivering, and Improving The Care.* St. Louis, MO: Beverly Cracom Publications; 1996.

Marcantonio ER, et al. Delirium symptoms in post-acute care: prevalent, persistent, and associated with poor functional recovery. *J Am Geriatr Soc.* 2003;51:4–9.

Simon S, LaBelle S, Littlehale S. Measuring quality with QMs. *Provider.* 2003;29:37–43.

Simon SE, Bergmann MA, Jones RN, Murphy KM, Orav EJ, Marcantonio ER. Reliability of a structured assessment for nonclinicians to detect delirium among new admissions to postacute care. *J Am Med Dir Assoc.* 2006;7:412–415.

Tait RC, Chibnall JT. Pain in older subacute care patients: associations with clinical status and treatment. *Pain Med.* 2002;3:231–239.

Von Sternberg T, et al. Post-hospital subacute care: an example of a managed care model. *J Am Geriatr Soc.* 1997;45:87.

Weinberg A. *Risk Management in Long-term Care—A Quick Reference Guide.* New York, New York: Springer; 1998.

Nursing Facility Care

Mary Pat Rapp ■ *Keith L. Rapp*

The current cohort of older Americans is a more robust group than in the past, and the prevalence of disability related to chronic disease is in decline. Despite improvements in the health of older people as a whole, the overall need for services provided by nursing facilities will rise. In the future, the medical needs of nursing facility residents will likely be more complex and require additional services from primary care practitioners, including physicians, nurse practitioners, clinical nurse specialists, and physician assistants. Nursing facilities already show a trend in the increasing percentage of residents who are not able to perform activities such as dressing and bathing independently. As shown in Figure 21-1, over a 20-year span, residents able to feed themselves declined from 67% to 53% and those able to dress themselves, from 30% to 13%.

The term *nursing facility* is inclusive of other commonly used terms, e.g., nursing home, long-term care facility, subacute care unit, or nursing home care unit. Nursing facilities are primarily free-standing in the community or are separate units in hospitals. Patients are usually referred to as residents. On the average, nursing facility residents have a median age of 85, three or more functional impairments, and six chronic illnesses. One-half are cognitively impaired with additional functional impairments and/or chronic illnesses. Most lack sufficient personal and financial support to remain in their homes. Payment for services rendered comes from Medicare Part A, Medicare Part B, Medicaid, Veterans Affairs, private insurance plans including long-term care insurance, and out-of-pocket. Skilled nursing facilities (SNF) are subsets of nursing facilities that receive payment for skilled nursing services under Medicare Part A. SNF services include rehabilitation therapies and/or skilled nursing care, such as intravenous therapy, wound care treatment for deep pressure ulcers, or close-monitoring posthospitalization in medically complex residents.

As shown in Figure 21-2, two populations are distinguished by length of stay and goals. Long-term residents stay more than 6 months and are either cognitively impaired, physically disabled, or both. Short-stay residents of less than 3 months duration are re-

covering from an acute illness, suffering from a terminal illness, or are medically unstable with a limited life expectancy. From 1985 to 2001, when payment structures for hospitalized older adults changed to encourage earlier discharges, trends in admissions demonstrate hospitals released the same percentage of residents to nursing facilities. However, in 1985, 18% of nursing facility residents admitted from hospitals were discharged to the community versus 30% in 2001. Today, more residents are being admitted for rehabilitation following surgery or acute illness and need a higher level of care for a shorter period of time.

Predictors of admission to a nursing facility include functional determinants, such as decline in strength and balance, and impairment in activities of daily living (ADL), especially in toileting, dressing, and eating. Medical conditions that contribute to functional decline include stroke, diabetes mellitus, and Parkinson's disease. For those older than 75 years of age, a decline in cognition is a consistent risk factor. Adequate caregiver support, both informal and formal, explains why many functionally dependent older adults are able to remain in community settings.

The purpose of this chapter is to help physicians, nurse practitioners, clinical nurse specialists, and physician assistants (hereafter practitioners) understand the nursing facility environment and principles of geriatric care adaptable to this special population. Regulatory issues that influence care processes, the role of nursing facility employees and consultants, and practical aspects of managing a nursing facility clinical practice are discussed.

REGULATORY ISSUES

Following extensive reforms developed with the 1987 Omnibus Budget Reconciliation Act, The Centers for Medicare and Medicaid Services (CMS) began enforcing the revised nursing facility regulations. In response to consumer complaints and known problems in the quality of care, new rules, including considerable federal

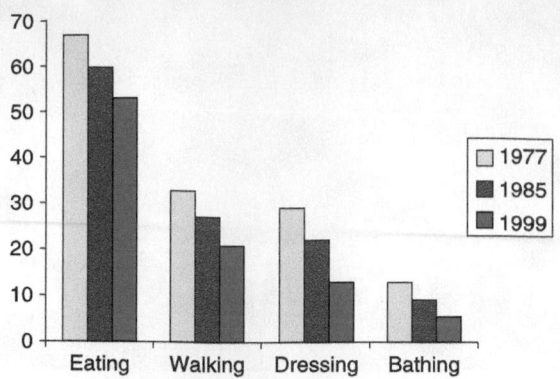

FIGURE 21-1. Decline in functional status in residents admitted to nursing facilities from 1977 to 1999. (NCHS. National Nursing Home Survey. 1999. http://www.cdc.gov/nchs/nnhs.htm.)

TABLE 21-1

Resident Assessment Instrument Trigger List
Delirium
Cognitive loss
Visual function
Communication
ADL functional/rehabilitation potential
Urinary incontinence and indwelling catheter
Psychosocial well-being
Mood state
Behavior problem
Activities
Falls
Nutritional status
Feeding tubes
Dehydration/fluid maintenance
Dental care
Pressure ulcers
Psychotropic drug use
Physical restraints

Minimum Data Set available at http://www.cms.hhs.gov/NursingHomeQualityInits/Downloads/MDS20MDSAllForms.pdf

and state oversight, emphasized process and outcomes with less emphasis on structural components. The federal rules for facility participation in Medicare and Medicaid services (commonly referred to as "F-Tags"), together with survey guidelines, clarify regulations, and mandate-specific outcomes and processes of care. By regulation, on-site surveys are federally mandated. They are unannounced, and noncompliance is associated with potential costly fines. State departments of health conduct surveys of quality of care under federal CMS contracts every 9 to 15 months. Additional on-site surveys occur sporadically based on consumer complaints.

Resident Assessment Instrument

F-Tag 272 stipulates that within 2 weeks of admission, the nursing facility must perform a standardized comprehensive assessment on each resident. Facilities use a federally developed and state-approved Resident Assessment Instrument (RAI) to accomplish this, and the resulting data guides care planning, state inspections, and reimbursement under Medicare Part A and, where applicable, Medicaid. The facility transmits the information electronically to the state regulatory and survey agency.

The RAI consists of the Minimum Data Set (MDS) the Resident Assessment Protocols (RAP), and the RAP Trigger List. The MDS screens residents for the 18 functional problems listed in Table 21-1. Noting a functional problem triggers a more in-depth assessment by the facility interdisciplinary team guided by the appropriate RAP.

An interdisciplinary plan of care based on this assessment must be completed by day 21 following admission. Each resident's MDS and care plan are updated quarterly and completed in entirety annually and when a significant change in condition occurs. For the purpose of the MDS, a significant change in condition is defined as a persistent improvement or decline in mood, behavior, or functional status. More frequent assessments are performed when residents are admitted for SNF care under Medicare Part A. These assessments are a specific responsibility of the facility, and require minimal physician input.

The Center for Health Systems Research and Analysis (CHSRA), the Nursing Home Quality Initiative (NHQI), and measurement experts have identified and validated quality indicators (CHSRA) and quality measures (NHQI) from the MDS. Using a national reporting mechanism, facilities and state surveyors review combined quality indicator/quality measure reports (Table 21-2) to identify potential problems in a facility. The quality indicators/quality measures

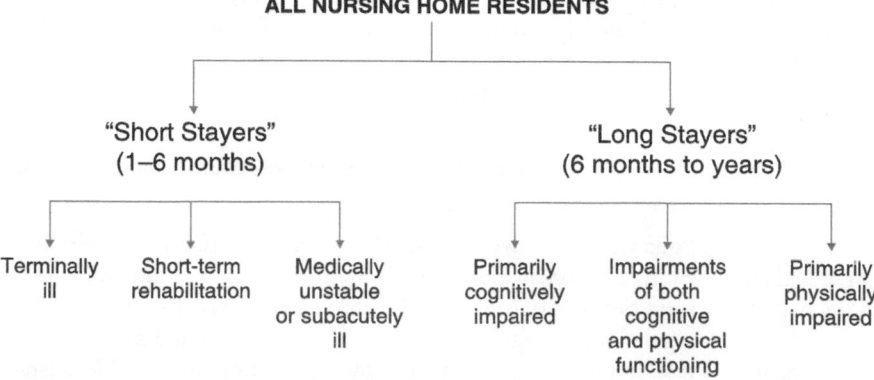

FIGURE 21-2. Types of nursing facility residents. (Revised with permission from Ouslander J, Osterweil D, Morley J. Medical Care in the Nursing Home. 2nd ed. New York, New York: McGraw-Hill; 1996.)

TABLE 21-2

Quality Indicators and Quality Measures Derived from the Minimum Dataset

Long-Stay Residents

Vaccinations

  Percent who were given the influenza vaccine during the flu season

  Percent who were assessed and given the pneumococcal vaccine

Accidents

  Incidence of new fractures

  Prevalence of falls

Behavior/emotional patterns

  Residents who have become more depressed or anxious

  Prevalence of behavioral symptoms affecting others

    All

    High risk

    Low risk

  Prevalence of symptoms of depression without antidepressant therapy

Clinical management

  Use of nine or more different medications

Cognitive patterns

  Incidence of cognitive impairment

Elimination/incontinence

  Low-risk residents who lost control of the bowels or bladder

  Residents who have/had a catheter inserted and left in their bladder

  Prevalence of occasional or frequent bladder or bowel incontinence
    without a toileting plan

  Prevalence of fecal impaction

Infection control

  Residents with a urinary tract infection

Nutrition/eating

  Residents who lose too much weight

  Prevalence of tube feeding

  Prevalence of dehydration

Pain management

  Residents who have moderate to severe pain

Physical functioning

  Residents whose need for help with daily activities has increased

  Residents who spend most of their time in a bed or in a chair

  Residents whose ability to move in and around their room got worse

  Incidence of decline in range of motion

Psychotropic drug use

  Prevalence of antipsychotic use in the absence of psychotic or related
    conditions

    All

    High risk

    Low risk

  Prevalence of antianxiety/hypnotic use

  Prevalence of hypnotic use more than two times in last week

Quality of life

  Residents who were physically restrained

  Prevalence of little or no activity

Skin care

  High-risk residents with pressure ulcers

  Low-risk residents with pressure ulcers

Short-Stay Residents

Postacute care measures

  Percent who were given the influenza vaccine during the flu season

  Percent who were assessed and given the pneumococcal vaccine

  Short-stay residents with delirium

  Short-stay residents who had moderate to severe pain

  Short-stay residents with pressure ulcers

Nursing Home Compare. http://www.medicare.gov/NHCompare

report identifies the facility's percentile rank on the items, where this rank can be compared with a group norm. Three items are considered sentinel events warranting closer evaluation: fecal impaction, dehydration, and pressure ulcer development in residents at low risk for pressure ulcers. When surveyors find evidence of noncompliance with regulations, deficiencies are cited and scored based on how many residents were affected and whether there was harm or immediate threat to resident safety. Depending on the scope and seriousness of the deficiencies, facility sanctions range from in-service education to termination of the Medicare and Medicaid contract with significant monetary fines.

In 2001, the Secretary of the Health and Human Services Department convened a group of nursing facility industry stakeholders to develop a plan to further improve the quality of care in nursing facilities. This activity became the Nursing Home Quality Initiative (NHQI), which currently monitors regulation and enforcement, communication with consumers regarding quality, community-based quality improvement programs, and collaboration to enhance knowledge and resources.

The NQHI collaborates with CMS to communicate information to consumers on the Nursing Home Compare Web site (www.medicare.gov/NHCompare). This site allows consumers to compare the quality of nursing facility care based on the quality indicators and quality measures. The Nursing Home Compare listing distinguishes between short-stay postacute care residents and long-stay chronic care residents. In addition to quality data, the Web site includes basic demographic information for each facility, nursing staff hours, and survey results. This public display of quality data is intended to stimulate nursing facilities to improve health care in order to be competitive (Wunderlich and Kohler, 2001).

A prospective payment system (PPS) based on 53 Resource Utilization Groups (RUG) is now used to determine reimbursement for skilled nursing care under Medicare Part A. Specific items from the MDS contribute to the RUG and the daily rate Medicare pays. Residents hospitalized for at least 3 days during the past 30 days are eligible for a potential 100-day benefit for skilled nursing care. Managed care organizations may waive the 3-day prior hospitalization requirement. The advent of this reimbursement system has resulted in a significant increase in the number of nursing facilities providing skilled nursing services. Regulatory requirements for visits by physicians are similar to requirements for long-stay residents in nursing facilities. In reality, residents who receive skilled nursing services usually need more attention from practitioners because of medical complexity or discharge planning issues.

NURSING FACILITY ATTENDING PHYSICIAN

Physicians working in a nursing facility environment manage and coordinate care for residents with multiple chronic medical and functional conditions. Goals are to cure when appropriate, restore and maintain function, and offer comfort. Most nursing facility physicians maintain an active office practice, care for hospitalized patients, and visit their residents in the nursing facility. This is especially true in rural health care environments. An increasing number of physicians are choosing to practice exclusively in nursing facilities. Positive rewards for the full-time nursing facility physician include flexibility in the hours worked and the ability to positively influence medical care delivery. Many physicians find that as they increase their time commitment to the facility, they are integrated into the facility culture and the work becomes more satisfying. This is particularly true of physicians with dual roles to provide direct patient care and facility medical direction.

Physicians with a part-time nursing facility practice typically devote 2 hours or less per week to nursing facility care. Physicians' perception of low reimbursement, excessive regulations, frequency of telephone calls from families, and extensive paperwork cause some physicians to hesitate to provide more time.

Nursing facilities often lack an organized medical staff typical of most hospitals. Although formal credentialing is usually not required, facilities often ask physicians to complete a medical staff application process to verify medical license and medical liability coverage. To encourage accountability, nursing facility administrators are required to ensure that physicians comply with the minimum standards for frequency of visits and quality of care set forth by federal and state regulations.

Which model of medical staff organization best benefits the resident and the facility is not clear. A closed medical staff comprising a few physicians practicing in a single nursing facility maybe associated with higher quality and intensity of care. One drawback is this limits choices for residents. Nursing facilities may be reluctant to limit the number of physicians on staff if the administrators perceive a potential decline in census because of a lack of physician referral resources. Data do not support the theory that facilities with a larger staff have either a higher census or better profitability. In fact, it appears that profitability is more closely linked to the quality of care, not the number of physician providers.

Providing medical care for nursing facility residents is intellectually stimulating and demands unique knowledge and practice skills. Although limited randomized controlled trials have produced adequate guidance in medical decision making, modifying the medical plan of care based on whether the resident has moderate to severe dementia, is physically frail, or has a limited life expectancy is a reasonable approach. Other considerations include the perceived quality life for the resident, the potential of any intervention to provide a positive benefit, risks, and costs. Physicians must also modify disease-specific management strategies. For example, dietary restrictions recommended for cardiovascular diseases and diabetes mellitus are not appropriate for undernourished residents suffering weight loss.

Medical care in a nursing facility requires an interdisciplinary team of social workers, nurses, physical therapist, pharmacists, and dieticians. Whether acting as the attending physician or medical director, physicians are an integral part of the interdisciplinary team and need to seek out and be receptive of input from the other disciplines.

Expectations of the attending physician are summarized in Table 21-3. According to F Tag 385, residents must be in the care of a physician who is expected to visit the resident in the facility unless specialized equipment is needed or a resident specifically requests an office visit. The physician visits and approves orders at least every 30 days for the first 90 days and then every 60 days thereafter. Qualified nurse practitioners, clinical nurse specialists, or physician assistants may substitute after the first required visit. For residents admitted under a Medicare Part A SNF benefit, the initial comprehensive assessment must be personally performed by the physician. This stipulation does not preclude these other practitioners from making a medically necessary visit prior to the physician's initial

TABLE 21-3

Role of the Attending Physician in the Nursing Facility

Assess new admissions within 30 days
Authorize admission orders in a timely manner
Contact the receiving institution or provider following transfer or discharge
Make periodic, on-site visits
• Visit every 30 days for the first 90 days and at least every 60 days thereafter
• Maintain informative, legible progress notes
• Periodically review and approve the overall plan of care
• During each visit evaluate the resident, talk with pertinent staff, and communicate with responsible parties as necessary
• Review the resident's current condition, status of episodic acute events since the last visit, diagnostic test results, and progress of interventions.
Ensure adequate coverage by alternate providers who will respond appropriately
Provide appropriate evidence-based care to residents
Provide appropriate, timely medical orders and documentation
Follow principles of appropriate conduct

Data from American Medical Directors Association Resolution and Position Statement: Role of the Attending Physician in the Nursing Home, Position Statement E03, March 2003.

comprehensive assessment. For residents without the SNF benefit, some states allow nurse practitioners, clinical nurse specialists, and physician assistants to substitute for all required physician visits. Regardless, medically necessary visits are allowed and are covered by Medicare (Table 21-4).

Visiting on a regular basis is encouraged whether it is daily, weekly, or on monthly schedules. Practice efficiency experts suggest physicians plan to see at least seven residents to make the site of service economically viable. The frequency of visits to the facility is determined by the number of residents under the care of the physician and the acuity. A physician planning well can care for 14 to 16 or more residents a day. Weekly visits permit conducting follow-up visits, attending to new problems, and seeing new admissions. When working with other practitioners who can visit weekly or more frequently, a physician may be able to deliver high-quality care with physician visits less than once a week. Facilities such as hospital-based SNF units or free-standing SNFs may warrant daily visits by practitioners. A balance between the physician and nurse practitioner or clinical nurse specialist visits assures that residents receive the benefits of both medicine and advanced practice nursing. Nurse practitioners, and particularly geriatric nurse practitioners, are well suited to manage syndromes such as falls, pressure ulcers, and weight loss as well as attend to the details of a monthly review of the plan of care. Table 21-5 clarifies approved delegation of physician tasks.

Because of the physician's intermittent presence, day-to-day contact is available via telephone. If allowed by state law and facility policy, standing orders or protocols maybe implemented for commonly occurring low-risk events such as skin tears (Figure 21-3). If weekly or more frequent visits are made, nurses may use nonurgent communication strategies, such as a communication manual to document follow-up concerns (Figure 21-4) and may store laboratory reports, dietary recommendations, and pharmacy reviews until the physician or other practitioner is in the building to address the issues. Structured progress notes and comprehensive assessments (Figures 21-5 and 21-6) are encouraged to ensure comprehensive data collection

TABLE 21-4

American Medical Directors Associations Statement on Medical Necessity

Primary care provider visits
- One visit per month for long-stay nursing facility resident
- One visit per week for short-stay skilled nursing facility care
- Initial comprehensive admission assessment
- Change in condition or instability that warrants an evaluation
- Follow-up visit to monitor the effect of therapy including pressure ulcer evaluation, psychotropic medications, or comfort measures for terminally ill
- Regulatory requirements
- Medical conditions including delirium or dementia with behavioral symptoms
- Need to address a concern expressed by resident, family, nursing, rehabilitation, or managed care

Consultation services
- The consultant possesses additional skills and/or knowledge
- The service is appropriate and aligned with known goals
- Care planning, treatment, and/or follow-up will be affected by the consultation

Diagnostic services
- Consider if the evaluation, management, and/or monitoring will change based on the results
- Evaluate the appropriateness of the service including the consequences of the results and whether acting on the results will improve the quality of life
- Determine whether the resident can tolerate the service safely

Therapeutic modalities
- There is a potential for functional improvement
- The provider can document goals and objectives of therapy
- Certain risks may be avoided by the intervention

Data from AMDA. White Paper on Determination and Documentation of Medical Necessity in Long Term Care Facilities. 2001. http://www.amda.com/library/ whitepapers/mednecwhitepaper.htm. Accessed January 29, 2004.

that is readily retrieved and meets or exceeds all regulatory requirements.

Nurse practitioners, clinical nurse specialists, and physician assistants are increasingly involved in nursing facility care. Whether employed by the nursing facility directly, a physician, or self-employed, their presence is noted in approximately 20% of facilities. Studies to

SKIN TEARS
- ☐ Cleanse wound with normal saline prior to any dressing application.
- ☐ Close the skin edges of the wound with adhesive skin closure tape (*steri strips*), if possible. Leave tape on until wound is healed.
- ☐ If steri strips are not used, apply topical dressings and continue until healed.
  - ☐ Polyurethane foam: *Flexan*, change q 3 days or when there is strike through discharge. If not available apply:
  - ☐ Transparent film: *Op Site*. Leave on until wound healed. May change prn if loose, or discharge seeps through. If not available apply:
  - ☐ Antibiotic ointment, *Dermagram ointment,* or *Dermagram spray*, cover with dry gauze. Change daily.
- ☐ Notify physician/NP of any skin tear wound that
  - ☐ Fails to show improvement in 5 days
  - ☐ Demonstrates erythema, discharge, edema, pain

Bibliography
Adv Ther 1996 Jan–Feb:13(1):10–9
Dermatol Surg 1995 Jul;21(7):583–90
J Trauma 1987 Mar;27(3):278–82
J Trauma 1990 Jul:30(7):857–65
Ostomy Wound Management 1999 Jun;45(6):22–4, 27–8

FIGURE 21-3. Management of Skin Tears. Geriatric Associates of America (GAA) Order Set. *(Used with permission from Geriatric Associates of America, PA.)*

date suggest that these practitioners working in concert with the primary care physician provide a higher level of care to nursing facility residents, enhance satisfaction with care, and decrease hospitalization rates while maintaining cost neutrality.

Nursing Facility Personnel

The nursing staff provides nearly all of the care provided to residents in nursing facilities. Nursing assistants receive at least 75 hours of training and must be certified within 4 months of employment. They provide the most basic resident care, including bathing, dressing, and eating assistance. Supervising the nursing assistants are the Licensed Vocational/Practical Nurses (LVN/LPN) that often serve as charge nurses and carry out physician orders as well as report changes in the resident's condition. The 1-year education and training for LPN/LVNs generally focuses on tasks and procedures oriented to acute care with less attention to the supervisory role in the nursing

TABLE 21-5

Physician Delegation of Tasks

	INITIAL REQUIRED VISIT*	INITIAL ORDERS	CERTIFICATION	RECERTIFICATION	SUBSEQUENT ORDERS
Skilled Nursing Facility (SNF): Medicare Part A					
NP, CNS, PA employed by the facility	May not perform	May not sign	May not sign	May not sign	May sign
NP, CNS not employed by the facility	May not perform	May not sign	May sign	May sign	May sign
PA not employed by the facility	May not perform	May not sign	May not sign	May not sign	May sign
Nursing Facility					
NP, CNS, PA employed by the facility	May not perform	May not sign	May not sign	N/A	May sign
NP, CNS, not employed by the facility	May not perform†	May not sign	May sign	N/A	May sign
PA not employed by the facility	May not perform†	May not sign	May sign	N/A	May sign

PA, physician assistant; NP, nurse practitioner; CNS, clinical nurse specialist.
*Initial visit is defined as first regulatory visit and must be performed within 30 days of admission.
†At the discretion of the states, the initial visit may be delegated to an NP, CNS, or PA.
Reprinted with permission from Rapp MP (2003). Opportunities for advance practice nurses in the nursing facility. J Am Med Dir Assoc, 4(6), 337–343.

Geriatric Associates of America, PA
Communication Log

Please indicate in this log any resident concerns you would like addressed during the time of the physician or nurse practitioner's next visit.

Resident Name _____

Station and Room Number _____ Date of occurrence _____

Nurse Signature _____

Concern/Assessment: _____

_____

_____

_____

_____

Physician/NP/CNS/PA initials _____ Date _____

FIGURE 21-4. Communication log. *(Used with permission from Geriatric Associates of America, PA.)*

facility setting. Facilities require a Registered Nurse (RN) to be on duty 8 hours daily, including weekends. The Director of Nurses (DON) manages nursing services and must be a RN. Registered nurses have an associate degree (2 years), a diploma (3 years), or a bachelor's degree (4 years). Descriptions of the key personnel in nursing facilities are noted in Table 21-6.

Practice Organization

Few nursing facilities utilize electronic medical records. Checklists and flowcharts are most often used to document routine nursing tasks. Facility nurses document vital signs and residents' general condition at least daily in the narrative nurse's notes for residents admitted under Medicare Part A SNF care. For long-stay residents, narrative documentation is limited to unusual occurrences or acute events. Physicians find the nurses' narrative notes a useful source of information. Many nursing facilities also document the resident's condition on a monthly summary form, and these forms help to track trends and response to medications. The plan of care maybe in the medical record or in a separate notebook at the nursing station. Diagnostic test results, consultant's reports, rehabilitation notes, social services records, and dietary consults usually remain in the chart for 1 year or more.

As physicians and practitioners monitor responses to medications and treatments, current daily documentation is found in other locations, usually on flowcharts in notebooks on medication and treatment carts. This documentation typically contains results of finger stick blood glucose testing, the frequency of as needed medications for pain or behavioral symptoms, behavioral monitoring for antipsychotic medications, monthly vital signs, monthly weights, treatments, and wound measurements. Daily or weekly blood pressures and pulses taken to monitor the response to antihypertensive medications or digitalis are found on the medication administration record. Automated blood pressure, temperature, and pulse oximetry equipment is usually located near the nurse's station. Other supplies and equipment to make the day more efficient are listed in Table 21-7.

The American Medical Directors Association (AMDA) suggests visiting long-stay residents monthly and short-stay SNF residents weekly. Physicians and practitioners could routinely plan to see one-fourth of the residents each week, allowing additional time to examine residents who have an acute change in condition, need additional follow-up from prior visits, or receive skilled nursing services. Fol-

lowing the same pattern for visits each month minimizes missing visits with residents. A list of residents by room number, with birth dates, the date of the last history and physical, date of the last physician visit, and a space to make comments assists in organizing the day.

New admissions and residents seen for a routine scheduled visit and those who have returned from the hospital since the last visit can be marked on the census sheet. When working with other practitioners, divide the work load in advance. One option is that in any one month, the physician makes 50% of the regulatory visits and the other practitioner the remaining. Some physicians prefer to conduct regulatory visits and utilize other practitioners for acute medically necessary visits. If functioning as a medical director, allocate time for that responsibility. Advance planning options that make the day go smoothly are shown in Table 21-8. Facility nurses are appreciative of physicians who are considerate of their time as nurses who make rounds also have other tasks, such as administering medications, performing treatments, or calling other physicians. Also, in respect of resident privacy, physician visits should occur in private rooms and not in the common areas.

Quality of Medical Care

As previously stated, practitioners are charged with periodically evaluating residents and reviewing the appropriateness of current medical plans of care (CMS, 2005). Specific evidence-based care processes guide the practitioners in evaluating and managing complex medical and functional problems. Using evidence-based quality indicators permits the practitioner to specifically identify care processes associated with improved outcomes, to evaluate the care against an accepted standard, and to guide future efforts to improve care and outcomes. The frequency of visits and mandated assessments of residents in the nursing facility affords the practitioner the opportunity to monitor the quality of ongoing assessments, care decisions, and outcomes of chronic care management.

For the nursing facility environment, a consensus panel of physicians, registered nurses, and a health systems methodologist adapted quality indicators from the Assessing Care of Vulnerable Elders (ACOVE) study. The consensus panel identified 11 medical conditions, 7 geriatric syndromes, and 6 quality of life parameters where the management approach differs significantly from that in a community setting. Examples are seen in Table 21-9, where each quality indicator was written as a two-part If–Then statement.

Geriatric Associates of America
History

Name: _____ _____ year old ☐ female ☐ male   **Birth Date:** _____

Present Medical History: Describe sequence of events that led up to admission to the facility, or summarize significant events in past year.

☐ New Admission ☐ Annual H&P ☐ Readmission, New MDS, ☐ Significant Change in Condition, New MDS ☐ Change in physician

Previous Illnesses

Past Surgical History: (Type and Year)

Family Medical History: _____

Smoking: _____ pack years. ☐ Still smokes ☐ Quit, year: _____

Alcohol history: ☐ Casual use ☐ Alcoholic ☐ None   Current use: ☐ None ☐ Occasional use

Allergies (reaction, if known)

Immunization dates: Flu _____ Pneumonia _____ Tetanus _____ TB reactivity ☐ neg ☐ pos ☐ unk

Preventive Care dates: Mammography _____ Pap _____ PSA _____ Prostate Exam _____ Other: _____

Present Social Status:

Marital Status: Married _____ times ☐ widow ☐ divorced ☐ spouse still living   Number of children locally _____

Total number of children involved: _____ Other:

Functional Status:

Ambulation ☐ Unassisted ☐ Assisted ☐ Cane ☐ Walker ☐ Wheelchair ☐ Bedfast <u>Transfer</u> ☐ Ind ☐ Dep

Continence   <u>Bladder</u> ☐ Continent ☐ Incontinent   <u>Bowel</u> ☐ Continent ☐ Incontinent

Basic ADL   <u>Dressing</u> ☐ Ind ☐ Dep   <u>Feeding</u> ☐ Ind ☐ Dep ☐ Artificial feeding

Vision ☐ Adequate for regular print ☐ Impaired, but can get around ☐ Severely impaired ☐ Correction

Hearing ☐ Adequate ☐ Minimal difficulty ☐ Moderate difficulty ☐ Uses amplifier ☐ No useful hearing

Usual Mental Status   ☐ Alert, oriented ☐ Alert, **dis**oriented, follows simple commands
                       ☐ Alert, **dis**oriented, **cannot** follow simple commands ☐ Not alert, comatose

Dementia   ☐ None ☐ Alzheimer's ☐ Multi infarct ☐ Uncertain ☐ Other _____

Most recent Folstein Mini Mental State Exam _____ /30   Date _____

Geriatric Depression Scale _____ /15   Date _____

Treatment status:

Advance Directives: ☐ Resident able/unable to participate in decision   If not, why not _____

Surrogate decision maker _____ Relationship _____

Decision: ☐ Do not attempt resuscitation ☐ Do not utilize artificial feeding ☐ Do not hospitalize except for comfort ☐

☐ Out of hospital DNAR ☐ Do not use intravenous hydration ☐ Do not use hypodermoclysis

☐ Full Code. Attempt resuscitation in event of cardiac or respiratory arrest

☐ Medical Power of Attorney for Health Care:

Designated Agent _____ Telephone Number ( ) _____

☐ Legal Guardian _____ Telephone Number ( ) _____

Hospital Preference/Hospital Physician: _____

Other physicians involved in the care, specialty and name:

Signature _____ Facility _____ Date _____

FIGURE 21-5. Example of a face sheet for the admission, annual, and change in condition comprehensive examination. The treatment status section is used to document discussions about intensity of care. *(Used with permission from Geriatric Associates of America, PA.)*

The quality indicators were chosen based on the evidence-based link between the care process and improved outcomes, the overall importance for improving care, the feasibility of measurement by medical record review or resident interview, and the ease of implementation in the average nursing facility. Practitioner assessment prevails over processes when medical conditions suggest the resident has advanced dementia or a poor prognosis with limited life expectancy. Electronic records set to trigger decision making, or simply carrying a notebook with the criteria, would facilitate guideline implementation.

ADDRESSING GERIATRIC SYNDROMES

Health Maintenance

Although preventive services are components of care and services, residents require to achieve and to maintain high level of physical, psychosocial, and functional well-being, screening for health maintenance in the nursing facility focuses on functional well-being. That

Geriatric Associates of America
Progress Note

Name_____   Facility_____

☐ Follow up visit ☐ New ☐ nursing ☐ family ☐ patient concern ☐ Readmission, no new MDS ☐ Change in physician ☐ Discharge Planning.

Reports from Nursing Staff _____

Progress in Rehabilitation Therapies _____

Reports from other Interdisciplinary Team Members _____

Consultant Reports _____

CC/HPI: Location, Quality, Severity, Duration, Timing, Context, Modifying factors, Associated signs and symptoms, OR interim history for 3or more chronic conditions. _____

_____

Meds reviewed : ☐ **Yes**_____

Diagnostic Tests reviewed: ☐ **Yes**_____

Review of Systems: Document specific abnormal and relevant negative findings

SKIN _____   GI/GU _____

HEENT _____   MSK _____

CV _____   NEURO _____

RESP _____   ☐ Unable to respond, unreliable historian

Exam: Describe specific abnormals.   ☒ **Check and/or describe relevant negatives**

System	Exam
Const	BP _____ / _____ P _____ R _____ T _____ Wt _____ % or lb loss_____
	☐ Awake, alert, appears stated age. Describe: Pain 0 1 2 3 4 5
HEENT	☐ PERRL, Sclera nonicteric, Conjunctiva pink ☐ TMs transluscent, ☐ Oropharynx moist, benign Describe
NECK	☐ No masses, ☐ Trachea midline, ☐ No thyromegaly. Describe
RESP	☐ No retractions, No use of accessory muscles. ☐ CTA bilaterally. Describe
CV	☐ RRR, ☐ No murmurs, No gallops, No rubs. ☐ No carotid, renal, femoral bruits. ☐ Pedal pulses = (B). ☐ No edema, no clubbing, no cyanosis, no lesions. Describe
BREAST	☐ No masses, no tenderness Describe:
ABD	☐ ABS x 4. Soft, non distended. ☐ No tenderness, no guarding, no rigidity. Describe
GU	☐ No masses, no erythema, no lesions. Decribe
LYMPH	☐ No adenopathy neck, axillae, groin Describe
MSK	☐ Steady gait. ☐ ROM intact, ☐ Good strength and tone, equal bilaterally. Describe
SKIN	☐ No lesions, rashes, ulcers. Describe
NEURO	☐ CN II-XII intact. ☐ DTRs intact. ☐ Cerebellar function intact. ☐ No cogwheeling. ☐ No tremor Describe
PSYCH	☐ Oriented to person, place, time. ☐ Mood and affect appropriate. Describe

Assessment

Presumptive diagnosis for new complaint or change in status

Stability of active conditions

Plan

Medications

Diet

Nursing Interventions; vital sign monitoring, skin care, etc.

Assessments by other disciplines

Consultants

Laboratory Tests

Discharge Planning

Signature _____   Date _____

FIGURE 21-6. Example of a progress note for the nursing facility. *(Used with permission from Geriatric Associates of America, PA.)*

is, screening for hearing and vision loss, depression, and insomnia may be more efficacious than screening for chronic disease or cancer. Components of prevention include vaccinations to prevent some infections, screening for chronic disease such as diabetes mellitus and thyroid disorders, medications to reduce complications of chronic illness, and counseling to make informed choices. For the physically frail or those with moderate dementia, bedside breast or prostate examinations and fecal occult blood testing maybe indicated after

TABLE 21-6

Key Nursing Facility Personnel

TITLE	ROLE	TRAINING
Certified Nursing Assistant	Provides most of the direct care for activities of daily living	At least 75 hours of training specific to caring for residents in a nursing facility
Charge Nurse	Supervises nursing assistants, carries out physician orders, contacts physician in a change in condition	Charge nurses are often LVN/LPNs and may be RNs
Director of Nursing	Coordinates and manages the nursing care	RN
MDS Nurse	Facilitates and/or completes the comprehensive assessment, the Minimum Data Set [MDS]	By regulation, an RN must coordinate completion of the MDS. Other licensed personnel may assist in completing the document
Medicare Coordinator	Screens new admissions and assists with discharges of residents admitted to the skilled nursing facility	RN or LVN/LPN
Inservice Coordinator	Orients new employees, helps existing employees maintain skills	RN or LVN/LPN. May have a dual role in the facility
Treatment Nurse	Administers topical medications, changes dressings, and may act as the pressure ulcer prevention coordinator	LVN/LPN, RN or RN with additional training in wound care such as a certified wound, ostomy, continence nurse
Restorative Nurses Aide	After physical and occupational therapy will continue restorative care to maintain function, e.g. ambulation	Certified nursing assistant, often one with at least one year experience. Reports to either nursing or physical therapy
Medication Aide	Administers oral and topical medications under the supervision of an RN	In some states, certified nursing aides with additional training in medication administration, may administer medications
Administrator	Financial manager	Bachelors Degree with post graduate certificate in Long-Term Care Administration
Admissions Coordinator	Coordinates admission documentation with families and residents. Frequently is the person families and residents ask to recommend an admitting physician	High school education or higher
Medical Records Coordinator	Organizes the medical record, thins charts, maintains lists of due dates for key functions e.g., care plan updates, MDS assessments, physician visits	High school education or degree in medical records coordination
Social Services	Provides medically related social services to attain or maintain the highest practicable physical, mental, and psychosocial well-being of each resident.	A facility over 120 beds must employ a full-time social worker with a bachelor's degree in social work or human services
Dietician	Identifies dietary needs, plans, and implements dietary programs	At a minimum a qualified dietician must be available as a consultant
Consultant Pharmacist	Reviews the drug regimen of each resident, must report any irregularities to the attending physician, and the director of nursing, and these reports must be acted upon	Bachelors degree or higher in pharmacy
Medical Director	Responsible for implementation of resident care policies and coordination of medical care in the facility	Licensed physician, may be certified as a medical director
Ombudsman	Citizen advocate for the residents and family	Part of the Older Americans Act, lay persons (often volunteers) are trained to solve problems in the facility

considering the consequences of a positive screening test. More invasive testing, including mammography, colonoscopy, and pelvic examinations, should be evaluated on an individual basis. Given the heterogeneous population in nursing facilities, guidelines for cancer screening and health maintenance need to take into account the residents physical and functional frailty, cognitive impairment, life expectancy, and known wishes.

Certain health maintenance activities have general acceptance and regulatory oversight. Screening for tuberculosis, annual dental and vision examinations, and medical care reviews are federally mandated whereas annual history and physical examinations, while widely accepted, are not. In accordance with F-Tag 334, nurs-

ing facilities offer residents various vaccines, and these include the trivalent-23 pneumococcal vaccine, an annual influenza vaccine, the varicella vaccine for the prevention of herpes zoster, and the tetanus booster every 10 years or the primary tetanus series.

General health maintenance activities occur on a regular basis. Residents are to be screened for cognitive deficits, depression, and gait and balance disturbances at least initially and as needed. In addition, reviewing residents' medications and assessing blood pressure, functional status, and evidence of pain, abuse and neglect are to be performed at each required visit, regardless of the resident's life expectancy and comorbidities. Recording the resident's weight should occur on required visits except for those residents with limited

TABLE 21-7

Pocket Tool Kit for Nursing Facility Visits
Stethescope
Pocket Oto-ophthalmascope
Cerumen spoon
Reflex hammer
Monofilament, 10 gram
Personal digital assistant
Drug reference
Medical calculations
Prescription pad
Bandage scissor
Mirror [to view heel ulcers]
Pen

TABLE 21-8

Organizing Your Clinical Work in the Nursing Facility
Obtain an update on the residents from the charge nurse
Ask the charge nurse to review the 24-hour reports since your last visit
Check any written communications for non-urgent events (Figure 21-4)
Review diagnostic tests, pharmacy recommendations and dietary requests
Locate blood glucose testing, weights, vital signs, etc.
Using your census sheet make note of pertinent information
Ask facility staff to take residents to their rooms where they will be seen
Talk to the resident and perform the appropriate exam
Document the history and physical exam at the bedside (Figure 21-5 and Figure 21-6)
When visits are complete retreat to a quiet place to review records, complete the progress note, confer with other members of the care team, write orders, and call families.
Sign consolidated orders
Complete discharge summaries
Respond to pharmacy alerts and recommendations
Respond to dietary requests
Sign telephone orders
Review orders with the charge nurse before leaving the unit

life expectancy. As a preventive measure for residents with a life expectancy of more than 2 years, screening for osteoporosis is recommended at least once. Usually, discussions on advance directives occur on admission and are updated as needed. Facility-based restorative nursing programs are effective to maintain resident participation in daily routine activities and to reduce the prevalence of decline in ADLs. In addition, physically frail residents find physical activity incorporating progressive resistance exercises to prevent muscle weakness helpful.

Little evidence exists to guide periodic laboratory monitoring. On admission, obtaining a complete blood count and albumin on admission is reasonable. Recommended disease-specific periodic laboratory testing is shown in Table 21-10. Estimating the creatinine clearance is helpful in choosing the correct dose for medications. Macrocytic anemia (vitamin B-12 and folate deficiency) and subclinical hypothyroidism are common conditions that are easily treated in nursing facility residents and warrant screening on admission and at least every 2 years.

Behavioral Symptoms

Dementia is the leading cause of institutionalization among older adults, and the prevalence among nursing facility residents is estimated at 50% or more. Although depression is the primary behavioral symptom in the early stages of dementia, it is usually not the primary cause for a nursing facility admission. Families and caregivers seek assistance more frequently in the moderate to later stages

when behavioral symptoms, including agitation, dysphoria, anxiety, apathy, and irritability, are most prevalent. Most aggressive or agitation behaviors are associated with providing assistance with ADLs and include grabbing, biting, kicking, scratching, or pulling hair. Other problematic behaviors are yelling, screaming, wandering, and insomnia. Less reported but still prevalent behaviors include verbal insults, racial slurs, sexual innuendoes, or inappropriate touching.

In terms of personal safety, nursing assistants are at greater risk of assault from aggressive residents than are LVN/LPNs and RNs as the nursing assistants perform most of the nursing duties. While the rate of assaults is declining, the nursing facility rate of 40 assaults per 10 000 workers exceeds that of any other industry. As aggressive behavior occurs frequently when nursing assistants administer intimate care, it maybe that the resident misinterprets personal care as an assault or invasion of privacy. Other factors associated with behavioral symptoms include a premorbid personality with aggressive behavior, delusional thinking, and neurological disorders.

Primary approaches to managing behavioral symptoms include nonpharmacological interventions or administering psychoactive

TABLE 21-9

Examples of Quality Indicators for the Management of Nursing Facility Residents		
TOPIC	**INDICATOR**	**COMMENTS**
Care planning (quality of life)	IF an older adult is admitted to a nursing facility THEN the documentation should demonstrate, or the resident/surrogate should report a discussion to establish goals of care. IF neither the resident nor family participates in planning goals of care THEN the reason should be clearly documented.	Feasible in the average community nursing facility
Calcium or vitamin D for osteoporosis (medical condition)	IF a resident has osteoporosis, THEN calcium or vitamin D supplements should be prescribed within one month of admission or new diagnosis of osteoporosis	Exclude if advanced dementia or poor prognosis
Malnutrition (Geriatric syndrome)	IF the nutritional status Resident Assessment Protocol has been triggered, THEN the presence or absence of malnutrition should be documented by the primary care provider.	

Data from Saliba D, Schnelle, JF. Indicators of the quality of nursing home residential care. J Am Geriatr Soc. 2002;50(8):1421–1430.

TABLE 21-10

Diagnostic Testing and Monitoring

PRACTICE	RECOMMENDED FREQUENCY	COMMENTS
Hemoglobin and hematocrit	Weekly if taking erythropoetin agent Monthly with iron replacement until Hb stabilizes, then every 3–6 months	Modified Diet in Renal Disease (MDRD) equation is recommended to screen for chronic kidney disease. Establish and document target hemoglobin
Ferritin	Baseline prior to starting erythropoetin agent or to differentiate iron deficiency anemia	Erythropoetin more effective with appropriate iron stores, ferritin >100. Ferritin < 20 associated with iron deficiency
PT/INR	Weekly until stable on warfarin, then monthly	Document duration of expected therapy
Electrolytes, renal function	Potassium prior to and after initiating ACE inhibitors, vancomycin or aminoglycosides Every 2–3 months if on diuretics.	Low salt diets may worsen hyponatremia. SSRIs are associated with SIADH in older adults
Estimated creatinine clearance	On admission or prior to medications dosing with known alterations based on function.	Many antibiotics Histamine-2 blockers Use Cockroft-Gault for medication dosing
ALT, AST	Baseline and every 6–12 months if taking > 4 g daily of acetaminophen or on statins or fibrates	Recommended frequency in F Tag 329
Albumin or pre-albumin	On admission to screen for under nutrition and periodically for change in condition or weight loss	Order pre-albumin to evaluate current protein stores and to monitor effect of supplemental nutrition
Thyroid function; TSH, T3, T4	After admission and medically stable, when symptomatic, and every 6–12 months if on therapy	TSH may be falsely elevated in acute illness
Vitamin B-12, folate	On admission if indicated and every 2 yrs	Defer if terminally ill.
Blood glucose Finger stick Hemoglobin A1c	QID if making dosage changes in anti-diabetic therapy. Thrice weekly morning and afternoon if stable Hemoglobin A1c every 3–4 months	Hb A1c < 8 may be associated with decreased morbidity and mortality with infections

ACE, angiotenin converting enzyme; SSRI, selective serotonin reuptake inhibitor; SIADH, syndrome of inappropriate antidurective hormone secretion; PT, prothombin time; INR, international normalized ratio.

medications and cholinesterase inhibitors. Examples of nonpharmacological interventions are using an unmet need approach, manipulating the resident's environment, and providing caregiver training. The unmet need approach assumes that all behavior has meaning, the aggressive behavior serves a purpose, and the behavior serves as some reward or consequence for the resident. Unmet need interventions investigate the antecedent, behavior, and consequence to assess the motivation behind the behavior and to design an approach specifically tailored for the resident.

For many residents, meaningful social engagement in the environment has a positive effect on loneliness, helplessness, and boredom. The challenge for the facility is manipulating the environment to find a balance between excessive stimulation and social isolation. One approach is to have residents with similar behaviors, symptoms, or degree of dementia residing on the same hall or unit. Residents in early stages of dementia who remain verbal and interact with their peers with a minimum of disturbing behaviors enjoy living where they can participate in social interaction.

Separating physically and verbally aggressive ambulatory residents from the physically frail provides a safer environment for residents who maybe passive targets of assaults. Security procedures for ambulatory residents prevent unsafe elopement while allowing maximal activity inside and outside the facility. Wandering behaviors that are problematic on a fully open unit are normalized and encouraged in a secure unit.

Residents with end-stage dementia have more labor-intensive needs for eating assistance, skin care, and mobility. To offset this, facilities often use staff from another unit during times of higher needs. For instance, staff from a unit where residents are more independent maybe available to assist with feeding residents who cannot feed themselves. Another environmental manipulation that is gaining in popularity is permanent assignments for all nursing facility staff. Behavioral symptoms maybe more easily managed and even diminish when the nursing assistants are assigned to the same residents everyday.

Caregivers may precipitate undesirable behaviors. For example, residents are more likely to react aggressively during bathing if caregivers speak negatively, are hurried, are disrespectful of privacy, or fail to give prompts or ask permission before spraying water. Bathing often becomes a battle to get residents clean regardless of their reluctance. Since the 1990s, the National Institutes of Health (NIH) has continuously funded two research teams to develop interventions to improve bathing. Using person-centered methods, ratings of over 500 videotaped baths found a 56% reduction in aggressive behaviors against caregivers, a 62% reduction in care recipient agitation, a 67% reduction in care recipient distress, and a 38% decrease in the proportion of bath time spent crying or screaming. Although not as extensively studied, it makes intuitive sense that similar person-centered approaches would be effective for other caregiving activities such as dressing and toileting.

Using pharmacological interventions to control behavioral symptoms is a common practice. Nearly 64% of nursing facility residents are given psychoactive medications including anxiolytics (17.1%), antidepressants (45.6%), antipsychotics (26.7%), or hypnotics (5.8%). Results are mixed on the efficacy of pharmacological interventions for controlling behavioral symptoms of dementia that include hallucinations, delusions, agitation, aggression, combativeness, and wandering. F-Tag 322 states that residents have the right to be free from chemical restraints imposed for purposes of discipline or convenience when such medication is not required to treat the resident's medical symptoms. Pharmacotherapy for behavioral symptoms should be limited to specific medical conditions including hallucinations, delusions, and other psychotic behaviors. Further in relation to pharmacotherapy, F-Tag 329 states that residents will not be given unnecessary drugs. Antipsychotic medications should be restricted for the treatment of specific medical conditions clearly documented in the resident's medical record. Planned behavioral interventions are expected when psychoactive medications are prescribed. Evaluation of the effectiveness of the interventions including medications and gradual dosage reductions is performed periodically. At least quarterly, reviewing the target symptoms, effect of the medication on the symptoms, changes in functional status, and medication-related adverse reactions will assist the facility in regulatory compliance. Gradual dose reductions should be attempted in two separate quarters of the first year unless clinically contraindicated. After the first year, a gradual dose reduction should be attempted annually unless clinically contraindicated.

Compared to giving a placebo, residents appear to gain little benefit from typical antipsychotic agents given to control chronic agitation or aggressive symptoms or for anticonvulsants used as mood stabilizers. Olanzapine and risperidone, as atypical antipsychotic agents, have been included in more trials and show modest benefit at the cost of a slight increased risk for stroke and all cause mortality. Because antidepressant agents are effective in reducing symptoms of depression, their use in nursing facilities is increasing.

Cholinesterase inhibitors, approved since 1996, are recommended for mild to severe Alzheimer dementia. The three most commonly prescribed agents are donepezil, rivastigmine, and galantamine. Memantine, a noncompetitive N-methyl-D-aspartate receptor antagonist, is the newest agent and was approved in 2003. As a class, these agents appear to improve or stabilize cognition, global functioning, activities in daily living, and moderate behavioral symptoms associated with Alzheimer dementia. In residents with moderate to severe dementia, donepezil and memantine as monotherapy are associated with improved cognition and stabilized function. Donepezil also improves and stabilizes behavioral symptoms. Adding memantine to donepezil as residents reach moderate to severe stages may improve cognition, ADL, and behavioral symptoms. The effects of these agents in clinical trials are modest in relation to placebo. None restore full cognition or functioning and regardless of the length of treatment or dose, the underlying neurological disorder will progress.

Although clinical guidelines on initiating pharmacotherapy for dementia exist, little information suggests when to terminate treatment. Treatment objectives in early stages of dementia include improving independence in ADLs and delaying admission to the nursing facility. However, these objectives need to change as dementia advances (Table 21-11). Some question the ethics of prescribing an expensive medication for a progressive, degenerative neurological disorder in an older adult not likely to live in the community again. Whether or not the use of these agents reduces hospitalizations or prevents pressure ulcers, unintended weight loss, infections, or other complications is not known.

Clinicians are divided on whether to continue therapy as long as the person is verbal and able to eat somewhat independently. For some, recognizing family members may be a sufficient criterion to continue therapy. For residents with moderate to severe Alzheimer dementia who tolerate donepezil, adding memantine maybe beneficial as long as treatment is compatible with previously stated wishes

TABLE 21-11

Treatment Objectives in Advanced Alzheimer's Dementia

OBJECTIVE	POTENTIAL MEANINGFUL OUTCOMES OF CHOLINESTERASE INHIBITORS
Stabilize cognition	Recognize family Continue to talk
Maintain function	Continue to eat independently
Stabilize behaviors	Facilitate bathing and continence care
Decrease caregiver stress	Reduce hitting, kicking, screaming and yelling.
Reduce utilization of healthcare resources	Reduce hospitalizations
Prevent complications of functional decline	Prevent pressure ulcers Prevent infections Maintain swallowing function

and known goals. A safe approach for treating behavioral symptoms with pharmacotherapeutic agents is to start with a cholinesterase inhibitor, add memantine and/or citalopram if behaviors escalate, and reserve the atypical antipsychotic agents as a last resort for documented psychotic behaviors.

Urinary Incontinence

Affecting slightly more than half of all nursing facility residents, urinary incontinence is an independent predictor for nursing facility admission and is associated with irritant dermatitis, pressure ulcers, falls, significant sleep interruptions, and urinary tract infections. Given that 82% of nursing facility residents require assistance or are dependent on caregivers for toileting assistance, it is not surprising that urinary incontinence is viewed as normal. The intent of F-Tag 315 is to ensure that incontinence is recognized, appropriately assessed, and managed so that the resident can achieve as normal a level of continence as practical. Physicians, geriatric advanced practice nurses, or certified continence nurses are valuable assets to the physical assessment team in identifying the cause and determining the appropriateness of bladder rehabilitation, toileting assistance, or check and change routines.

Residents who are only intermittently incontinent may benefit the most from an evaluation and management plan. For most residents with daytime continence as a goal, performing a focused physical examination that includes a rectal and genitourinary examination is reasonable. A cough test for stress incontinence, postvoid residual determination, urinalysis, and urine culture maybe helpful in guiding treatment in selected residents. Medical justification is required for indwelling catheters, including urinary retention or comfort in dying. As a cognitive screen, residents with advanced dementia who do not respond to their name or cannot state their name are unlikely to benefit from either a toileting program or bladder rehabilitation. Other incontinent residents should be given a 3- to 5-day trial of a systematic daytime toileting program such as prompted voiding. Bladder training is best reserved for ambulatory residents who are occasionally incontinent, are aware of the need to urinate, are able to learn and retain new information and are motivated to stay dry. Bladder training generally consists of teaching different techniques, including pelvic floor muscle exercises and scheduled voiding with systematic delay of voiding. Residents are taught distraction techniques to reduce urgency and delay toileting so that they can reach a goal to void continently every 2 to 4 hours during the day.

Toileting assistance programs may be resident-centered or caregiver-driven. Cognitively impaired residents who retain the ability to state their name or point to common objects respond favorably to prompted voiding. This resident-centered approach teaches the resident to recognize bladder fullness or the urge to void, to ask for assistance, and to accept or decline assistance when offered. Scheduled toileting depends on caregivers to toilet residents on a schedule that closely matches the resident's daily voiding pattern. Some residents may achieve daytime dryness without needing to wear incontinent briefs during the day. Residents who require two or more persons for assistance and are unable to respond to or consistently resist toileting assistance will need a schedule by which they are periodically checked for wet or soiled briefs and changed as necessary in order to maintain comfort and dignity.

Polypharmacy and Medication Errors

Medication-related adverse events are common in the nursing facility population. Factors that increase the risk of adverse consequences include complex medication regimens, the large number and types of medication used, physiological changes accompanying the aging process, and the resident's multiple comorbidities. Inappropriate prescribing and inadequate monitoring are the most common errors in medication management. The AMDA and the American Society of Consulting Pharmacists have identified the top 10 particularly dangerous drug interactions in nursing facilities, and this list is shown in Table 21-12.

The federal regulation F-Tag 428 states that the drug regimen of each resident is to be reviewed monthly by a licensed pharmacist. The pharmacist must report any irregularities to the attending physician and the director of nursing, who are to respond appropriately. The intent is to prevent or minimize adverse consequences that may impede residents reaching their highest level of functioning. According to F-Tag 329, each resident's drug regimen must be free from unnecessary drugs, which includes any drugs used in excessive dose (including duplicate therapy), for excessive duration, without adequate monitoring, without adequate indications for its use, or in the presence of adverse consequences. Following a few simple recommendations may reduce inappropriate prescribing and simplify the drug regimens (Table 21-13).

Common medication errors originating at the nursing facility include transcription errors, problems in drug administration, delay in obtaining medications, inadequate symptom management, and using as needed (prn) medications inappropriately. Asking the nurse to read orders before the physician leaves the building or to repeat a telephone order reduces transcription errors. Although most nursing facilities do not have pharmacies on site, facilities have policies and procedures to notify the attending physician or other practitioners if they encounter difficulties in obtaining medications promptly and may have an emergency medication supply. Practitioners can inquire about available antibiotics if urgent administration is required.

Following a few common procedures simplifies the drug regimen, encourages timely notification of a change in condition, and avoids adverse effects. Pain is more easily managed if analgesics are ordered around the clock. For convenience, many practitioners order a list of as-needed medications, where these include laxatives, mild analgesics, antipyretics, antitussives, topical antifungals, and antiemetics. Use of these medications, especially antipyretics in the absence of a documented infection, may result in a delay in notification of a significant change in condition and are best avoided. Limiting as needed medications to one mild analgesic for pain only and one laxative minimizes the problem. Regular laboratory assessment of drug levels, renal function, liver function, and blood counts is appropriate to monitor therapeutic responses and adverse effects of medications (see Table 21-10).

Falls

Falls are a cause of significant morbidity and liability in the nursing facility. Age-related changes, disease-specific pathology, and environmental factors contribute to falls. Falls maybe an atypical presentation of an acute change in condition, as a result of poor judgment, related to an adverse medication event or physical deconditioning. Osteoporosis, anticoagulation, and slowed reaction time contribute to the risk of serious injury, including bone fractures and subdural hematomas. Although totally eliminating falls is unrealistic, practitioners can significantly minimize falls and reduce the risk of serious injury.

Adopting a consistent approach to the management of falls across the spectrum of aging from the physically frail, the person with

TABLE 21-12

Top 10 Dangerous Drug Interactions in Nursing Facilities		
MEDICATION 1	**MEDICATION 2**	**ADVERSE EVENT**
Warfarin	NSAIDs such as ibuprofen, naproxen, COX-2 inhibitors	Potential for serious gastrointestinal bleeding
Warfarin	Sulfonamides such as trimethoprim/sulfamethoxazole	Increased effects of warfarin, with potential for bleeding
Warfarin	Macrolides such as clarithromycin, erythromycin	Increased effects of warfarin, with potential for bleeding
Warfarin	Fluoroquinolones such as ciprofloxacin, levofloxacin, ofloxacin	Increased effects of warfarin, with potential for bleeding
Warfarin	Phenytoin	Increased effects of warfarin and/or phenytoin
ACE inhibitors such as benazepril, captopril, enalapril, and lisinopril	Potassium supplements	Elevated serum potassium levels
ACE inhibitors such as benazepril, captopril, enalapril, and lisinopril	Spironolactone	Elevated serum potassium levels
Digoxin	Amiodarone	Digoxin toxicity
Digoxin	Verapamil	Digoxin toxicity
Theophylline	Fluoroquinolones such as ciprofloxacin, levofloxacin, ofloxacin	Theophylline toxicity

Data from the American Medical Directors Association; www.amda.com.

TABLE 21-13

Strategies to Avoid Medication Related Problems

POTENTIAL PROBLEM	RECOMMENDATION
Delay in obtaining medications	The nursing facility will have an "emergency drug box" If urgent administration of antibiotics is necessary, ask what is available at the facility
Inadequate symptom management	Prescribe pain medications around the clock
Delayed notification of change in condition	Limit prn medications to one over-the-counter laxative and acetaminophen for pain only Order acetaminophen for fever only during active illness and only for 2–3 days.
Inadequate monitoring for psychoactive medications	Utilize standardized tools to periodically evaluate depression, mental status, behavioral symptoms, e.g., Geriatric Depression Scale
Simplify the drug regimen	Utilize extended release medications Work toward once or twice a day dosing for all medications
Inadequate monitoring of medical conditions	Order weekly monitoring of blood pressure [antihypertensives], pulse [beta-blockers, digoxin], weight [megestrol acetate], monthly PT/INR [warfarin]
Duplicate medications	Specify the diagnosis for each medication. This may need to be written as a physicians order, e.g., "add diagnosis of seizure (resident is on phenytoin)" When original order is written put diagnosis after the drug, e.g., "warfarin for deep vein thrombosis"
Medications commonly over prescribed	Histamine—2 blockers, proton pump inhibitors: treat peptic ulcer disease or document gastroespophageal reflux disease Vitamin C and zinc: no good evidence for use in pressure ulcers Ferrous sulfate: rarely necessary more than once a day Multiple laxatives: choose one and order on a regular basis, stool softeners are generally ineffective

Data from the American Medical Directors Association; www.amda.com.

dementia, and to the individual who is dying, is reasonable. The AMDA suggests a structured interdisciplinary approach to falls including recognition, assessment, intervention, and assessment. A comprehensive approach to fall management ("The Fall Management Program") is available at www.medqic.org (under "Nursing Homes, Restraints, Tools").

A prior history of a fall is the single most potent predictor of future falls; fear of falling also imposes substantial risk. For newly admitted residents, interviewing the resident, family, or other caregivers is important in identifying these risk factors. Conditions that increase the risk for falls include chronic medical problems (such as cardiovascular disorders and degenerative joint disease), medications, impaired functional status, vision, dementia, and depression. Some conditions place residents at higher risk for severe injury in the event of any fall. These include anticoagulants that may cause excessive blood loss at a lower impact. Frequent fallers have a higher rate of significant injury as opposed to those who fall infrequently. Fractures of the hip, spine, and wrist are more common in persons who lack sufficient subcutaneous fat and muscle bulk to absorb the impact of a fall. Residents with visual impairment also are a higher risk for injurious falls. Most facilities contact the practitioner immediately after any fall, injurious or not. While the merits of immediate notification continue to be debated, residents who fall need a prompt nursing assessment for injury and then reassessment for at least 72 hours for any delayed appearance of injury. The AMDA recommends an additional interdisciplinary assessment to define the scope, frequency, causes, and complications of falls. Recurrent falls often have an identifiable cause. Falling maybe the presenting sign for a urinary tract infection, hypovolemia from dehydration, or postural hypotension following a medication adjustment. It is reasonable to rule out temporary conditions before assuming that a chronic condition such as dementia or Parkinson's disease is the cause.

Resident autonomy and safety are important aspects of fall management. Residents and families may accept some risk to maximize autonomy and promote dignity. Until recently, physical restraints were used to limit mobility. The intent of F-Tag 222, as shown in Table 21-14, is to promote the highest practicable well-being for each resident and to specifically prohibit physical restraints for discipline

---

TABLE 21-14

Physical Restraints

The resident has the right to be free from any physical or chemical restraints imposed for purposes of discipline or convenience, and not required to treat the resident's medical symptoms.

The intent of this requirement:
- assist the resident to attain and maintain highest level of function
- prohibit using restraints for discipline or convenience
- limit restraint use to medically indicated circumstances

A physical restraint is a device the resident cannot remove easily and restricts freedom of movement including leg restraints, arm restraints, hand mitts, soft ties or vests, lap cushions, and lap trays. Also:
- side rails that keep a resident from voluntarily getting out of bed
- sheets, fabric, or clothing used to restrict movement
- chairs with trays, tables, bars or belts, that the resident cannot remove easily
- placing a resident in a chair that prevents a resident from rising

Alternatives to Physical Restraints
- Restorative care to enhance strength for mobility
- Meaningful engagement in activities and interests
- Place the bed lower to the floor
- Soft floor mats next to the bed
- Monitoring devices to alert staff
- Frequent staff monitoring, hourly room rounds
- Consistent, frequent, assistance with toileting
- Call bells or visual reminders to ask for assistance, if appropriate

CMS. State Operations Manual: Appendix PP. 2006. http//cms.hhs.gov/manuals/ Downloads/som107ap_pp_guidelines_ltcf.pdf. Accessed March 12, 2007.

TABLE 21-15

Interventions to Prevent Falls in the Nursing Facility

INTERVENTION	STRATEGY
Exercise	Screen with "Get Up and Go Test"
	Physical therapy
	Restorative nursing programs
	Walk to dine, walk to commode, walk to the outside, etc.
	Emphasize mobility during daily care
	Group exercise activities
Sensory impairment	Screen for visual acuity and contrast sensitivity
	Wear corrective lenses
	Appropriate referral to ophthamology
Medication	Inform caregivers of dosage adjustments in medications, especially psychoactive medications, antihypertensives, diuretics, and antiepileptics
	Reduce the total number of medications
Footwear	Rubber sole, high collar, sturdy upper, and good fit
	Make shoes available within 24 hours of admission
Cognitive impairment technology	Redirection and diffusion for aggressive behaviors.
	Rigid hip protectors, if ambulatory
	Alarm systems
	Walkers and canes
	Scoop mattresses
	Split side rails, half rails, or no bed rails
	Raised toilet seat.
	Low beds with padded floor mats
	Close fit between bed mattress and any bed rail

Data from Bonner AF. Falling into place: a practical approach to interdisciplinary education on falls prevention in long-term care. Annals Long-Term Care 2006;14(6):21–29. Also see "The Fall Management Program"; www.medqic.org, (under Nursing Homes, Restraints, Tools).

TABLE 21-16

Nutrition

The facility must ensure that each resident
- Maintains acceptable parameters of nutritional status, such as body weight and protein levels, unless the resident's clinical condition demonstrates that this is not possible and
- Receives the appropriate diet when there is a nutritional problem

The intent of this regulation is to assure that the resident maintains acceptable parameters of nutritional status, taking into account the resident's clinical condition or other appropriate intervention, when there is a nutritional problem.

Managing Unintended Weight Loss
Obtain weight on admission and weekly for 4 weeks
Admission assessment
- Albumin
- Cholesterol
- Complete blood count
- Ideal body weight and body mass index
- Establish goals of care; cure, restoration, maintenance, or comfort.

Assess early when weight loss is identified

Interval	Significant Loss	Severe Loss
1 month	5%	Greater than 5%
3 months	7.5%	Greater than 7.5%
6 months	10%	Greater than 10%

Identify common or potentially reversible causes when weight loss occurs
- Adverse drug effects
- Complete blood count
- Comprehensive metabolic panel
- Thyroid stimulating hormones
- Fecal occult blood testing

CMS. State Operations Manual: Appendix PP. 2006. http://cms.hhs.gov/manuals/Downloads/som107ap_pp_guidelines_ltcf.pdf. Accessed March 12, 2007.

or convenience and limit restraint use to circumstances in which the resident has medical symptoms that warrant restraint use.

Physical restraints are associated with accelerated physical decline, depression, and anxiety, contribute to hip and knee contractures, and may contribute to falls and injuries rather than reduce them. Families may unrealistically ask that falls be prevented. Educating families about the steps to assess and reduce risk may be helpful. Examples of specific interventions are noted in Table 21-15. Monitoring the resident's response to the interventions allows practitioners to determine if the interventions are effective.

Altered Nutritional Status

Citizen advocacy groups, the community, and health care providers often equate weight loss to the quality of care in a nursing facility. While over half of nursing facility residents either gain or lose weight over 2 years, weight loss is most closely related to inadequate intake or altered utilization of nutrients. Nursing facilities are bound by federal regulation to maximize nutritional status for residents (Table 21-16). As weight changes that occur quickly may have significant negative consequences, federal guidelines mandate an assessment when a resident loses 5% or more of body weight in 30 days. Some facilities adopt a stricter parameter, intervening when a resident loses more than two pounds in 1 month. A significant unintended weight loss accompanied by protein–calorie malnutrition

often precedes worsening health status. Protein–calorie malnutrition increases susceptibility to infections and pressure ulcer risk, delays wound healing, and increases mortality from comorbidities. With the exception of weight gain due to fluid retention from heart failure, chronic kidney disease or liver failure, the outcomes for weight gain are usually favorable and do not require intervention.

As with other clinical practice guidelines, the AMDA recommends a systematic approach to the evaluation and management of altered nutritional status in nursing facility residents including recognition, an assessment based on appropriate goals, treatment, and ongoing monitoring. The registered dietician calculates the resident's ideal body weight and body mass index. Obtaining weekly weights for 4 weeks and ordering basic laboratory testing identifies most newly admitted residents at highest risk for under nutrition. Eating preferences and functional abilities are generally components of the admission interdisciplinary nutrition evaluation. If appropriate, a skilled clinician may perform a bedside eating evaluation (Table 21-17) to differentiate a swallowing disorder from other medical conditions. If a swallowing problem is identified, discussions with the resident or family lets practitioners determine if further testing falls within the goals of care.

Other conditions may precipitate nutritional problems, increase nutritional requirements, or mask potential nutritional problems.

TABLE 21-17

Bedside Eating Evaluation

Assess:
- oral cavity for ulcers, dental caries, poorly fitting dentures
- gag reflex, tongue movement
- ability to handle saliva
- ability to eat independently

Administer in order:
- thickened liquids; nectars, milkshakes
- pureed foods; pudding, yogurt, ice cream
- soft foods requiring chewing; cake, rice, bread
- firm texture foods; sliced meats, fruits
- clear liquids

Observe for:
- coughing before, during, or after swallowing
- multiple swallows with each portion
- frequent throat clearing
- hoarse or wet voice after swallowing
- drooling
- pocketing
- protruding tongue movements

Data from Taler G, Rapp MP, Brandt N, et al. Altered Nutritional Status: Clinical Practice Guideline. Columbia, MD: American Medical Directors Association; 2001.

TABLE 21-18

Medical Interventions for Altered Nutrition

- Identify under-nutrition at the time of admission
- Treat depression aggressively
- Reassess all medications
- Order regular diets
- Consult with dietician to increase the nutrient density of foods
- Order 2 kcal per cc liquid supplements with medication passes
- Consider a daily vitamin supplement

Managing artificial nutrition with tube feeding
- Tube feeding is consistent with resident advance directives
- Establish clear goals
- Discuss the probable lack of benefit for end stage dementia
- Withdraw tube feeding when goals are no longer met
- Consult with dieticians for calorie and fluid needs
- Order feedings for 16–20 hours a day to encourage out of bed activities

Data from Taler G, Rapp MP, Brandt N, et al. Altered Nutritional Status: Clinical Practice Guideline. Columbia, MD: American Medical Directors Association; 2001.

Nutritional requirements are increased in residents with pressure ulcers, healing surgical wounds, and infections. The consulting pharmacist can identify medications that alter taste, decrease appetite, precipitate dysphagia, or cause gastrointestinal complaints. Residents with agitation behavioral symptoms or movement disorders may need extra calories to maintain their weight. Infections may present with anorexia, malaise, or weight loss and should be ruled out.

A gradual, persistent weight loss is a more sensitive trigger for nutritional problems than the RAP and MDS. A common practice is to evaluate the resident's weight during each required visit and compare the current weight to that of the previous 3 to 4 months. It is helpful to establish notification parameters that identify residents who demonstrate an abrupt change in food and/or fluid intake as this frequently signals an acute condition or medication effect.

Treatment for weight loss is guided by the resident's goals and plan of care. Interventions may involve several disciplines, especially nursing, dietary, and medicine. As few residents return to earlier adult weights or regain weight lost during an acute event, stabilization at a lower weight may be appropriate. Facility interventions addressing the eating environment, tailoring meals for resident personal and cultural preferences, and providing adequate eating assistance are critical. Medical interventions listed in Table 21-18 are low cost and often effective.

Disease-specific diets for hyperlipidemia, heart failure, and diabetes mellitus are not as palatable as unrestricted diets and probably do not control symptoms in nursing facility residents. However, restricting protein in late-stage chronic kidney disease may delay the need for dialysis. A more effective dietary intervention is to increase the food's nutrient density by adding milk powder, butter, or oil. Offering liquid dietary supplements at time of medication increases the likelihood that these supplements will be consumed.

It is reasonable to address artificial nutrition and hydration early in the admission evaluation, at least annually and if a significant change in condition occurs. Family members may have unrealistic expectations regarding artificial nutrition and hydration, especially in dementia. Artificial nutrition and hydration has a limited effect on the natural course of dementia and further diminishes the resident's interaction in the facility environment. For persons in a persistent vegetative state, tube feeding extends life without an effect on functional status. Aspiration is a common problem with progressive dementia, and artificial nutrition does not reduce aspiration risk. Ongoing discussions with the family are necessary until the acute need for aggressive intervention is resolved, or the prognosis and goals are clearly understood. These conversations should be documented in the medical record.

Pressure Ulcers

Pressure ulcers are caused by external pressure usually due to in-bed immobility and out-of-bed inactivity. The intensity and duration of pressure interrupts blood flow over a bony prominence and causes tissue damage. Other risk factors include poor nutrition, impaired cognition, urinary and fecal incontinence, and friction and shear. Short-stay residents admitted for skilled nursing services are at the highest risk of developing a pressure ulcer, and this pressure ulcer usually develops within 3 weeks of admission. An acute change in the medical condition of a long-stay resident, such as an acute infection, is associated with an increased risk.

Topical treatment for pressure ulcers is based on the characteristics of the pressure ulcer, the treatment goals, cost, efficiency for nursing, and patient comfort. Limiting topical treatments to a facility-based formulary reduces variability and error in application. If allowed per facility policy and the state nursing practice, standing orders or protocols for Stage 1 and/or Stage 2 pressure ulcers facilitate prompt intervention (Figure 21-7). The "Tool Kit for Implementation of Clinical Practice Guidelines" from the AMDA is a valuable resource in developing a comprehensive pressure ulcer prevention and treatment program.

Palliative Care

Palliative care has become increasingly important in the nursing facility where currently 30% of persons admitted die within the first year, a number that is expected to increase as the population ages. Despite this reality, F-Tag 309 specifically states that each resident

PRESSURE ULCER TREATMENT PROTOCOL

The intent of this protocol is to provide registered nurses [RN] and licensed vocational nurses [LVN] with a procedure to follow to initiate treatment of a stage 1 or stage 2 pressure ulcer. The nursing staff may not deviate from this protocol without prior consultation with the physician or nurse practitioner.

Check the appropriate boxes in each section. When complete, place the form in the physician order section of the chart.

Assessment:
☐ Stage 1: Change in temperature, tissue consistency, and/or sensation in a defined area of persistent redness in lightly pigmented skin, or persistent red, blue, or purple hues in darker skin over an area prone to pressure ulcers
☐ Stage 2: Shallow, clean wound base with light to moderate exudates, color red to yellow
☐ Location _____
☐ Describe any pain associated with the pressure ulcer.

Treatment Orders:
☐ Cleanse with normal saline
☐ Apply a hydrocolloid dressing and change every 7 days and prn
☐ Observe and document daily that the dressing is intact and in place.

If there is pain:
☐ Acetaminophen 325 mg two tablets po or per tube twice a day until the ulcer heals
☐ Notify the physician or nurse practitioner if there is pain associated with the pressure ulcer is present and there are no treatment orders for pain

FIGURE 21-7. Pressure ulcer treatment protocol. Geriatric Associates of America (GAA) Order Set. *(Clinical Practice Guideline: Pressure Ulcer Therapy Companion. American Medical Director's Association 1999. Clinical Practice Guideline # 15: Treatment of Pressure Ulcers. Agency for Health Care Policy and Research 1994. Used with permission from Geriatric Associates of America, PA.)*

must receive care and services to attain or maintain the highest practicable physical, mental, and psychosocial well-being. The intent is to ensure residents receive optimal health care and do not deteriorate within the limits of a recognized pathology and the normal aging process. No F-Tag specifically addresses the quality of care in dying or dealing with symptoms such as pain or the emotional distress that may accompany the dying process. Although efforts have been made to use MDS items to predict death, there is neither a RAP for assessing a dying person nor is there currently a RAP for chronic pain.

The trajectory of dying occurs over months to years and can be characterized by exacerbations of chronic illnesses or a gradual global decline in health and function. Most often, an acute episode of illness such as a myocardial infarction, cerebral vascular accident, or pneumonia precedes death. In the absence of advance directives to the contrary, this acute event often precipitates a transfer to the hospital. Staff at nursing facilities are often more capable of caring for dying residents with as much if not more dignity and comfort than staff at hospitals. To help assure a resident's death according to their wishes, practitioners should discuss preferences (Figure 21-8). Improving palliative care in the nursing facility includes educating caregivers and families, managing the resident's pain, increased utilization of hospice services or palliative care plans, close attention to advance care planning, and better communication between the resident and family, staff, and physician.

MANAGING THE ACUTE CHANGE OF CONDITION

Nursing facility residents are at high risk for acute illness and hospitalization. Hospitalization is both costly and disruptive and exposes residents to risks of fragmented transitional care and iatrogenic complications, including delirium, malnutrition, pressure ulcers, and adverse drug reactions. Residents most frequently hospitalized are those with preexisting pulmonary and/or cardiovascular disease, diabetes mellitus, swallowing dysfunction, and genitourinary tract disorders. The most common admitting diagnoses are pulmonary conditions, urinary tract and skin infections, heart failure, and dehydration/malnutrition syndromes. The primary issues contributing to preventable hospitalization include lack of early recognition of change in condition, absence of an appropriate assessment by the nursing staff, a delay in notification of the change in condition to the medical provider, and lack of appropriate monitoring and follow-up by both nursing and medical provider when a change is recognized.

Determining the underlying cause of a change in condition enables the staff to assess the situation appropriately. The staff must know residents who are at highest risk of hospitalization, be aware that when the residents become ill, symptoms may differ from those in younger persons, and be able to evaluate whether or not the resident can be cared for at the facility. Atypical presenting signs and symptoms compromise early detection of an acute change in condition. As residents with cognitive or communication deficits do not often report physical complaints, common presenting signs, which includes sleepiness, lethargy, and fatigue, are frequently not recognized until the resident is moribund. Direct care staff may not have a mechanism to report observations or fail to appreciate the significance of early, subtle changes in condition. Personnel from other departments, such as dietary or housekeeping, who do recognize a change may assume they are not qualified to make such an observation and fail to report it. Practitioners responding to multiple nonurgent or notification-only calls often fail to respond appropriately to the urgency of the condition.

The F-Tag 157 states that a facility must immediately consult with the resident's physician in the event of an accident with injury, deterioration in health, a need to discontinue a treatment due to adverse consequences or start a new treatment, and request transfer or discharge resident to another level of care. The regulations allow for consultation prospectively for minor frequently occurring events, such as skin tears or noninjurious falls. Protocols, such as the example for skin tears (see Figure 21-3) developed in consultation with the nursing facility team and used to manage commonly occurring events, may reduce the burden of communication.

Due to their knowledge of residents ADL habits, nursing assistants are often the first to observe a change in condition. Nurse assistants utilizing an instrument (Figure 21-9) or procedure to facilitate reporting permits LVN/LPNs and RNs to assess, monitor, and convey the appropriate information to the practitioner. Once a change is reported, the LVN/LPN or RN verifies the report to determine the change's nature, severity, and possible cause. At a minimum, the LVN/LPN or RN personally obtains the vital signs, performs a pain assessment, verifies food and fluid intake, evaluates the level of consciousness and weakness, and reviews fall history. The LVN/LPN or RN can ask the nursing assistant about changes in elimination, behavioral symptoms, and the ability to perform ADLs. The next step is to determine the resident's stability and, based on the urgency of the symptoms, call the practitioner.

Palliative Care Form

The information on this form assists in documenting the reasons for palliative, or comfort care. The resident will continue to receive nursing, dietary, social, and medical services that will provide comfort.

Diagnoses to support the Palliative Care Plan

_____

_____

_____

The physician, nurse practitioner, or physician's assistant has identified conditions or procedures that may be unavoidable for the resident. The nursing facility staff will talk to you about the procedures that may be used to decrease the occurrence of these conditions.

☐ Weight loss
☐ Skin breakdown and/or pressure sores [bedsores]
☐ Dehydration
☐ Severe constipation
☐ Gradual or rapid loss of the ability to move about independently
☐ The resident may not be able to get out of bed
☐ An indwelling bladder catheter may be necessary for comfort
☐ Medications to control symptoms may be necessary including but not limited to narcotics for pain or breathing symptoms, anti-anxiety medications, and sleeping medications.

The nursing facility wants to understand what heroic measures you would like to avoid. At your request the nursing facility will follow your instructions for the procedures listed.

Specifically

☐ **DO NOT** Hospitalize unless symptoms cannot be controlled in the facility
☐ **DO NOT** Attempt cardiopulmonary resuscitation
☐ **DO NOT** Administer medications to cure a condition [antibiotics]
☐ **DO NOT** Use artificial nutrition [tube in the nose or stomach]
☐ **DO NOT** Use artificial hydration with fluids in the veins [intravenous or IV]
☐ **DO NOT** Use artificial hydration with fluids under the skin [hypodermoclysis]

Date

Date

Family Signature

Physician/Nurse Practitioner/Physician Assistant Signature

Comments by the Resident and/or Family [in the Resident/Family handwriting]

FIGURE 21-8. Palliative care form. This may be used to document advanced directive decisions. *(Used with permission from Texas Department of Aging and Disability Services.)*

Adopting a standardized mechanism for reporting information promotes accurate and timely communication. The SBAR (situation–background–assessment–recommendation) is one such process to enhance communication between practitioners and facility nurses (Figure 21-10). Editing the format for the facility to initiate the call serves as a reminder to the nurses to collect the appropriate assessment information. The mnemonic is easy to remember, familiar to both nurses and practitioners, and encourages communication of critical information.

Regardless of the severity of the change noted in the initial report, it is critical for the nurse to follow-up and monitor the resident for a period of time. Three days is usually sufficient to assess trends and changes in vital signs, including pulse oximetry, the level of alertness, and appetite and fluid intake. During this time, the practitioner may make a visit to further assess the situation and intervene appropriately.

Medical conditions that usually warrant hospitalization include acute abdominal pain with vomiting, chest pain not due to stomach pain or musculoskeletal pain, a fall with pain and signs of fracture, hypertension with systolic BP over 230 mm Hg, signs of stroke, vomiting blood, low blood pressure, tachycardia, or respiratory distress with rate over 28 and not relieved with oxygen, nebulizers, or suctioning. In the absence of these conditions, the practitioner ascertains whether or not the facility has adequate support for the resident to remain in the facility (Figure 21-11).

Acute Care/Nursing Facility Interface

Transitions between the hospital and the nursing facility are commonplace for residents with serious acute illnesses and exacerbation of chronic conditions. Relocation may lead to detrimental effects on residents, including delirium, adverse drug events, and undesirable

Early Warning Illness Report

Please answer these questions about your resident. If you answer **NO** to any of the following questions, please **tell the charge nurse as soon as possible**, no later than the end of your shift.

☐ Seems like herself/himself?
☐ Ate the same amount of food?
☐ Talked to you in usual way?
☐ Looked at you in usual way?
☐ Participated in usual leisure activity?
☐ ADL activity the same

Please check for the following...

☐ Nervous or Agitated
☐ Weak
☐ Drowsy or Tired
☐ Confused
☐ Need help with dressing, toileting, transfers

If any of these conditions seem **WORSE** than other days, or if she/he or anyone else tells you she/he had a health problem today **report it to the charge nurse as soon as possible!**

FIGURE 21-9. Early warning illness report. *(Adapted and used with permission from Boockvar K, Brodie HD, Lachs M. Nursing assistants detect behavior changes in nursing home residents that precede acute illness: development and validation of an illness warning instrument. J Am Geriatr Soc. 2000;48(9):1086–1091.)*

S

Situation

You are calling about [resident name] _____ at [facility] _____

Your name is _____

The residents code status is _____

The resident may be hospitalized   YES   NO

The problem you are calling about is _____

The vital signs are

BP _____/_____, Pulse _____, Respiration _____, Temperature _____

if appropriate

Pulse oximetry _____ %   ON oxygen, NOT on oxygen

How long has the resident used oxygen? _____

B

Background

How is the resident now?

   Like usual

   Sleepier

   More agitated or combative

   More confused

   In pain that is new or worse

   Stuporous, not responding

Have any new medications been ordered in the past week? _____

What medications does the resident take regularly? _____

A

Assessment

What do you think the problem is?

Does the problem seem to be cardiac, infection, respiratory, behavior, neurologic?

Is the resident getting worse?

How sick do you think the resident is? 0 1 2 3 4 5 [five is sickest]

Do you think something needs to be done right now?

R

Recommendation

I need to order XRAY, CBC, BMP, UA, C&S, PT/INR

I will order this medication _____

Is this resident taking warfarin [Coumadin]? YES   NO

Please continue to monitor the following _____/day for _____days

   Vital signs

   Pulse oximetry

   Intake and/or output

   Pain

Call back if _____

Is there anything else you think I need to order? _____

This patient needs to go to the hospital

Send to _____ hospital

Admit to Dr. _____

If this resident is on hospice and needs to go the hospital, please call the hospice nurse before sending the resident.

My name is _____

FIGURE 21-10. Receiving notification of change in condition. (Data from Permanente, K. SBAR Technique for Communication: A Situational Briefing Model. December, 2004. http://www.ihi.org/IHI/Topics/PatientSafety/SafetyGeneral/Tools/SBARTechniqueforCommunicationASituationalBriefingModel.htm. Accessed January 6, 2007.)

- Reporting mechanisms to ensure that changes in condition are reported appropriately
- Ability to start treatment, e.g., antibiotics, pain medication in a few hours
- Ability to start intravenous or hypodermoclysis therapy for hydration within 2 hours of the order
- Sufficient RN coverage to over see appropriate monitoring over 24 hours
- Sufficient RN staffing to ensure daily RN assessment until the acute change has resolved or stabilized
- Sufficient RN staffing to recognize and report possible complications of treatment within 24 hours of their identification

FIGURE 21-11. Criteria for managing an acute change in condition in the facility. (Data from Levenson S, Rapp MP, Barnett AM, et al. (2003). Acute Change in Condition in the Long Term Care Setting. Baltimore, MD: American Medical Directors Association; 2003.)

interventions. Effective communication and efficient transfer of information will ease the transition of nursing facility residents to and from the emergency department and hospital. The point of transfer for nursing facility residents to hospitals is usually the emergency department, where residents are admitted for evaluation of a change in condition frequently complicated by delirium, dehydration, and frailty.

Each setting presents a unique set of challenges for critical information exchange. Urban hospitals often depend on multiple medical disciplines to manage one admitted patient, and teaching hospitals regularly rotate medical residents and students each month. In the nursing facility, changes in administration, ownership, nursing leadership, and staff nursing further complicate communication between the hospital and the facility. Emergency departments (Figure 21-12) and nursing facilities (Figure 21-13) have different information

RESIDENT TRANSFER FORM

Name of Nursing Home: _____

Address: _____

Print only and answer each question (Please do not leave any blanks). Shaded areas may be completed prior to the date of the emergency and updated as needed.

Resident's Last Name:	First Name:	MI:	Sex: ☐ M ☐ F	Date of Birth: ___/___/___

Name of the unit/floor resident transferring from:	Phone number of that unit/floor:	Fax number of unit:

Attending Physician:	DNR orders: ☐ Yes ☐ No	Advance Directive sent: ☐ Yes ☐ No

Name Resident's Next of Kin/Health care power of attorney:	Phone number:	Next of kin notified: ☐ Yes ☐ No	Religion:

(Check if present)

Functional Status:

Disabilities:	Incontinence:	Impairments:	Mental Status ___ A ___ O	Independent	Assistance	Dependent
☐ Amputation	☐ Bladder	☐ Speech	Feeding	☐	☐	☐
☐ Paralysis	☐ Bowel	☐ Hearing	Bathing/Dressing	☐	☐	☐
☐ Contracture	☐ Saliva	☐ Vision	Transfer	☐	☐	☐
☐ Pressure Ulcer			Ambulation	☐	☐	☐

Behavior Issues:

Copy of the MAR with current medications (with in the last 24 hrs) highlighted. ☐ Yes ☐ No *(If no, list current medications below)*	Allergies:

Chief complaint(s) that bring(s) the patient to the Emergency Room (If altered mental status is the chief complaint, please describe behavior prior to the change). Date of onset/duration ___/___/___ .	Diagnosis:	Past Medical History:

Lab or other Test ordered prior to transfer or within 24 hrs: ☐ Yes (Send copy of results) ☐ No	Diet/Therapies:

Resident uses:			Sent with resident	
☐ Glasses	☐ Bladder Catheter	☐ Crutches	☐ Glasses	☐ Crutches
☐ Hearing aid	☐ Tracheostomy	☐ Walker	☐ Hearing aid	☐ Walker
☐ Dentures	☐ Ostomy	☐ Dialysis Access (describe) _____	☐ Dentures	☐ Other
☐ Feeding tube	☐ Cane	☐ Other (explain) _____	☐ Cane	_____

Name of MD/NP/PA who made the decision to send patient Beeper number	Physician's orders attached: ☐ Yes ☐ No

| Vital signs at the time of transfer:

T:_____ ; P:_____ ; R:_____ ; B/P:_____	Transport via: ☐ Ambulance ☐ Other (explain) _____

Signature of the Transfer Nurse:	Print Name:	Date of transfer: ___/___/___	Time of transfer: ___/___/___

ER Dispatch FAX #: ___/___/___ **(Cover letter required)**   Last revision: 3/21/02

ER Dispatch Phone #: ___/___/___ **(Phone notification of NH transfer to the ER. Call to be brief and to the point.**

Give patient name, NH name, and exact reason for patient transfer to the ER & ETA. Do not give a full report.

DNR = Do not Resuscitate; MAR = Medication administration record; NP = nurse practitioner; PA = physician assistant; NH = nursing home; ER = emergency room; ETA = estimated time of arrival.

DNR = Do not Resuscitate; MAR = Medication administration record; NP = nurse practitioner; PA = physician assistant; NH = nursing home; ER = emergency room; ETA = estimated time of arrival.

FIGURE 21-12. Resident transfer form. *(Used with permission from Davis MN, Brumfield VC, Smith ST, Tyler S, Nitschman J. A one-page nursing home to emergency room transfer form: what a difference it can make during an emergency! Ann Long Term Care. 2005;13(11):34–38.)*

When discharging nursing facility [NF] patients	Facts about NFs
1. Use a standardized Discharge Progress Note Form. 2. Complete all items. 3. Describe the hospital course fully. For a surgical patient, include any medical complications and any ICU stay. 4. Print your name and your phone number on the form in case the NF and attending physician need clarification from you.	1. The NF is home to residents who become hospital patients. 2. Nursing facilities **do not** have a pharmacy. **The NF will have to specially order an intravenous pole**. Do not discharge patients on the last minute or late in the day on Friday afternoon. Nursing facility physicians are not in the facility daily. They must verify your admission orders and the nurses must be able to read your orders. **Please write legibly.**
Be clear with your orders 1. Wound care: Specific treatment, frequency, and write legibly. 2. **If MRSA***, state location. 3. **If VRE***, state if colonized or not 4. For follow-up appointments with specialty clinics, indicate the reason for follow up. 5. **Be specific with range of motion and weight bearing status**. It is not enough just to order physical and/or occupational therapy.	**Who are the NF caregivers?** 1. Charge nurses and treatment nurses are licensed vocational/practical nurses [LVN/LPN]. 2. Frontline caregivers are nursing assistants. 3. There may be 2–3 registered nurses [RNs] in the entire facility and one of them does full time administration work. The average RN time for each resident per day is 5–6 minutes. 4. Medications are often administered by medication aides who have been nursing assistants for 6 months or more.
Please DO NOT 1. **Document "no rehabilitaton potential"; this can change.** 2. **Order sitters [NFs cannot afford this].** 3. **Order expensive medications or change antibiotics after the patient has been accepted by the NF without prior notification.**	*MRSA = methicillin resistant staph aureus *VRE = vancomycin resistant enterococcus

FIGURE 21-13. Pocket reference for hospital providers (interns, residents, hospitalists, nurse practitioners, physician assistants). *(Used with permission from Davis MN, Smith ST, Tyler S. Improving transition and communication between acute care and long-term care: a system for better continuity of care. Ann. Long Term Care. 2005;13(5):25–32.)*

needs on point of transfer. Processes including standardized forms and checklists can improve the bidirectional communication.

Infections

Diagnosing infections in nursing facility residents is difficult because of the limited availability of diagnostic tests, the variable assessment skills of the facility nurses, and lack of practitioners on site 24/7. Clinical presentation of illness in nursing facility residents is often subtle or atypical. Guidelines and standards appropriate to acute care or community-based settings may not be appropriate to the nursing facility. Provided there are no advance directives to the contrary, nursing facility residents suspected of an infection should be diagnostically evaluated and treated as is appropriate.

The most common infections among nursing facility residents are urinary tract infections, respiratory infections, skin and soft tissue infections, and gastroenteritis. The usual clinical clues to infection may or not be present, e.g., change in the characteristics of urine, fever, cough, and yellow sputum. Noted more often is a change in mental or cognitive function, falling, or an inability to perform usual activities in daily living. An indicator of pneumonia is that the resident may have tachypnea (> 25 breaths per min). In the absence of laboratory diagnostics, the respiratory rate effectively differentiates respiratory infections from urinary tract and soft tissue infections. Because of high mortality within 24 hours of presentation, blood cultures should not be performed in suspected bacteremia. As long as transfer is compatible with the plan of care admit residents to the hospital who are likely to have bacteremia.

Recommended criteria for recognizing fever in the nursing facility resident are (1) an oral temperature of 100°F (37.8°C) measured once or (2) an oral temperature of 99°F (37.5°C) on repeated measures (or an increase of 2°F (1.1°C) above baseline). As most facilities obtain vital signs providing a baseline, including temperature, at least monthly, either method should suffice.

Clinical evaluation of residents includes measuring vital signs and performing an initial assessment at the facility. Using the SBAR (see Figure 21-10), the nursing staff should communicate information regarding the resident's status to the practitioner on the same shift the assessment is made. The evaluation and management plan is documented and, if applicable, the rationale for with holding any diagnostic or treatment measures noted. Before administering antibiotics, practitioners should consider assessment parameters, diagnostic tests, and minimum criterion outlined in Table 21-19.

ROLE OF THE MEDICAL DIRECTOR

To ensure compliance with Medicare and Medicaid regulations under F-Tag 501, nursing facilities appoint a physician to serve as

TABLE 21-19

Management of Common Infections

INFECTION	SIGNS AND SYMPTOMS	DIAGNOSTIC TESTING	MINIMUM CRITERIA FOR ANTIBIOTICS
Urinary tract	Specific: Fever, dysuria, urgency, frequency, nocturia, increased incontinence Nonspecific: new or increased confusion, anorexia, functional decline	Urinalysis and if positive for pyuria, urine culture Complete blood count with differential	1. No indwelling catheter: acute dysuria alone or with fever plus one of the following; new or worsening urgency, frequency, suprapubic pain, gross hematuria, costovertebral angle tenderness, or urinary incontinence 2. With and indwelling catheter: fever, new costovertebral tenderness, rigors, or new onset delirium
Pneumonia	Respiratory rate >25, pulse oximetry < 90, cough, fever, purulent sputum, positive auscultory findings, or pleuritic chest pain	Pulse oximetry Chest radiograph Complete blood count with differential	1. Temperature >102°F (38.9°C) plus one of the following: respiratory rate >25 or productive cough 2. Temperature >100°F (37.9°C) and cough plus one of the following, pulse >100, delirium, rigors, respiratory rate >25 3. Afebrile with chronic obstructive pulmonary disease (COPD): new or increased cough with purulent sputum production 4. Afebrile without COPD: new cough with purulent sputum production and one of the following: respiratory rate >25 or delirium
Skin	Erythema, tenderness, warmth, new or increased swelling, new or increased pain, failure of wound to heal	Complete blood count with differential For pressure ulcer cultures, deep tissue sample via biopsy	New or increasing purulent drainage at the site or at least two of the following: fever >100°F (37.9°C), redness, tenderness, warmth, new or increased swelling at the site (pressure ulcers, vascular wounds, percutaneous gastrostomy or jejunostomy sites, tracheostomy sites)
Gastrointestinal	More than one isolated diarrhea stool, fever, abdominal cramps	1. No workup if there is low-grade fever, new-onset diarrhea, no clinical change, and no outbreak in the facility 2. If on antibiotics in the past 30 days, obtain *C.difficile* toxin assay 3. If no antibiotics recently and fever, abdominal cramps, bloody diarrhea, or white blood cells, obtain stool culture for other enteropathogens	Presence of diarrhea with fever >100°F (37.9°C) and the onset of delirium or rigors

Data from Loeb M, Bentley DW, Bradley S, et al. Development of minimum criteria for the initiation of antibiotics in residents of long-term-care facilities: results of a consensus conference. Infect Control Hosp Epidemiol. 2001;22(2):120–124.

medical director. Most medical directors are independent contractors who devote 2 to 4 hours weekly of administrative time to a particular facility. Although the regulations concerning a medical director's function are brief, the potential impact is significant. Key components of the medical director's role include implementation of resident care policies and coordination of medical care in the facility. The unique needs and perspectives of each nursing facility dictate how the medical director's role is operationalized. The medical director functions in a similar manner to the chief of the hospital medical staff and as such, participates in the development of policies and procedures relevant to medical care delivery, coordinates a medical quality improvement program, and represents the facility to the community.

The nursing facility medical director works closely with all disciplines and is constantly cognizant of the interplay between laws, ethics, regulations, and the organization of medical care. Medical directors perform most effectively when they report directly to the facility administrator and work collaboratively with the Director of Nursing. It is helpful to also have a line of communication with governance above the level of the administrator. A working relationship between the medical director and the medical staff ensures that quality standards set forth by the facility are instituted. The medical director is expected to be knowledgeable of current standards of care and proactively provide leadership while promoting adherence to standards.

As one of three required members of the nursing facility's quality assurance committee, the medical director meets at least quarterly with the facility administrator, DON, and any other appointed members. This committee reviews quality of care issues, develops strategies to improve quality, and provides a structure within the facility to correct negative outcomes and proactively enhance quality of care and quality of life for residents.

Certification for medical directors is offered through the American Medical Director's Association following completion of a formal course. However, as most medical liability insurance policies do not cover the role of the medical director, a physician acting as medical director should seek an alternate source if the nursing facility is not able to provide liability coverage. Further information regarding medical director responsibilities, certification requirements, and relevant policies and procedures are available through the AMDA.

SUMMARY

In summary, federal and state regulations serve to remind and guide practitioners regarding appropriate processes and expected outcomes of care. The approach to evaluating and managing syndromes (such as incontinence, pressure ulcers, falls, and weight loss) necessitates adaptation to the environment and differentiating the goals of care, where these goals often include maintenance, or comfort and palliation in addition to cure and restoration. Becoming familiar with the environment, learning to work with the interdisciplinary team, and managing the day-to-day practice efficiently facilitates establishing a successful satisfying nursing facility practice.

Unanswered questions and research for the future include studying collaborative models of care with physicians and nurse practitioners, clinical nurse specialists, and physician assistants. In addition, randomized controlled trials for pharmacological and nonpharmacological interventions for chronic illness and behavioral symptoms are needed as well as the need to know when to initiate and stop medications. In the future, a fully integrated electronic medical record may facilitate evaluation of medical care decisions which directly bears on the quality of care and quality of life.

FURTHER READING

AMDA. White Paper on Determination and Documentation of Medical Necessity in Long Term Care Facilities. 2001. http://www.amda.com/library/whitepapers/mednecwhitepaper.htm. Accessed January 29, 2004.

AMDA. Role of the Attending Physician in the Nursing Home. 2003. http://www.amda.com/governance/resolutions/e03.cfm. Accessed March 14, 2007.

Ayalon L, Gum AM, Feliciano L, Arean PA. Effectiveness of nonpharmacological interventions for the management of neuropsychiatric symptoms in patients with dementia: a systematic review. *Arch Intern Med.* 2006;166(20):2182–2188.

Bentley DW, Bradley S, High K, Schoenbaum S, Taler G, Yoshikawa TT. Practice guideline for evaluation of fever and infection in long-term care facilities. *J Am Geriatr Soc.* 2001;49(2):210–222.

Bergstrom N, Allman RM, Alvarez OM, et al. Treatment of pressure ulcers. (Vol. Publication No. 95-0652). Rockville, MD: U.S. Department of Health and Human Services, Public Health Service; 1994.

Birks J. Cholinesterase inhibitors for Alzheimer's disease. *Cochrane Database Syst Rev.* 2006;(1):CD005593.

Bonner AF. Falling into place: a practical approach to interdisciplinary education on falls prevention in long-term care. *Ann Long-Term Care.* 2006;14(6):21–29.

CMS. Investigative protocol, Guidance to surveyors: long term care facilities (No. 274). Washington, DC: U.S. Department of Health and Human Services; Centers for Medicare and Medicaid Services; 2005.

CMS. Nursing Home Quality Initiatives. 2005. Accessed March 12, 2007, from http://www.cms.hhs.gov/NursingHomeQualityInits/

CMS. Nursing Home Compare. 2006. http://www.medicare.gov/NHCompare/. Accessed March 12, 2007.

CMS. State Operations Manual: Appendix PP. 2006. http://cms.hhs.gov/manuals/Downloads/som107ap_pp_guidelines_ltcf.pdf. Accessed March 12, 2007.

Davis MN, Brumfield VC, Smith ST, Tyler S, Nitschman J. A one-page nursing home to emergency room transfer form: what a difference it can make during an emergency! *Ann Long Term Care.* 2005;13(11):34–38.

Davis MN, Smith ST, Tyler S. Improving transition and communication between acute care and long-term care: a system for better continuity of care. *Ann Long Term Care.* 2005;13(5):25–32.

Decker FH. *Nursing Homes, 1977–99: What Has Changed, What Has Not?* Hyattsville, MD: National Center for Heatlh Statistics; 2005.

Fama T, Fox PD. Efforts to improve primary care delivery to nursing home residents. *J Am Geriatrics Soc.* 1997;45:627–632.

Farley DO, Zellman G, Ouslander J, Reuben DB. Use of primary care teams by HMOS for care on long-stay nursing home residents. *J Am Geriatrics Soc.* 1999;47(138–144):139–144.

Franco KN, Messinger-Rapport B. Pharmacological treatment of neuropsychiatric symptoms of dementia: A review of the evidence. *J Am Med Dir Assoc.* 2006;7(3):201–202. [Epub 2006, Feb 2007].

Levy C, Epstein A, Landry L, Kramer A, Harvel J, Liggins C. Literature Review and Synthesis of Physician Practices in Nursing Homes. Washington, DC: U.S. Department of Health and Human Services; 2005.

Loeb M, Bentley DW, Bradley S, et al. Development of minimum criteria for the initiation of antibiotics in residents of long-term-care facilities: Results of a consensus conference. *Infect Control Hosp Epidemiol.* 2001;22(2):120–124.

NCHS. National Nursing Home Survey. 1999. http://www.cdc.gov/nchs/nnhs.htm. Accessed March 12, 2007.

Ness J, Ahmed A, Aronow WS. Demographics and payment characteristics of nursing home residents in the United States: A 23-year trend. *J Gerontol A Biol Sci Med Sci.* 2004;59(11):1213–1217.

Ouslander J, Osterweil D, Morley J. *Medical Care in the Nursing Home.* 2nd ed. New York, New York: McGraw-Hill; 1996.

Rader J, Barrick AL, Hoeffer B, et al. The bathing of older adults with dementia. *Am J Nurs.* 2006;106(4):40–48, quiz 48–49.

Rapp MP. Opportunities for advance practice nurses in the nursing facility. *J Am Med Dir Assoc.* 2003;4(6):337–343.

Saliba D, Schnelle JF. Indicators of the quality of nursing home residential care. *J Am Geriatr Soc.* 2002;50(8):1421–1430.

Saliba D, Solomon D, Rubenstein L, et al. Feasibility of quality indicators for the management of geriatric syndromes in nursing home residents. *J Am Med Dir Assoc.* 2004;5(5):310–319.

Saliba D, Solomon D, Rubenstein L, et al. Feasibility of quality indicators for the management of geriatric syndromes in nursing home residents. *J Am Med Dir Assoc.* 2005;6(3 Suppl):S50–S59.

Schamp R, Levy S, Bade P, et al. Health Maintenance in the Long-Term Care Setting: Clinical Practice Guideline. Columbia, MD: American Medical Directors Association; 2007.

Schnelle JF, Ouslander JG. CMS guidelines and improving continence care in nursing homes: The role of the medical director. *J Am Med Dir Assoc.* 2006;7(2):131–132. [Epub 2005 Dec 2007].

Staats DO, Beier M, Cantrell L, et al. Falls and Fall Risk: Clinical Practice Guideline. Columbia, MD: AMDA; 1998.

Taler G, Rapp MP, Brandt N, et al. Altered Nutritional Status: Clinical Practice Guideline. Columbia, MD: American Medical Directors Association; 2001.

Community-Based Long-Term Care and Home Care

Jennifer Hayashi ■ *Bruce Leff*

In 2007, an estimated 7 million older Americans needed long-term care due to functional impairment, usually as a result of chronic medical conditions and illnesses. Most of these people choose to remain in the community, and require services to help them stay in their homes rather than enter an institution. These services constitute what is generally known as community-based long-term care (CBLTC). As the population ages and the number of functionally impaired older adults increases, so will the need for CBLTC. Unfortunately, no coherent national policy drives CBLTC in the United States, which leaves a "system" that is inconsistent, decentralized, difficult to access, bewildering to navigate, and unable to fully meet the needs of many patients. Much of what is actually done to meet these needs is provided by unpaid family caregivers at great personal and economic cost. This chapter addresses CBLTC for older adults in the United States. We outline the semantic challenges in understanding the scope and nature of CBLTC and the heterogeneity of care models that comprise CBLTC, describe who receives, provides, and pays for it, and review the evidence for its effectiveness. We also discuss important public policy issues and identify emerging innovations and trends in CBLTC delivery.

SEMANTIC CHALLENGES OF CBLTC

The term "community-based long-term care" overlaps with several other terms in the medical and social sciences literature, including *home care, personal care services, home and community-based services, home visits, and house calls.* In general, these terms refer to nursing, personal care, or social services provided to older persons, with an explicit goal of filling unmet needs or maintaining them in the community. Most of this kind of care is provided by unpaid family members or friends, sometimes with support from a variety of formal caregivers. Home care may mean home-based rehabilitation or disease management after hospital discharge, preventive health interventions, geriatric assessment, primary care physician visits, or highly

technological care provided in individual patient homes. These services often overlap to such an extent that important aspects of a given intervention are not accurately reflected in a single label. For example, a program in which an interdisciplinary team provides comprehensive geriatric assessment followed by primary care home visits, inpatient management as needed, and continuing longitudinal care after hospital discharge does not fit neatly into any one category. Several forms of CBLTC integrate housing arrangements with personal and medical care, further blurring the distinction between CBLTC and institutional long-term care. Table 22-1 depicts the heterogeneity and scope of services and settings that fall under the rubric of community-based long-term care.

Home health care usually comes in two forms: unskilled and skilled care. Unskilled care refers to services provided by unpaid caregivers, usually female family members. The estimated 26 million informal caregivers in the United States provide 45% to 70% of all home care and CBLTC services at an estimated economic value of $196 billion—far greater than national spending on formal home care ($32 billion) and nursing home care ($83 billion). Skilled home health care refers to formal services delivered by professional providers, such as nurses or physical, occupational, or speech therapists. Medicare certifies and reimburses home healthcare agencies (HHAs) to provide this type of care when a patient is homebound and has a skilled need (see "Who Provides and Pays for CBLTC" later in the chapter). HHAs may also provide formal personal care services (bathing, dressing, etc.) under the Medicare home health care benefit while a patient is receiving skilled care. Although hospitalization is not required by Medicare to initiate home health care, postacute hospital skilled needs and rehabilitation are common reasons physicians refer patients for these services. For example, an older patient who suffers an acute exacerbation of chronic obstructive pulmonary disease may spend several days in bed (at home or in the hospital), and may need nursing to monitor her respiratory status and physical therapy to help her regain her baseline functional mobility. It is important to note that the effectiveness of skilled home care often

TABLE 22-1

Types of Community-Based Long-Term Care and Home Care

TYPE OF CBLTC	DESCRIPTION/SERVICES	FUNDING
CBLTC services provided at home		
Home health care	Home health agency or client provides and pays	Medicare or private long-term care insurance
Formal (agency or consumer-directed)	personnel	
Skilled care	Nursing, occupational and physical therapy	Private pay (if no skilled need)
Personal care	ADL assistance	"Cash and counseling" (Medicaid)
Informal	ADL/IADL assistance as needed	None/opportunity cost of caregivers
Physician house calls	Medical visits in patient's home	Medicare, private insurance, private pay
Preventive home visits	Health maintenance visits by health care providers (physicians, nurses, social workers) or trained "health visitors"	National insurance (Europe/UK), research grants (US)
Home-based geriatric assessment	Multidisciplinary evaluation of medical, social, functional, and cognitive issues	Variable depending on evaluator and context
Hospital at Home	Acute-level care at home with daily nurse/physician visits	Variable depending on system implementing the model
Case management	Disease-specific teaching and support provided by nurses	Medicare (as part of skilled care) or private insurance
CBLTC services requiring temporary or permanent relocation		
Program of All-Inclusive Care for the Elderly (PACE)	Comprehensive medical, functional, and social care for dually eligible, nursing home–eligible patients	Medicare and Medicaid capitated payments
Adult day care	Supervised congregate activities, 1–7 d/wk for	Private pay, Medicaid
Medical	several hours a day	
Social	Includes medication administration and basic monitoring	
	Limited to social interaction	
Assisted living	Apartment-style living with unskilled and/or skilled services available on-site	Long-term care insurance, private pay
Sheltered housing	"Senior apartments" with varying social services on site (e.g., friendly visitors, congregate meals, transportation)	Private pay, subsidized by federal and local governments
Adult foster care	Older adult who needs assistance or supervision moves in with "foster" family	Private pay, subsidized by federal and local governments
Group home	Group of adults who need assistance or supervision lives in one building with unskilled and/or skilled services available on site (can be similar to assisted living)	Private pay, subsidized by federal and local governments
Continuing care retirement communities (CCRCs)	Geographically localized and self-contained spectrum of living arrangements from independent housing to nursing home care	Private pay
Life care at home	Spectrum of care from minimal assistance to nursing home–level care provided in patient's own home	Private pay

relies on services provided by an informal caregiver who, if available, can implement a home exercise program, clean and dress pressure ulcers, or bathe, dress, and toilet a dependent patient.

Two related models of formal home medical care include physician house calls and hospital-at-home. Physician house calls, in which physicians (and, increasingly, nurse practitioners and physician assistants) provide ongoing longitudinal medical care at home, can play an important role in providing access to routine and urgent care for older adults who have difficulty getting to a medical office. Physician house call programs have been increasing in prevalence in recent years, though they are not yet widespread. Hospital-at-home is an emerging care model that provides hospital-level care in a pa-

tient's home as a substitute for an acute hospital admission. Other forms of CBLTC involve intermittent assessment and monitoring over time. Preventive home visits and home-based geriatric assessment typically aim to identify older adults in the community who have hidden risks for developing illness or functional decline, and modify those risks to prevent poor outcomes. Disease management targets patients known to have specific diseases or conditions that require significant care coordination, such as diabetes or heart failure, for formal support in managing those conditions, with the goal of delaying disease progression and avoiding hospitalization.

Still other forms of CBLTC entail temporary or permanent changes in location of care. Adult day care generally includes

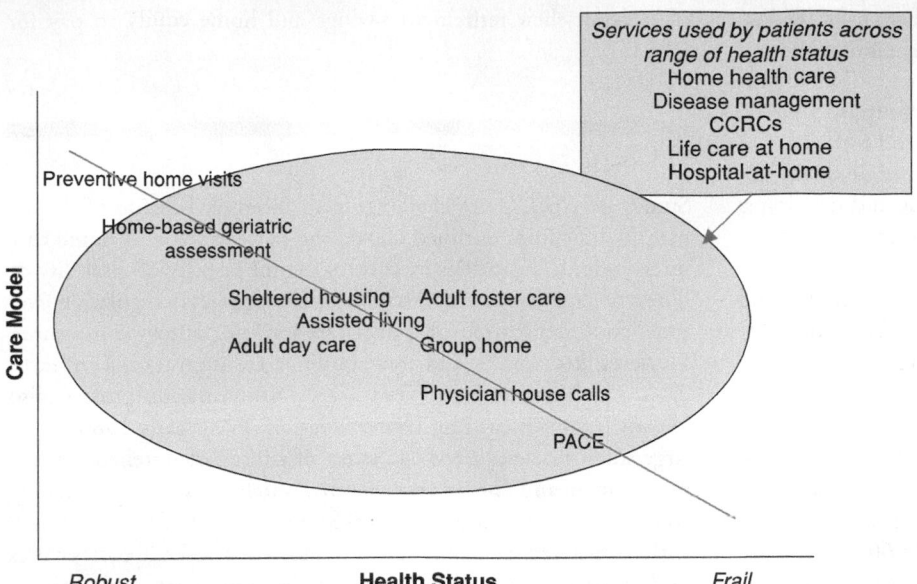

FIGURE 22-1. CBLTC continuum of care.

transportation to a day care center, and can provide both structured social activities and basic medical monitoring and treatment. The Program of All-Inclusive Care for the Elderly (PACE) relies heavily on a "day health center" in which dually eligible (i.e., Medicare and Medicaid eligible) nursing-home eligible participants receive comprehensive medical, hygienic, social, and rehabilitative care. For patients who cannot continue to live in their own homes, assisted living, sheltered housing (also known as senior apartments), adult foster care, and group homes all provide varying levels of functional assistance and access to some medical services. Continuing care retirement communities (CCRCs), as the name suggests, are self-contained organizations that allow people to move within the community to increasing levels of care as their needs dictate. At one end of the continuing care spectrum, a fully independent older adult lives in a single-family home or apartment, but over time may transition first to an assisted-living apartment, then to the skilled nursing facility within the same CCRC. There are several variations on this model, but most charge an entrance and monthly fee that provides lifelong care in the event that the participant develops some kind of functional impairment. Finally, some continuing care models, called life care at home, provide a similar range of care but do not require purchasers to move from their own homes.

This array of services and settings can be framed as a quasicontinuum of care services for older adults, as shown in Figure 22-1. While some forms of CBLTC are designed to address the needs of older adults through a variety of health or disease states, such as home health care, CCRCs or postacute disease management programs, others are targeted to specific populations based on levels of impairment or disability, such as preventive home visits or PACE. Again, many patients and programs do not fit neatly into a single category and patients do not usually move across the continuum in a straight line, as the use of services depends not only on the fit between the needs of an older adult and the care model, but also on the preferences of older adults and local availability of care models. For example, skilled home health care may be used by a healthy older adult after elective joint replacement surgery, or by a frail chronically ill patient recovering from a recent episode of community-acquired

pneumonia treated at home by a physician house call program. However, the concept of a continuum is a useful construct for organizing categories of CBLTC.

WHO RECEIVES CBLTC?

As Figure 22-1 demonstrates, CBLTC services may be used by older adults over a wide range of health status. Health maintenance strategies such as preventive home visits and geriatric assessment tend to target patients who are relatively robust and functionally independent, while PACE and physician house calls address the needs of patients who are more frail and impaired. CCRCs and life care at home explicitly transition patients from the robust state through functional decline. Postacute home health care, physician house calls, and hospital at home may be used by both robust and frail older adults in specific circumstances, but the primary intended users of most CBLTC remain those who have chronic and complex medical illness accompanied by some level of functional disability, and thus require care for a prolonged or even indefinite time. The likelihood of receiving formal care is lower for men, minorities, married individuals, those with lower socioeconomic status, and those who are less dependent for assistance with activities and instrumental activities of daily living.

WHO PROVIDES AND PAYS FOR CBLTC?

The role of unpaid informal caregivers cannot be overemphasized. The work they perform is not directly reimbursed or financially rewarded by the health care system. The indirect costs are enormous when lost wages, productivity, and future social insurance losses are calculated for caregivers who may sacrifice paid employment to provide informal care for a parent or other relative. For formal care, the provider varies with the type of CBLTC. In the most common model of home health care, a home health care agency (HHA) certified to provide care under Medicare reimbursement rules employs nurses, therapists, aides, and social workers, and assigns them to individual patient cases. A physician must certify that the patient is homebound and has a skilled need in order for a Medicare-certified HHA to provide care for a 60-day "certification period." By definition, a skilled need requires care that is part-time, intermittent, and must be provided by a person with special training (e.g., a nurse or therapist). Personal care assistance with ADLs such as bathing and dressing is covered during the certification period, but Medicare does not pay for it in the absence of a skilled need.

The HHA must catalog each patient's medical, functional, and socioeconomic characteristics in the Outcome and Assessment Information Set (OASIS), which then determines in the Prospective Payment System the Medicare reimbursement the agency will receive for the certification period. PPS was implemented in 2000 in response to a period of extraordinary growth in medical home health care expenditures in the 1990s, which was unfortunately accompanied by inefficient or even fraudulent fee-for-service (FFS) billing. A patient can be "recertified" for multiple 60-day periods as long as a skilled need exists. HHAs can also be privately paid by the care recipients. Additionally, an emerging "consumer-directed" or "cash and counseling" model allows selected patients to choose, train, and pay their personal care providers directly with designated state funds (usually from Medicaid programs), instead of using an agency as an intermediary. In these programs, care providers can be family members or other previously unpaid caregivers. This model has had positive results, showing increased patient empowerment and satisfaction, and fewer unmet needs.

Interdisciplinary teams are critical in coordinating and delivering care in home health care, home-based geriatric assessment, PACE, and home hospital (see Chapter 26). Such teams typically include physicians, although the physician role may vary in different settings depending on the medical complexity of the patient and the setting. For example, in PACE, the physician provides primary care services, manages acute illness during hospitalization, and coordinates the activities of the interdisciplinary team. In postacute and home rehabilitation care, the interdisciplinary team drives most of the management with a focus on restoring function and following up medical issues, with the physician acting largely in an administrative role. In hospital-at-home interventions, the physician actively manages acute illness at home, so that physician house calls complemented by close coordination of the interdisciplinary team are crucial in this setting. Improvements in Medicare reimbursement for physician house calls have contributed to a recent growth in academic and private sector house call programs.

Other forms of CBLTC rely less on physicians and more on specialized nurses or trained lay visitors. Disease management, postacute home health care, and medical day care are often based on protocols driven by nurses. Home-based geriatric assessment is usually performed by geriatric nurses or nurse practitioners and then discussed as needed with physicians, while preventive home visits have been successful in using "health visitors," or specially trained community residents, in screening for health risks. Medical care in ALFs, sheltered housing, and group homes is generally limited to medication administration and vital signs monitoring and may include relatively easy access to physicians when needed, such as domiciliary care visits or a clinic housed within a senior apartment building. A small number of older adults carry privately funded long-term care insurance, and in recent years, some businesses have added this option to their employee benefit packages. Ultimately, many people exhaust their retirement savings and home equity to pay for CBLTC.

IS CBLTC EFFECTIVE?

Studies of CBLTC are challenging to interpret because of the semantic difficulties outlined above, the heterogeneity of home care interventions, difficulties in controlling for severity of disability or illness of patients, patient attrition issues, changes in regulation over time, and examination of a disparate range of outcome measures. However, key studies and their findings are summarized in Table 22-2. The National Long Term Care Demonstration project (also known as the Channeling Demonstration) in the early 1980s was a large study that evaluated the effect of adding comprehensive case management and a broad array of other purchased services to existing community care networks. It served an extremely frail population with unmet service needs, but did not show overall cost savings or decrease hospitalization, nursing home placement, or functional decline. However, it did improve in-home care, unmet needs, and quality of life of patients and caregivers. This landmark study set a pessimistic tone for home care research: that home care may be preferred by patients and caregivers, but difficult to justify in terms of clinical and economic effectiveness. Similarly, the Social Health Maintenance Organization demonstration projects (S/HMO I and II) that expanded case management services within Medicare managed care organizations (MCOs) failed to demonstrate any patient care or cost advantages over usual managed-care practices, and in 2003 reverted back to standard Medicare MCOs.

On the other hand, two recent outcomes-based quality improvement (OBQI) Medicare demonstration programs collected, encoded, and transmitted patient-level health status information to provide a risk-adjusted outcome report, which was then used to implement action plans to change Medicare-certified home health care agency behaviors. Each demonstration agency focused on reducing rehospitalization rates and one other targeted outcome (e.g., functional status or medication self-management) based on its performance report. With over 260 000 patients in 73 home care agencies in 28 states, the OBQI intervention achieved a more than 20% reduction in hospitalization and a 5% to 7% improvement in other targeted outcomes. In addition, the comprehensive management strategies of PACE programs appear effective at reducing institutionalization of at-risk patients, and postacute hospital disease management programs for conditions such as congestive heart failure, deep venous thrombosis, and diabetes mellitus improve patient outcomes such as hospital readmissions and self-management skills. Finally, hospital-at-home experiments, especially those that substitute entirely for an acute hospital admission, have reduced total days in care and geriatric clinical complications such as confusion and incontinence, with health outcomes and health-related quality-of-life measures comparable to usual care.

The evidence on the effects of other CBLTC interventions is less consistent and may result from issues related to model design and targeting of models to the appropriate patient population. A recent meta-regression analysis on the effects of home visits to prevent adverse outcomes found a 24% risk reduction in mortality for "young-old" (younger than 80 years) rather than "old-old" (older than 80 years) populations, while multidimensional assessment was associated with better functional outcomes compared with single-clinician

TABLE 22-2

Evidence for Effectiveness of CBLTC

AUTHOR, YR	STUDY	SETTING	TARGETED POPULATION	MAJOR FINDINGS
Kemper, 1986	National Channeling Demonstration	United States	Frail older adults at risk of nursing home placement	Improved patient/caregiver quality of life, in-home care, and unmet needs No decrease in costs, hospitalization, nursing home placement, or functional decline
Thompson, 2002	SHMO I and II	U.S. Medicare HMOs	Frail older adults	No improvement in quality of care, institutionalization, or hospital utilization compared with usual capitated care
Shaughnessy, 2002	OBQI	Medicare-certified home health agencies	Homebound older adults with skilled needs	Reduced hospitalization and improved other targeted outcomes
Eng, 1997	PACE	Eleven PACE sites in 9 US states across United States	Dually eligible, nursing home–eligible frail older adults	Decreased hospital length of stay Fewer nursing home days Less outpatient subspecialist utilization Decreased polypharmacy No increase in mortality Cost savings of 5%–15% relative to nursing home
Abt Associates, 2001	PACE	Eleven PACE sites in 8 U.S. states	Dually eligible, nursing home–eligible frail older adults	Increased life expectancy Decreased use of NH/hospital Improved (self-rated) health status Improved satisfaction with care and with life in general Decreased Medicare costs Increased Medicaid costs
Naylor, 1999	Post-hospital disease management	Two urban U.S. academic hospitals	Older adults hospitalized for 1 of 8 medical or surgical diagnoses	Decreased readmission rate Lengthened time between discharge and readmission Decreased Medicare costs
Caplan, 1999	Hospital at home	Australia	Acutely ill older adults randomized to hospital admission or hospital-at-home services	Significantly reduced incidence of geriatric complications (confusion, falls, urinary and bowel problems)
Weissert, 1988	Home care	Systematic review	N/A	Targeting was uneven and best accomplished when accompanied by a mandatory nursing home preadmission-screening program Cost savings on institutional care did not offset costs of intervention Hospital use increased in some studies
Stuck, 2002	Preventive home visits	Meta-analysis	N/A	Functional decline reduced in trials using multidimensional assessment with follow-up and in trials with control group mortality in lowest tertile Nursing home placement reduced in trials with >9 home visits during follow-up Mortality reduced in younger (<77.5 yr) but not older populations (>80 yr)
Hughes, 2000	Team-managed home-based primary care	Veterans' Administration	Elderly veterans with CHF, COPD, terminal illness, or impairments in 2 or more ADLs	Increased patient and caregiver satisfaction but also increased overall costs
Hedrick, 1993	Adult day care	Veterans' Administration	Elderly veterans with dependency in one or more ADLs	Increased costs and use of home care without improving health outcomes or caregiver satisfaction

assessment (relative risk 0.76), and risk of nursing home placement decreased by 34% as the number of follow-up visits increased from <4 to >9. Similarly, some physician house call programs have been shown to reduce hospital or emergency department utilization, and a large Veterans Administration study demonstrated significant improvements in patient health-related quality of life and caregiver satisfaction for patients receiving team-managed home-based primary care. In an important VA study of adult day care, there was no difference in health outcomes between patients who attended adult day care in the VA or in the community and those who did not attend day care, except in a subgroup of intervention patients with severe disabilities who had lower nursing home, clinic, home care, pharmacy, and laboratory costs, while the rest of the intervention group had generally higher costs. As Table 22-2 indicates, an extensive home care literature includes a wide variety of interventions and target populations. While this heterogeneity creates significant difficulty in drawing conclusions about the effectiveness and cost-effectiveness of home care, the overall body of evidence suggests that specific models when appropriately targeted are probably effective.

This issue of targeting care to appropriate patient populations is a major determinant of the cost-effectiveness of specific interventions. A related factor that complicates discussions of cost-effectiveness is the notion of paid care inappropriately substituting for informal care at a cost to society, or the "moral hazard" or "woodwork" effect. In theory, if CBLTC services are made widely available, functionally impaired patients will "come out of the woodwork" to utilize them, even though most of these patients will never enter an institution even without using CBLTC. Thus, the cost of providing care will overwhelm the potential savings of avoiding institutionalization. As one expert notes, "if you spend too much it's hard to save money." Targeting services to patients who are at high risk for institutionalization is generally accepted as an important way to optimize cost-effectiveness, but no practical, precise, and accurate targeting tools have been developed and tested. A recent systematic review and analysis of predictors of nursing home placement, hospitalization, functional impairment, and mortality identified 22 risk factors that consistently predicted two or more of these outcomes, including three factors that predicted all four outcomes: worse non-ADL physical function, illness severity, and previous hospital use. These factors have not been validated prospectively. Cost-effectiveness also depends upon the economic features of the health systems in which various forms of CBLTC have been studied; findings from European programs in which the government is the payer for CBLTC, institutional LTC, and acute care are difficult to apply to the U.S. fee-for-service environment with multiple public and private payers and complex cost-shifting pressures.

INNOVATIONS

Recent technological and social advances have the potential to improve access to care, quality of care, and coordination of care for medically complex community-dwelling older adults. Telemedicine is a small but growing field with particular relevance to rural or home-bound populations with chronic diseases that cannot otherwise access specialized care; dermatology, ophthalmology, and wound care have been widely studied in small clinical trials and appear to allow accurate diagnosis and management through both real-time inter-

actions and "store-and-forward" applications in which clinical data including video images are collected and stored for later review by a clinician. Other specialties relying heavily on verbal interactions, such as psychiatry and neurology, appear to effectively diagnose and treat patients via interactive video conferencing. Similarly, home-based telemedicine interventions in chronic diseases probably enhance communication between patients and providers and facilitate closer monitoring of overall health when conducted in settings with specialized equipment and dedicated staff. Although the evidence is limited by methodologic variability, lack of comparison with in-person evaluation, and absence of clinical outcome measures, a recent systematic review by the Agency for Healthcare Research and Quality (AHRQ) concluded that in some situations, the use of telemedicine might be warranted even if the evidence is inconclusive, including "remote rural areas or other locations where medical care is not available locally and the patient is for whatever reason unable to travel to a setting where it can be obtained." Additional small or methodologically weak trials are unlikely to significantly add to the evidence base for telemedicine, and larger, well-designed comprehensive trials that include clinically meaningful outcome measures are needed in light of the increasing advocacy for health care payers to cover its use.

Like telemedicine, point-of-care diagnostic and therapeutic technology including electrocardiography, ultrasound, blood analysis, and intravenous treatment holds promise for health care delivery in home care and house calls. Wireless telephone and Internet applications that allow secure, high-speed broadband connections between portable electronic medical records (EMR) systems and acute care or office information systems can provide safe and seamless continuity of care with immediate data access and entry for providers caring for complex older patients with multiple medical issues, medications, sites of care, and consultants.

A third important innovation in caring for community-dwelling functionally impaired older adults is not based on technology, but on social, medical, and financial support. Medicaid waiver programs, authorized in section 1915(c) of the Social Security Act, allow states to shift funds for extensive home-based services for older or disabled people. Since much nursing home care is paid for by state-administered Medicaid programs, Medicaid has a major stake in financing CBLTC that can substitute for nursing home care without increasing costs, unmet needs, or adverse outcomes. Hence, 1915(c) waiver programs lower the income and asset thresholds for Medicaid, and provide a combination of traditional medical services (i.e. dental services, skilled nursing services) and nonmedical services (i.e. respite, case management, environmental modifications) with the goal of avoiding relatively expensive institutionalization for at-risk older adults with functional disabilities. Family members and friends may be providers of waiver services if they meet standard provider qualifications. Approximately 287 waiver programs are currently active in 48 states and the District of Columbia as government struggles to mitigate the costs of institutional care. A recent analysis showed that 58% of patients in these programs were elderly or disabled. A relatively small proportion of Medicaid waiver spending went toward this group (23.8% or $3.4 billion) compared with the amount expended on patients with mental retardation or developmental disability (74% or $10.5 billion).

Finally, a 2005 Medicare demonstration project, Care Management for High-Cost Beneficiaries (CMHCB), awarded 3-year contracts to several health care provider organizations across the nation to "test the ability of intensive management for high-cost beneficiaries with various medical conditions to reduce cost as well as improve quality of care and quality of life." These organizations are using a variety of care management tools such as increased provider availability (including physician house calls), structured chronic care programs, restructured physician practices, and expanded flexibility in care settings in an attempt to demonstrate overall cost savings and care improvement. Results from this demonstration should be available beginning in 2008.

TRENDS

Several emerging trends in CBLTC will undoubtedly affect the future health care of the aging U.S. population. Interdisciplinary team-based models of care providing medical care, nursing, and social work at home for older adults with multiple chronic illnesses, once seen only in academic medical centers, are being developed by private sector companies and hospitals. These teams focus not on single-disease management, but on coordination of care, integration of patient goals and preferences, and improvement of patient outcomes relevant to this particularly frail and vulnerable group. At the same time, an increasing number of physicians are withdrawing from the current Medicare fee-for-service system as the reimbursement schedule continues to decline relative to the costs and risks of medical practice. This "opting out" trend, combined with the already grave shortage of primary care physicians including geriatricians, may, over time, drive a demand-based shift toward private insurance, health savings accounts, and concierge practices, further depleting the supply of physicians. The current interest in "pay-for-performance" (P4P) is aimed primarily at discrete, disease-specific measures such as hemoglobin A1C levels, which are not consistently applicable to a frail geriatric population. A recent effort to establish performance standards for home-based primary care adapted the Assessing Care of Vulnerable Elders (ACOVE) quality indicators for ambulatory geriatric and nursing facility patients to create a comprehensive framework for quality evaluation and future comparative research. The care of medically complex older adults will also require evaluation of events such as hospital admissions, intensive care stays, or nursing home placement for high-cost populations. Health systems that care for these high-cost populations should receive support for lowering the overall costs rather than for documenting the results of specific elements of single-disease management programs or discrete quality indicators. Finally, the growing recognition that patient empowerment and involvement improves quality and satisfaction will ideally translate into systems that value, support, and pay informal family caregivers for their essential and indispensable work.

CONCLUSION

CBLTC is a varied collection of services aimed at allowing functionally impaired older adults to age in place according to their wishes. Although decades of research have resulted in some evidence of cost-effective benefit, this evidence is limited by semantic and methodological issues. Overall, CBLTC is effective when appropriately targeted; older adults continue to prefer living in the community over living in institutions, and social pressures from an aging generation will only increase demand for CBLTC in the future. The current fragmented system of CBLTC will be untenable in the coming years as the number of older adults with complex multimorbidity and functional disability increases. Emerging models of CBLTC including physician house calls, team-based primary care coordination, and population-based pay-for-performance hold promise for improving health care for these patients, although systematic barriers exist to their widespread implementation. Creative economic, technological, and clinical solutions that focus on quality and cost-effectiveness will be critical in reforming the system to affirm and fulfill the public trust.

FURTHER READING

1. Arno PS, Levine C, Memmott MM. The economic value of informal caregiving. *Health Aff.* 1999;18:182–188.
2. Caplan GA, Ward JA, Brennan AJ, et al. Hospital in the home: a randomized controlled trial. *Med J Aust.* 1999;170:156–160.
3. Carlson BL, Foster L, Dale SB, et al. Effects of cash and counseling on personal care and well-being. *Health Serv Res.* 2007;42:467–487.
4. Centers for Medicare and Medicaid Services (CMS) Web site, http://www.cms.gov/ Accessed 30 January 2007.
5. Eng C, Pedulla J, Eleazer GP, et al. Program of all-inclusive care for the elderly: an innovative model of integrated geriatric care and financing. *J Am Geriatr Soc.* 1997;45:223–232.
6. Grabowski DC. The cost-effectiveness of noninstitutional long-term care services: review and synthesis of the most recent evidence. *Med Care Res Rev.* 2006;63:3–28.
7. Hedrick SC, Rothman ML, Chapko M, et al. Summary and discussion of methods and results of the Adult Day Health Care evaluation study. *Med Care.* 1993;31:SS94–SS103.
8. Hersh WR, Hickam DH, Severance S, et al. Telemedicine for the Medicare population: update. Agency for Healthcare Research and Quality Report; 2006.
9. Hughes SL, Weaver FM, Giobbie-Hurder A, et al. Effectiveness of team-managed home-based primary care: a randomized multicenter trial. *JAMA.* 2000;284(22):2877–2885.
10. Kane RA. Expanding the home care concept: blurring distinctions among home care, institutional care, and other long-term-care services. *Milbank Quart.* 1995;73:161–186.
11. Kemper P, Brown RS, Carcagno GJ, et al. The evaluation of the national long term care demonstration: final report. Princeton, NJ: Mathematica Policy Research, Inc.; 1986.
12. Kitchener M, Ng T, Miller N, et al. Medicaid home and community-based services: national program trends. *Health Aff.* 2005;24:206–212.
13. Miller EA, Weissert WG. Predicting elderly people's risk for nursing home placement, hospitalization, functional impairment, and mortality: a synthesis. *Med Care Res Rev.* 2000;57:259–287.
14. Naylor MD, Brooten D, Campbell R, et al. Comprehensive discharge planning and home follow-up of hospitalized elders: a randomized clinical trial. *JAMA.* 1999;281:613–620.
15. Shaughnessy PW, Hittle DF, Crisler KS, et al. Improving patient outcomes of home health care: findings from two demonstration trials of outcome-based quality improvement. *J Am Geriatr Soc.* 2002;50:1354–1364.
16. Smith KL, Soriano TA, Boal J. National quality-of-care standards in home-based primary care. *Ann Intern Med.* 2007;146:188–192.
17. Stuck AE, Egger M, Hammer A, et al. Home visits to prevent nursing home admission and functional decline in elderly people: systematic review and meta-regression analysis. *JAMA.* 2002;287:1022–1028.
18. Thompson T. Evaluation results for the social/health maintenance organization II demonstration. *Report to Congress* 2002.
19. Weissert WG. One more battle lost to friendly fire—of if you spend too much it's hard to save money. *Med Care.* 1993;31:SS119–SS121.
20. Weissert WG, Cready CM, Pawelak JE. The past and future of home- and community-based long-term care. *Milbank Quart* 1988;66:309–388.
21. White AJ, Abel Y, Kidder D. Evaluation of the program of all-inclusive care for the elderly demonstration. Abt Associates; 2001.

Rural Aging

Kenneth Brummel-Smith

Over 51 million Americans live in areas classified by the U.S. Office of Management and Budget (OMB) as nonmetropolitan, or "rural." They comprise one-fifth of the U.S. population. The rural life holds great value in the history of the United States. For most of our country's history, rural living was practically the only way of life. Throughout the years, rural living has been seen as a noble and pure form of existence. Getting "back to the land" has long been viewed as a dream for many city dwellers. Unfortunately, when it comes to being old in a rural setting, there are many aspects which are not so sanguine.

Rural aging reflects many of the attitudes held toward older people in our society. Some, for instance, have questioned whether very high health care expenditures on persons at the end of life are worthwhile. Similarly, when viewed from an economic sense, rural residence is expensive for both society and individuals. The costs of distance, inefficiencies of spatial dispersion, and absence of economies of scale mean that health care has difficulties supplying specialty care and services. Forty years ago, William Myernick wrote that it does not make sense for society to expend resources in supporting small, dispersed, economically challenged communities. Yet the fact is older people make up a large percentage of the population of people living in rural settings.

The Kellogg Foundation conducted interviews with over 200 persons from different communities to assess views of rural living. Respondents viewed rural life as being primarily agricultural, as emphasizing family values with a strong sense of self-reliance, as having beautiful landscapes with animals and family farms, and as having a relaxed and friendly way of life. Interestingly, aging, or growing older and frailer, were not mentioned as common perceptions.

Rural life is also connected to prominent American values—the dual values of self-reliance and interdependence with one's neighbors, freedom from governmental control, a slower pace of living, and the back to nature philosophy. As will be discussed, a significant movement, or "in-migration" of older people back to rural areas is occurring in part because of these values. However, the long trend of younger people moving away from rural areas and poorer and sicker older people remaining also continues. What society may be facing in the next few decades is a population of primarily older people living in large portions of the country—a population made of two subgroups, healthy active and politically motivated baby boomers who have returned to the land, and a larger group of frail elders who have lived all their lives in that environment. This development will challenge health care service providers, as well as Medicare and Medicaid.

DEMOGRAPHY OF RURAL AGING

One of the problems in discussing rural aging is the definition of "rural." The two most frequently used definitions used in research and policy development are the U.S. Census Bureau's use of community size and density and the OMB's designation of counties as "nonmetropolitan." The U.S. Census Bureau defines as "urban" any incorporated city, town, village, or borough with a population of at least 2500 people. Any area not defined as urban is defined as rural. Previously, the OMB used the terms Metropolitan Statistical Areas and Nonmetropolitan Statistical Areas to categorize populations. Recently, the OMB released a new classification system using Core Based Statistical Areas (CBSA). These are areas with at least 10 000 people with adjacent territories that have a high degree of social and economic integration (Table 23-1). Those areas that do not meet CBSA numbers are called Outside Core Based Statistical Areas, which equates with rural living. This change has significant implications. First, it reduced the number of people living in nonmetropolitan areas from 55 million to 49 million. More importantly, the OMB definitions are used to assign eligibility and reimbursement for a number of federal programs, including Medicare. In addition, the two definitions do not overlap, creating difficulties in planning. As it is, most counties contain a mixture of rural and urban living.

TABLE 23-1

OMB Classifications of Rural and Urban Areas

Core-Based Statistical Areas
    Metropolitan—urbanized areas with a population of 50,000 or more
    Micropolitan—urban areas, population 10,000–49,999

Outside Core-Based Statistical Areas
    Rural

There are many myths about rural aging. Krout outlined many stereotypes of rural elders, including that they

live on farms and are a homogenous group,

are in better physical and mental shape because of hard work, good food, and living in the country,

are more active,

better able to take care of themselves and make ends meet,

are not homeless and have better housing,

are surrounded by large families who are available and willing to help,

have less need for health and social services, and

can get what they need in the local stores.

The realities of rural aging are far different and much more diverse. Rural populations are vastly different—rural Florida is not the same as rural Minnesota, or even rural Mississippi. Americans 65 years and older make up 12.4% of the total population. However, nonmetropolitan areas have a higher percentage of older people—14.6% compared to 11.9% in metropolitan areas. The reasons for greater concentration include (1) aging in place, (2) younger persons migrating out for better jobs, and (3) in-migration of older adults after retirement. The percentage of women and those who are widowed reflects similar numbers to the general population of metropolitan areas. Ethnic diversity is increasing, but the current cohort is less diverse than in urban areas. Whites comprise 92.4%, African-Americans 6.2%, Hispanics 2.6%, and less than 1% are American Indian, Alaska Native, or Asian.

Although poverty rates in rural areas are the lowest they have been since 1980, persistent poverty is predominantly a rural problem. Of the 382 counties with poverty rates greater than 20% since 1952, 95% are rural. Fourteen percent of the rural older population is poor, compared to 10.8% in urban areas, and 50% are considered low income versus 38% of urban elders. Socioeconomic status is probably the strongest factor affecting health and health care services so the implications of this fact cannot be overstated.

Another important aspect of aging that affects health care is the availability of caregivers. Nationally, one out of four families is providing assistance to an older family member. Informal caregiving is the primary source of long term care in this country, and that is certainly true for the rural population. Unfortunately, rural elders appeared to be trapped between their higher expectations for care from a family member, and the decreasing availability of younger family members. A larger percentage of rural elders receive assistance from "fictive kin"—friends and others in the rural community. This probably is a main contributor to the fact that long-term institutional care is more common in rural areas than urban areas.

Finally, an important dynamic in the demographics of rural aging is the resettlement of rural areas by retirees, which is termed "in-migration." In the 1970s, a net in-migration to rural areas followed decades of out migration. This was caused by a combination of some manufacturing jobs moving to more rural areas for cheaper land and labor and a "back-to-the-earth" movement following the tumultuous 1960s. Some of these residents are now the rural elders who have aged in place. However, this in-migration was short-lived, and in the 1980s, almost 2 million persons aged 20 to 29 years moved away from rural areas. More recently, wealthier and healthier elders have been moving back into rural areas after retirement, in order to seek a lower cost of living and the amenities afforded by recreational and cultural opportunities. A recent study of this development has revealed a number of interesting outcomes:

- Although in-migration encourages job growth, it does not increase per capita income or contribute to economic stability in host communities.

- Retired migrants contribute their fair share of taxes but they also bring added costs to rural governments with increased demands for public and health care services.

- Rural in-migration is likely to accelerate with the retirement of the baby boomers.

Less than 11% of the nation's physicians are practicing in rural areas. Over 20 million rural residents live in areas that have a shortage of physicians to meet their basic needs. The majority of physicians (54%) in rural areas are in the primary care specialties of family or general practice, general internal medicine, pediatrics, and obstetrics/gynecology, compared with 38% of metropolitan physicians. In 1995, there were 56,635 office-based physicians practicing in rural areas. Family physicians are far more likely to practice in rural areas than all other specialties.

However, maintenance of a rural practice has been difficult. Medicare does offer a 10% bonus payment to physicians practicing in Health Professions Shortage Areas. Yet many physicians do not make use of the bonus and some who are not eligible have used it extensively. A recent study of rural physicians in Florida revealed that many were considering dropping Medicare or some services because of reimbursement problems.

Like the rest of the country, rural America is aging. However, it started out being the primary place of living of older people. While rural living still reflects strongly held American values, the aging of rural society will create significant challenges for the provision of health care to a population that is already at-risk.

HEALTH STATUS OF RURAL ELDERS

Contrary to the myth of healthy, clean living older adults in the country, elders in rural areas have high rates of illness and disability. Populations living in rural areas have higher rates of heart disease, diabetes, hypertension, depression, emphysema, cancer, and arthritis than those in metropolitan areas. Some studies have shown diabetes to be 17% higher in rural areas. Compounding these high rates is the difficulties that older adults have in accessing specialist care and even primary care providers in some areas.

According to Rural Healthy People 2010, rural populations lag behind metropolitan populations in many health status indicators.

These include higher rates of heart disease, respiratory disease, diabetes, stroke, mental diseases, malnutrition, obesity, substance abuse, and cancer, as well as reduced rates of having insurance, and access to primary care. In addition, recommended screening practices also occur at lower rates.

While recent studies have documented a declining rate of disability among older Americans, the rate of frailty and dependency in activities of daily living (ADL) and instrumental activities of daily living (IADL) continues to be high in rural communities. Almost three-quarters (73%) of the rural older population has activity limitations, compared to approximately 50% in those living in metropolitan areas, and is also complicated by the relative lack of services, especially for rehabilitation. In addition, access to personal care by physical and occupational therapists, or in-home services are limited as well.

Higher rates of mental illness and substance abuse are particularly problematic in rural areas, where providers are few and special services are limited. The MoVIES Project, a 10-year prospective study of dementia in rural elderly showed that the incidence rates of Alzheimer's and other dementias was higher than in urban populations, with particularly high rates in men. Self-reported hopelessness, helplessness, worthlessness, and lethargy were reported at higher rates by older people in the National Health Interview Survey. Depression rates have been reported as high as 40% in women in rural areas, compared to 13% to 20% in urban older women. Rural Hispanic women have been found to rates of depression two times higher than white women.

Polypharmacy is always a risk in geriatrics but has special implications among rural elders. The use of multiple health care providers, who are often at great distance from one another, and limited access to pharmacies and knowledgeable pharmacists, makes polypharmacy even more risky for rural elders. In one study of falls among rural elders, four of five significant risk factors were drugs: analgesics, sedatives, antiarthritic medications, and antihypertensive medications.

Nutritional problems are very common among rural elders. Both overnutrition (obesity and overweight) and undernutrition are common (Table 23-2). In addition, rural elderly women consume lower amounts of recommended protein, vitamins A, C, E, B-6, B-12, riboflavin, and folate, as well as some minerals (calcium, phosphorus, and magnesium). Many rural elders consume a diet of low-nutrient value, including a high intake of bread, cereal, rice, pasta, fats, oils, and sweets. This pattern leads to high calorie consumption and low intake of essential vitamins and minerals. In addition, many older rural residents consume limited amounts of fruits and vegetables. In one study of 50-year-old and older residents in six rural communities, 45% ate less than one serving of fruit or vegetable juices per week, 33% consumed less than one serving of fruits, and 21% ate less than one serving of any vegetable per week. Substantial numbers of rural elders report not having enough to eat or not having enough money to purchase quality foods. Rural minorities are at substantially increased risk for food insecurity.

Options for improvement in nutrition for elders are food stamps and home-delivered meals. Unfortunately, a smaller percentage of rural elders participate in the food stamp program than urban older persons (7.9% vs. 9.4%) and the majority of elders get the minimum benefit (U.S. Department of Agriculture Web site). Similarly, home-delivered meals, such as Meals on Wheels Programs, are much less commonly located in rural areas.

ETHNIC AND MINORITY RURAL AGING

The well-known presence of health care disparities among ethnic groups is present, and in some cases, magnified in rural areas. For instance, African-Americans in rural areas are less likely to receive specialized medical care, to adhere to long-term preventive drug regimens, and are less likely to use more complex health care services. Unfortunately, there is little hard data on individual ethnic groups in rural settings because they have not been sufficiently studied.

Over 90% of rural African-Americans live in the South, and three-quarters of these live in just seven states (Louisiana, Mississippi, Alabama, Georgia, South Carolina, North Carolina, and Virginia). There are fewer home- and community-based services available to them, and consequently the rate of nursing home utilization is higher among rural African-Americans than those in urban areas.

Rural Hispanic elders have a higher prevalence of ADL and IADL deficits, and cognitive impairments than comparable non-Hispanic white elders. However, rural Hispanics are twice as likely as nonrural Hispanics to use nursing home care. Still, because over 60% of rural Hispanic elders were born outside the United States, their access to care is limited and they are often underserved. In part, this is due to lack of Medicare, lack of knowledge of available services, and language barriers. In addition, Hispanic elders have high expectations that their children will provide assistance when needed.

There are approximately 300,000 older American Indians and Alaskan Natives (AI/AN), according to the 2000 U.S. Census, which is 26% greater than 10 years before. There are 562 federally recognized tribes, who speak over 200 languages. Although American Indians live in all 50 states, approximately one-half of them live in three states: Oklahoma, California, and Arizona. Older American Indians have often lived their whole lives in one community. According to the Indian Health Service (IHS), the incidence of chronic diseases is increasing rapidly, substantially raising health care costs. Disability is extremely common among AI/AN elders with 30% having at least one ADL deficit (compared to 17% of whites).

Although there has been a movement toward independent and self-administered health care for many AI/AN tribes, the IHS continues to provide care to many older persons. However, funds have never been appropriated to the IHS for long-term care. Hence, most elders in need of LTC use tribal support, Medicaid and Administration on Aging funded services. Many go without services. There are only 20 tribally funded nursing homes in the United States. Many providers involved in caring for older American Indians and Alaskan Natives have been advocating for expansion of home and

TABLE 23-2

Percentage of Overweight and Obese Rural Elders (>65) by Selected States and Regions		
	OVERWEIGHT	**OBESE**
West Virginia	34	20
Pennsylvania	44	35
North Carolina	31	34.5
Mississippi delta	N/A	42.6

N/A, data not available.

community-based waivers through the state's Medicaid programs or funding at a national level.

RURAL HEALTH CLINICS

The federal government authorized Public Law 95-210, the Rural Health Clinic Services Act, in 1997, which assures Medicare and Medicaid reimbursement to certified clinics staffed by physician assistants (PAs) and nurse practitioners (NPs) working with physician supervision. The purpose of the rural health clinic (RHC) program is to increase primary care medical services in rural, physician-shortage areas by utilizing PAs and NPs. Financial stability was promoted by providing cost-based compensation for care of Medicare and Medicaid patients. RHC are now paid under a special prospective payment system designed for them. The program failed to thrive for 10 years until Congress made a series of changes that reduced burdensome paperwork, increased payment levels, and enhanced technical assistance and awareness. Modifications to state PA laws, such as relaxation of onsite supervision requirements and the delegation of prescriptive authority, have also contributed to the program's success. As a result, the number of certified RHCs has grown from less than 600 in 1990 to approximately 3600 in 2003.

Because of changes in the Medicare law authorizing Medicare Part B coverage for PAs and NPs in all practice settings, the original incentive for utilizing PAs and NPs was diminished. However, because an RHC gets reimbursed the same amount from Medicare and Medicaid regardless of whether the patient is seen by a mid-level provider such as a PA, NP, or a physician, the facility continues to have a strong incentive to utilize these practitioners whenever it is clinically appropriate.

RHCs care for large numbers of Medicare, Medicaid, and uninsured patients. A 2003 national survey revealed that approximately 56% of patient visits in RHCs are covered by Medicare or Medicaid and approximately 15% are uninsured. Unlike a fee-for-service practice where Medicare and Medicaid payment is based on the cumulative charges for all services provided, a RHC is paid on a clinic-specific, all-inclusive rate that is adjusted annually and, in a majority of cases, subject to a limit set by the government. Challenges continue including questions about reimbursement models, the requirement for use of Pas and NPs, and the impact of managed care programs.

RURAL HOSPITALS AND LONG-TERM CARE

Rural hospitals service nearly 54 million people, including 9 million Medicare beneficiaries. Like many hospitals, Medicare payments present some challenges. However, they also face other significant pressures—continued shortages of trained staff, rising health care liability premiums, and access to capital for investments in new technology or information systems. Rural hospitals are more at risk due to their small size, modest assets, and limited financial reserves. They also serve a higher percentage of Medicare patients since rural populations are typically older than average urban populations. Hence, Medicare margins are the lowest for rural hospitals, with the smallest hospitals having the lowest margins.

Rural hospitals have undergone many changes in the last two decades. With the advent of prospective payment in the 1980s, and managed care in the 1990s, many rural hospitals diversified by developing a variety of postacute services. These included in-hospital skilled nursing facilities and home health programs. Some also developed assistive living facilities and adult daycare programs. However, the Balanced Budget Act of 1997 decreased payments to rural hospitals for skilled nursing and home health services, so many of the hospitals reduced or closed down these programs. There have been, however, a number of other Medicare policy decisions that have supported rural hospitals in maintaining a diverse service line. This is important, as rural communities usually have only one health center (if at all). In addition, unlike urban communities where physicians now specialize in a site of practice (hospitalists, office, or nursing home) rural health care providers usually practice in all settings.

Because of these challenges, the federal government has developed some special programs to support rural hospitals. Critical Access Hospitals (CAH) are rural community hospitals (RCHs) that receive cost-based reimbursement. To be designated a CAH, a rural hospital must meet defined criteria. As of March 2006, there are 1279 certified CAHs located throughout the United States. A list of CAH can be viewed online at http://www.flexmonitoring.org/documents/CAHlist_current.xls.

The Rural Community Hospital Demonstration Program was created as part of the Medicare Modernization Act of 2003 to test the advisability and feasibility of establishing RCHs to provide Medicare-covered inpatient hospital services in rural areas. Medicare inpatient services are paid based on reasonable costs of providing such services to Medicare beneficiaries. After a period of time, the reimbursement process is modified to account for increased costs. In order to participate in the demonstration, the hospital must be located in a rural area, have fewer than 51 acute care beds, have 24-hour emergency care services available, and not be eligible for CAH designation. For this demonstration, hospitals had to be located in one of the 10 least densely populated States: Alaska, Idaho, Montana, Nebraska, Nevada, New Mexico, North Dakota, South Dakota, Utah, or Wyoming. Thirteen small rural hospitals in seven sparsely populated states are program participants.

The Social Security Act permits certain small, rural hospitals to enter into a swing bed agreement, under which the hospital can use its beds, as needed, to provide either acute or skilled nursing facility (SNF) care. Approximately 95% of rural hospitals operate swing beds. As defined in the regulations, a swing bed hospital is a hospital or CAH participating in Medicare that has CMS approval to provide posthospital SNF care and meets certain requirements. Medicare Part A (the hospital insurance program) covers posthospital extended care services furnished in a swing bed hospital. Swing bed facilities must be incorporated into the SNF prospective payment system by the end of a statutory transition period. CAHs with swing beds are exempt from the SNF PPS under more recent legislation. To qualify for SNF-level services, a beneficiary is required to receive acute care as a hospital inpatient for a medically necessary stay of at least 3 consecutive calendar days.

The Health Resource Services Administration has the Rural Hospital Performance Improvement (RHPI) project focuses on strengthening rural hospitals in the Mississippi delta as the cornerstone to preserving health care access. It is a source for technical expertise and business tools to help rural hospitals achieve performance improvement goals. The first contract in 2001–2004 yielded 71 applications and provided 59 consultations to small rural hospitals. Forty-six hospitals throughout the Delta Region have been served during

2004–2006 including 25 performance improvement assessments, 19 targeted consultations, and seven balanced scorecard consultations.

Nursing home care is the mainstay of long-term care services in rural areas. Home care and assisted living are far less common than in urban areas. Nearly 40% of the nation's nursing homes are in rural areas, and nursing home beds per 1000 population are higher than urban areas. However, skilled beds and special care units are less common. A large number of rural hospitals still offer a variety of postacute and long-term services. Approximately 50% of rural hospitals operate an SNF.

Rural hospitals are involved in operating home health agencies, though the number has been declining. Approximately 35% of CAH have home health programs. However, after the BBA of 1997, home health care in rural areas dropped by 26%, compared to a 19% decline in urban areas. Many rural hospitals are finding it difficult to maintain these programs and 52% of programs are operating at a loss. Those units that are part of a multihospital system tend to offer both skilled nursing unit services and home health at a higher rate than independent hospitals.

Integration of acute and long-term services has been promoted as a method to improve quality, reduce errors in transitions in care, and lead to reduced costs. Care integration is more difficult in rural areas for a number of reasons. Limited financial resources are the main hindrance. Rural hospitals do not operate high-volume, high reimbursement business lines, such as transplant or cardiac surgery programs. They also serve a larger proportion of Medicare and Medicaid clients. However, some states such as Wisconsin and Minnesota have developed successful integrated rural programs. Perhaps the quintessential integrated program is the Program of All-inclusive Care of the Elderly (PACE). This model uses capitated Medicare and Medicaid funding to provide services to nursing home eligible clients. The BBA of 1997 allowed the development of two rural PACE sites. Progress was initially slow, in part due to the $1 million to $2 million start-up costs for a PACE site. In 2005, the Center for Medicare and Medicaid Services announced $7.5 million in competitive grants to 15 rural health care provider organizations to support development of PACE across rural America. More on rural PACE programs can be found at www.npaonline.org.

TECHNOLOGY AND RURAL AGING

Because of the problems of distance, and the lack of providers, facilities, and economies of scale, technology holds great promise to expand the services provided to older adults living in rural areas. A wide variety of technologies exist for this use, and the technology is rapidly changing and becoming less expensive.

Interactive televideo can be used with telephone or special lines. A video camera, monitor, and connection system are all that is needed. Such a system can provide video and audio information, gathered by an in-home visiting nurse and projected to a consultant physician at a distant site. Real-time consultations can be made, or the data can be saved for later (asynchronous) interactions. The Telemedicine Research Center reported in 2004 that there were 88 telehealth networks across the United States providing over 85 000 patient-provider teleconsultations in 2003.

Telemedicine may be particularly useful when using interdisciplinary teams in rural geriatric care. NPs, PAs, and rehabilitation therapists can communicate with one another, and a physician to optimize care for frail older persons. Kansas University has been using telemedicine to enable speech and language pathologists to conduct swallowing evaluations from remote sites. It has also been used in rural nursing homes for monitoring and directing wound care. Comprehensive geriatric assessment has been conducted in rural areas using telemedicine to link with a geriatrician at a remote area.

Finally, it is particularly useful in home care, where a wide variety of health assessments, such as blood pressure, temperature, monitoring of heart and lung sounds, oximeters, spirometers, and laboratory determinations can be made. Patients of family caregivers can be trained to administer the assessments and transmit the results to treatment of team members. This is particularly useful in chronic disease management programs.

The use of the Internet will expand the options for telemedicine even more. Videos can be transmitted live or asynchronously. Web cameras are inexpensive and Voice over Internet Protocol (VoIP) allows audio transmission. The major obstacle is the speed of transmission but high-speed lines are being expanded into rural areas and a number of cell phone companies provide wireless transmission.

The challenges of instituting widespread use of interactive televideo medicine are numerous. They include limitations of reimbursement, the absence of or antiquated technical infrastructure, interstate telemedicine license questions, privacy concerns, and the fact that the present cohort of elders, and particularly those in rural areas are not particularly technologically savvy. However, in spite of these barriers, rural physicians who recognize the benefits to both themselves and to their patients ate likely to implement a telemedicine strategy when offered.

SUMMARY

Rural aging provides both significant challenges and special opportunities. The number of elders in rural settings is not likely to decline soon. Primary care physicians will always provide the bulk of care to older persons in rural areas. The advent of new technologies, particularly the Internet, should allow expansion of services and greater access to high-quality geriatric care.

FURTHER READING

American Hospital Association. http://www.aha.org/aha_app/issues/Rural-Health-Care/index.jsp. Accessed March 23, 2007.

Bradley DE, Longino CF. Demographic and resettlement impacts on rural services. In: Goins RT, Krout JA, eds. *Service Delivery to Rural Older Adults*. New York, New York: Springer; 2006.

Bryant LL, Shetterly SM, Baxter J, Hamman RF. Modifiable risks of incident functional dependence in Hispanic and non-Hispanic White elders: the San Luis Valley Health and Aging Study. *The Gerontologist*. 2002;42:690–697.

Chan L, Hart LG, Ricketts LC, Beaver SK. An analysis of Medicare's incentive payment program for physicians in Health Professional Shortage Areas, *J Rural Health*.2004;20:109–117.

Coburn AF, Bolda EJ. The rural elderly and long term care. In: Ricketts TC, ed. *Rural Health in the United States*. New York, New York: Oxford University Press; 1999:179–189.

Coburn AF, Loux SL, Bolda EJ. Rural hospitals and long-term care. In: Goins RT, Krout JA, eds. *Service Delivery to Rural Older Adults* New York, New York: Springer; 2006.

Colorado Governor Richard Lamm's speech in 1984 on older people's "duty to die." http://www-hsc.usc.edu/~mbernste/ethics.dutytodie.html. Accessed May 2, 2007.

Coward TR, Netzer JK, Peek CW. Older rural African-Americans. In: Coward RT, Krout JA, eds. *Aging in Rural Settings: Life Circumstances and Distinctive Features*. New York, New York: Springer; 1998.

Cravens DD, Mehr DR, Campbell JD, et al. Home-based comprehensive assessment of rural elderly persons: The CARE Project. *J Rural Health.* 2005;21:322–328.

Edmund S. The characteristics and roles of rural health clinics in the United States; A chartbook. Muskie School of Public Services, University of Southern Maine; January 2003.

Gamm LD, Hutchinson L, Dabney B, Dorsey A. Rural Healthy People 2010: A companion guide to Healthy People 2010. Texas A & M University System Health Science Center, School of Public Health, Southwest RuralHealth Research Center, College Station, TX; 2003.

Ganguli M, Dodge HH, Chen P, et al. Ten year incidence of dementia in a rural elderly U.S. community population: The MoVIES Project. *Neurology.* 2000;54:1109–1116.

Glasgow N. Rural/urban patterns of aging and caregiving in the United States. *J Family Issues.* 2000;21:611–631.

Goins RT, Mitchell J, Wu B. Service issues among rural racial and ethnic minority elders. In: Goins RT, Krout JA, eds. *Service Delivery to Rural Older Adults.* New York, New York: Springer; 2006.

Gunderson A, Menachemi N, Brummel-Smith K, Brooks R. Physicians who treat the elderly in Florida: trends indicating concerns. *J Rural Health.* 2006;22:224–228.

Indian Health Service. U.S. Department of Health and Human Services. Trends in Indian health. Washington, DC: U.S. Government Printing Office; 2001.

Isserman AM. In the national interest: defining rural and urban correctly in research and public policy. *Int Regional Sci Rev.* 2005;28:465–499.

Krout JA, ed. *Providing Community-based Services to Rural Elderly.* Thousand Oaks, CA: Sage Press; 1994.

Larson SL, Machlin SR, Nixon A, Zodet M. Chartbook #13: Health care in urban and rural areas, combined year 1998–2000. Rockville, MD: Agency for Healthcare Research and Quality. www.meps.ahrq.gov/papers/CB13_04-0050/CB13.htm.

Lethbridge-Cejku M, Schiller JS, Bernadel L. Summary health statistics for U.S. adults: National Health Interview Survey, 2002. Hyattsville, MD: National Center for Health Statistics; 2004.

Lewin ME, Altman S, eds. America's health care safety net: Intact but endangered. Washington, DC: Institute of Medicine, National Academy; 2000.

Liebman M, Propst K, Moore SA, et al. Gender differences in selected dietary intakes and eating behaviors in rural communities in Wyoming, Montana, and Idaho. *Nutr Res.* 2003;23:991–1002.

List of Critical Access Hospitals. http://www.flexmonitoring.org/documents/CAHlist_current.xls. Accessed March 24, 2007.

Longino CF, Smith MH. The impact of elderly migration on rural communities. In: Coward R, Krout JA, eds. *Aging in Rural Settings: Life Circumstances and Distinctive Features.* New York, New York: Springer; 1998.

Mitchell J, Mathews HF, Hunt LM, et al. Mismanaging prescription medications among rural elders: effects of socioeconomic status, health status and medication profile indicators. *Gerontologist.* 2001;41:348–256.

Mosley JM, Miller KK. What the research says about... spatial variations in factors affecting poverty. Rural Poverty Research Center, Research Brief 2004-1, 2004.

Myernick W. Needed: Appalacian ghost towns. *Appalac Rev.* 1967:14–20.

National Alliance for Caregiving/AARP. Family caregiving in the U.S.: Findings from a national study. Bethesda, MD: AARP; 1997.

Place JL. Workforce development and competency engancement. In: Bridging the health divide: The rural public health research agenda. Pittsburg, PA: University of Pittsburg Center for Rural Health Practice; 2004.

Redford L, Spaulding R. Transforming rural health care. The role of technology, In: Goins RT, Krout JA, eds. *Service Delivery to Rural Older Adults.* New York, New York: Springer; 2006.

Richardson DR, Hicks MJ, Walker RB. Falls in rural elders: an empirical study of risk factors. *J Am Board Fam Pract.* 2002;15:178–182.

Rogers CC. Changes in older population and implications for rural areas. Washington, DC: U.S. Department of Agriculture. Economic Research Service. Rural Development and Research Report No. 90, 1999.

Rowles GD. Foreward. In: Goins RT, Krout JA, eds., *Service Delivery to Rural Older Adults.* New York, New York: Springer; 2006.

Rural Assistance Center, http://www.raconline.org/info_guides/hospitals/cahfaq.php#whatis. Accessed March 24, 2007.

Rural Assistant Center. Information Guides: Rural Health Clinics Frequently Asked Questions. www.raconline.org/info_guides/clinics/rhcfaq.php.

Sharkey JR, Bolin JN. Health and nutrition in rural areas. In: Goins RT, Krout JA, eds. *Service Delivery to Rural Older Adults.* New York, New York: Springer; 2006.

Sharkey JR. Variations in nutritional risk among Mexican-American and non-Mexican American homebound elders who receive home-delivered meals. *J Nutr Elderly.* 2004;23:1–19.

Sharpe DL, Huston SJ, Finkle MS. Factors affecting nutritional adequacy among single elderly women. *Family Econ Nutr Rev.* 2003;15:74–82.

Shaughnessy PW. Changing institutional long-term care to improve rural health care. In: Coward RT, Bull CN, Kukulla G, Galliher JM, eds. *Health Services for Rural Elders.* New York, New York: Springer; 1994.

Spaulding RJ, Russo T, Cook DJ, Doolittle GC. Diffusion theory and telemedicine adoption by Kansas healthcare providers: Critical factors in telemedicine adoption for improved patient access. *J Telemedicine Telecare.* 2005;11(suppl): S1–S3.

Swenson CJ, Baxter J, Shetterly SM, et al. Depressive symptoms in Hispanic and non-Hispanic White rural elderly: The San Luis Valley Health and Aging Study. *Am J Epidemiol.* 2000;152:1048–1055.

Telemedicine Information Exchange. http://tie.telemed.org/default.asp. Accessed March 25, 2007.

U.S. Department of Agriculture. Economic Research Service. Briefing Room. Rural Population and migration: Rural elderly. Washington, DC: U.S. Government Printing Office; 2005.

U.S. Department of Agriculture. Elderly participation and the minimum benefit. www.fns.usda.gov/oane/MENU/Published/FSP/FILES/Participation/Elderly PartRates.pdf.

U.S. Department of Health and Human Services, Health Resources Service Administration, Rural Health Policy. http://deltarhpi.ruralhealth.hrsa.gov/. Accessed March 24, 2007.

W. K. Kellogg Foundation. Perceptions of rural America. 2001. www.wkkf.org/pubs/FoodRur/pub2973.pdf.

Wagner DL, Niles-Yokum KJ. Caregiving in a rural context. In: Goins RT, Krout JA, eds. *Service Delivery to Rural Older Adults.* New York, New York: Springer; 2006.

Waidmann TA, Lew-Ting CY. Disability trends among elderly persons and implications for the future. *J Gerointol Soc Sci.* 2000;55B:S298–S307.

Additional Resources

National Rural Health Association: www.nrharural.org

National PACE Association: www.npaonline.org

National Association of Rural Health Clinics: www.narhc.org/

Appropriate Approach to Prescribing

Paula A. Rochon ■ Jennifer Tjia ■ Sudeep S. Gill ■ Jerry H. Gurwitz

Prescribing for older patients offers special challenges. Older people take about three times as many prescription medications as do younger people, mainly because of an increased prevalence of chronic medical conditions among the older patient population. Taking several drugs together substantially increases the risk of drug interactions and adverse events. Many medications need to be used with special caution because of age-related changes in pharmacokinetics (i.e., absorption, distribution, metabolism, and excretion) and pharmacodynamics (see Chapter 8). For some drugs, an increase in the volume of distribution (e.g., diazepam) or a reduction in drug clearance (e.g., lithium) may lead to higher plasma concentrations in older patients than it does in younger patients. Pharmacodynamic changes with aging may result in an increased sensitivity to the effects of certain drugs, such as opioids, for any given plasma concentration. The pharmacokinetic and pharmacodynamic changes with aging are discussed in Chapter 8.

While a physician can usually do little to alter the characteristics of individual older patients to affect the kinetics or dynamics of drugs, the decision whether to prescribe any drug, the choice of drug, and the manner in which it is to be used (e.g., dose and duration of therapy) are all factors that are under control of the prescriber. This chapter discusses ways to optimize prescribing of drug therapy for older adults.

EPIDEMIOLOGY OF DRUG THERAPY

Writing a prescription is the most frequently employed medical intervention. Yet, creating optimal drug regimens that meet the complex needs of older persons requires thought and careful planning. Multiple factors contribute to inappropriate drug prescribing, including lack of adequate training of doctors in safe prescribing behavior and in prescribing for geriatric patients. Further, a lack of a routine use of safe medication prescribing behaviors such as checking drug allergies, double checking drug doses, adjusting doses for

renal impairment, and potential drug–drug interactions also contribute to prescribing errors. Avoidable adverse drug events (ADEs) are the most serious consequences of inappropriate drug prescribing. The possibility of an ADE should always be borne in mind when evaluating an elderly individual. A maxim from one wise geriatrician recommends: "In evaluating virtually any symptom in an older patient, the possibility of an ADE should be considered in the differential diagnosis." Advanced age, frailty, and increased drug utilization are all factors that contribute to an individual patient's risk for developing a drug-related problem. In the ambulatory setting, 25% of patients may have ADEs. When an ADE is identified in the ambulatory setting between 11% and approximately 25% are considered to be preventable. In the nursing home setting, the incidence is higher and approaches 10 ADEs per 100 resident-months, of which over half were preventable. These estimates are probably low because preventable ADEs were strictly defined and assumed that, in many cases, the prescription of the offending drug was indicated and the ADE was therefore not preventable. As many as 28% of hospital admissions among older patients result from drug-related problems. Up to 70% of these drug-related admissions are attributed to adverse drug reactions. Perhaps the most compelling explanation for the prevalence of ADE in older patients is that we lack methods for determining the harms associated with the multiple medications consumed simultaneously.

A random sample of 2590 noninstitutionalized older adults in the United States during the years 1998 and 1999 provides information on the use of prescription and over-the-counter medications in the community. This survey demonstrated that use of all medications (prescriptions, over-the-counter drugs, vitamins/minerals, and herbals/supplements) (Figure 24-1) and the use of prescribed drug therapies (Figure 24-2) increases dramatically with advancing age. The highest prevalence of medication use was among women aged 65 years and older. Among these women, 12% took 10 or more medications and 23% took at least five prescribed drug therapies. The use of a larger number of drugs is associated with an increased

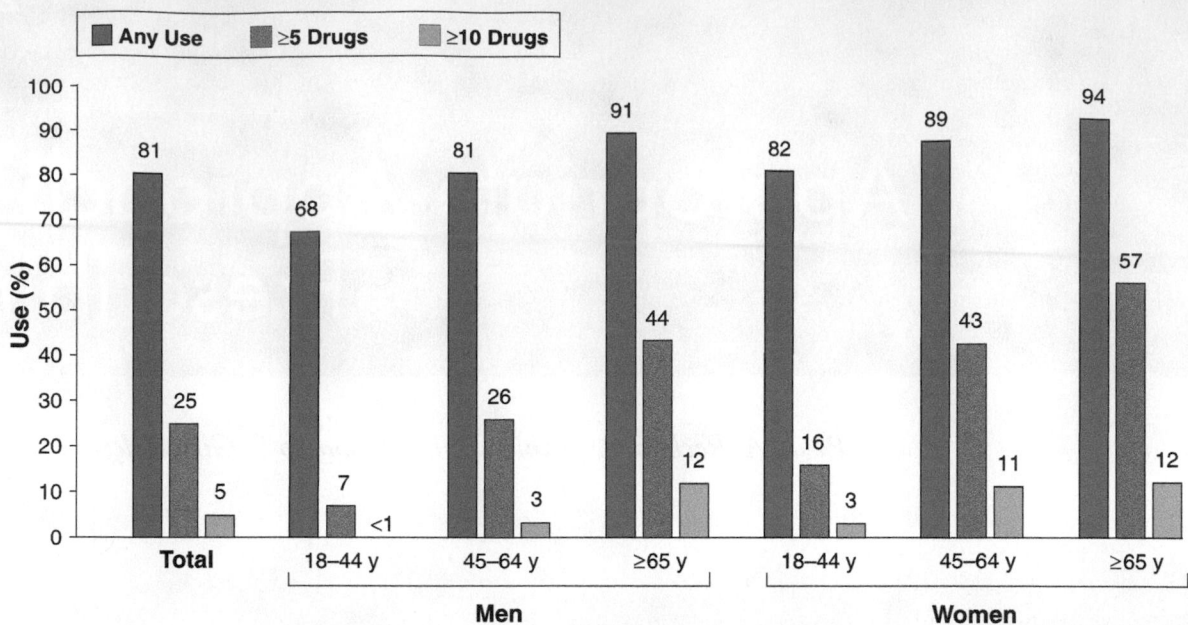

FIGURE 24-1. Use of medications during the preceding week, by sex and age. (Adapted from Kaufman DW, Kelly JP, Rosenberg L, et al. Recent patterns of medication use in the ambulatory adult population of the United States: the Slone survey. JAMA. 2002;287:337.)

likelihood of inappropriate prescribing, ADEs, and risk for geriatric syndromes including cognitive impairment, falls, hip fractures, and urinary incontinence. The widespread use of over-the-counter drug therapies indicates the importance of routinely inquiring about their use when evaluating a drug therapy regimen.

Herbal medicines are frequently used by older adults; physicians often do not question patients about such use. An estimated 14% of the U.S. population takes an herbal medicine or supplement such as ginseng, ginkgo biloba extract, and glucosamine. The use has increased from among adults who are 50 years of age or older, from 28% in 1991 to 39% in 1997. In one survey, almost 75% did not inform their physician that they were using unconventional treatments including herbal medicines. Herbal medicines may interact with prescribed drug therapies leading to adverse events, underscor-

ing the importance of routinely questioning patients about their use of these unconventional therapies. Examples of herbal–drug therapy interactions include warfarin in combination with ginkgo biloba extract leading to an increased risk of bleeding and serotonin-reuptake inhibitors in combination with St. John's Wort leading to serotonin syndrome in older adults.

MEASURING THE QUALITY OF DRUG PRESCRIBING IN OLDER PERSONS

Various criteria have been developed by expert panels in Canada and in the United States to assess the quality of medication use in elderly patient populations. The most widely used criteria employed

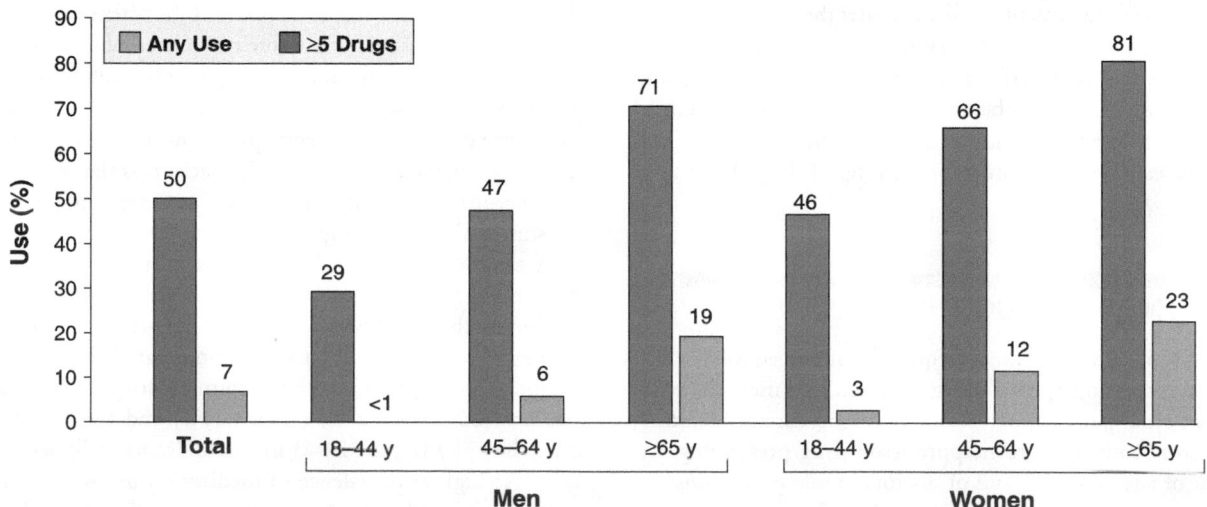

FIGURE 24-2. Use of prescription drugs during the preceding week, by sex and age. (Adapted from Kaufman DW, Kelly JP, Rosenberg L, et al. Recent patterns of medication use in the ambulatory adult population of the United States: the Slone survey. JAMA. 2002;287:337.)

for the assessment of inappropriate prescribing are based on the Beers criteria. These criteria were developed in 1991 by a consensus panel of experts in geriatric medicine, geriatric psychiatry, and pharmacology to evaluate inappropriate prescribing in nursing home residents. This expert group identified a list of medications considered inappropriate for older patients, either because they are ineffective or because they pose a high risk for adverse events. The list included long-elimination half-life benzodiazepines (e.g., diazepam) and hypoglycemic agents with long half-lives (chlorpropamide), antidepressants with strong anticholinergic properties (e.g., amitriptyline), and ineffective dementia treatments (e.g., cyclandelate). The Beers criteria were revised in 1997 and again in 2003 to make them more relevant to current prescribing issues and to generalize them beyond the nursing home setting. The 1997 revision recategorized the 33 medications deemed inappropriate according to the Beers criteria into three groups: (1) drugs that should always be avoided (e.g., barbiturates, chlorpropamide); (2) drugs that are rarely appropriate (e.g., diazepam, propoxyphene); and (3) drugs with some indications, but that are often misused (e.g., oxybutynin, diphenhydramine). The 2003 reorganization acknowledged that precise information to evaluate appropriateness may be lacking; two categories were generated: (1) medications or medications classes that should generally be avoided in persons 65 years or older because they are either ineffective or they pose unnecessarily high risk for older persons and a safer alternative is available and (2) medications that should not be used in older persons known to have specific medical conditions.

Use of drug therapies considered inappropriate according to the Beers criteria has been identified as an ongoing problem among community-dwelling older adults. The prevalence of inappropriate drug use remained steady between 1995 and 2000. Using the subset of the 20 drug therapies from the original Beers criteria that should be entirely avoided, 23.5% of community-dwelling older adults in the United States, as identified using the 1987 National Medical Expenditure Survey, were found to be taking one or more of the inappropriate medications. Three percent used at least one of the 11 drug therapies that the panel determined should always be avoided by older adults. Data from other surveys showed that the risk of hospitalization, emergency department visits, and death were greater for nursing home patients who had been prescribed potentially inappropriate medications.

The Health Care Financing Administration (now called The Centers for Medicare and Medicaid Services) expert consensus panel drug utilization review criteria have also been used to evaluate inappropriate prescribing in community-dwelling older adults. These criteria target eight prescription drug classes (i.e., digoxin, calcium channel-blockers, angiotensin-converting enzyme (ACE) inhibitors, histamine-2 receptor antagonists, nonsteroidal antiinflammatory drugs (NSAIDs), benzodiazepines, antipsychotics, and antidepressants) and focus on four types of prescribing problems: (1) use of an inappropriate dosage; (2) duplication of therapies; (3) potential for drug–drug interactions; and (4) inappropriate duration of therapy. Based on the criteria, almost 20% of 2508 community-dwelling older adults were found to be using one or more medications inappropriately. NSAIDs and benzodiazepines were the drug classes identified with the most frequent potential problems.

Unfortunately, the vast majority of medications that are commonly implicated in preventable ADEs are not identified by these widely used "bad drug" lists. Inappropriate prescribing is often more subtle, more pervasive, and often unrecognized. "Good drugs" prescribed in an inappropriate manner may be far more common and problematic. Very few drugs that cause difficulty for older adults are inherently bad. To address these concerns, a more comprehensive approach to evaluating the quality of pharmacologic care for older adults was developed by the Assessing Care of Vulnerable Elders (ACOVE) project. These include 12 quality indicators for appropriate medication use identified by Knight and Avorn. Table 24-1 describes each of the 12 indicators and summarizes the rationale for its need. These indicators start with the need to document the indication for a new drug therapy, to educate patients on the benefits and risks associated with the use of a new therapy, the need to maintain current medication lists in patient medical records, the importance of documenting response to therapy, and the need for a periodic review of drug therapies. In addition, these indicators specify seven drug therapies that either should not be prescribed for older adults (i.e., hypoglycemic agent chlorpropamide, drugs with strong anticholinergic properties, barbituates, and meperidine) or that warrant careful monitoring after they have been initiated (i.e., warfarin, diuretic, and ACE inhibitor therapy).

Underprescribing of potentially useful medications is at least as problematic as overprescribing of potentially harmful medications. Using a subset of ACOVE quality indicators and a sample of 372 vulnerable older adults in two managed care organizations, investigators determined the proportion of patients who met criteria for underprescribing potentially useful medications and overprescribing potentially harmful medications. Of nine quality indicators measuring the overprescribing of harmful medications, eight had a pass rate of 90% or greater. Of 17 quality indicators measuring the underprescribing of useful medications, only 1 had a pass rate of 90% or greater; eight had a pass rate of less than 60%. In another study, investigators found coexistence of both the inappropriate use of harmful medications and the under use of beneficial medications in 42% of study patients; 13% had neither. The complexity of safe and effective prescribing for older adults with multiple chronic conditions makes the determination of appropriate prescribing difficult to assess. Defining over- and underprescribing outside the context of individual measures of disease burden, total medication use, and preferences may be misleading and fraught with unintended consequences. These estimates of over- and underprescribing should, therefore, be interpreted cautiously.

PRESCRIBING CASCADES

A particularly concerning aspect of suboptimal medication use in older adults relates to the occurrence of prescribing cascades. A prescribing cascade begins when an ADE is misinterpreted as a new medical condition. An additional drug therapy is prescribed, and the patient is placed at risk for the development of additional ADEs relating to this potentially unnecessary treatment (Figure 24-3). Prescribing cascades and other risks associated with drug therapy are particularly important for older adults with multiple chronic diseases who are likely to be prescribed multiple drug therapies. Selected examples of prescribing cascades are described below.

Drug-Induced Parkinsonism

Among 95 new cases of Parkinson's disease from community-dwelling older adults referred to a geriatric medicine department

TABLE 24-1

Quality Indicators for Appropriate Medication Use in Older Adults

INDICATOR TITLE	DESCRIPTION	RATIONALE
Indication	When prescribing a new drug, the therapy should have a clearly defined indication documented in the medical record.	The medication may have been prescribed for an indication that was unclear or transient.
Patient education	When prescribing a new drug, the patient or caregiver should be educated about the optimal use of the therapy and the anticipated adverse events.	Education may improve adherence, clinical outcomes, and alert patients or caregivers to potential adverse events.
Medication list	Medical records (outpatient or hospital) should contain a current medication list.	Allows identification and elimination of duplicate therapies, corrects drug interactions, and streamlines the drug regimen to improve adherence.
Response to therapy	Every new drug prescribed on an ongoing basis (e.g., for a chronic condition) should have documentation of response of therapy within 6 months.	Provides a rationale for continuation of the therapy if effective, or change or discontinuation if ineffective.
Periodic drug review	Annual drug regimen review.	Provides an opportunity to discontinue unnecessary therapy or to add needed drug therapies.
Monitoring warfarin therapy	When warfarin is prescribed, international normalized ratio (INR) should be evaluated within 4 days and at least every 6 weeks.	Older adults are at high risk for drug toxicity that can be identified earlier if there is close monitoring for agents with a narrow therapeutic range.
Monitoring diuretic therapy	When a thiazide or loop diuretic therapy is prescribed, electrolytes should be checked within 1 week after initiation and at least annually.	Risk of hypokalemia because of diuretic therapy.
Avoid use of chlorpropamide as a hypoglycemic agent	When prescribing an oral hypoglycemic agent, chlorpropamide should not be used.	This therapy has a prolonged half-life that can result in serious hypoglycemia and is more likely than other agents to cause the syndrome of inappropriate secretion of antidiuretic hormone.
Avoid drugs with strong anticholinergic properties	Do not prescribe drug therapies with a strong anticholinergic effect if alternative therapies are available.	These therapies are associated with adverse events such as confusion, urinary retention, constipation, and hypotension.
Avoid barbituates	If older adult does require the therapy for control of seizures, do not use barbiturates.	These therapies are potent central nervous system depressants, have a low therapeutic index, are highly addictive, cause drug interactions, and are associated with an increased risk for falls and hip fracture.
Avoid meperidine as an opioid analgesic	When analgesia is required, avoid use of meperidine.	This therapy is associated with an increased risk for delirium and may be associated with the development of seizures.
Monitor renal function and potassium in patients prescribed angiotensin-converting enzyme inhibitors	If angiotensin-converting enzyme inhibitor therapy is initiated, potassium and creatinine levels should be monitored with 1 week of initiation of therapy.	Monitoring may prevent the development of renal insufficiency and hyperkalemia.

Data from Knight E, Avron J. Quality indicators for appropriate medications use in vulnerable elders. Ann Intern Med. 2001;135(Pt 2):703.

in the United Kingdom, more than half were found to have drug-induced Parkinsonism. Conventional antipsychotic medications such as haloperidol, prochlorperazine, and thioridazine were among the major drug therapies implicated.

The association between antipsychotic drug exposure and subsequent treatment of Parkinsonism was identified among 3512 adults aged 65 to 99 years who were enrolled in a Medicaid program and initiated on a drug therapy for the treatment of Parkinsonian symptoms. Patients dispensed a antipsychotic therapy in the 90 days prior to the initiation of anti-Parkinson's therapy were more than five times more likely to begin anti-Parkinson's therapy relative to control patients who were not dispensed antipsychotic therapy. Furthermore, a dose–response relationship was demonstrated.

Antipsychotic therapy is widely used in older adults for the management of behavioral problems associated with dementia. Antidopaminergic-related adverse effects associated with these agents have long been recognized, including the development of extrapyramidal signs and symptoms. This drug-related symptom may be potentially misdiagnosed as a new medical condition (i.e., Parkinson's disease). A recent study has demonstrated that even the newer

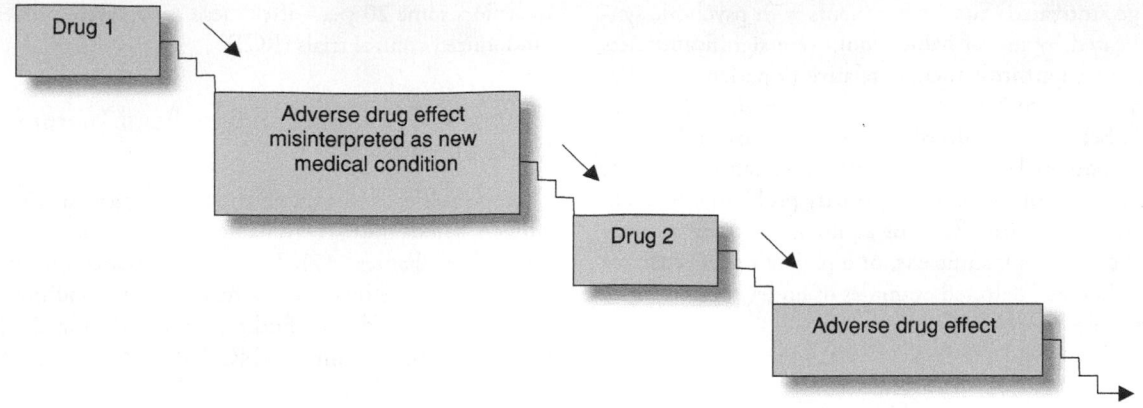

FIGURE 24-3. Prescribing cascade. *(Adapted from Rochon PA, Gurwitz JH. Drug therapy. Lancet. 1995;346:32.)*

"atypical" antipsychotics can be associated with Parkinsonism in a dose-related fashion. Patients who are placed on anti-Parkinsonian therapy then become vulnerable to the adverse events associated with this new therapy, including hypotension and delirium. A better approach is to discontinue or reduce the dose of the antipsychotic therapy. If an antipsychotic is deemed essential, it is prudent to select a therapy with a more favorable adverse effect profile and to use this therapy at the lowest feasible dose. Even newer agents have adverse effects at higher doses.

Drug-induced Parkinsonism has also been reported with other drug therapies, including metoclopramide. A case–control study of adults aged 65 years and older in the New Jersey Medicaid Program demonstrated that metoclopramide users were three times more likely to begin drug treatment for Parkinson's disease as compared with nonusers. Risk increased with increasing daily metoclopramide dose such that the odds ratio was 1.19 for up to 10 mg/day, 3.33 for 10 to 20 mg/day, and 5.25 for >20 mg/day. Thus, drug-induced Parkinsonism may lead to the initiation of anti-Parkinson drug therapy. Such drug-induced symptoms in an older person can be misinterpreted as indicating the presence of a new disease or be attributed to the aging process rather than to the drug therapy. This misinterpretation is particularly likely when the symptoms are indistinguishable from an illness, such as Parkinson's disease that is seen in greater frequency in older persons.

Acetylcholinesterase Inhibitors and Anticholinergic Therapy

Cholinesterase inhibitors (such as donepezil, rivastigmine, and galantamine) are often prescribed to manage the symptoms of Alzheimer's disease and related dementias. Through their effects on the autonomic nervous system, cholinesterase inhibitors can sometimes precipitate urge urinary incontinence. However, new-onset or worsening urge incontinence is also commonly seen as part of the natural history of dementia. Thus, clinicians may misinterpret incontinence in patients with dementia as an unavoidable progression of their underlying disease, when it may in fact represent a potentially reversible drug-related adverse event. A population-based cohort study demonstrated that cholinesterase inhibitor use was associated with an increased risk of receiving anticholinergic medications to manage urinary incontinence. This study suggests the use of anticholinergic drugs in patients with dementia may sometimes represent an unrecognized ADE related to cholinesterase inhibitor use. The use of anticholinergic drugs by older adults with dementia may expose them to anticholinergic adverse effects (such as urinary retention and postural hypotension) and may also dilute the benefits of cholinesterase inhibitor treatment.

Other prescribing cascade scenarios, such as the association between the use of hydrochlorothiazide therapy and the initiation of antigout therapy or the use of NSAID therapy and hypertension, have been identified. Many more potential prescribing cascades will become apparent as physicians carefully consider the relationship between the initiation of a new drug therapy, the adverse event profile of that therapy, and the development of a new medical condition. The increased recognition of similar prescribing scenarios hopefully will reduce the occurrence of inappropriate prescribing decisions.

UNDERUSE OF BENEFICIAL THERAPY

Prescribing strategies that seek to simply limit the overall number of drugs prescribed to older adults in the name of improving quality of care may be misdirected. For example, a patient with a myocardial infarction maybe prescribed three essential drug therapies: a beta-blocker, an ACE inhibitor, and acetylsalicylic acid. If this patient has elevated lipid levels and diabetes, three or more additional medications maybe required. Accordingly, many elderly persons may benefit from taking six or more essential medications. Under use of beneficial drug therapy by older adults may be associated with increased morbidity, mortality, and reduced quality of life. This suggests a need for a more complex model for assessing the quality and appropriateness of prescribing for older persons than simply counting the number of different medications that a patient is receiving. This complex model should be directed toward assessing the potential benefit versus harm of the patient's total medication regimen. One proposed model for the initiation or discontinuation of medications for older adults in late life considers remaining life expectancy, time until benefit will be achieved, the patient's goals of care and whether the medication can meet treatment goals. For example, if a patient's life expectancy is short and the goals of care are palliative, then prescribing a prophylactic medication requiring several years to realize a benefit may not be considered appropriate.

For patients of advanced age with multiple medical problems, secondary prevention may not be given a high priority. Among patients 65 years of age or older who have a chronic condition, unrelated diseases often go untreated. Similarly, patients with psychotic syndromes, as indicated by use of haloperidol, were significantly less likely to be dispensed arthritis therapy relative to patients without psychoses (18% relative to 27%, $p < 0.001$). While an understanding of the logic behind these decisions for individual patients remains uncertain, potential explanations for under treatment include "a belief that treatment of the patient's primary problem is enough; a judgment that the adverse effects of additional medications are too great and the benefits insufficient; or a patient's preference for taking fewer medicines." Selected examples of under prescribing of beneficial therapy are described below.

Example of Underuse of Beneficial Therapy: Hypertension

Despite the availability of guidelines to facilitate hypertension management, this condition is inadequately treated even when physicians are monitoring their patients in a clinic. For example, among 800 men with hypertension with a mean age of 65 years receiving care in Veterans Affairs outpatient clinics in New England, approximately 40% had a blood pressure of 160/90 mm Hg despite an average of more than six hypertension-related visits in a year. At visits in which a diastolic blood pressure of <90 mm Hg and a systolic blood pressure of >165 mm Hg were recorded, increases in the antihypertensive regimen occurred only 22% of the time. The Systolic Hypertension in the Elderly Person (SHEP) study demonstrated that treating isolated systolic hypertension in people 60 years of age and older reduced the risk of stroke by 36% ($p = 0.0003$) and also reduced major cardiovascular events relative to the placebo condition.

Example of Underuse of Beneficial Therapy: Beta-Blocker Therapy Postmyocardial Infarction

Studies demonstrate that older adults, including those at high-risk for poor outcomes, benefit from beta-blocker therapy postmyocardial infarction. The relation between beta-blocker use and subsequent mortality was evaluated among New Jersey Medicare recipients sustaining an acute myocardial infarction between 1987 and 1992. Among those dispensed beta-blocker therapy, mortality was decreased by 43% relative to nonrecipients of this agent (aRR = 0.57). In a sample of "ideal" beta-blocker therapy candidates in the Cooperative Cardiovascular Project's cohort of myocardial infarction survivors between 1994 and 1995, being discharged from hospital with a prescription for beta-blocker therapy was associated with a 14% mortality reduction (aRR = 0.86).

Withholding beta-blocker therapy maybe most harmful to seniors of advanced age and with potential contraindications to beta-blocker therapy. Among 201 752 seniors participating in the Cooperative Cardiovascular Project, patients at high-risk for beta-blocker-related complications (i.e., patients with heart failure, pulmonary disease, and diabetes) obtained substantial mortality reduction when prescribed beta-blocker therapy relative to those who were not prescribed this treatment. For example, patients with congestive heart failure treated with beta-blocker therapy had a 40% mortality reduction relative to nonrecipients. While it is impossible to eliminate unmeasured confounding as at least a partial explanation for this survival benefit in recipients versus nonrecipients, observational studies suggest continued under prescribing of beta-blocker therapy

to seniors some 20 years after these agents were proven effective in randomized control trials (RCTs).

Example of Underuse of Beneficial Therapy: Osteoporosis

Osteoporosis is a common condition, particularly among older women. Guidelines are available for the management of the condition (see Chapter 117). To treat osteoporosis, it must first be diagnosed. Despite increasing attention, this condition continues to be underdiagnosed. The findings obtained from the National Osteoporosis Risk Assessment (NORA) study illustrate this problem. The NORA study is a longitudinal observational study of more than 200 000 postmenopausal women to evaluate the relationship between bone mineral density and the risk for fractures. Ambulatory, postmenopausal women with no previous diagnosis of osteoporosis and not on osteoporosis therapy (i.e., bisphosphonate, calcitonin, or raloxifene) were eligible. Of the patients evaluated 39.6% were classified as having osteopenia and 7.2% with osteoporosis. Among the individuals with follow-up information at 1 year, those with osteopenia were almost twice as likely to develop a fracture relative to those with normal bone mineral density. Those older women with a diagnosis of osteoporosis were four times as likely to develop a fracture during the 1 year of follow-up relative to those with a normal bone mineral density. These findings suggest that undiagnosed low bone mineral density is very common in postmenopausal women and is associated with a high rate of fractures. Improved measures aimed at primary prevention in combination with better diagnosis could lead to better outcomes for older women.

Example of Underuse of Beneficial Therapy: Opioid Analgesia and Cancer Pain

Opioid analgesia reduces pain and improves quality of life for cancer patients. Underprescribing of analgesia for cancer pain means that older patients may suffer needless discomfort. Pain guidelines are available to assist physicians in managing pain associated with metastatic cancer. In a study of 1308 outpatients with metastatic cancer being followed by oncologists, 769 patients reported experiencing pain, which 62% described as being substantial. Furthermore, older patients were more likely than younger patients to report that their pain was not being adequately managed. Older persons may be at risk of undertreatment because of a reluctance to prescribe opioid analgesics to older cancer patients. If analgesics are prescribed, the dose may not be adequate to achieve pain control. Efforts to address underprescribing of beneficial therapy in the elderly population must focus on educating health care providers, improving the adherence to prescribed drug regimens by older patients, and reducing the financial barriers to access to essential medications.

Example of Underuse of Beneficial Therapy: Warfarin in Atrial Fibrillation

Warfarin is recommended in evidence-based guidelines for stroke prevention for older adults with atrial fibrillation, but is often inappropriately prescribed to older adults in long-term care setting. Among 429 residents of long-term care facilities with atrial fibrillation, 42% were prescribed warfarin therapy. Of the 83 older adults who were classified as being "ideal" candidates for warfarin therapy (i.e., no known risk factors for hemorrhage), only half (53%) were prescribed this therapy. Furthermore, international normalized ratio (INR) readings were often found to be either below or above the therapeutic range. In fact, INR values were maintained in the therapeutic range only 51% of the time, placing patients at unnecessary risk for an adverse event despite long-term care residents residing in a supervised setting.

The American Geriatrics Society and the ACOVE project introduced guidelines to address the need for a more systematic approach to decision-making regarding the use of warfarin for stroke prevention in frail older persons. The proposed strategy guides the consideration of appropriate use of warfarin therapy and encourages more frequent monitoring until INR is stable in older adults because of the increased risk of hemorrhage. More widespread use of specialized anticoagulation clinics in order to provide coordinated anticoagulation care may offer an option to improve the effectiveness and safety of warfarin therapy in this particularly high-risk group of patients.

SPECIAL CONSIDERATIONS REGARDING DRUG THERAPY IN THE LONG-TERM CARE SETTING

Long-term care residents include a disproportionate number of women, people of advanced age, and those with multiple medical problems, in particular dementia. Of all types of therapeutic interventions, medications are the most commonly used in the nursing home setting. The average U.S. nursing home resident uses six different medications; more than 20% use 10 or more different drugs, placing this group at increased risk of ADEs.

Antipsychotic Therapy in the Long-Term Care Setting

In long-term care facilities, excess use of antipsychotic therapy for the management of behavioral problems is an area of concern. Atypical antipsychotic medications are among the drugs most frequently associated with adverse events in long-term care facilities. Use is widespread and a study of 19,780 older adults with no history of major psychosis prior to long-term care admission found that antipsychotic therapy was prescribed for 24% within 1 year. Further, there is marked variation in the use of antipsychotic therapies in the nursing home. A study of antipsychotic therapy use in 47 322 residents of 485 provincially regulated nursing homes found that the mean rate of antipsychotic prescribing ranged from 20.9% in facilities with the lowest mean prescribing rates and 44.3% in facilities with highest mean prescribing rates. Compared with individuals residing in nursing homes with the lowest mean antipsychotic prescribing rates, those residing in facilities with highest rates were three times more likely to be dispensed an antipsychotic therapy irrespective of their potential clinical indication. There is recent evidence that the benefit from atypical antipsychotics for management of behavioral and psychological symptoms in Alzheimer's type dementia may be offset by the risk of ADEs. There is also evidence about the risk of death with both conventional and atypical antipsychotic medications warranting careful monitoring. Health Canada and the Food and Drug Administration have issued warnings about their use. Given these important safety concerns, use of antipsychotic therapy should generally be reserved for situations where the benefit outweighs the risk. Specifically, antipsychotic therapy is potentially indicated to manage psychoses and for situations where the behavioral problems pose a risk to the resident or others.

An Institute of Medicine report on improving the quality of care in nursing homes in the United States determined that excessive use of antipsychotic therapy was evidence of poor quality of care. Concern about overuse of antipsychotic therapy led to the introduction of guidelines and legislative action in the United States designed to reduce antipsychotic therapy use in long-term care. As a result of these U.S. federal regulations implemented in 1990, the indication for treatment with antipsychotic therapy now has to be documented, nonpharmacologic approaches must be tried first, and a record of gradual reduction of therapy has to be on file after 6 months of treatment. Following the institution of these federal guidelines, antipsychotic therapy in nursing homes decreased by 27% with no compensatory increase in use of other psychoactive medications.

Risk of Adverse Drug Events in the Long-term Care Setting

The occurrence of ADEs that may have been prevented is among the most serious concerns regarding suboptimal medication use in the nursing home setting. Few studies have systematically examined the incidence of ADEs in the nursing home population. A retrospective review of incident reports relating to adverse and unexpected events in an academically oriented, 700-bed, long-term care facility identified 50 reports of adverse drug reactions over a 1-year period. Skin rashes were the most frequently reported events, and antibiotics were the most commonly implicated medication category. The limited number of reports of drug-related events suggests that voluntary reporting systems in the nursing home setting lead to very low reporting rates of only a very narrow spectrum of events.

In recent cohort study of two academic long-term care facilities in Ontario and Connecticut over a 9-month period, drug-related incidents were detected by computer-generated signals from a computerized physician order entry system, clinical pharmacist investigators, and periodic review of medical record. Incidents were classified by physician reviewers according to whether they represented an ADE, and if so, the severity (significant, serious, life-threatening, and fatal) and preventability of the event. During this study 815 ADEs were identified (9.8 ADEs per 100 resident-months). Of these, 42% were judged preventable. Of all ADEs, 4 (<1%) were fatal, 33 (4%) were life-threatening, 188 (23%) were serious, and 590 (72%) were less serious.

In this study, residents using anticoagulants, atypical antipsychotic agents, diuretics, antiinfectives, and antiepileptics were at the greatest risk of ADE. Psychoactive drugs (i.e., antipsychotics, antidepressants, and sedatives/hypnotics), cardiovascular and anticoagulants were the most commonly implicated drug categories associated with the occurrence of preventable ADEs (Table 24-2). Confusion, oversedation, delirium, and hemorrhagic events were the most commonly identified preventable ADEs (Table 24-3). Errors resulting in preventable ADEs occurred most often at the stages of ordering and monitoring. Among the prescribing errors, the most common were wrong dose, wrong drug choice, and known drug interaction. Dispensing and administration errors were less commonly identified. Independent risk factors for experiencing a preventable ADE included using medications in several drug categories, including antipsychotic agents, anticoagulants, diuretics, and antiepileptic. Extrapolating

TABLE 24-2

Frequency of Adverse Drug Events and Potential Adverse Drug Events by Drug Class*

DRUG CLASS	ADVERSE DRUG EVENTS NO. (%) (n = 815)	PREVENTABLE ADVERSE DRUG EVENTS NO. (%) (n = 318)	NONPREVENTABLE ADVERSE DRUG EVENTS NO. (%) (n = 497)
Atypical and typical antipsychotics	110 (11)	52 (16)	58 (12)
Antibiotics/antiinfectives	106 (13)	5 (2)	101 (20)
Antidepressants	77 (9)	41 (13)	36 (7)
Sedatives/hypnotics	61 (8)	43 (14)	18 (4)
Anticoagulants	167 (21)	65 (20)	102 (21)
Antiseizure	40 (5)	22 (7)	18 (4)
Cardiovascular	195 (24)	98 (31)	97 (20)
Hypoglycemics	49 (6)	26 (8)	23 (5)
Nonopioid analgesics	26 (3)	16 (5)	10 (2)
Opioids	51 (6)	26 (8)	25 (5)
Antiparkinsonians	11 (1)	4 (1)	7 (1)

*Drugs in more than one category were associated with some events. Frequencies in each column sum to greater than the total number cited.
Adapted from Gurwitz, JH, Field TS, Judge J, et al. The incidence of adverse drug events in two large academic long-term care facilities. Am J Med. 2005;118:251.

TABLE 24-3

Frequency of Adverse Drug Events by Type*

TYPE	NUMBER (%) Adverse Drug Events (n = 815)	NUMBER (%) Preventable (n = 338)
Neuropsychiatric[†]	199 (24)	97 (29)
Hemorrhagic	159 (20)	53 (16)
Gastrointestinal	140 (17)	55 (16)
Electrolye/fluid balance abnormality	80 (10)	40 (12)
Metabolic/endocrine	64 (8)	35 (10)
Dermatologic	36 (4)	4 (1)
Cardiovascular	36 (4)	15 (4)
Extrapyramidal symptoms/ tardive dyskinesia	30 (4)	7 (2)
Fall without injury	21 (3)	11 (3)
Fall with injury	21 (3)	17 (5)
Infection	19 (2)	1 (<1)
Syncope/dizziness	16 (2)	8 (2)
Anticholinergic[‡]	9 (1)	3 (1)
Ataxia/difficulty with gait	9 (1)	5 (2)
Hematologic	8 (1)	3 (1)
Respiratory	6 (1)	4 (1)
Anorexia/weight loss	3 (<1)	2 (<1)
Functional decline[§]	3 (<1)	2 (<1)
Hepatic	1 (<1)	1 (<1)

*Adverse drug events could manifest as more than one type.
[†]Neuropsychiatric events include over sedation, confusion, hallucinations, and delirium.
[‡]Anticholinergic effects include dry mouth, dry eyes, urinary retention, and constipation.
[§]Adverse drug event manifested only as decline in activities of daily living without any other more specific type of event. Other types of events may have been associated with functional decline.
Adapted from Gurwitz, JH, Field TS, Judge J, et al. The incidence of adverse drug events in two large academic long-term care facilities. Am J Med. 2005;118:251.

from the results of this research, 1.9 million ADEs per year may occur among the 1.6 million U.S. nursing home residents and more than 40% maybe preventable. There are almost 86 000 fatal or life-threatening ADEs per year, of which 70% maybe preventable. Drug-related morbidity and mortality is an important area to target in efforts to both improve the quality of medical care for older persons and reduce the costs of health care for this population.

Failures in the design of systems of care often contribute to the occurrence of medical errors, as well as the injuries that result from some of those errors. Enhanced surveillance and reporting systems for ADEs occurring in the nursing home setting are required as are continued educational efforts relating to the optimal use of drug therapies in the frail elderly patient population. However, as Leape et al. (1995) concluded in regard to the occurrence of serious medication errors in the hospital setting, "preventive efforts that focus solely on the individual provider or which rely on inspection alone have limited impact. Analysis and the correction of underlying systems faults is much more likely to result in enduring changes and significant error reduction." Ordering and monitoring errors in the nursing home setting maybe particularly amenable to prevention strategies that use systems-based approaches. The benefits of such an approach to error reduction in the hospital setting that uses computerized order entry have been reported. For example, a computer-based decision aid reduced in-hospital inappropriate dosing of psychotropic medications for geriatric inpatients. Successes in the hospital setting pave the way for similar efforts in the nursing home setting aimed at reducing drug-related injuries and disability and improving the quality of care provided to the frail elderly patient population. At least one large Canadian academic long-term care facility has adopted a computerized order entry system with decision aids for prescribing to improve the quality of medication prescribing. Figure 24-4 is an example of the kind of decision support, which provides drug therapy dosing recommendations in patients with renal impairment.

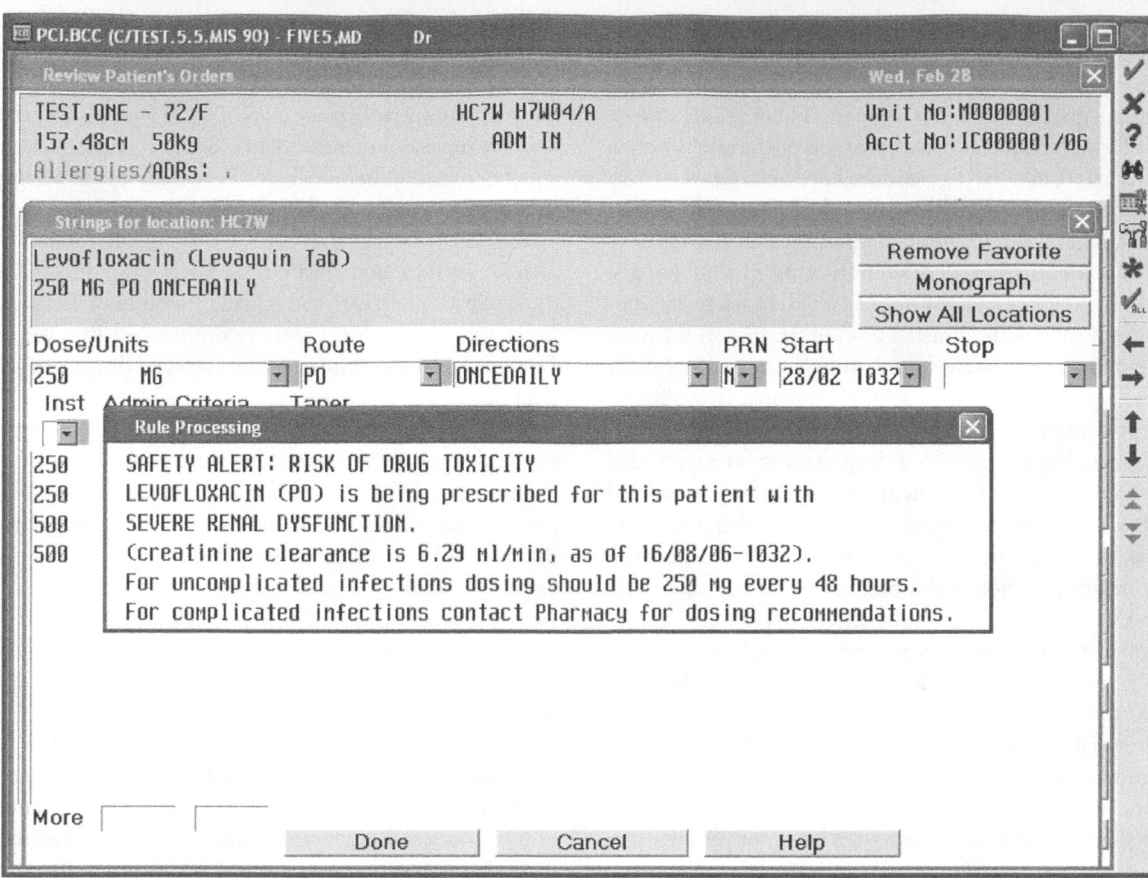

FIGURE 24-4. Example of computerized physician order entry.

DEFICIENCIES IN INFORMATION ABOUT DRUG THERAPY IN OLDER ADULTS

Selecting the right medication and the right dose to prescribe for an older person is difficult because so little evidence is available to guide choices. Decision-making often has to draw on information obtained from the experience of patients very different from those encountered in clinical practice, where patients often have several medical conditions and are taking more than one drug. The findings of clinical trials of treatments for conditions commonly affecting older people cannot directly be extrapolated to that age group, as older persons, particularly frail persons and those with multiple illnesses, have often been excluded from participation in such studies. This poses challenges to the adoption of clinical practice guidelines developed to improve the quality of health care for many chronic conditions. A review of clinical practice guidelines for nine common chronic diseases promulgated by national and international medical organizations found that most clinical practice guidelines did not modify or discuss the applicability of their recommendations for older patients with multiple comorbidities. Most did not comment on burden, short- and long-term goals, and the quality of the underlying scientific evidence, nor give guidance for incorporating patient preferences into treatment plans. But clinical practice guidelines have important implications for medication prescribing. This study describes an example where, if the relevant guidelines were followed, a hypothetical 79-year-old patient with osteoporosis,

osteoarthritis, type 2 diabetes mellitus, hypertension, and chronic obstructive pulmonary disease would be prescribed 12 medications. There are several ways in which the quality and availability of information about the use of drugs in older persons might be improved. These include enhancing the inclusion of older persons in drug trials, and using observational studies and systematic reviews to provide information to guide clinical decision making.

Inclusion of Older Persons in Clinical Trials

Approximately two decades ago, the United States Food and Drug Administration published "Guidelines for the Study of Drugs Likely to be Used in the Elderly." The guideline was intended to encourage routine and thorough evaluation in elderly populations of the effects of new drugs being proposed for federal approval so that physicians would have sufficient information to use such drugs properly in their older patients. The guidelines state "there is no good basis for the exclusion of patients on the basis of advanced age alone, or because of the presence of any concomitant illness or medication, unless there is a reason to believe that the concomitant illness or medication will endanger the patient or lead to confusion in interpreting the results of the study." In short, drug trials should include subjects that reflect the group that would eventually be prescribed the therapy.

Despite these guidelines, older adults continue to be underrepresented in clinical trials. For example, while almost 50% of older people report some form of arthritis, RCTs of NSAID therapy include few older people and hardly any older than age 85 years. National funding agencies, particularly the National Institutes of Health in the United States, have also developed guidelines to ensure that the trials they fund adequately represent women. These guidelines are very important for older adults because women outnumber men in the older age groups. While these guidelines have been received with enthusiasm, their impact on the inclusion of older women in clinical trials is less encouraging. For example, despite the fact that 80% of deaths caused by acute myocardial infarction occur in persons aged 65 years and older, older patients continue to be excluded from clinical trials. In a review of 214 randomized trials of treatments for acute myocardial infarction, 60% were found to exclude patients older than 75 years of age (Gurwitz et al., 1992). Similarly, it was found that women represented, on average, less than a quarter of participants in trials evaluating the benefit of drug therapy for myocardial infarction. In a comparison of the inclusion of elderly persons and women in trials of acute coronary syndromes (myocardial infarction, unstable angina, or acute coronary syndromes) published between 1966 and 1990 relative to those published between 1991 and 2000, trials with explicit age-related exclusion criteria were noted to decrease from 58% to 40% in more recent years. The inclusion of older patients (i.e., 75 years of age and older) increased from 2% between 1966 and 1990 to 9% between 1991 and 2000. The inclusion of women in these trials increased from 20% from 1966 to 1990 to 25% in the more recent years. However, this number remains below the number of women presenting with myocardial infarction. These findings suggest that federal guidelines have not yet met their expectation.

Using Alternative Study Designs to Study Drug-Related Risks and Benefits

Using alternative study designs as a complement to clinical trials may help to improve the quality and availability of information about the use of drug therapy by older persons. RCTs have long been considered the gold standard for evaluating the efficacy of a drug therapy. Ethical concerns may prevent the inclusion of the very impaired and the very old in RCTs and it maybe unrealistic to expect these studies to include adequate numbers of all relevant subgroups in the elderly population. In addition, there is mounting concern that such clinical trials are not the optimal way to evaluate ADEs in older adults. Drug trials are of relatively short duration. Drug-related problems that present months after initiating therapy may not be identified during the course of these relatively short trials. In general, drug trials focus on the efficacy of the therapy and give less emphasis to the potential risks associated with the use of the therapy. For example, in a survey of 192 randomized drug trials, the severity of clinical adverse events was adequately defined in fewer than 40% of the published trials. The amount of text devoted to the discussion of the adverse events was similar to that given to the listing of contributor's name and affiliations, suggesting underreporting of adverse events. Furthermore, the older persons included in RCTs have fewer comorbid illnesses than their age-matched peers. Thus, RCT results may not reflect the benefits or adverse effects of medications in frailer older persons or persons with multiple chronic illnesses.

Well-designed observational studies provide a promising approach for evaluating the relative risk and benefit of new drugs among subgroups of older persons who were not represented in clinical trials. Observational data may detect rare adverse events that become of major public health importance when a drug therapy is taken by very large numbers of people. For example, a study of adults 60 years and older from the Tennessee Medicaid program found that patients currently dispensed an NSAID were almost five times more likely as those not dispensed an NSAID to die from a peptic ulcer or a gastrointestinal hemorrhage. This study made an important contribution to alerting health care providers to important risks associated with commonly used therapy. Following the reporting of heart attacks, strokes, and deaths associated with the COX-2 inhibitor, rofecoxib (tradename: Vioxx), the Institute of Medicine Report of Reducing Medication Errors recommended that the United States Food and Drug Administration mandate drug manufacturers conduct postmarketing surveillance and risk assessments.

Observational data may also provide information about the benefits of drug therapy at doses that were not evaluated in clinical trials. The major RCTs demonstrating the benefit of beta-blocker therapy post myocardial infarction evaluated doses of beta-blocker therapy that are higher than those generally used in clinical practice. Using linked Ontario provincial databases, 10,991 myocardial infarction survivors were identified who were dispensed one of the evaluated beta-blocker therapies (i.e., atenolol, metoprolol, propranolol, or timolol). Almost 90% received a lower dose of a beta-blocker than have been evaluated in a clinical trial. Among 13,623 older myocardial infarction survivors in the province of Ontario, relative to those not dispensed beta-blocker therapies, the adjusted risk ratios for mortality were lower for all three doses (low, standard, or high) of beta-blocker therapy. In a study from the United States, myocardial infarction survivors dispensed beta-blocker therapy at doses less than half of that evaluated in clinical trials received substantial benefit from the therapy. These findings support the strategy of initiating beta-blocker therapy at low dose and titrating the dose as tolerated.

While there are many challenges in using observational data, careful attention to design and methodological issues maximize the likelihood of obtaining high-quality usable data. Inception cohorts using strict criteria ensure the identification of the populations at risk and the time of exposure. Risk-adjustment techniques enable the modeling of outcomes controlling for observed differences between exposed and unexposed groups. Despite their limitations, observational studies provide valuable information on the benefits and harms of medications when prescribed to actual patient in a real-world setting.

Systematic Reviews to Guide Therapeutic Decision Making

A systematic review provides another important source of information. Systematic reviews can be a useful way to organize and synthesize the vast amount of information available from clinical trials, which individually may include relatively small numbers of older people. By combining the information from older individuals obtained from a series of trials, useful information can be retrieved. Standardized reporting of trial data by age would make such analyses easier. The high-quality systematic reviews produced and maintained by the Cochrane Collaboration provide important information to improve the care of older adults with a specific medical condition. For example, in a systematic review of the evidence for pharmacotherapy for hypertension treatment in elderly persons, 15 hypertension trials involving 21 908 adults who were at least 60 years of age or older were evaluated. This review demonstrated that treating hypertension in elderly persons, at least the spectrum of elderly persons included in RCTs, reduces coronary heart disease and cerebrovascular morbidity and mortality. Systematic reviews can be used to summarize data and inform clinical decisions that clinicians have had to make empirically.

Better representation of older and frailer adults in clinical trials, the evaluation of the risks and benefits of drug therapy through the use of observational data, and the use of high-quality systematic reviews are examples of ways to improve the quality of information available to clinicians in making prescribing decisions for older patients. In the meantime, limitations on what is known about drug treatments for many common conditions in older persons suggest the need for special care in prescribing and extra caution in considering use of new products in older patients.

POLICY ISSUES RELATED TO DRUG THERAPY IN OLDER ADULTS

Cost-Related Adherence

A prescription maybe written but not filled, or filled and not taken regularly, because of financial considerations. The use of drug therapy has been shown to be directly related to coverage of drug costs. It is estimated that more than 40% of all Medicare enrollees in the United States had no coverage for outpatient drug expenditures prior to the implementation of the 2003 Medicare Modernization Act. In the United States, cost has been identified as an important reason that patients did not take medication that was prescribed by their health care provider. Specifically, among older adults, 13% of a national sample of 13 869 noninstitutionalized Medicare enrollees reported cost-related underuse of medications. Those in fair to poor health, with multiple comorbidities, and without coverage were most at risk.

Enhanced drug coverage for elderly persons may encourage the use of beneficial treatments. Among two groups of Medicare patients with heart disease, statins use ranged from 4.1% in those without coverage to 27% in those with employer-sponsored drug coverage ($p <.001$). Significant differences were also seen for use of relatively inexpensive beta-blocker therapy (20.7% vs. 36.1%; $p = .003$) and nitrates (20.4% vs. 38%; $p = .005$). This study suggests that older adults without drug coverage are less likely to be dispensed inexpensive life-saving drug therapy relative to those with drug coverage. Whether this difference is caused by the differences in drug coverage or to differences in characteristics of persons with and without such coverage is not clear.

Limited Manufacturing of Low-Dose Formulations of Recommended Drug Therapy

Limited manufacturing of low-dose formulations of drug therapy may make it more difficult for patients to take their prescribed drug therapy. Low-dose therapy is often recommended for older adults. For example, there is considerable evidence supporting the efficacy and greater safety of low doses of thiazide diuretic therapy in the treatment of hypertension in the older patient population. The Joint National Committee on Detection, Evaluation and Treatment of High Blood Pressure Guidelines (JNC VII) suggest starting antihypertensive therapy at low doses in all patients. Specifically, these guidelines suggest that therapy be initiated with a 12.5 mg dose of

TABLE 24-4

Five Steps of Medication Reconciliation

(1) Develop a list of current medications.
(2) Develop a list of medications to be prescribed.
(3) Compare the medications on the two lists.
(4) Make a clinical decision based on the comparison.
(5) Communicate the new list to the patient and appropriate caregivers.

Adapted from JCAHO Web site. http://www.jointcommission.org/SentinelEvents/ SentinelEventAlert/sea_35.htm.

a thiazide diuretic. Low doses of thiazide diuretics (e.g., 12.5 mg of hydrochlorothiazide) often produce as large an antihypertensive effect as larger doses, with a reduced risk of metabolic abnormalities. In fact, there is evidence that a dose of hydrochlorothiazide as low as 6.25 mg can be as efficacious in treating hypertension in many older patients, when combined with a low dose of another antihypertensive medication.

Medication Reconciliation

In the United States, the Joint Commission on Accreditation of Healthcare Organizations recently required accredited facilities to implement a system of medication reconciliation to reduce medication errors at transitions of care. Medication reconciliation is the process of comparing a patient's medication prescriptions to all the medications that the patient has been taking (Table 24-4). Patients, and responsible physicians, nurses, and pharmacists should be involved in the medication reconciliation process. This reconciliation is done to avoid medication errors such as omissions, duplications, dosing errors, or drug interactions. Changes in medication (different dose, discontinued therapies, additional therapies), common during transitions between hospital and nursing home or institutional setting and home, are a common source of medication errors and confusions. ADEs attributed to medication changes occurred in 20% of patients on transfer from hospital to a nursing home, occurring most commonly for patients being readmitted to the nursing home. One study found that discharged patients understood the potential side effects of their medications less frequently than their attending physicians believed. One Canadian multisite study found that 25% of 325 older adults experienced an ADE after discharge home from the hospital; half of these events were considered preventable. Medication reconciliation systems and processes have successfully reduced medication errors in many health care organizations. Pharmacy technicians at one hospital reduced potential ADEs by 80% within 3 months by obtaining medication histories of patients scheduled for surgery.

PRACTICAL APPROACH TO PRESCRIBING MEDICATIONS TO OLDER PERSONS

Review Current Drug Therapies

A periodic evaluation of the drug regimen that a patient is taking is an essential component of the medical care of an older person. Such a review may indicate the need for changes to prescribed drug therapy. These changes may include discontinuation of a therapy prescribed for an indication that no longer exists, substitution of a

TABLE 24-5

Practical Steps to Consider in Optimizing Drug Regimens for Older Adults

Review current drug therapy
Discontinue unnecessary therapy
Consider adverse drug events as a potential cause for any new symptom
Consider nonpharmacologic approaches
Substitute with safer alternatives
Reduce the dose

Modified from Rochon PA, Gurwitz JH. Drug therapy. Lancet. 1995;346:32.

required therapy with a potentially safer agent, reduction in dosage of a drug that the patient still needs to take, or an increase in dose or even addition of a new medication (Table 24-5). Randomized controlled trials examining the effect of medication reviews report mixed results. All studies reported that medication review leads to recommendations for different types of changes, including elimination of drugs, increasing the number of drugs, therapeutic substitutions, or better dosing. However, few reported statistically significant changes in patient drug use and drug expenditures. Studies that involved direct contact between the consulting pharmacist and the patient appeared to be more effective than interventions aimed at recommending drug changes to the patient's physician. One intervention study found that patients were resistant to reducing medications to recommended levels, particularly psychoactive drugs. To conduct a medication review, the physician should ask the patient to bring to the visit all the bottles of pills that they are using. For example, patients may not consider over-the-counter products, ointments, vitamins, ophthalmic preparations, or herbal medicines to be drug therapies. Patients need to be specifically told to bring these therapies to the visit. In addition, patients should be instructed to keep a complete, accurate, and up-to-date medication list including over-the-counter medications and herbal preparations. This list should be brought to every physician visit. A patient-generated list is particularly important as patients are prescribed medications from several physicians and receive their medications from several pharmacies. Although there are an increasing number of effective medications for preventing or controlling a range of illnesses and for alleviating many symptoms, several studies show that adherence decreases, and adverse medication effects increase, with the complexity of the medication regimen. The goal should thus be the simplest regimen that controls the patient's symptoms and illnesses, and optimizes disease prevention. A medication grid, which displays each medication with dosage and frequency, has been found effective at facilitating the reduction in medication complexity.

Discontinue Potentially Unnecessary Therapy

Physicians are often reluctant to stop medications, especially if they did not initiate the treatment and the patient seems to be tolerating the therapy. Sometimes, however, this exposes the patient only to the risks for an adverse event with limited or no therapeutic benefit. The use of chronic digoxin therapy among older adults with normal systolic function is one such example. Use of digoxin therapy by older adults is not without risk. Renal impairment that progresses over time or dehydration associated with a gastrointestinal or respiratory illness, or urinary tract infection, may predispose older adults to

digoxin toxicity. Often digoxin therapy has been prescribed for years for reasons that were not well documented. In a small study of 23 nursing home residents with normal sinus rhythm, normal ejection fraction, and no clinical evidence of heart failure, digoxin was discontinued in 14 residents. One patient developed a decreased ejection fraction (from 60% to 50%) and digoxin therapy was restarted even though the patient remained clinically asymptomatic. At 2 months following the discontinuation of digoxin therapy, all patients with digoxin therapy discontinued remained clinically stable. These findings suggest that digoxin can be safely discontinued in selected nursing home residents. Other investigators, however, have found that discontinuation of digoxin therapy in patients with impaired systolic function can have a detrimental effect.

Physicians should carefully consider whether the development of a new medical condition could be linked to an existing drug therapy before adding a new drug therapy to the patient's drug regimen. For example, tricyclic antidepressants such as amitriptyline are used for a variety of indications in elderly patients, from depression to the relief of chronic pain. The tricyclic antidepressants tend to have especially strong anticholinergic properties with the potential for side effects including constipation. A patient started on a strongly anticholinergic antidepressant may develop constipation. As a result, laxative therapy may be prescribed. A better alternative may be to discontinue the anticholinergic therapy.

Consider Nonpharmacologic Approaches

Physicians should limit prescribing of a new drug therapy to situations in which benefits clearly outweigh risks and to use drug therapy only after potentially safer alternatives have been attempted. For example, NSAIDs maybe extremely useful in treating patients with rheumatoid arthritis. However, the use of this medication to manage pain in older adults with osteoarthritis maybe inappropriate because safer options are available. Epidemiologic and clinical studies have characterized the adverse consequences of NSAID use in older persons, particularly the association between NSAID use and gastrointestinal bleeds and renal impairment. Thus, alternative approaches should be considered before NSAIDs are prescribed for indications such as osteoarthritis. Possible nonpharmacologic approaches, such as gentle exercise and weight reduction, may be beneficial alternatives to treatment with NSAIDs. When pharmacologic therapy is required, a drug therapy with a less-adverse event profile, such as acetaminophen, should be used.

Hypertension is another example of a condition for which nonpharmacologic treatments may be beneficial. Drug therapy is beneficial in reducing the risk of stroke and coronary heart disease associated with hypertension in older adults. However, use of drug therapy is associated with the potential for drug-related adverse events and can be costly, particularly when the therapy is required long-term. Nonpharmacologic approaches are an attractive option. The benefit of dietary sodium reduction and weight loss in the treatment of hypertension was recently examined. Three months following the intervention, a withdrawal of hypertension therapy was attempted and patients were followed for the combined outcome measure (i.e., occurrence of high blood pressure, treatment with an antihypertensive medication, or the occurrence of a cardiovascular event). Among 585 obese older adults, participants assigned to reduced sodium intake, weight loss alone, or to a reduced sodium intake and weight loss intervention were significantly more likely to remain free of an outcome relative to those participants assigned to usual care without a lifestyle intervention. This trial indicates restricting sodium intake and weight reduction are beneficial nonpharmacologic therapies for hypertension management in older adults.

Often when drug therapy is deemed necessary for the patient, a safer alternative to the current regimen is available. For example, if a patient is taking a long elimination half-life benzodiazepine such as diazepam and continued therapy is required, a shorter half-life agent may reduce risks associated with drug accumulation with repeated dosing especially in the context of age-related pharmacokinetic changes. Longer half-life agents are more likely to produce central nervous system adverse events such as daytime somnolence, confusion, and impaired motor coordination. The evidence remains inconclusive as to whether long-acting benzodiazepines are associated with an increased risk of hip fractures relative to shorter-acting preparations. Another study suggests that the benzodiazepine dose is a more important risk factor for hip fracture than the elimination half-life. Given this information, a prudent approach would be to avoid using both long elimination half-life and high doses of benzodiazepine therapy in older adults.

Reduce the Dose

Many ADEs are dose-related. A classic example of dose-related adverse events is the association between use of long elimination half-life hypnotic-anxiolytics, antipsychotics, and tricyclic antidepressants and the development of hip fracture. A dose-related association has been found for each class of drug. Many studies have illustrated dose-related ADEs. When prescribing drug therapies, it is important to use the minimal dose required to obtain clinical benefit.

SUMMARY

Optimizing drug therapy means achieving the balance between over prescribing of inappropriate therapy and underprescribing of beneficial therapy. Particular attention should be given to using all drug therapies only when required and at the minimum effective dose. Beneficial therapy should be prescribed when indicated. Financial pressures need to be recognized and strategies developed to make sure that older adults have access to drug therapies when needed. ADEs are common and system-level approaches need to be developed to minimize their impact.

FURTHER READING

Alla, J, Hebert R, Rioux M, et al. Efficacy of a clinical medication review on the number of potentially inappropriate prescriptions prescribed for community-dwelling elderly people. *CMAJ.* 2001;164:1291.

American Geriatrics Society Clinical Practice Committee. The use of oral anticoagulants (warfarin) in older people. *J Am Geriatr Soc.* 2002;50:1439.

Avorn J. Drugs and the elderly: wielding the double-edged sword. In: Avon J, ed. *The Medication Education Program.* Boston: Brigham and Women's Hospital Division of Pharmacoepidemiology and Pharmacoeconomics; 2003.

Bates DW, Leape LL, Cullen DJ, et al. Effect of computerized physician order entry and a team intervention on prevention of serious medication errors. *JAMA.* 1998;280:1311.

Beers M., Ouslander JG, Rollingher I, et al. Explicit criteria for determining inappropriate medication use in nursing homes residents. UCLA Division of Geriatric Medicine. *Arch Intern Med.* 1992;151:1825.

Beers MH. Explicit criteria for determining potentially inappropriate medication use by the elderly. An update. *Arch Intern Med.* 1997; 157:1531.

Boyd CM, Darer J, Boult C, et al. Clinical practice guidelines and quality of care for older patients with multiple comorbid diseases: implications for pay for performance. *JAMA.* 2005;294:716.

Bronskill SE, Anderson GM, Sykora K, et al. Neuroleptic drug therapy in older adults newly admitted to nursing homes: incidence, dose, and specialist contact. *J Am Geriatr Soc.* 2004;52:749.

Calkins DR, Davis RB, Reiley P, et al. Patient–physician communication at hospital discharge and patients' understanding of the postdischarge treatment plan. *Arch Intern Med.* 1997;157:1026.

Committee on the Assessment of the U.S. Drug Safety System. In: Baciu A, Stratton K, and Burke SP, eds. *The Future of Drug Safety: Promoting and Protecting the Health of the Public.* Washington, DC: The National Academies Press; 2007.

Eisenberg DM, Davis RB, Ettner SL, et al. Trends in alternative medicine use in the United States, 1990–1997: results of a follow-up national survey. *JAMA.* 1998;280:1569.

Eisenberg DM, Kessler RC, Foster C, et al. Unconventional medicine in the United States—prevalence, costs, and patterns of use. *N Eng J Med.* 1993;328:246.

Federman A, Adams AS, Ross-Degnan D, et al. Supplemental insurance and use of effective cardiovascular drugs among elderly Medicare beneficiaries. *JAMA.* 2001;286:1732.

Fick DM, Cooper JW, Wade WF, et al. Updating the Beers criteria for potentially inappropriate medication use in older adults: results of a US consensus panel of experts. *Arch Intern Med.* 2003;163:2716.

Food and Drug Administration: Guidelines for the study of drugs likely to be used in the elderly. Food and Drug Administration Centre for Drug Evaluation and Research; 1989.

Forman DE, Coletta D, Kenny D, et al. Clinical issues related to discontinuing digoxin therapy in elderly nursing home patients. *Arch Intern Med.* 1991;151:2194.

Forster AJ, Clark HD, Menard A, et al. Adverse events among medical patients after discharge from hospital. *CMAJ.* 2004;170:345.

Gandhi T, Weingart SN, Borus J, et al. Adverse drug events in ambulatory care. *N Eng J Med.* 2003;348:1556.

Garbutt JM, Highstein G, Jeffe DB, et al. Safe medication prescribing: training and experience of medical students and housestaff at a large teaching hospital. *Acad Med.* 2005;80:594.

Gill SS, Bronskill SE, Normand SL, Anderson GM, Sykora K, Lam K, Bell CM, Lee PE, Fischer HD, Herrmann N, Gurwitz JH, Rochon PA. Antipsychotic drug use and mortality in older adults with dementia. *Ann Intern Med.* 2007 Jun 5;146(11):775–86.

Gill SS, Mamdani M, Naglie G, et al. A prescribing cascade involving cholinesterase inhibitors and anticholinergic drugs. *Arch Intern Med.* 2005;165:808.

Gormley EA, Griffiths DJ, McCracken PN, et al. Polypharmacy and its effect on urinary incontinence in a geriatric population. *Br J Urol.* 1993;71:265.

Gottlieb SS, McCarter RJ, Vogel RA. Effect of beta blockade on mortality among high-risk and low-risk patients after myocardial infarction. *N Engl J Med.* 1998;339:489.

Goulding MR. Inappropriate medication prescribing for elderly ambulatory care patients. *Arch Intern Med.* 2004;164:305.

Gurwitz JH, Col NF, Avorn J. The exclusion of the elderly and women from clinical trials in acute myocardial infarction. *JAMA.* 1992;268:1417.

Gurwitz JH, Field TS, Harrold LR, et al. Incidence and preventability of adverse drug events among older persons in the ambulatory setting. *JAMA.* 2003;289:1107.

Gurwitz JH, Sanchez-Cross MT, Eckler MA, et al. The epidemiology of adverse and unexpected events in long-term care setting. *J Am Geriatr Soc.* 1994;42:33.

Gurwitz JH. Polypharmacy: a new paradigm for quality drug therapy in the elderly? *Arch Intern Med.* 2004;164:1957.

Gurwitz, JH, Field TS, Judge J, et al. The incidence of adverse drug events in two large academic long-term care facilities. *Am J Med.* 2005;118:251.

Hanlon JT, Schmader KE, Boult C, et al. Use of inappropriate prescription drugs by older people. *J Am Geriatr Soc.* 2002;50:26.

Health Canada. Endorsed Important Safety Information on ZYPREXA (olanzapine). 2004 [cited December 28, 2006]; Available from: http://www.hc-sc.gc.ca/hpfb-dgpsa/tpd-dpt/zyprexa_hpc_e.html.

Herings RM, Stricker BH, de Boer A, et al. Benzodiazepines and the risk of falling leading to femur fractures: dosage more important than elimination half-life. *Arch Intern Med.* 1995;155:1801.

Higashi T, Shekelle PG, Solomon DH, et al. The quality of pharmacologic care for vulnerable older patients. *Ann Intern Med.* 2004;140:714.

Holmes HM, Hayley DC, Alexander GC, et al. Reconsidering medication appropriateness for patients late in life. *Arch Intern Med.* 2006;166:605.

Jacox AD, Carr D, Payne R. New clinical-practice guidelines for the management of pain in patients with cancer. *N Engl J Med.* 1994;330:651.

Kaufman DW, Kelly JP, Rosenberg L, et al. Recent patterns of medication use in the ambulatory adult population of the United States: the Slone survey. *JAMA.* 2002;287:337.

Klarin I, Wimo A, Fastbom J. The association of inappropriate drug use with hospitalisation and mortality: a population-based study of the very old. *Drugs Aging.* 2005;22:69.

Knight E, Avron J. Quality indicators for appropriate medications use in vulnerable elders. *Ann Intern Med.* 2001;135(Pt 2):703.

Krumholz HM, Radford MJ, Wang Y, et al. National use and effectiveness of beta-blockers for the treatment of elderly patients after acute myocardial infarction. National Cooperative Cardiovascular Project. *JAMA.* 1998;280:623.

Lagnaoui R, Begaud B, Moore N, et al. Benzodiazepine use and risk of dementia: a nested case-control study. *J Clin Epidemiol.* 2002;55:314.

Lau HS, deBoer A, Beuning KS, et al. Validation of pharmacy records in drug exposure assessment. *J Clin Epidemiol.* 1997;50:619.

Leape LL, Bates DW, Cullen DJ, et al. Systems analysis of adverse drug events. *JAMA.* 1995;274:35.

Lenzer J. FDA warns about using antipsychotic drugs for dementia. [News roundup]. *BMJ.* 2005;330:922.

McCormick D, Gurwitz JH, Goldberg RJ, et al. Prevalence and quality of warfarin use for patients with atrial fibrillation in the long-term care setting. *Arch Intern Med.* 2001;161:2458.

Michels RD, Meisel SB. Program using pharmacy technicians to obtain medication histories. *Am J Health Sys Pharm.* 2003;60:1982.

Moawad M, Hassan W. Update in hypertension in the Seventh Joint National Committee Report and beyond. *Ann Saudi Medicine.* 2005;25:453.

Mulrow C, Lau J, Cornell J, et al. Pharmacotherapy for hypertension in the elderly, in *The Cochrane Library,* T.C. Collaboration, ed. The Cochrane Collaboration; 2002.

Paterniti S, Dufouil C, Alperovitch A. Long-term benzodiazepine use and cognitive decline in the elderly: the Epidemiology of Vascular Aging Study. *J Clin Psychopharmacol.* 2002;22:285.

Perri M 3rd, Menon AM, Deshpande AD, et al. Adverse outcomes associated with inappropriate drug use in nursing homes. *Ann Pharmacother.* 2005;39:405.

Peterson JF, Kuperman GJ, Shek C, et al. Guided prescription of psychotropic medications for geriatric inpatients. *Arch Intern Med.* 2005;165:802.

Redelmeier DA, Tan SH, Booth GL. The treatment of unrelated disorders in patients with chronic medical diseases. *N Eng J Med.* 1998;338:1516.

Rochon PA, Field TS, Bates DW, et al. Computerized physician order entry with clinical decision support in the long-term care setting: insights from the Baycrest Centre for Geriatric Care. *J Am Geriatr Soc.* 2005;53:1780.

Rochon PA, Gurwitz JH. Drug therapy. *Lancet.* 1995;346:32.

Rochon PA, Stukel TA, Sykora K, et al. Atypical Antipsychotics and Parkinsonism. *Arch Intern Med.* 2005;165:1882.

Rochon PA, Stukel TA.Bronskill SE., et al. Variations in nursing home antipsychotic prescribing rates. *Arch Intern Med.* 2007;167:676–683.

Rochon PA, Tu JV, Anderson GM, et al. Rate of heart failure and 1-year survival for older people receiving low-dose beta-blocker therapy after myocardial infarction. *Lancet.* 2000;356:639.

Schneider LS, Dagerman KS, Insel P. Risk of death with atypical antipsychotic drug treatment for dementia: meta-analysis of randomized placebo-controlled trials. *JAMA.* 2005;294:1934.

Schneider LS, Tariot PN, Dagerman KS, et al. Effectiveness of atypical antipsychotic drugs in patients with Alzheimer's disease. *N Eng J Med.* 2006;355:1525.

Sellors J, Kaczorowski J, Sellors C, et al. A randomized controlled trial of a pharmacist consultation program for family physicians and their elderly patients. *CMAJ.* 2003;169:17.

Siris ES, Miller PD, Barrett-Connor E, et al. Identification and fracture outcomes of undiagnosed low bone mineral density in postmenopausal women: results from the National Osteoporosis Risk Assessment. *JAMA.* 2001;286:2815.

Sorensen L, Stokes JA, Purdie DM, et al. Medication reviews in the community: results of a randomized, controlled effectiveness trial. *Br J Clin Pharmacol.* 2004;58:648.

Soumerai SB, McLaughlin TJ, Spiegelman D, et al. Adverse outcomes of under-use of Beta-blockers in elderly survivors of acute myocardial infarction. *JAMA.* 1997;277:115.

Soumerai SB, Pierre-Jacques M, Zhang F, et al. Cost-related medication nonadherence among elderly and disabled medicare beneficiaries: a national survey 1 year before the Medicare drug benefit. *Arch Intern Med.* 2006;166:1829.

Spinewine, A., Swine C, Dhillon S, et al. Appropriateness of use of medicines in elderly inpatients: qualitative study. *BMJ.* 2005;331:935.

Steinman MA, Landefeld CS, Rosenthal GE, et al. Polypharmacy and prescribing quality in older people. *J Am Geriatr Soc.* 2006;54:1516.

Systolic Hypertension in the Elderly Program Cooperative Research Group: Prevention of stroke by antihypertensive drug treatment in older persons with isolated systolic hypertension. Final results of the Systolic Hypertension in the Elderly Program (SHEP). *JAMA.* 1991;265:3255.

Topol EJ. Failing the public health—rofecoxib, Merck, and the FDA. *N Eng J Med.* 2004;351:1707.

Wagner AK, Zhang F, Soumerai SB, et al. Benzodiazepine use and hip fractures in the elderly: who is at greatest risk? *Arch Intern Med.* 2004;164:1567.

Wang PS, Schneeweiss S, Avorn J, et al. Risk of death in elderly users of conventional vs. atypical antipsychotic medications. *N Eng J Med.* 2005;353:2335.

Wenger NS, Solomon DH, Roth CP, et al. The quality of medical care provided to vulnerable community-dwelling older patients. *Ann Intern Med.* 2003;139:740.

Whelton PK, Appel LJ, Espeland MA, et al. Sodium reduction and weight loss in the treatment of hypertension in older persons: A randomized controlled trial of nonpharmacologic interventions in the elderly (TONE). *JAMA.* 1998;279:839.

Willcox SM, Himmelstein DU, Woolhandler S. Inappropriate drug prescribing for the community-dwelling elderly. *JAMA.* 1994;272:292.

Williams ME, Pulliam CC, Hunter R, et al. The short-term effect of interdisciplinary medication review on function and cost in ambulatory elderly people. *J Am Geriatr Soc.* 2004;52:93.

Zermansky AG, Petty DR, Raynor DK, et al. Randomised controlled trial of clinical medication review by a pharmacist of elderly patients receiving repeat prescriptions in general practice. *BMJ.* 2001;323:1340.

Complementary and Alternative Medicine

Joseph T. Hanlon ■ *Marc R. Blackman* ■ *Ronald M. Glick*

INTRODUCTION

Complementary and alternative medicine (CAM) modalities constitute a diverse group of consumer-driven medical and health care practices outside the realm of conventional medicine, which are yet to be validated using scientific methods. Considered as such, CAM practices are ever changing. Most CAM use is complementary, that is, as an adjunct to conventional practices, and only a minority is used as an alternative to mainstream medical care. A main tenet of CAM therapy is that it stimulates and strengthens the body's own natural defense systems to prevent and treat diseases. Thus, elderly as well as nonelderly individuals use CAM practices with the hope of improving wellness and for relief of symptoms attributable to chronic, "stressful," degenerative, or fatal conditions.

From a conceptual perspective, the panoply of CAM modalities can be divided into five major groupings: alternative medical systems, mind–body interventions, manipulative and body-based methods, energy therapies, and biologically based treatments (including dietary supplements) (Table 25-1). A dietary supplement is defined as: (1) a product that contains one or more of the following ingredients: vitamin, mineral, herb, botanical, amino acid, or a substance to increase total daily intake; (2) ingested orally; (3) not a conventional food or sold as a meal or diet, and (4) labeled as a dietary supplement (Food and Drug Administration (FDA) Web site).

In the United States, CAM practices are widely available (Table 25-2), but are largely unregulated. Among CAM practices, only five (acupuncture, chiropractic, massage, naturopathy, and homeopathy) are licensed in multiple states, whereas several others (art therapy, traditional Chinese medicine, reflexology) are licensed in only a few states, and still others (biofeedback, hypnosis) require only certification. Moreover, the scope of practice may vary from state to state (e.g., acupuncture). The American public spends more out-of-pocket for CAM practices than for all other health care needs. Most consumers believe that their health plans should pay for CAM

treatments, and an increasing number of insurers and Health Maintenance Organizations are now doing so.

The reasons for CAM use are multiple, but include dissatisfaction with conventional medicine because of its ineffectiveness in producing cures, cost, adverse effects, and depersonalization. CAM use also empowers the individual to take control over personal health decisions, and focuses on the individual's values, spiritual and religious philosophy, and beliefs regarding the nature and origins of illness. The fragmentation of care by busy specialists, and provision by CAM therapists of "touch, talk, and time," as well as media reports of dramatic results, all contribute to the increasing interest in CAM therapies.

CURRENT USE AND CONCERNS WITH CAM MODALITIES

In recent years, the use of CAM has steadily increased among adults of all ages. In the largest U.S. study to date, nearly 29% of 30 801 respondents to a 1999 National Health Interview Survey reported using at least one CAM modality in the prior year (Barnes, et al., 2004). This prevalence of CAM usage is somewhat less than that reported in other surveys. According to Eisenberg's (1998) follow-up of his earlier national survey, the probability of an adult American visiting a CAM provider increased by 30% during the 1990s, to 46.3% in 1997, accounting for approximately $27 billion in out-of-pocket expenses. It was estimated that nearly 60% of CAM use was not disclosed to health care providers. Alternative therapies were most frequently pursued for chronic conditions including back problems, anxiety, depression, and headaches. The therapies of escalating usage included botanicals, massage, vitamins, self-help group, folk remedies, energy healing, and homeopathy.

The use of dietary supplements in older adults is substantial. The Slone Survey reported that 40% of U.S. older adults take at least

TABLE 25-1

CAM Domains

Alternative medical systems	Complete systems that evolved independent of and often prior to conventional medicine, e.g., traditional systems • Traditional Chinese medicine • Ayurveda • Native American medicine • Homeopathy • Naturopathy
Mind–body interventions	Application of techniques designed to facilitate the mind's ability to affect one's body symptoms and functions. • Meditation or guided imagery • Dance, music, and art therapy • Prayer • Biofeedback
Biologically based treatments	Natural and biologically based practices, interventions, and products • Herbal therapies • Dietary supplements • Special diets • Orthomolecular therapies
Manipulative and body-based methods	Modalities based upon manipulation and/or movement of the body • Chiropractic • Osteopathic manipulation • Therapeutic massage
Energy therapies	Focus on energy fields believed to originate within the body or from other sources • Biofields (internal), e.g., reiki, qi gong, therapeutic touch • Bioelectromagnetic based (external), e.g., electroacupuncture, magnetic fields

one vitamin/mineral and one in seven older adults take at least one herbal supplement (Kaufman, et al., 2002). A study using data from the 2002 National Health Interview reported that 12.9% of the elderly reported the use of a herbal product in previous 12 months (Bruno, et al., 2005). The most common products used included glucosamine/condroitin, saw palmetto, ginkgo, and St. John's Wort.

The use of dietary supplements is of concern because the manufacturers are not responsible for proving efficacy or safety for these products before marketing (Anon, 2002). The FDA has however recommended that manufacturers stop selling several products due to concerns about toxicity (e.g., kava, ephedrine). They have also cautioned about drug interactions with St. John's Wort, a potent

TABLE 25-2

CAM Practitioners and Their Utilization

- *Chiropractic:* 55,000 licensed, $8 billion estimated market for services
- *Massage:* 1 million, 150,000–200,000 certified. $6 billion market.
- *Acupuncture:* 5000–8000 licensed (1000 MD's) $0.5–1 billion
- *Homeopathy* – 3000 (500 MDs), $0.2 billion
- *Naturopathy* – 1000–3000 licensed; $0.2 billion.

Source: The state of healthcare in America—1998 Business & Health.

TABLE 25-3

Potentially Clinically Significant Herbal–Drug Interactions

OBJECT DRUG	INTERACTING HERB	OUTCOME
Antidepressants	St. John's Wort	Serotonergic syndrome
Anticonvulsants	Shankpushpi	↓ Seizure threshold
Anticonvulsants	Wormwood	↓ Seizure threshold
Anticonvulsants	Gingko biloba	↓ Seizure threshold
Cyclosporine	St John's Wort	Transplant rejection
Digoxin	Hawthorn	↑ Digoxin activity
Digoxin	Siberian ginseng	↑ Digoxin levels
Digoxin	St John's Wort	↓ Digoxin levels
Indinavir	St John's Wort	↓ Indinavir levels
Theophylline	St John's Wort	↓ Theophylline levels
Warfarin	Gingko biloba	↑ Risk of bleeding
Warfarin	Dong quai	↑ Risk of bleeding
Warfarin	St. John's Wort	↓ Warfarin activity
Warfarin	Ginseng	↓ Warfarin activity

inducer of certain hepatic cytochrome P450 isoenzymes (Xie and Kim, 2005). Table 25-3 lists clinically important drug interaction with St John's Wort and other dietary supplements with prescription medications (especially narrow therapeutic range drugs) and their impact on patient outcomes (Xie and Kim, 2005; Holbrook, et al., 2005; Williamson, 2003; Tyagi, et al., 2003).

Recently, new FDA regulations have been passed regarding dietary supplements. As of December 2007, manufacturers will now be required to report serious adverse events to the FDA (Morrow, 2008). Moreover, starting June 2008, a new FDA rule will be implemented entitled "Current Good Manufacturing Practice in Manufacturing, Packaging, Labeling, or Holding Operations for Dietary Supplements." Essentially what this rule does is assure that what is on the label of a dietary supplement is what is contained in the product itself (Morrow, 2008).

USE OF CAM MODALITIES FOR DISORDERS OF THE ELDERLY PATIENT

While CAM modalities may be used for a number of conditions experienced by the elderly, evidence-based data supporting their use is limited. We describe in the following sections what is known for six common conditions, depression, anxiety, insomnia, osteoarthritis, dementia, and benign prostatic hypertrophy.

Depression, Anxiety Disorders, and Insomnia

Of the domains of CAM listed on Table 25-1, the modalities most commonly used for mental health conditions fall under the headings of biologically based treatments and mind–body interventions. Of the herbal agents and supplements, St. John's Wort or Hypericum is in (wide) use by the general population. Studies have shown only modest efficacy over placebo for mild–moderate depression and favorable side effect profile as compared to standard antidepressants Table 25-2 (Schulz, 2006). As mentioned previously, St. John's Wort can interact with numerous prescription medications. Consequently, this herbal product is best reserved for patients who are otherwise healthy with few other prescription medications.

A common measure that has made it into the lay media is the importance of the dietary balance between omega-6 and omega-3 fatty acids with the former being proinflammatory and seen as contributing to many health conditions including depression. Consequently, there has been a push to modify our diets with a reduction in red meats, fried foods, and trans-fats, all of which contribute to the omega-6 side of the equation. On the omega-3 side consumption of fish, using olive or canola oil for cooking, and eating nuts—particularly walnuts in moderation are seen as beneficial. There is a moderate level of evidence supporting a connection between this balance and depression, including the observation that dietary intake and blood concentrations of omega-6 over omega-3 correlates with the incidence of depression (Kiecolt-Glaser, et al., 2007). While the circumstantial evidence is strong, the clinical trial data is inconclusive (Severus, 2006). Nonetheless, the addition of a fish oil supplement is a reasonable measure as an adjunct in the treatment of depression or bipolar disorder. Pharmaceutical grade fish oil supplements concentrate the two essential fatty acids eicospentaenoic acid (EPA) and docosahexaenoic acid (DHA) while removing contaminants, particularly mercury. One thousand milligrams appears to be a safe dose at which there does not appear to be a significant concern of drug–drug interaction or platelet inhibition in most individuals.

Other supplements have been used or studied for depression. S-adenosylmethionine (SAM-e) has good support of efficacy (Mischoulon & Fava, 2002). However, given the dosage requirement of 800 to 1600 mg/day to see the effect, the cost is roughly 5 to 10 times higher than a generic selective serotonin reuptake inhibitor antidepressant (SSRI). This limits the potential utility of this agent, although it should be considered when patients do not tolerate an SSRI. Another agent, 5-hydroxytryptophan (5-HTP), is a direct serotonin precursor and has the potential to serve as a weak antidepressant itself or to augment the classical antidepressants (Turner, 2006). In clinical practice, this dietary supplement appears to have the advantage of fewer of the classical serotonin side effects (e.g., nausea, sexual dysfunction). One option is to use this well-tolerated agent as an adjunct (e.g., if someone continues with moderate anxiety symptoms or insomnia while being treated with an antidepressant). When using serotonergic medications in combination, it is prudent to advise patients as to the potential for serotonin syndrome, with physical or psychological symptoms of hyperarousal as well as cardiac symptoms such as tachycardia or palpitations.

Valerian root may work by being a benzodiazepine receptor agonist. Its use may have benefit for anxiety and insomnia but studies have not shown a consistent benefit over placebo (Taibi, et al., 2007). The most common patient complaint is of the bitter taste or aftertaste and mild dyspepsia. Melatonin appears to be a logical treatment for geriatric insomnia. Paralleling the drop-off in sleep efficiency and hours of sleep with age is the decline in production of melatonin by the pineal gland. Trials of melatonin, with a half-life ($t_{1/2}$) of just under 1 hour, find benefit for falling asleep. However, as a majority of insomnia patients have difficulty remaining asleep, the overall benefit on sleep patterns has been disappointing. In one study of insomnia in older adults 2 mg of a sustained-release form of melatonin was found to be of significant benefit to sleep (Wade, et al.,

2007). Sustained-release melatonin can be ordered from several nutritional supplement companies and 3 to 6 mg taken 1 to 2 hours before bed can be tried.

Mind–body approaches have been used extensively for mental health disorders as well as for chronic pain and other general health conditions that may have a stress-related component. Depression, anxiety, and insomnia are associated with a sympathetic nervous system predominant pattern. Mind–body approaches have been shown to result in a shift of autonomic reactivity to a more parasympathetic pattern. In geriatric medicine, in addition to the direct effects of these primary psychological conditions on quality of life, we are greatly concerned about the potential impact on general health, morbidity, and mortality. Some potentially helpful mind–body approaches are: yoga, meditation, rhythmic breathing, and biofeedback. These are not recommended in lieu of traditional therapies. Rather, as an adjunct, they can be of benefit for enhancing mood, decreasing anxiety, and improving sleep. In addition to benefit for mood, they may help with comorbid medical conditions such as hypertension or coronary heart disease. Mindfulness-Based Stress Reduction (MBSR) is a meditation-focused program that was developed by Dr. Jon Kabat-Zinn of the University of Massachusetts in the late 1970s. MBSR's central concept is the development of mindfulness, or present moment nonjudgmental awareness (Grossman et al., 2004). The program includes formal meditation practices such as body scan, sitting and walking meditation, and mindful movement (simple yoga) as well as mindfulness practices for coping with everyday life stressors. This 8-week program is currently taught worldwide. Mindfulness-Based Cognitive Therapy, a variant of MBSR, combines meditation practice with a cognitive-behavioral approach for individuals with recurrent depression in remission to help prevent future recurrences (Smith, et al., 2007).

There is moderate support in the traditional Chinese medicine (TCM) literature for the use of acupuncture in the treatment of insomnia, but this remains to be examined in a carefully designed randomized-controlled trial (RCT) (Kalavapalli & Singareddy, 2007). One commonality to seemingly different treatments, acupuncture and massage therapy, both have an impact on autonomic stress reactivity and result in a shift from sympathetic to parasympathetic predominance. This may explain the potential benefit of these modalities for anxiety symptoms, insomnia, and other hyperarousal states.

Several therapeutic modalities or practices fall outside of the realm of CAM but are included here because they are often omitted from the discussion. With greater recognition of the presence of seasonal affective disorder, the use of bright light therapy has come into common psychiatric practice and many insurance companies will cover the cost of the light boxes. Similarly, while we have always known that exercise is health-promoting, there is greater recognition of the mood-enhancing effect of aerobic exercise such as walking half-hour per day at a brisk pace (Motl, et al., 2005). Obviously for individuals whose mobility is limited, it can be helpful to find some other means of exercise, such as a pool aerobic class, arm ergometry, or seated exercise classes. Social isolation is seen as a major risk factor for cardiovascular and all-cause mortality as well as for depression and it goes without saying that isolation is a major concern for older adults. It may be that social interventions can have the greatest impact for many of our patients (Greaves & Farbus, 2006). Such interventions include CAM programs such as yoga or Tai Chi classes, but can also involve adult education, exercise—such as with Silver Sneakers programs or regular religious observance.

Osteoarthritis, Degenerative Disk Disease, and Chronic Pain

Glucosamine and chondroitin sulfate have been used extensively to treat knee osteoarthritis (OA) pain with a moderate level of literature support. An elegant multicenter study with over 1500 subjects examined the effects of glucosamine and chondroitin individually and in combination as compared with celocoxib versus a placebo finding no advantage of the supplements over placebo (Cleggl, et al., 2006). Compared to placebo, glucosamine and chondroitin sulfate were not significantly better in reducing knee pain. Concerns about the study include the placebo response rate as high as 60% and the use of gluosamine hydrochloride, given that all prior positive studies were of glucosamine sulfate. This leaves us without clear guidance from the literature, but if patients elect to try these agents it is advised to use glucosamine sulfate at 1500 mg and chondroitin sulfate at 1200 mg/day both divided into twice or thrice daily dosing, depending on the preparation. Additionally, patients should be advised to stick with the supplements for at least 3 months to see an effect.

SAM-e may be the unsung hero in the management of OA. In RCTs, SAM-e has demonstrated a comparable level of improvement in pain and functioning as nonsteroidal anti-inflammatory drug (NSAIDs), also showing a better side-effect profile with doses ranging from 400 to 1200 mg/day (Soeken, et al., 2002). As noted above, it also has the potential benefit of enhancing mood, which can be affected by OA pain.

While OA has classically been considered a noninflammatory disorder, mounting evidence supports the importance of inflammation in its pathogenesis. Elsewhere in the literature anti-inflammatory effects have been seen with omega-3 fatty acids and fish oil. While fish oil has shown a benefit for lupus and rheumatoid arthritis, the research on OA and degenerative disk disease (DDD) is very preliminary (Maroon & Bost, 2006). Nonetheless, fish oil supplementation may be a reasonable adjunct in the management of OA for several reasons: it is generally safe and well-tolerated; it offers the potential for a direct benefit for OA-related pain; it may result in a reduction of NSAID use, with concomitant decrease in adverse effects; and it has the potential to decrease comorbidities of chronic pain including cardiac disease and depression. Dosing recommendations are as noted above, using 1 gram combination of EPA and DHA of a concentrated pharmaceutical-grade fish oil supplement.

For years, we have been puzzled by the disparity between the apparent benefit of acupuncture for many chronic pain conditions noted in practice and in open trials versus the observation that RCTs did not support a significant difference over placebo. Many factors go into this discussion including the possibility that superficial needling commonly used as a control condition may have a physiological analgesic effect. Several recent well-designed RCTs have shown a significant benefit of acupuncture over control needling for knee osteoarthritis and stronger evidence is emerging supporting efficacy in low back pain and other chronic pain conditions (Berman, et al., 2004; Manheimer, et al., 2005; Witt, et al., 2005). Future studies are needed to confirm these findings, highlight specific acupuncture protocols that can be readily reproduced in clinical practice, and address the issue of durability of the treatment on pain and func-

tioning. While acupuncture is not likely to take the place of surgery, for patients electing a nonsurgical option, this treatment has the potential to decrease pain, increase functioning, and allow patients to limit NSAID and opioid medications.

Among older adults, pain is the most commonly cited reason for seeking CAM treatments and chiropractic is the most commonly used modality (Foster, et al., 2000). There is moderate support of the use of chiropractic manipulation for the treatment of low back pain with benefit for pain, functioning, and medical and indirect costs, although effects appear to be comparable to other interventions such as physical therapy and massage (Hurwitz, et al., 2006). Theoretically by alleviating nerve root pressure with manipulation, this modality could be beneficial for the radicular pain associated with cervical and lumbar spinal stenosis and this improvement is described widely in clinical practice. Unfortunately, chiropractic research is limited in the treatment of spinal stenosis or treatment of older adults in general. To their credit, many chiropractors have extended their practice from the passive manipulative treatment to include more active rehabilitation measures which can potentially help patients to recondition and maintain the enhanced range-of-motion.

Although the most visible changes for our patients with OA and DDD can be seen radiologically, it is quite common to have prominent secondary myofascial pain. Treatments directed at this component, including massage therapy and physical therapy involving stretching of the tight muscles, can result in a dramatic improvement. In addition to or in lieu of formal physical therapy, yoga classes can provide an interesting social setting in which participants experience a number of benefits including total body stretching, core stabilization, a mild aerobic workout, and relaxation response associated with the exercise and breathing techniques. It is important that the class be geared for older adults or that the instructor be knowledgeable in modifying activities for individuals with OA. Although Tai Chi is commonly discussed in the setting of prevention of falls, this approach can also provide similar benefits including core stabilization, stretching, aerobic activity, and relaxation.

As noted above, some of the benefit of yoga and Tai Chi relate to a mind–body effect. Meditation programs, specifically MBSR, have the potential to greatly help our patients experiencing chronic pain (Morone, et al., 2008). Pain has both sensory and affective components. Through mindfulness training and meditation practice, patients describe two significant changes. The mindful awareness can allow them to attend to the sensory component of the pain without this automatically eliciting a reactive affective response. Additionally, with this uncoupling of sensory and affective components, they describe that the common pain–stress cycle seems to be circumvented. Consequently, many describe greatly reduced pain intensity and associated distress, as well as improved function.

Dementia

The two most common types of dementia in the elderly are vascular and Alzheimer's disease. Ginkgo biloba extract, EGb 761, is widely used to increase memory and cognitive ability. There is a lack of convincing evidence that gingko may be beneficial for enhancing cognitive function for patients with both vascular and Alzheimer's dementia (Birks et al., 2007). Adverse effects of ginkgo biloba are generally mild. The NIH is currently sponsoring a large, multicenter study to examine the efficacy and safety of EGb 761 in the treatment of dementia caused by Alzheimer's disease.

Benign Prostatic Hyperplasia

Symptomatic benign prostatic hyperplasia (BPH) affects more than 40% of men older than 70 years of age. During the past several years, men have increasingly begun to self-treat this condition with the herbal compound *Serenoa repens*, known as saw palmetto. A recent meta-analysis that included patients with moderate benign prostatic hypertrophy who averaged 65 years of age and were studied for at least 3 months (Wilt, et al., 1998). Saw palmetto was found to be superior to placebo and to exhibit similar efficacy to the standard pharmacologic treatment. Few side effects were reported other than intermittent slight abdominal distress. However, the rigor of the experimental design of these trials has been questioned. Recently, a large, multicenter, NIH-sponsored clinical trial to assess the effect of saw palmetto extract in men with moderate to severe BPH was published (Bent, et al., 2006). They found that saw palmetto was not effective in treating BPH.

CONCLUSION

The escalating use of CAM modalities by the U.S. public, including the elderly population, and the paucity of information supporting the safety, efficacy, and mechanisms of action of these diverse modalities, argue strongly for increasing the scope and rigor of CAM-related research. To address important public health needs in the elderly population, including those who are underserved, it would seem prudent to investigate the basic biology and potential clinical utility of selected CAM modalities that may allay or attenuate a variety of a life "stressors," including depression, cognitive decline, chronic pain, musculoskeletal frailty, and sleep disorders. Of particular note is that the aforementioned conditions are disproportionately more problematic in older persons than in younger persons, often coexist in the same individual, and account for substantial use of one or more CAM modalities. Moreover, from a pathophysiologic perspective, each of these age-related stressors exhibits derangements in the interrelationships among endocrinologic, neurologic, and immunologic functions. Thus further research efforts might profitably be directed towards unraveling the interactions among these three important physiologic systems, particularly as they affect aged individuals.

Identifying an appropriate agenda for future CAM studies in the elderly population poses significant challenges. To select among the myriad CAM modalities that are currently being used by consumers, several considerations appear warranted, including the extent of use by aged persons; the public health importance of the diseases or conditions being treated; the quality and quantity of reported data, which allows for determination of whether to emphasize preclinical versus clinical studies; and the feasibility and cost of conducting the research. Integrating allopathic and CAM approaches in the design of the next generation of CAM studies represents another exciting yet daunting opportunity to advance the discipline of CAM in the twenty-first century.

FURTHER READING

Anon. Problems with Dietary Supplements. *Med Letter.* 2002;44:84–86.

Barnes PM, Powell-Giner E, McFann K, et al. Complementary and alternative medicine use among adults. United States 2002. *Adv Data.* 2004;343:1–19.

Bent S, Kane C, Shinohara K, et al. Saw palmetto for benign prostatic hyperplasia. *N Engl J Med.* 2006;354:5557–5566.

Berman BM, Lao L, Langenberg P, et al. Effectiveness of acupuncture as adjunctive therapy in osteoarthritis of the knee: a randomized, controlled trial. *Ann Intern Med.* 2004;141:901–910.

Birks J, Grimley EJ, Lee H. Ginkgo biloba for cognitive impairment and dementia. *Cochrane Database Syst Rev.* 2007:(2): Art. No. CD003120.

Bruno JJ, Ellis JJ. Herbal use among U.S. elderly: 2002 National Health Interview Survey. *Ann Pharmacother.* 2005;39:643–648.

Clegg DO, Reda DJ, Harris CL, et al. Glucosamine, chondroitin sulfate, and the two in combination for painful knee osteoarthritis. *N Engl J Med.* 2006;354:795–808.

Eisenberg DM, et al: Trends in alternative medicine use in the United States, 1990–1997: Results of a follow-up national survey. *JAMA.* 1998;280:1569. FDA Website: http://www.cfsan.fda.gov/~dms/diesupp.htm.

Foster DF, Phillips RS, Hamel MB, Eisenberg DM. Alternative medicine use in older Americans. *J Am Geriatrc Soc.* 2000;12:1560–1565.

Greaves CJ, Farbus L. Effects of creative and social activity on the health and well-being of socially isolated older people: outcomes from a multi-method observational study. *J Royal Soc Health.* 2006;106:134–142.

Grossman P, Niemann L, Schmidt S, Walach H. Mindfulness-based stress reduction and health benefits. A meta-analysis. *J Psychosom Res.* 2004;57:35–43.

Holbrook AM, Pereira JA, Labiris R, et al. Sysematic overview of warfarin and its drug and food interaction. *Arch Intern Med.* 2005;165:1095–106.

Hurwitz EL, Morgenstern H, Kominski GF, et al. A randomized trial of chiropractic and medical care for patients with low back pain: eighteen-month follow-up outcomes from the UCLA low back pain study. *Spine.* 2006;31:611–621.

Kaufman DW, Kelly JP, Rosenberg L, et al. Recent patterns of medication use in the ambulatory adult population of the United States: the Slone survey *JAMA.* 2002;287:337–344.

Kalavapalli R, Singareddy R. Role of acupuncture in the treatment of insomnia: a comprehensive review. *Complem Ther Clin Pract.* 2007;13:184–193.

Kiecolt-Glaser JK, Belury MA, Porter K, et al. Depressive symptoms, omega-6:omega-3 fatty acids, and inflammation in older adults. *Psychosomatic Med.* 2007;69:217–224.

Manheimer E, White A, Berman B, et al. Meta-analysis: acupuncture for low back pain. *Ann Intern Med.* 2005;142:651–663.

Maroon JC, Bost JW. Omega-3 fatty acids (fish oil) as an anti-inflammatory: an alternative to nonsteroidal anti-inflammatory drugs for discogenic pain. *Surg Neurol.* 2006;65:326–331.

Mischoulon D, Fava M. Role of S-adenosyl-L-methionine in the treatment of depression: a review of the evidence. *Am J Clin Nutrition.* 2002;76:1158S–1161S.

Morone NE, Greco CM, Weiner DK. Mindfulness meditation for the treatment of chronic low back pain in older adults: a randomized controlled pilot study. *Pain.* 2008;134:310–319.

Morrow JD. Why the United States still needs improved dietary supplement regulation and oversight. *Clin Parmacol Ther.* 2008;83:391–393.

Motl RW, Konopack JF, McAuley E, et al. Depressive symptoms among older adults: long-term reduction after a physical activity intervention. *J Behav Med.* 2005;28:385–394.

Schulz V. Safety of St. John's Wort extract compared to synthetic antidepressants. *Phytomedicine.* 2006;13:199–204.

Severus WE. Effects of omega-3 polyunsaturated fatty acids on depression. *Herz.* 2006;31Suppl 3:69–74.

Smith A, Graham L, Senthinathan S. Mindfulness-based cognitive therapy for recurring depression in older people: a qualitative study. *Aging Mental Health.* 2007;11:346–357.

Soeken KL, Lee WL, Bausell RB, et al. Safety and efficacy of S-adenosylmethionine (SAMe) for osteoarthritis. *J Fam Pract.* 2002;51:425–430.

Taibi DM, Landis CA, Petry H, et al. A systematic review of valerian as a sleep aid: safe but not effective. *Sleep Med Rev.* 2007;11:209–230.

Turner EH, Loftis JM, Blackwell AD. Serotonin a la carte: supplementation with the serotonin precursor 5-hydroxytryptophan. *Pharmacol Ther.* 2006;109:325–338.

Tyagi A, Delanty N. Herbal remedies, dietary supplements, and seizures. *Epilepsia.* 2003;44:228–235.

Wade AG, Ford I, Crawford G, et al. Efficacy of prolonged release melatonin in insomnia patients aged 55-80 years: quality of sleep and next-day alertness outcomes. *Curr Med Res Opin.* 2007;23:2597–2605.

Wlliamson EM. Drug interactions between herbal and prescription medicines. *Drug Safety.* 2003;26:1075–1092.

Wilt TJ, Ishani A, Stark G, et al. Saw palmetto extracts for treatment of benign prostatic hyperplasia: a systematic review. *JAMA.* 1998;280:1604–1609.

Witt C, Brinkhaus B, Jena S, et al. Acupuncture in patients with osteoarthritis of the knee: a randomised trial. *Lancet.* 2005;366:136–143.

Xie HG, Kim RB. St John's Wort associated drug interactions: short term inhibition and long term induction. *Clin Phamacol Ther.* 2005;78:19–24.

Team Care

Ellen Flaherty ■ *Kathryn Hyer* ■ *Terry Fulmer*

Geriatric interdisciplinary team care has been shown to be essential to manage the complex syndromes experienced by frail older adults. Providing comprehensive care to geriatric patients with multiple illnesses, disabilities, increased social problems, and fragmented care requires skills that no one individual possesses. Older adults are, therefore, best cared for by a team of health professionals. Outcomes associated with effective geriatric interdisciplinary team care include the improvement of functional status, perceived well-being, mental status, and depression. Geriatric interdisciplinary team care has also been shown to be cost effective by reducing patient readmission rates and numbers of physician office visits. Specialized interdisciplinary teams focusing on specific diseases such as congestive heart failure, stroke, or myocardial infarction have also demonstrated improved patient outcomes. The purpose of this chapter is to outline the benefits of interdisciplinary geriatric team care. The current and projected health care workforce shortage, coupled with the aging of the population dictate that care models be as efficient and effective as possible. Managing the complex syndromes experienced by frail older adults requires skills beyond the training of one discipline and multiple clinicians to communicate with each other regularly in order to coordinate services. These needs have resulted in the growth of geriatric interdisciplinary teams.

In 1993, the Pew Health Professions Commission predicted that health professionals would need 17 competencies to practice health care in 2005. Anticipating a shift toward population-based medicine, increasing use of technology, and managed care, the competencies included an emphasis on primary care, participation in coordinated care, involvement of patients and families in decision making, and ensuring cost effectiveness. While regulators and policy makers, almost a decade later, seem less enthralled with managed care, the forces driving managed care-increasing costs, concerns about cost effectiveness, and a focus on prevention have not slowed.

The Joint Commission on Accreditation of Healthcare Organizations stated that shared decision making and an interdisciplinary health care team approach are essential to reduce medical errors and to provide improved patient safety in all health care organizations in America. The Institute of Medicine of the National Academies made a similar plea in the *Quality Chasm* report, strongly urging that all health professionals receive interdisciplinary team training to ensure the delivery of patient-centered care. More recently, additional reports from the Institute of Medicine of the National Academies specifically point to the need for interdisciplinary care for geriatric patients.

In 1995, The American Geriatrics Society developed a position statement on interdisciplinary care for older adults, which supports the interdisciplinary care model for the following reasons:

1. Interdisciplinary care meets the complex needs of older adults with multiple, interacting comorbidities.

2. Interdisciplinary care improves health care processes and outcomes for geriatric syndromes.

3. Interdisciplinary care benefits the health care system as well as caregivers of older adults.

4. Interdisciplinary training and education effectively prepares providers to care for older adults.

Studies of the clinical effectiveness and cost effectiveness of teams generally demonstrate that patients are helped by an initial comprehensive geriatric assessment conducted by multiple disciplines. Team management and internal performance also seem to matter. In a study of the 26 Program of All-Inclusive Care for the Elderly (PACE) sites, teams that ranked themselves as performing better had patients with better 3- and 12-month outcomes in Activities of Daily Living (ADL) performance and better urinary incontinence rates. It appears that coordination of services, ability of team members to communicate well, and agreement from the multiple providers over how to implement complex care improve patient outcomes in both the short and the long terms. While there was no difference in mortality owing to team performance, changes in patient outcome were risk adjusted. Teams require management skills, leadership, and well-honed communication skills. Coordinating care, leading group discussions, and managing conflict are the key team skills that are discussed below.

Studies focusing on patient satisfaction have demonstrated that the presence of a team champion and the involvement of the physicians on the team are positively associated with greater perceived team effectiveness. Maintaining a balance among culture values of participation, achievement, openness to innovation, and adherence to rules and accountability also appeared to be important.

COLLABORATION AND THE IMPORTANCE OF "INTERDISCIPLINARITY"

Collaboration implies a process of shared planning, decision making, accountability, and responsibility in the care of the patient. In collaborative practice, providers work together. They demonstrate effective communication, trust, mutual respect, and understanding of others' skills. While skills and services may overlap, most skills and services are complementary and reinforce each other.

With advanced technology and the growth of community-based care, providers frequently provide home treatments or treatments in the nursing home that were previously delivered exclusively in the hospital setting. Monitoring older adults in these community settings requires good communication skills, because providers need to understand and correctly implement complex plans of care. It is crucial to recognize when to alert other providers of change in status. It is also important to learn what information other team members require to make decisions about treatment.

With the advent of managed care, there is an emphasis on efficiency and appropriate use of resources. Skills in coordinating care and being responsive to older adults increase in importance. Physicians, nurses, social workers, and other providers must recognize when referrals to other providers are necessary and know what outcome to expect. Understanding the skills of other health providers is increasingly important for all patients but is critical in the care of frail older adults.

Transitions from one health care setting to another are particular periods of risk for elders, and programs designed to smooth those transitions result in better patient outcomes. Patients have benefited from programs designed to improve the transition between hospital and home. A study in which nurse practitioners followed elders after hospital discharge for heart failure at home demonstrated the effectiveness of these clinicians in reducing rehospitalizations and improving the confidence and comfort of the caregiver at home.

For almost a decade, the John A. Hartford Foundation of New York City has supported an effort to incorporate team training into graduate medical, nursing, and social work education. The program, Geriatric interdisciplinary Team Training (GITT), has trained more than 1800 health care students and professionals across the country and developed training materials to encourage the development of effective geriatric teams. Two important principles were realized in the development of curriculum and programs. Effective teams require a structure and an understanding of group process, skills that can be taught and should continue to evolve during professional development. However, teams must focus on the outcome of the team process, the creation of an interdisciplinary care plan, or the management of the complex patient. While structure and process increase the efficiency of teams, assessing the team's effectiveness must be based on the outcome of team meetings and the ability of the team to address and improve the patient's and the family's needs.

To be effective in managing the complex care of older adults, team knowledge and skills must emphasize multidimensional geriatric assessment, interdisciplinary team care planning, maximization of self-care and function, self-determination in the care plan, and improving quality of life. Future health professionals providing care to older individuals will be expected to apply knowledge and skill in practice. Clinical care managers will need to evaluate providers on patient satisfaction, cost effectiveness, productivity, and quality of care. Geriatric teams of the future will be expected to identify individuals at greatest risk of functional limitations and manage groups of older persons with similar problems in a cost-effective manner. In this context, the task for educators of future health professionals and practice-based managers becomes one of ensuring that providers are knowledgeable about the principles and practices of team care.

According to the American Congress on Rehabilitation Medicine, a team is capable of achieving with patients what individuals who constitute the team cannot achieve in isolation. Simply forming a team comprised of several disciplines does not, however, guarantee that the team will function well or that the outcome of the process will be the desired one. Effective teaming as an interdisciplinary group requires structure, the use of agendas, agreement upon ground rules and process, attention to issues of leadership, communication, and respect for one another's expertise.

PRINCIPLES OF SUCCESSFUL TEAMWORK

To provide the important benefits of team care, team members must know their functions and how to interact to make the team effective. The essential elements of teamwork are coordination of services, shared responsibility, and communication. Effective teams must work across settings and have well-organized mechanisms to share information. Geriatric assessment is often shared among two or more providers who administer various tests and other components of the assessment. Because the focus of the team is on the older person, the team shares a common goal. Effective teaming requires rules to govern the team and team member behavior, plans to make meetings run efficiently, clarity about the skills and boundaries for the roles and responsibilities of each team member, team communication skills, and mechanisms for managing team conflict.

Teams and Team Member Rules

Team rules, both for team governance and for member behavior, are needed in the early stages of team development. Table 26-1 provides an overview of the eight principles of successful team work. Not having these rules is a primary cause of team problems later on and can slow or stop team development completely. Rules for team governance should include some or all of the following:

- Share a clear understanding by all members (and the larger organization within which it operates) about the overall purpose of the team and the goals for each meeting.
- Determine the composition of the team, including which disciplines are needed as members and the number of members (enough to get the job done; not so many that the work cannot

TABLE 26-1

Eight Principles of Successful Team Work

1. All team members share a common purpose and work together to establish explicitly stated patient care goals.
2. The patient and family are at the center of all team activities and are active team members.
3. The full scope of the professional capabilities of each team member is clearly understood by everyone on the team; professional roles are dynamic and are determined by the needs of the team, individual experience, and the knowledge and skills of team members.
4. All team members should contribute to team function through constructive individual behaviors, including rotating leadership.
5. There must be effective team communication across all work and care settings.
6. The team must have tools or strategies for the effective management of conflict.
7. The team should have explicit rules about participation and decision making.
8. The team must be adaptable, responding to new challenges and conditions as these develop over time.

get done). Allow the problem to define the composition of the team, not vice versa.

- Determine how often the team needs to meet and specify attendance requirements. (Is there a core team of physician, nurse, and social worker? Are other disciplines asked to participate on cases that require their expertise?)
- Identify time, place, and duration of team meetings.
- Determine a system by which cases are to be presented and by whom. Identify how care plans and action will be carried out and documented. (Is one member chosen to write down the care plan or does this responsibility rotate?)
- Identify opportunities or requirements for team building meetings and/or team training.
- Create mechanism for enforcing both governance and behavior rules through ongoing evaluation of the effectiveness of the meeting (if rules are made and not enforced, the team can quickly become ineffective and be a negative experience for everyone involved).

People are usually more willing to spend time and energy if there is a clear understanding of what is going to occur and why it is needed. The time spent with participants clarifying rules and getting a commitment for involvement will prevent team problems and support the development of an effective and efficient team.

While the above governance rules provide a structure for team interaction, behavior rules are also needed for each team. They can include some or all of the following:

- Ensure clear understanding by all team members of what an interdisciplinary team is and what members should bring to the group.
- Promote understanding and respect for others' expertise.
- Recognize the implications of idioms by the professionals involved. Learn how to articulate information clearly to others. (Do "client" and "patient" mean the same thing in different professional groups?) Health care goals will come from different perspectives and from different disciplines.

- Share information and expertise openly.
- Identify and follow a decision process when roles overlap. Resist setting rigid boundaries on roles. Instead, promote effective ways of sharing responsibilities and tasks.
- Define acceptable behavior (willingness to work with other professionals to develop a care plan, active participation, and respect for others' roles).

THE WELL-PLANNED MEETING

Teams with poorly planned and organized meetings become ineffective and inefficient. This cultivates negative attitudes toward teams and leads to poor attendance and less than enthusiastic participation by the team members. Elements essential to the structure of an effective meeting include the following:

1. Agenda (what do we expect to accomplish?).
2. Estimated timeline for completing agenda (reasonable time frames).
3. Establishment of meeting roles. Members can and should rotate the following roles but every meeting should include
   a. leader (calls meeting to order, has agenda, and sets expectations),
   b. timekeeper (keeps group on task),
   c. recorder (keeps track of agreements about the care plan and modifications and is responsible for recording changes to care plan).
4. Summary of agreements (recorder reports agreements).
5. Evaluation/reflection on team process (both team process and outcome of the meeting are discussed).

Suggested Structure for Regular Health Care Team Meetings

Creating a structure and format for health care team meetings standardizes the meeting process and assists in making teams more efficient and effective. By using a standard agenda, health care team members are more prepared for meetings and the flow of the meeting is predictable. Table 26-2 provides tips on how to facilitate a team meeting. Key elements are an agenda item, a timekeeper to encourage

TABLE 26-2

How to Facilitate a Team Meeting

1. Ensure that goals and objectives of the meeting are clear to all members.
2. Observe and value the participation of each member.
3. Acknowledge both verbal and nonverbal communication and address dysfunctional behaviors within the team.
4. Identify conflict, exploring thought processes that lead to differing conclusions.
5. Seek mutual understanding.
6. Assure shared decision making.
7. Suggest tools/techniques to enhance meeting flow, information gathering, decision making, and future planning.
8. Give constructive feedback.
9. Encourage team to evaluate its progress.

the group to stay on track, and a recorder who captures the group decisions and delineates the responsible person for specified tasks. Evaluating meetings is important and improves the quality of the structure and process, especially if evaluation is a routine part of the regularly scheduled meetings. The following format should work for most meetings:

1. Review meeting objectives to ensure that all members understand and are in agreement with the meeting objectives.

2. Review agenda and order of items. Add, reorder, or delete items as the group decides. Ensure that all team members agree with the agenda items.

3. Assign timekeeper, recorder, and leader roles. Confirm time intervals timekeeper will use to cue group.

4. Report follow-up from last meeting.

5. Discuss issues or patients as listed on the agenda.

6. Summarize action items from this meeting. Decide who will do what before the next meeting.

7. Decide what the objectives and agenda items will be for the next meeting.

8. Evaluate the meeting. Ask each member to evaluate the meeting. Evaluation can be written or verbal, but the questions should focus on: What did the team do well that it should continue doing? What could the team do differently to improve the meeting?

SKILLS OF DIFFERENT PROFESSIONALS ON TEAMS

Team members from different disciplines bring a unique set of skills (Table 26-3), but those skills also overlap. Understanding the skills and education of various team members contributes to respect but also allows team members to refer elderly clients appropriately to other professionals. Because each profession trains its members in a culture that reflects a common language, professional behaviors, values, and beliefs, disagreement between professionals may occur because of different expectations and language. Most professionals recognize the training of others and learn what other professionals do only after being in professional practice. Although a range of individuals serve as members of an interdisciplinary team in geriatrics,

TABLE 26-3

Helpful Questions in Eliciting Patient and Family Goals and Values
What are you expecting?
What do you most want to accomplish?
What is most important in your life right now?
What are you hoping for?
What do you hope to avoid?
What do you think will happen?
What are you afraid will happen?
What gives your life joy or meaning?
What would be left undone, if you were to die soon?

Data from Emanuel LL et al: Goals of Care. EPEC Participants Handbook. EPEC Project [Module 7]. Chicago, IL: American Medical Association; 1999:pM7.

the core professional members are typically the physician, nurse, social worker, and pharmacist. The extended professional members of the team might include nonphysician providers (nurse practitioners and physician assistants), physical therapist, occupational therapist, speech pathologist, dietitian, and psychologist or psychiatrist. The older patient and the patient's family are also important members of the team.

Knowledge about the preparation, expertise, and scope of practice affects individual team member performance, in that it can

- reduce tension that occurs around who is doing what;
- help members accept role overlap as necessary and positive;
- foster positive views toward the efforts of several disciplines; and
- increase the ability to solve problem beyond a single discipline.

EFFECTIVE TEAM COMMUNICATION

Communication is the foundation for all team functioning. It requires that all team members cooperate to establish ongoing communication with each other, with the patient, and with the family for the sole purpose of developing an integrated care plan that addresses each aspect of care.

Barriers to communication range from the lack of a shared language, born of differences in core values and terminology used by different disciplines, to systems and organizational barriers. Moreover, in a busy health care organization, a major hurdle is finding the time for a team meeting and developing methods for effective team communication. In an organization where care is being provided in multiple locations and settings, informal communication often occurs in hallways and elevators, and by telephone, voice mail, and e-mail. The provision of effective coordinated care requires the team to have a clear mechanism for the exchange of information. At the simplest level, this requires the time, space, and regular opportunity for members to meet and discuss patients. An ideal system for interdisciplinary team communication includes

- a well-designed record system;
- a regularly scheduled forum for members to discuss patient management issues;
- a regularly scheduled forum to discuss and evaluate team function and development, and to address related interpersonal issues;
- a mechanism for communicating with the external system (e.g., hospital administration) within which the team operates.

Effective communication also relies on listening, explaining perceptions, acknowledging, and discussing the differences and similarities in views, recommending appropriate treatment, and negotiating agreement. In our increasingly diverse workplaces, language and cultural barriers can exist among members of a team. These barriers can make it difficult for one member to understand the finer points in the meanings, intentions, and reactions of other team members. Our cultural heritage, our gender, our socioeconomic status, and our stage of life all influence our use of language and our perception of others. Some degree of cultural competency must be in place for team members to effectively communicate with each other as well as with patients and family members. Additional barriers to effective communication and teamwork can include

- lack of a clearly stated, shared, and measurable purpose;
- lack of training in interdisciplinary collaboration;
- role and leadership ambiguity;
- team too large or too small;
- team not composed of appropriate professionals;
- lack of appropriate mechanisms for timely exchange of information.

Even among team members of similar cultural backgrounds, members need to recognize and value the different competencies and approaches of different disciplines. People do not need to think the same to be unified. The key to team success is to value the differences on the team and use such diversity to achieve the team's common purpose.

VALUING DIVERSITY

Values are a major source of conflicting and competing communication patterns among health professionals. The education and training of health care professionals vary according to different modes and methods of practice. For example, a patient who is being seen by a team may have a problem with depression. A pharmacist might see a patient with no drug therapy, a social worker might see a patient who is socially isolated, and a physician might see a patient with possible dementia. Furthermore, if members of an interdisciplinary team do not possess at least a basic understanding of each other's knowledge and values, then it is likely that misunderstandings will result. For example, most physicians equate quality of life with mental status or freedom from mental impairment, while many nurses relate quality of life to physical strength, seeing, hearing, and having someone who cares.

The following tips may be helpful for valuing diversity on a team:

- Reasonable people can—and do—differ from each other. No two people are the same. Diversity among team members enhances creativity.

- Learn as much as you can from others. Learning the various backgrounds, cultures, and professional values of others can enrich your own skills and abilities.

- Evaluate a new idea based on its merits. Avoid evaluating ideas based on who submitted them or how closely these mirror your own personal preferences.

- Avoid comments and remarks that draw negative attention to a person's unique characteristics. Humor is a key factor in a healthy team environment but should never be used at the expense of another's identity or self-esteem.

Differences among team members should be honored and utilized to advance the goals of the team. Decision making and conflict resolution are also components of the communication process that must be acknowledged by teams. The group process must integrate openness and confrontation, support and trust, cooperation and conflict, sound procedures for solving problems and getting things done, and good communication. Establishing a planned process for decision making is essential. The process must also take resolution of conflicts into account, because conflict is inevitable.

TABLE 26-4

Common Approaches to Negotiation and Conflict Resolution

1. Welcome conflict and use it as potential for change. Address data, facts, assumptions, and conclusions.
2. Clarify the nature of the problem as seen by all parties.
3. Try to identify areas of agreement. Focus on common interests, not positions.
4. Deal with one problem at a time, beginning with the easier issues.
5. Listen with understanding. Reflect and clarify when communicating.
6. Brainstorm.
7. Use objective criteria when possible.
8. Invent new solutions where all parties gain.
9. Evaluate and review the problem-solving process after implementing the plan.

TEAM CONFLICT

Conflict is a natural and unavoidable part of human affairs, especially in such groups as interdisciplinary health care teams that seek to grow and develop. The various health professionals on a team have underlying differences in their modes and methods of practice that affect their relationships with each other, as well as with their patients. For example, various professionals may differ in their logic of geriatric clinical assessment or how to define a patient's problem.

Differences may be characterized by two different styles of practice. One, a "ruling-out problem" approach, systematically eliminates possibilities until only one problem and a corresponding solution remain. The other, a "ruling-in problem" approach, relies on expanding the range of professional view to encompass an increasingly long list of potential factors. For example, physicians are trained in diagnostic techniques that narrow the range of options, relying heavily on such objective data as laboratory tests in the process. Social workers, on the other hand, are taught to go beyond the narrow presenting problems to view it within larger, encompassing psychosocial issues, such as income, family relationships, and environment. In addition to the diverse professional perspectives, team members also have different personalities, which influence interactions among team members. Other factors that may lead to conflict in team care include scarce resources and organizational or professional changes that threaten guidelines for using conflict to promote interdisciplinary problem solving.

The discussion of different points of view promotes growth and development, which in turn leads to improved outcomes. This sort of discussion often leads to conflict, a natural and unavoidable part of human affairs. Successful resolution of conflict requires the ability to communicate effectively as well as to confront issues, not people, focusing on the search for win–win solutions in which both sides achieve a benefit. Table 26-4 lists common approaches to negotiation and conflict resolution.

EMPHASIZING CARE GOALS AND INTERDISCIPLINARY CARE PLANNING

The concept of goals is essential on at least two levels within interdisciplinary geriatric care teams. Teams are generally organized to achieve specific programmatic goals. Health care teams work with patients, families, and others to achieve patient-specific goals. For an interdisciplinary team to function effectively, the team's purpose and goals should be understood clearly and agreed on by all members. With the increasing cost consciousness in health care, the goals of teamwork and the products of interdisciplinary collaboration are of paramount importance. In managed care, the measurement of outcomes is an important and widely accepted way of demonstrating that adequate care is being provided. Goals established—whether long- or short-term—need to be feasible and take into account that interdisciplinary teams function in a variety of settings (e.g., home care, impatient) and that the team membership, types, and intensity of services provided vary. One step toward establishing goals is to have the team answer the questions, "What do we want to achieve with this patient?"

Interdisciplinary Care Planning

After programmatic goals are determined, team members next must agree on what they mean in reality. For example, if "improve patient outcome" is a goal used by a team, successful outcome will need to be defined case by case. The process of interdisciplinary team care planning is the means of achieving consensus on desired patient outcomes. One discipline might want to save the patient's life at all costs, while another discipline might want comfort and less aggressive medical care. For example, when a patient shows sings of confusion and an inability to care for self, a physician might want the patient hospitalized for the patient's own safety, while a social worker might want to bring social services or health care into the home first. These choices can keep the team in a conflict mode, without reaching a decision on the care plan unless the purpose and goals are clear and the patient or a surrogate is meaningfully involved in the decision about care.

An interdisciplinary team developing care plans and treatment goals for patients must be able to conceptualize patients broadly, incorporating all relevant information and knowing how different pieces of information relate. The ability of each discipline to add to the overall care plan will depend on team member's understanding of the linkages between the problems. A general treatment outcome goal of optimum health for the patient can be easily agreed on by team members, but the best means of obtaining that goal will be considered differently by the various disciplines represented on the team. Professionals will share their views of plan initiatives based on their professional knowledge or previous experience. This exchange will lead the team into areas that might not be considered if it were not for the team expertise available. Team members must communicate their own professional opinions, and all members need to respect the different kinds of expertise each brings to the group in order to optimize care planning.

For all the great effort put into developing a care plan, a plan cannot work unless the team has a system for documenting it and indicating clearly who will be responsible for what and by when. This documentation should be completed before the end of the meeting and available to all team members to remind them of their responsibilities. In addition, there must be in place a system (formal and informal) for communicating and continuing with the next steps of the care plan between team meetings. This is most often done informally with the different disciplines, talking with each other as needed.

SUMMARY

Good interdisciplinary care teams can enhance management of the complex syndromes experienced by older adults. Good teams require team members with excellent clinical skills who are schooled in the knowledge and skills of teaming. Good teaming does not happen by accident but is a function of well-developed team structure. This includes rules to govern the team and team member behavior, plans to make meetings run efficiently, clarity about the skills and boundaries for the roles and responsibilities of each team member, team communication skills, and mechanisms for managing team conflict. Fulfilling these requirements can lead to care goals and care planning that emphasizes the particular needs of an individual older adult. The demographic imperative and the workforce demand for the future necessitate fresh approaches to team care, as well as new research from which to build the science of efficient and effective team care.

FURTHER READING

American Congress on Rehabilitation Medicine. In: Long DM, Wilson NL, eds. *Houston Geriatric Interdisciplinary Team Training Curriculum.* Houston, TX: Baylor College of Medicine, Huffington Center on Aging; 2001.

Cassel C, et al., eds. *Mount Sinai Geriatric Interdisciplinary Team Training Resource Manual.* New York, New York: Mount Sinai School of Medicine; 2000.

Clark P. Values in health care professional socialization: implications for geriatric education in interdisciplinary teamwork. *Gerontologist.* 1997;37(4):441.

Clark PG. Quality of life, values, and teamwork in geriatric care: Do we communicate what we mean? *Gerontologist.* 1995;35:402.

Coleman EA, Berenson RA. Lost in transition: challenges and opportunities for improving the quality of transitional care. *Ann Intern Med.* 2004;141(7):553–556.

Drinka T, Streim J. Case studies from purgatory: maladaptive behavior within geriatric health care teams. *Gerontologist.* 1994;34(4):541.

Fisher K, et al. *Tips for Teams: A Ready Reference for Solving Common Team Problems.* New York, New York: McGraw-Hill; 1995.

Fulmer T, Hyer K, Flaherty E, et al. Geriatric interdisciplinary team training program: evaluation results. *J Aging Health.* 2005;17(4):443–470.

Grant RW, Finocchio LJ. *California Primary Care Consortium Subcommittee on Interdisciplinary Collaborative Teams in Primary Care. A Model of Curriculum and Resource Guide.* San Francisco: Pew Health Professions; 1995.

Harrington-Machkin DH. *Let's Meet: Team Meetings. The Team-Building Toolkit: Tips, Tactics, and rules for Effective Workplace Teams.* New York, New York: American Management Association; 1994:31.

Hyer K, et al., eds. *The GITT Curriculum Guide.* New York, New York: NYU GITT Resource Center; 2001.

Hyer K, et al., eds. *The GITT Implementation Manual.* New York, New York: NYU GITT Resource Center; 2001.

Institute of Medicine. *Health Professions Education: A Bridge to Quality.* Washington: National Academies Press; 2003.

Institute of Medicine. *Crossing the Quality Chasm: A New Health System for the 21st Century.* Washington: National Academies Press; 2001.

Long D, Wilson N, eds. *Houston Geriatric Interdisciplinary Team Training Curriculum.* Houston, TX: Baylor College of Medicine, Huffington Center on Aging; 2001.

Mezey M, et al., eds. *Ethical Patient Care: A Casebook for Geriatric Health Care Teams.* Baltimore: Johns Hopkins; 2002.

Mukamel DB, Temkin-Greener H, Delavan R, et al. Team performance and risk-adjusted health outcomes in the Program of All-Inclusive Care for the Elderly (PACE). *Gerontologist.* 2006;46(2):227–237.

Naylor MD, Brooten DA, Campbell RL, Maislin G, McCauley KM, Schwartz JS. Transitional care of older adults hospitalized with heart failure: a randomized, controlled trial. *J Am Geriatr Soc.* 2004;52:675–684.

O'Leary D. *Testimony on Medical Errors.* A statement before the Committee on Health, Education, Labor and Pensions, U.S. Senate and the Subcommittee on Labor, Health and Human Services, and Education of the Senate Committee on Appropriations; February 22, 2000.

Pew Health Professions Commission and California Primary Care Association. *Interdisciplinary Collaborative Teams in Primary Care: A Model Curriculum and Resource Guide.* San Francisco: Pew Health Professions Commission; 1995.

Qualls SH, Czirr R. Geriatric health teams: classifying models of professional and team functioning. *Gerontologist.* 1988;28:372.

Siegler EL, et al., eds. *Geriatric Interdisciplinary Team Training*. New York, New York: Springer; 1998:3.

Shortell S, Marsteller J, Lin M, et al. The role of perceived team effectiveness in improving chronic illness care. *Med Care*. 2004;42(11):1040–1048.

Walker P, et al. Building community: Developing skills for interprofessional health professions education and relationship-centered care. NLN Appointed Interdisciplinary Health Education Panel. *J Allied Health*. 1998;27(3):173.

Woodcock M, Francis D. *Teambuilding Strategy*. Brookfield, VT: Gower Publishing; 1994.

Internet Resources

The Great Lakes GITT. http://www.gitt.cwru.edu.

The Huffington Center on Aging at Baylor College of Medicine. http://www.hcoa.org/hgitt/.

The Mount Sinai School of Medicine GITT. http://www.mssm.edu/geriatric.

The NYU GITT Resource Center. http://www.gitt.org.

The University of California at Los Angeles. http://www.geronet.med.ucla.edu.

The University of Colorado Health Sciences Center. http://www.uchsc.edu.

Social Work

Ruth E. Dunkle ■ *Mary Catherine Dennis*

Social workers provide services to older patients across a continuum of care needs that range from supporting community living to providing palliative care services at the end of life. This occurs in many different health care arenas including institutional settings, such as acute care hospitals, chronic care settings, and nursing homes, as well as in patients' homes in the community. Social workers support and enhance the adaptive capacities of patients within their living environments and are knowledgeable about interviewing, assessment, and intervention in social problems faced by individuals, couples, families, and groups. Using negotiating skills, social workers mediate conflicts and obtain resources for clients and their families. Knowledge of group process makes social workers effective in forming natural helping networks and serving as members of interdisciplinary teams. Their expertise in coordinating services within a single organization or across different agencies or settings helps to ensure appropriate and adequate care for older patients.

While 76% of social workers in a health care settings work with older patients, not all social workers have specialized training in geriatrics. This is changing rapidly, primarily through training efforts sponsored by the Hartford Foundation's initiative established in 1999. Such training enhances social workers' awareness of older people's needs and subsequently leads to better quality of care by helping social workers provide the appropriate services at the right time. Proper care provided by gerontologically trained professionals including social workers can reduce the cost of care by 10% each year in hospitals, nursing homes, and patients' homes as well as improve psychosocial outcomes and reduce mortality.

This chapter describes the key roles for geriatric social workers, the practice issues they face, and the settings in which they work.

KEY ROLES FOR GERIATRIC SOCIAL WORKERS

The roles social workers play vary within health care settings (Tables 27-1 and 27-2). Social workers provide direct service to elders as well as facilitate linkages between service workers and agencies.

Direct Service Provision

Social workers meet face to face with patients and consumer groups to provide services as caseworkers, marital or family therapists, and group worker or educators. Individual casework and counseling services help elders who have mental health problems or need help with resolving issues in such areas as housing, finances, or interpersonal problems. Martial and family therapies include meeting with individual elders, with marital partners, as well as with groups of elders who are experiencing concerns related to their families. This could involve helping elderly grandparents be more effective in raising their grandchildren, aiding families in coping with an elderly parent with a dementing illness, or supporting elderly couples as they struggle with debilitating health problems, which strain the emotional resources necessary to maintain their marriage bonds. Group work services include support groups for elders with a variety of health concerns, such as those who have cancer, low vision, or early-stage dementia. Support groups have been particularly helpful to caregivers of patients with such diseases as Alzheimer's. These groups run by social workers help caregivers better understand the disease process and provide information that helps them deal with the problems of caregiving more effectively and thus improve the disease outcome. Groups also focus on self-help issues, where elders learn to deal with such problems as alcoholism or smoking. Psychotherapy groups work to resolve such concerns as abuse (as victim or perpetrator), depression, and marital problems. Social workers also work directly with older adults and their families as educators and disseminators of information. For instance, they provide educational sessions on caregiving, stress management, and various aspects of mental and physical health care.

Linkage Roles

Social workers link elderly individuals to the services they need. This may be because agencies are not meeting the older person's needs, because elders themselves lack knowledge of available resources or

TABLE 27-1

The Roles Social Workers Perform

ROLES	DESCRIPTION	EXAMPLES
Group worker	Social worker plans and conducts group activities for clients to help understand themselves better through a variety of methods; can be therapeutic, educational, social, or for support	Worker organizes a group for grandparents raising grandchildren to share information and provide support
Advocate	Social worker fights for, defends, and promotes patient's perspectives and rights	Social worker helps a patient destined for a nursing home receive home health care rather than be institutionalized
Case manager	Social worker assesses patient needs, connects patient to resources, and coordinates and oversees delivery and participation of services	The case manager coordinates the services. A patient might need rehabilitation therapy, psychotherapy, and home health care as well as transportation services
Educator	Social worker offers knowledge regarding health care information, processes, and procedures with patients and provides knowledge of patient with the team	In hospice, the social worker provides information regarding the dying process, pain management, stages of grief, and option for burial services
Discharge planner	Social worker prepares patient for next phases of departure from facility by designing a course of action	When patient leaves the hospital and goes home, the social worker may arrange transportation services, meal delivery, home care services, and assessment of home for safety
Therapist	Social worker engages clients in interpersonal interactions regarding client's behavior, feelings, attitudes, and perceptions	Social worker works with an older couple who is having marital problems resulting from stress of caregiving
Team member	Social worker collaborates with health professionals to provide efficient delivery of services	Social worker shares information with physicians and nurses and provides insight into the patient's cultural and personal life
Broker	Social worker connects patients to most relevant resources	Social work brokers help African-American elders overcome the racial and ethnic disparities they face in receiving health care, by building trust between the patient and health care professionals
Information and referral	Social worker has knowledge of community resources and offers connection to these agencies	Social worker has knowledge of respite care services and links caregiver of Alzheimer patient to the respite care agency
Mediator/arbitrator/ advocate	Social worker facilitates conflict resolution	The social worker advocates for the older patient in a guardianship hearing

TABLE 27-2

The Setting Where Social Workers Work and the Roles They Perform

SETTINGS	ROLES
Home	Support patients' adjustment to health status, provide emotional support, address barriers in access to medical care (i.e., transportation), provide education so that patient can make informed decisions, assess social support and referral to resources, and case management
Hospital	Assessment; discharge planning; prevention and treatment of mental and physical health; promotion of psychosocial health, advocacy in relation to aspects of human diversity; mediate between patients, families, and the health care team; group work; psychotherapy
Nursing home	Financial planning; psychosocial assessment and addressing emotional needs; care planning; mediation between residents, staff, and family; linking residents and families to resources
Assisted-living facility	Negotiate placement and transition, support in navigating decision-making and emotions regarding changes in autonomy, financial planning, and fostering communication
Senior center	Administration, program planning, case management, facilitate group and individual therapy, address life transitions, and organize advocacy groups
Dept of Public Welfare	Case management, oversee and evaluate programs, community outreach, advocacy, development of services, income assistance, protective services, support parents raising grandchildren
Community mental health setting	Perform client assessments, conduct support groups, provide emergency and crisis services to older mental health clients and their families; referral to other resources in the community such as adult day care, respite services, and partial day treatment programs
Hospice	Liaison between care settings; case manager; address psychosocial needs of families and patients; support for adjustment to setting, treatment, illness, and death; educator, advocate, broker, and mediator between family members, patient, and medical professionals; team member; information and referral; group worker; and counselor
Adult day care/ respite program	Assess clients' mental and physical abilities, plan and facilitate activities to maximize physical and cognitive functioning, facilitate support groups, provide information and support for Alzheimer's and other disease processes, and referral to community resources
Primary care	Plan and implementation of safety and illness prevention programs, identify social factors that support prevention of illness and cause of disease, provide emotional and social support, facilitate support groups around a specific disease or mental illness, and provide education, information, and referral

ability to access those resources, or because elders and their families need help in overcoming fears and concerns they might have about using services. For instance, family members who are struggling to provide home care to their mother with Alzheimer's disease may be reluctant to use a support or educational group of other family members in similar circumstances for fear of revealing the personal problems their mother faces. Social workers can help overcome these fears by helping family members realize that all families where a family member has a dementing illness face similar problems and have similar reactions to their circumstances. Social workers also work as case managers to help elders receive services in a timely fashion. In general, case management involves screening, assessment, care planning, implementation, monitoring, and reassessment to evaluate ongoing service needs. Case management meets a variety of goals in numerous settings. The social worker assesses the elder's problems and needs to determine eligibility for services as well as financial resources and links elders to the needed services. Family and friends may provide collateral information to help the social worker determine their capacity for support. Goals for a care plan are set by discussing the elderly patients' perception of their needs. Interventions are then designed to meet these goals. Resources are identified to this end. Subsequently, the social worker monitors the delivery of the services. When care is needed over a longer period of time, the needs of elders are reevaluated. Ultimately, an outcome evaluation is conducted to determine if the patient's goals were achieved.

Social workers also work as mediators and advocate for their clients/patients. As mediators, social workers determine the issues behind a conflict. Social workers facilitate family discussion of issues identified by the family and elders as important. For example, adult guardianship mediation can be used to discuss how the family can best help elders to preserve autonomy (or to maximize his/her greatest level of independent functioning). When advocating for their clients, social workers often form partnerships with lawyers to aid victimized elders who need legal redress. For example, social workers and lawyers can aid gays, lesbians, bisexuals, and transgendered (GLBT) elders who face housing and service delivery discrimination in accessing benefits to which they are entitled.

PRACTICE ISSUES WITH POPULATIONS SERVED

Geriatric social workers strive to meet the basic human needs of all elders, with a particular emphasis on those who are vulnerable owing to oppression and poverty. With health care provided in a myriad of public and private settings, the social worker acts as a broker, a mediator, and an advocate for clients.

This section reviews key populations served by social workers and the practice issues that come into play with elders in these groups.

Cultural Diversity

Social workers are uniquely situated to respond to the needs of older adults across racial–ethnic groups and sexual orientation because of their skills in training and cultural awareness in service delivery. Attention to cultural diversity includes sensitivity to differences in cultural history, language, values, religion, ethnicity, nationality, regionality, immigration status, and sexual orientation as well as recognition of within-group variation. For example, cultural assessment strategies are used to understand the clients' definition of

their problem. During the assessment process, social workers working with culturally diverse groups evaluate attitudes toward health care and the clients' belief about the causes of illness and benefit of health care services. As social workers attempt to understand the clients' problems, they evaluate the language skills, educational level, and degree of acculturation of the patients. In addition, determining which family member has the authority to make care decision is important for the health care professional to know. For females, in some cultures, a male decides how care proceeds. In Native American culture, generational standing comes into play in decision-making for care. The patient's use of language to label and categorize a problem, the availability and use of indigenous community resources, the decision-making involved in problem intervention strategies, and the patient's cultural criteria for determining problem resolution are important issues for the social worker and other health care workers to consider in working effectively with older patients and their families.

While there are common themes that are relevant to people of color, and other minority elders such as lesbians, bisexuals, and transgender persons, each group has its own cultural history relevant to care. Social workers identify barriers to seeking help, such as stigma, denial, and financial and access barriers resulting from service fragmentation and gaps in health care. For some older minorities, health problems are rooted in historic experiences of discrimination that prevent access to the social service system. Therefore, culturally specific interventions consider the unique background and resources of the individual. Initial contact with a patient requires understanding of the individual's identity, including their degree of acculturation, generational status, immigration/refugee status, as well as sexual orientation. Nonverbal cues may be more meaningful than verbal expressions. These may provide information about knowledge or problems and ways of handling them. Knowing the client's sense of ethnic identity, attitudes toward formal services, and service preferences helps the social worker sort out cultural values and traditions and family beliefs and practices relevant to care.

The Poor

While government programs such as Social Security, Medicare, unemployment insurance, and welfare have reduced the extent of poverty in the older population, it is still a significant problem, resulting, in part, from the cumulative effects of lifelong discrimination, particularly for elders of color, those older than 75 years, those residing in rural areas, and women. Underutilization of health and mental health services by elders in poverty makes these groups a target for social work intervention. One significant barrier to meeting the needs of elders in poverty is lack of knowledge about their problems and needs. Gerontological social workers are aware of the barriers that impede the development and delivery of appropriate services and are aware of formal as well as informal resources to aid elders in rural communities, women, and racial/ethnic minorities.

Immigrants and Refugees

Since the early 20th century, rising numbers of elders have arrived from South America and Asia. The majority of older immigrants to the United States has a median length of residence of 14 years and has close relatives who are U.S. citizens. The diversity in this population is reflected in race and ethnicity, as well as age, length of residence in the United States, English language proficiency, and reasons for immigration. These elders are more likely to live in households with extended family and nonfamily than are nonimmigrants and, if they come from developing countries, to live with their children. Families are central to the provision of care to their aging relatives. Demand for family caregiving often occurs in the context of limited coping resources, inadequate knowledge of services, misperceptions of eligibility requirements of government programs, and the elders' beliefs that children will be their care providers. Unfortunately, the multiple roles result in greater caregiving strain and increased neglect and abuse of elderly family members. Social workers educate elders and their families about the available services and how to obtain transportation and financial resources to access these services. More importantly, through a culturally competent assessment, social workers can identify negative attitudes toward formal services, culturally specific definition of illness and healing, and religiously acceptable perceptions of services for these families.

Abused and Neglected

The abuse or neglect of elders is often identified in a health care setting. Many types of mistreatment, such as physical abuse, sexual abuse, and neglect (including self-neglect), result in injury, pain, and physical and psychological impairment. Other types of abuse such as financial and identity theft are more difficult to detect. The assessment of mistreatment, which may require several contacts, involves an interview with the elder to review the risk of abuse and the elder's cognitive ability and level of independent functioning. While all states have mandatory or voluntary reporting laws, the elderly victim's willingness to receive help is voluntary. Social workers help in the assessment process for elder abuse by providing education about the nature of abuse and prevention strategies. Social workers can be instrumental in helping the elder recognize the power imbalance in abusive relationships and devise strategies for protection. The biggest challenge that health professionals face is identifying and helping abused or neglected elders who do not realize that they are victims of mistreatment.

Mentally Ill

The incidence of mental illness among the elderly ranges from 15% to 25% across all care settings. Approximately 4% receive assistance for their problems, with half of the help coming from primary-care physicians. Many elders are reluctant to seek help because of stigma, language barriers, or the lack of culturally appropriate services. Social workers work with a health care team to assess the mental health issues and to identify appropriate treatment and services. They can provide structured cognitive-behavioral, interpersonal, and problem-solving treatments that are effective mental health approaches, often in conjunction with prescribed medication. Pharmacological interventions and psychosocial treatments are both effective in the elderly.

Cognitively Impaired

Social workers are involved with the assessment of older adults with dementia and their caregivers. Such an assessment considers the client's social and medical history, including a physical and mental status examination, an assessment of the individual's living environment, a functional ability assessment of both instrumental activities of daily living and activities of daily living, social service needs and family dynamics, service and resource needs, legal issues such as power of attorney and health care proxy, advance care planning, and end-of-life planning. Social workers also play a variety of roles on the interdisciplinary team used when an elder and his/her family experience a dementing illness. In the early stages of the dementing illness, social workers can support the elder with dementia and provide cognitively stimulating programs. In some cases, the elder is able to plan for his/her own future physical and financial needs, which the social worker can facilitate. Social workers are also helpful to family members who are struggling with the acceptance of physical and emotional changes in their loved one as the dementing illness progresses. Finally, social workers may function as case managers for individuals experiencing cognitive impairment.

Older GLBT

This is often an invisible population, but one that has special needs and has experienced a history of discrimination leading to barriers in service delivery. Few organizations offer specialized services to GLBT patients or are sensitive to their needs. Unfortunately, stigma and hatred toward homosexuals limit access to services as well as the scope of available services provided to people in these populations. Without the protection of legal marriage, GLBT persons and their children do not have access to Social Security survivor benefits, employee health benefits, inheritance, or housing and hospital visitation. When confronted with institutional care, elders in these communities worry that their partnerships will not be honored. Social workers connect GLBT clients to services and service providers who do not discriminate against them and respect their identity. In addition, social workers help establish GLBT-friendly resources such as providing a list of physicians and elder-friendly living facilities and facilitating completion of power of attorney, advanced directives, and other health care documents to secure access to financial and health care decisions for GBLT partners.

Substance and Alcohol Abusers

This problem often is unrecognized by health care professionals as symptoms are often mistaken for other age-related problems such as depression and dementia. Risk factors for the substance and alcohol abuse include social isolation, living-alone, chronic pain, and a variety of losses such as retirement, widowhood, and mobility. Six percent to 11% of elders seen in health care settings show symptoms of alcoholism, and this increases to 14% in emergency departments and 20% in psychiatric settings. Treatment for these problems in older people is more successful than in younger adults. Social workers aid other health care professionals in assessing the problem and providing the necessary treatment. Social workers provide successful educational interventions with older patients who are not aware that they are consuming too much alcohol or misusing over-the-counter medications. Counseling can also aid the older person in changing their behaviors and reducing stress that leads to overuse of alcohol and medications. Counseling that uses motivational interviewing to help clients desire a change in their behavior has been effective with older people. Group and individual interventions using a cognitive-behavioral approach as well as self-help and psychoeducation groups are effective approaches to these problems. Social workers provide couples and family interventions, which also aid in reducing the stress that may trigger the overuse of alcohol and medications.

HIV/AIDS Victims

Many older people come into contact with HIV/AIDS either as patients with the disease or as caretakers for loved ones with this disease. Currently, approximately 10% to 12% of people with AIDS are older than 50 years, but, with treatments that prolong life, this is expected to increase. The isolation of elders with HIV/AIDS is greater than for younger people, as they are more likely to live alone. They are also more reluctant to seek social service and mental health support. This same resistance is evident with caretakers of persons infected with this disease as a result of concerns about being stigmatized, adding additional stress to the caregiving situation. Social workers can help identify elders with HIV and help improve access to services and social networks with older people who have HIV concerns. Social workers offer educational information about HIV as well as case management services that coordinate the raft of services that many patients with HIV and their families need, such as caregiver respite services, home health care and hospice care, individual and group supportive counseling, and financial assistance.

WHERE SOCIAL WORKERS PRACTICE

Social workers are employed in a variety of settings that older persons use for their health care. Several of the central practice arenas are reviewed below.

Nursing Homes

Social workers are employed in nursing homes of all sizes but when the size of the facility is 120 beds or larger, their employment is mandated under the Omnibus Budget Reconciliation Act of 1999. The number of elders using nursing homes has declined during the last 20 years because of a reduction in disability among elders as well as an increase in home health care and the expansion of assisted living facilities. Because these facilities are residences where people live, social workers have the responsibility of helping in all aspects of life, including the resident and their family, facility staff, and the overall institutional environment. Their assistance begins with the transition into the facility. Adjustment to a new living environment is faced by not only the older person but their family as well. The social worker provides direct services to residents and their families as part of an interdisciplinary team. They assess the psychosocial needs of the resident and aid in the development of a care plan under the government requirements of maintaining a Minimum Data Set. The Minimum Data Set is part of the U.S. federally mandated process for clinical assessment of all residents in Medicare or Medicaid-certified nursing homes. This process provides a comprehensive assessment of each resident's functional capabilities and helps nursing home staff (physicians, social workers, and nurses) identify health problems and develop strategies to address them. Social workers also facilitate psychosocial well-being among residents and their families, linking the resident and family members to services inside and outside the facility, helping with discharge planning for the elders who are discharged, and serving as advocates for appropriate care and treatment for all patients and their families. Because social workers are often the

only staff members focused on the psychosocial needs of residents and their families, they are in the best position to identify and address mental health issues. Often they complete the cognitive, mood, behavioral, and psychosocial portion of the Minimum Data Set and the resident assessment protocol and can readily identify the mental health needs of the residents.

Community Mental Health Facilities

Twenty percent of elders experience mental health disorders, and almost 70% of them live in the community. Unfortunately, older persons are underrepresented in community mental health facilities, as mental health symptoms are sometimes mistaken for issues of aging by family, friends, and health professionals. When elders seek treatment, they usually have more severe symptoms. Social workers are part of a team of mental health practitioners, which includes nurses, psychologists, and psychiatrists, who work in these settings. Social workers do client assessments, conduct support groups, provide emergency and crisis services to older mental health clients and their families, and refer these people to other resources in the community such as adult day care, respite services, and partial day treatment programs. They often provide therapeutic interventions in the form of brief psychotherapy and behavior modification to individuals or groups. They also provide indirect services through community education and consultations in long-term care facilities.

Hospitals and Health Care Facilities

Social work practice with older adults in health care settings is focused on adaptation and coping with chronic illness, adjustment to disability and physical limitation, decisions about end of life, compliance with medical regimens, wellness, long-term care, and quality of life. Social workers also provide mental health services that address depression, substance abuse, management of long-term mental health issues, cognitive deficits, suicide prevention, and adjustment to changes in life by patients and families.

In hospital settings, social workers are members of an interdisciplinary team (consisting of physicians, nurses, social workers, and chaplains, among others), providing services to patients and families regarding assessments of a patient's cognitive, emotional, and behavioral status, as well as social support network. Social workers counsel patients and families, assisting them in adjustment to illness and providing crisis intervention and connection to community resources. Additionally, social workers identify interpersonal aspects of patients' lives that contribute to positive outcomes in relation to their chronic illnesses, such as addressing obstacles to medical compliance and environmental and financial obstacles, by acquiring information and accessing support resources for geriatric patients. Social workers advocate for the cultural, language, sexual orientation, ethnicity, religious, class, and other aspects of diversity by affirming and addressing these aspects of patients' lives. Social workers also advocate on behalf of patients with the health care team when patients face barriers to receiving care. For example, social workers can aid in the care of abused and neglected elders by documenting and reporting instances of abuse and neglect and can testify in court with regard to these matters.

In acute care settings, where patient stays are very short, social workers focus on high-risk screening, brief counseling, bereavement services, discharge planning, collaboration, information, referral, follow-up, and emergency services on call programs. Social workers are typically assigned to specific medical or psychiatric departments in hospitals. Patients are screened to determine whether they need social work services. Need for services is also conveyed to other health care professionals by having social workers attend team meetings and discharge planning conferences, by referrals from nurses or physicians, or by requests from patients and families. A social worker's presence, when a diagnosis, death, or other unpleasant news is communicated, can ease shock and help individuals address the emotion loss and face forthcoming decisions. Additionally, the social worker can provide information regarding aspects of diseases, care options, and assistance in meeting the patient's needs.

Discharge planning is particularly important for older adults who are transitioning from the hospital to other facilities or their homes. Addressing older adults' needs during discharge is necessary, in order to allow the older adult the best possible scenario for recovery from illness. The social worker assesses caregiving needs, and availability of social supports, family support, and home and community environment, as well as financial supports when the patient leaves the hospital.

Hospice

Hospice social workers practice in a variety of end-of-life settings, such as palliative care centers in hospitals, nursing homes, assisted living facilities, outpatient practices, and residential hospice facilities, and in homes. Palliative care requires an interdisciplinary team, where the social worker is a crucial member providing psychosocial support and referral to resources, easing transitions between settings, and addressing issues of loss for patients and families.

The role of the social worker begins before patients enter into hospice or palliative care and continues with families and loved ones after end-of-life care ends. Social workers provide a variety of services to address the needs of patients, families, and caregivers in end-of-life care. Social workers in end-of-life care fulfill a variety of roles such as liaison, educator, mediator, advocate, broker, and counselor. As patients face debilitating illness in palliative care, social workers help with the transition between care facilities, assessing readiness for palliative care and beginning to address the emotional and psychological aspects of end of life. Social workers are pivotal in assessing and supporting patients, families, and caregivers in their psychological, spiritual, social, financial, and cultural needs at the end of life. Addressing loss in patients and families is essential, as individuals and families may have difficulty communicating and accepting their feelings regarding the losses they face. Identifying social support for patients and families is important, as they may reconcile their relationships with family and friends and find support in these relationships. Discord may arise when families are brought together at the end of life, and, therefore, social workers assist families to communicate and understand decisions that are made, emotions that are expressed, and relationships that are negotiated.

As an educator and mediator, the social worker provides information regarding the plan of care, the illness, and the process of dying; communicates with the heath care team; informs the patient of their rights; provides information regarding medical rights to accept or refuse medical interventions; and provides information regarding the grieving process for families and caregivers. Additionally, educating the health care team regarding the specific needs of a particular patient or family and providing information regarding cultural and spiritual accommodations that may be made are important aspects of hospice care. Social workers act as brokers for resources and services to address the needs of patients who are dying and their families, arrange services, facilitate communication among family members, provide services to fulfill last wishes, and provide assistance with funeral plan arrangements. As an advocate, the social worker supports and represents the patients' and families' needs, wishes, and desires to the health care team; recognizes the dying person as a social person during the end-of-life stages; and works toward fulfilling end-of-life wishes. As a counselor, a social worker addresses the psychological, emotional, and spiritual needs of the family in addressing losses, illness, and reconciling relationships. Also, grief support to families, friends, and caregivers is provided after death through individual counseling sessions with family members, support groups, grief camps for children, and formal ceremonies and services for families who have lost loved ones.

Home Care

Home care is a term that encompasses a variety of services, including home health agencies, homemakers, home health aides and assistance, medical equipment and supplies, visiting nurses, caregiver respite, and other medical services that are provided in the home. One agency may provide one or several of these services to older adults.

Social workers in home care address a wide range of issues that are similar to and unique from other settings. These fall into several areas including adaptation to illnesses and chronic conditions; decisions regarding end of life, dementia, and behavior management; caregiving; issues of abuse, neglect, and prescription drug misuse and handling theft; family discord; and connecting family members who live long distances from the older adult. In addition, financial management, addressing unsafe living conditions, connecting to resources to provide safe living quarters, social support, mental health, legal issues, and compliance to medical treatments are part of the social worker's job in home care for older people.

In order to address these diverse issues, home care social workers employ a case management approach, where interventions are crafted for individuals and their unique needs. Also considered in these situations are the families, caregivers, the environment, and the community resources that are available. Key aspects of these services include assessment, planning, management and coordination of resources, and advocacy. Social workers are equipped to communicate with older adults and assess their preferences, wishes, desires, emotional states, coping styles, needs, and cultural diversity issues involved in service delivery. When older adults continue living in their homes, social workers arrange and monitor services, such as meals on wheels or grocery deliveries. As caregivers are often involved, caregivers' burden is evaluated along with the need for respite services in case of illness or hospitalization. A holistic approach is employed, where psychological, spiritual, and cultural needs are met. For example, religious services can be arranged so that the older adult can continue practicing their faith.

Social workers provide a unique psychosocial perspective that allows for assessment and monitoring of older adults' ability to make decisions. Social workers can advocate on behalf of the older adult to the members of the home health team regarding termination of services and understand patients' perspectives and unique needs. Finally, social workers assist with discharge planning and transition from home to other medical providers when needed.

SUMMARY

Geriatric social workers are integral members in the health care team serving older patients. Their wide range of skill, as well as their knowledge of available services in a variety of settings, makes social workers valuable members of the team serving older patients.

FURTHER READING

Administration on Aging. *A Profile of Older Americans 2002.* Washington, D.C.: Administration on Aging. Available at: www.aoa.gov/prof/Statisitcs/profile/12-pf.asp.

Barranti C, Cohen H. Lesbian and gay elders: an invisible minority. In: Schneider R, Kropf N, Kisor A, eds. *Gerontological Social Work: Knowledge, Service Settings and Special Populations.* Chicago: Nelson-Hall; 1992.

Barry KL, Oslin DW, Blow FC. *Alcohol Problems in Older Adults: Prevention and Management.* New York, New York: Springer; 2001.

Beaulieu EM. *A Guide for Nursing Home Social Workers.* New York, New York: Springer; 2002.

Berkman B, ed. *Handbook of Social Work in Health and Aging.* New York, New York: Oxford Press; 2006.

Centers for Disease Control. AIDS among persons greater than or equal to 50 years, United States, 1991–1996. *Morb Mortal Wkly.* 1998;47(02):21–27.

Cowles LA. *Social Work in the Health Field. A Care Perspective.* 2nd ed. New York, New York: Haworth Social Work Practice Press; 2003.

Egan M, Kadushin G. The social worker in the emerging field of homecare. *Health Soc Work.* 1998;24:43.

Gelfand DE. *Aging and Ethnicity: Knowledge and Services.* 2nd ed. New York, New York: Springer; 2003.

Good RA. *Social Work Practice in Home Health Care.* New York, New York: Haworth Press; 2000.

Lee JS, Gutheil IA. The older patient at home: Social work services and home health care. In: Berkman B, Harootyan L, eds. *Social Work and Health Care in an Aging Society.* New York, New York: Springer; 2003:73.

Lum D. *Culturally Competent Practice: A Framework for Growth and Action.* Pacific Grove: Brooks/Cole; 1999.

Mizrahi T, Abramson JS. Collaborations between social workers and physicians: Perspectives on shared cases. *Soc Work Health Care.* 2000;26(3):1–2.

National Association of Social Workers. *NASW Guidelines for Social Work Practice in Healthcare Settings.* 2005. Available at: www.socialworkers.org/practice/standars/NASWHealthCareStandards.pdf.

Senior Action in a Gay Environment and Brookdale Center on Aging. *No Need to Fear, No Need to Hide: A Training Program for Inclusion and Understanding of Lesbian, Gay, Bisexual, and Transgender (LGBT) Elders in Long-Term Care Facilities.* New York, New York: Brookdale Center on Aging; 2003.

Sheldon FM. Dimensions of the role of social worker in palliative care. *Palliat Med.* 2000;14(6):491.

Merck Institute of Aging and Health. *The State of Aging and Health in America.* Washington, D.C.: The Gerontological Society of America; 2003.

Walsh K. *Social Workers in Hospice and Palliative Care Settings: End of Life Care.* NASW Practice Update, 2003. Available at: www.socialworkers.org/practice.

U.S. Department of Health and Human Services. *Mental health: Culture, Race, and Ethnicity: A Supplement to Mental Health: A Report of the Surgeon General.* DHHS Publication No. SMA01-3613. Rockville, MD: U.S. Department of Health and Human Services, Substance Abuse and Mental Health Services Administration; 2001.

U.S. Health Resources and Services Administration. *The AIDS Epidemic and the Ryan White CARE Act: Past Progress and Future Challenges 2002–2003.* Rockville, MD. Available at: http://hab.hrsa.gov/tools/progressreport/.

Self-Management of Health Behavior in Geriatric Medicine

W. Jack Rejeski ▪ *Lawrence R. Brawley* ▪ *Mary E. Jung*

INTRODUCTION

A significant development in medicine is the recognition that patients should be treated as active agents in their health care. Contemporary consumers show increased interest in becoming more personally involved in decisions about their health, as evidenced by the popularity of such resources as WebMD and the marketability of health-related products and services. In the context of the traditional office visit, self-management is an inevitable part of treatment, since patients ultimately decide when to initiate the process and to what extent they will adhere to recommended courses of action prescribed by health care professionals.

Geriatric medicine is no exception to this trend. A guiding assumption of this chapter is that older adults' self-management of health behaviors is central to understanding the etiology, treatment, and downstream consequences of illness, chronic disease, and disability. An appropriate model for 21st-century geriatric medicine will focus on creating a partnership between health care professionals and their patients and will require that health care professionals have a working knowledge of what motivates older adults to initiate health behaviors and the potential reasons for success or failure in self-management. The early sections of this chapter will define and provide a conceptual framework for self-management; later sections will review key studies in the area and offer guiding principles and suggestions for incorporating patient self-management into practice. Mastering this knowledge will enable geriatric health care professionals to deliver state-of-the-art care to their patients.

DEFINING SELF-MANAGEMENT

In 2003, Noreen Clark noted important distinctions among terms such as self-care, disease management, self-regulation, and self-management. Establishing clear definitions is an important first step

in ensuring that health care professionals understand how to integrate self-management with clinical practice.

Using Clark's distinctions as a guide, *self-care* involves actions taken by an older adult to maintain a desired health status without the interaction or assistance of a professional. Examples might include taking herbal supplements or participating in a yoga class at the YMCA independently, without any advice or monitoring by health care professionals.

Although self-care is important in the lives of older adults, in this chapter, we are interested in health behaviors that either do or should directly involve health care professionals. Such behavior falls under the rubric of either *disease management* or *self-management*. Clearly, older adults managing chronic disease and disability must frequently consult health care professionals and adhere to the various therapies they prescribe. Adherence implies that the older adults perceive that they have an active role in making decisions about, and carrying out, a particular regimen. It implies a collaborative relationship between patient and health provider. In contrast, compliance suggests an unquestioning and passive response by the patient and a provider–patient relationship that is one-way and top–down. Adherence has been shown to be better in promoting persistence and motivation than compliance, underscoring the necessity for collaboration in health care.

How, then, does disease management differ from self-management? *Disease management* involves both the health care system and the individual. At the system level, disease management refers to what the provider and health care system do to manage chronic disease and disability; for example, making available necessary services and prescriptions. At the individual level, disease management refers to the strategies implemented by patients and their families to manage both the disease and its consequences.

The individual level is the arena of *self-management* within disease management; it involves a partnership among the older adult, family and caregivers, and the health care professional. Ideally, the patient who self-manages effectively learns to use these human resources toward the goal of minimizing symptoms and optimizing function while living with the chronic disease or disability. In Clark's view, *self-regulation* refers to the way that patients derive strategies to handle their chronic disease; it is a process embedded in the larger context of self-management. While we agree that self-regulation is at the core of the self-management process, we contend that it will be strongly influenced by the health care provider. It should not be limited solely to patient-derived strategies, which are in the domain of self-care. In fact, the provider must educate patients about the self-regulation process if they are to understand and use it to manage their health behavior.

In summary, we define self-management as *a process that involves self-regulatory strategies taken by patients, who use their personal skills as well as those of health care professionals and supportive others to detect and manage their symptomatology and improve function.* While learning about and maintaining self-management of chronic disease require a partnership, the partners' responsibilities may vary over time, and the eventual goal is for the patient to achieve as much independence as possible. These partnerships must strive to help older adults acquire the self-regulatory skills essential to effective self-management of health behavior.

HEALTH BEHAVIORS EMBODIED IN SELF-MANAGEMENT

To explain self-management in geriatric medicine, we must clarify what is meant by health behavior. Generally speaking, older adults' self-management may involve three broad classes of health behavior: detection, promotion, and prevention. These behaviors must be distinguished because the motives and strategies to encourage each of them differ. Further, the extent of adherence to each class can be influenced by both positive (taking action) and negative (avoiding action) responses. Self-management encompasses both responses. For example, one older adult might attempt to adopt and maintain a therapeutic regimen of physical therapy for a frozen shoulder, yet another may decide not to go to the therapist to avoid the pain and discomfort of treatment. While avoidance by patients is rarely effective in managing symptoms in the long run and contributes to nonadherence, health care professionals must recognize that self-management does not always involve what they may view as the "correct" response.

Detection behavior, performed by the individual or the provider, provides information about the presence or absence of unhealthy or potentially unhealthy chronic conditions, for example older women performing breast self-examinations or health care professionals ordering mammograms. Promotion behavior is intended to maintain or improve an older adult's current state of relatively good health, for example healthy eating, regular exercise, and meditation when used proactively to manage stress. Often, health promotion behaviors do not involve the health care provider and are best conceptualized as part of self-care than self-management. On the other hand, prevention behavior is performed either to reduce or prevent the risk of future health problems or to facilitate recovery from a health event. Examples of preventive self-management include reducing saturated fat in the diet to lower cholesterol and the risk for cardiovascular disease (primary prevention) or engaging in exercise therapy to facilitate recovery following a myocardial infarction (secondary prevention) (Table 28-1).

TABLE 28-1

Examples of Self-Management Behaviors

DETECTION	PROTECTION	PROMOTION
Performing breast or testicular self-examination	Using sunscreen every day	Eating a healthy diet
Scheduling regular checkups with the dentist, optometrist, and physician	Flossing and brushing teeth each day	Exercising regularly
Checking blood pressure regularly	Getting an influenza shot	Meditating regularly to maintain a healthy state of psychological well-being
Testing home for safe radon and carbon monoxide levels	Wearing seat belt every time you drive	Maintaining a healthy social network

In geriatric medicine, health providers must encourage and actively facilitate older adults' development of self-management skills. They must also work to build the adherence of older adults toward desired detection, prevention, and promotion behaviors and thus strengthen and reinforce older adults' related self-confidence for managing those behaviors. Later in the chapter, we will discuss the research literature in self-management, which holds promise for successful collaborations between older adults and health care professionals in achieving these goals.

CONCEPTUAL FRAMEWORK FOR SELF-MANAGEMENT

Having defined self-management and discussed different classes of health behavior, the next logical step is to ask the following questions: What motivates older adults to engage in self-managing health behaviors? What causes success or failure in effective self-management? In answering these questions, we offer a conceptual framework that will serve two important roles. First, it will be used to examine evidence from research on self-management. What are the features of successful programs designed to promote self-management? What are important gaps in the knowledge? Second, it will provide health care professionals with a template for examining current practices or designing new initiatives that target self-management of health behavior for older adults.

Older adults engage in self-management in response to a conscious goal or to remove barriers in the path toward goals. For geriatric medicine, health-related goals most often stem from concerns related to detection or prevention behavior; that is, older adults want to identify and to alleviate or avoid a specific physical or psychological symptom/condition. If the symptom is new to them, then older adults' self-management behavior is frequently encouraged by a family member and begins with seeking a diagnosis.

However, in many instances, patients seek treatment for chronic disease, and a diagnosis is not needed. Here, prevention of the symptom becomes the goal. A common example among older adults is the pain associated with osteoarthritis. Quite often, they may not view pain management as self-management because they may perceive chronic pain as beyond their control. They believe that the health care provider has the sole remedy to fix their problem and prevent it in the future. For example, they might expect to obtain new medication or an increased dose of their current medication to alleviate arthritic pain. The physician's actions may reinforce this passive solution to the pain. The physician may feel that pain from osteoarthritis is rooted in some underlying pathology and that it is a biological problem and immediately rule out collaborative self-management. Such a decision and subsequent behavior either knowingly or unwittingly discourage self-management, reinforcing patients' notion that they have no role to play in treating their chronic condition. This example illustrates that both patients' understanding of their medical conditions and the behavior of health care professionals contribute to the motivation to self-manage health behavior. Active partnerships between patients and their health care professionals develop the motivation to take action and are essential in shaping patients' self-management behaviors.

Commonsense Model of Self-Regulation

Howard Leventhal and his colleagues have been instrumental in promoting a "commonsense" model of self-regulation for health behavior and have conducted considerable research on what motivates people to seek treatment. Their model also has relevance to adherence to self-management over time. A critical feature is its bottom-up, as opposed to top–down, organization. The focus begins with an older adult's perceptual experiences (feeling off-balance or weak) and physical symptoms (pain and fatigue)—the raw sensory experience that something is wrong. Moods and emotions related to this raw sensory experience as well as feelings of competence in being able to manage the problem are also important in determining higher-order reasoning, such as, "I'm in trouble and need help."

The model identifies five features of health events that motivate people to act: label/symptom, timeline, consequences, cause, and perceived control. The following scenario provides an explanation of how these features operate. Fred has noticed that he seems to have weakness and some mild discomfort in his upper legs when getting out of the car or rising from a kneeling or sitting position: the perceptual experience/symptom. Originally, he thought that these might be the result of an overuse injury, the inevitable effects of aging, or a complication related to the tension he has been experiencing with his younger son: the suspected cause. However, the symptoms have persisted for 8 weeks, and he long ago resolved the conflict with his son: the timeline. He has also noticed that friends of his age are not reporting this problem. He reasons that if aging were the cause, more of his friends would have the same symptoms. The symptoms are very frustrating because those have all but stopped him from working around the house and seem progressively worse because he now has discomfort when rising from his chair after watching TV. Consequently, Fred questions his original, suspected causes and now concludes and worries that he may have nerve damage in his spine or a musculoskeletal disease: loss of control.

Fred's initial cause-and-effect explanations of his symptoms are consistent with his personal reasoning about the relationship between stress and illness and age and illness and may have delayed his seeking treatment. However, when their duration and their absence among his peers suggest that these are not a normal problem of aging or stress, these become prompts to seek treatment. Leventhal and his group have found that, in addition to these five factors, fear is

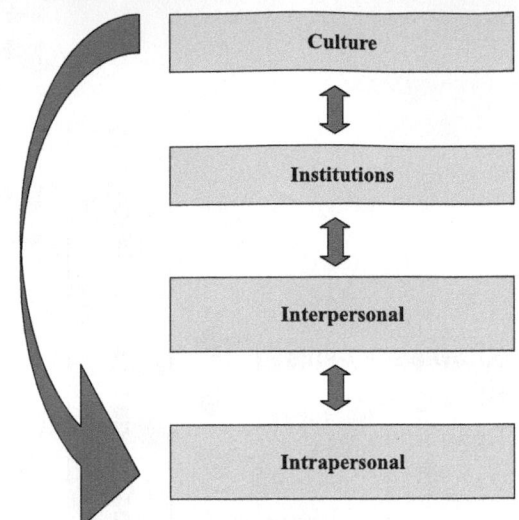

FIGURE 28-1. Multiple levels of influence that can affect older adult self-management.
Note that culture indirectly influences all levels in self-management but can especially influence the individual (intrapersonal) because of prevailing ageist stereotypes.

an important motive for action, but that without an action plan, fear does little to promote constructive behavior. For Fred, an action plan might consist of intending to call his physician tomorrow morning after breakfast to make an appointment for the following week.

Of course, older adults' commonsense models are not created in a vacuum; they are influenced by the social system. Individual health behavior is influenced by factors at interpersonal, institutional, and cultural levels, and our understanding of self-management has to be considered from a systems-based perspective (Figure 28-1).

Factors from multiple aspects of the system can both facilitate and inhibit older adults' actions. For example, a wife's insistence may result in her husband going for a prostate examination for potential detection of cancer (interpersonal influence). TV documentaries on the biology of aging may lead older adults to adopt a regimen of vitamin supplementation (institutional influence). Grown children may openly verbalize an emotional objection to their elderly parents seeking treatment for a symptom, being convinced that physicians are just trying to collect money on procedures for benign aches and pains, in effect "ripping off" Medicare (cultural influence). Other powerful cultural stereotypes in our society can discourage physical activity among older adults.

Symptoms do not always lead older adults to seek a solution, even when they are severe and persistent. In many instances, older adults self-manage their symptoms through avoidance. For example, a woman ignored rectal bleeding for more than a year until acute pain forced her to visit the emergency department, where colon cancer was diagnosed. She knew that something was seriously wrong long before this event, but she was afraid that once she went for a diagnosis, she would be hospitalized, and that would be the end of her life as she knew it. Such avoidance can also be triggered by older adults' beliefs about specific health behaviors. For example, older adults may have adopted stereotypes that support their position that they are too old to be physically active or that losing weight is unhealthy for them.

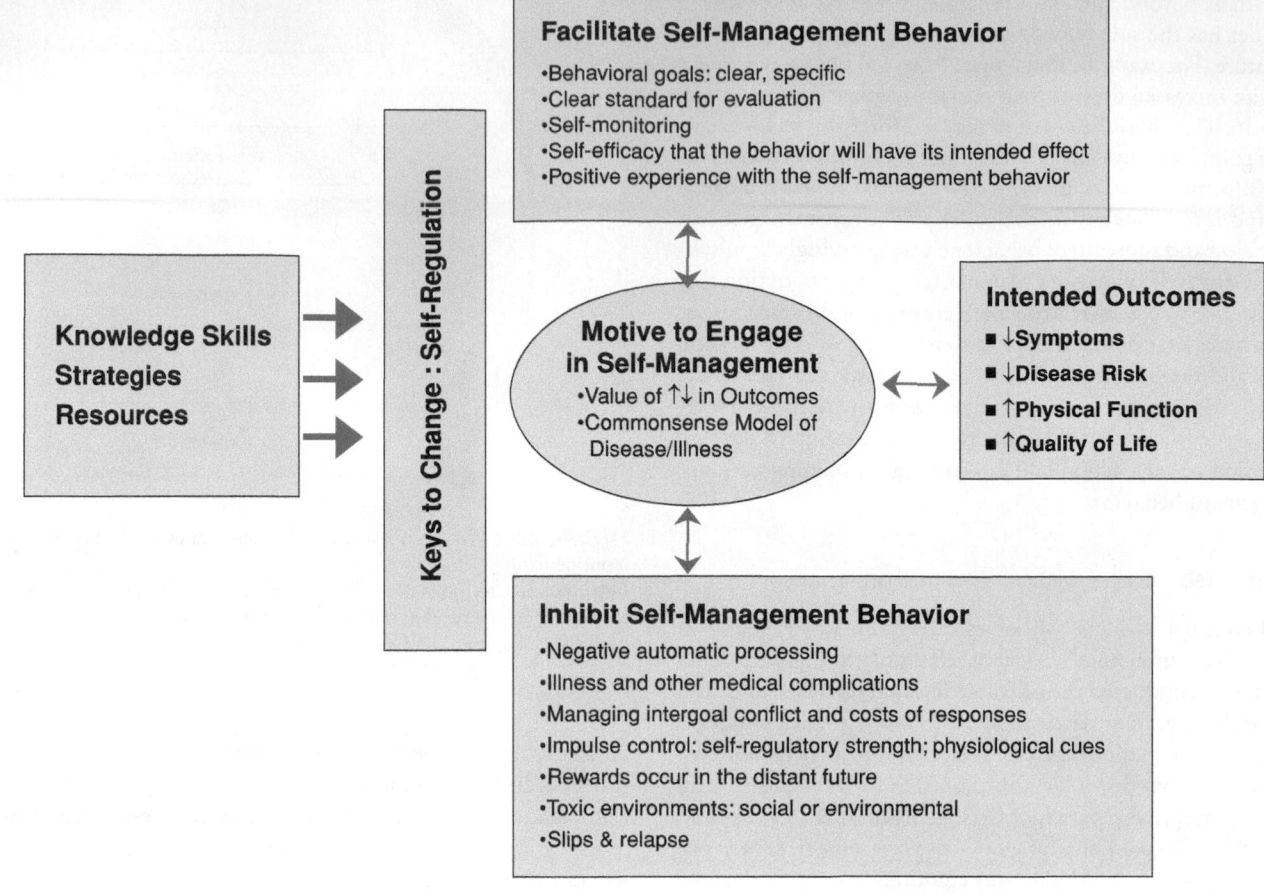

FIGURE 28-2. Blueprint for self-management.

Conceptual Framework for Understanding the Complexities of Self-Management

We will elaborate on three features in the following sections: (1) facilitating factors, (2) inhibitory factors, and (3) knowledge, skills, strategies, and resources (Figure 28-2).

Facilitating Factors in Self-Management

More than two decades of research in psychology have identified several factors that promote effective self-management of health behavior. Consider the following example. Helen is an obese, physically compromised older adult. She is frustrated by several consequences of her poor health, including the fatigue she experiences when moving, the loss of some of her functional independence, and a recent confirmation by her physician that she has type-2 diabetes. In collaboration with her physician, Helen decides to join a research study that is treating physical disability and diabetes in older adults using a combination of caloric restriction and increased physical activity. When she first enters the study, the intervention team evaluates her diet and activity patterns, and, based on these data, she and an interventionist together establish goals for modifying them over the next month. In addition, they discuss the importance of establishing weekly behavioral goals related to self-monitoring and evaluation of her progress. Together, they decide that, each month, Helen will time herself while walking four laps at the local YMCA track (~400 m)

and also record her fatigue on a simple 10-point scale (0 = no fatigue whatsoever and 10 = as tired as she has ever felt). Helen's progress and her confidence in being able to complete the prescription are checked weekly. Her goals are adjusted as necessary. On a monthly basis, Helen is asked to reflect on what she has done and to notice what effects, if any, the program is having on various aspects of her life (Table 28-2). As a result of this self-evaluation and a number of successes in pursuing the goals that she helped to set, Helen gained confidence in the skills necessary to make progress in changing her behavior. She could see the change happening as she engaged in these self-regulatory processes to manage her chronic health condition (see Table 28-2).

The scenario and the description provided in Table 28-2 illustrate how self-regulation generates effective self-management. The skills inherent in this process warrant repeating, since they are part of the tools that health care professionals must share with older adults in self-managing health behavior. They include:

1. setting clear, specific, and reasonably challenging goals for behavioral change;

2. monitoring personal behavior and how it influences reaching goals and the rate of change;

3. providing feedback and information on each health behavior goal that has been collaboratively established between the health care professional and the older adult;

TABLE 28-2

Factors that Promote Effective Self-Management

SELF-REGULATORY SKILL	EXAMPLE
Establishing proximal and distal goals	Helen and her HCP* discuss her current diet and activity patterns in order to develop realistic, challenging goals together. In addition to a long-term, monthly goal, weekly proximal goals are also created.
Self-monitoring progress toward goal	Helen writes down specifics about her diet and her exercise workouts each day. She also "tests" herself each month by walking around a track four times and seeing how much this tires her out.
Attaining feedback	Helen meets with her HCP weekly to discuss her log book. The HCP provides constructive feedback on how Helen is doing.
Self-evaluating progress toward goal	Helen looks back and reflects on her previous log entries to make note of any progress she is making toward her goals and whether she is noticing any changes in other areas of her life. She sees that it now takes less effort for her to walk around the track four times and that she can now ride the bike 10 min longer than she could 2 weeks ago. Both of these improvements are seen as progress toward her goal of increasing her physical activity level.
Making corrections to goal-directed behavior	The HCP helps Helen think of ways in which she can progress. She suggests, for example, that Helen work toward increasing her fruit and vegetable consumption gradually just as she has increased gradually the number of minutes of continuous physical activity. Helen brainstorms on practical tips that she can do to reach her short-term goals, such as buying precut vegetables and adding sautéed vegetables to all of her entrees.
Raising self-efficacy beliefs	Helen is encouraged to dote on the progress she has made—to see all of the workouts and positive changes she has made to her diet. This increases Helen's confidence in her abilities to successfully change her health behaviors, regardless of barriers that she encountered along the way.

*HCP, health-care professional.

4. self-evaluating progress related to the goal—collecting the older adults' personal judgments and emotional reactions about their pursuit of goals and making or not making progress;

5. correcting behavior as a result of feedback and self-evaluation, leading to more effective and persistent change in the direction of established goals;

6. encouraging belief in their ability to organize and to take actions associated with the specific circumstances that they are trying to change, in order to achieve specific goals. These beliefs foster the persistence necessary to increase behavioral change, despite the setbacks, difficulties, or rate of progress (self-efficacy beliefs).

The interaction of these multiple factors influences the success that older adults will have with health behavior change. However, their collaboration with health care professionals as their partners influences the entire self-regulatory process. The partners can make informed judgments about expectations and outcomes. In the example above, consequences could include not only Helen's reduced calorie consumption and increased walking but also compliments from family and friends, and the personal satisfaction with her own accomplishments. Regular reflection on progress (feedback) and comments about how it has affected life (outcome information) by both parties characterize a self-evaluative process and influence the desire of older adults to adhere to the collaborative prescription for change. The health care professional's comments about change in Helen's outlook and persistence and Helen's pleasure in being able to stick with reduced caloric consumption for more than a month jointly contribute to her self-efficacy (confidence) to adhere to their plan over the next month.

Inhibitory Factors in Self-Management

For some older adults, behavioral practices that reflect effective self-management of chronic disease are well learned and help to resist threats, such as competing behaviors and events. Many older adults consistently visit their physicians when they encounter novel physical symptoms, schedule screening examinations and vaccinations as recommended by health care professionals, and take recommended supplements and daily walks without fail. However, health care professionals must often ask older adults dealing with chronic disease or disability to adopt new remedial or preventive behaviors or to change dysfunctional patterns of behavior. Under such circumstances, a number of factors inhibit effective self-management.

Operating on Automatic Pilot Clearly, a major threat to self-regulation and effective self-management is operating automatically. The self-regulation needed to adopt a new behavior or to change an old pattern requires conscious control of thought and action. If an older adult behaves without thinking, opting for the easier, routine path that allows dysfunctional behavior, hope for change is futile. Why do older adults persist in automatic patterns? According to Walter Mischel's research, strong emotions, which are common in older adults, shut down their rational thinking and derail attempts at conscious behavior change. In our studies with older adults, these emotions have a variety of causes, including the frustration with failed treatments, the concern that they are a burden for their caregivers, and the acute illness or injury that disrupts the action plans that they use to self-manage their behavior change. The important lesson from Mischel's research is that self-management planning cannot ignore these emotions and their related causes.

In addition, decades of eastern writings and recent research in western psychology on mindfulness convincingly argue that North American society encourages automatic responding. Many individuals find it difficult to pay attention in the present moment to where they are headed and whether or not the direction of their path is consistent with what they value. It has been suggested that we have this difficulty because we spend much of our young and middle adult years striving to get somewhere or to complete the next task. This behavior pattern continues into old age. Some customary routines do not require that older adults consciously monitor what they are doing, and their inclination is not to alter what seems to be working for them in day-to-day situations. The problem, of course, is that many customary routines run counter to the strategies or prescriptions that health care professionals hope to make a part of older adults' health self-management: "I always have a doughnut with my coffee." More will be said about how health care professionals can counter the phenomenon of "operating on automatic pilot" later in the chapter.

Slips, Relapses, and Intergoal Conflict A second general threat to effective self-management is the occurrence of slips and relapses in behavior and intergoal conflict. The failure to remain true to personal goals is often distressing, and older adults are no exceptions to this experience. For this reason, slips and relapses often spark negative emotions, which contribute to giving up the adoption or maintenance of new self-regulatory behavior that can facilitate self-management. For example, Byrne, Cooper, and Fairburn conducted a qualitative study comparing obese women who were either successful or unsuccessful in maintaining weight loss after an initial intensive treatment. They found that relapse was related to (1) the failure to achieve weight goals and dissatisfaction with the weight achieved, (2) the tendency to evaluate self-worth in terms of weight and shape, (3) a lack of vigilant weight control, (4) a dichotomous (black-and-white) thinking style, and (5) the tendency to use eating to regulate mood. The theme that emerges is that relapse is often triggered by negative thoughts and feelings about self-management, which can arise from (1) unrealistic expectations about outcomes, (2) eliminating a behavior that is used to cope with life stress, or (3) having zero-tolerance for slips.

We have also found that slips in self-management are often related to competing events—intergoal conflict. A common example for older adults is vacation or family gatherings, which compete for time and priority with preventive actions. In these situations, self-management behavior takes a back seat and can even lead to negative thoughts, such as: "I just don't have time for this program on vacation," or "I don't like the feeling of guilt that I am suddenly experiencing; something's got to give." The black-and-white thinking style posits that vacation and active self-management of health behavior are incongruent. However, with the development of appropriate self-regulatory skills, the two goals need not be in conflict.

Toxic Environments Poor physical and social environments as well as lack of resources for effective self-management can interfere with diagnosis, prevention, and promotion. According to Marcia Ory and her colleagues, barriers often evolve from negative stereotypes related to six common myths of aging. These ageist stereotypes are reflected in the media and social and health care services. Expert witnesses who testified before the U.S. Senate Special Committee on Aging reported that the media and marketing depict older adults as helpless, feeble, and ineffective. In the realm of health care, Ory and her colleagues found that physicians tend to provide less aggressive treatments to older patients and that self-management programs typically target younger populations. Furthermore, behavioral and lifestyle interventions are believed to have only minimal impact on older adults, despite accumulating evidence to the contrary (Table 28-3).

TABLE 28-3

Popular Myths of Aging

	MYTH	REALITY
1	To be old is to be sick	Although chronic illnesses and disabilities do increase with age, the majority of older people are able to perform functions necessary for daily living and to manage independently until very advanced ages. The effects of population aging are mediated, in part, by declining disability rates.
2	You can't teach an old dog new tricks	Older people are capable of learning new things and continue to do so over the life course. This relates to cognitive vitality as well as the adoption of new behaviors.
3	The horse is out of the barn	The benefits of adopting recommended lifestyle behaviors continue into the later years. It is never too late to gain benefits from highly recommended behaviors, such as increasing physical activity.
4	The secret to successful aging is to choose your parents wisely	Genetic factors play a relatively small role in determining longevity and quality of life. Social and behavioral factors play a larger role in one's overall health status and functioning.
5	The lights may be on, but the voltage is low	While interest and engagement in sexual activities decline with age, the majority of older people with partners and without major health problems are sexually active, although the nature and frequency of their activities may change over time.
6	The elderly don't pull their own weight	The majority of older adults who do not work for pay are engaged in productive roles within their families and/or the community at large.

Costs and the Problems of Distant Benefits Research from multiple theoretical perspectives illustrates that the anticipated costs of behavior weigh heavily on the decision to seek or to persist with a treatment. For example, research has shown that the fear of a medical procedure, without a plan to deal with the fear, is a significant barrier to treatment. In our own work on lifestyle behavior, we find that negatively interpreted physical symptoms during activity are barriers to older adults' continued involvement with exercise programs, and having to eliminate favorite foods in caloric and fat restriction prescriptions for weight loss is, at times, difficult for older adults to accept.

Another common challenge for older adults is what researchers have described as temporal discounting or the delay of gratification necessary to reach some outcomes. Willingness to persist with treatment for weeks, and sometimes months, before any major outcome is realized may wane. Many older adults may be faced with delayed gratification both in achieving desired outcomes and in the heavy costs of day-to-day treatment. No wonder self-management can be perceived as complex and stressful and lead to avoidance or nonadherence.

Knowledge, Skills, and Strategies

The final component of our conceptual blueprint for self-management addresses the knowledge, skills, and strategies that

TABLE 28-4

Six Key Questions Concerning Traditional and Collaborative Care

QUESTION	TRADITIONAL CARE	COLLABORATIVE CARE
What is the relationship between patient and health professionals?	Professionals are the experts who tell patients what to do. Patients are passive.	Shared expertise with active patients. Professionals are experts about the disease and patients are experts about their lives.
Who is the principal caregiver and the problem solver? Who is responsible for outcomes?	The professional	The patient and professional are the principal caregivers; they share responsibility for solving problems and for outcomes.
What is the goal?	Compliance with instructions. Noncompliance is a personal deficit of the patient.	The patient sets goals and the professional helps the patient make informed choices. Lack of goal achievement is a problem to be solved by modifying strategies.
How is behavior changed?	External motivation	Internal motivation. Patients gain understanding and confidence to accomplish new behaviors.
How are problems identified?	By the professional, e.g., changing unhealthy behaviors.	By the patient, e.g., pain or inability to function; and by the professional.
How are problems solved?	Professionals solve problems for patients.	Professionals teach problem-solving skills and help patients in solving problems.

inform self-regulation and, in turn, promote effective forms of self-management. Knowledge about illness, chronic disease, and disability is important from at least two perspectives. First, patients must know about the origin and course of the disease itself. For example, it has been well documented that adults are better at managing diabetes when they understand the importance of self-monitoring their blood glucose level and have specific action plans to implement when values are below or above the target. Second, consistent with Leventhal's commonsense model of illness and disease, older adults' concepts of their health conditions must be explored and expanded. As we saw in Figure 28-1, important areas include (1) symptoms, (2) perceived causes, (3) anticipated consequences, (4) degree of perceived control over the process and course of the disease, and (5) the timeline for disease progression and achieving symptom management.

Skills and strategies refer to intervention methods that have been proven effective in promoting the self-regulation of positive and negative factors toward health behavior change. As we review selected examples from the literature, we will identify elements that are consistent markers of success and indicate how the methods fit into our self-management blueprint.

LESSONS FROM THE LITERATURE ON SELF-MANAGEMENT

Self-management is good medicine. If the huge benefits of these few habits were put into a pill, it would be declared a scientific milestone in the field of medicine. (Bandura A. Health promotion by social cognitive means. *Health Education & Behavior* 2004;31:143.)

Partnerships in Self-Management: A Description and Conceptual Rationale

A central position of this chapter that is reinforced in the contemporary literature on self-management is the importance of establishing partnerships between patients and health care professionals. An inherent quality of any effective self-management program is that the patient is an active partner in treatment. What is actually meant by the term partnership? How does traditional care differ from collaborative care? How do these two approaches influence the approach a health care professional should take to patient education? What is the conceptual significance of partnerships?

Traditional Versus Collaborative Patient Care

Bodenheimer and his colleagues have recently offered an excellent description of traditional and collaborative care paradigms in chronic disease management and explained the impact of this distinction on patient education. Table 28-4 identifies their six key questions about patient care together with answers based on each of these paradigms. Note that in a traditional medical model, patients tend to take a more passive role in the interaction with the health care professional. Health care professionals identify the problem, provide solutions, and expect that patients will comply with recommendations and prescriptions; noncompliance is viewed as a dysfunctional patient problem. In contrast, when partnerships are established in collaborative care, patients are allowed to define their problems, and patient and professional share responsibility for the creation of treatment plans. Health care professionals facilitate and guide rather than dictate treatment, and noncompliance is viewed as a shared problem to be solved. Indeed, in some instances, most obviously involving side effects from pharmacological therapy, noncompliance may be a wise and rational step, indicating that treatment plans should be either modified or expanded (see Table 28-4).

In suggesting that patients be allowed to help to define problems, we do not mean that they should supplant health care professionals as diagnosticians. Rather, health care professionals must listen carefully to what patients are saying about their health status and treatment. Consider the example of an older male patient in cardiac rehabilitation. His main concern was his impotence, not the condition of his heart. After considerable dialogue, close examination of his medications, and consultation with his cardiologist, his beta-blocker was changed. Within a very brief time, his erections improved, and his entire attitude toward treatment changed. He was now emotionally able and willing to consider how he could prevent further disease. In fact, what motivated him to exercise, take lipid-lowering medication, and watch his diet was the realization that the vessels that

TABLE 28-5

Contrasts Between Traditional and Collaborative Medicine

	TRADITIONAL PATIENT EDUCATION	SELF-MANAGEMENT EDUCATION
What is taught?	Information and technical skills about the disease	Skills on how to act on problems
How are problems formulated?	Problems reflect inadequate control of the disease	The patient identifies problems he/she experiences that may or may not be related to the disease
Relation of education to the disease	Education is disease specific and teaches information and technical skills related to the disease	Education provides problem-solving skills that are relevant to the consequences of chronic conditions in general
What is the theory underlying the education?	Disease-specific knowledge creates behavior change, which in turn produces better clinical outcomes	Greater patient confidence in his/her capacity to make life-improving changes (self-efficacy) yields better clinical outcomes
What is the goal?	Compliance with the behavior changes taught to the patient to improve clinical outcomes	Increased self-efficacy to improve clinical outcomes
Who is the educator?	A health professional	A health professional, peer leader, or other patients, often in group settings

served the penis were also subject to atherosclerosis. The benefit of listening to the patient's concerns and then collaborating on a solution provided huge gains in adherence to the traditional goals of cardiac rehabilitation. This process also contributed to his understanding of the system-wide impact of both disease and adherence on the rehabilitation prescription.

Traditional and collaborative medical care lead to different sets of goals and strategies for patient education. According to Bodenheimer and colleagues, the traditional model is delivered by health care professionals and reinforces patients' ability and need to follow "what the physician orders." By contrast, in a partnership model, education is synonymous with the concept of self-management (Table 28-5). Geriatric health care professionals are part of a larger network of services and individuals that promote the health of older adults. Thus, an important goal of geriatric medicine is to teach patients to leverage resources in their communities and within the health care system. Using such resources enables older adults to reach effective solutions for their current problems and compress their future disability, morbidity, and mortality into the last few months or years of life. This perspective is at the heart of what the healthy aging research network concluded: Healthy aging is most easily achieved when two sets of conditions are operating. The first is when physical environments and communities are safe and support the adoption and maintenance of attitudes and behavior known to promote health and well-being. The second is through the effective use of health services and community programs to prevent or minimize the impact of acute and chronic disease on function (see Table 28-5).

The Conceptual Importance of Partnerships in Health Care

Partnerships have immense significance to the development and maintenance of effective self-management and health in older adults for several reasons. First, older adults' commonsense models of their disease and illness play a key role in determining health behaviors. In the absence of a partnership between patients and their health-care professionals, these commonsense models go unnoticed. A recent paper by Halm and his associates illustrates the significance of such oversight among minority inner-city adults with persistent asthma. They found that many patients—53% of their sample—believed that they only had asthma when they were having acute symptoms.

The authors termed this phenomenon the no symptoms, no asthma belief. Men older than 65 years and those who had no consistent health care provider were most likely to hold this belief, which was related to lower use of flowmeters, poorer adherence to inhaled corticosteroids, and the belief that using inhaled corticosteroids in the absence of symptoms was less important. Rates of morbidity and mortality from asthma are highest among these minority inner-city populations.

The importance of partnerships is also supported by epidemiological studies, indicating that physician advice can strongly enhance older adults' desire and confidence in their ability to perform specific health behaviors. Many older adults choose not to discuss health-related self-care with physicians because they are unsure whether the physicians will approve of what they are doing. Thus, geriatricians are often unaware of whether or not their patients are in counseling or dieting or exercising or receiving other forms of health-related treatment, which severely compromises the process of self-management. When health care professionals engage their older patients as partners in a health care plan, discussions are more likely to be open and mutually enlightening.

Finally, through partnerships, health care professionals are in a good position to teach patients effective self-regulation of health behavior. Communication and buy-in occur when goals are clearly specified and action plans are articulated, monitored, and evaluated on a regular basis to enhance patients' motivation and confidence in various treatment regimens. The remainder of this chapter will demonstrate the promise that various programs of self-management have in encouraging health behavior. Although some of the research does not directly involve physicians, these programs work best when physicians understand and support their goals.

Chronic Disease Self-Management Program

Kate Lorig has published widely on the Arthritis Self-Management Program (ASMP), which has since evolved into a generic Chronic Disease Self-Management Program (CDSMP). ASMP and CDSMP are led by individuals with chronic health conditions who receive 20 hours of training, based on detailed manuals for group facilitation. ASMP is disease specific, emphasizing the management of arthritic pain. It is delivered in 2-hour group sessions (10–15 individuals), meeting once a week for 6 weeks. Major topics include

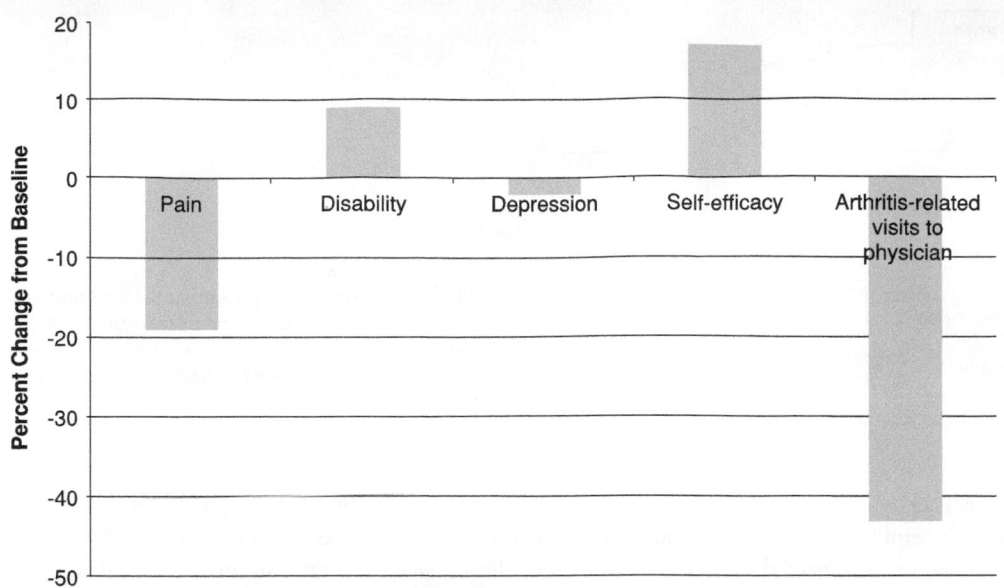

FIGURE 28-3. Twelve years of research on the Arthritis Self-Management Program. (Adapted with permission from Lorig K, Holman H. Arthritis self-management studies: a twelve-year review. Health Educ Q. 1993;20:17).

pain and stress management; exercise; problem solving; communication skills, especially for physician/patient interactions; nutrition; medications; and nontraditional treatments. CDSMP is designed to treat people who have a range of chronic diseases and is delivered in 2.5-hour sessions every week for 7 weeks. Topics include managing physical symptoms and negative emotions, exercise, problem solving and decision making, communication skills, nutrition, medication use, and the use of community resources. In both programs, leaders function as facilitators, rather than lecturers, actively engaging participants to develop personal goals and specific action plans for each week. Regular feedback is a crucial component, and the objective is to enhance patients' confidence in their ability to acquire specific behaviors or skills in each area of content.

Despite the limited time allotted to address such a broad range of complex health behaviors, data from randomized clinical trials of both ASMP and CDSMP have been encouraging. Figure 28-3 summarizes 12 years of research on ASMP, as reported by Lorig. Note that the 6-week ASMP interventions led to enduring positive changes in self-efficacy, level of pain, and frequency of physician visits (see Figure 28-3).

In a 6-month randomized trial of CDSMP, intervention patients experienced statistically significant increases in weekly minutes of exercise, frequency of cognitive symptom management, improved communication with physicians, and enhanced self-reported health, as compared to control patients. Other improvements favoring intervention patients were lower levels of health distress, fatigue, and disability, and fewer limitations in social/role activities. They also had fewer hospitalizations and days in the hospital. However, they did not differ from controls in their pain or physical discomfort, shortness of breath, or psychological well-being.

While self-efficacy beliefs appear to play an important role in the apparent success of ASMP and CDSMP, establishing proximal goals and providing feedback on goal attainment are also important. These latter steps help to create short-term incentives and to guide behavior in the desired direction. Moreover, to sustain efforts in the face of inevitable barriers and to assist with problem solving, the interventions encourage participants to enlist support from health care professionals, peer groups, and significant others.

Other Programs from Stanford University

The same self-regulation principles that facilitate self-management can be found in other types of interventions that employ an individual, as opposed to a group format, yet are designed to reach large segments of the population. One example of this approach is the case-management system for health care, originally developed by DeBusk and his colleagues at Stanford University-to modify and reduce coronary risk factors. The program is conducted by nurses who receive 80 hours of special training by multidisciplinary experts to deliver interventions for smoking cessation, exercise training, and dietary-drug therapy for hyperlipidemia. Scheduled interventions during a 1-year period include: (1) questionnaires that patients complete and then mail to the nurse case manager; (2) computerized progress reports mailed to patients, based on those questionnaires; (3) 14 nurse-initiated phone contacts; (4) four one-on-one patient visits to the nurse case manager; and (5) eight patient visits to the blood chemistry laboratory. Figure 28-4 illustrates the interdependence of physician, case manager (implementer), and patient using phone contacts and the computerized system to facilitate self-management. Note that the computerized system serves a dual role: one for data management and another in providing knowledge and information on self-regulatory skills that are essential to health behavior change (see Figure 28-4).

The initial study using this system was conducted on adults with a mean age of 57 years who were hospitalized for acute myocardial infarction. Patients were randomized to this treatment or usual care and then followed for 1 year. At the 1-year assessment visit, biochemically determined rates of smoking cessation were significantly higher in the case-managed group (70%) than in the usual care control group (53%), and on a treadmill test performed at 6 months, patients in the case-managed group had higher cardiovascular fitness. At 1 year, lipid-lowering drugs had been prescribed to ~80%

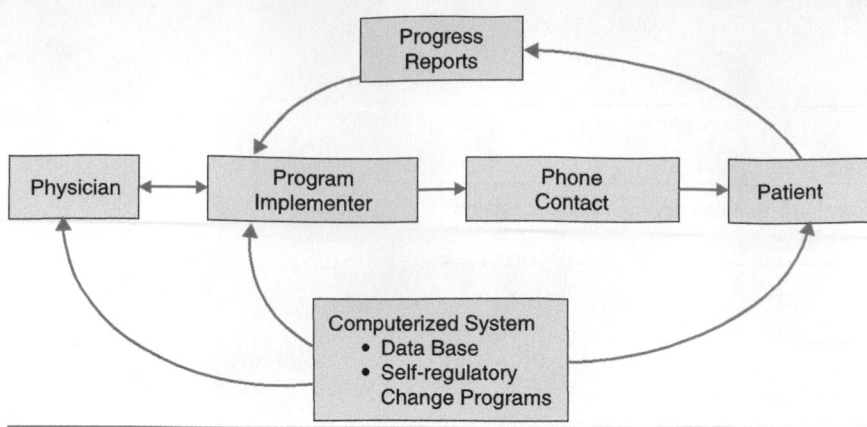

FIGURE 28-4. Case management model for coronary risk modification. (Adapted with permission from DeBusk RF, Miller NH, Superko HR, et al. A case-management system for coronary risk factor modification after acute myocardial infarction. Ann Inter Med. 1994;120:721.)

of patients in the case-managed group but only 21% in usual care. While corresponding differences in plasma cholesterol favored those in the case-managed group, patients in both groups experienced decreasing levels of dietary cholesterol and fat from baseline to the 1-year assessment.

Haskell and his colleagues at Stanford conducted a related study of risk reduction in middle-aged to older adults who had coronary atherosclerosis. Their study was a randomized trial with two groups: usual care and intensive risk management. Their trial design had an objective measure of disease progression and 4 years of follow-up. Patients were provided with short- and long-term goals and an individualized action plan for risk reduction. Progress was tracked, and short-term goals were adjusted using telephone and mail contacts as well as face-to-face clinic visits every 2 to 3 months across the 4 years of the study. The staff included experts in the content areas of interest, such as nutrition, exercise, smoking, and lipid management.

After 4 years of treatment, patients who were randomly assigned to usual care showed little or no change in study outcomes. By comparison, those in intensive risk management showed dramatic changes in their health, improving their cholesterol profile, lowering saturated fats, losing weight, increasing their physical activity, and improving the functional capacity of their cardiovascular system (Figure 28-5). This shift in health behavior was reflected in significant reductions in cumulative cardiac deaths at the 4-year assessment visit (Figure 28-6). As in the case management study by Debusk, at some point during the course of this study, 93% of those in the intensive risk management condition were placed on drugs for lipid management, compared to only 30% in the usual care condition. Since patients in both studies improved in areas unrelated to blood lipids, not all of the observed effects were contaminated by the introduction of lipid-lowering drugs into treatment. The superiority of results for the intervention groups in both studies implies that even drug therapy can be enhanced by being embedded in a program that establishes clear goals for therapy and provides more frequent evaluation of patients' health status (see Figures 28-5 and 28-6).

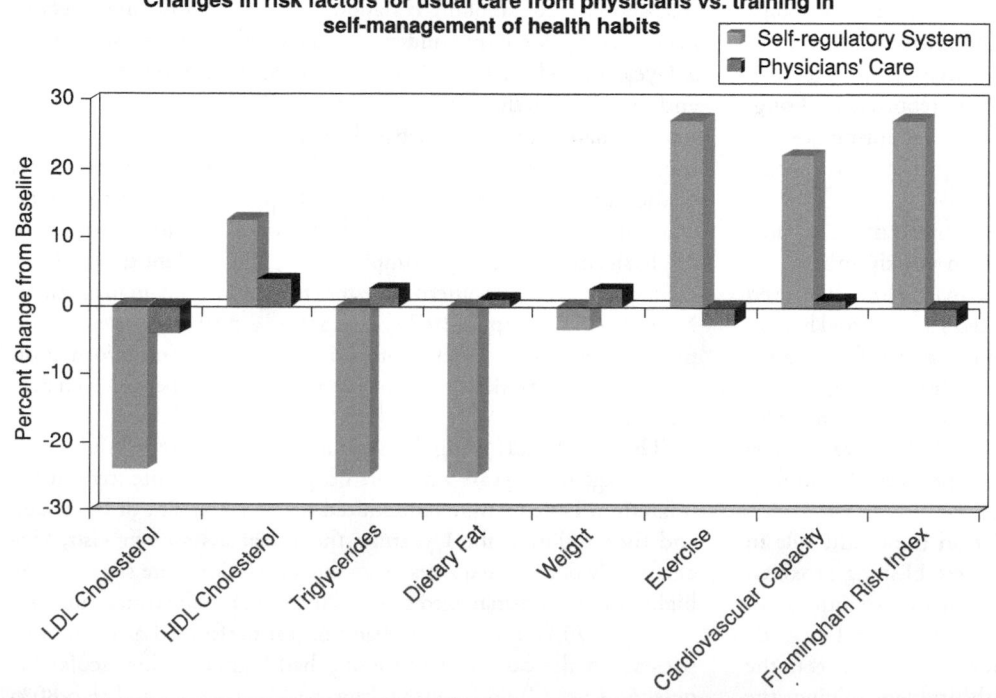

FIGURE 28-5. A comparison of a self-regulatory system for self-management with usual care. (Data from Haskell WL, Alderman EL, Fair JM, et al. Effects of intensive multiple risk factor reduction on coronary atherosclerosis and clinical cardiac events in men and women with coronary artery disease: the Stanford Coronary Risk Intervention Project (SCRIP). Circulation. 1994;89:975.)

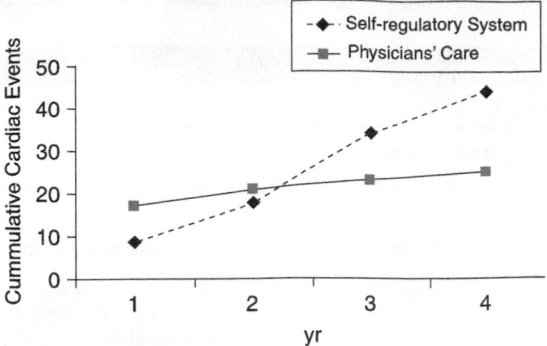

FIGURE 28-6. Four-year cumulative cardiac events with a self-regulatory intervention as compared to usual care. *(Data from Haskell WL, Alderman EL, Fair JM, et al. Effects of intensive multiple risk factor reduction on coronary atherosclerosis and clinical cardiac events in men and women with coronary artery disease: the Stanford Coronary Risk Intervention Project (SCRIP). Circulation. 1994;89:975.)*

One other study that deserves mention is a workplace project described by Bandura. Although it was not conducted on older adults, it underscores the potential value of social support in self-management. The goal of this project was to lower cholesterol in workers by reducing foods high in saturated fats. A nutritionist supervised the self-management system that was conceptually similar to the previously described programs conducted at Stanford. At the 3-month assessment, plasma cholesterol between those assigned to an experimental group dropped approximately 10 mg/dL as compared to a control group; however, this difference increased to ~17 mg/dL when spouses participated in the program (Figure 28-7). The effects of the intervention appear to have been compromised somewhat by the inclusion of individuals who had relatively low plasma cholesterol at the onset of the program (panel B, Figure 28-7). However, these data are worth mentioning because they suggest that self-managing lipids is particularly beneficial to those who need it most—those with more severe disease or disability (see Figure 28-7).

Individual Versus Group-Based Interventions

The work at Stanford and elsewhere indicates the benefits of incorporating groups into programs to instill self-management of health behavior for older adults when appropriate and possible. In our research, we have compared the effects of group-mediated cognitive-behavioral self-management among older patients who qualify for cardiac rehabilitation with a standard model. Both interventions involved center-based exercise therapy. In the standard therapy, patients met three times a week for exercise only. For the group-mediated cognitive-behavioral self-management treatment, patients met less often for exercise at the center, in order to promote home-based exercise, but, when they did exercise at the center, they also met afterward in small counseling groups, designed to provide the knowledge, motivation, self-regulatory skills, and resources, to be more physically active and to reduce self-perceived mobility disability (Table 28-6). At 3 months, after both groups had been heavily involved in their respective treatment plans, older adults who had been more compromised at entry into the study achieved greater reductions in self-perceived mobility disability under the group-mediated cognitive-behavioral condition than those who had been randomly assigned to standard exercise therapy (Figure 28-8). In addition, at 12 months, those in the group-mediated treatment group made greater improvements in their MET capacity (a measure of cardiovascular fitness), physical activity habits, and confidence to perform a timed walk test than those in standard treatment (see Figures 28-6 and 28-8).

This successful example shows that groups are useful in developing participants' self-regulatory skills. The group is developed to foster an active, collaborative learning of rehabilitation and self-regulation. Over the course of the group intervention, patients are encouraged to integrate the skills they learn and, with mutual input, test and evaluate their successes and failures in using these skills in their home-based activity. Belonging to a group whose members' goal is active involvement and collective change is a powerful agent that creates the impetus for, and, eventually, the practice of, effective self-management. The approach differs markedly from the use of

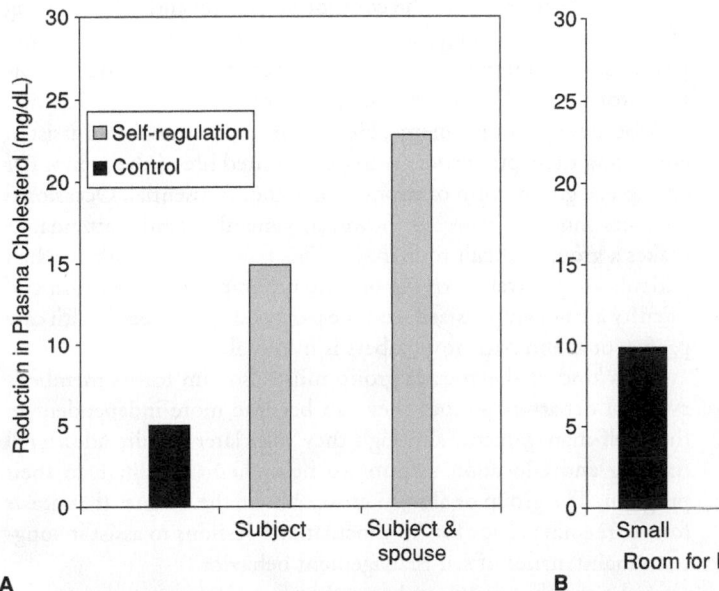

FIGURE 28-7. The effects of spouse support and the law of initial values on plasma cholesterol. *(Adapted with permission from Bandura A. Health promotion by social cognitive means. Health Educ Behav. 2004;31:143.)*

TABLE 28-6

Self-Regulatory Skills Taught in Group-Mediated Cognitive-Behavioral Interventions

WEEK IN PROGRAM	SELF-REGULATORY GOAL	EXAMPLE ACTIVITY
Week 1	Promote and develop group identity	Participants created and adopted group name.
Week 2	Learn how to self-monitor effort, symptoms, and behavior	Participants were taught how to log physical activity bouts and gauge perceived effort expended during the bout.
Week 3	Set individual and group goals	Participants were taught how to set specific, realistic, yet challenging goals for themselves and as a group.
Week 4	Planning how to exercise independently	Participants were paired with a "buddy" and asked to brainstorm solutions to possible barriers that one may encounter when attempting to exercise alone.
Week 5	Foster social support for individual and group goals	Each participant stated their individual goal to the group and indicated how it would help the group achieve the group goal, and fellow group members offered suggestions on how to attain that goal.
Week 6	Same as week 5, only for decreasing sedentary behaviors	
Week 7	Encourage self-reinforcement and self-evaluation	Participants were taught how to use self-reinforcement to achieve similar future goals.
Week 8	Increasing exercise independence	Participants worked in pairs to design individualized exercise plans for the next week.
Week 9	Recognition of environmental cues	Participants were asked to brainstorm on what cues they could use to facilitate their home-based activity.
Week 10	Develop coping strategies	Feedback was given by group members to each participant's report of success/failure with self-planned activity. Members were encouraged to suggest ways in which others could improve or avoid barriers encountered during the next week.
Week 11	Learn how to prevent and deal with relapses	The group identified signs of relapse and suggested strategies for overcoming relapse.
Week 12	Increasing self-efficacy	Participants were reminded of all the success and improvements and then created their first week of totally independent home-based activity, as well as a general plan for their first month of independent activity.

Note: All weekly plans were integrated such that goals were continually assessed and revised. From week 8 to 12, participants continued to plan and try their programs when away from the center. In summary, participants gradually weaned themselves from the group toward independent exercise.

the group as a simple forum of convenience, in order to deliver standard therapy to multiple participants where they primarily follow direction provided by a trained leader. Results from cancer research have shown that it is not group contact per se but how the group is leveraged that promotes effective self-regulation.

How can group potential for health care improvements be maximized? As Yalom noted in his classic text on the use of groups for psychological therapy, group cohesiveness must be developed. In the preceding example on cardiac rehabilitation, we used classic formative techniques to optimize the dynamics of these small groups ($n = 7$–10 members). Older adults who have chronic diseases have a common motivation for uniting in a group. Older adults best suited to groups are receptive to the concept of therapy and (1) discussing their disease, (2) learning from other members, (3) developing group goals, and (4) interacting with other members in practicing self-regulatory skills. Within this receptive context, group goal-setting and social support can emerge. Health care professionals can assist in enhancing these properties during the limited life of the group. For example, a group norm of strong attendance is essential. Occasional absences must be expected; however, general sporadic attendance makes a group difficult to manage. This failure is more likely when patients are passively carrying out their therapy, group mission and identity are not emphasized, and the partnership between health care professional and patient members is minimal.

This kind of therapeutic group must also aim for its members' eventual departure so that they can become more independent in their self-management, although they may later require additional training and education sessions to help them to adhere to their program. The group or alumni group can be the magnet that draws former members back for "re-inoculation" sessions to assist in long-term maintenance of self-management behavior.

Although the group can be used to foster self-management and the learning of self-regulatory skills, practitioners should be mindful

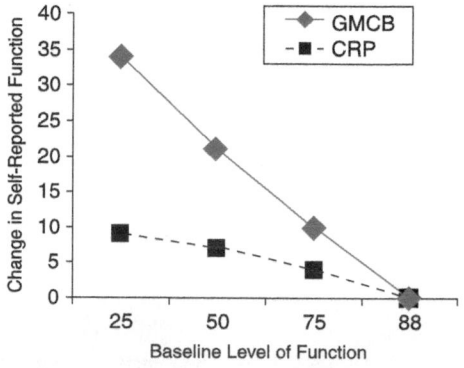

FIGURE 28-8. Three-month changes in self-reported physical function in traditional versus a group-mediated cognitive-behavioral intervention. (Adapted with permission from Rejeski WJ, Foy CG, Brawley LR, et al. Older adults in cardiac rehabilitation: a new strategy for enhancing physical function. Medicine and Science in Sports and Exercise. 2002;34:1705–1713.)

of caveats. First, as Bandura and others have noted, groups can create dependency, and older adults may quickly revert to their old ways when their group terminates. Cancer research suggests that if groups have no specific purpose other than to allow patients to meet with their peers, then the effects on self-management are nil.

Challenges to Active Self-Management

Heterogeneity in Health Status and Health Goals

Self-management programs frequently target chronic diseases, such as diabetes, asthma, COPD, or arthritis, which require managing medications and lifestyle in response to specific symptoms. In such instances, the outcomes of effective self-management are often clear and reinforcing to patients. They realize that their active involvement in disease management makes a difference. They experience increased confidence in managing their symptoms, and enhanced perceptions of personal control become a central part of their commonsense model of the disease process.

Unfortunately, this success does not come to everyone with a chronic disease. For example, if the disease or symptom becomes worse and/or they experience a considerable loss in function, older adults may perceive a loss of control that understandably inhibits the motivation for active self-management. Ample research has shown that when doubt surrounding the effectiveness of behavior is strong, the impetus either to expend effort on action plans or to pursue goals for change is weak.

Before we discuss possible solutions to such challenges, it is useful to recognize that goals exist in a hierarchy. In the current context, a common goal for older adults is "to maintain a healthy state." However, its pursuit is not necessarily conscious and active until it is threatened by either the loss of function or the emergence of physical symptoms. Once this occurs, then older adults are inclined to institute "do goals," such as taking medication to relieve symptoms or participating in physical therapy to improve their balance. Because such "do goals" are more specific than the global goal of a healthy state, their achievement requires an action plan or a sequence of steps to follow. If medication is prescribed, it may involve going to the medicine cabinet at a specific time of day, opening the bottle, and taking the medication as well as monitoring medication use and impact over time. In the case of physical therapy, it involves making appointments, scheduling transportation to the appointment, clarifying the physiotherapist's teaching of exercises for balance improvement, trying the exercises at home at a specific time of day, and monitoring the impact of the regimen on personal balance control.

Need to Change Health Goals as Health Declines

With a better understanding of goal hierarchy, we can propose ways to help older adults whose motivation to engage in self-management has been depleted. Scheier and Carver have emphasized that western culture frowns on giving up on goals, yet they argue that, in some contexts, goal disengagement is an important coping process. Aging inevitably presents some insoluble problems. Our physiological systems deteriorate, yielding predictable declines in mental and physical functioning. From a self-management perspective, detaching from an unrealistic goal allows the health care professional and patient to recalibrate less ambitious goals that still point the patient in the same persistent direction, while enhancing their sense of part-

nership. For example, a physical activity goal of 150 minute/week may be trimmed to 80 minute/week. Experts believe that following this principle of partial disengagement—moving from an unrealistic to a more realistic and achievable goal without totally abandoning a particular behavioral domain—is essential because it keeps the person engaged with life and may well delay the onset of further health problems.

Unfortunately, some circumstances may dictate total elimination of activities that provide older adults with a purpose for living. We have seen many older individuals with chronic diseases who eventually have to give up valued activities owing to a variety of impairments in the later stages of functional decline. In these instances, some older adults disengage and cope effectively by redirecting their energies into other domains, such as spirituality. In effect, they redefine or reprioritize their higher-order goals to accommodate their limited health state. Others fail to cope. They cling to old concepts, are unwilling to let go, and create suffering for themselves and their families. Indeed, contemporary research suggests that failing to disengage from past goals that are no longer feasible creates intense regret among older adults and predisposes them to depression and physical symptoms like constipation and skin disease. Health care professionals may be frustrated in attempting to pursue a partnership on a treatment path that is unacceptable to the patient.

Mindfulness-based interventions may be particularly beneficial in this realm of self-management for older adults, and they are being offered as part of hospital, outpatient, and community outreach programs. These interventions teach centering skills, designed around breathing, for controlling negative thoughts and emotion; they foster insights designed to promote acceptance of life experiences that are not subject to personal control. Although further discussion of this topic is beyond the scope of this chapter, interested readers may consult the end of chapter reference by Baer (Baer, 2006).

Evidence of Effectiveness of Interventions that Facilitate Self-Management

To date, several hundred studies have been conducted in the area of self-management. The set of adequately designed experiments is smaller. Chodosh et al. (2005) reviewed 53 randomized trials of chronic disease management programs for older adults. The authors concluded that programs targeting diabetes and hypertension produced clinically important benefits. However, determining which elements of the interventions were responsible for the observed effects proved impossible. Although this review did not find a beneficial effect of self-management in patients with osteoarthritis, a more focused literature review suggests a small but statistically significant effect on pain and function.

The results of self-management programs that target objective measures of physical disability among older adults with multiple chronic diseases are more encouraging. Several critical reviews have shown that strength training and walking programs produce robust improvements in physiological functioning and small-to-moderate clinical effects on various functional tasks, such as rising from a chair, climbing stairs, and walking 400 m. For example, in a recent study of adults older than 70 years who had compromised function at baseline, we demonstrated a clinically significant change in scores on the Short Physical Performance Battery (SPPB), a well-validated measure of physical functioning that includes very basic tests of balance, strength, and mobility disability (Figure 28-9). Other studies

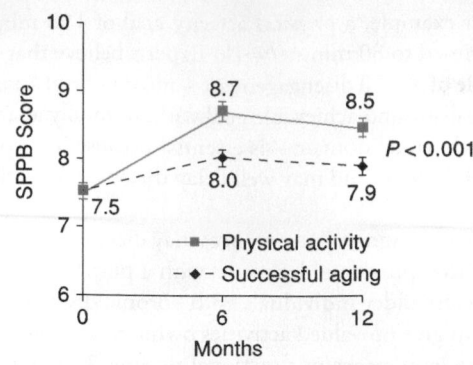

FIGURE 28-9. Comparison of a physical activity intervention with a successful aging intervention on SPPB scores. Means estimated from repeated measures ANCOVA adjusted for gender, field center, and baseline values. (Pahor M, Blair SN, Espeland M, et al. Effects of a physical activity intervention on measures of physical performance: results of the lifestyle interventions and independence for elders pilot (LIFE-P) study. J Gerontol A Biol Sci Med Sci. 2006;61A:1157.)

demonstrate that training older adults for balance has noticeable effects on preventing falls.

Thus, research findings on the topic of self-management vary considerably. Why do they differ so widely both within and between diseases? What conclusions can we draw for clinical practice?

First of all, the value of attributing clinical meaning to the strength of effects that are statistically averaged across studies, even after grouping them according to specific characteristics, such as tailored treatment or group versus individual treatment, is questionable. Among the many reasons for this concern, three stand out: (1) varying duration of intervention, from 6 weeks to 24 months; (2) targeting multiple outcomes; and (3) studying persons with a broad range of disease severity. These variable elements preclude making useful clinical generalizations. For example, we know from our extensive research in weight management that the intensity and duration of treatment are critical factors in the success of behavior change. Also, when studies target multiple outcomes, individual behaviors are rarely given the attention that is required for many participants to focus on their change. The clinical effectiveness of self-management on osteoarthritis pain is much greater in intensive studies of pain management than in short-term community programs that target multiple outcomes, such as the ASMP. While both programs have benefits, comparing them is not clinically appropriate; they are inherently different.

As for disease severity, both the chronic disease and the disability literature adduce good evidence that people with mild disease have less room for improvement in function than those with more severe disease or disability. Of course, for most health conditions, there comes a point where severity offers little room for hope, but this state represents only a minority of the older adult population. Reviews that include studies without controlling for the severity of patients' conditions are obviously misleading. Individuals who are severely ill or have disabilities require different treatments that may not be classified as self-management.

Perhaps more important for geriatric health care professionals is the clinical utility of the information presented both in this section dedicated to research and in the previous section on a conceptual blueprint for change. How does the geriatrician use the informa-

tion we have presented? Can specific principles and suggestions be proposed to optimize self-management in geriatric medicine?

PRINCIPLES AND SUGGESTIONS FOR INTEGRATING SELF-MANAGEMENT INTO GERIATRIC MEDICINE

How do health care professionals best promote self-management in the context of their own practices? Are particular target behaviors of interest? Choices will vary with resources and personnel. Several fundamental principles that have evolved from the evidence presented in this chapter can and should be common to all self-management programs for chronic health problems. In addition, health care professionals might want to consider targeting several specific types of behaviors (see also Chapter 9).

The Self-Management Partnership

A core principle in promoting effective self-management is establishing partnerships between health care professionals and their patients. Health care professionals can use the contrast noted between traditional and collaborative styles of interaction (see Table 28-1) as a guide to set concrete goals for themselves in establishing a consistent model of care with patients and then to formulate plans of action in conducting their practice. If these steps sound familiar, it is because these are identical to those we suggested earlier for patients. Because health care professional/patient interaction is bidirectional and bilateral, health care professionals should also examine their own behavior to ensure that they are contributing to, rather than detracting from, the partnership to promote self-management. The same factors that limit the patient's contribution to self-management also pose challenges for health care professionals trying to follow through on their own plans of action to contribute to the partnership's achievement of goals.

By definition, partnerships require cooperation between two or more people. An important facet of promoting partnerships in geriatric medicine is enlisting patients' support and educating them about the skills and commitment required of both parties. Clearly, a major challenge for health care professionals is that the common-sense model of medicine in our culture is one in which patients are relatively passive, expecting physicians and nurses to solve or to fix problems. While health care remains a problem-solving enterprise, the partnership model must (1) identify problems collaboratively; (2) specify options and choose a treatment together; (3) make detailed action plans; and (4) clarify for patients steps for evaluation, including feedback to the health care professional. Communication between health care professionals and patients should reinforce the patient's active role in health care, underscoring diverse behaviors that include adhering to medication regimens, monitoring symptoms, or altering lifestyle behaviors.

Fostering Collaboration

Meichenbaum and Turk's classic text (Meichenbaum and Turk's 1987; p. 187), *Facilitating Treatment Adherence: A Practitioner's Guidebook*, offers health care professionals the following practical advice to facilitate collaboration in self-management:

1. Ascertain the patient's preference for each aspect of the treatment regimen.

2. Assess the patient's previous experience with self-management.

3. Ensure that the patient has the requisite skills and resources for implementation.

4. Introduce change gradually over the course of several visits to learn together how the patient is doing.

5. Break complex tasks that require more demanding adherence into actions that can be handled sequentially.

6. Begin the collaboration with a step that can be readily accomplished to foster immediate patient control and direction.

7. Enlist support of family or other strong allies.

8. As the patient assumes an increasing level of self-management, gradually reduce the health care professional's role in order to foster greater patient responsibility.

All of these suggestions imply frequent, ongoing contact with patients, a necessary aspect of managing chronic disease. Physicians and nurses must carefully plan how they use contact time with patients to most efficiently build the collaboration.

With the exception of smoking, physicians are not aggressive in giving patients advice about lifestyles, despite the profound effect that changes in lifestyle behaviors have in accruing, preventing, and treating chronic disease and disability. For adults older than 65 years who report on their physician's guidance, only 31.3% are told to get more exercise, 41.5% are given advice to eat more fruits and vegetables, 38.2% are instructed to reduce their dietary fat, 25.5% are advised to reduce stress, and 82.8% are advised to stop smoking. These statistics only concern one of the most prevalent forms of physician behavior—providing advice—not teaching or actively changing patient behavior. The number of older adults who are assisted in self-managing lifestyle behaviors remains low. Incorporation of counseling on health behaviors into clinical encounters is discussed further in Chapter 9: Preventive Gerontology.

Implementing a Framework for Effective Self-Management

Self-management is heavily influenced by older adults' commonsense models of health-related problems and treatment options. When they are unclear about the meaning of their symptoms and conditions, they may experience anxiety and perhaps avoid important self-management behavior. Interpreting a symptom as "nothing to worry about—it's old age" can lead patients to be passive, and they may fail to take action that could prevent downstream morbidity. On the other hand, overreacting to the single occurrence of a symptom may result in overcompensation, for example resting, when a more helpful reaction should be increased activity. Clarifying and documenting the type, intensity, frequency, and duration of symptoms that older adults are experiencing should be a priority of any practice. These data should be updated on follow-up visits.

Any diagnosis should also be accompanied by information about both the disease/health state and the patients' role in managing the health event. Simply asking older adults whether or not they understand the problem they are encountering and then moving on if they answer affirmatively is insufficient for two reasons. First, they may be embarrassed to admit that they do not understand common disease states, such as hypertension or diabetes. Second, even if patients think

that they understand a specific diagnosis, components of their commonsense models may well be in error (see Figure 28-1) and detract from adherence to recommended and agreed-upon action. Health care professionals discussing self-management with older adults in relation to these diagnoses can underscore the importance of their partnership, using it as a platform for mutual understanding (1) to set concrete goals in specific areas, (2) to establish action plans, and (3) to discuss the importance and means of providing feedback about these action plans (Table 28-2).

Health care professionals should be able to link their older patients to resources in either their own network or the community that might be valuable in managing their health states. For example, someone who is obese and has elevated glucose should be referred for weight loss. Referrals should be proactive when possible; that is, if patients are receptive, health care professionals should arrange the initial contact with resource personnel. They must also be aware of whether or not patients have the economic means, time, and transportation required to take advantage of the proposed resources. This kind of matching and planning greatly increases the likelihood that older adults will follow-up on recommendations. Of course, health care professionals must monitor patients' progress with outpatient programs if they really are to function as active partners in self-management. However, as noted in Chapter 15, The Health Care System, these coordinating activities are not reimbursable under Medicare. This represents a significant barrier to health care professionals who wish to incorporate these important self-management activities into their practices.

Targets for Self-Management: General Practices

Health care professionals must specify behavioral targets and have concrete goals for self-management that patients can understand and accomplish. For example, a number of screening behaviors should be a part of every geriatric practice (see Chapter 9). These include colon screens, breast examinations, skin cancer screening, prostate examinations, bone mineral density, and physical disability. Without having specific action plans in place to ensure participation in these screenings, adherence rates will suffer. Here are some suggestions, based on the framework we proposed earlier:

1. Underscore the threat of electing not to be screened.

2. Schedule visits for patients, as opposed to simply suggesting that screening be completed.

3. Systematically monitor screening tests for each patient and be certain that feedback is provided immediately.

4. Schedule follow-up visits immediately when test scores are abnormal.

5. Display rates of participation in screening tests by patients in your practice in highly visible areas and set goals of 100% participation.

With older adults, take time to evaluate and advise on health behaviors, such as (1) caloric consumption, (2) healthy eating practices, (3) smoking behavior, (4) level of physical activity, and (5) depression/anxiety. Simply telling the patient, "You seem to be doing fine," might be well intended, but that feedback lacks clarity and may be deceiving. For example, when older adults have two comorbidities, they are at risk of future decline in functional independence. If they consider this risk normative, and the health care professional says they "seem to be doing fine," they may not try to do anything to

TABLE 28-7

The Short Physical Performance Battery (SPPB)

COMPONENT	SCORE RANGE	DESCRIPTION OF TASK
Balance tests	Either 0 (unable to hold for 10 s) or 1 (held for 10 s)	Side-by-side stand: participant stands with feet side by side and attempts to hold for 10 s without moving feet.
	Either 0 (unable to hold for 10 s) or 1 (held for 10 s)	Semi-tandem stand: participant stands with one side of heel touching the big toe of the other foot and attempts to hold for 10 s without moving feet.
	Either 0 (held for less than 3 s) or 2 (held for 10 s)	Tandem stand: participant stands with one heel directly in front of toes of other foot and attempts to hold for 10 s without moving feet.
Gait speed test	Between 0 (unable to do the walk) and 4 (took less than 4.82 s)	Participant walks 4 meters at their usual pace, while HCP times them with stopwatch.
Chair stand test	If cannot do, end test here. If can do, move to repeated chair stand test.	Participant folds arms across chest while sitting in a chair and then attempts to stand up without use of arms.
Repeated chair stand test	Between 0 (could not perform five in a row or took longer than 60 s to complete) and 4 (performed five in less than 11.19 s)	Participant folds arms across chest while sitting in a chair and attempts to stand up and sit back down as quickly as possible.

SPPB Score Between 0 and 12.

improve their condition. Feedback and guidance must be specific for individuals to understand their health status. General feedback can unintentionally reinforce a counterproductive commonsense model of older adults' health status. Patients can complete self-report tests, that evaluate their lifestyle behaviors either prior to their visits or while they are waiting to be examined. Results of these self-reports can provide a clearer picture for both partners and build the foundation for ongoing interaction that effective self-management requires.

Targets for Self-Management: Assessing and Acting on Physical Disability

Because the loss of mobility is such a catastrophic health event for older adults, brief assessments with specific recommendations promoting active lifestyles should be performed on a regular basis (see Chapters 11 and 115). Increased physical activity has preventive value not only for mobility loss but also in managing multiple health problems. According to data from the Centers for Disease Control and Prevention (CDC), physicians ask 56.6% of 65- to 79-year-old adults about their level of physical activity, decreasing to 38.9% of those ≥80 years old. Physicians only give 12.6% of adults, older than 65 years, assistance in structuring an exercise program. Moreover, even when assistance is given, no information is provided on how to successfully self-manage it, and systematic follow-up is poor.

Physicians report that they do not counsel patients because they lack practical tools, time, reimbursement, and confidence that it will trigger the desired behavior change.

There are some simple tools for assessing physical capacities of older adults (Chapters 11 and 115). One is the SPPB, which takes approximately 10 minutes, can be conducted by a nurse or trained volunteer, and involves three tasks: walking 4 meters, completing a simple chair-sitting exercise, and performing two very brief static balance tests. Results from this test have been shown to predict both morbidity and rates of nursing home admissions (Table 28-7 and Figure 28-10).

Our own research has found that SPPB test results have a motivational effect on older adults. Given this specific feedback, they are more responsive to receiving and seeking information about remedial physical activity to enhance their basic performance. Fortunately, an increasing number of community-based programs offer physical activity for seniors.

As a closing guide, we offer additional practical suggestions on how to maintain adherence from the classic textbook by Meichenbaum and Turk (pp. 244–251).

1. *Anticipate nonadherence:* There are a variety of reasons for nonadherence; some of which neither the health care professional nor the patient can control. Do not treat it as a sign of failure on your part or typecast older adults who struggle with self-management

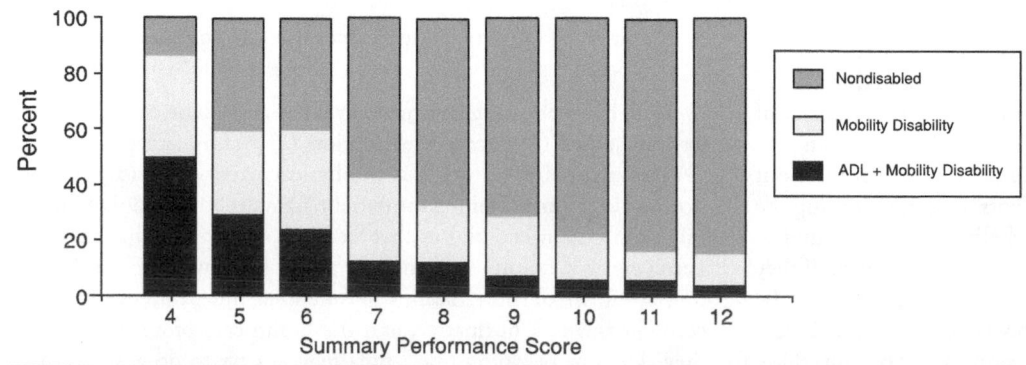

FIGURE 28-10. Disability status assessed 4 yrs later among those nondisabled at baseline based on baseline SPPS score. (Guralnik JM, Ferrucci L, Simonsick EM et al. Lower-extremity function in persons over the age of 70 as a predictor of subsequent disability. The New England Journal of Medicine. 1995;332:556–561.)

as nonadherers. Either response is destructive to the process of mutual problem solving.

2. *Consider self-management from the patient's perspective and establish a collaborative relationship:* Carefully study the inhibitory factors discussed earlier in this chapter. Understanding them can lead to a renewed appreciation of the challenges that patients face and result in renegotiating more realistic self-management goals. Meichenbaum and Turk remind us that: "*An acceptable regimen that is carried out appropriately is better than an ideal one that is ignored*" (p. 247).

3. *Be patient oriented:* Health care professionals should gain knowledge of their patients' commonsense understanding of their disease or functional problem and the proposed treatment. Listen carefully to what patients say and to what they do not say. For example, are patients really not listening when they say nothing? Perhaps they are embarrassed about their lack of understanding. In addition to clear instruction from the health care professional, patients should articulate their understanding of what the health care professional said.

4. *Customize treatment:* As part of self-management, the health care professional must be prepared to work with the patient to adjust and to modify standard protocols.

5. *Use family or significant other support:* Because other people can facilitate or hinder older adults' self-management, family and/or significant others must be included in the health care partnership. They should understand the chronic disease, the nature of the treatment, and the goals of self-management. The obvious benefit is their support for the approach being taken without eliminating or blocking the older adults' role in the self-management process.

6. *Provide accessibility and continuity of care:* If patients find difficulty gaining access to health care professionals, if your staff does not show the same interest and care as you, and if you do not draw on other health care professionals and community programs that could assist in treatment (for example, psychosocial specialists for depression; exercise rehabilitation specialists for older adults), self-management has a greater risk of failure. Developing an integrated, highly communicative group of health care professionals is essential for effective self-management, although challenging under the existing fragmented health care system and lack of reimbursement.

7. *Repeat everything and do not give up:* Intervention research in a variety of areas suggests that, for chronic problems, patients must

be "re-inoculated." Long-term maintenance requires repeating education and behavioral practice about treatment regimens and modifying the self-management approach to counter declines or lapses in adherence.

FURTHER READING

Baer RA. *Mindfulness-Based Treatment Approaches: Clinician's Guide to Evidence Base and Applications.* New York, New York: Academic Press; 2006.

Bandura A. Health promotion by social cognitive means. *Health Educ Behav.* 2004;31:143.

Bodenheimer T, Lorig K, Holman H, et al. Patient self-management of chronic disease in primary care. *J Am Med Assoc.* 2002;288:2469.

Bryant LL, Altpeter M, Whitelaw, NA. Evaluation of health promotion programs for older adults: an introduction. *J Appl Gerontol.* 2006;25:197.

Cameron LD, Leventhal H. *The Self-Regulation of Health and Illness Behaviour.* New York, New York: Routledge; 2003.

Chodosh J, Morton, SC, Mojica W, et al. Meta-analysis: chronic disease self-management programs for older adults. *Ann Intern Med.* 2005;143:427.

Clark NM. Management of chronic disease by patients. *Annu Rev Public Health.* 2003;24:289.

DeBusk RF, Miller NH, Superko HR, et al. A case-management system for coronary risk factor modification after acute myocardial infarction. *Ann Intern Med.* 1994;120:721.

Ersek ME, Turner JA, McCurry SM, et al. Efficacy of a self-management group intervention for elderly persons with chronic pain. *Clin J Pain.* 2003;19:156.

Glasgow RE, Eakin EG, Fisher EB, et al. Physician advice and support for physical activity. *Am J Prevent Med.* 2001;21:189.

Halm EA, Mora P, Leventhal H. No symptoms, no asthma: The acute episodic disease belief is associated with poor self-management among inner-city adults with persistent asthma. *Chest.* 2006;129:573.

Haskell WL, Alderman EL, Fair JM, et al. Effects of intensive multiple risk factor reduction on coronary atherosclerosis and clinical cardiac events in men and women with coronary artery disease: the Stanford Coronary Risk Intervention Project (SCRIP). *Circulation.* 1994;89: 975.

Lorig K, Holman H. Arthritis self-management studies: a twelve-year review. *Health Educ Q.* 1993;20:17.

Lorig KR, Holman HR. Self-management education: history, definition, outcomes, and mechanisms. *Ann Behav Med.* 2003;26:1.

Maes S, Karoly P. Self-regulation assessment and intervention in physical health and illness: a review. *Appl Psychol Int Rev.* 2005;54:267.

Meichenbaum D, Turk DC. *Facilitating Treatment Adherence: A Practitioner's Guidebook.* New York, New York: Plenum; 1987.

Pahor M, Blair SN, Espeland M, et al. Effects of a physical activity intervention on measures of physical performance: results of the lifestyle interventions and independence for elders pilot (LIFE-P) study. *J Gerontol.* 2006;61A:1157.

Rejeski WJ, Brawley LR, Haskell WL. Physical activity: preventing physical disablement in older adults. *Am J Prevent Med.* 2003;25(suppl 2).

Teresi JA, Ramirez M, Ocepek-Welikson K, et al. The development and psychometric analyses of ADEPT: an instrument for assessing the interactions between doctors and their elderly patients. *Ann Behav Med.* 2005;30:225.

Warsi A, LaValley MP, Wang PS, et al. Arthritis self-management education programs: a meta-analysis of the effect on pain and disability. *Arthritis Rheum.* 2003;48:2207.

Rehabilitation

Cynthia J. Brown ■ *Claire Peel*

DEFINING REHABILITATION

The purpose of rehabilitation is to restore some or all of a person's physical and mental capabilities that have been lost as a result of disease, injury, or illness and to help achieve the highest possible level of function, independence, and quality of life. The techniques and modalities used to achieve these goals are numerous and typically do not differ for younger versus older persons. However, rehabilitation outcomes and approaches are frequently different for the older adult. For example, most young adults experience a single acute event that results in disability. Older adults are more likely to have multiple comorbid conditions that, over time, result in disability. Even if the older persons have acute events, like a hip fracture or a stroke, their underlying comorbid conditions may impact on the outcomes of rehabilitation. Older patients may also have subclinical physical or cognitive comorbidities, which become evident when challenged by a new disability. For example, mild cognitive impairment may be first recognized during rehabilitation after a hip fracture, when the patient has difficulty learning how to use a new assistive device.

Goals of rehabilitation for older adults usually focus on recovery of self-care ability and mobility, while for younger persons reentering the work force or returning to school may be the goal. In general, recovery for older adults requires a longer period of time to achieve, and functional outcomes are usually worse when compared with younger adults. It is important to discuss rehabilitation goals with all patients and focus therapy toward achieving those goals. For example, older persons may have been avid golfers or fishermen, and return to this activity may be important for their quality of life. Rehabilitation efforts and goals of care may also be impacted by a person's values and beliefs about exercise and social roles. For example, if a patient has never cooked and does not believe that this is an important task to learn, taking the patient to the kitchen to learn how to prepare a meal may be viewed as a useless task. Participation by the patient and family in the development of the goals of rehabilitation is critical to achieve a successful outcome.

Disability is common in older persons and can have a significant impact on function and quality of life. In order to better understand the process of disablement, a variety of theoretical models have been explored and are presented below.

History of the Disability Framework

In an attempt to provide a framework for the discussion of the consequences of disease and injury, Nagi developed the first disablement model in the 1960s (Figure 29-1). The model uses four related yet distinct phenomena considered by Nagi to be the basis of rehabilitation and include active pathology, impairment, functional limitation, and disability. Active pathology was described as a disruption in the normal cellular function and the body's efforts to regain a normal state. Impairment, which usually results from active pathology, referred to an abnormality or loss at the tissue or organ level. Functional limitation described restrictions at the individual level, while disability described a physical or mental limitation in a social context. Nagi's view of disability was a product of the interaction between individuals and their environment. Importantly, individuals could have similar functional impairments that result in different patterns of disability, depending on the environment in which they function.

In 1980, the World Health Organization's (WHO) *International Classification of Impairments, Disabilities, and Handicaps* (ICIDH) was developed in Europe. Like Nagi's disablement model, the ICIDH characterized three distinct concepts related to disease and health conditions: impairments, disabilities, and handicaps. While the ICIDH was developed to classify function and disability, it failed to receive endorsement by the World Health Assembly. A major criticism of these early disablement models was that these presented the response to disease or illness as a static process with a linear progression through the disablement process. It was recognized that the interaction between disease and disability is more complex, particularly for older persons. Recognition of this complexity led to

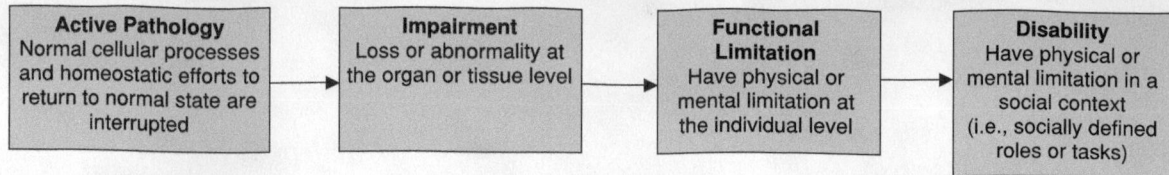

FIGURE 29-1. Schematic of the Nagi disablement model with definitions. The first disablement model was described by Nagi in the early 1960s. The initial disablement model focused on a linear progression to disability and has been replaced over time with new models such as the International Classification of Functioning, Disability, and Health (ICF). Importantly, the Nagi model was the first attempt to describe the process of disability. (*Jette AM. Toward a common language for function, disability, and health. Phys Ther. 2006;86(5):726.*)

significant dialogue within the rehabilitation community and to a major revision of the ICIDH.

In 2001, the WHO released the *International Classification of Functioning, Disability and Health* (ICF) (Figure 29-2), which attempted to incorporate, from a biological, personal, and social perspective, a biopsychosocial view of health. The ICF characterizes decreases in function as the consequence of a dynamic interaction between various health conditions and contextual factors. Health conditions are described as diseases, disorders, injuries, or aging. Contextual factors are divided into two categories: environmental factors and personal factors. Environmental factors include the physical, social, and attitudinal environment in which people live. These might include individual environment like furniture placement in the home or societal environment like policies regarding access to buildings. Personal factors are characteristics of the individual, which are not part of the health condition or illness. These might include gender, fitness, or coping styles. Listed across the center of the model are the three domains of human function: body functions and structures, activities, and participation. Body functions and structures are the physiologic functions and the anatomical parts of the body. The execution of a task or action by a person is an activity, while participation is the application to a real-life activity. For each of these three domains of human function, there are several levels on which

the function can be experienced. These include functioning at the level of the body or body parts and the level of the whole person and the whole person in their environment. Disability is defined as any decline at any of these levels.

Using the ICF model, we could describe an older woman who has a history of osteoarthritis of the knees and hypertension who presents to rehabilitation after a hip fracture. She lives alone in a second-floor apartment and has a daughter who lives at a distance 6 hours away. The patient has a large circle of friends and regularly attends social gatherings at the local senior center. Figure 29-3 demonstrates how this patient's problems might be placed in the ICF model, with the goal of generating hypotheses about the best treatment options. Important issues include not only improving the patient's strength and walking ability but also addressing where she will live after discharge and how to keep her active in her community. Understanding the relationships between the different components and addressing them is the key to a successful rehabilitation.

It is believed by many that the ICF framework has the potential to provide a standard disablement language, which could facilitate dialogue across disciplines. The ICF model attempts to reflect the interactions between different components of health and avoids the linear view of previous models. This framework also looks beyond

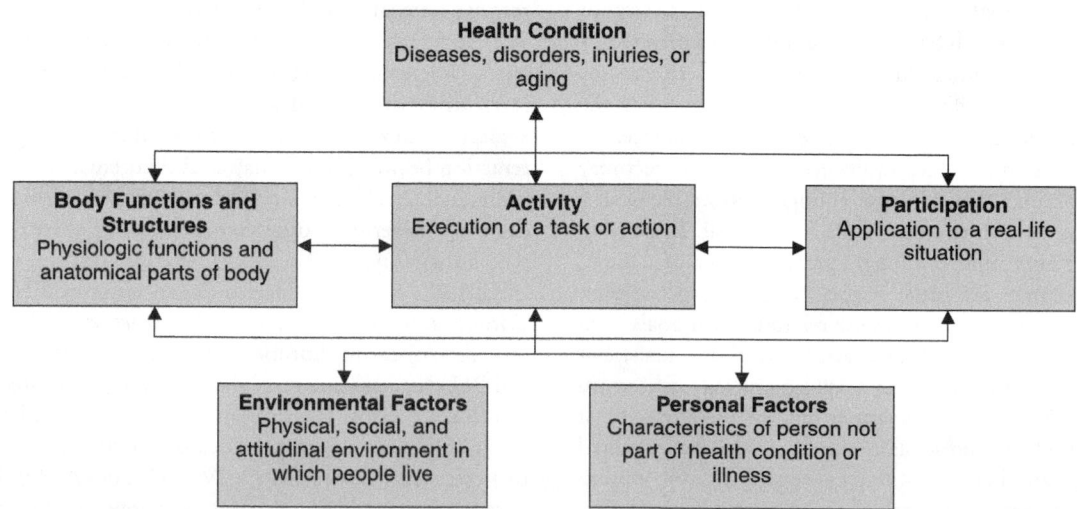

FIGURE 29-2. International Classification of Functioning, Disability and Health (ICF). The latest version of the ICF focuses on the interaction between various factors and the impact these factors have on health and functioning. Prior models focused on disability and portrayed the path to disability as a linear process. This model attempts to incorporate, from a biological, personal, and social perspective, a biopsychosocial view of health. (*Reprinted with permission of the World Health Organization. Towards a Common Language for Functioning, Disability and Health: ICF. Geneva, Switzerland. 2002.*)

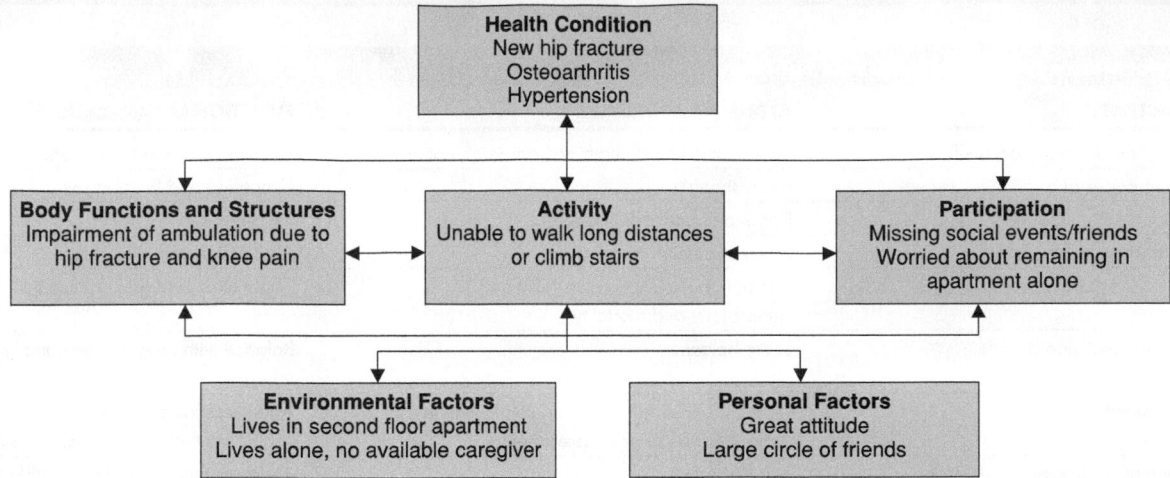

FIGURE 29-3. Using the ICF model to describe patient function. This figure demonstrates how a patient's problems might be placed in the ICF model with the goal of generating hypotheses about the best treatment options. In the case of this patient with osteoarthritis and new hip fracture, the ICF model illustrates how addressing where the patient will live after discharge and how to keep the patient active in the community are as important as improving the patient's strength and walking ability. Understanding the relationships between the different components and addressing them is the key to successful rehabilitation. *(Authors' own work using WHO ICF model.)*

disease and mortality to focus on how people live with their disabling conditions.

EVALUATION

Goals of Evaluation

An important goal of evaluation is to identify the cause of the disability for which rehabilitation is required. While there is frequently a final common pathway for many disabilities, the cause may impact on treatment and outcomes. For example, a person's walking difficulty could be caused by osteoarthritis of the knee or a meniscal tear. For the patient with osteoarthritis, an exercise program focused on strengthening the musculature around the knee has been demonstrated to decrease pain and improve the ability to walk. For the patient with a meniscal tear, surgical intervention may be a better option. Evaluation prior to rehabilitation is also important to identify comorbidities that may directly or indirectly affect rehabilitation outcomes. While the older person may have osteoarthritis causing limited walking ability, they may also have poor cardiac or pulmonary function that further limit walking ability. Another goal of evaluation is to determine the best site for rehabilitation to occur. Several settings are available, including an inpatient rehabilitation facility, a subacute nursing home, or a home. The appropriate setting is usually determined through evaluation of the disability and comorbid conditions that may affect rehabilitation. The next section outlines the evaluation process and focuses on creation of an individual treatment plan that addresses the patient's unique disabilities.

Disability-Oriented History and Physical Examination

During the initial evaluation, the history and physical examination can help characterize the disability and lead the clinician toward the most effective types of treatment. Determining if the functional decline occurred suddenly or has taken a more slowly progressive course may be very helpful in determining the cause of the disability. Symptoms associated with a given activity may also help narrow the cause to a specific organ system. For example, while the impairment may be difficulty in walking, the limitation could be caused by shortness of breath or pain with weight bearing. Differentiating the causal pathway, in this case pulmonary versus musculoskeletal, helps to refine the workup required and assists the provider in targeting the appropriate therapy. Functional status and residence prior to the illness or injury may also help guide expectations of rehabilitation.

Table 29-1 lists several brief screening maneuvers, which can be done in the physician's office when evaluating a patient for disability. These assessment tools can be used to quickly assess baseline functional status as well as monitor progress during rehabilitation. If these screening tests are positive, additional testing should be performed, as the screening tests are often not as accurate as more detailed maneuvers. A variety of standardized measures are available to further test function during basic and instrumental activities of daily living.

For example, lifting a heavy book overhead tests shoulder range of motion and strength. If a person is unable to achieve this task, additional range of motion and muscle testing should be done to isolate the cause of the difficulty.

Many of the screening tests listed have normative values and have been well validated for the geriatric population. The short physical performance battery includes three of the screening tests gait speed, timed chair stands and static balance with worse scores being associated with falls, nursing home placement, and mortality. The University of Alabama at Birmingham (UAB) Study of Aging Life-Space Assessment is a validated instrument that measures a person's mobility in the home and community during the month preceding the assessment. Importantly, the Study of Aging Life-Space Assessment goes beyond measuring the individual's ability to perform specific tasks by assessing the person's actual pattern of mobility, which may help identify factors other than physical impairment, such as emotional or socioeconomic factors, which might be limiting mobility.

TABLE 29-1

Physical Performance Tests Used to Assess Function

SCREENING ACTIVITY	ATTRIBUTE ADDRESSED	FUNCTIONAL IMPLICATION
Put a heavy book on an overhead shelf	Upper extremity strength and range of motion	Ability to perform housework
Grasp a piece of paper and resist its removal	Pinch strength	Grooming and feeding self
Write a sentence	Fine motor coordination	Feeding self
Timed rise to standing five times*	Lower extremity strength	Ambulation and stair climbing
Gait speed*	Dynamic balance, predicts falls, and morbidity and mortality	Ambulation and general function with ADLs
Standing balance*; feet side by side, semitandem and tandem	Static balance	Balance with progressively smaller base of support
Life space assessment†	Mobility within the home and community in the 4 weeks prior to assessment	Addresses factors in addition to physical function that might impair mobility
Rhomberg; standing with eyes closed and assess sway or loss of balance	Proprioception	Ability to balance without visual input

Authors' own work summarizing physical performance measures from *Studenski SA, Perera S, Wallace D, et al. Physical performance measures in the clinical setting. J Am Geriatr Soc. 2003;51(3):314; and †Peel C, Sawyer-Baker P, Roth DL, et al. Assessing mobility in older adults: the UAB Study of Aging Life-Space Assessment. Phys Ther. 2005;85:1008–1019.

In addition to the history and physical examination, an evaluation should include assessments of cognition, motivation, depression, social support, and financial resources, as these factors can have a significant impact on rehabilitation outcomes. A variety of validated assessment tools can be used to screen for cognition and depression, such as the Geriatric Depression Scale or the mini mental state examination. Assessment of current methods utilized by the patient for coping with disability, including use of assistive devices, level of assistance needed, and any limitation of activities, should also be explored.

Determining Rehabilitation Potential

Many factors influence the choice of who would benefit from rehabilitation and the success of those rehabilitation efforts. Assessment for rehabilitation potential needs to be done when the acute medical illness has resolved. A patient with a hip fracture and concurrent delirium may do poorly on initial assessment but, once the delirium clears, may progress nicely with rehabilitation. At times, the medical condition will need to be treated concurrently with rehabilitation efforts. After a prolonged ICU stay, a patient may have significant orthostatic hypotension, which will resolve as they regain the upright position during rehabilitation. Table 29-2 lists a variety of acute medical illnesses that might delay referral to rehabilitation until these are resolved.

Other determinants of rehabilitation benefit include motivation, cognition, and prior functional status. Comorbid illness may have a significant effect on rehabilitation efforts and may even cause a change in rehabilitation approaches. For example, a patient with chronic obstructive pulmonary disease (COPD) on home oxygen who falls and fractures a hip may not be able to tolerate more than 5 minutes of therapy at one time. The rehabilitation approach might be changed to include frequent walks of short duration by therapy and nursing, as opposed to an hour-long therapy session twice a day. Table 29-3 lists a variety of factors that might influence either the use of rehabilitation or the goals of the rehabilitation. In some cases, like terminal illness with a short life expectancy, the goals of

care may need to be addressed with the patient and family, and palliative care may be a more appropriate option. For other factors, like lack of motivation, well-defined patient-centered goals that are easily measured may help overcome this potential obstacle.

After careful evaluation, including a disability-oriented history and physical examination, assessment of factors that may impact on rehabilitation outcomes, and the development of goals with the team, including the patient and the family, we are ready for the final step prior to initiation of rehabilitation, choosing the site for rehabilitation. Determining the optimal setting in which rehabilitation

TABLE 29-2

Factors for Which Rehabilitation May Need to be Delayed Until Resolved

FACTOR OF INTEREST	REASON FOR POSSIBLE DELAY IN REHABILITATION
Delirium or altered level of consciousness	Unable to cooperate or learn
Hemodynamic instability	May make it unsafe to carry out certain types of exercise
Occult fracture and bony metastasis	Weight bearing or resistance exercise could worsen fracture or cause fracture
Acute infections (e.g., bladder infection and pneumonia)	May cause confusion, fatigue, and/or hypotension
Acute skin or joint infection	May cause fatigue, pain, and/or muscle splinting
Acute inflammatory disease (e.g., certain rheumatologic and neuromuscular conditions)	Resistive exercises may impair recovery
Acute orthopedic conditions	Joint instability may preclude use of certain exercises, and functional goals may be limited

Adapted from Hoenig H and Cutson T, Geriatric Rehabilitation. In: Principles of Geriatric Medicine and Gerontology, Ed. Hazzard WR, Blass JP, Halter JB, Ouslander JG, Tinetti ME. 5th edition, McGraw-Hill; 2003.

TABLE 29-3

Factors That May Influence the Success of Rehabilitation Interventions

Cognitive Impairment	Goals may be more limited. Take advantage of skills patient already has, use interventions that do not require carryover.
Disability has been present for many years	Goals may be more limited and directed to compensatory strategies or treatment of deconditioning.
Motivation is limited	Goals need to be well defined and reached in measurable steps.
Patient had prior rehabilitation for the same problem	Rehabilitation may be limited unless new functional decline has occurred.
Terminal illness	Intervention is directed toward reducing care giver burden and patient discomfort.
Severity of disability	Extremely mild disability may not require intervention. Extremely severe disability may have very limited potential for benefit.
Social and cultural circumstances	Absence of a caregiver, financial limitations, and cultural beliefs may preclude use of certain techniques or technologies.
Malnutrition	Unable to build muscle; rehabilitative interventions may be limited unless nutritional status is improved.

Adapted from Hoenig H and Cutson T, Geriatric Rehabilitation. In: Principles of Geriatric Medicine and Gerontology, Ed. Hazzard WR, Blass JP, Halter JB, Ouslander JG, Tinetti ME. 5th edition, McGraw-Hill; 2003.

should occur is based on many of the factors previously evaluated, as well as patient preference.

COMPONENTS OF REHABILITATION

The Organization of Rehabilitation

Settings for Care

A variety of settings are available, both inpatient and community based, in which to receive rehabilitation services. It is important for the provider to understand the range of available settings and the advantages and disadvantages of each setting. While the provider may be responsible for helping match the patient to the optimal setting, insurance and cost also play a role. Rehabilitation services are available through Medicare Part A on a time-limited basis. Patients must demonstrate that they are making progress with rehabilitation in order to qualify for services.

Inpatient rehabilitation is offered in rehabilitation centers and Medicare-skilled nursing facilities. In order to qualify as a Medicare-certified inpatient rehabilitation hospital, a certain percentage of all admitted patients must have at least one of 13 conditions, which include diagnoses like stroke, burns, and neurological disorders. Patients must be managed by an interdisciplinary team of skilled nurses and therapists, be seen daily by a physician, and have 24-hour rehabilitation nursing care. Rehabilitation is intensive with patients receiving a minimum of 3 hours of therapy daily. As the rehabil-

itation center offers 24-hour-a-day medical care, patients in need of close medical supervision during therapy can receive it. However, the patient must be able to tolerate the intensity of therapy provided, which may be difficult for the older patient.

Like the rehabilitation center, Medicare-approved skilled nursing facilities must provide 24-hour nursing care. While physicians must be available 24 hours a day, they are just supervising care and can visit the patients less frequently. Multidisciplinary care may not occur, although therapy services, dietary, pharmacy, and social services are available. There are no requirements for intensity or duration of therapy sessions, or any required case mix. This setting allows for a slower rehabilitation pace, which may be necessary for some older patients with multiple comorbid diseases. The availability of 24-hour nursing care is also a benefit for persons who are unable to care for themselves or who do not have caregivers at home.

Home health benefits for rehabilitation are also available through Medicare to patients who are defined as "homebound." This includes patients for whom leaving the home is difficult or who require help of another person to get out of the home. Part-time nursing and therapy services are available if prescribed by a physician, and these services must be recertified every 60 days. While the intensity of the rehabilitation is less and the nursing services are part time, many patients prefer rehabilitating in their own home. If the patient has the necessary support system, this can be an excellent option.

While a number of studies have examined the effect of the rehabilitation setting on outcomes, the results remain unclear. For patients with hip fracture, the setting of care does not appear to have an impact on outcomes. After a stroke, patients who are treated in inpatient rehabilitation hospitals or special stroke units are more likely to be discharged to home and with improved function. Ultimately, factors such as patient prognosis, level of medical and nursing care needed, and intensity of therapy the patient can tolerate will help determine the optimal setting for rehabilitation.

Rehabilitation Providers

An interdisciplinary team is often required to meet the complex rehabilitation needs of older patients. While team members have defined roles and functions, there is considerable overlap in the services provided. For example, while the physical therapist may focus on transfer and gait training, the occupational therapist may also encourage practice of transfers while performing self-care skills. In addition, there are different levels of education and licensure required for different providers. Table 29-4 outlines the types of rehabilitation providers and their usual methods of evaluation and treatment.

Key members of this interdisciplinary team are the patient and the family. An important component of chronic disease management is patient self-management, and patients must be active participants in the decision-making process. The team is responsible for establishing goals, in collaboration with the patient and the family, and developing a treatment plan to achieve those goals. In addition to teaching the patient, a key component of rehabilitation is training the caregiver or family. Specifically, caregivers must be taught how to assist with exercise programs ambulation and ADLs. The caregiver may need to know how to use adaptive equipment or even how to transfer the patient safely, if the patient is not independent with this task. Communication among all team members, including the patient and their family, is critical for success.

TABLE 29-4

Rehabilitation Providers and Typical Methods Used for Evaluation and Treatment

PROVIDER	PRIMARY METHODS OF EVALUATION AND TREATMENT
Physical therapist	• Assessment of joint range of motion and muscle strength • Assessment of gait and mobility • Provision of appropriate assistive devices • Exercise training to increase range of motion, strength, endurance, balance, coordination, and gait • Treatment with physical modalities (heat, cold, ultrasound, massage, and electrical stimulation)
Occupational therapist	• Evaluate self-care skills and other activities of daily living • Home assessment • Self-care skills training; recommendations and training in use of assistive technology • Fabrication of splints and treatment of upper extremity deficits
Speech therapist	• Assessment of all aspects of communication • Assessment of swallowing disorders • Treatment of communication deficits • Recommendations for alterations of diet and positioning to treat dysphagia
Nurse	• Evaluation of self-care skills • Evaluation of family and home care factors • Self-care training • Patient and family education • Liaison with community
Social worker	• Evaluation of family and home care factors • Assessment of psychosocial factors • Counseling
Dietician	• Assess nutritional status • Alter diet to maximize nutrition
Recreation therapist	• Assess leisure skills and interests • Involve patients in recreational activities to maintain social roles
Prosthetist	• Makes and fits prosthetic limbs
Orthotist	• Makes a variety of orthotics including braces, ankle–foot orthoses, splints, and shoe inserts • Assesses fit of orthotics

Revised and updated by authors. Twersky J, Hoenig H. Rehabilitation. In: Salerno J, ed. Geriatric Review Syllabus: A Core Curriculum in Geriatric Medicine. New York, New York: American Geriatrics Society; 1999:84.

Process of Care: Rehabilitation Interventions

A variety of interventions are available to treat physical impairments and disability. The selection of intervention strategy is determined by the results of the assessment. All interventions should either directly or indirectly lead to an improvement in function and/or quality of life. Major categories of interventions include (1) exercise/physical activity; (2) modalities including thermal agents, electrotherapy, and phototherapy; (3) adaptive aids such as walkers, canes, and devices to improve activities of daily living; and (4) orthotics (splints and braces) and prosthetics (artificial limbs).

Exercise/Physical Activity

General Principles of Exercise   Exercise, also referred to as physical activity, is the cornerstone of physical rehabilitation. Each exercise

prescribed for a patient should be related to achievement of a goal, and all goals should lead to improvement in function. For example, a common exercise for patients is elbow and shoulder flexion. Typical goals related to these exercises are feeding oneself, dressing oneself, or reaching over head to retrieve an item from a shelf. The expected functional outcome for each exercise should be shared with the patient and his/her family. The involvement of the patient and the family is important to maximize compliance.

In setting goals for exercise programs, it is important to consider any pathology that is present. If there is irreversible damage to the neuromuscular system, then the potential for improvement in muscle function is limited. Amyotrophic lateral sclerosis is an example of a pathology in which improvement in muscle function is limited. However, in most cases, decline in muscle strength results from a combination of pathology and deconditioning occurring secondary to inactivity. The deconditioning component is reversible, and therefore some improvement in muscle strength is possible.

A common question often asked is whether exercise is safe for older adults. The number of adverse events reported as a result of exercise in adults is relatively low, with adverse events being more common with vigorous exertion and in persons with atherosclerotic heart disease. To facilitate a safe response, close monitoring before exercise, during exercise, immediately after exercise, and 24 hours after exercise is important. In addition, prior to the initiation of an exercise program, it is important for medical conditions such as congestive heart failure and diabetes to be stable and under optimal medical management. Exercise should be supervised initially to assure appropriate changes in heart rate and blood pressure. There is an expectation that minor muscle soreness will occur with most types of exercise, and patients should be counseled to expect some discomfort. Some patients with osteoarthritis may actually experience a decrease in joint discomfort with exercise. Because increased activity typically has a positive effect on insulin resistance, patients with diabetes may experience a need for less medication to control blood glucose levels.

For exercise to cause a change in physical function, the body must be stressed greater than the usual stress of everyday life. Therefore, it is important that patients are challenged in their exercise programs. For example, when a patient achieves a specific goal, such as walking 30 m at 0.5 m/s, the goal needs to be increased to a greater distance and/or speed. In comparison to younger adults, older adults need a longer recovery time both during an exercise session (between bouts) and between sessions. Improvement may also take longer for older versus younger adults, which should be considered when setting timeframes for the achievement of goals.

There are many classification systems for types of exercise. In the following discussion, we will describe exercise types based on the anticipated outcome, including exercise to increase muscle strength, endurance, balance, flexibility, and motor control.

Exercise to Increase Muscle Strength   A typical exercise program to increase muscle strength involves movements performed against resistance. The resistance can be weights, rubber tubing or bands, or the person's own body weight. To achieve optimal results, the resistance should be 60% to 80% of the person's maximal lifting ability. For the majority of older adults who are starting an exercise program, it is wise to begin at a lower level (approximately 40%–50% of maximal capacity) until the person has mastered the movement patterns.

Sarcopenia refers to the age-related decline in muscle strength, which naturally occurs as we age. At approximately 50 years of age, individuals begin to experience a decline in muscle strength. This decline in muscle strength typically does not interfere with function until persons are 70 years or older. The cause of the decrease in muscle function is thought to be multifactorial and may include changes in muscle metabolism, endocrine alterations, and nutritional factors. One of the most effective treatments is high-intensity resistance exercise training.

Adequate muscle strength is essential to both balance and gait. A positive correlation has been shown between lower extremity muscle strength and gait speed, demonstrating that persons with higher levels of muscle strength walk faster. Balance is determined both by sensory input and by motor output. Even if sensory input is appropriate and the person senses as if they are falling, without adequate muscle strength, the individual will fall.

Bone density can be positively affected by exercises designed to increase muscle strength. Prior to initiating a program to increase muscle strength, it is important to know the individual's bone status, or the extent and location of osteoporosis and/or osteopenia. In persons with osteoporosis, the amount of resistance may need to be modified to avoid overstressing bones and causing a fracture.

Exercise to Increase Endurance Exercise programs, designed to increase endurance, involve continuous activity (such as walking, cycling, and stair stepping), usually performed for at least 20 minutes at an intensity that is 50% to 80% of one's maximal oxygen consumption. Older adults who are beginning a program may need to start with 5 to 10 minutes of continuous activity at a lower intensity. In fact, several sessions of shorter duration (i.e., 10 minutes) per day have shown similar benefits as one session of 30 minutes. To achieve benefits, endurance training needs to be performed three to five times per week. For older persons in rehabilitation programs who have physical limitations, the specific activities may need to be modified. For example, cycling may not be possible for a person who has significant hemiparesis after a stroke. Adaptations, such as securing the person's foot to the pedal, may allow the individual to exercise. Moving to another venue, such as a therapeutic pool, may be another option.

A benefit of endurance training is an increase in maximal oxygen consumption, which is defined as the amount of oxygen consumed while performing the maximal workload that one can perform for 2 to 3 minutes. Improving the maximal amount of work that a person can perform is not necessarily a direct benefit because daily activities are performed at submaximal, rather than maximal, levels of exertion. However, with an increase in maximal oxygen consumption, a given amount of submaximal work is performed at a lower percent of maximal oxygen consumption. Consequently, as a result of endurance training, submaximal work expressed as a percent of maximal oxygen consumption is lower. From a functional perspective, activities such as dressing, bathing, and performing housework can be performed with less fatigue and for longer time periods.

Endurance exercise has positive benefits for persons with hypertension, hypercholesteremia, and obesity. Regular endurance exercise has been shown to decrease resting blood pressure, resulting in either a decrease in the amount of or a need for medications. Although, endurance exercise often does not decrease total cholesterol, many studies have shown positive benefits for High Density Lipoprotein-cholesterol and triglyceride levels. For both treatment and prevention of obesity, endurance exercise is a key component of a successful program.

Endurance exercise also has benefits for cardiovascular and pulmonary diseases. For persons with angina, participation in a regular endurance exercise program produces an increase in the "anginal threshold," allowing persons to exercise at higher levels prior to the onset of angina. Persons with chronic pulmonary disease typically experience less breathlessness with activities, as a result of a regular exercise program. One of the most effective treatments for claudication is walking to the onset of pain, which ultimately produces an increase in the distance walked prior to the onset of claudication.

Exercise to Improve Balance Balance, defined as the ability to remain upright as the body's center of gravity shifts relative to the base of support, declines as people age. The somatosensory, visual, and vestibular systems contribute to our ability to maintain balance. Balance is an essential component to walking because walking involves a continuous shift of the body's center of gravity relative to the base of support.

Balance exercises are important for persons who have fallen or who are at high risk of falls. Exercises are prescribed that are appropriate for the individual's current level of function. For example, low-level exercises may involve standing and shifting one's center of gravity. As the person progresses, he/she may practice standing on one extremity or walking on a balance beam. Exercises performed with eyes closed force the use of the vestibular and somatosensory systems. Exercises performed on altered surfaces, such as foam or carpet, force the use of the visual and vestibular systems. For persons with a specific abnormality of the vestibular system, such as benign positional vertigo, there are specific exercises that often are helpful.

Flexibility Exercises The goal of flexibility exercises is to increase range of motion of a body part by increasing muscle length and/or joint motion. The most effective and safe approach is a prolonged, low-intensity stretch of the muscle/joint with limited motion. Having a sufficient amount of motion is important for many functional activities. For example, going up- and downstairs using a reciprocal gait pattern requires at least 90 degrees of knee flexion. Reaching overhead requires 120 to 150 degrees of shoulder flexion and abduction. In addition, sufficient range of motion at the hip and ankle is important for maintaining standing balance. Excessive range of motion, however, decreases stability and can lead to pain, decreased mobility, and falls.

Parkinson's disease is an example of a common condition in older adults in which flexibility exercises are important. Persons with Parkinson's disease assume a flexed posture, resulting in loss of cervical and thoracic extension. Prescribing exercises early in the course of the disease may prevent the severity of the postural abnormalities. Maintaining spinal extension is important to prevent compromise of respiratory capacity, and to minimize gait and balance disorders.

Task-Oriented Exercises to Improve Motor Control Older persons may lose their ability to perform tasks because of abnormal tone (spasticity) and/or muscle weakness. Task-oriented exercises are used to improve coordination and motor performance. Constraint-induced movement therapy (CIMT) is one method used to improve motor function. With constraint-induced movement therapy, the stronger, less affected extremity is "constrained" using a cast or mitt. The person is forced to use the affected extremity and practice tasks needed for daily living. This method typically involves participation in therapy for 4 to 6 hours per day. The approach is based on learning theory and assumes plasticity of the central nervous system with re-forming of neural connections after injury. A recent report of a multicenter randomized controlled trial reported greater improvements in upper extremity motor function in persons post stroke with constraint-induced movement therapy compared to conventional treatment.

A second method used to improve walking performance and balance is treadmill training with partial body support. A harness is connected to an overhead system, which is mounted on a treadmill. By providing partial weight support in combination with a speed-controlled treadmill, patients can perform a greater amount of task-specific practice compared to traditional methods of gait training. A recent review of treadmill training with and without body weight support after stroke concluded that there was insufficient evidence at this time to determine if this intervention was more effective in improving walking performance compared to conventional therapy.

Designing Exercise Prescriptions   Exercise should be prescribed in an individualized manner similar to prescriptions for medications. The components of an exercise prescription include mode (type of activity), frequency (number of times per day or week), intensity (level of exertion), and duration (time of each individual session). Sufficient research is not available to determine the ideal exercise prescription for older adults with the variety of comorbidities that are typically present. However, for some types of exercise, such as moderate- to high-intensity strength training, there is evidence that exercising every other day or every third day is optimal because of the need for recovery time. Because specific guidelines for persons with pathology are not available, pre- and postexercise monitoring is essential. Vital signs and blood glucose levels (if diabetes is present) need to be checked prior to and after exercise. Persons who are beginning an exercise program or increasing their current exercise level need to be asked how they are feeling 24 hours after exercise. Severe muscle soreness or general body fatigue are signs that the exercise stress was excessive.

Physical Modalities

Physical modalities that are often used with older adults include heat and cold agents, aquatic or pool therapy, electrotherapy, and phototherapy (monochromatic infrared energy—MIRE). For most of these agents, there is limited evidence of effectiveness as a sole intervention. However, when used in combination with other therapies, especially exercise therapy, these modalities can enhance the effectiveness of the overall intervention. The most common indication for use of physical modalities is pain management. Because older adults may have reduced mental status, or impaired circulation and sensation, using modalities in older adults requires caution. Educating patients and their families on the rationale for use of modalities is essential, especially if these are to be used in the home environment.

Thermal Agents (Including Aquatic Therapy)   Thermal agents include superficial and deep heating modalities and cryotherapy. Physiological effects of heat include increased blood flow and edema, increased extensibility of connective tissue structures, and decreased pain. Superficial modalities primarily increase the temperature of the skin and underlying subcutaneous tissue and include hot packs, heating pads, paraffin, and whirlpool baths. Superficial heat is beneficial for persons with osteoarthritis, rheumatoid arthritis, and conditions resulting in cervical and low-back pain. The most popular deep heating modality is ultrasound, a form of acoustical energy, which when absorbed by tissues is converted into heat. Ultrasound is often used for tissue contractures, tendonitis, and pain resulting from musculoskeletal disorders. Ultrasound should not be administered close to the brain, eyes, reproductive organs, pacemakers, or arthroplasties.

Cryotherapy includes cold packs, ice massage, cold water immersion, and vapocoolant sprays. Physiological effects of cold include cutaneous vasoconstriction, decreased nerve conduction velocity, decreased spasticity, and increased joint stiffness. Cold therapy provides short-term analgesia and often allows patients to move when movement otherwise would be too painful. Cold therapy should be avoided in persons with arterial insufficiency, impaired sensation, cold hypersensitivity, and Raynaud's disease.

Aquatic or pool therapy is an alternative to physical modalities and/or exercise on land. A therapeutic pool provides a combination of heat and buoyancy for support of upright activities. Patients with muscle weakness and pain often can walk and exercise in a therapeutic pool when movement on land is limited. Because total body heating produces significant vasodilation, patients with cardiac insufficiency may experience chest pain. All patients need to be careful exiting the pool because of the possibility of postural hypotension.

Electrotherapy   Electrotherapy can be used as an intervention for pain management, muscle activation, wound healing, and urinary incontinence. Transcutaneous electrical nerve stimulation (TENS), a popular treatment for pain, involves placing electrodes over peripheral nerves, nerve roots, or painful areas. The mechanism of action is unclear but probably involves the release of endogenous endorphins in the cerebrospinal fluid, which block pain by binding to opiate receptors. Adverse effects of TENS are minor and typically involve skin irritation secondary to sensitivity to the electrodes or gel. Contraindications to the use of TENS include persons with impaired sensation and/or cognition and persons with either a pacemaker or an implanted cardiac defibrillator. Studies have shown TENS to be effective in the geriatric population for persons with low-back pain, knee osteoarthritis, and carpal tunnel syndrome.

Neuromuscular stimulation is used to activate muscles addressing treatment goals in persons post stroke, spinal injury, or knee surgery. For persons post stroke, electrical stimulation can be used to enhance functional movement patterns, such as contraction of the anterior tibialis muscle to prevent foot drop during the swing phase of gait or contraction of the quadriceps at heel strike during gait. After knee surgery or injury, persons often "forget" how to contract the quadriceps muscle as a result of pain and/or joint effusion. Neuromuscular simulation can be used to "retrain" the quadriceps muscle counteracting atrophy that occurs with immobilization.

An important difference between normal muscle contraction and electrically induced muscle contraction is the order of recruitment of motor units. With normal muscle contraction, the smaller fatigue-resistant motor units are recruited first, followed by larger, fatigable motor units. With electrical stimulation, the larger-diameter fatigable fibers are recruited first. The consequence is that fatigue occurs fairly quickly with neuromuscular stimulation. Providing adequate rest periods and limiting the duration and frequency of contractions are strategies to lessen fatigue.

Electrotherapy used for wound healing involves application of electric current either directly to a wound or to the skin surrounding the wound. Electrical stimulation is approved for Medicare coverage for the treatment of stasis, arterial pressure, and diabetic ulcers that have not responded to conventional therapy. Animal and human studies have shown that electrical stimulation increases both DNA and collagen synthesis; directs epithelial, fibroblast, and endothelial cell migration into wound sites; inhibits the growth of some wound pathogens; and increases the strength of scar tissue. The effectiveness of electrical stimulation is demonstrated not only in case reports but also in randomized controlled trials, with the strongest evidence being demonstrated in the treatment of pressure ulcers.

Phototherapy (MIRE) Devices that deliver MIRE were approved by the FDA in 1994 to increase circulation and decrease pain. This treatment involves placing pads over the lower leg and foot. The pads contain diodes that emit light energy in the near-infrared spectrum (890-nm wave length). The typical treatment protocol involves 30-minute treatments, three times a week, for a total of 12 treatments. The infrared photo energy is thought to release nitric oxide from hemoglobin. Nitric oxide relaxes smooth muscle cells, dilating blood vessels and improving circulation.

MIRE recently has gained popularity for the treatment of peripheral neuropathy, with the goal to improve sensation and decrease neuropathic pain. Research studies are conflicting with one randomized controlled trial reporting that MIRE was no more effective than placebo in improving sensation. An interesting finding from this study was that both groups (treatment and placebo) showed significant improvements in plantar sensation. This finding may explain why noncontrolled studies have shown improvements in sensation using MIRE. Important implications of the demonstrated improvement in sensation shown in some studies are a lower incidence of falls and foot ulcers and an increase in activity level.

Adaptive Aids

Adaptive aids include devices that allow persons with physical limitations to participate in activities, such as basic and instrumental activities of daily living, with greater ease and/or less pain. Categories of adaptive aids include mobility aids to assist people to move around within their home and community, bathroom aids to assist with bathing and toileting, and self-care aids that assist with dressing, personal hygiene, cooking, and other activities. It is not unusual for older persons to have devices that they do not need, often as a gift from a friend or relative. The opposite also occurs when older persons need devices that are not prescribed. The devices described below need to be prescribed by a professional, and the patient and family or caregiver need to be instructed in their use. Devices that are used incorrectly can lead to falls and other adverse events. It is often helpful for the professional (typically a physical or occupational therapist) to make a home visit to assess whether the prescribed adaptive devices can be used safely in the patient's home.

Mobility Aids Canes are the most popular mobility aid for older adults because they are lightweight and easy to use when space is limited. Canes are used to decrease weight bearing (and pain) in an extremity with an arthritic joint and to improve balance. When adjusted to the proper height, the handle of the cane is at the level of the wrist when the arm is fully extended. Canes should be used in the hand on the side opposite of the involved extremity. The base of support is increased, which improves stability, and the patient can shift weight to the cane when weight bearing on the involved side. Many people will incorrectly use the cane in the hand on the

side of the involved extremity. The cane then acts as a brace for the involved extremity, producing an abnormal gait pattern and limiting range of motion of both the hip and the knee of the involved side. To achieve a normal gait pattern, patients are instructed to hold the cane in the hand opposite the involved extremity and advance the cane and the involved extremity simultaneously. Patients then swing thru with the uninvolved extremity while bearing weight on the cane and, to a lesser degree, the involved extremity. For stairs, patients are taught "up with the good and down with the bad." To ascend the stairs the uninvolved extremity is advanced up the stairs first, while the involved extremity and the cane remain on the lower step. To descend the stairs, the involved extremity and the cane are lowered first and then the uninvolved extremity descends to the same step. For persons with decreased sensation in the lower extremities, a cane can also provide proprioceptive input to the brain by transmitting information from intact proprioceptors in the hand.

Two major types of canes are straight canes and quad canes. Straight canes are usually made of aluminum or wood, with a variety of handles available. Quad canes are aluminum canes with a four-legged base. One advantage of a quad cane is that the cane does not fall if the person releases the handle. A disadvantage of some quad canes is that the base is too large to place on stairs, making stair climbing difficult.

Crutches are usually not used with older adults because a higher level of coordination and skill is required. The two major types of crutches are axillary and forearm crutches. If axillary crutches are used incorrectly, shoulder injury and/or axillary nerve damage can occur. Forearm crutches are more functional because a cuff secures the crutch on the patient's arm allowing use of the hand to manipulate objects. Crutches are usually used to provide bilateral support. However, a single crutch can be used instead of a cane if additional unilateral support is needed.

When a cane does not provide sufficient support, a walker usually is prescribed. Walkers provide bilateral support and are easier to use than crutches. Walkers should be adjusted so that the user maintains an erect posture and is not required to lean forward to reach the walker. There are several types of walkers that vary in stability and function. The standard four-point or "pick-up" walker provides the most stability. The walker is picked up with each step, requiring arm strength and endurance, and producing a slow walking speed. With a two-wheeled rolling walker, the person can use a more normal gait pattern and speed. Having two rather than three or four wheels provides more stability. A four-wheeled walker, called a "rollator," has hand brakes so that it can be locked when the user is standing up and sitting down. This type also has a platform seat for resting, and a basket for carrying objects. The rollator requires greater skill because of the use of the hand brakes. It is preferred for outdoor use because the wheels are larger and move easier over sidewalks and slightly rough terrain. A final option is the Merry Walker®, which provides the maximal amount of support. This type of walker includes front, side, and back bars, and a seat for resting. Merry Walkers® are larger and more difficult to manipulate in homes. They are often used in institutional settings for persons with severe balance and coordination deficits.

A wheelchair should be prescribed when the person can no longer walk safely or when walking endurance is low. The wheelchair allows the person to continue to do activities such as shopping that require extended periods of standing and walking. Quality of life is maintained and social isolation is avoided. Two main types of wheelchairs are manual and power chairs. There are many options available for customizing a chair for individual needs. In considering the optimal chair, both stability and mobility need to be considered. For example, a back height that is too high makes propelling the chair independently difficult, impairing mobility, whereas a back height that is too low may not provide adequate trunk support. There are a variety of manual wheelchairs available with many different features. The width of the seat can range from narrow to wide to accommodate larger persons. Removable arm rests and foot rests are available and make transfers easier and safer. Fixed foot rests are not recommended because they can contribute to falls. Consultation with the Occupational Therapist or Physical Therapist is recommended, as the therapist would know best how to order appropriate parts to maximize function.

Manual wheelchairs are lighter in weight than power chairs and are fairly easy to fold and load into a car for travel. Power chairs and scooters provide enhanced mobility outdoors and in the community. Most power chairs are difficult to maneuver in homes. In addition, a car carrier is needed for travel.

Prescribing a wheelchair for use is an important decision, and the advantages and disadvantages for each patient need to be considered. For patients who are able to walk, having a wheelchair may discourage walking, leading to decreased muscle strength and endurance and increasing the probability of falling. However, not prescribing a wheelchair as walking ability declines can negatively affect quality of life. Patients and families need to be counseled on appropriate use of a wheelchair based on their unique needs.

Table 29-5 illustrates some of the commonly prescribed types of canes, walkers, and power chairs and describes some of the benefits and risks of using the different mobility aids.

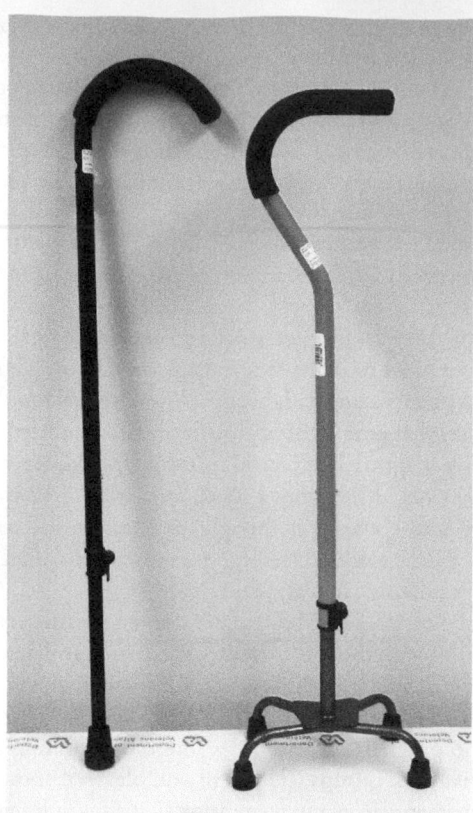

FIGURE 29-4. Canes (straight and quad). *(Photograph by David T. Gadbois.)*

Bathroom and Self-care Aids For many older adults with physical disabilities, the bathroom is a challenging and unsafe place. Devices are available for use in a typical home bathroom to make activities easier and safer. Grab bars located close to the toilet and shower or tub should be considered for all older adults. Many older adults have

difficulty rising from a regular toilet seat because of the low height. A raised toilet seat can be secured to a regular toilet. For persons who need more assistance, bedside commode chairs are available. Some bedside commode chairs have wheels, and can be rolled over a regular toilet. Tub benches are available for individuals who have difficulty getting out of a regular tub, and shower chairs are available for persons who cannot stand independently to take a shower.

Devices are also available to assist patients with activities of daily living. Occupational therapists can assist with identifying the most appropriate adaptive aids. Some examples for dressing include aids to assist with manipulating buttons, securing pants, and putting on/off shoes and socks. For eating, enlarged handles on utensils and modified plates are available. Having an appropriate aid often results in independence in performing a task versus needing to ask for assistance.

Electronic Devices (Environmental Control Units/Augmentative Communication Aids) Devices are available that use more sophisticated technologies to allow patients a greater degree of independence and enhanced communication. Environmental control units typically are used for patients with severe disabilities to allow turning on/off lights and controlling other electronic devices. Whatever voluntary motion is available is used to control the unit, usually through a joystick, mouth stick, or eye motion. Devices used to enhance communication include communication boards, voice amplifiers, and telephone adaptations. For strategies to enhance communication, consultation with a speech and language pathologist is recommended.

TABLE 29-5

Commonly Prescribed Mobility Aids		
TYPE	**EXAMPLE**	**DESCRIPTION**
Canes: straight and quad	Figure 29-4	• Easiest to use, provides the most mobility with walking • Provides unilateral support • Supports 15%–20% of body weight • May not provide sufficient support
Walkers: rolling and rollator	Figure 29-5	• Bilateral support • Supports more body weight than the cane • Gait is slower • More difficult to use on stairs and in smaller spaces
Power chairs: wheelchair and scooter	Figures 29-6 and 29-7	• Total body support • Provides community mobility but may be difficult to use in the home • May contribute to decline in strength and walking performance

Authors' own work summarizing the different available mobility aids. Photographs by David T. Gadbois.

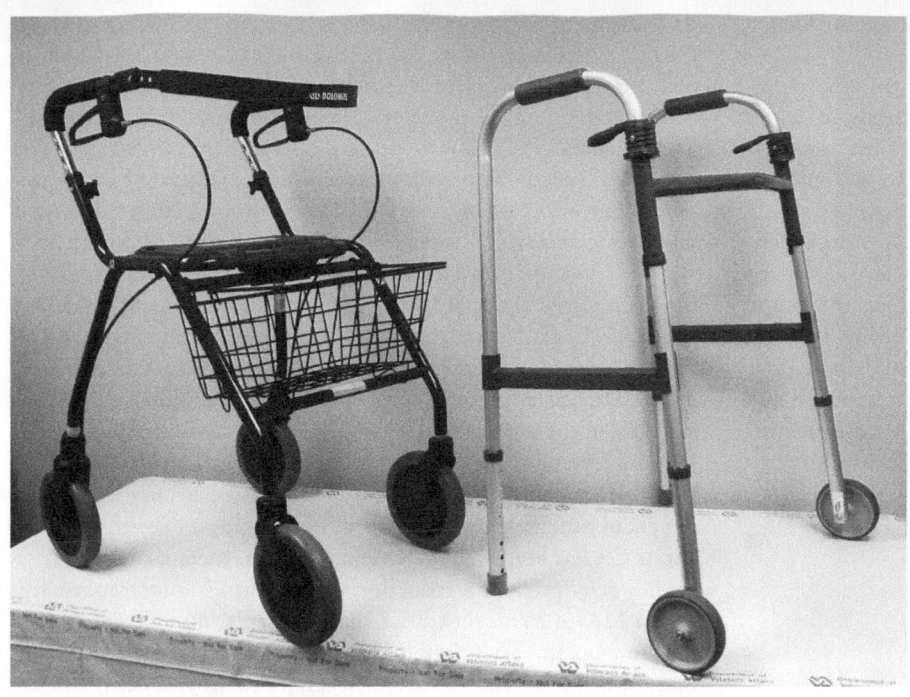

FIGURE 29-5. Walkers (rolling and rollator). *(Photograph by David T. Gadbois.)*

Orthotics and Prosthetics

Orthotics and prosthetics are external devices used to enhance function. Orthoses typically are used to either restrict or assist motion and are named according to the joints or body parts that are affected. For example, ankle–foot orthoses include the foot and ankle, and knee–ankle–foot orthoses extend from the thigh to the foot.

The most commonly used orthoses for older adults are foot orthoses and ankle–foot orthoses. Foot orthoses include shoe inserts and other devices placed inside the shoe. Inserts can be used to relieve pain or to protect insensitive feet. Examples of commonly used foot orthoses include heel spur cushions, scaphoid pads to correct flattening of the arches, and metatarsal pads to transfer weight from the metatarsal heads to the metatarsal shafts. Ankle–foot orthoses are used for patients with either weakness or paresis of dorsiflexors to prevent foot drop during gait. These orthoses can be made of plastic or metal. Plastic orthoses can be interchanged between shoes but do not provide as much support as metal orthoses. Appropriate

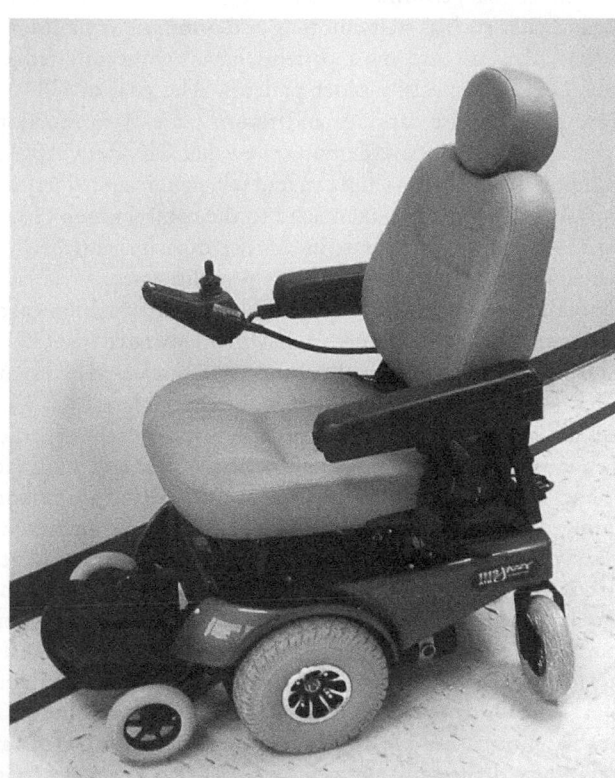

FIGURE 29-6. Power wheelchair. *(Photograph by David T. Gadbois.)*

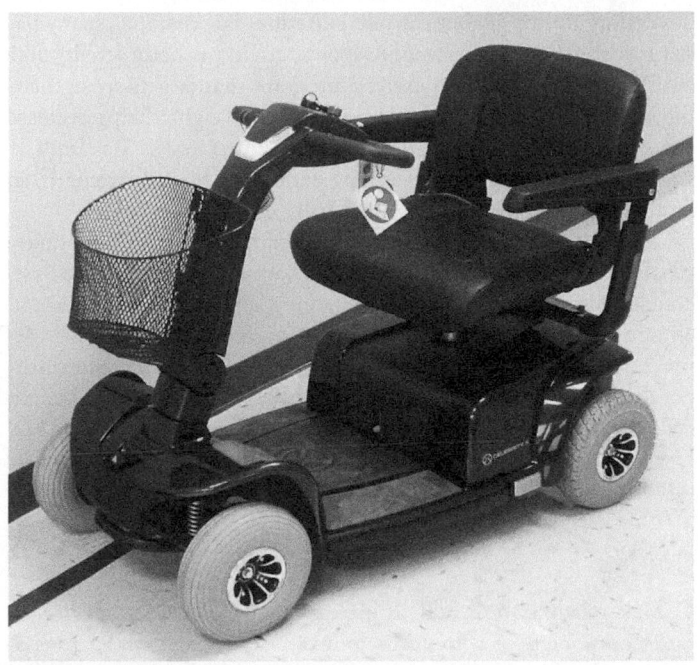

FIGURE 29-7. Power scooter. *(Photograph by David T. Gadbois.)*

use of foot and ankle orthoses can improve function by providing a safe, more comfortable gait.

Many older adults require prostheses because of amputation resulting from vascular disease. In prescribing prostheses for older adults, important considerations include ease of donning and doffing, stability during activities, and overall function. In persons with severe dementia or advanced cardiopulmonary disease, wearing a prosthesis may not be practical. Persons who are not independent in basic Activities of Daily Living (ADL) skills, such as transferring and dressing, typically are not good candidates for prosthetic use. To achieve the optimal outcome, the patient should be involved in a preprosthetic training program to improve strength and endurance. The physician should work closely with the physical therapist and prosthetist to assure that the prosthesis is evaluated for correct fit and that the patient receives training on use of the prosthesis.

SPECIFIC CONDITIONS TREATED WITH REHABILITATION

Pulmonary Rehabilitation

Patients with chronic respiratory diseases frequently experience disability owing to decreased exercise tolerance and symptoms like dyspnea and anxiety. The established benefits of pulmonary rehabilitation include improved exercise capacity, a decreased sensation of dyspnea, and overall improvement in quality of life. The cornerstone of most pulmonary rehabilitation programs is exercise, although other components may include education and behavioral modifications like energy-conservation techniques. As with other rehabilitation programs, pulmonary rehabilitation can occur in inpatient, outpatient, and home settings with equal success. Exercise programs are individually tailored to meet the patients' needs, and patients are usually encouraged to exercise three times a week or more to a level where they experience moderate dyspnea. Training regimens vary, depending on the goal of the rehabilitation. For example, many patients with COPD experience dyspnea with upper body activity, like bathing or grooming. An exercise program that targets strengthening of the arms with elastic bands or light weights helps decrease the dyspnea and work effort required for these tasks. Treadmill or track training will improve walking endurance but not strength, so a variety of training exercises are usually utilized.

The majority of studies have examined the benefit of pulmonary rehabilitation for patients with COPD, and a recent meta-analysis concluded that pulmonary rehabilitation showed both statistical and clinical improvements in dyspnea and disease-specific quality-of-life measures. Supervised programs offered greater benefit than unsupervised ones, and patients with severe disease appeared to benefit the most when compared to those with mild-to-moderate COPD. However, many questions still remain about what components are essential and how to best assess outcomes after rehabilitation.

Cardiac Rehabilitation

Cardiac rehabilitation (CR) is increasingly recognized as an important component of a multidisciplinary treatment strategy for patients with a history of myocardial infarction and stable angina and patients after coronary artery bypass graft (CABG) surgery. Many of the benefits of CR occur through the exercise component of these programs. Exercise training has been found to decrease coagulability, increase fibrinolysis, improve endothelial function by moderating inflammation, and improve endothelium-dependent vasodilation. These beneficial effects can be demonstrated by the reduction in C-reactive protein seen with exercise and the improvement in hyperemic myocardial flow after CR. Disability or functional decline is often associated with a variety of cardiac conditions, and participation in CR can improve fitness and reduce the signs and symptoms of exercise intolerance. This can lead to improved functional independence. In addition to exercise training, CR provides a structured environment for risk factor management through patient monitoring plus support of compliance and adherence. However, despite evidence of the beneficial effects, CR remains underutilized, with a 15% to 25% participation rate among eligible patients.

CR after acute myocardial infarction has been an important component of patient management for several decades. The survival benefit of CR has been well documented by two meta-analyses. These studies demonstrated a reduction of 20% to 24% total mortality, with a 22% to 25% reduction in cardiovascular mortality at 3 years of follow-up. Importantly, CR is a cost-effective way to reduce health care expenditures and recurrent hospitalizations and compares favorably with other well-established therapeutic interventions like cholesterol-lowering and CABG surgery. Older patients with coronary heart disease frequently have a greater severity of disease, with more left ventricular dysfunction and more medical comorbidities leading to decreased exercise tolerance and higher rates of disability. One of the most predictable benefits of CR is improved exercise capacity, making it an ideal therapy for older patients. One randomized controlled study of resistance training in older women with a disability who has a coronary heart disease documented improvement in functional performance, including household activities and endurance tasks such as stair climbing and 6-minute walk distance.

After CABG surgery, most patients have significantly reduced exercise capacity, especially older patients. The goal of CR is to improve peak exercise capacity and return patients to functional independence. Studies have demonstrated that CR after CABG reduces hospital readmissions and can lead to a significant reduction in cardiovascular events when compared to the control group (18.4% vs. 34.7%). The improvements in exercise capacity with CR have translated into a decrease in long-term mortality rates.

For patients with congestive heart failure, randomized clinical trials conducted during the last decade have demonstrated that CR can improve exercise tolerance, quality of life, and disease-related symptoms, without adversely affecting left ventricular function. While there is no consensus regarding the optimal exercise program, guidelines support the use of regular aerobic and/or strengthening exercises. Exercise training induces peripheral and central adaptations, including improvement in vasodilation among active muscle, decreased sympathetic nervous system activation, and increases in peak cardiac output, heart rate, and stroke volume. These adaptations lead to a reduction in the commonly observed exercise intolerance because of fatigue and dyspnea. Using peak oxygen consumption (VO2) to measure exercise capacity, improvements have ranged from 15% to 30%. Other common symptoms associated with heart failure such as shortness of breath, ability to perform activities of daily living, anxiety, depression, and general well-being have all been improved with CR. The magnitude of improvement has ranged from 15% to 50% for each of these variables, and improvements in quality of life can be seen as early as 2 months after initiation of the exercise program. In addition to improvements in symptoms and quality of life, reduction in mortality has also been demonstrated. Increased sympathetic nervous system activity and higher plasma and tissue cytokine concentrations are associated with worsening disease and poorer prognosis in patients with heart failure. Exercise training causes a down-regulation of these systems, with a resultant 28% reduction in total mortality and hospitalization and a 29% reduction in death rate. Prior to initiation of an exercise program, patients must be clinically stable with controlled fluid status for at least 3 to 4 weeks.

The literature demonstrates a beneficial effect of CR for a variety of cardiac diagnoses, including acute myocardial infarction, congestive heart failure, and after CABG surgery. Exercise training positively affects both the basic pathophysiology of coronary artery disease and the underlying disease process. This, in turn, minimizes the impact of disability, improves quality of life, and reduces mortality. Referral to CR increases the likelihood of participation and long-term compliance, which can have significant beneficial effects for the patient.

Peripheral Arterial Disease

Lower extremity peripheral artery disease is common in older persons, with a prevalence of 16% to 34% in patients older than 65 years. Studies have demonstrated that the optimal exercise rehabilitation program for improving the distance walked prior to the onset of claudication uses intermittent walking to the onset of pain. The increased distance achieved occurs through improvements in cardiopulmonary function, peripheral circulation, and walking economy. Improvements require an exercise program of at least 6 months duration to be effective. Treadmill walking has been shown to be more effective than strength training.

Amputation

In the United States, approximately 50 000 new major lower extremity amputations are performed each year. The majority of these amputations occur in patients older than 60 years, and peripheral vascular disease and diabetes mellitus account for more than 90% of these amputations. The estimated 5-year survival after amputation is 35% to 40%, and the risk of contralateral amputation in the subsequent 2 years can be as high as 20%.

During the initial postoperative period, goals include relieving pain, preventing medical complications, and preventing mobility problems, particularly muscle atrophy and contractures. Between 60% and 80% of persons undergoing a lower extremity amputation experience phantom limb pain. Approximately 10% of those who experience phantom pain rate the pain as severe enough to be disabling. Conflicting evidence exists regarding the success of adequate pain control preoperative or perioperatively on the incidence of phantom pain. However, there is little controversy regarding the importance of adequate pain control for persons undergoing amputation.

Common medical problems after amputation include poor wound healing, skin breakdown, and falls. Early mobilization with or without a prosthesis is critical for recovery of function. Older persons who already have decreased lean muscle mass are at risk of additional muscle atrophy. Joint contractures occur when patients spend significant periods of time sitting in a chair or a wheelchair and can have a negative impact on their ability to ambulate with a prosthesis. Initially after amputation, older persons are instructed in the basics of self-care and mobility and then discharged to home. Rehabilitation occurs later after healing of the amputation site and can occur in a rehabilitation facility, in the home, or as an outpatient.

For the older adult, comorbid conditions and premorbid functional status impact the success of the surgery and subsequent rehabilitation. Prior to surgery, the older person should be medically stable, with special attention being paid to cardiopulmonary status. Level of amputation should also be considered. The energy expenditure required for a transtibial amputee is much less than for a transfemoral amputee and may predict a person's ability to regain ambulatory ability. However, while preserving the knee joint may be beneficial, preoperative evaluation should carefully assess the risk and benefit of knee preservation to avoid surgical revisions and longer lengths of stay in the hospital.

Prosthesis use can decrease energy expenditure with transfers and ambulation and should at least be considered, irrespective of age. Firm criteria for prosthesis use do not exist. Some authors suggest using functional status, medical status, and ability to learn as potential markers of success with prosthesis training. These measures would certainly be useful when developing goals for the patient after amputation. A variety of lower limb prosthetic devices are available. To date, studies have not included a large enough sample of older persons to determine the optimal socket or foot design for this population. This determination should be made with the input of the patient, physician, prosthetist, therapists, and insurance company.

Stroke Rehabilitation

Rehabilitation after stroke begins once the patient is medically stable and initially focuses on prevention of medical complications like pressure ulcers or deep vein thrombosis, minimization of spasticity, encouragement of patients to resume self-care activities, and provision of emotional support to the patient and family. There appears to be a statistically significant and clinically important benefit from organized inpatient interdisciplinary rehabilitation in the postacute period. In several randomized controlled trials, either organized inpatient multidisciplinary rehabilitation or stroke unit care demonstrated improved outcomes, including reduced odds of death. Guidelines for the management of stroke were developed by Veterans Affairs and the Department of Defense and rate the quality of available evidence. The guidelines present algorithms for initial assessment as well as management after rehabilitation referral (http://stroke.ahajournals.org/cgi/content/full/36/9/e100).

Techniques used during stroke rehabilitation vary and are tailored to the needs and deficits of an individual patient. Strengthening and task-oriented approaches, like constraint-induced therapy, are common. Facilitation techniques that progress movement to higher-level control by suppressing primitive reflexes may also be used. The goal of therapy, no matter the approach, is improvement of function and quality of life.

After a stroke, patients may have a variety of impairments in addition to muscle weakness. Dysphagia places patients at risk of aspiration and can be silent in up to one-third of patients with dysphagia. Communication disorders including aphasia also occur in one-third of patients, with prognosis being worse for patients of advanced age, or with delayed treatment. During the first month after a stroke, the incidence of bladder incontinence is 50% to 70%, although it returns to levels seen in the general population by 6 months. Treatment can include timed voiding schedules and monitoring of postvoid residuals. Hemiplegic shoulder pain is also a common occurrence, affecting 34% to 84% of patients post stroke. Major risk factors include advanced age and changes in muscle tone, which occur after the stroke. Treatment involves proper positioning to avoid joint subluxation and early range of motion exercises to prevent contractures and spasticity. There is some evidence that electric stimulation can improve hemiplegic shoulder pain for up to 6 months after treatment. Depression is another frequent complication after stroke, one that can have a significant negative effect on rehabilitation. Incidence ranges from 15% to 70% depending on the study, and several antidepressant medications have been associated with improvement. An organized, interdisciplinary team approach helps to address these common sequelae after stroke.

Parkinsonism

Physical manifestations of parkinsonism include muscular rigidity, bradykinesia, postural instability, and gait disturbances. Muscle rigidity and bradykinesia are often manifested by difficulty initiating movement, which causes patients to have significant difficulty performing even simple activities of daily living. Owing to postural instability and gait disturbances, patients with parkinsonism are more likely to experience falls and are at risk of injury owing to slow reaction speed.

At this time, there are no guidelines or generally accepted rehabilitation techniques for persons with Parkinson's disease. Traditionally, therapy has focused on improving posture, range of motion, and gait. There is evidence that exercise programs including resistive and flexibility exercises can improve physical function. One meta-analysis demonstrated improvements in stride length, gait speed, and ADL performance with exercise. Another commonly used technique is an external cueing strategy where auditory pacing, use of a walking stick, or visual cues can help improve gait and decrease episodes of freezing for some patients. Because of the success of rhythmic cueing, studies are being done to explore the use of treadmill training as a method to improve the gait pattern of patients with parkinsonism. Early studies are promising, with a decrease in variability of stride length and swing time being seen. The long-term benefits of all the exercise interventions are still unknown.

Osteoarthritis and Total Joint Replacement

Osteoarthritis is the leading cause of impaired mobility in older persons because of the associated joint pain, muscle weakness, and atrophy. In persons with osteoarthritis of the knee, the severity of the knee pain is directly correlated with the degree of muscle weakness. Several randomized trials have demonstrated the efficacy of strengthening exercises to lessen pain and improve function. Weight loss combined with strengthening exercises was shown to be more effective than weight loss alone for improving function and reducing pain. If pain occurs with an exercise, that exercise should be avoided, and monitoring by a physical therapist during the initial rehabilitation period is reasonable. Osteoarthritis of the hip is less amenable to exercise, probably because improving strength in the ball and socket hip joint does not provide the same support as strengthening the hinged knee joint.

Total joint arthroplasty is the most common elective surgical procedure done in the United States. The primary indications for arthroplasty are mobility limitation and progressive pain, despite conservative treatments like exercise and use of mobility aids. After total joint replacement, the principal goal is to attain the highest level of functional independence possible. Rehabilitation after a total hip replacement focuses on strengthening exercises and gait training. In the early stages of recovery, patients are taught to avoid crossing their legs and flexing their hips more than 90 degrees, to decrease the risk of hip dislocation. Raised toilet seats are also recommended to prevent excessive hip flexion during the first few months after surgery. After total knee replacement, rehabilitation is focused on pain control, reduction of swelling, improving range of motion, and strengthening the muscles around the knee. Recovery from total knee replacement requires the patient work hard to attain and maintain range of motion during the first few months after surgery, which is distinct from hip replacement surgery.

Falls

A multicomponent strategy has been demonstrated in a series of randomized controlled trials to be highly effective in reducing falls in all older persons. These successful interventions have included strength and balance training as important components. In one meta-analysis, exercise programs alone have been demonstrated to reduce the risk of falling. Demonstrating a positive effect for environmental modifications has been more difficult, although a recent Cochrane analysis noted that two trials showed a reduction in falls with home hazard reduction.

Hip Fracture

Hip fractures are common, with approximately 95% being caused by falls. Excess mortality of 12% to 20% has been documented after hip fracture and as much as 80% of those who survive fail to regain their prior level of function. One year after hip fracture, half of the patients who had been independent with walking were no longer independent.

The initial rehabilitation efforts are focused on early mobilization to prevent complications of bed rest, like deconditioning and deep vein thrombosis. Post repair, decreased weight bearing on the fractured limb is standard and patients are taught to walk with an appropriate assistive device. The amount of weight that can be placed on the repaired limb depends on fracture stability. If possible, patients should be allowed to weight bear as tolerated as opposed to "touchdown" weight bearing, which is often difficult for older patients to achieve. A meta-analysis examining outcomes of rehabilitation after hip fracture demonstrated that there was no measurable difference between inpatient rehabilitation and subacute care. The goals of care are the same despite the setting and include lower extremity strengthening, gait and balance training, and assessment of fall risk factors, which might be modifiable.

Sarcopenia and Deconditioning

While there is considerable variation in the loss of muscle mass with aging, cross-sectional studies indicate that strength declines at a rate of 12% to 15% per decade after the fifth decade. This age-related loss of muscle strength and mass is termed sarcopenia. Sarcopenia leads to losses of muscle strength, power, and endurance, which are all critical to daily function. The decline in power output, or the ability to contract a muscle quickly, may also be related to an increased risk of falls, as well as difficulty with functional tasks.

A variety of factors appear to impact on the loss of strength, in addition to age. Reduction in anabolic hormones and local growth factors may also contribute to the observed decline. There appear to be gender differences in response to the same exercise program, with older women showing a blunted response to muscle fiber hypertrophy when compared to older men. The most effective resistance programs for older women occur twice a week, suggesting that older women required longer recuperation periods between bouts of resistance exercise. It has been suggested that, in addition to these factors, the frequently observed decline in physical activity may be a significant mediator in the recognized strength and muscle mass loss.

This decline in physical activity, or deconditioning, is often associated with acute illness or chronic disease. Patients with osteoarthritis may limit activity because of pain. As a result, they lose muscle mass and strength, making daily activities more difficult to accomplish. Over time, the patient will tend to perform fewer activities, as they continue to lose strength and endurance. Bed rest during acute care hospitalization can also lead to loss of strength and muscle mass, even after only a few days. The adverse outcomes associated with this low level of activity include functional decline and increased nursing home placement, even after controlling for severity of illness and comorbidities. Early mobilization has been demonstrated to improve functional outcomes for a variety of patients, including those with a hip fracture or pneumonia.

While no consensus exists regarding the optimal training program, numerous studies have demonstrated resistance exercises to be very beneficial in the treatment of sarcopenia and deconditioning. Increased muscle mass and strength occur with loading the muscle at 60% to 80% of one repetition maximum (1RM), two to three times a week. Some researchers also recommend that at least once a week low-intensity, high-velocity resistance training should be done to address the loss of power that occurs with sarcopenia.

Improvement in muscle strength and power through endurance exercise can reduce the difficulty older adults may experience in performing daily functional activities and may promote spontaneous additional physical activity. While sarcopenia owing to aging may not be reversible, other components of the observed decline in physical activity can be ameliorated with exercise.

Pain

For older persons, pain is common and frequently associated with adverse consequences such as depression, anxiety, and impaired ability to walk. In the community-dwelling older adults, 25% to 50% experience significant pain, and, in the nursing home, rates range from 45% to 80%. Having persistent pain may worsen the level of physical activity achieved, and the associated deconditioning can contribute to further pain and disability.

Many of the physical modalities, such as thermal agents (heat or cold) and electrotherapy, can be very beneficial in relieving pain.

There is evidence that participation in an exercise program can improve pain as well as improve function. The prescribed exercise program needs to be individualized for the patient and focused on improving range of motion, strength, and endurance. For additional information on pain management, the American Geriatrics Society has guidelines on the management of persistent pain in older persons (available at www.americangeriatrics.org/education/cp_index.shtml).

CONCLUSION

Because disability is common among older persons, rehabilitation is an important component of geriatric health care. Defining the cause or causes of disability will allow the rehabilitation team to provide treatment in the optimal setting for the individual patient. Much remains unknown about the most effective rehabilitation techniques for patients with multiple comorbidities; however, available literature supports the continued use of rehabilitation to improve function, independence, and quality of life for older persons.

FURTHER READING

American College of Sports Medicine. *Guidelines for Exercise Testing and Prescription.* 7th ed. Philadelphia, PA: Lippincott, Williams & Wilkins; 2006.

Aronow WS. Management of peripheral arterial disease of the lower extremities in elderly patients. *J Gerontol Series A Biol Sci Med Sci.* 2004;59:M172.

Clifft JK, Newton TS, Kasser RJ, et al. The effect of monochromatic infrared energy on sensation in patients with diabetic peripheral neuropathy: a double-blind, placebo-controlled study. *Diabetes Care.* 2005;28:2896.

Duncan PW, Zorowitz R, Bates B, et al. Management of adult stroke rehabilitation care: a clinical practice guideline. *Stroke.* 2005;36:e100. http://stroke.ahajournals.org/cgi/content/full/36/9/e100.

Frieden RA. The geriatric amputee. *Phys Med Rehabil Clin North Am.* 2005;16:179.

Gage H, Storey L. Rehabilitation for Parkinson's disease: a systematic review of available evidence. *Clin Rehabil.* 2004;18:463.

Harkless LB, DeLellis S, Carnegie DH, et al. Improved foot sensitivity and pain reduction in patients with peripheral neuropathy after treatment with monochromatic infrared photo energy – MIRE. *J Diabetes Complicat.* 2006;20:81.

Hill NS. Pulmonary rehabilitation. *Proc Am Thorac Soc.* 2006;3:66.

Hunter GR, McCarthy JP, Bamman MM. Effects of resistance training on older adults. *Sports Med.* 2004;34(5):329.

Jette AM. Toward a common language for function, disability, and health. *Phys Ther.* 2006;86(5):726.

Minor MAD, Minor SD. *Patient Care Skills.* 5th ed. Upper Saddle River, NJ: Pearson, Prentice Hall; 2006.

Moseley AM, Stark A, Cameron ID, et al. Treadmill training and body-weight support for walking after stroke. *Cochrane Database Syst Rev.* 2005;(4):CD002840. doi: 10.1002/14651858.CD002840.pub2.

Ojingwa JC, Isseroff RR. Electrical stimulation of wound healing. *Prog Dermatol.* 2002;36(4):1–11.

O'Sullivan SB, Schmitz TJ. *Physical Rehabilitation.* 5th ed. Philadelphia, PA: FA Davis Company; 2007.

Peel C, Sawyer-Baker P, Roth DL, et al. Assessing mobility in older adults: the UAB Study of Aging Life-Space Assessment. *Phys Ther.* 2005;85:1008–1019.

Perret DM, Rim J, Cristian A. A geriatrician's guide to the use of the physical modalities in the treatment of pain and dysfunction. *Clin Geriatr Med* 2006;22:331.

Shah MA. Rehabilitation of the older adult with stroke. *Clin Geriatr Med.* 2006;22:469.

Studenski SA, Perera S, Wallace D, et al. Physical performance measures in the clinical setting. *J Am Geriatr Soc.* 2003;51(3):314.

Williams MA, Ades PA, Hamm LF, et al. Clinical evidence for a health benefit from cardiac rehabilitation: an update. *Am Heart J.* 2006;152:835.

Wolf SL, Winstein CJ, Miller JP, et al. Effect of constraint-induced movement therapy on upper extremity function 3 to 9 months after stroke: the EXCITE randomized clinical trial. *JAMA.* 2006;296(17):2095.

Pain Management

Bruce A. Ferrell ■ *Susan L. Charette*

THE OLDER PATIENT IN PAIN

Pain is a common complaint among elderly persons. For ambulatory care visits, pain-related problems are more common than any other complaint. The intensity of pain often correlates with the severity of injury and indicates urgency for treatment. Unrelieved pain, pain that persists, or pain out of proportion to tissue damage, over time, often results in substantial disability and psychological distress.

Epidemiology studies of pain in general populations have suffered from the lack of standard definitions for what might be considered "significant" pain. Nonetheless, studies have suggested that the prevalence of pain in community-dwelling older persons may be as high as 25% to 56%. Sources of pain also vary from study to study. Prevalence of back pain has been reported from 21% to 49.5%; joint pain 20.5% to 71%; and headache 1.2% to 50% in persons older than 65 years. In general, the most common causes of pain in elderly persons are probably related to musculoskeletal disorders such as back pain and arthritis. Neuralgia is common, stemming from diseases such as diabetes, herpes zoster, and trauma such as surgery, amputation, and other nerve injuries. Nighttime leg pain (e.g., cramps and restless legs) is also common, as is claudication. Cancer, although not as common as arthritis, is a cause of severe pain. The distress of cancer pain has brought attention to the obligation that clinicians have to provide effective pain management especially near the end of life. Pain is also common in nursing homes. Between 45% and 80% of nursing home residents may have substantial pain. Many have multiple pain complaints and multiple potential sources of pain. Pain is associated with a number of negative outcomes in elderly people. Depression, decreased socialization, sleep disturbance, falls, adverse drug events, slow rehabilitation, and increased health care utilization and costs have all been associated with either the presence of pain or its treatment in older people. Older patients rely heavily on family and other caregivers near the end of life. For these patients and their caregivers, pain can be especially distressing. Caregiver strain and caregiver attitudes can have substantial impact on pain.

The approach to pain management is different in elderly versus younger persons. Older persons may underreport pain. They often present with concurrent illnesses and multiple problems, making pain evaluation and treatment more difficult. Elderly persons have a higher incidence of side effects to medications and higher potential for complications and adverse events related to many treatment procedures. Despite these challenges, pain can be effectively managed in most elderly patients. Moreover, clinicians have an ethical and moral obligation to prevent needless suffering and provide effective pain relief, especially for those near the end of life.

HOW AGING AFFECTS PAIN PERCEPTION

The effect of aging on pain perception has been a topic of interest for many years. Elderly persons often present with altered presentation of common diseases. For example, older persons have been observed to present with apparently painless myocardial infarction and painless intra-abdominal catastrophes. The extent to which these observations are attributable to age-related changes in pain perception remains uncertain. Anatomical studies, as summarized in Table 30-1, have observed some age-related changes in the nervous system that might alter pain perception. Some of these findings include decreased numbers of various pain receptors in the skin and other organs, altered nerve conduction, and some central nervous system changes that may affect sensory processing. Most of these studies were based on cross-sectional studies of animal and postmortem specimens, for which little or no data were actually available, or correlated with the premortem pain experiences.

Likewise, a large number of physiologic studies of pain perception also exist. These studies typically use a heat probe, electrical stimulation, or other methods to induce pain in volunteers in an effort

TABLE 30-1

Age-Related Changes in Pain Perception

COMPONENT	AGE-RELATED CHANGE	COMMENTS
Pain receptors	• 50% decrease in Pacini's corpuscles • 10%–30% decrease in Meissner's/Merkles disks • Free nerve endings—no age change	Few studies largely limited to skin
Peripheral nerves	• Myelinated nerves 　○ Decreased density 　○ Increase abnormal/degenerating fibers 　○ Slower conduction velocity • Unmyelinated nerves 　○ Decreased number of large fibers (1.2–1.6 μn) 　○ No change in small fibers (0.4 μn) 　○ Substance P content decreased	Evidence of change in pain function is lacking; findings are not specific to pain
Central nervous system	• Loss in dorsal horn neurons 　○ Altered endogenous inhibition and hyperalgesia • Loss of neurons in cortex, midbrain, and brainstem 　○ 18% loss in thalamus 　○ Altered cerebral-evoked responses 　○ Decreased catecholamines, acetylcholine, GABA, and 5HT 　○ Endogenous opioids—mixed changes 　○ Neuropeptides—no change	Findings not specific to pain

Data from Gibson SJ, Helme RD. Age differences in pain perception and report: a review of physiological, psychological, laboratory and clinical studies. Pain Rev. 1995;2:111–137.

to identify a pain threshold or pain tolerance level. These studies have shown mixed results, some showing increased, some showing decreased, and some showing no change in pain perception with aging in normal volunteers. Moreover, it has been difficult to conduct a formal meta-analysis using all of these studies because of flaws in many of these studies concerning sampling errors and methodological differences. In the final analysis, most investigators have concluded that actual age-associated changes in pain perception are subtle and probably not clinically significant.

On the other hand, elderly people often present with concurrent illness and sensory impairments that may mask pain complaints. Cognitive impairment, sensory neuropathies, and visual and hearing impairment, each may make communication of pain complaints more difficult and thus appear to be a perceptual problem. Elderly patients may be more stoic; they may expect pain with aging and fear diagnostic tests, other interventions, or the meaning of pain. These issues can make pain assessment and measurement much more difficult in older people.

CLASSIFICATION OF PAIN

Pain is quite variable in description, character, and intensity among individuals. For the purpose of understanding, predicting, and treat-ing pain, a variety of classification schemes have been used. For diagnostic purposes, it may be helpful to categorize pain as acute or persistent. The old term "chronic pain" is now considered obsolete, and the newer term "persistent" is used to reduce the common biases and negative stereotypes associated with the label "chronic pain patients" in the past. For treatment purposes, it may be more helpful to categorize pain as nociceptive versus neuropathic.

Acute Versus Persistent Pain

Acute pain is defined by a distinct onset, obvious cause, and short duration. Trauma, burns, infarction, and inflammation are examples of pathological processes that result in acute pain. Acute pain is often associated with autonomic nervous system signs, including tachycardia, diaphoresis, or elevation in blood pressure. The presence of acute pain usually indicates an acute injury or acute disease, and the intensity of acute pain often indicates the severity of injury or disease. Thus, acute pain should trigger an urgent search for an underlying cause that might be life-threatening or require immediate intervention. The effective management of acute pain is important to facilitate diagnostic tests. Preoperative pain management of acute pain makes anesthesia easier and postoperative pain control better. In some cases, management of acute pain can help prevent development of chronic pain syndromes.

Chronic pain is usually defined by its persistence beyond an expected time frame for healing, usually longer than 3 months. Intensity of chronic pain is often out of proportion to the observed pathology and associated with prolonged functional impairment, both physical and psychological. Autonomic signs are often absent. Underlying causes of chronic pain are often associated with chronic disease and are less remedial.

Chronic pain is often more difficult to manage in older patients because the underlying cause is less curable and many treatment strategies are short lived, difficult to maintain, or associated with long-term side effects. Chronic pain usually requires a multidimensional approach to treatment, including use of both analgesic drug and nondrug strategies with attention to sensory, emotional, and behavioral components of the pain experience.

Nociceptive Versus Neuropathic Pain

For treatment purposes, it may be helpful to identify the underlying mechanism of pain perception. Treatment aimed at specific pathophysiologic pain mechanisms may be more effective. Pain problems that result largely from stimulation of pain receptors are called nociceptive pain. Nociceptive pain may arise from tissue injury, inflammation, or mechanical deformation. Examples include trauma, burns, infection, arthritis, ischemia, and tissue distortion. Pain from nociception usually responds well to common analgesic medications.

Neuropathic pain results from pathophysiologic processes that arise in the peripheral or central nervous system. Examples include diabetic neuralgia, postherpetic neuralgia, and post-traumatic neuralgia (postamputation or "phantom limb" pain). In contrast to nociceptive pain, neuropathic pain syndromes are often persistent and difficult to treat. They may, however, respond to nonconventional analgesic medications such as tricyclic antidepressants and anticonvulsant drugs. For these syndromes, it is important to recognize them early and to begin treatment with adjuvant analgesic strategies before development of long-term complications of persistent pain including physical and psychological disability.

There are other physiological mechanisms of pain, including mixed nociceptive and neuropathic syndromes and pain syndromes of unknown mechanisms. Treatment for these is more problematic and often unpredictable. Examples include recurrent headaches and some vasculitic syndromes. Finally, psychologically based pain syndromes are those with psychological factors that play a major role in the pain experience. Examples include somatoform disorders and conversion reactions. These patients may benefit from specific psychiatric intervention, as traditional pain strategies are often ineffective.

CLINICAL EVALUATION OF PAIN

Pain assessment is the most important part of pain management. Any pain complaint that has an impact on physical function or quality of life should be recognized as a significant problem. Unfortunately, there are no objective biological markers of pain. The most accurate and reliable evidence for the existence and intensity of pain is the patient's description.

Pain History and Physical Examination

Assessment of pain should begin with a thorough history and physical examination to help establish a diagnosis of underlying disease and form a baseline description of pain experiences. The history should include questions to elicit: when the pain started, what events or illnesses coincided with the onset, where does it hurt (location), how does it feel (character), what are the aggravating and relieving influences, and what treatments have been tried. Past medical and surgical history is important to identify coexisting disease and previous experience with pain and analgesic use. The review of systems should probably focus on the musculoskeletal and nervous system because of the frequency of which these pain problems often occur in older persons. Any history of trauma should be thoroughly investigated because falls, occult fractures, and other injuries are common in this age group. Care must be taken to avoid attributing acute pain to preexisting conditions and recognize that chronic pain may fluctuate with time. Injuries from minor trauma and acute disease such as gout or calcium pyrophosphate crystal arthropathy can be easily overlooked. Finally, many older persons do not use the word "pain," but may refer to their problems as "hurting," "aching," or other descriptions. It is important to probe for and identify pain in the patient's own words so that references for subsequent follow-up evaluations are clearly established.

A physical examination should confirm any suspicions suggested by the history. Because of the frequency with which problems are often identified, the physical examination should probably concentrate on the musculoskeletal and nervous systems. Tender points of inflammation, muscle spasm, and trigger points should be palpated. Observation of abnormal posture, gait impairment, and limitations in range of motion may trigger a need for physical therapy and rehabilitation. Evidence of kyphosis, scoliosis, and abnormal joint alignments should be identified. A systematic neurological examination is also important to identify potential sources of neuropathic pain. Focal muscle weakness, atrophy, abnormal reflexes, or sensory impairments may indicate peripheral or central nervous system injury. Mottled skin in a denervated extremity, presence of a Charcot joint, orthostatic hypotension, impaired gastric emptying, or incontinence may indicate autonomic nervous system dysfunction that can imply sympathetically maintained pain or a complex regional pain syndrome.

Assessment of functional status is essential to identify self-care deficits and formulate treatment plans that maximize independence and quality of life. Functional status can also represent an important outcome measure of overall pain management. Functional status can be evaluated from information taken from the history and physical examination, as well as the use of one or several functional status scales validated in elderly people.

A brief psychological and social evaluation is also important. Depression, anxiety, social isolation, and disengagement are all common in patients with persistent pain. There is clearly a significant association between persistent pain and depression, even when controlling for overall health and functional status. Therefore, assessment should, at least, include a screen for depression. Psychological evaluation should also include consideration of anxiety and coping skills. Anxiety is common among patients with acute and persistent pain, which requires extra time and frequent reassurance from health care providers. Persistent pain often requires effective coping skills for anxiety and other emotional feelings that can be learned. For those with significant psychiatric symptoms, referral for formal psychiatric evaluation and management may be required. In these patients, cognitive-behavioral therapy, specific counseling, supportive group therapy, biofeedback, or some psychoactive medications may be necessary for developing and maintaining effective coping strategies as well as management of major psychiatric complications. Social networks should also be explored for availability and involvement of family and other caregivers. Family and informal caregivers are often involved and can have a substantial impact on overall pain management. Evaluation of caregivers is necessary when complicated or high-tech pain management strategies are contemplated, such as continuous analgesic infusions. Some pain management strategies can place substantial demands on caregivers, resulting in substantial caregiver stress. Needs for frequent transportation, administration of pain treatments, and technical training may result in substantial stress for nonprofessional caregivers, which can result in work absence and emotional and physical illness.

Pain Assessment Scales

A variety of pain scales are available to help categorize and quantify the magnitude of pain complaints. Results of these scales are helpful in documentation initially and periodically to maximize treatment outcomes. Results can be recorded in flow chart or graph, making it easy to identify stability or changes in pain over time. Since there are no "gold standards," the validity of pain scales relies largely on face value, correlation with other known scales (concurrent validity), correlation with pain-related constructs (convergence), and experience in many populations over several years.

Pain scales can be grouped into multi- and unidimensional scales. In general, multidimensional scales with multiple items often provide more stable measurement and evaluation of pain in several domains. Table 30-2 summarizes some of the multidimensional scales available. For example, the Brief Pain Inventory has been shown to capture pain in terms of intensity, location, and interference with activities. At the same time, multidimensional scales such as the McGill Pain Questionnaire are often long and time consuming and can be difficult to score at the bedside, making them difficult to use in a busy clinical setting. Table 30-1 provides a description of several available multidimensional scales for pain. For the last

TABLE 30-2

Multidimensional Scales for Pain Measurement

	DESCRIPTION	TARGET	VALIDITY	RELIABILITY	ADVANTAGES	DISADVANTAGES
McGill Pain Questionnaire	Subjects asked to identify words descriptive of individual pain from 78 words grouped in 20 categories; plus four other items (including a five-point word descriptive scale of pain intensity) at the moment [PPI] scored separately	All pain	Good	Good	Multidimensional, extensively studied over a long time; may discriminate between types of pain	Long, difficult to score
Short-form McGill Pain Questionnaire	15 words scored on Likert scale, plus a visual analog and PPI scales	All pain	Good	Good	Shorter than original McGill; not studied as deeply as original	May not discriminate between pain types
Wisconcin brief pain inventory	16-item scale; items scored separately	Cancer pain	Good	Good	Multidimensional	Studied largely in cancer pain
Memorial Sloan Kettering Pain Scale	Four-word descriptor scales	Cancer pain	Good	Good	Multidimensional	Studied largely in cancer pain
Geriatric pain measure	24-item questionnaire; 22 items scored dichotomously; two items scored 0–10	Ambulatory elderly	Good	Good	Multidimensional; tested in elderly	Limited experience; sensitivity to change unknown
Neuropathic Pain Scale	10 items each scored 1–10	Neuropathic pain			Specific for neuropathic pain	Individual item analysis may be more helpful than changes in total score
WOMAC	41 items in five domains: pain, stiffness, physical function, social function, and emotional function	Arthritis	Good	Good	Specific for arthritis	Difficult to use clinically
Roland and Morris Disability Questionnaire	24 items scored yes or no	Back Pain	Good	Good	Specific for back pain	May not be generalizable to other pain syndromes
Hurley Discomfort Scale	Designed to score discomfort behaviors in patients with severe Alzheimer's disease	Acute pain	Probably fair	Reasonable	Does not rely on self-report	Relies on behavioral observation
Osteoarthritis pain behavior observation system	Designed to score position, movement, and behavior among adults	Osteoarthritis of knee	Compared to 0–10 scale $r = 0.45$	Test–retest for more than 10 weeks $r = 0.53$	Does not rely on verbal ability	Limited to osteoarthritis of knee

Adapted from Ferrell BA. Pain. In: Osterweil D, Brummel-Smith, K, Beck JB, eds. Comprehensive Geriatric Assessment. New York, New York: McGraw-Hill, 2000:389.

10 years, data have been accumulating on some of these scales in older persons.

One example of a behavioral scale is the Hurley Discomfort Scale. This instrument was developed for the assessment of discomfort in patients with profound dementia. The scale consists of nine items scored by a trained examiner after observation the behavior of a non-communicative patient. Behavioral observations such as breathing, vocalization, facial expression, body language, and restlessness are scored on Likert scales. Testing of the scale has demonstrated reasonable reliability and stability over time. The scale requires some

TABLE 30-3

Unidimensional Scales for Pain Measurement

	DESCRIPTION	VALIDITY	RELIABILITY	ADVANTAGES	DISADVANTAGES
Visual analog	100-mm line; vertical or horizontal	Good	Fair	Continuous scale	Requires pencil and paper
Present pain intensity	Six-point 0–5 scale with word descriptors (subscale of McGill Pain Questionnaire)	Good	Fair	Easy to understand, word anchors decrease clustering toward middle of scale	Usually requires visual cue
Graphic pictures	Happy faces; others	Fair	Fair	Amusing	Requires vision and attention
Sloan Kettering pain card	Seven words randomly distributed on a card	Good	Fair	Ease of administration	Requires visual cue
Verbal 0–10 scale	"On a scale of 0 to 10, if 0 means no pain and 10 means the worst pain you can imagine, how much is your pain now?"	Good	Fair	Probably easiest to use	Requires hearing

Adapted from Ferrell BA. Pain. In: Osterweil D, Brummel-Smith K, Beck JB, eds. Comprehensive Geriatric Assessment. New York, New York: McGraw-Hill, 2000:390.

skill and experience to administer, which may be problematic for some clinical settings.

Unidimensional scales consist of a single item that usually relates to pain intensity alone. These scales are usually easy to administer and require little time or training to produce reasonably valid and reliable results. They have found widespread use in many clinical settings to monitor treatment effects and for quality assurance indicators. Table 30-3 describes some unidimensional scales that are commonly used, but a large number of variants that have similar characteristics and produce similar results are also available. Unidimensional pain scales often require framing the pain question appropriately for maximum reliability. Subjects should be asked about pain in the present tense (here and now). For example, the interviewer should frame the question: "How much pain are you having right now?" Alternatively, the interviewer can ask: "How much pain have you had over the last week?" or "On average, how much pain have you had in the last month?" The latter questions require accurate memory and integration of pain experiences over time, which may be more difficult for some older patients. Recent studies in those with cognitive impairment have shown that pain reports requiring recall are influenced by pain at the moment. Thus, it may be more useful to use unidimensional scales in this population to assess pain at the moment, much the way vital signs are used.

Pain Assessment in Those with Cognitive Impairment

Cognitive impairment, delirium, dementia, Alzheimer's disease, or stroke can present substantial challenges to pain assessment. Fortunately, it has been shown that pain reports from those with mild-to-moderate cognitive impairment are no less valid than other patients with normal cognitive function. Commonly available instruments, such as those in Table 30-3, are feasible for use in most patients with cognitive impairment. Patients with severe cognitive impairment may represent substantial challenges, for which no generalizable methods for pain assessment have been identified. Although it has been assumed that those in deep coma do not experience pain, it is not clear that such brain damage necessarily results in complete anesthesia. Patients with "locked-in syndrome" (having intact perception and cognitive function but no purposeful motor function and no means of communication) may suffer severely. Unfortunately, no reliable methods exist to assess pain in these individuals. Health

care providers must be aware of these situations and provide analgesia empirically, especially during procedures or for conditions known to be uncomfortable or painful. More often, the majority with severe cognitive impairment can and do make their needs known in simple yes or no answers communicated in various ways. For example, those with profound aphasia can often provide accurate and reliable answers to yes and no questions when confronted by a sensitive and skilled interviewer. For these patients, it is important to be creative in establishing communication methods for the purpose of pain assessment.

Although pain is an individual experience, the use of family and caregivers in the assessment of pain can sometimes be helpful. Among patients with cognitive impairment, the history is often only obtainable from family or close caregivers. Family and caregivers are an excellent source of qualitative information about general behavior, medication usage, and actions that seem to aggravate or reduce pain. Family and caregivers are, however, limited in their interpretation of events and behaviors. In fact, evidence suggests that proxies are not always very accurate or reliable in estimating pain intensity. Studies of elderly patients having cancer suggest that caregivers may overestimate pain intensity and distress. It is often distressing to family and other caregivers who feel helpless in managing severe pain. Both physicians and nurses may underestimate pain as well as provide inadequate pain medication. In the final analysis, family and close caregivers can be valuable sources of qualitative information, but they probably should not be relied on entirely for quantitative assessment of pain intensity or distress, especially among those patients able to communicate their pain experiences.

MANAGEMENT OF ACUTE AND PERIOPERATIVE PAIN

The treatment of acute pain relies largely on short-term use of analgesic medications and resolution of the underlying cause. A variety of nondrug strategies have also been shown to be helpful. The choice of analgesic medications and other strategies to be used may depend on the severity of pain, availability of technical equipment and expertise, expectations for resolution of underlying injury, and individual patient characteristics.

The most common approach to treating acute pain relies on the World Health Organization recommendations for choosing the potency of analgesic drugs based on the intensity of pain. Pain of mild intensity usually responds to nonopioid drugs, used alone or in combination with other physical and cognitive-behavioral interventions. Pain of moderate intensity often requires more intensive efforts such as weak opioids or low doses of more potent opioid drugs. Many of these drugs are compounded with nonsteroidal anti-inflammatory drugs (NSAIDs) or acetaminophen to achieve enhanced relief with only modest exposure to the risk and side effects of many potent opioids. Severe pain usually requires potent opioid analgesic medications given alone or in combination with other analgesic strategies. For severe trauma or postoperative pain, intermittent intravenous, continuous intravenous, or spinal anesthesia may provide faster and more continuous pain relief. Finally, when patients present with acute pain, even though establishing a diagnosis is a priority, symptomatic pain treatment should not be held while investigations are proceeding. It is rarely justified to defer analgesia until a diagnosis is made. In fact, a comfortable patient is better able to cooperate with diagnostic procedures.

Acute and postoperative pain is dynamic. Without treatment, sensory input from damaged tissue causes alterations in spinal cord neurons, which result in enhanced responses. Pain receptors also become more sensitive after injury. Studies have demonstrated long-lasting changes after brief painful stimuli. These observations may explain why long-standing pain is more difficult to suppress. Thus, patients should be encouraged to take pain medications continuously or to prevent pain before it becomes severe and requires higher doses of medication suppress. In general, it may be helpful to provide continuous analgesics initially, with intermittent or "prescribed-as-needed" doses reserved for breakthrough or intermittent pain as the injury resolves.

Aggressive pain prevention and control before, during, and after surgery can have both short- and long-term benefits. Good preoperative pain control has been shown to make postoperative pain easier to control. Postoperative patients who use analgesia via a continuous infusion pump with self-administered boluses for breakthrough pain report less pain and are more satisfied with their pain control. These patients use less medication, have fewer postoperative complications, and tend to be discharged earlier compared to similar patients who are given similar drugs on an intermittent or "as-needed" basis.

The importance of preoperative patient education cannot be overemphasized. Studies have shown that preoperative patient education and preparation dramatically enhance postoperative outcomes and improved pain management. Patients given complete information about specific procedures including detailed descriptions of expected discomfort postoperatively often have less pain, use less pain medication, and have earlier discharges.

MANAGEMENT OF PERSISTENT PAIN

The management of persistent pain often requires a multimodal approach of drug and nondrug pain management strategies. Although analgesic medications are the most common strategy employed, the concurrent use of cognitive-behavior therapy and other nondrug strategies may be essential to reduce long-term reliance on medications alone, which have substantial side effects when used on a long-term basis. Persistent pain management is often a labor-intensive ef-

fort. Not unlike the effort required during warfarin anticoagulation, pain management requires frequent monitoring and often requires frequent adjustments. Indeed, elderly patients with chronic pain benefit particularly from physicians, nurses, and restorative personnel who are able to employ an interdisciplinary approach to complex problems.

In general, persistent pain is more difficult to relieve than acute pain. Patients should be given an expectation of pain relief, but it is unrealistic to suggest or sustain an expectation of complete relief for some patients with persistent pain. The goals and trade-offs of possible therapies need to be discussed openly. Sometimes a period of trial and error should be anticipated when new medications are initiated and titration occurs. Review of medications, doses, use patterns, efficacy, and adverse effects should be a regular process of care. Ineffective drugs should be tapered and discontinued.

Economic issues are also important in the management of persistent pain. It is appropriate to consider economic issues and make balanced decisions while basic principles of assessment and treatment are followed. Health care professionals should be aware of the costs and economic barriers patients and families may encounter with the strategies often prescribed. These issues include lack of Medicare reimbursement for some strategies, limited formularies, delays in referrals in some managed care environments, delays from mail-ordered pharmacies, and limited availability of strong opioid medications in some pharmacies.

ANALGESIC MEDICATIONS

Any patient who has pain that impairs functional status or quality of life is a candidate for analgesic drug therapy. Analgesic medications are safe and effective in elderly people, but they carry a balance of benefits and burdens. For some classes of pain-relieving medications (opioids, for example), elderly patients have been shown to have increased analgesic sensitivity. However, elderly people are a heterogeneous population; thus, optimum dosage and known side effects are difficult to predict. Recommendations for age-adjusted dosing are not available for most analgesics. In reality, dosing for most patients requires beginning with low doses with careful upward titration, including frequent reassessment for dosage adjustments and optimum pain relief.

The least invasive route of drug administration should be used. Some drugs can be administered from a variety of routes such as subcutaneous, intravenous, transcutaneous, sublingual, and rectal. Most drugs are limited to only a few safe routes of administration, but new delivery systems are being created each year. The oral route is preferable because of its convenience and relatively steady blood levels produced. Significant drug effects are often seen in 30 minutes to 2 hours for most analgesics given orally, which may be a drawback in acute, rapidly fluctuating pain. Intravenous bolus provides the most rapid onset and shortest duration of action, which may require substantial labor, technical skill, and monitoring. Subcutaneous and intramuscular injection, although commonly used, has disadvantages of wider fluctuations in absorption and rapid falloff of action compared to oral routes. Transcutaneous, rectal, and sublingual routes are also more difficult to predict but may be essential for those with difficulty swallowing.

Timing of medications is also important. Fast-onset, short-acting analgesic drugs should be used for episodic pain. Medications for intermittent or episodic pain can usually be prescribed as needed. For continuous pain, medications should be provided around the clock. In these situations, a steady-state analgesic blood level is more effective in maintaining comfort. Most patients with continuous pain also need fast-onset short-acting drugs for breakthrough pain. Breakthrough pain includes (1) end-of-dose failure as the result of decreased blood levels of analgesic with concomitant increase in pain prior to the next scheduled dose; (2) incident pain, usually caused by activity that can be anticipated and pretreated; and (3) spontaneous pain, common with neuropathic pain that is often fleeting and difficult to predict.

The use of placebos is unethical in clinical practice, and there is no place for their use in the management of acute or persistent pain. Placebos, in the form of inert oral medications, sham injections, or other fraudulent procedures, are only justified in certain research designs where patients have given informed consent and understand that they may be receiving a placebo as a part of the research design. In research, placebos help identify and measure random or uncontrollable events that may confound results of some research designs. In clinical settings placebo effects are common, but they are neither diagnostic of pain nor indicative of a therapeutic response. The effects of placebos are short lived, and most patients eventually learn the truth, resulting in loss of patient trust and more needless suffering.

Acetaminophen

Acetaminophen is the drug of choice for elderly persons with mild-to-moderate pain, especially that of osteoarthritis and other musculoskeletal problems. As an analgesic and antipyretic, acetaminophen acts in the central nervous system to reduce pain perception. Although it may have some minor drug interactions (e.g., warfarin), given in a dose of 650 to 1000 mg four times a day, it remains the safest analgesic medication compared to traditional NSAIDs and other analgesic drugs for most patients. Unfortunately, acetaminophen overdose can result in irreversible hepatic necrosis. Therefore, the maximum daily dose should never exceed 4000 mg/day.

Nonsteroidal Anti-inflammatory Drugs

NSAIDs have analgesic activity both peripherally and centrally. They are potent inhibitors of prostaglandin synthesis, which have effects on inflammation, pain receptors, and nerve conduction and may have central effects as well. There are two major NSAID-sensitive cyclooxygenase enzymes (COX-1 and COX-2) synthesized in a variety of organs. COX-1 is present in most organ systems and plays a role in normal organ function such as gastric mucosal blood flow and barrier function, renal blood flow, hepatic blood flow, and platelet aggregation. COX-2, normally present in lower concentrations, is an inducible enzyme in response to injury or inflammation. Selective inhibition of COX-2 gives rise to analgesic and anti-inflammatory activity with less organ toxicity compared to the nonselective inhibition of both enzymes. Clinical trials have found COX-2 inhibitors to be similarly effective to traditional NSAIDs in terms of peak pain relief and total pain relief and in reducing joint inflammation in patients with arthritis. Safety profiles of these agents have shown a 50% reduction of gastrointestinal injury when used alone, but little data are available to support additional gastrointestinal injury

with concomitant use of proton pump inhibitors or mesoprostyl. On the other hand, patients taking some COX-2-specific inhibitors (specifically roficoxib) have been shown to increase the risk for cardiovascular events. Thus, patients at risk of cardiovascular events who are taking a COX-2-specific NSAID should also consider low-dose aspirin to offset this effect. Unfortunately, the COX-2 drugs remain expensive and the cost–benefit ratio remains controversial.

Nonspecific inhibitors of COX enzymes (most older NSAIDs) are still appropriate for short-term use in inflammatory arthritic conditions such as gout, calcium pyrophosphate arthropathy, acute flares of rheumatoid arthritis, and other inflammatory rheumatic conditions. They have also been reported to relieve the pain of headache, menstrual cramps, and other mild-to-moderate pain syndromes. These drugs can be used alone for mild-to-moderate pain or in combination with opioids for more severe pain. They have the advantage of being nonhabit forming. Individual drugs in this class vary widely with respect to anti-inflammatory activity, potency, analgesic properties, metabolism, excretion, and side-effect profiles. Moreover, failure of response to one NSAID may not predict the response to another. A disadvantage of NSAIDs (including COX-2-specific inhibitors) is that these all demonstrate a ceiling effect, that is, a level at which increase in dose results in no further increase in analgesia. A large number of NSAIDs are now available; however, there is no evidence to support a particular compound as the NSAID of choice. Several are available over the counter without a prescription. Table 30-4 lists COX-2 and other selected NSAIDs for pain.

High-dose NSAIDs for long periods of time should be avoided in elderly patients. Of major concern is the high incidence of adverse reactions in elderly patients, including gastrointestinal bleeding, renal impairment, and bleeding diathesis from platelet dysfunction. The concomitant use of mesoprostyl, histamine-2 receptor antagonists, proton pump inhibitors, and antacids is only partially successful at reducing the risk of significant gastrointestinal bleeding associated with NSAID use. Also, the side-effect profiles of gastroprotective drugs in this population must be weighed against their limited benefits. These gastroprotective medications do nothing to prevent the renal impairment and other side effects. For those with multiple medical problems, NSAIDs are associated with increased risk of drug–drug and drug–disease interactions. NSAIDs may interact with antihypertensive therapy. Thus, the relative risks and benefits of NSAIDs must be weighed carefully against other available treatments for older patients with chronic pain problems. For some patients, long-term opioid therapy, low-dose or intermittent corticosteroid therapy, or many other nonopioid analgesic drug strategies may have fewer life-threatening risks compared to long-term, high-dose NSAID use.

Opioid Analgesic Medications

Opioid analgesic medications act by blocking receptors in the central nervous system (brain and spinal cord), resulting in a decreased perception of pain. Many opioids also act similar to local anesthetics and have recently found widespread use in epidural anesthesia. Selected opioid analgesic medications are listed in Table 30-5. Opioid drugs have no ceiling to their analgesic effects and have been shown to relive all types of pain. Advanced age is associated with a prolonged half-life and prolonged pharmacokinetics of many

TABLE 30-4

Selected Nonsteroidal Anti-inflammatory Drugs for Pain*

DRUG	MAXIMIM DOSE	DESCRIPTION	COMMENTS
Celecoxib (Celebrex)	200 mg bid	Selective COX-2 inhibition; pain and anti-inflammatory activity similar to other NSAIDs	Less gastric toxicity; less platelet inhibition
Relafen (Nabumetone)	2000 mg/24 h (q 24 h dosing)	Partially COX-2 selective; gastric toxicity may be less; occasionally requires q 12 h dosing	Avoid maximum dose for prolonged periods
Aspirin	4000 mg/24 h (q 4–6 h dosing)	Prototype NSAID	Salicylate levels may be helpful in monitoring
Salsalate (Disalcid)	3000 mg/24 h (q 6–8 h dosing)	Hydrolyzed in small intestine to aspirin	Elderly may require dose adjustment downward to avoid salicylate toxicity; salicylate levels may be helpful in monitoring
Ibuprofen (Motrin by prescription; Advil, Nuprin, and others otc[†])	2400 mg/24 h (q 6–8 h dosing)	Gastric, renal, and abnormal platelet function may be dose dependent; constipation, confusion, and headaches may be more common in older persons	Avoid high doses for prolonged periods of time
Diclofenac (Voldaren and Cataflam)	50 mg tid	Nonspecific COX inhibitor	As for ibuprofen
Diflunisal (Dolobid)	1000 mg/24 h maximum dose Loading = 1000 mg, then 500 q 12 h; or 750 mg, then 250 mg q 8 h in small patients or frail elderly	Relatively good analgesic properties but requires loading dose	Dose may need downward adjustment for small patients or elderly who are frail
Sulindac (Clinoril)	400 mg/24 h (q 12 h dosing)	Same as ibuprofen	Same as ibuprofen
Naproxen (Naprosyn by prescription; Aleve and others otc[†])	1000 mg/24 h (q 8–12 h dosing)	Same as ibuprofen; may require a loading dose.	Same as ibuprofen
Choline magnesium trisalicylate (Trilisate)	5500 mg/24 h (q 12 h dosing)	Lower effect on platelet function	Salicylate levels may be helpful to avoid toxicity
Indomethacin (Indocin)	200 mg/24 h (q 8–12 h dosing)	Extremely high toxicity in frail elderly; should be reserved for acute inflammatory conditions (e.g., gout, etc.)	Keep dose to a minimum (25 mg q 8 h) and for short-term use only; avoid use for osteoarthritis or other noninflammatory problems
Ketorolac (Toradol)	IM[‡]—120 mg/24 h (30–60 mg loading dose; followed by half the loading dose, 15–30 mg q 6 h limited to not more than 5 days) PO[§]—60 mg/24 h (q 6 h dosing limited to not more that 14 days)	Substantial gastrointestinal toxicity as well as renal and platelet dysfunction; relatively high postoperative complications have been documented	Duration of treatment limited because of high toxicity; reduce dose in half for those <50 kg or >65 yrs of age

*A limited number of examples are provided. For comprehensive lists of other available NSAIDs and a host of brand names, clinicians should consult other sources.

[†]otc indicates over-the-counter or available without prescription.

[‡]IM, by intramuscular injection.

[§]PO, per oral route or by mouth.

opioid drugs. Thus, elderly people may achieve pain relief from smaller doses of opiate drugs than younger people.

Opioid drugs have the potential to cause cognitive disturbances, respiratory depression, constipation, and habituation in older people. Drowsiness, cognitive impairment, and respiratory depression associated with opioids should be anticipated when opioids are initiated and doses are escalated rapidly. These effects occur in a dose-dependent fashion and can be used to judge dose escalations. If patients have unrelieved pain with little drowsiness or cognitive impairment, doses may be safely escalated. Tolerance usually develops in a few days to these side effects, at which time, patients usually return to a fully alert status and baseline cognitive function. Until tolerance develops, patients should be instructed not to drive and

to take precautions against falls or other accidents. But once tolerance to these effects has developed, patients can return to normal activities including driving and other demanding tasks, despite high doses of opioid drugs. In fact, cancer patients are often observed to improve physical function once pain is adequately relieved on opioid analgesics.

Constipation is a side effect of opioid drugs to which older patients do not develop tolerance. The management of constipation usually includes increasing fluid intake, maintaining mobility, and use of cathartic medications. Some patients find relief with remedies like prune juice or other natural laxatives. Other patients may require more potent osmotic laxatives such as milk of magnesia, lactolose, or sorbitol. But for many patients opioid-induced constipation may

TABLE 30-5

Selected Opioid Analgesic Medications for Pain*

DRUG	STARTING DOSE (ORAL)	DESCRIPTION	COMMENTS
Morphine (Roxanol, MSIR)	30 mg (q 4 h dosing)	Short-intermediate half-life; older people are more sensitive than younger people to side effects	Titrate to comfort; continuous use for continuous pain; intermittent use for episodic pain; anticipate and prevent side effects
Oxymorphone (Opana)	10–20 mg (q 4 h dosing)	Slightly more potent than morphine	Caution in opioid-naïve patients; ? advantage over morphine
Codeine (plain codeine, Tylenol #3, other combinations with acetaminophen or NSAIDs)	30–60 mg (q 4–6 h dosing)	10% of codeine is metabolized to morphine, which is responsible for most analgesia; subject to genetic enzyme polymorphisms	10%–30% of patients cannot metabolize to morphine
Hydrocodone (Vicoden, Lortab, others)	5–10 mg (q 3–4 h dosing)	Toxicity similar to morphine; acetaminophen or NSAID combinations limit maximum dose	Constipation, nausea, and drowsiness may limit effectiveness
Oxycodone (Roxicodone, Oxy IR; or in combinations with acetaminophen or NSAIDs such as Percocet, Tylox, Percodan, and others)	20–30 mg (q 3–4 h dosing)	Toxicity similar to morphine; acetaminophen or NSAID combinations limit maximum dose; oxycodone is available generically as a single agent	Same as above
Hydromorphone (Dilaudid)	4 mg (q 3–4 h dosing)	Half-life may be shorter than morphine; toxicity similar to morphine	Similar to morphine
Sustained release morphine (MS Contin, Oramorph, and Kadian)	MS Contin—30–60 mg (q 12 h dosing) Oramorph—30–60 mg (q 12 h dosing) Kadian—30–60 mg (q 24 h dosing)	Morphine sulfate in a wax matrix tablet or sprinkles; MS Contin and Oramorph should not be broken or crushed; Kadian capsules can be opened and sprinkled on food but should not be crushed	Titrate dose slowly because of drug accumulation; rarely requires more frequent dosing than recommended on package insert; immediate release opioid analgesic often necessary for breakthrough pain
Sustained release oxymorphone (Opana ER)	5 mg q 12 h in opioid-naïve patients	Titrate 5–10 mg q12 every 3–7 days	Do not crush or chew
Sustained release oxycodone (Oxicontin)	15–30 mg (q 12 h dosing)	Similar to sustained release morphine	Similar to sustained release morphine
Methadone (Dolophine)	2.5–5 mg (q 12 h)	Oxidized by CP450 system; may have NMDA receptor activity; no toxic metabolites; highly lipid soluble; analgesic half-life shorter than serum half life	High risk for drug accumulation in elderly persons; titrate slowly every 3–5 days
Transderm fentanyl (Durgesic)	25 μg patch (q 72 h dosing)	Reservoir for drug is in the skin, not in the patch; equivalent dose compared to other opioids is not very predictable (see package insert); effective activity may exceed 72 h in older patients	Drug reservoir is in skin, not patch. Titrate slowly using immediate release analgesics for breakthrough pain; peak effect of first dose may take 18–24 h; not recommended for opioid-naive patients
Fentanyl lozenge on an applicator stick	Rub on bucal mucosa until analgesia occurs, then discard	Short half-life; useful for acute and breakthrough pain when oral route is not possible	Absorbed via bucal mucosa, not effective orally

*A limited number of examples are provided. For comprehensive lists of other available opioids, clinicians should consult other sources.

require potent stimulant laxatives such as senna or biscodyl. It should be remembered that stimulants should not be used until impactions have been removed and obstruction has been ruled out. Finally, some patients require regular enemas to ensure bowel evacuation during high-dose opioid administration for severe pain.

Nausea also occasionally complicates opioid therapy. Nausea from opioid medications may result from several mechanisms and may wane as tolerance develops. Traditionally, antiemetics such as prochlorperazine, chlorpromazine, and antihistamines have been the mainstay of treatment for nausea in younger patients. Low-dose haloperidol has also been used, anecdotally noting lower side-effect profile compared to other neuroleptic drugs. All of these agents have high side-effect profiles in elderly patients, including movement disorders, delirium, and anticholinergic effects. Thus, clinicians should choose antiemetic medications with the lowest side effects and continue to monitor patients frequently.

Tolerance is a pharmacologic phenomenon that occurs with many drugs. Tolerance is defined by diminished effect of a drug associated with constant exposure to the drug over time. For opioid drugs, tolerance is difficult to predict. In general, tolerance to drowsiness and respiratory depression occurs much faster than tolerance to analgesic properties of the drug. Previous reports that described tolerance among patients having cancer, resulting in the need for massive doses of morphine to achieve adequate analgesia, were probably misinterpreted because those patients also had rapidly advancing cancer. More recent studies of opioid managed arthritis pain have noted that tolerance was not often significant. In fact, some patients have been noted to remain on stable doses of opioids for many years without demonstrating significant tolerance to the analgesic effects.

Dependency is also a pharmacologic phenomenon associated with many drugs, including corticosteroids and beta-blockers. Dependency is present when patients experience uncomfortable side effects when the drug is withheld abruptly. Drug dependence requires constant exposure to the drug for some period of time, but it is difficult to predict. The minimum dose and time relationship between drug exposure and development of dependent withdrawal symptoms is not precisely known, but it appears to vary with individual opioid compounds. Symptoms associated with opioid withdrawal may include anorexia, nausea, diaphoresis, tachycardia, mild hypertension, and mild fever. Worsening symptoms may include skin mottling, gooseflesh, and frank autonomic crisis. Fortunately, these symptoms can be ameliorated easily by tapering opioids over a few days. In severe cases, clonidine given short term in titrated doses will usually control serious autonomic signs. It is important to remember that physiologic effects of opioid withdrawal are usually not life-threatening compared to serious withdrawal common with alcohol, benzodiazepine, or barbiturate withdrawal.

Addictive behavior is defined by compulsive drug use despite negative physical and social consequences and the craving for effects other than pain relief. Patients who are addicted often have erratic behavior that can be observed in a clinical setting in the form of selling, buying, and procuring drugs on the street, and the use of medication by bizarre means such as dissolving tablets for self intravenous administration. It is now clear that drug use alone is not the major factor in the development of addiction. Other medical, social, and economic factors play immense roles in addictive behavior. It is also important to not construe certain behaviors as necessarily addictive behaviors. Hoarding of medications, persistent or worsening pain complaints, frequent office visits, requests for dose escalations, and other behaviors associated with unrelieved pain has coined the term "pseudoaddiction." Laws, regulations, and unintentional behavior by prescribing clinicians may require patients to hoard medication and seek other physicians for additional help. In fact, true addiction is rare among patients taking opioid analgesic medications for medical reasons. This is not meant to imply that opioid drugs can be used indiscriminately, only that fear of addiction and side effects do not justify failure to treat pain in elderly patients, especially those near the end of life.

Other Nonopioid Medications for Pain

A variety of other medications not formally classified as analgesics have been found to be helpful in certain specific pain problems. The term "adjuvant analgesic drugs," although frequently used, is a misnomer in that some of these nonopioid drugs may be the primary pain-relieving pharmacologic intervention in certain cases. Table 30-6 provides some examples of nonopioid drugs that may help certain kinds of pain. The largest body of evidence available relates to the use of these drugs for neuropathic pain, such as diabetic neuropathies, postherpetic neuralgia, and trigeminal neuralgia. Tricyclic antidepressants, anticonvulsants, and local anesthetics are the most frequently used nonopioid analgesics for neuropathic conditions. In general, these drugs have had limited success in pain syndromes that are not associated with neuropathic mechanisms. Most reports have found that these agents are only partially successful. Typically, approximately 50% to 70% of patients have a measurable response, and of those most experience only partial relief. Thus, these drugs are often not panaceas and are rarely totally successful as single agents. One exception may be trigeminal neuralgia, where carbamazepine is probably the drug of choice. Usually these agents work better in combination with other traditional drug and nondrug strategies, in an effort to improve pain and keep other drug doses to a minimum. Failure of response to one particular class of drugs does not necessarily predict failure of another class of agents. In general, nonopioid medications for neuropathic pain should be chosen according to lowest side effects. Treatment should usually start with lower doses than recommended for younger patients, and doses should be escalated slowly based on known pharmacokinetics of individual drugs and appropriate knowledge of disease-specific treatment strategies. Unfortunately, most of the nonopioid medications for pain management have high side-effect profiles in elderly people. Thus, these medications often have to be monitored carefully.

Antidepressants have been the most widely studied class of nonopioid medications for pain. The mechanism of action for these drugs is not entirely known but probably has to do with interruption of norepinephrine and serotonin-mediated mechanisms in the brain. For neuropathic pain, the major effect of these drugs is not their mood-altering capacity, although this may also be helpful in those with concurrent major depression. More is probably known about tricyclic antidepressants than the other subclasses. A randomized placebo-controlled trial of amitriptyline, desimipramine, and fluoxitine indicated that desimipramine may be as effective as amitriptyline, but fluoxitine is no better than placebo for the treatment of diabetic neuropathy. Thus, desimipramine may be a better choice because it has a lower side-effect profile in elderly people than amitriptyline. Unfortunately, tricyclic antidepressants have been criticized for high anticholinergic side effects in elderly patients, which often limits their effectiveness.

The newer norepinephrine reuptake inhibitors (SNRIs) including venlafaxine and duloxetine have been shown to have modest effect on diabetic neuralgia, and duloxetine is FDA approved for use in diabetic neuropathy. Studies of these drugs have indicated small but statistically significant effect sizes.

Studies of the SSRIs, which may have lower side-effect profiles for elderly people, have not been shown effective for pain management. In fact, none have shown significant effect on pain despite being highly effective for depression.

It has been known for many years that some medications with antiepileptic activity may relieve the pain of trigeminal neuralgia (Tic Douloureux). Drugs such as dilantin, tegretol, and valproic acid may also help diabetic neuralgia and other neuropathic pains in some patients. In general, the usefulness of these drugs has been limited by their high side-effect profiles in elderly people and the fact that most patients respond only partially, making the overall risk/benefit ratio rather large in this population. Indeed, these drugs are not simple analgesics and should not be used for the relief of trivial aches and

TABLE 30-6

Selected Nonopioid Medications for Pain*

DRUG	DESCRIPTION	COMMENTS
Antidepressants: amytriptyline, desipramine, nortriptyline, and others	Older people are more sensitive to side effects, especially anticholinergic effects; desipramine, or nortriptyline are better choices than amytriptyline	Complete relief unusual; used best as adjunct to other strategies; start low and increase slowly every 3–5 days
Serotonin–norepinephrine uptake inhibitors (SNRIs): venlafaxine (Effexor) and duloxitine (Cymbalta)	Venlafaxine—25–37.5 bid or tid; titrate q 4 days Duloxitine—60 mg qd	Venlafaxine—taper gradually Duloxitine—do not crush or chew; taper gradually
Anticonvulsants: clonazapam and carbamazepine	Carbamazepine may cause leukopenia, thrombocytopenia, and rarely aplastic anemia; clonazepine side effects may be similar to other benzodiadapines in the elderly	Start low and increase slowly; check blood counts on carbamazepine
Gabapentin (also an anticonvulsant) Neurontin	Less serious side effects than other anticonvulsants	Start with 100 mg and titrate up slowly; tid dosing; monitor for idiosyncratic side effects such as ankle swelling, ataxia, etc.; effective dose reported 100–800 mg q 8 h
Pregabalin (Lyrica)	Similar to gabapentin. Start at 50 mg tid and gradually increase. Taper dose to discontinue	Side effects similar to gabapentin
Antiarrhythmics mexiletine (Mexitil)	Common side effects include tremor, dizziness, and paresthesias; may rarely cause blood dyscrasias and hepatic damage	Avoid use in patients with preexisting hear disease; start low and titrate slowly; monitor EKGs; q 6–8 h dosing
Local anesthetics: lidocaine (intravenous), lidocaine transdermal patch (Lidoderm), and capsiacin	IV lidocaine associated with delirium Transdermal patch has minimal systemic absorption Capsiacin depletes nerve endings of substance P	IV lidocaine may predict response to anticonvulsants and antiarrhythmics May apply up to three patches alternating 12 h intervals to improve pain, reduce denervation hypersensitivity, and decrease systemic absorption May take 2 weeks to peak effect
Tramadol (Ultram)	Partial opioid and serotonin agonist; more of a norepinephrine antagonist; may cause drowsiness, nausea, vomiting, and constipation	Has ceiling effect; dose >300 mg/24 h usually not tolerated because of nausea; q 4–6 h dosing
Muscle relaxants (blacofen, chlorzoxazone [Paraflex], and cyclobenzaprine [Flexaril])	Sedation; anticholinergic effects; abrupt withdrawal of baclofen may cause CNS irritability	Mechanism of action not precisely known; monitor for sedation and anticholinergic effects; taper baclofen on discontinuation
Substance P inhibitors (capsiacin) available otc; for topical use only	Burning pain during depletion of substance P may be intolerable by as many as 30% of patients; may take 14 days for maximum response; avoid eye contamination	Start with small doses; can be partially removed with vegetable oil
NMDA inhibitors: ketamine and dextromethorophan	N-Methyl-D-aspartate antagonists (NMDA) Ketamine: potent anesthetic Dextromethorophan: common cough suppressant	Ketamine only available IV Both may cause delirium
Drugs for osteoporosis: Calcitonin and bisphosphonates	Pain relief mechanisms unknown	Not effective on pain other than osteoporosis
Corticosteroids: Prednisone Dexamethazone	Decrease inflammation in many tissues	Classic corticosteroid side effects limit overall usefulness in chronic pain

*A limited number of examples are provided. For comprehensive lists of other available medications for pain, clinicians should consult other sources.

pains. Of recent interest has been the effectiveness of gabapentin for treatment of diabetic and postherpetic neuralgias. Clinical observations suggest that this agent has a significant analgesic effect on neuropathic pain with a much lower side-effect profile compared to other antiepileptic drugs and most antidepressants as well.

Several local anesthetics have also been shown to relieve neuropathic pain when administrated systemically, in addition to their known local anesthetic effects. Intravenous lidocaine has been found to sometimes predict the response to other anticonvulsant and systemically administered local anesthetics. Mexilitine, similar to lido-caine but active orally, has also shown some activity against neuropathic pain of diabetic neuralgia. Although this drug also has a high risk/benefit ratio, some studies have reported response rates at lower doses than are often recommended for cardiac arrhythmias.

Finally, chronic pain associated with osteoporosis has often been shown to improve with calcitonin. Most investigators of the effects of calcitonin on osteoporosis have reported anecdotally that pain improves significantly. These studies have not been designed as pain studies, and more sophisticated assessment of pain in these studies would be welcome, but results thus far are encouraging.

ANESTHETIC AND NEUROSURGICAL APPROACHES TO PAIN MANAGEMENT

A wide variety of anesthetic and neurosurgical approaches to pain are available, and some require highly specialized skills. Although it is beyond the scope of this chapter to review details of all of these techniques, a few deserve mention.

Trigger point injections have been used extensively for the treatment of myofascial pain syndromes. Myfascial pain with trigger points was first recognized more than 50 years ago. In a relatively high percentage of cases, trigger points may initiate a reflex mechanism that produces referred pain, tenderness, and muscle spasm. With local injection of the trigger point, followed by stretching and reconditioning of the muscles, the myofascial pain syndrome usually subsides. More recently, similar results have been obtained using ice massage or vapocoolant spray applied topically, followed by specific muscle stretching and physical therapy techniques. Nonetheless, for many myofascial pain syndromes, trigger point injection with dilute local anesthetics may be highly effective when combined with specific physical therapy.

Continuous drug infusions are highly effective for providing steady-state analgesic drug levels. Continuous infusions can be maintained by implantable pumps or external devices to deliver intravenous, subcutaneous, intrathecal, or epidural medications. Continuous infusions of opioid drugs have found widespread use in severe chronic cancer pain, especially among those near the end of life. Other uses have included continuous infusion of muscle relaxants for patients with severe muscle spasm from spinal injury, multiple sclerosis, or end-stage Parkinson's disease. The techniques are very expensive, but they are often reimbursed by third-party payers including Medicare. These issues have raised ethical concerns about the application of high-tech strategies for patients who might be equally well managed using oral medications that are not reimbursable. In general, these methods should be used only when oral medications become ineffective or the oral route of administration is no longer viable. More work needs to be done to justify these risky and expensive techniques that need to be carefully monitored in nursing homes, home care, and other low-tech long-term care settings.

NONDRUG STRATEGIES FOR PAIN MANAGEMENT

Nondrug strategies, used alone or in combination with appropriate analgesic medications, should be an integral part of the care plan for most elderly patients with significant pain problems. Nondrug strategies for pain management encompass a broad range of treatments and physical modalities, many of which carry low risks for adverse effects. Used in combination with appropriate drug regimens, these interventions often enhance therapeutic effects, while allowing medication doses to be kept low to prevent adverse drug effects.

Among the nondrug interventions, the importance of patient education cannot be overstated. Studies have shown that patient education programs alone significantly improve overall pain management. Such programs often include content about the nature of pain, how to use pain diaries and pain assessment instruments, how to use medications appropriately, and how to use self-help nondrug strategies. Whether conducted in groups or individually, education should be tailored for individual patient needs and level of understanding. Written materials and methods of reinforcement are important to the overall success of the program. Education on the use of heat and cold can be especially helpful for some patients.

Physical exercise is important for most patients with pain. A program of exercise can be tailored to most patients' needs and is extremely important for rehabilitation, and the maintenance of strength and endurance. Clinical trials of older patients with chronic musculoskeletal pain have shown that moderate levels of exercise (aerobic and resistance training) on a regular basis are effective in improving pain and functional status. Initial training for chronic pain patients usually requires 8 to 12 weeks, with supervision by a professional who can focus on the needs of older people with musculoskeletal disorders. There is no evidence that one form of exercise is better than another, so programs can be tailored for the individual's needs, lifestyle, and preference. Water aerobics may be especially helpful for older patients with arthritic pain. The intensity of exercise along with frequency and duration must be adjusted to avoid exacerbation of the underlying condition while gradually increasing and later maintaining overall conditioning. Stretching to relieve muscle spasm and prevent further muscle injury is another critical exercise intervention. It is important to remember that feeling better often gives rise to a false impression that the discipline of regular exercise is not necessary. Continued encouragement and reinforcement is often required. Unless complications arise, the program of exercise should be maintained indefinitely to prevent deconditioning and deterioration.

Psychological strategies have also been shown to be helpful for some with significant pain. Cognitive therapies are strategies aimed at altering belief systems and attitudes about pain and suffering. Cognitive therapies include various forms of distraction, relaxation, biofeedback, and hypnosis. Behavioral therapies are strategies aimed at enhancing healthy behaviors and discouraging abnormal behavior that is unpredictable and self-defeating. Cognitive therapy can be combined with behavioral approaches, and together they are known as cognitive-behavioral therapy. Cognitive-behavioral therapy, in its purest form, includes a structured approach to teaching coping skills, which might be used alone or in combination with analgesic medications and other nondrug strategies for pain control. Effective programs can be conducted by trained professionals with individual patients or in groups, and there is some evidence that the effect is enhanced with caregiver involvement. Although it may not be appropriate for those with significant cognitive impairment, there is evidence from randomized trials to support the use of cognitive-behavioral therapy for many patients with significant chronic pain.

Finally, a variety of alternative therapies are also used by many patients. Many patients seek alternative medicine approaches with and without the knowledge or recommendation of their physician or other primary-care provider. Alternative medicine approaches to chronic pain may include homeopathy, spiritual healing, or the growing market of vitamin, herbal, and natural remedies. Although there is little scientific evidence to support these strategies for pain control, it is important that health care providers not abandon patients or leave them with a sense of hopelessness.

FURTHER READING

AGS Panel on Persistent Pain in Older Persons. The management of persistent pain in older persons. *J Am Geriatr Soc.* 2002;50(5):205–224.

Hadjistavropoulos T, Herr K, Turk DC, et al. An interdisciplinary expert consensus statement on assessment of pain in older persons. *Clin J Pain.* 2007;23(1 suppl):S1–S43.

Miaskowski C, Cleary J, Burney R, et al. Cancer Pain Management Guideline Panel. *The Management of Cancer Pain in Adults and Children.* The American Pain Society; 2005.

Arthritis Pain Guideline Panel. *Guideline for the Management of Pain in Osteoarthritis, Rheumatoid Arthritis and Juvenile Chronic Arthritis.* The American Pain Society; 2002.

Gibson SJ, Weiner DK, eds. *Pain in Older Persons.* Seattle: IASP Press; 2002.

Ashburn MA, Lipman AG, Carr D, et al. *Principles of Analgesic Use in the Treatment of Acute Pain and Cancer Pain.* 5th ed. The American Pain Society; 2003.

Ferrell BA, Whiteman JE. Pain. In: Morrison RS, Meier DE, eds. *Geriatric Palliative Care.* New York, New York: Oxford University Press; 2003:205–229.

Dionne CE, Dunn KM, Croft PR. Does back pain prevalence really decrease with increasing age? A systematic review. *Age Ageing.* 2006;35:229–234.

Barkin RL, Barkin SJ, Barkin D. Propoxyphene (dextropropoxyphene): a critical review of a weak opioid analgesic that should remain in antiquity. *Am J Ther.* 2006;13:534–542.

Kuffner EK, Dart RC, Bogdan GM, et al. Effect of maximal daily doses of acetaminophen on the liver of alcoholic patients. *Arch Intern Med.* 2001;161:2247–2252.

Mahe I, Bertrand N, Drouet L, et al. Interaction between paracetamol and warfarin in patients: a double blind, placebo-controlled randomized trial. *Haematologica.* 2006;91:1621–1627.

Palliative Care

Audrey Chun ■ *R. Sean Morrison*

Our society is facing one of the largest public health challenges in its history—the growth of the population of older adults. Improvements in public health, the discovery of antibiotics, and advances in modern medicine have resulted in unprecedented gains in human longevity. For most Americans, the years after the age of 65 are a time of good health, independence, and integration of one's life's work and experience. Eventually, however, most adults will develop one or more chronic illnesses with which they may live for many years before they die. More than three-quarters of deaths in the United States result from chronic diseases of the heart, lungs, brain, and other vital organs. Even cancer, which accounts for nearly a quarter of U.S. deaths, has become a chronic, multiyear illness for many. For a minority of patients with serious illness (e.g., metastatic colon cancer), the time following diagnosis is characterized by a stable period of relatively good functional and cognitive performance, followed by a predictable and short period of functional and clinical decline. However, for most patients with advanced illness (e.g., heart or lung disease, dementia, stroke, neuromuscular degenerative diseases, and many cancers), the time following diagnosis is characterized by months to years of physical and psychological symptom distress, progressive functional dependence and frailty, considerable family support needs, and high health care resource use. Indeed, as the population continues to age, most physicians will be caring for chronically ill individuals whose medical care is characterized by high degrees of complexity, lengthy duration of illness, and intermittent acute exacerbations interspersed with periods of relative stability. Abundant evidence suggests that the advanced stages of disease for most are characterized by inadequately treated physical distress; fragmented care systems; poor communication between physicians, patients, and families; and enormous strains on family caregiver and support systems.

THE EXPERIENCE OF SERIOUS ILLNESS FOR PATIENTS AND THEIR FAMILIES

Whereas a century ago, most adults died suddenly as a result of an acute infection or accident, the leading causes of death today are chronic illness such as heart disease, cancer, stroke, and dementia. Accompanying this shift in the causes of death has been a corresponding change in the location of death. Whereas in the early part of the 20th century, most persons died at home, today, most Americans will die in an institution (57% in hospitals and 17% in nursing homes). The reasons for this shift in location of death are complex but appear to be related to health system and reimbursement structures that promote hospital-based care and provide relatively little support for needed home care and custodial care services. Whereas the majority of Americans will die in an institution, these statistics hide the fact that most of an older person's last months and years are still spent at home in the care of family members, with hospitalization and/or nursing home placement occurring only near the very end of life. National statistics also obscure the variability in the experience of dying. For example, need for institutionalization or paid formal caregiving in the last months of life is much higher among the poor and women. Similarly, persons suffering from cognitive impairment and dementia are much more likely to spend their last days in a nursing home compared to cognitively intact elderly persons dying from nondementing illnesses.

Multiple studies have demonstrated that the clinical care of older adults with serious and advanced illness is in need of improvement. Studies have suggested that the prevalence of significant pain in community-dwelling older adults may be as high as 56% and that almost one-fifth of older adults take analgesic medications on a regular basis. Similarly, it has been suggested that 45% to 80% of nursing home residents have substantial pain and that many of these patients have multiple pain complaints and multiple potential sources of pain. Available data also point to a high prevalence of nonpain symptoms in older adults with serious and chronic illness. In retrospective interviews with family members of patients who died of noncancer illnesses in the United Kingdom, 67% of patients experienced moderate-to-severe pain, 49% had trouble breathing, 27% reported nausea, 36% reported depression, and 36% reported sleep disturbances. Similarly, SUPPORT (Study to Understand Prognoses and Preferences for Outcomes and Risks of Treatments), a study of 9 105 seriously ill hospitalized adults, found that after 1 week in the hospital, among patients who could be interviewed, about one in two patients reported pain, nearly one in six reported moderate-to-severe pain at least half of the time, and nearly one in six patients with pain were dissatisfied with its control. In subanalyses of patients with heart failure, end-stage liver disease, lung cancer, and chronic obstructive pulmonary disease (COPD), more than 20% of patients consistently experienced severe dyspnea during the 6 months prior to death. A companion study to SUPPORT reported almost identical pain findings for a cohort of hospitalized patients aged 80 years and older and also noted a high prevalence of anxiety and depression in the last 6 months of life.

The burdens of serious and chronic illness extend beyond patients to their families and friends. SUPPORT found that more than one-third of patients needed a large amount of family caregiving, which was not adequately provided for by the health care system. Similarly, another study of just less than 900 caregivers of persons with advance illness reported that more than one-third of these caregivers reported substantial stress. Furthermore, 86% of these respondents stated that they needed more help than what they were currently receiving or could afford including assistance. These needs included transportation (62%), homemaking (55%), nursing (28%), or personal care (26%). Caregiving has also been shown to be an independent risk factor for death, major depression, and associated comorbidities.

PALLIATIVE CARE

Palliative care is interdisciplinary care focused on the relief of suffering and achieving the best possible quality of life for patients and their loved ones. It involves formal symptom assessment and treatment, aid with decision making and establishing goals of care, practical support for patients and their caregivers, mobilization of community support and resources to ensure secure and safe living environments, and collaborative and seamless models of care (hospital, home, nursing homes, and hospice). It *is offered simultaneously* with life-prolonging and curative therapies for persons living with serious, complex, and eventually terminal illness. Palliative care was recently approved as a subspecialty of internal medicine, family medicine, and seven other parent boards.

Perhaps because it is codified in the Medicare hospice benefit, palliative care, or more typically hospice, traditionally has been conceptualized as care that should be provided only at the end of life when treatments directed at the cure of disease and life prolongation are no longer effective. This artificial dichotomy (cure vs. comfort) ignores the fact that the overwhelming majority of older adults living with advanced chronic illness require both life-prolonging and palliative treatments and that the forced choice of cure versus comfort

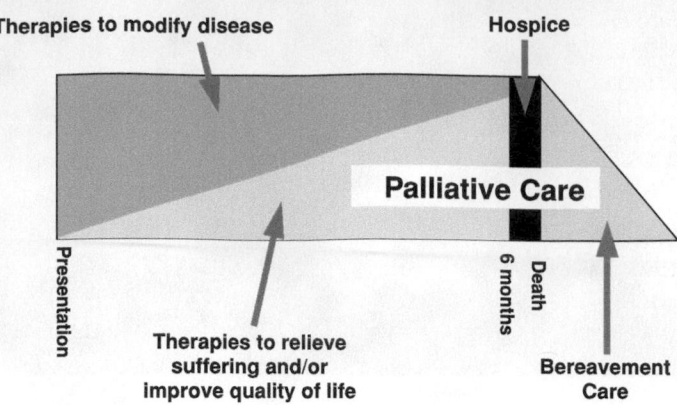

FIGURE 31-1. The integrated model of palliative care.

results not only in reflexive, burdensome, and costly life-prolonging treatments long after the time that these are beneficial to the patient, but also in preventable suffering during all stages of an advanced illness. For example, a frail 88-year-old woman with advanced heart failure, Parkinson's disease, diabetes, and deconditioning after hospitalization for pneumonia typically requires life-prolonging measures (medications for heart failure, oxygen, insulin, and antibiotics), preventive measures (influenza vaccinations), rehabilitation (home physical and occupational therapy to restore bed–chair mobility), and palliative care (setting goals of medical care; treatment of anxiety and depression; pharmacologic [psychostimulants] and nonpharmacologic [energy conservation therapies] management of fatigue; diuretics, oxygen, and opioids for breathlessness; and advance care planning and appointment of a health care proxy). Thus, the model of palliative care that patients and families require through the many-year course of illness, and the one promulgated in this chapter, is care focused on the simultaneous mix of beneficial (i.e., effective) life-prolonging treatments, palliation of symptoms, rehabilitation, and support for family caregivers, with the nature of these treatments varying in response to patient needs and preferences (Figure 31-1).

Palliative care for geriatric patients differs from what is usually appropriate in younger adults because of the nature and duration of chronic illness during old age. Specifically, the many-year duration of most geriatric chronic illnesses, the high prevalence of long-term functional and cognitive impairment, and the need for long-term caregivers are less common and rarely present in younger populations. Indeed, palliative care for younger adults is typically focused on the identification of symptoms associated with either a specific advanced terminal illness and its immediate manifestations or signs of poor prognosis/imminent death. Conversely, many of the characteristics of advanced old age (frailty, functional dependence, cognitive impairment, multiple comorbidities, and symptom distress) are multifactorial in etiology and are present for many years. In the frail elderly, disease-specific treatments may ameliorate or lessen the burdens of frailty, dependence, and symptom distress but are unlikely to eliminate them. Thus, palliative care for the elderly is most appropriately centered on the identification and amelioration of functional and cognitive impairment, development of frailty and dependence on caregivers, and the associated burden of symptom distress rather than, as is typical in advanced cancer and traditional hospice settings, identification of specific and advanced terminal illness and its immediate manifestations or signs of poor prognosis or imminent death. In response to the unique needs of older adults, we believe that palliative care is as integral a part of geriatric medicine as is the focus on function.

SYMPTOM ASSESSMENT AND TREATMENT

Successful approaches to the assessment and management of pain, many physical symptoms, and some psychological symptoms have been well established in controlled clinical trials. Effective symptom management requires the evaluation and treatment of underlying etiologies, when possible; therapies specifically targeted at symptoms; and frequent reassessment after therapies are initiated. Table 31-1 details standard treatment approaches for pain and other symptoms.

Pain

Despite major advances in the treatment of pain, studies continue to demonstrate undertreatment in the majority of patients and care settings. In addition to unnecessary suffering, studies suggest that untreated pain is associated with adverse outcomes, including delirium, atelectasis, and pneumonia; deconditioning; and impaired functional recovery.

Pain is the most common symptom experienced by those with advanced illness, and successful management requires three key components: routine and standardized assessment, appropriate analgesic prescribing and use of nonpharmacologic modalities; and expert management of opioid-related side effects. Although somewhat rudimentary, The World Health Organization's (WHO) analgesic ladder has traditionally been the framework most often cited for the management of malignant and nonmalignant persistent pain syndromes. Under the WHO analgesic ladder, patients rate their pain as mild (1–4 on a 10-point scale), moderate (5–6), or severe (7–10), and an analgesic is prescribed based on the patient's pain level: acetaminophen, a nonsteroidal anti-inflammatory agent, or a Cox-II inhibitor for mild pain; an opioid combination product (e.g., oxycodone/acetaminophen, hydrocodone/acetaminophen, and codeine/acetaminophen) for moderate pain; and a strong opioid (morphine, oxycodone, hydromorphone, and fentanyl) for severe pain.

Although the WHO ladder has been shown to be quite effective for the treatment of cancer pain in younger adults, recently, several expert panels and the American Geriatrics Society task force on persistent pain have recommended alterations to the WHO ladder. First, because of gastrointestinal and renal toxicities associated with nonsteroidal anti-inflammatory agents and the recent data on cardiovascular toxicity of Cox-II inhibitors, acetaminophen should be considered the medication of choice for older adults with mild pain. Nonsteroidal anti-inflammatory agents should be used with extreme caution and only in select patients with minimal risk factors (i.e., good renal function and no history of gastric ulcers or gastrointestinal bleeding). Patients with mild pain that persists despite maximal doses of acetaminophen should be started on a short-acting opioid and the opioid titrated until adequate pain relief is achieved. Once pain relief is achieved, consideration should be given to switching to a sustained-release opioid for ease of administration and to improve compliance. Second, combination products should be used with caution because of the danger of acetaminophen toxicity with dose escalation. Indeed, we recommend that combination products be avoided altogether and that patients who do not respond to acetaminophen for mild pain or present with moderate or severe pain be started immediately on a pure opioid (morphine and oxycodone) and the opioid titrated upward until adequate pain relief is achieved. Acetaminophen can be prescribed separately for additive/opioid sparing analgesia.

The choice of which opioid to use is driven largely by price and route of administration. Table 31-2 lists recommended starting doses for common opioids, equianalgesic doses, and the formulations of opioids currently available. For chronic or persistent pain, patients should be placed on a standing dose of a short-acting opioid, with the dosing interval being determined by the half-life of the drug (see Table 31-2). Patients should also receive "as-needed" opioids for breakthrough pain. This "breakthrough" or "prn" dose should be 10% of the total daily dose of the standing medication administered every hour as needed for an oral medication and every 15 to 30 minutes as needed for a parenteral medication. For uncontrolled pain, standing doses should be increased by 25% to 50% for moderate pain and by 50% to 100% for severe pain, with a corresponding increase in the breakthrough dose until adequate analgesia is achieved or intolerable side effects are present (see Table 31-2) Once a stable dose is reached and pain is well controlled, the patient can be switched to an extended-release oral or transdermal preparation. Given the difficulties with titrating sustained-release or transdermal preparations and the risk of opioid toxicity that can result if sustained release opioids are titrated too rapidly, we recommend that such preparations be used only after effective analgesia is achieved with a short-acting drug.

Neuropathic pain syndromes resulting from diabetes, spinal stenosis, side effects of chemotherapy or other medications, postherpetic neuralgia, or cancer are particularly resistant to treatment. Amitriptyline and other tricyclic antidepressants, although efficacious in some neuropathic pain syndromes and still considered first-line therapy by many, are poorly tolerated in older adults because of their anticholinergic properties and should only be used after other treatments have proven ineffective. Anticonvulsants such as gabapentin and local topical therapies such as transdermal lidocaine patches have both been shown to improve neuropathic pain in randomized controlled trials. Data with regards to selective seratonin reuptake inhibitors (SSRIs) and mixed norepinephrine/seratonin-reuptake inhibitors (e.g., venlafaxine) on neuropathic pain are mixed with some studies showing modest benefit and others showing no improvement over placebo. Finally, several studies have shown that high-dose opioids are effective in neuropathic pain syndromes and should be considered in patients who do not respond to therapies detailed above or for patients who experience dose-limiting side effects with these medications (e.g., sedation with gabapentin or anorexia with SSRIs).

Successful management of pain requires not only appropriate analgesics dosing but also expert management of opioid-related side effects. Table 31-3 lists common opioid side effects in older adults and approaches to their management. It is important to note that the majority of patients develop tolerance to almost all opioid-related side effects, with the exception of constipation. For example, tolerance to the respiratory depressive effects of opioids develops during 48 to 72 hours, tolerance to nausea typically occurs over a few days to a week, and tolerance to the cognitive side effects (sedation and mental cloudiness) occurs during 5 to 14 days. For patients who do not develop tolerance or for whom side effects are intolerable,

TABLE 31-1

Common Symptoms in Seriously Ill Older Adults

SYMPTOM	ASSESSMENT	TREATMENT RECOMMENDATIONS
Anorexia/cachexia	Assess whether symptom is owing to disease process or secondary to other symptoms (nausea and constipation). Determine if the patient is troubled by symptoms—often families, more than patients, are bothered by anorexia.	Pharmacologic approaches that have been shown to improve appetite and quality of life include corticosteroids, megestrol acetate, and the cannabinoids. Dexamethasone is advantageous in that it allows once-a-day dosing, has minimal mineralocorticoid properties, and may improve mood and energy. Megestrol acetate has been shown to be the most effective appetite stimulant with fewest side effects in randomized controlled trials for younger, but not older, adults.
Anxiety	Is there is excessive worry, restlessness, agitation, insomnia, hyperventilation, or tachycardia?	Supportive counseling and cautious use of benzodiazepines because of increased risk of delirium in older adults. Selective seratonin reuptake inhibitor (SSRIs) if life expectancy is greater than 2 months.
Constipation	Regular and routine assessment of constipation is critical, particularly for patients on opioids. Patients underreport constipation and life-threatening complications of fecal impaction, and perforation can develop quickly if regular bowel movements are not maintained.	With few exceptions, all patients on opioid therapy need an individualized bowel regimen. When an effective regimen is found, it must be continued for the duration of the opioid therapy. Most patients respond to a stool softener plus a stimulant. If dose escalation of the stimulant proves ineffective, addition of agents from alternate classes may be required. Agents available for the treatment of constipation are detailed below in order of suggested use. Additional recommendations are in Table 31-3. *Stool softeners* (ineffective alone and should be combined with other agents): docusate sodium and calcium docusate *Stimulant laxatives*: prune juice, senna, and bisacodyl *Osmotic laxative*: propylene glycol, milk of magnesia, and magnesium citrate Large-volume tap water enemas, high colonic enemas, or disimpaction may be needed in cases of severe constipation
Delirium	Are the symptoms acute with episodes of inattention? Is there disorganized thinking or an altered level of consciousness?	Identify underlying/reversible causes. Ensure an appropriately calm environment with caregivers/family at bedside. Prescribe haloperidol (0.5 mg every 4 h as needed, titrated to symptoms) or an atypical antipsychotic. Benzodiazepines should be avoided as they have been shown to worsen delirium.
Depression	Assess severity using validated instruments. The question "Are you depressed?" is a sensitive and specific question for patients with advanced illness. Reliable symptoms include feelings of helplessness, hopelessness, anhedonia, loss of self-esteem, worthlessness, persistent dysphoria, and suicidal ideation. Somatic symptoms are not reliable indicators of depression in this population of patients.	Supportive psychotherapy, cognitive approaches, behavioral techniques, and pharmacologic therapies have all been shown to be effective for treatment of depression in patients with advanced disease. Psychiatric consultation should be obtained in cases of severe depression. Patients should be asked specifically about suicidal ideation, and, if present, the reasons behind it should be carefully explored. Suicidal ideation often represents a measure of extreme distress in patients with advanced illness. Choice of pharmacologic therapy is often dictated by the patient's estimated life expectancy. Psychostimulants (e.g., methylphenidate and dextroamphetamine) provide rapid treatment of symptoms (within days) with minimal side effects. Increased energy, decreased fatigue, and improved well-being have been reported with the use of psychostimulants. SSRIs are highly effective but may require 3–4 weeks to take effect. The side-effect profile of tricyclic antidepressants (sedation, dry mouth, constipation, and orthostasis) is a relative contraindication to their use in patients with advanced illness.
Dyspnea	Assess severity using validated instrument. Treat reversible causes if possible.	*Oxygen*: Oxygen provides relief of dyspnea in circumstances of hypoxia but has also been shown to provide symptomatic relief in situations where hypoxia is not present. A cool breeze across the face (either from oxygen or a fan) has been shown to decrease breathlessness through stimulation of the V2 branch of the trigeminal cranial nerve. *Opioids*: Opioids have been demonstrated to significantly reduce breathlessness in randomized controlled trials without measurable reductions in respiratory rate or oxygen saturation. Effective doses are often lower than those used to treat pain, and tolerance has not been demonstrated to be a clinical problem. *Anxiolytics*: Anxiety and breathlessness are tightly intertwined. Anxiety may worsen breathlessness, and breathlessness may heighten anxiety. Benzodiazepines, reassurance, relaxation, distraction, and massage therapy may decrease anxiety and improve breathlessness.
Fatigue	Assess severity and treat reversible causes if possible (e.g., anemia, electrolyte imbalances, infection, and hypoxia)	*Pharmacologic therapy*: Corticosteroids (e.g., dexamethasone) and psychostimulants (e.g., methylphenidate and dextroamphetamine) *Nonpharmacologic therapies*: energy conservation, frequent naps, occupational therapy, and physical therapy

(continued)

TABLE 31-1

Common Symptoms in Seriously Ill Older Adults (*Continued*)

SYMPTOM	ASSESSMENT	TREATMENT RECOMMENDATIONS
Nausea	Assess severity and probable cause using validated instrument.	*Chemoreceptor trigger zone stimulation*: drugs (opioids, digoxin, estrogen, and chemotherapy agents), biochemical disorders (hypercalcemia and uremia), and toxins (tumor-produced peptides, infection, radiotherapy, and abnormal metabolites) Treatment: Butyrophones/phenothiazines (e.g., haloperidol and prochlorperazine), prokinetic agents (e.g., metoclopramide), serotonergic antagonists (e.g., ondansetron), and atypical neuroleptics (olanzapine) *Mechanical causes*: gastric irritation (drugs, alcohol, iron, mucolytics, expectorants, and blood), tumors (external compression, intestinal obstruction, constipation, liver capsule stretch, upper bowel, genitourinary, and biliary stasis, peritoneal inflammation, and cardiac pain), and gastric distension (opioid-induced stasis) Treatment: Antihistamines (e.g., diphenhydramine), serotonergic antagonists (e.g., ondansetron), prokinetic agents (e.g., metoclopramide), and cytoprotective agents (e.g., ranitidine and omeprazole) Treatment of delayed gastric emptying/squashed stomach: prokinetic agents (e.g., metoclopramide, and cisapride if not contraindicated) Treatment of nonsurgical bowel obstruction: Octreotide is effective both for nausea and for abdominal pain resulting from bowel obstruction *Intracranial processes*: increased central nervous system pressure and anticipatory nausea. Treatment: corticosteroids and benzodiazepines *Vestibular vertigo*: local tumors, opioids, and motion sickness Treatment: acetylcholine antagonists (transdermal scopalamine and meclizine)
Pain	Assess severity, location, character, precipitating, and alleviating factors using a validated instrument.	In general, pain medications should be administered on a standing or regular basis with "prn" or rescue doses available for breakthrough pain or pain not controlled by the standing regimen. Medications should be chosen based on patients' initial pain level, and, if pain remains uncontrolled, clinicians should advance to the next level. *Mild pain* (1–4/10): Begin acetaminophen or a nonsteroidal anti-inflammatory agent in select patients (those with normal renal function and minimal risk of gastrointestinal toxicity). Do not exceed 3 or 2 g/d for those with hepatic dysfunction. If pain is not controlled by acetaminophen, initiate opioid therapy. *Moderate pain* (-5–6/10): Begin a short-acting standing opioid (morphine or oxycodone) and titrate every several days by 25%–50% of the current dose until pain relief is achieved. Once pain is well controlled, consider switching to a sustained release oral opioid or transdermal fentanyl (see Table 31-2 for recommended starting doses and conversion guidelines). Rescue doses employing immediate release opioids should be 10% of the 24-h total opioid dose and given every hour (oral) or every 30 min (parenteral) as needed. Because of their potency, hydromorphone and oxymorphone should be used with extreme caution in older adults with moderate pain and in most cases reserved for patients already on standing opioid therapy or those in severe pain. Acetaminophen can be employed for additive and opioid-sparing analgesia. *Severe pain* (8–10/10): Begin a standing short-acting opioid (morphine sulfate, oxycodone, and hydromorphone) and titrate rapidly until pain relief is obtained or intolerable side effects develop. Strongly consider a parenteral opioid and titrate by 50%–100% of the dose every 30–60 min until pain is controlled. Long-acting opioids (sustained release morphine/oxycodone and transdermal fentanyl) should typically be started only after pain is well controlled and steady state is achieved. Rescue doses employing immediate release opioids should be 10% of the 24-h total opioid dose and given every hour (oral) or every 30 min (parenteral) as needed. Methadone should only be used by clinicians experienced in its use. All patients on opioids should be started on a bowel regimen. Adjuvant agents (corticosteroids, anticonvulsants, tricyclic antidepressants, and bisphosphonates) can be used depending on the pain syndrome and response to opioids.

Adapted with permission from Morrison RS, Meier DE. Palliative care. N Engl J Med. 2004;350:2582–2590.

TABLE 31-2

Opioid Analgesic Equivalences and Recommended Starting Dosed for Older Adults*

OPIOID AGONIST	IV/SQ/IM†	PO/RECTAL	RATIO IV:PO	DURATION OF EFFECT (h)	STARTING DOSE (ORAL)‡ (mg)	COMMENTS
Morphine	10	30	1:3	4	2.5–10	Oral liquid concentrated formulation recommended for breakthrough pain
SR morphine	NA	30	NA	8–12		Begin after stable dose obtained with short-acting opioid
Hydrocodone	NA	30	NA	4	2.5–10	
Oxycodone	NA	20	NA	4	2.5–7.5	Oral liquid concentrated formulation recommended for breakthrough pain
SR oxycodone	NA	20	NA	8–12		Begin after stable dose obtained with short-acting opioid
Oxymorphone	1	10	1:10	4	1–3	
SR oxymorphone	NA	10		12		
Hydromorphone	1.5	7.5	1:5	3–4	0.5–2	
Fentanyl§	0.2 (200 μg)	NA	NA	1–2		Transdermal fentanyl patch (μg/h) = IV fentanyl (μg/h). Duration of patch is 48–72 h and should be started only after initial dose determined by oral/parenteral opioids
Methadone¶				6–8		
Codeine**	130	200	1:1.5	4	30–60	

*If converting between opioids when pain is well controlled, decrease the dose of the new opioid by 25% to 50% to account for incomplete cross-tolerance. Rapid titration to achieve effective analgesia may be required in the first 24 hours.

†Intramuscular administration is strongly discouraged because subcutaneous administration is as effective and less painful.

‡Starting doses are adapted from the American Geriatrics Society Panel on Persistent Pain in Older Adults. *J Am Geriatr Soc.* 2002;50(6 suppl):S214–S215.

¶Breakthrough or "prn" doses of oral morphine for patients on the fentanyl patch are roughly one-third of the fentanyl patch dose (e.g., if a patient is prescribed a fentanyl patch 75 μg/h q 72 h, breakthrough dose of short-acting morphine is 25 mg q 1 h prn.

§Methadone has a complex pharmacokinetic and pharmacodynamic profile that makes equianalgesic dosing particularly difficult. Consultation with an experienced clinician is recommended before initiating or adjusting the dose of methadone.

**Codeine is highly emetigenic and its use is strongly discouraged.

Table 31-3 details strategies to manage the most common symptoms associated with opioids.

Finally, many physicians, patients, and families have concerns about physical and psychological (addiction) dependence. Almost all patients treated with opioids develop physical dependence, characterized by the presence of a withdrawal syndrome, if the medication is abruptly discontinued or the dose significantly reduced. For patients taking opioids, dependence can develop after only several days of therapy. For patients whose analgesic requirements are suddenly reduced (e.g., following a course of radiation therapy), tapering the opioid dose by 30% to 50% per day has been found to be a safe and effective strategy to avoid withdrawal symptoms.

Psychological dependence (addiction) is defined as the continued use of a medication despite harm to self or others. Studies to date suggest that the risk of addiction in patients treated with opioids for pain and without a history of substance abuse is extremely small (less than 1%). For patients with a life-threatening or terminal illness, concerns about psychological dependence should never inhibit appropriate analgesic prescribing. Persons with a history of substance abuse who require opioids for pain require specialized approaches to pain management. A description of these approaches is beyond the scope of this chapter.

Dyspnea

Dyspnea is the subjective experience breathlessness and is one of the most common and distressing symptoms experienced by pa-

tients with advanced illness. For example, 70% of patients with advanced cancer and more than 56% of those with advanced COPD report moderate-to-severe dyspnea. Treatment of dyspnea begins with treating the underlying etiology whenever possible (i.e., inhaled β_2 agonists and anticholinergics for COPD and diuretics, beta-blockers, and angiotensin-converting enzyme inhibitors in advanced heart failure). When disease-modifying therapies are not effective, a number of symptomatic treatments can significantly reduce breathlessness and improve patient comfort. These include oxygen, opioids, and anxiolytics (see Table 31-1).

Oxygen should clearly be utilized for breathlessness in the presence of hypoxia. However, even when hypoxia is not present, oxygen has been shown to be effective in reducing dyspnea by direct stimulation of the V2 branch of the trigeminal cranial nerve in the nares. When oxygen is not available, fans or positioning patients near an open window or door can be effective in reducing breathlessness.

Opioids remain the gold standard treatment for dyspnea. Opioids reduce breathlessness through several mechanisms. First, they diminish ventilatory response to hypoxia and hypercapnea, typically at doses lower than those required for pain control. Second, they act centrally to reduce the subjective sensation of breathlessness. Third, opioids reduce preload and can be particularly effective for patients with symptoms of volume overload associated with advanced heart or renal disease.

Finally, because dyspnea is often accompanied and exacerbated by anxiety, low-dose short-acting benzodiazepines such as lorazepam (0.5 mg every 6 hours) are often beneficial in reducing patient

TABLE 31-3

Management of Opioid-Related Side Effects	
Constipation	Almost a universal complication of opioid therapy and prophylactic laxatives are always indicated unless there is a clear contraindication. Maintain a high index of suspicion for bowel obstruction or fecal impaction. Rule out impaction with digital rectal examination or abdominal X-ray if clinically suspicious. Rectal disimpaction must occur before treating with an oral laxative. *Step 1:* Docusate 100 mg po tid plus senna 2 tabs qhs (can titrate up to 8 senna/d). *Step 2:* Add polyethylene glycol (17 g mixed with 8 ounces water/d). *Step 3:* If constipation persists for 3 or more days, add bisacodyl suppository (10 mg/24 h), docusate mini-enema qhs, fleet mineral oil retention enema, or sodium phosphate oral solution. If no results, consider a high colonic tap water enema.
Nausea	Opioid-induced nausea occurs in approximately 30% of patients. It is important to determine the etiology (gastric stasis/irritability, central irritation of the chemoreceptor trigger zone, or vestibular irritation) and choose a treatment based on the etiology. If nausea cannot be controlled, rotating to another opioid is often effective. See guidelines in Table 31-1 for treatment of nausea.
Sedation	Common at the start of therapy, but tolerance develops in the majority of patients. Psychostimulants can be useful at the beginning of treatment until tolerance develops. If sedation remains a problem, rotating to another opioid is often effective. See guidelines for psychostimulants in Table 31-1.
Myoclonus	Opioid rotation to a more potent opioid is often useful as metabolite accumulation is often implicated. Benzodiazepines are also useful if opioid rotation fails to resolve the symptom.
Pruritis	Rarely a problem with chronic opioid therapy. Antihistamines are commonly used although highly sedating and rarely effective. Opioid rotation is likely to be the most effective treatment. Case series report that ondansetron may be effective.
Respiratory depression	Although highly feared, respiratory depression is a very rare complication for patients on chronic opioid therapy owing to the development of tolerance. If respiratory status is compromised (less than 8 breaths/min) opioid reversal with naloxone is indicated. One ampule of naloxone (0.4 mg/mL) should be diluted in 10 mL of saline and injected at a rate of 1 mL every 2–3 min with careful observation of respiratory rate and level of consciousness until the respiratory rate returns to a normal rate. As the half-life of naloxone is only 30 min, patients should be frequently reassessed and additional naloxone administered as above. Patients on methadone commonly require a naloxone infusion as a result of the extended half-life of methadone.

suffering and breaking the cycle of anxiety–dyspnea–anxiety, which is commonly observed in patients with severe breathlessness.

Gastrointestinal Symptoms

Gastrointestinal symptoms such as nausea, vomiting, anorexia, and constipation are common in patients with advanced illness and are particularly prevalent in patients receiving opioids. As with all symptoms, the cause of these symptoms should be investigated and treatable conditions addressed. Nausea is a subjective feeling that is caused by stimulation of the gastrointestinal lining, chemoreceptor trigger zone, vestibular apparatus, or cerebral cortex. Table 31-1 details common etiologies of nausea and vomiting, details the primary neurotransmitters involved, and lists pharmacologic and nonpharmacologic approaches to treatment.

Anorexia, or loss of appetite, is usually more distressing for family members than for patients. Typically, anorexia is a reflection of the severity of underlying disease and usually cannot be permanently reversed. Approaches to the treatment of anorexia include educating patients and families as to the natural course of the disease process, providing favorite foods and nutritional supplements, encouraging small frequent meals, and determining if assistance with feeding is required. Patients should avoid gastric irritants like spicy food and milk and focus on foods that are enjoyed and easily digested. Although corticosteroids and progesterones (e.g., megestrol acetate) have been associated with increased appetite and sense of well-being in cancer and AIDS patients, there are few corresponding studies in

older adults. One study of megestrol acetate (400 mg/day) in nursing home residents was found to improve appetite but did not result in meaningful weight gain. Potential benefits of both classes of agents should be weighed against their known adverse effects. Corticosteroids can cause mood swings, sleep disturbances, hyperglycemia, edema, delirium, and myopathy. Progesterones have been associated with delirium, venous thromboembolism, and edema. Table 31-1 summarizes approaches to the treatment of anorexia.

Constipation presents both as a primary symptom and, often, as a consequence of other treatments (e.g., opioids, calcium-channel blockers, etc.). Before initiating any laxative treatment, patients should be assessed for the presence of fecal impaction and, if present, disimpacted with tap water or fleets enemas, manually, or with high colonic enemas if the former two approaches prove ineffective. All patients started on opioids should receive prophylactic stool softeners in combination with a stimulant laxative (e.g., senna and bisacodyl), unless contraindicated. Although most patients respond to this combination, persistent constipation (opioid-induced or primary) can be addressed by a trial of additional laxatives with a different mechanism of action such as an osmotic agent (e.g., polyethylene glycol) or regular enemas. Lactulose, although commonly prescribed, is relatively expensive and large volumes are needed to effectively treat constipation. Additionally, lactulose causes flatulence and abdominal cramping in about 20% of patients. Bulk agents (e.g., bran) should be avoided because they may precipitate obstruction in debilitated patient by forming a viscous mass in the setting of inadequate fluid intake.

Depression, Delirium, and Anxiety

Delirium in advanced disease is a marker of worsening illness and often associated with the last stages of life. Characterized by an acute change in cognition with variable degrees of inattention as well as disorganized thinking or an altered level of consciousness, delirium increases the need for higher levels of care and limits the opportunities to communicate and direct one's own care. For delirium near the end of life, haloperidol is recommended as first-line treatment owing to its multiple forms of administration and wide therapeutic window. Extrapyramidal effects are of less concern when used in the setting of limited life expectancy, and there is little evidence that the atypical antipsychotics are more effective than traditional antipsychotics in the treatment of terminal delirium. If symptoms of delirium are especially distressing, particularly in the final hours to days of life, sedating major tranquilizers such at chlorpromazine is highly effective and should be considered.

Patients with advanced illness should always be assessed for depression and anxiety. Asking "Are you depressed?" is a relatively sensitive and specific screen for depression in patients with advanced illness. For patients with a life expectancy greater than 2 months, SSRIs are the treatment of choice for both depression and anxiety because of their more favorable side-effect profile. For patients with more limited time, psychostimulants for depression and low-dose benzodiazepines for anxiety should be considered. Methylphenidate is probably the best choice for older adults, given its relatively short half-life. Therapy should be initiated at 2.5 to 5 mg twice a day (upon awakening and between noon and 2 PM) and titrated upward as tolerated. Although benzodiazepines have the potential for precipitating delirium and falls and can result in somnolence and cognitive impairment in some patients, these risks should be weighed carefully against the marked benefit that these medications can provide in reducing the distress of anxiety. Table 31-1 provides additional details about dosing and contraindications to these medications.

Fatigue

Fatigue is usually multifactorial in patients with advanced disease. Patients and families should be encouraged to promote energy conservation, and, indeed, explicit permission by the physician to rest and to nap is often required. Consultation with a physical therapist with palliative care experience—local hospice programs are often an excellent referral source—can be extremely useful in teaching patients and families techniques for energy conservation. Physicians and nurses should carefully evaluate and review patients' medications and discontinue those that might be contributing to fatigue (calcium channel-blockers, beta-blockers, anticholinergics, and antihistamines). Optimizing fluid and electrolyte intake should also be undertaken to minimize the effects of dehydration. As in the case of anorexia, communication and education about the role of underlying diseases are important in establishing realistic expectations for patients and their caregivers.

Pharmacologic management of fatigue involves primarily corticosteroids and psychostimulants. Corticosteroids may increase feelings of well-being and energy levels, but the effect typically wanes after 4 to 6 weeks. Psychostimulants such as methylphenidate can be used in debilitated patients, but side effects of tremulousness, anorexia, tachycardia, and insomnia can limit their use in some patients.

Last Hours of Life

The last hours of life often are marked by a constellation of symptoms that can be especially distressing for family members. Family education about expected symptoms such as delirium, excessive secretions, edema, and coma can help prepare families for the impending death, alleviate anxiety if these symptoms develop, and improve families' abilities to care for their loved ones in the last hours of life (Table 31-1). Aside from terminal delirium (discussed above) the presence of the "death rattle"—a gurgling sound caused by air moving through uncleared secretions in the trachea and vocal cords of a comatose patient—is perhaps the most distressing symptom experienced by families of dying patients. Education of family members as to the cause of the noise is critical. It is crucial to emphasize that the noise does not represent gasping or suffocation, and the patient is not experiencing suffering or breathlessness. Despite understanding its etiology, some families and caregivers still find this symptom distressing, and, in these situations, medications such as hyoscyamine, transdermal scopolamine, or atropine drops; positioning patients to the side; and reducing fluid intake can be employed to reduce or eliminate the "death rattle." If edema is present, therapies that can exacerbate edema, such as IV fluids, should be discontinued when at all possible. Skin care should continue with a focus on prevention of skin breakdown using lubricants and emollients rather than turning or repositioning, which can cause increased discomfort and pain. If pressure ulcers are present, efforts should be focused on pain management and minimizing discharge and odors rather than turning, repositioning, or active wound care directed at ulcer healing.

COMMUNICATION

Communication skills are essential to the relief of suffering and the practice of palliative medicine. Surveys of patients suggest that health care workers typically elicit fewer than half of patients' concerns and consistently fail to discuss patients' values, goals of care, and treatment decisions. Conversely, improved physician–patient communication, including advance care planning, is associated with decreased anxiety, improved patient well-being, higher satisfaction with providers and health care, and improved outcomes.

Essential components of communication in the setting of advanced illness have been identified. A qualitative focus group study of 137 providers, family members, and patients identified six themes of central importance in communicating with patients with advanced illness: talking honestly and in a straightforward way, being willing to talk about dying, giving bad news in a sensitive way, listening, encouraging questions, and being sensitive to patients when they want to talk about difficult issues such as death and dying. Specific interviewing techniques that include establishing eye contact, eliciting and clarifying disclosures, probing for emotional and psychological concerns, displaying empathy, and responding to distress have been shown to improve the detection of anxiety, depression, and other patient concerns in general medical and oncology practices. Protocols (Figure 31-2), based largely on expert opinion, qualitative data drawn from patient interviews, and data from studies detailed above, are available to guide discussions focused on establishing goals of medical care, communicating bad news including balancing hope with realistic expectations, and withholding and withdrawing medical treatments (including cardiopulmonary resuscitation and feeding).

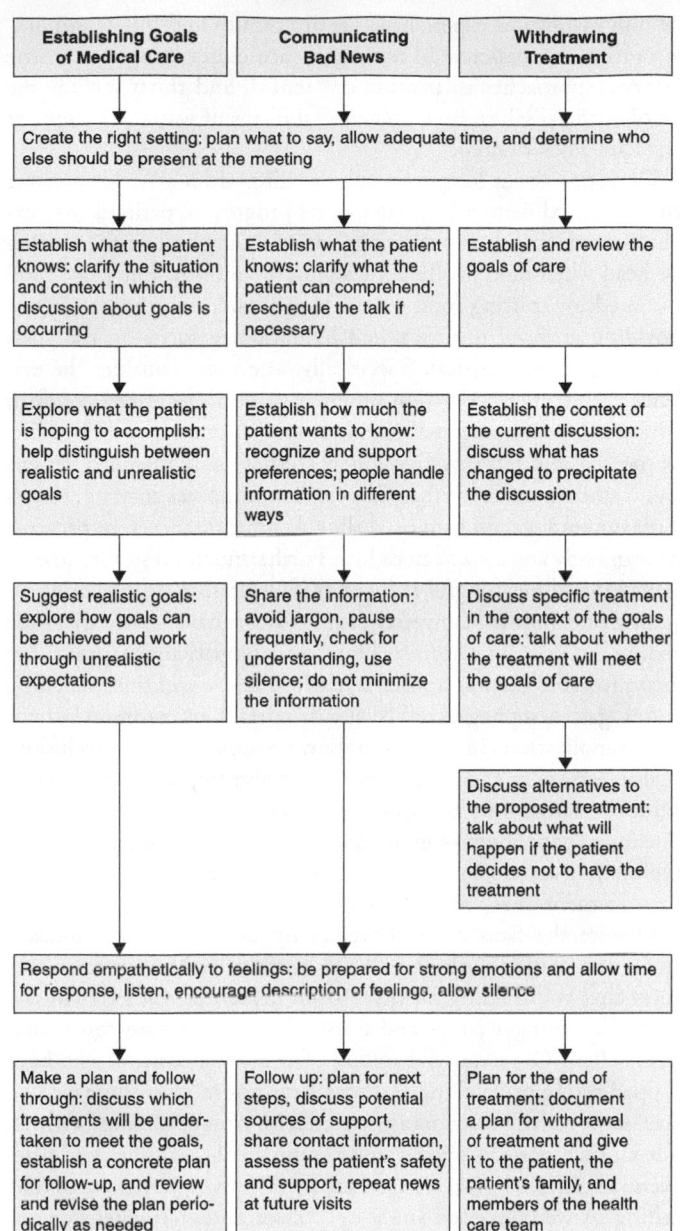

Establishing Goals of Medical Care	Communicating Bad News	Withdrawing Treatment
Create the right setting: plan what to say, allow adequate time, and determine who else should be present at the meeting		
Establish what the patient knows: clarify the situation and context in which the discussion about goals is occurring	Establish what the patient knows: clarify what the patient can comprehend; reschedule the talk if necessary	Establish and review the goals of care
Explore what the patient is hoping to accomplish: help distinguish between realistic and unrealistic goals	Establish how much the patient wants to know: recognize and support preferences; people handle information in different ways	Establish the context of the current discussion: discuss what has changed to precipitate the discussion
Suggest realistic goals: explore how goals can be achieved and work through unrealistic expectations	Share the information: avoid jargon, pause frequently, check for understanding, use silence; do not minimize the information	Discuss specific treatment in the context of the goals of care: talk about whether the treatment will meet the goals of care
		Discuss alternatives to the proposed treatment: talk about what will happen if the patient decides not to have the treatment
Respond empathetically to feelings: be prepared for strong emotions and allow time for response, listen, encourage description of feelings, allow silence		
Make a plan and follow through: discuss which treatments will be undertaken to meet the goals, establish a concrete plan for follow-up, and review and revise the plan periodically as needed	Follow up: plan for next steps, discuss potential sources of support, share contact information, assess the patient's safety and support, repeat news at future visits	Plan for the end of treatment: document a plan for withdrawal of treatment and give it to the patient, the patient's family, and members of the health care team

FIGURE 31-2. Communication protocols for delivering bad news, communicating goals of care, and withholding or withdrawing medical treatments. *(Reproduced with permission from Morrison RS, Meier DE. Palliative care. N Engl J Med. 2004;350:2582–2590.)*

Recently published data from cancer patients suggest that these protocols are effective in communicating information to both patients and caregivers in a sensitive manner and can be taught to trainees.

SYSTEMS OF CARE FOR THE SERIOUSLY ILL

The current reimbursement system fails to address many of the needs of seriously ill patients and their families. Medicare coverage is targeted to acute, episodic illness and is not equipped to respond to the long-term needs of the chronically ill. Patients with serious chronic illness typically make multiple transitions between care settings and require long-term care at home or in skilled nursing facilities, care

coordination as they traverse a fragmented system, prescription drug coverage, personal and custodial care needs, home infusion therapies, and transportation to physicians' offices and other health care settings. Medicare does not cover most of these aspects of care coordination. Although the Medicare hospice benefit covers comprehensive services; only patients who are certified by their physicians as within 6 months of the end of life and who are willing to forego coverage for certain life-prolonging treatments are eligible for this benefit. Thus, in reality, it is the minority of persons with life-threatening illness—those with predictable prognoses who are willing to give up life-prolonging efforts—who can benefit from this system.

For patients unable or unwilling to access the hospice benefit, Medicaid, a means-tested reimbursement system designed as a safety net for the poor, remains the only payment system that covers comprehensive care services. Since Medicaid eligibility is means tested, coverage is not an available option for most patients in most states. As a result, almost 26 million Americans provide an average of 18 or more hours of uncompensated personal care per week to a seriously ill homebound relative, which, using a conservative estimate of $8/hour, amounts to an annual figure of $194 billion dollars. SUPPORT found that 31% of families caring for patients with serious and chronic illness lose the majority of their family savings and 29% lose the major source of their family income. Families with significant care needs are more likely to take out a loan or mortgage, spend their savings, or obtain an additional job.

Fortunately, programs that coordinate care for complex patients are becoming increasingly available in many communities. Hospital palliative care programs providing comprehensive interdisciplinary palliative care are now present in greater than 30% of U.S. hospitals and greater than 70% of hospitals with more than 250 beds. These programs have been shown to improve clinical care, improve family satisfaction, and facilitate transitions from the acute care hospital to more appropriate care settings. Increasingly, nonhospice palliative care programs for ambulatory or homebound patients who are not eligible for or unwilling to access the Medicare hospice benefit are being established by hospitals, hospices (open access or bridge programs), or traditional home care agencies. Additionally, comprehensive multidisciplinary home care programs targeting frail older adults are available under both the Medicare and the Veteran's Administration programs. The Program of All Inclusive Care for the Elderly (PACE) is a capitated Medicare and Medicaid benefit for frail older adults featuring comprehensive medical and social services provided at adult day health centers, home, and/or inpatient facilities. Studies of PACE have demonstrated increases in advance directive completion rates and decreases in nursing home admissions, hospitalization rates, and hospital death. Similar programs of team-coordinated, home-based care exist within Virginia. Finally, geriatric home care programs that provide visiting physician and nursing services to homebound elders are available in select cities and communities throughout the United States.

CARE TRANSITIONS

Patients with chronic and serious illness undergo transitions across multiple care sites ranging from the home to ambulatory practices, acute hospital stays, rehabilitation admissions, nursing homes, and more. Both qualitative and quantitative studies suggest that transitions from one care site to another are associated with inadequate transfer information and follow-up, conflicting advice about disease management, and adverse drug events. Several recent studies suggest that transitions can be made safer for seriously ill older adults. One patient-centered care transition intervention, which included assistance with medication self-management, a patient-centered record owned and maintained by the patient, timely follow-up with primary or specialty care, and a list of "red flags" indicative of a worsening condition and instructions on how to respond to these, reduced recurrent hospital admissions. Other interventions, including hospital discharge checklists and pharmacy medication reconciliation, have been shown to improve patient safety during care transitions. Because transitions are such a vulnerable time for any patient, all providers should take responsibility for ensuring adequate information exchange and follow-up. Assistance for clinicians in managing transitions can be found at www.caretransistions.org.

SPECIAL ISSUES

Dementia

Identification of distressing symptoms in dementia patients can be especially challenging, given that the gold standard for pain and symptom assessment is patient self-report. Work by Ferrell and colleagues has shown that even patients with mild-to-moderate dementia can self-report symptoms and that such symptoms are as valid as those obtained from cognitively intact adults. In patients unable to self-report, behavioral signs such as agitation, withdrawal, tachypnea, vocalizations, grimacing, tense body posturing, and excessive sedation or changes in sleep–wake cycle patterns resulting from sleep deprivation can indicate untreated pain or other symptoms. Several behavioral scales have been developed for use in long-term care populations to aid clinicians in identifying pain and discomfort in dementia patients (Hurley Discomfort Scale, Feldt Checklist of Nonverbal Pain Indicators).

Pain should always be in the differential diagnosis for an unexplained behavior change in a dementia patient, and a time-limited trial of an analgesic medication should be considered if the source of the behavior is not clearly identified. Common and often undiagnosed sources of pain include osteoarthritis, contractures, pressure ulcers, fecal impaction, and neuropathy resulting from diabetes or spinal stenosis.

Artificial Hydration and Nutrition

In serious illness, anorexia and weight loss are common symptoms. As a result of the social, religious, and ethical values surrounding nutrition, the decision regarding initiation of artificial hydration and nutrition through tube feeds and/or IV therapy can be especially difficult for patients and their families. For patients who are actively dying, it is important to point out to both patients and families that artificial nutrition has not been shown to prolong survival and, indeed, may cause nausea, diarrhea, and electrolyte abnormalities. Artificial hydration, particularly when used in frail, hypoalbuminemic, and debilitated dying patients, can worsen discomfort by causing increased ascites, peripheral edema and anasarca, pulmonary edema, and excess secretions. Data from cognitively intact cancer patients who have voluntarily stopped eating and drinking suggest that that

the only symptoms experienced are dry mouth and thirst, and, importantly, such patients do not experience either hunger or gastric distress. Approaches to treating dry mouth and thirst include the use of artificial saliva, lip emollients, and sips of water, ice chips, or popsicles when desired.

Decisions about long-term tube feeding often arise for patients with advanced dementia. As dementia progresses, patients may exhibit behaviors such as pocketing food without swallowing, turning the head when food is offered, keeping the mouth shut when food is offered, or spitting food out. When considering the benefits of providing artificial nutrition and hydration, a focus on the goals of medical care is critical. Specifically, one must consider the evidence that artificial nutrition prolongs survival, improves comfort, reduces aspiration and malnutrition, and improves quality of life. Prospective and retrospective cohort studies using matched designs have found no evidence that tube feeding improves survival, results in meaningful weight gain or healing of pressure ulcers, or prevents the lean body and muscle mass loss. Furthermore, no studies to date have reported meaningful reductions in aspiration or infections including pneumonia. Conversely, some studies have shown that tube feeding can increase discomfort for dementia patients by producing uncomfortable gastrointestinal sensations and distention including nausea, gastroesophageal reflux, and diarrhea. Less common but not rare, complications include aspiration pneumonia, tube occlusion, local infection, and leaking. Finally, it is also important not to discount the discomfort and distress of placing a permanent external tube into a patient who can neither understand why such a device is in place nor understand or consent to the hospitalizations required if replacement or repair is necessary.

Despite the facts cited above, many caregivers and clinicians equate the withholding of artificial nutrition with starvation and worry that withholding nutrition from dementia will result in discomforting hunger pangs and thirst. Evidence to date contradicts these beliefs. Observational studies of dementia patients who have stopped eating or drinking and who have not received tube feeding have not revealed behaviors associated with pain or discomfort, and, indeed, such patients appear quite comfortable. Families and caregivers should also be aware that there are effective alternatives to tube feeding. A well-designed study by Volicer and colleagues demonstrated that feeding difficulties in advanced dementia patients can be successfully managed by an aggressive spoon feeding program, which includes verbal reminders, frequent small meals, specialized pureed diets, and appropriate feeding postures, and that survival in patients enrolled in this feeding protocol was equal to patients who received gastrostomy tube feeding.

In summary, although data from randomized controlled trials are not available, prospective cohort studies suggest that tube feeding in end-stage dementia is associated with neither increased survival nor comfort and that alternate measures of providing nutrition (e.g., careful and time-intensive spoon feeding) are effective interventions in the majority of patients.

Grief and Bereavement

Grief and bereavement is a normal response to the death of a loved one, and it is important to recognize that normal grief can persist for up to 6 months. Contrary to the traditional five-stage theory of grief developed by Kubler-Ross (denial–dissociation–isolation, anger, bargaining, depression, and acceptance), emerging evidence suggests that disbelief, yearning, anger, depression, and acceptance more accurately describe the experience of bereaved individuals. Whereas most of these feelings dissipate within 6 months of the death of a loved one, 10% to 20% of bereaved individuals may continue to experience such feelings beyond 6 months. Prolonged grief disorder (previously termed complicated grief) has been linked to poor physical and mental health outcomes as well as impairments within social, familial, and occupational domains and increased risk of suicide. Spouses are at particular risk of morbidity and mortality during this period. Short screening tools to identify prolonged grief disorder in bereaved individuals are now available (Inventory of Complicated Grief), as are effective therapies for individuals diagnosed with this disorder.

CONCLUSION

In summary, palliative care is an interdisciplinary care that is focused on relieving suffering and improving quality of life for patients and families living with chronic serious illness. It is neither end-of-life care nor hospice, and it is offered simultaneously with all other appropriate medical treatments. As the population continues to age and more and more persons are living with chronic illness, multiple comorbidities, and frailty, the need to incorporate palliative care into geriatrics will become even more pressing. Whereas the need for palliative care is perhaps greatest in older adults, the current evidence base to provide such care is relatively weak and based largely on expert opinion and studies from young adults. Considerable knowledge gaps exist with respect to the prevalence of pain and other symptoms in older adults; the association of pain and other symptoms on outcomes of function, independence, and quality of life; interventions directed at the assessment and treatment of pain and other symptoms and their effect on outcomes; and research instruments, designs, and analytic techniques to conduct the necessary research. Investment in research directed at helping older adults with serious and advanced illness live in comfort and with dignity over the course of the rest of their lives is critically needed.

FURTHER READING

The SUPPORT Principal Investigators. A controlled trial to improve care for seriously ill hospitalized patients. The study to understand prognoses and preferences for outcomes and risks of treatments (SUPPORT). *JAMA.* 1995;274:1591–1598.

Cassarett DJ, Inouye SK. Diagnosis and management of delirium near the end of life. *Ann Intern Med.* 2001;135:32–40.

Coleman E, Parry C, Chalmers S, Min S. The care transitions intervention. *Arch Intern Med.* 2006;166:1822–1828.

Covinsky K, Goldman L, Cook E, et al. The impact of serious illness on patients' families. *JAMA.* 1994;272:1839–1844.

Davis GF. Loss and the duration of grief. *JAMA.* 2001;285:1152–1153.

Emanuel EJ, Fairclough DL, Slutsman J, Emanuel LL. Understanding economic and other burdens of terminal illness: the experience of patients and their caregivers. *Ann Intern Med.* 2000;132:451–459.

EPEC. The EPEC Project: Education for Physicians on End of Life Care. Available at: http://www.epec.net/.

Finucane T, Christmas C, Travis K. Tube feeding in patients with advanced dementia: a review of the evidence. *JAMA.* 1999;282:1365–1370.

Fisher ES, Wennberg DE, Stukel TA, Gottlieb DJ, Lucas FL, Pinder EL. The implications of regional variations in Medicare spending. Part 1: the content, quality, and accessibility of care. *Ann Intern Med.* 2003;138:273–287.

Halasyamani L, Kripalani S, Coleman E, et al. Transition of care for hospitalized elderly patients—development of a discharge checklist for hospitalists. *J Hosp Med.* 2006;1(6):354–360.

Inouye SK, Bogardus ST Jr, Charpentier PA, et al. A multicomponent intervention to prevent delirium in hospitalized older patients [see comments]. *N Engl J Med.* 1999;340:669–676.

Maciejewski PK, Zhang B, Block SD, Prigerson HG. An empirical examination of the stage theory of grief. *JAMA.* 2007;297:716–723.

Morrison RS, Meier DE, eds. *Geriatric Palliative Care.* New York, New York: Oxford University Press; 2003.

Schulz R, Beach S. Caregiving as a risk factor for mortality: the Caregiver Health Effects Study. *JAMA.* 1999;282:2215–2219.

Morrison RS, Meier DE. Palliative care. *N Engl J Med.* 2004;350:2582–2590.

Quill TE. Perspectives on care at the close of life. Initiating end-of-life discussions with seriously ill patients: addressing the "elephant in the room." *JAMA.* 2000;284:2502–2507.

Shear K, Frank E, Houck PR, Reynolds CF III. Treatment of complicated grief: a randomized controlled trial. *JAMA.* 2005;293(21):2601–2608.

Steinhauser KE, Christakis NA, Clipp EC, McNeilly M, McIntyre L, Tulsky JA. Factors considered important at the end of life by patients, family, physicians, and other care providers. *JAMA.* 2000;284:2476–2482.

Steinhauser KE, Clipp EC, McNeilly M, Christakis NA, McIntyre LM, Tulsky JA. In search of a good death: observations of patients, families, and providers. *Ann Intern Med.* 2000;132:825–832.

Wenrich MD, Curtis JR, Shannon SE, Carline JD, Ambrozy DM, Ramsey PG. Communicating with dying patients within the spectrum of medical care from terminal diagnosis to death. *Arch Intern Med.* 2001;161:868–874.

Legal Issues

Marshall B. Kapp

The law regulates human relationships, both prospectively and retrospectively, in a wide variety of ways. To a large extent, the legal implications of medical practice are generic, in the sense that these apply to patients of all ages. Rules developed to deal with the care of younger adults apply with full force to older persons, whose rights do not diminish just because of advanced chronological age. However, a patient's advanced years may sometimes raise issues demanding particular attention by the involved participants in the professional/patient relationship. This chapter concentrates on several selected aspects in which the law influences the delivery of geriatric services through its impact on the recognition and enforcement of the respective rights and responsibilities of the parties, within the specific dynamics of an older patient/health care provider relationship.

OVERVIEW OF HEALTH CARE REGULATION

The U.S. Constitution establishes a federal system of government, under which health care delivery and other matters are regulated at the national (federal), state, and local levels. Under separation of powers principles, such regulation takes the form of constitutional (federal, state, and local) provisions, statutes enacted by elected legislatures, rules or regulations promulgated by executive branch administrative agencies like health or social service departments on the basis of authority conferred on the agency by the legislature via a statute, and common law doctrines created by the courts as a matter of public policy and prior case precedent. These various forms of regulation may impose specific or general duties on parties, may authorize but not require parties to act in specific ways, or may prohibit parties from engaging in particular conduct. Health care regulation may be directed at individual health professionals or at health care facilities, agencies, institutions, and other organizations.

Regulation of Health Professionals

One primary mechanism for regulating individual health professionals to assure adequate qualifications and acceptable conduct is licensure, which entails the requirement that an individual satisfy—on both an initial and a continuing basis—certain enumerated standards to be permitted to practice a particular profession. Professional licensure ordinarily occurs at the state level through statutes (such as state Medical Practice Acts or Nursing Practice Acts) and regulations promulgated by a state's licensing body (such as the Medical Board or Nursing Board) to implement the Practice Act. Licensure statutes and regulations limit certain activities to licensed professionals; engaging in those activities without prior state approval (in other words, practicing medicine or nursing without a valid license) subjects the wrongdoer to potential civil fines and even criminal sanctions.

Many statutory and regulatory requirements or prohibitions imposed on health professionals occur as conditions attached to payment for professional services under government insurance programs, especially Medicare and Medicaid. Professionals who treat patients covered by these government programs must satisfy the positive (e.g., "Thou shalt" maintain adequate patient records) or negative (e.g., "Thou shalt not" engage in self-referral) "strings" placed on the payment of public dollars to receive compensation for services rendered.

Another significant manner of health professional regulation under the civil law is tort liability in private lawsuits claiming malpractice; this form of regulation is discussed below. Particularly egregious behavior (such as patient abuse or billing fraud) may subject a health professional to criminal law punishments.

Regulation of Health Care Facilities and Agencies

Besides regulating individual health professionals, government additionally regulates provider facilities and agencies through licensure requirements, conditions attached to the receipt of compensation under public insurance programs including Medicare and Medicaid, criminal prohibitions on specific behaviors such as the filing of false claims, and civil liability for malpractice claims brought by or on behalf of individual patients. For example, Congress enacted the Nursing Home Quality Reform Act, codified at Title 42 U.S. Code §#1395i-3(a)-(h), as part of the Omnibus Budget Reconciliation Act (OBRA) of 1987, Public Law No. 100-203. This act, which has been amended several times subsequently, contains many of the recommendations proposed in a 1986 Institute of Medicine report that Congress had directed the Department of Health and Human Services to commission. OBRA 1987 amended the Social Security Act, Titles 18 (Medicare) and 19 (Medicaid), to require substantial upgrading in nursing home quality and enforcement. To implement this legislation, Department of Health and Human Services published a series of regulations, which have been codified at Title 42 Code of Federal Regulations Part 483. Violation of these regulations subjects nursing homes to a range of sanctions, up to decertification from participation in the Medicare and Medicaid programs.

STANDARDS OF CARE AND PROFESSIONAL LIABILITY IN GERIATRICS

Overview of Malpractice Liability

In a private civil lawsuit predicated on a theory of professional negligence, the plaintiff is required to establish four distinct elements by a preponderance of the evidence (Table 32-1). First, the patient/plaintiff has the burden of proving that the professional/provider defendant owed the patient an obligation defined by the appropriate standard of care. The existence of this duty ordinarily is established by showing that there existed, within the relevant time frame, a professional relationship between the patient and provider; that is, that the plaintiff was a patient of the provider for diagnostic and/or therapeutic purposes.

Second, the plaintiff must present sufficient evidence that the professional/provider breached or violated the appropriate standard of care within the professional relationship. The professional/provider does not guarantee particular results, let alone perfection. By the same token, however, it is not enough for professionals/providers to "do their best" if their conduct does not rise to the applicable level of care, even when the errors or omissions were unintentional (i.e., negligent). How the law determines the applicable level of professional care is discussed in the following section.

The third element that a medical malpractice plaintiff is required to prove is the occurrence of some financially compensable injury or damage. Besides special or economic damages that include such quantifiable items as lost income and past and future health care–related costs, plaintiffs may be awarded general or noneconomic damages for such things as pain and suffering, mental anguish, grief, and other emotional complaints. In recent years, juries have become much more willing to award substantial noneconomic damages to older patients claiming medical negligence. In very rare circumstances, punitive or exemplary damages may be awarded over and above compensatory damages, where the defendant's conduct has been not merely negligent, but actually reckless or malicious. For example, a jury might award punitive damages when it finds that a patient has developed serious pressure ulcers because of a hospital's or nursing home's demonstrated ongoing pattern of neglect.

The final component of proof in a professional malpractice lawsuit is the element of causation. To succeed, a plaintiff must persuade the jury, to a reasonable (not absolute) degree of medical certainty, that his or her injuries were the result of the defendant's negligence. A plaintiff must prove not only that the defendant's negligence was a "substantial factor" in bringing about the injury or that "but for" (*sine qua non*) the defendant's negligence the injury would not have happened, but further that there were no intervening, superceding (i.e., not reasonably foreseeable) forces that acted to break the chain of proximate or direct causation between the defendant's negligence and the patient's injury. For example, a physician might negligently fail to diagnose cancer in an older patient in a timely manner and the patient, on learning that cancer is at such stage that it cannot be treated effectively, commits suicide. Assuming the availability of effective treatment if the cancer had been properly diagnosed in a timely manner, representatives of the deceased patient may argue that "but for" the physician's negligence the death would not have taken place; however, the physician would respond that the patient's act of committing suicide was an intervening, superceding (i.e., not reasonably foreseeable) factor that disrupted the chain of proximate causation between the physician's negligence and the patient's injury.

Developing and Disseminating Standards of Care

Legal standards of care have been established mainly by the courts as a matter of common law on an incremental, case-by-case basis. State statutes, such as those containing professional licensure requirements, also help to define the required standards of care.

Under the traditional formulation, a professional who is accused of negligent acts or omissions in a medical malpractice claim is usually held to a standard requiring the professional to have and exercise that level of knowledge and skill ordinarily possessed and exercised by competent, reasonable professional peers (determined on a national rather than a local basis) in similar circumstances. Put differently, under long-standing tort principles of negligence, professionals have been judged legally according to the prevalent practice or custom of peer professionals in clinical circumstances like the situation that confronted the particular defendant in the case immediately before the court.

However, there is a significant current trend in many states to deviate from the traditional customary professional standard of care in favor of imposing more objective, external standards of "reasonableness" against which the professional's behavior is to be evaluated by the jury. An objective, evidence-based standard of reasonableness may exceed (i.e., require more knowledge and sophistication than) the prevailing customary practice within the professional community at the time in handling a specific clinical challenge presented by a patient. Thus, the state of the art in a particular area of care, required under a reasonableness standard, frequently may not be synonymous with and reflected in the current customary practice within the practitioner community. Courts adopting a reasonableness

---

TABLE 32-1

Elements of a Professional Negligence Claim

1. Duty owed by professional/provider to the patient
2. Breach or violation of duty
3. Damage or injury to the patient
4. Causal (both general and proximate) link between the professional/provider breach of duty and the injury suffered by the patient

TABLE 32-2

Proof of the Standard of Reasonable Care Under the Circumstances

1. Expert testimony about appropriate care
2. Professional codes of ethics
3. Medical journal literature
4. Textbooks (learned treatises)
5. *Physician's Desk Reference* (PDR) and pharmaceutical package inserts (PPIs)
6. Relevant statutes or regulations
7. Voluntary accreditation standards
8. Clinical practice guidelines or parameters

standard often recite the famous maxim of Judge Learned Hand: "Courts must in the end say what is required; there are precautions so imperative that even their universal disregard will not excuse their omission."

When a reasonableness standard is imposed on malpractice defendants, expert witnesses may be allowed to testify, and thereby educate the lay jurors, regarding the appropriate professional conduct under the circumstances. To establish what conduct would have been reasonable, the parties may also introduce other kinds of evidences to supplement the testimony provided by the expert witnesses (Table 32-2). Additional forms of evidence introduced for this purpose may include professional codes of ethics, medical journal literature, textbooks (learned treatises), the *Physician's Desk Reference* (PDR) and pharmaceutical package inserts (PPIs) pertaining to the correct use and dosage of prescription drugs, pertinent statutes or regulations, voluntary accreditation standards such as those of the Joint Commission on the Accreditation of Healthcare Organizations (JCAHO), and, of increasing importance, pertinent clinical practice guidelines or parameters.

Leaders in health care delivery and financing acknowledge (although frequently not in public) that a good deal of routine medical practice has long been predicated more on habit and inertia than on solid empirical evidence establishing clinical efficacy. Out of a concern about both the wasteful resource usage and the quality of patient care, in the last couple of decades professional organizations and specialty societies including the American Geriatrics Society and the American Medical Directors Association, governmental agencies led by the federal Agency for Healthcare Research and Quality (AHRQ), and individual institutions and agencies in the United States and elsewhere have engaged in a concerted movement to develop, collect, and disseminate to practicing clinicians a variety of evidence-based clinical practice guidelines or parameters to educate practitioners about whether a particular diagnostic or therapeutic intervention actually has been demonstrated to produce desired health benefits for patients. The Institute of Medicine has defined clinical practice guidelines as "systematically developed statements to assist practitioner and patient decisions about appropriate health care for specific clinical circumstances."

The legal ramifications of clinical practice guidelines or parameters continue to evolve. Nevertheless, there is a growing tendency for the courts to admit into evidence, on behalf of either side to a malpractice dispute (that is, for either inculpatory or exculpatory purposes), properly validated, scientifically supported contemporary practice parameters on the issue of the standard of care to be applied under any particular set of circumstances. This develop-

ment already has consequences, in that surveys show that plaintiffs' attorneys consider health professionals' compliance with or deviation from relevant practice parameters in making decisions about whether to initiate malpractice litigation at all and how to conduct settlement negotiations for claims that are pursued.

INFORMED CONSENT

Basics of Informed Consent

The informed consent doctrine originates with the ethical principle of autonomy or self-determination, especially regarding the physical integrity and dignity of one's own body. A health professional/provider may be held civilly liable, usually under a negligence theory but in rare cases under a battery or intentional tort theory, for subjecting a person to any diagnostic, therapeutic, or research-related intervention without that person's effective consent to the intervention. In their legal formulation, the substantive parts of the informed consent rule have evolved over time as a function of state common (judge-made) law. Moreover, the majority of states have, by now, enacted statutes and regulations spelling out a jurisdiction's specific details regarding informed consent, for clinical care generally and/or within particular settings such as nursing homes or public mental institutions.

For a patient's decision about whether to accept or reject a suggested medical intervention to be considered legally valid, three separate but interrelated elements must be present (Table 32-3).

First, the patient's participation in the decision-making process and the final decision(s) regarding intervention must be voluntary, as opposed to being unduly dictated by force, fraud, duress, or any other actual or perceived ulterior form of constraint or coercion. Second, the patient's agreement or disagreement with recommended interventions must be properly informed. The professional is obligated to disclose sufficient information about the proposed intervention to empower the patient to make a knowledgeable, intelligent consent or refusal. The third essential element of legally effective medical decision making is adequate capacity on the part of the patient to cognitively and emotionally understand and manipulate pertinent information about personal care.

In terms of the informed component of the informed consent doctrine, there are two competing standards for determining how much information about a proposed medical intervention must be

TABLE 32-3

Elements of Legally Valid Medical Decision Making

1. Voluntary
2. Informed
   a. Diagnosis or nature of the problem
   b. Expected benefits
   c. Risks
   d. Alternatives, including complementary and alternative interventions
   e. Risks and benefits of refusal
   f. Cost implications
   g. Level of uncertainty
3. Competent/capable decision maker

shared with the patient in advance. The medical custom or reasonable professional standard requires the disclosure of such information that an objective reasonable, prudent professional would disclose under similar circumstances. By comparison, the materiality or patient orientation standard compels the sharing of information that might make a difference (that is, might be material) in the decision-making process of a reasonable, average patient in similar circumstances. The different states are approximately evenly split between these two competing standards of information disclosure.

Under either the materiality or the reasonable professional standard, the basic components of information disclosure implicated by the professional's fiduciary or trust obligations to the patient include the following items: diagnosis or nature of the patient's medical problem; nature and purposes (the expected benefits) of the proposed interventions; reasonably foreseeable risks associated with the intervention, specifically, the likelihood of a risk materializing and the severity or gravity if it does occur; reasonable alternative interventions and their anticipated risks and benefits; and the reasonably foreseeable risks and benefits of not undergoing the proposed intervention. Other informational items that a health professional should seriously consider disclosing to the patient are: complementary and alternative medicine alternatives, which are increasingly popular with older individuals; cost ramifications to the patient of proposed alternatives; professional-specific information pertinent to the particular intervention (for instance, the professional's own track record with the particular intervention or any financial incentives the professional has regarding the patient's course of care); and the level of uncertainty within the medical community concerning the particular intervention.

Informed consent to a medical intervention may be implied or expressed. There are many situations in which a patient's permission to proceed with a medical intervention does not need to be put into words but, instead, may be implied from the context. This happens when, through demonstrative actions, the patient indicates a wish (or at least willingness) to undergo a specific intervention by voluntarily submitting to it in a manner that the health professional can reasonably rely on to conclude that the intervention has been authorized. Implied consent is appropriate for most routine, non-invasive, nonrisky kinds of medical interventions such as taking a patient's blood pressure or listening to the heart. Implied consent is not an exception to the general informed consent requirement, but just a different (created by behavior instead of words) form of permission.

Express consent (put into spoken or written words), by contrast, is more appropriate when the proposed medical intervention is intrusive and/or significantly more risky than ordinary, everyday life. With a small number of exceptions created by particular state statutes for designated kinds of interventions (such as testing for the HIV virus), express consent in the form of spoken rather than written patient words is quite legally adequate, as long as the consent is voluntarily and competently given on the basis of sufficient information being disclosed. However, for particularly intrusive or risky interventions, the professional/provider should consider documenting the patient's decision to consent or refuse by asking the patient to sign a separate written form, in addition to the professional making a progress note in the patient's medical record. Also, voluntary accreditation standards with which the provider complies, such as those of the JCAHO, may require the use of separate written consent forms for particular sorts of medical interventions.

TABLE 32-4

Components of Functional Assessment of Decisional Capacity

1. Ability to communicate decisions
2. Ability to give reasons for decisions
3. Reasons given are logical and factually accurate
4. Appreciation of ramifications
5. Comprehension of ramifications

Decisional Capacity Issues

Sometimes, a patient is not mentally and/or emotionally capable of assimilating pertinent information and engaging in a rational, voluntary decision-making process about the proposed and alternative medical interventions. Some older persons with dementia, depression, or other age-related mental disorders are so impaired that they fall into this category. When the patient personally lacks adequate decisional capacity, the health professional is not at all relieved of the duty to obtain informed consent but, instead, must work with someone else who is willing to act as a surrogate on the patient's behalf.

Assessing decisional capacity in older persons entails a functional inquiry. Among the basic questions to be posed are the following (Table 32-4): (1) Can the person make and communicate in an understandable form any decisions at all? (2) Is the person able to offer reasons for the choices made, indicating some degree of reflection and consideration? (3) Are the reasons given based on logical reasoning proceeding from factually accurate suppositions? (4) Can the patient appreciate the ramifications (that is, the likely risks and benefits) of the options outlined and the choices expressed, and the reality that these ramifications apply to that patient? (5) Does the individual, in fact, comprehend the practical implications of his or her choices?

A patient's present cognitive and emotional capacity should be evaluated on a decision-specific, rather than a global or all-or-nothing, basis. A patient may be capable of making some kinds of decisions, but not others; partial or limited capacity is quite possible even when total capacity is not. Moreover, capacity may fluctuate within a specific patient according to variables such as time of day, day of the week, physical location, acute and transient physical problems, other persons available to support or coerce the patient's choice, and medication reactions. Older individuals may be especially vulnerable to fluctuations in capacity induced by these factors. Some of these factors may be susceptible to manipulation by caregivers (for example, through changes in the timing of drug administration) so that discussions with the patient (rather than or in addition to the surrogate) about the care plan can take place under the most lucid circumstances possible.

Advance Health Care Planning as Prospective Decision Making

There are several legal mechanisms available to maximize a patient's medical autonomy. An older person (although these planning tools are available to any decisionally capable adult) may, while still competent, execute certain legal instruments to take steps to anticipate and prepare for eventual incapacity by voluntarily delegating or directing the exercise of future medical decision-making power. Although oral advance medical directives, theoretically, are completely legally valid, patients should be encouraged to execute written versions to maximize the likelihood that the directive will be ultimately respected by family members and health professionals. Organizational providers are required by the federal Patient Self-Determination Act to initiate discussions with competent patients about the availability of advance medical directive opportunities.

The durable power of attorney (DPOA) consists of a written document in which an individual (the principal) appoints an agent, or attorney-in-fact, to make various kinds of decisions for the principal. Each state has enacted one or more statutes that explicitly authorize the use of a DPOA for health care to empower an agent (including a nonfamily member) to make medical choices on a patient's behalf, should the patient later lose decision-making capacity. A DPOA may be immediate in nature, meaning that it comes into effect as soon as the agent is named. In a springing DPOA, on the other hand, the legal authority transfers (springs) from the patient to the agent only on the occurrence of some specified future event, like a declaration of the principal's incapacity by a designated number of examining physicians. The patient should be informed by attending health professionals when they have decided to act as though decision-making authority has sprung to the designated agent, so that the patient can utter a protest, if desired, to the agent's exercise of power.

The DPOA is a proxy directive, and hence distinguishable from a living will, which is an instruction-type directive. In an instruction directive, a presently competent patient documents his or her wishes regarding future medical treatment (e.g., "no extraordinary measures" or "keep me alive forever no matter what pain or expense") rather than naming an agent to make future treatment decisions in the case of eventual incapacity. The two kinds of legal devices are not mutually exclusive; indeed, patients may be encouraged to execute them in tandem because the living will can help an agent named under a DPOA to exercise the patient's substituted judgment (defined below) more accurately.

When a patient is decisionally incapable but has not previously executed an instruction or proxy directive, in a majority of states health professionals may rely on legislation empowering family members and enumerated other persons to make medical decisions for incapacitated persons. In states with such family consent statutes, the approved procedure usually consists of documenting unanimous agreement among the attending physician, specified relatives or others (listed in a stated order of preference), and sometimes consultant physicians as well.

When there is no valid proxy or instruction directive, family consent statute, or judicial precedent in one's jurisdiction authorizing the family to act as patient surrogate, or in those relatively uncommon situations in which family members strongly and irreconcilably disagree about the best course of care for their decisionally incapacitated loved one, judicial creation of a guardianship or conservatorship (nomenclature varies by jurisdiction) may be advisable to transfer decision-making power formally and definitively from an incapacitated patient to a single, specific surrogate. However, the official legal process (ordinarily entailing significant financial, time consumption, and emotional costs) should not be initiated unless and until less formal approaches, such as mediation or consultation with an Institutional Ethics Committee (IEC) or ethics consultation service, have been exhausted in an effort to reach a sufficient level of agreement among all the interested stakeholders. In a guardianship/ conservatorship case, professionals who have evaluated and/or treated the alleged incompetent person usually are called on to provide evidence to the court in the form of a written affidavit and/or live sworn testimony. Many jurisdictions have public or volunteer guardianship programs that operate to provide surrogate decision makers for individuals with substantially impaired cognitive and/or emotional capacity who have no suitable family members or other private parties to be appointed guardians for them.

In the past, a surrogate has been expected to make decisions consistent with the guardian's view, as a trust agent, of the patient's best interests. The more modern trend, however, is toward enforcement of a substituted judgment standard of proxy decision making, whenever it is realistically feasible. Under this latter approach, the surrogate is obligated to make those decisions that the patient would make, according to the patient's own preferences and values to the extent these can be accurately ascertained, if the patient were presently able to make and express his or her own competent decisions.

CONFIDENTIALITY

In the course of providing care, health professionals routinely are exposed to very private information about patients and their families. Professionals owe patients a fiduciary responsibility to hold in confidence all sensitive patient information entrusted to them as a consequence of the professional/patient relationship. This ethical obligation, predicated on the patient's important interest in protecting personal privacy and avoiding the social stigma and potential discrimination that breach of one's medical privacy might entail, is enforceable legally under both state and federal law.

State Law

Every state, both within its various state professional practice acts and in separate statutes pertaining to particular health care delivery settings, has legislatively enacted provisions pertaining to the confidentiality duties of health care professionals, institutions, and agencies. Often, state agencies have published accompanying regulations to implement these statutes. Moreover, a strong common law health care confidentiality doctrine has been forged by state court decisions rendered over time. Violation of state common law or the relevant statutory or regulatory requirements regarding the confidentiality of patient information may subject erring health professionals/providers to civil damage suits, brought by or on behalf of the patient whose privacy was improperly infringed; additionally, violation of state Practice Act provisions may subject the violator to administrative sanctions by the state, including license suspension or even revocation.

However, numerous exceptions to the general confidentiality rule have been recognized, either by the courts as part of the common law or embedded in state legislation or regulation (Table 32-5). The most prominent exception occurs when a patient, expressly or impliedly, voluntarily and knowingly waives, or gives up, the right to assert the confidentiality of particular information. These waivers take place daily to make information available to third-party payers (for instance, Medicare claims processors and private health insurers), quality of care auditors (such as JCAHO surveyors), and other public and private entities like health care surrogates authorized to make medical decisions on behalf of a decisionally incapacitated

TABLE 32-5

Exceptions to the Duty of Confidentiality

1. Patient permission (waiver)
2. Danger to others
3. Mandatory or permissive reporting statutes
4. Legal process (court order)
5. "Treatment, payment, and health care operations" (HIPAA)

patient. Also, because the modern delivery of health care most often is a team endeavor, each patient implicitly gives permission for the sharing of certain otherwise private pieces of information among the members of the treatment team. Internal information sharing of this nature is essential to optimal care, especially for accomplishing coordination and continuity of long-term care for older patients with disabilities. Indeed, failures in communication among the multiple providers involved in the care of a patient needing such coordination and continuity may form the basis for negligence liability claims when harm results.

Second, the usual confidentiality duty may be outweighed in situations of jeopardy to innocent, at-risk third parties, such as happens when a patient with serious sensory or cognitive impairments insists on continuing to drive an automobile or maintaining loaded firearms in the home for protection against intruders. Particular details regarding methods for the health professional to discharge the responsibility to report a credible threat of harm to public health or law enforcement authorities vary on the basis of state statutory and case law.

Third, the patient's reasonable expectation of privacy must give way when the health professional is mandated by state statute to report to enumerated public health or law enforcement authorities (e.g., Adult Protective Services [APS]) the professional's reasonable suspicion that certain conditions or activities have occurred or are occurring. Such reportable conditions or activities may include elder mistreatment or neglect (in many states including cases of self-neglect within that definition), domestic violence, infectious diseases, births, and deaths. Some states that have declined to mandate the reporting of particular situations to public authorities nonetheless encourage voluntary reporting; a few states have pursued this approach regarding cases of suspected elder abuse or neglect. Those states supply an incentive for voluntary reporting by expressly providing legal immunity against any form of civil or administrative liability for covered persons making good faith reports to public authorities. Mandatory and voluntary reporting statutes embody the state's exercise of either its inherent police power to protect and promote the general health, safety, welfare, and morals of the community or its *parens patriae* power to step up and safeguard individuals (such as persons with serious cognitive or emotional disabilities) who are not capable of protecting themselves. Further, a health professional may be compelled to reveal otherwise confidential information about particular patients by the force of legal process, namely, by a judge's issuance of a court order requiring such release. This is a possibility in any civil or criminal lawsuit involving a factual dispute about a patient's physical or mental condition. A court order (as opposed to a subpoena or subpoena *duces tecum*, which is issued simply as an administrative, nondiscretionary matter by the court clerk rather than by a judge) requiring one to produce personally identifiable patient information may overrule the state's provider/patient testi-

monial privilege statute that ordinarily would prohibit the provider from testifying in a legal proceeding regarding private patient information. Every state testimonial privilege statute provides for judicially compelled testimony on the part of the health professional when, for example, the patient has placed his or her own health condition and medical treatment in issue in a lawsuit. This could occur when, for instance, the individual challenges the allegations propounded by others about one's mental impairments made in a guardianship/conservatorship petition.

Federal Law

Particular Health Care Settings

There are a variety of federal statutes and regulations imposing on health professionals/providers' particular confidentiality obligations when care is provided within specific types of health care settings, including federal penal institutions, veterans affairs facilities, military institutions, federal community health centers, and facilities specializing in the treatment of persons having drug and alcohol addiction. Violation of these laws may result in substantial civil fines. Statutes and regulations setting the conditions for receipt of Medicare and Medicaid payments contain confidentiality provisions, set within general patients' rights standards, applicable specifically to nursing homes and home health agencies. Noncompliance with those provisions could trigger a range of regulatory sanctions, at the extreme including decertification of the facility or agency from participation in federal health care financing programs.

Health Insurance Portability and Accountability Act

Federal regulations, codified at Title 45, U.S. Code Parts 160 and 164, became effective in 2003 to implement the Health Insurance Portability and Accountability Act (HIPAA) of 1996 (Public Law No. 104-191, title XI, Part C). These regulations, published in the form of a Privacy Rule and a Security Rule, impose on covered health care entities (defined as any health providers who transmit any patient-related information electronically) an extensive set of requirements regarding the handling of personally identifiable medical information contained in patient records. These regulations impose severe criminal and civil sanctions for unauthorized disclosures of personal health information, although as of the beginning of 2007 the Department of Health and Human Services Office of Civil Rights had brought no enforcement action against any covered health entity for an HIPAA violation, despite the receipt of more than 23,000 complaints.

Substantively, HIPAA and its implementing regulations, in essence, codify preexisting state statutory and common law protections for patients, with the addition of provisions making it clear that patients now have the right to access the information contained in their own medical records. (Previously, state law had varied or was unclear regarding the issue of patient access to records.) HIPAA contains provisions authorizing covered entities to transmit personal health information to certain others for purposes of "treatment, payment, and health care operations" such as quality assurance or marketing. These and other exceptions explicitly contained in HIPAA basically track the preexisting state statutory and common law exceptions discussed in the previous section.

SUMMARY

Individual health care professionals and organizational providers serving older patients inevitably and continuously interact with laws and the legal system. This chapter has outlined a handful of the arenas in which this interaction is likely to occur. For advice in particular circumstances, especially pertaining to relevant state law, specialized legal consultation should be sought from knowledgeable attorneys in private practice, counsel and/or risk managers employed or retained by the health provider, the professional's or provider's liability insurance carrier, or an Institutional Ethics Committee.

FURTHER READING

American Bar Association Commission on Law and Aging and American Psychological Association. *Assessment of Older Adults with Diminished Capacity*. Washington, DC: Authors; 2005.

Berg JW, Appelbaum PS. *Informed Consent: Legal Theory and Clinical Practice*. New York, New York: Oxford University Press; 2001.

Brandl B, Dyer CB, Heisler CJ, et al. *Elder Abuse Detection and Intervention: A Collaborative Approach*. New York, New York: Springer Publishing Company; 2007.

Chiplin AJ Jr. Breathing life into discharge planning. *Elder Law J.* 2005;13:1–69.

Fisher AL, Hill R. Ethical and legal issues in antiaging medicine. *Clin Geriatr Med.* 2004;20:361–382.

Frolik LA. *The Law of Later-Life Health Care and Decision Making*. Chicago: ABA Publishing; 2006.

Frolik LA, Kaplan RL. *Elder Law in a Nutshell*. 4th ed. St. Paul, MN: West Law School Publications; 2006.

Jones CJ. Say what? How the Patient Self-Determination Act leaves the elderly with limited English proficiency out in the cold. *Elder Law J.* 2005;13:489–518.

Krohm C, Summers SK. *Advance Health Care Directives: A Handbook for Professionals*. Chicago: ABA Publishing; 2002.

Kwiencinski M. To be or not to be, should doctors decide? Ethical and legal aspects of medical futility policies. *Marquette Elder Advisor*. 2006;7:313–355.

Meisel A, Cerminara K. *The Right to Die: The Law of End-of-Life Decisionmaking*. 3rd ed. Frederick, MD: Aspen Publishers; 2006.

National Research Council. *Elder Mistreatment: Abuse, Neglect, and Exploitation in an Aging America*. Washington, DC: National Academies Press; 2003.

Post LF, Blustein J, Dubler NN. *Handbook for Health Care Ethics Committees*. Baltimore: Johns Hopkins University Press; 2007.

Quinn MJ. *Guardianship of Adults: Achieving Justice, Autonomy, and Safety*. New York, New York: Springer Publishing Company; 2005.

Reisman NR. Legal issues associated with the current and future practice of anti-aging medicine. *J Gerontol Med Sci.* 2004;59:674–681.

Spirituality

Timothy P. Daaleman

New information about linkages between religious and spiritual factors and health-related outcomes continues to be reported by both the popular media and the scientific community. From a cover story in *Newsweek*, to a case conference in *JAMA*, to a clinical trial of intercessory prayer published in *Lancet*, there is ongoing interest in the intersection of religion and spirituality with health and health care in the United States. Such a trend reflects America's overall fascination with spirituality—much of which lies outside of organized religion—so much so that some forecasters have projected a future view of health that places spiritual factors alongside physical, psychological, and social determinants.

This chapter provides an overview and framework for understanding the current phenomenon of spirituality and health, particularly as it relates to the care of older adults. The first section orients how religion and spirituality are defined and understood by several academic disciplines. The core part of the chapter outlines and illustrates a categorical approach to the study of spirituality that has been proposed by Bernard McGinn. The next segment briefly reviews the organization of spiritual care before the final section closes with a perspective that introduces some ideas about a spirituality of practice within a spirituality of place.

WAYS OF UNDERSTANDING RELIGION AND SPIRITUALITY

Religion and religiosity are generally understood in several ways: the totality of belief systems, an inner piety or disposition, an abstract system of ideas, and ritual practices. For communities of faith, religious doctrine and faith traditions provide a foundation for understanding the wide range of human experience in areas such as suffering, death, and relationships with God and others. The term spirituality, on the other hand, has multiple connotations and interpretations that are less easily defined; academic disciplines such as sociology, psychology, and theology have approached and con-

ceptualized spirituality in various ways. The social work literature, for example, operationalizes spirituality as a process of making sense of self and the world. Here spirituality is proposed as a condition of asking and answering major philosophical questions: who am I, why do I exist, what is my purpose, and how do I fit in the world? Several sociological perspectives resonate with this decidedly existential orientation. Spirituality is represented as that which promotes human agency, or the power that comes from within, in addition to an ongoing search to know our deepest selves and what is held to be sacred.

A psychological perspective is often used when considering spirituality's relationship with health or well-being, since theoretical or conceptual frameworks, which postulate a causal, mediating, or moderating relationship between variables of interest, can be employed. In this way of thinking, the characteristics of spirituality are presented as a web of plausible relationships, predominantly within the domain of well-being. The growing interest in positive psychology, for example, casts an individual's subjective experience in an optimistic light and often depicts spirituality as providing a foundation for adjustment, growth, and reaching one's human potential. A related approach, one that is especially relevant to older adults, considers spirituality within the framework of religiously based coping mechanisms.

The social and psychological sciences have contributed greatly to contemporary perspectives of spirituality; however, the roots of this concept lie within theological sources. Historians trace the etymology of spirituality to the spirit of God (*ruah*) in the Old Testament, which subsequently provided emphasis for the term "spirit" (*pneuma*) found in the New Testament. Despite the central place of this idiom in such foundational texts, the abstract word *spiritualitas* (spirituality) did not arise until the fifth century, here having a biblical meaning of a spiritual person, or one whose life is ordered or influenced by God. By the 12th century, spirituality was associated mainly with what pertained to the inner life of the soul. However, this usage of spirituality went into eclipse by the 18th and 19th centuries, largely because of Voltaire and other contemporary thinkers who wrote about spirituality in disparaging ways. The genesis of contemporary understandings regarding spirituality is linked with French Catholic writers who used the term in a devotional sense in the early part of the 20th century. As time progressed, spirituality gradually migrated into more academic and technical circles, predominantly within the Catholic tradition.

Current, generally more inclusive theological contexts consider spirituality in light of beliefs in God or a divine being, as well as the sociological, philosophical, and psychological manifestations of those beliefs. One representative viewpoint locates spirituality within the stories, practices, and beliefs that are developed within religious traditions and communities but that are ultimately carried into and worked out in ordinary and everyday life events. A more applied perspective—a white paper on professional chaplaincy—depicts spirituality as "an awareness of relationships with all creation, an appreciation of presence and purpose that includes a sense of meaning." Such representations shed light on how most Americans can consider themselves to be religious and/or spiritual, grasping these concepts as independent, although perhaps related, qualities of what it is to be human.

A CATEGORICAL APPROACH TO SPIRITUALITY

McGinn provides a categorical approach to spirituality, one that is useful to clinicians and other providers seeking to understand the multiple ways in which spirituality is manifested in care settings, as well as to investigators interested in developing better ways to study it. The three approaches—historical/contextual, anthropological/social scientific, theological/normative—are collectively holistic in scope, since these seek to capture the range of human experience. As a result, these are not mutually exclusive; more than one may be operational or applicable at a given time.

Historical/Contextual

A historical/contextual approach looks at the place of spirituality within the context of a shared lived history by a defined group, community, or population. Such an approach can lend insight into the current, accelerated interest and recognition of spirituality in health care circles by examining two parallel, patient-centered movements: end-of-life care and complementary and alternative medicine. Both movements may be viewed as an impetus to rehumanize a health care system in the United States, which has become increasingly impersonal, spiritually barren, and grounded in technology. The ongoing momentum to improve end-of-life care is understandably inclusive of spiritual factors, despite the lack of consistency in how spirituality is addressed in clinical settings.

Complementary and alternative medicine has also promoted rapprochement between spirituality and health care, yet also holds a conflicted perspective on the place of spirituality within its armamentarium. Studies that have examined the prevalence and patterns of complementary and alternative medicine usage vary in their assignment of alternative spiritual interventions—such as faith healing and prayer—as either a therapeutic modality or a conventional religious or spiritual ritual that is exclusive of complementary and alternative medicine. In 1993, a widely publicized survey on unconventional therapies found that 25% of respondents acknowledged

using prayer as a medical modality. A 5-year follow-up study by the same investigators documented an increase in the use of self-prayer and a prevalence of spiritual healing as a common therapy for anxiety, depression, and lung problems. In a subsequent analysis of this data set, one-third of U.S. adults surveyed were found to use prayer for health concerns, both for wellness and for illnesses characterized by painful or aggravating symptoms, nonspecific diagnoses, and limited treatment options such as depression, headaches, and back and/or neck pain. Respondents in this study who used prayer for their health concerns also reported high levels of perceived helpfulness, or efficacy.

For clinicians and other care providers, a historical/contextual approach can enhance a richer, more complete understanding of how patients view the relationship between their own spirituality, however defined, and their health and health care. Here it is important to appreciate and distinguish the various organizational and social contexts in which care is provided; care within a clinical setting is very different than care offered within a faith-based setting, or within the supportive environment of a religious or spiritual community. A historical/contextual perspective can facilitate spiritual assessments—the process of discerning an individual's spiritual needs and determining what resources are available to meet those needs—which have recently been recommended by the Joint Commission on the Accreditation of Healthcare Organizations (JCAHO) for all hospitalized patients.

Well-developed clinical skills are the soil for fruitful spiritual assessments: empathic and active listening; open-ended questioning; validating, restating, or clarifying information that the patient provides; and determining whether a directed physical or mental status examination is necessary. The 7×7 Model, developed by George Fitchett, is a useful tool that incorporates a multidimensional approach to a spiritual assessment, since it includes medical, psychological, and spiritual domains. The model encourages care providers to consider seven different areas: belief and meaning, vocation and obligations, experience and emotions, courage and growth, ritual and practice, community, and authority and guidance. Equally important, it provides a way for providers to effectively communicate with other spiritual caregivers, such as community clergy, hospital chaplains, family members, or other sources of spiritual support.

Anthropological/Social Scientific

An anthropological or a social scientific approach, according to McGinn, views spirituality as a basic element in human nature and experience. Such a viewpoint allows the spiritual to be distinguished ontologically from the social and psychological and provides for the study of spirituality by the human sciences. More than a century ago, Emile Durkheim's seminal work on the association between suicide rates and religious denominations in Europe ushered in the scientific study of the relationship between religion, spirituality, and health, which continues to this day. The pace of this research has accelerated in the last 20 years, and more than 1600 studies have been published in this area. For example, a series of articles in the late 1980s suggested that morbidity and mortality rates varied by religious denomination and that high levels of involvement with religious activities were associated with better overall health status.

Religion, and now spirituality, occupies a central place in the lives of older Americans. Popular polls report that religion is very important in the elderly; 67% of those aged 50 to 64 years, 79% of those aged 65 to 74 years, and 72% of those 75 years and older note that religion is very important. Longitudinal studies suggest that the relationship between age and the importance of religion is nonlinear; importance initially declines between early and middle adult life but increases as people enter old age. African-Americans and women report more strongly held religious and spiritual beliefs than whites and men, even after adjusting for age, level of education, marital status, family income, and region. Finally, attendance at religious and spiritual services is common among older adults, with 52% of those aged 65 to 74 years and 43% of those 75 years and older reporting participation within the last 7 days.

A field analysis of the literature on religion, spirituality, and health highlights several methodological and conceptual shortcomings in this area, but it also concludes that many studies investigating the relationship between church/service attendance and mortality are persuasive. Lynda Powell and colleagues provide a thorough review of this empirical evidence by examining 11 independent, longitudinal studies of the relationship between church/service attendance and mortality incidence. In representative, population-based studies, the strength of the relationship was a 30% reduction in mortality after adjustment for demographic, socioeconomic, and health-associated confounders, and a 25% reduction in mortality after adjustment for established risk factors. In their summary, the reviewers proposed several hypotheses for the protective impact that service attendance may have on mortality: (1) healthy lifestyle behaviors; (2) religious social support; (3) positive emotional experience; (4) modeling of positive and caring behaviors, attitudes, and beliefs; and (5) access to material, emotional, and social resources.

In light of empiric evidence, which is largely mixed, most Americans continue to hold positive attitudes and beliefs about the efficacy of spiritually related interventions (e.g., prayer) in healing, although many remain skeptical about the place of spirituality in clinical encounters. A *USA Weekend* poll reported that 79% of respondents believed that spiritual faith can help people recover from disease, but only 56% said that their faith had actually helped in their recovery. Eighty percent of people sampled in a *CBS News* poll believed that prayer helps healing, but only 34% agreed that prayer should be a standard part of medical care. One multisite survey study found that a small proportion of primary-care outpatients preferred that physicians address spiritually related matters during routine office visits. However, the study also reported that the context of the visit was important, since patients desired greater physician involvement with their spiritual and religious concerns when the severity of their illness increased (i.e., when hospitalized or near death).

Exploratory studies provide some illumination to the inconsistencies in these survey findings. When asked to describe spirituality in the context of well-being, patients in focus group interviews depicted positive thinking and self-efficacy beliefs, and agency beliefs or their use of power or influence. Agency beliefs are empowering beliefs, viewing individuals as active participants constructing their own life course through the actions that they take. Patients also outlined an ongoing process of finding meaning in the face of illness and of placing their illness experience within a larger life context. These qualitative data substantiate one conceptualization of spirituality as the capability to construct an empowering interpretative framework—an explanatory model so to speak—through which health, illness, and life events are viewed: a lattice of meaning and self-identity.

Yet if spirituality is somehow tied to individual systems of empowered meaning, what is the link between the lived experience of the patient and the larger culture that shapes the illness experience? Anthony Giddens provides a useful theoretical orientation for integrating the individual perspectives and social currents found in these surveys and narratives. Giddens posits that maintaining self-identity is an ongoing process of selecting and editing individual narratives amid a diversity of options and possibilities. Self-identity provides a sense of control or mastery in day-to-day activities, but, when there are threats to self-identity and personal meaning, individual biographies are reconfigured and reconstructed.

Consider the chronically ill older adult. The diagnosis and treatment confront this person , with the specter of a life-limiting illness, a functional limitation, or a compromised quality of life, all threats to self-identity. Here, spirituality may be understood in how such individuals begin to integrate their illness experience within their larger life course and how well meaning making empowers them to live their life. Yet this patient, and each one of us, arrives at such a point with a lifetime accumulated with beliefs, stories, and practices: our *background spiritualities*, according to John Shea. Many of these spiritualities will be linked with an identified religious or faith tradition, some will not. But all background spiritualities can be responsive to threats to self by offering beliefs, stories, and practices that provide a template for the ongoing creation of a personally meaningful world, a constructed empowered "reality" in the face of current illness. This constructed world is manifested by the recreated beliefs, stories, and practices that have been transformed by ongoing experiences: our *foreground spiritualities*, in Shea's way of thinking. More importantly, such a constructed world is contingent upon the social actions and interactions maintained in a larger social world, with family and friends and care providers.

Theological/Normative

If spiritualities—those beliefs, practices, and stories that respond to a shared human need for meaning—are generated from social actions and interactions, theological, ethical, and normative issues are never far off from the beliefs and values that guide human action and behavior. A theological or normative approach seeks to develop and establish criteria—either by philosophical consistency and cogency or by theological orthodoxy—for determining what may be considered to be "healthy" or "legitimate" spirituality. A Nazi or Satanic spirituality viscerally illustrates "unhealthy" spirituality; it is normatively discomforting despite how well such a belief system may be integrated, or how effectively it empowers its adherents.

The lived worlds of patients and providers intersect during care encounters, and both arrive with a lived history that is located in specific social and cultural frameworks. Larger cultural and social influences within and outside of the encounter are embedded within this activity. Factors such as race/ethnicity, social support, education, gender, and religion are parts of the scaffolding in the construction of a meaningful world as illness, disability, or death is faced. Faith traditions, for example, provide an important ethical foundation for decision making in related areas such as end-of-life care.

Moral imperatives are part of the fabric of care encounters, specifying what ought to be done to maintain health, avoid illness, and promote healing. Approaching spirituality from an ethical or normative perspective would consider how the intersecting spiritualities of patient and provider are negotiated. At the outset, any proposed model must be congruent with ethical principles that guide aspects of clinical practice, such as those found in medicine. However, the concept of power is at the forefront of ethically considering spirituality in care encounters. Howard Brody identifies several useful guidelines for power's ethical use. First, the provider and patient should use all of their power to affect a good patient outcome, which is determined by the patient's definition of the presenting problem and by the provider's contextual understanding of the patient's life course. Providers should also be supportive of the patient's own sense of power, as long as it is consistent with a good outcome and the patient's goals and interests. When a conflict arises between the patient's use of power and those ends, it should be handled with negotiation and persuasion and with concern for the patient's vulnerability.

Brody recommends that providers should share their power with patients by informing them about the nature and treatment of the disease, or the presenting problem. This interaction can be extended to include contextual interpretations that are generated, such as cultural scripts and illness trajectories that are conveyed to patients through clinical impressions, and by the recommendation of selected therapeutic interventions. For example, an encounter in which a patient discloses to have cancer and is hopeless, an assessment of a major depressive episode and consultation with a psychiatrist frames hopelessness in a traditional medical model. However, if hopelessness results in the patient declining treatment, another provider may view this as the beginning of a more active dying process and possibly recommend hospice care.

Implicitly or explicitly, providers wield power through their respective frameworks and in the selection of cultural scripts and illness trajectories that are presented to patients. The power wielded by such an interpretative and framing process can be minimized by offering more than one template. In each care encounter, patients may choose to either incorporate or discard proffered scripts as they construct or reconstruct their self-identity. The resultant clinical narratives are stories of a therapeutic activity facilitated and cocreated by the spiritualities of both patient and provider.

Ongoing clinical narratives that are cocreated by both patient and provider spiritualities can be therapeutic for providers as well. Older adults, especially those with chronic illness, can confront and perhaps threaten a provider's sense of self through their disability, serious illness, or death. Yet the spiritualities found in patient narratives can contribute to the ongoing construction of a provider's own self-identity, by presenting and affirming the human condition in its entirety. For some providers, spiritualities may be inclusive of practices that are common to patients, such as prayer, reflection, and self-awareness. For others, spiritualities may arise as philosophical or religious belief systems: beliefs that may be held or shared with their patients and beliefs that provide a foundation of purpose. However, for all providers, spiritualities that are brought forth by patient stories, and are woven into ongoing narratives, are responsive to a basic human desire of finding meaning in an integrated way.

THE ORGANIZATION OF HEALTH-RELATED SPIRITUAL CARE

The Institute of Medicine, the National Hospice and Palliative Care Organization, and the JCAHO advocate attention to the spiritual care of patients, despite ambiguity in how spirituality is understood in health care settings. In clinical arenas, physicians, nurses, and other health care workers are being called upon to assume greater responsibility for addressing and meeting the spiritual needs of their patients, tasks that have been traditionally assigned to pastoral care providers and clergy.

Investigations into the structure, process, and outcomes spiritual care have been limited to qualitative research and small survey studies, largely of nursing staff in long-term care. For example, one exploratory study of nurses described the spiritual care of dying nursing home residents using five themes: honoring the person's dignity, struggling with end-of-life treatment decisions, wishing to do more, personal knowledge of self as a caregiver, and intimate knowledge of the resident. Other survey studies of oncology nurses suggest that spiritual care involves several tasks: referring to pastoral care providers and clergy, acknowledging and supporting patients' spiritual or religious concerns, and being attentive to both patients and family members.

A recent multistate study of spiritual care at the end of life adds greater understanding to the organizational aspects of spiritual care. This report of 284 decedent residents, from a sample of 100 residential care/assisted living facilities and nursing homes, found that most residents (87%) nearing the end of life received assistance with their spiritual needs. Residents who received spiritual care were perceived to have had better overall end-of-life care by their family members, and the provision or facilitation of individual devotional activities was found to be an essential component of spiritual care. Other qualitative studies of family members and nurses caring for dying residents provide a richer understanding of what may constitute the practice of spiritual care. For example, one study reported that an intimate knowledge of the resident and the provision of spiritual comfort—largely through life review and shared devotional activities—were important to end-of-life care in nursing homes. Another report described a variety of caring behaviors by nursing staff, such as listening and answering questions and allowing family members to grieve, as integral parts of spiritual care.

The aforementioned multistate study also found that spiritual care delivered by facility staff, rather than clergy or chaplains, was a key care component; decedents who received care from staff had better overall perceived care. Care and support from the staff was more common in religiously affiliated facilities, which may have been owing to a self-selection among staff who chose to work in such an organizational setting. However, the influence of an organizational ethos, or a commonly held value and mission, which promoted spiritual care in religious facilities, may be more at play.

FUTURE DIRECTIONS: A SPIRITUALITY OF PRACTICE WITHIN A SPIRITUALITY OF PLACE

In *After Heaven*, Robert Wuthnow suggests that contemporary spirituality in the United States can be understood for the last 50 years as a movement from a spirituality of dwelling to a spirituality of seeking, and he introduces the idea of a practice-oriented spirituality. For older adults and their care providers, who dwell within and are major constituents of multiple organizations and communities—congregations of faith, acute care hospitals, senior centers, and long-term care facilities—a future challenge will be how to integrate a spirituality of practice within a spirituality of place.

One envisioned spirituality of place would be predicated on Peter Senge's work regarding the learning disciplines, as interpreted through Alasdair MacIntyre's idea of communities of virtue. Each of the learning disciplines described by Senge—systems thinking, personal mastery, mental models, building shared vision, and team learning—may be considered on three levels: practices, principles, and essences. Practices are the tasks and work involved in an organization, a primary focus of both individuals and groups. Senge's perspective theoretically represents a point of reference for organizational members, by helping individuals make sense of, and through which they are continually refining, their practices.

Essences are states of being or self-perceptions that come to be experienced spontaneously and naturally by individuals or groups with high levels of mastery in the disciplines. MacIntyre contributes to a complementary understanding of communities, which are formed in identified virtues, including the virtue of "just generosity." This way of thinking may contribute to the health of organizations, communities, and their members. Faith communities and health care organizations, for example, are particular and distinctive types of communities formed over time, with the virtue of "just generosity" as a commonly held virtue, embedded in the guiding principles and practices of learning organizations of virtue. As such, community members have the capacity to become formed in the practices of relatedness and caring and come to embody essences that contribute to the health of both members and the larger community.

A spirituality of practice would be grounded in the practice of narrative, where both patients and providers readily welcome spiritualities—the stories, beliefs, and practices—that reside outside of care encounters but are central to shared experiences of illness and health. A narratively based spirituality of practice can be the foundation to enlarge and sustain the inner life of both patient and provider by forming and nurturing essences: a self that arise spontaneously, authentically, and creatively. This is a normative and moral activity of spirituality, an activity that has the potential for laying the foundation for a greater and sustained therapeutic activity. And it is here where the purpose and goals—the principles—of care can be fashioned and refashioned.

A spirituality of practice embedded within a spirituality of place would be holy common ground, a place filled with a creative, transformative tension, generated by lives that are linked to a present moment but that are uncertain how the story will continue to unfold, and eventually end. In this way of believing, thinking, and relating, spirituality is embodied as caring within a much larger enterprise: authentic human interactions in which ongoing meaningful life stories—moments of incandescence, both human and divine—are cocreated, nurtured, and shared.

FURTHER READING

Brody H. *The Healer's Power*. New Haven, CT: Yale University Press; 1992.

Canda ER, Furman LD. *Spiritual Diversity in Social Work Practice: The Heart of Helping*. New York, New York: Free Press; 1999.

Daaleman TP. Religion, spirituality, and the practice of medicine. *J Am Board Fam Pract*. 2004;17:370–376.

Daaleman TP. Spirituality assessment. In: Murray JL, ed. *AAFP Home Study*. Kansas City, MO: American Academy of Family Physicians; 2005.

Daaleman TP, Williams CS, Hamilton VL, Zimmerman S. Spiritual care at the end of life in long-term care. *Med Care*. 2008;46:85–91.

Fitchett G, Handzo G. Spiritual assessment, screening, and intervention. In: Holland JK, ed. *Psycho-oncology*. New York, New York: Oxford University Press; 1998:790–808.

Giddens A. *Modernity and Self-Identity*. Stanford, CA: Stanford University Press; 1991.

Koenig HG, McCullough ME, Larson DB. *Handbook of Religion and Health*. New York, New York: Oxford University Press; 2001.

Macintyre A. *After Virtue: a Study in Moral Theory*. Notre Dame, IN: University of Notre Dame Press; 1984.

McGinn BG. The letter and the spirit: spirituality as an academic discipline. *J Soc Study Christ Spirituality*. 1993;1:1–10.

Pargament K. *The Psychology of Religion and Coping*. New York, New York: Guilford Press; 1997.

Powell LH, Shahabi L, Thoresen CE. Religion and spirituality. Linkages to physical health. *Am Psychol*. 2003;58(1):36–52.

Senge P. *The Fifth Discipline: the Art and Practice of the Learning Organization*. New York, New York: Doubleday; 1990.

Shea J. *Spirituality and Health Care, Reaching Toward a Holistic Future*. Chicago: The Park Ridge Center; 2000.

Wuthnow R. *After Heaven: Spirituality in America Since 1950*. Berkeley, CA: University of California Press; 1998.

Ethical Issues

Jason H. T. Karlawish ■ *Bryan D. James*

INTRODUCTION

The competent practice of geriatric medicine requires physicians and other clinicians to master both a body of knowledge about how to diagnose and treat geriatric health conditions and an ethic to apply this knowledge to the care of their patients. In general, the ethics of patient care focus on using the principles of respect for autonomy and beneficence. Perhaps, one of the most important mechanisms to apply these principles is informed consent: the voluntary choice of a competent patient. In these respects, geriatrics is just like fields such as cardiology and endocrinology, which have carved out a particular focus of research, education, and practice and share a common ethic to guide the care of patients.

However, geriatrics differs from other fields of medicine in a number of distinct and ethically substantive ways. Most fields are largely organized around an organ system, such as the gastrointestinal system, or around pathology, such as cancer. But geriatrics is organized around a group of persons defined by a label: the elderly. Being elderly does not simply equate to an organ system or pathology. Instead, it describes a stage in a life course, with an indeterminate beginning and features constructed out of a matrix of biological, social, political, and cultural conditions. For example, geriatric patients are often defined as persons aged 65 years and older. This age cutoff, while precise, is constructed out of the legislation that defines eligibility for state or federal retirement and health care benefits.

Of course, all medical practice is, in some manner, bound to social, political, and cultural conditions. For example, concepts of mental illness are influenced by concepts of what is "normal behavior." Geriatricians face the challenge of negotiating the fungible borders between illness and normal aging, and between living and dying. This means that mastery of the common ethic of medicine is necessary, but it is not sufficient. This chapter addresses the ethics of medicine focused on the care of elderly patients. The focus is an ethic that addresses the relationship between the patient and the clinician—informed consent—and particular issues in informed consent that are important for the competent practice of geriatric medicine: diagnostic disclosure, advance care planning, quality of life, refusal of treatment, withdrawal and withholding of treatment, and surrogate decision making. We will also discuss the conditions that underlie decisions: voluntariness and the system of care.

DECIDING WITH PATIENTS

The ethical foundation of making decisions with patients is informed consent: the voluntary choice of a competent patient following adequate disclosure of the relevant facts. Competency is an essential guiding principle to assure that clinicians strike a proper balance between protecting patient autonomy and promoting patient welfare. In other words, competency provides a tool to balance the two ethical principles of respect for autonomy and beneficence. A competent patient should be allowed to choose even if the choice is harmful or "goes against medical advice." In contrast, an incompetent patient is not allowed to choose. This denial of choice is not because the clinician objects to the patient's choice but because the patient cannot make a choice. Chapter 13 defines and discusses how to assess competency and decision-making capacity. The point of this section is to address three challenges in the practice of informed consent.

Informed consent originated largely from surgical cases whose essential theme is as follows. A patient suffers a harm after an intervention such as lower extremity paralysis after an aortic angiogram. The patient argues that when the intervention was agreed on the clinician did not inform about the chance of hemiplegia and had the clinician told about it, the patient would not have agreed to the intervention. From these surgical cases grew an ethical model of informed consent, applicable not only to surgical procedure but to all of medical practice.

The model is that a clinician provides the patient facts about the decision, verifies that the patient has adequate decision-making abilities to use these facts in making a decision, and then practices care based on the patient's choice. This model describes patients who desire information and control over the decision and want their care guided by their values. It is seen as a remedy to a clinician making unilateral decisions for patients based on the clinician's preferences and values, that is, paternalism.

Informed consent is a vital ethic to guide medical care. In certain kinds of decisions, informed consent is useful to facilitate decision making. These include a choice between interventions with very different kinds of risks and benefits (such as surgery vs. medical therapy vs. watchful waiting for prostate cancer), decisions that are highly personal and value laden (such as advance care planning, which is discussed in more detail below), and decisions that are not part of the formal physician–patient relationship (such as enrollment in research). As useful as informed consent is, there are at least three challenges to its practice.

First, informed consent may not be the ethic that a patient wants to follow. Specifically, many patients describe an asymmetry between their desire for information and their desire to make their medical decisions. In particular, elderly patients often indicate that they want their physician to give them information but they want the physician to make the decision. This asymmetry is often greatest in the case of decisions about the management of serious and life-threatening situations. In these cases, patients will describe decision making built on trust and identification with their physician.

The second challenge to the practice of informed consent is effectively communicating medical information. Much of medical information is probabilistic. This means that the occurrence of an event, such as a fall, is bounded by a chance. Such information can be expressed numerically using figures such as an odds ratio or percentage, or qualitatively using expressions such as "rare" or "likely." Each of these presents challenges to the practice of informed consent. People—both patients and clinicians—have difficulty with quantitative expressions. This numerical illiteracy means that people may misunderstand information. Related to this is the ambiguity of qualitative expressions such as "rare," which can mean 1% to one person and 0.001% to another. Finally, biases often influence people's decisions as well as clinicians' communication of information and, thus, should be addressed in the communication of information.

Related to the challenge of communicating medical information is a third challenge: Many patients have impairments in their cognition as a result of geriatric conditions such as dementia and delirium. These impairments can limit a patient's decision-making abilities, specifically the ability to understand, appreciate, and reason through information. Consequently, their capacity to make a decision is impaired to the degree that they are incompetent to make the decision. In these situations, the traditional model of informed consent simply cannot hold. The clinician has to talk to another person, commonly called a proxy or surrogate.

Table 34-1 summarizes these challenges to the practice of informed consent and for each challenge suggests strategies to address them. A general strategy is to reject a "consumer model" of informed consent wherein the patient is the "informed customer" and the clinician a kind of "service provider." A more useful strategy is one grounded in the relationship between physician and patient. In this relationship, doctor means "teacher" (from the Latin *doctore*) and consent means "to feel together" (from the Latin *con* plus *sentire*). Taken together, these concepts mean that the geriatrician's practice should recognize that patients, like students, have different kinds of learning needs and skills.

Some patients are quick studies who take charge of the task, while others need careful tutoring and even prompting. Some simply cannot be taught or do not want to be. In each of these cases, the goal is to create a shared understanding of the relevant facts and the patient's values. These skills are essential for all of medical decision making. The issue is not that some patients are more or less intelligent than others, but that some patients, even very intelligent ones, choose not to control decision making. Below, we discuss additional skills needed to address common challenges to making decisions with older patients: diagnostic disclosure; advance care planning; quality of life; refusing, withdrawing, and withholding treatment; and decisions at the end of life.

Disclosing a Diagnosis of Alzheimer's Disease

In the care of persons with Alzheimer's disease, diagnostic disclosure is an ethically and clinically challenging issue. On the side for disclosure is the argument that patients deserve the truth and to deny this information to them is to deny an adult's right to the truth. The argument against disclosure is that not all truth is good to tell, especially to a person who may be harmed by it. In ethical terms, these competing arguments square off as a dilemma between respecting the principles of autonomy versus beneficence and nonmaleficence. In short, is it better to be honest but risk cruelty or kind but risk paternalism? Two issues resolve this question: a person's capacity and desire to know the diagnosis and the moral challenge that Alzheimer's disease presents to the family of a person diagnosed with it.

One critical step in living with an illness is to understand and appreciate it. Understanding is about knowing the facts. In the case of a person with a chronic illness, it means knowing what the illness is, what stage the patient is at, what to expect in the future, and what can be done to maximize quality of life. In contrast, appreciation describes how well a person recognizes how facts apply to him- or herself. This ability is distinct from understanding because it refers to integrating knowledge into one's sense of self.

In the case of persons with Alzheimer's disease, several studies have shown that many persons with mild-stage Alzheimer's disease can understand information. Although they may not remember it, when taught, they are often able to provide a relatively accurate restatement of the facts when asked to summarize what they have learned. This information ranges from descriptions of clinical trials for Alzheimer's disease and treatments for Alzheimer's disease to issues such as voting.

Appreciation is a complex issue in persons with Alzheimer's disease. It is often mixed. A patient may appreciate one feature of the disease, but not another. In the case of appreciating Alzheimer's disease, there are at least three features: the diagnosis, the severity, and the prognosis. Studies examining appreciation show that patients may appreciate one of these features but not the other. That is, patients may be aware of their diagnosis, but not the severity and prognosis. Or, patients could be aware of the severity and prognosis of their cognitive problems, but not the diagnosis.

These findings suggest that to argue either for or against diagnostic disclosure as the standard of care for the class of persons with very mild-to-moderate Alzheimer's disease oversimplifies the issue. It treats the class of persons indiscriminately when, in fact, patients differ in ethically relevant ways: some know there is something wrong, see that it has gotten worse, and have even figured out or remembered

TABLE 34-1

Common Challenges to the Practice of Informed Consent in Geriatrics and Strategies to Address the Challenge

Challenge #1. A patient wants information but does not want to make own medical decisions

Address information needs

Find out what the patient does know: *"Can you tell me in your own words what you see as the options for your* [fill-in name of medical problem]*?"*

Find out what kinds of information the patient wants to know: *"What else is important for you to know about?"*

Verify that the patients have fulfilled their information needs: "What else [and then pause for a 15 second count]?"

Identify decision-making preferences

Ascertain the patient's decision-making preference. *"Patients are all unique. I want to make sure I do what is right for you. Is this the kind of decision you want to make on your own, with me, or leave it up to me?"*

Other strategies

Address issues that can impact on the legitimacy of the patient's trust. For example, identify and address conflicts of commitment and interest such as serving as a researcher and clinician, ownership of a facility the patient is referred to, and receiving speaking fees from a manufacturer of an intervention the patient is considering.

Challenge #2. Quantitative information is difficult to understand

Numerical illiteracy	In the rare instances when quantitative information is available, present it
Many people do not understand quantitative expressions very well.	using teaching aids such as graphics. For particularly complex decisions
Numerical indeterminacy	or decisions in which patient values significantly can influence the
People attach variable meanings to qualitative expressions of probability such as "rarely" and "likely."	importance of probabilities, use decision aids. Examples of such decisions include the care of low-grade prostate cancer.

Biases

Biases are unintended prejudices or distortions in the way people perceive reality that may introduce error into a decision. They affect both physicians and patients. Biases are best addressed by "debiasing" techniques. Once aware of the potential for the bias, the effective teacher explicitly shows the bias to the patient.

Availability bias—the most recent or salient event determines a person's estimate of the chance of the event.	Identify the availability bias by asking *"Do you know anyone else who faced this decision?"*
Framing bias—the description of event in positive (e.g., chance of cure is 95%) versus negative terms (e.g., chance of no cure is 5%) influences willingness to have the intervention.	The framing bias is best addressed by presenting both sides of probabilistic information. For example, of 100 persons, five will experience the event and 95 will not experience the event.
Representativeness Bias – the chance of an event is evaluated based on how much that event resembles a similar thing without attention to the chance of the event	The representativeness bias occurs when hoofbeats are taken to be the sounds of a zebra instead of a horse (except in Africa). People need to pay attention to the prior probability of an event.

Challenge #3. Patients may have cognitive impairments

The presence of a diagnosis such as dementia does not mean that a patient is not competent. It does increase the likelihood compared to patients who are not demented of being not competent.

Assess the patient's decision-making abilities (see Chapter 13). This skill should be applied to all patients, but in the care of cognitively impaired patients it requires careful practice.

---

that they were told that they have Alzheimer's disease, while others do not.

Diagnostic disclosure depends on the capacity of the persons to understand and appreciate the diagnosis, their expressed desire to know what is wrong, and the emotional and moral impacts that this knowledge may have. Decisions concerning disclosure should also account for the role of the caregivers and the power they hold over the patients. Table 34-2 describes a four-step approach a clinician can use to assess whether and how to disclose a diagnosis of Alzheimer's disease.

Advance Care Planning

Elderly patients often have chronic and ultimately fatal illnesses. The care of patients in the severe-to-terminal stages of these illnesses typically involves decisions that require tradeoffs between different kinds of symptoms, or quality versus quantity of life. The patients are often unable to make decisions. One strategy to make these difficult decisions is to make them in advance when the patient is competent. Advance care planning describes competent patients dis-

cussing and then documenting their preferences for future medical care. This preserves patients' self-determination even after they have lost decision-making capacity. The classic mechanism to do this is an advance directive.

An advance directive is a set of instructions indicating a competent person's preferences for future medical care should the person become incompetent or unable to communicate. Advance directives typically focus on the conditions of being terminal, comatose, or in a state of irreversible suffering. However, there is no reason why an advance directive cannot address periods of incapacity as a result of other conditions, such as the years spent in the moderate-to-terminal stages of dementia or a period of delirium that might follow a planned surgery. There is no reason as well why an advance directive cannot address decisions that are not necessarily tied to a terminal condition. For example, persons whose religious beliefs proscribe the receipt of blood products can have an advance directive that instructs health care providers not to give them a blood transfusion.

There are two types of advance directives: a living will and a durable power of attorney. These are described briefly in Table 34-3, and more in depth in Chapter 32 on legal issues. The Patient

TABLE 34-2

Steps to Disclose a Diagnosis of Alzheimer's Disease*

Step 1. Assess patients' awareness of their cognitive problems:
Are you having problems with your memory or thinking?
What about even a little problem?
Are you noticing problems with remembering a list of items? Remembering the date?
Among patients who have little or no awareness of cognitive problems, diagnostic disclosure is problematic and may need to be skipped.

Step 2. Assess the degree to which patients are bothered by these problems:
Do these problems bother you?
How do you cope with them?
The degree of patient distress over their symptoms helps to guide how they might cope with the diagnosis of Alzheimer's disease, and it also gauges their desire to know the cause of their cognitive problems.

Step 3. Assess patients' desire to know the cause of their memory problems:
Do you want to know what is causing these problems?
This question gives patients the opportunity to express their values about knowing the cause of their cognitive problems. The prior questions lead up to this question in a manner that makes this question relevant.

Step 4. Assess patients' understanding of Alzheimer's disease and their desire to know if they have that disease:
One common cause of memory problems is a disease called Alzheimer's disease. Have you ever heard of that disease? What do you know about it?
Would you want to know if you had that?
As with step 3, these questions give patients the opportunity to express their values about knowing the cause of their cognitive problems. Together with the prior questions, these give the patients several opportunities to not learn their diagnosis and these inform the physician about how well prepared the patients are to learn the diagnosis.

*At the end of these steps the clinician has patient specific data to guide whether to disclose the diagnosis of Alzheimer's disease.

Self-Determination Act (PSDA) is a federal law requiring health care facilities that receive Medicaid and Medicare funds (such as hospitals and nursing homes) to inform patients of their rights to execute advance directives. Many states have template forms based on the specifics of advance directive laws. An advance directive that does not strictly follow such a template is valid in most states. Persons may revoke or change their advance directive at any time. A physician who morally objects to a patient's advance directive may choose not to comply but must facilitate the patient's transfer to another physician.

At their debut, advance directives were hailed as the solution for unnecessary suffering at the end of life, potentially circumventing the inherent dilemma among conflicting views of the right way to care for frail, seriously ill, or dying patients. It was predicted that dilemmas between "the right to die" versus "the right to life" would be avoided because clinicians and patients would plan ahead. But evidence suggests that advance directives have not achieved this goal. Despite efforts to make advance directives more accessible to patients, overwhelming endorsement by major medical and law associations, and patient interest in the discussion of advanced care planning with their physicians, few patients have them. Even when patients do complete advance directives, evidence suggests that these actually may not assure that the patients' wishes are followed. A number of studies show that advance directives have little effect on resuscitation decisions or the use of medical treatments.

There are three major reasons why advance directives have not accomplished their intended goals. First, they have conceptual limitations. Living wills may seem to assure the strictest adherence to a patient's self-determination (e.g., *"I do not want a blood transfusion."*). However, they often apply only to specific scenarios such as "terminal illness" or a "persistent vegetative state." This limited scope means that they can often be the source of uncertainty in other scenarios or if there is disagreement about the patient's current state or prognosis. Living wills may not be specific enough to deal with certain clinical questions that arise. In contrast, a durable power of attorney allows for much greater flexibility, as the surrogate can make decisions should any unforeseen circumstance arise. However, surrogates' preferences may be at odds with the patient's preferences. This suggests that a durable power of attorney may not preserve a patient's true autonomous choice.

A second reason for the limited success is that advance directives fail to follow the patients when they are transferred from institution to institution (such as nursing home to hospital), and most clinicians do not know when their patients have completed advance directives.

A third reason is that patients may not see advance directives as an instrument to assure that their will is carried out. Only one-third of patients who have advance directives indicate that they expect them to be strictly followed. Instead, many patients regard their advance directive as a guide for their care and that decisions should also address what is in their best interests.

Advance directives are only effective in promoting patient control over treatment decisions if the patient, surrogates such as family, and health care professionals all have the same understanding of what the document says and how the patient wants it interpreted. Advance care planning is not intended simply to produce a document. Rather, it should be viewed as a process of discussion and feedback in which the clinician is able to elicit the values and preferences that are important to the patient, and the patient is able to understand, appreciate, and reason through the prognoses and treatment options. Furthermore, approaching advance care planning with a checklist of consent for specific treatments does not meet a patient's needs. Such discussions are valuable only as part of a broader discussion of the patient's values and experiences of the illness. Table 34-4 describes the steps in a discussion about end-of-life care and questions to achieve them. Table 34-5 lists useful questions to guide a discussion about advance care planning.

TABLE 34-3

Advance Directives

Living will
A document describing a patient's preferences for the initiation, continuation, or discontinuation of particular forms of treatment.

Durable power of attorney (DPA), a.k.a., health care proxy
A document that designates a surrogate (also called an "agent," "proxy," or "attorney-in-fact") to make medical decisions on a person's behalf should that person become unable to make a decision.

Recognized in some states: oral statements
Oral statements that arise in conversations with family, friends, and physicians are recognized ethically, and in some states legally, as advance directives, if properly charted in medical records.

TABLE 34-4

Steps to Follow in a Discussion About End-of-Life Care and Questions to Achieve Them

Step 1. Identify the patient's present concerns with attention to both the patient and the family.

What concerns you most about your illness?

How is treatment going for you? What about for your family?

What has been most difficult about this illness for you? What about for your family?

Step 2. Learn the patient's understanding about potential outcomes. Correct any misunderstandings of pertinent facts.

When you think about your illness, what is the best that could happen?

When you think about your illness, what is the worst that could happen?

Step 3. Identify patient's concerns about the future.

What are your hopes for the future?

What are your fears for the future?

As you think about the future, what matters most to you?

Step 4. Identify how the patient conceives quality of life.

If you were dying where would you want to receive medical care? At home? In a hospital? In a hospice?

What makes life worth living?

Step 5. Clarify vague terms.

What do you mean by "being a vegetable?"

Step 6. Identify a proxy decision maker.

If you were to become ill and could not speak for yourself like you are talking with me now, who would you want to speak on your behalf? Who do you trust?

Quality of Life

An overarching theme in discussions about the care of patients with chronic illness is quality of life. The term is often invoked as the best means to assess the outcomes of care or balance of the risks and benefits of treatment options. Quality of life is the substance of what is in the patient's best interests. There are many ways to measure it. These include utility measures such as time tradeoffs, functional measures such as the ability to perform basic activities of daily living, disease-specific measures, symptom severity, or a global measure.

TABLE 34-5

Guidelines for Successful Communication About Advance Care Planning

Treat advance care planning as an ongoing process, not a discrete event.

Shift focus away from completion of documents toward a discussion of values and preferences.

Do not just focus on specific treatments or likely scenarios. This can lead to a false specificity to the directive. Be sure to elicit patients' deeper values and goals and address the more common uncertainty of end-of-life decisions.

Elicit patients' emotions. Patients' emotions and concerns are very important when exploring their goals.

Do not dominate the conversation. Spend at least as much time listening to patients as talking.

Ensure that patients understand the implications of their stated preferences and that you understand their values.

Establish trust that everything possible will be done to meet the patients' goals and to respect how the patients want their autonomy respected.

Scales to measure quality of life are especially useful to guide decisions about how to treat groups of patients. For example, measures of function or global quality of life can inform the clinical significance of clinical trial results or to track the quality of care in a long-term care facility. Measures of quality of life can be useful in clinical practice as well. In clinical practice, these scales can help to assess the overall effect of care on a patient. In this setting, simplicity of measurement is essential. For example, a global rating—"How would you rate your overall quality of life? Would you say poor, fair, good, very good, or excellent?"—followed by an open-ended question to explain the choice is a useful way to determine how a patient is doing and what matters to the patient.

Refusing, Withdrawing, and Withholding Treatment

In the United States, patients have an ethical and legal right to refuse life-sustaining treatments including artificial nutrition and hydration. Surrogates have a similar right, but, in some states, they must achieve a standard of evidence to support that the decision reflects what the patient would have wanted. Specifically, in some states, strict evidentiary standards govern the decision about artificial nutrition. In other words, a surrogate cannot refuse or withdraw artificial nutrition based on what is in the patient's best interests but only on the basis of a well-documented substituted judgment. Geriatricians who practice in these states have a clear warrant to discuss these issues with patients and family members.

Some clinicians are comfortable accepting a patient's or surrogate's refusal of treatment before it is initiated, yet find themselves ethically opposed to withdrawing the treatment after it is initiated. The distinction between withholding and withdrawing treatment is understandable psychologically, but it lacks both ethical and legal justification. The concept of this distinction relies heavily on the feeling that withholding is an act of omission, not performing an action, while withdrawing is an instance of commission, performing an action. Withholding a procedure is often seen as wisely abstaining from subjecting the patient to an overly invasive intervention. Conversely, withdrawing a treatment already initiated can give the clinician a sense of responsibility for action bringing about the patient's death and can be regarded as an act of abandonment or breach of expectations or promises.

However, both starting and stopping treatment can be justified depending on the circumstances. Both can *cause* the death of a patient and both can *allow* the patient to die. In the cases of both withholding and withdrawing treatment according to a patient's wishes or best interests, it is the underlying illness that is the cause of death, not the clinician's actions. Moreover, the distinction's reliance on the difference between omission and commission is ambiguous. Withdrawing can happen through an omission such as not putting the infusion into a feeding tube, and withholding the next stage of treatment can be viewed as stopping treatment (i.e., withdrawing). Crimes and moral wrongs can be committed through omission as well as commission. The more important concern is whether a patient or proxy has granted an informed consent.

Euthanasia, Physician-Assisted Suicide, and Terminal Sedation

The physician's role at the end of life is no longer to cure or control the patient's illness but to provide adequate relief of pain and suffering.

Comprehensive palliative care is the standard of care for the dying. This includes adequate pain and symptom management, support for the patient and family, and the opportunity to achieve meaningful closure to life. Unfortunately, situations may arise in which standard management efforts fail to control pain and suffering. Sometimes patients may ask to die to relieve their suffering. At this point, the clinician's dual obligations of beneficence and nonmaleficence come into conflict. There are a number of options available to the geriatrician at this point, some of which are not accepted as the standard of care and are illegal in some states.

Euthanasia is the act of a physician ending the life of a patient having terminal illness or an incurable disease. The physician acts directly in bringing about the patient's death, such as injecting a lethal dose of drugs. This practice raises strong objections. When it is done to a noncompetent patient, it can be called "murder." When it is done to a competent patient, it remains controversial because many argue it violates core physician duties. Euthanasia is currently illegal throughout the United States. Physician-assisted suicide is the act of providing a lethal dose of medication to a patient to self-administer. Thus, the physician is a necessary instrument but does not actively take part in the ending of the patient's life. This practice is currently legal in only a handful of countries; in the United States, it is illegal in all states except for Oregon. Terminal sedation is the act of administering high-dose medication to relieve extremes of pain and suffering. As the name implies, the patient is sedated to unconsciousness (sedation), and this practice may hasten the death of the patient (terminal) by the impairment of respiratory function. Terminal sedation properly done is distinct from both assisted suicide and euthanasia. Medication doses are increased until sedation occurs (along with the possible risk of the hastening of death) only if nonsedating doses do not achieve pain relief. Also, the dose of medication is maintained but not increased once sedation occurs, and no further intervention, such as a muscle-paralyzing agent, is given to hasten the onset of death. The purpose of terminal sedation is *not* the death of the patient, but the relief of overwhelming physical suffering. The desired and expected benefit of pain relief is significant enough to warrant the risk of hastening death. Terminal sedation is legal throughout the United States.

DECIDING WITH OTHERS: SURROGATE DECISION MAKING

A common scenario in the practice of geriatric medicine is the following: The patient is not competent but either does not have an advance directive or has one but the directive is not a useful guide. This may be the case because the patient's condition does not meet the terms described in the directive (for example, the patient is not terminal) or the patient indicated that his or her best interests should be part of the decision. In these situations, who decides and how that person should decide invoke issues of surrogate decision making.

The immediate response of most clinicians is to talk to the patient's family. In some states, the law endorses this and describes an ordered list of the kinds of persons who can make decisions, such as the spouse, then adult children, then adult siblings, and so on. In some states, the family is proscribed from making certain kinds of decisions. For example, in New York, the family cannot withdraw or refuse artificial nutrition or hydration for a patient who lacks an advance directive that permits that. Finally, in the majority of states,

the law is simply silent as to who can make decisions for a noncompetent patient. This is the case in the vast majority of medical decisions, for example, the choice of treatments, or whether a patient can benefit from rehabilitation. In clinical situations in which the law does not direct medical practice (which is, fortunately, most of medicine), a physician should practice usual and customary medical practice. In the case of medical decision making for noncompetent patients, this means talking to the family.

In general, surrogates should be treated in much the same way as patients. However, there are unique conditions that guide surrogate decision making. Surrogate decision makers should use the patient's preferences to the extent that these are known. Using a patient's previously disclosed preferences to make medical decisions for that patient is called a substituted judgment. Substituted judgments are intended to preserve the patient's autonomy after the patient is not competent to make a choice. However, in many cases, the patient's preferences are unknown, or, because of significant changes in the patient's health and well-being, these are not relevant to the decision at hand. In these circumstances, the guide for surrogate decision makers becomes the patient's dignity and quality of life. This standard of decision making is called the best-interests standard, as the surrogate must assess the risks and benefits of various treatments and alternatives to treatment and choose the one that best maximizes the patient's quality of life.

Western bioethics argues that the best-interests standard should only be used when the patient's preferences are unknown or irrelevant to a particular decision. However, substituted judgments may not be legitimate expressions of patients' autonomous choices. Multiple studies have shown surrogate decision makers to be only slightly better than random chance at predicting patient preferences. This evidence has been used as evidence against the moral authority of surrogate decision makers. But this criticism, based on a strict focus on substituted judgments, misses the strengths of surrogate decision making. For many patients, their relationships with their loved ones are more important than specific decisions, and placing the process of end-of-life decision making within these relationships can offer a great sense of control. Many patients realize that they cannot anticipate every circumstance of dying, but they can assure that the people who love them and care for them will be there to make these difficult decisions when the patients no longer can. Patients generally want their surrogate decision makers to use their judgment rather than be bound by the specifics of living wills.

Surrogate decision making is among the most fulfilling challenges of geriatric medicine. Consider the case of Mrs. A with profound-stage Alzheimer's disease. Her husband and her daughter are faced with a tough choice about the management of recurrent aspiration pneumonia. One key strategy to effective decision making is to make sure that everyone shares a common story about the patient's diagnosis and prognosis. Open-ended questions are a useful way to determine how each person understands or misunderstands the progression and prognosis of the patient's illness. In addition, the clinician should screen for depression and related emotional disorders. These are common among caregivers of chronically ill people and can influence how they assess the patient's quality of life. The clinician should explain to a depressed caregiver how this can impact on how the caregiver perceives the patient's situation. One of the most common consequences of depression is that people fail to see options (in the extreme, this leads to suicidal ideation). Sharing the insight about the impact of depression on decisions may help the

TABLE 34-6

Guide to Facilitating Surrogate Decision Making

GUIDING PRINCIPLES	ETHICAL BASIS
Substituted judgment	Deciding based on patient's previously stated preferences. Ethical basis: autonomy.
Best interests	Deciding based on patient's dignity and quality of life. Ethical basis: beneficence. Usually used when patient preferences are unknown.
Combination	Patients often want loved ones to use their judgment rather than be bound by specifics of living will.
STRATEGIES	**REPRESENTATIVE QUOTES/OPEN-ENDED QUESTIONS**
Allow surrogate to narrate how the patient has come to this stage of illness and elicit his or her understanding of diagnosis and prognosis.	"I know you've been though a lot with [name of patient] Mrs. A., what's your understanding of how [he/she] got to this point and what is wrong now?"
Teach the decision makers about the expected clinical course of the patient's disease.	The following is an example of how to communicate the judgment that a patient is dying: "[Name of patient] has an incurable, progressive, and ultimately fatal disease. I can't say for certain when [she/he] will die of [his/her] Alzheimer's disease, but given its severity, we shouldn't be surprised when it does."
Screen for depression and related emotional disorders. Explain how these can impact decision making.	"Many people caring for a person like your relative feel sad and worry that this affects how they think about what to do for their relative. Is this something you've felt?"
Decisions should be based on (1) the patient's preferences and (2) a balance of the burdens and benefits of each option in terms of relieving suffering and maximizing dignity and quality of life.	"As you think about the options for your relative., a useful guide in making a choice is to focus on what [he/she] would have wanted, and to make sure that we maximize [his/her] dignity and quality of life."
Provide guidance on basis of existing data and clinical experience.	The following is an example of communication about enteral feeding in persons with neurogenic dysphagia: "For patients like your relative, feeding with a tube does not significantly reduce the risk for pneumonia. On the basis of my experience, a speech therapist can give us some useful hints on ways to feed her that will allow her to continue to eat by mouth."

family member to see the other side. Once there is a common understanding about the patient, it is useful to give the surrogates guidance on how to make the decision. A useful guide is to invoke simultaneously both the principles of substituted judgment and best-interests to assure that Mrs. A's preferences as well as quality of life are respected. These strategies and representative quotes and open-ended questions to guide surrogate decision making are listed in Table 34-6.

DECIDING TOGETHER: LIVING AND WORKING IN HEALTH CARE SYSTEMS

The issues discussed in this chapter largely address the ethics of interacting with patients and their proxies. Informed consent, instruments such as advance directives, and ethical and legal consensus on matters of refusing treatments (including nutrition and hydration) all have an implicit message: maximizing patient choice will maximize the quality of their care. However, attempts to maximize patient choice may do little to actually affect patient care. For example, the Study to Understand Prognoses and Preferences for Outcomes and Risks of Treatments, a 2-year trial, which randomly assigned 4804 seriously ill patients to either "usual care" or an intervention arm to promote communication between patients and clinicians, found no difference between the treatment and control groups in any of the following outcome measures: incidence and timing of do-not-resuscitate orders; patient–physician agreement on preferences for cardiopulmonary resuscitation; days in ICU, in coma, or in ventilated state before death; pain; and hospital resource use.

These results suggest that facilitating communication and disseminating information about options for care may not be sufficient to improve patient choice. Instead, we must be cognizant of the conditions that either enable or constrain a patient's ability to choose or for those choices to influence care. A host of institutional factors influence a patient's choices and the provision of care in adherence to these choices. In particular, the voluntariness of a choice can be limited. This is especially true in the care of patients with chronic illness because they develop a long-term interdependence with health care. Nursing homes are, perhaps, the best example of this. Here, the borders between where older persons live and receive health care are indistinct. In this kind of total institution, freedom of choice can be elusive. Instead, resources such as unoccupied nursing home beds, the number of area hospitals, and the institution's tacit culture and attitudes establish the boundaries of permissible choices.

The individual geriatrician who cares for patients may feel powerless in the face of institutional factors. Institutions are slow to change. When they do change, it is largely a political as opposed to a scientific process. And even when science is the chosen instrument of change, medicine's fascination with the randomized controlled trial as the "gold standard" to establish whether an intervention works leaves geriatricians in a bind. Much of geriatrics involves caring for complex patients. It is difficult to control for all factors and still measure clinically significant changes on meaningful end points. In addition, randomized trials are difficult to apply to interventions at the level of an institution. These difficulties include blinding/masking subjects and researchers and selecting what to randomize (the subjects, different wards, or the institution).

TABLE 34-7

Options for Improving Medical Care

1. *Implementing changes without measurement*
   Least desirable for obvious reasons: changed based on theory alone; no measurement of outcomes or definitive proof that change is an improvement.
   Example: Asking nursing home staff to get patients to make decision-specific living wills.
2. *Formal studies with experimental designs, i.e., randomized controlled trials (RCTs)*
   These forms of scientific investigation can lead to large-scale changes in medical care. However, these are often not useful for change at the local level. These require a large investment in resources—time, money, large sample sizes, and disruption of daily patient care—and these may not be feasible.
   Example: A randomized controlled trial of "usual care" versus an intervention with a trained nurse facilitator to improve communication, decision making, and treatment patterns (e.g., the Study to Understand Prognoses and Preferences for Outcomes and Risks of Treatments study).
3. *Quality improvement through plan–do–study–act (PDSA) cycles*
   Short, small-scale tests of change of procedure. Very useful for improving local systems with their own special conditions. Allows for small cycles of change based on measurement and reflection that can cumulatively lead to large-scale improvement. Quality improvement is particularly useful when the intervention has been shown to work, using techniques such as a randomized and controlled trial.
   Example: Staff at a long-term care facility jointly identify barriers to advance care planning; they then design interventions to address these barriers, and, after a cycle of intervention, they reassess rates of advance directive completion and discussions.

But there is a way to affect change in an institution that respects political realities as well as scientific rigor: quality improvement. In this model, a community such as a nursing home or an inpatient geriatrics unit sets clear goals, plans an intervention to achieve them, assesses the response, and reevaluates the intervention. This model of plan, do, study, and act can galvanize a system to change. Table 34-7 discusses how plan, do, study, and act cycles can be useful in the quality improvement of medical care systems.

CONCLUSION

The central focus of much of western Bioethics is a concern with equalizing the power between physician and patient. In this model, "paternalism" is a wrong, and ethical dilemmas are largely framed as a tension between autonomy and beneficence. Informed consent directs clinicians to "empower" their patients to be "informed consumers of health care." It is no accident that this ethic gained popularity in the free-market models of fee for service and man-aged health care. It is a useful way to conduct cosmetic medicine. But it is simply bizarre to consider an 83-year-old frail woman with mild dementia who resides in a nursing home as someone we should assume wants to be treated like a customer who makes medical decisions according to a hyperrational utility maximizing process of decision making. And yet, we cannot imagine that the values of a young clinician who sees her once a month and the culture of a busy and highly regulated long-term care facility should determine this woman's care. For these kinds of patients, the clinician and the system's duty is to promote the patient's independence guided by her abilities and values.

FURTHER READING

Albert SM, Logsdon RG. *Assessing Quality of Life in Alzheimer's Disease.* New York, New York: Columbia University Press; 2000.

Beauchamp TL, Childress JF. *Principles of Biomedical Ethics.* 4th ed. New York, New York, Oxford: Oxford University Press; 1994.

Berwick DM. Developing and testing changes in delivery of care. *Ann Intern Med.* 1998;128:651–656.

Bok S. Death and dying: euthanasia and sustaining life: ethical views. In: Reich WT, ed. *Encyclopedia of Bioethics.* Vol. 1. New York, New York: Free Press; 1978:268–278.

Cole TR. *The Journey of Life. A Cultural History of Aging in America.* New York, New York: Cambridge University Press; 1992.

Faden RR, Beauchamp TL. *Part III. A Theory of Informed Consent: A History and Theory of Informed Consent.* New York, New York: Oxford University Press; 1986:235–381.

Fischer GS, Arnold RM, Tulsky JA. Talking to the older adult about advance directives. *Clin Geriatr Med.* 2000;16:239–254.

Gunter-Hunt G, Mahoney JE, Sieger CE. A comparison of state advance directive documents. *Gerontologist.* 2002;42:51–60.

Kahneman D, Slovic P, Tversky A. *Judgment Under Uncertainty: Heuristics and Biases.* Cambridge: Cambridge University Press; 1982.

Karlawish JHT, Quill T, Meier DE. A consensus-based approach to practicing palliative care for patients who lack decision-making capacity. *Ann Intern Med.* 1999;130:835–840.

Karlawish JHT, Casarett D, Klocinski J, et al. The relationship between caregivers' global ratings of Alzheimer's disease patients' quality of life, disease severity and the caregiving experience. *J Am Geriatr Soc.* 2001;49:1066–1070.

Lo B, Quill T, Tulsky J. Discussing palliative care with patients. ACP-ASIM End-of-Life Care Consensus Panel. American College of Physicians-American Society of Internal Medicine. *Ann Intern Med.* 1999;130:744–749.

Lynn J, Arkes HR, Stevens M, et al. Rethinking fundamental assumptions: SUPPORT's implications for future reform. *J Am Geriatr Soc.* 2000;48:S214–S221.

Lynn J, De Vries KO, Arkes HR, et al. Ineffectiveness of the SUPPORT intervention: review of explanations. *J Am Geriatr Soc.* 2000;48:S206–S213.

Prendergast TJ. Advance care planning: pitfalls, progress, promise. *Crit Care Med.* 2001;29:N34–N39.

Puchalski CM, Zhong Z, Jacobs MM, et al. Patients who want their family and physician to make resuscitation decisions for them: observations from SUPPORT and HELP. Study to Understand Prognoses and Preferences for Outcomes and Risks of Treatment. Hospitalized Elderly Longitudinal Project. *J Am Geriatr Soc.* 2000;48:S84–S90.

Sehgal A, Galbraith A, Chesney M, et al. How strictly do dialysis patients want their advance directive followed? *JAMA.* 1992;267:59–63.

Snyder L, Caplan A. *Assisted Suicide. Finding Common Ground.* Bloomington: Indiana University Press; 2002.

Sulmasy DP, Terry PB, Weisman CS, et al. The accuracy of substituted judgements in patients with terminal diagnoses. *Ann Intern Med.* 1998;128:621–629.

Tulsky JA, Fischer GS, Rose MR, et al. Opening the black box: how do physicians communicate about advance directives? *Ann Intern Med.* 1998;129:441–449.

Perioperative Evaluation and Management

Preeti N. Malani ■ *Peter V. Vaitkevicius* ■ *Mark B. Orringer*

THE OLDER SURGICAL PATIENT

The progressive aging of the American population is challenging the surgical and medical communities with an expanding group of patients who will require surgical interventions much later in life. In coming years, our health care system will continue to be stressed by the need to provide surgical care that not only prolongs life but also promotes the greatest level of functional independence for older patients, without an excessive risk of complications. Among the most frequently performed surgical procedures in this age group are hip repairs, cataract extractions, coronary artery bypass grafting, cholecystectomies, and hernia repairs.

When factors influencing postoperative complications are examined, chronologic age remains an independent risk for adverse surgical outcomes. Advancing age is a marker for significant medical comorbidities that can complicate surgical procedures. The age-associated reduction in the capacity to adapt to stress, a progression in functional frailty, and the number of comorbid illnesses are better predictors than age alone for doing poorly with the rigors of surgery. In addition to increasing operative risk, these factors also prolong recovery times, promote postoperative functional declines, and increase the need for rehabilitation, nursing, and home care support after surgery. Therefore, a comprehensive review of each patient's medical, social, cognitive, and functional status is paramount. Whenever possible, the preoperative clinical assessment should include a discussion with the primary-care physician. The primary-care physician typically has the greatest experience with the patient and is often able to provide useful insights, such as history of developing delirium during hospitalizations, which prove useful in guiding the older patient through surgery. The availability of high-quality geriatric medical care is also essential. A lack of communication between the surgical and the medical providers is a frequent reason why important clinical issues are overlooked, concerns that may have an adverse impact on the older patient's perioperative care. Formal "co-management" approaches have emerged, which involve both medi-

cal and surgical specialists in the perioperative period and appear to improve overall quality of care, including decreased length of stay. The critical nature of the transition between in- and outpatient and subacute care has been recognized as an important area for quality improvement at many institutions.

Because the medical and surgical managements of older patients often overlap, a comprehensive review of the medical and surgical goals and any ethical implications should be routinely completed. The primary goal of surgery is to maximize the life span of these patients in a manner that ensures dignity, self-esteem, and independent function; limits suffering and pain; and occasionally palliates adverse clinical symptoms. To accomplish these goals, an ongoing dialogue between medical and surgical providers is essential.

HOW AGE INCREASES SURGICAL RISK

The effect of age on risk of surgery is reviewed in Chapter 37. An effort to identify reversible factors associated with perioperative morbidity in geriatric surgical patients is critical to improving surgical outcomes (Table 35-1). In patients older than 80 years, the most prevalent operative risk factors are a history of hypertension, coronary artery disease (CAD), impaired pulmonary function, and prior neurologic events. In one study of older patients, the only intraoperative event predicting a postoperative complication was the use of vasoactive agents. Twenty-five percent of these patients developed neurologic, cardiovascular, or pulmonary complications. Intraoperative events were less important than preoperative comorbidities in predicting adverse postoperative outcomes.

One example of how age increases operative risk is the age-associated changes in cardiac physiology. Primarily as a result of a loss of vascular compliance, the left ventricle demonstrates an increase in stiffness, impaired diastolic relaxation, and an increase in filling pressures. These changes make the ventricle less tolerant of shifts in intravascular volume. An acute increase in volume (e.g.,

TABLE 35-1

Physiological Changes of Aging and Effects on Perioperative Care

SYSTEM	CHANGE	SIGNIFICANCE
General	↓ Skeletal muscle mass ↓ Thermoregulation	Altered volume of distribution Potential drug toxicity Greater frailty ↓ Functional recovery
Skin	↓ Reepithelialization ↓ Dermal blood vessels	↓ Rate of wound healing
Cardiac	↑ Vascular stiffness ↑ Ventricular stiffness Conduction system degeneration Valvular degeneration ↓ Maximal heart rate Cardiopulmonary deconditioning ↑ Prevalence of coronary artery disease	↑ Blood pressure and ventricular vascular load Hypertension Ventricular hypertrophy ↑ Sensitivity to volume shifts ↓ Heart rate response ↑ Risk of high grade arteriovenous blocks ↑ Risk of myocardial ischemia
Pulmonary	↓ Elastic recoil ↑ Chest wall stiffness ↑ V/Q mismatch ↓ Airway protections	↑ Potential for respiratory failure, (e.g., sedative drugs) ↑ Risk of aspiration and infections
Renal	↓ Number of nephrons ↓ Decreased sodium and water excretion Prostatic hypertrophy	↓ Half-life of drugs cleared by the kidney ↑ Risk for fluid overload ↓ Retention and infection risk
Immune	↓ Immune function	↑ Risk of infections
Hepatic	↓ Blood flow ↓ Microsomal oxidation	↑ Half-life for drugs cleared by the liver
Endocrine	Insulin resistance Impaired insulin secretion	Hyperglycemia

from intravenous fluids administered during surgery) leads to a further increase in left ventricular filling pressures and could result in pulmonary congestion as a consequence of the age-related increase in diastolic stiffness. Conversely, an acute loss of intravascular volume, such as the third spacing of fluid or intraoperative blood loss, reduces preload to the stiffened ventricle and could produce a marked reduction in systolic blood pressure. CAD, a common comorbidity, increases the risk associated with these adverse age effects. Adding the intraoperative burden of myocardial ischemia to the already impaired diastolic relaxation leads to a further worsening of ventricular filling pressures and increases the risk of pulmonary edema.

Altered renal and hepatic drug metabolisms place the older patient at a greater risk of perioperative drug toxicities. A previously unrecognized disorder of cognitive function may cause an older person to decline substantially with the stress of surgery. Such a decline may present atypically, such as the development of an acute confusional episode or frank delirium. Adverse changes in cognitive function will often prolong a hospital stay and worsen clinical outcomes. Significant age- and disease-related reductions in skeletal muscle mass (sarcopenia) decrease the capacity of the older patient to make a functional recovery, possibly resulting in a discharge to a subacute or long-term care facility.

The older patient may be unable to adequately communicate concerns or clinical history to a health care provider. Therefore, to ensure the best possible surgical outcome for the older patient, it may be necessary to maximize the communication and exchange of data between the surgical team and the medical providers. Clinical programs that have fostered a closer relationship between the surgeon and the consulting internist or geriatrician have demonstrated a trend for better surgical outcomes and greater functional recoveries. Several groups within the academic community are promoting comprehensive programs to increase geriatric expertise in the surgical and medical specialties by direct education of the surgical and consulting teams in the principles of geriatric medical care. These efforts are likely to further improve operative outcomes for older patients.

In summary, because normal aging does not account for the bulk of operative risk, the clinician's task is to identify underlying illnesses in older surgical patients and assess their impact on perioperative risk. Teamwork and communication between the various services are critical to promoting the best possible understanding of the patient's clinical situation, helping to mitigate surgical risk.

SPECIFIC CONSIDERATIONS

Cardiac Complications

CAD is highly prevalent in older populations and remains the primary cause of death for the elderly patient. An estimated 25% to 30% of all perioperative deaths are attributed to cardiac causes. Because older adults are more likely to have significant CAD, these patients should be carefully screened for signs and symptoms of occult or overt disease. As previously noted, the age-associated increases in vascular and left ventricular stiffness result in a greater sensitivity to volume shifts. Age-related declines in the electrical conduction system place the elderly patient at a greater a risk of drug-induced bradycardia or high-grade atrioventricular blocks. A history of prior myocardial infarction or a low ejection fraction is associated with a greater risk of ventricular tachycardia.

Pulmonary Complications

With advancing age, the respiratory system demonstrates several changes in function, which may include a loss of pulmonary elastic recoil, decreased diffusion capacity, and reduced cough and gag reflexes, as a consequence of either neurological injury or respiratory muscle weakness. Postoperatively, it is common for older patients to experience atelectasis or frank aspiration. An estimated 14% of older patients will have a major pulmonary perioperative complication (pneumonia, pulmonary edema, or a pulmonary embolus), particularly after an abdominal or a cardiothoracic procedure. Postoperative pneumonia in older patients is associated with a 15% to 20% mortality rate and must be treated with aggressive respiratory therapy and appropriate antimicrobials. A detailed pulmonary and occupational exposure history prior to surgery can help predict impaired respiratory function. Because neurological events that may impair airway protection are occasionally subtle, obtaining a history of swallowing difficulties or prior aspiration may prompt an early start to postoperative interventions aimed at reducing aspiration risk.

Renal Complications

Renal function is reduced as a result of glomerular and tubular senescence. The progressive sclerosis of glomeruli that occurs with increasing age is typically hastened by comorbid conditions like hypertension, diabetes mellitus, and CAD. In the older patient, the serum creatinine often does not fully reflect the reduction in renal function. The age-associated reduction in skeletal muscle reduces creatinine production, so a reduced creatinine clearance is not always as apparent, even in the setting of diminished filtration. There is greater risk for volume and pH disturbances in the perioperative period because of baseline renal insufficiency. Medications and use of contrast dye can also contribute to renal toxicity.

Infectious Complications

Postoperative infectious complications represent a major source of morbidity and mortality for older adults. In addition, the development of a surgical site infection or other health care-acquired infection can substantially increase length of stay and associated health care costs. The extended use of indwelling devices, prolonged ventilation, and length of stay are important risk factors for postoperative infections. Infections associated with devices and prosthetic material can present unique treatment challenges. The treatment of significant infections often requires extended courses of parenteral and/or oral antimicrobial therapy, which can raise issues related to safety and tolerability of antimicrobial agents, including nephrotoxicity. Prolonged need for antimicrobials can also contribute to the development of *Clostridium difficile*-associated disease, which is frequently severe in older adults.

Functional Capacity

Functional impairment is an index of the severity of many chronic diseases, and its severity predicts operative risk to some degree.

For example, poor performance on a bicycle ergometer is a better predictor than the Goldman criteria of surgical outcomes and postoperative pulmonary complications. The metabolic demand of surgery and the physical immobility associated with recovery may promote further declines in strength and function. Not infrequently, a previously independent older adult can become so frail postoperatively that rehabilitative care is needed. Promoting clinical services that increase physical activity and rehabilitation during the surgical recovery process may improve the level of functional independence, shorten recovery times, and prevent readmissions. Postoperatively, the "transitional" care plan must be seamless. Some patients also benefit from referral to a formal cardiac rehabilitation program.

Emergency Surgeries

While emergency surgeries are associated with a higher overall death rate in all age groups, this finding is most apparent in older patients who have the highest rates as a consequence of a greater number of complications. The causes for the increased risk are multifactorial. The identical surgical disease in the elderly patient may present later in its course, and diagnosis can be delayed because of an atypical presentation. Also, the elderly patient may be treated later by surgeons wishing to correct the associated comorbidities prior to surgery. In the older patient, a delay in a needed nonemergent surgery may have a greater risk if there is a chance that the delay could result in an emergent procedure. Therefore, clinicians should be aware that if the time needed to optimize the patient for surgery is extended, an anticipated elective procedure could become a higher mortality emergent procedure.

Other Concerns

A neurologic event, such as a stroke, may increase the risk of aspiration by making it difficult to swallow, to move food through the esophagus, and to control respiratory secretions. Advancing age is also associated with a decrease in esophageal peristaltic wave amplitude, reduced tone of the lower esophageal sphincter, a greater incidence of hiatal hernias, delayed gastric emptying, and increased gastroesophageal reflux. All are factors that may increase the perioperative aspiration risk. Age-associated changes in the immune system are subtle but may contribute to a greater risk for infection from organisms that colonize the pulmonary and urinary tracts. Impaired glucose regulation and risk for stress hyperglycemia are common in this age group and may increase infection risks. Thus, careful monitoring to control blood sugars perioperatively may have important benefits. Pressure ulcers are another important postoperative complication (see Chapter 58). Age-related changes in mobility and sensation can contribute to breakdown of skin integrity. Aggressive preventative measures including frequent assessment and pressure unloading are essential aspects of postoperative management.

Taking the time to discuss the surgery with the older patients and their families promotes a clearer understanding of risk and benefits and will help to reduce the chance of false expectations with surgery. Incorporating the common geriatric care format of patient and family conferences in the surgical environment can be very helpful. In such discussions, it is often apparent that an older patient has a different outlook and acceptance of a specific level of care. Shorter-term goals, such as the quality, not quantity, of life may be most important. Additionally, the tolerance of surgery may be different than that of a younger person. The understanding that a longer time to recover may be necessary is often best communicated in this forum. It is also important to inform the patient and family that an intermediate-care program may be needed, such as a subacute care center, a rehabilitation unit, or the extended use of home care services.

Period of Risk

Anesthesia is generally considered a safe procedure in elderly patients, with a progressive decline in complication rates being observed in recent years (see Chapter 36). Preoperative risk factors are a better predictor of 7-day mortality than is the duration of anesthesia or the experience of the anesthesiologist. The type of anesthesia (e.g., spinal vs. inhalational) fails to predict outcomes once the preoperative risk factors are controlled. The greatest period of risk for complications remains the time after surgery, with half of adverse events occurring within 3 weeks of surgery.

PREOPERATIVE MANAGEMENT

History and Physical

The accurate assessment of risk begins with a detailed review of the clinical history and physical examination. This comprehensive review guides the patient along the various algorithms and directs the selection of preoperative testing. Underlying decline in cognitive function is an essential aspect of the risk assessment of the older patient and may reduce the validity of reported signs and symptoms. A discussion with family members should be sought if clinical data are unclear, cognitive impairment is profound, or the responses are misleading.

The assessment should include a review of physical function, cognitive ability, competency, availability of social support, and symptoms of depression. Cognitive impairment places the patient at an increased risk of perioperative delirium and a longer hospital course. Elderly patients should be screened for impairments using the mini-mental state examination or similar standardized screening instrument. An elderly patient with little family or social support who undergoes surgery is likely to have a protracted recovery period. Therefore, a preoperative evaluation by a social worker with experience in geriatric medicine is helpful in structuring a supportive network of resources that will reduce complications during the recovery process. Subacute nursing care facilities may play a particularly helpful role in advancing the frail older patient through the recovery process and back to independence. Many institutions have active geriatrics consult services, which can provide detailed guidance on discharge planning issues.

The physical examination can be altered by age and disease. For example, a systolic ejection murmur suggesting aortic stenosis may represent aortic valve sclerosis rather than a hemodynamically significant valvular stenosis. Additionally, markers of severe aortic stenosis, a diminished S2, or a delay in the carotid up-stroke may be less apparent in older patients. When the examination is uncertain, echocardiography and Doppler studies are warranted to establish an accurate cardiac diagnosis, particularly if the murmur is late peaking or radiating to the carotids.

Medications

The preoperative examination is an ideal time to review medication lists and to determine the overall benefit of these drugs for the patient. Aspirin, clopidogrel, nonsteroidals, and other antiplatelet drugs increase the risk of perioperative bleeding and, if not essential, should be held for a recommended 7 to 10 days. Drugs with anticholinergic properties, such as diphenhydramine or meclizine, are likely to increase the risk of perioperative delirium and should be held. Chronic benzodiazepine use is common and often under-recognized. These drugs should be tapered to reduce the risk of withdrawal symptoms when the patient is made NPO (nothing by mouth). Holding diuretics for 24 to 48 hours prior to surgery should be considered if these are not needed to treat excessive volume or symptoms of pulmonary congestion in patients with congestive heart failure.

Patients on antiepileptic, cardiovascular, and antihypertensive medications typically should take their medications on the morning of surgery with limited amounts of water. Abrupt discontinuation of beta-blockers and clonidine is associated with significant cardiovascular complications. Patients using these medications can be effectively managed with intravenous propranolol, metoprolol, or transcutaneous clonidine patches. Oral hypoglycemics are generally held the night prior to surgery, to reduce the risk of perioperative hypoglycemia. Insulin-treated diabetic patients typically receive half of their usual dose of intermediate-acting insulin on the morning of surgery and are typically given appropriate amounts of a 5% dextrose solution intravenously, based on blood glucose monitoring. Postoperative glucose above 250 mg/dL is safely managed with subcutaneous insulin or short-acting intravenous infusions of insulin, if hemodynamic instability is present (a cause of variable absorption of subcutaneous insulin). Recent data suggest that tight glucose control in the perioperative period may help decrease risk of surgical site infection, especially related to cardiac procedures. If tight glucose control is chosen, comanagement with a diabetes care team is recommended. Adrenal suppression resulting from chronic steroid use should be treated with stress doses of a steroid, typically 100 mg of hydrocortisone every 6 hours beginning the night prior to surgery and tapering to the maintenance dose in 3 to 5 days, as is permitted by their postoperative course.

Preoperative Assessment for Noncardiac Surgery

As 25% to 30% of perioperative deaths are attributed to cardiac causes, much of the risk assessment is focused on predicting these cardiac complications. The poor surgical performance of the older patient reflects the high prevalence of CAD, which is often subtle or even silent until the stress of surgery. The current American College of Cardiology and American Heart Association (ACC/AHA) guidelines are a rapidly applied algorithm, which is helpful in assessing risk and directing appropriate preoperative testing and management (Figures 35-1 to 35-3). The Coronary Artery Revascularization Prophylaxis trial used a randomized design to compare preoperative revascularization (either percutaneous coronary intervention or coronary artery bypass grafting) versus medical therapy in patients with stable coronary disease undergoing major vascular surgery. The results suggest that preoperative revascularization does not

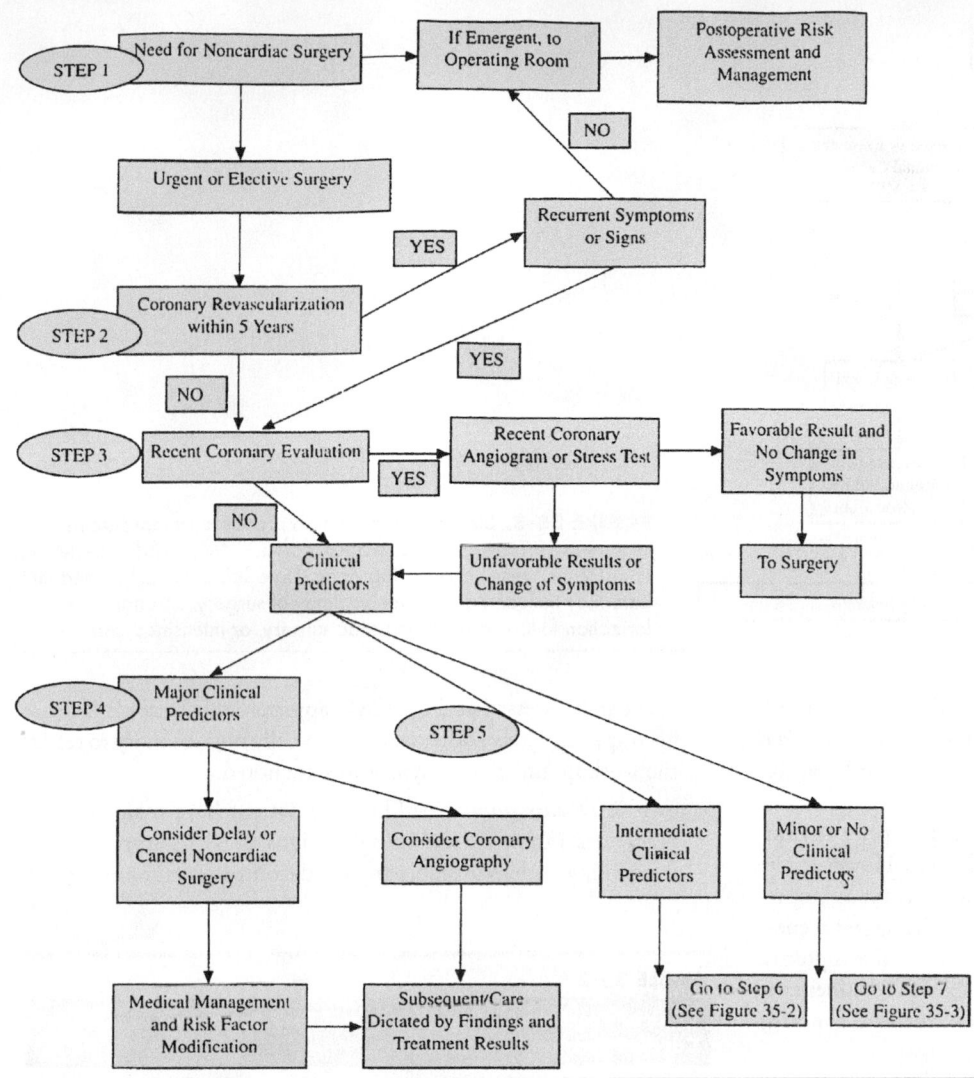

FIGURE 35-1. Stepwise approach to preoperative cardiac risk assessment.

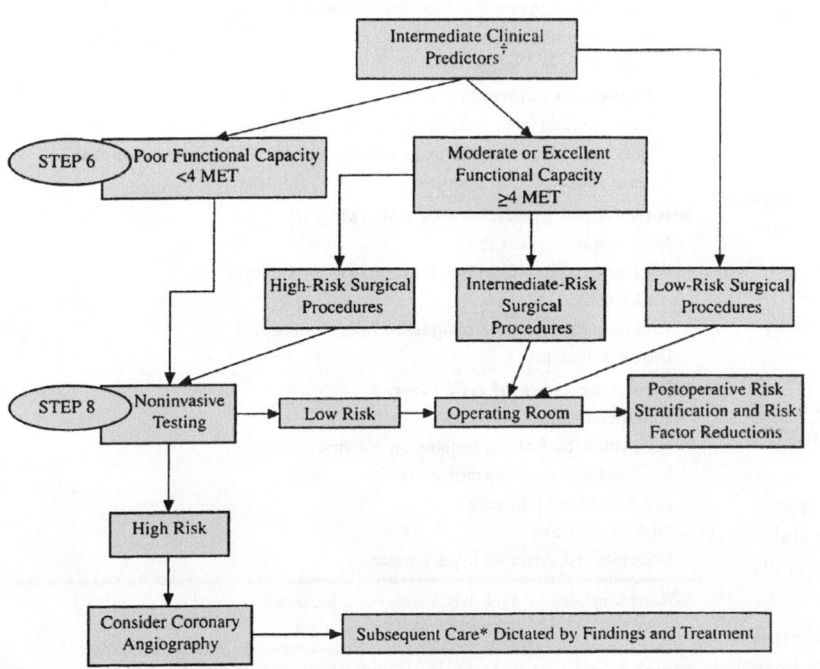

FIGURE 35-2. Stepwise approach to preoperative cardiac risk assessment. MET, metabolic equivalents of task. *Subsequent care may include cancellation or delay of surgery, coronary revascularization followed by noncardiac surgery, or intensified care. †See Table 35-2.

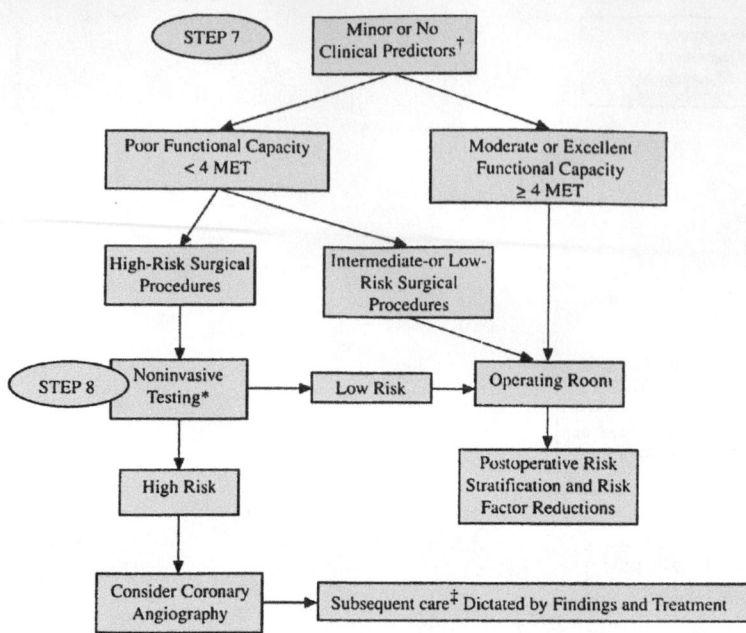

FIGURE 35-3. Stepwise approach to preoperative cardiac risk assessment. MET, metabolic equivalents of task. *Myocardial perfusion imaging or stress echocardiography. †See Table 30-2. ‡Subsequent care may include cancellation or delay of surgery, coronary revascularization followed by noncardiac surgery, or intensified care.

significantly alter long-term outcomes in terms of mortality as well as cardiac events. Based on these findings, a strategy of revascularization before elective vascular surgery in patients with stable cardiac symptoms is generally not recommended.

An in-depth review of the preoperative assessment prior to noncardiac surgery is beyond the scope of this chapter. However, the reader is encouraged to review the published guidelines for a comprehensive understanding of their appropriate use. The aggressiveness of the evaluation is determined by the patient's clinical symptoms. If a surgical emergency exists, appropriate testing and treatment are provided until the time of surgery. On occasion, medical concerns may require the cancellation of surgery.

The initial history, physical examination, and electrocardiogram are helpful in identifying potentially serious cardiac disease such as a prior myocardial infarction, angina, congestive heart failure, conduction abnormalities, or arrhythmias. It is essential to define the severity of the disease, its stability, and any prior treatments before surgery. Clinical factors that are significant tools in assessing risk are functional capacity, age, comorbidities, and the type of surgery. Vascular procedures or prolonged thoracic, abdominal, and head and neck surgeries are considered higher risk.

The benefit of the ACC/AHA guidelines is the stepwise strategy that uses clinical characteristics to define surgical risk in algorithmic tables (see Figures 35-1 to 35-3). Eight key questions help to direct the decision process down the flow chart and are briefly reviewed.

- *Step 1. Urgency of surgery:* If a patient has an immediate need for surgery, with a poor likelihood of survival without it, then it is best to provide medical management as needed and permit the surgery without delay (see Figure 35-1).

- *Step 2. Revascularization:* Have the patients had coronary revascularization in the past 5 years? If yes, have they remained stable or are they currently symptomatic? Further testing is generally not necessary if they have stable symptoms.

- *Step 3. Recent evaluation:* Has there been an evaluation of ischemic symptoms in the past 2 years? If yes, have the symptoms been

adequately assessed and the CAD appropriately treated? If it has been appropriately addressed, it is typically not necessary to repeat the workup, unless new symptoms are noted.

- *Step 4. Disease instability:* Does the patient have major clinical predictors (Table 35-2); unstable signs or symptoms that are concerning such as unstable angina, decompensated heart failure,

TABLE 35-2

Clinical Predictors of an Increased Risk for Perioperative Cardiovascular Events

Major clinical predictor of risk (Step 4)
Unstable coronary signs and symptoms
    Recent myocardial infarction* with ischemic risk by symptoms or testing
    Unstable or severe angina† (class III to IV)‡
Decompensated heart failure
Significant arrhythmias
    High-grade atrioventricular block
    Symptomatic ventricular arrhythmias with underlying heart disease
    Supraventricular arrhythmias with uncontrolled ventricular response
Severe valvular heart disease

Intermediate predictors of risk (Step 6)
Mild angina (class I to II)
Prior myocardial infarction by history or pathologic
    Q waves
Compensated or prior congestive heart failure
Diabetes mellitus

Minor predictors of risk (Step 7)
Advanced, age
LVH, LBBB, ST-T abnormalities on electrocardiogram
Rhythm other than normal sinus
Low functional capacity
History of stroke
Uncontrolled systemic hypertension

LBBB, left bundle-branch block; LVH, left ventricular hypertrophy.
* Recent myocardial infarction is ≥ 7 days but <30 days.
† May include stable angina in those who are very sedentary (e.g., nursing home patients).
‡ Canadian Cardiovascular Society class.

TABLE 35-3

Estimated Energy Requirements			

1 MET ⇩ 4 MET	Activities of daily living, self-care
	Eat, dress, toilet
	Walk indoors
	Walk 1 to 2 blocks on level ground
	  (2–3 mph)
	Do light work around the house such
	  as dusting or washing dishes
		4 MET ⇩ > 10 MET	Climb a flight of stairs or walk a hill
			Walk, level ground at 4 mph
			Run a short distance
			Do heavy work, scrubbing floors,
			  moving furniture
			Moderate exercise: golf, bowling,
			  dancing doubles, tennis, throwing
			  a ball
			Strenuous sports: swimming, singles
			  tennis, football

MET, metabolic equivalent of task.

symptomatic arrhythmias, and severe valvular heart disease; or a recent myocardial infarction? A yes answer to one of these concerns indicates a significant risk factor that may lead to a delay in surgery until symptoms are addressed and potential interventions are thoroughly considered.

- *Step 5. Intermediate risk:* Does the patient have intermediate clinical predictors of risk (see Table 35-2)?

- *Step 6. Functional capacity:* Patients lacking major risk factors but having intermediate predictors of risk and who have a moderate-to-excellent functional capacity can routinely undergo intermediate risk surgeries with a small probability of perioperative death or myocardial infarction (see Figure 35-2). Functional capacity is best assessed in metabolic equivalents of task (MET) and is helpful in predicting risk (Table 35-3). Noninvasive testing is considered for patients with a poor or moderate functional capacity when higher-risk surgery is planned, especially if two or more intermediate predictors are present. Perioperative and long-term cardiac risks are higher in patients unable to meet a four-MET level of exertion during most daily activities.

- *Step 7. Minor or no clinical predictors:* Noncardiac surgery is generally safe for patients lacking both major and intermediate predictors of risk and who have a moderate or excellent functional capacity (≥4 MET) (see Figure 35-3). Further testing is considered on an individual basis for patients without clinical markers but with a poor functional capacity who are facing higher-risk operations, especially those individuals with several minor clinical predictors who will undergo a vascular surgery. Table 35-4 lists examples of a given surgery's specific risks.

- *Step 8. Noninvasive testing:* The result of noninvasive testing can be used to determine further preoperative management, which may include further medication or revascularization.

These steps facilitate selecting the appropriate direction on the algorithms. Clinical situations not addressed by these protocols should be reviewed with a consultant cardiologist.

Other Cardiovascular Concerns

Hypertension

Severe hypertension should be controlled before surgery, as permitted by the clinical circumstances. Continuation of preoperative antihypertensive treatments throughout the perioperative period is critical, particularly if that agent is a beta-blocker or clonidine.

Valvular Disease

Indications for the evaluation and treatment of valvular heart disease are similar to those in the nonoperative setting. Symptomatic mitral or aortic stenosis is associated with significant perioperative risk, severe congestive heart failure, or shock. Patients could be considered for percutaneous valvotomy or valve surgery preoperatively. Symptomatic aortic or mitral regurgitant disease is typically of less risk during surgery, when managed with intensive medical therapy and monitoring. The patient with both severe valvular regurgitation and reduced left ventricular function is best managed with the assistance of a consultant cardiologist.

Perioperative Beta-Blockers

Beta-blocker therapy is recommended perioperatively for all patients at high risk of coronary events who are scheduled for noncardiac surgery, provided contraindications do not exist. When atenolol was

TABLE 35-4

Cardiac Event* Risk Stratified by Noncardiac Surgeries
High (cardiac risk >5%)
Emergent major operation, especially in the elderly patient
Aortic or major vascular procedure
Peripheral vascular
Prolonged surgeries with large volumen shifts and/or blood loss
Intermediate (cardiac risk <5%)
Carotid endarterectomy
Head and neck
Intraperitoneal and intrathoracic
Orthopedic
Prostate
Low† (cardiac risk <1%)
Endoscopic procedures
Superficial procedures
Cataracts
Breast

*Combined incidence of cardiac death and nonfatal myocardial infarction.
†Further perioperative cardiac testing is generally not required.

given intravenously or orally, beginning 2 days before surgery and continuing for 7 days after, the event-free survival at 6 months was higher in the atenolol group. Ideally, beta-blocker therapy should be initiated several days to weeks prior to surgery. The dose is adjusted to achieve a resting heart rate of no more than 60 beats per minute. The use of a shorter-acting agent may be preferable in the elderly patient because it permits greater flexibility in dose titration and allows the opportunity to stop the drug quickly, with less risk of sustained side effects such as symptomatic bradycardia. Beta-blocker therapy should be continued throughout the perioperative period.

Other Preventive Measures

The waiting period before an elective procedure can be used to promote activities that may enhance the recovery from surgery. Patients who receive exercise training twice a week, education, nurse-initiated telephone calls, and an offer to participate in postoperative cardiac rehabilitation have fewer days in the hospital, less time in the intensive care unit, and greater improvements in measures of quality of life. Many surgeons recommend preoperative physical conditioning by encouraging the patient to walk daily for 2 to 3 weeks prior to an elective surgery. This is often coupled with postoperative care plans that encourage early ambulation.

Patients with severe lung disease or who are debilitated should have an introduction to the proper use of incentive spirometry prior to surgery, to reduce the risk of pulmonary atelectasis and its associated complications. This is, perhaps, the most important element in reducing postoperative pulmonary complications, particularly when there is an aggressive education program that encourages the use of these devices in the weeks prior to an elective surgery. Aggressive efforts to promote smoking cessation prior to surgery should be encouraged. Reactive airway disease should be maximally treated with bronchodilators and possibly steroids prior to surgery.

Intravascular volume status is critical and should be optimized preoperatively. Volume contraction should be avoided because of the older patient's greater dependence on left ventricular preload to maintain cardiac output. Routine hemodynamic monitoring using invasive techniques may prevent a few complications, but its routine use remains highly controversial. The use of an intraoperative pulmonary artery catheter to optimize preload, afterload, and isotropic support is of benefit only in selected patients.

Deep venous thrombosis (DVT) is a vexing concern in the postoperative patient. Pulmonary emboli are still thought to be one of the leading causes of in hospital death and may account for one-third of the postoperative deaths of elderly patients. Procedures commonly performed in the older person, such as hip or knee replacement and urologic or gynecologic procedures, place the older patient at a high risk for this complication. For low-to-moderate-risk procedures, low-dose heparin subcutaneously or external pneumatic compression devices started immediately after surgery is recommended and should be continued until the time of discharge. For higher-risk surgeries, low-molecular-weight (LMW) heparin or warfarin should be considered as a means to prevent postoperative DVT.

Endocarditis remains a risk because of the higher prevalence of valvular disease in older patients. Oral, bowel, urinary tract, biliary, and pulmonary procedures may result in bacteremia and an increased risk for infection if significant valve disease exists. Use of central venous catheters is another important source of bacteremia.

The use of such devices should be minimized whenever possible. The AHA/ACC recommendations for endocarditis prophylaxis, as well as the preoperative assessment guidelines, can be reviewed at the following websites: www.americanheart.org and www.acc.org.

Do Not Resuscitate Orders

The need for surgery in patients with do-not-resuscitate (DNR) orders or concerns of medical futility may be an issue in some elderly patients. Unfortunately, many elderly patients still do not have discussions with their health care providers prior to a hospitalization concerning DNR status, even though this is often mandated. The Patient Self-Determination Act requires that hospitals and other health care facilities inform patients of their right to appoint a proxy or surrogate decision maker to act on their wishes regarding life-sustaining care should they become incompetent. Focused efforts by nurses, clinicians, and consultants to enhance communication can increase the use of advance directives. Debate exists about honoring these orders in the operating suite when a patient requests a DNR status and still must undergo surgery (e.g., percutaneous feeding tube). Surgery may hasten a death as the result of an unanticipated complication. Most of the immediate operative causes for a cardiac arrest are more treatable than the causes of an arrest in other clinical settings, such as the nursing home, because these may include correctable conditions such as oversedation, an arrhythmia, hypotension, pulmonary edema, or bleeding. It is a common practice to suspend a DNR order during the procedure and for 24 to 48 hours afterward. If a complication occurs, the patient is treated and the family or those with decision-making responsibilities are consulted. An evaluation of survivability is made and a decision to suspend or continue the interventions is discussed. This process is less clear when there is a concern that the surgical procedure is potentially medically futile (i.e., when a procedure would have only marginal benefit).

POSTOPERATIVE MANAGEMENT

Postoperative management includes the appropriate use of medications for pain, increasing mobilization, proper use of urinary catheters, the treatment and prevention of delirium, and anticoagulation use.

Pain Control

The American Geriatrics Society has published a comprehensive review of pain management in the elderly patient. This report notes that pain is undertreated in older patients because of the concern of using potent analgesics in older patients and a misconception that pain sensations are diminished in such patients. Postoperative patients should be regularly asked about the severity of their discomfort using analog scales, and analgesics should be given according to anticipated needs rather than "as needed." Simply scheduling pain medications is another useful approach. Comments on the management of persistent pain, medication dosing, and metabolism, as well as associated toxicities, are well summarized by the American Geriatrics Society's review of this topic.

Early Mobilization

Prolonged bed rest can adversely affect the elderly patient. Changes noted with prolonged immobility include a decrease in cardiac output and aerobic capacity, baroreceptor desensitization and orthostatic hypotension, skeletal muscle deconditioning, bone loss, hypercalcemia, joint contractures, constipation, incontinence, pressure sores, sensory deprivation, an increased risk for DVT, atelectasis, hypoxemia, and pneumonia. The earliest possible mobilization from bed is vital, helping to reduce the risk for complications. If the recovery process prevents full mobilization, then a physical therapy referral for range or motion exercises and the maintenance of an upright posture (chair) may reduce the frequency and severity of these complications.

Catheters

Postoperative urinary drainage is typically managed by an indwelling catheter but that predisposes to urinary tract infection and associated complications. Catheter use should be short, with a goal of prompt removal by the morning after surgery. If there is a concern for urinary retention or bladder distension, then intermittent catheterization should be considered. The use of a urinary catheter beyond 48 hours should be avoided, except when retention cannot be managed by other means. Patients requiring longer-term use of a urinary catheter should not be given prophylactic antimicrobials.

Postoperative Delirium (see Chapter 53)

An acute confusional state occur in 10% to 15% of older patients undergoing general surgery, 30% of cardiac surgery patients, and, in one study, up to 50% of hip fracture repairs. Making the correct diagnosis of delirium is important. Although the causes are numerous, it is often the result of a postoperative complication that may not be apparent. Delirium is also a marker for worse functional recovery, and older patients with in-hospital delirium are at risk of significant long-term reduction in cognitive function.

Delirium is often subtle and can easily be missed. Clinical factors key to the diagnosis are a rapid onset, a disturbed level of consciousness, decreased attention and environmental awareness, memory deficits, disorientation, perceptual disturbances, and evidence of a condition that contributes to its development. A history of dementia as well as prior delirium, advanced age, and a prior decline in cognitive function are risk factors for perioperative delirium. As a rule, delirium fluctuates and may not be evident during all visits. Nursing staff and family members are often the most reliable source for the serial assessments of an at-risk patient.

Delirium often compromises postoperative care and extends length of stay. Behaviors can often be controlled with environmental measures, such as a bedside sitter, increased visitations by family, orientation stimuli, minimizing abrupt relocations, and permitting patients to return to a more normal day–night cycle. If medically appropriate, the use of a sleep protocol is often helpful. Symptomatic control of agitation to prevent harm is occasionally needed. Unfortunately, no single drug has an accomplished record. High-potency antipsychotics such as risperidone, haloperidol, olanzapine, and quetiapine should be cautiously titrated to improve symptoms. Lower-potency drugs such as chlorpromazine and thioridazine should be avoided because of their anticholinergic and arrhythmogenic effects.

If delirium is secondary to alcohol withdrawal, short-acting benzodiazepines can be used with close monitoring for excessive sedation. Formal delirium prevention protocols can be helpful, especially in the intensive care unit setting.

Other Complications

Postoperative surveillance for myocardial ischemia, infarction, arrhythmias, and DVT should ideally lead to a reduction in mortality. Postoperative myocardial ischemia is the strongest predictor of cardiac morbidity. Anginal pain may be masked by narcotics or may be difficult to verbalize during recovery. Postoperative ST-segment changes are indicative of myocardial ischemia and are an independent predictor of events. Such changes are associated with a worse long-term survival. The optimal surveillance strategy for the diagnosis of postoperative ischemia or infarction has not been defined. Currently, no evidence supports the routine use of pulmonary artery catheter monitoring of ventricular performance. In patients without documented CAD, surveillance should be restricted to patients who develop signs or symptoms of cardiovascular dysfunction. In patients with high- or intermediate-risk surgical procedures, an electrocardiogram at baseline, immediately after surgery, and daily for the first 2 days appears to be the most cost-effective strategy. Cardiac troponin measurements should be part of the diagnostic plan for myocardial infarction detection, but additional research is needed to correlate outcomes to the magnitude of an isolated cardiac troponin elevation. As a rule, postoperative myocardial infarctions have a similar pathology to infarction occurring in a nonsurgical patient, the spontaneous thrombosis of the coronary artery. Therefore, when this complication occurs, an aggressive attempt at opening the infarct-related artery should be considered in the appropriate postoperative patient.

Postoperative arrhythmias are often caused by correctable noncardiac problems such as infection, hypotension, metabolic abnormalities (hypokalemia and hypomagnesemia), and hypoxia. Ventricular arrhythmias (frequent ventricular ectopic beats or nonsustained ventricular tachycardia) may occur in more than one-third of high-risk patients. Prophylactic use of antiarrhythmics other than beta-blockers is currently not justified. Sustained ventricular tachycardia with or without hemodynamic complications requires consultation with a cardiologist. Atrial fibrillation is common. Approximately 25% of elderly patients develop this rhythm. Age and the type of surgery are strong predictors for the development of atrial fibrillation. The prophylactic use of a beta-blocker and amiodarone has shown some benefit by reducing the frequency of this rhythm.

Hemoglobin levels often fall after major surgery. Many elderly patients will tolerate a hemoglobin level below 10 g/dL. Transfusions should be reserved for patients with symptoms and those with levels below 7 g/dL. Controlled trials of oral iron in hip fracture patients demonstrate a lack of benefit, and its routine use is not beneficial. If iron is given, once-daily dosing should be considered.

Cognitive decline has been noted following a variety of surgeries. The International Study of Postoperative Cognitive Dysfunction found that 26% of patients older than 60 years who had either intra-abdominal or orthopedic procedures had a significant decline in cognitive function 1 week after surgery. Risk factors included older age, greater use of anesthetics, and postoperative respiratory and infectious complications. In coronary artery bypass surgery, where the aorta is often cross-clamped and a bypass pump is used, embolization of both gas and particulates occurs. Central nervous system ischemic damage is often noted after these procedures. Postoperative infarcts are the likely cause of cognitive decline noted with cardiac surgery. Off-pump coronary artery bypass surgery seems to have a lower rate of short-term decline in cognitive function (21% vs. 29%), but similar decline is noted at 6 months (31% vs. 38%). The risk of further decline in cognitive function should be incorporated into the decision process for patients with underlying dementia who are not undergoing emergent or life-saving surgery. Finally, postoperative critical pathways involving regimens, including low-dose opiates, early extubation, and an emphasis on accelerated functional recovery, can be safely applied to older patients.

The management of anticoagulants prior to surgery is briefly summarized. For patients on chronic warfarin with an Int'l normalized ratio (INR) goal of 2.0 to 3.0, four scheduled doses should be withheld to allow the INR to normalize to less than 1.5 before surgery. If the INR is typically kept above 3.0, then longer periods without a warfarin dose may be required. The INR should be measured a day before surgery to ensure that it has reached an acceptable range. If the INR is excessive (>1.8), a small dose of vitamin K, 1 mg SQ, may be given. When the INR is <2.0 other prophylactic antithrombotic interventions should be considered.

Elective surgery is best avoided for a month following a DVT. If this is not possible, then LMW heparin should be given before and after the procedure while the INR is <2.0. LMW heparin should be stopped 6 hours before surgery; restarting it can be considered as soon as 12 hours after surgery, depending on the type of surgery and its result. Patients with a DVT on warfarin for 2 to 3 months need not be on heparin prior to surgery unless there are additional risks. LMW heparin should be given postoperatively until the INR returns to >2.0. Patients with a DVT on warfarin for more than 3 months may not need preoperative heparin. These patients should receive postoperative prophylaxis with LMW heparin until the INR returns to >2.0. These recommendations should be combined with mechanical prophylaxis (gradient compression stockings intermittent pneumatic compression). Elective surgery should be avoided in the first month after an arterial embolism.

SUMMARY

As our society ages, the need for surgical procedures of all types will continue to increase among older adults. Age alone is not a very good predictor of operative risk and should not be the sole criteria for deciding who should and who should not have surgery. However, age is associated with a higher prevalence of chronic diseases, which, in turn, are strong predictors of risk and are determinants of who might benefit from surgery and preoperative testing. The AHA and ACC have published revised algorithms, which are helpful in preoperative risk assessment. Perioperative care requires a careful medical evaluation and comprehensive postoperative observation that anticipates potential complications. Newer techniques related to minimally invasive surgery appear promising. Besides decreasing recovery time and postoperative pain, there is some suggestion that overall operative risk may be decreased. Future studies examining clinical outcomes of interest in older adults will be an essential component of evaluating the relative risks and benefits of new interventions.

FURTHER READING

AGS Clinical Practice Committee. The use of oral anticoagulation (warfarin) in older people. *J Am Geriatr Soc.* 2000;49:224.

AGS Panel on Persistent Pain in Older Patients. The management of persistent pain in older persons. *J Am Geriatr Soc.* 2002;50:S205.

Ang-Lee MK, Moss J, Yuan CS. Herbal medicines and perioperative care. *JAMA.* 2001;286:208.

Auerbach AD, Goldman L. B-Blockers and reduction of cardiac events in noncardiac surgery: scientific review. *JAMA.* 2002;287:1435.

Bonow RO, et al. ACC/AHA 2006 guidelines for the management of patients with valvular heart disease: a report of the American College of Cardiology/American Heart Association task force on practice guidelines (Writing committee to revise the 1998 guidelines for the management of patients with valvular heart disease). *J Am Coll Cardiol.* 2006;48:e1.

Eagle KA, et al. ACC/AHA guideline update on perioperative cardiovascular evaluation for non-cardiac surgery—2002. Available at either http://www.acc.org or http://www.americanheart.org.

Fleisher LA, Eagle KA. Lowering cardiac risk in noncardiac surgery. *N Engl J Med.* 2001;345:1677.

Lawrence VA, et al. Functional independence after major abdominal surgery in the elderly. *J Am Coll Surg.* 2004;199:762.

Lindenauer PK, et al. Lipid-lowering therapy and in-hospital mortality following major noncardiac surgery. *JAMA.* 2004;291:2092.

Lindenauer PK, et al. Perioperative beta-blocker therapy and mortality after major noncardiac surgery. *N Engl J Med.* 2005;353:349.

Makary MA, et al. Pancreaticoduodenectomy in the very elderly. *J Gastrointest Surg.* 2006;10:347.

McFalls EO, et al. Coronary-artery revascularization before elective major vascular surgery. *N Engl J Med.* 2004;351:2795.

Solomon DH, et al. The new frontier: increasing geriatrics expertise in surgical and medical specialties. *J Am Geriatr Soc.* 2000;48:702.

Spell NO III. Stopping and restarting medications in the perioperative period. *Med Clin North Am.* 2001;85:1117.

Young MH, Washer LL, Malani PN. Surgical site infections among older adults: epidemiology and management strategies. *Drugs Aging.* 2008;25:399.

Anesthesia

Jeffrey H. Silverstein ■ *G. Alec Rooke*

Perioperative management of the older adult is complex. Anesthetic care itself is challenging, and both preoperative preparation and postoperative care for older adults assume greater importance than for young, healthy adults. Ideally, care is based on a comprehensive plan that integrates the roles of the anesthesiologist, surgeon, geriatrician, primary caregivers, and medical specialists. This chapter provides an overview of the role of the anesthesiologist and anesthesia techniques in pre-, peri-, and postoperative care of the older adult, in order to improve communication with other professionals who provide care to this vulnerable population.

ANESTHESIA AND THE ANESTHESIOLOGIST

Anesthesia is the art and science of controlling physiologic processes in order to permit interventions on the body that would be intolerable owing to normal compensatory mechanisms. Surgery, which involves a direct assault on body tissues, is the standard paradigm for understanding anesthesia. Anesthesiologists perform other valuable services, including sedation for less invasive procedures, management of pain syndromes, and the provision of critical care. European anesthesiologists are also actively involved in emergency care. Anesthesia is based on an understanding of homeostatic mechanisms and their manipulation. *Homeostenosis*, the restricted range and capacity of homeostatic mechanisms associated with aging, provides a challenge to the anesthesiologist. In order to tailor appropriate anesthesia care for an older adult, the anesthesia team must be familiar with the effects of aging on multiple organ systems, particularly the heart, lungs, and brain, and must be familiar with physiologic changes of age, such as increase in body fat, decreased glomerular filtration, and reduced hepatic blood flow, which affect anesthetic drug action and duration.

PREOPERATIVE CARE OF THE OLDER SURGICAL PATIENT

Preoperative care can take place in multiple settings and can occur briefly or over a period of time. The most important goal of preoperative assessment is not the risk assessment, but the improvement of the patient's medical status prior to surgery and planning for the recovery process. The anesthesiologist provides care in a different time frame and uses a different approach than is typical for other specialties. The chief complaint usually takes the form of a request for anesthesia services for a specific operation. The anesthesiologist uses a vertical or systems-based approach, most clearly articulated by Stanley Muravchick (Figure 36-1). As part of this approach, the anesthesiologist assigns an American Society of Anesthesiologists physical status classification (Table 36-1). The American Society of Anesthesiologists score is a clinician's tool, not a predictor of perioperative risk, because, while the American Society of Anesthesiologists score correlates broadly with outcomes, it does not incorporate age or type of operation, both significant influences on outcomes.

In terms of ability to tolerate anesthesia and surgery, physiologic status is more important than chronological age. Aging is a highly variable process; young adults are more similar to each other physiologically than are older adults. While chronological age is insufficient to explain surgical outcomes, it has repeatedly been found to be associated with an increased risk of morbidity, mortality, and poor surgical outcomes. Age appears to be an important modifier of disease load, and the number of diseases (disease burden) appears to be the primary determinant of outcomes. Older adults with limited or low disease load have relatively lower risk of postoperative complications (Figure 36-2A), and the combination of high disease load and age is associated with extremely high rates of morbidity and

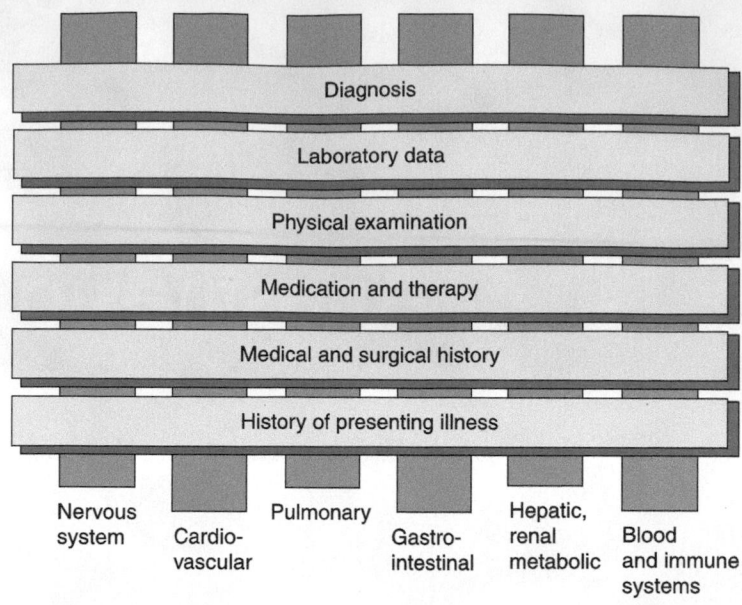

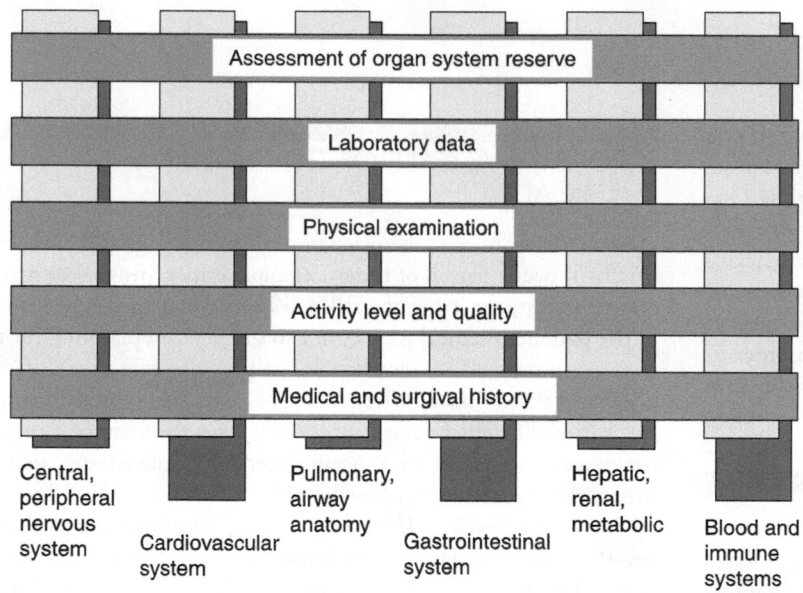

FIGURE 36-1. A. The traditional medical approach to diagnosis can be represented schematically as a series of horizontal techniques of inquiry (open bars) applied across the various organ systems (shaded bars) to consolidate data describing the status of different organs into a unified diagnostic group. B. An organ-system-based "vertical" approach to preoperative assessment of the elderly patient by anesthesiologists differs from the traditional diagnostic approach because it applies the various technique of inquiry (shaded bars) sequentially in each major organ system (open bars) in order to assess organ function and functional reserve. The primary objective of preoperative assessment should be evaluation of physical status, rather than the identification of specific underlying disorders. (Used with permission from Muravchick S: Geroanesthesia. Principles for Management of the Elderly Patient. St. Louis, Mosby, 1997, page 17–18.)

mortality (Figure 36-2B). In addition, aging is not uniform across organ systems, and some organ systems may have aged or have been affected by disease more than others. Since aging is so heterogeneous, a careful preoperative evaluation is extremely important in preparing the older adult for surgery.

TABLE 36-1

American Society of Anesthesiologists Physical Status Categories	
P1	A normal healthy patient
P2	A patient with mild systemic disease
P3	A patient with severe systemic disease
P4	A patient with severe systemic disease that is a constant threat to life
P5	A moribund patient who is not expected to survive without the operation
P6	A declared brain-dead patient whose organs are being removed for donor purposes

How and when the preoperative evaluation occurs is highly variable. Many modern surgical practices admit patients for major surgery on the day of the operation. In this scenario, the anesthesiologist must perform the preoperative evaluation and discuss the perioperative experience and anesthetic options with the patient in a tight time frame. Alternative approaches include preoperative clinics and telephone calls, which can provide important opportunities to develop an understanding of the patient's physical condition prior to the day of surgery.

The preoperative evaluation is an essential process in developing an anesthetic plan. Just as importantly, it provides an opportunity to answer questions for the patient and family. The most constructive of preoperative evaluations provide plans for minimizing risk in the perioperative period (i.e., before, during, and after surgery). As part of the evaluation, a general internist maybe consulted. Institutional policy and practices vary as to whether such input is required or even routine. A generalist's statement that the patient has been "cleared for surgery" is of limited value. Much more useful to the

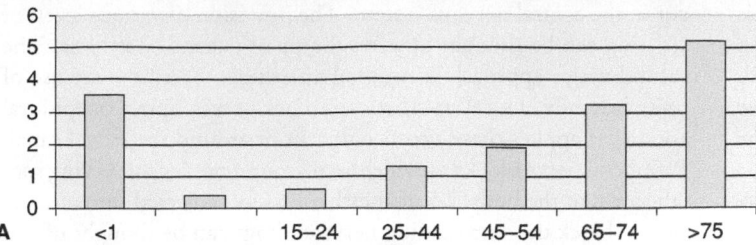

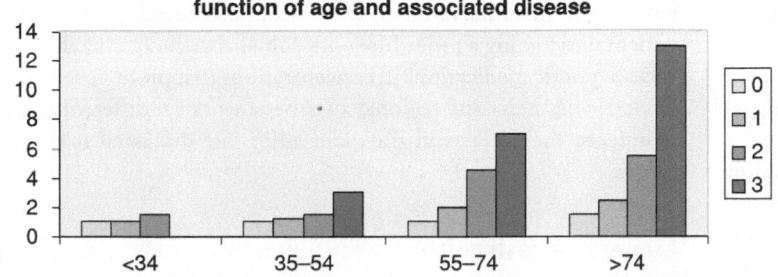

FIGURE 36-2. (A) Major anesthetic complications per 1000 related to age. (B) Major anesthesia complications per 1000 as a function of age and associated disease. Legend indicates the number of diseases identified (0 = no disease, 3 = 3 or more diseases). Note that the disease burden significantly increases the likelihood of major complications as patients age.

anesthesiologist and surgeon is a complete overview of the patient's medical condition, recent evaluations, and medications. The more the preoperative evaluator knows and understands, the less often the need for additional consultation. The best plan is based on good communication between the generalist and specialist physicians, the surgeon, the anesthesiologist, and the patient.

Preoperative management of significant medical problems should be determined. Medication regimens (such as anticoagulants, antidiabetic agents, and antiparkinsonian medications) require modifications and advance planning prior to surgery. Several members of the medical team can lead this effort, but the individual responsible should have a good understanding of the issues that need to be addressed and how they should be handled. Medication management protocols that have been jointly set by surgeons, anesthesiologists, and internists are often useful. When additional consultation is sought, the request should clearly define the issues that need to be addressed and the expected role of the consultant. The example shown in Figure 36-3 illustrates a reasonable delineation of the problem to be addressed. Anecdotally, an organized preoperative clinic can improve patient satisfaction and decrease the number of perioperative consults.

Risk assessment is a part of the preoperative process. Most of the time the objective of risk assessment is to decide how aggressive one should be in preparing the patient for surgery, rather than deciding that the surgical risk is too high. Risk assessment is most formalized in the form of the AHA/ACC guidelines for the evaluation of cardiac disease. The guidelines attempt to integrate severity of comorbid disease, exercise tolerance, and surgical severity into a rational plan, in order to determine who needs to enter an advanced evaluation process or to avoid diagnostic procedures with a risk greater than the proposed surgery itself. In fact, the AHA/ACC guidelines were originally developed specifically to limit the frequency of noninvasive cardiac testing, which has the potential to be used unnecessarily. It is important to remember that the AHA/ACC guidelines have never been formally tested, nor are they meant to supplant clinical judgment. Many medical problems in the older adult cannot be addressed using established guidelines so that decisions are based

on clinical judgment. The impact on postoperative outcomes of optimizing medical conditions prior to surgery is usually unknown. Typical conditions that might be optimized preoperatively, even if not seriously unstable, include high blood pressure, diabetes, reactive airway disease, and coronary artery disease. One of the best examples of medical optimization leading to improved outcome is the use of beta-blockade for patients with known or suspected coronary heart disease.

Sometimes internists and anesthesiologists disagree on preoperative management, often about whether or not planned diagnostic tests can be delayed until after the surgery. The consult shown in Figure 36-3 provides an example. In this case, atrial flutter is not a contraindication to surgery. Why should its evaluation delay surgery? Some would argue that if the tests provide useful information or lead to an intervention that improves the patient's status, then the patient will be better off having the tests done prior to elective surgery.

To: General Medicine Consult Service
From: General Surgery

Mr. DD is a 71 y/o man scheduled for resection of a recurrent dermatofibrosarcoma of the right clavicle. He has diet-controlled adult onset diabetes. He also has a history of a "racing heart" previously evaluated with a Holter 8 months ago revealing brief runs of asymptomatic atrial tachycardia. Today's EKG shows atrial flutter with variable block, and a ventricular rate of approximately 90. Please evaluate his arrhythmia and clear for surgery so anesthesia doesn't cancel him.

To: General Surgery
From: General Medicine Consult Service

The patient reports no new symptoms over the past several months. He describes some shortness of breath on exertion, but denies past or present angina, MI or symptoms of CHF. According to ACC guidelines, he has intermediate clinical predictors (diabetes) and is undergoing a low-risk surgical procedure.
Recommend:
1. Beta-blockade to limit the heart rate response to surgical stress.
2. Proceed with surgery.
3. Subsequent outpatient evaluation/treatment for his atrial fibrillation (Echocardiogram, TSH level, anticoagulation and a trial of cardioversion).
Thank you for this interesting consult.

FIGURE 36-3. An example of a consult request from a surgical service to a medical service.

In the example in Figure 36-3, an echocardiogram provides useful information, even if normal. If a test should be performed, it is reasonable to do it before surgery, unless surgical urgency dictates otherwise. Furthermore, if elective cardioversion is being considered, it should be done before surgery because heart rate control in the intra- and postoperative periods is more easily achieved when the patient is in sinus rhythm. As stated above, there is frequently little evidence upon which to base such judgment but coherent preoperative planning in an older adult can avoid confusion, surgical delay, and requests for emergent consultations that are rarely as complete as elective evaluations.

Geriatrician involvement improves perioperative care but is undervalued in most usual care settings. Comprehensive geriatric assessment (discussed in detail elsewhere) has a place in perioperative care because it is the best way to prevent geriatric-specific postoperative issues like delirium and pressure ulcers.

A unique part of the preoperative assessment of the older adult arises when a patient has a "do not resuscitate" order or other advanced care directives. Many patients have, in consultation with their primary-care physicians, elected to forgo resuscitative measures, because of fears that resuscitation will lead to poor outcome, or because they feel that resuscitation measures will be futile. These fears are supported by numerous studies that demonstrate that cardiac arrest in most settings carries a very poor prognosis, because arrests are usually unwitnessed and may be caused by advanced disease states. However, the operating room is a special setting in this regard. In contrast with other in-hospital cardiac arrests, cardiac arrests in the operating room carry a very favorable prognosis, because arrests are often because of reversible causes such as hemorrhage or drug effects, and because they are witnessed events where resuscitation is instituted within seconds. This means that, in the setting of surgery, a patient's DNR order must be reconsidered in light of the different prognostic implications of cardiac arrest during surgery. Some organizations have standing policies that DNR orders are rescinded in the operating room. The DNR may be reinstituted either upon a physician's order or automatically upon return to the ward. Regardless of the management plan, DNR orders require review and discussion with the patient. While the anesthesiologist should have such discussions with the patient, input from the patient's other physicians can be invaluable.

Sometimes a primary-care physician or consultant offers advice on anesthetic management as a part of the anesthesia preoperative referral. These recommendations are usually not helpful. Requests to avoid hypotension and hypoxemia are so obvious as to be unnecessary. Surgical clearance limited to local or regional anesthesia can create problems. These restrictions may not be based on clear evidence. Regional techniques have limitations (see section on "regional anesthesia"). Regional anesthetic techniques occasionally fail in the operating room, requiring an immediate alternative. In some cases, local anesthesia may be feasible, but not preferable, as a result of patient characteristics such as apprehension or positioning issues, or because adequate anesthesia would be difficult to achieve with local approaches alone.

ANESTHETIC METHODS AND THE OLDER ADULT

Anesthesiologists have developed two major approaches to the provision of anesthesia. The first is general anesthesia, based on the systemic administration of medications whose principal effects occur in the central nervous system. The provision of various levels of sedation can be thought of as a subtype of general anesthesia. The second major approach is regional anesthesia, based on the use of one of a family of local anesthetics to block nerves. Spinal or epidural anesthesia applies these agents either in or around the spinal canal. Peripheral nerve blocks provide them around nerves subserving specific areas of the body. Local anesthetic agents injected into areas of skin to block the surrounding nerve endings can be thought of as a form of regional anesthesia. The two main forms of anesthesia are not mutually exclusive. A patient undergoing general anesthesia may have a peripheral nerve block to control postoperative pain, and a patient undergoing a procedure with spinal anesthesia is likely to receive hypnotic medications in concentrations that produce sedation. General anesthesia and regional anesthesia work via different mechanisms, so their effects in the older adults are discussed separately below.

General Anesthesia

This section will review the goals of general anesthesia, principles of intraoperative care, types of anesthetic agents, and age-related special management issues. While unconsciousness is the most apparent distinguishing feature of general anesthesia, it has many other important effects. The cardinal features of general anesthesia are (1) lack of consciousness, including amnesia for events that occur under anesthesia, (2) analgesia or absence of pain, (3) lack of movement in response to painful stimuli, and (4) control of the reflex responses to painful stimuli. In the early years of anesthesiology, ether was found to provide all of these properties, although it did cause prolific vomiting following emergence and had a tendency to cause explosions in the operating theater. The observation that ether, a relatively simple molecule, produced an adequate anesthetic state, along with compelling physicochemical evidence suggesting that potency was linked to the length of the carbon chain of the anesthetic, led anesthesiologists to search for a single mechanism or receptor that was responsible for anesthesia. In subsequent years, it has become clear that anesthesia does not result from alterations of a single receptor, but that all available drugs with anesthetic properties have specific targets. General anesthesia results from alterations at multiple receptors and multiple drugs are almost always used to produce general anesthesia.

Intraoperative Anesthesia Care

Standard procedure for anesthetic care is to monitor the electrocardiogram, blood pressure, and oxygen saturation. When general anesthesia is undertaken, end-tidal carbon dioxide monitoring is required and temperature should be monitored for most procedures. Intravenous access with large-bore (18 gauge or larger for major surgery) catheters inserted into peripheral veins is almost universally required as part of anesthetic care. The induction of anesthesia is generally accomplished with intravenously administered hypnotic agents. The appropriate dosages of these agents are all decreased with aging. Maintenance of a patent airway and adequate ventilation are primary goals, usually attained via an endotracheal tube and positive pressure ventilation. In recent years, anesthesiologists have developed a variety of new airway devices, such as the laryngeal mask airway, as alternatives to endotracheal intubation. The choice of device and backup procedures varies with procedure and practitioner.

Spontaneous breathing is also a feasible and potentially desirable alternative to positive pressure ventilation.

Adjustment of the depth of anesthesia consumes a good deal of the anesthetic manipulations during surgery. How "deep" or "light" the patient is at any moment depends on the balance of drug effects and the surgical stimulus. Titration of the depth of anesthesia is typically a matter of balancing the tendency of the surgical stimulus to activate the brain and stimulate the sympathetic nervous system against the anesthetic's ability to depress brain activity and limit the stimulation of the sympathetic nervous system. Thus, a patient might be fully anesthetized one moment and then be inadequately anesthetized a moment later if the surgical (painful) stimulus suddenly increases. The effective depth of anesthesia can be monitored through a variety of methods. The primary approach for years has been to monitor blood pressure and heart rate. Hemodynamic signs of light anesthesia generally appear long before a patient has any chance of "waking up" or of having postoperative recall. A rise in blood pressure and/or heart rate is typically the first sign of light anesthesia and triggers an increase in the concentration of volatile gas (currently isoflurane, sevoflurane, or desflurane) concentration or administration of a small bolus of a fast-acting opioid such as fentanyl. A safe strategy is to keep blood pressure at or slightly lower than the patient's usual baseline, although this can be quite difficult to accomplish in older patients. The risk of awareness/recall is relatively remote under such circumstances.

Since depth of anesthesia is such a critical issue in perioperative care, and because it can change moment to moment, anesthesiologists have attempted for years to use electroencephalograms to define a brain-based measure of depth of anesthesia. Recently, devices have been developed that use advanced signal processing and computer miniaturization to provide a single number between 0 and 100 that indicates depth of anesthesia. When these devices have been applied to older adults, the findings suggest that the amount of anesthetic typically used to control blood pressure and heart rate frequently results in extremely deep anesthesia for the brain. Excessive depth of anesthesia has been proposed to contribute to poor outcomes. This important area requires further study and might be valuable in the clinical arena in the future.

Patient movement in response to a surgical stimulus, even if very slight, suggests an inadequate depth of anesthesia. Too light anesthesia can result in patient awareness and failure of amnesia. The amount of movement is usually subtle. Most slight movement does not imply such a light level of anesthesia as to result in awareness or recall. Movement cannot be used as an indicator of depth of anesthesia if a patient is paralyzed by neuromuscular blocking agents and common adjuvants for abdominal surgical cases or in cases where even minimal movement is surgically unacceptable. Unintentional excessively light anesthesia is most likely to occur when neuromuscular blocking agents produce muscle relaxation in the presence of lighter general anesthetic agents, such as nitrous oxide and opioids, with little or no potent gases. The electroencephalogram monitors described above have an unclear role in preventing awareness during surgery.

Anesthetic Agents

The pharmacokinetics and pharmacodynamics of the intravenous and volatile anesthetic agents are altered in the older adult, so that administration must be adjusted. A general rule of the thumb is that all drugs will have more dramatic and longer-lasting effects in older patients, although this is not universally true. The mechanisms vary with the drug but include changes in protein binding, decreases in initial volume of distribution, alterations in receptor sensitivity, and slowed renal or hepatic metabolism. The therapeutic effect of many intravenous anesthetic agents is not dissipated by metabolism, but by redistribution of the drug from the brain to the fat. These drugs are highly lipid soluble and cross membranes rapidly. On initial injection, the blood levels are very high but will fall as the drug is taken up into fat. The high initial blood levels will promote rapid transfer of the drug into highly perfused organs such as the brain. Even though fat serves as an almost limitless sink for lipid-soluble drugs, blood flow to fat is low and transfer of drug into fat takes time. Transfer time largely dictates the duration of a drug's clinical effect. As blood levels decrease, drug returns to the blood from the more vascular organs and is then transferred to the fat, dissipating the therapeutic effect. Substantial and/or prolonged administration of many drugs results in drug levels in fat that become high enough to sustain a (residual) blood level that has a therapeutic effect. From an anesthetic management viewpoint, the pharmacokinetic and pharmacodynamic changes of aging rarely present a major problem. Patient response to drugs is variable at any age, so, with the exception of induction, drugs are given in small doses and titrated to effect. The trend today in anesthesia practice is to use drugs that are short acting. These drugs either have shorter metabolic half-lives or redistribute to yield very low blood levels with minimal residual effects, or do both. For example, propofol and thiopental are equally effective induction agents and both are "short-acting" because these redistribute rapidly into fat. The residual blood levels of propofol, however, produce less residual sedation than occurs with thiopental, and propofol also has a shorter metabolic half life. These principles of drug pharmacokinetics apply to patients of all ages, but the ability to use drugs with rapid fat uptake, but minimal residual effects, is particularly helpful in older patients.

Hemodynamic Stability During Anesthesia

Hemodynamic stability is a core goal of anesthesia and one of the more challenging aspects of anesthetic care of the older adult. Many characteristics of aging contribute to the increased vulnerability of older adults to hemodynamic instability (Table 36-2). General anesthesia lowers the blood pressure in everyone. This effect is owing to decreased sympathetic tone, which, in turn, may lower heart rate, decrease systemic vascular resistance, and cause peripheral pooling of blood, which will lower cardiac preload. There is also some direct myocardial depression. These effects are exaggerated in older adults. Sympathetic nervous system activity commonly increases with age and so may be more reactive to stimuli than in young people. Chronic hypertension, common in older patients, further exaggerates the vascular response to changes in sympathetic nervous system activity. In particular, the aorta stiffens with age and typically results in left ventricular hypertrophy. Hypertrophy leads to a reduction in the rate of diastolic relaxation, which, in turn, diminishes early diastolic filling. Adequate ventricular preload becomes dependent on passive filling related to left atrial pressure and active filling related to atrial contraction. Both mechanisms must overcome the increased ventricular stiffness and both require a full atrium. Yet atrial blood volume is difficult to keep constant. Veins also stiffen with age. Venous stiffness reduces the capacity to buffer changes in blood volume, making

TABLE 36-2

Cardiovascular Aging and Anesthetic Implications

AGING-INDUCED CARDIOVASCULAR CHANGE	PHYSIOLOGICAL CONSEQUENCE	ANESTHETIC AND PERIOPERATIVE IMPLICATION
Loss of sinoatrial node cells and conduction system fibrosis	First-degree block and occasional sick sinus syndrome	Severe bradycardia when coupled with potent opioids
Stiff arteries	Systolic hypertension Impedance mismatching at end ejection, leading to myocardial hypertrophy and impaired diastolic relaxation	Labile blood pressure Diastolic dysfunction and sensitivity to volume status
Myocardial hypertrophy and connective tissue stiffening	Increased ventricular stiffness Ventricular filling dependent on a well-maintained atrial pressure	Failure to maintain filling causes an exaggerated decline in cardiac performance; excessive volume more easily increases filling pressures to congestive failure levels
Decreased beta-receptor responsiveness	Limited increases in heart rate and contractility in response to endogenous and exogenous catecholamines Impaired baroreflex control of blood pressure	Increased dependency on Frank–Starling mechanism to maintain cardiac performance. Labile blood pressure
Stiff veins	Decreased buffering of changes in body blood volume impairs ability to maintain constant atrial pressure	Changes in blood volume or body distribution of blood cause exaggerated changes in cardiac filling Hypovolemia more easily impairs cardiac performance, whereas hypervolemia more easily leads to symptoms of congestive failure
Increased sympathetic nervous system activity at rest and in response to stimuli	Basal vascular resistance more dependent on basal sympathetic nervous system	Hypotension from anesthetic blunting of sympathetic tone Increased blood pressure lability from changes in sympathetic tone in response to the surgical stimulus

atrial filling more sensitive to overall volume status as well as to the effects of the sympathetic nervous system on blood distribution. In consequence, older patients are more prone than young patients to both hypotension and hypertension during surgery.

Management of the inevitable swings in blood pressure can be a challenge. Alterations of blood pressure are particularly common during induction of anesthesia and the laryngoscopy/intubation sequence. Hypertension is usually managed by increasing the depth of anesthesia with more opioid and/or increasing the anesthetic gas concentration. Unfortunately, the surgical stimulus can increase or decrease faster than the depth of the anesthetic can be manipulated. One approach is to complement the anesthetic with beta-blockade to minimize the hemodynamic response to the surgical stimulus. Another approach is to use relatively high doses of opioid and relatively less volatile anesthetic. Opioids produce less intrinsic depression of blood pressure than do volatile anesthetics while preventing significant rise in blood pressure during surgery. If high-dose opioids are used to prevent the hemodynamic response to the surgical stimulus, the primary role of the volatile anesthetic is to produce unconsciousness, requiring approximately half the concentration of gas needed without opioids. An ultra-short-acting opioid, remifentanil, can be employed primarily for short cases that are accompanied by profound simulation in sensitive areas. High doses of moderate-duration opioids (e.g., fentanyl or morphine) are limited by residual respiratory depression, which can unacceptably depress ventilatory drive at the end of the surgery. Continuous use of ultrashort agents is not currently encouraged because of cost. Another approach is to use a limited amount of opioids compatible with the surgical procedure and then maintain the volatile anesthetic concentration high enough to block the hemodynamic response to the highest level of surgical stimulus. Such a strategy will minimize hypertension but will also make the patient more prone to hypotension at other, less stimulat-

ing, times of the surgery. Sometimes even the minimum level of anesthesia causes an unacceptable depression of blood pressure. In these circumstances, blood pressure must be actively supported. Volume administration can support blood pressure but is of limited utility in older patients. Volume may restore stroke volume but will not compensate for hypotension caused by severe bradycardia or a low vascular resistance. Bradycardia generally responds to glycopyrrolate, an anticholinergic drug that crosses the blood–brain barrier poorly and is presumably less likely to promote postoperative delirium than atropine. Ephedrine stimulates both alpha and beta-receptors and effectively raises pressure, but tachyphylaxis eventually develops and so it is not used for extended time periods. Phenylephrine, a pure alpha agonist, can be conveniently given as either a bolus or a low-dose infusion and effectively maintains blood pressure. On occasion, inotropic infusions (e.g., dopamine) are used, especially if bradycardia does not respond to anticholinergics or there is concern over baseline ventricular function. All pressors have potential adverse effects, of course, but serious problems from their use are infrequent.

Intravascular fluid therapy in older adults is a controversial topic. Much has been written, little has been proven, and clinical practice tends to be based more on habit than on science. Much of the science underlying the most standard anesthetic and surgical approach to volume replacement is based on studies undertaken in the 1960s and 1970s. As noted above, cardiovascular aging makes volume administration more difficult. The stiffness of the venous system exaggerates the response to a given volume excess or deficit. Well-anesthetized patients may appear hypovolemic during surgery as a result of the suppression of sympathetic nervous system activity. A common concern of the geriatric anesthesiologist is that large amounts of crystalloid used for blood pressure control may achieve what appears to be normovolemia during surgery, but, when surgery is over and postoperative pain restores sympathetic activity, that volume may shift back to the central circulation and create a volume overload. Recently, the basis for fluid administration has been questioned, and an alternative strategy that uses less fluid has been proposed. To date, this approach to fluid management has not been extensively tested or adopted in the United States. The recent literature on reduced fluid volume has not attended to the special issues of cardiovascular aging. Strategies that limit fluid administration frequently are attended by increased use of vasopressors (phenylephrine, norepinephrine, and vasopressin). Since traditional anesthesia care reserves vasopressor use for when fluid administration has failed to maintain perfusion, vasopressor use can be considered an ominous clinical sign that is frequently cited as an adverse consequence of limited fluid administration. In many cases, volume administration is unavoidable and there are no extant guidelines for managing fluid, particularly in older adults. There is also an extensive literature about the proper content of fluids; particularly comparing crystalloid to colloid solutions. There are no clear-cut guidelines for use in older adults.

Anesthesia and the Pulmonary System

Aging and general anesthesia have important effects on the respiratory system (Table 36-3). Closing capacity increases with age because of diminished airway tethering by connective tissue. General anesthesia enhances expiratory muscle tone and diminishes inspiratory muscle tone, thereby decreasing functional residual capacity. Sighs are suppressed. Atelectasis develops more easily because of the increased closing capacity, decreased functional residual capacity, and the loss of sighs. Atelectasis occurs in the great majority of patients undergoing general anesthesia. Mechanical ventilation disturbs the normal pattern of diaphragmatic breathing in the supine patient, altering normal ventilation/perfusion matching. Volatile anesthetics reduce the effectiveness of hypoxic pulmonary vasoconstriction. Both volatile anesthetics and the placement of an endotracheal tube diminish ciliary action of the respiratory tract, an effect that extends into the postoperative period. Opioids diminish the carbon dioxide ventilatory drive. Volatile anesthetics suppress the hypoxic ventilatory drive, even at the low concentrations present postoperatively. Particularly very frail patients are at increased risk of ventilatory failure postoperatively. The increase in body oxygen consumption during recovery from surgery may exceed the ventilatory reserve that is compromised by increased chest wall stiffness and decreased skeletal muscle mass. Finally, silent regurgitation and aspiration is more common in older patients. At-risk patients will be challenged postoperatively by drugs that may further depress the airway protective reflexes and impair gastric emptying. Aspiration is much more likely to occur postoperatively than intraoperatively. It is important to understand, however, that patients who suffer aspiration to a degree that causes clinical signs or symptoms will present with some evidence of dysfunction (e.g., hypoxia) within a few hours of the aspiration. It is unlikely that a patient will aspirate, have no consequences for many hours, and then develop a clinical problem that could be attributed to much earlier aspiration.

Intraoperative respiratory management of older patients is straightforward. Bronchospasm is probably the most common intraoperative untoward event. Bronchospasm usually resolves promptly with easily administered treatments. Volatile anesthetic gases themselves produce bronchodilation, and inhaled bronchodilator medications can be administered through the endotracheal tube. Atelectasis prevention strategies during the intraoperative period have been variously successful. Supplemental oxygen is freely used in the operating room, and all patients are monitored by pulse oximetry and frequently with expired gas analysis. This has allowed the anesthesiologist to ensure that all patients are well oxygenated and has markedly decreased the incidence of clinically significant hypoxemia in all age groups.

Most pulmonary problems do not manifest until after surgery. Some degree of hypercarbia is common for at least the immediate postoperative period, especially after considerable opioid administration. This finding usually means nothing more than the presence of good analgesia, so long as supplemental oxygen is administered and the patient can be watched carefully. Supplemental oxygen will likely be necessary for a longer period of time after surgery in older patients. Patients with tenuous respiratory function may need ventilatory support until they are past the acute recovery period. Pneumonia remains an important complication and the ability to prevent its development is limited. Deep breathing and vigorous coughing by the patient are thought to help prevent pneumonia, but postoperative pain may impair these maneuvers. Improved pain control may

---

TABLE 36-3

Pulmonary Aging and Anesthetic Implications

AGING-INDUCED PULMONARY CHANGE	PHYSIOLOGICAL CONSEQUENCE	ANESTHETIC AND PERIOPERATIVE IMPLICATION
Decrease in bony thorax elasticity	Stiff chest that is hard to move, increasing the work of breathing and making it more difficult to increase minute ventilation Increased residual volume	Increased risk of respiratory failure
Loss of muscle mass	Reduced strength to meet the increased minute ventilation requirements secondary to the metabolic demands after surgery	Increased risk of respiratory failure
Decreased lung parenchymal stiffness	Increased lung compliance Decreased "tethering" of small airways, leading to increased closing volume Impaired ventilation-perfusion matching	Increased risk of atelectasis, hypoxia, and pneumonia
Impaired airway-protective reflexes	More frequent aspiration	Increased risk of pneumonia and Adult Respiratory Distress Syndrome
Decreased central nervous system responsiveness	Decreased hypercapnic and hypoxic drives	Increased risk of hypoxia Greater sensitivity to anesthetic agents

be one mechanism by which epidural analgesia improves perioperative outcome (see section on "postoperative analgesia"). The role of silent aspiration in the development of postoperative pneumonia is unclear and warrants closer examination.

Regional Anesthesia

Regional anesthesia uses a family of pharmacologic agents with unique properties and a range of techniques designed to meet the needs of the surgical plan. This section will review agents first and then techniques. Local anesthetic agents reversibly inhibit the propagation of signals along nerves. When applied to a specific nerve or pathway in sufficient concentration, these agents produce anesthesia (loss of sensation) and paralysis (loss of muscle power). The currently used local anesthetics belong to one of two classes: aminoamide and aminoester local anesthetics. All of these medications are structurally related to cocaine but do not stimulate the sympathoadrenal system and, thus, do not produce hypertension or local vasoconstriction, nor do they have any abuse potential. Local anesthetics vary in their pharmacological properties. Field and nerve blocks are frequently performed using long-acting drugs such as bupivacaine. This often provides exceptional postoperative analgesia for up to 24 hours. The local anesthetic lidocaine is also used as a Class Ib antiarrhythmic drug. At higher doses, lidocaine and all local anesthetics are arrythmogenic. All agents have limited therapeutic windows, and overdosage can result in cardiac arrest and death. There are large variations in how aging alters the pharmacokinetics of local anesthetics, and aging per se accounts for less than 20% of variability. There is little suggestion that sensitivity to local anesthetics is altered by aging. Some forms of regional anesthesia can be combined with a light general anesthetic.

Regional anesthesia techniques include topical anesthesia (surface), infiltration, plexus block, epidural (extradural) block, and spinal anesthesia. As a rule, field and nerve blocks have minimal systemic effects unless there is an untoward event during placement, such as intravascular injection of the local anesthetic, or there is an allergic reaction to the drug. Many procedures, such as cataract surgery, can be accomplished with local anesthetic drops and no additional sedation. Blocks of specific nerves or nerve plexi are associated with anatomically specific side effects and complications. An interscalene block of the cervical plexus provides good anesthesia for operations on the shoulder. It may also result in anesthesia of the ipsilateral phrenic nerve, resulting in hemidiaphragmatic paralysis. An ipsilateral Horner syndrome may also be observed. Field blocks are often placed by the surgeon at the operative site prior to or at the conclusion of surgery.

Neuraxial blocks, including spinal and epidural anesthesia, are considered complete anesthetics; no other supplemental treatment is necessary, although sedation is often provided at the request of the patient or the surgeon. These blocks produce the greatest physiological effects and are presented here in more detail than other forms of regional anesthesia because their use in older adults is common. Spinal anesthesia differs from epidural anesthesia in the location of anesthetic administration, in the consequences of location of administration on type of nerve affected, and on the resulting clinical manifestations of treatment. With spinal anesthesia, the local anesthetic is injected into the cerebrospinal fluid, inside the dura and arachnoid, where it quickly diffuses into the spinal nerves. Inside the dura and arachnoid, spinal nerves have minimal connective tissue surrounding them so that the local anesthetic effectively blocks all nerve fibers, including motor, touch, and sympathetic nerves. The patient is, thus, provided not only anesthesia but also paralysis and sympathetic blockade. In contrast, an epidural anesthetic is typically administered through a catheter placed just outside the dura. In the epidural space, spinal nerves are covered with a thick connective tissue sheath, which slows the onset of anesthetic effect. By varying the concentration of the injected local anesthetic, nerve types can be differentially blocked. Differential blockade is important for postoperative analgesia, where partial blockade of pain fibers are desired, but touch and motor nerves are to be spared. Unfortunately, it is not possible to fully anesthetize pain fibers without also affecting the sympathetic nerves. When high concentrations of the local anesthetic will be used to achieve full anesthesia, all nerve types will be blocked.

The hemodynamic effects of neuraxial anesthesia stem from the blockade of sympathetic nerves. The hemodynamic response depends on many factors, including how many thoracic dermatomes of sympathetic fibers are affected and how much of a reflex response can be mounted via the vagus and any unblocked sympathetic fibers. In the case of spinal anesthesia, the sympathetic fibers may be at least partially blocked for many dermatomes above the level of sensory blockade, as defined by sharp–dull discrimination. It is not uncommon, therefore, to have a near-total sympathectomy with spinal anesthesia. The hemodynamic consequences can be dramatic. If one accepts the hypothesis that vascular resistance is increased with age because of increased sympathetic tone, then removal of that tone often results in a large decrease in vascular resistance (Figure 36-4). Pharmacologic sympathectomy in young adults results in a much

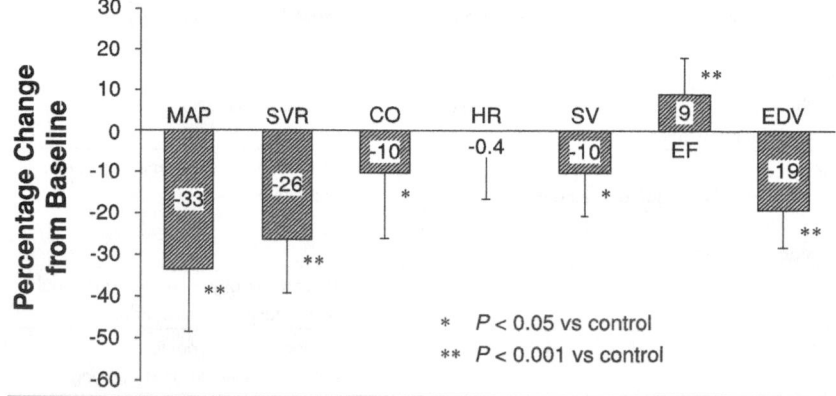

FIGURE 36-4. The hemodynamic response to high spinal anesthesia is shown in 15 elderly men with cardiac disease. The large decrease in mean arterial blood pressure (MAP) was primarily because of decreases in systemic vascular resistance (SVR) and not decreases in cardiac output (CO). Overall, heart rate (HR) did not change; therefore, the decrease in cardiac output was because of a decrease in stroke volume (SV). The decrease in left ventricular end-diastolic volume (EDV) did not cause a comparable decrease in stroke volume because the ejection fraction (EF) increased. *(Adapted with permission from Rooke GA, Freund PR, Jacobson AF. Hemodynamic response and change in organ blood volume during spinal anesthesia in elderly men with cardiac disease. Anesth Analg. 1997;85:99–105.)*

* P < 0.05 vs control
** P < 0.001 vs control

smaller decrease in vascular resistance but a similar decrease in cardiac output. In Figure 36-4, the sympathectomy also decreased left ventricular filling as blood volume shifted to the legs and mesentery. However, the increase in ejection fraction ameliorated much of what the decrease in preload would have otherwise been expected to do to stroke volume and cardiac output.

Many patients request sedation during surgery performed under a regional anesthetic, usually because they are not interested in being aware of the activities in the operating room. Small quantities of midazolam and fentanyl often suffice, but if higher levels of sedation are desired, typically a propofol infusion will be used. Interestingly, older patients commonly fall asleep during spinal anesthesia, even in the absence of any sedative medications. The mechanism behind this phenomenon is unknown but may involve the loss of sensory input to the brainstem. If sedative and analgesic drugs are used, the risk of airway obstruction increases. The combination of sedation plus spinal anesthesia, for example, produces more postoperative hypoxia than sedation or spinal anesthesia alone. With careful monitoring and skill in airway management, the risk of airway obstruction should be minimal. In unskilled hands, however, airway obstruction can rapidly lead to hypoxia and patient injury. This risk to the patient forms the basis for the recent JCAHO requirement that trained personnel must be present at procedures performed anywhere in the hospital whenever the patient is likely to be sedated to the point of drowsiness that requires verbal stimuli or worse to arouse. The requirements include assigning a person to the sole task of monitoring the patient.

Regional anesthetic techniques can be combined with general anesthesia. Combined general/regional anesthesia involves the provision of primarily a high thoracic epidural anesthetic with subsequent induction of general anesthesia with endotracheal intubation. This approach has been most extensively studied in Denmark in association with a fast-track approach to colonic surgery, which also includes rapid ambulation and food consumption (day of surgery) and early discharge (postoperative day 2). The advantages of the technique combine the ability to use considerably less general anesthetic with resulting rapid emergence, with the complete absence of pain, because the epidural is still active and will be used to manage postoperative pain. The main limitation of the technique is the added difficulty in maintaining blood pressure in the operating room. In addition, it is common to place an epidural catheter exclusively for postoperative pain control, which will only be activated at the end of surgery, i.e., it is not used as part of the anesthetic technique.

Regional Versus General Anesthesia

Many anesthesiologists prefer regional anesthesia over general anesthesia. There is something attractive to providing an anesthetic that just blocks nerves but spares direct effects to the brain and other vital organs. Markers of stress such as cortisol, catecholamines, and cytokines become elevated during and after surgery with a general anesthetic, while spinal and epidural anesthesia markedly attenuate these changes during surgery, and much of the attenuation will continue after surgery if epidural analgesia is continued postoperatively. The presumption has been that the reduction in stress would translate into a reduction in morbidity and mortality, but it has been surprisingly difficult to prove this hypothesis. Early studies centered around the benefits of postoperative analgesia via an epidural catheter typically infused with a dilute local anesthetic plus opi-

oid. These studies employed random group assignment but enrolled small numbers of patients (40–60 each). Perhaps because a high-risk population was recruited, several of the studies demonstrated lower mortality and morbidity with respect to cardiac and pulmonary complications. Other studies have demonstrated additional benefits of regional anesthesia, including less blood loss during hip replacement surgery, a decreased incidence of deep vein thrombosis and pulmonary emboli, and a reduction in early graft thrombosis in peripheral vascular surgery. Not all studies demonstrate consistent benefits, however.

In order to circumvent the problem of small patient enrollment, a meta-analysis has been performed on 141 studies that had employed randomized assignment to general anesthesia versus spinal or epidural anesthesia. In approximately half of the studies, the regional anesthetic was accompanied by a general anesthetic. When an epidural catheter was employed (75% of the neuraxial blocks), postoperative epidural analgesia was frequently employed. Thus, group comparison was somewhat muddled. Nevertheless, the results were strongly in favor of the regional technique with deaths from all causes reduced by 30%. Decreases in rates of myocardial infarction, pneumonia, and pulmonary embolism (but not stroke) were also demonstrated.

These encouraging results must be tempered by two prospective studies, each involving roughly 1000 patients randomly assigned to general anesthesia alone with parenteral opioids for postoperative analgesia versus combined general plus epidural anesthesia with postoperative epidural analgesia. In one study, the general plus epidural group demonstrated a decreased incidence of respiratory failure. The other study only found a lower incidence of adverse events in the subset of patients within the epidural group who were undergoing repair of an abdominal aortic aneurysm. Therefore, neither study found overwhelming evidence of improved outcome from the addition of epidural anesthesia/analgesia.

It is apparent, then, that the current evidence of the benefit of postoperative epidural analgesia is weak, as is the evidence of the superiority of neuraxial anesthesia over general anesthesia as the primary anesthetic technique. Nevertheless, better pain relief is usually achieved by regional techniques, and it is still possible that some medical benefits exist. Therefore, these techniques continue to be used, at least in selected circumstances. Given the difficulty in proving a difference in outcome between regional and general anesthesia, it would be surprising if any study could demonstrate a difference in mortality or major morbidity when comparing, for example, different types of general anesthesia. In the absence of compelling outcome data, whether to perform a regional or a general anesthetic depends on many factors. Carotid endarterectomies, for example, may be performed under either a local block with an awake patient or a general anesthesia. Experienced teams of surgeons and anesthesiologists can perform either of these techniques with excellent and equivalent results. Usually, a center chooses one or the other technique. Both the surgeon and the anesthesiologist must be comfortable working with the chosen technique. Patient physical limitations, including uncomfortable patient positioning for the surgery, may prevent the use of a pure regional technique. For example, total hip replacement surgery requires the patient to lie in a fixed position on their side for the entire procedure. Even with careful positioning and padding, the position can be uncomfortable if only the lower half of the body is anesthetized. Sometimes sedation is adequate to make the procedure tolerable, whereas other patients require sedation bordering on general anesthesia that requires a secured airway. The presence of coagulopathies or the use of preoperative anticoagulation may preclude the use or regional techniques, as a result of the risk of bleeding and, in the case of spinal or epidural anesthesia, the risk of epidural hematoma (see the section below on "postoperative analgesia"). Also, the patient must be willing to undergo the regional technique, which will invariably involve placing a needle somewhere into the body. Some patients will not accept needles under any circumstance unless they are totally asleep, but, for safety reasons, most blocks will not be performed under such conditions. Other patients may refuse regional techniques owing to prior bad experiences. There is also a common fear of paralysis following spinal anesthesia, which is, for the most part unfounded, representing an extremely unusual complication with multiple potential causes. On the other hand, many patients welcome the opportunity to avoid a general anesthetic and the attendant postoperative sedation and risk of nausea. There is little evidence to suggest that the choice of anesthesia has a significant impact on either cognitive abilities or the incidence of postoperative delirium. All anesthetics should be preceded by a thorough discussion with the patient about anesthetic options, including their benefits, disadvantages, and associated risks. This discussion is best carried out by an anesthesiologist, who is best able to recognize the characteristics of the patient and procedure that will determine which anesthetic options are appropriate, and to explain to the patient the important risks and benefits of each option. In many cases, the choice of anesthetic technique can include patient preference; therefore, it is important to provide patients with comprehensive information and involve them in the decision-making process.

POSTOPERATIVE ANALGESIA

The options for postoperative analgesia have expanded considerably in the past 15 years. Highlighted here are patient-controlled analgesia and peripheral nerve blocks.

Patient-Controlled Analgesia

Patient-controlled analgesia devices are programmable infusion pumps that can provide either basal infusion or controlled access on request (usually pushing a button) to an opioid preparation, which is maintained in a locked compartment. The device offers the patient the opportunity to obtain pain medication without having to wait for a busy nurse. The device also provides more smooth analgesia compared to intermittent administration, which produces a cycle of heavy sedation with the initial peak effect, followed by a period of alertness and reasonable analgesia, and ending with increasing pain and anxiety until the next dose comes due. Patient-controlled analgesia allows the patient to finely titrate the analgesia against the opioid side effects, including nausea, sedation, dysphoria, and itching. In recent years, patient-controlled analgesia has become a standard part of postoperative pain management, in which orders follow specific templates. Since there is a tremendous variability in pain tolerance and response among individuals in general, and older adults in particular, effective postoperative pain management programs require a knowledgeable individual to observe the patient on a regular basis, in order to adjust the device properly. While elderly patients are sensitive to the respiratory depressant effects of nar-

cotic agents, it is impossible to prescribe an age-specific approach to the use of postoperative opioids. Each patient is highly individual, and the therapeutic window for many analgesics is narrowed in the elderly.

Peripheral Nerve Blocks

Peripheral nerve blocks performed with long-acting local anesthetics provide up to 24 hours of postoperative analgesia. These blocks provide both significant advantages and risks. These are typically performed in a sedated, but awake and cooperative, patient prior to surgery. The most elaborate technique for postoperative analgesia is provided through indwelling catheters. Given the time involvement for catheter placement and management and the uncertainty of enhanced outcome, this technique is used selectively. Initially, epidural analgesia was nothing more than boluses of morphine through a lumbar catheter. Now the typical formula is low concentrations of both a local anesthetic and an opioid, which are infused continuously through a catheter placed at the dermatome most central to the incision, be it thoracic or lumbar in location. The quality of analgesia afforded by a well-managed epidural catheter is excellent and associated with high levels of satisfaction.

There are significant risks to epidural catheter use. The most common problem is failed placement. The next most common problem is inadvertent dural puncture. As epidural catheters are placed with large-bore needles, the risk of a spinal headache is relatively high. Fortunately, the risk of postdural puncture headache decreases with age. If a thoracic catheter is placed, dural puncture could also lead to direct spinal cord trauma. This complication is rare. The most feared complication is the development of an epidural hematoma. The epidural space has many veins that are occasionally punctured. Generally, any bleeding stops spontaneously and quickly, but if it does not, epidural hematoma may cause cord compression. Permanent paraplegia becomes likely, since the success of emergency laminectomy is poor once symptoms appear. Retrospective analysis of spinal and epidural anesthetics suggests that the intrinsic risk of paralysis is less than 1:150 000. Patients who have abnormal coagulation, however, are thought to be at greater risk. Most reports of epidural hematoma have been in patients who were anticoagulated when the block was performed or when heparin therapy was instituted less than an hour after the needle placement. The relative risk owing to anticoagulation is unknown, as all reports are anecdotal and do not include a denominator. In the case of epidural catheters, epidural hematomas develop almost as often on catheter removal as on insertion, so the catheter removal must be considered an at-risk event as well. There are case series reports on spinal or epidural block performed in anticoagulated patients, but the largest series involved 1000 patients and is too small to be meaningful despite a zero incidence of hematoma. Even subcutaneous heparin can provide enough anticoagulation to increase risk at its peak effect at around 2 hours after administration. Particularly distressing has been the high number of epidural hematomas reported in patients receiving low-molecular-weight heparin. Many of the hematomas developed after catheter removal. In response to these reports of epidural hematoma, it is recommended that any patient with an epidural catheter be given frequent neurologic checks if they receive anticoagulants (warfarin, heparin, and low-molecular-weight heparin). Guidelines for catheter placement and removal are given in Table 36-4.

TABLE 36-4

Guidelines for Epidural Catheters in Anticoagulated Patients*

MEDICATION	RECOMMENDATIONS
Warfarin	Do not place needle or remove catheter if prothrombin levels are therapeutic. Discontinuation of warfarin must be of sufficient duration to restore all prothrombin factors, not just factor VII. If warfarin is initiated prior to needle placement or catheter removal, check the prothrombin time even if only one dose of warfarin has been given.
Intravenous heparin	Do not place needle or remove catheter if partial thromboplastin time is elevated. Heparin therapy should not be initiated until at least 1 h after needle placement or catheter removal. Catheter removal should be preceded by heparin discontinuation for 2–4 h and evaluation of the coagulation status.
Subcutaneous (mini-dose) heparin	Needle placement and catheter removal is not contraindicated, but it may be wise to avoid doing so at the peak heparin effect at around 2 h after injection.
Low-molecular-weight heparin (LMWH)	Needle placement and catheter removal should occur at least 2 h before, and at least 10 h after, once-a-day LMWH therapy. Twice-a-day LMWH dictates holding one dose, and waiting 20–24 h after the last dose.
Nonsteroidal anti-inflammatory drugs	No evidence of increased risk.
Combination therapy	Little data, but risk may be increased, especially if low-molecular-weight heparin is one of the therapies.

*For full set of recommendations of the American Society of Regional Anesthesia Consensus Statement, see http://www.asra.com/items_of_interest/consensus_statements.

PERIOPERATIVE COMPLICATIONS

The most common surgical indicator of complications is morbidity and mortality within a defined period following a procedure, frequently 30 days. Hamel reported on 26 648 patients aged ≥80 years (median age 82 years) and 568 263 patients <80 years (median age 62 years) from the Veterans Administrations National Surgical Quality Improvement Program (NSQIP) database. Mortality is low (<2%) for many common procedures (transurethral prostatectomy, hernia repair, knee replacement, carotid endarterectomy, vertebral disc surgery, laryngectomy, and radical prostatectomy). The incidence of complications increases and the impact of complications on mortality and functional recovery increases with age. The presence of a complication increased mortality from 4% to 26%. Respiratory and urinary tract complications were most common.

Anesthetic risk is difficult to quantify separately from the risk of surgery, because few people receive an anesthetic in the absence of a surgical procedure. For healthy patients, the risk of death purely caused by the anesthetic has been estimated to be as low as 1 in 250 000. Such a figure is trivial in comparison to the 1 in 500 risk of death associated with surgery and anesthesia overall. Mortality is dependent on patient age and strongly influenced by the type of surgery. Even in patients older than 90 years of age, minor surgeries carry a near-zero 30-day mortality, but major abdominal, thoracic, and vascular surgeries are associated with a 20% to 30% mortality. Clearly, comorbid disease, the effects of surgical trauma, and presumably the anesthetic must interact in some way to increase risk. The mechanisms underlying increased risk are poorly understood but are presumed to be influenced by the interaction of age and comorbid disease on reduced physiological reserve. This reduced reserve is presumed to make the body less able to withstand the various stresses associated with surgery such as pain, a hypermetabolic state, and altered neuroendocrine hormones.

Course of Recovery and Common Perioperative Complications in Older Patients

The influence of age on the course of recovery after surgery has not been a focus of research but a recent study by Lawrence et al. provides valuable insights. Among geriatric patients who had undergone abdominal surgery, recovery of independence in basic activities of daily living took almost 3 months on average. Some measures, such as hand grip strength, had, on average, not returned to baseline even at 6 months. Since recovery from surgery involves patient effort, it is important for the patients to understand their own role in the recovery process and to have a realistic idea of how long it will be before they will feel like themselves again.

An exhaustive discussion of complications that may occur in association with anesthesia and surgery is beyond the scope of this chapter. Nevertheless, it is worth commenting on a few complications. The most feared complication from anesthesia is the loss of the ability to ventilate a patient with subsequent hypoxic injury. This type of complication has become rare, and there is nothing to suggest that these events are more common in elderly patients.

Pulmonary complications are most common in elderly surgical patients, with postoperative pneumonia carrying a 20% mortality rate. Gag reflexes are decreased in the elderly and easily impaired by sedative and analgesic medications. Unless an older adult is specifically assessed as needing prolonged mechanical ventilation following surgery, there is nothing to suggest an advantage delaying extubation based on age. The current practice is to return to spontaneous ventilation and avoid prolonged intubation. Programs to prevent the development of pneumonia have had mixed results to date.

Cardiac events have received intensive focus in the perioperative arena. The nature of perioperative risk has changed during the years, with full Q-wave infarctions becoming less common. The risk of myocardial infarction increases with the prevalence of coronary disease in the patient population examined. In a relatively high-risk group such as patients undergoing peripheral vascular surgery, the incidence of myocardial infarction is approximately 4% and congestive heart failure around 9%. Among patients with a prior history of myocardial infarction, a perioperative myocardial infarction is still associated with approximately 30% mortality. The most common time when myocardial infarctions and congestive heart failure are detected is 2 days after surgery. The use of perioperative beta-blockers for patients at risk of myocardial infarction is rapidly becoming a standard of care, and there is no reason to avoid beta-blockers solely on the basis of age.

Stroke is a less frequent, but feared, complication of surgery. Perioperative stroke occurs much more frequently than would be expected for the same population in the absence of surgery. The most common cause of stroke in medical patients is thromboembolism, and there is no indication that it is any different perioperatively. In all likelihood, the same changes that increase the risk of myocardial infarction are responsible for the increased risk of stroke. While perhaps widely assumed to be a contributor to surgical stroke risk, hypotension is not a likely cause of stroke in the setting of surgery and anesthesia. There are two main sequences of evidence for this assertion. The first rests on the timing of onset of stroke in the perioperative period, and the second rests on the lack of relationship between duration of hypotension and stroke. The vast majority of strokes occur after the patient recovers from anesthesia and has demonstrated an immediate postoperative unchanged neurologic examination. Intraoperative hypotension is certainly not uncommon in older patients, although it rarely is allowed to persist for long periods of time. It is unlikely that brief periods of intraoperative hypotension are associated with stroke. If brief periods of hypotension caused strokes, then extended periods should, too. Yet no study involving deliberate hypotension for control of blood loss has reported an associated stroke. The best such study, involving 235 patients with an average age of 72 years who were randomly assigned to have mean arterial pressure maintained between 45 and 55 mm Hg or 55 and 70 mm Hg during surgery, demonstrated no strokes. Of much greater concern than hypotension as a mechanism for stroke is atrial fibrillation and cardiac emboli, perhaps accentuated by hypercoagulability. The degree to which atrial fibrillation is a risk factor is not well understood, but it raises the issue of how to manage patients who take warfarin chronically for atrial fibrillation or artificial valves. Based on the low risk of stroke in the immediate few days surrounding surgery in the absence of anticoagulation, it seems statistically safe to stop warfarin 4 days before surgery. A heparin infusion does not need to be used unless the patient has a history of arterial embolus or deep vein thrombosis within the previous 3 months. Warfarin therapy should be reinstituted postoperatively as soon as feasible.

There are two neurocognitive syndromes, delirium and postoperative cognitive dysfunction (POCD), that emerge in the postoperative period most commonly in older adults. Postoperative delirium is a change in mental status that consists of the inability to focus, sustain, and shift attention that is accompanied by other cognitive symptoms (e.g., disorientation and episodic memory dysfunction), and/or perceptual disturbances (misinterpretations, illusions, or hallucinations). Delirium as an entity is discussed elsewhere in this text. There are two forms of delirium after anesthesia. Emergence delirium occurs early, during emergence from general anesthesia. Postoperative delirium on the other hand develops later, usually 24 to 48 hours after an otherwise uneventful recovery from surgery. The risk of postoperative delirium is higher in older adults. For any major general surgery, the incidence is approximately 9% but may be as high as 60% in select surgical populations (major orthopedic and cardiac procedures). In contrast to medical patients, surgical patients rarely have delirium on hospital admission. Approximately a third to a half of the cases of delirium in medical patients are present at admission to the hospital, while only 7% of patients with delirium associated with hip fracture were delirious on admission. The etiology of delirium in general, and in postoperative delirium in particular, remains unknown. Drugs such as meperidine and anticholinergics are potential contributors and should be avoided in the elderly, but the risk from opioids is not clear, especially when failure to use such drugs could lead to increased pain and decreased sleep.

One might expect general anesthesia to be a major risk factor for delirium, but multiple studies have all failed to demonstrate any differences in rates of delirium between general and regional anesthesia, even when careful monitoring of attention and cognitive function is performed. Delirium, if present at any time in the hospitalization, is associated with increased rates of complications, significantly prolonged hospital stay, and a decrease in function (e.g., ADLs) on hospital discharge. Aggressive management of geriatric patients can result in significant decreases in the incidence of postoperative delirium, as shown primarily by Edward Marcantonio in hip fracture patients (see section below on "integrated care"). Both the regular confusion assessment method (CAM) and the CAM-ICU can be used in the perioperative period to detect delirium. As with medical patients, some patients are hyperactive and aggressive, but many delirium patients are hypoactive and quiet, so monitoring programs are required to reliably detect postoperative delirium. Management resembles delirium prevention and care in other settings (see Chapter 53). POCD is defined as a measurable decline in performance on a battery of neurocognitive tests. POCD appears to be distinct from delirium but may prove to be related. For years, there have been anecdotal reports of cognitive decline following surgery and anesthesia. In 1998, a prospective study tested surgical patients before and at 1 week and 3 months after surgery. A matched set of control subjects not having surgery was selected and tested as well. At 3 months, 10% of the surgical patients had demonstrable cognitive decline, in comparison to only 3% of the control subjects. Subsequent follow-up of this cohort suggested that approximately 1% had a persistent deficit after 2 years. As neurocognitive testing is not routinely done prior to surgery, POCD is primarily a research finding. It appears to be primarily a problem of the elderly, in that incidence is minimal below 60 years of age. POCD is uncommon following minor surgery. POCD following cardiac surgery occurs at a higher rate, approaching 50% at discharge from the hospital. POCD following cardiac surgery had traditionally been attributed to the influence of cardiopulmonary bypass; however, a recent study showed similar levels of cognitive decline among patients undergoing coronary artery bypass with and without cardiopulmonary bypass. Thus, the cause of POCD for both cardiac and noncardiac surgery remains unknown. There are neither strategies to prevent POCD nor treatments once cognitive decline occurs.

MODELS OF COLLABORATIVE CARE FOR THE SURGICAL PATIENT

The most mature literature regarding the role of geriatricians in the care of surgical patients has been focused on patients with fractures of the upper femur. Heyburn and colleagues described four models that have been applied to hip fracture patients: the traditional model in which care is directed by the orthopedic surgeon and medical queries are directed to a consultant, the second is a variation in which multidisciplinary rounds with geriatricians and surgeons increase awareness of cross specialty issues, the third involves early postoperative transfer to a geriatric rehabilitation unit, and the fourth is combined orthogeriatric care in which the patient is admitted to a specialized ward where care is coordinated by geriatricians and orthopedic surgeons. There are clear advantages to patients from these models, the key factor being the implementation of the geriatric parts of the care plan. Marcantonio demonstrated the potential for a marked improvement in outcome in a randomized trial of proactive geriatric consultation based on a structured protocol for patients with hip fractures. The intervention reduced delirium by more than one-third. Some perioperative comprehensive geriatric assessment programs have cut down on length of stay. More complex programs such as the Hospital Elder Life Program are being evaluated for their impact on surgical patients.

CONCLUSION

Since there are more and more older adults, and since surgical procedures are increasingly feasible in complex older adults owing to technical and medical advances, the demand for anesthetic care of older patients is increasing. This care is intricate and carries real risks. Better preoperative preparation and postoperative care are likely to have a greater impact on outcomes than further advances in intraoperative anesthetic management, at least in the near future. The role of postoperative analgesia in improving outcomes and reducing the costs of medical care is still in its infancy. Optimal care of the older adult in the perioperative setting depends on the combined expertise of many specialties and an integrated, comprehensive approach.

FURTHER READING

ACC/AHA 2006 Guideline Update on Perioperative Cardiovascular Evaluation for Noncardiac Surgery. Focused update on perioperative beta-blocker therapy. *J Am Coll Cardiol.* 2006 Jun 6;47(11):2343–2355.

Bryson GL, Wyand A. Evidence-based clinical update: general anesthesia and the risk of delirium and postoperative cognitive dysfunction. *Can J Anaesth.* 2006;53:669–677.

Hamel MB, Henderson WG, Khuri SF, Daley J. Surgical outcomes for patients aged 80 and older: morbidity and mortality from major noncardiac surgery. *J Am Geriatr Soc.* 2005;53:424.

Heyburn G, Beringer T, Elliott J, Marsh D. Orthogeriatric care in patients with fractures of the proximal femur. *Clin Orthop Relat Res.* 2004;425:35–43.

Inouye SK, Bogardus ST, Jr, Baker DI, Leo-Summers L, Cooney LM, Jr. The Hospital Elder Life Program: a model of care to prevent cognitive and functional decline in older hospitalized patients. Hospital Elder Life Program. *J Am Geriatr Soc.* 2000;48:1697–1706.

Kearon C, Hirsh J. Management of anticoagulation before and after elective surgery. *New Engl J Med.* 1997;336:1506.

Klopfenstein CE, Herrmann FR, Michel JP, Clergue F, Forster A. The influence of an aging surgical population on the anesthesia workload: a ten-year survey. *Anesth Analg.* 1998;86:1165–1170.

Lakatta EG, Levy D. Arterial and cardiac aging: major shareholders in cardiovascular disease enterprises: part I: aging arteries: a "set up" for vascular disease. *Circulation.* 2003;107:139–146.

Lawrence VA, Cornell JE, Smetana GW. Strategies to reduce postoperative pulmonary complications after noncardiothoracic surgery: systematic review for the American College of Physicians. *Ann Intern Med.* 2006;144:596–608.

Lawrence VA, Hazuda HP, Cornell JE, et al. Functional independence after major abdominal surgery in the elderly. *J Am Coll Surg.* 2004;199:762–772.

Liu S, Carpenter RL, Neal JM. Epidural anesthesia and analgesia—their role in postoperative outcome. *Anesthesiology.* 1995;85:1474.

Mangano DT, Layug EL, Wallace A, et al. Effects of atenolol on mortality and cardiovascular morbidity after noncardiac surgery. *N Engl J Med.* 1996;335:1713.

Marcantonio ER, Flacker JM, Wright RJ, Resnick NM. Reducing delirium after hip fracture: a randomized trial. *J Am Geriatr Soc.* 2001;49:516–522.

Moller JT, Cluitmans P, Rasmussen LS, et al. Long-term postoperative cognitive dysfunction in the elderly: ISPOCD1 study. *Lancet.* 1998;351:857.

Muravchick S. *Geroanesthesia.* St. Louis: Mosby; 1997.

American Geriatrics Society. *New Frontiers in Geriatrics Research: An Agenda for the Surgical and Related Medical Specialties.* New York, New York: American Geriatrics Society; 2004.

Park WY, Thompson JS, Lee KK. Effect of epidural anesthesia and analgesia on perioperative outcome. *Ann Surg.* 2001;234:560.

Horlocker TT, Wedel DJ. Neuraxial block and low-molecular-weight heparin: balancing perioperative analgesia and thromboprophylaxis. *Reg Anesth Pain Med.* 1998 Nov–Dec;23(6 suppl 2):164–77.

Rodgers A, Walker N, Schug S, et al. Reduction of postoperative mortality and morbidity with epidural or spinal anaesthesia: results from overview of randomised trials. *BMJ.* 2000;321:1493.

Rooke GA, Freund PR, Jacobson AF. Hemodynamic response and change in organ blood volume during spinal anesthesia in elderly men with cardiac disease. *Anesth Analg.* 1997;85:99.

Rowe JW, Kahn RL. Human aging: usual and successful. *Science.* 1987;237:143–149.

Silverstein J, ed. *Anesthesiology Clinics of North America.* Philadelphia: W.B. Saunders; March 2000.

Silverstein JH, Rooke GA, Reves JG, McLeskey CH, eds. *Geriatric Anesthesiology.* 2nd ed. New York, New York: Springer; 2007.

Silverstein JH, Timberger M, Reich DL, Uysal S. Central nervous system dysfunction after noncardiac surgery and anesthesia in the elderly. *Anesthesiology.* 2007;106(3):622–628.

Tiret L, Desmonts JM, Hatton F, et al. Complications associated with anaesthesia – a prospective survey in France. *Can Anesth Soc J.* 1986;33:336.

Vandermeulen EP, Van Aken H, Vermylen J. Anticoagulants and spinal-epidural anesthesia. *Anesth Analg.* 1994;79:1165.

Vidan M, Serra JA, Moreno C, Riquelme G, Ortiz J. Efficacy of a comprehensive geriatric intervention in older patients hospitalized for hip fracture: a randomized, controlled trial. *J Am Geriatr Soc.* 2005;53:1476–1482.

Warner MA, Hosking MP, Lobdell CM, et al. Surgical procedures among those ≥90 years of age. *Ann Surg.* 1988;207:380.

Williams-Russo P, Sharrock NE, Mattis S, et al. Randomized trial of hypotensive epidural anesthesia in older adults. *Anesthesiology.* 1999;91:926.

Wu CL, Hsu W, Richman JM, Raja SN. Postoperative cognitive function as an outcome of regional anesthesia and analgesia. *Reg Anesth Pain Med.* 2004;29:257–68.

Surgical Outcomes

Emily Finlayson ■ *John D. Birkmeyer*

As the population ages, an increasing number of elderly patients become candidates for major surgery. According to the National Center for Health Statistics, the rate of hospital discharges for hip replacement in elderly people rose from 2.5 per 10,000 in 1970 to 72.5 per 10,000 in 2004 (http://www.cdc.gov/nchs/agingact.htm). Based on current rates of surgery and census projections, the number of elderly patients undergoing oncologic procedures is expected to increase by up to 51% by the year 2020.

Surgical risks in general are declining over time, and many assume that surgery for elderly patients is getting safer. Case series suggest that surgery can be performed with low morbidity and mortality in elderly people. For lung, esophageal, and pancreatic resection, single-center studies report operative mortality rates between 3% and 4% in very elderly patients. Case series are advocating bariatric surgery in obese patients older than 65 years, touting low morbidity and mortality rates.

Results from clinical series, however, may lead to unrealistic expectations about the safety of surgery in the elderly population, as many published studies have selection bias. Reports of operative mortality tend to represent experiences of high-volume, tertiary academic centers. It is well documented that for high-risk cancer surgery, high-volume surgeons and hospitals have superior outcomes. In addition, results from case series are more likely to be submitted and published if the observed mortality is low, resulting in a publication bias toward lower operative mortality. As a result, existing data generally yield unrealistic risk estimates.

This chapter examines operative risk in very elderly patients using "real-world" results from large databases. In addition, evidence will be reviewed about predictors of surgical outcomes in elderly patients—fatal surgical outcomes as well as functional status and independence after major surgery.

PREDICTORS OF OPERATIVE MORBIDITY AND MORTALITY

Age

In general, increasing age is associated with increased rates of morbidity, functional dependence, and mortality after surgery. Countless studies for several decades have documented that age predicts adverse outcomes after surgery. In a comprehensive analysis of more than 50,0000 patients undergoing noncardiac surgery in the Veterans Affairs National Surgical Quality Improvement Project (NSQIP) database, Hamel et al. found that age was an independent predictor of operative mortality, after adjusting for comorbidities. For all operations in aggregate, 30-day mortality was 2.8% for patients younger than 80 years compared with 8.2% in older patients. For colectomy, mortality was 6.4% in younger patients versus 11.9% in older patients. Similarly, younger patients undergoing elective hip replacement had much lower operative risk (1.3%) when compared to older patients (6.8%). In a single-center study, patients aged 80 years and older had a fourfold increase in risk of both operative mortality and discharge to nursing home after cardiac surgery. This finding persisted after adjustment for patient characteristics. Age is also a known independent predictor of deterioration in cognitive function after coronary artery bypass graft (CABG) surgery.

To assess the impact of age on mortality for a wide range of procedures frequently performed in the elderly, national mortality rates were examined using the Nationwide Inpatient Sample. The Nationwide Inpatient Sample is a large national database containing hospital discharge data for all payers. It is a sample of all U.S. nonfederal hospitals and contains data from approximately

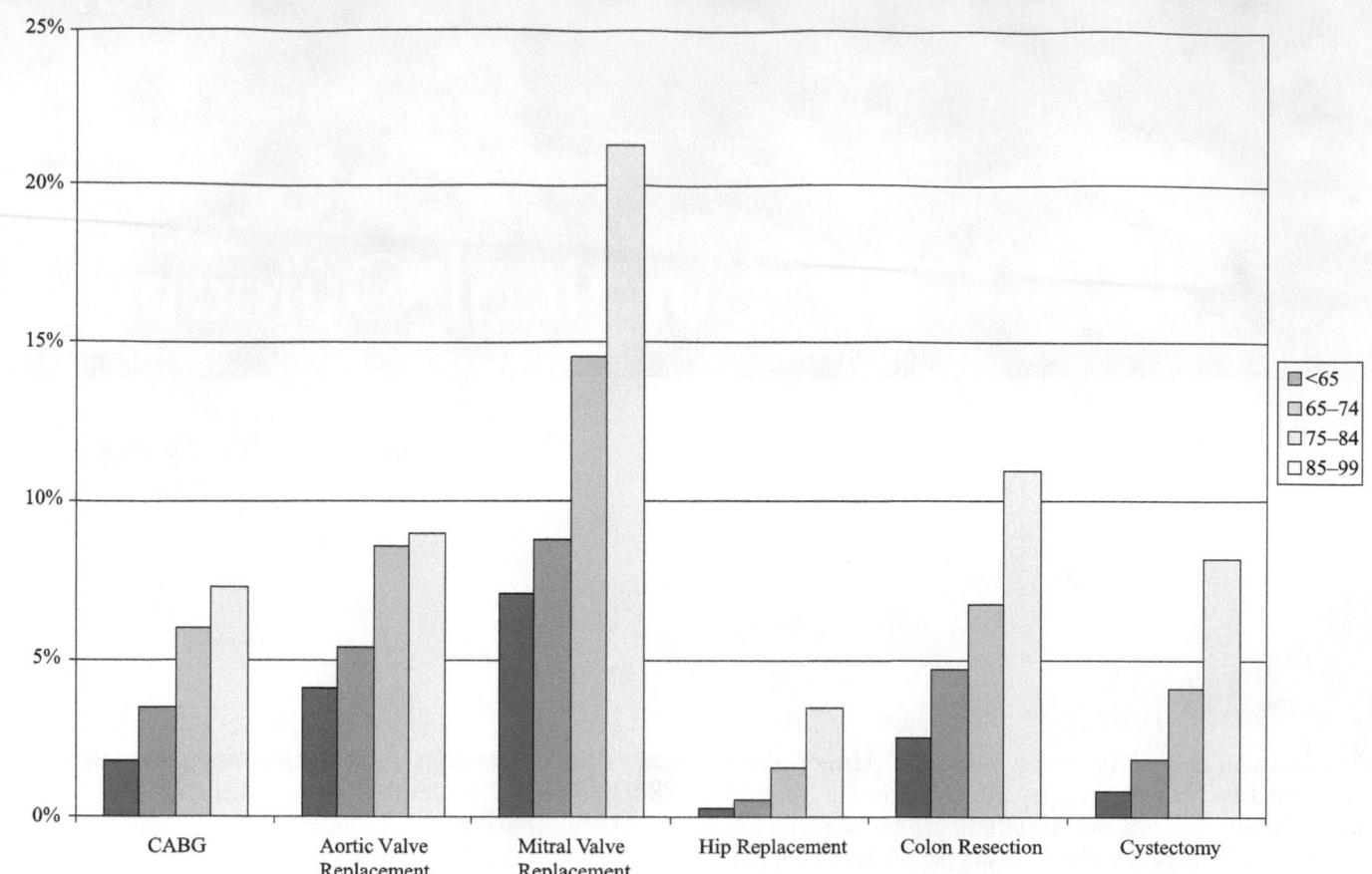

FIGURE 37-1. Operative mortality, by age. *(Unpublished data from the Nationwide Inpatient Sample (NIS), 2003. The NIS contains hospital discharge data for all payers from approximately 1000 hospitals in 22 states.)*

1000 hospitals in 22 states. Selected hospitals represent five strata of hospital characteristics: ownership control, bed size, teaching status, rural–urban location, and geographic region. Based on analysis of all discharges for CABG, mitral and aortic valve surgery, hip replacement, colectomy, and cystectomy in 2003 using ICD-9 procedure codes, operative mortality increased substantially with age for all six procedures (Figure 37-1). Operative mortality was highest for mitral valve replacement, ranging from 7% for patients younger than 65 years to 21% among patients aged 85 to 99 years. For CABG, aortic valve replacement, colon resection, and cystectomy, operative mortality rates among patients older than 85 years ranged from 7% to 11%. Operative mortality was low after hip replacement (0.2%–3%).

Comorbidity

The presence of medical comorbidities increases operative risk in all age groups. In general, with age, patients accumulate medical conditions. It is unclear whether age—as a risk factor for adverse outcomes after surgery—is primarily a proxy for increased comorbidity burden. The relative importance of age and medical comorbidities has been examined carefully in vascular surgery. While age is an independent predictor of mortality in vascular surgery, in multivariate analysis, cardiac, pulmonary, and renal dysfunction have a greater impact on mortality than age for abdominal aortic aneurysm repair,

lower extremity bypass, and amputation. In an analysis of noncardiac procedures, Hamel found that risks associated with selected comorbidities were the same in patients younger or older than 80 years. While it is well known that both age and comorbidity impact operative risk, the interaction between age and comorbidity in surgical outcomes has not been fully elucidated.

Functional Status and Cognitive Function

There is limited evidence that functional status is an important independent predictor of morbidity and mortality after surgery. In a comprehensive analysis of surgical outcomes after abdominal surgery in 24 patients older than 80 years, including physiologic, biochemical, and functional characteristics as well as surgical process measures, age, and activities of daily living score were two of three independent predictors of operative mortality. For gastrectomy, patients with partially dependent functional status are at higher risk of operative mortality than fully independent patients. Poor preoperative functional status has also been shown to predict neurologic and cardiac complications after major surgery in elderly patients.

Although cognitive impairment is common in older adults, the influence of cognitive function on clinical and functional outcomes of surgery in this population is largely unexplored. In one study, surgical patients with cognitive impairment were at higher risk of mortality than other general surgery patients (9.6% vs. 6.3%).

Frailty

Frailty is a common clinical syndrome in elderly patients characterized by decreased physiological reserve and vulnerability to stressors (see Chapter 52). The phenotype includes unintentional weight loss, self-reported exhaustion, grip weakness, slow walking speed, and low physical energy. Frailty appears to be an independent predictor of surgical complications in elderly patients. In one study, frailty was highly associated with postsurgical complications, while ASA score and Lee's Revised Cardiac Index score were not.

FUNCTIONAL OUTCOMES

Functional Status Outcomes

For frail older adults undergoing surgery, functional status is an essential outcome measure. Small changes in functional status after surgery are likely to have an important impact on the ability of such patients to care for themselves and live independently. In a study of 672 elderly patients admitted to the intensive care unit after general, vascular, or trauma surgery, activities of daily living scores decreased significantly at late follow-up, and 13% of patients lost their ability to live independently. For cardiac surgery, functional declines are even more dramatic. In a study of 191 patients aged 80 years and older, undergoing elective cardiac surgery, only 64% of late survivors were fully autonomous. Only the occurrence of a postoperative complication was a significant predictor of impaired postoperative autonomy.

Postoperative functional impairment is common and often protracted in elderly patients. In one study, elderly patients undergoing major open abdominal surgery had comprehensive postoperative functional assessments at 1, 2, and 6 weeks and 3 and 6 months. Mean functional recovery time ranged from 3 weeks for Folstein mini-mental state examination to 6 months for instrumental activities of daily living (Table 37-1). A substantial proportion of elderly patients did not return to baseline function after 6 months for instrumental activities of daily living, Medical Outcomes Study Short Form-36 Physical Component Scale, timed walk, and functional reach. In this study, preoperative physical conditioning and depression were important predictors of functional recovery after surgery.

TABLE 37-1

Mean Functional Recovery Time After Surgery	
FUNCTIONAL OUTCOME	**MEAN RECOVERY TIME**
Mini mental state examination	3 weeks
Activities of daily living	3 months
Instrumental activities of daily living	6 months
SF-36 Physical Component Scale	3 months
Functional reach	3 months
Timed walk	6 weeks

Adapted from Lawrence V, et al. Functional independence after major abdominal surgery in the elderly. J Am Coll Surg. 2004;199:762–772.

Cognitive Outcomes

Acute confusional state is common in older surgical patients in the postoperative period. The incidence of delirium ranges from 5% to 45% in elderly patients undergoing major surgery. Advanced age, hearing and visual impairment, dehydration, sleep deprivation, immobility, severe illness, preoperative narcotic use, and baseline mental status are independently associated with the development of postoperative delirium. Targeted interventions such as frequent reorientation, nonpharmacological sleep protocols, early mobilization, early use of visual and hearing aids, and volume repletion protocols can reduce the incidence of delirium in elderly hospitalized patients.

Long-term declines in cognitive function after cardiac surgery have been well studied. A meta-analysis of both cohort and randomized trials estimated neurocognitive dysfunction after CABG surgery to be 22% at 2 months after surgery, with a range from 14% to 47%. The mean age in most of these studies ranged from 54 to 64 years. Cognitive outcomes of elderly patients are likely to be substantially worse. Although there is some improvement in cognitive function after hospital discharge in CABG patients, one study with long-term follow-up suggested that cognitive function remains poor in this population, with a pattern of early cognitive improvement followed later by decline. Among 261 patients studied by Newman et al., the incidence of cognitive decline was 53% at discharge, 36% at 6 weeks, 24% at 6 months, and 42% at 5 years. Significant predictors of late cognitive decline were older age, fewer years of formal education, and the presence of cognitive decline at discharge.

Less is known about late cognitive outcomes after noncardiac surgery. In one study, noncardiac surgery was associated with long-term postoperative cognitive decline in elderly people, and the risk increased with age. Cognitive dysfunction occurred in 26% of elderly surgical patients at 1 week and in 10% at 3 months, compared to 3% in a control population. Similar to the findings in cardiac surgery, older age and less formal education were independent predictors of poor cognitive outcome.

Discharge Disposition and Independent Living

Discharge disposition after surgery can be considered a proxy for functional and cognitive outcomes. Functional limitations in the perioperative period often prevent older patients from being discharged to home after surgery. The very elderly are much more likely to require admission to a skilled care facility after surgery than their younger counterparts. In Michigan, 20% of elderly patients are discharged to a skilled care facility after cardiac surgery. Of those discharged to home, more than 30% are readmitted to the hospital or a skilled care facility. In the 2003 Nationwide Inpatient Sample database, age was associated with discharge to an extended care facility (i.e., rehab, nursing home, or another hospital) after CABG, valve replacement, hip replacement, colon resection, and cystectomy (Figure 37-2). Patients undergoing hip replacement in all age groups had a high rate of discharge to an extended care facility, but the likelihood of discharge to a facility increased dramatically with age, from 28% for patients younger than 65 years to 87% for patients older than 85 years. Over half of patients aged 85 years and older undergoing cardiac procedures were not discharged to home after surgery. Rates of discharge to a facility were nearly as high after colectomy and cystectomy in the oldest patients. This information is important for several reasons. First, elderly patients and their families need to

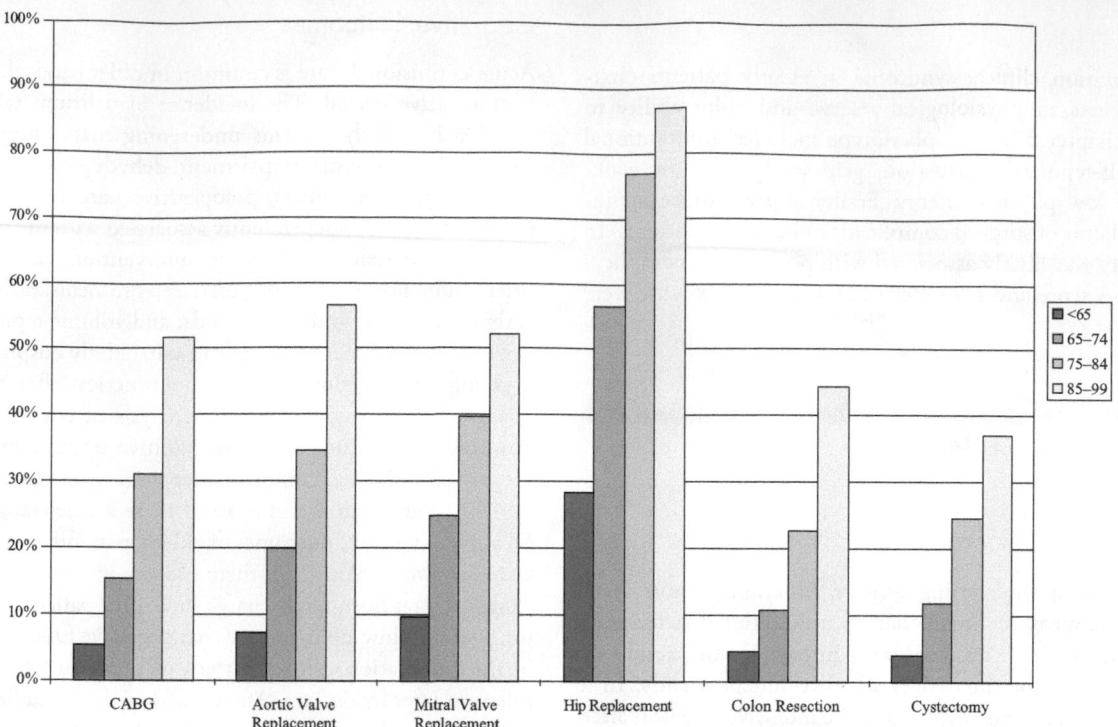

FIGURE 37-2. Rates of discharge to a facility, by age. *(Unpublished data from the Nationwide Inpatient Sample (NIS), 2003. The NIS contains hospital discharge data for all payers from approximately 1000 hospitals in 22 states.)*

have realistic expectations about recovery after major surgery when deciding whether to undergo an elective operation. Second, once the decision for surgery has been made, patients and caregivers need to anticipate the longitudinal needs of elderly patients in the recovery period.

LATE SURVIVAL AFTER CANCER SURGERY

There has been considerable debate about the appropriateness of major surgical resection in very elderly patients with cancer. As surgery is perceived as safer, there is more enthusiasm about offering high-risk cancer operations to elderly patients. Frail elderly patients, however, should be carefully evaluated preoperatively to assess their perioperative risks (see Chapter 35). Some of these patients have competing risks of mortality. These risks may make the risk–benefit tradeoff of a major surgical resection for cancer with a poor prognosis (e.g., pancreatic cancer) tip in favor of foregoing surgery. For many cancers, the use of surgery for "resectable" cancer declines with age. Analysis of the Surveillance, Epidemiology, and End Results database has shown that rates of surgical resection for breast, colon, and rectal cancer are high in all age groups. However, the likelihood of undergoing surgery for localized lung, liver, esophageal, or pancreatic cancer—higher-risk operations with a lower chance for cure—declines sharply with age. Whether decreased use of cancer-directed surgery in the elderly population is appropriate is unknown.

In addition to higher operative mortality rates, elderly cancer patients have substantially lower 5-year survival when compared to younger patients. A retrospective cohort study of octogenarians undergoing major resections for lung, esophageal, and pancreas cancer used the Surveillance and End Results-Medicare-linked database

(1992–2003) to measure late survival. Five-year survival in octogenarians was low for all three cancers: 11% after pancreatectomy, 18% after esophagectomy, and 31% after lung cancer resection. Survival among octogenarians with two or more comorbidities was substantially worse than those with fewer comorbid diagnoses—10% versus 14% for pancreatectomy (Figure 37-3), 15% versus 23% for esophagectomy (Figure 37-4), and 27% versus 37% for lung (Figure 37-5). These population-based outcomes after high-risk cancer surgery in octogenarians were considerably worse than typically reported in case series and in frequently cited survival statistics. Realistic information about long-term survival should be available to elderly patients and their caregivers to better inform clinical decision making—particularly in multimorbid patients.

SUMMARY

Surgical procedures are being performed with increasing frequency in elderly patients. Rates of surgery in this population are likely to skyrocket as the population ages. While advances in surgical technique and perioperative care are making surgery safer, morbidity and mortality rates in elderly patients remain substantially higher than in younger patients. In addition to common medical complications, elderly patients are at increased risk of sustained cognitive dysfunction and loss of independence after surgery. For elderly patients with cancer, survival benefits gained from surgical resection are not equivalent to those seen in younger patients.

Comprehensive risk assessment and realistic expectations about outcomes after a major surgery in elderly patients are essential for several reasons. In this age group, functional status and frailty need to be taken into consideration when estimating the risk of surgery.

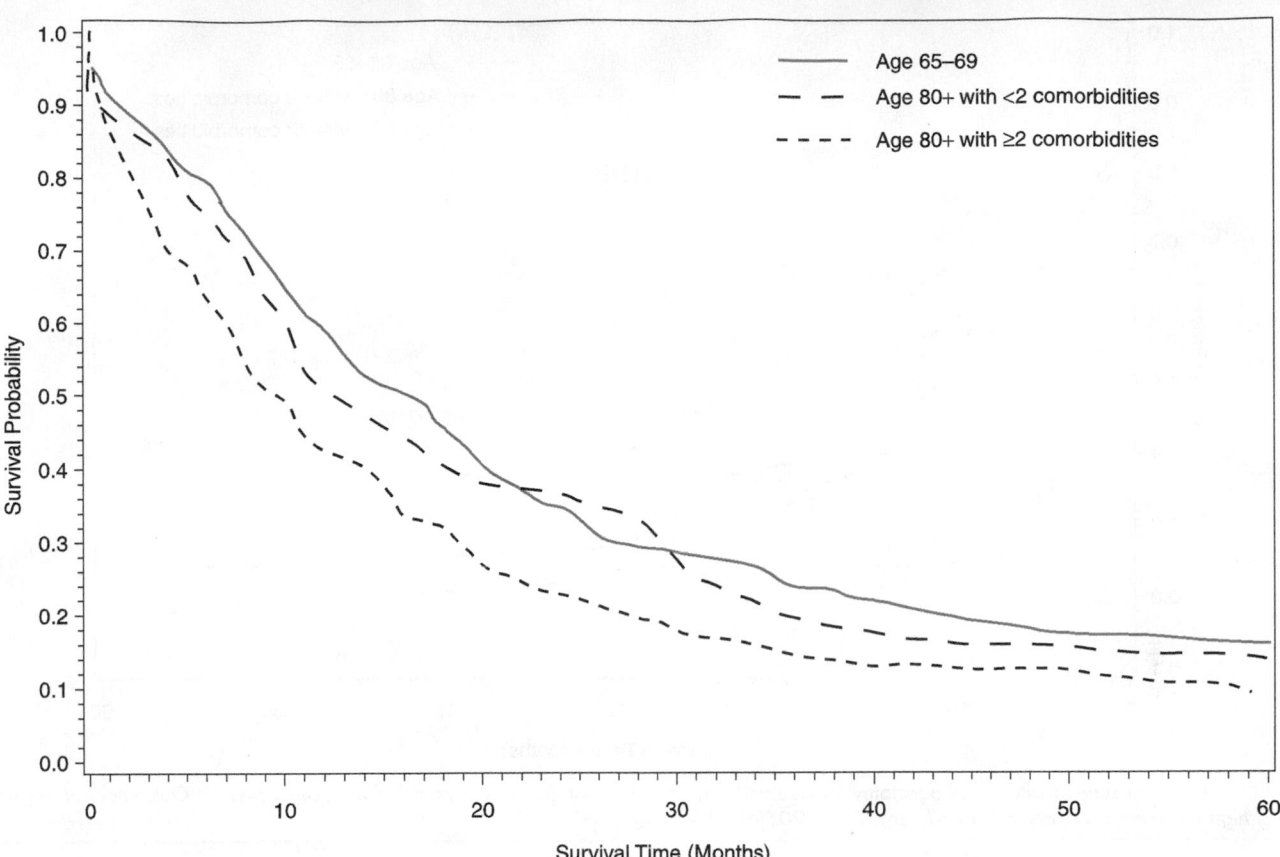

FIGURE 37-3. Five-year survival after pancreatic resection, by age and comorbidity count. *(From Finlayson E, Fan Z, Birkmeyer JD. Outcomes in octogenarians undergoing high risk cancer surgery. J Am Coll Surg. 2007;205(6):726–734.)*

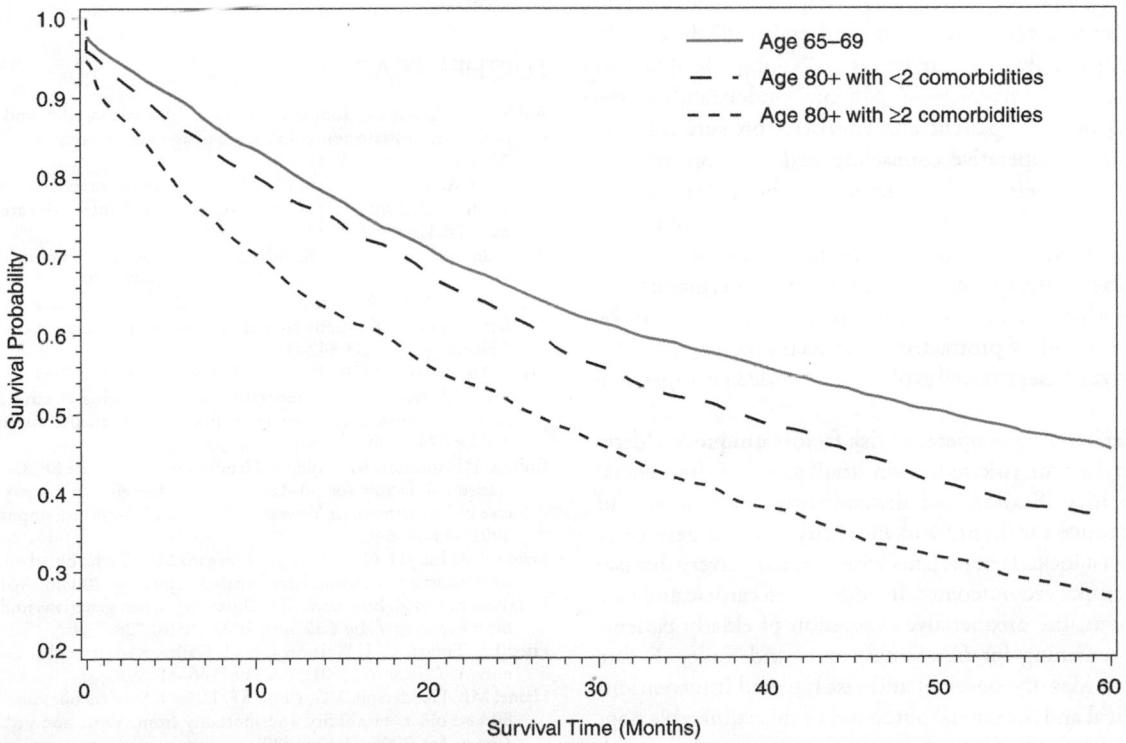

FIGURE 37-4. Five-year survival after lung surgery, by age and comorbidity count. *(From Finlayson E, Fan Z, Birkmeyer JD. Outcomes in octogenarians undergoing high risk cancer surgery. J Am Coll Surg. 2007;205(6):726–734.)*

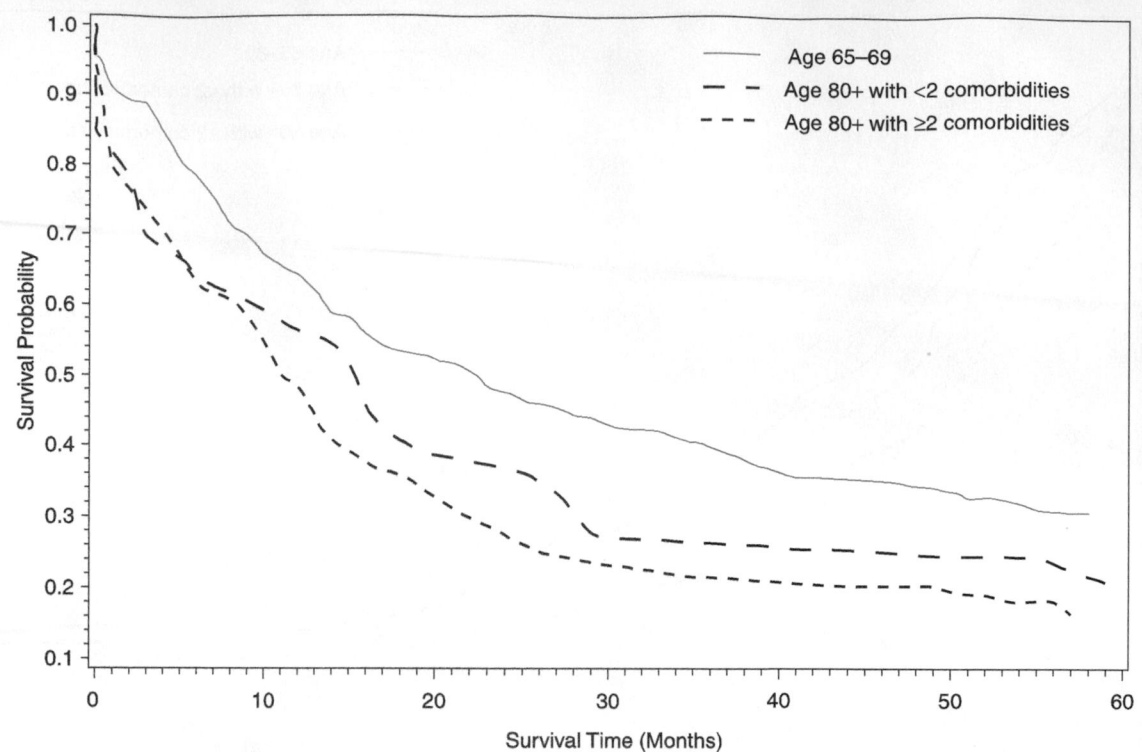

FIGURE 37-5. Five-year survival after esophagectomy, by age and comorbidity count. *(From Finlayson E, Fan Z, Birkmeyer JD. Outcomes in octogenarians undergoing high risk cancer surgery. J Am Coll Surg. 2007;205(6):726–734.)*

Toward this aim, more research is needed to improve risk stratification for this complex and diverse population. Although age strongly predicts morbidity and mortality after major surgery, it is only one of many risk factors. Complex interactions of age, functional status, cognitive status, and frailty likely explain what clinicians generally characterize as a "young" 85-year-old patient versus an "old" 85-year-old patient. Understanding the risk implications of these patient characteristics on surgical outcomes will inform preoperative counseling and decision-making. Elderly patients and their families should also be aware that, in addition to increased risk of mortality after surgery, many elderly patients may experience substantial functional decline and loss of independence after surgery—either temporary or permanent. It is important for elderly patients, caregivers, and physicians to be aware of the likelihood of protracted functional recovery in order to inform operative consent as well as plan for extended postoperative support.

A better understanding of operative risk factors unique to elderly people will also inform risk reduction strategies. In the general population, the identification and dissemination of processes of care shown to reduce morbidity and mortality after surgery (e.g., perioperative beta-blockade in patients with coronary artery disease) have resulted in improved outcomes. In addition to cardiac and pulmonary assessment, the preoperative evaluation of elderly patients should include screening for functional status and frailty. Future work is needed to identify, develop, and test targeted interventions to improve medical and functional outcomes in this vulnerable population of elderly patients. Once these interventions are identified, protocols can be developed by multidisciplinary teams of surgeons and geriatricians to standardize evidence-based preoperative evalua-

tion and perioperative care for elderly patients undergoing surgery. Through collaboration and dissemination of "best practices" in this vulnerable population, outcomes after surgery are likely to improve substantially.

FURTHER READING

Alibhai SM, Leach M, Tomlinson G, et al. 30-day mortality and major complications after prostatectomy: influence of age and comorbidity. *J Natl Cancer Inst.* 2005;97(20):1525–1532.

Bashour CA, Yared JP, Ryan TA, et al. Long-term survival and functional capacity in cardiac surgery patients after prolonged intensive care. *Crit Care Med.* 2000;28(12):3847–3853.

Bernstein GM, Offenbartl SK. Adverse surgical outcomes among patients with cognitive impairments. *Am Surg.* 1991;57(11):682–690.

Berry AJ, Smith RB, Weintraub S, Chaikof EL, et al. Age versus comorbidities as risk factors for complications after elective abdominal aortic reconstructive surgery. *J Vasc Surg.* 2001;33:342–353.

Brady AR, Fowkes FGR, Greenhalgh RM, Powell JT, Ruckley CV, Thompson SG. Risk factors for postoperative death following elective surgical repair of abdominal aortic aneurysm: results from the UK small aneurysm trial. *Br J Surg.* 2000;87:742–749.

Collins TC, Johnson M, Daley J, Henderson WG, Khuri SF, Gordon HS. Preoperative risk factors for 30-day mortality after elective surgery for vascular disease in Department of Veterans Affairs hospitals: is race important? *J Vasc Surg.* 2001;34:634–640.

Etzioni DA, Liu JH, O'Connell JB, Maggard MA, CY K. Elderly patients in surgical workloads: a population-based analysis. *Am Surg.* 2003;69:961–965.

Finlayson E, Fan Z, Birkmeyer JD. Outcomes in octogenarians undergoing high risk cancer surgery. *J Am Coll Surg.* 2007;205(6):726–734.

Fried LP, Tangen CM, Walston J, et al. Frailty in older adults: Evidence for a phenotype. *J Gerontol.* 2001;56A(3):M146–M156.

Hamel MB, Henderson WG, Khuri SF, Daley J. Surgical outcomes for patients aged 80 and older: morbidity and mortality from major noncardiac surgery. *J Am Geriatr Soc.* 2005;53:424–429.

Inouye SK, Bogardus ST, Charpentier PA, et al. A multicomponenet intervention to prevent delirium in the hospitalized older patients. *N Engl J Med.* 1999;340:669–676.

Jain NB, Guller U, Pietrobon R, Bond TK, Higgins LD. Comorbidities increase complication rates in patients having arthroplasty. *Clin Orthop Relat Res.* 2005;435:232–238.

Kirsch M, Guesnier L, LeBesnerais P, Hillion ML. Cardiac operations in octogenarians: perioperative risk factors for death and impaired autonomy. *Ann Thorac Surg.* 1998;66:60–67.

Lawrence VA, Hazuda HP, Cornell JE, et al. Functional independence after major abdominal surgery in the elderly. *J Am Coll Surg.* 2004;199:762–772.

Lightner AM, Glasgow RE, Jordan TH, et al. Pancreatic resection in the elderly. *J Am Coll Surg.* 2004;198:697–706.

Makary M, Takenaga R, Pronovost P, et al. Frailty in elderly surgical patients: implications for operative risk assessment. *J Surg Res.* 2006;130(2):212.

Masuo K, Kumagai K, Tanaka T, Yamagata K, Shimizu K. "Physiological" age as an outcome predictor for abdominal surgery in elderly patients. *Jpn J Surg.* 1998;28:997–1000.

Moller JT, Cluitmans P, Rasmussen LS, Houx P. Long-term postoperative cognitive dysfunction in the elderly: ISPOCD1 study. *Lancet.* 1998;351:857–861.

Nallamothu BK, Rogers MAM, McMahon LJ, Fries BE, Kaufman SR, Langa KM. Skilled care requirements for elderly patients after coronary artery bypass grafting. *J Am Geriatr Soc.* 2005;53(7):1133–1137.

Newman MF, Kirchner JL, Phillips-Bute B, et al. Longitudinal assessment of neurocognitive function after coronary-artery bypass surgery. *N Engl J Med.* 2001;344(6):395–402.

Sabel MS, Smith JL, Nava HR, Mollen K, Douglass HO, Gibbs JF. Esophageal resection for carcinoma in patients older than 70 years old. *Ann Surg Oncol.* 2002;9:210–214.

vanDijk D, Keizer AMA, Diephuis JC, Durand C, Vos LJ, Hijman R. Neurocognitive dysfunction after coronary artery bypass surgery: systematic review. *J Thorac Cardiovasc Surg.* 2000;120(4):632–639.

Nutrition and Aging

Dennis H. Sullivan ■ *Larry E. Johnson*

INTRODUCTION

Throughout life, nutrition is an important determinant of health, physical and cognitive function, vitality, overall quality of life, and longevity. The quantity and variety of available foods, as well as the meaningfulness of the social interactions provided by meals, are important to psychological well-being. The composition of the diet and the amount that is consumed are strongly linked to physiological function. When a well-balanced diet is not maintained, malnutrition may develop with consequent detrimental effects on health and well-being.

Malnutrition can have many manifestations. As outlined in Chapter 40, a diet that is deficient in one or more required nutrients (e.g., calories, protein, minerals, fiber, or vitamins) can lead to a state of nutritional deficiency. The greater the magnitude and duration of the nutritional deprivation and the more fragile the individual, the more likely nutritional deficits will produce noticeable body compositional changes, functional impairments, or overt disease. Even borderline dietary deficiencies can have important health consequences such as producing subtle organ system impairments, diminished vitality, or increasing the individual's susceptibility to disease. Protein and protein-energy undernutrition are two of the most common, frequently unrecognized, and potentially serious forms of nutritional deficiency. The prevalence of these conditions is particularly high among chronically ill older individuals and those in hospitals, nursing homes, and other institutional settings. Although there is a complex interrelationship between nutrition, disease, and clinical outcomes, protein and protein-energy undernutrition appear to be significant contributors to disease-related morbidity and mortality in these populations. At the other end of the spectrum, the persistent consumption of excess quantities of one or more nutrients can have similar untoward consequences. Forms of malnutrition that result from excess consumption include hypercholesterolemia, hypervitaminosis, and obesity. Studies indicate that obesity is the most common nutritional disorder of advanced age in western societies with a high prevalence among the noninstitutionalized free-living elderly. Many obese older individuals have other nutritional disorders. Among chronically ill or functionally debilitated obese older individuals, protein undernutrition is a common, serious, and frequently unrecognized problem that can develop for many reasons including an imbalanced diet, disease, and inactivity.

Recognizing and maintaining an optimally balanced diet is an important challenge, particularly as individuals age. The challenge is particularly great for older people who already are malnourished, especially if they have nutritional disorders that developed earlier in life, such as obesity, osteoporosis, or protein undernutrition. Even healthy individuals often fail to maintain an optimal diet owing to lack of knowledge, resources, or willpower. The process of aging can introduce other factors including acute and chronic disease, physical disabilities, social isolation, use of multiple medications, depression, impaired cognitive ability, and disregulation of appetite control that may contribute further to poor eating habits and the development or exacerbation of nutritional disorders. In turn, inappropriate dietary intake and poor nutritional status can impact the progression of many acute and chronic diseases such as coronary heart disease, cancer, stroke, diabetes, and osteoporosis, which are among the 10 leading causes of death in the United States. The 1988 Surgeon General's Report on Nutrition and Health noted that two-thirds of all deaths within the United States are because of diseases associated with poor diets and dietary habits.

Assessing the quality of the diet of elderly persons is critical to addressing issues relevant to their health and nutritional status. Such an assessment must be based on knowledge of what constitutes a balanced diet for a given individual. The goal of this chapter is to identify an approach to nutrition evaluation and management that takes into account the unique needs, limitations, and desires of each elderly individual. The chapter starts out by examining the interrelationship among nutrition, activity, disease burden, and health outcomes and then focuses on age-related changes in body composition, lifestyle, and appetite regulation that affect nutritional status and nutrient requirements. Also included is a discussion of specific dietary considerations related to optimal health requirements.

THE INTERRELATIONSHIP BETWEEN NUTRITION, ACTIVITY, AND DISEASE

Although nutrition is a vital component of good health, it cannot be evaluated in isolation. The relationship between nutrient intake and health is influenced by other factors, most notably activity level, disease burden, and advancing age. A basic understanding of these interrelationships is essential in order to assess the potential benefits and limitations of nutritional interventions.

Nutrition–Activity Interrelationship

Nutrition and physical activity are closely linked, each having vitally important and interacting effects on body composition, functional ability, and well-being. The balance between nutrient intake and physical activity is particularly important in determining muscle mass and strength, body fat content and distribution, and bone density and resilience. In recognition of the importance of the interrelationship between nutrition and activity on health, the U.S. Department of Agriculture (USDA) has released the MyPyramid food and activity guidance system. The MyPyramid symbol (Figure 38-1), which replaces the prior food pyramid, is designed to emphasize this interrelationship. The symbol is also designed to convey the message that variety, proportionality, moderation, gradual improvement, and personalization are all important in both diet and exercise prescriptions. Consumers can go to the MyPyramid Web site (www.mypyramid.gov) to learn more about this system and to obtain a detailed assessment and analysis of their current eating and physical activity habits.

To preserve existing muscle mass and strength, it is necessary to maintain both an adequate level of physical activity and a balanced diet that includes sufficient protein, energy, vitamins, and minerals to meet metabolic demands and prevent negative nitrogen balance (as discussed in detail below). It is not known precisely what level of physical activity is needed to prevent loss of existing muscle mass and strength in older adults. However, studies indicate that even a week or two of bed rest or similar degrees of activity restriction can result in noticeable loss of muscle mass, strength, and function even when the diet is adequate and the individual is otherwise healthy. In one study of 12 healthy, moderately active older adults, 10 days of voluntary total bed rest resulted in a 16% loss of strength and a 6% loss of skeletal muscle mass from the lower extremities. Muscle biopsies indicated that muscle protein synthesis declined by 30%. Despite the provision of a diet containing the recommended dietary allowance for protein, the participants remained in negative nitrogen balance throughout the study. In contrast, fat mass did not change. The combination of inadequate diet and inactivity can result in an even more rapid loss of muscle. In contrast, overfeeding does not prevent muscle atrophy associated with inactivity and may exacerbate the functional consequences since the excess nutrients are converted to fat.

To increase muscle strength, size, or endurance, the average daily level of exertion has to increase significantly. Aerobic exercises are most effective in improving the oxidative capacity of muscles and are the mainstay of endurance training. High-intensity, progressive resistance training, such as weight lifting, is needed to build strength and mass. Nutrition alone has never been demonstrated to be an effective method of repleting muscle mass, improving strength, or increasing endurance in frail older individuals who have experienced a recent loss of weight. Efforts at repletion should focus on both increasing nutrient intake and exercise. Based on studies of healthy elderly men, the combination of progressive resistance muscle strength training and a high protein diet (containing up to 1.6 g of protein/kg body weight/d) may be the most effective method of improving muscle mass.

Exercise can have an important effect on body fat content and distribution. In obese older individuals, exercise can play a synergistic role with caloric restriction in promoting weight loss and preventing further weight gain. With weight loss, visceral fat is mobilized at a rate two to five times that of other fat stores. Even when total body weight does not change, exercise can induce a significant decrease in intra-abdominal fat in both obese and nonobese individuals. The preferential mobilization of fat stores has important metabolic implications for the prevention or treatment of the insulin resistance syndrome, since it is predominantly excess visceral fat that is associated with the derangements of dyslipidemia, elevated fibrinogen, hyperinsulinemia, and hypertension.

Exercise and nutrition also play a critical role in maintenance of optimal bone density and strength. As discussed in Chapter 117, the nutrient needs of bone include the correct balance of protein and energy and adequate intake of vitamins and minerals, especially vitamin D and calcium. The amount of exercise that is needed for optimal bone health is not defined. However, it is known that people who exercise regularly have higher bone density than more sedentary age-, race-, and gender-matched controls. Randomized controlled trials involving postmenopausal women demonstrate that those assigned to progressive resistance muscle strength training or weight-loading aerobic exercise programs attain a 1% to 1.6% greater bone mineral density in both the lumbar spine and femoral neck region per year compared to the controls. It is also known that bed rest and weightlessness are associated with a rapid decline in bone mineral density. Consequently, osteopenia can develop despite an optimal diet if exercise or other weight bearing activities are not adequate. Because of its apparent beneficial effects on bone mineral density, exercise should be combined with an appropriate diet for both prevention and treatment of osteoporosis and fracture-related disability.

Having both direct and indirect effects on numerous metabolic processes within muscle, bone, and adipose tissues, exercise has a major impact on how nutrients are utilized by the body during health and illness. By inducing an increase in the mass and metabolic capacity of muscle, exercise affects energy expenditure, glucose metabolism, and size of protein reserves in a manner that counteracts some of the effects of aging and thus has important nutritional implications for individuals as they grow older. Total energy expenditure (TEE) represents the sum of basal energy expenditure, postprandial thermogenesis, and the energy expenditure of activity. Muscle represents not only the primary source of energy expenditure during physical activity, it is also the primary contributor to basal energy expenditure, which may represent 50% to 80% of TEE. With advancing age, there is a parallel decline in muscle mass and both basal and total daily energy expenditure that may be partially or fully accounted for by the fact that people tend to become more sedentary as they grow older. A study of master athletes demonstrates that men who maintain a vigorous weekly routine of weight training throughout

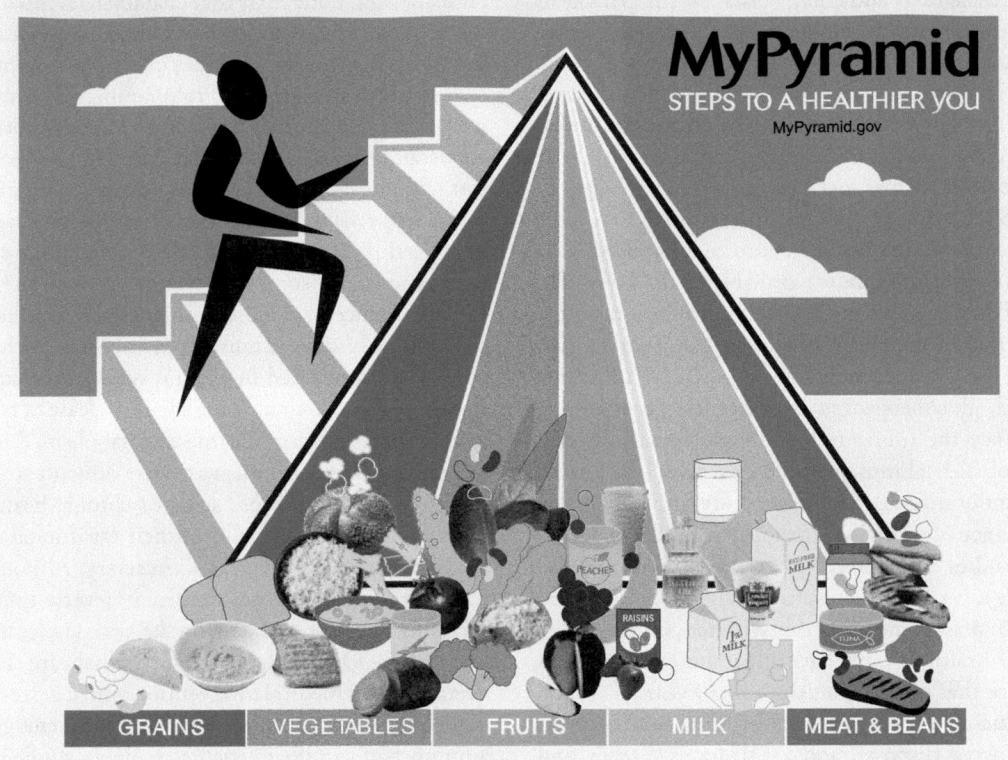

GRAINS Make half your grains whole	VEGETABLES Vary your veggies	FRUITS Focus on fruits	MILK Your calcium-rich foods	MEATS & BEANS Go lean with protein
Eat at least 3 oz of whole-grain cereals, breads, crackers, rice, or pasta every day

1 oz is about 1 slice of bread, about 1 cup of breakfast cereal, or 1/2 cup of cooked rice, cereal, or pasta | Eat more dark-green veggies like broccoli, spinach, and other dark leafy greens

Eat more orange vegetables like carrots and sweetpotatotes

Eat more dry beans and peas like pinto beans, kidney beans, and lentils | Eat a variety of fruit

Choose fresh, frozen, canned, or dried fruit

Go easy on fruit juices | Go low-fat or fat-free when you choose milk, yogurt, and other milk products

if you don't or can't consume milk, choose lactose-free products or other calcium sources such as fortified foods and beverages | Choose low-fat or lean meats and poultry

Bake it, broil it, or grill it

Vary your protein routine—choose more fish, beans, peas, nuts, and seeds |

For a 2000-calorie diet, you need the amounts below from each food group. To find the amounts that are right for you, go to MyPyramid.gov.

Eat 6 oz every day	Eat 2½ cups every day	Eat 2 cups every day	Get 3 cups every day; for kids aged 2 to 8, it's 2	Eat 5½ oz every day

Find your balance between food and physcial activity

- Be sure to stay within your daily calorie needs.
- Be physically active for at least 30 minutes most days of the week.
- About 60 minutes a day of physical activity may be needed to prevent weight gain.
- For sustaining weights loss, at least 60 to 90 minutes a day of physical activity may be required.
- Children and teenagers should be physically active for 60 minutes every day, or most days.

Know the limits on fats, sugars, and salt (sodium)

- Make most of your fat sources from fish, nuts, and vegetables oils.
- Limits solid fats like butter, stick margarine, shortening, and lard, as well as foods that contain these.
- Check the Nutrition Facts label to keep saturated fats, *trans* fats, and sodium low.
- Choose food and beverages low in added sugars. Added sugars contribute calories with few, if any, nutrients.

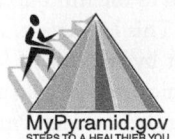

MyPyramid.gov
STEPS TO A HEALTHIER YOU

U.S Deparment of Agriculture
Centre of Nutrition Policy and Promotion
April 2005
CNPP-15

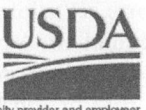

USDA is an equal opportunity provider and employeer.

FIGURE 38-1. MyPyramid.gov, U.S. Department of Agriculture, Center for Nutrition Policy and Promotion, April 2005, CNPP-15, http://www.mypyramid.gov

their lives have the muscle mass and energy capacity comparable to that of healthy 30-year-old males. Nonexercising older men have significantly less muscle mass than their younger counterparts.

Exercise-induced increases in muscle size or protein content result in greater body protein reserves, which can be critical to survival during episodes of nutritional deprivation that usually accompany profound physiologic stress such as that caused by trauma, sepsis, or other acute disease. Such acute physiologic insults trigger an acute inflammatory response that causes ketogenesis to be suppressed, leaving glucose as the primary energy source available to the body. The problem is invariably compounded by reduced nutrient intake that results as a consequence of the anorexia and gastrointestinal tract dysfunction induced by the inflammatory response. With nutrient intake suppressed, gluconeogenesis becomes the predominant source of glucose. Since the substrate for gluconeogenesis is provided by catabolism of skeletal muscle, lean body mass becomes an important determinant of survival. Once lean body mass falls below a critical level, the chance of surviving a serious acute illness diminishes dramatically. Studies conducted within the Warsaw Ghetto, hospital intensive care units, and other settings suggest that a loss of >40% of baseline lean mass is incompatible with life. Other studies indicate that very few healthy people have a lean body mass that is <70% of the mean for that of adults aged 20 to 30 years.

In addition to inducing muscle hypertrophy, exercise also affects insulin sensitivity, glucose disposal, and HDL levels directly and plays a synergistic role with diet in maintaining a healthy weight and a sense of well-being. These effects of exercise can be important adjuncts to good nutrition in the prevention and treatment of hypertension, diabetes, dyslipidemia, and osteoporosis.

Nutrition–Disease Interrelationship

There is a complex interrelationship between nutrition, health status, and clinical outcomes. Although a full discussion of this topic is beyond the scope of this chapter, it is important to emphasize several key points. First, nutrient requirements and the ability to metabolize select nutrients are influenced by many disease states. In addition, many diseases compromise the older individual's ability to consume adequate amounts of all nutrients. This can occur through a number of mechanisms including disease-induced suppression of appetite, alteration of the normal swallowing mechanism, maldigestion or malabsorption, and a loss of self-feeding ability.

The detrimental effects of disease on nutrient metabolism often become more pronounced with advancing age. This is particularly true of the many acute and chronic diseases that induce an inflammatory response, including acute and chronic infections, congestive heart failure, chronic pulmonary disease, cancer, end-stage renal disease, and rheumatoid arthritis. With advancing age, the inflammatory response often becomes dysregulated as indicated by persistently elevated serum concentrations of proinflammatory cytokines and other inflammatory mediators (Chapter 4). The proinflammatory cytokines include interleukin(IL)-6, IL-1(beta), tumor necrosis factor(TNF)-alpha, and possibly IL-8 and others. These cytokines function both as intermediaries and directly to induce many of the signs and symptoms associated with inflammation including weight loss. The proinflammatory cytokines have been implicated in the pathogenesis of many of the detrimental consequences of chronic inflammation including anemia, hypoalbuminemia, and cachexia. IL-1, IL-6, and TNF-alpha all contribute to the loss of skeletal muscle,

fat tissue, and bone mass that characterizes inflammation-associated cachexia. Although anorexia is almost always a contributing factor, the inflammation-induced loss of fat and lean mass is often refractory to nutrition support. Proinflammatory cytokines create a state of muscle catabolism by suppressing muscle protein synthesis and/or accelerating muscle protein breakdown independent of dietary factors. Additionally, the proinflammatory cytokines induce lipolysis while suppressing fat and liver lipoprotein lipase activity resulting in hypertriglyceridemia and a decrease in the availability of fat to be used as an energy source. As energy production from fat diminishes, the importance of glucose as an energy source increases. The amino acids derived from the muscle proteolysis are either converted to glucose or are consumed in hepatic synthesis of acute phase proteins. Additionally, cytokines stimulate the release of cortisol resulting in a further acceleration of the muscle catabolism. Since these potentially deleterious effects of disease can be difficult to predict, older individuals with one or more acute or chronic health problems should have frequent reassessments of their nutritional status and their nutritional care plan revised as necessary. Although nutrient intake may not be adequate to completely reverse inflammation-induced catabolism, a low nutrient intake will accelerate the development of cachexia. Optimally, good nutritional care should be part of the overall plan of medical intervention aimed at treating the underlying pathology as well as addressing protein and energy deficits. Although a number of specific nutrients are being studied to determine their value in counteracting inflammation-induced loss of lean body mass, there is not yet adequate evidence that any given dietary supplement is more effective than current standard dietary or nutrition support practices.

AGE–RELATED CHANGES THAT AFFECT NUTRITION

Changes in Body Composition

With advancing age, there are significant changes in body composition that affect the nutritional needs of an individual. Based primarily on cross-sectional studies, weight increases steadily in most people from age 30 to 60 years. An increase in total body fat accounts for a majority of this weight gain. After age 60, weight usually stabilizes, and then begins to decline. Improved survival of nonobese individuals during middle age and cohort effects may account for some of the decline in weight with age that is reported in the cross-sectional studies. However, weight maintenance becomes increasingly difficult in the advanced years of life. The incidence as well as the potential causes of weight loss increases with age, particularly beyond age 75.

Regardless of whether or not weight changes, advancing age is characterized by a progressive loss in lean body mass, a relative increase in fat mass, and a redistribution of fat from peripheral to central locations within the body. Based primarily on cross-sectional studies, it appears that all of these changes begin in the third decade and increase at an accelerated rate after age 65. This late accelerated phase may be a threshold effect brought about by the loss of lean body mass and the increased prevalence of chronic disease in old age. The loss of lean body mass consists predominantly of skeletal muscle, particularly type II or fast twitch fibers. Central lean body mass, such as the liver and other splanchnic organs, is relatively preserved. Some studies indicate that muscle mass may decline by up to 45%

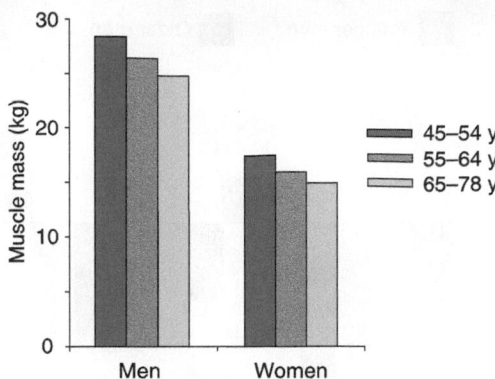

FIGURE 38-2. Declining muscle mass with increasing age. *(Reproduced with permission from Frontera WR, Hughes VA, et al. A cross-sectional study of muscle strength and mass in 45- to 78-yr-old men and women. J Appl Physiol. 1991;71:644.)*

between the third and eighth decade of life (Figures 38-2 and 38-3). The few longitudinal studies that have been reported indicate that the loss of muscle mass with age may be greater in men than women. However, this remains controversial.

The loss of muscle mass with age appears to be the result of multiple interrelated factors including age-related changes in metabolism, function, or structure of organ tissues, disease, medical therapeutics, heritability, and behavior and lifestyle choices of the individual. Notable age-related changes that appear to contribute to loss of muscle include a progressive loss of alpha motor units in the spinal column, a diminution in the intrinsic muscle protein synthesis capacity, and a decline in the production of multiple hormones including testos-

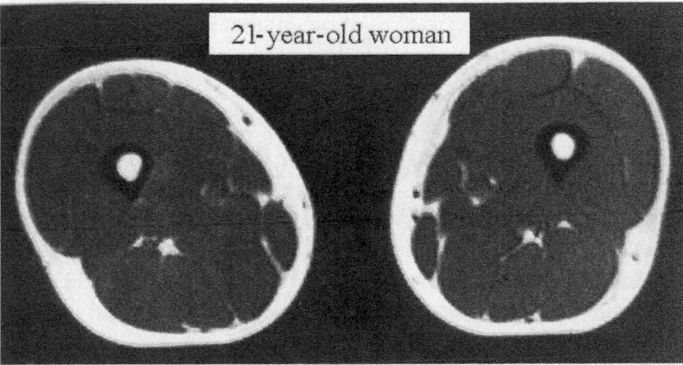

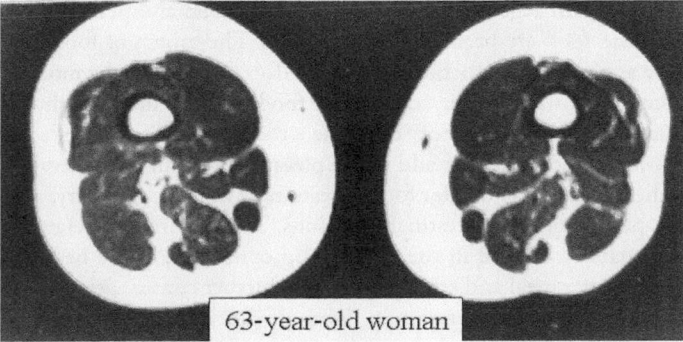

FIGURE 38-3. Cross-sectional computed tomography images of the midthighs of a younger and an older woman demonstrating the decline in muscle mass and relative increase in fat mass with age.

terone, estrogen, and the insulin-like growth factors. The decline in the intrinsic muscle protein synthesis capacity parallels and may be causally related to a loss of mitochondrial ATP production with advancing age. Other age-related changes detrimental to muscle include the increased production and delayed inactivation of catabolic mediators and a change in liver protein metabolism that may decrease the availability of amino acids to axial muscles. The decline in nutrient consumption and activity level that often accompanies advanced age are possibly modifiable contributors to the loss of muscle mass. Many diseases accelerate the age-related decline, particularly degenerative diseases of the central nervous system and those affecting any part of the motor pathway. An accelerated loss of muscle mass can occur when a serious illness requires treatment with steroids or other antianabolic drugs or is accompanied by low nutrient intake and the need for prolonged bed rest. In all individuals, the loss of muscle mass with age is closely linked with a reduction in muscle strength and exercise capacity, a decline in one causing further loss of the others. When exercise capacity falls below that required to comfortably perform basic activities of daily living, physical activity often becomes very limited, which causes a rapid acceleration of the downward spiral. The loss of muscle mass and exercise capacity is also linked to the development of coronary artery disease, diabetes mellitus, and other diseases that contribute further to the decline.

In parallel with the loss of lean body mass, there is an increase in the relative amount and the distribution of body fat with advancing age. Between the second and ninth decades of life, the percentage of body weight that is fat increases by 35% to 50% in females and to an even greater extent in males. In one cross-sectional study of 500 healthy individuals between the ages of 18 and 85 years, fat mass as a percentage of body weight increased across the age range of the sample from 33% to 44% in females and 18% to 36% in males. Whether or not total body weight changes, intra-abdominal (visceral) fat increases quantitatively and proportionally more than peripheral fat mass. In females, the accumulation of intra-abdominal fat accelerates at menopause and represents primarily a shift from peripheral sites. In males, the increase in intra-abdominal fat with age represents primarily an increase in total body fat mass. For a given waist circumference, older adults have greater visceral fat than young adults and men have greater visceral and less subcutaneous fat than women.

Numerous factors have been sited as potential contributors to the changes in adipose tissues with advancing age. Some studies suggest that much of this change can be accounted for by the reduction in both the quantity and oxidative capacity of skeletal muscle that also occurs during the same time interval. With advancing age, fat oxidation is reduced at rest, following a meal, and during exercise. This reduced rate of fat metabolism with age promotes accumulation of fat at both peripheral and central locations. The decline in total skeletal muscle mass that occurs with age correlates with, and may be responsible for, the decreased rate of metabolism of fat at rest. Likewise, the decline in maximal oxidative capacity of muscle may cause the reduction in fat metabolism with exercise. The decline in physical activity resulting from the loss of muscle with age contributes to the increase in intra-abdominal fat. Other factors that may also contribute to the increased intra-abdominal fat with age include declining testosterone in men, estrogen withdrawal or increased testosterone in females, the decline in growth hormone, increased resistance to leptin, and increased secretion of cortisol.

Weight cycling can also contribute to the relative increase in fat mass in some older adults. When older adults lose weight, particularly when this weight loss occurs in association with an acute illness, they usually experience a greater decline in lean compared to fat mass. Those individuals who later regain some or all of the lost weight usually gain predominantly fat mass. It is not known whether exercise, specialized diets, or anabolic agents would be effective in helping to restore lean body mass in these older adults. Given the high prevalence of illness-induced weight loss among older adults, this is an important area for further research.

Changes in Appetite and Energy Intake Regulation

Maintenance of a stable weight requires a steady balance between nutrient intake and energy expenditure. With advancing age, the metabolic, neural, and humoral pathways that normally maintain this delicate balance by regulating appetite and hunger begin to lose their compensatory responsiveness to changes in energy demands. Psychological, socioeconomic, and cultural influences and numerous disease processes further contribute to the disregulation. From the third to seventh decade of life, these factors integrate to create an imbalance usually favoring a tendency toward weight gain and increased fat deposition, at least in societies where food is plentiful and the physical demands of life are light. However, after age 70, the risk of losing weight increases steadily with each year of survival. This correlates with the findings from numerous studies that indicate that low dietary energy intake is common among both healthy and frail elderly people.

Impaired regulation of food intake has been observed in sedentary elderly men. As shown in Figure 38-4, young and older subjects gained similar amounts of weight during overfeeding. When allowed to resume a normal ad libitum diet, the young subjects decreased their energy intake and lost weight. In contrast, the elderly subjects failed to readjust their nutrient intake and at the end of the study remained above their starting weight. As shown in Figure 38-5, there were similar age group differences in the response to underfeeding.

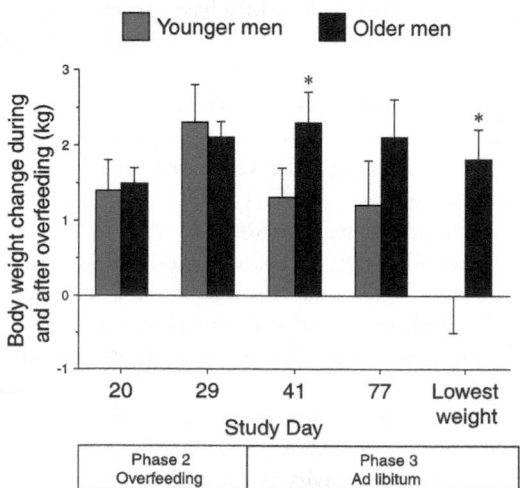

FIGURE 38-4. Body weight change during 21 days of overfeeding by 1000 kcal/d (phase 2) and a subsequent 46-d period of ad libitum diet (phase 3). Values are means (+SEM) for younger (n = 7) and older (n = 9) men. The asterisks indicate significance at P < 0.05 relative to the younger men. (Reproduced with permission from Roberts SB, Fuss P, et al. Control of food intake in older men. JAMA. 1994;272:1601.)

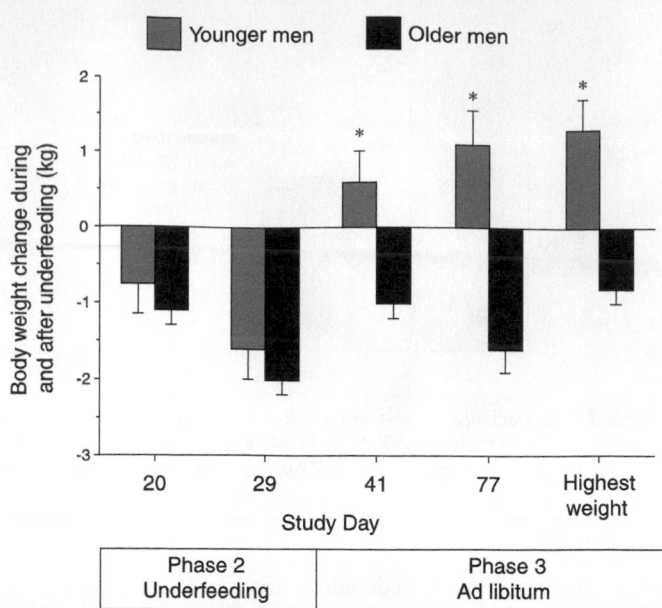

FIGURE 38-5. Body weight change during 21 days of underfeeding by 792 kcal/d (phase 2) and a subsequent 46-day period of ad libitum diet. Values are means (+ SEM) for younger and older men. The asterisks indicate significance at P < 0.001 relative to the younger men. (Reproduced with permission from Roberts SB, Fuss P, et al. Control of food intake in older men. JAMA. 1994;272:1601.)

The young and old subjects experienced similar amounts of weight loss during the intervention phase. However, the young men increased their nutrient intake and regained weight after returning to an ad libitum diet, whereas the elderly subjects did not. These findings suggest that a reduced ability to regulate food intake may contribute to the progressive loss of weight that many older individuals experience when their lives are disrupted by illness, psychological stress, or economic hardship.

Loss of Taste, Smell, and Appetite with Advancing Age

Numerous pathologic and age-related physiologic changes contribute to the difficulty older people have maintaining a balance between metabolic needs and nutrient intake. The look, smell, taste, and texture of food all contribute to the desirability of a meal and can serve to stimulate or inhibit further consumption. Normal sensory systems are therefore necessary for the full enjoyment of food and are important regulators of nutrient intake. The abilities to smell and taste food are particularly important. The aroma of food can serve as a powerful appetite stimulant. After food enters the mouth, aromatic substances released from the food circulate up through the nasopharynx to the olfactory cleft where they enhance taste. The sensations of smell and taste add to the pleasure of eating while serving as chemosensory signals for food digestion by triggering salivary, gastric, pancreatic, and intestinal secretions. The texture, temperature, and quantity of food in the mouth also contribute to the hedonic qualities of a meal and serve to promote further consumption.

A significant deterioration in sight, olfactory function, taste sensation, or ability to feel the temperature and texture of food in the mouth can have a deleterious effect on eating habits and the likelihood of maintaining an adequate diet. This becomes an important concern with advanced age. Even healthy older individuals

TABLE 38-1

Conditions That Can Suppress Appetite and Alter Olfactory Function

Nutritional	Infections
Zinc deficiency	Sinusitis
Niacin deficiency	Acute viral hepatitis
Vitamin B-12 deficiency	Upper respiratory tract viral infections
Head and neck	**Central nervous system**
Allergic rhinitis	Alzheimer's disease
Glossitis	Head trauma
Nasal polyps	Multiple sclerosis
Sjogren syndrome	Neoplasia
Dental problems	Parkinsonism
Radiation therapy	Korsakoff syndrome
Smoking	Cranial nerve lesions
Systemic diseases	**Endocrine**
Cirrhosis of the liver	Diabetes mellitus
Renal failure	Hypothyroidism
Cancer	Adrenocortical insufficiency
	Panhypopituitarism
Iatrogenic	
Laryngectomy	
Chemotherapy	

experience a modest deterioration in their ability to detect odors and to differentiate one odor from another. There is a similar pattern to the loss of taste. Compared to young people, older individuals who suffer from no diseases and take no medications have a moderately reduced ability (i.e., require greater concentrations) to both detect and to identify sweet, sour, salty, and bitter substances and amino acids such as glutamate salts. Elderly persons also have reduced ability to discriminate intensity differences and to recognize taste mixtures.

Much greater losses in taste and smell occur in association with medication usage and other health-related concerns. Tables 38-1 and 38-2 contain a representative listing of local, central nervous system, and systemic diseases; nutritional deficiencies; medications; surgical interventions; and environmental exposures (including smoking) that can cause appetite suppression and a loss of olfactory function

TABLE 38-2

Classes of Medications That Can Suppress Appetite and Alter Olfactory Function*

Antidepressants
Anti-inflammatories
Antihypertensives and other cardiac medications
Lipid-lowering drugs
Antihistamines
Antimicrobials
Antineoplastics
Bronchodilators and other asthma medications
Muscle relaxants
Drugs for the treatment of parkinsonism and dementia
Anticonvulsants
Vasodilators

*Numerous drugs in each category can alter appetite and olfactory function.

and taste sensation. Poor oral health and many diseases that decrease mastication, salivary flow, or ability to swallow can also lead to deterioration in taste and smell and adversely affect appetite. The grinding and mixing of food with saliva play important roles in the release of volatiles and in bringing substances in contact with taste receptors, while swallowing movements are essential to pump the released volatiles up to the olfactory cleft where they are perceived.

Gastrointestinal Tract and Postabsorptive Effects on Appetite

In addition to the special senses, there are various neural and humoral pathways within the gut that change with advanced age. Although controversial, some of these changes may contribute to the inability of many older individuals to adequately regulate food intake. Normally, stretch reflexes within the wall of the stomach play a key role in signaling the brain when adequate amounts of food have been ingested. Some investigators theorize that these reflexes become overly responsive in advanced age leading to early satiety and reduced food intake. Other investigations have revealed that gastric emptying is delayed with advanced age and that this may lead to slower absorption of carbohydrates, a reduction in insulin secretion, and a relative suppression of the hunger response. However, other studies have found postprandial insulin levels to be elevated in the elderly suggesting that it is the age-related change in the meal-induced pattern of insulin secretion that may be the more important determinant of food intake. There is also evidence that certain gastrointestinal hormones, such as cholecystokinin, contribute to the appetite dysregulation with advancing age. Both the amount of cholecystokinin released in response to a meal and its potency in producing early satiety are greater in old compared to younger individuals. A number of other hormones have also been linked to appetite control. These include ghrelin, a gastric peptide that has apparent orexigenic properties, and leptin, a hormone produced by adipose tissue that induces satiation at high serum concentrations. Whether age- or disease-related changes in the secretion of these and other hormones are causally related to the decline in nutrient intake and loss of weight seen in many frail older adults remains controversial.

Psychological, Socioeconomic, and Cultural Influences on Appetite

After the seventh decade of life, the importance of psychological, socioeconomic, and cultural factors to maintaining an adequate diet increases. Depression is a common, frequently unrecognized, and potentially treatable cause of a poor appetite and must always be considered when evaluating an older patient who is losing weight. A correct diagnosis is often difficult to make in the elderly, particularly when the individual suffers from other medical problems or dementia. Similarly, bereavement is associated with a lack of appetite. Poverty, lack of education, limited mobility, feeding dependency, and social isolation are also important risks. Some, though not all, studies of healthy adults have found that eating alone is associated with a lower energy intake than when eating with others and that the presence of family and close friends leads to greater nutrient intake than eating with less familiar individuals. Within institutional settings, particularly nursing homes, physical environment and ambience within the dining areas are known to affect appetite. Interventions to ameliorate the dining experience within nursing homes have been shown to improve nutrient intakes and promote weight gain.

Therapeutic diets (e.g., low salt or low cholesterol) are frequently prescribed in nursing homes, often to residents who are losing weight, even though they may add little or nothing to disease management. For these reasons, the American Dietetic Association has published a position statement suggesting that use of therapeutic diets in the nursing homes be restricted.

NUTRIENT REQUIREMENTS TO MAINTAIN HEALTH

Energy

Daily energy requirements per kilogram of body weight generally decline with age, dropping as much as 33% between the third and ninth decade of life. Male gender and chronic disease are associated with a greater rate of decline. However, a decrease in energy requirements with age occurs even among those who remain healthy. The primary reason for this decline is the loss of muscle mass that is nearly universal with advanced age. Muscle is much more metabolically active than adipose tissue. As muscle mass is lost, the ratio of fat to lean mass increases leading to a greater drop in basal metabolic rate (BMR) than predicted by the decrease in total body mass. With advanced age, there is also a slight decline in metabolic rate per kilogram of fat-free mass. This may relate to the age-related change in the ratio of high (e.g., muscle) to low (e.g., bone) metabolic rate tissues within the fat-free mass compartment. Because the BMR generally accounts for 60% to 75% of TEE, the end result of the muscle loss is a significant decline in TEE and thus in energy requirements. It is estimated that every 10-kg loss of skeletal tissue mass results in an approximate 150 kcal/d decline in basal energy expenditure.

A second mechanism accounting for the decline in energy requirements with age is a decrease in physical activity. Energy expenditure of physical activity (EEA) generally declines with age to the same extent as BMR, accounting for approximately 15% to 35% of TEE in the majority of elderly adults. However, EEA can range from 5% of TEE in those who are bedridden to 50% in highly active, physically fit older adults. Studies of free-living older adults demonstrate that the strongest independent predictors of EEA are maximum oxygen consumption, fat-free mass, and body mass. After adjustment for body composition, there are no significant differences in TEE, BMR, or EEA between males and females. Other studies indicate that lifestyle plays a big role in determining EEA of older people, just as it does in those who are younger. Although the increased prevalence of chronic disabling disease accounts for some of the decline in physical activity with advancing age, even healthy older adults tend to be more sedentary than younger individuals.

Many chronic diseases, including congestive heart failure, Parkinson disease, and Alzheimer dementia, are associated with an increase in BMR. However, these conditions have been found to be associated with a decreased TEE because of decreased energy of physical activity. Some chronic conditions may result in an increased TEE, although this remains controversial. Individuals with Alzheimer's disease who constantly pace would fall into this category, as would individuals with a constant tremor. Even when individuals appear to be rather sedentary, their TEE from physical activity may be greater than expected, particularly if they have certain disabilities such as neurologic disorders and amputations. These conditions sometimes result in a loss of neuromuscular energy efficiency and thus exceptional levels of energy expenditure are required to complete even basic activities of daily living.

Several different clinical methods of estimating the energy requirements of older adults have been validated with sophisticated energy expenditure measurement techniques, such as doubly labeled water studies. These estimates are reviewed in Chapter 40 and summarized in Table 40-2.

The decline in energy requirements with advancing age means that older persons need to consume less food in order to maintain their weight and customary activity level. This places the older individual at risk of developing protein and micronutrient deficiencies, since requirements for other nutrients do not decrease as much as energy. Consequently, it is important that older individuals increase their activity level and change their diet to protein and micronutrient rich foods in order to maintain their muscle mass and avoid obesity.

Protein

Because of the paucity of high-quality nutrition studies with adequate representation from older age groups, current recommendations for protein intake do not differentiate individuals older than 65 from those who are younger. Various panels have recommended protein requirements for healthy adults of 0.6 to 0.8 g per kg of body weight per day. However, the question of whether protein requirements change appreciably with advancing age continues to be debated. Based on their interpretation of available data, some recommend that protein intake for elderly adults should be 1.0 to 1.25 g/kg/d. Until better measurement techniques become available, it may not be possible to determine the protein requirements of older adults with any higher level of certainty.

Several metabolic methods have been used to estimate the protein requirement of older adults. However, because of the many concerns about the accuracy of these metabolic study techniques, some believe that epidemiologic methods should play a larger role in setting recommendations for protein intake. The amount of protein consumed by healthy adults who have a stable body composition could be included as a basis of the recommendation. In most studies of community-dwelling older adults, median protein intakes tend to exceed the RDA. However, the population variance is significant. One study found that healthy older community-residing individuals eating a self-selected diet in the United Kingdom were in equilibrium with daily intakes equivalent to 0.97 g/kg body weight. Another study found that homebound elderly people consuming their habitual dietary protein intake of 0.67 g/kg/d were in negative nitrogen balance.

Factors That Influence Protein Requirements

The protein requirements of an individual can change with time, being influenced by age, nonprotein content of the diet, activity level, medications, and health status. The energy content of the diet is particularly important. The protein intake required to maintain nitrogen balance increases with decreasing energy intake. Carefully conducted metabolic studies of healthy young males indicate that nitrogen balance can not be attained at any protein intake when total energy intake is less than 126 kJ/kg (30 kcal/kg). Although comparable data are not available for individuals older than 65, the importance of energy intake in older individuals is well recognized.

A negative energy balance usually precipitates a negative nitrogen balance, especially in individuals who are ill or who have a low level of activity. Whether progressive resistance muscle strength training, alone or in combination with a high protein diet, can prevent loss of lean body mass in older individuals during periods of voluntary caloric restriction and weight loss is being investigated. As a general rule, protein requirements increase with high levels of activity such as sustained high-intensity exercise.

Many disease states and medications can induce a catabolic state for protein by altering the normal balance between protein synthesis and degradation. Older individuals who are both confined to bed and have an injury, infection, or another acute inflammatory condition are at particularly high risk of developing a profoundly negative nitrogen balance that can lead to a rapid loss of lean body mass, particularly skeletal muscle mass. High doses of corticosteroids can have a similar effect. The amount of protein that needs to be consumed in order to minimize loss of lean body mass and optimize recovery from such disease states is often difficult to determine. In general, older hospitalized patients who are acutely ill or recovering from major surgery or trauma warrant a protein intake of 1.5 g/kg of body weight/d unless they have a condition that necessitates protein restriction such as renal or hepatic insufficiency. Chronically ill and bedridden older residents of long-term care institutions are also likely to have similarly high protein requirements.

The source of the dietary protein may be another important factor influencing protein requirements following illness. Although far more needs to be learned about this subject, current evidence suggests that a number of factors including the ratio of the various amino acids within a dietary protein may influence how effectively the protein can be utilized by the body. Several animal and laboratory-based human studies suggest that protein or amino acid supplements containing high concentrations of branched-chain amino acids such as leucine may be more effective than other dietary proteins in stimulating muscle protein synthesis, particularly in sedentary or chronically ill older adults.

Fat and Cholesterol

Fat serves as a key source of energy and essential fatty acids as well as a vehicle for transporting fat-soluble vitamins. Even when obesity and elevated cholesterol or triglycerides are a concern, fat intake should not fall below 10% of total energy requirements in order to allow for adequate absorption of fat-soluble vitamins (A, D, E, K) and to ensure that the requirements for the essential fatty acids are met. There are two main types of essential fatty acids, the omega-6 series, derived from linoleic acid (e.g., arachidonic acid and gamma-linolenic acid), and the omega-3 series, which could be derived from alpha-linolenic acid (from plant sources) or contained in certain cold water fish (e.g., eicosapentaenoic acid [EPA] and docosahexaenoic acid [DHA]). The essential fatty acids are required for the synthesis of cell membrane phospholipids and eicosanoids, which include prostaglandins, leukotriene, and hydroxy acids. Cell membrane phospholipids influence the biomechanical properties of the membranes and their membrane-bound receptors. The eicosanoids, derived predominantly from arachidonic acid and EPA, serve many functions including modulation of inflammation and host defenses. It is currently recommended that intake of the omega-6 linoleic acids be at least 1% of total food energy. Clinical deficiency of these essential fatty acids is rarely seen in adults since western diets generally

provide 8 to 15 g/d and adipose tissue provides a reserve of 0.5 to 1~kg. When a deficiency does develop, it is usually a result of profound cachexia or extensive small bowel disease or necrosis and the inadequate provision of nutrition support. Although current recommendations call for the omega-3 derivatives of alpha-linolenic acid to be at least 0.2% of total food energy, many nutritionists suggest higher intakes owing to their beneficial effects on lipid metabolism. Oils from a variety of cold water fish species including halibut, mackerel, herring, and salmon are high in the omega-3 fatty acids. Mediterranean fish, namely sardine, anchovy, and picarel, contain moderate amounts of omega-3 fatty acids. Several omega-3 fatty acid supplements are readily available in many stores, but these provide varying amounts of marine-based EPA and DHA. Alpha-linolenic acid, which serves as a precursor of EPA, is also a polyunsaturated omega-3 fatty acid and is found primarily in plant products such as soybeans, canola oil, flaxseed oil, and walnut oil. However, it is controversial as to how effectively humans can convert alpha-linolenic acid to EPA; some studies suggest that only 10% of alpha-linolenic acid is converted. Omega-6 fatty acids are abundant in many of the foods common to the average American diet including most vegetable oils, nuts, cereals, seeds, and legumes.

The optimal fat intake for older adults needs to be determined on an individual basis. Although coronary heart disease (CHD) remains the number one killer of older Americans, the importance of dietary fat after the age of 65 remains controversial. Recent studies indicate that total cholesterol (TC) may be as strong a risk factor for CHD in nondebilitated men and women older than 71 years as it is in middle-aged individuals. Since many healthy older adults in this age range have reasonably long life expectancies, they may benefit from dietary interventions designed to prevent coronary artery disease or its consequences (see Chapter 110). However, fat and cholesterol restricted diets probably do not have any beneficial effects in reducing CHD mortality and may have detrimental consequences in frail older individuals, especially those who are having problems maintaining their weight. Therefore, it seems prudent to adjust fat intake only in healthy older individuals who otherwise would not be adversely affected by such dietary restrictions.

Serum TC and low-density lipoprotein cholesterol are influenced by the ratio of unsaturated to saturated fats and the total amount of energy, fat, and cholesterol in the diet. The National Cholesterol Education Program (NCEP) recommends that all adults limit their total fat intake to 30% or less of total dietary energy, with saturated fatty acids providing 8% to 10%, polyunsaturated fatty acids up to 10%, and monounsaturated fatty acids up to 15% of total energy intake. Cholesterol intake should not exceed 300 mg/day. If elevated serum lipids remain a concern despite adherence to this diet for 3 months, further reductions in dietary fats (especially saturated and trans-fatty acids) are recommended. This is a reasonable recommendation for healthy older adults. However, few are willing to adhere to a diet that contains less than 25% to 30% fat. Even at this level of dietary restriction, the average TC reduction is in the range of 3% to 5% after 1 year. If greater reductions are indicated, other types of dietary modifications or drug therapy may be needed.

Some studies indicate that increasing the ratio of monounsaturated and polyunsaturated fat to saturated fat, without changing total fat intake may be beneficial. For this reason, some experts support the use of the Mediterranean-style diet, which promotes the use of flaxseed and olive oil and the avoidance of saturated fats. More recently, concern has been raised about the use of partially hydrogenated fats rich in trans-fatty acids, as these products have also been demonstrated to have an adverse effect on lipid metabolism. Although more study is needed before any special diet can be recommended, it is probably prudent to emphasize the use of natural fats derived from vegetable oils (both poly- and monounsaturated), nuts, and fish, while avoiding those from animal products and partially hydrogenated oils.

These guidelines may not be applicable to frail older individuals, especially those who are losing weight involuntarily, have a body mass index less than 20, or have disease conditions limiting their nutrient intake. Since fats have twice the energy content per gram as carbohydrates and protein, a diet high in fat may be necessary for such frail older individuals in order to meet their maintenance energy requirements or to replete deficits.

Carbohydrates

Recommendations for carbohydrate content of the diet are generally based on two considerations, the source of the carbohydrates and the energy requirements of the individual. Ideally, food sources should be rich in fiber (see section on "fiber content of diet below") and provide primarily complex carbohydrates rather than simple sugars. The amount of carbohydrates that should be included in the diet is usually determined by default. The energy, protein, and fat requirements of an individual are determined first. Carbohydrate requirements are then determined by subtracting the amount of energy supplied by protein and fat from the total energy requirements. Since protein requirements represent approximately 15% of the total energy content of the diet and fat ideally should be less than 30%, carbohydrates usually represent 55% to 70% of the total. When carbohydrates are excluded from the diet, energy requirements of the body are met by the incomplete oxidation of fatty acids, which leads to ketosis and often causes lethargy and depression. To prevent ketosis, at least 50 to 100 g of carbohydrates should be consumed each day.

Water

Although fluid requirements do not change appreciably with age in adults, people older than 65 years have a reduced ability to regulate their fluid intake and are much more likely than young adults to become dehydrated when their health status or environment changes. Aging is associated with a decline in the intensity of the thirst response to fluid deprivation, a delay in correcting the resulting increase in serum osmolarity, and a reduced ability of the kidneys to concentrate the urine despite an increase in serum vasopressin concentration. Chronic disease and injuries that cause a deterioration of cognitive or physical function increase the risk of dehydration further by altering the perception of thirst, reducing the ability to express the desire for water, or diminishing the capability to access and drink adequate amounts of fluids. When an acute febrile illness occurs in an older individual who is already physically or cognitively impaired, life-threatening dehydration can develop rapidly. This scenario occurs with alarming frequency in nursing homes. The failure of many health care providers, family members, and personal aid assistants to recognize the risk factors and early warning signs of dehydration contributes to the danger that a frail older individual will become severely dehydrated. Many older adults themselves do not recognize their risks and may inappropriately restrict their fluid intake, sometimes as a method of controlling incontinence. Prolonged exposure to elevated environmental temperatures, such as may occur during heat waves, may also precipitate profound dehydration.

Care must be taken to prevent dehydration by recognizing those at highest risk, especially older individuals with cognitive and physical deficits, swallowing problems, ongoing weight loss, diarrhea, fever, or poorly controlled diabetes, or receiving enteral feeding, diuretics, or laxatives. Maintenance water requirements range from 1500 to 2500 mL/d or approximately 30 mL/kg body weight/d. With a normal diet, this would equate to approximately 1 mL/kcal of food intake/d. Requirements increase with fever, activity, or prolonged exposure to elevated environmental temperatures. Those at high risk for developing dehydration should be given set prescriptions for fluid intake and have their fluid intake monitored closely. Whenever hydration status is in doubt, the subject should be weighed, orthostatic blood pressure reading recorded, and serum electrolytes, urea nitrogen, and creatinine checked. In some settings, it may also be appropriate to monitor urine output. Skin turgor is not a reliable indicator of hydration status and should not be used as such in the care of older subjects. Patients, family, and all health care staff, especially in nursing homes, need to be trained to recognize the importance of maintaining an adequate fluid intake at all times, and to carefully monitor intake if there is a change in mental status, activity level, or health status, or if fluid requirements increase, as occurs during heat waves.

Fiber

Dietary fiber is derived from structural components of plant cell walls and consists of plant polysaccharides and lignin, which are resistant to digestion by intestinal enzymes. Many professional health organizations recommend a diet containing 20 to 35 g of fiber a day or 10 to 13 g dietary fiber per 1000 kcal consumed. Dietary fiber may be associated with health benefits including a decreased rate of certain forms of cancer, diabetes, heart disease, and obesity. However, the average American diet is very low in fiber with consumption usually in the range of only 10 to 15 g daily.

There are two general categories of dietary fiber: water-insoluble fibers (cellulose, hemicellulose, and lignin) and water-soluble fibers (gum and pectin). Each category of fiber has a somewhat different spectrum of beneficial effects. Both types lower the energy density of the diet. The added bulk also has a short-term satiety effect, which helps control appetite and prevent overconsumption. Water-insoluble fiber has the further effect of holding water within the intestinal contents, which results in an increased fecal bulk, a decreased gut transit time, and a lower intraluminal pressure within the colon. These properties of water-insoluble fiber make it an important dietary component, since it reduces constipation and may help to prevent the formation of colonic diverticula. There is considerable controversy as to whether a high-fiber diet reduces the risk of colon cancer. Population-based studies demonstrate that intake of fiber-rich foods, which contain primarily insoluble fiber, is inversely related to the risks of developing both colon and rectal cancer. However, several short-term (less than 4 years) clinical intervention trials failed to find any benefit of a high fiber diet in reducing the incidence of recurrent adenomatous colon polyps or cancer. Until more definitive studies are available, the importance of fiber intake in preventing colon cancer will remain uncertain. Sources of insoluble fiber include fruits, vegetables, dried beans, wheat bran, seeds, popcorn, brown rice, and whole grain products such as breads, cereals, and pasta. Approximately two-thirds to three-fourths of the dietary fiber in typical mixed-food diets is water insoluble. There are many excellent Web sites that provide tables listing the soluble and insoluble fiber content of foods (e.g., http://www.wehealny.org/

healthinfo/dietaryfiber/fibercontentchart.html, http://www.md-phc.com/fiber/food.htm, http://www.mayoclinic.com/health/fiber/NU00033).

Water-soluble fiber increases the viscosity of intestinal contents, prolongs gut transit time, and decreases the rate of small intestinal absorption of carbohydrates and bile acids. These effects have important physiologic implications that can be used to advantage clinically. By slowing the rate of carbohydrate absorption, a high soluble-fiber diet appears to be effective in lowering the postprandial surge in the serum glucose, which may be beneficial in the treatment and prevention of diabetes. Through its effects on bile acid absorption, soluble fibers can lower TC and LDL cholesterol by 3% to 10%. The greatest decreases are attainable when initial blood cholesterol concentrations are elevated. Some studies demonstrate an inverse association between the total dietary fiber intake and the rate of fatal and nonfatal myocardial infarctions suggesting the possible importance of fiber in cardiovascular disease prevention. Most of these effects of soluble fibers were demonstrated using fiber concentrates. Comparable amounts of fiber can be obtained from food sources if the diet is carefully formulated. Fruits such as apples, oranges, pears, peaches, and grapes, vegetables, seeds, oat and rice bran, dried beans, oatmeal, barley, and rye are good sources of dietary soluble fiber. Diets that are high in fiber from food sources also provide essential micronutrients and nonnutritive compounds such as xenobiotics, antioxidants, and phytoestrogens that may have important health promoting consequences.

As a general rule, a diet rich in fresh fruits, vegetables, legumes, and whole-grain products is recommended. As portrayed in the USDA MyPyramid, this should include 2 to 3 servings of fruit, 3 to 4 servings of vegetables, and 6 or more servings of grains each day (Figure 38-1). Since most fruits and vegetables contain less than 2 g/serving total fiber and most refined grain products contain less than 1 g/serving, legumes, whole grains, and cereal brans should be substituted for other foods whenever possible in order to increase the amount of both kinds of fiber. Supplementing the diet with any of the commercially available concentrated fiber sources may be necessary, especially in the frail elderly. Concentrated sources of dietary fiber may also be helpful in the treatment of chronic constipation when a limited variety of food is available or the amount of food consumed is inadequate. A large increase in fiber intake over a short period of time may result in bloating, diarrhea, gas, and general discomfort. It is important to add fiber gradually over a period of several weeks to avoid abdominal problems. Fiber should always be taken with adequate fluid in order to avoid worsening constipation.

Vitamins and Minerals

Recommended Intakes

The Food and Nutrition Board of the US National Research Council, between 1997 and 2001, developed the Dietary Reference Intakes (DRIs), which updated and expanded the 1989 Recommended Dietary Allowances (RDAs) for vitamins and minerals. The new DRIs include separate intake recommendations for adults aged 51 through 70 years, and for adults older than 70 years. There are not enough scientific data to calculate requirements for all micronutrients, some of the recommendations already appear outdated, and any person with a medical disorder may need more or less than the RDA for some nutrients. Table 38-3 lists the recommended intakes for various vitamins, as well as the recommended Tolerable Upper Intake levels

TABLE 38-3

Adult Recommended Dietary Allowances and Tolerable Upper Limits for Selected Vitamins and Minerals

VITAMIN OR MINERAL	RECOMMENDED DAILY ALLOWANCE*	TOLERABLE UPPER LIMIT
Vitamin A (retinol)	900 μg (males) 700 μg (females)	3000 μg
Vitamin D	200 IU (age <50) 400 IU (age 51–70) 600 IU (age >70)	2000 IU
Vitamin E	15 mg 22 IU (natural vitamin E) 33 IU (synthetic vitamin E)	1000 mg
Vitamin K	120 μg (males) 90 μg (females)	†
Vitamin B-1 (thiamin)	1.2 mg (males) 1.1 mg (females)	†
Vitamin B-2 (riboflavin)	1.3 mg (males) 1.1 mg (females)	†
Niacin (nicotinamide)	16 mg (males) 14 mg (females)	35 mg
Vitamin B-6 (pyridoxine)	1.7 mg (males) 1.5 mg (females)	100 mg
Vitamin B-12 (cobalamin)	2.4 μg	†
Folic acid (folate)	400 μg	1000 μg
Vitamin C (ascorbic acid)	90 mg (males)‡ 75 mg (females)‡	2000 mg
Calcium	1200 mg	2500 mg
Selenium	55 μg	400 μg

*The recommended daily allowance is the recommended average daily intake that will fulfill the nutritional needs of most healthy adults. The tolerable upper limit (UL) is the highest level of daily nutrient intake that is likely to pose no adverse health risk in most people. As intake above the UL occurs, there is an increasing risk of adverse effects.
†Tolerable upper limit not yet determined.
‡Increase by 35 mg for smokers.

(ULs). Intakes of micronutrients that are lower than the UL usually pose little risk for toxic side effects in healthy people. The UL allows patients and health care workers to understand possible risks if large amounts of vitamins and minerals are consumed. Understanding and consuming the RDA for vitamins and minerals have reduced the risk for classic deficiency disorders (like scurvy and pellagra and beriberi, etc.), but the ideal intake of vitamins and minerals needed for optimum health, which may be higher than the RDAs or ULs, remains controversial. For example, new information regarding vitamin D suggests that much higher intakes than the current RDAs are necessary to reduce risk for osteopenia with aging. Any changes to the DRIs are controversial and have major medicolegal and financial implications for fortified foods and the supplement/health food industry.

Vitamin and Mineral Supplementation

Many older adults, including those who are healthy and living independently as well as those who are frail, ill, or institutionalized, are at risk for micronutrient deficiencies. Several population-based nutritional surveys demonstrate that community-dwelling older adults commonly consume as little as 50% of the RDAs for many vitamins. These findings reflect the fact that even healthy adults do not consistently consume recommended amounts of fortified dairy products and fruits and vegetables (see MyPyramid, Figure 38-1). Risk factors for poor intake, adverse drug–nutrient interactions, and nutrition-related diseases all increase as a function of age, and clinical (and subclinical) deficiencies of vitamins and minerals become more likely, particularly once frailty and the need for institutionalization occurs. The micronutrients most commonly deficient include vitamins C, D, E, B-12, thiamine (B-1), and folic acid, and the minerals calcium, magnesium, and zinc. Because of this, many nutritionists recommend that older adults add a general vitamin and mineral supplement to their diets, although the evidence for benefit remains weak. The least controversial recommendation is for one daily iron-free multivitamin–mineral tablet supplying the RDA for most micronutrients, since the cost is low and associated with no significant side effects. On the other hand, it remains unclear whether intakes of individual micronutrients above the RDA in selected populations are associated with significant health benefits or toxicity. High intakes of some micronutrients (such as vitamins A, D, and pyridoxine) are well known to cause toxicity, which may be so subtle and nonspecific that the harmful effects may not be easily diagnosed. High supplemental intakes of other vitamins or provitamins (like vitamin E and beta carotene), which had been thought to be risk free, have now been associated with adverse health consequences. Older adults should be counseled not to exceed the ULs (Table 38-3) for vitamin intake (see discussion of vitamin D, below as a possible exception), and to disclose all vitamin and mineral supplement use whenever medications are reviewed by any health professional. Any vitamin and mineral supplementation should always be part of an overall program of healthy nutrition (e.g., high fruit and vegetable and whole grain intake and reduced saturated and trans fat intake).

Vitamin B-12 (Cobalamin)

Low serum vitamin B-12 levels become more common with aging. Most recent population studies indicate that approximately 10% to 15% of older adults have vitamin B-12 deficiency. Thus, low levels do not represent normal aging. Pernicious anemia, an autoimmune disorder causing decreased gastric intrinsic factor production, is a rare cause of deficiency in the older adult. Cobalamin deficiency in older adults is more commonly caused by malabsorption of cobalamin in foods, usually owing to atrophic gastritis and hypochlorhydria (Table 38-4); supplemental B-12 in crystalline form is not affected by this and continues to be well absorbed. Stomach acid helps to remove the vitamin from food and make it bioavailable. There may be other causes for deficiency in older adults that are not yet known. Disorders that interfere with enterohepatic absorption (such as ileal disease or surgery) will lead to deficiency more rapidly than low intake does because the high efficiency of the enterohepatic vitamin B-12 reabsorption will be impaired and the vitamin may be lost in the stool.

Vitamin B-12 deficiency can present clinically with two relatively independent disorders. There is a hematologic disorder that causes macrocytosis and anemia. And there is a neurologic disorder that can cause a peripheral neuropathy, including paresthesias and numbness; spinal column lesions, including loss of vibration and position sense, sensory ataxia, limb weakness, orthostatic hypotension, and plantar extensor responses; and neuropsychiatric symptoms, discussed below (Vitamins and Cognition). These signs and symptoms of vitamin B-12 deficiency are nonspecific and common in many older adults with comorbid disorders. When there are several possible causes for the neurologic signs and symptoms, vitamin B-12 supplementation

TABLE 38-4

Causes of Vitamin B-12 Deficiency

Atrophic gastritis and hypochlorhydria
Chronic antacid use (histamine-2 blockers, proton pump inhibitors)
Gastric surgery
Ileal surgery
Diseases of the small intestine and terminal ileum: Crohn disease, sprue, malabsorption syndromes
Helicobacter pylori infection
Pancreatic insufficiency
Parasitic infections of the small bowel (e.g., fish tapeworm)
Bacterial overgrowth syndromes
Strict vegetarianism
Acquired immune deficiency syndrome (AIDS) and AIDS treatment (e.g., zidovudine)
Pernicious anemia
Possibly metformin

is usually accompanied by disappointedly little measurable neurologic or behavioral improvement. The older the patient and the more profound the signs and symptoms, the less likely the recovery. However, some patients may respond, especially if deficiency is relatively recent. Since patients with more severe hematologic signs often have less neurologic impairment, and vice versa, it is important to consider vitamin B-12 deficiency even if the patient lacks macrocytosis and anemia. Thus, screening all older adults for vitamin B-12 deficiency should be considered, and supplementation of all deficient patients is recommended.

Many patients with low normal vitamin B-12 serum levels (<350 pg/mL) have measurable biochemical abnormalities, including elevated methylmalonic acid (MMA) (>270 nmol/L) levels, which improve with supplementation. Although these patients often appear to be asymptomatic, it is probable that borderline serum vitamin B-12 levels represent an early preclinical deficiency state. If this is the case, current laboratory norms for vitamin B-12 are too low since they may not identify patients with early deficiency. Secondary tests for low B-12 status are also nonspecific; for example, MMA may also be elevated with renal failure, and homocysteine levels are also affected by folate and vitamin B-6 status. Other tests for vitamin B-12 deficiency, such as methylcitric acid or holotranscobalamin levels, may prove better (when used with vitamin B-12 blood levels), but are not yet readily available.

An approach to screening for vitamin B-12 deficiency and treatment guidelines are discussed in Table 38-5. Intramuscular or oral replacement is most common; alternative formulations (such as nasal gels) are more costly and have not been rigorously tested. There is no scientific basis for prescribing vitamin B-12 supplementation as a general tonic, and it is not recommended.

Folate (Folic Acid)

Folate deficiency is associated with general malnutrition (particularly associated with alcohol abuse) or with specific folate antagonists, such as methotrexate, phenytoin, sulfasalazine, primidone, phenobarbital, and triamterene. Like vitamin B-12 deficiency, it can present as a megaloblastic macrocytic anemia. Folate supplementation alone may improve the macrocytosis and anemia in vitamin

TABLE 38-5

Evaluation and Treatment of Vitamin B-12 Deficiency in Older Adults

1. Screen with a determination of serum vitamin B-12 level any older adult who is frail, has macrocytosis or neutrophil hypersegmentation with or without anemia, has peripheral neuropathy or a gait disorder, or has otherwise unexplained neuropsychiatric symptoms.

2. Any patient with a vitamin B-12 serum level less than 200 pg/mL (150 pmol/L) can be considered to have a deficiency. A serum level between 200 and 350 pg/mL (150–260 pmol/L) indicates a borderline deficiency.

3. Most older adults with a B-12 deficiency can be treated with supplementation without further investigation. Only in rare cases is it essential to prove that an older patient has pernicious anemia by testing for antibodies to intrinsic factor or performing a Schilling test. Assessing for infection by *Helicobacter pylori* is an additional option.

4. Most older adults with a borderline deficiency can also be treated with supplementation. If it is necessary to obtain further biochemical evidence that a borderline serum vitamin level represents a significant deficiency, the methylmalonic acid (MMA) level (serum or urine) can be determined before and after treatment. (An elevated MMA level should fall to normal with correct treatment.) Assessing for infection by *H pylori* is an additional option.

5. All patients with possible symptoms of vitamin B-12 deficiency should receive parenteral supplementation. This can be accomplished by giving several intramuscular shots (100–1000 μg) within several days to weeks and then continuing supplementation indefinitely with monthly injections. Any healthy patient whose deficiency was found incidentally and is otherwise asymptomatic can be given a trial of oral supplementation with 1 mg daily. These patients should have their serum vitamin B-12 level reassessed in a month to affirm absorption, and periodic (once or twice yearly) screening thereafter.

B-12 deficiency, without correcting the ongoing neurological disorder of vitamin B-12 deficiency, and may even cause a more rapid neurologic/cognitive deterioration. However, in patients with normal B-12 status, high folate intake is associated with protection from cognitive impairment. Although measures of both vitamin B-12 and folate status are often included in the evaluation of macrocytosis, low folate is a rare cause of this disorder. Fortification of grains with folic acid began in the United States in 1998 and has reduced the incidence of neural tube defects in developing fetuses. It was feared that this fortification (approximately 100 μg folate/d) would mask vitamin B-12 deficiency, although this has not been proven. Consumption of a diet rich in fruits and vegetables, along with fortified grains, continues to be recommended as the best source for folic acid, but folate in supplements is more bioavailable.

Folate status may be assessed by measuring serum folate if dietary intake (diet or vitamin supplementation) has not recently changed, or with erythrocyte (RBC) folate levels if there has been a recent change in diet (as after hospital admission). Homocysteine levels can be elevated in folic acid deficiency, but may also increase with renal insufficiency and with vitamin B-12 or vitamin B-6 deficiency.

Calcium, Vitamin D, and Bone Health

Osteopenia (loss of bone mass) is common in older adults and causes an epidemic of hip and vertebral fractures. One common cause is osteoporosis, a multifactorial disease that causes brittle bones (see Chapter 117). Another cause is osteomalacia, caused by vitamin D deficiency and inadequate calcium absorption. In older adults, osteoporosis and osteomalacia frequently coexist. Early symptoms of vitamin D deficiency include nonspecific musculoskeletal pain, particularly in the bones and muscles of the back, hips, legs, and shoulders, as well as proximal leg weakness. A very high proportion of middle-aged and older adults have inadequate vitamin D [25(OH)D] levels. Vitamin D status is best assessed by measuring both 25(OH)D and parathyroid hormone (PTH). Serum calcium, ionized calcium, phosphate, alkaline phosphatase, and 1,25(OH)D levels do not adequately identify vitamin D deficiency. Renal failure (GFR $\leq$ 60 mL/min) increases the risk for vitamin D deficiency. All persons receiving antiresorptive treatment for bone fracture protection and those on anticonvulsants, as well as those with a fat malabsorption syndrome, need assessment of their vitamin D status.

Bone mass usually peaks around age 30 and gradually declines thereafter, with an added rapid loss in women around menopause. It has been estimated that the majority of women after adolescence do not consume enough calcium. Daily intake of elemental calcium should be approximately 1000 to 1500 mg in most persons from adolescence onwards, and many persons, and particularly older adults, consume far less. In addition, calcium absorption declines with age. There are a variety of calcium sources. A cup of milk or cup of yogurt contains approximately 300 mg of calcium. Green vegetables contain some calcium, but they also contain other phytochemicals that interfere with calcium absorption. Therefore, calcium bioavailability from vegetables may be limited. Many persons will be unable to consistently obtain the recommended intake of calcium from natural sources, and will need to take calcium supplements. Some brands of orange juice and candy now contain added calcium. In pill form, calcium carbonate is least expensive, but should be consumed with food (although high fiber foods may reduce absorption somewhat). Some formulations, like calcium citrate, are better absorbed but cost more. Calcium supplements can increase constipation in some individuals. Persons who develop calcium oxalate kidney stones should not drastically limit their calcium intake, as dietary calcium can bind with and reduce food oxalate absorption and decrease risk of stone formation.

The level of vitamin D necessary for optimum bone health is uncertain, but PTH begins to rise (that is, secondary hyperparathyroidism begins) at 25(OH)D levels between 12 and 20 ng/mL (30–50 nmol/L). Frank deficiency is considered a 25(OH)D level <10 ng/mL (25 nmol/L), and desirable levels (to avoid hyperparathyroidism and reduce bone fractures) are >30–40 ng/mL (75–100 nmol/L). Optimal calcium intestinal absorption occurs in older adults at 25(OH)D levels above 34 ng/mL (85 nmol/L). A 25(OH)D level <20 ng/mL (50 nmol/L) in older adults is associated with greater risk of nursing home admission.

Vitamin D is available in two forms: ergocalciferol (vitamin D_2) and cholecalciferol (vitamin D_3). Vitamin D_2 may be used for fortification, but vitamin D_3 seems to be approximately two to three times more potent in raising 25(OH)D levels for longer periods of time, and this may be especially so in older adults. Thus, vitamin D_3, the form made naturally from sunlight exposure to skin, is the preferred supplemental form.

Vitamin D is required for calcium absorption, and vitamin D receptors in the intestine decrease with age. The capability of the skin to manufacture vitamin D when exposed to unfiltered sunlight (UV-B, not UV-A, radiation) also decreases with age, with darker skin pigmentation (blacks have a much higher prevalence of low vitamin D levels than whites), and with the recommended use of topical sunscreen, which reduces skin production of vitamin D by as much as 95%. In addition, in the winter in many parts of the United

States, the skin makes very little vitamin D. A cup of fortified milk or fortified orange juice is supposed to contain approximately 100 IU of vitamin D (some studies of fortified milk find a high proportion of samples to have much less or even none); unfortified milk has negligible amounts. Fatty fish, particularly salmon, also has vitamin D; of note, farmed salmon has approximately 25% of the vitamin D content found in wild salmon. Supplementation of vitamin D is often necessary in older adults. Fracture reduction in older adults requires supplementing both vitamin D and calcium.

The goal in supplementation is to raise the 25(OH)D level to more than 30 ng/mL (75 nmol/L); levels above 36 to 40 ng/mL (90–100 nmol/L) may be more beneficial, but this remains uncertain. This may require vitamin D intake substantially above the RDA and, perhaps, near or above the UL of 2000 IU daily. The 2005 Dietary Guidelines for Americans recommend older persons consume 1000 IU (25 μg) of vitamin D daily. There appears little risk for vitamin D toxicity at daily intakes up to 10 000 IU daily in persons not at risk for hypercalcemia (e.g., malignancy, sarcoidosis), despite the current RDA and UL. Vitamin D deficiency can be treated with an oral dose of 50,000 IU D_2/week for 8 weeks or 2,000 IU D_3/day for 6 months, and then checking 25(OH)D, PTH, and calcium levels. In individuals at high risk for vitamin D deficiency and fracture risk, it may be preferable to schedule high dose oral vitamin D_3 supplementation (e.g., 100,000 IU) three to four times a year; this also optimizes treatment adherence compared with daily medications. Persons taking glucocorticoids need vitamin D and calcium supplementation, but also need a bisphosphonate or intermittent PTH therapy for bone protection as well (see Chapter 117).

Vitamin D receptors are present on many different cell types, and vitamin D has many other roles beyond that in bone health: stimulates insulin production, improves myocardial contractility, modulates B and T lymphocytes, promotes TSH secretion, reduces age-related macular degeneration, and may improve periodontal health, muscle strength and muscle mass, falls risk, and physical performance in older adults. Chronically elevated PTH levels (caused by vitamin D deficiency) may be toxic to muscles and can cause adipogenesis within muscles. Current research is studying whether optimal intake of vitamin D, or vitamin D analogues, may decrease the risk for diabetes mellitus, inflammatory bowel disease, congestive heart failure, colon and prostate cancers, multiple sclerosis, and rheumatoid arthritis.

Preformed vitamin A intake (that is, not provitamin A carotenoids), at levels around twice the RDA and much less than the upper limit of toxicity, has been linked to an increased risk for osteoporosis and hip fracture. High-dose preformed vitamin A supplementation has been shown to improve morbidity and mortality in young children in developing countries so intakes above the RDA are common in this situation. More research is needed to determine whether this pediatric supplementation will subsequently be associated with decreased bone health.

Vitamin K also plays a role in normal bone metabolism. This is yet another reason to encourage eating green leafy vegetables (collards, broccoli, spinach, salad greens). Persons who are taking the anticoagulant coumadin, which interferes with vitamin K synthesis, should try to eat consistent amounts of green leafy vegetables from day to day to reduce fluctuations in coagulation times. A diet high in fruits and vegetables significantly reduces bone turnover and increases bone mineral content. High plasma homocysteine is associated with increased hip fracture risk in older adults.

SPECIFIC DIETARY CONSIDERATIONS FOR OPTIMAL HEALTH

Nutrients and Immunity

Malnutrition, particularly protein-energy undernutrition, is known to impair some aspects of immune status in older adults, including specific B and T cell-mediated functions and nonspecific immunity (polymorphonuclear cells and monocytes). Certain vitamins also appear to have a role in immune function. Several studies of vitamin B-6 supplementation of 2 to 50 mg/day have found that lymphocyte proliferative responses and IL-2 production increased in older adults. Supplementation of healthy older adults with 200 to 800 IU of vitamin E and 15 to 60 mg of beta-carotene has been found to increase delayed-type hypersensitivity responses and lymphocyte proliferative responses in some, but not all studies. Cell-mediated immunity may also decline in folate deficiency. It remains controversial whether ascorbic acid (vitamin C) deficiency plays a significant role in immune function. The evidence indicating that high doses of vitamin C reduce the incidence of viral infections or illness duration is very weak.

Multiple vitamin/mineral supplements may produce improvements in immune function if taken on a long-term basis. Several studies indicate that healthy older subjects who consumed a daily multiple vitamin/mineral supplement for 1 year experienced greater improvements in immune responsiveness, IL-2 production, and NK cell cytotoxicity than did nonsupplemented controls. In one study, there was a greater antibody response to influenza vaccination, a decreased incidence of infections, and less antibiotic use in the supplemented group. These improvements occurred even in those subjects who were very healthy and not vitamin deficient. In contrast, several studies with shorter treatment periods (2.5–4 months) failed to find an association between multiple vitamin usage among healthy older adults and either protection against common infections or immune status improvement.

Trace minerals also play a role in immune function. Zinc can affect immune function; however, no readily available measures of tissue zinc status are available. Serum zinc is not a good marker of tissue status; low serum zinc merely reflects low serum albumin. Older adults commonly have low zinc intakes, and low intake is correlated with poor immune function and tissue healing. However, high intakes (>100–150 mg/day zinc sulfate) may also depress immune status and copper absorption. Vitamin and mineral supplements can improve serum markers of antioxidant activity in nursing home residents, but after 2 years only supplementation of zinc (20 mg) and selenium (100 μg), but not vitamin supplementation, was found to decrease infections. There is evidence that selenium supplementation has beneficial effects on immune markers, lipoperoxidation, and erythrocyte sensitivity to hemolysis.

Vitamins and Cognition

Numerous vitamins have been linked to cognitive decline with advancing age and to the pathogenesis of Alzheimer's disease. The potential protective and adverse effects of antioxidants continue to be debated. According to one theory, the accumulated effects of oxidative stress contribute to the development of both Alzheimer's and vascular disease, which are common causes of dementia in older individuals. High intakes of alpha-tocopherol alone as a vitamin E supplement have not been found to affect cognition, but intake of mixed forms of alpha and other tocopherols from foods has been associated with slowing the rate of cognitive decline with aging. Cross-sectional data have also implicated a role for carotenoids in protecting against cognitive impairment, perhaps by decreasing small vessel disease in the brain.

There is an association between neurocognitive dysfunction (including cognitive impairment without dementia, Alzheimer's disease, and vascular dementia) and elevated plasma homocysteine. It is still uncertain whether elevated homocysteine and low folate and vitamin B-12 are a contributing cause of cognitive decline rather than a consequence of it. Randomized studies of vitamin B-12 and/or folate supplementation have shown a reduction in serum homocysteine and MMA concentrations; however, most have shown no beneficial effect on cognition for either healthy or cognitively impaired subjects, although one well-designed study found improvement in memory, information processing speed, and sensorimotor speed in healthy younger patients (aged 50–70 years) who received 800 μg of daily folate for 3 years compared with placebo.

A search for reversible causes of dementia has routinely included the assessment of folic acid and vitamin B-12 status. Vitamin B-12 deficiency can cause neuropsychiatric symptoms, including delirium manifesting as slowed thinking, depression, confusion, memory loss, and poorer language comprehension and expression that is difficult to differentiate from early Alzheimer's disease. Low serum folate is associated with atrophy of the cerebral cortex, perhaps as a result of hyperhomocysteinemia. A 3-year longitudinal study of nondemented persons older than 75 years found that those with low levels of either vitamin B-12 or folate on entry to the study had increased risk for developing Alzheimer's disease. There are very rare case reports of neuropathy associated with folate deficiency. Some studies find slowed mental processing, including poorer performance on mental status testing, and depressive symptoms (particularly impaired motivation and social withdrawal) in patients with folic acid deficiency. However, while deficiency of these vitamins is common in frail older adults with cognitive disorders, vitamin B-12 and folic acid supplementation rarely affects the course of slowly progressive cognitive decline.

Nutrition and Cardiovascular Disease

There is a growing body of evidence that nutrition plays an important role in cardiovascular disease (CVD) prevention (also see Chapter 110). Diets that are low in saturated fat, contain modest amounts of polyunsaturated fat, and include an abundance of fruits and vegetables are associated with a significantly reduced risk of cardiovascular events. As indicated in Chapter 110, the American Heart Association Step I diet is similar and is recommended for community-dwelling elderly people with dyslipidemia and increased risk for CVD. Others may benefit from a heart healthy type diet as well.

The so-called Mediterranean diet is another example. It is characterized by the use of olive oil as the principal source of fat, an abundance of fruits and vegetables, and a moderate consumption of Mediterranean fish such as sardine, anchovy, and picarel. No one component of this diet has been shown to be more important than another in terms of CVD prevention. The benefits of the various types of oils, especially those containing omega-3 essential fatty acids, have already been discussed. Various hypotheses have been suggested

to explain the beneficial effects of increased consumption of vegetables and fruits. There are probably multiple reasons including the fact that many vegetables and fruits are low in saturated fats and contain ample amounts of vitamins, dietary fiber, and plant polyphenols, a large group of natural antioxidants. In addition to their antioxidant properties, polyphenols have been shown to elicit several interesting effects in animal models and in vitro systems: they trap and scavenge free radicals, regulate nitric oxide, decrease leukocyte mobilization, induce apoptosis, inhibit cell proliferation and angiogenesis, and exhibit phytoestrogenic activity. Whether these properties of polyphenols are important in human nutrition or contribute to the role of fruits and vegetables in CVD protection remains to be determined.

Specific vitamins may also play a role in CVD prevention. Homocysteine is associated with thrombogenicity and vascular disease throughout the body. Folic acid (and, to a lesser extent, vitamin B-12, vitamin B-6, and riboflavin) can lower homocysteine levels. Following fortification of grains in the United States in 1998, homocysteine levels have declined in the general population. A meta-analysis found no benefit of antioxidant supplementation on restenosis after percutaneous transluminal coronary angioplasty. Studies are currently underway to determine whether specific vitamin therapy will reduce clinical endpoints of heart attack and stroke, although preliminary studies have not shown a protective effect. The role of iron (a prooxidant) in atherosclerosis is under study.

Antioxidants have been promoted as protective for CVD. Many epidemiologic observational studies have shown a lower rate of cardiac death in people who consume a diet rich in the antioxidant vitamins E and C, and carotenoids. High levels of serum carotenoids are associated with a lower risk of periventricular white matter lesions on magnetic resonance imaging, particularly in smokers. These studies are difficult to interpret as diets rich in antioxidants are also higher in fiber and lower in cholesterol and saturated fat, and people who consume large amounts of fruits and vegetables, or who take vitamin supplements often have healthier lifestyles. There may also be a gender difference in the interaction of antioxidant vitamins and atherosclerosis. Randomized clinical studies for primary prevention of CVD have not found that any single vitamin is consistently beneficial. In fact, some studies have found increased mortality with the use of supplemental beta-carotene and vitamin E. There is evidence that high supplemental vitamin E may increase risk for hemorrhagic stroke and all cause mortality. Overall, current evidence is insufficient to conclude that antioxidant vitamin supplementation reduces clinically significant oxidative damage in people, although large randomized studies in the United States and Europe are continuing.

Persons at risk for CVD may still wish to consume supplemental vitamins, but should be educated to modify other more clearly associated risk factors, such as smoking, hypertension, diabetes mellitus, saturated and trans fat intake, exercise, etc. Although the toxicity of antioxidant vitamins and most B vitamins is quite low, certain subgroups, such as smokers or persons with uncontrolled hypertension, may be at higher risk for side effects. For this reason, ULs should not be exceeded.

Micronutrients and Cancer

In observational epidemiologic studies, populations who consume foods highest in antioxidants (fruits and vegetables) have lower cancer rates. Similar to studies of antioxidants and CVD, it is difficult to determine whether these findings are because of the antioxidant nutrients or to other reasons. Nutritional studies of supplements for cancer prevention are difficult for many reasons, including the wide range of etiologies, unknown optimum age for intervention, the long time to achieve an effect, the effect of baseline nutritional status, and the possible role for various gene–nutrient interactions. Many studies or meta-analyses of studies have not found a benefit for antioxidant supplements. On the other hand, some clinical prevention trials using micronutrients have shown promising effects: selenium in lung, prostate, and colorectal cancer; vitamin A, beta-carotene, vitamin E, and selenium in stomach cancer; and vitamin E in prostate and colon cancer. In contrast, several studies have found an increased risk of lung cancer in some persons taking beta-carotene supplements (although in persons not taking high-dose supplements, there is an inverse association between cancer mortality and plasma carotene levels), and vitamins may impair the effectiveness of cancer therapy, perhaps by protecting cancer cells during radiation therapy. Fiber intake remains unproven to be protective against colon polyps or cancer. Any protective role for other nutrients (vitamin D analogues; calcium; phytonutrients like green tea, lycopene, and soy isoflavones) and special diets (e.g., the Mediterranean diet) remain under investigation.

It is very likely that people with cancer will try alternative therapies, including mega-vitamin and mineral supplements, and herbal or folk remedies. This should be discussed proactively with patients, from the very time that their cancer is detected, so that they can have the best information available to make their decisions and toxic side effects can be prevented.

Nutrition and Age-Related Eye Diseases

Evidence to support a protective effect of individual vitamins and minerals on age-related eye diseases is conflicting. A number of studies have suggested a possible role for zinc in preventing age-related macular degeneration, or in slowing its progression. Doses used have varied between 80 mg zinc oxide and 220 mg of zinc sulfate. At these pharmacologic doses, there is a risk for stomach upset, immune dysfunction, and impairment of copper absorption. The use of zinc and antioxidant vitamin supplementation (beta carotene, and vitamin C and E) in persons at higher risk for age-related macular degeneration may be beneficial and should be discussed with a retina specialist for appropriate dosing and to avoid toxicity. Studies in progress are evaluating lutein, zeaxanthin, omega-3 fatty acids, and lower doses of zinc. Smoking has been shown to be the strongest environmental risk factor for age-related macular disorders.

Critical assessment of related studies supports a diet rich in food antioxidants rather than vitamin supplements to possibly prevent age-related cataract. The Antioxidants in Prevention of Cataracts Study and Age-Related Eye Disease Study, using supplements of zinc with cupric oxide, beta-carotene, and vitamins C and E, did not find any reduction in cataract development and progression.

ASSESSMENT OF NUTRITIONAL STATUS

This topic is also discussed in Chapter 40.

Initial Screening Assessment

The risk of developing one or more nutritional disorders increases as a function of age, paralleling the age-associated increase in the prevalence of disease and disability that are often causally related to the development of protein, energy, and micronutrient deficiency states as well as obesity. Prevention and early intervention are the best approaches to keeping older individuals optimally nourished because many forms of malnutrition, particularly protein and energy undernutrition, are very difficult to reverse.

Providers should routinely screen their older patients to determine if they have or are at risk of developing nutritional problems. Ideally this should be done as part of a general health maintenance program that is automatically scheduled at least annually and whenever there is a change in the patient's health state. Like other screening instruments, the nutritional screen should use simple criteria, be relatively easy to complete, have relatively low attendant costs, and provide a valid assessment of nutritional risk with a reasonable degree of sensitivity and specificity. Components of the screening evaluation can be self-administered, completed by associate staff, or gleaned from other assessments including a routine history and physical examination. Individuals identified by the screen to be at risk of having or developing nutritional disorders should be scheduled for a more in-depth assessment.

For the purpose of the initial screening assessment, older individuals that have experienced a recent deterioration in their socioeconomic or health status should be considered at risk for the development of subsequent nutritional problems. For this reason, it is important to carefully assess for new health concerns and change in socioeconomic status as part of a nutritional screening assessment. Screening for alcohol abuse with the University of North Carolina's CAGE questionnaire or similar instrument can be included as part of the nutritional assessment.

Other known risk factors for the development of nutritional problems include a recent deterioration in physical or cognitive function and a change in the number or type of medications prescribed. Older patients who are hospitalized because of an acute illness or surgical problem are at very high risk of developing nutritional deficits prior to discharge. Prolonged bed rest, acute inflammation, and inadequate nutrient intake, which are common during hospitalization, rapidly lead to the depletion of both lean and total body mass, placing older patients at a high risk for subsequent mortality. For this reason, any hospitalization for an acute illness should be recognized as a nutritional risk factor and prompt a more in-depth assessment.

A careful weight history, possibly the most important and specific component of the nutrition screen, should be obtained from all older patients. If prior weights are available from the medical record, these should be utilized since patients often provide inaccurate accounts of their weight history. A weight loss of 5% or more within the prior 6 months or 10% or more within the prior 3 years should be considered indicative of a potentially serious nutritional problem unless the weight fluctuation can be ascribed with certainty to alterations in fluid balance. Numerous studies have demonstrated a direct correlation between the amount of weight that is lost and an increased risk of subsequent mortality (Figure 38-6). This is true even if the older individual states that he/she voluntarily lost the weight. Voluntary weight loss in frail older adults has been shown to have the same adverse implications as involuntary weight loss. This probably relates to the fact that few older individuals are successful in their efforts to volitionally lose weight and to keep the weight off while healthy. "Voluntary" weight loss is probably the result of underlying pathology in most older individuals.

As part of the general physical examination, a weight and height should be obtained. If significant kyphosis or scoliosis is present,

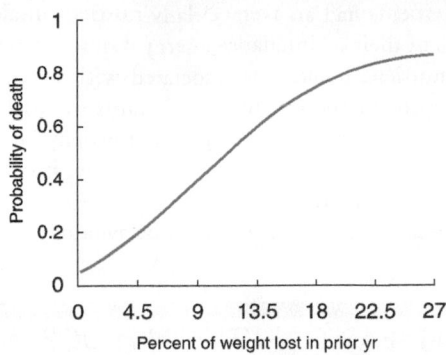

FIGURE 38-6. The relationship between the amount of weight that was lost in the prior year and the estimated risk of mortality within the subsequent year. Based on a study of 750 patients aged 65 and older discharged from an acute care hospital.

the patient's estimate of peak adult height can be utilized for current height. From the weight and height measurements, the patient's body mass index (BMI), weight as a percentage of ideal, and weight as a percentage of usual weight can be calculated as shown in Table 38-6. Signs of dry skin, thinning hair and nails, and other dermatological findings are very nonspecific findings and probably of no value in the nutritional assessment other than indicating the need for careful review of appetite and eating patterns. Since poor oral health may contribute to the development of nutritional problems, a careful oral examination is indicated.

Comprehensive Nutritional Assessment

Anthropometrics

Although poor reliability limits their usefulness for monitoring change over time, anthropometric measurements provide a prognostically important assessment of an older individual's nutritional status when skillfully obtained. While the skinfold measurements (biceps, triceps, suprailiac, subscapular, and midthigh) provide a rough indication of the adequacy of subcutaneous fat stores, arm and arm muscle circumferences are indicators of both muscle mass and subcutaneous fat. Numerous studies of individuals older than 65, conducted in a variety of clinical settings, have found an indirect correlation between both types of anthropometric measurements and an increased risk of subsequent mortality. Values below

TABLE 38-6

Formulas for Calculating Specific Weight Indices

$$\text{Body mass index} = \frac{\text{Weight (kg)}}{\text{height (m}^2)} = \frac{\text{Weight (lb)}}{\text{height (in}^2)} \times 706$$

Weight as a percentage of usual weight* = (current weight/ usual weight) × 100

IBW (males)† = 106 + (6 × [height (in) − 60])

IBW (females)† = 100 + (5 × [height (in) − 60])

Weight as a percentage of IBW = weight (lb)/IBW (lb) × 100

IBW, ideal body weight.
*Usual weight is weight before onset of illness or frailty; it may be the same as peak adult weight.
†To convert to kg, divide by 2.2.

the 10th percentile for age for any of these measures should prompt a careful assessment of both nutrient intake and functional status or activity level. The value of these measures in the assessment of obesity in older individuals is less clear. Because of the age-associated changes in body composition described previously, both BMI and the skinfold measurements may provide a poor indication of total body fat mass if there is significant intra-abdominal fat accumulation as often occurs with advanced age. Waist circumference and the waist to hip ratio are reasonably useful indicators of abdominal fatness. These measurements can be obtained easily in most clinical settings and provide a useful indication of nutritional status when viewed in conjunction with the other anthropometric measures. A waist-to-hip ratio greater than 1.0 in males and 0.8 in females or a waist circumference >40 inches (102 cm) in males and >35 inches (88 cm) in females are indicators of central obesity and an increased risk of diabetes and CVD.

Laboratory Assessment

Although serum albumin, transferrin, prealbumin, and cholesterol are commonly utilized as indicators of nutritional status, considerable caution must be exercised when interpreting the results of these serum measurements. With advancing age, it becomes increasingly difficult to differentiate the interrelated effects of natural aging, disease, and nutritive state on the physiological processes that determine the serum concentrations of these substances. Consequently, random determinations may have marginal clinical value. However, when used to supplement other data, these measurements often provide valuable clues as to the patient's nutritional status and prognosis and can help in guiding treatment decisions, including the need for nutritional support. Interpretation of these measures is aided by knowledge of what physiological and pathological factors influence their serum concentration.

Albumin. A random serum albumin, interpreted without regard to clinical context, has low sensitivity and specificity and only limited clinical utility as a nutritional indicator. While albumin synthesis decreases by 30% to 50% after only 24 to 48 hours of protein and energy deprivation, a decreased rate of albumin degradation and mobilization of albumin from the extravascular space may contribute to the maintenance of a normal serum albumin concentration. Conversely, a low albumin concentration has low specificity as an indicator of protein-energy undernutrition because acute stress, chronic inflammation, and other disease conditions can cause low serum albumin. This effect on the albumin concentration is probably mediated by cytokines (such as tumor necrosis factor and interleukin-6) that are believed to increase vascular permeability to albumin resulting in rapid loss of the normal concentration gradient between the intra- and extravascular space. The same cytokines also suppress albumin synthesis and may trigger an increased rate of albumin degradation. Prolonged hypoalbuminemia can be caused by advanced liver disease (cirrhosis), severe congestive heart failure, nephrotic syndrome, and protein-losing enteropathies. Since it is not currently possible to differentiate the effects of inflammation from those of nutritional deprivation, a low albumin indicates only that the patient is at risk for being undernourished. Serum albumin often does not increase with refeeding and should not be utilized as an indicator of the adequacy of nutritional support.

Transferrin. Like albumin, serum transferrin has relatively low sensitivity and specificity as a nutritional indicator even though its rate of production within the liver is also influenced by nutrient intake. Because its half-life of 8 days is considerably shorter than that of albumin, serum transferrin is a somewhat more sensitive indicator of early changes in nutritional status. However, the serum concentration responds much more sluggishly to changes in nutrient intake than that of other proteins, such as prealbumin. Iron deficiency, acute hepatitis, and estrogen all result in higher serum transferrin levels and may mask developing nutritional problems. In addition to nutritional deprivation, advanced liver disease (cirrhosis), nephrotic syndrome, cancer, and chronic infections often produce a sustained drop in the serum concentration. As is the case with albumin, transferrin is a negative acute phase reactant, meaning the serum concentration can drop precipitously in response to sepsis, major surgery, and other forms of acute severe physiological stress.

Prealbumin. The prealbumin level has moderate specificity as a nutritional indicator. Prealbumin (also known as transthyretin) has a half-life of 2 days and a much smaller volume of distribution compared to albumin. Like albumin and transferrin, prealbumin is a negative acute phase reactant. In response to systemic inflammation, liver production declines and the serum concentration drops rapidly. Low levels are also found in association with end-stage liver disease, iron deficiency, and nutrient deprivation. Renal failure and high-dose steroid therapy are associated with elevated prealbumin concentrations. Because of its relative short half-life, prealbumin is more sensitive to changes in nutrient intake and disease activity than are albumin or transferrin. With resolution of the inflammatory process, the serum concentration will climb rapidly to the normal range if nutrient intake is adequate.

Cholesterol. The serum TC concentration is also influenced by inflammation and other disease states and has very low sensitivity and specificity as a nutritional indicator. The importance of cholesterol is as a prognostic indicator. A total serum cholesterol value less than 160 mg/dL is often seen in association with chronic debilitating disease and is associated with an increased risk of subsequent mortality. Since such disease states often induce anorexia or give rise to other pathologies that limit food intake and eventually lead to nutritional deprivation, a low cholesterol should prompt a careful assessment of the older person's nutrient intake and ongoing weight history.

Assessment of Nutrient Intake

Although frequently difficult to obtain, a detailed nutrient intake assessment is often the most critically needed part of the nutritional assessment. In the outpatient setting where both over- and undernutrition may be a concern, a 24-hour recall or a 3-day food intake diary can be effective tools for estimating nutrient intake and identifying where dietary modifications need to be made, especially if a dietitian or comparably skilled health care provider gives the patient and the family adequate instructions on how to collect the needed data. The employment of more accurate methods of measuring nutrient intake is often necessary within hospitals and nursing homes. Several recent studies demonstrate that many older patients are maintained throughout their hospitalization on nutrient intakes that are far less than their estimated maintenance energy requirements. Contributing to the problem, the attending health care team often overestimates how much food the older patient is consuming. In one study, more than 20% of the nonterminally ill older

hospitalized patients had an average daily nutrient intake that was less than 50% of their maintenance energy requirements. This lack of adequate nutrient intake was associated with a significant deterioration in protein-energy nutritional status by discharge and a sevenfold increased risk of mortality. Low nutrient intake may be an even more widespread problem within nursing homes. Only by carefully monitoring each older individual's nutrient intake during their institutional stays can this problem be avoided.

COMMUNITY-BASED NUTRITION PROGRAMS FOR OLDER ADULTS

Federal, state, and local governments provide many programs designed to help meet the nutritional needs of older adults, particularly those with low incomes. Many of these programs are partially funded through the Administration on Aging (AoA) Elderly Nutrition Program (ENP). The program is designed to be a federal, state, and local partnership. For every $1 of federal funds provided for congregate nutrition services, $1.70 additional funding is leveraged; for every $1 of federal home-delivered funds, $3.35 additional funding is leveraged. The leveraged funds come from other sources including state, tribal, local, and other federal moneys and services, as well as through donations from participants. Nationally, total contributions amounted to $170 million.

The ENP provides for congregate and home-delivered meals and other nutrition services. These meals and services are provided in a variety of group settings, such as senior centers, faith-based settings, and schools, as well as in the homes of homebound older adults. These nutrition services help to address a number of problems faced by many elders, including poor diets, health problems, food insecurity, and loneliness. They include nourishing meals, as well as nutrition screening, assessment, education, and counseling, to ensure that older people achieve and maintain optimal nutritional status and to evaluate for diseases such as hypertension and diabetes. Through additional services, older participants learn to shop, plan, and prepare nutritious meals that are economical and enhance their health and well-being. The congregate meal programs provide older people with positive social contacts with other seniors at the group meal sites.

Meals served under the program must provide at least one-third of the RDAs established by the Food and Nutrition Board of the Institute of Medicine of the National Academy of Sciences, as well as the Dietary Guidelines for Americans, issued by the Secretaries of Departments of Health and Human Services and of Agriculture. In practice, the Elderly Nutrition Program participants are receiving an estimated 40% to 50% of required nutrients from meals provided by the program. The program currently provides congregate and home-delivered meals and other nutrition- and health-related services to approximately 7% of the older population, including an estimated 20% of the nation's poor elders.

FURTHER READING

Arts IC, Hollman PC. Polyphenols and disease risk in epidemiologic studies. *Am J Clin Nutr.* 2005;81:317S–325S.

Campbell WW, Crim MC, Dallal GE, et al. Increased protein requirements in elderly people: new data and retrospective reassessments. *Am J Clin Nutr.* 1994;60: 501–509.

Ewing JA. Detecting alcoholism: the CAGE questionnaire. *JAMA.* 1984;252: 1905–1907.

Frontera WR, Hughes VA, Lutz KJ, et al. A cross-sectional study of muscle strength and mass in 45- to 78-yr-old men and women. *J Appl Physiol.* 1991;71: 644–650.

Jula A, Marniemi J, Huupponen R, et al. Effects of diet and simvastatin on serum lipids, insulin, and antioxidants in hypercholesterolemic men: a randomized controlled trial. *JAMA.* 2002;287:598–605.

Mata LP, Ortega RM. Omega-3 fatty acids in the prevention and control of cardiovascular disease. *Eur J Clin Nutr.* 2003;57(suppl 1):S22–S25.

McGee M, Jensen GL. Nutrition in the elderly. *J Clin Gastroenterol.* 2000;30: 372–380.

National Research Council. *Recommended Dietary Allowances.* 10th ed. Washington, DC: National Academy Press; 1989.

Roberts SB, Fuss P, Heyman MD, et al. Control of food intake in older men. *JAMA.* 1994;272:1601–1606.

Roubenoff R. Sarcopenia and its implications for the elderly. *Eur J Clin Nutr.* 2000;54(suppl 3):S40–S47.

Schiffman SS, Graham BG. Taste and smell perception affect appetite and immunity in the elderly. *Eur J Clin Nutr.* 2000;54(suppl 3):S54–S63.

Sullivan DH. What do the serum proteins tell us about our elderly patients? *J Gerontal Med Sci.* 2001;56A(2):M71–M74.

U.S. Department of Agriculture, Center for Nutrition Policy and Promotion. April 2005. CNPP-15. http://www.mypyramid.gov/. (Accessed October 10, 2008).

Willett WC, Stampfer MJ. Clinical practice. What vitamins should I be taking, doctor? *N Engl J Med.* 2001;345:1819–1824.

Wolfe RR. The underappreciated role of muscle in health and disease. *Am J Clin Nutr.* 2006;84:475–482.

World Health Organization/Food and Agriculture Organization. Energy and protein requirements. *WHO Tech Rep Ser.* 1985;724:1–206.

Weight and Age: Paradoxes and Conundrums

Tamara B. Harris

The evaluation of weight in an older person is pathognomonic of the challenges of geriatric medicine, requiring integration of information on normative biologic change with age and past individual health behaviors to assess future risk. Although weight is one of the easiest clinical measures to obtain, the interpretation of weight in the geriatric patient and assessment of the need for intervention on weight is far more difficult. This chapter provides a rationale and recommendations for an approach to weight in older patients.

SHOULD THE HEALTH PRACTITIONER BE CONCERNED ABOUT WEIGHT IN AN OLDER PATIENT?

Body weight is an important contributor to health in old age. However, health practitioners are often skeptical about evaluating weight in older patients because it seems unlikely that this evaluation will change clinical treatment, except in the event of clear-cut weight loss. In practice, many of the health issues of old age are linked to weight. Clinically, weight stability is used as a sign of general health status. Weight is a contributor to the most problematic syndromes in geriatric medicine, particularly comorbidity contributing to hospitalization and physical and cognitive decline, and resulting health care costs. With the development of new drugs for symptomatic relief of weight-related conditions such as osteoarthritis and with extension to older persons of established preventive treatments for hypertension and hyperlipidemia, polypharmacy is increasingly a weight-related health issue as well. Caring for older patients involves dealing with weight-related issues on a daily basis, even if not explicitly recognized as such.

Apart from weight-related diseases, change in body composition with age, particularly the loss of muscle and bone and the increase in fat, may independently contribute to decline in functional status and loss of independence. Osteoporosis, a disease of loss of bone structure and quality, is an important risk factor for fracture. The loss of muscle with age, termed sarcopenia, is hypothesized to contribute to disability. The increase in fat mass with age may contribute as well. Adipose tissue is now known to produce multiple endocrine factors, including proinflammatory cytokines such as interleukin-6 (IL-6). IL-6 is associated with body fat, independent of weight-associated health conditions, and is also an independent risk factor for physical disability and death. Thus even accounting for body weight, change in body composition with age may independently contribute to risk.

Caloric restriction consistently promotes longevity in laboratory animals, even when restriction is instituted in adult life. Restricted animals are thinner and weigh less, reflecting their lower calorie intake, but lower weight alone does not completely explain the protection from disease and the survival advantage. Nonetheless, lower body weight appears to mediate fundamental physiological processes associated with health and longevity.

PREDICTING WEIGHT IN OLDER PEOPLE: NOTHING SPECIAL

Prediction of body weight from metabolic measures is similar in older and younger persons. Total energy expended daily reflects resting metabolic rate, the energy used for digestion (thermic effect of food), and physical activity. Doubly labeled water studies for total energy expenditure (a gold standard technique that uses CO_2 production to calculate activity over a specified period of time) suggest that, in the absence of acute illness, the same general principles of metabolism pertain. Total energy expenditure does, however, generally decline with age. Although lean mass is known to decrease with age, the change in energy expenditure mainly reflects lower levels of discretionary activity. Total energy expenditure for persons aged 60 to 69 years averages 2186 ± 42 kcal/day for women and 2715 ± 56 kcal/day for men, while for persons in their seventies, the total energy expenditure was 1885 ± 286 kcal/day for white women; 2324 ± 436 kcal/day for black men and 2521 ± 396 kcal/day for white men.

Decreased exercise activity coupled with a small average increase in caloric intake leads to the deposition of extra body weight over time (as little as a 1% excess caloric intake over expenditure daily for a year would result in an increase of approximately 2.5 pounds in that year). Controlled feeding studies in older and younger men suggest that appetite in older people may be relatively insensitive to imbalance between calories and energy output.

Recommendations for body weight do not vary by age or race. These recommendations are based primarily on the relationship between weight and mortality, but they also account for morbidity and some disability. Body mass index (BMI), weight in kilograms divided by height in meters squared (to increase the association of this measure with percent fat), is recommended as a measurement to follow for assessment of risk associated with weight. Normal weight is considered to be a BMI between 18.5 and 25; overweight, a BMI of 25 to 30; and obesity is defined as a BMI of 30 or more. Consideration of body fat distribution has also been advocated, primarily through measurement of waist circumference as an index of central adiposity. Although there are many studies supporting the addition of waist circumference as a measure of adiposity, there are currently no agreed on cutpoints that are clearly associated with clinical outcomes. As a result, the role of waist circumference in clinical practice is still unclear. Waist circumference may be clinically useful in identifying high-risk patients for evaluation of cardiometabolic factors or to follow as a response to weight loss.

The American Society for Nutrition and the Obesity Society convened a technical review panel to review the evidence regarding the health consequences of overweight and obesity in older persons. Review of published studies from 1966 to April 2005 led this group to the conclusion that overweight, obesity, and weight-related health conditions contribute to disability. The evidence was sufficiently strong that programs to address safe and effective weight loss in older persons were considered important. Obesity and overweight are particularly important as they contribute to age-related declines in physical activity and losses in strength and muscle mass. Thus the major motivation for addressing issues of weight in old age relate to disability and the loss of independence.

LIFETIME WEIGHT HISTORY: CURRENT WEIGHT AND RECENT WEIGHT CHANGE ARE NOT ENOUGH

Only a small proportion of people, probably less than 10% of the population, remain approximately at the same weight over their lifetime. Most people gain weight slowly over their lifetime. In Japanese American men participating in the Honolulu Heart Program, a lean and long-lived cohort, the average pattern of weight change with age was a steady increase from young adulthood to a plateau in late middle age with a decline in old age (Figure 39-1). However, the average disguises the heterogeneity in this pattern, as subgroups continue to gain and lose weight over the entire lifetime (Figure 39-2). This late life decline may be as long as 13 to 15 years, associated with many chronic conditions that increase risk of death in old age, including Alzheimer's disease. Longitudinal studies of weight from middle age to old age show that thinner older people were often heavier earlier in life. Conversely, among heavier older people, many have gained weight since middle age (Figure 39-3). Excessive weight gain early in life was associated with premature mortality. However, as treatment

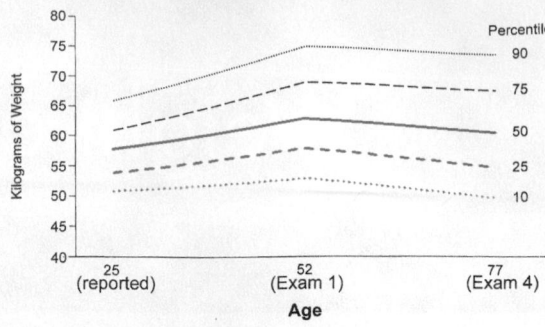

FIGURE 39-1. Lifetime weight patterns based on percentile distributions in 3611 Japanese American men from the Honolulu Heart Study cohort. Weight was measured at examination 1 (1965–1968) and at examination 4 (1992–1994); weight at age 25 yrs was reported at examination 1.

for weight-associated diseases improves, it is likely that more people who have had lifelong overweight or obesity will survive into old age, joining those persons who have more recently become overweight or obese.

As a result of the heterogeneity of such changes over a lifetime, the clinician should not assume the current weight is representative of a general lifelong pattern. Risk of disease, disability, and mortality in old age has been associated with change in weight from early adult weight (age 25 years) or from midlife, and with the difference between maximum and minimum weight. These two weight measures plus current weight and weight change over the prior 6 months constitute a reasonable weight history.

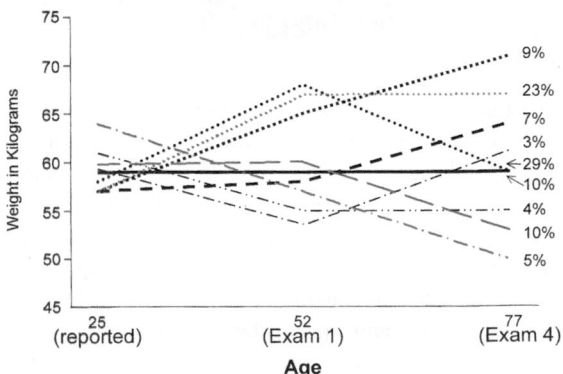

FIGURE 39-2. Weight patterns across the lifetime from age 25 yrs to old age based on 3611 Japanese American men in the Honolulu Heart Study cohort. Each line represents one of nine weight patterns over the lifetime, with the percentages on the right side of the figure indicating the frequency of each pattern. These patterns were determined by using weight at examination 1 as the base; the position of the line for age 25 yrs and examination 4 was based on whether weight at that time was less than, greater than, or within 5% of weight at examination 1. Ten percent of the men (solid line) were within 5% of their mean weight at examination 1 on reported weight at age 25 yrs and at examination 4. Twenty-nine percent had gained 5% or more from age 25 yrs and then lost at least that much, whereas 23% had gained 5% or more from age 25 yrs and maintained that weight.

Weight Pattern Groups within Tertiles of BMI at Exam 4
(Japanese-American Men)

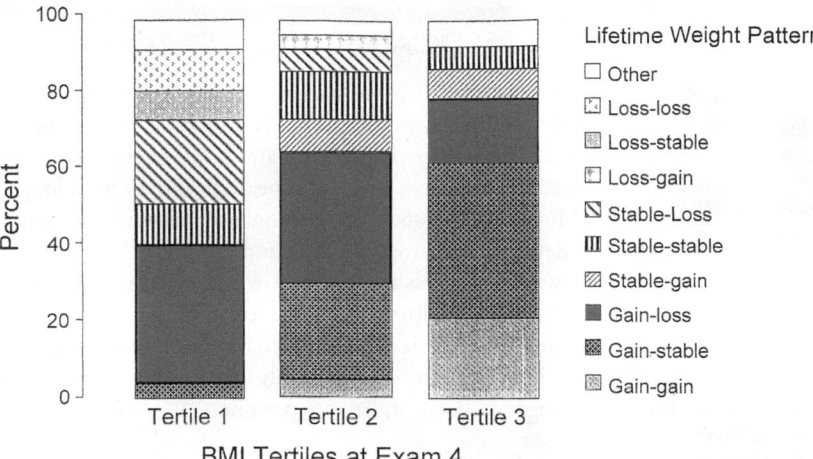

FIGURE 39-3. The weight patterns across the lifetime from Figure 39-2 are shown within each tertile of the population based on increasing body mass index as measured in old age at examination 4. The legend refers to the type of change between reported weight at age 25 yrs and measured weight at examination 1 and change between measured weight at examinations 1 and 4. Men in the lowest third of body mass index in old age had lost weight (the most common patterns are gain-loss and stable-loss), whereas men in the highest third of body mass index had generally gained weight over time (the most common patterns are gain-gain and gain-stable).

Weight loss is associated with a diverse set of factors including depression, cancer, pulmonary disease, and inflammatory arthritides. Weight loss may also be associated with diseases thought of as associated with overweight, including diabetes, coronary heart disease, and stroke, all of which may have a wasting phase. Stressful life events, such as care giving or deaths of significant others, may also play a role in either weight gain or loss. Periods of weight loss are important also as accelerators of loss in lean mass. The issue of weight loss in older people is reviewed in greater depth in Chapters 38 and 40.

ADIPOSITY

Even if weight is maintained constant over life, the body becomes relatively fatter with age, with increases in total fat and losses in lean mass and bone. Fat redistributes centrally with the growth of the visceral fat compartment reflected as an increase in waist circumference. In many tissues, including muscle and bone marrow, there is a gradual replacement of tissue by fat. At any weight then, older people will have relatively more fat, less muscle, and less bone than will younger people.

Gain in weight and increases in body fat are associated with metabolic and physiological alterations that affect health and level of physical function. Cardiovascular risk factors of blood pressure, lipids, and glucose reflect increased weight and fat. Higher levels of intraabdominal fat are associated with insulin resistance, which may cause metabolic abnormalities even in the absence of overt overweight. Intramuscular fat may also contribute to these metabolic abnormalities. Adipose tissue has the potential for paracrine effects by release of molecular factors that influence the metabolism of muscle cells.

Adipose tissue may also play an important role in the promotion of inflammation and its health-related effects. In the past, fat was regarded primarily as an energy storage tissue primarily active in production of sex steroids and glucocorticoid metabolism. However, adipocytes actively produce and secrete a number of hormones and proteins, termed *adipokines*, which may have both local and systemic effects. These factors include leptin, angiotensin, resistin, adiponectin, plasminogen-activator inhibitor 1, and the cytokines,

IL-6, and tumor necrosis factor alpha. Many of these substances have been associated with cardiovascular morbidity, disability, or risk of mortality. As the importance of these and other newly identified molecular metabolic regulators is identified for obesity, we may come to understand more about physiological function in old age. For instance, leptin is highly correlated with body fat even in old age, and was thought to primarily regulate fat mass. Leptin may also play a role in the regulation of bone metabolism and in the vascular system. Activated macrophages are present in adipose tissue and related to expansion of adipose depots. Subcutaneous adipose tissue may be less able to store excess lipid in obesity and in old age. As a result, ectopic growth of fat cells may occur in and around selected organs including muscle, liver, and heart.

An imbalance between calories and activity, however, is not the only explanation for body composition changing with age. Even master athletes who maintain a high level of physical activity tend to lose muscle mass with age, albeit at a slower pace than inactive people. Hormone changes with age including estrogen, testosterone, and growth hormone may contribute to change in body composition. Genetic factors likely contribute to body composition and change with age, interacting with behavioral factors even late in life. For instance, although sarcopenia is common in old age, both men and women with preserved muscle mass and little infiltrating fat can be identified, representing part of the spectrum of genetic predisposition to muscle loss with age. Cigarette smoking also affects weight and body composition. Smokers are generally thinner, as smoking is associated with increased metabolic rate coupled with decreased appetite; smokers tend to gain weight when they stop smoking. Paradoxically, current smokers have a relatively higher waist circumference, which suggests preferential deposition of intraabdominal fat.

STANDARDS FOR OVERWEIGHT AND OBESITY: RIGHT FOR OLDER PATIENTS?

Using current guidelines, overweight is common in both men and women, even in older people (Figures 39-4 and 39-5). Earlier data, using a slightly different cutpoint, show that the prevalence of obesity

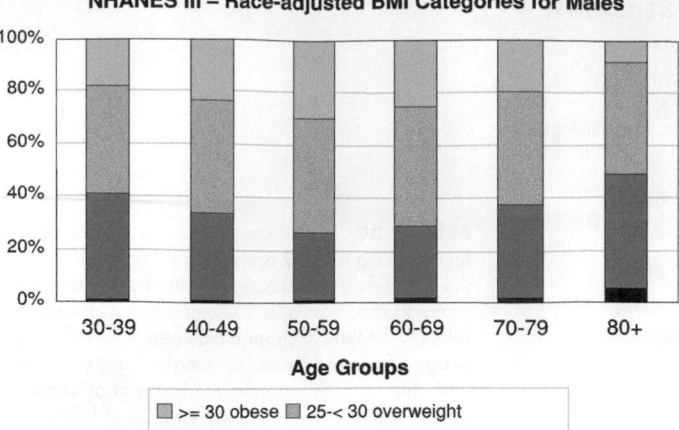

FIGURE 39-4. Data for body mass index (BMI) categories for noninstitutionalized U.S. males aged 30 yrs and older from the National Health and Nutrition Examination Survey (NHANES) III. With age, the proportion of obese people (BMI greater or equal to 30) increases and then decreases in old age, while the proportion in the normal weight category follows an opposite pattern, decreasing to middle age and then increasing with age. Of those aged 80 yrs or older, 5% are underweight and 8% are obese.

in old age was increasing over time, especially in men reflecting changes in the U.S. population.

There is controversy whether the same guidelines for weight should apply across all age groups or whether there should be age-specific guidelines liberalized for older people. While overweight consistently increases morbidity risk in old age, the data on mortality are less consistent, suggesting there may be a trade-off in risks. The data are discussed below; in terms of recommendations, the appropriateness of the guidelines for geriatric patients is likely health status specific. In healthier individuals, these guidelines are appropri-

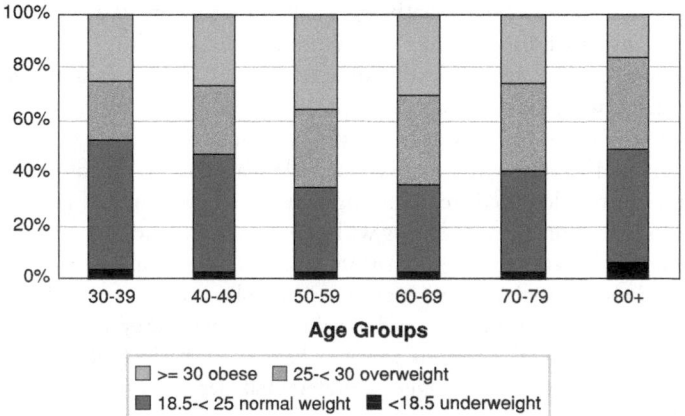

FIGURE 39-5. Data for body mass index (BMI) categories for noninstitutionalized U.S. females aged 30 yrs and older from the National Health and Nutrition Examination Survey (NHANES) III. With age, the proportion of obese people (BMI greater or equal to 30) increases into middle age. The proportion in the normal weight category decreases into middle age and then increases again in old age. Of those aged 80 yrs or older, 6% are underweight and 16% are obese.

ate and good clinical practice. In more frail older persons, different considerations are relevant.

RISKS ASSOCIATED WITH UNDERWEIGHT

Undernutrition is more likely an issue than overnutrition in frail elderly people. Undernutrition is associated with poor health and weight loss. Older people who are underweight are often found in situations of dependency at home, in hospitals, or in long-term care facilities. Risks associated with undernutrition are generally related to depletion of protein stores and are exacerbated by episodes of illness. These issues are reviewed in greater depth in Chapters 38 and 40. However, frailty can occur even in persons who are overweight or obese. Frailty is characterized by extreme debility and loss of function. While more commonly associated with weight loss, these findings can occur in heavier persons.

RISKS ASSOCIATED WITH OVERWEIGHT

Morbidity and Disability

Overweight in old age is associated with the same risk factors and diseases as in younger populations and, for many diseases, continues to have similar relative risks. Overweight is a major contributor to osteoarthritis of knees and hips. In postmenopausal women, overweight and weight gain are associated with risk of breast cancer, and with poorer outcomes for the cancer; overweight increases the risk of colon cancer. Coronary heart disease risk is increased in heavier older persons, particularly when weight change in earlier life is accounted for and overweight is associated with incidence of diabetes. Waist circumference, independent of level of weight, may also contribute to risk of diabetes and coronary heart disease. The diseases of overweight are exacerbated by weight gain. Thus, overweight remains an important risk factor for increased morbidity in old age. Given the association of overweight with these diseases, it is not surprising that disability risk is also associated with overweight, particularly in women. While disability risk is decreasing in normal weight persons aged 60 and older, there is now evidence that disability is increasing in those who are obese (Figure 39-6).

In terms of body composition, both fat and lean mass appear to influence function. The New Mexico Aging Study found that lower lean mass is associated with disability, while other studies suggest that higher fat mass primarily is associated with disability. These are surprising results given that improved functional outcomes are associated with increased strength and muscle mass. It is possible that heavier weight and greater body fat may contribute to disability risk over a wide range of body weight, but that muscle mass is associated with a threshold of risk such that only those individuals below that threshold will be affected. Some heavier individuals have relatively less muscle mass than expected on the basis of size, a situation described as sarcopenic obesity, but risk is likely attributed to body fat rather than muscle. The association of fatty infiltration into muscle with lower strength and physical performance has now been assessed by computerized tomography. Even accounting for body size, height, and other aspects of body composition, fatty infiltration into

Predicted Probability of Impairment by Obesity and Time

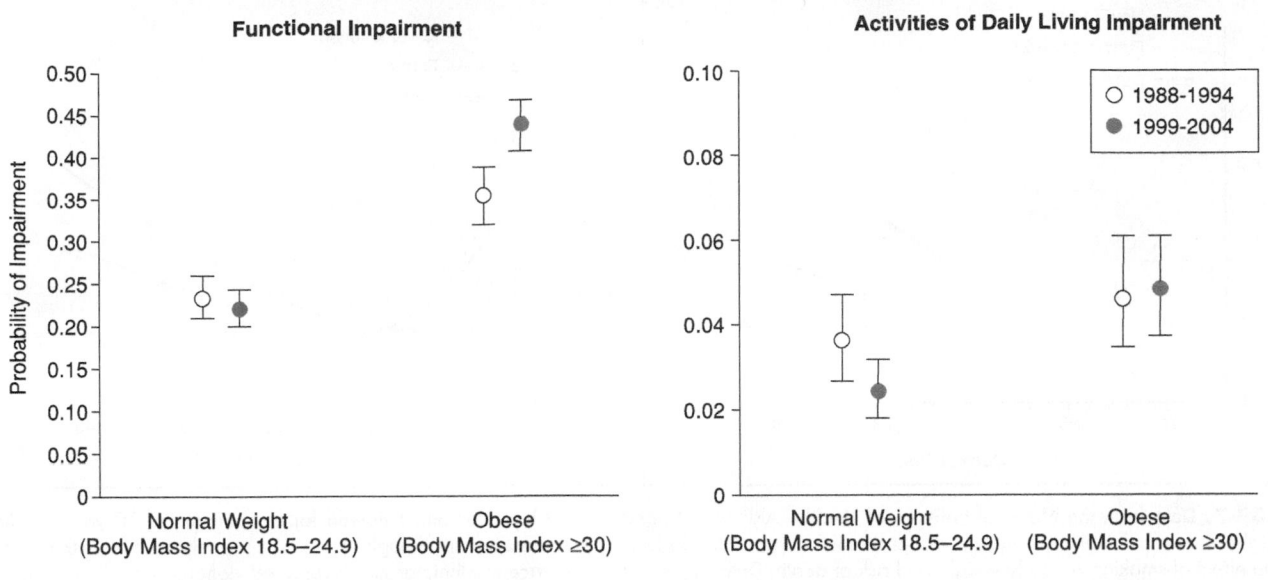

Values are adjusted for age, sex, race/ethnicity, education, and income. Error bars represent 95% confidence intervals. Note that y-axis of right figure indicates a much smaller probability range from 0 to 0.10 than the left figure.

FIGURE 39-6. These data from the National Health and Nutrition Examination (NHANES) III (1988–1992) and NHANES 1999–2004 show trends in functional impairment and activities of daily living disability over this time period by level of body weight. In persons aged 60 yrs and older with normal body weight, both forms of disability did not change over time, while the prevalence of functional impairment increased over time in obese persons. *(Data from Flegal KM, et al. Cause-specific excess deaths associated with underweight, overweight, and obesity. JAMA. 2007;298:2028.)*

muscle is associated with an increased risk of symptomatic functional decline, poorer physical function, and change in strength.

Mortality Risks

In younger populations, overweight is associated with risk of death. Some studies of older people are consistent with this result, particularly those studies in which midlife weight is used to estimate risk of death in old age or where those with significant weight loss are excluded, as in a cohort of over 500,000 persons recruited from the American Association of Retired Persons (Figures 39-7 and 39-8). However, most studies of weight and mortality in old age show a U-shaped association with increased risk associated with both lower and heavier weight. Other studies, particularly of people older than age 75 years, report either an increase in deaths, primarily in underweight individuals, or no relationship at all between weight and mortality. What might explain these results and should these studies affect the approach to the geriatric patient?

Several explanations may contribute to differing results among studies and between older and younger populations. In body weight studies, thinner persons are generally thought to be the relevant healthy contrast population. Cigarette smoking, which leads to thinner body habitus and also to increased risk of death secondary to smoking-related illnesses, tends to confound results in both younger and older populations. In addition, with increasing age, there are fewer healthy thin persons as a result of the usual age-associated gain in weight and to the tendency of individuals with chronic diseases to lose weight secondary to the illness. Therefore, in older age, those

who are ill and losing weight are overrepresented among the thinner populations and at increased risk of death. The critical factor contributing to risk of death may be low protein reserves. The loss of lean mass with age would exacerbate the risk in thinner people and the risk associated with thinness would increase with age, which is what is observed.

Among the heavier older people, there are at least theoretical protective benefits in terms of mortality risk with age. Heavier weight is associated with higher bone mineral density and with lower fracture risk. Heavier weight is associated with greater lean mass, and under catabolic stress, heavier weight may supply a functional nutritional reserve. Heavier weight is often associated with never having smoked, which may be an advantage in terms of pulmonary function; in addition, these individuals often had substantially thinner midlife weight. When risk of death in old age is estimated on the basis of weight in middle age, risk of death is consistently increased in the group whose middle age weight was heavier. Furthermore, it is clear that in old age, health appears to be associated with the ability to gain or maintain body weight in the face of physiologic stress.

The mortality risk in old age may relate to fat distribution rather than body fatness per se. Larger waist circumference is associated with increased risks of disease and mortality even when there is no increased risk observed with weight alone. Future studies using body composition should yield even better estimates.

However, without strong evidence supporting any of these hypotheses, there is no a priori reason to assume that the relationship between heavier weight and poor health outcomes should be different in old age, especially with regard to functional independence.

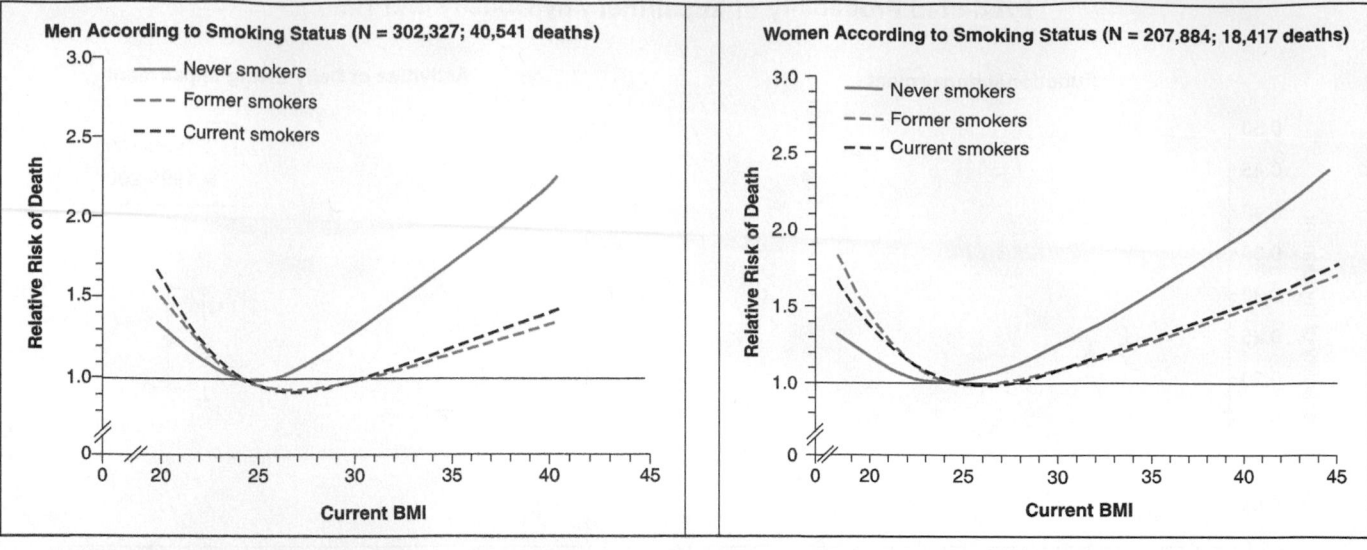

FIGURE 39-7. Data from the National Institutes of Health-AARP cohort aged 50 to 71 yrs old and followed for a maximum of 10 yrs. Men (left) and women (right) shown by smoking status in relation to their current BMI. Risks for never smokers are thought to most accurately estimate risk because they remove the effect of smoking on body weight and risk of death. Data adjusted for age, race or ethnic group, level of education, alcohol consumption, and physical activity.

The most important issue is to judge the weight of older persons in the context of their weight trajectory and their current health status.

INTERVENTIONS AND RECOMMENDATIONS

Body Composition

Regardless of level of weight, interventions to change body composition hold promise, although it is unclear at present which method will prove most effective. Ideally, these interventions would increase lean mass and decrease body fat, particularly visceral fat. Interventions attempted have included increased physical activity, which tends to decrease body fat with concomitant improvement in metabolic parameters associated with overweight, but has little effect on lean mass. Clinical trials for older patients with strength training have demonstrated increases in muscle mass, increased strength, and improvement in level of physical function. Whether these gains can be sustained over time and translated into programs applicable to larger, less-selected populations of older people is being tested. These studies have encouraged many older people to become involved in regular exercise and strength training. These interventions

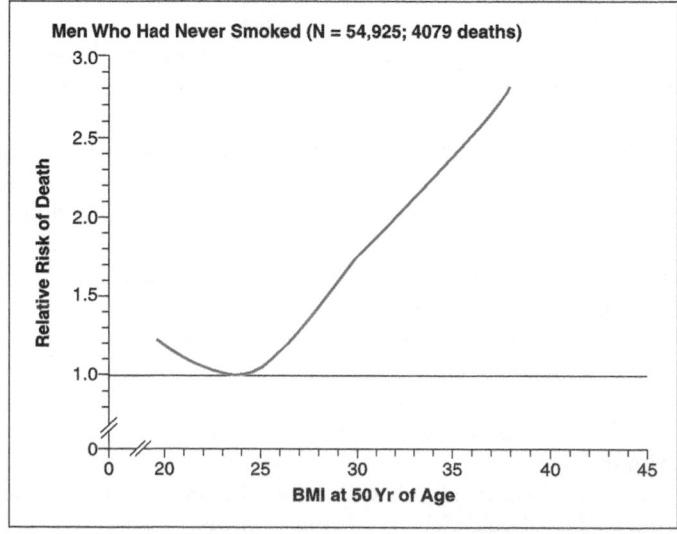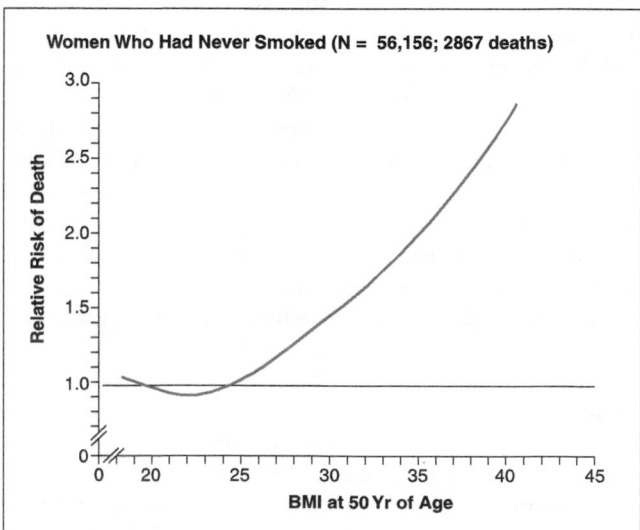

FIGURE 39-8. Data from the National Institutes of Health-AARP cohort aged 50 to 71 yrs old and followed for a maximum of 10 yrs. Men (left) and women (right) never smokers are shown in relation to their reported BMI at age 50. The risks for overweight and obesity are steeper, caused by BMI at age 50 yrs being less confounded by illnesses that might increase risk of death but cause weight loss. Data adjusted for age, race or ethnic group, level of education, alcohol consumption, and physical activity.

are reviewed in Chapter 114. Interventions to alter body composition by using various trophic factors and pharmacologic agents show promise but are also problematic. Trials of these agents, either alone or in combination with exercise or strength interventions, are likely to inform the next generation of efforts to control body fat and increase muscle mass and strength in old age.

Overweight and Weight Reduction

What should we counsel older patients about weight reduction? A history and physical examination related to weight should include a survey of weight-related health conditions, particularly those that are treatable with weight reduction, including hypertension, hyperlipidemia, type 2 diabetes, arthritis of the knees and hip, and peripheral vascular disease. A detailed weight history should be part of the initial evaluation of all geriatric patients and should include early adult weight, midlife weight, maximum and minimum weight, and recent weight change. In the absence of major cognitive impairment, reported weight history is reasonably accurate. Even in an overweight patient, recent unexplained weight loss should raise the need for a careful evaluation for contributory medical, psychological, or functional factors. Prevention of weight gain may be another consideration, particularly for older smokers who decide to quit or those who become disabled with diminished mobility. All older persons should be encouraged to participate in regular physical activity, including some resistance training and stretching. This can be tailored to the level of initial fitness and function, and can be adapted over time to reflect gains in capacity.

Overweight, accompanied by metabolic abnormalities or difficult-to-control symptomatic disease or polypharmacy, suggests the need for a weight-loss program. Will weight reduction benefit the older person? Short-term clinical trials of weight loss in older people show that weight loss can be achieved and results in improvements in hypertension, diabetes, and symptomatic relief of osteoarthritis of the knee. Most of the studies in which weight loss is associated with poor health outcomes are observational studies in which the weight loss was likely to be involuntary. In one of the few observational studies in which voluntary and involuntary weight loss could be differentiated, there was no increase in adverse outcomes with voluntary weight loss. In the absence of relevant long-term clinical trial data on outcomes with weight reduction, advice on weight loss should be guided by symptoms related to the overweight, anticipated short-term health benefits, and the general level of health status of the patient. In a patient on multiple medications for weight-related health conditions, weight reduction may be an important adjunct in weaning the patient off of the medications.

The goal of a weight reduction program should be to achieve a modest weight loss, resulting in improvement in the target weight-related health condition. Little is known about how to best achieve and maintain weight loss successfully in older adults. Efforts to increase physical activity and to decrease caloric intake are preferable to drug therapy for obesity and overweight. Drugs should be considered when it proves impossible to control the metabolic consequences of obesity (e.g., sustained hypertension or prolonged inadequate diabetic control) or under circumstances in which the obesity would constitute a major deterrent to approaching other health problems, for example, knee replacement surgery. The current set of drugs for weight reduction is limited, but active drug development is under way.

Greater numbers of clinical trials of weight loss are now focusing on older populations. Two trials have demonstrated that weight loss achieved through lifestyle interventions on energy restriction and increased physical activity improved glucose, lipids, and cytokine levels. In persons with knee osteoarthritis, a 6-month intervention of caloric restriction and exercise was associated with improvement in walking, stair climbing, and osteoarthritis symptoms. Despite the loss of lean mass as weight loss occurred, knee strength was maintained, suggesting that there may be compensatory effects from the exercise and weight loss to mitigate the loss of muscle (Figure 39-9). This mitigation of change in body composition by weight loss was supported by a 1-year trial using exercise as the primary cause of weight loss; weight loss was not associated with change in bone mineral density at key sites while caloric restriction alone, without exercise, decreased bone mineral density. These trials have been

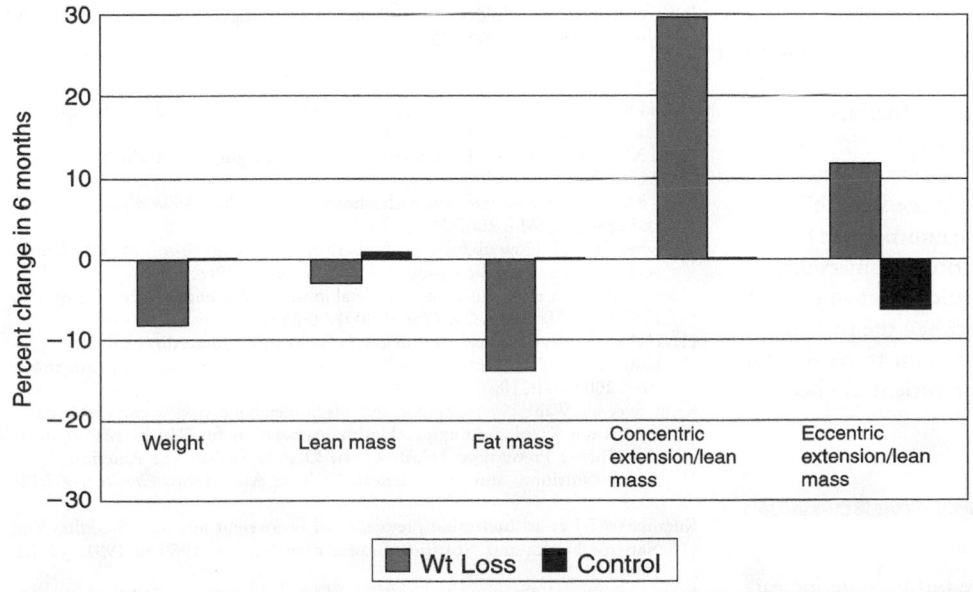

FIGURE 39-9. These data are adapted from the 6-month Physical Activity, Inflammation, and Body Composition clinical trial. The weight loss intervention (identified as "weight loss" group) had a weekly education class, a weight loss diet, and exercise sessions 3 days each week. The control group had bimonthly meetings and a newsletter. The data show that weight loss in this study did not result in loss of either eccentric or concentric strength.

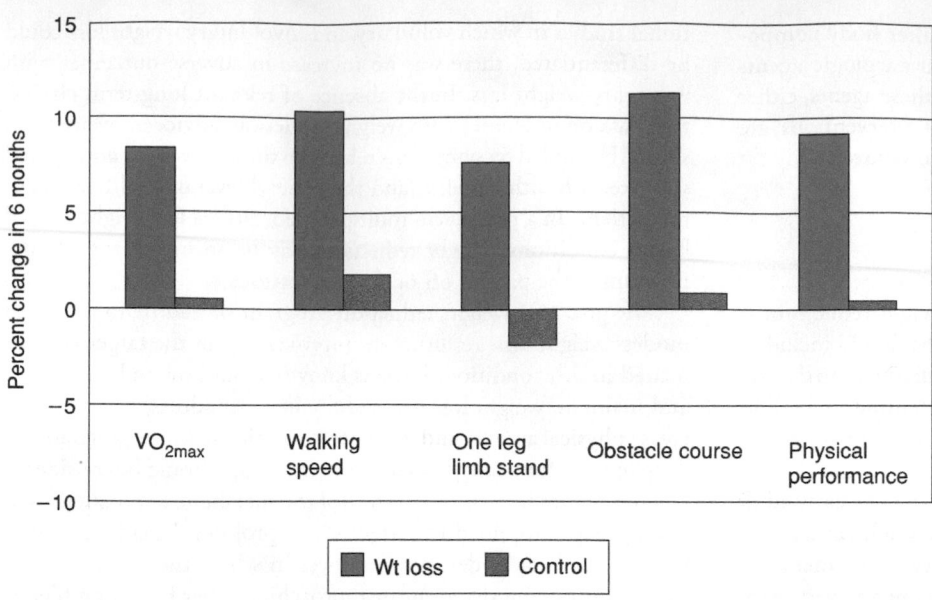

FIGURE 39-10. These data are adapted from a 6-month clinical trial for frail older persons aged 65 yrs and older with a baseline BMI of 30 or more. The weight loss intervention (identified as "weight loss" group) had a weight loss diet and participated in an exercise program. These data show that weight loss resulted in improvement in physical function by all measurements.

successfully extended to frail older persons, showing that weight loss and exercise training focused on endurance, balance, strength, and flexibility lead to better physical performance, self-reported function, and peak oxygen consumption (Figure 39-10).

If a weight reduction program is undertaken, whether by caloric restriction or by drug intervention, it is important to recognize that bone and muscle will be lost as part of this process. Older persons lose weight in similar proportions of fat and muscle as in younger people; however, because they start with less lean mass as a result of age-related changes in muscle and bone, continued losses may result in falling below thresholds of risk for fracture and loss of strength. Efforts should be made to preserve bone and muscle in the face of weight loss, including aerobic and resistance exercise components, or other short-term antiosteoporotic therapy. In addition, caloric restriction needs to be supplemented to insure adequate intake of nutrients and vitamins during a period of dieting.

The physician caring for older people also needs to identify particular times when older people are likely to be at high risk for loss of body weight, especially lean mass. These include major episodes of illness, whether inpatient or outpatient, that result in a significant period of bed rest or recuperation; changes in patterns of daily activities, such as retirement, caring for a sick spouse or friend, or minor injuries such as strains or sprains, that limit usual activity; or new medications that may prevent full activity secondary to sensory or cognitive effects including mild sedation or increased instability in balance. Encouragement of specific activities to return to the former baseline is desirable. These may include nutritional intervention, short-term physical therapy, change in medication, and an exercise prescription. It is likely far easier to intervene when the patient appears relatively healthy and can assist in a program to regain and stabilize body weight and mass than when the patient has become frail and in clear need of rehabilitation.

CONCLUSIONS

Weight concerns remain important in old age but become increasingly complex. There is no simple set of tables that give appropriate ideal weights for older people, especially considering that what may be ideal as a predictor of one outcome (e.g., mortality) may be quite different from what may be ideal for another outcome (functional ability). Further developments in the field will incorporate measurements of body composition and fat distribution as well as information about neuromodulation of weight to assist clinicians in rational management of this complicated problem. For the present time, most important is recognition and control of symptomatic weight-related health conditions and attention to precipitants of involuntary gains or losses in weight.

REFERENCES

Adams KF et al. Overweight, obesity, and mortality in a large prospective cohort of persons 50 to 71 years old. *N Engl J Med.* 2006;355:763.

Alley DE, Chang VW. The changing relationship of obesity and disability, 1988–2004. *JAMA.* 2007;298:2020.

Allison DB et al. Hypothesis concerning the U-shaped relation between body mass index and mortality. *Am J Epidemiol.* 1997;146:339.

Andres R et al. Impact of age on weight goals. *Ann Intern Med.* 1985;103:1030.

Baumgartner RN et al. Epidemiology of sarcopenia among the elderly in New Mexico. *Am J Epidemiol.* 1998;47:755.

Blanc S et al. Energy requirements in the eighth decade of life. *Am J Clin Nutr.* 2004;79:303.

Ensrud KE et al. Weight change and fractures in older women. Study of Osteoporotic Fractures Research Group. *Arch Intern Med.* 1997;157:857.

Flegal KM et al. Excess deaths associated with underweight, overweight, and obesity. *JAMA.* 2005;293:1861.

Flegal KM et al. Cause-specific excess deaths associated with underweight, overweight, and obesity. *JAMA.* 2007;298:2028.

Gallagher D et al. How useful is body mass index for comparison of body fatness across age, sex, and ethnic group? *Am J Epidemiol.* 1996;143:228.

Goodpaster BH et al. Attenuation of skeletal muscle and strength in the elderly: The Health ABC Study. *J Appl Physiol.* 2001;90:2157.

Hays NP et al. Effects of an ad libitum low-fat high-carbohydrate diet on body weight, body composition, and fat distribution in older men and women. *Arch Intern Med.* 2004;164:210.

Klein S et al. Waist circumference and cardiometabolic risk: a consensus statement from Shaping America's Health: Association for Weight Management and Obesity Prevention; NAASO, The Obesity Society; the American Society for Nutrition; and the American Diabetes Association. *Obesity.* 2007;15:1061.

Kuczmarski RJ et al. Increasing prevalence of overweight among US adults. The National Health and Nutrition Examination Surveys, 1960 to 1991. *JAMA.* 1994;272:205.

Losonczy KG et al. Does weight loss from middle age to old age explain the inverse weight mortality relation in old age? *Am J Epidemiol.* 1995;141:312.

Manini TM et al. Daily activity energy expenditure and mortality among older adults. *JAMA.* 2006;296;171.

McTigue KM et al. Obesity in older adults: a systematic review of the evidence for diagnosis and treatment. *Obesity.* 2006;14;1485.

Miller GD et al. Intensive weight loss program improves physical function in older obese adults with knee osteoarthritis. *Obesity.* 2006;14;1219.

Petersen KF et al. Mitochondrial dysfunction in the elderly: possible role in insulin resistance. *Science.* 2003;300;1140.

Stevens J et al. The effect of age on the association between body-mass index and mortality. *N Engl J Med.* 1998;338:1.

Villareal DT et al. Obesity in older adults: technical review and position statement of the American Society for Nutrition and NAASO, The Obesity Society. *Obesity Res.* 2005;13:1849.

Villareal DT et al. Effect of weight loss and exercise on frailty in obese older adults. *Arch Intern Med.* 2006;166:860.

Villareal DT et al. Bone mineral density response to caloric restriction-induced weight loss or exercise-induced weight loss. *Arch Intern Med.* 2006;166:2502.

Visser M et al. Reexamining the sarcopenia hypothesis. Muscle mass versus muscle strength. Health, Aging, and Body Composition Study Research Group. *Ann N Y Acad Sci.* 2000;904:456.

Wang X et al. Knee strength maintained despite loss of lean body mass during weight loss in older obese adults with knee osteoarthritis. *J Geron Med Sci.* 2007;62A:866.

Williamson DF et al. Prospective study of intentional weight loss and mortality in never-smoking overweight US white women aged 40–64 years. *Am J Epidemiol.* 1995;141:1128.

Malnutrition and Enteral/ Parenteral Alimentation

Jeffrey I. Wallace

MALNUTRITION

Definition

Protein-energy malnutrition (PEM), the primary focus of this chapter, is present when insufficient energy and/or protein is available to meet metabolic demands. PEM may develop because of poor dietary protein or calorie intake, increased metabolic demands as a result of illness or trauma, or increased nutrient losses.

Epidemiology

Maintenance of nutrition is an essential component of comprehensive geriatric care, particularly in the acute care setting where the presence of malnutrition is clearly associated with increased complications and other adverse health outcomes. Prevalence data, relying on a variety of measures of nutritional adequacy, suggest that deficiencies in macronutrients (protein-energy intake) and micronutrients (vitamins and minerals) are very common among older adults. National survey data indicate that 40% to 50% of noninstitutionalized older adults are at moderate to high risk for nutritional problems, and that up to 40% have diets deficient in three or more nutrients. Prevalence estimates in selected populations over 65 years old indicate that 9% to 15% of older persons seen in outpatient clinics, 12% to 50% of hospitalized elderly persons, and 25% to 60% of older persons residing in institutional settings have one or more nutritional inadequacies—with PEM being the most common. Physical and psychosocial factors that may lead to inadequate nutrition are listed in Table 40-1.

Energy intake does decline significantly with age, attributable to the decrements in lean body mass and physical activity that often accompany aging. A still greater reduction in caloric intake to levels that may be below daily requirements has been a consistent finding of nutritional surveys conducted among community-dwelling el-

derly people. In the most recent National Health and Nutrition Examination Survey (NHANES III), the mean daily energy intake of persons aged 70 years and older was approximately 1800 kcal/d for men and 1400/d kcal for women, and more than 10% of elderly people reported consuming less than 1000 kcal/d. Even if this limited energy intake met the caloric needs of less-active older adults, it is unlikely that all noncaloric nutrient needs (vitamins and minerals) would be met unless the diet was extremely diverse and rich in nutrients. Although micronutrient deficiencies are common when PEM is moderate to severe, it is the PEM that tends to have the greater clinical impact. Accordingly, this section focuses primarily on PEM, with particular attention to prevention and management of PEM in the acute care setting.

Poor nutritional status and PEM are associated with altered immunity, impaired wound healing, reduced functional status, increased health care use, and increased mortality. Despite the confounding effect of coexisting nonnutritional factors, many studies indicate that poor nutrition remains an independent source of increased morbidity and mortality after adjustment for nonnutritional factors. Similarly, the efficacy of nutritional support to improve outcomes in many circumstances is unproven, but data are accumulating suggesting that there are measurable benefits from interventions to correct or prevent nutritional deficits.

Pathophysiology

PEM may occur as a consequence of inadequate intake alone (e.g., starvation) or in association with disease-activated physiological mechanisms that affect body metabolism, composition, and appetite (i.e., cachexia). In the former (primary caloric deficiency state), the body adapts by using fat stores while conserving protein and muscle, and the resulting physiological changes are often reversible with resumption of usual intake and activity. Cachexia is marked by an acute phase response that is associated with elevated inflammatory mediators (e.g., tumor necrosis factor-α [TNF-α] and interleukin-6) and

TABLE 40-1

Factors Contributing to Inadequate Nutrition in Older Adults

Socioeconomic	Physiologic
Fixed income	Impaired strength/aerobic capacity
Reduced access to food	Impaired mobility/dexterity (arthritis, stroke)
Social isolation	Impaired sensory input (smell, taste, sight)
Inadequate storage facilities	Poor dentition/oral health
Inadequate cooking facilities	Malabsorption
Poor knowledge of nutrition	Chronic illness (via anorexia, altered metabolism)
Dependence on others	Alcohol
Caretakers	Drugs (e.g., SSRIs,* NSAIDs,† digoxin,
Institutions	opiates, levodopa, antibiotics, metformin, iron, others)
Psychological	**Acute Illness/Hospitalization**
Depression	Failure to monitor dietary intake and record weights
Bereavement	Failure to consider increased metabolic requirements
Anxiety, fear, paranoia	Iatrogenic starvation (e.g., NPO‡ for diagnostic tests)
Dementia	Delay in instituting nutritional support

*Serotonin reuptake inhibitors.
†Nonsteroidal anti-inflammatory drugs.
‡Nothing by mouth.

increased protein and muscle degradation that may not be readily reversed by refeeding. Although cachexia is usually associated with specific chronic disease conditions (e.g., cancer, infection), this state may develop in older persons without obvious underlying disease. To some extent, these physiological changes maybe adaptive. Thus, caution is necessary when devising strategies to halt the lean body mass loss and functional decline that often accompanies cachexia.

Presentation and Evaluation

Despite its apparent clinical importance, physician recognition of malnutrition is often lacking. Effective management of frail or ill older adults mandates an evaluation of nutritional status to better allow for early recognition of PEM and consideration of appropriate interventions. Assessment of nutritional status by standard anthropometric, biochemical, and immunological measures can be complex, as both nutrient intake and nonnutrition-related factors can affect these parameters. The use of such measurements (e.g., body mass index, skinfold thickness, muscle circumferences, serum concentrations of proteins, and lymphocyte counts) to detect the presence of poor nutrition is often advocated, but may not result in earlier or more effective intervention than can be achieved by a careful history and physical examination. The close monitoring of body weight, a readily obtainable measure that reflects imbalance between caloric intake and energy requirements, maybe the simplest and most reliable way to screen for malnutrition, particularly in the outpatient setting. Body weight should be recorded at all patient visits. Weight change should be expressed as a percentage of change from past to current weight, because proportional weight change helps account for variability in baseline weight and appears to be the most clinically relevant measure. Although weight gain caused by excessive energy

intake is a common form of malnutrition, only undernutrition and weight loss caused by deficits in energy balance are considered here. Weight loss of 5% or more of usual body weight, a degree that has been associated with increased morbidity and mortality in the outpatient setting, should prompt investigation. Illness-related weight loss exceeding 10% of preillness weight is associated with functional decline and poor clinical outcomes. Weight loss of 15% to 20% or more of usual body weight implies severe malnutrition.

In the hospital setting, where acute illness or injury often coexists with inadequate intake, alterations in nutritional parameters associated with PEM may develop rapidly. Elevated levels of inflammatory mediators appear to be responsible for the greater losses in lean body mass and the rapid declines in albumin that often accompany PEM in physiologically stressed patients. While serial weight measures remain clinically relevant, early detection and correction of PEM in acutely ill hospitalized patients is enhanced by determination of dietary intake relative to metabolic requirements. Although registered dietitians often provide this information, physicians should routinely monitor dietary intake and can readily estimate caloric and protein requirements using formulas presented in Table 40-2. Biochemical and immunological measures (e.g., albumin, prealbumin, transferrin, and lymphocyte counts) are useful adjuncts in the assessment of nutritional status and can provide prognostic information, but their lack of specificity limits their utility as markers of PEM. Anthropometric measures of fat stores (skinfolds) and muscle mass (midarm muscle area) may help in the assessment of PEM, but clinicians are generally not well versed in obtaining these measures and interrater variability can be high. Although less sensitive, clinical evaluation for loss of skin turgor and the presence of atrophy in hand interosseous or head temporalis muscles can help assess for losses in subcutaneous fat and muscle mass. Because all of these parameters maybe affected

TABLE 40-2

Estimation of Daily Energy and Protein Needs

I. Daily energy requirements (kcal/d)
   A. Quick estimate: maintenance 25–30 kcal/kg; stress 30–40 kcal/kg; sepsis 40–50 kcal/kg (tends to overestimate requirements for elderly and obese patients)
   B. Estimates based on resting metabolic rate (RMR, kcal/d):
      1. First estimate RMR (using either equation below)
         a. Harris–Benedict: $RMR_{women} = 655 + [9.5 \times wt(kg)] + [1.8 \times ht(cm)] - (4.7 \times age)$
            $RMR_{men} = 66 + [13.7 \times wt(kg)] + [5 \times ht(cm)] - (6.8 \times age)$
         b. Schofield: $RMR_{women} = [Wt (kg) \times 9.1] + 659$
            (age >60 yrs) $RMR_{men} = [Wt (kg) \times 11.7] + 588$
      2. Then multiply RMR by adjustment factor to estimate total energy requirement:
         Total daily energy requirement = RMR × 1.3 for mild illness/injury
                                        = RMR × 1.5 moderate illness/injury
                                        = RMR × 1.7–1.8 severe illness/injury
II. Daily protein requirements (g/d) (may overestimate if patient obese)

RDA healthy adult age 51 + yrs	0.8 g/kg
Minimally stressed patients	1.0 g/kg
Injury/illness	1.2–1.4 g/kg
Severe stress/sepsis	1.4–1.8 g/kg

by nonnutrition-related factors, an effective assessment of nutritional status requires synthesis of information provided from the dietary history, physical examination, and biochemical data. There are no definitive criteria for classifying degrees of PEM. However, when weight loss exceeds 20% of premorbid weight, serum albumin is less than 21 g/L, transferrin is less than 1 g/L, and total lymphocyte count is less than 800/μL, PEM is generally considered to be severe.

Assessment for Causes of Weight Loss

Initial management of patients with PEM and/or weight loss should include a thorough evaluation to identify underlying causes, and if found, to aggressively attempt to correct potentially remediable factors. In the acute care setting, the cause(s) of malnutrition are often readily evident, although depression maybe a contributing factor that is frequently overlooked. In contrast, reasons for poor nutrition and weight loss among community-dwelling elderly persons maybe multiple and not as readily discernible. Data available from studies on the causes of involuntary weight loss suggests that depression, gastrointestinal (GI) maladies (most often peptic ulcer or motility disorders), and cancer are the three most common causes of weight loss in older adults (Table 40-3). In these studies, when cancer was the cause of weight loss, the diagnosis was rarely obscure. Most diagnoses were readily made after standard evaluations that included a careful history and physical examination and basic screening tests (urinalysis, complete blood count, serum electrolytes, renal, liver and thyroid function tests, stool hemoccults, and a chest radiograph), with additional tests only as directed by signs and symptoms. If this initial basic evaluation is unrevealing (as the data in Table 40-3 suggests will occur in around 25% of cases), it is best to enter a period of "watchful waiting" rather than pursue more extensive undirected testing. A diagnostic algorithm (Figure 40-1) focusing first on verifying actual weight loss (patients may inaccurately report a history of weight loss) and then on whether caloric intake is adequate can help guide an appropriate workup.

Management

General Considerations

Older persons who are not meeting their protein and caloric requirements through oral intake should be considered for nutritional support. Table 40-4 outlines approaches to nutritional support and factors to consider in deciding whether to pursue specific interventions. The urgency for nutritional interventions relates to the degree of protein-calorie depletion at the time of diagnosis coupled with the expected magnitude and duration of inadequate nutrition. In the hospital setting, clinicians must consider that patients may have been suffering from PEM for some time prior to admission. Therefore, avoidance of delays in instituting appropriate nutritional support while waiting for improved intake is desirable. One approach is to intervene after a period of 5 to 7 days of severely limited intake, or for weight loss more than 10% of preillness weight in hospitalized patients. However, attempts should be made to prevent PEM rather than wait for this degree of PEM to develop because weight loss and undernutrition are associated with worse clinical outcomes and recovery of lost lean body mass is often difficult. This is particularly important in severe stress states (e.g., sepsis, major injury) where protein catabolism can lead to losses of lean body mass that approach

0.6 kg/d. In support of early intervention when the development of PEM is likely, a trial of enteral nutrition (EN) among patients with major injury found that early (within 24 hours) enteral feeding had clinical benefits over tube feeding started later in the course of hospitalization.

Patient Preference

The effect of the planned intervention on the patient's quality and/or quantity of life should be addressed before proceeding with nutritional support. Although nutritional support interventions may improve weight and other nutritional parameters, evidence demonstrating their ability to improve clinical outcomes is still limited, particularly when PEM is associated with serious (e.g., critically ill intensive care unit patients) or irreversible underlying disease (e.g., cancer). While most agree that efforts to improve nutrition, even in patients with serious underlying disease, are warranted, late in the course of disease appropriate palliative care may include, if not mandate, discontinuing such efforts. Determination of the care preferences of the patient and family is a critical component of the decision-making process. Patient and family counseling prior to implementing nutritional support should include a review of the interventions being considered and their potential for adverse, as well as beneficial, effects. Figure 40-2 shows an algorithm to help guide nutritional support decisions.

Enhancing Oral Intake

Nonpharmacological Although it is uncommon for elderly persons with PEM to be able to increase their food consumption sufficiently to correct their nutritional deficits, short trials of strategies to improve voluntary intake are reasonable for stable patients with mild PEM (no definitive criteria exist, but parameters consistent with mild-moderate PEM include weight 85–90% of premorbid weight, albumin 25–30 g/L, transferrin 1.5–2.0 g/L, total lymphocyte count 800 to 1200/μL). As previously outlined, underlying causative or contributing condition(s) to PEM should be considered and addressed. Strategies to help overcome anorexia and improve oral intake include assessing and meeting food preferences, providing frequent small meals and snacks, use of flavor-enhanced foods, and providing favorite high-calorie foods (i.e., sweets). Dietitians may aid greatly in these efforts.

High-calorie snacks and oral nutritionally complete supplements are generally recommended. Randomized trials provide some evidence that oral nutritional supplements can improve dietary intake, prevent or lessen weight loss, improve measures of immune function, and improve health outcomes of older adults with, or at high risk for, malnutrition. Higher-calorie "plus" variety nutritional supplements (1.5–2.0 kcal/mL) are preferred over standard (1 kcal/mL) formulas. Costs are only slightly higher, and because they deliver higher calorie content per milliliter ingested, patients need not drink as much volume to improve caloric intake. Supplements should be provided between, rather than with, meals as this appears to result in less compensatory decreases in food intake at mealtime, thereby more effectively increasing total daily caloric intake. However, even if total caloric intake is only marginally improved, the provision of energy from nutritionally dense supplement sources maybe beneficial because of improved micronutrient intake.

A standard multivitamin supplement should also be considered for all older adults with poor intake. Evidence suggests that

TABLE 40-3

Diagnostic Spectrum of Involuntary Weight Loss

	STUDY (STUDY SIZE)					
	Marton et al. **(N = 91)**	**Rabinovitz et al.** **(N = 154)**	**Huerta et al.** **(N = 50)**	**Lankisch et al.** **(N = 158)**	**Levine** **(N = 107)**	**Thompson et al.** **(N = 45)**
Study population	70% Inpatient	Inpatient	Inpatient	Inpatient	Outpatient	Outpatient
Weight loss definition*	≥5%/6mos.	≥5%/not stated	≥10%/6mos.	≥5%/6mos.	≥5%/6mos.	≥7.5%/6mos.
Mean age (range)	59 ± 17†	64 (27–88)	59 (18–83)	68 (27–92)	62 (17–91)	72 (63–83)
Gender (% male)	100%	45%	64%	44%	53%	33%
Diagnosis [n(%)]						
Neoplasm	18 (19%)	56 (36%)	5 (10%)	38 (24%)	6 (6%)	7 (16%)
Gastrointestinal	13 (14%)	26 (17%)	9 (18%)	30 (19%)	6 (6%)	5 (11%)
Psychiatric	8 (9%)	16 (10%)	21 (42%)	17 (11%)	24 (22%)	8 (18%)
Endocrine	4 (4%)	6 (4%)	5 (10%)	18 (11%)	5 (5%)	4 (9%)
Cardiopulmonary	13 (14%)	–	1 (2%)	16 (10%)	9 (9%)	–
Other medical diagnoses‡	16 (18%)	14 (9%)	4 (8%)	13 (8%)	17 (16%)	10 (22%)
Unknown	24 (26%)	36 (23%)	5 (10%)	26 (16%)	38 (36%)	11 (24%)

*Weight loss study definition: percent body weight lost per time interval in months.
†Mean age in yrs ± SD (age range not reported).
‡Neurologic, infectious, alcohol, medication, renal, inflammatory disease, multifactorial.

From Huerta G, Viniegra L. Involuntary weight loss as a clinical problem. Rev Invest Clin (Spanish). 41 (1):5, 1989. Lankisch PG, et al, Unintentional weight loss: diagnosis and prognosis. J Intern Med. 249:41, 2001. Levine MA. Unintentional weight loss in the ambulatory setting: Etiologies and outcomes. [Personal communication and abstract]. Clin Res 39(2):580A, 1991. Marton KJ, et al. Involuntary weight loss: diagnostic and prognostic significance. Ann Intern Med. 95:568, 1981. Rabinowitz M, et al. Unintentional weight loss in the ambulatory elderly. J Am Geriatr Soc. 39:497, 1991. Thompson MP, Morris LK. Unexplained weight loss in the ambulatory elderly. J Am Geriatr Soc. 39:497, 1991.

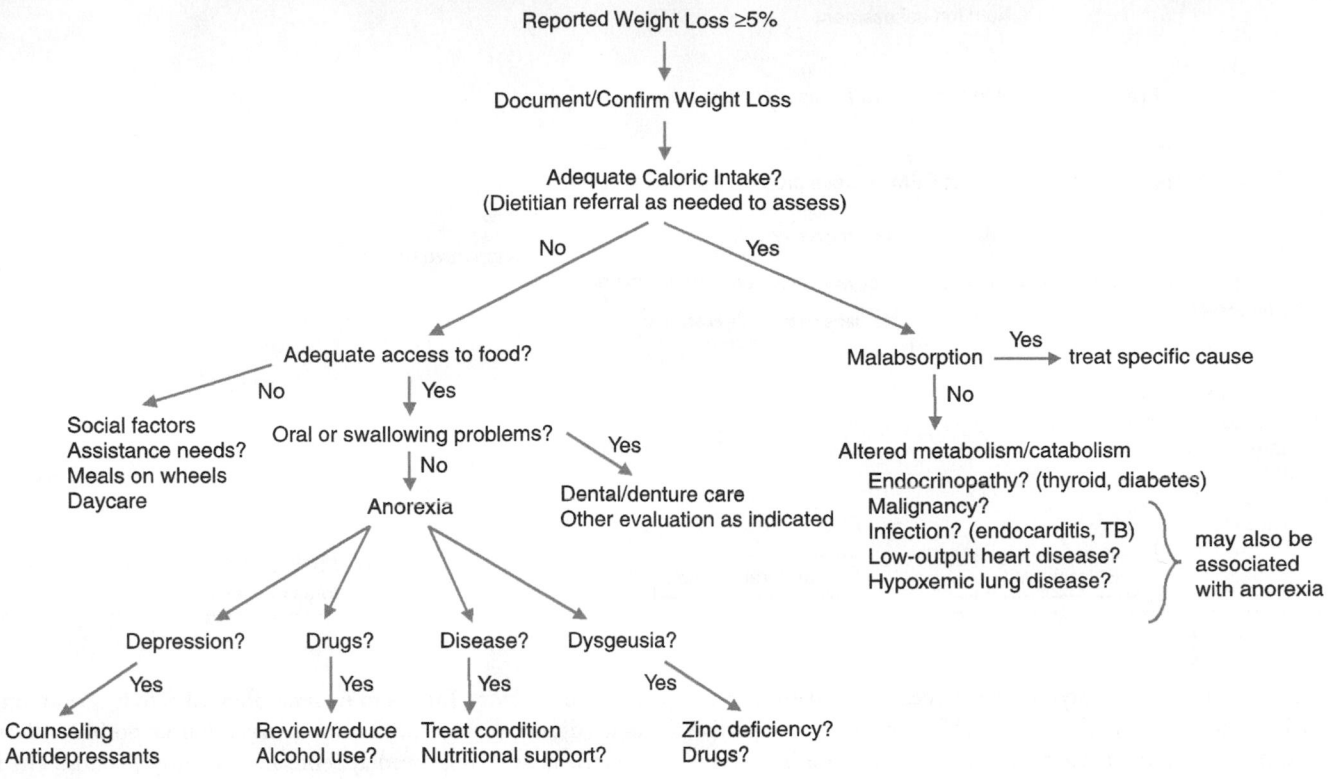

FIGURE 40-1. Weight loss evaluation algorithm.

improving micronutrition with multivitamins, particularly in malnourished or at-risk persons, can improve clinical outcomes (e.g., infection rates). Increased physical activity is an important adjunct that can improve appetite and sense of well-being, thereby leading to improved caloric intake, micronutrient, and functional status.

Drugs Pharmacologic approaches to stimulate appetite and promote weight gain maybe considered on an individual basis with the knowledge that the few agents (megestrol acetate [MA], dronabinol, cyproheptadine) that can improve intake in some patient populations (e.g., cancer, human immunodeficiency virus [HIV], anorexia nervosa) have not been shown to be effective in older adults and have the potential to cause important side effects. Further, the weight gain that has been observed with these agents has usually been small, dispro-

portionately fat mass, and not associated with improved function, quality of life, or decreased morbidity and mortality. MA and dronabinol have shown, at best, limited promise in relatively small studies conducted in nursing home patients. Also of note, in one small nursing home trial, MA did not increase food intake unless combined with increased mealtime feeding assistance. A head-to-head comparison trial in cancer patients found MA to be more effective than dronabinol in improving appetite and promoting weight gain. MA's mechanism of action may involve suppression of inflammatory cytokines (e.g., interleukin-6 and TNF-α), consistent with the observation that this agent appears most effective in persons with elevated cytokine levels (e.g., cancer or acquired immunodeficiency syndrome [AIDS] patients). If initiated, MA may not have a demonstrable effect on appetite for several weeks, but if no effect is seen by 8 weeks, MA should probably be discontinued. If positive effects are demonstrated without significant side effects, MA maybe continued for up to 12 weeks. Potential side effects include fluid retention, nausea, glucose intolerance, and venous thromboembolism. Treatment for more than 8 to 12 weeks can suppress the adrenal–pituitary axis, resulting in adrenal insufficiency and insufficient response to acute stressors. MA also appears to blunt the beneficial effects of progressive resistance exercise, consistent with an undesirable glucocorticoid-like catabolic effect. Only very preliminary data exists for dronabinol use in older adults. Although potential benefits of this agent include positive effects on pain, mood, and nausea, as well as appetite, further study is needed to clarify its efficacy and safety in this population. Delirium is the major side effect of concern from dronabinol.

If depression is felt to be a likely, or possible, contributing factor to poor intake, a trial of therapy is usually warranted. Selective serotonin reuptake inhibitors (SSRIs) are first-line antidepressant agents and improve appetite by improving depression. Mirtazapine and tricyclic

TABLE 40-4

Approaches to Implementing Nutritional Support	
AVAILABLE INTERVENTIONS	**FACTORS TO CONSIDER**
Enhance oral intake	Degree of baseline protein-calorie depletion
Frequent meals, snacks	Current intake relative to requirements
Enhance food flavor	Expected duration of
Provide favorite foods	inadequate nutrition
Protein-calorie supplements	Effect of intervention on clinical outcomes
Multivitamins	Potential benefits
Appetite stimulants	Potential adverse effects
Anabolic agents	Potential for reversibility
Enteral nutrition	Quality of life
Parenteral nutrition	Patient/family care preferences

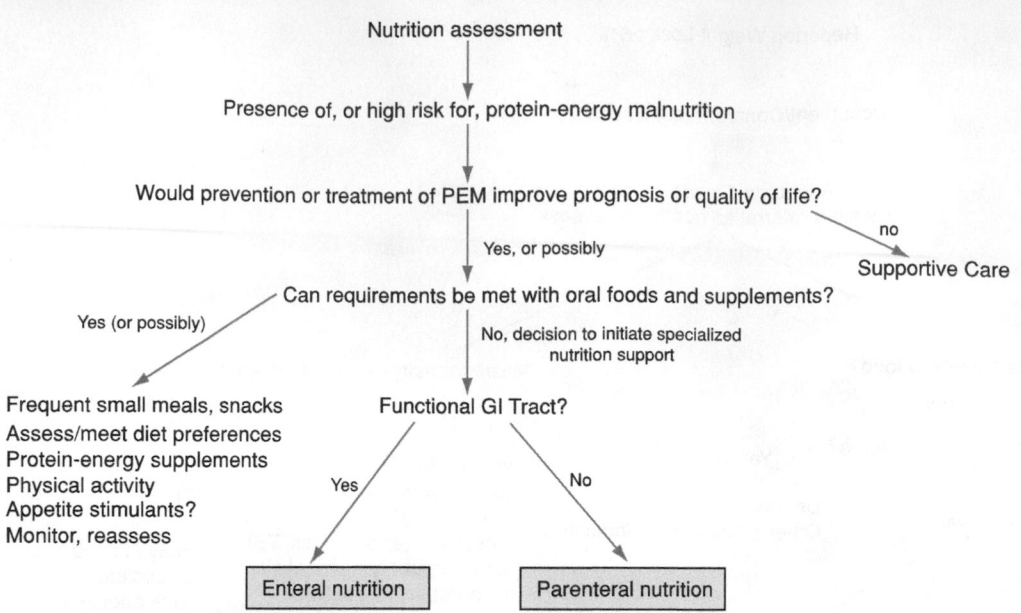

FIGURE 40-2. An algorithmic approach to nutritional support.

antidepressants (e.g., nortriptyline) have been claimed to increase appetite independent of effects on mood. However, one retrospective study did not find a difference between the effects of SSRIs versus tricylcic antidepressants on weight change.

Maintaining Lean Body Mass and Functional Status

Anabolic Agents Anabolic hormones (e.g., growth hormone, testosterone, oxandrolone) have received considerable attention in the search to find strategies to help preserve or increase lean body mass in patients with malnutrition and weight loss. Although adequate nutrition is essential for patients with weight loss, a physiologically stressed catabolic patient may lose significant lean body mass despite aggressive nutritional support (and the weight gain that does occur with nutritional support and appetite stimulants maybe primarily fat and water). A trial of growth hormone in 20 undernourished elderly patients did demonstrate a slightly faster weight gain but differences in weight after 4 weeks were no longer significant. The use of growth hormone in intensive care and congestive heart failure patients has yielded disappointing results with evidence of increased mortality. The cost, need for injection, and potential side effects of growth hormone further limit its clinical utility. Testosterone increases muscle protein synthesis mass and strength, and improvements in functional outcomes have been observed in small controlled trials in selected male populations (e.g., older men after knee replacement surgery, deconditioned older men on a Geriatric Evaluation and Management unit). Although testosterone might be considered in men with documented hypogonadism, its role in the setting of malnutrition and/or cachexia remains to be clarified. Oxandrolone, a synthetic anabolic agent with an increased anabolic to androgenic effect ratio, has shown some utility for patients with weight loss in association with AIDS/HIV or burns, and preliminary data also suggests benefit in patients with chronic obstructive pulmonary disease (COPD). This agent can cause hepatitis, hirsutism, and fluid retention, and is contraindicated in patients with breast or prostate cancer. Further research is needed to define the clinical role of oxandrolone as a pharmacological intervention to be used in combination with nutrition therapy in older adults.

Physical Activity Efforts to increase physical activity are an important adjunct to any nutritional intervention as positive effects of exercise include improved appetite and functional status. The benefits (and safety) of exercise in older populations are reviewed in Chapter 114.

NUTRITIONAL SUPPORT

Enteral Nutrition

Enteral nutrition is defined as the nonvolitional delivery of nutrients by tube into the GI tract. EN should be considered for patients with PEM, or at high risk for it, who cannot meet their requirements through oral intake. However, specific indications regarding if and when to provide EN are not clearly established other than use in patients with neurological dysphagia >1 week. EN requires a functional GI tract and is contraindicated in patients with inadequate bowel surface area, intestinal obstruction, or paralytic ileus. Purported benefits of enteral tube feedings relative to parenteral nutrition (PN) include the maintenance of GI structure and function, more physiological delivery and use of nutrients, less risk of overfeeding and hyperglycemia, and lower costs. Although these advantages maybe more theoretical than actual, EN is recommended when GI function is felt to be adequate. However, enteral and PN should not be considered mutually exclusive. For patients unable to fully meet their nutritional requirements through EN, a mixture of PN and EN is preferable to moving to PN alone.

Efficacy

EN can improve prognostically important intermediate nutritional parameters, but the effects of EN on clinical outcomes (e.g. functional status, medical complications, mortality) are unclear owing to limited and/or mixed data. EN is not often initiated until advanced undernutrition is present, which is a clear impediment to the potential positive effects of nutritional therapy. Several prospective studies, including a randomized, controlled trial among older under-nourished hip fracture patients, have suggested EN can improve both nutritional parameters and clinical outcomes (e.g., length of stay, infectious complications, and mortality). However, further study is needed to determine which elderly hospitalized patients might bene-fit most from aggressive nutritional support. In the interim, sufficient rationale exists to consider EN for patients who are undernourished or at risk for undernutrition and cannot meet their nutritional needs with oral intake.

Tube Placement

The route selected for tube feeding depends on the anticipated dura-tion of feeding, the potential for aspiration, and the condition of the GI tract (e.g., esophageal obstruction). Nasogastric or nasointestinal tubes provide the simplest approach for patients requiring relatively short-term EN (<30 days). Patient comfort is often problematic and tolerance is best when a small-diameter, soft feeding tube is used rather than a standard large-bore nasogastric tube. The use of longer specialized feeding tubes also allows the tube to reach beyond the pylorus into the small intestine, which is the preferred site of placement. Methods to promote passage of the tube past the pylorus and into the duodenum or jejunum include ensuring adequate tube length, having the patient lie on their right side, and prescribing metoclopramide. If these methods fail and the risk of aspiration is felt to be high, tube placement into the duodenum or jejunum can be performed under fluoroscopic guidance. After placement, the de-sired tube position should be verified radiologically before starting feedings and then tubes should be marked at their exit point to help identify if subsequent movement occurs.

Percutaneous tube placement (gastrostomy, gastrojejunostomy, jejunostomy) is indicated when long-term tube feeding is anticipated (>4 weeks). However, it may also be appropriately considered earlier, especially when EN is likely to exceed 2 weeks, because such a tube is better tolerated, allows more consistent nutrition delivery, and has less treatment failures than nasointestinal tubes. Percutaneous placement of a gastrostomy tube (G-tube) can be performed either endoscopically or under radiographic guidance. The risks of major complications with either procedure are generally low, but infection,

hemorrhage, and peritonitis have each been reported at rates of 1% to 3%. Insufficient data are available to clearly favor one method over the other in terms of safety and efficacy, but one meta-analysis suggested that radiologic placement had slightly higher success rates and slightly lower complication rates. Radiological placement does offer advantages in terms of ability to navigate tubes into the je-junum or past near-total proximal obstructions (e.g., head and neck or esophageal cancers that endoscopes cannot get past), whereas en-doscopic placement offers added diagnostic capabilities and possibly lower overall costs.

Tube feeding maybe associated with risk for aspiration pneumo-nia. However, most aspiration pneumonias are the result of difficulty in handling endogenous (oral or gastric) secretions rather than aspi-ration of material introduced through tube feeding. Thus it is not entirely surprising that although distal (postpyloric) feeding tube placement is generally advised, evidence is not definitive that such placement reduces rates of aspiration pneumonia (e.g., studies com-paring aspiration pneumonia rates in patients with gastrostomy vs. jejunostomy tubes have had mixed results). Postpyloric feeding may offer other advantages such as less gastric residual problems in per-sons with gastric dysmotility and reduced esophageal reflux symp-toms. Placement of feeding tubes directly into the jejunum maybe required for patients with abnormal or inaccessible stomachs (e.g., gastrectomy, duodenal obstruction). Although direct jejunostomy tube (J-tube) placement can be accomplished using percutaneous radiologic methods, a J-tube traditionally requires an open surgi-cal procedure and is often placed at the time of laparotomy when the need for prolonged nutritional support is anticipated. Endo-scopically placed G–J tubes and direct J-tubes tend to have smaller diameters and are more prone to clogging.

Formula Selection

Adult enteral formulas fall into one of the following categories: general use, high nitrogen, high nitrogen and high calorie, fiber-enriched, disease-specific, and elemental (Table 40-5). All consist of varying mixtures of protein (often casein), carbohydrate (often cornstarch), and fat (usually vegetable oils), and most do not con-tain lactose. Formula variability includes digestibility, availability of

TABLE 40-5

Approximate Composition of Standard and Disease Specific Enteral Nutrition Products

PRODUCT TYPE (BRAND EXAMPLES)	CALORIC DENSITY (kcal/mL)	PROTEIN (g/L)	PERCENT ENERGY FROM		
			CHO*	Fat	Protein
General use formula (Osmolite, Ensure, Jevity)	1.0	35–45	55%	30%	15%
High nitrogen (Promote, Replete, Sustacal)	1.0	62	50%	25%	25%
High nitrogen, high calorie (Nutren 1.5, "Plus" products†)	1.5	60	50%	35%	15%
Very-high nitrogen, very-high cal (Magnacal, Nutren 2.0)	2.0	70–80	45%	40%	15%
Renal disease					
Predialysis (Suplena, Amin-Aid)	2.0	20–30	50–75%	20–45%	5%
Dialysis (Nepro)	2.0	70	43%	43%	14%
Diabetes (Glucerna)	1.0	70	33%	50%	17%
Pulmonary disease (Pulmocare, NutriVent)	1.5	60–70	27%	55%	18%
Critical care (Alitraq, Impact)	1.0	50–70	55–65%	15–25%	20%
Gastrointestinal dysfunction/elemental (Vivonex, Vital HN)	1.0	40	75%	5%	20%

*Carbohydrate.
†For example, Ensure Plus, Resource Plus, Sustacal Plus.

nutrients, nutritional adequacy, viscosity, osmolality, and cost (costs tend to be substantially higher for disease-specific specialty formulas, and up to 10-fold higher for critical care and elemental specialty formulas). Isotonic general-use formulas with caloric densities of 1 to 1.2 kcal/mL, with or without added fiber, are usually the initial products of choice. Higher caloric density formulas (1.5–2.0 kcal/mL) maybe useful when volume restriction is paramount, but their higher viscosity increases the risk of tube clogging and their higher osmolalities increase the likelihood of diarrhea. Formulas with higher fiber content can be useful for preventing or decreasing tube-feed-related diarrhea.

Disease-specific/specialty formulas are available for patients with renal failure, liver failure, diabetes mellitus, pulmonary disease, GI dysfunction, and critical illness. Renal disease formulas are low in protein, low in electrolytes, and dense in calories to assist in fluid restriction. These formulas maybe useful before dialysis but are not necessary for most patients once on dialysis. Some formulas have been developed for diabetic patients, but use of a cheaper standard formula with adjustment in the glucose control regimen as necessary is adequate for most diabetic patients. Formulas for pulmonary patients have higher fat content, because energy utilization from fat results in less carbon dioxide production relative to the metabolism of carbohydrate energy sources. Although possibly useful for patients being weaned from ventilators, these formulas are of questionable clinical importance for most patients with chronic lung disease. Hepatic formulas have specific amino acid mixtures (high in branched-chain, low in aromatic amino acids) that are less likely to cause or exacerbate hepatic encephalopathy. They are indicated when, in spite of appropriate medical therapy, hepatic encephalopathy limits the delivery of adequate protein to a patient with liver disease.

A number of specialty formulations have been designed for critically ill patients and patients with decreased digestive and absorptive capacity. Some of these products are enriched with glutamine (an amino acid associated with improved nitrogen balance and gut barrier function as well as immune modulating effects when delivered parenterally) or arginine (an amino acid associated with improved nitrogen balance and immune function). However, a large trial of such "immunonutrition" in an intensive care unit (ICU) population failed to show any detectable clinical benefits. Thus, further study of potential beneficial effects of these amino acids in enteric formulas is needed before advocating increased use. In elemental formulas, carbohydrates are supplied primarily as oligosaccharides and proteins have been partially or fully hydrolyzed to free amino acids. Although they are promoted for patients with diminished ability to digest nutrients, it is uncommon for patients to be incapable of digesting and absorbing standard formulas unless they have significantly impaired GI function (assuming appropriate adjustments are made in rates of feedings, osmolality, and fiber content). Elemental diets can also cause, rather than reduce, diarrhea because of their high osmolality.

Administration Guidelines

After desired tube placement is confirmed, tube feeds can be started at a rate of 25 to 50 cc/hour. Isotonic formulas can be started at full strength, whereas elemental/hyperosmolar formulas are usually diluted to half strength to improve initial tolerance. Gastric residuals should be monitored every 2 to 4 hours until the desired rate, which should be based on estimates of the patient's total protein and energy needs (see Table 40-2), is established. Feeding rates can be advanced 25 cc every 8 to 12 hours based on individual tolerance. Feedings should be held if residuals are more than 1.5 times the hourly rate. Once daily requirements are reached, further adjustments to deliver nutrients primarily at night maybe desirable to allow more freedom of movement during the day (nocturnal feeds probably offer little benefit in terms of decreased satiety and improved intake during the day relative to continuous feeds). Larger-bore nasogastric and gastrostomy tubes allow for intermittent feedings without requirement of a pump. Although this offers convenience advantages and maybe more physiological, intermittent bolus feedings can increase the risk of diarrhea, vomiting, and aspiration pneumonia. Attention must also be paid to water and electrolyte requirements. Basal-free water requirements for hospitalized patients are 30 to 35 mL/kg per day, or about 1 cc/kcal delivered. Free water will need to be increased if excess fluid loss is occurring as a consequence of diarrhea, urinary, or increased insensible losses. For patients with fever, an additional 300 to 400 cc of water maybe needed for each degree centigrade of temperature elevation. Monitoring of weight and electrolytes can help clarify any necessary adjustments, with additional free water given in divided boluses three or four times a day.

Risks and Complications

Proper consideration of whether to proceed with EN entails an understanding of common adverse effects (Table 40-6). Nasogastric

TABLE 40-6

Adverse Effects of Enteral Nutrition and Management Approaches

ADVERSE EFFECTS	MANAGEMENT
Poor tolerance	Consider
Frequent self-extubation	Parenteral nutrition
Agitation	Percutaneous gastrostomy tubes
Pulmonary	Elevate head of bed $\geq$30°
Aspiration	Monitor gastric residuals, ↓ rate as needed
	Nasointestinal, G-J, J-tubes
Gastrointestinal	
Gastric retention	Low-fat formula, metaclopramide
Nausea/vomiting	Nasointestinal, G-J, J-tubes
Diarrhea	↓ Delivery rate, ↑fiber, antidiarrheals
Metabolic complications	
Hyperglycemia	Routine monitoring glucose, electrolytes
Fluid and electrolytes	Monitor weight, volume status, free water
Refeeding syndrome*	Monitor phosphate, magnesium, potassium
Mechanical problems	
Insertion site irritation/ infection	Local skin care
Tube plugging	Regular flushing, cola/cranberry flushes
G-tube, J-tube extubation	See text
Nasopharyngitis, sinusitis, local pain, epistaxis	Use small-bore flexible tube and avoid prolonged nasal intubation (>4–6 weeks)
Drug interaction considerations	
Tube feeds ↓ bioavailability (e.g., ciprofloxacin, azithromycin)	Hold feedings 15 min before and after medications
Frequent medications interrupt nutrition	Alternate medication routes (IV, IM, rectally, transdermal)

*Abrupt, often large drops in serum potassium, phosphorous, magnesium, which may accompany initiation of nutritional support in malnourished patients.

(NG) tubes are often not well tolerated, with patient agitation and self-extubation being particularly common among patients with cognitive impairment or delirium. The subsequent need for physical or chemical restraints can increase complications and appropriately dampen enthusiasm for NG tube feedings. Also, EN in actual practice often involves delayed and inadequate nutritional support because of frequent problems with tubes (e.g., self-extubation, plugging) or GI intolerance (e.g., high residuals, bloating, diarrhea). These factors may explain why attempts to provide elderly persons with EN are often abandoned after only a short course of therapy. Some have advocated an early switch to, or starting with, PN, particularly if patients are confused or delirious and the expected duration of therapy is short (1–2 weeks). If longer-term support is likely, early use of percutaneous gastrostomy tubes, which tend to be better tolerated by uncooperative or confused patients, maybe considered (along with a reevaluation of overall patient care preferences and goals before proceeding with this more invasive approach).

Pulmonary aspiration is a relatively common and serious complication of EN. Patients with gastric retention, decreased gag reflex, and altered levels of consciousness are at increased risk for aspiration, and mechanically ventilated patients should not be considered protected by the presence of an endotracheal cuff. The risk of aspiration can be reduced as outlined in Table 40-6. Gastric retention problems may respond to a change to a low-fat formula or to pharmacologic intervention with metoclopramide. Diarrhea is another GI problem that frequently complicates EN. When significant diarrhea occurs, infectious causes (particularly *Clostridium difficile*) must first be excluded. The possibility of intolerance to formulas with high osmolality or high fat content should also be considered. Interventions to reduce diarrhea include slowing the rate of infusions, diluting hypertonic formulas, increasing formula fiber content, and the use of antidiarrheal agents. In addition to the electrolyte abnormalities that can be caused by diarrhea, hyperglycemia, and other metabolic abnormalities may develop related to tube feedings. Potassium and phosphorous requirements can be very high in the first few days after nutritional support is started because of extracellular to intracellular shifts that accompany nutrient utilization, particularly among cachectic patients ("refeeding syndrome"). Fluid-retention problems are also not uncommon in older adults with impaired renal or cardiac function. To minimize these problems, monitoring protocols should include frequent evaluations of GI tolerance, daily weights, and daily monitoring of glucose and electrolytes (including phosphorus, calcium, and magnesium) until stable.

Increased problems with tube clogging often occur when more viscous higher-calorie formulas and medications (especially fiber and calcium supplements) are passed via small-bore (smaller than no. 10 Fr) catheters. Tube maintenance with regular flushing every 4 to 8 hours for patients on continuous feeds, and before and after the delivery of intermittent tube feeds or medications (with 30 cc warm water) can reduce clogging problems. When possible, give medications by mouth rather than by feeding tube. Use of cola, cranberry juice, or meat tenderizer in solution may help open clogged catheters. Another common mechanical problem is the replacement of gastrostomy or jejunostomy tubes that have fallen out. Feeding tube fistula tracts are generally not well established for at least 1 to 2 weeks after placement (and often substantially longer given malnutrition's effect on wound healing). Tubes that come out early (in the first 2–3 weeks after placement) require replacement by the original specialist. If the fistula tract is well established, patients or care providers should be able to gently replace tubes that have fallen out, and delay in doing so for more than 6 to 12 hours risks spontaneous closure of the tract. However, feeding should not be resumed until proper tube placement is radiologically confirmed.

Parenteral Nutrition

Parenteral nutrition (PN), the delivery of required nutrients by vein, is generally indicated to prevent the adverse effects of malnutrition in patients who are unable to obtain adequate nutrients by oral or enteric routes. However, specific indications regarding if and when to institute PN, as well as the utility of PN once instituted, have not been clearly delineated. In general, the decision to institute PN depends on the severity and expected course of the underlying disease(s) and the severity of preexisting and anticipated undernutrition. The duration of undernutrition that can be tolerated before adverse effects occur is not clear. Some expert opinion guidelines have suggested that to preserve nutritional status and prevent starvation-induced complications, PN should be considered for even well-nourished, minimally stressed patients who are anticipated to be unable to eat for more than 10 to 14 days. PN might also be considered to prevent starvation-induced complications in critically ill or severely stressed patients in whom enteric intake is precluded for 5 to 7 or more days. The decision to institute PN requires careful consideration of the patient's clinical condition and prognosis, clinical judgment about the patient's ability to tolerate undernutrition, and insight regarding patient care needs and preferences.

Efficacy

Evidence that PN can improve clinical outcomes is generally not robust. Limited data that PN can have beneficial effects comes primarily from the following settings: postoperative PN in patients with esophageal or gastric cancers; a randomized trial demonstrating that PN reduces complications in severely malnourished patients (defined in the reference study by a low nutritional risk index score, which generally was reached if weight loss exceeded 10% to 15% and albumin was <33 g/L, or, in the absence of weight loss, if serum albumin was <28 g/L) undergoing major elective surgery; and studies in selected patient populations that include bone marrow transplant recipients, malnourished critically ill patients, and patients with short bowel syndrome. There is a paucity of studies and many unanswered questions about the efficacy and safety of PN in elderly individuals. Furthermore, findings such as detrimental clinical outcomes with routine PN for cancer chemotherapy patients, along with the cost and invasiveness of PN, suggest that risks and benefits must be reviewed carefully for each patient. That PN maybe of some benefit when used in cancer patients who are severely malnourished affirms the importance of patient selection and the identification of clear goals of therapy before instituting PN.

Administration Guidelines

Intravenous Access Total parenteral nutrition (TPN), the delivery of all required nutrients by vein, requires the use of hypertonic solutions that can only be tolerated when delivered into large venous vessels, preferably into the superior vena cava. Because peripheral veins are limited to solutions containing lower concentrations of amino acids and dextrose (<10% dextrose), peripheral parenteral nutrition (PPN) usually cannot deliver nutrients in sufficient quantity to meet all requirements. The infusion of lipids can improve energy delivery and vessel tolerance to PPN, making PPN occasionally useful for short-term support or as adjunctive therapy for patients with limited tolerance of EN support. Central catheter placement has traditionally been accomplished via subclavian or internal jugular veins with associated operator-dependent risks of insertion complications that include pneumothorax, inadvertent arterial puncture, and hemorrhage. Central venous access for long-term use (weeks to months) can also be obtained via catheters advanced through peripheral vessels (usually median cubital, basilic, or cephalic veins). Such peripherally inserted central lines (PICCs) offer reduced risks of the aforementioned central placement complications and may have a reduced risk of infectious complications. Complications that maybe increased with PICCs include early mechanical phlebitis, catheter occlusions, and catheter tears, although the latter two problems can be minimized with proper line maintenance. One nonrandomized study of TPN delivered through PICCs versus through subclavian vein-inserted central catheters found no difference in complication rates and concluded that PICC lines can be used safely and effectively for TPN. Regardless of the placement method used, proper line position needs to be confirmed by x-ray before initiating TPN.

TABLE 40-7

"Average" TPN Formula Composition and Parameters for Daily Vitamin, Mineral, and Electrolyte Requirements

MACRONUTRIENTS*	
Protein	15%
Carbohydrate	55–65%
Fat	20–30%
MICRONUTRIENTS	
Vitamins	
Vitamin A	3300 IU
Vitamin D	200 IU
Vitamin E	10 IU
Thiamine (B-1)	6 mg
Riboflavin (B-2)	3.6 mg
Niacin (B-3)	40 mg
Pantothenic acid (B-5)	15 mg
Pyridoxine (B-6)	4 mg
Biotin (B-7)	60 μg
Folic acid (B-9)	600 μg
Cobalamin (B-12)	5 μg
Vitamin C	200 mg
Trace Elements	
Zinc	5 mg
Copper	1 mg
Chromium	10 μg
Manganese	0.5 μg
Selenium	60 μg
Electrolytes	
Sodium	60–150 mEq
Potassium	40–100 mEq
Chloride	Equal to sodium
Magnesium	16 mEq
Phosphorus	10–30 mmol
Calcium	10 mEq

*Percent of total calories.

TPN Composition Standard TPN solutions contain carbohydrate (dextrose) and protein (amino acid) concentrates, fat emulsions (soybean or safflower oil with egg phospholipids), micronutrients, and electrolytes. Knowledge of usual TPN formula composition can help provide a working framework (Table 40-7) but macronutrient and electrolyte content in particular must be individualized. Energy and protein content should be based on estimates of patient requirements (see Table 40-2). Electrolyte requirements are highly variable and often require adjustments as they are influenced by the patient's underlying disease (e.g., heart failure, renal dysfunction) and factors such as renal or GI fluid losses. Standard packages of vitamins and trace elements are added to TPN solutions daily to prevent the development of micronutrient deficiencies. Because patients on warfarin should not receive vitamin K, it is not included in standard vitamin packages and must be given separately in doses of 5 to 10 mg/wk.

The optimal proportions of fat and carbohydrate to meet energy needs are controversial. All standard formulas contain hypertonic glucose (10–70% dextrose before mixing), but because glucose tolerance declines with age, slow upward titration in delivery rates are necessary in older adults. Aggressive glucose monitoring and treatment is important as hyperglycemia is associated with increased infection risk, particularly when blood glucose exceeds 200 mg/dL. Glucose infusion rates should not exceed 5 mg/kg/min (about 500 g/d for a 70-kg person on continuous TPN) because the rate at which stressed patients can metabolize glucose as energy is limited. Overfeeding with glucose results in increased risks of hyperglycemia, increased carbon dioxide production, and the conversion of excess glucose calories into fat (which requires energy and contributes to fatty liver changes).

Lipids in the form of 10% to 20% fat emulsions are added to TPN as a source of concentrated energy and to supply essential fatty acids. Delivery of fat emulsions two to three times a week is usually adequate to prevent essential fatty acid deficiency. Fat emulsions are isotonic and are generally well tolerated, but patients occasionally develop hyperlipidemia and, less frequently, have allergic reactions (usually to the egg phospholipid component). Increasing the proportion of energy supplied by fat can reduce hyperglycemia and carbon dioxide production, but fat delivery should not exceed 2.5 g/kg/d (or 50–60% of nonprotein calories) to avoid possible adverse consequences associated with fat overload. The fat overload syndrome is characterized by hyperlipidemia with diffuse fat deposition that can cause organ and reticuloendothelial system dysfunction, impaired immune function, and increased risk of sepsis. Lipid formulations enriched with medium-chain triglycerides may have less potential for these side effects and improve nitrogen balance relative to long-chain triglycerides, but studies have not demonstrated consistent benefits and their proper role in nutritional support remains unclear.

TPN formulas with special amino acid compositions are available for patients with severe renal or hepatic disease. The renal formulas consist primarily of essential amino acids to allow delivery of necessary proteins while minimizing nitrogen loads. Their use should be restricted to predialysis renal failure patients. The hepatic failure formulas have increased ratios of branched chain amino acids to aromatic amino acids. They can reduce problems with hepatic encephalopathy, but because of their expense, they should be reserved for patients who develop hepatic encephalopathy with standard TPN formulas.

Formula Delivery Initial infusion rates should be at a rate of 25 to 50 cc/hour and increased every 8 to 12 hours as metabolic status allows until fluid and nutrition goals are met. At some institutions, carbohydrate, fat, and protein TPN components are mixed together into a single bag (total nutrient admixture or three-in-one formula). Although this simplifies administration, the admixed product is less stable, and concerns have been raised that the haziness imparted to the admixture by the lipids makes it difficult to detect problems that can occur with calcium and phosphorous precipitation (though inline filters should be routinely used to help prevent particulate matter safety problems). In most circumstances, daily TPN volumes are infused continuously over the full 24 hours. This allows slower delivery of carbohydrate (which can help reduce hyperglycemia) and the continuous flow may decrease the risk of catheter occlusion while avoiding interruptions that might lead to hypoglycemia. Shorter infusion schedules with brief periods off TPN (cyclic TPN) are occasionally desirable, but this is more of an issue for long-term TPN in the home care setting. Because TPN formulas (especially the lipid component) can suppress appetite, it maybe desirable to reduce or hold lipid emulsions for a few days to help improve intake prior to planned discontinuation of TPN.

Patient Monitoring and Complications Elderly persons receiving TPN should be monitored closely (Table 40-8). Table 40-9 details common complications and their prevention and/or treatment. Correction of dehydration and volume depletion can most readily be accomplished with standard intravenous fluids, which can be infused separately or added to TPN bags for convenience. Fluid overload can be managed by using higher concentrations of macronutrients to limit total volumes infused, with diuretics added as needed. Although insulin maybe added directly to TPN solutions as needed to control hyperglycemia, it is best to give intravenous insulin separately until caloric delivery and glucose control are stabilized. Intravenous insulin is preferred over subcutaneous insulin owing to the latter's potential for erratic absorption in malnourished patients. Infection and volume depletion need to be considered if hyperglycemia is a persistent problem. As with EN, potassium and phosphate must be monitored closely because they may drop precipitously after initiating TPN in malnourished patients. In most cases, electrolyte requirements stabilize within 1 week. The relative amounts of chloride (which can lead to metabolic acidosis) and acetate (which can be metabolized to bicarbonate and lead to metabolic alkalosis) can be adjusted as needed depending on the patient's acid–base balance. Patient monitoring should also include clinical (e.g., weight, functional status) and laboratory (e.g., albumin, prealbumin) assessment of the efficacy of nutritional support.

Infection of the access line is uncommon in the first 72 hours, so early fevers are usually a result of other causes. The risk of infection can be reduced with proper aseptic line care, and the line site should be monitored daily for erythema, tenderness, or discharge. Positive line cultures in the absence of other sources are usually an indication for line removal. The increased rates of sepsis that have been observed in some trials of TPN (and which possibly diminished the potential for TPN trials to demonstrate improved clinical outcomes) maybe related to overfeeding and hyperglycemia. Avoidance of hyperglycemia in particular may decrease the risk of TPN associated infections. Liver abnormalities that can occur with TPN include fatty liver with elevated liver function tests (often occurs early, maybe related to carbohydrate overfeeding, generally benign/reversible) and cholestasis (tends to occur later, after 3+ weeks). EN, even in small amounts, may reduce problems with cholestasis.

Special Issues

Comorbidity

Responses to nutritional support efforts may vary substantially owing to heterogeneity in underlying disease states associated with PEM (particularly the presence and severity of inflammatory/catabolic states). Limited data on the interaction between nutritional support and specific comorbid conditions and care settings include the following.

TABLE 40-9

TPN Complications and Potential Corrective Measures

CONDITION	PREVENTION/MANAGEMENT
Metabolic	
Fluid overload	Restrict fluid by ↑ macronutrient concentrations
Hyperglycemia	↓ Carbohydrate delivery (rate, concentration), insulin IV; consider ↑ proportion energy from fat
Hypoglycemia	Avoid sudden cessation/ interruption of TPN
Refeeding syndrome	Start/titrate TPN slowly, avoid overfeeding
Hypertriglyceridemia	↓ Fat infusion rates and/or frequency of lipids
Hyperchloremic metabolic acidosis	↑ Acetate/↓ chloride; consider renal/ gastrointestinal causes
Metabolic alkalosis	Consider renal/gastrointestinal causes; replete K+;↓ acetate
Respiratory (hypercarbia)	↓ Total calories, ↑ proportion energy from fat
Nonmetabolic	
Line infection	Single-lumen catheter; dedicated TPN line; aseptic line care; rule out other fever sources
Hepatic	
Steatosis/↑ LFTs	Avoid carbohydrate overfeeding; rule out other causes
Biliary (cholestasis)	Enteral feed if possible; rule out other causes
Catheter occlusion	Regular flushes; no line blood draws; urokinase

LFTs, liver function tests.

TABLE 40-8

Guidelines for Monitoring Patients on TPN

CLINICAL DATA	LABORATORY DATA
Vital signs three times per day until stable	Glucose chemsticks qid until stable
Daily weights	Daily: Electrolytes, glucose, creatinine, blood urea nitrogen, calcium, phosphorus, magnesium until stable, then twice weekly
Daily fluid input and output	
Daily line and skin inspection	Weekly: LFTs, albumin, CBC, PT, triglyceride
Efficacy of nutritional support	

CBC, complete blood count; LFTs, liver function tests (alanine and aspartate aminotransferase, alkaline phosphatase, bilirubin) PT, prothrombin time.

Hip Fracture As many as half of all older patients who present with hip fractures are malnourished. Undernutrition may directly contribute to hip fracture events via increased presence of osteoporosis, increased risk of falls as a consequence of reduced muscle mass and strength, and reduced fat to "cushion" a fall. A Cochrane Library review of 21 randomized trials of postoperative nutritional support (with oral supplements or EN) in hip fracture patients concluded that there is some evidence that oral supplements improve health outcomes (reduced combined outcome measure of mortality and medical complications), but nasogastric feedings were not well tolerated and did not improve mortality. The authors concluded that oral supplements maybe effective (although the evidence is still very weak) and that the benefits of nasogastric feeding are even less certain and should probably be reserved for very malnourished patients, with extremely poor intakes not responsive to oral supplementation.

Chronic Obstructive Pulmonary Disease Prevalence estimates of malnutrition in patients with COPD range from 20% to 70%. Increased inflammatory activity probably contributes to catabolic processes that combine with undernutrition to cause weight loss and loss of lean body mass. Although a meta-analysis concluded that energy supplementation does not have significant effects in patients with *stable* COPD, another review indicated that 10 of 12 randomized-controlled trials have noted positive effects of nutritional support (mostly oral supplements providing 400–1000 kcal/d) on anthropometric, immune, muscular strength, and respiratory function outcome measures. Given the relative low cost and potential for benefit, nutritional support might be considered for patients with COPD and evidence of PEM.

Nursing Home Care Setting Very high prevalence rates of PEM and weight loss have been documented in nursing home settings. Because conditions associated with reduced intake are common in nursing home residents (e.g., dental, chewing, swallowing problems, depression, cognitive impairment, and dependence on others for feeding), it is likely that the proportion of patients with PEM caused by reduced intake (without inflammatory/cachexia states) is higher than in hospitalized patients. In this setting, simple interventions, such as high-calorie snacks and nutritional supplements, can improve nutritional parameters and help to stabilize weight. Although it is not clear that improvements in these intermediate measures translate to improved clinical outcomes, such interventions are likely reasonable and appropriate for many nursing home residents.

Dementia Use of tube feeds in patients with advanced dementia is generally not advised. Observational studies suggest that tube feeding such patients does not improve nutritional status, decrease pressure sores or infections, reduce aspiration problems, or improve functional status or survival. Potential adverse effects of tube feeds in these patients include increased risk of aspiration, discomfort, and complications from tube placement, potential for increased pressure ulcers from increased urine and fecal output (and possibly increased use of restraints), and diminished quality of life from decreased interaction at mealtime and loss of gustatory pleasure from food intake. Although perhaps controversial in earlier stages of dementia, the lack of proven benefits combined with considerable potential for harm argues against the use of feeding tubes in patients with severe dementia who can no longer meet their nutritional requirements through oral intake.

FUTURE DIRECTIONS

An increased understanding of the physiologic mechanisms underlying appetite, inflammatory and other systemic responses to acute stressors, illness, and aging is leading to new approaches that may help to attenuate the adverse outcomes associated with undernutrition and cachexia. Such approaches are needed. Despite aggressive nutritional support, it is often difficult to lessen the catabolic effects that occur in response to illness or injury. Also, anthropometric measures suggest that when body weight does increase with nutritional support, gains are mostly in the form of fat and water, whereas greater increases in lean body mass might lead to better functional and overall clinical outcomes. Strategies under investigation to better prevent protein catabolism and/or promote anabolism include enriched delivery of certain macronutrients (e.g., glutamine, arginine, and omega-3 fatty acids) that may have positive immunomodulating action independent of their role as nutritional substrates. Glutamine, an important intermediate for many metabolic pathways and the primary fuel source for enterocytes and other rapidly dividing cells, is probably the best studied of these nutrients. Glutamine appears to enhance stress protein and attenuate inflammatory protein responses to acute stressors, effects that might improve outcomes in ill or elderly patients. Clinical trials with TPN solutions supplemented with glutamine have found improved nitrogen retention, decreased infections, and decreased hospital days. However, a trial of an enteral formula enriched with glutamine (and arginine, omega-3 fatty acids, and antioxidants) in a heterogeneous intensive care unit population did not detect beneficial effects. The role of immunonutrition in treating undernutrition and cachexia remains to be clarified.

Aging, acute, and chronic illnesses are associated with an increased production of catabolic cytokines. It is possible that blocking the production or activity of these cytokines can improve clinical outcomes. Agents with anticytokine activity that have the potential to be useful include inhibitors of TNF-α production (pentoxifylline and thalidomide), anti-TNF-α antibodies and TNF-α receptor blockers (eternacept, infliximab, adalimumab). However, a potential adverse effect is interruption of necessary TNF roles. To date, no convincing data exist for the utility of these drugs in patients with cachexia. Other approaches to weight loss and cachexia may focus on overcoming anorexia by modulating effects of peptides and cytokines involved in appetite and energy regulation such as ghrelin, neuropeptide Y, and leptin. Although promising, such strategies to increase appetite, anabolism, and/or decrease catabolism require further study to better define their efficacy and safety in various disease states before considering for clinical use.

FURTHER READING

Akner G, Cederholm T: Treatment of protein-energy malnutrition in chronic non-malignant disorders. *Am J Clin Nutr.* 2001;74:6.

Alibhai S, Greenwood C, Payette H: An approach to the management of unintentional weight loss in elderly people. *CMAJ.* 2005;172(6):773.

Avenell A, Handoll HH: Nutritional supplementation for hip fracture aftercare in older people. *Cochrane Database Syst Rev.* 2006;18;(4):CD001880.

Barringer TA, Kirk JK, Santaniello AC, et al: Effect of a multivitamin and mineral supplement on infection and quality of life: A randomized, double-blind, placebo-controlled trial. *Ann Intern Med.* 2003;138(5):365.

Fiatarone Singh M: Exercise comes of age: rational and recommendations for a geriatric exercise program. *J Gerontol Med Sci.* 2002;57A:M262.

Finucane T, Christmas C, Travis K: Tube feeding in patients with advanced dementia. *JAMA.* 1999;282:1365.

Heyland D, Novak F, Drover JW, et al: Should immunonutrition become routine in critically ill patients? *JAMA.* 2001;286:944.

Jeejeebhoy K: Total parenteral nutrition: Potion or poison? *Am J Clin Nutr.* 2001;74:160.

Koretz RI, Avenell A, Lipman TO, et al: Does enteral nutrition affect clinical outcome? A systematic review of the randomized trials. *Am J Gastroenterol.* 2007;102:412.

Kotler D: Cachexia *Ann Intern Med.* 2000;133:622.

Milne AC, Avenell A, Potter J: Meta-Analysis: Protein and Energy Supplementation in Older People. *Ann Intern Med.* 2006;144(1):37.

Morley JE: Weight loss in the nursing home. *J Am Med Dir Assoc.* 2007;8(4):201.

Reuben DB, Hirsch SH, Zhou K, et al: The effects of megestrol acetate for elderly patients with reduced appetite after hospitalization. *J Am Geriatr Soc.* 2005;53:970.

Rigler SK, Webb MJ, Redford L, et al: Weight outcomes among antidepressant users in nursing facilities. *J Am Geriatr Soc.* 2001;49(1):49.

Sullivan DH, Bopp MM, Roberson PK: Protein-energy undernutrition and life-threatening complications among the hospitalized elderly. *J Gen Intern Med.* 2002;17(12):923.

Thomas DR: Weight loss in older adults. *Rev Endocr Metab Disord.* 2005;6(2):129.

Volkert D, Berner YN, Berry E, et al: ESPEN Guidelines on enteral nutrition: Geriatrics. *Clin Nutr.* 2006;25(2):330.

Woodcock NP, Zeigler D, Palmer MD, et al: Enteral versus parenteral nutrition: A pragmatic study. *Nutrition.* 2001;17:1.

Yeh S, Lovitt S, Schuster MW: Pharmacological Treatment of Geriatric Cachexia: Evidence and Safety in Perspective. *J Am Med Dir Assoc.* 2007;8:363.

Zaloga GP: Parenteral nutrition in adult inpatients with functioning gastrointestinal tracts: assessment of outcomes. *Lancet.* 2006;367:1101.

Disorders of Swallowing

JoAnne Robbins ■ *Jacqueline Hind* ■ *Steven Barczi*

Demographic changes related to aging necessitate that clinicians have the resources to address eating and swallowing difficulties present in older adults. The capacity to effectively and safely eat or swallow is one of the most basic human needs and also can be a great pleasure. Therefore the loss of this capacity can have far-reaching implications. Many would argue that swallowing is one of the cardinal behaviors needed to sustain life. The process of swallowing requires orchestration of a complex series of psychological, sensory, and motor behaviors that are both voluntary and involuntary. Dysphagia refers to difficulty swallowing that may include oropharyngeal or esophageal problems. More specifically, there may be difficulty in oral preparation for swallowing and/or moving material from the mouth to the esophagus and from the esophagus to the stomach.

Although age-related changes place older adults at risk for dysphagia, an older adult's swallow is not inherently impaired. *Presbyphagia* refers to characteristic changes in the mechanism of swallowing of otherwise healthy older adults. Clinicians need to be able to distinguish among *dysphagia*, presbyphagia, and other related diagnoses such as globus hystericus to avoid overdiagnosis and overtreatment of dysphagia. Older adults can be more vulnerable and, with additional stressors such as acute illness and certain medications, they can cross over from having a healthy older swallow (*presby*phagia) to experiencing *dys*phagia. This chapter reviews the normal swallowing process and presbyphagia, as a healthy aging evolution, dysphagia outcomes, multidisciplinary approaches to diagnosing and managing dysphagia, and newly recognized rehabilitation strategies for dysphagia care.

IMPACT OF DYSPHAGIA

Dysphagia prevalence depends on the specific population sampled, with community-dwelling and more independent individuals having rates near 15%. Upward of 40% of people living in institutional settings such as assisted-living and nursing homes are dysphagic. With the projected growth in the number of individuals living in nursing homes, there is a compelling need to address dysphagia not only in ambulatory and acute care settings but also in long-term care settings.

The consequences of dysphagia vary from social isolation because of the embarrassment associated with choking or coughing at mealtime to physical discomfort (e.g., food sticking in the chest) to potentially life-threatening conditions. The more ominous sequelae include dehydration, malnutrition, and both overt and silent aspiration precipitating pulmonary complications. For the purposes of this chapter, aspiration is defined as the entry of material into the airway *below* the level of the true vocal folds. Silent aspiration refers to the circumstance in which a bolus comprising saliva, food, liquid, medication, or any foreign material enters the airway below the vocal folds *without* triggering overt symptoms such as coughing or throat clearing. Both overt and silent aspiration may lead to pneumonitis, pneumonia, exacerbation of chronic lung disease, or even asphyxiation and death. To gain a better understanding of the effect, these consequences have on older adults and the impact of dysphagia interventions, research in this area has aimed to develop more meaningful outcome measures. Assessments focused on pathophysiology, function, and health services are now being conducted to create more evidence-based practices in dysphagia care.

Insofar as dysphagia is a biomechanical disorder of bolus flow, signs of flow abnormality, using videofluoroscopy, have been well detailed. These include (1) the duration, direction, and completeness of bolus flow; (2) the duration and extent (range) of anatomic structural movements; and (3) the relationship between bolus flow and structural movements as well as between physiologic and anatomic parameters such as pressure generation and muscle/fat structure. More recently, the bulbar innervated swallowing mechanisms are being studied and are providing targets specific for novel treatment paradigms aimed at improving swallowing function. Other clinical outcomes of dysphagia have become important endpoints in assessing interventions that aim to make it possible for patients to eat and drink adequately and safely. These include measures of hydration,

TABLE 41-1

Summary Descriptions of Selected Tools for Assessing Eating and Drinking Function

TOOL	COMPONENTS
American Speech Language Hearing Association Scale (1996)	1. Oral versus nonoral 2. Need for supervision 3. Need for special techniques 4. Need for extra time
Rehabilitation Institute of Chicago Clinical Evaluation of Dysphagia (Cherney et al, 1986)	1. Oral versus nonoral 2. Need for and type of supervision 3. Need for special techniques 4. Type of diet 5. Episodes of choking
Amyotrophic Lateral Sclerosis Severity Scale (Hillel et al, 1989)	1. Oral versus nonoral 2. Type of diet 3. Time to eat 4. Patient symptoms 5. Choking
Dysphagia Disability Index (Silbergleit et al, in progress)	1. Emotional reactions 2. Time to eat 3. Need for compensations 4. Need for special food and liquid 5. Coughing 6. Choking 7. Other influences on behavior
Dysphagia Severity Rating Scale (Waxman et al, 1990)	1. Findings from videofluoroscopy 2. Oral versus nonoral 3. Time to eat 4. Consistency of food and liquid 5. Need for cueing and compensation
Functional Outcome Swallowing Scale (Salassa, 1997)	1. Findings from videofluoroscopy 2. Variety of medical consequences 3. Oral versus nonoral 4. Coughing, choking, and other symptoms
Functional Outcome Assessment of Swallowing (Wisconsin Speech and Hearing Association, 1996)	1. Percent oral and nonoral 2. Food/liquid consistency 3. Need for cueing 4. Need for strategies 5. Time to eat

Source: Adapted from McHorney CA, Rosenbeck JC: Functional outcome assessment of adults with oropharyngeal dysphagia. Semin Speech Lang 19 (3):235, 1998.

nutrition, aspiration episodes, and emotional sequelae. Other measures have been developed that target what and how dysphagic adults eat and drink. Most of these scales are directly applicable to older adults (Table 41-1). Additionally, pneumonitis, overt aspiration pneumonia, and additional forms of evidence of pulmonary damage are monitored. Nonetheless, it has been difficult to attribute mortality directly to dysphagia because it is often a secondary rather than a primary diagnosis.

Dysphagia profoundly influences quality of life (QOL). Patients with swallowing difficulties, especially those who relinquish oral eating, manifest significant changes in psychosocial status, functional status, and emotional well-being. Eating and drinking are social events that relate to friendship, acceptance, entertainment, and communication. As such, major adjustments in the process of feeding

and eating can lead to distressing responses such as shame, anxiety, depression, and isolation. Only recently have practical dysphagia-specific, comprehensive, QOL measures been developed. By monitoring functional outcomes in clinical practice, physicians and other health care providers may be able to better assess and adjust their treatment of dysphagia.

SWALLOWING PROCESS

Swallowing is an orchestrated activity that balances the competing behaviors of ingestion, speaking, and breathing. Approximately 30 oral and pharyngeal muscle pairs and multiple nerves must perform precisely on cue so that the upper aerodigestive tract is reconfigured from a mechanism that channels air for breathing and speaking (Figure 41-1) to a food-propelling mechanism that accomplishes ingestion (Figure 41-2). The four morphologic regions serving these purposes are the oral cavity, pharynx, larynx, and esophagus. Of these, the first three collectively are termed the upper aerodigestive tract because they also serve the airway-dependent functions of respiration and speech production. In humans, with our upright posture, it is the adjacent position of the anatomy for breathing to the anatomy for food passage that facilitates gravitational influences on food to flow into an unprotected airway. Such anatomy and physiology require precision to satisfy the delicate balance between swallowing physiology and breathing—each a life-sustaining

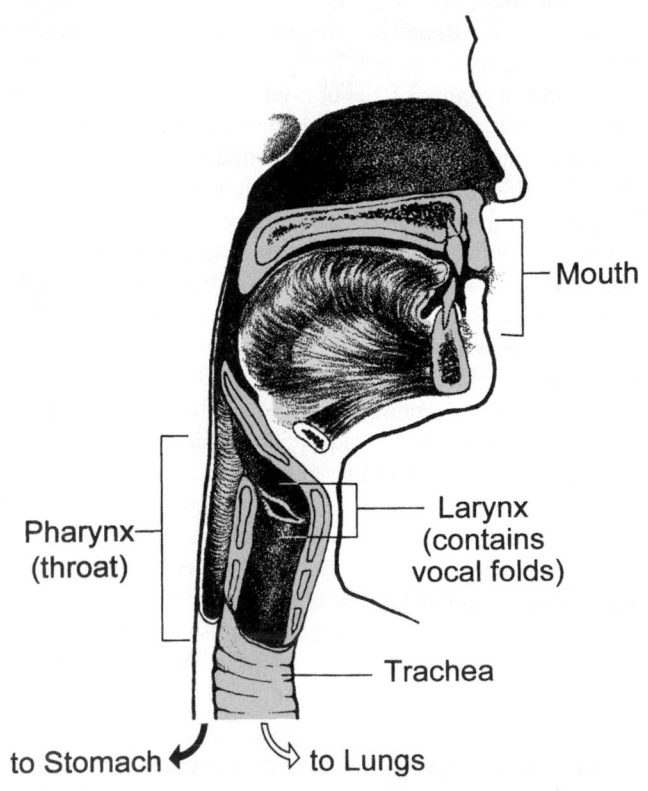

FIGURE 41-1. Aerodigestive tract channeling air for breathing from the nose and mouth through the open larynx into the lungs and back up and out. For speaking, air is channeled similarly, but the vocal folds vibrate to produce voice. *(Adapted with permission from Weihofen D et al. Shape. The Easy to Swallow, Easy to Chew Cookbook. New York, New York: John Wiley and Sons; 2002.)*

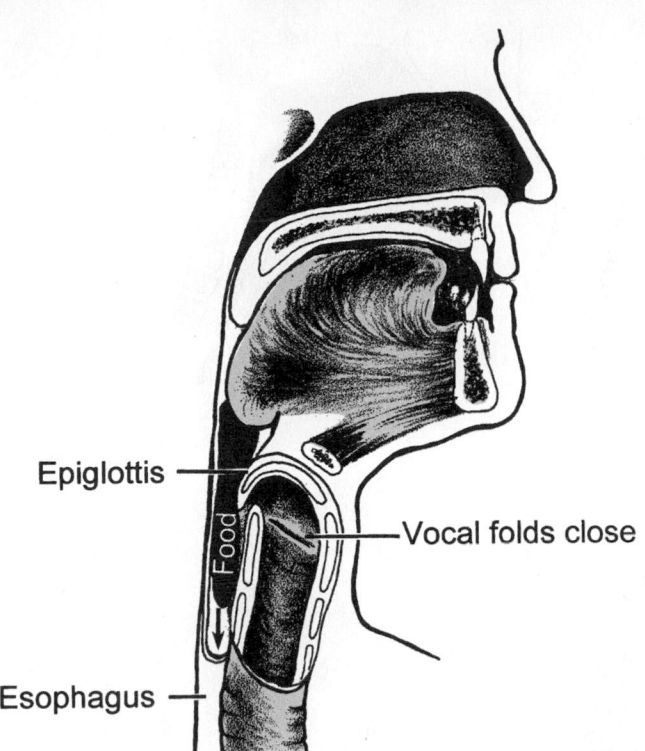

FIGURE 41-2. Aerodigestive tract reconfigured from an air channel to a food-propelling mechanism during swallowing. The tongue propels food into the throat; the epiglottis covers the larynx, which is the airway entrance; and the vocal folds close to protect the trachea and lungs from foreign material. *(Adapted with permission from Weihofen D et al. The Easy to Swallow, Easy to Chew Cookbook. New York, New York: John Wiley and Sons; 2002.)*

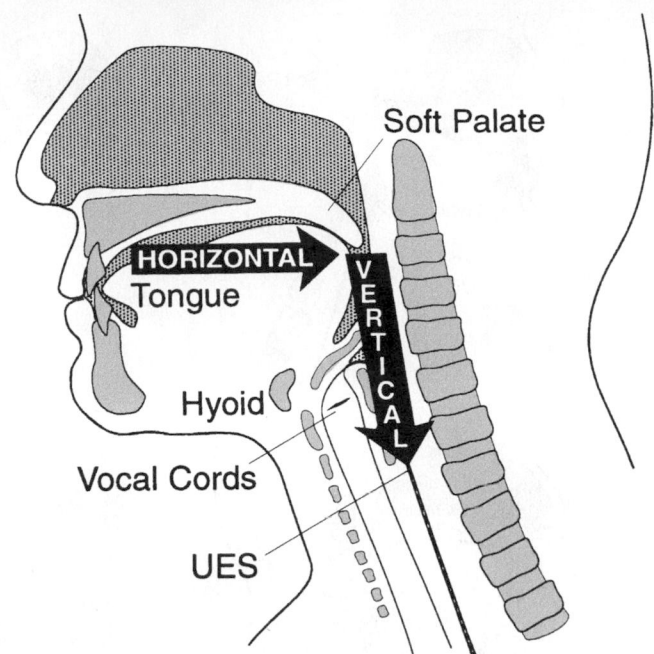

FIGURE 41-3. The oropharyngeal swallowing mechanism can be divided into two basic structural subsystems, horizontal and vertical, that mirror the direction of bolus flow. UES, upper esophageal sphincter. *(Adapted with permission from Robbins JA. Normal swallowing and aging. Semin Neurol. 1996; 16(4):309.)*

function that must occur during cessation of its counterpart. Thus, a basic understanding of the relationship between the anatomic components and the functional interaction of this mechanism is essential to an understanding of normal swallowing and the effects of age and age-related diseases on it.

Normal Swallowing

Swallowing is an integrated neuromuscular process consisting of a combination of volitional and relatively automatic movements. Although normal swallowing is usually conceptualized as a continuous sequence of events, the process of deglutition has been conveniently described as occurring in two, three, or four phases or stages. Moreover, the system engaged in swallowing can be divided into two basic structural subsystems, horizontal and vertical (Figure 41-3), that mirror the direction of bolus flow and the potential for gravitational influence on it.

Horizontal Subsystem

The oral cavity components comprise the horizontal subsystem. As such, this subsystem is involved in the initial, largely volitional, processing and transport phases of swallowing—the swallow preparatory phase and the oral transport phase. The swallow preparatory phase is characterized by food acceptance, containment, and manipulation. The lips and the buccal musculature act in complex patterns, varying the size and shape of the oral opening to allow acceptance and/or containment of food within the oral cavity. The process of

chemically changing the material requires that numerous labial and lingual glands secrete into the oral cavity an enzyme-rich fluid that maintains and lubricates the mucosa and is directly incorporated into the food. This textural manipulation of food and the mechanical formation of a bolus are accomplished largely by the tongue. The tongue positions the bolus between the teeth and moves in a complex three-dimensional chewing pattern if the bolus requires mastication. The moistening of the food in the oral cavity is essential for normal bolus transit and/or flow and clearance, particularly because gravity provides no assistance until the vertical phases of swallowing.

The oral transport phase comprises movement of the cohesive bolus (masticated if necessary) posteriorly (and horizontally when the subject is in a normal upright seated posture) to the inlet of the superior aspect of the vertical subsystem, the pharynx (Figure 41-4). The intrinsic tongue muscles change the shape of the tongue, forming grooves along its body and anterior and lateral seals to facilitate containment. The extrinsic tongue muscles change the position of the tongue within the oral cavity and assist in changing its shape (Figure 41-4A), and then progressively arching the tongue posteriorly to transport the bolus to the vertical subsystem (Figures 41-4B and C).

Vertical Subsystem

The pharyngeal and laryngeal components, in conjunction with the tongue dorsum, comprise the superior aspect of the vertical subsystem, where gravity begins to assist in the transport of the bolus. The anatomic juxtaposition of the entrance to the airway (laryngeal vestibule) and the pharyngeal aspect of the upper digestive tract demand biomechanical precision to ensure simultaneous airway

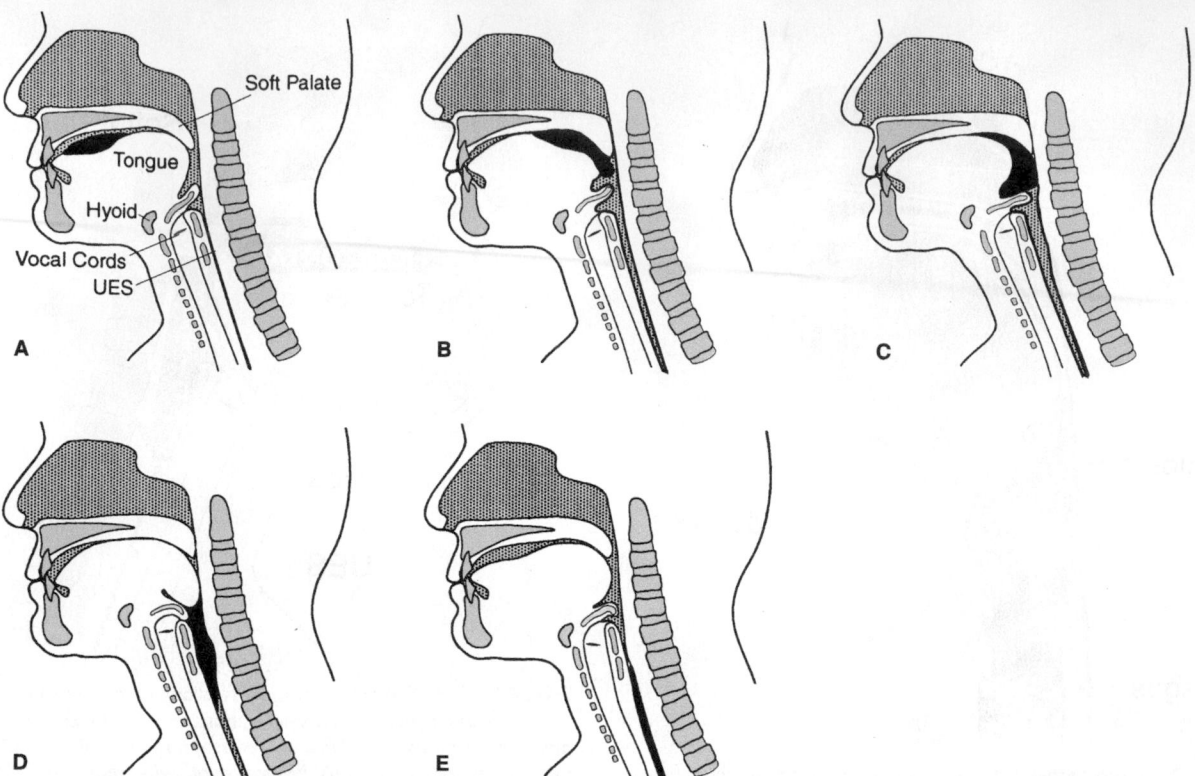

FIGURE 41-4. Lateral view of bolus propulsion during swallowing. (A) Voluntary initiation of the swallow by tongue "loading." (B) Bolus propulsion by tongue dorsum and UES opening anticipating bolus arrival. (C) Bolus entry into pharynx associated with epiglottal downward tilt, hyolaryngeal excursion, and UES opening. (D) Linguapharyngeal contact facilitating bolus passage through the pharynx and (E) UES closing and completion of oropharyngeal swallowing; then the entire bolus is in the esophagus. *(Adapted from Robbins JA: Normal swallowing and aging. Semin Neurol. 16(4):309–317, Dec., 1996.)*

protection and bolus transfer or propulsion through the pharynx. To this end, the pharyngeal transport phase is characterized by a sequence of rapid, highly coordinated neuromuscular events that cause pressure changes critical to bolus transport or transit in a safe, timely, efficient manner.

Linguapalatal contact sequentially moves the bolus against the posterior pharyngeal wall, contributing to the positive pressures imparted to the bolus and propelling it downward. Simultaneously, the pharyngeal constrictors begin to contract in a descending sequence, first elevating and widening the entire pharynx to engulf the bolus (Figure 41-4D and E), and clean up residue after swallowing is completed. A descending peristaltic wave then cleanses the pharynx of residue. Tight closure of the velopharynx during the pharyngeal transport phase provides a seal at the superior aspect of the vertical system, preventing nasal leakage of the bolus and contributing to the generation of high positive pressures, which are applied to the bolus.

Several mechanisms ensure the redundancy by which airway protection is accomplished. Three levels of sphincteric closure include (1) the aryepiglottic folds, (2) the false vocal folds, and (3) the true vocal folds, with closure of the true vocal folds (the lowest of the three sphincters) providing "the last line of defense" to prevent aspiration of invasive material. The hyolaryngeal complex is lifted upward and forward by the combined contraction of the suprahyoid muscles, thyrohyoid muscles, and pharyngeal elevators. This hyolaryngeal elevation and anterior movement, coupled with retraction of the tongue base, covers the laryngeal vestibule and diverts the bolus laterally around the airway. Timely relaxation and opening of the upper esophageal sphincter (UES) permits continuous vertical passage of the bolus into the esophagus. The UES functions as a mechanical valve. For it to open normally, four criteria must be met: (1) relaxation of muscle tone, (2) compliant tissue, (3) traction force provided by sufficient hyolaryngeal excursion, and (4) pulsion force imparted by the bolus. In normal swallowing, UES relaxation and opening occur prior to bolus arrival at the hypopharynx.

Neurophysiology of Oropharyngeal Swallowing

Historically, swallowing was largely viewed as a sequence of pharyngeal and esophageal events and was defined as reflexive. The findings from quantitative temporospatial studies on normal swallowing conducted in the last two decades, and current knowledge of the underlying neural substrates, have provided new insights into oropharyngeal swallowing, showing that it is a patterned response rather than a traditional reflex.

Sensorimotor control of swallowing requires the coordinated activity to be distributed across both the cranial and spinal nerve systems, including the peripheral nerves, their central nuclei, and their neural centers. More specifically, the neural control of swallowing involves five major components: (1) afferent sensory fibers contained in cranial nerves, (2) cerebral and midbrain fibers that synapse with the brainstem swallowing centers, (3) paired swallowing centers in

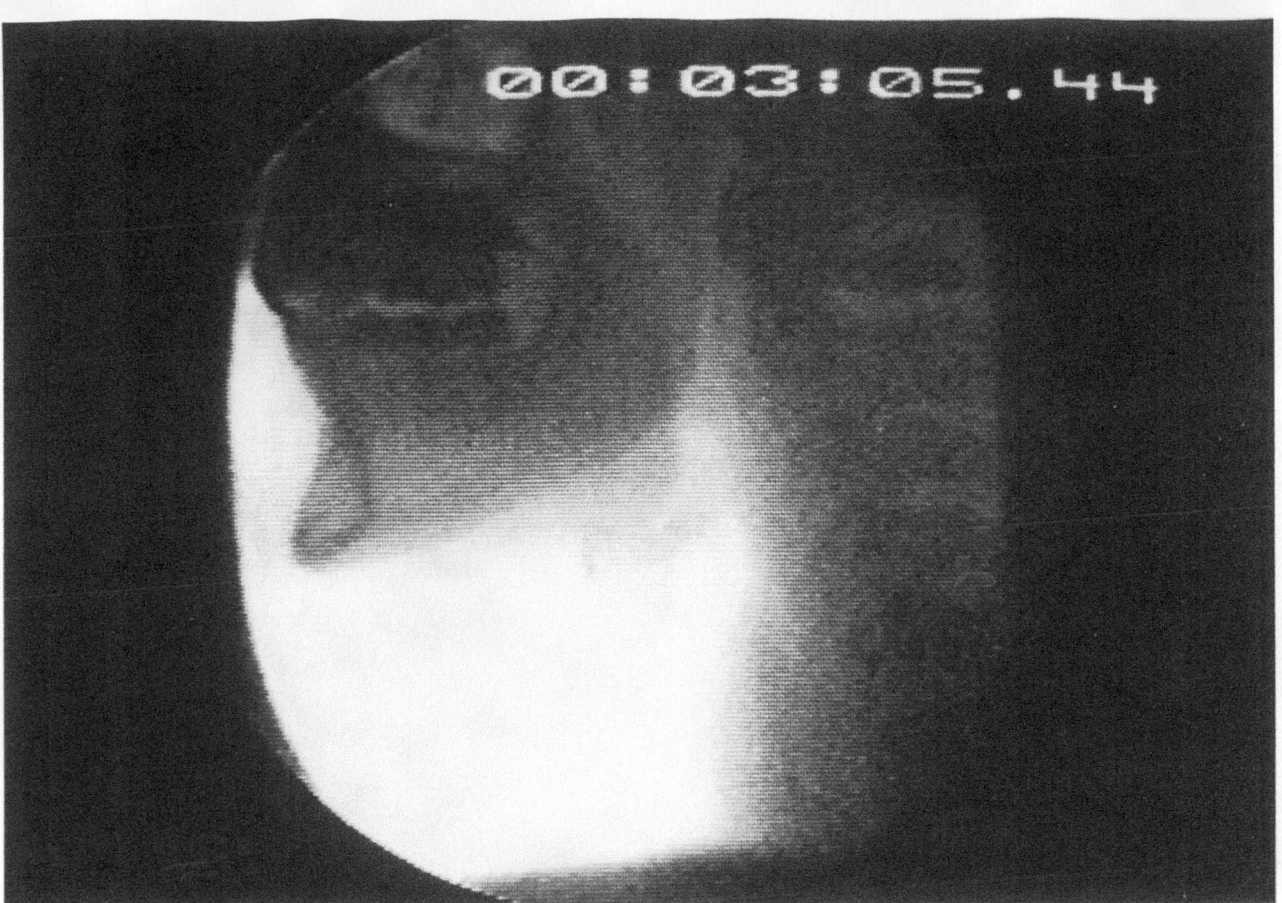

FIGURE 41-5. Healthy young swallowing documented with videofluoroscopy. (A) Bolus in oral cavity, ready to be swallowed. (B) Bolus appears as a "column" of material swiftly moving through the pharynx. (C) Oropharynx cleared of material when the swallow is completed. *(Adapted with permission from Robbins JA. Normal swallowing and aging. Semin Neurol. 1996; 16(4):309.)*

the brainstem, (4) efferent motor fibers contained in cranial nerves and the ansa cervicalis, and (5) muscle and end organs. Indeed, this neural network spans all levels of the neuraxis from the cerebrum superiorly to the brainstem and spinal nerves inferiorly and muscles and end organs at the periphery. This relatively diffuse network is designed to integrate and sequence both the volitional and automatic actions of swallowing.

Healthy persons depend on a highly automated neuromuscular sensorimotor process that intricately coordinates the activities of chewing, swallowing, and airway protection. To accomplish a normal swallow, which occurs in 2 seconds or less, the muscles of chewing interact with 26 pairs of striated pharyngeal and laryngeal muscles. The muscles involved in chewing include the masseters, temporalis, and pterygoids (innervated by cranial nerve V); the lip and buccal musculature, the orbicularis oris, and the buccinator (innervated by cranial nerve VII); and the intrinsic and extrinsic lingual muscles (innervated by cranial nerve XII). Optimal structural integrity and precise neural mediation result in continuous, rapid bolus flow from the mouth to the esophagus (Figure 41-5A, B and C) that accommodates variations in bolus size, texture, and temperature and the individual's intent to swallow, chew, or just hold the bolus in the mouth.

Research on swallowing neurophysiology over the past decade has begun to reveal complex underlying neural substrates that may pro-

vide an understanding of how willful control during the early stage of swallowing allows access to the patterned response. Behavioral and sensory interventions attempting to modify a response certainly have more treatment potential than if they are aimed at a reflex. Accessing mechanisms of neural plasticity, defined as the ability of the brain to change, is becoming a focus to elicit neuroprotection relative to aging effects or recovery from dysphagia following injury such as stroke.

SENESCENT SWALLOWING

Traditional thinking suggests that the causes of dysphagia are always disease-related, with direct or indirect damage to effector end-organ systems of swallowing. Research during the past decade has indicated that swallowing changes occur even with healthy aging. This work, with a focus primarily on the anatomy and physiology of the oropharyngeal swallowing mechanism, describes a progression of change that may put the older population at increased risk for dysphagia. This research is particularly relevant when an older healthy adult, whose functional reserve is naturally diminished, is faced with increased stressors such as central nervous system (CNS)-altering medications, mechanical perturbations (e.g., a nasogastric [NG] tube or a tracheostomy), or chronic medical conditions

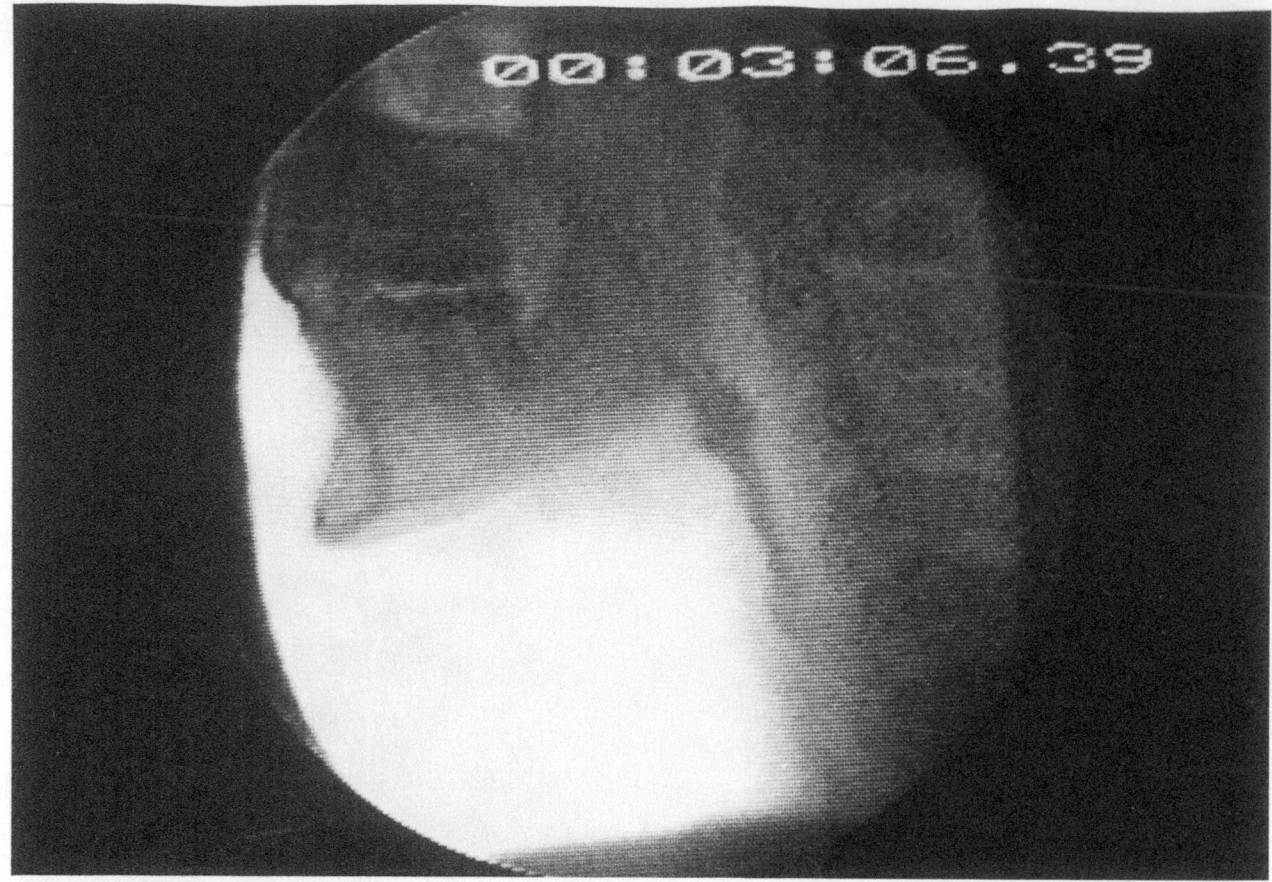

B

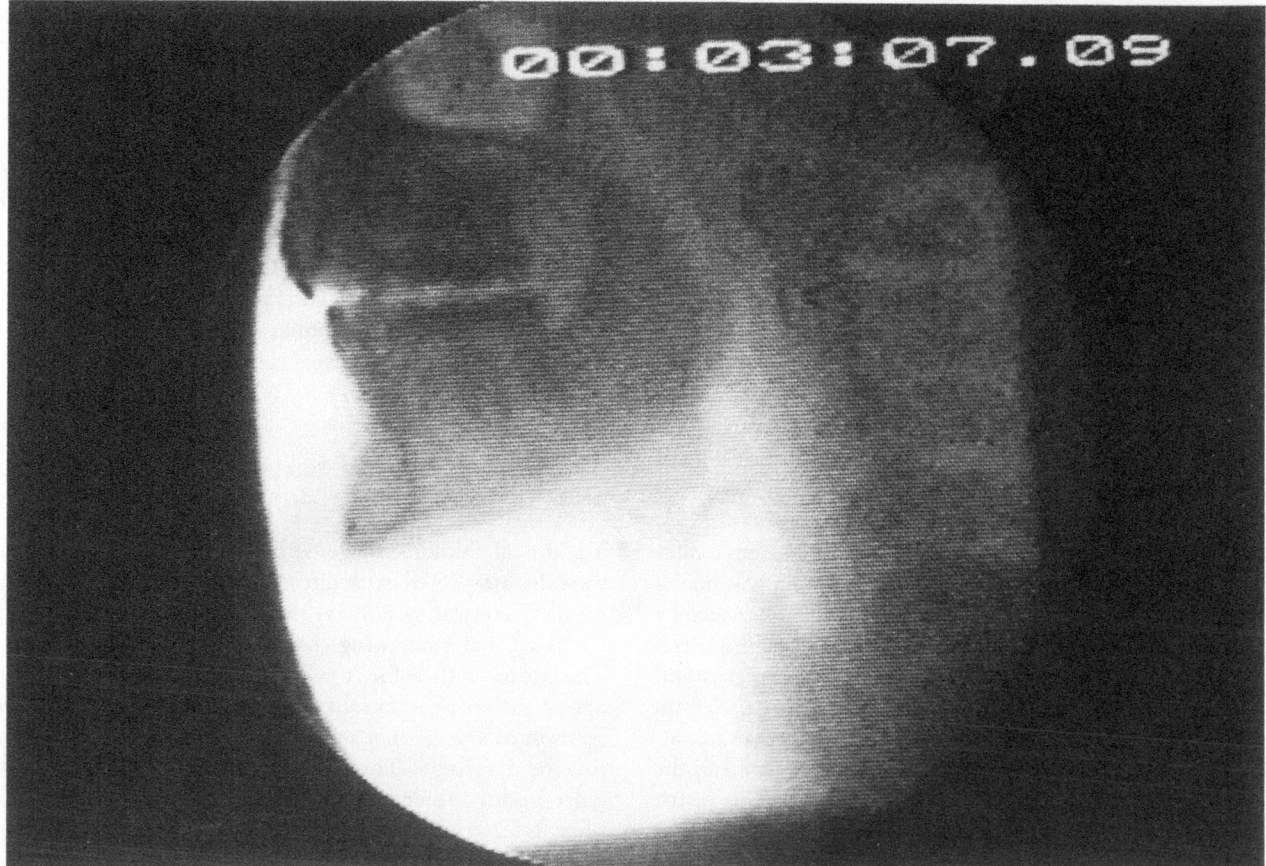

C

FIGURE 41-5. *(Continued)*

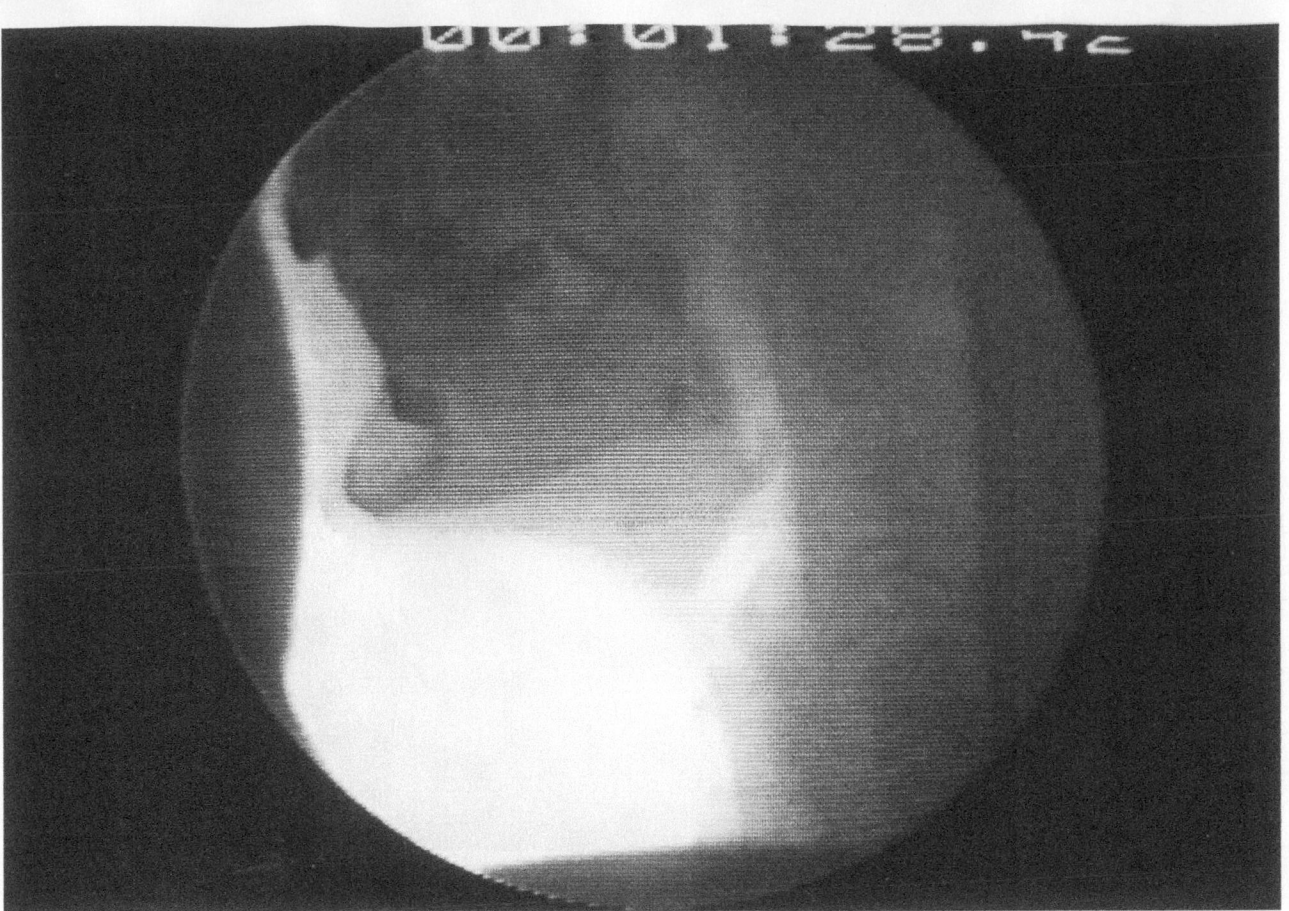

FIGURE 41-6. Healthy old swallowing documented with videofluoroscopy. (A) Bolus in mouth ready for swallowing. (B) Bolus pooled in vallecula and pyriform sinus during delayed onset of pharyngeal response. (C) Bolus cleared of material when the swallow is completed. *(Adapted with permission from Robbins JA. Normal swallowing and aging. Semin Neurol. 1996; 16(4):309.)*

(e.g., frailty) that might not elicit dysphagia in a less vulnerable individual. Translation of this work into clinical practice will provide safeguards against the overdiagnosis and overtreatment of dysphagia in the elderly population.

Age-Associated Changes in Swallowing

A major characteristic of older healthy swallowing is that it occurs more slowly. In people older than 65 years, the initiation of laryngeal and pharyngeal events, including laryngeal vestibule closure, maximal hyolaryngeal excursion, and upper UES opening, takes significantly longer than in adults younger than 45 years. Although the specific neural underpinning has not been confirmed, oral events may become uncoupled from the pharyngeal response. Thus, in older healthy adults, the bolus may remain adjacent to an open airway by pooling or pocketing in the pharyngeal recesses longer than in younger adults (Figure 41-6).

Aspiration and airway penetration are believed to be the most significant adverse clinical outcomes of misdirected bolus flow, as reflected in the high rates of pneumonia with increasing age and disease. However, airway invasion in healthy adults is commonly believed to be largely absent. The use of an eight-point scale (Table 41-2) that discretely quantifies the occurrence, the depth, and the person's reaction to airway penetration or aspiration found no significant difference between young (21- to 32-year-olds) and old

(63- to 84-year-olds) age groups in scale scores on three repeat swallows. However, when a greater number of swallows were performed, aspiration did occur in the older group, indicating fatigue or change in endurance as a possible factor that may relate in a very practical sense to eating meals.

Using simultaneous videofluoroscopy and manometry (manofluoroscopy) and a tube through the nasopharynx similar in size to a "garden variety" NG tube, a significant interaction was found for tube by age. That is, liquid penetrated the airway significantly more frequently when the tube was in place only in the *oldest* group of men and women (older than 70 years). Thus, it appears that under demanding conditions (e.g., endurance = demanding, or NG tube placement), older individuals are less able to compensate and are more at risk for aspiration. Findings such as these characterize presbyphagia or "old swallowing" which is *not* abnormal swallowing in the elderly population.

Age-related changes in the generation of lingual pressure also define presbyphagia. Healthy older individuals have reduced isometric tongue pressures compared with younger individuals. In contrast, the generation of maximal lingual pressure during swallowing (which requires submaximal pressures) remains "young" in magnitude but slows in the time necessary to achieve those "young" swallowing pressures. The relationship between maximum isometric pressure and peak swallowing pressures can be considered an indication of the functional reserve available for swallowing. As people get older,

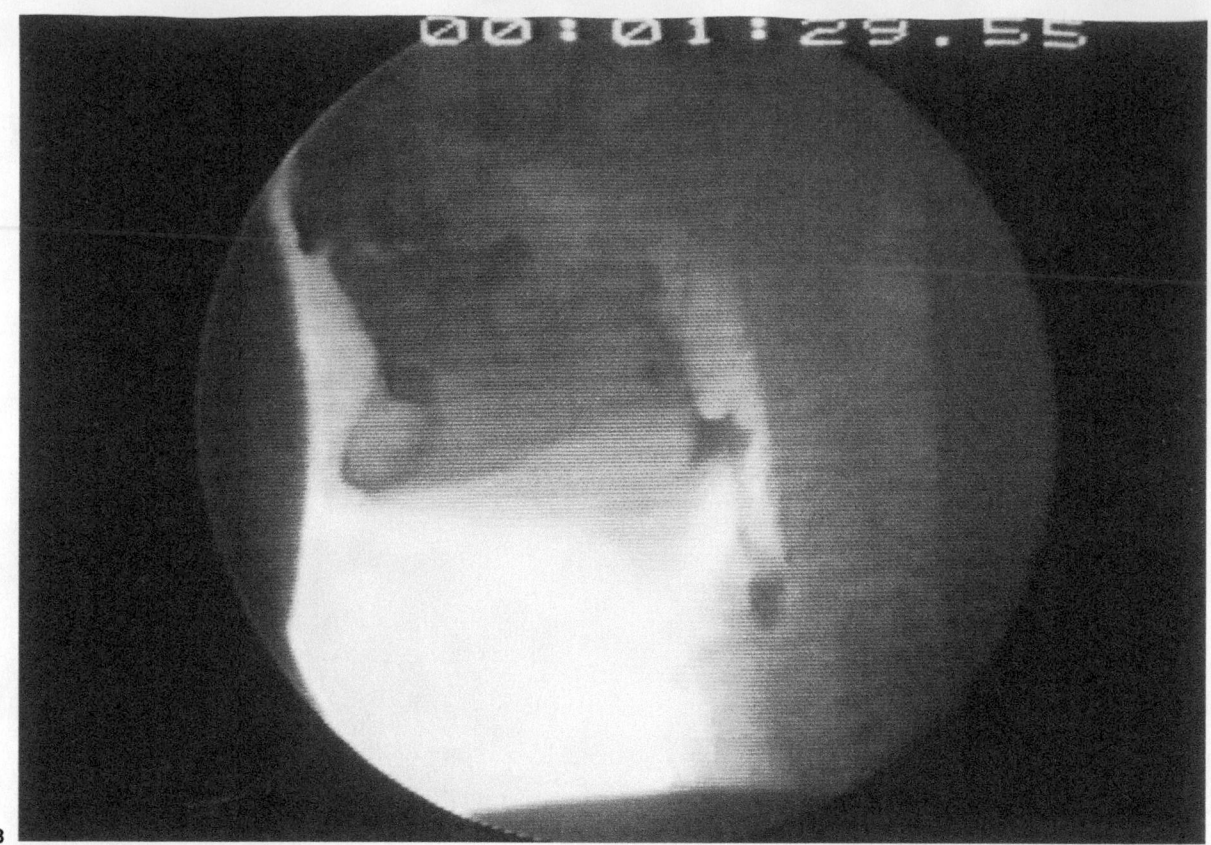

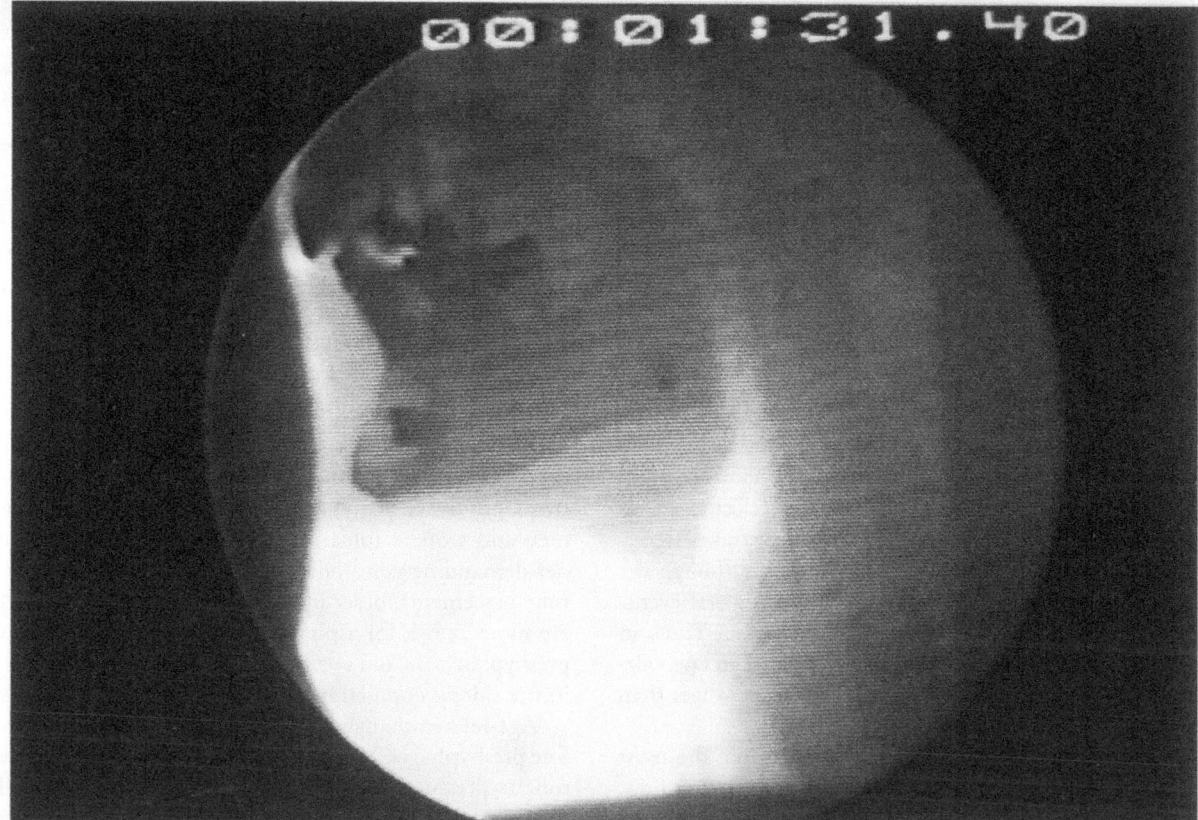

FIGURE 41-6. *(Continued)*

TABLE 41-2

Multidimensional Depth of Airway Invasion and Residue, Single-digit Scoring System for the Penetration-Aspiration Scale

CATEGORY	SCORE	DESCRIPTION
No penetration or aspiration	1	Contrast does not enter the airway
P E N E T R A T I O N A S P I R A T I O N	2	Contrast enters the airway, remains above vocal folds, no residue
	3	Contrast remains above vocal folds, visible residue remains
	4	Contrast contacts vocal folds, no residue
	5	Contrast contacts vocal folds, visible residue remains
	6	Contrast passes glottis, no subglottic residue visible
	7	Contrast passes glottis, visible subglottic residue despite patient's response
	8	Contrast passes glottis, visible subglottic residue, absent patient response

Rosenbek JC, Robbins JA, Roecker EB, Coyle JC, Woody GL: A penetration aspiration scale. Dysphagia, 11: 93–98, 1996.
Robbins JA, Coyle JC, Roecker EB, Rosenbek JC, Woody GL: Differentiation of normal and abnormal airway protection during swallowing using the penetration aspiration scale. Dysphagia, 14(4):228–232, 1999.

slower swallowing may allow time to recruit the necessary number of motor units required for pressures critical for adequate bolus propulsion through the oropharynx. However, fluids of low viscosity (e.g., water, tea), by their composition, are likely to move more quickly than the physiology to handle them safely and thus put older people at increased risk for aspiration.

Neurophysiological Correlates of Senescent Swallowing

Neuroimaging studies using cranial magnetic resonance imaging (MRI) in normal adults have shown a relationship between slower swallowing and an increase in the number and severity of periventricular white-matter hyperintensities (PVHs) in the brain, supporting the concept that voluntary control of swallowing is mediated by corticobulbar pathways traveling within the periventricular white matter. The occurrence and degree of PVHs increase with age and may explain, at least in part, the relatively asymptomatic decline in oropharyngeal motor performance observed in older people. Cerebral atrophy, a common finding in asymptomatic older individuals, may be another contributing factor to presbyphagia.

Changes in the periphery also occur with age and may be a function of changes in various sensory mechanisms or caused by muscle atrophy. Similar to the age-related loss of limb skeletal muscle, are the changes with age in fiber density, muscle tension, muscle strength, and muscle contraction in facial, masticatory, and lingual musculature. Rather than reflecting CNS deterioration, slowed swallowing

that remains coordinated and effective, as found in most healthy old people, may represent a compensatory strategy for achieving pressure-generation values that may be critical to successful bolus propulsion.

DIFFERENTIAL CONSIDERATIONS FOR DYSPHAGIA AND ASPIRATION

Etiologies

Older adults are at increased risk for developing dysphagia because of a number of age-associated phenomena. Several factors contribute to and several comorbid processes also increase the chances that older adults will suffer the adverse consequences of dysphagia—dehydration, malnutrition, and aspiration pneumonia. By targeting high-risk groups and intervening with acceptable compensatory and rehabilitative approaches, it is hoped that the ultimate burden of dysphagia on the geriatric population will decline.

A decreased physiologic reserve can combine with a number of age-related, disease-related, or iatrogenic changes to transform an at-risk individual into an older adult with dysphagia. The concept of homeostenosis, or decreased physiologic reserve, is being recognized as a crucial covariable with dysphagia. Frailty or sarcopenia may be outward manifestations of this poor reserve. Several anatomic or pathologic perturbations occurring throughout the orobuccal cavity, the laryngopharyngeal region, and the esophagus must also be acknowledged as important cofactors in the onset of dysphagia.

Age-Related Conditions

Age-related changes throughout the upper aerodigestive tract can influence swallowing integrity. Oral risks are also discussed in Chapter 42. During the oral phase, the food bolus may be inadequately prepared because of poor or absent dentition, periodontal disease, ill-fitting dentures, or inappropriate salivation caused by xerostomia. Musculoskeletal factors such as weakness of the muscles of mastication, arthritis of the temporomandibular joint or larynx, osteoporosis of the jaw, or changes in tongue strength and coordination of the oropharyngeal events can deter efficient swallowing. Sensory input for taste, temperature, and tactile sensation changes in many older adults. This disruption of sensory-cortical-motor feedback loops may interfere with proper bolus formation and timely response of the swallowing motoric sequence and detract from the pleasure of eating. Controversy exists regarding the predictive value of an absent gag reflex for aspiration, although many clinicians still use this criterion to screen for altered pharyngeal sensation. Davies and colleagues studied the gag reflex in 140 healthy young (mean: 27 years) and old people (mean: 76 years) and reported that 43% of the older group and 27% of the younger group had an absent gag while all but one had intact pharyngeal sensation.

Material can penetrate into the upper airway in normal individuals if the bolus is not properly prepared, if the timing of the swallow is delayed, or if the intake is too rapid. Important risk factors for aspiration include altered level of attention during feeding (e.g., delirium), altered sensory discrimination in the oropharynx, feeding problems, mechanical ventilation, and feeding tube placement. In the latter circumstance, the rate of tube feeding, the position of the patient,

TABLE 41-3

Neurological Disorders Causing Dysphagia

Stroke

Head trauma

Parkinsonism and other movement and neurodegenerative disorders

Progressive supranuclear palsy
  Olivopontocerebellar atrophy
  Huntington's disease
  Wilson's disease

Torticollis
  Tardive dyskinesia

Alzheimer's disease and other dementias

Motor neuron disease (amyotrophic lateral sclerosis)

Guillain-Barré syndrome and other polyneuropathies

Neoplasms and other structural disorders
  Primary brain tumors
  Intrinsic and extrinsic brainstem tumors
  Base of skull tumors
  Syringobulbia
  Arnold–Chiari malformation
  Neoplastic meningitis

Multiple sclerosis

Postpolio myelitis syndrome

Infectious disorders
  Chronic infectious meningitis
  Syphilis and Lyme disease
  Diphtheria
  Botulism
  Viral encephalitis, including rabies

Myasthenia gravis

Myopathy
  Polymyositis, dermatomyositis, inclusion body myositis, and sarcoidosis
  Myotonic and oculopharyngeal muscular dystrophy
  Hyper- and hypothyroidism
  Cushing's syndrome

Iatrogenic conditions
  Medication side effects
  Postsurgical neurogenic dysphagia
    Neck surgery
    Posterior fossa surgery
    Irradiation of the head and neck

TABLE 41-4

Warning Signs Associated With Dysphagia and Aspiration Risk

Decreased alertness or cognitive dysfunction
  Stupor, coma, heavy sedation, delirium, "sundowning," dementia, agitation
  Playing with food, inappropriate size of bites, talking or emotional lability during attempts to swallow

Changes in approach to food
  Avoidance of eating in company
  Increase in amount of food remaining on plate
  Special physical preparation of food or avoidance of foods of specific consistency
  Prolonged mealtime, intermittent cessation of intake, frequent "wash downs"
  Compensatory measures (head and neck movements)
  Laborious chewing, repetitive swallowing
  Coughing and choking on swallowing, increased need to clear throat

Manifestations of impaired oropharyngeal functions
  Dysarthria
  Wet, hoarse voice and other voice changes
  Dysfunction of focal musculature (facial asymmetries, abnormal reflexes or dystonia, dyskinesias or fasciculations)
  Drooling or oral spillage, pooling and pocketing of food
  Frequent throat clearing

Patient complaints or observations of
  Difficulty initiating a swallow
  Sensation of obstruction of bolus in the throat or chest
  Regurgitation of food or acid
  Inability to handle secretions
  Unexplained weight loss
  Impaired breathing during meals or immediately after eating
  Pain on swallowing
  Leakage of food or saliva from a tracheostomy site

altered intestinal transit times, and the ability of the patient to protect their airway all influence the occurrence of reflux and aspiration and are discussed in detail in Chapter 40. Gastroesophageal reflux caused by lower esophageal sphincter (LES) incompetence as well as intraesophageal reflux defined as material moving proximally within the esophagus prior to crossing the LES also predispose individuals to micro- or macroaspiration.

Age-Related Disease

Neurological and neuromuscular disorders are one of the principal risks for dysphagia (Table 41-3). Neurologic diseases rise in prevalence in older cohorts of the population. Stroke, brain injury, Alzheimer's disease, and other dementia syndromes, and parkinsonism all place older adults at increased risk for dysphagia with its incipient consequences.

Because cognitive function and/or communication may be impaired, it is important for the practitioner to note the warning signs associated with dysphagia and a risk of aspiration (Table 41-4). Between 50% and 75% of patients who have had a recent acute stroke develop eating and swallowing problems, with ensuing complications of aspiration developing in 50%, malnutrition in 45%, and pneumonia in 35%. Other delayed adverse consequences have also been reported, with up to 15% of patients who have suffered a cerebrovascular accident (CVA) developing pneumonia within 1 year of the acute insult. Brainstem or bilateral hemispheric strokes predictably produce dysphagia, but unilateral lesions also can contribute to dysphagia. Daniels and colleagues identified six clinical features associated with an increased risk for aspiration poststroke. These included (1) an abnormal volitional cough, (2) an abnormal gag reflex, (3) dysarthria, (4) dysphonia, (5) a cough following a trial swallow, and (6) a voice change following a trial swallow. The presence of any two of these findings had a sensitivity of 92% and a specificity of 67% in predicting that there would be penetration and aspiration of material as evidenced with videofluoroscopy.

A host of common problems involving the head and neck can directly damage the effector muscles of swallowing and increase the risk for dysphagia. Head and neck injury, carcinoma, complex infections, thyroid conditions, and diabetes are associated with age-related dysphagia. Although vertebral osteophytes are common, these bony growths alone rarely cause dysphagia. Dysphagia more commonly results from the presence of osteophytes in conjunction with neuromuscular weakness or discoordination. This can be caused by combinations of several underlying conditions or comorbidities such as diabetes, chronic obstructive pulmonary disease, congestive heart failure, renal failure, an immunocompromised status, and/or cachexia for which an individual no longer can draw an adequate reserve to effectively compensate.

Sometimes dysphagia can be a direct consequence of a treatment provided for another disease process. Health care interventions can result in drug-induced delirium, protracted hospital stays, and ultimately malnutrition. Indwelling NG tubes, airway intubation, and medication effects may all predispose a frail older adult with borderline airway protection to develop frank aspiration. Understanding the iatrogenic causes of dysphagia can alter medical practice and may reduce its incidence and complications.

Older adults are much more likely to be taking medications for multiple medical conditions. These medications can influence salivary flow, intestinal peristalsis, cognition, or psychomotor status, thereby interfering with normal oropharyngoesophageal function or altering airway protection. More than 2000 drugs can cause xerostomia or reduced salivary flow via anticholinergic mechanisms. The list is extensive and can include common antidepressants, antihistamines, antipsychotics, and antihypertensive agents. Likewise, a number of delirium-promoting therapies exist and similarly produce adverse consequences through either anticholinergic or other central mind-altering effects. Certain agents can directly relax the LES and increase acid reflux and esophageal problems. Finally several psychotropic drugs can produce delayed neuromuscular responses or extrapyramidal effects, thereby influencing the tongue and bulbar musculature. Table 41-5 provides a partial list of these agents and how they can contribute to dysphagia.

An altered level of attention and cognition may also produce special concerns with regard to safe eating and swallowing. As described elsewhere in this book, delirium is frequently underrecognized and undertreated in both hospital and institutional settings. In general, testing an inattentive adult for dysphagia results in the poorest evaluation. If swallowing is assessed during one of these episodes, aspiration is likely to occur. If a staff member at a hospital or nursing home feeds a patient during one of these intervals, the outcome may be disastrous.

Several different treatments can either directly or indirectly damage swallowing effector organs as described previously. Head and neck cancer surgeries, some spinal cord surgeries, thyroid surgeries, and any intervention that can jeopardize the recurrent laryngeal nerve may result in dysphagia. A number of chemotherapy and radiotherapy regimes can cause oropharyngeal injury. The prospective outcome of dysphagia should be incorporated into the risk–benefit discussions of these procedures.

Symptoms

Medical history plays a critical role in establishing a diagnosis of dysphagia (Table 41-6). A detailed history can elucidate the proper diagnosis in some dysphagic adults and is an important first step in

TABLE 41-5

Mechanisms by Which Common Medications Contribute to Dysphagia

Xerostomia

Anticholinergic effects
　Tricyclic antidepressants
　Antipsychotic agents
　Antihistamine drugs
　Antispasmodic drugs
　Antiparkinsonism drugs
　Antimetic drugs
Other mechanisms
　Antihypertensives (e.g., diuretics, calcium channel-blockers)

Reduction in esophageal and/or laryngeal peristalsis

Antihypertensive drugs (e.g., dihydropyridine calcium channel-blockers)
Antianginal drugs (e.g., nitrates)

Delayed neuromuscular responses

Drugs that promote delirium (e.g., anticholinergic agents, opiates, benzodiazepines)
Drugs that have extrapyramidal side effects (e.g., antipsychotic drugs)

Esophageal injury and/or inflammation

Drugs that relax the lower esophageal sphincter (e.g., calcium channel-blockers, nitrates)
Large pills that have incomplete esophageal transit

TABLE 41-6

Historical Data Used for Clinical Diagnosis of Dysphagia

Site or timing of impairment
　Oral (problems with chewing, bolus gathering, initiation of swallow)
　Pharyngeal (problem immediately on swallowing, choking after a long delay, suggestive of passage of residue from the pharynx into the larynx)
　Esophageal (seconds after swallow, behind chest bone)

Onset, frequency, and progression
　Duration, sudden onset related to a specific event (stroke, pill impaction, etc.), or gradual
　Frequency (constant, intermittent)
　Progression and severity (including more and more foods and impairing nutrition and hydration?)

Aggravating factors and compensatory mechanisms
　Food consistency (solids and/or liquids)
　Temperature
　Usefulness of sucking, turning, and tilting of head, and so on
　Intermittent, constant, or fatiguing symptoms

Associated symptoms
　Change in speech or voice
　Weakness; lack of control of musculature, particularly of the head and neck
　Choking or coughing
　Repetitive swallows or increased need to clear the throat
　Regurgitation (pharyngeal and nasal, or esophageal and gastric; immediately on swallow, or long delay, undigested food, putrefied or secretions?)
　Fullness/tightness in the throat (globus sensation)
　Pain, localized or radiating
　Odynophagia (pain on passage of bolus)

Ancillary symptoms and evidence of complications
　Loss of weight or loss of energy (including from dehydration)
　Change in appetite; attitude toward food, toward eating in company; preparation of foods
　Respiratory problems (cough, increased sputum production, shortness of breath, pneumonias and other respiratory infections)
　Sleep disturbances (secondary to secretion management or regurgitation)
　Changes in salivation (water brash or dry mouth)

the evaluation process. Recognizing the classic complaints associated with dysphagia and differentiating them from symptoms of common age-related diseases can be challenging. Nevertheless, a careful history may avert increased testing and potential iatrogenic complications in frail older patients. Dysphagia may also present in a more subtle fashion, without symptoms, but with recurring exacerbations of an underlying disease such as chronic obstructive pulmonary disease.

Patients may initially complain of difficulty swallowing liquids, solid food, or pills. Caregivers or nursing personnel may note such difficulties experienced by the patient including "pocketing" of pills within the oral cavity. The patient or the patient's observant family members may complain of the increased time needed to complete a meal. The patient or the practitioner may identify weight loss without any other localizing explanation. However, clinicians must distinguish these dysphagia or aspiration symptoms from a myriad of other common health problems that may mimic dysphagia in older adults. For example, in frail individuals, depression or early parkinsonism may be manifested solely by weight loss and slowed eating. Without a complete history, these patients may be sent for a dysphagia workup before an attempt is made to manage their "root problem."

Symptoms of esophageal dysphagia include food "hanging up" behind the sternum, neck pain, chest pain, and heartburn. This issue is also addressed in Chapter 91, which includes a discussion of esophageal disorders. A specific problem with solid food dysphagia suggests a mechanical obstruction. If the symptoms are intermittent, a lower esophageal ring may be present. If the symptoms are progressive, a peptic stricture or carcinoma is more likely. If there are difficulties in ingesting solids and liquids, a neuromuscular or dysmotility etiology must be considered.

SCREENING ACROSS A CONTINUUM OF CARE SETTINGS

Dysphagia evaluation varies depending on the clinical setting. The comprehensive diagnostic approaches available for hospitalized older patients with dysphagia may not be logistically feasible for bedbound nursing home residents. Likewise, interdisciplinary dysphagia teams are frequently available in academic settings or in larger hospital systems and less common in other settings. When such a team is not available, the responsibility for screening for swallowing problems falls on the primary provider or the hospital staff. Speech language pathologists, who are usually the swallowing therapists, are well trained to conduct bedside (also referred to as noninstrumental) examinations that include history taking, oral motor assessment, voice evaluation, and assessment of trial swallows. Prior to this referral though, clinicians can provide a focused secondary screening during their encounter with the patient. A number of attempts have been made to identify a simple screening tool for use in ambulatory clinics or at the patient's bedside. None of these approaches has proven altogether effective, but certain approaches warrant mention.

A 3-oz water swallow test can be performed at the bedside. The clinician auscultates over the patient's trachea before and after the water is swallowed. Overt coughing, choking, or a change in the character of breath sounds suggests aspiration. While this test identified 80% of poststroke patients in a rehabilitation unit who aspirated during a subsequent videofluoroscopic swallow study, in addition

to resulting false negatives, it provides no information for identifying the underlying pathophysiology of the swallow or for selecting specific interventions.

Because swallowing difficulties are very common in geriatric patients, some mechanism of primary screening should also take place within a primary care clinic setting. An example of a dysphagia screening form is provided in Table 41-7. Because swallowing is not something a patient usually mentions, it may be necessary to ask related questions until a particular word or phrase triggers an association with the patient's experience (e.g., swallowing, chewing, moving food to the throat, coughing, choking).

Many forms of comprehensive geriatric assessment now include nutritional screening, which can be used as a surrogate screening for dysphagia. Some geriatric clinics now incorporate questions about difficulties with eating or swallowing that are included in periodic screening questionnaires. The simple question, "Do you have difficulty swallowing food?" was reported to have 100% sensitivity and 75% specificity in detecting swallowing difficulties in patients with parkinsonism. Alternatively, a practitioner's recognition of the relationship among symptoms of weight loss, cough or respiratory decompensation, and dysphagia may serve as a start in addressing this common problem. Nonetheless, once dysphagia is suspected, a more complete assessment is necessary not only to validate its presence but also to define and construct a treatment plan that modifies the underlying sensorimotor pathophysiology.

TEAM APPROACH TO DYSPHAGIA

Interdisciplinary health care teams play a vital role in the care of complex older adults with dysphagia. This cross-disciplinary focus helps to address not only the medical but also the functional and psychosocial consequences of this problem. The team approach offers the stated advantage of a more efficient comprehensive assessment with shared responsibility for interventions and often makes timely consultation possible. The responsibilities of team members are often divided among disciplines and can include reviewing health issues, obtaining pertinent swallowing history, and an examination (which may include instrumental studies), providing education and counseling to the patient and to the family or the care provider, conducting psychosocial screening, and reviewing advance directives. Teams can be either formal or informal in composition. Core teams frequently include a speech language pathologist, a dietitian, and either a physician or a nurse practitioner.

Focused Assessment of Swallowing

A major function of the swallowing team is to perform a thorough assessment of the swallowing mechanism and its function. Most commonly, the speech language pathologist plays a major role, performing a two-part examination consisting first of a clinical (bedside) noninstrumental evaluation often followed by an instrumental assessment of swallowing. A brief description of both methods follows.

Noninstrumental Swallowing Assessment

The clinical evaluation is noninstrumental and although often referred to as a "bedside" procedure can be performed in a variety of environmental settings including an outpatient office. It usually

TABLE 41-7

Dysphagia Screening Form–University of Wisconsin and Madison GRECC

Patient Name: _____

Medical record # _____ or Social security # _____

Primary Diagnosis: _____

1. Do you have difficulty swallowing? Yes No   Chewing? Yes No
2. Do you have difficulty moving food/liquid out of your mouth into your throat to swallow? Yes No
3. Does food/liquid remain in your mouth after you finish swallowing? Yes No
4. Do you cough or choke when drinking or eating? Yes No
    If so, how often does this occur: Infrequently
                                                  Once a day
                                                  1 or more times per meal
5. Does food/liquid feel like it remains in your throat after you finish swallowing? Yes No
6. Does food/liquid feel like it stays in your chest (esophagus) after you finish swallowing or eating a meal? Yes No
7. Do you bring back up food or liquid after you've swallowed it? Yes No
    If so, how many minutes or hours after swallowing does it come back up?
8. Do you have any pain when swallowing? Yes No   If so, where?
9. Is your mouth dry? Yes No
10. Any difficulty swallowing your saliva? Yes No
11. Have you noticed any drooling? Yes No   Wet pillow in the morning? Yes No
12. Is it taking longer to eat a meal? Yes No
13. Do you eat everything you want to eat? Yes No
14. What have you stopped eating because of difficulty?
15. What type of foods are easiest for you to swallow:
    A. All kinds of foods
    B. Soft solids (e.g., pasta, soft vegetables)
    C. Pureed
    D. Liquids
16. Are you hungry? Yes No
17. Current weight: _____
    Occurrence of weight loss over past 3 months: Yes No
    If so, please specify amount: _____
18. Are you congested in your chest, throat, nose? Yes No
    How often do you have a head cold or chest cold?

involves four types of assessment: (1) history taking; (2) speech and voice assessment; (3) oral motor assessment; and (4) performance on trial swallows. The specific methods and measures preferred and most frequently used by clinicians when working with dysphagia of neurogenic origin, which is frequently the case in older patients, are shown in Table 41-8.

Although a noninstrumental assessment provides a breadth of information, it can only increase the suspicion of aspiration through findings such as increased secretions or a wet and/or gurgly voice quality. Given the possibility of silent aspiration as a result of decreased cognition or diminished sensation in older people, coughing and throat clearing, which are the characteristic signs of aspiration, may be absent. To rule out aspiration with an acceptable level of confidence, an instrumental assessment is often necessary. Moreover, effective dysphagia intervention relies on an accurate diagnosis of the specific pathophysiology. That is, the underlying movement disorder that results in disordered bolus flow in terms of direction, duration, and clearance, must be defined and remediated in order to eliminate or minimize the dysphagia. Most frequently, instrumental methods are necessary to clarify the aspects of the swallowing sequence that must be modified to effect safe and efficient bolus flow. Although clinicians must pursue a complete oropharyngeal and esophageal assessment of many dysphagic patients, this section focuses on oropharyngeal dysphagia and the reader is referred to Chapter 50 for a discussion of the esophagus.

Instrumental Examination

To obtain the most useful and valid representation of swallowing, an instrumental diagnostic test should

1. Depict soft tissues, air, fluid-filled cavities, and surrounding bone,
2. Produce clear images of functional changes in multiple planes and real time,
3. Allow viewing of the entire swallow,
4. Be noninvasive and risk-free,
5. Detect and quantify aspiration,
6. Allow objective and repeatable measurements, and
7. Estimate prognosis and treatment potential.

A variety of imaging methods are available for studying the swallow, including ultrasound, MRI, computed tomography scanning, and scintigraphy. The two most commonly used techniques are described in the following sections.

TABLE 41-8

Clinical and Bedside Swallowing Methods and Measures

History	Oral motor
Patient report of problem	Tongue strength/range of motion
Family report of problem	Lip seal/pucker
History of pneumonia	Jaw strength/lateralization
Type of neurological insult	Soft palate movement/symmetry
Nutritional status	Dysarthria
Gastrointestinal anomaly	Speech intelligibility
Structural abnormality	Oral apraxia
Previous surgery	Volitional cough
Other disease	Ability to follow directions
Medications	Management of secretions

Voice	Trial swallows
Breathiness	*Bolus Type:*
Harshness	Thin liquid
Wet/gurgly	Thick liquid
Strained/strangled	Puree
Overall dysphonia/aphonia	Solid
Resonance	*Swallowing-related events:*
	Oral transit estimate
	Estimate swallow duration
	Laryngeal elevation
	Voice quality after swallow
	Ability to feed self
	Swallows per bolus
	Spontaneous cough
	Estimate of penetration/aspiration
	Estimate of oral stasis
	Observation of meal

Source: Adapted from McCullough GH et al: Clinicians' preferences and practices in conducting clinical/bedside and videofluoroscopic swallowing examination in an adult/neurogenic population. Am J Speech Lang Pathol 8(2):149, 1999.

Oropharyngeal Videofluoroscopic Swallowing Evaluation

An oropharyngeal videofluoroscopic swallowing evaluation is most commonly used to assess the integrity of the oropharyngeal anatomy, swallowing physiology, and bolus flow. Structural abnormalities and mucosal lesions are identified by the barium that is swallowed and used to outline the soft tissue structures it passes. In this manner, webs, pharyngeal diverticula, masses, and other soft tissue anomalies are revealed. Structural anomalies such as postsurgically modified anatomy, scar tissue, and osteophytes can be elucidated by radiographic means. Perhaps, the two greatest strengths of the videofluoroscopic swallow evaluation are that the swallow is recorded in motion and preserved digitally or on videotape for replay.

This method permits viewing of the dynamic swallow. All oropharyngeal structures can be examined with regard to their contribution to the coordinated (or uncoordinated) swallow in terms of timing and range of motion. Their impact on bolus flow is made apparent. Therefore, the specific pathophysiology and its impact on bolus flow are clarified and can be targeted for treatment.

An oropharyngeal videofluoroscopic swallow study is not designed simply to determine if a patient is aspirating or even why a patient is aspirating or retaining residue. It is designed also to assist a clinician in determining if a patient can safely receive oral nourishment and allows for trials of proposed interventions to maximize efficacy and safety. During the study, the clinician often varies bolus characteristics sufficiently to be able to offer a diet recommendation (such as thickened liquid or semisolid). Additional recommendations may be simple postural adjustments, such as tucking the chin, which are shown under fluoroscopy to improve direction or efficiency of bolus flow.

Although videofluoroscopy is the instrumental method most commonly used to assess swallowing, it is limited in the following ways:

1. The amount of information obtained is restricted to a few minutes in an effort to limit radiation exposure.

2. The environment can be distracting for patients with cognitive deficits.

3. The material ingested is barium, not food, and may not simulate the swallow evoked when real food is used as a stimulus (taste, smell).

Despite these limitations and exposure to a small amount of radiation (equivalent to 2 years of natural background radiation or a set of dental x-rays), videofluoroscopy is preferred for the breadth of information it provides with regard to anatomy, physiology, bolus flow, and assessment of trial intervention.

In addition, a fluoroscopic examination can easily be extended to the esophagus when indicated. Merging of the videofluoroscopic swallow study directly into esophagraphy, which results in a distinct third test referred to as an oropharyngeal esophagram, may reveal anatomic or physiological findings for the referred sensation. Findings may include a Schatzki's ring, an esophagus-narrowing web or stricture, a delay in LES opening or esophageal stasis, or other esophageal etiologies for the dysphagia. Thus, an oropharyngeal esophagram permits a more organized, efficient, cost-effective process for professional personnel and for the patient. Most importantly, it optimizes the potential for comprehensive findings and facilitates immediate intervention.

Fiberoptic Endoscopic Evaluation of Swallowing

Fiberoptic endoscopic evaluation of swallowing (FEES) is second to videofluoroscopy in frequency of instrumental approaches used with elderly patients. It combines the traditional endoscopic examination, in which the flexible scope allows direct visualization of the nasal cavity, the entire nasopharynx, the oropharynx, the larynx, and the hypopharynx, with dynamic recording of swallowing. Although FEES permits only limited observation of the pharyngeal swallow because it is "whited out" or visually obliterated during swallowing caused by constriction of the anatomy, the method provides a valuable alternative to a noninstrumental clinical assessment. It is being used with increased frequency in long-term care facilities where videofluoroscopy is unavailable and also with bariatric patients or those who cannot be moved to radiology because of medical instability. Other advantages are its repeatability, the use of real food and fluid during the assessment, and its potential as a biofeedback tool.

In addition to limited visualization of the dynamic oropharyngeal swallow, the limitations of FEES involve risks related to endoscopy, which include nosebleed, mucosal injury, gagging, allergic reaction to the topical anesthesia, laryngospasm, and vasovagal response. Laryngospasm is reported most often as patients are being extubated or by a sudden flow of refluxed gastric contents. Aspiration of food or liquid also might trigger laryngospasm. Patients with a history of significant aspiration, patients who require supplemental oxygen, and patients with acute mental status depression may be at increased risk if they are functioning on the edge of adequate respiratory status and cannot tolerate the minor laryngopulmonary trauma caused by the endoscope. Finally, a vasovagal response, commonly manifested as fainting, is a fairly uncommon event but can be dangerous. The unlikely possibility of encountering an adverse reaction during a flexible endoscope examination must be balanced against the daily risks faced by patients with dysphagia.

DYSPHAGIA INTERVENTION

Dysphagia clinicians and researchers have historically felt most comfortable with physiologic outcomes (movement parameters such as range of motion) and the effect on bolus flow direction, duration, and clearance as indicators of the success of an intervention. Attitudes are changing as reflected by increased concern about QOL and the development of SWAL-QOL, a dysphagia-specific patient-centered QOL instrument. Through focus group methodology, SWAL-QOL was designed to represent the patient's perspective in measuring QOL attributable to dysphagia. The questionnaire, comprising 10 domains, is completed by patients in 10 minutes on an average.

The intent is for advances in QOL measurement such as SWAL-QOL to fill a void in dysphagia care, including understanding how variations in treatment affect the human experience of living with a swallowing difficulty and documenting the effectiveness of any given treatment in terms of both physiologic function and QOL. Once data are obtained clarifying how QOL varies with treatment, the dysphagia-specific tool can be used to facilitate decision making by patients and clinicians and to monitor the longitudinal course of individual patient treatment outcomes.

Treatment for dysphagia is usually compensatory, rehabilitative, or a combination of the two approaches. Compensatory interventions avoid or reduce the effects of impaired structures or neuropathology and resultant disordered physiology and biomechanics on bolus flow. Rehabilitative interventions have the capacity to directly improve dysphagia at the biological level. That is, aspects of anatomic structures (e.g., muscle) or neural circuitry are the targets of therapy that may have a direct influence on physiology, biomechanics, and bolus flow.

Compensatory Dysphagia Interventions

Traditionally, interventions for dysphagia in elderly patients are compensatory in nature and are directed at modifying bolus flow by targeting neuromuscularly induced pathobiomechanics or by adapting the environment. Compensatory strategies are believed by clinicians to be less demanding on the patient in terms of effort, and many of these strategies can be imposed on a relatively passive patient. A nonexclusive sampling of compensatory strategies includes postural adjustment, slowing the rate of eating, limiting bolus size, adaptive equipment, and the most commonly used environment adaptation, diet modification.

Postural Adjustments

Postural adjustments are relatively simple to teach to a patient, require little effort to employ, and can eliminate misdirection of bolus flow through biomechanical adjustment. A general postural rule for facilitating safe swallowing is to eat in an upright posture so that the vertical phase of the oropharyngeal swallow capitalizes on gravitational forces at work when the patient is sitting with the torso, and neck at a 90-degree angle to the horizon and the head in line with

the horizon. This posture also can assist in precluding early spillage of food or liquid from the horizontal oral phase into the pharynx and a potentially open airway as well as diminishing the probability of nasal regurgitation. A less obvious postural adjustment is useful for patients with hemiparesis. For this group of patients, a common strategy is a head turn toward the hemiparetic side, effectively closing off that side to bolus entry and facilitating bolus transit through the nonparetic pharyngeal channel. If the pathophysiologic condition is the uncoupling of the oral from the pharyngeal phase of the swallow, a simple chin tuck (45 degrees) reduces the speed of bolus passage, thereby giving the neural system the time it needs to initiate the pharyngeal and airway protection events prior to bolus entry. Other postural adjustments facilitate safe swallowing and are designed to specifically compensate for pathophysiologic conditions analyzed and treated by a swallowing clinician on referral for a swallowing assessment and treatment.

Food and Liquid Rate and Amounts

Although we live in a "fast food" society, older individuals and especially those with dysphagia take longer to eat. Eating an adequate amount of food becomes a challenge not only because of the increased time required to do so but also because fatigue frequently becomes an issue. Typically, smaller amounts per swallow are less likely to enter or block the airway, but in individuals who experience a sensory loss in the mouth or throat, larger amounts of food or liquid may be necessary to trigger a swallow. To promote a safe, efficient swallow in most individuals with swallowing and chewing difficulties, the following recommendations are useful:

- Eat slowly and allow enough time for a meal.
- Do not eat or drink when rushed or tired.
- Take small amounts of food or liquid into the mouth—use a teaspoon rather than a tablespoon.
- Concentrate on swallowing—eliminate distractions like television.
- Avoid mixing food and liquid in the same mouthful.
- Place the food on the stronger side of the mouth if there is unilateral weakness.
- Alternate between liquids and solids.
- Use sauces, condiments, and gravies to facilitate cohesive bolus formation and prevent pocketing or small food particles from entering the airway.

Adaptive Equipment

Eating and drinking aids can assist in placing, directing, and controlling the bolus of food or liquid and in maintaining proper head posture while eating. For example, modified cups with cutout rims (placed over the bridge of the nose) or straws prevent a backward head tilt when drinking to the bottom of a cup. A backward head tilt, which results in neck extension, should be avoided in most cases because when the head is tilted back, food and liquid are more likely to be misdirected into the airway. Spoons with narrow, shallow bowls, or glossectomy feeding spoons (spoons developed for moving food to the back of the tongue) are useful to individuals who require assistance in placing food in certain locations in the mouth. More importantly, these utensils and devices promote independence in eating and drinking. A speech pathologist or swallowing clinician can make suggestions regarding appropriate aids for optimizing swallowing safety and satisfaction. Occupational therapists are experts in the area of adaptive equipment and can be helpful in obtaining products that are often available only commercially.

Diet Modification

The most common compensatory intervention is diet modification, a totally passive environmental adaptation. Withholding thin liquids such as water, tea, or coffee, which are most easily aspirated by older adults, and restricting liquid intake to thickened liquids is almost routine in nursing homes in an attempt to minimize or eliminate thin-liquid aspiration, presumably the precedent to the long-term related outcome, which is pneumonia. Despite the huge impact these seemingly unappealing practices may have on patient QOL, they have been commonly implemented in the absence of efficacy data.

A large National Institutes of Health (NIH)-funded multisite, randomized clinical trial (RCT) was designed as two sequential RCTs to compare the efficacy of two of the most commonly prescribed dysphagia interventions: chin-down posture and thickened liquids (nectar and honey viscosity) for patients with Parkinson's disease (PD) and/or dementia in the short term and over a longer period of time. Seven hundred eleven patients were enrolled in a short-term arm of the study (Part I) in which each intervention was evaluated using videofluoroscopy to assess its effectiveness in preventing the primary outcome: immediate aspiration. In Part II of the study, the long-term follow-up, 515 patients were randomly assigned to use one of these common interventions for 3 months and were monitored for incidence of the primary outcome: pneumonia. The primary outcome of Part I showed that aspiration was significantly reduced with honey-thick liquids as compared with both nectar-thick and chin-down posture interventions. The primary outcome of Part II showed equal value in chin-down posture and thickened liquids in pneumonia prevention. Several secondary outcomes also are of great importance. Patients with dementia (with or without PD), regardless of intervention, had significantly greater incidence of pneumonia than patients with PD only. Patients who aspirated more frequently with all of the interventions during the videofluoroscopic evaluation of swallowing also were more likely to incur pneumonia during Part II. Of the individuals who did get pneumonia, those randomized to drink honey-thick liquids (defined as 3000 centipoise, which is very thick) for 3 months were hospitalized for an average of 13 days longer than patients drinking nectar-thick liquids (4 days) or those performing the chin-down posture (6 days) while drinking.

With the recent appearance of SWAL-QOL on the clinical scene, some of these ongoing practices can be evaluated from the patient's perspective as well as by the clinicians who, with good intent, recommend them. In the NIH RCT, significantly more patients who were cognitively intact reported preferring chindown posture with thin liquids over nectar or honey-thickened fluids. Between the thickened fluids, they found nectar more satisfactory, or pleasant to drink, than honey.

Additional diet modifications include a pureed diet, and a soft food diet in which the bolus maintains itself in a cohesive mass during transit but has more texture than the pureed diet. The use of sauces and gravies to minimize the formation of dry particles that may easily be misdirected into the airway is a common practice. Other strategies within this category as interventions are available, and the dietitian should work closely with the team to ensure that the safest diet is provided and that it is effective in maintaining adequate nutrition and hydration, while also acceptable to patients in order to insure compliance.

Knowing the Heimlich Maneuver

Educating care providers and family members about the signs of choking and the standard first-aid technique for clearing the airway, namely, the Heimlich maneuver, is essential. While the Heimlich maneuver can be self-administered, it is recommended that individuals with dysphagia eat in the company of someone who knows this first-aid technique. Family members should be trained in emergency techniques for clearing the airway.

Rehabilitative Dysphagia Interventions

Rehabilitative exercises are, by nature, more active and rigorous. Often a rehabilitative approach to dysphagia intervention is withheld from elderly patients because such a demanding activity is assumed to deplete any limited remaining swallowing reserve, thus potentially exacerbating dysphagia symptoms. Sufficient treatment efficacy data are unavailable, and so assumption-based patterns of practice prevail.

Although progressive resistance training appears to be safe and effective for limb musculature in older adults, such training has only begun to be systematically applied to the muscles of swallowing. A description of two different exercise regimens that are supported with efficacy data for improving swallowing-related function in the elderly follow.

One is a simple isotonic/isometric neck exercise performed over a 6-week period in which the patient simply lies flat on his back and lifts his head (keeping shoulders flat) for a specified number of repetitions. The improved physiologic outcome of UES opening that affects swallowing is speculated to result from strengthening the mylohyoid/geniohyoid muscle groups and possibly the anterior segment of the digastric muscle.

Another exercise regimen demonstrating effectiveness in older dysphagic patients comprises an 8-week isometric resistance exercise for the tongue and was shown in acute and chronic stroke patients to improve swallowing safety by reducing airway invasion, increasing lingual pressure generation both isometrically and during swallowing and increasing lingual structure, specifically volume or size, as measured via MRI. Such findings suggest that older, dysphagic individuals are able to benefit from rehabilitative exercises focused on bulbar-innervated head and neck musculature. The methods hold promise for not only influencing safe, efficient bolus flow with significant functional gains but also may restore health and improve QOL as well.

OPTIMIZING SWALLOWING AND RELATED HEALTH THROUGH PREVENTION

Medications

Minimizing medications that may, most often in combination, put a patient at risk for dysphagia is an important goal. Furthermore, pills are often described by patients as being difficult to swallow. Patients should be informed about medications that can be crushed, can be mixed with foods, or are available in liquid form. Pill-induced damage to the esophagus can occur if pills are taken when lying down or with inadequate amounts of liquid.

On the other hand, some medicines can enhance the swallow. For example, in parkinsonism, the timing of medication can be adjusted to decrease bradykinesia, thereby achieving the greatest effect in improving swallowing coordination at mealtimes.

Oral Hygiene

Poor oral hygiene is a risk factor for pneumonia, and aspiration of saliva, whether or not it is combined with food or fluid, can increase the likelihood of infection. Therefore, patients should be encouraged to perform oral hygiene several times a day and undergo periodic dental examinations. Furthermore, products to relieve oral dryness, as well as alcohol-free mouth care products, can be recommended.

TuBe or Not TuBe—Oral Versus Nonoral Intake

Oropharyngeal dysphagia is potentially life-threatening. In the older population, critical decisions often must be made that impact on the patient's safety, health, and QOL. Among these perplexing issues is the question of continuing oral intake or providing nonoral enteral or parenteral nutrition. This dilemma is also reviewed in Chapter 40.

Enteral nutrition, the delivery of nutritive products to the digestive system through nonoral means, is often selected for the temporary prevention of aspiration in acutely ill patients. It also is chosen for longer-term nutritive supplementation or permanent replacement in patients whose disease process results in confirmed or suspected swallowing-related aspiration or malnutrition and dehydration. In the case of the latter, older patients whose chronic disease processes are overlaid on a system with a reduced functional reserve for safe, sufficient swallowing, the clinician's impressions often direct decisions relating to tube feeding for weeks, months, or even years. Rabenek et al. wrote: "No explicit guidelines for percutaneous endoscopic gastrostomy (PEG) tube placement are available to guide clinical decision-making. In the absence of such guidelines, the decision to place a PEG tube focuses mainly on the patient's ability to take food by mouth." However, it would clearly be narrow and short-sighted to make decisions with such an impact solely on the basis of empirical swallowing abilities or even instrumental physiologic and bolus flow test results. For an issue that may be a critical source of a patient's sense of autonomy, self-respect, dignity, and QOL, swallowing ability is merely one factor in a decision-making formula that is yet to be determined. Unfortunately, the current situation remains as stated by Logemann: "An important decision is whether the patient should continue to be fed orally, or be placed on a nasogastric tube or given some type of gastrostomy or jejunostomy. At this time, there are no absolute guidelines the clinician can use to make the decision."

Therefore, both published evidence and the practitioner's own clinical experience must contribute to such decision making. One study involving an elderly population followed for 11 months documented the incidence of complications of tube feeding. At 2 weeks postintubation, 43% of patients fed by NG tube and 56% of those fed by gastric (G) tube had been diagnosed with aspiration pneumonia. Sixty-seven percent of patients fed by NG tube and 44% of those fed by G tube had become agitated and/or self-extubated, requiring restraints or sedative medications to maintain the integrity

of enteral nutrition. Late complications in patients in the NG tube group included a 44% incidence of aspiration pneumonia and a 39% incidence of self-extubation, whereas a 56% incidence of aspiration occurred in the gastrostomy group.

These data and others have led to comparisons between the outcomes of parenteral (intravenous) and enteral modes of feeding. Findings suggest advantages in safety and somewhat equivocal physiologic and clinical outcomes, whereas costs may be less for the latter mode.

In summary, while oropharyngeal dysphagia may be life-threatening, so are the alternatives, particularly for frail elderly patients. Therefore, contributions by all team members are valuable in this challenging decision-making process, with the patient's family or care provider's point of view perhaps being the most critical second, of course, to the competent patient, himself. The state of the evidence calls for more research, including RCTs in this area. Until (and perhaps after) these data are collected and have been analyzed, the many behavioral, dietary, and environmental modifications described in this chapter and being further refined are compassionate and, in many cases, preferred alternatives to the always present option of tube feeding.

FURTHER READING

Barczi SR, Sullivan P, Robbins J. How should dysphagia care of older adults differ? Establishing optimal practice patterns. *Semin Speech Lang.* 2000;21(4):347.

Cohen LG, Ziemann U, Chen R, et al. Studies of neuroplasticity with transcranial magnetic stimulation. *J Clin Neurophys.* 1998;15:305–324.

DePippo KL, Holas MA, Reding MJ. Validation of the 3 oz water swallow test for aspiration following stroke. *Arch Neurol.* 1992;49:1259–1261.

ECRI. *Diagnosis and Treatment of Swallowing Disorders (Dysphagia) in Acute-Care Stroke Patients.* Evidence Report/Technology Assessment 8. Prepared by the ECRI Evidence-Based Practice Center under contract 290-97-0020, AHCPR Publication 99-E024. Rockville, MD: Agency for Health Care Policy and Research; 1999.

Howard L, Malone M. Clinical outcome of geriatric patients in the United States receiving home parental and enteral nutrition. *Am J Clin Nutr.* 1997;66:1364.

Hudson HM, Daubert CR, Mills RH. The interdependency of protein-energy malnutrition, aging and dysphagia. *Dysphagia.* 2000;15:31.

Langmore SE. Risk factors for aspiration pneumonia. *Nutr Clin Pract.* 1999;14:S41.

Logemann J. *Evaluation and Treatment of Swallowing Disorders.* Austin, TX: Pro-Ed; 1998.

Logemann J, Gensler G, Robbins J, et al. A randomized study of three interventions for aspiration of thin liquids in patients with dementia or Parkinson's disease. *J Speech Lang Hear Res.* 2008;51:173–183.

Mitchell SL. The risk factors and impact on survival of feeding tube placement in nursing home residents with severe cognitive impairment. *Arch Intern Med.* 1997;157:327.

Rabeneck L, McCullough LB, Wray NP. Ethically justified, clinically comprehensive guidelines for percutaneous endoscopic gastronomy tube placement. *Lancet.* 1997;349:396.

Robbins J, Kays SA, Gangnon R, et al. The effects of lingual exercise in stroke patients with dysphagia. *Arch Phys Med Rehabil.* 2007;88(2):150–158.

Robbins J, Gangnon R, Theis S, et al. The effects of lingual exercise on swallowing in older adults. *J Am Geriatr Soc.* 2005;53:1483–1489.

Robbins J. The evolution of swallowing neuroanatomy and physiology in humans: A practical perspective. *Ann Neurol.* 1999;46:279–280.

Robbins JA, Nicosia M, Carnes M, et al. Lingual isometric and swallowing strength in the elderly: is intervention warranted? *Gerontology.* 1998;38:6.

Robbins J, Coyle J, Roecker E, et al. Differentiation of normal and abnormal airway protection during swallowing using a penetration-aspiration scale. *Dysphagia.* 1999;14:228.

Robbins J, Hamilton JW, Lof GL, et al. Oropharyngeal swallowing in normal adults of different ages. *Gastroenterology.* 1992;103:823.

Robbins J, Gensler G, Hind J, et al. Comparison of 2 interventions of liquid aspiration on pneumonia incidence: a randomized trial *Ann Intern Med.* 2008;148:509–518.

Ship JA, Duffy V, Jones JA, et al. Geriatric oral health and its impact on eating. *J Am Geriatr Soc.* 1996;44:456.

Zald DH, Pardo JV. The functional neuroanatomy of voluntary swallowing. *Ann Neurol.* 1999;46:281–286.

Oral Cavity

Jonathan A. Ship

The oral cavity serves three essential functions in human physiology: (1) the production of speech, (2) the initiation of alimentation, and (3) protection of the host. A discussion of oral–pharyngeal health and function throughout the human life span must consider the impact of any disturbance of these three functions on an older person's life.

In order to speak, process food, and protect the host from pathogens and trauma, many specialized tissues have evolved in the oral–facial region (Table 42-1). The teeth, the periodontium, and the muscles of mastication exist to prepare food for deglutition. The tongue occupies a central role in communication, and is also a key participant in food bolus preparation and translocation. Salivary glands provide a secretion with multiple functions. Saliva, in addition to lubricating all oral mucosal tissues to keep them intact and pliable, moistens the developing food bolus, permitting it to be fashioned into a swallow-acceptable form. All these tissue activities are finely coordinated, and a disturbance in any one tissue function can significantly compromise speech and/or alimentation and diminish the quality of a patient's life (Table 42-2).

The oral cavity is exposed to the external world and is vulnerable to a limitless number of infectious, traumatic, and environmental insults. Extensive mechanisms have evolved to protect the mouth and permit normal oral function. The oral cavity is richly endowed with sensory systems that contribute to the enjoyment of food and alert an individual to potential problems. These systems include mechanisms for taste (and its inextricable relationship with smell); thermal, textural, and tactile sensation; and pain discrimination. Also, saliva plays an important protective role and contains a broad spectrum of antiviral, antibacterial, and antifungal proteins that modulate oral microbial colonization. Other proteins maintain the functional integrity of the teeth by keeping saliva supersaturated with calcium and phosphate salts and provide the first role in repairing incipient caries (tooth decay) via a remineralization process.

The use of dental services among older cohorts has improved over the past 40 years in the United States. However, findings from several national surveys indicate that a significant proportion of the elderly population does not see a dental professional on a regular basis and may thus be at risk for developing severe oral medical problems. For example, patients of all ages report more physician visits per year than dental visits, and this difference increases with greater age. More than 25% of the U.S. population aged 65+ years has not seen a dental professional in the past 5 years. In addition, elderly persons who wear complete dentures are four times less likely to visit a dentist than are those with remaining teeth.

These trends may change, however, for several reasons. First, future cohorts of older persons will have experienced improved oral health earlier in life, which will result in more patient visits than previous older-aged cohorts. Second, dental insurance coverage and retirement assets are more available for older-aged dental care than for previous generations of retired individuals. Third, nearly one-third of the elderly population is edentulous, but the prevalence of edentulousness has been decreasing steadily for the past four decades. This has resulted in an increased retention of the natural dentition, and therefore dental caries and periodontal diseases will remain substantial oral health concerns for older individuals in the future.

Half of adults aged 55+ years in the United States wear an oral prosthesis (partial or full denture), and 60% of them report problems with their appliances. This includes oral–fungal infections, traumatic lesions, and alveolar bone loss, yet edentulous adults are less likely to see dentists than their dentate counterparts. Oral and pharyngeal cancers develop in both dentate and edentate older adults, especially individuals with long-term alcohol and tobacco use, and regular cancer screening examinations are essential to diagnose and treat these tumors at early stages. Therefore, adequate oral health care for the elderly people should include preventive dental treatment and increased availability and use of dental health services. Most oral diseases are preventable and treatable at every age.

Accordingly, physicians, nurses, and aides who care for older patients need either to recruit dental expertise routinely as part of the overall assessment or to familiarize themselves with the appearance of oral health and disease states. Patient well-being is optimized

TABLE 42-1

Oral Tissues and Their Functions

ORAL TISSUE	FUNCTION
Teeth	Mastication, bone regeneration
Periodontium	Mastication, bone regeneration, host defense
Salivary glands	Lubrication, buffering acids, antimicrobial activity, mechanical cleansing, mediation of taste, remineralization of teeth, oral mucosal repair
Taste buds	Taste, host defense
Oral mucosa	Host defense, mastication, swallowing, speech
Muscles of mastication and facial expression	Mastication, swallowing, speech, posture

TABLE 42-3

Oral–Pharyngeal Processes in Older Adults

PROCESS	HEALTHY OLDER ADULTS	MEDICALLY COMPLEX OLDER ADULTS
Taste	Unaffected	Diminished
Smell	Diminished	Diminished
Food enjoyment	Unaffected	Diminished
Salivary output	Unaffected	Diminished
Chewing efficiency	Slightly diminished	Diminished
Swallowing	Slightly diminished	Diminished

when nondentists detect oral disease and recommend preventive and interventive services. Similarly, dentists should refer patients to physicians for previously undiscovered or inadequately controlled medical problems (e.g., diabetes, hypertension, cardiovascular disease). Communication is critical between dental and medical practitioners regarding medically complex patients who may need individualized health care planning to maintain oral health at minimal risk.

This chapter focuses on specific oral tissues and their functions. It summarizes "normal" oral physiologic status in older adults and explains how common systemic diseases and their treatments may affect the oral tissues during aging (Table 42-3). It also briefly reviews the evaluation and management of oral disorders frequently encountered in the elderly population. Additional information on the diagnosis and treatment of these disorders is available in several comprehensive reviews cited in the reference section.

DENTITION

The loss of teeth has long been associated with aging. National health surveys in demonstrate that approximately one-third of Americans older than age 65 years are edentulous. Although the prevalence of edentulous adults has decreased dramatically over the past 50 years, the population older than age 65 years still has an average of 11 missing teeth. Advances in dental treatment, disease prevention, increased availability of dental care, and improved awareness of dental needs have resulted in significant gains in dental health.

Tooth loss is attributed to two major processes: dental caries (discussed below) and periodontal diseases (discussed in the next section). Caries affects the exposed dental surfaces, and periodontal diseases are confined to the supporting bony and ligamentous dental structures. With the current trends toward increasing tooth retention in aging populations, there is a correspondingly greater risk for the development of both of these disease entities.

A tooth consists of several mineralized and nonmineralized components supported by the periodontal ligament and the alveolar

TABLE 42-2

Clinical Manifestations of Oral Infections

DISEASE	ORAL MANIFESTATIONS
Dental and periodontal infections	
Dental caries	Soft to hard discolored defect on tooth surface
Gingivitis and periodontitis	Erythematous, edematous, and hemorrhagic gingiva, which may be accompanied by gingival recession and tooth mobility
Viral infections	
Primary herpes simplex infection	Clear to yellow vesicles that rupture and form shallow, painful ulcers on all mucosal surfaces; gingival tissues inflamed, edematous, and painful
Recurrent herpes simplex infection	Burning or tingling prodrome in lesion sites (lip, hard palate, attached gingiva); whitish-gray vesicles rupture to form painful ulcers, which then develop a crust
Herpes zoster	Unilateral vesicular eruptions in areas following the distribution of ophthalmic, maxillary, or mandibular divisions of trigeminal sensory nerves
Cytomegalovirus	Mononucleosis-like symptoms, petechial hemorrhages, enlarged salivary glands, pharyngotonsillitis
Fungal infections	
Pseudomembranous candidiasis	Soft, white or yellow plaques that can be wiped off to expose an underlying erythematous mucosa
Hyperplastic candidiasis	Leukoplakic or keratotic lesions that cannot be removed by scraping
Erythemic or atrophic candidiasis	Painful erythematous oral mucosal lesions; tongue appears "bald"; diffuse inflammation of denture-bearing areas
Angular cheilitis	Erythematous cracked or fissured lesions at the lip commissures
Salivary gland infections	
Acute sialoadenitis	Tender salivary gland swelling with purulent discharge on palpation of the gland duct
Chronic sialoadenitis	Recurrent, tender swellings of salivary gland progressing to a firm and atrophic gland

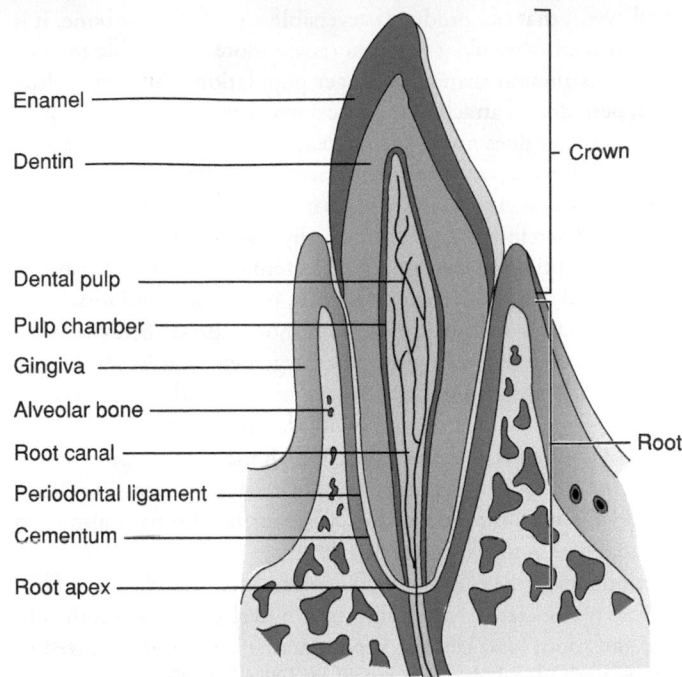

FIGURE 42-1. Dental, periodontal, and alveolar bone anatomy. (*From Ship JA, Heft M, Harkins S. Oral facial pain in the elderly. In: Lomranz J, Mostofsky DI, eds. Handbook of Pain and Aging. New York, New York: Plenum Press; 1997:1214.*)

bone (Figure 42-1). The outer dental structure is enamel and is the hardest, most mineralized component, consisting of ~90% hydroxyapatite. Enamel covers the coronal aspect of the tooth and is the first hard tissue exposed to caries-causing bacteria. Dentin constitutes the main portion of the tooth structure, extending almost the entire length of a tooth. It is covered by enamel on the crown and by cementum on the root. Cementum is the least mineralized of the three components (50%) and is the component most susceptible to caries-causing bacteria. The central, nonmineralized portion is the dental pulp, which houses the vascular, lymphatic, and neuronal supply to the tooth.

Tooth loss in children and young adults is caused predominantly by dental caries, whereas in middle-aged and older adults, periodontal diseases play a greater role in the loss of teeth. Longitudinal studies of generally healthy adult males have found that the principal cause of tooth extraction is dental caries. Furthermore, caries activity continues throughout life and is not a phenomenon confined to any single period.

There are two classifications of dental caries, depending on the dental surface affected. Coronal caries is characteristic of caries in young adults and children. This occurs when the enamel and dentin of the coronal portion of the tooth are affected. In older adults, if gingival recession or periodontal disease causes the root surfaces of the tooth to become exposed to the oral environment, root surface or cervical caries may occur.

The primary caries-causing microorganism is *Streptococcus mutans*; oral *Streptococcus, Actinomyces,* and *Lactobacillus* organisms are also associated with coronal and root surface lesions. These bacteria reside on the tooth surface in dental plaque, a soft, firmly adherent mass that contains bacteria, food debris, desquamated cells, and bacterial products. Acid production by plaque bacteria dissolves the

mineral content of the enamel, dentin, or cementum. The exposed protein constituents are destroyed by hydrolytic enzymes, and caries results. Dental plaque is considered a primary etiologic factor in dental caries, as well as a principal source of pathogenic organisms in periodontal diseases.

As a dentate individual gets older, there is susceptibility to coronal caries as a result of recurrent decay around existing restored surfaces, and the prevalence of root surfaces caries increases. For example, there is an 18-fold increase in the average number of tooth surfaces with root caries between persons aged 20 years and those aged 64 years (thus root caries often begins well before old age). There are many risk indicators for root surface caries: increased age, decreased exposure to fluoride, coronal caries, periodontal attachment loss, diminished oral–motor skills required for proper oral hygiene, and additional medical, behavioral, and social factors.

Studies in the United States reveal an increase in the mean number of decayed and restored teeth among older-aged dentate adults over the last 50 years. These trends probably reflect the increased retention of the natural dentition and a greater use of dental services by older adults; it is unlikely that they represent a true increase in dental caries activity. However, epidemiologic projections suggest that significant increases in the prevalence of root surface caries will occur in aging populations in the future.

For an older person with teeth, caries is a significant concern and may be a source of pain, infection, and malnutrition. Dental caries will appear as darkish lesions that frequently are associated with dental plaque (Figure 42-2) (Color Plate 7). Long-standing caries ultimately results in the destruction of the tooth with the possibility of a disseminated infection to the maxillofacial tissues and ultimately into the systemic circulation (septicemia). Once teeth have been destroyed from dental caries or periodontal disease, mastication, phonation, and deglutition may be perturbed. Also, social contact and nutritional status may be affected in a substantially edentulous aging individual.

The prevention of dental caries in an older adult is no different from that in a younger individual: fluoride, daily effective oral hygiene, and regular visits to dental professionals. Adult tooth surfaces can become resistant to decalcification and decay through repeated exposure to fluoride in water supplies, toothpaste, rinses, and gels. However, even resistant tooth surfaces can become carious when oral hygiene is inadequate and the mouth is exposed repeatedly to

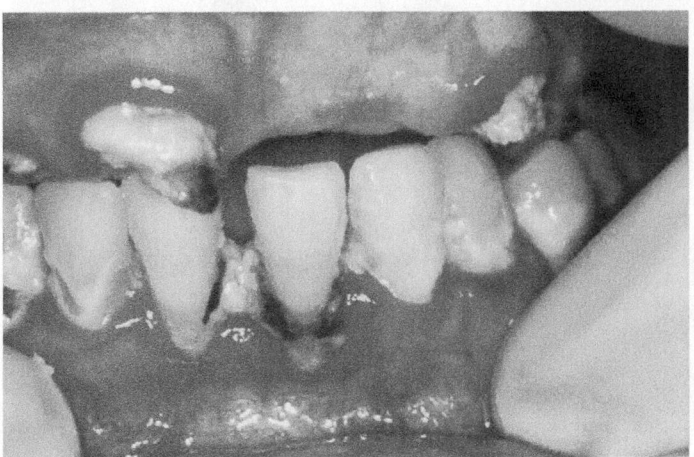

FIGURE 42-2. Severe dental caries and associated dental plaque.

fermentable carbohydrates. When detected early, caries can be debrided from a tooth, and the missing tooth structure can be restored with a wear-resistant, insoluble restorative material (e.g., amalgam or composite resin). Some restorative materials contain fluoride (glass ionomer cements) and can help reduce caries risk. Untreated dental caries, however, in most circumstances progress to severe or even total loss of tooth structure and possibly pain, abscess formation, cellulitis, and bacteremia. Replacements for lost teeth are available with removable prostheses (partial dentures) or fixed prosthodontic appliances (crowns, bridges, implants).

PERIODONTIUM

The periodontium consists of the tissues that invest and support the tooth. It is divided into the gingival unit (gums) and the attachment apparatus (cementum, periodontal ligament, and alveolar bony process) (see Figure 42-1). Gingivitis occurs when the gingival unit is inflamed. Periodontitis (or periodontal disease) exists when there is inflammation and an appreciable loss of the attachment apparatus as a result of the presence of pathogenic microorganisms. Microbial species (e.g., *Bacteroides, Fusobacterium, Prevotella, Actinobacillus, Capnocytophaga, Streptococcus*) cross the gingival epithelium and enter subepithelial tissues, where they activate specific host defense mechanisms. Eventually, this causes tissue destruction, including bone loss and tooth morbidity.

Certain periodontal changes occur in aging individuals. For example, cross-sectional studies demonstrate that older adults show an increase in dental plaque, calculus (calcified dental plaque), and the frequency of bleeding gingival tissues. Older persons also experience greater gingival recession and loss of periodontal attachment (Figure 42-3) (Color Plate 8). Longitudinal studies report that periodontitis is more prevalent and usually more extensive among black people, subjects with less education, those who have not seen a dentist recently, and those with gingivitis and certain pathogenic organisms. Currently, it is believed that periodontal disease proceeds through a series of episodic attacks rather than occurring as a slowly progressing continuous process. Furthermore, periodontal bone destruction results from an overly aggressive local immune reaction to the pathogenic organisms, triggering a cascade of cytokine and immuno-

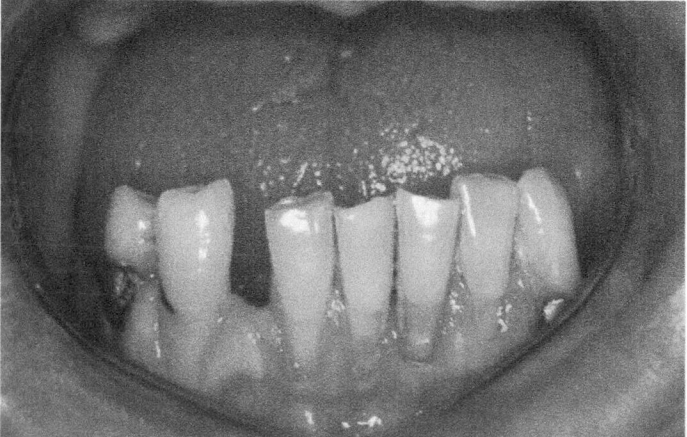

FIGURE 42-3. Gingival recession and loss of periodontal–alveolar bone attachment in an older adult.

logical events that can produce irreversible loss of alveolar bone. It is not known whether older age cohorts are more susceptible to periodontal destruction than are younger populations. Among healthy adults, periodontal attachment loss occurs at small increments in all age cohorts and does not occur in greater amounts in older healthy adults. However, many systemic diseases and therapeutic regimens commonly found in older individuals may affect adversely periodontal health. Therefore, an older medically compromised adult is especially susceptible to developing periodontal diseases and is at risk for associated dental–alveolar infections, pain, and tooth loss.

Several classes of medications commonly prescribed for older people are associated with gingival enlargement and hyperplasia, a condition that if left untreated predisposes to both caries and destructive periodontitis. The family of calcium channel-blockers can cause this unwanted drug side effect, which may require periodontal surgery for definitive treatment. The antiseizure medication phenytoin and the immunosuppressant cyclosporine also have also been associated with gingival enlargement.

Periodontal diseases have oral and systemic effects on health. They are directly associated with halitosis, gingival bleeding, tooth mobility, and tooth loss. Untreated periodontitis has been reported to interfere with blood glucose control in diabetic patients, and recent investigations suggest associations between cardiovascular disease and periodontitis after controlling for traditional risk factors such as weight, gender, tobacco use, age, and blood lipid levels. Gram-negative bacteria are implicated in the pathogenesis of periodontal disease, and colonization of the oropharynx with gram-negative bacilli predisposes a patient to pneumonia. Aspiration pneumonia can occur when oropharyngeal secretions are aspirated into the lungs, causing infection. Periodontal bacteria from the gingival sulcus in dentate individuals have been isolated from patients with pneumonia. Risk factors for aspiration pneumonia include older age, immunocompromised state, mechanical ventilation, feeding problems and/or feeding tubes, and deteriorating health status. Importantly, many debilitated older patients have received inadequate oral hygiene and are therefore highly susceptible to aspiration pneumonia.

For an older person with teeth, periodontal diseases can cause pain, difficulty with mastication, infection, and possibly social isolation. Gingivitis may be detected by the presence of erythematous and/or edematous gingival tissues with occasional hemorrhage, as well as halitosis. Gingival recession produces exposed dental root surfaces, a sign of periodontitis. This ultimately causes tooth mobility, a condition that necessitates definitive treatment. The systemic health of an already compromised individual may be further threatened by bleeding and suppurating gingiva, dental alveolar infections, and the potential transmission of oral bacteria via bacteremias and/or oral–pharyngeal secretions.

Treatment of gingivitis and periodontitis starts with regular oral hygiene in the form of toothbrushing and flossing after each meal. Electric toothbrushes and mechanical irrigation systems can assist older patients who have motor and/or cognitive disorders. Periodontal therapy ranges from local (e.g., dental prophylaxis, local debridement) to pharmacological (e.g., use of intrasulcular antimicrobial solutions, systemic low-dose doxycycline as an immunomodulator) to surgical techniques (e.g., debridement, excision of hyperplastic tissue), depending on the extent of periodontal infection and bony destruction. Numerous antimicrobial and anticollagenase pharmaceuticals have been approved for treatment as well: oral rinses (e.g., chlorhexidine 0.12%), subgingival antimicrobials (e.g., minocycline hydrochloride 1 mg microspheres), short-term antimicrobials (e.g., clindamycin 300 mg qid or metronidazole 400 mg tid for 7 to 10 days), or long-term anticollagenases (e.g., doxycycline 20 mg). While periodontal healing after surgery tends to be slower even in healthy older persons, the long-term results of periodontal therapy are indistinguishable from those in younger adults. The decision either to save the dentition and restore periodontal health or to extract teeth with moderate periodontal disease should be determined after all oral and systemic factors have been evaluated. Therefore, the health of a person, rather than age per se, should determine the extent of periodontal treatment.

SALIVARY GLANDS

There are three major pairs of salivary glands (parotid, submandibular, and sublingual) and numerous groups of minor glands (e.g., labial, palatal, and buccal), all of whose principal function is the exocrine production of saliva. Each gland type makes a unique secretion derived from either mucous or serous cell types, forming the fluid in the mouth termed *whole saliva*. Saliva includes many constituents that are critical to the maintenance of oral health. Its most important functions are lubrication of the oral mucosa, promotion of the remineralization of teeth, and protection against microbial infections. Although the role of saliva in digestion is limited, saliva helps prepare the food bolus for deglutition and is responsible for dissolving tastants and delivering them to taste buds.

It was previously thought that salivary output diminishes with increasing age. This was based on the clinical observation that older individuals frequently have a dry mouth and complain of xerostomia. However, investigations reveal that, in general, there is no substantial diminution in salivary production across the human life span in healthy adults. Thus, in the absence of complicating factors (e.g., certain systemic diseases, medications), there is no generalized age-related perturbation in the production of salivary fluid. In addition, there appear to be no significant alterations in the composition of saliva in older, healthy persons.

These physiologic findings contrast with the morphologic changes seen in aging salivary glands. Major salivary glands lose ~30% of their parenchymal tissue over the adult life span. The loss primarily involves acinar or fluid-producing components, while proportional increases are seen in ductal cells and in fat, vascular, and connective tissues. Because acinar components are primarily responsible for the secretion of saliva, it is not known why, in the presence of a significant reduction in the gland acinar volume, total fluid production does not diminish with increasing age. It has thus been deduced that salivary glands possess a functional reserve capacity that enables them to maintain fluid output throughout the human adult life span. There is evidence that with a reduced reserve capacity, additional burdens placed on aging salivary glands (e.g., anticholinergic medications) increase their vulnerability to functional decline. Therefore, salivary hypofunction and complaints of a dry mouth (xerostomia) should not be considered to be normal sequelae of aging but instead are indicative of a host of conditions and their treatments (Table 42-4). The most common etiology of salivary gland hypofunction is iatrogenic. Many medications taken by older persons reduce or alter salivary gland performance. In addition, radiation for head and neck neoplasms and cytotoxic chemotherapy can have direct and dramatic deleterious effects on salivary glands.

TABLE 42-4

Causes of Salivary Hypofunction in Older Adults

CATEGORY	EXAMPLES
Medications	Anticholinergics
	Antidepressants
	Antihistaminics
	Antihypertensives
	Anti-Parkinson's disease
	Anxiolytics
	Diuretics
Oncological therapy	Cytotoxic chemotherapy
	Head and neck radiotherapy
Oral conditions	Bacterial and viral infections
	Salivary gland obstructions
	Traumatic lesions
	Neoplasms
Other conditions	Alzheimer's disease
	Cerebrovascular accidents
	Dehydration
	Diabetes mellitus
	Late-stage liver disease
	Sjögren's syndrome
	Systemic lupus erythematosus
	Thyroid disorders (hyper and hypo)

The single most common disease affecting salivary glands is Sjögren's syndrome, an autoimmune exocrinopathy that occurs predominantly in postmenopausal women. Alzheimer's disease, diabetes, dehydration, rheumatoid arthritis, and cerebrovascular accidents may also affect salivary output. Several oral inflammatory and obstructive salivary gland disorders (e.g., bacterial infections, sialoliths, trauma, neoplasms) result in salivary dysfunction, as well as benign and malignant salivary tumors.

A clinician is likely to encounter many older patients with oral complaints related to salivary gland hypofunction. A brief clinical examination should include palpation of all major glands and inspection of the duct orifices to ensure patent glands. The application of a mild solution of citric acid or lemon juice to the tongue can help determine whether a patient's salivary glands will respond to a gustatory stimulus. Regardless of etiology, any of the major oral physiologic roles influenced by saliva (see Table 42-1) may be affected adversely. With impaired glandular output, increased dental caries will ensue rapidly, increasing the possibility of tooth loss. The oral mucosa becomes desiccated and cracked, leaving the host more susceptible to microbial infection (Figure 42-4) (Color Plate 9). Older adults experience difficulty in swallowing or speaking at length, pain (which may arise from either the teeth or the oral soft tissues), impaired denture use, altered taste, and diminished food enjoyment.

Treatment of salivary dysfunction starts with identification of the etiology. Medication-induced salivary problems can be eliminated by stopping unneeded drugs, modifying drug use and dose, or substituting one drug with another drug that has fewer anticholinergic side effects. Even when no reduction in the daily dose is recommended, the splitting of a dose into several smaller and more frequently taken doses may alleviate or diminish the sensation of oral dryness. To enhance salivary production, gustatory (sugar-free mints, candies), masticatory (sugar-free gums), and pharmacologic (pilocarpine

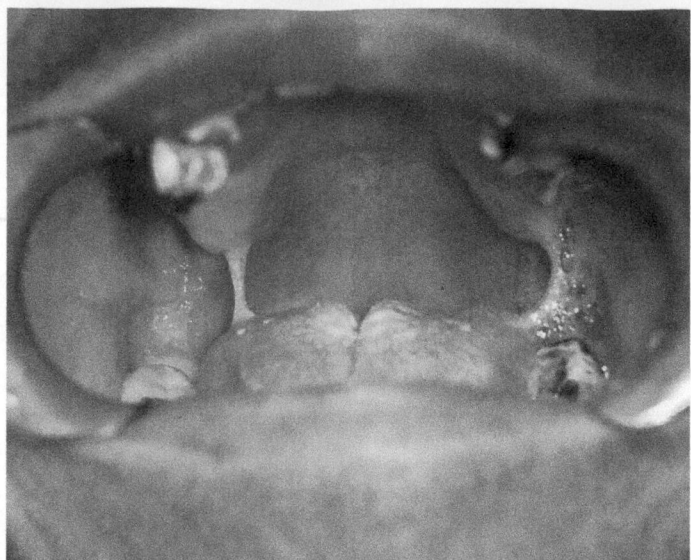

FIGURE 42-4. Dry mouth and salivary hypofunction caused by external beam radiotherapy used for tongue cancer. Remaining salivary output is viscous and difficult to swallow, caused by destroyed serous-producing salivary glands.

5 mg tid and qhs, cevimeline 30 mg tid) stimulants can be useful in a patient who has remaining salivary function. Salivary substitutes, rinses, and moisturizing gels can assist a patient who has little or no remaining salivary function. Prevention of dry-mouth problems is essential and can be achieved with the frequent use of sugarfree beverages, topical fluoride, and regular oral hygiene after meals. Removable prostheses must be kept clean and out of the mouth during sleeping hours. Frequent lubrication of the lips helps prevent lip cracking and infections.

SENSORY FUNCTION

Many reports suggest that food enjoyment, recognition, and sensory function decline as a function of age and that this can produce significant nutritional deficits. It has been suggested that there is a true anorexia (loss of appetite) associated with aging, although this is confounded by the many comorbidities that cause anorexia, and which are so common in elderly people, as well as other social and psychological factors that may reduce oral food and fluid intake. Perturbations in taste, smell, other oral sensory modalities can occur with age, and with dental/periodontal problems, increasingly reduce the rewards of eating, thus contributing to a diminished interest in food among many elderly persons.

The taste receptors of the human gustatory system are distributed throughout the oropharynx and are innervated by three cranial nerves: VII, IX, and X. It appears that the number of lingual taste buds does not diminish with age. The registration of a taste phenomenon is complex, because multiple factors are involved: gustation, olfaction, and central nervous system function. The ability to taste is often evaluated at two levels: (1) *threshold*, the most common measure, a "molecular-level" event, which reflects the lowest concentrations of a tastant that an individual can recognize as being different from water and (2) *suprathreshold*, a measure that is reflective of the ability to taste the intensity of substances at functional concentrations encountered in daily life. In addition to detection, recognition, and intensity, the normal sensation of taste involves a hedonic component: the degree of pleasantness.

Many earlier studies citing a higher frequency of taste complaints among older persons examined institutionalized individuals rather than healthy elderly people. It now appears that subjective reports of taste function among generally healthy, community-dwelling persons demonstrate that only modest changes occur with increased age, in comparison to studies revealing a threefold increase in the frequency of subjective complaints among older persons who take prescription medications. Objective threshold and suprathreshold evaluations of gustatory function in healthy older adults have been reported for all four taste qualities (sweet, sour, salty, and bitter), and in general, the decremental changes detected with increased age have been modest and taste-quality-specific. For example, the ability of older persons to detect salt decreases slightly with age, while no changes in the detection threshold for sucrose (sweet) are noted. The importance of medication usage and place of residence in the evaluation of taste dysfunction has been confirmed in clinical studies in which institutionalized persons and those using more prescription medications had significantly elevated taste thresholds.

Older individuals perform less well in the more complicated problems of flavor perception, food recognition, and food preference. This is probably a result of diminished olfactory performance rather than the modest changes that accompany taste function with aging. The available data on olfactory performance clearly indicates declines in thresholds, suprathreshold intensity judgments, and odor recognition in both men and women with increasing age. Among older adults, average thresholds are higher, the ability to perceive suprathreshold intensities is blunted, odor recognition is impaired, and the judgment of pleasantness is reduced compared with younger subjects. Moreover, longitudinal studies demonstrate that as people get older, recognition decrements become even more severe.

However, in the real world, people do not typically taste a single tastant in aqueous form and foods that contain solely olfactory cues are not consumed. Foods are chemosensory mixtures, and the most relevant but most difficult to obtain measures of gustatory and olfactory function involve the use of complex food analogs. In one study, younger subjects were significantly better than were elders at recognizing stimuli in blended food. However, when younger persons repeated the test with their nasal airways occluded, their performance dropped to the level of elderly individuals. One conclusion from this finding is that the daily life chemosensory functions of older individuals are handicapped by diminished olfactory performance. Moreover, it has been suggested that for many persons, the "anorexia of aging" can be reduced or reversed by adding flavor enhancers to foods.

Many other sensory cues (temperature, texture, pressure) participate in the experience of food enjoyment. Little research attention has been dedicated to these phenomena. One study demonstrated no age-related changes in the ability of subjects to distinguish fluids of varying temperatures and viscosities; however, a specific decline was observed in the perception of localized lingual pressure.

Normal chemosensory function cannot operate independently of good oral health. Numerous oral conditions can directly or indirectly affect smell and taste by altering the underlying biology of the taste or smell system or by introducing exogenous stimuli into the mouth or nose. Many oral conditions, including fungal/bacterial/viral infections, vesiculobullous diseases, salivary gland hypofunction, poorly

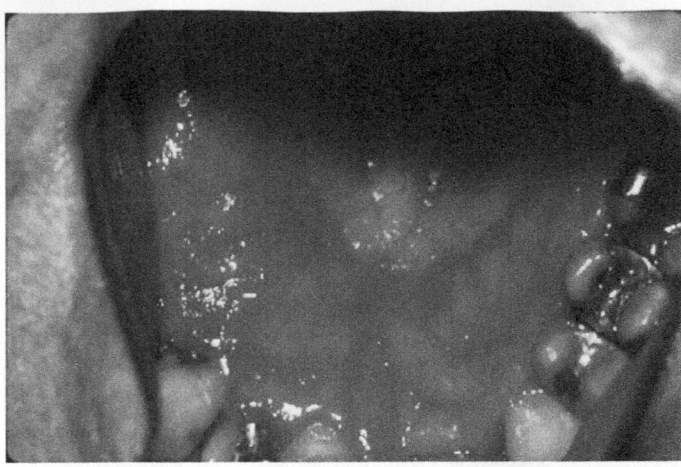

FIGURE 42-5. Asymptomatic erythematous candidiasis (denture stomatitis) caused by an ill-fitting oral prosthesis. This mycotic infection combined with a poorly fitting removable prosthesis contributes to impaired taste, smell, chewing, and swallowing.

fitting prostheses, and oral manifestations of systemic diseases, can cause chemosensory dysfunction. For example, inadequate removal of food particles can allow their breakdown or metabolic conversion by oral microorganisms to noxious, unpleasant substances. Periodontal diseases can result in accumulations of putrefied acidic materials that may leak into the oral cavity and alter taste sensation. Similarly, dental–alveolar bacterial infections with subsequent fistula formation may contribute continuously low levels of purulent matter in the mouth.

The complaint of a smell or taste problem may be indicative of a chemosensory disorder or could be the manifestation of an oral and/or systemic medical problem. For example, the sudden loss of either smell or taste may be a sign of brain tumor. Alternatively, gradual diminishment in food enjoyment may be related to multiple sources (e.g., a poorly fitting removable prosthesis, an oral fungal infection, decreased smell identification, a drug) (Figure 42-5) (Color Plate 10). Older subjects are more likely to have chemosensory complaints, but unfortunately those complaints are very poor predictors of olfactory dysfunction. A patient should be asked if he or she can specifically identify the four basic tastants and distinguish between different odorants; such patients can be given the University of Pennsylvania Smell Identification Test. A thorough multidisciplinary approach is required for a patient presenting with chemosensory complaints because of the wide range of potential oral, systemic, physiologic, cognitive, and pathologic factors that are involved in oral sensory functioning.

ORAL MUCOSA

The soft-tissue lining of the mouth may be characterized by three general types: (1) well-keratinized tissue with a dense layer of connective tissue and firmly attached to underlying bone (e.g., marginal gingiva, palatal mucosa), (2) slightly keratinized and freely movable tissue (e.g., labial and buccal mucosa, floor of the mouth), and (3) specialized mucosa (e.g., dorsum of the tongue). The primary function of the oral mucosa is to act as a barrier to protect the underlying structures from desiccation, noxious chemicals, trauma,

thermal stress, and infection. The oral mucosa plays a key role in the defense of the oral cavity.

Aging frequently is associated with changes in the oral mucosa similar to those in the skin, with the epithelium becoming thinner, less hydrated, and thus supposedly more susceptible to injury. The reasons for these changes (if they are normally a sequela of aging) are complex and include alterations in protein synthesis and responsiveness to growth factors and other regulatory mediators. Cell renewal (i.e., mitotic rates) and the synthesis of proteins associated with oral mucosal keratinization occur at a slower rate in aging individuals. Alternatively, the normal tissue architecture and patterns of histodifferentiation, which probably are dependent on complex interactions with the underlying connective tissue, do not display any changes with age. Overall, changes in the vascularity of oral mucosa probably contribute to an alteration in mucosal integrity because of reductions in cellular access to nutrients and oxygenation. Mucosal, alveolar, and gingival arteries demonstrate the effects of arteriosclerosis. Varicosities on the floor of the mouth and the lateral and ventral surfaces of the tongue (comparable to varicosities on the lower extremities) are also observable in geriatric patients.

The maintenance of mucosal integrity depends on the ability of the oral epithelium to respond to an insult. Insults can be caused by physical factors (eg, trauma), exposure to chemical or microbiological toxins, microbial infections, and oral and/or systemic conditions. Many studies have documented that the immune system undergoes a decline with age (see Chapter 3), and it is likely that this decline extends to mucosal immunity. Therefore, the oral mucosa may be more susceptible to transmission of infectious diseases as well as delayed wound healing. Similar findings have been reported for healing gingival tissues.

Cross-sectional studies have demonstrated that age per se has no effect on the clinical appearance of the oral mucosa. However, considerable evidence suggests that the use of removable prostheses has a potentially adverse effect on the health of the oral mucosa. The denture-bearing mucosa of aged maxillary and mandibular ridges shows significant morphologic changes. Ill-fitting dentures can produce mechanical trauma to the oral tissues (see (Figure 42-5) as well as cause mucosal hyperplasia. Oral candidiasis frequently is found on denture-bearing areas in an edentulous individual, often occurring with angular cheilitis (deep fissuring and ulceration of the epithelium at the commissures of the mouth). Therefore, the clinician should ask the patient to remove all removable prostheses before conducting an adequate oral examination.

Oral mucosal alterations in an older person are often a result of multiple oral and systemic factors (Table 42-5). Numerous medications have been associated with oral mucosal changes. For example, long-term use of antibiotics frequently results in oral candidal infections, while drugs with xerostomic side effects (see above) increase the potential for mucosal injury. Bisphosphonate drugs used for cancer metastasis and osteoporosis (primarily those administered IV, but possibly those delivered orally) have been associated with an unusual but severe destruction of oral mucosa and bone referred to as osteonecrosis. Drugs commonly used in older patients for arthritic conditions, hypertension, cardiac arrhythmias, seizures, and dementia are associated with lichenoid-like reactions. The withdrawal of a causative drug usually results in complete resolution of the lesion within 2 to 3 weeks, but if there is no clinical improvement, a definitive diagnosis should be obtained with a biopsy specimen.

TABLE 42-5

Conditions Associated with Oral Mucosal Changes

CLASSIFICATION	DISEASE/DISORDER	EXAMPLES
Oral conditions	Infections	Candidiasis, herpes simplex, herpes zoster
	Ulcerative conditions	Recurrent aphthous stomatitis
	Cancer	Oral squamous cell carcinoma
	Periodontal diseases	Gingivitis, periodontitis
	Prosthodontic problems	Poorly fitting dentures, denture stomatitis
	Salivary gland hypofunction	Dessicated oral tissues
	Food allergies	Lichenoid changes
	Trauma	Traumatic fibroma, mucocele
Systemic diseases	Dermatological disorders	Systemic lupus erythematosus, lichen planus, pemphigus vulgaris, cicatricial pemphigoid, erythema multiforme
	Endocrine disorders	Diabetes mellitus
	Neurologic disorders	Alzheimer's, Parkinson's, CVA
	Immunocompromising disorders	HIV, AIDS, rheumatoid arthritis
Medical therapies	Medications	Diuretics, calcium channel-blockers, antibiotics, antiseizures, immunomodulating drugs, bisphosphonates
	Radiotherapy	Head and neck radiotherapy
	Cytotoxic chemotherapy	Methotrexate, 5-FU, cyclosporin

AIDS, acquired immunodeficiency syndrome; CVA, cerebrovascular accident; 5-FU, 5-fluorouracil; HIV, human immunodeficiency virus.

Numerous oral mucosal disorders affect the elderly population, ranging from benign (e.g., recurrent aphthous ulcers and traumatic lesions) to malignant (e.g., squamous cell carcinomas) (Figure 42-6) (Color Plate 11). The diagnosis of mucosal diseases requires a detailed history and a thorough head and neck and oral examination, including all mucosal tissues. For vesiculobullous and erosive diseases, a simple three-item classification is helpful: (1) acute multiple lesions (e.g., erythema multiforme, herpes simplex, herpes zoster, allergic reaction), (2) recurring oral ulcers (e.g., recurrent aphthous stomatitis, traumatic ulcer), and (3) chronic multiple lesions (e.g., pemphigus vulgaris, mucous membrane pemphigoid, lupus erythematosus, lichen planus, dysplasia, squamous cell carcinoma). If a lesion does not resolve after 2 to 3 weeks, a tissue biopsy is required. For lesions that are suspected to be oral manifestations of autoimmune connective tissue disorders (e.g., pemphigus, pemphigoid, lichen planus), biopsies should also include specimens for direct immunofluorescence. If trauma from an injury or an ill-fitting denture is suspected, removal of the etiology should allow the lesion to heal. Many of these conditions have an immunological etiology, and therefore management strategies involve topical and/or systemic immunomodulating agents (Table 42-6).

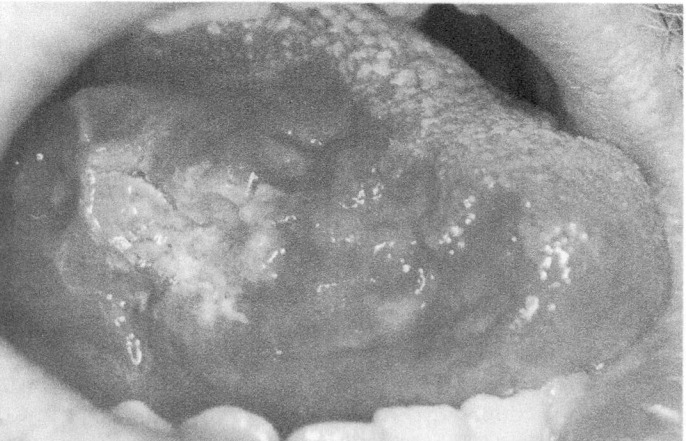

FIGURE 42-6. Squamous cell carcinoma of the right lateral border of the tongue. The lesion is characterized by unhealing erythematous, ulcerative, and leukoplakic regions, poorly defined margins, and regional lymphadenopathy.

TABLE 42-6

Treatment of Common Vesiculobullous and Erosive Diseases in Older Adults

MEDICATION	REGIMEN
Topical treatments[*†‡§]	
Fluocinonide gel 0.05%	Apply to affected regions tid and qhs
Triamcinolone acetonide in gel base 0.1%	
Clobetasol propionate gel 0.05%	
Oral rinses[†‡¶]	
Dexamethasone elixir 0.5 mg/5 mL	Rinse and spit 10 mL qid for 5 min
Diphenhydramine elixir 12.5 mg/5 mL	
Systemic medications[†**]	
Prednisone 5 mg	12 tabs qod × 2 days, decreasing by 2 tabs every other day
Azathioprine 50 mg	1 tab bid

*If extensive gingival lesions are present, use with a custom-fabricated tray.
†Oral candidiasis may result and concomitant antifungal therapy may be necessary.
‡Taper as indicated by clinical response.
§Can be combined in a 1:1 mixture with orabase.
¶Can be combined in a 1:1 mixture with sucralfate, kaopectate, or maalox.
**Dose and duration depend on severity of disease and concomitant systemic diseases. Azathioprine in combination with prednisone permits use of lower doses of prednisone.

The oral mucosal disease with the greatest potential morbidity and mortality is cancer. For example, 2.4% (more than 34 360 cases) of all cancers in 2007 in the United States were in the oral cavity and pharyngeal region, resulting in nearly 8000 deaths per year. The three greatest risk factors for developing oral cancer are age, alcohol, and tobacco use; nearly half of all oral cancers occur in persons older than 65 years of age. The average age at the time of diagnosis is approximately 60 years, and males are more than twice as likely to develop oral cancer as are females. While attempts to diagnose and treat oral cancer have improved in the last 30 years, 5-year survival rates have not improved dramatically, and the average 5-year survival rate is only ~50%.

Neoplasms may arise in all oral soft and hard tissues and in the oropharyngeal and salivary gland regions. The clinical appearance of an oral carcinoma is quite diverse (ulcerative, erythematous, leukoplakic, papillary) and may be innocuous as well as asymptomatic (see Figure 42-6). If a patient presents with an unusual and suspicious lesion with no readily apparent etiology (such as a denture sore), the patient should be referred to a specialist more familiar with the appearance of the oral mucosa. Any oral lesion that does not heal completely in 3 to 4 weeks after removal of suspected etiologies (e.g., ill-fitting denture) should undergo a diagnostic biopsy procedure. Importantly, carcinoma should be considered part of the differential diagnosis of any oral lesion.

The treatment of oral cancers involves oral, head, and neck surgery, radiotherapy, chemotherapy, or a combination of any of these three modalities, depending on the tumor's histopathology and stage. Before receiving definitive therapy, the patient should have a comprehensive oral examination so that focal areas of infection or potential infection (dental caries, periodontal disease, dental–alveolar infections, soft and hard tissues lesions) can be treated before surgery, radiotherapy, or chemotherapy. The patient must be educated about many potential risks: surgery-related sensory, esthetic, and functional problems; radiotherapy-induced mucositis, salivary gland hypofunction, and osteoradionecrosis; and chemotherapy-induced mucositis and immunosuppression.

MOTOR FUNCTION

The oral motor apparatus is involved in several routine yet intricate functions (speech, posture, mastication, and swallowing). Regulation of these activities may occur at three levels: the local neuromuscular unit, central neuronal pathways, and systemic influences. In general, aging is associated with changes in neuromuscular systems. Animal studies strongly suggest that age-associated deficiencies in motor function are not related to the composition and contractile function of skeletal muscles. Instead, these changes probably are related to other factors such as neuromuscular transmission and propagation of nerve impulses.

Studies of oral motor function have shown that some alterations in performance (mastication, swallowing, oral muscular posture, and tone) can be expected with increased age. These changes appear to be more common among predominantly edentulous persons than among those with a natural dentition. The most frequently reported oral motor disturbance in the elderly population is related to altered mastication, and even fully dentate older persons are less able to prepare food adequately for swallowing than are younger individuals. Older persons are more likely to be partially or completely edentulous than are persons in other age groups, and therefore the geriatric population is susceptible to altered chewing. It also has been reported that older persons tend to swallow larger-sized food particles than do younger adults. This suggests that there is a diminution in masticatory efficiency that can be further exacerbated among individuals with a compromised dentition (those with dental caries, periodontitis, missing teeth). Furthermore, older individuals may be more susceptible to aspiration pneumonia resulting from chewing and swallowing problems in addition to periodontal pathogens. In summary, the majority of research findings suggest that dentition, not age per se, has a direct influence on mastication.

After mastication, a food bolus is ready for swallowing. A thorough review of swallowing problems in older people is provided in Chapter 41. Normal aging has minor adverse effects on swallowing, although in a healthy older person, advanced age per se does not appear to cause any clinical dysfunction. However, a host of conditions common in the elderly population will cause clinically significant swallowing deficiencies. Salivary hypofunction (see earlier) impairs swallowing times and under severe conditions increases the likelihood of aspiration. Patients with neuropathies have been reported to have oral swallow times four- to sixfold longer than those in healthy controls, and these persons may not even be able to produce the recognizable characteristics of an oral swallow. Neurovascular conditions (e.g., cerebrovascular accidents, dementia, motor neuron disease) are likely to cause dysphagia and predispose a person to the danger of aspiration. Therefore, swallowing changes in older persons are usually caused by sensory, muscular, and neurologic deterioration.

The temporomandibular joint (TMJ) is located between the glenoid fossa and the condylar process of the mandible, and exhibits a functionally unique gliding and hinge-like movement. It is of particular interest to clinicians, for it is the focus of several craniofacial pain disorders. Using radiographic and postmortem evaluations, several studies have reported that various components of this joint undergo degenerative alterations with increasing age. However, research reports confirm that TMJ functional impairment is not a "normal" age-associated event. Conversely, many oral and systemic conditions commonly seen in the elderly population are linked with temporomandibular disorders (TMD). Orofacial pain in the elderly patient may be a result of a variety of problems of the cranio-mandibular-oral complex and other extraoral diseases, making diagnosis and treatment challenging and frequently requiring a multidisciplinary approach.

In general, two types of pathology are associated with the TMJ: articular, related to the joint itself, and nonarticular, pathology occurring in structures unrelated to the joint but causing similar or referred symptomatology. Several articular abnormalities common to all joints also affect the TMJ, including trauma, ankylosis, dislocation, and arthritis. Nonarticular disorders may result from a variety of clinical entities, including trigeminal neuralgia, headache, migraine, otitis, dental–alveolar pain/infection, and masticatory myalgia. Orofacial habits (e.g., jaw clenching and tooth grinding) and poor head and neck posture can produce muscle fatigue and subsequent spasm. Moreover, psychological conditions (stress and depression) can exacerbate underlying articular and nonarticular disorders. Clinically, the patient will present with pain in many regions: TMJ, temporal, cervical, or neck region, masticatory muscles, and the oral cavity. Diagnosis is also challenging since symptoms may occur primarily in any of these sites with regular, irregular, or no pain referred to the

TMJ region. Limited jaw opening (less than 40 mm from the maxillary central incisor to the mandibular central incisor) and pain on mastication or during jaw movements may be indicative of TMD. Treatment, as with other arthritic or muscular disorders, requires the elucidation of an appropriate diagnosis and ranges from conservative and reversible regimens (anti-inflammatories, analgesics, muscle relaxants, physical therapy, oral bite splints) to more invasive procedures for unresolved painful conditions (e.g., TMJ surgery).

The National Health Interview Survey indicates that older adults report considerable amounts of orofacial and TMJ pain. The estimated prevalence rates among adults 75 years and older were 1.2% for burning mouth pain, 1.6% for face pain, 3.4% for toothache, 3.9% for jaw joint pain, and 6.2% for oral sores. While toothaches, oral sores, and jaw joint pain decreased with age, face pain was age-independent, and burning mouth pain increased with age. Interestingly, similarly aged adults are approximately five times more likely to visit a physician than a dentist in a year. This finding suggests that people may be more likely to visit a physician even for orofacial problems and/or that a considerable number of older adults may not seek stomatological treatment from dentists for their pain.

Speech production is another function subserved by the oral structures, and it undergoes some changes with increasing age, including significant alterations in activities such as tongue shape and function during specific phoneme production and frequency variability. However, among healthy older persons, these changes do not compromise or alter speech in any perceptible way. Tongue strength undergoes decreases with age, even among healthy adults, yet tongue endurance is similar between younger and older persons. There are also age-associated alterations in intraoral and maxillofacial posture. Drooping of the lower face and lips in the elderly person results not only from the loss of supporting hard tissues, but also from a diminished tone of the circumoral muscles. The latter changes may elicit esthetic concerns and can lead to embarrassment from drooling or food spills caused by the inability of an older individual to close the lips competently while eating or speaking. Often, drooling caused by reduced circumoral muscle tone can result in complaints of excess salivation.

Significant oral motor disorders also may result from a number of therapeutic drug regimens, such as the frequent association of tardive dyskinesia with phenothiazine therapy. These dyskinesias may include diminished performance and speech pathoses as well as alteration in movement (chorea, athetosis).

SUMMARY

The health of the oral cavity and its ability to fulfill its function of communication, nutritional intake, and host protection can be impaired in older adults. Age alone does not appear to play a strong role in the impairments. Instead, oral and systemic conditions and their treatments with drugs, chemotherapy, and radiation compromise oral health and function. This will predispose an older person to develop oral microbial infections including dental caries and periodontal diseases, pain, salivary hypofunction, altered chemosensation, dysphagia, difficulty chewing and speaking, greater risk for disseminated systemic infections, and, importantly, a diminished quality of life. All health care providers should attempt to identify older persons at risk for developing oral diseases, be able to recognize existing oral diseases, and either treat or refer patients who have stomatological disorders.

FURTHER READING

Anusavice KJ. Dental caries: risk assessment and treatment solutions for an elderly population. *Compend Contin Educ Dent.* 2002;23(10 Suppl):12–20.

Atkinson JC, Grisius M, Massey W. Salivary hypofunction and xerostomia: diagnosis and treatment. *Dent Clin North Am.* 2005;49(2):309–326.

Chavez EM, Ship JA. Sensory and motor deficits in the elderly: impact on oral health. *J Public Health Dentistry.* 2000;60(4):297–303.

Ciancio SG. Medications: a risk factor for periodontal disease diagnosis and treatment. *J Periodontol.* 2005;76(11 Suppl):2061–2065.

Ettinger RL. The unique oral health needs of an aging population. *Dent Clin North Am.* 1997;41(4):633–649.

Ghezzi EM, Ship JA. Systemic diseases and their treatments in the elderly: impact on oral health. *J Public Health Dentistry.* 2000;60(4):289–296.

Greenberg MS, Glick M, Ship JA. *Burket's Oral Medicine: Diagnosis and Treatment.* 11th ed. Hamilton, Ontario: BC Decker; 2007.

Migliorati CA, Siegel MA, Elting LS. Bisphosphonate-associated osteonecrosis: a long-term complication of bisphosphonate treatment. *Lancet Oncol.* 2006;7(6):508–514.

Mioche L, Bourdiol P, Monier S, Martin JF, Cormier D. Changes in jaw muscles activity with age: effects on food bolus properties. *Physiol Behav.* 2004;82(4):621–627.

Musacchio E, Perissinotto E, Binotto P, et al. Tooth loss in the elderly and its association with nutritional status, socio-economic and lifestyle factors. *Acta Odontol Scand.* 2007;65(2):78–86.

Ship JA, Heft M, Harkins S. Oral facial pain in the elderly. In: Lomranz J, Mostofsky DI, eds. *Handbook of Pain and Aging.* New York, New York: Plenum Press; 1997: 321–346.

Ship JA, Pillemer SR, Baum BJ. Xerostomia and the geriatric patient. *J Am Geriatr Soc.* 2002;50(3):535–543.

Ship JA. *Clinician's Guide to Oral Health in Geriatric Patients.* 2nd ed. Hamilton, Ontorio: BC Decker; 2005.

Silverman S. *Oral Cancer.* 5th ed. Lewiston, NY: BC Decker; 2002.

Spielman AI, Ship JA. Taste and smell. In: Miles TS, Nauntofte B, Svensson P, eds. *Clinical Oral Physiology.* Copenhagen: Quintessence Publishing Co. Ltd; 2004:53–70.

Squier CA, Hill MW. *The Effect of Aging in Oral Mucosa and Skin.* Boca Raton, FL: CRC Press; 1994.

Terpenning M. Geriatric oral health and pneumonia risk. *Clin Infect Dis.* 2005;40(12):1807–1810.

Walls AW, Steele JG. The relationship between oral health and nutrition in older people. *Mech Ageing Dev.* 2004;125(12):853–857.

Yoshikawa M, Yoshida M, Nagasaki T, et al. Aspects of swallowing in healthy dentate elderly persons older than 80 years. *J Gerontol A Biol Sci Med Sci.* 2005;60(4): 506–509.

Assessment and Rehabilitation of Older Adults with Low Vision

Gale R. Watson

DEMOGRAPHICS

Many large, population-based, cross-sectional studies have documented the increase in prevalence of eye disease and visual impairment with increasing age, particularly in persons over the age of 75 years. U.S. population estimates indicate that more than 26 million people over the age of 40 years are affected with some type of visual disorder and that more than 4 million individuals in the U.S. aged 55 years or older are currently experiencing severe vision loss.

Estimates of the prevalence of visual impairment per 1000 persons in the United States demonstrate the significant increase in vision problems with age. A 2001 study estimated that 14% of persons aged 70 to 74 years have serious difficulty seeing, even with their spectacle correction, and this increases to 32% among persons aged 85 years or older. Centers for Disease Control and Prevention (CDC) and the National Centers for Health Statistics (NCHS) estimate the prevalence of severe visual impairment among persons 70 to 74 years of age at about 1% of the elderly population, but by age 85 years, nearly 2.5% of persons are severely visually impaired. After age 85 years, one in four older people cannot read a newspaper even with best-corrected vision.

Age-related visual impairment is not only challenging to the person in whom it develops, but also affects society as a whole. Medicare beneficiaries with coded diagnoses of vision loss have been shown to incur an additional $2.14 billion in 2003 in noneye-related medical costs, incurring significantly higher costs than those with normal vision. Additional eye-related costs per patient yearly are approximately $345 for those with moderate vision loss, $407 for those with severe vision loss, and $237 for those who are blind. Additional noneye-related costs per patient yearly are $2193, $3301, and $4443, respectively. Prevent Blindness America, a national volunteer eye health and safety organization, puts the medical loss for visual impairment at $5.48 billion for persons 40 years and older. Their number includes increased medical expenditures, as well as increased informal care days. They define informal care as unpaid care provided by people not living with the older person, and valued it according to minimum wage dollars. Health utility (distress, pain, depression, lack of mobility, social limitations) was converted into quality-adjusted life years and the total lost value for this factor was $10.5 billion. Thus, preventing vision loss among older persons is not only a medical imperative, but also an economic one.

Vision loss is reason enough for a decline in function among older persons, but vision loss has also been associated with cognitive decline, heart disease, arthritis, hypertension, falls and hip fracture, depression, reduced overall quality of life and mortality. Older visually impaired persons are twice as likely to have difficulty walking as do sighted peers, three times more likely to have difficulty getting outside, more than twice as likely to have difficulty getting in and out of a bed/chair, and three times more likely to have difficulty preparing a meal.

The most prevalent age-related causes of visual impairment in the United States are macular degeneration, diabetic retinopathy, glaucoma, and cataract. Approximately 60% of persons with visual impairments who are not institutionalized have one or more additional impairments. These include the loss of hearing, impaired mobility, decreased energy and stamina from respiratory and heart disease, and cognitive changes resulting from stroke or dementia. Vision loss has been ranked third, behind arthritis and heart disease, among the most common chronic conditions causing older persons to require assistance with activities of daily living (ADLs). Because the majority of people with visual impairments have useful vision, rehabilitation services and vision-enhancing techniques and devices offer opportunities to increase their visual and general functional capacity.

AGING AND LOSS OF VISION

Normal Age-Related Changes in Vision

Every older person experiences age-related changes in vision. Table 43-1 summarizes the age-related changes that cause functional declines for older persons. Decreased transmission of the ocular media, increased scatter in the cornea, lens, vitreous body, and retina as well as decreased pupil size are related to anatomic changes in the aging eye. The age-related changes discussed here are those that have the greatest impact on function in daily life. These common changes in vision function must be taken in account when considering the daily living, quality of life, and the design of facilities for all older persons.

The ability to accommodate for focus on visual targets from distance to near, which is dependent on a flexible crystalline lens and the ciliary muscle, is altered with age, beginning around age 45 years. During this change, an increasing amount of plus in a concave lens (usually prescribed in bifocal lenses or reading glasses) is required to boost the focusing power of the eye to compensate for the loss in refracting ability of the lens for near tasks.

The visual acuity of normally sighted older persons shows only a modest decrease under high-contrast conditions, but reducing the illumination of an acuity chart, reducing the contrast of the acuity chart, and/or adding surrounding glare, produces drastic age-related acuity losses, as compared to young observers. For example, in a sample of 900 older observers, for those at age 82 years, the median high-contrast visual acuity was 20/30, low-contrast high-luminance acuity was 20/55, low-contrast, low-luminance acuity was 20/120, and low-contrast acuity in glare conditions was 20/160. A young observer loses only about one line of acuity under similar conditions.

Because of anatomic changes in the eye and media, older persons are more sensitive to glare in the environment, more likely to experience disabling glare, and have reduced glare recovery time. This may have the most impact on activities such as walking outdoors or driving, but may also affect indoor activities as well, if very bright and dim environments are adjacent, such as restaurants, movie theaters, and atriums. Visual discomfort may arise because of glare, and disabling glare may hide important targets that must be viewed for the sake of safety. Glare sensitivity has been associated with motor vehicle accidents for older drivers.

Attentional visual field, the visual field area over which one can process rapidly presented visual information, declines with age. Unlike conventional measures of visual field that assess visual sensory sensitivity (such as static flashing lights), attentional visual field relies on higher-order processing skills such as selective and divided attention and rapid processing speed. Decreased attentional visual

TABLE 43-1

Normal Age-Related Changes in Vision

CHANGES	REASON	IMPLICATIONS FOR DAILY LIFE
Loss of accommodation	• Crystalline lenses lose flexibility • Ciliary muscles lose tone	Increasing inability to focus on close targets beginning around age 45 yrs. Plus lenses prescribed in a bifocal, reading glasses, or contact lenses; required to compensate for loss of accommodative ability.
Loss of low-contrast acuity	• Decreased transmission of ocular media • Decreased pupil size	Functional loss of acuity under glare or low lighting may cause small targets to be missed, bumping or tripping into low-lying objects.
Increased sensitivity to glare	• Increased light scatter in cornea, lenses, vitreous body, and retina	Discomfort even in low glare conditions such as cloudy days. High glare causes decreased acuity and difficulty in seeing targets in the environment. Sun lenses, hats, visors, and umbrellas provide more comfort outdoors; tinted lenses may be prescribed for indoors.
Increased difficulty with dark adaptation	• Losses in ocular transmittance and papillary miosis	Difficulty moving from bright to dim environments. Risk for stumbling or falling is greater under these circumstances. Fear of balance problems or falling may cause compensatory behaviors such as shuffling, reaching for hand-holds, etc. Change environmental lighting to avoid light/dim areas.
Loss of color discrimination	• Smaller pupil diameter, reduced light transmission through the lens, changes in photoreceptors and neural pathways	Difficulty detecting differences in dark colors and pastels; adding lamps or identifying matching colors near a sunny window helps.
Loss of attentional visual field	• Decline of higher order visual processes such as selective and divided attention and rapid processing speed	Risk factor for balance and mobility problems and vehicle crashes in driving. Training improves performance.
Increased difficulty with visual reading ability	• Related to attentional visual field and low contrast acuity and slower saccadic performance in eye movements.	Reading speed of older readers reduced by one-third that of younger readers; text navigation skills decline with age. Training improves performance.

field has been correlated to a greater incidence of driving accidents and is related to a greater risk for balance and mobility problems for normally sighted older persons. Attentional visual field can be improved with training, but such training is not widely available.

Visual reading ability decreases with age as well. The reading rate of older persons who are normally sighted and have good high-contrast visual acuity decreases by as much as a third of that of young readers. Accuracy of reading, however, can remain comparable to that of younger readers. Reading performance among older persons with good acuity (20/30) is highly correlated with attentional visual field; those with good reading performance into very old age also retain good attentional fields as well. Low-contrast visual acuity is also correlated with reading performance for this population; older persons with poor low-contrast acuity tend to read more slowly. Even when high-contrast acuity is good, older persons, especially the oldest old, are at risk for reading difficulties that may arise from a combination of reduced attentional visual field, slower saccadic performance in eye movements, and poor low-contrast visual acuity. Reading rate for normally sighted older adults with good high-contrast acuity and good comprehension skills can be improved with training. Training in reading efficiency that emphasizes improvements in eye movements for reading similar to those exercises used to improve reading for school children has given good results for this population. Such training, however, is not widely available.

Color discrimination is another aspect of vision that declines with advancing age. Persons who are older have greater difficulty detecting differences between dark colors such as brown, black, or navy, and also have difficulty with pastels. Loss of color vision in old age is related to smaller pupil diameter, reduced light transmission through the lens, and changes in photoreceptors and neural pathways.

Dark adaptation declines as a result of losses in ocular transmittance and pupillary miosis resulting from the aging process. Difficulty with dark adaptation can be limiting to older adults moving from light to dim environments and vice versa. The risk for stumbling or falling may be greater under these circumstances. The normally sighted older person may function as if severely visually impaired when first adjusted to a drastic change in illumination.

Although not related to a change in vision per se, care must be taken in providing refractive correction in spectacle form for geriatric patients. Multifocal spectacle lenses either in the form of bifocals or varifocals are commonly prescribed but are associated with a higher risk of "edge of step" accidents, and multifocal lens wearers are twice as likely to fall as single focus lens wearers. A large percentage of these falls are reported to occur outside the home, perhaps as a result of tripping or stumbling resulting from obstacles not seen in the near vision correction of the lower visual field. The bifocal portion of a spectacle correction provides additional dioptric power to provide vision at near distance for reading, etc. This means that objects outside this near-focal range such as steps, curbs, stairs, house cats, etc. are blurred and indistinct. This effect is greatest in older patients, as the need for extra dioptric power for near vision increases with age. Patients with multifocal correction are encouraged to tuck their chins and look over the top of the bifocal correction when moving so that they can look through the distance correction in the upper portion of the lenses, but head flexion significantly increases postural instability. Encouraging those who are at risk for falling to explore these issues with their eye care specialists can be an important aspect of falls prevention.

PREVALENT AGE-RELATED CAUSES OF VISUAL IMPAIRMENT

Age-Related Macular Degeneration

Functional vision loss because of age-related macular degeneration may include metamorphopsia (visual images appear distorted and wavy), relative scotomas, and result in dense central scotomas for those whose pathology progresses to visual impairment. Individuals with central scotoma usually develop a strongly preferred retinal locus (PRL) that performs as the primary fixation reference, although the patient may not always be aware that there is a scotoma present. The loss of central visual field results in loss of visual acuity and contrast sensitivity. The ability to use the PRL that develops for fixation may be difficult for many persons. The effects of macular degeneration on daily life include difficulty with reading print, inability to recognize faces (that can lead to reluctance to participate in social activities), difficulty with distance and depth cues (that adversely affect safe mobility), and loss of color and contrast sensitivity (that interfere with a variety of household and work/leisure tasks) (Table 43-2).

Diabetic Retinopathy

The progression of diabetic retinopathy includes macular edema that may cause blurred vision if the fovea is involved, retinal hemorrhages (and/or laser treatments), which may result in scattered central, peripheral, and/or midperipheral scotomas, and retinal detachment, which can cause larger areas of field loss if not reattached. Diabetic retinopathy can progress to total blindness. Loss of function can include decreased visual acuity, scattered field loss over the retina, metamorphopsia across the retina, increased sensitivity to glare, and loss of color and contrast sensitivity. If the fovea is lost to scotoma, then a PRL will develop. Vision fluctuations can be manifested over time as macular swelling increases or subsides, and can also be related to hemorrhage. Sudden vision loss is common following hemorrhage, with the patient describing episodes of smoky vision, a dropped veil over the eye(s), or seeing black or red strings across the field of view. Treatment and absorption of blood can improve acuity, though not usually to normal levels. The effects on daily life include difficulty reading print materials, difficulty recognizing faces, increased sensitivity to glare and light/dark adaptation, difficulty with distance and depth cues, loss of color and contrast sensitivity, and fluctuating vision.

Cataract

Age-related cataract is manifested by gradual opacity of the lens, which interferes with the passage of light, causing reduced visual acuity, light scatter, sensitivity to glare, altered color perception, and image distortion (straight lines appear wavy). Persons with cataracts may experience trouble with glare and loss of contrast, may have decreased acuity, and report areas of metamorphopsia or small scotomas in the visual field. When the cataract has begun to interfere with lifestyle, surgery may be performed to remove either the entire lens or the posterior portion. Correction for the removal of the lens

TABLE 43-2

Age-Related Causes of Visual Impairment

CONDITION	COMMON CLINICAL PRESENTATION	IMPLICATIONS FOR REHABILITATION
Macular degeneration	• Reduced visual acuity • Loss of central visual field and contrast sensitivity	Difficulty with tasks requiring fine detail vision such as reading, inability to recognize faces, distortion or disappearance of the visual field straight ahead, loss of color and contrast perception, mobility difficulties related to loss of depth and contrast cues.
Diabetic retinopathy	• Reduced visual acuity • Scattered central scotomas • Peripheral and midpheripheral scotomas • Macular edema	Difficulty with tasks requiring fine detail vision such as reading, distorted central vision, fluctuating vision, loss of color perception, mobility problems because of loss of depth and contrast cues.
Cataract	• Reduced visual acuity • Light scatter • Sensitivity to glare • Altered color perception • Loss of contrast sensitivity • Image distortion • Possible myopia	Usually remedied by lens extraction and implant, except in extreme cases. If not managed by implant, difficulty with detail vision, difficulty with bright and changing light, color perception, decreased contrast perception, some mobility problems caused by loss of perception of depth and distance, sensitivity to glare, and loss of contrast.
Glaucoma	• Degeneration of optic disk • Loss of peripheral visual fields	Mobility and reading problems because of restricted visual fields, people suddenly appearing in the visual field seen as "jack in the box."
Traumatic Brain Injury	• Loss of hemi/quadrant visual field, or paracentral scotoma • Possible visual neglect • Visual perceptual difficulties • Visual agnosia	Mobility and reading problems owing to visual field loss and spatial perceptual difficulties that reduce ability to drive, reach correctly, and execute eye movements related to reading, difficulty with visual and cognitive processing. Visual neglect may include inability to complete shaving and/or dressing. Difficulty completing other rehabilitation assessments and interventions because of neglected visual impairment.

is provided through intraocular lens implants, eyeglasses, or contact lens. Cataract surgery is the most common major surgical procedure done for persons older than age 65 years who are receiving Medicare. Cataract surgery with lens implantation is associated with improved objective and subjective measures of function in ADL, as well as improved levels of vision to normal acuity in most cases.

Glaucoma

Glaucoma is an increase in intraocular pressure caused by an abnormality in flow of aqueous fluid from the anterior chamber. It can cause a degeneration of the optic disk, loss of visual fields, and severe visual impairment. When left untreated, or if treatment is not successful, glaucoma results in a loss of peripheral fields and can lead to blindness. The effect of peripheral field loss on daily life is most problematic in safe ambulation. Because of field restrictions, the patients may not see objects in their path and may bump into objects that fall outside the field of view in any direction (street signs, tree branches, etc.). In addition, a person outside the patient's field of view may suddenly be seen as a "jack-in-the-box" and create a startle effect. Peripheral field loss may also create problems in reading and writing as only a small portion of the page can be seen at once.

Traumatic Brain Injury

Head injury to older adults such as cerebrovascular accident, falls, or automobile accidents resulting in traumatic brain injury can lead to visual impairment. Between 20% and 40% of stroke results in visual disorder that can inhibit cognitive functioning and may reduce the effectiveness of rehabilitation of traumatic brain injury. Visual field disorders can result from injury to the visual pathway anyway between the retina and the striate cortex. The optic chiasm is used as an anatomical landmark to differentiate between the peripheral (prechiasmatic) and the central (postchiasmatic) visual pathway. Unilateral injury to the prechiasmatic pathway affects the ipsilesional field only, but postchasmatic injury causes visual deficits in both monocular hemifields and are referred to as homonymous. Visual field disorders must be discerned by visual field measurement techniques called perimetry; patients are often unaware of them and do not report the defect, but may suffer from their effects, for example, bumping into objects, tripping, falling, being unable to read, etc. Vision can be completely lost in the missing field, or some vision function (for example, light detection) may remain. The most common visual field losses are hemianopsia (loss of half the visual field), followed by quadranopsia (loss of one quadrant) and paracentral scotoma (island of vision loss in the parafoveal region), and rarely results in central scotoma. Recovery of some visual field following injury may be spontaneous, and some patients learn spontaneously to adapt to visual field loss by oculomotor strategies; shifting gaze may reveal what is missing in the field of view of a street scene (such as an oncoming car) or the missing portion of a line of text. Systematic training in oculomotor adaptation and visual perceptual training can improve vision function and has limited ability to improve the visual field. Visual field loss may also be accompanied by visual neglect. Older adults with neglect may not spontaneously be able to attend to the neglected side. Traumatic Brain Injury (TBI) may also result in disorders of visual space perception, which affect reach (over- or underreaching for objects, knocking things over), driving (accidents resulting from inability to judge distance and depth), and reading (inability to plan and execute accurate eye movements). Visuospatial localization and orientation may be improved through training, but may not reach pre-TBI thresholds. Visual agnosia, a failure to visually recognize an object because of "mistaken identity," is a disorder that is based in both visual-perceptual and visual-cognitive functions.

Typically, misidentifications result from the incomplete or inappropriate use of object features such as size, shape, or color. Older adults with TBI may be unaware that they are ignoring other features that might assist with correct identification. Cognitive and/or communication disorders can make visual impairment more difficult to detect following TBI. Undetected or untreated visual impairment in TBI can limit the effectiveness of other rehabilitation (e.g., many cognitive and functional assessments use visual items that cannot be appropriately identified by older persons with TBI-related vision loss, visual motor assessments require eye–hand coordination). If TBI vision loss is not detected and treated to the extent possible, the examiner or therapist may get a false-negative impression of the level of TBI disability. In addition, the TBI patient will be frustrated and troubled unduly by participating in rehabilitation that does not simultaneously address the vision deficit.

ROLE OF THE GERIATRICIAN IN VISION REHABILITATION

After diagnosis and medical management of the patient's vision loss by an ophthalmologist, the geriatrician can play an important role in assuring that visually impaired persons receive rehabilitation services that are of high quality, are sought in a timely manner, and provide all the benefit that the patient might be able to derive from them.

A geriatrician can provide the following services for their patients related to vision rehabilitation:

1. A visual acuity evaluation. Current best practice includes the use of a logarithmic visual acuity chart.

2. A contrast sensitivity function evaluation. The Pelli–Robson chart is recommended for its ease of use and reliability.

3. A referral to a low-vision eye care specialist (ophthalmologist or optometrist) for the appropriate clinical low-vision evaluation and prescription of optical low vision devices for tasks the older person can no longer perform such as reading, writing, watching television, and recognizing street signs.

4. A referral to vision rehabilitation professionals for assessment and instruction of vision and magnification devices for literacy, ADLs, and safe travel. These therapists can also provide environmental analyses and teach the use of environmental cues.

5. Assistance to patients in preparing for rehabilitation by providing information and encouraging them to consider the goals they would like to achieve. The National Eye Institute: Visual Functioning Questionnaire-14 is a modified 14-item questionnaire that is effective in assessing the impact of vision loss on quality of life and is helpful in assisting patients in setting goals for rehabilitation.

6. Counseling or referral for coping with psychosocial issues related to visual impairment. Patients may not be forthcoming about these issues, so the physician must ask. Adjustment disorder and depression are associated with visual impairment for older persons. When patients are dealing with loss of independence and control, lowered self-esteem and strained social relations, counseling and/or psychotherapy may be recommended for both patients and family members.

7. Reinforcement of simple strategies, such as the use of saturated colors and contrast in the home environment, and the use of simple devices, such as sun lenses outdoors and brighter indoor environments.

8. Information to the patient and family about the variable nature of low vision, its effect on daily life tasks, and the variable nature of visual abilities according to fluctuations of light and contrast.

9. Sponsorship of, or referral to, support groups where older persons with vision loss and their families can discuss problems, coping, and rehabilitation strategies they have learned with other patients.

10. Assistance in community awareness efforts about the prevalence, treatment, and rehabilitation of visual impairment among older persons.

Patients likely to benefit from vision rehabilitation include those with reduced acuity of less than 20/50 in the better-seeing eye, central or peripheral field loss with intact visual acuity, reduced contrast sensitivity, glare sensitivity, and/or light/dark adaptation difficulties as well as those with traumatic brain injury. Candidates for cataract surgery with macular disease might also benefit from preoperative low-vision assessment and coincident rehabilitation training that enhances postoperative visual performance and satisfaction with a cataract procedure.

ADAPTATIONS OF CLINICAL AND FUNCTIONAL EVALUATIONS FOR OLDER ADULTS

The clinical and functional low-vision examinations for older persons should distinguish aging from treatable disease processes; focus holistically; be multidisciplinary and incorporate family and caregiver support; and identify and set realistic goals to improve functional status and quality of life.

In health care service, delivery to older adults with low vision, certain aspects of the examination sequence is adapted to accommodate these principles.

Case History Interview

Because most age-related visual impairments result in a central scotoma, most patient complaints will be related to the loss of acuity, loss of central visual field, and resultant decrease in contrast sensitivity and color sensitivity. Patient goals for rehabilitation will usually include reading, writing, ADLs such as meal preparation and household maintenance, management of glare and other illumination concerns, leisure activities, and safe independent movement and travel. If older persons also have specific health-related activities that require the use of vision (e.g. loading a syringe with insulin, changing an ostomy bag), these will be goals as well.

This information may be taken by a preexamination telephone interview to lessen the amount of time a first visit might require. Because low-vision rehabilitation requires a great deal of energy and motivation from the patient, it will be guided by their personal goals for rehabilitation and by those tasks that are difficult or impossible to perform because of low vision. In this regard, the intake interviewer may find that some education is necessary in order to set reasonable goals for low-vision treatment. Because most low-vision interventions are "task-specific," it is important to state treatment goals as specifically as possible.

Because of the nature of the older person's vision loss, professionals should become familiar with some of the courtesies and accessibility issues that assist in providing quality health care. Unless there is a problem with the person's hearing, always speak directly to the older adult with visual impairment. Allow the older adult to take your arm when moving from place to place in the environment, and use appropriate sighted guide techniques. If you are guiding a person with visual impairment on your arm, you are responsible for assuring that the path you are taking is wide enough to accommodate both of you. If the path is not wide enough (e.g. a crowded hallway), ask the person to step behind you, while still holding your arm with his other hand when walking. Say your name when first coming into the room, and tell the older adult when you are leaving the room. Do not leave the older adult with low vision standing alone in a hallway or room without a wall or furniture near to touch for orientation and balance. Avoid using directional cues that are visual in nature such as pointing or giving directional references that are unclear to those with low vision. For example, instead of saying, "take that chair over there," say, "take the red chair against the white wall to your immediate right."

Clinical Low-Vision Evaluation

The low-vision eye care specialist (who may be an ophthalmologist or an optometrist) must be flexible and adaptable to a variety of different environments, schedules, and communication styles. The conventional pattern of the low-vision examination will be followed including distance and near acuities; internal and external ocular health examination; retinoscopy; tonometry and slit-lamp biomicroscopy; ophthalmoscopy; ophthalmometry; determination of central and peripheral fields; color vision and contrast-sensitivity testing; glare testing; and near and distance testing of vision-enhancing devices, including optical, electronic, and nonoptical devices. For many older adults, especially those in long-term care facilities, a careful refraction and updating conventional spectacles may provide significant improvement in vision. Table 43-3 summarizes the aspects of the clinical low-vision examination.

Because of the nature of medical and long-term care service delivery to older adults, it is often necessary to take the low-vision examination and therapeutic intervention out of the office or clinical setting. There is a growing trend of providing low-vision services as a part of outpatient hospital care, comprehensive outpatient rehabilitation facilities, and long-term care facilities, such as nursing homes and private homes of older adults.

Nursing Homes

Despite the fact that an estimated 26% of persons in nursing homes have visual impairment, few nursing home residents receive low-vision care. For example, one study estimated only 25% of visually impaired patients at a long-term care facility who were in need of vision rehabilitation were referred by their attending ophthalmologists. Another study found that there was no difference in the referral rate for vision services for nursing home residents between those who complained about their vision and those who did not. Another study found that only 11% of all residents in 19 nursing homes had received eye examinations in the last 2 years. Providing information about vision and vision impairment to the nursing home staff is important for assisting residents in using their remaining vision effectively. Because stroke is another common medical condition requiring rehabilitation for older adults, it is important that the low-vision team work closely with those professionals who diagnose, treat, and rehabilitate older adults who have experienced cerebrovascular accident. A curriculum in low vision for in-service training for long-term care staff has been developed and is effective in increasing staff knowledge and positive outcomes for patients.

Hospital Settings

Low-vision care is routinely provided to older veterans in the hospital system of the Veterans Health Administration. In the Blind Rehabilitation Centers, the veteran who is legally blind is seen for up to 10 weeks of rehabilitation, including low vision rehabilitation. Preliminary results from a national outcomes study indicate positive outcomes and veteran satisfaction from these programs. The Veterens Health Administration (VHA) also provides low-vision services to veterans who have low vision but who are not legally blind. Recently, the VHA has expanded low-vision services and provided an additional $40 million in funding for clinical vision rehabilitation services closer to veterans' homes. Outcome studies of all VA vision rehabilitation services indicate that veterans who are provided low-vision services regain their ability to perform independent activities of daily living (IADLs) independently and become active community participants. Hospitals in the private sector are increasing services to older persons as a part of outpatient services, and low-vision rehabilitation is often provided.

Community Service Agency Settings

The Older Americans Act mandates the provision of supportive community resources for older adults. Some examples of community agency settings include senior centers, nutrition centers, senior clubs, adult daycare centers, and senior rehabilitation centers. These services may be contacted through the local telephone book yellow pages. For example, in Atlanta, the services are clustered in the BellSouth Yellow Pages under the heading, "Senior Services." The explanation of the local county services contracts is provided and a

TABLE 43-3

Clinical Low Vision Examination	
Settings	• Long-term care facilities
	• Individual's home
	• Community service agency
	• Rehabilitation center
Aspects of the examination	• Distance/near acuities
	• Internal/external health exam
	• Retinoscopy
	• Tonometry
	• Slit-lamp biomicroscopy
	• Ophthalmoscopy
	• Ophthalmometry
	• Central/peripheral fields
	• Color vision testing
	• Contrast-sensitivity testing
	• Evaluation of low vision
	• Devices (optical, nonoptical, and electronic)

contact number for each county is listed. Low-vision services might be provided onsite at these community service settings because of the prevalence of visual impairment among older adults.

Private Home Settings

Approximately 70% of the older population requiring long-term care reside in the community. Senior residential retirement centers have increased in number. Most frail older persons requiring care are living at home with family members, and not in long-term care facilities. Interactions with family members and caregivers become very important in these situations. It is crucial that family members and caregivers understand the sometimes contradictory nature of visual impairment; for example, visual performance varies widely under different levels of illumination and can decline if the older person is fatigued. Comorbid conditions such as dementia, mobility impairment, depression, etc. can affect how the older person uses vision or interprets visual images. Understanding the interaction of these factors will help the family in supporting the older adult achieve their goals for vision rehabilitation.

Functional Visual Assessment

Whenever possible, the functional assessment should take place in the older adult's daily environment. Specific goals stated by the older adult will guide the functional assessment to discover what visual target size, target distance, and visual skills are required to achieve that goal. For example, if the patient's goal is to read the newspaper again, the target size requires approximately 20/40 or better visual acuity with magnification, the target distance will be determined by the magnification device, and the visual skills required are precise fixation and saccades while maintaining the focal distance of the magnification device. The functional assessment can also uncover the need to address other goals, the need for environmental assessment and modification, and provide ongoing opportunities to educate the older adult and their significant others about vision and rehabilitation. Table 43-4 presents the key aspects of the functional vision assessment.

The functional low-vision assessment may be completed by a wide variety of rehabilitation professionals. Traditionally, the functional low-vision assessment of older persons has been provided by a low-vision therapist, a rehabilitation teacher for the visually impaired, an orientation and mobility specialist, or some other professional from the field of visual impairment. Now, as low vision is increasingly a part of hospital services and comprehensive outpatient rehabilitation facilities, the functional assessment may be provided by a rehabilitation nurse, an occupational therapist, or some other rehabilitation professional who has received specialized training in low vision.

Regardless of the background of the rehabilitation professionals, they should be well versed and experienced in basic optics of the eye, lenses and low-vision devices, methods of observation and evaluation of visual skills for all ADLs, the causes and functional implications of visual impairments, basic techniques of sighted guide and orientation and mobility, assessment of reading, assessment of the environment, and basic techniques of assessing and using technology such as low-vision devices (e.g., magnifiers, spectacles, monoculars) and electronic devices (e.g., Braille writer, Kurzweil reader, closed-circuit television system [CCTV]). The rehabilitation professional providing the evaluation may also be the rehabilitation therapist,

TABLE 43-4

Key Aspects of the Functional Visual Assessment

Functional visual acuities	Distance and lighting required for discriminating detail of objects in the environment
Functional visual fields	Ability to perceive objects in the environment in central and peripheral quadrants of the visual field at near and distance
Color/contrast discrimination	Ability to detect objects, their color, and contrast with the background at varying distances
Ocular motor skills	Ability to maintain fixation and move the eyes/head/body to fixate, scan, track, and localize targets in the environment
Visual perceptual skills	Ability to make sense of what is seen; recognize critical features, perceive part-to-whole relationships, figure-ground, etc.
Lighting	Analysis of the usefulness of environmental lighting; need for illumination and control
Use of visual and nonvisual cues	Availability and use of visual and nonvisual cues in the environment for task performance
Performance of activities of daily living and instrumental activities of daily living that are affected by vision	Observe for ability to perform, ease and speed of performance, comfort and stress level, safety

in which case they must be familiar with techniques of instructing visual–motor skills for all ADLs and IADL with and without low-vision and electronic devices, task analysis, teaching basic orientation and mobility, and teaching basic techniques of reading and writing with low-vision devices. The professional must also be familiar with tools and techniques that do not require the use of vision in order to assist the older person with low vision in developing other mechanisms for performance when using vision is not the safest or most efficient mechanism (e.g., slate and stylus that are used for writing Braille). This rehabilitation professional will work closely with the eye care specialist providing the clinical low-vision examination, and the low-vision team may also include a counseling professional and any other professionals who are providing care associated with the use of vision. Because many older persons are at risk for multiple impairments, this team may also include other physicians, such as a geriatrician or physiatrist, orthopedist, speech, physical, respiratory, and recreational therapists, other nurses, and technicians.

MANAGEMENT OF LOW VISION

Developing a Vision Rehabilitation Plan

The clinical low-vision examination and functional visual assessment culminates in a vision *rehabilitation plan* that summarizes the information obtained in the evaluations into clearly stated goals and objectives. If Medicare is funding the low-vision services, the plan will follow that format and requirements. In many cases, family members also may be involved. The implementation of the vision rehabilitation plan should emphasize a process using the principles of andragogy, or adult learning, that incorporate the older person's values, beliefs, attitudes, and life experiences.

Following the clinical examination and functional assessment, the low-vision team will recommend low-vision devices (including optical, electronic, nonoptical, and environmental modifications) that will be evaluated to assess their usefulness to the older adult. There should be additional focus on the rehabilitation program and its adaptation for older individuals. Successful use of low-vision devices is related to the intensity of the instructional program. Research shows that specialized therapy in the use of visual skills and low-vision devices improves the abilities of low-vision individuals who are older to a greater extent than do the services provided by eye care specialists alone.

Instruction and Guided Practice Using Remaining Vision and Low-Vision Devices

Working with a low-vision therapist will provide an opportunity for the older adult to develop the appropriate visual skills, as well as learn the benefits, limitations, and uses of low-vision devices, and apply principles of color, illumination, and contrast that make the environment as conducive as possible to the use of remaining vision. It is important to assist caregivers in understanding how remaining vision and low-vision devices aid the older adult in accomplishing visual tasks. Family members and caregivers can provide important social support in this regard, but must understand the process in order to be most helpful. In a study of visually impaired older veterans, a supportive caregiver was the most strongly correlated variable to continued use of low-vision devices 1 to 2 years after they were prescribed. If at all possible, low-vision devices should be loaned for use in the daily environment before they are prescribed to assure that they are useful.

Some aspects of instructing the use of vision and devices are particularly important when working with older persons with low vision. Because of the potentially devastating consequences of falling, the low-vision therapist must be certain to address safety issues related to using low-vision devices that will prevent falls. Nausea, dizziness, and other aspects of motion sickness are common side effects of using magnification, and reducing these effects is an important aspect of instruction. Monoculars and binoculars should be used as spotting devices only, and older adults must never attempt to walk while viewing through them. If the older person's goal is watching television or spectator sports, binoculars that are spectacle-mounted may be provided and the older person will use them only while seated.

Another factor to be explored in the use of low-vision devices for older adults is hand tremor. Hand tremor may be severe enough that handheld magnifiers or telescopes are not useful. The low-vision team may want to explore spectacle-mounted devices to avoid the difficulty of maintaining focus if hand tremor is problematic.

Postural support and ergonomic considerations are an important aspect to using devices for persons who are older. Because of the prevalence of back and neck pain, as well as limited stamina, it is important that the therapist be able to keep the older person as comfortable as possible. The low-vision therapist will evaluate and teach the use of appropriate ergonomic devices such as the appropriate chair and table, lumbar and cervical support, footstool, lamps, and reading stands.

Cognitive decline may limit the usefulness of low-vision devices for independent functioning; however, an additional goal can be added for rehabilitation—reducing caregiver burden. Assuring that vision rehabilitation includes ergonomic solutions for safe functioning by providing good lighting for ambulation and other visual tasks, judicious use of bold color and contrast for cuing activity and movement and use of simple devices for common activities (e.g., watching television, reading, getting a snack from the refrigerator).

Finally, illumination is an important aspect of the instruction. Most older persons need more light, but some may be extremely sensitive to light. An evaluation of a variety of lamps and overhead lighting situations is necessary, with the use of illumination controls that are individually recommended such as filters, absorptive lenses, hats with brims and pinhole glasses.

Low-Vision Devices

Low-vision devices are optical devices, electronic devices, lighting devices, ergonomic devices, and other tools that enhance the use of vision. Some devices, such as those optical devices that incorporate refractive correction, require special prescription. Others are more simple and straightforward in their assessment and recommendation, such as lamps, reading stands, or large-print books. During the clinical evaluation and functional assessment, the low-vision team will discover whether magnification, minification, or other nonoptical devices (such as large print books, lamps, reading stands, etc.) will be useful for enhancing the vision. Table 43-5 summarizes the types of devices available and their uses. Devices are prescribed based on the goals of the older person and most persons require instruction and practice in their use.

Magnification devices may be categorized as four types: relative distance, relative size, angular, and electronic. Relative distance magnification is provided by bringing the device to be viewed closer to the eyes. Often older adults who want to recognize someone will move more closely to the face they want to see, exhibiting this type of magnification. Spectacle-mounted magnifiers focus the target image, such as print for reading, at ranges closer than the older eye can accommodate, and allow very close distances to be maintained. These lenses must be prescribed by an eye care specialist experienced in low vision in order to incorporate the refractive correction of the older person when required. Typically, these devices require a close focal distance and a short depth of focus. Depending on the power and focal distance, they can be used for near tasks such as reading, writing, and viewing photographs.

Magnification may also be provided by stand or handheld magnifiers, which are often more familiar to older adults who may have used them previously for maps or coins. These devices do not require a close eye-to-lens distance, but the closer to the eye the lens is held, the wider the field of view. Some are available with built-in illumination, which overcomes the problem of illuminating the target the older adult is viewing. Handheld magnifiers require a steady hand to maintain focus and may be fatiguing to use for long periods. Older adults who use stand magnifiers must wear their bifocal correction for visual accommodation, as the lens is set slightly inside the true focal distance of the lens in order to provide a better optical image at the periphery of the lens.

Relative size magnification is used whenever a target to be viewed is made physically larger. Examples of this are phone dials with enlarged numbers or large print in magazines and newspapers.

TABLE 43-5

Low-Vision Devices

OPTICAL/ELECTRONIC DEVICES	TYPICAL USE
Stand or handheld magnifiers	Short-term reading or writing tasks such as checking a price tag or recipe, signing a check
Spectacle-mounted magnifiers	Long-term reading such as newspaper; used for writing in low powers
Handheld monoculars or binoculars	Traffic or street signs, spectator events
Spectacle-mounted monocular or binocular telescope	Television viewing, spectator events, possible driving Short-focus telescope can be used for cards, reading music, games, woodworking, etc.
Closed-circuit television system	Reading, writing, independent activities of daily living, with distance camera, can be used like a telescope
Field-expansion devices: • Reverse telescope • Field-expansion prisms • Hemianopic mirrors	Field expansion for ambulating or obstacle detection, identification, and/or avoidance Best with normal or near-normal acuity

NONOPTICAL DEVICES	TYPICAL USE
Lamps	Provide brighter illumination, primarily used as task lighting
Illumination control devices	Control glare, may increase contrast: sun lenses, hats, visors, colored filters
Handwriting implements	Felt-tip pens, bold-line paper, check- and letter-writing stencils, allow user to stay on line and write legibly
Posture and focal distance support	Upright reading stand, footstool, chair with arms and high back Cervical and lumbar support: provide comfort and allow user to read or write for a longer period
Large print	Large-print books and news, large phone dials, etc., to enhance visibility
Color/contrast aids	Brightly colored tape/paint for marking dials, edge of steps, etc., to enhance visibility and safety

Environments such as older adult high-rise apartments or condominiums and planned communities may also use enlarged signage, another example of relative size magnification.

Telescopic devices provide angular magnification by the use of a positive and negative lens in housing (galilean) or by the use of two positive lenses with an erecting prism (keplerian). Older adults may have used monoculars or binoculars in the past for sporting or other events, and may have developed basic skills in their use. Older adults use telescopic devices for identifying targets that are further away, such as street signs or television. The telescope may be handheld or may be mounted into spectacles for hands-free viewing. Mounted short-focus telescopes may be used for tasks that are closer, such as reading music from a stand or identifying cards on a table. Some older adults with visual impairment who meet visual and driving requirements may use miniature mounted telescopes for driving.

The CCTV is an example of electronic magnification. The CCTV provides a camera to focus on the visual task and the older adult sees the image projected onto a monitor. The visual task may be reading and writing from a desktop or the camera may be positioned for visual tasks at a greater distance such as seeing the minister and choir at church. The advantages of the CCTV include more magnification than any other device, a wider field of view, and contrast enhancement via reversed polarity. CCTV offers a mechanism for the development of new technologies such as miniaturization, head-worn devices, and contrast enhancement.

A variety of software and hardware packages have been developed that produce enlarged print as well as speech-out on a computer. Computer use in conjunction with CCTV can use multiple cameras to provide split-screen images for designing a workstation that simultaneously accesses computer, print viewing, word processing, and distance viewing.

Expanded field devices are helpful to older adults who maintain normal or near-normal acuity while experiencing decreased field of view, such as that caused by glaucoma or hemianopsias. Expanded field devices provide the ability to find targets by increasing the perceived view of a scene. For example, an older adult with restricted fields wishes to find the arriving and departing flight monitors in an airport. By using a field-expansion device, these monitors can be more easily located and the user then moves closer to them in order to read the information without the device. A reverse telescope functions similar to a peephole in a door, but with better optics. Another type of field-expanding device minifies in the horizontal meridian only. The visual field may also be expanded by the use of base-out prisms incorporated into spectacles. The base-out prism shifts the image in, allowing a small eye movement to see the expanded field. Small mirrors attached to spectacles may also be used for field expansion.

Nonoptical devices that enhance the use of vision may also enhance the use of optical and electronic devices. Illumination controls in the form of lamps, filters, absorptive sun lenses, and environmental lighting are of vital importance to visual functioning for older adults. Setting up kitchen and living room "workstations" for visual activities that include ergonomic considerations enhances the use of vision and all devices. Simple devices that use large features, large print, and the judicious use of bold color and contrast can enhance the vision and independence of older adults.

Instruction in the Use of Low-Vision Devices

A sequence of instructional procedures covers several areas:

- Use of visual skills without low-vision devices
- Use of visual skills with low-vision devices
- Use of vision and low-vision devices for individualized functional tasks that lead to the accomplishment of defined goals.

Instruction in the use of visual skills without devices covers fixation, spotting, localization, scanning, tracing, and tracking. Individuals with maculopathy (such as age-related macular degeneration or diabetic retinopathy) may require additional instruction in the development and maintenance of visual skills using the PRL.

Instruction in the use of visual skills with low-vision devices includes integrating unaided visual abilities with the unique demands of a low-vision device such as maintaining the focal distance or focusing the device, and adjusting eye and head movements to compensate for a restricted field of view through the lens. If the individual is using eccentric viewing (the use of a PRL other than the fovea), the instructor assures that the device selected allows the opportunity to maximize field and acuity in the eccentric position.

Reading and Writing with Low-Vision Devices

Reading is a task that is so fundamental to our society and so disrupted by age-related visual impairment that it is the primary goal for vision rehabilitation among older adults. Readers with low vision can develop visual skills that are well-adapted to reading if they receive appropriate intervention. Most readers develop a strongly PRL following the onset of central scotoma. The PRL is an area that will take over the function of fixation in an eccentric, nondamaged area of the retina. The reader may require instruction and practice in using the PRL for reading, especially because of the demands of using magnification to compensate for acuity loss. A Swedish study found that 71% of older adults with low vision could read the newspaper following rehabilitation, although at a 3-year follow-up that number had dropped to 48%. However, the number of fluent readers (70 words per minute or better) had increased from 41% to 48% over the 3-year period. These results indicate that those older adults with vision loss who persevere with rehabilitation strategies are able to continue improving their skills over time. In another study, persons with macular loss who had a PRL below the scotoma exhibited faster reading rates, and the size of the atrophic area in the macula was the predominant limiting factor in reading; the larger the atrophy, the lower the reading rate. Reading rate is also related to visual span (number of characters available in the field of view) and the reserves of acuity and contrast sensitivity provided by the visual system and low-vision device. Accuracy of word identification and comprehension of reading, however, can remain near normal for readers with macular loss despite their slow rates. Readers with low vision often supplement visual reading with speech output devices such as spoken computer programs and books on audiotape.

Older adults with low vision can write effectively using a combination of magnification devices, lighting devices, stencils (templates for checks, envelopes, letters, etc. that assure that writing is spatially correct), and pens that provide more visibility.

ENVIRONMENTS FOR OLDER PERSONS

The onset of visual impairment for older adults can make even the most familiar environment seem strange and hazardous. It is important that older adults be oriented to familiar and unfamiliar environments, and that the environment be as "user-friendly" as possible to increase independence and safety. There are a variety of rehabilitation techniques that assist in accomplishing this task. Table 43-6 presents the basic strategies.

Improving the Lighting

Most older persons require two to three times more light than do younger persons for the same tasks, but those with cloudy media (cataract, keratoconus, vitreous floaters, etc.) are more sensitive to glare. The challenge is to get enough light without creating glare,

TABLE 43-6

Ways to Make an Environment More Visually Accessible

Change the real or perceived size of objects to be viewed	For loss of detailed vision: • Increase size (large print) • Move closer (move chair closer to the television) • Use magnification For loss of peripheral fields with normal acuity: • Minify image (reverse telescope) • Move further away • Use field-enhancement devices such as mirrors
Improve lighting	Use appropriate environmental lighting to decrease glare and increase overall light level; use illumination controls such as sunlenses, hats with brims, visors, colored filters; use task lighting such as flex-arm lamps
Increase contrast between objects and background	Eliminate busy background patterns, mark down steps with contrasting color on risers; increase contrast between furniture, china, and background
Use bright, clear colors	Mark light switches, dials, etc. with colored tape; use large areas of bright color for discrimination of objects
Organize the environment for ease and safety	Doors completely open or closed, chairs under table when not in use, furniture against the wall, organize clothing for color and function, etc.
Consider alternative strategies that do not use vision	Use of other senses for task performance, such as audiotaped reading materials, use of long cane for safe travel, olfactory cues for doneness of food, etc.

which can be disabling. For example, the glare from a sunny window onto a waxed floor, tabletops, and glass could cause objects in the dining room of a senior community to be obscured. An older person with low vision might function as if blind in that environment and be unable to find a chair, recognize his friends, serve his plate, or even see the food in a buffet line.

In an environment that is conducive for the function of older persons, it is important to manage not only light, but also shadow, which can be conducive to function, for example, a triangular shadow at the end of a step indicates the height and depth of the step as well as how many steps are there. But shadow can also be hazardous, such as the shadow of a garden wall that obscures a sidewalk curb, causing a person to trip or fall.

Lighting is best if controllable, no matter what type it is. Most older persons with low vision will require task lighting that can be positioned closer to reading/writing material or craft activity. Because the intensity of light is inversely related to the square of distance from its source, adding light at ceiling height will not provide adequate task illumination for older viewers. Task lights must be used that can be positioned closely, and therefore flex-armed lamps are best in this regard.

There are a variety of different types of bulbs that are useful and recommended for older viewers with low vision.

• Fluorescent lighting spreads evenly, is inexpensive and energy efficient, but provides less contrast because of that evenness and produces less shadow. It is a harsh light and flickers and may be bothersome to some viewers, causing headache and eye strain. Covering or shading fluorescent bulbs or bouncing the light from the ceiling to the eye may be helpful.

- Incandescent light is easily directed and provides more contrast and shadow. But the light can pool, especially if provided by one bulb suspended from the ceiling, causing pinpoint glare or pools of light within relative darkness. Using multiple incandescent fixtures can eliminate this problem. Incandescent lamps are good for task lighting such as reading, sewing, or hobbies.

- Halogen light uses the glow of halogen gas, as well as the incandescent filament to create a brighter light. The light is more blue and therefore may require filtering. Ultraviolet or blue light may generate superoxide and hydroxide free radicals that may be related to damage in the eye. Although controlled clinical studies have not been done, blue light has been suggested as increasing risk of cataract and macular degeneration. Subsequent studies have not shown a correlation to visible light exposure and risk, but many rehabilitation services are cautious about "blue light hazard." An Australian study suggests that persons with less melanin (i.e., light-colored iris, fair skin) are at more risk from light.

- Neodymium oxide and incandescent bulbs are currently touted as "full-spectrum lighting." These bulbs emit fewer ultraviolet and infrared rays and provide a sharp drop in the emission of yellow light. The effect is a more vivid "true" color, similar to sunlight, so contrast is increased.

These types of lighting can be mixed to achieve effects that are most pleasing and comfortable for older people with low vision. A study exploring these types of lighting in reading lamps found strong preferences among older readers with low vision, but no differences in objective measures of reading performance based upon the type of light. Thus, informed reader choice should guide the selection of the type of light for older readers.

Light/dark adaptation is another aspect of environmental lighting that must be considered. Most older persons have difficulty traveling from bright areas to dim ones because their dark adaptation is not as efficient as in young adults. Persons with severely restricted field loss (e.g., advanced glaucoma) become functionally blind in dim lighting. Avoiding light/dark areas in the environment such as a bright dining room and dim hallway is helpful. When these areas are unavoidable, the older person could use illumination controls such as sunglasses or brimmed hats to assist with light/dark adaptation. Persons with severely restricted visual fields who are at risk for falling when ambulating at night may use lightweight, very bright, portable lamps with long battery life that have been designed for night hunters.

Increasing Contrast

Light/dark contrast is produced by the amount of light that is reflected from different surfaces (a light object is brighter than a dark one). A greater contrast between objects and their backgrounds make them easier to see. Therefore, providing an area of dark background and an area of light background in the bathroom, kitchen, and bedroom can help a person more easily identify possessions. For example, if a comb and brush are of light color, they may be kept on a dark tray. Most TV remotes are black, so they should be placed on a very light background. Similarly, marking the edge of stairs with contrasting colored tape makes each step more visible.

Using Color

The ability to identify colors, especially darks and pastels diminishes with age. Certain visual impairments, especially those that affect the cones, such as macular degeneration, also reduce color vision. However, bright, clear colors can be seen by most older persons with low vision. For example, yellow against navy blue is very visible, because it combines both color and contrast cues.

Using Organizational Strategies

Organization can be extremely helpful for the person with low vision. For example, always making sure that doors are completely open or completely closed, and placing chairs under the table when not used increases the safety of the environment. Organizing and labeling clothing by color and function in closets and drawers and organizing the kitchen can assist an older person in continuing to live independently. Learning new ways of performing daily tasks can make the loss of vision less of a problem in independent living. For example, retrieving a pair of spectacles that have fallen onto a light carpet might be difficult for some older adults. Learning a visual scanning pattern that begins at the site where the spectacles seem to have fallen and then continues in a circular pattern outward until they are found will assist in retrieving them.

Using color coding can be helpful as well. For example, chicken soup cans could be marked with wide yellow rubber bands, and tomato soup cans could be marked with wide red rubber bands. These markers could be quickly identified, avoiding the necessity for identifying the soup with a magnifier each time a can is retrieved from the cabinet. Brightly colored and nubby stick-on "dots" may be provided that provide both contrast and tactile cues for marking dials, buttons, and controls of appliances.

Alternative Strategies

Even when an older adult with low vision retains useful vision for a wide variety of tasks, it is sometimes helpful to use alternative techniques that do not require the use of vision because vision may not be the most efficient or safest way of accomplishing some tasks. For example, even though an older adult may have useful vision for walking, he may find it best to use a long white mobility cane in order to detect drop-offs, so that vision can be used to seek landmarks for orientation. An older adult with low vision may use speech output (a program that speaks symbols or words) for most computer word processing so that limited stamina for reading and writing may be used for reading mail, which must be done visually. A metal plate called a "flame-tamer" may be placed on the eyes of a gas stove in order to avoid burns in the kitchen. Knowledge of a wide variety of rehabilitation strategies and tools will assist older adults with low vision in developing a repertoire of techniques and devices that allows them to complete tasks safely, efficiently, and effectively.

Orientation to a new setting requires some basic alternative techniques that can be used anywhere. Some older adults may be able to use all of the techniques, some may only need one or two. It is important to remember not to rush the older adult in orientation, whether it is a long-term care facility or physician's office. These exercises

TABLE 43-7

Orientation to a New Setting for Older Adults with Vision Loss

Using a starting/ ending point	Begin at one starting/ending place in the room, such as the door. Have the older adult reach out and feel both sides of the doorway, then describe the contents of the room, while leading him around the room via sighted guide and trailing and allowing him to feel features. Give simple names to the walls using some feature of the wall (example, the wall to the right is the bed wall, the wall opposite is the window wall).
Using compass directions or clock face	Some older adults will be more familiar with compass directions. Using the same starting points as previously explained, use north wall, south wall, east wall, and west wall to name the four sides of the room. Proceed using compass directions as the way of finding and naming locations in the room. Use clock face numbers in a similar manner for those who can more easily understand them.
Using landmarks and cues	Use familiar landmarks for orientation to a new environment, for example, the smell of food is a landmark for the dining room. The audible hum and red glow of a soft-drink machine may be another landmark.

may be repeated as often as necessary. Teaching family members these techniques may be helpful when new environments come up in the future. Table 43-7 presents an overview of these techniques.

PSYCHOSOCIAL CONSIDERATIONS

Adaptation to Vision Loss

Anxiety and depression are common reactions to loss, and age-related visual impairment is complicated by the other losses associated with aging. There are two schools of thought on the timing of rehabilitation related to adaptation. Some rehabilitation professionals subscribe to a "loss theory" of psychological adjustment. This theory proposes that the person must "die" as a sighted person, and be "reborn" as a visually impaired person, incorporating the visual impairment into the sense of self. According to this theory, attempting rehabilitation would be fruitless until the process is complete. Others subscribe to the theory that anxiety and depression are related to a person's negative stereotypes about visual impairment and a lack of confidence and motivation to attempt rehabilitation, but that if rehabilitation is successful, depression and anxiety should be reduced.

Older adults may hold many negative stereotypes associated with visual impairment: increased helplessness, inhabiting a world of darkness, increased vulnerability to crime, the perception that use of devices mark them as different, or to be pitied. Older adults with low vision may attempt to pass as fully sighted in order to avoid having others project these negative stereotypes onto them. But attempting to pass as fully sighted may cause other difficulties. For example, older adults with low vision do not recognize faces well, and the lack

of a friendly hello when passing acquaintances may be interpreted as unfriendliness. Failure to use alternative techniques for identifying targets and moving in the environment may lead to falls, burns, or other safety hazards.

Support groups and peer counseling for older adults with low vision can be extremely helpful in coping with vision loss. Support groups may be found through local multiservice agencies for persons who are visually impaired or may be started by senior citizen's centers or other groups. Short-term professional counseling in conjunction with rehabilitation may be very helpful.

Family and Social Support

In a recent study of low-vision device use among veterans, most of whom were older males with macular degeneration, family support was the most powerful predictor of continued use of devices up to 2 years following their prescription. Providing information and support to family members who are experiencing the impact of an older member's vision loss can be powerful. Visual impairment is experienced by the entire family or caregiving system, not just by the older person, and both social and psychological concerns must be addressed. The loss of vision by one family member can disrupt roles in the family, create economic demands, and add stress when tasks previously performed by the older adult must be performed by someone else.

For family members who understand the functional implications of visual impairment, understanding the behavior of their older adult with low vision is easier. For example, understanding the effect of changing lighting conditions, the effects of glare, the adaptation times when traveling from dim light to bright and vice versa, can help explain behaviors like shielding the eyes, shuffling the feet, hesitation, fear of falling, and ceasing previously enjoyed activities. The fact that an older adult with restricted visual fields may pick up a dime from the floor, then bump into a partially open door seems contradictory, but is perfectly explained by the functioning field of view.

Assisting older adults with low vision in continuing social activities, such as hobbies, crafts, games, and traveling can aid them in maintaining important contacts with family and peers. Social support and contact is associated with less depression in older adults with low vision. Support groups can assist older adults with low vision in completing and using their rehabilitation, as well as facilitating adaptation to vision loss. Peer support, or mutual aid groups who meet regularly to share their concerns may be especially beneficial for older adults who may be overprotected, abused, or treated paternalistically by those who do not understand visual impairment or aging. Facilitating assertiveness for older adults with low vision is recommended because it is linked to less depression and more social support. Social skill training in assertiveness for older adults with low vision has been shown effective in decreasing depression, and deriving greater satisfaction in life.

FUNDING FOR LOW-VISION REHABILITATION

Traditionally, vision rehabilitation services have been funded through private pay, or through vocational rehabilitation services for individuals who were preparing for the work force. Funding for services to older adults with vision impairment has been a critical health care issue in the United States. Public funding for the Independent

Living Services for Older Individuals Who are Blind program under the Rehabilitation Act is minimal, with approximately $32.9 million allocated nationally in fiscal years 2006 and 2007. The funding remains at this level in the President's appropriations for 2008. These funds provide services in the traditional "blindness" system—state or private agencies for the visually impaired that are serving persons of all ages who have visual impairments.

Prior to 2002, only older veterans with low vision who served in the U.S. military and whose disability is service-connected had full access to comprehensive blindness and low-vision services through the Department of Veterans Affairs Medical Centers. However, most visually impaired veterans have age-related vision loss and their income is such that a copayment is required from them or from their private insurance carrier. Vision rehabilitation services were developed initially to meet the needs of blinded veterans returning from World War II. Young war-blinded men had few other medical problems, so efforts to rehabilitate them for the work force spawned the professions of orientation and mobility instructors, rehabilitation teachers for the blind, and low-vision therapists in order to meet their unique needs. This specialized "blindness and low-vision" rehabilitation was not considered part of the broader medical rehabilitation. Credentialing of vision-rehabilitation professionals developed separately from occupational or physical therapists, and their practice was autonomous, requiring neither medical referral nor supervision. As a result, many medical professionals are unaware of their services and do not understand the "blindness" rehabilitation system in which their practice began. The Department of Veterans Affairs model of service delivery in vision rehabilitation continues today in the same vein. Services are provided nationally by teams of professionals. Ophthalmologists or optometrists provide the medical eye care services, and the rehabilitation professionals are orientation and mobility specialists, rehabilitation teachers, and low-vision therapists. Recently the Department of Veterans Affairs appropriated $40 million to provide vision rehabilitation services in a continuum of care to patients who have low vision as well as those who are legally blind, in recognition that veterans are aging in place and require services close to home. The vision/blind rehabilitation service in this milieu is also unique in that prosthetic devices are included. Low-vision devices such as magnifiers, telescopes, binoculars, closed circuit television systems, computer equipment, etc. are dispensed according to VA policy at no cost to veterans as a part of the VA's commitment to vision/blindness rehabilitation services.

The rise in older adults with low vision has spurred Medicare to produce a national policy of reimbursement as well. In 2002, the Centers for Medicare and Medicaid Services (CMS) released a national program memorandum to alert the provider community that Medicare beneficiaries who are blind or visually impaired are eligible for physician-prescribed rehabilitation services from approved health care professionals on the same basis as beneficiaries with other medical conditions that result in reduced physical functioning. This memorandum was issued in response to the committee report accompanying the FY 2002 Labor/Health and Human Services/Education appropriations bill.

The memorandum further directed that the patient receiving services must have a potential for restoration or improvement of lost functions, and must be expected to improve significantly within a reasonable and generally predictable amount of time. The rehabilitation that is covered was short-term and intense; maintenance therapy was not covered. Applicable Health Care Common Procedural Coding System therapeutic procedures are outlined in the memorandum, as are applicable International Classification of Diseases (ICD)-9 codes that support medical necessity.

The effect of the program memorandum has been to increase the visibility of Medicare provisions for vision rehabilitation, but it is not a national coverage decision. Medicare carriers are not compelled by the memorandum to develop a Local Medical Review Policy as a result, and are still able to deny all claims that the local carrier does not deem medically reasonable or necessary.

In 2003, Congress authorized the Secretary of Health and Human Services to carry out a nationwide outpatient vision rehabilitation services demonstration project. The purpose of this demonstration project is to examine the impact of standardized national coverage for vision rehabilitation services in the home by physicians, occupational therapists and certified vision rehabilitation professionals. Medicare beneficiaries who are diagnosed with moderate to severe visual impairment may be eligible to receive covered vision rehabilitation services under this demonstration project. The demonstration covered services will only be available to Medicare beneficiaries who live in New Hampshire, New York City, Atlanta, Georgia, North Carolina, Kansas, and Washington state and must be prescribed by a qualified physician, such as an ophthalmologist or an optometrist who also practices in one of the specified demonstration locales. Eligible beneficiaries can be covered for up to 9 hours of rehabilitation services provided in an appropriate setting, including at home. Two notable aspects of this project are that (1) vision rehabilitation professionals are covered to provide services under the general supervision of the qualified physician (optometrist or ophthalmologist) and (2) for purposes of this demonstration, CMS is waiving the usual "incident to" rules in order to allow occupational therapists who are in private practice and certified vision rehabilitation professionals to provide services under general supervision of the physician. Neither the 2002 Medicare policy nor the 2003 Demonstration Project provides coverage for adaptive equipment (low-vision devices) as does the Department of Veterans Affairs.

FURTHER READING

Brabyn JA et al. The Smith–Kettlewell Institute longitudinal study of vision function and its impact among the elderly: an overview. *Optom Vis Sci.* 2001;78:264.

Elner SG. Gradual painless visual loss: retinal causes. *Clin Geriatr Med.* 1999;15:25.

Haegersrtrom-Portnoy G, Schnec M, Brabyn J. Seeing into old age: vision function beyond acuity. *Opom Vis Sci.* 1999;76:3.

Kendrick R. Gradual painless visual loss: glaucoma. *Clin Geriatr Med.* 1999;15:95.

Magione CM et al. Development of the "activities of daily vision scale," a measure of visual functional status. *Med Care.* 1992;30:1111.

National Eye Institute (NEI). *Vision Problems in the U.S.: Prevalence of Adult Vision Impairment and Age-Related Eye Disease in America.* Office of Science Policy and Legislation, National Eye Institute, National Institutes for Health. Bethesda, MD: Government Printing Office; 2002.

Schuchard RA, Fletcher DC. Preferred retinal locus: a review with applications in low-vision rehabilitation. *Ophthalmol Clin North Am.* 1994;7:243.

Silverstone B et al., eds. *The Lighthouse Handbook on Vision Impairment and Vision Rehabilitation.* New York, New York: Oxford University Press; 2000.

Valluri S. Gradual painless vision loss: anterior segment causes. *Clin Geriatr Med.* 1999;15:87.

Age-Related Changes in the Auditory System

Su-Hua Sha ■ *Andra E. Talaska* ■ *Jochen Schacht*

INTRODUCTION

The sense of hearing is unequalled by our other sensory modalities in terms of its sensitivity, dynamic range, and discrimination of the finest nuances in stimuli. It does serve us well through a part of our lifetime, but beginning in our forties (slightly earlier for men and later for women), our inner ears suffer the influence of aging in a very subtle yet progressive manner. Age-related hearing impairment (ARHI) affects most people aged 65 years and older and represents the predominant neurodegenerative disease of aging. Hippocrates had already noted deafness to be more prevalent among his elderly patients and in *The Comedy of Errors*, Shakespeare's elderly merchant, Aegeon, complains of his own "dull deaf ears." Thus, ARHI or presbycusis is not a disease of modern societies but has been accepted for centuries as one of Lord Byron's inevitable "woes that wait on age" that it still appears to be.

It was the New York otologist, St. John Roosa, who first drew the attention of his colleagues to hearing loss of the elderly as a medical condition. In 1885 he proposed the name presbycusis that he had coined from the Greek $\pi\rho\acute{e}\sigma\beta\upsilon\varsigma$, old man, and $\alpha\kappa o\acute{\upsilon}\epsilon\iota\nu$, to hear. Systematic studies of the anatomical pathology began in the late nineteenth century, leading by the 1930s to the realization that the decreased auditory acuity could be attributed to deterioration of the auditory sensory cells and the auditory nerve. These changes frequently affect the perception of the upper frequencies first, resulting in high-frequency hearing loss as a hallmark of presbycusis. However, age-related hearing loss is not a uniform condition, but a multifactorial one combining genetic predispositions with a plethora of lifetime insults to the hearing organ because, in all its versatility and efficacy, our sense of hearing is also uniquely vulnerable to environmental influences. These may include noise, chemicals, and solvents at the workplace, lifestyle (e.g., smoking), and leisure activities (from iPods to rock concerts and target shooting), diseases (e.g., diabetes, respiratory disorders), viral or bacterial infections, and even the adverse effects of the very medications designed to cure the diseases and infections. This spectrum of potential abuse of our auditory organ yields an exceedingly intricate etiology and pathology of hearing loss in the elderly. Age-related pathology of the central auditory system adds to the complexity of the problem. Presbycusis has been defined as "hearing impairment associated with various types of auditory dysfunction, peripheral or central, that accompany aging and that cannot be accounted for by extraordinary ototraumatic, genetic, or pathological conditions" but it is almost impossible in practice to separate the confounding factors from a "true" effect of aging. It has therefore often been debated whether presbycusis indeed exists in populations that are isolated from adverse environmental influences.

Animal models provide hope to resolve some of the basic mechanisms that underlie the deterioration of hearing and point to ways and means to delay or prevent presbycusis. By virtue of the availability of molecular and genetic information and of transgenic and knock-out animals, mice have become one of the preferred model animals although, as we shall point out later, caveats do apply here too. This review will illustrate the features of human presbycusis and draw on animal models to discuss its potential molecular basis.

Epidemiology of Age-Related Hearing Impairment

ARHI is the most frequent sensory impairment in the elderly and the prevalence of the disorder increases with age. In humans, as in most other species, age-related hearing loss begins at the high frequencies and progresses gradually into the lower speech range. Males suffer age-related hearing loss earlier than females, beginning in the late thirties to early forties while women will match the males' deficits in the later decades of their lives. Approximately 44% of people suffer from a significant hearing loss in their sixties; this number rises to 66% between the ages of 70 and 79 years, and skyrockets to 90% after age 80 years. With an increased life span of the population worldwide, especially in developed countries, the impact of ARHI will continue to increase in the future.

The individual rate of decline in hearing, however, is exceptionally variable and some people may maintain excellent hearing with "golden ears" late into life as a result of genetic traits that have yet to be elucidated. Superimposed on the gender differences, race apparently also plays a role, although whether this role is causative or correlative is unknown. One study of over 2000 elderly Americans aged 73 to 84 years found the incidence of high-frequency hearing loss that met their criteria to be 91.8% in Caucasian American men, 76.1% in African-American men, 74.2% in Caucasian American women, and 59.2% in African-American women. In addition to genetic differences, each group had tendencies toward particular risk factors, suggesting that the incidence of hearing loss across groups is presumably caused by a combination of genetic and risk factor diversity.

Risk Factors Modulating Age-Related Hearing Impairment

Genetics

Family history plays a role in predisposition to presbycusis. An analysis of hearing thresholds in sibling or parent/child pairs versus spousal pairs (control) in Framingham Heart Study patients found that the inherited genetic effects were significant. The predictive power of family history appeared stronger for females than males and stronger for "metabolic" type rather than sensory type hearing loss (see Schuknecht's classification of age-related hearing loss in section "Peripheral Pathology of Age-Related Hearing Impairment in Humans"). Overall, the study suggested that about 55% of the variance in age-related hearing loss can be ascribed to genetic factors. This influence is then modulated by external risk factors.

Environmental Factors

The great variation in the progression and severity of hearing loss has long led to the recognition of ARHI as a complex genetic disorder with environmental risk factors. Major environmental risk factors that may contribute to the manifestations of ARHI, briefly mentioned above, include exposure to excessive noise, ototoxic medications (primarily aminoglycoside antibiotics and anticancer agents of the cisplatin class), and industrial solvents. These environmental factors appear to damage the auditory system by oxidative injury and thus may aggravate the age-related changes in the auditory system. Animal experiments bear out the accelerating influence of these factors, which do not necessarily have to inflict damage by themselves. When mice at 3 months of age received a mild noise exposure causing only temporary threshold shifts, their hearing recovered to normal within 3 days. These mice, however, developed a significantly greater hearing loss with age than control animals.

Gender Differences and Hormonal Factors

Age-related hearing loss sets in earlier in males than in females, both in the human population and experimental animals. In the later decades of life, however, these differences diminish, suggesting that differences in hormonal levels between male and female contributes to onset of ARHI. Receptors for steroid hormones are indeed present in the cochlea. In support of a link between ARHI and hormonal levels, fluctuations in hearing thresholds have been observed during the menstrual cycle and estrogen therapy slowed the development of ARHI in postmenopausal women. Furthermore, in patients (and mouse models) with Turner syndrome who do not synthesize estrogen, ARHI sets in early. A correlative study in human saw a protective effect of elevated serum levels of aldosterone on auditory thresholds and an improvement of "hearing-in-noise" in older individuals. Aldosterone receptors in the inner ear influence the ionic homeostasis of inner ear fluids, which is essential for cochlear homeostasis and the transduction of sound.

Diabetes Mellitus

Both type I and type II diabetes promote hearing loss and cochlear pathology in humans and in animals. Deficits in several aspects of auditory function were significantly more pronounced in a group of people with type II diabetes aged 60 years or older compared with a group of age- and sex-matched controls and excluding those with other significant health problems or a history of hearing problems. Diabetes mellitus and associated deregulated blood glucose levels, in fact, exact a multitude of stresses on a cellular level, which could lead to loss of function in the delicately balanced hearing organ with time and age. Fundamentally, increased blood glucose levels leads to cellular hypoxia and build up of reactive oxygen species and other metabolic by-products, as well as changes in the collagen and microtubule structure of the cells. Also, the effects of diabetes on vasculature are profound, including atherosclerosis and vessel wall dystrophy. In the inner ear, which depends on the stria vascularis to carefully maintain the endocochlear potential, this could result in impaired sensory function and apoptosis.

Cardiovascular Disease

All conditions that affect the function of blood vessels such as hyperlipidemia, hypercholesterolemia, hypertension, hyperlipoproteinemia, and cardiovascular disease have been implicated in ARHI. Specifically, strial ARHI (see next section) appears to be aggravated because stria vascularis is most vulnerable to any restriction of blood flow. Just as in diabetes, any cardiovascular disease leading to vascular compromise will impair the function of this tissue and, by way of decreased endolymphatic potential, decrease the sensitivity of the cochlear organ to sound.

Lifestyle

Poor health habits with regard to exercise, smoking, and diet are also considered risk factors for ARHI based on data of population studies. Since some of these habits influence cardiovascular function and other potential risk factors for ARHI, it remains open how much lifestyle acts directly on the auditory organ or secondary to general health.

Psychology

Interestingly, adherence to negative stereotypes about the elderly, i.e., the concept in many societies that aging is met with an inevitable decline in function of all faculties, demonstrates as a predicting risk factor for ARHI. External stereotyping (the prevalence of stigmata with aging in the subject's culture) and negative internal perception (extent of internalization of these stigmata) acted as independent risk factors on hearing loss with age, and had a stronger impact than gender or race. This predicts an observable phenomenon wherein cultures with positive concepts of aging do not expect their elders' hearing to become enfeebled and, in fact, the incidence of ARHI is then lower. Here again, an influence on the auditory system maybe secondary to the effect of stigmata on general well-being.

Hearing Loss Basics: Frequencies and Sound Intensity

A significant hearing loss of any origin will eventually lead to difficulties in communication and a decreased awareness of the environment. In addition to the social isolation at all ages, subjects with early-onset presbycusis may suffer economic consequences from difficulties in employment or professional advancement. The question of what constitutes a significant hearing impairment is complex as it involves consideration of both the magnitude of sensitivity loss and the frequencies at which the loss occurs. Although the most convenient assessment criterion for age-related hearing loss is a subjective one—that is, posing the question, "do you have a hearing problem?" or a more elaborate questionnaire like the Hearing Handicap Inventory for the Elderly-Short (HHIE-S)— a more quantitative evaluation can be obtained by an audiogram (see section on "Functional Assessment of Hearing"). While there is not one set paradigm for classification of audiograms into handicapping and nonhandicapping hearing thresholds, the American Medical Association/American Academy of Otolaryngology—Head and Neck Surgery sets the bar at an average threshold shift (hearing loss) of 25 dB or above at frequencies between 500 and 3000 Hz.

What does a loss of 25 dB hearing acuity mean in practical terms? The bel or decibel scale of sound pressure ("intensity") is logarithmic, such that an increase in 3 bels (30 dB) confers approximately a doubling of the sound intensity ($10^{3/10} = 1.995$). Therefore, a reduction of sensitivity of 25 dB, as is required for some definitions of occupational hearing impairment, is considerable. In rough terms, a difference of 25 dB in threshold makes normal conversation equivalent to a whisper, and a whisper equivalent to silence (Table 44-1). The crying baby would still be heard—albeit subdued—but the leaves rustling in the forest or the crickets in summer would not be heard.

ARHI poses a specific problem as the hearing loss mostly sets in at the high frequencies. As a result, many with age-related hearing loss do not recognize their condition for a long time. The frequency spectrum of human hearing, at its best, ranges from about 60 Hz to 16 kHz. A hearing loss at the very high frequencies may not produce any communicative disadvantages since frequencies over 4 kHz contribute little to speech (Table 44-2). Even musical instruments have a limited range in their fundamental frequencies. Since the progression of ARHI is also gradual, the subject maybe unaware of the gradual loss of overtones in speech or instrumental music, which can extend two or three octaves higher than the fundamentals, i.e., to two or three times the frequencies.

Although basic hearing needs center on the 1000 to 2000 Hz range, higher frequency losses like those in ARHI cost the ability to discriminate between many words with f, p, k, s, t, th sounds (Table 44-2). For example, to a person with high-frequency hearing loss, "sick" and "thick" maybe difficult to differentiate, and "three socks" may sound like "free fox" unless the listener has developed the ability to read the speakers lips for more information. Such communication errors may seem trivial, but can cause enormous social disability when they happen in work situations or become cumulative.

TABLE 44-1

Typical Sound Levels	
dB	**SOUND**
15	Pin drop at close range
15–20	Rustling leaves, dripping faucet
35	Whisper
50–60	Normal conversation
60–70	Vacuum cleaner
70–90	Screaming child
85	*Safety limit for an 8-h workday*
100	*Safe for 15 min or less*
105–110	Gas engine mower, chain saw
110	Car stereo at maximum volume
110	*Safe for 1 min 29 s*
115	Maximum volume from an iPod
116	*Human body perceives low frequency*
120	Front row at a rock concert
120–130	Jet plane taking off
127	*High risk of tinnitus*
130–140	Gun shot from a hunting rifle
140	*Hearing deficit at exposures < 1 s*

Intensity levels of some familiar sounds can provide a guide to understanding the impact of hearing loss as discussed in the text. The comparison of these levels to safety standards also illustrates the potential impact of environmental noise exposure on the complex manifestations of presbycusis.
Safety levels are taken from DHHS (NIOSH) Publication No. 98–126 on Occupational Noise Exposure.

The high frequencies are also important for auditory discrimination in the presence of background noise. A common and often the first noticed signal of presbycusis is the "party effect" when an individual with good one-on-one communication experiences difficulties in speech perception in a noisy environment such as a

TABLE 44-2

Frequency Ranges of Common Sounds	
SOUND	**APPROXIMATE FUNDAMENTAL FREQUENCY RANGE (Hz)**
Guitar	82–1175
Truck engine	125–250
Dog's bark	200–300
Violin	196–4400
Soprano singer	200–1400
Most spoken consonants	250–500
Middle C of the musical scale	264
Spoken vowels	500–750
Crying baby	750–1000
Consonants: c, p, ch, g, h, sh	1000–2000
Telephone ring	3000–4000
Consonants: f, k, s, t, th	3000–8000
Birds chirping	4000–8000

In addition to these fundamental frequencies, most sources of sounds and musical instruments in particular, produce overtones that add to the richness of the sound. These overtones reach two to three times the fundamentals. Comparison of the frequencies to the classical pattern of high-frequency age-related hearing impairment illustrates the early impact on specific speech features and the quality of music appreciation.

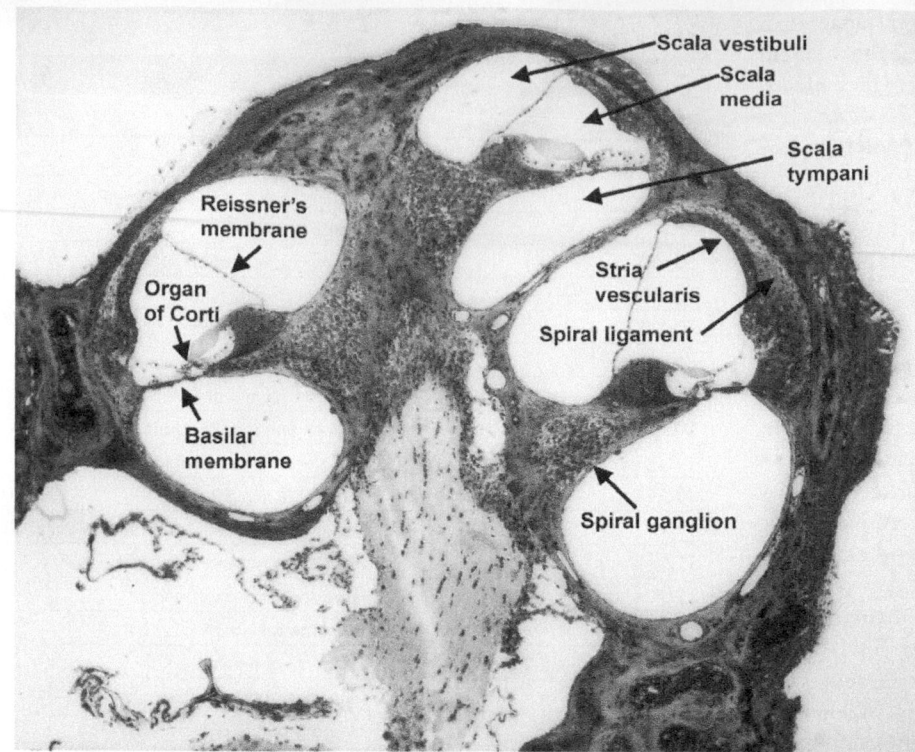

FIGURE 44-1. Anatomy of the cochlea. A low magnification light micrograph of a near midmodiolar cross-section illustrates the tissues and fluid-filled spaces of the 2½ turns of the mouse cochlea. As indicated in the upper turn, the fluid spaces are the scala tympani and scala vestibuli filled with perilymph, and scala media filled with endolymph. They are separated by the thin Reissner's membrane and the basilar membrane upon which the organ of Corti is located. When sound reaches the ear, the vibrations of the tympanic membrane (ear drum) are passed along the middle ear ossicles to the cochlea where they initiate a traveling wave in the fluids which, in turn, move the basilar membrane. The tectorial membrane, an acellular structure, rests on the stereocilia of the hair cells. Spiral ganglion neurons run from the organ of Corti where they make contact with the hair cells through the modiolus to the central auditory system. The stria vascularis and spiral ligament, tissues involved in setting up the ionic composition and high (+70–100 mV) potential of the endolymph, lie along the lateral wall of the cochlea.

restaurant, a party, or a conference. Audiological examinations routinely include frequencies up to 8000 Hz and would reveal the presbycusic changes although the individual may still be told by the audiologist that their hearing is "normal for the age."

Anatomy of the Auditory Periphery

Not only is age-related hearing loss shaped by many influences, it also shows a variety of morphological manifestations. The present framework for classifying age-related hearing loss was proposed by Schuknecht in 1964 based on the histopathology of human temporal bones. In order to understand its age-related changes, we should first sketch the structure of the mammalian auditory organ, the cochlea (Figure 44-1). Encased in bone, the tissues and fluids of the cochleae of different species coil "snail-like" for 2½ to 4½ turns and a total length of a few centimeters without any relationship to body size. A human cochlea, for example, extends for 33 mm in 2½ turns while the dimensions in the guinea pig are 20 mm and 4½ turns. The cochlea is tonotopically organized in all species, and high frequencies are processed in the base, low frequencies in the apex.

Several structures with distinctly different functions and susceptibility to environmental and age-related insults can be discerned within this membranous labyrinth and best seen in a midmodiolar section that transverses the length of the cochlea. The lumen of the cochlea is separated into three fluid-filled compartments by the basilar membrane and Reissner's membrane. Scala vestibuli and scala tympani contain perilymph, similar in composition to extracellular fluids. Scala media contains endolymph, unique among body fluids by its high concentration of K^+ and low Na^+, creating a large positive endolymphatic potential as a driving force for the transduction current, which is used by the sensory cells. Scala media is bounded laterally by spiral ligament and stria vascularis, the tissues that are responsible for maintaining endolymph. These tissues

are highly vascularized and provide most of the oxygen and nutrient supply to the cochlea. The organ of Corti (Figure 44-2), located on the basilar membrane, is the auditory end organ containing sensory cells and supporting cells. Sensory cells include the inner hair cells and three rows of outer hair cells, numbering several thousand in all species. The name "hair cell" is derived from the stereocilia that protrude from the apical end of the cells (Figure 44-3). Inner hair cells are the primary sensory cells that convert the mechanical acoustic input into receptor potential and release of neurotransmitter, triggering action potentials that are carried to the brain by the spiral

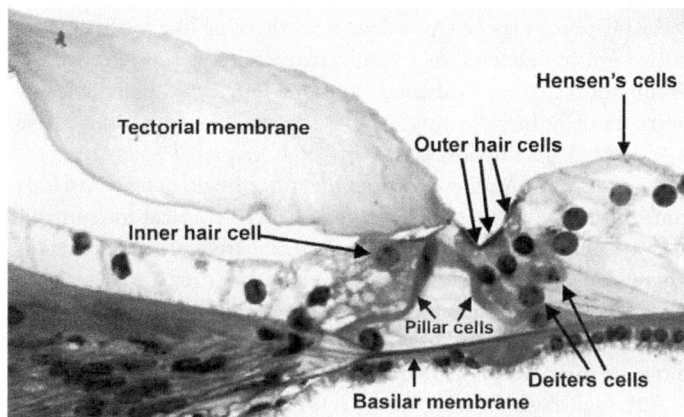

FIGURE 44-2. The organ of Corti. A cross section shows details of the mouse organ of Corti located on the basilar membrane. The sensory cells are arranged in one row of inner hair cells and three rows of outer hair cells. Inner hair cells are the primary transducers of sound and receive most of the afferent innervation of the spiral ganglion nerve. Outer hair cells amplify transduction and receive most of the efferent innervation. Supporting cells include Deiters', Hensen's, and pillar cells. The tectorial membrane does not extend to its full length because of preparation artifacts.

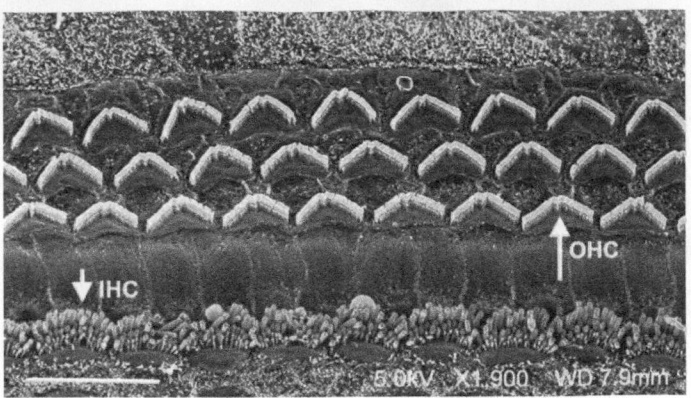

FIGURE 44-3. Hair cells and their stereocilia. A scanning electron micrograph of a "surface preparation" gives a top view of the organ of Corti, presenting the apical aspects of hair cells and supporting cells. The hair cells are clearly distinguished by their stereocilia, the white tufts arranged in linear (inner hair cells, IHC) and W-like (outer hair cells, OHC) form. In the process of sound transduction, the stereocilia are deflected by a shearing motion generated between the basilar membrane and the tectorial membrane, causing transduction channels to open and allow influx of potassium from the endolymph. This influx triggers a receptor potential and release of neurotransmitter (glutamate) at the synapse between the inner hair cell and the spiral ganglion nerve. Scale bar: 20 μm. (Scanning electron micrograph from mouse cochlea kindly provided by Dr. Andrew Forge, Institute of Laryngology and Otology, University College London, UK.)

ganglion neurons. Most of the afferent innervation by this auditory nerve converges on the inner hair cells. The major function of outer hair cells is to enhance the performance of the cochlea, particularly at low intensities of sound. They receive mostly efferent innervation from auditory centers in the brain. Supporting cells include the inner pillar, outer pillar, Deiters', Hensen and Claudius' cells, about whose function we know relatively little.

The cells in the sensory epithelium are highly differentiated. Hair cells, once lost, are not regenerated by other cell types in the mammal and replaced by permanent "scars" (Figure 44-4). Consequently, any damage to these cells leads to irreversible hearing loss.

Functional Assessment of Hearing

From a clinical functional aspect, pure tone audiometry, tympanometry, acoustic reflex measurements, and word recognition scores with behavioral tests are the most common and important methods for hearing assessment. Tympanometry and acoustic reflex (stapedius reflex) test the integrity of the middle ear while audiometry yields information about acoustic thresholds at distinct frequencies. Word recognition and behavioral tests explore more complex interactions

that involve both the auditory periphery and the central processing of the information. Auditory brainstem response (ABR) and otoacoustic emission measurements are passive sound-evoked responses and therefore most easily adapted to routine testing in animals, providing information on the integrity of the auditory pathway and outer hair cells, respectively. Some invasive methods, essentially limited to animal experimentation, such as recordings of cochlear microphonic potential (largely derived from outer hair cells), cochlear whole nerve action potential, and single unit recordings can be used to asses hair cell transduction and synaptic activity, the function of auditory afferent nerves, and individual neurons of the cochlear and vestibular nerves in experimental animals.

Peripheral Pathology of Age-Related Hearing Impairment in Humans

Schuknecht's classification of 1964 is still a valuable guideline today for the various forms of presbycusis although the framework has limitations. The broad categories of ARHI are as follows: (1) *Sensory* ARHI refers to a primary degeneration of hair cells of the organ of Corti that begins in the base, yielding an audiogram that is abnormal only at the high frequencies (Figure 44-5A). Current data suggest that ARHI in humans largely follows such a pattern of a high-frequency hearing loss. (2) *Neural* ARHI mainly reflects loss of afferent neurons while cochlear structures remain relatively normal, leading to a loss of word discrimination ability. In general, aging people lose afferent neurons only slowly and significant changes in the audiogram may require a loss of 90% of neurons. The incidence of neural ARHI is low and the existence of a purely neural ARHI is even controversial. As hair cells degenerate, secondary neuronal degeneration follows, so that the term "sensorineural" ARHI is favored over a separation of sensory and neural ARHI. (3) *Strial*, or *metabolic*, ARHI is caused by a degeneration of the stria vascularis (primarily a "flattening," reduction of volume) resulting in a decrease of the endocochlear potential. This decrease of the driving force for transduction affects the entire cochlea and therefore all frequencies. The audiogram shows a flat hearing loss (Figure 44-5B). Strial ARHI may account for 20% to 35% of ARHI according to Schuknecht, who also noted that strial ARHI tends to occur earlier in life than other forms. Others peg the incidence of this form of hearing loss much lower. Although Schuknecht did not include the spiral ligament in the hallmarks of strial ARHI, human and animal studies have tied strial pathology to that of the adjacent spiral ligament. (4) *Cochlear conductive* ARHI *or mechanical* ARHI is caused by changes in the stiffness of the basilar membrane. An audiogram of this type shows a linear decline of over 50 dB at all frequencies without degeneration of any cochlear cells or structures. Only a small portion

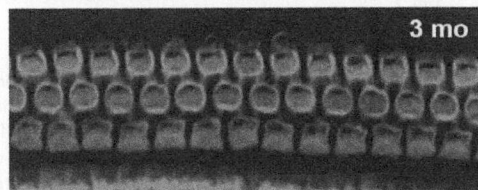
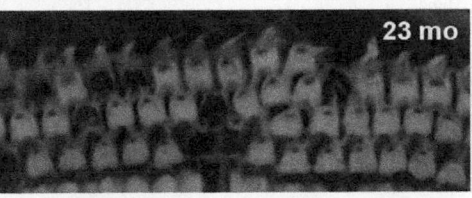

FIGURE 44-4. Loss of hair cells with age. Surface preparations of the mouse cochlea are stained with phalloidin to visualize F-actin, a major component of stereocilia and hair cells. Three rows of outer hair cells are complete and arranged in an orderly fashion in an animal of 3 months of age. At 23 months, the structure is disturbed and some cells are missing.

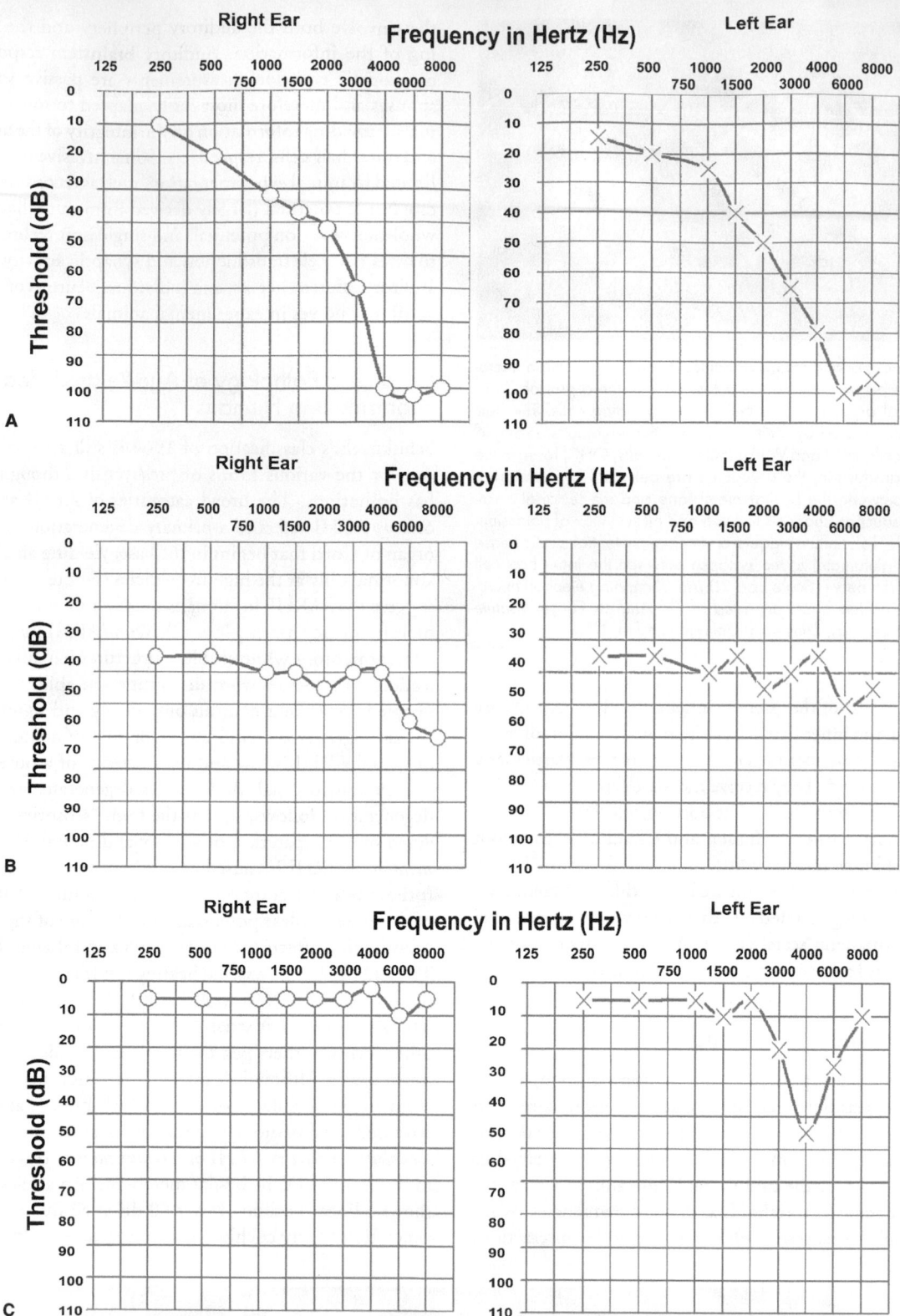

FIGURE 44-5. Audiograms of different forms of hearing loss. Pure-tone audiograms record the auditory thresholds, i.e., the minimal sound level necessary to elicit a response in the listener at specific frequencies. Typical audiograms cover the range from 250 to 8000 Hz and the increasing intensity of the sound is plotted downward on the y-axis. A normal ear (Figure 45-5c, right) would yield an audiogram with flat responses around 0 to 10 dB; if the threshold is increased in a subject, the curve drops lower. Thresholds of 25 to 30 dB constitute a subjectively noticeable impairment, 70 dB and above would make perception at this frequency difficult to impossible. (A) The sloping audiogram from a 62-year-old male shows progressive high-frequency hearing loss in both ears. Fundamental speech frequencies are moderately affected but the threshold of 65 dB at 3000 Hz renders speech discrimination in noise difficult. (B) The flat audiogram from a 64-year-old male shifted to higher thresholds is indicative of a "metabolic" presbycusis. (C) The audiogram from a 32-year-old male shows a sharply defined hearing loss of 45 dB only at 4 kHz in the left ear. Such a "notch" in the audiogram is typical for noise damage, here from target shooting or hunting.

of ARHI is estimated to fall into this category. (5) Mixed ARHI in which multiple forms of pathologies overlap. About 25% of cases may be of mixed pathology.

In evaluating age-related hearing loss, it is oftentimes difficult to determine the contributions of environmental influences that also damage the hair cells in the organ of Corti, such as exposure to noise, industrial solvents, or ototoxic medications. Aminoglycoside antibiotics (exemplified by streptomycin, gentamicin, kanamycin, and related drugs), in particular, destroy hair cells in a base-to-apex progression, causing an initial high-frequency hearing loss reminiscent of sensorineural presbycusis. Noise-induced hearing loss usually differs in its pattern as the site of cochlear damage relates to the frequency of the exposure. Furthermore, a fingerprint of noise trauma in hunters and shooters is a unilateral hearing deficit in the 4 kHz region (Figure 44-5C). Damage from industrial noise would be expected to be bilateral and show a broader area of hearing loss.

Central Auditory Aspect of Age-Related Hearing Impairment

Central auditory changes with aging can essentially be classified into two major types. The first is referred to as "peripherally induced central effects," which presents with changes in the cochlear nucleus driven by the decline of peripheral cochlear inputs that occur with age, typically starting with hearing loss at high frequencies. The other is referred to as "true aging" neurodegenerative changes in the brain. In this case, ARHI share similarities or common mechanisms with other central nervous system conditions of the aged such as Alzheimer's and Parkinson's diseases. Age-dependent changes in auditory structures include declines in the number of ventral cochlear nucleus and lemniscal nerve fibers.

The elderly often present with difficulties in speech recognition, rather than an inability to hear sound. Despite audiograms within the normal range, the subjects still require a stronger speech signal, particularly, in a noisy environment. These subjects may have deficits in processing sound in the higher auditory centers. Specific comprehension tests (e.g., a speech perception in noise (SPIN) test) can be used to diagnose such a condition.

Animal models have illuminated some central consequences of peripheral degeneration. Neurons with low thresholds for high-frequency tones (e.g., in the ventral inferior colliculus) cease to respond and the locations of frequency representation change. Synaptic connections may change in number, spontaneous activity, or their inhibitory or excitatory properties. Such changes do not bode well for a rehabilitation of the hearing impaired with, for example, cochlear implantation (see section on "Management of Age-Related Hearing Impairment"). The adult auditory system, however, shows surprising plasticity and electrical stimulation by implants can reverse some of the central changes.

Animal Models of Peripheral Age-Related Hearing Impairment

A large variety of species has been studied for age-related auditory pathology including chinchillas, guinea pigs, primates, dogs, and rodents. These species cover the range of cochlear pathologies, including organ of Corti, neural and strial degeneration, as is noted for humans, and the majority of animals show a complex mix of cochlear pathologies. Mongolian gerbils are considered a model for strial presbycusis, presenting with strial atrophy, decrease in the endocochlear potential, and decreased cochlear blood flow. Degeneration of spiral ganglion cells and fibrocyte vacuolization and interstitial edema in the spiral ligament are also observed. In cats and rats, the underlying pathology has been linked to a combination of hair cell loss and spiral ganglion cells. Recently, a strial type of hearing loss was also observed in the rat underscoring the fact that a singular "pure" type of hearing loss maybe rare in any species.

Mice have become favored for study of ARHI, because of availability of molecular and genetic information and of transgenic and knock-out animals. A caveat, however, is that each mouse strain differs significantly in its rate of hearing loss, ranging from those such as CBA and CAST, which exhibit minimal hearing loss by 18 months of age, to those such as C57BL/6 and DBA, which exhibit significantly accelerated hearing loss by approximately 8 and 3 months of age, respectively. The accelerated loss of hair cells and hearing found in C57BL/6 and BALB/cJ mice correlates with the presence of a recessive locus on proximal mouse Chr 10, the age-related hearing loss (Ahl) gene. The Cdh23[ahl] allele (cadherin 23 or otocadherin) promotes degeneration of the organ of Corti in the cochlear base and high-frequency hearing loss beginning after 1 year of age as shown in congenic B-6.CAST-Cdh23[ahl]. Furthermore, Cdh23[ahl] also promotes noise-induced hearing loss, suggesting a connection between noise and ARHI. Since BALB/cJ and C57/BL mice are genetic mutations, they may not reflect a normal biological aging process.

The CBA/J mouse loses hearing sensitivity late in its life span progressively from high frequencies to low. ARHI begins around 12 months of age and progresses slowly until 18 months after which point a more rapid rate of hearing loss is seen. The hearing loss at high frequencies is accompanied by loss of outer hair cells and a moderate degeneration of spiral ganglion cells. Since the CBA/J strain maintains a normal morphology of stria vascularis and normal endocochlear potential in aging, a sensorineural origin of the observed auditory deficits can be inferred.

Molecular Mechanisms of Age-Related Hearing Impairment in Animal Models

Recent work places "auditory aging" in animals—at least for sensorineural presbycusis—into the category of oxidant-stress related events. Reaction products of reactive oxygen species are elevated in the cochlea of the aging CBA/J mouse including markers for increased activity of hydroxyl radicals, peroxynitrite, and H_2O_2. At the same time, antioxidant defense systems including mitochondrial superoxide dismutase and apoptosis-inducing factor, both radical scavengers, decrease. Other suggestive evidence comes from heterozygous mice lacking superoxide dismutase. Age-related hearing loss developed earlier and with greater severity, as evidenced by increased hair cell loss following the canonical base-to-apex progression. The imbalance of oxidant stress in the cochlea then stimulates redox-regulated signaling pathways, leading to apoptotic and necrotic cell death. Strong support for the notion of oxidant stress as a contributing factor in cochlear aging comes from dietary manipulations in which antioxidants slow the progression of cochlear degeneration and hearing loss (see section on "Prevention of Age-Related Hearing Impairment").

Deletions in mitochondrial DNA are also an established indicator of cumulative oxidative damage to a tissue and have been observed in the aging cochlea. The mtDNA[4977] deletion is the most common

mutation, which affects cells' capacity for oxidative phosphorylation and appears to accumulate with age. A strong correlation exists
between these signs of free radical-inflicted injury and the hearing
ability of rats.

Vascular abnormalities are another pathological change with aging potentially affecting oxygen supply and mitochondrial respiration thus adding to oxidant stress in the inner ear. As a case in point,
suppression of cochlear blood flow promotes mitochondrial DNA
mutations and may impact hearing loss. In addition, reduction of
cochlear blood flow from age-related degeneration could lead to
a compromised function of the stria vascularis and an inability to
maintain cochlear homeostasis for the maintenance of transduction
currents and tissue integrity.

Genetic Contributions to Age-Related Hearing Impairment in Animal Models

The vast majority of known mouse models of genetic hearing loss exhibit sensory dysfunction soon after birth. Analysis of these models
has implicated a diverse array of genes required during early embryonic development and postnatal maturation of the auditory sensory
neuroepithelium. However, the utility of these models for understanding later-onset hearing loss is unclear. The few studies that
have directly examined the influence of genetic variation on later
hearing acuity in the mouse indicate that ARHI combines contributions from several genes in addition to environmental influences.
For example, the aforementioned Cdh23 gene locus modifies other
loci related to calcium metabolisms. Calcium is not only a second
messenger in homeostatic mechanisms but it is a universal signal
responsible for controlling a plethora of cellular processes, including cell death pathways. Calcium also plays a central role in mitochondrial function and a dysregulation of mitochondrial calcium
can impair energy metabolism and enhance free radical generation,
triggering further mitochondrial dysfunction, cytochrome c release,
and apoptotic pathways. Although it is has been postulated that
many genes will participate in the etiology of ARHI, little research
data are available on the identity of such genes. Some candidate
genes include a gene responsible for a carcinogen metabolizing enzyme, N-acetyltransferase 2 (NAT2), polymorphism, and a single-
nucleotide polymorphism within gene KCNQ4 that codes for a
potassium voltage-gated channel expressed in hair cells.

Prevention of Age-Related Hearing Impairment

As discussed above, several environmental and personal behavioral
factors are associated with the overall manifestations of ARHI.
Therefore, avoiding noise, ototoxins and smoking, regular exercising, and maintaining a healthy diet will aid in attenuating progressive
hearing loss as it will contribute to general health. The question as to
what extent interventive strategies can specifically delay ARHI cannot yet be conclusively answered but some data point to the general
concept that the rate of ARHI can be influenced.

"Augmented Acoustic Environment" is a concept to influence the
progression of presbycusis by exposure to controlled stimuli. This
environment could be created by an enhanced ambient acoustic
background or by delivery of specific stimuli through hearing aids.
Studies in mice, mostly on inbred strains with accelerated hearing
loss, confirm that the auditory system responds to such treatment
but not necessarily in predictable ways. While amelioration of some

forms of age-related changes was found, other effects were detrimental, leaving final judgment to future experimentation.

Dietary restriction has been widely used in aging studies and can
slow certain age-related physiological declines and extend longevity.
For the auditory system, results of such studies are inconclusive
and emphasize the point that organ-specific effects of a generalized
treatment are impossible to predict. Caloric restriction had positive
effects on the progression and magnitude of ARHI in rats but was
ineffective in rhesus monkeys. A comprehensive study of 15 mouse
strains brought every conceivable result from an apparent amelioration of the rate or severity of presbycusis to no effects and to an
acceleration of hearing loss. Such results indicate a major influence
of genotype on the outcome, cautioning that similar problems might
be encountered in presbycusis therapy in humans.

Antioxidant therapy in animal models, based on the premise that
oxidant stress is a contributor to ARHI, has shown promise but also
inconsistencies. Rats that were placed on vitamin supplementation
(vitamins C and E) shortly after birth outperformed their placebo
controls in hearing tests at old age. When the supplementation with
antioxidants (acetyl carnitine and lipoic acid) was started later in
life and upheld for 6 weeks, results were less convincing. Dogs, on
the other hand, fed an antioxidant diet (DL-α-tocopherol acetate, L-
carnitine, DL-α-lipoic acid, and ascorbic acid) for the final 3 years of
their life had better preserved auditory neurons. The key to success,
aside from a suitable combination of compounds, seems to be the
long duration of treatment.

Human studies corroborate the hypothesis that ARHI can be
manipulated by therapeutic intervention. Daily supplementation of
folic acid for 3 years affected the hearing of elderly participants.
There was a small but significant positive effect on low-frequency
hearing while changes in high-frequency hearing, the area normally
most afflicted by aging, were not affected by the treatment. Nevertheless, since low-frequency hearing is important for speech, the
result is encouraging. The underlying mechanism of this protection has yet to be established but the effect goes hand-in-hand with
controversial observations that patients with higher erythrocyte and
serum concentrations of folate maintain lower hearing thresholds.
It should be noted however that routine folic acid supplementation
of foods is not permitted in the Netherlands where the study was
carried out. Results may differ in countries where basic folate levels
in the population maybe higher.

Quite intriguingly, several surveys indicate alcohol consumption
as a possible modulator of ARHI. Moderate use of alcohol was associated with better hearing in the elderly, an effect in line with
observations that low alcohol intake can be beneficial for general
health. Heavy drinkers, in contrast, had a tendency toward more
pronounced high-frequency hearing loss.

Management of Age-Related Hearing Impairment

The major cause of ARHI is the loss of hair cells and cochlear neurons. Since hair cells, as mentioned, cannot regenerate, restoration
of normal hearing is not possible. The choice for rehabilitation of
ARHI is hearing aids. Digital hearing aids present a wide range
of user options and have advanced technologically in all aspects
including the tolerance of a noisy environment and improved cos-
metology. Hearing aids, individually tailored to a subject's audiogram, provide clearly increased hearing ability and speech discrimination (Figure 44-6). However, knowledge about the benefits and

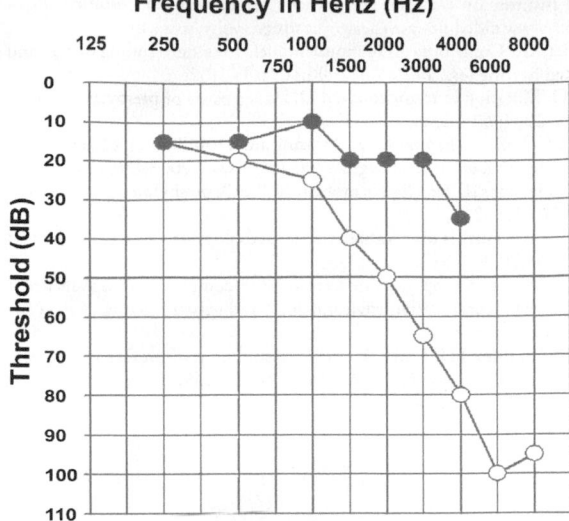

FIGURE 44-6. Typical effects of a hearing aid. The unaided audiogram (open circles) shows presbycusic high-frequency hearing loss. With hearing aids in place (closed circles), acuity is improved to near-normal levels for frequencies up to 3000 Hz. Note that low frequencies deliberately are not boosted and that rescue of the elevated thresholds at high frequencies is not possible.

acceptance of hearing aids is low. About one-half of elderly people who could benefit from a hearing aid never try; others are dissatisfied after short use and only 10% to 30% wear hearing aids. While rejection to a large extent depends on personal idiosyncrasies, health care, and cultural aspects, it can in some instances have a pathophysiological basis. "I can hear but I can't understand" may point to a central auditory deficit that cannot be easily corrected by enhancing the peripheral stimulus.

If the magnitude of the hearing loss exceeds the corrective capability of hearing aids, cochlear implants are recommended with increasing frequency to older subjects. Such "bionic ears" are indicated for persons with bilateral hearing loss and 50% or poorer word recognition. While a hearing aid essentially amplifies sound to the cochlea and therefore depends on remaining sensory cells, the cochlear implant bypasses the cochlea and stimulates the auditory nerve directly. To achieve an effective transformation to an electrical stimulus, the acoustic information needs to be preprocessed and delivered to the nerve via an electrode implanted into the cochlea. The success depends on appropriate coding paradigms and a healthy complement of cochlear nerve innervation. Since the degeneration of the cochlear nerve is slow in humans, much of the aging population presenting with presbycusis would be good candidates. The outcome of implantation is variable but almost all of the patients greatly improve speech perception and most even acquire the ability to carry on telephone conversations. Challenges that remain are speech recognition in unfamiliar contexts and the enjoyment of music.

Outlook

Age-related hearing loss is an exceedingly complex disease besetting an organ of even greater complexity. It appears to be a sequel to numerous morphological and molecular changes that befall the auditory system as we age, and which are being characterized with increasing acuity by basic and clinical research. Our understanding and ability to design interventive and curative therapies will much depend on advances into the molecular mechanisms of auditory pathologies.

Given the partial success of pharmacological protection, this approach should yield the first practical results. Appropriate agents for and timing of interventions will be explored in animal models, both independent of and tied into interventions in extending life span and general health. Gene therapy also shows promise as a possible strategy to protect hair cells. To date, research has successfully focused on prevention of hearing loss caused by acute trauma like drugs and noise. Such model systems can easily be applied to hearing loss from aging as the etiology of these insults can be strikingly similar to age-related sensorineural hearing loss. As the caveats in the preceding sections point out, we have to be careful in translating results from models to humans, and lengthy trials may prevent the immediate implementation of prospective solutions.

In the area of rehabilitation, technological advances of hearing aids and cochlear implants will improve not only speech recognition but also music appreciation, an area of difficult rehabilitation. A direct nerve implant, already successfully tested in an animal model, may replace the cochlear implant for better efficacy of stimulation and a wider range of frequency and intensity perception. The following generation of prostheses will bypass the cochlea and its nerve and stimulate higher auditory centers. Although clinical application of auditory midbrain implants is in its infancy, a handful of patients have already been treated. Such prosthetic therapy could prove advantageous for patients with massive degeneration of the auditory periphery and/or degeneration of the auditory nerve as in a severe neural type of ARHI.

Lastly, functional hair cell regeneration is the final frontier in the field. Recent studies have shown that cells in the organ of Corti, such as supporting cells, may mitose or transdifferentiate into hair cells if appropriately stimulated. The challenges, however, are highly complex: not only hair cells need to be (re)generated, they also have to be incorporated into the intricate cytoarchitecture of the cochlea and find their appropriate connections to the central auditory structures. Stem cell research may likewise provide new insights for replacement of hair cells and the regeneration of the auditory nerve.

Although presbycusis is not yet preventable or treatable, progress in basic and clinical research promises hope for the future. Most realistic in the near term seem protective pharmacological strategies to delay or attenuate age-related hearing impairment and improved rehabilitation through next-generation hearing aids and implants. A plausible clinical therapy for the regeneration of new and functional hair cells may, despite recent encouraging advance, still be decades away.

ACKNOWLEDGMENT

Dr. Schacht's and Sha's research on age-related hearing loss is supported by program project grant AG-025164 from the National Institute on Aging, NIH.

FURTHER READING

Durga J, Verhoef P, Anteunis LJ, Schouten E, Kok FJ. Effects of folic acid supplementation on hearing in older adults: a randomized, controlled trial. *Ann Intern Med.* 2007;146:1–9.

Frisina RD, Walton JP. Age-related structural and functional changes in the cochlear nucleus. *Hear Res*. 2006;216–217:216–223.

Gates GA, Cooper JC Jr, Kannel WB, Miller NJ. Hearing in the elderly: the Framingham cohort, 1983–1985. Part I. Basic audiometric test results. *Ear Hear*. 1990;11:247–256.

Helzner EP, Cauley JA, Pratt SR, et al. Race and sex differences in age-related hearing loss: the Health, Aging and Body Composition Study. *J Am Geriatr Soc*. 2005;53:2119–2127.

Jiang H, Talaska AE, Schacht J, Sha S-H. Oxidative imbalance in the aging inner ear. *Neurobiol Aging*. 2007;28:1605–1612.

Johnsson LG, Hawkins JE. Sensory and neural degeneration with aging, as seen in microdissections of the human inner ear. *Ann Otol Rhinol Laryngol*. 1972;81: 179–192.

Levy BR, Slade MD, Gill TM. Hearing decline predicted by elders' stereotypes. *J Gerontol B Psychol Sci Soc Sci*. 2006;61:P82–P87.

McFadden SL, Ding D, Salvi R. Anatomical, metabolic and genetic aspects of age-related hearing loss in mice. *Audiology*. 2001;40:313–321.

National Institute on Deafness and Other Communication Disorders. Presbycusis. http://www.nidcd.nih.gov/health/hearing/presbycusis.asp

Ohlemiller KK. Contributions of mouse models to understanding of age- and noise-related hearing loss. *Brain Res*. 2006;1091:89–102.

Pickles JO. Mutation in mitochondrial DNA as a cause of presbyacusis. *Audiol Neurootol*. 2004;9:23–33.

Rosenhall U, Karlsson Espmark AK. Hearing aid rehabilitation: what do older people want, and what does the audiogram tell? *Int J Audiol*. 2003;42(Suppl 2):2S53–2S57.

Schacht J, Hawkins JE. Sketches of otohistory. Part 9: presby[a]cusis. *Audiol Neurootol*. 2005;10:243–247.

Schuknecht HF. Further observations on the pathology of presbycusis. *Arch Otolaryngol*. 1964;80:369–382.

Van Eyken E, Van Camp G, Van Laer L. The complexity of age-related hearing impairment: contributing environmental and genetic factors. *Audiol Neurootol*. 2007;12:345–358.

Willott JF, Chisolm TH, Lister JL. 2001. Modulation of presbycusis: current status and future directions. *Audiol Neurootol*. 6:231–249.

Sex and Gender Across the Human Life Span

William R. Hazzard

John Anderson, My Jo *

> *John Anderson, my jo, John,*
> *When we were first aquent:*
> *Your locks were like the raven,*
> *Your bonie brow was brent.*
> *But now your brow is beld, John,*
> *Your locks are like the snaw;*
> *But blessings on your frosty pow,*
> *John Anderson, my jo.*
> *John Anderson, my jo,*
> *We clamb the hill thegither;*
> *And mony a cantie day, John,*
> *We've had wi' ane anither;*
> *Now we maun totter down, John,*
> *And hand in hand we'll go,*
> *And sleep thegither at the foot,*
> *John Anderson, my jo.*

> *Robert Burns, 1789*

Do you recall this poem above from your high school English literature course? I certainly do, for its romantic depiction of a couple's idealized journey together through this life and perhaps beyond. Little did I dream at the time that the central theme of this chapter would define a paradox that would provide a focus throughout my career in gerontology and geriatric medicine: women outlive men even as they experience greater levels of morbidity, health care utilization, and functional impairment throughout their lives.

A visit to almost any long-term care facility will prompt an obvious question from even the most casual observer: "Where are the men?" This chapter attempts to answer this intriguing question on the basis of both practical and theoretical considerations and extrapolate its conclusions and speculations to considerations of the health

and social care of the elderly in this century of an unprecedented "age wave" in America and the world at large.

The principal questions addressed in this chapter include:

- What is the magnitude of the sex differential in longevity in the United States?
- How universal is this differential among different populations? Among ethnic groups in the United States? Among different nations, especially by degree of socioeconomic development?
- Has this differential always existed? If not, when did it emerge? And why?
- Are there genetic determinants of this differential? Are these mediated by sex hormones? How do these change across the life cycle?
- What are the extragenital consequences of the sex differential in sex hormone physiology at various stages in the life cycle? What are these consequences, notably in the:
  - Nervous system?
  - Endocrine/metabolic system?
  - Immune system?
  - Cardiovascular system?
- What are the social, psychological, and behavioral implications of these differentials at various stages in the life cycle?
- What are the age-specific mortality rates of men and women (commonly expressed as the ratio between the two)—both all-cause and cause-specific?
- What are the age-specific morbidity rates in men and women—both all-cause (especially as expressed in functional status) and cause-specific?
- How do these differentials affect the lives of older persons, with specific implications for the duration and quality of life for elderly men and women? For the prevalence and duration of widowhood? For the health—physical, psychological, social, functional, and

*Joy.

financial—and social and living circumstances of elderly widows and widowers?

- Are these trends changing? If so, how and why? And if so, what are the implications of those changes for the lives of elderly Americans in the twenty-first century?

- Finally, on a more macro level, what are the planning and policy implications of those changes (with special reference to health care and long term care)?

DEFINITIONS

Throughout this chapter the following definitions are used, conforming to the recommendations of the Committee on Understanding the Biology of Sex and Gender Differences formed by the Board on Health Sciences Policy of the Institute of Medicine of the National Academy of Sciences as explicitly advanced in their landmark 2001 report, edited by Wizeman and Pardue, entitled *Exploring the Biological Contributions to Human Health: Does Sex Matter?*:

- *Sex:* The classification of living things, generally as male or female according to their reproductive organs and functions assigned by chromosomal complement.

- *Gender:* A person's self-representation as male or female, or how that person is responded to by social institutions based on the individual's gender presentation. Gender is rooted in biology and shaped by environment and experience.

It is noteworthy that simply to clarify use of the terms *sex* and *gender* was one of the principal recommendations of this report. As will become evident, this distinction is important in consideration of the central issues in this chapter wherein sex and gender interact dynamically across the lifespan. This is evident perhaps most dramatically during periods of exceptional rates of change, notably during adolescence and across the menopause, transitions that will be highlighted in the discussion that follows. For both sex and gender contribute significantly to the longevity, function, and quality of life of elderly Americans and both must be considered in responsible planning efforts for their health and social care in the twenty-first century.

HISTORY OF THE SEX DIFFERENTIAL IN LONGEVITY

The sex differential in longevity from birth in contemporary American society is currently over 5 years (Table 45-1). However, this differential has changed dramatically over the past century and continues to evolve. At the beginning of the twentieth century, when the United States was still a developing nation, the sex differential in human longevity was just 2 years, and the overall age-adjusted male:female mortality ratio was only 1:1 (Figure 45-1). Throughout the first 70 years of that century, the ratio climbed steadily (except for a brief decline to near unity during the period 1918 to 1919, which was attributable to the [still unexplained] greater female mortality during the influenza pandemic of that era). This continuous increase translated into a sex differential in expected longevity at birth that reached a maximum at 7.5 years during the period 1969 to 1971. During those seven decades, the nation experienced progressive and dramatic socioeconomic development, a series of cataclysmic wars, and major changes in the roles of men and women in society. The social

TABLE 45-1

Life Expectancy at Birth, Age 65, and Age 75 Yrs, United States, All Races, 1998

AGE	LIFE EXPECTANCY (YEARS)		DIFFERENCE (FEMALE MINUS MALE)	PERCENT PERCENT DIFFERENCE*
	Males	Females		
At birth	73.8	79.5	5.7	7
At 65 yrs	16.0	19.2	3.2	17
At 75 yrs	10.0	12.2	2.2	18

*Percent Difference equals (life expectancy for females minus life expectancy for males) divided by life expectancy for females.

Adapted from National Center for Health Statistics, 2000a Reprinted with permission from Institute of Medicine, *Exploring the Biological Contributions to Human Health: Does Sex Matter?* Washington, DC: National Academy Press; 2001.

progress of women in the post-World War II and Vietnam war era and the rise of the feminist movement led some cynics (mostly men) to predict that women would begin to suffer the health and mortality consequences of the lifestyles and social roles historically considered as "masculine" (the so-called "they'll get theirs" scenario). In this author's experience, all persons, both lay and professional, have strong opinions as to why women outlive men. These opinions, however, are more often rooted in personal biases than objective scientific consideration. To illustrate this point, a 1996 survey of more than 500 college-aged students confirmed a distinct sex difference in attribution of the sex differential in longevity: young males ascribed the difference to the traditionally greater physical labor of men and the less stressful life of women, while the females attributed it to better self-care and attention to health by women.

While there is very little evidence to support any of the predicted deterioration in health or longevity of women in the present climate of changing lifestyles and occupational status (women in the

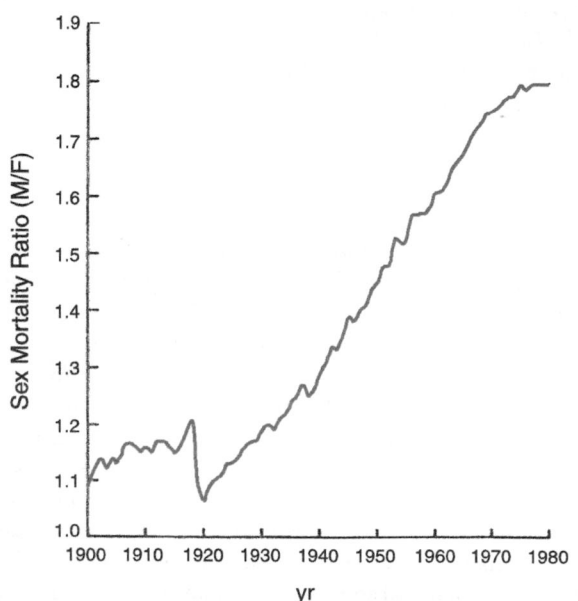

FIGURE 45-1. Gender mortality ratio (M/F), United States 1900–1980. Based on mortality rates age-adjusted to the 1940 total U.S. population. (*From Wingard DL. The sex differential in morbidity, mortality, and lifestyle. Ann Rev Public Health. 5:433, 1984.*)

TABLE 45-2

Average Life Expectancy at Given Ages for White Adults, United States, 1980, Presented by Gender

AGE	LIFE EXPECTANCY (YEARS)		MALE/FEMALE RATIO, %
	Male	Female	
At birth	70.7	78.1	90.5
At 60 yrs	17.5	22.4	78.1
At 65 yrs	14.2	18.5	76.8
At 70 yrs	11.3	14.8	76.4
At 75 yrs	8.8	11.5	76.5
At 80 yrs	6.7	8.6	77.0
At 85 yrs	5.0	6.3	79.4

Adapted from Wylie CM: Contrasts in the healths of elderly men and women: An analysis of recent data for articles in the United States. J Am Geriatr Soc. 1984;32:670.

TABLE 45-3

Genetic Factors That May Differentially Affect the Basic Biochemistry of Male and Female Cells

Female specific:
- Expression of some genes from both X chromosomes
- Defect in initiation or maintenance of X chromosome inactivation
- Changes in estrogen-responsive genes (e.g., the HER2 gene in breast cancer) in germ line or somatic cells

Male specific:
- X-chromosome-linked recessive mutations
- Expression of Y-chromosome-specific genes
- Changes in androgen-responsive genes in germ line or somatic cells

Reprinted with permission from Institute of Medicine, Exploring the Biological Contributions to Human Health: Does Sex Matter? Washington, DC: National Academy Press; 2001.

workforce generally experience considerably fewer health problems, seek medical attention substantially less often, and carry less mortality risks than women who are not employed), there can no longer be any doubt that the sex differential in longevity in America has begun to narrow and, in retrospect, has been doing so progressively over the past 30 years. Harbingers of this trend were apparent in mortality data from the late 1960s, when a plateau in the previous linear rise in the sex differential in age-specific death rates began to emerge (see Figure 45-1), and the absolute difference between the sexes in expected longevity subsequently began to decline (see Table 45-1). However, as this trend has continued, it has reflected a greater gain among males than females (compare Table 45-2 with Table 45-1), even as both sexes have experienced continuing moderate increases to unprecedented average longevity. Should this pattern continue, it will introduce an important change in demography of the aging population, as the sex differential progressively narrows. This will reduce the burden of widowhood on survivors and hence the vulnerability of those survivors, especially widows, to loss of independence and consequent institutionalization (discussed further below).

Nevertheless, a certain minimum sex differential in longevity appears to be a fundamental, perhaps immutable, principle of human gerontology. In America, this appears to hold true across ethnic groups with a broad range of average longevities. Nor is this phenomenon confined to the United States: the gap that developed in the United States in the twentieth century simultaneously emerged in all nations that underwent similar socioeconomic development (albeit with considerable variance in the magnitude of those changes; see Ory and Warner), with accompanying increases in average longevity of both sexes. Indeed, as detailed in the insightful review by Austad, women outlive men in 103 of the 104 demographic units tracked in the *United Nations Demographic Yearbook*, the lone recent exception being Bangladesh. These longevity increases are attributed principally to improvements in nutrition, education, housing, transportation, sanitation, public health, and health care, all leading to reductions in the diseases and conditions that predispose to the vastly premature deaths of infants and children. These developments also reduced the deaths of women of reproductive age associated with childbearing (including reduced numbers of pregnancies and deliveries). The same societies also generally experienced simultaneous advances in the status of women in general, a trend that appears to parallel reductions in premature mortality of women wherever it occurs (see Table 45-3 and concluding section).

WHEN DOES THE SEX DIFFERENTIAL IN MORTALITY BEGIN?

The sex differential in mortality (Figure 45-2) appears to begin at conception, when the ratio of male to female zygotes may be as high as 170 to 100 (for reasons that remain unclear, Y-bearing sperm are more likely to fertilize an egg than are sperm with the X-chromosome). Because of greater in utero male fetal death, however, by 10 to 12 weeks of gestation (as determined in abortuses), the gender ratio has declined to approximately 130:100. This decline in male survival continues throughout fetal life such that by birth this

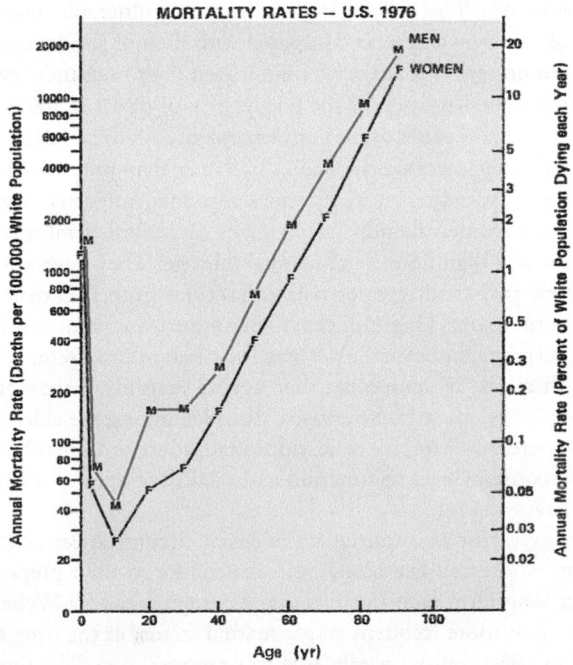

FIGURE 45-2. Mortality rates by gender, United States, 1976. *(Compiled from data presented in Gee EM, Veevers JE: Accelerating sex differential in mortality: An analysis of contributing factors. Soc Biol. 30:75, 1984).*

ratio has decreased yet further to 106:100 (see chapter by Neel in the volume edited by Ory and Warner).

This trend continues throughout the remainder of the human life span, albeit less dramatically with advancing age. And because the sex ratio of the population at every age reflects the cumulative survival of the sexes from each preceding birth cohort, the sex differential among survivors progressively favors females over males with every passing year of life. After the initial 6% excess of males over females at birth, the continued surplus of male deaths produces parity in numbers between the sexes during adolescence. However, at every age beyond that era, women outnumber men with an ever-growing sex disparity. This leads to a progressive rise in the ratio of women to men with advancing age, a pattern that appears to grow almost exponentially in old age, to a female:male ratio of approximately 3:2 among community-dwelling elderly persons older than age 85 years.

Somewhat paradoxically, this sex differential in the population grows with age in spite of a progressive narrowing in the gap in expected remaining longevity between the sexes, especially beyond middle age. This dwindles to little more than 2 years at age 75 years (see Table 45-2) and 1 year at age 85 years. Of practical utility to clinicians (e.g., in counseling aging couples), the ratio of remaining expected longevity between men and women remains relatively constant beyond middle age, stabilizing at approximately 80% (men compared with women) (see Table 45-1) even as the absolute difference narrows with each passing year of survival. Thus, a strategy designed to minimize the duration of widowhood should place special emphasis on survival of men through youth and middle age, the phases of life in which their greater vulnerability to premature death contributes most to the sex differential in longevity and protracted widowhood of their spouses.

By contrast with the situation among community-dwelling older persons, however, the sex ratio among residents of long-term care facilities (except, of course, those in the Veterans Affairs system) is far higher than 3:2. Ratios of 6:1 or 7:1 are not unusual in community nursing homes. This reflects in part the more vulnerable functional status of elderly women, as compared with men of similar age, and the common reality that they have outlived their husbands (even in nursing homes—in spite of the greater risk of death in the men in such facilities, measures of the performance of activities of daily living (ADLs) display lower average scores in female than male residents— one of many paradoxes raised in the sex/gender/longevity domain). Thus older women demonstrate greater musculoskeletal weakness and disability than do men of comparable age. They have more osteoporosis and are at greater risk to fractures from falls than their male counterparts. They also experience more urinary incontinence, an impairment that especially raises their risk of long-term institution utilization. Women older than age 85 years also have a greater prevalence of dementia, a pervasive disorder among the elderly that greatly increases their risk of institutionalization and often has devastating consequences to function and quality of life in the nursing home environment.

However, just as important, the social circumstances of elderly women, who often live alone, also contribute to their preponderance in long-term care institutions. As emphasized by Wylie, this reflects their more frequent single marital status: at the time of his review in 1980 approximately 80% of American men older than age 65 years were married, only 40% of women older than age 65 years were married, and the widow to widower ratio was 4:1, all figures that grew by each year of advancing age. Thus, given that for both sexes the person most likely to provide close and continuing support for a vulnerable older individual is the spouse, an elderly man who requires social and health care support to remain in the community is much more likely to have the help and companionship of his wife (who is also usually younger and more vigorous). However, an elderly woman who requires such support is much less likely to have an able spouse in attendance, often having outlived her husband, and she is a candidate for long-term institutional care unless alternative sources of social and health care support can be identified. Widowhood is the normative last phase of life for women: it often lasts more than a decade and is a reality that deserves serious consideration in responsible planning for the care and welfare of older persons for both individual couples and also as social policy.

This differential in caregiving needs and provision of care to elderly men and women is an example of how the terms *sex* and *gender*, as defined earlier, differ in a meaningful way: caregiving is culturally (as well as, arguably, genetically and hormonally) determined; the care provided by wives to their husbands represents an extension of their traditional and normative female nurturing role, a role that carries major implications for the care and welfare of aging persons, both male and female.

MECHANISMS OF THE BIOLOGICAL BASIS OF THE SEX DIFFERENTIAL IN LONGEVITY

The universal nature of the sex differential in mortality across ethnic and geographic lines suggests that this phenomenon may be rooted in the biology as well as the sociology of the human species. The nature and possible biological mechanisms of this differential have recently been concisely summarized by Federman. As recently reviewed by Austad, examples from comparative zoology suggest that the greater longevity of the female versus the male generally predominates in the animal world. An important and instructive caveat prevails here, however: to observe this differential, the environment must be sufficiently protected as to mitigate the harsher consequences of "survival of the fittest" according to strict Darwinian principles, circumstances that prevail in the wild as well as during more primitive stages of human evolution. This cushioned environment, in turn, will permit survival of both sexes to an age approaching the maximum lifetime potential (MLP) of any given species. This is notably the case in zoos, in which aged animals are protected from inimical forces such as predation and malnutrition, and there females generally outlive males. As noted by Austad, in arguably the nonhuman primate most closely resembling the human, the chimpanzee, in zoos or similar protected environments females typically live longer than males by 3 to 4 years, a difference representing about 10% of their MLP. In this example, however, this reflects a dramatic decrease in male survival during relative youth (4–7 years of age), with parallel rates of survival thereafter.

BASIC MOLECULAR GENETICS OF SEX DIFFERENCES (see Table 45-3)

The following systematic review of potential mechanism that mediate the sex differential in human longevity begins with the examination of the genetic platform of both sexes as concentrated in the sex chromosomes and upon which sex and gender dimorphism

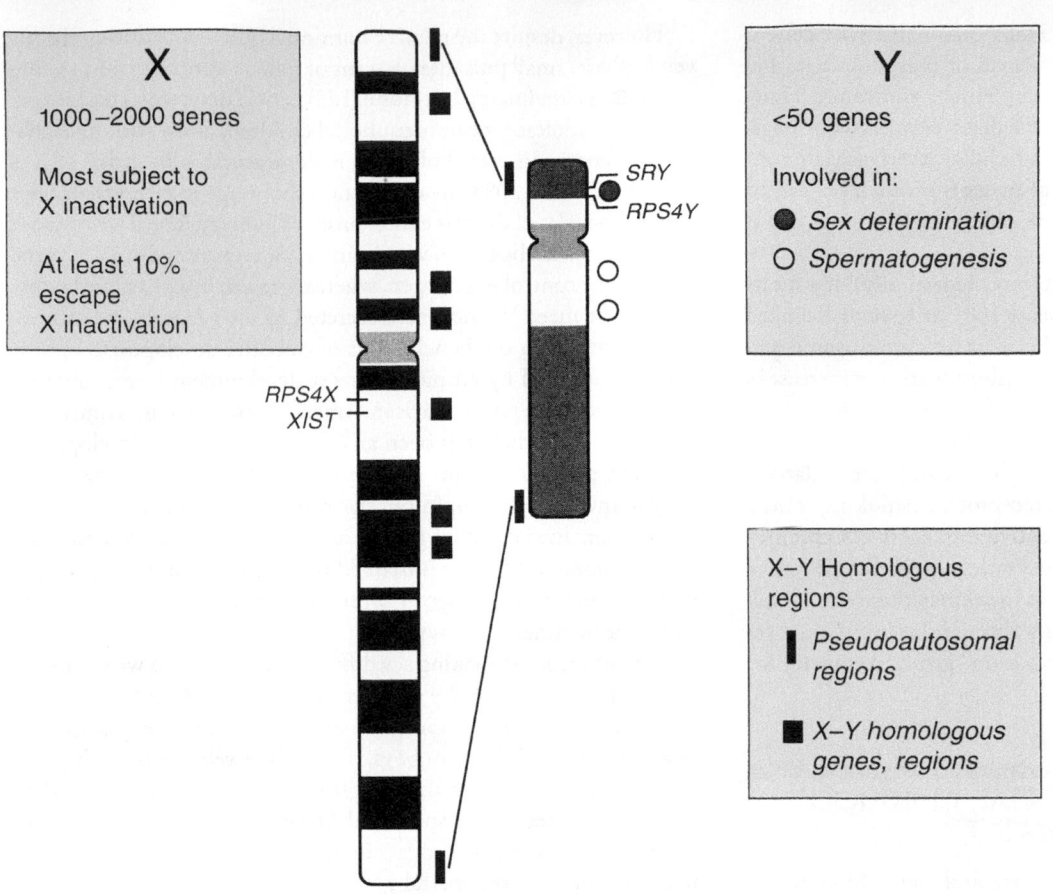

X
1000–2000 genes

Most subject to
X inactivation

At least 10%
escape
X inactivation

RPS4X
XIST

Y
<50 genes

Involved in:

● Sex determination

○ Spermatogenesis

SRY
RPS4Y

X–Y Homologous
regions

❙ Pseudoautosomal
regions

■ X–Y homologous
genes, regions

FIGURE 45-3. The human sex chromosomes. (Reprinted with permission from Institute of Medicine. Exploring the Biological Contributions to Human Health: Does Sex Matter? Washington, DC: National Academy Press; 2001.)

is played out across the life span and focus upon general biological regulators, notably levels of oxidative stress.

The sex chromosomes constitute but approximately 5% of the human genome (Figure 45-3). The Y chromosome is much smaller than the X chromosome and codes for only about two dozen different genes. Of those, the SRY gene determines development of the male gonadal phenotype, while spermatogenesis is related to a small number of other genes, mutation or deletion of which has been associated with certain cases of male infertility. Another class of Y chromosomal genes code for ribosomal proteins in Y-bearing cells (RPS4Y in Figure 45-3), while homologous genes on the X-chromosome code for those proteins in XX cells; thus certain ribosomal proteins throughout the organism differ between male and female cells. However, the functional consequences of these differences remain to be determined.

Male and female genomes differ in another important respect: females have twice the dose of X-chromosomal genes (i.e., "heterogametic"). This difference has led to the heterogametic sex hypothesis that the lack of a second X-chromosome in the male underlies at least a portion of his diminished longevity compared with the female. Here information from comparative zoology offers tantalizing mechanistic insight; for example, in the bird, the female has one long and one short sex chromosome and is thus the heterogametic sex (while the male has the two long ["Z"] sex chromosomes). According to the heterogametic hypothesis, male birds would be predicted to have a longevity advantage over females—which as cited by Austad is indeed the case for several species listed (budgerigars, zebra finches, and Japanese quail)—once again, however, explicitly specific to those raised in captivity.

In the human the X chromosome has approximately 160 000 DNA base pairs encoding an estimated 1000 to 2000 genes (see Figure 45-3). Only a few of these, the "pseudoautosomal," have homologues on the Y chromosome. Products of these genes, like those on the autosomes, play a role in virtually every aspect of cellular function, metabolism, development, and control of growth and turnover. Especially germane to this discussion are those that play specific roles in particular tissues at particular points in development, several of which have been demonstrated to play critical roles in gonadal differentiation.

The twofold increase in X-chromosomal genes in females is in general offset by X-chromosomal inactivation, a complex, carefully regulated process unique to female cells marked in each by one of the two X-chromosomes becoming heterochromatic (identifiable on microscopy as the Barr chromatin body in the nucleus of female cells). This process renders genes on the inactivated X-chromosome functionally silent. It occurs in every somatic cell of XX females but not in XY males. Thus, not only must XX cells maintain the state of cell-specific X-inactivation throughout life but also, because the same X-chromosome is not inactivated in every cell, XX females are "epigenetic mosaics." Not surprisingly, the process of X-inactivation is itself controlled by multiple factors, including genes. However, this may vary widely; in some families, sisters may show nearly identical patterns of X-inactivation, whereas in other studies of female identical twins, such patterns differ widely within twin pairs.

Directly germane to the focus of this discussion, female mosaicism underlies the dramatic sex difference in the severity and risk of death from diseases that are transmitted in a sex-linked recessive mode. For whereas a mutation in a gene on the X-chromosome will be expressed in every cell of an affected male, only half of the cells of the female will experience the consequences of that mutation, and her heterozygous state may carry no functional significance. However, given the rarity of X-linked recessive diseases with major physiologic consequences (e.g., classical hemophilia), the aggregate contribution of all the premature deaths of males from such sex-linked autosomal recessive diseases to the sex differential in longevity is miniscule.

Perhaps more relevant, however (at least theoretically), it appears that in cells grown in culture that at least 10% to 15% of X-linked genes appear to be expressed from the inactive chromosome and hence have "escaped" X-inactivation, contributing to a net increase in activated X-chromosomal gene products in females. This differential X-inactivation may have implications for vulnerabilities to certain diseases in affected individuals; for example, the suspected relationship between gastrin-releasing peptide receptor and smoking-related lung cancer, which is released by both active and inactive X chromosomes, with elevated levels hypothesized to lead to increased risk of lung cancer in women smokers. And, at the purely theoretical level, is X-inactivation maintained constantly throughout life? Could reactivation of the silenced X provide "back-up" genetic resiliency for women in later life?

SEX DIFFERENTIALS DURING FETAL, CHILDHOOD, AND ADOLESCENT DEVELOPMENT

All humans—XX, XY, or with an atypical sex chromosome configuration—begin development from a common starting point *in utero*, with similar, phenotypically female genitalia until 6 to 7 weeks of gestational age. After that point expression of the SRY gene on the Y chromosome in males induces development of the testes. At about 9 weeks, this results in the secretion of testosterone. This, in turn, as modulated by multiple genes (at least 70 on sex chromosomes and autosomes), results in the development of the reproductive tract and masculinization of the male fetus as expressed most notably in the genitalia and the brain. In the absence of testosterone, the female phenotype is expressed; ovarian hormones are not required for this development. Moreover, animal studies and research on human dizygotic twins have suggested that testosterone secreted by a male fetus can exert a masculinizing influence on adjacent female fetuses, with anatomic, physiologic, and behavioral consequences. Thus events during intrauterine life, especially the secretion of testosterone by the fetal testis, exert powerful and enduring effects on postnatal life.

During late fetal life and infancy, however, the hypothalamic–pituitary–gonadal axis is largely suppressed, giving rise to relative hormonal stability throughout childhood (the "juvenile pause"). Adolescence, the gradual coming of age that transpires during most of the second decade of life, is the next phase of development during which the sex and gender differentials in growth and behavior are dramatic. Within that phase, puberty constitutes the transitional period between the juvenile state and adulthood during which the adolescent growth spurt occurs, secondary sexual traits appear (producing the dramatic sexual dimorphism of adult men and women), sexual activity is commonly initiated, and profound psychological changes occur. This tends to be conceptualized as a series of changes arising from reactivation of the hypothalamic–pituitary–gonadal axis.

However, despite the relative hormonal quiescence during the juvenile phase, small pulsatile patterns of follicle-stimulating hormone (FSH) and luteinizing hormone (LH) can be detected as harbingers of coming adolescence in prepubertal children, and a striking eight-fold difference in estradiol levels is demonstrable in girls. This is associated with a 20% advancement in bone age in girls versus boys and maybe related to their earlier onset of puberty. The development of breasts, which begins in white girls at an average age of 10.6 years, is under the control of estrogen, whereas growth in axillary and pubic hair is influenced by androgens secreted by the adrenals and ovaries. The age at which the benchmarks of pubertal development appear is also influenced by ethnicity (breast development begins about a year earlier on average in African-American girls than in white girls). Whether or not there has been an earlier age of breast development in recent decades remains a subject of controversy. However, contrary to much popular opinion, the average age of menarche appears to have remained constant for at least the past four decades. In boys, the beginning of puberty is marked by an increase in testicular size, which begins at a mean age of approximately 11 years (in both white and African-American boys).

One of the most striking sex differentials associated with puberty is the earlier onset of the growth spurt in girls (Figure 45-4), in whom it may actually begin prior to breast development or growth of axillary or pubic hair. In boys, peak height velocity is reached approximately 2 years later than in girls, although boys are taller than girls at the onset of the spurt and finish, albeit later, with a mean height that is 12.5 cm (about 5 inches) greater. This differential reflects the greater prepubertal growth of boys and their taller status when their pubertal growth spurt takes off as well as their greater growth during the pubertal phase. The principal hormonal determinants of the growth spurt are growth hormone, insulin-like growth factor-1 (IGF-1) (hypothesis #3 in Table 45-3), and triiodothyronine in the prepubertal phase (accounting for 50% of the height increase during the subsequent pubertal phase), while estradiol is the main sex hormone involved in the pubertal phase in boys as well as in girls (the estrogen in boys arising principally by extragonadal conversion from testosterone).

Another hormonal feature of puberty is the phenomenon of adrenarche, which begins before age 8 years and is marked by progressive increases in adrenal androgen secretion and plasma dehydroepiandrosterone (DHEA) and DHEA-sulfate. Adrenarche is independent of the mechanisms that regulate the secretion of sex steroids from the gonads (gonadarche). Clinically adrenarche is signaled by the appearance of axillary and pubic hair and is considered premature when it occurs in white girls before age 7 years and in African-Americans before age 5 years. In contrast to the circumstance in boys, in whom premature adrenarche is a benign variant of normal puberty, in girls it is associated with a 10-fold increased risk of the polycystic ovary syndrome (PCOS) and its associated (and pathophysiologically important) features of ovarian hyperandrogenism and insulin resistance. These lead to an increased incidence of central obesity, type 2 diabetes, hypertension, and dyslipidemia (with a male-type pattern of higher low-density lipoprotein [LDL] and lower high-density lipoprotein [HDL] cholesterol levels prior to the era of the menopause), all cardinal features of the "metabolic syndrome." PCOS, which has been estimated to occur in as many as 10% of women, appears to attenuate the sex-specific relative immunity to cardiovascular disease (CVD) otherwise enjoyed by women. As such, its understanding may provide special insights

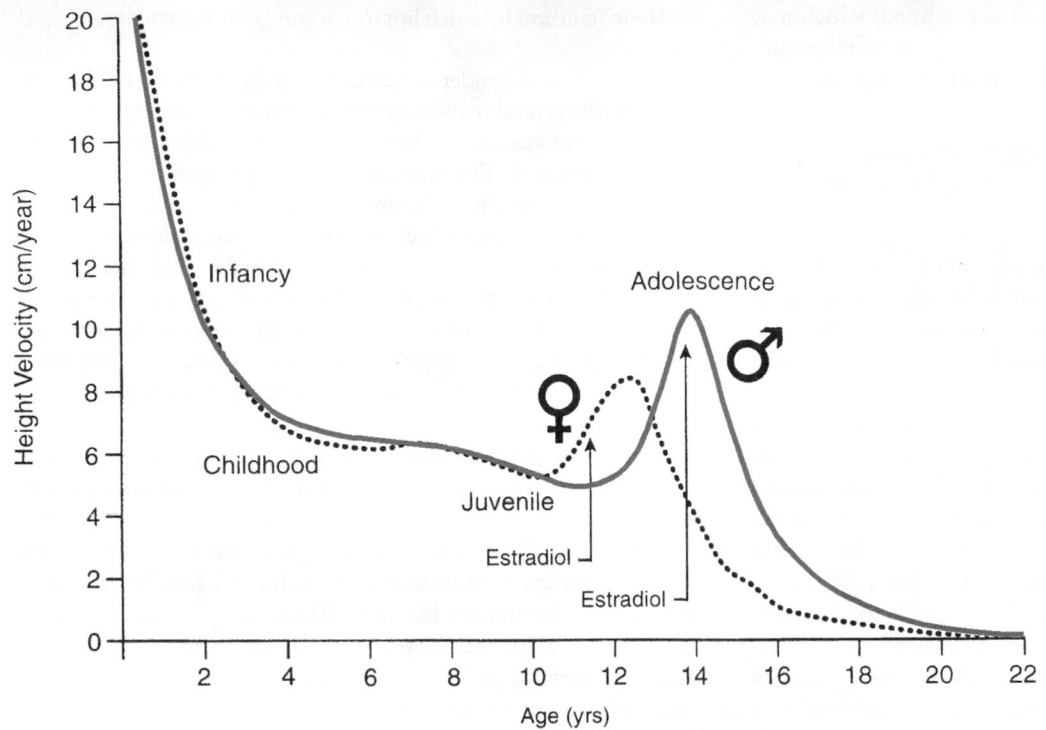

FIGURE 45-4. The relationship between age and height velocity through adolescence in human females and males. *(Reprinted with permission from Institute of Medicine. Exploring the Biological Contributions to Human Health: Does Sex Matter? Washington, DC: National Academy Press; 2001.)*

into the mechanism whereby men are at increased CVD risk, as compared with women, and the role of hormones, including insulin and sex hormones, in mediating that sex differential. Such insight may also provide opportunities to intervene with both behavioral and pharmacologic strategies to prevent premature CVD in men (and potentially in women as well, especially those with PCOS).

Of special relevance to the premise of this chapter that the sex differential in longevity originates in events in the life cycle long before old age, an intriguing body of evidence suggests that there is an association in girls between retarded in utero growth, the risk of premature adrenarche, and their subsequent development of PCOS; certain recent studies suggest that girls with antenatal growth retardation and low birth weights have fewer primordial ovarian follicles and a smaller uterus and ovaries at puberty and subsequent hyporesponsiveness to FSH, which may mediate (or at least be a marker for) the pathophysiology of PCOS. Thus, PCOS may be a classic example of a disorder of adolescence and adulthood that is programmed during fetal life but which holds important implications for health and longevity in middle and late life—as well as providing major insight into the general mechanism whereby nonandrogenized women enjoy longer (and more CVD-free) lives than their male counterparts.

These hormonal and physical changes at puberty also hold important implications for the sex differences in behavior during adolescence that are the subject of such intense contemporary public interest and concern. Some of these differences appear to proceed from the direct effects of gonadal hormones on the brains of adolescent boys and girls. For example, in studies of early adolescents, increasing levels of testosterone were associated with increasing aggression and social dominance in boys, while changes in estrogen levels correlated with changes in behavior patterns in girls during the pubertal transition. In various studies, certain behaviors appear to relate to absolute levels of sex hormones, others to the ratio of testosterone to estrogen, and still others to fluctuations in hormone levels. Still other studies reported changes in sex hormones in response to behaviors, such as increases in testosterone following athletic successes.

Such changes may have important, even life-altering, effects on the adolescents who experience them. Earlier maturation by girls, for instance, has been associated with social adjustment problems during puberty, earlier initiation of sexual activity and pregnancy, and later problems with eating disorders, depression, and substance abuse.

Boys may not have the same extent of social and behavioral problems, partly because of the recognition they receive from precocious physical strength and athleticism. However, there can be little doubt but that the risk-taking behavior of adolescent and young adult males contributes importantly to the stark contrast in mortality rates between young men and women (see below), and it seems logical to attribute such behaviors to hormonally mediated sex differentials across the adolescent transition. These become manifest not only in differentials mediated by sex in the sense of the definition urged by the Institute of Medicine report, but, importantly, also in how adolescents present themselves to the world and how its social institutions respond to them; that is, their gender manifestations. These issues are explored in depth in the provocative essay by Courtenay. Again the physical, psychological, behavioral, and social sex and gender differentials that present such stark contrasts during adolescence are rooted in the antecedent genetic, hormonal, and environmental lives of those boys and girls and also continue to modulate individual and group sex and gender differentials in health and longevity throughout adolescence and the remainder of the life span.

A practical consideration regarding the earlier maturation of girls than boys is also germane to the central theme of this chapter: that the duration of widowhood is an important determinant of the long-term care needs of elderly persons, especially women who have outlived their husbands. Because there is a normative sex differential in the age at marriage of bride and groom (generally about 2 years, likely reflecting the earlier maturation of females), this adds a commensurate period to the duration of widowhood, which may average nearly a decade (2–3 years difference in age at marriage plus approximately 5 to 6 years in the sex differential in longevity).

SEX MAY AFFECT REGULATION OF REDOX STATE AND OXIDATIVE STRESS

An attractive strategy in gerontological research examines mechanisms of homeostatic regulation that apply broadly across tissues and organ systems and which impact function across the life span. As such, they may converge with advancing age to become final common pathways that may mediate age-related comorbid diseases and ultimately frailty and demise in old age. One such mechanism that may contribute to the greater longevity of females is their reported superior regulation of redox balance and level of oxidative stress. As noted by Austad, this appears most evident in studies of rats (as apposed to mice), in which certain (notably the Wistar and Fischer 344) strains demonstrate substantially (ca. 16%) longer female longevity. Especially notable in this regard have been the reports from the laboratory of Vina, where studies of male (vs. female) rats demonstrated more oxidative DNA damage in isolated mitochondria. Yet more intriguing, these investigators reported that ovariectomy in females increased the production of oxygen-free radicals (hydrogen peroxide) in liver and brain mitochondria, an increase that was prevented by estrogen replacement. These findings were extended in measurement of endogenous mitochondrial antioxidant levels of glutathione peroxidase (mRNA and protein activity), which as predicted was higher in females than males. These authors interpreted these findings to attribute the greater longevity of female rats to attenuation of the age-related increase in reactive oxygen species (ROS) by estrogen, enhancing their antioxidant protection against age-related tissue damage. However, this provocative line of research clearly requires much further confirmation and investigation.

SEX AFFECTS NEURAL ANATOMY AND FUNCTION

Another fundamental strategy of gerontologic investigation looks to biological integrating systems for insights into the aging process. This strategy examines how changes in those systems with aging render the organism progressively more vulnerable to insults from the environment in a stochastic cascade that limits survival of the individual and determines average and maximum longevity of a given species. Hence, consideration of the determinants of the sex differential in longevity (as well as of the causes of morbidity at various stages of the life cycle) have focused upon modulation of the neural, endocrine, and immune systems by sex hormones across the life span and how these might explain that differential.

As introduced in the immediately preceding sections and well-summarized in the 2003 Institute of Medicine report, fundamental differences in genetics and physiology between males and females result in important differences in neural anatomy and circuitry as well as in cognition and behavior at all points across the life span. While these differences begin during fetal life, they are amplified and modulated continuously at each age and each stage in a fashion that interacts dynamically with the environment, including sex and gender-sensitive interactions between children and their parents and other aspects of the different "male/masculine" and "female/feminine" cultures in which boys/men and girls/women develop and live.

These sex and gender differences can increasingly be demonstrated in the central nervous system and brain as investigative techniques in neuroanatomy, physiology, and neural imaging become more sophisticated. The brain is increasingly appreciated as an endocrine organ, too, with behavioral and anatomical consequences of exposure to hormones, including sex steroids, especially testosterone (e.g., greater aggression in male than in female mice). Such exposures are also being examined in relation to the gender identity of children. For example, case studies report that certain children with an XY-karyotype raised as girls because of mutilated or ambiguous genitalia may ultimately develop a male gender identity, presumably because of their intrauterine testosterone exposure. This challenges the belief that individuals are born with the potential to develop either male or female gender identity as determined by the sex of rearing.

Other sex differences in human behavior are also becoming increasingly documented in studies of males and females at various stages across the human life span. Many have focused on childhood play behavior and related activities and interests, personality (such as aggression and interest in babies), nonverbal communication, and cognitive abilities. These differences carry over into adult life and notably in patterns of health and health care. Here there are well-documented sex differences in frequency of visits to health professionals, use of complementary medicine, both higher in women than men, and incidence and course of certain mental disorders, notably depression, also substantially more frequent in women, as contrasted with substance abuse, notably of tobacco and alcohol, which is far more common in men. Underscoring the confounding of such behavioral differences by cultural definitions of what constitutes behavior appropriate to one's gender, such contrasts in health status and behavior have been hypothesized to represent gender-"appropriate" responses to a common pathophysiology of depression in women versus men.

These sex differences also apply to cognition, differences that are more marked at the extremes of the distribution of any given ability. In general, women more often demonstrate greater abilities in the verbal domain: verbal fluency, speech production, the ability to decode a language, spelling, and perceptual speed and accuracy. Suggestive of a hormonal basis of such abilities, these variations in performance, especially verbal skills, have been observed in women across the menstrual cycle; for example, during the preovulatory phase, when estrogen levels are high, women have demonstrated deterioration in spatial abilities, while manual coordination and skills in articulation improved.

Women also generally excel in fine motor skills. Men, on the other hand, more frequently demonstrate better performance on tests of spatial and quantitative abilities, as well as gross motor strength. These sex differences may be reflected in the performance of certain tasks highly relevant to certain conditions common in old age (e.g., dementia), because women typically perform better than men in tests of working memory of both verbal and nonverbal information. Mathematical abilities of males are greatest at the highest levels of performance (e.g., boys outperform girls on the mathematics SATs by 2:1 at a score of 500 and above, 5:1 at 600 and above, and 17:1 at 700 and above). However, such differentials are confounded by the important contribution of experience to performance on such tests, and because boys are enrolled in advanced mathematics courses far more often than girls, their superior performance, especially at the highest levels, may reflect that exposure more than their sex, gender, or sex hormone physiology (a general caveat for interpreting all such studies).

Recent technologic imaging advances are translating these descriptive studies into visual images of differential performance in cognitive tasks between men and women. For example, functional magnetic resonance imaging (fMRI) studies of cerebral blood flow during performance of certain activities have revealed differences between the sexes: men typically rely upon the left inferior frontal gyrus (Broca's area) to carry out phonologic processing, while women generally employ both left and right frontal gyri (extrapolated perhaps to why women may experience less loss of speech function than men after a stroke involving the left frontal gyrus).

Another area of differential neural function with major implications for health and function of women versus men across the life span that was a focus of the Institute of Medicine report is the reported increased perception of pain by women (Table 45-4). This bears much further investigation but clearly impacts morbidity in old age and the care of the elderly. Not only are older persons preponderantly women but women also have a greater prevalence of many of the disorders listed in Table 45-4, the management of which commonly falls into the domain of the geriatric clinician.

SEX AFFECTS IMMUNE FUNCTION

Just as there is a general "domino hypothesis" of aging and longevity regarding general physiological regulation across the life span, there is an analogous hypothesis regarding the immune system and aging: involution of the thymus, which begins at puberty, is associated with a progressively reduced thymic cellular output that leads to fewer naïve T cells contributing to the peripheral T-cell pool. In the steady state, the number of T cells within that pool is held constant within narrow limits by homeostatic mechanisms. These induce the proliferation and extend the survival of resident T cells to fill niches left by declines in naïve T cells. According to this hypothesis, however, with the passage of time (and perforce aging), as T-cell population is maintained constant through proliferation, increasing proportions of T cells come to reach their replicative limit. This, in turn, renders the organism vulnerable to infections and certain cancers as the immune response to those challenges progressively fails. Relevant to the theme of this chapter, comparison of sex differences in life span and death rates at each age from infectious and parasitic diseases suggests that the immune system works more efficiently and is effective longer in females than males (implying in turn that thymic involution occurs at a more rapid rate in males).

This sex differential applies more to the adaptive than the innate immune system (granulocytes and their products). The adaptive system includes activation and suppression of T and B lymphocytes, macrophages, and dendritic cells; secretion of their cytokine products; production of immunoglobulin antibodies; and activation of the complement and coagulation systems. As a general rule, although the sex differential in these functions is relatively narrow, estrogens upregulate and androgens downregulate these systems. Accordingly, modest variation in these functions can be seen at various phases of the menstrual cycle. In general, these differences have been sufficiently subtle as to present a challenge to providing mechanistic insights through research. And whereas studies of animals in controlled circumstances have demonstrated that males are more susceptible to infections with parasites, bacteria, fungi, and viruses than females, this has not been clearly demonstrable in humans, in whom the sex differentials in such infections have generally been attributed to sex differentials in exposures rather than in a sex differential in the individual's response to those exposures.

In contrast to the relatively subtle hypothesized greater vulnerability of males to infections, the far higher risk of females to diseases of autoimmune origin stands out as a major cause of the greater morbidity of women than men from these afflictions across the adult life span (summarized in Table 45-5). Indeed, as well-summarized and

TABLE 45-4

Sex Prevalences of Some Common Painful Syndromes and Potential Contributing Causes

FEMALE PREVALENCE	MALE PREVALENCE
Head and neck	
Migraine headache with aura	Migraine without aura
Chronic tension headache	Cluster headache
Postdural puncture headache	Posttraumatic headache
Cervicogenic headache	Paratrigeminal syndrome*
Tic douloureux	
Temporomandibular disorder	
Occipital neuralgia	
Atypical odontalgia	
Burning tongue	
Carotodynia	
Temporal arteritis	
Chronic paroxysmal hemicrania	
Limbs	
Carpal tunnel syndrome	Thromboanglistis obliterans[†]
Raynaud's disease	Hemophilic arthropathy[‡]
Chilblains	Brachial plexus neuropathy
Reflex sympathetic dystrophy	
Chronic venous insufficiency	
Piriformis syndrome	
Peroneal muscular atrophy[†,¶]	
Internal organs	
Esophagitis	Pancoast tumor[§,**]
Gall bladder disease**	Pancreatic disease
Irritable bowel syndrome	Duodenal ulcer
Interstitial cystitis	
Proctalgia fugax	
Chronic constipation	
General	
Fibromyalgia syndrome	Postherpetic neural
Multiple sclerosis, T[††]	
Rheumatoid arthritis, T	
Acute intermittent prophyria[‡]	
Lupus erythematosus, T	

*Raeder's syndrome.
[†]Buerger's disease.
[‡]Sex-linked inheritance is a potential contributory cause.
[¶]Charcot–Marie–Tooth disease.
[§]Bronchogenic carcinoma.
**Lifestyle is a potential contributory cause.
[††]T, autoimmune.
Berkley and Holdcroft (1999). Sex prevalence information is mainly from Merskey and Bogduk (1994) and was cross-checked by using MedLine and other search sources. Reprinted with permission from Institute of Medicine, *Exploring the Biological Contributions to Human Health: Does Sex Matter?* Washington, DC: National Academy Press; 2001.

TABLE 45-5

Female/Male Ratios Associated with Common Autoimmune Diseases

DISEASE	FEMALE:MALE RATIO
Hashimoto thyroiditis	10
Primary biliary cirrhosis	9
Chronic active hepatitis	8
Graves' hyperthyroidism	7
Systemic lupus erythematosus*	6
Scleroderma	3
Rheumatoid arthritis	2.5
Idiopathic thrombocytopenic purpura*	2
Multiple sclerosis	2
Autoimmune hemolytic anemia	2
Pemphigus	1
Type I diabetes*	1
Pernicious anemia	1
Ankylosing spondylitis	0.3
Goodpasture nephritis/pneumonitis	0.2

*Age specific.

Not all disease are predominant in females.

Reprinted with permission from Institute of Medicine, Exploring the Biological Contributions to Human Health: Does Sex Matter? Washington, DC: National Academy Press; 2001.

referenced in the Institute of Medicine report, autoimmune diseases may well constitute the prototypical domain of greatest contrast between the sexes and hence provide unique insights into mechanisms of the sex differential in many other diseases as well as in overall morbidity and longevity. However, research to date demonstrates great complexity in the determinants of the sex differential in this domain as well, with sex differentials in exposure at different stages of the life cycle and of hormonal modulation (including that related to pregnancy in females) playing important roles. Especially germane to the sex differential in health and function across the life span, because those autoimmune diseases with greatest female preponderance arise in young adulthood and generally carry over throughout the remainder of life (e.g., rheumatoid arthritis), the contribution of those disorders to the greater lifelong morbidity of women and their greater burden of chronic illness in old age is substantial. However, as is proving to be the case in most diseases that differ by sex, the role of sex hormones in their pathophysiology and management is not clear; for example, many of the autoimmune diseases appear to be ameliorated during pregnancy and not aggravated by female hormone replacement therapy (HRT). Thus a simple, cohesive theory to explain the sex disparity is lacking, and caution is urged in attributing the difference in both auto- and isoimmune functions to either physiological or pharmacological effects of the sex hormones.

SEX AFFECTS SEX HORMONE PHYSIOLOGY ACROSS THE ADULT LIFE SPAN

Review of the changes in sex hormone physiology across the adult life span is distributed among several other chapters in this textbook, notably, regarding the aging of the endocrine system (Chapter 65), menopause (Chapter 99), male HRT (Chapter 103), and female

HRT for osteoporosis prevention and treatment (Chapter 75). These chapters focus on aspects with implications for the aging process and approaches to HRT as part of a strategy to mitigate some of the age-associated declines in physical and functional status.

Female HRT is also addressed in the present chapter in the section devoted to that subject as related to thromboembolism and CVD, cancer, and gall bladder disease. For details of other aspects of sex hormone physiology such as reproductive function, the reader is referred to standard textbooks of endocrinology (e.g., *Williams Textbook of Endocrinology*, 9th ed.) Suffice it to summarize here that such changes are likely to influence the physiology and pathophysiology of human aging across the entire adult life span. Such differentials in sex hormone physiology are also likely to underlie much of the sex differential in longevity, as well as the health status of elderly adults in cumulative, complex patterns in multiple organ systems and diseases of those organs. However, it must be stressed that sex differences in the physiology of sex hormone regulation and the attributed effects of those differences on the function, health, and longevity of men and women cannot be not legitimately extrapolated to HRT (for either women or men), which differs from physiologic hormone regulation both quantitatively and qualitatively. Attempts to obviate the changes in sex hormone physiology with aging through HRT remains a controversial approach in both sexes, an "antiaging" strategy that lacks consistent validation through rigorous research and evidence-based practice. Indeed, a lesson of history learned once again in the early termination of the Women's Health Initiative (WHI) (see below) is that HRT—as with all such hopeful gerontologic interventions—must be formally tested in randomized clinical trials (RCTs) before any such treatment can be recommended for widespread clinical use. Furthermore HRT, especially using the regimens employed in the WHI, is currently quite definitely not recommended for this purpose.

SEX DIFFERENTIAL IN LONGEVITY

An empirical approach to the sex differential in human longevity begins with inspection of the sex ratio in longevity from all causes across the life span in the United States. This displays a bimodal pattern, with a peak ("spike") of approximately 3:1 at age 20 years and a plateau ("dome") of approximately 2:1 in late middle age (and a decline toward unity in old age). A similar pattern is seen in nearly all developed nations (although the ratios under the spike and plateau/dome vary by country), with the late sex mortality ratio being notably higher (and more in a dome-like configuration) and the sex differential in longevity growing, not declining in the nations of Eastern Europe and the former Soviet Union, where male mortality rates are increasing at an alarming rate. Perhaps providing insight to the genesis of this "spike and dome" configuration, it seems germane to note that this pattern emerged in the United States and these other nations in the twentieth century in parallel with their socioeconomic development as well as their involvement in major military conflicts.

To pursue the possible mechanisms of the evolution of the sex longevity disparity at the next level of inquiry, the sex ratio for the top 12 causes of death in 1980 (Table 45-6 and Figure 45-5) can be reviewed. This exercise reveals that men have a higher age-adjusted death rate than do women for nearly all causes. Diabetes is the one clear exception to this rule: men and women are at virtually identical age-adjusted mortality risk (i.e., diabetes nullifies the otherwise

TABLE 45-6

Gender-Specific Mortality Rates and Gender Differentials for the 12 Leading Causes of Death, United States, 1980*†

CAUSE	AGE-ADJUSTED MORTALITY RATE		GENDER RATIO (M:F)	ABSOLUTE GENDER DIFFERENCE (M:F)	% OF DIFFERENCE
	Males	Females			
Diseases of the heart	280.4	140.3	1.99	140.1	40.7
Malignant neoplasms	165.5	109.2	1.51	56.3	16.3
Respiratory system	59.7	18.3	3.43	41.4	12.0
Cerebrovascular diseases	44.9	37.6	1.19	7.3	2.1
Accidents	64.0	21.8	2.93	42.2	12.2
Motor vehicle	34.3	11.8	2.90	22.5	6.5
Other	29.6	10.0	2.96	19.6	5.7
Chronic obstructive pulmonary disease	26.1	8.9	2.93	17.2	5.0
Pneumonia and influenza	17.4	9.8	1.77	7.6	2.2
Diabetes mellitus	10.2	10.0	1.02	0.2	0.1
Cirrhosis of the liver	17.1	7.9	2.16	9.2	2.7
Atherosclerosis	6.6	5.0	1.32	1.6	0.5
Suicide	18.0	5.4	3.33	12.6	3.7
Homicide	17.4	4.5	3.86	12.9	3.7
Certain causes in infancy	11.1	8.7	1.27	2.4	0.7
All other causes	98.5	63.5	1.55	35.0	10.1
All causes	777.2	432.6	1.79	344.6	—

*Rank based on number of deaths.
†Per 100,000, direct standardization to the 1940 total US population.
Calculated from data from the National Center for Health Statistics, 1983.

powerful reduction in all-cause mortality enjoyed by women versus their male counterparts especially in the pre/perimenopausal period). However, such inspection also readily allows grouping of those causes of death into ones that are frequent in adolescence and young adulthood—notably, those related to violence and the risks of a youthful lifestyle—and those that are prevalent in middle and old age, the chronic and progressive "degenerative" diseases of complex etiology that increasingly dominate the practices of primary care physicians and geriatricians. In the first group, neurobehavioral gender differentials clearly appear causative—"macho" behavior involving considerable risk constituting the most obvious factor increasing male vulnerability. There is increasing acknowledgment that such behavior is determined at least in part by hormonal factors, although modulation—exaggeration or dampening—by sociocultural forces is clearly also important (i.e., sex plus gender issues). This risk-taking behavior also extends to sex differentials in drug abuse and sexual

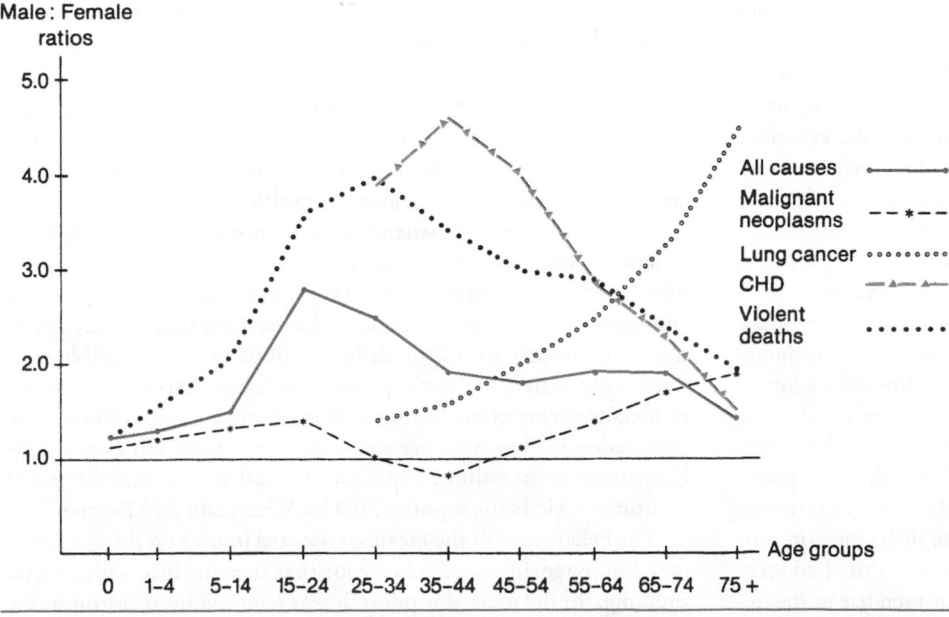

FIGURE 45-5. Sex mortality ratios for specific causes of death by age in the United States according to World Health Organization (WHO) statistics *(World Health Statistics Annual: Vital Statistics and Causes of Death.* Geneva: World Health Organization; 1986). CHD, coronary heart disease. *(Reprinted with permission from Johnasson S. Longevity in women. In: Douglas P, ed. Heart Disease in Women. Philadelphia: Davis; 1989:8.)*

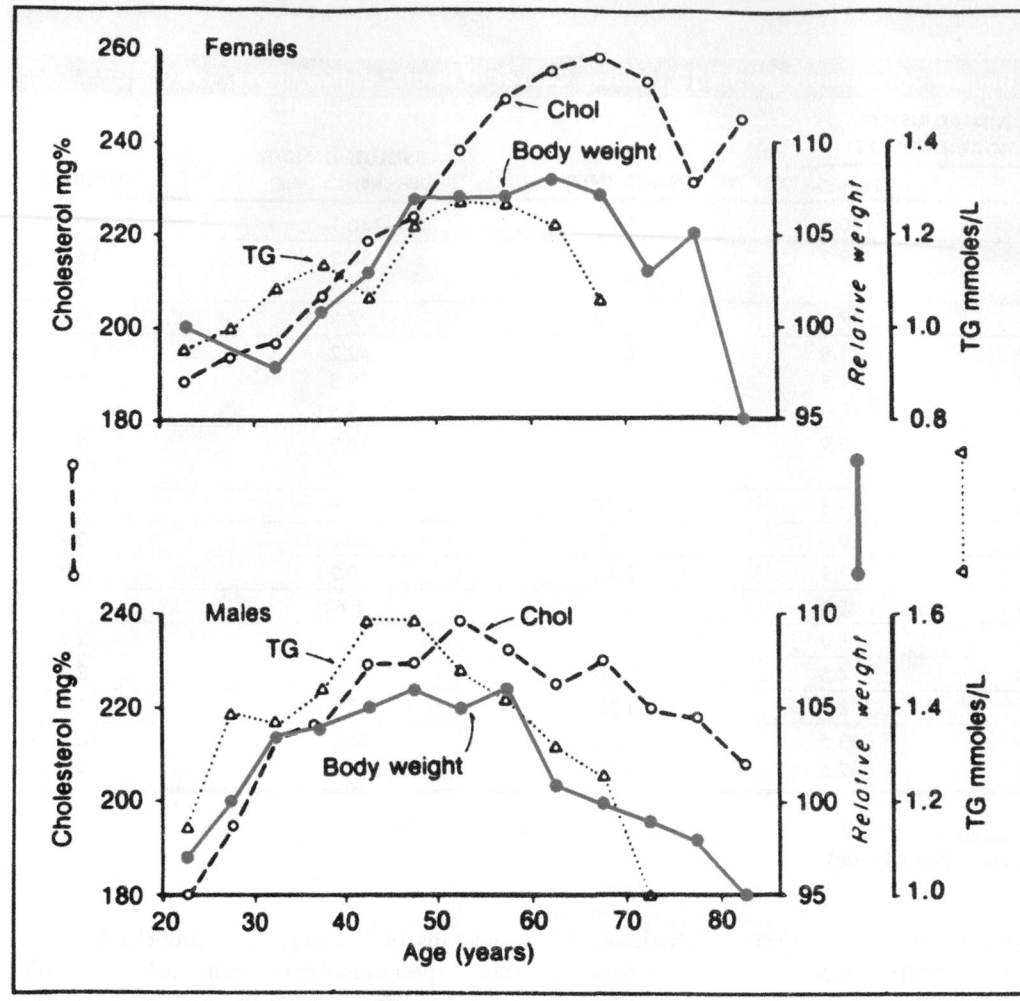

FIGURE 45-6. Median plasma cholesterol (Chol), triglyceride (TG), and relative body weight values as a function of age in Tecumseh (cholesterol and relative weights) and Stockholm (TG) community studies. *(Reprinted with permission from Williams RDH, ed. Textbook of Endocrinology, 5th ed. Philadelphia: Saunders; 1974.)*

practices, with consequences that could have a dramatic impact on the sex differential in longevity especially if the human immunodeficiency virus (HIV) epidemic continues to affect more men than women (see Chapter 87). However, narrowing in the sex differential in HIV-related deaths has recently become apparent as the viral infection spreads to women by heterosexual contact and intravenous drug abuse and through more effective antiviral treatment, HIV has become more of a chronic disease. Indeed, HIV disease is now the fastest-growing cause of death in young American women, while men from earlier cohorts are now experiencing chronic, especially metabolic and CVD accelerated by side effects of retroviral agents.

The causality of the diseases clustered under the plateau of greater male mortality in late life, which in the aggregate account for approximately 90% of the sex differential in longevity (see Figure 45-6 from Ory and Warner), is more complex and certain to prove multifactorial. An attractive hypothesis, advanced principally by social scientists, has, as with the spike in youth, focused on behavioral–cultural factors. Men in western societies have traditionally adopted lifestyles with greater risk to their health throughout mid-life: more miles driven, more cigarettes smoked, less focus on health promotion, disease prevention, and early detection. Men also historically have made fewer visits to physicians and taken fewer prescription drugs. Indeed, as reported by Courtenay, these differences in attitudes and health behaviors that undermine men's health often serve as signifiers of masculinity and instruments that men use in the ne-

gotiation of social power and status. Put another way, denial of their vulnerability to disease and death is part of the masculine tradition and gender identity, an attribute that presents a cultural and behavioral barrier to effective strategies of "preventive gerontology" for men (see Chapter 6).

This barrier is especially imposing to boys/men of lower socioeconomic and vocational strata, who have less access to the advantages enjoyed by males in the higher strata, which include greater positive reinforcement of healthy behaviors that positions of economic and social power bring (including greater access to health care and control over time and schedule). These phenomena have tended to confound the issue of sex/gender and health, introducing an intriguing paradox: women experience greater morbidity (often reported in terms of numbers of encounters with the health care system), but men have higher mortality rates at every age. The bases for these sex and gender differentials in health behavior have been widely investigated (although with little definitive outcomes and notably relatively little correlation with quantitative biomarkers of disease risk or measurements of sex hormone physiology or effects). These have been reviewed elsewhere (see especially chapters by Wingard and by Nathanson in the volume edited by Ory and Warner and the recent Institute of Medicine report edited by Wizemann and Pardue).

The behavior with the greatest potential impact on the sex differential in longevity—and a behavior that remains flux—is cigarette smoking. To illustrate this point, it was reported by Waldron in the

Ory and Warner volume that mortality in middle-aged nonsmoking men exceeds that in nonsmoking women by only 30%, as compared with a male excess of greater than 120% for the total population studied (put another way, nonsmoking men and smoking women have more equal age-adjusted mortality rates). Cigarette smoking became fashionable in the United States in the twentieth century, and until recently, was predominantly a masculine habit—men started earlier in life and smoked more heavily than women. This behavioral sex differential was reinforced by incentives that encouraged cigarette smoking by servicemen during the World Wars of that era. The clear parallel between increases in male cigarette smoking and the rising sex ratio in mortality in the twentieth century would seem causally related. Review of the sex ratios in mortality from the leading causes of death in America (see Table 45-6) strongly suggests that the historical sex differential in cigarette smoking constituted a major factor in the majority of such causes, notably vascular disease, both coronary heart disease (CHD) and stroke, cancer, especially lung cancer, and nonmalignant lung disease. Indeed, it was estimated by consensus at the NIA conference that produced the volume by Ory and Warner that the historical sex differential in cigarette smoking behavior might account for as much as 4 years of the 7-year U.S. sex differential in longevity at birth when it reached its peak in 1970.

In this context, it is relevant to examine more recent trends in cigarette smoking in both sexes and parallel trends in mortality rates from diseases related to smoking. Cigarette smoking reached its peak prevalence and intensity in the United States shortly after World War II, when nearly half of the adult population was smokers. At that time not only did more men than women smoke, but also heavy cigarette use was far more prevalent in men. From that time until the present, cigarette smoking has declined progressively in the United States (although recent reports disclose that this trend is slowing, especially in younger persons and notably in younger women). The beginning of this decline closely paralleled the release of the first Surgeon General's Report on Smoking and Health in 1963, the first clear public statement linking cigarette smoking with lung cancer and other feared diseases. Initially, the decline in smoking appeared to be greater in men than women, but by the late 1960s, women were also giving up smoking at a comparable rate. The decline has been most notable among those older than age 35 years in both sexes. When the decrease in CHD mortality first received public attention in the early 1970s (the "epidemic" having reached its peak at the time of the Surgeon General's report), a significant proportion of that reduction was attributed to the decline in cigarette smoking. This decline, which has continued to the present (albeit at a diminishing rate), has generally been equivalent as expressed in relative (percentage) terms in both genders. However, because the previous absolute levels of CHD mortality were far greater in men, their absolute decrease in CHD deaths has been greater. In parallel fashion, because the level of cigarette smoking in men was far higher, their absolute reduction in cigarette consumption has been greater (see especially the chapter by Nathanson in the volume edited by Ory and Warner). Hence, recent trends show a decrease in the difference in the number of CHD deaths in men versus women, in parallel with the decrease in the number of cigarettes smoked by men as compared with women. That women are as vulnerable as men to the untoward effects of cigarette smoking—given the lag between exposure to tobacco carcinogens and the onset of lung cancer—is evident in the narrowing of the historical sex differential in lung cancer, which surpassed breast cancer as the most common cause of cancer-related death in women in the 1980s (see Figure 45-5), as well as in other smoking-related diseases, such as chronic obstructive lung disease and peptic ulcer disease. However, these trends appear likely to stabilize as cigarette smoking rates become equivalent in both sexes, and both men and women, especially those of higher income and educational levels, have adopted healthier lifestyles in response to the widespread public health educational campaigns against cigarette smoking.

THE SEX DIFFERENTIAL IN ATHEROSCLEROSIS

Review of the sex differential in the leading causes of death (see Table 45-6) clearly places atherosclerosis and its clinical consequences—CHD, cerebrovascular disease, aortic aneurysm, and peripheral arterial disease—at the center of any consideration of the sex/gender gap in longevity: in the aggregate, these diseases account for more than 40% of the total (Figure 45-6). Moreover, it has been estimated that elimination of all atherosclerotic disease could add up to 10 years to average longevity beyond age 65 years in the United States, raising the mean age at death to nearly 85 years (a popular estimate of the maximum possible average human longevity according to the essays by Fries and by Olshansky et al.). Furthermore, by deferring death among men to beyond middle age, when the sex ratio is highest, a reduction in ages at death between marriage partners (and a decrease in duration of widowhood) would be important by-products.

SEX DIFFERENTIAL IN CARDIOVASCULAR DISEASE RISK FACTORS

Although sex differentials may exist in the most basic aspects of atherogenesis (e.g., arterial intimal integrity, vasomotor response, lipoprotein uptake, or other aspects of arterial wall biology—see Chapter 34), evidence for all such possibilities, albeit intriguing, must at present be considered preliminary. A more practical approach is to review sex differentials in the traditional atherosclerosis risk factors across the life span during stages as defined in general and convenient terms by this author: childhood and adolescence (infancy to age 25 years); middle age (ages 25–75 years, conveniently bisected at age 50 years [approximately the age of menopause for women] into first and second halves); and old age (older than age 75 years).

Here population studies suggest at least subtle differences at each stage that provide a pathophysiologic basis for earlier clinical expression of CVD in men. These studies demonstrate that sex differentials begin in childhood and adolescence, as well documented in the Bogalusa community studies led by Berenson (which also demonstrated early atherosclerosis in the arteries of adolescents killed in vehicular accidents in that community). In middle age, blood pressure, both median systolic and diastolic, is lower in women than men during the first half (25–50), beyond which a crossover occurs such that hypertension (especially isolated systolic hypertension) is more common in older women than men. Regarding control of blood glucose levels, glucose tolerance tests applied to population samples (e.g., in Tecumseh) demonstrate a pattern of change in efficiency of glucose disposal with age also favoring women until midlife, with convergence between the sexes beyond middle age. This carries over into an overall age-adjusted excess male prevalence of diabetes of greater than 10%, a disparity still evident in old age. Regarding median levels of blood lipids (cholesterol and triglyceride), these change with age in a biphasic pattern, increasing in both sexes (albeit at a lower rate in women) until the midpoint of middle age, when a plateau is reached, and declining thereafter (see Figure 45-6). Except for the abrupt increase in cholesterol levels in women older than age 50 years (the "postmenopausal overshoot"), these changes in lipids, blood pressure, and glycemic control in the first half of middle age are in general correlated with and maybe mediated by gains in relative body weight, which normatively continue until the middle of middle age, when a plateau is reached (although adiposity may continue to accrue, it is offset by decreases in lean body mass). A decline in median relative body weight during old age ultimately follows, perhaps signaling the onset of frailty and terminal decline (the continued increases in blood pressure and blood glucose beyond middle age require a different explanation).

Close inspection of such curves reveals patterns that are subtly different between men and women, the middle-aged weight plateau being achieved approximately a decade later in women than in men (during their sixties rather than their fifties). Thus, a slower accretion of weight and a later achievement of peak weight in women than men may at least partly explain the more favorable CVD risk profile of women prior to age 50 years and their relative infrequency of clinical CVD prior to that age, a benefit that may carry over into the succeeding postmenopausal era by virtue of the slower rate of atherogenesis to that point.

A sex differential in regional patterns of midlife weight gain is another possible explanation of the lower CVD risk in women (see also Chapter 92). Beyond adolescence, women prototypically gain more adipose mass about the hips and buttocks (producing "lower body," "pear-shaped," or "gynoid" obesity), whereas adult men prototypically add fat about the waist (leading to "upper body," "apple-shaped," or "android" obesity). The latter pattern confers extra CVD risk, exaggerating the known interaction between relative body weight and the traditional risk factors in population studies such as in Framingham. Moreover, those atypical women who develop upper-body obesity—especially those with hyperandrogenism and the PCOS—have CVD risk profiles resembling those of men, and they are at substantially increased risk of type 2 diabetes (presumably because of increased insulin resistance and compensatory hyperinsulinism) and its attendant increased risk of atherosclerosis and its complications.

These phenomena are coming under increasing scrutiny in the present, accelerating worldwide pandemic of obesity afflicting both men and women. This advancing wave of progressive obesity is not only lowering the age of the onset of type 2 diabetes to young adulthood and even childhood but also threatens to negate continuing advances in average longevity of both sexes. With its associated, pathophysically important increase in insulin resistance, this trend also calls increasing attention to the "metabolic syndrome" as a major risk profile associated with premature atherosclerotic cardiovascular disease (ASCVD) and other sequelae of diabetes, hypertension, and dyslipidemia. Here, however, the disproportionate accumulation of visceral (central, upper body) adiposity by men especially in the first half of mid-life (25 to 50 years) would appear to place them at continuing disadvantage compared with women in ASCVD risk as well as overall longevity as this epidemic progresses.

Additional insight into the role of sex hormones in mediating the sex differential in atherosclerosis may be afforded by inspection of the sex ratio in cardiovascular mortality across the adult life span (see Figure 45-5). After the peak in this ratio is reached in the premenopausal era, there occurs a major, progressive decline with advancing age, from nearly 5:1 at age 35 years to but 1.2:1 at age 85 years (it never drops below unity). Viewed from another perspective, women enjoy an approximately 10-year relative immunity to CVD, as compared with men (the rate in women ages 55–65 years, for instance, is equivalent to that in men ages 45–54 years). Consideration of this delay in women reaching equivalent CVD mortality risk as men is important in resolving an apparent paradox in popular media presentations on population aging and especially the wave of post-World War II female baby boomers currently passing through the menopause and contemplating HRT (see discussion on HRT below). Whereas at any given age women are at lower risk to CVD mortality than are men, CHD remains the leading cause of death in women beyond reproductive age. However, because of their greater longevity, and survival to an age of high risk, the percentage of women dying of CHD ultimately equals that of men (nearly 50% in both sexes). Moreover, because with advancing age, the population becomes progressively skewed toward surviving women, the annual numbers of women who succumb to CHD death may actually come to exceed those in men. As death rates from CHD progressively decline (unless nullified by increasing obesity and the metabolic syndrome), those deaths will occur in older and older persons (already the majority of CHD events occur in Medicare recipients, older than the age of 65 years), and cardiology will focus on progressively older patients and especially older women.

ROLE OF SEX HORMONES IN MEDIATING THE SEX DIFFERENTIAL IN CORONARY HEART DISEASE RISK

Population studies such as those from Framingham, which have reported a higher prevalence of CHD in pre- versus postmenopausal women of comparable age, suggested a physiologic role for sex hormones (specifically estrogen and progesterone) in mediating the sex differential in CHD between women and men. Other population studies, such as those of the Lipid Research Clinics in the early 1970s, carefully examined average cholesterol levels (total, LDL, and HDL) in males and females (more of whom were taking HRT) between childhood and old age (Figure 45-7). These studies revealed that average lipid levels are equivalent between the sexes until puberty. However, at that point (and in parallel with the Tanner stage of pubertal development) HDL concentrations begin to decline in boys, and average levels of HDL remain relatively stable at lower concentrations in men than women (by approximately 10 mg/dL) from the twenties through the seventies. This suggests that this gap is principally attributable to an HDL-lowering effect of testosterone in men. This hypothesis is supported by studies of the effect of testosterone replacement in hypogonadal men, which suppressed HDL levels. This hypothesis has also received direct experimental support in studies of normal men rendered hypogonadal with a gonadotropin-releasing hormone (GnRH) agonist, in whom HDL levels rose (a rise that could be prevented with simultaneous testosterone administration). However, this consequence of testosterone therapy is not a pure androgenic effect, because a substantial fraction of testosterone is converted to estrogen by aromatase in various tissues. Consistent with this mixed effect, treatment with testosterone with coadministration of aromatase inhibitors results in a greater decrease in HDL levels. Moreover, androgenic anabolic steroids, which are incapable of conversion to estrogen, invariably produce a profound suppression

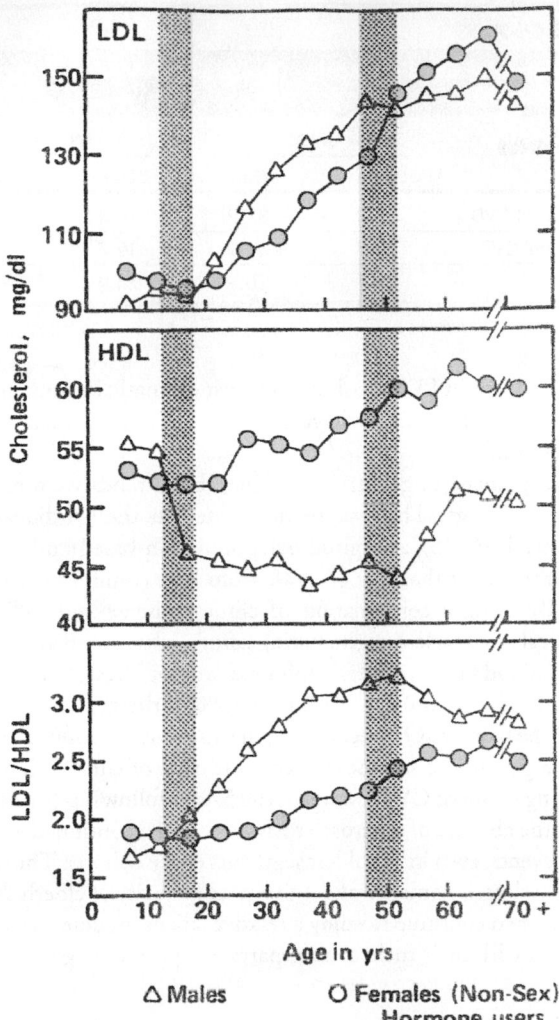

FIGURE 45-7. Median North American population high-density lipoprotein (HDL) cholesterol, low-density lipoprotein (LDL) cholesterol, and the ratio between the two versus age in white subjects. *(Data from The Lipid Research Clinics. Population Studies Data Book. vol. 1. The Prevalence Study. DHHS (NIH); 1990;80:1527.)*

of HDL levels: experimental studies of women given such agents for osteoporosis or endometriosis have demonstrated a 50% reduction in total HDL levels, ominously especially marked (85%) in the more antiatherogenic HDL2 subfraction.

On the other side of the coin, prospective studies of HDL levels in women followed across the menopause (Chapter 99) have also disclosed a slight average decline (especially in HDL2) coincident with ovarian failure. This suggests at least a mild effect of endogenous estrogen in raising HDL and specifically HDL2.

With regard to LDL, whereas mean levels rise in both sexes between puberty and the menopause (perhaps attributable to increasing adiposity), they remain substantially lower in women than men until the menopausal era, when they rise significantly, average levels in postmenopausal women actually coming to exceed those in men of comparable age. These trends in women seem most likely to be attributable to the physiological effects of estrogen in premenopausal women and the lack of estrogen beyond the menopause.

The net effect of these changes in lipid levels across the adult life span produces a more favorable pattern in women than men at all stages, with the lower HDL levels in men overriding the higher

LDL levels in postmenopausal women as to associated CHD risk. However, the sex differential in the LDL:HDL ratio (a convenient single index of lipid-associated risk) is greatest in the premenopausal era, when the sex differential in CHD is also the greatest, declining following menopause in parallel with the declining magnitude of that differential.

However, the mechanism of these putative effects of endogenous, physiologic sex hormones on plasma lipids remains largely conjectural, since there is a notable lack of association between plasma levels of those hormones and plasma lipoprotein concentrations in either population-based or carefully controlled metabolic investigations. Further investigations may reveal correlations with mechanistic implications for atherogenesis beyond lipoprotein metabolism, as suggested in analyses of the American Atherosclerosis Risk in Community (ARIC) cohort study by Golden et al. However, these may prove counterintuitive. In the ARIC study of carotid atherosclerosis, for example, intimal–medial thickening was inversely related to testosterone levels in postmenopausal women.

Thus mechanistic conclusions to date are largely extrapolated from results of pharmacologic interventions, which at best produce but a caricature of the effects of endogenous sex hormones and their physiologic regulation. Perhaps the most insightful of these on a population basis were the same Lipid Research Clinic Prevalence studies (Figure 45-8). Compared to women not taking hormone supplements, in premenopausal women taking oral contraceptives, average LDL levels were higher, while HDL concentrations were equivalent. However, closer examination of the data revealed that women

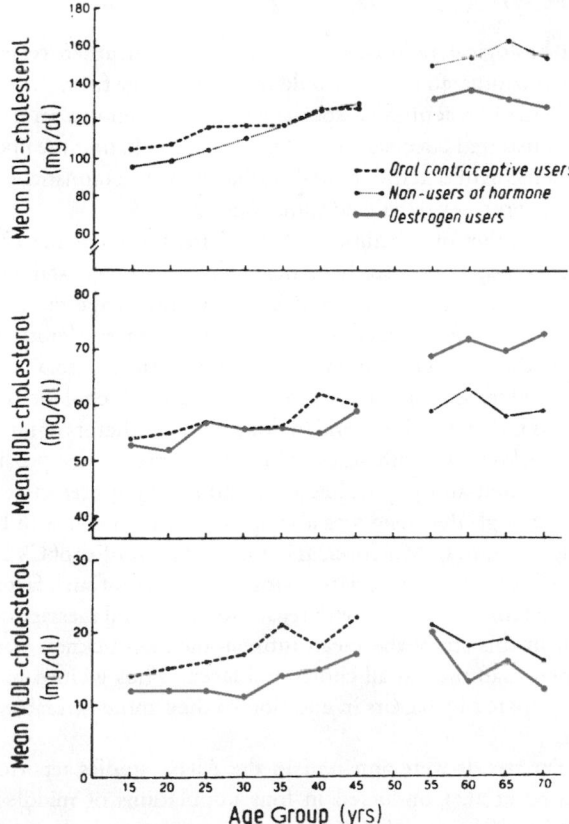

FIGURE 45-8. Plasma lipoprotein cholesterol levels in users and nonusers of oral contraceptives and estrogens. *(Reprinted with permission from Wallace RB, et al. Altered plasma lipid and lipoprotein levels associated with oral contraceptives and oestrogen use. Lancet. 2:11, 1979.)*

consuming contraceptives with more powerful androgenic progestational components had lower HDL than those taking contraceptives containing less androgenic progestins. In the postmenopausal women taking HRT (in that era, almost all ingesting unopposed conjugated equine estrogens (CEEs) in a dose of 1.25 mg/day) average LDL levels were lower and HDL levels clearly higher than in women not taking estrogens.

These population studies have been widely confirmed in the intervening decades. Furthermore, careful metabolic studies of postmenopausal women such as those reported by Applebaum-Bowden et al. have quantitatively documented the powerful effects of exogenous (oral) estrogen in both lowering LDL levels and raising HDL (and selectively HDL2) levels.

Other studies have identified multiple additional mechanisms by which exogenous HRT in postmenopausal women might sustain their relative immunity to CHD. Indeed, for several decades, observational population studies suggested that the changes in lipid levels seen with HRT were insufficient to account for the degree of relative protection enjoyed by women who took such preparations. Studies at the mechanistic level reported beneficial effects of estrogens in decreasing arterial wall LDL uptake, perhaps retarding LDL oxidation and hence its atherogenic potential, and protecting against the paradoxical vasoconstrictive effects of such agents as acetylcholine in the presence of atherosclerosis (likely mediated by enhanced NO synthesis by arterial endothelial intimal cells induced by estrogen).

SEX DIFFERENTIAL IN ATHEROSCLEROTIC CARDIOVASCULAR DISEASE

Thus a biological rationale for a slower rate of atherogenesis in women as compared to men would seem to emerge from their more favorable CVD risk profile, especially in the premenopausal era, and the demonstrated effects of sex hormones in mediating the lipoprotein dimension of that differential—albeit clearly demonstrable only with exogenous sex steroid administration.

Other studies of subclinical atherosclerosis, such as the 15-year prospective population study of the middle-aged men and women of Tromso, Norway, as reported by Stensland-Bugge et al., have confirmed a sex differential in progression of atherosclerosis as reflected in ultrasound measurements of carotid artery intimal–medial thickness. Here age, blood pressure, total and HDL cholesterol, and body mass index were independent long-term predictors of intimal–medial thickness in both sexes, while triglycerides were predictive only in women and physical activity and smoking predictive only in men (though the trend was also apparent in women with heavy smoking exposures). Moreover, as in many other studies of CVD risk factors, CVD risk was associated with the number of such factors in a stepwise fashion. Of note with regard to the central message of this chapter, in this study the mean intimal–medial thickness was less in women than men at all cholesterol levels. Thus women may be relatively spared by factors in addition to their more favorable lipid profiles.

Similar trends were apparent in the ARIC studies reported by Chambless et al. Conducted in four populations of middle-aged subjects (45–64 years of age) over an 11-year period, these studies demonstrated that increased carotid intimal–medial thickness was associated with baseline diabetes, (diminished) HDL-cholesterol, pulse pressure, white blood cell count, and fibrinogen levels, as well

TABLE 45-7

Prevalence of Cardiovascular Disease in the Cardiovascular Health Study

PREVALENCE (%)	MEN		WOMEN	
	Blacks	Whites	Blacks	Whites
Any clinical CVD	37.2	37.2	36.4	28.2
Subclinical CVD	43.7	41.9	39.7	41.3
Neither	19.1	20.9	24.9	32.5

CVD, cardiovascular disease.

as with changes in LDL-cholesterol (most dramatic in women passing through menopause), triglycerides, and new-onset diabetes and hypertension.

Most germane to geriatric medicine, these trends seem to carry over into old age. This was demonstrated in the Cardiovascular Health Study (CHS), a longitudinal, population-based study of men and women older than age 65 years from four communities (Table 45-7). By using a combination of clinical disease and indices of subclinical atherosclerosis (including carotid ultrasound and ankle-brachial blood pressure index), this epidemiologic research disclosed detectable, significant CVD in up to 80% of the men, but in only 67% of the women. Of special note, in this study, subclinical disease carried a prognostic significance equal to that of clinical disease in predicting incident CVD events in the 5-year follow-up (while conversely, the absence of atherosclerosis predicted a continued low risk of such events, even in the oldest segments of the cohort). Thus, even as atherosclerosis comes to affect the great majority of elderly Americans, women continue to enjoy a relative, albeit modest, protection compared with their male counterparts of equivalent age.

FEMALE HORMONE REPLACEMENT THERAPY

Despite the biological plausibility of an important role for sex steroids in mediating the relative immunity of women to CVD and the clear effect of exogenous HRT in sustaining and even magnifying the putative role of endogenous estrogen in conferring more favorable lipid profiles, this does not translate into HRT being recommended for postmenopausal women for either primary or secondary prevention of CVD. As with all studies based upon epidemiologic associations, these must be confirmed in formal clinical trials before such recommendations can be justified. The recent dramatic change in the trend toward widespread postmenopausal HRT is perhaps the most compelling case in point, as well-summarized in the reviews by Manson and Martin and the landmark report from the WHI Writing Group.

At the time these reports were released around 2002, it was estimated that approximately 38% of U.S. postmenopausal women were using HRT. This was not only for relief of menopausal symptoms, where the benefit continues to remain clear, but also in the belief that such therapy would reduce the burden of several chronic diseases in the remaining over one-third of their lives spent in the postmenopausal state. Such putative benefits included reductions not only in CVD, but also all cancer, osteoporosis (see Chapter 75)—where the benefit also continues to remain clear—and even risk of cognitive impairment (although associated increased risks of breast cancer, thromboembolism, and gall bladder disease gave pause to many women contemplating HRT). This hopeful, pleiotropic preventive intervention strategy was increasingly embraced by an "age wave" cohort of midlife baby boomers, notably the more highly educated and health-conscious women from higher socioeconomic strata who were more likely to receive such supplements. Their enthusiasm for HRT was buttressed by numerous (more than 40) clinical and observational epidemiologic studies that reported substantially less CVD in women taking HRT. As reviewed earlier, such benefit from HRT is biologically plausible, estrogen-exerting effects at multiple levels from the genome to whole populations that, on balance, might support their widespread use in postmenopausal estrogen replacement (as reviewed by Mendelsohn and Karas). RCTs confirmed that oral estrogen reduces LDL cholesterol by 10% to 14% and increases HDL cholesterol by 7% to 8%. Estrogen was also shown to favorably affect other indices of CVD risk: lipoprotein levels were reduced, LDL oxidation inhibited, and plasminogen-activator inhibitor-1 (PAI-1) levels decreased. However, other indices appear to be adversely affected: triglyceride levels rise; coagulation is promoted through increases in factor VII, prothrombin fragments 1 and 2, and fibrinopeptide; and—perhaps most germane to CVD in old age—C-reactive protein (CRP), a marker of immune system activation, is increased (specifically by oral [but not trans-cutaneous] HRT). Thus at the level of basic biology, a mixed scorecard in support of HRT for CVD prevention was being assembled even as more and more postmenopausal women elected to take such agents as the WHI was being designed and initiated (Table 45-8).

However, the wisdom of this trend began to engender skepticism among professionals and the lay public alike when the results of the Heart and Estrogen/Progestin Replacement Study (HERS) were reported in 1998 by Hulley et al. HERS was a 4-year RCT of HRT in the secondary prevention of CVD, which compared continuous daily CEE (Premarin) combined with medroxyprogesterone acetate (MPA; Provera) versus placebo in 2673 women with established CHD. This study demonstrated no overall effect of the HRT on coronary death rate and nonfatal myocardial infarction. In the first year of the trial, however, there was a 50% *greater* incidence of coronary events in the women taking HRT. Nevertheless, by the termination of the study this had abated, and even a trend toward a later benefit of HRT appeared to emerge in years 3 through 5, suggesting a biphasic pattern of response to the hormones. During subsequent unblinded follow-up, however, this possible later benefit did not prove sustained. Thus after 6.8 years, neither net benefit nor increased risk of HRT for secondary prevention of CHD was apparent. This disappointing outcome was subsequently echoed in the Estrogen Replacement and Atherosclerosis (ERA) secondary prevention trial of estrogen either alone or in combination with progestin on angiographically quantified coronary atherosclerosis: here too no net effect was seen. Subsequently, a review of 22 primary prevention trials of HRT, albeit mostly small and of short duration, also failed to disclose net benefit.

Subsequently the impact of these limited trials, especially as related to the potential for primary CHD prevention, was overwhelmed in 2002 when the first principal results of the WHI RCT of the effect of HRT on all-cause and cause-specific morbidity and mortality were released. This arm of the WHI was a large, community-based, placebo-controlled, RCT of continuous oral CEE (0.625 mg/day) plus MPA (2.5 mg/day). Involving 16 608 postmenopausal women with intact uteri aged 50 to 79 years (average age 63 years, including 21% older than age 70 years) recruited to 40 clinical centers in 1993 to 1998, the study had a planned duration of 8.5 years. The primary favorable targeted outcome was CHD (nonfatal myocardial infarction and CHD deaths), with invasive breast cancer as the primary adverse predicted outcome. A global index was also developed reflecting these two primary outcomes plus stroke, pulmonary embolism, endometrial cancer, colon cancer, hip fracture, and death from other causes.

After just 5.2 years of average follow-up, the study was terminated prematurely because the test statistic for invasive breast cancer exceeded the stopping boundary and the global index statistic indicated that the risks exceeded the benefits of the HRT (Figures 45-9 and 45-10). The estimated hazard ratios (HRs) and nominal 95% confidence intervals (CIs) (in parentheses) included CHD 1.29 (1.02–1.63); breast cancer 1.26 (1.00–1.59); stroke 1.41 (1.07–1.85); pulmonary embolism 2.13 (1.39–3.25); colorectal cancer 0.63 (0.43–0.92); endometrial cancer 0.83 (0.47–1.47); hip fracture 0.66 (0.45–0.98); and death as a result of other causes 0.92 (0.74–1.14). The corresponding HRs and CIs for composite outcomes were: total CVD (arterial and venous), 1.22 (1.09–1.36); total cancer, 1.03 (0.90–1.17); combined fractures, 0.76 (0.69–0.85); total mortality, 1.02 (0.82–1.18); and global index, 1.15 (1.03–1.28). Absolute excess risks per 10 000 person-years attributable to the combination HRT were 7 more CHD events, 8 more strokes, 8 more cases of pulmonary embolism, and 8 more invasive breast cancers, while absolute risk reductions per 10 000 person-years were 6 fewer colorectal cancers and 5 fewer hip fractures. The absolute excess risk of events in the global index was 19 per 10 000 person-years. The WHI writing group concluded that "this regimen should not be initiated or continued for primary prevention of CHD."

Subsequent analyses reported in 2004 evaluated the effect of treatment of 10 739 trial participants with prior hysterectomy treated with CEE alone in the same 0.625 mg/day dosage for an average of 6.8 years. This disclosed no significant effect of the estrogen on hazard ratios for: CHD, 0.91 (0.75 to 1.12); pulmonary embolism, 1.34 (0.87 to 2.06); or colorectal cancer, 1.08 (0.75 to 1.55), while providing suggestive benefit for breast cancer, 0.77 (0.59 to 1.01) and confirming reduced incidence of hip fracture, 0.61 (0.41 to 0.91). Results for composite outcomes with CEE alone suggested no effect on: total CVD, 1.12 (1.01 to 1.24); total cancer, 0.93 (0.81 to 1.07); total mortality, 1.04 (0.88 to 1.22); and the global index, 1.01 (0.91 to 1.12), while total fractures were reduced, 0.70 (0.63 to 0.79). For the outcomes significantly affected by CEE, there was an absolute excess risk of 12 additional strokes and an absolute risk reduction of 6 fewer hip fractures per 10 000 person-years.

This important addendum to the initial, "blockbuster", counterintuitive report from WHI illustrates the dynamic, continuing, and no doubt still incomplete nature of the substantive reports that will continue to emanate from this landmark study. In this particular instance, it is tempting to deduce that the different outcomes from combined CEE and MPA regimen in the initial report and the less ominous findings from the CEE alone substudy must be attributable to the MPA, a progestational and weakly androgenic component in the combination regimen. However, it is important to bear in mind that the participants in the CEE-alone trial had all undergone hysterectomy, and those who have had that procedure are unlikely to be similar in health and socioeconomic parameters, which confounds such a simplistic interpretation. Furthermore, the unexpected relative protection (and clearly without the increased risk of breast cancer) found with CEE–MPA in the initial report is

TABLE 45-8

Benefits and Risks of Postmenopausal Hormone-Replacement Therapy (HRT)

VARIABLE	EFFECT	BENEFIT OR RISK		SOURCE OF DATA
		Relative	Absolute	
Definite benefits				
Symptoms of menopause (vasomotor, genitourinary)	Definite improvement	>70–80% decrease		Observations studies and randomized trials
Osteoporosis	Definite increase in bone mineral density; probable decrease in risk of fractures	2–5% increase in bone density; 25–50% decrease in risk of fractures	172 fewer hop fractures (402 vs. 574) per 100 000 woman-years	Observation studies and limited data from randomized trials
Definite risks				
Endometrial cancer	Definite increase in risk with use of unopposed estrogen; no increase with use of estrogen plus progestin	Increase in risk by a factor of 8–10 with use of unopposed estrogen* for >10 yrs; no excess risk with combined estrogen-progestin	Excess of 46 cases (52 vs. 6) per 100 0000 woman-years of unopposed estrogen use (>10 yrs of use); no excess with use of combined therapy	Observational studies and randomized trials
Venous thromboembolism	Definite increase in risk	Increase in risk by a factor of 2.7	Secondary prevention: excess of 390 cases per 100 000 woman-years; primary prevention: excess of 20 cases per 100 000 woman-years	Heart and Estrogen/Progestin Replacement Study Observational studies
Probable increase in risk				
Breast cancer	Probable increase in risk with long-term use (>5 yrs)	Overall increase in risk by a factor of 1.35 with HRT use of >5 yrs	Excess of 20 cases per 10 000 women using HRT for 5 yrs; 60 excess cases after 10 yrs of use; 120 excess cases after 15 yrs of use	Meta-analysis of 51 observational studies
Gallbladder disease	Probable increase in risk	Increase in risk by a factor of 1.4	Excess of 360 cases per 100 000 woman-years	Heart and Estrogen/Progestin Replacement Study
Uncertain benefits and risks Cardiovascular disease				
Primary prevention	Could range from net benefit to net harm	Uncertain	Uncertain	Observational studies and randomized trials†
Secondary prevention	Probable early increase in risk	Uncertain	Uncertain	Observational studies and randomized trials
Colorectal cancer	Possible but unproven decrease in risk	20% decrease	24 fewer cases (96 vs. 120) per 100 000 woman-years	Observational studies
Cognitive dysfunction	Unproven decrease in risk (inconsistent results)	Uncertain	Uncertain	Observational studies and randomized trials

*The term "unopposed estrogen" refers to the use of estrogen without medroxyprogesterone acetate.

†Observational data suggest a decrease in risk of 35 to 50 percent, whereas randomized trial data show no effect or a possible harmful effect during the first 1 or 2 yrs of use. Most studies have assessed conjugated equine estrogen alone or in combination with medroxyprogesterone acetate.

Reproduced with permission from Manson JE, Martin KA: Postmenopausal hormone replacement therapy, N Engl J Med. 2001;345:34.

counterintuitive regarding the effect of estrogen on this important outcome.

An additional dimension from the WHI study of CEE–MPA of special interest to physicians caring for elderly persons was a substudy focused upon the effect of the combined hormone therapy on cognitive function, the Women's Health Initiative Memory Study (WHIMS). Analogous to the hope for HRT engendered by observational epidemiological cohort studies that suggested reduced inci-

dence of dementia (and Alzheimer's disease) in women taking HRT, this substudy examined a substantial fraction (4894) of the WHI participants to test the hypothesis that this HRT regimen would reduce decline in cognitive function as assessed by Modified Mini Mental State Examinations (MMMSEs). Contrary to the predicted effect, more women in the estrogen–progestin group (6.7%) experienced a substantial and clinically important *decline* in MMMSE (25% or more) compared with placebo (4.8%). Thus, as with CHD

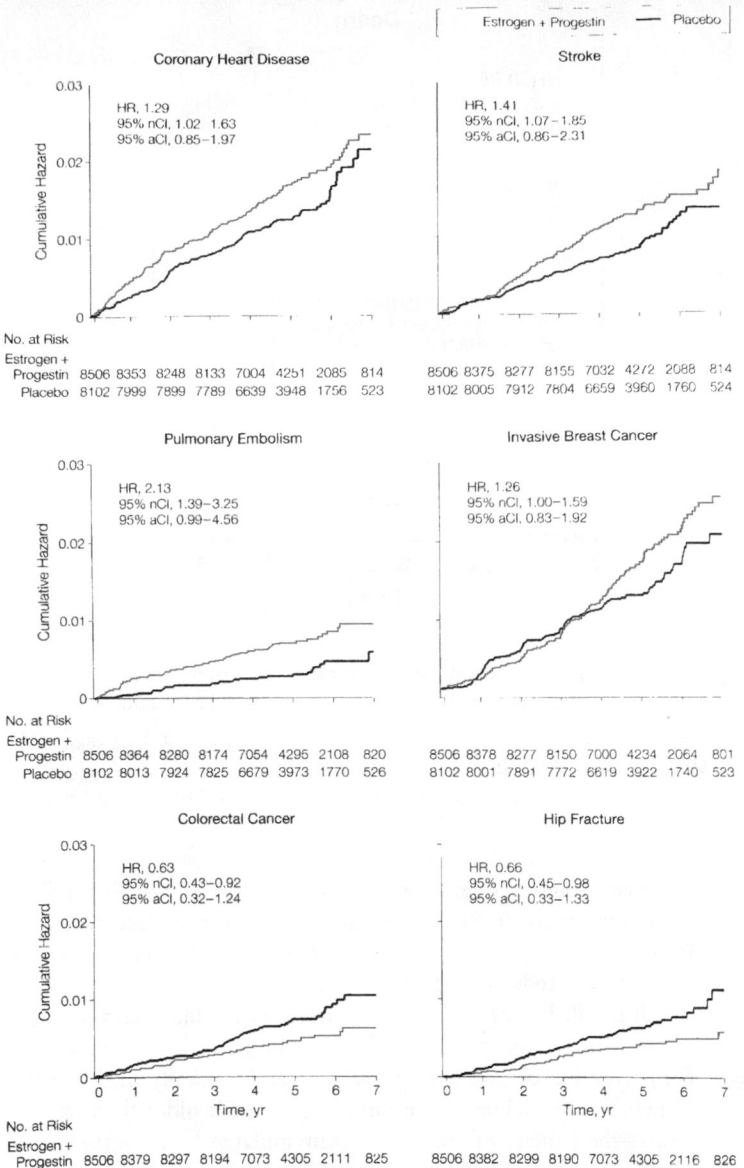

FIGURE 45-9. Kaplan–Meier estimates of cumulative hazards for selected clinical outcomes of the Women's Health Initiative randomized controlled trial. *(Reproduced with permission from Rossouw JE, et al. Writing Group for the Women's Health Initiative Investigators: Risks and benefits of estrogen plus progestin in healthy postmenopausal women. Principal results from the Women's Health Initiative randomized controlled trial. JAMA. 288:321, 2002.)*

prevention, the WHIMS demonstrated an unpredicted adverse outcome, and hence postmenopausal combined HRT could not be justified in a strategy to reduce cognitive decline or prevent dementia, including Alzheimer's disease.

Thus for both primary and secondary prevention of CHD (or dementia), combination HRT cannot presently be recommended, especially in the form of continuous treatment with CEE and MPA in a woman with an intact uterus. Nor do these studies engender enthusiasm for the use of CEE alone to prevent CHD in postmenopausal women after hysterectomy. However, individualized regimens for women at increased risk for, for example, colon cancer or osteoporosis, may be prescribed. And doubtless many women will elect at least short-term HRT for control of menopausal symptoms; some may even choose long-term treatment because of strongly held beliefs as to the long-term benefits of HRT (and perhaps especially estrogen alone in the posthysterectomy state).

Nevertheless, these largely unanticipated results had a rapid, profound impact on the prevalence of HRT in postmenopausal women in the United States and worldwide. The conservative, almost nihilistic conclusions published by the writing group have met with skepticism and at most grudging acceptance by longtime proponents of HRT and especially perhaps by gynecologists and reproductive endocrinologists. As to the focus of this chapter, these outcomes have served to highlight the paradox that is one of its central features: while pre-menopausal women clearly enjoy a major relative immunity to CHD, the exogenous replacement of the hormones that putatively mediate that protection in the postmenopausal state appears not only ineffective but downright hazardous. Consequently post-WHI research by determined researchers has increasingly sought to resolve this enigma, especially as related to the peri- and postmenopausal era when a myriad of symptoms, vasomotor in particular, cause women to seek relief through estrogen replacement in spite of WHI (which was not sufficiently powered to focus in this era).

Thus the relative immunity to CHD enjoyed by women, especially premenopausally, continues to suggest that a regimen of postmenopausal HRT more accurately reflecting premenopausal female hormone physiology might provide enduring benefits to women over their remaining life span. Indeed, the discrepancies between

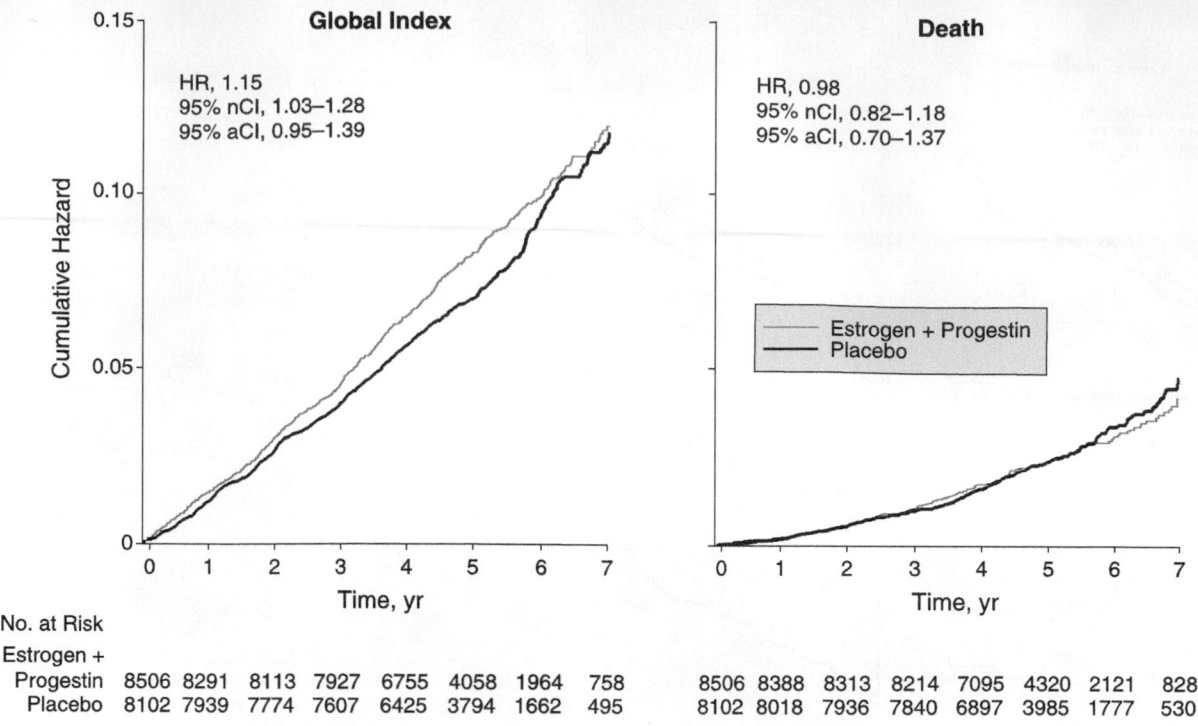

FIGURE 45-10. Kaplan–Meier estimates of cumulative hazards for global index and death, Women's Health Initiative randomized controlled trial. (Reproduced with permission from Rossouw JE, et al. Writing Group for the Women's Health Initiative Investigators: Risks and benefits of estrogen plus progestin in healthy postmenopausal women. Principal results from the Women's Health Initiative randomized controlled trial. JAMA 288:321, 2002.)

endogenous physiology and exogenous HRT suggest that important mechanistic insights might be provided by careful examination of the differences. For example, current research in atherosclerotic CVD is focusing on the role of inflammation in the pathogenesis of this disease, with special emphasis on the CRP and other proinflammatory markers even as potential mediators. Here research suggesting contrasting effects of oral versus transcutaneous or vaginal estrogens are especially intriguing, as reported for example by Modena et al. Oral estrogens, subject to magnification of their effect on hepatic metabolism by their "first pass" exposure, induce increases in CRP, while transdermal estrogens, which enter the systemic circulation directly, actually suppress CRP levels in healthy postmenopausal women.

Finally, this area of intense interest to gerontologists who consider the entire life span as the domain of their investigation and concern will endure as a focus of important research to unravel the principles as well as the paradoxes that underlie the sex and gender determinants of longevity and morbidity across the life span. The WHI itself will continue to generate important studies germane to resolution of this conundrum. Recently, for instance, Manson and her coworkers reported findings regarding coronary artery calcification from the substudy of CEE-alone. This disclosed significantly lower calcification scores (an important index of coronary artery atherosclerosis) in the women assigned to the CEE (vs. placebo) arm, especially those who adhered to their assigned CEE by 80% or more. Similarly supportive of continued HRT for perimenopausal women and as buttressed by findings from more basic research in nonhuman primates, a more finely grained analysis of the WHI-CEE substudy by Rossouw et al. in 2004 reported a potential benefit of the oral estrogen on heart disease among participants 50 to 59 years of age (the study was terminated, however, before a statistically significant

advantage could be demonstrated). And more recently, this possibility is being tested in RCTs of similar regimens in subjects recruited in the perimenopausal years. So the story is far from complete and will continue to bear watching in the years to come.

All in all, however, at least for the present, long-term, combination estrogen–progestin HRT cannot be generally recommended for prevention of postmenopausal CVD. Specifically in the realm of geriatric medicine—for example, in women older than age 75 years—the paucity of current or contemplated future research regarding HRT for CHD prevention seems certain to make this an area of uncertainty for the indefinite future and render the taking of HRT by elderly women distinctly uncommon.

PREDICTING THE FUTURE: THE SEX DIFFERENTIAL IN LONGEVITY IS DECLINING

By the end of the 1960s, the progressive rise in the sex differential in average American longevity that marked the first seven decades of the twentieth century had begun to abate (see Figure 45-2). Subsequently, this trend has converted to a clear and progressive decline in the differential (see Table 45-2), even as the expected longevity of both sexes continues to rise (albeit at a slower rate in women than in men). Thus by the advent of the twenty-first century, the United States (and other developed countries) were entering the fourth and final, "posttransitional" stage of convergence in longevity by sex hypothesized.

The reasons for this convergence remain uncertain and controversial. As suggested earlier in this chapter, these are perhaps most focused in the narrowing sex ratio in cigarette smoking exposure in the past four decades and hence in the various disease risks attributable to such an exposure. Of the factors, CVD contributes the greatest proportion of that decrease: the decline in CHD in the United States in both sexes during that interval has been continuous and cumulatively profound. In the ARIC surveillance study of more than 360 000 men and women aged 35 to 74 years in the four communities as reported by Rosamund et al., for example, the reduction in CHD applied both to hospital admissions and deaths caused by CHD both in and out of the hospital. Between 1987 and 1996, the age-adjusted CHD mortality rate fell 3.2% in men (CI 2.0–4.3) and 3.8% in women (CI 1.9–5.6). However, this produced a somewhat greater reduction in the absolute number of such deaths in men than women (adjusted for age) because of the greater risk in men at the beginning of the study. The reductions in both hospitalizations and in-hospital mortality were consistent with earlier studies of national data that attributed declines in CHD mortality equivalently to improved population preventive strategies and risk factor profiles as well as more effective treatment of CHD once clinically manifest. It should also be noted, however, that these reductions were more evident in the earlier years of the ARIC study, 1987 to 1991, than subsequently. This raises the question as to whether the decline in CHD will continue indefinitely or whether and when a floor effect will be observed, below which further decreases may not be possible, especially in an aging population.

FUTURE OF THE SEX DIFFERENTIAL IN LONGEVITY AND ITS IMPLICATIONS FOR GERIATRIC MEDICINE AND GERONTOLOGY

Population health data in the United States and worldwide suggest that these CHD benefits accruing especially to men extend to other causes of death as well as to overall mortality rates, and indeed, longevity.

This raises the more general issue as to whether the greater advances in longevity among men than women in the past three decades reflect greater relative improvements in health behaviors and medical interventions in men over that time span or the reality that women are approaching the upper limit of the average potential longevity of the human species, the "barrier to immortality" described by Fries as 85 ± 4 years (recently modified to 85 ± 7 years, with a preterminal phase of "compressed morbidity" of 2–3 years).

Regardless that the sex differential in longevity in the United States is declining is no longer a subject of debate. This is clearly evident in Tables 45-1 and 45-2 (the latter continuing to document this narrowing trend since the last edition of this textbook). Projecting these trends forward has suggested that the sex differential in United States longevity will decline to only 2.2 years by 2025 in the United States, a trend that will be replicated in most industrialized nations and attributed principally to diminishing rates of vastly premature death in men (in the 25- to 59-year age group). Perhaps the most encouraging aspect of this progressive narrowing in the sex/gender longevity gap to gerontologists and geriatricians are its implications for institutional long-term care services in the upcoming decades. As men live longer, couples can expect to live independently together longer, the duration of widowhood will decline, and the need for long-term care services will decrease accordingly. There is already mounting evidence that this hopeful sequence of events has begun. Even as the number of persons most likely to require such services continues to increase (notably those older than age

85 years), American nursing home bed capacity has for decades been at a plateau. Nor is this trend confined to the United States. Other nations at comparable levels of socioeconomic development (e.g., Sweden and Australia) are experiencing a similar relative decline in long-term institutional care. Careful deconvolution of the curves of decline in per capita nursing home utilization by elderly citizens has fractionated these trends into multiple components, including those that reflect improved health and reduced age-adjusted disability of the population as well as the development of noninstitutional alternatives to nursing home care. These encouraging trends continue in the early twenty-first century, especially in the United States, where serial studies of aging populations have disclosed progressive decrements in disability among the elderly, especially those older than age 80 years, as well as declining mortality rates for both sexes in this age group. Importantly, such studies have suggested that the greater longevity gains in men than women in recent decades may well be the predominant factor contributing to the decline in nursing home utilization, particularly in the 1990s.

This optimistic trajectory is also likely to continue well into the twenty-first century in developed nations. This prediction is reinforced by the association between enhanced longevity of both sexes and increased educational level, and because the cohort of elderly citizens with low levels of educational attainment born in the first half of the twentieth century will be succeeded by later cohorts with higher average educational levels. This might also disproportionately favor men, given the relationship between attained educational level and the adoption of more healthy lifestyles in both genders and the probability that men of higher educational level (and often higher socioeconomic status) seem especially likely to embrace health attitudes and behaviors (such as decreased cigarette smoking) and effective management of CVD and other risk indices consistent with the practice of effective "preventive gerontology" (see Chapter 9). Or to put it otherwise, since men have been traditionally so disadvantaged in longevity by their "macho" image and behaviors, they will disproportionately benefit by relaxation of that attitude as gaps in educational and socioeconomic status and the health behaviors of men and women become more closely approximated in developed nations in this current century.

Thus the poetic dream of Robert Burns that serves as the preamble to this chapter may yet become reality in a future wherein average longevity of both sexes might approach the MLP of our species.

Nevertheless, given the evidence and theoretical projections gathered to date, as a gerontologist, geriatrician, and endocrinologist, I would predict that because of fundamental and immutable biological differences between the sexes, women will always outlive men. However, in the steady state, the gap will be substantially narrower than at present—perhaps 2 to 3 years (the estimate of Kranczer for the year 2025), and the average duration of widowhood for married women will remain at least that long.

Thus, in the early twenty-first century, presented by Lopez in the volume edited by Ory and Warner (see Table 45-3) America and other developed nations may be entering the hypothesized fourth and final, steady-state, posttransitional stage in the evolution of the sex differential in longevity.

FURTHER READING

Applebaum-Bowden D, Mchean P, Steinmetz A, et al. Lipoprotein, apolipoprotein, and lipolytic enzyme changes following estrogen administration in postmenopausal women. *J Lipid Res*. 1989;30:1895.

Austad SN. Why women live longer than men: sex difference in longevity. *Gend Med.* 2006;3:79.92.

Berenson GS, Srinivasan ER, Bao W, et al. Association between multiple cardiovascular risk factors and atherosclerosis in children and young adults. *N Engl J Med.* 1998;338:1650.

Borras C, Goombin J, Vina T. Mitochondrial oxidant generation is involved in determining why females live longer than male. *Front Bio Sci.* 2007;12:1002–1013.

Chambless LE, Folsom AR, Davis V, et al. Risk factors for progression of common carotid atherosclerosis: The Atherosclerosis Risk in Communities Study. *Am J Epidemiol.* 2002;155:38.

Cheitlin MD, Gevstenblith G, Hazzard WR, et al. Do existing databases answer clinical questions about geriatric cardiovascular disease and stroke? *Am J Geriatr Cardiol.* 2001;10:207.

Courtenay WH. Constructions of masculinity and their influence on men's well-being: a theory of gender and health. *Soc Sci Med.* 2000;50:1385.

Federman D. The biology of human sex differences. *N Engl J Med.* 2006;354:1507–1514.

Fries JF. Aging, natural death and the compression of morbidity. *N Engl J Med.* 1980;303:130.

Golden SH, Maguire A, Din J, et al. Endogenous postmenopausal hormones and carotid atherosclerosis: a case control study of the atherosclerosis risk in communities cohort. *Am J Epidemiol.* 2002;155:437.

Grady D, Herrington D, Bittner V, et al. Cardiovascular disease outcomes during 6.8 years of hormone therapy: Heart and Estrogen/Progestin Replacement Study follow-up (HERS II). *JAMA.* 2002;288:49.

Hodis HN, Mack HN, Lobo RA, et al. Estrogen in the prevention of atherosclerosis. *Ann Intern Med.* 2001;135:939.

Hulley S, Grady D, Bush T, et al. Randomized trial of estrogen plus progestin for secondary prevention of coronary heart disease in postmenopausal women: Heart and Estrogen/Progestin Replacement Study research group. *JAMA.* 1998;280:605.

Humphrey LL, Chan BK, Sox HC, et al. Postmenopausal hormone replacement therapy and the primary prevention of cardiovascular disease. *Ann Intern Med.* 2002;137:273.

Kranczer S. Continued United States longevity continues. Metropolitan Insurance Companies. *Stat Bull.* 1999;80:20.

Manson JE, Hsia J, Johnson KC, et al. Estrogen plus progestin and the risk of coronary heart disease. *N Engl J Med.* 2003;349: 523–534.

Manson, JE, Allison MA, Rossouw JE, et al. Estrogen therapy and coronary-artery calcification. *N Engl J Med.* 2007;356:2591–2602.

Mendelsohn MM, Karas RH. The protective effects of estrogen on the cardiovascular system. *N Engl J Med.* 1999;340:1801.

Modena MG, Bursi F, Fantini G, et al. Effects of hormone replacement therapy on C-reactive levels in healthy postmenopausal women: comparison between oral and transdermal administration of estrogen. *Am J Med.* 2002;113:331.

Olshansky SJ, Carnes BA, Cassel C, et al. In search of Methuselah: estimating the upper limits to human longevity. *Science.* 1990;250:634.

Ory MG, Warner HR, eds. *Gender, Health, and Longevity.* New York, New York: Springer; 1990.

Rosamund WD, Folsom AR, Chambless LE, et al. Coronary heart disease trends in four United States communities. The Atherosclerosis Risk in Communities (ARIC) study 1987–1996. *Int J Epidemiol.* 2001;30(Suppl 1):S17.

Rossouw, JE, Prentice RJ, Manson JE, et al. Postmenopausal hormone therapy and risk of cardiovascular disease by age and years since menopause. *JAMA.* 2007;297:1465–1477.

Stensland-Bugge E, Bonaa KH, Joakimsen O, et al. Sex differences in the relationship of risk factors to subclinical carotid atherosclerosis measured 15 years later: the Tromso study. *Stroke.* 2000;31:574.

Wallace JE. Gender differences in beliefs of why women live longer than men. *Psychol Rep.* 1996;79:587.

Wingard DL. The sex differential in morbidity, mortality, and lifestyle. *Ann Rev Public Health.* 1984;5:433.

Wizemann T, Pardue ML, eds. *Exploring the Biological Contributions to Human Health: Does Sex Matter?* Washington, DC: National Academy Press; 2001.

Writing Group for the Women's Health Initiative. Risks and benefits of estrogen plus progestin in healthy postmenopausal women. Principal results from the Women's Health Initiative randomized controlled trial. *JAMA.* 2002;288: 321.

Women's Health Initiative Steering Committee. Effects of conjugated equine estrogen in postmenopausal women with hysterectomy. *JAMA.* 2004;291:1701–1712.

Wylie CM. Contrasts in health of elderly men and women: an analysis of recent data for articles in the United States. *J AM Ger Soc.* 1984;32:670.

Menopause and Midlife Health Changes

MaryFran R. Sowers

The profile of female geriatric patients will be changing considerably over the next decade. A substantial number of women born during the baby boom following World War II are at or beyond midlife, resulting in an increasing number of women who will be seeking treatment for symptoms associated with menopause and for chronic conditions that have their origin in midlife (see Chapter 5 for details on demographics). Further, the cohort of U.S. women who are now at midlife is unique. More than three-quarters are in the workforce; more than one-third have college degrees; and family composition has changed remarkably as evidenced by the number of live births that have declined by almost half.

For many of these women, the midlife, which encompasses the menopausal transition, will be a significant milestone and a harbinger of their health status and their interaction with health care systems for the ensuing decades. Thus, it is important to understand the events of the menopause transition and that these events are likely to affect health, the perception of health, and the perception of the contribution of the health care provider to health maintenance.

The initiation of the menopause transition (that time from active reproduction to the cessation of significant estrogen secretion because of the depletion of functional ovarian follicles) is an ill-defined period that commences with the onset of menstrual irregularity or skipped menses and ends 12 months following the final menstrual period (FMP). The median age at FMP is currently estimated to be 51.4 years. The menopause itself is the permanent cessation of menses and is clinically diagnosed following 12 continuous months of amenorrhea.

This geriatrics textbook includes a chapter on menopause because exposure to declining levels of ovarian hormones appears to modify risk factors associated with the development of debilitating diseases and health concerns of the geriatric patient. Furthermore, the menopause transition may represent an optimal time for clinical intervention. These clinical interventions can address two potential patient groups: (1) the 12% to 25% of women who already have some evidence of disability (see the physical limitations section) and

for whom active interventions are critical and (2) the majority of women who are not disabled and are open to information about preventive care, risk factor screening, and maybe seeking care for menopausal symptoms.

PHYSIOLOGICAL BASIS OF REPRODUCTIVE AGING

Aging of the female reproductive system is unique because the timeframe for the permanent cessation of menses has changed little over time, while the average life expectancy of women now extends to more than 30 years after the FMP. Further, women have a finite period of reproductive capacity. Unlike men, who usually retain reproductive capacity throughout their lifetime, women are born with a set number of primordial follicles, whose depletion begins prior to birth (Figure 46-1). At menopause, when a woman's ovarian reserve is depleted, the number of available follicles recruited to form preovulatory follicles has dwindled to a point where ovarian-based hormones, including estrogens and progesterone, are no longer predictably produced. A progressively greater rise in gonadotropin, such as follicle stimulating hormone (FSH), is observed with the diminution of the follicular pool and the increasing nonresponsiveness in regulation of hormone secretion.

It is likely that changes in lipid, bone, or immunological functioning, among others, are related to those marked changes in estradiol and FSH concentrations during the menopause transition and occur when the hormone changes around the FMP are most pronounced. The Michigan Study of Women Across the Nation (SWAN) evaluated FSH values in relation to time and identified that there was an accelerated rise in FSH levels between 5 and 2 years prior to the FMP. FSH levels further accelerated from 2 years prior to 1 year after the FMP; thereafter, the FSH levels tended to plateau (Figure 46-2).

Because of the complexity and the cost of measuring these hormone-driven menopausal transition events in the clinical setting, progress through the transition is frequently estimated with

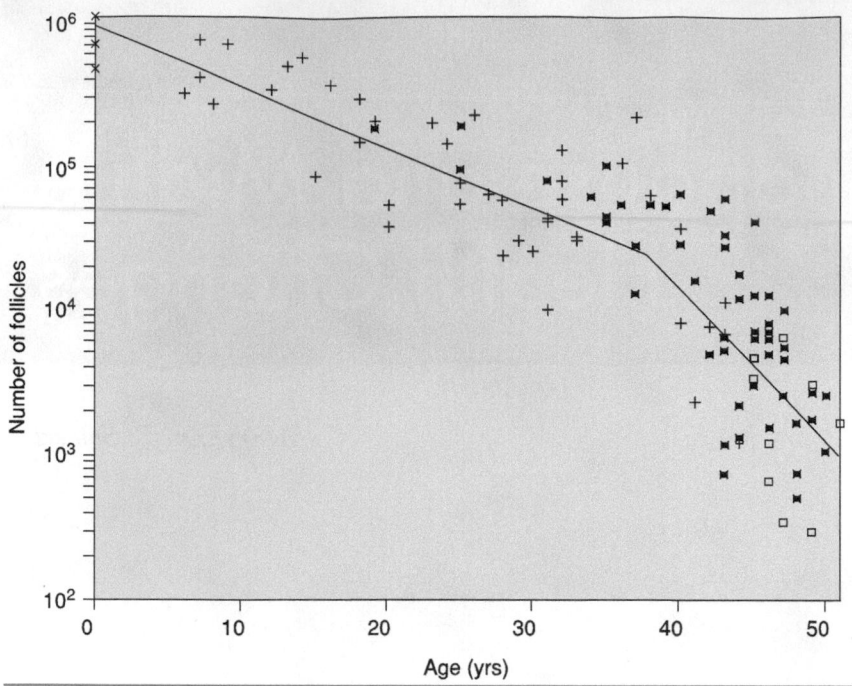

FIGURE 46-1. Biexponential model of declining follicle numbers in pairs of human ovaries from neonatal age to 51 yrs old. Data were obtained from the studies of Block (1952, 1953) (X, n = 6; +, n = 43), Richardson et al. (1987) (□, n = 9) and Gougeon (1987) (*, n = 52). *(Faddy MJ, Gosden RG, Gougeon A, et al. Accelerated disappearance of ovarian follicles in mid-life: implications for forecasting menopause. Human Reprod. 7:1342–1346, 1992. With permission from Oxford University Press.)*

menstrual cycle characteristics. In 1996, the World Health Organization suggested definitions of the stages describing the transition to natural menopause. A broader and simpler staging system, including earlier stages of reproductive aging and later stages of postmenopause, was proposed at the International Stages of Reproductive Aging Workshop (STRAW). The STRAW staging definitions are based primarily on bleeding changes with the acknowledgment that discriminating hormone levels, specifically FSH, would add precision when sufficiently described (Table 46-1).

Based on menstrual calendar diary data of women undergoing the menopause transition, cycle lengths in excess of 60 days are a sensitive indicator of an impending FMP. This represents a pragmatic marker for use by patient and clinician alike in characterizing the menopause status of the woman. Further, these timeframes are consistent with our understanding that there are two follicle pools, one recruitable pool in which follicles, when stimulated, are immedi-

ately available for growth and a second pool of follicles insensitive to gonadotropin signals. The growable pool is refreshed approximately every 60 to 90 days. As the follicle supply decreases, the growable pool of follicles can no longer replenish itself to those numbers seen in mid-reproductive life. As the follicle reserve becomes critically diminished and few remaining responsive follicles are present, menstrual cycles become more irregular and are more likely to be anovulatory.

Aging of the reproductive system is frequently only considered in the context of the ovary; however, it actually involves all three levels of the reproductive axis—the brain, pituitary, and the ovary. While the hypothalamus and pituitary play extensive roles in all aging processes, the exact mechanisms by which gonadotropin releasing hormones (GnRH) change with age with respect to biosynthesis, transport, release, and receipt of feedback from neurotransmitters or steroids is incompletely understood. The total numbers of GnRH neurons

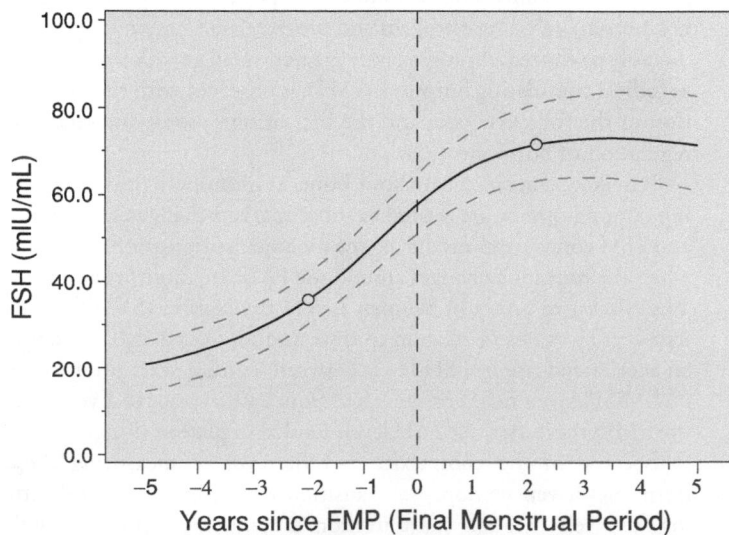

FIGURE 46-2. Average FSH values (with 95% confidence intervals from bootstrapping) in relation to final menstrual period (FMP). *(Sowers M, Zheng H, Tomey K et al. Changes in body composition in women over six yrs at mid-life: ovarian and chronological aging. J Clin Endocrin Metab. 2007;92:895–901. Copyright 2007, The Endocrine Society.)*

TABLE 46-1

Comparison of the Definition of Reproductive Stages and the Transition to Menopause: WHO and STRAW

World Health Organization (WHO)

Natural Menopause
The permanent cessation of menstruation resulting from the loss of ovarian follicular activity. It is recognized after 12 consecutive months of amenorrhea, for which there is no other pathological or physiological cause. An adequate independent biological marker for the event does not exist.

Perimenopause
The period when the endocrinological, biological, and clinical features of menopause begin through the first year after the menopause.

Menopausal Transition
The period of time before the final menstrual period (FMP) when variability in the menstrual cycle is usually increased.

Premenopause
The period ambiguously referred to as either the 1 to 2 yrs immediately before the menopause or the whole of the reproductive period prior to the menopause. It is recommended that this term be used consistently in the latter sense to encompass the entire reproductive period up to the FMP.

Induced Menopause
The cessation of menstruation following either surgical removal of both ovaries or iatrogenic ablation of ovarian function.

Simple Hysterectomy
At least one ovary is conserved. It is used to define a distinct group of women in whom ovarian function may persist for a variable period after surgery.

Postmenopause
The period dating from the FMP, regardless of whether the menopause was induced or spontaneous.

Premature Menopause
Menopause that occurs at an age less than two standard deviations below the mean estimated for the reference population. In the absence of reliable population estimates, 40 yrs is frequently used as an arbitrary cut-off point.

Stages of Reproductive Aging Workshop (STRAW)

Reproductive Stage
The period from menarche to the beginning of the perimenopause.

Menopausal Transition
The time of an increase in follicle-stimulating hormone and increased variability in cycle length, two skipped menstrual cycles with 60 or more days of amenorrhea or both. The menopausal transition concludes with the final menstrual period (FMP) and the beginning of postmenopause.

Postmenopause
Begins at the time of the FMP, although it is not recognized until after 12 months of amenorrhea.

Sources: World Health Organization. Research on the Menopause in the 1990s: Report of a WHO Scientific Group. Geneva: World Health Organization; 1996:12–14. WHO Technical Report Series No. 866; Soules MR, Sherman S, Parrott E et al. Executive Summary: Stages of Reproductive Aging Workshop (STRAW). Fertil Steril. 76:874–878, 2001.

do not appear to be the critical factor in determining reproductive senescence. Rather, changes in intermittent hormone secretion (i.e., luteinizing hormone (LH) or FSH) or glycoprotein free α-subunit (FAS) in pre- versus postmenopausal women result in a change in gonadotropin levels, characterized as a change in their pulse amplitude and, possibly, their pulse frequency. These changes in pulsatile release may reflect an unappreciated aging process or a greater insensitivity to feedback during the menopause transition.

In the aging hypothalamus, dopamine secretion into the portal vasculature declines and, with aging, the stimulatory action of estrogen is absent. In addition to dopamine, it is thought that norepinephrine, acting primarily through the α-adrenergic receptor, stimulates GnRH release, a process that declines with aging. This aging phenomena may explain why some of the symptoms commonly associated with the menopause transition (including potential cognitive changes) are more likely to reflect chronological change while other symptoms, such as vasomotor symptoms, appear to be more reflective of the events of change in ovarian hormone concentrations.

Disaggregating Menopause Symptoms and Chronological Aging

The onset or exacerbation of a constellation of symptoms, including vasomotor problems, vaginal dryness and other sexual symptoms, urine leakage, changes in skin, fatigue, and problems with sleeping, negative mood, and decline in cognitive acuity, is frequently attributed to the menopause. Further, many women choose to begin hormone replacement therapy in an effort to combat these menopausal symptoms and to replace the endogenous hormones that have been declining. These symptoms are described below in relation to their development, frequency, and degree of bother during the menopause transition and, when relevant, the effect of hormone therapy (HT).

MENOPAUSE SYMPTOMS AND CLINICAL FEATURES

Vasomotor Symptoms

Vasomotor symptoms, including hot flashes, cold sweats, or night sweats, have been consistently associated with the menopause transition, occurring to some degree in more than 70% of women during midlife, with more than 50% of women reporting their presence for more than five years. Vasomotor symptoms are defined physiologically as a disruption in the hypothalamic central thermoregulation, causing the core body temperature to change by at least 0.2 degrees Celsius. In SWAN, the pattern of increasing perimenopausal hot flashes compared to the premenopause was consistent among African-American, Japanese, and Hispanic women. More vasomotor symptoms are found in those with increasing body mass index (BMI), current smoking status, baseline depression, and premenstrual symptoms. In a study evaluating symptom constructs in more than 500 Caucasian women, increasing frequency and amount of bother from vasomotor symptoms and sexuality were predicted by the transition from a premenopause to a postmenopause state over time. Low estradiol concentrations and higher FSH concentrations were significantly predictive of having vasomotor and sexual symptoms, but not other symptoms commonly identified with the menopause transition including urinary leakage and negative moods. Consistent with the findings from SWAN, this study found that higher BMI and current smoking behavior were highly related to increased bother with many symptom constructs, but especially vasomotor symptoms.

Sleep Disturbances

Investigators at the 2005 National Institute of Health (NIH) State-of-the-Science Conference, Management of Menopause-Related Symptoms, reported that sleep problems are identified by 16% to 42% of premenopausal women, 39% to 47% of perimenopausal women, and 35% to 60% of postmenopausal women. Although aging, in general, is associated with decrements in sleep quality, gender differences in sleep disturbances that emerge at midlife suggest that the increase in sleep difficulties may not be simply an aging effect. However, the majority of published studies are limited by small sample sizes, cross-sectional data, and limited assessments of sleep and menopausal status. In the SWAN multiethnic sample of 12 603 Caucasian, African-American, Chinese, Japanese, and Hispanic women, aged 40 to 55 years, almost 40% reported difficulty in sleeping. Age-adjusted rates for difficulty in sleeping were highest in the late perimenopause (45%) and in women with surgical menopause (48%). Menopausal status was associated with greater difficulty in sleeping, even following adjustment for age, race/ethnicity, vasomotor and psychological symptomatology, self-perceived health status and health behaviors, arthritis, and education, all factors that were also associated with sleeping difficulty (Table 46-2).

Factors that might trigger acute sleep disturbances during the menopause transition may include the onset and exacerbation of vasomotor symptoms, rate of changing hormone levels (especially FSH), and increases in symptoms of stress associated with acute and chronic ongoing life events. There is considerable overlap between sleep disturbances and vasomotor symptoms. A study by Dzaja et al. found that 68% to 85% of symptomatic menopausal women have vasomotor symptoms and 51% to 77% report insomnia.

In some studies comparing HT users and nonusers, HT users report more sleep disturbances suggesting that preexisting sleep disturbances influence the association between HT and the exacerbation of sleep disturbances. In a longitudinal study, Matthews et al. found that twice as many incident sleep complaints (28%) occurred among HT users compared to nonusers (14%). The greater increase in sleep problems among women who used HT may have been because of the preexisting characteristics of the women or to particular HT formulations or doses.

Worsening sleep during the menopausal transition is important because this sleep is associated with decreases in quality of life and poorer work performance. Persistent insomnia has been associated with an increased incidence of mood and anxiety disorders. Further, subjective sleep complaints and polysomnography-described sleep disruptions are associated with many negative health outcomes, including susceptibility to upper respiratory tract infections, immunosuppression, cardiovascular disease (CVD), and stroke and their attendant health care costs.

Sexuality Dysfunction (also see Chapter 47)

Sex steroids are postulated to affect sexual function (desire, arousal, orgasm, and pain) either directly through their neurohormonal effects on pain or desire or indirectly by maintaining the anatomic competence that allows arousal to occur. Atrophic changes in the vagina, including a decrease in lubrication accompanying sexual arousal, thinning of the endothelium, and loss of rugation, which are associated with dyspareunia have been well described. Because the menopausal transition is a time of significant change in sex steroid hormones and in sexual function, it has been speculated that the menopause leads to a diminution in sexual functioning, apart from the simultaneous potential effects of normal aging. However, the evidence linking sexual function to individual endogenous hormones or changes in hormones over time remains largely circumstantial.

The few large longitudinal studies of sexual functioning and menopause suggest that domains of sexual functioning change differentially, over time with some changes resulting from aging and others from menopause. The most consistent decrements in sexual functioning have been associated with rising FSH concentrations rather than declines in estradiol, androgens, or dehydroepiandrosterone sulfate (DHEAS). In SWAN, with more than 3000 African-American, Caucasian, Chinese, Hispanic, and Japanese women, testosterone and higher FSH were associated with the desire domain, higher FSH with less arousal and lower estradiol with the pain domain, consistent with findings in the Melbourne Women's Midlife Health Program (MWMHP) and the Massachusetts Women's Health Study. The negative association of estradiol with vaginal coital pain is consistent with the described effects of estrogens on vaginal integrity and the utility of estrogen treatment for vulvo-vaginal atrophy. SWAN has reported that testosterone was positively associated with sexual desire among women with a partner, but the differences in testosterone levels among women within different desire categories are small and all within the midportion of the normal testosterone

---

TABLE 46-2

Adjusted Odds Ratio for Reporting Difficulty Sleeping by Menopausal Status, All Women vs. Women Without Vasomotor Symptoms, Study of Women's Health Across the Nation, 1995–1997

MENOPAUSAL STATUS	ALL WOMEN ($n = 11\,222$)		WOMEN WITHOUT VASOMOTOR SYMPTOMS ($n = 7338$)	
	Odds Ratio	95% CI	Odds Ratio	95% CI
Premenopausal	1.00	Reference	1.00	Reference
Early perimenopause	1.11	0.99–1.24	1.10	0.96–1.26
Late perimenopause	1.33	1.07–1.65	1.40	1.01–1.92
Natural postmenopause	1.21	1.03–1.43	1.26	1.01–1.58
Surgical postmenopause	1.55	1.25–1.92	1.19	0.87–1.62
Postmenopause with hormones	1.12	0.95–1.31	1.03	0.83–1.27

Adapted from Table 3 in Kravitz HM, Ganz PA, Bromberger J, et al. Sleep difficulty in women at midlife: a community survey of sleep and the menopausal transition. Menopause. 10:19–28, 2003.

range for women. FSH has not been postulated to have a direct role in sexual function but to be an indirect marker of gonadal function; however, its association with sexual function domains argues for an expanded view that incorporates neuroendocrine signaling into the study of complex sexual behavior.

While concurrent annual serum reproductive hormone levels and change in those concentrations over time have been associated with major domains of sexual function during the menopausal transition, the magnitude of these associations is consistently modest. Favorable outcomes in sexual functioning are much more strongly associated with having a partner and emotional satisfaction with the relationship than the most prominent hormone values. Other highly important factors included increasing age of the woman, poor health status, smoking behavior, and body size.

Depressed Mood

Throughout the life span, women are two times more likely than men to suffer from depression. A number of factors, including hormones, reproductive factors, genetics, biology, and societal or cultural norms may increase the propensity for depressed mood in women. The menopause transition may represent a period of heightened risk for the development of clinically significant depressive symptoms based on the increasingly variable and declining estradiol concentrations. The risk is reportedly greater for women regardless of preexisting symptoms. Further, while estrogen therapy was thought to promote improvement in depressive symptoms, the controversial findings from the Women's Health Initiative (WHI) have led to additional questions about the hypothesis that sex steroids and their changes during the menopause are an explanatory factor in depression and mood disorders.

The report from the NIH State-of-the-Science Conference concluded there is limited evidence about mood symptoms in the menopause transition. In studies where hormone concentrations have been related to measures of depressed symptomology, change in FSH and LH levels are the more consistent predictors, whereas change in estradiol and testosterone levels have been substantially less predictive. Further, in general, stages of the menopause transition have not been predictive of mood changes. The gonadotropins, FSH, and LH have not been studied for their direct role in affect and mood, but are considered indirect markers of gonadal function;

however, their more consistent association with mood argues for expanding the view to incorporate other aspects of neuroendocrine signaling.

While the natural menopause may or may not be associated with depressed mood, other attributes associated with the menopause (vasomotor symptoms, insomnia, and other sleep disorders) appear to have a greater impact on presentation with depressed mood. Additionally, other factors including BMI, smoking behavior, stress, and relationship problems, which can change during the menopause transition period, are important factors in depressed mood.

Cognition and Memory

Memory complaints are common in the menopausal transition, but the implications of these complaints for subsequent cognitive decline and dementia are yet to be defined. In SWAN, approximately 30% of 12 000 women aged 40 to 55 years reported perceived forgetfulness in the previous 2-week period. Sixty-two percent of responses by 230 women, aged 40 to 60 years, to a series of open-ended questions in the Seattle Midlife Women's Health Study (SMWHS) indicated memory changes over a median 24-month period. A cross-sectional study of 1270 Chinese midlife women (58% premenopausal, 27% perimenopausal, and 15% postmenopausal) noted that the Trail Making Test, a test of motor speed and visual acuity, significantly declined with the progression of menopausal status. In contrast, the MWMHP evaluated episodic verbal memory (a word list recall task) cross-sectionally in 326 women aged 52 to 63 years (majority postmenopausal) and concluded that memory was similar across the menopausal transition phases. Both SMWHS and the MWMHP have identified an association between memory problems and depressed mood, suggesting that depressed mood might confound the associations of cognition and menopause-related biological and sociological changes.

Longitudinal data about cognitive changes during the menopausal transition have come from a SWAN substudy in which a subgroup of 868 premenopausal and early perimenopausal women, aged 42 to 52 years, were assessed annually for an average of three years in working memory (Digit Span Backwards) and perceptual speed (Symbol Digit Modalities Test). In the test for perceptual speed (the ability to quickly and accurately compare objects and patterns), there was a significant decrease over time in postmenopausal women and slight increases among perimenopausal women (Table 46-3).

TABLE 46-3

Adjusted Estimated Rate of Change per Year in Cognitive Score by Menopausal Status, Study of Women's Health Across the Nation, 1996–2001				
COGNITIVE TEST	**MENOPAUSAL STATUS**	**ADJUSTED ESTIMATED RATE OF CHANGE PER YEAR**	**95%**	**CI**
Digit Span Backwards	Premenopausal	0.17	0.03,	0.30
	Early perimenopausal	0.19	0.09,	0.28
	Late perimenopausal	0.20	–0.14,	0.54
	Postmenopausal	0.03	–0.26,	0.33
Symbol Digit Modality Test	Perimenopausal	0.52	0.05,	0.98
	Early perimenopausal	0.34	0.01,	0.67
	Late perimenopausal	1.51	0.35,	2.66
	Postmenopausal	–1.13	–2.11,	–0.15

Adapted from Table 4 in Peyer PM, Powell LH, Wilson RS, Everson-Rose SA, et al. A population-based longitudinal study of cognitive functioning in the menopausal transition. Neurology. 61:801–806, 2003.

Whether HT can enhance cognitive performance is controversial. The benefits of HT have been identified in some studies on measures of perceptual speed, fluency, spatial, and articulatory/motor functioning. However, other studies have failed to identify a relationship between postmenopausal estrogen use and cognition. Further, the Women's Health Initiative Memory Study (WHIMS), a substudy of the Women's Health Initiative (WHI) trial, found a slight decline, not improvement, in cognitive function among late postmenopausal women assigned to HT compared to placebo.

Cardiovascular Disease Risk

It has been hypothesized that loss of estradiol with the menopause transition is associated with a greater risk for CVD in women following menopause. This hypothesis evolved and was supported by studies comparing age-specific heart disease rates of men and women, observational studies of women with early age at natural menopause or surgical menopause, and studies of women using HT. While one study suggested that for each year of delay in menopause, there was a 2% decrease in CVD mortality risk, other studies have failed to identify a statistically significant association of menopausal age to CVD risk. Thus, studies of menopause and CVD risk have yielded inconsistent results, particularly those focused on natural menopause and the age at menopause. The findings from the WHI trial, in which the use of hormone preparations was associated with greater risk of heart disease events, further calls into question whether estrogen

status is too simplistic a physiological explanation for the variation in heart disease risk in women compared to men.

Atherosclerosis in the abdominal aorta is more likely to occur among women who have a bilateral oophorectomy or experience early natural menopause than among premenopausal women. Heightened risk for CVD among women with bilateral salpingo oophorectomy has been observed, especially when it occurs relatively early and without HT. An early natural menopause is also associated with heightened risk for CVD; however, statistical adjustments for other cardiovascular risk factors such as age and smoking status can eliminate the association of age at natural menopause and CVD.

SWAN has considered the contribution of the menopause transition to four axes associated with CVD (lipids, blood pressure hemodynamics, carbohydrate metabolism, and hemostatic/inflammatory factors). Representative intermediate markers of three of these axes are shown in Figure 46-3. LDL-C and insulin levels appear to increase across the menopause, while PAI-1 levels tend to fall.

Because both menopause and lipid levels are highly correlated with age, it remains uncertain whether lipid changes at the time of menopause are independent of age effects. Observational studies have been limited in their ability to accurately adjust for the effects of age independent of menopause, since few have followed women throughout the entire menopause transition. Some studies have suggested an independent effect of menopause while others have concluded that elevations in LDL-C and decreases in HDL-C are related to aging rather than menopause per se. However,

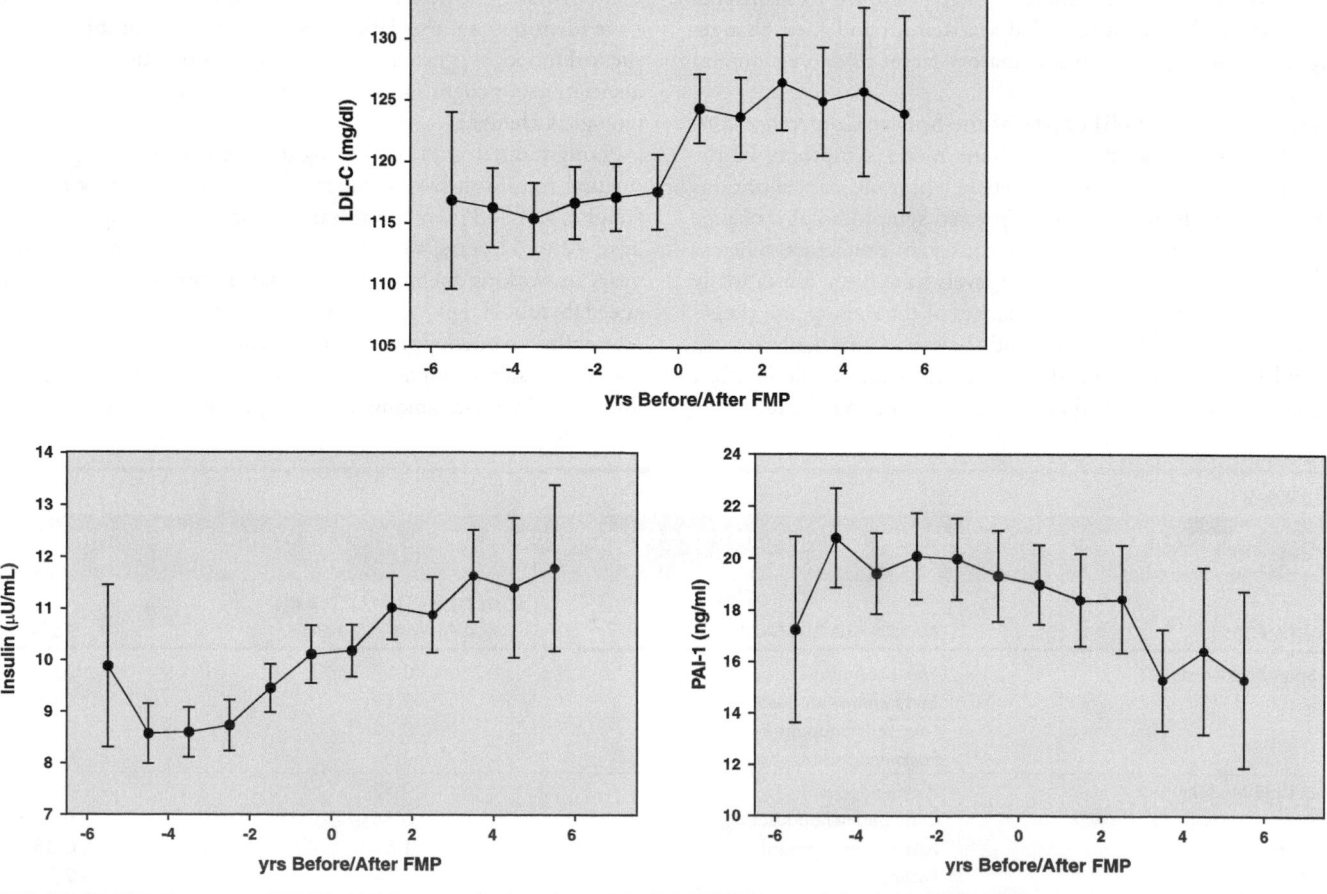

FIGURE 46-3. Change in mean LDL-C (top), mean systolic blood pressure (top right), mean insulin (bottom left), and mean PAI-1 (bottom right)—measures of three axes of cardiovascular disease risk—across the menopause transition, Study of Women's Health Across the Nation. Data represent measures taken approximately 6 yrs before through 6 yrs after the final menstrual period (FMP) for a total of 2336 observations in 722 women.

in SWAN, a longitudinal study across the menopause transition, menopause status-related changes were greater than aging-related changes for total cholesterol and LDL-C, whereas the magnitude of change for HDL and triglycerides were apparently less sensitive to the menopause-related changes. Increases in total cholesterol and LDL-C during menopause are gradual and occur late in the transition. In the MWMHP and SWAN, for reasons yet unknown, HDL increases slightly in the year prior to menopause, a trend that is then offset by a similar decrease in the year following the FMP. The Pittsburgh Healthy Women Study compared the magnitude of change in risk factors from premenopause to 5 years postmenopause and correlated those changes with carotid disease measured 5 to 8 years after the menopause. Increases in LDL-C and triglycerides and declines in HDL-C were greater during the perimenopause; that is, changes were more pronounced between the premenopausal and first year of postmenopausal evaluations than between the first and fifth years of postmenopausal evaluations. These findings reinforce the idea that understanding the lipid changes during the perimenopause defines a potential time frame for both early prevention and intervention activities that could affect the health of the aging woman.

Limited studies of hemostatic factors (i.e., plasminogen activator indicator-1 (PAI-1), tissue plasminogen activator t(pa), C-reactive protein (CRP), Factor VII or fibrinogen) have reported little or no effect of stages of the menopausal transition, defined by irregularity in menstrual bleeding. Androgens or sex hormone binding globulin (SHBG) are more likely to be associated with measures of hemostatic factors than the estrogens. Additionally, higher FSH concentrations were associated with higher Factor VII-c and t(PA) and negatively associated with hemostatic CRP (hsCRP) and fibrinogen concentrations. Clearly, the role of the menopause in relation to CVD-related risks remains to be more clearly elaborated.

Diabetes Risk

While there is a marked increased in diabetes prevalence during the time of the menopause transition, there is limited evidence that this is a direct consequence of the changes during the menopause transition (although there maybe an indirect association). In SWAN, the incidence of diabetes was 2% to 3% per year, with substantial variation within the race/ethnic groups. There are two factors that may be important contributors to diabetes incidence during the menopause transition. First, obesity, particularly central obesity, increased markedly during the transition period (see "Obesity and Body Composition"), and central or visceral obesity is associated

with an increased risk of diabetes. A second element that is altered with the menopause transition is the relative amount of androgen in relation to estrogen. With the relatively stable production of adrenal androgens and the diminished production of ovarian estrogen, there is a shift in the androgen:estrogen ratio. Whether this shift is actually associated with an increased risk of diabetes, and the degree of altered ratio that might be required to generate the increased risk, is an area of active investigation.

Obesity and Body Composition

The role and impact of obesity and body composition (lean, fat mass, and skeletal muscle mass) during the menopause are poorly documented. Longitudinal changes of body composition during the menopausal transition from one study are shown in Table 46-4. Among the 543 pre- or perimenopausal women at study entry, there was a 0.6% (~0.5 kg) annual increase in weight, which was a relative 6-year increase of 3.4%. There was an annual increase of 0.7% in BMI (~0.2 kg/m^2) and a relative 6-year increase of 4%. There was a 1.6% (~0.57 kg) increase in fat mass for a relative 6-year increase of 10%. There was a 1% (~0.9 cm) annual increase in waist circumference, representing a 6-year increase of 6%. Annual measurements of lean mass did not change across the 6-year time period.

This longitudinal study also found that increasing levels of FSH were associated with increasing fat mass and waist circumference, before and after adjusting for baseline age, baseline fat mass, or baseline waist circumference. Increasing FSH was associated with increasing fat mass, and decreasing lean mass and skeletal muscle mass across the 6-year timeframe. While waist circumference continued to increase during the transition, approximately 1 year after FMP, the rate of increase slowed. Women continued to gain fat mass, and no point was identified at which the rate of change increased or decreased. These body size changes take on new relevance as current research increasingly identifies that adipose tissue functions as an endocrine organ, secreting a variety of cytokines including leptin, adiponectin, resistin, PAI-1, tumor necrosis factor (TNF)-α, and interleukin (IL)-6 with immunological, vascular, and metabolic actions.

Bone Loss

It is common wisdom that the immediate postmenopause is a time of accelerated bone loss; in a sample of white women followed prospectively for 16 years, radial bone loss in the perimenopause to 5 years

TABLE 46-4

Estimates of Body Composition Changes with Time from Statistical Models with Body Composition Measures as the Dependent Variables and Time as the Linear or Curvilinear Independent Variable(s)

BODY SIZE/COMPOSITION MEASURES	ANNUAL CHANGE	RELATIVE 6-YEAR CHANGE	ABSOLUTE CUMULATIVE 6-YEAR CHANGE
Weight (kg)	0.6% (~0.5 kg)	3.4%	2.9 kg
Height (cm)	−0.064 cm	0.24%	−0.38 cm
BMI (kg/m^2)	0.7% (~0.2 kg/m^2)	4%	1.2 kg/m^2
Waist (cm)	1% (~0.9 cm)	6.2%	5.7 cm
Fat mass (kg)	1.6% (~0.57 kg)	10.1%	3.4 kg
Skeletal muscle mass (kg)	−0.18% (~0.04 kg)	−1.06%	−0.23 kg

Sowers M, Zheng H, Tomey K, et al. Changes in body composition in women over six years at mid-life: ovarian and chronological aging. J Clin Endocrin Metab. 2007;92:895–901. Copyright 2007, The Endocrine Society.

postmenopause was reportedly 2.4% to 2.6% per year compared to 0.4% to 1.9% per year in the 5 to 11 years postmenopause. However, few studies have examined bone mineral density (BMD) change prospectively during the menopausal transition, incorporating information about hormone patterns and bleeding patterns. Several studies, including SWAN, the Michigan Bone Health and Metabolism Study, and the MWMHP now indicate that bone loss commences prior to the menopause and that the acceleration in remodeling deficit is related to rise in FSH in the perimenopause. Initial cross-sectional reports from the MWMHP showed that FSH levels were incrementally higher among Caucasian women classified as pre-, peri-, and postmenopausal, and that BMD levels were progressively lower for each of the three groups. In SWAN, BMD levels were 2.5% lower in those pre- and early perimenopausal women with FSH levels greater than 26 mIU/mL; these same women had greater n-telopeptide levels, indicating increasing bone resorption. Moreover, SWAN studies indicated that information about baseline FSH values and subsequent FSH values were predictive of the amount of BMD change over a corresponding 4-year period (Figure 46-4). Estradiol concentrations were not predictive of rate of bone loss although women with estradiol levels less than 35 pg/mL had significantly lower BMD. In another study of 231 women, aged 32 to 77 years, with multiple measures of sex steroids and BMD, bone loss was associated with lower estrogen and SHBG, but FSH change was not evaluated.

Postmenopausal bone loss has been attributed to a state of relative estradiol deficiency, so it may appear incongruous that FSH concentrations were more predictive of bone loss during the transition than were estradiol values. There is limited reason to believe that FSH is acting directly on bone through receptors or by nongenomic means. Since FSH serves as a proxy measure of ovarian dynamics involving estradiol, FSH values may better characterize ovarian status and its changes than would estradiol values.

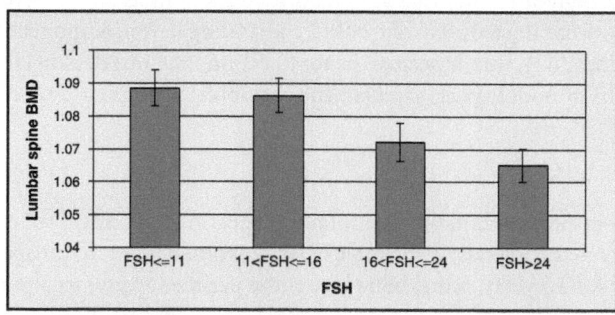

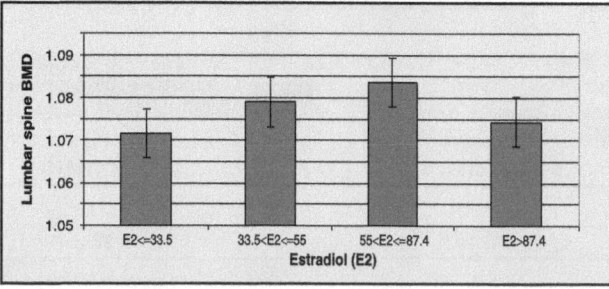

FIGURE 46-4. Adjusted least square means of lumber spine bone mineral density (BMD) by varying levels of FSH (top) and Estradiol (bottom), Study of Women's Health Across the Nation. Measures were adjusted for ethnicity, study site, BMI, and physical activity.

Thus, there is growing evidence from longitudinal studies that bone loss begins earlier than thought, accelerates in the late perimenopausal period, and continues into the early postmenopausal period. The rate of loss appears to decelerate approximately 10 years after the FMP. There are marked individual differences in the rate of bone loss, and risk factors contributing to this wide variation are yet to be fully characterized. More research is needed to evaluate the predictive value of measures of bone microarchitecture to consider the predictive values of biochemical markers of bone turnover in relation to perimenopausal bone loss and to address rates of bone loss in determining subsequent fracture risk.

Physical Function

Geriatricians are familiar with the role of physical function assessment in elderly people, but increasing information suggests that 12% to 25% of newly menopausal women already have substantial functional limitations. The long-term implications for physical limitations for women in the fifth through the seventh decades have not been evaluated. Women are more likely than men to report a physical limitation, for reasons that are poorly understood, although there is evidence that these are probably true reflections of increasing disability. It has been hypothesized that the period of the menopause transition could represent the time of initiation and exacerbation of functional limitations because of the increasing prevalence of diabetes, less favorable lipid profile, decline in sensory function including hearing and vision, and greater propensity to obesity (Figure 46-5).

A 10-item physical function measure (MOS SF-36) provided evidence of a relatively high prevalence of physical limitations in 16 063 women, aged 40 to 55 years, at the seven nationwide SWAN sites. Nine percent of the more than 16 000 interviewees reported substantial functional limitation (difficulty in climbing one flight of stairs, walking one block, or bathing/dressing one's self) while 11% of the interviewees reporting some degree of functional limitation. As shown in Table 46-5, menopausal status was associated with greater risk of physical limitation among postmenopausal women or HT users, compared to premenopausal women, after statistical adjustment for age, difficulty in paying for basics, and being obese.

Two other studies, including women of menopausal transition age, have identified that female participants are more likely to have functional limitations than men, have a greater rate of decline in physical function than men, and are less likely to recover from disability than men. While there is an increased risk of functional limitations with changes during the menopause transition, these risks are dwarfed by those observed in women who report difficulty in paying for basics such as food, housing, and medical care.

Two longitudinal studies of performance-based measures of functioning suggest that two groups are vulnerable to decrements in physical function. In Michigan SWAN and the Michigan Bone Health and Metabolism Study, those women who had transitioned to the postmenopause, as well as women with surgical menopause (both without HT), took a longer time to walk short distances, ascend and descend stairs, and had less reach in comparison to pre- and perimenopausal women, after statistical adjustment for age, time in study, smoking status, and BMI. Gait studies indicated a slower walking velocity in these menopausal women (both natural and surgical).

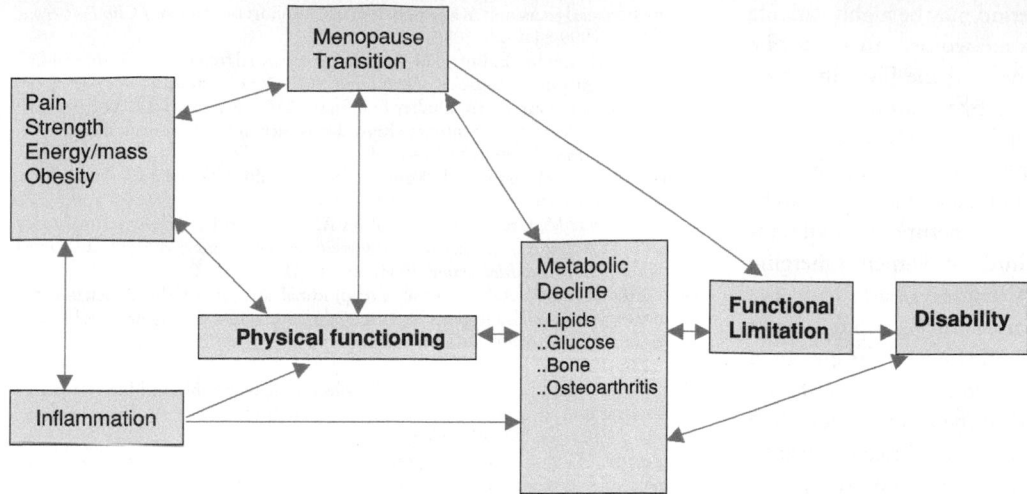

FIGURE 46-5. Conceptualization of the development of functional limitations at midlife in women. *(Adapted from Figure 1 of Sowers M, Pope S, Welch G et al. The Association of Menopause and Physical Functioning in Women at Midlife. J Am Geriatr Soc. 49:1485–1492, 2001.)*

Osteoarthritis

Between the ages of 40 and 55 years, the incidence of x-ray-defined osteoarthritis of the knee (OAK) increases 2% to 3% per year. There has been a long-term debate as to whether estrogen interacts favorably to sustain the collagen associated with cartilage in women. As identified in the section below on skin, collagen loses its flexibility as fibrillar cross-links develop. Limited studies have compared prevalence of OAK in those with and without HT use. However, there are well-known differences in women prescribed hormones, such as smoking behavior and body size, which are risk factors for the development and progression of osteoarthritis.

One study has found that women at the midlife who developed x-ray-defined OAK had greater odds of having lower baseline endogenous estradiol levels during the early follicular phase, even following adjustment for age, BMI, and physical activity. In addition, women who developed OAK had greater odds of having low levels of the estrone metabolite, 2-hydroxyestrone. Since viable interventions for OAK are restricted to joint replacement, the menopause may be a time in which there should be substantial focus on preventive strategies.

Skin and Collagen

During the menopause transition, notable changes occur in skin that not only include the esthetic associations with increasing wrinkling, sagging, and thinness, but also health-related associations such as change in collagen, elastin, and water content, atrophy, and change in wound-healing responsiveness.

Sebum production decreases with the menopause transition, diminishing the barrier to insensible water loss and leading to an increased frequency of dry skin. Additionally, there are declines in collagen, particularly type III, and elastin levels that make skin less resilient and 10% to 20% thinner. Notably, skins that are richly colored with melanin are intrinsically protected from the impact of photoaging. This may explain the lower prevalence of atrophy, dry skin, and wrinkling observed in women of African descent.

Atrophy of the skin is associated with a prolonged time required for wound contraction and wound healing as well as impaired formation of granulation tissue. Because this more fragile skin is associated with the menopause transition, careful suturing is required to prevent skin tears.

Hormone replacement, including topical application of estradiol cream, has been used therapeutically to treat conditions of the aging skin. Additionally, transdermal estrogen delivery systems have been used to avoid the first-pass hepatic metabolism of oral exogenous estrogen replacements. While effective, these methods may have their own adverse effects including allergic/inflammatory reactions.

CONCLUSIONS

The endocrine, sociological, and physiological changes that accompany menopause occur over 8 to 10 years, although the actual

TABLE 46-5

Level of Physical Functioning Limitation or Substantial Limitation in Reference to No Physical Limitation in 16 063 of the SWAN Cross-Sectional Study in Women Aged 40–55 Yrs				
MENOPAUSE STATUS	**SOME LIMITATION**		**SUBSTANTIAL LIMITATION**	
Premenopausal	1.00	Reference	1.00	Reference
Perimenopausal	1.10	(0.95, 1.28)	1.73	(1.46, 2.06)
Natural postmenopause	0.95	(0.77, 1.16)	2.67	(2.21, 3.24)
Surgical postmenopause	1.27	(1.06, 1.52)	3.39	(2.84, 4.05)
HT use	1.57	(1.31, 1.88)	2.33	(1.90, 2.87)

Modified from Table 4 of Sowers M, Pope S, Welch G, et al. The Association of Menopause and Physical Functioning in Women at Midlife. J Am Geriatr Soc. 49:1485–1492, 2001.

duration of the menopausal transition period may be highly variable among individual women. At least in some women, there may be a period of time spanning 2 to 4 years around the FMP in which changes are more pronounced as indicated by variation in levels of FSH, amount of bone loss, and changes in lipid levels. There is substantial between-woman variability during the transition period and greater understanding of that variation is an area of active research.

Vasomotor symptoms are a hallmark of the perimenopausal transition, experienced by more than two-thirds of women. Emerging studies suggest that possible risk factors include greater body size and smoking behavior. Studies from community samples suggest that vasomotor symptoms have a substantial effect on the quality of life of approximately 10% of women. Further, the impact of the vasomotor symptoms may not be restricted to the actual events; their contribution to other conditions, such as disrupted sleep or exacerbation of mood disorders, may have substantial effect on the quality of life.

Ovarian aging appears to be associated with alterations in lipids, bone, and body composition. Thus, the midlife is a time of small but significant changes in a number of systems, including glucose, insulin, lipids, sleep patterns, bone, and joints. Weight gain in midlife is small on an annual basis, but cumulative changes over midlife can be quite substantial and have important effects on other systems. Collectively, these changes are associated with decrements in physical functioning in both natural and surgical menopause.

It is likely that the coming generations will have higher expectations about quality of life, including those that ensue from the menopausal transition, because they are better educated, more often in the labor force, and have smaller families relative to previous generations. Midlife is an optimal time to consider a reorientation to disease prevention and health promotion by the geriatric health care team.

FURTHER READING

Avis NE, Zhao X, Johannes CB, Ory M, Brockwell S, Greendale GA. Correlates of sexual function among multi-ethnic middle-aged women: results from the Study of Women's Health Across the Nation (SWAN). *Menopause.* 2005;12:385–398.

Block E. Quantitative morphological investigations of the follicular system in women. Variations at different ages. *Acta Anat.* 1952;14:108–123.

Block E. A quantitative morphological investigation of the follicular system in newborn female infants. *Acta Anat.* 1953;17:201–206.

Burger HG, Dudley EC, Hopper JL, et al. Prospectively measured levels of serum follicle-stimulating hormone, estradiol, and the dimeric inhibins during the menopausal transition in a population-based cohort of women. *J Clin Endocrinol Metab.* 1999;84:4025–4030.

Dennerstein L, Dudley E, Burger H. Are changes in sexual functioning during midlife due to aging or menopause?. *Fertil Steril.* 2001;76:456–460.

Do KA, Green A, Guthrie JR, Dudley EC, Burger HG, Dennerstein L. Longitudinal study of risk factors for coronary heart disease across the menopausal transition. *Am J Epidemiol.* 2000;151:584–593.

Dzaja A, Arber S, Hislop J, et al. Women's sleep in health and disease. *J Psychiatr Res.* 2005;39:55–76.

Ford K, Sowers M, Crutchfield M, Wilson A, Jannausch M. A longitudinal study of the predictors of prevalence and severity of symptoms commonly associated with menopause. *Menopause.* 2005;12:308–317.

Gold EB, Colvin A, Avis N, et al. Longitudinal analysis of the association between vasomotor symptoms and race/ethnicity across the menopausal transition: study of women's health across the nation. *Am J Public Health.* 2006;96:1226–1235.

Gold EB, Sternfeld B, Kelsey JL, et al. Relation of demographic and lifestyle factors to symptoms in a multi-racial/ethnic population of women 40–55 years of age. *Am J Epidemiol.* 2000;152:463–473.

Gougeon A, Chainy GBN. Morphometric studies of small follicles in ovaries of women at different ages. *J Reprod Fertil.* 1987;81:433–442.

Guthrie JR, Ebeling PR, Hopper JL, Dennerstein L, Wark JD, Burger HG. Bone mineral density and hormone levels in menopausal Australian women. *Gynecol Endocrinol.* 1996;10:199–205.

Harlow SD, Cain K, Crawford S, et al. Evaluation of four proposed bleeding criteria for the onset of late menopausal transition. *J Clin Endocrinol Metab.* 2006;91:3432–3438.

Henderson VW, Guthrie JR, Dudley EC, Burger HG, Dennerstein L. Estrogen exposures and memory at midlife: a population-based study of women. *Neurology.* 2003;60:1369–1371.

Kershaw EE, Flier JS. Adipose tissue as an endocrine organ. *J Clin Endocrinol Metab.* 2004;89:2548–2556.

Meyer PM, Powell LH, Wilson RS, et al. A population-based longitudinal study of cognitive functioning in the menopausal transition. *Neurology.* 2003;61:801–806.

NIH State-of-the-Science Conference Statement on Management of Menopause-Related Symptoms. *NIH Consens State Sci Statements.* 2005;22:1–38.

Research on the menopause in the 1990s. Report of a WHO Scientific Group. *World Health Organ Tech Rep Ser.* 1996;866:1–107.

Richardson FJ, Senikas V, Nelson JF. Follicular depletion during the menopausal transition: evidence for accelerated loss and ultimate exhaustion. *J Clin Endocrinol Metab.* 1987;65:1231–1237.

Soules MR, Sherman S, Parrott E, et al. Stages of Reproductive Aging Workshop (STRAW). *J Womens Health Gend Based Med.* 2001;10:843–848.

Sowers M, Pope S, Welch G, Sternfeld B, Albrecht G. The association of menopause and physical functioning in women at midlife. *J Am Geriatr Soc.* 2001;49:1485–1492.

Sowers M, Zheng H, Tomey K, et al. Changes in body composition in women over six years at mid-life: ovarian and chronological aging. *J Clin Endocrinol Metab.* 2007;92:895–901.

Sowers MR, Jannausch M, McConnell D, et al. Hormone predictors of bone mineral density changes during the menopausal transition. *J Clin Endocrinol Metab.* 2006;91:1261–1267.

Sowers MR, McConnell D, Jannausch M, Buyuktur AG, Hochberg M, Jamadar DA. Estradiol and its metabolites and their association with knee osteoarthritis. *Arthritis Rheum.* 2006;54:2481–2487.

Sexuality, Sexual Function, and the Aging Woman

Stacy Tessler Lindau

INTRODUCTION

Until recently, little has been known about women's sexuality in later life. Negative societal attitudes about aging, sexuality among older people, and women's sexuality in particular, present a significant barrier to scientific inquiry and medical attention to older women's health concerns. Proven interventions for promoting female sexual well-being or treating women's sexual problems are not widely available. Public health attention to older women's sexuality is virtually nonexistent.

The 2005–2006 National Social Life, Health and Aging Project (NSHAP), funded by the National Institutes of Health, provides the first population-representative, baseline data on sexuality among older women and men in the United States and informs many of the insights presented in this chapter. The study enrolled a national probability sample of 3005 community-residing men and women aged 57 to 85 years (75.5% weighted response rate), with oversampling of African-American, Hispanic, and men in the 75- to 85-year-old age group. About half the respondents were male, half were female, and they were divided approximately equally across three age strata: 57 to 64, 65 to 74, and 75 to 85 years. Respondents participated in a face-to-face questionnaire covering social, psychological, and health domains, including detailed information on sexual relationships and functioning. It is the first comprehensive, population-based study of older women's sexuality.

This chapter first locates older women's sexuality in a sociodemographic context, describes sexual activity, behaviors and problems experienced by women in later life, reviews physiological changes that affect sexual functioning as women age, and recommends a clinical approach to evaluation, prevention, and treatment of sexual problems common among older women. Older women, and their sexual relationships, are very heterogeneous. Generalizations made in this chapter, based on population data from the NSHAP study and findings from other sources, are rooted in statistical norms but should not be interpreted as a normative prescription for older women's sexuality.

Interactive Biopsychosocial Model

The interactive biopsychosocial model (IBM) provides a conceptual framework for understanding the relationship between sexuality and health throughout the life course (Figure 47-1). To the degree that medicine attends to matters of sexuality, the orientation is largely negative. The medical model approach to understanding sexuality focuses on sexual dysfunction as a problematic consequence of aging, disease, or treatment. Occasionally, medical texts suggest that older patients' complaints about sexual problems, particularly male erectile difficulties, may herald serious underlying disease and ought not be ignored. While clinically valid, this narrow conceptualization of sexuality defies its multidimensional nature and limits understanding of the meaning of sexuality for health.

A broader framework, as defined by the IBM, conceptualizes a bidirectional relationship between sexuality and health. Sexual behavior can result in health problems, such as sexually transmitted infection, victimization, and, in younger women, unwanted pregnancy. Aging, physical and mental health problems, surgeries, and medications can cause sexual dysfunction. The IBM acknowledges this reciprocal relationship between sexuality and health but incorporates the possibilities that sexuality may also be health-promoting and that aging, or even illness, may confer advantages for sexual life.

In this model, health comprises biological, psychological, and social components and is conceptualized as jointly produced by a woman in conjunction with her spouse or other intimate partner. Joint production of health means that both partners of the couple contribute assets (or liabilities) to the "health endowment," and these assets and liabilities impact the health of the other. The hourglass shape symbolizes the dynamic nature of both health and intimate relationships over time. Clinically, this model can be used as a

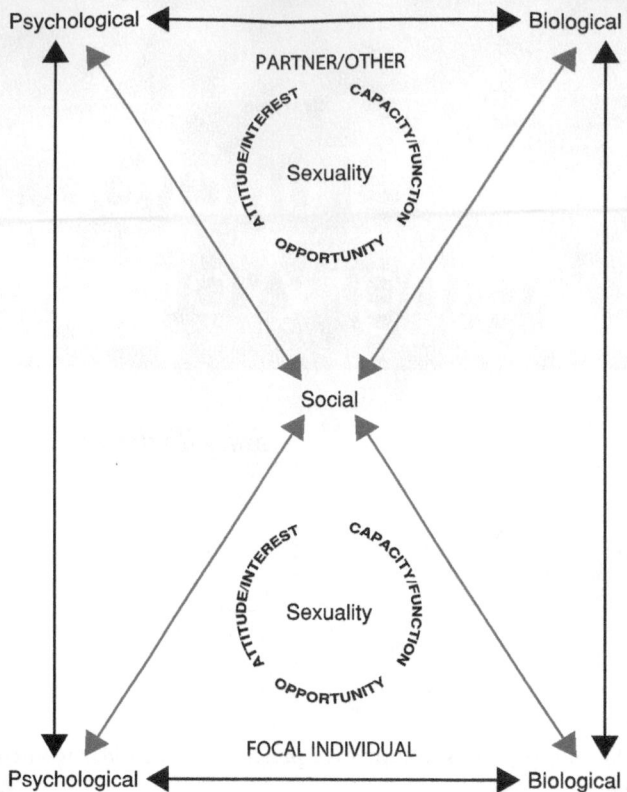

FIGURE 47-1. The Interactive Biopsychosocial Model. *(Adapted from Lindau ST, Laumann EO, et al. Synthesis of scientific disciplines in pursuit of health: the Interactive Biopsychosocial Model. Perspect. Biology Med. 46(3 Suppl):S74–S86, 2003.)*

mnemonic for the broad domains of inquiry pertinent to assessing a patient's sexual history and reminds the clinician of the importance of ascertaining the presence, and health, of the patient's intimate partner.

SOCIODEMOGRAPHIC CONTEXT OF OLDER WOMEN'S SEXUALITY

Sexuality in later life for most, but not all, people occurs in the context of a long-term marital relationship. For men, aging is largely a partnered experience. Men are significantly more likely than women to have a spouse or other romantic partner in later life and to be engaging in a satisfying sexual relationship, even despite a high prevalence of erectile difficulties. As a result of greater longevity, women, in contrast, are much more likely to experience aging, illness, and death without their life partner (Figure 47-2).

Still, many older women regard sexuality as important for health and relationships and, among those with a spousal or other intimate relationship, many engage in regular sexual activity. Women tend to be less satisfied with sex in later life than their male counterparts and also report a high frequency of sexual problems including low desire, vaginal dryness, and difficulty experiencing orgasm. An older married woman is often healthier and more vital than her spouse and commonly assumes a caregiver role, which can interfere with the romantic dynamic of the relationship. Physical health problems, medications, and medical treatments affect the sexual lives of older

couples; older heterosexual adults with a spouse or other intimate partner who are not sexually active most commonly attribute this to the male partner's health problems.

Sexuality is widely valued by older adults, even those without a partner, as an important aspect of health and life. In his 2001 report, the U.S. Surgeon General, David Satcher, acknowledged that "Sexuality is an integral part of human life... Sexual health is inextricably bound to physical and mental health... (it) is not limited to the absence of disease or dysfunction, nor is its importance confined to just the reproductive years..." Although some aspects of aging are regarded as detrimental to sexual life, older women also identify ways in which aging is beneficial for sexuality (Table 47-1).

Lack of formal sexuality education combined with widely restrictive social, religious, and cultural practices around female sexuality during much of the twentieth century have influenced the current generation of older women's sexual expectations throughout their life. As a result, many report that they have never discussed nor would they initiate discussion of sexual matters with anyone, including their spouse. Most older women report that they have never spoken of sexual matters with a physician, yet feel that sexuality is an appropriate issue for physicians to address and that the physician, rather than the patient, should initiate the discussion (Table 47-2). Gender and age differences between women and their physicians can also present barriers to communication about sexual matters. In addition, older women perceive physicians to be poorly trained to deal with patients' sexual concerns and that physicians presume older women to be asexual or disinterested (Table 47-2).

Aging of the baby boomers, the generation of the sexual revolution, is expected to increase demand for medical attention to sexual matters over the next several decades. Although male longevity is expected to increase, older women will continue to outnumber older men through 2050; this presents a significant gender disparity in the opportunity for formation of new sexual relationships in later life and, in some cases, results in multiple women sharing a single male partner. Little is known about the implications and consequences of nonmonogamy in later life, but health assessment of older women, as discussed in detail below, should include questions to ascertain sexual activity, number of current sexual partners, and partner monogamy as this information may be relevant to risk for sexually transmitted disease (STD) and/or psychological well-being.

Sexuality in Long-Term Care Institutions

Although older women's sexuality has largely been a taboo subject, residential institutions for elderly people have long recognized that sexual expression and desire continue even among individuals affected by dementia, frailty, and other life-threatening illness. Dementia, mental illness, and some medications, including dopaminergic medications such as those used to treat Parkinson's disease, can result in sexual disinhibition or hypersexuality, sometimes directed at nursing home staff. The U.S. federal and many state governments declare a right to privacy for residents of nursing homes or elder care institutions; protection of privacy for sexual expression by institutionalized elders is not explicitly guaranteed by the government and therefore relies on individual institutions and providers to respect privacy and maintain individuals' sexual dignity.

Some responsive institutions have addressed this problem by providing private rooms for residents and by training staff to understand and accept elder sexuality in a respectful manner. Sometimes,

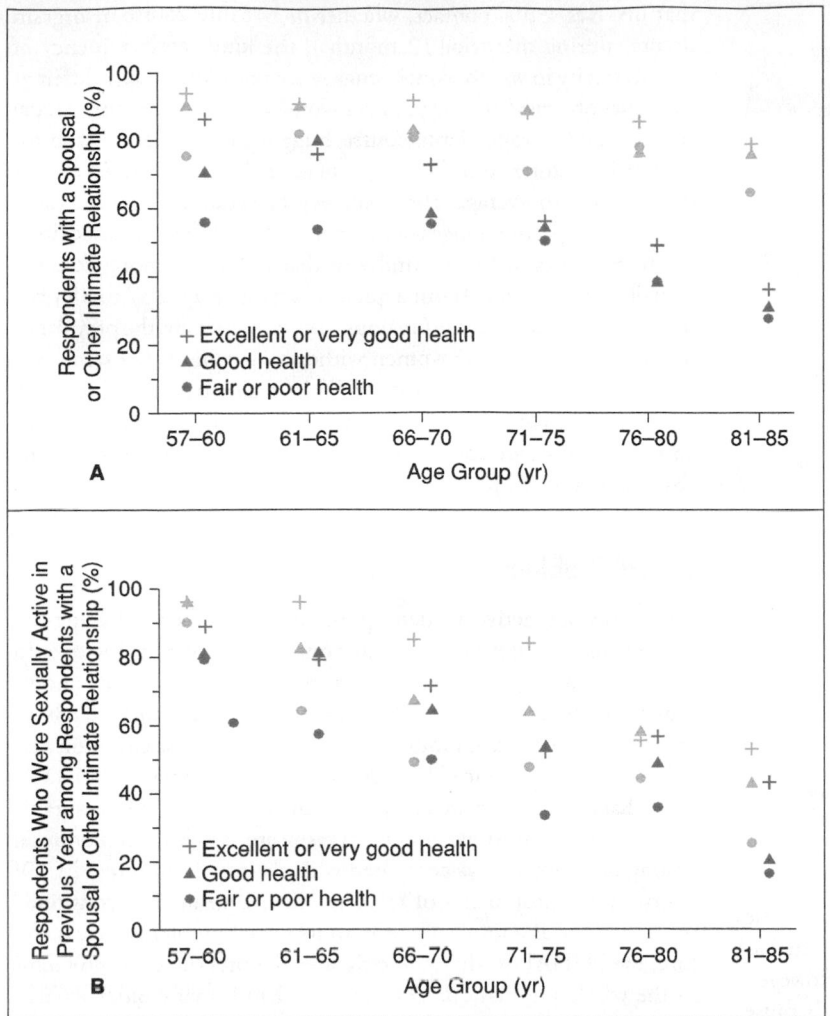

FIGURE 47-2. Prevalence of relationships and sexual activity by age and health status. Panel A shows the percentage of survey respondents who were in a spousal or other intimate relationship. Panel B shows the percentage of respondents who were sexually active in the previous year among those with a spousal or other intimate relationship. Blue symbols denote men, red symbols women, plus signs respondents who reported being in excellent or very good health, triangles respondents who reported being in good health, and circles respondents who reported being in fair or poor health. *(Adapted from Lindau ST, et al. A study of sexuality and health among older adults in the United States. N Engl J Med. 2007;357(8):762–774.)*

sexual relationships form among older residents with dementia who have, but may not remember, a community-residing spouse. Likewise, community-residing spouses may initiate new intimate relationships while maintaining involvement with and commitment to their institutionalized spouse. The implications of these relationships for health and integrity in later life are a growing reality, but poorly understood and often a cause of distress for families. Sexual exploitation and abuse of older women living in residential facilities (and in the community) is poorly documented, but vulnerability is heightened by cognitive impairment, which can interfere with a woman's ability to consent to sexual relations.

SEXUAL ACTIVITY, BEHAVIOR, AND PROBLEMS

Sexual Partnership

The NSHAP study provides the first comprehensive population-representative data on sexual activity, behavior, and problems experienced by community-residing women (and men) aged 57 to 85 years in the United States. For older women, sexual activity is largely determined by availability of a sexual partner. Among women aged

TABLE 47-1

Older Women's Views on Sexuality and Aging

Effects of aging on sexuality	Beneficial	Partners know each other better; decreased sexual inhibition; more time; fewer distractions; know own body
	Detrimental	Less intense physical sexual response; increased inhibition because of poor body image; societal prejudice; need for secrecy
Effects of sexuality on aging	Beneficial	Better circulation; form of exercise; feeling of youthfulness or completeness; security of not being alone; pride in body; optimistic outlook on life; indicative of good general health; happiness/endorphins; physical release; physical outlet; alleviates arthritic pain
	Detrimental	Worry about transmitting or contracting infection; lost status as respected elder if sexually active

Based, in part, on qualitative work by S. T. Lindau funded by the John A. Hartford Foundation, 1993.

TABLE 47-2

Older Women's Perceptions about Barriers to Discussing Sex with a Physician

Why patients don't discuss sex
- Patients "don't know what they don't know"
- Patients feel intimidated
- Feel that it might be disrespectful to physician
- Feel uncomfortable discussing sex with male physician
- Feel uncomfortable discussing sex with younger physician
- Worry that difference in sexual orientation between patient and physician will threaten relationship
- Think physicians not capable of or interested in discussing sex, so no value in raising the issue

Why physicians don't discuss sex
- Physicians assume older people are not interested in talking about sex or having sex
- Physicians "look upon us as their parents"
- Physicians don't know enough to feel qualified to talk about sex
- Physicians assume someone else is dealing with these issues
- Physicians are focused on treating older people for illness rather than maintaining health and quality of life
- They don't have time
- Physicians have their own hang-ups about sex
- Physicians are embarrassed to talk about sex with older female patients
- Physicians' religious beliefs interfere

Based, in part, on qualitative work by S. T. Lindau funded by the John A. Hartford Foundation, 1993.

57 to 64 years, about 85% have a current spouse or other romantic or intimate partner. Nearly all of these relationships are reported as heterosexual, monogamous, and involve sexual activity. However, the proportion of women with a partner declines with age, because of earlier male mortality, and by age 85 years, only about 40% of women have a partner, and fewer than 20% engage in sexual relations.

As compared with younger women, those 57 years and older report fewer total sexual partners over the lifetime. In the NSHAP study, 5% of women reported ever having a female sexual partner and only 5 women (0.3%) reported currently being in a relationship with another woman. Although data on lesbian relationships at older ages are very limited, estimates from the younger population suggest that women in this study may have underreported same-sex relationships. Additionally, qualitative research and clinical experience reveals cases of older women choosing or demonstrating receptivity to female partners for the first time in later life. Some women explain this as a choice caused by the scarcity of men and others are fulfilling a lifelong interest. Most sexually active older women report that their relationships are monogamous. However, women with nonmarriage partners are significantly more likely to report that their partner has had other sexual partners during the relationship. In the NSHAP study, nearly 1 in 10 married women and twice as many nonmarried women with a sexual partner believed that their current partner had other sexual partners during the relationship.

Sexual Activity

Among those who are sexually active (defined in the NSHAP study as engaging in "any mutually voluntary activity with another person

that involves sexual contact, whether or not intercourse or orgasm occurs" during the prior 12 months), the kinds and frequency of sexual activity in which women engage are not substantially different from that observed among younger women. Most commonly, sexual activity involves vaginal intercourse, hugging, kissing, or other forms of sexual touching, and about 45% of sexually active women engage in oral sex. On average, the frequency of sexual activity for those with a sexual partner ranges between monthly and two to three times per month. Again, this is similar to that observed among younger sexually active adults. About a quarter of women aged 57 to 85 years report masturbating in the previous year. Interestingly, the prevalence of masturbation among women without a partner is the same as it is among women with a partner. This is also true for older men (50% report masturbating) and suggests that older adults maintain an individual desire for sexual pleasure and/or release, even in the absence of a sexual partner.

Sexual Problems

Among sexually active women, approximately half report having one bothersome sexual problem; almost one-third report having two. In contrast to older men whose sexual problems are heavily concentrated around erectile difficulties, older women are more likely to have sexual problems in multiple domains. The most common sexual problems experienced by older women are summarized in Table 47-3. Lack of interest in sex, pain with intercourse, unpleasurable sex, and inability to experience orgasm are much more common among older women as compared with their male counterpart. Of course, some proportion of sexually inactive women discontinued sexual activity as a result of bothersome sexual problems and, therefore, the NSHAP study underestimates the prevalence of problems in the whole population. On the other hand, many older women engage in sex despite bothersome problems. The explanation for this is unknown: the rewards or gains of sexual engagement may outweigh these negative experiences, some women may obligatorily participate in sex, others may lack the ability to refuse.

TABLE 47-3

Most Common Sexual Problems Experienced by Older Women*

	PERCENTAGE BY AGE GROUP[†]		
	57–64	**65–74**	**75–85**
Lacked interest in sex (n = 504)	44	38	49
Difficulty lubricating (n = 495)	36	43	44
Unable to climax (n = 479)	34	33	38
Pain during intercourse (n = 506)	18	19	12
Sex not pleasurable (n = 498)	24	22	25
Anxious about performance (n = 500)	10	12	10
Avoided sex because of problems (n = 357)	34	30	23

*Among those of 1550 women surveyed in the National Social Life, Health and Aging Project who reported having sex in the last 12 months, as indicated by the number of respondents in each row.
[†]Estimates (means) are weighted to account for differential probabilities of selection and differential non-response. Asked only of those who reported at least one sexual problem.

Problems related to sexuality in later life, including female sexual dysfunction, can result from sexually transmitted infection, trauma, and sexual violence or abuse. These topics are discussed below. Sexual dysfunction, including clinical diagnosis and treatment, is discussed in more detail later in this chapter.

Sexually Transmitted Infection

Data from the National Health and Nutrition Examination Survey (NHANES) and NSHAP provide the only U.S. population prevalence of sexually transmitted infections among older women. Overall, prevalence of most infections in the general population is very low, although it maybe higher in some elder residential communities or geographic regions with high concentrations of sexually active older adults (e.g., Florida and Hawaii in the United States), or in other subpopulations. STD prevalence among older adults is likely underestimated because of lack of uniform tracking systems and underidentification in the clinical setting. One study showed that physicians are more likely to counsel older African-American and married women about human immunodeficiency virus (HIV) and other STDs, but the majority of older women report that a physician has never initiated such discussion.

Viral infections, including genital herpes simplex virus (HSV) and human papillomavirus (HPV), are among the more prevalent STDs found in older women. HSV-2 seroprevalence among men and women 70 years and older based on NHANES III data (1988–94) was 28%, but women had a higher overall prevalence than men and rates were much higher among blacks (74%) and Mexican Americans (45%). High-risk, or oncogenic, HPV (HR-HPV) prevalence among women aged 57 to 85 years, based on 2005–2006 NSHAP data was 6% and did not vary significantly across age or racial/ethnic groups. The prevalence of this sexually transmitted infection is similar to that documented by NHANES for women aged 50 to 59 years and calls into question age-based eligibility criteria for screening and prevention strategies, including implementation of HPV vaccination.

While there is evidence for new infection in later life as a result of sexual transmission, and infection of sexual partners by infected older women occurs, the majority of incident infections occur earlier in life and either persist or are latently expressed. HR-HPV is an important factor in cervical dysplasia and cancer, a leading cause of female cancer death in the world. In the United States, about 20% of cervical cancer cases, but more than a third of cervical cancer deaths, occur in women aged 65 years and older. Most screening and prevention strategies, including HPV vaccine, use age-based eligibility criteria that largely exclude older women.

Although data are very limited and likely underestimate prevalence (as explained above), population incidence estimates of other STDs among older women are lower than 1% for *Chlamydia trachomatis*, *Neisseria gonorrhea*, and Syphilis. U.S. population data on *Trichomonas vaginalis* among older women are not available; late twentieth century data from Danish and Chinese epidemiological studies indicate that very few cases occur among women older than 60 years. Changes in the cervical epithelium caused by loss of estrogen in older women may account for reduced susceptibility to some infections such as HPV and Chlamydia.

The vast majority of cases of HIV/AIDS in the United States and the world occur among people younger than age 50 years. However, the rate of new HIV infection among older women in the United States, particularly those of minority racial and ethnic groups, has been increasing over the last several years, due mostly to transmission by heterosexual sex. Prolonged survival of individuals infected with HIV in their fourth and fifth decades primarily accounts for increasing prevalence of HIV and AIDS in the United States among older adults. Of all prevalent HIV infections in the United States, 10% to 13% are estimated to occur among people aged 50 years and older. In 2002, 25% of Americans diagnosed with HIV/AIDS after the age of 55 years were women. Public health messages regarding HIV/AIDS prevention and detection have not targeted older women, and physicians rarely offer HIV counseling or testing to this group.

STD prevention strategies have not been well-tested for older adults. Few older women, including those in nonmarital sexual relationships, report using condoms. Condom use by older couples to prevent STDs may be compromised by similar knowledge, communication, behavioral, and cultural barriers experienced by younger couples and by changes in male and female physiology that occur with age. A condom is best applied when the penis is fully erect, but for some older men, full erection may not occur until after coitus is initiated. For women, increased susceptibility to condom-induced vaginal irritation or abrasion may result from vaginal dryness and/or atrophy caused by estrogen depletion.

Counseling women with new or multiple sexual partners warrants attention to prevention of STDs including discussion of barrier methods such as male and female condom and the dental dam (for oral sex) (Figure 47-3). Couples receptive to using condoms should be taught proper application, encouraged to use foreplay to encourage full penile erection and maximal female arousal before penetration, and consider water-based lubricants (oil-based lubricants or vaginal medications can reduce condom effectiveness) to reduce vaginal and vulvar friction. Condoms with spermicide are not necessary for postreproductive age women and should be avoided because they have a shorter shelf-life and have been associated with urinary tract infection in younger women. Male and female condoms and dental dams are for one-time use only.

Sexual Trauma, Violence, and Abuse

Early life events, including sexual trauma in the form of abuse, exploitation, genital injury, and rape, can have lasting effects on sexuality and health that persist into later life. Estimates of lifetime intimate partner violence among older women indicate that 20% to 26% of women are victims; nearly 40% in one study reported that this was severe, including forced sex or sexual contact. In the NSHAP study, 9% of women aged 57 to 85 years reported a lifetime history of forced sex (which may or may not have been with an intimate partner); of these, nearly 40% reported that the most recent event occurred at or younger than age 19 years and 16% reported that the most recent event occurred after age 40 years. Sexual dysfunction, particularly conditions such as vaginismus, dyspareunia, inability to experience orgasm, lack of pleasure with sex, and disturbing fantasies are more common among women with a history of sexual trauma, violence, or abuse. In conjunction with medical treatment and/or physical therapy, psychotherapy including cognitive-behavioral techniques and strategies used for treatment of posttraumatic stress can be effective in helping women at any age cope with sexual violence and experience positive sexual relationships.

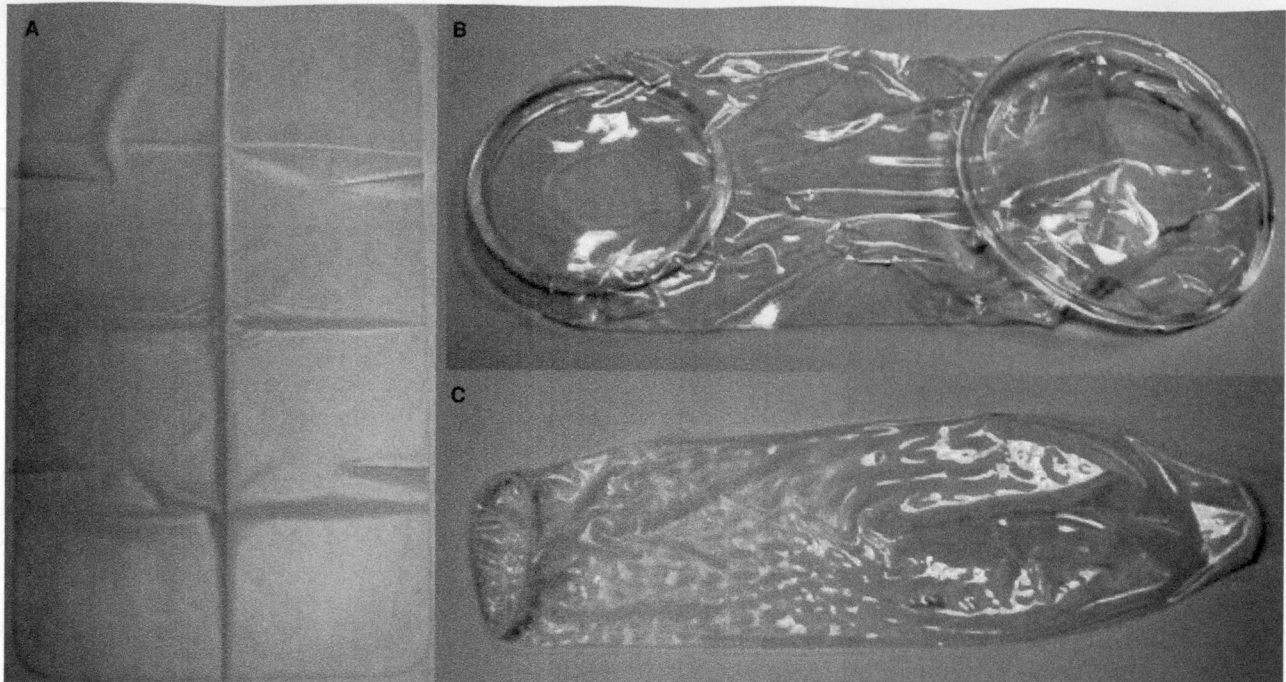

FIGURE 47-3. Dental dam, female condom, and male condom. (A) Latex dental dam. (B) Latex female condom. (C) Latex male condom.

Elder mistreatment, or abuse, discussed in Chapter 60, can also involve sexual abuse but is not limited to an intimate partner. In fact, lack of a spouse or other partner, cognitive impairment, and institutionalization are risk factors for female sexual abuse and rape in later life. Very little is known about how commonly older women experience sexual violence or abuse, but few older women report that a physician has ever asked questions to ascertain sexual victimization. Screening questions for identifying intimate partner violence in the clinical setting are summarized in Table 47-4 and should be part of routine assessment of the older woman.

Consideration of intimate partner violence and sexual abuse in the acute or emergency care settings should be given, particularly when a woman presents with physical injury, vague symptoms (especially recurrent visits), acute mental status changes, and/or is accompanied by a partner or other individual who interferes with the patient's interaction with health care providers.

FEMALE SEXUAL RESPONSE CYCLE

The female sexual response cycle provides one simplified framework for understanding and remembering domains of sexual problems experienced by women. The Masters and Johnson model of the female sexual response cycle, based on physiologic research initiated in the 1960s with a convenience sample of local sex workers, other volunteers, and patients presenting for treatment of sexual problems or contraception, remains the most widely represented model in medical textbooks and the foundation for the Diagnostic and Statistical Manual definitions for sexual dysfunction. This traditional, linear model describes four phases of human sexual response: excitement, plateau, orgasm, and resolution (sex therapist Helen Singer-Kaplan modified this in 1979 to include orgasm, excitement, and desire) and illustrates notable differences in female as compared with male sexual physiology (Figure 47-4A).

According to Masters' and Johnson's work, the female sexual response is more variable than that of males and orgasm maybe single and peak-like, as in men, more gradual or undulating, and/or repetitive during a single sexual encounter. The typical male sexual response is described as much more uniform, peaking in a single orgasm, and includes a latency period during which a subsequent orgasm cannot occur. Arousal for women tends to require tactile stimulation, otherwise known as foreplay; for younger men, visual stimulation plays an important role in arousal but this can abate with age. Many women require direct clitoral or periclitoral stimulation before, during, and/or following intercourse (which may involve penile–vaginal, penile–anal, oral, or manual penetration) in order to experience orgasm. This maybe particularly important for older women engaging in vaginal intercourse with male sex partners because of reduction in the firmness and fullness of the male erection in later life. A longer duration to orgasm in older men maybe realized by some couples as better synchrony of the arousal phase and more frequent experience of simultaneous orgasm.

The pattern of female sexual response may vary across time within a single relationship or with different sexual partners, although little is known empirically about the physiology of the female sexual response cycle in later life or in the context of very long-term (several decades or more) relationships. Psychoemotional changes, and changes in physical appearance with age, including appearance of the vulva and breasts, can negatively or positively affect an older woman's feeling of attractiveness, and can influence her interest in sex. Some women indicate less psychological inhibition about physical appearance with age, or improvement with age, both of which can be sexually liberating.

TABLE 47-4

Measurement Tools to Assess Intimate Partner Violence

MEASURE	CHARACTERISTICS	CONTENT
Women's Experience with Battering (WEB) Scale	10 items 1 = (strongly disagree) to 6 = (strongly agree)*	• My partner made me feel unsafe even in my own home • I felt ashamed of the things my partner did to me • I tried not to rock the boat because I was afraid of what my partner might do • I felt like my partner kept me a prisoner • My partner could scare me without laying a hand on me • I hid the truth from others because I was afraid not to • I felt owned and controlled by my partner • My partner made me feel like I had no control over my life • My partner had a look that went straight through me and terrified me
Behavioral Risk Factor Surveillance Survey (BRFSS)	5 items yes/no response scale[†]	*Sexual* • Now I want to ask you about forced sex involving vaginal, oral, or anal penetration. Has an intimate partner ever forced you to participate in a sex act against your will? • Has an intimate partner ever threatened, coerced, or physically forced you into any sexual contact that did not result in intercourse or penetration? *Physical* • Has an intimate partner ever hit, slapped, shoved, choked, kicked, shaken, or otherwise physically hurt you? *Psychological* • Have you ever been frightened for your safety, or that of your family or friends because of the anger or threats of an intimate partner? • Has an intimate partner ever put you down, or called you names repeatedly, or controlled your behavior?

*WEB scores equal to or higher than 20 (range 10–60) is an indicator of exposure to abuse.

[†] Any woman who answered "yes" to any of the BRFSS questions for their most recent partner is classified as having "any abuse."

Adapted from Bonomi AE, Thompson RS, Anderson M, et al. Ascertainment of intimate partner violence using two abuse measurement frameworks. Injury Prevention. 12(2):121–124, 2006.

Changes in men's sexual response that occur with age can affect female partners both physically and psychologically. As men age, the sexual response becomes more similar to that of women (a phenomenon some refer to as "feminization of the male sexual response cycle"). Tactile stimulation and foreplay are increasingly important for older male arousal, duration to erection and orgasm is longer, and latency (or the refractory period) between orgasms is increased. Because few older men or women are aware of this phenomenon, these changes are often perceived as abnormal, cause unnecessary anxiety and shame, and can strain both members of a couple. Some couples cease sexual activity as a consequence and most do not seek medical help.

Building on the pioneering work of Masters and Johnson, Basson proposed a widely referenced intimacy-based, cyclical model of the female sexual response that incorporates the quality and duration of the relationship as well as the psychoemotional component of female sexuality (Figure 47-4B). In older and younger women, sexual desire may occur before or following sexual arousal. This model emphasizes the role of intimacy in generating female sexual desire and suggests that lack of intimacy and unsatisfying sexual encounters can raise the threshold for interest and arousal in a subsequent sexual encounter. Rather than linear and discrete, the phases of the female sexual response are described by Basson as variably overlapping in a way that "blends mind and body."

Early experimental work suggests that each of these models applies to some women. A survey of nurses (published in 2007) with a response rate of 23% found that the Basson model may resonate most for women with sexual problems. Further empirical characterization of the physiology and psychosocial aspects of the female sexual response cycle in later life, including how it might fluctuate within relationships over long durations of time, across relationships, and with aging, is needed both to inform women's expectations and the clinical approach to older women's sexuality.

FEMALE SEXUAL PHYSIOLOGY IN LATER LIFE

Effects of senescence on the endocrine, neurovascular, musculoskeletal, genitourinary, and gastrointestinal systems are particularly salient to sexual function in later life. More global changes in physical appearance, sensory function (hearing, vision, olfaction, taste, and tactile sensation), cognitive function and memory, and body aromas such as scent, breath, and genital odor can also affect sexual engagement and enjoyment. The female sexual response involves a complex and highly interconnected series of physiologic events connecting mind and body. Disruptions or changes in any of these physiologic systems caused by age-related changes, physical or mental illness, or medication use can alter the sexual response and the ability of a woman to derive pleasure and satisfaction from her sexual encounters.

Endocrine System

Loss of estrogen as a result of menopause is a dominant physiologic event that can affect many aspects of older women's sexual

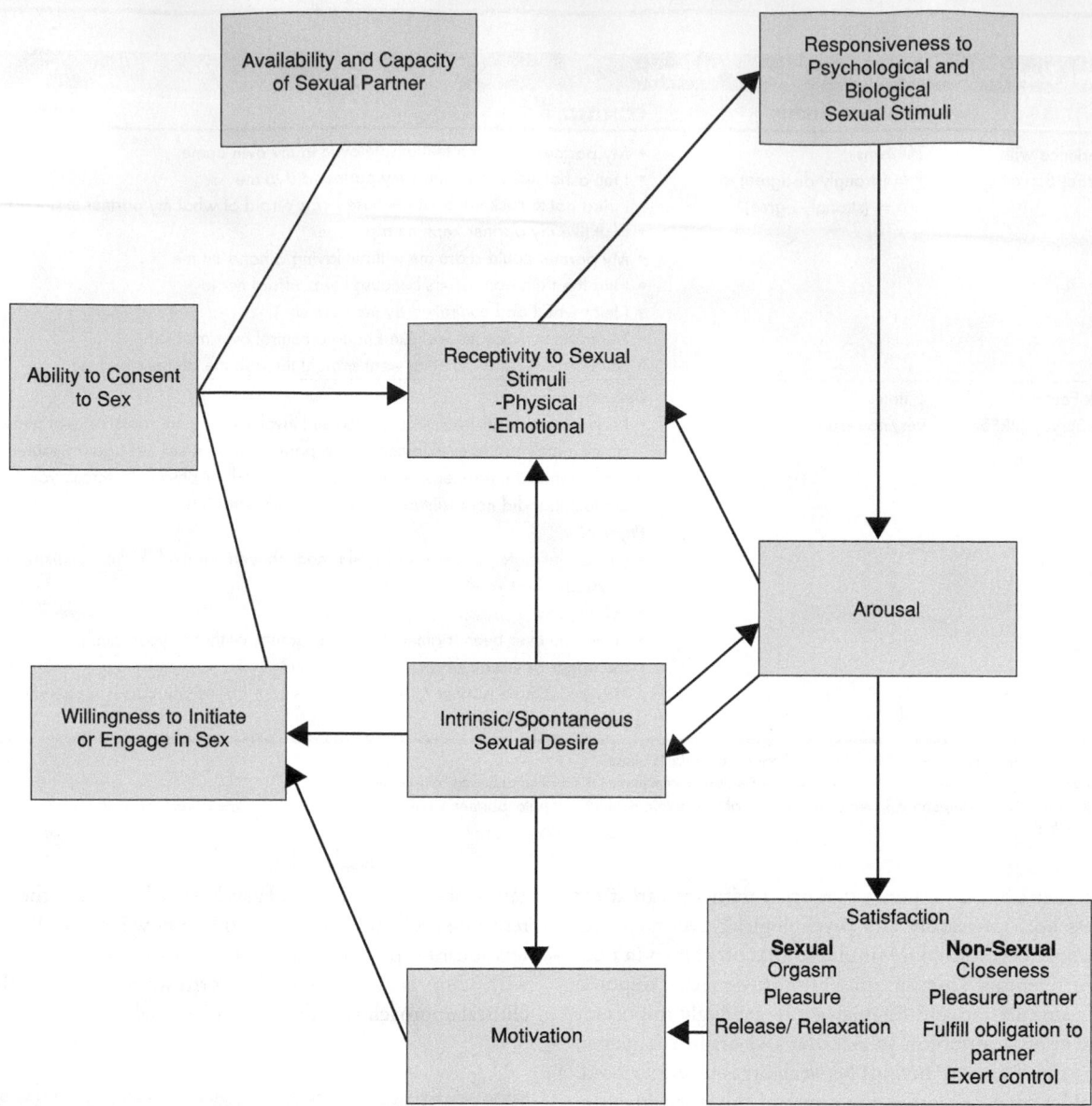

FIGURE 47-4. Models of female sexual response cycle. Female sexual response cycle a, b, c refer to three different sexual response patterns found in females. Model of the partnered female sexual response highlighting features pertinent to older women. *(Data from Basson R. The female sexual response: a different model. J Sex Marital Ther. 26(1):51–65, 2000.)*

function. Despite extension of the human life span, the age of menopause has not changed. Women can live a third or more of life in menopause: the median age of natural menopause in the United States is about 51.3 years and average female life span is 80.4 years. Surgical menopause occurs when a woman undergoes bilateral oophorectomy (or loses ovarian function as a result of other interventions such as chemotherapy or radiation) prior to natural menopause. In the NSHAP study, about 1 in 5 U.S. women aged 57 to 85 years report a history of surgical menopause. Women who have undergone bilateral oophorectomy, pre- or postmenopause, also experience an abrupt and irreversible loss of androgen production.

Estrogen is important for maintaining skin, subcutaneous, mucosal (vaginal, bladder, and rectal) and musculoskeletal integrity, the vaginal microenvironment (pH balance and microflora), vascular flow to the vagina and clitoris via regulation of nitric oxide synthase expression, and sensory perception. Over time, in the genital tract, low estrogen results in vaginal dryness, loss of epithelial cell glycogen, shortening of the vagina, narrowing of the introitus, thinning of the labia, and diminution of the fat pad underlying the mons pubis (Table 47-5). Loss of vaginal acidity results from glycogen depletion and can increase propensity for vaginitis. Urinary and fecal incontinence can be exacerbated by estrogen depletion and inhibit social and sexual relationships as well as sexual function. Maintenance of sexual activity in later life appears to offset some of these local genital changes, in part by maintaining flexibility of the vulvovaginal tissues, pelvic floor musculature, and pelvic joints. Additionally, sexual activity and other forms of physical contact may mitigate estrogen-related

TABLE 47-5

Age-associated Anatomical and Physiological Changes in the Vagina.

Narrowing of vaginal barrel
Epithelium loses glycogen content and normal bacterial flora
Pathogenic bacteria often replace lactobacillus, resulting in atrophic vaginitis
Decreased lubrication results in dryness
Reduced vaginal blood flow
Vaginal pH increases from 4.5–5.5 to 7.0–7.4
Atrophy of vaginal mucosa
    Pale color
    Loss of vaginal folds

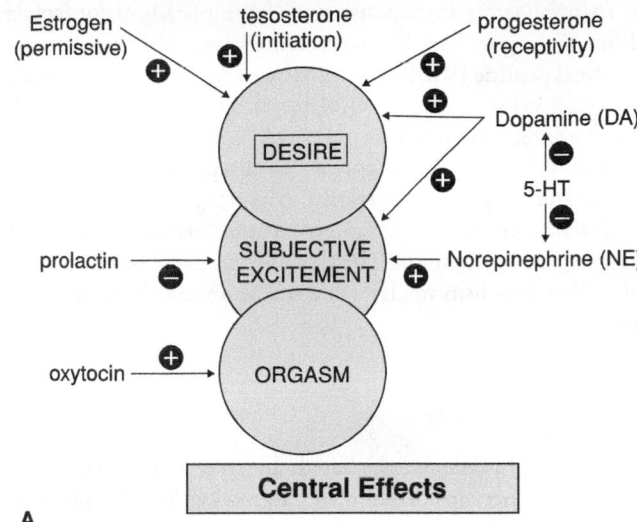

A

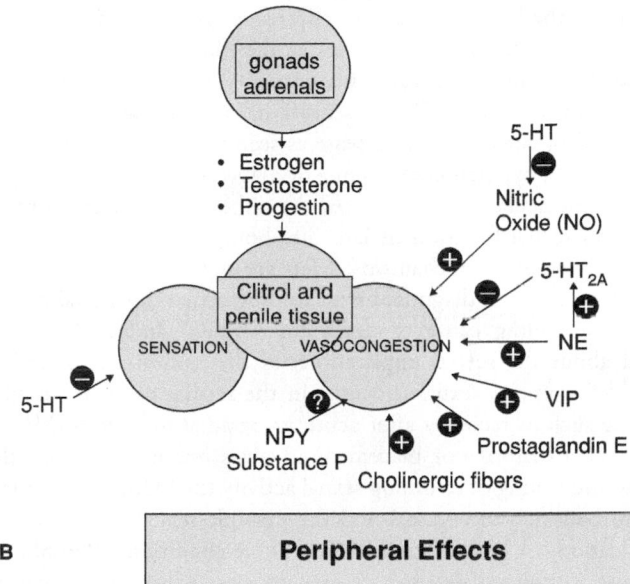

B

FIGURE 47-5. Central and peripheral effects on sexual function. + indicates a positive effect. – indicates a negative effect. VIP, vasoactive intestinal polypeptide; 5-HT, serotonin (5-hydroxytryptamine); NPY, neuropeptide Y; NE, norepinephrine. (Clayton AH. Sexual function and dysfunction in women. Psychiatr Clin North Am. 26(3):673–82, 2003.)

decline in sensory perception and function with age and may play a role in female attractiveness. Largely owing to highly publicized findings from the randomized, controlled hormone therapy trials of the U.S. Women's Health Initiative Study (comparing use of combination equine estrogen alone or in combination with progesterone to placebo among postmenopausal women aged 50 to 79 years at baseline), a minority of women currently use prolonged estrogen therapy for treatment of menopausal symptoms or preservation of sexual function.

Testosterone, along with dehydroepiandrosterone (DHEA), plays an important role in female libido, arousal, genital sensation, and orgasm. Loss of testosterone can exacerbate vaginal mucosal atrophy, thinning of pubic hair, and may compromise an older woman's sense of general well-being. Although female androgen insufficiency as a treatable condition or syndrome is controversial, testosterone therapy for low libido has been shown to be effective in clinical trials involving women with bilateral oophorectomy or total loss of ovarian function as well as postmenopausal women on estrogen therapy (estrogen reduces bioavailable testosterone by increasing sex hormone binding globulin production). However, the U.S. Food and Drug Administration (FDA) has not approved a testosterone patch for this indication. Use of testosterone or DHEA to treat female sexual dysfunction is currently off-label in the United States and most countries and requires close monitoring for side effects. Although rare, irreversible deepening of the voice and growth of facial hair may occur with testosterone use.

Figure 47-5 summarizes central and peripheral hormonal mediators of sexual function (also see Chapter 107). Understanding centrally mediated neuroendocrine changes that occur with senescence is an active area of discovery, focused heavily on understanding cognitive pathophysiology. In women and female animal studies, interest in the cascade of neuroendocrine events resulting in menopause has been similarly driven by an effort to understand the role of sex hormones and hormone therapy in neuroplasticity and degeneration, as well as by efforts to treat female infertility. Application of this knowledge to female sexual function in later life, particularly sex differences in endocrine regulation of the sexual response cycle is nascent.

Aside from its peripheral effects, described above, estrogen plays an important central role both via direct membrane receptor activity and modulation of neurotransmitters. Estrogen appears to exert

neurotrophic and neuroprotective activity in the brain that mitigate against hypothalamic damage that occurs with age. Estrogen also interacts with serotonin and norepinephrine metabolism, which may explain the role of estrogen depletion in sleep, mood, memory and, through these and no doubt other mechanisms, the female sexual response cycle in later life.

The hypothalamic-pituitary-adrenal (HPA) axis mediates the human physiologic stress response and, of course, is the pathway or pacemaker through which sex hormonal regulation occurs. The loss of temporality and pulsatility in HPA neural signaling is a key event in menopause; the dynamics of HPA function over the portion of the life span following menopause, and the implications for female sexual functioning in later life are much less well-defined. Vasoactive intestinal peptide (VIP), now recognized to play a role in female sexual arousal via vasocongestion of the clitoral tissue, also signals time of day information for central GnRH regulation. Rhythmic synthesis of VIP in the brain appears to disappear by middle age in women and maybe an important triggering event in the loss of hypothalamic-pituitary-ovarian access coordination required for ovulation and menstruation. The peripheral effects of changes in central VIP metabolism for later life sexual arousal in women are unknown.

Neurovascular System

Neurovascular physiology, mediated by the sympathetic and parasympathetic nervous systems and a growing list of nonadrenergic/noncholinergic neurotransmitters (e.g., nitric oxide, VIP, nonadrenergic noncholinergic (NANC) is particularly important for the arousal and orgasm phases of the female sexual response cycle. Arousal involves vascular engorgement of the genitopelvic organs, including the labia, vagina, and clitoris, lengthening, dilation and lubrication of the vagina, retraction of the clitoral hood, and tumescence of the clitoris. Microvascular integrity is important for genital sensation and orgasm. Clitoral sensation, in particular, can be compromised by microvascular disease as seen in chronic smokers and women with hypercholesterolemia or diabetes.

Cardiovascular disease caused by atherosclerosis can impair women's sexual function in later life both through psychological and physiological mechanisms. Men are significantly more likely than women to be diagnosed with cardiovascular disease (although it is the leading cause of death for women) and to be counseled about the sexual implications of this condition. Attention to older women's sexual concerns in the setting of cardiovascular disease such as recovery after acute myocardial infarction (MI) or pacemaker/defibrillator placement involves reassurance about the safety and timing of resuming sexual activity (including intercourse, masturbation, and orgasm) and the possible sexual side effects of medications or devices used to treat these conditions. Phosphodiesterase inhibitors are used in men to treat neurovascular causes of erectile dysfunction; similar effectiveness has not been found in women. The only U.S. FDA-approved device for treatment of female sexual dysfunction, the Eros Therapy™ (UroMetrics) clitoral pump, may assist some women with microvascular disease in experiencing improved clitoral sensation, vaginal lubrication, and orgasm.

Musculoskeletal System

Parity, childbirth-related injury, pelvic or lower extremity trauma, obesity, and sedentariness can compromise the integrity of the vulvar, pelvic floor, and lower extremity musculature. Effective contraction and relaxation of the peri-introital, perineal, and pelvic floor muscles is important for penetration, arousal, orgasm, and the relaxation phase following orgasm. Loss of flexibility of hip muscles and compromised stability and mobility of hip joints commonly experienced by women with arthritis or hip fracture can interfere with sexual functioning in later life. Skeletal changes in the hips and vertebrae caused by loss of bone density, osteoporosis, vertebral compression and fracture, and arthritis can make vaginal penetration, particularly using "missionary" (female supine with hips and knees flexed) position difficult and maybe accommodated by use of alternative sexual positioning such as side-lying or sex without vaginal penetration. Prevention and treatment of these conditions with attention to maximizing musculoskeletal strength and flexibility can improve overall physical functioning and help preserve sexual capacity for aging women. Endorphin release associated with pleasurable sexual activity may help alleviate musculoskeletal pain.

Genitourinary System

Changes in the genitourinary system are heavily influenced by postmenopausal loss of estrogen. The urethral orifice can become everted and sensitive to friction, which may cause pain during penetration. Laxity in the pelvic tissues can result in prolapse of the uterus and vaginal walls (i.e., cystocoele, rectocoele, enterocoele). Cervical contact with sexual penetration can cause an "electric shock" or otherwise painful sensation during vaginal intercourse and limits the depth and force of penetration; cervical prolapse that is visible at the introitus or procidentia (prolapse through the vagina) can make vaginal intercourse very difficult physically and psychologically. Urinary incontinence is common, and commonly goes untreated, for older women and loss of urine during intercourse, particularly with orgasm, can also cause physical and psychological discomfort with sex and avoidance of sex. Pessaries maybe used to reduce prolapse and treat urinary incontinence; some, such as ring pessaries, are designed for compatibility with intercourse but should be removed and cleaned following intercourse. Procedures to treat pelvic organ prolapse and urinary incontinence may improve sexual functioning for some women, but colpocleisis (partial or total surgical closure of the vagina to treat prolapse) is largely prohibitive for penetrative vaginal sex.

Gastrointestinal System

Gastrointestinal changes with aging that are most relevant to female sexual function include incontinence of stool and flatus, hemorrhoids, and borborygmy. Anal incontinence typically results in cessation of sexual activity and can be very socially isolating. Hemorrhoids can be exacerbated by sexual activity, particularly anal intercourse, and may result in bleeding during or following sex. Borborygmy can be controlled to some degree by timing of meals in relation to symptoms. Older women who have ceased and/or who wish to resume sexual activity after a hiatus should be screened and evaluated for both urinary and anal incontinence and treated in order to prevent embarrassing or painful sexual experiences that can be very detrimental to her sexual self-image and function.

FEMALE SEXUAL DYSFUNCTION

Use of terms like "dysfunction," "normal," and even "healthy," in relation to human sexuality requires caution and has been criticized, particularly in the feminist and recent psychology literatures. For example, what is a normal level of sexual desire for older women? Is celibacy unhealthy? Few older women report same-sex partners, so is lesbianism abnormal? Is a distressing sexual difficulty a "dysfunction" or a "normal" response to unhappy circumstances in a relationship? Critiques are rooted in a painful history of sexual discrimination, particularly in the United States, and partially in medical history; as recent as the early 1990s, female sexual dysfunction could be diagnosed as a sexual problem experienced by a woman even if it was only troublesome to her partner. In addition, skeptics of the "medicalization" of female sexuality question how "normal" or "functional" sexuality can be defined as the absence of problems, given the high prevalence of sexual problems in the population.

Diagnostic Classification of Female Sexual Dysfunction

The current Diagnostic and Statistical Manual IV–TR classification of female sexual dysfunction stipulates that the problem is persistent or recurrent and causes marked personal distress or interpersonal difficulty. The 2nd International Consensus of Sexual Medicine (2003) adopts a similar classification approach for clinical diagnosis of sexual dysfunction (Table 47-6). Although many validated tools, such as the Female Sexual Function Index and the Sexual Function Questionnaire, can be used to assist clinical diagnosis of female sexual dysfunction (these are generally more relevant for younger women), parallel tools have not been widely validated for use in population studies, particularly of older women. Consequently, population estimates of sexual dysfunction from the NSHAP study (illustrated in Figure 47-6) and others are useful for quantifying the baseline prevalence of sexual problems in later life, or even bothersome sexual problems, but should not be expected to translate into population rates of female sexual dysfunction, clinically defined.

Causes of Female Sexual Dysfunction

Causes of female sexual dysfunction in later life can be primary, such as hypoactive sexual desire disorder, or secondary. Secondary causes can be related to the IBM model referred to previously and include (1) interpersonal and personal psychological factors including depression and substance use, (2) biological factors including a wide spectrum of illnesses, injuries, physical disabilities, and their medical and surgical treatments (note that earlier life illnesses such as cancer and cancer treatment have been shown to have long-lasting effects on sexual function in survivors), and (3) social factors. The patient's psychosexual history and her current partner's physical and mental health, medication, and substance use and sexual function must also be investigated in order to gain a full picture of the patient's sexual functioning and to appropriately tailor therapeutic interventions. Common medications affecting older women's sexual function are summarized in Table 47-7.

Sexual History—Talking and Communication about Sexual Problems

The NSHAP study and several other surveys including older women, even those who are not sexually active, indicate that patients are widely receptive to physician initiation of discussion about sexual problems. If appropriately addressed, patients are not offended; to the contrary, inquiring about this aspect of a woman's history and health can signal that the physician respects her as a vital and whole person. Table 47-8 lists several questions that can be incorporated into a routine geriatrics encounter and should be tailored to the individual's needs. Questions to assess sexual dysfunction when identified are ideally addressed to the individual and the couple and are summarized in Table 47-9. Identification of the level of personal distress caused by each problem can be assessed informally by asking "How much does this problem bother you?" and can be noted as a lot, somewhat, or not at all (a validated instrument, the Derogatis Female Sexual Distress Scale (2002) is useful, particularly for research purposes). The clinician should also document whether the problem is lifelong or acquired and situational or generalized, as these features are important for diagnosis and treatment.

Clinical Management of Female Sexual Dysfunction

A growing, but nascent, evidence base for treatment of female sexual problems (few studies include women older than 65 years) limits the strength of recommendations for management. Treatment of most sexual problems seems to benefit from an interdisciplinary approach, involving psychology, medical evaluation and consideration of medical or surgical treatment, and in some cases, physical therapy. Unfortunately, cost can be prohibitive, particularly for mental health services, which are generally poorly covered by Medicare and private insurance plans. The summary presented here draws heavily on recommendations by Basson (2005) from the international committee convened by the Foundation of Urological Disease (2002–03) and accepted with revisions by the Second International Consensus of Sexual Medicine (2003). It aims to give primary care providers initial treatment options. Where available and affordable, referral to a specialist with experience in treatment of female sexual dysfunction maybe optimal. The International Society for the Study of Women's Sexual Health (http://isswsh.org) and the Society for Sex Therapy and Research (http://www.sstarnet.org/) are useful online resources. Psychotherapy, including couples' and sex therapy, cognitive-behavioral approaches, and sensate focus techniques have long been implemented for treatment of female sexual dysfunction and can be adapted to the needs of older women and couples.

Dyspareunia

Dyspareunia, or pain with intercourse, is a common problem for older women, and many cease sexual activity as a consequence. Thinning of the vaginal mucosa, prolapse of the pelvic organs, and shortening of the vagina caused by loss of estrogen or surgery (by age 60 years, approximately one in three of U.S. women have undergone hysterectomy) in addition to deconditioning resulting from infrequent or prolonged abstinence from sex, can contribute to this problem in older women. Skeletal pain caused by arthritis, vulvar skin conditions, and neurogenic pain can also cause dyspareunia. Management involves treatment of the underlying condition and may include cognitive-behavioral therapy. Vaginal estrogen therapy to address atrophy and pelvic physical therapy including transvaginal pelvic floor massage show clinical benefit in many cases.

TABLE 47-6

Female Sexual Dysfunction Definitions

SEXUAL DYSFUNCTION	DSM-IV-TR	BASSON (2005)
Sexual desire/ interest disorder	"Sexual aversion disorder"—Persistent or recurrent extreme aversion to, and avoidance of, all (or almost all) genital sexual contact with a sexual partner. "Hypoactive sexual desire disorder"—Persistently or recurrently deficient (or absent) sexual fantasies and desire for sexual activity. The judgment of deficiency or absence is made by the clinician, taking into account factors that affect sexual functioning, such as age and the context of the person's life.	Feelings of sexual interest or desire, sexual thoughts or fantasies, and responsive desire are absent (or diminished). Motivating reasons or incentive for attempting to become sexually aroused are scarce or absent. The lack of interest is beyond the normative lessening that may occur with life cycle and relationship duration.
Sexual arousal disorder	Persistent or recurrent inability to attain, or to maintain until completion of the sexual activity, an adequate lubrication-swelling response of sexual excitement.	"Subjective sexual arousal disorder"—Absent or markedly reduced subjective sexual arousal (feelings of excitement, pleasure) from any type of stimulation. Vaginal lubrication and other signs of physical response still occur. "Genital arousal disorder"—Absent or impaired genital sexual arousal: minimal vulval swelling or vaginal lubrication from any type of sexual stimulation, and reduced sexual sensation from caress of the genitalia. Subjective sexual excitement still occurs from nongenital sexual stimuli. "Combined Sexual Arousal Disorder"—Absent or markedly reduced subjective sexual arousal (feelings of excitement, pleasure) from any type of stimulation, and absent or impaired genital sexual arousal (vulvar swelling, lubrication). "Persistent sexual arousal disorder"—Spontaneous, intrusive and unwanted genital arousal (tingling, throbbing) when sexual interest or desire is absent. Any awareness of subjective arousal is typically but not invariably unpleasant. The arousal is unrelieved by orgasm(s), and the feelings persist for hours or days.
Orgasmic disorder	Persistent or recurrent delay in, or absence of, orgasm following a normal sexual excitement phase. Women exhibit wide variability in the type or intensity of stimulation that triggers orgasm. The diagnosis of Female Orgasmic Disorder should be based on the clinician's judgment that the woman's orgasmic capacity is less than would be reasonable for her age, sexual experience, and the adequacy of sexual stimulation she receives.	Despite self-report of high sexual arousal, orgasm from any kind of stimulation is lacking, markedly diminished in intensity or considerably delayed.
Vaginismus	Recurrent or persistent involuntary spasm of the musculature of the outer third of the vagina that interferes with sexual intercourse.	Persistent or recurrent difficulties in allowing vaginal entry of a penis, finger or any object, despite the woman's expressed wish to do so. There is often (phobic) avoidance; anticipation, fear or experience of pain; and variable involuntary contraction of pelvic muscles. Structural or other physical abnormalities must be ruled out or addressed.
Dyspareunia	Recurrent or persistent genital pain associated with sexual intercourse in either a male or a female.	Persistent or recurrent pain with attempted or complete vaginal entry or penile–vaginal intercourse

Adapted from Basson R. Women's sexual dysfunction: revised and expanded definitions. CMAJ. 172(10):1327–1333. 2005.
American Psychiatric Association 2000. (DSM-IV-TR) Diagnostic and Statistical Manual of Mental Disorders, 4th ed. Washington, DC: American Psychiatric Press, Inc.

Vaginismus

Treatment of vaginismus, another condition that can occur in women who have been abstinent for prolonged periods, is best accomplished in conjunction with behavioral therapy that allows a woman to gain comfort and control with penetration. A period of nonsexual genital and peri-introital self-touch followed by gradu-ated vaginal dilator or insertion therapy that can involve the patient and her partner can easily be instructed. Under appropriate circumstances in the office setting, including a chaperone if necessary, guided practice by the patient with the dilators and a handheld mirror can also be accomplished.

Dilators can be used with water-based vaginal lubricant or vegetable oil to facilitate passage and should be used with caution in

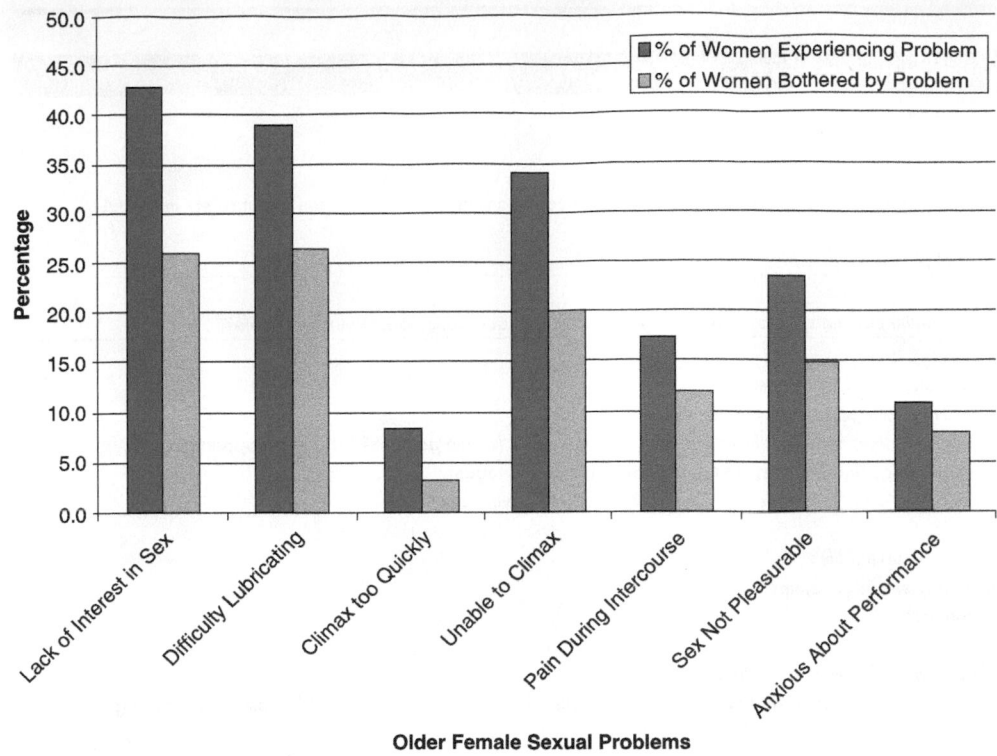

Older Female Sexual Problems

FIGURE 47-6. Sexual Problems among Older Women[a,b,c]
[a]Estimates are weighted to account for differential probabilities of selection and differential non-response.
[b]Among those of 1550 women surveyed in the National Social Life, Health and Aging Project who reported having sex in the last 12 months.
[c]Asked only of those who reported at least one sexual problem.
Adapted from Lindau ST et al. A Study of Sexuality and Health Among Older Adults in the United States. *New England Journal of Medicine.* 2007;357:762–64.

women with recent hysterectomy so as not to perforate the vaginal cuff. Vaginal estrogen therapy prior to or in conjunction with dilation maybe appropriate in women with severe atrophy. Dilator kits can be purchased from a medical supplier or directly by patients via the Internet and typically cost between US $40 to $150. Use over a several-week period, on a daily basis for 15 to 30 minutes, in a reclining position under relaxed conditions, followed by washing of the dilator with a gentle soap and warm water should be instructed.

Periodic assessment by the clinician should occur to ensure safe and hygienic use and to promote progress. Women who use pessaries for treatment of urinary incontinence or pelvic organ prolapse and those who have undergone vaginal, vulvar, bladder, or colorectal surgery or anogenital radiation, may benefit from consultation with a gynecologist or urologist prior to initiating dilator therapy.

Orgasmic Disorder

Management depends heavily on whether the disorder is lifelong or acquired and situational or generalized. Because many older women, particularly 75 years and older do not masturbate (and may never have), ability to assess orgasmic ability maybe limited. Encouragement to self-stimulate either manually or with a vibrator, a technique sometimes used with younger women, must take into account the older woman's experience and attitudes about masturbation. Psychotherapy to assess psychological issues and attitudes regarding orgasm and to complement physical interventions maybe necessary. Education about vulvar anatomy, the role of the clitoris in orgasm, and variations in female orgasm maybe therapeutic for some women. Women with arousal disorders also typically do not experience orgasm so evaluation of arousal should be included in women with this complaint.

Persistent Sexual Arousal Disorder

This rare condition can disproportionately affect older women and may relate to a new onset seizure disorder. Consideration of brain imaging and referral may be necessary. Management strategies are uncertain, but physician awareness of the condition, if communicated to the patient, can itself be reassuring particularly for older women who may feel extremely embarrassed and stigmatized.

TABLE 47-7

Medications Associated with Sexual Problems in Older Women

Cardiovascular and Antihypertensive Medications
  Beta adrenergic blockers
  Clonidine
  Digoxin
  Spironolactone
Psychoactive Medications
  Amphetamines and related anorexic drugs
  Antipsychotics
  Barbiturates
  Benzodiazepines
  Lithium
  Selective serotonin reuptake inhibitors
  Tricyclic antidepressants
Histamine H2 – receptor blockers
Narcotic analgesics
Gonadotropin releasing hormone agonist
Ketoconazole
Phenytoin sodium

TABLE 47-8

Sexual History-Taking and Sexual Education in the Routine Geriatrics Encounter

Context:

Ensure privacy

Communicate comfort and matter-of-fact attitude

Educate patient about how typical changes in sexuality that can occur with age and specific health conditions/treatments; educate about safety in sexual relationships

If proxy required or requested, educate and engage that person

Transition:[a]

"To round out my understanding of your health (or your health concerns) today, may I ask you a couple of questions about your sexual life?"

Questions:

"Do you currently have a spouse or other romantic, intimate, or sexual partner?"

"How many partners have you had in the last year?" "Does your partner have other sexual partners?"

"Is your partner male or female?" "Have your partners been male, female or have you had both male and female partners?" This is an opportunity to communicate non-judgmentalism about same-sex relationships and openness to the possibility of non monogamy.

"When is the last time you had sex?" If no longer having sex, ask: *"What are the reasons you stopped having sex?"*

"Are you satisfied with your sexual life?"

"Do you have any worries or difficulties with regard to your sexual life?"[b]

"How's your partner's health?" "Is your partner having any sexual problems?"

"Has anyone ever forced you to have sex or sexual contact?"[c]

If new partner, or concern about risk factors:

"Have you and your partner been tested for sexually transmitted infections, including HIV/AIDS?"

Educate about testing, inform about confidential versus anonymous testing and meaning of test results. Plan follow-up visit to provide post-test counseling.

"Do you use condoms to prevent sexually transmitted infection?" Educate about barrier methods for STD prevention.

Conclusion:

If no problems identified or patient not sexually active: *"I want to encourage you to feel comfortable talking with me about any sexual concerns should they arise."*

If problem(s) identified: *"I'm concerned about the problem you're having. Would you and your partner be willing to return (or be referred) to discuss this further?"*

[a] Not always necessary, but can be useful if no other obvious transition. The screening sexual history can easily flow out of questions to ascertain the home setting, such as "Who lives at home with you?," and "Are you safe in your home?"

[b] If the patient responds yes, the clinician could then pursue the line of questions summarized in Table 8 or defer to a subsequent visit (see Conclusion).

[c] If yes or risk factors, pursue questions summarized in Table 4.

TABLE 47-9

Questions to Asses Sexual Dysfunction in Primary Care Setting

WHO	QUESTIONS
Individual Partner (alone) –interview patient and partner alone, if permission from patient to interview partner	1. Clarify this partner's view of the problem(s) and how this partner thinks they are coping. 2. Review this partner's sexual response to self-stimulation. 3. Ask about the interviewee's past partnered sexual experiences and their positive and negative aspects. 4. Determine a developmental history: any losses or traumas, and how he or she coped. 5. Inquire if the partner ever experienced sexual, emotional or physical abuse, whether as a child or as an adult.
Couple	1. Ask the couple to explain their sexual problem(s) in their own words. 2. Establish duration of problems; generalized or situational 3. Determine the context of the sexual problems including relationship quality. 4. How is the erotic context? What frequency of sex is expected or attempted? Are there concerns about safety from STDs or privacy? Adequacy of partner's sexual skills? Is there mutual communication about sexual needs? 5. Determine the rest of the sexual response for each partner. 6. Inquire how each partner has reacted to the problem(s). 7. Note any previous treatment(s), their compliance and benefit. Clarify why the couple is seeking help now, and assess their motivation to make changes.

Adapted From: Basson R. Women's sexual dysfunction: revised and expanded definitions. CMAJ 2005;172(10):1327–33. Permission pending.

Medical Therapy for Sexual Desire/Arousal Disorders and Dyspareunia

Although there are currently no FDA-approved medical treatments for female sexual dysfunction, androgen therapy is being used off-label in some cases for treatment of sexual desire/interest disorder in a subset of women with bilateral oophorectomy or those taking oral estrogen (which can reduce bioavailable testosterone by increasing sex hormone binding globulin levels). Treatment of depression can improve sexual desire and interest, but some antidepressants, particularly selective serotonin reuptake inhibitors (SSRIs), can inhibit sexual interest. Bupropion has been used in combination with SSRIs to offset this side effect and appears to be effective for some women.

Off-label use of phosphodiesterase inhibitors has also been implemented for women with genital arousal disorder (a very small subset of women with sexual dysfunction). Tricyclic antidepressants and anticonvulsants are being used by some practitioners for treatment of vulvovestibulitis (a cause of dyspareunia), but these should be used with caution because of central nervous system side effects that maybe exaggerated in older women, particularly those taking other medications. Funding for intervention research in the area of female sexual dysfunction comes primarily from pharmaceutical sources supporting clinical trials of small numbers of young, healthy subjects followed for brief periods. Building an evidence base is a necessary step to offering safe and effective medical, psychological, and other treatments for female sexual dysfunction in later life. More than a dozen drugs for treatment of female sexual dysfunction, particularly sexual desire/interest disorder, are currently in preclinical and clinical trials.

CONCLUSION

Older women comprise more than half the population of older adults in the United States and will outnumber older men until 2050. Despite this, many aspects of older women's health are neglected by researchers and clinicians, including sexuality. Sexual and intimate relationships in later life can promote health and well-being and sustain a basic human need. Many older women engage in sexual relationships despite sexual problems and pain, others discontinue sex caused by problems that could be treated. Physicians caring for older women can positively impact their patient's sexual functioning and overall well-being by initiating and fostering an open and ongoing dialogue about sexual matters in the context of healthy aging or in relation to medical conditions and their treatments. Research is needed to establish trajectories of older women's sexuality with aging and to provide an evidence base for diagnosis and treatment of female sexual dysfunction in later life.

FURTHER READING

American Psychiatric Association. *Diagnostic and Statistical Manual of Mental Disorders (DSM-IV-TR)*. 4th ed. Washington, DC: American Psychiatry Press, Inc.; 2000.

Aylott J. Sexuality in care homes: expression or oppression? *Nursing Resident Care.* 2000;2(9):433–435.

Bachmann GA, Leiblum SR. The impact of hormones on menopausal sexuality: a literature review. *Menopause.* 2004;11(1):120–130.

Basson R, Berman J, Burnett A, et al. Report of the international consensus development conference on female sexual dysfunction: definitions and classifications. *J Urol.* 2000;163(3):888–893.

Basson R. Women's sexual dysfunction: revised and expanded definitions. *CMAJ.* 2005;172(10):1327–1333.

Bonomi AE, Anderson ML, Reid RJ, et al. Intimate partner violence in older women. *Gerontologist.* 2007;47(1):34–41.

Calvet HM. Sexually transmitted diseases other than human immunodeficiency virus infection in older adults. *Clin Infect Dis.* 2003;36(5):609–614.

Dima MQ, Alexander GC, Conti RM, Johnson M, Schumm P, Lindau ST. *JAMA.* 2008;300(24):2867–2878.

Masters W, Johnson, V. *Human Sexual Response.* Boston: Little, Brown and Company; 1966.

Lindau ST, Laumann EO, Levinson W, Waite LJ. Synthesis of scientific disciplines in pursuit of health: the Interactive Biopsychosocial Model. *Perspect Biol Med.* 2003;46(3 Suppl):S74–S86.

Lindau ST, Leitsch SA, Lundberg KL, Jerome J. Older women's attitudes, behavior, and communication about sex and HIV: a community-based study. *J Womens Health (Larchmt).* 2006;15(6):747–753.

Lindau ST, Schumm P, Laumann, EO, Levinson W, O'Muircheartaigh C, Waite L. A National Study of Sexuality and Health Among Older Adults in the U.S. *N Engl J Med.* 2007;357(8):762–774.

Lindau ST, Gavrilova N, Anderson D. Sexual morbidity in very long term survivors of genital tract cancer: a comparison to national norms. *Gynecol Oncol.* 2007:413–418.

Lindau ST, Drum ML, Gaumer E, Surawska H, Jordan JA. "Prevalence of high-risk human papillomavirus among older women". *Obstet Gynecol.* 2008;112(5):979–989.

Quirk FH, Heiman JR, Rosen RC, Laan E, Smith MD, Boolell M. Development of a sexual function questionnaire for clinical trials of female sexual dysfunction [see comment]. *J Women Health Gender-Based Med.* 2002;11(3):277–289.

Rehman HU, Masson EA. Neuroendocrinology of female aging. *Gender Med.* 2005; 2(1):41–56.

Rosen R. Female sexual dysfunction: industry creation or under-recognized problem? *BJU Int.* 2003:3–4.

Sand M, Fisher WA. Women's endorsement of models of female sexual response: the nurses' sexuality study. *J Sexual Med.* 2007;4(3):708–719.

Satcher D. *The Surgeon General's Call to Action to Promote Sexual Health and Responsible Sexual Behavior.* US Department of Health and Human Services; July 9, 2001.

Valanis BG, Bowen DJ, Bassford T, Whitlock E, Charney P, Carter RA. Sexual orientation and health: comparisons in the women's health initiative sample. *Arch Family Med.* 2000;9(9):843–853.

World Health Organization. *Defining Sexual Health: Report of Technical Consultation on Sexual Health.* Geneva 28–31 January, 2002.

Gynecological Disorders

Karen L. Miller ■ *Tomas L. Griebling*

In the United States, women comprise 60% of the older population, so that geriatricians need a working knowledge of gynecologic care, including cancer screening, symptom evaluation, and assessment of incidental findings. After first presenting suggestions for a gynecological history and physical examination in an older woman, this chapter addresses findings and issues in the order they would be approached on a physical examination. Following this, evaluation and management of some common gynecological issues are presented. Management of incontinence with pessaries is included in this chapter, but other incontinence issues are dealt with in Chapter 59. Gynecological care encompasses management of benign breast disease, which is also included in this chapter. Hormone replacement therapy (HRT) is discussed primarily in Chapters 46 and 47, but discontinuation and topical therapies are addressed here.

GYNECOLOGICAL HISTORY

A gynecologic history (Table 48-1) should include age of menarche and menopause, use of hormone replacement (indication, type, route, dose, timing of onset in regards to menopause, duration), current sexual activity, new sexual partners, past gynecological or urogynecologic procedures and their indications, number of pregnancies carried beyond 20 weeks, exposure to diethylstilbestrol (DES), Papanicolaou (pap) smear frequency and results in the past 10 years, mammographic screening in the past 5 years, breast cancer, gynecologic cancers, and history of pelvic irradiation. If urogynecological procedures were performed, note whether the symptoms were resolved, and whether they recurred. Important family history includes gynecological and other malignancies.

DES was first synthesized in 1938, and until as late as 1971 was employed to reduce pregnancy complications. Women ranging in age from 50 to over 100 years could have received DES during pregnancy. These women have an increased risk of breast cancer, but

not of other gynecological malignancies. DES exposure in utero increases the risk of adenocarcinoma of the cervix and vagina mainly in adolescence and the third decade. These women are just beginning to enter geriatric age. The older ones in this cohort (age 40 years and above) have shown an increased incidence of breast cancer compared to women not exposed in utero, so continued surveillance is warranted. Current recommendations are to follow age-appropriate screening guidelines.

Additional information that is sometimes relevant includes total parity (spontaneous or induced abortions, preterm deliveries, term deliveries), route of deliveries (vaginal or cesarean), obstetrical trauma, and past contraception used (especially hormonal). The older a cohort of women, the less the association of current urogynecologic disorders with obstetrical history. Therefore exact knowledge of parity, route of delivery, highest birth weight, or use of forceps have little bearing on understanding etiologies and planning nonsurgical management in advanced age.

The gynecological review of symptoms should include breast pain or lump, nipple discharge; pelvic pain; vaginal bulge, pressure, discomfort, discharge, or bleeding; vulvar irritation, lumps, or rashes; irritative voiding symptoms (frequency, urgency, dysuria), urinary and fecal incontinence or urgency; difficulty voiding or defecating; sexual activity; and sexual abuse.

PHYSICAL EXAMINATION

Breast examination should be performed annually (see Table 48-1). Pelvic examination recommendations for older women vary. Specific utility or cost-effectiveness of the pelvic examination apart from cervical cancer screening in older women has not been studied. Oftentimes despite a negative review of systems, problems are remembered by the patient during the pelvic examination. It may be that the more frail or cognitively impaired the patient, the more important the examination because of a lack of reporting ability. The American

TABLE 48-1

Gynecological Periodic Examination

	COGNITIVELY INTACT	COGNITIVELY IMPAIRED*
Preventive services	Mammography annually (or biennially) until reduced life expectancy Cervical cytology annually if risk factors, triennially if no risk factors 　(Upper age limit disputed, no limit per ACOG, age 70 per ACS)	Mammogram more useful than pap smear. (Shorter lead time for breast cancer.)
History	Hormones: menarche, menopause, past and current hormone use Breast complaints: pain, lump, nipple discharge Vulvovaginal irritation, bulge, bleeding, discharge Urinary issues: incontinence, frequency, urgency, hesitancy, nocturia Defecation issues: Constipation, incontinence (gas, liquid, solid) Sexual practices, contacts, satisfaction, abuse	Current hormone use Staining of brassiere or clothing Apparent discomfort in perineal area Toileting practices, pad use Defecation frequency, stool consistency Sexual behavior
Physical examination	Breast examination annually Pelvic examination every 1 to 3 yrs 　External genitalia/perineum: architecture, integument 　Urethra: meatus visibility, condition 　Bladder: tenderness, fullness 　Vagina: integument, discharge 　Cervix: lesions, growths 　Uterus: size 　Adnexa: palpability, mass	Breast examination annually if tolerated Annual inspection of external genitalia is potentially useful. Initial internal examination is worthwhile, but subsequent examinations may have lower benefit except for fecal impaction.

ACOG, American College of Obstetricians and Gynecologists; ACS, American Cancer Society.

*Considerations in the cognitively impaired (moderately to severe impairment) are suggestions from clinical experience (Level D evidence).

College of Obstetricians and Gynecologists (ACOG) recommends an annual pelvic examination in asymptomatic patients. Some chronic conditions have a medical indication for annual reexamination, such as lichen sclerosus. Because of Medicare regulations excluding payment for preventive care, patients with lichen sclerosus, pelvic organ prolapse, and other chronic conditions should be educated that they need the pelvic examination annually because of their condition, not for a "routine pap smear."

Breast examination includes axillary, supraclavicular, and infraclavicular lymph nodes. During the abdominal examination, the inguinal lymph nodes should be assessed. Performance of the pelvic examination in older women requires more patience, ingenuity, leg positioning, and speculum variety than in younger women. Use of additional assistants or a central foot rest may allow the patient to be examined in the dorsal lithotomy position. Both genital inspection and internal bimanual examination can also be performed in the lateral decubitus position, albeit with less certainty about the bimanual palpation of internal organs and assessment of pelvic organ prolapse. Examination in the standing position may be necessary to demonstrate the extent of prolapse. If the examination needs to be performed in a bed, the patient's hips can be elevated on an upside-down bed pan covered with a folded towel or on a stack of towels to allow speculum insertion.

Typical age-related changes of the external genitalia include decreased fat content of the mons pubis and labia majora and diminished pubic hair. Vulvar structures include a right and left labium majus, a right and left labium minus, and the clitoris. The labia minora meet anteriorly to form the clitoral hood at the distal end of the clitoris. Each of these structures should be noted upon examination. The clitoris may be prominent because of a predominance of androgen relative to estrogen, or it may be obscured by labial fusion. The urethra may not be easily visualized if it has receded into the vaginal canal from atrophy or is obscured by fused labia. Lifting the labia anteriorly without lateral stretching will usually allow meatus visualization without undue pain. "Perineum" refers to the entire vulva, perineal body, and anus, that is, the approximate boundary of the pelvic outlet, through which the urogenital ducts and rectum pass. However, it is also used to indicate the area between the anus and posterior part of the external genitalia, especially in lay publications and Medicare documents. These areas should be inspected and their neurological status examined. Sensation to light touch in the labia majora and perianal regions correspond to the lower lumbar (L4–L5) and sacral (S2–S4) dermatomes. Altered sensation, including asymmetry, may be associated with voiding, defecatory, or sexual dysfunction.

Speculum examination is facilitated by having an adequate variety of specula, including very narrow with normal length. Pediatric specula are appropriately narrow but usually too short to reach the cervix or vaginal apex. Lubrication with water or water-soluble lubricating jelly applied to the introitus or sides of the speculum eases insertion. If the patient is tender, 2% lidocaine jelly applied to the introitus, especially the posterior fourchette, will reduce sensation within 2 to 3 minutes. This is particularly useful for cognitively impaired women. If a pap smear is to be obtained, the jelly can be wiped away with a cotton swab. The vaginal walls should be inspected as the speculum is withdrawn whenever possible.

Bimanual examination is usually performed first with two fingers in the vagina, then with one in the vagina and one in the rectum. More information is obtained with the vaginal hand than the abdominal hand. Assess the size, orientation, and mobility of the cervix and uterus (if present), support of the vaginal apex, presence of any pelvic organ prolapse, and identification of any mass lesions. Rectal sphincter tone should be assessed, and the bulbocavernosus reflex can be tested if neurologic impairments are a consideration. Any palpable mass warrants additional evaluation. The presence and characteristics of stool in the rectal vault should be noted as this may be a clinical sign of constipation or other significant defecation disorder. A stool occult blood test may also be obtained. This requires changing gloves before the rectal examination if any bleeding occurred with speculum insertion or pap smear.

ISSUES AND CONDITIONS BY ANATOMICAL APPROACH

Benign Breast Disease

The breast is a complex structure subject to many pathological conditions, including ones affecting skin, muscle, nerves, ligaments, vasculature, and mammary ducts and alveoli. While numerous studies address the epidemiology of breast cancer and cancer precursors, little is known about the epidemiology of benign breast disease, especially in older women. Whereas fibrocystic changes in breast tissue are present asymptomatically in over half of older women, the prevalence of symptoms constituting "benign breast disease" is unknown. These usually present as a lump, pain, nipple discharge, or inflammation.

Breast Lump

Physical examination of the breast should not be completely supplanted by mammography, which can be negative in the setting of palpable tumors. Evaluation of a lump includes not only a description of the size, position, and character of the lump, but also documentation of pertinent negatives, such as lymph nodes, skin changes, and nipple discharge. All lumps should be evaluated by a surgeon or breast specialist, and a diagnostic mammogram should be obtained. Whether the mammogram is done before or after the surgeon sees the patient depends on the physicians and systems involved. If the patient complains of a lump not palpated by the physician, additional consultation is in order. If both the patient and physician agree that now there is no palpable abnormality, the patient should be asked to return in 2 months for reassessment.

Breast Pain

Breast pain is common and rarely indicative of dangerous pathology. It may be unilateral or bilateral, intermittent or persistent, and may or may not be associated with exogenous hormone therapy. Only half of women with significant breast pain seek medical attention. An important aspect of the history is the impact of the pain, such as inability to hug grandchildren, or awakening at night. Causes of pain originating in breast structures include fibrocystic disease, duct ectasia, trauma, sclerosing adenosis, and stretching of Cooper's ligaments. Cancer uncommonly presents with breast pain, and mastalgia is not an indication for a diagnostic mammogram. However, surgical consultation is occasionally in order for focal persistent pain. Many conditions can be perceived as breast pain, such as costochondritis (Tietze's syndrome), cervical radiculopathy, intercostal neuralgia, thrombophlebitis of the thoracepigastric vein (Mondor's disease), herpes zoster, angina, cholecystitis, and hiatal hernia. Physical examination maneuvers to differentiate breast from chest wall pain include palpating the breast between both hands rather than putting pressure on the chest wall, and examination in the lateral recumbent position. If history and physical examination are benign, and mammographic screening for cancer is current, the patient can be offered reassurance and/or analgesics.

Nipple Discharge

Breasts always have the potential to secrete fluid, particularly if a woman has lactated previously. History and physical examination of nipple discharge should determine whether it is spontaneous or expressed, unilateral or bilateral, and involves single or multiple ducts. The color of the discharge and the presence of any mass should also be noted. Whereas unilateral, single-duct, spontaneous, bloody discharge holds the most concern, bilateral expressed discharge from multiple ducts does not indicate breast cancer. Many times the situation is between these two clear-cut extremes. A thick grumous or purulent discharge may indicate duct ectasia (dilated lactiferous ducts with inspissated secretions) or subareolar abscess. Duct ectasia is also the most common cause of blood-stained discharge from multiple ducts. If the discharge is white, an evaluation for hyperprolactinemia is in order, although this is rare in older women. Eczematous and other skin conditions may imitate nipple discharge. Most cases of spontaneous discharge necessitate referral.

Breast Inflammation

Inflammatory conditions intrinsic to the breast include duct ectasia, fat necrosis, foreign body, Mondor's disease, radiation, and inflammatory carcinoma. Extrinsic conditions that may present with breast inflammation include metastatic lung cancer, Wegener's granulomatosis, sarciodosis, and other skin diseases. Evaluation and referral will depend on the specific presentation.

Vulva

Examination of the Vulva

Age and estrogen deficiency may lead to loss of vulvar architecture, especially of the labia minora. Bartholin's glands are located in the inferior (dorsal) aspect of each labium majus. Any mass, cystic or solid, in the area of the Bartholin's gland should be referred to a specialist for additional evaluation. Usually these are excised to rule out carcinoma. Cherry angiomata and epithelial inclusion cysts on the labia are common and not concerning. Asymmetrical pigmented lesions should be noted and considered for either biopsy or follow-up examination.

Benign Conditions of the Vulva

Literally hundreds of disorders involve the vulva, generally falling into categories of infections, neoplasia, and dermatoses, which may reflect systemic disorders. Establishing clinically useful and pathologically appropriate nomenclature of vulvar disorders is challenging, and classification changes are not infrequent. The most recent classification of dermatoses by the International Society for the Study of Vulvovaginal Disease relies primarily on histologic morphology (Table 48-2). The vulva is more sensitive to allergens and irritants than other skin sites. Estrogen deficiency rarely causes symptoms, but may increase vulvar susceptibility to trauma, irritation, and secondary infection. A patient with "atrophic vaginitis" unresponsive to estrogen usually has a vulvar dermatologic condition. A very

TABLE 48-2

Classification* of Vulvar Dermatoses: Pathological Subsets and their Clinical Correlates

Spongiotic pattern
   Atopic dermatitis
   Allergic contact dermatitis
   Irritant contact dermatitis

Acanthotic pattern (formerly squamous cell hyperplasia)
   Psoriasis
   Lichen simplex chronicus
     Primary (idiopathic)
     Secondary (superimposed on lichen sclerosis, lichen planus, or other)

Lichenoid pattern
   Lichen sclerosus
   Lichen planus

Dermal homogenization/sclerosus pattern
   Lichen sclerosus

Vesiculobullous pattern
   Pemphigoid, cicatricial type
   Linear IgA disease

Acantholytic pattern
   Hailey-Hailey disease
   Darier's disease
   Papular genitocrural acantholysis

Granulomatous pattern
   Crohn's disease
   Melkersson-Rosenthal syndrome

Vasculopathic pattern
   Aphthous ulcers
   Behçet's disease
   Plasma cell vulvitis

*2006 International Society for the Study of Vulvovaginal Disease classification.

important part of the history is exactly what preparations, cleansing agents or routines a woman has employed to treat symptoms. Atopic, allergic contact, and irritant contact dermatitis may be caused by soaps, feminine hygiene products, or urine. A minor irritation can potentially be exacerbated into a severe irritant vulvitis with almost any topical preparation. Secondary infections with yeast and bacteria frequently occur whenever there is epithelial compromise, and must be treated along with the underlying condition. Ointments have fewer additives than creams and often cause less irritation.

Inflammatory Dermatoses of the Vulva

Benign inflammatory disorders of the vulva may be difficult to recognize, even by dermatologists, because the warm, moist, frictional environment alters the otherwise typical appearance of these entities. The lichenoid pattern dermatoses, lichen sclerosus and lichen planus, involve inflammation and disruption of basal epidermis.

Lichen sclerosus areas are typically white, bilateral, and relatively symmetrical with sharply demarcated borders, but may assume any configuration. White with a parchment-like surface is the most common appearance, but areas may be pink or red. With more advanced cases, vulvar architecture is lost. Labia minora may not be identifiable. The labia may be agglutinated anteriorly. A biopsy to confirm the diagnosis is helpful. The malignant potential of lichen sclerosus is debated, but may be as high as 4% to 5%. Areas should be inspected at least annually. Treatment is necessary only to control symptoms,

most commonly pruritus. Regimens vary, generally involving aggressive topical steriods for a few weeks with each symptomatic flare, then steroid tapering, then a nonsteroid maintenance regimen. One option is to use clobetasol proprionate 0.05% ointment daily or bid for 1 to 2 months, then reduce the schedule over the next 1 to 3 months. Women often erroneously believe less medication is better, and should be encouraged to continue the steroids as prescribed until the itching is completely under control. Maintenance therapy probably reduces the frequency of symptomatic flares. Petroleum jelly, solid vegetable shortening, or other bland barrier ointment should be applied daily. When symptoms recur, steroids are reinitiated. Vaginal stenosis may occur in severe lichen sclerosus cases. Steroids, estrogen cream, dilators, and occasionally surgery may be useful to treat dyspareunia and sexual dysfunction.

New-onset autoimmune disorders of the vulva are uncommon in older women, but should be considered in the differential diagnosis of vulvar ulcers or rashes. Lichen planus may be associated with localized or generalized inflammation, which can be severe enough to cause introital stenosis. Other considerations include Zoon's disorder (plasma cell vulvitis), Behçet's disease, Crohn's disease, aphthous ulcers, and Hailey-Hailey disorder (fragile and inflamed vulvar and axillary skin). Thickened epithelium is no longer called squamous hyperplasia, but is divided into psoriatic and lichen simplex chronicus categories. Psoriatic lesions of the genitalia do not exhibit the silver appearance seen elsewhere on the body, and are more often simply erythematous. There is usually a personal or family history of psoriasis. Lichen simplex chronicus may be primary or superimposed on other dermatoses. Medium to high-potency steroids are administered until symptoms are controlled, then maintenance therapy may be instituted.

Ulcerations and Infections of the Vulva

The differential diagnosis of genital ulceration includes a wide variety of sexually transmitted diseases, the most common of which in the United States is herpes simplex virus (HSV). A primary infection is usually associated with lymphadenopathy, vaginal discharge, urinary frequency, and painful ulcers on the labia and cervix. The incubation period is 2 to 12 days. Lesions clear in 2 to 3 weeks. Symptoms improve more quickly with the use of antiviral agents (e.g., acyclovir, famciclovir, valacyclovir). Frequent recurrences may require suppressive therapy. Immune suppression, including very advanced age, is a risk factor for HSV infection in the absence of sexual contact and for herpes zoster. Zoster of the S3 dermatome may inhibit detrusor function, and inability to void may be the presenting complaint. Condyloma acuminata may occur at any age, usually in association with human papillomavirus (HPV) from a new sexual contact. Biopsy of any raised lesion is appropriate if the diagnosis is in doubt.

Cancer of the Vulva

Vulvar cancer is the fourth most common malignancy of the female genital tract, accounting for 3% of all cases. The incidence of invasive vulvar cancer rises steadily with age, reaching 12 per 100 000 per year over age 80 years. Pruritus, pain, and a palpable lesion are typical presenting complaints, but particularly frail older women may not be aware of even a large lesion. Many women delay evaluation, leading to a worse prognosis (Table 48-3). Any focal, raised, irregular, or pigmented lesion warrants biopsy, which may be performed

TABLE 48-3

Estimated 5-Year Gynecological Cancer Survival by Disease Stage

CANCER TYPE	STAGE I	STAGE II	STAGE III	STAGE IV
Endometrial*	54–88%	40–76%	22–57%	12–18%
Ovarian	80–90%	65–70%	30–59%	17%
Cervical	80–95%	74–77%	46–52%	20–29%
Vulvar	85%	69%	40%	22%
Vaginal	74%	50%	32%	0–18%

*Includes clinical and surgical staging.
Data summarized from FIGO Annual Report. J Epid Biostat. 6:1, 2001.

by the primary care physician without fear of causing spread. The most common vulvar malignancies are squamous cell carcinoma and malignant melanoma.

The incidence of vulvar carcinoma in situ increased 400% from 1973 to 2000, predominantly in women younger than 65 years. This parallels the increase in exposure to HPV. By contrast, the incidence of invasive vulvar cancer increased only 20% during this time. While HPV is the most common cause of vulvar carcinoma in situ and invasive vulvar cancer in younger women, only about half of invasive cancers are caused by HPV in women aged older than 65 years. The remainder may be associated with poor Langerhans cell function alone.

Vulvar intraepithelial neoplasia (VIN) is used to describe histologic findings of squamous dysplasia and squamous cell carcinoma in situ. This is usually considered a premalignant lesion, although there is some controversy about this. Identified risk factors include cigarette smoking and HPV exposure. The most common presenting symptom is generalized pruritus of the vulva. Multifocal lesions are common, and treatment is often performed with carbon dioxide laser ablation of the lesions. Multiple treatments may be needed and close clinical follow-up is indicated to evaluate for recurrence. The presence of high-grade VIN near invasive vulvar carcinomas is usually associated with a poor overall prognosis.

Malignant melanoma of the vulva is rare. However, melanoma should be considered as a possible diagnosis in any patient with pigmented vulvar lesions. This is particularly important if the lesion has increased in size or has irregular borders or coloration. Biopsy is indicated for any such lesion.

Wide local excision may suffice for some early cancers and may be used palliatively in frail women. Radical vulvectomy with inguinal lymphadenectomy, radiation, and chemotherapy may be employed depending on cancer stage and the patient's overall health status.

Urethra

A urethral caruncle typically appears as a protuberant red area at the urethral meatus in the six o'clock position. This represents a prolapse of the urethral mucosa that may be associated with loss of support of the periurethral fascia. Most caruncles are asymptomatic and do not require any evaluation or treatment. Caruncles are caused by estrogen deficiency, and symptoms of bleeding or pain can be relieved by topical estrogen. If symptoms persist, excision or cauterization may be performed.

Vagina

Vaginal Atrophy

Vaginal atrophy secondary to hypoestrinism includes thinning of the epithelium, loss of rugae, elasticity and distensibility, increase in subepithelial connective tissue and vaginal pH (>4.5), and reduction in vaginal secretions. Lactobacilli are fewer and potential pathogens greater in number, predisposing to urinary tract infections and vaginidities. Atrophic "vaginitis" is poorly defined apart from simple atrophy, but should be diagnosed if there are bothersome symptoms (dyspareunia, irritative voiding symptoms) or signs (telangiectasias, petechiae, inflammation, discharge). A maturation index would reveal 60% to 100% parabasal cells, but is not necessary for the diagnosis.

The preferred treatment remains low dose intravaginal topical estrogen, which can be administered via ring (Estring®), tablet (Vagifem®), or cream (Premarin®, Estrace®). The ring lasts 3 months and releases 6 to 9 mcg estradiol daily, of which roughly 10% may be absorbed. Tablets are given nightly for 2 weeks, then twice a week. Serum estradiol rises initially, then remains within the postmenopausal range. Each gram of estrogen cream contains the equivalent of one standard oral or transdermal daily dose. Premarin has 0.625 mg of conjugated equine estrogens per gram, and Estrace has 100 mcg of estradiol per gram. The amounts needed to treat atrophic vaginitis are much smaller than the lowest doses measurable on the applicator, but unless a woman has an extremely strict reason to avoid estrogen, using one-quarter to one-half gram twice weekly approximates an appropriate dose. With all these low doses, progestins to prevent endometrial hyperplasia are not usually needed, and the standard of care is to not prescribe them. However, it should be kept in mind that the amount of systemic estrogen absorbed from vaginal preparations varies considerably between individuals, and endometrial growth from these low-dose preparations could occur. Any brown or red discharge necessitates endometrial evaluation. Breast cancer patients who take aromatase inhibitors may achieve higher serum estradiol levels, and any estrogen preparation should be given only after consultation with an oncologist.

Nonestrogen therapies are far less effective in reducing dyspareunia and irritative voiding symptoms, but may provide significant benefit. Vaginal moisturizers, such as Replens®, should be used daily to maintain epithelial moisture and vaginal pH. In addition, vaginal lubricants may be used for intercourse. Frequent sexual activity helps maintain supple tissues.

Vaginitis, Vaginosis, Vaginal Discharge

Vaginitis, vaginosis, and vaginal discharge may be separate from or associated with vulvar disorders. Inquiry should be made as to color, odor, pruritus, staining of underwear, use of pads, hygienic products and practices employed, and recent sexual contacts. Microscopy with both saline and potassium hydroxide is preferable, but empiric therapy is initiated in some cases. With saline microscopy epithelial cells (e.g., copious, mature, parabasal, clue cells), polymorphonuclear leukocytes, motile flagellates, and yeasts (blastospheres or mycelium) should be noted. Addition of potassium hydroxide lyses cell membranes and better reveals hyphae, as well as releases amine odor in the case of bacterial vaginosis. Measurement of pH is less helpful in postmenopausal women not taking estrogen since atrophy causes a rise in pH, but a low pH (<4.5) may help identify a yeast infection.

Asymptomatic white discharge with copious epithelial cells but few leukocytes may be simply desquamation, typically in association with either estrogen therapy or recent replacement of externalized vaginal prolapse. Microscopy shows copious epithelial cells and few polymorphonuclear cells. If the patient is not bothered, no further evaluation is necessary. If the discharge is thick, copious, malodorous, pruritic, irritating, or otherwise symptomatic, its etiology must be sought.

Thick, clumpy white discharge with inflammation of the vaginal mucosa is typical of a vaginal yeast infection, usually accompanied by vulvar pruritus. These are less common in postmenopausal than premenopausal women, but occur commonly with estrogen or antibiotic therapy, diabetes mellitus, and immune suppression. Yeasts are normal vaginal flora for up to 50% of women. Symptomatic infections occur as a result of complex host inflammatory response, pathogen virulence, and/or epithelial integrity reasons. *Candida albicans* accounts for 80% to 90% of cases. Microscopy reveals budding yeast and hyphae in roughly half the cases. If yeast infection cannot be confirmed, a culture should be sent. Opinions vary as to whether empiric treatment should be given. Occasional (fewer than four per year) infections in uncomplicated patients can be treated with any of the wide variety of oral and topical antimycotic agents available. Because of polypharmacy issues, topical (intravaginal) therapy is preferred. Oral medication may be better for women with very sensitive skin, and if vaginal treatment is uncomfortable or impractical. Recurrent infections may require 2 to 4 weeks of therapy. Prolonged therapeutic regimens have not been sufficiently studied, and are given according to practitioner preference and experience, such as a topical azole for 7 to 14 days, or fluconazole 150 mg orally every 3 days for three doses. Some women improve after weekly maintenance therapy for 6 months.

Thin, malodorous discharge without pruritus may indicate bacterial vaginosis, a polymicrobial overgrowth of anerobic bacteria. This is a bacterial colonization (vaginosis) rather than an inflammatory condition (vaginitis). It is more common in postmenopausal women not using estrogen than those on hormone replacement. Diagnosis is established with three of the following findings: thin, grayish-white discharge, pH >4.5, release of odor with the addition of potassium hydroxide (positive whiff test), and more than 20% clue cells on wet mount. Usual treatment for symptomatic patients is either metronidazole gel 0.75% or clindamycin cream 2%. Asymptomatic patients do not require treatment in the absence of planned vaginal surgery. However, if odor is noted on examination, patients often admit to having wondered about it. Recurrence rates are high, even when oral metronidazole is used.

Purulent vaginal discharge without evidence of a pathogen may be associated with vulvovaginal lichen planus or desquamative inflammatory vaginitis. Desquamative inflammatory vaginitis is a poorly understood entity associated with inflammation, high epithelial turnover (many parabasal cells), and Gram-positive cocci. Affected patients have usually tried several unsuccessful antimicrobial therapies. Both of these disorders can be difficult to treat, and generally warrant referral to a gynecologic specialist. The inflammation may cause extreme vulvar tenderness and vaginal stenosis. Topical steroids are given intravaginally, usually achieving substantial relief, but ongoing management will be needed.

If purulent malodorous discharge is persistent, the vagina should be thoroughly examined for evidence of an enterovaginal fistula. Endometritis also causes a thick malodorous discharge, which is often bloody. Even without blood, such discharge can be a sign of endometrial cancer and necessitates an office biopsy.

Trichomonas vaginalis is an uncommon finding in older women, but should be considered in the presence of vaginal discharge plus pruritus. If trichomoniasis is present, the patient and her partner(s) should be screened for all other sexually transmitted diseases. *Neisseria gonorrhea* and *Chlamydia trachomatis* can be detected with nucleic acid amplification testing of a urine sample. Current recommendations for detection and treatment of sexually transmitted diseases are maintained on the Web site of the Centers for Disease Control and Prevention (www.cdc.gov/std/default.htm).

Cancer of the Vagina

Vaginal cancer accounts for only 1% or less of female genital tract cancers. Metastatic disease of the vagina is more common than primary vaginal cancer, notably from cancers of the endometrium, cervix, vulva, ovary, breast, rectum, and kidney. The most common primary vaginal cancer is squamous cell carcinoma, but adenocarcinoma, sarcomas, melanomas, and others do occur. Vaginal squamous cell carcinoma is often preceded by cellular changes and development of vaginal intraepithelial neoplasia, which is associated with concomitant cervical or vulvar neoplasia in about 50% of cases.

Risk factors for primary vaginal cancer are the same as those for cervical cancer (see below). The incidence is higher in women who have had prior gynecologic cancer, particularly cervical, and those who have undergone radiation therapy. In women who are not sexually active, these cancers may grow asymptomatically for an extended period, but eventually present with bleeding, discharge, pain, or symptoms involving extension to urinary or rectal structures. As many as 20% of vaginal cancers are detected as a result of screening for cervical cancer. Only half are in the upper one-third of the vagina. Inspection of vaginal walls during speculum withdrawal as well as attentive vaginal palpation during the bimanual examination is important. Surgery is the primary treatment for small localized tumors, but radiation is the mainstay of treatment for most vaginal cancers. Chemotherapy is advocated in some situations.

Cervix

Examination of the Cervix

The border between squamous and columnar epithelia (squamocolumnar junction) is the most common site of cervical neoplasia. It is usually visible in young but not older women. Cysts near the cervical os are almost invariably Nabothian cysts. These are not true cysts, but are areas where the squamous cells have covered the glandular epithelium, trapping mucus. They do not require biopsy or treatment. Any lesion whose benignity is uncertain should be further investigated with referral or biopsy. A pap smear is not an appropriate screening test if an abnormality is present.

Cervical Cancer Screening

The most common consideration regarding older women and cervical cancer screening is the age at which to discontinue pap smears. Although screening has dramatically decreased the toll of cervical cancer, the age-adjusted incidence and death rates among U.S. women aged 65 years or older are higher than among younger women. Higher mortality is caused by later stage at diagnosis, as well as less aggressive therapy. Among white women, the incidence of cervical cancer women peaks at age 35 to 45 years (15 per 100 000), remains relatively flat through age 65 years, and then declines. Among African-American and other minority women, the incidence continues to rise with age, reaching 30 per 100 000 at age 85 years and above. Thus, although cervical cancer is relatively uncommon in older women, the risk should not be minimized, especially in minority women.

Most major health care organizations with the exception of ACOG recommend discontinuation of routine pap smears after age 65 or 70 years if the woman has been appropriately screened in the previous 10 years. Discontinuation presupposes that the physician keeps an accurate history of risk factors for cervical cancer, although the relevance of many of these factors to older women is uncertain. A higher risk for cervical cancer is potentially present in women having had an abnormal pap smear (especially within the past 3 years), a history of cervical or vaginal cancer, a history of moderate to severe intraepithelial neoplasia, a weakened immune system, a history of sexually transmitted disease (including HPV), onset of intercourse when younger than 16 years, more than five lifetime sexual partners, and exposure to DES *in utero*. While "multiple" sexual partners is frequently listed as a risk factor, exposure to one new sexual partner in advanced age is not addressed. Because of a less active "transformation zone" of the cervix, older women may be less susceptible to acquiring HPV, but this is unknown. It must be assumed that any older women with a new partner may be at risk and should reinitiate pap smear screening. Women in whom screening information is not available should also be screened. The use of HPV DNA testing in older women has not been evaluated. Its utility for primary screening, evaluating an atypical pap smear, or triage is unknown. Although most guidelines recommend three annual pap smears for previously unscreened women, in older women the chance of a significant abnormality in the 2 years following one normal pap smear is low. Prior to discontinuation of screening, a patient should ideally have three normal pap smears within 10 years.

Cytologic screening of women who have undergone a total hysterectomy (*corpus et cervix uteri*) is not recommended unless the hysterectomy was performed for cancer or the woman was exposed to DES in utero. However, some older women are not aware their hysterectomy was subtotal (*corpus uteri* only). Furthermore, cancers of the vaginal "cuff" (apex) do occur. Therefore, while not recommended, intermittent vaginal cuff pap smears potentially benefit the individual patient. Women with a history of vulvar cancer, vaginal cancer, cervical or uterine cancer, or DES exposure *in utero* should continue regular cytological screening. If a hysterectomy was performed, it may be appropriate to discontinue screening after three negative pap smears within 10 years.

Cancer of the Cervix

Cervical cancer is the third most common gynecological malignancy diagnosed in the United States. Although it can occur in any age group, the disease is most commonly diagnosed in patients in the fifth and sixth decades of life. The overall incidence of cervical cancer does not differ between women who have undergone prior supracervical hysterectomy (cervix left in situ) and those with an intact uterus.

Three-fourths of cervical cancers are squamous cell carcinoma. Adenocarcinoma, adenosquamous, and clear cell carcinoma comprise most of the rest. Exposure to HPV, particularly HPV subtypes 16 and 18, is associated with an increased risk of cervical cancer. While HPV is the etiologic agent in most if not all cervical cancers in younger women, an unknown number of cancers in older women are not HPV-related. Nonsquamous cell cancers have higher mortality rates. Having had one normal pap smear reduces the risk of squamous cell more than adenocarcinoma. Studies differ on whether age is associated with worse survival after adjusting for confounders.

Symptoms of cervical cancer are variable and depend on tumor stage. Vaginal bleeding, postcoital bleeding, and pain are common presenting symptoms. Early tumors are usually silent and may be diagnosed only by physical examination and pap smear screening.

Radial hysterectomy is the primary treatment for patients with cervical cancer in its early stages. In general, surgery is well-tolerated, even in older women, and age has not been identified as a significant risk factor for perioperative complications. Radiation therapy is the primary treatment of locally advanced disease and adjunctive treatment for many surgically managed cases. Radiation and chemotherapy are also used for palliation in women with metastatic disease, although the overall prognosis is poor.

Uterus

Benign Conditions of the Uterus

The postmenopausal uterus shrinks in size. Leiomyomata also shrink postmenopausally. If the uterus is enlarged and it is unknown whether this is stable, pelvic ultrasound and gynecologic consultation should be considered. The endometrium is usually a sterile environment, protected from vaginal flora by cervical mucus. Endometritis is uncommon, but may occur even in the absence of uterine manipulation or exposure to known pathogens. It is usually associated with a purulent discharge, but bleeding may be the predominant symptom. An endometrial biopsy can establish the diagnosis, as well as rule out cancer.

Cancer of the Uterus

Uterine tumors can begin in either the endometrium or the myometrium. Endometrial cancers are relatively common, but most myometrial tumors are benign.

Endometrial Neoplasia

Endometrial cancer is the most commonly diagnosed malignancy of the female genital tract. Approximately 36 000 new cases are diagnosed annually in the United States, and it represents the fourth leading cancer among American women. Several risk factors for endometrial cancer have been identified including nulliparity, prolonged exposure to unopposed estrogens, and obesity. These risk factors apply primarily to adenocarcinoma, associated with prolonged unopposed estrogen. The less common serous carcinomas usually arise from atrophic endometrium and tend to be aggressive.

The most common presenting symptom for endometrial cancer is postmenopausal vaginal bleeding. Any patient who presents with abnormal vaginal bleeding should be evaluated as discussed below. Only 35% to 50% of patients with endometrial cancer will have abnormal findings in pap smear alone. Office endometrial biopsy should be performed. Initial screening pelvic ultrasonography instead of biopsy is acceptable, but the few cases of endometrial cancer arising in a thin endometrium and missed on sonography are usually of the more aggressive serous type. Therefore obtaining a tissue sample is preferable. No guidelines have been established to govern the evaluation of severely impaired women, such as those residing in long-term care. Because limited radiation therapy may palliate symptoms while not causing undue treatment burden, it is wise in most cases to obtain a tissue diagnosis via office biopsy, even if sedation is required.

The primary treatment for endometrial cancer is hysterectomy and bilateral salpingo-oophorectomy, usually with tumor debulking. Radiation therapy and/or chemotherapy are often indicated as adjunctive therapy or in women who are too frail to undergo surgery. The role of laparoscopic surgical techniques is still evolving. It is possible that laparoscopic and robotic technology may eventually lessen the impact of surgical therapy. Prognosis depends on the stage of disease and grade of tumor, with overall 5-year survival estimated at 65%. Age is associated with a worse prognosis, in many cases because of comorbidity, late diagnosis, and lack of aggressive treatment.

Myometrial Neoplasia

The most common myometrial tumor is the benign uterine fibroid. These can be single or multiple, and can range in size from very small lesions, which do not cause significant symptoms, to large bulky tumors, which can cause abdominal and pelvic pain. Hysterectomy remains the primary form of therapy, but many other techniques are evolving, most notably uterine artery embolization. However, in the absence of hormone therapy, a leiomyoma should not grow and become symptomatic, so any such enlargement is suspicious for cancer.

Malignant lesions of the myometrium include leiomyosarcoma and other sarcomatoid tumors. These do not typically cause bleeding in early stages, and may only be detected by the presence of an enlarging uterus or pelvic mass. They are typically aggressive tumors with high metastatic potential. Surgery is usually indicated and adjuvant chemotherapy and radiation may be utilized. Extension of tumor beyond the confines of the uterus is associated with a very poor prognosis.

Adnexa

Evaluation of the Adnexa

Postmenopausal ovaries normally become atrophic and almond-sized. Any adnexal mass palpated in an older woman raises suspicion for a tumor and requires further investigation, usually starting with imaging. Each imaging modality offers advantages and disadvantages, and it should be kept in mind that each occasionally gives misleading information. Transvaginal sonography is the preferred initial technique to evaluate the uterus and adnexa, sometimes with Doppler sonography. Computed tomography (CT) describes ovarian masses less well, but offers a comprehensive evaluation of the pelvis, such as differentiating adnexal structures from bowel and uterus, ruling out abscesses, and detecting lymphadenopathy. Magnetic resonance imaging (MRI) visualizes reproductive organs well, and better defines uterine pathology in many cases. If an adnexal mass is found incidentally on a CT scan, a pelvic ultrasound usually

provides additional useful information. However, if found on MRI, sonographic imaging may be unnecessary.

Adnexal Cysts

Ultrasonography can differentiate solid and cystic masses. Simple cystic ovarian lesions are common, and are most often benign. CA 125 is elevated with any peritoneal irritation and usually in women with epithelial ovarian causes and should be checked if a mass is found. A simple, unilocular ovarian cyst less than 5 cm in diameter with a negative CA 125 has a very low chance of being malignant. In some cases, such a cyst may be followed with sonography and CA 125 levels every 3 to 6 months. A complex cystic lesion (multilocular or having solid components on ultrasound) indicates an ovarian neoplasm, which may be benign or malignant. Any mass greater than 5 cm in diameter or with any complexity should be referred immediately for surgical consultation.

Cancer of the Ovary

Ovarian cancer is the second most common malignancy of the genital tract in the elderly women. Its peak incidence occurs between the ages of 50 and 70 years. Specific risk factors include nulliparity, prolonged exposure to estrogen, and mutation of the BRCA-I and BRCA-II genes. Ovarian neoplasms may grow to a considerable size asymptomatically. Because ovarian cancer begins silently, the diagnosis is most commonly made at stage III or stage IV disease. The 5-year survival rate for stage IV disease is less than 20% (see Table 48-3). Initial symptoms are often vague and may include abdominal pain, bloating, gastrointestinal complaints, or a palpable mass, and are usually associated with advanced disease. In retrospect, most ovarian cancer patients have had symptoms for several months before their cancer is diagnosed. Therefore, ordering a pelvic ultrasound to investigate vague lower abdominal complaints is reasonable. Current screening tests of asymptomatic women, pelvic ultrasonography and serum tumor markers, have a low overall yield and are of limited value except in high-risk patients.

Surgical therapy with tumor debulking is the primary treatment for ovarian cancer. Adjuvant chemotherapy may be administered either systemically as an intravenous infusion, or via direct intraperitoneal administration. Intraperitoneal administration may be helpful to deliver higher doses of medication to the affected areas, but both forms of therapy can be associated with significant chemotherapy-related morbidity. Immunotherapy and biologic response modifiers such as interferon and the interleukins may be helpful in some patients.

Cancer of the Fallopian Tube

Primary cancers of the fallopian tube are rare. The two most common histologic types include serous and endometrioid tumors. Other types of mullerian carcinomas are less common. Mutations of the BRCA-I and BRCA-II genes may be associated with an increased risk for fallopian tube malignancies. Infections including nontuberculous salpingitis may mimic symptoms of fallopian tube malignancy. The symptoms are similar to those seen with ovarian cancers and include abdominal pain and distension. Diagnosis can be difficult and is often delayed because symptoms may be vague and often do not present until the disease has progressed outside the fallopian tube. These are often aggressive tumors with a poor overall prognosis.

COMMON CLINICAL ISSUES

Gynecological Malignancies

Multiple studies have shown that older women have worse cancer survival primarily owing to late detection and nonaggressive therapy. Older women do well with surgery, radiation therapy, and chemotherapy. Treatment paradigms are changing rapidly with advances in medications, surgical techniques, and epidemiological knowledge. For instance, many tumors formerly treated with only surgery and/or radiation now respond to chemotherapeutic agents. Indications for tumor debulking have expanded. For optimal outcomes, it is critical that the correct initial surgery be performed, rather than having the patient undergo an initial diagnostic or partially therapeutic surgery and then later be referred to a cancer center. Therefore, gynecological cancer treatment is usually best when a gynecologic oncologist is consulted early in the course of care.

Vaginal Bleeding

Initial Approach to Vaginal Bleeding

Abnormal vaginal bleeding may occur in as many as 20% of women aged 65 years or older. History should include any sources of estrogen and other hormones. Most bleeding is uterine, predominantly from endometrial atrophy. Even if a likely cause is found, other sources must always be ruled out, including hematuria, hematochezia, vulvovaginal pathology, and trauma (Table 48-4). Examination of the patient who presents with vaginal bleeding generally begins with the breast and abdomen, including axillary, supra- and infraclavicular, and inguinal lymph nodes. External genitalia, vagina, and cervix should be carefully inspected and a pap smear obtained. Bimanual examination should evaluate uterine size, adnexal masses, and mobility of gynecological organs. Rectal examination should evaluate for neoplasms, hemorrhoids, and induration or nodularity in the posterior cul-de-sac (pouch of Douglas).

Endometrial Evaluation for Vaginal Bleeding

Uterine bleeding is associated with hyperplasia or neoplasia in 22% of postmenopausal women. Office biopsy is the standard endometrial evaluation. A pelvic ultrasound offers additional and separate information, but is not requisite if the biopsy is negative. An ultrasound should be obtained before or several days after the biopsy to avoid artifact. A thin (<5 mm) endometrium on ultrasound usually rules out endometrial neoplasia, but the false-negative rate is up to 4%. Outpatient hysteroscopy, sonohysterography, and MRI are other potential screening modalities.

Genital Prolapse and Incontinence

Genital organ prolapse can be a very bothersome condition for many older women. This may include prolapse of organs from

TABLE 48-4

Differential Diagnosis of Vaginal Bleeding in Older Women

Uterus (*corpus uteri*)	Endometrial atrophy
	Endometritis
	Endometrial polyp
	Endometrial hyperplasia
	Endometrial cancer
	Endometrial proliferation from estrogen-secreting ovarian tumor
	Myometrial cancer
Cervix (*cervix uteri*)	Polyp
	Cervicitis
	Cancer
Vagina	Vaginal atrophy
	Vaginal infection
	Vaginal cancer
	Vaginal trauma
	Foreign body
Vulva	Ulcerations, excoriations
	Cancer
Urinary tract	Urethral caruncle
	Urethral mucosal prolapse
	Hematuria
Gastrointestinal tract	Rectal polyp
	Hemorrhoids
	Hematochezia
Other	Metastatic spread from non-gynecologic primary tumors
	Oviduct cancer
	Endometriosis
Systemic illness	Coagulation disorder
	Hepatic cirrhosis
Iatrogenic	Anticoagulation
	Estrogen therapy

the vagina (cystocele, rectocele, enterocele) or prolapse of the rectum. Evaluation and treatment of prolapse depends on the involved anatomy and the degree of symptoms experienced by the patient (Table 48-5).

Evaluation of Genital Prolapse

The presence of prolapse is only important if it is causing symptoms of bulge, pressure, discomfort, or the patient is experiencing bladder or rectal symptoms. Rarely ulcerations will be detected by examination of an asymptomatic patient, but usually the patient will have mentioned discomfort, bleeding, or discharge. Pelvic organ prolapse has been graded by many different systems over the past century. "POP-Q" is the current standard. Knowing an exact extent of the prolapse, the grade or stage, is useful for planning surgical therapy and following a patient over time for progression. The exact nature (anatomic abnormality) may also be important if urinary or intestinal symptoms are present. Otherwise, exact descriptions are unnecessary, and it is adequate to note whether the vaginal wall(s) extend above (within the vagina), a little below, or far below the introitus. The usual reference point for "introitus" is the hymeneal ring, but any such description will suffice.

TABLE 48-5

Evaluation and Management of Genital Tract Prolapse

History
  Bulge, pressure or pain
  Bleeding or discharge
  Urinary frequency or incontinence
  Difficulty initiating or completing voiding
  Constipation
  Need to elevate or support for micturition or defecation

Physical examination
  Ulcerations or abrasions
  Above or below hymen/introitus with maximal Valsalva
  Anterior vaginal wall, posterior wall, apex
  Urethral support/mobility

Postvoid residual

Management
  Estrogen cream for ulcerations
  Barrier cream/ointment to protect mucosa
  Truss (strong elastic support)
  Pessary
  Surgery
    Major vaginal reconstruction
    Vaginal obliterative procedure (colpocleisis)

Any external prolapse should be inspected for epithelial abrasions. These are often painful, and may bleed if extensive or deep. Topical estrogen is used initially to promote healing. Barrier ointments can be helpful in treating local irritation and abrasions. Reduction of the prolapse is also important to help prevent and treat abrasions.

If there is uncertainty about the type of prolapse, anterior vaginal wall (typically a cystocele) can be differentiated from posterior vaginal wall (rectocele or enterocele) prolapse with a single-blade speculum. The speculum is inserted to first depress the posterior vaginal wall, then removed, then reinserted to elevate the anterior vaginal wall, and having the patient Valsalva or cough. Many older women cannot generate adequate pressure with Valsalva or even with cough, and the only way to determine the extent of prolapse is to examine them in the standing position.

A cystocele is a weakness of the anterior vaginal wall fascia such that the bladder descends toward or outside the vaginal opening. Cystoceles may or may not be associated with stress urinary incontinence. A large cystocele may be associated with a large postvoid residual (PVR), which implies a weak detrusor muscle. An elevated PVR does not imply potential renal damage in women as it may in men, because there is usually no significant outlet obstruction and urine storage and voiding occurs as a low-pressure system, even in the presence of a cystocele. However, a truly obstructed outlet may occur after incontinence surgery, and this history should be sought. Some women may need to manually reduce (elevate) the cystocele in order to initiate or complete micturition.

A rectocele is a protrusion of the rectum through the posterior vaginal wall caused by weakness of the perirectal fascia. Patients may experience difficulty with defecation including the need to strain and the need to "splint" (press on or support) the rectovaginal wall. An enterocele is a herniation of small bowel and peritoneum through the apical vagina or between the uterosacral ligaments and the rectovaginal space. It is the only true hernia among the various forms of prolapse. Enterocele is more common in women who have un-

dergone hysterectomy, but may be present in any posterior vaginal wall prolapse, and rarely in anterior vaginal wall prolapse.

Uterine prolapse may result from defects in support from the cardinal or uterosacral ligaments. The vagina may be entirely everted, which is typically called procidentia (*procidentia uteri*) if the uterus is present, and complete vaginal vault eversion if there is no uterus. An uncommon complication of this condition is hydroureter and hydronephrosis caused by ureteral kinking at insertion into the bladder. This is more likely if the uterus is present. If no therapy is planned, screening with serum creatinine or a renal ultrasound may be indicated to exclude obstructive uropathy.

Rectal prolapse may be associated with significant pain, bleeding, or problems with defecation. A history of both constipation and fecal incontinence is common. Examination reveals an extrusion of rectal tissue outside of the anus. Careful examination should be performed to determine if the prolapse can be reduced. Rectal prolapse that cannot be manually reduced has an increased risk of incarceration with subsequent tissue necrosis. Patients with rectal prolapse should be referred to a colorectal surgeon or gastroenterologist for additional evaluation and management.

Management of Genital Prolapse

Management of prolapse disorders may be surgical or nonsurgical. The main conditions necessitating definitive treatment or referral to a specialist are nonhealing ulcerations, bleeding, elevated PVRs causing recurrent urinary tract infections, and hydronephrosis. If the patient is not significantly bothered and there are none of the above complications, she can be reassured and managed conservatively. Application of estrogen cream once or twice weekly is advisable for preventive care. On nonestrogen days, application of a topical barrier cream such as solid vegetable oil may be helpful. Large ulcerations require more intensive therapy initially. Some patients find comfort using a supporting elastic panty.

Pessary insertion is straightforward, but good management requires a variety of sizes and types for fitting, appropriate follow-up, and good patient education. Most patients can learn to remove and reinsert their own pessaries. Many women benefit from surgical correction. Patients with burdensome problems who are frail or "afraid of surgery" should still be referred to a specialist (gynecologist, urogynecologist, female urologist) because some surgical options are far less extensive than others.

Procedures generally fall into "reconstructive" and "obliterative" categories. Colpocleisis, a procedure that essentially closes off the vagina, is simple and effective with a very low prolapse recurrence rate of but is only appropriate for women who do not and will not have vaginal intercourse. Rectal prolapse is usually treated surgically with either reduction and fixation of the rectum or excision of the prolapsed portion of the rectum. Treatments to prevent chronic constipation are indicated to help prevent recurrence.

Pessaries for Genital Prolapse

Pessaries are intravaginal devices that are designed to reduce pelvic organ prolapse. This concept has been used for thousands of years, and there are references to pessary-like devices in the Egyptian hieroglyphs. Pessaries are particularly useful in women who may not be candidates for surgical prolapse repair. They can also be used to determine the response to prolapse reduction, which can help identify patients who might benefit from surgical repair.

Pessaries come in a wide variety of shapes and sizes. Selection is based on patient anatomy and the experience and preference of the health care provider who is fitting the pessary. If a pessary is correctly fit, the patient generally will not feel the device when it is in place. A pessary that is too large may cause pain and may be difficult to insert or remove. A pessary that is too small may not stay in position and will have a tendency to fall out with ambulation or strenuous activity. Topical estrogen and antibiotic creams are often used with the pessary to help prevent infection and tissue erosion. The pessary should be removed periodically and physical examination performed to look for signs of tissue irritation or erosion. If the patient is unable to remove the pessary herself, she must be seen by a nurse or practitioner every 1 to 3 months, depending on the epithelial integrity and amount of vaginal discharge. Neglected pessaries may cause odor, discharge, vaginal wall erosion, and fistula formation. They may also be asymptomatic for many years, such that a cognitively impaired woman will have forgotten that she has a pessary. This is an additional reason that pelvic examination may benefit those with cognitive impairment.

Pessaries for Urinary Incontinence

Pessaries may also be used to treat stress urinary incontinence. There are pessaries designed specifically for this purpose. These typically have a small "button" or increased width under the urethra designed to provide additional support. This increases the urethral resistance to elevated abdominal pressure. Rarely women may need to remove the pessary in order to void, but usually voiding is not obstructed. Incontinence pessaries may inform those who wish to test whether surgical therapy to increase urethral outlet resistance might be successful. A variety of urethral plugs and caps have also been designed for this purpose. Although many of these other devices have shown good efficacy in clinical trials, patients often find them difficult to use, and compliance is generally low.

Pelvic Pain and Dyspareunia

While some practitioners consider "pelvic pain" to refer only to disorders associated with viscera, disorders associated with the lumbosacral back, buttocks, hip, perineum, or abdomen are commonly considered in the differential diagnosis and management of pelvic pain. Pain is considered chronic if symptoms have persisted for more than 3 months. History should include not only the usual location, quality, duration, etc., but also symptoms related to bladder and rectum. After the initial visit, it is useful to repeat a careful physical examination at subsequent appointments. It is typical for physical findings to change somewhat, and reexamination helps clarify the source(s) of pain.

Abdominal and Myofascial Pain

Evaluation of pelvic pain begins with abdominal and musculoskeletal examination, including the lower back, sacroiliac joints, hips, and abdominal wall musculature. A common but often-overlooked cause of pain is myofascial "trigger points." The history associated with myofascial pain may be vague and inconsistent. The pain may be sharp, burning or dull, exacerbated with exercise or not, and inconsistent in its diurnal pattern. Examination reveals point tenderness that persists or increases when the patient raises her shoulders off the examination table (Carnett's test). This tensing of abdominal muscles guards intra-abdominal structures, but not the abdominal wall itself.

Vulvar Pain, Vaginal Pain, and Dyspareunia

Vulvar pain may be secondary to a specific disorder (inflammation, infection, neoplasm, or neurological disease), or may be present in the absence of any clinically identifiable disorder, which is called vulvodynia. It may be unilateral or bilateral and constant or sporadic. The term "vestibulitis" is often inaccurate, and is not currently used by the International Society for the Study of Vulvovaginal Disease. Rather, pain with touch limited to the vulvar vestibule is termed vestibulodynia. Vulvodynia may be referred pain from pelvic myalgia or spine or hip abnormalities. Herpes zoster and postherpetic neuralgia should be considered in unilateral cases.

Careful single-digit or cotton swab palpation superficially and deeply on the labia, perineum, and around the vaginal vestibule will allow localization of the pain, and may distinguish allodynia (an exaggerated sensitivity to light touch) from hyperalgesia (increased response to a painful stimulus). Areas of erythema should be noted. If vulvodynia is present, referral to gynecological specialist may be useful. A bland barrier ointment such as petroleum jelly or solid vegetable oil applied daily or twice daily may improve symptoms. This works best as long-term preventive therapy. Topical estrogen cream may also be of long-term benefit.

Unlike the vulva, the vagina is rarely a source of pain unless the patient is sexually active. Vaginal pain may be associated with the epithelium, the muscles and supporting tissues, or intraperitoneal pathology. Examination should proceed slowly and sequentially, inspecting then palpating the side, anterior, and posterior vaginal walls before reaching the vaginal apex. For atrophic vaginitis, the best treatment is topical estrogen (see above). Small doses are given more frequently in the first 2 to 4 weeks, after which very low maintenance doses usually suffice. Symptoms improve within the first month, but mucosal remodeling continues for over a year. If, however, the patient is already taking standard estrogen placement, topical estrogen is of unlikely benefit and consultation may be needed. Sexual function and dysfunction are addressed in Chapter 42.

Pain Associated with Reproductive Organs

If abdominal tenderness is present, only the vaginal hand should initially examine the internal pelvic organs. The uterus and adnexa should be moved with only the vaginal hand before the abdomen is palpated. The uterus and adnexa uncommonly cause pain in older women. Tenderness in these structures should be further evaluated. Endometriosis, hemorrhagic ovarian cysts, and ovarian torsion are rarely issues in older women. Diverticulitis should always be considered.

Interstitial Cystitis

A history of pain associated with urgency, frequency, and/or nocturia should prompt further evaluation for painful bladder syndrome or interstitial cystitis (IC), especially in association with a tender anterior vaginal wall. The exact etiology of IC is unknown. Theoretical causes include an autoimmune response, direct chemical irritants or inflammatory mediators in the urine, and defects in the epithelial barrier layer of the bladder. IC is typically a diagnosis of exclusion.

Other conditions that should be considered include bladder cancer or carcinoma in situ, bladder stones, and urinary tract infection. The presence of significant symptoms of urinary urgency, frequency, and pain in the absence of these other conditions should prompt consideration of IC as a potential diagnosis.

Cystoscopy with hydrodistension of the bladder under anesthesia is usually used to confirm the diagnosis of IC. Patients typically have a reduced bladder capacity and mucosal lesions including petechial hemorrhages and ulcerations that are visible after hydrodistension. Patients may be treated for painful bladder syndrome without cystoscopic confirmation of IC, but in older persons, it is wise to rule out other pathology. Bladder wash cytology and biopsies are used to help exclude a malignancy as the cause of symptoms.

Treatment for IC includes dietary modification with avoidance of bladder irritants such as caffeine, carbonated beverages, spicy foods, and alcohol. Medical therapies include antihistamines, antispasmodics, and anticholinergic medications. Low-dose tricyclic antidepressant medications are often used for this purpose, although they must be used with caution in elderly patients because of the significant risk of side effects. Pentosan polysulfate is a low molecular weight heparin derivative that is administered orally. It is excreted in the urine and is thought to help rebuild the glycosaminoglycan layer of the bladder. Intravesical therapies may also be used with direct administration of medications into the bladder. Surgical therapy is generally avoided because symptoms may recur even after removal of the bladder.

Hormone Replacement Therapy

The use of HRT after menopause is controversial and fraught with a potential for more complications than benefits in geriatric-aged women. At this time, no useful and clear outcomes other than vasomotor symptoms, atrophic vaginitis, and osteoporosis prevention and treatment guide our administration. Nonetheless, estrogen has neurotrophic and neuroprotective effects, and HRT investigations in the elderly should continue. Any use of HRT in the elderly will probably evolve toward lower doses. Women require lower estrogen doses to achieve the same biological effects as they age.

In women aged 65 years or older, HRT should not be initiated, and the issue in this age group is often how to discontinue therapy without suffering menopausal symptoms. Many older women can simply discontinue long-term HRT abruptly with minimal symptomatology. If vasomotor symptoms, insomnia, irritability, short-term memory loss, or excess fatigue occur, estrogen can be tapered as slowly as necessary. Potential tapering schedules are innumerable, typically reducing the dose 25% to 50% every 3 to 12 months. If complete discontinuation is then a problem, omitting one dose per week (of oral medication) every 1 to 2 months may be more tolerable. Transdermal estradiol is available in extremely low doses, including 14 mcg patches, which can facilitate the final tapering. If a woman needs to suddenly discontinue estrogen but not progestin, such as with venous thrombosis, progestins effectively eliminate hot flashes. Medroxyprogesterone acetate 30 mg/day or megestrol acetate 20 to 40 mg/day may be required. After several months, this can be discontinued with fewer symptoms.

If an older patient has new vasomotor symptoms without recent estrogen discontinuation, the symptoms are not "menopausal" as the patient may believe. History should include onset, timing during the day, associated factors, all medications and supplements used, and her symptoms at the time of menopause. Estradiol levels can occasionally be beneficial in interpreting symptoms or enhancing patient comprehension.

SUMMARY

Numerous gynecological issues occur in older women. Because of a usual reluctance to discuss these matters, physicians should specifically ask about any problems (see Table 48-1). Pelvic examination may detect unanticipated problems in their early stages, or detect significant current problems in the cognitively impaired. Early diagnosis and treatment of gynecological disorders can improve quality of life and longevity for many older women.

FURTHER READING

American College of Obstetricians and Gynecologists. Cervical cytology screening. ACOG Practice Bulletin Number 45. Washington, DC: American College of Obstetricians and Gynecologists; 2003.

Carr PL, Rothberg MB, Friedman, RH, et al. "Shotgun" versus sequential testing. Cost-effectiveness of diagnostic strategies for vaginitis. *J Gen Intern Med.* 2005;20:793.

Coker AL, Du XL, Fang S, Eggleston KS. Socioeconomic status and cervical cancer survival among older women: findings from the SEER-Medicare linked data cohorts. *Gynecol Oncol.* 2006;102:278–284.

Cooper SM, Wojnarowska F. Influence of treatment of erosive lichen planus of the vulva on its prognosis. *Arch Dermatol.* 2006;142:289.

FIGO Annual Report. *J Epidemiol Biostat.* 2001;6:7–173.

Hatasaka H. The evaluation of abnormal uterine bleeding. *Clin Obstet Gynecol.* 2005;48:258–273.

Judson PL, Habermann EB, Baxter NN, Durham SB, Virnig BA. Trends in the incidence of invasive and in situ vulvar carcinoma. *Obstet Gynecol.* 2006;107:1018–1022.

Kendall A, Dowsett M, Folkerd E, Smith I. Caution: vaginal estrogen appears to be contraindicated in postmenopausal women on adjuvant aromatase inhibitors. *Ann Oncol.* 2006;17:584.

Lidor A, Ismajovish B, Confino R, David MP. Histopathological findings in 226 women with post-menopausal uterine bleeding. *Acta Obstet Gynecol Scand.* 1986;65:41–43.

Lynch PJ, Moyal-Barrocco M, Bogliatto F, Micheletti L, Scurry J. 2006 ISSVD classification of vulvar dermatoses. Pathologic subsets and their clinical correlates. *J Reprod Med.* 2007;52:3–9.

Moroney JW, Zahn CM. Common gynecologic problems in geriatric-aged women. *Clin Obstet Gynecol.* 2007;50:687–708.

Moyal-Barracco M, Lynch PJ. 2003 ISSVD terminology and classification of vulvodynia: a historical perspective. *J Reprod Med.* 2004;49:772.

Ozalp S, Tanir HM, Gurer H. Gynecologic problems among elderly women in comparison with women aged between 45–64 years. *Eur J Gynaecol Oncol.* 2006;27:179–181.

Sarnelli R, Squartini F. Fibrocystic condition and "at risk" lesions in asymptomatic breasts: a morphologic study of postmenopausal women. *Clin Exp Obstet Gynecol.* 1991;18:271–279.

Sawaya GF. Should routine screening Papanicolaou smears be done for women older than 65 years?. *Arch Intern Med.* 2004;164:243–245.

Sharp HT. Myofascial pain syndrome of the abdominal wall for the busy clinician. *Clin Obstet Gynecol.* 2003;46:783–788.

Summers PR, Hunn J. Unique dermatologic aspects of the postmenopausal vulva. *Clin Obstet Gynecol.* 2007;50:745–751.

Surveillance, Epidemiology, and End Results (SEER) Program (www.seer.cancer.gov) SEER*Stat Database: Incidence—SEER 13 Regs Limited-Use, Nov. 2006 Sub (1992–2004), National Cancer Institute, DCCPS, Surveillance Research Program, Cancer Statistics Branch, released April 2007, based on the November 2006 submission.

Swift S. Current opinion on the classification and definition of genital tract prolapse. *Curr Opin Obstet Gynecol.* 2002;14:503–507.

Tabor A, Watt HC, Wald NJ. Endometrial thickness as a test for endometrial cancer in women with postmenopausal bleeding. *Obstet Gynecol.* 2002;99:663–670.

Willhite LA, O'Connell MB. Urogenital atrophy: prevention and treatment. *Pharmacotherapy.* 2001;21:464.

Sexuality, Sexual Function, Androgen Therapy, and the Aging Male

J. Lisa Tenover

Sexuality is a basic human need that exists throughout life in one form or another and is a significant component to quality of life of many older individuals. Although 70% of adult patients in a large sample study considered sexual matters to be an appropriate topic for a general clinician or geriatrician to discuss, sexual problems are noted in less than 2% of primary care physicians' notes. It is not easy to find physicians and other health care providers who are knowledgeable about sexuality in general and sexuality among the aging population in particular. Sexuality and sexual function in the aging female is addressed in Chapter 47. Sexuality, sexual function, and dysfunction in the aging male will be addressed in the first part of this chapter, with the second part being devoted to androgen replacement therapy in the older man.

SEXUALITY AND SEXUAL FUNCTION IN OLDER MEN

Sexual Behaviors

Idealized societal concepts of older people do not include sex or the facility for sexual function. A poll conducted by the National Council on Aging, regarding attributes of people aged 65 years or older, reported that older persons were frequently thought of as being "warm and friendly" (74% of respondents) or "wise from experience" (70% of respondents), but being "sexually active" was only attributed to older persons by 5% of the survey respondents. Yet epidemiologic studies of sexuality and aging, such as the Duke Longitudinal Studies, the Massachusetts Male Aging Study, and, most recently, the University of Chicago study, report many older adults are sexually active. Sexual expression can encompass many forms, including sexual intercourse, oral sex, masturbation, intimacy, physical appearance, erotic stimuli (reading, movies) and fantasies (daydreams), but most study data involve the first three components.

Figure 49-1 depicts the prevalence of male sexual activity with a partner based on a probability sampling of 3000 U.S. adults aged 57 to 85 years. The likelihood of sexual activity with a partner declined with age, but nearly 39% of men aged 75 to 85 years reported sexual activity with a partner within the previous 12 months, with 54% of these sexually active 75- to 85-year-old men reporting sex at least two to three times a month.

In addition to partner availability, there are other factors that affect sexual activity in older adults. Health status has a strong influence. Diseases such as arthritis, especially when it involves the hips and pelvis, can affect sexual positions, endurance, and comfort. Urinary incontinence, with or without the need of urinary catheters, or the presence of ostomies can affect body image and may raise physical barriers to sexual activity. Chronic diseases, such as diabetes, stroke, or cardiovascular disease also will have significant impact, especially with regard to erectile function in the aging male, as will be discussed later. The effect of self-reported health status on the prevalence of sexual activity is shown in Figure 49-1. Older men across all age ranges who reported excellent or good health were more likely to be sexually active than men with fair or poor health. Medications also may have an impact on the level of sexual activity and function, particularly for men, as many medications can impact erectile function; this will be discussed in detail later in the chapter.

Changes in Male Sexual Physiology with Age

Overall there is a gradual slowing of sexual physical response time as men age. It takes more time to achieve sexual arousal, complete the sexual act, and become rearoused for further sexual activity. Table 49-1 lists the specific changes in the male sexual response cycle with age. Some of the changes have been shown to be impacted, at least in part, by low testosterone levels, while others are unaffected by hormone levels. The aging male may need reassurance that slowing of the sexual response is normal and predictable in order to avoid the fear and anxiety that may ensue without such information. Lengthening

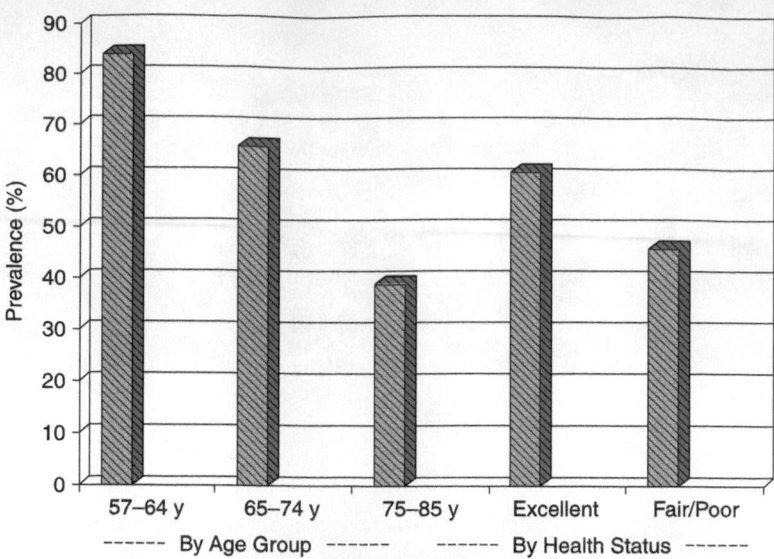

FIGURE 49-1. Prevalence of male sexual activity with a partner in previous 12 months as obtained from a survey of a probability sample of 3000 U.S. adults aged 57 to 85 yrs. Data are presented by age group and self reported health status. *Data from Lindau ST, Schumm LP, Laumann EO, et al. A study of sexuality and health among older adults in the United States. N Engl J Med 357:762, 2007.*

of the period of foreplay is one approach to adapting to these normal aging changes.

The Aging Male Homosexual

In the United States, there are about 3.5 million gay people aged 60 yrs and older. Older homosexual men have similar sexual problems as older heterosexual men, but may suffer additional problems of stress while trying to find a partner, especially if their living situation changes and they move into assisted living facilities or nursing homes. Specific organizations that address issues of aging gay and bisexual persons have formed across the country. Examples include Senior Action in the Gay Environment (SAGE) in the New York City area or Gay and Lesbians Older and Wiser (GLOW) in Ann Arbor, Michigan.

Unprotected sex occurs in approximately 10% of older homosexuals. Compared to younger homosexual men, older homosexual men get tested less often for sexually transmitted diseases, including testing for acquired immunodeficiency syndrome (AIDS). The incidence of AIDS is increasing in older men. Education about safe sex practices is important in the older population. Older males with a history of anal sex need to be regularly examined for anal cancer, as the prevalence increases in such persons.

TABLE 49-1

Changes in the Male Sexual Response Cycle with Age

Lengthening of the excitement phase (plateau)
Decreased penile rigidity*
Longer interval to ejaculation phase (plateau)
Fewer and less forceful contractions of the urethra
Lower ejaculatory volume
Less well defined sense of impending orgasm*
Shortening of the ejaculatory event and orgasmic phase*
Increased occurrence of resolution without ejaculation*
More rapid detumescence
Lengthening of the refractory period

---

*Aspects which may be affected by testosterone levels.

Older male homosexuals should be encouraged to get advanced directives for health and to specifically designate their Durable Power of Attorney for Healthcare. This should facilitate the ability of their partners to make their health decisions.

Sex in Long-Term Care

Persons who live in nursing homes frequently have no opportunity for a private, social, or sexual life. Federal regulations issued in 1978 provide some right to privacy, but it is limited to married couples and to nursing homes that participate in federal Medicare and Medicaid programs. Specifically, the regulations state that (1) the nursing home residents have the right to share a room with their spouse when married residents live in one facility and both spouses consent and (2) the residents have the right to privacy during a visit with their spouse. These regulations are not uniformly enforced, however, and the majority of long-term care staff possess minimal understanding about how to deal with the sexuality of their nursing home residents. Education programs for nursing staff are important.

Additional barriers to sexual expression in long-term care include lack of a partner and physical or mental illness. Issues surrounding romantic liaisons between two unmarried residents in a nursing home can be especially problematic. Deciding about the competency of a cognitively impaired individual to consent to sexual interactions and the objection of adult children to a parent's romantic liaison are just two examples of issues that can arise.

Sex and Dementia

Issues of sexuality are especially complex for those individuals who have cognitive impairment, as the diagnosis of dementia does not in itself determine in which domains a person is capable of making decisions. Some men with dementia become impotent, but others remain quite interested and capable, and a few older men with dementia become hypersexual. Physicians of demented male patients need to ask the spouse about sexual issues, as the wife may be embarrassed to reveal sexual difficulties. If the problems are placed in the context of dementia, it can assist with discussion of coping strategies.

TABLE 49-2

Major Categories of Sexual Dysfunction in Older Men

#1	Erectile dysfunction (ED)
#2	Low desire (libido)
#3	Performance anxiety and other psychological problems
#4	Inability to climax

Nonsexual ways of expressing intimacy, such as touching, holding hands, and massages, might be suggested.

SEXUAL DYSFUNCTION IN THE AGING MALE

Categories of Male Sexual Dysfunction

Table 49-2 lists the major categories of sexual dysfunction in older men. Erectile dysfunction (ED) is the most prevalent of these categories. Erectile dysfunction (also called impotence) is defined as the inability to obtain and sustain a penile erection adequate for intercourse. Erectile dysfunction is not a result of aging per se, in that healthy older men do not lose the capacity for erections and ejaculation. However, it is a common problem for the aging man. Severe erectile dysfunction is estimated to be present in 20 million men in the United States. In the Massachusetts Male Aging Study, a community-based study of middle aged and older men, the reported incidence of any erectile dysfunction was 55% for men at age 60 years, and 65% for men at 70 years; the prevalence of total erectile dysfunction at age 70 years was 15%. In the University of Chicago study, about 45% of men aged 65 to 74 years reported having some erectile dysfunction.

Libido, the enthusiasm for sex, or sexual desire, is dependent on learned responses, general health-related quality of life, and, to some extent, serum testosterone levels. As will be discussed later in this chapter, testosterone levels decline in men with normal aging and some men may reach levels that are low enough to affect libido. However, testosterone replacement studies in hypogonadal men suggest that the level of testosterone needed to maintain libido is likely below the serum "normal" range for most men.

Performance anxiety is common in older men and often a result of equating masculinity with speed and magnitude of sexual activity. A man may become so preoccupied by his performance that his confidence and sexual capacity lessen, leading to erectile dysfunction. Depression and psychosocial stresses also are prevalent in older men and contribute to sexual problems. "Widower's syndrome," a condition in which a man fails to achieve erection after the death of spouse, is a reported entity.

Inability to reach climax or to resolve without ejaculation can occur. In the University of Chicago study, this occurred in about 16% in the 57- to 64-year age range, but increased to 33% in men aged 75 years and older.

Erectile Dysfunction

Physiology

To better understand how diseases and medications impact erectile function, it is important to have at least a cursory understanding of the physiology of penile erection. An erection of the penis is obtained in three ways: through local sensory stimulation of the penile shaft and glans penis, through visual or auditory stimuli, and spontaneously during rapid eye movement (REM) sleep. As men age, erection becomes more dependent on physical stimulation of the penis and less responsive to visual and other nongenital stimulation.

When the penis is flaccid, there is alpha-adrenergic-mediated vasoconstriction of arterioles and sinusoidal spaces of the corpora cavernosa. During erection, parasympathetic input results in vasodilatation, which leads to an increase in arterial blood flow and pressure in the cavernosal sinusoids, resulting in occlusion of the venous outflow system and penile erection. A number of neurotransmitters play a role in this process. Nitric oxide is released by penile endothelial cells and cavernous sinus nerves during sexual stimulation. This release of nitric oxide, along with other agents such as prostaglandins E1 and E2 and vasoactive intestinal peptide (VIP), results in smooth muscle relaxation within the corpora, which leads to an erection.

Etiologies

Table 49-3 lists the major etiologies of erectile dysfunction. The prevalence of the specific etiology depends on the type of reporting center (primary care, urology, endocrinology). Vascular disease, which includes both atherosclerotic arterial occlusive disease and corpora cavernosa venous leak, is the most common cause of erectile dysfunction across referral centers. The likely mechanism is that penile hypoxia leads to replacement of corpora smooth muscle by connective tissue, which results in impaired cavernosal expandability and inability to compress subtunical venules. Risk factors for vascular erectile dysfunction include the presence of diseases and habits associated with atherosclerosis, such as diabetes mellitus, hypertension, hyperlipidemia, and smoking. Trauma and Peyronnie's disease can exacerbate the potential for corpora venous leakage. The penis is a high blood flow system during erectile function, so erectile

TABLE 49-3

Major Etiologies of Erectile Dysfunction

Vascular disease
    Atherosclerotic arterial occlusive disease, corpora venous leak
Neurologic disease
    Neuropathy, cord injury, stroke, multiple sclerosis, temporal lobe epilepsy, Parkinson's disease
Diabetes mellitus
    Both vascular and neurologic effects
Other systemic diseases
    Renal failure, COPD
Hormonal
    Hyper- and hypothyroidism, hypercortisolemia, severe hypogonadism
Urologic
    Lower urinary tract systems (LUTS) caused by BPH
Surgery/trauma
    Prostate cancer surgery, Peyronnie's disease
Lifestyle
    Obesity, smoking, heavy alcohol use
Medications
Psychogenic
    Depression, anxiety

dysfunction maybe an early sign of vascular inadequacy on the basis of atherosclerosis. Men who present with erectile dysfunction of vascular etiology are at very high risk of developing other vascular diseases, such as angina, myocardial infarction, or stroke, within 2 years of their diagnosis of erectile dysfunction. This risk remains even when controlled for current smoking or family history of myocardial infarction. Therefore, men with erectile dysfunction of suspected vascular etiology should be provided with appropriate screening and treatment for cardiovascular disease. Men with uncontrolled hypertension can develop erectile dysfunction as well, and erectile dysfunction can improve when the blood pressure normalizes. Men with mild to moderate hypertension need not restrict themselves sexually, but because systolic blood pressure can increase significantly with sexual activity, those with uncontrolled or severe hypertension should postpone sexual activity until blood pressure is controlled.

Neurological diseases, such as peripheral neuropathy, spinal cord injury, stroke, multiple sclerosis, temporal lobe epilepsy, and Parkinson's disease all can cause erectile dysfunction. In men who develop multiple sclerosis, about half of them present initially with erectile dysfunction. In these men, erectile dysfunction maybe present for some amount of time, then disappear, and reappear at the next exacerbation. Men with stroke-related erectile dysfunction also tend to have ejaculatory problems.

Diabetes mellitus is the most common single disease to cause erectile dysfunction. The pathophysiology involves neuropathic, angiopathic, and general vascular changes. Although the severity of hyperglycemia has been suggested as a predictor of erectile dysfunction, there is little relation to the likelihood of erectile dysfunction in older men treated with oral agents or those needing insulin. Age, duration of diabetes, and other diabetic complications appear to be better predictors of erectile dysfunction than degree of hyperglycemia. Sometimes erectile dysfunction is the first symptom of diabetes mellitus, so all men who present with newly diagnosed erectile dysfunction should be evaluated for undiagnosed diabetes.

Significant other systemic diseases that can cause erectile dysfunction are renal failure and chronic obstructive pulmonary disease (COPD). Chronic renal failure impacts erectile function through effects on the vascular system and via the development of autonomic neuropathy. In addition, many men with end-stage renal disease are severely hypogonadal. Neither hemodialysis nor testosterone replacement in men with renal failure have been shown to improve erectile dysfunction. Men with COPD and low PaO_2 have decreased cavernosal nitric oxide. Oxygen therapy may improve erectile function in some men with COPD.

Both hypercortisolemia and hyper- and hypothyroidism have been associated with hypoactive sexual desire and erectile dysfunction. Hypothyroidism also is associated with delayed ejaculation, with a prevalence of up to 64%; normalization of thyroid function frequently leads to improvement. Hyperthyroidism is associated with a 50% prevalence of premature ejaculation, which also improves with normalization of thyroid function.

Many studies have shown a clear association of erectile dysfunction with aging, but there have been no consistent correlations of erectile dysfunction in older men with low serum testosterone levels. In the Massachusetts Male Aging Study, where serum testosterone levels were measured throughout the study duration, of the men with no erectile dysfunction at baseline who were then followed up 8 years later, 16% developed erectile problems. Of the men who developed erectile dysfunction, 22% were in lowest tertile for serum testosterone levels, but 12% were in highest tertile. Other studies in healthy older men have shown that testosterone levels may correlate with sexual desire, but not with erectile function or coitus frequency.

Erectile dysfunction and lower urinary tract symptoms (LUTS), occurring as the result of benign prostatic hyperplasia (BPH), have significant effects on each other. Treatment of one can often improve the other. Both LUTS and erectile dysfunction are prevalent in the older male and frequently coassociate, contributing to diminished quality of life. Epidemiologic studies have shown strong associations between LUTS and erectile dysfunction, with a temporal relationship in onset and cessation and a dose response. A study in older men who had both erectile dysfunction and LUTS and were treated with the phosphodiesterase-5 (PDE-5) inhibitor, sildenafil, for 12 weeks, reported that both erectile function and LUTS symptoms improved with the sildenafil treatment.

While transurethral resection of the prostate (TURP) for BPH seldom results in erectile dysfunction, surgery for prostate cancer is more extensive and results in some degree of erectile dysfunction in about 60% of men. Nerve sparing surgery offers a greater chance of preserving sexual potency. In addition, penile rehabilitation with PDE-5 inhibitors immediately after surgery helps prevent complete erectile dysfunction. Peyronnie's disease, in which fibrosis of the corpora occurs, also can lead to erectile problems.

A number of lifestyle factors have been associated with the development of erectile dysfunction. Obesity alone is associated with a 20% increased risk of developing erectile problems. Although men with obesity often have low serum total testosterone levels, their free testosterone levels usually are normal, making hypogonadism an unlikely cause for obesity-associated erectile dysfunction. Often, however, obese men have elevated serum estrogen levels owing to the conversion of androgens to estrogens in adipose tissue. Improving obesity can improve erectile function. Smoking also can cause erectile dysfunction, both from direct effects of nicotine on penile smooth muscle and from longer term effects on accelerating atherosclerosis. High levels of alcohol consumption are associated with erectile dysfunction, but moderate to low alcohol use has been associated with a lowering of the risk of erectile dysfunction. Physical activity alone, regardless of weight, can improve or delay development of erectile dysfunction.

A large number of medications have produced adverse drug events reports involving male sexual dysfunction, usually erectile dysfunction. These medications are listed in Table 49-4. By and large, the effects on sexual function are medication class effects based on mechanisms of action. It is unlikely that medications would precipitate symptomatic erectile dysfunction in a man who had absolutely no erectile problems prior to initiating the medication, but for men with mild preexisting erectile dysfunction, these medications may precipitate clinically significant erectile problems. Sometimes, when relying on adverse drug event reports in the absence of large randomized trials, conclusions regarding the potential of a medication to impact sexual function maybe exaggerated or incorrect. For example, although the 5-alpha reductase inhibitor, finasteride, has been reported to cause erectile dysfunction, analysis of the prospective quality of life data from the large Prostate Cancer Prevention Trial showed finasteride had no significant effect on sexual function.

A few comments about some of the medications listed in Table 49-4 are warranted. Among the diuretic antihypertensives, hydrochlorothiazide has frequently been reported to be associated with

TABLE 49-4

Medications Associated with Male Sexual Dysfunction

Antihypertensives
  Central acting agents (reserpine, clonidine, alpha-methyldopa)
  Diuretics (thiazides; spironolactone)
  Beta-blockers (especially propranolol)
  Alpha adrenergic blockers
  Hydralazine
  Verapamil

Cardiac medications
  Nitrates
  Some antiarrhythmics

Psychotropic agents
  Antidepressants
  Antipsychotics
  Benozodiazepines
  Lithium

Addictive medications
  Opiates

Other agents
  Cimetidine
  Famotidine
  Digoxin
  Many cancer chemotherapeutics
  Phenytoin
  Ketoconazole
  Clofibrate
  Metoclopramide
  5-alpha reductase inhibitors
  St. John's Wort

erectile problems, yet analysis of the large NHANES database for evaluation of the effect of medication exposure on erectile dysfunction using multivariate analysis showed that the use of thiazides was not associated with erectile dysfunction. Among the beta-blockers, propronolol is the one most associated with erectile dysfunction, and erectile problems are more often seen with the higher beta-blocker dosages. Among the antidepressants, both tricylic antidepressants and serotonin reuptake inhibitors are associated with erectile dysfunction. Mirtazapine, bupropion, and citalopram have been reported to cause somewhat fewer negative sexual side effects. Many benzodiazepines, including those used to counteract insomnia, are associated with exacerbation of erectile dysfunction, but sleep deprivation alone can induce sexual dysfunction.

Evaluation of Sexual Dysfunction

The first step in evaluation of sexual dysfunction is often the most difficult: eliciting the information that the patient has sexual dysfunction. Screening for sexual dysfunction can be done by asking a brief question or two about sexual activity in all patients and can legitimize the topic for conversation. Examples of possible screening questions include: "Are you satisfied with your sexual activity?"; "How has your illness affected your sex life?", if the patient has a chronic illness; or "Many of my male patients your age have noticed some change in their sexual function; how about you?"

If sexual dysfunction is discovered during screening, then a more extensive sexual and health history and physical examination are warranted. A careful history from the man's sexual partner can be helpful as well. If psychological or couples' problems exist, or if the patient is depressed, these should be treated before pursuing the direct management of other problems, such as erectile dysfunction. As noted earlier, an evaluation for general vascular disease and for diabetes, as well as a medication evaluation, should be done.

Treatments for Erectile Dysfunction

The initial step in the treatment approach to erectile dysfunction is to identify reversible causes and then to change them if possible. This includes making alterations in a medication regimen, facilitating smoking cessation and weight loss, and encouraging physical exercise. If there is evidence for a significant psychological component to the erectile dysfunction, couples counseling or treatment for depression, if appropriate, are warranted.

Table 49-5 lists the current medical treatments for erectile dysfunction. Vacuum erection devices consist of a vacuum cylinder connected to a pump to create controlled negative pressure, and one or more constriction rings that go at the base of the penis after vacuum-induced engorgement has occurred. Intercourse occurs with rings in place, but the ring should not be left on for more than 30 minutes. Erection satisfactory for intercourse occurs in 75% to 90% of the users. Overall satisfaction rate is 65% to 70% if the method is chosen and used, but only about 12% of men select the vacuum device as an initial choice of therapy. Side effects or reasons for dissatisfaction include pain, inconvenience, and premature loss of rigidity. There are few contraindications to its use, but if on anticoagulants, these devices should be used with care.

Penile prosthetic implants are either semirigid/noninflatable or inflatable. Designs have improved over the last decade, and the 5-year failure rates for the inflatable prosthesis are now about 5%. Infection is the most significant complication and varies from <1% to 16%.

Erection predominantly requires arterial dilation and venous sinusoidal relaxation, facilitated by alpha adrenergic blockade and smooth muscle relaxation via mechanisms involving nitric oxide, prostaglandin E1 (PGE1), acetylcholine, or VIP. Nitric oxide activates guanylate cyclase in smooth muscle cells, leading to a rise in cGMP, which leads to muscle relaxation. cGMP is degraded in the

TABLE 49-5

Current Medical Treatment Options for Erectile Dysfunction

Vacuum erection devices
Penile prosthetic implants
Medications
  Intracavernous injections
    Papaverine (PDE inhibitor) + phentolamine (alpha adrenergic blocker)
    Alprostadil (PGE1)
  Transurethral
    Alprostadil (PGE1)
  Oral
    Alpha adrenergic blockers
      Yohimbine, phentolamine
    PDE-5 inhibitors
      Sildenafil, vardenafil, tadalafil
  Testosterone

penis predominantly by PDE-5. Major medications approved for use in the United States for treating erectile dysfunction are PGE1, PDE-5 inhibitors, or alpha adrenergic blockers. Delivery methods for these medications are by intracavernous injections, transurethral, or oral.

Intracavernous injections with PGE1 or a PDE inhibitor, with or without an alpha adrenergic blocker have efficacy of 65% to 90%. Side effects include mild local pain (10% to 15%), penile fibrosis, prolonged erections, and rhinitis. PGE1 can also be delivered via urethral insertion, followed by vigorous penile massage to assist with medication delivery. Reported efficacy is between 45% and 65% and side effects include mild pain, minor urethral bleeding, dizziness, and lowered blood pressure.

The main oral therapies for erectile dysfunction are the PDE-5 inhibitors, sildenafil, vardenafil, and tadalafil. Reported efficacy is variable, ranging from 45% to 90%. There are no good data to support one PDE-5 inhibitor as more efficacious than another. None of these medications are totally specific for the PDE-5 enzyme, but vardenafil is a little more specific than the other two, so there is a lower incidence of visual "blue haze" with this agent. Tadalafil has the longest half-life of the three medications. Side effects of these agents are primarily related to their effects on lowering blood pressure, which can lead to events such as myocardial infarction and stroke in susceptible patients. Oral alpha adrenergic blockers, such as yohimbine or phentolamine, have been used to treat erectile dysfunction, but with low efficacy (10% to 20%).

Testosterone and Male Sexual Dysfunction

The human male requires at least a minimal amount of testosterone for normal sexual behavior. Profoundly hypogonadal young and middle-aged adult men need testosterone to restore both libido and normal erectile function, but serum levels of testosterone that need to be achieved in order to restore full sexual function are low and often below the normal serum testosterone range. There are, however, men with very low serum testosterone levels and no overt sexual dysfunction and men with complete erectile dysfunction who have high serum testosterone. Decreased libido is considered the most prominent symptom of low testosterone and can impact erectile function. Using low libido as a screening for low testosterone, however, is not very sensitive. In the Massachusetts Male Aging Study, assessment of the association of low testosterone with low libido demonstrated that the two were significantly associated when evaluated on a population level, but decreased libido was not a strong predictor of testosterone level in an individual man. If a man had low libido, the positive predictive value that he also would have a low serum testosterone level (<300 ng/dL) was only about 23%.

Testosterone works in the brain to affect sexual interest, but it also has effects in the penis. Testosterone can increase the level of penile nitric oxide synthetase, leading to an increase in nitric oxide and the vasodilatory cascade. It also may have direct effects on other penile neurotransmitters. A meta-analysis of studies of erectile dysfunction and testosterone treatment in nonelderly adult men demonstrated that the prevalence of low testosterone as a reversible cause of erectile dysfunction was only 1% to 35%, and studies that showed an improvement in libido with testosterone treatment often did not show an improvement in erectile dysfunction. There have been several placebo-controlled studies in which men with erectile dysfunction and low testosterone levels, who initially did not respond therapeu-

tically to a PDE-5 inhibitor, when given testosterone in addition to the PDE-5 inhibitor then did show improved erectile function. This suggests that testosterone's direct effects in the penis may synergize with PDE-5 inhibitors to improve erectile function in some men.

There have been only a few trials of testosterone replacement in older men in whom sexual function was assessed, in most cases as secondary or tertiary study outcomes. In seven of the most recent studies of testosterone replacement in which aspects of sexual function were measured and at least some men were 65 years and older, three studies reported improvement in libido or morning erections with testosterone therapy, while four studies reported no changes in any aspects of sexual function with testosterone therapy.

In summary, testosterone replacement therapy is not the primary treatment for the majority of older men with erectile dysfunction, but maybe beneficial in some older men in whom decreased libido is a significant complaint or serum testosterone levels are very low. In addition, testosterone therapy can be used as adjunctive therapy for hypogonadal men who have failed PDE-5 inhibitor therapy alone.

ANDROGEN REPLACEMENT THERAPY IN OLDER MEN

When an older man presents with decreased libido and/or erectile dysfunction, androgen deficiency is considered a potential cause. However, androgens have effects on a broader range of organs and physiologic functions than those involved with sexual function. Testosterone levels decline with normal aging, a decline that may parallel changes in muscle, bone, and other androgen-responsive tissues. This has led to the concept that replacing androgens, mainly testosterone, in testosterone-deficient older men might prevent, stabilize, or even reverse some of the detrimental target-organ changes seen with aging.

Androgen Physiology and Changes with Aging

A further discussion of this topic appears in Chapter 107. Nearly all testosterone, which is the most plentiful androgen in the human male, circulates in blood bound to two proteins, albumin and sex hormone-binding globulin (SHBG); only about 1% to 2% of testosterone circulates totally free in plasma. Testosterone is tightly bound to SHBG, whereas its affinity for albumin is weak. Because of the strong affinity of testosterone for SHBG, the portion of plasma testosterone not bound to SHBG is often called *bioavailable* testosterone. Bioavailable testosterone best correlates with parameters such as bone mineral density and sexual function in older men, and is predictive for the development of frailty in inner-city African-American males. It is not known, however, if non-SHBG (*bioavailable*) testosterone is the component of testosterone that is truly bioavailable to every androgen target organ; for example, testosterone bound to SHBG maybe available to the prostate.

Not all target organ effects of testosterone are the result of the steroid directly, but maybe the result of one of its metabolites. Testosterone can be converted to 17 beta-estradiol through the action of an aromatase enzyme. In men, the majority of estrogen is felt to come from the action of an aromatase enzyme in adipose tissue rather than from direct production by the testis. Testosterone also can be converted, via a 5-alpha-reductase, to dihydrotestosterone (DHT), which is the predominant androgen in some organs, such as the prostate. Although some DHT is found in serum, most of the effects of DHT at the target-organ level are felt to be caused by its local formation from testosterone. Both testosterone and DHT affect target organs through their interaction with the same intracellular androgen receptor.

Figure 107-4 and Table 107-9 in Chapter 107 summarize age-related changes in the hypothalamic-pituitary-testicular axis. Serum levels of total testosterone, free testosterone, and bioavailable testosterone, but not DHT, decline with aging in many normal men. Both cross-sectional and longitudinal studies demonstrate these age-related changes. Most data on testosterone levels and age are from studies where the men were predominantly Caucasian of western European descent. Some smaller cross-sectional evaluations of men of African-American or Asian descent, however, suggest that these ethnic groups also may demonstrate age-related testosterone decline. Figure 49-2 demonstrates the longitudinal effects of aging on total testosterone and free testosterone index (total testosterone/SHBG) as determined from 890 men in the Baltimore Longitudinal Study of Aging (BLSA). There is an average testosterone decline of 1.24 nmol/L/decade of age beginning at about 30 years of age.

While age alone has a strong predictive value for lower plasma testosterone levels, concomitant disease such as diabetes mellitus, liver disease, or hemochromatosis can contribute. Certain medications also have been associated with lower testosterone levels, including ketoconazole, cimetidine, and glucocorticoids. Only some men

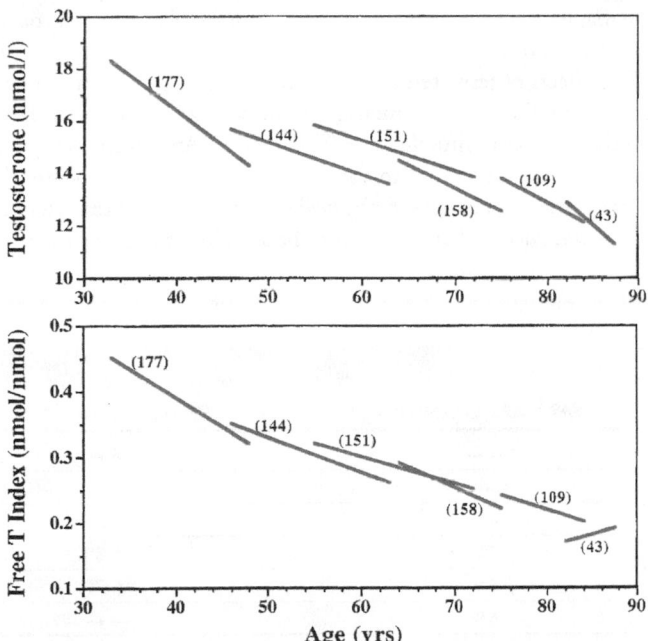

FIGURE 49-2. Longitudinal effects of age on plasma total testosterone levels and free testosterone index in men from the Baltimore Longitudinal Study of Aging. Each linear segment represents the data from a cohort, designated by age in decades, who were studied longitudinally (minimum of 4 yrs). For each cohort, the slope of the line equals the mean of the individual slopes, with the numbers in parentheses representing the number of men in that cohort. *Reprinted with permission from Harman SM, Metter EJ, Tobin JD, et al. Longitudinal effects of aging on serum total and free testosterone levels in healthy men. J Clin Endocrinol Metab. 86(2):724, 2001. Copyright © The Endocrine Society.*

will develop testosterone levels as they age that are low enough to cause obvious hypogonadism. The prevalence of "late onset" hypogonadism in the older male population is uncertain, largely because there is no agreement on how to define testosterone deficiency in this age group. There is no target-organ change, physiologic finding, or symptom that readily assists with this definition, and in general, serum LH levels are not helpful. Unlike the thyroid hormone axis, where an elevated serum thyroid-stimulating hormone level can establish the diagnosis of hypothyroidism, serum LH levels in most older men, even those men with quite low testosterone levels, are usually within the "normal" range for young adult men. It is possible that a single cutpoint for serum level of testosterone cannot define hypogonadism for all older men; the desired level of testosterone that maximizes target-organ effects may vary by the androgen target organ of interest, as well as being different among individuals.

Defining Hypogonadism in Older Men

In 2004, the Institute of Medicine (IOM) published a report on the current state of knowledge about the potential risks and benefits of testosterone therapy in older men and made recommendations about the need for additional clinical studies. This IOM report recognized that there were a limited number of studies, especially placebo-controlled randomized trials, of testosterone therapy in older men and that the assessments of risk and benefits have been limited, making for uncertainties as to the value of such therapy. The IOM concluded that clinical studies further evaluating the risks and benefits of testosterone replacement therapy in older men could ethically be conducted, and that studies targeting efficacy of such therapy for specific clinical endpoints were needed. The IOM targeted for this research those areas in which there are not currently safe and effective treatment options: weakness and frailty, sexual dysfunction, cognitive dysfunction, and well being and quality of life.

The American Academy of Clinical Endocrinology, the Endocrine Society, the American Society of Andrology, and the International Society of Andrology have all now published clinical guidelines for diagnosis and treatment of testosterone deficiency in adult men. Within these guidelines are included some recommendations related to late onset hypogonadism. All the societies have agreed that late onset hypogonadism should not be just a biochemical diagnosis, but must include age-related pathology or symptoms that would warrant treatment. All the societies, as well as the IOM, also have agreed that total testosterone levels are the appropriate initial test for hormonal evaluation. In these guidelines, cut-off values for serum total testosterone levels, above which older men are not likely to have testosterone deficiency, vary from 200 ng/dL (6.9 nmol/L) up to 346 ng/dL (12 nmol/L). A number of the clinical trials of testosterone therapy in older men have enrolled men with serum total testosterone levels higher than these current recommendations.

The signs and symptoms that might be related to low serum testosterone levels in older men are listed in Table 49-6. These are based on extrapolation from the clinical syndrome of androgen deficiency in young men. All the listed signs and symptoms are nonspecific and could be indicators of many other diseases that are common in an aging male, making the diagnosis of late onset hypogonadism less than straightforward.

TABLE 49-6

Signs and Symptoms Possibly Related to Testosterone Deficiency in Older Men

Reduced muscle mass
Increased visceral fat
Low bone mineral density
Loss of libido
Fatigue; diminished physical or work performance
Decreased energy, motivation, aggressiveness
Depression, dysphoria, or irritability
Vasomotor symptoms
Poor concentration and memory
Sleep disturbance

Testosterone Therapy Effects on Specific Target Organs

Bone

The IOM report did not recommend pursuing additional studies of testosterone therapy for treatment or prevention of male osteoporosis, largely because they felt that other efficacious therapies are available. Nonetheless, long standing testosterone deficiency is a known risk factor for male osteoporosis, and testosterone is known to be anabolic for bone. The studies of androgen replacement therapy in older men, which have evaluated an effect on bone have all utilized testosterone as the treatment androgen. This may be important, since testosterone is converted to estradiol in vivo, and older men receiving testosterone often show a substantial increase in plasma estradiol levels. Since bioavailable estradiol has been shown to be a better predictor of bone mineral density in older men than any component of testosterone, it is possible that the effects of testosterone replacement on bone in older men could be mediated through its conversion to estradiol.

The published studies of testosterone replacement in older men, which have evaluated bone related outcomes have lasted from 3 to 36 months, with the shorter studies measuring biochemical parameters of bone turnover and the longer studies evaluating bone mineral density. Some, but not all, of the studies enrolled older men who were osteoporotic at baseline. In general, the studies showed that the rate of bone degradation is slowed by testosterone replacement and bone mineral density increases. Whether positive effects on bone density can be maintained over longer periods of time than have been studied and what might be the optimal level of testosterone replacement to achieve the maximal benefit for bone are both currently unknown. There are as yet no data on the effect of testosterone replacement therapy on fracture rates in older men.

Body Composition and Strength

Sarcopenia, the loss of muscle mass with age, leads to decreased muscle strength and a decline in physical function. Testosterone is known to have anabolic effects on muscle, through alterations in intramuscular gene expression. Testosterone therapy can lead to an increase in muscle mass. Whether increases in muscle mass will then translate to improvement in muscle strength and improvement in physical function are key to its therapeutic potential in the older individual. There have been at least 15 clinical studies in older men in which fat mass and/or muscle mass have been evaluated in older men during androgen therapy. Table 49-7 summarizes the body composition changes that have been observed in these clinical trials. Changes in body composition with testosterone therapy have occurred consistently: a decline in body fat, an increase in lean body mass (predominantly muscle mass), or both. The magnitude of the changes in both muscle mass and fat mass in older men appear similar in magnitude to that seen with testosterone replacement in young hypogonadal men.

The effects of testosterone replacement therapy on strength and physical function in older men have not been as consistent as have been the changes in muscle mass (Table 49-8). Androgen therapy in older men appears to lead to variable increases in muscle strength. The magnitude of changes in physical performance with testosterone therapy was far less than that would be seen in response to physical

TABLE 49-7

Testosterone Effects on Body Composition in Older Men

LENGTH OF TREATMENT (mo)	TOTAL mg T GIVEN	FAT MASS CHANGE*	LEAN MASS CHANGE*
6	920	→←	→←
3	1200	—	→←
3	1300	→←	↑ 3%
6	1300	↓ 7%	↑ 3%
6	ND	↓ 4%	↑ 7%
9	ND	↓ 6%	→←
12	1800	↓ 7%	↑ 2%
12	ND	↓ 4%	↑ 2%
6	2400	↓ 4%	↑ 7%
5	2500	↓ 7%	↑ 7%
5	6000	↓ 8.5%	↑ 8%
36	6570	↓ 14%	↑ 4%
18	7800	↓ 14%	↑ 5%
5	12,000	↓ 13%	↑ 11%
36	12,480	↓ 17%	↑ 8%

*Trend and mean percentage change; ND, no data; →←, no change; ↓, decrease; ↑, increase.

TABLE 49-8

Testosterone Effects on Strength and Physical Function in Older Men

LENGTH OF TREATMENT (mo)	TOTAL mg T GIVEN	STRENGTH LE*	STRENGTH UE*	FUNCTION
1	400	↑	—	—
2	800	—	↑	↑
6	920	→ ←	—	→ ←
3	1150	→ ←	—	→ ←
3	1200	→ ←	→ ←	—
3	1300	—	→ ←	—
3	ND	↑	—	—
12	1825	→ ←	—	—
12	ND	→ ←	—	—
6	2400	↑	—	—
5	2500–12 000	↑	—	—
12	5200	—	↑	—
36	6570	→ ←	—	→ ←
36	12 480	→ ←	↑	↑

*UE, upper extremity; LE, lower extremity; ND, no data; → ←, no change; ↓, decrease; ↑, increase.

exercise. Studies are now underway to evaluate whether testosterone therapy and exercise training maybe synergistic in improving muscle strength and physical function in older men.

The clinical significance of the fat mass changes with testosterone therapy remains to be delineated. Fat mass loss with testosterone therapy is primarily subcutaneous fat, not visceral fat. Quantitative data on effects of testosterone therapy on insulin sensitivity are lacking, and fasting insulin, glucose, C peptide, or HBA1C are not changed with testosterone therapy in older men. Therefore, whether testosterone replacement therapy will have any impact on metabolic syndrome in older men remains uncertain.

Mood

Young men with profound testosterone deficiency have symptoms of dysphoria, fatigue, and irritability, all of which improve with normalization of testosterone levels. There is also some epidemiologic support for a relationship between low androgen serum levels and dysphoria or depression in older men. Studies of middle-aged men with depression and low serum testosterone levels have shown no improvement in depression scales with testosterone treatment alone, but for those men treated with an antidepressant and testosterone, depressive symptoms were better than with just antidepressant treatment alone.

There have been no studies of the efficacy of testosterone replacement therapy in depressed elderly men. In older men who were not depressed, there have been at least seven blinded controlled clinical trials, which have evaluated effect on mood; only one of these studies reported any change with testosterone replacement. Another five blinded controlled studies of testosterone therapy in older men evaluated aspects of quality of life by various scales, and none of these reported a change with testosterone therapy.

Cognition

Cross-sectional studies of older men have found an association of higher serum total testosterone levels with higher scores on some cognitive tests. In the BLSA, a higher baseline free testosterone index correlated with better scores on visual and verbal memory at baseline and a slower decline of visual memory after 10 years of follow-up. A higher baseline free testosterone index, after adjustment for a number of risk factors, also was correlated with 26% reduction in risk for development of Alzheimer's dementia at 10 years.

To date, there have been eight randomized controlled clinical trials evaluating cognitive function with testosterone replacement therapy in older men without significant cognitive deficits at baseline. Four of these studies involved men with low or low-normal baseline total testosterone and the other four enrolled men with normal baseline total testosterone levels. Half of the studies in each category showed some improvement on aspects of cognition such as visuospatial memory, total memory, or verbal memory, and half of the studies reported no detectable effect of testosterone on cognitive test scores. No consistent effect of testosterone replacement has been observed in older men with dementia, but only small numbers of patients have been studied thus far.

Cardiovascular System

Compared with premenopausal women, men have a higher incidence of cardiovascular disease and mortality. Whether this sexual dichotomy is because of a protective effect of estrogens in premenopausal women or whether androgens have a detrimental impact on the cardiovascular system in men is not yet known. Epidemiologic studies have demonstrated that low, rather than high, serum testosterone levels are associated with an increased risk of cardiovascular disease in older men. Therefore, testosterone replacement in older men could be beneficial, detrimental, or neutral with regard to the cardiovascular system. Factors associated with risk for cardiovascular disease that might be affected by sex steroids include serum lipoprotein levels, vascular tone, platelet and red-blood-cell clotting parameters, and direct atherogenesis. There are currently no data on the effects of testosterone therapy in older men on many of these parameters. Testosterone therapy may decrease platelet aggregation or positively affect vasomotor tone, but more data are needed.

TABLE 49-9

Potential or Reported Adverse Effects of Testosterone Replacement Therapy in Older Men

Liver toxicity (oral androgens only)
Fluid retention
   Peripheral edema
   Exacerbation of hypertension
   Worsening of congestive heart failure
Breast tenderness or gynecomastia
Exacerbation of sleep apnea
Development of polycythemia
Exacerbation of benign or malignant prostate disease
Increased risk of cardiovascular disease
   Effects on clotting
   Effects on vasomotor tone
   Effects on rate of atherogenesis

The effects of testosterone therapy on serum lipoprotein levels in older men have been more extensively investigated. In general, parenteral testosterone therapy has led to a decrease in total and low-density lipoprotein cholesterol levels, a decrease in lipoprotein(a) levels, and no change or a small decrease in high-density lipoprotein cholesterol levels. These changes in serum cholesterol levels with testosterone therapy were generally modest, and the ultimate impact on cardiovascular disease is unknown.

Adverse Effects of Testosterone

Table 49-9 lists potential or reported adverse effects of testosterone therapy in older men. Liver toxicity, although known to occur with oral methylated agents, has not been seen with parenteral forms of therapy. Fluid retention is possible, especially during the first few months of therapy, but is not as dramatic as in the case of oral anabolic steroids. Testosterone replacement therapy in older men does not appear to cause peripheral edema or exacerbation of hypertension, but there was one reported case of exacerbation of congestive heart failure in a study in which very high doses of testosterone were used. Nearly all the studies of testosterone replacement therapy in older men have enrolled relatively healthy men. In chronically ill, frail, elderly men, fluid retention might pose more of a concern. Tender breasts or gynecomastia occurs in a small number of older men receiving testosterone therapy, perhaps because of the relatively greater increase in serum estradiol levels (as compared with serum testosterone levels) that occurs with the therapy. Testosterone supplementation has been reported to exacerbate sleep apnea, but this adverse effect has not been found uniformly.

Testosterone replacement therapy in older men often increases red blood cell mass and hemoglobin levels. In a meta-analysis of testosterone replacement trials in older men, there was a nearly four-fold relative risk of developing a hematocrit level over 50%. The increases in hemoglobin and hematocrit seen in older men with testosterone therapy are much larger than those usually observed when young hypogonadal men are given testosterone replacement. In some cases in which polycythemia has developed in older men, it has been necessary to either terminate therapy or decrease the dose of testosterone used. While the coexistence of sleep apnea and ele-

vated body mass index seems to contribute to the development of polycythemia in certain older men, this has not been the case for many of the men studied. Methods of testosterone replacement that give a more uniform level of testosterone within the physiologic range throughout the dosing period appear to have less of an effect on red blood cell mass.

Androgens have a role in promoting both BPH and prostate cancer. Androgen deprivation therapy has been used in the treatment of both these disorders, but the exact mechanism by which testosterone supplementation may promote prostate disease in older men is not known. Both the Massachusetts Male Aging Study and the BLSA have reported no relationship between serum testosterone levels and subsequent development of symptomatic BPH. The BLSA did report that a higher free testosterone at baseline increased the risk of detectable prostate cancer during an average 18.5-year follow-up, with relative risk of 2.59 (CI 1.28–5.25).

A number of testosterone replacement studies in older men have evaluated serum levels of prostate-specific antigen (PSA), prostate size, or functional prostate parameters. The large majority of these studies have reported no significant change in PSA serum levels or other prostate parameters. A meta-analysis of adverse events from 19 double-blind, placebo-controlled testosterone replacement trials in middle-aged and older men has been published. These studies represented a total of 651 men who received testosterone, and at least seven of these studies had treatment duration of 1 year or more. Rates of prostate cancer, the number of prostate biopsies performed, and a rise in PSA to greater than 4 ng/mL or a PSA increase of more than 1.5 ng/mL over baseline were numerically higher in men on testosterone compared to placebo, but none of the individual prostate parameters were significantly different between the testosterone and placebo treatment groups. However, the rate of all prostate events combined was higher in the testosterone therapy groups compared to placebo, with those men receiving testosterone having a 1.8-fold higher likelihood of having some "prostate event."

Since both prostate cancer and BPH are diseases with long natural histories, and the observation time for testosterone therapy in older men is limited to less than 2200 man-years, the long-term effects of testosterone supplementation on the prostates of older men is still of concern. Screening for prostate cancer prior to initiation of testosterone therapy, especially in older men, is mandatory, and periodic monitoring of PSA levels and digital rectal examinations of the prostate should be done while men are on testosterone therapy.

Testosterone Preparations for Replacement Therapy

The testosterone delivery systems that are currently available in the United States for use in replacement therapy are: long-acting injectable testosterone esters, such as testosterone enanthate or cypionate; transdermal patches; transdermally applied gels; or buccal patch (Table 49-10). The 17-alkylated testosterone oral preparations, although available, are not recommended for male hormone replacement because of hepatoxicity and unfavorable alterations in serum lipoprotein profiles that occur with their use. All preparations of testosterone should be efficacious for replacement therapy if adequate serum testosterone levels are achieved, so selecting the specific preparation will depend on patient preference with regard to acceptability, dosing regimen, and cost, as well as possible adverse effects related to the specific preparation (Table 49-10).

TABLE 49-10

Testosterone Delivery Preparations Available in North America: Recommended Dosing in Older Men and Potential Specific Advantages and Disadvantages

PREPARATION	RECOMMENDED INITIAL REGIMEN	ADVANTAGES	DISADVANTAGES
Oral 17-alkylated testosterone	Not recommended*		
Injectable esters Testosterone enanthate or cypionate (100–200 mg/cc)	75 mg IM/wk or 150 mg IM/2 wks	Reliable delivery Good dosing flexibility Low cost	Widely variable serum T levels over dosing period Mood swings Significant increase in hemoglobin Increase in serum estradiol levels Pain at injection site
Implantable pellets	225 mg/4–6 mo	May last up to 6 months Steady serum T levels	Local site infection Extrusion of pellet Significant increase in hemoglobin Poor dosing flexibility
Transdermal patch (2.5 or 5 mg)	5 mg patch/d	Easy self application Steady serum T levels	Dermatitis at application site Limited dosing adjustment Poor absorption in some patients
Transdermal gel (2.5- or 5-g packets, or pump; 5-g gel delivers 5 mg/day)	5 mg/day	Good dosing flexibility Easy self application Steady serum T levels Invisible	Occasional skin irritation Poor absorption in some patients Mildly elevated serum DHT levels
Buccal (30 mg adherent tab)	30 mg q 12 h	Easy self application Not transdermal	Gingival irritation Poor adhesion No dosing flexibility

*Not recommended because of increased incidence of hepatoxicity and unfavorable alternation in lipoprotein profiles.

The injectable esters deliver reliable testosterone serum levels, offer a wide range of dosing, and are relatively low in cost, especially if the patient or a family member can give the intramuscular injections. The disadvantages of injectable esters include the necessity for intramuscular injection, with possible discomfort at the injection site, and the large variation in serum testosterone levels over a single dosing period. Especially with the 2- and 3-week dosing regimens, supraphysiologic testosterone levels occur within the first few days after injection, and levels then fall below the normal range just prior to the next dose. This may result in mood swings and significant increases in hemoglobin and estradiol levels, and this is the reason why an every 3-week dosing regimen is not recommended. Since testosterone metabolism slows with aging, the recommended initial dose of injectable testosterone for older men is lower than that used in younger adults.

The pellet formulation delivers relatively stable serum testosterone levels for periods up to 6 months. However, it requires a skin incision and trocar to implant, site infection or extrusion of the pellet are possible, and there is no significant dosing flexibility.

The transdermal patch is easy to apply and provides physiologic levels of serum testosterone throughout most of the 24-hour dosing period. The disadvantages of transdermal patch include possible local skin irritation and limited dosing adjustment (the patch comes in two sizes and can not be cut). The testosterone gels are also easy to apply, deliver physiologic serum testosterone levels, and offer more dosing flexibility than the patch, because less than a full packet (or pump dose) can be applied. Disadvantages of the gel include its cost, production of mildly elevated serum DHT levels, and some occasional skin irritation. It is important to note that a small percentage of men are unable to achieve normal serum testosterone levels with *any* transdermal preparation. In that case, the injectable esters, the pellet, or the buccal formulation must be used. The disadvantages of the buccal preparation include gingival irritation and loss of the patch as a result of poor adhesion.

FURTHER READING

Araujo AB, Mohr BA, McKinlay JB. Changes in sexual function in middle-aged and older men: longitudinal data from the Massachusetts Male Aging Study. *J Am Geriatr Soc.* 2004;52:1502.

Bacon CC, Mittleman MA, Kawachi I, et al. Sexual function in men older than 50 years of age: results from the Health Professional Follow-up Study. *Ann Intern Med.* 2003;139:161.

Calof OM, Singh AB, Lee ML, et al. Adverse events associated with testosterone replacement in middle-aged and older men: a meta-analysis of randomized, placebo-controlled trials. *J Gerontol Med Sci.* 2005;60A:1451.

Francis ME, Kusek JW, Nyberg LM, et al. The contribution of common medical conditions and drug exposures to erectile dysfunction in adult males. *J Urol.* 2007;178:591.

Hajjar RR, Kamel HK. Sex and the nursing home. *Clin Geriatr Med.* 2003;12:575.

Harman SM, Metter EJ, Tobin JD, et al. Longitudinal effects of aging on serum total and free testosterone levels in healthy men. *J Clin Endocrinol Metab.* 2001;86(2):724.

Jain P, Rademaker AW, McVary KT. Testosterone supplementation for erectile dysfunction: results of a meta-analysis. *J Urol.* 2000;164:371.

Lindau ST, Schumm LP, Laumann EO, et al. A study of sexuality and health among older adults in the United States. *N Engl J Med.* 2007;357:762.

Liverman CT, Blazer DG. *Testosterone and Aging, Clinical Research Directions.* Washington, DC: National Academies Press; 2004.

McVary K. Lower urinary tract symptoms and sexual dysfunction: epidemiology and pathophysiology. *BJU Int.* 2006;97(Suppl. 2):23.

Moffat SD, Sonderman AB, Metter EJ, et al. Free testosterone and risk for Alzheimer's disease in older men. *Neurology.* 2004;62:188.

Moinpour CM, Darke AK, Donaldson GW, et al. Longitudinal analysis of sexual function reported by men in the Prostate Cancer Prevention Trial. *J Natl Cancer Inst.* 2007;99:1025.

Ottenbacher KJ, Ottenbacher ME, Ottenbacher AJ, et al. Androgen treatment and muscle strength in elderly men: a meta-analysis. *J Am Geriatr Soc.* 2006;54:1666.

Shabsigh R, Kaufman JM, Steidle C, et al. Randomized study of testosterone gel as adjunctive therapy to sildenafil in hypogonadal men with erectile dysfunction who do not respond to sildenafil alone. *J Urol.* 2004;172:658.

Sadovsky R. The role of the primary care clinician in the management of erectile dysfunction. *Rev Urology.* 2002;4(Suppl 3):S54.

Seftel AD. Erectile dysfunction in the elderly: epidemiology, etiology and approaches to treatment. *J Urol.* 2003;169:1999.

Shores MM, Moceri VM, Sloan KL, et al. Low testosterone levels predict incident depressive illness in older men: effects of age and medical morbidity. *J Clin Psychiatry.* 2005;66:1.

Thomas DR. Medications and sexual function. *Clin Geriatr Med.* 2003;19:553.

Thompson IM, Tangen CM, Goodman PJ, et al. Erectile dysfunction and subsequent cardiovascular disease. *JAMA.* 2005;294:2996.

Benign Prostate Disorders

Catherine E. DuBeau

DEFINITIONS

Many terms are used to describe benign prostate disease, and often interchangeably. Precision is important, however, because the conditions overlap only partially (Figure 50-1). Benign prostatic hyperplasia (BPH) is a histological condition characterized by benign proliferation of stromal and/or epithelial prostate tissue. Benign prostate enlargement (BPE) occurs in about half of men with BPH, and is quantified by milliliters of prostate tissue. Bladder outlet obstruction (BOO) occurs in only a subset of men with BPE. Older men often have voiding symptoms (urgency, frequency, nocturia, slow stream, hesitancy, incomplete emptying, postvoiding dribbling, and incontinence), which maybe related to BPH, BPE, BOO, age-related physiologic changes in the lower urinary tract, or comorbid conditions and medications. Therefore, voiding symptoms are best described by the nonspecific term lower urinary tract symptoms (LUTS).

EPIDEMIOLOGY AND NATURAL HISTORY

Early autopsy and epidemiological studies demonstrated a marked rise in prevalence of BPH and BPE with age, especially during the sixth and seventh decades, and a similar relationship between age and "clinical BPH" (LUTS and BPE on examination) (Figure 50-2). Overall, 28% to 35% of older men without previous prostate surgery have moderate to severe LUTS. More recent data from longitudinal epidemiological studies and placebo arms of treatment trials confirm that the incidence of benign prostate disease gradually and variably increases with age until the ninth decade (Figure 50-3). Only weak correlations exist between BPE, BOO, and LUTS, suggesting that their relationships are nonlinear and complex.

Some data suggest that African-American men have a higher risk of benign prostate disease urinary retention, and BPE/BOO surgery, possibly because they have higher levels of 5α-reductase and larger prostate transitional zone volume (see section "Pathophysiology"). The very limited available data suggest that Hispanic men have similar risk of BPH and characteristics of BPE as non-Hispanic white men. Asian men generally have lower rates of benign and malignant prostate disease, although this may differ by country of origin.

Progression of benign prostate disease is defined as worsening LUTS, acute urinary retention (AUR), and/or the need for surgical treatment. LUTS can vary significantly over time, and abate as well as progress. In a prospective cohort of men with moderate LUTS, by 1-year symptoms had improved in 16% and worsened in only 24%, and at 4 years, symptoms were only mild in 13%, unchanged in 46%, and worse in 41% (Figure 50-4). The incidence of AUR in men with LUTS and benign prostate disease is low: in a meta-analysis including 6100 moderately symptomatic men, the incidence of AUR was 13.7 per 1000 patient-years in all men and considerably higher in men aged ≥70 years or taking anticholinergic agents (34.7 per 1000 patient-years). Higher baseline prostate-specific antigen (PSA) levels are associated with greater risk of AUR and surgery; 7.8% of men with PSA levels up to 1.3 ng/mL develop AUR and/or require surgery by 4 years, compared with 12.6% of men with PSA levels 1.4 to 3.2 ng/mL, and 19.9% with PSA levels 3.3 to 12 ng/mL. Change in PSA over time (PSA velocity), however, is not associated with AUR or surgery. As PSA is strongly correlated with prostate volume, it is not surprising that higher volumes (>30 to 40 mL by ultrasound) are associated with worsening LUTS and AUR. Other factors that increase AUR risk include previous episode(s) of retention, baseline postvoiding residual volume (PVR) greater than 100 mL, worsening LUTS, and failure to respond to alpha-blocker treatment.

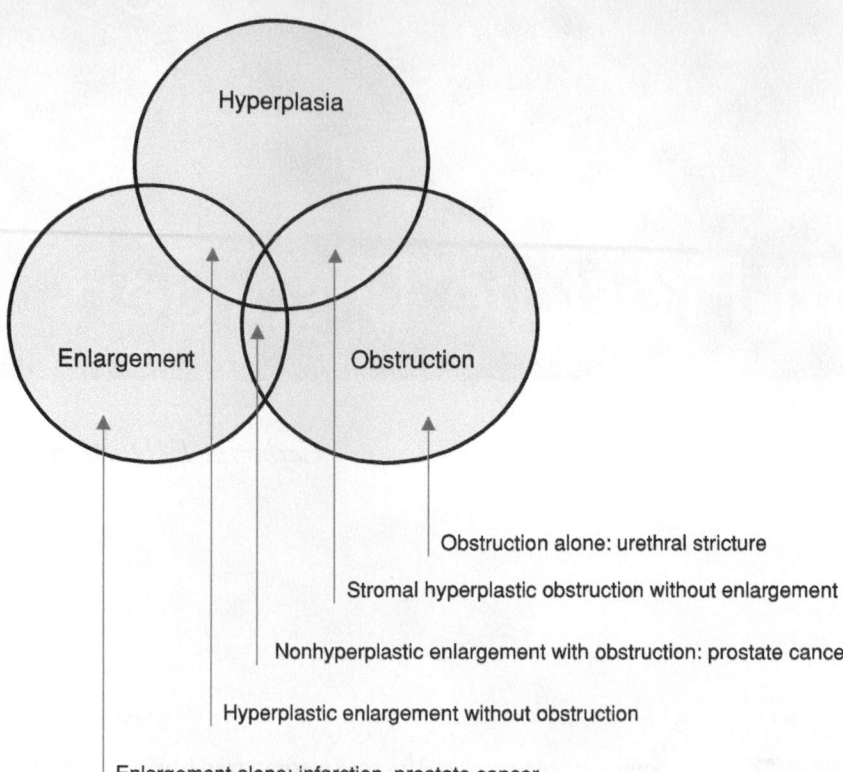

Obstruction alone: urethral stricture

Stromal hyperplastic obstruction without enlargement

Nonhyperplastic enlargement with obstruction: prostate cancer

Hyperplastic enlargement without obstruction

Enlargement alone: infarction, prostate cancer

FIGURE 50-1. Examples of incomplete concordance between benign prostatic hyperplasia, benign prostatic enlargement, and bladder outlet obstruction.

PATHOPHYSIOLOGY

Hyperplasia

Prostate hyperplasia occurs when prostate cell proliferation exceeds programmed cell death (apoptosis) as a result of stimulated cell

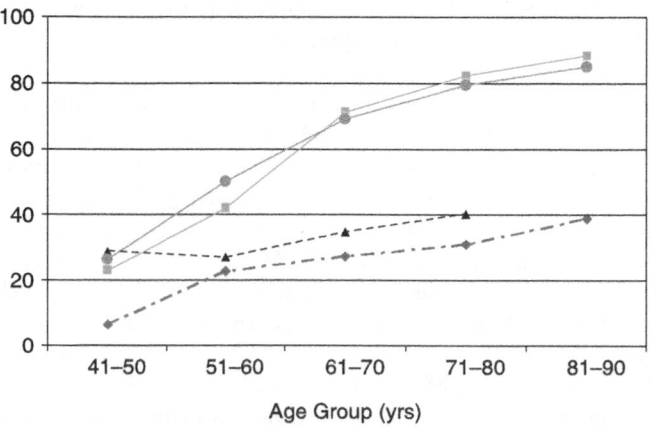

FIGURE 50-2. Autopsy evidence of prostate hyperplasia (percent of prostates, solid line with ■), mean weight (mL) of all prostates (dashed line with ◆), mean weight of prostates with hyperplasia (dashed line with ▲), and percent of men with lower urinary tract symptoms (solid line with o). Data from Berry SJ, Coffey DS, Walsh PC, Ewing LL. The development of human benign prostatic hyperplasia with age. J Urol. 132:474–479, 1984; Guess HA, Arrighi HM, Metter EJ, Fozard JK. Cumulative prevalence of prostatism matches the autopsy prevalence of benign prostatic hyperplasia. Prostate. 17:214–216, 1990.

growth, inhibition of apoptosis, or both. BPH occurs predominantly in the prostatic periurethral transitional zone, unlike prostate cancer, which tends to occur in more peripheral areas. BPH and prostate cancer are genetically distinct, and one is not a risk factor for the other.

The development of stromal and epithelial hyperplasia in BPH is androgen- and aging-dependent, and involves numerous paracrine and autocrine factors. The trophic androgen for prostate growth is dihydrotestosterone, produced from testosterone within the prostate by the enzyme 5α-reductase (thus the utility of 5α-reductase inhibitors for treatment). In the absence of 5α-reductase, even high serum levels of testosterone will not cause BPH. Additional factors supporting prostate cell growth include inflammatory cytokines (e.g., interleukin-8), autocrine cytokine growth factors, and neuroendocrine cell products. Stromal–epithelial interactions regulating proliferation also involve interactions between androgens, estrogens, and stimulatory and inhibitory peptide growth factors (e.g., fibroblast growth factor-2, transforming growth factor-β). Other regulatory factors include nitric oxide (nitric oxide synthetase levels are low in BPH), vitamin D, and local autonomic innervation and activity. Thus the development of BPH is the end result of numerous pathways involved in regulating sympathetic activity, androgen–estrogen balance, and smooth-muscle proliferation.

The divergence in prevalence between BPH, BPE, BOO, and LUTS results from many lower urinary tract factors (Table 50-1). In addition, numerous medical conditions, medications, and functional impairment may cause or worsen LUTS independent of prostate disease (see Chapter 59).

Risk Factors

Factors associated with the development of benign prostate disease include age, physical inactivity, high meat and fat intake (especially

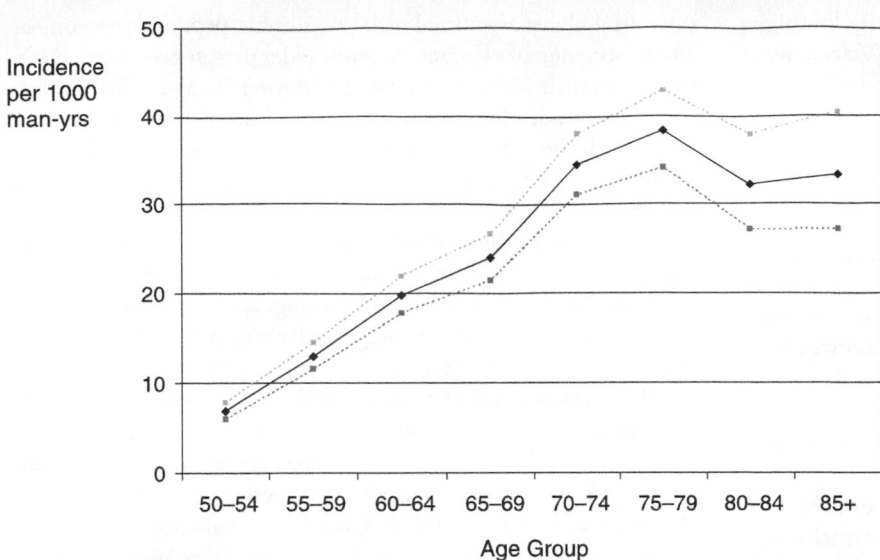

FIGURE 50-3. Incidence per 1000 man-years of BPH, as defined by LUTS plus a clinical diagnosis of BPH, medical therapy for BPH, or surgical treatment for BPH during follow-up. *Data from: Verhamme KMC, Dieleman JP, Bleumink GS, et al. Triumph Pan European Expert Panel. Incidence and prevalence of lower urinary tract symptoms suggestive of benign prostatic hyperplasia in primary care—the Triumph project. Eur Urol. 42:323–328, 2002.*

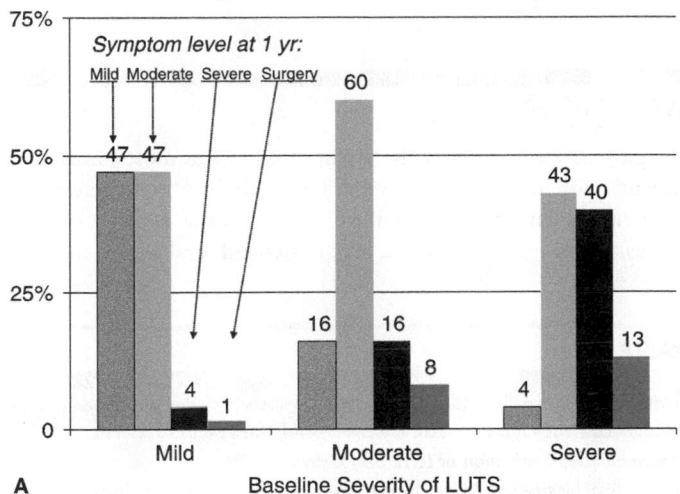

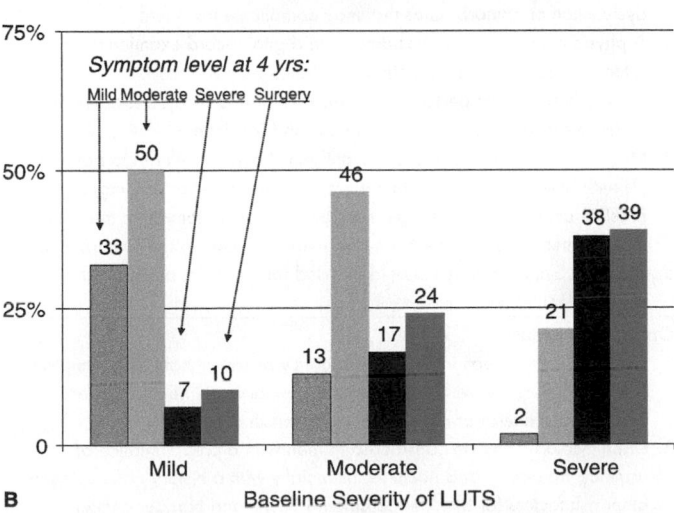

FIGURE 50-4. Natural history of LUTS. From a prospective study of 500 men, data available on 371 at 4 yrs. Baseline distribution of LUTS severity was mild 12%, moderate 49%, and severe 13%. (Symptom levels at (A) 1 yr and (B) 4 yrs. Bars indicate percent of men at follow-up with mild (white), moderate (gray), or severe (dark gray) LUTS or needing surgery (black). *Data from Barry MJ, Fowler FJ Jr, Bin L, Pitts JC 3rd, Harris CJ, Mulley AG Jr. The natural history of patients with benign prostatic hyperplasia as diagnosed by North American urologists. J Urol 157:10–14, 1997.*

TABLE 50-1

Lower Urinary Tract Factors Underlying the Divergence in Prevalence Between BPH, BPE, BOO, and LUTS

FACTOR	IMPACT
Ratio of stromal to epithelial hyperplasia (stromal proliferation predominates in 50%, glandular in 25%, and mixed in 25%)	Stromal glands tend to be smaller, more symptomatic, and have worse symptomatic outcomes to prostatectomy
Location of BPH nodules	Adenomas which occuring predominantly in central transitional and periurethral zones of the prostate, predispose to prostatic urethra compression. Adenomas in the median lobes may compress the bladder base without causing BOO.
Fibroelastic properties of prostate capsule	Altered compliance may increase urethral compression in the absence of mechanical BOO.
α-Adrenergic innervation of prostate	Increased number of α-adrenergic receptors promotes smooth-muscle contraction.
Variability in detrusor muscle structure and function	Detrusor contractility can be affected by BPE/BOO-associated increased connective tissue infiltration; smooth-muscle hypertrophy and disintegration; decreased autonomic neuronal number; and conversion from predominantly β-adrenergic (inhibitory) to α-adrenergic (stimulatory) responsiveness.
Detrusor overactivity	Detrusor overactivity (DO) is found in about two-thirds of men with BOO. Causality unclear as DO occurs in normal asymptomatic older men and women. DO resolves in up to two-thirds of men after TURP, yet tends to persist in the very elderly.
Atherosclerotic disease	May cause detrusor ischemia leading to impaired contractility, and acute BOO from prostate infarction.

BPH, benign prostatic hyperplasia; BPE, benign prostatic enlargement; BOO, bladder outlet obstruction; LUTS, lower urinary tract symptoms; TURP, transurethral resection of the prostate.

polyunsaturated fats), diabetes, high insulin levels, obesity, low high-density lipoprotein levels, and arteriovascular disease. Vasectomy is not a risk factor and the data on smoking are inconclusive.

NOCTURIA

Nocturia is defined as voiding at least once during the normal hours of sleep. As many as 80% of older men have nocturia, which is the most bothersome of all of the LUTS associated with benign prostate disease. The three main causes of nocturia are LUT pathophysiology, nocturnal polyuria, and sleep disturbance (Table 50-2). The latter two causes are especially important in older men because of the many age-related changes, comorbid conditions, and medications that can cause them.

Nocturnal polyuria is defined as the excretion of one-third or greater of the daily (24-hour) urine output during normal sleeping hours. Older persons are prone to nocturnal polyuria, possibly caused by higher nocturnal atrial natriuretic peptide levels and/or altered secretion of vasopressin. Some older person may excrete 50% or more of their 24-hour urine output during the night. For this reason, one episode of nocturia is considered normal in older persons and even the best treatment may not be able to completely eliminate nocturia. Another cause of nocturnal polyuria is peripheral edema (Table 50-2); edema fluid mobilizes when the patient reclines, leading to increased urine output. Sleep apnea is an underappreciated cause of nocturnal polyuria; apnea should be suspected when the patient or his partner report loud snoring, apneic periods, excessive daytime sleepiness, and morning headaches, and in men who are obese and/or have hypertension.

When aroused owing to primary sleep disorders, patients may sense their bladder volume (which tends to be higher at night) and get up and void, and report these episodes as "nocturia." Common causes of sleep disturbance in older persons include age-related changes in sleep architecture (see Chapter 55); pain (e.g., from arthritis), depression, restless leg syndrome, gastric reflux, pulmonary and cardiac diseases, dementia, and the effects of many medications.

EVALUATION

Benign prostate disease maybe asymptomatic, but most commonly presents with LUTS; other symptoms include urinary retention, recurrent urinary tract infections, or hematuria (from prostatic varices). Table 50-3 lists the recommended evaluation in men

---

TABLE 50-2

Causes of Nocturia

1. Nocturnal polyuria
   a. Age-related delay in urine excretion
   b. Fluid intake
      i. Late afternoon and evening intake
      ii. Caffeine
      iii. Alcohol
   c. Peripheral edema
      i. Venous insufficiency
      ii. Congestive heart failure
      iii. Medications
         1. Gabapentin
         2. Pregabalin
         3. Thiazolidinediones
         4. Nonsteroidal anti-inflammatory agents
         5. Pyridine calcium blockers (e.g., nifedipine)
   d. Medical conditions
      i. Obstructive sleep apnea
      ii. Uncontrolled diabetes mellitus
2. Sleep disturbance
   a. Insomnia
   b. Depression
   c. Congestive heart failure
   d. Obstructive sleep apnea
   e. Pain (e.g., arthritis)
   f. Restless leg syndrome
   g. Medications
      i. Stimulants
      ii. Beta-blockers
      iii. Steroids
      iv. Thyroxine
      v. Selective serotonin reuptake inhibitors antidepressants
      vi. Withdrawal from alcohol, narcotics, benzodiazepines
3. Lower urinary tract dysfunction
   a. Decreased functional bladder capacity
      i. Detrusor overactivity
      ii. Increased postvoiding residual volume
         1. Impaired contractility
         2. Outlet obstruction

TABLE 50-3

2006 American Urological Association Guideline on the Management of Benign Prostatic Hyperplasia

Recommended Evaluation of LUTS Suggestive of BPH

1. Medical history should be done to identify other causes of voiding dysfunction or comorbidities that may complicate treatment.
2. A physical examination, including both digital record examination and a focused neurological examination, should be performed.
3. Urinalysis should be performed by dipstick or microscopic examination of the sediment to screen for hematuria and infection.
4. Measurement of prostatic specific antigen should be offered to patients (1) with at least a 10-year life expectancy and for whom a diagnosis of prostate cancer would change management, or (2) for whom the PSA measurement may change the management of their voiding symptoms.
5. The AUA Symptom Index should be used for the initial assessment of each patient.

Optional Components

1. Other validated measures of the frequency or severity of LUTS, symptom bother, interference with daily activities, urinary continence, sexual function, or general or disease-specific measures of quality of life.
2. Urine cytology may be considered in men with a predominance of urgency, frequency and nocturia, especially with a history of smoking or other risk factors for bladder carcinoma in situ and bladder cancer.
3. Following the initial evaluation, measurement of postvoiding residual (PVR) and urine flow rate maybe appropriate. They are usually not necessary in men managed with watchful waiting or medical therapy. However, they may be helpful in patient with a complex medical history or prior failure of BPH therapy, and in those desiring invasive therapy.

Adapted from AUA Guideline on the Management of Benign Prostatic Hyperplasia, 2006 Update. Chapter 1: diagnosis and treatment recommendations. Available at: http://www.auanet.org/guidelines/bph.cfm Accessed June 27, 2007.

TABLE 50-4

American Urological Association Symptom Index

1. Incomplete emptying: Over the past month, how often have you had the sensation of not emptying your bladder completely after you finished urination?

Not at all	Less than 1 time in 5	Less than half of the time	About half of the time	More than half of the time	Almost always	Your score
0	1	2	3	4	5	

2. Frequency: Over the past month, how often have you had to urinate again less than 2 hours after you finished urinating?

Not at all	Less than 1 time in 5	Less than half of the time	About half of the time	More than half of the time	Almost always	Your score
0	1	2	3	4	5	

3. Intermittency: Over the past month, how often have you found that you stopped and started again several times when you urinated?

Not at all	Less than 1 time in 5	Less than half of the time	About half of the time	More than half of the time	Almost always	Your score
0	1	2	3	4	5	

4. Urgency: Over the past month, how often have you found it difficult to postpone urination?

Not at all	Less than 1 time in 5	Less than half of the time	About half of the time	More than half of the time	Almost always	Your score
0	1	2	3	4	5	

5. Weak stream: Over the past month, how often have you had a weak stream?

Not at all	Less than 1 time in 5	Less than half of the time	About half of the time	More than half of the time	Almost always	Your score
0	1	2	3	4	5	

6. Straining: Over the past month, how often have you had to push or strain to begin urination?

Not at all	Less than 1 time in 5	Less than half of the time	About half of the time	More than half of the time	Almost always	Your score
0	1	2	3	4	5	

7. Nocturia: Over the past month or so how many times did you get up to urinate from the time you went to bed until the time you got up in the morning?

None	1 time	2 times	3 times	4 times	5 times	Your score
0	1	2	3	4	5	

ADD UP THE SCORES FOR THE TOTAL AUA SCORE =

Quality of Life Due to Urinary Symptoms: If you were to spend the rest of your life with your urinary condition just the way it is now, how would you feel about that? (circle)

Delighted	Pleased	Mostly Satisfied	Mixed	Mostly Dissatisfied	Unhappy	Terrible

Adapted from Barry MJ, et al. The American Urological Association symptom index for benign prostatic hyperplasia. J Urol. 148:1549–1557, 1992.

presenting with LUTS suggestive of benign prostate disease from the American Urological Association (AUA) 2006 Guideline on the Management of Benign Prostatic Hyperplasia. The sections below highlight aspects of the evaluation especially relevant to older men.

History

The evaluation of older men with LUTS closely parallels that of older persons with urinary incontinence (UI; see Chapter 59). The history should include the onset, progression, and associated factors for the common LUTS (slow stream, urgency, nocturia, etc.), and quantification of LUTS using the AUA Symptom Index (see below). Distinguishing between "irritative" and "obstructive" LUTS is not useful, because the terms are poorly specific and does not correlate with symptom bother, severity, or physiologic measures. Older men always should be evaluated for causes of LUTS other than prostate disease. The history and review of systems should question patients about hematuria, dysuria, and pelvic pain (rare in benign prostate disease, more suggestive of infection, bladder stone, prostate or bladder cancers); episodes of urinary retention; cardiac symptoms (regarding possible congestive heart failure in patients with nocturia); bowel and sexual function; type and amount of fluid intake (in relationship to frequency and nocturia symptoms); and sleep disturbance. All medications (including nonprescription drugs) must be reviewed, with a focus on drugs that can decrease detrusor contractility (anticholinergics, calcium channel-blockers), diuretics, drugs that can cause pedal edema (see Table 50-2), and α-adrenergic agents.

American Urological Association Symptom Index

The American Urological Association Symptom Index (AUASI) quantifies the severity of BPH-associated LUTS on a scale 0 to 35; scores of 0 to 7 indicate mild symptoms, 8 to 19 moderate, and 20 to 35 severe (Table 50-4). An additional question, not tallied in the total score, assesses disease-specific quality of life impact. The similar International Prostate Symptom Score (IPSS) is widely translated and identically scored. A change in AUASI of ± 5 points has an 80% probability of indicating a true clinical change. The threshold for clinical change varies with symptoms severity (minimum perceptible difference is 2 points for AUASI <20 and 6 points for AUASI ≥20). Any magnitude of change, however, may be caused by interval changes in comorbidity and medications and not prostate disease.

Other Measures of LUTS and Quality of Life

There are a variety of other measures of LUTS and their impact. Some of the more widely used are the International Consultation on Incontinence Questionnaire (ICIQ) male module (ICIQ-MLUTS) and the BPH Impact Index. To assess sexual function, the Derogatis Interview for Sexual Functioning-Self Report and the International Index of Erectile Function can be used. Depending on the patient's symptoms, other potentially useful scales are the Incontinence

Impact Questionnaire and ICIQ Urinary Incontinence Short Form; and UI-specific and general quality of life measures e.g., ICIQ-LUTSqol, Urogenital Distress Inventory, Urge Impact Scale, SF-12.

The impact of LUTS on quality of life is critical to evaluate because it is the primary determinant of treatment. Quality-of-life impact may include interference with daily activities, work, sleep, and sexual function; worry, embarrassment, and impaired self-esteem; and physical discomfort. Patients' perception of bother may be independent of LUTS severity, and bother from an individual symptom may be more important than from all symptoms. Determining a patient's most bothersome symptom can help target evaluation and treatment; for example, nocturia is often extremely bothersome, yet many prostate-specific treatments are not very effective for it.

Physical Examination

Given the many medical causes of LUTS in older men a complete physical examination is required and should include evaluation of cognition, function, and mobility. The neurological examination should include the bulbocavernosus reflex, anal wink, and perineal sensation to assess sacral nerve integrity. Digital rectal examination (DRE) should be done to assess prostate nodularity, rectal tone, masses, and stool impaction. DRE is not accurate for assessing prostate volume, even when performed by specialists, because BPH adenomas can occur in the anterior and median lobes that are inaccessible to rectal palpation. Prostate volume is not associated with BOO, and is important only for decisions regarding surgical approach for prostatectomy. Although higher volume is associated with disease progression, it should not be routinely assessed for this purpose because accurate measurement requires ultrasound.

Laboratory Tests

Only urinalysis is needed in routine assessment. As noted in the AUA guideline, PSA should be offered *only* to men with at least a 10-year life expectancy, or for whom PSA measurement and/or a diagnosis of prostate cancer would change management (see Chapter 96). Serum creatinine is not required because of the extremely low prevalence of renal insufficiency in men with LUTS. Vitamin B-12 level may be considered in men with a high PVR because of the association of vitamin B-12 deficiency with peripheral neuropathy and detrusor underactivity.

Postvoiding Residual and Urine Flow Rate

PVR is not needed in the initial evaluation, especially in men with mild-moderate LUTS who can be managed with watchful waiting or medical therapy. PVR is small in randomly selected community men (75th percentile, 35 mL). In a large trial of men with moderate LUTS, the baseline mean PVR was 110 ± 74 mL. PVR correlates modestly with prostate volume, but is not significantly associated with age, AUASI, quality-of-life indices, BOO, or the need for invasive therapy.

PVR should be considered in men with coexistent neurological disease, impaired renal function, bladder-suppressant medications (anticholinergics, opiates, calcium channel-blockers), or who have failed empiric therapy. Inability to pass a urethral catheter for PVR measurement is more likely a result of sphincter spasm than BOO;

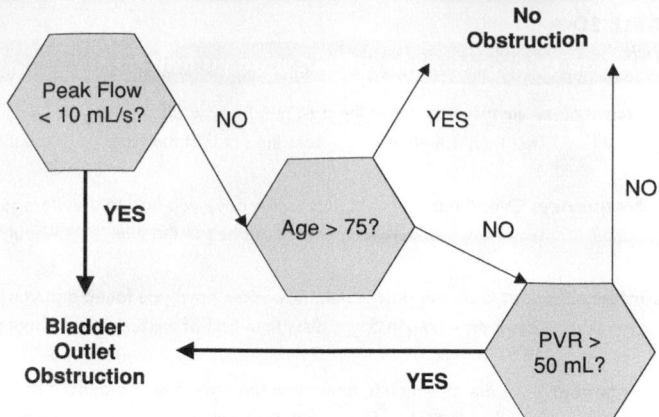

FIGURE 50-5. Algorithm for the clinical diagnosis of bladder outlet obstruction in older men with LUTS. PVR, postvoiding residual volume. *Adapted from DuBeau CE, Yalla SV, Resnick NM. Improving the utility of urine flow rate to exclude outlet obstruction in men with voiding symptoms. J Am Geriatr Soc. 46:1118–1124, 1998.*

this can be overcome using intraurethral lidocaine jelly and patient relaxation. Older men tend to have a larger PVR in the morning, which can increase within-patient PVR variability.

Urine peak flow rate measurement is commonly used in urologic practice, but is not routinely required. Low urine flow rates result from either impaired detrusor contractility, BOO, and/or a low bladder volume. Peak flow rate is very sensitive for BOO (peak flow >12 mL/s with voids ≥150 mL excludes BOO), but low flow rates are nonspecific. PVR, peak flow rate, and age can be combined in an algorithm to diagnose BOO with a sensitivity of 90% (vs. 55% for flow rate alone) and specificity of 43% (63% in men aged >75 years) (Figure 50-5).

Bladder Diaries (Frequency–Volume Charts)

Although not specified by the AUA guideline, bladder diaries can be very helpful to determine if polyruria contributes to frequency and/or nocturia symptoms (Table 50-5). To complete the diary, the patient records the time and volume of all voids (continent and incontinent). Several studies (albeit primarily in women) confirm that bladder diaries are reliable and valid, especially when done for 3 days.

Specialized Testing

Urodynamic Studies

Urodynamic studies are not needed in the initial evaluation of men with LUTS, especially for those manageable with watchful waiting or medical therapy. Even for men considered for surgery, the AUA guideline considers urodynamics, cystoscopy, and prostate ultrasound optional. Urodynamics should be considered: (1) for frail older men (especially those with Parkinson's disease or spinal cord injury) who desire surgical treatment, in order to exclude conditions such as detrusor hyperactivity with impaired contractility; and (2) for men who have failed empiric therapy and further management is desired. The urodynamic tests to evaluate LUTS are cystometry and pressure-flow study. Cystometry measures bladder pressure during

TABLE 50-5

Use of a Bladder Diary in the Evaluation of LUTS and Nocturia

DATE	TIME	VOLUME VOIDED (mL)	ARE YOU WET OR DRY?	AMOUNT OF LEAKAGE	COMMENTS
4/5	3:05 pm	240	Dry		
	6:10 pm	210	Dry		Beer with dinner
	8:15 pm	150	Dry		
	10:20 pm	150	Dry		
	10:30 pm	45	Dry		Went to bed
4/6	3:15 am	270	Wet	Tablespoons	
	5:50 am	300	Dry		
	7:40 am	120	Dry		Coffee
	9:50 am	60	Dry		
	11:20 am	90	Dry		
	12:50 pm	120	Dry		
	1:40 pm	120	Dry		
	3:35 pm	90	Dry		
	6:00 pm	90	Dry		
	8:40 pm	215	Dry		
	10:25 pm	180	Dry		Went to bed
4/7	1:00 am	240	Dry		
	3:50 am	400	Dry		Almost didn't make it
	5:20 am	200	Dry		
	8:00 am	180	Dry		Coffee
	11:15 am	90	Dry		
	4:00 pm	120	Dry		

Bladder diary of 75-year-old man with LUTS and bothersome nocturia. Shaded portions are the nighttime urine output (from time of sleep up to and including first morning void). The diary demonstrates nocturnal polyuria ranging from 720 to 1200 mL. On 4/6, nocturnal polyuria constituted 60% of the 24-hour urine output (1200/[1200 + 785]). The diary also demonstrates the common finding of lower voided volumes during the day compared tonight (60–240 mL vs. 45–400 mL). Even with the higher functional bladder volume at night, the volume of polyuria insures that he would have to awaken to void at least three times (1200 mL/400 mL = 3 voids) Thus, the evaluation of this patient should first focus on possible non-LUT causes of nocturnal polyuria.

Adapted from DuBeau CE, Resnick NM. Evaluation of the causes and severity of geriatric incontinence: a critical appraisal. Urol Clin N Amer, 18:243–256, 1991.

filling to determine detrusor stability (vs. overactivity), contractility, and compliance. The standard for diagnosing BOO is pressure-flow study, which simultaneously measures flow rate versus bladder pressure during voiding.

Other Tests

Cystoscopy is needed only in men with hematuria (especially those with risk factors for bladder carcinoma such as smoking), positive cytology, or pelvic pain; it should not be used to diagnose BOO. Renal ultrasound may be considered in men with new renal impairment, yet even in this group, hydronephrosis is usually only found in men with PVR >150 mL.

MANAGEMENT

Making Treatment Decisions

Treatment decisions must be patient-centered because benign prostate disease has variable impact on patients and only a small absolute risk of morbidity. No treatment prolongs life or guarantees durable cure, and watchful waiting and lifestyle changes provide relief with little risk for many men. Only the small minority of men with hematuria, significant renal impairment, hydronephrosis, re-

current urinary tract infections, retention, and large PVR (e.g., over 200 mL) require immediate referral to a urologist. Issues to discuss in making management decisions include symptom severity and quality of life impact; their risk for disease progression; preferences for immediate versus delayed symptom improvement; likely treatment outcomes and adverse effects; short- and long-term costs; and ability to comply with long-term monitoring. Providers should offer guidance in tailoring treatment so that men are supported in—and not burdened by—decision making. There are video and print decision aids to help both patients and providers weigh treatment risks and benefits. Men with nocturia should be offered prostate-specific medical and invasive therapy *only* after treatment of any contributing polyuria and/or sleep disturbance.

Multiple medical problems, frailty, and short life expectancy need not preclude treatment of benign prostate disease. The broad range of available therapies permits tailoring to the desired immediacy of symptom relief, avoidance of specific adverse effects, and patient comorbidity. Noninvasive treatment is possible in care settings where adequate clinical monitoring and medication adjustment are possible. Assisted-living residents will require either community or inpatient skilled nursing after surgical interventions. Across settings, surgery may not be desirable for men at high risk for in-hospital functional and cognitive decline.

Treatment decisions of course include the efficacy, durability, and associated adverse effects of therapy. Table 50-6 summarizes outcomes for the major therapies based on meta-analyses and

TABLE 50-6

Outcomes from Therapy

TREATMENT	CHANGE IN AUASI			CHANGE IN AUASI QoL QUESTION SCORE			MORBIDITY						
Length of follow-up (months)	3–9	10–16	>16	3–9	10–16	>16							
Watchful Waiting													
	−1.0	−0.5											
Medical Therapy													
Alpha Blockers							Asthenia	CV	Dizzy	GI	OH	ENT	ED*
Alfuzosin	−4.4			−1.1			4%	1%	5%	10%	2%	6%	3%
Doxazosin	−5.1	−5.6		−1.3	−1.5		15%	2%	13%	10%	9%	8%	4%
Tamsulosin	−4.6	−7.5		−1.4			7%	8%	12%	11%	11%	11%	4%
Terazosin	−6.2	−6.0		−1.7	−1.4		12%	2%	15%	5%	18%	6%	5%
5-alpha reductase inhibitors													
Finasteride	−3.4	−3.4	−2.37				2%		5%	6%	7%	9%	8%
Placebo	−2.4	−2.3	−1.0	−0.7	−0.7		2%		5%	6%	1%	6%	4%
Minimally Invasive Therapy													
							AUR	UI	UTI	I-LUTS	Ejac-ED*	Repeat Rx	
UroLume® Stent	−11.5	−12.4	−13.2	−1.3			6%	25%	11%	92%		10%	
Thermal therapies													
Prostaton® version 2.5 TUMT	−8.8			−1.3			15%		9%	74%	16–1%		
Targis® TUMT	−10.1			−2.2	−2.4	−2.3	6%		9%		5%–NA	16%	
Transurethral needle ablation (TUNA)	−11.5			−3.1	−2.7	−2.4	20%	1%	17%	3%	4–3%	23%	
Surgical Therapy													
							AUR	UI	UTI	I-LUTS	Ejac-ED	Repeat Rx	
TURP	−14.7	−14.8	−13.5	−3.4	−3.3	−3.0	5%	3%	6%	15%	65–10%	5%	
HoLEP	−17.8	−17.9					8%	1%	1%	6%	59–3%	1%	
Laser coagulation	−17.0	−20.0	−18.4	−3.22			21%	1%	9%	66%	17–6%	7%	
Transurethral incision	−11.9	−15.2	−10.8		−3.7	−3.7	6%	2%	5%	99%	18–13%	14%	
Laser vaporization	−13.4	−14.1	−14.2	−4.0	−1.7		13%	3%	9%	36%	42–7%	8%	
Open prostatectomy			−10.1				1%	6%	8%		61–NA	1%	
Watchful waiting	−1.0	−0.5					3%	2%	0%		NA–21%	55%	

AUASI, American Urological Association Symptom Index; QoL, quality of life; CV, cardiovascular; Dizzy, dizziness; GI, gastrointestinal; OH, orthostatic hypotension; ENT, nasal congestion; ED, erectile dysfunction and impotence; AUR, acute urinary retention; UI, urinary incontinence; UTI, urinary tract infection; I-LUTS, postoperative irritative LUTS; Ejac-ED, ejaculatory disorders and erectile dysfunction; Repeat Rx, secondary procedure necessary; TUMT, transurethral microwave thermotherapy; TURP, transurethral resection of the prostate; HoLEP, holmium laser enucleation of the prostate, TUIP, transurethral incision of the prostate, NA, not available.

*Percentages represent ejaculatory disorders and erectile disorders.

Data from Roehrborn CG, O'Connell JD, Barry MJ, et al. *American Urological Association Guideline on the Management of benign prostatic hyperplasia (BPH). Update, 2006.*

systematic reviews. Figure 50-6 shows the suggested treatment algorithm.

Nonpharmacological Management

Watchful Waiting

The natural history of benign prostate disease and the large placebo effects seen in randomized controlled treatment trials support the use of watchful waiting as a specific intervention. Men most appropriate for watchful waiting have mild to moderate LUTS, are comfortable with this approach, and can be reliably followed. Clinicians should be "watchful" and not passive in following these patients, with regular follow-up, instruction in voiding hygiene, and behavioral approaches to decrease LUTS (see Chapter 59), counseling to avoid medications that can cause retention (e.g., over-the-counter "cold" tablets containing α-agonists and antihistamines), and careful monitoring for men on anticholinergics or calcium channel-blockers.

Unhurried voiding without straining may help with bladder emptying. Addition of an afternoon loop diuretic may help reduce nocturia in men with nocturnal polyuria if other approaches have failed. A pilot study of the efficacy of a patient self-management program comprising education and reassurance, lifestyle modifications, and behavioral interventions was encouraging, and results of a randomized trial are forthcoming.

In the largest randomized trial of watchful waiting versus transurethral resection of the prostate (TURP) (*n* = 556 men with moderate LUTS), TURP had significantly greater symptom improvement at 3 years yet the watchful waiting results were not trivial (mean decrease in symptom score 66% and 38%, respectively). One-third of men on watchful waiting crossed-over to TURP, but absolute failure rates with watchful waiting were low (urinary retention 2.9%, PVR >350 mL 5.8%, worsening LUTS 4.3%). There were no significant differences in sexual function, general well-being, or social activities. The improvement in LUTS was less in men with the least symptom bother, especially after TURP. In the Medical

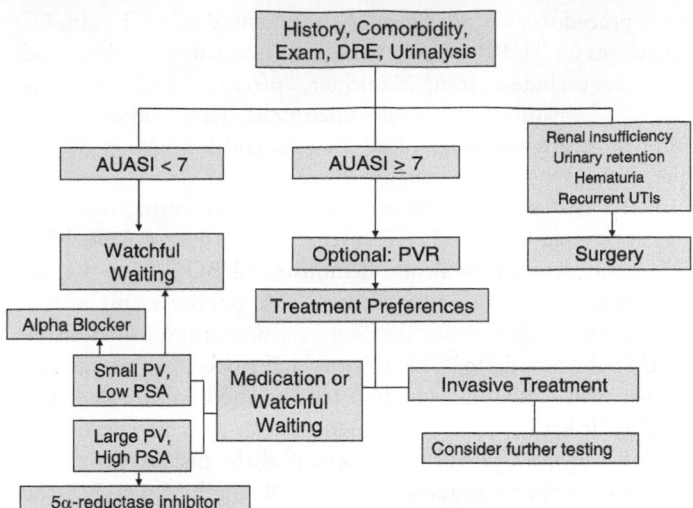

FIGURE 50-6. Algorithm for treatment of symptomatic BPH. PVR, postvoiding residual volume; UTI, urinary tract infection; AUASI, American Urological Association Symptom Index; PV, prostate volume; PSA, prostatic-specific antigen. (*Adapted from the American Urological Association Guideline on the Management of benign prostatic hyperplasia (BPH); Marberger M. Drug insight: 5α-reductase inhibitors for the treatment of benign prostatic hyperplasia. Nat Clin Pract Urol. 3:495–503, 2006.*)

Therapy of Prostatic Symptoms (MTOPS) trial, only 17% of men in the placebo (watchful waiting) arm had "clinical progression" at 4 years, and 80% of these cases were considered "progression" because of AUASI increase of ≥4 points.

Medications

Alpha-Adrenergic Blockers

Alpha$_1$-selective adrenergic blockers reduce BPH-related LUTS by several proposed mechanisms: decreased contractility of prostatic tissue, capsule, and urethra; increased apoptosis caused by higher levels of tumor growth factor-β; and improved vascular flow to the detrusor. Currently available agents are prazosin (1 to 2 mg twice daily), terazosin (2 to 10 mg daily), doxazosin (4 to 8 mg daily), tamsulosin (0.4 to 0.8 mg daily), and alfuzosin (10 mg daily). Time to onset of action is 2 to 4 weeks. Randomized controlled trials show no significant differences in LUTS reduction between these agents. Efficacy is greater in men with more severe LUTS, and appears durable, although most long-term data are from open label trials. Alpha-blockers do not prevent urinary retention and are not very effective in reducing nocturia.

Side effects most commonly include asthenia, headache, dizziness, and more significantly orthostatic hypotension; all are more prevalent with higher doses. For all of the agents, withdrawal rates in published trials are 10% to 15%, and may be higher in clinical practice. Tamsulosin is the only agent selective for the α_{1A}-receptor and the only one associated with retrograde ejaculation and a high risk of intraoperative floppy iris syndrome during cataract surgery. To prevent the latter complication, special surgical approaches are necessary and men taking tamsulosin should alert their ophthalmologist. The impact of stopping tamsulosin preoperatively is unclear, as some cases occurred months after discontinuation. Tamsulosin also has the lowest risk of orthostatic hypotension. Alfuzosin should be taken within 1 hour of a meal to maximize bioavailability. Terazosin

and doxazosin have significantly higher rates of dizziness, orthostasis, and treatment withdrawal than tamsulosin. Orthostatic hypotension is more likely in men with hypertension, regardless of any hypertension treatment. Slow titration from minimal starting doses and nighttime dosing help mitigate first-dose hypotension. Alpha blockers should *not* be used as first-line antihypertensive agents in men with LUTS and hypertension. Men with diastolic dysfunction or taking other antihypertensives need to be carefully monitored, and men treated with doxazosin especially should be monitored for congestive heart failure. Concomitant use of phosphodiesterase type 5 inhibitors for erectile dysfunction can cause potentially dangerous hypotension with all alpha blockers except tamsulosin.

5-α Reductase Inhibitors

The 5-α reductase inhibitors (5-αRIs) finasteride and dutasteride decrease prostate size by blocking the 5-α reduction of testosterone to dihydrotestosterone, the active androgen for prostate growth. 5-αRIs decrease prostate volume over 6 months by a maximum of 30%. 5-αRIs have a slow onset of action, with no significant decrease in LUTS until 6 to 10 months; they should not used when men want rapid symptom improvement or life expectancy is short. Lifetime use is necessary to prevent recurrent BPE and LUTS, raising the potential for higher lifetime treatment costs. In one study, finasteride was more cost-effective for men with moderate LUTS than watchful waiting (up to 3 years) and TURP (up to 14 years), but cost-effectiveness decreased over time.

The PLESS trial (Proscar® Long-term Efficacy and Safety Study) established the disease-modifying effects of 5-αRIs in men with moderate to severe LUTS and BPE. Finasteride decreased the incidence of AUR (absolute risk reduction [ARR] 5% [95% CI 10–5%], number needed to treat [NNT] 26–49), and prostatectomy (ARR 4% [95% CI 7–3%], NNT 18–31). Risk reduction was apparent by 1 year and was greatest in men with large glands (prostate volume > 58 mL and/or PSA ≥1.4 ng/mL). Sexual dysfunction with finasteride was 8% greater than placebo (absolute difference).

Although 5-αRIs maintain or even increase serum testosterone levels, they can cause adverse sexual effects including decreased libido (6%) and impotence (8%). A subanalysis of PLESS found no effect of finasteride on bone density over 4 years. Finasteride decreases PSA levels by 40% to 60% in the first year. When prostate cancer screening is appropriate for men given 5-αRIs, PSA should be monitored and if it remains stable or rises, biopsy is necessary. In the Prostate Cancer Prevention Trial, finasteride lowered prostate cancer rates (25% relative reduction, 20% absolute), but high-grade tumors more common (37% vs. 22% with placebo). Considerable debate continues about the implications of this finding for long-term 5-αRI treatment, but results from a forthcoming similar trial with dutasteride may provide more answers.

Combination Therapy

Because of their different mechanisms of action, combination treatment with alpha-blockers and 5-αRIs have the potential for additive benefit. The pivotal Medical Therapy of Prostate Symptoms (MTOPS) study randomized nearly 3000 men with moderate LUTS to placebo, doxazosin, finasteride, or both with a mean follow-up of 4.5 years. The primary outcome was "clinical progression," not LUTS reduction. At 1 year, only doxazosin (alone or in combination) was significantly more effective than placebo, but at 5 years, finasteride was more effective than doxazosin, and combination therapy more effective than either finasteride or doxazosin alone (albeit with high withdrawal rates and adverse effects). Men with baseline prostate volume >40 mL and/or PSA >4 ng/mL benefited the most from combination therapy. Disease progression was associated with rising PSA and prostate volume during the trial in men on placebo or doxazosin, but not finasteride or combination therapy. The Symptom Management After Reducing Therapy (SMART) trial evaluated whether the efficacy of short-term combination therapy could be maintained with a 5-αRI alone. After 24 weeks of dutasteride ± tamsulosin, stopping tamsulosin caused increased symptoms only for men with severe baseline LUTS. Additional data will come from the CombAT trial (Combination of Advodart® and Tamsulosin), which will follow men at high risk for progression over 4 years.

Another approach combines alpha blockers with antimuscarinic bladder relaxants for men with more severe frequency, urgency, and/or urge UI. In a 12-week trial of tamsulosin and extended-release tolterodine, ($n = 979$, 25% aged ≥70 years) 80% of men on combined therapy had subjective improvement, versus 71% with tamsulosin alone, 65% with tolterodine, and 62% with placebo. AUR occurred in only 3 men on placebo, 2 on tolterodine, and 2 on combination therapy. Other studies have demonstrated the safety of using antimuscarinic agents in men with LUTS.

Phytotherapy

Plant-derived compounds that have been used to treat BPH-related LUTS, especially outside of the United States, include saw palmetto, β-sitosterols, and cernilton. Most phytotherapy trials suffer from short-term treatment (typically 4 to 24 weeks) and lack of standardized preparations. Although a Cochrane systematic review concluded that saw palmetto significantly improved LUTS and decreased nocturia, in a recent 1-year trial saw palmetto had the same AUASI and quality of life outcomes as placebo among men with moderate to severe LUTS. Cochrane meta-analyses also have concluded that β-sitosterols and cernilton significantly reduce LUTS, but the source trials were heterogeneous and small. Phytotherapeutic agents have few reported side effects, but long-term data are lacking.

Emerging Therapies

Several agents that act on neurotransmitters and trophic factors other than alpha adrenergic systems and androgens are under active investigation. In early trials, phosphodiesterase type 5 inhibitors decreased LUTS but did not affect flow rate, and intraprostatic injection of botulinum toxin-A decreased prostate size. There are no data yet on effect size and duration, impact on other outcomes and disease progression, and adverse effects. A randomized trial of the calcitriol analog BXL-353 is underway.

SURGERY

Transurethral Resection of Prostate

TURP remains the standard surgical treatment for benign prostate disease because it has the best evidence for robust and durable symptom improvement. The advent of new surgical and minimally invasive procedures has not diminished its central role. The absolute indications for TURP are high grade BOO, urinary retention (medical causes excluded), recurrent urinary infections, hydronephrosis, recurrent hematuria, and renal impairment. These indications account for nearly one-third of all TURPs, and for 50% to 60% of operations in men older than age 80 years.

TURP is superior to watchful waiting in preventing worsening LUTS, elevated PVR, and AUR over 5 years (10% vs. 21%, NNT 9). Men with urodynamically demonstrated BOO have the best symptomatic outcomes, but quality of life improves only in men with severe LUTS. Efficacy declines over time, from 87% decrease in LUTS at 3 months to 75% at 7 years, and reoperation rates average 1% per year. Symptom reduction tends to be lower in older men (<80%). It has been difficult to demonstrate the cost-effectiveness of TURP in the United States because of the marked geographic variability in operation rates, charges, and length of stay. Whether TURP prevents late detrusor decompensation from BOO is unclear, and the true proportion of men at risk is unknown.

Adverse effects of TURP include retrograde ejaculation (74%); erectile dysfunction (14%, and increases with age); immediate surgical complications (12%); UI (5%); bleeding requiring transfusion (2%); failure to void; and infection. In one trial, there was no difference in erectile dysfunction and UI rates between TURP and watchful waiting. Men over age 80 years have higher rates of complications (early 30% to 40%, late 13% to 22%), reoperation (4% per year), and perioperative mortality (2% to 3% vs. 0.4%); but no change in long-term survival. Many of the studies in elderly men, however, did not adjust for increased comorbidity.

Laser Prostatectomy

Laser surgery has the advantage of being an outpatient procedure, with outcomes similar to TURP. In one randomized controlled trial, TURP was superior to noncontact lasers in improving LUTS and quality of life at 7 months, but outcomes were equivalent at 1 year. The sole 5-year study found higher reoperation rates with laser (38%) despite a TURP reoperation rate (16%) higher than nearly any other study. Laser procedures require longer postoperative catheterization and cause more infections and urethral irritation than TURP. Side effects vary by technique, and can include impotence, retrograde ejaculation, increased urgency and frequency, UI, and bladder neck stricture.

Several laser systems are available, and some have already been abandoned for lack of efficacy. Holmium laser enucleation of the prostate (HoLEP) is mainly used for men with AUR with significant BPE. It provides results similar to TURP with less bleeding and shorter recovery time, but the technique can be more difficult to learn. Initial studies suggest that HoLEP may produce more durable results than other laser surgeries. Photoselective vaporization of the prostate also has similar efficacy as TURP, with less bleeding and a shorter recovery; it appears to work better for smaller prostates. Transurethral evaporation of the prostate is used less frequently. Because of poor efficacy and high adverse events, Ng:YAG lasers (used in visual laser ablation of the prostate, contact laser ablation, and interstitial coagulation systems) are seldom used today.

Open Prostatectomy

Men with very large prostate volume (>60 mL) require open prostatectomy (via an abdominal or perineal approach) because the operative time needed for TURP in these cases significantly increases perioperative complications. Open procedures account for ≤5% of prostatectomies, and some surgeons prefer to perform an "incomplete" TURP to avoid the morbidity of abdominal or perineal surgery. In retrospective studies, open prostatectomy has lower reoperation rate and mortality than TURP, but these analyses did not adequately control for the higher age and comorbidity in TURP patients or the secular trend of decreasing TURP mortality.

Minimally Invasive Procedures

Prostate Incision

Transurethral incision of the prostate (TUIP) is a technically simpler procedure used in men with small glands (<30 mL). TUIP is done local anesthesia with shorter operation time and less bleeding than TURP. TUIP has similar symptomatic efficacy to TURP at 1 year. In a select case series, at two years only 8% of TUIP patients had required a subsequent TURP. TUIP has the potential to be a safe and effective alternative for obstructed older men with smaller prostates who have high operative risk and have failed noninvasive treatment.

Thermotherapy

Transurethral needle ablation (TUNA) employs transurethrally placed radiofrequency needles to heat prostate tissue, causing coagulation necrosis and a tissue defect. Symptomatic efficacy is smaller and less durable than with TURP, and no studies compare TUNA to other procedures, medical therapy, or watchful waiting. Transurethral microwave thermotherapy is a related outpatient procedure that requires repeated treatments. Symptomatic improvement is typically modest, and in short-term trials is inferior to TURP, sham procedures, and terazosin. The future of these procedures is uncertain.

Stents

Urethral stents to facilitate voiding should be reserved for high risk patients with recurrent AUR who are unfit for surgery or for whom long-term indwelling catheterization is undesirable. Permanent absorbable stents are complicated by encrustation, pain, and infection, and failure rates run 20% to 30%. Nonabsorbable temporary stents are complicated by migration, UTI, stricture, and encrustation.

PREVENTION

Data on risk and protective factors suggest that increased physical activity, a diet low in meat and fat and high in vegetables and micronutrients, and moderate alcohol consumption may prevent or slow the progression of benign prostate disease. Weight loss for obese men, glycemic control in diabetes, and treatment of high cholesterol also may be important. However, there are no intervention trials to support these suggestions.

FURTHER READING

Barry MJ. Evaluation of symptoms and quality of life in men with benign prostatic hyperplasia. *Urology.* 2001;58:25.

Barry MJ, Link CL, McNaughton-Collins MF, McKinlay JB. Boston Area Community Health (BACH) Investigators. Overlap of different urological symptom complexes in a racially and ethnically diverse, community-based population of men and women. *BJU Int.* 2008;101:45–51.

Blake-James, Rashidan A, Ikeda U, Emberton M. The role of anticholinergics in men with lower urinary symptoms suggestive of benign prostatic hyperplasia: a systematic review and meta-analysis. *BJU Int.* 2006;99:85–96.

Bouza C, Lopez T, Magro A, Navalpotro, Amate JM. Systematic review and meta-analysis of transurethral needle ablation in symptomatic benign prostatic hyperplasia. *BMC Urol.* 2006;6:14–17.

Chuang U-C, Chancellor M. The application of botulinum toxin in the prostate. *J Urol.* 2006;176:2375–2382.

Crawford EF, Wilson SS, McConnell JD, et al. Baseline factors as predictors of clinical progression of benign prostatic hyperplasia in men treated with placebo. *J Urol.* 2006;175:1422–1427.

Donovan JL, Peters TJ, Neal DE, et al. A randomized trial comparing transurethral resection of the prostate, laser therapy, and conservative management for lower urinary tract symptoms associated with benign prostatic enlargement: the ClasP study. *J Urol.* 2000;164:65.

Flanigan RC, Reda DJ, Wasson JH, Anderson RJ, Abdellatif M, Bruskewitz RC. 5-yr outcome of surgical resection and watchful waiting for men with moderately symptomatic BPH: VA cooperative study. *J Urol.* 1998;160:12.

St Sauver JL, Jacobson DJ, Girman CJ, Lieber MM, McGree ME, Jacobsen SJ. Tracking of longitudinal changes in measures of benign prostatic hyperplasia in a population based cohort. *J Urol.* 2006;175:1018–1022.

Kaplan SA, Roehrborn CG, Rovner ES, Carlsson M, Bavendam T, Guan Z. Tolterodine and tamsulosin for treatment of men with lower urinary tract symptoms and overactive bladder. *JAMA.* 2006;296:2319–2328.

Marberger M. Drug insight: 5α-reductase inhibitors for the treatment of benign prostatic hyperplasia. *Nat Clin Pract Urol.* 2006;3:495–503.

Marks LS, Roehrborn CG, Andriole GL. Prevention of benign prostatic hyperplasia disease. *J Urol.* 2006;176:1299–1306.

McConnell JD, Bruskewitz R, Walsh P, et al. The effect of finasteride on the risk of acute urinary retention and the need for surgical treatment among men with benign prostatic hyperplasia. Finasteride Long-Term Efficacy and Safety Study Group. *N Engl J Med.* 1998;338:557–563.

McConnell JD, Roehrborn CG, Bautista OM, et al. The long-term effect of doxazosin, finasteride, and combination therapy on the clinical progression of benign prostatic hyperplasia. *N Engl J Med.* 2003;349:2387–2398.

O'Leary MP. Treatment and pharmacological management of BPH in the context of common comorbidities. *Am J Man Care.* 2006;12:S129–S140.

Madersbacher S. Stents for prostatic disease: any progress after 25 years? *Eur Urol.* 2006;49:212–214.

Patel AK, Chapple CR. BPH: treatment in primary care. *BMJ.* 2006;333:535–539.

Roehrborn CG, O'Connell JD, Barry MJ, et al. American Urological Association Guideline on the Management of benign prostatic hyperplasia (BPH). Update, 2006. http://www.auanet.org/guidelines/bph.cfm Accessed July 25, 2007.

Weiss JP, Blaivas JG. Nocturia. *J Urol.* 2000;163:5–12.

Wilson LC, Gilling PJ. From coagulation to enucleation: the use of lasers in surgery for benign prostatic hyperplasia. *Nat Clin Pract Urol.* 2005;2:443–448.

Yap TL, Brown CT, Emberton M. Self-management in lower urinary tract symptoms: the next major therapeutic revolution. *World J Urol.* 2006;24:371–377.

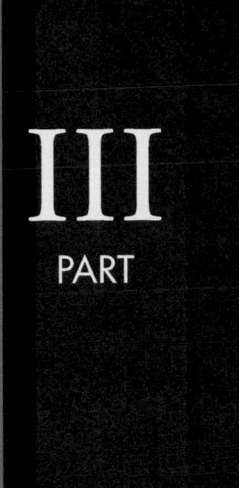

GERIATRIC SYNDROMES

Aging and Homeostatic Regulation

George A. Kuchel

"Besides more or less obvious physical changes in old age, physiological investigation may reveal increasing limitation of the effectiveness of homeostatic devices which keep the bodily conditions stable."

Walter Bradford Cannon (1871–1945)

BACKGROUND

Elderly patients present the clinician with many unique challenges. Many of these issues are fully discussed in chapters that address care of older adults in the context of individual organ systems and diseases (Chapters 61 to 130). However, some of the most common, debilitating and costly clinical problems seen in geriatrics are extremely challenging because they defy conventional medical wisdom by crossing traditional organ- and discipline-based boundaries. Termed "geriatric syndromes," conditions such as frailty (Chapter 52), delirium (Chapter 53), falls (Chapter 54), sleep disorders (Chapter 55), dizziness (Chapter 56), syncope (Chapter 57), pressure ulcers (Chapter 58), incontinence (Chapter 59), and elder mistreatment (Chapter 60) are discussed individually. Nevertheless, given the central importance of these diverse conditions to the practice and science of geriatric medicine, it is also important to address their common features.

In addition to being highly prevalent in the frail elderly, geriatric syndromes also exert a substantial impact on quality of life and disability. Moreover, these are complex multifactorial conditions in which large numbers of underlying and provocative risk factors involving different organ systems interact in influencing ultimate clinical presentation, course, and outcome. These unusual features present important challenges for the clinician since the patient's chief complaint may point away from, rather than toward, the specific pathologic condition, which actually underlies the change in health status. At times, the two processes may involve distinct and distant organs with a disconnect between the site of the underlying insult and the site highlighted by the resulting clinical symptom. For example, when an infection involving the urinary tract precipitates delirium, it is the altered neural function in the form of cognitive and behavioral changes, which permits the diagnosis of delirium and which determines many functional outcomes.

Grouping distinct conditions together as geriatric syndromes also highlights those common features that may help in the development of innovative clinical and research strategies. One of the primary goals of geriatric medicine has been to maintain functional independence in frail older adults, addressing the common paradox of an older patient who is able to maintain usual function under basal conditions, yet decompensates when exposed to seemingly minor challenges. In fact, the clinical dilemma of a frail older adult who is at significant risk of delirium, falls, or incontinence can be restated within a homeostatic framework. Viewed in this manner, function is determined by a complex balance between underlying physiology and health; the nature, number, and intensity of the challenges being experienced, as well as overall physiological plasticity expressed as the effectiveness of relevant homeostatic mechanisms. This approach has several advantages, above all, permitting a collaborative dialogue between investigators conducting more descriptive research and those interested in the study of mechanisms.

HOMEOSTASIS IN A HISTORICAL CONTEXT

The term homeostasis was first coined by Claude Bernard in the mid-nineteenth century and is now extensively used in the medical literature. Unfortunately, it is often forgotten that homeostasis has always referred to the body's attempts at maintaining an internal constancy, which is required for optimal function. Far from reflecting physiologic "stasis," effective homeostasis actually requires that all relevant compensatory mechanisms remain suitably vibrant, responsive, and well-calibrated. During the twentieth century, it became increasingly clear that overall health status, as well as many individual disease processes may impair an individual's ability to appropriately respond to common homeostatic challenges. The recognition that aging can also exert a measurable impact on homeostatic mechanisms came later, but is not recent, as illustrated by the 1932 quote preceding this chapter from the great physiologist Walter Cannon. Finally, in the modern era, several events have greatly impacted upon our understanding of homeostasis. In an extension of the concept of homeostasis, Yates has introduced the term homeodynamics to emphasize the concept that the resiliency of living organisms requires a dynamic interplay of multiple regulatory mechanisms rather than a constancy of the internal environment. Advances in basic research have also permitted investigators to explore homeostatic principles at the level of subcellular processes ranging from gene expression to protein turnover. Most recently, some of the limitations inherent in purely reductionist studies have led to a trend toward systems biology, emphasizing an integration of relevant homeostatic processes from the level of individual cells to tissues and organisms. Moreover, it is now possible to begin defining mechanisms in a manner which reflects the multifactorial and systemic nature of typical geriatric conditions or syndromes.

HOMEOSTATIC REGULATION IN OLD AGE

General Considerations

Physiological systems responsible for maintaining homeostatic regulation may control variables as divergent as body temperature, blood pressure, intracellular calcium, or serum cortisol. At the same time, even among distinct systems, it is possible to observe shared common physiological principles by which they all exert homeostatic control (Table 51-1). With these considerations in mind, a number of investigators have sought to identify unifying and preferably specific "fingerprints" by which aging affects homeostatic control within different physiologic systems.

Systemic Patterns of Change

Homeostenosis of old age has been viewed as a diminished capacity to respond to various homeostatic challenges. Even healthy older adults may exhibit homeostenosis when exposed to a cold or hot environment, on rapidly assuming the upright posture, and while responding to an acute fluid challenge or hypovolemia. Traditionally, these deficits were attributed to a loss of physiologic reserve, an appealing, yet somewhat ill-defined concept emphasizing static (e.g., losses in neuronal numbers, declines in glomerular filtration rate) rather than dynamic explanations. In an effort to better define physiological factors responsible for the dynamic nature of stability in old age, disease, and frailty, Lipsitz has instead focused on categories of relevant complexity that decline with aging. For example, study of aged bone and brain demonstrates evidence of declining complexity in terms of trabecular or neuronal architecture. Other examples of declining complexity involve physiological processes such as narrowing of auditory frequency responsiveness, decreased long-range correlations in time series data such as blood pressure measurements, as well as increased randomness or stochastic activity in terms of cardiac intervals. It has been proposed that such alterations in dynamics of physiologic systems contribute to functional decline and frailty.

TABLE 51-1

Common Features of Homeostatic Dysregulation in Old Age

CONCEPT	EXAMPLES
Homeostenosis	Diminished capacity to respond to varied homeostatic challenges such as changes in ambient temperature, orthostasis, fluid load or dehydration
Diminished physiological reserve	Increased homeostatic vulnerability as a result of a critical loss in numbers of neurons or a decline in glomerular filtration rate
Loss of complexity	Declines in bone or neuronal architecture; narrowing of hearing frequency responses or loss of long-range correlations in blood pressure readings
Enhanced variability	Greater inter- and intraindividual variability in sympathetic activity or blood pressure readings
Higher basal activity	Basal sympathetic activity is elevated in older adults
Excessive response to stressors	Sympathetic responses to common challenges are excessively large and prolonged
Diminished end-organ responsiveness	Ability of peripheral catecholamines to increase heart rate via β-adrenergic receptors or to mediate arterial vasoconstriction via α-adrenergic receptors is decreased.
Loss of negative feedback	Ability of corticosteroids to downregulate activity of the hypothalamic-pituitary-adrenal system via negative feedback is diminished
Allostatic load	Increased biological burden in terms of estimates of cumulative exposure exacted by attempts to adapt to life's demands predicts future mortality, as well as declines in cognitive and physical function

However, changes in complexity should not be confused with those involving variability. These are two distinct concepts, with aging often having distinct and at times directly opposite, effects on complexity and variability. For example, aging *increases* interindividual and intraindividual variability in blood pressure measurements, while long-range correlations involving the complexity of these readings *decrease* with aging. Finally, proponents of the concept of allostatic load have used population-derived measurements (e.g., blood pressure, waist–hip ratio, cholesterol, glycosylated hemoglobin, cortisol, catecholamines, and DHEA-S) as an estimate of cumulative physiologic burden exacted on the body through attempts to adapt to life's demands.

Alterations in Specific Homeostatic Mechanisms

In addition to systemic perspectives of homeostasis, there has also been a growing interest in uncovering specific homeostatic mechanisms that are impaired in old age. For example, markers of sympathetic activity such as peripheral norepinephrine (NE) levels are elevated in older adults under basal conditions. At the same time, a variety of different stimuli (see below) result in an elevation in peripheral NE levels, which is both enhanced and prolonged in older adults. Another common feature is a decline in end-organ responsiveness of many, but not all, receptors to their relevant ligand in the form of a neurotransmitter or hormone. Finally, decreased tissue responsiveness translates in many cases to lessened effectiveness of negative feedback mechanisms as shown for a number of hormones, including corticosteroids.

Reconciling Different Views of Homeostatic Dysregulation

Many different aspects of homeostatic dysregulation in old age have been emphasized in published studies, often in support of a specific concept or theory. Nevertheless, common unifying principles can sometimes be identified. For example, research conducted using simple gene circuits has shown that negative feedback loops enhance the complexity and stability of such systems, permitting more precise and rapid responses to homeostatic challenges. Thus, declines in negative feedback demonstrated for many mammalian homeostatic systems could also contribute to some of the other commonly described features of homeostatic dysregulation in old age and frailty. Moreover, a marker of "allostatic load" such as peripheral cortisol, is not only a predictor of future cognitive and functional impair-

ment, but can also contribute to neuronal cell death involving hippocampal cells involved in cognition, while also contributing to a decline in the ability of cortisol to downregulate its own synthesis and release.

SPECIFIC HOMEOSTATIC CHALLENGES

General Considerations

As discussed earlier, under normal basal conditions, many older adults are able to maintain their usual level of function even in the presence of a large number of health problems. However, once exposed to additional challenges, the same individuals may experience rapid and at times even catastrophic declines in their health status and functional independence. A growing understanding of normal homeostatic mechanisms has led many investigators to conduct studies evaluating the impact of aging on such responses. Table 51-2 provides an overview of our current understanding of the impact of aging on the ability to effectively respond to specific homeostatic challenges in terms of the most relevant biomarkers or physiological measurements. However, it must also be noted that aging

TABLE 51-2

Impact of Aging on Physiological Responses to Specific Homeostatic Challenges

HOMEOSTATIC CHALLENGE	SELECTED BIOMARKERS UNDER BASAL CONDITIONS	IMPACT OF AGING ON RESPONSE TO SPECIFIC CHALLENGE	CHAPTERS
"Fight or flight" challenge or mental stress	—Norepinephrine ↑ —Epinephrine N.C. —Sympathetic neural recordings ↑ —Cortisol levels N.C.	Enhanced and prolonged ↑ in norepinephrine levels, sympathetic neural activity and cortisol levels	7, 70, 107
Decreased ambient temperature	—Temperature N.C. —Metabolic rate ↓	—Sensation of cold ↓ —Shivering intensity ↓ —Thermogenesis ↓ —Vasoconstriction ↓	
Elevated ambient temperature	—Temperature N.C.	—Sweating responses ↓ —Vasodilatation ↓ —Ability to raise cardiac output ↓	
Orthostasis, meals, and hypovolemia	—Blood pressure N.C.	—Hypotension risk ↑ with frailty, comorbidity and concurrent challenges	57, 74, 88
Hyperglycemia and hypoglycemia	—Fasting glucose N.C. or small ↑	—Glucose clearance ↓ —Response to hypoglycemia N.C. or small ↓	107, 109
Fluid challenge and dehydration	—Serum sodium N.C. —Osmolarity N.C. —Osmolality N.C.	—Ability to retain Na+ in salt depletion ↓ —Ability to excrete Na+ in salt loading ↓	88
Bladder outlet obstruction	—Detrusor contractility mildly ↓	—Ability to raise detrusor pressure ↓ —Likelihood of detrusor decompensation with muscle degeneration and fibrosis ↑	55
Major burns and trauma		—With comorbidity favorable outcome ↓	37, 68
Altered physical activity		—Extent and speed of deconditioning ↑ —Extent and speed of gains in muscle mass and strength ↓	29, 37, 114, 115
Anticholinergic medications		—Xerostomia, cognitive problems, constipation, urinary retention ↑	8, 53, 55, 63
Antidopaminergic medications		—Rigidity, poverty of movement ↑	63, 66
Neuronal degeneration		—Compensatory neuronal plasticity ↓	61

may influence some of these measurements under basal conditions. Moreover, since some of these topics are discussed in far greater detail elsewhere in this book, relevant chapter numbers are also provided. Finally, when evaluating the large body of literature that supports the information provided in Table 51-1, several overarching principles must be kept in mind. First, while animal studies largely support results of human research, occasional discrepancies have been noted. Thus, all summary findings in Table 51-1 are based on human research. Second, clinicians deal with older adults who represent the full spectrum of health, comorbidity, disability, and frailty. Nevertheless, in order to attribute a specific physiological change to aging, it is important to make a distinction between changes that are caused by confounding illness from those associated with usual or successful aging. With these considerations in mind, most of the changes reported in Table 51-1 can be attributed to normal aging, with common geriatric illnesses often enhancing such vulnerability. In many cases, it remains unknown whether individuals who age particularly well or successfully also exhibit these changes.

"Fight or Flight Response"

When confronted with a stressful situation, animals and humans respond in a fairly predictable fashion involving a series of predetermined responses collectively referred to as the fight or flight response. Although thought to have evolved as a response to the risk of attack by a predator, in the context of our patients, such responses are more commonly be activated during mental stress for any reason (Chapter 7, Psychosocial Disorders; Chapter 70, Mood Disorders), while caring for an ill or disabled spouse (Chapter 7, Psychosocial Disorders; Chapter 65, Dementia) or during bereavement (Chapter 7, Psychosocial Disorders; Chapter 31, Dying Patient). Stress results in the activation of hypothalamic and brainstem neurons, leading to increased stimulation of sympathetic preganglionic neurons, which regulate cardiac and adrenal medullary function. Stress also promotes the release of corticotropin-releasing factor, which in turn increases ACTH release. All of these events result in both local and systemic release of corticosteroids and catecholamines, which are ultimately responsible for mediating most of the clinical features of the response to stress (Chapter 107, Aging of the Endocrine System and Selected Endocrine Disorders). The above sequence of reactions can ultimately influence a broad range of systemic functions ranging from cardiac performance, energy metabolism, as well as immune and inflammatory responses. Under basal conditions, the overall sympathetic nervous system (SNS) activity appears to be increase with aging.

This basal activity increase is manifested in the form of increased sympathetic nerve activity on microneural recordings, elevated basal plasma NE, and less consistently epinephrine (E) levels, while basal cortisol levels do not appear to be altered with aging. In contrast, both systems demonstrate somewhat similar patterns of dysregulation in old age with enhanced and prolonged responsiveness following exposure to varied challenges. For example, assuming the upright posture, an oral glucose meal, insulin infusion, isometric exercise, and mental stress all result in enhanced elevation of peripheral NE levels in older subjects, while cortisol responses to surgical stress are also increased. Moreover, demonstrated deficits in terms of decreased negative feedback have been proposed as being major contributors to exaggerated SNS and hypothalamic-pituitary-adrenal (HPA) axis activation with aging. For example, the ability of clonidine or elevated blood pressure to downregulate SNS activity via central nervous system (CNS) α2-receptors or baroreceptor activation, respectively, is impaired in old age. This is in addition to well-described declines in the ability of peripheral catecholamines to increase heart rate via β-receptors or to mediate arterial vasoconstriction via α-adrenergic receptors. Similarly, the ability of circulating corticosteroids to downregulate HPA activity via hypothalamic receptors is also diminished in old age.

Lowered Ambient Temperature

Epidemiology

Older adults are less able to adjust to extremes of low temperature. Hypothermia has historically received greatest attention in the United Kingdom, at least in part as a result of a tendency to maintain lower indoor ambient temperatures in the winter than is the custom in the United States. Some of this earlier British literature described hypothermia among 3.6% of individuals 65 years and older admitted to the hospital, with nearly 10% of community-dwelling older adults found to demonstrate evidence of borderline hypothermia. Nevertheless, recent literature has demonstrated a significant prevalence of hypothermia in North America. U.S. CDC statistics point to the fact that hypothermia-related deaths may also occur in sunbelt states and illustrate the importance of advanced age, chronic medical conditions, substance abuse, and homelessness as contributing risk factors. Moreover, a number of individual case series have highlighted the need to remain vigilant to the development of hypothermia among frail and immobile residents of air conditioned long-term care facilities. Concerns have also been raised about the role played by medications, which may enhance the risk of hypothermia.

Pathophysiology

While basal body temperature remains unaltered with aging, older adults are less able to sense and respond to cold challenges when exposed to lowered ambient temperatures. Relevant mechanisms include a decreased sensation of cold, as well as declines in shivering intensity, thermogenesis, and vasoconstriction. Such changes may be related to both physiologic declines associated with aging or with specific diseases. For clinical purposes, hypothermia is generally defined as a body core temperature of less than 35°C (95°F), obtained using tympanic, rectal, or esophageal probes. Nonetheless, significant clinical consequences may occur outside of the boundaries of these definitions. Moreover, the development of frank hypothermia depends on a balance between the severity and length of the cold exposure and an individual subject's ability to sense and mount an effective response to such a challenge. Ultimately, aging, frailty, comorbidity, and diseases may all contribute to determining an individual's specific vulnerability.

Normal body temperature is regulated by the thermoregulatory center, which controls heat loss and heat generation by regulating sweating, blood vessel tone, as well as shivering and nonshivering (chemical) thermogenesis. Older adults demonstrate evidence of deficits in both afferent and efferent thermoregulatory pathways. For example, a diminished sensitivity to changes in environmental temperature may have both physiologic and behavioral consequences. As a result, already compromised compensatory mechanisms may be overwhelmed by the fact that older individuals may be less likely to seek suitable shelter or clothing in the cold. Declines in shivering thermogenesis may be particularly catastrophic in older adults, given the importance of these mechanisms in normal responses to the cold. Other contributing physiological risk factors for hypothermia include deficient autonomic mechanisms with a decreased vasoconstrictor response, which is more common among older adults with orthostatic hypotension, as well as decreased ability of β-adrenergic stimuli to effect thermogenesis. Of course, decreases in lean body mass with a lower metabolic rate also enhance the vulnerability of older adults. Absence of fat mass may also provide frail older adults with less insulation against heat loss.

A large number of potentially reversible factors also need to be considered. For example, malnutrition, hypothyroidism, hypoglycemia, as well as immobility and decreased physical activity may all contribute to decreased thermogenesis. Medications, which have been linked to hypothermia, include alcohol, phenothiazines, barbiturates, benzodiazepines, opioids, and general anesthetics, as well as more recent antidepressants and neuroleptics. Central thermoregulatory control may also be affected by hypothalamic neural injury following anoxic, vascular, traumatic, or malignant lesions. Severe sepsis, especially in frail older adults, can occasionally overwhelm host defenses, resulting in a blunted and even paradoxical response to infection with hypothermia. The association of infection with hypothermia is generally viewed as a poor prognostic sign and is felt to reflect altered hypothalamic regulatory function. Finally, a clinician's approach to hypothermia is incomplete without an assessment of the cognitive, social, and economic factors, which may result in self-neglect, poor judgment, or lack of financial resources to provide for adequate heating.

Clinical Presentation

Early manifestations of hypothermia may be subtle and nonspecific. Moreover, older adults may become hypothermic even without exposure to extremely cold temperatures. Thus, a high index of suspicion is essential, as is a thermometer capable of recording very low temperatures. Early hypothermia (core temperatures of 32°C to 35°C or 90°F to 95°F) can be associated with fatigue, lethargy, apathy, slow gait, slurred speech, confusion, and cool skin. Challenging the diagnosis is the nonspecific nature of these symptoms and signs, combined with the finding that some hypothermic older patients may not complain of feeling cold and may not shiver. With more advanced hypothermia (core temperatures of 28°C to 32°C or 82°F to 90°F), skin becomes cold and cyanotic, while hypopnea and altered consciousness first become apparent. Bradycardia, as well as atrial and ventricular arrhythmias, represent common cardiac abnormalities. These cardiac events, combined with volume contraction resulting from fluid redistribution, as well as cold-induced water and solute diuresis contribute to the risk of hypotension and cardiovascular collapse in these individuals. Altered consciousness may progress to coma with slowing of neurological reflexes and sluggishness of pupillary responses. Finally, with core temperatures below 28°C (82°F), individuals may be mistaken for dead since they may be unresponsive and apneic, with very cold skin, ventricular fibrillation, absent neurologic reflexes, as well as fixed and dilated pupils. Individuals who have survived early cardiovascular complications of severe hypothermia, are at risk for pneumonia, aspiration, pulmonary edema, pancreatitis, gastrointestinal hemorrhage, acute renal failure, and intravascular thrombosis. Abnormal J (Osborne)

waves may follow each QRS on the electrocardiogram (ECG). These relatively specific changes disappear as temperature returns to normal. Much less specific ECG changes include bradycardia, prolongations of P-R interval, QRS complex, and QT segment, as well as atrial fibrillation, premature ventricular contractions, and ventricular fibrillation. ECG changes may mimic those seen with acute myocardial ischemia or infarction. Finally, hypothermic individuals may also suffer from hypothyroidism. Not only do myxedema coma and hypothermia share some clinical features, but hypothyroism may contribute to the development of hypothermia. On occasion, a history of previous thyroid disease, a surgical scar in the thyroid region, or a delay in the relaxation phase of deep tendon reflexes may provide the only clues.

Treatment

Emergency Care Severe hypothermia represents a medical emergency. If outdoors, such individual need to be immediately moved away from severe cold, wet clothing must be removed and warmed blankets applied. Early cardiac monitoring is essential since even minor stimuli can trigger significant dysrhythmias. Procedures such as chest compression or pacemaker placement should be avoided as long as a heartbeat is detectable and patient is breathing spontaneously. In individuals who are asystolic or in ventricular fibrillation, resuscitation should be pursued. Since a cold heart may be relatively unresponsive to drugs or electrical stimulation, such efforts must be pursued aggressively and need to include warmed intravenous fluids (e.g., 5% dextrose normal saline without potassium).

General Support Severe hypothermia is associated with a mortality exceeding 50%. These figures worsen further with advanced age and with associated comorbidity. As a result, such patients require close supportive care in an intensive care unit. Such supportive care must include treatment of contributing conditions such as infection, hypoglycemia, and hypothyroidism. Clinicians need to have a high index of suspicion for infection in hypothermic older adults, administering broad spectrum antibiotics without waiting for results of confirmatory cultures. When administering thyroid hormone for suspected hypothyroidism, corticosteroids may also be required in order to avoid inducing adrenal insufficiency. While ECG monitoring is necessary, central lines should be avoided, given cardiac irritability in these subjects. Pharmacodynamic and pharmacokinetic properties of many commonly used drugs may become dramatically altered in hypothermic patients, creating therapeutic challenges. Such drugs may accumulate as metabolism is delayed and as ever increasing doses are administered because of a lack of response at lower temperatures, causing potential problems as responsiveness to accumulated doses of these medications increases during body warming. Since insulin is ineffective at temperatures below 30°C (86°F), it should not be administered at low temperatures. Volume depletion as well as hypoxemia needs to be corrected. Intubation may be required and blood gases should be monitored. Nevertheless, rewarming strategies may need to be undertaken immediately following stabilization, since cardiac arrhythmias, acidosis, fluid, and electrolyte disorders may be resistant to treatment until body core temperatures are raised.

Rewarming For patients who are only mildly hypothermic (core temperatures of 32°C to 35°C or 90°F to 95°F), passive rewarming techniques using insulating materials and transfer to a warm environment generally suffice. For such individuals, active external rewarming using electric blankets, warm mattresses, hot water bottles, or warm water baths are generally not necessary. Moreover, such treatment can be associated with significant risk as warmth-induced peripheral vasodilatation may precipitate hypovolemic shock in vulnerable individuals.

For individuals in more severe hypothermia (core temperatures under 32°C or 90°F), active core rewarming becomes necessary. A variety of techniques are available, with peritoneal dialysis rewarming representing the most practical solution in most institutions. Mediastinal lavage involves a major surgical procedure, while extracorporeal circulation requires special equipment and carries risks of hypotension and heparin-induced hemorrhage. Gastric lavage using balloons filled with warm fluid is simple, yet rate of warming may be slow and pharyngeal irritation may induce arrhythmias. Peritoneal dialysis with rapid instillation and removal of warm (40°C or 104°F) potassium-free dialysate can provide for safe core warming within six to eight fluid exchanges.

Raised Ambient Temperature

Epidemiology

Heat stroke is a major public health problem with nearly 4780 U.S. deaths attributed to extreme heat between 1979 and 2002. Recent heat waves in the United States (e.g., Chicago) and abroad (e.g., France) have graphically illustrated the tremendous vulnerability of older adults to excessively high temperatures. Given a growing awareness of the need to be vigilant for the development of hyperthermia in institutional settings, nursing home cases have fortunately become more rare. Nevertheless, older adults living in the community, especially those who are frail, suffer from disabilities and live alone are at great risk. In addition to the risk of heatstroke, hyperthermia also contributes to excessive cardiac mortality and morbidity. Older women appear to be at a particularly high risk of dying during a heat wave.

Pathophysiology

As in the case of hypothermia, heatstroke represents an example of homeostatic decompensation in which older adults' deficient or sluggish compensatory mechanisms are unable to maintain normal body temperature in the face of increased environmental temperature. Excess mortality in older adults during heat waves may be attributed to heat-provoked cardiac events or to primary thermoregulatory failure. In recent years, there has been a growing awareness that heatstroke is a form of hyperthermia, which is associated with an excessive systemic inflammatory response contributing to multiorgan dysfunction. Impairments of thermoregulatory systems may occur at a number of different levels and, as in the case of hypothermia, may result from aging or from associated comorbidity and diseases. Sweating responses to thermal, pharmacologic, and chemical stimuli are reduced with aging, representing a significant contributor to homeostatic decompensation by older adults faced with significant heat challenges. Moreover, older adults require higher body core temperatures before compensatory sweating mechanisms are activated. During times of heat stress, younger individuals depend on being able to increase their skin heat loss by shunting blood flow from core toward peripheral blood vessels. In older individuals, the extent and speed of these important compensatory homeostatic mechanisms is impaired as a result of decreased cardiac output and a diminished vasodilatation of peripheral blood vessels. However, some of the above changes may also be the result of occult cardiac disease or physical deconditioning. For example, maximum oxygen uptake appears to be a much more important predictor of sweat rate and forearm flow during exercise than is chronological age. Moreover, with increased physical activity, older adults are able to improve some of these physiological responses to heat challenge toward those seen in younger individuals. Finally, as for hypothermia, presence of significant comorbidity, medications, as well as social and environmental factors may further place older adults at risk of homeostatic decompensation during heat waves. For example, decreased mobility or impaired judgment caused by dementia or psychiatric illness may keep some older adults from seeking assistance and from taking sensible precautions such as removal of heavy clothing and increasing fluid intake. Moreover, air conditioning may not be an option for individuals living on a fixed income. Common chronic conditions such as congestive heart failure, diabetes mellitus, COPD, and alcoholism further enhance the risk of heatstroke. Anticholinergic agents used for urge incontinence, depression, or behavioral problems may also contribute to hyperthermia by inhibiting normal sweating mechanisms, while diuretics may lead to hypovolemia.

Clinical Presentation

Earliest warnings of thermoregulatory failure or heat exhaustion may be subtle and nonspecific. In addition to a feeling of warmth, such individuals may also present with a sense of lethargy, weakness, dizziness, anorexia, nausea, vomiting, headache, and dyspnea. Frank heatstroke is defined clinically as a core body temperature above 40°C (105°F) that is accompanied by hot, dry skin, and major central nervous system abnormalities, which may include delirium, convulsions, and coma. Nonneurologic multiorgan dysfunctions are also common and may include congestive heart failure, cardiac arrhythmias, hepatic necrosis, hypokalemia, respiratory alkalosis, metabolic acidosis, and hypovolemic shock. Rhabdomyolosis, disseminated intravascular coagulation, and acute renal failure may occur in older adults, but are more common in exertional heatstroke typically seen in younger athletes.

Treatment

Heatstroke is a medical emergency, requiring prompt and aggressive therapy. Rapid cooling is essential since its pathophysiology involves thermoregulatory failure rather than a reset thermostat point. Field management must include removal of clothing, cooling the patient's skin with cold water or ice packs, and transfer to cooler setting. Cool intravenous fluids should be considered, but oral hydration may lead to aspiration. Other effective cooling techniques include ice-water baths, cold water gastrointestinal lavage, or the administration of cool water followed by warm air to promote evaporation. Irrespective of the technique chosen, speed is of the essence with careful continuous monitoring in order to prevent hypothermic overshoot. Careful fluid balance management and cardiovascular monitoring are also essential. However, given the high prevalence and mortality associated with heatstroke, preventive measures are extremely important. Above all, vulnerable older adults, as well as their families and neighbors must be educated as regards both the seriousness of this problem and commonsense strategies, which can help reduce its toll.

Orthostasis, Meals, and Hypovolemia

An ability to appropriately respond to the challenge of assuming the upright posture is absolutely critical to remaining independent. Under normal conditions, significant or symptomatic orthostatic hypotension is rare among healthy older adults (Chapter 57, Syncope). However, aging does blunt the ability of older individuals to defend against more major hemodynamic challenges, especially among frail individuals, in the presence of significant comorbidity and following exposure to multiple provocative factors (Chapter 88, Disorders of Fluid Balance; Chapter 74, Aging CVS). The presence of hypertension increases the risk of hypotension by decreasing baroreceptor sensitivity and ventricular compliance beyond declines observed in normal aging. Use of hypotensive medications, as well as the presence of diseases such as for example diabetes mellitus, aortic stenosis, and Parkinson's disease, are all important risk factors. Some risk factors can be synergistic as seen with a modest diuretic-induced sodium depletion, which can induce orthostatic hypotension in previously well-compensated healthy old adults. Similarly, while meal ingestion induces only negligible and asymptomatic blood pressure changes in most healthy older adults, frail elderly nursing home residents may develop symptomatic postprandial hypotension, which may even contribute to altered mental status and syncope.

Hyperglycemia and Hypoglycemia

Aging has been shown to be associated with glucose intolerance. Even in healthy individuals who do not meet criteria for diabetes mellitus or for impaired glucose tolerance, aging is associated with a dramatic slowing in the return of glucose levels back to normal following a glucose ingestion. In contrast, most healthy older adults are able to respond adequately to hyperglycemia. Nevertheless, diabetes, malnutrition, medications, as well as a number of comorbidities may significantly attenuate older adults' ability to recover from a hypoglycemic episode (Chapter 107, Aging Endocrine System; Chapter 109, Diabetes).

Fluid Challenge and Dehydration

When given a major water challenge, older adults tend to have greater difficulty in appropriately diluting their urine. While less well studied, declines in GFR (glomerular filtration rate) tend to compromise the ability of the aged kidney to deal effectively with a sodium load.

Difficulties with water disposal can predispose older individuals to develop hyponatremia, while decreased capacity to adapt to increased salt load may contribute to dependent edema, nocturia, hypertension, and congestive heart failure. The aged body's capacity to prevent dehydration is also affected. Aging is associated with a decreased sensation of thirst even in the setting of significant dehydration. Moreover, aging is associated with a delay in the time required for the kidney to appropriately concentrate urine in response to sodium restriction. Large numbers of medications, as well as the presence of significant comorbidity, can further enhance the clinical impact of these aging-related changes (Chapter 88, Disorders of Fluid Balance).

Bladder Outlet Obstruction

Bladder outlet obstruction is a relatively common complication of benign prostatic hyperplasia and older men with this problem are much more likely to develop urinary retention with detrusor decompensation than are their younger counterparts. Normally, during a compensatory phase, bladder emptying is maintained with an increased bladder muscle mass, mostly caused by hypertrophy of individual muscle cells. During a subsequent decompensation phase, the bladder undergoes muscle loss, collagen infiltration, and axonal degeneration. Aging appears to increase the likelihood of detrusor decompensation, with its associated degenerative changes (Chapter 55, Incontinence).

Major Burns and Trauma

For any given total percentage of body surface burned, advanced age contributes to a measurable decrease in survival. Such systemic vulnerability has been attributed to a combination of progressive reductions in the function of many organs, together with simultaneous reductions in varied homeostatic capabilities and functional impairments associated with specific disease states. In spite of remarkable improvements in the perioperative care of older adults, older individuals have significantly worse outcomes that their younger counterparts following burns, road traffic injuries, and head trauma. While more research is needed, this differential vulnerability may be related to the catastrophic nature of these events, as well as underlying vulnerabilities and presence of significant comorbidity (Chapter 68, Brain Trauma; Chapter 37, Surgery).

Altered Physical Activity

Older adults are particularly vulnerable to the loss of function and the development of individual adverse events following bed rest. With immobilization, muscle mass can be lost at a rate of up to 5% a week, which together with disruptions in subcellular muscle structure, can result in losses in muscle strength, which may approach 40% by 6 weeks. When unloaded, aged muscle cells are more likely to atrophy or to degenerate via apoptotic mechanisms. Strategies, which can diminish the impact of bed rest, include opting for minimally invasive surgery whenever possible, rapid mobilization following surgery or injury, exercise, nutritional supplementation, as well as efforts to decrease offending medications and to address relevant comorbidity. Increased physical activity represents an extremely attractive option since contrary to conventional wisdom, even frail institutionalized older adults are able to benefit from exercise, experiencing significant benefits in terms of muscle mass, muscle performance, and improvements in relevant homeostatic mechanisms (Chapter 29, Rehabilitation; Chapter 114, Exercise; Chapter 115, Mobility).

Anticholinergic Medications

While systematic literature is lacking, older adults appear to be highly sensitive to anticholinergic effects of commonly used medications including altered cognitive function, dry mouth, constipation, and urinary retention. Some of this vulnerability can be attributed to the presence of underlying disease or preclinical pathology. For example, subjects with Alzheimer's disease develop new learning deficits at lower scopolamine doses than do age-adjusted normal controls, while the presence of detrusor underactivity predisposes older adults to develop urinary retention when treated with anticholinergic agents. However, aging in itself contributes to an enhanced anticholinergic vulnerability as shown by the presence of an augmented and prolonged inhibition of stimulated parotid flow rate in healthy older adults following exposure to an intravenous anticholinergic drug (glycopyrrolate). Increased blood–brain permeability in old age and in the setting of specific diseases has been proposed as one mechanism that could mediate an augmented vulnerability to develop cognitive or other CNS problems with anticholinergic medications. Other relevant contributing mechanisms include a decreased homeostatic capacity with declines in both numbers and complexity of relevant cellular elements, as well as an aging-associated loss in the ability of muscarinic receptors to be upregulated when exposed to anticholinergic agents (Chapter 8, Pharmacology; Chapter 53, Delirium; Chapter 55, Incontinence; Chapter 63, Psychoactive Drugs).

Antidopaminergic Medications

Older adults often develop extrapyramidal side effects when given neuroleptic agents with potent antidopaminergic properties. Interestingly, adverse events such as acute dystonia are relatively rare in old age, while others including rigidity, poverty of movement, and tardive dyskinesia appear to be more common in old age. In many cases, early or preclinical Parkinson's disease may render individuals more vulnerable to pharmacological disruption of relevant CNS dopaminergic circuits. Moreover, aging-associated declines in numbers and function of CNS dopaminergic neurons, as well as a decreased capacity to compensate for additional losses by upregulation of dopaminergic receptors or by neuronal plasticity involving surviving dopaminergic fibers, are also likely to contribute to the loss of such homeostatic mechanisms (Chapter 63, Psychoactive Drugs; Chapter 66, Parkinson's Disease).

Neuronal Degeneration

Past dogma has held that aging is associated with a significant, progressive, and inevitable decline in all categories of neurons. In recent years, this pessimistic view has been greatly modified with evidence of selective neuronal vulnerability, as well as dramatic demonstrations of the brain's continued plasticity throughout the lifespan. The observation that specific neurons and neural circuits are vulnerable to aging- and disease-associated declines, while others are quite resistant, has raised considerable hope for the development of physiologically sound interventions, which could help maintain normal neural function into old age. First, evidence of selective neural vulnerability raises the possibility of developing interventions designed to specifically target the most vulnerable cellular elements. Second, many decades of research have demonstrated the presence of neuronal plasticity, in particular collateral sprouting, the formation of new nerve terminals by intact nerve cells, which represents a compensatory homeostatic mechanism with the potential of maintaining normal function following declines in neural circuits, which are similar and in near proximity. Collateral sprouting involving peripheral and central nerve cells tends to decline in old age, yet the ability of modifiable factors such as hormonal levels and nerve activity or experience to influence this category of neural plasticity raises hope

for the development of effective interventions (Chapter 61, Aging Brain).

ACKNOWLEDGMENT

GAK would like to acknowledge the contribution of Dr Itamar Abrass who authored CH. 124, Disorders of Temperature Regulation in the previous edition.

FURTHER READING

Ahn AC, Tewari M, Poon CS, Phillips RS. The limits of reductionism in medicine: could systems biology offer an alternative? *PLoS Med.* 2006;3(6):e208.

Bloomfield SA. Changes in musculoskeletal structure and function with prolonged bed rest. *Med Sci Sports Exerc.* 1997;29(2):197–206.

Bouchama A, Knochel JP. Heat stroke. *N Engl J Med.* 2002;346(25):1978–1988.

Burke SN, Barnes CA. Neural plasticity in the ageing brain. *Nat Rev Neurosci.* 2006;7(1):30–40.

Cannon WB. The aging of homeostatic mechanisms. In: Cannon WB, ed. *The Wisdom of the Body.* New York, New York; W.W.Norton & Co. 1932:202–215.

Carpenter RH. Homeostasis: a plea for a unified approach. *Adv Physiol Educ.* 2004; 28(1–4):180–187.

Collier TJ, Lipton J, Daley BF, et al. Aging-related changes in the nigrostriatal dopamine system and the response to MPTP in nonhuman primates: diminished compensatory mechanisms as a prelude to parkinsonism. *Neurobiol Dis.* 2007;26(1):56–65.

Collins KJ, Dore C, Exton-Smith AN, Fox RH, MacDonald IC, Woodward PM. Accidental hypothermia and impaired temperature homoeostasis in the elderly. *Br Med J.* 1977;1(6057):353–356.

Collins KJ, Exton-Smith AN. 1983 Henderson Award Lecture. Thermal homeostasis in old age. *J Am Geriatr Soc.* 1983;31(9):519–524.

Crutcher KA. Aging and neuronal plasticity: lessons from a model. *Auton Neurosci.* 2002;96(1):25–32.

Danzl DF, Pozos RS. Current concepts: accidental hypothermia. *N Engl J Med.* 1994;331:1756–1760.

Deschenes MR, Britt AA, Chandler WC. A comparison of the effects of unloading in young adult and aged skeletal muscle. *Med Sci Sports Exerc.* 2001;33(9):1477–1483.

Dharmarajan TS, Manalo MG, Manalac MM, Kanagala M. Hypothermia in the nursing home: adverse outcomes in two older men. *J Am Med Dir Assoc.* 2001;2(1):29–33.

Dickstein DL, Kabaso D, Rocher AB, Luebke JI, Wearne SL, Hof PR. Changes in the structural complexity of the aged brain. *Aging Cell.* 2007;6(3):275–284.

Donaldson GC, Keatinge WR, Saunders RD. Cardiovascular responses to heat stress and their adverse consequences in healthy and vulnerable human populations. *Int J Hyperthermia.* 2003;19(3):225–235.

Douglas A, Morris J. It was not just a heatwave! Neuroleptic malignant-like syndrome in a patient with Parkinson's disease. *Age Ageing.* 2006;35(6):640–641.

Epstein M, Hollenberg NK. Age as a determinant of renal sodium conservation in normal man. *J Lab Clin Med.* 1976;87(3):411–417.

Evans E, Rendell M, Bartek J, et al. Thermally-induced cutaneous vasodilatation in aging. *J Gerontol.* 1993;48(2):M53-M57.

Feller I, Flora JD, Jr, Bawol R. Baseline results of therapy for burned patients. *JAMA.* 1976;236(17):1943–1947.

Fiatarone MA, O'Neill EF, Ryan ND, et al. Exercise training and nutritional supplementation for physical frailty in very elderly people. *N Engl J Med.* 1994; 330:1769–1775.

Fox RH, Woodward PM, Exton-Smith AN, Green MF, Donnison DV, Wicks MH. Body temperatures in the elderly: a national study of physiological, social, and environmental conditions. *Br Med J.* 1973;1(5847):200–206.

Fried LP, Storer DJ, King DE, Lodder F. Diagnosis of illness presentation in the elderly. *J Am Geriatr Soc.* 1991;39(2):117–123.

Ghezzi EM, Ship JA. Aging and secretory reserve capacity of major salivary glands. *J Dent Res.* 2003;82(10):844–848.

Goligorsky MS. The concept of cellular "fight-or-flight" reaction to stress. *Am J Physiol Renal Physiol.* 2001;280(4):F551-F561.

Gosling JA, Kung LS, Dixon JS, Horan P, Whitbeck C, Levin RM. Correlation between the structure and function of the rabbit urinary bladder following partial outlet obstruction. *J Urol.* 2000;163(4):1349–1356.

Grande F, Visscher MB. *Claude Bernard and Experimental Medicine.* Schenkman Cambridge, MA; Publishing Company, Inc. 1967.

Heat-related mortality—Arizona, 1993–2002, and United States, 1979–2002. *MMWR Morb Mortal Wkly Rep.*2005;54(25):628–630.

Hof PR, Morrison JH. The aging brain: morphomolecular senescence of cortical circuits. *Trends Neurosci.* 2004;27(10):607–613.

Hypothermia-related deaths—United States, 1999–2002 and 2005. *MMWR Morb Mortal Wkly Rep.* 2006:17;55(10):282–284.

Inouye SK, Studenski S, Tinetti ME, Kuchel GA. Geriatric syndromes: clinical, research, and policy implications of a core geriatric concept. *J Am Geriatr Soc.* 2007;55(5):780–791.

Jacobs DG. Special considerations in geriatric injury. *Curr Opin Crit Care.* 2003;9(6):535–539.

Jacobsen SJ, Jacobson DJ, Girman CJ, et al. Natural history of prostatism: risk factors for acute urinary retention. *J Urol.* 1997;158(2):481–487.

Jansen ASP, Nguyen XV, Karpitskiy V, Mettenleiter TC, Loewy AD. Central command neurons of the sympathetic nervous system: basis of the fight-or-flight response. *Science.* 1995;270:644–646.

Kay GG, bou-Donia MB, Messer WS, Jr., Murphy DG, Tsao JW, Ouslander JG. Antimuscarinic drugs for overactive bladder and their potential effects on cognitive function in older patients. *J Am Geriatr Soc.* 2005;53(12):2195–2201.

Khan S, Plummer M, Martinez-Arizala A, Banovac K. Hypothermia in patients with chronic spinal cord injury. *J Spinal Cord Med.* 2007;30(1):27–30.

Kilbourne EM, Choi K, Jones TS, Thacker SB. Risk factors for heatstroke. A case–control study. *JAMA.* 1982;247(24):3332–3336.

Kilbourne EM. Heat-related illness: current status of prevention efforts. *Am J Prev Med.* 2002;22(4):328–329.

Kilbourne EM. The spectrum of illness during heat waves. *Am J Prev Med.* 1999;16(4):359–360.

Kohan AD, Danziger M, Vaughan ED, Jr, Felsen D. Effect of aging on bladder function and the response to outlet obstruction in female rats. *Urol Res.* 2000;28(1):33–37.

Kuchel GA, Cowen T. The aged sympathetic nervous system. In: Hof PR, Mobbs CV, eds. *Functional Neurobiology of Aging.* San Diego, CA: Academic Press; 2001:929–939.

Kuchel GA, Hof PR. *Autonomic Nervous System in Old Age.* Basel: Karger Press; 2004.

Lee WY, Cameron PA, Bailey MJ. Road traffic injuries in the elderly. *Emerg Med J.* 2006;23(1):42–46.

Leeuwenburgh C, Gurley CM, Strotman BA, Dupont-Versteegden EE. Age-related differences in apoptosis with disuse atrophy in soleus muscle. *Am J Physiol Regul Integr Comp Physiol.* 2005;288(5):R1288-R1296.

Lipsitz LA, Fullerton KJ. Postprandial blood pressure reduction in healthy elderly. *J Am Geriatr Soc.* 1986;34(4):267–270.

Lipsitz LA, Goldberger AL. Loss of 'complexity' and aging: potential applications of fractals and chaos theory to senescence. *JAMA.* 1992;267:1806–1809.

Lipsitz LA. Dynamics of stability: the physiologic basis of functional health and frailty. *J Gerontol A Biol Sci Med Sci.* 2002;57(3):B115-B125.

Mattson MP, Magnus T. Ageing and neuronal vulnerability. *Nat Rev Neurosci.* 2006;7(4):278–294.

McGill V, Kowal-Vern A, Gamelli RL. Outcome for older burn patients. *Arch Surg.* 2000;135(3):320–325.

Mercer JB. Cold—an underrated risk factor for health. *Environ Res.* 2003;92(1):8–13.

Norman AB, Battaglia G, Creese I. Differential recovery rates of rat D2 dopamine receptors as a function of aging and chronic reserpine treatment following irreversible modification: a key to receptor regulatory mechanisms. *J Neurosci.* 1987;7(5):1484–1491.

Okazaki K, Kamijo Y, Takeno Y, Okumoto T, Masuki S, Nose H. Effects of exercise training on thermoregulatory responses and blood volume in older men. *J Appl Physiol.* 2002;93(5):1630–1637.

Pedigo NW Jr. Pharmacological adaptations and muscarinic receptor plasticity in hypothalamus of senescent rats treated chronically with cholinergic drugs. *Psychopharmacology (Berl),* 1988;95(4):497–501.

Phillips PA, Rolls BJ, Ledingham JG, et al. Reduced thirst after water deprivation in healthy elderly men. *N Engl J Med.* 1984;311(12):753–759.

Reuler JB. Hypothermia: pathophysiology, clinical settings, and management. *Ann Intern Med.* 1978;89(4):519–527.

Richardson D, Tyra J, McCray A. Attenuation of the cutaneous vasoconstrictor response to cold in elderly men. *J Gerontol.* 1992;47(6):M211-M214.

Rowe JW, Kahn RL. Human aging: usual and successful. *Science.* 1987;237:143–149.

Rowe JW. Health care of the elderly. *N Engl J Med.* 1985;312(13):827–835.

Scremin G, Kenney WL. Aging and the skin blood flow response to the unloading of baroreceptors during heat and cold stress. *J Appl Physiol.* 2004;96(3):1019–1025.

Seeman TE, McEwen BS, Rowe JW, Singer BH. Allostatic load as a marker of cumulative biological risk: MacArthur studies of successful aging. *Proc Natl Acad Sci USA.* 2001;98(8):4770–4775.

Semenza JC, Rubin CH, Falter KH, et al. Heat-related deaths during the July 1995 heat wave in Chicago. *N Engl J Med.* 1996;335(2):84–90.

Shannon RP, Wei JY, Rosa RM, Epstein FH, Rowe JW. The effect of age and sodium depletion on cardiovascular response to orthostasis. *Hypertension.* 1986;8(5):438–443.

Smolander J. Effect of cold exposure on older humans. *Int J Sports Med.* 2002;23(2):86–92.

Sullivan-Bolyai JZ, Lumish RM, Smith EW, et al. Hyperpyrexia due to air-conditioning failure in a nursing home. *Public Health Rep.* 1979;94(5):466–470.

Sunderland T, Tariot PN, Cohen RM, Weingartner H, Mueller EA, III, Murphy DL. Anticholinergic sensitivity in patients with dementia of the Alzheimer type and age-matched controls. A dose–response study. *Arch Gen Psychiatry.* 1987;44(5):418–426.

Taylor JA, Kuchel GA. Detrusor underactivity: clinical features and pathogenesis of an underdiagnosed geriatric condition. *J Am Geriatr Soc.* 2006;54(12):1920–1933.

Testa JA, Malec JF, Moessner AM, Brown AW. Outcome after traumatic brain injury: effects of aging on recovery. *Arch Phys Med Rehabil.* 2005;86(9):1815–1823.

Yates FE. Complexity of a human being: changes with age. *Neurobiol Aging.* 2002;23(1):17–19.

Yates FE. Self-organizing systems. In: Boyd CAR, Noble R, eds. *The Logic of Life—The Challenge of Integrative Physiology.* New York: Oxford University Press; 1993:189–218.

Yu HJ, Levin RM, Longhurst PA, Damaser MS. Effect of age and outlet resistance on rabbit urinary bladder emptying. *J Urol.* 1997;158(3 Pt 1):924–930.

Frailty

Linda P. Fried ■ *Jeremy D. Walston* ■ *Luigi Ferrucci*

FRAILTY IS AT THE CORE OF GERIATRIC MEDICINE

The cornerstone, even raison d'etre, of geriatric medicine concerns the identification, evaluation, and treatment of frail older adults and prevention of loss of independence and other outcomes for which they are at risk. The proportion of frail within the older population is high and will increase with the aging of society. A focus on frailty has been a consistent theme in geriatric theory and practice. In 1990, Fretwell stated "frailty in an individual (is) defined as an inherent vulnerability to challenge from the environment." Because of the high-risk status of frail older adults, geriatric medicine seeks to intervene in frail patients to prevent or minimize illness and dependency. In 1992, a conference on the physiologic basis of frailty agreed that controversy on definition and limited understanding of etiology hindered preventive strategies. In 1993, W. Bortz stated that "A major threat to active life expectancy is the development of frailty.... Despite absence of easy categorization, there is no question as to the immense participation of frailty in both individual and composite morbidity and mortality. Recognizing this pervasive impact on well-being, it is strange to note the lack of critical insight that attends it." Baltes and Smith observed that the oldest old, those in the "fourth age" after 85 years (in developed countries), are particularly biologically vulnerable and frail and have compromised ability to tolerate stressors. As a result, their well-being is increasingly dependent on the use of extrinsic compensations to maintain life and autonomy, because there is such diminished ability to compensate physiologically. These observations frame the conceptual understanding that aging is associated with increased likelihood of frailty, and that older persons have reduced physiological reserve than younger persons and these changes are likely independent of disease. Over the past 15 to 20 years since the statements above, we have attained increasing clarity about the definition and characteristics of frailty and its import and etiology, and a new basis for prevention and interventions. This chapter seeks to synthesize this knowledge.

Geriatric medicine has found the concept of frailty compelling for several reasons (Table 52-1). First, frail individuals are perceived to constitute those older adults at highest risk for a number of adverse health outcomes, including disability, dependency, institutionalization, falls, injuries, acute illness, hospitalizations, slow or incomplete recovery from illness and/or hospitalization, and mortality.

Additionally, they have compromised ability to tolerate hospitalization or invasive procedures and are at high risk of related complications.

Second, frail older adults are thought to be a subset in high need of health care and community and informal support services, as well as long-term care. These special needs were the main basis for the development of comprehensive geriatric assessment and creation of specific geriatric systems for care delivery as optimal clinical approaches to decreasing preventable adverse outcomes for frail older adults. The provision of care for this increasing subgroup of frail individuals is a critical clinical and public health concern. Although some decry the increased costs anticipated as the numbers of frail older adults increase, others, particularly in geriatric medicine, propose that redesign of health care delivery to optimize outcomes in these vulnerable older adults will lead to a health care system specifically tailored to chronic care delivery and, if so, less costly. The ability of the health care system to care effectively for those who are frail, and even to prevent frailty, will depend on our ability to grow a geriatrically expert, adequately sized clinical work force, and to provide appropriate economic incentives, recognizing that caring for frail older people requires exceptional skills and is extremely time-consuming.

Third, the prevalence of frailty is high, with estimates ranging from 10% to 25% of persons aged 65 years and older, with as many as 30% to 45% of those aged 85 years and older identified as frail. Such estimates are based on clinical perceptions of a notable change in vulnerability, health status, and clinical appearance with age in a substantial subset of older adults that is not explained by disease alone. These changes are often reported by family and friends of patients, as well as clinicians, when they describe the patient as

TABLE 52-1

Frailty is at the Core of Geriatric Medicine

1. Frail older persons are at risk for multiple adverse health outcomes, including
   a. Medical instability
   b. Disability, dependency
   c. Institutionalization
   d. Injuries
   e. Falls
   f. Acute illness
   g. Hospitalization
   h. Health care resources utilization
   i. Slow or incomplete recovery from illness and/or hospitalization
   j. High risk of iatrogenesis and side effects from medical interventions
   k. Mortality
2. The prevalence of frailty increases dramatically with age.
3. Frailty is manifested as an impaired ability to cope with challenges in health and reduced ability to regain a stable health status, possibly related to reduced functional reserve. Severity of frailty spans from subclinical to a clinical stage to impending death.
4. In aging individuals, the variability in health and functional status is explained less and less by the effect of clinically evident or even subclinical diseases. Older age is associated with increased vulnerability to multiple diseases with no evident pathogenetic connections. Such global vulnerability is not explained by changes in recognizable risk factors.
5. Frail older persons require intensive and multidimensional continuous care and have high need of community and informal support services. These care needs necessitate a shift in the deployment of heath care resources.
6. Geriatrics is a medical specialty particularly skilled in care of frail older adults.

"appearing" frail. This condition includes a composite image of loss of muscle mass, weakness, slowed pace of movement, decreased activity and engagement, and possibly unexplained weight loss—often in combination. This clinical characterization is supported by an extensive literature summarized by Ferrucci et al. (Table 52-2).

Fourth, it is thought that the increased risk of adverse outcomes associated with frailty is a result of an increased vulnerability to stressors itself caused by a decreased ability to maintain homeostasis when the individual is stressed. Stressors can be intrinsic, such as infection, or extrinsic, such as change in environment. There is some evidence to suggest that, in addition to those who already appear frail clinically, a subset of older individuals have subclinical frailty, i.e., have increased vulnerability to adverse outcomes in the face of stressors but without the clinical stigmata of frailty or any of its outcomes. Further, some clinical reports indicate that there is a subset of older adults with advanced frailty stigmata and significant outcomes, particularly disability or dependency, who have lost reserves and resilience to a point that they have a very high likelihood of dying within 6 to 12 months, and are quite unlikely to respond to therapies, including rehabilitative therapies. These differentiations of vulnerability—with or without the clinical appearance of frailty and its sequelae—are consistent with the idea of a continuum of frailty among older adults as a core component underlying the heterogeneity of health status observed with increasing age (Figure 52-1).

This continuum of frailty incorporates what is thought clinically to be a distinct causal pathway to disability, with frailty being a major etiologic risk factor independent of disease (Figure 52-2).

Note that the causal pathway from frailty to disability has not been considered in the conceptualization of the causal pathway to disability proposed by the World Health Organization and the Institute of Medicine, which map the effect of specific diseases and impairments. In contrast, conceptually, a survey in six U.S. academic centers and one in Great Britain indicated that 98% of geriatricians (both faculty and postdoctoral fellows) thought that frailty and disability were separate, but causally related, conditions; 90% of the

TABLE 52-2

Reported Components of the Frailty Syndrome

REFERENCE	MOBILITY	STRENGTH	BALANCE	MOTOR PROCESSING	COGNITION	NUTRITION	ENDURANCE	PHYSICAL ACTIVITY
Winograd CH et al.	X				X	X		X
Ory MG et al.	X	X	X		X		X	
Pendergast DR et al.		X	X	X			X	
Rockwood K et al.					X			X
Tinetti ME et al.	X	X						
Gill TM et al.	X		X					
Campbell AJ et al.		X	X	X	X	X	X	
Dayhoff NE et al.		X	X					
Strawbridge WJ et al.	X				X	X		
Chin APMJ et al.						X		X
Vellas B et al.		X				X	X	X
Brown M et al.	X	X	X	X				
Fried LP et al.	X	X				X	X	X
Saliba D et al.	X							

Ferrucci L, Guralnik JM, Studenski S, et al. Designing Randomized, Controlled Trials aimed at preventing or delaying functional decline and disability in frail, older person: a consensus report. J Am Ger So. 2004;52:625–634.

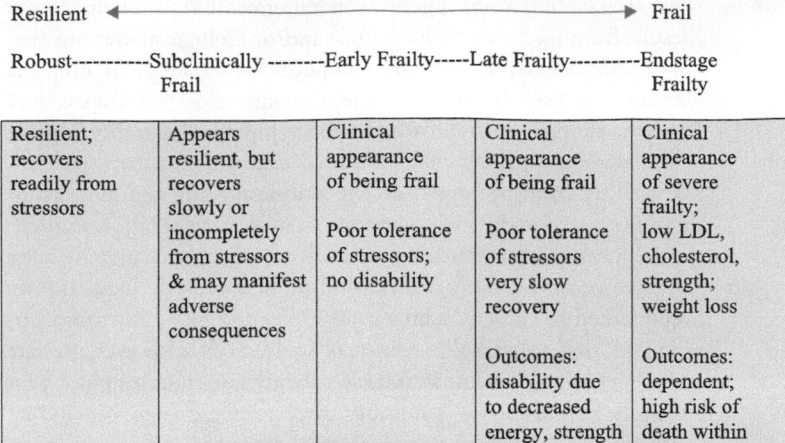

Resilient ◄———————————————► Frail

Robust———————Subclinically————————Early Frailty———Late Frailty——————Endstage
                Frail   Frailty

| Resilient; recovers readily from stressors | Appears resilient, but recovers slowly or incompletely from stressors & may manifest adverse consequences | Clinical appearance of being frail

Poor tolerance of stressors; no disability | Clinical appearance of being frail

Poor tolerance of stressors; very slow recovery

Outcomes: disability due to decreased energy, strength | Clinical appearance of severe frailty; low LDL, cholesterol, strength; weight loss

Outcomes: dependent; high risk of death within 12 months |

FIGURE 52-1. Continuum of resilience/frailty in older adults.

geriatricians interviewed thought that frailty caused disability (of which 40% thought that this was usually or always the case), while 88% thought that disability caused frailty (of which 13% thought that this was usually or always the case) (Table 52-3). These close and bidirectional relationships likely cause frequent co-occurrence of frailty and disability and the conceptual confusion of the two.

Increasingly, frailty is thought distinguishable from disability (as an outcome) and comorbidity, although there are overlapping co-prevalences (Figure 52-3).

A fifth reason that the concept of frailty has had saliency for geriatricians is the mounting evidence that there is a decrease with age in the ability of disease alone to explain the increased variation in health status, outcomes, or response to therapy. Measures of subclinical organ system changes and physical functional and cognitive variables, rather than presence or absence of diseases, are the most powerful predictors of longevity and functional outcomes. For example, in the Cardiovascular Health Study, physiological and functional measures, rather than diseases, were significant predictors of 5-year mortality, with the exception of congestive heart failure. In analyses from the Canadian Study of Health and Aging and the Gothenburg H-70 Cohort Study, Rockwood et al. demonstrated that deficit accumulation, from a list of 40 to 51 symptoms, signs, and disabilities as well as diseases, predicts mortality in a linear fashion in relation to a baseline count of deficits, with all deficits weighted equally. In the InCHIANTI study, slow walking speed (<0.8 m/s) was as strong a predictor of mortality as a diagnosis of malignant cancer. Thus, nosologically defined diseases, alone or in combination, are not sufficient to explain functional outcomes in older persons, suggesting that a disease-independent, age-related alteration accounts for the progressively higher variability in health, impairments, prognosis, and outcomes with aging. This condition, if not equivalent to frailty as defined above, is certainly reminiscent of this condition. Age-related frailty may explain why older age is associated with the increased variability in response to treatments, both in terms of

effectiveness and risk of side effects, not explained fully by disease status. The increased risk of iatrogenesis is likely a product of the altered reserves and associated physiologic vulnerabilities that are components of frailty.

Sixth, with increasing age, there is a concurrent, increased susceptibility to multiple chronic diseases that is not explained by "classic" risk factors. This increased susceptibility with no evident pathogenetic connections in risk between the multiple diseases could be related to the progressive collapse of the regulatory network of biological signals aimed at maintaining the homeostatic equilibrium. For example, there is evidence that old age is associated with a low grade, chronic proinflammatory state, which also appears to be causally related to frailty (see further). Physiologic dysregulation with aging in this and many other systems may lead both to aggregate loss of reserves and vulnerability and to disease-specific manifestations such as atherosclerosis. Such associations could lead to correlation between frailty and disease, which does not indicate a true causal association. In some instances, frailty maybe the terminal stage of selected chronic diseases. Overall, as represented by Figure 52-3 and Table 52-3, frailty, comorbid disease, and disability are overlapping, causally related, but distinct entities.

Seventh, given the discussion above, it would appear that frailty is a condition of impending deterioration in health and functional status that requires immediate attention to prevent disability and other associated outcomes. It requires substantial clinical expertise

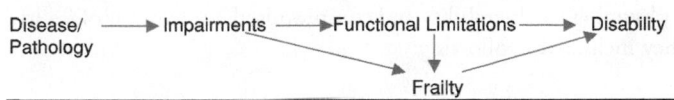

FIGURE 52-2. Causal pathway to disability. *Adapted from multiple sources.*

TABLE 52-3

Geriatricians' Position on the Relationship Between Frailty and Disability (N = 62)

QUESTION	RESPONSE		
		Yes (%)	
	No (%)	Sometimes	Usually/Always
Are frailty and disability the same?	97.5	2.5	—
Is disability a cause of frailty?	12.5	75.0	12.5
Is frailty a cause of disability?	10.0	50.0	40.0

From Fried LP, Ferrucci L, Darer J, Williamson JD, Anderson G. Untangling the concepts of disability, frailty, and comorbidity: implications for improved targeting and care. J Gerontol A Biol Sci Med Sci, 59(3):255–263, 2004.

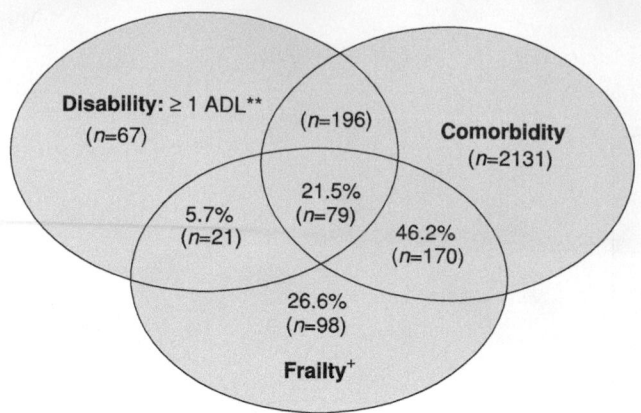

FIGURE 52-3. Venn diagram displaying extent of overlap of frailty with comorbidity (≥2 diseases) and ADL disability in people 65 and older participating in the Cardiovascular Health Study.
Total represented 2762 subjects who had comorbidity and/or disability and/or frailty. N of each subgroup indicated in parentheses. + Frail: overall n = 368 frail subjects (both cohorts). *Comorbidity: overall n = 2576 with 2 or more out of the following 9 diseases: myocardial infarction, angina, congestive heart failure, claudication, arthritis, cancer, diabetes, hypertension, COPD. Of these, 249 were also frail. **Disabled: overall n = 363 with an ADL disability: of these 100 were frail. *From Fried LP, et al: Frailty in older adults: Evidence for a phenotype. From Fried LP, Tangen CM, Walston J, et al. Frailty in older adults: evidence for a phenotype. J Gerontol A Biol Sci Med Sci. 56;M146–M156, 2001.*

to both recognize those who are frail and/or vulnerable, and accurately diagnose and effectively intervene to prevent adverse outcomes or frailty itself. Because of the complexity of presentation, attendant vulnerabilities, and multiple health problems likely to be concurrently present, health care in frail older people needs to be skilled, intensive, and continuous to be effective and, therefore, is intrinsically more expensive. Current U.S. health care models are driven, however, by a unique focus on disease diagnosis and a primary organization for acute, event-driven care, with reimbursement for care heavily driven by specific diagnostic categories. This approach does not permit addressing effectively the complexity of care issues, nor the specialized care required when frailty is also present, or for frailty in the absence of disease. In regards to the former, for example, care for a patient with a hip fracture is erroneously considered the same, regardless of age or frailty status of the individual, with reimbursement the same as well. However, expert geriatric care for a frail older patient with a hip fracture has a greater real cost of caring and likely commensurate benefit. Redesign of care and reimbursement to match the needs of such patients will likely lead to improved care outcomes and potentially decreased overall costs. Overall, postulating the existence of age-related frailty addresses and incorporates all of the issues above, assuming that frailty can be operationalized and recognized in clinical practice.

WHAT IS FRAILTY?

There is strong consensus among geriatricians and gerontologists that frailty is a clinical state of increased vulnerability and decreased ability to maintain homeostasis that is age-related and centrally characterized by declines in functional reserves across multiple physiologic systems. This vulnerability is age-related and also related to, but distinct from, disability and disease states (see Table 52-3 and

Figures 52-2 and 52-3). There is general agreement as well that frailty results from underlying physiologic and/or biologic alterations that are age-associated and maybe compounded by single or multiple diseases, or even be an end-stage outcome of severe disease. Key systems thought to be involved in development of frailty include musculoskeletal, hormonal, immune, and inflammatory systems, with likely contributions from the autonomic and central nervous systems. Sarcopenia, or loss of muscle mass with aging, is thought to be a central manifestation of frailty. In fact, a change in body composition with a progressive decline in lean body mass, mostly represented by muscle, is an almost obligatory manifestation of aging and, past a threshold severity, of frailty itself. However, the rate of age-associated decline in muscle strength and muscle mass is profoundly modulated by a number of physiologic factors including inflammation, hormones, neurological integrity, nutritional status and physical activity, along with other contributors. It is noteworthy that the multiple physiologic systems that affect sarcopenia are also thought to contribute to generalized dysfunction that is aging-related, an issue well beyond sarcopenia itself. This is consistent with the theory proposing that it is the aggregate dysregulation of many systems that results in the vulnerability and clinical presentation of frailty more than the dysregulation of any one system.

One way to understand frailty is by comparison with the traditional concept of disease. Traditionally, diseases are defined by symptoms, signs, and pathophysiologic mechanisms. Specific diseases impair selected aspects of the homeostatic equilibrium that is essential for life. A large variety of stressors continuously challenge the homeostatic equilibrium and facilitate the emergence of diseases. Health is characterized by a perfect equilibrium between stressors and homeostatic mechanisms (Figure 52-4A). Diseases emerge when specific physiological system(s) or anatomical structure(s) are impaired and pose an entropic challenge that cannot be fully counteracted by homeostatic mechanisms. This is typical of young and middle age, where diseases are stochastic, somewhat "rare" events that often target a specific mechanism (Figure 52-4B). For example, a brain hemorrhage is unlikely to occur in a healthy, young individual unless there is clear cause (malignant hypertension, aneurysms etc). In old age, this can more easily result from a combination of multiple processes that include both strong entropic challenges and thinning of the mechanisms that maintain the homeostatic equilibrium (Figure 52-4C). Under the assumption that homeostatic mechanisms are general, it is more difficult with aging to recognize a specific pathophysiological mechanism for each disease and clinical presentation maybe atypical. As a result, treatment of specific diseases one by one is less likely to be successful. Understanding the causes of derangement of the homeostatic mechanisms and possibly correcting them is more likely to be beneficial than targeted treatment or a specific system. According to this interpretation, prevention in old age may need to be focused on reinforcing homeostatic mechanisms rather on risk factors for specific diseases. This is compatible with the idea that change in nutrition and exercise are the only interventions that have been shown to prevent disability.

There are several dominant theories as to the underlying causes of physiologic vulnerability and compromised homeostasis of frailty. They include the following:

1. Frailty comes from accumulation of potentially unrelated diseases, subclinical dysfunctions, and disability across organs, parts, and systems of the body. This approach has been posited by Rockwood and colleagues, who have operationalized this theory in

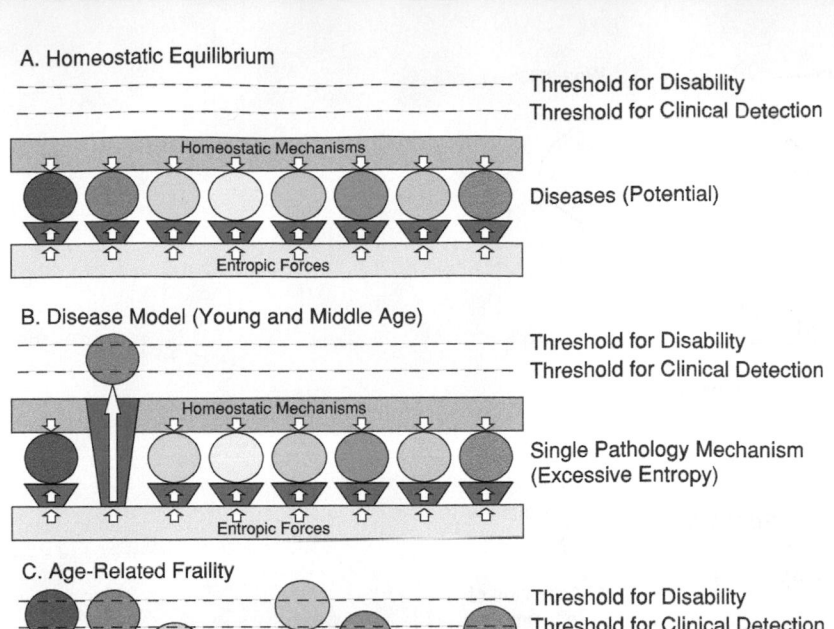

A. Homeostatic Equilibrium

Threshold for Disability
Threshold for Clinical Detection

Homeostatic Mechanisms

Diseases (Potential)

Entropic Forces

B. Disease Model (Young and Middle Age)

Threshold for Disability
Threshold for Clinical Detection

Homeostatic Mechanisms

Single Pathology Mechanism
(Excessive Entropy)

Entropic Forces

C. Age-Related Frailty

Threshold for Disability
Threshold for Clinical Detection

Risk Accumulation and Homeostatic
Mechanisms Disfunction

Entropic Forces

FIGURE 52-4. Diseases in young and old age. Homeostatic equilibrium is maintained by robust function and interconnections between multiple physiologic systems (A). When one system is dysregulated or impaired, as in a specific disease, disability can result in the specific areas of function affected by the disease (B). The derangement of general homeostatic mechanisms characteristic of frailty induces a multiple systems impairment which emerges clinically as frailty as well as development of multiple diseases and complex patterns of disability (C).

terms of a summary of all potential deficits present in an individual (symptoms, signs, diseases, geriatric conditions, laboratory abnormalities, disabilities); a simple count of all such deficits assessed has been shown to predict mortality. This approach indicates that a summary measure of deficit accumulation across many different types of health conditions at many levels (functional, clinical, physiological) predicts risk of mortality. Inferentially, frailty is an intermediary, almost latent, construct that is the summary effect of all of these deficits on homeostatic reserves; the number of deficits leads to a dose–response relationship with mortality, presumably through this intermediary mechanism.

2. Frailty is a unique pathophysiological process: This theory posits that frailty can be characterized as a primary defect, which involves the diminution of physiologic function and, eventually, breakdown of homeostatic mechanisms. This could result from alterations in a range of basic biological mechanisms, which then lead to dysregulation of multiple physiologic systems. These systems are known to mutually affect each other, providing a rich network of homeostatic regulation and ability to compensate, to a degree, if any one system is impaired. This redundant network, with intact function within and between systems, underlies reserves and resiliency to stressors (Figure 52-5A). Dysregulation of multiple systems with aging, and decreased effectiveness of interconnections (Figure 52-5B) could lead to depletion of reserves and compromised ability to maintain homeostasis in the face of stressors. Ultimately, this could lead to a negative spiral of declining function. Basic biological systems involved may well include those that maintain a stable production, distribution, and utilization of energy, while key physiologic systems include hormones, immune, inflammatory, and neurological processes. Decreased energy available would diffusely affect multiple physiological systems, leading to compromised function both within and between systems. Further, decreased availability of energy

could underlie decline in physical function, especially in tasks requiring endurance (Figure 52-6). A similar scenario could occur as a result of other basic biological alterations with aging, such as shortened telomeres or excessive free radical damage. Alternatively, or additionally, frailty may result from a progressive loss of complexity in the function of individual physiologic systems and in their regulation of homeostatic responses, leading to both chronic over- or underfunction.

The complexity of the homeostatic network in a healthy organism allows rapid and flexible adaptations to different types and intensities of internal and external perturbations. The more specific the response, the more rapid and efficient the adaptation. With aging, the range of adaptive strategies may progressively become limited, up to the point that the normal state of redundancy is lost and any perturbation is addressed with a more limited number of stereotypic

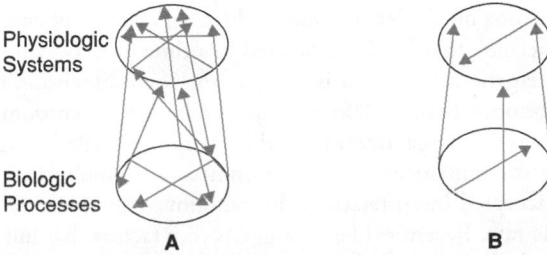

Physiologic
Systems

Biologic
Processes

A   B

FIGURE 52-5. Conceptual summary of interconnections between biologic and physiologic systems that comprise a stable homeostatic system, with rich network that offers redundancy and reserves. (A) Robust interconnections between these systems, as indicated by multiple arrows. (B) Many fewer arrows, signifying decreased function of different systems and weakened interconnections, threatening homeostasis. *From Fried LP, Hadley EC, Walston JD, et al. From bedside to bench: research agenda for frailty. Sci Aging Knowledge Environ. 2005(31):pe24, 2005.*

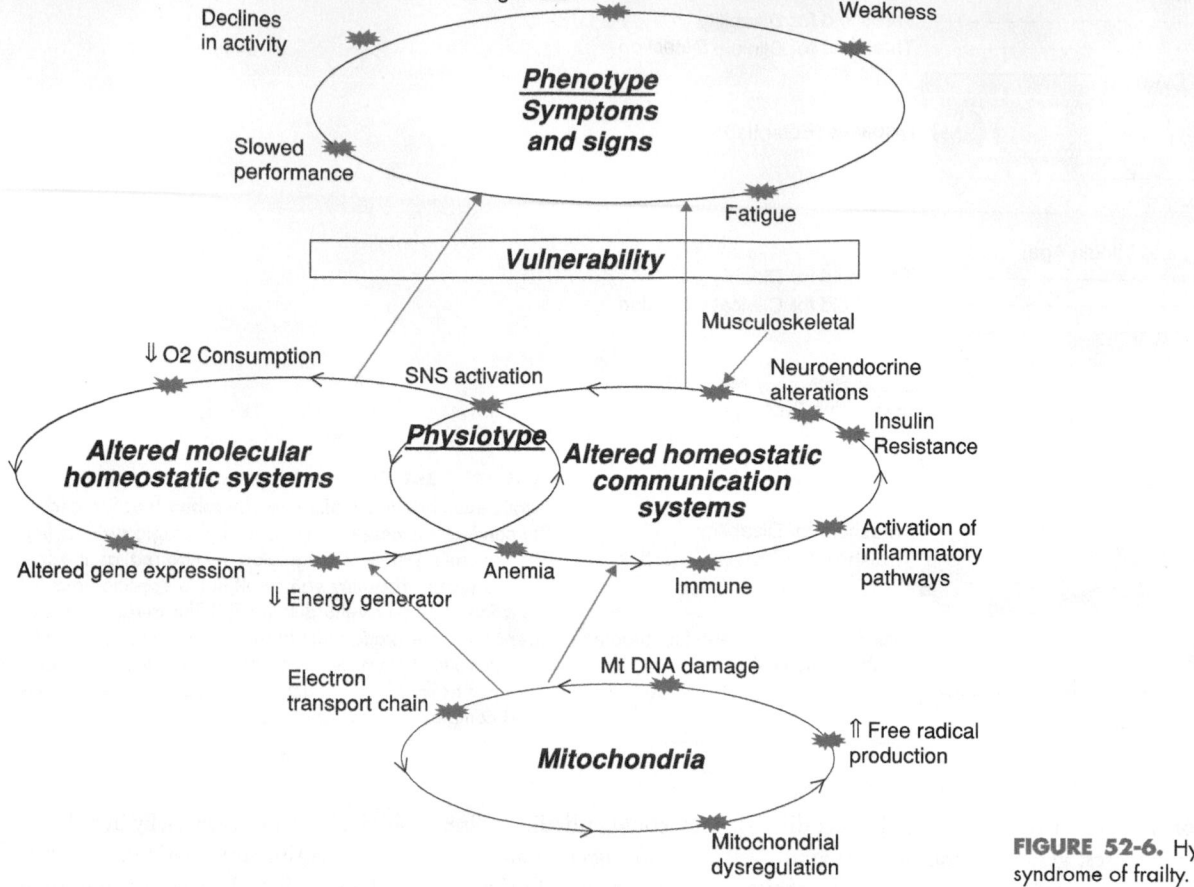

FIGURE 52-6. Hypothesized levels of the syndrome of frailty.

responses. For example, heart rate can decrease or lose the more complex modulations in the frequency domain typically seen in healthy, younger individuals. Similarly, altered energetics could lead to compromised networks and adaptive responses; the former are graphically suggested by the decreased number of arrows linking different physiological and biological systems in Figure 52-5B, compared with Figure 52-5A. Both types of processes could underlie dysfunctions in many physiologic systems, as well as in the communication between systems. Other mechanisms may also be at issue.

Building on a scientific paradigm of frailty previously proposed by Buchner et al. and Fried and Walston, Ferrucci and Ruggiero have further developed the theory regarding the existence of an energetic pathway to frailty. This theory is summarized in Figure 52-7. The box on the left represents the total amount of energy, or ATP molecules, that can be generated in a time unit. Because most of the energetic metabolism is aerobic, the total dimension of the box can be operationally defined as maximum oxygen consumption (MVO$_2$max). A large amount of this energy is needed simply to maintain the human machine in a homeostatic equilibrium. In a broadly accepted interpretation, this amount of energy is the basal metabolic rate. Recent evidence suggests that factors that influence basal metabolic rate include not only physiological factors but also pathological components. On top of the "minimum requirement for homeostasis," which is a function of age, sex, body composition, and physical activity, we need to consider, especially in an older person, an extra quota of energy required to balance the unstable homeostasis caused by pathology. We may call this extra energy "homeostatic effort." Theoretically, in a healthy individual, the "homeostatic effort"

is negligible but increases rapidly with health status deterioration. There is evidence that the "homeostatic effort" is a risk factor for mortality. The remaining energy in the "box" is used for cognitive and physical activities. This maybe highly diminished if the "homeostatic effort" is high.

Within the range of energy that is used for physical activity, with increasing workload the individual starts experiencing fatigue. The threshold at which fatigue develops is influenced by a number of still undefined factors, which certainly include biological (inflammation, oxidative stress, hormones, anabolic metabolism), psychological, and physiological factors. Efficiency of movement (or, analogously, the efficiency of thinking) also affect the amount of workload that the individual can accomplish before feeling fatigue. Whether the threshold is low or high conditions the level of physical activity in daily life. If fatigue develops for small workloads, the individual is likely to be sedentary. On the contrary, if a high level of workload can be handled without much feeling of fatigue, then the individual will be more physically active.

In the long term, a sedentary state reduces the total amount of energy that can be generated (shrinks the box), thereby triggering a vicious cycle that leads to progressive, accelerated decline in physical function (Figures 52-7 and 52-8). In this model, an active lifestyle is the best preventive strategy to frailty.

A complementary, potentially related theory considers the clinical implications of energy dysregulation in terms of both homeostatic instability and resulting manifestations, including low muscle strength, reduced exercise tolerance, slowed motor speed, further decreased physical activity, increased fatigue, or "exhaustion." Note

Vicious Cycle of Energetic Fraility

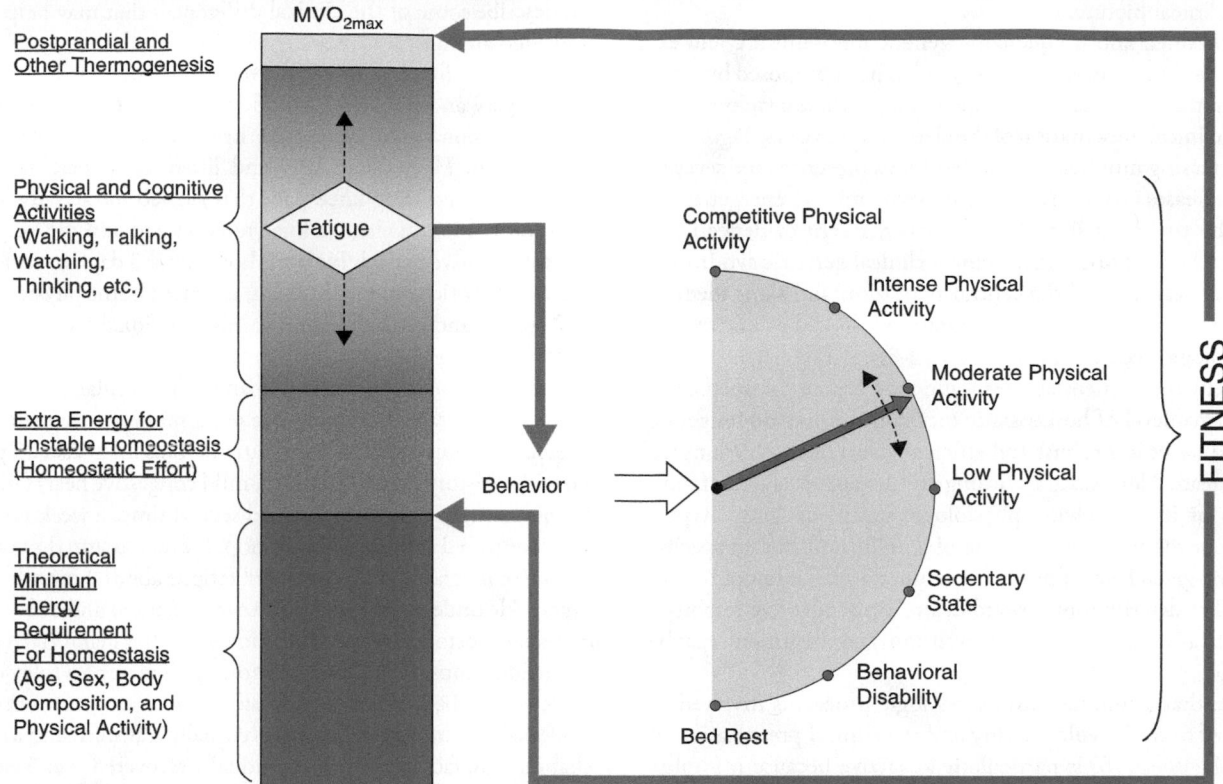

FIGURE 52-7. Vicious cycle of energetic frailty.

that the accelerated loss of muscle can be masked by a parallel increase in fat mass, leading to the condition of sarcopenic obesity. In terms of etiology, note that the proposed dysenergetic origin of frailty is consistent with the fact that many of the genetic diseases associated with mitochondrial DNA mutations emerge with clinical manifestations concentrated at the level of muscle and the central nervous system. The consequences of decreased energy can be exacerbated in catabolic states and in the common situation of anorexia of aging, both leading to decreased nutritional intake out of proportion to the level of energy expenditure through activity. These

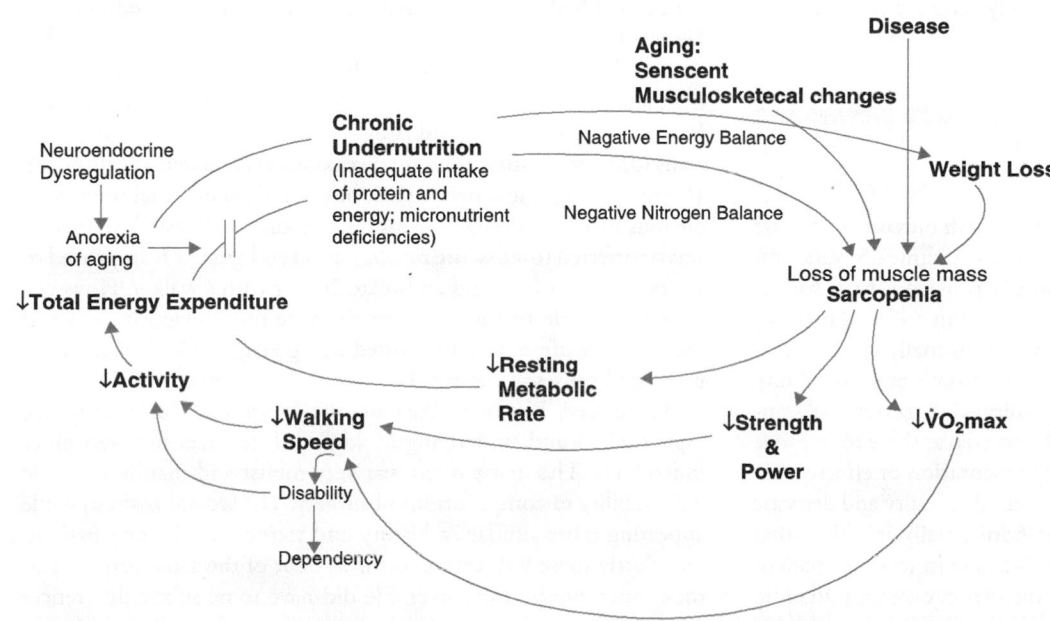

FIGURE 52-8. A vicious cycle of frailty, resulting from dysregulated energetics as well as altered physiologic functioning, intra- and intersystem. *From Fried LP, Tangen CM., Walston J, et al. Frailty in older adults: evidence for a phenotype. J Gerontol A Biol Sci Med Sci. 56;M146–M156, 2001.*

scenarios would compound the dysregulation of energetics above, adding further loss of lean body mass and, if severe enough, weight loss to the clinical picture.

Thus, a defined and unique pathogenetic mechanism could explain the clinical presentation of frailty. It has been proposed by Fried and Walston that dysregulated energetics may initiate a vicious cycle involving a clinical presentation of the elements above (see Figure 52-8), with increasing numbers of manifestations present as the severity of frailty increases, which is driven by dysregulated energetics, as supported by the discussion above. Further, recent evidence from Bandeen-Roche supports frailty being a clinical geriatric syndrome, whereby a critical mass of the central symptoms and signs identify it, not any one, and the clinical presentation is linked to underlying pathophysiology (see Figures 52-6 and 52-8).

Ultimately, the homeostatic response may become so inefficient that the normal level of homeostatic mechanisms may no longer be possible and other less robust and efficient states of equilibrium are selected instead. Note that, according to this approach, the frailty phenotype, or its underlying physiologic status, or "physiotype," may represent the best possible state of equilibrium in that specific person at any given level of physiologic function, an attempt to prevent a spiral of deterioration toward death. Since adaptive responses can theoretically be improved, prevention and treatment maybe possible.

The idea that a unique pathophysiologic process is involved in the genesis of both the vulnerability and the clinical presentation of frailty (see Figure 52-6) is particularly attractive because it implies that diagnosis of frailty as a distinct clinical entity is possible based on a finite number of criteria (signs, symptoms, test results, etc.). In addition, and perhaps more important, if prevention and treatment are possible, then diagnostic criteria can provide a basis for targeting persons who already show clinical manifestations and may lead to the ability to identify those in a subclinical stage. Targeting interventions to those with clinical manifestations could have a goal of reducing consequences of frailty or causing its remission. Targeting those at earlier stages, such as those vulnerable to stressors or with excessive and unopposed oxidative stress as a cause of homeostatic dysregulation, could have the benefits of frailty prevention as well as decreased adverse outcomes and potentially reduced susceptibility to disease.

HOW CAN FRAILTY BE IDENTIFIED IN CLINICAL PRACTICE?

Given the marked vulnerability to adverse health outcomes of those who are frail, it is critically important to have clinically valid approaches to recognizing frailty. This would provide a basis for incorporating intentional approaches to prevention and treatment of frailty into clinical care. To date, there are no formally agreed-upon diagnostic criteria that identify the biological state of vulnerability underlying frailty, or clinical evident frailty. Recognition of standardized clinical approaches is a critical next step as these to improve screening and targeting of care and implementation of effective interventions to decrease premature or preventable frailty and decrease adverse outcomes associated with frailty. Additionally, it is likely that frail older adults are the subset most vulnerable in terms of patient safety issues. Application of geriatric principles of care for frail older adults to situations that could compromise safety maybe a highly effective approach to prevent adverse events.

Clinical scenarios are illuminating. We present here three clinical case histories that reflect the heterogeneity observed in older adults, and describe some of the clinical differences that may help identify those who are most frail (see Figure 52-1).

Case 1: The first case involves a very robust older man who underwent surgery and did very well. He was 75 years old, had a history of hypertension, mild congestive heart failure, and chronic knee osteoarthritis. He walked daily and lifted some weights, but had experienced increasing knee pain that slowed his activity level. He was admitted for an elective knee replacement and did very well in the postoperative period. He went home after 3 days on anticoagulation and narcotic pain medications, tolerated home physical therapy for 2 weeks, and returned close to his functional baseline within a month.

Case 2: In the second case, a man with a similar clinical history exhibited vulnerabilities to adverse outcomes following surgery that differentiated him from the first patient. This man, also 75 years old and with a history of hypertension, mild congestive heart failure, and chronic knee osteoarthritis, walked several times a week for exercise and volunteered at a hospital gift shop. He had to stop these activities because of increasing knee pain and fatigue about 2 months prior to surgery. He underwent elective knee replacement and did well in the immediate postoperative period. However, after being given narcotic pain medications, he became delirious, pulled out his foley catheter, and fell out of bed. He refused all physical therapy interventions and developed incontinence. He was eventually transferred to a subacute rehabilitation facility, where he gradually recovered over 3 weeks. He was then transferred to home and required 3 more weeks of physical therapy. After 3 months, he approached his previous functional baseline, but still described fatigue and inability to do as much as he did before.

Case 3: An obviously frail, vulnerable older man without known medical illness had a series of adverse events near the end of life. He was 83 years old and had lived alone since his wife died 5 years earlier. He had a history of hypertension, compensated congestive heart failure, and a fall with fracture of left hip 3 years earlier. He did most of his own activities of daily living, but was not able to get out in the community anymore because of fatigue and fear of falling. He had minimal activity and almost no planned exercise. He was found on the floor by a neighbor when it was noticed that he had not been outdoors to get his morning newspaper. The patient reported that he had simply fallen and was too weak to get up. In the emergency room and subsequent hospitalization, the physicians identified diffuse muscular weakness and elicited a history of a 10 pound weight loss over a year, but found no other laboratory or obvious medical etiology for his decline and weakness. The patient was transferred to subacute rehabilitation and gradually improved to the point where he could ambulate 20 feet with a walker. However, he was not able to care for himself as he did previously, and was therefore transferred to an assisted living facility. He died there, of undefined causes, 3 months later.

These case histories illustrate the continuum of frailty (see Figure 52-1) and underlying biological differences between older individuals. The first patient was very robust and manifested little vulnerability to complications of surgery. The second patient, while appearing quite similar in history and stamina to the first patient, was clearly more vulnerable to the stressor of the same surgery and took much longer to recover. He did have some subtle differences from the first patient, in that he was fatigued for a period of time before the surgery, in addition to having knee pain. Finally, the third patient was overtly frail, with diffuse weakness, fatigue, low activity and energy, and weight loss. Verdery and others have proposed that, past a certain point in severity, frailty is a predeath phase that is irremediable (see Figure 52-1). Consistent with this, the third patient died 3 months after discharge.

These case histories suggest that frailty is, in fact, a continuum, ranging from latent physiological alterations to a clinically apparent syndrome without, and then with, resulting disability. There is now substantial theory that a "physiotype" of underlying alterations in physiological systems occurs (as above), with the consequent development of a clinical presentation, or "phenotype," past a certain level of severity of global dysfunction (see Figures 52-6 and 52-8). This latent physiotype may become clinically or phenotypically apparent when vulnerable systems decompensate in the face of stressors.

STANDARDIZED APPROACHES DEVELOPED TO ASCERTAIN FRAILTY

Several approaches have been developed to identify those who are frail. One, developed by Rockwood and colleagues, described above, creates a summary measure of deficit accumulation across many different types of health conditions at many levels: functional, clinical, and physiological. It was designed to quantifying the theorized impact of aggregate disease and illness burden. The investigators have shown that increasing numbers of conditions present are associated with a stepwise increase in mortality risk. Inferentially, they theorize that the aggregate physiological effect of these multiple conditions is "frailty." This approach has the two main disadvantages: the number of parameters to be collected makes it unsuitable for clinical utilization and, second, it does not offer a unifying theory as to etiology that might guide prevention and treatment.

A second approach posits, consistent with discussion in the prior section, that there is a distinct pathophysiology to frailty with a syndromic clinical presentation. Several groups have proposed related approaches, building on the observation of characteristic signs and symptoms of people who are "frail." In 1999, Paw et al. posited that inactivity and malnutrition were two major determinants of frailty that jointly provide strong prediction of the adverse outcomes of frailty. In the Zutphen Elderly Study, they found the combination of inactivity (less than 210 mins of physical activity per week, among walking, bicycling, hobbies, gardening, odd jobs, and sports) and weight loss (more than 4 kg over 5 years) identified 6% of this cohort of older men as "frail," and predicted slow walking speed, and greater disability and mortality. By necessity, these authors used weight loss over 5 years, but identified this as a limitation to sensitivity and suggested use of weight loss over the last year instead. Overall, the authors claim that this approach offers a simple, inexpensive, and effective screening for identifying a frail population.

In 1998, Fried and Walston proposed that there were a few major presenting symptoms and signs of frailty, and that these were interrelated in a vicious cycle, or feed-forward loop, resulting from dysregulated energetics (see Figure 52-8), with declines in strength, energy, walking speed, physical activity, and weight loss (over 1 year), all interrelated and presenting cardinal manifestations of a clinical syndrome of physical frailty.

This proposal was subsequently operationalized by defining the frail as those with a critical mass of clinical manifestations, i.e., three or more. This definition has been validated (face, criterion, construct, predictive) in more than five population-based studies

as identifying those at high risk of disability, falls, hospitalization, hip fracture, and mortality. Further, this frailty phenotype has been shown to have characteristics of a medical syndrome, in which the multiplicity of signs and symptoms present identifies those who are frail more than any one or two. Risk of adverse outcomes is more strongly associated with the constellation of presentations than with any one or two and no specific cluster of criteria carry distinguishable risk. This approach to characterizing frail older adults is based on the theory of a discrete syndrome with specific definable causes, both biological and environmental. By this definition of frailty, prevalence is 7% overall in community-dwelling men and women aged 65 years and older, and increases with increasing age from 3% in those 65 to 74 years up to 25% in those 85 years and older. There is a twofold higher prevalence in African-American older adults, compared to whites, at each age group 65 years and older. Using this definition, there is now evidence as to the natural history of frailty, indicating it is a dynamic but generally chronic, progressive condition, with 43% transitioning to states of greater frailty over 18 months, while 23% transitioned to states of lesser frailty, and almost no one transition from frail to being nonfrail. Further, initial presentations of frailty are most likely to be decreased strength or slow walking speed, which then predict development of additional manifestations, consistent with the hypothesis of a cycle of frailty (Xue et al., personal communication). Those with one or two manifestations are at twofold higher risk of progressing to three, four, or five over 3 years, thus suggesting they are prefrail. There is now strong evidence for the association of this clinical phenotype with dysregulation in number of physiologic systems. Thus, with this approach, frailty can be thought about in terms of a core phenotype manifesting a syndrome, with definable outcomes and recognized etiology. Ongoing research aims to define the physiological alterations and the ultimate biological causes of frailty (see Figures 52-6 and 52-8).

As stated by Bergman, the underlying assumption of an operational definition of a syndrome, based on symptoms, is that domains used for the diagnosis do not represent all possible manifestations of the syndrome; rather, they constitute the important domains that can be easily and reliably measured and together maximize specificity of the diagnosis. Because many components of the pathological process are associated with each other, it is not necessary to require the presence of all of them to make the diagnosis. Consistent with this, these authors suggest that the phenotype described above, with distinct, standardizable measures and criteria for definition, built on biologic theory, validated with diagnostic criteria that are strongly age-related, lends itself for use in screening, diagnosis, and as a basis for prevention and treatment of frailty; the components are summarized in Table 52-4.

A disadvantage of this particular definition, however, is that assessment requires approximately 10 to 15 minutes: to weigh a patient, measure grip strength and walking speed, and to ask two questions regarding "exhaustion" and a physical activity questionnaire. Studenski and others advocate that measurements of walking speed and possibly strength should be considered geriatric "vital signs" and assessed regularly in clinical settings. If this is implemented generally in clinical practice, then the time-consuming part of this assessment is determining physical activity level; methodological work is needed to develop a more parsimonious approach to screening physical activity than current questionnaires offer.

An alternative approach has been proposed for clinical characterization of patients as frail and using clinical judgment particularly to measure change over time clinically and/or in response to treatment.

TABLE 52-4

Components of Frailty Phenotype as Initially Operationalized in CHS (Three or More Components Present Indicate Frailty)				
GRIP STRENGTH*	**WALK TIME**	**EXHAUSTION**	**PHYSICAL ACTIVITY (LEISURE)**	**WEIGHT LOSS**
	≥6–7 s to walk 15 ft	"Everything I did was an effort." or "I could not get going."	Men (kcal/week): <383 Women (kcal/week): <270	>10 lb in past yr

Cut-Off for Grip Strength (kg) Criterion for Frailty	
Men	
BMI ≤24	<29
BMI 24.1–26	<30
BMI 26.1–28	<30
BMI >28	<32
Women	
BMI ≤23	<17
BMI 23.1–26	<17.3
BMI 26.1–29	<18
BMI >29	<21

*Grip strength, stratified by gender and body mass index (BMI) quartiles.

A clinical global impression of change in physical frailty has been developed by Studenski and colleagues to represent the clinician's perspective on clinically meaningful change resulting from interventions on physical frailty, e.g., exercise, nutrition, medications, and multifactorial approaches. This measure records clinician judgment regarding the domains of intrinsic frailty (strength, balance, nutrition, stamina, physical activity, neuromotor function, and mobility) plus appearance, medical complexity, perceived health, healthcare utilization, and outcomes of frailty (physical disability in basic, instrumental, and advanced functions; emotional status; and social status). Its goal is to create a reference point for defining the magnitude of change in simple objective measures in order to eventually measure effects of interventions to prevent or treat frailty, integrating clinical meaning with traditional measurement properties. Evaluation of the measure indicates content and face validity, feasibility, reliability, and acceptability to clinicians, and classification by severity of frailty. Ability to measure change is not yet determined. This global frailty measure can be completed by the clinician in less than 10 minutes per patient.

POTENTIAL USES OF AN OPERATIONAL DEFINITION OF FRAILTY

It would appear that enough theoretical and evidenced-based research has been done to establish an operational definition of frailty. We suggest here why having an initial standardized definition of frailty is so important. First, clinically, this would provide a starting point of a standardized, validated approach to identifying geriatric patients at high risk of multiple health-related outcomes, including disability and death. Further, there is evidence that such screening could help identify the patients at high risk of complications after acute illnesses and injuries, and most at risk of delayed or blocked recovery or functional decline after a stressful medical intervention, whether a hospitalization, surgical procedure, or chemotherapeutic agent. With the development of expanded research on this area, screening could also offer a basis for prognostication essential to

therapeutic decision-making and potentially for hospice eligibility for those with advanced frailty.

There is already initial evidence that introducing frailty into prognostic algorithms is more predictive of adverse outcomes than staging criteria established by clinical specialties. For example, assessment of frailty contributes substantially to prediction of mortality in older patients with upper gastrointestinal bleeding and characterizing those at risk of dependency after hospitalization. As frail patients are likely to be highly vulnerable to adverse outcomes of medications, environmental hazards, surgery, or "patient safety"-related issues, screening could help focus clinical attention and target preventive care to this high risk group. Further, use of a standardized definition of frailty in clinical care would provide a basis for developing appropriate levels of reimbursement for clinicians caring for this high-risk group that requires time-intensive care for extended time periods. Such expert geriatric care maybe shown to optimize appropriate resource use and, through this, potentially decrease costs of care for this population. Finally, a standardized measure of frailty would offer a basis for screening and identification of participants in randomized, controlled clinical trials aimed at prevention or treatment of frailty and/or its major consequences.

Frail older individuals who are not yet disabled and those with early disability who are at high risk of progression are most likely to benefit from interventions to prevent disability and therefore, represent ideal candidates for clinical trials that target these outcomes. Ironically, a substantial proportion of older persons with frailty, as well as comorbidity, are often excluded from clinical trials. As a result, the effectiveness of most new treatments for chronic diseases that typically affect older persons, particularly medications, has historically been established in individuals substantially healthier than age-matched persons in the general population. Thus, when these new medications are utilized in older or frail persons, who often have the greatest need for new therapeutic agents, unexpected side effects commonly emerge and the benefits evidenced in the original trials may not occur or be relevant in this population. In these complex patients, it is critical to know if the intervention has improved, or at least slowed, decline in functioning.

Conducting a clinical trial in the frail population is far more complex than doing the same trials in younger and healthier individuals: we suggest eligibility criteria based on a multistage process, and implementation of strategies to improve retention and compliance and monitor their effectiveness. Estimation of cost and sample size should contemplate high dropout rates and interference by competing outcomes. In spite of the difficulty, it should be recognized that research in this subgroup is essential to the advancement of geriatric medicine.

Overall, we propose that the screening criteria already validated could provide a starting point for a standardized definition of frailty. Only by implementation of a standardized definition can ongoing research serve as a basis for refinement and broad improvements of these same criteria.

EVIDENCE AND THEORY REGARDING THE PATHOGENESIS OF FRAILTY AND IMPLICATIONS FOR TREATMENT

Building on the discussion above and Figures 52-6 through 52-8, there is now evidence of the syndromic nature of frailty, and that there are inputs at multiple levels including (1) biologic, (2) altered physiological functions in homeostatic systems and altered communications systems, and then (3) a clinical presentation that appears to be the outcome of these multiple changes and constitutes a constellation of presentations that are interrelated in themselves and likely involved in a vicious cycle of dysregulated energetics. The aggregate impact of dysfunction at multiple levels is thought to result in compromised ability of the organism to maintain homeostasis and the vulnerability to stressors manifested by frail older adults. This section summarizes evidence to date at each level in Figure 52-6 and discusses the systems biology of frailty as a complex system. It draws primarily from the Women's Health and Aging Studies (WHAS), the Cardiovascular Health Study, and the InCHIANTI Study, which have all utilized the CHS frailty phenotype in Figure 52-8 and Table 52-4. This section then is followed by a section, which discusses the implications of this evidence in terms of potential treatments.

The clinical phenotype of frailty is based on proposed interrelationships of declines in strength, performance, energy, activity, and weight loss (see Figure 52-8). It is well established that sarcopenia contributes to altered production and utilization of energy. With loss of muscle mass and decreased muscle function, there is a decline in muscle strength and exercise tolerance. The latter can be validly represented by the concept of "fatigue" or "exhaustion." Although it directly relates to the amount of physical work the individual can produce, "fatigue" or "exhaustion" may also directly result from altered cellular production or consumption of energy. Further, there is evidence that declines in strength and exercise tolerance predict both slower walking speed and further decreases in physical activity. In a subset of older adults, who maybe frail (although that is not yet demonstrated), there is a mismatch between inadequately low food intake and inadequately high energy expenditure through physical activity (even at low levels), resulting in further loss of muscle and, in cases extremely severe cases, weight loss. These interconnections support the concept of a "cycle" of frailty. There is now evidence that this cycle has a natural history of chronic progression that often begins with declines in strength and/or walking speed, which

then predicts declines in physical activity. However, when strength, walking speed, and physical activity are all impaired, then the system rapidly progresses toward frailty.

A number of physiologic systems at abnormal levels have been shown to be associated with the frailty phenotype above. These include sarcopenia and higher fat deposits in muscle, low testosterone, insulin, DHEA-S, and IGF-1, higher levels and blunted diurnal variation of cortisol, insulin, elevated proinflammatory markers (i.e., IL-6 and C-reactive protein [CRP]), elevated markers of blood clotting, anemia, low micronutrient levels (especially total carotenoids, beta carotene, and lutein/zeaxanthin), decreased immune function (with decreased T cell proliferation and altered cytokine production), and decreased heart rate variability. Further, the severity of abnormality within each system and, particularly, the number of systems at abnormal levels are associated with the presence and severity of frailty (see Figures 52-4 to 52-6). Frail older women are more likely to have two or more micronutrient deficiencies and low daily energy intake of 21 kcal/kg or less, along with low intake of protein, vitamins D, E, C, and folate. Thus, circulating antioxidants are low in those who are frail compared to nonfrail. It is beyond the scope of this chapter to review the physiology of each system.

These systems are themselves interrelated, affecting each other as well as the clinical presentation. New evidence indicates that the risk of frailty is highly associated with multiple systems at abnormal levels, significantly more than any one system described above. The multiplicity of systems at abnormal levels is the hallmark of frailty. In spite of overwhelming evidence that age and frailty affect multiple physiological parameters in parallel, most research on biomarkers of aging is based on single measures. As schematically shown in Figure 52-9, it is generally assumed that decline in one parameter can be fully corrected by replacement, restoring the individual to the improved trajectory of "normal aging." This is the rationale for replacement of testosterone or estrogen. Unfortunately, but not completely

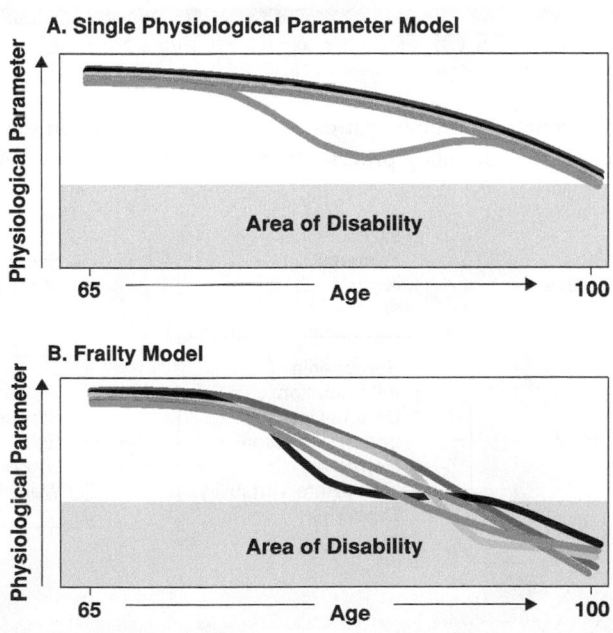

FIGURE 52-9. Dysregulation of one physiological system, as may be the norm in a specific disease (A) is the exception in frailty, where multiple physiologic systems are dysregulated (B). The implications of this finding for potential therapies is discussed in the text.

unexpectedly, this approach has met with little success. Results of trials of testosterone and estrogen replacement are somewhat disappointing. An alternative hypothesis that may explain the partial failure of this approach, exemplified in Figure 52-9, is that multiple parameters decline together, as the organisms attempts to obtain different states of equilibrium during the aging process. This interpretation implies that only by examining at multiple parameters at the same time will we be able to identify effective interventions. The condition when only one hormonal axis is dysfunctional is probably different from the multihormone dysregulation and may respond to different therapeutic approaches.

One hallmark of frailty is the dysregulation of homeostatic or communications systems, at both the molecular and physiological level (see Figure 52-6). As mentioned previously, declines in hormones important in muscle mass maintenance such as IGF-1 and DHEA-S, and increases in afternoon cortisol levels and in inflammatory and clotting markers, point toward the immune and neuroendocrine systems as likely candidates as the physiological source of this dysregulation (Figures 52-6 and 52-10). Theories of basic aging provide in part a molecular explanation for some of these changes. For example, increased oxidative stress generated in mitochondria is likely to set in motion many processes that can impair physiology. Further, declines in energy production (ATP) can lead to less efficient signal transduction and protein transcription and translation in many cells, which in time leads to alterations in biological systems. In addition, free radicals themselves damage mitochondrial DNA, which in turn will lead to even less efficient energy production and greater increases in oxidative stress. This process may lead to increasing DNA and protein damage, as well as direct transcription of inflammatory mediators, which are strongly associated with frailty. Although much work remains to be done in this area, physiological association studies are providing clues as to where these investigations should focus.

BIOMARKERS OF FRAILTY AND HOMEOSTATIC DYSREGULATION

An intriguing hypothesis that emerges from recent data in the literature is that the aging process affects multiple physiological systems in parallel (harmonically, see Figure 52-9) because the signaling network that maintains a stable homeostasis and adequate distribution/utilization of energy becomes progressively less efficient and less able to adapt to stress. Although all elements of this homeostatic network have not been identified, some indications as to the most critical components have begun to surface. The primary elements required for energy generation are provided by nutrition (in this context, oxygen is considered a nutrient) and constitute the input of the system. The output of the network is energy expenditure, which is mostly accounted for by resting metabolic rate and physical/cognitive activity. The production of energy during aerobic metabolism generates reactive oxygen species (ROS; oxidative stress) that are scavenged by antioxidant mechanisms. A dynamic stability of the internal environment is maintained by the combined effects of hormones and the autonomic nervous system. Finally, the integrity of the "self" is maintained by the immune system through inflammatory processes. Although these homeostatic systems are traditionally addressed in medicine as compartmentalized physiological systems, it is becoming clear that they belong to the same signaling network and function in a very integrated way.

Researchers have proposed that accumulated damage in the homeostatic network maybe captured by measuring signaling molecules freely circulating in the bloodstream. We have already mentioned the importance of studying multiple hormone dysregulation in older patients. It has been recently demonstrated that serum levels of single hormones such as testosterone, DHEA-S, and IGF-1 are only weak predictors of metabolic syndrome, frailty, and mortality. Evidence in support of the hypothesis that aging is associated with dysregulation of different components of the homeostatic network is emerging rapidly, especially for biomarkers of inflammation and nutritional status. Through studying the relationship between and among elements of this paradigm, we will better understand the age-related pathway to frailty and progressive disability.

Aging and frailty are associated development of a mild proinflammatory state, indicated by increased levels of proinflammatory markers. It has been demonstrated that, among nondisabled older persons, those in the highest IL-6 tertile are at high risk of developing disability over a 4-year follow-up. Older persons with elevated IL-6 and high CRP had higher mortality and there is some evidence that a short-term increase in IL-6 is a strong, independent predictor

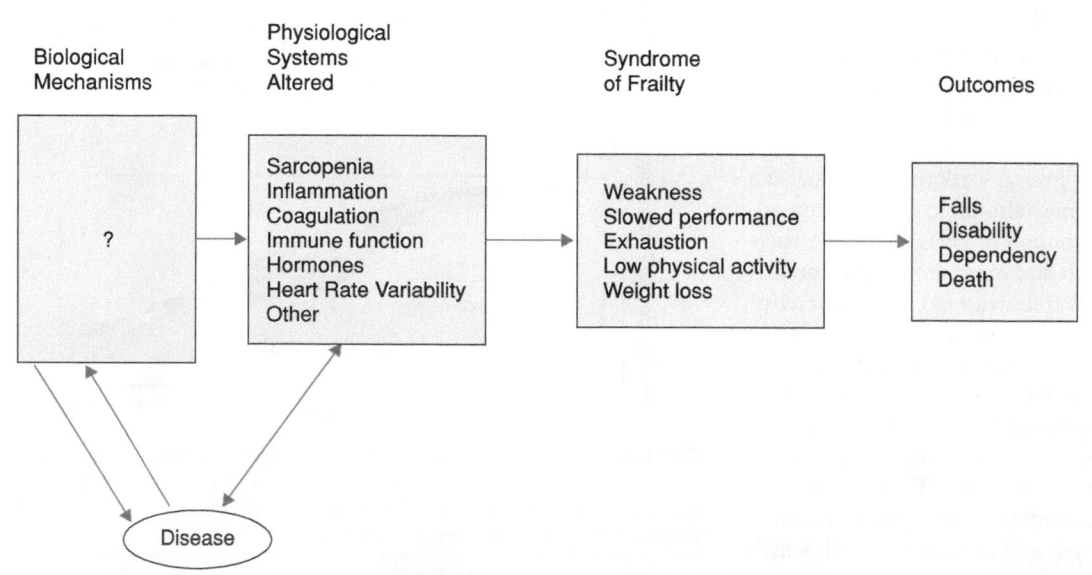

FIGURE 52-10. Model pathway of frailty.]

of mortality. Additionally, some studies suggest that the causal link between inflammation and disability is accelerated sarcopenia. In accordance with this hypothesis, there is increasing evidence that inflammation is involved in the pathogenesis of age-related muscle wasting, perhaps by the up-regulation of the NF-κB activation of the ubiquitin proteasome pathway. Adiposity appears to play an important role in the inflammatory process, and, possibly, the onset of sarcopenia. Studies have suggested that inflammatory cytokines produced by adipose tissue, especially visceral fat, accelerate muscle catabolism and may contribute to the vicious cycle that initiates and sustains sarcopenic obesity and may lead to frailty in older persons. There is cogent evidence of a connection between inflammation and frailty, but whether the link between these two conditions is completely explained by the effect of inflammation on sarcopenia is unclear. Inflammatory states also affect energy availability, hematologic, and hormonal status.

Emerging data suggest that quantitative and qualitative undernutrition is an important, and perhaps reversible, cause of frailty and disability in older persons. Oxidative stress is a major mechanism implicated in the pathogenesis of sarcopenia; aging muscle shows increased oxidative damage to DNA, protein, and lipids. Carotenoids quench free radicals, reduce damage from ROS, and appear to modulate redox-sensitive transcription factors such as NF-κB that are involved in the upregulation of IL-6 and other proinflammatory cytokines. A recent but robust literature suggests that inadequate intake of antioxidant and anti-inflammatory nutrients (in particular selenium, vitamin E, carotenoids, and polyunsaturated fatty acids (PUFAs)) contribute to sarcopenia and decline in physical function in older persons. In the InCHIANTI baseline evaluation, plasma alpha-tocopherol, but not gamma-tocopherol, was significantly correlated with knee extensor strength and lower extremity performance. Intake of vitamin C and beta-carotene were significantly correlated with knee extensor strength, and vitamin C was significantly associated with lower extremity performance. In addition, low selenium level was independently associated with poor muscle strength and higher mortality. In the WHAS, low selenium level was a risk factor for mortality and future increase in inflammatory markers, and in conjunction with low vitamins B-6 and B-12, was an independent risk factor for mortality. Low alpha-tocopherol was an independent correlate of frailty and poor cognitive function. Both in WHAS and InCHIANTI, low carotenoids was an independent risk factor for accelerated decline of muscle strength and incident disability. Thus, deficient intake of multiple nutrients is an independent correlate of frailty, even after adjusting for total energy intake.

Examining the many overlaps between the different components of the homeostatic network, it is disappointing to realize that most studies to date have somewhat arbitrarily dismantled and deconstructed a perfectly integrated architecture. This approach stems, in part, from following the epidemiological paradigm of studying "risk factors to predict outcomes" or, more generally, "independent and dependent variables." It is now apparent that the traditional epidemiological approach is inadequate to capture the multiple and often reciprocal interrelationships between events and processes. This methodology was developed in the context of studying cardiovascular disease and cancer, with the basic assumption that "exposure" to one or more risk factors increases the probability of an "event" to occur. This perspective is so ingrained that establishing a temporal relationship between the risk factor and the event is considered a necessary step for determining causality. There are at least two reasons why this model is inadequate for studying the aging process and for

investigating compensation, homeostasis and frailty in particular: (1) For all practical purposes, many of the events and processes we study occur at the same time. For example, inflammation is followed by a modification of iron metabolism, hormone levels, cardiovascular reactivity, oxidative stress, and autonomic activity within seconds. In this context, demonstrating that "baseline inflammation predicts changes in iron metabolism" in the context of a longitudinal study is very unlikely. The system that maintains stable homeostatic and maximal function is redundant and its elements are connected by complex, nonlinear interactions. For example, although increased IL-6 is usually considered a negative event, it maybe in reality an unsuccessful attempt to compensate for deteriorating health status. This alternative hypothesis is compatible with most data in the literature, but is seldom discussed. In the end, to completely explicate the complexity of the physiology and pathology of homeostasis, new epidemiologic paradigms and statistical methodology must be developed.

An essential but still unanswered question should be addressed to further understand the mechanisms that lead to frailty in old age. Why is such a high level of complexity required to guarantee a stable homeostasis? Is the level of complexity an indicator of weakness or robustness? Complex physiological dynamics enable an organism to rapidly respond to internal and external perturbations. The complex dynamics underlying healthy physiological control systems probably serve an important purpose: they enable an organism to mount a focused adaptive response in order to perform a specific task or overcome an external stress. Therefore, baseline system complexity should predict one's ability to mount a response. Because the response is, by definition, singular and directed at overcoming a stress, it should be less complex than the baseline condition. Lipsitz and Goldberger have conducted extensive theoretical and empirical work indicating that aging and disease are associated with a loss of complexity in a variety of fractal-like anatomic structures and dynamics of many integrated physiological processes. Such progressive loss of complexity implies loss of adaptive capacity. In fact, less complex systems respond to stress with less specific, stereotyped responses that are less effective and efficient. Researchers have suggested that such loss of complexity maybe reversible with interventions such as exercise that can restore healthy dynamics in multiple physiological systems.

TREATMENT AND PREVENTION OF FRAILTY

Diagnosis, treatment, and prevention of frailty can be considered in terms of our current understanding of frailty and according to each of the levels described in Figures 52-6 and 52-10 and the sections above. The first premise of evaluation is to identify vulnerable, frail individuals before the adverse outcomes for which they are at risk occur. Such a clinical approach should involve careful identification of secondary frailty resulting from latent, undertreated, or end-stage disease such as congestive heart failure, which could be causing a catabolic state and weight loss or decreased nutritional intake. A number of diseases which cause wasting are responsive to therapy, including congestive heart failure, diabetes, thyroid disease, tuberculosis, and other chronic infections, undiagnosed cancer, and inflammatory conditions such as temporal arteritis. Psychological conditions such as depression, psychosis, and grief—as well as dementia—can also present in this manner.

Whether or not frailty results from underlying disease, focus should be placed on the prevention of related adverse outcomes (see Table 52-1 and Figure 52-10), including falls, delirium, and disability. Evaluation should also include screening for factors that may exacerbate vulnerability for these outcomes, such as medications, hospitalization, surgery, or other stressors, with intervention as indicated. Outpatient geriatric assessment and intervention, with patient-centered goal-setting, family and/or caregiver involvement, and regular follow-up by a geriatrically expert team would help facilitate the identification of problems that would benefit from intervention. Such longitudinal, continuous care has been demonstrated to slow functional decline and reduce symptoms and adverse outcomes in frail older adults.

If disease has been ruled out as the cause of frailty, and thus frailty appears to be the primary condition, a goal should be to institute supportive interventions early. These include targeting the environmental provocations that can trigger or accelerate manifestations of frailty, especially low activity, inadequate nutrition, and catabolic medications. The goal of this intervention would be prevention of muscle loss and improvement in strength and energy. Much of the focus of future research in this area will likely focus on populations where specific deficiencies or increased requirements are recognized.

Attention to maintaining strength and nutritional intake may include prescription of regular exercise, potentially with additional nutritional supplementation if indicated. Screening of frail individuals should evaluate factors such as depression that may contribute to decreased activity or food intake. There is now good evidence indicating that resistance exercise to increase strength of a frail older adult has potential from both a preventive and a therapeutic point of view. In very frail nursing home patients, aged 72 to 98 years, Fiatarone et al. showed that progressive resistance exercise training over a 10-week period improved strength, gait velocity, stair-climbing power, and spontaneous physical activity. Greatest benefit from this resistance (strengthening) exercise program was seen in those who were initially weak but without severe muscle atrophy, i.e., a group with more recent onset of weakness. These findings indicate benefit from exercise for even the most frail, while suggesting that improvement is greatest if declines in strength are caught earlier rather than later. Note that, in this randomized, controlled trial, nutritional supplementation was only effective if added to exercise training; used by itself, it did not lead to increased muscle mass, strength, or functional improvements.

At the other end of the spectrum, primary prevention of frailty through regular strength training also has good potential. In one study of 40 postmenopausal women aged 50 to 70 years, high-intensity strength training exercise 2 days per week led to increased bone mineral density in the femoral neck and lumbar spine, plus significantly improved muscle mass, muscle strength, and dynamic balance in those receiving training, compared to controls. In addition, as with the nursing home patients engaging in resistance exercise (above), the exercise group increased their energy expenditure 27% in activities outside of the intervention itself, compared with the controls who decreased their energy expenditure by 25%. Thus, resistance training appeared to improve a number of risk factors for frailty, as well as for osteoporotic fractures. Evans has also reported that high-intensity strength training has highly anabolic effects in the elderly population. He reported a 10% to 15% decrease in nitrogen excretion at the initiation of such training, which persisted for 12 weeks. That is, progressive resistance training improved nitrogen balance. As a result, older patients performing resistance training had a lower mean protein intake requirement than did sedentary

subjects. In contrast, aerobic exercise causes an increase in protein requirements. Overall, exercise training appears to improve muscle mass and strength and resulting functional performance. It is notable that increases in strength with high-intensity strength training are substantially greater than those seen to date with growth hormone, while increases with growth hormone do not appear to translate into functional improvements.

Preservation of fat-free mass and prevention of sarcopenia should help prevent the decrease in metabolic rate described in association with frailty. Maintenance of strength should facilitate maintenance of exercise tolerance directly and also because those with improved strength appear to engage spontaneously in more activity. In prevention of frailty, this appears to be a critical stage, both to prevent the downward cycle of frailty and the development of disability. Otherwise, with declining exercise tolerance, activities of daily living start to take up larger proportions of VO_2 max, with highly sedentary older adults requiring as much as 90% of their VO_2 max to carry out basic self-care tasks.

The role of nutritional supplementation is less well defined. In the trial by Fiatarone of resistance exercise and nutritional supplementation in frail nursing home patients, total energy intake did not increase in those exercising (without nutritional supplementation) or in those receiving nutritional supplementation but not exercise, compared to controls. This was the case even though this population had a marginal nutritional intake at baseline. Only with both exercise and nutritional supplementation did energy intake increase; these people gained weight but not fat-free mass, however.

CONCLUSION

For geriatric medicine, studying frailty and establishing an operational definition that allows its implementation in clinical practice is an opportunity, a need, and a responsibility. To make explicit the value of geriatric medicine, the fundamental difference between using a whole patient-centered approach compared to the disease-centered approach should be demonstrated in terms of health outcomes. Understanding and operationalizing frailty in clinical practice maybe a key to reaching this goal. Frailty is also an opening that allows a view into the complexity of events that cause susceptibility and loss of function in older individuals. Through this opening, it maybe possible to identify new targets for interventions that, in the future, may reduce the burden of morbidity and disability in this vulnerable portion of the older population.

FURTHER READING

Baltes PB, Smith J. New frontiers in the future of aging: from successful aging of the young old to the dilemmas of the fourth age. *Gerontology.* 2003;49(2):123–135.

Bortz WM II. The physics of frailty. *J Am Geriatr Soc.* 1993;41(9):1004–1008.

Brown M, Sinacore DR, Binder EF, et al. Physical and performance measures for the identification of mild to moderate frailty. *J Gerontol A Biol Sci Med Sci.* 2000;55A:M350–M355.

Buchner DM, Wagner EH. Preventing frail health. *Clin Geriatric Med.* 1992;8:1–17.

Campbell AJ, Buchner DM. Unstable disability and the fluctuations of frailty. *Age Ageing.* 1997;26:315–318.

Chin APMJ, Dekker JM, Feskens EJ, et al. How to select a frail elderly population? A comparison of three working definitions. *J Clin Epidemiol.* 1999;52:1015–1021.

Dayhoff NE, Suhrheinrich J, Wigglesworth J, et al. Balance and muscle strength as predictors of frailty among older adults. *J Gerontol Nurs.* 1998;24:18–27.

Disability in America: toward a national agenda for prevention. In: Pope AM, Tarlov AR, eds. Committee on a National Agenda for the Prevention of Disabilities, Institute of Medicine Washington, DC: National Academy Press; 1991.

Fried LP. Conference on the physiologic basis of frailty. *Aging.* 1992;4:251–252.

Fried LP, Ferrucci L, Darer J, Williamson JD, Anderson G. Untangling the concepts of disability, frailty, and comorbidity: implications for improved targeting and care. *J Gerontol A Biol Sci Med Sci.* 2004;59:M255–M263.

Fried LP, Kronmal RA, Bild D, et al.; for the Cardiovascular Health Study Collaborative Research Group. Risk factors for five-year mortality in older adults: The Cardiovascular Health Study. *JAMA.* 1998;279:585–592.

Fried LP, Hadley EC, Walston JD, et al. From bedside to bench: research agenda for frailty. *Sci Aging Knowledge Environ.* 2005;2005(31):pe24.

Fried LP, Tangen CM, Walston J, et al. Frailty in older adults: evidence for a phenotype. *J Gerontol Med Sci.* 2001;56;M146–M156.

Gill TM, Williams CS, Richardson ED, et al. Impairments in physical performance and cognitive status as predisposing factors for functional dependence among nondisabled older persons. *J Gerontol A Biol Sci Med Sci.* 1996;51A:M283–M288.

Ory MG, Schechtman KB, Miller JP, et al. Frailty and injuries in later life: the FICSIT trials. *J Am Geriatr Soc.* 1993;41:283–296.

Pendergast DR, Fisher NM, Calkins E. Cardiovascular, neuromuscular and metabolic alterations with age leading to frailty. *J Gerontol.* 1993;48(spec no.):61–67.

Rockwood K, Fox RA, Stolee P, et al. Frailty in elderly peoplean evolving concept. *Can Med Assoc J.* 1994;150:489–495.

Rockwood K, Mitnitski A, Song X, Steen B, Skoog I. Long-term risks of death and institutionalization of elderly people in relation to deficit accumulation at age 70. *J Am Geriatr Soc.* 2006;54(6):975–979.

Ruggiero C, Ferrucci L. The endeavor of high maintenance homeostasis: resting metabolic rate and the legacy of longevity. *J Gerontol A Biol Sci Med Sci.* 2006;61(5):466–471.

Saliba D, Elliott M, Rubenstein LZ, et al. the vulnerable elders survey: a tool for identifying vulnerable older people in the community. *J Am Geriatr Soc.* 2001;49:1691–1699.

Strawbridge WJ, Shema SJ, Balfour JL, et al. Antecedents of frailty over three decades in an older cohort. *J Gerontol B Psychol Sci Soc Sci.* 1998;53B:s9–s16.

Tinetti ME, Inouye SK, Gill TM, et al. Shared risk factors for falls, incontinence, and functional dependence. Unifying the approach to geriatric syndromes. *JAMA.* 1995;273:1348–1353.

Vellas B, Gillette-Guronnet S, Nourhashemi F, et al. Falls, frailty and osteoporosis in the elderly: a public health problem. *Rev Med Interne.* 2000;21:608–613.

Walston J, Hadley EC, Ferrucci L, et al. Research Agenda for Frailty in Older Adults: Towards a Better Understanding of physiology and Etiology. *J Am Geriatr Soc.* 2006;54(6):991–1001.

Winograd CH, Gerety MB, Brown E, et al. Targeting the hospitalized elderly for geriatric consultation. *J Am Geriatr.* 1988;36:1113–1119.

Delirium

Sharon K. Inouye ■ *Michael A. Fearing* ■ *Edward R. Marcantonio*

Delirium, defined as an acute disorder of attention and global cognitive function, is a common, serious, and potentially preventable source of morbidity and mortality for hospitalized older persons. It occurs in 14% to 56% of such persons and represents the most frequent complication of hospitalization for this group. With the aging of the U.S. population, delirium has assumed heightened importance because persons aged 65 years and older presently account for more than 49% of all days of hospital care. Delirium complicates hospital stays for at least 20% of the 12.5 million patients 65 years of age or older who are hospitalized each year and increases hospital costs by $2500 per patient, so that $6.9 billion (in 2004 U.S. dollars) of Medicare hospital expenditures are attributable to delirium. Importantly, substantial additional costs linked to delirium accrue after hospital discharge because of the increased need for institutionalization, rehabilitation services, closer medical follow-up, and home health care. Delirium often initiates a cascade of events in older persons, leading to a downward spiral of functional decline, loss of independence, institutionalization, and ultimately, death. These statistics highlight the importance of delirium from both clinical and health policy perspectives. In fact, a recent consensus panel identified delirium as among the top three target conditions for quality-of-care improvement for vulnerable older adults. With its common occurrence, its frequently iatrogenic nature, and its close linkage to the processes of care, incident delirium can serve as a marker for the quality of hospital care and provides an opportunity for quality improvement.

DEFINITION

The definition of and diagnostic criteria for delirium continue to evolve (Table 53-1). The standardized criteria for delirium that appear in the American Psychiatric Association's *Diagnostic and Statistical Manual of Mental Disorders, Fourth Edition, Text Revision* (DSM-IV-TR) remain the current diagnostic standard. Expert consensus was used to develop these criteria, however, and performance characteristics such as diagnostic sensitivity and specificity have not been reported for DSM-IV criteria. A standardized tool, the Confusion Assessment Method (CAM), provides a brief, validated diagnostic algorithm that is currently in widespread use for identification of delirium. The CAM algorithm relies on the presence of acute onset and fluctuating course, inattention, and either disorganized thinking or altered level of consciousness. The algorithm has a sensitivity of 94% to 100%, specificity of 90% to 95%, and high interrater reliability. Given the uncertainty of diagnostic criteria for delirium, a critical area for future investigation is to establish more definitive criteria, including epidemiologic and phenomenologic evaluations assisted by advances in functional neuroimaging and other potential diagnostic marker tests.

EPIDEMIOLOGY

Most of the epidemiological studies of delirium involved hospitalized older patients, in whom the highest rates of delirium occur. Reported rates vary based upon the subgroup of patients studied and the setting of care (e.g., hospital, intensive care, surgical). Previous studies estimated the prevalence of delirium (present at the time of hospital admission) at 14% to 24% and the incidence of delirium (new cases arising during hospitalization) at 6% to 56%. The rates of delirium in high-risk hospital venues, such as the intensive care unit and posthip fracture settings, range from 70% to 87% and 15% to 53%, respectively. Delirium occurs in up to 60% of patients in nursing homes or postacute settings, and in up to 83% of all patients at the end of life. The rates of delirium in all older persons presenting to the emergency department in several studies have ranged from 10% to 30%. While less frequent in the community setting, delirium is an important presenting symptom to emergency departments and community physicians, and often heralds serious underlying disease. Delirium is often unrecognized; previous studies have documented that clinicians fail to detect up to 70% of affected

TABLE 53-1

Diagnostic Criteria for Delirium

Diagnostic and Statistical Manual (DSM-IV) Diagnostic Criteria

A. A disturbance of consciousness (i.e., reduced awareness of the external environment) with reduced ability to focus, sustain, or shift attention.

B. A change in cognition (such as memory deficit, disorientation, language disturbance) or the development of a perceptual disturbance that is not better accounted for by a preexisting dementia.

C. The disturbance develops over a short period of time (usually hours to days) and tends to fluctuate over the course of a 24-hour period.

D. Evidence from the history, physical examination, or laboratory findings that the disturbance is caused by an underlying organic condition or is the direct physiologic consequences of a general medical condition or its treatment.

The Confusion Assessment Method (CAM) Diagnostic Algorithm*

Feature 1. Acute onset and fluctuating course

This feature is usually obtained from a reliable reporter, such as a family member, caregiver, or nurse, and is shown by positive responses to these questions: Is there evidence of an acute change in mental status from the patient's baseline? Did the (abnormal) behavior fluctuate during the day, that is, tend to come and go, or did it increase and decrease in severity?

Feature 2. Inattention

This feature is shown by a positive response to this question: Did the patient have difficulty focusing attention, for example, being easily distractible, or have difficulty keeping track of what was being said?

Feature 3. Disorganized thinking

This feature is shown by a positive response to this question: Was the patient's thinking disorganized or incoherent, such as rambling or irrelevant conversation, unclear or illogical flow of ideas, or unpredictable switching from subject to subject?

Feature 4. Altered level of consciousness

This feature is shown by any answer other than "alert" to this question: Overall, how would you rate this patient's level of consciousness (alert [normal], vigilant [hyperalert], lethargic [drowsy, easily aroused], stupor [difficult to arouse], or coma [unarousable])?

*The ratings for the CAM should be completed following brief cognitive assessment of the patient, for example, with the Mini-Mental State Examination. The diagnosis of delirium by CAM requires the presence of features 1 and 2 and of either 3 or 4.

Source: Modified with permission from American Psychiatric Association: Diagnostic and Statistical Manual of Mental Disorders, Fourth ed. Text Revision. Copyright 2000 American Psychiatric Association and Inouye SK, vanDyck CH, Alessi CA, et al. Clarifying confusion: the confusion assessment method. A new method for detection of delirium. Ann Intern Med. 113:941, 1990.

patients across all of these settings. Furthermore, the presence of delirium portends a potentially poor prognosis; hospital mortality rates in patients with delirium range from 22% to 76%, as high as mortality rates associated with acute myocardial infarction or sepsis. Following hospitalization, the one-year mortality rate associated with cases of delirium is 35% to 40%.

ETIOLOGY

The etiology of delirium is usually multifactorial, like many other common geriatric syndromes, such as falls, incontinence, and pressure sores. Although there may be a single cause of delirium, more commonly, delirium results from the interrelationship between patient vulnerability (i.e., predisposing factors) and the occurrence of noxious insults (i.e., precipitating factors). For example, patients

who are highly vulnerable to delirium at baseline (e.g., such as patients with dementia or serious illness) can experience acute delirium after exposure to otherwise mild insults, such as a single dose of a sedative medication for sleep. On the other hand, older patients with few predisposing factors (low baseline vulnerability) would be relatively resistant, with precipitation of delirium only after exposure to multiple potentially detrimental insults, such as general anesthesia, major surgery, multiple psychoactive medications, immobilization, and infection (Figure 53-1). Moreover, based on predictive models of delirium, the effects of multiple risk factors appear to be cumulative. Clinically, the overall importance of the multifactorial nature of delirium is that removal or treatment of one risk factor alone often fails to resolve delirium. Instead, addressing many or all of the predisposing and precipitating factors for delirium is often required before the delirium improves.

Predisposing Factors

Predisposing factors for delirium include preexisting cognitive impairment or dementia, advanced age, severe underlying illness and comorbidity, functional impairment, male gender, depression, chronic renal insufficiency, dehydration, malnutrition, alcohol abuse, and sensory impairments (vision or hearing) (Table 53-2). Preexisting cognitive impairment, or dementia, is a powerful and consistent risk factor for delirium demonstrated across multiple studies, and patients with dementia have a two- to fivefold increased risk for delirium. Moreover, up to half of delirious patients have an underlying dementia. Nearly any chronic medical condition can predispose to delirium, ranging from diseases involving the central nervous system (e.g. Parkinson's disease, cerebrovascular disease, mass lesions, trauma, infection, collagen vascular disease), to diseases outside the central nervous system, including infectious, metabolic, cardiac, pulmonary, endocrine, or neoplastic etiologies. Independent predisposing risk factors for delirium at the time of hospital admission validated in a predictive model include severe underlying illness, vision impairment, baseline cognitive impairment, and high blood urea nitrogen (BUN):creatinine ratio (used as an index of dehydration). Predictive risk models that identify predisposing factors in populations such as surgical patients, cancer patients, and nursing home residents, have recently been developed and aid in the understanding of baseline patient characteristics contributing to delirium risk.

Precipitating Factors

Major precipitating factors identified in previous studies include medication use (see section on "Drug Use and Delirium"), immobilization, use of indwelling bladder catheters, use of physical restraints, dehydration, malnutrition, iatrogenic events, medical illnesses, infections, metabolic derangement, alcohol or drug intoxication or withdrawal, environmental influences, and psychosocial factors (see Table 53-2). Decreased mobility is strongly associated with delirium and concomitant functional decline. The use of medical equipment and devices (e.g., indwelling bladder catheters and physical restraints) may further contribute to immobilization. Major iatrogenic events occur in 29% to 38% of older hospitalized adults (three to five times the risk when compared with adults younger than 65 years old). Examples include complications related to diagnostic or therapeutic procedures, allergic reactions, and bleeding caused

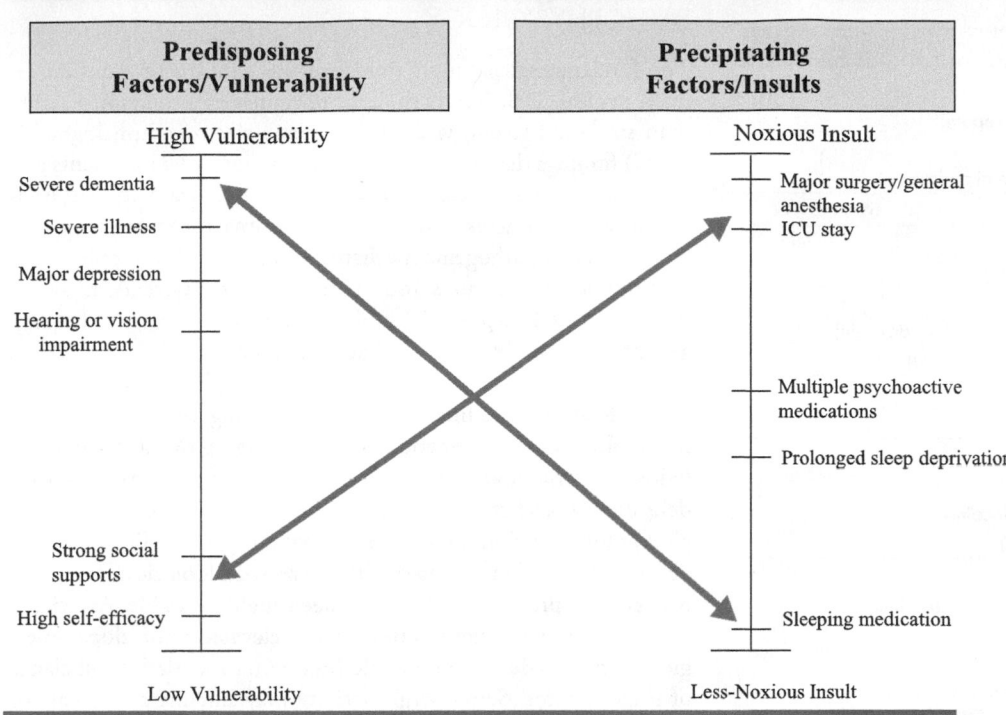

FIGURE 53-1. Multifactorial model for delirium. The etiology of delirium involves a complex interrelationship between the patient's underlying vulnerability or predisposing factors (*left axis*) and precipitating factors or noxious insults (*right axis*). For example, a patient with high vulnerability, such as with severe dementia, underlying severe illness, hearing or vision impairment, might develop delirium with exposure to only one dose of a sleeping medication. Conversely, a patient with low vulnerability would develop delirium only with exposure to many noxious insults, such as general anesthesia and major surgery, ICU stay, multiple psychoactive medications, and prolonged sleep deprivation. (*Adapted from Inouye SK. Delirium in hospitalized older patients. Clin Geriatr Med. 475, 1998.*)

by over anticoagulation. Many of these events potentially are preventable. Disorders of any major organ system, particularly renal or hepatic failure, can precipitate delirium. Occult respiratory failure has emerged as an increasing problem in elderly patients, who often lack the typical signs and symptoms of dyspnea and tachypnea. In older adults, acute myocardial infarction and congestive heart failure may present with delirium or "failure to thrive" as the cardinal feature, and minimal or none of the usual symptoms of angina or dyspnea. Occult infection, caused by pneumonia, urinary tract infection, endocarditis, abdominal abscess, or infected joint, is a particularly noteworthy cause of delirium because older patients may not present with leukocytosis or a typical febrile response. Metabolic and endocrinologic disorders, such as hyper- or hyponatremia, hypercalcemia, acid–base disorders, hypo- and hyperglycemia, and thyroid or adrenal disorders, may also contribute to delirium. The precipitating factors for delirium in hospitalized older patients that have been validated in a predictive model include use of physical restraints, malnutrition, more than three medications added during the previous day (more than 70% of these were psychoactive drugs), indwelling bladder catheter, and any iatrogenic event. The presence of these independent factors contributes to delirium risk in a predictable and cumulative manner, yet each risk factor is potentially modifiable.

Drug Use and Delirium

In 40% or more of delirium cases, use of one or more specific medication contributes to its development. While medications often incite delirium, they are also the most common remediable cause of delirium. A broad array of medications and their metabolites can lead to delirium; the most common are those with known psychoactive effects, such as sedative hypnotics, anxiolytics, narcotics, H_2-blockers, and medications with anticholinergic activity (Table 53-3). In previous studies, use of any psychoactive medication was associated with a fourfold increased risk of delirium, while use of two or more psychoactive medications was associated with a fivefold increased risk. Sedative–hypnotic drugs are associated with a 3- to 12-fold increased risk of delirium; narcotics with a threefold risk; and anticholinergic drugs with a 5- to 12-fold risk. The incidence of delirium, similar to other adverse drug events, increases in direct proportion to the number of medications prescribed, because of the effects of the

TABLE 53-2

Predisposing and Precipitating Factors for Delirium

Predisposing factors
- Dementia or underlying cognitive impairment
- Severe illness
- Comorbidity
- Depression
- Vision and/or hearing impairment
- Functional impairment, inactivity
- Volume depletion
- Chronic renal insufficiency
- Structural brain abnormality or previous stroke
- History of alcohol abuse
- History of delirium
- History of falls
- Advanced age
- Baseline use of psychoactive drugs
- Male gender
- Malnutrition

Precipitating factors
- Psychoactive drugs
- Immobilization
- Indwelling bladder catheters
- Physical restraints
- Dehydration
- Poor nutritional status
- Iatrogenic complications
- Intercurrent medical illnesses
- Major surgical procedure
- Metabolic derangements (electrolytes, glucose, acid–base)
- Infections
- Hypoxia
- Alcohol or drug intoxication or withdrawal
- Sensory deprivation
- Sensory overload
- Pain
- Emotional stress, bereavement
- Prolonged sleep deprivation

TABLE 53-3

Drugs Associated with Delirium

Sedatives/hypnotics
 Benzodiazepines (especially flurazepam, diazepam)
 Barbiturates
 Sleeping medications (diphenhydramine, chloral hydrate)

Narcotics (especially meperidine)

Anticholinergics
 Antihistamines (diphenhydramine, hydroxyzine)
 Antispasmodics (belladonna, Lomotil)
 Heterocyclic antidepressants (amitriptyline, imipramine, doxepin)
 Neuroleptics (chlorpromazine, haloperidol, thioridazine)

Incontinence (oxybutynin, hyoscyamine)
 Atropine/scopolamine

Cardiac
 Digitalis glycosides
 Antiarrhythmics (quinidine, procainamide, lidocaine)
 Antihypertensives (beta-blockers, methyldopa)

Gastrointestinal
 H_2-antagonists (cimetidine, ranitidine, famotidine, nizatidine)
 Proton pump inhibitors
 Metoclopramide (Reglan)
 Herbal remedies (valerian root, St. John's Wort, kava kava)

medications themselves, as well as to the increased risk of drug–drug and drug–disease interactions. Recent studies provide compelling evidence that suboptimal medication management, ranging from inappropriate use to overuse of psychoactive medications, occurs commonly in older adults in the hospital and in community settings, and suggests that many cases of delirium and other related adverse drug events may be preventable. As the number of prescription and over-the-counter drugs consumed by the older population increases, review of potentially problematic medications will remain an important step in the search for predisposing factors in the patient with delirium.

Relationship between Delirium and Dementia

While delirium and dementia are highly interrelated, the nature of their relationship remains poorly examined. The contribution of delirium itself to permanent cognitive impairment or dementia remains controversial; however, previous studies document that at least some patients postdelirium never recover their baseline level of cognitive function. Thus, delirium and dementia may represent two ends along a spectrum of cognitive impairment with "chronic delirium" and "reversible dementia" falling along this continuum. Dementia is the leading risk factor for delirium, and fully two-thirds of cases of delirium occur in patients with dementia. Moreover, studies have shown that delirium and dementia are both associated with decreased cerebral metabolism, cholinergic deficiency, and inflammation, reflecting their overlapping clinical, metabolic, and cellular mechanisms. Delirium can alter the course of an underlying dementia, with dramatic worsening of the trajectory of cognitive decline, resulting in more rapid progression of functional losses and worse long-term outcomes. In follow-up studies, patients with dementia in whom delirium develops have worse outcomes than those with dementia alone, including worsened cognitive function and increased rates of hospitalization, institutionalization, and death.

PATHOPHYSIOLOGY

The fundamental pathophysiological mechanisms of delirium remain unclear. Delirium is thought to represent a functional rather than structural lesion, with characteristic electroencephalographic (EEG) findings demonstrating global functional derangements and generalized slowing of cortical background (alpha) activity. The leading current hypotheses view delirium as the final common pathway of many different pathogenic mechanisms, resulting from dysfunction of multiple brain regions and neurotransmitter systems. Evidence from EEG, evoked-potential studies, and neuroimaging studies suggest predominantly right-sided abnormalities in delirium localized to the prefrontal cortex, thalamus, basal ganglia, temporoparietal cortex, fusiform, and lingual gyri. Studies using x-ray computed tomography (CT) or magnetic resonance imaging (MRI) have found lesions or structural abnormalities in the brains of patients with delirium. Several studies of cerebral blood flow (CBF) using single photon emission computed tomography (SPECT) found that delirium is mostly associated with decreased blood flow. However, results from previous studies have been highly variable. Associated neurotransmitter abnormalities involve elevated brain dopaminergic function, reduced cholinergic function, or a relative imbalance of these systems. Serotonergic activity may interact to regulate or alter activity of these other two systems, and serotonin levels may be either increased or decreased. Extensive evidence supports the role of cholinergic deficiency. Acetylcholine plays a key role in consciousness and attentional process. Given that delirium is manifested by an acute confusional state often with alterations of consciousness, it is likely to have a cholinergic basis. Anticholinergic drugs can induce delirium in humans and animals, and serum anticholinergic activity is increased in patients with delirium. Physostigmine reverses delirium associated with anticholinergic drugs, and cholinesterase inhibitors appear to have some benefit even in cases of delirium that are not induced by drugs. The stress response associated with severe medical illness or surgery involves sympathetic and immune system activation, including increased activity of the hypothalamic–pituitary–adrenal axis with hypercortisolism, release of cerebral cytokines that alter neurotransmitter systems, alterations in the thyroid axis, and modification of blood–brain barrier permeability. Age-related changes in central neurotransmission, stress management, hormonal regulation, and immune response may contribute to the increased vulnerability of older persons to delirium. The description of delirium as "acute brain failure"—involving multiple neural circuits, neurotransmitters, and brain regions—suggests that understanding delirium may help to elucidate the essential underlying mechanisms of brain functioning.

PRESENTATION

Cardinal Features

Acute onset and inattention are the central features of delirium. Determining the acuity of onset requires accurate knowledge of the patient's prior cognitive status. Pinpointing the origin and time course of changes in mental status often entails obtaining historical information from another close observer, such as a family member, caregiver, or nurse. Typically with delirium, the mental status changes occur over hours to days, in contrast to the changes that occur with dementia, which present insidiously over weeks to months. Another key feature is the fluctuating course of delirium, with symptoms tending to wax and wane in severity over a 24-hour period. Lucid intervals are characteristic, and the reversibility of symptoms within a short time can deceive even an experienced clinician. Inattention is manifested as difficulty focusing, maintaining, and shifting attention or concentration. With simple cognitive assessment, patients may display difficulty with straightforward repetition tasks, digit spans, or recitation of the months of the year backward. Delirious patients appear easily distracted, experience difficulty with multistep commands, cannot follow the flow of a conversation, and often perseverate with an answer to a previous question. Additional major features include a disorganization of thought and altered level of consciousness. Disorganized thoughts are a manifestation of underlying cognitive or perceptual disturbances, and can be recognized by disjointed and incoherent speech, or an unclear or illogical progression of ideas. Clouding of consciousness is typically manifested by lethargy, with a reduced awareness of the environment that may show diurnal variation. Although not cardinal elements, other frequently associated features include disorientation (more commonly to time and place than to self), cognitive impairments (e.g., memory and problem-solving deficits, dysnomia), psychomotor agitation or retardation, perceptual disturbances (e.g., hallucinations, misperceptions, illusions), paranoid delusions, emotional lability, and sleep–wake cycle disruption.

Tools for Evaluation of Delirium

Table 53-4 describes the most widely used instruments for identification of delirium, along with their performance characteristics. These include CAM, the Delirium Rating Scale (DRS), the Delirium Symptom Interview (DSI), and the Memorial Delirium Assessment Scale (MDAS). Each instrument has strengths and limitations, and the choice among them depends on the goals for use. Notably, the evaluation for the CAM has been adapted recently as the CAM-ICU for nonverbal or intubated patients. In addition, the DRS–Revised-98 version allows more refined measurements of delirium severity over a broad range of symptoms. An adapted version of the CAM is also being included as the delirium screening tool in the ongoing national test of the new version of the Minimum Data Set (MDS Version 3.0). The Minimum Data Set is a standardized resident assessment that is completed on every person admitted to a Medicare certified nursing home in the United States.

Forms of Delirium

The clinical presentation of delirium can take two main forms, either hypoactive or hyperactive. The hypoactive form of delirium is characterized by lethargy and reduced psychomotor functioning, and is the more common form in older patients. Hypoactive delirium often goes unrecognized and carries an overall poorer prognosis. The reduced level of patient activity associated with hypoactive delirium, often attributed to low mood or fatigue, may contribute to its misdiagnosis or underrecognition. By contrast, the hyperactive form of delirium presents with symptoms of agitation, increased vigilance, and often concomitant hallucinations; its presentation rarely remains unnoticed by caregivers or clinicians. Importantly, patients can fluc-

tuate between the hypoactive and hyperactive forms—the mixed type of delirium—presenting a challenge in distinguishing the presentation from other psychotic or mood disorders. Moreover, recent recognition of partial or incomplete forms of delirium has brought attention to the persistence of symptoms among older patients, particularly during the resolution stages of delirium, when manifestation of the full syndrome may not be apparent. Partial forms of delirium also adversely influence long-term clinical outcomes.

PROGNOSIS

Delirium is an important independent determinant of prolonged length of hospital stay, increased mortality, increased rates of nursing home placement, and functional and cognitive decline—even after controlling for age, gender, dementia, illness severity, and baseline functional status.

Delirium has long been thought to be a reversible, transient condition. Recent research on the duration of delirium symptoms, however, provides evidence that delirium may persist for much longer than previously recognized. In fact, delirium symptoms generally persist for a month or more; as few as 20% of patients attain complete symptom resolution at 6-month follow-up. In addition, those patients with extant cognitive impairment may experience greater deleterious effects than comparable patients without dementia. The chronic detrimental effects are likely related to the duration, severity, and underlying cause(s) of the delirium, in addition to the baseline vulnerability of the patient.

EVALUATION

The acute evaluation of delirium centers on three main tasks that occur simultaneously: (1) establishing the diagnosis of delirium; (2) determining the potential cause(s) and ruling out life-threatening contributors; and (3) managing the symptoms. Delirium is a clinical diagnosis, relying on astute observation at the bedside, careful cognitive assessment, and history taking from a knowledgeable informant to establish a change from the patient's baseline functioning. Identifying the potentially multifactorial contributors to the delirium is of paramount importance, because many of these factors are treatable, and if left untreated, may result in substantial morbidity and mortality. Because the potential contributors are myriad, the search requires a thorough medical evaluation guided by clinical judgment. The challenge is enhanced by the frequently nonspecific or atypical presentation of the underlying illness in older persons. In fact, delirium is often the *only* sign of life-threatening illness, such as sepsis, pneumonia, or myocardial infarction in older persons. Recently, The Royal College of Physicians has established national guidelines to aid in the prevention, treatment, and management of delirium in older people (www.rcplondon.ac.uk/pubs/books/pdmd/index.asp). These guidelines highlight both the importance of delirium in the aged, and the need for better recognition and treatment of delirium.

History and Physical Examination

A thorough history and physical examination constitute the foundation of the medical evaluation of suspected delirium. The first step in evaluation should be to establish the diagnosis of delirium

TABLE 53-4

Sample Instruments Used to Evaluate Delirium

DESCRIPTION	DOMAINS	VALIDATION	REFERENCE STANDARD	RELIABILITY	FEASIBILITY
Confusion Assessment Method (CAM) Nine operationalized delirium criteria scored according to CAM algorithm. Shortened version uses four criteria. Based on observations made during interview with MMSE, by trained lay or clinical interviewer.	• Onset/course Attention Organization of thought • Level of consciousness Orientation • Memory • Perceptual problems Psychomotor behavior • Sleep—wake cycle	Sensitivity = 0.94–1.0 (n = 26 delirious patients) Specificity = 0.90–0.95 (n = 30 controls without delirium) Convergent agreement with four other cognitive measures Ability to distinguish delirium and dementia verified	Geropsychiatrists' diagnoses based on clinical judgment and DSM-III-R criteria	Interrater: K = 1.0 overall	Observer-rated: 10–15 min for cognitive testing and completion of rating
CAM–ICU (CAM adaptation) Uses four CAM criteria. Cognitive assessment adapted for use only in nonverbal or ventilated patients.	• Onset/course Attention • Organization of thought • Level of consciousness	Sensitivity = 0.93–1.0 Specificity = 0.98–1.0 (n = 91 patients)	Delirium expert clinicians' ratings based on DSM-IV criteria	Interrater: K = 0.96 overall	Observer-rated: <5 min for cognitive assessment and completion of rating
Delirium Rating Scale (DRS) Ten-item rating, with additive score 0 to 32, designed to be completed by a psychiatrist after complete psychiatric assessment. Useful to rate severity.	• Onset/course Cognitive status • Perceptual problems • Delusions • Psychomotor behavior • Emotional lability • Sleep—wake cycle • Physical disorder	No overlap in scores between delirious group (n = 20) and three control groups: demented (n = 9), schizophrenic (n = 9), and normal (n = 9). Convergent agreement with two other cognitive measures. Ability to distinguish delirium and dementia verified	Consult-liaison psychiatrist's diagnosis based on DSM-III criteria	Interrater: intraclass correlation coefficient = 0.97	Observer-rated: based on lengthy interview and detailed assessment (time not specified)
Delirium Symptom Interview (DSI) Includes interview with brief cognitive assessment and rating scale for 7 symptom domains of delirium, by trained lay or clinical interviewer.	• Course • Organization of thought • Level of consciousness • Orientation Perceptual problems • Psychomotor behavior • Sleep–wake cycle	Sensitivity = 0.90 Specificity = 0.80 (n = 30 "cases", 15 noncases, 3 borderline, 2 disagreements by psychiatrist and neurologist). Ability to distinguish delirium and dementia not tested	Psychiatrist's and neurologist's assessments based on presence of any 1 of 3 "critical symptoms" (disorientation, disturbance of consciousness, or perceptual disturbance)	Interrater: K = 0.90 overall	Observer-rated part; 15+ min for interview, plus additional time for completion or rating (not specified)
Memorial Delirium Assessment Scale (MDAS) Ten-item scale, with additive score 0 to 30 using cognitive testing and behavioral observations, by experienced mental health professionals. Designed to rate delirium severity, not for screening or diagnosis.	• Level of consciousness • Orientation • Memory • Digit span • Attention Organization of thought • Perceptual problems Delusions • Psychomotor behavior • Sleep–wake cycle	Sensitivity = 0.82 Specificity = 0.75 (with score = 10; n = 33: 17 delirium, 8 dementia, 8 other psychiatric)	Consult-liaison psychiatrist's diagnosis using DRS, MMSE, and Clinician's Global Rating of delirium severity	Interrater: intraclass correlation coefficient = 0.92 overall	Observer-rated in part; 10+ min for administration

DSM-III, *Diagnostic and Statistical Manual of Mental Disorders*, 3rd ed.; DSM-III-R, *Diagnostic and Statistical Manual of Mental Disorders*, 3rd ed. rev.; DSM-IV, *Diagnostic and Statistical Manual of Mental Disorders*, 4th ed.; MMSE, Mini-Mental State Examination.
K = Kappa coefficient; n = number of subjects.
Modified with permission from Inouye SK, vanDyck CH, Alessi CA, et al. Ann Intern Med. 113:941, 1990; Ely EW, Inouye SK, Bernard GR, et al. JAMA. 286:2703, 2001; Trzepacz PT, et al. Psychiatry Research 23:89, 1988; Albert MS, Levkoff SE, Reilly C, et al. J Geriatr Psychiatr Neurol. 5:14, 1992; Breibart W, Rosenteld B, Roth A, et al. J Pain Symptom Manage. 153:231, 1997.

through careful cognitive assessment and to determine the acuity of change from the patient's baseline cognitive state. Because cognitive impairment may easily be missed during routine conversation, brief cognitive screening tests, such as the Mini-Mental Status Examination and the CAM, should be used. The degree of attention should be further assessed with simple tests such as a forward digit span (inattention indicated by an inability to repeat five digits forward) or recitation of the months of the year backward. A targeted history, focusing on baseline cognitive status and chronology of recent mental status changes, should be elicited from a reliable informant. In addition, such historical data as intercurrent illnesses, recent adjustments in medication regimen, the possibility of alcohol withdrawal, and pertinent environmental changes may point to potential precipitating factors of delirium.

The physical examination should include a detailed review that focuses on potential etiologic clues to an underlying or inciting disease process. Vital sign assessment is important to identify fever, tachycardia, or decreased oxygen saturation, each of which may point to specific disease processes. Auscultatory examination may suggest pneumonia or pulmonary effusion. A new cardiac murmur or dysrhythmia may suggest ischemia or congestive heart failure. Gastrointestinal examination should focus on evidence of an acute abdominal process, such as occult bleeding, perforated viscus, or infection. Patients with delirium may also demonstrate nonspecific focal findings on neurologic examination, such as asterixis or tremor, although the presence of any new neurologic deficit should raise suspicion of an acute cerebrovascular event or subdural hematoma. As previously mentioned, in many older patients and in those with cognitive impairment, delirium may be the initial manifestation of a serious new disease process. Therefore, attention to early localizing signs on serial physical examinations is important.

A complete medication review, including over-the-counter medications, is critical, and any medications with known psychoactive effects should be discontinued or minimized whenever possible. Because of pharmacodynamic and pharmacokinetic changes in aging adults, these medications may cause deleterious psychoactive effects even when prescribed at customary doses and with serum drug levels that are within the "therapeutic range."

Laboratory Tests and Imaging

Notwithstanding the growing recognition of geriatric syndromes such as delirium, there is little evidence-based research that assesses the predictive value of laboratory and other diagnostic testing in the evaluation of delirium. Consequently, laboratory evaluation should be guided by clinical judgment, taking into account specific patient characteristics and historical data. An astute history and physical examination, medication review, focused laboratory testing (e.g., complete blood count, chemistries, glucose, renal and liver function tests, urinalysis, oxygen saturation), and search for occult infection should help to identify the majority of potential contributors to the delirium. Obtaining additional laboratory testing such as thyroid function tests, B-12 level, cortisol level, drug levels or toxicology screen, syphilis serologies, and ammonia level should be based on a patient's distinct clinical presentation. Further diagnostic workup with an electrocardiogram, chest radiograph, and/or arterial blood gas determination may be appropriate for patients with pulmonary or cardiac conditions. The indications for cerebrospinal fluid examination, brain imaging, or EEG remain controversial. Their overall

diagnostic yield is low, and these procedures are probably indicated in less than 5% to 10% of delirium cases. Lumbar puncture with cerebrospinal fluid examination is indicated for the febrile delirious patient when meningitis or encephalitis is suspected. Brain imaging (such as CT or MRI) should be reserved for cases with new focal neurologic signs, with history or signs of head trauma, or without another identifiable cause of the delirium. Of note, some neurologic symptoms are associated with delirium, including tremor and asterixis. EEG, which has a false-negative rate of 17% and a false-positive rate of 22% for distinguishing between delirious and nondelirious patients, plays a limited role and is most commonly employed to detect subclinical seizure disorders and to differentiate delirium from nonorganic psychiatric conditions.

Differential Diagnosis

Distinguishing a long-standing confusional state (dementia) from delirium alone, or from delirium superimposed on dementia, is an important, but often difficult, diagnostic step. These two conditions can be differentiated by the acute onset of symptoms in delirium, with dementia presenting much more insidiously and by the impaired attention and altered level of consciousness associated with delirium.

The differential diagnosis of delirium can be extensive and includes other psychiatric conditions such as depression and nonorganic psychotic disorders (Table 53-5). Although perceptual disturbances, such as illusions and hallucinations, can occur with delirium, recognition of the key features of acute onset, inattention, altered level of consciousness, and global cognitive impairment will enhance the identification of delirium. Differentiating among diagnoses is critical because delirium carries a more serious prognosis without proper evaluation and management, and treatment for certain conditions such as depression or affective disorders may involve use of drugs with anticholinergic activity, for example, which could exacerbate an unrecognized case of delirium. At times, working through the differential diagnosis can be quite challenging, particularly with an uncooperative patient or when an accurate history is unavailable, and the diagnosis of delirium may remain uncertain. Because of the potentially life-threatening nature of delirium, however, it is prudent to manage the patient as having delirium and search for underlying precipitants (e.g., intercurrent illness, metabolic abnormalities, adverse medication effects) until further information can be obtained.

Algorithm for the Evaluation of Altered Mental Status

Figure 53-2 presents an algorithm for the evaluation of altered mental status in the older patient. The initial steps center on establishing the patient's baseline cognitive functioning and the onset and timing of any cognitive changes. Chronic impairments, representing changes that occur over months to years, are most likely attributable to a dementia, which should be evaluated accordingly (see Chapter 65). Acute alterations, representing abrupt deteriorations in mental status, occur over hours to weeks, although they may be superimposed on an underlying dementia. They should be further evaluated with cognitive testing to establish the presence of delirium. In the absence of notable delirium features (see "Presentation" earlier in this chapter), subsequent evaluation should focus on the possibility of major depression, acute psychotic disorder, or other psychiatric disorders (see Chapters 70 to 72).

TABLE 53-5

Differential Diagnosis of Altered Mental Status

CHARACTERISTIC	DELIRIUM	DEMENTIA	DEPRESSION	ACUTE PSYCHOSIS
Onset	Acute (hours to days)	Progressive, insidious (weeks to months)	Either acute or insidious	Acute
Course over time	Waxing and waning	Unrelenting	Variable	Episodic
Attention	Impaired, a hallmark of delirium	Usually intact, until end-stage disease	Decreased concentration and attention to detail	Variable
Level of consciousness	Altered, from lethargic to hyperalert	Normal, until end-stage disease	Normal	Normal
Memory	Impaired commonly	Prominent short- and/or long-term memory impairment	Normal, some short-term forgetfulness	Usually normal
Orientation	Disoriented	Normal, until end-stage disease	Usually normal	Usually normal
Speech	Disorganized, incoherent, illogical	Notable for parsimony, aphasia, anomia	Normal, but often slowing of speech (psychomotor retardation)	Variable, often disorganized
Delusions	Common	Common	Uncommon	Common, often complex
Hallucinations	Usually visual	Sometimes	Rare	Usually auditory and more complex
Organic etiology	Yes	Yes	No	No

PREVENTION

Primary prevention—preventing delirium before it develops—is the most effective strategy for reducing delirium and its associated adverse outcomes, which range from functional disability to longer lengths of hospital stay, institutionalization, and death. Table 53-6 describes well-documented delirium risk factors and tested preventive interventions to address each risk factor. A controlled clinical trial demonstrated the effectiveness of a delirium prevention strategy targeted toward these risk factors. The selection of risk factors was based upon their clinical relevance and the degree to which they

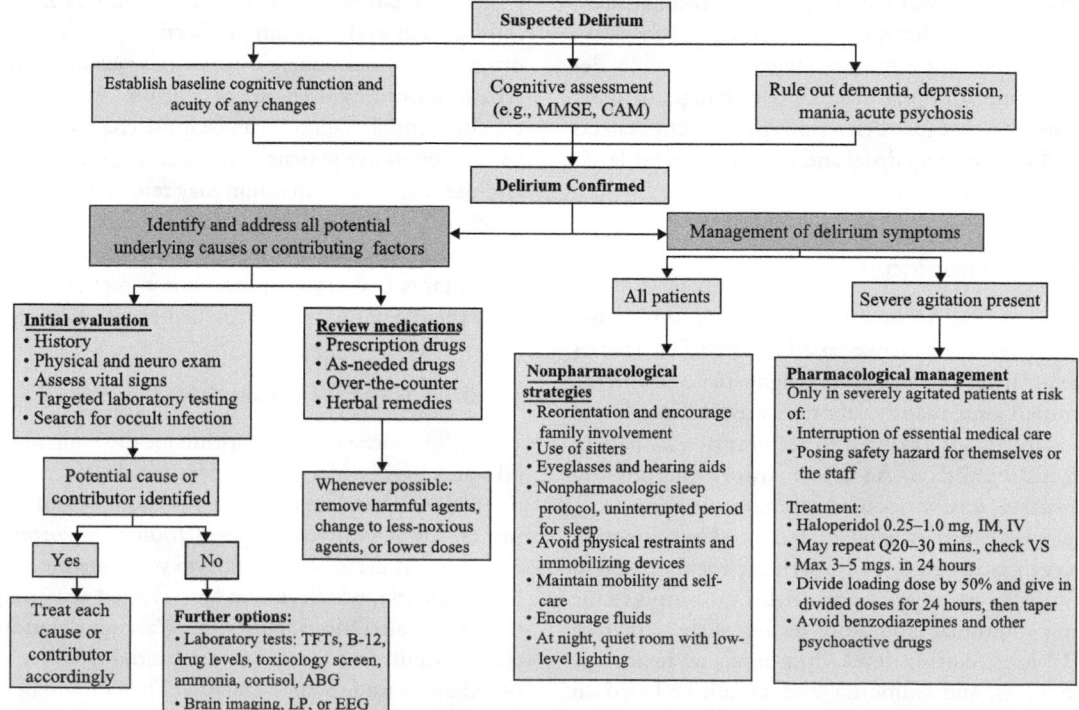

FIGURE 53-2. Flowchart for evaluation of suspected delirium in an older person. ABG, arterial blood gas; B-12, cyanocobalamin for vitamin B-12 level; CAM, Confusion Assessment Method; EEG, electroencephalography; LP, lumbar puncture; MMSE, Mini-Mental State Examination; neuro exam, neurologic examination; TFT, thyroid function tests (e.g., T4, thyroid index, thyroid-stimulating hormone); VS, vital signs. (Adapted from Inouye SK. Delirium and other mental status problems in the older patient. In: Goldman L, Bennett JC, eds. Cecil Textbook of Medicine, 21st ed. Philadelphia: WB Saunders; 2000:18.)

TABLE 53-6

Delirium Risk Factors and Tested Interventions	
RISK FACTOR	**INTERVENTION PROTOCOL**
Cognitive impairment	• Orienting communication, including orientation board • Therapeutic activities program
Immobilization	• Early mobilization (e.g., ambulation or bedside exercises) • Minimizing immobilizing equipment (e.g., restraints, bladder catheters)
Psychoactive medications	• Restricted use of PRN sleep and psychoactive medications (e.g., sedative–hypnotics, narcotics, anticholinergic drugs) • Nonpharmacological protocols for management of sleep and anxiety
Sleep deprivation	• Noise-reduction strategies • Scheduling of nighttime medications, procedures, and nursing activities to allow uninterrupted period of sleep.
Vision impairment	• Provision of vision aids (e.g., magnifiers, special lighting) • Provision of adaptive equipment (e.g., illuminated phone dials, large-print books)
Hearing impairment	• Provision of amplifying devices; repair hearing aids • Instruct staff in communication methods
Dehydration	• Early recognition and volume repletion

Modified with permission from Inouye SK, Bogardus ST Jr., Charpentier PA, et al. N Engl J Med. 340:669, 1999.

TABLE 53-7

Preventive Interventions after Hip Fracture	
RISK FACTOR	**INTERVENTION**
Hypoxia	• Supplemental oxygen • Raise systolic blood pressure • Transfusion to Hematocrit >30%
Fluid/electrolyte imbalance	• Restore serum sodium, potassium, glucose • Treat fluid overload or dehydration
Pain	• Around-the-clock acetaminophen • Low-dose morphine, oxycodone for break-through pain
Psychoactive medications	• Minimize benzodiazepines, anticholinergics, antihistamines • Eliminate drug interactions and redundancies
Bowel/bladder dysfunction	• Treat constipation • Discontinue urinary catheter by postoperative day 2, screen for retention or incontinence
Poor nutrition	• Provide dentures, assistance • Supplements or enteral nutrition
Immobilization	• Early mobilization (out of bed postoperative day 1) • Physical therapy

Postoperative complications	• Monitor and treat for:
	  Myocardial ischemia
	  Atrial arrhythmias
	  Pneumonia
	  Pulmonary embolus
	  Urinary tract infection

Sensory deprivation	• Use glasses and hearing aids • Provide clock and calendar • Provide radio and soft lighting
Treatment of agitation	• Diagnostic work-up • Reassurance, family presence, sitter • If pharmacologic management necessary, use haloperidol

Modified with permission from Marcantonio ER, Flacker JM, Wright RJ, et al. J Am Geriatr Soc. 49:516, 2001.

could be modified by employing practical and feasible interventions. Compared with standard care, implementation of these preventive interventions resulted in a 40% risk reduction for delirium in hospitalized older patients.

The Hospital Elder Life Program (HELP; www.hospitalelderlifeprogram.org) represents an innovative strategy of hospital care for older patients, designed to incorporate the tested delirium prevention strategies and to improve overall quality of hospital care. Programs such as HELP underscore the importance of an interdisciplinary team's contributions to the prevention of delirium. For example, trained volunteers and family members can play roles in daily orientation, therapeutic recreation activities, and feeding assistance. Physical rehabilitation experts and nurses can assist with mobilization and the incorporation of daily exercises to prevent functional decline. Dietitians can help to maximize appropriate caloric intake and oral hydration in acutely ill patients. Consultant pharmacists, chaplains, and social workers also may provide specialized expertise to address patient care issues pertinent to individuals at risk for delirium.

Proactive geriatric consultation has been demonstrated to reduce the risk of delirium posthip fracture by 40% in a randomized controlled trial. The targeted multicomponent consultation strategy focused on 10 domains, namely, adequate brain oxygen delivery, fluid/electrolyte balance, pain management, reduction in psychoactive medications, bowel/bladder function, nutrition, early mobilization, prevention of postoperative complications, appropriate environmental stimuli, and treatment of delirium (Table 53-7). The recommendations were carried out with good adherence (77%)

and provided a feasible and effective approach to address a leading complication of hip fracture surgery. Although not yet tested, this multicomponent approach is likely to be effective at reducing the risk of delirium in high-risk patients other than those with posthip fracture repair.

At least eight additional recent studies have examined preventive delirium interventions in controlled trials. These studies have applied multifactorial interventions (six studies) or educational strategies targeted toward healthcare staff (two studies), and have demonstrated reductions in delirium rates and/or duration. Multifactorial interventions consisted of staff education strategies combined with the administration of individually tailored treatment and management of patients with delirium. Educational interventions sought to increase awareness and knowledge of delirium among medical staff, in hopes of improving assessment, prevention, and management strategies of patients with delirium. Regarding different care and rehabilitation settings, a recent controlled trial found that home rehabilitation after acute hospitalization in the elderly was associated with lower risk of delirium, and greater patient satisfaction, when compared with the hospital setting. Taken together, results from controlled trials suggest that 30% to 40% of cases of delirium may actually be preventable and that prevention strategies should begin in the preoperative period.

On a larger scale, preventive efforts for delirium will require system-wide changes and large-scale shifts in local and national policies and approaches to care. Recommended changes include routine cognitive and functional assessment on admission of all older patients; monitoring mental status as a "vital sign"; education of physicians and nurses to improve recognition and heighten awareness of the clinical implications; enhanced geriatric physician and nursing expertise at the bedside; incentives to change practice patterns that lead to delirium (e.g., immobilization, use of sleep medications, bladder catheters, and physical restraints); and creation of systems that enhance high-quality geriatric care (e.g., geriatric expertise, case management, clinical pathways, and quality monitoring for delirium). Implementing these changes will impact not only on delirium, but will result in high-quality hospital care more generally.

MANAGEMENT

Pharmacological Management

The recommended management approach for all delirious patients begins with nonpharmacologic strategies (see "Nonpharmacological Management" and "Nonpharmacological Sleep Protocol" later in this chapter), which usually result in successful symptom amelioration. In selected cases, such strategies must be supplemented with a pharmacologic approach, usually reserved for patients in whom delirium symptoms would result in interruption of needed medical therapies (e.g., mechanical ventilation, central lines) or may endanger the safety of the patient or other persons. However, prescribing any drug requires balancing the benefits of delirium management against the potential for adverse medication effects because no drug is ideal for the treatment of delirium symptoms. Sometimes the decision to prescribe may be influenced by other members of the clinical team, the family, or caregivers. All interested parties should understand that the choice of almost any medication may further cloud the patient's mental status and obscure efforts to monitor the course of the mental status change. Consequently, any drug chosen should be initiated at the lowest starting dose for the shortest time possible.

Neuroleptics

In general, neuroleptics are the preferred agents of treatment, with haloperidol being the agent in most widespread use, whose effectiveness has been established in a randomized clinical trial. Haloperidol is available in parenteral form and is associated with less postural blood pressure changes and fewer anticholinergic side effects compared with thioridazine; however, high-potency antipsychotics such as haloperidol are associated with a higher rate of extrapyramidal side effects and acute dystonias. The intravenous route can be used when parenteral administration is required, which results in a rapid onset of action and a short duration of effect, whereas oral or intra-

muscular use is associated with a more optimal duration of action. The recommended starting dose is 0.5 to 1.0 mg haloperidol orally or parenterally. The dose may be repeated every 30 minutes after the vital signs have been rechecked and until sedation has been reached. The clinical end point should be an awake but manageable patient, a goal that can be achieved by following the general geriatric prescribing principle, "start low and go slow." Most older patients naïve to prior treatment with a neuroleptic should require a total loading dose of no more than 3 to 5 mg of haloperidol. A subsequent maintenance dose consisting of one-half of the loading dose should be administered in divided doses over the next 24 hours, with doses tapered over the ensuing several days as the agitation resolves.

Other Pharmacological Approaches

Benzodiazepines (e.g., lorazepam) are not recommended as first-line agents in the treatment of delirium because of their increased propensity to cause oversedation and to exacerbate acute mental status changes. However, they remain the treatment of choice for delirium caused by seizures and alcohol- and medication-related withdrawal syndromes. While other drugs have been advocated for use in treatment of delirium, their use has been evaluated only in case series or uncontrolled studies and is not recommended. These drugs include the newer atypical antipsychotic agents, procholinergic agents (such as donepezil), and serotonin receptor antagonists (such as trazodone). While the newer antipsychotic drugs (such as risperidone, olanzapine, and quetiapine) have the potential for fewer sedative and extrapyramidal effects, they may be less effective for controlling delirium symptoms and have not yet been evaluated in randomized clinical trials. Moreover, official warnings have been issued regarding the increased mortality associated with use of atypical antipsychotics in dementia patients.

Nonpharmacological Management

Nonpharmacological approaches are the mainstays of treatment for every delirious patient. These approaches include strategies for reorientation and behavioral intervention, such as ensuring the presence of family members, use of sitters, and transferring a disruptive patient to a private room or closer to the nurse's station for increased supervision. Orienting influences such as calendars, clocks, and the day's schedule should be prominently displayed, along with familiar personal objects from the patient's home environment (e.g., photographs and religious artifacts). Personal contact and communication are critical to reinforce patient awareness and encourage patient participation as much as possible. Communication should incorporate repeated reorientation strategies, clear instructions, and frequent eye contact. Correction of sensory impairments (i.e., vision and hearing) should be maximized as applicable for individual patients by encouraging the use of eyeglasses and hearing aids during the hospital stay. Mobility and independence should be promoted; physical restraints should be avoided because they lead to decreased mobility, increased agitation, and greater risk of injury. Patient involvement in self-care and decision-making should also be encouraged. Other environmental interventions include limiting room and staff changes and providing a quiet patient care setting with low-level lighting at night. An environment with decreased noise allowing for an uninterrupted period for sleep at night is of crucial importance in the management of delirium. This may require unitwide changes in the coordination and scheduling of nursing and medical procedures, including medication dispensing, vital sign recording, and administration of intravenous medications and other treatments. Hospital-wide changes may be needed to ensure a low level of noise at night, including minimizing hallway noise, overhead paging, and staff conversations.

Nonpharmacological Sleep Protocol

Nonpharmacological approaches for relaxation and sleep can be effective for management of agitation in delirious patients and for prevention of delirium through minimization of psychoactive medications. The nonpharmacological sleep protocol includes three components: (1) a glass of warm milk or herbal tea, (2) relaxation music or tapes, and (3) back massage. This protocol was demonstrated to be feasible and effective. Use of the protocol reduced the use of sleeping medications from 54% to 31% ($P < .002$) in a hospital environment.

SPECIAL ISSUES

Nursing Home Setting

The patient population in nursing homes can be divided into two distinct groups: postacute patients who receive short-term rehabilitative care in nursing homes after an acute hospitalization, and long-term care patients who reside in nursing homes as a result of severe cognitive and functional impairments. Both are high-risk groups for delirium, though the epidemiology differs between the two populations.

For the postacute population, persistent delirium after an acute hospitalization is the major issue. A recent study demonstrated that 16% of new admissions to postacute care met full CAM-criteria for delirium, while another 50% demonstrated signs of subsyndromal (partial) delirium. Patients with delirium on admission to postacute care experience more complications such as falls, have higher rehospitalization rates, and higher mortality. Delirium among postacute patients is also persistent—of those admitted with delirium, over 50% are still delirious 1 month later. Persistence of delirium prevents functional recovery in the postacute setting; only those patients whose delirium cleared within 2 weeks of admission recovered to their prehospitalization functional status. Persistent delirium is also associated with higher mortality.

The long-term care population represents a high-risk group for delirium, with a high prevalence of dementia and functional impairments. In these individuals it is incident, rather than prevalent delirium, which is the primary concern. Large-scale epidemiological studies of delirium in these patients have not been performed, but data from the Minimum Data Set suggest that incident delirium is common in this population, and frequently heralds the onset of an acute illness that results in hospitalization and/or death.

Interventions for delirium in the nursing homes are challenging. First, because of the high prevalence of dementia in both postacute and long-term care populations, case identification can be challenging. This is compounded in the postacute population by a lack of knowledge of the patient's baseline cognitive state. Poor nursing staffing ratios, high turnover, and competing concerns make attention to delirium challenging in this setting. Nonetheless, these patients represent among the most vulnerable of all elders, and further attention to delirium in this setting is warranted.

Palliative Care Setting

Management of delirium at the end of life poses particular challenges. Because delirium occurs in more than 80% of patients at the end of life, it is considered nearly inevitable in the terminal stages by most hospice care providers and may serve as a predictor of approaching death. Establishing the goals of care with the patient and family is a crucial step, including discussions about the potential causes of the delirium, intensity of medical evaluations considered appropriate, and the need for titration between alertness and adequate control of pain and agitation. For example, some patients may wish to preserve their ability to communicate as long as possible, while others may focus on comfort perhaps at the expense of alertness. Physicians must be cognizant that even in the terminal phase, many causes of delirium are potentially reversible, and may be amenable to interventions (e.g., medication adjustments, treatment of dehydration, hypoglycemia, or hypoxia) that may improve comfort and quality of life. However, the burdens of evaluation (e.g., invasive testing) or treatment (e.g., reduction in narcotic dose) may not be consistent with the goals for care. In all cases, symptom management should begin immediately, while evaluation is underway. Nonpharmacological approaches should be instituted in all patients, with pharmacological approaches for selected cases. Haloperidol remains the first-line therapy for delirium in terminally ill patients. In end-of-life care, there is a lower threshold for the use of sedative agents. Sedation may be indicated as an additional therapy for management of severe agitated delirium in the terminally ill patient, which can cause considerable distress for the patient and family. Because sedation poses the risks of decreased meaningful interaction with family, increased confusion, and respiratory depression, this choice should be made in conjunction with the family according to the goals for care. If sedation is indicated, an agent that is short-acting and easily titrated to effect is recommended. Lorazepam (starting dose 0.5 to 1.0 mg po, IV, or SQ) is the recommended agent of choice.

Ethical Issues

In a condition characterized by acute fluctuations in attention and decision-making capacity, delirium presents formidable challenges to the ethical care of afflicted patients (see Chapters 13 and 34). Recent research has highlighted the importance of determining and appropriately documenting cognitive impairment prior to initiating nonemergent treatments. Cognitive assessments in patients with suspected delirium help to ensure that appropriate surrogate decision makers (e.g., family members or caregivers) are involved in representing a patient's wishes, and understanding the risks and benefits of procedures and treatments. Because the patient may exhibit periods of lucidity in delirium, there may be times during which the informed consent process can and should involve the patient. Following resolution of an acute delirium episode, the clinician should be cognizant of ongoing subclinical manifestations of delirium, or partial forms of delirium, which may be important for considerations of both the long-term management and decision-making capacity of the patient.

FURTHER READING

Albert MS, Levkoff SE, Reilly C, et al. The delirium symptom interview. *J Geriatr Psychiatry Neurol.* 1992;5:14.

Alsop DC, Fearing MA, Johnson K, et al. *J Gerontol Med Sci.* 2006;61A:1287.

Amador LF, Goodwing, JS. Postoperative delirium in the older patient. *J Am Coll Surg.* 2005;200:767.

American Psychiatric Association. *Diagnostic and Statistical Manual of Mental Disorders,* 4th ed., Text Revision. Washington, DC: American Psychiatric Association; 2000.

American Psychiatric Association. Practice guideline for the treatment of patients with delirium. *Am J Psychiatry.* 1999;156(5 Suppl):1.

Breitbart W, Marotta R, Platt MM, et al. A double-blind trial of haloperidol, chlorpromazine, and lorazepam in the treatment of delirium in hospitalized AIDS patients. *Am J Psychiatry.* 1996;153:231.

Breibart W, Rosenfeld B, Roth A, et al. The Memorial Delirium Assessment Scale. *J Pain Symptom Manage.* 1997;13:128.

Creditor MC. Hazards of hospitalization of the elderly. *Ann Intern Med.* 1993;118: 219.

Ely EW, Inouye SK, Bernard GR, et al. Delirium in mechanically ventilated patients: validity and reliability of the confusion assessment method for the intensive care unit (CAM-ICU). *JAMA.* 2001;286:2703.

Inouye SK. Delirium in older persons. *N Engl J Med.* 2006;354:1157.

Inouye SK, vanDyck CH, Alessi CA, et al. Clarifying confusion: the confusion assessment method. A new method for detection of delirium. *Ann Intern Med.* 1990;113:941.

Inouye SK, Viscoli CM, Horwitz RI, et al. A predictive model for delirium among hospitalized elderly persons based on admission characteristics. *Ann Intern Med.* 1993;119:474.

Inouye SK, Charpentier PA. Precipitating factors for delirium in hospitalized elderly persons: predictive model and inter-relationship with baseline vulnerability. *JAMA.* 1996;275:852.

Inouye SK, Bogardus ST Jr, Charpentier PA, et al. A clinical trial of a multicomponent intervention to prevent delirium in hospitalized older patients. *N Engl J Med.* 1999;340:669.

Marcantonio ER, Flacker JM, Wright RJ, et al. Reducing delirium after hip fracture: a randomized trial. *J Am Geriatr Soc.* 2001;49:516.

Marcantonio ER, Rudolph JL, Culley D, et al. Serum biomarkers for delirium. *J Gerontol Med Sci.* 2006;61A:1281.

Naughton BJ, Saltzman S, Ramadan R, et al. A multifactorial intervention to reduce prevalence of delirium and shorten hospital length of stay. *J Am Geriatr Soc.* 2005;53:18.

Tabet N, Hudson S, Sweeney V, et al. An educational intervention can prevent delirium on acute medical wards. *Age Ageing.* 2005;34:152.

Trzepacz PT, van der Mast RC. The neuropathophysiology of delirium. In: Lindesay J, Rockwood K, Macdonald A, eds. *Delirium in Old Age.* Oxford: Oxford University Press; 2002:51.

Trzepacz PT, Mittal D, Torres R, et al. Validation of the Delirium Rating Scale–Revised-98: Comparison with the Delirium Rating Scale and Cognitive Test for Delirium. *J Neuropsychiatry Clin Neurosci.* 2001;13:229.

Falls

Mary B. King

DEFINITION

Falls are common in older persons. A fall injury is costly in terms of morbidity, loss of physical function and independence, and mortality, as well as health care utilization. Falls have not always been recognized as a serious health problem. Prior to the 1940s, a fall was considered an unpredictable event that could not be prevented. In the past 20 years, however, research studies have shown the incidence and consequences of falls, revealed their multifactorial etiology, and demonstrated that they can be prevented by treating the factors that increase an older person's risk of falling. Effective treatment requires a multidisciplinary approach. Perhaps because of this, fall prevention is not widely practiced in clinical settings outside of specialized geriatric assessment clinics; thus, falls remain an undertreated public health issue.

This chapter addresses nonsyncopal (Syncope is discussed in Chapter 57) falls—unintentional events in which a person comes to rest on the floor or ground that are not caused by loss of consciousness, stroke, seizure, or overwhelming force. Falls in three different settings—the community, skilled nursing facilities, and hospitals—are discussed; reasons for falling and, therefore, interventions differ by site.

INCIDENCE AND CONSEQUENCES OF FALLS

Incidence and Prevalence of Falling

Approximately 35% to 40% of persons age 65 years and over fall in a given year; half of persons who fall do so more than once. The incidence increases steadily after age 60 years; approximately 50% of persons aged 80 years and older fall in a year. Women are more likely to fall than men. More than half of all falls in the community happen at home. The rates for falls in skilled nursing facilities and hospitals are almost three times that for community-dwelling elders, and are estimated at 1.5 falls per bed per year.

Fall Injuries

Incidence of Fall Injuries

Although young children and athletes also have a high incidence of falls, older persons are at high risk of injury with a fall because of age-related changes such as slow reaction time, impaired protective responses, and comorbid diseases such as osteoporosis. As a result, serious fall injuries, including fractures, lacerations, serious soft-tissue injuries, and head trauma, occur in 5% to 15% of falls in the community. Injury rates are higher, from 10% to 25% of falls, in institutional settings. Approximately 8% of persons aged 65 years and older visit an emergency department because of a fall-related injury each year; almost half of these persons are admitted to the hospital for treatment. In 2003, 1.8 million older persons were treated in an emergency department for nonfatal fall injuries. Fractures, most commonly of the hip, pelvis, femur, vertebrae, humerus, hand, forearm, leg, or ankle, occur in approximately 3% of falls. Conversely, falls account for 87% of all fractures and for more than 95% of hip fractures in this group. Falls are the second leading cause of brain and spinal cord injury in older adults. According to data from 2001 to 2005, the annual rates of nonfatal injuries are about 48% higher for women than men (Figure 54-1).

Hip Fractures

Hip fractures are probably the most dreaded fall-related injury, as approximately half of older persons who sustain a hip fracture cannot return home or live independently after the fracture, and up to 20% die within a year of the fracture. Between 1993 and 2003, the age-adjusted hospitalization rate for hip fractures initially increased, then

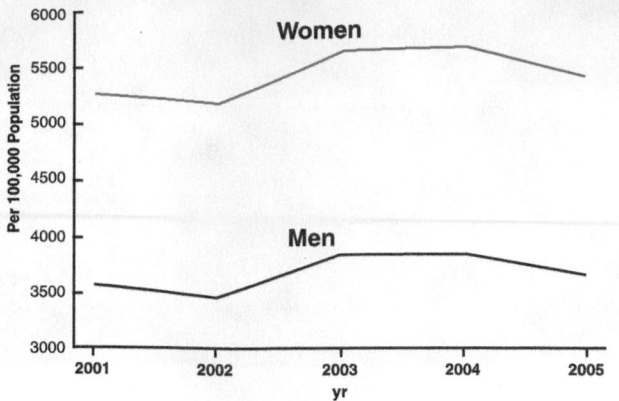

FIGURE 54-1. Age-adjusted nonfatal fall injury rates among men and women aged 65 yrs and older, United States. Rates are per 100,000 people, age-adjusted to the 2000 U.S. population. *(Redrawn from Centers for Disease Control and Prevention, National Center for Injury Prevention and Control. Web-based Injury Statistics Query and Reporting System (WISQARS), 2005. Available at: www.cdc.gov/ncipc/wisqars.)*

declined, with an overall rate of 775.5 per 100,000 people in 2003. The incidence of hip fracture is higher for women than men, but there was a decline of 20.8% in the hospitalization rate for hip fractures in women between 1993 and 2003, while that for men has remained the same.

Death

In the United States, unintentional injury is the fifth leading cause of death in persons age 65 years and older; falls are the cause of two-thirds of the deaths resulting from injuries in this age group. In 2003, approximately 13 700 older persons died as the result of a fall. The age-adjusted death rate from falls increased significantly between 1993 and 2003, and men in this age group continue to have a significantly higher fatality rate than women (Figure 54-2).

Other Consequences of Falling

Falls are costly for older persons, both in terms of health care dollars and in loss of physical function and independence. Fall-related in-

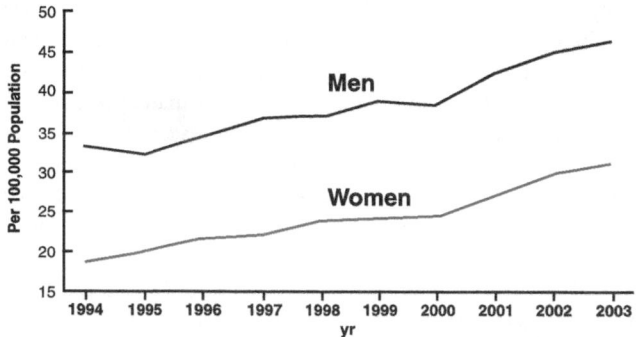

FIGURE 54-2. Age-adjusted fatal fall injury rates among men and women aged 65 yrs and older, United States. Rates are per 100,000 people, age-adjusted to the 2000 U.S. population. *(Redrawn from Centers for Disease Control and Prevention, National Center for Injury Prevention and Control. Web-based Injury Statistics Query and Reporting System (WISQARS), 2005. Available at: www.cdc.gov/ncipc/wisqars.)*

juries account for approximately 6% of all health care expenses for persons aged 65 years and older in the United States. Falls also take a toll on an older person's independence and quality of life. Falls account for approximately 20% of restricted activity days in older people—more than for any other health condition. In addition to immediate curtailment of activity, older persons who have a fall injury may restrict activity for several months or longer after the injury because of residual physical impairment or because of fear of falling again. Older persons are often unable to get up from the ground or floor after a fall, resulting in long lies with the risk of pneumonia, dehydration, and rhabdomyolysis. Fear of falling occurs in at least 50% of those who fall, and leads to restriction of activities in 10% to 25%. Finally, falls and fall injuries are a major determinant of nursing home placement.

ETIOLOGY OF FALLS AND FALL INJURIES

A fall occurs when a person's center of gravity moves outside of their base of support and insufficient, ineffective, or no effort is made to restore balance. Classification schemes have been developed to explain how falls occur. One such scheme classified falls according to cause, namely extrinsic, or as a consequence of slips, trips, and other environmental factors that perturbed balance; intrinsic, or as a consequence of deficits in balance, mobility, cognitive or sensory function; nonbipedal falls, such as falling out of bed; or nonclassifiable falls. Falls have also been classified by most likely immediate cause, including environmental factors, balance or gait disorder, drop attack, dizziness, or postural hypotension. However, while observation may suggest that one factor predominates, more often it is the interaction of multiple factors that results in a fall (Figure 54-3). Intrinsic, personal characteristics, in conjunction with pharmacologic and behavioral factors, can alter resting balance or affect an older person's postural responses to challenges posed by the environment, or posed simply by movements such as transfers or walking.

Risk Factors for Falling

Age-Associated Changes and Chronic Diseases

Prospective and retrospective community- and nursing home-based studies in the past 15 years have identified a number of factors that increase an older person's risk of falling. Table 54-1 lists the most commonly identified factors. Studies show that the risk of falling increases with the number of risk factors a person has (Figure 54-4).

Age greater than 80 years, need for assistance with activities of daily living, and previous falls, indicate risk for future falls. While these characteristics cannot be modified, they serve as indicators for clinicians to pay increased attention to the presence of other, treatable risk factors for falls. The most important modifiable intrinsic risk factors for falls are balance, strength, and gait impairments. Impairment in these areas may be caused by a number of sensory, neurological, or musculoskeletal diseases, in addition to deconditioning as a result of lack of activity, age-related changes, and medication effect.

Postural Control
Balance, or postural control, is dependent upon the integration of visual, vestibular, and proprioceptive input by the central nervous system to effect an appropriate postural response to

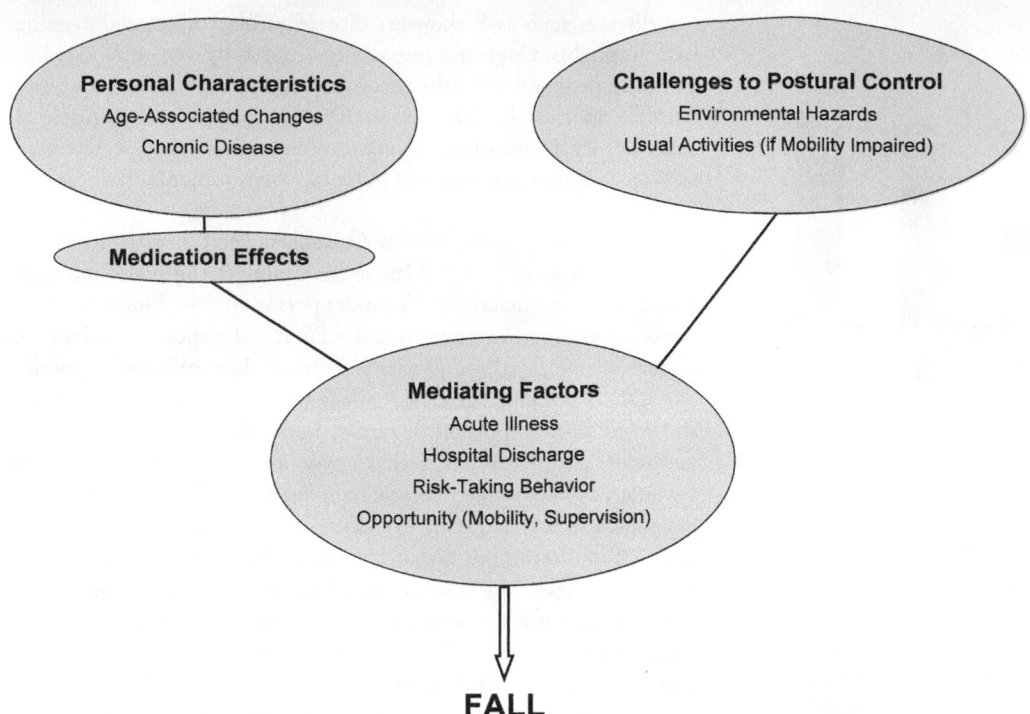

FIGURE 54-3. Interactions among intrinsic, pharmacologic, environmental, and situational factors that affect risk of falling in older persons. *(Modified with permission from King MB, Tinetti ME. Falls in community-dwelling older persons. J Am Geriatr Soc. 43:1146, 1995.)*

control the movement of the center of mass over the base of support, the feet. With quiet standing, there is little movement of the center of mass. The area over the feet within which a person is able to lean decreases with age. Fall risk has been linked to mediolateral instability; clinically this can be tested by the ability to stand in tandem

stance or on one leg, both of which reduce the mediolateral base of support. The effect of impaired performance of static balance tasks may be manifested in activities such as walking and transferring. Persons who experience difficulty with standing balance tasks may walk more slowly and therefore spend a greater percentage of the gait cycle in more stable double stance with a wider base of support. Maintaining balance during body movements requires a reaction to restore the person's displaced center of mass over the base of support. A loss of balance may be caused by the speed or magnitude of displacement, an inability to quickly detect the displacement because of sensory impairment, slowing of central nervous system integration of sensory information into a motor response, or muscle weakness or joint pain, causing an inadequate or ineffective response. Older persons take compensatory steps at lower levels of balance disturbance than young adults, but may have less effective stepping responses (multiple steps, difficulty controlling lateral stability) with greater challenges to balance. Older persons are slower than young adults in initiating reaching reactions to break a fall or grasp a handrail.

Sensory Input   Sensory modalities that provide afferent input for balance responses include vision, hearing, proprioception, and vestibular function. Vision is affected by age and disease. While decreased visual acuity may be important, impaired contrast sensitivity (the ability to detect edges) and depth perception have been found to be the most significant visual risk factors for falls. Multifocal lenses, commonly worn by presbyopic older persons, are problematic because the lower, near-vision lenses impair distance depth perception in the lower visual field where tripping hazards would be seen. Cataracts, glaucoma, and macular degeneration affect vision and are common diseases in older persons. There is some evidence that first-cataract surgery can reduce fall risk. Hearing loss is found in more than 50% of older people, and can affect perception of and orientation to the environment. Vestibular function changes with age and with diseases affecting the inner ear. Impaired vestibular function

TABLE 54-1

Results of Univariate Analysis of Most Common Risk Factors for Falls Identified in 16 Studies* that Examined Risk Factors			
RISK FACTOR	**SIGNIFICANT/ TOTAL[†]**	**MEAN RR-OR[‡]**	**RANGE**
Muscle weakness	10/11	4.4	1.5–10.3
History of falls	12/13	3.0	1.7–7.0
Gait deficit	10/12	2.9	1.3–5.6
Balance deficit	8/11	2.9	1.6–5.4
Use of assistive device	8/8	2.6	1.2–4.6
Visual deficit	6/12	2.5	1.6–3.5
Arthritis	3/7	2.4	1.9–2.9
Activities of daily living (ADL) impairment	8/9	2.3	1.5–3.1
Depression	3/6	2.2	1.7–2.5
Cognitive impairment	4/11	1.8	1.0–2.3
Age >80 yrs	5/8	1.7	1.1–2.5

*See source for study references.

[†]Number of studies with significant odds ratio or relative risk ratio in univariate analysis/total number of studies that included each factor.

[‡]Relative risk ratios (RR) calculated for prospective studies. Odds ratios (OR) calculated for retrospective studies.

Modified with permission from Anonymous. Guideline for the prevention of falls in older persons. American Geriatrics Society, British Geriatrics Society, and American Academy of Orthopaedic Surgeons Panel on Falls Prevention. J Am Geriatr Soc. 49:664, 2001.

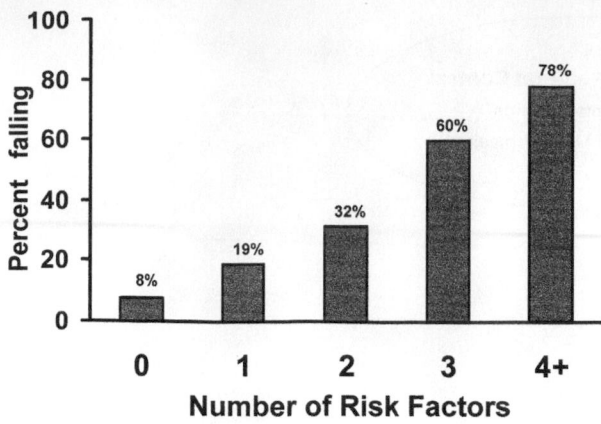

A

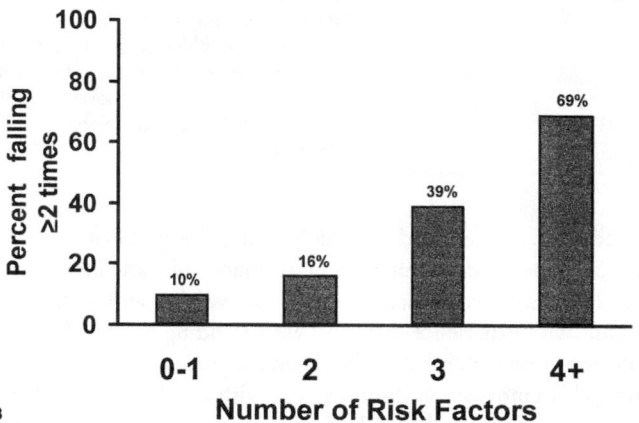

B

FIGURE 54-4. The risk of falling increases with the number of risk factors present, both for single and recurrent falls. (A) Occurrence of falls, according to the number of risk factors, in a study of 336 persons older than age 75 yrs living in the community. Risk factors included sedative use, cognitive impairment, lower-extremity disability, palmomental reflex, foot problems, and balance/gait abnormalities. *(Adapted with permission from Tinetti ME, Speechley M, Ginter SF. Risk factors for falls among elderly persons living in the community. N Engl J Med. 319:1701, 1988. Copyright ©1988 Massachusetts Medical Society. All rights reserved).* (B) The proportion of subjects who fell more than two times increased with number of risk factors in a study of 325 community-dwelling persons older than age 60 yrs who had fallen in the previous year. Risk factors were difficulty standing up from a chair, difficulty with tandem walk, arthritis, Parkinson's disease, more than three falls or a fall with injury in the previous year, and white race. *(Data from Nevitt MC, Cummings SR, Kidd S, et al. Risk factors for recurrent nonsyncopal falls. A prospective study. JAMA 261:2663, 1989. Copyright ©1989, American Medical Association. All rights reserved.)*

can lead to loss of balance when there is decreased visual input as a consequence of disease, or as a result of environmental factors, such as movement in the dark. Mechanoreceptors in apophyseal joints and peripheral nerves provide proprioceptive input and may be affected by age, degenerative joint disease, cervical disorders such as spondylosis, or peripheral neuropathy. Proprioceptive dysfunction can result in loss of balance on uneven ground or in situations, such as walking in the dark, where there is decreased visual input.

Central Processing Central nervous system processing of sensory input to initiate a postural response may be affected by neurolog-

ical diseases such as Parkinson's disease, stroke, or normal pressure hydrocephalus. Cognitive impairment caused by dementia may impair judgment and affect the perception and interpretation of sensory stimuli, resulting in falls even without the presence of a muscle or gait disorder. Depression may increase fall risk because of decreased concentration or awareness of potential environmental hazards.

Musculoskeletal Impairments Musculoskeletal impairments increase the risk of falling. Muscle mass and strength decline with age, disease, and inactivity. The older person may no longer be capable of generating the strength and accuracy of response to a balance disturbance (e.g., tripping) that is required. Loss of lower-extremity strength, in particular ankle dorsiflexor strength, has repeatedly been shown to be an important determinant of fall risk. Weakness of hip abductors and adductors may decrease an older person's ability to maintain balance while stepping to avoid a fall. Musculoskeletal diseases such as osteoarthritis can cause pain, deformity, and limited range of motion in joints, particularly in the back, hips, knees, and feet that increase the risk for falls. Upper body arthritis or muscle weakness can affect an older person's ability to break the impact of a fall, increasing the risk of injury such as a fracture. Foot problems, such as calluses, bunions, long nails, or joint deformity, can affect balance by compensatory strategies as a consequence of pain or impaired sensory input.

Postural Hypotension Postural hypotension, which may result in instability, occurs in 10% to 30% of community-dwelling older persons aged 65 years and older. A drop in systolic blood pressure of 20 mmHg or more with change in position from lying to standing may be medication-related, caused by dehydration, or a result of age-associated changes or diseases that affect autonomic control of vascular tone. Postprandial hypotension may be suspected in persons complaining of dizziness or who fall after getting up from, or soon after, a meal.

Medications

Several studies show that the use of four or more prescription and nonprescription medications increases the risk of falling. Older persons often take more than four medications each day because of multiple chronic diseases, multiple prescribing physicians and consultants, accumulation of medications over time, lack of understanding about how to take medications, and demand for medications based on advertising. Medications may cause postural instability by their expected effects on cognitive functioning, fluid and electrolyte balance, or blood pressure, or by adverse effects. Observational data in multiple studies demonstrate an increased risk of falls with anticonvulsants and any psychotropic medication use, including sedative/hypnotics, antidepressants, short- or long-acting benzodiazepines, or neuroleptics. In addition, a meta-analysis of observational studies of cardiac and analgesic drug use showed a weak association between falls and the use of class IA antiarrhythmic medications, digoxin, and diuretics. The risk of an adverse drug event increases with the number of medications taken, such that a person taking nine or more medications has 3.3 times the risk of an adverse event as compared to someone taking four or fewer medications. Fatigue, altered mental status, somnolence, dizziness, and impaired balance, listed as side effects of many medications, are also risk factors for falls.

Acute Illness and Hospital Discharge

Time-related or situational factors also may result in impaired balance by augmenting already present risk factors for falls. Acute illness, such as pneumonia or exacerbation of congestive heart failure, may present as a fall in a frail older person because of altered mental status, postural hypotension, or weakness. Older persons are also vulnerable after treatment in the emergency department or after hospitalization because of the illness that caused their admission, deconditioning, or medication effects. The risk of a fall in older persons recently discharged from the hospital and receiving home care is about fourfold higher than that for others in the community during the first 2 weeks after discharge.

Challenges to Postural Control

Extrinsic risk factors for falls include environmental hazards that, in concert with intrinsic factors, increase susceptibility to falls. Because more than half of older persons' falls occur at home, studies have examined the contribution of environmental factors to fall risk. While no particular hazard has been implicated in falls, home safety remains a concern. There are checklists available to use in reviewing home safety; Table 54-2 summarizes areas at home that should be checked. Environmental factors that did not pose a safety risk previously become hazardous to an older person with declining balance and mobility (e.g., transfers in and out of a bathtub).

Opportunity to Fall

Additional factors contributing to fall risk are an older person's risk-taking behavior and opportunity for a fall. Older persons with impaired balance or strength may do activities that are beyond their capabilities—such as climbing on a chair or counter to reach high cabinets, hanging curtains, rushing to answer the telephone—because of poor judgment, a desire to maintain independence, or lack of family or friends to help. Persons who are confined to bed or have close supervision are less likely to fall because of lack of opportunity to do so. Fear of falling is frequently seen in older persons, both in those who have fallen and in those with limited mobility who have not yet fallen. Fear may lead to destabilizing compensatory strategies when walking or transferring, such as reaching to hold on to furniture, which increase the risk of falling.

Risk Factors for Fall Injury

Osteoporosis

Injury with a fall is dependent upon factors in addition to those for falling. The presence of osteoporosis increases an older person's risk of fracture. A decrease of one standard deviation in femoral neck bone mineral density increases the risk of hip fracture 2.7 times. Low body mass index and low weight increase the force of impact with a fall because of lack of cushioning effect of muscle and subcutaneous tissue (see Chapter 117, Osteoporosis).

Characteristics of the Fall

The force of a fall and direct impact on a bone increase the likelihood of injury, particularly of fracture. Factors that increase the force of a fall include falling from a greater height, such as on stairs; not attempting to break the fall (e.g., by reaching for furniture); and landing on a hard surface. Falling sideways or directly onto the hip increases the likelihood of hip fracture; falling forward onto an outstretched wrist increases the likelihood of a Colles' fracture.

FALL PREVENTION IN COMMUNITY-DWELLING OLDER PERSONS

Trials of Interventions to Prevent Falls

Trials to reduce the incidence of falls have varied in their approach. Investigators have either focused on improving a single factor or multiple factors. Study participants either have been unselected or have been screened for the presence of risk factors. To date, the most successful strategies have been those targeted at older persons at risk or who have fallen, those designed to intervene on multiple risk factors, to be of longer duration or greater intensity, or to be individually tailored to treat risk factors. The involvement of more than one health care discipline in the intervention, including nursing, occupational and physical therapy, and physicians, has also been effective.

TABLE 54-2

Checklist of Measures to Improve Safety in and Around the Home

Outside
  Repair uneven pavement, cracked sidewalks
  Install railings for outdoor steps
  Use adequate lighting
  Keep shrubbery trimmed near walks

Inside
  Floors
    Remove throw rugs
    Use nonskid carpet backing; tack down or tape carpet edges
    Avoid wax or use nonskid wax
    Mark high thresholds with reflective tape
    Remove clutter and furniture from traffic areas
    Keep electrical and telephone cords near walls, out of walkways
    Make sure that telephone can be reached from floor, or have emergency call device
  Lighting
    Adjust to decrease glare
    Have adequate lighting from bedroom to bathroom at night
    Have lights with switches at top and bottom of stairways
  Stairways
    Install railings on both sides, extending full length of stairs
    Make sure railings are secure
    Ensure stairs have nonskid surfaces and are free of clutter
    Mark top and bottom step with reflective tape
  Bathroom
    Install grab bars in bath and next to toilet if mobility impaired
    Use rubber mat in bath or shower
    Install raised toilet seat if needed
  Kitchen
    Keep food, dishes within easy reach
    Do not use cupboards that are too high or too low

Single Interventions

A number of interventions have been designed to reduce the incidence of falls by improving balance and strength through home or group exercise. The more successful programs generally have been those in which participants were selected for impairments in balance, strength, or mobility; the exercise program was intensive, well-supervised, and sustained over at least 10 weeks; and the program included exercises to improve balance. A meta-analysis of seven of the Frailty and Injuries: Cooperative Studies of Intervention Techniques (FICSIT) trials that studied the effect of exercise on fall risk in older persons showed that, while exercise in general reduced fall risk by 10%, balance exercise reduced the incidence of falls by 17%. In one of the FICSIT studies, practicing Tai Chi C'uan to improve balance significantly reduced the subsequent incidence of falls.

Several studies have examined the effect of modifying the home environment to reduce falls, but there is insufficient evidence that correcting home hazards reduces falls or fall injuries. There was one randomized controlled trial of psychotropic medication withdrawal that was effective in reducing falls. Other trials of single interventions have produced results of questionable effectiveness. Educational programs for older persons about fall risk factor modification have not been effective by themselves in preventing falls.

Multifactorial Interventions

Several studies employing a multidisciplinary, multifactorial approach to risk factor reduction in community-dwelling older persons have been published, and more are being completed. Effective components of these studies include exercise programs, reduction in the number and dosage of medications, treatment of postural hypotension and other cardiovascular disorders, and treatment of visual impairment. One strategy that has been successful has been a combination of assessment and treatment in the home by a nurse, and/or a physical or occupational therapist, and medical risk factor assessment and treatment in an outpatient office setting. Modification of the home environment to improve home safety as part of a multifactorial intervention has been of equivocal or no efficacy. None of the intervention studies has had enough participants to show a reduction in fall injuries.

Strategy for Decreasing Falls and Fall Injuries

The most effective fall-prevention programs require coordination of efforts by several health care disciplines to treat the older person who is at risk for falls. The strategy is first to screen for fall risk, and then to perform a thorough assessment and create a treatment plan for those who are likely to fall in the future.

Screen for Fall Risk

All older persons seen for routine medical care should be screened for fall risk by asking, at least once a year, if they have fallen. They should be observed getting up from a chair and walking across a room for difficulty with the activity, unsteadiness, or use of an assistive device. Fall risk assessment is included in Center for Medicare and Medicaid's new Patient Quality Reporting Initiative. If there is no history of falls and no problem with balance, mobility, or gait, then no specific fall risk assessment is necessary (Figure 54-5). However, in all healthy older adults, routine vision and hearing screening, regular review and reduction, when possible, of medications, screening for and treatment of osteoporosis, exercise prescription, and discussion of home safety, can aid fall prevention.

Multifactorial Assessment

If there is a history of one or more falls, or if the person has problems with mobility or gait, then a more detailed fall risk assessment is warranted (see Figure 54-5). Other potentially high-risk times are during acute illness, after hospital or emergency department discharge, or after introduction of new medications. Determination of risk factors for falls is within the capability of the primary care provider; it requires a systematic approach and a plan of treatment that often requires coordination among several different specialties and disciplines. Referral to a geriatric specialist with resources to coordinate multidisciplinary care may be the most effective way to accomplish fall risk assessment and treatment. The assessment should include history taking and medication review, physical examination, including physical performance testing, and, when indicated, assessment of the home environment. It is important to look for all possible contributing factors, as the concept of risk reduction is to treat as many factors as possible to lessen the likelihood of a fall.

The medical history should focus on information about physical function, mobility, use of an assistive device such as a cane or walker, performance of activities of daily living, previous falls and fractures, and acute or chronic medical problems. If the person has fallen, details of fall circumstances, including setting and activity at the time of the fall, can help determine specific risk factors for future falls. A list should be made of the dose and frequency of all medications that the older person actually takes, including over-the-counter medications. This can be done by "brown bag" review of medications in the office, or, if the older person is eligible for visiting nurse services, by a nurse in the home.

Aspects of the physical examination that pertain to fall risk are: checking for postural blood pressure changes (lying, then standing after 3 mins); pulse (looking for cardiac arrhythmias and appropriate response to positional change); hearing and visual acuity screening; and examination of joints for range of motion and evidence of arthritis, and of the feet for deformity and painful lesions. A neurologic examination should include mental status testing, cranial and peripheral nerve function, reflexes, muscle strength, and cerebellar and sensory function. Tests of functional gait and balance maneuvers during usual activities are part of a fall risk assessment (Table 54-3). The Timed Up and Go Test can be done in less than 1 minute in an office setting and has high sensitivity and specificity in predicting fall risk. Other measures, such as the Performance-Oriented Mobility Assessment, give more specific information about balance, gait, and mobility impairment, but take longer to perform and are best used for assessment prior to a rehabilitative program. Laboratory testing is determined by the history and physical examination, and may include a complete blood count, fasting blood glucose, electrolytes, blood urea nitrogen (BUN) and creatinine, thyroid-stimulating hormone (TSH), B-12 level, and levels of medications such as digoxin and anticonvulsants. Testing for osteoporosis will determine the need for medication to improve bone density (to reduce risk of fracture). Radiographs, such as cervical spine films, and computed tomography or magnetic resonance imaging of the brain, are only indicated if diseases that would be diagnosed by these tests are suspected.

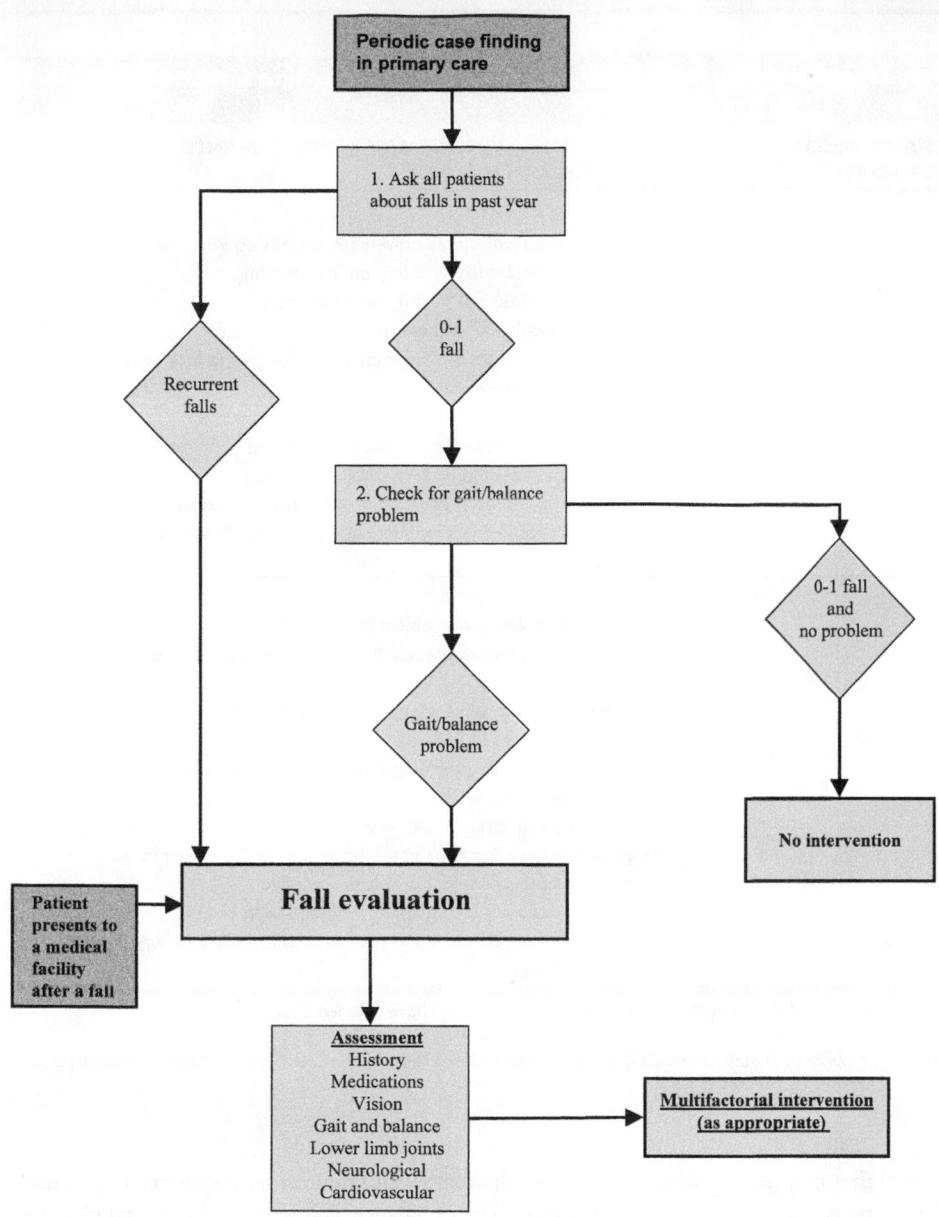

FIGURE 54-5. Algorithm summarizing screening, assessment, and management of falls. *(Modified with permission from Anonymous. Guideline for the prevention of falls in older persons. American Geriatrics Society, British Geriatrics Society, and American Academy of Orthopaedic Surgeons Panel on Falls Prevention. J Am Geriatr Soc. 49:664, 2001.)*

Multidisciplinary Treatment

Once the older person's risk factors for falls have been determined, an individually tailored, multidisciplinary treatment plan can be put in place. The key components of such a plan include one or more of the following: (1) exercise and training to improve deficits in balance, mobility, and strength; (2) correction of sensory deficits (vision, hearing, vestibular and proprioceptive function); (3) evaluation and treatment of postural hypotension; (4) review and reduction of medications; (5) treatment of foot problems; and (6) environmental modification and use of adaptive equipment, if indicated. Although education is not effective as a single intervention, it is a key component of the treatment plan. The older persons and their caregivers need to understand the importance of falls, the multifactorial nature of fall risk, and the strategies for fall prevention. Table 54-4 summarizes possible interventions for factors that contribute to falling.

Physical therapy, with instruction in exercises to improve balance and mobility, is an important part of the fall prevention strategy. Progressive exercises under the guidance of a physical therapist can help the older person improve confidence and reduce fear of falling. Older persons can also be taught how to get up from the floor in order to prevent a long lie as a result of a fall.

Other strategies for older persons with limited mobility include wearing an emergency call device in order to summon help or to have a telephone within reach in case of a fall. Treatment of osteoporosis can reduce the likelihood of a fracture with a fall. The use of hip protectors in the community setting has not been shown to be effective in reducing the incidence of falls or hip fractures.

Falls in Skilled Nursing Facilities

The general approach to fall-risk evaluation and treatment in nursing home residents is the same as with older people living in the community, although the relative importance of individual risk factors for falls in each setting differs. While most community-dwelling elderly persons have as their goal to increase function and maintain independence, nursing home residents and their family members

TABLE 54-3

Observation of Position Changes, Balance Maneuvers, and Gait Components Used in Daily Activities that Indicate Fall Risk if Not Performed Adequately

MANEUVER	MEASURE(S) IN WHICH IT IS A COMPONENT	OBSERVATION: ABNORMALITY IN PERFORMANCE THAT INDICATES FALL RISK
Position change or balance maneuver		
Getting up from a chair*	A,B	Does not get up with single movement; pushes up with arms or moves forward in chair first; unsteady on first standing
Sitting down in a chair*	A,B	Plops in chair; does not land in center of chair
Withstanding pull back at waist	A	Moves feet; begins to fall backward; grabs object for support
Side-by-side standing with eyes open	A	Feet not touching side by side; moves feet; begins to lose balance or grabs object for support
Semitandem, tandem standing	C	Cannot maintain stances for 10 s (same as above)
Standing on one leg	A	Cannot maintain stance for 5 s (same as above)
Bending over	A	Unable to bend over to pick up small object (e.g., pen) from floor; grabs object to pull up on; requires multiple attempts to arise
Neck turning	C	Moves feet; grabs object for support; complains of vertigo, dizziness, or unsteadiness
Gait component or maneuver		
Gait initiation	A,B	Hesitates; stumbles; grabs object for support
Step height (raising feet with stepping)	A,B	Does not clear floor consistently (scrapes or shuffles); raises foot too high (more than 2 in.)
Step continuity	A,B	After first few steps, does not consistently begin raising one foot as other foot touches floor
Step symmetry	A,B	Step length not equal (pathologic side usually has longer step length—problem may be in hip, knee, ankle, or surrounding muscles)
Path deviation	A,B	Does not walk in straight line; weaves side-to-side
Turning	A,B	Stops before initiating turn, staggers; sways; grabs object for support
Stepping over obstacles	A	Unable to step over obstacles or loses balance
Gait speed	A	Unable to increase walking speed without losing balance
	B	Takes longer than 10 s to stand up from chair, walk 3 m, turn, walk back to chair and sit

Maneuvers that are components of physical performance tests are indicated as follows: A, Performance-Oriented Mobility Assessment; B, Timed Up and Go Test; C, other maneuvers.
*Use hard, armless chair.

Modified with permission from Tinetti ME and Ginter SF. Identifying mobility dysfunctions in elderly patients. JAMA. 259:1190, 1988. Copyright ©1988 American Medical Association. All rights reserved.

and caregivers must weigh the risk of decreased safety that may accompany independent mobility, particularly as frailty increases.

The focus of fall risk assessment and treatment in skilled nursing facilities is to find the least-restrictive means by which the resident can move safely. Because it is less likely that personal risk factors as a result of age and chronic disease can be modified sufficiently to prevent falls, and because the opportunity for observation and supervision is greater in the nursing home setting, more emphasis should be placed on improving individual patient safety within the environment.

Evaluation

A careful assessment of risk factors for falls is important for all residents on admission, at yearly examinations, with a significant change in condition, or after a fall. The history may be difficult to obtain owing to cognitive impairment, and may require input from family members or caregivers. Specific symptoms such as dizziness, foot or joint pain, weakness, or decreased sensation, if elicited, may indicate acute or chronic diseases that contribute to fall risk. As in community-dwelling older adults, the physical examination should include checking for postural changes in blood pressure, screening for cognitive, vision, and hearing impairments, examination of car-

diovascular, musculoskeletal, and neurological systems, and examination of the feet. Tests of balance, transfers, and gait, and observation for proper use of assistive devices are also part of the evaluation. Laboratory testing may be of help in diagnosing or evaluating specific chronic diseases.

Pharmacologic and situational factors play a key role in fall risk in the nursing home. Risk assessment should include regular medication review and reduction, if possible. Medication use, particularly of psychotropic medications, is an important contributor to fall risk in this setting, and this is a factor that potentially can be modified. Because of the prevalence of chronic disease, nursing home residents are likely to be on more than four medications, and may be less able to identify symptoms of adverse reactions to drugs, such as fatigue and dizziness, that increase risk of falling. Early recognition of acute illnesses, such as urinary tract infection or pneumonia, which are likely to begin with symptoms of impaired cognition or mobility, can lead to treatment and preventive measures to keep the older person from falling.

After a fall, there may be greater opportunity to get accurate information about fall circumstances and to evaluate the resident because of closer supervision by health care professionals in this setting as compared to the community. Symptoms of dizziness may suggest postural hypotension or medication effect; symptoms or

TABLE 54-4

Multidisciplinary Treatment of Factors Contributing to Fall Risk

FACTOR CONTRIBUTING TO FALL RISK	TREATMENT
Age-Associated or Caused by Chronic Disease	
Impaired balance, gait, mobility	
Neurologic disease, with impaired strength, sensation, balance, gait, tone, and/or coordination	M: Diagnose and treat specific disease (e.g., Parkinson's disease, stroke, normal pressure hydrocephalus) R: Physical therapy; balance and gait training; correct walking aid E: Home safety assessment; appropriate adaptations (e.g., high, firm chairs, raised toilet seats, grab bars in bathroom)
Dementia, with impaired gait, apraxia	M: Diagnose and treat specific disease; minimize centrally acting medications R: Supervised exercise and walking S: Evaluate home safety; need for supervision

Musculoskeletal disease
    Muscle weakness
    Arthritides with back/joint deformity causing postural instability
    Feet: pain, deformity
	M: Diagnose and treat specific diseases; referral to podiatry, if indicated, for foot care
	R: Physical therapy with muscle strengthening exercises, balance, and gait training; correct walking aid; correct footwear
	E: Home safety assessment; appropriate adaptations

Sensory impairment	
Vision: acuity, accommodation, contrast sensitivity	M: Referral for refraction; cataract extraction R: Balance and gait training E: Home safety assessment with attention to good lighting
Hearing: spatial disorientation, balance impairment, distorted environmental signals caused by decreased auditory input	M: Cerumen removal; audiologic evaluation with hearing aid if appropriate
Vestibular dysfunction: spatial disorientation at rest; balance impairment especially with head or body turning	M: Avoid vestibulotoxic drugs; surgical ablation R: Habituation exercises E: Good lighting (increased reliance on visual input); home safety assessment
Proprioceptive: cervical disorders; peripheral neuropathy; spatial disorientation during position changes or while walking on uneven surfaces or in dark	M: Diagnose and treat specific disease (e.g., spondylosis, B-12 deficiency, diabetes mellitus) R: Physical therapy; balance and gait training; correct walking aid E: Good lighting (increased reliance on visual input); appropriate footwear; home safety assessment
Impaired perception or concentration	
Dementia: impaired judgment, problem solving	See "Dementia" above
Depression: poor concentration or awareness?	M: Watch for adverse medication effects E: Home safety assessment
Postural hypotension	
Impaired cerebral blood flow leading to fatigue, weakness, postural instability; syncope if severe	M: Diagnose and treat specific diseases; review medications and reduce/eliminate offending ones; adequate salt and water intake R: Graded pressure stockings; dorsiflexion and hand flexion exercises prior to arising
Total number and dose of medications	
Taking ≥ 4 medications	M: Regular review and reduction, when possible, of number and dose of medications, including nonprescription medications; consider nonpharmacologic treatments; start medications low and increase slowly
Specific medications Sedatives, antidepressants, neuroleptics, diuretics, antihypertensives, antiarrhythmics, anticholinergic medications	
Other	
Change in dose; new medications	
Situational and Environmental Factors	
Onset of acute illness	M: Diagnose and treat specific diseases; close supervision of mobility
Hospital or emergency department discharge	M: Review medications and doses; look for adverse effects of new medications; evaluate balance, mobility R: Physical therapy if indicated E: Home safety assessment S: Assess need for increased supervision
Risk-taking behavior	S: Assess need for increased supervision or community services R: Recommend avoiding only clearly hazardous and unnecessary activities (e.g., climbing on chairs); balance and gait training E: Home safety assessment
Environmental hazards	E: Home safety assessment

E, environmental; M, medical; R, rehabilitative; S, social services/case management.

signs of acute infection, myocardial infarction, heart failure, or stroke may be elicited. The time and location of the fall may give clues as to the most effective intervention. A fall in the hallway after lunch may indicate postprandial hypotension; a fall in the bathroom near bedtime when nursing staff are helping other residents may indicate the need for scheduled toileting or greater supervision at that time. Examination of footwear and condition of assistive devices may also lead to interventions to prevent future falls.

Treatment

Multifactorial Approach

As in community fall prevention and risk reduction, a multifactorial approach is most effective in the nursing home setting; however, the risk factors targeted may be different. Because poor balance and decreased mobility are such important predictors of falls, interventions have been designed specifically to address these impairments. However, while studies have shown that it is possible to improve balance and strength with exercise in nursing home residents, these improvements have not resulted in fewer falls. Multidisciplinary interventions that have been effective included education of patient care staff, ensuring environmental safety, fitting and repair of assistive devices, reduction of psychotropic medications, instruction in safe transfers and walking, exercise classes, and the use of hip protectors. Maintaining a safe environment is of great importance in the nursing home setting, as environmental factors play a larger role in fall risk for patients with impaired mobility and cognition. Attention should be paid to floors, removing clutter, unstable furniture such as rolling tray tables, and lighting. Beds should be low enough so that the resident can sit with knees bent to 90 degrees and feet on the floor. Use of half-rails can improve safety and aid in transfers in and out of bed. Chairs should be firm, with arms. Bathrooms should be equipped with rails and, if appropriate, raised toilet seats.

Alternatives to Restraints

Since the 1990s, there have been widespread efforts to reduce the use of physical and chemical restraints and to find alternatives to prevent falls in nursing home residents. The use of restraints has not been shown to decrease the incidence of fall injuries. Bed and chair alarms to alert caregivers that residents are getting up are alternatives to restraints for fall prevention. Low beds and mats placed on the floor next to the bed reduce the risk of injury with a fall. Additional alternatives to restraint use to reduce fall risk include structured group activities to increase supervision of at-risk residents, scheduled toileting, particularly before and after meals, and attention to the safe use of assistive devices.

Hip Protectors

In the setting of a skilled nursing facility, ambulatory older persons at risk for falls also are likely to have osteoporosis. Treatment of risk factors for falls and osteoporosis are not sufficient to prevent all falls and fractures, particularly in residents who have low bone density. One option for treatment is the use of hip protectors, which attenuate the force of a fall on the hip. Those studied most extensively consist of foam or plastic pads placed inside pockets on a stretchy undergarment so that the protectors lie over the greater trochanter of each hip.

The undergarment is designed to be fairly easy to wear without affecting walking or sitting. Initial research indicated that, when worn, hip protectors significantly reduced the incidence of hip fractures. However, as more studies have been done, the evidence supporting the use of hip protectors has become weaker. Their use in the nursing home setting is marginally beneficial in reducing hip fractures. Compliance with hip protectors is problematic because of difficulty pulling the undergarment up or down for toileting, discomfort, poor fit, skin irritation, or lack of perceived risk for hip fracture.

HOSPITAL FALLS

Research on prevention of falls and fall injuries in the hospital setting has been problematic. Trial design is difficult because of short patient stays, the variation in case mix and staffing in different units in a hospital, and lack of control patients or units. Studies have utilized multifaceted interventions, such that it is difficult to evaluate the effectiveness of individual components. An insufficient number of randomized, controlled trials preclude making evidence-based recommendations concerning the evaluation of fall risk and prevention of falls and fall injuries in the hospital setting, other than that a multifaceted approach appears to reduce the incidence of falls. However, fall prevention is a focus for hospitals as well as hospital regulatory agencies, and best practice nursing guidelines have been published.

Fall prevention requires hospital administrative support and the ongoing attention of staff through multidisciplinary review and revision of patient care. Individual units may vary in their approach because of differences in patient mix and staffing. The components of a fall prevention program should include: (1) risk factor assessment and identification of patients at risk for falls; (2) individualized care plans for fall prevention; (3) evaluation of incident falls; and (4) revision of the care plan after a fall as appropriate to prevent further falls. Communication of falls risk among care providers and to patients and their families is an essential element of a hospital fall prevention program.

Risk Factor Assessment

Patients at risk for falls in the hospital are those with chronic or acute cognitive impairment; weakness and difficulty with balance, transfers, or gait; need for frequent toileting because of urinary frequency, incontinence, or diarrhea; medication use; history of a previous fall at home or, more significantly, in the hospital; fear of falling; depression; dizziness; functional impairment; environmental factors; and advanced age. Various assessment tools have been created to identify patients at risk for falls; however, risk screening tools may perform better in some hospital unit settings than others. Performing a fall risk screen on a patient at least daily can serve as a reminder of fall risk for nursing personnel caring for the patient.

Preventive Measures

Once a patient is screened as being at risk for falls, many hospitals use markers in the chart, on the patient's wristband, and/or in the patient's room to designate fall risk and to communicate that risk to caregivers. Standard preventive strategies are used, such as keeping the call bell within reach, the bed in the lowest position, and the room uncluttered. Strategies to address specific risk factors are employed, such as physical therapy to improve gait and balance; scheduled toileting for those with elimination issues; use of low beds, half-rails on the bed, and nonskid footwear for patients with mobility problems; and increased supervision for patients with cognitive impairment or delirium. The use of physical restraints in acute care settings should be avoided as there is no evidence that restraints prevent falls in these patients, and restraints may increase the risk of injury.

Evaluation of Falls and Revision of Care Plan

When a patient falls, unit personnel should note the circumstances and outcome of the fall, as well as contributing factors and functional assessment. The physician evaluating the person who falls should note associated symptoms (e.g., dizziness, confusion, incontinence, palpitations, weakness); perform a physical examination, including assessment for postural hypotension, new neurological deficit, and trauma; a medication review to reduce or eliminate possible contributing medications; and appropriate laboratory and radiological studies. This information can be used to revise the nursing plan of care as well as medical treatment.

Communication of fall risk to all hospital personnel taking care of the patient is important; it is also important for patients and their families to be made aware of fall risk in the hospital setting and the plan of care that is in place to decrease that risk. At discharge, fall risk should be communicated to the skilled nursing facility or home care agency that will be providing further care.

AREAS FOR FUTURE RESEARCH

Although much is now known about falls and their consequences, there are still questions about what the best, most cost-effective interventions are to prevent falls and fall injuries. Within the current U.S. health care system, care is not coordinated among different providers and disciplines and is aimed more at treatment rather than prevention of disease. Given these constraints, studies need to be done of fall prevention in community practice settings. Research studies of interventions that have been successful generally have targeted older persons at risk for falling; yet more needs to be learned about who will benefit most from fall prevention efforts, particularly in nursing home and hospital settings. The most effective treatment of specific impairments, such as visual problems, dementia, and cardiovascular disease, to reduce falls needs further investigation.

CONCLUSION

Falls are common in older persons, and are costly in terms of injury, loss of function, and health care costs. There is now evidence that multidisciplinary programs aimed at reducing multiple risks for falls are effective in preventing falls in a community research setting. The evidence is less compelling for nursing home and hospital falls. Screening for fall risk, careful assessment of older persons who have fallen or have mobility impairment, and oversight of an individualized, multidisciplinary risk reduction plan are important components of the care of geriatric patients.

FURTHER READING

Anonymous. Guideline for the prevention of falls in older persons. American Geriatrics Society, British Geriatrics Society, and American Academy of Orthopaedic Surgeons Panel on Falls Prevention. *J Am Geriatr Soc.* 2001;49:664.

Gillespie LD, Gillespie WJ, Robertson MC, et al. Interventions for preventing falls in elderly people (Cochrane Review). *The Cochrane Library,* Volume 4, 2006. Oxford: Update Software.

Leipzig RM, Cumming RG, Tinetti ME. Drugs and falls in older people: a systematic review and meta-analysis: I. Psychotropic drugs. *J Am Geriatr Soc.* 1999;47:30.

Leipzig RM, Cumming RG, Tinetti ME. Drugs and falls in older people: a systematic review and meta-analysis: II. Cardiac and analgesic drugs. *J Am Geriatr Soc.* 1999;47:40.

Lyons RA. Modification of the home environment for the reduction of injuries (Cochrane Review). *The Cochrane Library,* Volume 4, 2006. Oxford: Update Software.

Mahoney J, Sager M, Dunham NC, et al. Risk of falls after hospital discharge. *J Am Geriatr Soc.* 1994;42:269.

National Center for Injury Prevention and Control, Centers for Disease Control and Prevention (CDC). http//www.cdc.gov/ncipc/ Last accessed September 2007.

Nevitt MC, Cummings SR, Kidd S, et al. Risk factors for recurrent nonsyncopal falls. A prospective study. *JAMA.* 1989;261:2663.

Oliver D, Connelly JB, Victor CR, et al. Strategies to prevent falls and fractures in hospitals and care homes and effect of cognitive impairment: systematic review and meta-analyses. *BMJ.* 2007;334:82.

Parker MJ, Gillespie WJ, Gillespie LD. Hip protectors for preventing hip fractures in the elderly (Cochrane Review). *The Cochrane Library,* Volume 4, 2006. Oxford: Update Software.

Perell KL, Nelson A, Goldman RL, et al. Fall risk assessment measures: an analytic review. *J Gerontol Med Sci.* 2001;56A:M761.

Podsiado D, Richardson S. The timed "Up & Go": a test of basic functional mobility for frail elderly persons. *J Am Geriatr Soc.* 1991;39:142.

Resnick B. Preventing falls in acute care. In: Mezey M, Fulmer T, Abraham I, Zwicker DA, eds. *Geriatric Nursing Protocols for Best Practice.* 2nd ed. New York, New York: Springer; 2003:141–164.

Rubenstein LZ, Josephson KR, Robbins AS. Falls in the nursing home. *Ann Intern Med.* 1994;121:442.

Tinetti ME, Speechley M, Ginter SF. Risk factors for falls among elderly persons living in the community. *N Engl J Med.* 1988;319:1701.

Tinetti ME. Preventing falls in elderly persons. *N Engl J Med.* 2003;348:42.

Sleep Disorders

Mairav Cohen-Zion ■ *Sonia Ancoli-Israel*

INTRODUCTION

Over the past several years, much research has focused on normal age-related changes in sleep as a function of aging. However, in addition to these common changes, aging is also associated with an increase in sleep complaints and chronic sleep disturbances, resulting in poorer daytime functioning and increases in health care usage. This chapter reviews sleep and sleep disorders in order adults, including information on presentation, etiology, pathophysiology, evaluation, and management of sleep-related issues.

CHANGES IN SLEEP WITH AGING

Approximately 50% of community-dwelling elderly persons complain of some form of sleep difficulty. Subjective and objective reports show that when compared to their younger counterparts, older adults take longer to fall asleep, have lower sleep efficiency (defined as the amount of sleep given the amount of time in bed), have more nighttime awakenings, wake up earlier than they would like in the morning, and require more daytime naps (Table 55-1). Polysomnographic (PSG) sleep recordings have confirmed these findings, showing that despite older adults spending more time in bed, they have a harder time getting to sleep, get overall less sleep, and have more nighttime awakenings, resulting in reduced sleep efficiency. It is not surprising then that Multiple Sleep Latency Tests (MSLTs), objective measures assessing daytime sleepiness via PSG-recoded napping opportunities, indicate that older adults are significantly sleepier throughout the day than are younger adults.

One central question raised by researchers in the field is whether these age-related changes represent a decrease in the need for sleep or a decrease in the ability to sleep. Although this question is still being debated and there is no clear consensus on whether there is a reduced need for sleep, there is clearly a reduced ability to sleep

in this population. As discussed in this chapter, sleep difficulties in this population are associated with several factors, including specific sleep disorders, changes in the endogenous circadian clock, medical and psychiatric illness, and medication intake (Table 55-2). Recent developments in sleep research have identified several effective treatments for many of these sleep difficulties. Given the high prevalence of sleep complaints and sleep disorders in this population and the link between insufficient sleep and heightened levels of morbidity and mortality, there is a clear need for increased awareness, assessment, and treatment of these sleep disturbances.

SLEEP-DISORDERED BREATHING

Definition

Sleep-disordered breathing (SDB) is characterized by respiratory events, including hypopneas (partial respiration) and/or apneas (complete cessation of respiration), during sleep. These respiratory events occur repeatedly over the course of the night with each respiratory event lasting a minimum of 10 seconds. The number of apneas per hour of sleep is called the apnea index (AI) and the number of apneas and hypopneas per hour of sleep is called the apnea–hypopnea index (AHI; also sometimes called the respiratory disturbance index [RDI]). Clinical diagnosis of SDB is traditionally given when a patient has an AHI of 10 to 15.

The cessations in breathing in SDB lead to repeated arousals from sleep, as well as to reductions in blood oxygen levels over the course of the night, which result in nighttime hypoxemia.

Epidemiology

SDB is more common in older than younger adults and among nursing home patients, specifically elderly with dementia, when

TABLE 55-1

Sleep Complaints of Older Adults
Spend too much time in bed
Spend less time asleep
Increase in number of awakenings
Increase in time to fall asleep
Less satisfied with sleep
Significant increase in daytime sleepiness
Napping more often and longer

TABLE 55-3

Potential Age-Dependent Risk Factors in Sleep Disordered Breathing
Increased body mass index (central obesity)
Decreased muscle tension
Changes in airway anatomy
Increased airway collapsibility
Decreased thyroid function
Decreased lung volume

compared to those elderly living independently. Table 55-3 summarizes several potential age-dependent risk factors in the development of SDB. The prevalence of SDB varies by severity level or AHI. Approximately 2% to 4% of middle-aged men and women (age 30 to 60 years) have an AHI ≥ 5, compared to 32% to 81% of older adults (age 60+ years). With increasing AHI, these percentages are slightly lower, with 19% to 62% of older adults having an AHI ≥ 15 and up to 24% having an AHI ≥ 20. In addition, within the older population, SDB is more common in men than in women and in patients with hypertension, and may be more severe in elderly people in the African-American than in the Caucasian population.

Pathophysiology

There are three types of apneic events: central, obstructive, and mixed. Central events are a result of a dysfunction of the respiratory neurons. Obstructive events are caused by anatomic obstruction of the upper airways despite respiratory effort. Mixed events are a combination of central and obstructive components.

Presentation

The cardinal symptoms of SDB are snoring and excessive daytime sleepiness. It is often one or both of these two symptoms that motivate the patient to seek evaluation and treatment of this sleep disorder. Additional symptoms may include insomnia, nocturnal confusion, and cognitive deficits, such as difficulty with concentration and memory.

Approximately 50% of regular snorers suffer from some degree of SDB and snoring may be an early precursor to SDB. Snoring is reflective of the airway collapse and is a component of the breathing cessation during an apneic event. It may be extremely loud, being heard all over the house. Often bed partners have moved into separate bedrooms. While not all snoring is associated with sleep apnea,

TABLE 55-2

Factors Contributing to Sleep Disturbances in Older Adults
Circadian rhythm changes
Primary sleep disturbances (e.g. SDB, PLMS)
Medical illness (e.g., hyperthyroidism, arthritis)
Psychiatric illness (e.g., depression, anxiety disorders)
Multiple medications
Dementia
Poor sleep hygiene habits

SDB, sleep disordered breathing; PLMS, periodic leg movements in sleep.

snoring alone is associated with increased risk of ischemic heart disease and stroke.

The excessive daytime sleepiness seen in SDB is associated with sleep fragmentation or repeated nighttime awakenings, which frequently follow the apneic events, and with the nocturnal hypoxia. Daytime sleepiness may manifest as being unable to stay awake or falling asleep at inappropriate times during the day. Patients with excessive daytime sleepiness secondary to untreated SDB may fall asleep while reading, watching television, or at the movies, while in conversation with a group of friends, or while driving. Daytime sleepiness can be a very debilitating symptom, causing social and occupational difficulties, reduced vigilance, and cognitive deficits, including decreased concentration, slowed response time, and memory and attention difficulties. These symptoms may be particularly relevant to older adults who are at an increased risk of developing such symptoms with aging or already suffer from some initial cognitive impairment. SDB may therefore unnecessarily further exacerbate these cognitive deficits.

SDB is often associated with other serious health problems, including hypertension and cardiac and pulmonary disease, which can then lead to increased risk of mortality. Recent research indicates that even those patients with only five events per hour of sleep are at greater risk for developing hypertension. While cause and effect between SDB and cardiovascular disease has not yet been determined, increasing SDB has been associated with increased risk of developing cardiovascular diseases, including hypertension, coronary artery disease, and stroke.

Upon initial evaluation, sleep complaints such as snoring and/or gasping and excessive daytime sleepiness may be suggestive of SDB. The assessment should begin with a thorough sleep history from the patient, including information on daytime behavior. Because the patient is often unaware of (or not disturbed by) the loud snoring or cessations in breathing during the night, it is helpful to have the patient's bed partner present at the assessment interview. The clinician should examine the patient's airway and throat to check for obstruction of the airway. The medical history should include information on history of hypertension and any cardiac or pulmonary problems. The clinician should also collect information on recent weight gain or obesity (excess fatty tissue may contribute to airway obstruction), smoking history (may irritate oropharynx and/or nicotine may affect central nervous system), alcohol intake, and intake of any sedating medications (may result in airway relaxation thus facilitating obstruction). Although patients with SDB are often overweight, it may be less strong a predictor of the presence or absence of SDB in the older population. Thus evaluation of the older patient of normal or even slender weight should not be overlooked.

If the clinician suspects SDB, the patient should be referred for an overnight PSG recording in a sleep disorders clinic, or for ambulatory monitoring of sleep and respiration in the patient's home. Based on the results of the objective recording, recommendations for treatment can be suggested.

Management

Pharmacologic treatments for SDB are ineffective; however, there are several effective nonpharmacologic treatments that have become first-line treatment of SDB.

Positive Airway Pressure

The gold standard for treatment for SDB is positive airway pressure. There are several types of devices that provide positive airway pressure, including continuous positive airway pressure (CPAP), bilevel positive airway pressure (BiPAP), and auto-CPAP. CPAP is composed of a nose mask, which is connected via a hose to a machine that provides continuous air pressure. The air pressure acts as a splint to maintain the opening of the upper airway, thereby preventing the obstruction or collapse of the airway. The degree of air pressure (traditionally, 5 to 20 cm H_2O) is set individually for each patient at the sleep laboratory and is dependent on the patient's AHI or the severity of the patient's SDB. CPAP alleviates all snoring and most of the apneic events, repeated awakenings, and nighttime hypoxemia in these patients. This intervention is also very effective in the reduction of daytime sleepiness and has been shown to improve cognitive performance.

BiPAP was designed to allow for the variation in positive airway pressure during expiration and inspiration. The device looks and acts similarly to CPAP but rather than providing continuous airway pressure, the BiPAP device has reduced expiratory positive airway pressure (EPAP) when compared to the inspiratory positive airway pressure (IPAP). The BiPAP prevents the obstruction of the airway by using lower EPAP levels when compared to CPAP. At this time, there are no data to suggest that BiPAP is more effective than CPAP, however some reports suggest better compliance with BiPAP, possibly because of its more gentle approach, when compared to CPAP.

The auto-CPAP was designed to allow for the overnight variability in airway pressure, which is adjusted automatically depending on the extent of airway obstruction, which may fluctuate with specific sleep stages and body position. In contrast to the constant airway pressure in traditional CPAP, this device adjusts for periods of reduced obstruction by providing lower airway pressure, while providing greater airway pressure with increases in obstruction. To date, no studies suggest increases in compliance with the auto-CPAP when compared to other positive airway pressure devices.

Clinicians should be aware of possible poor patient compliance, however, these devices are recommended for nightly use and are a long-term management approach. The addition of a humidifier to some units reduces the discomfort and possible nasal irritation associated with the use of these devices. Clinicians should not assume that elderly patients cannot tolerate CPAP; one study has shown the extent of dementia, older age, and AHI severity are not associated with compliance, rather only the presence of depression seems to be linked with poor long-term compliance.

Surgical Interventions

There are several different surgical approaches for the treatment of SDB, including (1) nasal reconstruction, which corrects nasal valve collapse, septal deviations, and turbinate hypertrophy; (2) uvu-lopharynpalatoplasty (UPPP), which corrects pharyngeal obstruction by removal of pharyngeal tissue, including soft palate, uvula, tonsillar pillars, and tonsillar tissue; (3) laser-assisted uvulopharyn-palatoplasty (LAUP), which has the same standard procedure as UPPP, but uses a laser to remove the pharyngeal tissue; (4) genioglossus advancement, which corrects by the forward advancement of the insertion of the tongue (usually in conjunction with UPPP or LAUP); and (5) hyoid myotomy, which corrects hypopharyngeal obstruction by suspending the hyoid bone to the superior edge of the larynx (usually in conjunction with UPPP or LAUP).

The surgical approach or combination of approaches (including nonsurgical) chosen for an individual patient is decided on a case-by-case basis and is dependent on the location and the type of obstruction present. Depending on the choice of surgical approach, the effectiveness of the intervention in reducing AHI varies from 48% to 72% and depends on the severity of the SDB and the obstruction. Surgical methods should be approached with caution in the elderly patient, as the effectiveness of the treatment may be lower and their recovery may be longer and more difficult.

Oral Appliances

Oral devices are appropriate for the management of milder forms of obstructive sleep apnea and snoring. The two most common oral devices are the tongue-retaining device (TRD) and the mandibular advancement device (MAD). These oral appliances are anchored on the patient's teeth or gums and work by moving the tongue or the mandibular forward, thereby preventing obstruction at the hypopharyngeal level. Depending on the type of device used, the effectiveness of this approach in decreasing AHI and increasing blood oxygen saturation levels varies from 40% to 81%. Clinicians need to be aware of possible side effects, including pain or discomfort in the temporomandibular joint or short-term occlusion abnormalities when removing the appliance, which occurs in an estimated 30% of patients. Newer devices can be used with dentures, which make them particularly appropriate for use in the older patient.

Diet and Lifestyle

There are several dietary and lifestyle factors that can exacerbate SDB, such as obesity, alcohol intake, and smoking. Obesity is a common problem in patients with obstructive sleep apnea, as the additional fatty tissue often results in the obstruction of the upper airways. These patients will benefit significantly from weight loss, which sometimes dramatically reduces or even eliminates apneic events.

Alcohol and certain medications, such as sedative-hypnotics, narcotics, and barbiturates, have a depressant effect on the upper airway musculature and may exacerbate SDB. Furthermore, given the usually high number of prescriptions taken by older patients, clinicians should be diligent when prescribing sedating medications, particularly to those older patients who are at higher risk for SDB. Smoking is also associated with exacerbation of SDB. Although the mechanism is not fully understood at this time, several theories have been suggested, including irritation of oropharynx by cigarette smoke and the possible effect of nicotine on the central nervous system.

For patients with mild SDB, positional SDB, or positional snoring, body position during sleep may account for many of the respiratory events in these cases. The supine position is associated with the majority of the positional apneic events, which are likely a result of the relaxation of the anterior neck and oropharyngeal structures while in this position. A simple behavioral technique for dealing with positional apnea is to place a tennis ball in a pocket sewn to the back of a night shirt, thereby deterring the patients from sleeping on their back and preventing positional respiratory events.

In general, treatment of SDB in the elderly depends on (1) the severity of the condition, (2) the extent of daytime symptoms, and (3) the presence of other comorbid medical conditions, such as hypertension, cardiac disease, or cognitive deficits. Decision to treat should be made on a case-by-case basis and age of the patient should not be a factor in making this assessment.

PERIODIC LIMB MOVEMENTS IN SLEEP/RESTLESS LEGS SYNDROME

Definition

Periodic limb movements in sleep (PLMS) is characterized by clusters of repeated leg (or sometimes arm) jerks that occur approximately every 20 to 40 seconds over the course of the night. These clusters of movements last on an average 0.5 to 5 seconds and cause repeated brief awakenings. The number of limb movements followed by arousals per hour of sleep is called the periodic limb movement index (PLMI). Clinical diagnosis of PLMS is typically given when a patient has a PLMI >5.

Another disorder, often comorbid with PLMS, and believed to be more disruptive, is restless leg syndrome (RLS). RLS is characterized by dysesthesia in the legs, usually described by patients as "a creeping crawling sensation" or as "pins and needles," which can only be relieved with vigorous movement. These sensations often occur in the evening or whenever the patient is in a restful, relaxed state. About 90% of patients with RLS also have PLMS, but only about 20% of PLMS patients suffer from RLS.

Epidemiology

The prevalence of PLMS increases significantly with age and is estimated at 45%, compared to 5% to 6% in younger adults. Despite this increase in prevalence, the severity of the condition does not worsen with age. The prevalence of RLS increases with age as well. There is no known gender difference in PLMS, however RLS is twice as common in older women than men.

Pathophysiology

The exact mechanisms underlying PLMS and RLS are not fully understood; however, current hypotheses suggest possible dysfunction of the dopamine system. These theories are derived from the therapeutic effects of dopamine agonists in RLS and PLMS. Recent studies have also suggested that the pathophysiology of RLS might involve iron homeostatic dysregulation, as ferritin levels in the cerebrospinal fluid are lower in these patients.

Presentation

The most common complaints of patients with PLMS are sleep initiation insomnia, sleep maintenance insomnia, and excessive daytime sleepiness. Patients may or may not be aware of leg kicks or jerks. Some may complain simply of having difficulty falling asleep or staying asleep with no knowledge that they kick. Often, bed partners may be aware of the leg movements and may have moved into separate beds. Many patients with PLMS also suffer from RLS and therefore may also complain of discomforting sensations in their legs during the day.

Evaluation

Patients are often unaware of the multiple nighttime awakenings and the associated sleep loss, therefore it is often helpful to have the patient's bed partner present at the assessment interview. An accurate diagnosis of PLMS can only be made by recording limb movements and associated arousals. This can be accomplished via an overnight PSG recording in the sleep disorders laboratory, or in the home with unattended monitoring. Additionally, several actigraphic devices, placed on the ankle, have been validated against PSG for measurement of PLMS.

The diagnosis of RLS is based on the patient's report of uncomfortable sensations in the legs, which are only relieved by movement. Patients with symptoms of RLS should be assessed for anemia, iron deficiency, uremia, and peripheral neuropathy prior to treatment.

Management

There is some discussion about the significance of PLMS and whether it does in fact constitute a sleep disorder. However, the treatment for PLMS and RLS is the same (Table 55-4). Currently, the first-line treatment for PLMS/RLS consists of dopamine

TABLE 55-4

Pharmacological Treatment of PLMS/RLS			
CLASS	GENERIC	BRAND	DOSE
Dopaminergic agents	Ropinirole	Requip	1.5–4 mg
	Pramipexole	Mirapex	0.25–0.75 mg
	Carbidopa/Levodopa*	Sinemet	25/100–25/250 mg
Benzodiazepines	Clonazepam	Klonopin	0.25–2 mg
	Tempazepam	Restoril	15–30 mg
Opiate agents	Codeine	Tylenol #3/#4	30–60 mg (codeine)
	Propoxyphene hydrochloride	Darvon	65–135 mg

*Off-label.

agonists, as they reduce or eliminate both the limb jerks and the associated arousals. There are two medications approved by the Food and Drug Administration (FDA) for the treatment of RLS: ropinirole and pramipexole. However, carbidopa/levodopa, has also been shown to be effective. Shifting of limb movements from the nighttime to the daytime may occur with treatment and therefore continued evaluation is needed.

Less effective drugs for these conditions in the elderly include benzodiazepines (e.g., clonazepam, temazepam), which decrease the number of arousals, but do not significantly reduce the number of limb movements; opioids, which decrease the number of limb movements, but do not always decrease the number of arousals; gabapentine, and iron supplements. Long-acting benzodiazepines are contraindicated in patients with SDB and as PLMS is often comorbid with SDB, clinicians should be cautious when prescribing long-acting benzodiazepines. Clinicians should also be aware of possible daytime sedation, particularly in elderly persons, resulting from these longer-acting medications.

CIRCADIAN RHYTHMS SLEEP DISORDERS

Definition

Circadian rhythms refer to 24-hour biological rhythms that control many physiologic functions, such as endogenous hormone secretions, core body temperature, and the sleep–wake cycle. These rhythms originate in the suprachiasmatic nucleus (SCN) in the anterior hypothalamus, which houses the internal circadian pacemaker. Circadian rhythms are synchronized to the 24-hour day by other internal rhythms (e.g., hormone secretions), as well as by external zeitgebers (literally time-givers or cues), the most powerful being bright light. The sleep–wake cycle is primarily entrained by internal rhythms, such as core body temperature and the endogenous melatonin cycle, and the external light/dark rhythm, which asserts its effect on the sleep–wake cycle via the retinohypothalamic visual pathway. For example, as core body temperature drops, melatonin secretions increase and individuals start feeling sleepy; as core body temperature rises and melatonin drops, individuals begin waking up.

As people age, several factors may make circadian rhythm less entrained and thereby result in weaker or more disorganized sleep–wake rhythms. Such changes may include (1) slow degeneration of the SCN with age, (2) progressive reduction in endogenous melatonin secretion during the night, and (3) decreased sensitivity to external cues, or alternatively external cues such as bright light may be lacking or weak in older adults. Considerable data have shown that older persons are exposed to significantly less bright light than their younger counterparts. Healthy older adults receive on average only 60 minutes of bright light a day (>2000 lux), whereas elderly demented patients living in the community receive on average 30 minutes of bright light a day (>2000 lux), and demented nursing home patients receive on average no light >2000 lux and only 10 minutes of bright light >1000 lux a day. All these issues may add to the weakening of the sleep–wake circadian rhythm, resulting in more nocturnal awakenings, less consistency of sleep–wake cycles, and heightened daytime sleepiness.

Another common circadian rhythm change in older age is the shifting, or advancing, of the sleep–wake cycle. This circadian rhythm disorder is called advanced sleep phase syndrome (ASPS), a condition in which the sleep–wake rhythm and the core body temperature rhythm are advanced, as compared to those of younger adults. Older adults with ASPS get sleepy in the early evening and wake up in the early morning hours, in part because the core body temperature is dropping earlier in the evening (perhaps at about 7:00 P.M. or 8:00 P.M.) and rising about 8 hours later, at about 3:00 A.M. or 4:00 A.M.

Epidemiology

Prevalence of ASPS is approximately 1% in middle-aged adults. Although the prevalence in older adults is known to increase, the exact percentage has not been established. This may be partly because these patients have learned to function with the changes in their circadian clocks, and therefore do not present for treatment.

Pathophysiology

Changes in the sleep–wake cycle are likely caused by changes in the core body temperature cycle, decreased light exposure, and environmental factors. Recent research suggests there may also be a genetic component.

Presentation

The overall weakening of the circadian rhythm in older age may also result in increased awakenings during the night. The most common complaints of patients with ASPS are being sleepy early in the evening and waking up too early in the morning. If patients with ASPS went to bed as their core body temperature was dropping, for example, around 7:00 P.M. or 8:00 P.M., they would have little difficulty falling asleep and would sleep for a full night, about 8 hours. As explained above, this would result in their waking up somewhere between 3:00 A.M. and 4:00 A.M. An additional problem results when these patients, despite their physiological changes, prefer to maintain more "normative" or "acceptable" sleep–wake schedules, thereby delaying their bedtimes; however, as a result of the phase advance of their circadian rhythm, they continue waking up at the earlier morning times, thereby reducing their time in bed and their nightly sleep duration. A second scenario involves patients falling asleep while reading or watching television in the early evening, and subsequently having difficulty falling asleep, but still awakening in the early morning hours. This significant sleep loss can result in daytime sleepiness, often resulting in daytime naps.

Evaluation

As symptoms of ASPS may mimic symptoms of sleep-maintenance insomnia, the two highly common conditions in the elderly, clinicians may have difficulty distinguishing between the two disorders. However, in order to implement the correct treatment, appropriate evaluation is imperative. When assessing for ASPS, the clinician should obtain an extensive sleep history and at least 1–2 weeks of sleep diaries (Table 55-5), which can be sent to the patient several weeks prior to their treatment. If possible, the patient should also wear a wrist actigraph for 3–7 days, allowing for the objective

TABLE 55-5

Sample Sleep Diary

Name: _____   Date: _____ to _____

	Monday	Tuesday	Wednesday	Thursday	Friday	Saturday	Sunday
1. Bed time							
2. Time taken to fall asleep (after lights off)							
3. Number of nighttime awakenings							
4. Wake-up time							
5. Time out of bed (morning)							
6. Total sleep time (night only)							
7. Total wake time (night only)							
8. Nap time (if any)							
9. Medication (time/dosage)							
10. Alcohol (time/dosage)							
11. How was your sleep last night?*							
12. How tired were you in the morning?							

*1 = excellent to 5 = very poor; 1 = not tired to 5 = very tired.

examination of the shifting of the sleep–wake cycle. If these assessments suggest early evening sleepiness and early evening bedtimes along with early morning awakenings, the clinician should suspect ASPS.

Management

As shifting of the circadian rhythm is a common and expected development in older age, patients should be educated that ASPS is not a medical disorder and does not necessarily need to be treated. Treatment is dependent on the extent of the discomfort the ASPS has on the day-to-day life of the individual patient. Patients often complain that their waking hours are no longer consistent with societal norms, causing them to be awake (or asleep) when those around them are not.

Nonpharmacologic therapies, focusing on strengthening and entrainment of the sleep–wake rhythm, are the treatments of choice for patients with ASPS, particularly bright-light therapy.

Bright-Light Therapy

As bright light is the most influential external zeitgeber on the sleep–wake circadian system, it is not surprising that it is also the most appropriate and effective treatment for circadian rhythm disturbances. By increasing light exposure during specific times of the day, it is possible to advance or delay the sleep–wake circadian rhythm. Specifically, exposure to bright light in the early morning will strengthen and advance the rhythm (i.e., patient will become sleepier earlier), whereas exposure to bright light in the late afternoon or early evening will delay the rhythm (i.e., patient will become sleepier later in the day allowing them to stay alert longer). Exposure to bright light will not only shift the sleep–wake circadian rhythm but will also shift related rhythms such as core body temperature and endogenous melatonin.

To delay the advanced sleep–wake rhythm, patients with ASPS should be exposed to bright light for approximately 2 hours a day during the late afternoon to early evening. The best source of bright light is sunlight, therefore patients should attempt to spend time outdoors in the late afternoon. Because the mechanism of the light is primarily through the eyes, sunglasses should not be worn during this time; however they should be worn in the morning hours to avoid having rhythms advance even more or canceling out the afternoon light exposure. Normal room light is not generally bright enough to shift rhythms. Therefore, if the patient is unable to spend 2 hours a day outdoors, another option is a special commercially available "light box," which provides a minimum of 2500 lux light exposure, which has been shown to improve sleep consolidation in institutionalized elderly.

RAPID EYE MOVEMENT SLEEP BEHAVIOR DISORDER

Definition

Rapid eye movement (REM) sleep behavior disorder (RBD) is characterized by a dissociated state during which complex motoric behaviors occur, most likely resulting from an intermittent lack of skeletal muscle atonia that is typically present during REM sleep. RBD usually occurs during the second half of the night, when REM is more prevalent. Nighttime behaviors in RBD include vigorous and complex body movements and actions, such as walking, talking, and eating.

Epidemiology

The prevalence of RBD is unknown. However, recent reports suggest elderly men may be at higher risk for developing RBD.

Pathophysiology

To date, the etiology of RBD remains unknown. Some reports suggest that acute RBD is associated with the intake of tricyclic antidepressants, fluoxetine, and monoamine oxidase inhibitors, and withdrawal from alcohol or sedatives. In contrast, chronic RBD has been associated with narcolepsy and other idiopathic neurodegenerative disorders such as dementia and Parkinson's disease.

Presentation

Patients engage in complex motoric behaviors over the course of the night and may be unable to recollect these actions in the morning. Some patients' recollections of their dreams suggest these nighttime activities and movements may be the acting out of patient dreams, made possible by the lack of muscle atonia during REM sleep. At times, movements may be violent and may harm the patient and/or the patient's bed partner.

Evaluation

Assessment of RBD should include a complete sleep history. Because patients may be unaware of their behaviors over the course of the night, bed partners should also be interviewed. Clinicians should acquire simultaneous overnight PSG and video recording of nighttime behavior in order to examine whether there is a link between REM sleep and the complex behaviors exhibited by the patients. When examining the PSG, clinicians should be attentive to any marked unusual elevations in muscle tone and/or limb movements in the electromyogram (EMG) recording, specifically during REM sleep, when they usually rare.

Management

Pharmacological Interventions

To date, there have been only a few reports of pharmacologic treatments for RBD, with promising initial results. Currently, clonazepam is the most prescribed pharmacological treatment for RBD. Clonazepam acts by inhibiting nighttime motoric movements, without directly affecting muscle tone. It has been shown to result in cessation (partial or complete) of abnormal body movements during the night in about 90% of RBD patients. If the medication is stopped, all symptoms return. Patients may complain of excessive daytime sleepiness because of this drug's long half-life. If clonazepam is contraindicated, several alternative drugs have shown some positive effects in RBD, including tricyclic antidepressants, dopaminergic agents, and melatonin.

Lifestyle

Clinicians should educate RBD patients and their bed partners on making changes in bedtime/sleeping routines and environment, in order to make the bedroom safer and to decrease the potential for injurious behavior during the night. For example, heavy curtains should be placed on bedroom windows, and doors and windows should be locked at night if there is risk of the patient wandering out of bed during the night and engaging in complex behaviors. If the patient is extremely active or violent during the night, heavy or breakable objects should be removed from the vicinity of the bed, and if needed, patients may want to sleep on a mattress placed on the floor to avoid falling off the bed and/or hurting themselves or their bed partners.

INSOMNIA

Definition

Insomnia is a complaint of low quantity and/or poor quality sleep, resulting in a sense of nonrestorative sleep. There are several different types of insomnia, including sleep onset insomnia (an inability to initiate sleep), sleep maintenance insomnia (an inability to maintain sleep throughout the night), early morning insomnia (awakening early in the morning with an inability to return to sleep), and pathophysiologic insomnia (behaviorally conditioned insomnia associated with maladaptive behaviors). Although older adults can suffer from any of the types of insomnia, the most common complaints in the elderly are of sleep maintenance insomnia and early morning insomnia.

Insomnia is also classified based on the length of time the complaint has persisted, with transient insomnia lasting only a few days prior to (or during) a brief stressful experience, short-term insomnia lasting a few weeks during an extended period of stress and adjustment, and chronic insomnia lasting several months to years, which may have begun following a discrete event, but continues even after the antecedent event is no longer relevant. In many cases of chronic insomnia, the inability to sleep may have become a conditioned response and may be associated with poor sleep hygiene.

Epidemiology

The prevalence of insomnia is greater in older than younger adults, with a prevalence of 40% to 50% for chronic sleep onset or sleep maintenance insomnia, and an incidence of about 5%. Women report more insomnia complaints than men.

Pathophysiology

There are multiple factors that may play a causal role in the development of insomnia. Insomnia is most commonly co morbid with medical, psychiatric, or psychosocial conditions, and/or secondary to the treatment of these conditions. Medical illnesses common in the elderly population, such as arthritis, cardiovascular disease, pulmonary disease, chronic pain disorders, and other illnesses associated with physical discomforts, are often associated with insomnia. Major life changes, such as retirement and death of loved ones, can also lead to insomnia. These psychosocial and environmental factors may cause or exacerbate psychiatric and/or sleep difficulties. Depression and anxiety disorders are therefore among the most common comorbid conditions associated with sleep disturbances in the elderly person. Only about 7% of incident insomnia cases in older adults are not related to one of these conditions. In addition, a linear relationship exists between the number of these illnesses and insomnia in older adults.

Polypharmacy has become increasingly common in elderly patients, particularly those suffering from multiple medical and psychiatric conditions. Pharmacologic treatments for these conditions often exert either sedating or alerting properties, however these sleep effects are rarely taken into consideration. For example, alerting or stimulating drugs (Table 55-6), when taken late in the day, may

TABLE 55-6

Effect of Common Drugs Taken by Older Adults	
SEDATING	**ALERTING**
Hypnotics	Alcohol/nicotine
Antihypertensives	CNS stimulants
Antihistamines	Thyroid hormones
Antpsychotics	Bronchodilators
Antidepressants	Corticosteroids
	Beta-blockers
	Calcium channel-blockers

TABLE 55-7

Sleep Hygiene Rules for Older Adults
Check effect of medication on sleep and wakefulness
Avoid caffeine, alcohol, and cigarettes after lunch
Limit liquids in the evening
Keep a regular bedtime–waketime schedule
Avoid naps or limit to 1 nap a day, no longer than 30 min
Spend time outdoors (without sunglasses), particularly in the late afternoon or early evening
Exercise

cause difficulty falling asleep at night. On the other hand, sedating drugs (see Table 55-6) taken early in the day may lead to excessive daytime sleepiness and daytime napping behavior, which may contribute to sleep onset insomnia or may further exacerbate and maintain the existing insomnia. Therefore it is not the aging process per se that causes insomnia, rather it is the co-occurring conditions and their treatment, which may underlie the higher prevalence of insomnia with increasing age.

Presentation

Complaints of insomnia may vary significantly from patient to patient. Apart from the inability to sleep at various periods of the night (early, middle, or late), patients often complain of excessive daytime sleepiness, leading to daytime napping and decreased mental functioning.

Evaluation

Evaluation of insomnia should begin with a thorough medical, psychiatric, and sleep assessment, and a review of recent medication intake (including time of medication ingestion). The clinician should also request 1 to 2 weeks of sleep diaries (and/or actigraphic recordings) in order to obtain an exact description of the nature of the insomnia. In addition, the clinician needs to collect information on the characteristics, onset, duration, and severity of the insomnia, as well as on any factors that may contribute to the sleep condition, such as sleep hygiene practices, diet, alcohol intake, and smoking history.

Management

There are several behavioral and pharmacological interventions and lifestyle changes that may aid in the management of insomnia. Overall, given the high number of medications prescribed and known changes in rates of metabolism and elimination in this population, clinicians should attempt to implement behavioral treatments prior to pharmacologic interventions.

Nonpharmacological Interventions

Nonpharmacological treatments include cognitive-behavioral treatments (CBT) and educational approaches. These treatments attempt to change the inappropriate or maladaptive behaviors associated with sleep and are particularly effective in cases of psychophysiological insomnia where the initial cause of the insomnia may no longer be present.

Many nonpharmacological interventions have been shown to be highly effective in reducing insomnia, producing short-term and long-term positive changes in sleep habits, as well as the subjective perception of better sleep. Below are examples of the most common nonpharmacologic interventions.

Sleep Hygiene Sleep hygiene is an educational approach designed to give insomniacs, as well as the general population, a list of guidelines on how to maintain healthy sleep–wake routines. Poor sleep habits are associated with a reduction in nighttime sleep quality and difficulties with alertness during the day. When the clinician is collecting the patient's sleep history, information should also be collected on any disruptive nighttime or daytime behaviors that may be affecting the patient's sleep. Table 55-7 summarizes sleep hygiene rules specifically adapted for older adults. Sleep hygiene rules can also be incorporated with other treatments for sleep difficulties.

Stimulus-Control Therapy Stimulus-control therapy was developed for the management of psychophysiological insomnia. Patients often have negative associations with the bedroom environment, leading to arousal. These associations can be redefined for the patient by associating the sleep environment with positive and calming cues, thereby promoting sleep.

Stimulus-control therapy is designed to break any preexisting associations between the bed (and bedroom) and wakefulness, which are often the result of maladaptive classical conditioning. It requires patients to stop all in-bed activities other than sleep and only go to bed when feeling tired enough to fall asleep. Patients should avoid any stimulating or arousing activities prior to bedtime, such as watching television, reading exciting books, or watching the alarm clock. If the patient cannot fall asleep within 20 minutes, they should get out of bed (and get out of bedroom if possible) and return to bed only when they feel tired enough to be able to fall asleep. This pattern continues until the patient is able to fall asleep within the 20-minute limit.

For a regular sleep period to develop, the patient should wake up and get out of bed at the same time everyday (including weekends). Napping behavior should be avoided, so that the need for sleep can accumulate. However, some modification is possible in the case of older adults who may be allowed to nap during the day (if absolutely necessary), but for no longer than 30 minutes in the early part of the day, so as not to interfere with sleep onset. These rules should be followed when first attempting to fall asleep in cases of

TABLE 55-8

Instructions for Stimulus-Control Therapy for Older Adults

1. Patient should only go to bed when tired or sleepy
2. If unable to fall asleep within 20 min, patient should get put of bed (and bedroom if possible). While out of bed, do something quiet and relaxing.
3. Patient should only return to bed when sleepy
4. If unable to fall asleep within 20 min, patient should again get out of bed
5. Behavior is repeated until patient can fall asleep within a few minutes
6. Patient should get up at the same time each morning (even if only a few hours of sleep)
7. Naps should be avoided

TABLE 55-9

Instructions for Sleep Restriction Therapy for Older Adults

1. Calculate the average amount of time in bed per night reported by patient
2. Patient is only allowed to stay in bed for this amount of time plus 15 min
3. Patient must get up at the same time each day
4. Daytime napping should be strictly avoided
5. When sleep-efficiency has reached 80% to 85%, patient can go to bed 15 min earlier
6. This procedure should be repeated until patient can sleep for 8 h (or period needed for a good night's sleep)

sleep onset insomnia or upon each awakening for patients with sleep maintenance insomnia. Table 55-8 summarizes the instructions for stimulus control therapy. Patients may resist this method because it may require significant effort on their part and may initially reduce the sleep period and increase daytime sleepiness. Therefore, to increase compliance when recommending this method, the clinician should explain the underlying theory behind this approach, and review possible initial discomforts.

Sleep-Restriction Therapy Sleep-restriction therapy was developed in response to the clinical observation that patients with sleep difficulties often spend a significant amount of time in bed unsuccessfully attempting to fall asleep. This inability to fall asleep in an appropriate amount of time results in anxiety and frustration, which, over time, can lead to the development of psychophysiological insomnia. In addition, spending too much time in bed can lead to fragmented sleep. This method is designed to reduce the amount of time the patient spends awake in bed, thus increasing sleep efficiency. As described above, sleep efficiency is defined as the amount of time asleep given the amount of time in bed. Ideally, an older adult's sleep efficiency will be 85% or greater.

Sleep-restriction therapy requires the patient to fill out sleep logs for 1 to 2 weeks. Based on these sleep logs, the average amount of time the patient sleeps a night is calculated. The patient is only allowed to spend this amount of time, plus 15 minutes, in bed each night for the following week. For example, if the patient reports sleeping an average of only 5 hours a night, the patient is only allowed to be in bed 5 hours and 15 minutes. Although this reduction in time in bed causes an initial reduction in time spent asleep and possible sleep deprivation, it is likely to lead to shorter sleep onset and sleep consolidation in the long run. Patients should also wake up at the same time each day and avoid daytime napping. In our example, if the patient's normal time to awaken is 6:00 A.M. and they estimate they sleep for only 5 hours, they would not be allowed to go to bed until 12:45 A.M. Once sleep efficiency has reached 85%, the time allowed to spend in bed at night is increased by 15 minutes at the start of the night, so that now the patient would go to bed at 12:30 A.M. This pattern is repeated until the patient is in bed, able to sleep 8 hours, or the number of hours that affords the patient a good night's sleep.

To increase compliance, clinicians should help the patient understand the underlying theory behind this method and educate them on some initial difficulties they should expect, such as initial sleep loss and daytime sleepiness. Table 55-9 summarizes the instructions for sleep-restriction therapy.

Cognitive-Behavioral Therapy CBT for insomnia involves educational, behavioral, and cognitive components. The educational component involves encouraging the patient to determine which factors might be predisposing, precipitating, or perpetuating the insomnia. The therapist explains that CBT is effective by eliminating the perpetuating factors with behavioral and cognitive strategies. The behavioral component involves the behavioral techniques described above. The cognitive component deals with the maladaptive thoughts or dysfunctional beliefs that the patient has about insomnia.

In an 8-week double-blind treatment longitudinal outcome study, CBT, a long-acting benzodiazepine (temazepam), a combined CBT/temazepam condition, and a placebo condition were compared in a sample of older adults. Compared to baseline, all three active treatments reduced night wakings at posttreatment, however only CBT alone and CBT/temazepam were associated with continued improvement at 3-, 12-, and 24-month follow-up interviews. In addition, one study found that even two 25-miunte CBT sessions for insomnia are effective in reducing nocturnal awakenings, which may be a more practical approach in the primary care setting. The NIH 2005 State-of-the-Science conference on insomnia concluded that CBT is the most effective treatment for insomnia. CBT has been found to be as effective as prescription medications for brief treatment of chronic insomnia, and, in contrast to medications, the effects may last well beyond the termination of treatment. There is no evidence that CBT treatment produces adverse effects. In sum, although pharmacologic treatments may be of more immediate help, particularly in the acute treatment phase, in order to maintain long-term clinical gains, nonpharmacological or combined approaches are more effective.

Pharmacological Interventions

Historically, multiple classes of medications have been used to treat insomnia, such as antidepressants, antihistamines, antipsychotics, and sedative-hypnotics. The 2005 NIH State-of-the-Science Conference on Insomnia concluded that (1) all antidepressants have potentially significant adverse effects, raising concerns about the risk–benefit ratio, (2) barbiturates and antipsychotic medications have significant risks, and thus their use in the treatment of chronic insomnia cannot be recommended and (3) there is no systematic evidence for efficacy of antihistamines, yet there are significant concerns about risks with these agents. The NIH conference also concluded that while the older benzodiazepines are safe in the short-term treatment of insomnia, the frequency and severity of adverse effects are much lower with the newer nonbenzodiazpines.

TABLE 55-10

Novel Nonbenzodiazepines Approved for Insomnia Treatment by the Food and Drug Administration				
GENERIC	BRAND	DOSE (mg)	TYPE OF INSOMNIA	HALF-LIFE (h)
Zaleplon	Sonata	5–20	Sleep-onset	1
Zolpidem	Ambien	5–10	Sleep-onset	2.5–3
Zolpidem MR	Ambien CR	6.25–12.5	Sleep-onset and sleep maintenance	2.8
Eszopicolone	Lunesta	1–3	Sleep-onset and sleep maintenance	6
Remelteon	Rozerem	8	Sleep onset	1–2.6

Clinicians should exercise caution when prescribing hypnotics to older adults, and often pharmacologic management of insomnia should be accompanied by cognitive-behavioral approaches (see above). If a hypnotic medication is needed for an older patient, clinicians should consider several issues: (1) prescribing the lowest-effective dose, (2) using hypnotics with shorter half-lives, and (3) evaluating possible effects on SDB and daytime alertness and performance. In general, longer-acting hypnotics are contraindicated in this population, as these medications have several sleep-related side-effects, such as changes in sleep architecture (i.e., reduction in delta or deep sleep), morning hangover effects, leading to excessive daytime sleepiness, poor motor coordination, and visuospatial problems, which may be particularly pronounced in the elderly.

If after careful consideration, the best course of treatment is a sleep medication, the approach to consider would be the newer FDA-approved selective shorter-acting nonbenzodiazepine hypnotics (Table 55-10). These novel medications have been repeatedly shown to be the most effective and safest approach for the treatment of insomnia in older adults. One additional FDA-approved drug, ramelteon, a melatonin agonist, has also been shown to be effective in the treatment of sleep-onset insomnia in elderly (see Table 55-10). Successful treatment is dependent on choosing the correct hypnotic and is based on the specific type of insomnia complaint, e.g., sleep onset difficulty versus repeated nighttime awakenings (see Table 55-10) and the time available to the patient to devote to sleeping in bed.

SPECIAL ISSUES

Sleep in Institutionalized Elderly Patients and Neurodegenerative Disorders

The sleep of older adults living in nursing homes is known to be extremely disturbed, particularly in those suffering from neurodegenerative disorders such as Alzheimer's disease, Parkinson's disease, Huntington's disease, and some other forms of dementia. Persons with dementia may be more susceptible to sleep disorders as a consequence of the disease processes, causing permanent damage to brain areas regulating sleep. In addition, progression and severity of the dementing condition has been associated with more sleep disturbances. A common reason for the institutionalization of an elderly person is frequent nocturnal awakenings with wandering and confusion.

Sleep disturbances affect elderly persons with neurodegenerative disorders differently than they affect "healthy" older adults. For example, Alzheimer's disease patients suffer from progressive increases in the duration and frequency of nocturnal awakenings, increases in daytime napping, and decreases in slow-wave sleep and REM sleep, when compared to healthy older adults. Nursing home patients often suffer from severely fragmented sleep, often to the extent that there is not a single hour in a 24-hour day that is spent fully awake or asleep. Many of the coping strategies summarized in Table 55-11 are also relevant to patients suffering from neurodegenerative disorders, particularly the need for significant light exposure during the day, increasing daytime activity and exercise, and decreasing the need for daytime napping.

Environmental factors in the nursing home may also contribute to the reduction in the quality of sleep. In the nursing home, noise and light exposure occurs intermittently throughout the night and contributes to the disruption of sleep for the patients. Patients in the nursing home spend a significant amount of the 24-hour day in bed, leading them to rapidly cycle between sleep and wake during this time. Changes in sleep hygiene and the sleep environment of nursing home patients may greatly improve the sleep quality in this population. Table 55-11 summarizes a list of strategies for dealing with sleep–wake disturbances in the institutionalized elderly patient. The purpose of these strategies is to help both patients and nursing home staff reduce the nighttime disturbances in the sleeping environment, while promoting stronger and more defined sleep–wake cycles.

It was previously mentioned that older adults have higher rates of SDB than do younger adults. Research also shows that patients suffering from neurodegenerative disorders and patients living in

TABLE 55-11

Sleep Hygiene Rules for Nursing Homes Patients
Limited the amount of time in bed, particularly during the day
Limited naps to 1 h once a day, early in the afternoon
Keep regular sleep–wake schedule (if possible similar to prior home routine)
Keep regular meal schedule (if possible patients should not eat in bed)
Avoid caffeinated beverages and food
Limit nighttime noise
Ensure that patient rooms are as dark as possible during the night
Ensure that patient environment is brightly lit during the day
Encourage exercise appropriate for each patient
Match roommates on sleep–wake behavior
Assess patients for possible sleep problems and initiate specific treatment
Check medications for sedating/alerting effects

nursing homes suffer from an even higher prevalence of SDB. One theory postulates this increased risk for SDB in elderly individuals with specific progressive dementias may be caused by the degeneration of brainstem areas managing various sleep-regulated autonomic functions (e.g. respiration). Recent reports also suggest a possible relationship between SDB and exacerbation of cognitive impairments in older adults with dementia. Consequently, clinicians should be even more attentive to symptoms of SDB in this population.

SUMMARY

Sleep in the older adult may become poorer and more fragmented over time. In healthy older adults, sleep complaints are relatively rare; however, older patients with medical and/or psychiatric illnesses are significantly more likely to suffer from chronic insomnia. The aging process per se does not seem to underlie the increase in sleep disturbances in this population; rather they seem to be associated with a host of physical and psychological illnesses, medication use, circadian rhythm disturbances, and other primary sleep conditions (e.g., SDB). In order to commence appropriate treatment, differential diagnosis of these sleep conditions and their underlying causes are imperative when evaluating this population. Treatment plans should also address the primary medical/psychiatric conditions (if present) including medication regimens, and any other sleep conditions. Nonpharmacological therapies are often effective. When drug treatment is used, short acting agents are preferred. In sum, comprehensive evaluation and treatment management approaches will likely result in improved daytime functioning and higher quality of life in this population.

ACKNOWLEDGMENT

This work was supported by NIA AG08415, NCI CA112035, CBCRP 11IB-0034, NIH RR00827, and the Research Service of the Veterans Affairs San Diego Healthcare System.

FURTHER READING

Aloia MS, Ilniczky N, Di Dio P, Perlis ML, Greenblatt DW, Giles DE. Neuropsychological changes and treatment compliance in older adults with sleep apnea. *J Psychosom Res.* 2003:54;71–76.

Ancoli-Israel S, Gehrman PR, Martin JL, et al. Increased light exposure consolidates sleep and strengthens circadian rhythms in severe Alzheimer's disease patients. *Behav Sleep Med.* 2003;1:22–36.

Ancoli-Israel S, Richardson GS, Mangano R, Jenkins L, Hall P, Jones WS. Long-term use of sedative hypnotics in older patients with insomnia. *Sleep Med.* 2005;6:107–113.

Ayalon L, Ancoli-Israel S, Stepnowsky C, et al. Treatment adherence in patients with Alzheimer's disease and obstructive sleep apnea. *Am J Geriatr Psychiatry.* 2006;14(2):176–180.

Dew MA, Hoch CC, Buysse DJ, Monk TH, et al. Healthy older adults' sleep predicts all-cause mortality at 4 to 19 years of follow-up. *Psychosom Med.* 2003;65:63–73.

Foley DJ, Ancoli-Israel S, Britz P, Walsh J. Sleep disturbances and chronic disease in older adults: Results of the 2003 National Sleep Foundation *Sleep in America* Survey. *J Psychosomatic Res.* 2004;56:497–502.

Littner M, Kushida C, Anderson WM, et al. Standards of Practice Committee of the American Academy of Sleep Medicine. Practice parameters for the dopaminergic treatment of restless legs syndrome and periodic limb movement disorder. *Sleep.* 2004;27:557–559.

NIH State of the Science Conference Statement on Insomnia. Manifestations and Management of Chronic Insomnia in Adults, June 13–15, 2005. *Sleep.* 2005;28:1049–1058.

Ondo WG, Restless Legs Syndrome. *Neurol Clinics.* 2005;23(4):1165–1185.

Quan SF, Katz R, Olson J, et al. Factors associated with incidence and persistence of symptoms of disturbed sleep in an elderly cohort: the cardiovascular health study. *Am J Med Sci.* 2005;329:163–172.

Shahar E, Whitney CW, Redline S, et al. Sleep-disordered breathing and cardiovascular disease: cross sectional results of the Sleep Heart Health Study. *Am J Respir Crit Care Med.* 2001;163:19–25.

Dizziness

Aman Nanda ■ *Richard W. Besdine*

DEFINITION

Dizziness is a broad term used to describe various abnormal sensations arising from perceptions of the body's relationship to space or of unsteadiness. Dizziness has been arbitrarily defined on the basis of duration as acute (present for less than 1 or 2 months) or chronic (present for more than 1 or 2 months). The differential diagnosis of acute dizziness is similar in younger and older persons and management of acute dizziness is not qualitatively different in older persons as compared to younger adults, with the possible exception that recovery maybe more prolonged in older adults. This chapter focuses on chronic dizziness.

EPIDEMIOLOGY

The prevalence of dizziness ranges from 4% to 30% in persons aged 65 years or older, and more commonly is reported by women than men. In one study of persons aged 65 years and older, the likelihood of reporting dizziness increased by 10% for every 5 years of increasing age.

Chronic dizziness is associated with a number of comorbid conditions, including falls, functional disability, orthostatic hypotension, syncope, and strokes. In older persons, chronic dizziness can cause significant adverse effects on a person's quality of life. In one prospective study of older persons with dizziness, after 2 years of follow-up, older persons with dizziness were more likely to become disabled than were those who were not, although mortality was no different. In another study, 197 older persons with chronic dizziness reported poor health-related quality of life, most notably in relation to limitations in the physical and emotional dimensions. Chronic dizziness is also associated with fear of falling, worsening depressive symptoms and self-rated health, and decreased participation in social activities.

PATHOPHYSIOLOGY

Dizziness is a sensation of postural instability or imbalance. Dizziness can be difficult to diagnose, specifically in older persons, in whom it often represents dysfunction in more than one body system. Maintenance of balance and equilibrium is complex, achieved by integration of sensory information obtained from vestibular, proprioceptive, visual, and auditory systems by the cerebral cortex and cerebellum, leading to appropriate balance-maintaining responses. Abnormal function in any one or a combination of these systems may result in imbalance and the sensation of dizziness.

The vestibular system maintains spatial orientation at rest and during acceleration. Elements of the vestibular system and its connecting pathways include the semicircular canals, utricle, saccule, vestibular nerve, vestibular nuclei, vestibulospinal tracts, and vestibulocerebellar pathways. Diseases affecting this system and producing dizziness include Ménière's disease, benign paroxysmal positional vertigo (BPPV), recurrent vestibulopathy, labyrinthitis/vestibular neuronitis, acoustic neuroma, and drug toxicity (especially aminoglycosides). Age-related changes have also been reported in the sensory (hair) cells in the semicircular canals, saccule, and utricle.

The proprioceptive system consists of mechanoreceptors in the joints, peripheral nerves, and posterior columns, and multiple central nervous system (CNS) connections. Proprioception contributes to equilibrium by providing information about changes in body position, and helping mediate the body's response to position change. Common disorders include peripheral neuropathy associated with diseases such as diabetes or vitamin B-12 deficiency and cervical degenerative disorders. The few data on age-related changes in proprioception have been conflicting with one study reporting a substantial decline in joint position sense with aging, while another found no major changes.

Vision provides important information about spatial orientation, and is relied upon particularly when vestibular and/or proprioceptive function is impaired. Common ocular diseases include cataracts, macular degeneration, and glaucoma. Age-related visual changes include decrease in each of visual acuity, dark adaptation, contrast sensitivity, and accommodation (see Chapter 43). Hearing also provides spatial clues, but to a lesser extent than vision. Impairment in hearing, common in older persons, maybe secondary to age-related changes or to disease processes (see Chapter 44).

The cerebral cortex and cerebellum, along with their synaptic networks, integrate information and supply the musculoskeletal system with information for appropriate responses. Because of multiple and complex connections, essentially any CNS disorder can lead to imbalance, which may manifest as dizziness.

PRESENTATION

Dizziness is described using many names, including vertigo, lightheadedness, dysequilibrium, giddiness, wooziness, and spinning. The sensation of dizziness is commonly categorized as vertigo, dysequilibrium, presyncope, and other. In addition to these four types, another category, mixed dizziness, is a combination of two or more of the above types. Mixed dizziness is the most common type of dizziness reported by older persons.

Vertigo

Vertigo refers to a sensation of spinning, in which the individual perceives movements of the environment in relation to the body (objective vertigo) or vice versa (subjective vertigo). Vertigo is often assumed to result from disorders of the vestibular system and its connecting pathways although other causes of dizziness such as cervical disorders may present as vertigo as well.

Dysequilibrium

Dysequilibrium refers to feelings of unsteadiness or imbalance primarily involving the lower extremities or trunk rather than the head. The person often expresses the feeling that they are about to fall. Dysequilibrium results mostly from disorders of the proprioceptive system, musculoskeletal weakness, or cerebellar disease.

Presyncope

Presyncope is a feeling of lightheadedness or impending faintness or the sensation that one is about to pass out. Presyncope usually results from hypoperfusion of the brain; cardiovascular causes (including vasovagal disorders) are common causes in older persons.

Other and Multifactorial

Often the sensation does not fit any of the above three types. The patient may describe "whirling," "tilting," "floating," and other nonspecific sensations. Furthermore, the correlation between sensations and organ systems is not as consistent among older persons as younger persons. Thus, the sensation reported does not have diagnostic specificity in older patients.

In addition, although dizziness maybe a symptom of one or more discrete diseases, multifactorial etiologies of dizziness are common in older persons. Chronic dizziness is associated with risk factors such as angina, myocardial infarction, arthritis, diabetes, stroke, syncope, anxiety, depressive symptoms, impaired hearing, and polypharmacy. In a population-based study of community-dwelling older persons, the factors that were independently associated with dizziness included anxiety, depressive symptoms, impaired hearing, the use of five or more medications, postural hypotension, impaired balance, and a past history of myocardial infarction. Almost 70% of patients with five or more of the above risk factors reported dizziness, whereas only 10% of patients with none of these factors reported dizziness. These findings suggest that chronic dizziness, at least in a subset of older persons, maybe a geriatric syndrome that is the result of the accumulated effect of multiple coexisting risk factors and diseases.

As presented in the following section, dizziness maybe the presenting complaint of a discrete disease or the results of contributing multiple factors.

ETIOLOGY

Discrete Diseases Causing Dizziness

Vestibular Disorders

Vestibular diseases have been reported in anywhere from 4% to 71% of older persons with dizziness. The most common vestibular disorders causing chronic dizziness in older persons are Ménière's disease, BPPV, recurrent vestibulopathy, the effects of ototoxic medications, and acoustic neuroma.

Ménière's Disease　Ménière's disease, also called endolymphatic hydrops, is reported in 2% to 8% of older patients with dizziness. It is a debilitating disorder of the inner ear, consisting of a triad of recurrent episodic vertigo, tinnitus, and fluctuating sensorineural hearing loss. A sensation of fullness in the inner ear is common. Episodes of true vertigo usually last for 1 to 24 hours. The patient may complain of nausea, vomiting, and headaches during the episodes. The exact cause is unknown, but the pathology is characterized by excess endolymph within the cochlea and vestibular labyrinth. The disease is unilateral in a majority of patients; men and women are affected equally. In a 14-year follow-up study, the episodes of vertigo disappeared in 50% of patients and improved in 28%, while hearing in the affected side was absent in 48% and impaired in 21% of the patients.

Benign Paroxysmal Positional Vertigo　BPPV has been reported to be the cause of dizziness in 4% to 34% of cases. In this condition, patients report sudden-onset, episodic vertigo, often associated with nausea and/or vomiting, precipitated by changes in the position of the head, such as rolling over in bed, getting in and out of bed, or bending forward to pick something up. It is classically accompanied by rotational nystagmus. In most cases, the etiology is unknown, although some patients have a history of head injury or viral neurolabyrinthitis. BPPV results from freely moving particulate matter within the posterior semicircular canal. These particles most likely are dislodged otoconia, which are tiny calciferous granules that make up part of the receptor mechanism in the otolithic apparatus. It is postulated that movement of these free-floating particles cause alteration in the endolymphatic pressure, resulting in episodes of vertigo and nystagmus. In one study, researchers reported that otoconia undergo degenerative changes, which may lead to their dislodgment from the utriculus. A definitive diagnosis of BPPV can be made by the Dix–Hallpike test described under "Evaluation" later in this chapter.

Recurrent Vestibulopathy Recurrent vestibulopathy is an idiopathic disorder characterized by recurrent episodes of vertigo without auditory or neurological symptoms or signs. The vertigo usually lasts from 5 minutes to 24 hours. It is differentiated from Ménière's disease by the absence of auditory symptoms. Over 8.5 years of follow-up, spontaneous recovery was reported in 62% of patients. The diagnosis was changed to Ménière's disease or benign positional vertigo in 14% and 8% of patients, respectively.

Acoustic Neuroma Acoustic neuroma, also known as cerebellopontine angle tumor, is a benign tumor of the eighth cranial nerve, and is reported in 1% to 3% of older persons with dizziness. Clinical features include tinnitus and progressive unilateral sensorineural hearing loss, particularly for the higher frequencies. Patients complain more often of a feeling of unsteadiness rather than of true vertigo. Patients with large tumors may also complain of occipital headache, diplopia, paresthesias in trigeminal or facial nerve distribution, and/or ataxic gait.

Central Nervous System Disorders

The frequency of cerebrovascular disease ranges from 4% to 70% among older persons with dizziness. Patients with transient ischemic attack (TIA) or stroke involving vertebrobasilar distribution commonly present with dizziness, along with diplopia, or dysarthria, numbness, or weakness. Dizziness rarely is a presenting symptom in patients with anterior or posterior cerebral artery ischemia or with internal carotid artery disease. The patient may complain of either a rotatory or nonrotatory dizziness along with other neurologic symptoms and signs. A number of specific stroke syndromes present with dizziness, including cerebellar infarction and posterior lateral medullary artery infarction, also known as Wallenberg's syndrome.

Other central nervous disorder causes of dizziness include Parkinson's disease and basilar artery migraine. The latter is rare in older persons.

Psychiatric Disorders

Anxiety, depression, obsessive-compulsive disorder, panic disorder, and other psychiatric conditions are among the most common causes of chronic dizziness in young adults. In older persons as well, psychiatric conditions are often associated with dizziness. Common psychiatric conditions causing or contributing to dizziness in older persons include depressive and anxiety disorders. Recent studies show that depressive symptoms are associated with symptoms of dizziness, while, conversely, persons who have chronic dizziness are at increased risk of depression, suggesting a reciprocal relationship between dizziness and depressive symptoms among older persons.

Cervical Disorders

Disorders of the cervical spine as a cause of dizziness in older persons have been reported in the range of 0% to 57%. Patients with cervical dizziness usually present with vague lightheadedness or vertigo associated with turning of the head. Both vascular and proprioceptive mechanisms have been proposed to explain cervical dizziness.

Obstruction of the vertebral arteries is thought to be the most common vascular mechanism of cervical dizziness. One hypothesis suggests that in the presence of atheromatous narrowing of one vertebral artery, rotation of the head may cause sufficient obstruction of the contralateral vertebral artery to produce ischemia of the brainstem. Another hypothesis suggests that turning the head or neck results in compression of adjacent vertebral artery by a strategic osteoarthritic spur, causing a transient disruption of the blood flow.

Degenerative changes in the cervical spine may cause dizziness because of impairment of the cervical proprioceptive mechanoreceptors. These receptors provide information for postural control via the vestibulospinal tract. The patient may present with decreased range of motion and radicular pain in the neck upon movement, as well as dizziness.

Systemic Causes

Hypothyroidism, anemia, electrolyte imbalance, hypertension, coronary artery disease, congestive heart failure, and diabetes mellitus are commonly found in patients with dizziness, although the frequency of dizziness as a symptom of each is low. Studies have found an independent association between dizziness and a history of hypertension, angina, myocardial infarction, and diabetes mellitus. Systemic disorders may contribute to instability or dizziness by affecting the sensory, central, or effector components. These systemic disorders may also cause decreased cerebral perfusion or oxygen delivery, fatigue, or confusion, each of which may subsequently lead to a sensation of instability or dizziness. Chapter 57 discusses cardiovascular disorders that can cause dizziness as well as syncope.

Orthostatic Hypotension

Orthostatic hypotension is a primary or contributing cause in 2% to 15% of older persons with dizziness. There is a long list of causes of orthostatic hypotension (see Chapter 57). Although there is no consensus on the definition of orthostatic hypotension in older adults, commonly noted criteria include a 20 mm Hg drop in systolic blood pressure, a 10 mm Hg drop in diastolic blood pressure, or typical symptoms associated with any drop in blood pressure after standing from a supine or sitting position. Another entity reported in literature is postural dizziness, in which patients complain of dizziness on standing from a supine position but have no drop in blood pressure. In these studies, a subset of patients who have orthostatic blood pressure changes do not complain of dizziness, suggesting that orthostatic changes in blood pressure maybe asymptomatic, while, conversely, all dizziness with postural changes may not be caused by a drop in blood pressure. Vestibular dysfunction is thought to account for the postural dizziness not accompanied by postural blood pressure drops.

Postprandial Hypotension

Another important entity to consider in older persons is postprandial hypotension. Postprandial hypotension is defined as a decrease in systolic blood pressure of 20 mm Hg or more in a sitting or standing posture within 1 to 2 hours of eating a meal; dizziness often is a symptom. In a recent study, the effects of postprandial hypotension and orthostatic hypotension were found to be additive but not synergistic, suggesting that the two entities have different patho-physiological mechanisms. Possible etiologies of postprandial hypotension are discussed in Chapter 57.

Medications Contributing to Dizziness

Many classes of drugs can cause or contribute to dizziness. Commonly used examples include antihypertensives, antiarrhythmic agents, anticonvulsants, antidepressants, anxiolytics, antibiotics (aminoglycosides, macrolides, and vancomycin analogs), antihistamines, nonsteroidal antiinflammatory agents, and over-the-counter cold and sleep preparations. These agents cause dizziness through different mechanisms. Antihypertensive agents can cause dizziness simply by lowering blood pressure to a level at which the postural drop in pressure becomes symptomatic. Calcium channel-blockers, nitrates, and hydralazine are common offenders. Loop diuretics such as furosemide can cause dizziness by ototoxicity and/or volume depletion. Antiarrhythmics, anticonvulsants, and anxiolytics are responsible for dizziness through their effects on the CNS. Tricyclic antidepressants, antihistamines, and cold preparations cause dizziness via their anticholinergic properties. Antibiotics (e.g., aminoglycosides, macrolides, and vancomycin analogs), nonsteroidal anti-inflammatory agents, and loop diuretics cause dizziness through ototoxicity, especially in the presence of impaired renal function, which decreases their clearance. The aminoglycosides are especially hazardous because of their toxicity to both the kidney and the vestibular system.

Apart from risks conferred by specific toxicity of drugs, studies have also reported an association between dizziness and the number of medications taken, independent of the effect of comorbid diseases.

EVALUATION

Evaluation of dizziness can be a complex and challenging task for clinicians. The differential diagnosis is broad and the literature offers no evidence-based clinical practice guidelines. Optimal care requires the identification and treatment of the condition or combination of conditions causing dizziness when possible. If treatable conditions cannot be found, then the objective becomes maximum symptomatic improvement of dizziness. Based on these objectives and on the available evidence, a stepwise approach is recommended for the evaluation of chronic dizziness, proceeding from careful history and physical examination to screening laboratory tests. A targeted battery of more elaborate and expensive tests is indicated only when routine evaluation suggests a specific disease entity and the results of these tests are likely to influence the management. For the majority of older persons in whom a routine evaluation does not suggest a single discrete cause, the clinician should try to focus on identifying various factors (Table 56-1) that might be contributing to dizziness, some of which are likely to be modifiable. When etiology is multifactorial, identifying and treating one or more contributing factors may improve, if not eliminate, the dizziness.

History

Patients should be asked to describe the feelings of dizziness in their own words, supplemented by directed questions. Older patients often describe a vague sensation, such as "whirling," or "giddiness,"

or a combination of sensations. Before physicians ask leading questions, patients should be encouraged to describe symptoms in their own words. In one retrospective chart review study of 310 older patients, charts documenting patients' dizziness symptoms in their own words were more likely to have a clinical diagnosis compared to charts without such documentation. Narrowing the differential diagnosis can often occur following a careful history. Determining whether the attacks are episodic or continuous may help in identifying a specific disease. For example, patients with Ménière's disease or BPPV will usually have episodic dizziness, the latter precipitated by specific movements, while psychogenic dizziness is usually continuous. Frequency and duration of dizziness also should be determined. Episodic dizziness lasting less than 1 minute suggests BPPV, 5 to 120 minutes suggest TIA or migraine, while episodes longer than 120 minutes suggest Ménière's disease or recurrent vestibulopathy. One should also ask about any precipitating factors of dizziness, such as missing a meal, drinking alcohol, taking a medication, standing from a lying position, rolling over in bed, changing the position of the head or neck such as looking up or from side to side, bending forward to pick something up, micturition, or defecation. Any relationship between the onset of dizziness and meals should be sought, because postprandial hypotension is common, especially in frail older persons. The patient should also be asked about any symptoms associated with dizziness. For example, patients with Ménière's disease often will complain of tinnitus, fullness in ear, and fluctuating hearing loss. Patients with vertebrobasilar involvement may complain of double vision, dysarthria, or sudden blackouts. Patients with cervical arthritis may also complain of associated pain in the neck on movement. The clinician should also ask about comorbid conditions such as anemia, cardiac diseases, or diabetes, which may contribute to dizziness. One should look for symptoms suggestive of depression or anxiety disorders; use of screening instruments can be helpful (see Chapter 70). Finally, all medications, including over-the-counter medications, should be reviewed as potential contributors to dizziness.

Physical Examination

The clinician should perform a focused physical examination (see Table 56-1), keeping in mind the complex pathophysiology and broad differential diagnosis of dizziness. The examiner should look for spontaneous nystagmus on cranial nerve testing. The nystagmus is vertical in central lesions and horizontal or rotatory in peripheral lesions. The nystagmus of central lesions is not suppressed by visual fixation; in peripheral lesions, nystagmus can be suppressed by visual fixation. One should also test for near and distant vision. The ear examination should include both a hearing test (Whisper Test or audioscope) and an otoscopic examination to rule out cerumen impaction or any structural abnormalities. Blood pressure and heart rate should be assessed both in supine and standing positions to rule out orthostatic hypotension after at least 5 minutes of quiet lying. One should examine the neck for local tenderness and restrictions in the range of movement, which can result from cervical arthritis. One should also consider that the patient might voluntarily restrict the range of neck movement in order to minimize dizziness secondary to vestibular dysfunction; such patients may respond well to vestibular rehabilitation.

A neurologic examination should include cranial nerves, the motor and sensory systems, and gait and balance. In the cranial nerve

TABLE 56-1

Possible Contributors to Chronic Dizziness

CONTRIBUTOR	HISTORY	EXAMINATION	POSSIBLE CAUSES	POTENTIAL INTERVENTIONS
Vision	Use of bifocals or trifocals	Abnormalities in near/distant acuity; contrast sensitivity; depth perception	Cataract; glaucoma; macular degeneration; perceptual difficulties with glasses	Appropriate refraction; consider avoiding bifocals or trifocals when walking; drugs for glaucoma; surgery; good lighting without glare
Hearing	Deafness in one or both ears; difficulty hearing in social situations	Abnormal findings with Rinne's test, Weber's test, Whisper Test, or audiometry	Presbycusis; otosclerosis	Hearing aid; surgery (for otosclerosis); hearing rehabilitation; listening devices
Vestibulocochlear system	True vertigo, worse in dark or with specific head positions; tinnitus; history of aminoglycosides, furosemide, aspirin use; ear surgery; ear or mastoid infections	Nystagmus (horizontal or rotary nystagmus suggests a peripheral vestibular disorder; vertical nystagmus suggests a central disorder); decreased neck range of motion; decreased hearing; abnormal Hallpike maneuver; abnormal vestibular testing	Drug toxicity; previous infections, tumor (e.g., acoustic neuroma); previous surgery; vascular (e.g., brain stem infarct); benign positional vertigo; Ménière's disease	Avoid toxic drugs and long-term vestibular suppressants; remove earwax; vestibular rehabilitation; surgery
Peripheral nerves	Worse in dark or on uneven surfaces or inclines	Decreased neck range of motion; signs of radiculopathy or myelopathy; clumsiness with fine motor tasks; mild spastic gait; increased tone	Spondylosis; degenerative or inflammatory arthritis	Treatment of underlying disease; cervical or balance exercises; appropriate assistive device; consider surgery in selected cases
Cerebral hypoperfusion	Presyncope; near fainting	Postural hypotension; signs of underlying disease	See causes for syncope in Chapter 57; cardiovascular and pulmonary diseases; anemia	Treatment of underlying disease
Postprandial hypotension	Symptoms within 1 h of eating	Hypotension after meals	Postprandial hypotension	Small meals; avoid exertion after meals; avoid hypotensive drugs near meals; have caffeine with meals
Postural hypotension	Near fainting—worse when getting up, walking, exercising; complaints consistent with predisposing diseases; maybe asymptomatic; history of predisposing drugs	Blood pressure and heart rate; signs of predisposing diseases	Drugs, volume/salt depletion; deconditioning; Parkinson's syndrome; diabetes; autonomic dysfunction	Treatment of salt and water repletion; reconditioning exercises; ankle pumps or hand clenching; slow rising; elevate head of bed; graduated stockings; lowest effective dosage of essential contributing drugs
Cardiac dysfunction	Variable, depending on specific etiology	Cardiac auscultation, ECG, echocardiography	Cardiac arrhythmias, valvular lesions, myocardial ischemia, myxoma, hypertrophic cardiomyopathy	Variable, depending on specific etiology
Brainstem	Any sensation (e.g., vertigo, near fainting, wooziness); transient neurological symptoms (e.g., slurred speech, visual change, one-sided weakness); symptoms on looking up	Findings maybe transient or fixed; ataxia	Transient ischemic attack; brainstem infarct; vertebrobasilar insufficiency	Low-dose aspirin; assistive device if ataxic
Metabolic diseases	Symptoms of underlying disease	Signs of underlying disease	Any metabolic disease, (e.g., thyroid disorders, diabetes)	Treatment of underlying disease

(continued)

TABLE 56-1

Possible Contributors to Chronic Dizziness *(Continued)*

CONTRIBUTOR	HISTORY	EXAMINATION	POSSIBLE CAUSES	POTENTIAL INTERVENTIONS
Medications				
Past	Vestibulocochlear symptoms (see above)	See above under vestibulocochlear system	See above under vestibulocochlear system	See above under vestibulocochlear system
Current	Confusion; fatigue; weakness; dizziness often vague, maybe constant	May have postural hypotension	Specific: nitrates, beta-blockers, antidepressants, antipsychotics, anticholinergics; vestibular depressants, benzodiazepines, others General: total number and dose of all drugs	Eliminate, substitute, or reduce specific offending drugs if possible; reduce all other drugs to lowest effective dose possible; remember over-the-counter drugs
Depression, anxiety	Constant dizziness; multiple somatic complaints; poor concentration; positive results on anxiety or depression screening; vegetative complaints (sleep, appetite)	See Chapter 70	Depression, anxiety	Thorough consideration of risks and benefits of antidepressant drug; counseling

Adapted from Beers MH, Berkow R, eds. The Merck Manual of Geriatrics. 3rd ed. Whitehouse Station, NJ: Merck Research Laboratories; 2000:181.

examination, the examiner should look for diplopia, dysarthria, or facial paresthesia to rule out vertebrobasilar involvement. An absence of corneal reflex may suggest acoustic neuroma, especially if accompanied by unilateral hearing loss, tinnitus, and cerebellar signs. The presence of cogwheel rigidity and bradykinesia is suggestive of Parkinsonism. Although most of the abnormalities detected in the balance examination are not specific, the presence of a positive Romberg's sign with the eyes closed is suggestive of an abnormality of proprioception and/or the vestibular system. A wide-based stance, a worsening of the gait with the eyes closed, and an improvement in gait with minimal handheld assistance of the examiner, in combination, suggest a proprioceptive deficit.

In addition to the history and physical examination, clinicians can also perform certain provocative tests at the bedside or in the office, which may help in detecting abnormalities of the vestibular system.

Provocative Tests

These tests include the Dix–Hallpike maneuver, head-thrust, postheadshake, and stepping tests. The Dix–Hallpike test establishes the diagnosis of BPPV (Figure 56-1). In this test, the patient is asked to sit on an examination table with the head rotated 45 degrees to one side. The patient is then asked to fix their vision upon the examiner's forehead. The examiner, while holding the patient's head firmly in the same position, moves the patient from a seated to a supine position with the head hanging below the edge of the table. If the ipsilateral ear is affected, then this maneuver will result in vertigo and nystagmus. If present, the direction, latency, duration of nystagmus, and duration of vertigo should be noted. The diagnostic criteria for BPPV are (1) vertigo accompanied by a rotatory nystagmus; (2) a latency of 1 to 5 seconds between the completion of the maneuver and the onset of vertigo and nystagmus; (3) paroxysmal nature of the vertigo and nystagmus (lasting for 10 to 20 seconds); and (4) fatigability, which is a decrease in the intensity of the vertigo and nystagmus with repeated testing.

The head-thrust and postheadshake tests can help in determining if the vestibuloocular reflex (VOR) is intact. The VOR helps maintain visual stability during head movement. It functions according to the information relayed by the vestibular nucleus to the sixth cranial nerve nucleus in the pons, as well as to the third and fourth cranial nerve nuclei in the midbrain through the median longitudinal fasciculus. The head-thrust test requires the patient to fix the vision on the examiner's nose, while the head is quickly turned approximately 10 degrees to the left or right. If the VOR is intact, the eyes will stay fixed to the target. But in patients with a vestibular defect, the eyes move with the head away from the target before a corrective saccade back to it. For instance, head thrusts to the left in patients with left-sided vestibular lesions will cause a slipping away of the pupils from the target followed by a corrective movement, whereas head thrusts to the right will produce a normal visual response.

Using Frenzel lenses to eliminate fixation of vision, the postheadshake test calls for the head to be rotated for approximately 10 seconds, either passively by the examiner or actively by the patient at a frequency of approximately 2 Hz in the horizontal plane, after which the examiner checks for nystagmus. If there is a unilateral peripheral vestibular lesion, a horizontal nystagmus will result; the fast phase will usually beat away from the side of the lesion. With central lesions, the nystagmus maybe vertical.

Unterberger originally introduced the stepping test, later modified by Fukuda. A positive stepping test suggests a lesion in the vestibular or vestibulospinal system. In this test, the patient stands at the center of a circle, which is divided into sections with lines intersecting at 30-degree angles. Blindfolded, the patient is asked to stretch out both arms at 90 degrees to the body and then to flex and raise high one knee and then the other, and to continue stepping in place at a normal walking speed for a total of 50 or 100 steps. The blindfolded patient marches and the examiner watches for deviation from the straight line. If there is a unilateral vestibular lesion or acoustic neuroma, a gradual rotation of the body (more than 30 degrees) toward the affected side will occur.

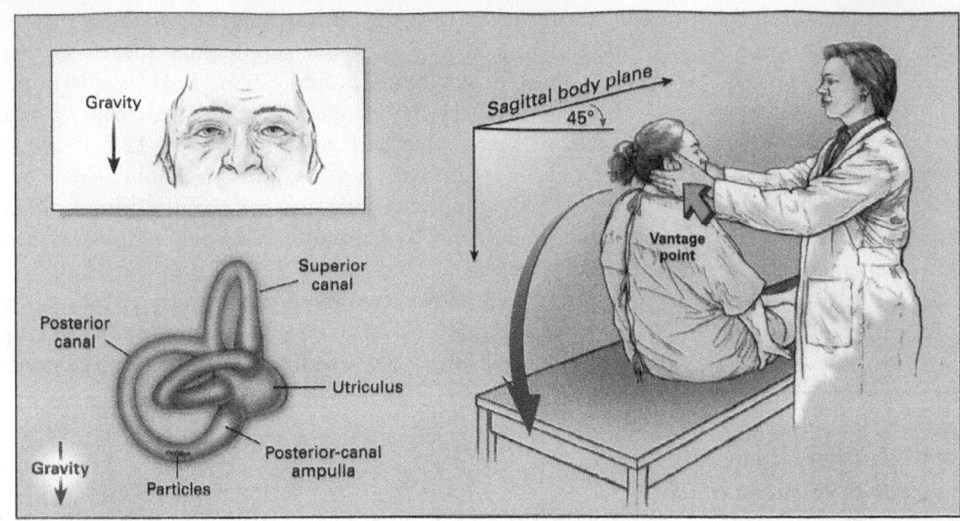

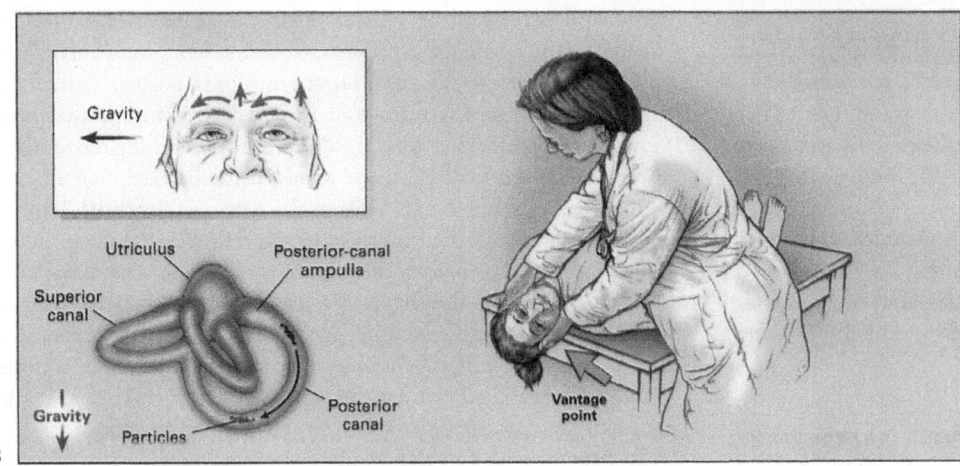

FIGURE 56-1. Dix–Hallpike test. *(Furman JM, Cass SP. Benign paroxysmal positional vertigo. N Engl J Med. 341:1590, 1999. Copyright ©1999 Massachusetts Medical Society. All rights reserved.)*

These tests are more useful in detecting unilateral than bilateral vestibular dysfunction. Upon finding any abnormalities, one can proceed with specialized vestibular function tests such as electronystagmography (ENG) and rotational chair test described under "Laboratory Tests." Clinicians must be aware that compensatory mechanisms may mask a vestibular deficit when these tests are used in patients with longstanding vestibular loss. There are no data addressing the specificity or sensitivity of these tests in older persons.

Laboratory Tests

There is no standardized approach for laboratory testing for patients with chronic dizziness. However, a modest baseline battery of tests should be done in all elderly persons with chronic dizziness to rule out common modifiable contributors to dizziness. Thus, a hematocrit, basic metabolic panel, thyroid function tests, and vitamin B-12 levels should be done in all patients to rule out anemia, diabetes, azotemia, hypothyroidism, and vitamin B-12 deficiency.

Further testing should be tailored to the situation. Audiometry should be done in patients with a history of fluctuating or gradual hearing loss. An audiogram will reveal sensorineural loss in both Ménière's disease and acoustic neuroma; the hearing loss will be greater in lower frequencies in Ménière's disease and in higher frequencies in acoustic neuroma, often unilaterally as opposed to presbycusis, which usually results in bilateral high-frequency hearing loss.

An electrocardiogram is indicated if there is a suspicion of myocardial infarction or cardiac arrhythmia. Holter or event monitoring, or tilt table testing, is indicated only in selected patients with unexplained syncope (see Chapter 57).

In patients with a suspicion of cervical osteoarthritis, radioimaging of the cervical spine can be considered, but the frequency of false-positives is great. Neuroimaging is needed when a stroke or cerebellopontine tumor is suspected. Magnetic resonance imaging (MRI) is preferred over computed tomography scans because of its greater sensitivity, particularly for lesions in the brainstem. Routine MRI is unlikely to reveal specific causes of dizziness. In one study of MRI in patients with dizziness, there were no significant differences in structural abnormalities found in the brain or neck in patients with versus without dizziness. Doppler studies or a magnetic resonance angiogram maybe needed to detect vertebrobasilar insufficiency.

Abnormalities of the peripheral vestibular system can be evaluated by performing special tests, such as ENG including caloric testing, a rotational chair test, and computerized posturography. These tests can provide data that help confirm history and physical examination data. However, abnormalities are common in older persons without dizziness, so a positive test is often nonspecific and nondiagnostic.

In ENG, movements of the eyes (nystagmus) are recorded in the form of tracings with the help of electrodes placed around the eyes. These electrodes record changes in scalp potential produced by the corneal-retinal potential in response to visual and vestibular stimuli, which can be either spontaneous or provoked by caloric stimuli of warm and cold water in the external ear canal. In caloric testing, each ear is stimulated first with warm water (111°F [44°C]) and then with cold water (86°F [30°C]), each instilled over 30 seconds. When vestibular function is normal, the temperature change will result in nystagmus, but there will be decreased or no response in an ear on the side of peripheral vestibular disorder. The caloric test assesses the symmetry of vestibular function and is useful in detecting unilateral vestibular lesions. However, patients with bilateral vestibular loss or patients in whom caloric testing cannot be performed should undergo rotational chair testing.

A rotational chair test, in addition to quantifying the extent of lesions in patients with bilateral peripheral vestibular loss, also helps reveal the degree of peripheral or central vestibular dysfunction. In this test, the patient is seated on a chair in a dark room, and eye movements are recorded when the chair is rotated at different frequencies.

Computerized posturography evaluates the ability of the patient to maintain balance in response to individual or combinations of visual, vestibular, or proprioceptive stimuli while standing on a platform that can be perturbed in three dimensions. This test maybe helpful in providing additional confirmatory data when there is a suspicion of peripheral vestibular pathology, but ENG and rotational chair testing are equivocal. In addition, computerized posturography maybe the only positive test in the case of central vestibular and extravestibular CNS pathology. Posturography also maybe helpful in determining which patients with dizziness are likely to benefit from vestibular rehabilitation.

MANAGEMENT

Clinicians often feel frustrated in managing patients with dizziness. As discussed in the previous section, the goal should be to identify and treat modifiable factors either causing (single condition causing) or contributing to (multiple conditions contributing) dizziness. In many patients with chronic dizziness, a single specific diagnosis maybe elusive in the presence of multiple factors contributing to dizziness. In these patients, instead of focusing on a single diagnosis-oriented approach, the examiner should try to identify and treat as many of these contributing or causative factors as possible, recognizing that some may not be modifiable. The result of such an approach usually is a decrease in the disability associated with dizziness.

Systemic disorders such as anemia, metabolic derangements, vitamin B-12 deficiency, and thyroid abnormalities should be corrected. Correction of vision and hearing deficits is very important. Anxiety and depression should be treated, recognizing the dilemma that most antidepressants also cause dizziness. Medications potentially contributing to dizziness, including over-the-counter medicines, should be identified and either withdrawn or reduced. The ideal approach should be to stop a potentially offending medication rather than adding new ones.

Pharmacological Therapy

Drugs commonly used as vestibular suppressants include antihistamines (e.g., meclizine), anticholinergic agents (e.g., scopolamine), and benzodiazepines (e.g., diazepam). Vestibular suppressants are more effective when used for acute episodes of dizziness than for chronic dizziness. Many vestibular suppressants themselves may cause dizziness. Scopolamine should not be used in elderly persons because of its anticholinergic side effects. Meclizine, a weak antihistaminic agent, is usually given in doses of 12.5 to 25 mg three times daily as needed. These medications should be used only temporarily as their prolonged use may compromise central and peripheral adaptation and thus, paradoxically, prolong the dizziness. Benzodiazepines may at times, however, be indicated as a long-term vestibular suppressant in persons with severe unilateral lesions who are not surgical candidates. In one study, selective serotonin reuptake inhibitors were found to be effective in treating chronic dizziness associated with anxiety.

Vestibular Rehabilitation

Vestibular rehabilitation plays an important role in managing patients with peripheral or central vestibular causes of dizziness by enhancing the adaptation of the vestibular system. Vestibular rehabilitation has been shown to improve symptoms, postural instability, and dizziness-related handicap in patients with chronic dizziness. Vestibular rehabilitation consists of exercises combining movements of eyes, head, and body designed to stimulate the vestibular system. At first, these exercises may worsen the dizziness, but with continued practice and gradual increase in the frequency, these exercises improve dizziness, probably through central adaptation and habituation. These exercises also may help patients alleviate anxiety and fears in performing various activities. Improvement is usually seen after 6 to 8 weeks of vestibular rehabilitation. Patients should perform these exercises initially under the supervision of a trained specialist such as a physical therapist and later independently at home.

In patients with cervical dizziness, physical therapy can substantially decrease the frequency and severity of dizziness and neck pain, and can improve postural stability. Some patients may benefit from cervical collars or cervical traction.

Patients suffering from BPPV can be treated by performing one of two bedside maneuvers, Epley's canalith repositioning procedure, or Brandt's and Daroff's exercises. Epley's canalith repositioning procedure (Figure 56-2) is performed to move free-floating particles from the posterior semicircular canal into the utricle of the labyrinth by the effects of gravity, thereby eliminating fluctuation of the endolymphatic pressure in the semicircular canals. In this five-position procedure, the patient is asked to sit on a table and a vibrator is applied to the ipsilateral mastoid process. Next, the patient is made to lie down supine on the examining table with the head rotated 45 degrees toward the affected ear and hanging below the edge of the table, similar to the Dix–Hallpike test. This position will induce vertigo. Once the vertigo subsides, the head is rotated 45 degrees to the opposite side, which may induce vertigo again. Then the head and body are rotated further in the same direction until the head is facing downward. Subsequently, while holding the head in the same position, the patient sits up. Finally, the head is turned forward with the chin down by about 20 degrees. The examiner holds the head in each of these positions for approximately 10 to 15 seconds or until the vertigo subsides. The patient should be told not to lie flat for the next 24 to 48 hours. Alternatively, a cervical collar can be used to prevent loose particles from sliding back to the posterior semicircular canals. There are no data to support these recommendations. These maneuvers can be performed without using the vibrator although

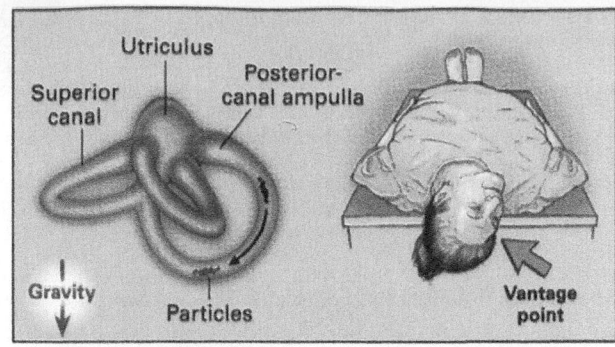

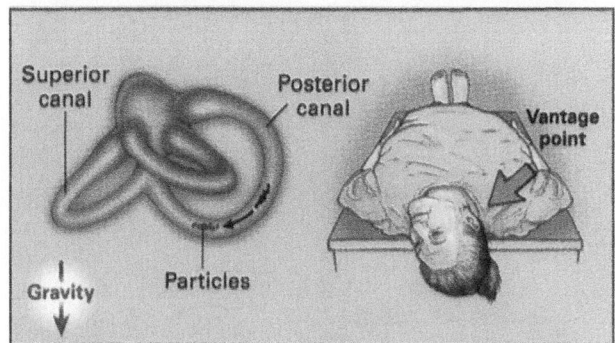

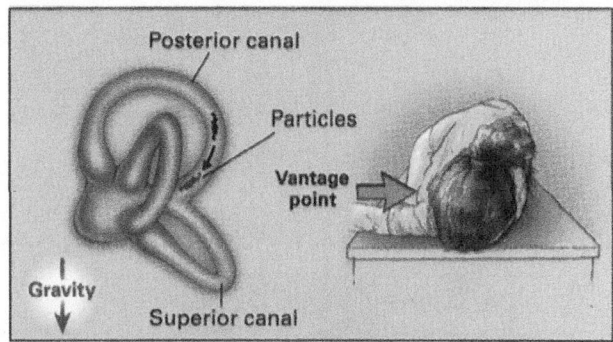

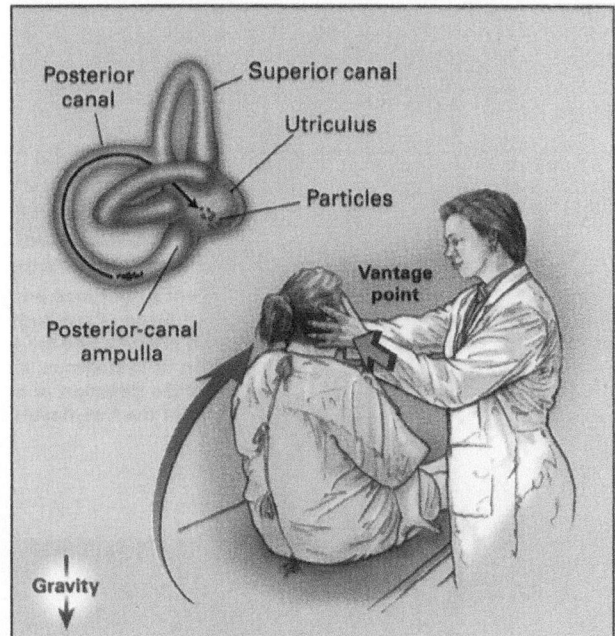

FIGURE 56-2. Epley's canalith repositioning procedure. *(Furman JM, Cass SP. Benign paroxysmal positional vertigo. N Engl J Med. 341:1590, 1999. Copyright © 1999 Massachusetts Medical Society. All rights reserved.)*

the results are said to be not as good. This maneuver can be repeated at weekly intervals until vertigo ceases and the Dix–Hallpike test is negative.

Brandt's and Daroff's exercises can be used in patients who cannot keep their heads upright for 24 to 48 hours as recommended in Epley's maneuver. The patient can do the exercises at home without the presence of a physician or therapist. These exercises probably work by habituation. The patient is asked to sit on the edge of the bed with eyes closed and to rotate the head horizontally by approximately 45 degrees. The patient then lies down on the side opposite to the direction of head rotation and waits for at least 30 seconds or until the vertigo has resolved. The movement is then repeated in the opposite direction. Patients can repeat these exercises every 3 hours and can stop them 2 to 3 days after becoming symptom-free. Improvement usually occurs after 1 to 2 weeks of exercises.

Surgery

Surgery is reserved for a small group of patients who fail pharmacologic treatment or vestibular rehabilitation, or who have cerebellopontine angle tumors. Patients with uncontrolled Ménière's disease can have a transmastoid labyrinthectomy, or partial vestibular neurectomy, or endolymphatic sac decompression. Very rarely, patients with BPPV who do not respond to repeated canalith repositioning procedures may benefit from disabling of the semicircular canal either by singular neurectomy or by occluding the posterior semicircular canal.

PATIENT EDUCATION

Patient education plays a very important role in the management of chronic dizziness. Understanding the basic pathophysiology of dizziness often alleviates associated anxiety. Education also helps patients to modify activities appropriately, thus encouraging patients to cope actively with their dizziness. While most patients need to be advised to be more active, some should be told to avoid looking up or bending down, when these motions clearly precipitate cervical dizziness attacks. Home modifications to reduce neck extension can include storing commonly used items on lower shelves. When orthostatic hypotension is present, patients should be instructed to rise slowly from a supine or sitting position. They should also flex their hands and feet a few times before standing and should never try to walk while feeling dizzy. They should avoid over-the-counter medications such as sleeping pills and cold and allergy medicine, and should ingest a sufficient amount of water.

FURTHER READING

Colledge N, Lewis S, Mead G, et al. Magnetic resonance brain imaging in people with dizziness: a comparison with non-dizzy people. *J Neurol Neurosurg Psychiatry.* 2002;72(5):587.

Colledge NR, Barr-Hamilton RM, Lewis SJ, et al. Evaluation of investigations to diagnose the cause of dizziness in elderly people: a community-based controlled study. *BMJ.* 1996;313:788.

Colledge NR, Wilson JA, Macintyre CC, et al. The prevalence and characteristics of dizziness in an elderly community. *Age Ageing.* 1994;23:117.

Davis LE. Dizziness in elderly men. *J Am Geriatr Soc.* 1994;42:1184.

Ensrud KE, Nevitt MC, Yunis C, et al. Postural hypotension and postural dizziness in elderly women. *Arch Intern Med.* 1992;152:1058.

Hsu LC, Hu HH, Wong WJ, et al. Quality of life in elderly patients with dizziness: analysis of the short-form health survey in 197 patients. *Acta Oto-Laryngologica.* 2005;125(1):55.

Jonsson R, Sixt E. Landahl S, et al. Prevalence of dizziness and vertigo in an urban elderly population. *J Vestibul Res.* 2004;14(1):47.

Kao A, Nanda A. Williams CS, et al. Validation of dizziness as a possible geriatric syndrome. *J Am Geriatr Soc.* 2001;49:72.

Katsarkas A. Dizziness in aging. A retrospective study of 1194 cases. *Otolaryngol Head Neck Surg.* 1994;110:296.

Kwong EC, Pimlott NJ. Assessment of dizziness among older patients at a family practice clinic: a chart audit study. *BMC Family Practice.* 2005;6(1):2.

Lawson J, Fitzgerald J, Birchall J, et al. Diagnosis of geriatric patients with severe dizziness. *J Am Geriatr Soc.* 1999;47:12.

Norre ME, Beckers A. Benign paroxysmal positional vertigo in the elderly. Treatment by habituation exercises. *J Am Geriatr Soc.* 1988;36:425.

Sloane PD, Baloh RW. Persistent dizziness in geriatric patients. *J Am Geriatr Soc.* 1989;37:1031.

Sloane PD, Coeytaux RR, Beck RS. Dizziness: state of the science. *Ann Intern Med.* 2001;134:823.

Staab JP, Ruckenstein MJ. Chronic dizziness and anxiety; effect of course of illness on treatment outcome. *Arch Otolaryngol Head Neck Surg.* 2005;131:675.

Tinetti ME, Williams CS, Gill TM. Health, functional, and psychological outcomes among older persons with chronic dizziness. *J Am Geriatr Soc.* 2000;48:417.

Tinetti ME, Williams CS. Gill TM. Dizziness among older adults: a possible geriatric syndrome. *Ann Intern Med.* 2000;132:337.

Walker MF, Zee DS. Bedside vestibular examination. *Otolaryngol Clin North Am.* 2000;33(3):495.

Yardley L, Donovan-Hall M. Smith HE, et al. Effectiveness of primary care-based vestibular rehabilitation for chronic dizziness. *Ann Intern Med.* 2004;141:598.

Syncope

Rose Anne Kenny

DEFINITION

Syncope (derived from the Greek words, "syn" meaning "with" and the verb "koptein" meaning "to cut" or more appropriately in this case "to interrupt") is a symptom defined as a transient, self-limited loss of consciousness, usually leading to falling. The onset of syncope is relatively rapid, and the subsequent recovery is spontaneous, complete, and usually prompt.

EPIDEMIOLOGY

Syncope is a common symptom, experienced by up to 30% of healthy adults at least once in their lifetime. Syncope accounts for 3% of emergency department visits and 1% of medical admissions to a general hospital. Syncope is the seventh most common reason for emergency admission of patients older than 65 years. The cumulative incidence of syncope in a chronic care facility is close to 23% over a 10-year period with an annual incidence of 6% and recurrence rate of 30%, over 2 years. The age of first faint, a commonly used term for syncope, is less than 25 years in 60% of persons, but 10% to 15% of individuals have their first faint after age 65 years.

Syncope because of a cardiac cause is associated with higher mortality rates than syncope from other causes irrespective of age. In patients with a noncardiac or unknown cause of syncope, older age, a history of congestive cardiac failure, and male sex are important prognostic factors of mortality. It remains undetermined whether syncope is directly associated with mortality or is merely a marker of more severe underlying disease. Figure 57-1 details the age-related difference in prevalence of benign vasovagal syncope (faint) compared to other causes of syncope.

PATHOPHYSIOLOGY

The temporary cessation of cerebral function that causes syncope results from transient and sudden reduction of blood flow to parts of the brain (brain stem reticular activating system) responsible for consciousness. The predisposition to vasovagal syncope starts early and lasts for decades. Other causes of syncope are uncommon in young adults, but much more common as people age.

Regardless of the etiology, the underlying mechanism responsible for syncope is a drop in cerebral oxygen delivery below the threshold for consciousness. Cerebral oxygen delivery, in turn, depends on both cerebral blood flow and oxygen content. Any combination of chronic or acute processes that lowers cerebral oxygen delivery below the "consciousness" threshold may cause syncope. Age-related physiological impairments in heart rate, blood pressure, cerebral blood flow, and blood volume control, in combination with comorbid conditions and concurrent medications account for the increased incidence of syncope in the older person. The blunted baroreflex sensitivity with aging is manifested as a reduction in the heart rate response to hypotensive stimuli. Older adults are prone to reduced blood volume owing to excessive salt wasting by the kidneys as a result of a decline in plasma renin and aldosterone, a rise in atrial natriuretic peptide, and concurrent diuretic therapy. Low blood volume together with age-related diastolic dysfunction can lead to a low cardiac output, which increases susceptibility to orthostatic hypotension and vasovagal syncope. Cerebral autoregulation, which maintains a constant cerebral circulation over a wide range of blood pressure changes, is altered in the presence of hypertension and possibly by aging; the latter is still controversial. In general, it is agreed that sudden mild to moderate declines in blood pressure can affect cerebral blood flow markedly and render an older person particularly vulnerable to presyncope and syncope. Syncope may thus result either from a single process that markedly and abruptly decreases

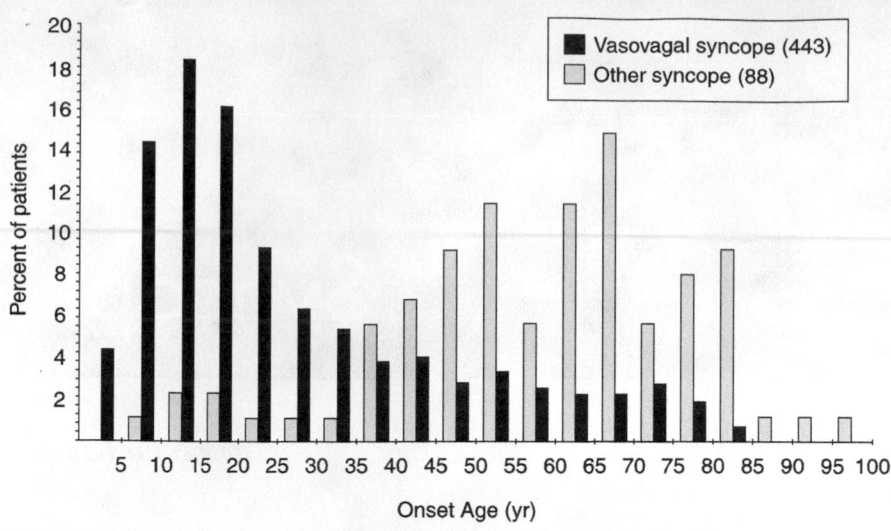

FIGURE 57-1. Comparison of ages of first syncope in 443 patients with vasovagal syncope and 88 patients with syncope of other known causes.

cerebral oxygen delivery or from the accumulated effect of multiple processes, each of which contributes to the reduced oxygen delivery.

Multifactorial Etiology

Up to 40% of patients with recurrent syncope will remain undiagnosed despite extensive investigations, particularly older patients who have marginal cognitive impairment and for whom a witnessed account of events is often unavailable. Although diagnostic investigations are available, the high frequency of unidentified causes in clinical studies may occur because patients failed to recall important diagnostic details, because of the stringent diagnostic criteria used in clinical studies or, probably most often, because the syncopal episode resulted from a combination of chronic and acute factors rather than from a single obvious disease process. Indeed, a multifactorial etiology likely explains the majority of cases of syncope in older persons who are predisposed because of multiple chronic diseases and medication effects superimposed on the age-related physiologic changes described above. Common factors that, in combination, may predispose to or precipitate syncope include anemia, chronic lung disease, congestive heart failure, and dehydration. Medications that may contribute to, or cause, syncope are listed in Table 57-1.

Individual Causes of Syncope

Common causes of syncope are listed in Table 57-2. The most frequent individual causes of syncope in older patients are neurally mediated syndromes including carotid sinus syndrome, orthostatic hypotension, and postprandial hypotension as well as arrhythmias including both tachyarrhythmias and bradyarrhythmias. These disease processes are described in the next section. Disorders that may be confused with syncope and that may, or may not, be associated with loss of consciousness are listed in Table 57-3.

PRESENTATION

The underlying mechanism of syncope is transient cerebral hypoperfusion. In some forms of syncope, there may be a premonitory period in which various symptoms (e.g., light-headedness, nausea,

TABLE 57-1

Drugs That Can Cause or Contribute to Syncope

DRUG	MECHANISM
Diuretics	Volume depletion
Vasodilators	Reduction in systemic vascular resistance and venodilation
Angiotensin-converting enzyme inhibitors	
Calcium channel-blockers	
Hydralazine	
Nitrates	
Alpha adrenergic blockers	
Prazosin	
Other antihypertensive drugs	Centrally acting antihypertensives
Alpha methyldopa	
Clonidine	
Guanethidine	
Hexamethonium	
Labetalol	
Mecamylamine	
Phenoxybenzamine	
Drugs associated with torsades de pointes	Ventricular tachycardia associated with a prolonged QT interval
Amiodarone	
Disopyramide	
Encainide	
Flecainide	
Quinidine	
Procainamide	
Sotalol	
Digoxin	Cardiac arrhythmias
Psychoactive drugs	Central nervous effects causing hypotension; cardiac arrhythmias
Tricyclic antidepressants	
Phenothiazines	
Monoamine oxidase inhibitors	
Barbiturates	
Alcohol	Central nervous system effects causing hypotension; cardiac arrhythmias

TABLE 57-2

Causes of Syncope

Reflex Syncopal Syndromes
- Vasovagal faint (common faint)
- Carotid sinus syncope
- Situational faint
  - acute hemorrhage
  - cough, sneeze
  - gastrointestinal stimulation (swallow, defecation, visceral pain)
  - micturition (postmicturition)
  - postexercise
  - pain, anxiety
- Glossopharyngeal and trigeminal neuralgia

Orthostatic
- Aging
- Antihypertensives
- Autonomic failure
  - Primary autonomic failure syndromes (e.g., pure autonomic failure, multiple system atrophy, Parkinson's disease with autonomic failure)
  - Secondary autonomic failure syndromes (e.g., diabetic neuropathy, amyloid neuropathy)
- Medications (Table 57–1)
- Volume depletion
  - Hemorrhage, diarrhea, Addison disease, diuretics, febrile illness, hot weather

Cardiac Arrhythmias
- Sinus node dysfunction (including bradycardia/tachycardia syndrome)
- Atrioventricular conduction system disease
- Paroxysmal supraventricular and ventricular tachycardias
- Implanted device (pacemaker, ICD) malfunction drug-induced proarrhythmias

Structural Cardiac or Cardiopulmonary Disease
- Cardiac valvular disease
- Acute myocardial infarction/ischemia
- Obstructive cardiomyopathy
- Atrial myxoma
- Acute aortic dissection
- Pericardial disease/tamponade
- Pulmonary embolus/pulmonary hypertension

Cerebrovascular
- Vascular steal syndromes

Multifactorial

TABLE 57-3

Disorders Commonly Misdiagnosed as Syncope

Transient ischemic attacks (TIA) of carotid or vertebrobasilar origin

Hypoglycemia and other metabolic disorders

Some forms of epilepsy

Alcohol and other intoxications

Hyperventilation with hypocapnia

---

individuals and in those with cognitive impairment. The postrecovery period may be associated with fatigue of varying duration.

Syncope and falls are often considered two separate entities with different etiologies. Recent evidence suggests, however, that these conditions may not always distinctly be separate. In older adults, determining whether patients who have fallen have had a syncopal event can be difficult. Half of syncopal episodes are unwitnessed and older patients may have amnesia for loss of consciousness. Amnesia for loss of consciousness has been observed in half of patients with carotid sinus syndrome who present with falls and a quarter of all patients with carotid sinus syndrome irrespective of presentation. More recent reports confirm a high incidence of falls in addition to traditional syncopal symptoms in older patients with sick sinus syndrome and atrioventricular conduction disorders. Thus, syncope and falls may be indistinguishable and may, in some cases, be manifestations of similar pathophysiologic processes. The presentation of specific causes of syncope is presented in the following sections.

EVALUATION

The initial step in the evaluation of syncope is considering whether there is a specific cardiac or neurologic etiology or whether the etiology is likely multifactorial. The starting point for the evaluation of syncope is a careful history and physical examination. A witness account of events is important to ascertain when possible. Three key questions should be addressed during the initial evaluation: (1) Is loss of consciousness attributable to syncope? (2) Is heart disease present or absent? (3) Are there important clinical features in the history and physical examination, which suggest the etiology?

Differentiating true syncope from other 'nonsyncopal' conditions associated with real or apparent loss of consciousness is generally the first diagnostic challenge and influences the subsequent diagnostic strategy (Table 57-3). A strategy for differentiating true and nonsyncope is outlined in Figures 57-2 and 57-3. The presence of heart disease is an independent predictor of a cardiac cause of syncope, with a sensitivity of 95% and a specificity of 45%.

Patients frequently complain of dizziness alone or as a prodrome to syncope and unexplained falls. Four categories of dizzy symptoms—vertigo, dysequilibrium, light-headedness, and others—have been recognized (see Chapter 56). The categories have neither the sensitivity nor specificity in older, as in younger, patients. Dizziness, however, may more likely be attributable to a cardiovascular diagnosis if associated with pallor, syncope, prolonged standing, palpitations, or the need to lie down or sit down when symptoms occur.

Initial evaluation may lead to a diagnosis based on symptoms, signs, or ECG findings. Under such circumstances, no further evaluation is needed and treatment, if any, can be planned. More commonly, the initial evaluation leads to a suspected diagnosis (Figure 57-3), which needs to be confirmed by directed testing. If a diagnosis is confirmed by specific testing, treatment may be initiated. On the other hand, if the diagnosis is not confirmed, then patients are considered to have unexplained syncope and should be evaluated following a strategy such as that outlined in Figure 57-2. It is important to attribute a diagnosis, if possible, rather than assume that an abnormality known to produce syncope or hypotensive symptoms is the cause. In order to attribute a diagnosis, patients should have symptom reproduction during investigation and preferably

---

sweating, weakness, and visual disturbances) offer warning of an impending syncopal event. Often, however, loss of consciousness occurs without warning. Recovery from syncope is usually accompanied by almost immediate restoration of appropriate behavior and orientation. Amnesia for loss of consciousness occurs in many older

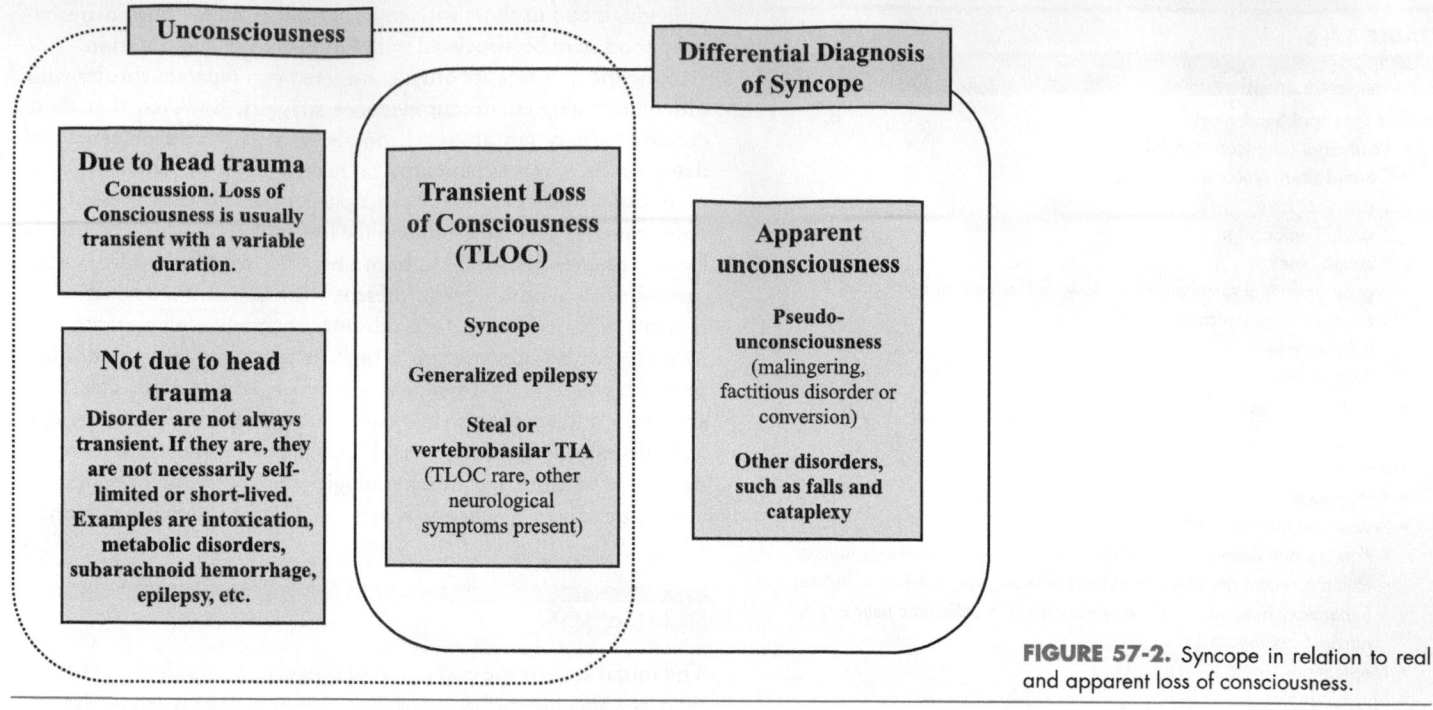

FIGURE 57-2. Syncope in relation to real and apparent loss of consciousness.

alleviation of symptoms with specific intervention. It is common for more than one predisposing disorder to coexist in older patients, rendering a precise diagnosis difficult. In older persons, treatment of possible causes without clear verification of attributable diagnosis may often be the only option.

An important issue in patients with unexplained syncope is the presence of structural heart disease or an abnormal ECG. These findings are associated with a higher risk of arrhythmias and a higher mortality at 1 year. In these patients, cardiac evaluation consisting of echocardiography, stress testing, and tests for arrhythmia detection

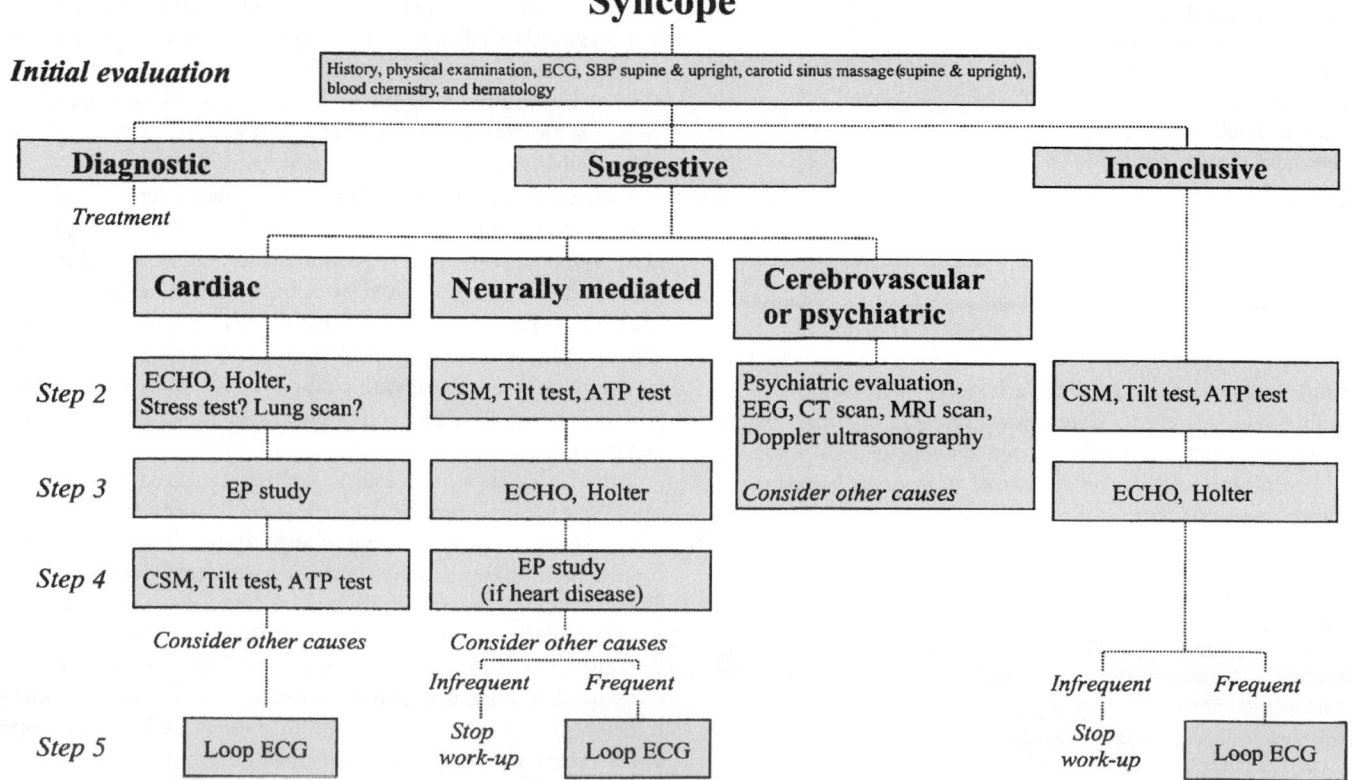

FIGURE 57-3. An approach to the evaluation of syncope for all age groups. ATP test, adenosine provocation test; CSM, carotid sinus massage; ECHO, echocardiogram; EEG, electroencephalogram; EP study, electrophysiologic study; ECG, electrocardiogram.

such as prolonged electrocardiographic and loop monitoring or electrophysiological study is recommended. The most alarming ECG sign in a patient with syncope is probably alternating complete left and right bundle branch block, or alternating right bundle branch block with left anterior or posterior fascicular block, suggesting trifascicular conduction system disease and intermittent or impending high-degree AV block. Patients with bifascicular block (right bundle branch block plus left anterior or left posterior fascicular block, or left bundle branch block) are at high risk of developing high-degree AV block. A significant problem in the evaluation of syncope and bifascicular block is the transient nature of high-degree AV block and, therefore, the long periods required to document it by ECG.

In patients without structural heart disease and a normal ECG, evaluation for neurally mediated syncope should be considered. The tests for neurally mediated syncope consist of tilt testing and carotid sinus massage.

The majority of older patients with syncope are likely to have a multifactorial etiology and thus both predisposing and precipitating causes should be sought in the history, examination, and laboratory evaluation (Tables 57-1 and 57-2), particularly if the initial evaluation does not suggest an obvious single cause.

The evaluation and management of cardiac arrhythmic causes of syncope such as supraventricular and ventricular tachycardia, atrioventricular conduction disorders, and bradyarrhythmias are addressed in Chapter 79. The presentation, evaluation, and management of other common etiologies of syncope are presented in the following sections. These etiologies may occur as the sole cause of a syncopal episode or as one of multiple contributing causes.

ORTHOSTATIC HYPOTENSION

Pathophysiology

Orthostatic or postural hypotension is arbitrarily defined as either a 20 mm Hg fall in systolic blood pressure or a 10 mm Hg fall in diastolic blood pressure on assuming an upright posture from a supine position. Orthostatic hypotension implies abnormal blood pressure homeostasis and is a frequent observation with advancing age. Prevalence of postural hypotension varies between 4% and 33% among community living older persons depending on the methodology used. Higher prevalence and larger falls in systolic blood pressure have been reported with increasing age and often signify general physical frailty. Orthostatic hypotension is an important cause of syncope, accounting for 14% of all diagnosed cases in a large series. In a tertiary referral clinic dealing with unexplained syncope, dizziness, and falls, 32% of patients older than 65 years had orthostatic hypotension as a possible attributable cause of symptoms.

Aging

The heart rate and blood pressure responses to orthostasis occur in three phases: (1) an initial heart rate and blood pressure response, (2) an early phase of stabilization, and (3) a phase of prolonged standing. All three phases are influenced by aging. The maximum rise in heart rate and the ratio between the maximum and the minimum heart rate in the initial phase decline with age, implying a relatively fixed heart rate irrespective of posture. Despite a blunted heart rate response, blood pressure and cardiac output are adequately maintained on standing in active, healthy, well hydrated, and normotensive older persons because of decreased vasodilatation and reduced venous pooling during the initial phases and increased peripheral vascular resistance after prolonged standing. However, in older persons with hypertension and cardiovascular disease receiving vasoactive drugs, these circulatory adjustments to orthostatic stress are disturbed, rendering them vulnerable to postural hypotension.

Hypertension

Hypertension further increases the risk of hypotension by impairing baroreflex sensitivity and reducing ventricular compliance. A strong relationship between supine hypertension and orthostatic hypotension has been reported among unmedicated institutionalized older persons. Hypertension increases the risk of cerebral ischemia from sudden declines in blood pressure. Older persons with hypertension are more vulnerable to cerebral ischemic symptoms even with modest- and short-term postural hypotension, because the threshold for cerebral autoregulation is altered by prolonged elevation of blood pressure. In addition, antihypertensive agents impair cardiovascular reflexes and further increase the risk of orthostatic hypotension.

Medications

Drugs (Table 57-1) are important causes of orthostatic hypotension. Ideally, establishing a causal relationship between a drug and orthostatic hypotension requires identification of the culprit medicine, abolition of symptoms by withdrawal of the drug, and rechallenge with the drug to reproduce symptoms. Rechallenge is often omitted in clinical practice in view of the potential serious consequences. In the presence of polypharmacy, which is common in the older person, it becomes difficult to identify a single culprit drug because of the synergistic effect of different drugs and drug interactions. Thus, all drugs should be considered as possible contributors to orthostasis.

Other Conditions

A number of nonneurogenic conditions are also associated with postural hypotension. These conditions include myocarditis, atrial myxoma, aortic stenosis, constrictive pericarditis, hemorrhage, diarrhea, vomiting, ileostomy, burns, hemodialysis, salt losing nephropathy, diabetes insipidus, adrenal insufficiency, fever, and extensive varicose veins. Volume depletion for any reason is a common sole, or contributing, cause of postural hypotension, and, in turn, syncope.

Primary Autonomic Failure Syndromes (see also Chapters 66 and 67)

Three distinct clinical entities, namely, pure autonomic failure, multiple system atrophy or Shy–Drager syndrome, and autonomic failure associated with idiopathic Parkinson's disease are associated with orthostatic hypotension. Pure autonomic failure, the least common condition and a relatively benign entity, was previously known as idiopathic orthostatic hypotension. This condition presents with orthostatic hypotension, defective sweating, impotence, and bowel disturbances. No other neurological deficits are found and resting plasma noradrenaline levels are low. Multiple system atrophy is the most common and has the poorest prognosis. Clinical manifestations include features of dysautonomia and motor disturbances because of striatonigral degeneration, cerebellar atrophy, or pyramidal lesions. Additional neurological deficits include muscle atrophy, distal sensorimotor neuropathy, pupillary abnormalities, restriction of ocular movements, disturbances in rhythm and control of breathing, life threatening laryngeal stridor, and bladder disturbances. Psychiatric manifestations and cognitive defects are usually absent. Resting plasma noradrenaline levels are usually within the normal range, but fail to rise on standing or tilting.

The prevalence of orthostatic hypotension in Parkinson disease rises with advancing years and with the number of medications prescribed. Cognitive impairment, in particular abnormal attention and executive function, is more common in Parkinson disease with orthostatic hypotension suggesting a possible causal association with hypotension including watershed lesions. Orthostatic hypotension in Parkinson disease can also be owing to autonomic failure and/or to side effects of anti-Parkinsonian medications.

Secondary Autonomic Dysfunction

Autonomic nervous system involvement is seen in several systemic diseases. A large number of neurological disorders are also complicated by autonomic dysfunction, which may involve several organs leading to a variety of symptoms in addition to orthostatic hypotension including anhidrosis, constipation, diarrhea, impotence, retention of urine, urinary incontinence, stridor, apneic episodes, and Horner syndrome. Among the most serious and prevalent conditions associated with orthostasis caused by autonomic dysfunction are diabetes, multiple sclerosis, brain stem lesions, compressive and noncompressive spinal cord lesions, demyelinating polyneuropathies (Guillain–Barre syndrome), chronic renal failure, chronic liver disease, and connective tissue disorders.

Presentation

The clinical manifestations of orthostatic hypotension are owing to hypoperfusion of the brain and other organs. Depending on the degree of fall in blood pressure and cerebral hypoperfusion, symptoms can vary from dizziness to syncope associated with a variety of visual defects, from blurred vision to blackout. Other reported ischemic symptoms of orthostatic hypotension are nonspecific lethargy and weakness, suboccipital and paravertebral muscle pain, low back ache, calf claudication, and angina. Several precipitating factors for orthostatic hypotension have been identified including speed of positional change, prolonged recumbency, warm environment, raised intrathoracic pressure (coughing, defecation, micturition), physical exertion, and vasoactive drugs.

Evaluation

The diagnosis of orthostatic hypotension involves a demonstration of a postural fall in blood pressure after active standing. Reproducibility of orthostatic hypotension depends on the time of measurement and on autonomic function. The diagnosis may be missed on casual measurement during the afternoon. The procedure should be repeated during the morning after maintaining supine posture for at least 10 minutes. Sphygmomanometer measurement will detect hypotension, which is sustained. Phasic blood pressure measurements are more sensitive for detection of transient falls in blood pressure.

Active standing is more appropriate than head-up tilt because the former more readily represents the physiological alpha adrenergic vasodilation because of calf muscle activation. Once a diagnosis of postural hypotension is made, the evaluation involves identifying the cause or causes of orthostasis mentioned above.

Management

The goal of therapy for symptomatic orthostatic hypotension is to improve cerebral perfusion (Table 57-4). There are several nonpharmacological interventions, which should be tried in the first instance. These interventions include avoidance of precipitating factors for low blood pressure, elevation of the head of the bed at night by at least 20 degrees and application of graduated pressure from an abdominal support garment or from stockings. Medications known to contribute to postural hypotension should be eliminated or reduced. There are reports to suggest benefit from implantation of cardiac pacemakers, in a small number of patients, by increasing heart rate during postural change. However, the benefits of tachypacing on cardiac output in patients with maximal vasodilatation are short lived, probably because venous pooling and vasodilation dominate. A large number of drugs have been used to raise blood pressure in orthostatic hypotension, including fludrocortisone, midodrine, ephedrine, desmopressin, octreotide, erythropoeitin, and nonsteroidal anti-inflammatory agents. Fludrocortisone (9-alpha fluhydrocortisone) in a dose of 0.1 to 0.2 mg, causes volume expansion, reduces natriuresis, and sensitizes alpha adrenoceptors to noradrenaline. In older people, the drug can be poorly tolerated in high doses and for long periods. Adverse effects include

TABLE 57-4

Management of Orthostatic Hypotension in Older Persons

Identify and treat correctable causes
Reduce or eliminate drugs causing orthostatic hypotension (see Table 57–1)
Avoid situations that may exacerbate orthostatic hypotension
Standing motionless
Prolonged recumbency
Large meals
Hot weather
Hot showers
Straining at stool or with voiding
Isometric exercise
Ingesting alcohol
Hyperventilation
Dehydration
Raise the head of the bed to a 5- to 20-degree angle
Wear waist-high custom-fitted elastic stockings and an abdominal binder
Participate in physical conditioning exercises
Controlled postural exercises using the tilt table
Avoid diuretics and eat salt-containing fluids (unless congestive heart failure is present)
Drug therapy
Caffeine
Fludrocortisone
Midodrine
Desmopressin
Erythropoeitin

hypertension, cardiac failure, depression, edema, and hypokalemia. Midodrine is a directly acting sympathomimetic vasoconstrictor of resistance vessels. Treatment is started at a dose of 2.5 mg three times daily and requires gradual titration to a maximum dose of 45 mg/day. Adverse effects include hypertension, pilomotor erection, gastrointestinal symptoms, and central nervous system toxicity. Side effects are usually controlled by dose reduction. Midodrine can be used in combination with low-dose fludrocortisone with good effect. Desmopressin has potent antidiuretic and mild pressor effects. Intranasal doses of 5 to 40 μg at bedtime are useful. The main side effect is water retention. This agent can also be combined with fludrocortisone with synergistic effect. The drug treatment for orthostatic hypotension in older persons requires frequent monitoring for supine hypertension, electrolyte imbalance, and congestive heart failure. One option for treating supine hypertension, which is most prominent at night, is to apply a nitroglycerine patch after going to bed, remove it in the morning and take midodrine ± fludrocortisone 20 minutes before rising. This is effective provided that the older person remains in bed throughout the night. Nocturia is therefore an important consideration. In order to capture these coexistent diurnal BP variations of supine hypertension and morning orthostasis, 24 hour ambulatory BP monitoring is the preferred investigation for the management of postural hypotension. Postprandial hypotension caused by splanchnic vascular pooling often coexists with orthostatic hypotension in older patients.

CAROTID SINUS SYNDROME AND CAROTID SINUS HYPERSENSITIVITY

Pathophysiology

Carotid sinus syndrome is an important, but frequently overlooked cause of syncope and presyncope in older persons. Episodic bradycardia and/or hypotension resulting from exaggerated baroreceptor mediated reflexes or carotid sinus hypersensitivity characterize the syndrome. The syndrome is diagnosed in persons with otherwise unexplained recurrent syncope who have carotid sinus hypersensitivity. The latter is considered present if carotid sinus massage produces asystole exceeding 3 seconds (cardioinhibitory), or a fall in systolic blood pressure exceeding 50 mm Hg in the absence of cardioinhibition (vasodepressor), or a combination of the two (mixed).

Epidemiology

Up to 30% of the aged healthy population have carotid sinus hypersensitivity. The prevalence is higher in the presence of coronary artery disease or hypertension. Abnormal responses to carotid sinus massage are more likely to be observed in individuals with coronary artery disease and in those on vasoactive drugs known to influence carotid sinus reflex sensitivity such as digoxin, beta-blockers, and alpha methyldopa. Other hypotensive disorders such as vasovagal syncope and orthostatic hypotension coexist in one-third of patients with carotid sinus hypersensitivity. In centers that routinely perform carotid sinus massage in all older patients with syncope, carotid sinus syndrome is the attributable cause of syncope in 30%. This frequency needs to be interpreted within the context that these centers evaluate a preselected group of patients who have a higher likelihood of

carotid sinus syndrome than the general population of older persons with syncope. The prevalence in all older persons with syncope is unknown.

Carotid sinus syndrome is virtually unknown before the age of 50 years; its incidence increases with age thereafter. Males are more commonly affected than females, and the majority have either coronary artery disease or hypertension. Carotid sinus syndrome is associated with appreciable morbidity. Approximately half of patients sustain an injury, including a fracture, during symptomatic episodes. In a prospective study of falls in nursing home residents, a threefold increase in the fracture rate in those with carotid sinus hypersensitivity was observed. Indeed, carotid sinus hypersensitivity can be considered as a modifiable risk factor for fractures of the femoral neck. Carotid sinus syndrome is not associated with an increased risk of death. The mortality rate in patients with the syndrome is similar to that of patients with unexplained syncope and the general population matched for age and sex. Mortality rates are similar for the three subtypes of the syndrome.

The natural history of carotid sinus hypersensitivity has not been well investigated. In one study, the majority (90%) of persons with abnormal hemodynamic responses, but without syncopal symptoms, remained symptom free during a follow-up over 19 ± 16 months while half of those who presented with syncope had symptom recurrence. More recent neuropathological research suggests that carotid sinus hypersensitivity is associated with neurodegenerative pathology at the cardiovascular center in the brain stem. Why some persons with carotid sinus hypersensitivity develop syncope as a consequence and others remain asymptomatic is not clear.

Presentation

The syncopal symptoms are usually precipitated by mechanical stimulation of the carotid sinus such as head turning, tight neckwear, neck pathology, and by vagal stimuli such as prolonged standing. Other recognized triggers for symptoms are the postprandial state, straining, looking or stretching upward, exertion, defecation, and micturition. In a significant number of patients no triggering event can be identified. Abnormal response to carotid sinus massage (see below) may not always be reproducible, necessitating repetition of the procedure if the diagnosis is strongly suspected.

Evaluation

Carotid Sinus Massage

Carotid sinus reflex sensitivity is assessed by measuring heart rate and blood pressure responses to carotid sinus massage (Figure 57-4). Cardioinhibition and vasodepression are more common on the right side. In patients with cardioinhibitory carotid sinus syndrome, more than 70% have a positive response to right-sided carotid sinus massage either alone or in combination with left-sided carotid sinus massage. There is no fixed relationship between the degree of heart rate slowing and the degree of fall in blood pressure.

Carotid sinus massage is a crude and unquantifiable technique and is prone to intra- as well as interobserver variation. More scientific diagnostic methods using neck chamber suction or drug-induced changes in blood pressure can be used for carotid baroreceptor activation, but are not validated for routine clinical use. The recommended duration of carotid sinus massage is from 5 to

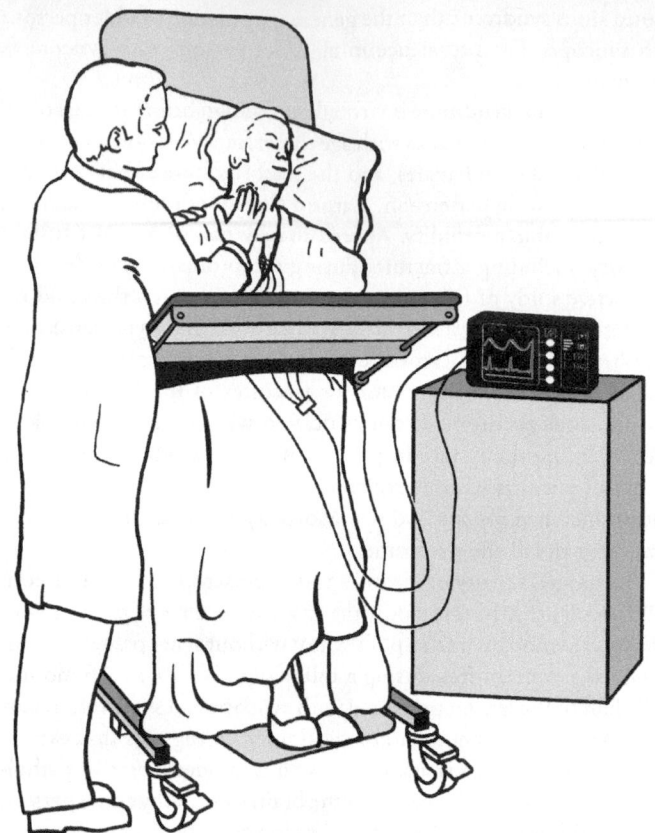

FIGURE 57-4. Procedure for carotid sinus massage while upright.

10 seconds. The maximum fall in heart rate usually occurs within 5 seconds of the onset of massage (Figure 57-4).

Complications resulting from carotid sinus massage include cardiac arrhythmias and neurological sequelae. Fatal arrhythmias are extremely uncommon and have generally only occurred in patients with underlying heart disease undergoing therapeutic rather than diagnostic massage. Digoxin toxicity has been implicated in most cases of ventricular fibrillation. Neurological complications result from either occlusion of, or embolization from, the carotid artery. Several authors have reported cases of hemiplegia following carotid sinus stimulation, often in the absence of hemodynamic changes. Complications from carotid sinus massage, however, are uncommon. In a prospective series of 1000 consecutive cases, no patient had cardiac complications and 1% had transient neurological symptoms that resolved. Persistent neurological complications were uncommon, occurring in 0.04%. Carotid sinus massage should not be performed in patients who have had a recent cerebrovascular event or myocardial infarction.

Symptom reproduction during carotid sinus massage is preferable for a diagnosis of carotid sinus syndrome. Symptoms reproduction may not be possible for older patients with amnesia for loss of consciousness. Spontaneous symptoms usually occur in the upright position. It may thus be worth repeating the procedure, with the patient upright on a tilt table, even after demonstrating a positive response when supine. This reproduction of symptoms aids in attributing the episodes to carotid sinus hypersensitivity especially in patients with unexplained falls who deny loss of consciousness. In one-third of patients, a diagnostic response is only achieved during upright carotid sinus massage.

Management

No treatment is necessary in persons with asymptomatic carotid sinus hypersensitivity. There is no consensus, however, on the timing of therapeutic intervention in the presence of symptoms. Considering the high rate of injury in symptomatic episodes in older persons as well as the low recurrence rate of symptoms, it is prudent to treat all patients with a history of two or more symptomatic episodes. The need for intervention in those individuals with a solitary event should be assessed on an individual basis, taking into consideration the severity of the event and the patient's comorbidity.

Treatment strategies in the past included carotid sinus denervation achieved either surgically or by radioablation. Both procedures have largely been abandoned. Dual chamber cardiac pacing is the treatment of choice in patients with symptomatic cardioinhibitory carotid sinus syndrome. Atrial pacing is contraindicated in view of the high prevalence of both sinoatrial and atrioventricular block in patients with carotid sinus hypersensitivity. Ventricular pacing abolishes cardioinhibition, but fails to alleviate symptoms in a significant number of patients because of aggravation of a coexisting vasodepressor response or the development of pacemaker-induced hypotension, referred to as pacemaker syndrome. The latter occurs when ventriculoatrial conduction is intact as is the case for up to 80% of patients with the syndrome. Atrioventricular sequential pacing (dual chamber) is thus the treatment of choice and because this maintains atrioventricular synchrony, there is no risk of pacemaker syndrome. With appropriate pacing, syncope is abolished in 85% to 90% of patients with cardioinhibition.

In a recent report of cardiac pacing in older fallers (mean age of 74 years), who had cardioinhibitory carotid sinus hypersensitivity, falls during 1 year of follow-up were reduced by two-thirds in patients who received dual chamber systems. Syncopal episodes were reduced by half. More than half of the patients in the aforementioned series had gait abnormalities and three-quarters had balance abnormalities, which would render individuals more susceptible to falls under hemodynamic circumstances, thus further suggesting the multifactorial nature of many falls and syncopal episodes.

Treatment of vasodepressor carotid sinus syndrome is less successful owing to poor understanding of its pathophysiology. Ephedrine has been reported to be useful, but long-term use is limited by side effects. Dihydroergotamine is effective but poorly tolerated. Fludrocortisone, a mineralocorticoid widely used in the treatment of orthostatic hypotension, is used in the treatment of vasodepressor carotid sinus syndrome with good results, but its use is limited in the longer term by adverse effects. A recent, small, randomized, controlled trial suggests good benefit with midodrine (an alpha agonist).

VASOVAGAL SYNCOPE

Pathophysiology

The normal physiologic responses to orthostasis, as described earlier, are an increase in heart rate, rise in peripheral vascular resistance (increase in diastolic blood pressure), and minimal decline in systolic blood pressure, to maintain an adequate cardiac output. In patients with vasovagal syncope, these responses to prolonged orthostasis are paradoxical. The precise sequence of events leading to vasovagal syncope is not fully understood. The possible mechanism involves a sudden fall in venous return to the heart, rapid fall in ventricular volume, and virtual collapse of the ventricle because of vigorous ventricular contraction. The net result of these events is stimulation of ventricular mechano-receptors and activation of Bezold–Jarisch reflex leading to peripheral vasodilatation (hypotension) and bradycardia. Several neurotransmitters, including serotonin, endorphins, and arginine vasopressin, play an important role in the pathogenesis of vasovagal syncope possibly by central sympathetic inhibition, although their exact role is not yet well understood.

Healthy older persons are not as prone to vasovagal syncope as younger adults. Owing to an age-related decline in baroreceptor sensitivity, the paradoxical responses to orthostasis (as in vasovagal syncope) are possibly less marked in older persons. However, hypertension, atherosclerotic cerebrovascular disease, cardiovascular medications, and impaired baroreflex sensitivity can cause dysautonomic responses during prolonged orthostasis (in which blood pressure and heart decline steadily over time) and render older persons susceptible to vasovagal syncope. Diuretic or age-related contraction of blood volume further increases the risk of vasovagal syncope.

Presentation

The hallmark of vasovagal syncope is hypotension and/or bradycardia sufficiently profound to produce cerebral ischemia and loss of neural function. Vasovagal syncope has been classified into cardioinhibitory (bradycardia), vasodepressor (hypotension), and mixed (both) subtypes depending on the blood pressure and heart rate response. In most patients, the manifestations occur in three distinct phases: a prodrome or aura, loss of consciousness, and postsyncopal phase. A precipitating factor or situation is identifiable in most patients. Common precipitating factors include extreme emotional stress, anxiety, mental anguish, trauma, physical pain or anticipation of physical pain (e.g., anticipation of venesection), warm environment, air travel, and prolonged standing. The commonest triggers in older individuals are prolonged standing and vasodilator medication. Some patients experience symptoms in specific situations such as micturition, defecation, and coughing. Prodromal symptoms include extreme fatigue, weakness, diaphoresis, nausea, visual defects, visual and auditory hallucinations, dizziness, vertigo, headache, abdominal discomfort, dysarthria, and paresthesias. The duration of prodrome varies greatly from seconds to several minutes, during which some patients take actions such as lying down to avoid an episode. Older patients may have poor recall for prodromal symptoms. The syncopal period is usually brief during which some patients develop involuntary movements usually myoclonic jerks, but tonic–clonic movements also occur. Thus, vasovagal syncope may masquerade as a seizure. Recovery is usually rapid, but older patients can experience protracted symptoms such as confusion, disorientation, nausea, headache, dizziness, and a general sense of ill health.

Evaluation

Several methods have evolved to determine an individual's susceptibility to vasovagal syncope such as Valsalva maneuvers, hyperventilation, ocular compression, and immersion of the face in cold water. However, these methods are poorly reproducible and lack correlation with clinical events. Using the strong orthostatic stimulus of head-upright tilting and maximal venous pooling, vasovagal syncope can be reproduced in a susceptible individual. Head-up tilting as a diagnostic tool was first reported in 1986 and since then validity of this technique in identifying susceptibility to neurocardiogenic syncope has been established. Subjects are tilted head up for 40 minutes at 70 degrees. Heart rate and blood pressure are measured continuously throughout the test. A test is diagnostic or positive if symptoms are reproduced with a decline in blood pressure of greater than 50 mm Hg or to less than 90 mm Hg. This may be in addition to significant heart rate slowing. As with carotid sinus syndrome, the hemodynamic responses are classified as vasodepressor, cardioinhibitory, or mixed. The cardioinhibitory response is defined as asystole in excess of 3 seconds or heart rate slowing to less than 40 beats/min for a minimum of 10 seconds.

The sensitivity of head-up tilting can be further improved by provocative agents that accentuate the physiological events leading to vasovagal syncope. One agent is intravenous isoprenaline, which enhances myocardial contractility by stimulating beta adrenoreceptors. Isoprenaline is infused, prior to head-up tilting, at a dose of 1 μg/min and gradually increased to a maximum dose of 3 μg/min to achieve a heart rate increase of 25%. Though the sensitivity of head-up tilt testing improves by approximately 15%, the specificity is reduced. In addition, as a result of the decline in beta receptor sensitivity with age, isoprenaline is less well tolerated, less diagnostic, and has a much higher incidence of side effects. The other agent that can be used as a provocative agent and is better tolerated in older persons is sublingual nitroglycerin, which, by reducing venous return caused by vasodilatation, can enhance the vasovagal reaction in susceptible individuals. Nitroglycerin provocation during head-up tilt testing is thus preferable to other provocative tests in older patients. The duration of testing is less, cannulation is not required, and the sensitivity and specificity are better than for isoprenaline.

Because syncopal episodes are intermittent, external loop recording will not capture events unless they occur approximately every 2 to 3 weeks. Implantable loop recorders (Reveal; Medtronic) can aid diagnosis by tracking brady- or tachyarrhythmias causing less frequent syncope. To date, no implantable BP monitors are available with the exception of intracardiac monitors, which are not recommended for diagnosis of a benign condition such as vasovagal syncope.

Management

Avoidance of precipitating factors and evasive actions, such as lying down during prodromal symptoms, have great value in preventing episodes of vasovagal syncope. Withdrawal or modification of culprit medications is often the only necessary intervention in older persons. Doses and frequency of antihypertensive medications can be tailored by information from 24-hour ambulatory monitoring. Older patients with hypertension who develop syncope—either orthostatic or vasovagal—while taking antihypertensive drugs, present a difficult therapeutic dilemma and should be treated on an individual basis. There is some evidence that captopril may benefit such patients. Beta-blockers and disopyramide have now been shown to have negative effects on postural blood pressure changes.

Many patients experience symptoms without warning, necessitating drug therapy. A number of drugs are reported to be useful in alleviating symptoms. Fludrocortisone (100–200 μg/d) works by its volume expanding effect. Recent reports suggest that serotonin antagonists such as fluoxetine (20 mg/day) and sertraline hydrochloride (25 mg/day) are also effective although further trials are necessary to validate this finding. Midodrine acts by reducing peripheral venous pooling and thereby improving cardiac output and can be used either alone or in combination with fludrocortisone but with the caution. Elastic support hose, relaxation techniques (biofeedback), and conditioning using repeated head-up tilt as therapy have been adjuvant therapies. Permanent cardiac pacing is beneficial in some patients who have recurrent syncope owing to cardioinhibitory responses.

POSTPRANDIAL HYPOTENSION

The effect of meals on the cardiovascular system was appreciated from postprandial exaggeration of angina, which was demonstrated objectively by deterioration of exercise tolerance following food. Postprandial reductions in blood pressure manifesting as syncope and dizziness were subsequently reported, leading to extensive investigation of this phenomenon. In healthy older subjects, systolic blood pressure falls by 11 to 16 mm Hg, and heart rate rises by 5 to 7 beats/min 60 minutes after meals of varying compositions and energy content. However, the change in diastolic blood pressure is not as consistent. In older persons with hypertension, orthostatic hypotension, and autonomic failure, the postprandial blood pressure fall is much greater and without the corresponding rise in heart rate. These responses are marked if the energy and simple carbohydrate content of the meal is high. In the majority of fit as well as frail older persons, most postprandial hypotensive episodes go unnoticed. When systematically evaluated, postprandial hypotension was found in more than one-third of nursing home residents.

Postprandial physiological changes include increased splanchnic and superior mesenteric artery blood flow at the expense of peripheral circulation and a rise in plasma insulin levels without corresponding rises in sympathetic nervous system activity. Vasodilator effects of insulin and other gut peptides, including neurotensin and VIP contribute to hypotension. The clinical significance of a fall in blood pressure after meals is difficult to quantify. However, postprandial hypotension is causally related to recurrent syncope and falls in older persons. A reduction in simple carbohydrate content of food, its replacement with complex carbohydrates or high protein, high fat, and frequent small meals are effective interventions for postprandial hypotension. Drugs useful in the treatment of postprandial hypotension include fludrocortisone and indomethacin, octreotide and caffeine. Given orally along with food, caffeine prevents hypotensive symptoms in fit as well as frail older persons, but should preferably be given in the mornings as tolerance develops if it is taken throughout the day.

SUMMARY

Syncope is a common symptom in older adults caused by age-related neurohumoral and physiological changes plus chronic diseases and medications that reduce cerebral oxygen delivery through multiple mechanisms. Common individual causes of syncope encountered by the geriatrician are orthostatic hypotension, carotid sinus syndrome, vasovagal syncope, postprandial syncope, sinus node disease, atrioventricular block, and ventricular tachycardia. Algorithms for the assessment of syncope are similar to those for young adults, but the prevalence of ischemic and hypertensive disorders and cardiac conduction disease is higher in older adults and the etiology is more often multifactorial. A systematic approach to syncope is needed with the goal being to identify either a single likely cause or multiple treatable contributing factors. Management is then based on removing or reducing the predisposing or precipitating factors through various combinations of medication adjustments, behavioral strategies, and more invasive interventions in select cases such as cardiac pacing, cardiac stenting, and intracardiac defibrillators. It is often not possible to clearly attribute a cause of syncope in older persons who frequently have more than one possible cause, and pragmatic management of each diagnosis is recommended.

FURTHER READING

Alboni P, Brignoli M, Menozzi C. The diagnostic value of history in patients with syncope with or without heart disease. *J Am Coll Cardiol.* 2001;37:1921–1928.

Allan LM, Ballard CG, Allen J, et al. Autonomic dysfunction in dementia. *J Neurol Neurosurg Psychiatry.* 2007;78:671–677.

Aronow WS. Heart disease and aging. *Med Clin North Am.* 2006;90:849–862.

Benditt DG, van Dijk JG, Sutton R, et al. Syncope. *Curr Probl Cardiol.* 2004;29:152–229.

Brignole M, Alboni P, Benditt D, et al. Guidelines on management (diagnosis and treatment) of syncope—update 2004. *Europace.* 2004;6:467–537.

Brignole M, Alboni P, Benditt DG, et al.; The task force on Syncope, European Society of Cardiology. Guidelines on management (diagnosis and treatment) of syncope—Update 2004. Executive Summary. *Eur Heart J.* 2004;25:2054–2072.

Chen LY, Shen WK, Mahoney DW, et al. Prevalence of syncope in a population aged more than 45 years. *Am J Med.* 2006;119:1088e1–7.

Ganzeboom KS, Mairuhu G, Reitsma JB, et al. Lifetime cumulative incidence of syncope in the general population: a study of 549 Dutch subjects aged 35–60 years. *J Cardiovasc Electrophysiol.* 2006;17:1–5.

Guidelines for the prevention of falls in older persons. American Geriatrics Society, British Geriatrics Society Panel on Falls Prevention. In preparation.

Kenny RA, O'Shea D, Parry SW. The Newcastle protocols for head-up tilt table testing in the diagnosis of vasovagal syncope, carotid sinus hypersensitivity, and related disorders. *Heart.* 2000;83:564–569.

Kenny RA, O'Shea D. Falls and syncope in elderly patients (editorial). *Clin Geriatr Med.* 2002;18:13–14.

Kenny RA, Richardson DA, Steen N, et al. Carotid sinus syndrome: modifiable risk factors for non-accidental falls in older adults. *J Am Coll Cardiol.* 2001;38:1491–1496.

Kerr SR, Pearce MS, Brayne C, et al. Carotid sinus hypersensitivity in asymptomatic older persons: implications for diagnosis of syncope and falls. *Arch Intern Med.* 2006;166:515–520.

Miller V, Kalaria RN, Slade JY, et al. Tau accumulation in central baroreflex nuclei in carotid sinus syndrome. *Neurobiol Aging.* In press.

Nath S, Kenny RA. Syncope in the older person: a review. *Rev Clin Gerontol.* 2005;15:219.

Parry SW, Kenny RA. Drop attacks in older adults: systematic assessment has a high diagnostic yield. *J Am Geriatr Soc.* 2005;53:74–78.

Parry SW, Steen IN, Baptist M, et al. Amnesia for loss of consciousness in carotid sinus syndrome: implications for presentation with falls. *J Am Coll Cardiol.* 2005;45:1840–1843.

Sheldon RS, Sheldon AG, Connolly SJH, et al. Age of first faint in patients with vasovagal syncope. *J Cardiovas Electrophysiol.* 2006;17:49–54.

Sun BC, Hoffman JR, Mangione CM, et al. Older age predicts short-term, serious events after syncope. *J Am Geriatr Soc.* 2007;55:907–912.

van der Velde N, van den Meiracker AH, Pols HA, et al. Withdrawal of fall-risk-increasing drugs in older persons: Effect on tilt-table test outcomes. *J Am Geriatr Soc.* 2007;55:734–739

van Dijk N, Boer MC, De Santo T, et al. Daily, weekly, monthly and seasonal patterns in the occurrence of vasovagal syncope in an older population. *Europace.* 2007;9:823–828.

Pressure Ulcers

Barbara M. Bates-Jensen

DEFINITION

Pressure ulcers are areas of local tissue trauma, usually developing where soft tissues are compressed between bony prominences and any external surface for prolonged time periods. A pressure ulcer is a sign of local tissue necrosis. Pressure ulcers are most commonly found over bony prominences subjected to external pressure. The most common locations are sacrum, ischial tuberosities, trochanters, and heels with sacral and heel sites most frequent. Pressure exerts the greatest force at the bony tissue interface; therefore, there may be significant muscle and subcutaneous fat tissue destruction underneath intact skin. Other terms for pressure ulcers include bedsore or decubitus ulcer, both of which imply development only in those confined to bed. Since the major causative factor is pressure, and because pressure ulcers occur in positions other than just lying down, pressure ulcer is the preferred term.

EPIDEMIOLOGY

The incidence and prevalence of pressure ulcers are high in all health-care settings. Among hospitalized older patients, the prevalence of pressure ulcers is estimated at 15%. Among patients expected to be confined to bed or chair for at least 1 week, the prevalence of stage II and greater pressure ulcers is as high as 28%, and the incidence during hospitalization ranges between 8% and 30%. Pressure ulcers generally occur within the first 2 weeks of hospitalization (the first 5 days in critical care units), and of those patients with an ulcer, more than half develop them after admission.

Pressure ulcers represent a significant health concern for those in nursing homes, rehabilitation systems, and for special populations. The incidence of new lesions varies widely by clinical situation: the highest rates are found among orthopedic populations (9–19% incidence) and quadriplegics (33–60% incidence). Among nursing homes, prevalence estimates vary from 2.3% to 28%. Incidence is similarly diverse with reports of 2.2% in a database study of a large corporate nursing home chain to 24% in a prospective observational study of 255 nursing home residents in multiple settings. As many as 20% to 33% of persons admitted to nursing homes have a stage II or greater pressure ulcer. Pressure ulcer development among new residents admitted ulcer-free during the initial 4 weeks of nursing home residence is 11% to 14%. Twenty-two percent of those residents admitted ulcer-free develop ulcers within 2 years of residence. African Americans demonstrate a higher incidence of pressure ulcers and more severe pressure ulcers compared to Caucasians in nursing homes with incidence rates reported as 0.56 per person year compared to 0.35 per person year for Caucasians. Incidence of stage II to IV pressure ulcers are nearly two times higher among African Americans than Caucasians. Further, pressure ulcer-associated mortality is higher among blacks than among whites.

Rehabilitation facilities present special concerns related to pressure ulcer development, because patients in these facilities have conditions that limit mobility, such as spinal cord injury, traumatic brain injury, cerebral vascular accident, burns, multiple trauma, or a chronic neurological disorder. Prevalence rates range from 12% to 25%. Individuals with spinal cord injury are at higher risk for pressure ulcer development, with incidence rates reported at 20% for those undergoing spinal surgery, increasing to 30% to 40% over 1 year's time. Prevalence of pressure ulcers in spinal cord injury persons is also high with reports of 33% to 40% during acute rehabilitation and for those living in the community, with recurrence rates up to 40% after an ulcer heals. In the community, the prevalence of pressure ulcers is 6% to 9% in home health-care settings, and 1.6% in outpatient clinic settings. In the home health setting, 20% of the pressure ulcers develop in the first week after admission, and the incidence increases 10% each week through week 4. Of those who develop a pressure ulcer, 50% develop the ulcer within 24 days after admission to home health services.

MORBIDITY ASSOCIATED WITH PRESSURE ULCERS

Pressure ulcers can lead to pain and disfigurement. Of those persons with pressure ulcers who are able to report pain, across nursing homes, home health, and hospital settings, 87% report pain with dressing changes, 84% report pain at rest, and 42% report pain both at rest and during dressing changes. Further, 18% of those persons reporting dressing change wound pain report pain at the highest level (e.g., "excruciating"). Yet, only 6% of those persons reporting pressure ulcer pain receive any medication for pain. There is some evidence that a higher proportion of persons with stage III or IV ulcers report ulcer pain compared to those persons with stage II ulcers and they report more severe pain than those with stage II pressure ulcers.

Septicemia is the most severe complication from pressure ulcers. The incidence of bacteremia from pressure ulcers is approximately 1.7 per 10 000 hospital discharges. When the pressure ulcer is the source of bacteremia, overall mortality is 48%. Further, septicemia is reported in 40% of pressure ulcer-associated deaths. Clinicians should be aware that transient bacteremia occurs after pressure ulcer debridement in as many as 50% of patients. Other infectious complications of pressure ulcers include wound infection, cellulitis, and osteomyelitis. Infected pressure ulcers are one of the most common infections found in skilled nursing facilities, and are reported in 6% of residents. Of note, pressure ulcers are typically colonized with $\geq 10^5$ organisms/mL of normal skin flora. Although $\geq 10^5$ organisms/mL of normal skin flora can cause local infection in intact skin and impair wound healing in flaps and skin grafts, chronic wounds such as pressure ulcers may bear microbial growth at this level for prolonged periods without noticeable clinical manifestations of infection and with evidence of healing. Among patients with nonhealing or worsening pressure ulcers, 26% of ulcers have underlying bone pathology consistent with osteomyelitis, 88% are colonized with *Pseudomonas aeruginosa* species, and 34% with *Providencia* species. The presence of either *P aeruginosa* or *Providencia* species should not be considered typical colonization. Infected pressure ulcers also can serve as reservoirs for infections with antibiotic-resistant bacteria.

Prolonged hospitalization, slow recovery from comorbid conditions, and increased death rates are consistently observed in elderly individuals who develop pressure ulcers in both hospitals and nursing homes. The death rate among bed- and chair-bound patients who develop a pressure ulcer during hospitalization is 60% 1 year after discharge, whereas the death rate for patients who do not develop a pressure ulcer is 38%. In addition, failure of an ulcer to heal or improve has been associated with a higher rate of death in nursing home residents. Nursing home residents whose pressure ulcer healed within 6 months show a lower mortality rate (11% vs. 64%) than residents with ulcers that did not heal within 6 months. It is unclear how pressure ulcers lead to death. The link between pressure ulcers and mortality may be related to an unidentified causal pathway, to pressure ulcers as a marker for coexisting morbidity in frail, sick patients, or to the association between fatal sepsis and pressure ulcers as cause of death. Whatever the link, pressure ulcers are reported as a cause of death among 114 000 persons per year (age-adjusted mortality rate of 3.8 per 100 000 population).

Pressure ulcers have become a quality issue for all areas of health care. Pressure ulcer incidence and severity are used as markers of quality care by regulators in long-term care facilities, home care agencies, and acute care hospitals. As a result, pressure ulcers are on the national agenda for improving quality. The Institute for Healthcare Improvement's 5 Million Lives Campaign lists preventing hospital-acquired pressure ulcers as one of 12 interventions that if implemented would dramatically improve the quality of American health care by protecting patients from harm. The Institute of Medicine's report, *Priority Areas for National Action: Transforming Health Care Quality*, outlines 20 priority areas for improving health-care quality, and preventing pressure ulcers in frail older adults is one of these 20 priority areas. In 2003, the National Quality Forum endorsed 30 "safe practices" that should be universally utilized in applicable health care settings to reduce the risk of harm resulting from processes, systems, or environments of care. This list includes the practice of evaluating each patient upon admission, and regularly thereafter, for the risk of developing pressure ulcers. The Department of Health and Human Services' health goals for the nation, *Healthy People 2010*, identified a 50% decrease in the prevalence of pressure ulcers in nursing homes as a part of the nation's health agenda and reducing pressure ulcers in high-risk residents is a top priority for the Medicare Quality Improvement Organization's 9th scope of work, as well as for a multiorganization campaign to advance excellence in nursing home care initiated in 2007. This emphasis on pressure ulcers across the spectrum of health care settings highlights the importance of the condition for clinicians. Pressure ulcers have also received attention in the courtroom. Organizations have been prosecuted for negligence related to pressure ulcer care and development, and, in a landmark case, one health-care facility operator was found guilty of manslaughter for a resident's death related to improper care for her pressure ulcers.

PATHOPHYSIOLOGY

Pressure ulcers are the result of mechanical injury to the skin and underlying tissues. The primary forces involved are pressure, shear, friction, and moisture. Pressure is the perpendicular force or load exerted on a specific area, causing ischemia and hypoxia of the tissues. High-pressure areas in the supine position are the occiput, sacrum, and heels. In the sitting position, the ischial tuberosities exert the highest pressure, and the trochanters are affected in the sidelying position. As the amount of soft tissue available for compression decreases, the pressure gradient increases, thus, most pressure ulcers occur over bony prominences where there is less tissue for compression and the pressure gradient within the vascular network is altered.

The changes in the vascular network allow an increase in the interstitial fluid pressure, which exceeds the venous flow. This results in an additional increase in the pressure and impedes arteriolar circulation. The capillary vessels collapse, and thrombosis occurs. Increased capillary arteriole pressure leads to fluid loss through the capillaries, tissue edema, and subsequent autolysis. Lymphatic flow is decreased, allowing further tissue edema, and contributing to the tissue necrosis.

Pressure, over time, occludes blood and lymphatic circulation, causing deficient tissue nutrition and accumulation of waste products, as a result of ischemia. If pressure is relieved before a critical time period is reached, a normal compensatory mechanism, reactive hyperemia, restores tissue nutrition and compensates for compromised circulation. If pressure is not relieved, the blood vessels collapse and thrombose. The tissues are deprived of oxygen, nutrients, and waste removal. In the absence of oxygen, cells use anaerobic pathways for metabolism and produce toxic by-products. The toxic by-products lead to tissue acidosis, increased cell membrane permeability, edema, and eventual cell death.

Tissue damage may also be owing to reperfusion and reoxygenation of the ischemic tissues or postischemic injury. Oxygen is reintroduced into tissues during reperfusion following ischemia. This triggers oxygen-free radicals known as superoxide anion, hydroxyl radicals, and hydrogen peroxide, which induce endothelial damage and decrease microvascular integrity.

Pressure is the greatest at the bony prominence and soft tissue interface, and gradually lessens in a cone-shaped gradient to the periphery. Thus, although tissue damage apparent on the skin surface may be minimal, the damage to the deeper structures can be severe. In addition, subcutaneous fat and muscle are more sensitive than the skin to ischemia. Muscle and fat tissues are more metabolically active and, thus, more vulnerable to hypoxia with increased susceptibility to pressure damage.

PRESENTATION

The first clinical sign of pressure ulcer formation, blanchable erythema, presents as discoloration of a patch or flat, nonraised area of the skin larger than 1 cm. This discoloration presents as redness or erythema that varies in intensity from pink to bright red in light-skinned patients. In dark-skinned patients, the discoloration appears as deeper normal ethnic pigmentation; a purple or blue–gray hue to the skin. Other characteristics include slight edema and increased temperature of the area. The beginning clinical indicators of pressure ulceration all relate to the signs of inflammation in the tissues. This beginning stage of damage is transient if the pressure is relieved. If pressure is not relieved, the damage can progress.

Nonblanchable erythema involves more severe damage to underlying tissues and is commonly the first stage of pressure ulceration (stage I pressure ulcer). The color of the skin is more intense. It varies from dark red to purple or cyanotic in both light- and dark-skinned patients. Dark-skinned patients exhibit deepening of normal skin color, a purple or gray hue to the skin, and changes in skin texture, with induration and an orange-peel appearance. Skin temperature is cool compared with healthy tissues, and the area may feel indurated. This stage of tissue destruction is also reversible, although tissues may take 1 to 3 weeks to return to normal.

The result of further deterioration in the tissues is evidenced as the epidermis is disrupted with subepidermal blisters, crusts, or scaling present (stage II pressure ulcer). If properly treated, the situation may resolve in 2 to 4 weeks. The early pressure ulcer is superficial, with indistinct margins and a red, shiny base, and reflects continued tissue insult and progressive injury. It is usually surrounded by erythema. If not dealt with aggressively, the lesion may progress to a chronic, deep ulcer. Superficial ulcers also may begin at the skin surface as the result of friction and moisture on the skin, the effects of both are increased with pressure. While superficial ulcers may progress to deeper ulcers, many deep ulcers do not originate at the skin surface; they begin at the bony prominence and soft tissue interface, and spread to involve the skin structures.

The chronic, deep, full-thickness ulcer usually has a dusky red wound base and does not bleed easily. It is surrounded by blanchable or nonblanchable erythema or deepening of normal skin tone, induration, and warmth. Undermining, or pocketing, and tunneling may be present with a large necrotic cavity. Eschar formation may be a result of larger vessel damage below skin surface from shearing forces. Eschar is the formation of an acellular dehydrated compressed area of necrosis, usually surrounded by an outer rind of blanchable erythema. Eschar formation indicates a full-thickness loss of skin.

ASSESSMENT

Assessment involves screening for risk of developing pressure ulcers, assessment of the severity of the tissue damage (staging), and evaluation of ulcer healing over the course of treatment.

Risk Assessment

Pressure ulcer development is related to multiple factors, with immobility or severely restricted mobility being the most important risk factor for all populations and a necessary condition for the development of pressure ulcers. A study of geriatric patients, who were monitored for movements using devices on the bed, showed that individuals with greater than 50 movements a night did not develop pressure ulcers compared to 90% of individuals with 20 or fewer spontaneous body movements at night who developed a pressure ulcer.

Incontinence, malnutrition, impaired mental status, and altered sensation or response to pain and discomfort are all risk factors with strong relationships to pressure ulcer development in prospective studies. Fecal incontinence has a more powerful relationship to pressure ulcer development than urinary incontinence. Other risk factors include dry skin, increased body temperature, decreased blood pressure, and advanced age. Identification of age as a risk factor may be related to the concomitant chronic diseases more prevalent in older persons or the age-associated changes in the skin that may play a role in this increased risk.

For practitioners to intervene cost-effectively, a method of screening for risk of developing pressure ulcers is necessary. Use of a risk assessment tool is a screening mechanism to identify those persons at risk of developing pressure ulcers in multiple health-care settings. Risk assessment is recommended in clinical practice guidelines for pressure ulcers. The purpose in identifying patients at risk for pressure ulcer development is to allow for appropriate use of resources for prevention. The use of a risk assessment tool allows targeting of interventions to specific risk factors for individual patients. There is, however, limited evidence to support a direct link between use of risk assessment tools and decreased incidence of pressure ulcers. Multifaceted prevention interventions that have included use of risk assessment tools have shown decreased pressure ulcer incidence levels from 13% to 23% preintervention to 2% to 5% postintervention. The outcome, however, cannot be solely attributed to use of risk assessment tools. Use of risk assessment tools is linked to increased documentation of prevention interventions and may be better than use of clinical judgment alone. While there is no study that provides definitive evidence linking risk assessment directly with pressure ulcer prevention, there is a relationship between conducting risk assessment and initiating preventive interventions leading to decreased pressure ulcer incidence.

Pressure ulcer risk assessment should be performed on admission to the health-care setting and at periodic intervals thereafter. In acute care hospitals, risk assessment should be repeated every 48 hours. Those persons admitted to intensive or critical care units should have risk assessment conducted on admission and if determined at risk, daily thereafter. In home health settings, risk assessment should be conducted weekly for the first 4 weeks with every other week reassessments thereafter depending on patient condition and frequency of home visits. Nursing home residents should be reassessed for pressure ulcer risk status weekly for the first 4 weeks following admission followed by quarterly assessments.

The most commonly used risk assessment tools are the Norton Scale and the Braden Scale for Predicting Pressure Sore Risk. The Norton Scale is the oldest risk assessment instrument. Developed in 1961, it consists of five subscales: physical condition, mental state, activity, mobility, and incontinence. Each parameter is rated on a scale of 1 to 4, with the sum of the ratings for all five parameters yielding a total score, ranging from 5 to 20. Lower scores indicate increased risk, with a score of or below 16 indicating "onset of risk" and scores 12 and below indicating high risk for pressure ulcer formation.

The Braden Scale was developed in 1987 and is composed of six subscales: sensory perception, moisture, activity, mobility, nutrition, and friction and shear. All subscales are rated from 1 to 4, except for friction and shear, which is rated from 1 to 3. The subscales may be summed for a total score, with a range from 6 to 23. Lower scores indicate lower function and higher risk for developing a pressure ulcer. The cutoff score for hospitalized adults is considered to be 16, with scores of 16 and below indicating at-risk status. In older patients, some have found cutoff scores of 17 or 18 to be better predictors of risk status. Levels of risk are based on the predictive value of a positive test. Scores of 15 to 16 indicate mild risk, with a 50% to 60% chance of developing a stage I pressure ulcer; scores of 12 to 14 indicate moderate risk, with a 65% to 90% chance of developing a stage I or II lesion; and scores below 12 indicate high risk, with a 90% to 100% chance of developing a stage II or deeper pressure ulcer.

Specific prevention strategies should be targeted to risk factors identified in individual patients. In those persons in whom prevention is not successful, the continued monitoring of risk status may prevent further tissue trauma at the wound site and development of additional wound sites.

Assessment of Pressure Ulcer Stage

Pressure ulcers are commonly classified using grading or staging systems based on the observable depth of tissue destruction. The stage is determined on initial assessment by noting the deepest layer of tissue involved. The ulcer is not restaged unless deeper layers of tissue become exposed. The initial method of classifying pressure ulcers was a pathology-based classification system intended to simplify communication for health-care professionals, provide a mechanism for identification of pressure ulcers, and suggest a broad guide for determining whether operative care was needed. Each grade of pressure ulceration was defined by the anatomic limit of soft tissue damage that could be observed. The numeric classification system suggested an orderly evolution of pressure ulceration. However, it is unknown if all pressure ulcers heal or deteriorate in a linear fashion.

The most commonly used staging system is the National Pressure Ulcer Advisory Panel's (NPUAP) classification system describ-

ing four stages of pressure ulcers. The NPUAP staging system was slightly revised in 2007 and Table 58-1 presents definitions for the four pressure ulcer stages. As part of the staging classification revisions, the NPUAP has also suggested criteria for deep tissue injury (DTI), which is tissue damage that does not fit into the classic four pressure ulcer stages. DTI presents as purple, blue, or black areas of intact skin. These lesions commonly occur on heels and the sacrum, and signal more severe tissue damage below the skin surface. DTI lesions reflect tissue damage at the bony tissue interface, and may progress rapidly to large tissue defects.

Assessment of Pressure Ulcer Healing

Routine pressure ulcer assessment is the base for maintaining and evaluating the therapeutic plan of care. Initial assessment and follow-along assessments at regular intervals to monitor progress are necessary to determine the effectiveness of the treatment plan. Assessment of ulcer status should be performed weekly and whenever a significant change is noted in the wound. Assessment should not be confused with monitoring the ulcer at each dressing change. Monitoring can be performed by less skilled caregivers; however, assessment should be performed on a routine basis by trained clinicians. At a minimum, the ulcer should be assessed for location, depth and stage, size, and wound bed description such as necrotic tissue, exudate, wound edges for undermining and tunneling, and presence or absence of granulation and epithelialization.

There are two research-based pressure ulcer assessment tools for evaluating wound status and healing, the Pressure Sore Status Tool (now called the Bates-Jensen Wound Assessment Tool [BWAT]) (Figure 58-1) and the NPUAP's Pressure Ulcer Scale for Healing tool (PUSH) (Figure 58-2). Clinical practice guidelines, expert panels, and federal nursing home guidelines recommend standardized assessment of pressure ulcers, and many groups are beginning to recommend use of a standardized tool for pressure ulcer assessment. One prospective study showed improved pressure ulcer healing outcomes when a tool was used for standardized pressure ulcer assessment and interventions were tied to the assessment.

The PUSH tool incorporates surface area measurements, exudate amount, and surface appearance. The clinician measures the size of the wound, using length and width to calculate surface area and chooses the appropriate size category of ten categories. Exudate is evaluated as none (0), light (1), moderate (2), and heavy (3). Tissue type is rated as closed (0), epithelial tissue (1), granulation tissue (2), slough (3), and necrotic tissue (4). Each of the three items is scored, then the three subscores can be summed for a total score. The PUSH tool offers a quick assessment to predict healing outcomes, but assessment of additional wound characteristics may still be needed in order to develop a treatment plan for the pressure ulcer.

The BWAT, developed in 1990 and revised in 2001, evaluates 13 wound characteristics using a 5-point numerical rating scale, and rates them from best (scored as 1) to worst (scored as 5) possible (see Figure 58-1). Characteristics include: size, depth, edges, undermining or pockets, necrotic tissue type and amount, exudate type and amount, surrounding skin color, peripheral tissue edema and induration, granulation tissue, and epithelialization. Similar to the PUSH tool, once characteristics have been scored, they can be summed for a total score (range 13 to 65). The total score differentiates between early pressure ulcers (stage I and II) and stage III and IV ulcers with mean total scores of 23 versus 32 respectively. A 1-week improvement

TABLE 58-1

National Pressure Ulcer Advisory Panel, 2007 Pressure Ulcer Staging Classifications

PRESSURE ULCER STAGE	DEFINITION AND CLINICAL DESCRIPTION
Stage I	Intact skin with nonblanchable redness of a localized area usually over a bony prominence. Darkly pigmented skin may not have visible blanching; its color may differ from the surrounding area. The area may be painful, firm, soft, warmer, or cooler as compared to adjacent tissue. Stage I may be difficult to detect in individuals with dark skin tones. May indicate "at risk" persons (a heralding sign of risk).
Stage II	Partial-thickness loss of dermis presenting as a shallow open ulcer with a red pink wound bed, without slough. May also present as an intact or open/ruptured serum-filled blister. Presents as a shiny or dry shallow ulcer without slough or bruising. This stage should not be used to describe skin tears, tape burns, perineal dermatitis, maceration, or excoriation.
Stage III	Full-thickness tissue loss. Subcutaneous fat may be visible, but bone, tendon, or muscle is not exposed. Slough may be present, but does not obscure the depth of tissue loss. May include undermining and tunneling. The depth of a stage III pressure ulcer varies by anatomical location. The bridge of the nose, ear, occiput, and malleolus do not have subcutaneous tissue and stage III ulcers can be shallow. In contrast, areas of significant adiposity can develop extremely deep stage III pressure ulcers. Bone/tendon is not visible or directly palpable.
Stage IV	Full-thickness tissue loss with exposed bone, tendon, or muscle. Slough or eschar may be present on some parts of the wound bed. Often include undermining and tunneling. The depth of a stage IV pressure ulcer varies by anatomical location. The bridge of the nose, ear, occiput, and malleolus do not have subcutaneous tissue and these ulcers can be shallow. Stage IV ulcers can extend into muscle and/or supporting structures (e.g., fascia, tendon, or joint capsule) making osteomyelitis possible. Exposed bone/tendon is visible or directly palpable.
Unstageable	Full-thickness tissue loss in which the base of the ulcer is covered by slough (yellow, tan, gray, green, or brown) and/or eschar (tan, brown, or black) in the wound bed. Until enough slough and/or eschar is removed to expose the base of the wound, the true depth, and therefore stage, cannot be determined. Stable (dry, adherent, intact without erythema or fluctuance) eschar on the heels serves as "the body's natural (biological) cover" and should not be removed.
Suspected Deep Tissue Injury	Purple or maroon localized area of discolored intact skin or blood filled blister due to damage of underlying soft tissue from pressure and/or shear. The area may be preceded by tissue that is painful, firm, mushy, boggy, warmer or cooler as compared to adjacent tissue. Deep tissue injury may be difficult to detect in individuals with dark skin tones. Evolution may include a thin blister over a dark wound bed. The wound may further evolve and become covered by thin eschar. Evolution may be rapid, exposing additional layers of tissue even with optimal treatment.

in the total score demonstrates a positive predictive value of 65% (sensitivity 61%; specificity 52%) for achieving 50% wound healing within a 6-week time period. Both the PUSH tool scores and the BWAT tool scores are highly correlated, and use is based on provider preference.

In general, pressure ulcer healing is accelerated during the initial 3 months after development. In both partial- and full-thickness pressure ulcers, reduction in size after 1 to 2 weeks of therapy has been shown to be predictive of healing outcomes. Clinical practice guidelines suggest pressure ulcers should show evidence of improvement within 2 to 4 weeks after initiating appropriate treatment, and if no improvement is evident, the treatment plan should be re-evaluated. Improvement rates for stage III and IV ulcers are slower than stage II ulcers with 75% of stage II wounds healing in 60 days, while only 17% of stage III or IV ulcers heal in the same time period.

MANAGEMENT

Local Treatment

Pressure ulcer management includes debridement of necrotic tissue, adequate wound cleansing, and application of appropriate topical therapy. Wound debridement is necessary to reduce the necrotic tissue burden, decrease risk for infection, and promote granulation tissue formation. Benefits of debridement also may include removal of senescent fibroblasts and nonmigratory hyperproliferative epithelium, and stimulation of blood-borne growth factor production. Debridement is not indicated for dry eschar presenting on the heel or when the pressure ulcer presents on an ischemic limb.

Five methods of debridement (e.g., surgical or sharp, mechanical, autolytic, enzymatic, biosurgical) are available. Choice of debridement method is currently based on clinician preference and availability rather than any specific evidence. Clinical practice guidelines on pressure ulcer treatment recommend wound debridement with surgical or sharp debridement for extensive necrosis or when obtaining a clean wound bed quickly is important and more conservative methods (autolytic and enzymatic) for those in long-term care or home care environments. Adequate wound debridement is essential to wound bed preparation and healing.

Sharp debridement involves use of a scalpel, scissors, or other sharp instruments to remove nonviable tissue. It is the most rapid form of debridement, and it is indicated over other methods for removing thick, adherent, and/or large amounts of nonviable tissue and when advancing cellulitis or signs of sepsis are present. Healthcare professionals who use sharp debridement must demonstrate their competency in sharp wound debridement skills and meet licensing requirements. One multicenter, randomized, controlled trial comparing the effects of topical growth factor versus placebo on

BATES-JENSEN WOUND ASSESSMENT TOOL

NAME

Complete the rating sheet to assess wound status. Evaluate each item by picking the response that best describes the wound and entering the score in the item score column for the appropriate date. If the wound has healed/resolved, score items 1, 2, 3, & 4 as = 0.

Location: Anatomic site. Circle, identify right **(R)** or left **(L)** and use "**X**" to mark site on body diagrams:

___	Sacrum & coccyx	___	Lateral ankle
___	Trochanter	___	Medial ankle
___	Ischial tuberosity	___	Heel Other Site

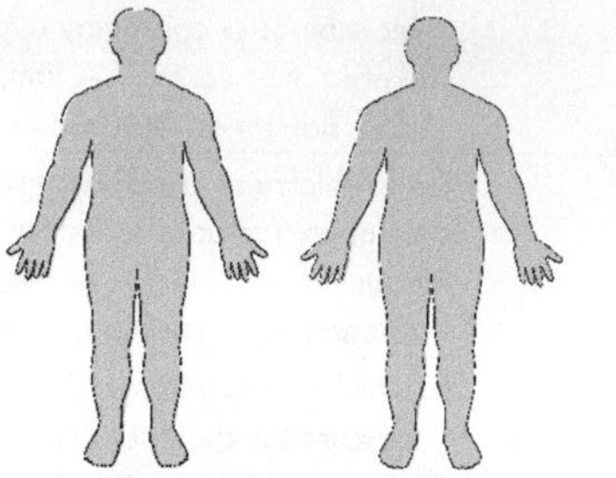

Shape: Overall wound pattern; assess by observing perimeter and depth. Circle and <u>date</u> appropriate description:

___	Irregular	___	Linear or elongated
___	Round/oval	___	Bowl/boat
___	Square/rectangle	___	Butterfly Other Shape

Item	Assessment	Date Score	Date Score	Date Score
1. Size*	*0 = Healed, resolved wound 1 = Length × width <4 sq cm 2 = Length × width 4–<16 sq cm 3 = Length × width 16.1–<36 sq cm 4 = Length × width 36.1–<80 sq cm 5 = Length × width >80 sq cm			
2. Depth*	*0 = Healed, resolved wound 1 = Nonblanchable erythema on intact skin 2 = Partial thickness skin loss involving epidermis &/or dermis 3 = Full thickness skin loss involving damage or necrosis of subcutaneous tissue; may extend down to but not through underlying fascia; &/or mixed partial & full thickness &/or tissue layers obscured by granulation tissue 4 = Obscured by necrosis 5 = Full thickness skin loss with extensive destruction, tissue necrosis or damage to muscle, bone or supporting structures			
3. Edges*	*0 = Healed, resolved wound 1 = Indistinct, diffuse, none clearly visible 2 = Distinct, outline clearly visible, attached, even with wound base 3 = Well-defined, not attached to wound base 4 = Well-defined, not attached to base, rolled under, thickened 5 = Well-defined, fibrotic, scarred, or hyperkeratotic			
4. Under-mining*	*0 = Healed, resolved wound 1 = Nonepresent 2 = Undermining <2 cm in any area 3 = Undermining 2–4 cm involving <50% wound margins 4 = Undermining 2–4 cm involving >50% wound margins 5 = Undermining >4 cm or tunneling in any area			
5. Necrotic Tissue Type	1 = Nonevisible 2 = White/grey nonviable tissue &/or nonadherent yellow slough 3 = Loosely adherent yellows lough 4 = Adherent, soft, black eschar 5 = Firmly adherent, hard, black eschar			
6. Necrotic Tissue Amount	1 = None visible 2 = <25% of wound bed covered 3 = 25% to 50% of wound covered 4 = >50% and <75% of wound covered 5 = 75% to 100% of wound covered			
7. Exudate Type	1 = None 2 = Bloody 3 = Serosanguineous: thin, watery, palered/pink 4 = Serous: thin, watery, clear 5 = Purulent: thin or thick, opaque, tan/yellow, with or without odor			

FIGURE 58-1. Bates-Jensen Wound Assessment Tool.

Item	Assessment	Date Score	Date Score	Date Score
8. Exudate Amount	1 = None, dry wound 2 = Scant, wound moist but no observable exudate 3 = Small 4 = Moderate 5 = Large			
9. Skin Color Surrounding Wound	1 = Pink or normal for ethnic group 2 = Bright red &/or blanches to touch 3 = White or grey pallor or hypopigmented 4 = Dark red or purple &/or nonblanchable 5 = Black or hyperpigmented			
10. Peripheral Tissue Edema	1 = No swelling or edema 2 = Nonpitting edema extends <4 cm around wound 3 = Nonpitting edema extends >4 cm around wound 4 = Pitting edema extends <4 cm around wound 5 = Crepitus and/or pitting edema extends >4 cm around wound			
11. Peripheral Tissue Induration	1 = None present 2 = Induration, <2 cm around wound 3 = Induration 2–4 cm extending <50% around wound 4 = Induration 2–4 cm extending >50% around wound 5 = Induration >4 cm in any area around wound			
12. Granulation Tissue	1 = Skin intact or partial thickness wound 2 = Bright, beefy red; 75% to 100% of wound filled &/or tissue overgrowth 3 = Bright, beefy red; <75% & >25% of wound filled 4 = Pink, &/or dull, dusky red &/or fills 25% of wound 5 = No granulation tissue present			
13. Epithelialization	1 = 100% wound covered, surface intact 2 = 75% to <100% wound covered &/or epithelial tissue extends >0.5 cm into wound bed 3 = 50% to <75% wound covered &/or epithelial tissue extends to <0.5 cm into wound bed 4 = 25% to <50% wound covered 5 = <25% wound covered			
	TOTAL SCORE			
	SIGNATURE			

WOUND STATUS CONTINUUM

| 1 | 5 | 9 | 13 | 15 | 20 | 25 | 30 | 35 | 40 | 45 | 50 | 55 | 60 |

Tissue Health Degeneration   **Healed**   **Wound Regeneration**   **Wound**

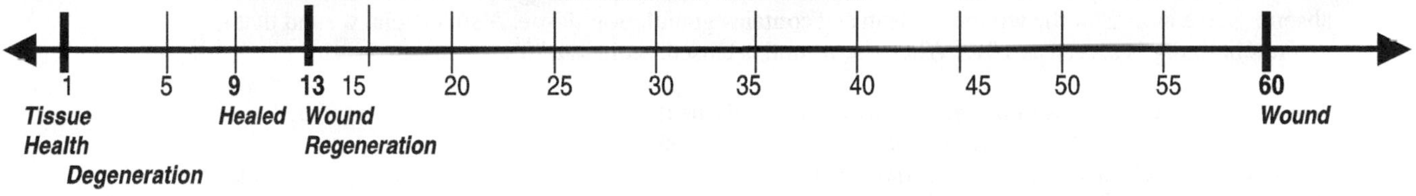

Plot the total score on the Wound Status Continuum by putting an **"X"** on the line and the date beneath the line.
Plot multiple scores with their dates to see-at-a-glance regeneration or degeneration of the wound.

2001Barbara Bates-Jensen

FIGURE 58-1. (Continued)

healing noted that independent of treatment effects, centers that used sharp debridement more frequently experienced better healing rates than those that used sharp debridement less frequently. Sharp debridement is rapid, but is also considered nonselective as viable tissues may be inadvertently removed along with necrotic tissue.

Mechanical debridement involves the use of wet-to-dry dressings, whirlpool, lavage, or wound irrigation. Wet-to-dry gauze dressings continue to be used for debridement, despite the significant disadvantages of increased time/labor for application/removal of the dressings, removing viable tissue as well as nonviable tissue, and pain. This method of debridement should be used cautiously, as it can traumatize new granulation tissue and epithelial tissue, and adequate analgesia should be administered when this method is employed.

Enzymatic debridement involves applying a concentrated, commercially prepared enzyme to the surface of the necrotic tissue, in the expectation that it will aggressively degrade necrosis by digesting devitalized tissue. There are three enzyme ointments available in

PUSH Tool 3.0

Patient Name:_____ Patient ID#:_____

Ulcer Location: _____ Date:_____

DIRECTIONS:

Observe and measure the pressure ulcer. Categorize the ulcer with respect to surface area, exudate, and type of wound tissue. Record a subscore for each of these ulcer characteristics. Add the subscores to obtain the total score. A comparison of total scores measured over time provides an indication of the improvement or deterioration in pressure ulcer healing.

Length	0	1	2	3	4	5	
	0 cm²	<0.3 cm²	0.3–0.6 cm²	0.7–1.0 cm²	1.1–2.0 cm²	2.1–3.0 cm²	
x Width		6	7	8	9	10	Subscore
		3.1–4.0 cm²	4.1–8.0 cm²	8.1–12.0 cm²	12.1–24.0 cm²	>24 cm²	
Exudate Amount	0	1	2	3			Subscore
	None	Light	Moderate	Heavy			
Tissue Type	0	1	2	3	4		Subscore
	Closed	Epithelial Tissue	Granulation Tissue	Slough	Necrotic Tissue		
							Total Score

Length x Width: Measure the greatest length (head to toe) and the greatest width (side to side) using a centimeter ruler. Multiply these two measurements (length x width) to obtain an estimate of surface area in square centimeters (cm²). Caveat: Do not guess! Always use a centimeter ruler and always use the same method each time the ulcer is measured.

Exudate Amount: Estimate the amount of exudate (drainage) present after removal of the dressing and before applying any topical agent to the ulcer. Estimate the exudate (drainage) as none, light, moderate, or heavy.

Tissue Type: This refers to the types of tissue that are present in the wound (ulcer) bed. Score as a "4" if there is any necrotic tissue present. Score as a "3" if there is any amount of slough present and necrotic tissue is absent. Score as a "2" if the wound is clean and contains granulation tissue. A superficial wound that is reepithelializing is scored as a "1". When the wound is closed, score as a "0".

    4 - Necrotic Tissue (Eschar): black, brown, or tan tissue that adheres firmly to the wound bed or ulcer edges and may be either firmer or softer than surrounding skin.
    3 - Slough: yellow or white tissue that adheres to the ulcer bed in strings or thick clumps, or is mucinous.
    2 - Granulation Tissue: pink or beefy red tissue with a shiny, moist, granular appearance.
    1 - Epithelial Tissue: for superficial ulcers, new pink or shiny tissue (skin) that grows in from the edges or as islands on the ulcer surface.
    0 - Closed/Resurfaced: the wound is completely covered with epithelium (new skin).

Version 3.0: 9/15/98
©National Pressure Ulcer Advisory Panel

FIGURE 58-2. National Pressure Ulcer Advisory Panel Pressure Ulcer Scale for Healing tool. © *National Pressure Ulcer Advisory Panel.*

---

the United States, collagenase, papain-urea, and papain-urea with chorophyllin. Some of the effects noticed with enzymatic agents have been attributed to autolysis. Enzymatic ointments have yielded consistently positive results for their efficacy in wound debridement. Debridement with enzymatic ointments is faster than with autolysis, and more conservative than sharp debridement.

Autolytic debridement is the process of using the body's own mechanisms to remove nonviable tissue. Maintaining a moist wound environment allows collection of fluid at the wound site, which allows enzymes within the wound fluid to digest necrotic tissue. Autolytic debridement typically involves adequate wound cleansing to wash out the partially degraded nonviable tissue. It is more effective than wet-to-dry gauze dressings, as it selectively removes only the necrotic tissue and therefore protects healthy tissues. Autolytic debridement may be slower to achieve a clean ulcer bed than other methods.

Biosurgery is the fifth method of debridement. Biosurgery is the application of maggots (disinfected fly larvae, *Phaenicia sericata*) to the wound typically at a density of 5 to 8 per square centimeter. Comparative controlled studies evaluating the use of maggot therapy for pressure ulcer debridement have shown a higher proportion of complete debridement in maggot-treated wounds versus standard debridement therapy (80% vs. 48%, respectively). Biosurgery may not be acceptable to all patients, and may not be available in all areas.

Pressure ulcer cleansing at each dressing change is recommended in clinical practice guidelines on pressure ulcer treatment. However, there is evidence that antiseptic solutions such as 5% mafenide acetate (Sulfamylon solution), 10% povidone with 1% free iodine (Betadine), 0.25% sodium hypochlorite ("half strength" Dakin's solution), 3% hydrogen peroxide, and 0.25% acetic acid have varying effects on wound healing parameters as well as antimicrobial management in an animal wound model yet, how this affects human wounds is unclear.

Use of antiseptic and antimicrobial solutions for cleansing *clean* pressure ulcers is not indicated based on in vitro studies of the toxicity of topical wound cleansers. Findings from in vitro studies have not been confirmed in human wounds. Use of antiseptic and antimicrobial solutions for cleansing pressure ulcers with *necrotic* debris should be employed thoughtfully with attention to the solution chosen, the characteristics of the microorganisms present in the wound, and duration of use (e.g., course of therapy for 2 weeks with evaluation for continuation at that time).

In general, if an ulcer contains necrotic debris or is infected, then antimicrobial activity is more important than cellular toxicity. The chemical and mechanical trauma of wound cleansing should be balanced by the dirtiness of the wound. For wounds with large amounts of debris, more vigorous mechanical force and stronger solutions may be used, while for clean wounds, less force and physiologic solutions such as normal saline should be used.

Topical therapy for pressure ulcers should be provided using moist wound healing dressings. Randomized controlled trials as well as several comparative studies provide compelling support for use of moist wound healing dressings instead of any form of dry gauze dressings (e.g., wet to dry or dry gauze dressing, impregnated gauze dressing) for persons with pressure ulcers. Moist wound healing allows wounds to re-epithelialize up to 40% faster than wounds left open to air. Controlled trials suggest that the use of occlusive dressings such as transparent films and hydrocolloid dressings improves healing of stage II pressure ulcers. These dressings are changed every 3 to 5 days, which allows wound fluid to gather underneath the dressing, facilitating epithelial migration. Moderate evidence exists to specifically support use of hydrocolloid dressings for pressure ulcer care in stage III/IV pressure ulcers. One multicenter, randomized trial demonstrated faster healing in stage III/IV pressure ulcers when treated sequentially with calcium alginate dressings followed by hydrocolloid dressings versus nonsequentially with hydrocolloid dressings. However, the relative merits of different categories of moisture retentive dressings versus another remain unclear. Table 58-2 presents general characteristics of moisture retentive dressing categories.

Surgery

Surgical treatment of pressure ulcers includes primary closure, a variety of approaches to skin grafts and myocutaneous flaps, and removal of underlying bony prominences. In patients with large infected pressure ulcers, more aggressive procedures such as amputation and hemicorporectomy are sometimes required. Surgical complication rates (including dehiscence, infection, necrosis, and hematoma) for both younger paraplegic patients and nonparaplegic elders are as high as 50%, and pressure ulcer recurrence at the same site has been reported ranging from 30% to 70%. Thus, the long-term outcomes have not been ideal even though 70% to 80% of surgically treated pressure ulcers are healed upon discharge from the hospital. Further, while recurrence of pressure ulcers at the same site is lower for elders (40%) compared to younger paraplegic patients (more than 70%), 30% of elders develop new ulcer sites, and mortality in elders ranges from nearly 50% to 68%.

Thus, the benefits of surgical closure for pressure ulcer are uncertain. In addition to questions about the efficacy of surgical intervention, geriatric patients present with multiple chronic diseases and conditions that may make them less than ideal surgical candidates or affect rehabilitation efforts after surgery.

There is some evidence supporting use of negative pressure wound therapy (NPWT) in large stage III and IV nonhealing pressure ulcers with poor granulation tissue or excess exudate. Several clinical practice guidelines and panels have recommended use of NPWT with large stage III and IV pressure ulcers that have failed to improve with standard care with moist wound healing. A case series of 10 patients with stage IV pressure ulcers treated with NPWT showed greater than 50% average reduction in wound volume and depth (55% and 61%, respectively) over 4 weeks.

Drugs

Pharmacologic interventions for pressure ulcers focus on antibiotics and pain management. Antibiotics may be systemic or local. Clinicians should institute systemic antibiotics for patients exhibiting signs and symptoms of systemic infection such as sepsis or cellulitis with associated fever and an elevated white blood cell count. Systemic antibiotics should be initiated for osteomyelitis or for the prevention of bacterial endocarditis in persons with valvular heart disease and who require debridement of a pressure ulcer. Because of the high mortality of sepsis associated with pressure ulcers despite appropriate antibiotics, broad-spectrum coverage for aerobic gram-negative rods, gram-positive cocci, and anaerobes is indicated pending culture results in patients with suspected bacteremia. Ampicillin–sulbactam, imipenem, meropenem, ticarcillin–clavulanate, piperacillin–tazobactam, and a combination of clindamycin or metronidazole with ciprofloxacin, levofloxacin, or an aminoglycoside are appropriate choices for initial antibiotic therapy. Vancomycin may be required for methicillin-resistant *Staphylococcus aureus*. Prolonged silver release topical dressings have been shown to be effective for pressure ulcers colonized with methicillin-resistant *S aureus*. The most effective strategy for preventing infection and dealing with existing infection is adequate debridement of necrotic tissue. In patients with signs and symptoms of systemic infection and in those who are septic, the appropriate debridement method is surgical debridement.

Topical antibiotics are most appropriate for stage III or IV ulcers when there is evidence of local infection such as erythema surrounding the wound, failure to improve with adequate treatment, or friable granulation tissue. A 2-week trial of a topical antibiotic, such as silver sulfadiazine, can be considered for clean pressure ulcers that are

TABLE 58-2

General Characteristics of Moisture Retentive Dressing Categories

DRESSING CATEGORY	DEFINITION	USES	NOTES
Composite Dressings	Combine one dressing group with another to address wound characteristics. For example, gauze/foam and transparent film dressing properties, hydrocolloid and alginates, etc.	Absorbent (depends on combination of dressings used in the composite) Wicks away excess moisture Nonadherent to wound bed Use depends on the combination of dressings used in the composite	• Some may be difficult to apply • If nonadherent to wound bed then requires secondary dressing to hold in place • Can be confusing to caregivers as combines various dressing category properties.
Transparent Film Dressings	Polyurethane and polyethylene membrane film coated with a layer of acrylic hypoallergenic adhesive. Moisture vapor transmission rates (MVTR) vary	Appropriate for partial-thickness wounds Promotes epithelialization Semipermeable Bacterial barrier Autolysis Wound visible Protects against friction Self adhesive	• May reinjure area on removal • Nonabsorbent so can lead to wound edge maceration • Tendency to remove prematurely • Indicated for minimal exudate, does not absorb drainage • Not indicated for moderate to heavy exudate.
Hydrocolloids Regular or thin wafers, paste, granules	Gelatin, pectin, carboxymethylcellulose in a polyisobutylene adhesive base with a polyurethane or film backing	Absorbs low to moderate wound fluid, Autolysis Thermal insulation Bacterial barrier Reduces pain Translucent to opaque Easy to apply Controls odor (until dressing removed) Impermeable to semipermeable	• Not indicated for heavy exudate, limited absorbent abilities when used alone • Use with other products increases absorbent abilities • Odor on removal • Regular wafers are opaque, thin wafers allow some wound visualization • Edges may melt down and stick to linens • Some difficult to remove • Possible sensitivity to adhesive backing • Use with close supervision on immunosuppressed and diabetic patients, extensive burns, infected lesions
Hydrogels Sheets, wafers Amorphous gels Impregnated gauze	May or may not be supported by a fabric net, high water content, varying amounts of gel-forming material (glycerin, copolymer, water, propylene glycol, humectant)	Absorbs low to moderate drainage Autolysis Nonadhesive, may have adhesive borders Semipermeable or impermeable depending on backing Thermal insulation Reduces pain Conformable Carrier for topical medication	• Can dry out • May macerate surrounding tissues • Requires secondary dressing or tape to keep in place • Does not cause reinjury upon removal • Cooling effect can help relieve wound pain • Candidiasis may present from inappropriate usage
Wound Fillers (Exudate absorbers) Beads, flakes Pastes, powders	Consists of copolymer starch, dextranomer beads or hydrocolloid paste that swell on contact with wound fluid to form gel, dextranomers, polysaccharides, starch, natural polymers, and colloidal particles	Moisture retentive Absorptive (moderate to large) Useful to fill cavities, pockets, undermining Can be used with topical medications	• Nonadhesive • Requires a secondary dressing to hold in place • May have burning sensation on application • May have odor • Some require mixing • Some require wound irrigation for nontraumatic removal
Alginates Ropes, pads, wafers	Calcium–sodium salts of alginic acid (naturally occuring polymer in seaweed)	Absorptive (moderate to large) Useful to fill cavities, pockets, undermining Moisture retentive Can use with topical medications or on infected wounds Reduces pain Thermal insulation	• Nonadherent, requires secondary dressing to hold in place • Hemostatic properties • May require wound irrigation for removal • No reinjury on removal • May dry out, should not be used on wounds with low exudate.

(Continued)

TABLE 58-2

General Characteristics of Moisture Retentive Dressing Categories (Continued)

DRESSING CATEGORY	DEFINITION	USES	NOTES
Foams Wafers (thick or thin), pillows, composite dressings with thin film covers, available with surfactant impregnated or charcoal layer	Inert material that is hydrophilic and nonadherent, modified polyurethane foam	Absorptive (moderate to large) Autolysis Can be used with topical medications & on infected wounds Conformable Thermal insulation	• Nonadhesive unless used with composite dressing • Requires tape or secondary dressing to hold in place • Nontraumatic removal • Opaque • Waterproof, inert
Hydrofibers Pads, wafers, ropes	Soft nonwoven pad or ribbon dressings made from sodium carboxymethyl-cellulose fibers, similar absorbent material used in hydrocolloid dressings	Absorptive (moderate to large) Autolysis Thermal insulation Reduces pain	• Nonadherent, requires secondary dressing to hold in place • Hemostatic properties • May require wound irrigation for removal • No reinjury on removal

not healing after 2 to 4 weeks of optimal management. Use of a prolonged silver release dressing may also be appropriate in this situation. On the other hand, clinicians should not use povidone–iodine, iodophor, sodium hypochlorite, hydrogen peroxide, or acetic acid as topical therapies on *clean* pressure ulcers. These antiseptic agents have been shown to be toxic to fibroblasts and to impair wound healing in in vitro laboratory studies, and how these solutions affect human wounds is unclear. There is no evidence for using prolonged silver release dressings in routine management of healing pressure ulcers.

There is limited evidence to guide clinicians on appropriate management of pressure ulcer related pain. The pressure ulcer alone may not require routine pain medication, but medication prior to procedures is essential. Lower levels of pain may be manageable with appropriate wound dressing choice and topical wound analgesia. Nonpharmacological techniques useful for noncyclic and cyclic wound pain associated with procedures (e.g., debridement, dressing changes) include use of distraction (e.g., talking to the patient while performing the procedure), allowing the patient to call a "time-out" during the procedure, allowing the patient to control and participate in the procedure. Pharmacological strategies for wound pain include providing opioids and/or nonsteroidal anti-inflammatory drugs 30 minutes prior to the procedure and afterwards, and administering topical anesthetics or topical opioids using hydrogels as a transport media. Two options have been successful for use in chronic wound pain, EMLA cream and diamorphine gel. EMLA cream (eutectic mixture of lidocaine 2.5% and prilocaine 2.5%) reduces debridement pain scores in chronic venous ulcers, and may have a vasoactive effect cutaneously. Use of EMLA cream in venous ulcers has been associated with a reduction in pain scores (measured on a 100 mm scale) of 20.6 mm. Low-dose topical morphine (diamorphine) has been used in several small, randomized, placebo controlled studies to successfully control pressure ulcer related pain.

Nutrition

Multiple studies have demonstrated a relationship between different markers of malnutrition (e.g., serum albumin level, dietary protein intake, inability to feed self, and weight loss) and pressure ulcer formation. Other studies have demonstrated that the severity of the pressure ulcer is associated with the severity of the malnutrition. Although it seems intuitive, it has proven difficult to define a causal relationship between malnutrition and pressure ulcer development. Modest evidence exists to support providing nutritional support to persons at risk for pressure ulcers with relative reduction in pressure ulcer incidence of 25%. There is some evidence that use of high-protein nutritional supplements (24–25% protein) improves pressure ulcer healing, and the goal should be to provide 30 to 35 kcal/kg/d and 1.25 to 1.5 g/kg of protein daily. However, provision of nutritional supplementation by tube-feeding to persons with pressure ulcers has not achieved positive results. No evidence exists for use of supplemental vitamins or minerals (e.g., vitamin A, E, C, zinc, arginine) in persons with pressure ulcers and no coexisting specific vitamin/mineral deficiency to improve pressure ulcer healing. Persons with pressure ulcers or at risk of developing pressure ulcers who also demonstrate malnutrition should have a nutritional assessment to identify deficits and nutrition support as indicated. A daily multivitamin and mineral supplement that provides recommended daily allowances of vitamins and minerals is recommended for persons with suspected nutritional deficiencies.

PREVENTION

Pressure ulcer prevention involves scheduled turning and repositioning programs, use of support surfaces to reduce/relieve pressure, nutritional support (discussed above), and general skin care. Prevention interventions should be implemented for persons at risk for pressure ulcer development and those with existing pressure ulcers as part of the treatment plan.

Patients at risk for pressure ulcers that are unable to move independently should be placed on scheduled repositioning programs. The recommended time interval for full change of position or turning while in bed is every 2 hours, depending on the individual patient profile and the use of support surfaces. Pressure-reducing support surfaces (e.g., foam, air, gel-filled mattress overlays, low-air-loss therapy devices) may reduce the frequency of repositioning required in some patients. One controlled clinical trial evaluating the effects of four different turn intervals in conjunction with standard hospital mattress versus a pressure reduction support surface found differences in pressure ulcer incidence. The four turn intervals evaluated were: 2 hours on standard mattress (2 h), 3 hours on standard mattress (3 h), 4 hours on pressure reducing surface (4 h), 6 hours on pressure reducing surface (6 h) and a control group with usual care (no specified turning schedule). Over 4 weeks, 838 geriatric nursing home residents were evaluated. Although there was no difference in the incidence of stage I pressure ulcers or erythema, stage II pressure ulcer incidence was significantly decreased in the 4 h group compared to all other groups (3% compared to 20%, no turns; 14.3%, 2 h; 24.1%, 3 h; and 15.9%, 6 h).

Repositioning patients to avoid placing pressure on bony prominences, in particular the malleolus and trochanter. To avoid placing pressure on the trochanter and outer malleolus, position the patient at a 30-degree side-lying position (e.g., 30-degree angle to the support surface) instead of the commonly used 90-degree side lying position, which increases tissue compression over the trochanter and malleolus. Maintain the head of the bed at the lowest degree of elevation consistent with medical conditions, and limit the amount of time the head of the bed is elevated. This will decrease exposure of the sacral area to shearing forces that may predispose to deep-tissue injury. Use of footboards and pillows under the lower legs to prevent sliding and to maintain position, are also helpful in reducing shear effects on the skin when in bed.

There are techniques to make turning patients easier and less time-consuming. Turning sheets, draw sheets, and pillows are essential for passive movement of patients in bed. Turning sheets are useful in repositioning the patient to a side lying position, and draw sheets are used for pulling the patient up in bed and help to prevent dragging the patient's skin over the bed surface. Pillows should be used to position patients with minimal tissue compression between the medial knees, the medial malleolus, and the heels. Place pillows between the knees, between the ankles, and under the heels as well as behind the back and under the arms for comfort.

Similar approaches are useful for patients in chairs. Full-body change of position involves standing the patient and resitting them in the chair. Observation of the patient when sitting is also important, because patients who slide out of the chair are at high risk for shear injury. Use of footstools and the foot pedals on wheelchairs and appropriate 90-degree flexion of the hip (may be achieved with pillows, special seat cushions, or orthotic devices) can help in preventing chair sliding. Attention to proper alignment and posture is essential. Individuals at risk for pressure ulcer development should avoid uninterrupted sitting in chairs and should be repositioned every hour. The rationale behind the shorter time is the extremely high pressure generated on the ischial tuberosities in the seated position. When possible, individuals should be taught to shift weight every 15 minutes while seated.

Pressure reducing/relieving support surfaces should be initiated for beds and chairs of persons determined at risk for developing pressure ulcers. Use of pressure reducing support surfaces instead of standard hospital mattresses results in relative reduction in pressure ulcer incidence of 60%. Additionally, clinicians should advocate for use of support surfaces in the operating room to reduce postoperative pressure ulcer incidence. Use of pressure reduction support surfaces such as mattress overlays (e.g., foam, gel, or alternating air pads) or low-air-loss therapy is appropriate for many patients at risk for pressure ulcers or with stage I or II pressure ulcers. However, for persons with existing pressure ulcers, use of air-fluidized therapy may improve healing rates. One retrospective, multisite, comparison study showed faster healing of existing pressure ulcers with air-fluidized therapy compared to both pressure reduction support surfaces and low-air-loss therapy (mean healing rate of 5.2 cm^2/wk for the air-fluidized surface group compared to 1.5 cm^2/wk for pressure reduction support surface group and 1.8 cm^2/wk for low-air-loss therapy group). In addition, the odds of showing improvement in pressure ulcers are more than five times greater when air-fluidized therapy and 4 hour repositioning is implemented compared to alternating air mattresses and 2 hour repositioning in hospitals. Although air-fluidized therapy increased the odds of ulcer improvement, only 12% of hospitalized patients achieved healing of the largest pressure ulcer. In nursing home residents, a randomized, controlled trial suggests that pressure ulcer areas decrease three times faster when low-air-loss beds are used compared with conventional care. Additional controlled trials are needed to define the optimal repositioning schedules for patients on a variety of support surfaces.

Providing topical preparations to eliminate or reduce the surface tension between the skin and the bed linen or support surface will assist in reducing friction-related injury. Use of appropriate techniques when moving patients so that skin is not dragged across linens will lessen friction-induced skin breakdown. Patients who exhibit voluntary or involuntary repetitive body movements (particularly of the heels or elbows) require stronger interventions. Use of a protective film, such as a transparent film dressing or a skin sealant; a protective dressing, such as a thin hydrocolloid; or protective padding will help to eliminate the surface contact of the area and decrease the friction between the skin and the linens. Even though heel, ankle, and elbow protectors do nothing to reduce or relieve pressure, they can be effective aids against friction.

General skin care should include routine skin inspection, incontinence assessment and management, and skin hygiene interventions to maintain skin health. Routine skin inspection should occur daily with particular attention to bony prominences. Reddened areas should not be massaged. Massage can further impair the perfusion to the tissues. The skin should be evaluated for dryness and cracking, use of moisturizers can be helpful. Attention should also be focused on gentle handling to prevent skin tears. Incontinence assessment and management with scheduled toileting or prompted voiding programs and for those unresponsive to these programs, check and change schedules are important. Prompt cleansing after incontinent episodes with warm water and gentle cleansers and use of protective ointments and creams help maintain perineal skin health. Table 58-3 presents general prevention interventions directed at risk factors for pressure ulcer development.

SPECIAL ISSUES

Some patients will benefit most from a palliative care approach. Palliative pressure ulcer care means that the goals are comfort and limiting the extent or impact of the pressure ulcer but without the intent of healing. Palliative care may be indicated for terminally ill patients such as those with end-stage cancer or in the terminal stages of other diseases. Institutionalized older adults with multiple comorbidities or older adults with severe functional decline may also benefit from palliative care. Palliative pressure ulcer care includes adequate debridement of necrotic tissue, identification and treatment of infection, provision of moist wound healing with management of exudate and odor, and prevention interventions. Prevention should

TABLE 58-3

Pressure Ulcer Prevention Interventions	
RISK FACTOR	**PREVENTION INTERVENTONS**
Immobility	Scheduled repositioning programs, use of pressure reduction/relief surfaces in bed and chairs.
Inactivity, limited mobility	Use of trapeze bars for self-movement in bed, encourage ambulation, rehabilitation as appropriate.
Decreased sensory perception	Scheduled repositioning programs, verbal reminders to move/reposition, use of pressure reduction/relief surfaces in bed and chairs.
Malnutrition	Nutritional assessment to determine deficits, nutritional supplementation (high protein) and daily multivitamin if indicated and appropriate to goals.
Excess moisture and incontinence	Scheduled toileting or prompted voiding programs if responsive, routine check and change programs with pads and adult briefs for persons who do not respond to scheduled toileting or prompted voiding, use of skin creams and ointments for protection from moisture.
Friction and shearing	Use of trapeze bars for those with upper body strength, turn sheets & draw sheets for moving in bed, use of cornstarch or lubricants to limit friction between surfaces, thin film or dressings, and pads over bony prominences subject to friction, use of footboards to help prevent sliding while in bed.
Dry skin	Use warm water, gentle cleansers, and limited force for cleansing when soiled and for routine bathing, lubricate and moisturize dry skin, inspect skin daily paying particular attention to bony prominences, avoid massage of reddened areas.

still consist of use of pressure reducing support surfaces and attention to scheduled repositioning, although time frames may be adjusted or lengthened to ease the burden on the patient. Providing pain medication 30 to 40 minutes prior to repositioning activity and use of positioning devices may help those with pain on movement.

SUMMARY

Pressure ulcers are chronic wounds and as such, require patience and diligence by clinicians. Many pressure ulcers never heal, and most require long periods of treatment with slow progress. Partial-thickness stage II pressure ulcers are more likely to heal than full-thickness stage III or IV pressure ulcers. In fact, stage II pressure ulcers are 5.2 times more likely to heal in 6 months than stage IV pressure ulcers. Among nursing home residents, up to 75% of stage II wounds heal within 60 days, while only 17% or fewer full-thickness pressure ul-

cers heal in the same time period. The best healing rate reported even after 6 months of treatment is 59%. Thus, identification of persons at risk for developing pressure ulcers and aggressive prevention interventions to actively avoid ulcer development is essential. Prevention includes screening for risk with risk assessment tools and implementing targeted prevention interventions based on identified risk factors. Scheduled repositioning programs, use of pressure reduction support surfaces, and assessment and management of nutrition are key prevention strategies. More research is needed to define optimal turning intervals for various support surfaces and to better elucidate the effect of nutrition interventions on both preventing pressure ulcers and healing pressure ulcers.

For those persons who do develop pressure ulcers, clinicians should provide appropriate treatment during early ulcer stages to capitalize on healing progress in the initial 3 months. Adequate debridement of necrotic tissue, identification and treatment of infection, and providing a moist wound environment are the key tenets of appropriate pressure ulcer care. All preventive and therapeutic interventions, and progress of the ulcer, should be carefully documented in the medical record. Unfortunately, no intervention or combination of interventions has demonstrated the ability to completely eliminate pressure ulcers. Thus, even as we develop more refined and specific screening, detection, and prevention interventions, it is likely we will continue to see pressure ulcers in all health-care settings. The guidelines presented in this chapter should provide a foundation for developing a successful approach to both those at risk for pressure ulcer development and those with existing pressure ulcers.

FURTHER READING

Allman RM, Goode PS, Patrick MM, et al. Pressure ulcer risk factors among hospitalized patients with activity limitation. *JAMA*. 1995;273:865–870.

Bates-Jensen B. The Pressure Sore Status Tool a few thousand assessments later. *Adv Skin Wound Care*. 1997;10(5):65–73.

Bates-Jensen BM, MacLean CH. Quality indicators for the care of pressure ulcers in vulnerable elders. *Journal of the American Geriatrics Society*. 2007:55 Suppl 2:S409–416.

Cuddigan J, Ayello EA, Sussman C, eds. *Pressure Ulcers in America: Prevalence, Incidence, and Implications for the Future*. Reston, VA: National Pressure Ulcer Advisory Panel; 2001.

National Pressure Ulcer Advisory Panel. Cuddigan J, Ayello EA, Sussman C (Eds.). *Pressure Ulcers in America: Prevalence, Incidence, and Implications for the Future*. Reston, VA: NPUAP. 2001

National Pressure Ulcer Advisory Panel. *Pressure Ulcer Definition and Stages*. NPUAP; 2007. http://www.npuap.org/documents/PU_Definition_Stages.pdf. Last accessed March 3, 2007.

Niazi ZB, Salzberg CA. Operative repair of pressure ulcers. *Clin Geriatr Med*. 1997;13:587–97.

Redelings MD, Lee NE, Sorvillo F. Pressure ulcers: more lethal than we thought? *Adv Skin Wound Care*. 2005;18:367–372.

Stotts NA, Rodeheaver GT, Thomas DR, et al. An instrument to measure healing in pressure ulcers: development and validation of the Pressure Ulcer Scale for Healing (PUSH). *J Gerontol Med Sci*. 2001;56A:M795–9.

Thomas DR, Goode PS, Huber Tarquine P, Allman RM. Hospital-acquired pressure ulcers and risk of death. *J Am Geriatr Soc*. 1996;44:1435–40.

Thomas DR. Issues and dilemmas in the prevention and treatment of pressure ulcers: a review. *J Gerontol Med Sci*. 2001;56A:M328–M340.

Incontinence

Theodore M. Johnson II ■ *Joseph G. Ouslander*

DEFINITION AND EPIDEMIOLOGY

Defined as the complaint of any involuntary leakage of urine, urinary incontinence is a common and bothersome condition in elderly persons. The prevalence of incontinence increases with age and with increasing frailty, and is 1.3 to 2.0 times greater in older women than in older men. Among community-dwelling older women, the prevalence of any urinary incontinence is approximately 35%; among older men, it is approximately 22%. The prevalence of daily urinary incontinence in older community-dwelling persons is approximately 12% for women and 5% for men. The prevalence approaches 60% among nursing home residents. Incontinence ranges in severity from occasional episodes of dribbling small amounts of urine to continuous urine leakage with concomitant fecal incontinence. In addition, many older people who do not "leak urine" still may have bothersome lower urinary tract symptoms such as urgency, frequency, and nocturia that require changes in lifestyle and/or the use of pads.

Physical health, psychological well-being, social status, and the costs of health care can all be adversely affected by incontinence. Urinary incontinence can be cured or greatly improved, especially in those who have adequate mobility and mental functioning. Even when not curable, incontinence can always be managed to allow for more patient comfort, make life easier for caregivers, and minimize costs of caring for the condition. Because many elderly patients are embarrassed to discuss their incontinence and may not be aware that treatment is available, it is essential for specific questions about incontinence to be included in periodic assessments and for incontinence to be noted as a problem (Table 59-1). This chapter briefly reviews the pathophysiology of incontinence in older persons and provides detailed information on the evaluation and management of this condition.

PATHOPHYSIOLOGY AND CLASSIFICATION

Continence requires effective functioning of the lower urinary tract, adequate cognitive and physical functioning, motivation, and an appropriate environment (Table 59-2). Anatomic and physiologic aspects of the lower urinary tract, as well as functional, psychological, and environmental factors, contribute to the pathophysiology of incontinence in older persons. Normal urination is a complex process; the neurophysiology of urination remains incompletely understood. Proper bladder filling and emptying are influenced by higher centers in the brainstem, cerebral cortex, and cerebellum. The brainstem facilitates urination and the cerebral cortex exerts a predominantly inhibitory influence. Additionally, the loss of the central cortical inhibitory influences over the sacral micturition center from diseases such as stroke can produce incontinence in older patients. Even in the absence of specific, overt neurological lesions, poor bladder control has been shown to be associated with inadequate activation of the orbitofrontal cortex. Disorders of the brainstem and suprasacral spinal cord can interfere with the coordination of bladder contraction and urethral relaxation. Interruptions of the sacral innervation can cause impaired bladder contraction and problems with continence.

At the most basic level, urination is governed by a reflex centered in the sacral micturition center. During normal bladder filling, afferent pathways (via somatic and autonomic nerves) carry information on bladder volume to the spinal cord. Motor output is adjusted accordingly (Figure 59-1). Sympathetic tone closes the bladder neck and inhibits parasympathetic tone (thus relaxing the dome of the bladder); somatic innervation maintains tone in the pelvic floor musculature (including striated muscle around the urethra). Voluntary pelvic floor muscle contracture also leads to inhibition of parasympathetic tone. For bladder emptying, sympathetic and somatic tones diminish, and parasympathetic, cholinergically-mediated impulses

TABLE 59-1

Asking About Urinary Incontinence

Questions about incontinence should be open-ended and phrased in language easily understood by the patient:

"Tell me about any problems you are having with your bladder?"

"Tell me about any trouble you are having holding your urine (water)?"

If the responses to the above questions are negative, following up with questions may be helpful:

"How often do you lose urine when you don't want to?"

"How often do you wear a pad or other protective device to prevent urinary accidents?"

Adapted from Fantyl JA, Newman DK, Colling J, et al. Urinary Incontinence in Adults: Acute and Chronic Management. Clinical Practice Guideline No. 2, 1996 Update. Rockville, MD: U.S. Dept of Health and Human Services, Public Health Service, Agency for Health Care Policy and Research; 1996. AHCPR publication 96–0682.

cause the bladder to contract. Normal urination is a dynamic process, requiring the coordination of several physiologic processes. Under normal circumstances, as the bladder fills, bladder pressure remains low (≤ 15 cm H_2O). The bladder volume at first urge to void is variable, but generally occurs at between 150 and 350 mL; normal bladder capacity is 300 to 600 mL. When normal urination is initiated, the detrusor contracts and detrusor pressure increases until it exceeds urethral resistance (which lowers immediately prior to bladder contraction). Urine flow occurs. If at any time during bladder filling, total bladder pressure exceeds outlet resistance, urinary leakage occurs. Transmitted intra-abdominal pressure alone by coughing or sneezing may cause leakage in someone with low outlet resistance pressure or urethral sphincter weakness. Alternatively, the bladder can contract involuntarily and cause urinary leakage.

Basic Causes

Urologic, neurologic, psychological, and functional factors may contribute to incontinence. As is the case for a number of other common geriatric problems, multiple disorders often interact to cause urinary incontinence. Determining the cause or causes facilitates proper management. Overall, aging is associated with increasing incontinence. The prevalence of stress incontinence likely does not

TABLE 59-2

Requirements for Continence

Effective lower urinary tract function

Storage
   Accommodation by bladder of increasing volumes of urine under low pressure
   Closed bladder outlet
   Appropriate sensation of bladder fullness
   Absence of involuntary bladder contractions

Emptying
   Bladder capable of contraction
   Lack of anatomic obstruction to urine flow
   Coordinated lowering of outlet resistance with bladder contractions

Adequate mobility and dexterity to use toilet

Adequate cognitive function to recognize toileting needs

Motivation to be continent

Absence of environmental and iatrogenic barriers

Adapted from Kane RL, Ouslander JG, Itamar B, et al. Essentials of Clinical Geriatrics. 5th ed. New York, New York: McGraw-Hill; 2003.

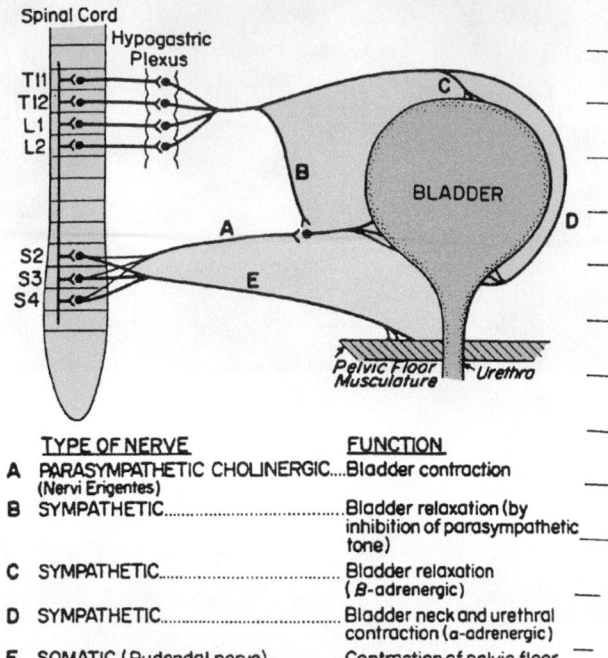

	TYPE OF NERVE	FUNCTION
A	PARASYMPATHETIC CHOLINERGIC (Nervi Erigentes)	Bladder contraction
B	SYMPATHETIC	Bladder relaxation (by inhibition of parasympathetic tone)
C	SYMPATHETIC	Bladder relaxation (β-adrenergic)
D	SYMPATHETIC	Bladder neck and urethral contraction (a-adrenergic)
E	SOMATIC (Pudendal nerve)	Contraction of pelvic floor musculature

FIGURE 59-1. Peripheral nerves involved in micturition. *(Reprinted with permission from Kane RL, Ouslander JG, Itamar B, et al. Essentials of Clinical Geriatrics. 5th ed. New York, New York: McGraw-Hill; 2004.)*

increase in women, while the prevalence of urge incontinence and mixed stress–urge incontinence does increase.

Several age-related changes can contribute to the development of urinary incontinence. In general, residual urine volume following voiding is greater with increasing age. While a decline in functional bladder capacity has been associated with advanced age, this may be because of the higher prevalence of involuntary bladder contractions and detrusor overactivity in older persons. Involuntary bladder contractions are found in 40% to 75% of elderly incontinent patients, but also in 5% to 10% of elderly continent women and in up to one-third of elderly men with no or minimal urinary symptoms. Detrusor overactivity has been associated with specific anatomical findings (protrusion junctions and ultra-close abutment of detrusor muscle cells) on bladder biopsy. While involuntary bladder contractions do not always result in urinary incontinence, when combined with impaired mobility, these contractions likely account for a substantial proportion of incontinence in elderly functionally disabled patients. Aging is also associated with a decline in bladder outlet and urethral resistance pressure in women. While there is a recognition that laxity of pelvic structures associated with prior childbirths (either via vaginal deliveries or Caesarean section) may result in a greater risk of future incontinence, the association between parity and incontinence is weak in women older than 65 years. Additionally, in older populations, poor vaginal support is more closely associated with obstructive urinary symptoms than with urinary leakage and urgency. Obesity, deconditioned muscles, and hysterectomy predispose women to future development of incontinence. Racial or ethnic characteristics are likely important; white women are more likely, as a group, to have stress urinary incontinence than are African-American women.

Older men with prostatic enlargement may have decreased urine flow rates and detrusor motor instability. Aging is also associated with higher rates of nocturia, which may in part be related to higher urine production at night (see Chapter 88). Many older individuals of both genders have impaired bladder contractility, often in combination with detrusor hyperactivity (a condition termed *detrusor hyperactivity with impaired contractility,* or DHIC). These individuals have evidence of widespread muscle degeneration on detrusor muscle biopsy.

Acute and Reversible Causes

The distinction between acute (or reversible) forms of incontinence and persistent (or established) incontinence is clinically important although not always distinct. *Acute incontinence* refers to those situations in which the incontinence is of sudden onset, usually related to an acute illness or an iatrogenic problem, and subsides once the illness or medication problem has been resolved. *Persistent incontinence* refers to incontinence that is unrelated to an acute illness and persists over time. Several of the reversible factors discussed below also can contribute to persistent forms of incontinence.

The potentially reversible causes of urinary incontinence are outlined in Table 59-3. These causes include impaired ability (or willingness) to reach a toilet, conditions that affect the lower urinary tract, conditions that cause or contribute to polyuria, and iatrogenic factors. Because of urinary frequency and urgency, many older persons, especially those limited in mobility, carefully arrange their schedules (and may even limit social activities) in order to be close to a toilet. Thus, an acute illness can precipitate incontinence by disrupting this

delicate balance. Hospitalization, with its attendant environmental barriers (such as bed rails), and the delirium and immobility that often accompany acute illnesses in older patients can contribute to acute incontinence. Acute incontinence in these situations is likely to resolve with resolution of the underlying acute illness. In a substantial proportion of patients, incontinence may persist for several weeks after hospitalization and should be further evaluated.

Fecal impaction is a common problem in both acutely and chronically ill elderly patients. Impaction may cause mechanical obstruction of the bladder outlet that can prevent adequate bladder emptying and cause reflex bladder contractions induced by rectal distension. Relief of a fecal impaction can lead to resolution of urinary, as well as fecal, incontinence. Urinary incontinence with a high postvoid residual should be considered in any patient who suddenly develops urinary incontinence. Immobility; anticholinergic, narcotic, calcium channel blocking, and beta adrenergic medications (Table 59-4); and fecal impaction can all precipitate incontinence with a high postvoid residual in an older patient. In addition, urinary retention may be an acute manifestation of an underlying process causing spinal cord compression or occur after a stroke.

Inflammation of the lower urinary tract may precipitate or exacerbate incontinence. Atrophic vaginitis and urethritis are common among older women, and can cause dysuria, urgency, and frequency that can contribute to incontinence. Physical signs include patchy erythema and increased vascularity of the labia minora and

---

TABLE 59-3

Reversible Conditions That Cause or Contribute to Urinary Incontinence in Older Persons

CONDITION	MANAGEMENT
Conditions affecting the lower urinary tract	
Urinary tract infection (symptomatic with frequency, urgency, dysuria, etc.)	Antimicrobial therapy (not for asymptomatic bacteriuria)
Atrophic vaginitis/urethritis	Topical estrogen
Postprostatectomy (incontinence will often resolve during first yr)	Behavioral interventions Avoid further surgical therapy until it is clear condition will not resolve
Stool impaction	Disimpaction; appropriate use of stool softeners, bulk-forming agents, and laxatives if necessary; implement high fiber intake, adequate mobility and fluid intake
Drug side effects (see Table 59–4)	Discontinue or change therapy if clinically appropriate. Dosage reduction or modification (e.g., flexible scheduling of rapid-acting diuretics) may also help
Increased urine production	
Metabolic (hyperglycemia, hypercalcemia)	Better control of diabetes mellitus; therapy for hypercalcemia depends on underlying cause
Excess fluid intake	Reduction in intake of diuretic fluids (e.g., caffeinated beverages)
Volume overload	
Venous insufficiency with edema	Support stocking Leg elevation Sodium restriction Diuretic therapy
Congestive heart failure	Medical therapy
Impaired ability or willingness to reach a toilet	
Delirium	Diagnosis and treatment of underlying cause(s) delirium (see Chapter 53)
Chronic illness, injury, or restraint that interferes with mobility	
	Regular toileting Use of toilet substitutes Environmental alterations (e.g., bedside commode, urinal)
Psychological	Remove restraints if possible Appropriate pharmacologic and/or nonpharmacologic treatment

Fantyl JA, Newman DK, Colling J, et al. Urinary Incontinence in Adults: Acute and Chronic Management. Clinical Practice Guideline No. 2, 1996 Update. Rockville, MD: U.S. Dept of Health and Human Services, Public Health Service, Agency for Health Care Policy and Research; 1996. AHCPR publication 96–0682.

TABLE 59-4

Medications That Can Potentially Affect Continence	
TYPE OF MEDICATION	**POTENTIAL EFFECTS ON CONTINENCE**
Diuretics	Polyuria, frequency, urgency
Anticholinergics	Urinary retention, overflow incontinence, stool impaction
Psychotropics	
Antidepressants	Anticholinergic actions, sedation
Antipsychotics	Anticholinergic actions, sedation, immobility
Sedative–hypnotics	Sedation, delirium, immobility, urethral muscle relaxation
Narcotic analgesics	Urinary retention, fecal impaction, sedation, delirium
Alpha adrenergic blockers	Urethral relaxation
Alpha adrenergic agonists	Urinary retention
Angiotensin-converting enzyme inhibitors	Cough precipitating stress incontinence
Beta adrenergic agonists	Rarely may contribute to urinary retention
Calcium channel-blockers	May contribute to urinary retention
Alcohol	Polyuria, frequency, urgency, sedation, delirium, immobility
Caffeine	Polyuria, bladder irritation

Adapted from Kane RL, Ouslander JG, Itamar B, et al. Essentials of Clinical Geriatrics. 5th ed. New York, New York: McGraw-Hill; 2003.

vaginal epithelium, petechiae and friability, and urethral erythema often with an inflamed caruncle (dark or bright red epithelium usually at the inferior aspect of the urethra). Topical estrogen therapy, as discussed under "Drug Treatment" later in this chapter, may be helpful in older women with these findings. Acute urinary tract infection also can precipitate or exacerbate incontinence. However, urine loss

among older patients with *chronic* incontinence, especially frail nursing home residents, with otherwise asymptomatic bacteriuria (with or without pyuria) does not appear to improve when the bacteriuria is eradicated. These patients, therefore, should not be treated with antibiotics because of the costs and risks unless the incontinence is new or acutely worsened.

Diuretics (especially rapid-acting loop diuretics) and conditions that cause polyuria, including hyperglycemia and hypercalcemia, can precipitate acute incontinence. Patients with volume-expanded states, such as those with congestive heart failure and lower extremity venous insufficiency, may have polyuria at night, which can contribute to nocturia and nocturnal incontinence. As is the case in many other conditions in geriatric patients, a wide variety of medications can play a role in the development of incontinence in elderly patients (see Table 59-4). Whether the incontinence is acute or persistent, the potential role of these medications in causing or contributing to a patient's incontinence should be considered. When feasible, stopping the medication, switching to an alternative, or modifying the dosage schedule can be beneficial and may be the only necessary treatment for incontinence. In addition to medications, drinking caffeinated beverages can cause urinary frequency and urgency, which may precipitate incontinence.

Persistent Incontinence

Table 59-5 lists the clinical definitions and common causes of persistent urinary incontinence. These types can overlap with each other, and an individual patient may have more than one type simultaneously. Three of these types of incontinence—stress, urge, and overflow—result from one or a combination of two basic abnormalities in lower genitourinary tract function:

1. failure to store urine, caused by a hyperactive or poorly compliant bladder or by diminished outflow resistance; and/or

TABLE 59-5

Basic Types and Causes of Persistent Urinary Incontinence		
TYPE	**DEFINITION**	**COMMON CAUSES**
Stress	Involuntary loss of urine (usually small amounts) with increases in intra-abdominal pressure (e.g., cough, laugh, exercise)	Weakness of pelvic floor musculature and urethral hypermobility Bladder outlet or urethral sphincter weakness Postprostatectomy sphincter weakness
Urge	Leakage of urine (variable but often larger volumes) because of inability to delay voiding after sensation of bladder fullness is perceived	Detrusor hyperactivity, isolated or associated with one or more of the following: Local genitourinary condition such as tumors, stones, diverticuli, or outflow obstruction CNS disorders such as stroke, dementia, parkinsonism, spinal cord injury
Mixed (stress & urge)	Combination of above	
Functional	Urinary accidents associated with inability to toilet because of impairment of cognitive and/or physical functioning, psychological unwillingness, or environmental barriers	Severe dementia and other neurological disorders Psychological factors such as depression and hostility
High postvoid residual (Formerly referred to as "Overflow")	Leakage of urine (usually small amounts) resulting from either mechanical forces on an overdistended bladder resulting in stress leakage or from other effects of urinary retention on bladder and sphincter function contributing to urge leakage	Anatomic obstruction by prostate, stricture, cystocele Acontractile bladder associated with diabetes mellitus or spinal cord injury Neurogenic (detrusor–sphincter dyssynergy), associated with multiple sclerosis and other suprasacral spinal cord lesions Medication effect (see Table 59-4)

Adapted from Kane RL, Ouslander JG, Itamar B, et al. Essentials of Clinical Geriatrics. 5th ed. New York, New York: McGraw-Hill; 2003.

2. failure to properly empty the bladder, caused by a poorly contractile bladder or by increased outflow resistance.

Stress incontinence is common in elderly women, especially in ambulatory clinic settings. The symptoms of stress incontinence are very specific: leakage coincident with increases in intra-abdominal pressure caused by coughing, sneezing, laughing, or exercising. Stress incontinence may be infrequent and involve very small amounts of urine. It may need no specific treatment in women who are not bothered by it; on the other hand, it may be so severe and/or bothersome that it renders the person housebound. Among women, it is most often associated with weakened supporting tissues, resulting in hypermobility of the bladder outlet and urethra and caused by lack of estrogen, obesity, previous vaginal deliveries, and/or surgery. Some women, generally those who have had previous lower urinary tract surgery, have intrinsic urethral weakness with failure of the urethra to coapt and prevent urine loss. These patients tend to have severe incontinence and occasionally have constant wetting. Stress incontinence is unusual in men, and it mainly occurs following transurethral surgery for benign conditions or after surgical or radiation therapy for lower urinary tract malignancy when the anatomic sphincters are damaged.

Urge incontinence can be caused by a variety of lower genitourinary and neurologic disorders (see Table 59-5). This type of incontinence is characterized by a sudden strong desire to void, accompanied by a fear of leakage, and followed by urine loss. The amount of urine lost is variable and largely dependent on sphincter function and the ability of the patient to abort a bladder contraction. Urge incontinence, when it occurs along with urinary urgency, daytime urinary frequency, and nocturia, has been called "*wet* overactive bladder". Urge incontinence is most often, but not always, associated with involuntary bladder contractions. Some patients have a poorly compliant bladder without involuntary contractions (e.g., interstitial cystitis or following irradiation). A subgroup of elderly incontinent patients with detrusor hyperactivity also has impaired bladder contractility, emptying less than one-third of their bladder volume with involuntary contractions on urodynamic testing. These patients may be predisposed to significant urinary retention and may require training to learn to completely empty their bladder with voiding.

There has been a recommendation *against* the usage of the term "overflow incontinence" in favor of terms such as *acute* or *chronic urinary retention* and (either stress or urge) *incontinence with a high post-void residual*. *Acute retention of urine* is "a painful, palpable or percussable bladder, when the patient is unable to pass any urine"; and *chronic retention of urine* is where the patient has a "nonpainful bladder, which remains palpable or percussable after the patient has passed urine... (and) the patient may be incontinent." A high postvoid residual can result from anatomic or neurogenic obstruction to urinary outflow, a hypotonic or acontractile bladder, or both. The most common causes include prostatic enlargement, diabetic neuropathic bladder, and urethral stricture. Low spinal cord injury and anatomic obstruction in women (caused by pelvic prolapse and urethral distortion) are less common causes of overflow incontinence in older patients. Several types of drugs also can contribute to this type of persistent incontinence (see Table 59-4). Some patients with suprasacral spinal cord lesions (e.g., multiple sclerosis) develop detrusor–sphincter dyssynergy and consequent urinary retention, which must be treated similarly to overflow incontinence; in some instances, a sphincterotomy is necessary.

Functional incontinence results when an elderly person is unable or unwilling to reach a toilet on time. Recognizing and removing these barriers to continence are critical. Factors such as inaccessible toilets and psychological disorders also can exacerbate other types of persistent incontinence. Patients with incontinence that appears to be predominantly related to functional factors also may have abnormalities of the lower genitourinary tract, most commonly detrusor overactivity. In some patients, it can be very difficult to determine whether the functional factors or the genitourinary factors predominate without a trial of specific types of treatment.

Many older patients have more than one type of incontinence. Most common are combinations of urge and stress incontinence (often called *mixed incontinence*) among older women and a combination of urge and functional incontinence among nursing home residents. In addition, many older patients have a syndrome of "overactive bladder," which results in bothersome urinary urgency, frequency, and nocturia, but may be continent. These patients should be assessed and treated similar to patients with symptoms of urge incontinence.

EVALUATION

Federal clinical practice guidelines, including an older guideline developed by the Agency for Health Care Policy and Research (now the Agency for Healthcare Research on Quality), and the Resident Assessment Instrument for nursing homes (which includes a section on continence in the Minimum Data Set and a Resident Assessment Protocol on continence and catheter management) recommend a basic diagnostic evaluation. This evaluation includes a history (which can be enhanced by a bladder record), a physical examination, a urinalysis, and a postvoid residual determination (PVR). The recommendation to obtain a PVR in all older patients with incontinence is controversial, and a reasonable approach may to do this procedure only in patients at risk for urinary retention (see below). A number of other diagnostic studies are indicated in selected patients (Table 59-6). Figure 59-2 summarizes the recommended diagnostic evaluation of incontinent older patients.

The objectives of the basic evaluation are threefold:

1. To identify potentially reversible conditions that might be contributing to the incontinence (see Table 59-3).

2. To identify conditions that require further diagnostic tests and/or referral for gynecologic or urologic evaluation.

3. To develop a management plan; this may include referral for further evaluation or a therapeutic trial of behavioral and/or pharmacologic therapy.

In patients with the sudden onset of incontinence (especially when associated with an acute medical condition and hospitalization), the potentially reversible causes of acute incontinence (see Table 59-3) can be ruled out by a brief history, a physical examination, and basic laboratory studies including urinalysis, culture, and tests for serum glucose or calcium, if indicated.

The history should focus on the characteristics of the incontinence, on current medical problems and medications, and on the impact of the incontinence on the patient and caregivers. The incontinence should be characterized in terms of frequency, timing, and amount of leakage; and symptoms of voiding difficulty including hesitancy, intermittent stream, and straining to void. Symptoms of

TABLE 59-6

Components of the Diagnostic Evaluation of Persistent Urinary Incontinence*

All Patients
- Focused history (a bladder record may be helpful in some patients)
- Targeted physical examination
- Urinalysis
- Postvoid residual determination†

Selected Patients
- Laboratory studies
  - Urine culture
  - Urine cytology
  - Blood glucose, calcium
  - Renal function tests
- Renal ultrasound
- Gynecologic evaluation
- Urologic evaluation
- Cystourethroscopy
- Urodynamic tests
  - Simple
    - Observation of voiding
    - Cough test for stress incontinence
    - Simple (single channel) cystometry
    - Urine flowmetry (for men)
  - Complex
    - Multichannel cystometrogram
    - Pressure-flow study
    - Leak point pressure
    - Urethral pressure profilometry
    - Sphincter electromyography
    - Videourodynamics

*See also Table 59–7.

†The recommendation for a postvoid residual determination in all incontinent elderly patients is controversial (see text).

Adapted from Kane RL, Ouslander JG, Itamar B, et al. *Essentials of Clinical Geriatrics.* 5th ed. New York, New York: McGraw-Hill; 2003.

urge versus stress incontinence should be sought, recognizing that symptom history does not perfectly predict subtype of urinary incontinence. Bladder records, such as the one shown in Figure 59-3, can be helpful in characterizing symptoms, as well as in following the response to treatment. The physical examination includes abdominal, rectal, and genital examinations, as well as an evaluation of lumbosacral innervation. The abdominal examination is insensitive for an elevated postvoid residual or chronic urinary retention, but gross bladder distention (e.g., ≥500 mL) can usually be detected. In acute urinary retention, the distended bladder is a firm, midline mass that emanates from the pelvis and is dull to percussion. In gross distention with either acute or chronic retention, the superior margin of the bladder is often identifiable by either palpation or percussion.

The pelvic examination in women includes inspection for significant prolapse, signs of inflammation suggestive of atrophic vaginitis, and a cough test to detect stress incontinence. The latter is best done in the standing position while the patient has a comfortably full bladder, but not a strong sense of urgency. The patient should be positioned over a pad or towel next to a commode and then should be asked to cough forcefully. Leakage simultaneously with coughing documents stress incontinence; delayed leakage (e.g., after 3 seconds) or the initiation of voiding generally indicates a cough-induced bladder contraction. The cough test for stress incontinence has excellent specificity and interrater reliability, but poor sensitivity.

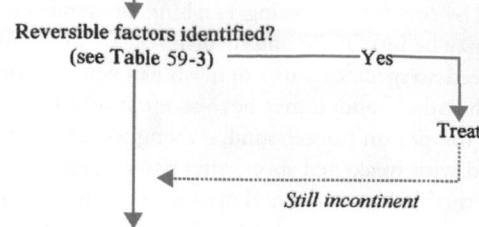

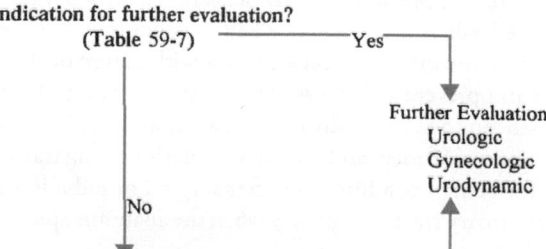

FIGURE 59-2. Summary of assessment of geriatric urinary incontinence.

Special attention during the examination should be given to mobility and mental status, because impairments may be either causing the incontinence or interacting with urologic and neurologic disorders to worsen the condition. Patients with nocturia or nocturnal incontinence should be examined for signs of congestive heart failure or venous insufficiency with edema.

Urinalysis should be performed to look for signs of infection, hematuria, and glucosuria. Clean urine specimens are often difficult to obtain from frail incontinent patients, but can be performed reliably without first resorting to in-and-out catheterization. For men who cannot void spontaneously, a condom-type catheter can be used after cleaning the penis to collect a specimen that accurately reflects bladder urine. While there is a clear relationship between acute symptomatic urinary tract infection and incontinence, the relationship between asymptomatic bacteriuria and incontinence is controversial. In nursing home populations, there is no benefit to treating bacteriuria in patients with chronic, stable incontinence. For patients in other settings, it is difficult to make clear recommendations. For the initial evaluation of incontinence among noninstitutionalized incontinent patients, it is reasonable to initially eradicate the bacteriuria and observe the effect on the incontinence.

BLADDER RECORD

Day: _____ Date: _____ / _____
month   day

INSTRUCTIONS:

1) In the 1st column make a mark every time during the 2-hour period you urinate into the toilet

2) Use the 2nd column to record the amount you urinate (if you are measuring amounts)

3) In the 3rd or 4th column, make a mark every time you accidentally leak urine

Time Interval	Urinated in Toilet	Amount	Leaking Accident	or	Large Accident	Reason for Accident*
6–8 am						
8–10 am						
2–4 pm						
4–6 pm						
6–8 pm						
8–10 pm						
10–12 pm						
Overnight						

Number of pads used today: _____

*For example, if you coughed and have a leaking accident, write "cough". If you had a large accident after a strong urge to urinate, write "urge".

FIGURE 59-3. Example of a bladder record for ambulatory care settings. (Reprinted with permission from Kane RL, Ouslander JG, Itamar B, et al. Essentials of Clinical Geriatrics. 5th ed. New York, New York: McGraw-Hill; 2004.)

A determination of postvoid residual should be performed to exclude significant urinary retention. Neither the history nor the physical examination is sensitive or specific enough for this purpose in geriatric patients. Although performing a PVR on all patients may not be necessary, patients at risk for retention should have this procedure. This includes diabetic patients, patients with neurological disorders, patients with symptoms of voiding difficulty or a history of urinary retention, and patients on anticholinergic medications. The PVR determination can be done by portable ultrasonography if equipment is available. To be accurate, the PVR determination should be done within a few minutes of a spontaneous continent or incontinent void. PVR values of less than 100 mL in the absence of straining to void generally reflect adequate bladder emptying in geriatric patients, whereas PVR values greater than 200 mL are abnormal; values in between must be interpreted in the context of other patient symptoms.

Clinical practice guidelines do not recommend that all incontinent elderly patients undergo a complex urologic, gynecologic, or urodynamic evaluation. Many patients can be treated with a trial of behavioral and/or drug therapy after the initial evaluation is completed and potentially reversible factors are addressed. Table 59-7 lists examples of criteria for referring incontinent geriatric patients for further urologic, gynecologic, and/or urodynamic evaluations. Among men, a noninvasive measurement of urinary flow rate can be very helpful in excluding obstruction and/or bladder contractility problems. Many urologists and continence clinics that see elderly men have such devices.

MANAGEMENT

Several therapeutic modalities are used in managing incontinent patients (Table 59-8). Special attention should be paid to the management of acute incontinence, which is common in elderly patients in acute care hospitals. A common approach to elderly incontinent patients in acute hospitals is indwelling catheterization. In some instances, this practice is justified by the need for accurate measurement of urine output during the acute phase of an illness. In many instances, however, it is unnecessary and poses a substantial and unwarranted risk of catheter-induced infection and may prolong immobilization. Although other procedures may be more difficult and time-consuming, making toilets and toilet substitutes accessible and combining this accessibility with some form of scheduled toileting is a more appropriate approach. Using launderable or disposable and highly absorbent bed pads and undergarments may be more costly than catheters, but results in less morbidity than catheter use. All the factors that can cause or contribute to a reversible form of incontinence (see Table 59-3) should be attended to in order to maximize the potential for regaining continence.

TABLE 59-7

Examples of Criteria for Referral of Incontinent Geriatric Patients for Further Urologic, Gynecologic, or Urodynamic Evaluation

CRITERIA	DEFINITION	RATIONALE
History		
Recent history of lower urinary tract or pelvic surgery or irradiation	Surgery or irradiation involving the pelvic area or lower urinary tract within the past 6 months	A structural abnormality relating to the recent procedure should be sought
Recurrent symptomatic urinary tract infections	Three or more symptomatic episodes in a 12-month period	A structural abnormality or pathologic condition in the urinary tract predisposing to infection should be excluded
Physical Examination		
Marked pelvic prolapse	A prominent cystocele that descends the entire height of the vaginal vault with coughing during speculum examination	Anatomic abnormality may underlie the pathophysiology of the incontinence, and selected patients may benefit from surgical repair
Marked prostatic enlargement and/or suspicion of cancer.	Gross enlargement of the prostate on digital examination; prominent induration or asymmetry of the lobes.	An evaluation to exclude prostate cancer may be appropriate.
Postvoid Residual		
Difficulty passing a 14-French straight catheter	Impossible catheter passage, or passage requiring considerable force or a large, rigid catheter	Anatomic blockage of the urethra or bladder neck may be present
Postvoid residual volume ≥200 mL	Volume of urine remaining in the bladder within a few minutes after the patient voids spontaneously in as normal a fashion as possible	Anatomic or neurogenic obstruction or poor bladder contractility may be present
Urinalysis		
Hematuria	Greater than 5 red blood cells per high-power field on microscopic exam in the absence of infection	A pathologic condition in the urinary tract should be excluded
Therapeutic Trial		
Failure to respond to adequate trials of behavioral and/or pharmacologic therapy	Persistent symptoms that are bothersome to the patient after adequate trials of behavioral and/or drug therapy	Urodynamic evaluation may help guide specific therapy

Adapted from Kane RL, Ouslander JG, Itamar B, et al. Essentials of Clinical Geriatrics. 5th ed. New York, New York: McGraw-Hill; 2003.

Management should be guided by the type of incontinence, and more importantly by patient and/or family preferences. Patients should be carefully questioned about the degree of bother the incontinence is causing, and how much risk and cost they are willing to undertake to treat it. Supportive measures are critical in managing all forms of incontinence and should be used in conjunction with other, more specific treatment modalities. Education, environmental manipulations, appropriate use of toilet substitutes, avoidance of iatrogenic contributions to incontinence, modifications of diuretic and fluid intake patterns (especially caffeine), treatment of constipation, and good skin care are all important.

Specially designed incontinence undergarments and pads can be very helpful in many patients, but they must be used appropriately. Although they can be effective, several caveats should be raised:

1. garments and pads are a nonspecific treatment;

2. many patients are curable if treated with specific therapies, and some have potentially serious factors underlying their incontinence that must be diagnosed and treated;

3. patients often prefer more specific incontinence therapy designed to restore a normal pattern of voiding and continence;

4. incontinence garments and pads are expensive and rarely covered by third-party payers.

To a large extent, the optimal treatment of persistent incontinence depends on identifying the type or types. Table 59-9 outlines the primary treatments for the basic types of persistent incontinence in the geriatric population. Each treatment modality is briefly discussed below.

Behavioral Interventions

Many types of behavioral interventions have been described for the management of urinary incontinence. These are either **patient dependent** (i.e., require adequate function and motivation of the patient), in which the goal is to restore a normal pattern of voiding and continence, or **caregiver dependent**, which can be used for functionally disabled patients, in which the goal is to keep the patient and the environment dry. Table 59-10 summarizes these interventions. The patient-dependent interventions generally involve the patient's continuous, self-monitoring use of a record such as the one depicted in Figure 59-3. In several studies, behavioral therapies have been shown to be equivalent to drug therapy, with approximately three-fourths of patients reporting improvement. Frequently, these behavioral interventions are a preferred treatment modality by the patients.

To be successful, patient-dependent interventions require a functional, motivated patient capable of learning and practice. These interventions also require a skilled, enthusiastic trainer and frequent patient contact, though positive results can be achieved by motivated patients who are self-directing their behavioral treatment with assistance of a pamphlet or book. Pelvic floor muscle (Kegel) exercises can be effective in men and women for the treatment of urge, stress, mixed stress–urge incontinence, and incontinence following prostatectomy. These exercises consist of repetitive contractions of the pelvic floor muscles. These exercises can be taught by brief verbal or written instructions, or instruction provided by having a patient squeeze the examiner's inserted finger during a vaginal or rectal examination (without doing a Valsalva maneuver, which is opposite

TABLE 59-8

Treatment Options for Geriatric Urinary Incontinence

Behavioral Interventions (see Table 59–10)
Patient-dependent
  Pelvic muscle exercises
  Bladder training
  Bladder retraining
  Adjunctive techniques
    Biofeedback
    Electrical stimulation
    Vaginal cones
Caregiver dependent
  Scheduled toileting
  Habit training
  Prompted voiding

Drugs (see Table 59–12)
Bladder relaxants
Alpha agonists
Alpha antagonists
Estrogen
Periurethral Injections

Surgery
Bladder neck suspension (retropubic suspension or sling procedure)
Removal of obstruction or pathologic lesion
Sacral neuromodulation

Mechanical Devices
Urethral plugs
Artificial sphincters
External penile clamps

Nonspecific Supportive Measures
Education
Modifications of medication intake
Avoid caffeine
Use of toilet substitutes
Environmental manipulations
Garments and pads

Catheters
External
Intermittent
Indwelling

Adapted from Kane RL, Ouslander JG, Itamar B, et al. Essentials of Clinical Geriatrics. 5th ed. New York, New York: McGraw-Hill; 2003.

TABLE 59-9

Primary Treatments for Different Types of Geriatric Urinary Incontinence

TYPE OF INCONTINENCE	PRIMARY TREATMENTS
Stress	Pelvic muscle (Kegel) exercises
	Other behavioral interventions
	Alpha adrenergic agonists (none are approved for use in the United States)
	Periurethral injections
	Surgical bladder neck suspension
Urge	Bladder training
	Bladder relaxants
Functional	Behavioral interventions (caregiver dependent)
	Environmental manipulations
	Incontinence undergarments and pads
High postvoid residual	Surgical removal of obstruction
	Intermittent catheterization (if practical)
	Indwelling catheterization

Adapted from Kane RL, Ouslander JG, Itamar B, et al. Essentials of Clinical Geriatrics. 5th ed. New York, New York: McGraw-Hill; 2003.

Once these muscles are strengthened, and better muscle control is achieved, the patient must be taught to use the exercises in everyday life under circumstances that precipitate the incontinence in order for them to be effective. A pelvic floor muscle contraction can be done coincidence with a cough, laugh, or sneeze to assist with stress incontinence; and used in rapid serial contractions to abort detrusor contractions associated with urinary urgency. Pelvic floor muscle exercises have also been shown to be effective in certain situations to prevent urinary incontinence and, if done preoperatively, will allow a more rapid return to continence in the postoperative period.

Other forms of patient-dependent interventions include bladder training and bladder retraining. Bladder training involves the educational components taught during biofeedback, without the use of biofeedback equipment. Patients are taught pelvic muscle exercises and strategies to manage urgency and are taught to use bladder records regularly. There is some evidence that these techniques are as effective as biofeedback in a selected group of cognitively intact, motivated elderly patients. Bladder retraining as described here is used primarily after a period of temporary bladder catheterization. Table 59-11 is an example of a bladder-retraining protocol. This protocol is applicable to patients who have had an indwelling catheter for monitoring of urinary output during a period of acute illness or for treatment of urinary retention with overflow incontinence. Such catheters always should be removed as soon as possible, and this type of bladder-retraining protocol should enable most indwelling catheters to be removed from patients in acute care hospitals as well as some residents in long-term care settings. A patient who continues to have difficulty voiding after 1 to 2 weeks of such a bladder-retraining protocol should be examined for other potentially reversible causes of voiding difficulties. When difficulties persist, a urologic referral should be considered to rule out correctable lower genitourinary pathologic conditions.

The goal of caregiver-dependent intervention such as scheduled toileting, habit training, and prompted voiding is to prevent incontinence episodes rather than to restore a normal pattern of voiding and complete continence. Highly motivated caregivers and cooperative

of the intended effect). Once learned, the exercises should be practiced many times throughout the day (e.g., three sets of 15–20 contractions building up from 3 seconds to 10 seconds in duration). Computer-assisted or manual biofeedback can be especially helpful for teaching patients who bear down (increasing intra-abdominal pressure) when attempting to contract pelvic floor muscles. Biofeedback involves the use of bladder, rectal, or vaginal pressure or electrical activity recordings, or the examiner's finger in the vagina or rectum with a hand placed on the abdomen, to train patients to contract pelvic floor muscles while leaving the abdominal muscles relaxed. Electrical stimulation, introduced either vaginally or rectally, and magnetic stimulation have also been used to help identify and train muscles in the management of stress incontinence and inhibit involuntary bladder contractions in patients with urge incontinence. The applicability of pelvic floor electrical or magnetic stimulation is somewhat limited because of equipment needs and that it may not be acceptable to many older patients in the United States.

TABLE 59-10

Examples of Behavioral Interventions for Urinary Incontinence

PROCEDURE	DEFINITION	TYPES OF INCONTINENCE	COMMENTS
Patient-Dependent			
Pelvic floor muscle (Kegel) exercises	Repetitive contraction and relaxation of pelvic floor muscles with use in everyday situations that precipitate leakage	Stress and urge	Requires adequate function and motivation; biofeedback often helpful for teaching
Bladder training	Use of education, bladder records, pelvic muscle, and other behavioral techniques	Stress and urge	Requires trained therapist, adequate cognitive and physical functioning, and motivation
Bladder retraining	Progressive lengthening or shortening of intervoiding interval, with intermittent catheterization used in patients recovering from overdistension injuries with persistent retention	Acute (e.g., postcatheterization with urge or overflow, poststroke)	Goal is to restore normal pattern of voiding and continence; requires adequate cognitive and physical function and motivation
Caregiver-Dependent			
Scheduled toileting	Routine toileting at regular intervals (scheduled toileting)	Urge and functional	Goal is to prevent wetting episodes; can be used in patients with impaired cognitive or physical functioning; requires staff or caregiver availability and motivation
Habit training	Variable toileting schedule based on patient's voiding patterns	Urge and functional	Goal is to prevent wetting episodes; can be used in patients with impaired cognitive or physical functioning; requires staff or caregiver availability and motivation
Prompted voiding	Offer opportunity to toilet every 2 hours during the day; toilet only on request; social reinforcement; routine offering of fluids	Urge, stress, mixed, functional	Same as above; 25–40% of nursing home residents respond well during the day, and can be identified during a 3-day trial

Adapted from Kane RL, Ouslander JG, Itamar B, et al. *Essentials of Clinical Geriatrics.* 5th ed. New York, New York: McGraw-Hill; 2003.

patients are essential for these interventions to be successful on an ongoing basis. Scheduled toileting involves putting the patient on the toilet at regular intervals, usually every 2 hours during the day and every 4 hours during the evening and night regardless of the presence or absence of the patient's expressed desire to void. Habit training involves a schedule of toileting that is individually modified according to the patient's pattern of continent voids and incontinence episodes. *Prompted voiding* is a behavioral protocol that involves focusing the patient's attention on his or her bladder by asking if the patient is wet or dry, asking (prompting) the patient to attempt to void (up to three times) every 2 hours during the day, toileting the patient if he or she responds positively, giving personal interaction as a social reward for attempting to toilet and maintaining continence, and offering fluids routinely. Between 25% and 40% of nursing home residents respond very well to daytime prompted voiding, and these responders can be identified by carrying out a 3-day trial of the intervention. Care for incontinence at night should be individualized. Routine incontinence care can be very disruptive to sleep. Because older people tend to awaken frequently at night, one way to individualize toileting is to check on the patient every hour or two, and only prompt to toilet when the patient is found awake.

Drug Treatment

Table 59-12 lists the drugs used to treat incontinence. Better data for efficacy in older patients are now available for some drugs. In general, carefully selected older research participants have been able to achieve roughly equivalent efficacy from drug treatment compared to their younger counterparts. Drug treatment should generally be prescribed in conjunction with one or more behavioral interventions.

For urge incontinence, antimuscarinic drugs with anticholinergic and bladder smooth-muscle relaxant properties are used. These drugs are available in immediate release, controlled release, and topical preparations. Most studies suggest a reduction of 60% to 70% in the frequency of incontinence episodes with drug therapy in selected older adults. While different drugs are likely equivalent on average, a particular patient who does not respond to one drug (either because of lack of efficacy or presence of adverse effects) may benefit from a trial on a different agent within the category. These drugs may have bothersome systemic anticholinergic side effects, especially dry mouth and constipation. They should be used carefully in patients with glaucoma and severe gastroesophageal reflux. Antimuscarinic agents may rarely precipitate urinary retention in some patients; men with some degree of outflow obstruction, diabetic patients, and patients with impaired bladder contractility are at the highest risk and should be followed carefully. For older men with overactive bladder symptoms (with or without urinary incontinence), alpha adrenergic antagonists may likely be a better choice for first-line drug therapy. Antimuscarinic bladder relaxants may also be used as single drug therapy in men, and the combination of an antimuscarinic and an alpha antagonist may be more effective in many older men. Patients with Alzheimer's disease must be followed for the development of drug-induced delirium when placed on antimuscarinic medications because of their anticholinergic effects, although it is unusual. Studies suggest that cognitive impairment, especially of memory and learning are associated antimuscarinic drug therapy. The results of these studies should not, however, preclude a treatment trial in this patient population when they make frequent attempts to toilet yet remain incontinent. The use of long-acting antimuscarinic drugs for urge incontinence has become commonplace, but it is

TABLE 59-11

Example of a Bladder-Retraining Protocol

Objective: To restore a normal pattern of voiding and continence after the removal of an indwelling catheter.

1. Remove the indwelling catheter (clamping the catheter before removal is not necessary)
2. Treat urinary tract infection if present
3. Initiate a toileting schedule. Begin by toileting the patient:
   a. Upon awakening
   b. Every 2 hours during the day and evening
   c. Before getting into bed
   d. Every 4 hours at night
4. Monitor the patient's voiding and continence pattern with a record that allows for the recording of:
   a. Frequency, timing, and amount of continent voids
   b. Frequency, timing, and amount of incontinence episodes
   c. Fluid intake pattern
   d. Postvoid catheter volume
5. If the patient is having difficulty voiding (complete urinary retention or very low urine outputs, e.g., ≤240 mL in an 8-hour period while fluid intake is adequate):
   a. Perform bladder ultrasonography or in-and-out catheterization, recording volume obtained, every 6 to 8 hours until residual values are ≤200 mL
   b. Instruct the patient on techniques to trigger voiding (e.g., running water, stroking inner thigh, suprapubic tapping) and to help completely empty bladder (e.g., bending forward, suprapubic pressure, double voiding)
   c. If the patient continues to have high residual volumes after 3 to 4 weeks, consider urodynamic evaluation
6. If the patient is voiding frequently (i.e., more often than every 2 hours):
   a. Perform postvoid residual determination to ensure the patient is completely emptying the bladder
   b. Encourage the patient to delay voiding as long as possible and instruct the patient to use techniques to help completely empty bladder
   c. If the patient continues to have frequency and nocturia, with or without urgency and incontinence:
      (1) Rule out other reversible causes (e.g., urinary tract infection medication effects, hyperglycemia, and congestive heart failure)
      (2) Consider trial of bladder relaxant if postvoid residuals are low

Adapted from Kane RL, Ouslander JG, Itamar B, et al. Essentials of Clinical Geriatrics. 5th ed. New York, New York: McGraw-Hill; 2003.

important to recognize that the cheaper, immediate release preparations are equally efficacious, but require more frequent dosing and have a higher incidence of bothersome side effects (particularly dry mouth).

Drug treatment for stress incontinence is less efficacious than is drug treatment for urge incontinence, and no drug is approved for this indication in the United States. Stress incontinence drug treatment involves a combination of an alpha agonist and topical estrogen therapy (in women). Pseudoephedrine is now the most commonly used oral agent for stress incontinence. Duloxetine, a drug approved for depression in the United States, also has alpha adrenergic effects on the lower urinary tract through a spinal cord mechanism, and is approved for the treatment of stress incontinence in several countries. Drug treatment is appropriate for motivated patients who (1) have mild to moderate degrees of stress incontinence, (2) do not have a major anatomic abnormality such as a large cystocele, and

(3) do not have a contraindication to alpha agonists drug therapy, such as poorly controlled hypertension. Previous data on the use of oral estrogen for urinary incontinence, using hormonal replacement dosages, had shown equivocal benefits. More recent studies have shown, for either opposed or unopposed oral conjugated estrogen therapy, an increased risk for previously continent women of developing and worsening of incontinence. Other forms of oral estrogen (estradiol) and topical estrogen are still used, either chronically or on an intermittent basis (i.e., 1- to 2-month courses), and may be effective for the treatment of irritative voiding symptoms and urge incontinence in women with atrophic vaginitis and urethritis. Although no specific topical treatment regimen has been shown to be more effective than others, therapy usually involves 0.5 to 1 g of vaginal cream nightly for 1 to 2 months and then a maintenance dose two or three times per week or a controlled, slow-release vaginal ring. Several months of therapy are often necessary to observe therapeutic benefit.

Many elderly women have symptomatically and urodynamically a combination of both urge and stress incontinence. If urge incontinence is the predominant symptom, a combination of estrogen and bladder relaxant would be appropriate. Behavioral interventions are also an effective approach for women with mixed incontinence.

Drug treatment in the setting of chronic urinary retention or urinary incontinence with high postvoid residual, with either a cholinergic agonist or an alpha adrenergic antagonist, is usually not efficacious. Although alpha adrenergic blockers and 5-alpha reductase inhibitors are useful for treatment of symptoms suggestive of benign prostatic hyperplasia, they may not obviate the need for surgical intervention or requirement for catheter drainage in patients with bladder outlet obstruction who have chronic urinary retention or urinary incontinence with high postvoid residuals (i.e., residuals consistently greater than 200–300 mL).

Surgical Approaches

Surgery is a well-established treatment for stress urinary incontinence. Surgery should be considered for elderly women with stress incontinence and for women with a significant degree of pelvic prolapse associated with stress incontinence or incontinence with urinary retention who are unresponsive to nonsurgical treatment. As with many other surgical procedures, patient selection and the experience of the surgeon are critical to success. Any woman being considered for surgical therapy should have a thorough evaluation, including urodynamic tests, before undergoing the procedure. In general, surgical treatment is designed to correct urethral closure problems and to remedy defects in support of the urethra–vesicular angle. Newly modified techniques of bladder neck suspension, tension-free vaginal tapes, and the use of periurethral collagen injections can be done with minimal risks. Periurethral injections appear to be most appropriate for women with intrinsic urethral weakness. Two or more sessions of injections are usually necessary to maintain effectiveness. Many elderly women with severe incontinence associated with intrinsic urethral weakness require a sling procedure rather than a simple bladder neck suspension. Men with stress urinary incontinence (and usually with continuous urinary leakage) can be treated with the implantation of an artificial urinary sphincter (or other similar mechanical device designed to reversibly block urine outflow in the penile urethra). Newer "sling" procedures have been used in men, also.

TABLE 59-12

Drugs Commonly Used in the United States To Treat Urinary Incontinence

DRUGS	DOSAGES	MECHANISMS OF ACTION	TYPE OF INCONTINENCE	POTENTIAL ADVERSE EFFECTS
Antimuscarinic and antispasmodic agents	In general, reduced dosages for renal and hepatic impairment			
Oxybutynin (Ditropan, immediate release, available as generic)	2.5–5.0 mg tid	Increase bladder capacity; diminish involuntary bladder contractions	Urge or mixed with urge predominant	Anticholinergic (dry mouth, blurry vision, elevated intraocular pressure, delirium, constipation)
Darifenacin (Enablex)	7.5–15 mg qd			Anticholinergic, lower dose if reduced hepatic function
Oxybutynin (extended release) (Ditropan XL)	5–30 mg qd (most often 10 mg qd)			Above, but with less dry mouth
Patch (Oxytrol)	3.9 mg qd	Patch applied twice weekly		
Solifenancin (Vesicare)	5–10 mg qd			Anticholinergic, lower for severe renal impairment or reduced hepatic function
Tolterodine (Detrol LA)	4 mg qd			Above, but with less dry mouth
Trospium chloride (Sanctura)	20 mg bid			20 mg once daily qhs with severe renal impairment
Alpha adrenergic agonists				
Pseudoephedrine (Sudafed)	30–60 mg tid	Increase urethral smooth-muscle contraction		Headache, tachycardia, elevation of blood pressure
Estrogens				
Topical	0.5–1.0 g per application	Strengthen periurethral tissues	Urge associated with atrophic vaginitis	
Vaginal ring (Estring) (estradiol acetate)	One ring every 3 months			
Alpha adrenergic antagonist				
Doxazosin (available as generic, or Cardura)	1–8 mg qhs	Relax smooth muscle of urethra and prostatic capsule	Urge incontinence associated with prostatic enlargement	Postural hypotension, dizziness, lowers blood pressure
Terazosin (available as generic, or Hytrin)	1–10 mg qhs			Same as above
Prazosin (Minipress)	1–2 mg tid			Same as above
Alfuzosin (Uroxatral)	10 mg qhs			Less effects on blood pressure
Tamsulosin (Flomax)	0.4–0.8 mg qd			Less effects on blood pressure (when used at 0.8 mg dose, greater blood pressure effects)

Adapted from Kane RL, Ouslander JG, Itamar B, et al. Essentials of Clinical Geriatrics. 5th ed. New York, New York: McGraw-Hill; 2004.

While surgical approaches have previously been considered only for stress incontinence, there are recently developed approaches for the treatment of urge incontinence that remains unresponsive to medical and behavioral treatment. Newer approaches include sacral nerve neuromodulation, where a two-stage operation involving general anesthesia and implantation of a pacemaker-like generator near the hip and sacral leads to stimulate the pudendal and sacral nerves. The procedure can be a safe, effective, and durable treatment, though cure rates for older adults and those with multiple medical comorbidities have been lower than in younger, healthier populations. Also, the use of botulinum toxin A for refractory urge incontinence has proven effective in several randomized, double-blinded, controlled studies, though this indication has not yet been approved by the U.S. Food and Drug Administration. Botulinum toxin A is accomplished via cystoscopic injections into multiple bladder sites under direct visualization. Benefit is believed to be because of an effect on both efferent and afferent pathways, and early trial results suggest that the therapy lasts 6 months and is equally effective in older and younger age groups.

Surgery may be indicated in men in whom incontinence is associated with outflow obstruction. Men may have either chronic urinary retention, or acute urinary retention that is *precipitated* (use of an anticholinergic drug, recent instrumentation, or alpha agonist drug) or *spontaneous*. Those who have had complete acute urinary retention requiring mechanical drainage, and particularly those with *spontaneous* retention, are likely to have another episode within a short period of time and should be evaluated for a prostatic resection, as should men with incontinence associated with enough residual urine to be causing recurrent symptomatic infections or hydronephrosis. In men who do not meet these criteria, the decision should be based on weighing carefully the degree to which the symptoms bother the patient, the potential benefits of surgery (obstructive symptoms often respond better than irritative symptoms), and the risks of surgery (which may be minimal with newer prostate resection techniques).

MECHANICAL DEVICES, UNDERGARMENTS, CATHETERS, AND OTHER SUPPORTS

Three basic types of catheters and catheterization procedures are used for the management of urinary incontinence: external catheters, intermittent straight ("in-and-out") catheterization, and chronic indwelling catheterization. External catheters generally consist of some type of condom connected to a drainage system. Improvements in design and observance of proper procedure and skin care when applying the catheter decrease the risk of skin irritation, as well as the frequency with which the catheter falls off. Existing data suggest that patients with external catheters are at increased risk of developing symptomatic infection compared to incontinent adults depending upon absorbent pads or diapers. External catheters should be used only to manage intractable incontinence in male patients who do not have urinary retention and who are extremely physically dependent. An external catheter for use in female patients is available commercially, but is not widely used.

Intermittent catheterization can help in the management of patients with urinary retention and overflow incontinence. The procedure can be carried out by either the patient or a caregiver and involves straight catheterization two to four or more times daily, depending on residual urine volumes. The goal is to keep residual urine volume generally less than approximately 300 to 400 mL. In the home setting, the catheter should be kept clean (but not necessarily sterile). Studies conducted largely among younger paraplegic patients show that this technique is practical and reduces the risk of symptomatic infection compared with the risk associated with chronic catheterization. Self-intermittent catheterization is also feasible for elderly female outpatients who are functional and willing and able to catheterize themselves. The technique may be especially useful following removal of an indwelling catheter in a bladder-retraining protocol (see Table 59-11). However, elderly nursing home residents, especially men, may be difficult to catheterize. Anatomic abnormalities commonly found in the lower urinary tracts of elderly patients may increase the risk of infection because of repeated straight catheterizations. In addition, using this technique in an institutional setting, which may have an abundance of organisms relatively resistant to many commonly used antimicrobial agents, may yield an unacceptable risk of nosocomial infections. Using sterile catheter trays for these procedures would be very expensive. Thus, it may be extremely difficult to implement such a program in a typical nursing home setting.

Chronic indwelling catheterization, when used for periods of months to years, has been shown to increase the incidence of a number of complications, including chronic bacteriuria, bladder stones, periurethral abscesses, and even bladder cancer. Elderly nursing home residents managed by this technique, especially men, are at relatively high risk of developing symptomatic infections. The limited evidence available to date does not suggest that routine changing of indwelling catheters is warranted, though this is a common practice. Given these risks, it seems appropriate to recommend that the use of chronic indwelling catheters be limited to certain specific situations

TABLE 59-13

Indications for Chronic Indwelling Catheter Use

Urinary retention that
    Is causing persistent overflow incontinence, symptomatic infections, or renal dysfunction
    Cannot be corrected surgically or medically
    Cannot be managed practically with intermittent catheterization

Skin wounds, pressure sores, or irritations where incontinent urine contributes to excessive moisture and results in poor healing

Care of terminally ill or severely impaired for whom bed and clothing changes are uncomfortable or disruptive

Patient preference

Adapted from Kane RL, Ouslander JG, Itamar B, et al. Essentials of Clinical Geriatrics. 5th ed. New York, New York: McGraw-Hill; 2004.

(Table 59-13). When indwelling catheterization is used, certain principles of catheter care should be observed in an attempt to minimize complications (Table 59-14). In situations where there is reduced urinary output, increased leakage around the catheter, or increased pain, it is important to perform an abdominal and genital examination to make certain the catheter is in the bladder and not obstructed. In these situations, it is often necessary to replace the catheter.

In men with postprostatectomy urinary incontinence who are not a candidate for or do not desire surgical therapy, an external penile clamp for compression of the urethra may be a useful adjunctive therapy. Patients must be able to monitor and remove the clamp every two hours. Some women with urinary incontinence and pelvic prolapse may respond well to use of a vaginal pessary, which is a device to slow the progression of prolapse by adding support to the

TABLE 59-14

Key Principles of Chronic Indwelling Catheter Care

SUMMARY OF MAJOR RECOMMENDATIONS

Category I. Strongly Recommended for Adoption
Educate personnel in correct techniques of catheter insertion and care
Catheterize only when necessary
Emphasize hand washing
Insert catheter using aseptic technique and sterile equipment
Secure catheter properly
Maintain closed sterile drainage
Obtain urine samples aseptically
Maintain unobstructed urine flow

Category II. Moderately Recommended for Adoption
Periodically re-educate personnel in catheter care
Use smallest suitable bore catheter
Avoid irrigation unless needed to prevent or relieve obstruction
Refrain from daily meatal care with povidone–iodine solution as this may result in an increased infection rate
Do not change catheters at arbitrary fixed intervals

Category III. Weakly Recommended for Adoption
Consider alternative techniques of urinary drainage before using an indwelling urethral catheter
Replace the collecting system when sterile closed drainage has been violated
Spatially separate infected and uninfected patients with indwelling catheters
Avoid routine bacteriologic monitoring

Wong ES, Hooton TM. Guideline for prevention of catheter-associated urinary tract infections. http://www.cdc.gov/ncidod/dhqp/gl_catheter_assoc.html. Accessed March 22, 2007.

vagina and increasing tightness of the tissues and muscles of the pelvis. Pessaries are made of rubber, plastic, or silicone, and come in a variety of types. Conclusive trials about which devices are better than others, or how well the devices compare to other treatments have not yet been reported. The ideal device would be easy to insert, be of low cost, have few adverse effects, and would control leakage. Often patients need to be individually fitted with the device.

There are a variety of available absorbent products and undergarments that can help patients contain leakage, including disposable inserts, reusable and single-use adult diapers, and disposable underwear. Additionally, there are pads that can protect beds and/or chairs. Controlled studies have been performed comparing one type to another, and criteria for success of these devices revolve around fit, odor control, cost, and ability to hold urine. More frequent changing of pads is expensive and inconvenient, but frequently helps control odor. Less frequent changing leaves skin wetter and likely more vulnerable to friction and abrasion. Most consumers select products by trial and error and are unaware of the range of products and services available. These products are available at drug stores, supermarkets, and medical supply stores.

In general, older adults want general information on urinary incontinence and sources of help. There are multiple consumer advocacy groups for those with incontinence that are dedicated to improving the lives of patients with urinary incontinence, e.g., the National Association for Continence (www.nafc.org), and the Simon Foundation (www.simonfoundation.org) that provide educational materials, reviews of available products, and links to researchers and manufacturers who provide incontinence materials.

FECAL INCONTINENCE

Fecal incontinence is less common than urinary incontinence. Its occurrence is relatively unusual in elderly patients who are continent of urine. Thirty to fifty percent of elderly patients in institutional settings with frequent urinary incontinence, however, also have episodes of fecal incontinence. This coexistence suggests common pathophysiologic mechanisms.

Defecation, like urination, is a physiologic process that involves smooth and striated muscles, central and peripheral innervation, coordination of reflex responses, mental awareness, and physical ability to get to a toilet. Disruption of any of these factors can lead to fecal incontinence.

The most common causes of fecal incontinence are problems with constipation and laxative use, neurologic disorders, and colorectal disorders (Table 59-15). In patients who are fed by enteral tubes, hyperosmotic feedings can precipitate diarrhea and fecal incontinence. Diluting the feedings or using slow continuous infusion is sometimes helpful. Constipation is extremely common in elderly persons and, when chronic, can lead to fecal impaction and incontinence. The hard stool (or scybalum) of fecal impaction irritates the rectum and results in the production of mucus and fluid. This fluid leaks around the mass of impacted stool and precipitates incontinence. Constipation is difficult to define; technically, it indicates fewer than three bowel movements per week, although many patients use the term to describe difficult passage of hard stools or a feeling of incomplete evacuation. Poor dietary and toilet habits, immobility, and chronic laxative abuse are the most common causes of constipation in elderly persons. Appropriate management of constipation prevents

TABLE 59-15

Causes of Fecal Incontinence

Fecal impaction
Constipation
Laxative overuse or abuse
Hyperosmotic enteral feedings
Neurologic disorders
Dementia
Stroke
Spinal cord disease
Colorectal disorders
Diarrheal illnesses
Diabetic autonomic neuropathy
Rectal sphincter damage

fecal impaction and resulting fecal incontinence. The management of constipation is discussed thoroughly in Chapter 93.

Fecal incontinence is sometimes amenable to biofeedback therapy, although many elderly demented patients are unable to cooperate. For those patients with end-stage dementia, a program of alternating constipating agents (if necessary) and laxatives in a routine schedule (such as giving laxatives and enemas three times a week) is effective in controlling defecation in many patients with fecal incontinence. Functionally dependent patients should be toileted regularly after a meal to take advantage of, or possibly regain, the gastrocolic reflex. Experience suggests that these measures should permit management of even severely cognitively impaired patients. As a last resort, specially designed incontinence undergarments are sometimes helpful in managing fecal incontinence and preventing skin irritation and other complications.

FURTHER READING

Brown JS, Vittinghoff E, Wyman JF, et al. Urinary incontinence: does it increase risk for falls and fractures? Study of Osteoporotic Fractures Research Group. *J Am Geriatr Soc.* 2000;48:721–725.

Burgio KL, Locher JL, Goode PS, et al. Behavioral versus drug treatment for urge urinary incontinence in older women: a randomized controlled trial. *JAMA.* 1998;280:1995–2000.

Goode PS, Burgio KL, Locher JL, et al. Effect of behavioral training with or without pelvic floor electrical stimulation on stress incontinence in women: a randomized controlled trial. *JAMA.* 2003;290:345–352.

Griffiths D, Derbyshire S, Stenger A, et al. Brain control of normal and overactive bladder. *J Urol.* 2005;174:1862–1867.

Hendrix SL, Cochrane BB, Nygaard IE, et al. Effects of estrogen with and without progestin on urinary incontinence. *JAMA.* 2005;293:935–948.

Holroyd-Leduc JM, Straus SE. Management of urinary incontinence in women: clinical applications. *JAMA.* 2004;291:996–999.

Holroyd-Leduc JM, Straus SE. Management of urinary incontinence in women: scientific review. *JAMA.* 2004;291:986–995.

Johnson TM II, Kincade JE, Bernard SL, et al. Self-care practices used by older men and women to manage urinary incontinence: results from the national follow-up survey on self-care and aging. *J Am Geriatr Soc.* 2000;48:894–902.

Kane RL, Ouslander JG, Itamar B, et al. *Essentials of Clinical Geriatrics.* 5th ed. New York, New York: McGraw-Hill; 2004.

Kaplan SA, Roehrborn CG, Rovner ES, et al. Tolterodine and tamsulosin for treatment of men with lower urinary tract symptoms and overactive bladder: a randomized controlled trial. *JAMA.* 2006;296:2319–2328.

Ouslander JG. Management of overactive bladder. [see comment]. *N Engl J Med.* 2004;350:786–799.

Thom DH. Variation in estimates of urinary incontinence prevalence in the community: effects of differences in definition, population characteristics, and study type. *J Am Geriatr Soc.* 1998;46:473–480.

Wagner TH, Hu TW. Economic costs of urinary incontinence in 1995. *Urology.* 1998;51:355–361.

Elder Mistreatment

Mark S. Lachs

DEFINITIONS

In the broadest context, *elder mistreatment* subsumes a variety of activities perpetrated upon an older person by others. Some proposed strategies for defining or classifying elder mistreatment have been based on the type of abuse (e.g., physical vs. verbal abuse), motive (e.g., intentional vs. unintentional neglect), perpetrator relationship (e.g., family vs. paid caregiver), and setting (e.g., community vs. nursing home). There is as yet no universally agreed definition or classification of elder mistreatment. Nonetheless, the clinician attempting to care for a victimized older person or to understand the spectrum of elder mistreatment will encounter several thematically similar definitions. For example, the older Americans Act of 1975 defines elder abuse as "the willful infliction of pain, injury, or mental anguish." This definition has been adopted, and/or modified, by many state protective service agencies that investigate cases of abuse. A more recent and encompassing definition created by an expert panel convened by the National Academy of Sciences adopted the definition that elder mistreatment in all its forms involves *a trusting relationship between an older person and another individual in which that trust is violated in some way.* Table 60-1 lists other representative definitions and examples of elder mistreatment. Whatever definition is employed, a consistent and important feature of elder mistreatment, and other forms of family violence, is that multiple types of mistreatment, such as physical and verbal abuse, neglect, and financial exploitation frequently coexist in the same abuser–victim dyad.

Virtually all experts, clinicians, and reasonable laypersons will agree that egregious instances of physical violence such as punching, hitting, slapping, or assaulting an older person with a gun or other weapon are elder abuse. The most contentious definitional (and clinical) area relates to elder neglect, because the term neglect immediately implies that a caregiving obligation—such as providing food, medicines, or care—has not been met. This, in turn, raises difficult questions that must, with clinical judgment and experience, be considered in the context of the older adult's environment. For ex-

ample, what are reasonable community standards for the frequency of bathing an assaultive spouse with Alzheimer's disease? Does that standard change if the designated caregiver also suffers from chronic diseases that preclude perfect hygiene for their impaired family member? What if this inadequate care enables the "victim" to live at home long after other families would have considered nursing home placement? Who exactly is the responsible caretaker, especially when multiple adult children are available to assume that role, but only one has "stepped up" because of birth order or some other arbitrary circumstance? And is it fair to label that adult child an "elder neglector" when caregiving becomes physically or psychologically impossible?

These difficult questions also highlight the fact that clinicians caring for elder abuse victims often find themselves working closely with alleged perpetrators of abuse and neglect, as these individuals are often the primary caregivers.

EPIDEMIOLOGY

However it is defined, elder mistreatment is common. Over the past 15 years, several prevalence studies have been conducted in different countries. These studies have used primarily self-report for case finding and validated family violence scales for case definition (typically an adopted version of the conflicts tactics scale, a common employed instrument used in all forms of family violence). The methodology assumes that all families have conflict, and that it is how that conflict is addressed or resolved that is the measurable and relevant aspect of mistreatment. Using this methodology, Pillemer and Finkelhor conducted the most commonly cited study in the United States. Surveying residents of metropolitan Boston by telephone, the investigators calculated a prevalence of 32 per 1000 population (i.e., 3.2% of the 2010 individuals surveyed reported having been victims of elder mistreatment at least once since turning age 65 years). In this study, cases of abuse exceeded cases of neglect. In the subsequent 20 years that have followed, most studies in western societies have

TABLE 60-1

Representative Definitions of Elder Mistreatment

MISTREATMENT CATEGORY	DEFINITION	EXAMPLES
Physical abuse	Acts of violence that may result in pain, injury, impairment, or disease	? Pushing, striking, slapping, force-feeding ? Incorrect positioning ? Improper use of restraints or medications ? Sexual coercion or assault
Neglect	The failure to provide the goods or services necessary for optimal functioning or to avoid harm	? Withholding of health maintenance care ? Failure to provide physical aids such as eyeglasses, hearing aids, false teeth ? Failure to provide safety precautions
Financial or material abuse	The misuse of the elderly person's income or resources for the financial or personal gain of a caretaker or advisor	? Denying the older person a home ? Stealing money or possessions ? Coercing the older person into signing contracts
Psychological or verbal abuse	Conduct that causes mental anguish	? Verbal berating, harassment, or intimidation ? Threats of punishment or deprivation ? Treating the older person like an infant ? Isolating the older person from others
Violation of a trusting relationship	Meant to encompass all forms of abuse in that all forms involve the older person relying on and trusting another party, who through acts of omission or commission, violates that trust, without regard to intent.	

Data from Aravanis SC, Adelman RD, Breckman D, et al. Diagnostic and treatment guidelines on elder abuse and neglect. Archives of Family Medicine 1993;2:371.

produced a remarkably stable and similar prevalence in the 2% to 5% range. Recently, the World Health Organization has embarked on a coordinated series of studies addressing prevalence and screening across several countries. This effort indicates growing worldwide interest in elder abuse.

A less-consistent epidemiologic picture emerges when one attempts to discern risk factors for elder mistreatment from the literature (Table 60-2). The most consistent findings relate to the relationship of the abuser to victim; most studies report that spouses and adult children are the most common perpetrators. Studies also show that when adult children are the abusers, sons and daughters are often equally implicated. At least one study found daughters to be the more common abuser. These findings must be viewed cautiously in that women are far more likely to be the de facto or designated care providers to frail older adults and are, therefore, more "at risk" for being accused of mistreatment should caregiving fall short of any arbitrary standard.

The most discordant literature is in the area of victim risk factors. Here the literature has produced inconsistent findings with respect to gender, functional disability, cognitive impairment, social network, and a variety of other factors proffered by elder abuse theorists. A particularly contentious area has been spawned by the "dependency theory" of mistreatment, which holds that mistreatment occurs when the victim becomes inordinately dependent upon the caregiver for a variety of medical and nonmedical needs. Again, studies show an inconsistent relationship between functional disability and elder mistreatment. In fact, a more consistent finding in the literature is the converse—the perpetrators are often dependent upon the victims for financial support and housing. Characteristically, an adult child unable to achieve independence is reliant on the older person for these needs.

The disparate findings probably derive from two major factors. The first is the methodologic quality of the studies, which have been highly variable and rife with susceptibility and other biases. The

TABLE 60-2

Possible Risk Factors for Elder Mistreatment

FACTOR	MECHANISM
Victim's poor health and functional disability	Disability reduces elder's ability to seek help and/or defend self.
Cognitive impairment	Aggression toward caregiver and disruptive behaviors resulting from dementia precipitate abuse. Higher rates of abuse have been found among patients with dementia.
Abuser deviance	Abusers likely to abuse alcohol or drugs and to have serious mental illness, which, in turn, leads to abusive behavior.
Abuser dependency	Abusers are very likely to depend on the victim financially, for housing, and in other areas. Abuse results from relative's (especially adult children's) attempts to obtain resources from the elder.
Living arrangement	Abuse much less likely among elders living alone. A shared living situation provides greater opportunities for tension and conflict that generally precede abusive incidents.
External stress	Stressful life events and chronic financial strain decrease the family's resistance and increase likelihood of abuse.
Social isolation	Elders with fewer social contacts more likely to be victims.
	Isolation reduces the likelihood that abuse will be detected and stopped. In addition, social support can buffer against the impact of stress.
History of violence	Particularly among spouses, prior history of violence in the relationship may be predictive of elder abuse in later life.

Reprinted with permission from Lachs MS, Pillemer K. Current concepts: abuse and neglect of elderly persons. N Engl J Med. 1995;332:437.

second relates to the heterogeneous nature of elder abuse cases. Elderly protective services workers and clinicians experienced in elder mistreatment know that the term elder mistreatment subsumes many situations—abusive spousal relationships that have "aged," caregivers to dementia patients who lash out in frustration, and physically abusive adult children with poorly managed mental health or substance abuse problems, are but a few examples. Epidemiologic studies that attempt to discern risk factors without acknowledging this reality probably are measuring an "average" effect, thus possibly missing important sets of risk factors among subgroups of abused or neglected elderly populations.

Whatever risk factors are identified in previous and future research should not foster a complacency wherein an absence or paucity of such factors causes the clinician to lower his or her guard. Elder mistreatment crosses all ethnic and socioeconomic boundaries. A high index of clinical suspicion is paramount for identification.

PATHOPHYSIOLOGY

Theories of elder mistreatment abound; three deserve detailed treatment here, because they may have clinical relevance with regard to the types of interventions contemplated in confirmed cases of mistreatment. The most commonly cited theory contends that family violence is a learned behavior; abused children grow up to potentially abuse not only their children, but also perhaps spouses and their parents. This is sometimes referred to as the transgenerational violence theory of mistreatment.

The dependency theory of mistreatment holds that abuse is fostered by situations in which victims have a degree of functional and/or cognitive disability that results in activities of daily living impairment and overwhelming care needs. Closely associated with this paradigm is another theory—that of the "stressed caregiver."

The psychopathology of the abuser theory shifts focus away from the victim and argues that elder mistreatment is firmly rooted in mental health problems of the abuser. Examples include personality disorders, poorly or undertreated schizophrenia, alcoholism, and other substance abuse problems.

Discerning the underlying causes of elder mistreatment is essential in fashioning an intervention plan (see "Management" later in this chapter).

PRESENTATION

For a variety of reasons, the identification of elder mistreatment is one of the most difficult clinical challenges in geriatric medicine. First, many highly prevalent chronic diseases in older adults may have clinical manifestations that mimic abuse. If elder abuse is present, the clinician may ascribe those findings to chronic disease rather than family violence. Conversely, the clinician may erroneously attribute findings from another disease to elder mistreatment. Second, the setting in which an elder mistreatment evaluation occurs is often quite challenging. The environment may be hurried (e.g., the emergency department). The presence of the suspected abuser only adds pressure to what is already likely to be a stressful encounter. Lastly, the competent identification and management of mistreatment propel the clinician into a world that he or she is likely to be unfamiliar with—a world that includes mandatory reporting statutes, adult protective service workers, and a criminal justice system with a vocabulary that is foreign to many medical professionals. Given these educational, emotional, and systemic obstacles, it is not surprising that elder mistreatment often is missed or unreported in the context of "customary care."

Elder abuse forensics is a recent area of intense interest. Of particular interest has been whether there are diagnostic and/or clinical signs and symptoms of abuse presentations, either during life or at autopsy that enables clinicians to opine definitively that abuse exists as in cases of child abuse (e.g., shaken baby syndrome). So far such studies have not been fruitful. For example, one group of investigators undertook a detailed longitudinal study of spontaneous bruising in older people; observers could not accurately date bruises by color (a long held belief in elder abuse evaluation). Additionally, many older subjects were unaware of bruising, a good proportion of which were spontaneous. This "negative" study should not be viewed as disappointing. Such painstaking work is needed to move the field forward with scientific rigor.

Without such markers, clinicians need to consider elder mistreatment in the differential diagnosis of many or most of the clinical presentations they encounter. Fractures may result from osteoporosis or force or both. Depression may be related to neurotransmitter imbalances or a hopeless abusive environment. Malnutrition may be the result of any number of chronic illnesses inexorably worsening, or from the withholding of sustenance.

Dramatic injuries or neglect pose no particular diagnostic challenge. Fractures, burns, contusions, and lacerations, in concert with a credible history, immediately lead to the diagnosis. At the other extreme, subtle presentations that mimic chronic disease are highly challenging. Examples include chronic diseases that frequently decompensate despite a care plan and adequate resources (e.g., repeated emergency department visits for congestive heart failure or chronic obstructive pulmonary disease exacerbation). Indeed, because elder mistreatment can be defined so broadly, there are very few presenting signs or symptoms in the geriatric patient for which elder mistreatment is not in the differential diagnosis.

Many instruments have been devised for the screening or evaluation of elder mistreatment, but they are not applicable to all settings and have not been validated against an external standard. Such a standard would be difficult to create. Rather, they can serve as useful "checklists" for a thorough evaluation. Table 60-3 suggests a system-by-system approach. The importance of heightened awareness cannot be overemphasized in considering the diagnosis. Frequently, clues about potential mistreatment come from ancillary staff members (e.g., office reception staff) or home care nurses who observe the abuser–victim dyad away from the health care provider. A general sense that something is amiss in the patient's environment such as caustic interaction between parties, poor hygiene or dress, frequently missed medical appointments, or failure to adhere with a clearly designated treatment strategy can all be important clues.

The patient and the alleged perpetrator should be interviewed separately and alone. Although there is an emerging consensus that patients of all ages should be routinely screened for family violence, an optimal strategy or instrument has not emerged. Patients should be asked candidly and calmly about the etiology of any unexplained injuries or other findings. Often patients are at first unwilling to speak candidly about being an elder abuse victim for reasons of embarrassment, shame, or fear of retribution from the perpetrator who is frequently a caregiver.

Interview of the suspected abuser is a tricky and potentially dangerous undertaking. On the one extreme, elder abusers who are

TABLE 60-3

Clinical Manifestations of Potential Mistreatment with Recommended Assessment	
TARGET	**ASSESSMENT**
History from elder	Interview patient alone; directly inquire regarding physical violence, restraint use, or neglect; ascertain precise details about nature, frequency and severity of events.
	Assess functional status (amount of dependence with activities of daily living [ADL]).
	Determine who the designated caregiver is if ADL disability is present.
History from abuser	Potential abuser should also be interviewed alone; this interview is best done by professionals with experience in this area; avoid confrontation in the information-gathering phase. Interview other sources if possible.
	Assess recent psychosocial factors (e.g., bereavement, financial stresses)
	Ascertain caregiver understanding of patient's illness (e.g., care needs, prognosis, etc.)
	Elicit caregiver's explanations for injuries or physical findings
Behavioral observation	Withdrawal
	Infantalizing of patient by caregiver
	Caregiver who insists on providing the history
General appearance	Hygiene
	Cleanliness and appropriateness of dress
Skin/mucous membranes	Skin turgor, other signs of dehydration; multiple skin lesions in various stages of evolution
	Bruises, decubiti; evidence of care for established skin lesions
Head and neck	Traumatic alopecia (distinguishable from male pattern alopecia on the basis of distribution)
	Scalp hematomas
	Lacerations, abrasions
Trunk	Bruises, welts; shape may suggest implement (e.g., iron/belt)
Genitourinary	Rectal bleeding
	Vaginal bleeding
	Decubiti, infestations
Extremities	Wrists or ankle lesions suggest restraint use or immersion burn (stocking/glove distribution)
Musculoskeletal	Examine for occult fracture, pain; observe gait
Neurological/psychiatric	Thorough evaluation to assess focality of neurological deficits
	Depressive symptoms, anxiety
Mental status	Formal mental status testing (e.g., Mini-Mental State Examination); cognitive impairment suggests delirium or dementia and plays a role in assessing decision-making capacity
	Psychiatric symptoms including delusions and hallucinations
Imaging	As indicated from the clinical evaluation
Laboratory	
	As indicated from the clinical evaluation (drug levels)
	Albumin, blood urea nitrogen, and creatinine toxicology
Social and financial resources	Determine whether there are other members of social network available to assist the elder; financial resources
	These resources are crucial in considering interventions that include alternate-living arrangements and home services

Reprinted with permission from Lachs MS, Pillemer K. Current concepts: abuse and neglect of elderly persons. N Engl J Med. 1995;332:437.

presented with an empathetic, nonjudgmental ear to describe their stresses and actions will sometimes describe their situations at great length and in great detail. On the other hand, all forms of domestic abuse share a pattern wherein abusers gain and control access to their victims. An elder abuser graphically confronted with allegations of mistreatment may move to sequester a frail victim in such a way that a frail isolated older adult loses access to critically needed medical and social services. Whenever possible, assistance from providers skilled in elder abuse evaluation and management should be enlisted to assist in such undertakings.

MANAGEMENT

Elder abuse is morbid and mortal. In one longitudinal study, victims had a threefold risk of death and nursing home placement compared to nonabused controls, even after adjusting for many risk factors

for these outcomes, including comorbidity. Thus, intervention is critical.

Unfortunately, there are no randomized trials of reasonable quality addressing interventions for elder mistreatment. The clinician confronted with a confirmed case of elder abuse is best served by a resourceful approach that combines experience, clinical judgment, and local resources. One relatively new and noteworthy trend is the creation of large multidisciplinary groups who convene regularly to discuss cases of mistreatment, not only for the purpose of planning intervention, but also to consider case-by-case forensics, cross train disciplines, and provide general support to one another in this difficult field. Again, however, there is no evidence-based evaluation of this strategy.

Whatever the approach to intervention, a dogmatic or algorithmic strategy to address all elder mistreatment cases is likely misguided. A rigid, inflexible approach ignores the enormous heterogeneity of the entity, including the type(s) of mistreatment being concurrently perpetrated, the underlying mechanisms, patient co-morbidities, caregiver burden issues, and the available resources (both familial and community) that can be brought to bear on the issue. A more sensible approach may be the multipronged strategy increasingly used to treat other geriatric syndromes that have multi-factorial etiologies. The paradigm may be a useful one in that elder mistreatment can be likened to geriatric syndromes. That is, there may be multiple "host" and environmental contributors; decompensation may be accelerated by other medical and social problems; and some of the contributors may be more remediable than others. The elder physical abuse victim with severe chronic obstructive pulmonary disease and an abusive schizophrenic child-caregiver will need an entirely different series of interventions than the spouse with progressive dementia who has suffered life-long domestic violence that is now worsening.

The first step in confronting any confirmed case of family violence is ensuring the safety of the victim. First, the immediate threat of danger to the victim should be ascertained. Even if there is no immediate threat, a *safety plan* is critical in the management of all forms of family violence (Table 60-4). What are the specific steps the victim should take if the perpetrator of mistreatment becomes acutely violent? Options include calling the local police department, accessing shelters, emergency department use/hospital admission, or

respite care in some evolved systems of long-term care. Additionally, in most states, cases of elder abuse must be reported to adult protective services agencies. This typically results in a home visit to adjudicate the veracity of such a report. State protective service agencies vary widely with respect to their caseloads and available resources; ideally a coordinated approach that brings to bear their expertise and resources in collaboration with the physician and multidisciplinary team produces the best response.

However, the safety plan paradigm will have limited utility in many cases of elder mistreatment because of victim frailty and/or cognitive impairment that limits the use of self-protective behaviors. Frequently, clinicians find themselves in the predicament of caring for an elder mistreatment victim who lacks capacity. Here the likely intervention will involve the appointment of a guardian in collaboration with adult protective service agencies or other elder social service programs in the community that serve such functions. In such a proceeding, the clinician's role is to provide objective evidence that documents the lack of decision-making capacity. The clinician may also have a role in ensuring the alleged perpetrator of mistreatment does not become the guardian.

One of the most frustrating situations for professionals working with victims of family violence is the individual who retains decision-making capacity, but insists on remaining in an abusive environment. Here the clinician's role is to educate the patient about the tendency of family violence to escalate and to review the safety plan created. The clinician should also explain to the patient that even if services are refused, the physician remains an important and available resource, should the situation change.

In general, the physician who suspects elder abuse would do well to employ the same creative strategies he or she uses to manage a variety of clinical problems in older adults. There may be local social services agencies in the community who provide an array of services such as meals on wheels or friendly visit. These services could represent a new resource for the patient, but also additional "eyes and ears" to ascertain what the home situation is like. A local adult day care referral might also enable a more detailed ongoing evaluation of a client while decompressing a stressful caregiving situation. A financial management program for the patient with cognitive impairment can shed light on the possibility of financial exploitation. The physician need not diagnose elder abuse while these useful services are being proffered.

TABLE 60-4

Safety Plan for Victims of Elder Mistreatment or Other Victims of Family Violence with Capacity Who Insist on Remaining in an Abusive Environment	
TIME FRAME	**ACTIVITY**
Prior to violent or abusive episode	Recognize patterns that lead to abusive behavior (e.g., abuser alcohol use).
	Determine who in the social network is available to assist when such an episode occurs through explicit conversations with neighbors, friends, other relatives.
	Be aware of elder domestic violence programs, shelters, and other resources in the local community available to assist; know their contact numbers.
	Have essential resources readily available if the patient needs to leave quickly (e.g., money, ATM cards, credit cards, driver's license, keys, identification, social security card, other important documents).
	Practice implementing safety plan (e.g., mock 911 call). Consider creating a "code" with a friend or neighbor so that the patient can communicate danger in the presence of the abuser.
During violent or abusive episode	Implement safety plan quickly and with discretion.
	Consider appeasing abuser briefly (if this does not cause a danger) so that safety plan may be implemented.
	Use of self-protective behaviors such as a weapon should be considered with the utmost caution.
After violent or abusive episode	Recognize that family violence is a chronic problem that usually recurs and escalates.
	Change locks as soon as possible.
	Strongly consider order of protection.
	Let neighbors and landlord know that abusive individual no longer lives in the home.

SPECIAL SITUATIONS

Elder mistreatment may also occur in institutional settings. The physician and nurse have roles in detecting these cases as well. Substantial regulatory safeguards have been progressively enacted since the 1970s to protect residents of long-term care facilities. These safeguards include mandatory criminal background checks of all employees, ombudsman programs to adjudicate complaints of mistreatment, and components of the omnibus budget reconciliation act of 1987, which includes residents' rights provisions (e.g., minimization of restraints). In some contexts, the failure to create or follow a reasonable plan of care for the long-term care residents may be viewed as abusive or neglectful.

While the focus of elder abuse in long-term care has been on staff abuse of residents, this is probably far less common than in decades past when regulatory scrutiny was lacking. Recently, resident on resident abuse has been identified as a far more common and pervasive problem among nursing home residents. Although there are no prevalence data on the phenomenon, several indirect lines of evidence suggest that it is highly prevalent. For example, more than 50% of nursing aides in long-term care report the personal experience of being physically hit by a resident in the previous year, typically in the course of providing direct care. Given that the prevalence of dementia and associated behavioral disturbance in long-term care facilities is high, it stands to reason that behavior of this type occurs frequently between residents.

Another recent area of interest has been abuse and neglect that occurs in long-term care environments other than nursing homes (e.g., assisted-living and board and care environments), because these facilities generally are under considerably less regulation. Interest in abuse in assisted-living facilities has also grown in recent years as much sicker patients begin to inhabit these institutions; many believe the higher acuity and generally lower levels of staff and supervision are a dangerous admixture in which abuse and neglect are more likely to occur. No data yet exist on the prevalence of abuse, or on the type of abusers, in these settings.

Physicians and other care providers have an important role in the detection of these institutional cases, because they may see potential manifestations of nursing home elder mistreatment in facilities or emergency departments as part of providing customary care. Physicians who suspect institutional abuse have an obligation to immediately report their suspicions to the nursing home ombudsman in their state. A complete list of reporting contact information can be found at http://www.elderabusecenter.org/default.cfm?p=statehotlines.cfm.

SUMMARY

Elder mistreatment is a prevalent problem with many potential manifestations. The epidemiology of injuries and other clinical findings is not completely understood, but this does not preclude the clinician from taking an active role in its detection and management. Studies show elder mistreatment victims to be at substantial independent risk of death and quality-of-life decline. The syndrome should be afforded the same vigilance that health care providers devote to other "traditional" medical problems in geriatrics.

FURTHER READING

Bonnie J, Wallace RB, eds. *Elder Mistreatment: Abuse, Neglect, and Exploitation in an Aging America.* Washington, DC: National Academy of Sciences Press; 2003.

Lachs MS, Pillemer K. Current concepts: abuse and neglect of elderly persons. *N Engl J Med.* 1995;332:437–443.

Lachs MS, Pillemer KA. Elder abuse. *Lancet.* 2004;304:1236–1272.

Lachs MS, Williams C, O'Brien S, et al. Risk factors for reported elder abuse and neglect: a nine-year observational study. *Gerontologist.* 1997;37:469–474.

Lachs MS, Williams CS, O'Brien S, et al. The mortality of elder mistreatment. *JAMA.* 1998;280:428–432.

Leonard R, Tinetti ME, Allore HG, et al. Potentially modifiable resident characteristics that are associated with physical or verbal aggression among nursing home residents with dementia. *Arch Intern Med.* 2006;166:1295–1300.

Pillemer K, Finkelhor D. The prevalence of elder abuse: a random sample survey. *Gerontologist.* 1988;28:51–57.

Tomoko ST, Leonard R, Pontikas J, et al. Resident-to-resident violent incidents in nursing homes. *JAMA.* 2004;291:591–598.

Wiglesworth A, Mosqueda L, Burnight K, et al. Findings from an elder abuse forensic center. *Gerontologist.* 2006;46:277–283.

World Health Organization. *Missing Voices: Views of Older Person on Elder Abuse. A survey of eight countries.* WHO Monograph 2004.

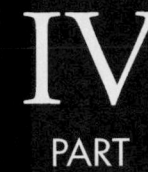

IV

PART

ORGAN SYSTEMS AND DISEASES

Cellular and Neurochemical Aspects of the Aging Human Brain

Mark P. Mattson

Many cellular and molecular aspects of brain aging are shared with other organ systems, including increased oxidative damage to proteins, nucleic acids and membrane lipids, impaired energy metabolism, and the accumulation of intracellular and extracellular protein aggregates. However, as a result of the molecular and structural complexity of neural cells, which express approximately 50 to 100 times more genes than cells in other tissues, there are age-related changes that are unique to the nervous system. For example, complex cellular signal transduction pathways involving neurotransmitters, trophic factors, and cytokines that are involved in regulating neuronal excitability and plasticity are subject to modification by aging. This chapter describes cellular and molecular changes that occur in the brain during aging and how such changes may predispose neurons to degeneration in disorders such as Alzheimer's disease (AD), Parkinson disease (PD), and Huntington disease (HD).

STRUCTURAL CHANGES IN THE AGING BRAIN

All of the major cell types in the brain undergo structural changes during aging. These changes include nerve cell death, dendritic retraction and expansion, synapse loss and remodeling, and glial cell (astrocytes and microglia) reactivity. Such structural changes may result from alterations in cytoskeletal proteins and the deposition of insoluble proteins such as tau and α-synuclein inside of cells and amyloid in the extracellular space. Alterations in cellular signaling pathways that control cell growth and motility may contribute to both adaptive and pathological structural changes in the aging brain.

Cytoskeletal and Synaptic Changes

The cell cytoskeleton consists of polymers of different sizes and protein compositions. The three major types of polymers are actin microfilaments (6 nm in diameter); microtubules (25 nm in diameter), comprising of tubulin; and intermediate filaments (10–15 nm in diameter), which are made of specific intermediate filament proteins that are different in different cell types (e.g., neurofilament proteins in neurons and glial fibrillary acidic protein in astrocytes). To regulate the processes of filament assembly and depolymerization, and to link the cytoskeleton to membranes and other cell structures, neurons and glial cells employ an array of cytoskeleton-associated proteins. For example, neurons express several microtubule-associated proteins (MAPs) that are differentially distributed within the complex architecture of the cells; MAP-2 is present in dendrites but not in the axon, whereas tau is present in axons but not in dendrites. While there are no major changes in the levels of the most abundant cytoskeletal proteins with aging, there are changes in the cytoskeletal organization and in posttranslational modifications of cytoskeletal proteins. For example, increased amounts of phosphorylated tau occur in some brain regions, particularly those involved in learning and memory (e.g., hippocampus and basal forebrain). In addition, there is evidence that calcium-mediated proteolysis of MAP-2 and spectrin (a protein that links actin filaments to membranes) is increased in some neurons during aging. Oxidation of certain cytoskeletal proteins is suggested by studies demonstrating their modification by glycation and covalent binding of the lipid peroxidation product 4-hydroxynonenal (see "Free Radicals and the Aging Brain" later in this chapter). A consistent feature of brain aging in humans and laboratory animals is an increase in levels of glial fibrillary acidic protein, which may represent a reaction to subtle neurodegenerative changes.

Synapses are dynamic structural specializations where neurotransmission and other intercellular signaling events occur. There is considerable evidence for synaptic "remodeling" in the brain as we age, which is likely related to changes in dendritic arbors and neuronal numbers. For example, there may be decreases in synaptic numbers in some brain regions, but these may be offset by increases in the size of the remaining synapses. In other brain regions, no loss of synapses can be discerned.

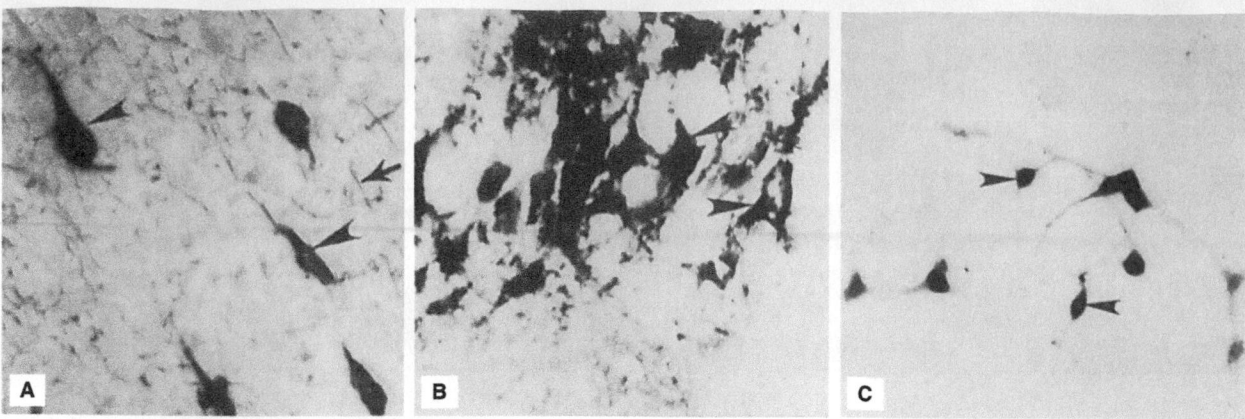

FIGURE 61-1. Neuronal cytoskeletal pathology in Alzheimer's disease is mimicked in experimental systems by insults that increase intracellular calcium levels and induce oxidative stress. (A) Section of hippocampal tissue from an AD patient immunostained with an antibody against the microtubule-associated protein tau. Note strong staining of degenerating "tangle-bearing" neuronal cell bodies (*arrowheads*). (B) Section of hippocampus from an adult rat that had been administered the seizure-inducing excitotoxin kainate 6 hours previously. The section was immunostained with an antibody against the microtubule-associated protein tau. Note strong staining of degenerating neurons (*arrowheads*). (C) Human embryonic cerebral cortical neurons in culture that were left untreated (control) or were exposed for 2 hours to a calcium ionophore. Cells were then stained with an antibody against ubiquitin, a stress-responsive protein present in degenerating neurons in AD.

In contrast to usual aging, striking alterations in the neuronal cytoskeleton and synapses occur in neurodegenerative disorders such as AD, PD, and HD. Neurofibrillary tangles are filamentous accumulations of tau protein that form in the cytoplasm of degenerating neurons (Figure 61-1). Neurons with tangles have a decreased number of microtubules and often exhibit accumulations of MAP-2 and tau in the cell body. Tau is excessively phosphorylated in neurofibrillary tangles, which may result from reduced phosphatase activity as a consequence of oxidation or covalent modification by lipid peroxidation products. In PD, structures called Lewy bodies form in neurons and comprise abnormal accumulations of neurofilaments, with associated MAPs (particularly MAP-1b) and actin-related proteins such as gelsolin. In amyotrophic lateral sclerosis (ALS), lower motor neurons are filled with massive accumulations of neurofilaments that concentrate in proximal regions of the axon. While the specific molecular events involved in formation of the cytoskeletal alterations in different neurodegenerative disorders have not been established, there is increasing evidence for major roles of aberrant elevation of intracellular calcium levels and increased oxidative stress. Conditions that elevate intracellular calcium levels (e.g., exposure to glutamate or calcium ionophores) and induce oxidative stress (e.g., exposure to Fe^{2+} and amyloid β-peptide [$A\beta$], or expression of mutant Cu/ZnSOD) can elicit changes in the cytoskeleton in experimental animal and cell culture models that are similar to those seen in the human disorders (Figures 61-1 and 61-2).

Synapse loss occurs in neurodegenerative disorders and is strongly correlated with clinical symptoms. Accumulating data suggest that

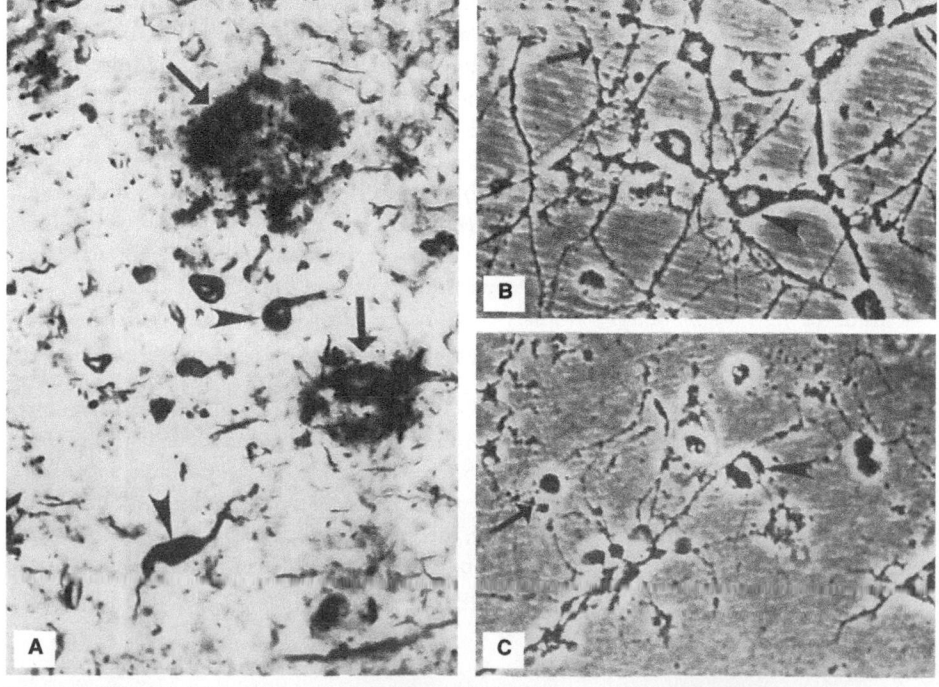

FIGURE 61-2. Histologic and experimental evidence that amyloid deposition plays a role in the neurodegenerative process in Alzheimer's disease. (A) Section of hippocampal tissue from an AD patient immunostained with an antibody against the microtubule-associated protein tau. Note strong staining of degenerating "tangle-bearing" neuronal cell bodies (*arrowheads*) and neurites associated with amyloid plaques (*arrow*). (B and C) Phase-contrast micrographs of cultured rat hippocampal neurons that had been exposed for 24 hours to amyloid β-peptide ($A\beta$) alone (B) or in combination with corticosterone (C). Note that neurites in the culture exposed to $A\beta$ alone are beginning to exhibit signs of damage (*arrow*), while the neuronal cell bodies still appear undamaged (*arrowhead*). Corticosterone exacerbated the damage to neurons exposed to $A\beta$. (See Goodman et al. *J Neurochem.* 1996;66:1836.)

synaptic degeneration, resulting from excitotoxic events localized to synapses, may initiate the neuronal death process in AD, PD, HD, and stroke. Glutamate receptors are highly concentrated in postsynaptic dendritic spines, which represent sites of massive calcium influx during normal physiologic synaptic transmission. Age-related decreases in energy availability and increases in oxidative stress, and disease-specific alterations such as Aβ accumulation in AD and trinucleotide expansions of the huntingtin protein, may render synapses vulnerable to excitotoxic injury (see below).

Vascular Changes

As in other organ systems, vessels that supply blood to the brain are vulnerable to age-related atherosclerosis and arteriosclerosis, which render the vessels susceptible to occlusion or rupture (stroke), a major cause of disability and death in the elderly population. Reduced brain perfusion in the absence of overt stroke may play a role in age-related cognitive dysfunction. Decreased cerebral blood flow occurs with advancing age and is accompanied by declines in cerebral metabolic rate for oxygen and glucose use. Age-related changes in cerebral vasculature are generally similar to those that occur in vessels elsewhere in the body and are therefore likely to result from common cellular and molecular changes, including oxidative damage to vascular endothelial cells and an inflammatory response in which macrophages may penetrate the blood–brain barrier (Figure 61-3).

Age-dependent cerebral vascular changes are strongly linked to heart disease and hypertension. Interestingly, apolipoprotein E polymorphisms are linked to increased risk of both atherosclerosis and AD, with the apolipoprotein E4 increasing the risk. This association suggests that age-related vascular changes may make an important contribution to the neurodegenerative process in AD. Finally,

important transport functions of cells (endothelial cells and astrocytes) that comprise the blood–brain barrier may also be impaired in the aging brain and more so in AD. Many of the same behavioral and dietary approaches now recognized to forestall cardiovascular disease may also forestall cerebrovascular disease; these include engaging in physical and mental activities, a low calorie intake, and a high antioxidant intake.

Amyloid Accumulation

Aβ is a 40- to 42-amino-acid peptide that arises from a much larger membrane-spanning β-amyloid precursor protein (APP). During normal aging, and to a much greater extent in AD, Aβ forms insoluble aggregates (plaques) in the brain parenchyma and vasculature (Figure 61-4).

Amyloid plaques accumulate most heavily in brain regions involved in learning and memory processes such as the hippocampus and entorhinal cortex. In AD, the accumulation of Aβ in the brain is correlated with the amount of neuronal degeneration and with the severity of cognitive impairment. Although the cause(s) of the majority of cases of AD is unknown, some AD cases are caused by mutations in APP, presenilin-1, or presenilin-2; mutations in each

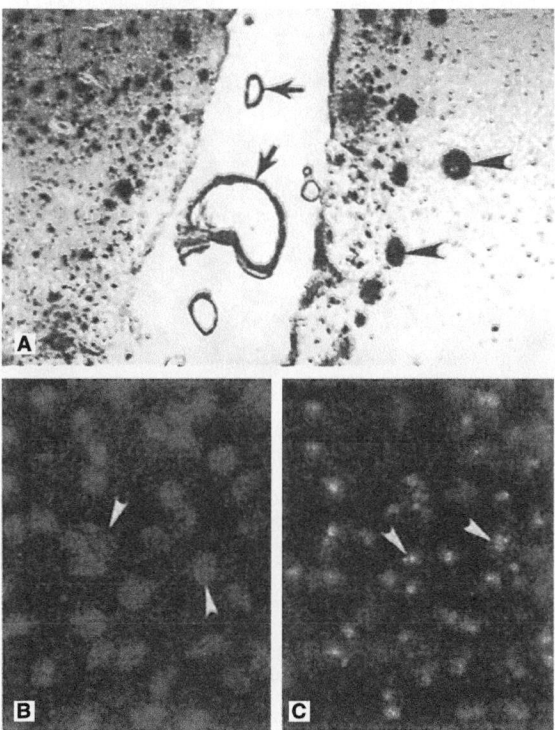

FIGURE 61-4. Amyloid deposits in the brain parenchyma and cerebral vessels: evidence that amyloid damages vascular endothelial cells. (A) Section of hippocampal tissue from an AD patient. The section was immunostained with an antibody against amyloid β-peptide (Aβ). Note numerous Aβ deposits of various sizes in the brain parenchyma (*arrowheads* point to large plaques) and cerebral blood vessels (*arrows*). (B and C) Cultured vascular endothelial cells were exposed for 24 hours to saline (B) or Aβ (C), and were then stained with the fluorescent deoxyribonucleic acid (DNA)-binding dye HOECHST 33342. The nuclear DNA in cells not exposed to Aβ exhibits the normal diffuse uniform distribution, while the chromatin in the cells exposed to Aβ exhibits condensation and fragmentation consistent with apoptotic death. (*Adapted from Blanc EM, Toborek M, Mark RJ, et al. Amyloid β-peptide disrupts barrier and transport functions and induces apoptosis in vascular endothelial cells. J Neurochem. 1997;68:1870.*)

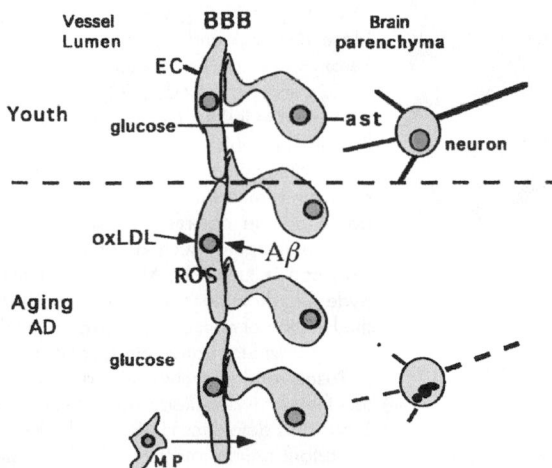

FIGURE 61-3. Adverse effects of aging and Alzheimer's disease on endothelial cells and the blood–brain barrier. Vascular endothelial cells (EC) and associated astrocyte (ast) processes form the blood–brain barrier (BBB), which plays important roles in transporting nutrients (e.g., glucose) into the brain, while at the same time preventing movement of toxic substances and blood cells such as macrophages (MP). With aging, and more so in AD, oxidative damage to endothelial cells results from exposure to oxidized LDL and amyloid β-peptide (Aβ). Oxidative stress impairs transport functions of the EC and promotes penetration of MP into the brain parenchyma. Such compromise of the vasculature results in reduced nutrient availability to neurons and inflammatory processes that promote degeneration of neurons.

of these proteins result in increased production of self-aggregating neurotoxic forms of Aβ. Aβ can be neurotoxic, and can increase neuronal vulnerability to metabolic, excitotoxic, and oxidative insults. The sequence of events involved in Aβ-induced neuronal injury and death may involve induction of membrane lipid peroxidation, which generates a toxic aldehyde called 4-hydroxynonenal that covalently modifies proteins involved in maintenance of cellular ion homeostasis and energy metabolism, including the plasma membrane Na^+/K^+ and Ca^{2+} ATPases (adenosine triphosphatases), glucose transporters, and glutamate transporters. This may lead to excessive elevation of intracellular calcium levels, mitochondrial dysfunction, and a form of cell death called apoptosis. In addition to its likely involvement in the neurodegenerative process, Aβ may also disrupt neurotransmitter signaling pathways. For example, Aβ impairs coupling of muscarinic acetylcholine receptors to their downstream GTP (guanosine triphosphate)-binding effector protein, an action that likely contributes to the well-established deficits in cholinergic signaling pathways in AD. Finally, Aβ may also contribute to vascular damage and inflammatory processes in the aging brain.

FREE RADICALS AND THE AGING BRAIN

A free radical is any molecule with an unpaired electron in its outer orbital; in biological systems, oxygen-based molecules are the predominant free radical species (Figure 61-5). A major oxyradical in cells $O_2^{-\cdot}$ is superoxide ($O_2^{-\cdot}$), which is generated during the mitochondrial electron transport process; superoxide dismutases (Mn-SOD and Cu/ZnSOD) eliminate $O_2^{-\cdot}$ by converting it to hydrogen peroxide (H_2O_2). H_2O_2 can be converted to hydroxyl radical (OH•) via the Fenton reaction, which is catalyzed by Fe^{2+} and Cu^+. Peroxynitrite ($ONOO^-$) arises from the interaction of nitric oxide (NO) with $O_2^{-\cdot}$; calcium influx is a major stimulus for NO production. While OH• and $ONOO^-$ can cause direct damage to proteins and deoxyribonucleic acid (DNA), their major means of damaging cells is by attacking fatty acids in membranes and initiating a process called lipid peroxidation. Studies of aging have provided compelling evidence that there is an increase in production and accumulation of oxyradicals in essentially all tissues in the body during the aging process, including in the brain.

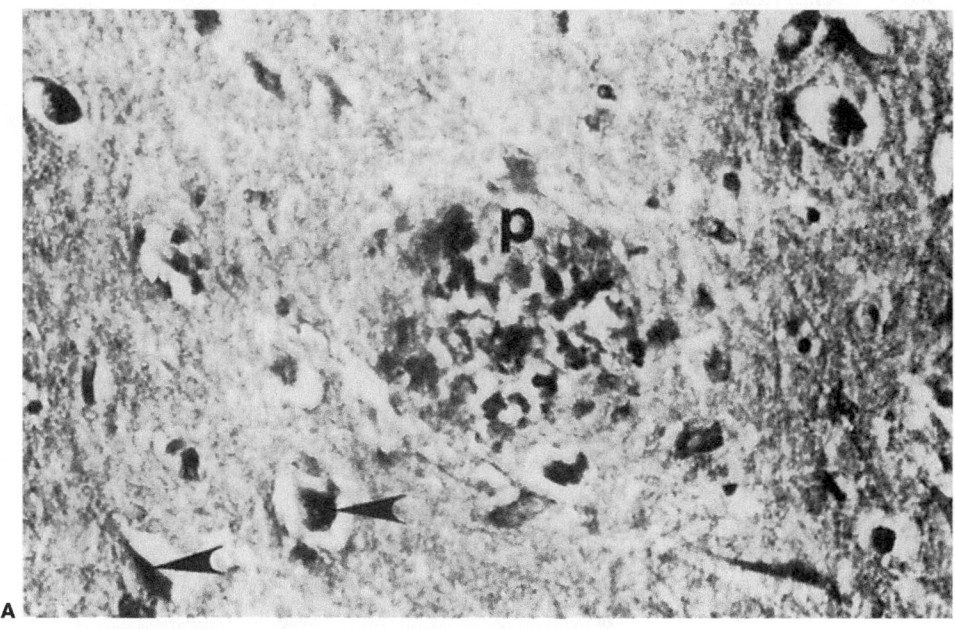

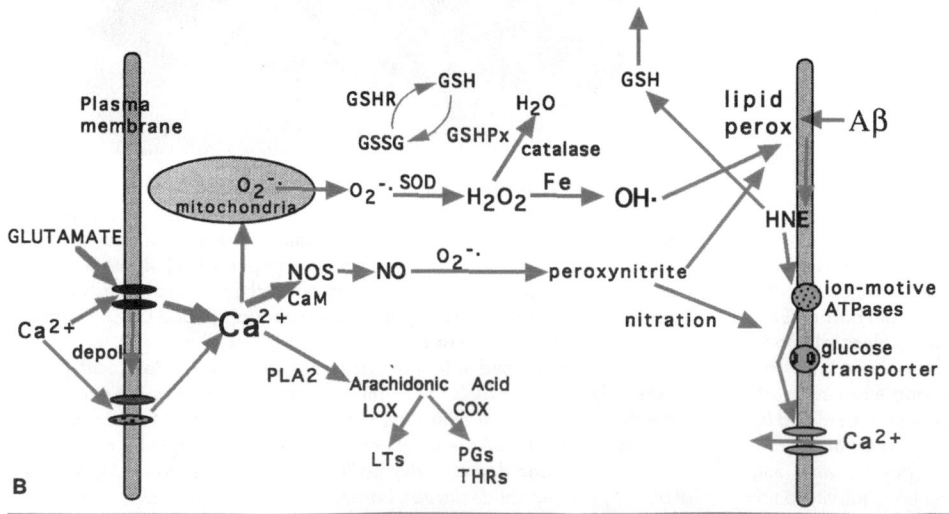

FIGURE 61-5. Possible sources of oxidative stress contributing to dysfunction and degeneration of neurons in aging and Alzheimer's disease. (A) Section of hippocampal tissue from an AD patient. The section was immunostained with an antibody that recognizes lipid peroxides that are by-products of membrane lipid peroxidation. Note immunoreactivity associated with neuritic plaques (p) and neurofibrillary tangles (*arrowheads*). (B) The major cellular source of reactive oxygen species in neurons is mitochondria where $O_2^{-\cdot}$ is generated during the electron transport process. The superoxide dismutase enzymes (SOD) convert $O_2^{-\cdot}$ to H_2O_2. Fe^{2+} catalyzes the production of OH• from H_2O_2, while glutathione peroxidase (GSHPx) and catalase detoxify H_2O_2. Peroxynitrite can be formed by the interaction of $O_2^{-\cdot}$ with nitric oxide (NO). Both OH•, and peroxynitrite induce membrane lipid peroxidation (MLP), which may occur in the plasma membrane, mitochondrial membranes, and endoplasmic reticulum (ER) membranes. During aging and in age-related neurodegenerative disorders, agents such as amyloid β-peptide (Aβ) can induce MLP. MLP liberates the aldehyde 4-hydroxynonenal (HNE), which impairs the function of membrane transporters (glucose and glutamate transporters, and ion-motive ATPases) and ion channels, and thereby alters their activities. Reduced glutathione (GSH) binds and detoxifies HNE, thereby serving an important neuroprotective role. The antiapoptotic gene product Bcl-2 may act, in part, by suppressing MLP in plasma, mitochondrial, and ER membranes. Elevation of intracellular calcium levels, as induced by glutamate, promotes oxyradical production and MLP by inducing NO and $O_2^{-\cdot}$ production, and by activating phospholipases resulting in production of arachidonic acid, which is then acted upon by cyclooxygenases (COX) and lipoxygenases (LOX). *(Modified from Mattson MP. Trends Neurosci. 1997;20:395.)*

Lipid Peroxidation

Levels of lipid peroxidation products such as lipid peroxides and 4-hydroxynonenal are significantly elevated in the brain parenchyma and cerebrospinal fluid in AD (see Figure 61-5). Immunohistochemical analyses of brain tissue from AD and PD patients, and spinal cord tissue from ALS patients, using antibodies directed against 4-hydroxynonenal adducts revealed increased levels of 4-hydroxynonenal in association with degenerating neurons and neuritic plaques suggesting a role for this aldehyde in the neurodegenerative process. Studies of cell culture and animal models of AD and ALS show that lipid peroxidation can impair the function of the plasma membrane glucose and glutamate transporters and renders neurons vulnerable to excitotoxicity and apoptosis. Administration of antioxidants such as vitamin E to cultured cells and transgenic mice expressing mutations that cause AD or ALS can retard the neurodegenerative process, suggesting a causal role for lipid peroxidation in these diseases.

Protein Oxidation

Levels of protein oxidation, measured as protein carbonyls, are significantly elevated in the brains of aged rodents, and such age-associated protein oxidation can be prevented by administration of antioxidants. Studies of membrane structure have provided evidence for oxidation-related alterations in membrane protein conformation in old rodents. Studies of brain tissues of patients with AD and PD have revealed increased levels of protein oxidation in vulnerable brain regions and, in particular, in degenerating neurons. Oxidation of proteins impairs their function and is therefore a likely contributor to age-related cellular dysfunction and neuronal degeneration. Progressive addition of sugar residues to many different proteins occurs during the aging process. This process, called glycation, may promote oxidative stress in cells. Two proteins that have been shown to be heavily glycated in AD are $A\beta$ and tau, the major components of plaques and neurofibrillary tangles, respectively.

DNA Damage

Very little nuclear DNA damage occurs in the nervous system during usual aging, but DNA damage may contribute to the pathogenesis of neurodegenerative disorders. Damage to nuclear DNA in striatum of HD patients, and in hippocampus and vulnerable cortical regions of AD patients, has been documented. Specifically, levels of 8-hydroxyguanosine are increased. This DNA damage may be caused by oxyradicals, with hydroxyl radical and peroxynitrite being the major culprits. Progressive oxidative damage to mitochondrial DNA occurs during aging, and may be exacerbated in neurodegenerative disorders. Mitochondrial DNA is particularly prone to damage because this organelle is the site where the vast majority of free radicals are generated and because cells do not possess effective systems for repair of damaged mitochondrial DNA. Damage to mitochondrial DNA can lead to failure of electron transport and reduced adenosine triphosphate (ATP) production. Moreover, the important calcium sequestering function of mitochondria may be compromised as the result of age-related DNA damage, which may increase neuronal vulnerability to excitotoxicity and apoptosis.

Mechanisms that Promote Oxidative Stress in Aging and Neurodegenerative Disorders

Mitochondria-derived oxyradicals are likely to play a central role in the cumulative oxidative damage to various cellular constituents that accrues with aging. Age-related impairments in energy availability and metabolism may contribute to an acceleration of oxyradical production with aging. The importance of mitochondrial oxyradical production in aging, in general, is underscored by recent studies of the mechanism whereby caloric restriction extends life span in rodents and nonhuman primates. Levels of cellular oxidative stress (as indicated by oxidation of proteins, lipids, and DNA) are decreased in many different non-neural tissues of rats and mice maintained on a calorie-restricted diet (30–40% reduction in calories). Recent studies suggest that levels of oxidative stress are also reduced in the brains of calorie-restricted rodents. The current dogma for the underlying mechanism is that reduced mitochondrial metabolism because of reduced energy availability results in a net decrease in mitochondrial ROS production over time, and hence less radical-mediated cellular damage. Thus, one factor contributing to brain aging is simply the constant production of oxyradicals and resultant progressive damage to cellular components.

In addition to the oxyradical damage that accrues with usual aging, there are specific initiators of oxidative stress that appear to play key roles in different age-related neurodegenerative disorders. For example, in AD the increased generation and accumulation of $A\beta$ may be a pivotal event that enhances oxidative stress in neurons. There is evidence that increased levels of Fe^{2+} in the substantia nigra plays a role in the degeneration of dopaminergic neurons in PD. The damage to neurons in the brain of individuals who had a stroke is the result of a combination of factors including excessive calcium influx and the presence of blood components such as Fe^{2+} and thrombin. In HD, the presence of trinucleotide repeats in the huntingtin protein may induce oxidative stress in striatal neurons by a yet-to-be-determined mechanism.

ALTERATIONS IN ENERGY METABOLISM AND MITOCHONDRIAL FUNCTION IN THE AGING BRAIN

During the aging process, changes that occur in cerebral blood vessels, as well as in the neural cells themselves, appear to result in reduced energy availability to neurons. These age-related changes may be accelerated in several different neurodegenerative disorders including AD and PD.

Cerebral Metabolism

Reduced glucose use, and changes in enzymes involved in energy metabolism, may occur during normal aging, but are not dramatic. Studies of aging rodents document decreases in glucose and ketone body oxidation, oxygen consumption, local cerebral glucose use, and glycolytic compounds (e.g., fructose-1,6-diphosphate). Additional studies show that brain cells in older animals exhibit increased vulnerability to metabolic stresses. Incorporation of glucose into amino acids declines in the brains of aging mice, and older people are much more vulnerable to metabolic encephalopathy than are young people. In contrast to normal aging, activities of several enzymes involved in energy metabolism are severely reduced in AD brain tissues. Three such enzymes, which are involved in mitochondrial oxidative metabolism, are the pyruvate dehydrogenase complex, the α-ketoglutarate dehydrogenase complex, and cytochrome c oxidase. These defects may result from age-associated oxidative damage to the DNA encoding these enzyme systems and/or reduced activity of the proteins in these systems.

Another factor that may contribute to reduced neuronal energy metabolism is impairment of the function of glucose transporter proteins in neuronal membranes. Studies of postmortem brain tissues of patients with AD document reduced levels of glucose transporters, and experimental studies of cultured hippocampal neurons and synaptosomes show that insults relevant to the pathogenesis of

AD (exposure to Aβ and oxyradical-generating agents) can impair glucose transport (Figure 61-6). Impairment of glucose transport and mitochondrial dysfunction would be expected to lead to ATP depletion and render neurons vulnerable to excitotoxicity.

Mitochondrial Function

Age-related structural changes in synaptic mitochondria have been reported and include a decrease in numbers and increase in size. During normal aging, levels of mitochondrial protein synthesis are unchanged. However, decreases in synthesis of specific mitochondrial proteins that are components of the electron transport chain occur in aging rodents. Damage to mitochondrial DNA progressively increases in somatic cells during the aging process, with the most pronounced damage occurring in postmitotic cells such as neurons. Mitochondrial dysfunction has been linked to several neurodegenerative disorders (Figure 61-7). In PD, there are marked decreases in complex I and α-ketoglutarate dehydrogenase activities. Exposure of cultured dopaminergic neurons to insults relevant to the pathogenesis of PD (e.g., MPTP and Fe^{2+}) cause mitochondrial dysfunction. In AD, cytochrome c oxidase and α-ketoglutarate dehydrogenase activity levels are markedly reduced in vulnerable brain regions. Interestingly, mitochondrial deficits are also observed in non-neuronal cells, including platelets and fibroblasts, of AD patients. When mitochondria from platelets of AD patients are introduced into cultured neuroblastoma cells, levels of oxidative stress are increased suggesting an important contribution of mitochondrial alterations to the increased oxidative stress present in neurons in AD brain. Mitochondrial alterations in neurons have been documented in studies of mouse models of AD (APP and presenilin mutant mice), PD (α-synuclein mutant mice), HD (huntingtin mutant mice), and stroke (middle cerebral artery occlusion).

NEURONAL ION HOMEOSTASIS IN THE AGING BRAIN

Among the properties of neurons that set them apart from many other cell types is their excitability, which is regulated by a complex array of neurotransmitters and ion channels. Neurons express voltage-dependent sodium channels, as well as multiple types of calcium and potassium channels that are differentially expressed among neuronal populations, and are segregated in different cellular compartments (e.g., L-type calcium channels in the cell body, N-type calcium channels in the dendrites, and T-type calcium channels in presynaptic terminals). In addition, neurons possess ion-motive ATPases that play critical roles in re-establishing ion gradients following neuronal stimulation. A variety of age-related alterations in electrophysiological parameters of neurons has been described in rodents and, in some cases, in humans, including increased thresholds for induction of action potentials in cranial nerves, increased after hyperpolarizations in hippocampal neurons, and impaired long-term potentiation of synaptic transmission in the hippocampus. Moreover, a generalized decrease in neuronal inhibition appears to occur during the aging process.

The calcium ion plays fundamental roles in regulating neuronal survival and plasticity in both the developing and adult nervous system. Calcium mediates the effects of neurotransmitters and

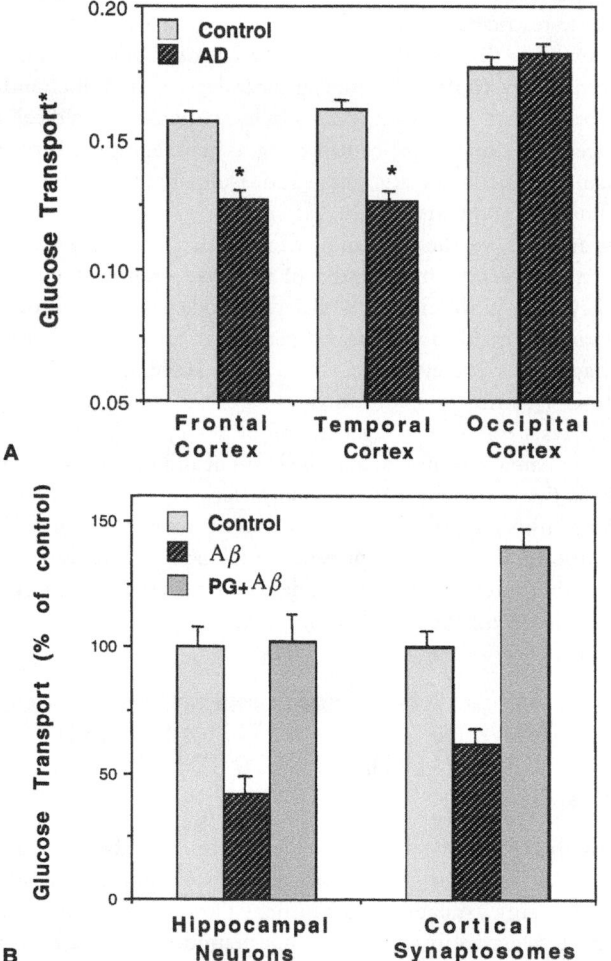

FIGURE 61-6. Evidence for reduced glucose transport in Alzheimer's disease. (A) Levels of glucose uptake into different brain regions of the patients with Alzheimer's disease and age-matched control subjects were quantified by dynamic positron emission tomography using [^{18}F]-fluorodeoxyglucose. Values are the rate constant K_1 expressed in mL/g/min and reflect glucose transport across the blood–brain barrier and into brain cells. *$p \leq 0.05$ compared to corresponding value for control subjects. (B) Cultured embryonic rat hippocampal neurons, or cortical synaptosomes from adult rats, were pretreated with vehicle or the antioxidant propyl gallate (PG), and were then exposed for 2 hours to saline (control) or Aβ. Glucose transport was quantified. Note that Aβ caused a decrease in glucose transport, and that PG blocked the effect of Aβ. (Part A data from Jagust et al. J Cereb Blood Flow Metab. 1991;11:323. Part B data from Mark et al. J Neurosci. 1997;17:1046, and Keller et al. J Neurochem. 1997;69:273.)

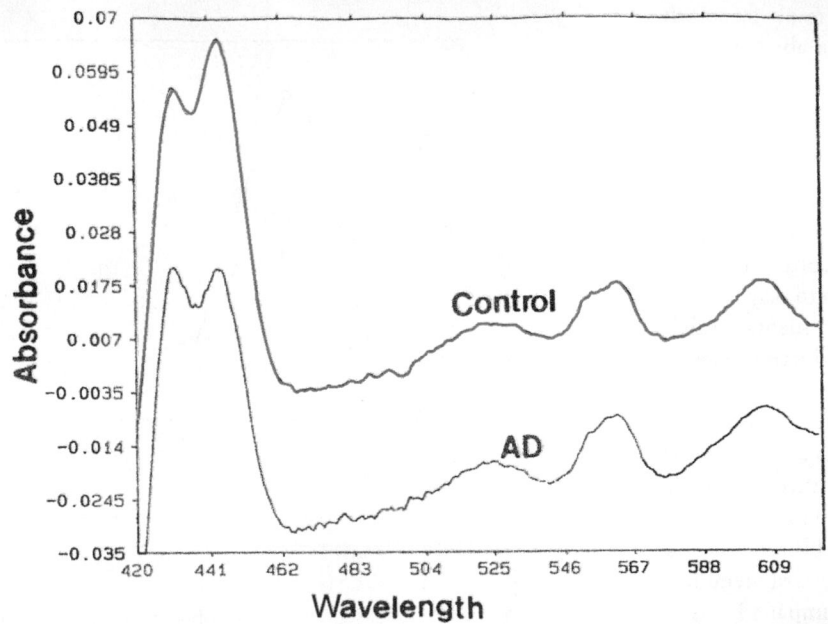

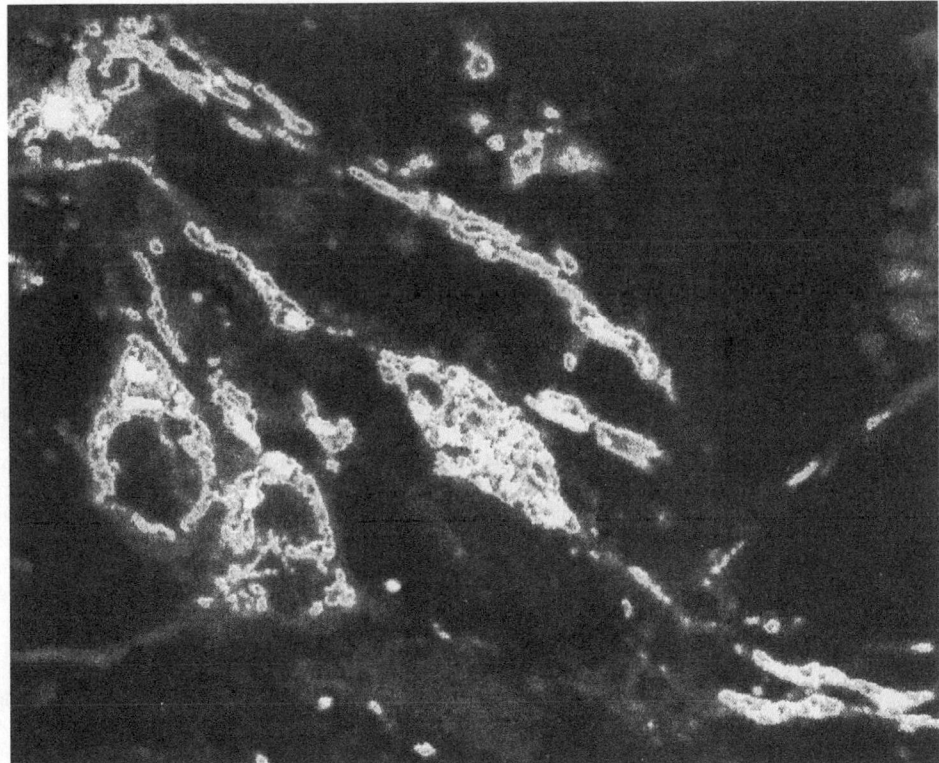

FIGURE 61-7. Evidence for mitochondrial dysfunction neurodegenerative disorders. (A) Reduced-oxidized difference spectra in isolated brain mitochondria from control and Alzheimer's disease (AD) patients. The spectra reflect levels of electron transport function in the mitochondria. Note reduced levels of cytochromes b, c_1, and aa_3 in mitochondria from the AD patients. (B) Confocal laser scanning microscope image of mitochondrial reactive oxygen species levels (dihydrorhodamine 123 fluorescence) in cultured rat hippocampal neuron that had been exposed to amyloid β-peptide for 4 hours. Note high levels of fluorescence in mitochondria indicating the presence of extensive mitochondrial oxidative stress. *(Part A adapted from Parker et al. Neurology. 1994;44:1090. Part B Mark et al. Brain Res. 1997;756:205.)*

neurotrophic factors on neurite outgrowth, synaptogenesis, and cell survival in many different regions of the developing nervous system, and in the adult nervous system, calcium regulates neurotransmitter release from presynaptic terminals and postsynaptic changes associated with learning and memory processes. Aging may result in decreases in the activity of the plasma membrane calcium ATPase and in levels of calcium-binding proteins, while increasing calcium influx through voltage-dependent channels and increasing the activation of calcium-dependent proteases. The factors that promote impaired calcium homeostasis in neurons in aging and age-related

neurodegenerative disorders likely include increased levels of oxidative stress and metabolic compromise (see above).

NEUROTRANSMITTER SIGNALING IN THE AGING BRAIN

A number of alterations in different neurotransmitter systems have been documented in studies of aging rodents, and in analyses of brain tissues from humans with age-related neurodegenerative disorders. While some of these alterations likely result from neuronal degeneration, others appear to occur in the absence of cell injury.

Cholinergic Systems

Acetylcholine is employed as a neurotransmitter in select populations of neurons in the brain, prominent among which are basal forebrain neurons that innervate widespread regions of neocortex and to the hippocampus; these cholinergic neurons are known to play key roles in learning and memory processes in humans and rodents. Deficits in one or more aspects of cholinergic signal transduction may occur with aging including choline transport, acetylcholine synthesis, acetylcholine release, and coupling of muscarinic receptors to their GTP-binding effector proteins. Cholinergic deficits are much more severe in patients with AD and also differ qualitatively from the changes observed during normal aging. Particularly striking is a reduced ability of muscarinic agonists to activate GTP-binding proteins in cortical neurons (Figure 61-8). Increased levels of membrane lipid peroxidation in neurons may contribute to impaired cholinergic signaling; for example, $A\beta$, Fe^{2+}, and the lipid peroxidation product 4-hydroxynonenal can impair coupling of muscarinic receptors to the GTP-binding protein G_{q11} (see Figure 61-8).

Dopaminergic Systems

Very prominent reductions in both pre- and postsynaptic aspects of dopaminergic neurotransmission occur during brain aging. Decreases in dopamine levels and dopamine transporter levels in the striatum occur with advancing age, and there is an age-related decrease in levels of D_2 receptor-binding sites in striatum. As with cholinergic signal transduction, there also appears to be an age-related impairment of coupling of dopamine receptors to their GTP-binding effector proteins. The contribution of oxidative stress to changes in dopaminergic signaling has not been established, although the prominent role of oxyradicals in the pathogenesis of PD argue that similar oxidative processes contribute to dopaminergic dysfunction during normal aging. These changes in dopaminergic signaling likely play a role in age-related deficits in motor control and may explain the fact that the elderly are susceptible to extrapyramidal effects of dopamine receptor antagonist drugs.

Monoaminergic Systems

Norepinephrine and serotonin are the major monoamine neurotransmitters in the brain. Noradrenergic neurons are located primarily in the locus ceruleus and serotonergic neurons in the raphe nucleus; both types of neurons project to widespread regions of cerebral cortex. There are several subtypes of receptors for norepinephrine, which each couple to GTP-binding proteins. There are also several subtypes of serotonin receptors, some of which couple to GTP-binding proteins and others of which are ligand-gated ion channels. There appear to be increased levels of norepinephrine with aging in some brain regions, while levels of α_2-adrenergic receptors may decrease in cerebral cortex with advancing age. Levels of serotonin may decrease in the striatum, hippocampus, and cerebral cortex. Age-related decreases in levels of evoked serotonin release and of serotonin binding sites have been reported, and may contribute to affective disorders such as depression.

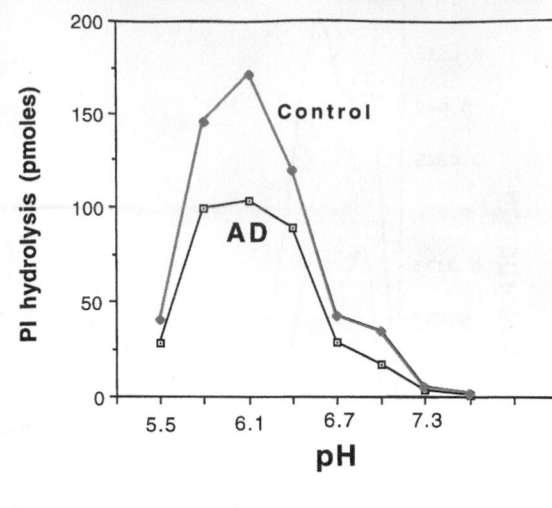

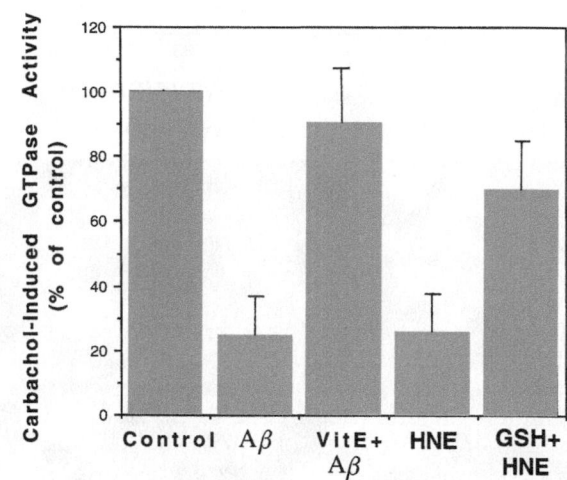

FIGURE 61-8. Impact of oxidative stress and Alzheimer's disease on muscarinic cholinergic signal transduction. (A) Levels of [^{3}H]-PI hydrolysis induced by GTPγS plus carbachol (muscarinic acetylcholine receptor agonist) in membranes from brains of AD patients and age-matched controls. Note reduced levels of ligand-induced PI hydrolysis in the membranes from the AD patients. (B) $A\beta$ and membrane lipid peroxidation impair coupling of muscarinic receptors to the GTP-binding protein G_{q11} in cultured cerebral cortical neurons. Cultured rat cortical neurons were exposed for 3 to 4 hours to vehicle (control), $A\beta$, vitamin E (VitE) plus $A\beta$, 4-hydroxynonenal (HNE), or glutathione ethyl ester (GSH) plus HNE. Membranes were then isolated and levels of carbachol-induced GTPase activity were quantified. Note that $A\beta$ and HNE impaired coupling of the muscarinic receptors to the GTP-binding protein, and that the antioxidants vitamin E and GSH attenuated the impairments. (Part A adapted from Jope et al. Neurobiol Aging. 1997;15:221. Part B data from Kelly et al. Proc Natl Acad Sci U S A. 1996;93:6753, and Blanc EM et al. Amyloid β-peptide disrupts barrier and transport functions and induces apoptosis in vascular endothelial cells. J Neurochem. 1997;68:1870.)

Amino Acid Transmitter Systems

The amino acid glutamate is the major excitatory neurotransmitter in the human brain. Glutamate stimulates inotropic receptors that flux calcium and sodium; excessive activation of ionotropic glutamate receptors may play a role in the degeneration of neurons in several age-related disorders including stroke, AD, PD, and HD. Levels of ionotropic glutamate receptors were reported to decrease with aging, but these decreases may be the result of degeneration of the neurons expressing the receptors. The contribution of dysfunction of glutamatergic transmission, in the absence of neuronal death, to age- and disease-related deficits in brain function is unknown. The major inhibitory neurotransmitter in the human brain is γ-aminobutyric acid (GABA). Relatively little information is available concerning the impact of aging on GABAergic systems, although levels of glutamate decarboxylase and GABA-A binding sites may be decreased. Interestingly, GABAergic interneurons are typically spared in various neurodegenerative disorders including AD.

NEUROENDOCRINE CHANGES IN THE AGING BRAIN

A variety of age-related alterations in neuroendocrine systems has been documented. Of particular importance for human brain aging and neurodegenerative disorders are changes in levels of steroid hormones, particularly glucocorticoids and estrogens. There is considerable evidence for age-related alterations in the diurnal regulation of circulating glucocorticoid levels, and an increase in the mean level. Moreover, regulation of the hypothalamic–pituitary–adrenal axis is altered in AD patients, such that plasma levels of glucocorticoids are increased. Increased levels of glucocorticoids, including those induced by physiological or psychological stress, can increase the vulnerability of hippocampal neurons to injury and death induced by ischemic and excitotoxic insults, suggesting that glucocorticoids may have a negative impact on the outcome of both acute (e.g., stroke) and chronic (e.g., AD) age-related neurologic disorders. Estrogen (17β-estradiol) may have a beneficial effect on brain aging. Epidemiologic studies suggest a reduced risk of AD in postmenopausal women who take estrogen replacement therapy (Figure 61-9), and elderly women who take estrogens perform better on cognitive tasks. Animal and cell culture studies have shown that 17β-estradiol can protect neurons from being damaged and killed by insults relevant to ischemia and AD including glucose deprivation, exposure to Aβ, and expression of AD-linked presenilin mutations (see Figure 61-9).

IMMUNOLOGIC FACTORS IN BRAIN AGING

While the blood–brain barrier limits access of circulating lymphocytes to neurons in the brain, it is becoming increasingly evident that the brain is by no means devoid of immune responses. The brain possesses resident immune effector cells called microglia that may respond to age- and disease-related neurodegenerative processes. Some data suggest that a decline in peripheral immune function during aging may lead to an autoimmune-like phenomenon in the brain wherein microglia are activated. Inflammatory processes are associated with, and contribute to, the neurodegenerative process in AD and other age-related neurodegenerative disorders; these include activation of microglia in the affected brain regions, increased local cytokine production in association with the neuropathological changes, and activation of components of the complement cascade system. Moreover, epidemiological and clinical data suggest that anti-inflammatory agents may suppress the development of AD. Collectively, the emerging data suggest a role for chronic inflammatory reactions in the pathogenesis of at least some neurodegenerative disorders.

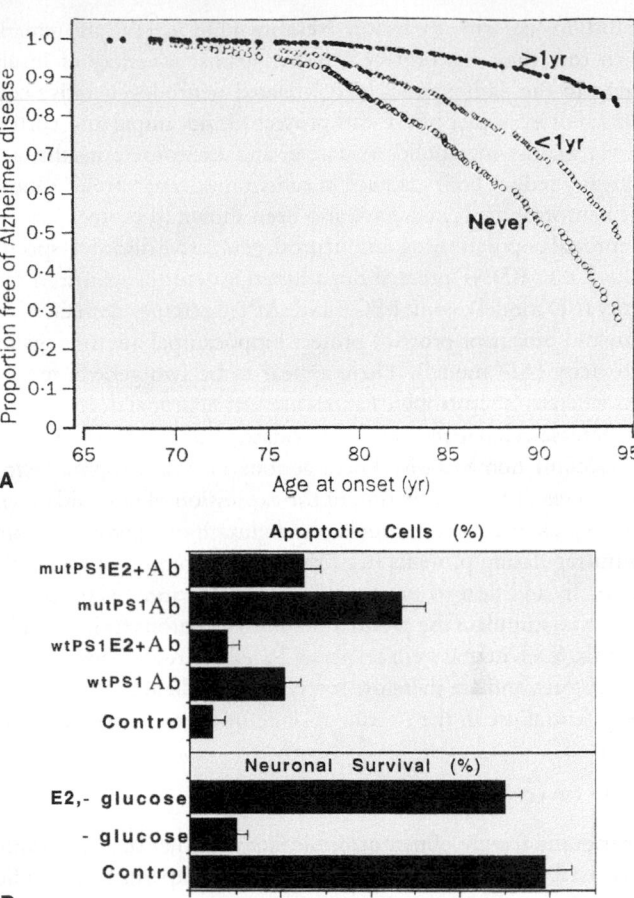

FIGURE 61-9. Estrogen protects women against Alzheimer's disease, and protects cultured neurons against genetic and environmental factors linked to Alzheimer's disease. (A) Plot of proportion of the study group free of Alzheimer's disease as a function of age in postmenopausal women receiving estrogen replacement therapy more than 1 yr, less than 1 yr, or not at all. (B) The lower portion of the graph shows data from cultured rat hippocampal neurons that were deprived of glucose (−glucose) for 24 hours in the absence or presence of 17β-estradiol (E2); control cultures were not deprived of glucose. The percentage of neurons surviving was quantified. Note that 17β-estradiol largely prevented neuronal death. The upper portion of the graph shows data from cultured PC12 cells overexpressing either wild-type presenilin-1 (wtPS1) or mutant presenilin-1 (mutPS1). Cultures were exposed to either Aβ alone or in combination with 17β-estradiol (E2); control cultures were not exposed to Aβ. The percentage of cells undergoing apoptotic cell death was quantified. Note that apoptosis was enhanced in cells expressing mutant PS-1, and that 17β-estradiol largely prevented the apoptosis. (Part A adapted from Tang et al. Lancet. 1996;348:429. Part B adapted from Goodman et al. J Neurochem. 1996;66:1836.)

NEUROTROPHIC FACTORS IN THE AGING BRAIN

Neurotrophic Factors Counteract Age- and Disease-Related Neurodegeneration

Cells in the nervous system produce a variety of proteins that serve the function of promoting neuronal survival and growth, and protecting the neurons against injury and death. Examples of such "neurotrophic factors" include nerve growth factor, basic fibroblast growth factor (bFGF), brain-derived neurotrophic factor (BDNF), and insulin-like growth factor. Neurotrophic factors are remarkable in that they can protect neurons against a variety of insults relevant to the pathogenesis of age-related neurodegenerative conditions. For example, bFGF can protect hippocampal and cortical neurons against metabolic, oxidative, and excitotoxic insults, and can greatly reduce brain damage in rodent models of stroke. One or more neurotrophic factors have also been shown to protect particular neuronal populations against neurodegenerative disorder–specific insults. Thus, BDNF protects dopaminergic neurons against MPTP toxicity (PD model), while bFGF and sAPP (secretory domain of the β-amyloid precursor protein) protect hippocampal neurons against Aβ toxicity (AD model). There appear to be two general mechanisms whereby neurotrophic factors prevent neuronal degeneration; they increase cellular resistance to oxidative stress and stabilize cellular calcium homeostasis. These actions of neurotrophic factors appear to result from induction of the expression of antioxidant enzymes (e.g., superoxide dismutases and glutathione peroxidase) and calcium-regulating proteins (e.g., the calcium-binding protein calbindin). In addition to preserving existing neurons, neurotrophic factors may stimulate the production of new neurons from so-called stem cells. Such neural stem cells may be able to replace lost or damaged neurons, and are therefore receiving considerable attention for their potential use in the treatment of neurodegenerative disorders.

"Use It or Lose It"

An intriguing feature of neurotrophic factors is that their expression is increased by activity in neuronal circuits. Experimental studies in cell culture and in vivo show that such activity-dependent production of neurotrophic factors plays a major role in promoting neuronal survival and neurite outgrowth. Rearing of rodents in an "intellectually enriched" environment results in expansion of dendritic arbors and increased numbers of synapses in hippocampus and certain regions of cerebral cortex. Moreover, epidemiologic data suggest that humans with "active" minds have a reduced risk for developing AD as they age. When taken together with data showing that neurotrophic factors can protect brain neurons against insults relevant to usual brain aging and neurodegenerative disorders (oxidative, metabolic, and excitotoxic insults), these findings suggest a "use it or lose it" scenario of brain aging in which brain activity induces expression of neurotrophic factors that, in turn, promote neuronal growth and plasticity (Figure 61-10).

GENETIC FACTORS IN BRAIN AGING AND NEURODEGENERATIVE DISORDERS

Longevity Genes

Individuals inherit two apolipoprotein E alleles, of which there are three isoforms (E2, E3, and E4). The E2 allele has been linked to increased life span and reduced incidence of AD; this "longevity gene" may act, in part, by reducing atherosclerotic processes in the vasculature. Another possible longevity gene is that encoding an isoform of angiotensin-converting enzyme, although its mechanistic links to aging are unclear. Finally, the multigene major histocompatability system appears to influence life span, and may act by sustaining functions of the immune system.

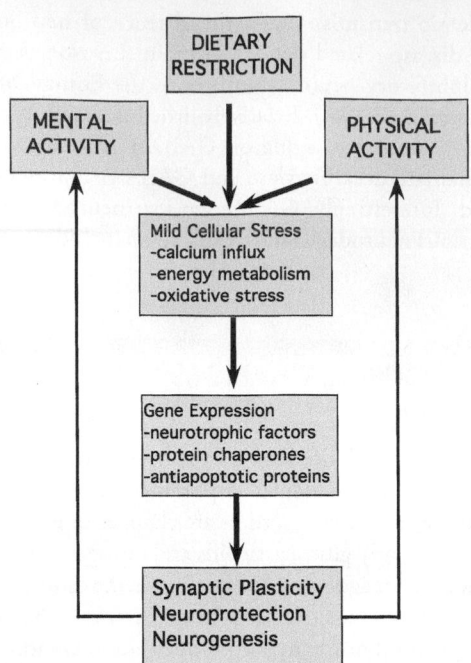

FIGURE 61-10. Mechanisms whereby dietary restriction and mental and physical activities promote successful brain aging. Dietary restriction and stimulation of activity in neuronal circuits by mental and physical activities induce mild stress in neurons as the result of reduced energy availability, calcium influx, and oxidative stress. The neurons respond to the stress by upregulating the expression of genes that encode proteins that promote neuronal plasticity and survival including neurotrophic factors, heat shock proteins, and antiapoptotic proteins. These changes increase the resistance of neurons to age-related diseases by promoting synaptic plasticity, cell survival, and neurogenesis.

Disorder-Specific Genes

Considerable progress has been made in identifying genetic factors that play roles in AD. Three different genes have been identified in which mutations cause early-onset autosomal dominant familial AD (Figure 61-11). Mutations in the APP gene on chromosome 21 are located immediately adjacent to the Aβ sequence. Expression of mutant APP in cultured cells and transgenic mice results in an increase in production of Aβ and a decrease in production of sAPPα. The increase in Aβ may promote plaque formation and associated neurotoxicity. The decrease in sAPPα levels may also play an important role in the neurodegenerative consequences of APP mutations, because sAPPα normally promotes neuronal survival and plasticity and can protect neurons against excitotoxic and oxidative injury. The two other genes causally linked to early onset familial AD are called presenilin-1 (PS-1) and presenilin-2 (PS-2). PS-1 is located in chromosome 14 and PS-2 is located in chromosome 1. PS-1 and PS-2 are integral membrane proteins localized in the endoplasmic reticulum of neurons throughout the brain. Studies of cultured cells and transgenic mice expressing PS-1 mutations have shown that the mutations increase Aβ production and sensitize neurons to death induced by metabolic and oxidative insults. The pathogenic action of presenilin mutations may involve perturbed regulation of endoplasmic reticulum calcium.

Some cases of PD are inherited and have an early age of disease onset. Mutations in several different genes have been shown to cause inherited PD including α-synuclein (PARK1), LRRK (PARK8;

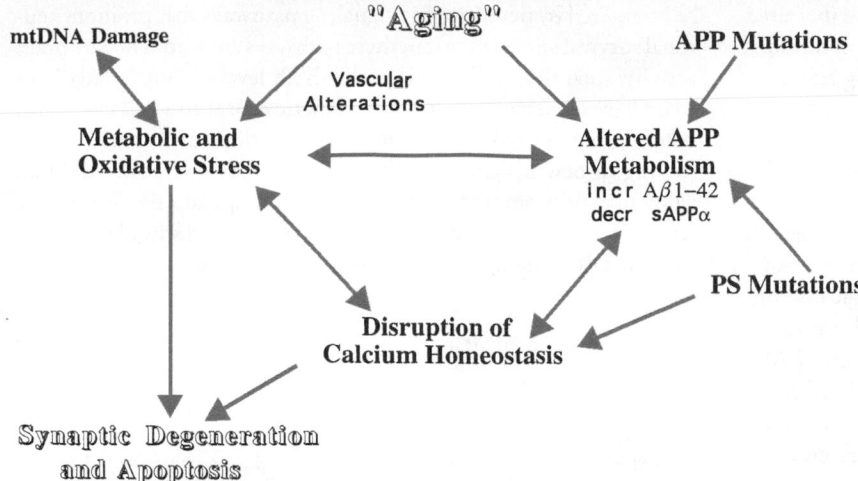

FIGURE 61-11. Interactions of aging and genetic factors in the pathogenesis of neurodegenerative disorders: Alzheimer's disease as an example. The aging process is associated with increases in cellular oxidative stress and metabolic impairment. Metabolic and oxidative stress disrupt neuronal calcium homeostasis and promote excitotoxic synaptic degeneration and apoptotic cell death. Mutations in the β-amyloid precursor protein (APP) and presenilins (PS) result in altered proteolytic processing of APP, increased production of amyloid β-peptide (Aβ1–42) and decreased sAPPα production. The result of these mutations is impaired calcium homeostasis and increased age-related oxidative stress. Vascular alterations contribute to reduced energy availability to neurons and increased oxidative stress. (Data from Mattson Mol Cell Biol. 2000;1:120.)

leucine-rich repeat kinase 2) and UCHL1 (PARK5; ubiquitin C-terminal hydrolase L1), Parkin (PARK2), DJ-1 (PARK7) and PINK1 (PARK6; PTEN induced putative kinase 1). Mutations in the gene encoding the mitochondrial serine protease HTRA2 (PARK13; high temperature requirement A2) have also been linked to PD in several families. Impaired proteasomal degradation of α-synuclein and mitochondrial dysfunction are key alterations caused by the different PD-causing mutations.

Several age-related inherited neurodegenerative conditions are caused by trinucleotide repeats in specific genes. The best known such disorder is HD in which polyglutamine repeats in the huntingtin gene promote degeneration of neurons in the caudate/putamen and cerebral cortex. Other examples include spinal and bulbar muscular atrophy, fragile X syndrome, spinocerebellar ataxia type 1, and Machado–Joseph disease. Trinucleotide repeat mutations do not follow strict rules of mendelian inheritance, as they are unstable and change size in successive generations. The mechanism(s) whereby expansions of trinucleotide repeats cause neuronal degeneration has not been established, but recent findings suggest roles for protein aggregation and oxidative stress. ALS is a disorder in which lower motor neurons in the spinal cord, and to a lesser extent neurons in the motor cortex, degenerate resulting in progressive paralysis. A small percentage of cases of ALS are caused by mutations in the gene encoding the antioxidant enzyme Cu/ZnSOD, which appear to alter the properties of the enzyme so that it produces hydroxyl radical and peroxynitrite. Finally, several "predisposition" genes have been identified in which polymorphisms or mutations increase the risk for developing one or more age-related neurodegenerative disorders. For example, inheritance of the E4 allele or mutations in the mitochondrial DNA encoding cytochrome c oxidase increase the risk for AD.

DIETARY FACTORS IN BRAIN AGING AND NEURODEGENERATIVE DISORDERS

It recently became evident that diet can affect one's risk of age-related neurodegenerative disorders. In particular, emerging findings indicate that several dietary risk factors for prominent age-related diseases including cardiovascular disease, cancer, and diabetes are also risk factors for AD, PD, and stroke.

Calorie Intake

The only known means of increasing the life span of rodents and nonhuman primates is by decreasing their calorie intake; both maximum and mean life span can be increased by up to 40%. The average life span of humans is certainly decreased by overeating, although it remains to be determined whether maximum life span can be increased. Epidemiologic data suggest that individuals with a low calorie intake are at a reduced risk for AD and PD. Biochemical markers of aging and deficits in learning, memory, and motor function are retarded in rodents maintained on dietary restriction. Recent studies show that neurons in the brains of rats and mice maintained on dietary restriction are more resistant to dysfunction and death in experimental models of AD, PD, HD, and stroke. The mechanism whereby caloric restriction increases the resistance of neurons to the adverse effects of aging is by stimulating the expression of genes that promote neuronal plasticity and survival (see Figure 61-10). These genes include those that encode neurotrophic factors such as BDNF and nerve growth factor, protein chaperones such as heat shock protein-70, and glucose-regulated protein-78. Thus, the benefits of dietary restriction may result from a hormesis mechanism akin to the beneficial effects of physical exercise on skeletal muscle and blood vessels.

Folic Acid (Homocysteine)

It was recognized long ago that folic acid deficiency can cause abnormalities in the developing nervous system. Subsequently, it was shown that people with low levels of folic acid tend to have elevated levels of homocysteine and that this condition is associated with increased risk of cardiovascular disease and stroke. Homocysteine is produced during metabolism of methionine, and folic acid plays an important role in removing homocysteine via remethylation. Epidemiological findings suggest that people with elevated homocysteine levels may be at increased risk of AD and PD. Animal studies support a cause–effect relationship between elevated homocysteine levels and neuronal vulnerability to neurodegenerative disorders. For example, hippocampal neurons of APP mutant mice (AD model), and substantia nigra dopaminergic neurons in mice given MPTP (PD model), exhibit increased vulnerability to degeneration when maintained on a folic acid-deficient diet. By increasing homocysteine levels, folic acid deficiency may promote accumulation of

DNA damage by inhibiting DNA repair. In neurons, the increased DNA damage can trigger apoptosis, particularly under conditions of increased oxidative or metabolic stress, as occur during aging.

Antioxidants

Neurons are clearly subjected to increased levels of oxidative stress during normal aging, and more so in neurodegenerative disorders. It is therefore reasonable to consider the possibility that dietary antioxidants might promote successful brain aging. Epidemiologic findings support a protective effect of antioxidants in fruits and vegetables against stroke, and possibly AD. Studies of animal models of AD, PD, HD, stroke, and ALS have documented beneficial effects of some antioxidants. Positive effects have been reported for several commonly used dietary supplements, including vitamin E, creatine, and ginkgo biloba. However, the effects of such antioxidants are relatively subtle compared to the quite striking neuroprotective effects of dietary restriction.

Stimulatory Phytochemicals

Epidemiological findings suggest that individuals who regularly consume vegetables and fruits have a lower risk of developing an age-related neurodegenerative disorders compared to those who eat few such plant products. Several phytochemicals have been reported to enhance neuronal plasticity and survival in studies of animal models of neurodegenerative disorders. Examples include sulforaphane, curcumin, resveratrol, and allicin. Instead of functioning as direct antioxidants, many of these beneficial phytochemicals may stimulate mild adaptive stress responses that result in increased production of antioxidant enzymes, neurotrophic factors, and other protective proteins in neurons. The possible therapeutic benefits of several such stimulatory phytochemicals are currently being tested in human subjects with age-related neurological disorders.

CONCLUSION

Structural changes occur in the brain during aging and appear to be compensatory responses to adverse changes in cellular metabolism that occur during the aging process. There are several biochemical processes that may predispose neurons to dysfunction and death in aging and neurodegenerative disorders. At the cellular and molecular levels these changes include, increased levels of oxidative stress, impaired mitochondrial function, and energy metabolism, and dysregulation of neuronal calcium homeostasis. Disease-specific initiators of neuronal degeneration are being identified and include increased production of Aβ and reduced production of sAPPα in AD; trinucleotide repeat expansions in HD and related disorders; and dopamine- and Fe^{2+}-mediated free radical production in PD. As in many other organ systems, untoward changes in blood vessels may contribute greatly to age-related declines in cell function and tissue damage in the brain. A role for chronic inflammatory processes involving microglial activation is implicated in the pathogenesis of some neurodegenerative disorders. Neurodegenerative cascades may

be countered by neurotrophic signaling pathways that promote neuronal survival and adaptation; these pathways are stimulated by brain activity, such that individuals with a high level of "intellectual" activity have a reduced risk for AD. Genetic causal and risk factors for neurodegenerative disorders are being identified and characterized, leading to new insights into disease pathogenesis. Successful brain aging may be promoted through dietary manipulations with dietary restriction and supplementation with folic acid and stimulatory phytochemicals being the most notable.

FURTHER READING

Bertoni-Freddari C, Fattoretti P, Paoloni R, Caselli U, Galeazzi L, Meier-Ruge W. Synaptic structural dynamics and aging. *Gerontology*. 1996;42:170–180.

Blanc EM, Toborek M, Mark RJ, Hennig B, Mattson MP. Amyloid β-peptide induces cell monolayer albumin permeability, impairs glucose transport, and induces apoptosis in vascular endothelial cells. *J Neurochem*. 1997;68:1870–1881.

Blass JP. Metabolic alterations common to neural and non-neural cells in Alzheimer's disease. *Hippocampus*. 1993;3:45–53.

Bowling AC, Beal MF. Bioenergetic and oxidative stress in neurodegenerative diseases. *Life Sci*. 1995;56:1151–1171.

Dai Q, Borenstein AR, Wu Y, Jackson JC, Larson EB. Fruit and vegetable juices and Alzheimer's disease: the Kame Project. *Am J Med*. 2006;119:751–759.

de la Torre JC. Cerebromicrovascular pathology in Alzheimer's disease compared to normal aging. *Gerontology*. 1997;43:26–43.

Disterhoft JF, Moyer JR, Jr., Thompson LT. The calcium rationale in aging and Alzheimer's disease. Evidence from an animal model of normal aging. *Ann N Y Acad Sci*. 1994;747:382–406.

Dustman RE, Emmerson RY, Shearer DE. Life span changes in electrophysiological measures of inhibition. *Brain Cogn*. 1996;30:109–126.

Evans DA, Burbach JP, van Leeuwen FW. Somatic mutations in the brain: relationship to aging? *Mutat Res*. 1995;338:173–182.

Finch CE, Cohen DM. Aging, metabolism, and Alzheimer's disease: review and hypotheses. *Exp Neurol*. 1997;143:82–102.

Jucker M, Ingram DK. Murine models of brain aging and age-related neurodegenerative diseases. *Behav Brain Res*. 1997;85:1–26.

Kalaria RN, Harshbarger-Kelly M, Cohen DL, Premkumar DR. Molecular aspects of inflammatory and immune responses in Alzheimer's disease. *Neurobiol Aging*. 1996;17:687–693.

Landfield PW. Nathan Shock Memorial Lecture 1990. The role of glucocorticoids in brain aging and Alzheimer's disease: an integrative physiological hypothesis. *Exp Gerontol*. 1994;29:3–11.

Markesbery WR. Oxidative stress hypothesis in Alzheimer's disease. *Free Radic Biol Med*. 1997;23:134–147.

Mattson MP. Apoptosis in neurodegenerative disorders. *Nat Rev Mol Cell Biol*. 2000;1:120–129.

Mattson MP. Cellular actions of β-amyloid precursor protein, and its soluble and fibrillogenic derivatives. *Physiol Rev*. 1997;77:1081–1132.

Mattson MP, Cheng A. Neurohormetic phytochemicals: Low-dose toxins that induce adaptive neuronal stress responses. *Trends Neurosci*. 2006;29:632–639.

Mattson MP, Duan W, Lee J, Guo Z. Suppression of brain aging and neurodegenerative disorders by dietary restriction and environmental enrichment: molecular mechanisms. *Mech Aging Dev*. 2001;122:757–778.

Mattson MP, Geddes JW, eds. The aging brain. *Adv Cell Aging Gerontol*. 1997;2:1.

McEwen BS, Gould E, Orchinik M, Weiland NG, Woolley CS. Oestrogens and the structural and functional plasticity of neurons: implications for memory, ageing and neurodegenerative processes. *Ciba Found Symp*. 1995;191:52–66.

Morrison JH, Hoff PR. Life and death of neurons in the aging brain. *Science*. 1997;278:412–419.

Rao MS, Mattson MP. Stem cells and aging: expanding the possibilities. *Mech Aging Dev*. 2001;122:713–734.

Riedel WJ, Jolles J. Cognition enhancers in age-related cognitive decline. *Drugs Aging*. 1996;8:245–275.

Sohal RS, Weindruch R. Oxidative stress, caloric restriction, and aging. *Science*. 1996;273:59–63.

Wisniewski T, Frangione B. Molecular biology of brain aging and neurodegenerative disorders. *Acta Neurobiol Exp (Wars)*. 1996;56:267–279.

Zielasek J, Hartung HP. Molecular mechanisms of microglial activation. *Adv Neuroimmunol*. 1996;6:191–122.

Cognitive Changes Associated with Normal and Pathological Aging

Suzanne Craft ■ *Brenna Cholerton* ■ *Mark Reger*

"Age does not depend upon years, but upon temperament and health. Some men are born old, and some never grow so. "

Tyron Edwards

"A man is as old as his arteries."

Thomas Sydenham

The dogma that aging brings inevitable cognitive decline is being challenged by studies of the rapidly expanding oldest segment of our society, adults older than 60 years. Although some aspects of cognition are affected by aging, many changes in cognition previously considered the unavoidable consequence of brain senescence may instead result from incremental insults on brain function associated with aging-related medical conditions. The detection of such changes, which may stabilize or even reverse with appropriate intervention, and their differentiation from the cognitive changes associated with neurodegenerative disease or other neurological disorders is a critical task. The primary goal of this chapter is to describe changes in various cognitive abilities that occur with normal aging and with common age-related medical and neurological conditions.

THE EFFECTS OF NORMAL AGING ON COGNITIVE FUNCTION

General Intellectual Functioning

Intelligence is generally measured by summing the scores on a variety of verbal and performance subtests. Studies of aging have consistently shown that subtests measuring verbal abilities remain stable with normal aging. In contrast, subtests that require nonverbal creative thinking and new problem solving strategies show a slow decline with age. Crystallized abilities (information and skills gained from expe-

rience) remain relatively intact with aging, while fluid intelligence, which involves flexible reasoning and problem solving approaches, declines. Numerous studies have documented this general pattern in both cross-sectional and longitudinal research designs. Below, we review the literature on the effects of normal aging on specific cognitive functions (Table 62-1).

Attention

Attention involves the ability to focus on one or more pieces of information (auditory or visual) long enough to register and make meaningful use of the data. Attention requires both simple and complex immediate processing and provides a foundation for working memory and other cognitive functions. Sustained attention, or vigilance, entails attending to one type of information over a period of time. After controlling for reaction time and sensory changes, sustained attention and strategies for maintaining vigilance do not appear to change significantly with age. Divided attention, or the ability to concentrate on more than one piece of information at a time, may worsen with age, though research in this area has produced mixed results. Increased distractibility (difficulty blocking out irrelevant or salient stimuli), decreased use of effective strategies, and reduced processing speed may be responsible for some of the noted declines in divided attention. Pronounced impairment of attention is not typical of normal aging, however, and a complete evaluation of medical and psychosocial issues is warranted for individuals who demonstrate such changes. Attention can be negatively impacted by perceptual or sensory changes, illness, chronic pain, certain medications, and psychological disturbance (in particular, depression and anxiety), all of which are common in an older population. As the ability to effectively attend is a requisite for nearly all other cognitive functions, it is important to identify the cause/s of attentional impairment whenever possible and to implement any changes in medications or treatment that may help to resolve these problems.

TABLE 62-1

Cognitive Effects of Normal Aging

	PRESERVED COGNITIVE FUNCTIONS	COGNITIVE FUNCTIONS SHOWING DECLINE
General intellectual functioning	Crystallized, verbal intelligence	Fluid, nonverbal intelligence, speed of information processing
Attention	Sustained attention, primary attention span	Divided attention (possibly)
Executive function	"Real world" executive functions	Novel executive tasks
Memory	Remote memory, procedural memory, semantic recall	Learning and recall of new information
Language	Comprehension, vocabulary, syntactic abilities	Spontaneous word finding, verbal fluency
Visuospatial skill	Construction, simple copy	Mental rotation, complex copy, mental assembly
Psychomotor functions		Reaction time

Executive Functions

Executive functions include the ability to control and direct behavior, make meaningful inferences and appropriate judgments, plan and carry out tasks, manipulate multiple pieces of information at one time (working memory), complete complex motor sequences, and solve abstract and complex problems. Neuropsychological test performance on executive tasks declines slightly with age, and several current theories posit that deficits in working memory and executive function underlie many age-related changes in cognition. Neurocognitive tasks that require response inhibition, such as the Wisconsin Card Sort Test, Stroop Color–Word Test, and Brown–Peterson Distractor Test, may be affected.

Alternatively, many have suggested that a reduction in cognitive processing speed rather than executive function per se may be, at least in part, responsible for decreased performance on executive tasks. It should be noted that changes in the executive system that occur with normal aging are much less severe than the deficits associated with dysexecutive syndromes, including those caused by stroke, heavy and prolonged alcohol use, head injury, and some neurodegenerative diseases. In fact, successful aging appears to produce little impact on "real world" executive functions requiring planning and executing multiple tasks. Thus, it is important to assess an individual's actual functional abilities in addition to performance on neuropsychological tests of executive function.

Memory

Memory changes are perhaps the most common cognitive complaints reported by older adults. Patients often wonder if their subjective concerns reflect normal age-related changes, or some pathological condition. For patients with a family history of Alzheimer's disease or other dementia, even minor memory failings can cause significant anxiety. One of the difficulties in answering such questions lies in the complex nature of the memory process. Different forms of memory are invoked when learning new information (declarative memory), recalling prior life events (remote memory), recalling general knowledge not tied to a specific event (semantic memory), and remembering procedures for performing tasks such as riding a bicycle (procedural memory). In addition, some conditions result in modality-specific deficits, differentially affecting verbal or visual memory.

A number of models describe the different stages or processes involved in forming and recalling memories. One example, the modal model, describes memory processes in terms of sensory memory, short-term (working) memory, and long-term memory. First, when a patient senses and attends to a given stimulus, a large amount of information is briefly held in sensory memory. Information is then rehearsed or manipulated in short-term or working memory. Although many factors are involved in determining what information is transferred to long-term storage, sufficient rehearsal is a common requirement for successful transfer. Thus, it is clear that when a patient complains of memory changes, additional information is required to make sense of the problem.

Although it is true that some older adults continue to demonstrate memory performances comparable to young adults, on average even healthy older adults do show changes in some aspects of memory. For example, when a large group of healthy, nondemented elderly subjects was followed over a 7-year period, a general memory factor showed significant decline with time. Other studies have attempted to describe which aspects of memory change with healthy aging. In general, older adults without significant illness demonstrate increased difficulty learning new information compared to younger cohorts. When older adults are given repeated chances to practice learning new information, they demonstrate a slower learning curve and a lower total amount learned.

Although healthy older adults may retain slightly less information after a delay than do younger adults, this effect is less pronounced than the slowed learning rate. For delayed memory tests, patients are generally asked to recall information 15 to 60 minutes after the initial exposure. Although patients recall less information at the delay with age, they generally retain a stable proportion of the information that they initially learned. In general, longitudinal studies of aging show only small declines in delayed memory with age, particularly on tests of visual memory. Some older adults also appear less likely to use cognitive strategies to aid memory than younger subjects. This may be owing to generational differences in learning style. However, it may be significant because the use of memory strategies (i.e., grouping vegetables and clothing items for easier recall) reduces the age effect observed on free recall tests.

A number of memory processes do not appear to change with successful aging. Remote memory, that is recall of events that occurred in the distant past, remains relatively intact, as does sensory memory. In addition, while elderly patients often have medical problems that limit physical movement, procedural memory appears to be unaffected by healthy aging. Lastly, semantic memory, such as vocabulary and general information about the world, remains largely unchanged by aging until very late in life.

Longitudinal studies have consistently shown that as groups age, the variability in cognitive performance increases. Overall, studies of healthy aging suggest that there are some statistically significant declines in memory in late life. However, the memory functions of patients who age successfully are typically adequate for the demands of independent living.

Language

Language abilities incorporate multiple levels of processing, and general language functions tend to remain relatively stable with increasing age. Some linguistic abilities, however, particularly those involving language output, show reliable declines in older adults. As with other cognitive functions, there are multiple potential intervening factors, including trauma, illness, and sensory disruption, that may lead to more severe changes in the language functions.

Language Comprehension

Language comprehension involves discerning the simple and complex rules of language and incorporating both visual and auditory information into a meaningful concept; language comprehension is generally associated with few age-related impairments. The ability to recognize basic word structure and word representation is typically measured using "lexical-decision" tasks (in which letters are rapidly presented and the person is asked to identify whether or not it is a word), and simple word reading tasks. While some studies have suggested an inverse relationship between performance on these tasks and age, it is generally believed that such changes are the result of decreased reaction time and processing speed rather than the ability to comprehend word structure and meaning. In addition, there is some indication that the level of lexical processing changes slightly with age, in that older adults tend to rely more on word recognition than do younger adults, while ignoring other factors such as word length. Phonological understanding of language does not appear to change significantly with age, although hearing loss may appear to reduce auditory comprehension. Overall, it is generally accepted that language comprehension remains relatively intact throughout the lifespan.

Language Production

Basic syntactic abilities do not appear to change significantly with advancing age, although minor repetitions, longer pauses, and an increased use of pronouns and other vague words while speaking have been noted. Additionally, a recent longitudinal study suggests a decline in spoken grammatical complexity during the eighth decade of life. The authors note, however, that there is high interindividual variability throughout the lifespan in terms of syntactic aptitude.

Semantic abilities involve aptitude with naming and retrieving long-stored information. There is a steady increase in vocabulary knowledge throughout middle adulthood, and such knowledge typically remains stable in the later years. A frequent complaint from older adults, however, involves the "tip-of-the-tongue" phenomenon, in which there is a notable struggle with spontaneous word finding. In contrast to the dysnomia that often accompanies dementia, however, such changes appear to result primarily from difficulties retrieving rather than storing information, and thus there is usually a marked improvement when cues are given. Verbal fluency, the rate at which a person can spontaneously produce words belonging to a single phonemic or semantic category, also appears

to change somewhat with age. Multiple research findings support a decrease in semantic fluency ("name all the animals you can") while phonemic fluency ("tell me as many words as you can that begin with the letter F") generally remains stable. In terms of strategy, it has been suggested that younger adults tend to produce more words and to change categories more frequently than do older adults on semantic fluency tasks, while older subjects generate the same amount of words but more "clusters" on tasks of phonemic fluency. Thus, older subjects likely rely more on structural word knowledge than on word meaning.

Visuospatial Skills

Visuospatial skills are commonly tested by constructional tasks in which patients are asked to draw figures or assemble objects. In general, as patients age, they become slower at completing visuospatial tasks. However, as noted, one of the more consistent findings in the field is that normal aging is associated with general slowing of psychomotor and cognitive speed. Therefore, performance on tests of visuospatial functioning is often confounded by slowing. Some studies have attempted to separate the effects of the two domains. For instance, after controlling for processing speed and executive functioning, the effects of age on the commonly used Wechsler Block Design test were dramatically reduced. Similarly, an 11-year follow-up of elderly subjects analyzed both speed and quality of performance (errors) on a parallelogram test. As expected, speed declined with age, but the quality of the performance actually improved significantly. This body of literature suggests that declining speed contributes to some of the findings that report visuospatial processing deficits in normal aging.

Speed does not appear to account for all of the visuospatial changes observed in healthy aging, however. Mental rotations of objects or spatial coordinates, accurate copy of complex geometric designs, and mental assembly of objects typically worsen with age even when unlimited time is allowed to perform such tasks. Furthermore, when speed is included in scoring, some studies have reported disproportionate slowing on visuospatial tasks compared to verbal tasks. Overall, some studies may exaggerate the visuospatial decline observed in normal aging because of the role speed plays in many tasks used to assess visuospatial function. However, abstract spatial abilities may decline with age, even when speed is controlled.

Psychomotor Functions

An age-associated increase in reaction time, related to both a general reduction in the speed of cognitive processing and to changes in peripheral motor skills, has been consistently reported. Age-related declines in brain dopamine activity and periventricular white matter changes may be associated with reduced cognitive speed and basic motor functions. As a result, performance on tests requiring speed and quick reaction to stimuli is likely to decline. As previously noted, increased psychomotor speed and reaction time are believed to underlie many of the age-related changes noted on neurocognitive testing, particularly tasks involving perceptual speed, attention, and working memory. In addition, changes in psychomotor functions can be associated with changes in real world tasks, such as driving. As a result, it is important to monitor the manner in which physical changes are impacting an individual's level of safety in performing daily activities.

COGNITIVE EFFECTS OF COMMON AGE-RELATED MEDICAL CONDITIONS

In the following section we review cognitive symptoms associated with common diseases affecting older adults. A summary of these symptoms is presented in Table 62-2.

Cardiovascular Disease

In addition to increasing the risk for developing stroke and/or vascular dementia, cardiovascular disease potentially jeopardizes cognitive function via multiple mechanisms.

Cognitive impairment subsequent to coronary artery bypass graft (CABG) surgery has been reported in up to 80% of patients, and older age significantly increases the risk for development of such complications. A wide range of cognitive deficits, including problems with attention and concentration, processing speed, memory, and visuospatial function, has been noted in patients immediately following surgery. Initial reports suggested that postoperative cognitive function stabilizes or even improves after a period of approximately 12 months in those patients who demonstrate initial decline. However, recent longitudinal data provide evidence that such patients are at high risk for continued cognitive deterioration 5 years postsurgery. For example, one study found that 42% of patients showed a significant decline in one or more areas of cognitive function 5 years postsurgery, including verbal and visual memory, attention and concentration, and general cognition. Notably, post-CABG neurocognitive status is related to overall quality of life, and current recommendations underscore the importance of closely monitoring cognitive status in the years following cardiac surgery.

Hypertension

Essential hypertension has been associated with cognitive impairment independent of secondary disease or organ damage, particularly in older patients. Potential cognitive effects of primary hypertension include reductions in mental status, slowed reaction time, reduced attention and vigilance, weakened executive function, poor verbal fluency, and impaired visual organization and construction. Memory functions, including spatial recall, verbal recall, and word recognition, may also be affected in some hypertensive patients. In addition, secondary effects of hypertension may lead to an increased risk for cognitive decline in older age. For example, uncontrolled hypertension potentiates the development of subcortical white matter lesions, and adversely impacts cerebral blood flow and energy substrate delivery. While there is currently debate concerning the extent to which hypertension and related subcortical effects overtly impact cognition, recent findings suggest that hypertension is a significant risk factor for dementia, and treating hypertension reduces this risk. In particular, mid-life hypertension increases the risk of later-life cognitive impairment. Interestingly, blood pressure often declines in the period immediately preceding the onset of Alzheimer's disease, and it has been suggested that low blood pressure in persons of advanced age may compromise brain function as a result of hypoperfusion. In particular, aggressive sudden lowering of blood pressure in older adults with long-term hypertension may potentially interact with their chronically upregulated cerebral vascular resistance and induce cerebral hypoperfusion. Thus, careful monitoring of blood pressure and gradual titration of medication regimens is of particular importance. Additional interest has been focused on the question of whether different methods of treating hypertension may confer particular protective effects on cognition. A recent epidemiologic study observed a reduced risk of dementia associated with the use of potassium-sparing diuretics. However, no adequately controlled, randomized trials have been conducted to definitively answer this question.

Nutritional Deficiency

Older adults are at considerable risk for nutritional deficiencies as a consequence of poor diet and malabsorption syndromes. Much research in this area has focused on deficiencies of B vitamins. A recent meta-analysis concluded that reduced folate levels may be associated with lowered cognitive function and increased risk of Alzheimer's disease; however, the accumulated evidence did not support a similar relationship for B-12 and B-6. Some studies have suggested that supplementation may improve cognitive performance in deficient individuals.

B vitamins play an important role in homocysteine metabolism. Homocysteine is an independent risk factor for cerebrovascular and cardiovascular disease. In patients with both Alzheimer's disease and vascular dementia, elevated plasma homocysteine levels have been reported, and recent studies suggest that homocysteine levels are related to cognitive function in normal aging. Reduced performance on tests of mental status, nonverbal pattern abstraction, construction, and processing speed are reported in patients with high plasma homocysteine. Given that plasma homocysteine and folate levels are inversely related, it is conceivable that such cognitive deficits are related to reduced folate rather than to increased homocysteine per se. Recent data suggest, however, that homocysteine increases the risk for cognitive decline independent of both folate levels and other vascular risk factors.

Type 2 Diabetes Mellitus

Much attention has been given to the rampant epidemic of type 2 diabetes mellitus (T2DM) in older adults, a trend thought to be largely attributable to obesity and physical inactivity. Current prevalence estimates suggest that 20% of adults older than 65 years are afflicted with T2DM. The negative impact of T2DM on multiple medical systems is well known. The clear impact of T2DM on cognitive function in older adults is less-widely known, but accruing evidence demonstrates that these patients show pronounced impairment in attention and verbal memory when compared to healthy age-matched adults, and show accelerated cognitive decline over time. Complex attentional impairment is most common, involving the inability to handle multiple streams of information or attend to information in the face of competing stimuli. Verbal memory deficits typically affect the ability to encode new verbal information. The magnitude of such impairment may vary from subtle subjective complaints to pronounced impairment that interferes with daily activities and may interfere with the patient's ability to adhere to complex treatment regimens. The mechanisms causing attentional and memory impairments are likely multifactorial and include vascular factors, as described above, in addition to the potential negative effects of hyperglycemia and glucose toxicity thought to cause oxidative injury. Recent work also suggest that insulin resistance, independent

TABLE 62-2

Possible Cognitive Effects of Common Age-Related Medical Conditions

	SYMPTOM COURSE	INCREASED RISK FOR DEVELOPING DEMENTIA?	MEMORY	ATTENTION	EXECUTIVE FUNCTIONS	LANGUAGE	VISUOSPATIAL FUNCTION	PSYCHOMOTOR FUNCTION	BEHAVIOR
Cardiac surgery	Symptom onset immediate after surgery, improvement noted in first year, then further decline possible in some patients	AD, VaD	Verbal and visual memory deficits possible several years after surgery	Reduced attention	Variable	No significant changes noted	May lead to impaired visual organization and construction	Reduced reaction time, general slowing	Depression common after surgery
Hypertension	May improve with antihypertensive treatment	AD, VaD	Verbal and visual recall and recognition deficits in some patients	Reduced attention and vigilance	Impairment in working memory and other executive function	Reduced verbal fluency	May lead to impaired visual organization and construction; more likely with comorbid diabetes	Reduced reaction time, general slowing	Variable
Diabetes	May improve with insulin or insulin-sensitizing agents	AD, VaD, PD	Verbal memory impairment related to deficits in encoding new information	Reduced complex attention, simple attention variable	Impairments in abstract reasoning and concept formation	No significant changes noted	Variable, more likely with comorbid hypertension	No significant changes noted	Depression common
COPD	May improve with oxygen therapy	AD, VaD	Verbal and visual memory deficits	Reduced attention	Impairment in abstract thinking	No significant changes noted	No significant changes noted	Reduced reaction time, general slowing	Depression common
Sleep apnea	May improve with CPAP treatment	Unknown	Verbal and visual memory deficits	Reduced attention	Impairment in general executive function; esp. working memory	No significant changes noted	No significant changes noted	Reduced reaction time, general slowing	Depression and irritability related to sleep disruption
Nutritional deficiency	May improve with supplementation, although effects of low vitamin B-12 may persists	Wernicke–Korsakoff syndrome	Recall deficits	Reduced attention	Impairment in abstract thinking	No significant changes noted	Nonverbal pattern abstraction, construction impaired in high homocysteine	Reduced processing speed in patients with high homocysteine	Variable
Hypothyroidism	May improve with thyroid treatment, although some patients do not return to baseline	AD	Recall deficits, intact recognition	Variable	Variable	No significant changes noted	Reduced visuospatial function	Reduced reaction time, general slowing	Depression

AD, Alzheimer's disease; COPD, chronic obstructive pulmonary disease; PD, parkinsonian dementia; VaD, vascular dementia; CPAP, continuous positive airway pressure.

of hyperglycemia, may have negative consequences on brain systems mediating memory and attention. This intriguing possibility has implications for therapeutic approaches to treating T2DM, suggesting that strategies focused on improving insulin sensitivity may be preferable to those focused on augmenting insulin levels. Successful treatment of T2DM has been shown to improve cognitive function. The importance of treating and preferably preventing T2DM has been underscored by recent findings that it is a risk factor for various forms of neurodegenerative disease, including Alzheimer's disease, vascular dementia, and Parkinson disease.

Oxygen Deprivation

Chronic Obstructive Pulmonary Disease

Emphysema and chronic bronchitis obstruct airflow, resulting in hypoxemia and hypercapnia. Cognitive dysfunction is commonly observed in chronic obstructive pulmonary disease, although the specific skills affected appear to be broad and diffuse. Deficits in verbal and visual memory, attention, abstraction, psychomotor speed, information processing speed, and IQ have all been reported. These changes in cognition appear to be caused by hypoxemia. The decrease in arterial oxygen partial pressure correlates with neuropsychological impairments, and most studies indicate that oxygen therapy results in modest improvements in cognition. Depression is also common in chronic obstructive pulmonary disease and must be considered as another cognitive risk factor.

Obstructive Sleep Apnea

The prevalence of obstructive sleep apnea (OSA) increases in geriatric populations. Many patients remain unaware of the disorder and report associated symptoms only when specifically queried. Cognitive changes in OSA can be diverse, but generally include attention, concentration, executive functioning, verbal and visual learning, and working memory. Tests of global functioning have also revealed differences compared to healthy elderly without OSA. There is debate regarding whether the cognitive deficits are caused by hypoxia, hypersomnolence, or both. However, severity of hypoxemia appears to relate to cognitive functioning, and continuous positive airway pressure treatment improves cognitive functioning in many patients.

Thyroid Dysfunction

There are a number of thyroid disorders that result in hypo- or hyperthyroidism. Hypothyroidism appears to be associated with cognitive changes. Deficits may be observed in visuospatial skills, psychomotor speed, and memory. There is some evidence that the memory deficits are related to retrieval rather than immediate recall or learning; thus, disproportionately better performance may be observed on tests of cued or recognition memory than on free recall tests. Thyroid replacement therapy frequently improves cognitive functioning, although skills may not return to baseline levels in some patients. Hyperthyroid episodes may result in cognitive changes that last for many years. Symptoms may include attention and executive functioning deficits, and memory impairment. Hyperthyroid dementia is less common than in hypothyroidism, and is also generally less severe. The evidence supporting cognitive deficits in adults with subclinical thyroid disease is equivocal. Thyroid hormone abnormalities

occur in a large proportion of patients with dementia. Therefore, levels should be routinely monitored as a treatable contributor to cognitive decline.

Depression

Depression is an increasingly common problem in older adults, with prevalence estimates ranging from 11% to 30%. Multiple situational risk factors for depression in older age include the loss of social support, death of family members and close friends, changing social roles, and physical limitations. Depressive symptoms, including lack of initiation, impaired executive function, cognitive slowing, poor attention and concentration, and mild memory impairment can mimic early signs of dementia and may potentially lead to misdiagnosis and/or lack of appropriate medical intervention. As depression is a potentially reversible cause of cognitive impairment, the differential diagnosis between depression and dementia is vital when evaluating elderly patients. Factors that are useful in discriminating between depression and dementia include the clinical course of symptoms, relationship to a specific crisis or stressful event, history of previous psychiatric problems, quality of effort, and level of impaired processing on cognitive evaluation (Table 62-3).

Recent findings suggest that late-onset depression is an independent risk factor for the development of neurodegenerative diseases, such as Alzheimer's disease and vascular dementia, and some hypothesize that depression may actually represent a preclinical phase of progressive dementia. In patients with early cognitive loss, depressive symptoms may represent realistic self-evaluation of such decline and/or may coincide with actual changes in neuroendocrinological status. In the absence of predisposing situational factors, late-onset affective disorders are quite rare. Subcortical vascular ischemic changes are frequently noted in patients with new-onset depression in late life, and such patients frequently have vascular risk factors such as hypertension, cardiovascular disease, and diabetes. For such cases, cognitive ability and independent functional status must be carefully evaluated, and an in-depth qualitative analysis of depressive symptoms may be useful. Major depressive disorder is associated with a range of affective, cognitive, and vegetative symptoms, while depressive symptoms in early dementia are more likely to include cognitive and motivational symptoms (e.g., poor concentration, lack of initiation) in the relative absence of central affective disturbance. Continued monitoring of the cognitive status of depressed elderly patients is essential in order to rule out progressive cognitive decline.

Medications

A number of medications have the potential to cause both subtle cognitive changes and alterations in overall mental status, particularly in the elderly. Medications known to adversely affect cognitive status include opiates and opioid-like analgesics, benzodiazepines, anticonvulsants, antipsychotic and antidepressant medications, antiparkinsonian agents, central nervous system stimulants, antihistamines and decongestants, and certain cardiovascular medications. A variety of other medications, particularly those that readily cross the blood–brain barrier, may impact cognitive function in certain individuals. In addition, drug interactions in older adults can lead to more serious physiological and cognitive consequences than those observed in younger adults, and adverse medication interactions are more likely to occur in an older population. As a result, changes in

TABLE 62-3

Depression Versus Alzheimer's Disease

	DEPRESSION	ALZHEIMER'S DISEASE
Symptom History		
Onset	Distinct, often related to a specific traumatic event or loss	Insidious onset
Progression	Rapid	Slow
Patient's description of symptoms	Detailed	Few details
Psychiatric symptoms/history		
Depressive symptoms	Affective, vegetative, cognitive	Cognitive, some vegetative
Psychiatric history	History of one or more depressive episodes usual	May or may not have a history of depression
Cognition		
Effort on testing	Often poor	Usually effortful
Memory		
Recent	Recall improves with cuing/recognition	Impaired, recall does not improve with cuing/recognition
Remote	May be impaired, may have memory "gaps"	Not impaired until late in disease
Procedural	May be impaired	Not impaired
Attention/concentration	Impaired	Impaired
Language	Assisted by semantic strategies	Unable to use semantic strategies

cognitive status must be carefully evaluated in light of a patient's current medication profile.

Certain medications may in fact enhance cognitive function in older adults and aid in the prevention of cognitive decline. The cholinesterase inhibitors donepezil, rivastigmine, galantamine, and tacrine have been shown to stabilize and even improve general cognitive function in some patients with Alzheimer's disease. Medications currently being evaluated for potential reduction of risk for cognitive decline in both healthy aging and dementia include statins, Nonsteroidal Antiinflammatory Drugs (NSAIDs), antioxidant vitamin supplements, and estrogen replacement therapy.

Delirium

Older adults are at a significantly increased risk for developing delirium, particularly following surgery or in response to medication changes or interactions. Delirium is a reversible condition that can be distinguished from most neurodegenerative diseases by a rapid onset of symptoms that include significant disorientation and disturbance in consciousness, reduced awareness of the environment, and attention deficits. While recent memory is generally impaired, altered consciousness is the primary indicator of delirium. Hallucinations, delusional thinking, and other disturbed thought processes may also be present. Delirium usually resolves quickly, but may persist for several weeks. It should also be noted that postoperative delirium may signify the presence of a beginning dementia. A primary concern is to identify and treat the underlying cause while providing a supportive and nonthreatening environment for the patient.

NEURODEGENERATIVE DISEASE

The following section reviews the cognitive and behavioral profiles associated with common neurodegenerative disorders (Table 62-4). Early identification of such disorders, many of which are diagnosed solely on these parameters, has become increasingly important owing to potential therapies that may delay disease progression.

Alzheimer's Disease

Alzheimer's disease (AD), the most prevalent of the primary neurodegenerative disorders, causes profound progressive cognitive and functional impairments. While confirmatory diagnostic procedures require histopathologic evaluation at autopsy, probable AD may be diagnosed on the basis of a thorough clinical assessment. The most widely accepted diagnostic standards for probable AD are the National Institute of Neurological and Communicative Disorders and Stroke (NINCDS) and the Alzheimer's Disease and Related Disorders Association (ADRDA) criteria, and include the following: (1) dementia as noted on clinical examination and established by neuropsychological testing, (2) significant impairment in two or more areas of cognition, (3) progressive memory decline, and (4) absence of other medical or psychiatric conditions, including delirium, as the cause for memory impairment. Current debate surrounds the value of an almost purely exclusionary diagnosis, and as a result potential cerebrospinal fluid markers (elevated beta amyloid or tau proteins), structural and functional changes on brain scan, and genetic factors are under close scrutiny for their potential diagnostic utility. In the absence of such tools, however, the current conventional diagnostic criteria are considered to be reasonably accurate, particularly when the evaluation is comprehensive and includes a complete medical and psychosocial history, medical evaluation, and neurocognitive testing.

Patient History

A complete medical and psychosocial history is a vital component of any dementia assessment. Such a history should be obtained both from the patient and a reliable informant, preferably someone who has regular contact with the patient and who has an adequate opportunity to observe patient's daily functional abilities. Typically, a patient in the earliest stages of AD will not exhibit deficits in basic self-care. However, more complex daily tasks, including driving, finances, shopping, and other chores and activities, are likely to be affected. A gradually progressive course and insidious onset of

TABLE 62-4

Early Cognitive Symptoms Associated with Different Dementia Types

	SYMPTOM ONSET	PROGRESSION RATE	Recent	MEMORY		
				Recognition Intact?	Remote Intact?	Procedural Intact?
Alzheimer's disease (AD)	Insidious	Steady, gradual	Significantly impaired declarative recall	N	Y	Y
Vascular dementia (VaD)	May be insidious or acute	Stepwise or gradual	Possible deficits	Y	Y	Y
Frontotemporal dementia (FTD)	Insidious	Steady, rapid	Relatively preserved	Y	Y	Y
Primary progressive aphasia (PPA)	Insidious	Steady, varied	Preserved recall, may score poorly on verbal memory tests	Y	Y	Y
Parkinson disease (PD)	Insidious	Varied	Possible deficits	Y	Y	N—possible impairments
Dementia with Lewy bodies (DLB)	Insidious	Steady, gradual	Mild impairment, less than AD	Variable	Y	Y
Progressive supranuclear palsy (PSP)	Insidious	Steady, gradual	Mild impairment, less than AD	Variable	Y	Y
Persistent alcohol dementia	Deficits persist after d/c alcohol use	May worsen over time	Impairment on recall, not more than other functions	Variable	Y	Y
Wernicke–Korsakoff syndrome	Acute (initial phase)	Steady, gradual (chronic phase)	Significant impairment on declarative recall relative to other deficits (semantic memory spared)	N	N	Variable
Prion disease	Insidious	Steady, rapid	Nonspecific impairments reported	Y	Y	Y
Normal pressure hydrocephalus (NPH)	Insidious	Varied, potentially reversible	Not prominently impaired	Y	Y	Y
Human immunodeficiency virus (HIV)	Usually later in the disease course	Varied	Variable	Variable	Y	Y
Neurosyphilis	Many years after initial infection	Varied, potentially reversible	Variable	Variable	Y	Y

ATTENTION	EXECUTIVE FUNCTIONS	LANGUAGE	VISUOSPATIAL FUNCTION	PSYCHOMOTOR FUNCTION	BEHAVIOR
Intact primary span; impaired selective/divided attention	Mildly impaired working memory, response inhibition, general problem-solving	Semantic organizational abilities significantly impaired, mild anomia	Simple construction intact, complex visual reasoning impaired	If present, symptoms are mild	Depression common
Intact primary span; impaired selective/divided attention	Significantly more impaired than AD and relative to performance on verbal memory tasks	Verbal fluency impaired	Relatively preserved, although may be affected by executive impairments	Slowing, possible discrete motor problems depending on distribution of vascular changes	Depression common
Intact primary span; impaired selective/divided attention	Impaired across a range of executive functions	Verbal fluency impaired	Relatively preserved, although may be affected by executive impairments	May exhibit ideational apraxia	Significant behavioral changes: apathy/blunting, disinhibition, lack of insight, etc.
Preserved	Preserved	*Nonfluent PPA:* Anomic aphasia, poor articulation, dysarthria, relatively preserved comprehension; *Fluent PPA:* Impaired comprehension, anomia, intact speech rate & prosody	In semantic dementia, may have visual agnosia	*Nonfluent PPA:* Buccofacial apraxia	Changes unlikely
Intact primary attention span, impaired selective/divided attention	Difficulty planning/shifting set	Verbal fluency, mechanical aspects of speech impaired	May be impaired	Resting tremor, bradykinesia, rigidity, postural instability, shuffling gait	Depression common, may exhibit hallucinations/delusions, less common than DLB
Significant fluctuations in attention	Variable	Variable; fluency may be impaired	Impaired construction, copy, visuospatial planning and problem-solving	May exhibit a range of parkinsonian symptoms	Hallucinations, delusions, depression
Impaired selective/divided attention	Impaired across a range of executive functions	Verbal fluency impaired	May be impaired	Vertical supranuclear gaze palsy, postural instability	Apathy, disinhibition
Impaired sustained attention	Abstraction, mental flexibility, perseveration, confabulation, impaired judgment, reduced ability to care for self	Perserved	Visual scanning, visuospatial organization impaired	May exhibit cerebellar tremor, impaired gait	Apathy, depression
Impaired across all attentional functions	Similar profile to persistent alcohol dementia	Preserved	Visual scanning, visuospatial organization impaired	Impaired gait, abnormal reflexes, other movement abnormalities	Personality change prominent feature, inappropriate behavior
Nonspecific impairments reported	Reduced problem solving ability	Generally preserved	Generally intact	May exhibit impaired reflexes and coordination	Apathy, emotional lability, impaired sleep, appetite loss
Primary deficits in attention	Nonspecific impairments in executive function reported	Generally preserved	Generally intact	Wide-based gait or other balance disturbance, urinary incontinence	May present with a confusional state
Nonspecific impairments reported	Nonspecific impairments in executive function reported	Generally preserved	Generally intact	Generally intact	Depression common
Variable	Variable	Generally preserved	Generally intact	May be ataxic	Hallucinations, delusions, personality change, mood disturbance

cognitive symptoms is a hallmark of the AD, and thus a careful history regarding the nature and timing of symptom onset and progression must be obtained. An inventory of all current medical concerns, past major medical problems, and medications must be evaluated in order to rule out conditions that may be either causing cognitive problems or influencing their expression.

Medical Examination

An important goal of the medical evaluation is to exclude the presence of medical conditions that may be responsible for the observed cognitive deficits. It is critical to investigate potentially reversible causes of dementia such as uncontrolled liver or kidney disease, adverse reactions to medications, and delirium. Laboratory blood tests can aid in ruling out systemic illnesses or organ malfunction. Structural brain scans are used to evaluate major cerebrovascular events, tumors, normal pressure hydrocephalus, and other neurologic conditions, while functional brain scans identify patterns of activity that may be useful in classifying dementia type.

Neuropsychological Assessment

Neuropsychological assessment of cognitive function not only provides confirmatory evidence for cognitive impairment, but may also aid in clarification of dementia type. Given the extensive variation in rate of AD progression among patients, regular neuropsychological examinations can also provide information regarding an individual's rate of progression and remaining cognitive strengths. Perhaps one of the most valuable assets of neuropsychological evaluation is the sensitivity of the tests to early cognitive decline. While there has been debate regarding the usefulness of providing an early AD diagnosis, it is generally accepted that such a diagnosis will allow the patients to avail themselves of current and emerging therapies, as well as to make decisions regarding health care, finances, and legal issues while still competent. In a typical neuropsychological evaluation, patients are given tests that sample a variety of domains of cognitive function. Results are compared to normative data based on age, and also to an individual's estimated premorbid abilities (based on educational and occupational background and performance on tests that tend to remain stable over time). Pattern analysis of test results, in combination with data from the patient history and medical evaluation, is then used to generate diagnostic possibilities. The following sections discuss cognitive impairment patterns typical in patients with AD.

Memory. The hallmark of AD, and most often the first cognitive symptom of the disorder, is anterograde amnesia, evidenced by difficulty with learning new information. Deficits are noted in declarative memory as a result of prominent impairment in information encoding, retrieval, and in particular, storage of new material. Patients are likely to exhibit deficits in recent episodic recall, and they or their caregivers often report misplacing items, forgetting recent events or conversations, and frequently repeating questions or statements. In contrast to impaired episodic recall and difficulty learning new information, procedural memory is rarely impaired, and remote memory remains relatively intact until later stages of the disease.

In order to adequately evaluate short-term memory loss and establish a pattern of impaired retrieval, neuropsychological evaluations include tests of both immediate and delayed verbal and visual recall. Tests such as the Folstein Mini Mental Status Examination

(MMSE) and other diagnostic screening instruments assess general mental status and orientation, but are not adequate for a comprehensive understanding of memory impairment. To satisfactorily assess a person's true memory ability, Zec recommends using tasks that are high in cognitive demand, that exceed the primary memory span (such as story recall and list learning tasks that include at least 10 items), and that have a recognition component. On neuropsychological examination, verbal and visual free immediate and delayed recall and recognition are significantly impaired in patients with AD relative to same-age peers, and patients typically exhibit a high number of intrusion errors and repetitions. Semantic recall is generally the most predominantly impaired, and thus verbal recall tasks are often the most sensitive to early memory loss.

Attention and Executive Function. Certain aspects of attention and concentration are often impaired early in the disease process, and recent research has supported that it may in fact be one of the earliest abilities affected in AD. While patients with AD are likely to have relatively intact simple attention (e.g., primary memory span), tests requiring selective and divided attention are likely to be impaired, particularly as task demands increase. This pattern of performance strongly supports the presence of a deficit in working memory (the ability to simultaneously attend, process, and respond to multiple pieces of information) early in the disease process, and a converging body of evidence supports a primary executive component in AD.

In addition to problems on tasks of complex attention and working memory, patients are likely to exhibit mild deficits in response inhibition, evidenced by intrusion errors and perseverative responses, on neuropsychological testing. Deficits in abstract reasoning, general problem solving ability, and making appropriate judgments are also commonly noted. In assessing for judgment and abstraction, patients may be asked the meaning of proverbs (e.g., "you can lead a horse to water but you can't make it drink"), and are often given hypothetical situations in which they must decide an appropriate course of action (e.g., "what would you do if you were in a crowded shopping mall and saw smoke and fire?"). On these tasks, even patients in their early stage of AD may provide incorrect or inappropriate responses.

Language. Semantic processing is considered the primary language deficit in AD, and is present in more than half of all patients with AD at the time of diagnosis. Word finding problems are commonly reported in both AD and normal aging, but patients with AD have more severe deficits and are more likely to produce a significantly higher number of semantic paraphasias and circumlocutions. Patients are generally impaired on tasks of confrontational naming, and, unlike changes that occur with normal aging, are not likely to be assisted by cues. Syntactic processing, in contrast to semantic processing, is typically unaffected in mild AD. For example, patients with early AD can typically process even complex sentences at the same level as their healthy counterparts, and generally remain unimpaired on repetition and fluent speech. Verbal fluency tasks are particularly useful in evaluating both semantic and syntactic processing. Semantic, or category fluency (e.g., "tell me as many animals as you can") is generally impaired disproportionately to syntactic, or phonemic fluency (e.g., "tell me as many words that begin with the letter___") in AD. While decreased information processing and working memory may impair an AD patient's responses on certain syntactic processing tasks, and comprehension and intelligible speech are likely to decline slowly as the disease advances, patients who present first with nonfluent aphasia or impaired comprehension should be carefully evaluated for other conditions.

Visuospatial Function. Deficits in visuospatial abilities are frequently seen in patients with AD, although they generally appear later than memory and language deficits. Patients may become lost in familiar places (e.g., grocery store) or while driving. Eventually, disorientation may lead to confusion in one's own home and subsequent wandering behavior. Early deficits, however, are more likely to involve visuospatial problem solving. Neuropsychological tests commonly used involve comparing simple construction or copying, typically not impaired early in the disease, to complex visual reasoning. The presence of constructional apraxia early in the disease may indicate greater pathology in visual processing areas of the brain and has been associated with more rapid symptom progression. In general, more complex drawing tasks, such as three-dimensional figure copy, may be more precise measures of the most common early visual spatial deficits in AD than simple copying tasks.

Motor Function. While motor dysfunction has not been typically considered to be a defining symptom of AD, recent research suggests that patients with AD may display impairments in gait, motor speed, and general level of activity even in the mild stages of the disease. In addition, converging evidence provides support for greater overlap between AD and Lewy body dementia, making motor changes such as tremor or gait disturbance more likely in these patients. Importantly, there have been reports of gait disturbance in patients taking cholinesterase inhibitors, a factor that should be carefully monitored when prescribing these medications.

Patients with AD may also exhibit mild ideomotor and ideational apraxia (deficits in skilled movements) as a result of concrete responses, lack of sufficient external cues, or a disruption in conceptualization ability. However, moderate to severe apraxia is not generally present until later stages of the disease. Incorporating an apraxia assessment into a dementia evaluation is useful, however, particularly for excluding other disorders that may initially present with more severe skilled movement disorders.

Behavioral Changes

As mentioned previously, depression is common in patients with AD, and may manifest as apathy, indifference, poor initiation, or emotional lability. Irritability, agitation, and paranoid ideation are also common in AD, and may worsen with disease progression, prompting wandering behavior and aggressive outbursts. Repetitive and aimless behavior may also increase as the disease progresses. More severe psychotic symptoms, such as hallucinations and severe delusions, have been reported in some patients with early AD, but are typically rare in the absence of coexisting disorders. Given the wide range of behaviors that may be exhibited in an AD patient, it is imperative that the patient's family be provided with ample dementia education, that they have access to social support, and that they possess the coping skills necessary to provide adequate care.

Awareness of Deficits

Patients in the early stages of AD typically vary in their level of deficit awareness. Whatever the starting point, deficit awareness declines with disease progression. Even when patients do acknowledge their cognitive decline, however, such awareness may not be "complete" as a result of deficits in executive function. For example, patients may be unable to translate cognitive problems into functional problems, and as a result may not understand how their deficits affect certain activities, such as driving, cooking, and finances. Again, providing the patient's caregivers with access to education can increase the likelihood that patients will comply with physician recommendations to limit certain unsafe behaviors.

Variant AD Presentations

While most often the primary early deficit in AD involves recent memory, there are several reported cases of variant forms of AD that involve primary deficits in language, visuospatial function, or central executive function. In such cases, differential diagnoses including frontotemporal dementia, primary progressive aphasia, Lewy body dementia, and others must be carefully considered prior to assigning a diagnosis of AD.

Mild Cognitive Impairment

The term "mild cognitive impairment" (MCI) has been used to describe cognitive impairment in aging that does not meet the criteria for dementia and that is not the result of a known medical condition. Petersen and colleagues have proposed a set of criteria used to diagnose MCI that includes the following: (1) subjective memory concerns, (2) objective impairment in memory on neuropsychological testing, (3) absence of dementia, and (4) absence of functional complaints. Longitudinal research suggests that 80% of those diagnosed with MCI will go on to develop AD within 5 to 8 years, and will convert at a rate of approximately 10% to 15% per year compared to general population conversion rates of 1% to 2%. The term "amnestic" MCI is currently used to differentiate between isolated impairment in memory versus impairments in other cognitive functions. Given the above noted conversion rates, it is proposed that amnestic MCI may actually be a preclinical stage of AD, while nonamnestic MCI may represent early onset of other forms of dementia, including frontotemporal, Lewy body, and vascular dementias (Figure 62-1). Neuropsychological assessment can be particularly useful in distinguishing between normal age-related changes and MCI.

Vascular Dementia

The constructs of vascular dementia (VaD) and vascular cognitive impairment are undergoing rapid development. One evolving view describes vascular cognitive impairment as an umbrella term that subsumes the condition of VaD. Progress in achieving a coherent nosology is hindered by the likely heterogenous nature of these conditions, which complicates efforts to identify characteristic cognitive profiles. According to NINDS–AIREN criteria, six vascular "subtypes" ascribe dementia to multiple large infarcts, strategic single infarcts, small vessel disease, hypoperfusion, hemorrhage, or miscellaneous vascular insult. It is likely that dementia caused by small vessel disease is the most common form of VaD and provides the most uniform pattern of cognitive impairment. Cognitive profiles of these patients at early stages typically reveal executive function deficits, reduced verbal fluency, and slowing, with preservation of cued memory and an absence of intrusions. Depression, irritability,

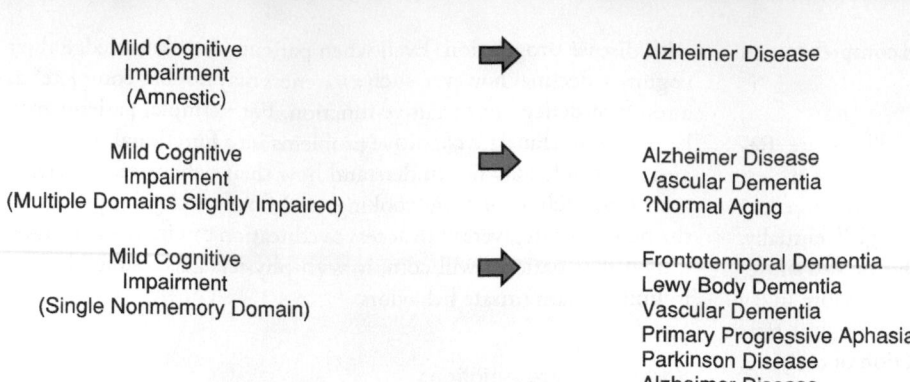

FIGURE 62-1. Heterogeneity of the term "mild cognitive impairment." (Reproduced by permission of Petersen R, Doody R, Kurz A, et al. Current concepts in mild cognitive impairment. Arch Neurol. 2001;58:1987. Copyright 2001 American Medical Association.)

and lack of initiative are also common. Difficulty in differentiating VaD from AD occurs in part because current criteria for dementia require memory impairment, and impairment in one additional cognitive domain. For adults with VaD, memory impairment may not occur until later in the disease process; thus, these patients have more progressed dementia and greater cognitive impairment at the time of diagnosis. A review of studies differentiating between early-stage AD and VaD found that the latter group had more pronounced deficits in executive function on tests such as the Wisconsin Card Sorting tests and the executive function scale of the Mattis Dementia Rating Scale than did adults with AD. Interestingly, performance between the two groups was similar on tests of selective attention and working memory such as the Trail-Making Test and Stroop Color–Word Interference test. In contrast, patients with VaD had better performance than patients with AD on tests of verbal learning and story recall, such as the California Verbal Learning Test and the Logical Memory subtest of the WMS-R, with fewer intrusions. It is important to note that as both VaD and AD progress, the cognitive profiles become more similar, so that differentiating mid-stage disease is very difficult. In addition, recent neuropathological studies have shown that many patients previously diagnosed with VaD caused by presence of vascular risk factors such as diabetes, hypertension, and radiologic evidence of ischemia have prominent AD pathology as well. Prevalence estimates of the co-occurrence of AD and VaD range from 20% to 40% of patients with dementia. Few studies have attempted to differentiate between mixed AD/VaD and either form of dementia on a neuropsychological basis, although it has been suggested that mixed dementia most closely resembles VaD from a cognitive perspective. Vascular pathology increases the likelihood that patients with neuropathological AD will show significant cognitive impairment. Finally, cognitive profiles for other forms of VaD such as multiple large vessel or single strategic infarcts are highly idiosyncratic, depending on lesion location and volume.

Frontotemporal Dementia

Frontotemporal dementia (FTD) is a diagnostic category that has been used to describe a number of conditions including Pick disease, progressive aphasia, semantic dementia, behavioral disorder and dysexecutive syndrome, familial chromosome 17-linked frontal lobe dementia, FTD of the non-Alzheimer type, and other histopathological classifications. FTD has been estimated to account for 3% to 20% of dementia cases. Prototypical symptoms of FTD include personality change and slowly progressive executive dysfunction. Patients often present with behavioral disturbance that includes disin-

hibition, a lack of conformity to social norms, perseveration, emotional blunting, and a lack of insight. Neuropsychological testing generally reveals impaired selective and divided attention, difficulty shifting mental set, poor abstraction, and impaired verbal fluency. Perseverative errors are common. Spatial skills are relatively preserved, except when organizational skills are required for completion of the task. Unfortunately, the MMSE is not very helpful in diagnosing early FTD since many patients score within normal limits.

Both the personality changes and cognitive dysfunction observed at early stages of FTD exceed those seen in normal aging. The most difficult differential diagnosis is between FTD and AD. Age of onset for FTD is typically in the late 50s or early 60s, although exceptions are observed. Therefore, on average, patients with FTD show symptoms around a decade earlier than patients with AD. As with AD, patients with FTD show insidious onset of symptoms with a gradual progression. Although comparisons of AD and FTD groups do not always reveal significantly different cognitive profiles, in general, patients with FTD show relatively spared memory performance in comparison to their executive and language functioning, especially when memory cues are provided. Apraxia is also more common than in AD. Often a multidisciplinary approach may be most helpful in the differential diagnosis since studies indicate that up to 75% of pathologically confirmed patients with FTD also appear to meet clinical criteria for probable AD.

Primary Progressive Aphasia

Primary progressive aphasia (PPA) has been described as the fifth most common cause of dementia. The diagnosis of PPA requires isolated language dysfunction for 2 years, with all other areas of cognition remaining largely intact, and the absence of radiological evidence of cerebrovascular or other neurological injury that would account for the aphasia. In the initial stages of PPA, anomia is inevitably present consisting of impaired object naming, impaired word finding, or both. Two broad categories of PPA are defined by the presence of additional language impairment. Nonfluent PPA is characterized by labored articulation, occasional dysarthria, dyscalculia and buccofacial apraxia, with preserved comprehension except for complex sentences with embedded clauses. In fluent PPA (also called PPA with verbal semantic comprehension deficits), word-finding pauses may still be evident, although speech rate and prosody are largely preserved. Comprehension is impaired, and patients may have difficulty both with naming objects and with pointing to objects when given their names. They are still able to demonstrate the use of such objects appropriately, however, reflecting intact knowledge of object meaning. As the disease progresses, speech becomes empty and paraphasic. A related condition, semantic dementia, is diagnosed when fluent PPA is accompanied by impairment in visual recognition of objects, and the semantic meaning of both words and objects is lost. Patients with semantic dementia display prominent visual agnosias and can no longer demonstrate object use accurately.

Because anomia and other language deficits may occur in a number of neurodegenerative conditions, the differential diagnosis of PPA rests on the clear demonstration that nonlinguistic cognitive and behavioral functions are intact for the first 2 years of the disease. The examiner must carefully determine whether poor performance on memory and other nonlanguage tests is caused by language deficits such as impaired comprehension of instructions. The onset of PPA is typically in the fifth or sixth decade of life, and its rate of progression varies greatly. As the disease progresses, however, other cognitive functions become impaired, as does the patient's ability to carry out functional activities, thus, making a diagnosis of mid-stage PPA difficult, at best. Differential diagnosis is also complicated by the heterogenous etiologies of PPA. The majority of patients have nonspecific focal atrophy of perisylvian language areas. A subgroup has AD-like pathology although not in brain regions typically associated with AD. Another subgroup have FTD and/or Pick pathology, although not the flagrant behavioral and executive function deficits of typical Pick disease.

Lewy Body Disease

Although the following diseases have a number of different neuropathological features, a common shared characteristic is the presence of Lewy bodies, abnormal intracytoplasmic inclusion deposits, on neuropathological examination.

Parkinson Disease

At its early stages, Parkinson disease (PD) can be difficult to differentiate from normal aging. Most patients initially present with a resting tremor. Other cardinal symptoms include bradykinesia, rigidity, and postural instability. Patients may also present with a shuffling gait, masked facies, and depression. Although there has been significant variability across estimates of the frequency of dementia in PD, it appears that approximately one-third of these patients develop dementia. Relatively healthy elderly patients can present with a number of these symptoms for unrelated problems. For instance, essential tremors are not uncommon and patients with arthritis often show slowed motor movements.

Typically, even nondemented patients with PD show slight cognitive deficits across a range of cognitive domains that are often conceptualized as executive dysfunction. PD with dementia is usually characterized by visuospatial deficits, attentional impairment, difficulty planning or shifting to a new stimulus, slowed information processing speed, and mildly impaired memory recall. Memory impairment is most frequently attributable to a retrieval deficit since recognition is generally intact. Procedural learning may be impaired, a pattern atypical in normal aging or in AD. Some language skills are intact, such as vocabulary, while others that tap additional cognitive domains, such as verbal fluency, are impaired. Mechanical aspects of speech are often impaired as well. Although PD has been characterized as a subcortical dementia to distinguish it from cortical dementias such as AD, this characterization has been criticized more

recently and may serve simply as a gross depiction of the cognitive profile.

Dementia with Lewy Bodies

According to consensus criteria for probable dementia with Lewy bodies (DLB), cognition must be carefully assessed. A progressive cognitive decline, usually over the course of a number of years, must be observed to a degree that it disables the patient. In addition, the patient must show some combination of fluctuations in attention, recurrent visual hallucinations, or spontaneous parkinsonism. Many patients may also present with other psychotic symptoms, neuroleptic sensitivity, and a history of falls and syncopal attacks. Based on these criteria, the differential diagnosis between DLB and PD is obviously difficult. At this time, the differential diagnosis is based purely on the timing of the onset of the cognitive symptoms. A patient with PD who develops cognitive symptoms after 1 year of motor symptoms is classified as "Parkinson disease with dementia." Earlier cognitive symptoms indicate DLB.

The differential diagnosis between DLB and AD can also be difficult. The presence of visual hallucinations in patients with MMSE scores greater than 20 is highly suggestive of DLB. Neuropsychological studies have identified typical cognitive profiles that may aid in diagnosis. In DLB, patients have more difficulty than patients with AD in copying complex designs, assembling pieces of an object, or completing other tasks requiring visuospatial skills. In contrast, AD subjects generally show significantly more impairment on delayed recall tasks than patients with DLB. Patients with DLB have attentional skills that are generally equivalent to those of patients with AD; however, patients with DLB exhibit significant attentional fluctuations. As a result, evaluating attention over time is more helpful than the overall severity of attention problems in the differential diagnosis. The clinical overlap of the two diseases may be related, in part, to the pathological overlap of the diseases. Neuropathological studies indicate that the majority of DLB cases have Alzheimer pathology (especially plaques) and that Lewy bodies are common in patients with AD. Finally, these cognitive profiles are most evident early in the course of the diseases. As the diseases progress, all cognitive functions become impaired and neuropsychological testing is less helpful for diagnosis.

Progressive Supranuclear Palsy

Progressive supranuclear palsy (PSP) is less common than PD. Although Lewy bodies are found in only the minority of PSP cases, PSP is frequently misdiagnosed as PD. A core feature of the disorder is vertical supranuclear gaze palsy, although this symptom may not present early in the course of the disease. Patients also present with postural instability, and falls are often seen shortly after onset. Cognition is characterized by mental slowing and executive dysfunction. Memory impairments are observed, but they are not as severe as in AD. Language functions resemble those seen in PD. Visual spatial deficits and increased apathy are also observed.

Alcohol-Related Dementia

Recent epidemiological analyses suggest that mild to moderate alcohol use reduces the risk for developing certain dementias, including AD and VaD. Chronic and profound alcohol use, however, can have a negative effect on cognition and may exacerbate the cognitive symptoms of other dementias and brain injuries. Poor nutrition (thiamine deficiency in particular) resulting from alcohol abuse is a primary contributor to the onset of cognitive problems. In addition, liver disease itself can interfere with thiamine regulation in the brain and may be a factor in the multiple cognitive and motor impairments associated with long-term alcohol use. Chronic alcoholics are often impaired on neurocognitive tests even following a period of abstinence, and many continue to show cognitive deficits indefinitely.

Persistent Alcohol Dementia

Alcohol dementia involves impairment in more than one area of cognitive function that persists after the patient stops drinking for a period of time. Visuospatial problem solving deficits and executive problems, including apathy, decreased judgment, and reduced interest in self-care, are prominent in these patients. Memory problems, in particular anterograde amnesia, are also common, but are generally not more impaired than other cognitive domains, and recognition is often intact. Typical neuropsychological sequelae include impairments on tasks requiring visual scanning, visuospatial organization, perceptual-motor speed, sustained attention, abstraction, and mental flexibility, while language functions are generally preserved. Perseveration and confabulation are common indicators of impaired executive function in the responses of patients with chronic alcohol use. It is also noteworthy that chronic alcohol use may potentiate the onset of AD, and produce a clinical picture of conjoint cognitive deficits.

Wernicke–Korsakoff Syndrome

The most severe neurological outcome of heavy and prolonged alcohol use, and the result of critical malnutrition, is Wernicke–Korsakoff syndrome. In contrast to patients with persistent alcohol dementia, patients with Wernicke–Korsakoff exhibit an acute symptom onset, often beginning with a grave confusional state, nystagmus, and significant ataxia. During this phase, symptoms progressively and rapidly worsen if treatment (immediate thiamine replacement) is not applied. This phase is almost always followed by a chronic and progressive stage that is associated primarily with impaired frontal and cerebellar functions. Unlike persistent alcohol dementia, patients with Korsakoff have significant impairments in memory relative to other cognitive effects, and memory impairment includes both retrograde and anterograde amnesia for episodic events, frequently with prominent confabulation. In contrast to AD, semantic memory is relatively spared in the Korsakoff patient. Patients show a characteristic gradient of remote memory impairment, with better recall for remote events and progressively reduced recall of recent events. As with persistent alcohol dementia, executive dysfunction and visuospatial impairments are also significant symptoms of the syndrome. Cerebellar atrophy and peripheral nerve damage lead to impaired gait, decreased or abnormal reflexes, and other movement abnormalities in these patients.

Prion Diseases

The prion diseases are a group of rare fatal spongiform encephalopathies that result from mutations and polymorphisms in the prion protein gene (PrP), causing rapid neurodegeneration. These diseases, of which Creutzfeldt–Jakob is the most well known, produce a profound and quickly progressive dementia, and may be sporadic, familial, or infectious. Sporadic cases are the most common, and are generally diagnosed in people in their 60's, with a typical age range between 40 and 80. Early cognitive signs of the prion diseases are usually vague and nonspecific, such as poor memory, concentration, and problem solving. Initially, there are also often psychiatric symptoms, including apathy, emotional lability, impaired sleep, and appetite loss. Early frank neurological symptoms are not common, but as the disease progresses, hyperreflexia, impaired coordination, changes in saccadic eye movements, and incontinence may occur. Given the early vague symptoms and dearth of neurological symptoms, patients are not likely to present for evaluation until they are in the more moderate to advanced stages, which can occur in a matter of months. Diagnosis typically involves measuring electroencephalographic changes, hyperintensities on magnetic resonance imaging, and abnormal 14-3-3 protein deposits in the cerebrospinal fluid. The most common differential diagnoses include depression, AD, and LBD.

Normal Pressure Hydrocephalus

Normal pressure hydrocephalus is a potentially reversible progressive dementia that makes up approximately 6% of the dementia cases. Abnormalities in the production, absorption, or flow of CSF result in ventricular dilatation. Patients may present with a triad of clinical symptoms that include gait or balance disturbance, urinary incontinence, and cognitive deficits. Unlike most other dementias, cognitive symptoms often present later in the course. This can make early clinical diagnosis difficult since gait abnormalities and incontinence have a variety of etiologies in geriatric populations. Radiographic evidence and intraventricular pressure measurement aid in the diagnosis. When cognitive deficits are present, they are most frequently observed in executive functioning. Although many subjects may have subjective memory complaints, memory deficits are not a prominent early symptom, and some memory declines are attributable to attention problems, which are more common.

When treated, a ventriculoperitoneal shunt is usually used to divert CSF for better absorption. However, surgery in geriatric populations always involves added risks, and the benefits of shunt surgery remain unclear. A wide variety of success rates have been reported, with better outcomes often reported after shorter follow-up periods. Patients with the full triad of symptoms appear to respond best to shunt surgery. Gait problems show the most frequent improvement, while cognitive function improves in the fewest patients. Recently, findings from a 5-year follow-up of normal pressure hydrocephalus patients with and without shunt surgery showed that at the 6-month assessment, 83% of the shunt cases improved in gait and 46% improved in memory. Of surviving shunt cases 5 years after surgery, 39% remained improved in gait, and fewer than 10% continued to show improvements on cognitive tests. Results suggested that outcomes may be improved in younger patients.

Human Immunodeficiency Virus

Although there is often the perception that geriatric patients are not at risk for HIV infection, the CDC reported that 10% of all HIV cases in the United States are in patients 50 years of age or older, and these numbers are expected to grow. The earliest cognitive areas affected are usually speed of information processing, attention, and motor speed. A subgroup of patients progresses to HIV-associated dementia, which is usually characterized by impairments in executive functioning, psychomotor speed, and memory.

Neurosyphilis

Neurosyphilis is an advanced syphilitic infection that may present with hallucinations, delusions, mood disturbance, personality change, strokes, ataxia, or cognitive decline. Deficits are observed in short-term memory and mental status with progressive cognitive decline in all areas of functioning. Although neurosyphilis is often classified as a reversible dementia, there is only limited evidence to support cognitive benefits with treatment. The onset of dementia in neurosyphilis often occurs several decades after contraction of the disease. Although screening procedures remain controversial, neurosyphilis should be considered in a differential diagnosis of dementia of unclear etiology in geriatric patients.

CONCLUSIONS

We have greatly furthered our understanding that age-related medical conditions not considered classically neurological in nature can nevertheless impact the central nervous system and thereby affect cognition. This knowledge has led to the realization that many of the changes in cognition previously thought to be unavoidable concomitants of normal aging are in fact preventable and in some cases even reversible. The deleterious consequences of not treating such disorders has become evident, given that many common diseases such as type 2 diabetes and hypertension appear to be risk factors for dementia. In turn, early identification of dementia or the prodromal condition mild cognitive impairment will become critical as therapeutic options for delaying disease progression proliferate. Careful characterization of cognitive status through neuropsychological assessment can provide the clinician with essential information to determine whether the patient is experiencing symptoms that warrant concern or further treatment. As the field of geriatrics approaches the goal of controlling or even preventing endemic late-life chronic diseases, it will become increasingly clear that the cognitive changes that occur with healthy aging are fewer than we thought, that they are more subtle in nature, and that they should not affect our ability to have rich, active lives into our eighties and beyond.

FURTHER READING

Anstey K, Christensen H. Education, activity, health, blood pressure, and apolipoprotein E as predictors of cognitive change in old age: a review. *Gerontology.* 2000;46:163–77.

Ballard C, Holmes C, McKeith I, et al. Psychiatric morbidity in dementia with Lewy bodies: a prospective clinical and neuropathological comparative study with Alzheimer's disease. *Am J Psychiatry.* 1999;156:1039–1045.

Bowler J, Steenhuis R, Hachinski V. Conceptual background to vascular cognitive impairment. *Alzheimer Dis Assoc Disord.* 1999;13(s3):S30–S37.

Burke D, MacKay D. Memory, language, and ageing. *Phil Trans R Soc Lond.* 1997;352:1845–1856.

Calvaresi E, Bryan J. B vitamins, cognition, and aging: a review. *J Gerontol B Psychol Sci.* 2001;56:P327–P339.

Collinge J. Prion diseases of humans and animals: their causes and molecular basis. *Annu Rev Neurosci.* 2001;24:519–550.

Elias P, Elias M, D'Agostino R, et al. NIDDM and blood pressure as risk factors for poor cognitive performance: the Framingham study. *Diabetes Care.* 1997;20:1388–1395.

Grossman M. Frontotemporal dementia: a review. *J Int Neuropsychol Soc.* 2002;8:566–583.

Laursen P. The impact of aging on cognitive function. An 11-year follow-up study of four age cohorts. *Acta Neurol Scand.*1997;S172:7–86.

Luszcz M, Bryan J. Toward understanding age-related memory loss in adulthood. *Gerontology.* 1999;45:2–9.

Malec J, Ivnik R, Smith G. Neuropsychology and normal aging: the clinician's perspective. In: Parks RW, Zec RF, Wilson RS, eds. *Neuropsychology of Alzheimer's Disease and Related Disorders.* New York, New York: Oxford University Press; 1993.

McKhann G, Drachman D, Folstein M, et al. Clinical diagnosis of Alzheimer's disease: report of the NINCDS-ADRDA work group under the auspices of Department of Health and Human Services Task Force on Alzheimer's Disease. *Neurology.* 1984;34:939–944.

Mesulam M. Primary progressive aphasia. *Ann Neurol.* 2001;49:425–432.

Newman M, Kirchner J, Phillips-Bute B, et al. Longitudinal assessment of neurocognitive function after coronary-artery bypass surgery. *N Engl J Med.* 2001;344:2874–2881.

Petersen R, Doody R, Kurz A, et al. Current concepts in mild cognitive impairment. *Arch Neurol.* 2001;58:1985–1992.

Reaven G, Thompson L, Nahum D, et al. Relationship between hyperglycemia and cognitive function in older NIDDM patients. *Diabetes Care.* 1990;13:16–21.

Savolainen S, Hurskainen H, Paljarvi L, et al. Five-year outcome of normal pressure hydrocephalus with or without a shunt: predictive value of clinical signs, neuropsychological evaluation, and infusion test. *Acta Neurochir.* 2002;144:512–523.

Saxton J, Munro C, Butters M, et al. Alcohol, dementia, and Alzheimer's disease: comparison of neuropsychological profiles. *J Geriatr Psychiatry Neurol.* 2000;13:141–149.

Storey E, Slavin M, Kinsella G. Patterns of cognitive impairment in Alzheimer's disease: assessment and differential diagnosis. *Front Biosci.* 2002;7:e155–e184.

Zekry D, Hauw J-J, Gold G. Mixed dementia: epidemiology, diagnosis, and treatment. *J Amer Geriatr Soc.* 2002;50:1431–1438.

Psychoactive Drug Therapy

Bruce G. Pollock ■ *Todd P. Semla* ■ *Christina E. Forsyth*

INTRODUCTION

In this chapter, we focus on the use of psychotherapeutic medications in the elderly, including the antidepressant, psychostimulant, antipsychotic, mood stabilizer, and anxiolytic medications that are used to treat the psychiatric disorders of late life, including major depression, anxiety, and the psychosis and behavioral disturbances that frequently accompany Alzheimer's disease (AD) and related disorders.

Mood and behavioral disturbances are of particular concern in the elderly. Late-life depression, including major depressive disorder and dysthymia, affects 5% to 12% of older adults. These rates are consistent with those in younger adults; however, the elderly face a disease profile that is more chronic and treatment resistant with an element of cognitive impairment. Frequently, depression in elderly, community dwelling individuals remains unidentified and untreated. Depression occurring past age 60 is likely distinct from that which occurs in younger age groups. It has been associated with significant vascular disease as evidenced in the imaging literature, and with low testosterone levels in older dysthymic men. This idiosyncratic disease profile may account for treatment resistance. For example, structural abnormalities in frontal white matter have been linked to a poorer remittance of depressive symptomatology.

Late-life depression leads to further deterioration in quality of life, as well as increasing risk for dementia and suicide. Depressed elders suffer greater rates of disability, mortality, and nursing home placement. Furthermore, when depression co-occurs with other medical or psychiatric illness, it negatively alters the disease process. For example, cardiac mortality is increased in depressed patients with unstable angina, postmyocardial infarction, or congestive heart failure, and comorbid anxiety impairs interpersonal function and leads to greater severity of physical symptoms. Consequently, the effects of depression result in greater strain on an already overburdened health care system.

Anxiety disorders are also highly prevalent in older adults, between 2% and 19% in community dwelling elders, with the most common forms being generalized anxiety disorder (GAD) and phobias. Anxious symptomatology not meeting criteria for a clinical diagnosis is experienced by a further 20% of elderly individuals. Late-life anxiety can co-occur with physical illness, depression, or side effects of medication use. Risk factors for anxiety in elders include cognitive and physical impairments, economic difficulties, and social segregation.

Older anxious individuals experience greater physical disability and cognitive impairment, as well as reduced ability to carry out activities of daily life. Quality of life is diminished and risk of mortality and coronary artery disease (particularly in men) is greater when anxiety is present in later life. Anxious elders are prone to excessive use of medical services, with anxiety disorders comprising 38% of mental health claims as compared to 21% for affective disorders.

Behavioral instability, including agitation, aggression, and psychosis, also appears frequently in late-life, especially when associated with dementia. Approximately 2% to 5% of elderly individuals 60 years of age or older suffer from dementing illnesses, while 15% to 40% of those older than 85 develop dementia. At some point in the course of dementia, most nursing home and community dwelling patients experience behavioral dysfunction and/or psychosis. For example, studies indicate that 10% to 70% of dementia patients experience psychotic symptoms. In a 4-year study, primary psychosis in patients with AD was reported to occur in 51% of patients. Across samples of AD patients, delusional symptoms, frequently related to theft or suspicion, can present in as many as 50% of patients. Hallucinations, typically related to phantom boarder syndrome (the belief that another person is in one's home), can involve either visual or auditory stimuli, and have been reported in 5% to 15% of dementia patients.

Alterations of personality can develop early in the course of illness. Such changes include depression, apathy, irritability, emotional withdrawal, and disinhibition (e.g., wandering, aggression, repetitive calling out or screaming). More severe reactions associated with frustration can include angry or violent outbursts. Such psychopathology can be particularly troublesome for caregivers. Patients may become stubborn, combative, or neglectful of activities essential to daily life. As such, many caregivers are compelled to institutionalize their loved ones. Both in long-term care residents and community dwelling elderly, patients experiencing behavioral or psychological symptoms of dementia (BPSD) are at increased risk for mortality. Incidence of increased extrapyramidal symptoms (EPS) and greater cognitive decline has also been associated with BPSD. The use of psychotropic medications to treat these conditions is second only to the use of cardiovascular medications among older patients, including the frail and chronically ill elderly. Nearly one in five community dwelling elders and 47% of nursing home residents were found to be taking regular psychotropic medications. However, the basic pharmacokinetic and clinical evidence base underlying this use is limited. In fact, most psychiatric medications have been tested only in younger and healthier patients, prior to their release.

There are indications that this limited knowledge base can compromise care in elders. In an acute geriatric medical unit, a recent study found that the prevalence of adverse drug reactions (ADRs) was 16% on admission for those patients taking appropriate medications and that 66% of admissions were preceded by at least one inappropriate medication. In the long-term care setting, psychoactive medications (antipsychotics, antidepressants, and sedative/hypnotics) and anticoagulants were the most common medications associated with ADRs, and neuropsychiatric events were the most common manifestations of preventable ADRs. There is also evidence that commonly used antidepressants may have limited efficacy and more adverse effects in the oldest old and frail elderly, and that the atypical antipsychotic agents often used for the treatment of the psychotic and aggressive symptoms in dementia may lead to cerebrovascular events and increased mortality in nursing home residents.

As with other medications, the treatment of older patients with psychotropics is also complicated by age-associated pharmacokinetic and pharmacodynamic changes, which are exacerbated by illness and their concomitant potential for drug–drug interactions and poor adherence. An additional complication for psychotropics is the lack of diagnostic precision and pathophysiologic understanding of what is being treated. Psychotropic treatment is based on treating symptoms that have a heterogeneous etiology. The strategy for drug discovery in psychiatry has relied upon the serendipitous observation of symptomatic benefit of a known drug, study of the mechanisms of that compound, and efforts to develop similar compounds with improved efficacy and tolerability. The limitations of this approach are evident in the treatment of "psychoses" in dementia, as if it were the same disorder as schizophrenia in younger patients. Similarly, depression appearing later in life may be associated with ischemic injury or associated with the development of AD. For currently available psychotropics, there have been few studies of their "real world" comparative effectiveness. One example is the recently published Clinical Antipsychotic Trials of Intervention Effectiveness-Alzheimer's Disease (CATIE-AD), which found an unfavorable risk to benefit ratio for use of atypical antipsychotic medications in patients with AD. It is also difficult to demonstrate efficacy when there is variability in drug exposure. The recent use of population pharmacokinetic methodologies in elderly psychiatric patients treated with antidepressants or antipsychotics is beginning to demonstrate the extensive interindividual differences in drug clearance for these medications.

ANTIDEPRESSANTS

Selective Serotonin Reuptake Inhibitors

The selective serotonin reuptake inhibitors (SSRIs) are considered first-line pharmacotherapy for late-life depression. These drugs act on the serotonergic system by blocking the reuptake of this neurotransmitter. In comparison with other antidepressants, the SSRIs generally have a more favorable side effect profile and are well tolerated. They are also markedly safer than tricyclic antidepressants in overdose. Over 30 randomized, placebo-controlled, clinical trials with more than 5000 older patients with SSRIs have been conducted. These studies have included patients with a variety of psychiatric and medical illnesses including mild cognitive impairment, dementia, minor depression, schizophrenia, cardiovascular and cerebrovascular disease, or other medical conditions. SSRIs have received substantial attention in the treatment of anxiety in younger adults, however, only a single placebo-controlled trial and two open label studies have suggested efficacy in anxious elderly patients. Limited evidence supports the efficacy of SSRIs in treating dementia related behavioral disturbances, such as agitation, disinhibition, delusions, and hallucinations.

Although there is similar efficacy between each of the SSRIs, citalopram, escitalopram, and sertraline have better pharmacokinetic profiles, are less of a risk for drug–drug interactions, and appear not to interfere with cognition. As such, these drugs are preferable to fluvoxamine, fluoxetine, or paroxetine. In the elderly, starting dosages are administered in one daily dose, and are half the amount administered in younger populations (Table 63-1). Dosages can be doubled after a week of use. Fluvoxamine is the only SSRI that should be given according to a twice-daily dosing regimen.

Fluoxetine

The first SSRI to become available on the market in 1988 was fluoxetine. This drug ushered in a new era of treatment, providing an alternative to the tricyclic antidepressants. In geriatric patients, fluoxetine has demonstrated superiority as compared to placebo, and is as efficacious as amitriptyline, doxepin, escitalopram, paroxetine, sertraline, and trimipramine. Dosage recommendations for the elderly indicate starting at 10 mg/day, which can be increased every 14 days by 10 mg to a maximum of 40 mg/day. This SSRI and its active metabolite norfluoxetine have mean half-lives of 4.6 and 9.3 days, respectively, rendering it an unfavorable choice for older adults. Fluoxetine and norfluoxetine inhibit the enzyme CYP2D6, and to a lesser extent CYP1A2 and CYP3A4. Thus, it is crucial to consider interactions with other medications metabolized by these enzymes to avoid drug accumulation and toxicity (Table 63-2).

Sertraline

Sertraline was the second SSRI introduced, and is more specific in its effects on the inhibition of serotonin (5-hydroxytryptamine,

TABLE 63-1

Antidepressant Oral Dosages and Side Effects

CLASS/ MEDICATION	INITIAL DOSE (mg)	MAX DOSE (mg)	RISK FOR DRUG INTERACTION	SIDE EFFECTS
Selective serotonin reuptake inhibitors				
Citalopram	10–20 qam	40 qd	Low	EPS, hyponatremia, GI distress, sexual dysfunction, slight weight gain
Escitalopram	10 qd	20 qd	Low	GI distress, sexual dysfunction, slight weight gain
Fluoxetine	10 qd	40 qd	High	Insomnia, slight anticholinergic effects, GI distress, sexual dysfunction, slight weight gain
Paroxetine	10 qd	40 qd	Moderate	GI distress, sexual dysfunction, moderate weight gain, minimal sedation, withdrawal symptoms
Paroxetine CR	12.5 qd	50 qd		
Sertraline	25–50 qd	200 qd	Low	Sexual dysfunction, slight weight gain
Serotonin norepinephrine reuptake inhibitors				
Duloxetine	20 qd or bid	60 qd or 30 bid	Low	GI distress, dry mouth, urinary hesitancy
Venlafaxine IR	25–50 bid	75–225 total bid	High	GI distress, minimal sedation, headaches, sexual dysfunction, serotonin syndrome, SIADH, hyponatremia, withdrawal symptoms, adrenergic effects, dose-dependent hypotension, ECG changes, arrhythmia, acute ischemia, EPS
Venlafaxine XR	75 qam	75–225 qd		
Other second-generation antidepressants				
Bupropion IR	37.5–50 bid	75–150 bid	Moderate	Slight GI distress, slight sexual dysfunction; CYP2B6 inhibitors: risk for seizure, gait disturbance, falls, psychosis
Bupropion SR	100 qd	150 bid		
Bupropion XR	150 qd	300 qd		
Mirtazapine	15 qhs	45 qd	Low	Mild anticholinergic events, hypotension, high sedation, slight sexual dysfunction, serotonin syndrome, increased appetite
Preferred tricyclic antidepressants				
Desipramine	10–25 qhs	50–150 qd	High	Therapeutic serum level ≥115 ng/mL; mild anticholinergic events, hypotension, slight GI distress, sedation, sexual dysfunction, slight weight gain
Nortriptyline	10–25 qhs	75–150 qd	High	Therapeutic window 50–150 ng/mL; anticholinergic events, hypotension, sedation, sexual dysfunction, slight weight gain

qd, once daily; bid, twice daily; qhs, once before bedtime; CR, controlled release; IR, immediate release; XR, extended release; SR, sustained release; EPS, extrapyramidal symptoms; GI, gastrointestinal (e.g., nausea, vomiting, diarrhea, constipation); SIADH, syndrome of inappropriate secretion of antidiuretic hormone; ECG, electrocardiogram.
Adrenergic effects: dry mouth, constipation, increased ocular pressure, cardiovascular difficulties, agitation.

5HT) reuptake than fluoxetine. Its effects on the reuptake of norepinephrine and dopamine are modest. Sertraline is more effective than placebo, and is comparable to amitriptyline, fluoxetine, fluvoxamine, imipramine, nortriptyline, and venlafaxine in treating late-life depression. It is tolerated more favorably than imipramine and venlafaxine and demonstrates greater cognitive improvement than nortriptyline or fluoxetine. Dosing in elderly patients is typically initiated at 25 mg or 50 mg, with increases occurring after 7 days to a daily maximum of 200 mg. This SSRI does require titration, with one study of frail nursing home patients noting an average maintenance dose of 77 mg/day. Although sertraline is a mild inhibitor of CYP2D6, its minimal effects translate to lower risk for drug interactions.

Paroxetine

Evidence supports that paroxetine is as effective in depressed geriatric patients as amitriptyline, bupropion, clomipramine, doxepin, fluoxetine, imipramine, and nortriptyline. Again, this SSRI demonstrates superiority to placebo; however, in a study of very old long-term care patients with minor depression, paroxetine resulted in greater cognitive impairment as compared to placebo. Mirtazapine has displayed marginal efficacy over paroxetine in one double-blind, randomized

trial. Paroxetine elicits fewer side effects compared to the tricyclic nortriptyline. A starting dose of 10 mg/day is recommended for geriatric patients. After 1 week, dosing can increase by 10 mg to a maximum of 40 mg/day. Dose titration from 20 mg to 30 mg results in median half-life changes (30 hours and 38 hours, respectively), as well as changes in steady state concentrations (46 ng/mL and 80 mg). Paroxetine can be given by controlled release tablets at an initial dose of 12.5 mg/day and titrated each week up to a maximum of 50 mg/day. This drug is another potent inhibitor of CYP2D6, and thus the metabolic activity of concomitant medications must be examined prior to administration of paroxetine.

Citalopram and Escitalopram

The majority of published trials examining citalopram in depressed older individuals include those with concomitant dementia or cognitive impairment. Escitalopram is the S-enantiomer of racemic citalopram. Only one randomized, controlled trial has evaluated escitalopram in late-life depression. Citalopram has demonstrated greater efficacy over placebo in depressed elderly without dementia, and similar efficacy as amitriptyline, and venlafaxine. While citalopram has been associated with lower remission rates than nortriptyline, it is much better tolerated. In the single study comparing escitalopram,

TABLE 63-2

CYP450 Isozyme Substrates and Inhibitors

CLASS/MEDICATION	1A2	2A6	2B6	2C19	2C8/9	2D6	2E1	3A4
Selective serotonin reuptake inhibitors								
Citalopram	-	0	-	++/-	0	+/-	0	++
Escitalopram	0	0	0	++	0	-	0	++
Fluoxetine	+/--	0	+/-	+/--	++/-	++/---	+	+/-
Fluvoxamine	++/---	0	-	---	-	++/-	0	-
Paroxetine	-	0	--	-	-	++/---	0	-
Sertraline	-	0	+/--	++/--	+/-	++/--	0	+/--
Serotonin norepinephrine reuptake inhibitors								
Duloxetine	++	0	0	0	0	++/--	0	0
Venlafaxine	0	0	-	+	+	++/-	0	++/-
Other second-generation antidepressants								
Bupropion	+	+	++	0	+	+/-	+	+
Mirtazapine	++/-	0	0	0	+	++	0	++/-
Preferred tricyclic antidepressants								
Desipramine	+	--	--	0	0	++/--	-	--
Nortriptyline	+	0	0	+	0	++/-	-	+
Atypical antipsychotics								
Aripiprazole	0	0	0	0	0	++	0	++
Clozapine	++/-	+	0	+/-	+/-	+/-	-	++/-
Olanzapine	++/-	0	0	-	-	+/-	0	-
Quetiapine	0	0	0	0	0	+	0	++
Risperidone	0	0	0	0	0	++/-	0	+/-
Ziprasidone	+	0	0	0	0	-	0	++/-
Anticonvulsant mood stabilizers								
Carbamazepine	---	0	---	---	+/---	0	0	++/---
Valproic acid	0	+	+	+/-	+/-	-	+	-
Anxiolytics								
Buspirone	0	0	0	0	0	+	0	++

0, No metabolism; +, Minor substrate; ++, Major substrate; -, Weak inhibitor; --, Moderate inhibitor; ---, Strong inhibitor.

fluoxetine, and placebo, both active drugs were well tolerated. However, neither was more efficacious in reducing depressive symptoms beyond placebo. Geriatric dosage recommendations for citalopram indicate a starting dose of 10 mg or 20 mg, which can be increased after 7 days to a maximum of 40 mg/day. For patients taking other medications, citalopram is an excellent choice as it is neither significantly affected by, nor does it affect, the CYP450 system. However, in older patients, the half-life of citalopram is increased, while availability and clearance are decreased. Those patients with mild to moderate renal function experience a 17% reduction in citalopram clearance.

Side Effects and Safety

Side effects are a particular concern in the elderly, especially in the oldest old, frail, or medically ill. SSRIs have received significant attention in the treatment of patients with ischemic heart disease, congestive heart failure, and immediately postmyocardial infarction. Evidence shows no increased cardiac risk, with no effects of SSRIs on blood pressure, cardiac conduction or arrhythmias. Patients with bradycardia or those taking β-blockers may, however, experience a further reduction in heart rate. Though the SSRIs are well tolerated in the geriatric population, caution should be exercised. Following initial treatment some patients may experience gastrointestinal (GI) difficulties (e.g., nausea), and there is slight potential for GI

or postsurgical bleeding. This may be a result of decreased platelet activation affecting platelet aggregation to prolong bleeding time. GI bleeding is also a concern when using SSRIs in conjunction with nonsteroidal anti-inflammatory medications (NSAIDs) or low-dose aspirin. Concomitant use, or use within 3 to 4 weeks of cessation, of monoamine oxidase inhibitors (MAOIs) can lead to the potentially fatal serotonin syndrome. Hyponatremia, especially in those patients with borderline sodium levels, is a possible consequence of SSRI use and should be assessed especially early in treatment or if there is a change in cognitive status.

While Parkinson's patients are able to tolerate SSRIs, EPS may be caused by SSRI use in some elderly patients. Antidepressant use is associated with risk for falls and hip fractures, and prolonged use of SSRIs may affect bone metabolism leading to risk of fragility fractures. Risk for suicide in the first month of SSRI treatment has been demonstrated in the elderly; however, there is a significant decrease in suicidal ideation in patients taking SSRIs versus placebo. This suggests that there may be a particular subgroup more susceptible to an unusual SSRI response.

Other Antidepressants

For those elderly patients who are unresponsive to, or are unable to tolerate the use of, SSRIs, medications such as bupropion, duloxetine, mirtazapine, or venlafaxine may be used as second-line therapy.

In younger patients, these medications exhibit favorable side-effect profiles; however, the controlled data are limited thus caution must be exerted when administering these agents to the elderly.

Bupropion

Nonresponders to SSRIs, or those elderly depressed patients who cannot tolerate SSRIs, may be given bupropion on its own or in augmentation to another medication. For example, bupropion is favored in those patients experiencing nausea, diarrhea, severe fatigue, or sexual dysfunction with SSRI use. This antidepressant is well tolerated in medically ill patients, including those with heart disease, those that smoke, and patients with neuropathic pain. Bupropion has demonstrated similar efficacy as imipramine and paroxetine in depressed elders. Starting dose recommendations for older patients are 37.5 mg of immediate release tablets twice daily, or 100 mg daily of the sustained release tablets. Increases consistent with initial dosages can be made every 3 to 4 days up to a maximum of 450 mg/day. However, evidence supports that the elderly may respond at doses up to 150 mg/day in divided administration. Bupropion should be avoided in patients with, or at risk for, seizure disorders or psychotic symptoms. Although seizures are not frequent in those patients taking sustained-release bupropion, case reports have demonstrated the onset of psychosis with bupropion possibly owing to its action on the dopaminergic system. This mechanism of action may also account for the association between bupropion use and gait disturbance and falls. In older adults, the half-life of bupropion is increased and it inhibits CYP2D6 moderately. It is metabolized by CYP2B6, thus medications inhibiting this isozyme (e.g., fluoxetine, paroxetine) may increase bupropion's adverse effects.

Duloxetine

Efficacy and tolerability of duloxetine in young adults are supported by several randomized, controlled trials in patients with major depression, pain associated with diabetic neuropathy, and stress urinary incontinence. In the elderly, duloxetine has been efficacious in the treatment of depression and associated pain symptoms as compared to placebo. Duloxetine inhibits both serotonin and norepinephrine reuptake, and aging does not seem to affect its pharmacokinetic profile. Initial doses are typically 20 mg/day in either single or divided doses. Increases can be made to a maximum of 60 mg/day in either one to two doses per day. Duloxetine has a moderate ability to inhibit CYP2D6 and CYP3A4. Although it is reported to have minimal effects on heart rate and blood pressure in healthy young adults, duloxetine's action on norepinephrine may have greater implications for older patients with heart disease. In the absence of further evidence of the safety of this newer antidepressant in the treatment of the elderly, duloxetine should be used cautiously.

Mirtazapine

By blocking α_2 autoreceptors, mirtazapine enhances noradrenergic and specific serotonergic transmission. Patients who do not tolerate SSRIs because of sexual dysfunction, tremor, or severe nausea may respond well to mirtazapine. This drug has also shown success in the treatment of depressed oncology patients receiving chemotherapy. Mirtazapine has demonstrated similar efficacy in the treatment of late-life depression to low-dose amitriptyline and marginal superi-

ority to paroxetine, yet no placebo-controlled trials have been published. As a result, mirtazapine is regarded as a third-line treatment following intolerance of, or nonresponse to, SSRIs or venlafaxine. Its concurrent use with other SSRIs raises concerns owing to the risk for serotonin syndrome in older adults. Furthermore, cognitive impairment in the elderly taking mirtazapine is another concern, possibly because of antihistaminergic and sedative effects. Two trials including healthy subjects taking this drug have reported driving impairments, and in demented elderly patients delirium has resulted. Drug–drug interactions are of minimal concern when taking mirtazapine, as it has little effect on the CYP450 system.

Venlafaxine

Venlafaxine is another serotonin–norepinephrine reuptake inhibitor. Geriatric trials of this antidepressant have included patients with atypical depression, dysthymia, and poststroke depression. Studies also show the utility of venlafaxine in the treatment of late-life GAD or chronic pain. However, higher doses of venlafaxine (i.e., 225 mg/day or greater) are required in the treatment of pain to activate its antinociceptive effects via its action on adrenergic mechanisms. Meta-analyses data indicate that venlafaxine may be as efficacious as SSRIs in the treatment of depression in younger adults and have benefits to remission rates above that of the SSRIs. Such benefits may be further enhanced in woman 50 years of age or older. Published randomized, controlled trials of venlafaxine including depressed geriatric patients demonstrate that it is as efficacious as citalopram, clomipramine, dothiepin, nortriptyline, and sertraline, and is superior to trazodone. These studies found venlafaxine to be less well tolerated than sertraline, but as tolerable as citalopram and dothiepin, with superior tolerability over clomipramine, nortriptyline, and trazodone.

Venlafaxine's effects on the serotonergic system occur at lower doses. However, its effects on norepinephrine neurotransmission result from higher doses. In younger individuals, dosages as high as 225 mg or more per day may be required, though these doses may elicit adverse reactions in a geriatric population. Patients may experience a similar side-effect profile as with SSRI use, including GI distress, headaches, sexual dysfunction, serotonin syndrome, the syndrome of inappropriate antidiuretic hormone secretion, and hyponatremia. Symptoms associated with the discontinuation of venlafaxine may also occur, regardless of drug preparation type. In addition, side effects associated with the adrenergic system can occur, such as dry mouth, constipation, increased ocular pressure, cardiovascular difficulties, and agitation. Hypertension results in a dose-dependent fashion, with hypotension, electrocardiographic changes, arrhythmia, and acute ischemia also possible when taking venlafaxine. Experts discourage the use of venlafaxine in patients with heart disease, and recommend close cardiac monitoring for patients on higher dosages. While venlafaxine has minimal effect on the CYP450 system, it is metabolized by CYP2D6. Thus, poor 2D6 metabolizers or patients taking other drugs inhibiting this isozyme may have higher concentrations of venlafaxine. Venlafaxine should only be considered after nonresponse to SSRIs has been established.

Tricyclic Antidepressants and Monoamine Oxidase Inhibitors

Once widely prescribed for the treatment of depression, tricyclic antidepressants (TCAs) have largely been supplanted by SSRIs as the treatment of choice. TCAs have been studied in numerous randomized, placebo-controlled, and comparator trials. Though these studies demonstrate the efficacy of TCAs in treating late-life depression, most do not account for optimal dosing strategies using plasma level monitoring. MAOIs have also shown antidepressant effects similar to TCAs. Both of these drug classes require significant efforts to prevent associated adverse events, many of which can be severe and toxic. As such, TCAs and MAOIs are considered third- and fourth-line treatments of geriatric depression.

Common side effects of the TCAs include sedation, orthostatic hypotension (leading to dizziness, falls, and fractures), and anticholinergic effects such as dry mouth, blurred vision, constipation, confusion, and delirium. Nortriptyline, a secondary amine TCA, is better tolerated in the elderly and has a lower tendency to result in orthostasis, falls, and anticholinergic effects. This TCA has an established therapeutic window, the optimal serum plasma level resulting in efficacy (50–150 ng/mL) or toxicity ($\geq$300 ng/mL), which allows for more accurate and effective dosing. Two open trials of nortriptyline have found this medication to be effective in treating depression in the elderly. Three randomized, comparator trials found that nortriptyline was as efficacious as paroxetine and sertraline in alleviating geriatric depression; however, paroxetine was better tolerated than the TCA, and sertraline was associated with better cognitive improvement. Starting doses are usually 10 mg to 25 mg before bedtime. Plasma levels are taken within 5 to 7 days, and linear dosage adjustments can be made up to target plasma levels of 50 to 150 ng/mL. Though nortriptyline is preferred to the tertiary TCAs (i.e., amitriptyline, clomipramine, doxepin, imipramine), it is still associated with anticholinergic effects. Cardiovascular events are also a significant concern with tricyclics as even slight overdoses can result in lethal heart block or arrhythmia. Patients with ischemic heart disease should not be given TCAs as risk for sudden cardiovascular death is increased.

MAOI use in elderly populations is infrequent. While these medications are associated with fewer cardiac and anticholinergic side effects, serious hypo- and hypertension or serotonergic crisis may result from the concurrent intake of other medications or foods containing tyramine. Thus, it is crucial for patients taking MAOIs to adhere to strict dietary restrictions, inform all health care providers of MAOI use, and have their blood pressure monitored. Any signs of headache, stiff neck, nausea, or vomiting require an evaluation of blood pressure; if blood pressure is elevated, immediate medical attention is required. Though very rarely used in the elderly owing to adverse events and dietary restrictions, phenelzine is the preferred MAOI as it has received the most study in geriatric patients and has been shown to treat late-life depression. Recently, a transdermal patch form of selegiline has also been approved by the Food and Drug Administration (FDA) to treat major depression. However, there is very limited geriatric experience with this medication and dietary restrictions are still recommended for higher dosages.

PSYCHOSTIMULANTS

Methylphenidate

Methylphenidate is a controlled substance used for the treatment of attention deficit disorder and for the management of the som-

nolence symptoms of narcolepsy. Some data indicate that depressed elderly with concomitant medical complications may have symptomatic benefit with acceptable tolerability. In particular, it may improve symptoms of apathy and anergia that often occur with depression or dementia. Using methylphenidate with an SSRI could potentiate its antidepressant effects; however, more systematic data are still required. Side effects associated with methylphenidate may be of particular concern in a geriatric population, such as anxiety, psychosis, anorexia, and hypertension. Drug interactions with warfarin are also concerning, as methylphenidate may decrease the metabolism of anticoagulants.

ANTIPSYCHOTICS

Atypical antipsychotic medications are first-line drugs in the treatment of psychotic symptoms associated with many late-life etiologies, but particularly in dementia. Studies examining medication use in long-term care facilities suggest that as many as 30% to 50% of elderly residents are prescribed an antipsychotic. Available evidence suggests that these agents may be efficacious in geriatric populations to alleviate schizophrenia, delirium, and the BPSDs. However, issues of the safety and tolerability of antipsychotics in elders remain a concern.

Conventional Antipsychotics

The first antipsychotics were introduced in the 1950s. Generally, all of the typical antipsychotics share similar rates of efficacy. However, side-effect profiles can vary. This class of medications has been shown to treat BPSDs; although placebo response rates were also high. Yet early studies have found EPS (e.g., dystonia, parkinsonism, akathisia, tardive dyskinesia) to be a significant adverse reaction associated with the conventional antipsychotics, even when administered at moderate doses. In a study comparing low and moderate doses of haloperidol to placebo, moderate doses of the antipsychotic were more effective in treating psychosis and psychomotor agitation, but again were associated with greater instances of EPS. In a comparison of perphenazine to citalopram and placebo, the antipsychotic was comparable in efficacy to citalopram and superior to placebo; however, the SSRI had a more favorable side-effect profile. Similar results were demonstrated in a comparison of citalopram and risperidone, where both medications successfully reduced symptoms of agitation and psychosis in hospitalized patients with dementia, yet citalopram was associated with significantly fewer adverse events. Nonetheless, further studies are required before the utility of antidepressant treatments in alleviating BPSDs in nondepressed patients can be recommended. Currently, the use of atypical antipsychotics is preferred to that of the typical antipsychotics in treating BPSDs.

Atypical Antipsychotics

In comparator trials of atypical and typical antipsychotics, olanzapine and risperidone have demonstrated comparable or greater efficacy and tolerability over promazine or haloperidol in elderly patients with BPSDs, schizophrenia, or delirium. Notable was the lower incidence of milder EPS with use of the atypical agents. Older patients have also been found to be at much greater risk of tardive dyskinesia

COLOR PLATES

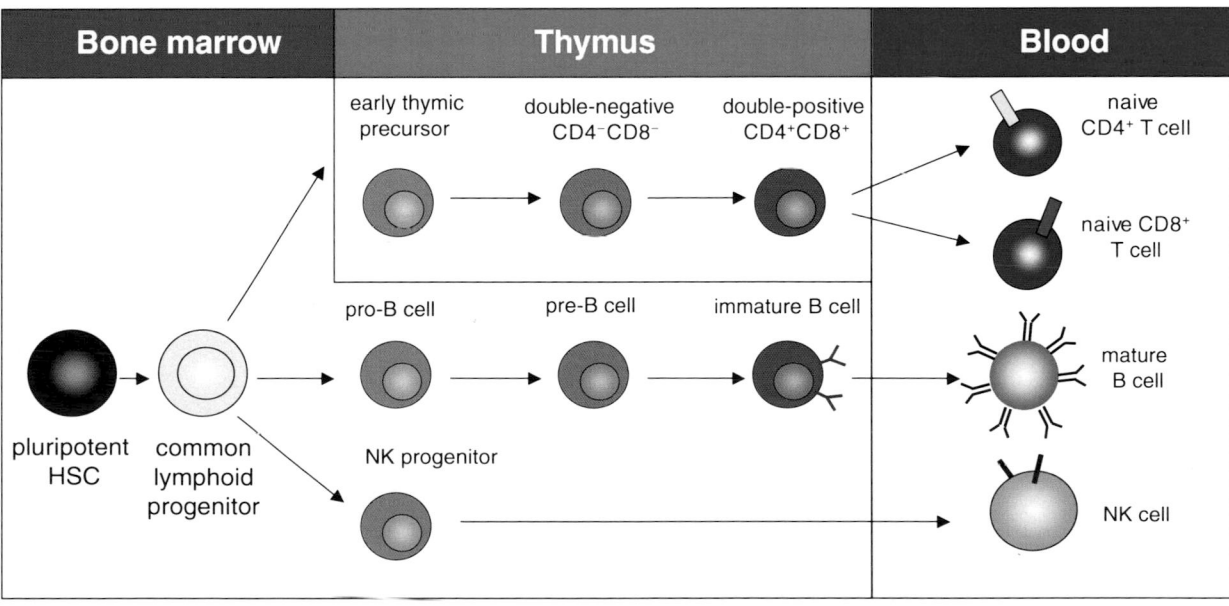

Color Plate 1. Maturation of lymphoid cells. Maturation of T cells takes place in the thymus, whereas B cells and NK cells undergo maturation in the bone marrow. All mature lymphocytes migrate into the periphery and can be found in blood.

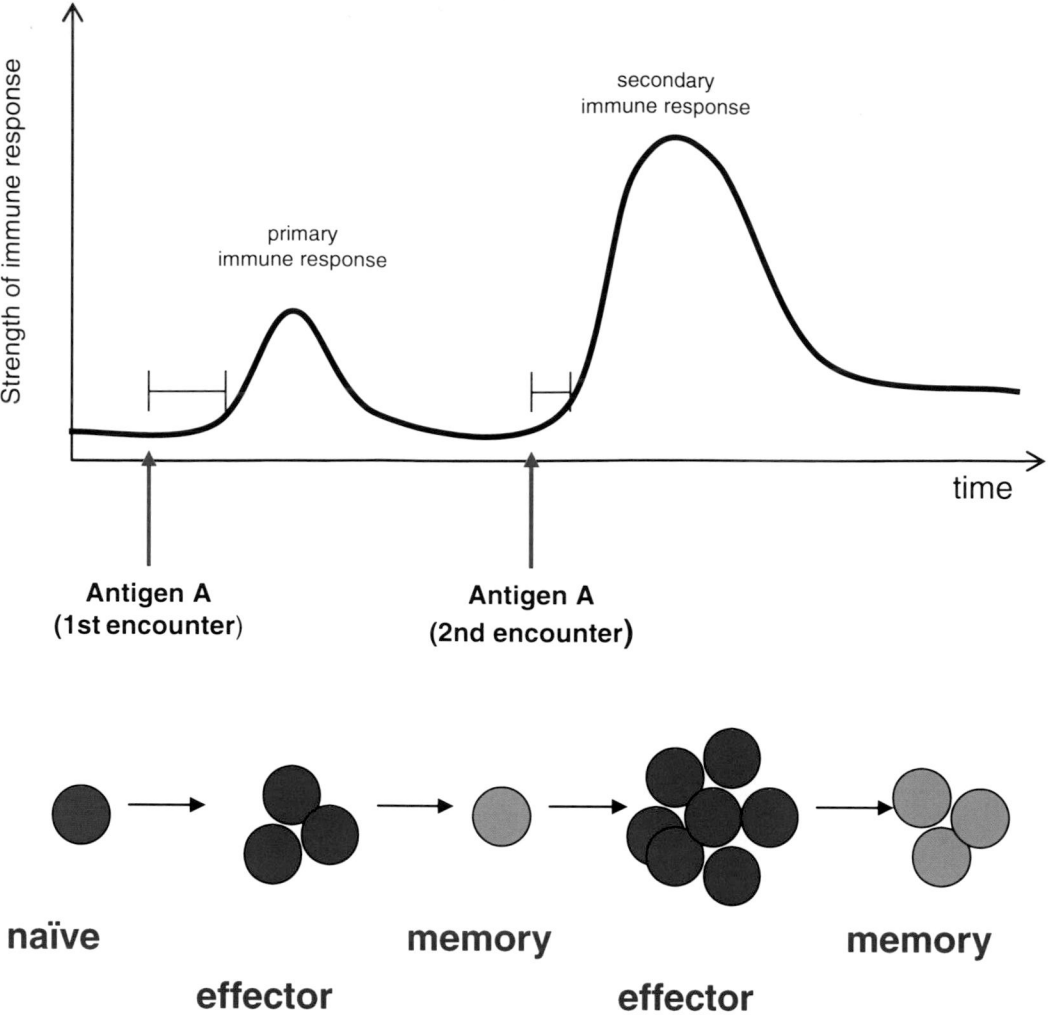

Color Plate 2. Primary and secondary immune response. The upper panel shows a schematic depiction of the strength of the immune response as measured, e.g. by antibody titers or numbers of effector T cells. The secondary immune response after repeated encounter with the same antigen is faster and more pronounced compared to the primary immune response. After repeated stimulation with the same antigen immune responses are sustained at a higher level. The lower panel depicts the expansion and differentiation of lymphocytes in the course of primary and secondary immune responses. Naïve cells differentiate into effector cells after encountering their antigen. Most effector cells are eliminated by apoptosis after clearance of the pathogens. Few cells remain in the body as long-lived memory cells and are able to quickly and efficiently differentiate into effector cells in case of a second contact with the same antigen. After clearance of the pathogens, most effector cells are again eliminated; however, more long-lived memory cells are generated.

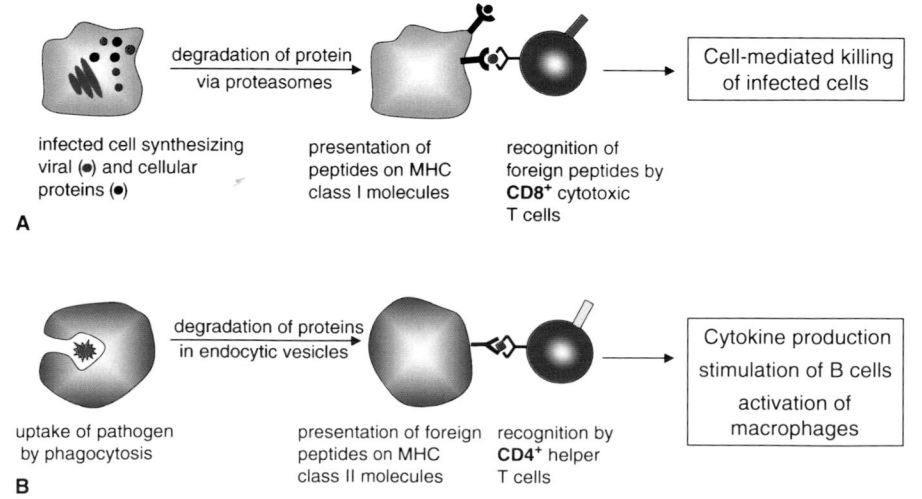

Color Plate 3. Processing and presentation of antigens via MHC class I or class II. (A) Synthesized proteins are degraded via proteasomes and presented on MHC class I molecules. CD8+ cytotoxic T cells recognize foreign peptides and mediate killing of infected cells. (B) Pathogens are internalized by antigen presenting cells; proteins are degraded in endocytic vesicles and presented on MHC class II molecules. CD4+ helper T cells recognize foreign peptides and stimulate B cells and macrophages.

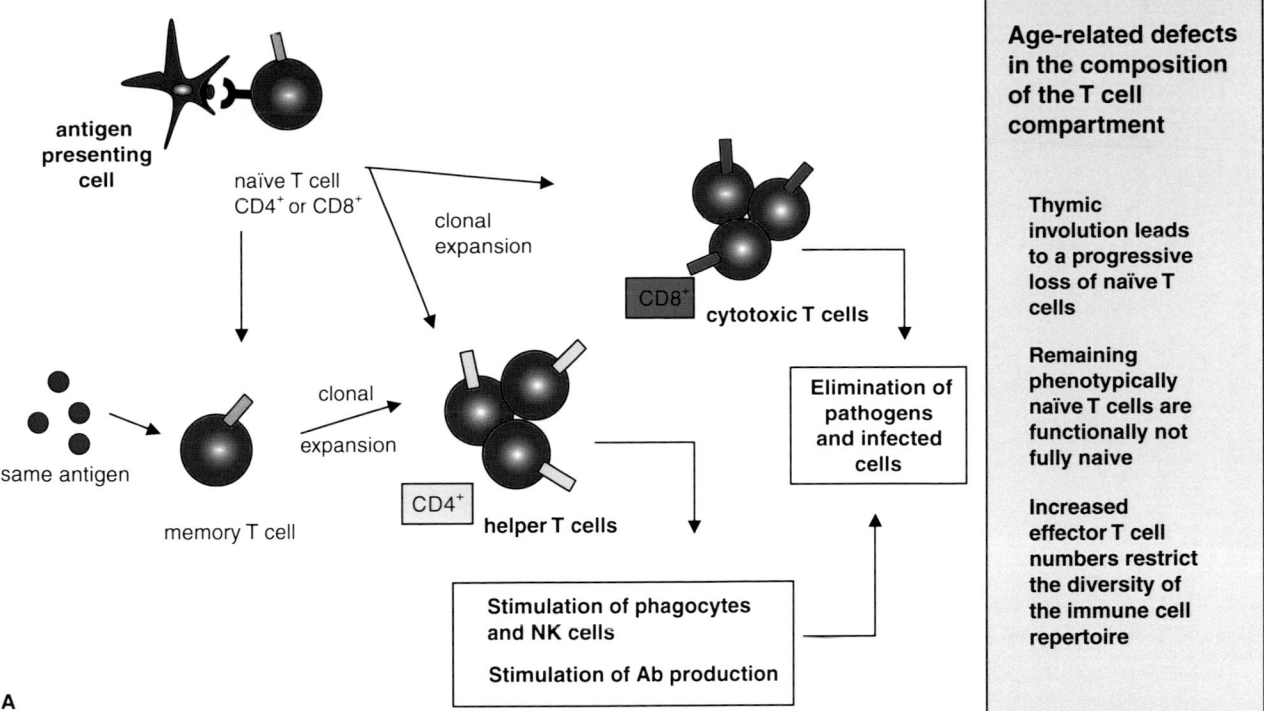

A

Age-related defects in the composition of the T cell compartment

Thymic involution leads to a progressive loss of naïve T cells

Remaining phenotypically naïve T cells are functionally not fully naive

Increased effector T cell numbers restrict the diversity of the immune cell repertoire

Color Plate 4. Schematic representation of adaptive immune responses and age-related changes. (A) Antigen presenting cells present foreign peptides to naïve T cells, which expand and differentiate into memory and effector T cells. CD8$^+$ cytotoxic T cells directly eliminate infected cells. CD4$^+$ helper T cells stimulate phagocytes and NK cells and are crucial for the induction of antibody production. Thus they indirectly contribute to elimination of pathogens and infected cells.

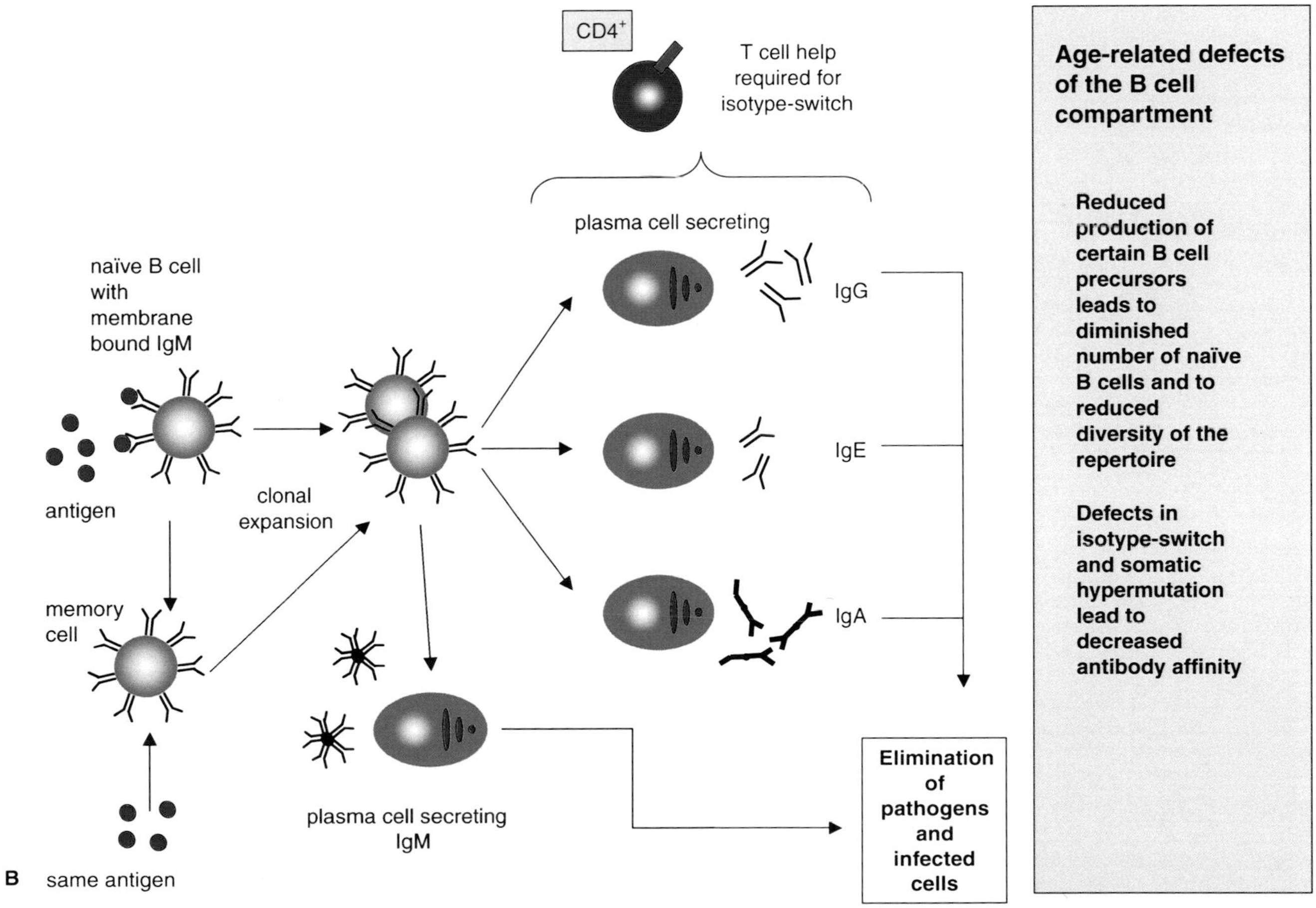

Age-related defects of the B cell compartment

Reduced production of certain B cell precursors leads to diminished number of naïve B cells and to reduced diversity of the repertoire

Defects in isotype-switch and somatic hypermutation lead to decreased antibody affinity

Color Plate 4. (*Continued*) (B) Antigens bind to the membrane-bound antibodies on naïve B cells which expand and differentiate into memory and effector B cells, which are called plasma cells and secrete antibodies. Contact with T helper cells and stimulation by cytokines leads to recombination events in the genes encoding for heavy chains of antibodies. Depending on the stimulus IgG, IgE or IgA antibodies are generated and secreted in order to eliminate pathogens.

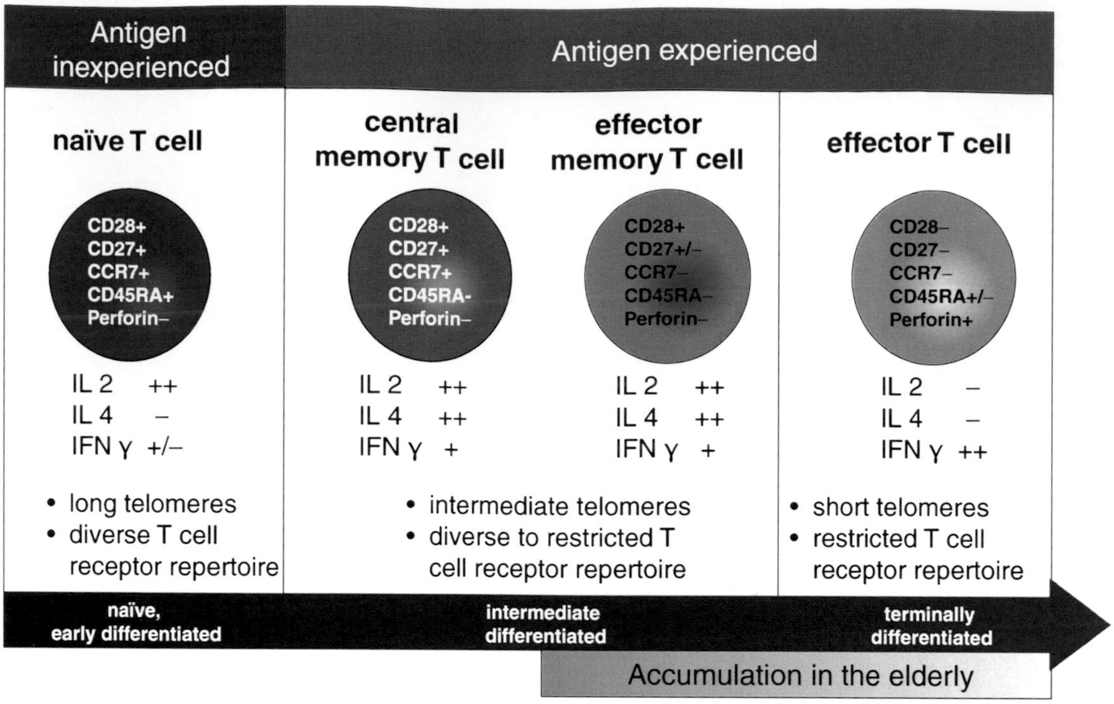

Color Plate 5. Characteristics of different T cell subsets upon differentiation. Antigen inexperienced (naïve) and antigen experienced (memory and effector) T cells are shown with respect to their surface marker expression, telomere length, and T cell receptor repertoire. Central memory and effector memory T cells can be distinguished within the memory compartment. Effector memory and effector T cells accumulate in the elderly.

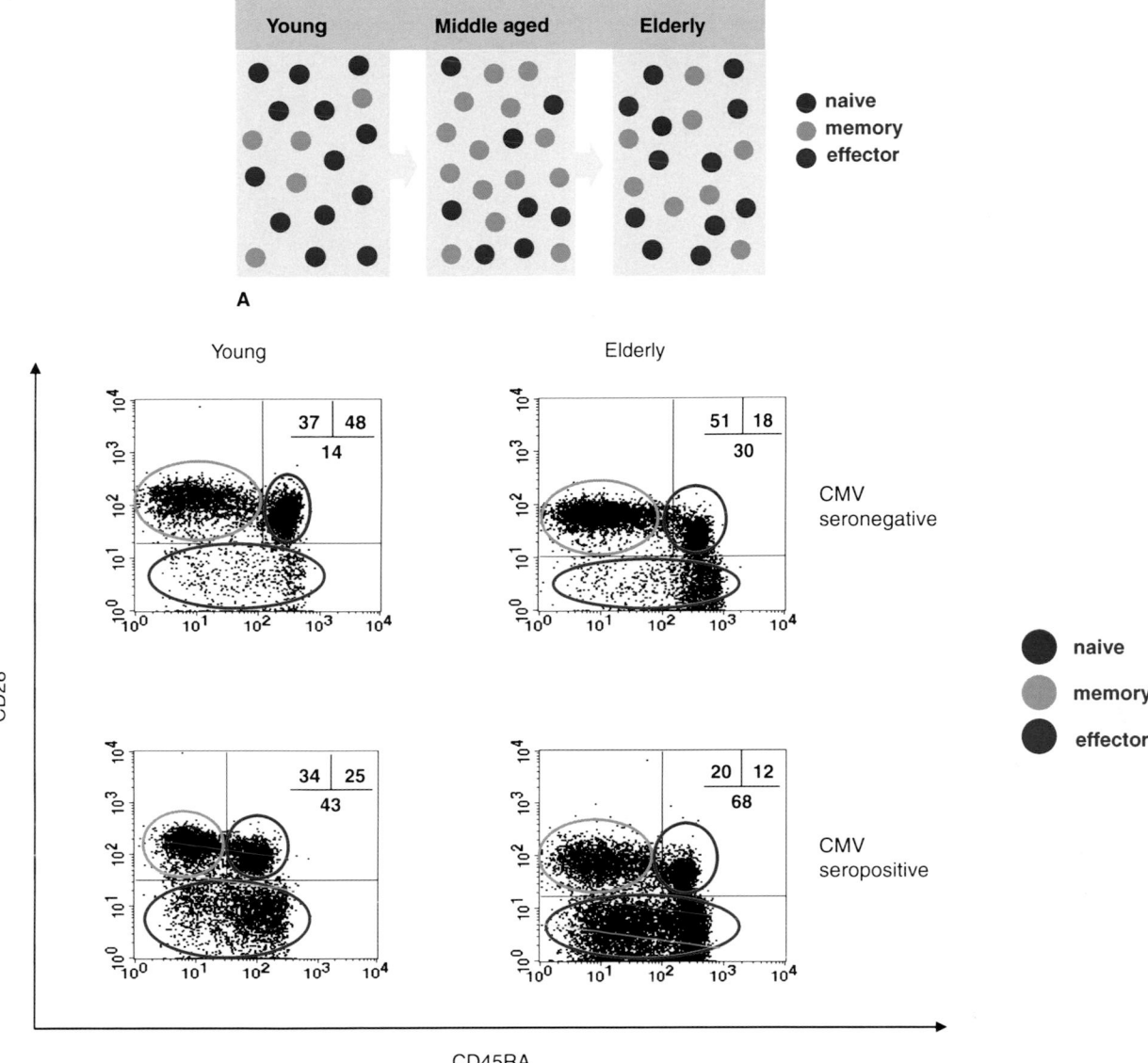

Color Plate 6. Age-related changes of the composition of the T cell compartment and influence of latent CMV-infection. (A) Schematic representation of changes in the quantitative distribution of naïve (blue), memory (black), and effector (gray) T cells in peripheral blood. (B) Representative FACS data are shown for young and old CMV-negative and CMV-positive donors. Naïve, memory, and effector CD8+ T cells are defined by expression of CD45RA and CD28 and are highlighted in blue, black, or gray respectively. Percentages of the individual subsets are depicted in the upper right corner. With increasing age the percentage of naïve cells decreases, whereas effector T cells accumulate. CMV-seropositivity significantly enhances these changes. *Reprinted with modifications from Almanzar G, et al. Long-term cytomegalovirus infection leads to significant changes in the composition of the CD8+ T cell repertoire, which may be the basis for an imbalance in the cytokine production profile in elderly persons J Virol. 2005;79:3675. With permission from the American Society for Microbiology.*

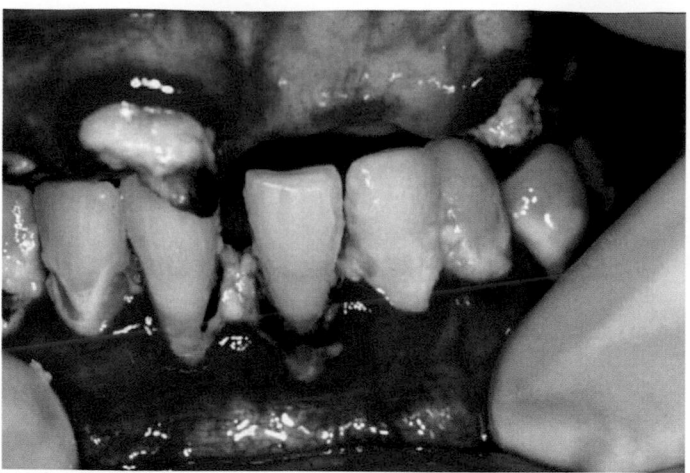

Color Plate 7. Severe dental caries and associated dental plaque.

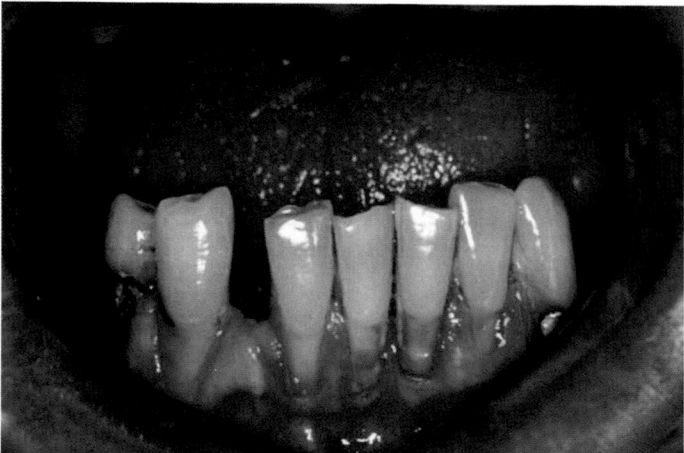

Color Plate 8. Gingival recession and loss of periodontal–alveolar bone attachment in an older adult.

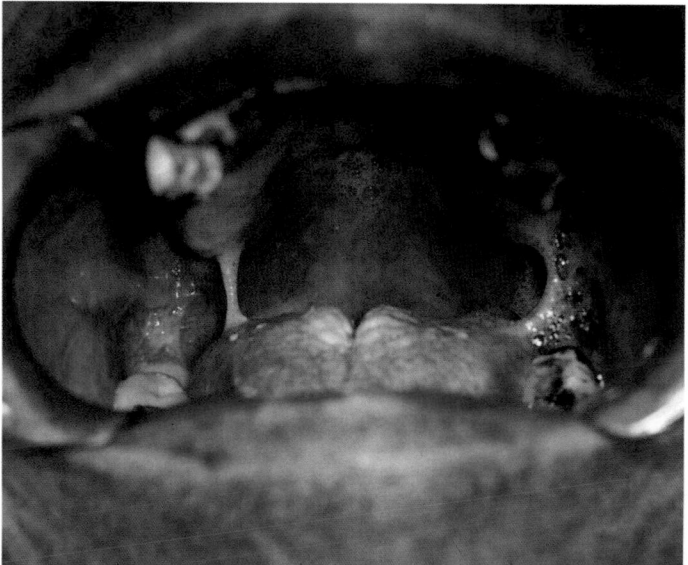

Color Plate 9. Dry mouth and salivary hypofunction caused by external beam radiotherapy used for tongue cancer. Remaining salivary output is viscous and difficult to swallow, caused by destroyed serous-producing salivary glands.

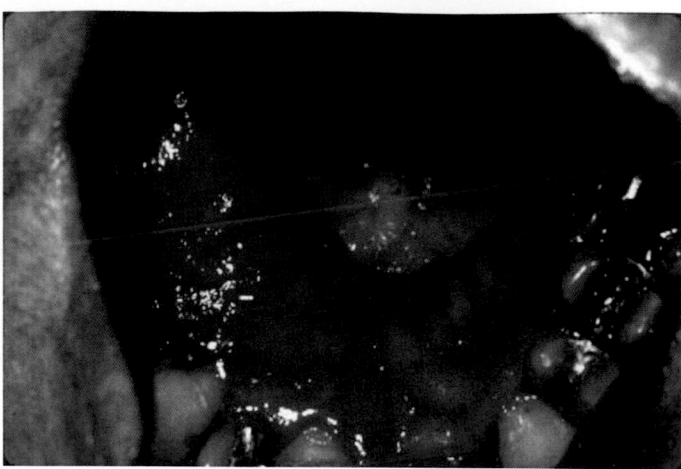

Color Plate 10. Asymptomatic erythematous candidiasis (denture stomatitis) caused by an ill-fitting oral prosthesis. This mycotic infection combined with a poorly fitting removable prosthesis contributes to impaired taste, smell, chewing, and swallowing.

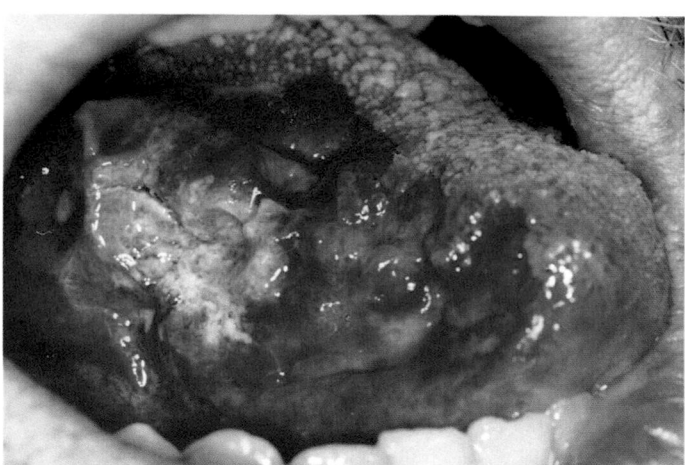

Color Plate 11. Squamous cell carcinoma of the right lateral border of the tongue. The lesion is characterized by unhealing erythematous, ulcerative, and leukoplakic regions, poorly defined margins, and regional lymphadenopathy.

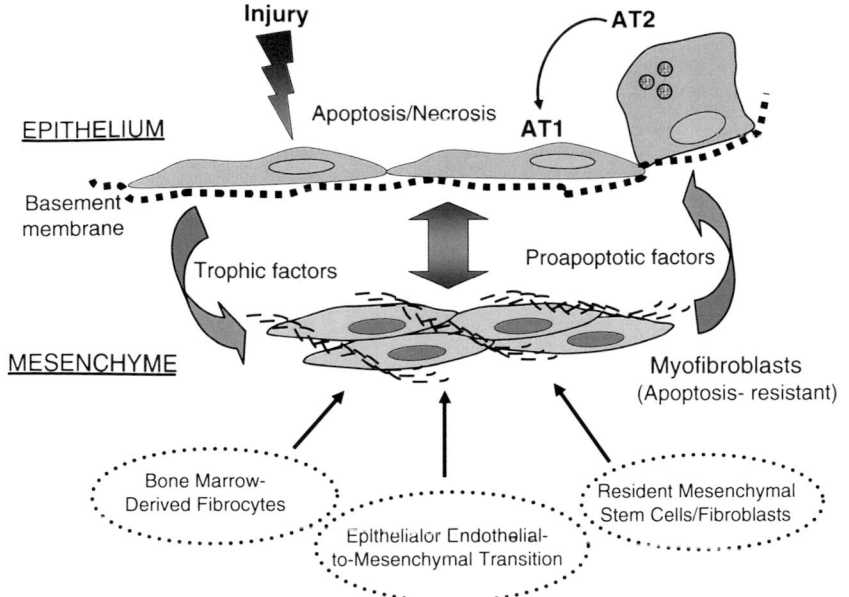

Color Plate 12. Epithelial–mesenchymal interactions in idiopathic pulmonary fibrosis (IPF). Current concepts on the pathogenesis of IPF suggest that repetitive alveolar epithelial injury result in aberrant or dysregulated repair responses with ensuing fibrosis. Alveolar type 1 (AT1) cells maybe more susceptible to injury/apoptosis, and alveolar type 2 (AT2) progenitor cells normally serve to reconstitute the alveolar epithelium by differentiating into AT1 cells. Recent studies suggest that AT2 cells in IPF may undergo epithelial–mesenchymal transition. Other potential sources of activated mesenchymal cells (myofibroblasts) include circulating fibrocytes and resident mesenchymal stem cells. Myofibroblasts, under the influence of trophic factors such as transforming growth factor-β1 acquire resistance to apoptosis. Additionally, activated myofibroblasts are capable of secreting soluble/diffusible factors such as angiotensin peptides, oxidants, and Fas ligand, which further contribute to impaired reepithelialization and unremitting fibrogenesis.

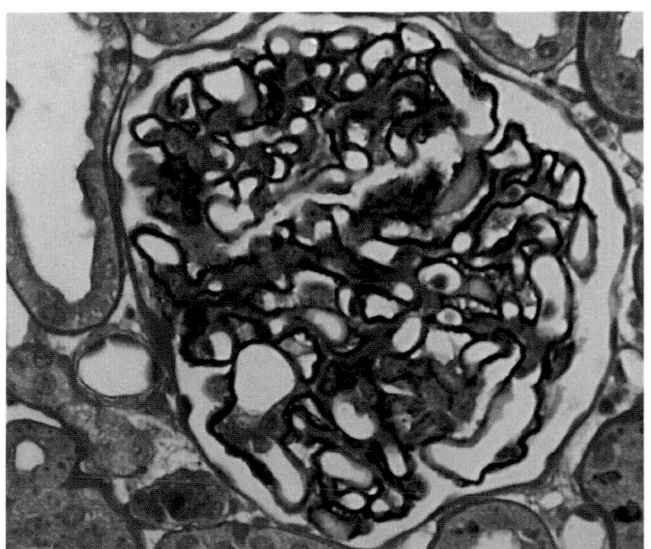 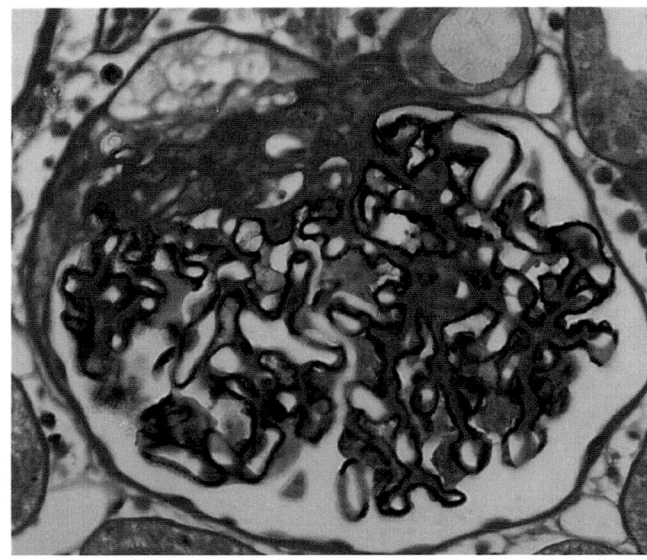

Color Plate 13. Renal glomeruli from a 24-month Fischer 344 rat stained with a podocyte marker, GLEPP1, and counterstained with PAS. Left panel: normal glomerulus showing normal architecture of the glomerular tuft. Right panel: age-related glomerulosclerosis showing normal cellular architecture replaced by extracellular matrix and adherence to Bowman's capsule.

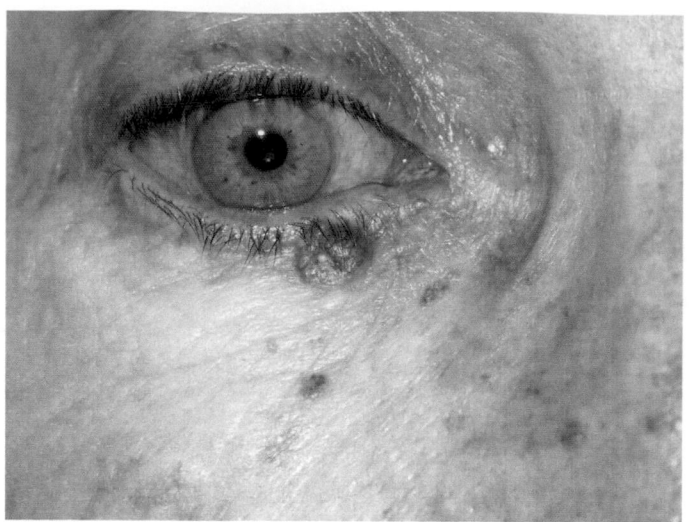

Color Plate 14. Nodular BCC on the lower eyelid. Small pearly papule with telangiectatic blood vessel visible at superior aspect of lesion.

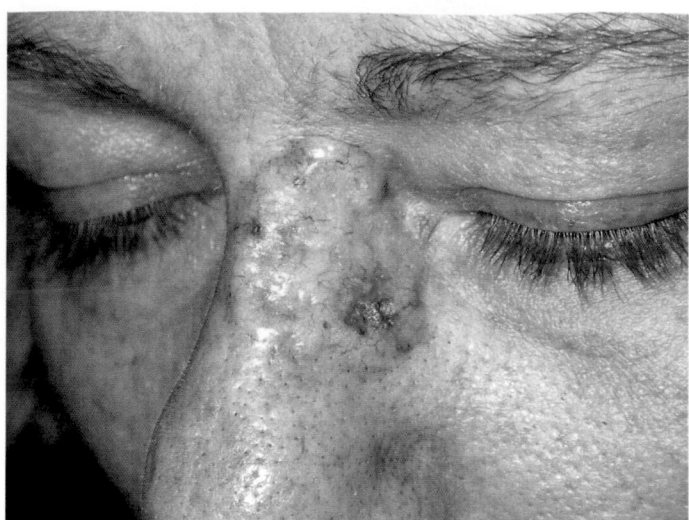

Color Plate 16. Aggressive BCC. Note the very subtle clinical features with an indurated plaque with telangiectasia present. This lesion is likely to have wide subclinical extension present.

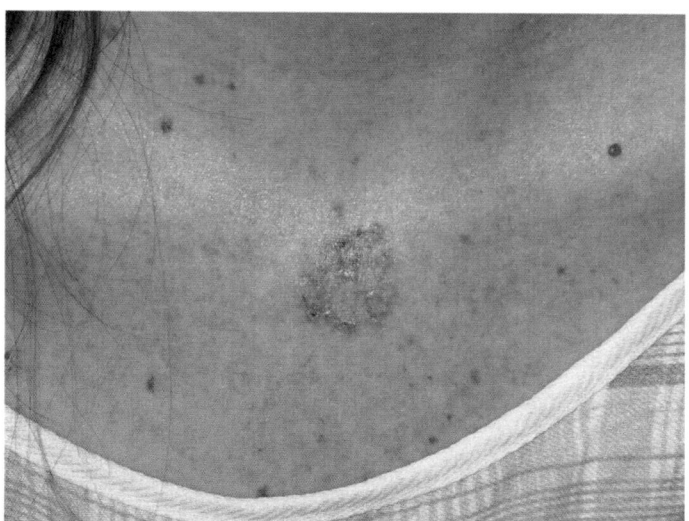

Color Plate 15. Superficial BCC occurring on the chest. Pink, flat lesion with slightly raised scaly borders.

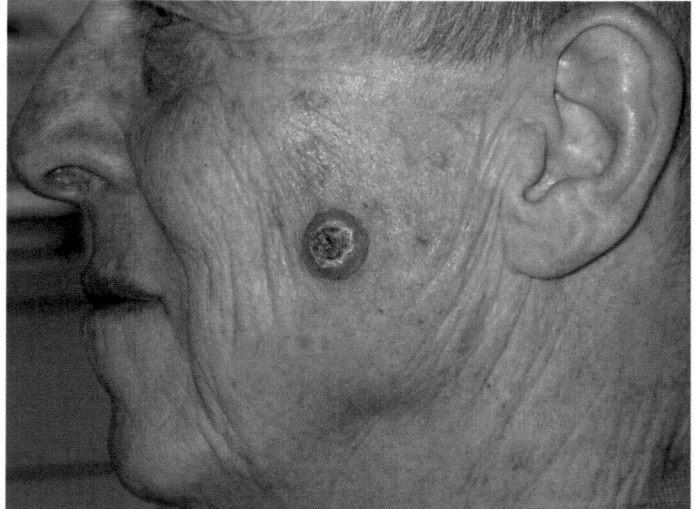

Color Plate 17. Invasive SCC on the cheek. Large ulcerated nodule with central core filled with hyperkeratotic material.

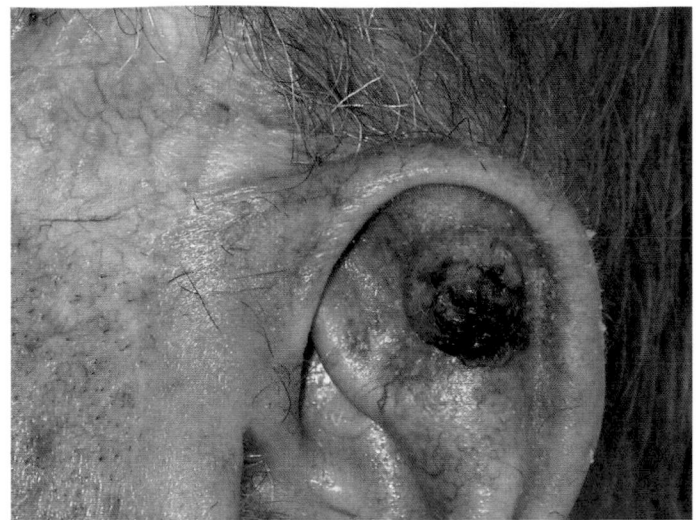

Color Plate 18. Invasive SCC on the ear. Ulcerated crusted lesion on the ear associated with a high risk of regional metastasis.

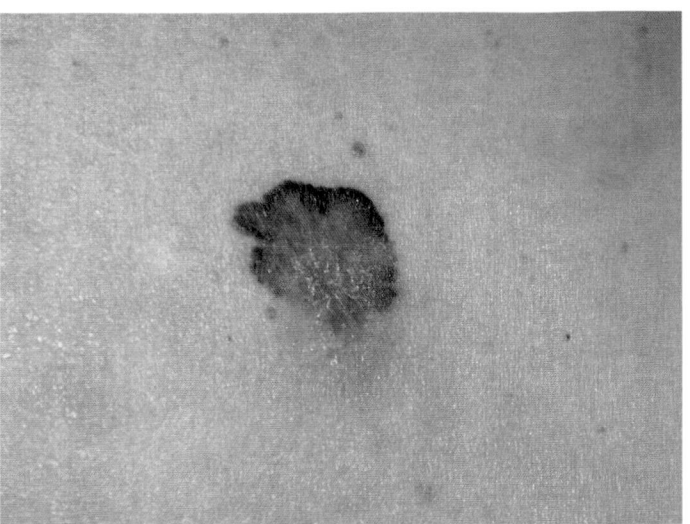

Color Plate 20. Superficial spreading melanoma showing all of the ABCD features. Breslow depth 3.5 mm.

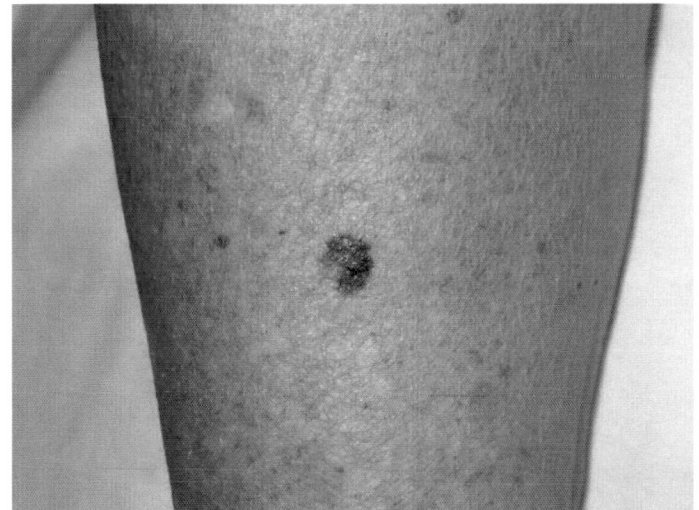

Color Plate 19. Early superficial spreading melanoma. Note asymmetry and irregular border.

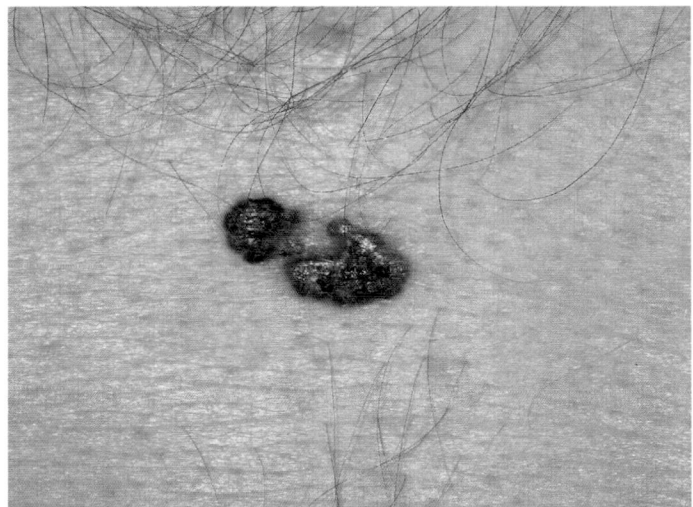

Color Plate 21. Superficial spreading melanoma. Breslow depth 1.1 mm.

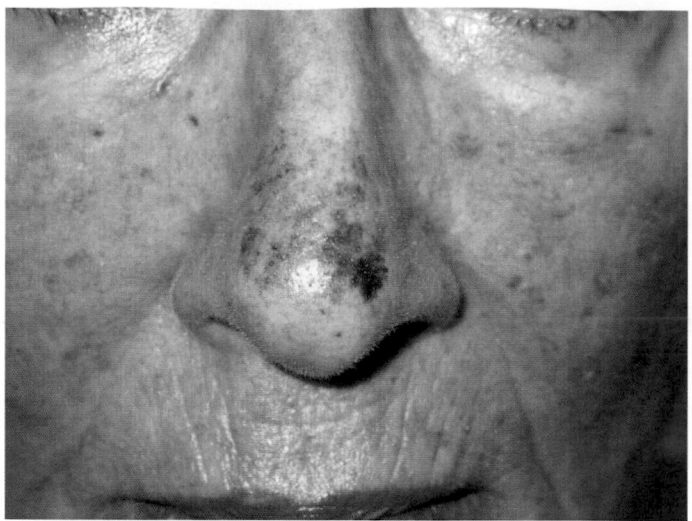

Color Plate 22. Lentigo melanoma (melanoma in situ) on the dorsum of the nose. Irregularly pigmented flat macule that had been slowly enlarging over a number of years.

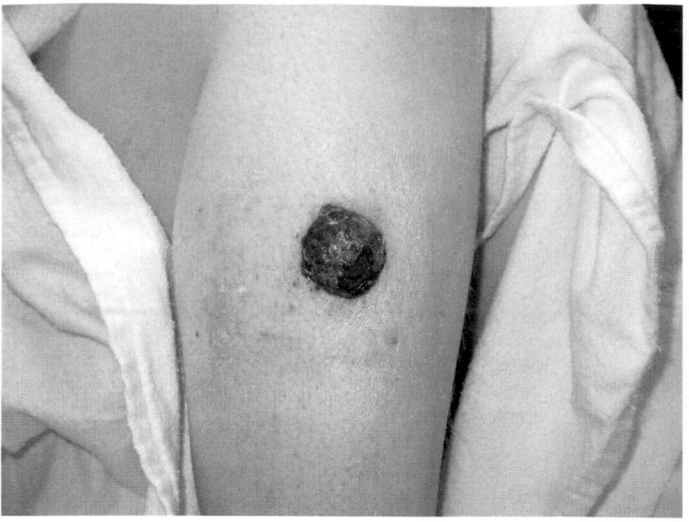

Color Plate 23. Large nodular melanoma. Breslow depth 11.5 mm with ulceration associated with 45% 5-yr survival (stage IIc).

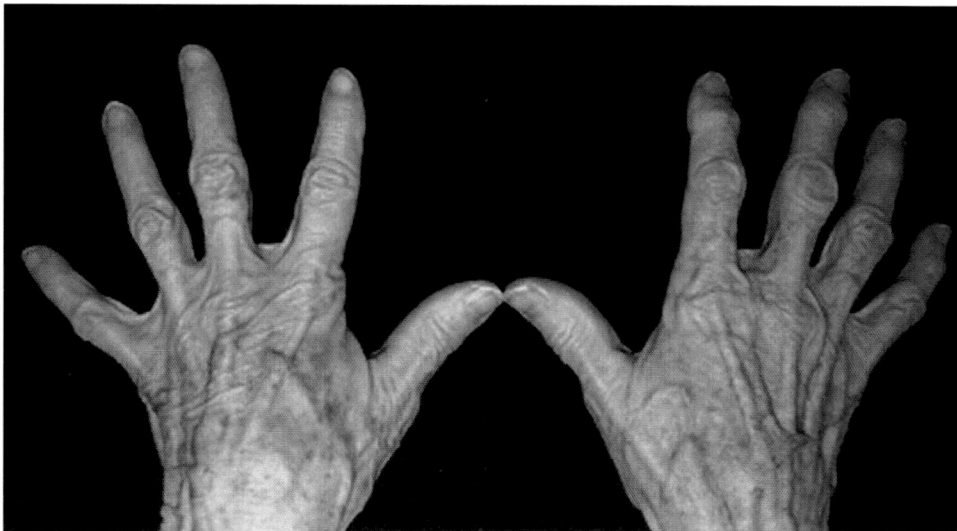

Color Plate 24. The features of bony prominence and deformity typical of hand OA are depicted here with Heberden's nodes of the distal and Bouchard's of the proximal interphalangeal joints of the fingers.

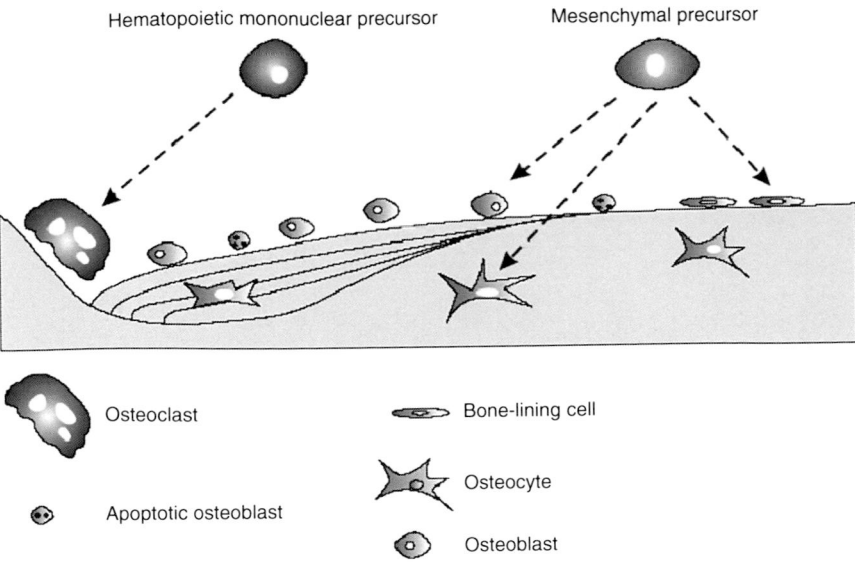

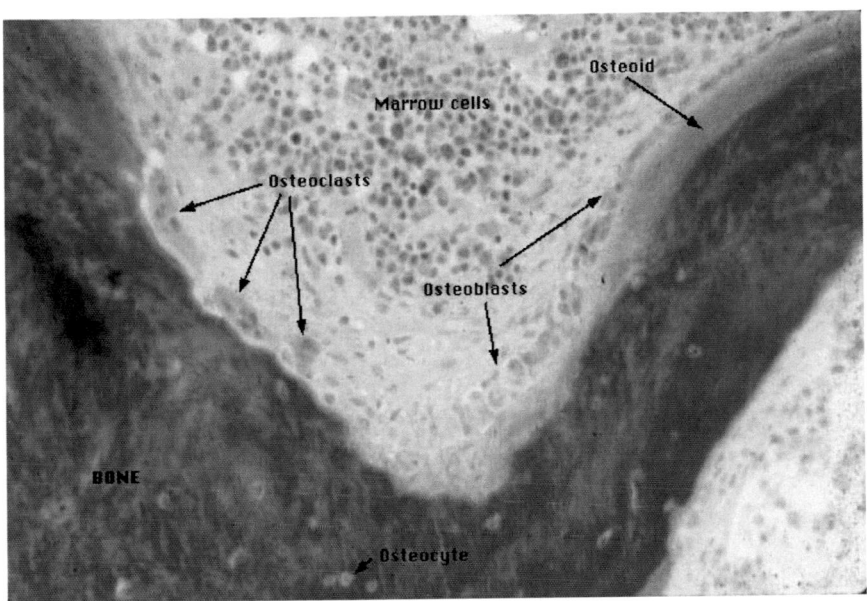

Color Plate 25. The cellular components of bone turnover. (A) Bone cell formation: After the expression of specific transcription factors, mesenchymal precursors differentiate into osteoblasts. In contrast, osteoclasts differentiate from mononuclear precursors and will act as bone-resorbing cells in the bone multicellular unit (BMU). After the completion of bone resorption, osteoclasts die by apoptosis and are replaced by active osteoblasts, which are responsible for the formation of new bone. Finally, osteoblasts end as either lining cells or as osteocytes embedded into the osteoid, or die by apoptosis. (B) Basic multicellular unit (BMU—also known as bone metabolic unit): Large multinucleated osteoclasts resorb bone on the left. Osteoblasts cascade into the resorption pit, laying down osteoid (unmineralized bone). The turquoise stain reflects mineralized bone. *(From Chan GK, Duque G. Age-related bone loss: old bone, new facts. Gerontology. 2002;48:62–71 [Figure 117-1A]; and Dr. Susan M. Ott http://courses.washington.edu/bonephys [Figure 117-1B].)*

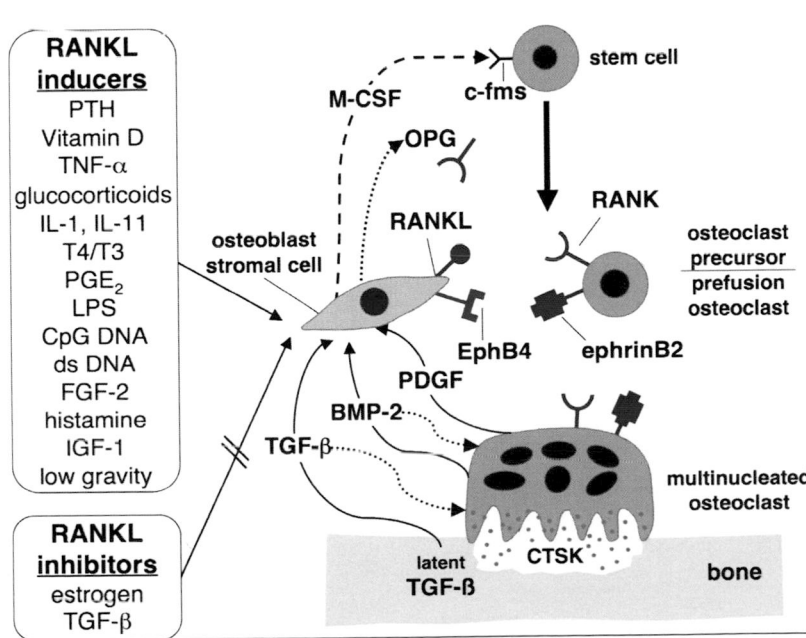

Color Plate 26. Osteoblast–osteoclast coupling and the regulation of RANK ligand expression. Osteoblast production of M-CSF and RANKL play critical roles in the differentiation and activation of osteoclasts. M-CSF acts to maintain monocytic stem cell survival, and subsequently RANKL acts to commit the cell toward osteoclast differentiation, fusion, polarization, and activation. EphB4 and ephrinB2 interact both to limit osteoclast activity and stimulate osteoblast differentiation. TGF-β acts only upon release from the extracellular matrix after osteoclastic resorption, which is mediated in large part by the excretion of CTSK. M-CSF, macrophage colony stimulating factor; RANKL, RANK ligand; TGF-β, transforming growth factor-β; BMP-2, bone morphogenetic protein-2; PDGF, platelet-derived growth factor; CTSK, cathepsin K. *(Adapted from Duque G, Troen BR. Understanding the Mechanisms of Senile Osteoporosis: New Facts for a Major Geriatric Syndrome. J Am Geriatr Soc. 2008;56:935–941).*

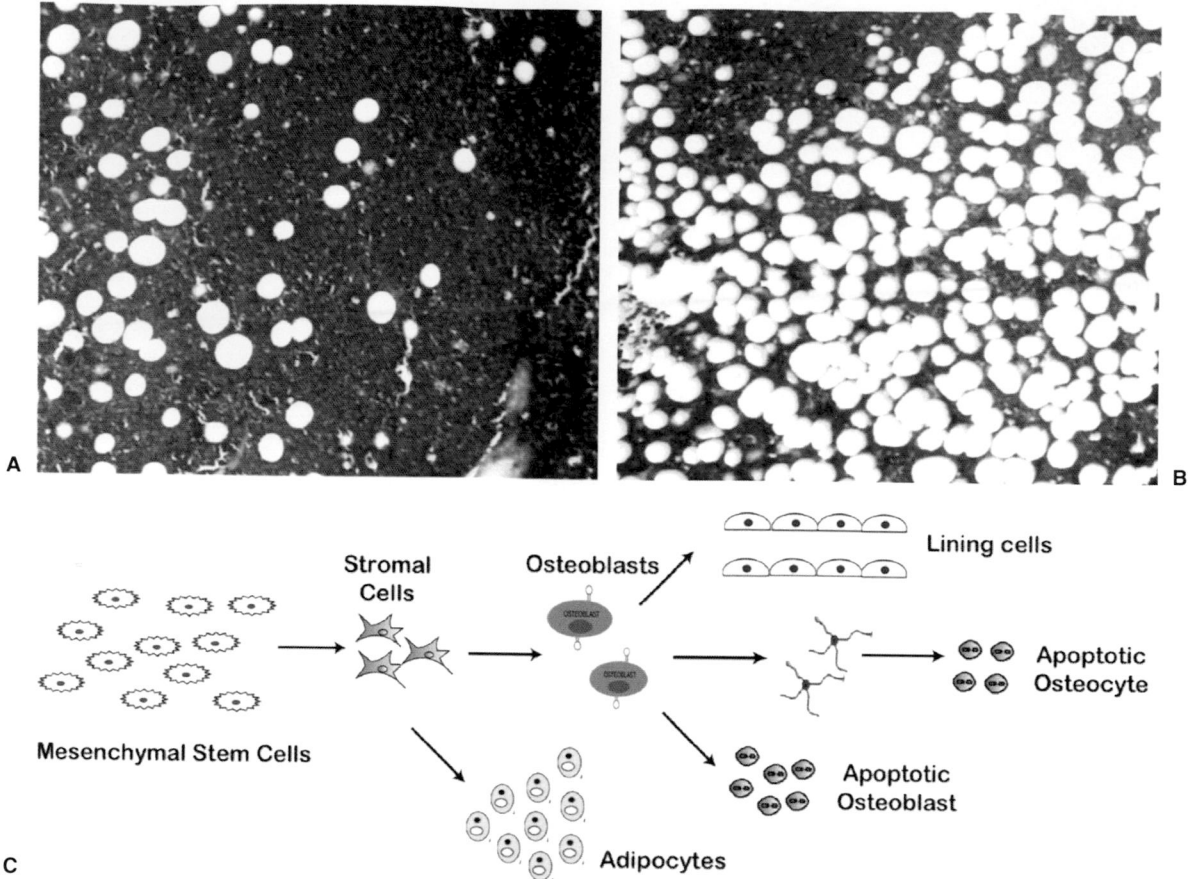

Color Plate 27. Cellular changes in senile osteoporosis. The panel on the right shows the much higher levels of bone marrow fat in the iliac crest of an 85-yr-old subject (A) compared with a 38-yr-old one in the panel on the left (B). There is also a marked reduction in the amount of hematopoietic tissue. (C) Changes in the confluence of mesenchymal stem cells (MSC) accompanied by a reduction in osteoblastogenesis result in the formation of fewer active osteoblasts in the bone multicellular unit. In addition, increasing levels of adipogenic differentiation leads to smaller numbers of differentiated osteoblasts. Finally, increasing osteoblast apoptosis reduces the number of active osteoblasts in the bone multicellular units.

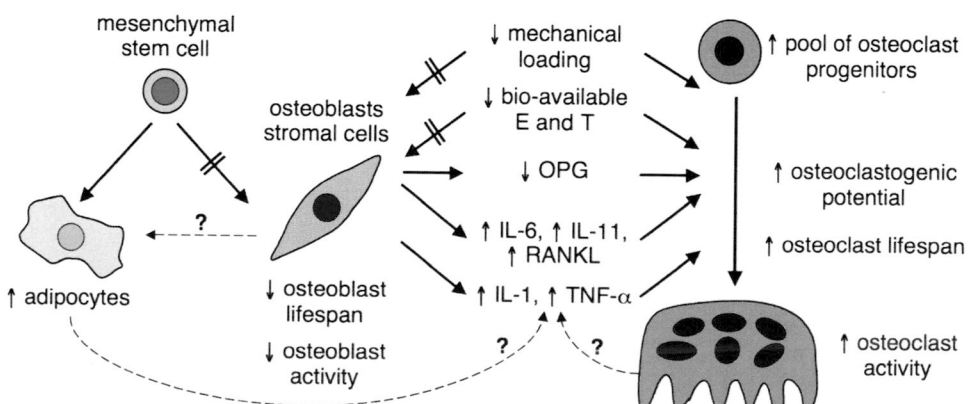

Color Plate 28. Changes in osteoblast–osteoclast interactions with aging. Aging predisposes to more adipogenesis and less osteoblastogenesis. In addition, transdifferentiation from osteoblasts to adipocytes may occur. Reduced physical activity/mechanical loading and decreased levels of bioavailable estradiol and testosterone exert diminished effects on osteoblasts (depicted by the arrows with the hatches), resulting in decreased osteoblast secretion of osteoprotegerin (OPG) and increased expression and secretion of RANKL, IL-1, IL-6, IL-11, and TNF-α. In turn, these compounds directly stimulate greater osteoclast formation and activity. The reduced OPG also permits greater binding of RANKL to RANK, which further facilitates increased osteoclastogenesis and resorption. (Adapted from Troen BR. Molecular mechanisms underlying osteoclast formation and activation. Exp Gerontol. 2003;38(6):605–614.)

TABLE 63-3

Atypical Antipsychotic Dosages, Half-Life and Side Effects

MEDICATION	DOSE (mg/day)	CLEARANCE (HALF-LIFE)	SIDE EFFECTS
Aripiprazole	Start 10–15 qd; max 30	75–96 hrs	Sedation (limited geriatric data)
Clozapine	25–150 qd	Mean 12 hrs	Excessive sedation, seizure, anticholinergic effects, agranulocytosis, orthostatic hypotension, sustained tachycardia, weight gain, high risk of diabetes mellitus and dyslipidemia
Olanzapine	2.5–10 qd	Mean 30 hrs	Sedation, dose-dependent anticholinergic effects, gait disturbance, orthostatic hypotension, high risk of weight gain, hyperglycemia, diabetes mellitus, risk of cerebrovascular events, dose-dependent EPS, EEG abnormality
Quetiapine	25–800 qd or total bid	3–6 hrs	Sedation, orthostatic hypotension, moderate risk of weight gain, diabetes mellitus, and dyslipidemia
Risperidone	0.25–1 qd or total bid	Mean 20 hrs	Orthostatic hypotension, dose-dependent EPS, tardive dyskinesia, hyperprolactinemia, risk of cerebrovascular events, weight gain, moderate risk of diabetes mellitus and dyslipidemia, moderate EEG abnormality, mild sedation, rare cognitive effects
Ziprasidone	20 total bid	7 hrs	Prolongation of QTc interval (limited geriatric data)

qd, once daily; bid, twice daily; EPS, extrapyramidal symptoms; EEG, electoencephalography; QTc, QT (cardiac output) corrected for heart rate.
Anticholinergic effects: dry mouth, blurred vision, constipation, confusion.

when treated with conventional antipsychotics. Cognitive difficulty in dementia is typically treated using cholinesterase inhibitors, such as donepezil, rivastigmine, or galantamine; these medications are safe to use concurrently with atypical antipsychotics. In selecting a particular medication from this class, it is prudent to consider both the clinical profile of the patient as well as the side effects common to that medication (Table 63-3).

Clozapine

The first atypical antipsychotic approved for use by the FDA was clozapine. It is a partial agonist of the $5HT_{1A}$ receptor, has a high affinity for the dopaminergic type 4 (D_4) receptor, and is a strong antagonist at adrenergic, cholinergic, muscarinic, and histaminergic receptor sites. Clozapine is indicated for the treatment of schizophrenia in younger adults, and is highly efficacious with relatively no risk for the development of tardive dyskinesia. Two case series provide evidence that moderate dosages of clozapine may provide symptomatic relief for elderly patients with primary psychotic diagnoses, and a randomized, comparator trial of clozapine and chlorpromazine supports these results. Lower dosages of clozapine (e.g., 12.5–50 mg/day) are suggested as safe and efficacious in the treatment of drug-induced psychosis in Parkinson's patients. There are no double-blind, placebo-controlled trials evaluating the efficacy or tolerability of clozapine in the treatment of BPSDs.

Data from retrospective reviews and case studies have found this atypical agent to be moderately effective, but not without significant side effects. Clozapine levels increase in a dose- and age-dependent fashion and levels may be attenuated in women. Adverse events are numerous with this drug, and range from minor to severe and potentially fatal. Common side effects include excessive sedation, and seizure; anticholinergic effects include dry mouth, constipation, and cognitive impairment. Agranulocytosis is a potentially serious and life-threatening adverse event that occurs in 0.38% of patients. Intensive hematological monitoring is required, especially in an elderly population. Orthostatic hypotension is another side effect that increases the risk for falls and fractures in older patients. Thus,

the side-effect profile of clozapine limits its utility in the treatment of late-life etiologies. Its use in demented elderly patients should be restricted to instances where other antipsychotics fail to produce relief.

Risperidone

Risperidone is a strong antagonist of $5HT_2$, D_2, adrenergic α_1 and α_2 receptors, a mild histaminergic H_1 antagonist, and has little effect at cholinergic receptor sites. Geriatric evidence including various conditions is the most extensive with risperidone. Several randomized, placebo-controlled trials; randomized, comparator trials (with haloperidol, promazine and olanzapine, or olanzapine); and uncontrolled or case studies have indicated that BPSDs are treated safely and effectively with risperidone. Risperidone has shown further success in the safe and efficacious treatment of schizophrenia in older adults as compared to olanzapine and in a randomized, open-label study, where patients were switched from a typical antipsychotic to either risperidone or olanzapine. Uncontrolled data including elderly schizophrenic patients and those with other psychotic disorders demonstrate similar results, as does an evaluation of a long-acting injectable preparation of risperidone in older schizophrenics.

Delirium in late-life has been shown to respond to risperidone, and risperidone is well tolerated, as indicated by a randomized, comparison trial with haloperidol and additional supportive uncontrolled reports. Yet conflicting case studies suggest the occurrence of risperidone-induced delirium. Risperidone's safety and efficacy, even at low doses, have not been clearly established in patients with drug-induced psychosis in Parkinson's disease or Lewy bodies dementia; some of these data suggest an aggravation of parkinsonism. The use of risperidone in these etiologies should be approached prudently and with careful monitoring. Furthermore, while evidence supports the use of risperidone in young bipolar patients, there is a paucity of data regarding risperidone for older bipolar patients. In this case, mood stabilizers are the preferred line of treatment. When severe mania or mania with psychosis co-occurs, a mood stabilizer is typically combined with risperidone, olanzapine, or quetiapine.

Risperidone, and its active metabolite 9-hydoxyrisperidone (paliperidone), appear to increase in concentration at certain dosages in an age-dependent manner. As such, in older demented patients dosages should range between 0.5 and 2 mg/day; initial doses can start at 0.5 mg and titration should be slow. In elderly patients without dementia, dosages should be initiated at 0.25 to 0.5 mg/day, increasing by 0.5 mg increments every 7 days to a maximum below 4 mg/day. Since the half-life of risperidone ranges from 20 to 22 hours, once daily dosing is acceptable. A common initial side effect is orthostatic hypotension, and EPS can occur in a dose-dependent manner. Tardive dyskinesia has been reported in patients with dementia taking an average dose of risperidone at 0.96 mg daily (SD 0.56 mg); however, the persistence of these symptoms one year later was quite low. Risperidone is the atypical antipsychotic most associated with hyperprolactinemia, but leads to moderate abnormalities in electroencephalography (EEG), and its limited affinity for muscarinic receptors results in rare effects on cognition. Mild sedation has also been reported. Weight gain, diabetes, or dyslipidemia are more likely to occur with use of risperidone than with aripiprazole or ziprasidone; however, these side effects appear more frequently when taking the atypical agents clozapine or olanzapine than risperidone.

Paliperidone is the most recently approved atypical antipsychotic for the treatment of schizophrenia in North America. Its action, efficacy, and safety are expected to be similar to that of risperidone, as it is risperidone's active metabolite. Furthermore, as a metabolite, hepatic impairment or metabolism by CYP2D6 should not impact paliperidone's clearance; however, renal function could affect clearance rates. The extended release formulation of paliperidone can be given once daily, which may be beneficial to patients with compliance difficulties. Geriatric evidence is limited to three small trials, but do not include patients with dementia, thus caution must be exercised when attempting treatment in this group.

Olanzapine

The use of olanzapine in geriatric patients has also received extensive examination. This atypical agent inhibits various receptor sites, with a high affinity for $5HT_{2A/2C}$, and milder effects at $D_{4/3/2/1}$, H_1, muscarinic acetylcholine, and α_1 receptors. Randomized, placebo-controlled trials and randomized, comparator trials (with haloperidol, promazine and risperidone, and risperidone) have demonstrated that olanzapine can safely and effectively treat BPSDs. As well, elderly schizophrenic patients have seen effective and tolerable benefits from olanzapine treatment in two randomized, comparator trials each, with haloperidol and risperidone. A large randomized, controlled trial found olanzapine and haloperidol to be similarly efficacious in the treatment of late-life delirium. Yet evidence from other controlled trials suggests cognitive worsening in demented patients receiving olanzapine, and case reports indicate the occurrence of olanzapine-induced delirium. Olanzapine's efficacy and tolerability are again uncertain in treating drug-induced psychosis in Parkinson. This agent did not reduce symptoms of psychosis beyond placebo, but did result in a worsening of parkinsonism and activities of daily living. Another randomized study found no difference between the efficacy of olanzapine and clozapine, and more toxicity with the former atypical antipsychotic. Furthermore, while a few open trials or case series have been positive, many have demonstrated that olanzapine can exacerbate motor symptoms in patients with Parkinson's or Lewy body dementia. Geriatric data regarding the utility and

safety of treating bipolar disorder with olanzapine have not been established; although this agent is effective and tolerable in younger bipolar adults and those with other mood disorders. Thus, caution must be exercised when using olanzapine in conditions other than late-life schizophrenia or to treat BPSDs.

Dosing in patients with schizophrenia, mood disorders, or BPSD can be initiated at 2.5 mg/day with clinically indicated titration up to 5 to 10 mg daily. Response should be evaluated for at least a week before doses are increased. The daily dosing schedule is made possible by olanzapine's mean half-life of 30 hours, and it is well absorbed with no effect of food intake. A 2004 consensus conference, examining available data including younger patients with psychotic or mood disorders taking olanzapine and clozapine, found that these agents demonstrated the highest diabetes risk, most risk for weight gain, and dyslipidemia as compared to other atypical antipsychotics. However, metabolic risks may be different for elderly patients, particularly in the presence of dementia. Sedation and gait disturbance are the most common complaints associated with olanzapine; however, dose-dependent EPS do occur, as well as orthostatic hypotension, typically above geriatric doses of 5 to 10 mg daily. EEG abnormalities have been reported with use of this agent. Other reported effects include constipation (institutionalized dementia patients), dose-dependent decreased efficacy (patients with BPSD), differential cognitive effect versus risperidone (elderly schizophrenics and dementia patients), cognitive decline (AD patients), and delirium. These adverse reactions may be associated with olanzapine's antagonism of the muscarinic receptor. Higher concentrations of olanzapine can be associated with greater risk for side effects and are of concern in elderly patients, women, nonsmokers, and those taking medications that inhibit CYP1A2 (e.g., fluvoxamine or ciprofloxacin). Olanzapine should not be considered a first-line therapy in geriatrics where cognitive impairment, constipation, diabetes, diabetic neuropathy, dyslipidemia, obesity, xerophthalmia, or xerostomia are of concern.

Quetiapine

This atypical antipsychotic works to inhibit $5HT_{1A/2}$, $D_{2/1}$, H_1, α_1 and α_2 receptors. As with olanzapine, quetiapine has a higher affinity for the serotonergic receptors than the dopaminergic sites. Furthermore, quetiapine has no effect on cholinergic, muscarinic, or benzodiazepine receptors. Quetiapine has been found to be efficacious in the symptomatic treatment of BPSDs, elderly patients with primary psychotic disorders, dementia, and delirium. Although, in four trials including patients with dementia or parkinsonism, quetiapine failed to significantly alleviate agitated or psychotic behaviors above placebo, with one trial demonstrating greater cognitive decline in patients treated with quetiapine. Evidence from published studies examining quetiapine in drug-induced psychosis and Parkinson's disease generally supports the efficacy and tolerability of this medication. However, one double-blind trial does report a high drop-out rate in patients taking quetiapine. Nonetheless, the positive data in patients at high risk for EPS indicate quetiapine is a first-line option for elderly Parkinson's or Lewy body dementia patients, and those with tardive dyskinesia.

Initiation of quetiapine can cause somnolence, and though most patients adjust to this relatively fast, quetiapine should be started at doses as low as 25 mg before bedtime. Maximum dosages can range between 25 and 800 mg daily. Generally, elderly patients are maintained around 100 mg/day, as the lower clearance rates in older adults can result in higher concentrations of this agent. Its short half-life of 3 to 6 hours may necessitate a twice-daily dosing regimen. Complaints of sedation and dizziness can be combated with a slower dose titration, and the risk for EPS is relatively low. Quetiapine and risperidone have similar risk for causing weight gain, diabetes, or dyslipidemia, but the risk for these side effects is greater with use of clozapine or olanzapine.

Aripiprazole and Ziprasidone

Aripiprazole and ziprasidone were approved by the FDA in 2002 and 2001, respectively. Aripiprazole acts as a partial D_2 agonist, though at increased concentrations, typical in elders, more complete dopaminergic inhibition results; while ziprasidone has a high affinity for dopaminergic, serotonergic, and alpha-adrenergic receptors, and little affinity for muscarinic and histamine receptors. These atypical antipsychotics have limited impact on glucose, lipids, and weight, and their lack of effect on the muscarinic receptor means limited propensity to impair cognition. As such, aripiprazole and ziprasidone show potential for the treatment of psychosis in the elderly. However, geriatric data are limited with these medications. A single randomized, placebo-controlled trial of aripiprazole to treat BPSDs has shown minimal efficacy in reducing psychosis on secondary outcome measures; and the average dose of 10 mg/day was well tolerated. The long half-life of this agent in younger adults (75–96 h) could also be a concern in the elderly. Similarly, evidence for the oral preparation of ziprasidone in older patients is limited to a published case series and a pharmacokinetic examination. Use of intramuscular ziprasidone has been reported in two studies, with no aversive cardiovascular or EEG effects observed. Concern regarding the potential of ziprasidone to prolong the QTc interval may limit its use in elderly patients with cardiovascular disease. Both of these atypical antipsychotics should be used as second-line treatments in the absence of further geriatric data in a variety of conditions.

Side Effects and Safety

Elderly patients are more susceptible to the side effects associated with antipsychotics, such as sedation, cardiac effects which include tachycardia and orthostatic hypotension, anticholinergic effects including dry mouth, blurred vision, constipation and urinary retention, neuroleptic malignant syndrome with hyperpyrexia, autonomic instability, pigmentary retinopathy, weight gain, allergic reactions, and seizures. Orthostatic hypotension, which can lead to falls and fractures in elders, is a likely consequence with low-potency typical antipsychotics such as chlorpromazine and thioridazine, and atypical agents like clozapine, risperidone, olanzapine, and quetiapine. Anticholinergic effects are most common with low-potency conventional antipsychotics and clozapine. Tardive dyskinesia and EPS are also of particular concern in the elderly; the low-potency atypical agents are less prone to causing EPS when compared to similar doses of high-potency typical antipsychotics (e.g., haloperidol). While, approximately half of patients aged 60 to 80 taking typical agents experience EPS or tardive dyskinesia. Elderly patients require doses of antipsychotics that are lower than those used in younger adults to try to limit the emergence of side effects.

According to published reports and an FDA issued warning, the rate of death in elderly patients with BPSD treated with atypical antipsychotics is close to double that seen in patients randomized to treatment with placebo (i.e., 2.6% mortality with placebo vs. 4.5% with atypicals over 12 weeks), though the absolute risk of mortality is low. Risk of sudden cardiac death in patients taking antipsychotics is also increased, with thioridazine users at particular risk. Some studies have challenged whether the atypical agents lead to reduced incidence of falls or EPS as compared to typical antipsychotics, especially when higher drug dosages are involved. Typical antipsychotics may demonstrate decreased risk for cerebrovascular events, venous thromboembolism, or pancreatitis; yet several meta-analytic and pharmacoepidemiologic studies have suggested these drugs have similar or increased risk to atypicals for diabetes mellitus, cerebrovascular events, stroke, or death. In light of the lack of consensus with regard to the safety of antipsychotics and paucity of data concerning alternate drug classes, clinicians must consider individualized risk–benefit analysis when providing care for patients. For treatment of agitation/psychosis in dementia, it was estimated from a meta-analysis of placebo-controlled studies with atypical antipsychotics that the number needed to treat is approximately 7 to 12 and the number needed to harm is between 44 and 118. In treating a particular disorder, it is also important to consider the strength of the data available for that condition for each drug, as well as the associated side-effect profiles of those drugs.

MOOD STABILIZERS

Randomized, controlled trials of mood stabilizers including geriatric patients are severely lacking. This class of medications is considered to be high-risk because of their potential for toxicity, serious adverse events, and interactions with other drugs. However, lithium continues to be prescribed for the treatment of bipolar disorder in elders. Whether lithium should be utilized as a first-line mood stabilizer or to treat mania in elderly patients remains to be determined. Anticonvulsants have also been prescribed to combat the agitation often associated with dementia.

Lithium

Lithium carbonate has been demonstrated as an effective acute and preventative treatment of mania in older patients. However, the use of lithium in elders necessitates special care. Renal function declines with age and as such so does the clearance of lithium by the kidneys. This increases the older adult's sensitivity to side effects and increases risk for toxicity. Also contributing to the toxicity of lithium in the elderly are common medical conditions such as renal dysfunction, hyponatremia, dehydration, and heart failure. Renal clearance is further complicated by use of thiazide diuretics, angiotensin-converting enzyme inhibitors, and NSAIDs. Thus, lower serum levels of lithium should be maintained in elderly patients. Serum levels should be measured 12 hours after dosing (150–600 mg once daily) with safe and efficacious measurements being 0.4 to 0.8 mmol/L (mEq/L).

Common side effects of lithium use include nausea, fine tremor in the hands, and urinary frequency. Neurological side effects indicating toxicity can include course tremor, slurred speech, ataxia, confusion, and drowsiness. Toxicity can develop at levels between 1.5 and 2 mmol/L in adults, and in the elderly can manifest with levels as low as 1.0 mmol/L; the lower range of the former serum level

TABLE 63-4

Drug-Interactions with Lithium

CLASS/MEDICATION	TOXICITY RISK
Acetylcholinesterase inhibitors	ACEI/ARBs: lithium toxicity Toxicity via sodium depletion
Carbamazepine	Neurotoxicity (ataxia, tremors, nausea, vomiting, diarrhea, tinnitus)
Calcium channel-blockers (e.g., diltiazem, verapamil)	Neurotoxicity
Haloperidol	Neurotoxicity; encephalopathy (results in irreversible brain damage)
Diuretics	Decrease in renal clearance leading to toxicity
MAOIs	Fatal malignant hyperpyrexia
Methyldopa	Neurotoxicity
Metronidazole	Lithium toxicity (rare) NSAIDs: Lithium toxicity
Phenothiazines	Neurotoxicity
Phenytoin	Lithium toxicity
SSRIs	Neurotoxicity (particularly fluoxetine and fluvoxamine)
Sibutramine	Serotonin syndrome
Tricyclic antidepressants	Neurotoxicity

ACEI, Antiotensin converting enzyme inhibitor; ARB, Angiotensin receptor blocker; MAOI, Monamine oxidase inhibitor; NSAIDs, Nonsteroidal antiinflamatory agent.

has been associated with delirium, and levels below the latter have resulted in cognitive impairment in older adults. Lithium toxicity necessitates immediate medical attention as it can result in death or persistent neurological dysfunction. Regular monitoring of electrolytes and electrocardiogram results should be completed, in addition to measurements of lithium levels in the elderly. Lithium-induced renal impairment should be monitored via checks of serum creatinine and urine osmolality, and lithium-induced hypothyroidism should be monitored via thyroid-stimulating hormone concentrations every 6 months. Drug interactions affecting renal clearance must also be considered to avoid toxicity (Table 63-4).

Anticonvulsants

Bipolar disorder can be treated using anticonvulsants as opposed to lithium. Bipolar patients with dysphoria or rapid cycling may actually respond better to anticonvulsants than lithium. Secondary mania, defined as mania occurring in the presence of dementia or other neurological illness, may similarly respond well to anticonvulsants.

Valproate

Valproate's anticonvulsant activity is thought to be mediated by increasing concentrations of gamma-aminobutyric acid (GABA) in the central nervous system. Case studies have shown tolerability of valproate by elderly bipolar patients and geriatrics with dementia related agitation. However, four placebo-controlled trials challenge this evidence by demonstrating that valproate did not relieve agitation symptomatology in dementia beyond placebo. Valproate is prepared

in several mutually exclusive formulations: valproic acid, divalproex sodium, and an extended-release preparation. Divalproex sodium is most commonly recommended, with doses initiating at 250 mg twice daily. Titrations can be made up to a maximum of 500 to 2000 mg/day in two or three divided doses. Efficacious and tolerable serum levels are between 200 and 700 mmol/L (35–100 mg/mL). Common dose-dependent side effects include sedation, nausea, weight gain, hand tremor, reversible elevations in liver enzymes and blood ammonia levels, and thrombocytopenia, which is a particular concern manifesting at lower drug levels in elderly patients. Liver failure or pancreatitis may also occur in rare instances. Metabolism of valproate initially occurs via mitochondrial β-oxidation, with minor metabolism occurring via the CYP450 system. Administering valproate in conjunction with carbamazepine, lamotrigine, diazepam, phenobarbital, or primidone increases these drug's concentrations. Concomitant use of valproate with carbamazepine, lamotrigine, topiramate, or phenytoin decreases valproate levels. Valproate works synergistically with fluoxetine and erythromycin, causing its effects to be amplified.

Carbamazepine

This drug inhibits the repetitive activation of sodium channels and works well to reduce seizures. In young patients, carbamazepine has been found to treat mania both acutely and as a preventative measure. In patients with dementia, this medication has also demonstrated efficacy in reducing agitated and aggressive symptomatology versus placebo. In elderly patients, serum levels of carbamazepine beyond 38 mmol/L (9 mg/L) are associated with higher risk for side effects, including nausea, dizziness, confusion, ataxia, neutropenia, hepatotoxicity, leucopenia, agranulocytosis, and drug interactions. Carbamazepine clearance is reduced with age. It is primarily metabolized by CYP3A4, and those medications that inhibit this isoenzyme (e.g., macrolide antibiotics, antifungals, some antidepressants) can lead to toxic concentrations of carbamazepine. Conversely, those medications that induce CYP3A4 (e.g., phenobarbital, phenytoin, and carbamazepine) will lower concentrations of drugs metabolized by this isoenzyme.

Gabapentin and Pregabalin

Gabapentin has a mild side-effect profile and works to reduce symptoms of anxiety and neuropathic pain. Trials have not established the efficacy of this medication in treating patients with bipolar disorder or dementia, though it is used clinically in these populations. It is eliminated exclusively via renal excretion. Renal impairment can result in ataxia, involuntary movements, disorganized thinking, excitation, and excessive sedation. In elderly patients, initial dosages are recommended at 100 mg twice daily. Pregabalin is the potent successor to gabapentin. No geriatric evidence is available using this drug, though its pharmacokinetic profile is favorable and it may have use in the treatment of neuropathic pain in older adults.

Lamotrigine

The FDA has granted approval for the use of lamotrigine in the preventative treatment of the depressive, manic, or mixed episodes of bipolar disorder. In elderly bipolar patients, lamotrigine has demonstrated superior efficacy versus placebo. Dosing in the elderly begins at 25 mg daily for 2 weeks. For the following 2 weeks, 50 mg is administered daily. The next titration is maintained at 100 mg/day for 7 days. Dosages can then be increased up to 200 mg daily. However, in patients also taking valproate, lamotrigine's titration schedule is reduced and target dosages are halved since valproate increases lamotrigine levels. Though lamotrigine does not appear to increase weight, common side effects in the elderly include excessive drowsiness, headaches, and rashes. Any sign of rash or hypersensitivity related to lamotrigine use should result in its discontinuation and immediate evaluation of the patient. While rare, severe rashes such as Stevens–Johnson syndrome or toxic epidermal necrolysis have occurred in 0.3% of adults. Reducing the dose titration of lamotrigine can lessen the risk for rashes.

ANXIOLYTICS

Benzodiazepines and Nonbenzodiazepine Hypnotics

Anxiety and insomnia in the elderly are frequently treated using benzodiazepines. However, the pharmacokinetic properties of these drugs must be taken into consideration as the rate of metabolism in the elderly is significantly slowed. Thus, the half-lives of benzodiazepines are far longer resulting in the accumulation of medication and an increased likelihood of adverse events. As such, intermediate acting benzodiazepines (e.g., lorazepam) are preferred when treating anxiety in older adults; although SSRIs and venlafaxine are increasingly prescribed. A meta-analysis examining the published studies of sedative-hypnotics in the elderly suggests that the significant adverse effects associated with benzodiazepines far outweigh the relatively minimal, short-term benefits. Side effects can include incidence of excessive daytime sedation, risk of falls and hip fractures, and impairments of cognition and psychomotor performance, even when doses are low. Chronic use of benzodiazepines in high doses followed by abrupt discontinuation can lead to symptoms of withdrawal, including anxiety, insomnia, tremor, tachycardia, delirium, psychosis, or seizure. Elderly patients experiencing heavy snoring (suggestive of sleep apnea), dementia, or concurrent use of other sedatives or alcohol should not be administered a benzodiazepine. Lorazepam and oxazepam do not affect the CYP450 isozymes and are not associated with drug interactions. Oxazepam exhibits variability in absorption making lorazepam the favored sedative. Lorazepam is administered in low dosages of 0.5 mg/day and should not exceed 2 mg daily.

Buspirone

The anxiolytic buspirone does not lead to sedation, is not addictive, and is tolerated well by anxious elders. It is a partial agonist of the $5HT_{1A}$ receptors with no affinity for the benzodiazepine/GABA receptors, and may be particularly useful in treating GAD in geriatric patients that are susceptible to falls, confusion, or chronic lung disease. A disadvantage of buspirone is that its onset of anxiolytic action may not be evident for 1 to 3 weeks following initial dosing. This drug may also lead to dizziness, headache, and nervousness. Initial dosages of buspirone are at 5 mg three times per day. Increases by 5 mg can be made weekly to a maximum daily dose of 60 mg/day. The pharmacokinetic profile of buspirone is similar in young and old adults, as well as between genders. However, concurrent use of verapamil, diltiazem, erythromycin, or itraconazole will elevate concentrations of buspirone, and concomitant administration of SSRIs can lead to serotonin syndrome.

SUMMARY

As with other classes of drugs, the use of psychoactive agents in older patients is complicated by comorbid medical illness and concomitant use of multiple medications. Consequently, geriatric patients experience more adverse events with psychoactive medications, which tend to be more serious than those in younger groups. Health care practitioners must consider individual patient risk to benefit (efficacy) regarding the use of psychoactive agents in geriatrics. Additionally, health specialists must take into account specific side effect profiles associated with potential medications and determine safety of use with other agents a patient may be taking. The detrimental effects of depression, anxiety, or psychosis in late-life on activities of daily living, cognition, institutionalization, and mortality cannot be ignored. These disorders further complicate concurrent physical ailments in patients and increase burden to the health care system. Although efficacy data are limited, clinical anecdotal and study data indicate that many elders are able to maintain an improved quality of life with the use of psychoactive agents. While psychotropic use in the elderly can be challenging, drug therapy can be an important tool in combating many debilitating behavioral and psychiatric illnesses.

FURTHER READING

Aparasu RR, Mort JR, Brandt H. Psychotropic prescription use by community-dwelling elderly in the United States. *J Am Geriatr Soc.* 2003;51(5):671–677.

Bigos KL, Bies RR, Pollock BG. Population pharmacokinetics in geriatric psychiatry. *Am J Geriatr Psychiatry.* 2006;14(12):993–1003.

Dalton SO, Sorensen HT, Johansen C. SSRIs and upper gastrointestinal bleeding: what is known and how should it influence prescribing? *CNS Drugs.* 2006;20(2):143–151.

Gurwitz JH, Field TS, Harrold LR, et al. Incidence and preventability of adverse drug events among older persons in the ambulatory setting. *J Am Med Assoc.* 2003;289:1107–1116.

Juurlink DN, Mamdani MM, Kopp A, et al. The risk of suicide with selective serotonin reuptake inhibitors in the elderly. *Am J Psychiatry.* 2006;163:813–821.

Laroche ML, Charmes JP, Nouaille Y, et al. Is inappropriate medication use a major cause of adverse drug reactions in the elderly? *Br J Clin Pharmacol.* 2007;63:177–186.

Looper KJ. Potential medical and surgical complications of serotonergic antidepressants. *Psychosomatics.* 2007;48(1):1–9.

Lotrich FE, Pollock BG. Aging and clinical pharmacology: implications for antidepressants. *J Clin Pharmacol.* 2005;45:1106–1122.

Lotrich FE, Pollock BG, Kirshner M, et al. Serotonin transporter genotype interacts with paroxetine plasma levels to influence depression treatment response. *J Psychiatry Neurosci.* 2008;33(2):123–130.

Mauri MC, Volonteri LS, Colasanti A, et al. Clinical pharmacokinetics of atypical antipsychotics: a critical review of the relationship between plasma concentrations and clinical response. *Clin Pharmacokinet.* 2007;46(5):359–368.

Mottram P, Wilson K, Strobl J. Antidepressants for depressed elderly. *Cochrane Database Syst Rev.* 2006;(1):CD003491. doi:003410.001002/14651858: CD14003491.

Pollock BG, Mulsant BH, Rosen J, et al. A double-blind comparison of citalopram and risperidone for the treatment of behavioral and psychotic symptoms associated with dementia. *Am J Geriatr Psychiatry.* 2007;15:942–952.

Reuben DB, Herr KA, Pacala JT, Pollock BG, Potter JF, Semla TP. *Geriatrics At Your Fingertips.* 9th ed. New York, New York: The American Geriatrics Society; 2007.

Schneider LS, Dagerman KS, Insel P. Risk of death with atypical antipsychotic drug treatment for dementia: meta-analysis of randomized placebo-controlled trials. *J Am Med Assoc.* 2005;294(15):1934–1943.

Schneider LS, Tariot PN, Dagerman KS, et al. Effectiveness of atypical antipsychotic drugs in patients with Alzheimer's disease. *New Engl J Med.* 2006;355(15):1525–1538.

Sink KM, Holden KF, Yaffe K. Pharmacological treatment of neuropsychiatric symptoms of dementia: a review of the evidence. *J Am Med Assoc.* 2005;293(5):596–608.

Snowdon J, Day S, Baker W. Current use of psychotropic medication in nursing homes. *Int Psychogeriatr.* 2006;18(2):241–250.

Spina E, Scordo MG. Clinically significant drug interactions with antidepressants in the elderly. *Drugs Aging.* 2002;19(4):299–320.

Wortelboer U, Cohrs S, Rodenbeck A, et al. Tolerability of hypnosedatives in older patients. *Drugs Aging.* 2002;19:529–539.

Young RC, Gyulai L, Mulsant BH, et al. Pharmacotherapy of bipolar disorder in old age: review and recommendations. *Am J Geriatr Psychiatry.* 2004;12(4):342–357.

Cerebrovascular Disease

Eric Edward Smith ▪ *Ferdinand Buonanno* ▪ *Aneesh Bhim Singhal* ▪ *J. Philip Kistler*

Although cerebral vascular disease is the third leading cause of death in the United States after heart disease and cancer, it remains the single most important cause of disability. One of several pathologic processes that either lead to occlusion or rupture of an extra- or intracranial artery or vein produces the clinical manifestation of cerebral vascular disease in terms of primary ischemic stroke, transient ischemic attacks (TIAs), and/or primary hemorrhagic stroke. With either TIA or primary ischemic or hemorrhagic stroke, the prelude to acute, chronic, or preventive therapy is precise diagnosis. The diagnostic formulation must not only establish that the clinical entity is an ischemic stroke or TIA, or a hemorrhagic stroke, but also must localize and characterize the precise arterial or venous pathologic process causing the stroke, as well as elucidate the nature of the spared collateral circulation (Figures 64-1 and 64-2). This chapter focuses on identifying this pathological process as the pivot on which hinge rational medical and/or surgical treatments or preventive strategies. For both primary ischemic and/or primary hemorrhagic stroke, as for TIAs, the precise pathophysiologic process divides logically into specific stroke or TIA subtypes.

ISCHEMIC STROKE OR TIA SUBTYPE

Pathophysiology and Clinical Presentation

It is important to recognize that ischemic stroke and/or TIAs share the same pathophysiological causation in terms of the underlying arterial pathology. The terms "stroke" and "TIA" are no more a diagnosis that dictates a specific therapeutic strategy than are the terms "fever" and "abdominal pain." Just as the primary care physician would treat the pneumococcal pneumonia giving rise to the fever, or the pancreatitis giving rise to abdominal pain, so should the underlying arterial pathophysiology of the ischemic stroke or TIA be the focus of a treatment strategy. The term "cerebral vascular accident"

should be discarded and the terms "TIA" and "ischemic stroke" should be complemented by terms defining their pathophysiologic subtype. Primary ischemic stroke and TIA conveniently divide into four subtypes: (1) large artery atherothrombotic (15%); (2) embolic (57%—cardiac, ascending aorta, or unknown source); (3) small vessel lacunar (25%); and (4) other (3%), such as arterial dissection, venous sinus occlusion, and arteritis. The percentages of the various ischemic stroke or TIA subtypes or pathophysiologic cause identified in the National Institutes of Health (NIH) Stroke Databank vary with different ethnic population groups. African-Americans are at relatively higher risk of lacunar stroke and atherothrombotic stroke, particularly that portion of atherothrombotic stroke caused by intracranial arterial atherosclerosis.

When transient or sustained focal neurological symptoms or signs develop in a patient, the history, physical examination, and neurologic examination suggest that it is a stroke, and may even suggest the pathophysiological subtype. This presumed pathophysiologic TIA or stroke subtype diagnosis requires immediate noninvasive assessment of the extra- and intracranial arterial system, focusing on the arteries supplying the suspected symptomatic arterial territory. This includes the large arteries from the aortic arch to the locus of ischemia or infarct. The "parent" artery pathology, or lack thereof, then confirms the subtype, namely, large artery atherothrombotic, embolic, small vessel disease, or other. Often an embolus has fragmented and migrated, leaving the parent vessel patent, or it may have entered a branch of the parent vessel not shown in the scheme outlined in Figure 64-2. In that case, embolism is suggested only by the specific territory of the infarction. When a small infarction occurs in the territory of a single penetrating vessel deep in the brain (as might arise from the basilar artery, the middle cerebral artery stem, or the arteries of the circle of Willis), a small vessel lacunar stroke is diagnosed. To confirm the clinically suspected presumed pathophysiological diagnosis, computed tomography (CT) scanning alone in the acute or subacute phase is inadequate. CT has nearly perfect sensitivity for acute intracerebral hemorrhage (approaching 100%)

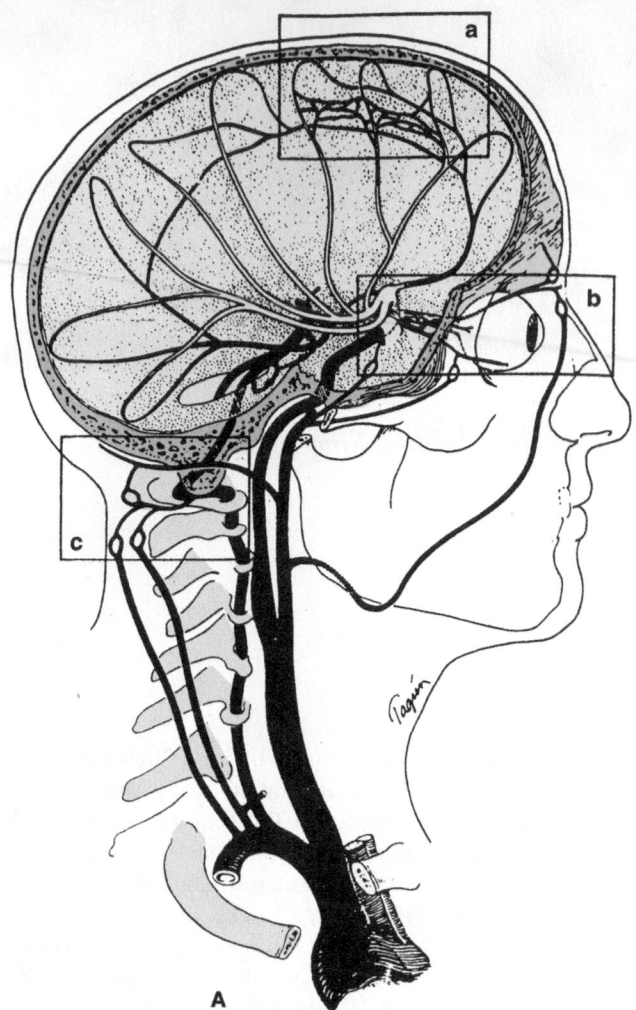

A

FIGURE 64-1. (A) Arrangement of the major arteries of the right side carrying blood from the heart to the brain. Also shown are vessels of collateral circulation that may modify the effects of cerebral ischemia (a, b, and c). Not shown is the circle of Willis, which also provides a source for collateral circulation. *a.* The anastomotic channels between the distal branches of the anterior and middle cerebral artery, termed borderzone or watershed anastomotic channels. Note that they also occur between the posterior and middle cerebral arteries and the anterior and posterior cerebral arteries. *b.* Anastomotic channels occurring through the orbit between branches of the external carotid artery and ophthalmic branch of the internal carotid artery. *c.* Wholly extracranial anastomotic channels between the muscular branches of the ascending cervical arteries and muscular branches of the occipital artery that anastomose with the distal vertebral artery. Note that the occipital artery arises from the external carotid artery, thereby allowing reconstitution of flow in the vertebral from the carotid circulation. *(Part A courtesy of C. M. Fisher, MD.)*

and good sensitivity for acute subarachnoid hemorrhage (approximately 90%). Sensitivity for ischemic infarction in the acute setting is, however, much lower. Ischemic infarction may not be demonstrable by noncontrast CT for 12 to 14 hours after symptom onset; additionally, infarction involving only the cortical surface supratentorially, or infarction in the posterior fossa, can often be obscured by bone artifact. Therefore, contrast CT angiography, magnetic resonance imaging (MRI) with MR angiography, and/or carotid duplex Doppler and transcranial Doppler, should be obtained to outline the parent vessels (Figure 64-2), before specific treatment based on the pathologic process can be devised. Only with precise knowl-

edge of the parent vessel pathology, or its absence, can therapy be properly addressed—whether it be thrombolytic, anticoagulant, or antiplatelet, interventional intra-arterial, or surgical. The following sections outline each of the four ischemic stroke and TIA subtypes, and intracerebral and subarachnoid hemorrhage, in terms of their pathophysiological process and clinical presentation. A discussion of a focused diagnostic approach to confirm that clinically presumed diagnosis follows. Based on the particular TIA or stroke subtype and its causative pathological process, acute, subacute, and preventive management strategies can then be addressed.

Large Vessel, Atherothrombotic Stroke/TIA Subtype

Atherothrombotic cerebral vascular disease accounts for only 15% of all ischemic infarcts in the NIH Stroke Databank. The atheromatous process occurs in strategically focal locations with predilection for four extra- and intracranial arterial locations (Figure 64-2): (1) the internal carotid artery origin, (2) or its siphon portion, (3) the middle cerebral stem, and (4) the vertebrobasilar junction. Although the origin of the common carotid artery and the vertebral arteries also are sites of atheromatous disease, they are less-often implicated in stroke or TIA. At each of the sites of predilection, two mechanisms are responsible for causing the stroke or TIA: (1) atherothrombotic plaque with clot formation that either occludes the vessel and gives rise to an embolic fragment that occludes a more distal vessel, that is, artery-to-artery embolus, or thrombus that propagates into a distal vessel; or (2) the atherothrombotic process might occlude or narrow the vessel to such a degree that distal flow is diminished and not compensated via the circle of Willis, that is, low-flow stroke or TIA. Generally, both artery-to-artery embolism and low-flow stroke occur when the vessel is narrowed by the atheromatous process to a degree that decreases pressure across the arterial segment, that is, producing a 70% or greater diameter stenosis, or frank occlusion. A TIA is said to occur if symptoms clear within an arbitrarily set time of 24 hours. In artery-to-artery embolic events, symptoms may last for shorter periods of time, and in low-flow transient ischemic events they may last only minutes to as long as an hour or more. Often, artery-to-artery or low-flow transient ischemic events may be associated with an MRI-proven area of infarction, notwithstanding resolution of the symptoms. When symptomatic stroke ensues in this setting, it is because the artery-to-artery embolic fragment lodges in an intracranial vessel with inadequate distal collateral supply, or because the clot propagates and occludes the vessel. A dramatic example of the latter occurs with internal carotid artery origin occlusion and propagation of the clot distally into the middle cerebral stem (Figures 64-1 and 64-2).

Low-flow stroke or TIA occurs less often from a cervical lesion because the circle of Willis provides distal collateral circulation. However, low-flow stroke or TIA occurs more often with atheromatous disease in the distal vertebral or in the basilar arteries. Similarly, the frequency of low-flow stroke or TIA increases when the atheromatous process is in the middle cerebral stem and compromises the ability of the circle of Willis to provide sufficient collateral flow. In 70% of the population, the circle of Willis is incompetent, with one or more of the connecting arteries atretic or functionally inadequate (Figure 64-2); in this circumstance, low-flow TIA or stroke may arise from atherothrombosis at the internal carotid artery origin or in its petrous or siphon portions.

Because of the advent of thrombolytic therapy, acute stroke diagnosis and management strategies differ significantly from those for

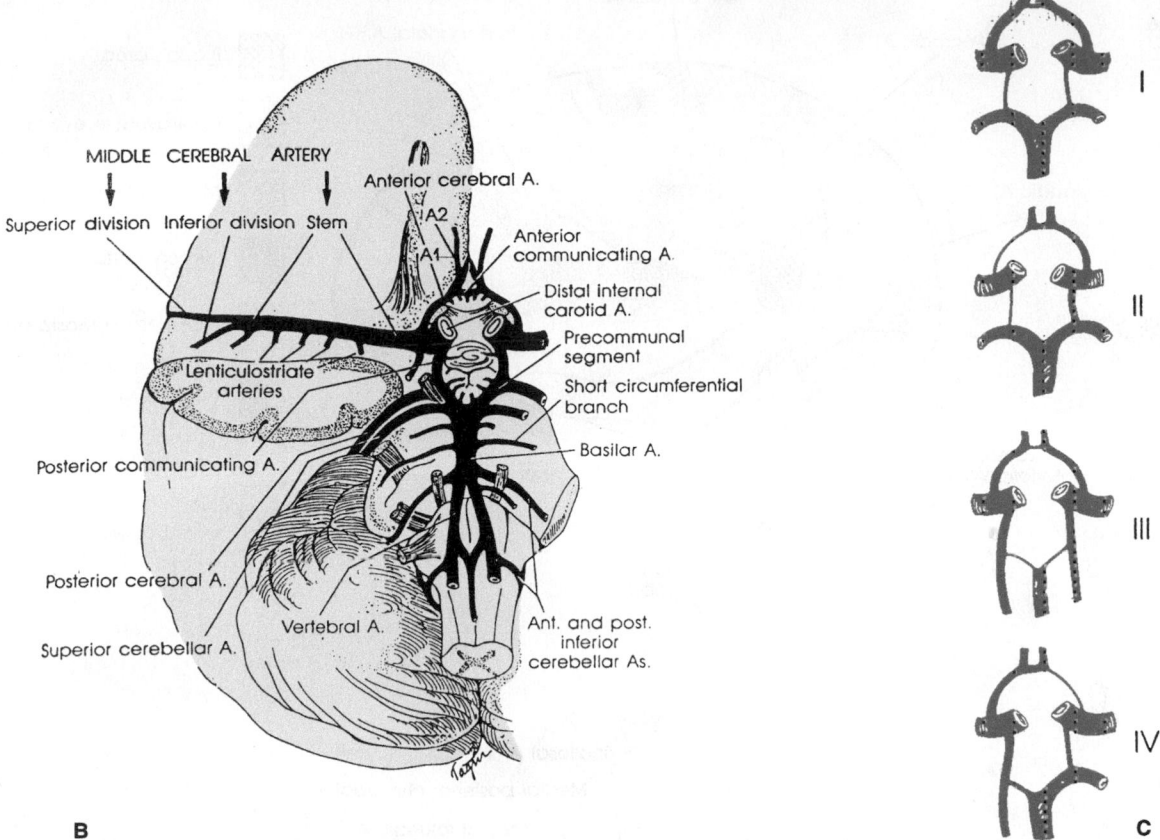

FIGURE 64-1. *(Continued)* (B) Diagram of the brainstem, cerebellum, inferior right frontal lobe, and temporal lobe transected. Principal branches of the vertebral basilar arterial system are pictured. Small branches of the vertebral and basilar artery that penetrate the medulla and pons are not pictured. The stem of the middle cerebral artery with its small, deep-penetrating lenticulostriate arteries and the circle of Willis with its small, deep-penetrating branches, are shown. (C). Roman numerals I, II, III, and IV represent some of the possible variations of the circle of Willis caused by atresia of one or more of its arterial components.

subacute stroke or TIA. Acute treatment strategies for all subtypes of ischemic stroke are discussed at the end of this section. In subacute stroke or TIA, the evaluation and management are best directed in relation to the specific pathophysiological subtype, as outlined in the sections that follow.

Atherothrombotic Disease of the Anterior Cerebral Circulation (Origin of the Internal Carotid Artery, Its Major Branches, and the Common Carotid Artery). In this arterial territory, atheroma occurs most often at the bifurcation of the common carotid artery, and usually begins on the posterior wall of the internal carotid artery origin.

• *Internal carotid artery*: Most often, atheroma at the origin of the internal carotid artery becomes symptomatic after it has narrowed the lumen by 70%, leaving a residual lumen diameter of 1.5 mm—the point where the pressure begins to drop across the stenosis, allowing both embolic or low-flow ischemic TIA and stroke to occur. Embolism from thrombus forming in an ulcerated crater may occur at 50% to 70% stenosis, but it is much less common, and very rarely occurs with lesser degrees of stenosis. Artery-to-artery embolism can also occur if the atheromatous process occludes the internal carotid artery origin forming a thrombus at the site. At times, the occluding thrombus may also propagate without embolization, reaching the ophthalmic artery

origin and producing monocular blindness, or extending even more distally to the middle cerebral artery origin and producing a devastating, total, middle cerebral territory stroke.

The symptoms of the artery-to-artery embolism are variable, depending on the distal branch in which the embolism lodges, and the degree of distal collateral flow. The middle cerebral artery territory is the most often affected. The exact clinical manifestations depend on the precise location of the ischemia, whether in the territory of the ophthalmic artery, the middle cerebral artery, or the anterior choroidal artery. Transient monocular blurring or blindness, often with a shade lowering or telescopic effect, points to ischemia in the *ophthalmic artery* territory. Symptoms associated with ischemia in the other territories are discussed, in their respective sections, below.

Low-flow symptoms caused by internal carotid artery origin stenosis are less common than artery-to-artery embolism, and occur only if two conditions exist: (1) the lesion has to be hemodynamically significant, that is, severe enough to provoke a drop in pressure across the lesion, which is a situation supervening at a residual lumen diameter <1.5 mm and (2) collateral flow distally through the circle of Willis or external carotid artery ophthalmic routes is inadequate, leading to a low-pressure state either in the middle cerebral artery or in one or both of the anterior cerebral arteries. If there is internal carotid artery occlusion and little distal collateral flow then a complete middle

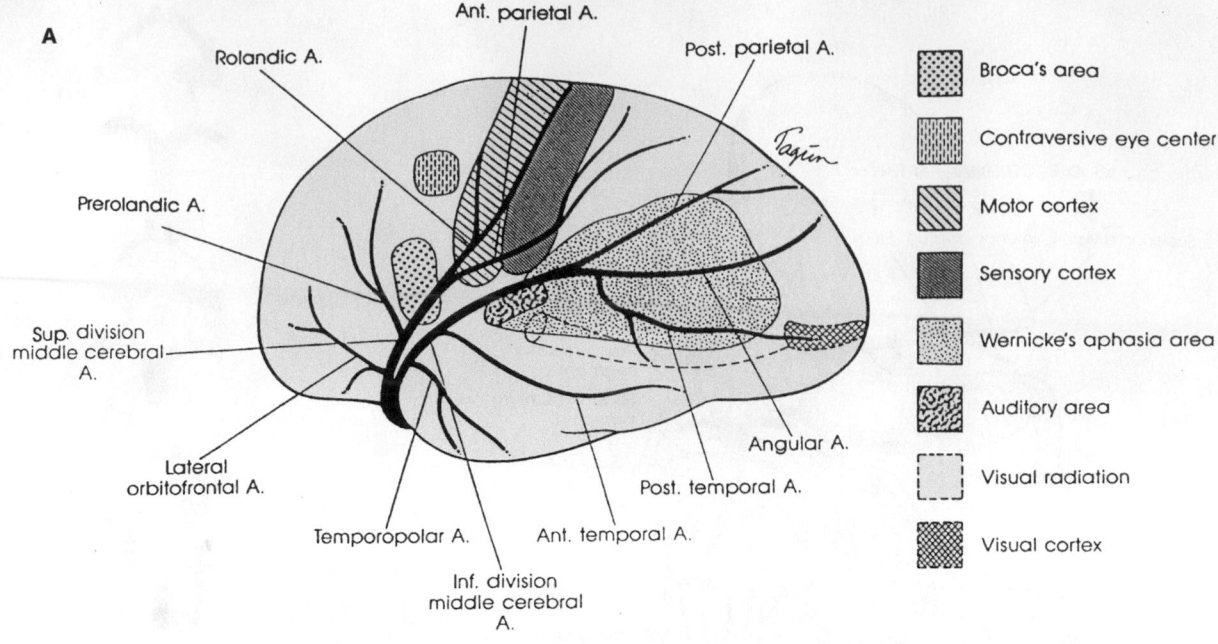

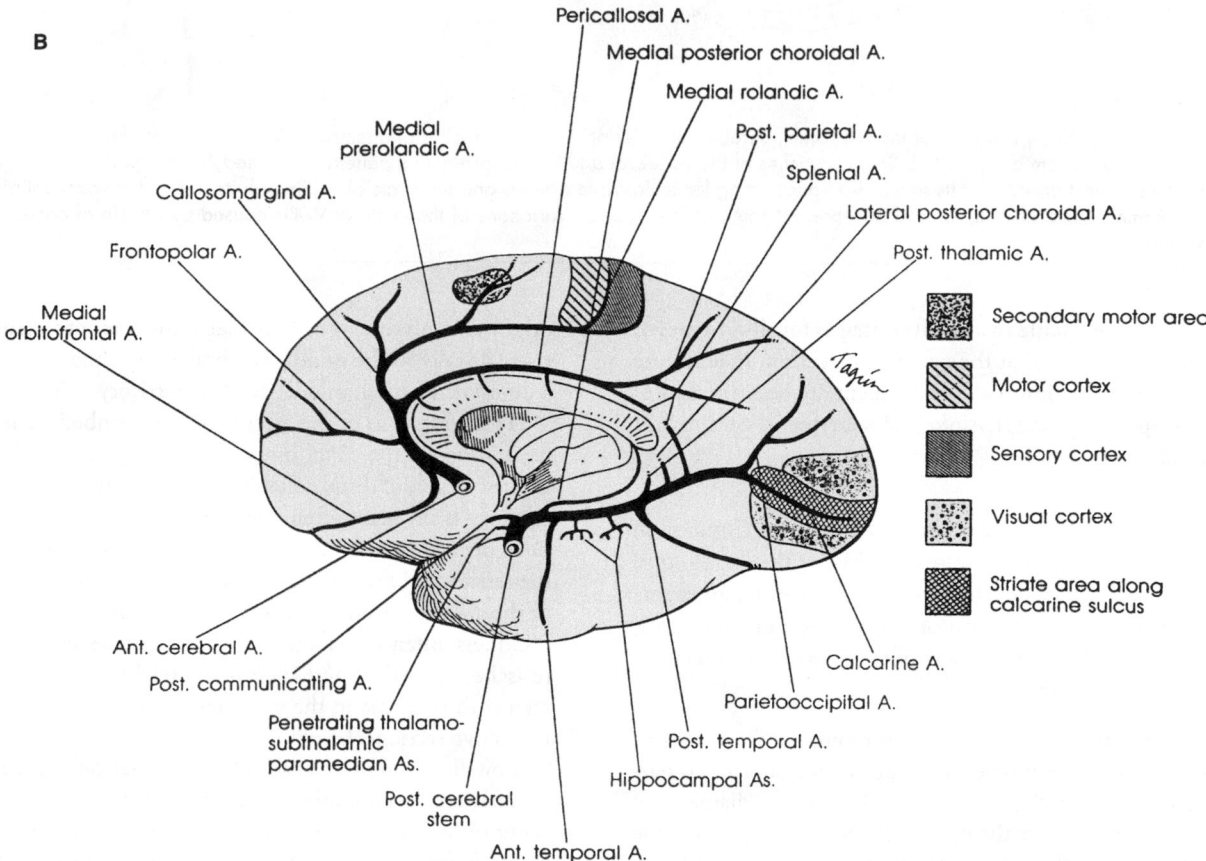

FIGURE 64-2. (A) Diagram of a cerebral hemisphere, lateral aspect, showing the branches and distribution of the middle cerebral artery and the principal regions of cerebral localization. Note the bifurcation of the middle cerebral artery into a superior and inferior division. (B) Diagram of a cerebral hemisphere, medial aspect, showing the branches and distribution of the anterior cerebral artery and the principal regions of cerebral localization. *(Courtesy of C. M. Fisher, MD.)*

cerebral syndrome may result. The posterior cerebral artery (PCA) territory may also be vulnerable to low flow when this artery arises directly from the internal carotid artery, that is, a "fetal PCA." If the circle of Willis is complete, then occlusion of the internal carotid artery can be asymptomatic if it does not have an associated embolic or propagated thrombotic component.

Atheromatous disease in the internal carotid artery siphon occurs less often, but shares the same type of physiologic mechanisms for TIA and stroke as seen with atheromatous disease of the internal carotid artery origin. By contrast, middle cerebral stem atheromatous lesions mainly cause low-flow TIA or stroke. Emboli to the middle cerebral artery branches from that source occur less frequently and tend to be small. Common carotid origin stenosis rarely causes symptoms, but when they occur, they are most commonly caused by embolism to a distal intracranial artery.

- *Middle cerebral artery*: Middle cerebral artery territory symptoms may conveniently be divided into those involving the stem territory (M1 segment; see Figure 64-2) and those symptoms resulting from ischemia in the superior or inferior territory division or one of their cortical surface branches (Figures 64-1 and 64-2). When the stem of the middle cerebral artery is occluded by thrombosis of an ulcerated atheromatous plaque or artery-to-artery embolism, a complete middle cerebral artery syndrome may occur. It produces a complete hemiplegia equally involving the face, arm, hand, leg, and foot because of the ischemia in the small penetrating (lenticulostriate) arteries that arise from the middle cerebral stem supplying the basal ganglia and internal capsule. Eye deviation toward the ischemic hemisphere occurs when either hemisphere is affected. In addition, ischemia in the upper and lower division cortical surface branches of the middle cerebral artery gives rise to global or partial aphasia (dominant hemisphere) or to neglect and apractognosia (nondominant hemisphere). Which cortical surface structures are involved depends on the level of occlusion and degree of cortical surface collateral flow (Figure 64-1). Smaller emboli cause single superior or inferior branch of the middle cerebral artery syndromes, or partial branch syndromes. In the superior division, these might result in unilateral hand, hand and arm, or hand, arm, and shoulder weakness, unilateral face weakness, or expressive aphasia. Inferior division branch embolic syndromes include difficulty with reading, writing, auditory comprehension of language, or fluent aphasic speech with no limb weakness. Paraphasic errors abound in both inferior and superior division syndromes. Neglect of the left visual hemifield occurs most noticeably in nondominant syndromes, but may also occur on the right with dominant syndromes.

Low-flow syndromes occur when the internal carotid artery occlusion is not supported by adequate collateralization distally. They include recurrent transient brief episodes of hip and shoulder weakness, arm and leg weakness, speech trouble, and face or tongue numbness or weakness, many of which are similar, that is, stereotyped. Cortical surface infarcts secondary to low flow tend to occur in the distal field of the middle cerebral artery branches, before they anastomose with the anterior or posterior cerebral artery cortical surface branches, or in the distal field of the lenticulostriate penetrating arteries, affecting the deep white matter of the corona radiata.

- *Anterior cerebral artery*: Anterior cerebral arteries divide into two segments: part of the circle of Willis (A1 or stem) and the post-

communal (A2) segment distal to the anterior communicating artery (Figure 64-1). The A1 segment gives rise to several deep penetrating arteries that supply the anterior limb of the internal capsule, the anterior perforate substance, medullar anterior hypothalamus, and posterior part of the head of the caudate nucleus. Infarction in these territories is more often caused by an embolus than by local atheromatous disease. If the A2 segments of both right and left anterior cerebral arteries arise from a single anterior cerebral artery A1 segment, a normal anatomic variant, then symptoms occur in both hemispheres and include bilateral leg weakness. The most common symptoms of A2 segment occlusion are foot and leg weakness, and incontinence; occasionally—when both A2 segments are affected—abulia, gait apraxia, and forced grasping may also occur.

- *Anterior choroidal artery*: This artery arises from the internal carotid artery and supplies the posterior limb of the internal capsule and its posterolateral white matter, through which pass some of the geniculocalcarine fibers. The complete clinical syndrome consists of contralateral hemiparesis, hemianesthesia, and hemianopia. However, because this territory is also supplied by penetrating vessels of the middle cerebral artery stem and the posterior communicating and posterior choroidal arteries, syndromes with minimal deficits occur and patients frequently have an excellent recovery.

- *Common carotid artery*: All of the neurologic symptoms of internal carotid artery stenosis or occlusion can occur with common carotid artery thrombosis or an atherothrombotic lesion occurring at its origin. But the occurrence of transient ischemia or ischemia stroke arising from disease in the common carotid artery is far less than that of the internal carotid artery. Bilateral common carotid occlusions can cause faintness on arising, recurrent loss of consciousness, bilateral dim vision, headache, atrophy of the iris, pericapillary arteriovenous malformations, rubeosis iridis, optic atrophy, and claudication of the jaw muscles. They are associated with an incomplete aortic arch syndrome and have been associated with various combinations of carotid, subclavian, and innominate stenosis or occlusion.

Atherothrombotic Disease of the Posterior Cerebral Circulation: Vertebrobasilar and Posterior Cerebral Arteries and Their Branches. As seen in the anterior circulation, atherosclerosis has a predilection for certain parts of the posterior circulation—most frequently, the distal vertebral artery and the lower- to mid-basilar artery (Figure 64-1).

- *Vertebral and posteroinferior cerebellar artery*: An occlusion of the distal vertebral or its major branch, the posteroinferior cerebellar artery (PICA), may be caused by either atherothrombosis or by embolism from a proximal artery or the heart. An occlusion of either artery produces infarction in the lateral medulla. Atherothrombotic vertebral artery stroke is often heralded by TIA or minor stroke before the larger, completed stroke. The symptoms and signs vary, but the most frequent include vertigo, nausea and vomiting, hoarseness, dysphagia, ipsilateral facial numbness associated with impaired sensation of pain and heat over the ipsilateral face and contralateral arm and leg, ipsilateral Horner syndrome, and ipsilateral limb ataxia. The PICA also supplies the posteroinferior cerebellum that may become infarcted if collateral circulation from the superior cerebellar artery is inadequate.

The infarct resulting from vertebral occlusion does not differ anatomically from that produced by PICA occlusion, except for a greater involvement of the restiform body in the latter. Nevertheless, involvement of the cerebellum does not appreciably alter the clinical picture, except in cases where cerebellar edema formation increases the pressure in the posterior fossa enough to result in progressive obtundation and death. Although cerebellar edema can be treated with osmotic agents such as mannitol, surgical decompression may be necessary.

- *Basilar artery*: TIA usually heralds atherothrombotic basilar artery occlusion and the consequent accompanying devastating brainstem infarction. The symptoms of a TIA in the territory of the distal vertebral and the basilar artery are more varied than in the carotid-middle cerebral territory because of the many different neuronal structures involved. Moreover, brainstem TIAs may be caused by disease of either of the small penetrating branches of the basilar or vertebral artery or of the basilar or vertebral arteries themselves. The penetrating branch disease may be atherothrombotic, involving the proximal origins of these small branch vessels, or lipohyalinotic, involving the small vessels deeper in the brainstem (see "Lacunar stroke/TIA subtype" later in this chapter). In general, small vessel disease is less threatening than disease of the basilar trunk. Therefore, when brainstem TIA or acute stroke occurs, it is extremely important to determine whether the problem lies in the basilar artery or in one of its smaller branches. Disease of a basilar branch produces unilateral infarction, whereas disease of the basilar artery itself usually causes bilateral infarction. Transient dizziness associated with diplopia, dysarthria, and numbness around the mouth strongly indicate the presence of basilar insufficiency. Other important symptoms occurring less often include a general profound feeling of weakness of the entire body, staggering, and/or a feeling of propulsion. Bilateral signs such as gaze paresis or internuclear ophthalmoplegia associated with ipsilateral sensory loss or weakness signify ischemic infarction in both sides of the pons, and therefore exclude single penetrating branch disease as the culprit.

  Many branch syndromes have been described; others await clinical correlation. Syndromes of unilateral brainstem infarction typically involve some combination of ipsilateral signs of the head and face, from involvement of cranial nerve nuclei or their fascicles, and contralateral signs in the limbs, from involvement of ipsilateral crossed long tracts, such as the corticospinal tract or spinothalamic tract. In both instances, that is, symptomatic disease of the basilar artery proper or its branches, the neurologic deficit may fluctuate, and usually is of low-flow type; artery-to-artery embolic TIA occur, but much less often, usually from embolism to the small basilar branches from a proximal or distal vertebral atheromatous lesion. In the case of an artery-to-artery embolic TIA or minor stroke, the events are single and the symptoms are less likely to fluctuate.

- *Major basilar branches—anteroinferior cerebellar artery, superior cerebellar artery, posterior cerebral artery*: These major artery branches of the basilar artery produce their own distinct pathophysiologic syndromes. They are most often caused by artery-to-artery embolism from an atherothrombotic source within the proximal basilar artery or the proximal or distal vertebral artery. Less often, an aortic or cardiogenic source is found. Rarely, primary atherothrombotic occlusion at their origins is the cause of the stroke or TIA.

  - *Superior cerebellar artery*: Occlusion of the superior cerebellar artery results in one or more of the following symptoms: ipsilateral cerebellar ataxia (caused by ischemia of the middle and/or upper cerebellar peduncle, or dentate nucleus); nausea and vomiting; dysarthria and contralateral loss of pain and temperature sensation over the extremities, body, and face (caused by ischemia of the spinal and trigeminal thalamic tract); and ataxic tremor of the ipsilateral upper extremity. Horner syndrome, partial deafness, and palatal myoclonus may occur rarely. Partial syndromes occur frequently.

  - *Anteroinferior cerebellar artery*: Occlusion of the anteroinferior cerebellar artery produces variable degrees of infarction because the size of this artery varies inversely with that of the PICA. The territory it supplies usually includes the lateral midpons, middle cerebellar peduncle, cerebellum, and the labyrinth and cochlea. The principal symptoms may include ipsilateral deafness, facial weakness, vertigo (whirling dizziness), nausea, vomiting, nystagmus, tinnitus, deafness, cerebellar ataxia, Horner syndrome, and paresis of conjugate lateral gaze. The opposite side of the body loses pain and temperature sensation. An occlusion close to the origin of the artery may cause cortical spinal tract signs.

  - *Paramedian and short circumferential branches of the basilar artery*: Occlusion of one of the 5 to 7 short circumferential branches of the basilar artery affects the lateral two-thirds of the pons and/or middle or superior cerebellar peduncle, whereas occlusion of one of the 7 to 10 paramedian branches of the basilar artery affects a wedge-shaped area on either side of the medial pons. Many brainstem syndromes with cranial nerve abnormalities and crossed hemiplegia have been given eponyms; others await description.

  - *Posterior cerebral artery*: Arising from the bifurcation of the top of the basilar artery, each posterior cerebral artery divides into two segments, each with its distinct clinical pathophysiologic syndrome: (1) the proximal precommunal segment, beginning at the top of the basilar artery and going to the posterior communicating artery takeoff, gives penetrating branches to the subthalamus, thalamus, and midbrain, (2) the postcommunal segment, beginning at the posterior communicating artery takeoff, supplies the medial inferior temporal lobe and the medial occipital lobe distally. Twenty percent of the time, one or both of the right or left posterior cerebral artery precommunal (P1) segments are atretic. In that case, the postcommunal (P2) segment is then supplied by the internal carotid artery via the posterior communicating artery. The majority of ischemic syndromes, TIA, or stroke, result from embolism (artery-to-artery, cardioaortic, or unknown source) to the pre- and postcommunal segments and/or one of their branches. Primary atherothrombotic disease of the posterior cerebral artery is much less common.

    - *Precommunal posterior cerebral artery syndromes* include midbrain, subthalamic, and thalamic signs that vary depending on whether the embolus occludes the top of the basilar area, the right or left posterior cerebral artery precommunal segment, that is, the stem, or the penetrating artery branches of the precommunal segment. Coma and quadriplegia, resulting from infarction of the reticular activating system and bilateral corticospinal tracts within the midbrain, are the consequence of a devastating top of the basilar occlusion. But, otherwise, branch syndromes abound, usually with third nerve and contralateral motor or sensory findings. There is a normal anatomic variant in which a single large medial mesencephalic artery, the artery of Percheron, penetrates upward to supply both sides of the subthalamus as well as part of the midbrain. Occlusion of this artery results in bilateral ptosis, paralysis of upgaze, and decreased consciousness, caused by involvement of the periaqueductal gray and the mesencephalic reticular formation. When only a single penetrating precommunal artery territory is involved, small vessel lacunar disease results (see "Lacunar or Small Vessel Disease" later in this chapter).

- *Postcommunal posterior cerebral artery syndromes* include cortical branches to the medial inferior temporal lobe, giving rise to memory loss and delirium, and branches to the medial occipital lobe, giving rise to homonymous visual field defects. Distal field border zone ischemia of the posterior cerebral and middle cerebral arteries give rise to visual impairment syndromes that include inability to recognize faces or pictures or to put items in a picture together to form an object (Balint syndrome).

Lacunar Stroke/TIA Subtype (Small Vessel Disease)

As defined by C. Miller Fisher through fastidious brainstem serial section, lacunar infarct results from an occlusion of a small single penetrating artery arising from the circle of Willis, the middle cerebral stem, the basilar artery, or either distal vertebral arteries. These penetrating arteries vary in size from 100 to 400 microns in diameter, rendering the infarct size finite from 0.5 to 1.5 cm in diameter, and usually no more than 3 cm in the longest dimension. The cause is lipohyalinotic narrowing or occlusion in the mid- or distal part of the artery or atherothrombotic lesion at its origin; embolism is rarely the cause. Lacunar strokes account for 25% of all strokes in the NIH Stroke Databank. These strokes cause recognizable clinical syndromes that evolve over hours to days, and may be preceded by transient symptoms (lacunar TIAs). The location of the ischemia determines the nature and severity of the symptoms. Recovery occurs often within days, but in some with especially strategically placed infarcts, significant disability is persistent.

The most common lacunar syndromes are the following:

- *Pure motor hemiparesis* from an infarct in the posterior limb of the internal capsule or basis pontis. The face, arm, leg, foot, and toes are equally paretic or plegic, but with no sensory deficit. The weakness may be intermittent (TIA), progress in a stepwise manner, or appear abruptly. The progression may result in a complete hemiplegia. Improvement almost to normal occurs in many cases.

- *Pure sensory stroke* from an infarct in the ventrolateral thalamus. This type of infarct produces face, arm, and leg sensory involvement with numbness, tingling, and loss of pain and temperature. The patient generally recovers but often is left with a sensory sensation that is abnormal. On rare occasions, an intolerable pain syndrome with dysesthesia occurs in the involved extremities some months afterwards (Dejerine–Roussy syndrome).

- *Ataxic hemiparesis* from an infarct in the basis pontis caused by an infarct in the basis pontis or corona radiata near the genu of the internal capsule.

- *Dysarthria–clumsy hand syndrome* caused by lacunar infarction of the genu of the internal capsule or, less frequently, the corona radiata or the paramedian rostral pons, with resulting mild contralateral arm ataxia or arm weakness, and dysarthric speech.

When multiple, lacunar infarctions may produce bilateral pyramidal and corticobulbar motor system signs, dysarthria, and a slowed abulic mental state with emotional lability, that is, pseudobulbar palsy. Such presentations have, however, become rare in today's era of effective antihypertensive therapy.

Careful attention to antihypertensive, diabetic, and dyslipidemic therapies offer the best form of prevention. In all lacunar stroke or TIA, it is essential to ascertain that the large arteries at the base of the brain giving rise to the penetrating small arteries, that is, the basilar artery, the middle cerebral artery stem, or the posterior cerebral artery stem, are not, in themselves, harboring a thrombus threatening their occlusion and causing the lacunar syndrome (see "Evaluation and Therapeutic Strategies" below).

Embolic Stroke/TIA Subtype

In this pathophysiologic stroke/TIA subtype the embolic fragment occluding the intracranial vessel, leading to the ischemia or infarction is derived from the aortic arch, the heart, or an unknown source (cryptogenic stroke), rather than from a local arterial source in the extra- or intracranial arteries, such as atherothrombosis or dissection.

Embolic strokes are diagnosed when a sudden or stuttering neurologic deficit appears in the territory of a large intracranial artery at the base of the brain or in one of its major branches, and the extra- or intracranial arterial supply to the ischemic zone does not have a detectable significant stenotic or thrombotic occlusive lesion as detected by ultrasonography, MRI, or CT angiographic imaging. In some cases, the embolic fragment may be seen, on imaging, to occlude the vessel or a distal branch. In other cases, the suspected embolic material is not visualized because it has already been dissolved by the endogenous fibrinolytic system, but not before significant ischemia has occurred. When the above definition of embolic stroke is used, it accounts for fully 60% of all strokes in the NIH Stroke Databank.

It is most convenient, for determining appropriate preventive therapy, to divide these types of emboli into treatment categories. First, those commonly accepted cardiac source emboli where anticoagulant therapy is standard of practice. Second, commonly accepted cardiac source emboli where anticoagulant therapy is contraindicated, as in bacterial endocarditis or atrial myxoma. Third, those possible cardioaortic sources that can only be diagnosed by transthoracic echocardiogram or transesophageal echocardiogram, in which debate exists as to the best therapy, be it anticoagulant, antiplatelet, or cardiointerventional. Fourth, those truly cryptogenic strokes in which a possible or definite cardiac and aortic source is excluded (Table 64-1). Within all of the source categories above, the level of activity of the hemostatic system may be a significant determinant in the incidence of local thrombus formation and embolism. Therefore, in addition to careful evaluation of the heart, evaluation of the hemostatic system, as well as exclusion of a primary arterial source of

TABLE 64-1

Embolic Stroke Classification

Cardiac source is definite: anticoagulant therapy generally considered
  standard of practice.
  Left ventricular thrombi
  Left atrial thrombi
  Rheumatic valvular disease
  Mechanical prosthetic valves
  Atrial fibrillation
  Nonbacterial thrombotic endocarditis

Cardiac source is definite: anticoagulation considered hazardous.
  Bacterial endocarditis
  Atrial myxoma

Cardiac source is possible: synonyms in the literature include "unknown
  source," "cryptogenic stroke"—these diagnoses are made by transthoracic
  or transesophageal echocardiogram. The efficacy of antiplatelet versus
  anticoagulant therapy is uncertain.
  Mitral annular calcification
  Left ventricular dysfunction and dilated cardiomyopathy
  Postmyocardial infarction with or without left ventricular aneurysm or thrombi
  Left atrial spontaneous echo contrast
  Patent foramen ovale
  Atrioseptal aneurysm
  Valvular strands

Ascending aortic atheromatous disease: mobile plaque 4 mm or greater.

Truly unknown-source embolic stroke.

embolism, is essential in order to plan appropriate pathophysiology-based treatment.

The clinical presentation of embolism in the anterior and posterior cerebral circulation is similar to that of artery-to-artery embolism, and was discussed in the preceding section. The nature and severity of the symptoms depend entirely on the location of the embolic fragment occluding the artery and the spared collateral circulation to its cerebral territory. The artery occluded, in turn, depends on the size of the embolic fragment and the extracranial artery it enters. In the case of an embolic fragment ending in the vertebral artery, it may migrate, stop, and then migrate again, leaving a trail of infarcted tissue from the cerebellum and lower brainstem to the upper brainstem, thalamus, and temporal and occipital lobes. Embolic fragments that enter the middle cerebral stem often disperse to branches of the superior and inferior division of the middle cerebral artery, giving rise to a patchy infarct in the deep or basal lenticulostriate arterial territory, and in the cortical surface branch territories.

In every case of embolic stroke, embolism from an infected heart valve should be considered because of the devastating consequences if not detected. Subacute bacterial endocarditis may have a very subtle presentation. A normal erythrocyte sedimentation rate at the time of the initial evaluation is a quick means of excluding it.

Patent Foramen Ovale and Embolic Stroke. Patent foramen ovale (PFO) is the consequence of failure of complete closure of the atrial septum primum and septum secundum immediately following birth, thereby leaving a communication between the right atrium and left atrium. PFO has been associated with stroke in epidemiologic studies, which show its prevalence is doubled in younger persons with otherwise cryptogenic embolic stroke. Stroke may be more common in those with PFO because the atrial communication pro-

vides a channel by which a venous embolism can pass from the right side to the left side of the heart with the potential for subsequent cerebral embolism (so-called "paradoxical embolism"). Alternately, the PFO may itself be the source of thrombus formation with subsequent embolism. The PFO may be identified by transthoracic echocardiography with injection of agitated saline; transesophageal echocardiography offers increased sensitivity. Transcranial Doppler ultrasound can also be used to detect the presence of right-to-left shunting by documenting the passage of agitated microbubbles into the cerebral circulation following a peripheral venous injection; it has equal or greater sensitivity than transthoracic echocardiography and can be used to guide the cardiac evaluation.

There is considerable controversy regarding the significance and therapeutic implications of PFO in stroke, both because of a lack of clinical trials and because PFO is common even in persons without stroke (15–20% of asymptomatic normal individuals have a PFO). Preventive therapy with aspirin or warfarin has been used, as well as invasive strategies to physically occlude the PFO, mostly using endovascular devices rather than cardiac surgery. One study identified the coexistence of an atrial septal aneurysm as an additional risk factor for recurrent stroke; however, it is unclear whether this should affect the therapeutic strategy. If a PFO is identified, the patient should be screened for the presence of deep venous thrombosis, which would itself be an indication for a period of anticoagulation. The significance of identifying PFO in elderly patients with "traditional" risk factors is unclear. A subgroup analysis of the Warfarin versus Aspirin Recurrent Stroke Study (WARSS), enrolling mostly patients older than 60 years with vascular risk factors, found that, among the subgroup with PFO, there was no difference in recurrent stroke among those on warfarin compared to those on aspirin.

Other Causes of Cerebral Infarction

Although other causes of cerebral infarction account for only 3% of all stroke in the NIH Stroke Databank, they are extremely important because their precise pathophysiologic diagnosis can lead to effective treatment.

Dissection of the cervical cerebral arteries is, by far, the most common cause of stroke in this category subtype. Generally, dissection begins at the point where the internal carotid artery enters the petrous bone, approximately 1 cm distal to the origin of the internal carotid artery, or in the vertebral artery as it transverses the foramen transversarium. The dissections divide the media and adventitia, or the media and intima, and clot forms in the division. Thrombus may form in the arterial lumen if it is compromised or occluded. Trauma, either severe or trivial, may be cause of the dissection, but Valsalva maneuvers with coughing and vomiting, weight-lifting, contact sports, or chiropractic manipulations are other recognized associations. Spontaneous dissections, without clear antecedent, are not uncommon. Dissections occur at all ages, but are a frequent cause of stroke in school-aged children or young adults. The clinical hallmark of carotid dissection is a Horner syndrome, which occurs in 50% of instances. Headache, cervical pain, or pain behind the eye occurs frequently. Carotid artery-to-artery embolism or low-flow infarction syndromes occur, just as they do for atherothrombotic disease of the internal carotid artery. Similar pathophysiologic circumstances exist for vertebral artery dissections; with them, cervical spine pain and occipital headache are the suggestive symptoms. The most common site of infarction in vertebral dissection is the lateral medulla, with or without concomitant involvement of a PICA territory. Dizziness, ataxia of gait, nausea and vomiting with a unilateral Horner syndrome, and ipsilateral face numbness with contralateral body numbness are the hallmark symptoms. Occasionally, diplopia and a hoarse voice are evident. Artery-to-artery emboli arising from a thrombus at the site of dissection in the vertebral artery may migrate to distal branches of the basilar artery, producing brainstem, cerebellar, or thalamic infarction. Although not proven by randomized clinical trial, our experience suggests that immediate anticoagulation with intravenous heparin, followed by 4 to 6 months of anticoagulant therapy with warfarin, using a target international normalized ratio (INR) of 2.0 to 3.0, is helpful in preventing recurrent or worsening stroke.

Fibromuscular dysplasia typically occurs in the extracranial carotid artery. On angiography, it looks like a ruffled sock. It is rarely symptomatic unless it becomes hemodynamically significant; then, both embolic or low-flow TIA or stroke can occur. Generally, antiplatelet therapy is used for prevention, but no clinical trial evidence exists in its support. Anticoagulant therapy and interventional arterial therapy are other possible options after symptoms have occurred.

Infectious arteritis caused by bacterial or syphilitic infection is no longer a common cause of cerebral thrombosis. Arteritis may rarely follow herpes zoster, particularly if the ophthalmic division is involved. Cerebral arteritis may rarely accompany certain systemic vasculitides, including polyarteritis nodosa or Wegener granulomatosis. Necrotizing granulomatous arteritis, or primary angiitis of the central nervous system, involves the distal small branches (less than 2 mm diameter) of the main intracranial arteries and produces small ischemic infarcts in the brain, optic nerve, and spinal cord. There is no systemic involvement. This rare disease is often relentlessly progressive. There may be cerebrospinal fluid pleocytosis. In some cases, glucocorticoid therapy (prednisone, 40–60 mg/day) has been helpful, as has immunosuppressive therapy (e.g., cyclophosphamide). Idiopathic giant cell arteritis involving the great vessels arising from the aortic arch (Takayasu syndrome) may, on occasion, cause carotid or vertebral thrombosis; nevertheless, it is an infrequent cause of the aortic arch syndrome in the western hemisphere.

Temporal arteritis is a relatively common affliction of elderly persons, in which the external carotid system—particularly the temporal arteries—is the site of a subacute granulomatous infiltration with an exudate of lymphocytes, monocytes, neutrophilic leukocytes, and giant cells. Usually, the most severely affected parts of the artery become thrombosed. Headache or facial pain is the chief complaint. The inflammatory nature of the illness is indicated by one or more of the following: fever, slight leukocytosis, increased erythrocyte sedimentation rate, and anemia. Systemic manifestations include anorexia, loss of weight, malaise, and polymyalgia rheumatica. Occlusion of the branches of the ophthalmic artery results in blindness of one or both eyes. Occasionally, an ophthalmoplegia caused by involvement of extrinsic ocular muscles occurs. In some cases, an arteritis of the aorta and its major branches, including the carotids, subclavian, coronary, and femoral arteries, has been found at postmortem examination. Significant inflammatory involvement of the intracranial arteries is rare, but strokes occur occasionally on the basis of occlusion of the internal carotid, middle cerebral, or vertebral arteries. The diagnosis depends on the finding of a tender thrombosed or thickened cranial artery and demonstration of the lesion in a biopsy specimen. The hallmark symptom is transient blindness. When that occurs in patients older than age 50 years, a sedimentation rate with a fibrinogen level and complete blood count should be done urgently. Corticosteroids may bring striking relief and prevent blindness. Prednisone is most often used, beginning with large daily doses of 80 to 100 mg/day and then tapering over 2 to 4 weeks using the sedimentation rate as a guide.

Moyamoya disease is a poorly understood occlusive disorder involving large intracranial arteries, especially the distal internal carotid artery, and the stem of the middle cerebral artery, as well as the anterior cerebral artery. The lenticulostriate arteries develop a rich collateral network around the middle cerebral occlusive lesion giving the impression of a puff of smoke ("moyamoya" in Japanese) on cerebral angiography. Other collaterals include transdural anastomoses between the cortical surface branches of the middle cerebral artery and the scalp arteries. The disease mainly occurs in the Oriental population, but should be suspected when TIAs or stroke occur in children or young adults. Its etiology is unknown; although it has been associated with sickle cell disease, cranial radiation, neurofibromatosis type I, and Downs' syndrome, many cases are idiopathic. There have been few pathologic studies; they suggest that hyalinotic fibrous type material is associated with the arterial narrowing and microaneurysm formation. The best treatment is not known. Although no formal study has been performed to determine the optimal treatment of patients with symptoms of ischemia or infarction, aspirin or other antiplatelet agents have often been used. Anticoagulation is not recommended in all symptomatic cases, but rather on a case-by-case basis. The use of antiplatelet and anticoagulant drugs must be balanced against the risk of hemorrhage (both intraparenchymal and subarachnoid) from rupture of the small, fragile anastomotic channels, or from rupture of the microaneurysms occurring in the perforating arteries from the circle of Willis. In the case of hemorrhage, of course, hematoma evacuation and ventricular drainage may be indicated. A variety of surgical revascularization procedures has been proposed to improve collateral flow and prevent brain infarction and hemorrhage: cervical sympathectomy, omentum transplantation, superficial temporal artery–middle cerebral artery bypass, or encephaloduroarteriosynangiosis.

Reversible cerebral vasoconstriction syndrome has been noted in patients with severe "thunderclap" headache, often recurrent, and fluctuating neurologic symptoms and signs. Brain imaging can be normal or show cerebral infarction, hemorrhage, or transient brain edema. The etiology is unknown. Eclampsia, the postpartum period, head injury, migraine, and sympathomimetic and serotonergic drugs have all been associated with this entity. Conventional contrast angiography is the only definitive means of establishing the diagnosis although newer imaging techniques such as CT angiography and MR angiography are proving useful. Cerebrospinal fluid is normal in most cases. The disease is self-limited and, with adequate supportive care, partial or complete recovery occurs in the majority of cases. The headaches and arterial vasoconstriction usually resolve within a few weeks. There is no proven therapy to prevent neurological deterioration. Vasodilators such as nimodipine, a calcium channel blocking agent, or intravenous nitroglycerin might be considered. Maintenance of normal systemic arterial pressure and adequate hydration seems important on empirical grounds.

Cerebral autosomal dominant arteriopathy with subcortical infarcts and leukoencephalopathy (CADASIL) is a rare primary arteriolopathy affecting small penetrating vessels to the basal ganglia, thalamus, and cerebral white matter. The disease is caused by a variety of mutations in the *Notch3* gene. The typical clinical symptom complex includes late-onset migraine with aura, recurrent stroke and/or TIAs, neuropsychiatric problems such as depression, bipolar disease, or subcortical dementia with pseudobulbar features occurring in persons between 40 and 50 years of age. Cerebrospinal fluid examination and cerebral angiography are normal. There is no specific treatment to date. The diagnosis can be made by genetic testing with sequencing of the *Notch3* gene. Cerebral, leptomeningeal, or skin biopsy with demonstration, by electron microscopy, of typical osmophilic granular deposits in or around the vascular smooth muscle cells of the tunica media and basal lamina matrix is also diagnostic.

Binswanger subcortical leukoencephalopathy, now rare, is a syndrome seen with advanced small-vessel hypertensive disease. Diffuse vascular lesions are seen in the subcortical layers of the cerebral hemispheres and there is widespread white matter demyelination. Usually affecting individuals around 50 years of age, it is characterized by fluctuations in mood and consciousness, perhaps even seizures; a dementia may be an early and prominent symptom preceded or accompanied by symptoms and signs of one or more small vessel infarctions. Confusional states, memory difficulties, and abulia are prominent, and sometimes accompanied by focal cortical–subcortical deficits such as aphasia, apraxia, or neglect. Focal neurological deficits, or uni- or bilateral limb signs may lead to a pseudobulbar state; gait difficulties are prominent. There is often evidence of vascular compromise in other body districts.

Binswanger disease must be differentiated from disorders with prominent subcortical white matter involvement on CT or MRI; these include hypertensive encephalopathy, cerebral amyloid (congophilic) angiopathy, CADASIL, normal pressure hydrocephalus, and Alzheimer's disease.

Hematological diseases such as acute and chronic leukemia, essential and secondary thrombocytosis, thrombocytopenia, and sickle cell disease, can be complicated by ischemic or hemorrhagic stroke. Hypercoagulable states such as the deficiency of protein C, protein S, or antithrombin III, are extremely rare causes of stroke, but are often included in the evaluation of stroke in the young.

Finally, stroke can ensue during the course of a severe attack of migraine, especially migraine with aura ("migraine-induced stroke"). It is often difficult to distinguish whether the patient developed a migraine-induced stroke, a stroke-induced headache, or had the coincidental occurrence of stroke and migraine. Since migraine-induced stroke is a diagnosis of exclusion, a thorough evaluation is required to exclude other potential causes, both common and uncommon, before making this diagnosis.

Evaluation

The initial history and physical is the hallmark of the evaluation to obtain a presumed pathophysiological stroke or TIA subtype diagnosis. The initial electrocardiogram and blood work should include a sedimentation rate as a screen for subacute bacterial endocarditis. In addition, the standard complete blood count, platelet count, prothrombin time, partial thromboplastin time, and general chemistry examination is essential. None of those laboratory assessments should interfere with the urgent timing of neuroimaging and ultrasound studies. Special clotting studies are not essential urgently, but are often useful when a hypercoagulable state is suspected or when there is embolism of uncertain origin. Such studies could include assessment of protein C, protein S, and antithrombin 3, antiphospholipid antibodies, factor V Leiden mutation, and prothrombin 20210 A gene mutation. The screen of thyroid function with a thyroid-stimulating hormone has helped us in identifying clinically inapparent hyperthyroidism, a condition that may be associated with atrial fibrillation or hyperlipidemia. In the initial blood evaluation, cardiac enzymes are also essential to rule out an associated myocardial infarction.

The pathophysiological stroke subtype, inferred from the history and physical examination, should then be urgently confirmed by imaging evaluation of the brain and the suspected arterial lesion. Noncontrast head CT is, for most centers, the initial component of the imaging evaluation that allows rapid exclusion of hemorrhage, but does not usually define the area of infarction and, of course, does not demonstrate the arterial pathology. The next urgent step, therefore, is imaging of the cerebral large arterial system with CT angiography (CTA), MR angiography (MRA), or transcranial Dopper ultrasound.

CTA is an extremely rapid, accurate way of identifying the pathology in the parent vessel from the origin of the aortic arch to the ischemic zone distal to the great vessels at the base of the brain (vessels shown in Figure 64-1B). This technique can be combined with *CT-perfusion* imaging, in which a contrast bolus is tracked, by serial scanning, as it passes through the tissue and the results deconvoluted into a map of perfusion times. Although CTA provides excellent definition of the arterial system, it is not good at defining acute infarction. In particular, CT scanning is insensitive to recent infarcts of less than 12 hours duration and small cortical surface embolic infarct and infarcts in the posterior fossa, because of beam-hardening artifact from the closely approximated bones of the skull.

MRI and MRA are the best ways of identifying infarcts accurately in terms of their extent and location, but do not offer as good resolution of the arterial system as conventional transfemoral angiography or CT angiography. Susceptibility sequences identify subacute hemorrhagic infarcts and small areas of chronic hemorrhage that might be associated with small vessel diseases such as amyloid angiopathy or hypertensive vasculopathy. MRA, especially when enhanced with gadolinium, can outline the parent vessel pathology from the arch all the way through to the branches of the major vessels at the base of the brain. Gadolinium should be avoided, however, in patients with renal dysfunction because of rare reports of subsequent nephrogenic fibrosing dermopathy. *MR perfusion weighted imaging* can, in an analogous way to CT-perfusion imaging, identify areas of perfusion delay that indicate tissue at risk of progression to infarction. The disadvantage of MRI imaging is the time it takes for the scan to be obtained. In addition, because of the small head diameter of the imaging system, there is a significant claustrophobic effect in approximately 10% of patients. These disadvantages decrease its efficacy in hyperacute stroke state, where the most urgent issue is elucidating the nature of the arterial pathology of the parent vessel leading to the ischemic infarct and the exclusion of hemorrhages, tasks that CT and CT angiography perform admirably.

Neurosonology tests include *carotid duplex Doppler* and *transcranial Doppler* assessment of the extra- and intracranial arterial system. *Carotid duplex Doppler* allows assessment of flow at the bifurcation of the common carotid artery, including flow in the proximal internal carotid artery; in addition, flow in the middle portion of the vertebral artery can be assessed to identify more proximal or distal obstructive lesions. *Transcranial Doppler* allows assessment of flow of the intracranial carotid artery and flow in the ophthalmic artery through the transorbital approach. The transtemporal approach permits assessment of flow in the middle, anterior, and posterior cerebral artery stems. The occipital foramen magnum approach easily and reliably allows determination of flow in the distal vertebral arteries and in the basilar artery. These ultrasound studies allow for immediate evaluation of the stroke or TIA presumed subtype and are important in the identification all four ischemic stroke subtypes. They can identify the presence and severity of an obstructive lesion in the parent vessel as well as identify the presence of collateral flow to the ischemic zone. Their disadvantage is that, on some occasions, the parent vessel of interest escapes examination. Nevertheless, in atherothrombotic stroke, often the severity and location of the atherothrombotic parent vessel lesion and the nature of the spared collateral flow can be identified. In addition, in an embolic stroke, migration and lysis of an embolism in a parent vessel can be noted by detecting normal flow in that vessel. In lacunar small-vessel stroke, the diagnosis can be supported by the identification of normal flow in the parent vessel to the penetrating artery that is suspected of being occluded. In dissection of the carotid or vertebral artery extracranially, obstruction of flow proximally in the vessel can be identified if the dissection is severe enough to affect flow distally. In cases of temporal arteritis, the pathology can be suspected by duplex ultrasound of the temporal artery. These neurosonology tests allow for ease in following these arterial lesions in terms of their progression or resolution. These tests have the advantage of being simple, can be used by the physician similar to the cardiologist's stethoscope examination, and are highly portable. We use these tests to identify acutely the suspected arterial lesion, but always confirm with neuroimaging studies. We then use neurosonology tests to follow the progression of the arterial pathology subacutely and chronically. The quantification of carotid artery atheromatous disease and its progression is an especially important use of carotid duplex Doppler combined with transcranial Doppler.

Cardiac Evaluation

Cardiac evaluation, in addition to an electrocardiogram, cardiac enzymes, and sedimentation rate acutely obtained, should include, on a subacute basis, cardiac ultrasonography and cardiac rhythm monitoring when an embolism is considered in the differential diagnosis. A cardiac evaluation, including echocardiography, should therefore also be considered in patients with lacunar stroke based on evidence that, uncommonly, small vessel lacunar strokes are caused by emboli. Echocardiography generally starts with transthoracic echocardiogram but, in cases where the diagnosis is not obvious, transesophageal echocardiogram is considered, especially when the obvious diagnostic source is important in deciding a precise preventive treatment. Contrast echocardiography or contrast transcranial Doppler ultrasonography can easily identify patients who have a PFO. Cardiac rhythm monitoring on a portable basis is very helpful if atrial fibrillation or other cardiogenic arrhythmias are to be considered. Only then can precise therapeutic preventive strategies be planned.

Therapeutic Strategies for Ischemic Stroke

With the acute onset of neurological deficits suggesting ischemia, the essential therapeutic goal is to prevent worsening and to try to facilitate or reestablish blood flow to the ischemic zone. The therapeutic strategy should always be guided by pathophysiology, whether presumed (history and physical) or confirmed (history, physical, and positive neuroimaging or neurosonology confirmatory diagnostic study). The diagnosis should include not only one of the four ischemic stroke or TIA subtypes noted earlier, but also the presence or absence of pathology in the parent vessel supplying the ischemic

zone and the extent of the spared collateral flow to it. The time of onset to treatment determines the therapeutic options. Three phases exist: (1) the hyperacute (1–3 hours) to acute (3–12 hours) phase, (2) the subacute phase, and (3) the preventive phase.

After the pathophysiological diagnosis has been determined and the patient has been evaluated for therapies designed to facilitate or reestablish cerebral perfusion and prevent subsequent strokes, further management efforts are directed at preventing common complications, such as deep venous thrombosis and aspiration pneumonia, and assisting with neurological recovery through rehabilitation.

Hyperacute/Acute

In this hyperacute/acute phase, the goal is to open the occluded parent artery. For patients in whom treatment can be initiated within 3 hours of symptom onset, intravenous recombinant human tissue plasminogen activator (Activase), at a dose of 0.9 mg/kg with 10% given as an immediate bolus and the remainder infused over 1 hour, has been shown to reduce stroke-related disability. In the pivotal NINDS rt-PA trial, patients treated with recombinant tissue plasminogen activator (rt-PA) had a 12% greater absolute chance of a good outcome, defined as minimal or no stroke-related disability. This benefit was present despite a 6% risk of intracranial hemorrhage in the rt-PA group, of which more than half were fatal. There is incomplete evidence regarding which stroke pathophysiologic subtypes respond best to rt-PA; posthoc analysis of the trial did not show statistical evidence that the treatment effect varied by presumed stroke subtype, although the power to detect differences was modest.

Because of the risks of hemorrhage, the decision to give rt-PA should be based on an individual assessment of the benefits and risks for the specific individual, with careful attention to the treatment inclusion and exclusion criteria. Patients with well-established CT evidence of infarction should not be treated. Those with early CT signs of infarction, such as loss of differentiation of the cortical ribbon from the underlying white matter in greater than one-third of the middle cerebral artery territory, have a worse prognosis from stroke and may not warrant treatment in all cases. Patients expected to have an excellent outcome may not warrant treatment because of the overall excellent prognosis. The decision not to give rt-PA should be made carefully, however, because data suggest that some patients with mild or improving stroke may have stroke recurrence or extension. The ability to predict which patients will have subsequent worsening is, unfortunately, limited. There has been concern about treatment of the elderly because age may be a risk factor for rt-PA related hemorrhage; however, the trial data show that this increased risk does not outweigh the potential benefit in elderly persons. Age is not an exclusion criterion to rt-PA use at our institution; the oldest subject we have treated was 99 years of age. Intravenous rt-PA is best administered by experienced stroke teams with expert neuroradiologic consultation available 24 hours a day. The Joint Commission on Accreditation of Hospital Organizations (JCAHO) now offers an accreditation program to certify hospitals as "primary stroke centers", which includes documentation of competency in administering rt-PA.

Intra-arterial approaches to therapy have been employed, in selected centers, in patient with moderate to severe neurological deficits within 6 to 8 hours of stroke onset. Patients with a basilar thrombus up to 12 hours after stroke onset are also sometimes treated because in the posterior circulation, particularly the brainstem and cerebellum, a rich collateralization can delay the progression to infarction for longer periods of time. Intra-arterial therapy is sometimes used after intravenous rt-PA in cases where there was no immediate response to the intravenous rt-PA because of persistent arterial occlusion. Intra-arterial treatment options include direct administration of thrombolytics, wire manipulation, angioplasty or stenting, or clot retrieval. Most of these approaches have not been proven effective in a randomized trial. Observational studies suggest, however, that they may be able to achieve recanalization of arterial occlusions of the proximal branches of the circle of Willis. Intra-arterial infusion of prourokinase was shown to produce better outcomes than placebo in the Prolyse in Acute Cerebral Thromboemboblism II (PROACT-II) study, but the evidence was not sufficient to prompt the United States Food and Drug Administration (FDA) to grant approval for the drug. More recently, the FDA has approved the Concentrics device for retrieval of intracranial thromboemboli within 8 hours of symptom onset. The efficacy of this device in reducing stroke-related disability has, however, never been tested in a controlled trial, therefore its role in therapy remains controversial.

Intravenous and low-molecular-weight heparins, as well as heparin-like anticoagulants, have been tested in a number of clinical trials with conflicting results. Reflecting this, current guidelines acknowledge that the benefit of using heparin for acute stroke, in any clinical setting, is uncertain. On the other hand, it is possible that heparin could prevent clot propagation in the parent vessel (although clot lysis is unlikely), or prevent early recurrent stroke especially from a high-risk arterial source. Intravenous heparin has been used in five common clinical settings. First, in large-vessel atherothrombotic disease to prevent clot propagation from the atherothrombotic locus, or to prevent further embolization from the atherothrombotic site. Second, in embolic stroke from a cardiac or aortic source where the embolus remains in the stem of the middle cerebral artery, the internal carotid artery or the basilar artery, that is, one of the parent vessels, and the deficit is submaximal, that is, the deficit could worsen if the embolus propagates as a thrombus. Third, in lacunar stroke, it is occasionally given when the motor weakness is relentlessly progressive. Its efficacy has not been very high in this setting in our hands. Fourth, it is likely of benefit in patients who have carotid or vertebral artery dissections, or sinovenous thrombosis; only in the latter setting has the efficacy of heparin been proven in a randomized trial. Many centers, including ours, use heparin in the acute setting of arterial dissection in order to prevent clot propagation and artery-to-artery embolus. Fifth, in patients with a high-risk cardioembolic source or arterial source of embolism, it may reduce the risk of early recurrent stroke. Heparin is associated with an increased risk of hemorrhagic transformation of ischemic stroke, and this risk is greater when the infarct volume is large. The risk of hemorrhage is, however, much lower than with rt-PA. In our practice, heparin is not given if the stroke is large (greater than one-third of the middle cerebral artery territory or the complete posterior cerebral artery territory), particularly if the stroke involves the deep penetrating branches to the basal ganglia. In patients who have received thrombolytics, heparin should not be given within 24 hours of treatment.

Subacute

Surgical therapeutic options can be considered in this subacute phase. Urgent carotid endarterectomy may be considered if the patient has a severe carotid stenosis with an inadequate collateral supply through the circle of Willis or the external carotid artery ophthalmic system. In this setting, the resultant stroke can be devastating, while emergency endarterectomy can be highly effective. Carotid endarterectomy for mild to moderate stroke or TIA in the territory of the internal carotid artery has also been proven effective, by the North American Symptomatic Carotid Endarterectomy Trial (NASCET) study, for patients with both 70% to 99% stenosis and 50% to 69% stenosis. But severe stroke in the middle cerebral artery territory in which further worsening would only be minimal, that is, the deficit is almost maximal, is not appropriate for endarterectomy in the subacute phase. If the patient improves in rehabilitation to the point where worsening of the deficit would be problematic, then endarterectomy can be reconsidered. If low-flow stroke is not the issue, surgery can be planned in patients with mild to moderate deficits on an elective basis after careful consideration of the cardiomedical status. The surgical benefit for patients with symptomatic moderate stenosis was statistically significant but small, with only 1.5% absolute risk reduction per year, and therefore surgery should only be considered in centers with low perioperative rates of surgical morbidity. The decision to perform carotid endarterectomy for symptomatic moderate carotid stenosis should be made on an individual basis, taking into account the patient's surgical risk, center-specific perioperative complication rate (which should be less than 2%), and the patient's life expectancy. Because the surgical risk occurs "up-front" during the perioperative period, the benefit from surgery accrues with increased years of life. For the elderly, the risks and benefits must be carefully weighed. When there is symptomatic severe stenosis (70–99% luminal narrowing) the surgical benefit is, by contrast, quite high, and most patients will benefit from surgical rather than medical management.

Carotid stenting has recently gained ground as an alternative to endarterectomy. Advantages include shorter hospital stay, lack of a neck incision, avoidance of general anesthesia, and a lower incidence of cranial neuropathy as a complication. However, two recent randomized trials, in patients with symptomatic carotid stenosis, showed that stenting was inferior to endarterectomy with higher rates of serious periprocedural complications. Stenting is still an option for patients at high risk for complications from endarterectomy, including those with medical comorbidities, unfavorable neck anatomy, and postendarterectomy restenosis. Additional trials, incorporating newer technologies to prevent stent-related embolization, may yet expand the indications for stenting.

Hemicraniectomy may be considered when progressive cerebral edema in the nondominant hemisphere becomes severe enough to compromise cerebral perfusion or cause brain herniation. This operation can prevent herniation and death by relieving intracranial pressure, but is unlikely to restore significant neurological function because it is typically performed in the setting of extensive brain infarction. A pooled analysis of three small trials confirms that hemicraniectomy prevents severe dependency or death. Observational studies suggest very poor outcomes in patients older than 65 years, and it is generally not used in elderly persons.

Preventive

There are two important aspects of preventive therapy. First, the control and prevention strategies related to the primary risk factors for all stroke subtypes and, second, preventive strategies directed toward the specific stroke or TIA subtype in the particular patient.

Preventive Strategies for Controlling Primary Risk Factors. Treatment of hypertension is, by far, the most important aspect of risk factor control. Achieving and maintaining blood pressure treatment targets are probably more important than proposed class effects of the drugs. Control of lipids is also important. Following the Third Report of the National Cholesterol Education Program Expert Panel on Detection, Evaluation, and Treatment of High Blood Cholesterol in Adults (ATPIII) guidelines for prevention of MI, the primary goal is lowering the low-density lipoprotein (LDL). Risk factor adjustment including diet, exercise, weight reduction, cessation of smoking, and diabetes management are all important first steps. Hydroxymethylglutaryl coenzyme A (HMG-CoA) reductase inhibitors ("statins") are associated with reduction in the risk of stroke, as well as reduction in the risk of MI. The recent Stroke Prevention with Atorvastatin to Reduce Cholesterol Levels (SPARCL) trial showed that, among patients with large vessel atherothrombotic or lacunar stroke subtypes and LDL >100 mg/dL, high-dose atorvastatin (80 mg every day) was superior to placebo in reducing subsequent stroke. Our practice is to treat all patients with large vessel atherothrombotic or lacunar stroke with statins to lower the LDL to less than 100 mg/dL.

Preventive Therapy Directed Toward the Specific Stroke/TIA Subtype. Therapy directed toward preventing the specific stroke subtypes consists of two aspects: (1) antiplatelet versus anticoagulant therapy and (2) surgical strategies.

- *Anticoagulant versus antiplatelet therapy*: Anticoagulant therapy is accepted as standard of practice in the cardiac conditions outlined in Table 64-1; but only in the case of atrial fibrillation has this treatment been proven by randomized clinical trial. The INR goal is 2 to 3, except in certain prosthetic valvular conditions, where an INR of 2.5 to 3.5 is recommended. Warfarin anticoagulation is contraindicated in infective endocarditis and in left atrial myxomatous syndromes because of associated cortical surface mycotic and myxomatous aneurysm with the risk of hemorrhage. In all other possible causes of cardioaortic embolism, as in cases of cryptogenic embolism, debate exists as to the efficacy of anticoagulant therapy. Aspirin or other antiplatelet agents have been prescribed in lieu of anticoagulant therapy, but their efficacy also has not been proven by randomized clinical trials. Stroke and TIA subtypes were not identified in those studies in which aspirin was compared to placebo or to another antiplatelet agent for the secondary prevention of recurrent stroke or TIA after a previous minor primary stroke or TIA. One study in which the primary and secondary stroke subtypes were accurately identified was the Warfarin Aspirin Recurrent Stroke Study (WARSS), which compared the efficacy of warfarin to aspirin in secondary stroke prevention. When all of the stroke subtypes were combined, there was no difference in the risk of stroke with warfarin compared to aspirin. When the data for primary individual stroke subtype were analyzed in terms of secondary stroke prevention, there was a trend in favor of anticoagulant therapy for patients with cryptogenic embolism. For patients with symptomatic intracranial stenosis, warfarin was also recently shown in a randomized trial to be no more effective than aspirin in preventing recurrent stroke. However, when there are recurrent cerebrovascular events on antiplatelet agents, which are common in the setting of high-grade intracranial stenosis, our practice is to then consider anticoagula-

tion, as well as to consider whether intracranial angioplasty with stenting should be performed. In addition, we manage carotid or vertebral dissection with warfarin. The INR goal in all of these conditions is 2 to 3. Generally, for dissection, we continue the warfarin for 6 months; then if ultrasonographic evidence or noninvasive neuroimaging evidence suggests the arteries are open and symptom-free, we switch to aspirin. If the artery has not healed, then one must consider whether to continue warfarin for a period of time and repeat the noninvasive imaging or, at some point, consider switching to aspirin.

Recent studies have compared the efficacy of aspirin to other antiplatelet agents, typically without consideration of the pathophysiologic stroke subtype. Two randomized trials show that the combination of aspirin with sustained release dipyridamole at a dose of 200 mg twice daily (marketed as Aggrenox) confers an absolute risk reduction of 1% to 1.5% per year compared to aspirin alone. This must be balanced against a risk of throbbing headache that led to higher drop out rates in the aspirin plus dipyridamole group. Clopidogrel was shown in a randomized trial to be slightly better than aspirin (0.5% absolute risk reduction per year) in preventing a combined endpoint of stroke, coronary events and peripheral vascular disease; when stroke endpoints alone were considered, the difference was no longer significant. Three large trials have looked at the combination of aspirin and plavix for chronic prevention of cardiovascular diseases and found that the combination has a relatively high rate of bleed complications compared to single agent therapy, without better efficacy. This combination should, therefore, be avoided except in specific circumstances where the benefit is well accepted, such as following arterial stenting.

- *Surgical therapy*: Carotid endarterectomy is the only widespread surgical therapy available in ischemic stroke. Two clinical settings apply, with different criteria: (1) symptomatic disease and (2) asymptomatic disease. The efficacy of carotid endarterectomy for symptomatic disease is high when there is a 70% to 99% stenosis, but modest when there is a 50% to 69% stenosis. Urgent carotid endarterectomy is also discussed in the section on subacute surgical therapies. Precise assessment of the degree of severity of the stenosis and its effect intracranially is extremely helpful when determining the urgency of timing of surgery. In addition, an image through CTA or MRA is also helpful in identifying the pathology not only in the internal carotid artery origin, but also in the arteries distally and in the arteries providing collateral flow. Neither CTA nor MRA can quantify the degree of stenosis when it becomes hemodynamically significant as well as carotid duplex Doppler and transcranial Doppler. There now exist 100% specific criteria noted by transcranial duplex Doppler for identifying such a lesion.

- *Asymptomatic carotid stenosis*: The clinical utility of endarterectomy or stenting for asymptomatic carotid stenosis and which patients should be treated remain controversial. Two large randomized trials have now reported that endarterectomy is superior to medical therapy for prevention of new stroke. Both of these studies enrolled patients with moderate degrees of stenosis, as low as 60%. Naturally, the event rates in the trials were extremely low. Both trials showed similar modest risk reductions in the surgical group, indicating that the surgical benefit, although statistically significant, is marginal.

Because of the relatively small surgical benefit, patient selection and low perioperative complication rates are essential in order to realize a benefit from endarterectomy for asymptomatic lesions. Younger persons accrue more benefit from surgery because of longer life expectancy. Surgery should be avoided in patients with poorly controlled cardiac or pulmonary conditions, and in those with a short life expectancy. We additionally will use information about the degree of stenosis and status of collateral flow. This despite the fact that asymptomatic endarterectomy trials did not find a correlation between the degree of stenosis and the risk of stroke. The low event rates in those trials probably gave too little power to properly identify this relationship, however. By contrast, natural history studies and the modern symptomatic endarterectomy trials point out that symptoms (low-flow transient ischemia or embolic ischemia, transient or permanent) most often occur as a result of internal carotid artery origin stenosis that is severe enough to produce a pressure drop across it. This occurs between 70% and 75% residual lumen diameter reduction or 1.5 mm actual residual lumen diameter. Duplex Doppler assessment of flow at the bifurcation of the common carotid artery and transcranial Doppler assessment of distal internal carotid artery, ophthalmic artery, and middle, anterior, and posterior cerebral artery stem flow can accurately identify such lesions. Confirmation by CTA and/or MRA eliminates the need, except in rare instances, for conventional intra-arterial angiography and its risks.

Our data from transcranial Doppler and duplex ultrasound studies suggest that a stenosis with a residual luminal diameter of 1.5 mm (i.e., 70–75% stenosis) represents the point at which a pressure drop across the stenosis occurs in most patients; that is, the point at which the stenotic lesion at the origin of the internal carotid artery becomes hemodynamically important. When the stenosis has hemodynamic consequences, the collateral flow through the ophthalmic artery or through the circle of Willis is called into play. If collateral flow is not adequate, low-flow TIAs and infarcts develop. If collateral flow is adequate, patients should remain free of low-flow symptoms (TIA or stroke).

Our concern is that reduced flow in the internal carotid artery, supplemented by good collateral flow distally, may promote the formation of thrombi at the origin of the internal carotid artery; such thrombi may embolize or propagate distally to cause sudden stroke. We, therefore, recommend surgery for asymptomatic patients whose lesions have progressed to this point, that is, those with stenosis of 70% to 75% or more. We identify such lesions on the basis of our 100%-specific criteria for hemodynamic importance, based on duplex and transcranial Doppler ultrasonography, combined with MRA or CTA. Because of the absence of clinical trials that have definitively assessed the surgical benefit for varying degree of stenosis, with adequate statistical power, we feel that this approach is warranted.

- *Carotid artery stenting compared to carotid artery surgery*: Transfemoral angiography with endovascular angioplasty and stenting of internal carotid artery plaque is emerging as an alternative to carotid endarterectomy. Stenting is attractive because it is associated with shorter hospital stay, allows avoidance of general anesthesia, and is not associated with the cranial nerve injury complications that sometimes complicate endarterectomy. A significant concern, however, is the risk of distal embolization of thrombus or fragments of atheroma dislodged during either arterial access, balloon inflation, or stent deployment. An evolving array of embolization protection devices, deployed distal to the stent, is designed to limit this risk.

Three randomized trials have recently addressed whether stenting can produce results as good as endarterectomy. All of the trials used a noninferiority design, that is, that stenting is not worse than endarterectomy. Two trials, Endarterectomy versus Angioplasty in Patients with Symptomatic Severe Carotid Stenosis (EVA-3S) and Stent-Supported Percutaneous Angioplasty of the Carotid Artery versus Endarterectomy (SPACE), showed that, in patients with symptomatic >60% internal carotid artery stenosis, stenting was worse than endarterectomy with regard to 30-day rates of major complications such as stroke and myocardial infarction. By contrast the Stenting and Angioplasty with Protection in Patients at High Risk for Endarterectomy (SAPPHIRE) trial, which included only patients who were deemed poor operative candidates for endarterectomy, showed equivalency between stenting and endarterectomy, with slightly lower complication rates in the stenting group. Long-term outcomes are not yet available from any of the trials.

At this time we do not see any clinical situation in which carotid stenting is clearly superior to endarterectomy. For symptomatic lesions that are poorly amenable to surgery, because of poor anatomical factors or medical comorbidities, stenting is a reasonable, possibly safer, alternative. Patients with asymptomatic stenosis and complex, difficult to treat lesions, or severe medical comorbidities, should have neither stenting nor surgery, based on the high periprocedural complication rates from the SAPPHIRE trial. There is a need for additional trials in symptomatic patients that incorporate the newer generation embolization protection devices, which were mostly not used in the EVA-3S and SPACE trials. Additionally, information on long-term stroke risk by stroke subtype, and the risk of in-stent restenosis, is needed before the role of carotid stenting in routine clinical practice can be fully defined. Until that information is available, good surgical candidates should be treated with endarterectomy, rather than stenting, except in the context of clinical trials.

Treatment and Prevention of Complications of Stroke

Common medical complications of stroke include aspiration pneumonia, deep venous thrombosis, and pulmonary embolism. When in-dwelling bladder catheters are used, then urinary tract infection is an additional concern. All stroke patients with evidence of dysarthria, aphasia, cough, or aspiration should have a formal evaluation of swallowing before being allowed to take food, liquid, or medicines by mouth. Some patients may require placement of a percutaneous gastrostomy feeding tube, which, in most cases, can be removed in 1 to 2 months when the ability to swallow improves. Deep venous thrombosis can be prevented by the administration of subcutaneous heparin or the use of pneumatic compression boots, followed by ambulation as soon as possible.

Patients with stroke-related disability should be evaluated by specialists in physical therapy, occupational therapy, or speech therapy as appropriate. A substantial number of patients may benefit from inpatient rehabilitation following the acute hospital stay. There is evidence from observational studies that patients treated in dedicated stroke units, with experienced physician, nursing and rehabilitation staff, have better outcomes than patients treated in general medical or surgical wards.

Stroke recovery may require 6 months to a year, or even longer, because of the slow nature of neuroplastic changes following brain injury. Late complications of stroke include spasticity, contracture, pressure ulcers, shoulder joint dislocation, and depression. The injection of botulinum toxin in affected muscles has been shown to improve symptoms of stroke-related spasticity.

INTRACRANIAL HEMORRHAGE

Intracranial hemorrhages are classified according to site of origin. The diagnosis, treatment, and secondary prevention of intracranial hemorrhage depend on the assessment of the underlying specific pathophysiology, analogous to the way in which ischemic stroke diagnosis and treatment depend on identifying the ischemic stroke subtype. There are four locations of origin: intracerebral, subarachnoid, subdural, and epidural. Subdural and epidural hemorrhages are predominantly traumatic and not related to an acute vascular event, and are not considered a form of hemorrhagic stroke. This section will therefore be concerned with intracerebral hemorrhage (ICH) and subarachnoid hemorrhage. ICH may be further divided by location into lobar ICH (arising in the cortex or at the junction of the cortex and the white matter) and deep ICH (arising in the deep hemispheric portions of the brain, including the basal ganglia, thalamus, brainstem, and cerebellum).

Intracerebral Hemorrhage

Deep Hemispheric Hemorrhage

Hypertension is by far the major cause of hemorrhages in deep brain locations. The favored sites are (1) the putamen and adjacent internal capsule, (2) the thalamus, (3) the pons, and (4) the cerebellum. A penetrating artery arising from the middle cerebral stem, basilar artery, or circle of Willis is generally the source of the hemorrhage. These same vessels are also frequently affected by lipohyalinosis and, when occlusion occurs rather than rupture, give rise to lacunar infarction.

Recently, a single family has been reported with a mutation in the *COL4A1* gene, encoding for type IV collagen α1, and deep ICH not associated with hypertension. Other features of this disease include migraine with aura, retinal arteriolar tortuosity with retinal hemorrhage, and infantile hemiparesis.

Each of the four sites of ICH produces a characteristic clinical syndrome. For *putaminal hemorrhage*, the eyes are deviated conjugately to the side of the hemorrhage and there is a contralateral hemiplegia. Stupor is evident at the onset in most cases. *Thalamic hemorrhage* has a similar clinical state unless the mass effect is directed downward; in that case, the eyes deviate downward and inward. Unequal pupils and skewed deviation with the eye on the side opposite the hemorrhage being displaced inferiorly and medially is also seen. *Pontine hemorrhage* produces deep coma, quadriplegia, decerebrate rigidity, and impairment of horizontal eye movements with pinpoint pupils. *Cerebellar* hemorrhage presents with vomiting and instability of gait; these may be the only signs. However, forced deviation of the eyes to the opposite side or ipsilateral sixth nerve palsy may be noted. Less frequent ocular signs include blepharospasm, involuntary closure of one eye, and skew deviation. Dysarthria may also occur. Babinski signs and bifacial weakness occur late. Hemiparesis or hemiplegia is not part of the clinical picture until coma has set in from increased pressure in the posterior fossa.

CT scan has excellent sensitivity for ICH and is the mainstay of diagnosis. There are no clinical signs or symptoms specific for ischemic stroke compared to hemorrhagic stroke, making CT mandatory in all cases. CT angiography, MRA, or conventional angiography can exclude the presence of an associated arteriovenous malformation, and T2-weighted MRI can detect the classical "popcorn" appearance of cavernous malformation. Older patients with a history of hypertension and hemorrhages in a typical location do not need angiographic assessment. Younger patients and those with an atypical appearing hemorrhage should, by contrast, have angiography. Hemorrhages in the basal ganglia that are contiguous, inferiorly, with the subarachnoid space should be investigated with angiography to exclude the presence of a middle cerebral artery bifurcation aneurysm. When hemorrhages occur in atypical locations or in the absence of a history of hypertension, our practice is to also obtain an MRI in 3 to 6 months, following ICH resorption, to screen for an underlying lesion such as a vascular malformation or tumor. Additional acute laboratory assessment should include platelet count, prothrombin time, and partial thromboplastin time. The history, physical examination, and imaging should exclude secondary causes of hemorrhage such as coagulopathy, brain tumor, aneurysm rupture, and hemorrhagic transformation of ischemic infarction.

The size and location of the hematoma determine the treatment and prognosis. Supratentorial hematomas >5 cm in diameter have a poor prognosis. Infratentorial hematomas >3 cm in size are generally fatal if they are in the pons. Other factors associated with poor prognosis are the presence of intraventricular blood and worse level of consciousness at presentation.

For cerebellar hemorrhages, neurosurgical consultation is essential because early hematoma evacuation can be life saving. In general, hemorrhages larger than 3 cm in diameter, and smaller hematomas associated with depressed consciousness or brainstem signs (other than nystagmus or ataxia), should be surgically evacuated. For other locations, surgical evacuation is controversial. The Surgical Trial for Intracerebral Hemorrhage (STICH) trial failed to find a benefit for surgical evacuation over medical management. Even so, we consider surgical evacuation or hemicraniectomy for nondominant hemisphere deep ICH accompanied by decreasing level of consciousness caused by increasing mass effect.

General supportive care should be provided. Accumulation of cerebral edema can be problematic by causing raised intracranial pressure (ICP). Osmotic agents including mannitol can be used to lower ICP, but are generally considered temporizing therapy, gaining time while preparing for surgery. Obstructive or communicating hydrocephalus should be treated by external ventricular drainage of cerebrospinal fluid followed, if necessary, by insertion of a permanent ventricular drainage shunt. Seizures may occur and, if the patient is at risk of deterioration from raised ICP, our practice is to administer preventative anticonvulsants, although this practice has not been evaluated in controlled trials.

Lobar Hemorrhage

Lobar hemorrhages occur spontaneously in the supratentorial white matter and cerebral cortex of all lobes of the brain. The manifestations are dependent on the area of white matter and cortex that are involved. Headache is sometimes present and may be most severe near the location of the hemorrhage. If the hemorrhage is large, then depressed consciousness may be present. The symptoms usually evolve over minutes or hours, in contrast to embolic ischemic stroke where the onset of symptoms is abrupt. A precise cause of lobar ICH is found in a significant number of cases: amyloid angiopathy and vascular malformations are the most common; metastatic disease is less frequent, but well known. Some proportion of lobar ICH are likely caused by hypertension. Lobar ICH is more readily accessible for surgical evacuation because of their superficial location. A subgroup analysis of the STICH trial showed a benefit for surgery, compared to initial conservative management, for ICH <1 cm from the cortical surface. At our institution, we consider, on an individual basis, surgical evacuation for nonmoribund lobar ICH patients who are deteriorating from mass effect caused by hematoma expansion or the accumulation of perihematomal edema.

Cerebral Amyloid Angiopathy. A cause of both single and recurrent lobar hemorrhages in the elderly population, amyloid angiopathy is diagnosed conclusively only by postmortem demonstration of amyloid in the media of cortical and leptomeningeal arterioles and capillaries. But the clinical history of repeated supratentorial lobar hemorrhages and the demonstration of small, 1- to 2-mm areas of hypointensity on MRI susceptibility pulse sequences, indicative of prior small asymptomatic hemorrhages, strongly suggest the diagnosis. These small, silent hemorrhages may be the cause of recurrent focal symptoms sometimes seen in these patients. A clinical–pathological correlation study suggests that cerebral amyloid angiopathy is the cause of approximately 70% of primary lobar ICH in persons aged >55 years. Sporadic amyloid angiopathy is caused by the deposition of beta-amyloid only in the cerebral arteries, without systemic amyloidosis. Extremely rare mendelian causes of cerebral amyloid angiopathy have been discovered and are caused by mutations in the BRI2 gene or the genes encoding the amyloid precursor protein, cystatin, transthyretin, prion protein, or gelsolin.

Other than avoidance of anticoagulants, treatment options remain elusive. There is a high recurrence rate of 10% to 14% per year in sporadic lobar ICH, mostly caused by cerebral amyloid angiopathy, which is significantly higher than the recurrence rate of 2% to 4% per year observed in survivors of deep ICH. Careful control of associated hypertension, if present, seems prudent.

A small number of cases are associated with vascular or perivascular inflammation that frequently responds to a pulse of steroids, although late relapses may occur. Cerebral amyloid angiopathy-associated inflammation typically presents with cognitive impairment, seizure or focal neurological signs rather than hemorrhagic stroke. Asymmetric white matter and gray matter hyperintensities, often with small silent hemorrhages on susceptibility sequence, are observed on MRI. Biopsy is usually indicated to exclude other causes of vasculitis.

Lobar Hemorrhages Caused by Metastatic Disease. Cerebral metastases, particularly malignant melanoma, may give rise to hemorrhage. Usually, the metastases are multiple and can easily be demonstrated by MRI or CT scanning, both with contrast.

Vascular Malformations

Increasingly recognized with advances in neuroimaging techniques, vascular malformations are classified into four types: venous malformations, capillary telangiectasias, arteriovenous malformations, and cavernous malformations or angioma. Vascular malformations may cause hemorrhage in either deep or lobar locations.

Venous malformations, also known as venous angiomas or developmental venous anomalies, consist of anomalous veins that, while not associated with arterial feeders, nevertheless provide functional venous drainage, and are usually asymptomatic.

Capillary telangiectasias are small, often punctate, lesions composed of small clusters of dilated capillaries with normal intervening parenchyma. Small capillary telangiectasias in basal ganglia areas or in the brainstem are usually asymptomatic (i.e., discovered at autopsy), but may rarely rupture and produce a hematoma.

Arteriovenous malformations and *cavernous malformations* are clinically significant because of their potential for producing hemorrhage and neurologic deficits.

Arteriovenous malformations consist of a tangle of abnormal vessels forming an abnormal communication between the arterial and venous systems. Most are developmental arteriovenous fistulas in which the constituent blood vessels enlarge and grow with the passage of time. They vary in size from a small blemish a few millimeters in diameter to a huge mass of tortuous channels composing an arteriovenous shunt of sufficient magnitude to raise the cardiac output. Hypertrophic dilated arterial "feeders" approach the main lesion and then disappear into a network of thin-walled blood vessels, which are the source of rupture. Some (perhaps 10%) may harbor berry aneurysms. Arteriovenous malformations occur in all parts of the brain, brainstem, and spinal cord, but larger ones are most frequently located in the hemispheres.

The chief clinical symptoms and signs are headache, seizures, and findings associated with rupture. When headache occurs (without bleeding), it may be hemicranial and throbbing, like migraine, or diffuse. A hemiplegia may accompany a headache, resembling the syndrome of hemiplegic migraine. Focal seizures that become generalized occur in approximately 30% of cases and are sometimes difficult to control with antiepileptic drugs. In half of the cases, arteriovenous malformations manifest with an ICH. In most of these cases, the hemorrhage is mainly intraparenchymal with a small amount of spillage into the subarachnoid space. Blood is usually not deposited in the basal cisterns, thus symptomatic vasospasm is rare. When the hemorrhage occurs, it may be large leading to death or small, giving rise to focal symptoms. Large supratentorial arteriovenous malformations may be associated with an audible bruit. The bruit is sometimes even self-audible, particularly when the malformation involves the dural vessels (also called arteriovenous dural fistula). Headache at the onset of the rupture is common, and it may be difficult to distinguish it from the headache present in nonruptured arteriovenous malformations.

Cavernous malformations represent approximately 10% of all intracranial vascular malformations. Located within the brain parenchyma, without site of predilection, they are composed of thin-walled, dilated vessels, like a mulberry, devoid of intervening normal brain, and often surrounded by a ring of hemosiderin, a residuum of prior hemorrhages. Cavernous malformations may be multiple in as many as 3.6% of patients; in some families, multiple cavernous malformations are inherited as an autosomal dominant trait. Three gene loci have recently been identified: CCM1 (caused by mutation of the *Krit1* gene), CCM2 (caused by mutations of the *Malcavernin* gene), and CCM3 (caused by mutations of the *PDCD10* gene).

The symptoms of cavernous malformations are similar to those of arteriovenous malformations: seizures, headaches, or neurologic deficits associated with rupture. Hemorrhages are usually small and circumscribed, but on occasion can be quite large, or clinically devastating because of their critical location, for example, in the pons. The reported risk of symptomatic hemorrhage varies widely across studies, from as low as 1% per year to as high as 20% per year. The hemorrhages are typically less disabling than primary ICH but, when there are multiple recurrences, are often associated with progressive neurological disability.

The management of patients with vascular malformations is best accomplished by an experienced team approach consisting of neurosurgeons and physicians who can consider both surgical and endovascular approaches, sometimes in combination. Radiosurgical obliteration may also be an option in some cases (i.e., deep, inaccessible lesions associated with repeated hemorrhages or progressive neurologic deficits). Each case requires a unique approach that takes into account the extent and location of the vascular malformation, and the feasibility and safety of the various therapeutic approaches.

Subarachnoid Hemorrhage

By far the most common cause of atraumatic subarachnoid hemorrhage is rupture of a berry aneurysm. Other less common causes include blood dyscrasia or leukemia, tumors (such as ependymoma or meningioma, glioblastoma, renal cell, or metastasis), peripheral vascular malformation or, rarely, venous sinus disease or meningitis.

Ruptured saccular "berry" aneurysms occur at the branch points of the arteries at the base of the brain and, following rupture, give rise to subarachnoid hemorrhage, or sometimes ICH. Histological examination shows interruption of the internal elastic lamina with an aneurysmal outpouching that appears like a berry. Although they are usually single, they can be multiple in 15% to 20% of cases. The most common sites are the anterior communicating artery, the junction of the posterior communicating artery with the internal carotid artery, the middle cerebral stem bifurcation, the top of the basilar artery bifurcation, the origin of the major branches of the basilar artery, and at the origin of the PICA. Intracranial aneurysms can be associated with coarctation of the aorta and are more common in autosomal domination polycystic kidney disease.

Prodromal symptoms and signs, prior to rupture, occur in as many as a third of cases. These symptoms may include headache, diplopia, or blurred vision. Pinpoint pain behind the eye with or without a third nerve palsy is the most common and indicates the presence of an aneurysm at the posterior communicating artery–internal carotid artery junction. It represents a medical emergency. Juxtaclinoid aneurysms compress the optic nerve, leading to amblyopia. Supraclinoid aneurysms can be confused with suprasellar tumors, sometimes producing a hypothalamic syndrome. Aneurysms in the vertebrobasilar system can produce occipital headaches and cerebellar or long-tract signs as well as cranial nerve deficits.

Once rupture occurs, the clinical syndromes are best divided into the *hemorrhage onset syndrome* and the *delayed onset syndrome*. *The hemorrhage onset syndrome* consists of a sudden, severe headache with or without loss of consciousness. Nausea and vomiting invariably occur on awakening. If the hemorrhage ruptures into the brain substance, stupor and focal signs appear that relate to the site of the rupture. Anterior communicating artery aneurysmal rupture produces a quiet, slowed or retarded abulic state with a crural paresis, or hemiplegia predominating in the leg, while middle cerebral bifurcation aneurysms rupture into the brain substance and often produce a faciobrachial hemiparesis, with aphasia if the dominant hemisphere is involved. *Delayed clinical syndromes* mainly consist of re-rupture syndromes, hydrocephalus, and the syndromes resulting from cerebral vasospasm. *Re-rupture* is most frequent during the first 72 hours after the initial rupture. Early surgical intervention or intra-arterial obliteration now precludes many re-ruptures. *Fever* (≥38°C) in the absence of a discernible infective etiology is common in subarachnoid hemorrhage, and in some instances, may be confused with a florid meningitis. *Hydrocephalus* may be acute in the first day or two after the subarachnoid hemorrhage and might require ventricular drainage. Delayed hydrocephalus presents several days to weeks after the subarachnoid hemorrhage and may require ventriculoperitoneal shunting. Worsening stupor is a sign of both early and delayed hydrocephalus. *Cerebral vasospasm* usually develops between days 4 and 14 following the subarachnoid hemorrhage. Its location and severity have been related to the extent and location of the subarachnoid blood, with thick clot typically present around the artery developing spasm. In 30% of cases, the spasm is severe enough to give rise to ischemic symptoms and infarction may ensue. In middle cerebral stem spasm, the resulting infarction may cause devastating edema. The extent and location of blood in the basal cisterns, postoperatively, may suggest the patients who will have severe enough vasospasm to develop signs of ischemia or infarction.

Management of the patient with subarachnoid hemorrhage from a ruptured berry aneurysm should focus on: (1) medical stabilization, with aggressive treatment of elevated blood pressure and good supportive neurocritical care; (2) early operation or endovascular coiling, in nonmoribund patients, to prevent re-re-rupture; and (3) prevention and treatment of delayed ischemia caused by vasospasm. The International Subarachnoid Aneurysm Trial (ISAT) showed that, for aneurysms equally accessible for surgical clipping or endovascular treatment with detachable coils, the endovascular strategy was associated with less death or dependency at 1 year. Volume expansion and blood pressure elevation together with calcium channel-blockers are often used to prevent symptomatic ischemia from vasospasm. Oral nimodipine, 60 mg given every 4 hours, has been shown in multiple clinical trials to reduce mortality and the incidence of delayed ischemia. For refractory cases local intra-arterial infusion of vasodilators such as nicardipine, or angioplasty of the affected arteries, may alleviate arterial stenosis caused by vasospasm.

Because of the above complications and the highly technical neurosurgical and endovascular approaches that are available for obliterating the aneurysm, as well as the specialized neurointensive care required, the patient should be managed in a center capable of carrying out these maneuvers.

FURTHER READING

Amarenco P, Bogousslavsky J, Callahan A, et al. High-dose atorvastatin after stroke or transient ischemic attack. *N Engl J Med.* 2006;355(6):549–559.

Atrial Fibrillation Investigators. Risk factors for stroke and efficacy of antithrombotic therapy in atrial fibrillation. Analysis of pooled data from five randomized controlled trials. *Arch Intern Med.* 1994;154(13):1449–1457.

Barnett HJ, Taylor DW, Eliasziw M, et al. Benefit of carotid endarterectomy in patients with symptomatic moderate or severe stenosis. North American Symptomatic Carotid Endarterectomy Trial Collaborators. *N Engl J Med.* 1998;339(20):1415–1425.

Boston Area Anticoagulation Trial for Atrial Fibrillation Investigators. The effect of low-dose warfarin on the risk of stroke in patients with nonrheumatic atrial fibrillation. *N Engl J Med.* 1990;323(22):1505–1511.

Brott T, Bogousslavsky J. Treatment of acute ischemic stroke. *N Engl J Med.* 2000;343(10):710–722.

Brott TG, Brown RD Jr, Meyer FB, Miller DA, Cloft HJ, Sullivan TM. Carotid revascularization for prevention of stroke: carotid endarterectomy and carotid artery stenting. *Mayo Clin Proc.* 2004;79:1197–1208.

Can U, Furie KL, Suwanwela N, et al. Transcranial Doppler ultrasound criteria for hemodynamically significant internal carotid artery stenosis based on residual lumen diameter calculated from en bloc endarterectomy specimens. *Stroke.* 1997;28(10):1966–1971.

Choi JH, Mohr JP. Brain arteriovenous malformations in adults. *Lancet Neurol.* 2005;4(5):299–308.

Einhaupl KM, Villringer A, Meister W, et al. Heparin treatment in sinus venous thrombosis. *Lancet.* 1991;338(8767):597–600.

Fisher CM. Lacunar strokes and infarcts: a review. *Neurology.* 1982;32(8):871–876.

Furlan A, Higashida R, Wechsler L, et al. Intra-arterial prourokinase for acute ischemic stroke. The PROACT II study: a randomized controlled trial. Prolyse in Acute Cerebral Thromboembolism. *JAMA.* 1999;282(21):2003–2011.

Halkes PH, van Gijn J, Kappelle LJ, Koudstaal PJ, Algra A. Aspirin plus dipyridamole versus aspirin alone after cerebral ischaemia of arterial origin (ESPRIT): randomised controlled trial. *Lancet.* 2006;367(9523):1665–1673.

Kern R, Ringleb PA, Hacke W, Mas JL, Hennerici MG. Stenting for carotid artery stenosis. *Nat Clin Pract Neurol.* 2007;3:212–220.

Kistler JP. Cerebral embolism. *Compr Ther.* 1996;22(8):515–530.

Kistler JP. Strategic location of large-vessel atherothrombotic cerebral vascular disease. *Arch Neurol.* 1999;56(11):1329–1330.

Mas JL, Arquizan C, Lamy C, et al. Recurrent cerebrovascular events associated with patent foramen ovale, atrial septal aneurysm, or both. *N Engl J Med.* 2001;345(24):1740–1746.

Mohr JP, Thompson JL, Lazar RM, et al. A comparison of warfarin and aspirin for the prevention of recurrent ischemic stroke. *N Engl J Med.* 2001;345(20):1444–1451.

National Institute of Neurological Disorders and Stroke rt-PA Stroke Study Group. Tissue plasminogen activator for acute ischemic stroke. *N Engl J Med.* 1995;333:1581–1587.

Qureshi AI, Tuhrim S, Broderick JP, Batjer HH, Hondo H, Hanley DF. Spontaneous intracerebral hemorrhage. *N Engl J Med.* 2001;344:1450–1460.

Suwanwela N, Can U, Furie KL, et al. Carotid Doppler ultrasound criteria for internal carotid artery stenosis based on residual lumen diameter calculated from en bloc carotid endarterectomy specimens. *Stroke.* 1996;27(11):1965–1969.

Dementia Including Alzheimer's Disease

Cynthia M. Carlsson ■ *Carey E. Gleason* ■ *Luigi Puglielli* ■ *Sanjay Asthana*

Alzheimer's disease (AD) is the most common neurodegenerative disorder projected to afflict more than 13 million Americans and 81 million individuals worldwide in the next 40 to 50 years. The disease is characterized by progressive cognitive and behavioral deficits accompanied by diffuse structural abnormalities in the brain. AD is associated with significant morbidity and mortality and is currently among the 10 most common causes of death in the United States. Unfortunately, the devastations of AD affect both the patient and caregivers, and involve numerous aspects of human life including physical, socioeconomic, psychological, functional, and quality of life. In addition, caring for patients with AD places heavy financial burden on patients, families, and the health care system at large. In the United States, the average annual cost of managing a patient with AD varies between $18,400 and $36,000, while, as a nation, we spend close to $100 billion each year to care for patients with AD. Similar data are reported from other countries as well. In the United Kingdom, more than $8 billion or 0.6% of the gross domestic product is spent each year to care for patients with cognitive impairments. Recognizing the enormity of the burden of AD, international collaborations between clinicians, researchers, policy makers, patient advocacy groups, the media, and many others have increased public awareness of the global impact of the disease and have laid the foundation for the development of effective preventive and therapeutic strategies as well as improvements in care management for patients with AD.

Recent advances in biomedical research have provided critical knowledge related to the pathobiology of AD and mechanisms underlying neuronal plasticity and death. While current therapies work mainly to slow the inevitable progression of the disease, these newly identified mechanisms now serve as targets to develop effective novel therapies that could either delay or preferably arrest the progression of AD. Moreover, treatment strategies are being developed for primary prevention of AD, especially for individuals at increased risk for the disease. The present chapter includes information on the major aspects of AD, including the pathology, epidemiology, clinical presentations, diagnosis, management, and potential neuroprotective therapies. Details related to non-Alzheimer types of dementia are discussed in Chapter 67.

GENETICS OF ALZHEIMER'S DISEASE

Alzheimer's disease is characterized by progressive cognitive and behavioral deficits accompanied by diffuse structural abnormalities in the brain. The common symptoms of the disease include memory loss, confusion, impaired judgment, personality changes, disorientation, and loss of language skills. Based on the onset of symptoms, AD is normally divided into two groups: early- (<60 years) and late-onset (>60 years). Early-onset, also called familial AD (FAD), accounts for approximately 3% of all the cases and has to date been linked to mutations in the genes for the amyloid precursor protein (APP; gene name *APP*) on chromosome 21, presenilin 1 (PS1; gene name *PSEN1*) on chromosome 14, and presenilin 2 (PS2; gene name *PSEN2*) on chromosome 1. Among these genes, more than 160 different mutations have so far been identified, accounting for approximately 40% of all cases of FAD. Most of the mutations (~140) are found in the *PSEN1* gene, while the remaining are almost equally split between *APP* and *PSEN2*. FAD is characterized by early onset (from mid 30s to mid 50s) of cognitive symptoms, but is clinically indistinguishable from late-onset AD.

Late-onset AD (LOAD), also called sporadic AD, accounts for close to 97% of all cases of AD and to date has not been linked with any mutations. Aging is the single most important risk factor for LOAD. Additionally, LOAD has been associated with many other environmental and genetic risk factors, including hypercholesterolemia and other vascular risk factors, history of head trauma, and low educational attainment. Among the genetic risk factors, the $\varepsilon 4$ allele of the apolipoprotein E (*APOE*) gene on chromosome 19 is the only polymorphism consistently found associated with LOAD in both case–control and genetic studies. The *APOE* gene exists as three major alleles ($\varepsilon2$, $\varepsilon3$, and $\varepsilon4$) that encode three different ApoE isoforms: ApoE2, ApoE3, and ApoE4. Interestingly, these isoforms only differ in amino acid sequences either at position 112 and/or 158: E2 (cysteine 112, cysteine 158), E3 (cysteine 112, arginine 158), and E4 (arginine 112, arginine 158). The inheritance of the $\varepsilon4$ allele confers a major risk for developing AD, while the $\varepsilon2$ allele confers protection. For example, presence of one copy of the $\varepsilon4$ allele increases risk of AD by fourfold, whereas inheritance of two copies enhances the risk by almost ninefold. However, unlike genetic mutations associated with FAD, the presence of *APOE4* (or other polymorphisms) is neither necessary nor sufficient to cause AD. Even though the first report of an association between *APOE4* and AD was published over a decade ago, the precise molecular mechanism(s) underlying this association still remain elusive. It is currently unknown if the *APOE4* allele influences the rate of production, clearance, or aggregation of amyloid β-peptide or whether it influences cholesterol metabolism and inflammation that reportedly play a major role in the pathobiology of AD.

In addition to *APOE4*, more than 40 other polymorphisms have been associated with increased risk for LOAD. However, none of these associations has been uniformly confirmed in every population-group studied to date.

NEUROPATHOLOGY OF ALZHEIMER'S DISEASE

The neuropathological hallmarks of AD include amyloid plaques, neurofibrillary tangles, and amyloid angiopathy accompanied by diffuse loss of neurons and synapses in the neocortex, hippocampus, and other subcortical regions of the brain (Figure 65-1). The predominance of the amyloid plaques versus neurofibrillary tangles or

amyloid angiopathy can differ from one patient to another. However, the neuronal/synaptic loss is a constant feature and eventually the direct cause of dementia. Interestingly, the distribution of the disease pathology seems to follow a region-specific pattern with the amyloid plaques more prevalent in the neocortex and the neuronal/synaptic loss more prevalent in the hippocampus, posterior cingulate, and corpus callosum areas of the brain closely involved with memory formation and higher cortical activities. The amyloid angiopathy is often observed in the "classical" LOAD, but seems to be more prevalent in a small subgroup of FAD (Dutch E693Q and Iowa D694N mutations in the *APP* gene). Finally, AD brains are also characterized by a diffuse and widespread invasion of reactive astrocytes, mostly concentrated in the hippocampus and around areas of neuronal loss; however, this is not specific to AD and can be observed in other neurodegenerative disorders associated with inflammatory and neurotoxic insults.

The dominant component of the plaque core is amyloid β-peptide (Aβ) organized in fibrils of approximately 7 to 10 nm intermixed with nonfibrillar forms of the peptide (Figure 65-1). The most characteristic form of the amyloid plaque, the "neuritic plaque", is characterized by a dense core of aggregated fibrillar Aβ, surrounded by dystrophic dendrites and axons, activated microglia, and reactive astrocytes. In addition, diffuse deposits of Aβ, likely representing a prefibrillary form of the aggregated peptide, are found without any surrounding dystrophic neurites, astrocytes, or microglia. These diffuse plaques can be found in limbic and association cortices, as well as in the cerebellum.

The other neuropathological hallmark of AD is a neurofibrillary tangle (NFT) found exclusively in the cytoplasm of neurons (Figure 65-1). The tangles appear as paired, helically twisted protein filaments composed of highly stable polymers of cytoplasmic

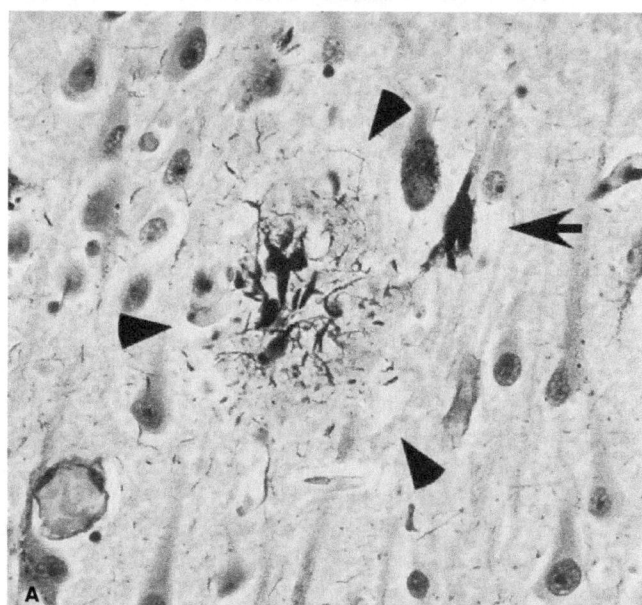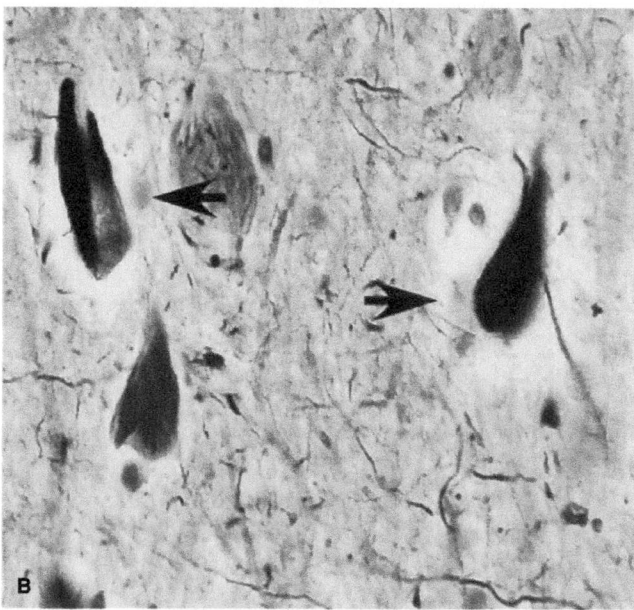

FIGURE 65-1. Small section of the neocortex from a patient with Alzheimer's disease showing two classical neuropathological lesions of the disease. (A) The modified silver staining shows one dense senile (amyloid) plaque indicated by three arrowheads. The plaque consists of aggregated extracellular deposits of Aβ fragments surrounded by silver-positive dystrophic neuritis. The arrow indicates a neuron containing neurofibrillary tangles, which appear as dark masses of abnormal filaments occupying most of the cytoplasm. (B) The image shows higher magnification of two neurons containing neurofibrillary tangles (indicated by arrows). *(Photograph courtesy of Shahriar Salamat, MD, PhD, University of Wisconsin School of Medicine and Public Health, Department of Pathology and Laboratory Medicine.)*

proteins called tau. Tau comprises a group of alternatively spliced proteins found in the cytoplasm that possess either three or four microtubule-binding domains and can assemble with tubulin, thus helping the formation of cross bridges between adjacent microtubules. Tau proteins can be phosphorylated in multiple sites and the degree of phosphorylation is inversely correlated with binding to microtubules. As a result, highly phosphorylated tau proteins dissociate from microtubules and polymerize into filaments forming NFTs. In addition to AD, the abnormal accumulation of filamentous tau is observed in frontotemporal forms of dementia, progressive supranuclear palsy, corticobasal degeneration, and Pick disease. Contrary to prior belief, tau proteins themselves can cause dementia, and multiple mutations in the *tau* gene have been found in frontotemporal dementia with parkinsonism. The possible role of tau proteins in the pathogenesis of AD and their potential interaction with Aβ are still unclear and are discussed in the section below.

PATHOBIOLOGY OF ALZHEIMER'S DISEASE

Amyloid Precursor Protein Processing and Generation of Aβ

Aβ is a 39 to 43 amino acid hydrophobic peptide proteolytically released from a much larger precursor, the amyloid precursor protein (APP). The generation of Aβ from APP (Figure 65-2) requires the sequential recruitment of two enzymatic activities: β-secretase, also called BACE1 (beta-site APP cleaving enzyme 1), and γ-secretase, a multimeric protein complex containing presenilin, nicastrin, Aph-1, Pen-2, and CD147. The β cleavage is the rate-limiting step and occurs before the γ cleavage. It liberates a large N-terminal fragment of the protein (sβAPP) that is released in the extracellular milieu and a small (~12 kDa) membrane-anchored fragment called β-APP-CTF (or C99). The release of the large N-terminal domain allows subsequent γ cleavage, and liberation of Aβ and the signaling of active intracellular domain of APP (Figure 65-2). Generation of Aβ40 and Aβ42 results from γ cleavage of Aβ at positions 40 and 42, respectively. The release of Aβ in the extracellular milieu is followed by oligomerization and aggregation in the form of fibrils and amyloid plaques. Additionally, small Aβ aggregates are also found in the soma of the neurons suggesting that the Aβ fragments can escape secretion and aggregate in the intracellular environment.

The molecular mechanisms underlying the toxicity of Aβ are still being investigated and currently incompletely understood. However, recent research seems to indicate that small Aβ aggregates (oligomers), which represent the "preplaque" neurotoxic species of Aβ, act as the proximate cause of neuronal injury and synaptic loss associated with AD. Additionally, the C-terminal tail of APP can undergo further processing at amino acid 664 of APP695 liberating two small cytosolic fragments, Jcasp (from aa. 649 to 664 of APP695) and C31 (containing the last 31 amino acids of the C-terminus of APP, from aa. 665 to 695). Both these fragments are generated only after γ cleavage, require caspase-mediated processing of APP, and can activate proapoptotic pathways in a variety of cellular systems.

It is widely known that, although the major source of Aβ, APP exerts several important functions in the nervous system. APP com-

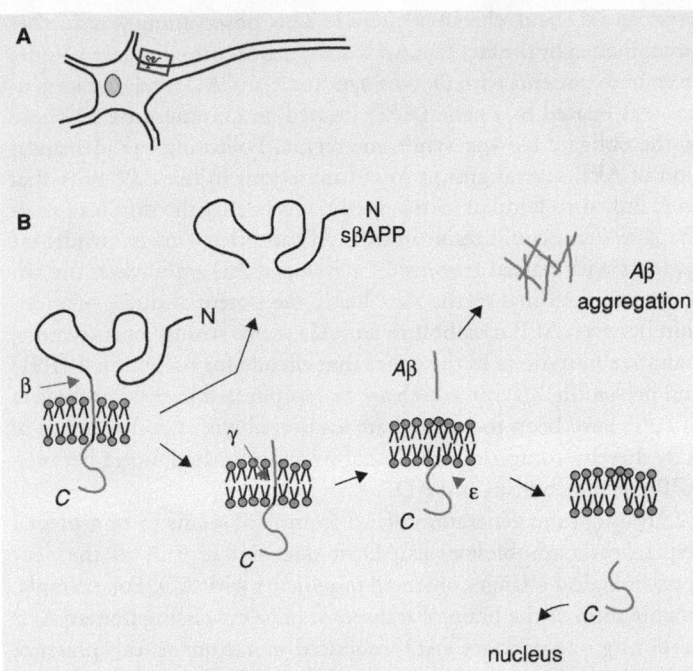

FIGURE 65-2. Generation of amyloid β-peptide (Aβ) from amyloid precursor protein (APP). APP is a type 1 membrane protein with a large extracellular domain, a single membrane-spanning domain, and a short cytoplasmic tail. The Aβ region of APP (in yellow) includes the first 12 to 14 amino acids of the membrane domain. (A) Shows a schematic image of APP on the cell-surface of a neuron, whereas (B) provides a closer view of APP processing. The initial enzymatic step for the generation of Aβ requires proteolysis of APP at β site (amino acid 1 of the Aβ region). This event liberates a large N-terminal fragment (sβAPP) that is rapidly secreted into the extracellular *milieu* and a small C-terminal fragment (β-APP-CTF) of 99 amino acids (also called C99). The removal of sβAPP most likely induces a conformational change that allows subsequent cleavage by γ-secretase. Once generated, the Aβ peptides aggregate in the brain in the form of plaques. Further cleavage of β-APP-CTF at the site liberates the signaling active APP intracellular domain (AICD). In addition to the above β/γ pathway, APP can also be cleaved at the α site (between amino acids 16 and 17 of the Aβ region) precluding the generation of Aβ.

prises a group of ubiquitously expressed proteins that are generated from one single gene by differential splicing, resulting in three major isoforms of 695, 751, and 770 residues. The first isoform (APP695) is highly abundant in neurons and differs from the others in the absence of a 56-amino-acid domain that is homologous to the Kunitz-type of serine protease inhibitors. Among others, some of the important proposed normal functions of APP include serving as a cell-surface receptor, growth factor, protease inhibitor, cell–cell interaction molecule, coreceptor/partner in the endocytic/lysosomal network, coagulation inhibitor factor, cell-surface scaffold protein, kinesin-interacting molecule for axonal transport, and transcription factor.

Aβ: Pivotal Role in the Pathogenesis of Alzheimer's Disease

The most critical clinical link between Aβ and AD came from the observation that patients with Downs' syndrome (trisomy 21) had a higher propensity of developing a clinical and pathological phenotype resembling AD, thereby suggesting a potential association between AD and chromosome 21. This observation was further strengthened by the fact that Aβ was the major component in plaques from both patients with Downs' syndrome and AD, and that its genesis was related to a gene (*APP*) located on chromosome 21, close to the obligate Downs' syndrome region. Following the identification of APP, several groups found mutations in the *APP* gene that were linked to familial forms of AD. Given that the duplication of the *APP* locus could result in early AD and that Downs' syndrome patients with partial trisomy 21 developed AD only when the trisomy was proximal to the *APP* locus, the potential direct relationship between APP metabolism and AD seems strong. Furthermore, causative mutations in the genes that encode for presenilin 1 (PS1) and presenilin 2 (PS2), which are also implicated in the metabolism of APP, have been found and are associated with familial forms of AD, thereby conferring additional strength to the linkage between APP/Aβ metabolism and AD.

Although the generation of Aβ from APP seems to be a pivotal step in the pathobiology of AD, it does not explain all the neuropathological changes observed in patients with AD. For example, examination of the brain of transgenic mice expressing human APP harboring one or more FAD-associated mutations reveals presence of amyloid plaques and some synaptic loss and cognitive deficits, but absence of tau pathology and astrocytosis. This suggests that additional biochemical/molecular events are required to develop the full pathological spectrum of AD. To circumvent this issue, several new animal models have been generated where human APP is accompanied by additional genes. These genes include the *presenilins* (harboring FAD-associated mutations), *tau*, and *ApoE*. Recently, several transgenic mice models harboring three or five FAD-associated mutations (respectively called 3X and 5X mice) in two or more genes have been generated. All of these models demonstrated that Aβ is an essential element for the development of AD-like neuropathology and revealed a close relationship between Aβ and the phosphorylation/aggregation state of tau. However, none of the mouse models fully reproduce the classical AD-phenotype; thereby again suggesting that Aβ seems to be necessary but not sufficient to produce the entire spectrum of AD neuropathology.

Transgenic mice expressing the human microtubule-associated protein tau develop the typical tau-related pathology found in individuals suffering from frontotemporal dementia with parkinsonism; however, they do not develop amyloid plaques suggesting that tau is not required for the formation of plaques. Crossing these mice with APP transgenic mice potentiates tau-related pathology and neuronal loss but does not aggravate plaque pathology suggesting that Aβ acts upstream of tau in the classical AD-phenotype. However, studies from patients with AD, mouse models, and ex vivo cellular systems indicate that Aβ and tau can interact synergistically, thereby fostering their respective aggregation and neuronal loss. The true relationship between Aβ and tau is more complex than previously thought and likely involves additional molecular and biochemical pathways acting upstream of both Aβ and tau in the AD brain.

The recent identification of the gene that encodes BACE1, the rate-limiting enzyme in the biosynthesis of Aβ, prompted the generation of "knock-out" mice that lack BACE1. Crossing these mice with the APP mutant mice models revealed that elimination of β cleavage of APP is sufficient to resolve many aspects of AD pathology, including the synaptic impairment and cognitive phenotype of the animals. Moreover, these approaches indicated that BACE1 rep-

resents a viable target for development of effective treatment strategies for AD, given that disruption of BACE1 does not result in a strong phenotype in the mouse. Overall, there is extensive evidence from laboratory research that Aβ plays a major role in the pathogenesis of AD; however, there are likely additional, yet unidentified, molecular pathways that contribute to the overall pathobiology of AD.

EPIDEMIOLOGY AND RISK FACTORS FOR ALZHEIMER'S DISEASE

Alzheimer's disease is the most common cause of dementia in older adults, currently affecting more than five million Americans and more than 24 million individuals around the world. Unless effective preventive strategies are identified, it is anticipated that the prevalence of AD will double every 20 years. Of note, the United Nations predicts that the major rate of increase in the prevalence of AD will likely occur in developing countries like India and China that may not possess all the essential resources, public health support system, or medical expertise to care for patients with AD.

There is clear evidence that a number of risk factors significantly enhance the overall risk for developing AD. These risk factors relate to both genetic and nongenetic markers, and are discussed below.

Aging

Aging is the single most important and validated risk factor for AD. The projected increase in AD prevalence in the coming decades is in part related to recent increases in the average human life span. Almost all of the epidemiological studies indicate that the incidence of AD increases with aging. For example, in the year 2000, the age-specific distribution of patients with AD was 5% between the ages of 65 and 74 years, 18% between the ages of 75 and 84 years, and 45% above the age of 85 years. Additionally, age-associated increases in the amount of amyloid plaques and NFTs in the brains of older persons further underscore a strong relationship between aging and AD pathology. Although not clearly understood, converging findings from recent research provides some clues concerning the potential molecular pathway(s) underlying the association between aging and AD. This pathway acts downstream of the insulin-like growth factor 1 receptor (IGF1-R) and plays a major role in determining both the lifespan and age-associated diseases. In general, activation of IGF1-R signaling accelerates aging and shortens lifespan, while a partial block—as achieved with either genetic or biochemical approaches—delays aging, extends lifespan, and, most importantly, delays the progression of many age-associated diseases, including AD and type 2 diabetes mellitus. Recent biochemical and genetic studies have delineated a precise molecular pathway involving IGF1-R, neurotrophin signaling, BACE1, and APP metabolism, suggesting that pharmacological approaches aimed at IGF1-R signaling might help delay the progression as well as onset of AD.

Aging and IGF1-R signaling are both associated with cerebrovascular dysfunction, which, emerging evidence supports, may play a key role in the development of AD. An increased exposure time to age-dependent vascular risk factors or an interaction between aging and vascular risk factors may in part account for the effects of aging on the pathobiology of AD. Thus, targeting treatment of vascular risk factors may ameliorate some of the age-associated risk for AD.

APOE Genotype

Late-onset AD is the most common form of the disorder, accounting for more than 90% of all AD cases. Although early-onset AD has strong genetic links, many cases of LOAD are seen in individuals without any clear genetic predisposition. A common polymorphism in the apolipoprotein E (*APOE*) gene is the major determinant of risk in families with LOAD. Of the three common allelic forms (*APOE2*, *APOE3*, and *APOE4*), *APOE4* is associated with up to fourfold increased risk of developing AD among individuals with at least one *APOE4* allele. However, *APOE4* genotype is neither necessary nor sufficient for the development of AD. *APOE4* allele may contribute to AD by influencing processes related to the development of AD, including altering the rate of production, clearance, or aggregation of amyloid β-peptide and/or influencing cerebral cholesterol metabolism and inflammation. Currently, routine genetic testing for LOAD is not recommended. Recent estimates based on twin studies suggest that nearly 50% of LOAD cases may be related to *APOE* allele and other unidentified genetic factors.

Gender

Although controversial, there is some evidence that AD is more common among women. Specifically in the population-based studies published to date, more than half reported a greater risk of AD in women, while the others found no difference. It is generally believed that the discrepant findings between various studies are likely owing to several important reasons, including methodological differences and a failure to account for the potential gender-related variability in education, occupation, and lifestyle variables that can directly affect the risk of AD. Some data support that estrogen deficiency following menopause may contribute to the development of AD; however, the effects of estrogen replacement therapy on cognition remains controversial.

Hypercholesterolemia and Vascular Risk Factors

There is mounting evidence that midlife vascular risk factors are associated with an increased risk of AD in later life. In epidemiological studies, hypercholesterolemia, hypertension, hyperhomocysteinemia, obesity, diabetes mellitus, and elevated inflammatory markers have all been associated with enhanced risk of developing AD. Furthermore, *APOE4* allele is related to abnormal cholesterol metabolism suggesting that the increased risk for AD associated with this genotype may be partially mediated through dysregulation of cholesterol. The cholesterol–AD connection is further supported by results from animal studies showing that hypercholesterolemia stimulates the amyloidogenic pathway of APP leading to increased production and deposition of Aβ. Conversely, decreased levels of cholesterol produce the opposite effect reducing the production and deposition of Aβ. Not only do some vascular risk factors appear to influence Aβ metabolism, but conversely, soluble Aβ has been shown to induce dysfunction in cerebral vessels of rats and in cultured endothelial cells. As both Aβ deposition and cerebrovascular dysregulation are two early findings in preclinical AD pathology, these processes most likely work synergistically to accelerate neuronal degeneration. Although the evidence supporting an association between vascular disease and AD is increasing, it is presently unclear whether treating these modifiable vascular risk factors will affect the development or progression of AD. Clinical trials are currently underway to evaluate the potential role of treating these risk factors in preventing or delaying AD progression.

The fact that cerebrovascular diseases such as vascular dementia and cerebral amyloid angiopathy (CAA) share common risk factors with AD supports that their pathologic mechanisms are related. A clear separation between vascular forms of dementia and classical AD based on cognitive impairment is extremely difficult. Typical patients with vascular dementia have a history of vascular disease and show a more pronounced impairment in executive function with only mild memory deficits. The presence of white matter hyperintensities and lacunar infarcts demonstrated by MRI constitutes an important criterion to support the diagnosis of vascular dementia. However, only 2% to 3% of patients with dementia fulfill the diagnostic criteria of pure vascular dementia. In contrast, a large group of patients show an overlapping phenotype with subcortical white matter changes, hypoperfusion, microinfarcts, and amyloid angiopathy. These patients tend to progress into classical AD and will show some degree of amyloid plaques and tau aggregates at autopsy, together with microglia and astrocytic proliferation. CAA is characterized by abnormal accumulation of fibrillar Aβ (especially Aβ40) in the walls of meningeal and cortical arterioles, venules, and capillaries. The damaged vessels undergo spontaneous rupture, and the patients often present with subcortical white matter changes and microhemorrhages. An autosomal dominant form of CAA is caused by a point mutation in the APP gene (Dutch-type) and is a form of FAD. Understanding the overlapping pathologic mechanisms among AD, vascular dementia, and CAA may help to identify common targets for disease-modifying therapies.

Head Trauma

Several epidemiological studies have indicated that a history of severe or repeated head trauma is a risk factor for cognitive decline and AD. The majority of patients develop AD, although a minority might manifest dementia of Parkinson disease and depression. Neuropathological examination of the brain from patients with a history of head trauma generally reveals changes of diffuse amyloid plaques together with tau pathology, inflammatory response, and loss of cholinergic neurons. A smaller number of patients show diffuse α-synuclein reactivity, Lewy body–type aggregates, and loss of dopaminergic neurons resembling Parkinson disease. In animals, pathological changes following experimental head trauma reveal transient upregulation of BACE1 together with increased generation of Aβ. These features are accompanied by tau hyperphosphorylation and increased caspase-mediated cleavage of APP. Thus, head trauma may lead to AD by triggering accelerated neurodegeneration.

Depression

Depression is a common psychiatric condition in the elderly and widely reported to present with symptoms of cognitive and functional impairment, commonly grouped into the clinical entity of *pseudodementia*. Furthermore, more than 30% of patients with AD develop depression during the course of their illness, and might present with the symptoms of depression as the first clinical manifestation of underlying AD. Thus, a better understanding of the potential relationship between depression and AD is of pivotal clinical significance. Although not confirmed universally, there is converging evidence from several studies that a history of depression can increase the risk of AD later in life. Findings of a recent meta-analysis and metaregression analysis involving 20 retrospective and prospective studies supported an increased risk of AD in patients with prior history of depression. The pooled odds ratio for developing AD in this analysis was 2.03 for case–control and 1.90 for cohort studies. To date, the precise mechanism(s) underlying the association between depression and enhanced risk for AD is unknown. However, several potential mechanisms have been proposed, including elevated levels of cytokines observed in both patients with AD and depression, increased association of vascular risk factors with the pathobiology of AD as well as depression, and the potential role of *APOE4* allele in enhanced risk for both AD and depression. Clearly, more research is necessary to better understand the biological basis of increased risk of AD in patients with a history of depression.

Education and Ethnicity

There is some evidence, albeit controversial, from epidemiological studies that higher education may protect against the development of AD. Individuals with elementary level education might be at an increased risk of developing AD, compared to those with high school and college education. Of note, these findings have not been substantiated by all studies and need to be systematically evaluated in larger epidemiological studies. The exact mechanism underlying the neuroprotective effects of higher education is currently unknown; however, based on the "use it or lose it" theory there is suggestion that individuals with higher education might have more neurons to lose before they cross the threshold of developing dementia.

It is generally presumed that AD affects all ethnic groups equally. However, there is some recent evidence that the disease might be more prevalent in certain ethnic groups. In a population based study in the Washington Heights and Inwood communities of New York City, the cumulative incidence of AD was increased twofold among individuals of African-American and Caribbean Hispanic origin. This ethnicity-based incidence of AD did not change following corrections for differences in the number of years of education, or a history of diseases like hypertension, diabetes mellitus, and cardiovascular disease. Although not universally confirmed, other studies also support these findings. In a study in Houston, both the incidence and prevalence of AD were higher among African-Americans and Hispanics than retirees of Caucasian origin. Although speculative, it is possible that the increased risk of AD among the above ethnic groups may be because of a higher incidence of comorbid vascular and cardiovascular diseases and a higher prevalence of *APOE4* genotype.

CLINICAL PRESENTATIONS OF ALZHEIMER'S DISEASE

The most common symptoms of AD include cognitive deficits and functional impairments. These deficits progress over time and eventually result in loss of activities of daily living, frequently necessitating admission to nursing homes and leading to eventual death. The majority of patients with AD initially present with slowly progressive memory impairments; however, in up to 40% patients the initial presentation might involve nonmemory symptoms like lan-guage impairments, symptoms of depression, personality changes, extrapyramidal manifestations, and visuospatial deficits. These patients are very likely to be misdiagnosed and require comprehensive evaluation by a physician with special expertise in dementia.

Typical Clinical Presentation of AD

Slowly progressive memory loss for recent events is the most common clinical presentation of AD. Patients with AD frequently have problems remembering recent conversations, dates, appointments, and may misplace items at home. Many patients are not aware of these deficits and are brought to medical attention by their family members or friends. The memory deficits of AD are generally differentiated from those caused by normal aging by the fact that these deficits are progressive and interfere with daily living activities. Cognitive changes associated with healthy aging, although frustrating, are caused by age-associated decline in mental processing speed and difficulty learning new material. However, these changes are not associated with alterations in day-to-day function. Memory loss leading to a change in functional status is not a part of normal aging and warrants further evaluation.

The second most common clinical presentation of AD is impairment in language function. Seen in up to 40% to 50% patients, these impairments generally start with word-finding problems followed by paraphasic errors and circumlocution. These initial deficits lead to expressive aphasia accompanied later with receptive and global aphasia. Unfortunately, given the impairments in communication, patients with AD having significant language impairments generally progress rapidly and have a poor prognosis.

Impairments in executive function are common early deficits in AD, leading to poor judgment, organization, reasoning and abstract thinking, and resulting in inability to complete complex demanding tasks. Deficits in concentration and attention are other common symptoms seen in patients with AD. These impairments lead to tangential tendencies, disorientation, and an inability to successfully complete daily tasks. Persons exhibiting deficits in visuospatial abilities may have problems with driving, dressing, using eating utensils, and walking.

As the disease progresses, changes in personality are commonly seen in patients with AD and may include increased passivity, lack of interest, restlessness, and overactivity. More than 30% of persons with AD develop symptoms of depression, which may be the first clinical presentation of the disease. Early signs of depression in patients with AD include changes in behavior, loss of appetite, alterations in sleep, social withdrawal, and a decline in physical function. Sundowning, or worsening of behavior and cognitive symptoms in the evening, is also common in patients with AD and may be because of changes in circadian rhythm from loss of sunlight.

In the later stages of the disease, individuals may have increased confusion, dysphagia, poor gait, and repeated falls. In some patients with AD, disruptive behaviors may increase with aggression, agitation, and physical or verbal hostility; in others, these behavioral symptoms lessen with disease progression. The majority of patients become increasingly frail and dependent for self-care and activities of daily living with many patients developing bowel and bladder incontinence. Persons in the late stages of AD may become immobile and bed-bound, which increases their risk of developing pressure sores, malnutrition, and dehydration. The most common causes of death in patients with AD include pneumonia, urinary sepsis, dehydration, pressure sores, fractures, and malnutrition. The median survival period from the time of diagnosis to death generally varies between 8 and 10 years, although some patients, especially those with FAD, die earlier.

Atypical Clinical Presentations of Alzheimer's Disease

It is widely reported that between 20% and 40% of patients with AD will initially present with atypical features of the disease. Unfortunately, these patients are commonly misdiagnosed with either a personality or related disorder, and may need to be evaluated by a specialist. As noted earlier, one of the common atypical presentations of AD is impairment in language. These patients are frequently misdiagnosed as having suffered a stroke. The other atypical presentation of AD includes prominent extrapyramidal manifestations. Between 5% and 10% of patients with AD might initially present with features resembling Parkinson disease, consisting of mild rigidity of extremities, hypokinesia, and expressionless face. However, these patients generally do not present with the classical Parkinsonian tremors and do not respond well to dopaminergic drugs. Another atypical feature of AD, seen in approximately 10% patients with AD, includes symptoms of behavioral disinhibition. These patients may make socially unacceptable remarks, become increasingly difficult to live or work with, and may be misdiagnosed with a personality disorder. Finally, less than 5% patients with AD present with symptoms of Balint syndrome, consisting of visual agnosia and ataxia, and complaints of inability to see.

Overall, it is important to recognize that AD can present itself with varied clinical features, and while memory impairment is a critical component of the disease, it is not the only clinical manifestation. Atypical clinical presentations of AD are common and should be evaluated by a physician with special expertise in dementia. Clearly, a misdiagnosis of AD has major serious adverse consequences including emotional, occupational, social, and financial.

DIAGNOSIS OF ALZHEIMER'S DISEASE

Diagnosis of AD involves a comprehensive medical, psychiatric, and neurological evaluation of a patient with cognitive impairment. To date, there is no clinical, laboratory, genetic, or neuroimaging investigation that can definitively diagnose AD. Thus, the diagnosis of AD is largely based on clinical evaluation. In specialized centers, there is up to 10% to 15% chance that the diagnosis of AD could be incorrect; in a general practice environment, an incorrect diagnosis may be made in approximately 30% to 40% of cases, especially if the initial presentation of disease is atypical. Definitive diagnosis of AD can only be made on neuropathological examination of the brain following death.

While the differential diagnoses for AD are extensive (Table 65-1), in usual practice making a clinical diagnosis of AD involves differentiating whether a patient's memory complaint is related to normal aging, mild cognitive impairment (MCI), delirium, depression, or a true dementia such as AD. Differentiating between these various conditions is critical for identifying whether or not the memory complaint is part of a progressive neurodegenerative disorder and for choosing appropriate treatment strategies. An algorithm for approaching the patient with memory complaints is shown in Figure 65-3, integrating various established diagnostic criteria.

TABLE 65-1

Differential Diagnosis for Alzheimer's Disease

Depression	AIDS (HIV)
Delirium	Chronic meningitis
Dementia with Lewy bodies	Encephalitis
Vascular dementia	Progressive multifocal leukoencephalopathy
Frontotemporal dementia	Neurosyphilis
Progressive supranuclear palsy	Lyme disease
Corticobasilar degeneration	Prion diseases (Creutzfeldt–Jakob disease,
Parkinson disease dementia	bovine spongiform encephalopathy)
Normal pressure hydrocephalus (NPH)	Drugs
	Alcohol
Huntington disease	Heavy metal toxicity
Alcoholic dementia	Hepatic encephalopathy
Binswanger disease	Wilson disease
CADASIL (cerebral autosomal dominant arteriopathy with subcortical infarcts and leukoencephalopathy)	Metabolic–endocrine disorders
	Uremia
	Central nervous system vasculitis
Mass lesions (neoplasms, subdural hematomas)	Nonvasculitic autoimmune inflammatory meningoencephalopathies
Seizures	
Vitamin B-12 deficiency	
Thiamine deficiency	

While a decline in mental processing speed and difficulty learning new material may be seen with normal aging, MCI is considered to be a predementia condition. Seen in up to 15% to 20% of older adults, MCI was originally characterized as a stage of memory impairment beyond normal aging in which other cognitive domains were preserved and daily function remained intact. Original criteria for MCI are outlined in Table 65-2. Findings from several epidemiological studies have indicated that between 12% and 15% of persons each year with MCI will progress to AD or other forms of dementia. MCI criteria have now been expanded to include both patients with memory impairment (amnestic MCI, with single vs. multiple cognitive domains affected) and those in whom memory function is intact, but other cognitive domains are impaired (nonamnestic MCI, single vs. multiple domain). Persons with amnestic MCI are more likely to progress to AD, whereas those with nonamnestic MCI may be more likely to progress to other forms of dementia, such as frontotemporal dementia, dementia with Lewy bodies, or vascular dementia. A history of intact functional status is a critical distinguishing feature between MCI and early AD and requires careful history-taking and collaborative history from family and/or friends.

Delirium is associated with an acute or subacute onset of fluctuating cognitive dysfunction and can be caused by a wide variety of medical conditions and medications. In patients with delirium, a careful history frequently can tease out the temporal relationship between the onset of potentially reversible cognitive symptoms and contributing underlying medical problems or medications. Depression may cause "pseudodementia" by leading to impaired concentration and attention, thus, affecting an individual's ability to attend to tasks on cognitive testing. Dementia is differentiated from the

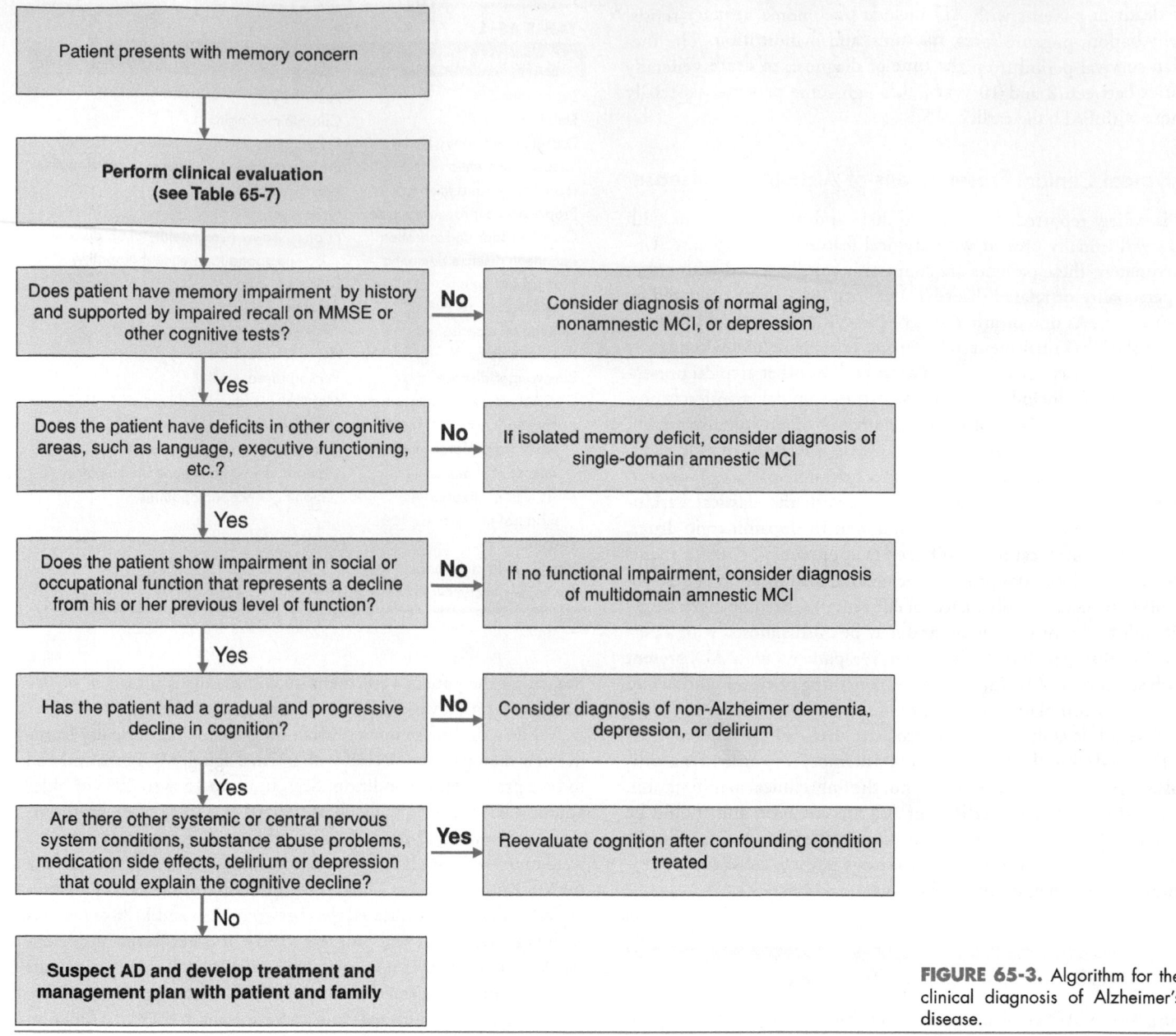

FIGURE 65-3. Algorithm for the clinical diagnosis of Alzheimer's disease.

above-mentioned conditions in that it is a progressive, irreversible process that causes impairment in two or more cognitive domains (such as memory, language, and executive functioning) to the degree that it impairs social or occupational performance. Such changes in cognitive function cannot be attributed to delirium or depres-

TABLE 65-2
Original Criteria for Mild Cognitive Impairment
Memory complaint, qualified by an informant
Memory impairment for age and education
Preserved general cognitive function
Intact social and occupational function
Not demented

Data from Petersen RC, Smith GE, Waring SC, et al. Mild cognitive impairment: clinical characterization and outcome. Arch Neurol. 1999;56(3):303–308.

sion. Diagnostic and Statistical Manual of Mental Disorders, Fourth Edition (DSM-IV) criteria for dementia are listed in Table 65-3. Once a diagnosis of dementia is suspected, the clinician must differentiate between various causes of dementia, discern if it is multifactorial, and decide if there is any reversible component to the cognitive loss that can be addressed.

AD is the most common form of dementia in the United States, accounting for 50% to 90% of all dementia cases. Dementia with Lewy bodies, vascular dementia, and frontotemporal dementia are other common forms of dementia (Table 65-4). Details of the clinical and pathological features of these dementias are covered in Chapter 67. Differentiating AD from other causes of memory loss can help clinicians choose effective therapies, anticipate behavior changes and other potential complications, and provide patients and caregivers information on prognosis. AD is characterized by a gradually progressive decline in memory and other cognitive abilities to the degree that it impairs social or occupational performance. These cognitive

TABLE 65-3

DSM-IV Diagnostic Criteria for Dementia

A. The development of multiple cognitive deficits manifested by both:
1. Memory impairment (impaired ability to learn new information or to recall previously learned information)
2. One (or more) of the following cognitive disturbances:
   a. Aphasia (language disturbance)
   b. Apraxia (impaired ability to carry out motor activities despite intact motor function)
   c. Agnosia (failure to recognize or identify objects despite intact sensory function)
   d. Disturbance in executive functioning (i.e., planning, organizing, sequencing, abstracting)
B. The cognitive deficits in Criteria A1 and A2 each cause significant impairment in social or occupational functioning and represent a decline from a previous level of functioning.
C. The deficits do not occur exclusively during the course of a delirium.

American Psychiatric Association. Task Force on DSM-IV. Diagnostic and Statistical Manual of Mental Disorders: DSM-IV. 4th ed. Washington, DC: American Psychiatric Association; 1994.

deficits must represent a decline from a previous level of functioning. The diagnosis of AD is a clinical diagnosis, with the only "gold standard" being autopsy confirmation. The most widely used diagnostic criteria for the disorder include DSM-IV criteria and the National Institute of Neurological and Communicative Disorders and Stroke–Alzheimer's Disease and Related Disorder Association (NINCDS-ADRDA) criteria (Tables 65-5 and 65-6).

In many cases, a clinical diagnosis of AD can be made in a primary care office setting using a careful history, a focused physical examination, cognitive screening tools, and appropriate laboratory data (Figure 65-3 and Table 65-7). A careful history should include collaborative information from the patient, family, caregivers, and/or friends. A patient's baseline level of functioning may be estimated based on educational background as well as occupational history, including

TABLE 65-5

DSM-IV Diagnostic Criteria for Dementia of the Alzheimer Type

A. The development of multiple cognitive deficits manifested by both:
1. Memory impairment (impaired ability to learn new information or to recall previously learned information)
2. One (or more) of the following cognitive disturbances:
   a. Aphasia (language disturbance)
   b. Apraxia (impaired ability to carry out motor activities despite intact motor function)
   c. Agnosia (failure to recognize or identify objects despite intact sensory function)
   d. Disturbance in executive functioning (i.e., planning, organizing, sequencing, abstracting)
B. The cognitive deficits in Criteria A1 and A2 each cause significant impairment in social or occupational functioning and represent a decline from a previous level of functioning.
C. The course is characterized by gradual onset and continuing cognitive decline.
D. The cognitive deficits in Criteria A1 and A2 are not caused by any of the following:
1. Other central nervous system conditions that cause progressive deficits in memory and cognition (e.g., cerebrovascular disease, Parkinson disease, Huntington disease, subdural hematoma, normal-pressure hydrocephalus, brain tumor)
2. Systemic conditions that are known to cause dementia (e.g., hypothyroidism, vitamin B-12 or folic acid deficiency, niacin deficiency, hypercalcemia, neurosyphilis, HIV infection)
3. Substance-induced conditions
E. The deficits do not occur exclusively during the course of a delirium.
F. The disturbance is not better accounted for by another Axis I disorder (e.g., major depressive disorder, schizophrenia).

American Psychiatric Association. Task Force on DSM-IV. Diagnostic and Statistical Manual of Mental Disorders: DSM-IV. 4th ed. Washington, DC: American Psychiatric Association; 1994.

TABLE 65-4

Clinical Features of Common Dementias

TYPE OF DEMENTIA	ALZHEIMER DISEASE	VASCULAR DEMENTIA	DEMENTIA WITH LEWY BODIES	FRONTOTEMPORAL DEMENTIA
Must first meet diagnostic criteria for dementia (see Table 65-3)				
TYPICAL COURSE	Gradually progressive	Stepwise deterioration	Progressive cognitive decline with fluctuating cognition, attention, and alertness	Insidious onset and gradual progression
COGNITIVE SYMPTOMS	Memory impairment plus one or more areas of cognitive deficit	Memory impairment plus two or more areas of cognitive deficit	Fluctuating cognitive symptoms May have prominent visuospatial/constructional impairment on cognitive testing	Early decline in social interpersonal conduct (frontal lobe predominance) or language skills (temporal lobe predominance) May not exhibit memory loss symptoms until later in illness
OTHER ASSOCIATED SYMPTOMS/ SIGNS		Focal neurological signs and evidence of relevant cerebrovascular disease by brain imaging	Recurrent visual hallucinations Parkinsonism motor features Recurrent falls Syncope Neuroleptic sensitivity Delusions	Early impairment in regulation of personal conduct Early emotional blunting Early loss of insight

TABLE 65-6

NINCDS-ADRDA Criteria for Clinical Diagnosis of Alzheimer's Disease

The criteria for the clinical diagnosis of PROBABLE Alzheimer's disease include:

Dementia established by clinical examination and documented by the Mini-Mental Test, Blessed Dementia Scale, or some similar examination, and confirmed by neuropsychological tests;

Deficits in two or more areas of cognition;

Progressive worsening of memory and other cognitive functions;

No disturbance of consciousness;

Onset between ages 40 and 90, most often after age 65; and

Absence of systemic disorders or other brain diseases that could account for the progressive deficits in memory and cognition.

The diagnosis of PROBABLE Alzheimer's disease is supported by:

Progressive deterioration of specific cognitive functions such as language (aphasia), motor skills (apraxia), and perception (agnosia);

Impaired activities of daily living and altered patterns of behavior;

Family history of similar disorders, particularly if confirmed neuropathologically; and

Laboratory results of:

Normal lumbar puncture as evaluated by standard techniques;

Normal pattern or nonspecific changes in EEG, such as increased slow-wave activity, and

Evidence of cerebral atrophy on CT with progression documented by serial observation.

Other clinical features consistent with the diagnosis of PROBABLE Alzheimer's disease, after exclusion of causes of dementia other than Alzheimer's disease, include:

Plateaus in the course of progression of the illness;

Associated symptoms of depression, insomnia, incontinence, delusions, illusions, hallucinations, catastrophic verbal, emotional, or physical outbursts, sexual disorders, and weight loss; other neurologic abnormalities in some patients, especially with more advanced disease and including motor signs such as increased muscle tone, myoclonus, or gait disorder;

Seizures in advanced disease; and

CT normal for age.

Features that make the diagnosis of PROBABLE Alzheimer's disease uncertain or unlikely include:

Sudden, apoplectic onset;

Focal neurologic findings such as hemiparesis, sensory loss, visual field deficits, and incoordination early in the course of the illness; and

Seizures or gait disturbances at the onset or very early in the course of the illness.

Clinical diagnosis of POSSIBLE Alzheimer's disease:

May be made on the basis of the dementia syndrome, in the absence of other neurologic, psychiatric, or systemic disorders sufficient to cause dementia, and in the presence of variations in the onset in the presentation, or in the clinical course;

May be made in the presence of a second systemic or brain disorder sufficient to produce dementia, which is not considered to be the cause of the dementia; and

Should be used in research studies when a single, gradually progressive severe cognitive deficit is identified in the absence of other identifiable cause.

Criteria for diagnosis of DEFINITE Alzheimer's disease are:

The clinical criteria for probable Alzheimer's disease and

Histopathologic evidence obtained from a biopsy or autopsy.

Classification of Alzheimer's disease for research purposes should specify features that may differentiate subtypes of the disorder, such as:

Familial occurrence;

Onset before age of 65;

Presence of trisomy-21; and

Coexistence of other relevant conditions such as Parkinson disease.

Adapted from McKhann G, Drachman D, Folstein M, et al. Clinical diagnosis of Alzheimer's disease: report of the NINCDS-ADRDA Work Group under the auspices of Department of Health and Human Services Task Force on Alzheimer's Disease. Neurology.1984;34(7):939–944.

detailed information on the highest level tasks associated with each vocation. In persons who have not worked outside the home or who are retired, questions on hobbies, household management, and other volunteer activities will provide important information on the patient's previous level of functioning. Changes in the person's ability to carry out these tasks should then be ascertained, and the degree to which these impairments affect daily functioning should be documented. Questions about changes in daily functional activities will help the clinician isolate problem areas representing functional decline.

Ascertaining the time course over which the memory symptoms developed is important, as AD is characterized by a gradually progressive decline in cognitive function occurring over years. Frequently, an inciting event that disrupts coping skills, such as a hospitalization or the death of a spouse, will draw the attention of family members

to a person's memory problems. The family may give a history of an acute onset of memory impairment following the inciting event, but careful questioning may identify memory problems preceding that time period and point to a gradually progressive course.

Additional information on safety should be obtained, including inquiries on medication management, kitchen fires, driving, wandering, financial scams, use of power tools, and hunting or other use of firearms. A review of systems should include questions on depression, tremors, rigidity, falls, dysphagia, urinary incontinence, stroke or transient ischemic attack symptoms, waxing and waning level of consciousness, and visual hallucinations.

A past medical history of cardiovascular disease and associated risk factors, coronary artery bypass surgery, head injury, seizures, depression, Parkinson disease, and heavy alcohol use may help guide the clinician in making a diagnosis. A careful substance use and

TABLE 65-7

Evaluation of the Patient with Memory Concerns

History of memory loss symptoms
- Time course of memory decline
  (gradually progressive, stepwise, or fluctuating)
- Past and present function at higher level tasks
  (including work history, hobbies, daily household tasks such as financial management)
- Safety concerns
  (driving, medication management, kitchen safety, use of firearms or heavy equipment, wandering)
- Other associated symptoms
  (depression, sleep disturbance, tremors, rigidity, falls, urinary incontinence, stroke or TIA symptoms, visual hallucinations)

Past medical and psychiatric history
- Vascular risk factors
- Strokes
- Coronary artery bypass surgery
- Alcohol and other drug use
- Seizures
- Head injury/loss of consciousness
- Parkinson disease or Parkinsonism
- Depression, anxiety, or other psychiatric illness

Medication review
- Prescription and nonprescription medications
- Association of onset of cognitive symptoms with medication use

Social history
- Family and other social support
- Education and occupation history, including responsibilities associated with occupation
- Hobbies and other daily activities

Family history
- Alzheimer's disease of other neurodegenerative disorder, strokes, depression

Physical examination
- General appearance, attention, cooperation level, mood, affect, speech
  Neurological examination:
  - Motor strength
  - Sensory examination
  - Coordination
  - Gait
  - Cranial nerves, including extraocular movements
  - Muscle tone/rigidity/cogwheeling
  - Resting or intention tremors
  - Deep tendon reflexes
  Vascular examination:
  - Carotid bruits
  - Cardiac examination
  - Other evidence of significant vascular disease (diminished pulses, abdominal bruits, etc.)

Cognitive testing

Laboratory testing
- Vitamin B-12
- Electrolytes
- Liver enzymes
- Red blood cell folate
- Thyroid-stimulating hormone
- Complete blood count
- Homocysteine
- Cholesterol panel

Neuroimaging (CT or MRI)

Other tests to consider (based on clinical suspicion)
- Lumbar puncture for cerebrospinal fluid collection
- Electroencephalogram (EEG)

medication history should be obtained, including specific questions regarding use of alcohol and common over-the-counter anticholinergic medications that can worsen memory, such as antihistamines.

The physical examination should include assessment of general appearance, such as level of attention and cooperation, psychomotor slowing, affect, hygiene, and speech pattern. A neurological examination should screen for focal deficits, increased muscle tone, cogwheeling, rigidity, or tremors. A detailed review of a comprehensive mental status and neurological examination in older adults is described in Chapter 12. Cardiac arrhythmias, carotid bruits, or abdominal or femoral bruits may suggest a predisposition to vascular dementia.

Cognitive testing can be readily performed in the primary care clinic setting using screening tests such as the Mini-Mental State Examination, the Clock Draw Test, and category fluency. In adults with high baseline cognitive functioning, however, these tests may be normal in the presence of obvious functional impairment necessitating referral to a neuropsychologist for more detailed testing. In those with lower educational levels, these cognitive screening tests may suggest impairment, but the history may not suggest any changes in functional status. Thus, it is critical to use age- and education-adjusted norms, and integrate historical information on baseline function to decide if further neuropsychological testing is warranted or if abnormal testing may actually represent the person's baseline status. In addition, screening for depression is a critical part of a memory assessment. Any suspicion of mood disturbances can be evaluated with a screening tool such as the Geriatric Depression Scale (GDS). These cognitive and affective screening tools can be easily administered by a variety of health care personnel, allowing for their use in a busy clinic setting.

Laboratory data can assist in identifying factors that may be contributing to cognitive decline. Rarely do these factors alone account for the overall cognitive changes that lead to the presentation of a patient with significant memory loss symptoms. Nevertheless, treating such factors may improve cognitive symptoms in patients with severe laboratory abnormalities, numerous comorbid illnesses, or in whom there is an underlying neurodegenerative process. Recommended laboratory tests include vitamin B-12, thyroid stimulating hormone (TSH), electrolytes, complete blood count, liver enzymes, homocysteine, red blood cell folate levels, and a cholesterol panel. If symptoms are atypical or if there are specific risk factors, then a serologic test for syphilis may be performed. In some European countries, routine assessment of cerebrospinal fluid (CSF) for β-amyloid and tau levels is done as part of the clinical evaluation. In the United States, CSF collection is usually reserved for ruling out Creutzfeldt–Jakob disease or other conditions such as normal pressure hydrocephalus (NPH). In most cases, it is recommended that some form of neuroimaging be obtained. Typical findings for AD on neuroimaging can range from a fairly normal scan to diffuse cerebral atrophy. A computed tomography (CT) of the head without contrast is usually sufficient to evaluate for significant cerebrovascular disease, brain tumors, subdural hematoma, or NPH. Magnetic resonance imaging (MRI) can provide more information if lacunar infarcts are suspected. In persons with suspected seizure disorder or Creutzfeldt–Jakob disease, an electroencephalogram (EEG) may be considered. Although positron emission tomography (PET) scans are used frequently in research settings, they are not yet advocated for regular use in clinical practice.

If a patient does not meet the criteria for AD yet clinical suspicion remains, either more detailed neuropsychological testing or repeat testing in 6 months may clarify the diagnosis as the symptoms progress. Persons with suspected MCI should be reassessed on an annual basis as 12% to 15% of individuals with this diagnosis progress to dementia each year. If the symptoms or course of the disease are atypical for AD, the level of functional decline is out of proportion to neuropsychological testing results, or if there are significant behavioral issues that need to be addressed, then referral to a geriatrician, neurologist, or psychiatrist with expertise in dementia is recommended.

Future Diagnostic Tools

Novel diagnostic tools are continually being investigated for use in the diagnosis of AD. Many of these tools are still mainly used in research settings, but are under continued study to evaluate their role in clinical practice. Current investigations are focusing on how to best identify biomarkers with strong relationships to clinically relevant outcomes in AD that could be used not only for diagnosis, but also for identifying asymptomatic persons at risk for AD. Neuroimaging modalities have shown great promise in documenting not only the late effects of neuronal damage in AD (regional and global cerebral atrophy), but also in identifying earlier in vivo pathology (such as in

vivo amyloid imaging on PET) and the functional consequences of such pathology (activation patterns on functional MRI). CSF levels of $A\beta$ and tau have been shown to predict risk for progression to AD in older adults and persons with MCI. With the recent advances in the safety and acceptability of lumbar punctures, CSF markers may eventually find their way into the clinical diagnostic workup of preclinical AD. Some blood and CSF inflammatory markers have also shown some value in predicting risk of cognitive decline. Future research is focusing how these biomarkers may be used in combination with cognitive tests to identify who is at greatest risk for AD, who would benefit most from preventive therapies, and how effective these therapies are in modifying the underlying disease process in asymptomatic individuals.

MANAGING PATIENTS WITH ALZHEIMER'S DISEASE

Managing patients with AD involves a comprehensive, multidisciplinary team approach including presentation of the diagnosis, initiation of medical therapy, assessment and treatment of concomitant depression and/or behavioral concerns, development of a social support network, education of patients and caregivers, provision of caregiver support, and initiation of appropriate safety measures. While not all medical centers have access to multidisciplinary team resources, effective care can still be given by focusing on providing established medical treatment, identifying a few strategies to maintain patient safety and providing basic education and caregiver support.

Presenting the Diagnosis

Presenting the diagnosis of AD to a patient is difficult, as it may generate significant emotional responses from the patient and their family and trigger fear of the future. Frequently, patients and family members suspect the diagnosis before it is presented, but how they respond to the news depends on personal coping mechanisms, cultural influences, family dynamics, and their preconceived understanding of AD. Clinicians may help patients and families adjust to this diagnosis by using an empathetic, yet honest approach and by providing them with educational and support resources, including those provided by agencies such as the Alzheimer's Association and the National Institute on Aging Alzheimer's Disease Education and Referral (ADEAR) Center. In addition, the clinician should emphasize the goals of diagnosing AD in order to take steps to protect the patient's memory, delay the progression of the disease, and to maintain the person's safety. In general, it is recommended to tell both the patient and family the diagnosis using the term "Alzheimer's disease", thus, providing patients and families with a starting point for education. Encouraging both persons with the disorder and caregivers to utilize resources such as local support groups and the Alzheimer's Association is an important part of the patient management plan.

Treatment of Cognitive Symptoms

Acetylcholinesterase inhibitors (AChEIs) are the mainstay of therapy for AD, and until several years ago, were the only medications approved in the United States for the treatment of AD. AChEIs increase the levels of the neurotransmitter acetylcholine in neuronal synapses, thereby enhancing cholinergic activity in the affected brain regions.

TABLE 65-8

FDA-Approved Medications for the Treatment of Alzheimer's Disease*

MEDICATION	INDICATION	AVAILABLE FORMULATIONS	DOSE RANGE AND TITRATION
Cholinesterase inhibitors			
Donepezil (Aricept®)	Mild to severe AD	5 and 10 mg tablets 5 and 10 mg oral disintegrating tablets	Tablets or oral disintegrating tablets: 5–10 mg once daily at bedtime May be taken with or without food Begin at 5 mg once daily at bedtime for 4–6 wk then increase to 10 mg daily as tolerated Effective dose: 5–10 mg daily
Galantamine (Razadyne® and Razadyne® ER)	Mild to moderate AD	4, 8, and 12 mg immediate-release tablets 4 mg/mL immediate-release oral solution 8, 16, and 24 mg extended-release capsules	Immediate-release tablets or oral solution: 4–12 mg twice daily Should be taken with meals Begin at 4 mg twice daily for 4–6 wk then increase to 8 mg twice daily for 4–6 wk then 12 mg twice daily as tolerated Extended-release capsules: 8–24 mg once daily Should be taken in the morning with food Begin at 8 mg once daily for 4–6 wk then increase to 16 mg once daily for 4–6 wk then 24 mg once daily as tolerated Effective dose: 16–24 mg daily
Rivastigmine (Exelon®)	Mild to moderate AD	1.5, 3, 4.5, and 6 mg capsules 2 mg/mL oral solution 4.6 mg/24 h and 9.5 mg/24 h patches	Capsules or oral solution: 1.5–6 mg twice daily Should be taken with meals Oral solution may be taken directly or mixed with beverage Begin at 1.5 mg twice daily for 2–4 wk then increase to 3 mg twice daily for 2–4 wk then 4.5 mg twice daily for 2–4 wk then 6 mg twice daily as tolerated Patch: Begin at 4.6 mg/24 h patch daily for 4–6 wk then increase to 9.5 mg/24 h patch daily as tolerated Effective dose: 6–12 mg daily
N-methyl-D-aspartate (NMDA) receptor antagonist			
Memantine (Namenda®)	Moderate to severe AD	5 and 10 mg tablets 4-wk titration pack 2 mg/mL oral solution	Tablets or oral solution: 10 mg twice daily May be taken with or without food Begin at 5 mg once daily for 1 wk then increase to 5 mg twice daily for 1 wk then 10 mg in the morning and 5 mg in the evening for 1 wk then 10 mg twice daily as tolerated (available in a 4-wk titration pack) Effective dose: 20 mg daily

*Information obtained from product inserts.

Although 18% to 48% of persons may experience improvements in cognition after taking these medications, the majority of patients do not have any noticeable improvement, but instead experience a plateau or slowing of their rate of cognitive decline. This lack of noticeable improvement has led to controversies regarding the benefit of using cholinesterase inhibitors. However, given the chronic nature of AD, delaying the progression of cognitive decline may lead to improvements in quality of life, reduced caregiver burden, and reduced economic cost associated with long-term care.

Four AChEIs have been approved for use in the United States by the Food and Drug Administration (FDA). These medications include tacrine (Cognex®), donepezil (Aricept®), rivastigmine (Exelon®), and galantamine (Razadyne®). Excessive gastrointestinal side effects have made use of tacrine less favorable given the improved safety and tolerability profiles noted with the newer agents. Dosing

recommendations for the commonly used AChEIs are shown in Table 65-8. In general, the most common adverse effects associated with AChEI use are nausea, anorexia, and diarrhea. Gastrointestinal side effects may be alleviated by taking the medications with food. Sleep disturbances are also common, and may improve with altering the dosing schedule.

While used for many years in Europe, the United States' FDA-approved memantine (Namenda®) for use in moderate to severe AD in 2003. Memantine is an uncompetitive N-methyl-D-aspartate (NMDA) receptor antagonist. At high concentrations, memantine can inhibit mechanisms related to learning and memory, but at lower concentrations, it can preserve or enhance memory in animal models of AD. Memantine can protect against the excitotoxic destruction of cholinergic neurons and may inhibit β-amyloid production. In persons with moderate to severe AD, memantine slows the progression of cognitive decline either alone or when used in conjunction with AChEIs. In addition, studies support that use of memantine showed better outcomes on measures of cognition, activities of daily living, global outcome, and behavior and was well tolerated. While early trials show promising results, additional studies are needed before memantine can be recommended for early stages of AD. In most circumstances, it is appropriate to add this medication to cholinesterase inhibitor therapy in persons with moderate to severe AD. Current prescribing recommendations for memantine are shown in Table 65-8. In persons who do not tolerate cholinesterase inhibitors, memantine may be used as first-line therapy. With use of either AChEIs or memantine, clinicians should educate families on what to expect with use of the medications, namely that they work to delay the progression of the disease and not to significantly improve their cognition. Consideration should be given to the modest expected benefit and cost of both medications per month.

Disease-Modifying Therapies

Currently there are no FDA-approved disease-modifying therapies available, but research is making progress in identifying pathways that could serve as targets for such therapies. A variety of agents targeting β-amyloid metabolism are in various stages of development, including Aβ immunotherapy, agents inhibiting Aβ fibrillization and reducing soluble Aβ, selective amyloid lowering agents (SALAs), and β- and γ-secretase inhibitors. In addition, potential disease-modifying agents with known cardiovascular benefits, such as statins and omega-3 fatty acids, are currently being studied in large clinical trials.

While clinical trials have not conclusively shown that treating vascular risk factors delays the development or progression of AD, aggressive treatment of vascular risk factors in many patients with memory complaints, including those associated with AD, may be warranted. Vascular risk factor modification has known cardiovascular benefits that may lead to reduction of coronary artery bypass grafting, cerebrovascular disease, and stroke—factors strongly linked to cognitive decline. Trials are underway to clarify if vascular risk factor reduction and improved cerebral perfusion modify the course of AD. Until the completion of such trials, clinicians should follow established cardiovascular prevention guidelines for patients presenting with memory complaints, taking into account the patient's comorbid illnesses, quality of life, treatment costs, and life expectancy.

Preventive Strategies

Currently there are no established preventive therapies for AD. Evidence supports that future therapies that either delay or prevent the onset of AD may need to be started in midlife in high-risk populations in order to significantly influence the onset and course of the disease. As the underlying pathologic changes that eventually lead to clinical AD begin decades before the onset of symptoms, primary prevention trials with conversion to AD as their primary outcome may prove costly and time-consuming. Integrating biomarkers with strong relationships to clinically relevant outcomes into such primary prevention trials may allow for earlier identification of disease-modifying effects of potential preventive therapies. Given the multifactorial nature of AD, future preventive strategies will most likely target a variety of mechanisms related to disease progression, similar to that used in cardiovascular disease prevention. Some potential prevention therapies currently under investigation include vascular risk factor modification, anti-inflammatory medications, antioxidants, lifestyle interventions such as exercise, social engagement, and cognitive stimulation, and novel compounds targeting Aβ metabolism.

Behavioral Management

AD is frequently associated with behavioral disturbances that include agitation, emotional or physical outbursts, and sexual inappropriateness. Such behaviors may be more distressing to family and caregivers than the actual memory decline. Such behaviors may be managed by nonpharmacologic as well as pharmacologic interventions. Nonpharmacological therapies should be explored and exhausted before using pharmacologic therapy, unless the person's agitation threatens his or her safety or living situation. Addressing physical pain or other medical symptoms or distressing situations that could be contributing to agitation is key prior to any pharmacologic intervention. Identifying and correcting physical or emotional stressors may alleviate agitation. Potential medication side effects should be considered to see if they are contributing to agitation symptoms. After nonpharmacologic measures have been tried, consideration may be given to use of low-dose atypical antipsychotics taking into account potential risks associated with these medications. Selective serotonin reuptake inhibitors (SSRIs) may reduce symptoms of sexual inappropriateness. Wandering symptoms typically do not respond to pharmacologic therapy. Taking patients for a walk or giving them busy tasks to do may help reduce wandering. Frequently, it is the behavioral changes associated with AD and other dementias that are most distressing to family members and provide the greatest challenge for primary care physicians who are managing the care of persons with AD. Referral to a multidisciplinary memory disorders clinic is appropriate for patients with significant behavioral concerns. More information is dedicated to this topic in Chapter 73.

Safety Management

Reviewing common safety concerns in persons with dementia may help identify significant risks and provide an opportunity for educating family members and caregivers on what areas to monitor closely and what safeguards they can take to protect the person with AD. Some patients may require further evaluation to assess driving safety, which can be done through occupational or physical therapy departments or local driving schools. Pill boxes or other similar medication planners may facilitate correct administration of medications and allow family or caregivers to help in setting up the medications properly. Other safety concerns such as proper use of the stove, woodworking equipment, hunting rifles, etc. should be discussed and appropriate supervision arranged.

Caregiver Support

Evidence is accumulating that the effects of AD are felt not only by the patient but also by the caregivers. Caregivers have increased depression, missed work, and health problems compared to those not caring for a family member with dementia. Use of respite services from family, friends, neighbors, and local adult day centers may allow for caregivers to take the appropriate time needed to maintain their own health and social connections.

End-of-Life Care

Upon diagnosis of AD, many patients and families have questions as to what to expect in the years ahead. As the rapidity of progression of AD may depend not only on genetic and environmental factors but also comorbid medical conditions, the course of decline can be difficult to predict in some persons. Once on medical treatment for AD and when all potentially reversible contributing factors have been addressed, obtaining repeat cognitive testing will give the clinician an idea of the trajectory of decline of the individual and help inform the family on what to expect in the years ahead. Providing information early in the disease course on end-of-life planning may help smooth this difficult transition later in the disease. Use of respite services and home health aides or family members may help the person with AD stay in the home longer. If the social network of the patient cannot support the patient as the care needs increase, then nursing home placement frequently is necessary. Involving hospice can help with symptom management late in the course of the illness. Involvement in Alzheimer support groups can provide support during the unique grieving process related to dementia, as family and caregivers watch the cognitive and personality transformations in their family member with AD.

SUMMARY

Alzheimer's disease is the leading cause of dementia worldwide and, unless effective preventive strategies are identified, is expected to significantly increase in prevalence in the coming decades as the population ages. The diagnosis of AD remains a clinical diagnosis that requires careful history-taking, a physical examination, and cognitive testing to document a decline in cognitive and functional abilities. Ancillary laboratory and neuroimaging can help differentiate between various causes of memory loss and different types of dementia. Treatment for AD involves not only pharmacologic therapy with cholinesterase inhibitors and NMDA antagonists, but also careful assessment of safety, behavioral concerns, and education for the patient, family, and other caregivers. While preventive therapies have not yet been established, newly identified mechanisms of disease pathobiology are being targeted to develop effective novel therapies that could either delay or preferably arrest the progression of AD. Future research may help identify persons at highest risk for AD and develop treatment strategies targeting multiple mechanisms underlying the pathobiology of AD.

FURTHER READING

American Psychiatric Association. Task Force on DSM-IV. *Diagnostic and Statistical Manual of Mental Disorders: DSM-IV.* 4th ed. Washington, DC: American Psychiatric Association; 1994.

Doody RS, Stevens JC, Beck C, et al. Practice parameter: management of dementia (an evidence-based review). Report of the Quality Standards Subcommittee of the American Academy of Neurology. *Neurology.* 2001;56(9):1154–1166.

Hardy J. A hundred years of Alzheimer's disease research. *Neuron.* 2006;52:3–13.

Hebert LE, Scherr PA, Bienias JL, et al. Alzheimer's disease in the US population: prevalence estimates using the 2000 census. *Arch Neurol.* 2003;60(8):1119–1122.

Iadecola C. Neurovascular regulation in the normal brain and in Alzheimer's disease. *Nat Rev Neurosci.* 2004;5(5):347–360.

Jellinger KA. Head injury and dementia. *Curr Opin Neurol.* 2004;17:719–723.

Lee VMY, Goedert M, Trojanowski JQ. Neurodegenerative tauopathies. *Annu Rev Neurosci.* 2001;24:1121–1159.

McKhann G, Drachman D, Folstein M, et al. Clinical diagnosis of Alzheimer's disease: report of the NINCDS-ADRDA Work Group under the auspices of Department of Health and Human Services Task Force on Alzheimer's Disease. *Neurology.* 1984;34(7):939–944.

Petersen RC, Smith GE, Waring SC, et al. Mild cognitive impairment: clinical characterization and outcome. *Arch Neurol.* 1999;56(3):303–308.

Puglielli L. Aging of the brain, neurotrophin signaling, and Alzheimer's disease: is IGF1-R the common culprit? *Neurobiol Aging.* 2008;29:795–811.

Puglielli L, Tanzi RE, Kovacs DM. Alzheimer's disease: the cholesterol connection. *Nat Neurosci.* 2003;6:345–351.

Selkoe DJ. Cell biology of protein misfolding: the examples of Alzheimer's and Parkinson's diseases. *Nat Cell Biol.* 2004;6:1054–1061.

Tanzi RE, Bertram L. Twenty years of the Alzheimer's disease amyloid hypothesis: a genetic perspective. *Cell.* 2005;120:545–555.

Thal DR, Del Tredici K, Braak H. Neurodegeneration in normal brain aging and disease. *Sci Aging Knowledge Environ.* 2004;2004:pe26.

Thal LJ, Kantarci K, Reiman EM, et al. The role of biomarkers in clinical trials for Alzheimer's disease. *Alzheimer Dis Assoc Disord.* 2006;20(1):6–15.

Parkinson's Disease and Related Disorders

Stanley Fahn

DISTINGUISHING BETWEEN PARKINSON'S DISEASE AND PARKINSONISM

The syndrome of parkinsonism must be understood before understanding what is Parkinson's disease (PD). Parkinsonism is defined as any combination of six specific, independent motoric features: tremor at rest, bradykinesia, rigidity, loss of postural reflexes, flexed posture, and the freezing phenomenon (where the feet are transiently "glued" to the ground). Not all six of these cardinal features need be present, but at least two should be before the diagnosis of parkinsonism is made, with at least one of them being tremor at rest or bradykinesia. Parkinsonism is divided into four categories (Table 66-1). PD or primary parkinsonism will be the principal focus of this chapter; not only as it is the one that is most commonly encountered by the general clinician, it is also the one on which much research has been expended and the one we know the most about. The great majority of cases of primary parkinsonism are sporadic, but in the last decade, several gene mutations have been discovered to cause PD (Table 66-2). Whether genetic or idiopathic in etiology, the common denominator is that this group of primary parkinsonism is not caused by known insults to the brain (the main feature of secondary parkinsonism) and is not associated with other motoric neurological features (the main feature of Parkinson-plus syndromes). The uncovering of genetic causes of primary parkinsonism has shed light on probable pathogenic mechanisms that may be a factor in even the more common idiopathic cases of PD. It may even turn out that many of the idiopathic cases will be linked to gene mutations, discoveries yet to be made. Although the term "idiopathic PD" has been applied to primary parkinsonism, the fact that there are known genetic causes should encourage us to adopt the term "primary parkinsonism" rather than "idiopathic parkinsonism."

Three of the most helpful clues that one is likely dealing with a category of parkinsonism other than PD would be (1) a symmetrical onset of symptoms (PD often begins on one side of the body), (2) a lack of a substantial clinical response to adequate levodopa therapy, and (3) the absence of rest tremor. The presence of any of these features does not necessarily exclude the diagnosis of PD, but the likelihood that the cause belongs to another category of parkinsonism is high. The clinical features suggesting a diagnosis favoring the other parkinsonian disorders and not PD are listed in Table 66-3. One common misdiagnosis is tremor owing to essential tremor, which can even be unilateral, although it more commonly is bilateral. Helpful in the diagnosis is that the tremor caused by PD is a rest tremor, whereas essential tremor is not present at rest, but appears with holding the arms in front of the body and increases in amplitude with intention activity of the arm, such as with handwriting or performing the finger-to-nose maneuver.

PD begins insidiously and gradually worsens. Symptoms, such as rest tremor, can be intermittent at the beginning, becoming present only in stressful situations. Patients with PD can live 20 or more years, depending on the age at onset; the mortality rate is approximately 1.5 times that of normal individuals of the same age. Death in PD is usually because of some concurrent unrelated illness or owing to the effects of decreased mobility, aspiration, or increased falling with subsequent physical injury. The Parkinson-plus syndromes typically progress at a faster rate and often cause death within 9 years. Thus, the diagnosis of PD is of prognostic importance, as well as of therapeutic significance, because it almost always responds to at least a moderate degree to levodopa therapy, whereas the Parkinson-plus disorders do not. While it may be difficult to distinguish between PD and Parkinson-plus syndromes in the early stages of the illness, with disease progression over time, the clinical distinctions of the Parkinson-plus disorders become more apparent with the development of other neurological findings, such as cerebellar ataxia, loss of downward ocular movements, and autonomic dysfunction (e.g., postural hypotension, loss of bladder control, and impotence).

There are no practical diagnostic laboratory tests for PD, and the diagnosis rests on the clinical features or by excluding some of the other causes of parkinsonism. The research tool of fluorodopa

TABLE 66-1

Classification of the Parkinsonian States

Primary parkinsonism (Parkinson's disease)
  Sporadic
  Known genetic etiology (see Table 66–2)

Secondary parkinsonism (environmental etiology)
  Drugs
    Dopamine receptor blockers (most commonly antipsychotic medications)
    Dopamine storage depletors (reserpine)
  Postencephalitic
  Toxins—Mn, CO, MPTP, cyanide
  Vascular
  Brain tumors
  Head trauma
  Normal pressure hydrocephalus

Parkinsonism-plus syndromes
  Progressive supranuclear palsy (PSP)
  Multiple system atrophy (MSA)
  Cortical–basal ganglionic degeneration (CBGD)
  Diffuse Lewy body disease (DLBD)
  Parkinson–dementia–ALS complex of Guam
  Progressive pallidal atrophy

Heredodegenerative disorders
  Alzheimer's disease
  Wilson disease
  Huntington disease
  Frontotemporal dementia on chromosome 17
  X-linked dystonia-parkinsonism (in Filipino men; known as lubag)

positron emission tomography measures levodopa uptake into dopamine nerve terminals, and this shows a decline of approximately 5% per year of the striatal uptake. A similar result is seen using ligands for the dopamine transporter, either by positron emission tomography or by single photon emission computed tomography; these ligands also label the dopamine nerve terminals. All these neuroimaging techniques reveal decreased dopaminergic nerve terminals in the striatum in both PD and the Parkinson-plus syndromes, and do not distinguish between them. A substantial response to levodopa is most helpful in the differential diagnosis, indicating presynaptic dopamine deficiency with intact postsynaptic dopamine receptors, features typical for PD.

TABLE 66-3

Criteria to Exclude the Diagnosis of Parkinson's Disease in Favor of Another Cause of Parkinsonism

	LIKELY DIAGNOSIS
History of:	
Encephalitis	Postencephalitic
Exposure to carbon monoxide, manganese, or other toxins	Toxin-induced
Recent exposure to neuroleptic medication	Drug-induced
Onset of parkinsonian symptoms following:	
Head trauma	Posttraumatic
Stroke	Vascular
Presence on examination of:	
Cerebellar ataxia	OPCA, MSA
Loss of downward ocular movements	PSP
Pronounced postural hypotension not because of concurrent medication	MSA
Pronounced unilateral rigidity with or without dystonia, apraxia, cortical sensory loss, alien limb	CBGD
Myoclonus	CBGD, MSA
Falling or freezing of gait early in the course of the disease	PSP
Autonomic dysfunction not because of medications	MSA
Excessive drooling of saliva	MSA
Early dementia or hallucinations from medications	DLBD
Dystonia induced with low-dose levodopa	MSA
Neuroimaging (MRI or CT scan) revealing:	
Lacunar infarcts	Vascular
Capacious cerebral ventricles	NPH
Cerebellar atrophy	OPCA, MSA
Atrophy of the midbrain or other parts of the brainstem	PSP, MSA
Effect of medication:	
Poor response to levodopa	PSP, MSA, CBGD, Vascular, NPH
No dyskinesias despite high-dose levodopa	Same as above

CBGD, cortical–basal ganglionic degeneration; DLBD, diffuse Lewy body disease, also called dementia with Lewy bodies; MSA, multiple system atrophy; NPH, normal pressure hydrocephalus; OPCA, olivo-ponto-cerebellar atrophy, which can be one form of MSA.

TABLE 66-2

Genetic Forms of Primary Parkinsonism

NAME	GENE SYMBOL	PROTEIN	CHROMOSOME
Autosomal Dominant Transmission			
PARK1/PARK4	SNCA	α-synuclein	4q21.3
PARK5	UCH-L1	Ubiquitin C-terminal hydrolase-L1	4p14
PARK8	LRRK2	Leucine rich repeat kinase 2	12p11.2–q13.1
	GBA	β-glucocerebrosidase	1q21
Dopa-responsive dystonia		GTP cyclohydrolase 1	14q22.1–q22.2
Autosomal Recessive Transmission			
PARK2	PRKN	Parkin (ubiquitin ligase)	6q25.2–q27
PARK6	PINK1	PTEN-induced kinase 1 (PINK1)	1p35–p36
PARK7	DJ-1	DJ-1	1p36
PARK9	ATP13A2	ATPase	1p32
Tyrosine hydroxylase deficiency			11p11.5

The development of dementia in a patient with parkinsonism remains a difficult differential diagnosis. If the patient's parkinsonian features did not respond to levodopa, the diagnosis is likely to be Alzheimer's disease, which can occasionally present with parkinsonism. If the presenting parkinsonism responded to levodopa, and the patient developed dementia over time, the diagnosis could be either PD dementia (PDD) or diffuse Lewy body disease (DLBD), also known as dementia with Lewy bodies. The nosologic distinction is less of substance and more of useful categorization. The term PDD is used if the symptoms of PD have been present for at least 1 year before dementia develops. The term DLBD is used if the symptoms of PD have been present less than 1 year before onset of dementia, or if dementia presents with the onset of parkinsonism. A major feature of PDD and DLBD is the presence of hallucinations. Without hallucinations, other types of dementias should be considered, including vascular disease, Alzheimer's disease, and frontotemporal dementia. DLBD is a condition where Lewy bodies are present in the cerebral cortex as well as in the brainstem nuclei. The heredodegenerative disease, known as frontotemporal dementia, is an autosomal dominant disorder caused by mutations of the *tau* gene or the *progranulin* gene on chromosome 17; the full syndrome presents with dementia, loss of inhibition, parkinsonism, and sometimes muscle wasting. PDD is associated with aging and increased duration of PD. The prevalence of PDD is approximately 20%, but the likelihood of developing dementia eventually in a patient with PD is much greater, with the highest estimate around 78%.

Some adults may develop a more benign form of PD, in which the symptoms respond to very low-dose levodopa, and the disease does not worsen severely with time. This form is usually caused by the autosomal dominant disorder known as dopa-responsive dystonia, which typically begins in childhood as a dystonia. But when it starts in adult life, it can present with parkinsonism. There is no neuronal degeneration. The pathogenesis is because of a biochemical deficiency involving dopamine synthesis. The gene defect is for an enzyme, GTP cyclohydrolase 1, required to synthesize the cofactor for tyrosine hydroxylase activity, the crucial rate-limiting first step in the synthesis of dopamine and norepinephrine. Infantile parkinsonism is caused by the autosomal recessive deficiency of tyrosine hydroxylase, another cause of a biochemical dopamine-deficiency disorder. Young-onset PD—less than 40 years of age, but some use a cut-off of 50 years—usually worsens more slowly than those with older onset. But these young-onset patients are more likely to develop motor complications from levodopa therapy (see below).

PATHOLOGY OF PARKINSON'S DISEASE AND PARKINSON-PLUS SYNDROMES

Parkinson's disease and the Parkinson-plus syndromes have in common a degeneration of substantia nigra pars compacta dopaminergic neurons, with a resulting deficiency of striatal dopamine caused by loss of the nigrostriatal neurons. Accompanying this neuronal loss in the nigra is an increase in glial cells and a loss of the neuromelanin in the nigra, because neuromelanin is normally contained in the dopaminergic neurons. In PD, intracytoplasmic inclusions, called Lewy bodies, are usually present in many of the surviving neurons. It is recognized today that not all patients with PD have Lewy bodies, those with a homozygous mutation in the *parkin* (PARK2) gene,

mainly patients with young-onset PD, have nigral neuronal degeneration without Lewy bodies. Lewy bodies contain many proteins, including the fibrillar form of the protein α-synuclein. Immunostaining for α-synuclein is utilized today as the most sensitive histologic method to detect Lewy bodies. Recent research has shown that Lewy neurites (α-synuclein fibers in axons) first appear in the medulla and the olfactory bulb, and over time become present in a rostral manner up the brainstem, from medulla to pons to midbrain, and then into the thalamus and cerebral cortex. Thus, Lewy neurites (and Lewy bodies) do not start in the substantia nigra, which is located in the midbrain. There are no Lewy bodies in the Parkinson-plus syndromes.

A pathological feature of multiple system atrophy (MSA) is the presence of inclusions in oligodendroglia; these inclusions also contain α-synuclein. PSP and CBGD contain tau filaments, and these two diseases share similar clinical features, especially in the late stages of these diseases. PSP shows neurofibrillary tangles in the substantia nigra and other nuclei, while CBGD shows ballooned neurons, especially in areas of the cerebral cortex.

CAUSE AND PATHOGENESIS OF PARKINSON'S DISEASE AND PARKINSON-PLUS SYNDROMES

Other than known genetic causes of PD (Table 66-2), the etiology of these disorders remains unknown. Alterations in the *tau* gene have been implicated for PSP and CBGD. Three of the identified genes causing PD (*PARK1, PARK2, PARK5*) point to an impairment of protein degradation with a build-up of toxic proteins that cannot be degraded via the ubiquitin–proteasomal pathway. This has led to the concept that perhaps most, if not all, cases of sporadic PD have an impairment of protein degradation. While PARK1 represents mutations in the gene for α-synuclein, triplications and duplications of the chromosomal area for the *α-synuclein* gene (*PARK4*) also cause PD, indicating that accumulation of wild-type α-synuclein, and not just gene mutations of this protein are capable of causing neurodegeneration. A heterozygotic mutation in the gene for the lysosomal enzymes, β-glucocerebrosidase and a lysosomal ATPase (PARK9), indicates that faulty degradation of substrates can be an important pathogenic factor. One gene (*PARK6*) is involved with mitochondrial function, suggesting impaired energy metabolism can lead to PD. *PARK7* is a gene for a protein that fights oxidative stress; thus supporting the notion that increased oxidative stress can be a risk factor for PD.

The most common gene mutation causing PD is PARK8, especially the G2019S mutation; approximately 5% of familial cases and up to 2% of nonfamilial cases have this mutation. There is ethnic disproportion of specific mutations in the *LRRK2* gene. The G2019S mutation is highly prevalent in North African Arabs, Portuguese, Spanish, and Ashkenazi Jews. In the Chinese, the G2385R mutation is the most common. LRRK2 is a complex protein with several functional domains, and mutations in any of them can lead to PD. It is not clear how such mutations cause the disease.

Because accumulated α-synuclein can cause porosity in the synaptic vesicle membrane, resulting in an outward leakage of stored dopamine, the increased cytosolic dopamine can auto-oxidize to form oxyradicals, such as dopamine quinone, to cause cell damage. Other pathogenic mechanisms being considered are (1) damage to the protein degradation properties of lysosomes leading to protein accumulation and aggregation; (2) other effects from oxidative stress, such as the reaction of oxyradicals with nitric oxide to form the highly reactive peroxynitrite radical; (3) impaired mitochondria leading to both reduced ATP production and accumulation of electrons that aggravate oxidative stress, with the final outcome being apoptosis and cell death; and (4) inflammatory changes in the nigra producing cytokines that augment apoptosis. These concepts on pathogenesis are leading researchers to test agents that affect these potential mechanisms in an attempt to reduce the rate of neurodegeneration in PD.

EPIDEMIOLOGY AND CLINICAL FEATURES OF PARKINSON'S DISEASE

Although PD can develop at any age, it is most common in older adults, with a peak age at onset around 60 years. The likelihood of developing PD increases with age, with a lifetime risk of approximately 2%. A positive family history doubles the risk of developing PD to 4%. Twin studies indicate that PD with an onset before the age of 50 years is more likely to have a genetic relationship than for patients with an older age at onset.

The early symptoms and signs of PD are rest tremor, bradykinesia, and rigidity; these are related to progressive loss of nigrostriatal dopamine. These signs and symptoms result from dopamine deficiency and are usually correctable by levodopa and dopamine agonists. As PD progresses over time, non-dopamine-related symptoms develop, such as flexed posture, the freezing phenomenon, and loss of postural reflexes; these do not respond well to levodopa therapy. Moreover, increasing bradykinesia that is not responsive to levodopa can appear as the disease worsens. All these intractable symptoms lead to disability.

While the motor symptoms of PD dominate the clinical picture, and even define the parkinsonian syndrome, many patients with PD have other complaints that have been classified as *nonmotor*. These include bradyphrenia (slowness in mental function), decreased motivation and apathy, dementia (discussed above), fatigue, depression, anxiety, sleep disturbances (fragmented sleep and REM sleep behavior disorder), constipation, bladder and other autonomic disturbances (sexual, gastrointestinal), and sensory complaints. Sensory symptoms, including pain, numbness, tingling, and burning, in the affected limbs occur in approximately 40% of patients.

PRINCIPLES OF THERAPY

Parkinson-plus syndromes respond poorly to medications, so the emphasis here is on the treatment of PD. Certain principles serve as guidelines.

Neuroprotective Therapy

So far no drug or surgical approach has unequivocally been shown to slow the rate of progression of PD, but if any drug could be proven to delay the progression of the disease process, it should be incorporated early. Two drugs that have suggested evidence in the ability to slow the rate of clinical worsening are selegiline and rasagiline; both are irreversible MAO-B inhibitors with a propargylamine moiety in their chemical structure, which has been found to suppress apoptosis.

Encourage Exercise to Keep the Patient Mobile

An active exercise program encourages the patients to participate in their own care, allows muscle stretching and full range of joint mobility, and enhances a better mental attitude toward fighting the disease. One of the nonmotor symptoms of PD is the tendency to being passive with decreased motivation. Encouraging activity helps fight these symptoms. Studies in rodents have shown that those in enriched cages allowing exercise have slowed degeneration of dopamine neurons following toxin injections into those neurons, supposedly because of exercise leading to an increase in brain tropic factors.

Individualize Therapy

No two patients are identical; each presents with a unique set of symptoms, signs, response to medications, and a host of social, occupational, and emotional problems that need to be addressed. The treatment of PD, therefore, needs to be individualized. One takes into account the severity of the patient's symptoms, the degree of functional impairment, the expected benefits and risks of available therapeutic agents, and the age of the patient. Younger patients are more likely to develop motor fluctuations and dyskinesias from levodopa, while older patients are more likely to develop confusion, sleep–wake alterations, dementia, and psychosis.

Deep Brain Stimulation

Stereotaxic surgical implantation of electrodes with stimulation of the subthalamic nucleus has been shown to reduce motor symptoms of PD, especially bradykinesia, tremor, and rigidity. These are the same symptoms that respond to levodopa. The dopa-nonresponsive symptoms of PD also do not respond to deep brain stimulation (DBS). The best candidates for DBS are younger patients with a very good response to levodopa, but with the uneven response of motor fluctuations and dyskinesias. DBS can provide a smoothing out of the clinical response and allows a reduction of medications.

MEDICAL THERAPY OF PARKINSON'S DISEASE

Treatment of patients with PD can be divided into three major categories: physical (and mental health) therapy, medications, and surgery. Physical exercise is mentioned above, and should be implemented as soon as the diagnosis is made, but it is useful in all stages of disease. In the early stages of the disease, the joints should be fully stretched to compensate for the tendency of the patient to have a reduced range of motion. In advanced stages of PD, formal physical therapy is more valuable by keeping the joints from becoming frozen, and by providing guidance how best to remain independent in mobility, particularly with gait training. Medications are the mainstay of therapy, but DBS can be appropriate for selected patients as described above.

Dopamine replacement therapy is the major medical approach to treating PD, and a variety of dopaminergic agents are available (Table 66-4). The most powerful drug is levodopa, the immediate precursor of dopamine. Levodopa, an amino acid, can enter the brain, whereas dopamine is blocked by the blood–brain barrier. Levodopa is usually administered combined with a peripheral decarboxylase inhibitor

TABLE 66-4

Dopaminergic Agents

Dopamine precursor: levodopa

Peripheral decarboxylase inhibitors: carbidopa, benserazide

Dopamine agonists: pramipexole, ropinirole, rotigotine, apomorphine

Catechol-O-methyltransferase inhibitors: tolcapone, entacapone

Dopamine releaser: amantadine

Peripheral dopamine receptor blocker: domperidone

MAO type B inhibitor: selegiline, Zydis selegiline, rasagiline

(carbidopa and benserazide) to prevent formation of dopamine in the peripheral tissues, thereby increasing levodopa's bioavailability and also markedly reducing gastrointestinal side effects. The brand name Sinemet is a combination of carbidopa and levodopa; the brand name Madopar is a combination of benserazide and levodopa. Such combination drugs are available in standard (i.e., immediate-release) and extended-release formulations. The former allows a more rapid and predictable "on," and the latter allows for a slightly longer plasma half-life, but with a slower and less predictable "on." The combination of the two release formulations can be administered in an attempt to smooth out and extend plasma levels of levodopa. One brand of carbidopa/levodopa is Parcopa that dissolves in the patient's mouth and enters the stomach via swallowing saliva. Its usefulness is for patients who have swallowing difficulties or who need to take a dose of carbidopa/levodopa quickly without delay in a search for liquid to swallow with a tablet. Although its pharmacokinetic profile is similar to a swallowed tablet of carbidopa/levodopa, many patients believe Parcopa works more quickly.

Although levodopa is the most effective drug to treat the symptoms of PD, approximately 60% of patients develop troublesome complications of disabling response fluctuations ("wearing-off" effect) and dyskinesias after 5 years of levodopa therapy, and younger patients (less than 60 years of age) are particularly prone to develop these problems even sooner. Thus, younger patients are often started with a dopamine agonist rather than levodopa (see below).

It should be pointed out that it is not safe to discontinue levodopa suddenly, such action can induce the neuroleptic-like malignant syndrome of fever, sweating, rigidity, and mental confusion and obtundation.

Besides being metabolized by aromatic amino acid decarboxylase (commonly known as dopa decarboxylase), levodopa is also metabolized by catechol-O-methyltransferase (COMT) to form 3-O-methyldopa. Two COMT inhibitors are available: entacapone and tolcapone. These agents extend the plasma half-life of levodopa with only slightly increasing its peak plasma concentration, and can thereby prolong the duration of action of each dose of levodopa. Their clinical indication is to help reduce motor fluctuations, i.e., increase "on" time and reduce "off" time. Because they enhance levodopa's efficacy, these agents can increase dyskinesias and the dosage of levodopa may need to be lowered.

Entacapone is very short acting, and each 200 mg tablet is taken simultaneously with levodopa; entacapone has been combined with carbidopa/levodopa into a single tablet, known as Stalevo. Tolcapone (100 and 200 mg tablets) is more potent and has a longer duration of action; it is taken three times daily. But it is encumbered with a greater likelihood to cause diarrhea and hepatic toxicity. Liver function must be monitored and the drug stopped if abnormal liver chemistries are seen. Tolcapone is therefore given only if entacapone has been found to be ineffective in controlling motor fluctuations.

After levodopa, the next most powerful drugs in treating PD symptoms are the dopamine agonists. Several of these are available. The ergot compounds of pergolide, bromocriptine, and cabergoline have the potential to induce fibrosis (cardiac valvulopathy and retroperitoneal, pleuropulmonary, and pericardial fibrosis), so these agents are not recommended; indeed pergolide has been withdrawn from the U.S. market. Pramipexole and ropinirole appear to be equally effective at therapeutic levels. Dopamine agonists are more likely than levodopa to cause hallucinations, confusion, and psychosis, especially in the elderly. Thus, it is safer to utilize levodopa in patients older than 70 years. On the other hand, clinical trials have shown that dopamine agonists are less likely to produce dyskinesias and the wearing-off phenomenon than levodopa. But these trials also showed that levodopa provides greater symptomatic benefit than do dopamine agonists. Other problems more likely to occur with dopamine agonists than levodopa are sudden sleep attacks, including falling asleep at the wheel; daytime drowsiness; ankle edema; and impulse control problems such as hypersexuality and compulsive gambling, shopping, and eating.

The newest dopamine agonist is rotigotine, applied via a dermal patch to the upper torso or arms. Rotigotine penetrates the epidermis and dermis and enters the subcutaneous fat where it slowly enters the blood stream. The skin patch is applied once daily, usually after the morning shower, and is removed the next day before the shower; a new patch is applied to a different surface of the skin to reduce the chance of a rash, a common adverse effect. Absorption is steady over 24 hours, and three dose strengths (four in Europe) are available: 2, 4, and 6 mg/day (plus 8 mg/day in Europe). It is useful for those with swallowing difficulties and may help smooth out motor fluctuations and nocturnal akinesia, when the last prebedtime dose of levodopa does not last throughout the night. It is less potent than the other dopamine agonists, but its milder action may offer fewer adverse effects such as mental and behavioral side effects.

Apomorphine may be the most powerful dopamine agonist, but it needs to be injected subcutaneously (or taken sublingually in Europe). It is used to provide faster relief to overcome a deep "off" state.

Amantadine has several actions; it has antimuscarinic effects, but more importantly, it can activate release of dopamine from nerve terminals, block dopamine uptake into the nerve terminals, and block glutamate NMDA receptors. Its dopaminergic actions make it a useful drug to relieve symptoms in approximately two-thirds of patients, but it can induce livedo reticularis, ankle edema, visual hallucinations, and confusion. Its antiglutamatergic action is useful in reducing the severity of levodopa-induced dyskinesias, and in fact, is the only known effective antidyskinetic agent. The dose of amantadine for its anti-PD effect is usually 100 mg twice daily, but its antidyskinetic effect requires higher dosages, usually 300 to 400 mg/day. Unfortunately, the antidyskinetic effect tends to lessen over time. The elderly do not tolerate amantadine well because of mental adverse effects of confusion and hallucinations. Domperidone is a peripherally active dopamine receptor blocker and is useful in preventing gastrointestinal upset from levodopa and the dopamine agonists. It is not available in the United States, but is available in other countries. Monoamine oxidase type B (MAO-B) inhibitors (selegiline, rasagiline, and Zydis selegiline) offer mildly effective symptomatic benefit and are without the hypertensive "cheese effect" seen with MAO-A inhibitors, and therefore can be used in the presence of levodopa therapy. Although there has been considerable debate about possible protective benefit with selegiline, recent studies evaluating its long-term use indicate that selegiline is associated with less freezing of gait and with a slower rate of clinical worsening compared to placebo-treated subjects. These benefits appear to be separate from its mild symptomatic dopaminergic effect, because all subjects were receiving the symptomatic benefit from concurrent levodopa therapy. Rasagiline is currently undergoing a large clinical trial to test its neuroprotective effect. Selegiline, but not rasagiline, is metabolized to L-amphetamine and methamphetamine. Zydis selegiline is a formulation of selegiline that dissolves under the tongue and is absorbed via the oral mucosa directly into the blood stream, thereby by-passing the gut and liver and not generating the amphetamines. All these drugs can reduce the severity of motor fluctuations with levodopa. They are more likely, however, to increase dyskinesias.

Nondopaminergic agents (Table 66-5) are useful to treat both motor and nonmotor symptoms in PD. Antimuscarinic drugs have been widely used since the 1950s, but these are much less effective than the dopaminergic agents, including amantadine. Because of sensitivity to memory impairment and hallucinations in the elderly population, antimuscarinics should be avoided in patients older than 70 years. They can reduce the severity of tremor. Antihistaminics have mild anticholinergic properties and can serve as alternatives to antimuscarinic drugs in the elderly population. Another alternative agent is the tricyclic amitriptyline, because it also has anticholinergic properties. Muscle relaxants can sometimes reduce muscle tightness and cramping, and might help overcome "off" dystonia and peak-dose dystonia that patients on levodopa therapy sometimes develop. Coenzyme Q10 is currently being tested in a controlled clinical trial to determine if it has protective effects.

Because depression is common in patients with PD, and often precedes the motor symptoms of PD, this mood disturbance needs to be vigorously addressed; the tricyclics and selective serotonin reuptake inhibitors are useful antidepressants. It is not certain if one type of antidepressant class of compounds is superior to the other in treating the depression accompanying PD. If insomnia is a problem for the patient, using an antidepressant that is also a soporific can be doubly advantageous, such as amitriptyline given at bedtime.

The benzodiazepines can reduce anxiety and stress, and therefore are useful to decrease parkinsonian tremor that is exacerbated by stress. Diazepam is usually well tolerated and does not exacerbate parkinsonian symptoms. Lorazepam and alprazolam are other agents in this class of drugs.

Psychosis induced by levodopa and the dopamine agonists can usually be controlled by quetiapine and clozapine without worsening the parkinsonism. Other antipsychotic agents are more likely to worsen the parkinsonism, therefore, they should be avoided. Clozapine is more effective than quetiapine, but because clozapine treatment requires weekly white blood cell counts, quetiapine should be tried first. Both drugs are soporific and bedtime dosing is helpful to also overcome insomnia. Patients with PD often have no problem falling asleep, but they have frequent arousals (sleep fragmentation), and if they have trouble returning to sleep, a short-acting drug, such as zolpidem, taken when trying to fall back to sleep can be helpful. REM sleep behavior disorder (RBD) is common in patients with PD and MSA, and often precedes the appearance of these disorders. RBD is manifested by patients moving about while dreaming, i.e., acting out their dreams. Normally, dreaming in REM sleep is associated with muscle paralysis, and this is lost in RBD. The bed-partner is the one usually disturbed by the patient with RBD; the patients are unaware that they are thrashing and kicking in their dreams. Clonazepam taken at bedtime is an effective drug to overcome this problem. Excessive daytime sleepiness, due either to disrupted nighttime sleep or to drowsiness from medications (dopamine agonists and levodopa), can sometimes lessen with the administration of modafinil.

Cognitive decline and frank dementia can be helped to a limited and modest degree with centrally active cholinesterase inhibitors, donepezil and rivastigmine, which have undergone clinical trials in PDD. Orthostatic hypotension in PD can be owing to the disease (or to MSA) or to the medications, particularly levodopa, dopamine agonists, and antidepressants. Fludrocortisone and midodrine can overcome this symptom to some extent. Restless legs syndrome (RLS) is common in patients with PD, possibly induced by levodopa therapy, which is known to augment symptoms in patients with RLS (without concomitant PD) who had been placed on levodopa or dopamine agonists. Since RLS can cause nocturnal sleep disturbance, this symptom is worth enquiring about when patients complain of a restless sleep at night. The typical symptom of RLS is an uncomfortable feeling of discomfort in the legs (like crawling ants under the skin) late in the evening or night. Walking around relieves this symptom. Bedtime dose of a dopamine agonist or, if that fails, an opioid can provide effective relief.

TABLE 66-5

Nondopaminergic Agents

Parkinsonian motor symptoms:
   Antimuscarinics: trihexyphenidyl, benztropine
   Antihistaminics: diphenhydramine, orphenadrine
   Antiglutamatergics (to reduce dyskinesia): amantadine
   Muscle relaxants: cyclobenzaprine, diazepam, baclofen
   Mitochondrial enhancer: coenzyme Q10

Nonmotor symptom control:
   Depression: selective serotonin reuptake inhibitors, tricyclics, ECT
   Anxiety: benzodiazepines—diazepam, lorazepam, alprazolam
   Psychosis (hallucinations, paranoïa): clozapine, quetiapine
   Insomnia: quetiapine, zolpidem, benzodiazepine, mirtazapine
   REM sleep behavior disorder: clonazepam
   Excessive daytime sleepiness: modafinil
   Dementia: donepezil (Aricept), rivastigmine (Exelon)
   Orthostasis: fludrocortisone, midodrine (ProAmatine)
   Restless legs: dopamine agonists, opioids (e.g., propoxyphene, oxycodone)

MOTOR COMPLICATIONS OF LEVODOPA THERAPY

Many patients on levodopa therapy develop motor complications (Table 66-6). Response fluctuations usually begin as mild wearing-off, which can be defined as when an adequate dose of levodopa does not last at least 4 hours. Typically, in the first couple of years of treatment, there is a long-duration response so that the timing of doses of levodopa is not important. Over time, the long-duration

TABLE 66-6

Pattern of Development of Response Fluctuations, Dyskinesias, and Other Complications

Dyskinesias (chorea and dystonia)
    Peak-dose dyskinesias
    Diphasic dyskinesias (beginning and end-of-dose dyskinesias)

Fluctuations
    Wearing off
    Delayed "ons"
    Dose failures
    Sudden, unpredictable "offs" (on-offs)
    Early morning "off" dystonia
    "Off" dystonia during day

Alertness
    Drowsy from a dose of levodopa
    Reverse sleep–wake cycle

Behavioral and cognitive
    Vivid dreams
    Benign hallucinations
    Malignant hallucinations
    Delusions
    Paranoia
    Confusion
    Dementia

response becomes lost, and only a short-duration response occurs; patients then develop the wearing-off phenomenon. The "offs" tend to be mild at first, but over time become deeper with more severe parkinsonism; simultaneously, the duration of the "on" response becomes shorter. Eventually, some patients develop random, sudden "offs" in which the deep state of parkinsonism develops over minutes rather than tens of minutes, and they are less predictable in terms of timing with the dosings of levodopa. Many patients who develop response fluctuations also develop abnormal involuntary movements, i.e., dyskinesias.

Treatment of the "Wearing-off" Phenomenon

The wearing-off phenomenon, when mild, may be ameliorated slightly with the addition of selegiline (introduced as 5 mg daily, and increasing to 5 mg twice daily, as necessary) or rasagiline (0.5 mg once daily, and increasing to 1 mg once daily, as necessary). Both MAO-B inhibitors potentiate the action of levodopa, and their introduction can induce confusion and psychosis, particularly in the elderly. A lower dose of levodopa may be necessary. Sinemet CR (continuous release carbidopa/levodopa) can also be effective in patients with mild wearing-off, and one can gradually switch from standard carbidopa/levodopa to Sinemet CR, or use the combination of both immediate- and extended-release formulations. Because it takes more than an hour for a dose of continuous release medication to become effective, most patients will require simultaneous standard immediate release carbidopa/levodopa to obtain an adequate response. One can attempt to utilize standard carbidopa/levodopa alone, giving the doses closer together, but ultimately most patients will develop progressively shorter durations of effectiveness from these doses. So, patients could require as many as six or more doses per day, and then, eventually, dose failures owing to poor gastric emptying often develop.

Dopamine agonists, which have a longer biological half-life than levodopa, can also be used in combination with standard Sinemet or Sinemet CR. The addition of a dopamine agonist tends to make the "off" state less severe when used in combination with carbidopa/levodopa. The addition of a dopamine agonist, however, will likely increase dyskinesias; in this situation the dosage of levodopa would need to be reduced. Rotigotine (Neupro Dermal Patch) might be helpful to reduce mild wearing-off.

Catechol-O-methyltransferase inhibitors (COMTIs) have been found useful for treating wearing-off. Because of entacapone's short half-life, it is given with each dose of carbidopa/levodopa, and is equally effective as rasagiline in reducing the amount of daily "off" time. For those patients who have "offs" at a specific time of day, entacapone can be strategically given just with the dosage of carbidopa/levodopa that precedes this "off" period. Tolcapone, which can be tried if entacapone fails to provide adequate benefit, is taken three times daily with biweekly monitoring of the patient's liver enzymes. A typical dose of tolcapone is to start with 100 mg tid with an increase to 200 mg tid possible should the need arise. Because tolcapone can increase dyskinesia, using 50 mg tid on initiation of treatment for patients who already have dyskinesia is a more gentle approach. The COMTIs are effective immediately, which is a distinct advantage.

Behavioral or sensory "offs" can also occur as do motor "offs," often in the absence of any motor "off," which means a return of parkinsonism. Behavioral and sensory "offs" tend not to be easily recognized, because visibly the treating physician sees no motor changes. Behavioral/sensory "offs" can consist of pain, akathisia, depression, anxiety, dysphoria, or panic, and usually a mixture of more than one of these. Sensory "offs," like dystonic "offs" are extremely poorly tolerated. It is often the presence of one of these sensory and behavioral phenomena, more so than motoric parkinsonian or dystonic "offs," that drives the patient to take more and more levodopa, turning the patient into a "levodopa junkie."

Treatment of Levodopa-Induced Dyskinesias

Levodopa-induced dyskinesias are involuntary movements and occur in two major forms—chorea and dystonia. Choreic movements are irregular, purposeless, nonrhythmic, abrupt, rapid, unsustained movements that seem to flow from one body part to another. Dystonic movements are more sustained, twisting contractions. Many patients probably have a combination of chorea and dystonia. Dystonia is a more serious problem than chorea, because it is usually more disabling.

Peak dose dyskinesias occur when the plasma concentration of levodopa is at its peak, and the brain concentration of levodopa and dopamine is too high. Reducing the individual dosage can resolve this problem. But the patient may need to take more frequent doses at this lower amount, because reducing the amount of an individual dose also reduces the duration of benefit. More frequent dosing of levodopa tends to lead to delayed "ons" and dose failures eventually. A simple approach is to add amantadine, which suppresses the severity of dyskinesias, possibly because of its antiglutamatergic action. Start with a dose of 100 mg bid and increase up to 200 mg bid if necessary. Another approach is to add or substitute higher doses of a dopamine agonist while lowering the dose of carbidopa/levodopa. Dopamine agonists are less likely to cause dyskinesias, and therefore can usually be used in this situation quite safely. But adding the agonist while maintaining the levodopa dosage will usually result in an increase of dyskinesias. If lowering the dose of levodopa results in more severe "off" states, then the agonists become more important. Sinemet CR is not helpful, because there is the danger of increased dyskinesias at the end of the day as the blood levels become sustained from frequent dosings of this extended release form of levodopa. Once dyskinesias appear with Sinemet CR, they last for considerable duration of time because of the slow decay in the plasma levels. In some patients, peak-dose chorea and dystonia occur at subtherapeutic doses of levodopa, and lowering the dose will render a patient even more parkinsonian. Such patients are candidates for deep brain stimulation (see below under Surgical Therapy).

Diphasic dyskinesias are dyskinesias that occur at the beginning and end of dose, not during the time of peak plasma and brain levels of levodopa. They tend to affect particularly the legs with a mixture of chorea and dystonia. Because the mechanism is unclear, treatment of diphasic dyskinesias is difficult. In this situation one should use a dopamine agonist as the major pharmacologic agent with supplementary levodopa.

"Off" dystonia and painful "off" cramps could be listed in both "dyskinesias" and "fluctuations," because these dystonias occur when the patient is "off." Dystonic spasms, therefore, can be either a sign of levodopa overdosage, as in peak-dose dyskinesias, or occur when the plasma level of levodopa is low, such as in early morning before the first dose of levodopa. "Off" dystonia can occur anytime when the patient is "off," but most commonly in the early morning hours upon awakening and when the last prebedtime dose of levodopa has worn off. Usually, the dystonia manifests as painful foot and toe cramps, which are relieved when the next dose of levodopa begins to take effect. Preventing "offs" is the best way to control these painful dystonias. An effective treatment is to use a dopamine agonist as the major pharmacologic agent with supplementary levodopa. Here the rotigotine dermal patch can be particularly useful, by keeping a steady pharmacokinetic level of active drug throughout the day and night. Baclofen has also been reported to benefit some patients. Bedtime Sinemet CR may be useful to prevent early-morning dystonia, but some patients need to set the alarm early to take a dose of standard carbidopa/levodopa in the middle of the night and then fall back to sleep and awaken at their usual time.

TREATMENT OF NONMOTOR FEATURES

In addition to PD having motor features, a number of nonmotor problems can also occur as complications from dopaminergic therapy. Mental changes of psychosis, confusion, agitation, hallucinations, paranoid delusions, and excessive sleeping are probably related to activation of dopamine receptors in nonstriatal regions, particularly the cortical and limbic structures. Elderly patients and patients with concomitant dementia are extremely sensitive to small doses of levodopa. But all patients with PD, regardless of age, can develop psychosis if they take excess amounts of levodopa as a means to overcome "off" periods.

If hallucinations are mild and not frightening, treatment can begin with the addition of quetiapine, starting with 25 mg at bedtime. The dose should be increased steadily until the hallucinations are brought under control. If quetiapine is ineffective or if the hallucinations are frightening, clozapine needs to be initiated instead of quetiapine, because clozapine is more effective than quetiapine. The

reason clozapine is not the first drug of choice in dopaminergic-induced hallucinations is because clozapine causes agranulocytosis in approximately 1% to 2% of patients. Patients must have their blood counts monitored weekly for this potential complication, and then discontinue the drug if leukopenia develops. Both quetiapine and clozapine often cause drowsiness, so bedtime dosing is recommended. Quetiapine can cause falling, and clozapine, seizures with high doses. The dosing regimen for clozapine is similar to that for quetiapine. Quetiapine and clozapine are labeled as "atypical antipsychotics," because they usually do not induce or worsen parkinsonism, and therefore can be used in patients with PD. Of the other antipsychotic drugs, olanzapine ranks next as being "atypical," but this drug will worsen PD, most atypical are quetiapine and clozapine. All the other antipsychotics, regardless if they had in the past been considered to by "atypical," actually are not, for they all worsen PD.

If the psychosis is severe or if the patient is in an acute delirious state, hospitalization is necessary, with immediate initiation of high doses of clozapine, and some reduction in anti-PD medication. These medications could even be withdrawn temporarily to overcome the psychosis, but this should be done stepwise over a 3-day period to avoid the neuroleptic-malignant-like syndrome that could occur with sudden withdrawal of levodopa.

If hallucinations are mild and the patient can be treated as an outpatient, and the patient does not respond well or tolerate quetiapine and clozapine, then the physician needs to reduce one or more anti-PD medication. All antiparkinson drugs have the potential to induce psychosis, so the less efficacious drugs should be withdrawn first. Accordingly, COMT inhibitors, MAO-B inhibitors, amantadine, anticholinergics, and dopamine agonists should be withdrawn in that order, reserving levodopa as the most effective agent.

An altered sleep–wake cycle of drowsiness during the daytime, particularly after a dose of levodopa, and insomnia at night are fairly common in the elderly and often accompany cognitive decline. If a patient becomes drowsy after each dose of medication, reducing the dose may correct this problem. If the patient is generally drowsy during the daytime and remains awake at night, this makes it difficult for the care provider. It is important to get the patient onto a sleep–wake schedule that fits with the rest of the household. Efforts must be made to stimulate the patient physically and mentally during the daytime and force him/her to remain awake, otherwise he/she would not be able to sleep at night. At night, the patient should then be drowsy enough to be able to sleep. If this fails, it may be necessary to use stimulants in the morning and sedatives at night in order to reverse the altered state. This should be done in addition to prodding the patient to remain awake during the day. Modafinil can sometimes be helpful to overcome daytime drowsiness, and one or two doses in the morning and early afternoon can be employed. Drugs such as methylphenidate and amphetamine are usually also well tolerated by patients with PD, and can be considered if modafinil fails. A 10-mg dose of either of these two drugs, repeated once if necessary, may be helpful. To encourage sleep at night, a hypnotic may be necessary in addition to using daytime stimulants. It should be noted that strong sedatives, such as barbiturates, are poorly tolerated by patients with PD. Milder hypnotics, such as benzodiazepines and zolpidem, are usually taken without difficulty. Taking advantage of the soporific effects of quetiapine, clozapine, mirtazapine, and amitriptyline is a good strategy if a patient can also benefit from their other actions of antipsychotic or antidepressant.

Orthostatic hypotension can be caused by levodopa, dopamine agonists, and other drugs taken by the patient, such as tricyclic antidepressants. These other drugs should be discontinued. If orthostatic hypotension remains, it can sometimes be managed by using support stockings, NaCl, midodrine (ProAamatine), and fluodrocortisone (Florinef), but often the dose of levodopa needs to be reduced.

Constipation is common in PD. It may be further aggravated by anticholinergics. Besides changing dietary habits by increasing intake of more fiber and dried fruits, polypropylene glycol (Mira-Lax) can be effective. For those who have bloating because of suppression of peristalsis when they are "off", keeping them "on" with levodopa is beneficial.

Depression is a common nonmotor symptom in PD, probably related to the reduction of all brain monoamines in this disease. Depression must be treated, not only for its own sake, but because its presence interferes with a good response to antiparkinson drugs. It often responds to selective serotonin reuptake inhibitors, such as fluoxetine, sertraline, and paroxetine, and those agents like nefazodone and venlafaxine that inhibit both serotonin and norepinephrine. It is not clear if any antidepressant is superior to any other, including the tricyclic antidepressants, such as amitriptyline, nortriptyline, and protriptyline. Because of its anticholinergic and soporific effects, amitriptyline can be useful for these properties as well as for its antidepressant effect. Protriptyline, on the other hand, has no anticholinergic effect and can be useful when this property is not needed. Electroconvulsive therapy can be effective in patients with severe, intractable depression, and it can sometimes transiently improve the motor symptoms of PD as well.

Impulse control problems have emerged in the last few years as a complication of dopamine agonists that had not been recognized previously. These consist of behavioral changes such as compulsive gambling, shopping, and eating, and hypersexual desire. Although infrequent, these can be serious problems. So far, the only remedy has been to reduce the dose of the dopamine agonists or stop them altogether.

SURGICAL THERAPY

Surgery for PD is becoming increasingly available as deep brain stimulation has evolved along with a better understanding of basal ganglia physiology. Stereotaxic DBS has replaced the older technique of lesioning in the brain, because the latter is more risky for inducing permanent neurological deficits. With DBS, the parameters of stimulation, such as voltage and frequency, can be adjusted, and the electrodes could be removed if required. However, DBS is more costly, and frequent adjustments of the stimulators are usually needed. The location of the stereotaxic target is a major factor that needs to be individualized for each patient. The subthalamic nucleus (STN) is the favored target, because this reduces bradykinesia and tremor, allowing for a reduction of levodopa dosage, thus reducing the severity of dyskinesias as well. The internal segment of the globus pallidus is a more satisfactory target for controlling choreic and dystonic dyskinesias, which in turn would allow a higher dose of levodopa to be used to control the major symptoms of PD. The thalamus, particularly the ventral intermediate nucleus, is the target most successful for controlling tremor, but this target does not eliminate bradykinesia as well as the STN does, so the thalamus is not a preferred choice today. Surgical procedures for patients with PD are best performed at specialty centers with an experienced team of a neurosurgeon, neurophysiologist to monitor the target during the operative procedure, and neurologist to program the stimulators. The patient needs close follow-up to adjust the stimulator settings to their optimum. Patients with cognitive decline should not have DBS, because cognition can be further impaired. Also, intractable symptoms of freezing of gait, loss of postural reflexes, and falling are not benefited. The major benefits of STN stimulation are those symptoms that respond to levodopa. Adverse effects include surgical complications, mechanical problems with the stimulator and leads to the electrodes, infections attacking any of the inserted hardware, and neurologic and behavioral changes. The latter include troubles with speech, dystonic postures, depression, suicide attempts, and cognitive decline. The best candidates are younger patients who can tolerate the penetration of the brain and who have uncontrollable motor fluctuations and dyskinesias.

FURTHER READING

Chaudhuri KR, Healy DG, Schapira AH. Non-motor symptoms of Parkinson's disease: diagnosis and management. *Lancet Neurol.* 2006;5:235–245.

Deuschl G, Schade-Brittinger C, Krack P, et al. German Parkinson's Study Group, Neurostimulation Section. A randomized trial of deep-brain stimulation for Parkinson's disease. *N Engl J Med.* 2006;355(9):896–908.

Klein C, Schlossmacher MG. Parkinson's disease, 10 years after its genetic revolution: multiple clues to a complex disorder. *Neurology.* 2007;69(22):2093–2104.

Krack P, Batir A, Van Blercom N, et al. Five-year follow-up of bilateral stimulation of the subthalamic nucleus in advanced Parkinson's disease. *N Engl J Med.* 2003;349(20):1925–1934.

Langston JW. The Parkinson's complex: parkinsonism is just the tip of the iceberg. *Ann Neurol.* 2006;59(4):591–596.

Miyasaki JM, Shannon K, Voon V, et al. Quality Standards Subcommittee of the American Academy of Neurology. Practice Parameter: evaluation and treatment of depression, psychosis, and dementia in Parkinson's disease (an evidence-based review): report of the Quality Standards Subcommittee of the American Academy of Neurology. *Neurology.* 2006;66(7):996–1002.

Pahwa R, Factor SA, Lyons KE, et al. Quality Standards Subcommittee of the American Academy of Neurology. Practice Parameter: treatment of Parkinson's disease with motor fluctuations and dyskinesia (an evidence-based review): report of the Quality Standards Subcommittee of the American Academy of Neurology. *Neurology.* 2006;66(7):983–995.

Palhagen S, Heinonen E, Hagglund J, et al. Swedish Parkinson's Study Group. Selegiline slows the progression of the symptoms of Parkinson's disease. *Neurology.* 200625;66(8):1200–1206.

Weintraub D, Siderowf AD, Potenza MN, et al. Association of dopamine agonist use with impulse control disorders in Parkinson's disease. *Arch Neurol.* 2006;63(7):969–973.

Other Neurodegenerative Disorders

Victor Valcour ■ *Bruce Miller*

Alzheimer's disease (AD) is the most common neurodegenerative disorder encountered by the practicing geriatrician. However, a sizable number of other neurodegenerative diseases will be seen in a typical practice, rendering a working knowledge of these disorders critical for practicing clinicians. This chapter provides an overview of the more common neurodegenerative disorders with emphasis on those that influence behavior and cognition early in the course. We begin by reviewing the clinical approach to neurodegenerative cognitive disorders and then review the clinical presentation, epidemiology, and examination findings of the more common neurodegenerative syndromes. We attempt to link clinical presentation to anatomy and neuropathology whenever possible.

APPROACH TO THE EVALUATION OF COGNITIVE AND BEHAVIORAL DISORDERS IN ADULTS

The evaluation of neurodegenerative disorders is multifaceted, requiring careful attention to the cognitive, behavioral, and motor history combined with a comprehensive neurological examination aiming to identify the brain regions involved. Isolating anatomy in patients who present with slowly progressive neurodegenerative disorders greatly facilitates the determination of the correct diagnosis.

Emphasis should be placed on the earliest presenting symptoms, whether cognitive, behavioral, or motor in origin. These early features may be critical to the identification of the pathological substrate. As diseases progress, signs and symptoms merge between the different disorders, making diagnosis more difficult. An early history of repeated falls, for example, should warrant concern for progressive supranuclear palsy (PSP) or vascular dementia; although most dementias are associated with basal ganglia involvement later in their disease course, diminishing the value of falls for diagnosis. Likewise, inappropriate behavior and disinhibition are commonly seen in patients with advanced dementia syndromes regardless of disease etiology. However, when these findings are a prominent presenting feature in the relative absence of amnestic symptoms, frontotemporal dementia (FTD) should be considered more likely.

Cognitive histories should be comprehensive, and must include evaluation of memory, language, visuospatial function, executive functioning, and attention (Table 67-1). The comprehensive history should probe for autonomic symptoms and sleep patterns, with emphasis on symptoms associated with disorders of rapid eye movement (REM) sleep behavior and sleep apneas.

The assessment of behavioral symptoms can be particularly helpful and sometimes critical in non-Alzheimer's neurodegenerative disorders. FTD is the most common cause of dementia in patients younger than the age of 60 years. Behavioral symptoms or personality change are commonly the presenting symptoms of this disorder (see Table 67-4 and discussion later in this chapter). When evaluating for change in personality, the clinician should gain an understanding of premorbid character. The emergence of predominant behavior and personality changes in the absence of episodic memory and perceptual complaints localizes disease to the frontal or anterior temporal lobes.

The neurological examination is a critical component to the assessment of neurodegenerative disorders and typically confirms the clinical impression obtained from the history. The motor examination identifies both pyramidal and extrapyramidal signs as well as features characteristic of FTD, dementia with Lewy bodies (DLB), corticobasal degeneration (CBD), and PSP. Examination of cranial nerves includes an assessment of eye movements and range of gaze. Abnormalities in vertical gaze with a preserved oculocephalic reflex are a characteristic finding in PSP while horizontal gaze abnormalities are more typical of CBD. Abnormalities in saccadic eye movements can be seen in a number of neurodegenerative disorders. Saccadic movements are tested by asking the patient to focus on an object in front of them (such as a pen tip held by the examiner) then to quickly refocus on an item in their peripheral field (such as the examiner's finger) while the examiner watches carefully for saccadic latency (delay in initiation of movement), incomplete saccades (gaze

TABLE 67-1

Assessment of Major Cognitive Domains in Neurodegenerative Disorders

Memory: repetitive statements, misplacing items, missed appointment or medications, recalling recent/remote events

Language: speech fluency, comprehension, reading, writing, articulation, word-finding, content of speech, output, spelling

Visuospatial: getting lost, driving, object perception, completing household repairs, parking

Executive: planning, flexibility/rigidity in thinking, organization, multistep tasks

Motor: gait, falls, tremor, dysphagia, weakness, handwriting, coordination

Autonomic: light-headedness, bowel/bladder function, impotence, hypotension

palsy), and interrupted/jerky saccadic movement. Saccades should be tested in all four directions. Ocular pursuit is tested by having the patient track an object, such as the examiner's finger, in both horizontal and vertical directions.

The combination of cognitive history, behavioral history, and neurological examination, with emphasis on earliest symptoms should sufficiently narrow the diagnosis to few neurodegenerative disorders, and in many cases, identify one highly suggested disease. Confirmatory imaging and laboratory work, and standard laboratory tests to exclude treatable etiologies of cognitive impairment can then be completed (Table 67-2).

DISORDERS ASSOCIATED WITH ALPHA-SYNUCLEIN DEPOSITION

Dementia with Lewy Bodies

The precise role of alpha-synuclein in health and disease is not fully understood. High concentrations of alpha-synuclein in synaptic regions suggest a role in synaptic plasticity. In DLB, alpha-synuclein accumulates with the brain stem, basal ganglia, and cortex, resulting in a progressive neurodegenerative cognitive and motor disorder. The prevalence of DLB is still uncertain and the coassociation of Lewy body and AD pathology is extremely common in aging dementia populations. Indeed, even with classical AD associated with

TABLE 67-2

Some Laboratory Tests Commonly Used in the Evaluation of Cognitive Disorders

Chemistries, including liver function tests and renal function tests

Complete blood count

Vitamin B-12

Homocysteine

Methylmalonic Acid

Syphilis serology

HIV

Thyroid function

apolipoprotein E4 genotype, more than 50% of subjects show Lewy bodies and genetic disorders that predispose to Lewy bodies often show the coassociation of Aβ-42. Based on autopsy studies, DLB is widely underdiagnosed.

The reported mean onset of disease is 75 years of age with a range from 50 to 80 years and a slight predominance of DLB in men compared to women. The clinical and pathological overlap between DLB and AD and with Parkinson disease dementia (PDD) is well-recognized, resulting in some diagnostic challenges. Accurate diagnosis has clinical implications as patients with DLB compared to AD tend to have more favorable responses to cholinesterase inhibitors and patients with DLB often have sensitivity to neuroleptic medications.

The characteristic features of DLB are cognitive impairment with profound fluctuation, spontaneous Parkinsonism, and visual hallucinations that are often complex. The typical neuropsychological profile differs somewhat from that of AD. DLB often involves greater parietal-occipital lobe deficits and lesser medial temporal lobe deficits. This manifests in testing as better performance on episodic memory tasks, and recognition memory when compared to AD patients. Invariably, memory becomes impaired over time. Combined cortical and subcortical deficits are common and deficits in attention are a core feature of the disease.

The degree of cognitive fluctuation can be so profound as to effect MMSE scores up to 50% from day-to-day. However, eliciting a history of fluctuation can be difficult and is inconsistently reported by caregivers. Clinicians should consider several different approaches, including questions focused on marked alteration in attention, staring spells, daytime sleepiness, and episodes of incoherent speech. On occasion, the fluctuation can be so severe as to result in emergency room evaluation for a transient ischemic attack (TIA) or delirium. Several structured scales exist to assist in assessment of fluctuation, including the One Day Fluctuation Assessment Scale and the Clinical Assessment of Fluctuation.

A common feature of neurodegenerative disorders with alpha-synuclein pathology is REM sleep behavior disorder (RBD) defined as vivid and often frightening dreams that are frequently acted out verbally or motorically. RBD occurs in 85% of DLB cases, compared to 15% of Parkinson disease patients and 60% of patients with multiple system atrophy (MSA). In the DLB diagnostic criteria, RBD is considered a suggestive feature. Autonomic dysfunction is also common and can be profound. When REM behavior occurs in association with severe autonomic symptoms, MSA rather than DLB should be considered. Unexplained loss of consciousness is another supportive feature of DLB and significant depressive symptoms occur in up to 40% of cases.

About two-thirds of DLB cases will exhibit visual hallucinations, misperceptions or, less frequently, delusional misidentification. When delusional misidentification, such as mistaking the spouse, friend, or relative as an impostor, occurs as the first symptoms of a dementia, DLB is highly likely. The visual hallucinations of DLB can be vivid, with distinct colors and the inclusion of human figures and animals. In contrast to the hallucinations sometimes seen with more advanced AD, visual hallucinations occur early in DLB. In one pathology-based study, visual hallucinations corresponded to a greater number of Lewy bodies in the anterior/inferior temporal lobes and to larger deficits in acetylcholine. Visual hallucinations often respond to boosting brain acetylcholine with cholinesterase inhibitors.

Spontaneous Parkinsonism is a hallmark feature of DLB, occurring in up to 70% of cases. Common findings include bradykinesia, axial greater than appendicular rigidity, postural instability, slowed response times, and hypomimia. In contrast to Parkinson's disease, the Parkinsonism of DLB is typically bilateral and less frequently includes tremor. Parkinsonism rarely occurs in isolation as an early finding in DLB although early features of the cognitive syndrome are commonly overlooked. Response to levodopa treatment is less frequent than the response seen in Parkinson disease; however, efficacy data may be biased. Clinicians are more likely to avoid such drugs in DLB patients for fear of adverse effects or aggravations of hallucinations.

Parkinsonism contributes substantially to the disability in DLB and alters the clinical course. Mean survival among postmortem confirmed cases of DLB is 10 years, with a rate of disability at approximately 10% per year, often exceeding that of Parkinson's disease. Cases of rapid progression to death in 1 to 2 years have been described. Risk factors for higher mortality include older age, hallucinations, greater degrees of fluctuation, and neuroleptic sensitivity.

Diagnostic criteria for DLB assist in identification of disease and are particularly useful for research purposes (Table 67-3). In the revised schema, core features include prominent fluctuation, recurrent visual hallucinations, and spontaneous features of Parkinsonism such as rigidity, bradykinesia, and hypomimia. Supportive and suggestive features are also defined. To meet diagnostic criteria for probable disease, two core features or the combination of one core feature and one supportive feature are required. If suggestive features are present in the absence of core features, the term possible DLB is used.

The pathological hallmark of DLB is the presence of neuronal spherical intracytoplasmic inclusions of alpha synuclein, termed Lewy bodies (Figure 67-1). The Lewy bodies seen in DLB are very similar in appearance to those that are seen in Parkinson's disease; however in DLB, the distribution extends beyond the substantia

---

TABLE 67-3

McKeith Criteria for DLB*

Central features
Progressive cognitive decline with functional impairment
Prominent memory impairment may not occur early but is usually evident with progression
Deficits in attention, executive functioning, and visuospatial ability may be prominent early

Core features
Fluctuating cognition with prominent variations in attention and alertness
Recurrent visual hallucinations
Spontaneous parkinsonism

Suggestive features
REM sleep behavior disorder
Neuroleptic sensitivity
Low dopamine transporter uptake in the basal ganglia (SPECT, PET)

Supportive features
Repeated falls
Transient, unexplained loss of consciousness
Severe autonomic dysfunction
Systematized delusions
Depression
Hallucinations in nonvisual modalities
Relative preservation of medial temporal lobe structures on CT/MRI
Generalized low uptake on SPECT/PET with reduced occipital activity
Abnormal MIBG scintigraphy
Prominent slow wave activity on EEG with temporal lobe transient sharp waves

*Probable DLB requires two core features or one core feature and at least one suggestive feature. Possible DLB requires one or more suggestive features. Probable DLB should not be based on suggestive features alone. MIBG (metiaodobenzyl guanidine scintigraphy).
Adapted from McKeith IG, Dickson DW, Lowe J, et al. Diagnosis and management of dementia with Lewy bodies: third report of the DLB Consortium. Neurology. 65(12):1863–1872, 2005.

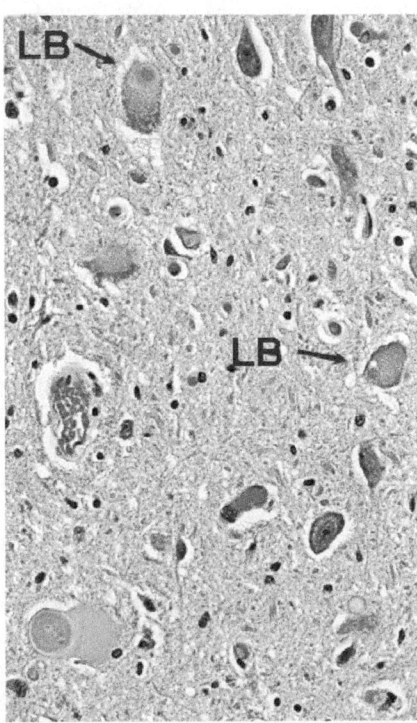 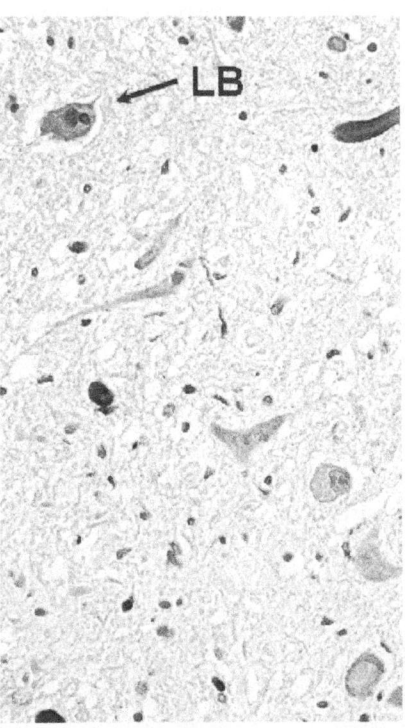

FIGURE 67-1. Lewy bodies (LB) seen with hematoxylin and eosin staining (left) and alpha-synuclein staining (right).

nigra and locus coeruleus to involve the neocortex and limbic system. Cortical Lewy bodies lack the typical dense core with pale halo appearance that is seen in Parkinson's disease. Other intraneuronal aggregates of alpha-synuclein (Lewy neurites), cortical senile plaques, sparse tau pathology, and spongiform change are all described in DLB. MSA is the third neurodegenerative disease with prominent alpha-synuclein pathology.

Currently, imaging studies do not add substantially to differentiating DLB from other neurodegenerative disorders and are only included as supportive in diagnostic criteria. Structural MRI often identifies less atrophy of the medial temporal lobes in cohorts of DLB compared to AD and variably identifies greater atrophy in the basal ganglia structures and the dorsal midbrain. In group studies, single photon emission computed tomography (SPECT) with ^{99m}Tc-hexamethylpropyleneamine oxime (HMPAO) tends to show decreased regional cortical brain activity in parietal-occipital regions of DLB compared to AD patients. DLB patients exhibit decreased dopamine transport in the putamen and caudate by dopaminergic SPECT and decreased postganglionic sympathetic cardiac innervation by I-metaiodobenzyl guanindine (MIBG) SPECT imaging. However, the modest performance characteristics of these tests limit their clinical utility.

The clinical course of DLB is often faster than that seen in AD and a drop of 4 to 5 points on MMSE per year is not unusual. Patients with DLB should be treated with cholinesterase inhibitors. Often this results in responses that exceed those seen in AD. Social stimulation and physical exercise to maximize balance and strength should be recommended. Symptomatic treatment with levodopa can be used, if indicated for Parkinsonian symptoms. Patients should be advised to avoid anticholinergic medications, including many common over-the-counter cold remedies. RBD, if severe, can be treated with clonazepam. Atypical neuroleptic medications should be cautiously considered only if intolerable behavioral disturbances emerge.

Parkinson's Disease Dementia

The temporal relationship between the onset of dementia and the development of Parkinsonism is the primary clinical feature distinguishing DLB from Parkinson's disease dementia (PDD). In PDD, cognitive deterioration occurs in well-established Parkinson disease, typically a decade after motor systems are identified. In contrast, research criteria for DLB require cognitive symptoms that predate Parkinsonism by 12 months; although this "1 year rule" is often difficult to apply in the clinical setting. This temporal distinction is debatably arbitrary as many believe the two disorders represent different points in the spectrum of the same disease and abnormalities in alpha-synuclein accumulation underlie both disorders.

Approximately one-third of older Parkinson's disease patients will develop sufficient cognitive symptoms during the course of their illness to impair function. In pure PDD, the prominent findings include motor and psychomotor slowing, decreased response times, and alterations in concentration and attention. The recognition that medications used to treat Parkinson's disease can affect cognition and the understanding that, as a result of age, a substantial number of Parkinson's patients will develop concurrent AD results in a scenario where cognitive symptoms in this population can be multifactorial. Possible predictors for dementia in Parkinson disease include older

age at onset of motor symptoms, bradykinesia, nontremor prominent PD, bilateral onset of motor signs, and declining response to levodopa. Depression and visual hallucinations may increase risk as well. Patients with DLB typically exhibit a faster clinical decline than do patients with PDD.

Multiple System Atrophy

MSA is a sporadic disease marked by degeneration of multiple neurological systems and resulting in relentlessly progressive clinical course. Death typically occurs within 6 to 10 years with an estimated 10-year survival of 40%. Relatively infrequent, the incidence is estimated to be 0.6/100 000 person-years or between 1.86 and 4.9 per 100 000 population. The incidence increases to 6/100 000 person-years among patients older than 50 years of age. The mean age of onset is 54 years. While currently speculated to have a combination of environmental and genetic predispositions, neither has been definitively established. Epidemiological studies suggest a potential risk associated with exposure to pesticides. MSA is about three times more frequent in men than women and limited epidemiological data suggest that it may be less frequent among smokers.

The term MSA was first used in 1969 and encompasses diseases previously labeled as striatonigral degeneration (now termed MSA-P for Parkinsonism), Shy-Drager syndrome, and olivopontocerebellar degeneration (now termed MSA-C for cerebellar). The MSA subtypes are indicative of the predominant neurological component involved. Patients with prominent orthostatic features tend to have decreased survival. Several derivations of diagnostic consensus statements exist with mixed sensitivity.

The presenting symptoms of MSA are variable and include cerebellar findings, autonomic failure, pyramidal findings, and Parkinsonism. Parkinsonism (MSA-P) is prominent in the majority of cases (80%) with cerebellar symptoms (MSA-C) more prominent in about 20% of cases. The more common presenting Parkinsonian features are akinesia, rigidity, and postural (rather than rest) tremor. Autonomic symptoms precede motor symptoms in most cases. Gait instability is common; but falls occur less frequently in early stages than in PSP. In early stages, MSA can mimic Parkinson's disease but more symptoms evolve within 5 years. Gait ataxia, limb kinetic ataxia, and dysarthria are the more frequent presenting symptoms in patients with cerebellar-dominant MSA. The dysarthria caused by cerebellar dysfunction has a characteristic appearance of jerky, intermittently explosive, and slurred output often associated with poor separation of syllables.

Autonomic symptoms include orthostasis, erectile dysfunction, constipation, and urinary incontinence. While orthostasis is common, syncope occurs infrequently. Diagnostic criteria for the orthostatic component of MSA require a 30 mm Hg drop in systolic blood pressure; although in practice, a 20 mm Hg drop in systolic blood pressure or 10 mm Hg drop in diastolic blood pressure is thought to be significant in the absence of appropriate increased heart rate. Occurrence of symptoms suggestive of MSA in an individual younger than 30 years of age or in an individual with a family history of similar disease should raise suspicion for alternative diagnoses.

Most MSA patients complain of sleep problems, commonly sleep fragmentation (53%), early waking (33%), and insomnia (20%). As with other synucleinopathies, RBD is common, occurring in up to 60% of MSA patients. Nocturnal stridor and obstructive sleep

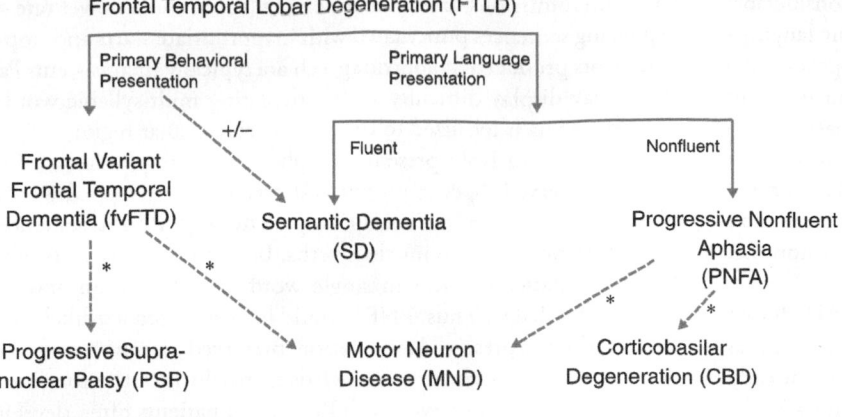

FIGURE 67-2. Frontotemporal lobar degeneration and potential associations to other neurodegenerative syndromes.

apnea are also frequent in MSA. Stridor is associated with decreased survival and risk of sudden death.

Brain MRI changes occur in some patients but lack sensitivity and specificity for definitive diagnosis. These findings include hypointensity and atrophy of the putamen on T2-weighted images with a slit-like marginal hypointensity just lateral to the putamen on axial images. A characteristic "hot cross bun" sign has been described in the pons and middle cerebral peduncles thought to be caused by degenerative changes in pontocerebellar fibers. This finding lacks sensitivity and is sometimes seen in Parkinson's disease limiting specificity. Atrophy of the brainstem, middle cerebellar peduncles, and cerebellum may also be seen. Volumetric analyses of the striatum and brainstem where atrophy is very severe in MSA-P but not simple Parkinson's disease demonstrate some promise in discriminating these two disorders. Electromyography (EMG) abnormalities at the anal sphincter can be seen in MSA; although the clinical utility for distinguishing MSA from Parkinson's disease in early stages of disease has not been established.

The hallmark pathology of MSA is cell loss, gliosis, and glial inclusions in multiple neurological systems including the spinal cord and cortex. Prominent abnormalities are also seen in the basal ganglia, substantia nigra, and olivopontocerebellar pathways, as suggested by the terminology, with anatomy reflecting symptoms. On gross inspection, the putamen is shrunken and displays a green-grey discoloration that can appear cribiform when disease is severe. As with DLB and PD, there is an accumulation of alpha-synuclein as half-moon-, oval-, or conical-shaped argyrophilic glial cytoplasmic inclusions.

Treatment is generally symptomatic with about one-third of patients responding to levodopa in the early stages of the disease. Patients should be encouraged to sleep in a lateral decubitus rather than supine position to minimize airway obstruction. Use of positive airway pressure devices should be considered. Invasive means of controlling stridor and apneas have included tracheotomy, but should be approached cautiously within the full context of ethical and quality of life considerations. RBD may respond to low-dose clonazepam at night. Labile blood pressures may develop and should raise concern when symptomatic. Avoiding alcohol, heaving meals, or straining at micturition and defecation is recommended. Elastic stockings and elevating the head of the bed may provide some relief. Pharmacological approaches designed to increase sympathetic

tone (midodrine) or volume expansion (fludrocortisone) may be required. Patients with MSA-C tend to maintain function for a longer period of time than those with MSA-P.

NEURODEGENERATIVE DISORDERS ASSOCIATED WITH TAU, PROGRANULIN, OR TDP-43 PATHOLOGY

Frontotemporal Lobar Degeneration Syndromes

Frontotemporal lobar degeneration (FTLD) includes the clinical syndromes of frontal variant FTD (FTD), progressive nonfluent aphasia (PNFA), and semantic dementia (SD). Recent evidence indicates that FTLD is closely related to several other neurodegenerative disorders: CBD, PSP, and motor neuron disease (Figure 67-2).

The core anatomical feature of FTLD is the focal, often asymmetric cortical degeneration of frontal and anterior temporal regions with general sparing of posterior cortical structures. The resultant brain atrophy can be severe, sometimes described as "knife-edge" and the brain can weigh as low as 750 g (Figure 67-3). Patients present with a primary behavioral or language deficit that typically corresponds to the region of greatest brain atrophy and dysfunction. Patients presenting with primary behavioral deficits most commonly

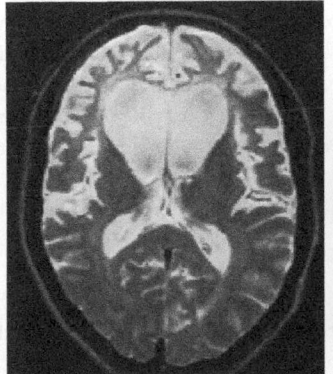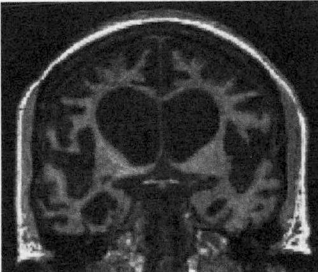

FIGURE 67-3. T2-weighted axial (right) and T1-weighted coronal (left) brain MRI in a 59 yr-old woman with pathology-confirmed Pick's disease.

have frontal variant FTLD (FTD). This can overlap considerably with the two syndromes that present with predominant language deficits, PNFA, and semantic dementia (SD), with the greatest degree of overlap seen with SD. FTD and SD each encompass about 40% of the FTLD syndromes. The neuropathological basis for approximately one-half of these diseases is the abnormal accumulation of tau protein. Recent scientific advances have identified abnormalities in the manufacture of progranulin and TDP-43 protein and are likely to clarify the pathology in the vast majority of non-Tau cases.

Many FTLD patients are misdiagnosed as having AD during life. In addition to changes in personality and behavior, features that should alert physicians to the possibility of FTLD include early abnormalities in social conduct, loss of sympathy and empathy for others, repetitive motor behaviors, or hyperorality. When cognitive testing is completed, suspicion should be raised when abnormalities in executive functioning occur in the absence of prominent amnestic complaints or cognitive features localizing to posterior structures, such as problems with calculations and visuospatial tasks. FTLD is the most common form of dementia, in patients younger than 60 years of age.

Patients who present with isolated language symptoms that exist for at least 2 years in the initial stages of cognitive decline are termed to have primary progressive aphasia (PPA). As a group, patients with PPA have left greater than right atrophy of the perisylvian region, the anterior temporal lobes, and the basal ganglia. Inferior parietal lobule atrophy has also been described. When carefully dissected based on anatomic, symptomatic, and linguistic parameters, it is evident that PPA may be the presenting syndrome of a number of diseases, most frequently PNFA, SD, and a logopenic variant of AD. As the syndrome progresses, patients presenting with PNFA may also develop CBD or PSP and less commonly amyotrophic lateral sclerosis (ALS). Thus, careful attention to the development of motor symptoms is necessary. The emergence of artistic behavior has been described in some patients with primary language difficulty.

Efforts to distinguish various PPA syndromes from each other may have clinical ramifications. Based on apolipoprotein epsilon 4 expression in clinical studies, it appears likely that the logopenic variety of PPA is a language presentation of AD; although pathological confirmation of this correlation is lacking. As the term implies, these patients have decreased speech output. They typically have slow speech with impaired syntactic comprehension and naming. The logopenic variety is associated with short-term phonological memory deficits. These patients exhibit profound echoic memory deficits manifested as forgetting portions of longer phrases during repetition tasks. As pathological studies become available, if confirmed to be AD in etiology, these patients may be amenable to treatment with cholinesterase inhibitors or emerging amyloid-directed treatment strategies.

Progressive Nonfluent Aphasia

Patients with progressive nonfluent aphasia (PNFA) typically have apraxic, labored speech with errors in grammar, and difficulty with more complex syntax. Speech apraxia is the inability to produce speech caused by difficulty in programming the sensorimotor commands for the positioning and movement of muscles used to produce speech. This leads to difficulty with initiation of speech, sound sub-

stitutions, omissions, transpositions of syllables, and a slower rate of expressing sentences punctuated with inappropriate starts and stops. The errors produced in apraxic speech are typically inconsistent. Patients may display difficulty with articulating multisyllabic words. Speech apraxia is localized to the left anterior insular region.

Anomia is variably present and phonemic paraphasias are frequently observed. Speech output is decreased and dropped words, often articles such as "the" occur. In patients with PNFA, sentences tend to be richer for nouns than verbs. In contrast to patients with SD, these patients maintain single word comprehension and semantic knowledge. Thus, PNFA would be considered less likely in a patient who has preserved articulation, preserved grammar, and who displays deficits in semantic knowledge. Insight into the condition can be exquisitely preserved with PNFA and patients often develop depression. Behavioral problems are uncommon in early stages of disease.

The evaluation of brain MRIs in 11 patients with PNFA using voxel-based morphometry (VBM) identified regions of atrophy that are typically asymmetrically left-dominant with preferential involvement of the inferior frontal lobe, the insular region, and the caudate. Hypometabolism of the left frontal region can be observed on FDG positron emission tomography (PET).

Semantic Dementia

In contrast to patients with PNFA, patients with SD have fluent speech that is grammatically accurate; but they exhibit the hallmark loss of semantic knowledge. Semantic memory is encyclopedic knowledge of people, objects, facts, and words. Unlike episodic memory, these types of memories are not linked to time or space. Thus, these patients typically do not remember where or when they learned these facts. Eventually individuals lose all knowledge about the fact or word and exhibit features of a multimodality agnosia. Therefore, even when they are provided with the name of the object, the object is not recognized. Early in the disease patients are often aware of word-finding difficulties, but are unaware of comprehension difficulties. Semantic paraphasias are frequent, with supraordinate substitutions of words and common use of nonspecific grouping words such as "stuff" and "things." Repetition and prosody are preserved as is syntax and verb recognition.

Patients with SD also display surface dyslexia manifest by difficulty pronouncing irregularly spelled words, such as "gnat," "heir," or "pint," when pronunciation does not follow standard phonological rules. On neuropsychological testing, patients with SD have difficulty with category fluency and confrontational naming, particularly with low-frequency words. Often, SD patients have difficulty naming famous people. In contrast to AD, many SD patients have greater deficits for remote compared to recent memory, when memory deficits become involved.

Of all the PPA syndromes, SD has the greatest propensity to include behavioral problems, which are included as supportive evidence in diagnostic criteria. As with FTD, the behavioral issues seen with SD often involve hyperorality, disinhibition, and aberrant motor behavior. Diagnostic criteria include behaviors such as loss of sympathy and empathy, narrowed preoccupations, and parsimony (excessive frugality, stinginess). Rigidity in thinking can be striking. SD patients can develop compulsions and have been described to have visual hypervigilance, such as recognizing a subtle hair out of place on an examiner or a coin on the street. They may exhibit difficulty in the interpretation of emotions, particularly negative emotions such as sadness, anger, and fear. Emergence of behavioral symptoms correlates with duration of illness, but can also be an early finding. The presence of early behavioral issues in a patient with a PPA syndrome should alert to the possibility of SD.

Anatomic studies may explain why SD patients often exhibit behavioral abnormalities. While SD usually begins in the anterior left temporal lobe, it typically spreads anteriorly to involve the frontal regions. Eventually it spreads to the right medial frontal lobe, the right orbitofrontal lobes, and the right insular region, areas associated with behaviors such as disinhibition and apathy. The absence of behavioral problems in the logopenic variety of PPA and in PNFA may be caused by the general sparing of these same structures in those diseases.

Patients with SD often have ubiquitin-positive, tau-negative inclusions at autopsy. Up to one-third of the patients will also have amyloid plaques. In one small series, the presence of plaques was associated with the absence of behavioral symptoms. The existing overlap in neuropathologies may be because of a lack of sensitivity in our diagnostic acumen, whereby some patients with PPA syndromes have AD.

Frontal Variant Frontotemporal Dementia

FTD presents with the insidious onset of change in personality and inappropriate behaviors. The mean age of onset is in the mid-fifties. Most commonly, symptoms include disinhibition, poor impulse control, loss of sympathy or empathy for others, and socially inappropriate behaviors (Table 67-4). Patients can develop stereotyped behaviors, defined as repetitive, invariant behaviors that lack purpose. Examples include counting, pacing, organizing, or the repetitive use of catch phrases. Socially inappropriate activities can include shoplifting and other criminal behavior, public urination, offensive

TABLE 67-4

Behavior Symptoms Seen in Frontal Variant FTD

Antisocial behavior
Apathy
Change in beliefs (hyperreligiosity, change in attitude)
Cravings (sweets, weight gain)
Criminal behavior (theft, assault, public urination)
Delusions
Disinhibition
Euphoria (inappropriate jocularity)
Hyperorality (oral exploratory behavior in late disease)
Hypersexuality (offensive statements, masturbation)
Impotence and decreased sexual drive
Impulsivity
Loss of empathy (coldness, self-centered)
Obsessive-compulsive behavior
Perseverative behavior
Poor insight
Stereotyped behavior (counting, pacing, repetitive use of catch phrases)

speech, and public masturbation. Perseveration is common. Cravings for sweets are often observed. When associated with the decreased sense of satiety that can occur, large and unhealthy amounts of weight gain result. Hyperorality and oral exploratory behavior can occur.

Patients with FTD are often misdiagnosed as having psychiatric illness. Delusions can occur, often with bizarre or grandiose overtones. Patients exhibit lack of empathy and can have a cold, blunted affect. When the anterior cingulate and medial frontal lobes are involved, apathy can be particularly prominent. Some patients undergo large changes in their beliefs and attitudes, including religious sentiments. In contrast to AD, depression is uncommon in FTD.

Neuropsychological testing demonstrates abnormalities in executive functioning and working memory with general sparing of visuospatial skills and verbal memory. Consequently, the MMSE score can be quite high even among patients with marked functional disability. FTD patients also display problems with set-shifting, concept formation, and abstract reasoning. They may demonstrate disinhibition, impulsivity, and poor judgment during testing. These behaviors can falsely lower verbal memory scores. When closely scrutinized, poor scores on such tests are accompanied by frequent intrusions of novel words and endorsement words that were not part of the original list learned (false positives on recognition testing).

Behavioral symptoms are a common late finding in most dementia syndromes. Thus the emergence of behavior and personality symptoms in a patient with well-established dementia should be looked upon with caution when considering a change in diagnosis to FTD. The importance of first symptom (often the presenting symptom) in the evaluation of patients with neurodegenerative disorders cannot be overstated.

Patients with FTD will typically have profound, usually bilateral, frontal lobe atrophy, with symptom presentation that matches anatomy. Thus, patients with right greater than left frontal atrophy have more severe behavioral symptoms. Stages of atrophy have been described with the earliest stage involving only mild atrophy of the orbital and superior medial frontal lobes and hippocampus. As disease progresses, the anterior frontal and temporal cortices and basal ganglia are increasingly involved. The severity of atrophy increases as disease advances. SPECT and FDG PET techniques have been used to differentiate FTD from AD with PET receiving Food and Drug Administration (FDA) approval for this indication. Both SPECT and FDG PET demonstrate bilateral frontal hypometabolism/perfusion in patients with FTD.

Pick's Disease

Pick's disease is a pathologic diagnosis and occurs in the minority of clinical cases presenting with signs and symptoms of FTLD. First described in 1892 by a German neurologist, Arnold Pick, the pathological hallmark of Pick's disease are agyrophilic cellular inclusions known as Pick bodies and swollen achromatic neurons termed Pick cells. This is invariably associated with loss of large pyramidal neurons, resulting in a spongiform histological appearance with selective atrophy of the frontal and anterior temporal lobes. Pick bodies are localized to the limbic cortex, paralimbic cortex, and predominantly the ventral aspect of the temporal lobe. The pre- and postcentral gyri are notably spared. The largest concentration of Pick bodies is found in the hippocampus and amygdala. Pick bodies are composed of randomly arranged tau filaments. In AD, tau pathology (neurofibrillary tangles) can spare the dentate gyrus; however, in Pick's disease, this region is heavily involved.

Other FTLD Neuropathologies

FTLD is associated with tau pathology in about half of cases. The tau gene product has six isoforms, half of which result in three microtubule binding repeats (3Rt) and the other half result in four microtubule repeats (4Rt). Pick's disease is usually associated with 3Rt although there is great variability. PSP and CBD, in contrast, are associated with 4Rt. The clinical features and neuropathology of PSP and CBD are described later in this chapter.

Among FTLD cases that do not stain for tau protein, the histopathology will typically indicate a variable pattern of neuronal loss and gliosis without characteristic features such as neurofibrillary tangles or Pick bodies. Historically, the term dementia lacking distinctive histology (DLDH) has been employed; however, new discoveries led to the reclassification of many such cases to FTLD-U (ubiquitin) and it remains unclear if the DLDH diagnostic classification will be archived. FTLD-U may account for over 50% of all nontau FTLD cases. In these cases, neuronal inclusion bodies with prominent ubiquitin staining are seen in the absence of other characteristic features. These inclusion bodies stain negative for tau and are localized throughout the neocortex and within anterior horn cells. This pathology has been identified in patients with and without concurrent motor neuron disease.

A number of proteins have been identified within the ubiquitin inclusions of FTLD-U including neurofilament, p62, HSP70, and, most recently, the TAR DNA-binding protein (TDP)-43. It is estimated that TDP-43 captures up to 50% of the cases previously categorized as DLDH. Additionally, there is overlap between FTLD and hippocampal sclerosis. In a series published from the Mayo clinic, 70% of patients with hippocampal sclerosis showed FTD pathology.

Our understanding of the genetics of FTLD is evolving. Early research revealed a mutation in the microtubule-associated protein tau (MAPT) found in patients with a familial form of FTD associated with Parkinson's disease (FTDP-17). Recently, a mutation in the progranulin (PRGN) gene (close to the tau gene) was identified and four differing classes of mutation have since been described. This mutation appears to account for up to 11% of sporadic and 25% of familial FTD cases. To date, the pathological characterization of this mutation and the clinical phenotype remain incompletely described. In one series of two families, the onset of disease ranged from 35 to 75 years and the clinical findings were variable, including language impairment, behavioral changes, or Parkinsonism.

Other isolated cases of FTLD-related mutations have been described, including valosin-containing protein gene (VCP) and charged multivesicular body protein 2B (CHMP 2B). Patients with the VCP mutation develop a rare disease with inclusion body myopathy, early Paget's disease of bone, and FTD (IBM-PDB-FTD).

Treatment of FTLD

Treatment approaches for FTLD are generally aimed at symptom management as there are no solid data regarding disease-modifying approaches. Potential treatments that deserve further investigation include memantine and possibly lithium, based on small nonran-
domized trials or tissue models. Selective serotonin reuptake inhibitor (SSRI) medications may be beneficial for behavioral symptoms, including carbohydrate craving and compulsions. If delusions are problematic, atypical neuroleptics can be considered. There is no theoretical basis for the use of cholinesterase inhibitors, which could aggravate agitation. Attention to caregiver issues is important as the stressors often differ from those seen in typical AD. The different social and behavioral issues presented to FTLD compared to AD caregivers and the younger age of both patients and caregivers in FTLD can result in a feeling of isolation in typical AD support groups.

AMYOTROPHIC LATERAL SCLEROSIS (ALS, LOU GEHRIG'S DISEASE)

ALS was first identified in 1869 by the French neurologist, Jean-Martin Charcot who described a progressive neurodegenerative disease with mixed upper and lower motor neuron signs and symptoms. The disease's name is derived from myelin pallor identified in the lateral aspects of the spinal cord representing axonal degeneration from upper motor neurons as they descend to the limbs. In the United States, the disease is best known as Lou Gehrig's disease, named after the famous baseball player who died of the disease in 1941. It occurs with an incidence of approximately 1 to 2/100 000 patients each year with a nearly 2:1 male to female predominance. About 5000 people develop ALS annually. As with FTLD, peak incidence occurs in mid-life; however disease can be seen in advancing ages.

ALS in inherited in an autosomal-dominant manner in up to 10% of cases. In 2% of cases, risk has been traced to a mutation in Cu/Zn superoxide dismutase 1 (SOD1). Most cases are sporadic and the etiology remains elusive. Intriguing small clusters of cases have been described, including a recent case report involving three amateur Italian soccer players. The neuropathology of ALS includes neuronal cytoplasmic inclusions of a ubiquinated protein, most commonly seen in lower motor neurons. Recently, these inclusions were shown to contain the 43-kDa TAR DNA-binding protein (TDP-43), the same protein that has been identified in FTLD-U. This finding is consistent with a previously recognized association between ALS and FTD. In this study, TDP-43 immunoreactivity was seen in all case of sporadic ALS and all cases of familial ALS that did not have an identified SOD1 mutation.

Patients with ALS typically present with complaints of weakness in one or more limbs, resulting in unexplained tripping or dropping of items. Clumsy fine finger movements lead to difficulty with tasks such as buttoning clothes or writing. Patients often complain of cramping. Bulbar symptoms such as speech slurring, difficulties with swallowing, and hoarseness occur in many patients. Bulbar symptoms are presenting symptoms in about 25% of cases and more commonly occur in older patients. Patients may complain of difficulty chewing or swallowing. Up to 45% of patient will develop a pseudobulbar affect characterized by episodes of uncontrolled laughter or crying, often in inappropriate settings. Many patients have symptoms of a slowly progressive behavioral syndrome including apathy, lack of insight, and loss of empathy.

The neurological examination identifies both upper and lower motor neuron abnormalities. Muscle atrophy is seen, usually in the hands and often noted at the thenar or hypothenar eminence. Fasciculations and weakness are noted as lower motor neuron findings.

Upper motor neuron findings include mild spasticity, hyperreflexia, and abnormal plantar responses. EMG is diagnostic for ALS.

The clinical course is relentlessly progressive with only a 50% survival at 3 years. Mild muscle weakness progresses to inability to walk, difficulty with speaking, and dysphagia. The FDA has approved riluzole for treatment of ALS, which extends survival and delays the need for ventilation support. Treatment is otherwise directed at symptom control and quality of life. This is best achieved with a multidisciplinary approach, including ancillary services such as physical therapy, respiratory therapy, and social work.

CORTICOBASAL DEGENERATION

Asymmetric Parkinsonism, often with a rigid akinetic arm, is the prototypical finding in CBD. Many patients will report a "useless" arm or gait problems. While speech or behavior concerns less often represent the first symptoms, this presentation does occur and CBD should be considered in any patient with symptoms consistent with FTLD, particularly those who present with PNFA. Occasionally, language will be the only symptom for the first 2 years of the disease, rendering CBD a potential diagnosis in patients presenting with PPA syndromes.

The mean age of disease onset for CBD is in the mid-sixties. A few series suggest that women may be more commonly affected than men. CBD is generally sporadic in occurrence; although familial cases have been described in association with both tau and progranulin mutations. Many cases are not correctly diagnosed during life.

In one series, common early findings included unilateral limb rigidity (75%), bradykinesia (71%), and postural instability (45%). The asymmetric Parkinsonism of CBD can be severe and usually involves the upper more than the lower extremities. As disease progresses, other limbs become involved. Severe upper limb dystonia typically results in internal contracture of the limb with the fingers clutching the thumb with flexion at the wrist. An alien limb phenomenon sometimes occurs with the limb not only levitating, but often hooking onto clothing or grabbing other body parts and behaving as if it were no longer under the control of the patient. On occasion, the alien limb will conflict with actions of the other hand. Simple levitation of the lower extremity is described as well, but is less specific to CBD. Focal reflex myoclonus that is typically present first in the fingers, then in the hand, can be elicited with distal percussion.

Concurrent cortical sensory loss is seen without deficits to peripheral sensory modalities. This is discriminated by testing for agraphesthesia, agnosia, or problems with two-point discrimination. Bilateral limb apraxia is common and apraxia of opening or closing the eyes can occur. Close evaluation of eye movements will often reveal saccadic latency with normal velocity, often in the horizontal plane. Supranuclear vertical gaze palsy can occur.

In one study, dementia was identified in about one-third of patients with CBD; however, this likely underestimates the frequency of cognitive features as nearly all had some manifestation of impairment in higher cortical function. Typically, cognitive impairment manifests with abnormalities that localize to the frontal and parietal lobes such as difficulty in executive functioning, calculations, and visuospatial ability. Behavioral problems are common and include depression (nearly three-quarters of patients), apathy, irritability, and agitation. Falls and dysphasia are also common. Constipation and urinary urgency occur.

CBD shares many neuropathological abnormalities with FTD and PSP, suggesting the possibility that they represent a spectrum of similar diseases linked by underlying tau pathology. Ballooned neurons throughout the neocortex associated with neuronal loss and astrocytic tau-staining plaques are the diagnostic histological features of CBD. Unlike Pick's disease, the distribution of ballooned neurons is extensive and involves both the primary sensory and motor regions. Pick bodies are absent. Commonly, the superior frontal lobes and the parietal lobes are most heavily affected and are reflected in patterns of neuropsychological testing. Secondary degeneration of the corticospinal tracts occurs. Grossly, asymmetric atrophy of the parasagittal superior frontal gyrus and superior parietal lobule are common, with relative sparing of the temporal and occipital regions.

The treatment of CBD is symptomatic as disease-altering therapies are not known. Levodopa is beneficial in the minority of patients. Muscle relaxants and physical therapy with range of motion exercises can be useful. Clonazepam may be instituted for myoclonus. There is no theoretical basis for the use of cholinesterase inhibitors in this disease.

PROGRESSIVE SUPRANUCLEAR PALSY

PSP, also referred to as Steele-Richardson-Olszewski syndrome, is a progressive neurodegenerative disease with prominent extrapyramidal motor findings and supranuclear ocular abnormalities. Patients with PSP present to both movement disorder clinics, resulting from motor abnormalities, and behavioral clinics, resulting from cognitive or psychiatric symptoms. The frequency of PSP in the general population is around 1 in 100 000, increasing to 7 in 100 000 among people older than 55 years. Diagnosis typically occurs in the sixth to seventh decade of life. There are only a few published reports of familial cases, suggesting that an autosomal dominant gene plays only a small role in the disease.

The initial descriptions of PSP emphasized abnormalities in movement with nearly all patients exhibiting early gait abnormalities and 60% presenting with falls as the first manifestation of disease. Patients often pivot with turns and have a tendency to fall backwards. Increased tone (axial more than appendicular) and dysphagia (affecting 46% in the first 5 years) are other common motor findings while bradykinesia is seen in only about a quarter of autopsy-proven cases. Spastic dysarthria results in slurred speech. Ultimately patients become mute.

Eye movement abnormalities are the hallmark feature of the disease, with vertical supranuclear palsy a critical feature for diagnosis. While vertical gaze palsy can be upward or downward, downward gaze palsy has greater specificity for PSP. The oculocephalic reflex for vertical movement is preserved early in disease despite the vertical gaze palsy. Square wave jerks, and both latency and hypometria of eye movements are often seen, typically greater with command (saccadic movements) rather than to pursuit. A decreased blink rate and a furred brow can be noticed when interviewing the patient.

The cognitive features of disease are variably described in early disease but are often present when sought. They are commonly identified if neuropsychological testing is completed, but are often overlooked in the clinical setting of frequent falls and prominent movement abnormalities. The pattern of cognitive dysfunction is characterized by abnormalities localizing to the frontal and temporal lobes and subcortical structures. Thus, slowing of cognitive performance and below expectation performance in verbal fluency and executive functioning tasks are often documented, typically with retained verbal and visual memory performance. Behavioral symptoms of apathy, compulsions, perseveration, and utilization behavior are common features. This pattern of neuropsychological and behavioral findings is similar to what is seen in FTD, consistent with the findings that the pathology of the two entities overlap considerably.

Treatment of PSP is focused on control of symptoms. Occupational therapy to address speech and visual limitations can be successful. Prevention of falls is critical, but often challenging as impulsivity and lack of insight can limit the effectiveness of therapeutic interventions. Levodopa can be helpful in some patients with PSP, but eventually loses its efficacy. Survival is between 6 and 10 years at the time of diagnosis.

SPINOCEREBELLAR ATAXIA SYNDROMES

Spinocerebellar ataxias (SCA) are a heterogeneous group of disorders with prominent, progressive cerebellar involvement. The current classification system corresponds to the order to which gene mutations have been identified. A comprehensive database, including scientific reviews and a listing of laboratories, that will evaluate for mutations is available at www.geneclinics.org.

The SCA genetic mutations that have been identified to date are associated with expansion of repeated trinucleotides and are inherited in an autosomal-dominant manner. However, penetrance can vary greatly. The length of the polyglutamine repeat appears to be a major determinant of age for disease onset in an inverse manner. Genetic analyses are estimated to identify only 40% to 60% of familial and less than 25% of sporadic cases. The likelihood that a gene mutation will be identified decreases with older age (>40 years of age). The prevalence of SCAs is between 1 and 4/100 000 with variation by region caused by founder effects [SCA 2 (Cuba), SCA 3 (Azores), and SCA 10 (Mexico)]. These disorders most commonly present in the third decade of life with some presenting in youth; however, the range of age extends into older ages for many SCAs.

Phenotypic overlap is common in SCA syndromes; however, progressive cerebellar disability often presenting early in disease is a common feature. SCA syndromes often affect the noncerebellar portions of the nervous system, particularly as the disease progresses, with neuropathology identified in the brainstem, basal ganglia structures, and cortex. Such clinical symptoms include oculomotor features (SCA 1, 2, 3), retinopathy (SCA 7), seizures (SCA 10, 17), peripheral neuropathy (SCA 1, 2, 3, 4, 8, 18, 25), or cognitive and behavioral deterioration (SCA 17, dentatorubrul pallidoluysian atrophy [DRPLA]).

Other neurodegenerative disorders should be considered in patients with progressive cerebellar dysfunction, including mitochondrial diseases, Huntington's disease, leukodystrophies, Frederick's ataxia, MSA, prion disease, and the premutation associated with Fragile X syndrome. Paraneoplastic processes should be considered in patients presenting with subacute cerebellar dysfunction. While scattered clinical reports describe benefits for some SCAs, treatment is generally aimed at symptom management, physical and occupational therapy, and genetic counseling.

CONCLUDING REMARKS ON NON-ALZHEIMER'S DISEASE NEURODEGENERATIVE DISORDERS

Scientific advances have remarkably altered our understanding of non-AD neurodegenerative disorders in the past decade; however, large gaps remain. In many cases, neuropathology can now be identified facilitating the process of linking disease syndromes by pathological substrate and supporting an in-depth understanding of disease. In such cases, clinical researchers can than begin to accurately describe the clinical presentation of pathology-proven cases to provide clinicians with clues to neuropathology. When combined with emerging noninvasive diagnostic tools, such as PET imaging with novel ligands such as the Pittsburg compound B, which binds to the protein in amyloid plaques, we can achieve the ultimate goal of promoting pathology-driven treatment approaches.

FURTHER READING

Belfor N, Amici S, Boxer AL, et al. Clinical and neuropsychological features of corticobasal degeneration. *Mech Ageing Dev.* 2006;127(2):203–207.

Gorno-Tempini ML, Dronkers NF, Rankin KP, et al. Cognition and anatomy in three variants of primary progressive aphasia. *Ann Neurol.* 2004;55(3):335–346.

Kumar-Singh S, Van Broeckhoven C. Frontotemporal lobar degeneration: current concepts in the light of recent advances. *Brain Pathol.* 2007;17(1):104–114.

Lippa C, Duda J, Grossman M, et al. for the DLB/PDD Working Group. DLB and PDD boundary issues: diagnosis, treatment, molecular pathology, and biomarkers. *Neurology.* 2007;68(11):812–819.

Manto MU. The wide spectrum of spinocerebellar ataxias (SCAs). *Cerebellum.* 2005;4(1):2–6.

McKeith IG, Dickson DW, Lowe J, et al. Diagnosis and management of dementia with Lewy bodies: third report of the DLB Consortium. *Neurology.* 2005;65(12):1863–1872.

Miller B, Hou C. Portraits of artists: emergence of visual creativity in dementia. *Arch Neurol.* 2004;61(6):842–844.

Rampello L, Butta V, Raffaele R, et al. Progressive supranuclear palsy: a systematic review. *Neurobiol Dis.* 2005;20(2):179–186.

Rosen H, Allison S, Schauer G, Gorno-Tempini M, Weiner M, Miller B. Neuroanatomical correlates of behavioral disorders in dementia. *Brain.* 2005;128(Pt 11):2612–2625.

Traumatic Brain Injury

Sterling C. Johnson

Traumatic brain injury (TBI) is common among the elderly mainly through the association with falls. TBI in the elderly presents special issues for the clinician to consider in the management of these patients, including a higher risk of poor recovery and physiatric and neuropsychiatric comorbidity. This chapter will review the epidemiology of TBI, mechanisms of injury, features on brain imaging, cognitive and psychosocial outcomes, and postacute management, with particular attention to research and practice with geriatric patients.

EPIDEMIOLOGY

TBI is craniocerebral trauma associated with decreased consciousness, cognitive or neurologic abnormalities, skull fracture, or intracranial injuries. More than 5.3 million Americans have disabilities related to TBI. With approximately 1.6 million incident cases per year, resulting in 1.2 million emergency department visits, 290 000 hospitalizations, and 51 000 deaths, TBI is a common cause of morbidity and mortality. Approximately 444 per 100 000 population are evaluated in the emergency department for TBI. In adults older than 85 years, the incidence of TBI-related emergency department evaluations is more than double the average (see Figures 68-1 and 68-2 for age breakdown). The annual incidence of hospitalized trauma or death is 101 per 100 000. The incidence of mild TBI across all ages (not resulting in hospitalization or death) is 392 TBI-related emergency department visits per 100 000 population.

The economic consequences of TBI are alarming. The annual costs of TBI are approximately $60 billion. Estimates for the cost of lifetime care for a person with severe TBI range between $600 000 and $1.9 million. These estimates do not account for lost income of the patients, and time and lost earnings of family members who care for patients with TBI. Nor do these include the opportunities these victims have lost and their reduced quality of life.

ETIOLOGY

The older patient may have a number of age-related existing risk factors or conditions that increase vulnerability to both TBI and unfavorable outcome. These risks include, but are not limited to, cognitive slowing/impairment, orthopedic/mobility issues, visual acuity, balance difficulty, and neurologic and cardiac diseases. These issues increase risk for falls and motor vehicle accidents, the two major etiologies for TBI. These and other etiologies of injury are categorized in Figure 68-3. It is estimated that 28% to 36% of TBI are because of falls, followed by motor vehicle accidents (19%), being struck by or against an object (18%), assault (10%), others (11%), and unknown (10%). In the general population, men are twice as likely to sustain TBI as women, although this difference is negligible in the elderly.

Falls

Up to 60% of nursing home residents fall each year as do one-third of older adults in the community. It is significant to note that approximately half of all TBIs in the elderly are attributable to falls. In addition to being the most common mechanism of TBI, falls produce the highest rates of TBI hospital admissions. People aged 65 to 74 years are three times as likely to be hospitalized from a TBI-related fall as young adults. The risk ratio doubles for ages 75 to 84 years (7.6 relative risk) and doubles again for adults 85 years and older (16.4 relative risk). Similarly, the length of hospital stay is longer in the older adult, and the likelihood of being discharged to home is poorer. In adults older than 85 years, the rate of home discharge is 30%; for patients aged 75 to 84 years, the rate is 41%; at age 65 to 74 years, the rate is 54%; and in adults younger than 65 years the rate of home discharge is 86%.

Because falls account for the majority of injuries, an assessment of risk for falls is an important part of the geriatric evaluation. Risks

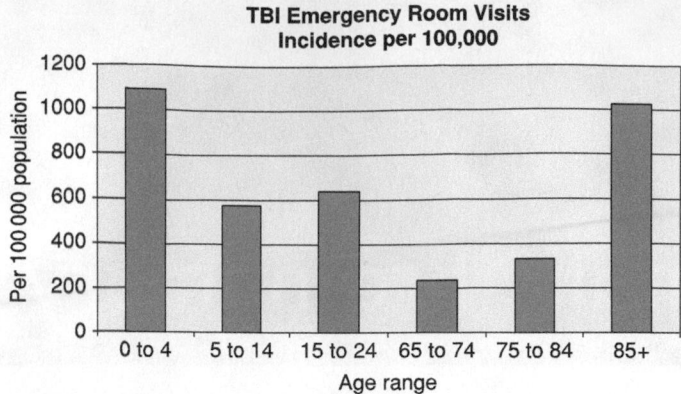

FIGURE 68-1. Incidence of emergency department (ER) visits with a TBI-related ICD-9 coding. Adults older than 85 yrs have high rates of TBI-related ER visits as do infants and toddlers. *(This graph is derived from Jager TE, Weiss HB, Coben JH, Pepe PE. Traumatic brain injuries evaluated in U.S. emergency departments, 1992–1994. Acad Emerg Med. 2000;7(2):134–140.)*

such as the following should be considered: chronic neurological, sensorial, or musculoskeletal disease; alcohol use, acute illness and delirium, episodic hypotension, and potential medication effects; as well as activity and environmental risks. More on falls and their prevention are covered in another chapter.

Motor Vehicle Accident

Motor vehicle accident is the most common etiology of injury in the young adult. In the older adult, motor vehicle accident is the second most frequent etiology. Collisions are often at lower speeds but may still result in substantial injury. Key risks for motor vehicle accident include visual acuity and cognitive ability, particularly in the domain of attention—distractibility.

Mortality

TBI-related death in the elderly is increasing. A CDC study found that for persons older than 75 years, the rate is 60 per 100 000 population. Falls, firearms, and motor vehicles were the most common causes. In hospitalized elderly patients with TBI, the rate of mortal-

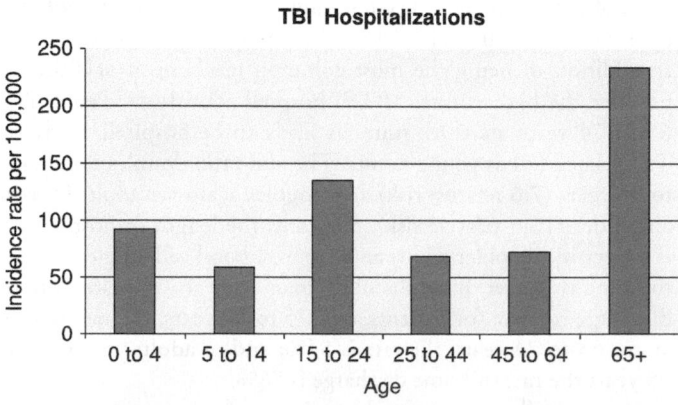

FIGURE 68-2. When TBI occurs in the older adult, it results in greater rate of hospitalization compared with other age groups.

Incidence by injury type

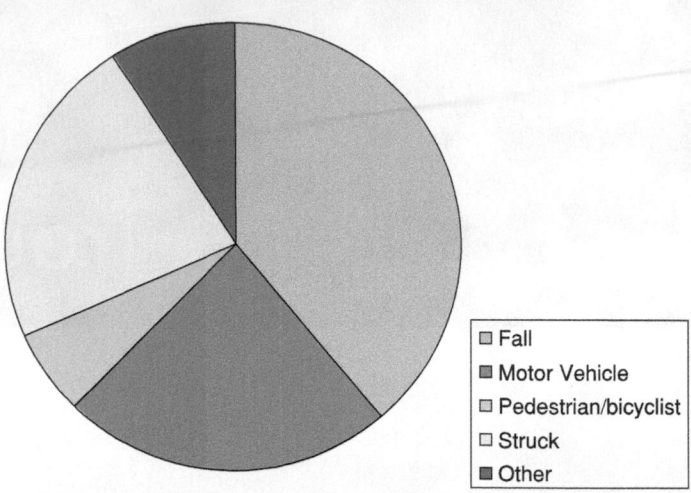

- ☐ Fall
- ■ Motor Vehicle
- ☐ Pedestrian/bicyclist
- ☐ Struck
- ■ Other

FIGURE 68-3. Etiology of TBI. Falls and motor vehicle accidents are the main causes of injury across all ages.

ity is high for subdural hematoma (33%), followed by contusions (25%) and diffuse axonal injury (11%).

TYPES OF BRAIN INJURY

The circumstances, location, severity, and outcomes after brain injury are quite variable, although, some broad categorizations can be made regarding the mechanisms of injury (Table 68-1). Gennarelli indicates that there are two principal mechanisms of primary brain tissue damage in TBI: contact and acceleration/deceleration. Contact-related injury is the result of the head coming in forceful contact with an object (such as the floor or windshield), or contact between the brain and the inner surface of the skull. Contact injuries tend to result in cerebral contusions and hematoma at the point of contact. Not infrequently *contra coup* lesions occur opposite to the site of contact as the brain rebounds from the initial impact against the skull. Acceleration/deceleration injuries are the result of tensile shearing and straining forces acting on the tissue at the sudden moment of the impact. Such forces may tear blood vessels surrounding the brain, resulting in epidural or subdural hematoma or in

TABLE 68-1

Traumatic Brain Injury Mechanisms
Primary injury
Skull fracture
Cortical contusions and arachnoid–pial layer lacerations
Intracranial hematoma
Diffuse axonal injury
Diffuse microvascular injury
Cranial nerve injury
Secondary injury
Hypoxia and ischemia
Edema
Increased intracranial pressure
Infection

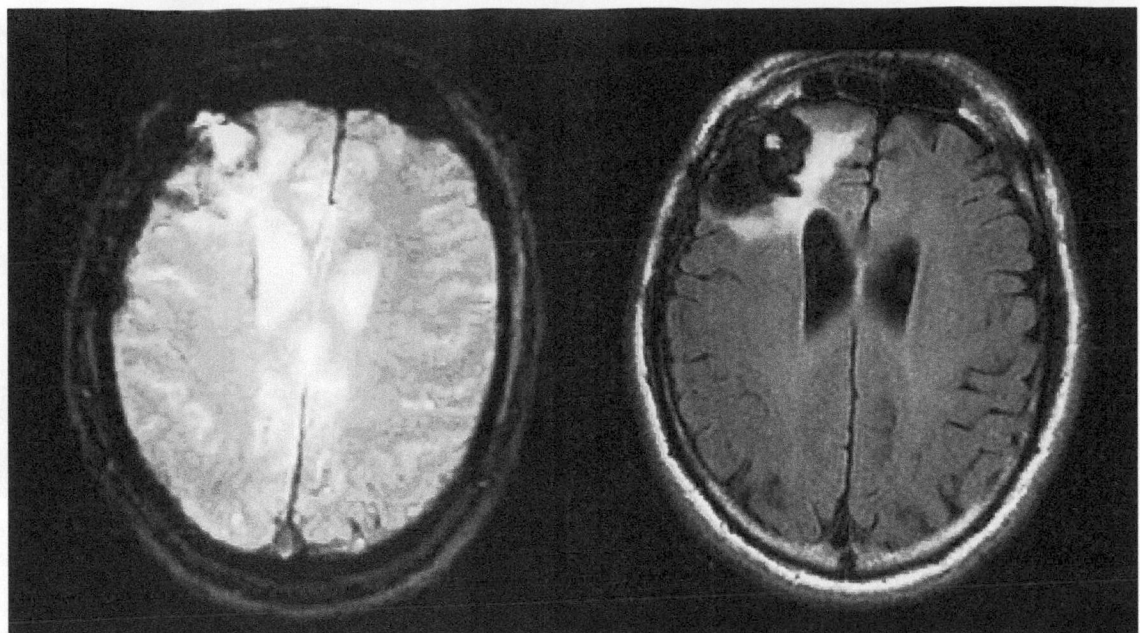

FIGURE 68-4. A 52-yr-old male 14 months post injury. The patient was involved in a low-speed motor vehicle accident and sustained a skull fracture with right frontal epidural and subdural hematomas (that were subsequently evacuated surgically) and right frontal contusions. The T2*-weighted scan in the left panel is negative for diffuse axonal injury. The image on the right is FLAIR T2 and highlights the right frontal lesion with associated gliosis and encephalomalacia around the edges.

widespread (diffuse) shearing of axons and microvasculature within the brain, which is termed diffuse axonal injury. The incidence of hematoma is very common in elderly patients with TBI, as a result of the fact that the proportion of brain volume to cranial volume is significantly smaller in the older adult, and the microvasculature is more brittle. These two factors may combine to yield more brain movement within the cranium at impact and higher incidence of hematoma owing to strain on the vessels, even with seemingly mild impact.

Focal effects of trauma can be observed in variable locations throughout the brain, depending on the specifics of the injury. However, contusions are more frequently observed in the polar, inferior, and lateral frontal and temporal lobes. For example, the lesion in Figure 68-4 is large, but focal to the frontal lobe. Another mechanism for the increased rate of contusions in these areas is actual movement of the brain over the bony anterior and middle fossa and forward motion frontal impact sustained in motor vehicle accidents.

Extra-axial hemorrhages (epidural, subdural, and subarachnoid hematomas) are common in TBI, particularly in the elderly, and the presence of hemorrhage may impact the quality of outcome. A classic lucid period may be described in which the patient exhibits an impact-related alteration in consciousness, followed by a period where consciousness is regained, followed by secondary deterioration of consciousness as the hematoma evolves. Elderly have a higher rate of secondary hematoma even though the initial impact/injury may be mild. On computed tomography imaging, an epidural hematoma is an extra-axial biconvex ovoid mass of blood. Its biconvex shape is caused by blood accumulation in the epidural space, compressing the dura mater onto the brain, causing mass effect. Acute subdural hematoma involves blood accumulation between the dura and brain parenchyma. On computed tomography, subdural hematoma has a characteristic crescent shape. The inner boundary of subarach-

noid hematoma is more irregular—characterized on imaging with blood accumulation that conforms to the sulcal and gyral pattern of the brain. Between 40% and 80% of patients with acute subdural hematoma have an initial Glasgow Coma Scale (GCS) in the severe range (8 or less). In severe cases of high-speed or penetrating injury, lacerations of the meninges may be present, owing to depressed skull fracture or rotational forces of the injury or from the penetrating object.

The diffuse effects of moderate-to-severe TBI can be seen throughout the white matter, indexed on gradient-echo MRI by small punctate hypointensities reflecting paramagnetic hemosiderin in the parenchyma, caused by microvascular shearing (Figure 68-5).

Secondary injury from diffuse axonal injury may involve a cascade of events, including defective axonal transport, swelling, and separation of proximal and distal segments of the axon for more than 12 to 24 hours. Further secondary injury may result from increased intracranial pressure, causing increased hypoxia and ischemia, and poorly regulated, excitotoxic release of glutamate and other excitatory neurotransmitters.

Severity of Injury

The GCS was developed by Jennett and Teasdale in 1974 and is still in wide use today to characterize the depth of coma, a major indicator of injury severity. The GCS is scaled from 3 to 15 (Table 68-2), with 3 being completely nonresponsive and 15 being completely alert, oriented, and following commands. Often the patient is necessarily intubated in the field, making an accurate assessment of GCS difficult.

Duration of loss of consciousness and duration of posttraumatic confusion are also important markers of injury severity, which may help predict eventual outcome (see outcomes section below). Guidelines to appraise injury severity are given in Table 68-3.

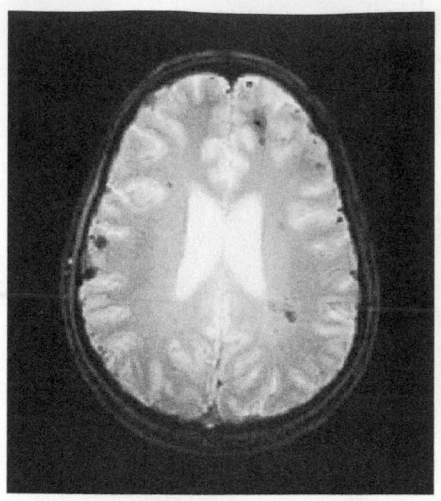 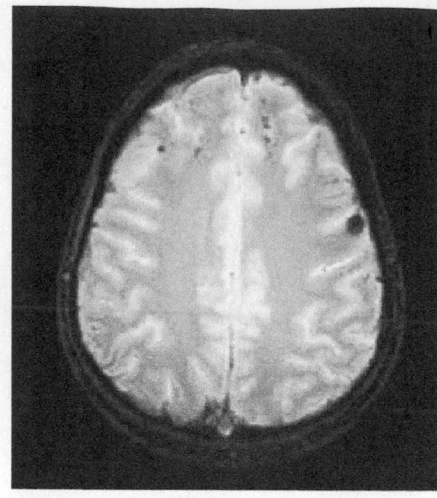 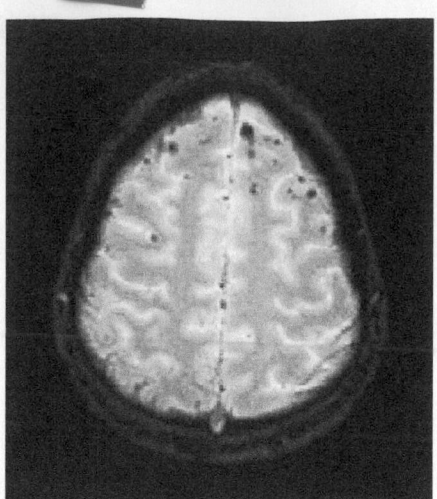

FIGURE 68-5. Diffuse axonal injury. The patient was involved in a high-speed motor vehicle accident 3 months prior to this scan. The patient's initial GCS at the scene was 5 and 3 following intubation. After 24 hours, the GCS was 7. At 3 weeks postinjury, the GCS was 11. By 4 weeks, the patient's GCS was finally at 15. Day of injury imaging indicated a small left frontal epidural hematoma, left frontal contusions, and prominent diffuse axonal injury. This gradient-echo T2*-weighted axial series of images highlights areas of hemosiderin deposition, a blood byproduct containing iron, and therefore results in punctuate areas of signal loss (dephasing) on the image. The multifocal pattern of hemosiderin suggests microvascular shearing and diffuse axonal injury. The multifocal lesions mainly appear at gray–white matter junctions.

OUTCOMES

TBI may result in a variety of adverse outcomes along several overlapping dimensions, including dependence, cognitive outcome, neuropsychiatric outcome, psychosocial outcome, and medical comorbidity. There are several factors that affect these various outcomes after TBI (Table 68-4), including characteristics of the injury and characteristics of the patient. These factors may interact. For example, an older patient in the prodromal phase of Alzheimer's disease (AD) may exhibit progressive symptomatology of AD, which may have been instigated by the TBI but cannot readily be attributed to brain injury alone. This concept is especially relevant to age-associated brain disorders in the elderly. Studies of people at risk of AD indicate that amyloid deposition and neuronal loss may occur

gradually and be fairly asymptomatic until a certain threshold is reached. A brain injury, even if mild, may be sufficient to lower the threshold. Additional information on this topic is provided in the section on dementia and TBI below.

Global TBI Outcome and Age

TBI can result in long-standing cognitive, personality/emotional, and interpersonal deficits that often interfere with successful rehabilitation, resumption of employment and other activities, interpersonal relations, and quality of life. A common finding is that elderly have *poorer* global outcome from the injury than their younger counterparts with similar injuries. The Glasgow Outcome Scale (GOS), a simple five-point scale ranging from death to good recovery (Table 68-5), is the predominant outcome instrument for global outcome. However, this measure is quite course—and there is considerable variability at the best outcome. Despite its limitations, this scale has been used in the largest number of patients and trials. In a recent pooled analysis of the International Mission for Prognosis and Clinical Trial (IMPACT) data involving more than 8700 patients with GOS outcome scores, results indicated that age is one of the most powerful prognostic indictors of GOS outcome, as is acute GCS motor score, pupil response, and computed tomography findings. In the case of severe injury, the chance of a GOS good recovery is

TABLE 68-2

Glasgow Coma Scale		
Best eye response (E)	Spontaneous	4
	To speech	3
	To pain	2
	None	1
Best motor response (M)	Obeys commands	6
	Localizes to pain	5
	Withdraws from pain	4
	Flexion response to pain	3
	Extensor response to pain	2
	None	1
Best verbal response (V)	Oriented and coherent	5
	Confused conversation	4
	Inappropriate words	3
	Incomprehensible sounds	2
	None	1

Total = E+M+V (3–15).

TABLE 68-3

Characterizing Injury Severity			
SEVERITY	GCS	LOC	PTA
Mild	13–15	<30 min	<24 h
Moderate	9–12	½–72 h	1 d to 1 week
Severe	8 or less	>72 h	>1 week

GCS, Glasgow Coma Scale; LOC, loss of consciousness; PTA, posttraumatic amnesia.

TABLE 68-4

Factors Influencing Outcome

Injury parameters
  Severity of injury (GCS, length of coma)
  Comorbid injury
  Location and extent of brain tissue injury
  Secondary brain injury; ICP/swelling, excitotoxicity, and hypoxia
  Physics and speed of the impact

Subject parameters
  Age
  Sex
  Genetic risk for neurocognitive disease
  Preinjury personality and cognitive status
  Social support
  Access to care
  Access to social and rehabilitation services

unlikely in the geriatric patient. Three studies have found that among patients older than 65 years who sustained severe injury (GCS >8), none exhibited a good recovery on the GOS. Another study found that only 6% of patients older than 65 years exhibit good recovery after severe TBI. A fifth study suggested that good recovery was possible after severe injury if the patient regained consciousness within 72 hours. Even when the injury is mild or moderate, the elderly have poorer GOS outcome.

With regard to rehabilitation outcomes, an important study of TBI model systems data found that patients older than 55 years experienced a doubling in the length of rehabilitation stay and associated costs, while only attaining half the rate of functional recovery of their younger counterparts. These patients also had greater cognitive impairments at discharge and higher rates of nursing home placement.

TABLE 68-5

Glasgow Outcome Scale

OUTCOME	SCALE	DESCRIPTOR
Death	1	
Vegetative state	2	Unable to interact with environment; unresponsive.
Severe disability	3	Conscious, but dependent—in need of supervision/assistance every day as a result of physical and cognitive impairments. Ranges from total dependency to assistance with one or more ADLs.
Moderate disability	4	Independent but with a disability. Basic ADLs are intact, but the patient is impaired in occupational and/or social functioning. Able to work in a supported environment.
Good recovery	5	The patient has mild to no residual deficits and has the capacity to resume independent occupational and social activity.

ADLs, activities of daily living.

Less research has been done with fine-tuned neuropsychological assessment of outcome, and studies tend to be much smaller. A review of major cognitive domains that are affected in TBI follows.

Executive Dysfunction

The selective vulnerability of the frontal and temporal lobes to injury gives rise to a preponderance of neuropsychological deficits involving frontal systems, including executive functions, working memory, speed of processing, episodic memory, and aspects of personality. All have been shown to be related to severity of injury. The precise definition of executive function is itself a matter of debate and some confusion. The executive functions are those that promote self-directed action. Self-monitoring, self-regulation, inhibition, introspective reflection, decision making, and planned and goal-directed activity are executive functions. Working memory and attentional capacity such as imperviousness to distraction and sustained attention are necessary components, but not sufficient by themselves for executive function. However, these capacities are conveniently operationalized into a quantifiable psychometric instrument (such as digit span, n-back, or serial 7s), and there is a great deal of research on these components of executive function. Executive functions and components are best assessed with a comprehensive neuropsychological evaluation, although some bedside tests such as clock draw, verbal fluency, and digit span, and go–no go tests may be useful to get a feel for the extent of the problem.

Speed of Processing

Speed of information processing is one of the most frequently observed deficits after TBI. For example, one study found patient's reaction time in a simple motor choice paradigm to be significantly slower than that of matched young adults. Another study assessed speed of information processing and attention in a group of 60 patients with severe TBI and controls. When speed of processing was statistically controlled, differences between patients and controls in focused and divided attention became nonsignificant, suggesting that slowed information processing was accounting for most of the difference. A similar finding was observed for planning and flexible problem solving in patients with severe TBI in the chronic stage of recovery. When speed was controlled, performance was equivalent between patients and controls. A factor analysis of a battery of neuropsychological test scores in survivors of TBI indicated that the most prominent factor was decreased perceptual and motor speed. Speed of processing also declines with age, and thus the older patient with TBI may have unusually slow cognitive processing speeds, which may greatly limit their range of activities and quality of social interactions.

Attention/Distractibility

The ability to allocate attention between multiple tasks and working memory are affected in TBI. For example, Baddeley's original model of working memory, which has been frequently proposed to help explain executive difficulties, states that a central executive process or supervisory attentional system within the prefrontal heteromodal cortex regulates the allocation of limited attentional resources. This system appears to be facilitated by D2 dopamine networks within the dorsolateral frontal lobe and is particularly vulnerable to trauma through either direct contact (contusion to the lateral frontal lobe) or disconnection via acceleration/deceleration injuries.

Memory Dysfunction

Memory complaints from patients are extremely common following TBI, and measured impairment seen on neuropsychological tests is frequently observed, including difficulty at the encoding or acquisition stage, as well as difficulty in retrieval of information. Whether these complaints and deficits are secondary to the more salient attentional, processing speed and executive deficits or whether these are a primary result of hypoxic and excitotoxic injury to the hippocampus is still somewhat unresolved and may vary depending on the nature and severity of the injury.

Personality/Emotional Functioning

The personality changes accompanying TBI vary depending on the injury location, severity, and preinjury personality factors. Prigatano has summarized the literature in detail on this point. Common overlapping descriptors of personality in patients with TBI include irritability/anger, impatience, impulsivity, poor social judgment, inappropriate social behavior, rapid mood swings, loss of drive, fatigability, and/or depression. Major ways of relating to the world following TBI have been described as "childishness" (self-centered behavior, insensitivity to others, or immature behaviors), "helplessness/dependence" (requiring supervision and inability to make important decisions or set goals), and "lack of insight/awareness" of any of the above difficulties. These patterns frequently overlap and have been collectively labeled "frontal lobe personality."

Self-Awareness

TBI results in very abrupt changes that may not be easily, and often only slowly, accommodated into one's stable sense of self. Characteristics of impaired self-awareness can be varied depending on injury location and severity. Acutely, patients with TBI may be unaware that they have deficits from the injury. Later, the patient may admit to some deficits but fail to appreciate the impact of these deficits on daily functioning. Prigatano et al. found that patients with TBI frequently underestimated their behavioral limitations, abnormalities in social interaction, and emotional dyscontrol when compared to a family member's rating of the patient's abilities, while more objective criterion-based competencies such as ADLs, laundry, and shopping may be areas where the patient's insight is more accurate. Critically, a syndrome of impaired self-awareness will significantly complicate or impede the rehabilitation process or treatment adherence, since patients may not perceive the need for such treatments. Damage to the anterior prefrontal regions (behind the forehead) has been associated with impaired self-awareness for social interaction, judgment, and planning. These are the very areas that are commonly injured in TBI.

NEUROPSYCHIATRIC OUTCOME

One recent study compared 120 adults with TBI between the ages of 18 and 65 years to a group of 45 adults older than 65 years. Psychiatric symptoms were assessed 1 year later. The study found that the younger group had double the proportion with psychiatric

disorders (32%) compared to the older group (16%). Further, the younger group was more likely to experience irritability and sleep difficulty, while the older group was more likely to experience poor memory, dependence, and slowness of thinking. This finding is consistent with prior research, indicating that aging with TBI may predispose patients to higher incidence of psychiatric symptoms later in life. Prevalence of major depression is higher (18% prevalence), as is memory difficulty (75%), concentration (53%), personality changes (65%), and increased social isolation (68%).

TBI AND SUBSEQUENT BRAIN ATROPHY AND COGNITIVE AGING

Previous neuroimaging research has demonstrated that TBI results in diffuse cerebral atrophy and that these changes can be observed within months of injury. However, the brain continues to undergo changes over the next year or longer, which are beyond the rates of normal aging (Figure 68-6). However, limited research has been conducted on patients further post injury. Furthermore, the effect of TBI on cerebral integrity during the aging process is not well understood. Studies in normal aging have demonstrated that gray matter volume peaks in adolescence and then decreases over time. In contrast, it has been suggested that white matter volume peaks much later, between the ages of 40 and 50 years. Since diffuse axonal injury affects white matter, one might expect TBI prior to accumulation of maximal white matter to alter its normal trajectory as the brain ages.

It is well accepted that aging results in gradual cognitive decline in many domains. One of the questions that needs to be addressed is whether TBI accelerates normal age-related cognitive decline (a rate of aging by TBI interaction). No studies have directly addressed this, but some studies have begun to approximate an answer. A 2006 study examined cognitive outcome after 30 years in 61 patients with TBI. The study found that older subjects showed significantly greater cognitive decline over the follow-up period. Whether the

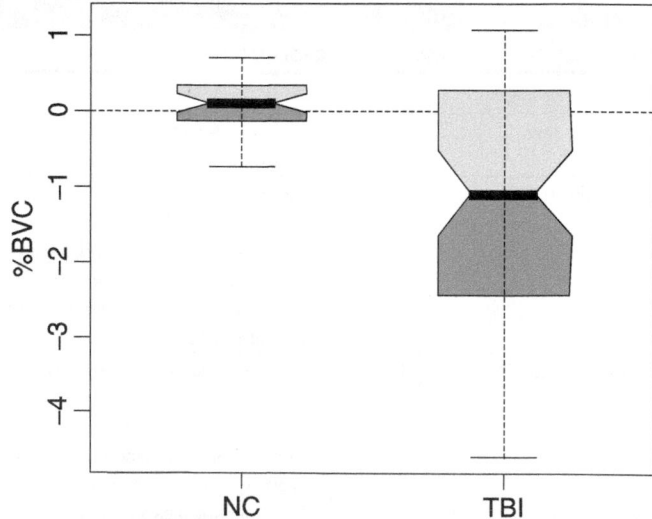

FIGURE 68-6. Patients with TBI show significant decline in global brain volume, here termed percent brain volume change or %BVC, more than a 1-yr interval, while matched controls do not. The notches in the box plot are the 95% confidence interval. The mean, fifth, 25th, 75th, and 95th percentiles are also shown.

rate of change exceeded the rate of change associated with normal aging was not directly assessed. The cognitive areas that exhibited the greatest declines were mental arithmetic, visuospatial reasoning, and immediate memory.

DEMENTIA AND TRAUMA

Dementia is defined as loss of cognitive functions in multiple domains, one of which is memory, which are severe enough to impair occupational or social functioning. Head trauma is an etiology of dementia and is designated as such in the Diagnostic and Statistical Manual of Mental Disorders-IV. After a single injury, dementia, if present, is expected to be nonprogressive. In the elderly, neural loss because of TBI may serve as a "stressor" to a preexisting asymptomatic neurodegenerative process such as AD.

Does Trauma Increase the Risk of AD?

The single greatest risk factor for dementia is age. The apolipoprotein (APOE) gene and other genes increase the risk of dementia, as does neurological history such as trauma. The APOE gene may play a role in multiple age-related diseases. APOE is lipid transporter, and the gene coding for APOE has three alleles: e2, e3, and e4. By far, the most common allele is e3. Persons with the e4 allele (approximately 15% of the general population) are at higher risk of dementia and cerebral vascular diseases, while e2 may be somewhat protective. The risk of dementia in TBI survivors has not always been clear-cut, but when studies include APOE status, the risk becomes somewhat clearer. For example, one large study of 236 community-dwelling older adults found that TBI by itself was not associated with risk of AD, while APOE4 was associated with a twofold increase. However, patients with APOE4-positive TBI had a 10-fold increased risk for AD. Elderly with APOE4 may also have a longer length of coma and earlier age of onset of dementia than non-APOE4 carriers. Another study examined patients with TBI at 6 months postinjury and found that patients with the APOE4 allele were twice as likely (57% vs. 27%) to have outcomes of 1 to 3 on the GOS (death, vegetative state, or severe disability).

Two related concepts of brain vulnerability are of interest here in explaining individual differences in decline to subsequent dementia. *Brain reserve* and *cognitive reserve* address the lack of measurable cognitive decline in the presence of brain disease or age. *Brain reserve* posits that, in the presence of tissue compromise, some brains have greater capacity to rely on spared heteromodal neurons and pathways to compensate in several possible ways, including activation of latent pathways and formation of new synapses. *Cognitive reserve* posits that age and disease-related declines may be protected against by higher premorbid cognitive ability and resources; those that are higher functioning premorbidly may have a greater repertoire of cognitive compensatory strategies to draw upon postinjury or may simply have farther to decline before testing in the impaired range.

POSTACUTE MANAGEMENT OF GERIATRIC PATIENTS WITH TBI

The geriatric patient post TBI presenting in the clinic may have difficulty with mobility and pain and have several less obvious problems including cognitive impairment, mood, anxiety and comportment-related issues, and decreased social and physical inactivity. A careful comprehensive assessment is warranted.

Neuropsychological Assessment

Cognition decline and affective dysfunction are not specific to TBI and may, in fact, co-occur in several neurological diseases and medical conditions. Neuropsychological evaluation may be helpful in making the differential diagnosis. Such an evaluation will identify cognitive profiles that are indicative of specific diagnoses and will identify patterns of strengths and weaknesses in order to inform and help maximize the effectiveness of treatments. Such an evaluation may also help prevent a misdiagnosis of Alzheimer dementia.

Neuropsychiatric Disturbances

Behavioral disturbances can have a negative impact on cognitive functioning, relationships with family and significant others, treatment compliance and motivation, and reintegration into the patient's social community. Common neuropsychiatric sequelae are provided in Table 68-6. A thorough clinical interview with the patient and with one or more other sources such as a spouse and adult child is important, in order to identify neuropsychiatric issues. Collateral sources are important because the patient may give an unreliable history and may have inaccurate insight into the extent of deficits and their effects on others in the patient's life.

When treatable neuropsychiatric disorders are present, it is important to try alternatives to medication when possible. Patients with TBI may be particularly prone to side effects and exaggerated and paradoxical responses to medications. Geriatric patients with TBI are even more vulnerable to adverse responses. Environmental changes may be helpful in some cases, such as increasing social engagement for depressed patients or reducing stressors in the environment that may be adding to agitated behavior. Supportive counseling may be tried for treatment of depression and anxiety. When psychotropic medication is warranted, the drug should be started with the lowest possible dose and titrated up. It has been shown that benzodiazepines

TABLE 68-6

Neuropsychiatric Sequelae
Dementia as a result of trauma; risk for Alzheimer's disease
Posttraumatic confusion
Isolated cognitive disorders: Aphasia, apraxia, amnesia, anosognosia, and executive function
Compartment disorders: Apathy, disinhibition, paranoia, irritability, and lability
Affective disorders: Depression or mania
Anxiety disorders: PTSD, panic, generalized anxiety, and obsessive
Psychotic disorders: Hallucinations and/or delusions
Sleep disorders: Insomnia and hypersomnia
Fatigue

and traditional antipsychotic medications hamper recovery in the geriatric patient, so alternatives with less sedating properties are preferred.

Depression in the elderly patient with TBI has a 30% to 77% prevalence rate. Studies have suggested that demographic (such as marital status and socioeconomic status) or injury characteristics (such as time since injury) are unrelated to postinjury depression. Both a more severe injury and a preinjury psychiatric history do predict postinjury depressive symptoms. Suicide risk is much higher in older adults with TBI, and suicidal ideation should be assessed. Anxiety disorders postinjury are also common. Post-Traumatic Stress Disorder (PTSD) is the most frequent with prevalence rate of 20% to 30%; generalized anxiety disorder and panic disorder are also common. Identification and treatment of these neuropsychiatric sequelae of TBI may contribute greatly to rehabilitation outcome, interpersonal dynamics with family and care providers, and community integration.

Pain

TBI may cause neuropathic pain as a result of CNS injury as well as nociceptive pain resulting from tissue damage. The older patient may have preexisting conditions such as arthritis that augment their discomfort. Physical modalities such as ice, heat, activity, and comfortable positioning are preferable interventions, followed by non-narcotic analgesics. For neuropathic pain, newer anticonvulsants may be advantageous.

FURTHER READING

Alexander S, Kerr ME, Kim Y, Kamboh MI, Beers SR, Conley YP. Apolipoprotein E4 allele presence and functional outcome after severe traumatic brain injury. *J Neurotrauma*. 2007;24(5):790–797.

Bigler ED. Structural imaging. In: Silver JM, McAllister TW, Yudofsky SC, eds. *Textbook of Traumatic Brain Injury*. Washington, DC: American Psychiatric Publishing Inc.; 2005:79–106.

Bigler ED, Blatter DD, Anderson CV, et al. Hippocampal volume in normal aging and traumatic brain injury. *Am J Neuroradiol*. 1997;18(1):11–23.

Blatter DD, Bigler ED, Gale SD, et al. MR-based brain and cerebrospinal fluid measurement after traumatic brain injury: correlation with neuropsychological outcome. *Am J Neuroradiol*. 1997;18(1):1–10.

Cruise CM, Sasson N, Lee MH. Rehabilitation outcomes in the older adult. *Clin Geriatr Med*. 2006;22(2):257–267; viii.

Flanagan SR, Hibbard MR, Riordan B, Gordon WA. Traumatic brain injury in the elderly: diagnostic and treatment challenges. *Clin Geriatr Med*. 2006;22(2):449–468; x.

Frankel JE, Marwitz JH, Cifu DX, Kreutzer JS, Englander J, Rosenthal M. A follow-up study of older adults with traumatic brain injury: taking into account decreasing length of stay. *Arch Phys Med Rehabil*. 2006;87(1):57–62.

Gennarelli TA, Graham DI. Neuropathology. In: Silver JM, McAllister TW, Yudofsky SC, eds. *Textbook of Traumatic Brain Injury*. Washington, DC: American Psychiatric Publishing Inc.; 2005:27–50.

Handel SF, Ovitt L, Spiro JR, Rao V. Affective disorder and personality change in a patient with traumatic brain injury. *Psychosomatics*. 2007;48(1):67–70.

Himanen L, Portin R, Isoniemi H, Helenius H, Kurki T, Tenovuo O. Longitudinal cognitive changes in traumatic brain injury: a 30-year follow-up study. *Neurology*. 2006;66(2):187–192.

Jager TE, Weiss HB, Coben JH, Pepe PE. Traumatic brain injuries evaluated in U.S. emergency departments, 1992–1994. *Acad Emerg Med*. 2000;7(2):134–140.

Kim E. Elderly. In: Silver JM, McAllister TW, Yudofsky SC, eds. *Textbook of Traumatic Brain Injury*. Washington, DC: American Psychiatric Publishing Inc.; 2005:495–508.

Mosenthal AC, Livingston DH, Lavery RF, et al. The effect of age on functional outcome in mild traumatic brain injury: 6-month report of a prospective multicenter trial. *J Trauma*. 2004;56(5):1042–1048.

Murray GD, Butcher I, McHugh GS, et al. Multivariable prognostic analysis in traumatic brain injury: results from the IMPACT study. *J Neurotrauma*. 2007;24(2):329–337.

Ownsworth T, Fleming J, Strong J, Radel M, Chan W, Clare L. Awareness typologies, long-term emotional adjustment and psychosocial outcomes following acquired brain injury. *Neuropsychol Rehabil*. 2007;17(2):129–150.

Prigatano G. *Principles of Neuropsychological Rehabilitation*. New York, New York: Oxford; 1999.

Rutland-Brown W, Langlois JA, Thomas KE, Xi YL. Incidence of traumatic brain injury in the United States, 2003. *J Head Trauma Rehabil*. 2006;21(6):544–548.

Stern Y. Cognitive reserve and Alzheimer's disease. *Alzheimer Dis Assoc Disord*. 2006;20(3 suppl 2):S69–S74.

Stevens JA, Corso PS, Finkelstein EA, Miller TR. The costs of fatal and non-fatal falls among older adults. *Inj Prev*. 2006;12(5):290–295.

Thompson HJ, McCormick WC, Kagan SH. Traumatic brain injury in older adults: epidemiology, outcomes, and future implications. *J Am Geriatr Soc*. 2006;54(10):1590–1595.

Zasler ND, Katz DI, Zafonte RD. *Brain Injury Medicine*. New York, New York: Demos; 2007.

Epilepsy

Ilo E. Leppik

DEFINITION OF EPILEPSY AND SEIZURES

There is currently a debate within the medical community regarding the precise definition of epilepsy. In the past, it was accepted that a person should not be diagnosed as having epilepsy until that individual had two or more seizures. However, with current diagnostic tools, brain pathology can be readily identified, and studies have shown that persons with certain conditions, such as stroke or brain tumor, have a high probability of having more seizures after a single seizure. As a result, many epileptologists, including prominent members of the ILAE (International League Against Epilepsy), are proposing that epilepsy be defined as a condition of the central nervous system predisposing to seizures. Thus, a single seizure associated with specific pathology would be sufficient to initiate treatment to prevent further seizures. This is of particular importance to the geriatrician because many persons with seizures in this age group have identifiable brain pathology.

Seizure classification is based on the functional anatomy of the brain. The smallest seizures are termed simple partial seizures. These do not involve loss of consciousness, and the manifestation of the seizure reflects the function of the area of brain from which these originate. Thus, clonic activity of the right hand (minor motor seizure) originates from an epileptogenic zone in the left motor cortex. Simple partial seizures can be motor, sensory, visual, olfactory, or psychic (de ja vue; brief panic). Because patients are alert during these seizures, they are able to remember what happened. This history can be of great value in localizing the area of brain from which the seizures originated. Complex partial seizures usually originate from the temporal lobes. During the seizure, a person will perform automatic activities such as lip smacking, unbuttoning, wandering aimlessly, or other semipurposeful behaviors. Because memory is mediated by the temporal lobes, persons have no memory for the event. A simple partial seizure can evolve into a complex partial seizure, and both can excite the whole brain and evolve into a generalized tonic-clonic

seizure (convulsion; "Grand Mal"). Persons with these seizures are described as having localization-related epilepsy, and most elderly have this type of epilepsy.

INCIDENCE AND PREVALENCE OF EPILPESY AND USE OF AEDs

Incidence in Community-Dwelling Elderly

Until a few decades ago, epilepsy was mostly a disorder of children. However, as the population of persons older than 65 years has increased, the demographics have changed dramatically. The incidence of epilepsy (new cases per 100,000) in the United States and developed countries now forms a U-shaped curve (Figure 69-1). The incidence of epilepsy is higher in the elderly than in any other age group and rises with each decade after the age of 55 years. Because of the rapid growth in their numbers and their propensity to develop epilepsy, elderly persons will represent an increasingly large group of patients needing expert care for this disorder. In the United States, approximately 181,000 persons developed epilepsy in 1995, and approximately 68,000 of these were older than 65 years. Similar high incidence rates have been reported from the Netherlands, and in Finland new cases of epilepsy in elderly now outnumber those in children.

Prevalence in Community-Dwelling Elderly

An estimate of the prevalence of epilepsy (active cases in a population) can be from a study of veterans. Of a total of 1,130,155 veterans 65 years and older identified from the national database of 1997–1999, 20,558 (1.8%) were identified as having epilepsy by having an ICD-9-CM code representative of this condition. Approximately

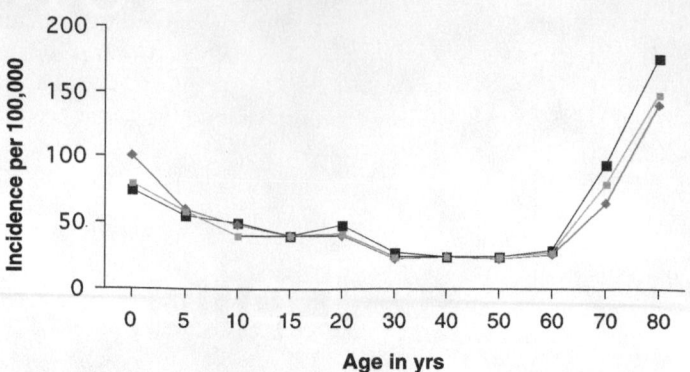

FIGURE 69-1. Age-specific incidence of epilepsy by gender in Rochester, MN, during 1935–1984. *(Constructed from data in Hauser WA. Seizure disorders: the changes with age. Epilepsia. 1992;33(suppl 4):S6–S14.)*

TABLE 69-1

Categorization of Elderly with Epilepsy		
Young old healthy EH	Middle old healthy EH	Old old healthy EH
Young old multiple medical problems EMMP	Middle old multiple medical problems EMMP	Old old multiple medical problems EMMP
Young old frail FE	Middle old frail FE	Old old frail FE

80% were receiving one antiepileptic drug (AED), and 20% were being treated with two or more. Phenytoin was used as monotherapy by almost 70%, whereas phenobarbital was used as monotherapy by approximately 10%. Another 5% were using phenobarbital in combination, mostly with phenytoin. Carbamazepine (CBZ) was used by just more than 10%, and newer AEDs (gabapentin and lamotrigine [LTG]) were used by less then 10% (levetiracetam was not available at the time of the survey). Smaller studies of AED used in community-dwelling elderly patients who are non-veteran administration (VA) patients have found a similar distribution of AED use with phenytoin, by far the most widely used AED in the United States in this population. Studies from Europe show a much different pattern of AED use, with CBZ or phenobarbital being used more frequently than phenytoin. There is no evidence upon which to base this pattern of use; hopefully studies will be done in elderly to delineate the best treatments.

Prevalence in Nursing Home Elderly

Recently, a surprisingly high rate of AED use in nursing homes has been identified, with cross-sectional studies indicating that as many as 10% of all nursing home residents are being prescribed an AED. In one study, phenytoin was used by 6.2% of the residents, followed by CBZ (1.8%), phenobarbital (1.7%), clonazepam (1.2%), valproic acid (0.9%), and all other AEDs combined (1.2%); these percentages exceed 10.5% owing to AED polytherapy. In approximately 6%, the indication is seizure or epilepsy. AEDs such as valproate and CBZ are often used for modification of behavior. If these results are extrapolated to the approximately 1,500,000 elderly residents in U.S. nursing homes (NHs) in 2000, then as many as 150,000 people were likely to have been receiving an AED. Of note, this prevalence in nursing homes is approximately five times that of AED use in the community-dwelling elderly. But the most striking difference between community-dwelling elderly and the nursing home population is the finding that the younger residents are much more likely to be prescribed an AED than the oldest. Analysis by subdivision into those 65 to 74 years of age ("young old"), those 75 to 84 years of age ("middle old"); and those 85 years or older ("old") and further subdivisions by the elderly healthy (EH) who have epilepsy, the elderly with multiple medical problems (EMMP), and the frail elderly, usually in nursing homes (FE), as shown in Table 69-1, are useful in analyzing results and deciding on therapy.

A sample from one nursing home study had the following age group distribution: young old 15%, middle old 36%, and old old 49%. Age was inversely related to AED use. Of the young old, 23.7% were prescribed an AED, 16.4% for seizure indication, and 7.3% for other indications. In the middle old, 12.2% had an AED, 8.3% for seizure and 3.9% for other, whereas the old old had only 5.8% use, 3.7% for seizure and 2.1% for other (Figure 69-2). This finding was unexpected and is just the opposite of the rate of epilepsy in the community. The reason for this reversed pattern is not known but may be related to the severity of the medical conditions in the younger nursing home residents.

Prevalence at Time of Admission to Nursing Homes

In a study of admissions using a longitudinal design to explore AED use at the time of admission, approximately 8% of the admissions group used one or more AEDs at entry, and among these, greater than half had an epilepsy/seizure disorder indication. This demonstrates that the prevalence of epilepsy is approximately three to four times higher in this cohort than in the general community and that these persons have a high rate of developing epilepsy just prior to nursing home entry.

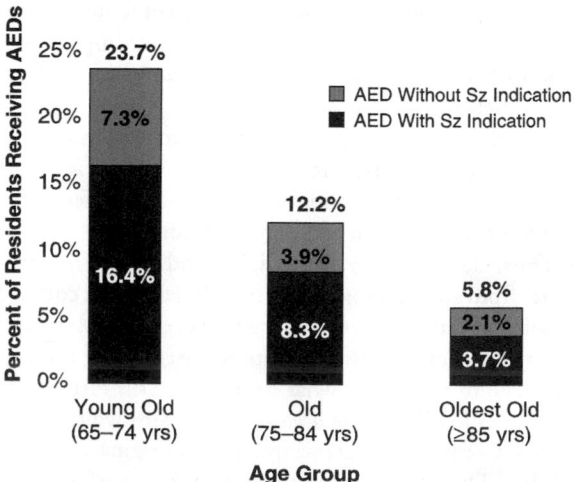

FIGURE 69-2. AED use among nursing home elderly by age group and seizure indication. Young old are much more likely to be treated with an AED than the old old, the inverse of what is observed in community-dwelling elderly. *(Constructed from data from Garrard J, Cloyd J, Gross C, et al. Factors associated with antiepileptic drug use among elderly nursing home residents. J Gerontol A Biol Sci Med Sci. 2000;55:M384–M392.)*

Incidence After Admission to Nursing Homes

The study of prevalence at admission also included a follow-up cohort ($n = 9516$) of those in the admissions group who were not using an AED at NH entry. This cohort was followed up for 3 months after their individual admission dates or until NH discharge, whichever occurred first. Among this group, 3% had an AED prescribed within 3 months of admission. Indications associated with the initiation of AEDs during this period included epilepsy/seizure (1%) and manic depression or other psychiatric diagnoses (2%); a crude estimate of the incidence would be 600/100,000 per 3 months, compared to the approximately 160/100,000 in the community-dwelling elderly. Thus, many persons admitted without a diagnosis of epilepsy are diagnosed as such after entry, and the incidence of newly diagnosed epilepsy within the nursing home far exceeds that in other populations.

These studies demonstrate that, in addition to epilepsy incidence being higher in the elderly overall, there is acceleration in the incidence prior to entry to a nursing home, and an even higher incidence after admission. The causes of this have not been studied but clearly as the individual becomes frailer, the probability of developing seizures and or epilepsy increases.

CAUSES

In the elderly, the most common identifiable cause of epileptic seizures is a previous stroke, which accounts for 30% to 40% of all cases. Approximately 10% of persons with a stroke will have a seizure within the first few months, and the overall incidence rises to approximately 20% by 2 years. Hemorrhagic strokes are more likely to produce seizures than ischemic stokes. Sometimes a transient ischemic attack (TIA) will produce seizures whose pattern is similar to the deficit of the TIA, but the clue is that seizures usually last only a few minutes. Brain tumor, head injury, and Alzheimer's disease are other major causes. However, in a large number of cases, the precise cause cannot be identified and the etiology is labeled cryptogenic (crypt = hidden; genic = cause).

DIAGNOSIS

History

A clear distinction must be made between epileptic seizures, those arising from brain pathology, and nonepileptic seizures, those in which a seizure is caused in a normal brain by some alteration in physiology, such as hypoxia. Thus, other causes of seizures, such as cardiac insufficiency, metabolic conditions, convulsive syncope (micturation syncope and cough syncope), and additional conditions must be eliminated before it can be concluded that the event was an epileptic seizure. The evaluation after a singe seizure must, therefore, be comprehensive. A thorough history must be obtained, focusing on events of the last day or so, to identify any precipitating or provoking factors. Epileptic seizures are usually unprovoked. An electrocardiogram (EKG) to rule out cardiac conditions is essential. Laboratory tests for metabolic disorders should be done. A review of prescription drugs, over-the-counter agents, and natural product use must be obtained. Many natural products designed to simulate weight loss or improve memory may have proconvulsant properties. Withdrawal from benzodiazepines or alcohol can provoke seizures, and methamphetamine and cocaine may cause convulsions. A drug screen should be considered.

CT and MRI Scans

Structural studies to explore for intracerebral hemorrhage, brain tumor, and encephalomalacia should be done. A CT scan is appropriate as the initial emergency study. Because its modality is x-rays, it is effective in detecting tissue contrasts. Thus, it is effective for detecting blood, areas of encephalomalacia, and calcified lesions. However, the MRI is much more sensitive for detecting subtle changes in brain tissue and should be done if obvious pathology is not detected by the CT scan. Glial tumors are often not well visualized by CT, nor are small changes in the hippocampus.

Electroencephalogram

An electroencephalogram (EEG) serves many useful roles in the diagnosis of epilepsy. A person with epilepsy has abnormal electrical discharges in between seizures (interictal activity). These can be detected by an EEG, just as abnormalities can be found on an EKG in between clinical cardiac events. The interictal patterns can confirm the presence of physiologically abnormal brain, thus cementing the diagnosis of an epileptic as opposed to a nonepileptic seizure. In addition, it can identify the epileptogenic region, providing additional clues to the etiology. Also, the degree of interictal activity can provide a clue as to the severity of the epilepsy. It is recommended that an EKG rhythm strip be obtained during an EEG to help identify artifacts and provide additional evidence to exclude a cardiac cause for the seizure.

TREATMENT

Deciding to Treat

After a single seizure, the decision to initiate treatment with an AED must be made on the basis of assessing the risk for additional seizures. Given the risks associated with additional convulsions, there is probably a greater urgency to treat. In an elderly person with a history of stroke or an identified CNS lesion, a single seizure would meet the newer proposed definition of epilepsy as a condition of the central nervous system predisposing to seizures, and treatment is warranted. A more complicated decision arises when the evaluation of a single seizure does not identify CNS pathology and the EEG is negative. In these cases, a more intensive search for nonepileptic seizures must be performed, and treatment may reasonably be deferred until a second seizure occurs. In addition, the elderly population is heterogeneous, and broad statements about elderly may not be relevant to each individual patient. Treatment in the elderly carries more risks than in younger persons because they may experience more side effects, have a greater risk for drug interactions, and be less able to afford the costs of medications. In addition to their use in epilepsy, AEDs are prescribed for a variety of other disorders affecting the elderly, including pain and psychiatric disorders. As a cause of adverse reactions among the elderly, AEDs rank fifth among all drug categories. Unfortunately, very little research has been done in this vulnerable population, and only general recommendations can be made at this time.

Clinical Pharmacology of AEDs in the Elderly

Drug concentration at the site of action determines the magnitude of both desired and toxic responses. The unbound drug concentration in serum is in direct equilibrium with the concentration at the site of action and provides the best correlation with drug response. Three of the major AEDs (valproic acid, phenytoin, and CBZ, respectively) are highly bound, and binding is frequently altered. Thus, for these AEDs, measurement of unbound (free) levels many be important to avoid errors in therapy.

The age-related physiological changes that appear to have the greatest effect on AED pharmacokinetics involve protein binding and the reduction in liver volume and blood flow. Reduced serum albumin and increased α1-acid glycoprotein (AAG) concentrations in the elderly alter protein binding of some drugs. By the age of 65 years, many individuals have low normal albumin concentrations or are frankly hypoalbuminemic. Albumin concentration may further be reduced by conditions such as malnutrition, renal insufficiency, and rheumatoid arthritis. The concentration of AAG, a reactant serum protein, increases with age; further elevations occur during pathophysiological stress such as stroke, heart failure, trauma, infection, myocardial infarction, surgery, and chronic obstructive pulmonary disease. Administration of enzyme-inducing AEDs also increases AAG. When the concentration of AAG rises, the binding of weakly alkaline and neutral drugs such as CBZ to AAG can increase, causing higher total serum drug concentrations and decreased unbound drug concentrations. Because of the complexity of confounding variables and the lack of correlation between simple measures of liver function and drug metabolism, the effect of age on hepatic drug metabolism remains largely unknown.

Renal clearance is the major route of elimination for a number of the newer AEDs. It is well known that an elderly person's renal capacity decreases by approximately 10% per decade, but this also is highly dependent on the general state of health.

Despite the theoretical effects of age-related physiological changes on drug disposition and the widespread use of AEDs in the elderly, few studies on AED pharmacokinetics in the elderly have been published. The available reports generally involve single-dose evaluations in small samples of the young old (65–74 years). There is a lack of data regarding AED pharmacokinetics in the oldest old (>85 years), individuals who may be at greatest risk of therapeutic failure and adverse reactions.

Variability of AED Levels in Nursing Homes

Studies have shown that in compliant patients, the variability of AED concentrations over time is relatively small. One study of phenytoin showed that in younger institutionalized patients, the variability between serial measurements over time was in the order of 10%. In the same study, compliant clinic patients had variability of approximately 20%. Approximately 5% of this can be accounted for by measurement instrument variability, although laboratories not following rigid quality control standards may have a much larger variability. The remainder of the variability arises from day-to-day alterations in

absorption and metabolism or differences in AED dose content. The variability for CBZ and valproate is in the order of 25%, possibly because of their shorter half-lives and, thus, increased variability from sampling times. An analysis of serial phenytoin levels from nursing home patients across the United States who had no change in dose, no change in formulation, and no additions of other medications found that some had a difference of two- to threefold from the lowest to the highest. Interestingly, some had very little fluctuation. Similar but less severe fluctuations were observed for CBZ and valproate. These findings suggest that the elderly frail nursing home residents may have much greater variability in absorption of drugs. Factors, which contribute to this, must be identified and strategies developed to minimize this phenomenon.

Clinical Trials of AEDs in the Elderly

All major AEDs have an FDA indication for use for the seizure types most likely to be encountered in the elderly. However, there are little data relating specifically to these drugs in the elderly, and those that are available have been limited to community-dwelling elderly. One post hoc study of the veteran administration hospital (VAH) cooperative study of CBZ and valproate found that elderly patients often had seizure control associated with lower AED levels than seen in the younger subjects. However, side effects were also observed at levels lower than those seen in younger. This suggests that the elderly need a different "therapeutic range" than those quoted for younger adults. A multicenter, double-blind, randomized comparison between LTG and CBZ in elderly patients (mean age 77 years) with newly diagnosed epilepsy in the United Kingdom showed that the main difference between the groups was the rate of drop out as a result of adverse events, with a rate for LTG of 18% compared to a rate of 42% for CBZ. The VA Cooperative Study in the United States, an 18-center, parallel, double-blind trial on the use of gabapentin, LTG, and CBZ in patients 60 years or older, found that efficacy did not differ, but the main finding favoring the two newer AEDs was tolerability.

Choosing an AED for the Elderly

At the present time, there are little data regarding the clinical use of AEDs in the elderly. The paucity of information makes it very difficult to recommend specific AEDs with any confidence that the outcomes will be optimal. A drug choice optimal for the EH group may not be appropriate for the EMMP or FE group, owing to differences in pharmacokinetic or pharmacodynamic properties among these groups. Phenytoin is still the most commonly used AED in both community-dwelling and nursing home elderly in the United States, although expert opinion may disagree with this practice. In the next section, discussion is based first on the most commonly used AEDs for which there are more data (often negative) and then on an alphabetical review of the newer AEDs. A summary of the properties of most AEDs is in Table 69-2.

Phenytoin

It is effective for localization-related epilepsies and, thus, has an efficacy profile appropriate for the elderly. Phenytoin has a narrow therapeutic range, is approximately 90% bound to serum albumin, and undergoes saturable metabolism, which has the effect of producing

TABLE 69-2

AEDs Used for Treatment of Epilepsy in the Elderly

DRUG	PROTEIN BINDING (%)	ELIMINATION	COMMENTS
Carbamazepine	75–85	Hepatic CYP 3A4/5	Levels increased by erythromycin, propoxyphene, and grapefruit juice Decreases levels of calcium channel-blockers (dilitiazem and verapamil) Decreases effect of warfarin Decreases tricyclic antidepressant levels
Gabapentin	<10	Renal	Elimination correlates with creatinine clearance No drug interactions
Lamotrigine	55	Hepatic–glucuronide conjugation	Levels decreased by inducing agents—carbamazepine, phenytoin, some hormones, and others yet to be determined Levels increased by vaproate
Levetiracetam	<10	Renal	Very water soluble; IV formulation available No drug interactions
Phenobarbital	50	Hepatic Renal	Induces metabolism of many drugs Very sedative IM and IV available
Phenytoin	80–93	Hepatic CYP 2C9 CYP 2C19	Protein binding decreased with reduced serum albumin and renal failure Decreases levels of calcium channel-blockers (dilitiazem and verapamil) Complicated interaction with warfarin Decreases tricyclic antidepressant levels Interacts with diabetes and arthritis medications Decreases effectiveness of cancer chemotherapy IV formulation available. Fosphenytoin can be given IM or IV
Valproic acid	87–95	Hepatic Multiple pathways	Protein binding decreased in elderly Inhibits glucuronidation and may increase levels of lamotrigine and other drugs Decreases platelet function IV formulation available

large changes in serum concentrations, with small changes in dose or absorption. The binding of phenytoin to serum proteins correlates with the albumin concentration. A number of studies have also shown that phenytoin metabolism appears to be reduced in the elderly. Thus, in the elderly, an initial daily dose of 3 mg/kg may be appropriate, rather than the 5 mg/kg/d used in younger adults. This 3 mg/kg dose is only 160 mg/day for a 52-kg woman, or 200 mg/day for a 66-kg man. As a result of the high protein binding of phenytoin, unbound phenytoin concentrations are a better indicator of efficacy and toxicity than total concentrations. Measurement of unbound phenytoin concentrations is recommended for elderly patients who have: (1) decreased serum albumin concentration, (2) total phenytoin concentrations that are more than 15 mg/L, (3) a low total concentration relative to the daily dose, or (4) total concentrations that do not correlate with the clinical state, such as apparent toxicity. A range of 5 to 10 mg/L total may be more appropriate as a therapeutic range for the elderly because of decreased protein binding and increased sensitivity to side effects.

Phenytoin has many drug–drug interactions and should be used cautiously in patients with EMMP receiving other medications. Selective serotonin reuptake inhibitor (SSRI) antidepressants may inhibit the cytochrome 2C family of P450 enzymes responsible for metabolizing phenytoin. Fluoxetine and norfluoxetine are more potent inhibitors of this enzyme, followed by sertraline and paroxetine. The latter two SSRI antidepressants may prove to be a safer choice in the elderly. Coumadin has a very strong and complicated interaction with phenytoin and concomitant use should probably be avoided.

Phenytoin has some effects on cognitive functioning, especially at higher levels. In addition, phenytoin may cause imbalance and ataxia. In a study of elderly, among the various lifestyle, demographic, and health factors, which contributed to an increased risk, phenytoin was the only drug that was associated with a significant increase in fractures. However, this study could not determine if this was caused by falls from ataxia or seizures or was an effect of bone changes. In spite of its limitations, phenytoin is the least expensive major AED. This and its long record of use may account for it presently being the most widely used AED in the United States.

Carbamazepine

It is effective for localization-related epilepsies and, thus, has an efficacy profile appropriate for the elderly. Two studies of new-onset epilepsy in elderly found it to be as effective as LTG, but it had a higher incidence of side effects.

Apparent clearance of CBZ has been reported to be 20% to 40% lower in the elderly as compared to adults. Decreases in clearance result in a prolonged elimination half-life. These changes in CBZ pharmacokinetics indicate that lower and less frequent dosing in elderly patients may be appropriate.

CBZ has some significant drug–drug interaction with medications that inhibit the cytochrome P450 enzyme, CYP 3A4. Among the inhibitors are erythromycin, fluoxetine, ketoconazole, propoxyphene (Darvon), and cimetidine (Tagamet). At least one food (grapefruit juice) has been identified to interact with CBZ, causing increases in CBZ serum concentrations. Patients with EH will need to be cautioned about these and should be instructed to inform the physician whenever they are beginning a new medication, including over-the-counter medications. Many other drug interactions occur, so CBZ is one AED which will need to be used cautiously in patients with EMMP receiving other medications. CBZ can also induce the CYP 3A4 system, reducing the effectiveness of other drugs.

CBZ may cause imbalance and ataxia. It is possible that patients with EMMP, especially those with CNS disorders, may be more sensitive to these effects. One of the major concerns with CBZ is its effect on sodium levels. The hyponatremia associated with CBZ is more pronounced as a person becomes older. This may become more problematic if a person is on salt restriction or a diuretic. Because of the mild neutropenia associated with CBZ use in younger adults, the effects of this AED on hematopoietic parameters in the elderly will need to be studied. CBZ is also known to affect cardiac rhythms and should be used cautiously, if at all, in persons with rhythm disturbances. CBZ is a moderately priced drug and should not present a significant cost issue.

Valproate

This drug has both antiseizure properties and behavioral control effects. Valproic acid, like phenytoin, is associated with reduced protein binding and unbound clearance in the elderly. As a result, the desired clinical response may be achieved with a lower dose than usual. A nationwide elderly nursing home study showed that valproic acid dose and total valproic acid concentrations decrease within the elderly age groups. If the albumin concentration has fallen or the patient's clinical response does not correlate with total drug concentration, measurement of unbound drug should be considered. Because of its effects on mood stabilization, it may be especially appropriate for elderly with a dual diagnosis.

Phenobarbital

This AED is effective for localization-related epilepsies and is the least expensive of all of the AEDs. However, its side effects of worsening of cognition and depression make it an undesirable drug for the elderly, especially in the nursing home setting.

Gabapentin

It is effective for localization-related epilepsies. It is not metabolized by the liver, but rather renally excreted; therefore, there are no drug–drug interactions. Thus, it may be especially useful in patients with EMMP. There is a reduction of renal function with advancing age, so doses may need to be adjusted in patients with both EH and EMMP. Levels must be monitored after initiation and doses adjusted accordingly. However, gabapentin does appear to have some sedative side effects, especially at higher levels, and the elderly may be more sensitive to this problem.

In the elderly its half-life may be longer because of decreased renal elimination. Because gabapentin is effective in treating neuralgic pain, it would be additionally beneficial for someone suffering from both epilepsy and pain.

Lamotrigine

LTG is effective for localization-related epilepsies. It is primarily metabolized by the liver using the glucuronidation pathway, not the P450 system, and this pathway may be less affected by age. Based on a study of 150 elderly subjects, the dropout rate owing to adverse events was lower with LTG (18%) than with CBZ (42%). LTG subjects had fewer rashes (LTG, 3%; CBZ, 19%) and fewer complaints of somnolence: 12% for LTG and 29% for CBZ. LTG clearance is increased by approximately two to three times with coadministration of phenytoin and CBZ, whereas LTG clearances decrease twofold when valproic acid is coadministered.

Levetiracetam

It has been approved as adjunctive therapy for partial-onset seizures in adults. It is extremely water soluble. This allows rapid and complete absorption after oral administration. Levetiracetam is not metabolized by the liver and, thus, is free of nonlinear elimination kinetics, autoinduction kinetics, and drug–drug interactions. Lack of protein binding (<10%) also avoids the problems of displacing highly protein-bound drugs and the monitoring of unbound concentrations. Lack of drug interactions would make it useful for treating elderly patients with epilepsy, EMMP.

Levetiracetam also appears to have a favorable safety profile. It was initially studied as a potential agent for treating cognitive disorders in the elderly, and thus a considerable amount of data regarding its tolerability in this age group are available.

Pregabalin

This drug is related to gabapentin but is more potent with doses generally one-fifth those of gabapentin needed for therapeutic effect. Its absorption also appears to be more predictable because of the lower amounts needed for being transported across the intestinal system. Although it may prove to be a favorable AED for the elderly, its cost and lack of experience may limit its use.

Dosing of AEDs in the Elderly

Compliance is a potential challenge in the elderly because of multiple medications, memory problems, and visual problems. In general, once- or twice-daily dosing is preferable, and even the AEDs with short half-lives in younger adults can be given less often in elderly. Reducing staff time spent administering multiple daily doses of medication to many patients may reduce errors and cost. In general, the elderly need lower doses than younger persons because (1) metabolism is slower and the same dose could give higher levels and (2) the elderly may need lower levels for seizure control and avoidance of toxicity.

Alternative Routes of Administration

All of the commonly used AEDs have liquids or suspensions available. These were developed primarily for pediatric use, but these can be used if a person has difficulty swallowing pills or capsules. These can also be administered by way of a nasogastric tube. Blood levels should be monitored if switching from one formulation to another to assure that adequate levels are being maintained.

Unfortunately, few AEDs are available for intramuscular (IM) or intravenous (IV) use. Phenytoin for IV infusion has a pH of 12, contains 40% propylene glycol, and can cause venous sclerosis, hypotension, and cardiac arrhythmias. It cannot be given IM. A much safer and better-tolerated phenytoin prodrug, fosphenytoin, is available and can be given IM or IV. Of the other AEDs, Phenobarbital can be given IM or IV, but valproate and levetiracetam have only IV indications.

Drug Interactions with Non-AEDs

Concomitant medications taken by elderly patients can alter the absorption, distribution, and metabolism of AEDs, thereby increasing the risk of toxicity or therapeutic failure. Comedications are frequently used by patients in nursing homes receiving AEDs (Table 69-3). No data are available for elderly outpatients. Calcium-containing antacids and sucralfate reduce the absorption of phenytoin. The absorption of phenytoin, CBZ, and valproate may be reduced significantly by oral antineoplastic drugs that damage gastrointestinal cells. In addition, phenytoin concentrations may be lowered by intravenously administered antineoplastic agents. The use of folic acid for treatment of megaloblastic anemia may decrease serum concentrations of phenytoin, and enteral feedings can also lower serum concentrations in patients receiving orally administered phenytoin.

Many drugs displace AEDs from plasma proteins, an effect that is especially serious when the interacting drug also inhibits the metabolism of the displaced drug. Several drugs used on a short-term basis (including propoxyphene and erythromycin) or as maintenance therapy (such as cimetidine, diltiazem, fluoxetine, and verapamil) significantly inhibit the metabolism of one or more AEDs that are metabolized by the P450 system. Certain agents can induce the P450 system or other enzymes, causing an increase in drug metabolism. The most commonly prescribed inducers of drug metabolism are phenytoin, phenobarbital, CBZ, and primidone. Ethanol, when used chronically, also induces drug metabolism. The interaction between antipsychotic drugs and AEDs is complex. Hepatic metabolism of certain antipsychotics such as haloperidol can be increased by CBZ, resulting in diminished psychotropic response. Antipsychotic medications, especially chlorpromazine, promazine, trifluoperazine, and perphenazine, can reduce the threshold for seizures. The risk of seizures is directly proportional to the total number of psychotropic medications being taken, their doses, any abrupt increases in doses, and the presence of organized brain pathology. The patient with epilepsy taking antipsychotic drugs may need a higher dose of antiepileptic mediation to control seizures. In contrast, central nervous system depressants are likely to lower the maximum dose of AEDs that can be administered before toxic symptoms occur.

CONCLUSIONS

The incidence of epilepsy is higher in the elderly than in any other age group, and, with the increasing number of elderly, the prevalence of epilepsy will be greater in older adults. Nursing homes have a much higher incidence and prevalence of epilepsy than community-dwelling elderly. Doses and blood levels generally need to be lower in the elderly for best outcome. The FE in nursing homes may have much greater variability in blood levels over time with stable doses with the older AEDs. Newer ones have not been studied. Of the newer AEDs, gabapentin, LTG, and levetiracetam are the most widely researched and used and have advantages such as less protein binding and fewer drug interactions. Cost may be one barrier to more extensive use. Much more research is needed, however, to determine the best treatments for the EH, EMMP, and FE cohorts.

FURTHER READING

Bach B, Hansen JM, Kampmann JP, Rasmussen SN, Skovsted L. Disposition of antipyrine and phenytoin correlated with age and liver volume in man. *Clin Pharmacokinet.* 1981;6:389–396.

Birnbaum A, Hardie NA, Leppik IE, et al. Variability of total phenytoin serum concentrations within elderly nursing home residents. *Neurology.* 2003;60:555–559.

Birnbaum AK, Hardie NA, Conway JM, et al. Valproic acid doses, concentrations, and clearances in elderly nursing home residents. *Epilepsy Res.* 2004;62:157–162.

Bourdet SV, Gidal BE, Alldredge BK. Pharmacologic management of epilepsy in the elderly. *J Am Pharm Assoc (Wash).* 2001;41(3):421–436.

Brodie MJ, Overstall PW, Giorgi L. Multicentre, double-blind randomized comparison between lamotrigine and carbamazepine in elderly patients with newly diagnosed epilepsy. The UK Lamotrigine Elderly Study Group. *Epilepsy Res.* 1999;37(1):81–87.

Cloyd JC, Lackner TE, Leppik IE. Antiepileptics in the elderly. Pharmacoepidemiology and pharmacokinetics. *Arch Fam Med.* 1994;3:589–598.

Cramer JA, Leppik IE, DeRue K, Edrich P, Kramer G. Tolerability of levetiracetam in elderly patients with CNS disorders. *Epilepsy Res.* 2003;56:135–145.

Cusack BJ. Drug metabolism in the elderly. *J Clin Pharmacol.* 1988;28:571–576.

Dong X, Leppik IE, White J, Rarick J. Hyponatremia from oxcarbazepine and carbamazepine. *Neurology.* 2005;65(12):1976–1978.

Epilepsy Foundation of America. *Epilepsy, a Report to the Nation.* Landover, MD: Epilepsy Foundation of America; 1999.

Garrard J, Cloyd J, Gross C, et al. Factors associated with antiepileptic drug use among elderly nursing home residents. *J Gerontol A Biol Sci Med Sci.* 2000;55:M384–M392.

Garrard J, Harms S, Hardie N, et al. Antiepileptic drug use in nursing home admissions. *Ann Neurol.* 2003;54:75–85.

Hauser WA. Seizure disorders: the changes with age. *Epilepsia.* 1992;33(suppl 4):S6–S14.

Kemper P, Murtaugh CM. Lifetime use of nursing home care. *N Engl J Med.* 1991;324:595–600.

Lackner TE, Cloyd JC, Thomas LW, et al. Antiepileptic drug use in nursing home residents: effect of age, gender, and comedication on patterns of use. *Epilepsia.* 1998;39:1083–1087.

Leppik IE. *Contemporary Diagnosis and Management of the Patient with Epilepsy.* 6th ed. Newtown, PA: Handbooks in Healthcare; 2006.

Mattson RH, Cramer JA, Collins JF, et al. Comparison of carbamazepine, phenobarbital, phenytoin, and primidone in partial and secondarily generalized tonic-clonic seizures. *N Engl J Med.* 1985;313:145–151.

TABLE 69-3

Frequently Used Comedications in Nursing Homes with Potential Pharmacokinetic or Pharmacodynamic Interactions with AEDs

DRUG CATEGORY	% USE WITH AEDs
Antidepressants	18.9
Antipsychotics	12.7
Benzodiazepams	22.4
Thyroid supplements	14.0
Antacids	8.0
Calcium channel-blockers	6.9
Warfarin	5.9
Cimetidine	2.5

Perucca E. Berlowitz, Birnbaum A, Cloyd JC, Garrard J, Hanlon JT, Levy RH, Pugh MJ. Pharmacological and clinical aspects of antiepileptic drug use in the elderly. *Epilepsy Res* 2006:68(Suppl 1):S49–S63.

Pugh MJV, Cramer J, Knoefel J, et al. Potentially inappropriate antiepileptic drugs for elderly patients with epilepsy. *J Am Geriatr Soc.* 2003;52:417–422.

Rowan AJ, Ramsay RE, Collins JF, et al. New onset geriatric epilepsy: a randomized study of gabapentin, lamotrigine, and carbamazepine. *Neurology.* 2005; 64(11):1868–1873.

Sillanpaa M, Kalviainen R, Klaukka T, Helenius H, Shinnar S. Temporal changes in the incidence of epilepsy in Finland: nationwide study. *Epilepsy Res.* 2006; 71(2–3):206–215.

Late-Life Mood Disorders

Dan G. Blazer

INTRODUCTION

Among the mood disturbances, depression is the most frequent cause of emotional suffering in older adults. Depression decreases the quality of life of the elderly, increases functional decline, and, when severe, is associated with a shortened life expectancy. Bipolar disorder, although much less frequent, can be most burdensome to the elderly and a difficult management problem for the clinician. Therefore, the diagnosis and treatment of mood disorders are among the most important and challenging tasks facing the geriatrician and other health-care providers.

During the past few years, a significant effort has been generated to better understand these common and frequently disabling maladies. We have learned much about the causes of late-onset depression. The evidence base for therapy has increased dramatically for both major depression and bipolar disorder. This chapter begins by first exploring current case definitions. Next, both clinical and community-based epidemiological studies are examined so that the reader appreciates the burden of depression across multiple settings. This is followed by extant evidence that informs us of the origins of late-life depression from a biopsychosocial perspective. The chapter concludes with a review of current therapies for depressed older adults. These therapies range from medications and electroconvulsive therapy (ECT) to family interventions.

THE SUBTYPES OF LATE-LIFE MOOD DISORDERS

Although clinicians frequently disagree about exact case definitions of late-life mood disorders, the most cogent subtypes are presented below, subtypes relevant to clinical practice. Naturally, clinicians encounter frequent overlap of subtypes. For example, the acute and usually self-limiting episodes of major depression may be accompanied by chronic and less severe mood disturbances, such as dysthymia.

In addition, the symptoms of late-life mood disorders often overlap with other psychiatric and physical disorders. Therefore, these case definitions or subtypes may be more useful for coding and communication than for actual patient care. These do remind the clinician, however, of the variation in symptom presentation and the necessity to tailor treatment strategies to the individual.

Major depression is the "bread and butter" diagnosis for moderate-to-severe, yet self-limited, mood disorders in late life. To be diagnosed with major depression according to the *Diagnostic and Statistical Manual of Mental Disorders*, fourth edition (DSM-IV), the older adult should exhibit most of the time for at least 2 weeks one or both of two core symptoms—depressed mood and/or lack of interest or pleasure in usual activities—along with four or more of the following symptoms: a feeling of worthlessness or inappropriate guilt, a diminished ability to concentrate or make decisions, fatigue, psychomotor agitation or retardation, insomnia or hypersomnia, significant decrease or increase in weight or appetite, and recurrent thoughts of death or suicide ideation. See Table 70-1 for a description of how the symptoms of major depression may vary with older adults compared to younger adults.

Although not a current diagnosis in DSM-IV, *minor, subsyndromal, or subthreshold depression* is a useful diagnosis for older adults with clear yet less severe depressive symptoms than those with major depression, and criteria are presented in the Appendix of DSM-IV. The diagnosis of minor/subsyndromal/subthreshold depression can be made in at least two ways. First, to meet criteria in DSM-IV, subjects must experience one of the core symptoms for major depression plus one to three additional symptoms. Another means by which the diagnosis of minor depression can be made is to administer a symptom screen for depression (such as the Center for Epidemiologic Studies Depression Scale). If the subject scores 16 or higher on this scale (a score that signifies clinically significant depressive symptoms) yet does not meet criteria for major depression, then the diagnosis of minor/subsyndromal/subthreshold depression can be made.

TABLE 70-1

Diagnostic Criteria for Major Depression and Description of How Symptoms May Vary Compared to those in Younger Adults

SYMPTOM	DESCRIPTION
Depressed mood and/or lack of interest or pleasure in usual activities	The older adults may be more likely to express a loss of pleasure than to specifically complain of depression
Feelings of worthlessness or inappropriate guilt	Less common in older adults than in younger adults
Diminished ability to concentrate or make decisions	Often manifested as a complaint of memory problems—adults of all ages with moderate-to-severe depression complain of problems with concentration and memory, but depressed elders, in contrast to younger adults, exhibit impairment on psychological testing even when they do not have a comorbid dementing disorder
Fatigue	Common regardless of age
Psychomotor agitation or retardation	Older persons may exhibit either of these symptoms
Insomnia or hypersomnia	Older persons rarely, if ever, exhibit hypersomnia—a symptom that is much more common in adolescence and young adults
Significant decrease or increase in weight or appetite	Older adults rarely gain weight or experience an increase in appetite during a depressive episode
Recurrent thoughts of death or suicidal ideation	Although thoughts of death are not uncommon in older adults, suicidal ideation among depressed elders is less frequent than among the depressed who are younger

Dysthymic disorder is usually less severe than major depression but much longer lasting than either major depression or minor depression. To meet criteria for dysthymic, the older patients must experience moderate symptoms of depression for at least 2 years or longer. Although dysthymic disorder rarely has its onset in late life, it frequently persists from midlife into late life.

Depression in the elderly, as noted above, is often *comorbid* with both physical and psychiatric conditions, especially among the oldest old. Elders suffering from myocardial infarction and other cardiovascular conditions, diabetes, hip fracture, urinary incontinence, kidney disease, and stroke are more likely to suffer from depression than the general population of elders. When depression is comorbid with physical health problems, the clinician must distinguish between symptoms that are appropriate to the physical condition and those that either may be exaggerated or are not typical of the physical health problem. For example, an older person with cardiovascular disease may experience difficulty sleeping. If the sleep disturbance is to be considered a signal of depression, then the sleep problem should not simply represent the difficulty sleeping experienced by, for example, a person with shortness of breath or angina.

Depression is also frequently present among older adults with dementing disorders, such as Alzheimer's disease and vascular de-

mentia. The assessment of depressive symptoms in patients with dementia is problematic. One problem is the overlap between symptoms of depression and those that are the behavioral or emotional manifestations of the underlying dementia syndrome. For example, apathy and social withdrawal occur frequently in dementia and mild cognitive impairment. On the other hand, patients suffering from dementia are less likely to experience other symptoms, such as psychomotor agitation. Nevertheless, patients with dementia are no less likely to endorse a depressed mood. Given the frequency of depressive symptoms in Alzheimer's disease, some investigators and clinicians have proposed a "*depression of Alzheimer's disease.*" To meet criteria for this syndrome, patients must first be diagnosed with dementia of the Alzheimer's type and exhibit at least three depressive symptoms such as depressed mood, anhedonia, social isolation, poor appetite, poor sleep, psychomotor changes, irritability, fatigue or loss of energy, feelings of worthlessness, and suicidal thoughts.

Episodes of major depression in late life can be of either *early onset* (that is, the first episode occurs before the age of 60 years and the current episode represents a relapse) or *late onset* (the first episode occurs after the age of 60 years). The symptoms of the depressive episode rarely differentiate early versus late onset. Nevertheless, a careful history may reveal factors that are associated with an earlier-onset disorder, such as long-standing personality disorder, a family history of psychiatric illness, or significant psychosocial stressors, such as a difficult employment history. One variant of late-onset depression is vascular depression, a subcategory of depression owing to vascular lesions in the brain. Vascular depression can be diagnosed only with the assistance of brain imaging. Nevertheless, elders experiencing this variant reveal more problems with verbal fluency, psychomotor speed, and especially executive cognitive functioning. Executive functioning is characterized by an ability to plan ahead, initiation, and perseveration.

Psychotic depression across the life cycle is much less frequent than nonpsychotic depression, yet is relatively more common in late life than earlier in life. For example, psychotic depression may be diagnosed in between 20% and 45% of hospitalized depressed elderly patients. Symptoms of late-life psychotic depression include a depression associated with delusions or hallucinations. These delusions or hallucinations may be "mood congruent" (delusions or hallucinations whose content is entirely consistent with the depressive themes of inadequacy, guilt, disease, death, and nihilism) or "mood incongruent" (the content of the delusions or hallucinations did not involve these depressive themes). As noted below, psychotic depression frequently will only respond to aggressive therapy such as electroconvulsive treatment.

Bipolar disorder is much less frequent than a unipolar major depression in late life. In addition, symptoms do not typically present with the classic cluster (i.e., hyperactivity, decreased sleep, flight of ideas, grandiose delusions, and hypersexuality). Mania may present with the predominant symptom of paranoia and fragmentation of ideas. A syndrome of reversible cognitive impairment, which appears much like an Alzheimer's type of dementia, can also be seen. The symptoms include confusion, agitation, and incomprehensible loud verbalizations. Yet another presentation of bipolar disorder is irritability and anger without evidence of an elated affect. Finally, bipolar disorder may present as a "dysphoric mania." These patients experience agitation and sleep problems but do not express feelings of elation or grandiosity but rather an uncomfortable "depressed" mood.

THE EPIDEMIOLOGY OF LATE-LIFE MOOD DISORDERS

The frequency of clinically significant depressive symptoms among community-dwelling older adults in most studies ranges from approximately 8% to 16%. Depressive symptoms may be more frequent among Latinos than among Caucasians and African-Americans. Major depression is more common among women compared to men, a difference that persists into late life. Depressive symptoms are more frequent among the oldest old, yet the higher frequency is generally explained by factors associated with aging, such as a higher proportion of women (women experience a higher frequency of depressive symptoms than men), increased physical disability, increased cognitive impairment, and lower social economic status. Overall, the frequency of depressive symptoms is no higher among older adults than among adults in young adulthood or midlife. Depressive symptoms, as assessed by usual screening instruments, are somewhat less frequent in African-Americans and more frequent among Latinos.

The prevalence estimates of major depression in the community are quite low, ranging from 1% to 4% overall with a higher prevalence among women, yet with no significant racial or ethnic differences. The frequency of bipolar disorder in community populations is low regardless of age (less than 0.5%). On psychiatry inpatient units, however, the frequency of mania in older adults may be as high as 5% overall and 9% of the persons having a mood disorder. Dysthymic disorder and minor depression are somewhat more frequent (4–6% for dysthymic disorder and 4% for minor depression). The frequency of major depression in hospitalized older adults on medical and surgical services usually ranges between 10% and 12%; in long-term care facilities between 10% and 15% experienced major depression. Between 5% and 10% of older adults visiting primary-care providers meet criteria for a diagnosis of major depression. Clinically significant depressive symptoms among hospitalized patients ranged between 20% and 25%, and as high as 35% of older adults in long-term care facilities experience the symptoms. Therefore, the burden of mood disorders is much higher in inpatient and long-term care facilities than found in the community.

THE OUTCOME OF MOOD DISORDERS IN LATE LIFE

Data from a 6-year follow-up of community-dwelling elderly in the Netherlands estimate that approximately 23% of subjects diagnosed with major depression recovered and remained recovered, 44% experienced a fluctuating course, and 33% experienced persistent and moderate-to-severe depressive symptoms. Data from a long-term study of major depression in a clinical setting reveal similar results. Thirty-one percent recovered and remained well, 28% experienced at least one relapse but recovered, 23% recovered only partially, and 17% experienced persistent depressive symptoms throughout the 6 years of follow-up. Predictors of partial remission include comorbidity, major depression and dysthymia, poor social support, and functional limitations.

Many factors adversely influence the outcome of late-life depression. In turn, late-life mood disorders can complicate the course of comorbid problems. For example, depression is a major cause of weight loss in late life, and weight loss can adversely influence the outcome of many chronic medical illnesses. In turn, depression increased the risk for heart failure, a decrease in bone mineral density, and the prognosis of persons experiencing a myocardial infarction. Depression is also associated with disability over time. Disability is also a risk for depression. Physical disability among the depressed can lead to a higher number of negative events, the restriction of social leisure activities, isolation, and reduced quantity and quality of social support. Severe depression associated with cognitive decline, even if the cognitive impairment remits, is a risk for Alzheimer's disease.

Nonsuicide mortality is a significant adverse outcome resulting from severe late-life depression. Both severity and duration of depressive symptoms increase the risk for mortality in elderly population studies. Even so, the causes of higher mortality rates in older adults may not be secondary to depressive symptoms themselves but rather factors associated both with depression and mortality, such as older age, medical comorbidity, smoking, and body mass index as well as chronic diseases and functional impairment.

Suicide frequency increases for white men, with peaks reaching rates as high as 62 per 100 000 in the 65 years and older age range. In contrast, suicide rates among elderly women are lower than for women in midlife. Persons attempting suicide are more likely to be widows (widowers), to live alone, to perceive their health status to be poor, to experienced poor sleep quality, to lack a confidante, and to experience stressful life events such as interpersonal problems in one's marriage. Suicidal ideation is high among older adults, ranging from 5% to 10% (usually expressed as a wish to not live longer, not active suicidal intent).

Suicide rates in the United States have declined in recent years, reversing earlier trends. From 1987 to 2002, the rates among older persons declined from 21.7 to 15.6 per 100 000. This decline mirrors the lower rates in the 45 to 64 years age group documented during the late 1970s. These two declines suggest a so-called period effects rather than cohort effect. Namely, events during the 1970s and 1990s could be operating to buffer the negative impact of depression and other factors that may increase risk for suicide in the elderly. For example, the stock market created wealth and more economic security for many Americans during the 1990s. A more controversial explanation is that the introduction of selective serotonin reuptake inhibitors (SSRIs), prescribed to more than 10% of older adults in the United States may have reduced the burden of depression such that suicide rates decreased.

ORIGINS OF LATE-LIFE MOOD DISORDERS

Biological Origins

Older adults appear to be at greater risk of major depression biologically, such as depression resulting from vascular changes, even though the frequency of depression is either lower or similar to that among younger adults. Older adults may therefore be protected psychologically because of factors such as cumulative wisdom and perhaps relatively protected from social risk. Genetic influences appear to account for less than 20% of the variance in total depression scores in twin studies, a minimal contribution compared to other factors. Most hypothesized genetic markers for late-life depression have not been substantiated in controlled studies. Even so, some unique possibilities of mutations or polymorphisms are being investigated for their contribution to late-life depression. For example, a rare disease, CADASIL (cerebral autosomal-dominant arteriopathy with subcortical infarcts and leukoencephalopathy), results from a mutation in the notch 3 gene. Depression is one of the initial symptoms of this condition.

Underactivity of serotonergic neurotransmission has been the focus of much research on the pathophysiology of depression in younger adults. Although serotonin activity (specifically receptor binding) decreases dramatically throughout midlife, there is less decrease from midlife to late life. Given that enhancement of serotonin neurotransmission has been a key to the development of antidepressant medications, these findings are of importance to the pathophysiology of late-life depression, although the specifics of the mechanisms have yet to be worked out. Polymorphisms in the serotonin transporter gene may influence antidepressant response to SSRIs. A single-nucleotide polymorphism in the rate-limiting enzyme of neuronal serotonin synthesis has been identified. This functional single-nucleotide polymorphism in older adults has been found to be associated with a significant decrease in response to SSRI antidepressant therapy.

Depressive symptoms can lead to increased cortisol secretion, which, in turn, inhibits neurogenesis, leading to hippocampal volume loss, which, in turn, may mediate the core symptoms of depression. Early-life stress may produce a permanent hypersensitivity to stress, with the production of ongoing HPA dysregulation, and, with repeated episodes of major depression plasticity, may decrease, giving rise to permanent damage. As described above, a vascular-based depression has been proposed, resulting from cortical ischemic events. These ischemic events are documented via magnetic resonance imaging (MRI) as white matter hyperintensities. The symptoms of vascular depression resemble those of frontal lobe syndromes secondary to structural abnormalities in areas associated with the limbic–cortical–striatal–palatal–thalamic–cortical pathways.

The hereditary predisposition to manic episodes is significant, regardless of age. Yet this predisposition does not appear to be as great in late life compared to earlier in the life cycle, especially for first-onset bipolar disorder. Despite the biologic predisposition to developing late-onset bipolar illness, life events can also contribute to the onset of manic episodes. More than half of persons who experience late onset of mania report a life event severe enough to disrupt usual activities of daily living. Clinicians should be especially vigilant in reviewing medications and their patients to present with manic episodes. Corticosteroids, levodopa, decongestants, bronchodilators, thyroid replacement, and antidepressant medications all can contribute to the onset of a manic episode. Finally, traumatic head injuries are thought to contribute to bipolar disorder as well.

Psychological Origins

A number of psychological factors have been suggested as contributing causes to depressive symptoms and disorders in the elderly. Older patients with personality disorders do not recover from depression as quickly, nor do they experience as long the remission as those without. One reason is that personality styles often modify the way in which the older adult adjusts to stressful events, such as medical illnesses.

Cognitive distortions have also been proposed as potential causes of late-life depression. The cognitive–behavioral psychotherapies (described below) are based on this theory. Specifically, older adults may overreact to life events or misinterpret these events and, therefore, exaggerate the negative outcome. For example, the older adult may ruminate excessively about a negative event or catastrophize the event. A frequent cause of ruminating or catastrophizing is family conflicts or perceived slights from family members (the basis of interpersonal psychotherapy as described below). Self-efficacy and a higher sense of mastery, in contrast, are associated with fewer depressive symptoms.

Social Origins

A number of social factors have been associated with late-life mood disorders, including stressful life events, bereavement, chronic stressors or daily hassles, socioeconomic status, and social support. Investigators have found a strong association between more severe stressful events, such as bereavement or life-threatening illness and major depression. Older adults lacking confidence are especially vulnerable to such stressful events. Stressful events, however, may be attenuated among older people for at least two reasons. First, the elderly usually gain experience through the life cycle that prepare them to manage the impact of such an event. This increased capacity for managing stressful events assumes that the older adult is cognitively intact and functions at a relatively normal level. In addition, older adults often have anticipated the events that confront them. For example, the death of a spouse for an 80-year-old woman may be a tragic but not an unanticipated event. She has seen many of her peers experience similar losses. Following the loss of a loved one, depression is more frequent but it is not the usual outcome. Older persons exposed to chronic strain are also at greater risk of developing depression. The most common and frequently studied example of such strain is caregiving (especially for demented). Financial strain has also been associated with increased frequency of depressive symptoms. In general, socioeconomic disadvantage and the perception that one's basic financial and tangible needs (such as adequate housing) are inadequate have been associated with a higher frequency and persistence of depressive symptoms.

Social support has long been associated with protection against the onset and persistence of depressive symptoms. The most robust relationship between social support and depression is the perception that one's social network and interactions with network members are limited or negative. Adequate social support, on the other hand, can modify the negative impact of stressful events and other risk factors for depression. For the most part, older adults perceive their support to be adequate (and therefore when support is perceived to not be adequate, clinicians should be especially attentive).

Given that the frequency of depression in the elderly is no higher than at other stages of the life cycle, yet biological risk for depression may be increased, some have suggested that psychological factors may modify the biological and social risk for depression. One example of a psychological factor modifying a biological risk is "wisdom." Wisdom is a nebulous concept, yet may be loosely defined as an expert knowledge system concerning the fundamental and practical aspects of life, such as a knowledge and ability to judge both the meaning and the conduct of life. Investigators have suggested five characteristics of wisdom: a rich factual knowledge, a rich procedural knowledge (that is, having an ability to assess, for example, what strategies might best solve a given problem), lifespan contextualization (that is, learning to integrate life experiences), relativism of values and life priorities (that is, a tolerance for differences in one's sociocultural environment), and a recognition and ability to manage uncertainty.

THE DIAGNOSTIC WORKUP OF LATE-LIFE MOOD DISORDERS

The diagnosis of late-life mood disorders derives primarily from a careful history (see Figure 70-1). The clinician should focus on not only present symptoms but also past history (especially history of previous episodic symptoms similar to those presenting at the time of the interview). Family history, medication history, recent life events, changes in social and economic status, and recent physical problems will inform the clinician of not only the diagnosis but also potential causes of the mood disorder. The diagnosis of depression can be made in older adults without comorbid disorders, using the diagnostic criteria for major depression in DSM-IV-TR. Yet, as outlined in Table 70-1, older adults are less likely to endorse a depressed mood,

rarely report weight gain (a symptom that is frequent among depressed younger adults), rarely complain of excess sleeping, are less likely to express feelings of worthlessness or inappropriate guilt, and are less likely to report suicidal thoughts.

Screening scales, such as the Geriatric Depression Scale and the Center for Epidemiologic Studies-Depression Scale, can complement the history and provide screening in busy clinics, especially primary-care clinics. Screening for depressive symptoms should be supplemented with screening for cognitive functioning using scales such as the Mini-Mental State Examination. Screening in primary care is critical, for not only is the frequency of depression high but suicidal ideation may range from 1% to 5% of all older adults attending a clinic. The success of screening in primary clinics, however, is mixed for busy physicians. These physicians, although accepting the responsibility for treating older adults with mood disorders, often perceived their clinical skills as inadequate. One reason for these feelings of inadequacy is that uncomplicated major depression makes up only approximately 15% of those depressed persons receiving

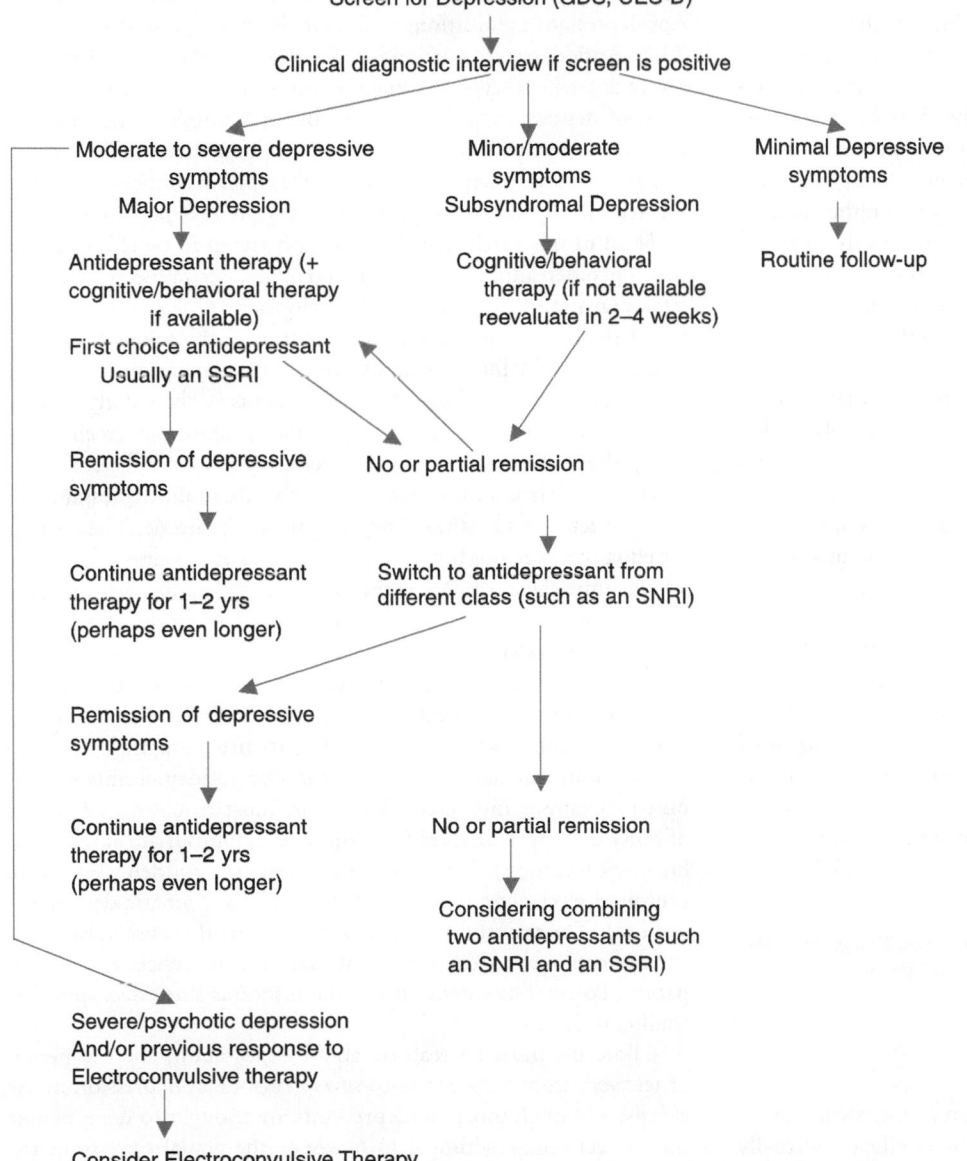

FIGURE 70-1. The diagnosis and treatment of depression in the elderly.

TABLE 70-2

Diagnostic Workup of the Depressed Older Adult

ROUTINE DIAGNOSTIC TESTS	ELECTIVE DIAGNOSTIC TESTS
Screen for depressive symptoms using commonly used symptom screening scales such as the Geriatric Depression Scale or the Center for Epidemiologic Depression Scale	Magnetic resonance imaging can be used to establish the diagnosis of subcortical white matter hyperintensities, a clue to the presence of a vascular dementia
The key to the diagnosis of late-life mood disorders is a thorough present and past history and mental status examination	Screens for vitamins and minerals, such as vitamin B-12 and folate deficiency, when deficiency is suspected
Cognitive function can be evaluated by administering a brief cognitive screen such as the Mini-Mental Status Examination	Polysomnography is used infrequently in routine diagnostic workups for late-life mood disorders but may be used when a sleep abnormality cannot be explained
Laboratory tests can be used to screen out comorbid medical conditions that may contribute to the depressive disorder or that may provide baseline data for the prescription of antidepressant medications	T_3 and T_4 as well as TSH may be ordered to rule out undiagnosed thyroid dysfunction

primary care. Recent studies have suggested that the effectiveness of treating late-life depression in primary care can be significantly augmented by case managers who maintain close contact with mental health professionals.

Clinicians should be aware of potential bias in the diagnostic process. For example, older men are less likely to be referred to primary-care physicians or mental health specialists for symptoms of depression. Older men are also less likely to endorse core depressive symptoms and to have received prior depressive treatment. The discomfort felt by depressed older men is more likely to present more as somatic symptoms and interpersonal stress rather than in emotional terms. In other words, men may be less likely to recognize their feelings. They also are less likely to accept a diagnosis of depression and perhaps therapy, if the diagnosis is made. Some symptoms of depression may be endorsed more frequently by older adults who are both depressed and cognitively impaired. The symptoms include greater emotional withdrawal and psychomotor retardation. The cognitively impaired depressed, however, are probably no less likely to endorse a depressed mood than those without cognitive impairment.

Laboratory tests are ordered primarily to augment the history and physical examination, for there is no biological marker for most subtypes of late-life depression. The one exception is vascular depression, where the presence of subcortical white matter hyperintensities on magnetic resonance imaging assists in the diagnosis. Routine laboratory tests, especially a chemistry screen and an electrocardiogram, should be obtained when antidepressant medications are prescribed. Elective tests include thyroid screens for undiagnosed thyroid dysfunction, polysomnography if significant sleep abnormalities cannot be explained, vitamin B-12 and folate assays when vitamin deficiency is suspected, and magnetic resonance imaging to establish the diagnosis of vascular depression (Table 70-2).

TREATMENT OF LATE-LIFE MOOD DISORDERS

Biological Therapies

Antidepressant medications are the foundation for the treatment of moderate-to-severe late-life depression. In terms of efficacy, virtually all antidepressant medications are equal (see Figure 70-1). There-

fore, the choice of an antidepressant medication is usually based on side effects that the clinician wishes to avoid. For this reason, the SSRIs have become the treatment of choice. Nevertheless, collision should recognize that these medications are not without side effects. Antidepressant medications and their doses are presented in Table 70-3. Antidepressants are most effective in treating moderate-to-severe depression (typically major depression). For less severe symptoms of depression, antidepressant therapy coupled with counseling/psychotherapy has not proven to be of great benefit. Perhaps for this reason, a number of alternative therapies have been described for depression, such as St. John's wort (*Hypericum perforatum*).

Most of the SSRIs have been demonstrated to be efficacious in treating older adults, including fluoxetine, sertraline, paroxetine, citalopram, and fluvoxamine. Escitalopram is probably an effective drug, but it has not been demonstrated efficacious in clinical trials, specifically for the elderly. Other new-generation antidepressants that have been shown to be efficacious in the elderly include mirtazapine, venlafaxine, and bupropion. Duloxetine, recently entering the market, has not been specifically proven effective in the elderly. Clinicians should not neglect the older antidepressants for some patients, such as nortriptyline and desipramine. These drugs are equally efficacious but, in many elders, cause adverse side effects, which limit their use. Nevertheless, some elders do well on these older drugs, and, if they respond without adverse side effects, there is no reason to switch to the newer agents.

Side effects of the antidepressant medications vary by category (and no category is without side effects). The SSRIs may lead to agitation, insomnia, gastrointestinal disturbances, weight loss, sexual dysfunction, and elevated levels of tricyclic antidepressants if combined therapy is instituted. A rare but most troubling side effect of SSRI therapy is SIADH (syndrome of inappropriate antidiuretic hormone secretion). This syndrome can emerge, suddenly leading to profound electrolyte imbalance (specifically a dramatic decrease in sodium). The tricyclic antidepressants frequently cause anticholinergic effects such as dry mouth, urinary incontinence, and constipation. Postural hypotension is a more serious side effect, possibly leading to falls.

Clinicians must be realistic about expectations for the period of recovery from a moderate-to-severe episode of depression in the elderly. Although most antidepressants are thought to demonstrate their effectiveness within 4 to 6 weeks, the actual time from the beginning of therapy to the subjective report by the patient that

TABLE 70-3

Pharmacotherapy for Late-Life Depression

ANTIDEPRESSANT	STARTING DOSE (mg)	AVERAGE DAILY DOSE (mg)	SIDE EFFECTS
Tricyclics			
Nortriptyline	25	25–100	Anticholinergic effects (such as dry mouth, constipation, and urinary retention),
Desipramine	25	25–100	postural hypotension, and possible cognitive dysfunction
SSRIs			
Paroxetine	10	10–40	Agitation, insomnia, gastrointestinal disturbances, SIADH, weight loss, sexual
Sertraline	50	50–200	dysfunction, and elevated blood levels of tricyclics
Fluoxetine	10	10–40	
Citalopram	10	10–20	
Escetalopram	10	10–20	
Other antidepressants			
Trazodone	50		Sedation and priapism
Buproprion	75		Agitation and insomnia
Venlafaxine	37.5		Nausea, vomiting, headache, and hypertension
Mirtazapine	7.5		Sedation and weight gain
Duloxetine	40		Orthostatic hypotension, nausea, and hypertension

they truly feel "back to normal" may take months and even up to a year in severe depression. Although biological symptoms may abate fairly quickly, such as sleep problems, the subjective sense of well-being and interest in life take much more time to return to normal. One reason is that the depressed persons when recovering require some time to reintegrate into their usual life activities and are often hesitant to return to past activities after a prolonged episode of depression.

Antipsychotic medication is the first-line treatment for acute agitated behavior in the manic patient. The drugs of choice are the new-generation (or atypical) antipsychotic medications. Olanzapine (5–10 mg) and risperidone (2–4 mg) are most frequently used among older adults. These newer agents, in contrast to the older antipsychotic agents, such as haloperidol, have become treatment of choice primarily because of fewer extrapyramidal side effects. Nevertheless, these newer agents can lead to weight gain and especially in a propensity toward diabetes mellitus.

Lithium carbonate has been the cornerstone for the prevention of the current manic and depressive episodes in bipolar disorder, yet the drug does present potential significant toxicity in late life. The usual dose is 300 to 600 mg daily. In younger adults, the normal range for a lithium level is between 0.8 and 1.2 mEq/L. In older adults, lithium can be maintained in the range of 0.4 to 0.6 mEq/L. Renal status of the older adults should be determined before lithium therapy is instituted by obtaining a chemistry screen. If compromised renal function is suspected, then a 24-hour creatinine clearance can be obtained.

Given the potential for side effects with lithium, antiepileptic medications have been used frequently to treat older adults with bipolar disorder. Valproic acid (400–800 mg/day) is the preferred agent by most clinicians. Gastrointestinal problems are the major side effect limiting use of this drug. Other agents that have been prescribed for prevention of manic episodes include carbamazepine (200–600 mg/day), clonazepam (0.5–1.5 mg/day), lamotrigine (100–200/d), and gabapentin (900 mg/day).

Clinicians face challenges in treating depressed older adults who do not respond to antidepressant medication. Older adults with

psychotic symptoms and who have responded previously to ECT do not respond well to antidepressants but often do respond to a second course of ECT. Although the response of older adults experiencing depression may be slightly less optimal than with young adults, some suggest that ECT is actually a superior treatment in late life compared to midlife. A higher percentage of moderately to severely depressed older adults receive ECT compared to younger adults primarily because older adults are more likely to be treatment resistant to antidepressant therapy. Memory problems persist as the primary adverse reaction to ECT, although these problems are usually transient and clear within a few weeks following treatment. A new procedure could replace ECT for older adults, namely, repetitive transcranial magnetic stimulation. The advantage of transcranial magnetic stimulation is that it does not require anesthesia and does not produce a seizure. Finally, exercise has been shown to be effective in treating mild-to-moderate symptoms of depression (but is not a treatment that can replace antidepressant therapy for moderate-to-severe depression). ECT may also be effective in bringing about a remission of a severe and pharmacologically resistant episode of mania.

Psychological Therapies

A number of psychotherapies have been explored in the treatment of late-life depression, especially cognitive/behavioral therapy and interpersonal psychotherapy. These therapies, unlike more long-term and subjective approaches to therapy (such as psychodynamic therapy), can be manualized and can be administered by clinicians with Masters-level training. Cognitive/behavioral therapy is an educational approach to therapy during which the therapist focuses on thoughts expressed by the patient that may perpetuate depression. The goal of therapy is to teach the older adult that these thought patterns can be changed. One approach to reversing these negative thoughts is by using a daily record of thoughts and then "stepping back" and examining the rational response to these thoughts (thoughts are usually precipitated by an adverse event). For example, an older woman may wait for a call on a Sunday night from her daughter and the call does not come. She may feel sad and abandoned, thinking that her daughter does not love her anymore. Upon a rational reflection, however, she recognizes that her daughter may have been busy during the evening and by late evening does not wish to disturb her mother and will call the following evening. Interpersonal psychotherapy is a therapy similar to cognitive/behavioral therapy, which focuses on four areas thought to cause or maintain depression: grief (such as the death of a loved one), role transitions (such as movement to a retirement community), interpersonal deficits (such as a propensity to express anger inappropriately), and interpersonal disputes (such as a conflict with a neighbor). Through an educational approach, older adults are instructed to implement adaptive means for confronting each of these problems.

A combination of psychotherapy and pharmacotherapy has been demonstrated to be more effective in bringing a depressive episode into remission, as well as preventing recurrence during the first year following remission. Recent studies, however, suggest that pharmacotherapy is, by far, more valuable than combined therapy in preventing recurrence during longer periods of time. The Improving Mood Promoting Access to Collaborative Treatment (IMPACT) study was developed to test whether placing a health specialist in a primary-care physician's office in order to influence the use of combined therapy is more effective than usual care in reducing the burden of late-life depression. Older adults in the treatment group (compared to the control group) were less likely to express suicidal ideation, to experience reduction in depressive symptoms, and to experience less functional decline.

Working with the Family of the Depressed Older Adult

Therapy for the depressed older adult almost always involves some interaction with the family. Family members usually accompany the older adult to the office, and the depressed elder rarely prohibits the physician from discussing the depressed mood with the family member. And the physician should take advantage of this opportunity. Initially, the family can provide valuable additional information about the duration, severity, qualitative differences they witness in the depressed elder compared to her/his usual state, and information about life events that may have contributed to the depressive episode. The physician also can address issues of concern to the family. When the physician takes time to discuss care with the family, hospitalization may be avoided and acute changes in behavior during the course of therapy may alert the clinician to problems such as adverse side effects from medications.

Families often can benefit from an explanation of symptoms that the elder is experiencing, for they are not accustomed to their loved one, for example, sitting all day in a chair. They also can benefit from guidance regarding how to manage behaviors. For example, how far should the family push the patient to become more physically active or engage in social activities? Finally, families should be educated about the risk for suicide. Families can help reduce suicide risk by restricting the behavior of the depressed elder, such as limiting access to medications, removing weapons from the house, or limiting driving to times when someone else is in the automobile. At the same time, families should be assured that there is no absolute method to prevent suicide and that the best the clinician and family can do is reduce suicide risk.

Evaluating and Managing Suicidal Risk in the Depressed Older Adult

When working with the depressed older adult, evaluation and management of suicidal risk are critical. Asking the older adult about suicidal ideation or behavior is of value but cannot be relied on as the best means for evaluation. The physician can ask a series of questions to determine increased risk:

1. Do you feel that life is worth living?

2. Have you ever thought about harming yourself? (Ask question #3 if the answer is yes.)

3. If you were to attempt to harm yourself what means would you use?

4. Have you ever tried to harm yourself?

If the older adult has considered a specific means for harming himself/herself (such as taking pills or shooting oneself) then the risk is increased.

Of greater value, however, in the evaluation of risk for suicide is the accumulation of known risk factors. In other words, the best evaluation for suicidal risk parallels the evaluation for risk of chronic disease events such as a myocardial infarct. A person is at greater risk of a myocardial infarct if the person has high cholesterol, is overweight, has a history of heart disease in the family, has diabetes, does not exercise, and so forth. Older adults are at greater risk of suicide if they are male, are in late-late life, are Caucasian, have lower income, are socially isolated, are divorced or widowed, are bereaved, are suffering from a comorbid medical illness, are diagnosed with depression in the past, are abusers of alcohol, and have a history of previous suicide attempts. Some clinicians believe that developing a suicidal contract (the patient agrees not to harm herself/himself until the clinician is contacted to discuss the emotional pain) prevents suicide. This is not the case, although a suicide contract may reduce risk somewhat.

If the physician determines that the older adult is at significant risk of suicide, then hospitalization is imperative. Acute suicidal risk is usually short-lived and therefore hospitalization for a few days is sufficient to both implement a comprehensive program of treatment and "ride out" the time of greatest risk. During hospitalization, privileges can be gradually increased and the patient gains confidence to return to the usual activities. Once the patient is discharged from the hospital, medication should not be prescribed in sufficient quantity that filling one prescription would provide the patient with enough medications to make a serious suicide attempt by overdose.

FURTHER READING

Alexopoulos G, Meyers B, Young R, Campbell S, Silbersweig D, Charlson M. 'Vascular depression' hypothesis. *Arch Gen Psychiatry.* 1997;54:915–922.

Baltes P, Staudinger U. Wisdom: a metahuerastic (pragmatic) to orchestrate mind and virtue toward excellence. *Am Psychol.,* 2000;55:122–136.

Beekman A, Geerlings S, Deeg D, et al. The natural history of late-life depression. *Arch Gen Psychiatry.* 2002;59:605–611.

Blazer D. *Depression in Late Life.* 3rd ed. New York, New York: Springer; 2002.

Blazer D. Depression in late life: Review and commentary. *J Gerontol Med Sci.* 2003;58A:249–265.

Blazer D, Burchett B, Service C, George L. The association of age and depression among the elderly: an epidemiologic exploration. *J Gerontol Med Sci.* 1991;46:M210–M215.

Blazer D, Hybels C. Origins of depression in later life. *Psychol Med.* 2005;35:1241–1252.

Hybels C, Blazer D, Steffens D. Predictors of partial remission in older patients treated for major depression: the role of comorbid dysthymia. *Am J Geriatr Psychiatry.* 2005;13:713–721.

McKeown R, Cuffe S, Schulz R. US suicide rates by age group, 1970–2002: an examination of recent trends. *Am J Public Health.* 2006;96:1744–1751.

Pinquart M, Duberstein P, Lyness J. Treatments for later-life depressive conditions: a meta-analytic comparison of pharmacotherapy and psychotherapy. *Am J Psychiatry.* 2006;163:1493–1501.

Post F. *The Significance of Affective Symptoms at Old Age.* London: Oxford University Press; 1962.

Radloff L. The CES-D Scale: a self-report depression scale for research in the general population. *Appl Psychol Measures.* 1977;1:385–401.

Reynolds C, Frank E, Perel J, et al. Nortriptyline and interpersonal psychotherapy as maintenance therapies for recurrent major depression: a randomized controlled trial in patients older than 59 years. *J Am Med Assoc.* 1999;281:39–45.

Reynolds CR, Dew M, Pollock B, et al. Maintenance treatment of major depression in old age. *N Engl J Med.* 2006;354:1130–1138.

Schulz R, Drayer R, Rollman B. Depression as a risk factor for non-suicide mortality in the elderly. *Biol Psychiatry.* 2002;52:205–225.

Unutzer J, Katon W, Callahan CM, et al. Collaborative care management of late-life depression in the primary care setting. *J Am Med Assoc.* 2002;288:2836–2845.

Yesavage J, Brink T, Rose T. Development and validation of a geriatric depression screening scale: a preliminary report. *J Psychiatr Res.* 1983;17:37–49.

Zhang X, Gainetdinov R, Beaulieu J, et al. Loss-of-function mutation in tryptophan hydroxilae-2 identified in unipolar major depression. *Neuron.* 2005;45:11–16.

Schizophrenia

Danielle L. Anderson ■ *Peter V. Rabins*

DEFINITION

Schizophrenia is a pervasive, debilitating disease characterized by positive symptoms of hallucinations, delusions, and thought disorder (also referred to as psychosis), and negative symptoms of chronic social dilapidation. Emil Kraepelin first distinguished schizophrenia (then termed dementia praecox) from bipolar psychosis more than 100 years ago, by contrasting the long-term deteriorating course of delusions and hallucinations characteristic of schizophrenia to the intermittent course of bipolar illness. Schizophrenia remains a clinical diagnosis made on the basis of the individual's psychiatric history and mental status examination, as no laboratory or imaging studies can validly diagnose it.

Inclusion Criteria

Schizophrenia is described in the fourth edition of the *Diagnostic and Statistical Manual of Mental Disorders* as two or more of the following symptoms active for a minimum of 1 month's duration (unless adequately treated) as well as the continuing presence of a symptom for 6 months: delusions, hallucinations, disorganized speech, disorganized behavior, and negative symptoms along with a significant disturbance of the individual's functioning that results in disturbances in occupation, social interaction, or the management of one's self-care. These symptoms of schizophrenia can be characterized as either positive or negative.

Positive Symptoms

The positive symptoms of schizophrenia consist of abnormalities of sensory experience and cognitive processing. These manifest as hallucinations, delusions, bizarre behavior, or formal thought disorder. *Hallucinations* are perceptions in the absence of physical stimuli. In schizophrenia, auditory hallucinations usually predominate, but, in patients with late-onset schizophrenia, olfactory, visual, tactile, or gustatory hallucinations may be present. In schizophrenia, the hallucinated voices are described as coming from outside the person's head and providing a running commentary on the patient's behavior. At times, these speak directly to the individual or converse with each other. Voices that tell the individual what to do are referred to as command hallucinations.

Delusions are fixed, false, idiosyncratic beliefs and consist of ideas and beliefs that are persecutory, bizarre, or grandiose. The idea that the person is being controlled by outside forces is common.

Bizarre behavior may be observed in the person's appearance (odd/inappropriate layering of clothing) or in their aggressive, agitated or repetitive/stereotyped behavior (for example, flipping the light switch multiple times or repeated closing and opening the door). *Formal thought disorder* includes illogical or incoherent speech in the absence of aphasia. It manifests as tangentiality, loose associations (a lack of logical connection between sentences), or derailment (the sudden loss of train of thought).

Negative Symptoms

The negative symptoms of schizophrenia result in a decline in the person's baseline social, interpersonal, and volitional activity. People with schizophrenia often have a diminished range of facial expression, a phenomenon termed affective flattening; poor eye contact, and decreased expressive gesturing. Spontaneous speech decreases and speech latency increases. Individuals with schizophrenia become less social and form few close relationships with others. As the disease progresses, avolition and apathy become common and impair work and school performance, grooming, and hygiene.

Clinical Course

Schizophrenia often has a prodromal period during which individuals become socially awkward and isolative. Negative symptoms emerge, and work or school performance gradually declines. Positive symptoms and bizarre, disorganized behavior then manifest more overtly. For example, people with schizophrenia frequently speak and laugh when they are by themselves, symptoms that are thought to represent patients' responses to internal stimuli such as hallucinations. The negative symptoms often result in a lowered socioeconomic status, leading to unemployment, estrangement from family members, and even homelessness.

Exclusion Criteria

Schizophrenia is not the only cause of hallucinations and delusions. For this reason, patients presenting with psychotic symptoms need to be fully evaluated and all other potential causes of these ruled out before a diagnosis of schizophrenia is made. The presence of prominent mood symptoms during the psychotic episode indicates the likelihood of a mood disorder or schizoaffective disorder. The presence of hallucinations or delusions with subacute onset of fluctuating disturbance of consciousness and attention suggests a delirium. In the elderly, psychosis often occurs in the setting of dementia; the presence of memory loss and either aphasia, apraxia, agnosia, or loss of executive function should raise the possibility of dementia, since individuals with schizophrenia generally remain oriented to their surroundings. Hallucinations and delusions can also be induced by exogenous substances (e.g., medications, illicit drugs, and toxins) or general medical conditions such as seizure disorder, brain tumor, and encephalitis.

Associated Symptoms

Abnormal psychomotor activities such as rocking, pacing, immobility, or repetitive stereotyped behaviors can impair social functioning. Hallucinations can impair concentration owing to the distraction produced by aberrant experiences. Demoralization and anhedonia, a loss of interest and enjoyment in activities, may also be found. Mortality is increased in schizophrenia; 28% of the increase in early death is attributed to suicide and 12% to accidents. The prognosis is worse in patients with impaired insight into their illness.

Age of Onset (Table 71-1)

Early Onset

The lifetime prevalence of schizophrenia is 1%. Although schizophrenia occurs with equal frequency in men and women, the age of onset is earlier in males, with a peak age of onset between 10

TABLE 71-1

Differences Between Early- and Late-Onset Schizophrenia

	EARLY ONSET	LATE ONSET
Age of onset	Teens–early adult	Fifth decade or later
Family history of schizophrenia	Frequently a positive family psychiatric history	Rare
Gender	Equal prevalence between men and women	Predominantly women
Symptom type	Negative and positive	Mostly positive symptoms; thought disorder rare
Prognosis	Poor	Moderate

and 25 years. Women have a bimodal age distribution with a first peak between 25 and 35 years and another peak in late middle age. The disease tends to have a more severe course in males with greater predominance of negative symptoms, and females tend to retain their social and premorbid function. However, patients with early-onset schizophrenia who live into late life usually have a many-year history of illness with prominent negative symptoms and an inability to live independently.

Late Onset

A consensus of international experts has identified two diagnostic forms of late age disease: late-onset schizophrenia, with onset after the age of 40 years, and very-late-onset-schizophrenia-like psychosis, with onset after the age of 60 years.

Schizophrenia beginning after the age of 40 years is characterized by prominent positive symptoms, but fewer negative symptoms than early-onset schizophrenia. However, thought disorder is rare in the late-onset condition. In addition, individuals with late-onset schizophrenia are less likely to have a family history of schizophrenia than those with early onset and are more likely to be female. Compared to the cognitive deficits seen in early-onset patients, late-onset illness is characterized by relatively intact learning, abstraction, and cognitive flexibility. Very-late-onset schizophrenia frequently occurs in the setting of sensory impairment (decreased auditory acuity and low vision states) and social isolation. It is important to note that late-onset schizophrenia is responsive to lower levels of antipsychotics than early-onset schizophrenia.

DIFFERENTIAL DIAGNOSES

Mood Disorders

Mood disorders include both major depressive disorder and bipolar affective disorder. In both, depressive episodes characterized by a loss of vital sense (a sense of physical discomfort, sleep disorder, appetite loss, poor self-attitude (lack of self-confidence, self-blame, and guilt), and sad mood. Bipolar affective disorder differs from major depressive disorder in that those affected also experience manic episodes. Although psychosis is not required for diagnosis, it can occur during either severe depressive or manic episodes.

One important distinction between psychosis in mood disorders and schizophrenia is that in the psychosis of mood disorders, symptoms are present only during severe mood episodes and resolve when the mood disturbance resolves. Although those with schizophrenia may experience mood symptoms during the course of their illness, psychosis is the dominant feature that persists regardless of mood disturbance. Another clinically useful distinction is that the delusions of mood disorder are congruent with the patient's mood state. For example, in mania, grandiose delusions accompany euphoric or elevated mood, while, in depression, self-blaming, self-deprecating, and guilty delusions parallel a sad mood.

Schizoaffective Disorder

Schizoaffective disorder is similar to schizophrenia in that psychotic symptomatology is prominent and may persist between episodes, but there is also a prominent disturbance in mood. Thus, the diagnosis of schizoaffective disorder requires a period of psychosis, lasting at least 2 weeks in the absence of any mood disturbance. However, criteria for a mood disorder must also be met for a predominant portion of the active and residual periods of the disease.

Dementia

Twenty percent to 30% of individuals with dementia experience hallucinations, and 30% to 40% develop delusions during the course of their illness. The cognitive deficits reflect a drop from the individual's prior level of functioning and cause impairment in activities of daily living. In the case of Alzheimer's dementia, the most common form of dementia, the onset is gradual, typically begins with memory deficits, and progresses to death over the course of 10 years. Although schizophrenia may include cognitive deficits, these are less severe than in dementia and progress more slowly.

Delirium

Delirium is characterized by an acute or subacute onset of cognitive impairment and a disturbance of attention and cognition. Fluctuation over the course of the day is common. Misperceptions of environmental stimuli, referred to as illusions, and visual hallucinations are also common. Delirium is usually because of a toxic, metabolic, or infectious disorder that needs identification and treatment in order to resolve. Delirium's acute onset and fluctuating cognitive deficits distinguish it from schizophrenia.

Delusional Disorder

Delusional disorder is characterized by a single, prominent delusion, which is described as "nonbizarre," that is, plausible, and has been present for at least a month. The individual with delusional disorder usually remains fully functional apart from the dysfunction that results directly from the delusion. The negative symptoms found in schizophrenia are absent in delusional disorder, and the individual with delusional disorder behaves normally when the delusion is not being acted upon or discussed.

Substance-Induced Psychotic Disorder

Hallucinations and delusions may be a result of intoxication or withdrawal of substance use. Sedatives (barbiturates and benzodiazepines), alcohol, and stimulants (amphetamines and cocaine) are common causes. These are not seen in withdrawal from opiates.

Schizophreniform Disorder and Brief Psychotic Disorder

The criteria to fulfill schizophreniform and brief psychotic disorder are the same as in schizophrenia, except for shorter illness durations than schizophrenia. Schizophreniform disorder lasts between 1 and 6 months, while brief psychotic disorder lasts anywhere from 1 day to 1 month. Social and occupational impairment is not required in these disorders.

Ictal Psychosis

Schizophrenia-like psychosis occurs in complex partial seizures, particularly those of the temporal lobe. A nonconvulsive status epilepticus can rarely mimic schizophrenia, but the symptoms are present only hours to days. Automatisms of the mouth and lips and eye fluttering can be seen. In these cases, an EEG will show active seizure activity. Psychosis also occurs postictally and following a flurry of seizures lasting an average of 70 hours. A seizure disorder is often present at least 10 years before the manifestation of interictal psychosis. Postictal suppression may be seen on EEG.

ETIOLOGY

Genetic

First-degree relatives of individuals with schizophrenia have a 10 times greater risk of developing schizophrenia than the general population, and twin studies show higher concordance rates among monozygotic twins than dizygotic twins. Nonetheless, monozygotic twins are 50% discordant, suggesting that environmental factors contribute as well. The heterogeneity of the disorder suggests that multiple genetic loci contribute a vulnerability to schizophrenia. Genetic vulnerability plays less of a role in late-onset schizophrenia.

Developmental

Persons born in the winter and early spring are more likely to develop schizophrenia than those born in late spring and summer. While no clear explanation for this has emerged, potential hypotheses include seasonal variability in diet or higher rates of prenatal virus exposure at different times of the year. Observational studies suggest that a complicated fetal history may predispose to the development of schizophrenia. This suggests a potential etiologic role for maternal exposure to influenza virus during pregnancy, perinatal hypoxia from obstetric complication, nutritional deprivation in utero, and autoimmune processes in the pregnant mother.

Brain structural abnormalities found in schizophrenia include a larger right temporal horn and third ventricle as well as decreased amygdala, hippocampus, and parahippocampal gyrus volumes. These changes are felt to represent a reduced synaptic density. Since synaptic density is maximal at the age of 1 years and decreases until adolescence, one etiologic theory postulates that synaptic pruning is excessive in schizophrenia and leads to the emergence of symptoms during late adolescence and early adulthood. Neuronal disorganization within the hippocampus has also been found and has been suggested to represent that disorganization may be the result of impaired neuronal migration during development.

TREATMENT

Antipsychotics

Typical Antipsychotic

The first antipsychotic, chlorpromazine, was originally developed as an antihistamine and found by chance in the 1950s to reduce psychotic symptoms in individuals with schizophrenia. The primary mechanism of action of antipsychotic drugs is believed to be D2 dopamine receptor blockade in the mesolimbic dopamine pathway, which travels from the ventral tegmental area of the midbrain to the nucleus accumbens. Since all neuroleptic drugs effective for schizophrenia cause D2 blockade, overactivity of the mesolimbic dopamine pathway is hypothesized as a necessary element in the development of the positive symptoms of schizophrenia. However, D2 blockade is not specific to the mesolimbic pathway, and antipsychotic drugs also block three other dopamine pathways, thought to cause many of the observed side effects of these drugs. Dysfunction of the mesocortical pathway traveling from the ventral tegmental area of the brainstem to the cortex is thought to be responsible for the negative and cognitive deficits found in the disorder. Dopamine blockade of the nigrostriatal dopamine pathway projecting from the substantia nigra to the basal ganglia, a part of the extrapyramidal nervous system that modulates motor movement, causes symptoms similar to those found in Parkinson's disease (increased muscle tone with cogwheel rigidity, shuffling gait, masked facies, and resting tremor). These are referred to as extrapyramidal symptoms. Extrapyramidal symptoms are especially impairing in the elderly, since the resultant shuffling gait may lead to falls in an already susceptible population. A decrease of dopamine in the basal ganglia is thought to cause *akathisia*, a severe feeling of restlessness, accompanied by pacing, shifting weight from foot to foot when asked to stand still, and difficulty remaining seated, and *dystonia*, persistent (tonic) involuntary contractions of muscles, most commonly of the neck and tongue. Dystonia is less common in the elderly but may present as lateral flexion at the hips ("Pisa syndrome"). Another side effect of neuroleptics that can become persistent and disabling is *tardive dyskinesia*, thought to result from the upregulation of dopamine postsynaptic receptors in the nigrostriatial pathway leading to persistent, repetitive, abnormal movements of the tongue, face, and lips. Choreoathetoid movements of the limbs, head, or trunk can also develop. The elderly, females, and individuals with brain injury are more susceptible to tardive dyskinesia. Tardive dyskinesia may resolve weeks or months after discontinuation of the medication, but often persists.

The final dopamine pathway is affected. Dopaminergic neurons from the hypothalamus project into the pituitary gland in the tuberoinfundibular pathway and inhibit the secretion of prolactin. As a result, neuroleptics can elevate prolactin levels and cause galactorrhea. In postmenopausal women, neuroleptics can cause an increased rate of bone demineralization.

Antipsychotics also affect muscarinic-cholinergic, alpha 1 adrenergic, and histaminergic receptors. Histaminergic blockade causes weight gain and sedation. Sedation, blurred vision, dry mouth, and constipation result from blockade of the muscarinic-cholinergic receptors. Alpha 1 adrenergic inhibition causes dizziness, drowsiness, and orthostatic hypotension. Since all of these increase susceptibility to falls and hip fractures, frequent monitoring in elderly patients is crucially important.

Atypical Antipsychotics

The atypical or second-generation antipsychotics antagonize serotonergic receptors in addition to dopamine receptors. These are thought to be more effective against the negative symptoms of schizophrenia and may cause less extrapyramidal symptoms. However, recent studies have shown a 1% to 2% increase in mortality in the elderly with dementia who are taking drugs in this class. The mechanism by which this occurs is not known, and it is uncertain whether this pertains to elderly individuals with schizophrenia.

Better cognition, social interaction, and fuller affect are reported with the use of atypical antipsychotics in younger individuals, but whether this is true of the elderly is not known.

Currently, there are six atypical antipsychotics available for clinical use. Although these are all considered atypical, these vary in their side-effect profiles and receptor affinities (Table 71-2). There is increasing concern over metabolic syndrome as a potential side effect of antipsychotics. Therefore, patients taking atypical antipsychotic drugs should be monitored for high blood pressure, obesity, high cholesterol, and insulin resistance. Patients taking olanzapine may be at higher risk than those taking other atypicals.

Neuroleptic malignant syndrome (NMS) is a life-threatening complication, which may occur with either typical or atypical antipsychotics. It is characterized by severe muscle rigidity and

---

TABLE 71-2

Commonly Used Pharmacotherapeutic Agents for Schizophrenia

ANTIPSYCHOTIC	STARTING DOSE (mg)	USUAL DOSE RANGE (mg/day)	PREDOMINANT SIDE EFFECTS	RECOMMENDED MONITORING
Haloperidol	0.25	0.5–4	EPS, TD, and dystonia	Monitor for EPS
Clozapine	6.25–12.5 bid	25–150	Agranulocytosis (1%–2%), sedation, tachycardia, decreased seizure threshold at doses greater than 600 mg, and sialorrhea	Weekly granulocyte counts, enforced by manufacturer
Risperidone	0.25–0.5 qd	0.25–3	Hypotension, sedation, and EPS	Monitor for EPS
Olanzapine	2.5 qd	2.5–10	Sedation, weight gain, and metabolic syndrome	Cholesterol and fasting blood sugar level every 6 months
Quetiapine	12.5–25 qd	25–200	Sedation and postural hypotension	Orthostatic blood pressures with dose increases
Ziprasidone	20 qd	40–80	QTc prolongation and cataracts	EKG at baseline and after dose increase, yearly ophthalmologic examination
Aripiprazole	5	5–15	Hypotension	

EPS, extrapyramidal symptoms; TD, tardive dyskinesia; EKG, electrocardiogram.
Note: Monitoring for all antipsychotics should include monitoring for EPS, weights, cholesterol, and fasting blood sugar level every 6 months for metabolic syndrome.

autonomic instability typified by elevated temperature, tachycardia, and elevated or labile blood pressure. Mutism, changing levels of consciousness (as seen in delirium), elevated white blood cell count, incontinence, and dysphagia may also be seen. Creatinine phosphokinase levels are raised when muscle rigidity is present. NMS is felt to result from the abrupt decrease in dopamine from neuroleptic use. Management of this syndrome includes stopping the neuroleptic drug, protecting the kidneys from muscle breakdown products with intravenous fluids, supportive medical measures, and, occasionally, administration of the dopamine agonists bromocriptine or dantrolene.

Psychosocial Treatments

Individuals with schizophrenia obtain benefit from psychosocial intervention in addition to drug therapy. To combat noncompliance, education and support should be given to individuals with schizophrenia as well as their family members. Supportive and behavioral therapy can be offered. Vocational and social skill training may be used to promote independence and quality of life.

NONPSYCHOTIC DISORDERS THAT CAN BE CONFUSED WITH SCHIZOPHRENIA

Charles Bonnet Syndrome

Charles Bonnet syndrome is a condition in which vivid visual hallucinations and generally good insight into the false nature of these hallucinations occur in the setting of poor vision. There is an absence of delusions. The poor vision, usually central, results from conditions such as macular degeneration or cataracts. If vision improves, the hallucinations often remit. Often the visions seen are figures or objects that are diminutive in size, termed Lilliputian hallucinations. Patients with this condition often do not report their hallucinations to health-care providers for fear of being labeled crazy.

Delusional Parasitosis (Ekbom Syndrome)

Delusional parasitosis is a condition in which the affected individual has a delusion of infestation by parasites. The individual visits multiple physicians with this complaint, is unshaken by negative test results, and often brings in skin scrapings and nail clippings as proof. Patients may try to kill the parasites by pouring kerosene, rubbing alcohol, insecticide, or other irritants over their skin. Some may physically pick or scrape at themselves. This condition will sometimes respond to antipsychotics.

Diogenes Syndrome

Diogenes syndrome is a condition of self-neglect. The affected individual tends to live in domestic squalor and be socially withdrawn. A tendency to hoard items (syllogomania) with no clear purpose may also be present. These individuals are reluctant to seek treatment, resist help when it is offered, and may remain undetected for years.

Hallucinations in Grief

Hallucinations commonly occur during the grief reactions of deceased loved ones. Patients report that they hear the voice of a loved one or see them pass by. This is more appropriately termed an illusion, as it usually consists of misinterpretation of stimuli. However, true hallucinations may occur and are even socially normative in some cultures.

Organic Delusional Disorder

Organic delusional disorder is characterized by a delusion that is the result of a metabolic, toxic, or neurologic abnormality. This disorder has a wide range of delusional content as well as potential causes (e.g., HIV, seizure disorder, brain damage, drug use, Alzheimer's, and Huntington's). Sudden onset, association with physical symptoms characteristic of the disorder, lack of a typical course, and lack of personal or familial psychiatric history suggest a nonpsychiatric etiology and should prompt further evaluation.

FURTHER READING

American Psychiatric Association. *Diagnostic and Statistical Manual of Mental Disorders, Fourth Edition, Text Revision.* Washington, DC: American Psychiatric Association; 2000.

Anderson D, Pankow L, Luchins D. The possible role of vision rehabilitation in the treatment of visual hallucinations in the elderly. *Topics Geriatr Rehabil.* 2004;20(3):204–211.

Brown S. Excess mortality of schizophrenia. A meta-analysis. *Br J Psychiatry.* 1997; 171:502–508.

Howard R, Rabins PV, Seeman MV, et al. Late-onset schizophrenia and very-late-onset schizophrenia-like psychosis: an international consensus. The International Late-Onset Schizophrenia Group. *Am J Psychiatry.* 2000;157(2):172–178.

Kaplan HI, Sadock BJ. *Kaplan and Sadock's Synopsis of Psychiatry: Behavioral Sciences, Clinical Psychiatry.* 8th ed. Baltimore: Williams and Wilkins.

Neugebauer R. Accumulating evidence for prenatal nutritional origins of mental disorders. *JAMA.* 2005;294(5):621–623.

Rabins PV, Aylward E, Holroyd S, et al. MRI findings differentiate between late-onset schizophrenia and late-life mood disorder. *Int J Geriatr Psychiatry* 2000;15:954–960.

General Topics in Geriatric Psychiatry

Mustafa M. Husain ■ *Shawn M. McClintock* ■ *Kip E. Queenan* ■ *Aaron Van Wright* ■ *Rajbir Bakshi*

SUICIDE

Elderly individuals account for a significant proportion of death by suicide in the United States. Recent statistics from the Centers for Disease Control (CDC) indicated that 14.6 persons per 100,000 aged 65 years or older died by suicide, with the highest risk group being males aged 85 years or older. Within that group, the rate of suicide was 51 per 100,000. Although the overall suicide rate in the elderly population has slightly decreased since 1999 (15.9 per 100,000), nonetheless, death by suicide remains a significant concern.

Factors Associated with Suicide

The majority of suicides occur within the context of a mood disorder with the remainder related to some form of psychiatric disorder including substance abuse, personality pathology, or schizophrenia. In the general population, risk factors for suicide include living in a rural area, owning firearms, and unemployment. For elderly adults, the risk factors vary based on age- and health-related issues. Table 72-1 outlines the risk factors for suicide as well as protective factors that may decrease the possibility of suicidality in elderly patients. With relation to depressive episodes, there is inconclusive evidence discerning between whether late onset (after age 60 years) or early onset, or prior or current depressive episodes are associated with increased risk.

Suicide is a complex construct with both biological and psychological etiologic factors. While there is limited information regarding biological components of suicide, the serotonergic system has consistently been implicated in suicide through mechanisms separate from affective disorders. Hydroxyindoleacetic acid, a serotonin metabolite, is significantly associated with suicide. Lower concentrations of hydroxyindoleacetic acid have been found to correlate strongly with suicide lethality, that is, patients with lower concentrations of hydroxyindoleacetic acid have been found to make more lethal suicide attempts. Regarding serotonin receptors, there tends to be an abnormality in the prefrontal cortex of patients who completed suicide, as evidenced by decreased presynaptic serotonin transporter sites. Also, compared to patients with no suicidal tendencies, patients with suicidal tendencies have increased serotonergic neurons in the dorsal raphe nucleus. The noradrenergic system has also been implicated in suicide, with research showing high noradrenalin levels in the prefrontal cortex and lower levels in the brainstem. In examining the dopaminergic system, while it has been found to be abnormal in patients with depression, there is too little research to conclude its association with suicide. Thus, research is required to further elucidate the psychiatric contributions to suicide as well as understand the connectivity between psychological, biological, and social factors.

Evaluation and Assessment

Evaluating and assessing suicide may be difficult in geriatric patients, as they may be prone to not discuss those feelings and thoughts. As such, the role of the clinician is to form a strong, trusting bond with the patient in order to comprehensively assess suicidal ideation, intent, and plan of action. The evaluation is an integral part of the treatment process, as it opens up discussion between the patient and clinician, thereby allowing prevention through decreasing access to available means of suicide, building trust, facilitating a supportive therapeutic relationship, and tailoring treatment interventions.

To increase the reliability of the interview, structured suicidal assessment scales can be used. A commonly used scale is the Scale for Suicide Ideation, which is a 19-item clinician-rated measure that assesses suicidal thoughts and behaviors for the prior 7 days and for the worst points in life as determined by the patient. The Scale for Suicide Ideation thoroughly measures many components of suicide, including suicidal plan, behavior, preparation for attempt, and

TABLE 72-1

Risk and Protective Factors Related to Elderly Suicide

RISK FACTORS	PROTECTIVE FACTORS
• Increased pessimism	• Perceived social support
• Increased helplessness	• Feeling useful
• Initial week of admission to inpatient unit	• Realistic outlook
• Discharge week from inpatient unit	• Positive future outlook
• Prior affective disorder	• Achieving goals
• Current affective disorder	• Close interpersonal relationships
• Medical comorbidity	• Successful adjustment to aging
• Functional disability	

TABLE 72-2

PROSPECT* Recommended Guidelines and Management Techniques for Working with Patients with Suicide

Guidelines while working with patients with suicidal ideation
- Be attentive
- Stay calm and nonthreatening
- Provide the patient with space and time to vent
- Be collaborative, use a team approach
- Be willing to say the word "suicide"

Management techniques for patients with high risk
- Directly assess the frequency and content of suicidal ideation and risk factors
- Explore the initial problem
- Have the patient describe reasons for and against suicide
- Assess the patient's access to means
- Provide the patient with education regarding depression including its etiology, prognosis, and treatment
- Decide how to manage an increase in suicidal ideation through either a formal contract or some other formality
- Provide education regarding alcohol and illicit substances and encourage their discontinuation
- Meet with the patient weekly at minimum if suicidal ideation is present
- Write prescriptions for no more than 1 week until suicidal risk has decreased
- Provide family education regarding suicide, including how to appropriately respond to the patient and assuring the living environment is safe (i.e., remove firearms)
- Provide supportive and collaborative interaction with the patient

At each treatment assess hopelessness, suicidal ideation, and substance abuse

*PROSPECT, Prevention of Suicide in Primary Care Elderly: Collaborative Trial.
Data from Brown GK, Bruce ML, Pearson JL. High-risk management guidelines for elderly suicidal patients in primary care settings. Int J Geriatr Psychiatry. 2001;16:593–601.

anticipation of attempt. Also, a recent scale developed specifically for use in an elderly population is the Geriatric Suicide Ideation Scale. The Geriatric Suicide Ideation Scale is a 66-item multidimensional measure of suicide in geriatric patients, which assesses four factors including suicide ideation, death ideation, loss of personal and social worth, and perceived meaning of life. This measure will require further study given its newness, but, thus far, it has strong psychometric properties, is easy to administer, has standardized administration and scoring procedures, and is sensitive to suicide detection.

Just as important as clarifying risk factors, within the assessment it will be of utility to identify protective factors. Protective factors (see Table 72-1) are adaptive for the patient and help to decrease the potential suicide completion. For example, research has found that having a positive future orientation, which involves constructively thinking about the future, generating positive future outcomes, identifying and nurturing goals, and identifying reasons for living, can help decrease suicide. Although Table 72-1 lists those protective factors that have been identified in elderly patients, it is essential to enquire and assess for patient-specific protective factors, which could include hobbies, prior therapeutic treatments, and high self-worth. Once identified, protective factors should be reinforced by the clinician in order to become concrete within the patient, which may aid in the treatment process.

Management and Treatment

Managing and treating geriatric patients with suicidal tendencies initially involves three steps. The first is to diagnose and treat the current psychiatric disorder. The second step is to assess the suicidal intent and lethality with an emphasis on prevention. And the third is to construct a specific treatment plan tailored to the patient. Guidelines for managing suicide in adults were provided by the American Psychiatric Association's (APA) practice guidelines for the assessment and treatment of patients with suicidal behavior.

For elderly adults, specific guidelines for treating and managing suicide were provided from the Prevention of Suicide in Primary Care Elderly: Collaborative Trial (PROSPECT). The primary goal of PROSPECT, a National Institute of Mental Health-funded, randomized, controlled trial, was to assess the effectiveness of an intervention (treatment by a psychiatric specialist) in preventing and reducing suicidal ideation and behavior. The study found that the intervention, relative to treatment as usual (with additional screening), was effective in decreasing suicidal ideation and depressive symptoms. Table 72-2 shows the PROSPECT general recommendations

for working with patients with suicide as well as management techniques for patients at high risk.

Many geriatric patients who are suicidal are usually seen by their primary-care physician, and, as such, it is important for their physician to be knowledgeable of suicidal signs and symptoms and treatment strategies. Many of the patients with suicidal ideation may also present with depression; thus, psychiatric treatment may commence with an antidepressant, psychotherapy, or a combination of both. Using cognitive behavior techniques to help the patient reframe his/her thoughts, constructing positive future orientations, and developing adaptive coping strategies may help to mitigate the risk of suicide. Overall, suicide is a significant risk in elderly adults, but, with proper care including comprehensive assessment, development and implementation of patient-specific treatment, and ongoing effective management, the risk of suicide may be lessened.

ANXIETY DISORDERS IN THE ELDERLY

The most common anxiety disorders in late life are generalized anxiety disorder and phobias. Agoraphobia without panic disorder has been described as occurring late in life, but obsessive compulsive disorder and panic disorder are generally thought to persist from earlier adulthood when present. Anxiety disorders in the elderly are commonly associated with depression. Studies looking at nursing home populations have found a prevalence ranging from 9.9% to 13.2%. It has also been shown that the presence of depression and anxiety can significantly impact the well-being of nursing home patients. Posttraumatic stress disorder (PTSD) has also been described in the elderly.

Treatment Options for Anxiety

Commonly used medications for anxiety spectrum conditions include selective serotonin reuptake inhibitors, other antidepressants, and benzodiazepines. As anxiety and depression are so commonly comorbid conditions, pharmacological treatment with antidepressants is often helpful for both conditions.

Benzodiazepine use in the elderly may be associated with some unique concerns. The indication for these drugs is similar to that for the general adult population. Studies have shown that their use is often more common in the institutional setting, and the actual indication for use is often something other than an anxiety disorder. When using benzodiazepines in the elderly, it is important to remember that pharmacological properties are influenced by age, and agents with longer half-lives and active metabolites are more likely to cause adverse events. Studies have shown that the elderly are more sensitive to the sedating effects of benzodiazepines on the central nervous system. Other adverse events documented have included dependence, cognitive impairment, paradoxical agitations, and psychomotor impairment and falls.

Posttraumatic Stress Disorder

PTSD in the elderly has been discussed in the literature, often in the setting of natural disaster and veterans of war. More than 50% of male veterans are predicted to be older than 65 years by the year 2020. Symptoms of PTSD may occur shortly after the event or may not develop until many years later. There is often a history of previous trauma in individuals with PTSD, and life stressors can bring about a relapse of symptoms. Treatment involving psychotherapy and psychopharmacology is similar to the general adult population, and studies looking at differences are lacking. However, anxiety disorders may impact the treatment outcomes for patients who are depressed. One study examining older adults in an outpatient setting showed a slower response to treatment in geriatrics with comorbid PTSD. Nonetheless, treatment can be effective and will require appropriate diagnosis and management.

LATE-LIFE PSYCHOTIC DISORDERS

Psychosis is a mental disorder often marked by a law of contact with reality and may affect individuals at any age. Geriatric healthcare specialists face a particular challenge in the management of psychosis in the older patient. One of the most disenfranchised groups in health care is the elderly with psychotic disorders. The impact of psychotic disorders in the elderly is significant in both financial costs and quality of life. With national health-care costs skyrocketing, the impact on families, caregivers, and the patients' quality of life is immeasurable. Psychotic episodes increase the risk of hospitalizations and mortality. Behavioral disturbances, are common in psychotic illness and may pose a significant threat to the safety of the elderly patient and those around them.

Clinical Presentation

The psychotic older person in a distressed state is likely to present first to a primary-care physician or geriatrician, rather than seek mental health services. As the primary-care clinician sorts through the history, the clinician may detect something odd in the nature of the person's complaints. For instance, the history may reveal a heightened suspiciousness toward family, children, or neighbors. Patients may feel that people are stealing from them or trying to control them. The patient's paranoia may further limit access to in-home attendants, visiting nurses, and other social service professionals. Fears of loss of autonomy and loss of mental and physical capacity can culminate in a frank paranoia. In one of the more familiar clinic scenarios, persons may present to their primary-care physician with vague somatic complaints. Upon further questioning, older persons may blame their symptoms on some implausible occurrence such as a noxious gas being pumped into their home by forces or people often unknown.

Psychosis in the older person can be a symptom of either an acute or a chronic illness. Acute psychotic symptoms are often the sequelae of a general medical condition such as infection, trauma, metabolic abnormality, on medication side effect. The psychotic symptoms in these instances noted may be more accurately described as being part of a delirium. Chronic or persistent psychotic symptoms may be consistent with a DSM-IV diagnosis. There are two distinct categorizations. The first is a primary diagnosis of psychosis including a delusional disorder, mood disorder with psychotic features, or schizophreniform illness. The second category includes psychosis as a specified feature of a dementia or because of a chronic general medical condition, such as a head trauma, Parkinson's disease, and a seizure disorder. Most of the further discussion in this section will cover psychosis in the elderly related to more persistent symptomatology. Often these psychotic episodes are diagnosed as part of a late-onset schizophrenia, schizophrenia-like illness or part of a dementia.

Epidemiology and Terminology

The onset of schizophrenia typically occurs in the late teens to early twenties. In adults younger than 60 years of age, the yearly incidence of schizophrenia is approximately one in 10 000 individuals, with a lifetime risk of 0.8. A minority of the population first experience psychotic symptoms in their later years. The majority of these older individuals with late-onset psychosis are diagnosed with schizophrenia. There are different ages of onset used to define early- and late-onset manifestations of psychotic illness. Swiss psychiatrist Manfred Bleuler's studies of late-onset schizophrenia involved individuals who developed the illness after the age of 40. Most of the subsequent English studies used an onset after the age of 60. The latter group is often referred to as having very-late-onset schizophrenia.

The term "*paraphrenia*" is used interchangeably with late-onset schizophrenia. Paraphrenia was a term used to identify a true *late-onset* schizophrenia as being different from a chronic schizophrenia of *early onset*. Physician Emil Kraeplin originally used paraphrenia to describe an illness in which the patient experiences suspiciousness, frank paranoia, and possible hallucinations but tends not to suffer significant deterioration as seen with negative symptomatology. Late-onset schizophrenia tends to be associated less with deterioration of personality and affect, which may increase the chance of achieving a good treatment response and better prognosis.

Risk and Comorbidity

Several comorbid conditions are linked with schizophrenia. Some of the conditions include depressive disorders, cognitive impairment, obsessive-compulsive disorder, aggressive disorder, and substance abuse. Each of these entities may have profound negative effects on treatment effectiveness and overall progress. Specific numerical breakdowns in the literature show depression as having 25% prevalence in schizophrenia. Obsessive-compulsive disorder has a 3.5% to 15% probability of occurrence in schizophrenia. Substance abuse is subdivided with 35% of the schizophrenic population using alcohol, 20% using cocaine, 15% using marijuana, 3% using heroin, and 70% to 90% using nicotine. In the nicotine addicted, nicotine use typically increases p450 enzyme activity, resulting in the need for upward dose adjustment in some neuroleptic medications to achieve therapeutic effect. Concerning aggression, there is a five- to sixfold higher probability for violence in patients with schizophrenia.

Moreover, the presence of sensory deficits and female gender seems to increase the risk of developing late-life psychosis. Sensorineural hearing loss has documented ties to the development of psychosis in the elderly adults. In addition, patients with late-onset schizophrenia are more likely to be women, with women having more severe positive psychotic symptoms (i.e., systemic persecutory delusions) and less severe negative symptoms (i.e., affective flattening and social withdrawal).

Psychosis in Dementia

Psychotic symptoms often present within the course of a dementing illness. The symptoms may vary widely from case to case and may only appear intermittently throughout the illness course. The psychosis of a dementia may pose serious problems for the caregiver. Approximately 50% of patients experience delusions or hallucinations within the first 3 years after a clinical diagnosis of Alzheimer's dementia. Paranoid delusions are often the most common psychotic symptoms to appear in Alzheimer's dementia, with visual hallucinations being second, followed by a lower incidence of auditory hallucinations. The patient with Alzheimer's dementia may provide a history of seeing people or animals moving freely throughout their home. Charles Bonnet syndrome is an example of this type of visual hallucination seen in Alzheimer's dementia. The patient with Alzheimer's may describe seeing people who are fully realized often, except for some unusual feature. These unusually perceived hallucinatory objects may appear to float from place to place or may be abnormally smaller in stature (Lilliputian). The patient with dementia may suffer other disturbances in perception, which involve disorientation to time and space. Reduplicative paramnesia is a curious phenomenon seen in some patients with dementia. It is a delusional belief that the person's present environment has either been duplicated or been moved from another location. The patient may strongly insist that the current hospital room is located in the patient's hometown or even connected to the patient's home in some physical way. This may often be considered as confusion or simple disorientation, but, in fact, it is a form of delusional misidentification.

Treatment Considerations

When approaching a patient with psychosis of unknown history, the clinician should first rule out a physical or systemic illness, including drug intoxication, neurological or vascular events, metabolic abnormalities, systemic infections, sepsis, and postoperative states. These conditions can cause delirium, complicate diagnosis, and impede timely treatment of psychotic symptoms. Remission of the psychosis will likely depend on adequate treatment of the underlying acute medical illness.

Once it is determined that the patient with psychosis is medically stable, the clinician may administer treatment using both nonpharmacologic and pharmacological methods. In the nonpharmacological approach, it is important to establish a working rapport. A good working rapport with the older patient who is paranoid may prove difficult, but establishing good rapport can result in reaching a more favorable treatment outcome. There is usually no need to confront patients about their psychotic or delusional symptom. The clinician and the patient can respectfully disagree about the source of the problem and still work together to maximize the patient's ability to function.

The most comprehensive treatment plans use pharmacological approaches in conjunction with nonpharmacological ones. The atypical antipsychotics (e.g., olanzapine, risperidone, and ziprazidone) have been the drugs of choice for the past few years. These typically have fewer of the side effects associated with the older antipsychotics (e.g., haloperidol, chlorpromazine, and thioridazine) such as tardive dyskinesia, dystonic reactions, parkinsonian symptoms, and anticholinergic and orthostatic hypotensive effects.

However, atypical antipsychotics should be used more cautiously for a number of reasons. There is an increased risk of developing type II adult-onset diabetes and dyslipidemias with atypical antipsychotic use. Recently, the Food and Drug Administration (FDA) issued a public health advisory that cautions about the use of atypical antipsychotics in the older patients with dementia for treatment of behavioral disturbances and agitation. The FDA stated that atypicals are associated with an increase in mortality (mostly owing to cardiac events and pneumonia). For example, atypical antipsychotics have been found to be associated with increased rates of mortality in patients with Alzheimer's disease. However, a Finnish study showed no associated increase in mortality with atypicals in the elderly patient with dementia. Thus, additional analysis of the data concerning safety and efficacy of these drugs is warranted. As a result of mixed findings, some clinicians have returned to using small doses of the first-generation antipsychotics, while others continue to use atypicals, and follow metabolic markers (i.e., fasting glucose, lipid profiles, and weight) on a monthly basis for the initial visits, then every 8 to 12 weeks during the stable dosing and maintenance phases.

ALCOHOL AND SUBSTANCE USE IN THE ELDERLY

The consumption of alcohol is common in American culture. The use of alcohol has been linked to many contrasting facets of the human experience such as social activities and religious rituals. It has also had its place in sometimes harmful rites of passage and patterns of self-destructive behaviors. Because of the ubiquitous nature of the alcoholic substance, it tends to illicit very different attitudes from health-care professionals than other potential substances of abuse. When considering these cultural issues and attitudes regarding the geriatric population in a medial setting, the existence of alcoholism can sometimes be overlooked simply because the elderly are often not considered to be alcoholics.

Geriatric Substance Abuse Prevalence

Research in the area of geriatric substance abuse is a relatively new area of interest. Even though abstinence is the most common drinking pattern among the elderly, recent data suggest that there is still a need for concern. Studies of community-dwelling older adults show prevalence estimates of problem drinking in 1% to 15% of individuals. Males tended to drink more and were more likely to have problem drinking. For example, one outpatient study found that 8.6% of geriatric patients with mental illness meet criteria for alcohol dependence. When examining lifetime prevalence, the numbers were even higher, with one study of short-term rehabilitation nursing home patients showing that 49% of individuals had a diagnosis of alcohol dependence at some time in their life, and 18% had active symptoms in the prior year. One hypothesis suggests that the number of elderly patients with substance dependence may increase in the near future. People who are currently in their thirties, forties, and fifties grew up between 1950 and 1970, which was a time of increased substance use and dependence, a factor that could contribute to elderly substance abuse. Substance use may continue or may resurface in this population, as it faces the stressors typically associated with late life including loss of a loved one, retirement, and loss of independence.

Diagnosis and Classification

A proper history is essential to diagnosing alcohol dependence. All patients should be initially asked how much alcohol they drink and whether or not they are an everyday drinker. It is often helpful to ask in a nonjudgmental fashion and reiterate that this information is very important to their medical evaluation and necessary to provide good treatment. A particularly useful and popular validated screening tool for use in the medical setting is the CAGE questionnaire. The CAGE questionnaire has four component questions represented by the four letters of the name: (1) Have you tried to Cut down on your drinking? (2) Are you Annoyed when asked to stop drinking? (3) Do you feel Guilty about your drinking? (4) Do you need and Eye-opener drink when you get up in the morning? The CAGE questionnaire focuses on the diagnosis of alcohol dependence. It, in and of itself, is not complete in evaluating a patient but can provide a useful starting place. Further history obtained can include a history of medical illness related to alcohol use, recent social stressors, and a family history of substance dependence. Medical evaluation into medical consequences of alcohol use can also be helpful.

When defining a pattern of alcohol consumption, it is important to distinguish two things: problem/at-risk drinking and dependence. For persons aged 65 years and older, at-risk drinking is considered to be more than seven standard drinks per week or more than three drinks per occasion. A standard alcoholic drink is defined as 1.5 ounces of 80 proof (40%) alcohol (e.g., vodka), 4 to 5 ounces of wine, or 12 ounces of beer. The multitude of different containers that alcohol is available in and the accuracy of the history can make it difficult to accurately estimate use. At-risk drinking, even in the absence of psychological dependence, can be concerning, as it may lead to acute injury and trauma and long-term medical and social complications. In mental health care, dependence is a disorder of substance use defined by the DSM-IV-TR as the presence of three or more of the following symptoms in a given year: withdrawal; tolerance; spending more time obtaining, using, or recovering from the substance; using more or longer than intended; unsuccessful attempts to control use; and continued use despite psychological and/or physical problems caused by the use.

Therapeutic Interventions

In the early stages of treatment, it is important to determine if an individual is at risk of alcohol withdrawal, a potentially life-threatening complication of discontinuing alcohol consumption. This can occur clinically in the settings as someone seeking help for at-risk drinking or dependence, or in the acute care or institutional setting when the individuals no longer have access to their usual supply of alcohol. Symptoms of alcohol withdrawal can include tremor, restlessness, elevated pulse and blood pressure, delirium, and/or seizure. The acute symptoms of withdrawal generally peak by 72 hours after the last drink consumed and can require treatment for up to 7 days (or longer if delirium is present). The course of withdrawal is often worse in individuals with a history of previous withdrawal and multiple comorbid medical problems. The elderly are more likely to have withdrawal symptoms for a longer period of time, but there is no evidence that being elderly alone puts one at risk of a more complicated course or a longer duration of treatment. Proper management of withdrawal is a critical first step in treatment and includes medical assessment and stabilization, pharmacologic treatments, and proper vitamin supplementation (including the proper use of thiamine supplementation to prevent the development of Wernicke–Korsakoff syndrome). Wernicke–Korsakoff syndrome is a brain disorder caused by alcohol-associated thiamine deficiency, which can result in memory impairment, hallucinations, changes in vision, and/on loss of muscle coordination.

Benzodiazepines are the agents of choice to treat and prevent alcohol withdrawal. Their cross tolerance at the type A gabba-aminobutyric acid receptors with ethanol is likely the basis for this. Barbiturates have been used effectively in the past but now have largely been abandoned because of their less favorable side-effect profile and lack of controlled evidence-based studies. When choosing a benzodiazepine for use in alcohol withdrawal, it is important to consider the half-life of the drug and the route of metabolism. In the elderly, an agent that is shorter acting and less extensively metabolized by the liver can sometimes be more favorable, as long as the medication is dosed appropriately to the half-life. This can be important to prevent the buildup of multiple CNS active metabolites that may increase the chance of oversedation, especially in patients with multiple medical comorbidities. Chlordiazepoxide, diazepam, lorazepam, and oxazepam are all commonly used agents in adults. Lorazepam and oxazepam are both metabolized via glucuronidation in the liver to inactive metabolites that are renally excreted, making them favorable shorter-acting agents in persons with functional liver insufficiency and intact renal functioning.

Once patients with at-risk consumption or dependence are identified and acute therapies initiated, the implementation of brief interventions has been shown to be cost-effective ways of further directing treatment. These have been studied in the general adult population extensively, and there have also been two studies in the geriatric population. Types of interventions included brief (10–15 minutes) counseling visits and telephone follow-ups. Older adults have been shown to be good candidates for treatment, especially when age-appropriate care is provided. There are limited data on randomized treatment outcomes. In one recent study, 1652 patients older than

50 years were admitted to a rehabilitation center for the treatment of alcohol dependence. The center used treatment programs designed to cater to older adults and found postdischarge rates of abstinence similar to that of middle-aged adults.

Clinical Approach and Management

When working with patients who suffer from alcohol and other substance disorders, it is important to keep some practical approaches in mind. Motivational interviewing approaches have been shown to be more effective in leading to reduced intake than more confrontational approaches that are common in the medical setting. Motivational interviewing itself is a specific therapeutic intervention, but its philosophy and techniques can be applied to brief interactions in any setting. It emphasizes the use of empathetic listening and encouraging patient-directed discussions about making behavior changes, rather than simply providing instructions to the patient. This process of beginning a discourse on change (referred to as "change talk") can be effective in leading to patients initiating changes in their behavior. It is helpful to begin such interactions with an assessment of whether or not the patients feel that their drinking is a problem and, if so, how confident they are to make a change. This may help identify early barriers to change. Other techniques include exploring the benefits and drawbacks to both changing and not changing, presenting the patient with data (i.e., laboratory results and standards of at-risk drinking), and correcting false perceptions. This is not meant to imply that persons should be vague or superficial in their expression of concern, but merely that the approach taken can lead to distinctly different results. Such techniques have been applied to other situations as well, including smoking cessation and medication compliance.

Treating addiction with medication is a new area of growth. For many years, the only available pharmacologic intervention was disulfiram. Its use in the elderly has been rare because of its potential for adverse events. More recently, naltrexone has been approved by the FDA for the treatment of alcohol dependence. It has mainly been studied in the general adult population, but one study of veterans aged 50 to 70 years showed similar results, with improvement in relapse to heavy drinking. The most recent medication to be approved for the treatment of alcohol withdrawal is acamprosate, but it has not been studied so far in the elderly.

Mental health comorbidity with substance dependence is common. Older alcoholics frequently have comorbid depression and may be at a greater risk of suicide. Alcohol abuse or dependence has also been shown to be higher in patients with cognitive impairment. It is also important to consider when mental health referrals would be warranted.

Other Addictive Substances and Treatment

Outside of alcohol and nicotine, the abuse and dependence of other addictive substance in the elderly has mainly been found to be prescription medications such as opiate analgesics and benzodiazepines. However, elderly adults have also been found to abuse illicit substances including marijuana, cocaine, amphetamines, and other stimulants. Again, because of the general misperception that elderly adults do not abuse illicit substances, there is a dearth of information in this arena.

There is a growing problem of misuse of prescription drugs in the elderly, and one estimate suggests that by 2020 the nonmedical use of prescription drugs will increase to 2.7 million. Presently, one in four elderly adults uses a medication with some abuse potential. Factors that are associated with drug use in the elderly are female gender, social isolation, past history, and exposure to addictive substances. Patients with complex medical histories or with a history of dependence are at higher risk of developing benzodiazepine dependence, which may increase with age. Not all patients using benzodiazepines will become psychologically dependent on them, but it has been documented that tolerance decreases with age and they will likely be physiologically dependent on them (i.e., at risk of withdrawal if the medication is abruptly discontinued). It is important to remember to discuss issues of abuse, dependence, and withdrawal when providing informed consent for medication use.

PERSONALITY PATHOLOGY IN THE ELDERLY

With the advent of the International Society for the Study of Personality Disorders and subsequently the *Journal of Personality Disorders*, interest and research in personality pathology has increased. Historically, personality disorders (PDs) were governed by psychodynamic theories and explanations; however, with changes in theory and practice, PDs have been explained and understood from other perspectives. For example, biological research with twin studies suggests that approximately 40% to 60% of the variance in personality is genetic.

The majority of PD research has taken place in the context of younger individuals from infancy to adulthood, with little examination of elderly adults. Many reasons have precluded a thorough investigation into geriatric PDs, including professional disagreement in valid diagnosis measures, problems in DSM-IV-TR nosology, and the difficulty associated with obtaining a comprehensive psychiatric history from the elderly patient. The latter difficulty is most problematic, as PDs are established based on lifelong behavior patterns. However, assessing PDs in geriatric patients could aid in the development of appropriate treatment algorithms and increase the knowledge of age-associated personality changes.

Personality Disorder Classification

According to the DSM-IV-TR, PDs are categorized into three distinct clusters based on similarities. Cluster A (odd and eccentric) consists of the paranoid, schizoid, and schizotypal PDs; cluster B (dramatic, emotional, and erratic) contains the antisocial, borderline, histrionic, and narcissistic PDs; and cluster C (anxious and fearful) includes the avoidant, dependent, and obsessive-compulsive PDs. This categorization has received criticism as a result of limited validity, meeting criteria for multiple PDs, and limited diagnostic utility.

Diagnosing elderly patients with an Axis II diagnosis can be difficult because of comorbid medical and psychiatric diagnoses, neurocognitive impairment, and psychosocial changes. Without an accurate longitudinal history, which is the basis for monitoring personality development and change, a reliable PD diagnosis could be difficult to make, as there would be limited evidence regarding personality formation, adaptation, rigidity, and associated impairment.

Prevalence

The prevalence of PDs in elderly patients has been found to vary depending on hospitalization status. In community residents, the rate was found to range between 2.8% and 13%, between 5% and 33% for elderly outpatients, and between 7% and 61.5% for elderly inpatients. In a meta-analytic review of 16 studies between the years of 1980 and 1997, an overall prevalence rate of 20% was found for all PDs in persons aged 50 or older.

The two clusters of PDs that elderly patients tend to fall into are cluster A (i.e., schizoid) and cluster C (i.e., obsessive-compulsive), and very rarely do elderly patients present with PDs in cluster B (i.e., histrionic). Cluster B disorders tend to dissipate, whereas clusters A and C tend to remain stable or increase as people age. For example, in an empirical study assessing PDs in five different age groups using a self-reported personality check list, patients 50 years and older reported more schizoid and obsessive-compulsive PDs relative to younger cohorts.

The majority of PDs are diagnosed in elderly patients with major affective disorders; however, caution must be taken as PDs should not be diagnosed within the context of an Axis I disorder such as major depressive disorder or bipolar disorder.

Age-Associated Personality Changes

Personality tends to form from infancy to young adulthood and then begins to remain stable throughout adulthood, with fluctuations depending on various traits or mood states. Trait characteristics are considered to be consistent, reliable determinants of human behavior, which occur regardless of state. State characteristics are those behaviors that are modified (i.e., over- and underexpressed) based on changes in state such as mood or environment.

As people age, personality characteristics may be expressed differently because of environmental, interpersonal, social, functional, or medical changes. In regard to the big five personality traits (neuroticism, extraversion, openness, agreeableness, and conscientiousness), older adults tend to show an increase in agreeableness and conscientiousness and a decrease in neuroticism and openness. Older individuals have been found to be less impulsive and risky and more inhibited. However, there tends to be high stability of earlier personality traits owing to underlying genetic components, with some variability in personality being an adaptive and protective quality. Personality changes, though, can also be a foreshadowing of complications. For example, there is some evidence to support that significant changes in personality may be an indication or a consequence of an organic pathology such as frontotemporal dementia or an aneurism.

Treatment Strategies

There exists no evidenced-based treatment for elderly patients with personality pathology. Treatment for elderly patients with PDs may involve a collaborative team approach that uses a biopsychosocial paradigm. As PDs may be more common among geriatric patients with a major affective disorder, treatment of the mood disorder will be paramount, in order to help alleviate the accompanying PD. However, in general, patients with PDs may be difficult to treat because of noncompliance with treatment recommendations or possible treatment resistance. Nonetheless, based on the associated functional, social, and overall impairment, treatment strategies may include supportive psychotherapy, psychiatric medication management, and a focus on activities of daily living. These treatment regimens may help to remit the PD and the comorbid mood disorder in turn, increasing the quality of life and functionality of geriatric patients.

FURTHER READING

Abrams RC, Horowitz SV. Personality disorders after age 50: a meta-analytic review of the literature. In: Rosowsky E, Abrams RC, Zweig RA, eds. *Personality Disorders in Older Adults.* Mahwah: Lawrence Erlbaum Associates; 1999:55–68.

American Psychiatric Association. *Diagnostic and Statistical Manual of Mental Disorders.* 4th ed, text revision. Washington, DC: American Psychiatric Association; 2000.

American Psychiatric Association. Practice guidelines for the assessment and treatment of patients with suicidal behaviors. *Am J Psychiatry.* 2003;160(suppl 11): 1–60.

Bouchard TJ, Loehlin JC. Genes, evolution, and personality. *Behav Genet.* 2001;31:243–273.

Brown GK, Bruce ML, Pearson JL. High-risk management guidelines for elderly suicidal patients in primary care settings. *Int J Geriatr Psychiatry.* 2001;16:593–601.

Flint AJ. Management of anxiety in late life. *J Geriatr Psychiatry Neurol.* 1998;11:4.

Kosten TR, O'Connor PG. Management of drug and alcohol withdrawal. *N Engl J Med.* 2003;348:1786–1795.

Lautenschlager NT, Forstl H. Personality change in old age. *Curr Opin Psychiatry.* 2007;20:62–66.

Mann JJ. Neurobiology of suicidal behaviour. *Nat Rev Neurosci.* 2003;4:819–828.

Oslin DW, Slaymaker VJ, Blow FC, et al. Treatment outcomes for alcohol dependence among middle-aged and older adults. *Addict Behav.* 2005;30:1431–1436.

Owens GP, Baker DG, Kasckow J, et al. Review of assessment and treatment of PTSD among elderly American armed force veterans. *Int J Geriatr Psychiatry.* 2005;20:1118–1130.

Saitz R. Unhealthy alcohol use. *N Engl J Med.* 2005;352:596–607.

Simoni-Wastila L, Yang HK. Psychoactive drug abuse in older adults. *Am J Geriatr Pharmacother.* 2006;4:380–394.

Smalbrugge M, Pot AM, Jongenelis L, et al. The impact of depression and anxiety on well being, disability and use of health care services in nursing home patients. *Int J Geriatr Psychiatry.* 2006;21:325–332.

Van Alphen SPJ. The relevance of a geriatric sub-classification of personality disorders in the DSM-V. *Int J Geriatr Psychiatry.* 2006;21:205–109.

Young RC. Evidenced-based pharmacological treatment of geriatric bipolar disorder. *Psychiatr Clin North Am.* 2005;28:837–869.

Management of Agitation in Dementia

Marcella Pascualy ■ *Eric Petrie* ■ *Lucy Y. Wang* ■ *Suzanne B. Murray* ■ *Elaine Peskind*

INTRODUCTION

Dementia affects at least 10% of patients older than 60 years and more than a third of patients older than 80 years. It is estimated that, by the year 2030, 14 million Americans will have Alzheimer's disease (AD), the most common disease underlying late-life dementia and the leading cause of nursing home placement in the elderly.

Neuropsychiatric behavioral symptoms are frequent in patients with dementia. It is estimated that between 61% and 92% of patients with AD will develop disruptive agitation during the course of their illness. Agitation is characterized by excessive verbal and motor behaviors, which suggest that the patient is distressed. Disruptive agitation includes such behaviors as hitting, biting, screaming, constant requests for attention, repetitive vocalizations, verbal threats, and forced motor activity like pacing. In 20% to 30% of cases, agitation is accompanied by psychotic symptoms such as hallucinations and delusions.

Agitation adversely affects quality of life for both the patient and the caregiver. More than 70% of caregivers consider the management of disruptive agitated behaviors to be the most challenging aspect of the caretaking process. Along with sleep disturbances, it is the major precipitant of institutionalization. In the nursing home setting, the management of agitation requires a high caretaker-to-patient ratio, further increasing the public health burden of this costly disease, which is presently estimated at $100 billion per year.

PATHOPHYSIOLOGY

The effects of AD on brain function and a number of neurotransmitters may contribute to the pathophysiology of neuropsychiatric behavioral symptoms in AD. In a fluorodeoxyglucose-positron emission tomography study mapping psychosis in AD, hypometabolism in the right prefrontal cortex was associated with delusions. Single photon emission computed tomography studies in patients with AD, with aggressive behaviors, demonstrated abnormalities in the right anterior medial temporal region.

Changes in a number of neurotransmitter systems likely contribute to the pathophysiology of agitation in AD. There is severe loss of cholinergic neurons in the basal forebrain nucleus basalis of Meynert and reductions in choline acetyltransferase (the synthetic enzyme for acetylcholine with a corresponding cholinergic deficit). In large clinical trials of acetylcholinesterase inhibitors (AChEIs; drugs that inhibit the enzymatic breakdown of acetylcholine and act to ameliorate the cholinergic deficit), there was a decreased incidence of emergent behavior problems in mild–moderate AD and a reduction in these behaviors in moderate–severe AD. These findings suggest that a subsyndromal "anticholinergic delirium" may contribute to the development of neuropsychiatric behavioral symptoms in AD. A caveat is that persons with severe disruptive agitated behaviors were excluded from trials of AChEIs. The role of AChEIs in the treatment of disruptive agitated behaviors is discussed below.

Loss of serotonergic neurons in the dorsal raphe nuclei results in a deficit state, which may be associated with depressive symptoms, irritability, and anxiety. Loss of dopaminergic neurons in the substantia nigra is variable, but there is little evidence for loss of dopaminergic function in AD.

Despite severe loss of neurons in AD in the locus ceruleus, the nucleus of origin of noradrenergic neurons, central nervous system (CNS) noradrenergic function is increased. Cerebrospinal fluid novepinephine (NE) concentrations in the later stages of AD (when disruptive agitation is common) are elevated compared to age-matched controls. Administration of the alpha-2 antagonist drug yohimbine (which increases CNS noradrenergic outflow) acutely precipitated disruptive agitation in community-dwelling patients with mild-to-moderate AD who had no previous agitation or other behavior problems. Postmortem brain tissue studies in AD have demonstrated both upregulation of tyrosine hydroxylase (the rate-limiting synthetic enzyme for NE) in surviving locus ceruleus

TABLE 73-1

Assessment of the Agitated Patient

Clearly define and document the problem

↓

Assess the impact on the caregiver

↓

Perform medical work-up: rule out delirium

↓

Rule out primary psychiatric disorder

neurons and upregulation of postsynaptic alpha-1 receptors. Upregulated postsynaptic beta-adrenergic receptors may also contribute to behaviorally relevant increased noradrenergic responsiveness.

ASSESSMENT OF THE AGITATED PATIENT
(see Table 73-1)

Clearly Define and Document the Problem

Disruptive agitation is a middle- to late-stage phenomenon in AD. As in the careful approach to any medical symptom in late life, it is important to first define and quantify the specific problem behavior in order to elucidate the etiology and intervene effectively. It is essential to clearly characterize and document the nature and frequency of the disruptive behavior so that a baseline record is established. This will serve as a frame of reference to determine whether subsequent interventions have been beneficial. Defining in detail the aberrant behavior frequently requires interviewing several caregivers to obtain an accurate appraisal of the problem. Specifically, ask if the patient has been aggressive or assaultive toward the caregiver. Often, caregivers are embarrassed to give an accurate history of the agitated behavior because they feel that they have tolerated more than they should have. They also may feel embarrassed for the patient. Ask the caregivers if they feel that they are at risk of being harmed. In questioning the caregiver, one needs to identify any events or situations that may precipitate or aggravate the behavior, e.g., disruption in the patient's daily routine, being left alone, or being exposed to new and unfamiliar situations. It is important to determine whether the agitated patient is experiencing psychotic symptoms, such as auditory or visual hallucinations or delusional thinking, which may be contributing to the behavioral disturbance. Affective and anxiety disorders must also be considered in the differential diagnosis. A survey of the patient's sleep pattern is useful to ensure that sleep disturbance (e.g., caused by inadequately treated pain, poor sleep hygiene, or sleep apnea) is not the cause of day- or nighttime agitation. Uncontrolled or inadequate pain management is a frequent cause of agitation at any time. Occult medical illnesses (e.g., urinary tract infections, pulmonary infections, hypoxia, and electrolyte imbalances) may also be precipitants of disruptive agitation in AD.

The following is a list of useful questions for caregivers when assessing the agitated patient:

1. Can you tell me what happens when the patient becomes agitated?
2. Has the patient been aggressive or assaultive? Do you fear that you or the patient will be injured?
3. What is the frequency of the behavior? How many times per day/per week does the agitated behavior occur?
4. How long do the episodes last?
5. What is happening immediately before the behavior begins? Can you link the behavioral disturbance with any particular activity, like bathing, dressing, eating, or dispensing medications? Does it happen only when certain people approach the patient? Does it happen during particular times of the day or night?
6. Has the patient appeared sad or anxious to you? Does the patient seem to be experiencing psychotic symptoms like hallucinations or paranoid delusions when the behavior occurs?
7. How are you managing this behavior? How does the patient respond to these interventions?

Assess the Impact on the Caregiver

It is especially important to evaluate the impact of the patient's behavior on the well-being of the caregiver. When combined with the physical, emotional, and financial demands of caring for someone with dementia, a behavior that by itself may not seem that distressing or frequent can overwhelm the caregiver who then becomes the one in need of care and support. Often, the caregiver is also elderly and frail. Caregivers often neglect their own physical and emotional health. Careful listening to the caregiver is valuable because it serves to identify these issues and having someone understand their problem also provides support to the caregiver. This helps to establish a positive therapeutic alliance, which greatly increases the likelihood that the caregiver will comply with subsequent treatment recommendations.

Interventions that will reduce care burden should also be considered. Such interventions may include having patients attend adult daycare centers for a few hours to days a week or recruiting family members to participate in assisting with care, thereby allowing caregivers respite and time to attend to their own emotional and other needs. The caregiver should receive a referral to the local chapter of the Alzheimer's Association, which can provide support services and information about community resources, respite care facilities, and caregiver support groups. These interventions are particularly helpful because these will reduce caregiver burden and may prevent or delay institutionalization. Caregivers who perceive themselves as "more burdened" tend to consider themselves less healthy, report a history of poor interactions with the patient, and describe the patient as having a greater number of agitated behaviors. A referral of the caregiver to individual psychiatric treatment may be advisable and helpful. If there is concern or evidence of neglect and/or abuse, further investigation is warranted and a referral to an adult protective agency may need to be considered.

Medical Workup: Rule Out Delirium

Delirium is a common cause of agitation in patients with dementia owing to their advanced age and underlying brain pathology. It is important to remember that signs and symptoms of delirium, which may manifest as acute changes in cognition and/or an acute onset or increase in agitated behaviors, may be the only indicators of an underlying systemic illness. Therefore, a high index of suspicion for delirium and underlying medical condition(s) is necessary when assessing the patient with dementia who is agitated.

The fundamental features of delirium are fluctuating disturbances of attention and level of consciousness that usually develop over a short period of time. The etiology of delirium tends to be multifactorial. Common causes of delirium include systemic medical illnesses, electrolyte disturbances, and medication or substance intoxication or withdrawal.

It is particularly difficult to diagnose delirium in the context of dementia because both disorders have several features in common. Shared features include evidence of cognitive impairment such as memory disturbances, language deficits, disorientation, perceptual abnormalities (including hallucinations), and agitation. Medically healthy elderly patients with dementia, however, are alert, without disturbances in level of consciousness. Typically, their cognitive deficits have developed insidiously and progress slowly. In contrast, in patients with deliriums, the level of consciousness fluctuates and cognitive deficits usually develop acutely. For example, in AD one can generally expect, on average, a three-point per year drop in the Mini-Mental State Examination score. If a patient with AD exhibits a sudden deterioration in cognitive function and/or a larger drop in Mini-Mental State Examination score, an explanation for this decline must be pursued and delirium needs to be considered in the differential diagnosis.

The following approaches are often valuable in assessing the patient having delirium in the nursing home or inpatient setting. Careful reading of the nursing staff's progress notes will often highlight changes in the patient's level of consciousness. The medication list should be systematically reviewed, and any recent medication changes should be noted. It is important to consider whether medication dosages are appropriate for the elderly, to investigate the possibility of drug–drug interactions, and to identify medications with anticholinergic side effects, a common culprit in delirium (Table 73-9). The use and frequency of prn or "as-needed" medications should be determined, especially for psychoactive medications such as sedative hypnotics, antipsychotics, and analgesics.

The assessment of the patient having delirium also requires a physical and neurological examination and laboratory studies to rule out systemic medical problems such as infection, congestive heart failure, electrolyte imbalance, or endocrine diseases. A careful workup may reveal a urinary tract infection or an occult carcinoma as the cause for the delirium and agitation. Once the underlying cause is corrected, the patient's mental status and behavior should return to baseline. Short-term, low-dose, intravenous haloperidol in the hospital setting or an oral atypical antipsychotic in the outpatient setting should be considered for management of significant agitation in the context of delirium. It is important to recognize, however, that recent studies have shown that persistence of delirium is common and resolution may require weeks to months.

Rule Out Primary Psychiatric Disorders

Recurrence or exacerbation of a primary psychiatric illness like schizophrenia, bipolar disorder, major depressive disorder, or panic disorder in the patient with a history of one or more of these disorders may explain current psychotic, affective, or anxiety symptoms. These episodes may present with atypical features in the patient who has now developed dementia. As the onset of bipolar disorder in old age is extremely rare, symptoms suggestive of a first episode of mania or hypomania should prompt a workup for causes other than bipolar disorder, such as delirium or partial-complex seizures. Appropriate

medication treatment should be instituted, starting at geriatric doses and slowly titrating up with close attention to the development of side effects and potential worsening of cognition.

Depression

Although estimates of the prevalence of major depression in AD vary widely, it is clear that depressive signs and symptoms are common. Depression has been associated with an increased risk of dementia and AD, but it is unclear whether it represents a true risk factor or is, instead, a prodromal symptom of incipient dementia. In either case, depression itself can further impair cognitive functioning and causes excess cognitive disability in the patient with dementia. This can make it more difficult for patients with dementia to process and judge events, thereby causing their responses and reactions to be more impaired and unpredictable. In the context of a severe depression, the patient may develop psychotic symptoms and psychomotor changes that can be mistaken for a worsening dementia or delirium. However, in our clinical experience caring for patients with AD, this is a rare occurrence. Apathy and language impairment complicate the diagnosis of depression in dementia. Apathy is the commonest early behavior change in AD and is not helpful in distinguishing between dementia and depression. In the middle to late stages of dementia, patients often have language deficits, which may limit their ability to give information regarding their mood state. The best indicators of depression in patients with dementia are persistent saddened mood, tearfulness, and depressed appearance. Vegetative signs such as sleep, energy, and appetite disturbance are less reliable. Knowledge of a past history of depression may be helpful in identifying patients at increased risk of a recurrence. An antidepressant trial is a reasonable diagnostic strategy in difficult to discern cases—a low index of suspicion for depression in the patient with dementia is appropriate.

Anxiety Disorders

Anxiety disorders are relatively common in the elderly and are usually accompanied by agitation. Rates for anxiety disorders in this age group are high, between 15% and 20%, and tend to go unrecognized. The most common anxiety disorders include phobias, generalized anxiety disorder, and panic disorder. An exacerbation of preexisting posttraumatic stress disorder may also be responsible for symptoms of anxiety and agitation in patients with dementia. Traumatic memories and dissociative/reexperiencing episodes ("flashbacks") may become more frequent and intense and difficult to distinguish from current events in patients with dementia because of their cognitive impairments (e.g., disorientation, short-term memory loss, impaired executive function, and confusion) and the fact that long-term memories for distant events are generally intact until late-stage dementia. For this reason, inquiring about a history of trauma exposure is often helpful when evaluating the patient with dementia who is agitated. Other disorders associated with anxiety symptoms in elderly patients with dementia include depression and Parkinson's disease. Given the high rates of anxiety disorders in the elderly, clinicians should actively consider these diagnoses in the patient with dementia who is agitated.

Psychotic Symptoms

Psychotic symptoms occur in approximately 20% to 30% of patients with AD and often contribute to the development of disruptive agitation. Delusions tend to be more common than hallucinations in AD; hallucinations (particularly visual hallucinations) are more common in patients with Lewy body pathology. Delusions in the patient with AD are often cognitively based. Memory deficits may lead to delusional beliefs that misplaced objects have been stolen. Symptoms of agnosia (failure to recognize the identity of objects or persons despite intact perceptual abilities) may result in a number of misidentification syndromes: that the identity of a person has somehow changed, that a person has been replaced by an imposter (Capgras syndrome), or that the patients' houses are not their homes. Less commonly, patients may develop the delusion that their spouses have been unfaithful or that the patients are being poisoned. Such delusions may cause distress for both patient and caregiver. Hallucinations are more likely to be visual than auditory and tend to occur more frequently in the moderate-to-severe stages of AD. In many instances, the hallucinatory experiences are unobtrusive and do not cause distress to the patient, so medication intervention is not warranted. The presence of visual hallucinations early in the course of dementia suggests presence of Lewy body pathology. The presence of hallucinations has been associated with increased cognitive decline, institutionalization, and mortality. Systematized, grandiose, nihilistic, or bizarre delusions are uncommon and should alert the clinician to the development or recurrence of another psychiatric disorder, such as late-life schizophrenia, delusional disorder, or major depression with psychotic features.

MANAGEMENT OF AGITATION (see Table 73-2 and Table 73-3)

Identify Target Symptoms

Certain behaviors respond better to medication intervention than others. In general, auditory hallucinations, delusions, irritability, uncooperativeness with care, physically aggressive behaviors, and forced motor activity such as pacing tend to respond better to medication intervention. Repetitive, nonaggressive behaviors such as aimless wandering, repetitive vocalizations, and hoarding are less responsive. Some behaviors may be more effectively targeted by utilizing distraction, modifying the patient's environment, or modifying the caretaker's mode of interaction with the patient. Patients who wander need to be provided with a safe environment in which to do so.

TABLE 73-2

Management of the Agitated Patient
Identify target symptoms
↓
Set realistic goals
↓
Nonpharmacological intervention
↓
Pharmacological intervention
↓
Reevaluate need for continued intervention

TABLE 73-3

Management of Major Psychiatric Symptoms	
PREDOMINANT NEUROPSYCHIATRIC SYMPTOMS	**CONSIDER**
Psychotic symptoms	Antipsychotic (haloperidol, risperidone, olanzapine, and quetaipine)
Dangerous aggression	Adrenergic antagonist Antipsychotics Short-acting benzodiazepine (only short term and in case of emergency)
Hypomanic symptoms	Valproic acid Carbamazepine
Prominent mood or anxiety symptoms or irritability	Selective serotonin reuptake inhibitor

Set Realistic Goals

It is important to remember that the primary reason to treat disruptive agitation is to relieve suffering in the patient. However, realistic goals on the part of the clinician and caregiver are necessary, particularly with respect to the likelihood of response of the target behaviors to the intervention. It should be stated clearly that the goal of treatment is to decrease the frequency and severity of the agitated behaviors. Total eradication of the disruptive behaviors is only occasionally achieved and often represents an unrealistic expectation. The preferred therapeutic goal is to achieve sufficient improvement so that the quality of life of the patient and the caregiver is enhanced and that, for patients in the home setting, institutionalization is forestalled.

Therapeutic Interventions

Nonpharmacological Interventions

It is important to institute nonpharmacological management first, if possible, in order to minimize the possible adverse effects of psychotropic medications in elderly patients and to optimize the likelihood of a positive response. Nonpharmacological interventions address potential psychosocial and/or environmental reason(s) for the development of agitation. There are three main theoretical models of psychosocial contributions to the etiology of behavioral disturbances associated with dementia: the *"unmet" psychosocial needs model, the reduced stress-threshold model, and the behavioral/learning model.*

The "unmet needs" model emphasizes the identification and resolution of underlying needs that are believed to be causing the inappropriate behavior. These may include sensory deprivation, boredom, loneliness, pain, and the need to empty bladder or bowel. Commonly described interventions include appropriate sensory stimulation, good lighting, provision of sensory aids (e.g., eyeglasses and hearing aids), a safe place to wander, social interactions, pain control, and frequent toileting.

The reduced stress-threshold model is based on the assumption that, because their impaired cognition limits their ability to process and cope with environmental stimuli (e.g., sound, light, and motion), patients with dementia have a lower threshold at which these stimuli become overwhelming, resulting in symptoms of disruptive agitation. The primary intervention in this model is to reduce the level of environmental stimulation with which patients with dementia have to contend, with the expectation that this will decrease their level of agitation.

The behavior/learning model assumes that there is a connection between antecedents, behavior, and reinforcement that has been learned. In this model, disruptive agitated behaviors are learned through reinforcement by caregivers, who provide attention when problem behaviors occur. A modification of the usual intervention (reinforcement) is required to change the behavior. For example, caregivers should be encouraged to provide attention and positive emotional responses to desired behaviors and attempt not to respond to problem behaviors, in the hopes of increasing the former and extinguishing the latter.

These models are not mutually exclusive, and several of them can be applied concurrently, depending on the specific behaviors and precipitating circumstances.

Educating caregivers about the nature of neuropsychiatric behavioral symptoms of dementia can be a useful first step. It may be helpful to explain to the caregiver that it is common for patients with dementia to be repetitive, to wander, to misplace items, and to accuse others of stealing because of their memory deficits and impaired reasoning ability. This may prevent the caregiver from interpreting these behaviors as reflecting intentional stubbornness or disruptiveness, thereby making it easier for the caregiver to tolerate these challenging behaviors and eliminate the need for pharmacological intervention.

In instituting nonpharmacological management, it is useful to first appraise current interventions, supporting those who have been successful and discouraging others who are ineffective or appear to aggravate the problematic behavior. As noted above, there is value in identifying circumstances that precipitate or exacerbate the agitation. It is particularly common for patients with dementia to become agitated if their routine is disrupted, if the environment is too stimulating, or if they are approached by strangers or relatives they do not recognize or who they believe are trying to harm them. Avoiding or minimizing these situations is often the best intervention. Patients who are cognitively impaired also tend to become agitated when others are trying to help them during activities of daily living (particularly bathing, dressing, and toileting), so allowing the patient to remain as independent as possible in these activities is important. Examples include person-centered showering (an intervention focused on resident comfort and preferences) and the towel bath (an in-bed bag bath method in which the resident remains covered at all times), which have been shown to be effective methods of reducing agitation, aggression, and discomfort during bathing. A patient who has difficulty dressing but still preserves some abilities may benefit from having clothing and shoes that use Velcro fasteners rather than buttons, zippers, or laces. Similarly, providing utensils with large handles and/or cutting food into bite-size portions may allow patients to continue to feed themselves. Some patients become agitated when they are asked to take their medications, so crushing the pills and diluting them in juice may avoid this source of agitation. Liquid forms of medications are also helpful in patients with swallowing difficulties who are at risk of aspiration. Other types of interventions that have shown some effectiveness in reducing agitation include exercise training, aromatherapy, pet therapy, and music therapy. Given the relative poor response rates in the treatment of agitation, it is important to be "creative" and develop individualized interventions whenever possible.

Since patients with AD gradually become aphasic, it is essential to use simple and clear language and use visual cues to improve communication and minimize frustration. Caregivers should be reminded to approach patients with dementia from the front to avoid startling them. They should stay at more than an arm's length away to prevent being injured. One should also be cautious when bending down to talk to a patient in a wheelchair, who may respond by hitting or kicking. Instituting predictable routines, eliminating unnecessary stimulation and novelty, maximizing the patients remaining abilities, and approaching the patient cautiously can all help reduce episodes of agitation.

The issue of wandering and getting lost, with the attendant increased risk of physical harm and death, is of extreme concern to caregivers and often precipitates institutionalization. Although unattended patients have higher rates of getting lost, many patients who get lost are in the presence of a caregiver or are living in a professional care setting. Therefore, caregivers need to be made aware that all persons with dementia are at risk of becoming lost, even if the individual has never wandered in the past. While signs on doors may help to orient patients and the use of safety alarms and difficult-to-open key latches may decrease the likelihood of the patient getting lost, continuous supervision is the best preventive measure. To facilitate the location of patients with dementia who do become lost, the Alzheimer's Association administers the nationwide "safe return" program that provides patients with identification bracelets, necklaces, or clothing tags and offers 24-hour assistance in locating lost patients.

Pharmacological Interventions

If a general medical cause for agitation has been ruled out and nonpharmacological interventions have been unsuccessful, psychotropic medications need to be considered. Unfortunately, there is no pharmacological regimen with proven good efficacy. In many instances, it is necessary to institute a period of trial and error before an effective medication intervention is identified for the individual patient.

Historically, nursing home residents have been overprescribed psychotropic medication and have been left on them indefinitely. Antipsychotics are the third most frequently used class of drugs in skilled nursing home facilities. The use of psychotropic and sedative medications in the nursing home setting is now regulated by the Omnibus Budget Reconciliation Act (OBRA-1987). The OBRA establishes guidelines for the use of psychoactive medications in the nursing home setting. OBRA regulations allow antipsychotic use only for psychotic symptoms or in dementia for dangerous symptoms. The use of hypnotics is restricted to 7 days of continuous use. The need for continued pharmacologic intervention needs to be periodically reviewed, and polypharmacy should be avoided.

Antipsychotics

Antipsychotics have traditionally been the cornerstone for treatment of agitation in dementia. Until fairly recently, "conventional" or "typical" antipsychotics were widely used. However, the "atypical" antipsychotics have recently gained popularity because of their improved side-effect profile and tolerability, and their usage in the elderly has increased markedly since their introduction into the market. Antipsychotics are used "off-label" for the management of agitation in dementia; these are not approved by the U.S. Food and Drug

Administration (FDA) for the treatment of behavioral symptoms in patients with dementia.

Efficacy

Two meta-analyses including 12 randomized clinical trials (RCTs) and two additional RCTs evaluating conventional antipsychotics have shown modest efficacy and significant adverse side effects. A slight benefit for haloperidol with aggression was found. In this same study, six RCTs of atypical antipsychotics were analyzed, and the authors concluded that risperidone and olanzapine had the best evidence for what was described as modest efficacy. In a Cochrane meta-analysis of nine studies, the authors found that there was significant improvement in aggression with risperidone and olanzapine and significant improvement in psychosis with risperidone.

The Clinical Antipsychotic Trials of Intervention Effectiveness was a multicenter effectiveness trial of atypical antipsychotics in patients with agitation and psychosis associated with AD who resided in the community. The study enrolled 421 participants. The study demonstrated that the response to atypical antipsychotic therapy was no greater than that achieved by placebo (improvement was observed in 32% of patients assigned to olanzapine, 26% of patients assigned to quetiapine, 29% of patients assigned to risperidone, and 21% of patients assigned to placebo). In addition, the adverse effects offset the modest improvements. A caveat to these conclusions is that Clinical Antipsychotic Trials of Intervention Effectiveness was designed to study the effectiveness of atypical antipsychotic treatment in community-dwelling patients with AD. It is unclear if these results also apply to nursing home patients with more severe dementia and behavioral impairment.

Mortality Risk and Antipsychotics

In April 2005, the FDA completed a meta-analysis of 17 placebo-controlled trials (only four studies were in the public domain) of aripiprazole, olanzapine, quetiapine, and risperidone and found the risk of mortality to be 1.6 to 1.7 times greater in treated versus untreated elderly patients with dementia, primarily owing to cardiovascular or infectious causes. The FDA reported, in a public health advisory that prompted a "black-box" warning, that the use of all second-generation ("atypical") antipsychotic medications for the treatment of behavioral symptoms in elderly patients with dementia is associated with increased mortality. Although the FDA findings were confirmed in an independently conducted meta-analysis, four observational studies did not replicate the finding of increased mortality with atypical antipsychotic treatment. In summary, atypical psychotics and possibly typical antipsychotics may be associated with a small increased risk of death.

Cerebrovascular Adverse Events and Antipsychotics

The evidence regarding increased cerebrovascular adverse events (mainly stroke, transient ischemic episodes, and cases of loss of consciousness or syncope), associated with the use of typical and atypical antipsychotic drugs is conflicting. A positive association was initially found in a pooled analysis of 11 RCTs, mainly nursing home clinical trials of risperidone and olanzapine for patients with dementia, performed by regulators who had access to unpublished data. A larger number of subjects with vascular and mixed dementias were included in the risperidone studies compared with the olanzapine studies, which likely accounted for the increased incidence of cerebrovascular adverse events in the risperidone group. When serious cerebrovascular adverse events like stroke were examined separately, the relative risk of risperidone treatment was not significantly higher than placebo. Other large observational administrative health database studies have also failed to demonstrate an increased risk of stroke in elderly patients treated with risperidone or olanzapine. In summary, pooled RCTs suggest an increase in cerebrovascular adverse events with olanzapine and risperidone; this may not include an increased rate of serious events such as strokes. Further studies are needed to confirm these findings.

Antipsychotics and Mortality in Patients with Dementia with Possible Lewy Body Pathology

Demented patients with Lewy body pathology experience more frequent and severe extrapyramidal motor symptoms as side effects of typical and atypical antipsychotic medications. In the most recent consensus criteria for the clinical diagnosis of dementia with Lewy bodies, "neuroleptic sensitivity" constitutes a "suggestive" feature, which, in the presence of one or more "core" features (i.e., dementia, parkinsonian motor signs, visual hallucinations, fluctuating attention, and alertness), supports a diagnosis of probable dementia with Lewy bodies. Neuroleptic sensitivity in patients with dementia with Lewy bodies has been associated with increased mortality in several studies. Therefore, instituting antipsychotic treatment in patients with symptoms of Lewy body pathology should be avoided whenever possible. When necessary, quetiapine in the preferred antipsychotic agent because of its low propensity for causing extrapyramidal motor symptoms and efforts should be made to limit administration to the lowest effective dose.

In summary, given the modest efficacy and the risk for significant and serious adverse effects, antipsychotics should only be used when nonpharmacologic interventions have failed and other pharmacologic interventions have been considered.

Other Side Effects of Antipsychotics

Elderly patients are at increased risk of developing troublesome adverse effects of antipsychotic medications, including extrapyramidal motor symptoms, sedation, tardive dyskinesia, and metabolic syndrome. Peripheral anticholinergic effects, such as dry mouth, constipation, and urinary hesitancy can complicate the care of the elderly patient with dementia. Central anticholinergic effects can worsen impairment of memory and other cognitive abilities and induce delirium. Oversedation and pseudoparkinsonism can increase the risk of falls and complications such as fractures and head injury. The clinician also needs to be alert to the development of antipsychotic-induced akathisia, an uncomfortable urge to move about that can increase pacing and other agitated behaviors. Low-potency antipsychotics, such as chlorpromazine and thioridazine, carry the added risk of orthostatic hypotension and cardiac toxicity and should be avoided.

In summary, given the modest positive efficacy found with antipsychotics and the increased risk of mortality, these should be prescribed only for patients with significant psychotic symptoms that are disturbing to the patient and/or aggressive behaviors that may result in harm to the patient or others. However, it is also important

TABLE 73-4

Selective Serotonin Reuptake Inhibitors—Dosages in the Elderly		
DRUG	STARTING DOSE (mg)	RANGE (mg)
Citalopram (Celexa®)	10	10–40
Escitalopram (Lexapro®)	5	5–20
Fluoxetine (Prozac®)	5	5–60
Paroxetine (Paxil®)	10	10–40
Sertraline (Zoloft®)	12.5–25	25–100

Each patient should be carefully assessed and dosing adjusted accordingly.

TABLE 73-6

Atypical Antidepressants—Dosages in the Elderly		
DRUG	STARTING DOSE	RANGE (mg)
Bupropion (immediate release) (Wellbutrin®)	75–100 mg every morning or twice daily	150–450
Bupropion (XL) (Wellbutrin XL®)	100–150 mg every morning or twice daily	150–450
Trazodone* (Desyrel®)	12.5–25 mg every evening	50–200

Each patient should be carefully assessed and dosing adjusted accordingly.
*Trazodone is used for sleep although it is FDA approved for depression only.

not to undertreat, because appropriate antipsychotic medication use can reduce patient distress or decrease potentially harmful behaviors. Maintaining a common sense approach where one weighs both benefits and risks in a collaborative process involving the patient's caregiver(s) will greatly facilitate the provision of good patient care. If medication treatment is deemed necessary, low-dose atypical antipsychotics are recommended. The general rule in dosing is to start low and go slow, *but* go up as necessary until symptoms improve or side effects intervene Table 73-7. In dementia with features of Lewy body pathology and in Parkinson's disease, quetiapine is the preferred agent because of its low incidence of extrapyramidal motor side effects. Patients and families should be clearly informed of the potential risks of antipsychotic treatment, including increased mortality, and detailed documentation of such discussions recorded. If the patient responds favorably, periodic attempts should be made to lower or discontinue the medication to see if continued treatment is necessary for control of the original target symptoms.

Antidepressants

A recent review of five RCTs of antidepressants (sertraline, fluoxetine, citalopram, and trazodone) showed *no efficacy* for treatment of agitation, with the exception of one study that found patients treated with citalopram had improvement in the total behavioral score. The study did not separate psychotic from aggressive behaviors, so it is unclear if citalopram would be effective in patients with psychotic symptoms alone.

Because these have a relatively benign side-effect profile, selective serotonergic reuptake inhibitors (SSRIs) are considered the agents of choice for depressive and anxiety disorders in dementia (Table 73-4). One study in patients with AD found that sertraline was superior to placebo in reducing depressive symptoms. The atypical antidepressants, such as venlafaxine, mirtazepine, and bupropion, have been less well studied in this population (Tables 73-5 and 73-6). Two multicenter trials with citalopram demonstrated efficacy in the management of depressive symptoms in patients with AD with mild side effects.

Pharmacological properties are important in selecting among SSRIs for elderly patients. In the elderly patient, the development of common SSRI side effects, particularly nausea, diarrhea, and anorexia, can be problematic because of subjective discomfort as well as the increased potential for deleterious effects from weight loss in this often frail population. Fluoxetine is often poorly tolerated in the elderly, even at low doses, because its prominent activating effects and the long half-lives of fluoxetine and its primary metabolite, nor-fluoxetine, complicate dosage adjustment. Paroxetine suffers from relatively greater anticholinergic side effects compared to other SSRIs. Sertraline offers the advantage of a relatively short elimination half-life. SSRIs also exert prominent effects on the activities of hepatic microsomal enzyme systems that metabolize other medications. This requires careful attention to the potential for drug–drug interactions. Citalopram has the fewest such effects and may be preferred in patients on multiple medications for physical illnesses. However, it is important to consider that SSRIs are also highly protein bound and may competitively inhibit protein binding and thereby alter the pharmacodynamic effects of other medications. This is particularly important in the case of medications that have a low therapeutic index, like warfarin.

Trazodone, a serotonergic antidepressant with prominent alpha-1 blocking activity and sedative properties, has been used by clinicians for the control of agitation and sleep disturbance. However, its potent alpha-adrenergic blocking activity can cause orthostatic hypotension and priapism. The only RCT that evaluated trazodone in the management of agitation in dementia showed no benefit over placebo.

Because tricyclic antidepressants (e.g., nortriptyline and desipramine) have significant anticholinergic side effects and may cause

TABLE 73-5

Serotonin Norepinephrine Reuptake (SNRI) and Mirtazapine—Dosages in the Elderly		
DRUG	STARTING DOSE	RANGE
Venlafaxine (SNRI) (Effexor®)	18.75–37.5 mg every morning or twice daily	75–150 mg twice daily
Venlafaxine extended release (SNRI) (Effexor XR®)	37.5 mg every morning or twice daily	75–100 mg twice daily
Duloxetine (SNRI) (Cymbalta®)	10–20 mg every morning or twice daily	20–60 mg once to twice daily
Mirtazapine* (Remeron®)	7.5–15 mg every morning evening	15–60 mg every evening

Each patient should be carefully assessed and dosing adjusted accordingly.
*Available as rapidly dissolving sol-tab preparation.

TABLE 73-7

Antipsychotics—Dosages in the Elderly

DRUG	STARTING DOSE (mg)	RANGE* (mg)
Olanzapine (Zyprexa®)	2.5	5–10
Quetiapine (Seroquel®)	12.5–25	25–200
Risperidone (Risperdal®)	0.25–0.5	0.5–4
Ziprasidone (Geodon®)	10	10–100
Aripiprazole (Abilify®)	2.5–5	10–15
Haloperidol† (Haldol®)	0.25–1	0.5–4

Each patient should be carefully assessed and dosing adjusted accordingly.
*Administer lower doses at night and divide higher doses throughout the day.
†The intravenous route is preferred for delirium in the hospital setting as a result of lower incidence of extrapyramidal symptoms.

orthostatic hypotension and cardiac rhythm disturbances, their use in the elderly is discouraged. Treatment of neuropathic pain in the elderly is probably better treated with anticonvulsants rather than low-dose tricyclics for this reason.

Anticonvulsants (see Table 73-8)

The effectiveness of mood stabilizers in controlling irritability, aggression, impulsivity, and mood instability in bipolar disorder prompted their use in patients with dementia who are agitated. As is true for the use of most agents in this clinical context, the use of anticonvulsants in based mainly on case reports. Large, well-controlled RCTs have not supported their efficacy for treating disruptive agitation in dementia.

Carbamazepine

The development of oversedation, confusion, and ataxia limits the use of carbamazepine in the elderly. Carbamazepine has been investigated in two small RCTs for its impact on agitation and aggression in dementia with mixed results. An additional recent randomized multisite trial in 51 nursing home patients with dementia and agitation showed improvement in all agitation measures compared to placebo. Side effects were significantly greater in the carbamazepine group compared to placebo. Of note, carbamazepine carries a "black-box" warning for hematologic toxicity, and its propensity for inducing hepatic drug-metabolizing enzymes makes it problematic.

Valproate

Valproate is extensively used in the treatment of bipolar affective disorder. Initially, case studies/series suggested possible efficacy in the treatment of agitation related to dementia. Subsequent rando-

TABLE 73-8

Anticonvulsants—Dosages in the Elderly

DRUG	STARTING DOSE	RANGE
Divalproex sodium (Depakote®)	10–15 mg/kg bid or tid 125 mg bid	Target trough level: 45–100 μg/mL
Carbamazepine (Tegretol®)	100 mg bid, increase by 100–200 mg every 2–4 d	400–1200 mg bid Blood level: 4–12 μg/mL

TABLE 73-9

Medications with Anticholinergic Activity

Amantadine (Symadine®)
Benztropine (Cogentin®)
Digoxin (Lanoxin®)
Diphenhydramine (Benadryl®)
Dipyridamole (Persantine®)
Furosemide (Lasix®)
Hydroxyzine (Vistaril, Atarax®)
Meclizine (Dramamine®)
Metoclopramide (Reglan®)
Oxybutinin (Ditropan®)
Prochlorperazine (Compazine®)
Ranitidine (Zantac®)
Scopolamine (Transderm-V®)
Theophylline (Aerolate®)
Tricyclic antidepressants
Antipsychotics

mized trials failed to show benefit with respect to primary outcome measures of agitation. A meta-analysis of three RCTs investigating valproate showed no efficacy for either short- or long-acting preparations.

Gabapentin

A small case series of gabapentin as a treatment for agitation associated with dementia showed mixed results as far as effectiveness. In addition, adverse events, including gait instability and sedation, were significant. These limited data do not support the use of gabapentin in dementia.

In summary, the evidence does not support the use of valproate for treatment of agitation in dementia, and there is insufficient evidence to support the use of carbamazepine or gabapentin. The use of anticonvulsants in the treatment of agitation in the demented elderly patient may have a role on a case-by-case basis, especially if they have failed other treatments. When utilizing these medications, a low-dose approach is recommended to avoid serious side effects. Hematologic toxicity and drug interactions are particularly concerning for carbamazepine, considering that many elderly patients with dementia are on multiple medications. Valproate, even at low dose, causes significant sedation. The lack of proven efficacy in randomized controlled trials should be considered when contemplating the use of these medications in this population.

Acetylcholinesterase Inhibitors

Two meta-analyses and six additional RCTs of AChEIs (tacrine, donepezil, galantamine, and rivastigmine) for the treatment of neuropsychiatric symptoms in dementing disorders have been published. Five of these studies showed statistically significant, albeit modest, benefits. Whether the behavioral responses are secondary to cognitive improvement is unclear. Based on these data, the AChEIs may have a role in the treatment of behavioral symptoms in patients with AD and other dementias, including vascular dementia and Lewy body spectrum dementia.

The theorized reason for efficacy in this broad range of dementia types lies in neuropathologic evidence for a common pathology of cholinergic neuronal degeneration, which is likely to contribute to both cognitive and behavioral symptoms. AChEIs counteract this by inhibiting acetylcholinesterase, an enzyme that breaks down acetylcholine in the synaptic cleft, resulting in a relative increase in intrasynaptic acetylcholine for stimulation of both postsynaptic nicotinic and muscarinic receptors.

Donepezil, rivastigmine, and galantamine are generally well tolerated; the most common side effects are gastrointestinal disturbances, including nausea, vomiting, and diarrhea. Anecdotal evidence suggests that severity of gastrointestinal side effects may be attenuated when AChEIs are coadministered with memantine. AChEIs are contraindicated in patients with severe asthma or obstructive pulmonary disease, bradycardia (resting heart rate <50), cardiac conduction abnormalities, or peptic ulcer disease.

In summary, AChEIs should be considered in the treatment approach for patients with dementia who are agitated. Although the full treatment effects on behavioral symptoms have not been fully elucidated, the known benefit in delaying cognitive symptom progression, the modest improvement of neuropsychiatric symptoms seen in clinical trials, and the tolerable side-effect profile of these medications make them reasonable tools for addressing agitation. However, it should be made clear that AChEIs are a long-term strategy for reducing disruptive agitated behaviors; these are not an appropriate approach for acute management of severe disruptive agitation.

Antiadrenergic Approaches

As noted earlier, enhanced behavioral responses to NE in AD may contribute to the pathophysiology of disruptive agitation. Because it is not clear which postsynaptic adrenergic receptor class (beta-adrenergic, alpha-1 adrenergic, or both) might mediate the expression of disruptive agitation, we have developed pilot data using the beta-adrenergic antagonist propranolol and the alpha-1 adrenergic antagonist prazosin.

We previously demonstrated that propranolol (mean dose 10 ± 5 mg/day) was superior to placebo on total Brief Psychiatric Rating Scale scores and Clinical Global Impression of Change (CGIC), and propranolol was well tolerated. However, behavioral (but not antihypertensive or bradycardiac effects) of propranolol appeared to dissipate with long-term treatment in several patients, thus limiting drug effectiveness. In these latter patients and in those medically ineligible for inclusion in the propranolol study, open-label low-dose prazosin (1–5 mg/day) appeared even more effective than propranolol, was well tolerated, and positive effects were sustained for at least 6 to 12 months of follow-up.

Eleven patients with advanced AD or AD/CVD who had severe disruptive agitation for at least 1 month (i.e., physically aggressive behavior, resistiveness to care, verbally abusive behavior, pacing, and/or nighttime restlessness/thrashing in bed) were treated open label with prazosin (1–5 mg/day). Prazosin was started at 1 mg qhs for 2 days to avoid "first-dose" hypotension and increased by 1 mg/day every 5 days. Other psychotropic medications were held constant. All patients were without delirium and were medically stable. Before and after 8 weeks of treatment, subjects were rated by a research psychiatrist with input from the nursing home staff on the CGIC regarding frequency and severity of disruptive agitated behaviors and its impact on patient function and demands on staff. Nine of 11 patients were rated as "markedly improved" or "moderately improved" on the CGIC. Among them, five had no or minimal improvement during treatment with an atypical antipsychotic (olanzapine, risperidone,

or quetiapine). The other two patients were rated on the CGIC as between "moderately improved" and "minimally improved." Nursing home staff and the patients' primary-care physician elected to continue maintenance prazosin after the 8-week point in 10 of the 11 patients. There were no cardiovascular or other troublesome adverse events. These open-label data suggest that the alpha-1 adrenergic antagonist prazosin may be a promising treatment for disruptive agitation in dementia. A placebo-controlled trial is currently underway.

Benzodiazepines

Benzodiazepines have a limited role in the management of agitated behavior in dementia. Their use should be circumscribed only to emergency situations in which severe agitated behavior places the patient or others at risk of injury and has proven unresponsive to systematic trials of alternative medications. Under these circumstances, patients may benefit from a time-limited trial of a short-acting benzodiazepine, like lorazepam, oxazepam, or temazepam. These medications are preferred to long-acting preparations because these do not accumulate with repeated dosing and because their metabolism is not affected by age and liver disease. In contrast, long-acting benzodiazepines, such as diazepam, should be avoided because the parent agent and its active metabolites have extremely long half-lives, which lead to accumulation. Low-dose lorazepam is our preferred choice. All benzodiazepines may worsen cognitive functioning and increase the likelihood of falls and fractures.

Gonadal Hormones

The utility of hormonal treatments for agitation in patients with dementia is still being clarified. It has been theorized that increasing estrogen activity or decreasing androgen activity in patients with aggressive dementia can reduce problematic behaviors. Consistent with this theory, several case reports have suggested that estrogen administration or the use of gonadotrophin-releasing hormone agonists (leuprolide and goserelin) in men may be beneficial. Small randomized placebo-controlled trials of estrogen treatment have yielded mixed results. One study that included both men and women favored the estrogen arm, whereas another study that included only men found no significant differences from placebo. This second study also observed "rebound" aggressive behavior in subjects whose estrogen was discontinued upon completion of the study. There are several case reports of high-dose estrogen, decreasing aggressive behavior in women with severe dementia. Progestin preparations such as Depo-Provera have been reported to control sexually inappropriate behavior in men with dementia. Given the mixed results of previous studies, further research is needed to determine the value of this treatment approach.

General Guidelines for the Selection of Pharmacological Interventions

The recommended strategy for effective yet safe and tolerable treatment is to add or change only one medication at a time, thereby making the source of improvement, deterioration, or emergence of side effects more easily apparent. Always start at recommended geriatric doses and titrate up slowly.

Several clinical guidelines are helpful when choosing a psychoactive agent for the treatment of agitation. Patients with AD who are agitated, who have not responded to nonpharmacologic interventions, should be placed on an AChEI. If psychotic symptoms such as hallucinations or paranoid delusions are a prominent feature, an antipsychotic is a good first choice. Physically aggressive behavior, uncooperativeness with care, and forced motor activity may respond to the alpha-1 adrenergic antagonist prazosin. If the clinical presentation is marked by dangerous aggression, a benzodiazepine may be required acutely but only for short-term use and then an antipsychotic or prazosin should be considered. An SSRI may be useful in the presence of prominent mood or anxiety symptoms and/or irritability. A trial of gonadal hormones including antiandrogen approaches may be beneficial for male patients exhibiting inappropriate sexual behaviors. The need for continued pharmacologic management of disruptive agitation in the nursing home setting must also be reviewed periodically, weighing risks and benefits, keeping in mind that these behaviors often are episodic in nature and may change or even disappear over the course of the dementing illness, particularly in the very late stages of the disease, when patients may no longer exhibit any behaviors. Justification for the chosen intervention must clearly be documented on an ongoing basis.

CONCLUSION

The management of the elderly patient with AD who is agitated and other dementing disorders requires a comprehensive biopsychosocial approach. Nonpharmacological interventions should always be instituted first. If the symptoms persist and are distressing to the patient or are potentially harmful, then careful deliberation—weighing risks and benefits—should be carried out before initiating pharmacological management, particularly with antipsychotics. It is also important to keep in mind that these behaviors often are episodic in nature and may change or even disappear over the course of the dementing illness regardless of interventions. In many cases, a combination of both nonpharmacological and pharmacological interventions is necessary in order to decrease symptoms, improve quality of life, and delay institutionalization.

FURTHER READING

Coen RF, et al. Behaviour disturbance and other predictors of caregiver burden in Alzheimer's disease. *Int J Geriatr Psychiatry.* 1997;12:331–336.

Coffey CE, Cummings JL. *Textbook of Geriatric Neuropsychiatry.* Washington, DC: American Psychiatric Press Inc. 1994.

Cohen-Mansfield J. Nonpharmacologic interventions for inappropriate behaviors in dementia: a review, summary, and critique. *Am J Geriatr Psychiatry.* 2001;9: 361–381.

Cohen-Mansfield J, et al. Agitation in elderly persons: an integrative report of findings in a nursing home. *Int Psychogeriatr.* 1992;4:221–240.

Elrod R, et al. Effects of Alzheimer's disease severity on cerebrospinal fluid norepinephrine concentration. *Am J Psychiatry.* 1997;154:25–30.

Forbes DA, et al. Nonpharmacological management of agitated behaviours associated with dementia. *Geriatr Aging.* 2005;8:26–30.

Gill SS, et al. Atypical antipsychotic drugs and risk of ischaemic stroke: population based retrospective cohort study. *BMJ.* 2005;339:445.

Gottfries CG, et al. Treatment of depression in elderly patients with and without dementia disorders. *Int Clin Psychopharmacol.* 1992;6(suppl 5):55–64.

Medicines and Healthcare Products Regulatory Agency. Summary of clinical trial data on cerebrovascular adverse events (CVAEs) in randomized clinical trials of risperidone conducted in patients with dementia: March 9, 2004. Available at: http://medicines.mhra.gov.uk. Accessed September 6, 2005.

Mega MS, et al: The spectrum of behavioral changes in Alzheimer's disease. *Neurology.* 1996;46:130–135.

Peskind ER, et al. Effects of Alzheimer's disease and normal aging on cerebrospinal fluid norepinephrine responses to yohimbine and clonidine. *Arch Gen Psychiatry.* 1995;52:774–782.

Peskind ER, et al. Propranolol for disruptive behaviors in nursing home residents with probable or possible Alzheimer's disease: a placebo-controlled study. *Alzheimer's Dis Assoc Disord.* 2005;19:23–28.

Pollock BG, et al. Comparison of citalopram, perphenazine, and placebo for the acute treatment of psychosis and behavioral disturbances in hospitalized, demented patients. *Am J Psychiatry.* 2002;159(3):460–465.

Rosen HJ, et al. Neuroanatomical correlates of behavioural disorders in dementia. *Brain.* 2005;128:2612–2625.

Russo-Neustadt A, Cotman CW. Adrenergic receptors in Alzheimer's disease brain: selective increases in the cerebella of aggressive patients. *J Neurosci.* 1997;17:5573–5580.

Schneider LS, et al. Effectiveness of atypical antipsychotic drugs in patients with Alzheimer's disease. *N Engl J Med.* 2006;355:1525–1538.

Schneider LS, et al. Risk of death with atypical antipsychotic drug treatment for dementia. *JAMA.* 2005;294:1934–1943.

Sink KM, et al. Pharmacological treatment of neuropsychiatric symptoms of dementia: a review of the evidence. *JAMA.* 2005;293:596–608.

Teri L, et al. Treatment of agitation in AD: a randomized, placebo-controlled clinical trial. *Neurology.* 2000;55(9):1271–1278.

Teri L, et al. Exercise plus behavioral management in patients with Alzheimer's disease: a randomized controlled trial. *JAMA.* 2003;15:2015–2022.

Thorgrimsen L, et al. *Cochrane Database Syst Rev.* 2003;(3):CD003150. doi: 10.1002/14651858.CD003150.

US Food and Drug Administration. 5 FDA Public Health Advisory: deaths with antipsychotics in elderly patients with behavioral disturbances; April 2005.

Wilkinson D, et al. Donepezil in vascular dementia: a randomized, placebo-controlled study. *Neurology.* 2003;61:479–486.

Wooltorton E. Risperidone (Risperdal): increased rate of cerebrovascular events in dementia trials. *CMAJ.* 2002;167:1269.

Wynn ZJ, Cummings JL. Cholinesterase inhibitor therapies and neuropsychiatric manifestations of Alzheimer's disease. *Dement Geriatr Cogn Disord* 2004;17: 100–108.

Effects of Aging on Cardiovascular Structure and Function

Dalane W. Kitzman ■ *George Taffet*

PRINCIPLES OF AGING BIOLOGY PERTINENT TO THE CARDIOVASCULAR SYSTEM

As the aging process begins after maturation, deteriorative, regenerative, and compensatory changes develop over time and result in diminished physiological reserve capacity and an increased vulnerability to challenges, particular disease, and, as a result, a decrease in the ability to survive. Importantly, aging itself does not result in disease; however, it does lower the threshold for the development of disease and can intensify and accelerate the effects of disease once initiated. The increased vulnerability with age to external or internal challenges is one of the tenets of geriatrics and gerontology and is called homeostenosis.

These concepts are particularly relevant to aging of the human cardiovascular system, especially older persons living in developed countries. In these populations, it is particularly important to screen for clinical and subclinical disease, particularly atherosclerosis, as well as to consider other cultural and environmental factors that are distinct from aging yet can mimic aging effects. These can manifest in human populations studies as cohort and period effects, can be subtle or overt, and are easily confused with aging. It has been proposed that a true age-related change should be absent in young persons, increase with age, be universally present in very old persons, and not be related to any known, definable disease.

In some early human aging studies, subjects with clinical and subclinical disease were not excluded, leading to an overestimation of the effects of aging on the cardiovascular system. Coronary atherosclerosis is highly prevalent in western societies and is one of the important disorders that can be occult and can significantly affect cardiac function. Systemic arterial hypertension is even more common. Therefore, reasonable screening for these two most common disorders is prudent to separate aging from disease.

In addition to the effects of subclinical disease, there are additional effects of physical inactivity. Humans and many animals become increasingly sedentary as they age. For example, rats given free access to a running wheel will run 20 km per week when they are young, but this decreases to less than 7 km per week when approaching the age of 23 months. Many older people are even less active. Another increasingly important life-style-related factor relatively new to civilization is obesity. Adipose tissue owing to excess caloric intake has numerous effects involving nearly all physiological systems, including cardiovascular, and obesity increases substantially with age. Thus, the changes that are seen in an older population reflect the combination of all these factors, period, cohort, lifestyle, and disease-related changes, as well as the biological effect of age itself. It is often challenging to precisely separate and discern, both qualitatively and quantitatively, the latter from the former. However, awareness of the important nuances of normal aging can help avoid most errors.

AGING OF THE VASCULATURE

Age Changes in Arterial Structure

With age a number of ultrastructural changes occur in the aorta, and all appear to contribute to increased stiffness. Elastin becomes fragmented in the internal elastic lamina and media perhaps because of inappropriate activation of matrix metalloproteinases. Calcification of the media is also seen. Collagen increasingly becomes cross-linked, making a stiff matrix, especially in the subendothelium.

Irregularities in size and shape of endothelial cells are seen at areas of turbulence, and high cellular turnover occurring at those sites suggest that replicative or cellular senescence may be occurring at those sites. Further evidence of this "in situ" replicative senescence may be provided by manipulations that inhibit telomere shortening. In endothelial cells with persistently long telomeres, age-associated abnormalities may be significantly reduced.

The aortic lumen diameter increases with age, as do vessel length and wall thickness. Because the aorta is fixed proximally and distally, the increase in length results in the tortuous, ectatic, and rightward-shifted aorta seen often on chest X-rays of older persons.

Angiogenesis is impaired in the old vascular tree in response to ischemia or chemical signals. Explants of arteries from old animals have decreased spouting of microvessels and decreased vascular invasion of implants. There is no deficit of smooth muscle cell proliferation, but endothelial cell proliferation is impaired. The impact on this is uncertain because neovascularization of myocardial infarcts or dermal wounds, which may be a bit slower in old rats, is ultimately similar for young and old rats.

Functional Changes of Aging Arteries

The older conduit artery may be less responsive to vasoactive substances. For example, nitric oxide (NO) is a vasorelaxor and (at least in the rodent) contributes to the balance that dictates resting arterial tone. Aortic strips isolated from older animals have higher NO synthase activity but produce less NO. Old aortas will relax appropriately when exposed to direct NO donors (nitroprusside) but are less responsive to agents whose effects are mediated by NO such as acetylcholine. Similarly, forearm arterial blood flow is increased less in older individuals in response to acetylcholine compared to younger and athletically active older individuals. As NO is produced from circulating arginine, with age a relative increase in arginase (a scavenging enzyme that competes for arginine) results in reduced arginine availability for the endothelium, explaining the relatively poor efficacy of arginine supplementation. Isoform-specific arginase inhibitors are not yet available, but genetically induced decreases in Arginase protein attenuate age-related changes in arterial function, making this a promising area for research. Again, the response to direct acting agents is the same in old and young. While the reasons for this paradox remain unclear, the net result is that the old artery is contracted and, again, stiffer.

Old arteries are also tonically contracted by an age-related increase in receptors to endothelin-1 and circulating levels of this potent vasoconstrictor. This results in a decreased maximum response to added endothelin in older persons. Exercise training appears to decrease basal endothelin-1 levels and restore its responsiveness.

Arterial wall stiffness can be measured noninvasively as pulse wave velocity (PWV), augmentation index, distensibility, and systolic and pulse blood pressure. PWV increases twofold from age 20 to 80 years, independent of blood pressure. A stiffer artery wall allows pressure to reflect from periphery to the heart while the aortic valve is still open, increasing the load on the heart, and thus PWV is a physiologically relevant parameter. Augmentation index, another measure of the impact of aortic stiffness, increases fourfold over that same age range, contributing to the increase in systolic pressure that occurs with age. For men in the Framingham study, systolic BP increased 5 mm Hg per decade until the age of 60 years; then the slope shifted to 10 mm Hg per decade. For women, systolic BP started lower but shifted to the higher slope earlier. Over the same age range, diastolic BP increases a little and then decreases, so overall it remains unaltered (80 in men, 70–80 in women). Older athletes have lower systolic pressures and PWVs than sedentary old people, but young people were still better than the old athletes. In fact, PWV correlates inversely with maximum oxygen consumption (VO_{2max}) in healthy people of all ages. VO_{2max} is strongly associated with measures of

vessel stiffness, particularly PWV, which may be a true contributor to the age-related decline in exercise capacity via a number of mechanisms, including increased load on the left ventricle as well as altered peripheral blood flow distribution. However, this has not been fully explored.

As noted above, at least one mechanism for the increase in arterial stiffness involves nonenzymatic glucose cross-links between vessel collagen molecules. ALT-711 (alagebrium) is a prototypical cross-link breaker and is effective in decreasing PWV and augmentation index as measures of vessel stiffness in older primates and people. Interestingly, plasma advanced glycosylation end products correlate with PWV in normals and hypertensives.

The net result of these changes is reduced compliance and increased impedance, leading to increased systolic blood pressure and little, if any, effect on diastolic blood pressure.

Aging and Atherosclerosis

In addition to the changes in the matrix, old smooth muscle cells appear to be less differentiated and proliferate more readily. In studies of smooth muscle cells isolated from young and old rat aortas, the freshly isolated old cells grew more rapidly and migrated more rapidly in comparison to those isolated from the young rat. The smooth muscle cells appear to have polyploidy, which may be another marker of dedifferentiation. While atherosclerosis is not a normal age-related change, especially in species other than man and possibly pigs, the higher propensity to proliferate may increase the probability of developing atherosclerosis if the environment is right.

It is important to understand that age-related changes in large arteries are different from atherosclerosis. First, atherosclerosis is essentially unique to western man; it has been difficult to reproduce the complicated plaque characteristic of advanced disease in humans, in animal models including genetically engineered mice. Atherosclerosis is heterogeneous compared to the age-related changes that occur quite uniformly throughout the conduit arteries. Atherosclerosis leads to a compromise of the vessel lumen compared to the relative dilation of the large vessels with age. The severity of atherosclerosis is related to blood turbulence and shear stress, whereas age-related changes have no such localization. Atherosclerosis clearly has an inflammatory component; none of the activation of white cells typical of atherosclerosis is seen in the age-related process. Cholesterol is a cofactor in atherosclerosis; it has no clear-cut role in age-related changes. Together, age-related changes are termed arteriosclerosis, but regrettably this term is often misused to indicate atherosclerosis, leading to confusion.

Nevertheless, it is clear that the functional and structural changes in the large arteries make the older person or animal at high risk of atherosclerosis, given the proper setting. If older rabbits are switched to atherogenic diets, the resulting lesions are more severe after an interval than young rabbits exposed for a similar duration. Thus, the aged arterial wall provides a more fertile ground for atherosclerosis to occur. And because both atherosclerosis and diabetes mellitus also increase large artery stiffness, these disease processes are multiplicative with age in increasing PWV, systolic blood pressure, and pulse pressure and their ultimate effects on the heart.

The impact of aortic stiffening and its clinical manifestations, increased systolic blood pressure and widened pulse pressure, are well appreciated. In addition to the recognition that increased systolic blood pressure and widened pulse pressure are risk factors for stroke, renal failure, and heart disease, the more rapid propagation of pressure waves by the stiff aorta may induce left ventricular (LV) hypertrophy and early fibrosis within the myocardium via increased load, as well as altered ventricular–vascular coupling. If the PWV is high enough, early pressure wave reflections return while the aortic valve is still open, increase workload, and induce hypertrophy. Importantly when the pressure waves return later (as in the young), these may improve coronary artery perfusion by increasing the pressure in the proximal aorta.

AGING CHANGES IN THE HEART

Substantial changes occur with aging in myocardial composition, cardiac structure, and cardiovascular function at rest and during exercise. The changes in anatomy are summarized in Table 74-1.

Changes in Myocardial Composition

Myocite hypertrophy

Cardiomyocyte hypertrophy has been recognized and seen as a part of the response to the pressure reflections and increased afterload described above. However, this should be interpreted in light of the clear evidence that the heart is renewing itself, continuously repopulated from stem cell population resident and/or sequestered in the bone marrow. The cellular hypertrophy associated with age may mark depletion of the process, as the youngest cells, those most recently differentiated into cardiomyocytes, are thought to be the smallest and in the mouse heart the heterogeneity of myocyte size increases dramatically with age. Interestingly, the largest cells are also the most vulnerable to stress.

Myocyte Degeneration

The loss of myocytes with age is greater than the ability to repopulate the heart, and loss is by both apoptosis and necrosis. The total number of cardiomyocytes may be reduced across the lifespan by 50% in healthy human and animal hearts. As above, those cardiac myocytes that remain are increased in size and are much more variable in size. Nearly universal findings in hearts from elderly individuals are focal basophilic degeneration, a result of abnormal glycogenolysis, and lipofuscin, a "wear and tear" pigment, which results in a macroscopic darkened appearance to the aged myocardium, which has been termed brown atrophy. Lipofuscin occupies up to 10%

TABLE 74-1

Normal Age-Related Changes in the Anatomy of the Heart

- Increased heart weight, LV mass, and LV wall thickness; mild hypertrophy
- Fibrosis, collagen accumulation in the myocardium
- LV cavity size decreases, shortening of long axis, rightward shift and dilatation of the aorta, dilation of left atrium, and senile septum
- Calcific and fatty degeneration of valve leaflets and annuli
- Coronary artery dilation and calcification
- Conduction system: fibrosis and loss of specialized cells and fibers; 75% of pacemaker cells in sinoatrial node lost; fibrosis of A-V node and left anterior fascicle

of myocardial volume in very elderly hearts. While profound, these changes are not detectable by routine diagnostic techniques, such as cardiac ultrasound, and their functional significance is not currently known.

However, older cardiomyocytes are intrinsically stiffer. This may be the contribution of active stiffness in part because of an increased leak of calcium from the SR with age, as well as passive stiffness as a result of viscoelastic changes within the cell. Each mitochondrion has its own genome, with relatively sparse ability to correct mutations. A number of investigators report that MitoDNA deletions may increase with age. The implications of this finding remain uncertain, as the number of mitochondria per myocyte is approximately 1000.

Nowhere is cellular dropout more impressive than in the sinoatrial node. The volume of the sinoatrial node decreases with age. The number of pacemaker cells is reduced (90% by the age of 70 years), with most volume replaced by fat. More modest cellular losses occur at the A-V node, and minimal changes are present in distal conduction system. The dropout of sinoatrial nodal cells is accompanied by a decrease in the slow, L-type calcium channel that is critical to initiation of depolarization. The sensitivity of the older sinoatrial node to calcium channel-blockers appears to increase in the older guinea pig pacemaker.

Connective Tissue

Diffuse foci of fibrosis are seen microscopically in the myocardium owing to an increase in interstitial collagen. The fibrous tissue appears in a delicate pattern, unlike the patches of fibrosis seen after acute injury, such as that seen after myocardial infarction. The fibrosis does not appear to be related solely to either ischemia or hypertension, although both of these disorders accelerate the process. Quantitatively, collagen content essentially doubles in the old rat heart. These changes may partly underlie age-related alterations in Doppler diastolic filling, which are discussed later.

Senile Cardiac Amyloid

Amyloid deposition is seen to varying degrees in the majority of hearts from persons older than 90 years but is uncommon before the age of 60 years. It is easily recognized at autopsy, particularly along the left atrial endocardium. Its significance is incompletely understood but might also contribute to LV diastolic stiffness seen by Doppler.

Adiposity

With aging, there is deposition of adipose, particularly in the right ventricular epicardium and the atrioventricular groove. This is most pronounced in women and in the obese. These observations from autopsy studies correlate with the well-known epicardial and pericardial fat stripes that superficially mimic pericardial effusion on echocardiography. In the Framingham study, the incidence and size of the echocardiographic clear spaces in the area of the pericardium increased significantly with age and were seen in the posterior as well as anterior regions. Previously thought to be an inert epiphenomenon, emerging data suggest that this adipose infiltration within the myocardium and grossly in the epicardium may have consequences for cardiac function, not surprising, given accumulating data indicating that adipose cells are metabolically and hormonally active and can generate a range of factors including cytokines. This is an exciting area of research.

Changes in Cardiac Structure

Mass

In an autopsy study of 765 normal hearts evenly distributed by age and gender from age 20 to 99 years from subjects without a history of hypertension or evidence of significant coronary atherosclerosis, indexed mean heart weight in men was not age related and was consistently greater than in women. For women, however, the indexed mean heart weight increased significantly with age. This interaction of gender and age was confirmed in a study in 111 healthy subjects using 2-D guided M-mode echocardiographic measurements of LV mass. Furthermore, in seminal work by Gardin et al., when data from healthy men and women were combined, echocardiographic LV mass was found to increase 15% from age 30 to age 70 years. These age and gender trends in echocardiographic LV mass were confirmed more recently by Gardin et al. with an analysis of data from the Cardiovascular Health study (CHS), an NHLBI-funded population-based, observational cohort study of more than 5000 persons aged ≥65 years.

Not surprisingly, there is a substantial impact of body size, particularly weight and lean body mass, on LV mass. In a healthy subgroup of participants in CHS, when weight was adjusted for, there was an approximately 1 g/yr increase in LV mass from age 65 to 80 years. In the healthy subgroup of the Framingham study, when obese persons were excluded, there was a minimal influence of age on LV mass.

Ventricular Wall Thickness

In the large autopsy study described above, right and left ventricular free wall thicknesses remained relatively constant with age, while ventricular septal thickness increased with age for both men and women. However, wall thickness measurements at autopsy may not correlate well with those made in living subjects, where measurements can be made in systole and diastole. In most echocardiographic studies of healthy subjects, mild age-related increases in both ventricular septal and LV free wall thickness have been found in women and men.

A frequent finding at autopsy and on echocardiograms of persons without apparent heart disease is mild disproportionate thickness of the basal ventricular septum. This has also been called sigmoid ventricular septum and senile septum. This finding may be the result of hypertension rather than biological aging. It has potential clinical relevance in that it can confound to some degree the diagnosis of hypertrophic cardiomyopathy in elderly patients.

Chamber Size

There is disagreement in the literature of the effect of aging on chamber size. Some investigators have found a decrease in LV internal diastolic and systolic dimensions with age, by echocardiography in live subjects or direct measurement in autopsy studies. Others have shown no age-related change in LV size.

Most echocardiographic and autopsy studies have found a significant age-related increase in left atrial size in subjects without apparent cardiovascular disease, with an increase in left atrial dimension between ages 30 and 70 years. The cause of age-related left atrial dilation is unknown, but it may have consequences for specific disorders that are common in the elderly, such as atrial fibrillation.

Aorta

A uniform finding in all studies, including large population-based studies such as the Framingham study, has been a substantial age-related increase in aortic diameter, particularly the aortic root. The degree of change, 22% between age 30 and 70 years, is sufficient that nomograms for aortic root diameter should probably be adjusted for age. The thickness of the aortic wall also increases significantly with age, probably independent of atherosclerosis, and the pulsatility (compliance) of the aorta decreases. These changes are most discernible by ultrasound with transesophageal and intravascular echocardiography.

Valves

The cardiac valves undergo several significant age-related changes. When measured directly at autopsy, the thicknesses of normal aortic and mitral leaflets increase, particularly along the closure margins. This is associated microscopically with collagen deposition and degeneration, lipid accumulation, and focal dystrophic calcification in the leaflets and annuli.

In those subjects most affected, this is recognized clinically and echocardiographically as aortic valve sclerosis, valve thickening without significant hemodynamic dysfunction. In the CHS study, this was found in 26% of participants and was related to male gender and hypertension. The relationship between these presumably age-related degenerative changes and the development of clinical aortic stenosis is incompletely defined. It was found in CHS that echocardiographically defined aortic sclerosis was independently associated with a 1.5-fold increased risk of cardiovascular mortality, calling into serious question whether this should be considered a normal age-related change.

Although not normal, age-related degenerative calcification of an otherwise normal-appearing tricuspid aortic valve may apparently result in progressive aortic stenosis and is currently the most common cause of aortic stenosis requiring valve surgery. The relationship between expected, near-universal age-related thickening and mild calcification of the aortic valve leaflets and the development of degenerative calcific aortic stenosis in a subset of elderly persons is unclear.

Microscopic deposits of calcium accumulated in the mitral annulus are expected with aging. However, gross mitral annular calcification should generally be considered a disease process. Relatively little is known about the true natural history of mitral annular calcification. It has been reported to be present in up to 40% of hearts from women older than 90 years, and there is a large (4 to 1) female predominance. Echocardiographically, it is often associated with modest degrees of mitral regurgitation but rarely with stenosis. A high incidence of atrioventricular block and bundle branch block has been described.

The circumferences of all four cardiac valves, measured at autopsy, increase with age in normal hearts from women and men, and this appears to be associated with collagen degeneration and lipid accumulation in the valve annuli. This is most notable for the semilunar valves than the atrioventricular valves. In the case of the aortic annulus, this normal age-related dilatation has been confirmed in living subjects with echocardiography.

It is likely that annular dilatation contributes to the age-related increase in valvular regurgitation documented by Doppler in healthy, normal, asymptomatic subjects. By the age of 80 years, 90% of apparently healthy subjects had multivalvular regurgitation, and the aortic valve was affected earliest and to the greatest extent. The degree of valvular regurgitation caused by normal aging is always trivial or mild, central, and associated with normal (for age) appearing leaflets.

As in aortic stenosis, there is an association between this normal age-related change and an important cardiovascular disorder. Age alone is the strongest risk factor for isolated severe aortic regurgitation, and idiopathic dilatation of the aortic annulus is the most common cause of aortic regurgitation in patients undergoing aortic valve surgery. This disease may be an exaggeration of an expected age-related degenerative change exacerbated by systemic hypertension, and there is most likely an additional, contributing factor as yet unidentified.

An interesting, although unanswered, question is whether these normal age-related changes in the cardiac valves, individually or collectively, increase the risk for infective endocarditis.

Pericardium

Wavy bands of collagen bundles comprise the normal pericardium. The straightening of these wavy bands allows a degree of distensibility when pericardial pressure or volume increases acutely. With aging, these bands of collagen become straighter and the pericardium becomes thicker. This causes the pericardium of older subjects to be stiffer. The significance of this aging change is unknown, but it could impact diastolic compliance in the elderly. As discussed above, the degree of epicardial and pericardial fat increases with age, particularly in women and obese persons, and the resultant echolucent spaces seen on echocardiography can superficially mimic a pericardial effusion.

Atrial Septum

The atrial septum thickens and becomes stiffer with advancing age, probably owing to fatty infiltration and fibrosis. This causes the atrial septum to become less mobile with phasic respiration. This phenomenon is helpful in echocardiographic diagnosis. The finding of a thinned, hypermobile atrial septum by echocardiography in an elderly person should raise the suspicion of fenestrated atrial septal aneurysm, patent foramen ovale, or atrial septal defect and lead to careful color Doppler and a peripheral venous injection of agitated saline contrast. An exaggerated form of the age-related fatty infiltration is found essentially exclusively in older patients and is called lipomatous hypertrophy of the atrial septum. It can mimic the appearance of an intracardiac tumor but is recognizable by its characteristic dumbbell shape.

A probe-patent foramen ovale is seen in approximately 35% of normal hearts younger than 30 years and in 20% by age 80 years. While paradoxical embolism is usually considered in the context of an atypical stroke in a person younger than 55 years, it likely is a contributor, although of unknown proportion, to strokes among the elderly. Because of this, injection of venous agitated saline contrast, a relatively benign procedure, is often used as an adjunct to echocardiographic imaging in older patients referred with atypical stroke.

Coronary Arteries

With aging, the coronary arteries tend to become more dilated and tortuous, possibly because of hemodynamic drag. Coronary collaterals may also increase in number and size with age, but it is not clear whether this is independent of atherosclerosis. While atherosclerosis is always considered a disease process, Mönckeberg's medial calcification (arteriosclerosis) probably represents an age-related degenerative process. It is a nearly universal finding in the very old and is independent of gender. In the peripheral vasculature, it may contribute to the age-related elevation in systemic systolic blood pressure and arterial impedance. A syndrome often seen in elderly patients and those with end-stage renal failure is the triad of cardiac calcifications involving the aortic cusps, mitral annulus, and coronary arteries, called the senile calcification syndrome. In these older persons, no evidence of altered calcium metabolism has been found, and, although a relationship with elevated serum cholesterol levels has been described, the etiology is not known.

Overall Appearance

It has been stated that a characteristic geometric configuration is imparted to the elderly heart by these age-related changes, particularly those observed in the cardiac chambers: shortening of the long-axis dimension, a mild decrease in the internal systolic and diastolic LV dimensions, dilatation and rightward shifting of the aortic root, and dilatation of the left atrium. These changes, as well as the mild regional calcification seen in the aortic and mitral valve annuli, are so characteristic that these can be used as clues to help detect the age group of patients during blinded readings of echocardiograms.

Changes in Cardiac Function with Age at Rest

Since there are significant changes in the anatomy of the cardiovascular system, discussed above, and since aging is accompanied by significant changes in function in most other organ systems, one would expect alterations in cardiac physiology as well. Several important age-related changes have already been discussed briefly above, including changes in valvular function and the potential anatomic substrates for altered diastolic function. While the effect of age on cardiac function has long been a topic of research efforts, only recently have studies been able to be performed using adequately robust techniques combined with appropriately defined reference populations. However, it is still true that little information is available regarding how these changes in function impact on the epidemiology, presentation, diagnosis, prognosis, and therapy of cardiovascular disease. Changes with age in cardiovascular function are summarized in Table 74-2.

Most studies of cardiovascular function at rest show either no substantial change in cardiac output, stroke volume, heart rate, and ejection fraction with aging or mild-to-moderate and significant increases in systemic and pulmonary arterial blood pressure, with

TABLE 74-2

Normal Age-Related Changes in Cardiovascular Physiology

- Peak cardiac output declines
- Peak heart rate declines
- Peak ejection fraction declines
- LV stiffness increases and diastolic relaxation decreases
- Valvular regurgitation develops
- Prolongation of PR, QRS, and QT; left axis deviation
- Arteries stiffen and aortic impedance increases
- Systolic blood pressure increases

resultant increases in left and right ventricular afterload as shown in Table 74-3.

Heart Rate and Rhythm

There is no change in resting heart rate with adult aging. However, as will be discussed further later in the section on exercise, there is a clear and marked decrease in maximum heart rate in response to exercise that is highly predictable and can easily be estimated by a simple equation. For men, (220 – age) predicts the target maximum predicted heart rate for exercise testing. Women have lower peak heart rate in youth and more gradual fall in maximum; thus, a correction factor of 0.85 is often used.

The age-related change in heart rate is perhaps the most substantial change in cardiac function, both in magnitude and in consequence. Although its mechanism(s) are not fully understood, a number of studies have been performed. In the presence of the beta-adrenergic antagonist, propranolol, and the parasympathetic antagonist, atropine, given to ablate both sympathetic and parasympathetic input to the heart, the intrinsic heart rate is seen. Intrinsic heart rate decreases by 5 to 6 beats/minute each decade of age so that the resting heart rate in an 80-year-old is not much slower than the intrinsic heart rate. This means that, at rest, the parasympathetic nervous system is not actively slowing the heart, and, as would be expected, the increase in heart rate after atropine is less than half that in the young.

There is also decreased response to sympathetic agonists. Administration of isoproterenol to healthy young and old people demonstrated that the chronotropic effects of this sympathomimetic agent were markedly attenuated in the old. At doses that increased heart rate by 25 beats/minute in young healthy males, heart rate increased by only 10 beats/minute or less in older persons.

Further supporting the decline in maximal heart rate as a primary age-related biological change is that it cannot be significantly modified by even vigorous exercise training, suggesting that it is not a secondary consequence of an age-related decline in physical activity level. Also, it does not appear to be caused by inadequate sympathetic stimulation, as serum norepinephrine and epinephrine are increased rather than decreased at rest in normal elderly. Further, with stress or exertion these catecholamines increase even more than in young persons under similar stress.

Perhaps as a direct reflection of the decreased parasympathetic nervous system input and decreased responsiveness to what autonomic input is present, there is a significant decrease in heart rate variability. Heart rate variability is a measure of the variations in instantaneous heart rate (or RR interval). This results in a decrease

in complexity, which may not seem important in itself but correlates with the decrease in physiological reserve. Any loss of complexity may then render the older persons or animals less likely to tolerate challenges to their homeostasis. Furthermore, the loss of complexity with age occurs in a number of physiologic systems and is forestalled by interventions like exercise training, which improve robustness.

In highly screened older people to exclude potential confounding effects of disease, the prevalence of atrial premature beats reaches 88% on 24-hour ambulatory monitoring. Because there is no association with cardiac risk over the next decade with the presence of even frequent atrial premature beats (APBs), this is thought not to reflect subclinical coronary artery disease. At exercise testing, isolated ventricular ectopic beats occurred in more than half of highly screened elders older than 80 years. Therefore, this increase in ectopy of both atrial and ventricular origin is thought to be normal aging process.

Diastolic Function

Increased LV stiffness associated with aging using invasive techniques was first described in young and old beagles. Ten years later, similar findings were identified by invasive techniques in humans. In between these two developments, there was the advent of spectral Doppler echocardiography, which greatly expanded our ability for noninvasively assessing LV diastolic filling. All studies, including the large population-based databases from the Framingham study and the CHS, have uniformly found that diastolic LV filling is substantially altered in older normal subjects. In addition, similar changes with aging are found in rats, dogs, and mice.

The age-related changes in the pulsed Doppler diastolic transmitral flow pattern that have been observed in humans are reduced early (E) and increased late atrial (A) flow velocities and decreased E/A ratio. Klein et al. expanded these findings by documenting an age-related increase in early deceleration time and isovolumic relaxation time, important parameters that were not included in many previous papers or in the population-based studies. The finding of a normal age-related change in early deceleration time may be particularly relevant, since this parameter predicts intrinsic LV chamber stiffness. In addition, the report by Klein et al. showed that similar age-related changes take place in pulmonary venous flow, with increased peak systolic flow velocity, decreased diastolic flow velocity, increased peak atrial reversal flow velocity, and increased percentage of forward flow in systole.

It is well known that these Doppler indexes of diastolic filling may be altered early in the course of a variety of disorders that are common and sometimes unrecognized in the elderly and are significantly influenced by a number of physiological variables, including LV mass and chronotropic, inotropic, and loading states, which may also be altered by aging. Thus, it had been questioned whether the age-related alterations in Doppler diastolic filling indexes were simply secondary to these or whether they occurred independent of cardiovascular disease and other confounding physiological variables. In a study of old and young healthy volunteers, rigorously screened for cardiovascular disease, comprehensive Doppler echocardiography, radionuclide ventriculography, and invasive measurements of right heart and left atrial pressures were performed. The old and young subject groups were closely matched for LV mass, volumes, ejection fraction, and end-systolic wall stress; left atrial size and heart rate; and right atrial, pulmonary arterial, pulmonary capillary wedge, and systemic arterial pressures. Despite this, there persisted the characteristic

TABLE 74-3

Effect of Age on Cardiovascular Function at Rest

INVESTIGATOR	n	GENDER	AGE RANGE (yr)	METHOD BP CO	CHANGE PER DECADE					
					HR (b/min)	CO (L/min)	CI (L/min m²)	SV (mL)	SVR (U)	SBP/DBP (mm Hg)
Granath (1964)	42	M	16–83	IA F	−0.6	−0.39	−	−5.2	+1.23	+5.0/−0.2
Higginbotham (1986)	24	M	20–50	IA F	+0.1	−0.30	−0.21	−6.1	+1.30	+3.0/−0.7
Kitzman (1989)	86	M + F	20–73	IA F	0.0	−0.29	−0.15	−4.0	+1.38	+4.2/−0.6
Cournand (1945)	13	M	21–52	F	0.0	−0.60	−0.30	−7.2	−	−
Brandfonbrener (1955)	67	M	19–86	DD	−2.1	−0.51	−0.23	−5.2	−	−
Julius (1967)	54	M + F	18–69	IA DD	−	−0.39	−	−6.2	+1.26	+3.3/−0.6
Conway (1971)	27	M + F	20–65	IA DD	−1.3	−0.30	−	−2.0	+1.57	+9.7/+2.7
Davidson (1990)	47	M + F	24–69	IA TD	+0.9	−0.32	−0.09	−5.0	+0.59	+2.3/−2.7
Kuikka (1982)	69	M	6–78	RD	−	−	−0.25	−	−	−
	79	F	−	−	−	−	−0.19	−	−	−
Leithe (1984)	16	M + F	24–70	RD	+1.8	−	−0.21	−	+0.53	−
Rodeheffer (1986)	65	M	25–80	EGNA	−0.7	+0.14	+0.11	+3.4	−	−
Shannon (1991)	16	M + F	<27–>74	AUT EGNA	+0.9	+0.15	+0.06	+1.1	+0.40	−
Luisada (1980)	84	M	20–89	IC	+1.8	−0.21	−0.21	−3.9	−	−
	48	F	−	IC	+0.4	−0.39	−0.08	−6.2	−	−
Vargas (1982)	17	M + F	<31–>71	OB IC	+3.6	−0.32	−	−8.8	+1.33	+8.4/+3.0
Smith (1987)	41	M	20–69	AUT IC	+0.6	−0.13	−0.06	−4.3	+0.780	+1.7/+1.6
Hainsworth (1988)	64	M + F	20–80	AUT SB	−0.6	−0.33	−0.18	−4.5	+2.33	+5.7/+2.5
Lewis (1938)	100	M	40–89	R	+0.1	−0.12	−0.03	−2.1	+1.67	+10.3/+0.7
Ogawa (1992)	27	M	23–62	OB R	+0.6	−	−	−	−	+1.4/−0.3
	28	F	20–72	OB R	−0.8	−	−	−	−	+3.1/+2.0
Fleg (1995)	121	M	22–85	EGNA	−1.8	−	−0.1	+1.7	0.6	+3/1
	79	F	22–86	EGNA	−1.8	−	−0.1	−1.4	0.4	+3.0
Beere (1999)	23	M	21–74	IA F	−2.1	−0.29	−	−2.4	+1.8	+6.9/+1.4

AUT, automatic; BP, blood pressure; CI, cardiac index; CO, cardiac output; DBP, diastolic blood pressure; DD, dyedilution; EGNA, equilibrium gated nuclear angiography; f, female; F, direct. Fick method: HR, heart rate; IA, intra-arterial; IC, impedance cardiography; M, male; n, number of subjects; OB, observer; R, rebreathing technique; RD, radioisotope dilution; SB, single. Breath technique: SBP, systolic blood pressure; SI, stroke index; SV, stroke volume; SVR, systemic vascular resistance; SVR, systemic vascular resistance index; TD, thermodilution; -, not available.

Adapted/updated from Kitzman DW. Aging in the heart. In: Developments in Cardiology, GL Freeman, ed. Orland, W.B. Saunders 1994, pp 3–16.

age-related alterations in Doppler LV filling. In univariate and multivariate regression analyses, peak early and atrial flow velocities were not related to any of the potentially confounding variables measured once age was taken into account. A complementary study showed that even though substantial changes in Doppler filling patterns were inducible by gravitationally induced alterations in LV load, filling patterns in elderly subjects were still distinguishable from those of young subjects. Taken together, these studies suggest that an altered Doppler diastolic LV filling is a primary, biologic effect of aging, intrinsic to the aged human heart, and not explicable by other physiological and pathological changes that frequently accompany the aging process and reflect a true alteration in LV diastolic function.

Since normal healthy elderly are expected to have an altered pattern of Doppler LV filling, what then should be considered abnormal? First, the large population-based databases have yielded important data that have been underappreciated and are significantly underused in current practice. In the CHS, among subjects aged 65 to 100 years, with no indicators of cardiovascular disease, the upper and lower 95% confidence limits for the E/A ratio included 0.65 to 1.45 for women and 0.64 to 1.56 for men. Similar results were found in a smaller group of healthy elderly subjects in the Framingham study. Therefore, findings obtained in elderly patients during basal conditions that fall outside this range should be considered abnormal, regardless of age. Second, the pattern of LV filling is helpful. Certain patterns, such as the pseudonormalized and restrictive patterns, can be more easily discerned from normal and can be more specific for disease when found in the elderly than in younger patients, because these differ more from the expected pattern. The more recent introduction of mitral annulus tissue Doppler has significantly boosted the ability to assess LV diastolic function noninvasively because the annular velocity measures are relatively load dependent. As would be expected, based on the above study, age alters the tissue Doppler velocities as well. Unfortunately, age-related normative reference data are relatively sparse.

In isolated papillary muscles from older rat hearts, the change in pattern of contraction and relaxation is clearly seen: slower force generation and relaxation with no change in peak force. In addition, the inotropic and lusitropic (facilitating relaxation) responses to sympathetic stimulation are also decreased with age. Cardiac contraction and relaxation are dictated by calcium fluxes. For contraction a small amount of calcium enters the cells via the slow L-type calcium channels and stimulates the release of 10- to 20-fold more calcium from the sarcoplasmic reticulum (SR). Active relaxation includes the calcium reuptake by the cardiac SR after contraction and extrusion from the cell by the Na–Ca exchanger and the sarcolemmal Ca pump. Ninety percent of calcium cycles in and out of SR. Calcium reuptake into the SR is decreased by almost 50% in old hearts from rats and mice, and the content of the SR Ca ATPase pump is decreased in old human hearts as well. This slows cardiac relaxation and results in smaller stores in the SR for release in the next contraction. To a small extent, compensation occurs in other calcium fluxes in that the SL Ca ATPase activity is increased in old rat hearts.

The significance of these age-related alterations in diastolic filling has not been fully established. An atrial gallop (S4) is a normal finding on physical examination in those older than 75 years, a manifestation of the increased contribution of left atrial systole to ventricular filling. Brain natriuretic peptide (BNP) elaboration and release by the left ventricle also increases mildly with age, a possible reflection of altered diastolic function with age; however, it may also reflect known age-related reduction in renal clearance of the peptide. Altered diastolic filling may play a role in reduced exercise capacity seen in normal older subjects, the lower threshold for expression of diastolic heart failure, and the poorer prognosis in older patients with heart failure.

Gene therapy, increasing the content of the SR Ca ATPase has markedly improved the function of old rat hearts. The age-related changes in diastolic function can also be modified and improved by exercise training. In old rats trained on treadmill for 1 to 2 months improved SR calcium uptake and cardiac relaxation to that seen in young sedentary rats. Similarly, changes in early filling, which is dependent on active relaxation, are also seen in humans after 6 months of endurance training. In addition, recent data suggest that humans who put themselves on a diet comparable to the caloric restriction diets have better diastolic function than age-matched controls, corroborating experiments in experimental animals. While this approach may not be highly practical, only 5 years of caloric restriction is needed to produce the change.

Systolic Function

In healthy humans, no age-related changes in measurable, overall LV contractility, assessed by the ejection fraction, fractional shortening, or mean velocity of circumferential fiber shortening, have been reported in those studies in which it has been measured. Wall motion abnormalities should not be considered normal, even in the very elderly. In CHS, the prevalence of unexpected wall motion abnormalities, in the absence of history and symptoms of coronary heart disease, was 0.4% in women and 0.5% in men.

The contraction and relaxation of the older left ventricle are not uniform. In older people, segments of the heart have started to relax while others are still contracting. As LV pressure must be low before filling can start, this prolonged contraction shortens the time available for filling to occur.

Age-related alterations in several Doppler measures of aortic outflow have been demonstrated. Aortic peak flow velocity, time–velocity integral, and acceleration are reduced with advancing age. While these hemodynamic factors relate to LV systolic performance, these are also substantially affected by afterload, which is known to increase with aging.

A recent report suggests that the inotropic (contractility) as well as lusitropic (diastolic function) responses to dobutamine decrease.

Possible Implications of the Age-Related Changes in Resting Cardiovascular Function

As noted in the introduction, aging decreases one's ability to tolerate challenges to homeostasis. This is most evident in the cardiovascular system. For example, the mortality and probability of developing heart failure after a myocardial infarction increase dramatically with age. While, clearly the pathogenesis of atherosclerosis and the myocardial infarction itself is not normal aging, the response to the systemic challenges produced by the infarction may well be impaired because of the aging process. Consistent with this, there is an age-related increase in mortality after experimental infarction in mice and rats. We suggest that homeostenosis, the depletion of reserves, may be the cost of invoking compensatory mechanisms just to maintain homeostasis.

Similarly, acute hypertension is poorly tolerated in the old. Old (18 months) and adult (9 months) rats had afterload increased by constriction of the aorta. Immediate early response gene signals were attenuated in the old rats. Decreased skeletal actin expression after pressure overload was present, and skeletal actin expression precedes cardiac actin expression in most models of hypertrophy. Atrial natriuretic peptide stimulates excretion of water and sodium by the kidney. Atrial natriuretic peptide (ANP) is only expressed by the atria in normal young hearts, but ANP is a marker of stress and compensation when seen in the ventricles. In the old rat, ANP is elevated in the ventricles at baseline and could not be further stimulated after additional stress. This suggested that the hypertrophy response was already invoked as part of aging in the older rats and was therefore not available to respond to the acute stress.

While the normal heart is unlikely to ever be exposed to ischemia, ischemic preconditioning is adaptation of the young heart that is not present in the old heart. Young hearts, if repeatedly exposed to brief episodes of ischemia, tolerate longer episodes well with less resultant damage, by possibly increasing levels of heat-shock proteins, opening ATP-gated potassium channels, stimulating the TNF-alpha cascade, and activating antioxidant enzymes. Old hearts cannot make this adaptation, perhaps contributing to the increased mortality after myocardial infarct in the old, but exercise training, caloric restriction, and certain growth factors mitigate it.

The responsiveness is decreased to some cardioactive drugs, including atropine, dobutamine, and other beta-adrenergic active agents. These agents may require higher doses to reach a desired effect in the old. Congestive heart failure becomes increasingly common, reaching a prevalence of more than 10% and being the most common reason for hospitalization of Medicare beneficiaries. The syndrome of heart failure with normal ejection fraction, the most common form among older persons, is likely facilitated by the above and below discussed age-related changes in diastolic function and myocardial composition additive to the arterial and myocardial changes caused by hypertension and other diseases.

Age-related changes in vessels and the heart do not by themselves produce disease, but, because of the changes in compliance, systolic hypertension is incredibly common. Finally compensation for these changes makes the old CVS more prone to decompensation in response to other insults.

Effect of Age on the Cardiovascular Response During Exercise

If aging affects cardiovascular performance even at rest or with moderate stress, such as dobutamine infusion, one would expect this to be magnified and become even more apparent during exercise. This is indeed the case. Exercise capacity can be quantified objectively by measurement of maximal oxygen consumption (Vo_{2max}) during exercise. It is solidly established that normal aging is inescapably accompanied by a reduction in Vo_{2max}. While the age at which this decline begins is unclear, it is probably variable and begins early in adult life. The reduction in Vo_{2max} is independent of gender and changes in body size. The magnitude of the decline is approximately 3% to 8% per decade and can be modified but not completely halted or reversed by exercise training.

A study from the Baltimore Longitudinal Study on Aging (BLSA) in 1988 showed results that the authors interpreted as showing a decline at the lowest part of this range (3%) and attributed the majority of this change to loss of muscle mass. In addition, an oft-cited study

in 1984 using subjects from the BLSA and subsequent reviews and commentaries have implied that these cross-sectional estimates for the age-related decline in Vo_{2max} were probably substantial overestimates of the true longitudinal decline and that declines in multiple measures of exercise cardiac function, including cardiac output, were relatively modest or were even preserved with aging. However, such conclusions were at substantial variance with all other studies performed before and since as shown in Table 74-4, and this difference was attributed to rigorous screening. However, a subsequent report from the BLSA in 2005, which examined a large number of subjects, both sedentary and well condition by training, during a 7.9-year period of follow-up showed that, in actuality, the decline in exercise capacity (Vo_{2max}) among older persons was actually more accelerated and greater in magnitude than all previous estimates. In addition, another subsequent report from the BLSA in 1995 showed that, in contrast to the original study in 1984, both men and women do, indeed, have substantial age-related declines in exercise cardiac output, accompanying and contributing to a 40% decline in Vo_{2max}. This is in accord with all other reports from other studies. Thus, there is now uniform agreement that aging, even in the absence of any identifiable disease, is associated with substantial declines in overall cardiovascular performance and reserve capacity, including maximal cardiac output.

By the Fick principle for oxygen, only a limited number of factors could be responsible for a decline in Vo_{2max}. The following equations are pertinent to this discussion:

$$VO_2 = \text{cardiac output} \times \text{arteriovenous oxygen difference}$$
$$\text{Cardiac output} = \text{stroke volume} \times \text{heart rate}$$
$$\text{Stroke volume} = \text{end-diastolic volume} - \text{end-systolic volume}$$

The arteriovenous oxygen difference (AVO) is determined by a number of noncardiac factors, including peripheral vascular and skeletal muscle mass and metabolic function. Thus, if Vo_{2max} declines with aging, there must be a decline in peak cardiac output or AVO or both during exercise.

Measurement of cardiac output in healthy human subjects during exercise is challenging methodologically. Investigators have used a variety of techniques, including direct Fick (probably the most reliable), dye dilution, equilibrium-gated radionuclide angiography, and gas rebreathing (Table 74-4). Each of these methods uses a number of variables to derive the cardiac output measurement. Direct measurement of AVO by oximetry, however, is quite accurate and reliable. Most investigators who have measured AVO during maximal exercise have documented no difference or increased AVO in elderly compared with young subjects. By simple algebra, this suggests that the age-related decline in Vo_{2max} must be because of reduced cardiac output. This has, indeed, been the finding reported by virtually all investigators.

The largest modern published study that used invasive techniques in order to directly measure all components of the Fick equation in healthy human subjects over a substantial age range was reported by Higginbotham et al. The subjects had a very low probability of coronary disease as they were all aged ≤ 50 years, were asymptomatic volunteers, and had normal electrocardiograms and radionuclide angiograms during exercise. Yet even over the short age range observed by Higginbotham et al., maximal cardiac output, measured by the Fick technique, declined significantly. These healthy subjects had the expected age-related decline in Vo_{2max} and heart rate. Stroke volume was calculated by dividing cardiac output by heart rate. Cardiac

TABLE 74-4

Effect of Age on Cardiovascular Function During Maximal Exercise*

INVESTIGATOR	n	GENDER	AGE RANGE (yr)	EXERCISE TEST	METHOD BP CO	Vo2 (mL/min)	Vo2 (mL/kg/min/)	CHANGE PER DECADE						
								HR (b/min)	CO (L/min)	CI (L/min/m²)	SV (mL)	AVO (mL/L)	SVR (U)	SBP/DB (mm Hg)
Granath (1964)	39	M	16–83	CY, supine	IA	−124	—	−5.6	−1.12	—	−3.5	+0.12	—	—
	15	M		CY, sitting	F	−117		−5.0	−1.12		−4.6	+1.79	—	—
					IA									
					F									
Hossack (1982)	98 (12)*	M	20–73	TR	F	−290	−4.6	−10.7	−1.35	−0.82	−2.2	+1.79	—	+8.0/+1.3
	104 (11)	F	20–70	—	F	−191	−4.4	−6.0	−0.53	−0.6	−0.9	—	—	—
Higgenbotham (1986)	24	M	20–50	CY, sitting	F		−3.1	−11.2	−1.32	−0.9	—	+0.07	—	—
Kitzman (1989)	82	M + F	20–72	CY, sitting	IA F	−200	—	−10.0	−1.50	−0.75	−5.0	+0.02	+1.41	+7.5/+1.2
Julius (1967)	54	M + F	18–69	CY, sitting	IA DD	−235	—	−9.0	−1.26	−0.72	−2.9	−0.55	+1.34	+9.0/+1.2
Conway (1971)	27	M + F	20–65	CY, sitting	IA DD	−125	—	−7.3	−0.97	—	−2.0	−0.23	+1.44	+16.0/+6.0
Rodeheffer (1984)	61	M + F	25–79	CY, sitting	EGNA	—	—	−0.5	−0.5	−0.3	+3.4	—	+0.4	+3.3/+2.0
Miyamura (1973)	147	M	17–54	CY	R	−272	−3.8	−2.4	−1.40	—	−6.5	−4.64	—	—
Ogawa (1992)	27	M	23–68	TR	R	−240	−3.6	−4.6	−1.0	—	−2.8	−0.36	—	—
	28	F	20–72	TR	R	−200	−3.0	−4.0	−0.7	—	−1.2	−0.31	—	—
Fleg (1995)	121	M	22–85	TR	EGNA	—	—	−9.0	—	−0.36	+2.0	—	0.3	+1.2/+3.0
	79	F	22–86	TR	EGNA	—	—	−5.0	—	−0.52	−1.7	—	+0.9	—
Beere (1999)	23	M	21–74	CY	IA F	−142	−2.6	−8.7	0.77	—	+0.9	−0.35	+0.63	+2.6/1.2

AVO, arteriovenous oxygen difference; CY, cycle; TR, treadmill; Vo2, oxygen uptake; n, number of subjects with invasive measurements.

*For other abbreviations, see Table 77-3.

Adapted/updated from Kitzman DW. Aging in the heart. In: Developments in Cardiology, GI Freeman, ed. Orland, W.B. Saunders 1994, pp 3–16.

output was measured by a gold standard technique, using the blood samples from systemic and pulmonary arteries along with measured Vo_2, and was confirmed by another high-fidelity technique, thermodilution by indwelling pulmonary catheter. They found that stroke volume, ejection fraction, and end-diastolic volume were unchanged with aging or showed a slight downward trend. Thus, the well-established age-related decline in maximal heart rate was translated into reduced maximal cardiac output, since stroke volume was unchanged. Similar results have been obtained by others in groups of older human subjects, both men and women, and in beagles. Furthermore, an invasive study confirmed those results in a group of older (age 66 years) versus younger (age 28 years) healthy subjects, as shown in Figure 74-1. These data indicated that both cardiac output and systemic AVO were reduced in older versus young healthy subjects and contributed to their 28% age-related reduction in Vo_{2max}.

Thus, the reduced Vo_{2max} and exercise capacity seen with aging are caused predominantly by reduced exercise cardiac output. That the heart should be responsible for the age-related exercise limitation is not surprising, since it has been observed that the skeletal muscles have a greater capacity for work than can be supported by the cardiac output. The primary mechanism of the age-related decline in exercise cardiac output is primarily the age-related reduction in maximal heart rate. Reduced maximal exercise heart rate appears to be a universal observation and to meet the criteria for a basic biological aging phenomenon. Its mechanism is unclear but may be related, in part, to an age-related decline in beta-adrenergic sensitivity.

Although reduced maximal heart rate is the primary mechanism for reduced maximal exercise cardiac output and oxygen consumption in elderly subjects, younger subjects in whom exercise heart rate is limited, either by congenital complete heart block or by beta-adrenergic blockade, stroke volume is increased and partially compensates for the reduced heart rate via the Frank-Starling response (increased end-diastolic volume). The effect of aging on end-diastolic volume and the Frank-Starling mechanism during exercise is not clear, since repeated studies from one group using invasive techniques described above show no change with aging and studies from another group suggest end-diastolic volume at peak exercise increases with aging and another showed no change. However, regarding peak exercise stroke volume, most studies show that older subjects have shown either no change or a modest decline in stroke volumes at maximal exercise with aging compared to younger subjects, including in women in the BLSA. An age related decline in Frank-Starling reserve would be consistent with observations suggesting increased LV diastolic stiffness owing to aging.

A lower stroke volume in the elderly could be because of higher end-systolic volume as well as lower end-diastolic volume. LV end-systolic volume was higher and ejection fraction was lower at peak exercise in older than in younger subjects in most studies in which these were measured. Thus, systolic LV function reserve is reduced with aging as well. Reduced stroke volume could also result partially from increased afterload, since systolic blood pressure, aortic impedance, and systemic vascular resistance are higher during exercise in old than in young healthy subjects. When afterload is taken into account, maximal stroke work is fairly similar in young and old subjects.

In evaluating elderly patients for coronary heart disease, particularly with radionuclide angiography, it should be recognized that in healthy elderly the LV ejection fraction does not increase as much from rest to peak exercise as it does in young healthy subjects. In fact, a flat response in elderly men and a mild decline in elderly women

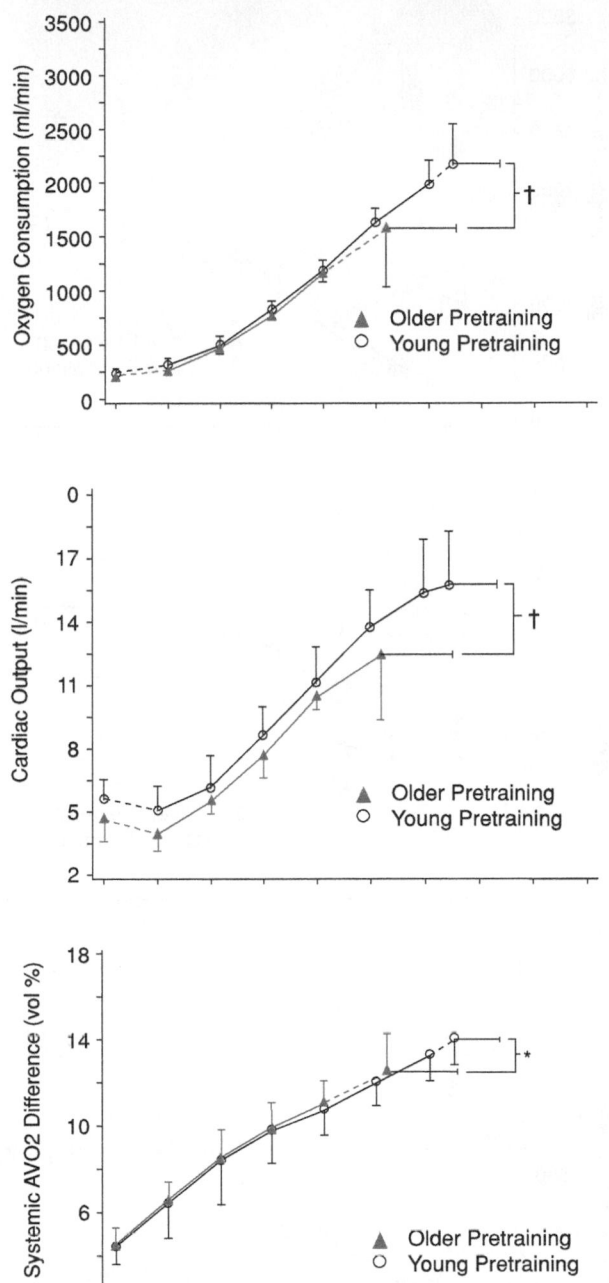

FIGURE 74-1. Oxygen consumption by expired gas analysis, cardiac output by the direct Fick technique, and systemic arteriovenous oxygen difference by direct oximetry at supine rest (SR), upright rest (UR), and during maximal exercise in younger and older healthy volunteers. Note that there are substantial and significant reductions in older compared to younger subjects in all measures, including maximal cardiac output †p<0.01 *p<0.05. (Modified from Beere PA, Russell SD, Morey MC, et al. Circulation. 1999;100;1085–1094.)

should be considered normal. However, it is important to note that development of wall motion abnormalities would not be considered normal, even in the presence of a mild nonspecific decline in ejection fraction.

There has been less information regarding peripheral cardiovascular function with aging, including systemic arterial function, which is required to efficiently deliver oxygenated blood to working muscle,

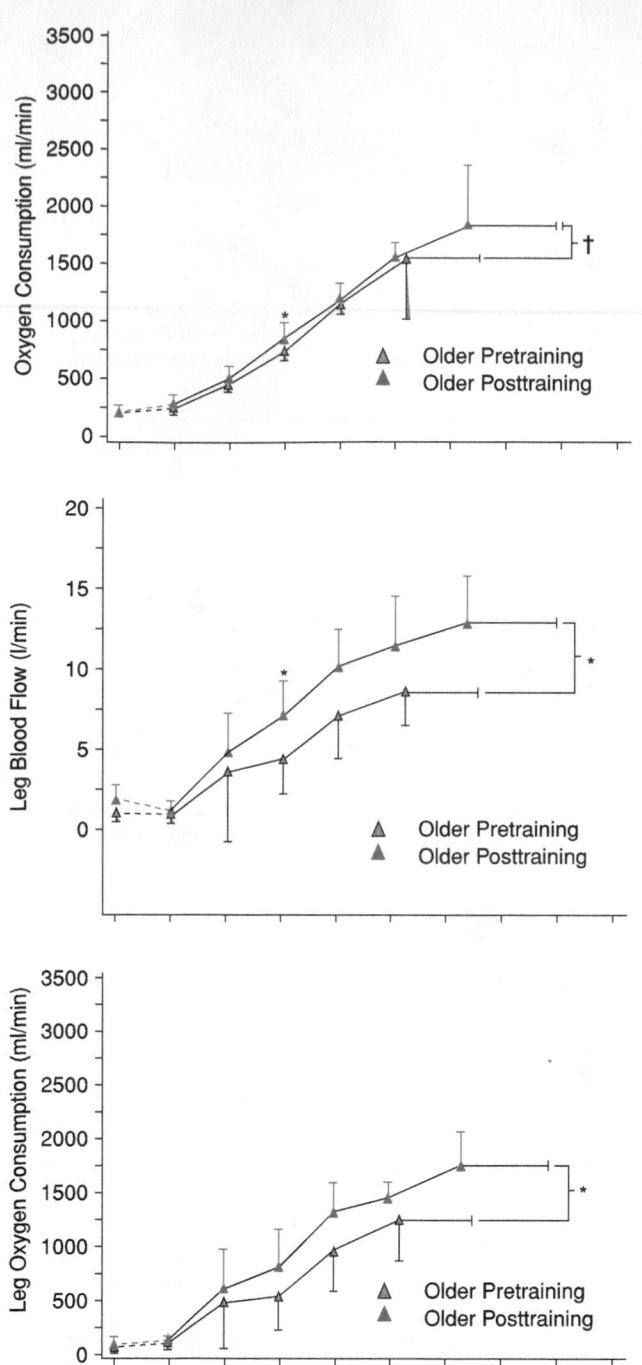

output, older men have reduced exercise leg blood flow. The study also repeated the detailed measurements of central and peripheral cardiovascular functions following exercise training. Their results confirmed the findings of a number of previous investigators that exercise training can improve Vo2max by 15% or more and thereby "reverse" some of the age-related decline in physical work capacity. Furthermore, they found that the primary mechanism of improvement in exercise capacity following training in older subjects was a large improvement in leg arterial blood flow.

SUMMARY

Normal aging is accompanied by substantial alterations in anatomy and physiology of the heart and vasculature. There are declines in most aspects of cardiovascular function, including both cardiac output and blood flow distribution, and these create significantly reduced reserve capacity, which becomes more apparent during exercise and stress.

The age-related alterations in the anatomy and physiology of the heart and vasculature likely have varying degrees of significance. Some may not have functional significance and are essentially epiphenomena of aging. Others, such as aortic sclerosis, ventricular septal thickening, and attenuated cardiac function response during exercise, may simulate disease. Some findings, which are associated with age and are prevalent in elderly hearts, such as senile amyloid and calcified mitral annulus, are likely part of poorly understood disease processes rather than owing to aging. With currently available information, it is not always possible to distinguish the effects of aging from the effects of disease, particularly in very elderly hearts. However, it is reasonable to propose that many of the age-related changes discussed may lower the threshold for clinical disease and, thus, predispose to a variety of cardiovascular disorders in the elderly, including congestive heart failure, hypertensive hypertrophic cardiomyopathy, valvular stenosis and regurgitation, systolic hypertension, supraventricular arrhythmias, and conduction disturbances. Awareness of these age-related changes, as well as the principles of aging biology in general, will help investigators avoid potential errors in research study design or interpretation and help clinicians tailor intelligently treatments to the older patient.

Because these age-related declines in cardiovascular and exercise performance are modifiable and have been shown to be partially preventable and reversible with exercise training, maintaining regularly scheduled physical activity and conditioning is a potentially important strategy to mitigate the potential adverse effects of aging on cardiovascular function.

FIGURE 74-2. Leg blood flow measured by indwelling catheter, and leg oxygen consumption by expired gas analysis during supine rest (SR), upright rest (UR), and during exercise in older healthy volunteers before and after aerobic exercise training. After exercise training, there is a 28% improvement in maximal body oxygen consumption, and this is accompanied by a 50% improvement in leg arterial blood flow and leg oxygen consumption during exercise $^\dagger p<0.01$. $^*p<0.05$ *(Modified from Beere PA, Russell SD, Morey MC, et al. Circulation. 1999;100;1085–1094.)*

FURTHER READING

Aviv H, et al. Age dependent aneuploidy and telomere length of the human vascular endothelium. *Atherosclerosis.* 2001;159(2):281–287.

Avolio AP, et al. Effects of aging on changing arterial compliance and left ventricular load in a northern Chinese urban community. *Circulation.* 1983;68(1):50–58.

Avolio AP, Clyde KM, Beard TC, et al. Improved arterial distensibility in normotensive subjects on a low salt diet. *Arteriosclerosis.* 1986;6:166–169.

Bharati S, Lev M. The pathologic changes in the conduction system beyond the age of ninety. *Am Heart J.* 1992;124(2):487–496.

Bonow RO, Vitale DF, Bacharach SL, Maron BJ, Green MV. Effects of aging on asynchronous left ventricular regional function and global ventricular filling in normal human subjects. *J Am Coll Cardiol.* 1988;11:50–58.

Cooper LT, Cooke JP, Dzau VJ. The vasculopathy of aging. *J Gerontol Biol Sci.* 1994;49:B191–B196.

and working muscle itself. The study by Beere et al. extended prior work by using a pediatric thermodilution pulmonary artery catheter inserted into the femoral vein, in order to acquire the best available measures of leg blood flow, oxygen consumption, and AVO. Their findings indicated that, in addition to reduced peak exercise cardiac

Craft N, Schwartz JB. Effects of age on intrinsic heart rate, heart rate variability, and AV conduction in healthy humans. *Am J Physiol.* 1995;268:H1441–H1445.

Davidson WR Jr, Fee EC. Influence of aging on pulmonary hemodynamics in a population free of coronary artery disease. *Am J Cardiol.* 1990;65:1454–1458.

Davis KM, Fish LC, Minaker KL, Elahi D. Atrial natriuretic peptide levels in the elderly: differentiating normal aging changes from disease. *J Gerontol A Biol Sci Med Sci.* 1996;51:M95–M101.

DeSouza CA, et al. Regular aerobic exercise prevents and restores age-related declines in endothelium-dependent vasodilation in healthy men. *Circulation.* 2000;102(12):1351–1357.

Ford GA. Ageing and the baroreceptor. *Age Ageing.* 1999;28:337–338.

Jones MR, Ravid K. Vascular smooth muscle polyploidization as a biomarker for aging and its impact on differential gene expression. *J Biol Chem.* 2004;279(7):5306–5313.

Katzel LI, Sorkin JD, Fleg JL. A comparison of longitudinal changes in aerobic fitness in older endurance athletes and sedentary men. *J Am Geriatr Soc.* 2001;49:1657–1664.

Kitzman DW. Normal age-related changes in the heart: relevance to echocardiography in the elderly. *Am J Geriatr Cardiol.* 2000;9:311–320.

Kitzman DW, Edwards WD. Mini-review: age-related changes in the anatomy of the normal human heart. *J Gerontol.* 1990;45:M33–M39.

Lakatta EG. Cardiovascular system. In: Masoro EJ, ed. *Aging: Handbook of Physiology.* New York, New York: American Physiological Society; 1995.

Lakatta EG, Sollott SJ. Perspectives on mammalian cardiovascular aging: humans to molecules. *Comp Biochem Physiol.* 2002;132:699–721.

Lee TM, Su SF, Chou TF, Lee YT, Tsai CH. Loss of preconditioning by attenuated activation of myocardial ATP-sensitive potassium channels in elderly patients undergoing coronary angioplasty. *Circulation.* 2002;105:334–340.

Levy WC, Cerqueira MD, Abrass IB, Schwartz RS, Stratton JR. Endurance exercise training augments diastolic filling at rest and during exercise in healthy young and older men. *Circulation.* 1993;88:116–126.

Li Z, Cheng H, Lederer WJ, Froehlich J, Lakatta EG. Enhanced proliferation and migration and altered cytoskeletal proteins in early passage smooth muscle cells from young and old rat aortic explants. *Exp Mol Pathol.* 1997;64(1):1–11.

Liu L, Azhar G, Gao W, Zhang X, Wei J. Bcl-2 and Bax expression in adult rat hearts after coronary occlusion: age-associated differences. *Am J Physiol.* 1998;275:R315–R322.

Longobardi G, Abete P, Ferrara N, et al. "Warm-up" phenomenon in adult and elderly patients with coronary artery disease: further evidence of the loss of "ischemic preconditioning" in the aging heart. *J Gerontol A Biol Sci Med Sci.* 2000;55:M124–M129.

Matsushita H, et al. eNOS activity is reduced in senescent human endothelial cells: preservation by hTERT immortalization. *Circ Res.* 2001;89(9):793–798.

Nichols WW. Clinical measurement of arterial stiffness obtained from noninvasive pressure waveforms. *Am J Hypertens.* 2005;18(1 Pt 2):3S–10S.

Nichols WW, O'Rourke MF. *McDonald's Blood Flow in Arteries.* 4th ed. New York, New York: Oxford University Press; 1998.

Nitahara JA, Cheng W, Liu Y, et al. Intracellular calcium, DNAase activity and myocyte apoptosis in aging Fischer 344 Rats. *J Mol Cell Cardiol.* 1998;30:519–535.

Novelli M, et al. Effects of life-long exercise on circulating free fatty acids and muscle triglyceride content in ageing rats. *Exp Gerontol.* 2004;39(9):1333–1340.

Olivetti G, Melissari M, Capasso JM, Anversa P. Cardiomyopathy of the aging human heart, myocyte loss and reactive cellular hypertrophy. *Circ Res.* 1991;68:1560–1568.

Olsen H, Vernersson E, Lanne T. Cardiovascular response to acute hypovolemia in relation to age. Implications for orthostasis and hemorrhage. *Am J Physiol Heart Circ Physiol.* 2000;278:H222–H226.

Rivard A, Fabre J-E, Silver M, et al. Age-dependent impairment of angiogenesis. *Circulation.* 1999;99:111–120.

Spagnoli LG, et al., Aging and atherosclerosis in the rabbit. 1. Distribution, prevalence and morphology of atherosclerotic lesions. *Atherosclerosis.* 1991;89(1):11–24.

Tanaka H, Monahan KD, Seals DR. Age-predicted maximal heart rate revisited. *J Am Coll Cardiol.* 2001;37:153–156.

Vaitkevicius PV, Fleg JL, Engel JH, et al. *Circulation.* 1993;88:1456–1462.

Vaitkevicius PV, et al. A cross-link breaker has sustained effects on arterial and ventricular properties in older rhesus monkeys. *Proc Natl Acad Sci USA.* 2001;98(3):1171–1175.

vanderLoo B, et al. Enhanced peroxynitrite formation is associated with vascular aging. *J Exp Med.* 2000;192(12):1731–1744.

Wang M, et al. Aging increases aortic MMP-2 activity and angiotensin II in nonhuman primates. *Hypertension.* 2003;41:1308–1316.

White N. The relationship of the degree of coronary atherosclerosis with age in men. *Circulation.* 1950;1:645.

Aging and Atherosclerosis

Susan Cheng ■ *Susan M. Bell* ■ *Susan J. Zieman*

Atherosclerosis confers an illness burden on the general population larger than that associated with any other disease process. With advancing age, the incidence and prevalence of coronary, cerebral, and peripheral arterial disease (PAD) and aneurysmal formation are higher and their severity is more pronounced. Thus, cardiovascular disease (CVD) outcomes are worse in older compared to younger adults. Although age is the most powerful independent risk factor for CVD, the mechanisms by which aging predisposes to atherogenesis are only now becoming elucidated, as are specific strategies to optimally prevent and treat atherosclerotic disease in older adults.

Research to date, spanning from basic science to epidemiology, suggests that aging potentiates atherosclerosis through a combination of factors (Figure 75-1). First, specific biological changes associated with aging increase vulnerability to atherosclerosis. Second, increasing age lengthens the time of exposure to known CV risk factors and modifies their effects. Finally, older individuals have increased comorbidities, which may contribute to or exacerbate the severity of atherosclerosis, particularly conditions that create or maintain a proinflammatory biologic milieu.

The clinical manifestations of atherosclerotic disease are more varied and severe in older compared to younger adults. Multiple etiologic factors have variable effects on the aging vasculature over a lifetime (Figure 75-2). Thus, vascular aging plays a primary and prominent role in predisposing older individuals to atherogenesis. This chapter highlights how vascular aging, in addition to both traditional and nontraditional risk factors, can enhance and accelerate the development of atherosclerosis in older adults.

VASCULAR AGING

It is a common misconception that vascular aging is synonymous with the development of atherosclerosis. Although the majority of individuals older than 60 years have clinically significant (>75%) coronary stenoses on autopsy, at least 25% of this age group will have only mild or no significant coronary plaque burden. Yet, age-associated vascular changes, and the cellular and molecular factors that underlie their development, do increase the vulnerability of older arteries to atherogenesis (Table 75-1).

The basic structure of the arterial blood vessel consists of three layers, each separated by a distinct elastic membrane. The intima is the innermost layer and consists of a monolayer of endothelial cells resting on a basement membrane made up of collagen and other extracellular matrix (ECM) molecules. The media consists primarily of smooth muscle cells (SMCs) on the background of an elastin-rich skeleton of ECM. Collagen, elastin, glycoproteins, and proteoglycans constitute the ECM. The outermost layer, the adventitia, contains a loose array of collagen fibrils as well as the vasa vasorum (blood vessels supplying the vasculature itself), nerve endings, fibroblasts, and mast cells.

Arterial structure changes with increasing age, but not in ways that necessitate atherogenesis. Morphologic changes associated with aging can include increased vessel diameter, intima-media thickening, SMC and collagen hypertrophy, fibrosis, and arterial wall calcification. In the absence of other predisposing factors, these progressive changes are age dependent but occur at varying rates in different individuals. Similar arterial alterations are seen prematurely in transplanted hearts and in a variety of vasculidities.

True atherosclerosis, by definition, requires the presence of an atheroma covered by a thin fibrous cap. An atheroma is a focal collection in the intima of foam cells (macrophages that have engulfed lipoproteins), proliferative SMCs (which have migrated from the media), and ECM. Postmortem studies of young Korean War soldier causalities revealed that the initial stages of atheroma formation can occur early in life.

Three major intertwining themes highlight how the biology of vascular aging predisposes to atherosclerosis (see Figure 75-1). First, *exposure* to various physical and metabolic stresses over time can alter normal pathways and processes. Second, progressive *accumulation* of metabolic byproducts can adversely affect arterial structure

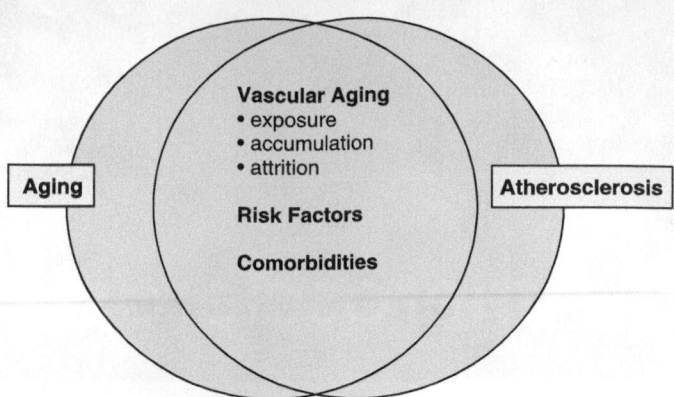

FIGURE 75-1. Schematic view of the intersection and overlap between aging and atherosclerosis.

and function. Finally, time-dependent *attrition* of the basic arterial constituents and adaptive and reparative mechanisms of the arteries can lead to their dysfunction and, in turn, promote atherogenesis. This section details each of these themes.

Exposure

Although biologic and chronologic ages are not necessarily equivalent, especially pertaining to vascular biology, the vector of time is inherent to the aging process (Figure 75-2). As such, chronic exposure to specific stresses over time contributes significantly to age-related pathology. These stresses include repeated exposure to both pulsatile and sheer forces on a mechanical level and ongoing oxidative stress at the molecular level. Stress-induced vascular changes ensue and, in some individuals, accelerate atherosclerosis.

Sheer stress over time provokes vascular injury, particularly at vessel bifurcations and curves, where atheromas tend to form. Endothelial cells subjected to chronic sheer stress can physically deform and display altered intracellular activity. Specifically, laminar sheer stress upregulates endothelial nitric oxide synthase (eNOS), the enzyme that produces nitric oxide (NO). Although sheer stress increases with age, overall eNOS activity is lower in aged compared to younger rats and contributes to impaired endothelium-dependent vasorelaxation. Cytokine-stimulated inducible-NOS activity, which raises NO levels, may create more negative feedback effect on eNOS than on inducible NOS. Age-related endothelial dysfunction is characterized by the decreased ability of smaller arteries to dilate in response

to increased blood flow. Endothelial dysfunction in healthy older adults improves with exogenous nitrate administration, suggesting impairment, in part, of endogenous NO production. Endothelial cells play a key role in nearly every step of the atherosclerosis process, including plaque formation, platelet adhesion and aggregation, cellular migration, and proliferation. Thus, their dysfunction plays a key role in atherosclerosis. In a vicious cycle, atherosclerosis further impairs endothelial cell function (Figure 75-3).

Similar to shear stress, chronic biomechanical stress can also affect endothelial function by activating mechanoreceptors, thereby converting physical stimuli to biochemical signals. In vitro, endothelial cells exposed to repeated pulsatile stress have diminished eNOS expression and Akt and NO signaling. Pulsatile stretch also stimulates vascular SMC hypertrophy and proliferation. Such exposed SMCs synthesize ECM components in a disorganized fashion. Mechanical stretch also activates matrix metalloproteinases (MMPs), some of which are proliferative while others are destructive. Imbalanced activation of MMP subtypes creates adverse vascular remodeling, including fibrosis, which increases arterial stiffness and decreases elasticity, further exacerbating sheer and pulsatile stresses (Figure 75-3).

At the molecular level, augmented oxidative stress, measured by reactive oxidant species (ROS), is a constituent of both vascular aging and atherogenesis. Since its conception in 1950s, the free radical theory of aging has contended that metabolic production of oxidants, especially ROS, results in a wide array of adverse reactions involving nucleic acids, proteins, and lipids. Cumulative exposure to toxic oxidative effects leads to progressive cellular and tissue dysfunction and eventual disease and death. ROS are implicated in every step of atherogenesis, and this relationship is magnified in older vessels owing to ROS augmentation (Figure 75-4). Lipid oxidation is also accelerated by ROS and, in turn, stimulates many atherogenic steps including inflammatory cell activation, SMC, monocyte and macrophage growth factor release, reduction of eNOS-regulated platelet activity, metalloproteinase formation, cytokine release, and renin–angiotensin activation. Accordingly, oxidized low-density lipoprotein (LDL) facilitates vulnerable plaque rupture. Conversely, oxidized LDL receptor blockade inhibits atherogenesis.

Accumulation

With aging, the time vector permits accumulation of metabolic byproducts in the vascular wall, which creates adverse structural

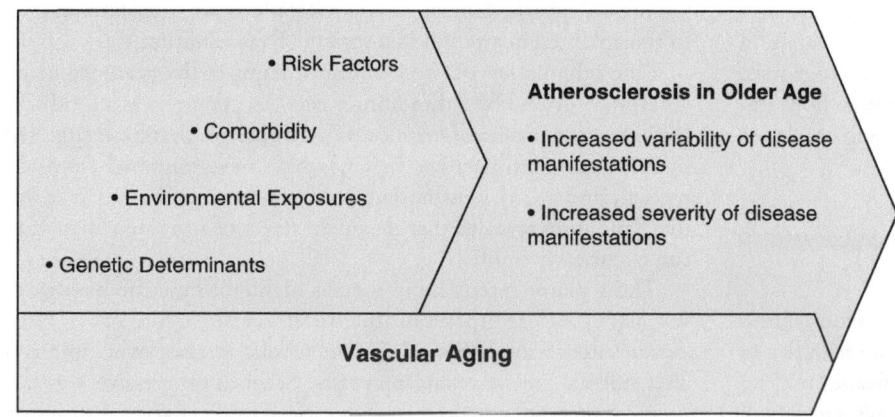

FIGURE 75-2. Contributors to the development of atherosclerosis interact with vascular aging to increase the variability and severity of disease manifestation in older age.

TABLE 75-1

Common Underlying Pathologies of Vascular Aging and Atherosclerosis

LAYER	MOLECULAR	CELLULAR	STRUCTURAL	DYNAMIC
Endothelium	• ↑ROS • NOS uncoupling • ↓Total and free NO • ↑Adhesion molecule expression	• ↓Angiogenesis • Endothelial cell senescence • Progenitor cell senescence	• ↑Permeability	• ↓Vasoreactivity • ↑Susceptibility to sheer stress
Intima	• ↑ROS • ↑MMP levels and activity • ↑Adhesion molecule expression • ↑Nitrite and nitrate • ↑ACE activity • ↑AT-II activity • ↑TGF-β	• ↑SMC proliferation • SMC senescence	• ↑Thickness (from SMC proliferation and matrix deposition) • ↑Luminal diameter • Basement membrane permeability	• ↑Susceptibility to mechanical stress
Media	• ↑ Interleukins • ↑Advanced glycation end products • ↑Collagen • ↓Elastin (calcification and fragmentation) • ↑Fibronectin • ↑Glycosaminoglycans	• ↑SMC proliferation and migration • SMC hypertrophy • SMC senescence • Fibroblast senescence (resistance to apoptosis)	• ↑Thickness • ↑Luminal diameter • Collagen cross-linking • Elastin breakage • ↑Collagen fibrils • Fibrosis	• ↑Stiffness • ↓Elasticity and compliance

ROS, reactive oxygen species; NOS, nitric oxide synthase; NO, nitric oxide; MMP, matrix metalloproteinases; ACE, angiotensin converting enzyme; AT-II, angiotensin II; TGF-β, transcription growth factor beta; SMC, smooth muscle cell.

and metabolic sequelae. The prototypical example is accumulation of oxidized lipids in the bloodstream and their subsequent incorporation into atheromas. With time, the arterial wall also accrues increased amounts of normal and dysfunctional collagen, as well as broken and frayed elastin fibrils caused by elastase enzyme upregulation. Additionally, recurrent inflammatory processes result in vascular fibrosis. These alterations decrease arterial compliance to

pulsatile flow, thicken the intima, and increase vascular permeability. Disruption in membrane permeability facilitates SMC proliferation and migration from the media to the intima as well as transit of immune and inflammatory cells that stimulate atherogenesis.

Progressive accumulation of advanced glycation end products (AGEs) also contribute significantly to CV structural and functional pathology over time. AGEs result from irreversible nonenzymatically formed bonds between glycated proteins. Time and high glucose concentration drive this reaction forward such in aging and diabetes. Long-lived proteins (collagen) are most susceptible to glycation over time and, once cross-linked, are less susceptible to routine hydrolysis and thus accumulate.

Structurally, AGE cross-linked arterial collagen is less compliant and contributes to age-associated central vascular stiffness. Similarly, AGE cross-linked myocardial collagen fibrils in the heart result in ventricular stiffness. In addition to their vascular structural impact, AGEs quench NO, stimulate ROS formation, facilitate inflammatory molecule and cell recruitment, and promote fibrosis. These alterations predispose the arterial wall to atherosclerosis. Receptors for AGE (RAGE) are located on endothelial cells, SMC,

↑SMC hypertrophy
↑SMC proliferation
↑MMP activation

ECM Changes
↑collagen→ ↑vascular stiffness
↓elastin → ↓vascular elasticity

↑Sheer Stress
↑Pulsatile Stress

• Endothelial injury
• Endothelial dysfunction

Accelerated Atherosclerosis

FIGURE 75-3. Chronic exposure of the arterial wall to sheer and pulsatile stresses leads to both vascular aging and accelerated atherosclerosis.

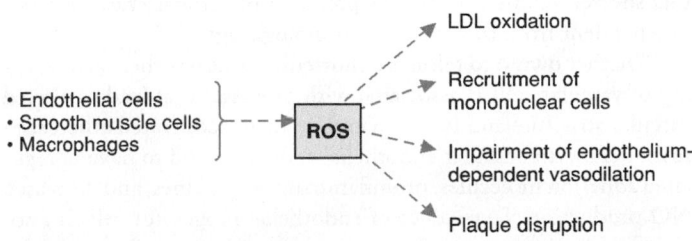

FIGURE 75-4. Reactive oxygen species are involved in almost every step of atherosclerosis.

macrophages, and blood cells. AGE–RAGE attachment modulates a cascade of molecular events, resulting in vascular inflammation, fibrosis, vascular permeability, and altered NO signaling. Thus, time- and age-dependent accrual of AGEs, especially in diabetics, likely contributes significantly to age-associated increased endothelial dysfunction, vascular wall thickening, arterial stiffening, inflammation and fibrosis, restenosis, and atherogenesis. Clinical manifestations include isolated systolic hypertension (ISH), elevated pulse pressure (PP), left ventricular hypertrophy, delayed early diastolic relaxation, and atherosclerotic disease. LDL apoproteins are also a target of AGE, resulting in decreased LDL receptor uptake, more LDL oxidation, and increased susceptibility to macrophage engulfment, all leading to the formation of foam cells and atherosclerotic plaque.

Attrition

The third age-related component predisposing to atherosclerosis is the reduced ability of reparative or compensatory biologic processes to appropriately adapt to the age-associated structural, dynamic, and molecular alterations. One hallmark of aging is cellular aging, also known as cellular senescence. Although the precise definition of cellular senescence is debated, it generally describes the irreversible arrest of the replicative cycle of a cell such that it no longer divides. The number of cell divisions in an organism is related to the organism's expected longevity. In addition to exhibiting a flattened and enlarged morphology, senescent cells express a specific set of genes, including negative regulators of the cell cycle such as p53 and p16. Cells with shorter life spans have been cultured from individuals with premature aging syndromes such as Werner syndrome and Hutchinson–Gilford progeria syndrome, both of which are characterized by very early-onset atherosclerosis. Recent studies suggest that cellular aging also plays an important role in the development of age-related diseases in general.

Senescent forms of endothelial progenitor cells and vascular endothelial cells, which have been found in atherosclerotic plaques, are likely facilitators of atherogenesis. Factors that predispose these vascular cells to premature aging are numerous and involve the attrition of basic cellular constituents and molecular mechanisms. These factors include telomere dysfunction, faulty DNA repair systems, dysregulation of the insulin/Akt pathway, and altered angiotensin II signaling (Figure 75-5). Telomere dysfunction is of particular interest, since telomeres act as protective caps at the ends of chromosomes and are involved in cellular replication pathways. Shorter telomere length, a marker of cell turnover, has been associated with endothelial dysfunction, elevated PP, and the presence of traditional CV risk factors as well as clinically significant atherosclerotic disease. There are now data from at least one large clinical trial (WOSCOPS) showing that shorter telomere length is a predictor of coronary heart disease, independent from the effect of chronologic age.

Whether owing to telomere shortening and/or other factors, aging of vascular cells is associated with processes that lead to altered vascular structure and function and, in turn, accelerated atherosclerosis. Senescent vascular endothelial cells are found to have upregulated adhesion molecules, proinflammatory cytokines, and decreased NO production. Senescence of endothelial progenitor cells is associated with decreased angiogenesis and impairment of the complex vascular repair system intended to attenuate the chronic vascular injury and inflammation that leads to atherosclerosis. Targeting the

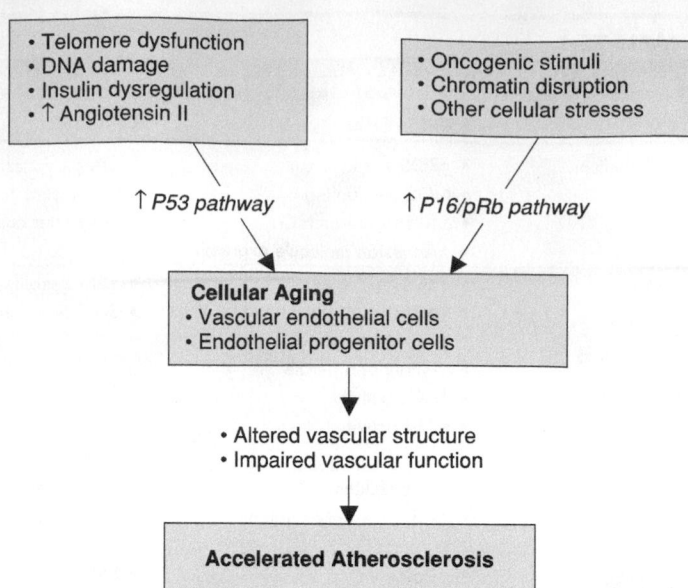

FIGURE 75-5. Attrition of basic cellular constituents and mechanisms leads to cellular aging, which, in turn, predisposes to premature or accelerated atherosclerosis.

mechanisms underlying vascular cellular senescence could represent new approaches to treating atherosclerosis in the future.

Summary

Vascular aging is characterized by specific structural and functional alterations that do not necessitate, but often potentiate, atherosclerosis (Table 75-1). Vascular aging changes result from ongoing exposure to physical and metabolic stresses, accumulation of metabolic byproducts, and attrition of basic cellular constituents and mechanisms that manifest as cellular senescence. Excess function or dysfunction of similar molecular pathways and cell types underlie vascular aging and atherosclerosis: endothelial cells, NO, ROS, SMC, AGE, and elements of the glucose metabolism pathway. Further elucidation of mechanisms that propagate vascular aging and its vulnerability to atherogenesis will facilitate development of interventions that could curtail both processes.

RISK FACTORS FOR VASCULAR PATHOLOGY IN OLDER ADULTS

The age-related arterial structural and functional alterations that predispose older vessels to atherogenesis are heterogeneous across individuals and populations. This variability is influenced largely by the presence or absence of CV risk factors and comorbidities. Prolonged exposure to traditional CV risk factors over time impacts atherogenesis in older adults; diagnosing and modifying these risk factors early in life can reduce and prevent CV events in individuals up to 85 years of age. Since factors such as comorbidities, survivor bias, birth cohort effect, and long-term risk modification affect the potency of traditional and nontraditional risk factors in much older age, data regarding risk reduction in the very old are limited.

Traditional Risk Factors

Hypertension

Age-associated increased central arterial stiffness results in hypertension being the most prevalent traditional risk factor in older adults: the lifetime risk of a 50-year-old developing hypertension is 90%. More than 80% of women and 69% of men older than 75 years are classified as hypertensive, and yet they have the lowest rates of control. Unlike in younger patients, who predominately have elevated diastolic blood pressures (DPBs), more than 60% of patients with hypertensions older than 65 years have ISH as defined by a systolic blood pressure (SBP) $\geq$140 mm Hg and a DBP <90 mm Hg. As individuals age, the CV risk index shifts from diastolic to systolic to pulse pressure (PP = SBP – DBP). This underscores the age-related difference in etiology (ISH is a manifestation of the vascular aging changes described in the previous section).

Although sphygmomanometry of the brachial artery is the most traditional noninvasive method to assess blood pressure, this technique does not fully characterize the age-related changes in central arterial stiffness. Brachial blood pressure measured this way represents an amalgamation of both small- and large-vessel properties. Accordingly, several noninvasive surrogate measures have been developed to assess central arterial pressure, including pulse wave velocity, carotid augmentation index, and estimated central pressures calculated by a generalized transfer function from applanation tonometry of a peripheral artery. These central artery stiffness surrogates are associated with increased CV risk, including myocardial infarction, stroke, renal disease, heart failure, and mortality. Ambulatory and nocturnal blood pressure results showing wide blood pressure variation also pose risk for adverse CV outcomes.

The importance of noninvasively determined central aortic pressure and its reduction was highlighted in The Conduit Artery Functional Endpoint (CAFÉ) study, which demonstrated discrepancies between two antihypertensive agents (amlodipine and atenolol) on CV outcomes despite similar brachial arterial cuff pressure changes. Improved CV outcomes associated with amlodipine compared with atenolol were coupled to an amlodipine-related reduction in estimated aortic stiffness.

Hypertension, itself, promotes vulnerability to atherosclerosis. This is especially true of the increased pulsatility associated with ISH. In response to increased perpendicular and parallel pressures on the arterials wall, vascular SMC hypertrophy and collagen accumulate. As discussed above, increased pulsatility on an endothelial cell with reduced capacity to stretch, such as in a stiff vessel, results in diminished NO signaling. Thus, hypertension exacerbates endothelial dysfunction and predisposes the endothelium to atherogenesis. As vascular collagen accrues in response to increased wall pressure so does AGE cross-linking, which, in turn, further thwarts vascular compliance in a viscous cycle. In this manner, hypertension and the excess forces it delivers to the older vascular wall accelerate vascular inflammation, AGE cross-linking, SMC hypertrophy, inflammatory cell migration, fibrosis, ROS production, apoptosis, and MMP stimulation, all of which predispose to atherogenesis.

Dyslipidemia

Longitudinal studies report that total cholesterol (TC) and LDLs decrease with increasing age. The relationship of TC to CV risk is additionally confounded by survival bias and the J-shaped correlation between TC and mortality. The CV risk of higher TC is offset by the increased total mortality associated with lower TC. However, TC remains predictive of incident CV events after controlling for levels of albumin, serum iron, and comorbidities. Observational studies show that a high TC/HDL ratio, high triglycerides (TG), and low HDL are all predictive of CV events in older women. Data from the Women's Health Study supports that high-sensitivity c-reactive protein (CRP) also adds predictive value to CV events in older women. In the Honolulu Heart Study, a longitudinal cohort study of adults older than 65 years, TC and LDL-C were only weakly associated with myocardial infarction, stroke, and all-cause mortality. In another large observational study, high HDL-C was associated with a decrease risk of ischemic stroke in men. Although it has not been formally studied, elevated TC, LDL, and triglycerides likely still increase the risk for further development of CVD in older adults with known CVD.

Altered Glucose Metabolism

The most common form of diabetes in the elderly, type II, is manifested not only by a hyperglycemic environment but also by metabolic abnormalities, insulin resistance, and insulin deficiency. In addition to the toxic effects of hyperglycemia, other factors likely impact the vasculature, as demonstrated by the increased coronary disease found in prediabetic patients with insulin resistance. The exact mechanism behind the increased vulnerability of diabetics to atherosclerosis is difficult to elucidate because of an inability to produce small animal models without confounding risk factors and the intimate link with dyslipidemia.

Insulin resistance and deficiency lead to the continuous hyperglycemia that fuels the stepwise production of AGEs and consequent increased vascular stiffening. Hyperglycemia also fuels production of ROS, promotes endothelial dysfunction, and increases SMC and MMPs. A diabetic mouse model confirms that induction of diabetes leads to unstable atherosclerotic plaques that are reduced with insulin therapy.

Smoking

The high incidence of atherosclerotic disease among smokers is well documented, contributing to 30% of attributable risk in strokes and 36% in first myocardial infarction. In fact, 11% of worldwide CV deaths are attributable to smoking. This risk is restricted not only to active smokers but also to second-hand smoke exposure. The prevalence of smoking decreases with age but remains a significant risk factor for atherosclerosis. Although continued smoking in patients older than 70 years has a higher relative risk for death or MI than each previous decade, older adults are far less likely to be given advice on smoking cessation. The exact contributing toxins are difficult to isolate in studies as more than 4000 chemicals exist in cigarette smoke, but the driving force appears to be via chronic vascular inflammation and oxidative stress. Chronic cigarette smokers display endothelial dysfunction leading to increased superoxide production through Nicotinamide Adenine Dinucleotide Phosphate (NADPH) oxidase and elevated xanthine oxidase transcription and activity. Despite upregulated NO production, NO levels are diminished because of ROS production and NO scavenging. Cigarette smoke promotes inflammation with elevated leukocyte counts, CRP, IL-6, and increased expression of I-CAM1, E-Selectin, and P-Selectin. Monocytes of smokers show increased adherence to endothelial cells and increased oxidized LDL, as represented by high oxLDL antibodies that promote atherosclerotic plaque formation. In aged individuals, current smoking appears not to correlate with adverse CV events; however, pack/years and lifetime smoking exposure does appear to correlate and may be reflected by high CRP levels in healthy elderly individuals with lifetime exposure.

Nontraditional Risk Factors

Chronic Renal Disease

Accelerated atherosclerosis in chronic renal disease is likely multifactorial and self-perpetuating with renal artery stenosis (RAS) as an ideal model of an atherogenic consequence as well as an accelerator or further CVD. As renal insufficiency progresses, activation of the renin–angiotensin–aldosterone system results in vasoconstriction, and sodium retention and sympathetic activity exacerbate hypertension and end-organ damage. Interestingly, increased angiotensin II activity is seen within atherosclerotic lesions and via stimulating macrophages, and adhesion cell expression contributes to plaque formation and eventual rupture. Moreover, stimulation of vascular endothelial growth factor (VEGF) and Platelet derived growth factor (PDGF) at the RNA level leads to arterial wall remodeling, changes in ECM composition, and induction of a prothrombotic state. Elevated aldosterone, via stimulation of NADPH oxidase and ICAM-1, can increase oxidative products, a mechanism by which angiotensin converting enzyme (ACE)-I and angiotensin receptor blockers (ARBs) may counteract atherosclerosis.

Renal insufficiency is associated with a marked increase in CVD among individuals with end-stage renal disease. The risk is 10-fold that of individuals with a normal creatinine. All-cause CV morbidity and mortality is even increased in individuals with elevated creatinine, even at low levels or near normal levels. Serum creatinine as a measure of renal function is limited, especially in older adults. Cystatin C is a new serum test and a more robust and validated predictor of renal insufficiency in the elderly. Cystatin C levels identify those at an earlier preclinical state of renal dysfunction and are associated with increased myocardial infarction, stroke, and heart failure risk. Another potential link between end-stage renal disease and CVD is a low circulating endogenous secretory receptor for AGEs, which predicts CV mortality.

Biomarkers Associated with Atherosclerosis

Interest has grown in novel markers as additive factors in atherosclerotic disease across the age spectrum. Whether these biochemical substances cause atherosclerosis or are simply markers of the overall inflammatory status of the host is difficult to separate. One such marker, CRP, has been investigated broadly as a predictor of outcomes. Prospective studies show increased events with elevated levels of high-sensitivity CRP. In men and women older than 65 years, regardless of other risk factors as assessed by Framingham scores, elevated CRP is associated with increased 10-year risk of coronary heart disease and augments the predictive value of those in high- and intermediate-risk groups. In patients aged 50 to 75 years, CRP levels were elevated in patients with ultrasound-confirmed carotid

atherosclerotic disease but not in those with cerebral small vessel disease by magnetic resonance imaging (MRI).

Serum homocysteine increases with age and is a strong independent risk factor for CVD, especially in younger individuals. As accelerated atherosclerosis involves enhanced collagen synthesis, smooth muscle proliferation, and increased lipoprotein oxidation, one mechanism is likely inflammation. Accordingly, high levels of acute-phase reactants correlate with homocysteine levels. In older subjects, IL-6 levels, but not other markers of inflammation, predict levels of homocysteine. Combined elevations of CRP and homocysteine are significantly associated with history of MI, heart failure, and CVD.

Depression and Social Isolation

Social isolation and depression are more prevalent and may play a prominent role in CVD in older adults. Morbidity and mortality following myocardial infarction are higher in aged individuals with depression than in those who are not. Similarly, accelerated atherosclerosis has been linked to distrust and depression, yet the mechanism is not fully understood. In persons aged 45 to 84 years free of clinical CVD, those with higher measured scores of cynical distrust, major depression, and stress have higher inflammatory markers CRP, IL-6, and fibrinogen levels, which highlights a potential common mechanism between depression and CVD.

Frailty

The phenotype of frailty encompasses low physical activity, weight loss, weakness, poor exercise tolerance, and slowness, and its severity is strongly associated with incident CVD. Patients meeting frailty criteria have a sixfold greater risk of death, and frailty is an independent mortality risk factor in persons without previous clinical atherosclerotic disease. Linking back to inflammatory mechanisms as a driver of atherosclerosis, frail individuals have increased hsCRP and IL-6 levels. Whether this relationship is cause or effect is unknown, as decreasing these markers in frail individuals does not appear to reduce adverse outcomes.

Obesity

Obesity has been reclassified as a major modifiable CV risk factor by the American Heart Association, concomitant with evidence that the U.S. childhood obesity epidemic may underlie the first reduction in life expectancy in recent history. In the general population, obesity and increased BMI are associated with a higher incidence of CV events. However, isolated BMI measurements are less predictive of CV events in the elderly than are central obesity, measured by waist–hip circumference, the metabolic syndrome, and insulin resistance. With increasing obesity, the ability of adipose tissue to store deposited fat is exceeded and the excess is stored in abdominal viscera, which is not primarily designed for this function. In addition to fat storage, adipose tissue acts as an endocrine organ producing and regulating steroid hormones and their influence on lipid profiles. Additionally, adipose tissue is a source of immune modulators, cytokines, and adipocytokines, the levels of which are markedly augmented in obesity. Adipocytokines including leptin, resistin, and adiponectin, as well as classic inflammatory markers IL-6 and TNF, invoke a proinflammatory state. Mechanistically, the proinflammtory affects of leptin include enhancing angiogenesis, impairing vascular distensibility, increasing platelet aggregation, and hence stimulating thrombus formation. Conversely, adiponectin appears to protect against atherogenesis and inflammation. Excessive obesity also predisposes the individual to hepatic steatosis, which along with insulin resistance alters glycogen pathways and lipid composition, which promotes atherogenesis. Levels of nonesterified fatty acids are increased with insulin resistance and contribute to endothelial dysfunction and oxidative stress, key steps in plaque formation.

Autoimmune Disease

Atherosclerosis is multifactorial, but as chronic inflammation emerges as a core mechanism, the high incidence of atherosclerotic disease in those with chronic autoimmune disease is understandable. Accelerated atherosclerosis may accompany systemic lupus erythematosus (SLE), rheumatoid arthritis, antiphospholipid syndrome (APL), systemic sclerosis, and vasculitidies such as Wegener's granulomatosis. Of these, rheumatoid arthritis, SLE, and APL are the most extensively investigated, and the correlation between CVD and these disorders contributes to the secondary later mortality peak, which is rising as more efficacious treatment has improved outcomes in the earlier active disease phase. The extent of increased attributable CV risk parallels the autoimmune disease duration, severity (measured by systemic inflammatory markers), extra-articular manifestations, and the long-term use of corticosteroids. Many of the activated components in autoimmune diseases, such as macrophages, T cells, cytokines, autoantibodies, and autoantigens, play a central role in atherogenesis. In the joints of patients with rheumatoid arthritis, damaged cartilage contains an abundance of adhesion cells, MMP, and cytokines. The relationship between SLE and premature CVD is highlighted in young women, who are otherwise unlikely to exhibit advanced atherosclerosis. Accordingly, patients with SLE with and without clinical CVD have evidence of central arterial stiffening, as evidenced by faster pulse wave velocities, than those without SLE. The vascular effects of autoimmune disorders are likely synergistic with vascular aging, as patients who are older at the time of SLE diagnosis have a higher risk of incident CVD.

Although not a chronic inflammatory condition by itself, APL is a prothrombotic state characterized by venous and arterial thrombus formation. The syndrome is characterized by high anticardiolipin antibody (aCL) levels and the autoantigen that aCL is most commonly directed to is B2GPI. Along with high oxLDL antibodies in APL, elevated aCL levels are associated with increased MI, cardiac death, and significant coronary artery stenosis compared with controls. The combination of aCL attracting monocytes into the arterial wall and the acceleration of oxLDL into macrophages promoted by B2GPI antibodies promotes atherosclerotic plaque formation. The impact of autoimmune diseases on atherosclerosis emphasizes their consideration as a CV risk equivalent.

Impact of Other Aging Organs

Age-associated changes of other organ systems and hormones greatly influence the hemodynamics and functioning of the vasculature of an older adult. The reduced compliance of stiffer central arteries creates greater fluctuations in blood pressure in response to changes in blood volume. Thus, alterations in systems controlling intravascular volume contribute greatly to increased blood pressure lability with aging. These changes are often magnified by age-associated reduc-

tions in beta-adrenergically driven cardiac chronotropy and inotropy, as well as alterations in homeostatic-regulating systems such as thirst and baroreflexes.

Volume-Regulating Hormones

Serum levels of aldosterone, angiotensin II, vasopressin, and renin diminish with increasing age. These changes manifest clinically as labile blood pressure to intravascular volume challenges. Salt sensitivity also increases with age, which may further challenge the reduced levels of volume-regulating hormones, creating an exaggerated hypertensive and edematous response to foods and medication or leading to salt and fluid retention.

Renal Aging

Glomerular filtration rate declines by approximately 8 cc/minute/decade with normative aging. Additionally, the older kidney has less ability to reabsorb free water and sodium in the distal tubules. The aging kidney also declines in size and blood flow. Reductions in renin and aldosterone impact further on volume regulation. These alterations contribute to intravascular volume shifts in the older adult, which manifest as wide alterations in blood pressure of the noncompliant vascular system.

Iatrogenic Contributors

Medications

Commonly used medications in older patients can inadvertently increase atherogenesis and CV risk. The impact of corticosteroids on the vasculature is multifactorial including weight gain, increased visceral adiposity, hypertension, dyslipidemia, hyperglycemic states, and predisposition to the metabolic syndrome. Additionally, hormone replacement therapy and COX-2 inhibitors, two classes widely used in older adults, are associated with increased CV risk. These medications are associated with thrombosis, fluid retention, and hypertension and thus, have been marked with warnings or removed from the market.

Radiation

As the detection and treatment of cancers improve, more cancer survivors treated with radiation are reaching advanced age. Anterior chest and neck radiations, especially for treatment of Hodgkin's lymphomas and local breast cancers, increase CV risk via radiation injury to arterial vessels in the treatment field. The incidence of coronary revascularization, carotid stenosis, and valve replacement is higher than expected in patients with a history of radiotherapy; the earlier in life the radiation, the more significant the CV risk. Common sites of radiation-related atherosclerotic disease included the left main, left anterior descending and right common coronaries and subclavian and carotid arteries. The mechanism of accelerated atherogenesis appears related to the acute inflammation following the radiation and subsequent neutrophil and cytokine infiltration. As the vessels, repair and remodel, fibrosis and scarring also enhance microvascular ischemia. Interestingly, increased CVD and events are also seen in atomic bomb survivors, the disease extent reflecting total radiation exposure. Techniques to reduce the dose and increase the focus of radiation therapy have reduced the incidence of radiation-associated CVD over the past decade.

Summary

Traditional CV risk factors continue to be important in older age and, in some cases, carry even higher risk than in younger age owing to their length of exposure. In addition, many nontraditional risk factors are increasingly important in older adults. Overall, CV risk factor profiling is more complex with older age as common risk profiling tools (Framingham Risk Score, European ProCam Risk Score, and Reynolds Risk Score) have limited ability to accurately predict CV risk beyond 80 years of age. Providers should be aware that these risk-profiling methods are generated using primarily middle-aged cohorts; although CV risk is most influenced by age, these do not account for the increasing variability of risk factors in older age groups. Risk-profiling models specific for older adults need to be developed.

CLINICAL IMPLICATIONS OF VASCULAR AGING AND ATHEROSCLEROSIS

Atherosclerosis manifests clinically as coronary artery disease, cerebrovascular disease, aortic atheromatous as aneurysmal lesions and peripheral arterial disease. In older adults, the clinical presentation of these CV conditions can be nontraditional, and, especially in those accustomed to debility, the severity of the impairment is often underestimated or downplayed. Atherosclerotic disease may often be occult or insidious and not recognized by the patients, their family, or their provider. Clinical presentation may also be altered by cognitive abilities or lack of usual stressors such as exercise or immobility from musculoskeletal and/or neurological deficits. For these reasons and as CVD prevalence increases with age, the diagnosis should be considered even for vague symptoms such as confusion, atypical pain, lethargy, and shortness of breath.

The physiologic changes imparted by a stiff central vasculature (increased pulsatility, left ventricular hypertrophy, impaired early left ventricular diastolic filling, increased afterload, and diminished coronary perfusion) increase the vulnerability to atherosclerosis and worsen its consequences by reducing cardiac reserve. Thus, stressor such as blood pressure lability to alterations in intravascular volume or tachycardia (from dehydration, fever, hyperthyroidism, arrhythmias, or deconditioning) can easily provoke symptoms or events in older adults. The central-stiffness-induced coronary perfusion pressure reduction, in addition to left ventricular hypertrophy, diminishes myocardial perfusion, resulting in ischemia often in the absence of discrete coronary lesions. Further, increased left ventricular pressures from augmented afterload exacerbate left atrial and pulmonary pressures, which lower the dyspnea threshold.

Isolated Systolic Hypertension

ISH is the clinical manifestation of both the vascular aging changes and/or the atherosclerosis of the older central arterial system. As previously noted, the vicious cycle of structural and dynamic arterial wall changes drives increased pulsatility and sheer stress, which further promotes vascular damage, inflammation, ROS accumulation, and endothelial dysfunction and vice versa. This pathology underlying older hypertensive adults with ISH and their vasculature is often reflected in their inability to respond to traditional antihypertensives designed to reduce peripheral vascular tone, as compared to younger hypertensive, and highlights the need for novel therapeutics that target these age-associated alterations. There is now an abundance of data confirming that treatment of ISH results in reduction of CV events including MI, heart failure, strokes as well as renal failure, total mortality, and dementia.

Heart Failure with Preserved Systolic Function

More than half of older heart failure patients presenting with symptomatic heart failure have a preserved ejection fraction, and the majority of these individuals are female. The pathogenesis of heart failure with preserved ejection fraction (HFPEF) is controversial but is likely based on long-standing hypertension, left ventricular hypertrophy (LVH) intrinsic ventricular stiffness, and impaired early diastolic relaxation. The myocardium of the left ventricle hypertrophies in response to increased ventricular afterload imposed by an increased aortic diameter, decreased aortic compliance, and the early reflected pulse wave. In addition to LVH, isovolumic relaxation of the ventricle is prolonged, encroaching on diastole. Thus, increased central arterial stiffness exacerbates impaired early diastolic relaxation and filling. At rest, the ventricular and central vascular functions of the older adult remain fairly energetically coupled. Normally, ventricular–vascular coupling implies that the heart is functioning at maximum metabolic efficiency and can maintain blood pressure and cardiac output in a physiologic range. However, in the older adult, as both the myocardium and the central vasculature stiffen, the CV reserve mechanisms are challenged by stressors, resulting in labile blood pressure at higher cardiac work. Characteristics associated with the clinical presentation of HFPEF include female sex, older age, relative obesity, anemia, and renal insufficiency. Factors that can trigger an exacerbation of HFPEF are similar to those that can trigger systolic heart failure. However, HFPEF may be more afterload and preload dependent, necessitating tight blood pressure control as a part of long-term management.

Coronary Artery Disease (See Chapter 76)

On presentation with acute coronary syndrome, the age of a patient is one of the most powerful predictors of outcome, with more than 60% of myocardial deaths occurring in those older than 75 years, which may be attributed to confounding factors including the atypical presentation and absence of characteristic EKG changes often seen in this group. Aged individuals often present later, and in a more compromised state with shortness of breath. Additionally, comorbidities, frailty, and renal insufficiency worsen the outcome. Older patients are at higher risk of complications from antiplatelet, anticoagulant thrombolytic, and revascularization, therapies but clinical trials demonstrate that aggressive treatment in this cohort reduced morbidity and mortality. Management of acute atherosclerotic disease in older patients is not often addressed by evidence-based guidelines owing to the underrepresentation of older adults in clinical trials.

Cerebrovascular Disease (See Chapter 64)

Atherosclerotic cerebrovascular disease is a significant cause of morbidity and mortality in aged individuals and of a major social cost because of disability. Presenting complaints range from classical hemiplegic stroke to vascular dementia that is often silent until significant cognitive disease is reported. Clinically occult cerebrovascular disease is common in elderly individuals, especially in those with orthostatic hypotension and hypertension independent of other risk factors.

Renovascular Disease

Approximately 90% renal artery stenosis (RAS) is caused by atherosclerosis, often characterized by plaque extending from the aorta into the renal artery lumen, creating an ostial lesion. The prevalence of RAS increases with age, especially in the setting of risk factors such as hypertension. Kidney atrophy and ischemic changes may result from progressive occlusion of renal blood flow or by microthromboembolism from unstable prothrombotic plaques. Progressive renal dysfunction, increased sympathetic nervous system activity by the ischemic kidney, and augmentation of the renin–angiotensin–aldosterone system can exacerbate preexisting essential hypertension, resulting in recurrent flash pulmonary edema in the absence of cardiac ischemia. This vicious hypertensive and shear stress cycle in unilateral RAS can also damage the contralateral kidney, resulting in rising creatinine, which signifies more than 60% reduction in nephron function. This risk of unilateral RAS evolving into bilateral renal disease is high and may progress to end-stage renal failure. Atherosclerotic RAS may account for up to 15% of elderly patients admitted to the hospital with ischemic nephropathy leading to end-stage renal disease.

Aneurysms

Abdominal aortic aneurysms are most commonly found incidentally on examination or imaging. Determining the timing of surgery is extremely important in older patients, as the mortality associated with repair of ruptured aneurysms is significantly higher in patients older than 80 years compared with those younger than 80 years. Despite this, fact elective abdominal aortic aneurysm repair is often delayed or avoided in this cohort because of perceived elevated surgical risk. Accordingly, recommendations for repeat screening in patients with already diagnosed atherosclerotic disease are well established. Regarding the pathophysiology, increased MMP activity and decreased tissue inhibitor of MMPs are found in abdominal and thoracic atherosclerotic aneurysms compared with nonatherosclerotic lesions.

Peripheral Arterial Disease

Prevalence of peripheral vascular disease in individuals older than 55 years is estimated at 16.9% in men and 20% in women (WHO) and is linked to symptomatic and asymptomatic CVD, smoking, and hypertension. Both objectively diagnosed PAD and symptomatic claudication increase with age. Interestingly, the trend to asymptomatic disease in the elderly is again found with the prevalence of PAD quite high but the corresponding prevalence of intermittent claudication at a much lower level. With chronic ischemia of the extremities, there may be evidence of dry skin changes, poor nail growth, and ischemic ulcers characteristically distal but may occur at the heel and ankle in immobile individuals. A large number of markers including homocysteine, TG, lipoprotein, and ApoA/B in patients up to 84 years of age have been investigated; however, CRP and HDL-C seem to have the strongest prognostic value in peripheral arterial disease.

Reduced Exercise Capacity

Exercise capacity, reflected by maximum oxygen consumption, declines with increasing age even after adjustment for estimated total body muscle mass. Studies of healthy older volunteers in the Baltimore Longitudinal Study of Aging have confirmed this phenomenon and investigated possible etiologies. Impaired cardiac output is a significant contributor, in addition to decreased respiratory and peripheral muscle reserve possibly related to deconditioning. Cardiac output is the product of heart rate and stroke volume, and the expected increase in both of these indices with exercise is blunted in aging. The decreased heart rate response is primarily caused by decreased beta-adrenergic sensitivity. The decreased stroke volume response is likely caused by multiple factors, including reduced myocardial contractility, increased vascular afterload from arterial stiffening, and arterial–ventricular load mismatch. Not surprisingly, this blunted stroke volume response in aging is even further impaired in the setting of exercise-induced silent myocardial ischemia evidenced by electrocardiogram.

DETECTION AND DIAGNOSIS

Advances in CV technology have enhanced our ability to detect and diagnose atherosclerosis at earlier stages of the disease process in adults of all ages. As the age-associated atherosclerotic burden continues to grow, diagnosing and managing CVD will consume a significant proportion of health care resources. Therefore, healthcare providers should be aware that newer technologies currently add only incrementally to traditional approaches used to diagnose atherosclerosis in adults both young and old. This section provides a brief overview of currently available approaches and their utility in older populations.

Stress Testing

The exercise treadmill test remains appropriate for diagnosing clinically important CAD in older adults who are not physically limited by noncardiac comorbidities and who have normal electrocardiograms. The ability to perform an adequate treadmill test declines with age; only a quarter of individuals older than 75 years achieve a maximal predicted effort. Causes may include reduced beta-adrenergic responsiveness, conduction disease, and decreased vascular compliance. Furthermore, the specificity of an ECG-positive treadmill stress is lower in older age as false positives from LVH increase. Despite these limitations, a good exercise tolerance in very old adults is associated with a favorable long-term prognosis, regardless of other findings.

Individuals who cannot exercise require the use of pharmacologic stress agents such as dobutamine, dipyridamole, or adenosine. Dobutamine, a beta-agonist, is often successful at inducing heart rate goals in older adults. Dipyridamole and adenosine, potent vasodilators, are used to assess distribution of vascular perfusion with stress. Both agents are as well tolerated in older adults as dobutamine. Dobutamine echocardiography may be more sensitive than adenosine echocardiography in assessing the presence and severity of CAD, but a positive adenosine echo often represents more severe disease.

Single-photon nuclear imaging or echocardiographic imaging is often used in pharmacological stress tests and especially for individuals with baseline ECG abnormalities, which are frequent in older adults. The ability of a normal nuclear stress result to predict low event rates is time limited, requiring repeat evaluation in older patients with recurrent or changing symptoms. Nuclear imaging is also subject to false-negative results in "balanced three-vessel disease." Likewise, the ability of echocardiography to image the lateral wall is limited and can produce false-negative results in this territory for individuals of any age.

Computed Tomography

Two types of computed tomography (CT) scanning currently used to detect atherosclerosis are electron-beam CT (EBCT) and multidetector CT (MDCT). The EBCT method uses relatively little radiation and can quickly assess coronary anatomy. EBCT is primarily used to quantify the presence of coronary artery calcium (CAC). High CAC scores correlate with histological plaque and to the number of stenosed vessels on invasive angiography. Furthermore, a high CAC score adds additional risk to the Framingham risk stratification, particularly in those with intermediate risk. However, CAC does not predict plaque stability, and EBCT cannot detect noncalcified plaques. Moreover, high CAC scores are widespread in older populations and do not correlate well with the clinical significance of the lesion. Thus, the use of EBCT to assist in differentiating between quiescent and clinically significant coronary disease in older adults is very limited.

The MDCT method uses more radiation than EBCT and images the heart in thinner slices to provide higher resolution and identify the presence of noncalcified as well as calcified plaques. Compared to invasive angiography, a 16-slice MDCT can detect hemodynamically relevant coronary stenoses with 90% sensitivity and specificity. However, 5% to 15% of the coronary circulation in a given study cannot be evaluated as a result of poor image quality. Factors that affect MDCT image quality include motion artifact of the heart, particularly at high heart rates, and the presence of severe CAC. Given the increased CAC in older adults, the ability of MDCT to evaluate for obstructive or hemodynamically significant lesions in older adults may be diminished compared to younger subjects. The combination of MDCT and single-photon nuclear imaging allows the process of acquiring anatomic and functional information in a single study. This technology has yet to be evaluated in large populations but may offer an important advantage over current modalities in the evaluation of older individuals who are more likely than their younger counterparts to have complex coronary anatomy.

Magnetic Resonance Imaging

Using cardiac MRI to image atherosclerosis offers the advantage of avoiding contrast dye and ionizing radiation. In addition, MRI is capable of isolating atheroma and identifying specific components of the plaque, such as the fibrous cap, calcifications, the lipid-rich necrotic core, and intraplaque hemorrhage. MRI can identify disruptions of the plaque–lumen interface such as those associated with fibrous cap rupture or ulceration. However, current MRI technology suffers from extensive variability of image quality owing to the time required to acquire images, the ability to account for cardiorespiratory motion, and limited spatial resolution. Limited penetration depth, in favor of better resolution, also affects the ability of MRI to evaluate plaques in larger vessels such as the aorta. For this reason, transesophageal MRI has been developed to optimize MRI of the aorta.

Vascular Studies

In addition to CT and MRI, investigational modalities to detect atherosclerosis of the peripheral circulation include carotid ultrasonography, ankle–brachial index (ABI), and brachial reactivity testing. Detecting large or symptomatic atherosclerotic lesions, such as plaque or aneurysm, in the aorta or other large vessels is straightforward, whether by CT or MRI or ultrasound. However, smaller asymptomatic or subclinical atherosclerotic lesions may be more difficult to detect.

Carotid ultrasound remains the cornerstone to detect flowlimiting or obstructive plaques for evaluation of cerebrovascular disease. This technology also measures intima-media thickness (IMT) at various sites around the common carotid bifurcation point. Increased carotid IMT represents subclinical atherosclerosis and is associated with adverse CV events. Conversely, reduction in carotid IMT with statin therapy is associated with risk reduction. Advanced age is very strongly associated with increased carotid IMT, and the degree to which this relationship reflects vascular aging versus atherosclerosis is unknown. In addition, the measurement of carotid IMT can vary widely between imaging operators and is presently not widely used outside of clinical research studies.

Perhaps one of the most overlooked modalities for assessing the presence and severity of atherosclerosis is the ABI. Traditionally used in the diagnosis and evaluation of PAD, ABI is the ratio of Dopplerrecorded SBP at the ankle divided by the SBP in the arm. Individuals without clinically significant PAD typically have an ABI greater than 1.00, while an ABI <0.90 is 90% sensitive and 95% specific for angiographically present PAD. Individuals with low-normal ABIs have a higher prevalence of CAC on CT and increased carotid IMT on ultrasound. Clinically diagnosed PAD carries higher risk for MI, stroke, and death, but even a low ABI alone is associated with increased CV morbidity and mortality. The ABI should be interpreted with caution, since its relationship with clinical atherosclerotic events is not linear. In fact, individuals with ABI >1.30 can also have increased CV risk. The degree to which higher ABIs represent upper extremity PAD (e.g., subclavian) out of proportion to lower extremity PAD (e.g., iliac, femoral, and popliteal) is unclear.

Another modality to identify the presence of atherosclerosis is brachial artery reactivity testing. Endothelial dysfunction may be one of the earliest detectable manifestations of atherosclerosis. Brachial artery reactivity testing detects endothelial dysfunction by measuring arterial vasodilatation in response to increased blood flow, or flow-mediated dilation. Changes in brachial artery blood flow and diameter are assessed before and immediately after blood vessel occlusion with a cuff using either high-resolution B-mode Doppler ultrasound or MRI. Endothelial dysfunction can predict CV events, even after adjusting for the presence and extent of morphologic atherosclerosis. Limitations to brachial artery reactivity testing include variations in flow-mediated dilation measurements and a lack of standardized approaches to interpreting measurements.

STRATEGIES TO PREVENT, RETARD, AND REGRESS VASCULAR AGING AND ATHEROSCLEROSIS

Novel Drug Targets

Elucidation of novel biochemical pathways, which contribute to vascular aging and atherosclerosis in older adults, has resulted in the design of novel targets for therapeutic intervention to reduce and ideally prevent the burden of atherosclerosis and its associated pathology. Pharmaceutical agents that block the formation of AGE have proved efficacious in decreasing vascular stiffness and nephrosclerosis, but clinical trials were halted owing to adverse drug effects. Preclinical studies with AGE cross-link breakers support their ability to reduce age-associated ventricular and vascular stiffness and reduce and prevent atherosclerotic plaques. Clinical trials with alagebrium chloride, an AGE cross-link breaker, demonstrate a significant reduction in total vascular compliance and left ventricular mass and improve endothelial dysfunction and early left ventricular diastolic filling. These strategies emphasize a shift in the focus of hypertension treatment from dynamic peripheral vasoconstriction to structural targets previously thought to be irreversible. Development of RAGE antagonist remains in the preclinical phase, but administration of these drugs are associated with significant reductions in endothelial-mediated vessel injury response and reduction in vascular inflammation and oxidative stress. Tetrahydrobioterin, an agent that "recouples" NOS dimers to a functional molecule, shows promise in improving endothelial dysfunction and reducing age-associated vascular stiffness. Other potential drug targets, which exploit age-associated changes, include inhibitors of the elastase enzyme and strategies to augment no activity such as arginase blockade.

Pleiotropic Effects of Available Therapies

ACE-I/ARB

Large clinical trials demonstrate the potential for ACE inhibitors to exhibit beneficial effects on morbidity and mortality beyond blood pressure lowering. Likewise, ARBs as well as ACE inhibitors specifically lower CV risk of type II diabetes. Both ARBs and ACE inhibitors also appear to increase insulin sensitivity through different mechanisms. ACE inhibitors do so via the bradykinin pathway. ARBs induce activity of peroxisome proliferator-activated receptor, a nuclear hormone receptor that plays an important role in regulating insulin sensitivity.

Statins

The pleiotropic effects of statins have beneficial effects on both vascular aging and atherosclerosis. Statins can improve endothelial function in individuals with hypercholesterolemia, atherosclerosis, smoking, and type II diabetes. These favorable endothelial effects are attributed to their ability to lower LDL cholesterol, downregulate eNOS, and exert antioxidant activity. With regard to atherosclerosis, statins contribute to plaque stability via fibrosis and MMP reduction and exhibit a powerful anti-inflammatory effect that can be reflected in lower CRP and adhesion molecule levels. Statins may even contribute to the differentiation and recruitment of endothelial progenitor cells as well as modulate immune mechanisms involved in atherogenesis.

Exercise

Despite the proven benefits of physical activity across all age groups, older adults are less likely than younger adults to be referred for exercise training. Although many older adults may be physically limited by non-CV comorbidities, older individuals can benefit significantly from any form of exercise program in which they can participate (e.g., aerobic, resistance, or flexibility training). In fact, exercise has a directly beneficial physiological impact on vascular changes associated with aging. Although these adaptations may be somewhat limited in areas of the vasculature affected by frank atherosclerosis, physical activity can both prevent and even reverse endothelial dysfunction in older adults. Subsequent improvements in vascular tone can manifest as significant lowering of blood pressure even beyond that achieved by antihypertensive medication alone. Indeed, the beneficial effects of exercise are likely pleiotropic. In addition to a lower blood pressure, older adults with coronary disease who participate in an exercise rehabilitation program can achieve improved lipid profiles, increased glucose tolerance, and also decreased measures of depression and anxiety.

SUMMARY AND TAKE HOME POINTS

Aging is the most potent risk factor for atherosclerotic disease, and, in turn, atherosclerosis is responsible for a dominant portion of the chronic illness burden in older adults. Research to date reveals that the relationship between aging and atherosclerosis is complex and multifaceted. Nevertheless, it is apparent that vascular aging plays a central role and involves numerous biologic processes that greatly enhance the development of atherosclerosis. In concert with vascular aging, traditional and nontraditional risk factors manifest in increased number and with greater magnitude in older individuals. Furthermore, exposure to non-CV illness and iatrogenic contributors potentiate the development and progression of atherosclerotic disease through a variety of mechanisms over the course of a lifetime. As a result, the clinical presentations of atherosclerosis in older compared to younger individuals are more varied as well as more severe. Newer imaging modalities for detecting and diagnosing atherosclerosis are being refined for widespread use. Novel therapies to target vascular aging and atherosclerosis are being tested. Yet, the most powerful reduction in atherosclerotic disease results for early recognition and risk factor modification. Traditional and readily available therapies are vastly underused in older patients with CVD, and this should be emphasized to patients and providers, as evidence-based guidelines for older patients with CVD continue be developed.

FURTHER READING

Chan SY, Mancini GB, Kuramoto L, Schulzer M, Frohlich J, Ignaszewski A. The prognostic importance of endothelial dysfunction and carotid atheroma burden in patients with coronary artery disease. *J Am Coll Cardiol.* 2003;42:1037–1043.

Faxon DP, Creager MA, Smith SC Jr, et al. Atherosclerotic Vascular Disease Conference: executive summary: Atherosclerotic Vascular Disease Conference proceeding for healthcare professionals from a special writing group of the American Heart Association. *Circulation.* 2004;109:2595–2604.

Franklin SS, Larson MG, Khan SA, et al. Does the relation of blood pressure to coronary heart disease risk change with aging? The Framingham Heart Study. *Circulation.* 2001;103:1245–1249.

Galis ZS, Khatri JJ. Matrix metalloproteinases in vascular remodeling and atherogenesis: the good, the bad, and the ugly. *Circ Res.* 2002;90:251–262.

Gill TM, DiPietro L, Krumholz HM. Role of exercise stress testing and safety monitoring for older persons starting an exercise program. *JAMA.* 2000;284:342–349.

Goldschmidt-Clermont PJ, Creager MA, Losordo DW, Lam GK, Wassef M, Dzau VJ. Atherosclerosis 2005: recent discoveries and novel hypotheses. *Circulation.* 2005;112:3348–3353.

Harman D. Aging: a theory based on free radical and radiation chemistry. *J Gerontol.* 1956;11:298–300.

Lakatta EG. Arterial and cardiac aging: major shareholders in cardiovascular disease enterprises: parts I–III. *Circulation.* 2003;107:139–146, 346–354, 490–497.

Lakatta EG. Arterial and cardiac aging: major shareholders in cardiovascular disease enterprises: part III: cellular and molecular clues to heart and arterial aging. *Circulation.* 2003;107:490–497.

Lee PY, Alexander KP, Hammill BG, Pasquali SK, Peterson ED. Representation of elderly persons and women in published randomized trials of acute coronary syndromes. *JAMA.* 2001;286:708–713.

Minamino T, Miyauchi H, Yoshida T, Tateno K, Kunieda T, Komuro I. Vascular cell senescence and vascular aging. *J Mol Cell Cardiol.* 2004;36:175–183.

O'Rourke MF, Nichols WW. Aortic diameter, aortic stiffness, and wave reflection increase with age and isolated systolic hypertension. *Hypertension.* 2005;45:652–658.

Peng X, Haldar S, Deshpande S, Irani K, Kass DA. Wall stiffness suppresses Akt/eNOS and cytoprotection in pulse-perfused endothelium. *Hypertension.* 2003;41:378–381.

Redfield MM, Jacobsen SJ, Borlaug BA, Rodeheffer RJ, Kass DA. Age- and gender-related ventricular-vascular stiffening: a community-based study. *Circulation.* 2005;112:2254–2262.

Samani NJ, Boultby R, Butler R, Thompson JR, Goodall AH. Telomere shortening in atherosclerosis. *Lancet.* 2001;358:472–473.

Shoenfeld Y, Gerli R, Doria A, et al. Accelerated atherosclerosis in autoimmune rheumatic diseases. *Circulation.* 2005;112:3337–3347.

Staessen JA, Gasowski J, Wang JG, et al. Risks of untreated and treated isolated systolic hypertension in the elderly: meta-analysis of outcome trials. *Lancet.* 2000;355:865–872.

Walston J, McBurnie MA, Newman A, et al. Frailty and activation of the inflammation and coagulation systems with and without clinical comorbidities: results from the Cardiovascular Health Study. *Arch Intern Med.* 2002;162:2333–2341.

Zieman SJ, Kass, DA. Inhibitors of advanced glycation endproduct cross-linking: therapeutic potential in the management of cardiovascular disease. *Drugs.* 2004;64(5):1–12.

Zieman SJ, Melenovsky V, Kass DA. Mechanisms, pathophysiology, and therapy of arterial stiffness. *Arterioscler Thromb Vasc Biol.* 2005;25:932–943.

Coronary Heart Disease

Eric D. Peterson ■ *Shahyar M. Gharacholou*

Data from the National Center for Health Statistics have noted that the life expectancy at birth in the United States reached a record high of 77.5 years in 2003, attributable, in part, to the decline in mortality from heart disease during the past three decades. Despite this, coronary heart disease (CHD) remains the leading killer of both men and women in the United States. More than 80% of CHD deaths occur in persons older than 65 years of age. In addition, 37% of recognized acute myocardial infarctions (MIs) occur in those older than 75 years of age, and, although these account for roughly 6% of the U.S. population, 60% of all MI-related deaths affect elderly patients 75 years of age or older.

The diagnosis, management, and posthospitalization care of elderly patients with CHD involve interplay of patient heterogeneity, comorbid conditions, functional status, drug pharmacology, and biological differences. This complexity is compounded by extrapolation of "evidence-based care" obtained from cardiovascular trials from which older patients were poorly represented. Given these characteristics, an adopted approach to cardiac care of elderly patients often requires developing a *patient-centered* plan of care and incorporating an individual's own goals and health expectations in the care decision process. While the term "elderly" has been used in the literature, no specific guideline to the care of elderly patients with CHD attributes a particular level of evidence to specific age. This chapter will reference specific age groups reported in the medical literature as available, bearing in mind that one's chronologic age may be a poor surrogate for one's overall health status.

PREVALENCE

The spectrum of CHD includes asymptomatic (or subclinical) CHD, chronic stable angina pectoris, unstable angina, and acute MI. Statistically, the first manifestation of CHD is an acute MI in 40% of cases and sudden death in 10% to 20% of cases. In the United States, the prevalence of overt CHD increases in a curvi-

linear fashion with advancing age in both men and women (Figure 76-1). Similarly, the annual rate of first heart attack rises with age in all race and gender subgroups. Furthermore, despite the fact that women typically have a 10-year lag in developing CHD as compared to men, the majority of patients with CHD ≥75 years of age or older are women because they typically have a longer lifespan.

It should also be realized that overt CHD represents just the tip of the coronary disease iceberg and a great number of elderly patients have asymptomatic, subclinical disease. Researchers for the Cardiovascular Health Study examined the prevalence of both clinical and subclinical cardiovascular disease in a large community-dwelling Medicare population by using a composite measure of MI on electrocardiogram (ECG) or echocardiography and abnormal carotid artery wall thickness or ankle–brachial blood pressure index and found that disease frequency increased from 22% in women aged 65 to 70 years to 43% in those aged 85 years or older. Similarly, the frequency of subclinical vascular disease in men increased from 33% to 45% in these age groups, respectively.

EFFECTS OF AGING ON THE CARDIOVASCULAR SYSTEM

The development of CHD is multifactorial and can be influenced by genetic predisposition and comorbid conditions such as diabetes, as well as environmental and lifestyle determinants such as diet, smoking, and physical exercise. Not surprisingly, as these factors vary among individuals, one's likelihood for developing CHD also varies. While it is often believed that CHD is inevitable with advancing age, autopsy studies have found that 40% of those persons in their nineties will not have occlusive coronary disease.

With this patient-to-patient variability noted, certain cardiovascular changes are seen more commonly with advancing age, and the aging process confers important physiological considerations in elderly patients. Diastolic heart failure, "heart failure with preserved

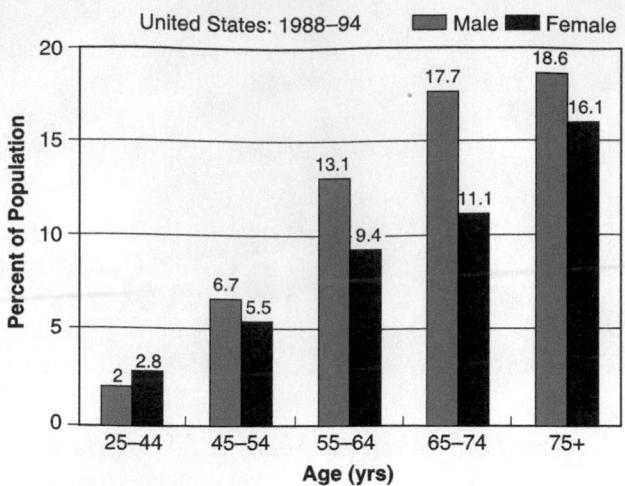

FIGURE 76-1. Estimated prevalence of coronary heart disease by age and sex. *(Adapted with permission from Vargas et al. Cardiovascular Disease in the NHANES III. Ann Epidemiol 1997;7:523.)*

ejection fraction," accounts for up to 50% of heart failure in patients older than 70 years of age and often coexists with vascular disease, contributing to significant morbidity and mortality. The exact mechanism of diastolic heart failure continues to remain controversial, but altered left ventricular end-diastolic pressures and increased pulmonary venous pressures can result in symptoms of dyspnea and signs of pulmonary edema. This disease process occurs with a higher prevalence in elderly patients with a history of hypertension and atrial fibrillation. Recent observational data suggest that rehospitalization or 1-year survival mirrors that of systolic heart failure, challenging earlier assumptions that diastolic heart failure might be a more benign condition. In parallel, arterial stiffening in elderly patients results in isolated systolic hypertension and widened pulse pressures, factors previously associated with increased cardiovascular events. The aging of the vasculature often heralds blunted responses to protective vasodilatory mediators and progressive endothelial dysfunction. This endotheliopathy results in increasing numbers and severity of atherosclerotic plaques (Figure 76-2). The composition of these lesions also changes with age, with reduction in the soft lipid core and an increase in calcification and fibrosis. While more

advanced calcified plaques are actually less likely to rupture, the sheer increase in lesion numbers leads to an increased overall likelihood for CHD events in the elderly patient.

PRESENTATION

The elderly are much less likely than younger patients to present with "classic" exertional chest heaviness. Instead, older patients more often complain of a vague feeling of dyspnea, abdominal pain, fatigue, confusion, or malaise that may be misinterpreted as consequences of aging or other comorbid illness. Findings from the Global Registry of Acute Coronary Events, a large, prospective, multinational registry of acute coronary syndromes (ACSs), demonstrated that patients presenting with atypical symptoms were less likely to receive appropriate cardiac medications, undergo cardiac catheterization, and were at higher risk of in-hospital morbidity and mortality. The elderly can also have an impaired ischemia warning system, which delays their CHD presentation. In a series of patients with CHD undergoing treadmill testing, researchers found that patients aged >70 years took more than twice as long as their younger counterparts to report anginal symptoms after ECG-documented ischemia was noted. In the Worcester Heart Attack Study, patients 75 years of age and older had the longest prehospital delay of any age group, many outside the critical 6-hour window for fibrinolytic therapy. The Rapid Early Action for Coronary Treatment study quantified delay time as an additional 14 minutes for every 10-year increment in age, beginning with the age of 30 years. The significant prehospital delay among elderly patients is likely multifactorial and includes considerations such as atypical presentation, medical comorbidities, previous experiences within the health-care system, socioeconomics, access to care, and cognitive and functional impairments.

Difficulty in recognizing symptoms contributes to later presentation for acute CHD events in the elderly. In fact, studies show that more than two-thirds of patients with MI, >65 years of age, fail to reach an emergency department within 6 hours after the onset of their symptoms. Major predictors of a delay in MI presentation include advanced age, female sex, diabetes mellitus, and social isolation. Importantly, delays in MI presentation have strong prognostic implications and are closely associated with poorer outcomes in elderly patients. Thus, clinicians should proactively discuss with their

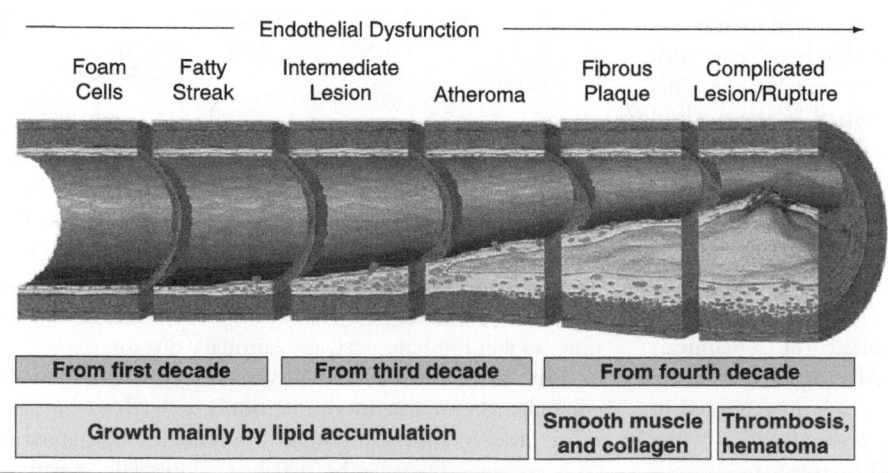

FIGURE 76-2. Atherosclerosis timeline.

patients that cardiac symptoms can vary widely and they should seek rapid medical attention if potential ischemic symptoms occur.

DIAGNOSTIC EVALUATION

Given its prevalence and often atypical presentation in the elderly, clinicians must harbor a high index of suspicion for CHD in order to make the correct diagnosis. In taking a thorough clinical history, with emphasis on prior cardiovascular disease history, clinicians must pay close attention to assessing a patient's major cardiac risk factors (smoking, hypertension, diabetes mellitus, and lipid status), as well as any symptoms suggestive of CHD. Eliciting the temporal course of these symptoms is also important. Patients with new, progressive, or refractory symptoms typically require an expedited—and possibly inpatient—evaluation, in contrast to those patients with chronic stable symptoms. Physicians should also assess the impact of symptoms on the patient's functional status and overall quality of life, as these issues may alter preferences for invasive testing and/or need for coronary revascularization.

A systematic approach to the physical examination with awareness of age-related changes in the cardiovascular system may improve diagnostic accuracy and provide further clues to the presence of CHD. After evaluation of the patient's general appearance, blood pressure assessment with an appropriately fitting sphygmomanometer, one that encircles at least 80% of the arm, and examination of pulses in the extremities should be performed. Some older patients develop calcific vascular disease, and pseudohypertension may be observed. This becomes an important distinction when further titration of antihypertensive medications may predispose the patient to symptoms of cerebral hypoperfusion. Diminution of the femoral pulses or brachial–femoral delay may suggest the presence of atherosclerotic aortoiliac disease, and these findings may accompany observed dermatological changes with lower extremity hair loss. Performing ankle–brachial indices remains a useful and sensitive screening tool for identifying patients with peripheral vascular disease, a known risk factor for increased cardiovascular events. The cardiac examination may include signs of left- or right-sided heart failure (pulmonary edema, displaced point of maximal impulse, an S_3, or peripheral edema) or characteristic murmurs of valvular heart disease. Once a thorough history and physical has been completed, further diagnostic evaluation should be based on the patient's symptoms as outlined below.

Asymptomatic Elderly Patients

For the asymptomatic elderly individual, risk factors, particularly blood pressure and lipid screening, should be measured as recommended for all aged patients in the Joint National Committee on Detection, Evaluation and Treatment of High Blood Pressure (JNC) VII and National Cholesterol Education Program (NCEP)—Adult Treatment Panel (ATP) III guidelines, as the elderly continue to remain the population with the lowest rates of blood pressure control. Obtaining a baseline ECG is also reasonable in the initial patient evaluation because of the high prevalence of "silent" MIs in the elderly population. This information should be summarized into a composite risk assessment using one of the multiple standardized indexes such as the Framingham Risk Score (http://www.nhlbi.nih.gov/about/framingham/riskabs.htm).

Patients with low CHD risk (10-year CHD risk <5%) can generally be reassured without further testing, with a plan for reevaluation of their risk factors in 5 years. In contrast, patients at high risk (10-year CHD risk >20%) should receive aggressive risk factor intervention to the same degree as if they had already experienced an overt CHD event. Patients with intermediate risk (10-year CHD risk, 5–20%) may benefit from further testing to clarify their CHD risk. In these intermediate patients, laboratory studies such as homocysteine, lipoprotein (a), B-type natriuretic peptide, and C-reactive protein have been proposed as means of identifying those at higher risk and in need of more aggressive risk-factor modification. Recently, this "multimarker" strategy was evaluated in a study of the Framingham Offspring cohort. The findings suggested that for outcomes of death or first major cardiovascular events, multimarker scoring added only a small increase to conventional risk factors in the ability to classify risk. Therefore, the role of biomarkers to aid in risk stratification of patients who are ambulatory remains an area of ongoing research, and its implications for clinical practice have yet to be clearly elucidated. Beyond the standard history, physical examination, and simple laboratory tests, further diagnostic testing (carotid ultrasound, treadmill testing, echocardiography, or electron-beam computed tomography) in the asymptomatic elderly patient to detect occult or subclinical CHD remains controversial and is not generally recommended.

Chronic Stable Angina in the Elderly Patient

Elderly patients with symptoms suggestive of CHD should undergo a similar assessment of their likelihood for obstructive coronary disease based on algorithms that take into account symptom characteristics, including angina type (nonanginal, atypical, or typical), its course (stable, progressive, or unstable), and its duration. This initial assessment of a patient's "pretest probability of disease" should then guide further diagnostic testing. In particular, clinicians need to be cognizant that, according to Bayesian theory, the predictive value of a test is influenced by the disease prevalence in the population tested. For example, clinicians may interpret a negative stress test in a high-risk elderly woman (pretest probability of disease 80%) as "ruling-out" the presence of CHD, whereas this patient's post-test likelihood remains more than 60% (Table 76-1). For these reasons, elderly patients with high pretest likelihood for coronary disease should be considered for direct referral for cardiac catheterization (if revascularization is an appropriate option). At the other extreme, patients with a low pretest probability for CAD ≤20% (i.e., no risk factors, normal ECG, and very atypical symptoms) can often be followed clinically and/or be assessed for other etiologies of their symptoms (gastrointestinal, pulmonary, musculoskeletal, etc.). Elderly patients with an intermediate pretest probability for CHD (between 20% and 70%) are those in whom stress testing tends to have its greatest impact on clinical decision making.

When a stress test is indicated, current guidelines still recommend standard exercise ECG as the test of choice for most patients. These tests provide very important prognostic information (including exercise duration and hemodynamic response), as well as electrocardiographic indications of ischemia (ST depression). Elderly patients, however, frequently experience difficulty with traditional stress testing because of deconditioning or comorbid illness or disability and may benefit from modified exercise protocols with lower starting levels and slower stage progression. Alternatively, for patients who

TABLE 76-1

Influence of Age on Predictive Value of Stress Testing (Bayes Theorem)

HISTORY	AGE (yr)	PRETEST LIKELIHOOD OF SIGNIFICANT CAD* (%)	TREADMILL TEST†	POSTTEST LIKELIHOOD OF SIGNIFICANT CAD (%)
Female, typical CP ↑ Lipids	45	30	Positive	56
			Negative	16
	75	80	Positive	92
			Negative	63
Female, atypical CP No RF	45	5	Positive	12
			Negative	3
	75	35	Positive	62
			Negative	18

CP, chest pain; RF, risk factors; CAD, coronary artery disease.
*Based on CAD risk nomogram for predicting significant CAD.
†Sensitivity of treadmill test = 68%, specificity = 77%.

cannot exercise sufficiently, one can use a pharmacologic-based stress test (dobutamine, adenosine, or dipyridamole).

In elderly patients with baseline ECGs abnormalities (resting ST depression, left bundle branch block, left ventricular hypertrophy with strain, or paced rhythms), imaging modalities, such as nuclear perfusion or stress echocardiography, are required. While these modalities significantly add to the cost of the test, these improve the diagnostic accuracy beyond stress ECG alone and provide information as to the location and extent of coronary disease. The published sensitivity and specificity for stress echocardiography and nuclear imaging (80–90% for each) are nearly identical in most series. Thus, the choice between the two should be based on local availability and expertise.

The use of cardiac catheterization in the elderly patient needs to be based on its potential risk–benefit ratio. While cardiac catheterization has become commonplace and relatively safe in contemporary practice, vascular injury, bleeding, MI, stroke, and even mortality can result, albeit rarely. Advanced age increases these risks slightly; however, the risk to life remains <0.2%, and the risk of other serious adverse events is <0.5%, even in those aged ≥75 years. Placing a patient even at minimal risk, however, is not worthwhile if the information obtained from a catheterization is unlikely to impact treatment decisions. For example, a cardiac catheterization may have limited impact on the management of an elderly patient who is not a candidate for coronary revascularization, based on medical comorbidity, cognitive decline, or personal preference.

ACUTE CORONARY SYNDROMES

The pathophysiology of the ACS involves atherosclerotic plaque rupture, platelet activation/aggregation and embolization, endothelial dysfunction, inflammation, and thrombus formation. If the clot completely occludes the vessel, the patient suffers an acute MI, and an injury pattern (e.g., ST elevation) is often seen on the ECG. In contrast, patients with plaque rupture can also form a nonocclusive thrombus, resulting in subendocardial ischemia. These patients often have an acceleration of chest pain symptoms (unstable angina) and may have more subtle changes on the ECG (e.g., flipped T waves or ST depression). There is some evidence that plasma levels of procoagulation markers and coagulation factors are elevated in

elderly patients, but it remains unclear whether these findings alone are responsible for increased thrombotic tendencies in the elderly or alter risk when accompanied by other traditional risk factors for thrombotic events.

There are also significant proportions of elderly patients who develop ACS secondary to exacerbations of chronic comorbid conditions or acute medical illnesses. These include sepsis, acute blood loss or chronic anemia, pneumonia, pulmonary embolism, chronic obstructive pulmonary disease, congestive heart failure, dysrhythmias, or hypertensive urgencies. A recent retrospective study demonstrated that approximately 30% of patients present with an acute noncardiac condition concomitant with an MI, contributing to increased in-hospital mortality and variations in receipt of cardiac medications and invasive cardiac therapies. These "secondary" ACSs usually occur in the context of increased myocardial oxygen demand or hemodynamic stress in patients with underlying coronary artery disease and represent a substantial number of cases.

Elderly patients who present with ischemic-type symptoms, which are rapidly progressive, severe, and refractory or which occur at rest, should be immediately transferred to an emergency care setting for further evaluation. Initial testing for myocardial damage should consist of an ECG and cardiac biomarkers (troponin [I or T] and/or creatinine kinase isoforms [CK-MB]). Some patients will have clear ST elevation, making the diagnosis of ST-segment elevation MI (STE MI) straightforward. In others, however, the ECG may be nondiagnostic and the diagnosis often being confirmed by elevations and temporal trends of cardiac biomarkers, with or without accompanying EKG changes. These patients are classified as having non-ST-segment elevation ACS (NSTE ACS).

PROGNOSIS

Multiple studies have shown that once CHD is manifested, the risk of morbidity and mortality increases steadily with age. In two very large randomized trials of patients having with ST elevation, age was the single strongest predictor of both short- and long-term mortality, with the risk of death increasing 6% with each year after 65 years of age. In another large registry population, patients aged 65 to 74 years admitted for an MI were four times more likely to die during the hospitalization than those aged 55 or younger. This risk rose to greater than 10 times higher for patients aged ≥85 years. Elderly patients are also much more likely to suffer complications from their MI, including heart failure, cardiogenic shock, cardiac rupture, atrial fibrillation, stroke, acute renal insufficiency, and pneumonia. Finally, patients aged ≥75 years were three times more likely to be discharged to a nursing facility after an acute MI than those aged 65 to 69 years.

The reasons for increasing MI mortality and morbidity as a function of advancing age are multifold. Elderly patients have less cardiac reserve and more comorbid illness (e.g., pulmonary, renal, and cognitive impairments), limiting their ability to compensate for cardiac events. Also, as noted above, the elderly often present with "secondary" MIs where the cardiac event is a complication of another potential mortal primary process (i.e., sepsis), leading to high mortality. Finally, the elderly patients with MI present later, often receive less aggressive medical care, and undergo fewer potentially life-saving invasive procedures than younger patients.

Acute Coronary Syndrome Therapies

Fibrinolysis and Primary Angioplasty in Elderly Patients

The primary objective in the management of patients with STE MI is to provide early reperfusion therapy with either pharmacological means (i.e., fibrinolysis) or percutaneous intervention with balloon angioplasty. Numerous studies have confirmed that reperfusion therapy (fibrinolytic therapy or primary angioplasty) in patients presenting with acute STE MIs improves survival if performed in a timely fashion. An overview of the major thrombolytic trials from the Fibrinolytic Therapy Trialists' Collaborative Group, a meta-analysis that included more than 58 000 patients, demonstrated a 15% relative risk reduction in death for patients 75 years of age or older with STE MI or bundle branch block treated with fibrinolytics. Despite elderly achieving a smaller relative reduction in death than younger patients, the trend toward absolute benefit in terms of lives saved with fibrinolytics was threefold greater in patients older than 75 years of age compared with those younger than 55 years.

In addition, an adjusted observational analysis from two studies using the Cooperative Cardiovascular Project database reported that patients aged ≥75 years actually had higher 30-day mortality with fibrinolysis than with standard medical therapy. Interestingly, in the one analysis that looked at 1-year outcomes, this early treatment risk in the very elderly reversed itself, and those treated with lysis actually had better survival rates after this interval (OR 0.84, 95% CI 0.79–0.89).

The possible therapeutic benefits of thrombolysis must be weighed carefully against the risks, especially in the elderly. Data from the Fibrinolytic Therapy Trialists' meta-analysis showed that patients aged >70 years had nearly a threefold higher relative risk of intracranial hemorrhage, the most feared complication in the postlytic period, after fibrinolysis than those aged <60 years. Bearing this in mind, clinicians should realize that intracranial hemorrhage is a rare event and the absolute risk of this complication after fibrinolysis in those >70 years remains between 0.7% and 2.1% in major trials and nearing 3% in those older than 85 years of age. The risk factors for intracranial hemorrhage include low body weight, elevated blood pressures, facial or head trauma, and dementia. Dementia was found in one trial to significantly increase the risk for intracranial hemorrhage by threefold.

In contrast with these mixed results for fibrinolysis, reperfusion for STE MI with timely percutaneous transluminal coronary angioplasty (PTCA) is almost universally associated with improved outcomes in all age groups. For example, a recent randomized study of primary PTCA versus thrombolysis in patients with STE MI showed a 40% relative risk reduction for death, MI, and stroke in patients treated within 3 hours of presentation with PTCA. Primary PTCA in treatment of MI in the elderly is also supported by a series of observational analyses. In the Cooperative Cardiovascular Project analysis, acute PTCA was associated with lower 30-day and 1-year mortality when compared to no therapy or thrombolysis among elderly patients with acute MI.

The only caveat to the successes of primary PTCA in elderly patients was seen in a trial of patients with very-high-risk MI whose course was complicated by cardiogenic shock (i.e., hypotension and signs of poor tissue perfusion). In one trial, those randomized to primary PTCA had significantly higher survival rates; however, this effect was age dependent, and those >75 years had actually had much higher mortality risk with PTCA.

Antiplatelet Therapy

There is very strong evidence supporting the long-term benefits of aspirin in patients at risk of CHD. The Antithrombotic Trialists' Collaboration, which performed a meta-analysis of aspirin trials and included more than 135 000 patients, identified a 25% risk reduction in cardiovascular events and noted that similar benefits were maintained in the older-aged patients. In the Physician's Health Study of 44 000 men without known CHD, those randomized to aspirin had a 44% lower risk for subsequent MI versus those taking placebo. Observational data from the Nurse's Health Study suggest similar benefits of aspirin for primary CHD prevention in women. These and other studies have led to the recommendation to treat all patients older than 40 years of age with one or more CHD risk factors with daily aspirin. Although the exact aspirin dose continues to be debated, evidence has suggested that efficacy of aspirin is not increased at doses greater than 150 mg/day, with higher doses increasing the risk for bleeding.

Clopidogrel, a thienopyridine that inhibits ADP-dependent platelet aggregation, was found to add incremental benefit to aspirin therapy in the setting on NSTE ACS by affording a 20% relative risk reduction in cardiovascular death, MI, or stroke in the Clopidogrel in Unstable angina to prevent Recurrent Events trial. The study found similar benefits in elderly patients; nevertheless, registry data suggest that the in-hospital use of clopidogrel in elderly patients after MI remains low. The use of clopidogrel is recommended as an alternative to aspirin in the small subset of patients who are aspirin allergic. Patients who require long-term dual-antiplatelet therapy or oral anticoagulation with warfarin are advised to take a reduced aspirin dose of 81 mg daily.

Intravenous glycoprotein IIb/IIIa inhibitors have also been demonstrated to provide incremental value in patients with high-risk ACS (including ST-segment abnormalities and positive troponin) when used in combination with aspirin and heparin. For example, the Platelet Glycoprotein IIb/IIIa in Unstable Angina: Receptor Suppression Using Integrilin Therapy trial noted a significant overall reduction in death or nonfatal MI (14.2% vs. 15.7%; $P = 0.04$) in patients who were treated with eptifibatide versus placebo. These benefits were also seen in patients aged 70 to 79 years. However, among those aged 80 years or older, benefit was not observed and an associated increase in bleeding events was identified. These later findings suggest the importance of appropriate dosing of these agents in the elderly. In particular, the small molecule glycoprotein IIb/IIIa inhibitors (eptifibatide or tirofiban) are renally cleared; therefore, dosing reductions are often needed in elderly patients. Overall, glycoprotein IIb/IIIa inhibitors appear to have a role in appropriately selected elderly patients presenting with acute MI who are likely to undergo cardiac catheterization. Further research to identify dosing considerations specific to elderly patients and its safe and efficacious application to a heterogeneous elderly population will be needed.

Antithrombin Therapy

Clinical trials of ACS have demonstrated reduction of cardiovascular events with the use of antithrombotic therapies, and these findings have been extended to the elderly population, making their use a class 1 recommendation by the ACC/AHA. Despite this, registry data reflect a decrease in use of antithrombotic therapy in elderly patients when compared to their younger counterparts. Unfractionated heparin, in conjunction with antiplatelet therapy, is associated with significant reduction in death or MI in patients with ACS, but important considerations involving their use are necessary as aged patients are more often susceptible to overdosing, reflected by an elevated partial thromboplastin time, and bleeding. The use of low-molecular-weight heparin for ACS has also been supported by evidence from clinical trials, with some suggestion of improved clinical outcomes, when compared with unfractionated heparin. Subgroup analyses of these studies have demonstrated a greater relative benefit in elderly patients treated with low-molecular-weight heparin, but concerns remain over the dosing of low-molecular-weight heparin in elderly patients, as these therapies are renally cleared and have been associated with excessive dosing and bleeding complications, which have translated to increased adverse events. There remains an ongoing need to further characterize and understand the efficacy and safety of antithrombotic therapies in elderly patients with ACS.

Beta-blockers

Beta-blocker therapy has demonstrated benefit in reducing cardiovascular events and mortality in patients with post-MI. A meta-analysis of 25 randomized control trials showed a 25% reduction from beta-blockers in all-cause mortality and reinfarction in patients with prior MI. Data from an adjusted observational analysis demonstrated that elderly patients receiving beta-blockers following acute MI had a 33% reduction in 1-year mortality compared with those not treated. These long-term benefits are even more remarkable in patients having CHD with chronic heart failure and depressed left ventricular function. Beta-blockers decrease myocardial oxygen demand and improve coronary blood flow and are essential medications in the care of elderly patients with chronic angina.

While beneficial, elderly patients are often vulnerable to drugs with hypotensive actions and have altered responses to beta-blockers owing to conduction system deterioration and diminished adrenergic tone. Additionally, a recent trial found that early use of beta-blockers in patients with MI could worsen risks for congestive heart failure and result in poorer outcomes. Thus, medications should be administered and titrated with caution in elderly patients along with a review of potential drug–drug interactions.

Secondary Prevention Strategies

Medical therapy can play a key role in reducing the morbidity and mortality of CHD in all aged patients. In fact, as elderly patients with CHD face higher overall risk, the benefits of intervention in absolute terms actually tend to rise with age and the corresponding "number needed to treat" for these therapies fall. Secondary prevention therapies are aimed at reducing the recurrence of cardiovascular events in patients with prior MI. These therapies are targeted toward aggressive control of known traditional risk factors, such as hypertension, hyperlipidemia, and tobacco cessation.

Ongoing research has demonstrated that the renin–angiotensin–aldosterone system is a key determinant in hypertension, inflammation, atherosclerosis, and, ultimately, increased cardiovascular events. ACE inhibitors have strong support as safe and effective treatment of hypertension. They have also been shown to improve survival in patients having post-MI with depressed heart function, heart failure, and large anterior MIs. Most recently, the Heart Outcomes Prevention Evaluation study extended the benefits of ACE inhibitors to nearly all patients with either known CHD or who were at high risk of CHD. In Heart Outcomes Prevention Evaluation study, patients with CHD and other patients with high CHD risk (e.g., diabetes plus one or more cardiac risk factor) were randomized to 10 mg of ramipril daily versus placebo. After 5 years, treated patients had 26% lower risk of CHD death than those who were not treated. Rates of MI, congestive heart failure, stroke, renal dysfunction, and even development of diabetes were lower in the ACE-treated patient group. The treatment effects of ACE inhibition were greater in those patients aged ≥65 years than in younger patients. Current guidelines suggest consideration of ACE inhibitors in all patients having CHD with depressed ventricular function, diabetes, or hypertension. Some experts have suggested that these drugs be considered in all patients with known CHD regardless of other risk factors or left ventricular dysfunction, yet there remains conflicting evidence from clinical trials regarding this issue. Angiotensin receptor blockers (ARBs), similar to ACE inhibitors, are designed to produce antihypertensive and anti-inflammatory effects within the cardiovascular system, and recent studies demonstrate that these agents translate to decreased cardiovascular events. Several randomized control trials have shown that the ARBs can slow the progression of nephropathy in patients with diabetes and microalbuminuria in a fashion similar to ACE inhibitors. Overall, the data favor the use of established ACE inhibitors for primary and secondary prevention of cardiovascular events, with the consideration of ARB substitution in patients who are intolerant of ACE inhibitors (most commonly from troublesome cough). Patients who experience angioedema secondary to ACE inhibitor therapy should not be prescribed ARBs because of the risk of cross-reactivity. When used in elderly patients, however, one should carefully monitor serum electrolytes and creatinine, as these drugs can cause decreased renal function and hyperkalemia.

There are several classes of drugs marketed for lowering serum cholesterol. These include fibrates, bile acid sequestrants, niacin, fish oil, and the HMG-CoA (hydroxymethylglutaryl coenzyme A) reductase inhibitors (statins). Of these, statins have the most evidence supporting their efficacy in primary and secondary CHD prevention. A meta-analysis done with pooled data from five large statin randomized control trials—two primary prevention and three secondary prevention studies—showed an average 31% relative risk reduction in coronary events and 29% relative risk reduction in coronary deaths. Unfortunately, of these five trials only one included patients aged ≥65 years and none included patients older than 75 years of age. Thus, the question of whether lipid lowering benefited the very elderly remained inconclusive until the recent Heart Protection Study.

The Heart Protection Study trial randomized more than 20 000 patients aged 40 to 80 years with known CHD or high-risk profiles to 40 mg of simvastatin daily or placebo. After 5 years, patients on simvastatin had a 16% relative risk reduction in cardiovascular deaths and 22% relative risk reduction in major cardiovascular events relative to placebo. Most importantly, the benefit of lipid-lowering therapy was independent of age and persisted among those in their middle eighties. Consistent with the results of this recent study, the NCEP guidelines for lipid-lowering therapy do not include age cutoffs or age-specific treatment recommendations. While lipid-lowering drugs are generally safe in elderly patients, routine monitoring of liver function studies are recommended.

Intensive lipid-lowering therapy in the post-MI period to prevent recurrent cardiovascular events has demonstrated benefit in elderly patients. In a post hoc analysis of the Pravastatin or Atorvastatin Evaluation and Infection Therapy-Thrombolysis in Myocardial Infarction (PROVE IT-TIMI 22) trial, elderly patients 70 years of age and older were found to derive greater benefit than younger counterparts in terms of reduction in cardiovascular events. In addition, the results suggested that if the NCEP optional LDL goal of less than 70 mg/dL were achieved, one could prevent four times as many events in the elderly as compared with the younger cohort. The benefits of statin therapy beyond lipid lowering alone—the so called pleiotropic effects—remain areas of ongoing investigation and suggest mechanisms of plaque stabilization, anti-inflammatory effects, and improvement in endothelial function as potential contributors to the overall cardiovascular benefit of these agents.

Post-MI Testing

The post-MI period requires not only the initiation and continuation of the evidence-based medical therapies already reviewed but also further assessment of an individual's risk for future cardiovascular events. Care guidelines recommend that all those diagnosed with an MI should have an assessment of both left ventricular function (via echocardiography or other means) and coronary disease severity. In patients with NSTE ACS, the two options for assessment of post-MI risk are routine angiography with revascularization for all patients who have no contraindications or a conservative strategy

of medical therapy with patient selection for angiography based on symptoms or demonstrable ischemia on investigation ("ischemia-driven" approach). While in the past it had been suggested that "early invasive" (cardiac catheterization) and noninvasive (stress testing) approaches represented equivalent strategies, recent clinical trials suggest that the early invasive approach might be preferable for patients at increased risk of recurrent cardiovascular events. With the introduction of contemporary trials, the Treat Angina with Aggrastat and Determine Cost of Therapy with an Invasive or Conservative Strategy-Thrombolysis in Myocardial Ischemia/Infarction (TACTICS-TIMI)-18 trial randomized patients with unstable angina/NSTE ACS to one or the other of these strategies and found that those in the early invasive arm (within 48 hours) had nearly 20% lower rates of death, nonfatal MI, or rehospitalization at 6 months than conservatively treated patients. Interestingly, the successful enrollment of elderly patients (40% of patients were 65 years of age or older) allowed the identification of a 44% relative risk reduction in 30-day death or nonfatal MI among patients 65 years or older (invasive 5.7% vs. conservative 9.8%; $P < 0.05$) and a 56% relative risk reduction in patients older than 75 years of age (invasive 10.8% vs. conservative 21.6%; $P < 0.05$) with the early invasive strategy, findings consistent with a greater benefit in the elderly relative to younger patients.

CORONARY REVASCULARIZATION

A major challenge in the care of elderly patients with CHD is related to who should be considered a candidate for coronary revascularization. In younger patients, randomized clinical trials have simplified this decision-making process by identifying subgroups in which PTCA or coronary artery bypass graft (CABG) surgery improves survival and/or quality of life beyond medical therapy. However, patients older than 75 years were generally not represented in these pivotal trials. Instead, clinicians and patients must rely on a careful comparison between the acute procedural risks and potential long-term benefits.

Procedural mortality rates following revascularization procedures rise dramatically and progressively with advancing age. Figure 76-3 displays the risks for in-hospital mortality following angioplasty and CABG from 123 991 patients in the National Cardiovascular Network Revascularization database. From these data, it is clear that age-associated risk in procedural mortality is not strictly linear but rises more rapidly beyond the age of 75 years. Additionally, at any age, patients with CABG face two- to threefold higher mortality risks than do patients receiving angioplasty. However, technological advances have led to improved procedural success rates and lower

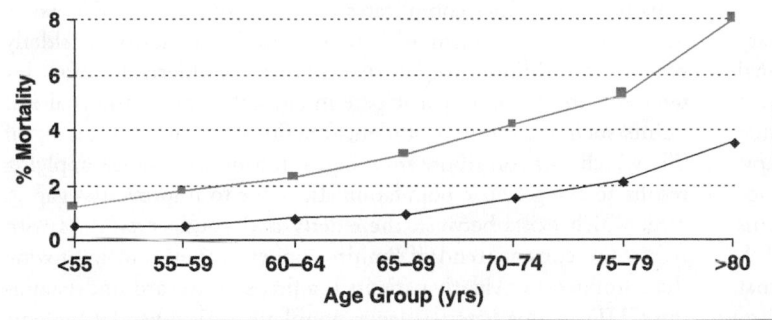

FIGURE 76-3. In-hospital mortality following coronary artery bypass surgery and angioplasty by patient age (National Cardiovascular Network Registry 1994–1998).

risks for both procedures. Thus, despite the fact that procedures were performed on patients with higher risk, the risk of death after CABG in patients aged 65 years or older in the Society for Thoracic Surgery database declined nearly 20% between 1990 and 1999 and now rests at just above 4%. The Society for Thoracic Surgery has devised risk models that can be used to guide the impact of patient risk factors on operative morbidity and mortality and can be used in patient management. The web-based risk calculator can be found at http://www.sts.org.

Nonfatal procedural complications (stroke, MI, and renal failure) also rise in a curvilinear fashion with age and are higher in patients with CABG relative to those undergoing angioplasty. Of major importance to many elderly patients are the procedural risks of stroke and loss in mental acuity. Patients with CABG aged 75 years or older have a reported 3% to 6% incidence of permanent overt stroke as compared with a <1% incidence for angioplasty. Additionally, by using highly sensitive neurocognitive testing, Newman and colleagues found that up to 50% of patients of all ages undergoing CABG had measurable impairments in neurocognitive function at hospital discharge. Although half of patients with initial impairment recovered by 6 months, cognitive deficits reappeared in many of them during long-term follow-up and portended an impaired functional status. However, one recent study that compared cognitive ability after CABG to angioplasty and age-matched controls noted no meaningful clinical deterioration of cognitive performance between groups. Similarly, the initial enthusiasm of improving neurocognitive outcomes by performing off-pump CABG versus traditional on-pump CABG has been tempered by findings from a recent randomized trial, which demonstrated comparable cognitive outcomes between the two groups, although long-term follow-up has yet to occur. While increasing age is generally a major risk factor for procedural complications or mortality, it is not the only factor to consider. For example, by using published risk models, one can stratify an octogenarian's likelihood for mortality with CABG from 2% to 3% for a "healthy" patient without other comorbidities, to greater than 30% for the patient with multiple risk factors such as diabetes or preexisting cerebrovascular disease.

As with reperfusion therapy, the risks of revascularization must be balanced against the potential benefits in terms of prolonged survival, improved functional outcomes, or both. The Alberta Provincial Project for Outcomes Assessment in Coronary Heart Disease registry examined the care and outcomes of more than 6000 patients aged 70 to 79 years who underwent cardiac catheterization. Compared with medical therapy, those receiving CABG or PTCA had significantly higher adjusted 4-year survival rates (CABG 87%, PTCA 84%, medical therapy 79%, $P < 0.001$). These survival benefits of revascularization also held for octogenarians and increased in all aged patients in proportion with the number of diseased vessels and the degree of left ventricular dysfunction. Results from the Alberta Provincial Project for Outcomes Assessment in Coronary Heart Disease registry have been confirmed in other observational analyses. Together, these studies strongly suggest that elderly patients with multivessel coronary disease have higher survival rates if treated with PTCA or CABG than if they are treated with medical therapy.

Beyond survival, there is also a growing body of literature to support the notion that PTCA and CABG also reduce angina symptoms and improve functional outcomes of elderly patients with CHD. Initially, these results were reported in observational studies that adjusted for treatment-selection issues, as well as other baseline clinical factors. Most recently, similar results have been validated in the Trial of Invasive Versus Medical Therapy in Elderly Patients with Chronic Symptomatic Coronary Artery Disease trial. The Trial of Invasive Versus Medical Therapy in Elderly Patients with Chronic Symptomatic Coronary Artery Disease study randomized 305 patients with chronic angina, aged 75 years or older, to diagnostic catheterization (followed by coronary revascularization as appropriate) or optimized medical therapy with intervention only for those with refractory symptoms. Of those randomized to catheterization and intervention as appropriate, 74% underwent CABG or PTCA, while almost 33% of the conservative management arm crossed over to revascularization by 6 months. Patients in the early revascularization arm had significantly greater improvement in their symptoms and almost all aspects of functional status and quality of life when compared with medically treated patients. However, clinical end points in the trial were mixed, with a higher 6-month mortality rate but a lower incidence of nonfatal MI in the early invasive arm. While this randomized study was limited in sample size and presented several methodological challenges, its results do provide further support for the consideration of revascularization in the very elderly patient with CHD. While we await more representative randomized trials, the ACC/AHA guidelines stipulate that age should not be used as the sole criterion to rule out consideration of revascularization and that complex medical and surgical interventions have an adjunctive role in the care of elderly patients when in accordance with available scientific evidence and with the wishes of the patient.

SPECIAL CONSIDERATIONS

Underrepresentation in Clinical Trials

Clinical trials should closely approximate treated populations to increase applicability, yet almost all of the national treatment guidelines have been based on trials performed predominately in younger patients, and elderly patients have been routinely and greatly underrepresented. For example, up to 60% of cardiovascular clinical trials performed prior to 1990 explicitly excluded elderly patients. Even among recent studies (i.e., those published since 1995), fewer than 50% of studies enrolled a single patient aged 75 years or older. Patients older than 75 years comprise approximately 9% of the population enrolled in clinical trials of ACS therapies, but account for more than 37% of patients treated for ACS in the community. This age difference is reflected in the greater average age of patients treated for ACS in the community compared to trial populations, highlighting the known fact that patients treated for ACS in the community often have greater comorbidity and are at greater disease-related risk. This practice further complicates the interpretation of trial results when these are obtained with small samples of healthier, elderly patients. In addition, studies suggest that the elderly are often interested and willing to participate in clinical research and trial end points such as symptom burden, functional status, and quality of life, which can contribute meaningful information when applying results to the geriatric population. In order to improve the gap in care, which exists between the elderly and younger patients with ACSs, the current trend of limiting age exclusions and improving the enrollment of elderly patients is a first step toward understanding CHD in this heterogeneous population. Beyond the biologic

TABLE 76-2

Key Differences in Elderly Patients

Cardiovascular
- Greater multivessel CHD
- Diastolic heart dysfunction
- Arterial stiffness, systolic hypertension, and endothelial dysfunction
- Increased conduction system disease

General health
- Medical comorbidity
- Cognitive and functional impairment
- Atypical symptoms of disease

Social
- More social isolation
- Hearing and visual impairments
- Limited or fixed financial resources
- Less formal education
- Different health-care expectations

Drug related
- Polypharmacy
- Altered drug metabolism
- Different body composition
- Altered volume of distribution

Biologic
- Anemia
- Altered coagulation and fibrinolytic proteins
- Elevated markers of inflammation

and cardiovascular changes observed with aging, fundamental ethical concerns are at the core of the patient–physician relationship, with particular emphasis on efforts to preserve individual autonomy and adhere to the doctrine of "do no harm." The recognition of important differences between younger and older patients is at the foundations of providing patient-centered and effective care for the elderly (Table 76-2).

Renal Function and Pharmacology

Consistently, an individual's renal function remains a powerful predictor of cardiovascular morbidity and mortality. In the Cooperative Cardiovascular Project, renal dysfunction predicted adverse outcomes among an elderly post-MI population, such that 1-year mortality was 24% if serum creatinine was below 1.5 mg/dL and 66% if creatinine was above 2.5 mg/dL. The pitfalls attributed to using the serum creatinine as a surrogate for renal function are often compounded in the elderly. For example, most laboratories often report the result of a serum creatinine of 1.2 mg/dL as "normal." However, when one considers that the sample is from an 85-year-old Caucasian female who weighs 125 pounds, using the Cockcroft–Gault formula, the estimated glomerular filtration rate is below 30 mL/min, consistent with severe renal impairment, and would necessitate dosing adjustments for many pharmacological agents. Consistent with recommendations from the Panel on Acute Coronary Care in the Elderly, the creatinine clearance should be calculated on all patients 75 years of age or older who present with an ACS. In addition, the clinician should remain cognizant of changes in the creatinine clearance during the index hospitalization and after discharge, as several medications prescribed may have an impact on renal function. From the Global Registry of Acute Coronary Events study, a 10 mL/minute decrease in creatinine clearance had the same impact on in-hospital mortality as a 10-year increase in age. The role of renal dysfunction in the management of elderly patients with ACSs cannot be overemphasized, as this entity plays a pivotal role at the interface of pharmacological management.

Cardiovascular drugs are among the most commonly prescribed therapies in elderly patients, and altered pharmacokinetics (i.e., drug distribution and metabolism) are frequently observed in elderly patients as a consequence of decreased lean body mass and volume of distribution. Combined, these factors lead to higher drug concentrations and prolonged half-lives. A drug's pharmacodynamics (i.e., the effect of a drug on a target cell) can be considerably altered with age. For example, increased calcification of the cardiac conduction system can increase an elderly patient's sensitivity to atrioventricular nodal blocking agents and lead to profound bradycardia. Comorbid illness and frailty can also influence drug selection and safety. For instance, a frail elderly person may have a higher risk of falling, which can markedly increase the likelihood of bleeding complications with anticoagulants. Finally, polypharmacy is often a serious issue in the elderly and can lead to life-threatening drug–drug interactions and poor compliance because of confusion over medications and/or prohibitive costs. It has been estimated that 25% of older patients have had at least one adverse drug reaction and that drug reactions are responsible for 3% to 10% of all hospital admissions in the elderly. Geriatricians have the adage, "start low, go slow," in recognition of polypharmacy, altered drug distribution and clearance, and adverse drug reactions common among the elderly.

Patient Preferences

Beyond physiological and pharmacological issues, cardiac treatment plans need to consider the patients' overall health, as well as their health preferences and willingness to accept risk. While some elderly individuals engage in very active, independent lives well into their advanced years, others are frail and suffer from disabling physical and/or mental illnesses. Beyond this variability in health and functional status, there is great diversity in the health values of elderly patients. Some consider illness and disability to be inevitable and have no interest in extensive medical or surgical intervention. However, many elderly patients favor longevity if coupled with good cognitive ability and lack of neurological disability. In hospital settings, many elderly patients feel vulnerable and abdicate medical decision making to family or physicians, who are being entrusted to act in the patient's best interest. It is incumbent on physicians caring for elderly individuals to attempt to directly elicit the elderly patient's treatment goals, while providing the patient with the necessary information regarding potential risks and benefits of each treatment option.

Social/Economic Issues

Finally, in devising a rational treatment plan for the elderly cardiac patients, physicians must consider the patient's social and economic situation. Transportation issues, which are a major limitation for many elderly persons, can disrupt close office follow-up. Many elderly patients live on fixed incomes and may not realize or acknowledge that they cannot afford multiple cardiac medications. Hearing and visual deficits may impair health communication and comprehension. Prior negative experiences within the health-care

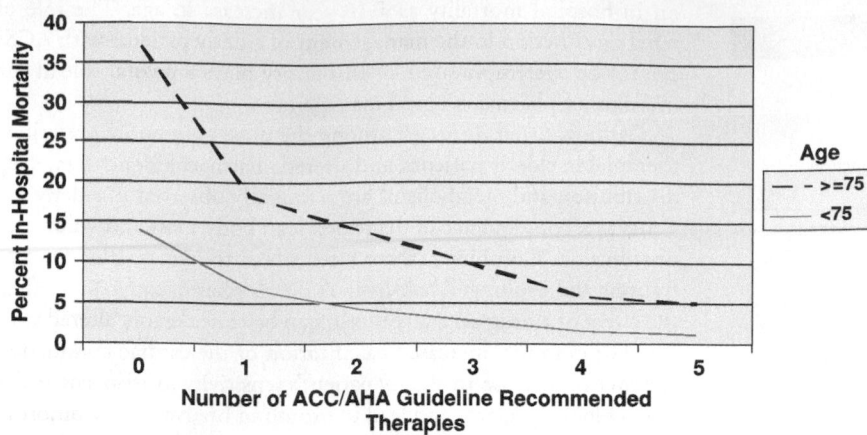

Adjusted in-hospital mortality among older and younger patients

Age
- - >=75
— <75

FIGURE 76-4. Evidence based care in elderly patients. Adherence to ACC/AHA guidelines improves outcomes. (Adapted from Alexander et al. Evolution in Cardiovascular Case For Elderly Patients With Non-ST-Segment Elevation Acute Coronary Syndromes: Results From the CRUSADE National Quality Improvement Initiative. J Am Coll Cardiol. 2005;46:1479, with permission.)

system may impact an elderly patient's willingness to receive care on subsequent occasions. The elderly population typically has fewer college graduates, and they are less likely to be connected to important sources of information and support. The health of an ailing spouse can also substantially impact on an elderly caregiver's personal health. Recently, one study found that the survival of a caregiving partner after hospitalization or death of a spouse was associated with an increased risk of death in the caregiver, particularly for the first 30 days. Although not thoroughly studied, clinicians must be aware of these fundamental issues and understand that additional time and attention are necessary to ensure proper communication during the physician–patient encounter.

SUMMARY

Despite remarkable advances in prevention and treatment, CHD remains a major health problem for the elderly in terms of morbidity and mortality. As our population ages, the need for high-quality, well-informed cardiac care for patients aged ≥75 years will increase. Opportunities for improvement in care are highlighted by the fact that, given their greater age-related risks, older patients benefit as much, if not more, from existing therapies as do younger patients. However, the care of CHD in the elderly takes place within the context of their multidimensional health status and requires awareness of atypical presentations of ACS, altered pharmacokinetics of therapy, and underlying cognitive and functional status. Bearing this in mind, evidence continues to demonstrate that many treatment paradigms applied to younger patient groups are appropriate when treating very elderly patients, and adherence to ACC/AHA guidelines for ACS translates into better outcomes (Figure 76-4). Similarly, the durability of coronary artery revascularization over medical therapy for multivessel CHD in elderly patients has shown reduction in morbidity and mortality over time. The observation that cardiovascular trials have shifted to include broader enrollment of elderly patients and gather information beyond traditional endpoints will undoubtedly impact the evidence base of geriatric cardiology. The identification of physiological frailty through performance measures may offer additional risk assessment of elderly patients before complex medical therapy or revascularization is undertaken. This information could potentially identify a cohort of patients who may

benefit from a geriatric intervention program before or after hospitalization or revascularization. Finally, studies must focus on relative safety and efficacy in medical or procedural interventions when reporting results on elderly patients. There are significant challenges in this complex area of cardiovascular care, but redirecting efforts to a patient-centered model, while balancing risk versus benefit of selected strategies, may provide additional opportunity to both improve current care practices and limit harm and disability.

FURTHER READING

Alexander KP, Roe MT, Chen AY, et al: Evolution in cardiovascular care for elderly patients with non-ST-segment elevation acute coronary syndromes. Results from the CRUSADE national quality improvement initiative. J Am Coll Cardiol. 2005;46:1479.

Alexander KP, et al. Acute coronary care in the elderly: a statement for healthcare professionals from the acute cardiac care subcommittee, council of clinical cardiology. American Heart Association. Circulation. 2007;115:2549.

American Heart Association. 2002 Heart and Stroke Statistical Update. Dallas, TX: American Heart Association; 2002. Available at: www.americanheart.org/statistics/medical.html.

Antithrombotic Trialists' Collaboration. Collaborative meta-analysis of randomized trials of antiplatelet therapy for prevention of death, myocardial infarction, and stroke in high risk patients. BMJ. 2002;324:71.

Antman EM, Anbe DT, Armstrong PW, et al. ACC/AHA guidelines for the management of patients with ST-elevation myocardial infarction: executive summary: a report of the ACC/AHA Task Force on Practice Guidelines. J Am Coll Cardiol. 2004;44:671.

Batchelor WB, Anstrom KJ, Muhlbaier LH, et al. Contemporary outcome trends in the elderly undergoing percutaneous coronary interventions: results in 7,472 octogenarians. J Am Coll Cardiol. 2000;36:723.

Berger AK, Schulman KA, Gersh BJ, et al. Primary coronary angioplasty vs. thrombolysis for the management of acute myocardial infarction in elderly patients. JAMA. 1999;282:341.

Bhatia RS, Tu JV, Lee DS, et al. Outcome of heart failure with preserved ejection fraction in a population-based study. N Engl J Med. 2006;355:260.

Braunwald E, Antman EM, Beasley JW, et al. ACC/AHA guideline update for the management of patients with unstable angina and non-ST-segment elevation myocardial infarction: a report of the American College of Cardiology/American Heart Association Task Force on Practice Guidelines (Committee on the Management of Patients With Unstable Angina). J Am Coll Cardiol. 2002;40:1366.

Brieger D, Eagle KA, Goodman SG, et al.; for the GRACE Investigators. Acute coronary syndromes without chest pain, an underdiagnosed and undertreated high-risk group: insights from the Global Registry of Acute Coronary Events. Chest. 2004;126:461.

Cannon CP, Weintraub WS, Demopoulos LA, et al.; for the TACTICS-TIMI 18 Investigators. Comparison of early invasive and conservative strategies in patients with unstable coronary syndromes treated with the glycoprotein IIb/IIIa inhibitor tirofiban. N Engl J Med. 2001;344:1879.

Cheitlin MD, Gerstenblith G, Hazzard WR, et al. Do existing databases answer clinical questions about geriatric cardiovascular disease and stroke? Am J Geriatr Cardiol. 2001;10:207.

Christakis NA, Allison PD. Mortality after the hospitalization of a spouse. *N Engl J Med.* 2006;354:719.

Cohen HJ, et al. A controlled trial of inpatient and outpatient geriatric evaluation and management. *N Engl J Med.* 2002;346:905.

Eagle KA, Guyton RA, Davidoff R, et al. ACC/AHA guidelines for coronary artery bypass graft surgery: executive summary and recommendations. A report of the American College of Cardiology/American Heart Association Task Force on Practice Guidelines (Committee to Revise the 1991 Guidelines for Coronary Artery Bypass Graft Surgery). *Circulation.* 1999;100:1464.

Ernest CS, Worcester MU, Tatoulis J, et al. Neurocognitive outcomes in off-pump versus on-pump bypass surgery: a randomized controlled trial. *Ann Thorac Surg.* 2006;81:2105.

Expert Panel on Detection, Evaluation, and Treatment of High Blood Cholesterol in Adults. Executive summary of the third report of the National Cholesterol Education Program (NCEP) Expert Panel on Detection, Evaluation, and Treatment of High Blood Cholesterol in Adults (Adult Treatment Panel III). *JAMA.* 2001;285:2486.

Ferrario CM, Strawn WB, et al. Role of the renin–angiotensin–aldosterone system and proinflammatory mediators in cardiovascular disease. *Am J Cardiol.* 2006;98:121.

Fibrinolytic Therapy Trialists' (FTT) Collaborative Group. Indications for fibrinolytic therapy in suspected acute myocardial infarction: collaborative overview of early mortality and major morbidity results from all randomized trials of more than 1000 patients. *Lancet.* 1994;343:311.

Fuster V, Badimon L, Badimon JJ, et al. The pathogenesis of coronary artery disease and the acute coronary syndrome. *N Engl J Med.* 1992;326:242.

Gibbons JG, Balady GJ, Beasley JW, et al. ACC/AHA guidelines for exercise testing: executive summary: a Report of the ACC/AHA Task Force on Practice Guidelines (Committee on Exercise Testing). *Circulation.* 1997;96:345.

Gibbons RJ, Chatterjee K, Daley J, et al. ACC/AHA/ACP-ASIM guidelines for the management of patients with chronic stable angina: executive summary and recommendations: a report of the ACC/AHA Task Force on Practice Guidelines (Committee on Management of Patients With Chronic Stable Angina). *Circulation.* 1999;99:2829.

Goff DC, Feldman HA, McGovern PG, et al.; for the Rapid Early Action for Coronary Treatment (REACT) Study Group. Prehospital delay in patients hospitalized with heart attack symptoms in the United States: the REACT trial. *Am Heart J.* 1999;138:1046.

Goldberg RJ, Yarzebski J, Lessard D, et al. Decade-long trends and factors associated with time to hospital presentation in patients with acute myocardial infarction: the Worcester Heart Attack Study. *Arch Intern Med* 2000;160:3217.

Graham MM, Ghali WA, Faris PD, et al. Survival after coronary revascularization in the elderly (APPROACH). *Circulation.* 2002;105:2378.

Greenland P, Smith SC, Jr, Grundy SM. Improving coronary heart disease risk assessment in asymptomatic people: role of traditional risk factors and noninvasive cardiovascular tests. *Circulation.* 2001;104:1863.

Gregoratos G. Clinical manifestations of acute myocardial infarction in older patients. *Am J Geriatr Cardiol.* 2001;10:345.

Hasdai D, Holmes DR, Jr, Criger DA, et al.; for the PURSUIT Trial Investigators. Age and outcome after acute coronary syndromes without persistent ST-segment elevation. *Am Heart J.* 2000;139:858.

Heart Protection Study Collaborative Group. MRC/BHF Heart Protection Study of cholesterol lowering with simvastatin in 20,536 high-risk individuals: a randomized placebo-controlled trial. *Lancet.* 2002;360:7.

Hoyert DL, Heron MP, Murphy SL, et al. *Deaths: Final Data for 2003. National Vital Statistics Reports.* Vol. 54, No. 13. Hyattsville, MD: National Center for Health Statistics; 2006.

Kandzari DE, Granger CB, Simoons ML, et al.; for the GUSTO-I Investigators. Risk factors for intracranial hemorrhage and nonhemorrhagic stroke after fibrinolytic therapy. *Am J Cardiol.* 2004;93:458.

Kausik KR, Bach RG, Cannon CP, et al.; for the PROVE IT-TIMI 22 Investigators. Benefits of achieving the NCEP optional LDL-C goal among elderly patients with ACS. *Eur Heart J.* 2006;27:2310.

Krumholz HM, Radford MJ, Wang Y, et al. National use and effectiveness of β-blockers for the treatment of elderly patients after acute myocardial infarction: Nation Cooperative Cardiovascular Project. *JAMA.* 1998;280:623.

LaRosa JC, He J, Vupputuri S, et al. Effects of statins on risk of coronary disease: a meta-analysis of randomized controlled trials. *JAMA.* 1999;282:2340.

Lee PY, Alexander KP, Hammill BG, et al. Representation of elderly persons and women in published randomized trials of acute coronary syndromes. *JAMA.* 2001;286:708.

Lichtman JH, Fathi A, Radford MJ, et al. Acute, severe noncardiac conditions in patients with acute myocardial infarction. *Am J Med.* 2006;119:843.

Mari D, Mannucci PM, Coppola B, et al. Hypercoagulability in centenarians: the paradox of successful aging. *Blood.* 1995;85:3144.

Mehta RH, Rathore SS, Radford MJ, et al. Acute myocardial infarction in the elderly: differences by age. *J Am Coll Cardiol.* 2001;38:736.

Mittelmark MB, Psaty BM, Rautanariu PM, et al. Prevalence of cardiovascular diseases among older adults: the Cardiovascular Health Study. *Am J Epidemiol.* 1993;137:311.

Newman MF, Kirchner JL, Phillips-Bute B, et al.; for the Neurological Outcome Research Group and the Cardiothoracic Anesthesiology Research Endeavors Investigators. Longitudinal assessment of neurocognitive function after coronary-artery bypass surgery. *N Engl J Med.* 2001;344:395.

Pasquali SK, Alexander KP, Peterson ED. Cardiac rehabilitation in the elderly. *Am Heart J.* 2001;142:748.

Pryor DB, Shaw L, McCants CB, et al. Value of the history and physical in identifying patients at increased risk for coronary artery disease. *Ann Intern Med.* 1993;118:81.

Purser JL, Kuchibhatla MN, Fillenbaum GG, et al. Identifying frailty in hospitalized older adults with significant coronary artery disease. *J Am Ger Soc.* 2006;54:1674.

PURSUIT Trial Investigators. Inhibition of platelet glycoprotein IIb/IIIa with eptifibatide in patients with acute coronary syndromes. *N Engl J Med.* 1998;339:436.

Rosengart TK, Sweet JJ, Finnin E, et al. Stable cognition after coronary artery bypass grafting: comparison with percutaneous intervention and normal controls. *Ann Thorac Surg.* 2006;82:597.

Ryan TJ, Antman EM, Brooks NH, et al. 1999 update: ACC/AHA guidelines for the management of patients with acute myocardial infarction: executive summary and recommendations: a report of the ACC/AHA Task Force on Practice Guidelines (Committee on Management of Acute Myocardial Infarction). *Circulation.* 1999;100:1016.

Santopinto JJ, Fox KAA, Goldberg RJ, et al.; for the GRACE Investigators. Creatinine clearance and adverse hospital outcomes in patients with acute coronary syndromes: findings from the global registry of acute coronary events (GRACE). *Heart.* 2003;89:1003.

Scheifer SE, Gersh BJ, Yanez ND III, et al. Prevalence, predisposing factors, and prognosis of clinically unrecognized myocardial infarction in the elderly. *J Am Coll Cardiol.* 2000;35:119.

Shlipak MG, Heidenreich PA, Noguchi H, et al. Association of renal insufficiency with treatment and outcomes after myocardial infarction in elderly patients. *Ann Intern Med.* 2002;137:555.

Smith SC Jr, Dove JT, Jacobs AK, et al. ACC/AHA guidelines for percutaneous coronary intervention (revision of the 1993 PTCA guidelines) - executive summary. A report of the American College of Cardiology/American Heart Association Task Force on Practice Guidelines (Committee to Revise the 1993 Guidelines for Percutaneous Transluminal Coronary Angioplasty). *Circulation.* 2001;103:3019.

The Heart Outcomes Prevention Evaluation (HOPE) Study Investigators. Effects of an angiotensin-converting-enzyme inhibitor, ramipril, on cardiovascular events in high-risk patients. *N Engl J Med.* 2000;342:145.

The Joint National Committee on Prevention, Detection, Evaluation, and Treatment of High Blood Pressure. The seventh report of the Joint National Committee on Prevention, Detection, Evaluation, and Treatment of High Blood Pressure. *Hypertension.* 2003;42:1206.

The TIME Investigators. Trial of invasive versus medical therapy in elderly patients with chronic symptomatic coronary-artery disease (TIME). *Lancet.* 2001;358:951.

Wang TJ, Gona P, Larson MG, et al. Multiple biomarkers for the prediction of first major cardiovascular events and death. *N Engl J Med.* 2006;355:2631.

Wei JY. Age and the cardiovascular system. *N Engl J Med.* 1992;327:1735.

White HD, Kleiman NS, Mahaffey KW, et al. Efficacy and safety of enoxaparin compared with unfractionated heparin in high-risk patients with non ST-segment elevation acute coronary syndrome undergoing percutaneous coronary intervention in the Superior Yield of the New Strategy of Enoxaparin, Revascularization and Glycoprotein IIb/IIIa Inhibitors (SYNERGY) trial. *Am Heart J.* 2006;152:1042.

Williams MA, Fleg JL, Ades PA, et al. Secondary prevention of coronary heart disease in the elderly (with emphasis on patients ≥75 years of age). An American Heart Association scientific statement from the Council on Clinical Cardiology Subcommittee on Exercise, Cardiac Rehabilitation, and Prevention. *Circulation.* 2002;105:1735.

Yusuf S, Zhao F, Mehta SR, et al.; for The Clopidogrel in Unstable Angina to Prevent Recurrent Events (CURE) Trial Investigators. Effects of clopidogrel in addition to aspirin in patients with acute coronary syndromes without ST-segment elevation. *N Engl J Med.* 2001;345:494.

Valvular Heart Disease

Nikhila Deo ■ *Niloo M. Edwards*

AORTIC STENOSIS

Etiology

Aortic stenosis is present in 2% to 9% of older patients and is the leading clinically significant valvular disorder in the elderly. The etiologies for aortic stenosis in this age group include calcification of a normal tricuspid aortic valve, calcification of a congenital bicuspid valve, and rheumatic valve disease.

Aortic stenosis in 90% of patients older than 65 years is caused by calcification of a tricuspid valve. The causes of aortic valvular calcification are unclear, although the process bears many similarities to atherosclerosis; both diseases are characterized by lipid deposition, inflammation, neoangiogenesis, and calcification. Even though the bicuspid aortic valve is the most common adult congenital cardiac anomaly and is present in approximately 2% of births, only one-third will progress to aortic stenosis with valve degeneration most frequently presenting in the fourth to sixth decade of life. Thus, it is not a major cause of aortic stenosis in the elderly. Similarly, rheumatic disease similarly presents earlier in life and often in association with mitral valve disease.

Clinical Presentation and Diagnosis

Aortic stenosis has a long asymptomatic period of latency, when the only finding is a harsh, late-peaking, crescendo–decrescendo systolic murmur that radiates to the carotids and is best heard over the right, second interspace: The second heart sound (S_2) may be paradoxically split. Characteristically, aortic stenosis is associated with "pulsus parvus et tardus": meaning the patient has a weak and diminished pulse with a late upstroke that is most easily noted in the carotids. However, these characteristic physical findings may be less obvious both in the elderly, because of the ef-

fects of aging on the vascular bed, and when the ventricle starts to fail.

The American Heart Association recommends evaluation of early systolic, midsystolic grade 3 or greater, late systolic, or holosystolic murmurs with echocardiography. Older patients may present with ominous murmurs owing to aortic valve sclerosis without significant valvular stenosis. Aortic stenosis is graded as mild, moderate, or severe (Table 77-1).

On average, the rate of progression of disease has been estimated at an increase in jet velocity of 0.3 m/s/yr with an associated reduction in valve area of 0.1 cm²/yr. Despite these average rates of disease progression, the rate for any one individual is difficult to predict; therefore, asymptomatic patients with mild-to-moderate disease should be followed on a regular basis.

Aortic sclerosis is defined as aortic valve thickening without outflow tract obstruction. This pathology is present in 25% of patients older than 65 years and 48% of those older than 75 years; it is associated with male gender, hypertension, smoking, diabetes mellitus, and lipid abnormalities. The rate of progression to frank stenosis is not clear, but the Cardiovascular Health Study has identified an increased incidence of adverse cardiovascular outcomes in patients with sclerotic valve even when corrected for other cardiovascular risk factors. The mechanism for this association is unclear, and there are currently no guidelines for intervention.

Older patients slated for valve replacement should undergo preoperative coronary artery angiography. Measurement of the transvalvular gradient can aid in the diagnosis if there is a question about the severity of the stenosis; however, it is not recommended as a tool for assessment of the severity of disease in the asymptomatic patient, or if the noninvasive studies are consistent with the physical findings.

Impaired platelet function and decreased levels of Von Willebrand factor are also associated with severe aortic stenosis, and 20% of patients may present with epistaxis or ecchymoses; interestingly both abnormalities will resolve with valve replacement.

TABLE 77-1

Echocardiographic Findings in Aortic Stenosis			
	MILD	MODERATE	SEVERE
Aortic valve area (cm²)	>1.5	1.0–1.5	<1.0
Velocity (m/s)	<3	3–4	>4
Mean gradient (mm Hg)	<25	25–40	>40

Patients with aortic valve stenosis also develop compensatory left ventricular hypertrophy, which can be seen both on echocardiogram and on electrocardiogram. The ventricular hypertrophy produces coronary malperfusion with subendocardial ischemia. These hypertrophied ventricles are also more sensitive to ischemic injury. Elderly females are prone to develop excessive ventricular hypertrophy, which may contribute to the higher perioperative morbidity and mortality in this cohort of patients.

Although aortic stenosis has a long latency, once symptoms develop the progression to death is rapid. The three classic symptoms are angina, syncope, and heart failure (Table 77-2). While sudden death occurs in 3% to 5% of patients with aortic stenosis and may be considered a fourth symptom group, this is rarely seen in asymptomatic patients. Unfortunately, the elderly often move into the symptomatic phase of aortic stenosis undetected because of the overlap of these major symptom constellations with other changes associated with aging.

Two-thirds of patients present with angina, which may be caused by concomitant coronary artery disease, although 40% of patients with severe aortic stenosis will present with angina without significant coronary artery disease. The most likely etiology for angina in the absence of coronary artery disease is subendocardial ischemia and the increased oxygen demands of the hypertrophied ventricle together with decreased coronary flow reserve. Untreated patients with aortic stenosis and angina have a 50% 5-year survival.

In the elderly, syncope is often caused by aortic stenosis. Syncope in this setting may be caused by inadequate cardiac output to meet demands, by dysfunctional left ventricular baroreceptor response, or by arrhythmias and is associated with a 50% 3-year mortality without valve replacement.

Aortic valve stenosis presenting with congestive heart failure carries the worst prognosis: 50% mortality at 2 years if not treated with valve replacement. The typical symptoms include paroxysmal nocturnal dyspnea, orthopnea, and dyspnea on exertion, which may be associated with signs of peripheral edema, pulmonary edema, and rales. Thickening of the left ventricle owing to aortic stenosis as well as the changes associated with aging both lead to diastolic dysfunction, consequently the older patient with aortic stenosis is more dependent on atrial contraction for ventricular filling. There-

TABLE 77-2

Aortic Stenosis Symptoms	
SYMPTOM	50% MORTALITY (yr)
Angina	5
Syncope	3
Failure	2

fore, these patients often present with exacerbated or new onset of symptoms if they develop atrial fibrillation.

Management

Asymptomatic Patients

Survival of asymptomatic patients is the same as age-matched individuals without aortic stenosis; however, given the significant decline in survival once symptoms develop, it is essential to consider surgical intervention and to confirm the absence of symptoms in the patient who does not appear symptomatic. If a careful history fails to elicit symptoms and the patient has severe aortic stenosis, exercise testing may be considered. Exercise testing in symptomatic patients is not indicated and should not be performed because of the high risk of complications.

Patients who are asymptomatic by history but who on exercise testing develop symptoms or fail to generate a 20 mm Hg increase in blood pressure or develop ST-segment abnormalities have a 19% 2-year symptom-free survival compared with 85% 2-year symptom-free survival for patients who do not manifest these abnormalities on exercise testing. Exercise testing may elicit symptoms in as many as a third of patients thought to be asymptomatic by history alone. Close supervision and prompt termination of the study at any decline in blood pressure, significant ST-segment depression, or onset of arrhythmia are strongly advocated. On average, the probability of a patient with severe aortic stenosis remaining symptom free at 5 years is only 50%, which has prompted some to recommend earlier surgery while the patient is "younger" and in better health to undergo valve replacement.

If the patient is truly asymptomatic, continued frequent routine monitoring is reasonable, but patient should be instructed to report any development of chest pain, tightening, or pressure; syncope, lightheadedness, or dizziness; and any sign of congestive heart failure. Monitoring should include annual or biannual echocardiograms for patients with severe aortic stenosis, every 1 to 2 years for patients with moderate aortic stenosis and echocardiograms every 3 to 5 years if the stenosis is mild, although echocardiograms should be performed as needed if the patient develops symptoms. Patients who are demonstrated to be symptom free do not need to have their activity restricted and may participate in exercise.

Medical Management

Once patients develop symptoms the patient should be considered for valve replacement. However, if the patient is asymptomatic or not a candidate for surgery, consideration should be given to medical management, even though there is no demonstrated survival advantage. Medical management includes antibiotic prophylaxis for endocarditis, antihypertensive management, and possibly statins. Although antihypertensive therapy with angiotensin-converting enzyme inhibitors and beta-blockers is warranted for the patient with hypertension, these should be initiated with caution in the elderly.

The American Heart Associate guidelines states that "patients who develop symptoms require surgery, not medical therapy"; nonetheless, every patient should be assessed based on their individual risks and benefits before advocating valve replacement. Given the similarities in histopathology between atherosclerosis and aortic stenosis, early retrospective studies suggested that statin therapy might retard the rate of progression of aortic valvular stenosis; however, a more recent randomized prospective study has not demonstrated a benefit to statins over placebo. Currently, there is no documented medical treatment that will delay or reverse aortic valvular stenosis; therefore, any treatment other than surgery should be considered palliative care.

Percutaneous Aortic Valvuloplasty

Balloon valvuloplasty is not a substitute for surgery but is a useful tool in the treatment armamentarium for temporary palliation of symptoms for nonsurgical candidates or as a bridge for patients with hemodynamically unstable aortic stenosis. The procedure uses transvalvular balloon inflations to crack the calcified aortic valve; unfortunately, the maximum enlargement rarely exceeds 1.0 cm^2 (severe-to-moderate aortic stenosis), carries a 10% risk of complications, and results in restenosis within 6 months to a year. One-year actuarial mortality is 35% to 50%, which is not better than untreated aortic stenosis, but it can result in significant relief of symptoms and improvement in quality of life.

On a more optimistic note, clinical studies are currently underway to explore deployment of percutaneously placed aortic valves. At this time, the data are too limited to determine the risks and durability of this procedure.

Surgical Management

The development of symptoms is a clear indication for valve replacement. Current American Heart Association recommendations are listed in Table 77-3. Aortic valve replacement is recommended for all symptomatic patients because of the improvement in both symptoms and survival. Moreover, since there is an increased risk of sudden death, replacement should be performed as soon as feasible after the development of symptoms. Age alone is not a contraindi-

cation to surgery, and to date numerous studies have demonstrated outcomes in elderly similar to those seen in younger patients. For example, as in younger patients, mortality in the elderly ranges from 3% to 4% to as high as 24%. On average, mortality for older patients in retrospective studies reportedly varies between 9% and 12%. The variability in published studies is the result of both patient selection and the definition of "older patient"—which varies from cohorts aged 65 to 80 years. Medicare outcomes data for 142,000 patients older than 65 years demonstrate a perioperative mortality of 8.8% and only 6.0% mortality in high-volume centers.

Predictors of mortality in this patient population include emergent surgery, right heart failure, severity of symptoms (NYHA class IV), renal insufficiency, female gender, depressed left ventricular function, associated coronary bypass, or mitral valve surgery. Consistent with most studies is the finding that emergent surgery increases the surgical risk substantially. This is often the result of a failure to refer the patient for elective surgery because it is "too risky," but reconsidering the patient as a suitable surgical candidate when the patient is critically ill and the medical options have dwindled to none. Unfortunately the result is a self-filling prophecy that older patients will not do well with surgery. A European study of older patients with aortic stenosis provocatively demonstrated that 41% of patients older than 70 years were not offered surgery despite severe valve stenosis and symptoms; these findings were corroborated in a second study of 1200 patients from 92 centers in 25 countries. In this study, 33% of patients older than 75 years with severe symptomatic aortic stenosis were denied valve replacement.

Although many studies have found that concomitant coronary artery bypass or mitral valve surgery increases the surgical risk, there is clear support for performing concomitant aortic valve replacement for any patient with severe aortic stenosis, who is undergoing any other cardiac surgical procedure, regardless of symptoms. Similarly, in patients with moderate stenosis, it is "accepted practice" to replace the aortic valve at the time of other cardiac surgery. Simultaneous valve replacement in patients with mild aortic stenosis undergoing heart surgery is more controversial, although an argument can be made for concomitant replacement in patients with mild stenosis but moderate-to-severe valve calcification.

TABLE 77-3

American Heart Association Recommendations for Valve Replacement in Aortic Stenosis

Indications for valve replacement in aortic stenosis
- Symptomatic patients with severe aortic stenosis
- Patients with severe aortic stenosis undergoing coronary artery bypass surgery (CABG)
- Patients with severe aortic stenosis undergoing other valvular or aortic surgery
- Patients with severe aortic stenosis and left ventricular dysfunction (ejection fraction less than 50%)

Considerations for valve replacement in aortic stenosis
- Patients with moderate aortic stenosis undergoing CABG
- Patients with moderate aortic stenosis undergoing other valvular or aortic surgery

Possible indications for valve replacement in aortic stenosis
- Asymptomatic patients with severe aortic valve stenosis with abnormal exercise testing
- Patients with mild aortic stenosis, with moderate-to-severe valve calcification who are undergoing coronary artery bypass surgery
- Severe asymptomatic stenosis in patients with a high likelihood of progression
- Critical aortic stenosis (valve area <0.6 cm², mean gradient >60 mm Hg, jet velocity >5.0 m/s) if the operative mortality is less than 1.0%

AORTIC INSUFFICIENCY

Etiology

Aortic insufficiency is seen in 20% to 30% of individuals older than 65 years. Most often the valvular regurgitation is mild and is caused by aortic valve sclerosis or root dilatation as a result of hypertension or atherosclerosis. Other important causes of valvular insufficiency include ascending aortic dissection and endocarditis. Similar to aortic stenosis, there is a long latency period during which the patient is asymptomatic. However, even asymptomatic patients with normal left ventricular function have a 0.2% incidence of sudden death and will progress to symptomatic disease at a rate of approximately 3.5% per year and develop either left ventricular dysfunction or symptoms at a rate of approximately 6% per year. Once patients develop left ventricular dysfunction, more than 25% each year will progress to symptomatic disease and, once symptomatic, the mortality rate for aortic regurgitation is more than 10% per year.

TABLE 77-4

Partial List of Eponymous Signs of Aortic Insufficiency

EPONYM	PHYSICAL FINDING
Austin–Flint murmur	Low-pitched mid-diastolic rumble
Becker sign	Accentuated retinal artery pulsation
Corrigan pulses	Rapidly rising and falling pulse to palpation
de Musset sign	Bobbing of head
Duroziez sign	To-and-fro femoral artery murmur with compression
Gerhard sign	Pulsatile spleen
Hill sign	Higher BP in lower than upper extremity
Mayne sign	Decrease in blood pressure with arm elevated
Mueller sign	Pulsatile uvula
Quincke sign	Pulsatile nail beds
Rosenbach sign	Pulsatile liver
Traube sign	Double femoral artery pulse sound
Sherman sign	Dorsalis pedis pulse prominent in patients older than 75 yr
Watson's water hammer pulse	Bounding peripheral pulse

The five identified risk factors for the development of left ventricular dysfunction, symptoms, or death include age, left ventricular end-systolic dimension/volume, left ventricular end-diastolic dimension/volume, and left ventricular ejection fraction with exercise. Each year 19% of patients with end-systolic size greater than 50 mm develop left ventricular dysfunction and symptoms or die. The rate of development of these same end-points was 6% per year for patients with end-systolic size between 40 and 50 mm.

Clinical Presentation and Diagnosis

The findings and eponyms associated with aortic insufficiency are a delight to lovers of medical trivia (Table 77-4); however, the most obvious physical findings are those of a diastolic murmur and a widened pulse pressure. Echocardiography provides both diagnostic confirmation and assessment of the severity of valve regurgitation; it also allows evaluation of both the valve and the aortic root as well as an assessment of left ventricular function and dimension. It is an excellent modality for monitoring left ventricular size and function, although these parameters can also be followed by cardiac magnetic resonance imaging or radionuclide angiography. Exercise testing may be reasonable for asymptomatic patients who wish to initiate an exercise regimen, but the results have not been consistently useful in predicting outcomes for asymptomatic patients with normal resting cardiac function.

Patients may present with angina or signs and symptoms of congestive heart failure. Surgery is indicated for patients who develop either angina or signs of congestive heart failure, since the mortality for patients with angina is more than 10% per year and for heart failure is more than 20% per year. Medical management in symptomatic patients results in poor outcomes even if the left ventricular function is normal. Patients older than 75 years are more likely to develop either symptoms or ventricular dysfunction at earlier stages of the disease and have a poorer prognosis once they develop ventricular dysfunction. Concomitant coronary artery disease should be ruled out by angiography in any older patient considered for valve replacement surgery.

Management

Medical Management

The medical management of aortic insufficiency is best achieved with vasodilators that reduce afterload and wall stress and, perhaps, ameliorate left ventricular dysfunction. Since symptomatic disease carries such a poor prognosis without surgery, medical management is primarily indicated for patients who are not surgical candidates because of comorbidities, to preoperatively optimize hemodynamics, or for asymptomatic hypertensive patients with normal ventricular function. Conflicting data exist as to the benefits of hydralazine, ACE inhibitors, and calcium channel-blockers, which suggests that vasodilator therapy is not indicated for asymptomatic, normotensive patients with normal ventricular function. However, once symptoms or ventricular dysfunction develops, the patient should be considered and evaluated for surgery.

The absence of data indicating that exercise contributes to the progression of aortic insufficiency would suggest that the asymptomatic patient with normal left ventricular function may participate in the full range of physical activities, with the exception of isometric exercises, which are contraindicated. However, it is prudent to exercise test patients to the anticipated level of activity to assess tolerance prior to initiating an exercise regimen.

Patients with aortic regurgitation should have regularly scheduled follow-up. Mild regurgitation with normal ventricular function can be followed clinically on an annual basis with biennial or triennial echocardiograms; more severe valvular regurgitation should be followed with annual or even biannual echocardiograms depending on the presence of ventricular dilatation (60 mm). Asymptomatic patients with more severe dilatation (>70 mm) should be followed with echocardiograms every 4 to 6 months because the likelihood of developing symptoms or ventricular dysfunction is as high as 20% per year.

Surgical Management

Surgery is not indicated for asymptomatic patients with normal ventricular function and minimal ventricular dilatation regardless of the severity of valvular regurgitation; however, once symptoms or left ventricular dysfunction develops in patients with severe aortic regurgitation, the patient should be considered for surgery (Table 77-5). Although significantly better than medical management, patients with severe left ventricular dysfunction have a high operative mortality (at least 10%) and a lower postoperative survival; therefore, asymptomatic patients should be closely followed for the development of left ventricular dysfunction.

In older patients with severe compensated aortic insufficiency, the onset of symptoms can be hard to ascertain, since mild dyspnea on exertion and fatigue often mimic the effects of aging. However, once ventricular dysfunction develops, the older patient is more likely to have continued postoperative ventricular dysfunction and symptoms, as well as decreased postsurgical survival. Therefore, in patients without comorbidities that contraindicate surgery, an earlier commitment to surgery carries a better overall prognosis.

If the patient is asymptomatic but the left ventricular end-diastolic dimension exceeds 75 mm, surgery should be considered because of the high risk of sudden death. Although the surgical treatment of asymptomatic patients with severe aortic regurgitation and left ventricular dilatation is controversial, if surgery is planned based

TABLE 77-5

Recommendations for Surgery in Aortic Insufficiency

Indications for valve replacement in aortic insufficiency
- Symptomatic patients with severe aortic regurgitation
- Asymptomatic patients with severe aortic regurgitation and left ventricular ejection fraction less than 50%
- Patients with severe aortic regurgitation undergoing other cardiac surgical procedures

Considerations for valve replacement in aortic insufficiency
- Asymptomatic patients with severe aortic insufficiency, normal left ventricular function and dilated ventricles—LVEDD >75 mm

Possible indications for valve replacement in aortic insufficiency
- Patients with moderate aortic insufficiency undergoing other cardiac surgical procedures
- Asymptomatic patients with severe aortic regurgitation, normal cardiac function, and left ventricular dilatation greater than 70 mm, in conjunction with progressive dilatation and decreased exercise capacity

on ventricular size or function, two consecutive studies should confirm the findings. Certainly consideration for surgery in the asymptomatic elderly patient should be carefully considered, if not avoided until symptoms develop.

MITRAL STENOSIS

Etiology

The overwhelming majority of mitral stenosis is caused by rheumatic heart disease; other etiologies are rare and include left atrial thrombus, left atrial myxomas, and other tumors. Therefore, this valvular disease tends to occur in the younger patient and is rarely seen in the elderly, although the number may be increasing. In developed countries, most patients present in their forties and fifties, although some studies note that a third of their patients are older than 65 years. Only 60% of patients presenting with mitral stenosis recall a history of rheumatic fever, which causes thickening and calcification of the leaflets and cordae as well as shortening of the cordae and fusion of the commissures. This results in a decrease of the mitral valve orifice, which normally measures 4.0 to 5.0 cm^2. The disease progresses very slowly, and it is estimated that the mitral valve area decreases by 0.09 to 0.32 cm^2 per year. When the valve area is reduced to 2.5 to 1.5 cm^2, patients start to develop symptoms. Significant valvular disease lags the development of rheumatic fever by 20 to 40 years; however, once symptoms start, the 10-year survival is only 50% to 60%. Patients who are asymptomatic or with minimal symptoms have an 80% survival for 10 years, with as many as 60% of patients having no progression of symptoms. However, once significant symptoms develop, the 10-year survival is as low as 0% to 15%. Patients with severe pulmonary hypertension usually live less than 3 years, and most patients will die from progressive pulmonary hypertension, congestive heart failure, systemic embolic, pulmonary emboli, or infection.

Clinical Presentation and Diagnosis

Most often, mitral stenosis presents with new-onset atrial fibrillation or an embolic event, sometimes patients come to medical attention because of fatigue or dyspnea and rarely because of hemoptysis or hoarseness. The onset of atrial fibrillation can result in pulmonary edema and death. On physical examination, an opening snap may be noted to the first heart sound associated with a diastolic rumble.

Evaluation of patients with suspected mitral stenosis includes an echocardiogram, both to confirm the diagnosis and assess the severity of the disease as well as to assess therapeutic options. Patients are deemed to have mild mitral stenosis if the valve area is greater than 1.5 cm^2, moderate if the valve area is 1.0 to 1.5 cm^2, and severe if the mitral valve area is less than 1.0 cm^2. Additionally, pulmonary pressures should be assessed, since these are helpful in grading the severity of the disease.

Management

Medical Management

It should be emphasized that medical management cannot reduce a mechanical narrowing like mitral stenosis; however, increasing diastolic filling time by slowing heart rate may be helpful in patients in sinus rhythm and exertional symptoms. Often, medical regimens include a beta-blocker or calcium channel blocker to reduce heart rate and increase diastolic fill time, as well as sodium restriction and a diuretic to ameliorate pulmonary edema. Additionally, patients with mitral stenosis should receive antibiotic prophylaxis for endocarditis for high-risk procedures (Tables 77-6 and 77-7). Asymptomatic patients should be followed closely for the development of symptoms, at which time they should be assessed by echocardiogram.

A substantial number of patients (30–40%) will present with atrial fibrillation, especially the older patient. Both age and left atrial size are predictive of the development of atrial fibrillation. Unfortunately, the development of atrial fibrillation carries a more guarded prognosis, since only 25% of patients with atrial fibrillation will survive 10 years compared to 46% of those who remain in sinus rhythm. Treatment for atrial fibrillation includes anticoagulation,

TABLE 77-6

Endocarditis Prophylaxis Procedures

	ENDOCARDITIS PROPHYLAXIS IS RECOMMENDED	ENDOCARDITIS PROPHYLAXIS IS NOT REQUIRED
Respiratory procedures	• Oral surgery including tonsillectomy and adenoidectomy • Respiratory tract surgery involving mucosal surfaces • Rigid bronchoscopy	• Intubation • Flexible bronchoscopy
Gastrointestinal procedures	• Esophageal procedures—sclerotherapy and dilatation • Biliary tract surgery or instrumentation—ERCP • Gastrointestinal surgery or procedures that violate the intestinal mucosa	• Transesophageal echocardiogram • Endoscopy without mucosa violation
Genitourinary procedures	• Prostate surgery • Urethral instrumentation—including dilatation	• Transvaginal surgery • Urethral catheterization in uninfected patient

TABLE 77-7

Prophylactic Antibiotic Recommendations		
	ANTIBIOTIC	**DOSAGE**
Standard	Amoxicillin	2.0 g PO 1 h before procedure
Penicillin	Clindamycin	600 mg PO 1 h before procedure
allergic	Cephalexin	2.0 g PO 1 h before procedure
Unable to take oral medicines	Ampicillin	2.0 g IV or IM 30 minute before procedure
and Penicillin allergic	Clindamycin	600 mg IV 30 minute before procedure
	Cefazolin	1.0 g IV or IM 30 minute before procedure

TABLE 77-8

Risk of Percutaneous Mitral Valvuloplasty	
COMPLICATION	**PERCENT RISK**
Left ventricular perforation	0.5–4.0
Systemic embolization	0.5–3.0
Myocardial infarction	0.3–0.5
Death	1.0–2.0

rate control, and electrical or chemical cardioversion, especially if associated with hemodynamic instability. Patients who remain in atrial fibrillation for more than 24 to 48 hours are at increased risk of embolic complications and should be promptly anticoagulated. Electrical cardioversion may be used but only after confirming the absence of a left atrial thrombus by echocardiogram; if a thrombus is present, treatment may include 3 weeks of anticoagulation, followed by confirmation of the absence of thrombus by repeat echocardiography and subsequent defibrillation. In this setting, transesophageal echocardiography is often the diagnostic tool of choice.

Atrial fibrillation often becomes refractory to treatment; should the patient develop paroxysmal or permanent atrial fibrillation, long-term anticoagulation is warranted. Certainly patients with either prior emboli or left atrial thrombus should be anticoagulated regardless of rhythm. Systemic emboli may occur in as many as 20% of patients; again age (and atrial fibrillation) is predictive of embolization. Paroxysmal and persistent atrial fibrillations as well as prior embolic events increase the risk of recurrent embolization; therefore, anticoagulation is indicated.

Older patients, patients with atrial fibrillation, and patients with prior history of emboli are at high risk for systemic embolization, which is as high as 20% in patients with mitral stenosis. Therefore, anticoagulation is recommended for mitral stenosis patients with atrial fibrillation, previous emboli, or left atrial thrombus. Additionally, warfarin may be appropriate for mitral stenosis patients with large left atria (greater than 55 mm), especially in conjunction with "smoke" or spontaneous contrast on echocardiogram.

Exercise is not contraindicated in asymptomatic patients with mild mitral stenosis. In patients with more severe stenosis, exercise is often limited by symptoms; therefore, exercise regimens for patients with more symptomatic or severe disease should be individually tailored.

Percutaneous Mitral Valvuloplasty

Percutaneous mitral valvuloplasty is successful in selected patients and often doubles the valve area with a substantial decrease in valve gradient. The selection of patients best suited for this treatment option is determined by echocardiographic assessment of the valve, which is based on leaflet mobility, subvalvular apparatus, leaflet thickening, and the presence of calcium. The lowest scores are assigned to valves with the greatest leaflet mobility, the least subvalvular thickening, the most normal leaflet thickness, and the least calcium

deposition; patients with these valve characteristics (lowest scores) are predicted to have the best response to balloon valvuloplasty. The majority of patients (90%) will see symptomatic relief, with a freedom from valve-related complications or death of between 50% and 65% at 7 years and as high as 80% to 90% in patients with favorable (low) pre-procedural echocardiographic scores.

Symptomatic patients or patients with pulmonary hypertension, those with favorable echocardiographic mitral valve scores and without atrial thrombi, should be referred for mitral valvuloplasty. The risks for percutaneous mitral valvuloplasty are low (Table 77-8); therefore, even patients with less favorable echocardiographic scores who are at high surgical risks may be considered candidates for this percutaneous approach. However, this approach is contraindicated in patients with moderate-to-severe mitral regurgitation and/or the presence of left atrial clot. Unfortunately, older patients (older than 65 years) have a lower success rate, higher incidence of complications, and shorter duration of symptom relief with this approach.

Surgical Management

As a result of the success of balloon valvuloplasty in patient with favorable valve morphology, surgery is usually indicated only if the patient has failed percutaneous intervention or if the valve characteristics make it unfavorable for balloon valvuloplasty. Patients with mitral stenosis in conjunction with moderate or severe mitral regurgitation are best treated surgically, as are patients with left atrial thrombus, which has not resolved despite an appropriate period of anticoagulation. Since balloon valvuloplasty requires a significant level of expertise and the outcomes are related to experience, the American Heart Association recommends surgery if this experience is not available.

Patients with mild symptoms, severe pulmonary hypertension, and moderate-to-severe mitral stenosis may also benefit from surgery if balloon valvuloplasty is not appropriate or available; similarly, patients with recurrent systemic emboli despite therapeutic anticoagulation may benefit from surgical intervention if ineligible for percutaneous treatment (Table 77-9). Notably, surgery is not recommended for patients with isolated mild mitral stenosis.

The surgical options include open repair with commissurotomy or valve replacement with either a mechanical or a bioprosthetic valve. The surgical risk increases with decreased preoperative functional status, age, cardiac function, pulmonary hypertension, and the presence of coronary artery disease. Operative mortality can be as high as 20% in the older patient with significant comorbidities and pulmonary hypertension; nonetheless, it is not recommended to wait until the patient becomes severely symptomatic (NYHA IV), since this results in a substantial increase in the surgical risk. Conversely, surgery should be considered despite severe symptoms, since

TABLE 77-9

Surgical Recommendations for Mitral Stenosis

Indications for valve replacement in mitral stenosis
- Symptomatic patients who are unable to undergo balloon valvuloplasty (owing to unavailability, contraindications, or unfavorable valve score)
- Symptomatic patients with moderate or severe stenosis and moderate or severe mitral regurgitation

Considerations for valve replacement in mitral stenosis
- Mildly symptomatic patients with severe mitral stenosis and severe pulmonary hypertension if ineligible for balloon valvuloplasty

Possible indications for valve replacement in mitral stenosis
- Patients with recurrent emboli despite anticoagulation

both quality of life and survival are exceedingly poor without surgical intervention.

MITRAL REGURGITATION

Etiology

The causes of mitral valve regurgitation can be divided into two broad categories: functional or organic. Organic regurgitation is caused by problems with the valve leaflets, the cordae, the papillary muscles, or the mitral annulus. The most common cause of organic valvular regurgitation include mitral valve prolapse, rheumatic heart disease, endocarditis, and coronary artery disease.

Mitral valve prolapse is present in 1% to 2.5% of the population and can occur either spontaneously or as a familial disorder; the latter is associated with a low but significant incidence of sudden death, presumably owing to ventricular arrhythmias. Acute mitral regurgitation, which can occur as a consequence of endocarditis or ruptured cordae or owing to a ruptured papillary muscle, is poorly tolerated because of the sudden volume overload and will present with shock and/or respiratory distress because of pulmonary edema. Chronic mitral regurgitation is better tolerated but, when severe, especially in association with a flail leaflet, is associated with a 7% per year mortality. A common cause of chronic mitral regurgitation in the elderly is myxomatous mitral valve disease. Patients with severe mitral valve regurgitation and a low ejection fraction have a poor prognosis; patients with ejection fractions less than 50% have a 32% 10-year survival, compared to 70% 10-year survival for patients with ejection fractions greater than 60%; even patients with borderline normal ejection fractions between 50% and 60% have decreased 10-year survival of only 53% if not corrected.

Clinical Presentation and Diagnosis

Patients with mitral valve prolapse may present with palpitations, atypical chest pain, dyspnea, easy fatigue, or panic attacks. Cessation of caffeine, tobacco, alcohol, and other stimulants may help control the anxiety in some patients. Acute mitral regurgitation presents either with shock or with respiratory distress, while more chronic regurgitation presents with dyspnea on exertion, pedal edema, and other signs of chronic volume overload and congestive heart failure.

Physical examination reveals a systolic ejection murmur, which is best heard at the apex of the heart with radiation to the axilla. As with other cardiac valvular problems, the diagnosis is best confirmed and quantified by echocardiogram. This study allows assessment of severity of regurgitation, putative cause of the valve dysfunction, as well as assessment of left ventricular ejection fraction. Patients without organic causes for mitral regurgitation should be assessed, based on patient history, for other etiologies such as coronary artery disease.

Management

Medical Management

Asymptomatic patients with organic moderate mitral regurgitation may be followed with annual echocardiograms; however, asymptomatic patients with organic severe regurgitation should probably undergo exercise testing to confirm the absence of symptoms or limitations and if truly asymptomatic should undergo restudy by echocardiogram every 6 to 12 months. The asymptomatic patient with organic mitral regurgitation, a normal ejection fraction without pulmonary hypertension, or left ventricular dilation may exercise without restriction.

Medical management consists mostly of control of hypertension, with vasodilators and diuretics. Once symptoms develop, either from atrial fibrillation or from volume overload, if the patient is not a surgical candidate, treatment is focused on the treatment of the symptoms as well as preload reduction. Endocarditis prophylaxis is recommended for all patients with mitral valve prolapse and patients with moderate or severe organic mitral regurgitation.

Surgical Management

The surgical options consist of either repair or replacement (Table 77-10). All patients should be considered with an eye to repairing the valve because of the marked improvement in survival, left ventricular function, and the avoidance of long-term anticoagulation with valve repair compared to valve replacement. Although

TABLE 77-10

Surgical Recommendations for Mitral Regurgitation

Indications for valve repair or replacement in mitral regurgitation
- Patients with mild-to-severe symptoms and severe mitral regurgitation and normal left ventricular size and function
- Asymptomatic patients with severe regurgitation and decrease left ventricular function (<60%) or ventricular dilatation (>40 mm)
- Acute mitral regurgitation

Considerations for valve repair or replacement in mitral regurgitation
- Asymptomatic patients with severe regurgitation and normal left ventricular size and function IF the valve can be repaired with a high degree of certainty
- New-onset atrial fibrillation in asymptomatic patients with severe regurgitation with normal left ventricular size and function
- Pulmonary artery hypertension in asymptomatic patients with severe regurgitation with normal left ventricular size and function

Not indicated for valve repair or replacement in mitral regurgitation
- Asymptomatic patients with severe regurgitation with normal left ventricular size and function when repair is unlikely
- Mild or moderate mitral regurgitation

durability of repair is excellent with freedom from reoperation equaling that of valve replacement (7%–10% at 10 years), the freedom from reoperation is dependent on the adequacy of the repair, whether the repair involved the anterior or the posterior valve leaflets, and whether cordal replacement was necessary. Patients with isolated posterior leaflet pathology are more likely to have long-term success compared to patients with anterior or bileaflet repairs.

Mitral replacement when necessary should strive to retain as much of the mitral valve apparatus as possible. Preservation of these structures results in improved left ventricular function, exercise tolerance, and survival. The choices for mitral valve replacement include bioprosthetic or mechanical valves. Bioprosthetic valves in the mitral position are not as durable as a bioprosthetic valve in the aortic position; however, this family of valves avoids the risks of lifelong anticoagulation. Conversely, a mechanical valve has the advantage of durability but requires a commitment to lifetime anticoagulation.

Mitral valve repair or replacement is indicated for all patients with symptoms (NYHA Class II–IV) and severe regurgitation even in the face of normal cardiac size and function. Asymptomatic patients benefit from surgical intervention if they develop atrial fibrillation, pulmonary hypertension, left ventricular dysfunction (ejection fraction <60%), or dilation (>40 mm). In patients with atrial fibrillation, an intraoperative maze or modified maze procedure combined with suture closure of the left atrial appendage should be considered, in order to reestablish sinus rhythm and possibly reduce the risk of systemic embolization, respectively. Once left ventricular dysfunction develops, patient survival even after repair or replacement is compromised; therefore, patients who are asymptomatic, with normal left ventricular size and function, should be followed closely, and, if necessary, exercise testing should be considered to confirm the absence of symptoms. Surgical intervention may be warranted for asymptomatic patients with severe mitral regurgitation with none of the noted indications for surgery if and only if the mitral valve can be repaired.

Operative mortality varies based on procedure. Mitral valve repair is associated with a 2% perioperative mortality compared to 6% for valve replacement. Patients with ischemic and functional mitral regurgitation do much worse than the patients with organic regurgitation. A study of 292 patients older than 70 years demonstrated an in-hospital mortality of 0.7% for mitral repair compared to 13.9% for replacement. Operative mortality is higher for the elderly, with the risk of mortality for valve replacement being as high as 14%, although repair carries a lower mortality. A recent paper comparing cohorts of patients older than 75 years, between 65 and 75 years and younger than 65 years, demonstrated an increased operative risk for the older patients, but restoration of life expectancy following surgery is the same for older as for younger patients. Although current data would suggest no improvement in survival by performing a concomitant mitral repair with coronary artery bypass, nonetheless there may be an improvement in postoperative symptoms.

GENERAL CONSIDERATIONS

Endocarditis Prophylaxis

Although there is surprising dearth of data supporting or refuting the use of antibiotic prophylaxis for patients with valvular disease,

TABLE 77-11

Anticoagulation for Prosthetic Valves

	MECHANICAL VALVE	BIOPROSTHETIC VALVE
Aortic	INR 2.0–3.0 Aspirin 75–325 mg daily	INR 2.0–3.0 *for 3 months* Aspirin 75–100 mg daily
Aortic with risk factors*	INR 2.5–3.5 Aspirin 75–325 mg daily	INR 2.0–3.0 Aspirin 75–100 mg daily
Mitral	INR 2.5–3.5 Aspirin 75–325 mg daily	INR 2.0–3.0 *for 3 months* Aspirin 75–100 mg daily
Mitral with risk factors*	INR 2.5–3.5 Aspirin 75–325 mg daily	INR 2.5–3.5 Aspirin 75–100 mg daily

*Risk factors: Atrial fibrillation, prior thromboembolism, LV dysfunction (ejection fraction <30%), and hypercoagulable condition.

the American Heart Association recommends antibiotic coverage for a variety of dental and surgical procedures.

Prophylactic antibiotics are recommended for patients with any valve replacement or repair and for patients with native valve abnormalities (Table 77-12). Patients at risk of endocarditis should be covered for all dental procedures and for other contaminated invasive procedures (a partial list is provided in Table 77-6).

Standard antibiotic prophylaxis is orally administered, penicillin based, and given 1 hour before the procedure (see Table 77-7).

Anticoagulation

Anticoagulation has a significant associated morbidity—particularly in the older patient. Consequently, the need for anticoagulation plays a pivotal role in the choice of valve. Patients with mechanical valves require lifelong anticoagulation, while patients with bioprosthetic valves are often anticoagulated for only 3 months (Table 77-11). If there is no contraindication to antiplatelet therapy, aspirin is also recommended for all patients with valve replacement.

Recommended INR for patients with mechanical aortic valves is between 2.0 and 3.0; however, if the patient has a history of prior thromboembolism, LV dysfunction, atrial fibrillation, or hypercoagulability, the INR should be maintained between 2.5 and 3.5. Patients with mechanical mitral valves should have their INR

TABLE 77-12

Indications for Endocarditis Prophylaxis

Patients for whom endocarditis prophylaxis is recommended
• Patients with any prosthetic valve—either mechanical or bioprosthetic
• Patients who have had valve repair procedures
• Patients with abnormal native valves—e.g., bicuspid aortic valve
• Mitral valve prolapse with clinical findings of regurgitation or leaflet abnormalities by echocardiogram

Endocarditis prophylaxis is not required
• Mitral valve prolapse without regurgitation or abnormal leaflets
• Aortic valve sclerosis if jet velocity <2.0 m/s
• Physiological mitral regurgitation with normal valve leaflets
• Physiological tricuspid regurgitation with normal valvular apparatus
• Physiological pulmonary valve regurgitation with normal valvular apparatus

maintained between 2.5 and 3.5. Patients with bioprosthetic valves are often anticoagulated (INR 2.0–3.0) for the first 3 months following implantation.

The risk of thromboembolism for anticoagulated patients with mechanical valves is approximately 1% to 2% per year. The risk is lower in bioprosthetic valves (0.7%) compared to mechanical valves, and lower in patients with aortic prosthetic valves compared to mitral valves, regardless of the type of prosthetic valve implanted.

Hemorrhagic complications are more likely if the INR is greater than 5.0. Patients with an INR between 5 and 10 can be treated by holding warfarin and administration of 1 to 2.5 mg of oral vitamin K. However, the INR should be monitored daily until the INR is below 5, at which time warfarin can be reinitiated at adjusted doses. Of note, it is often harder to manage anticoagulation in the older patient as a result of the numerous other medications that these patients are often taking and the high incidence of warfarin cross-reactivity with other medications. An acute reduction in the INR for patients who are suffering from bleeding complications may be achieved by administering intravenous fresh frozen plasma. Vitamin K can also help reduce a dangerously high INR, but it will make reanticoagulation difficult.

Sometimes temporary cessation of anticoagulation in patients with mechanical valves is medically necessary. Patients with mechanical aortic valves (without risk factors) can have warfarin held 48 to 72 hours preoperatively and restarted within 24 hours following surgery without the need for bridging heparin anticoagulation. However, patients with mechanical mitral or mechanical aortic valves and high-risk factors should be bridged with heparin when the INR falls below 2.0. The heparin may be held 4 to 6 hours before surgery and restarted as soon as possible when the immediate postoperative risk of bleeding allows. For emergent procedures, it is preferable to administer fresh frozen plasma to reverse the effects of warfarin, since the administration of vitamin K will make reanticoagulation difficult and increases the risk of a hypercoagulable state.

Prosthetic Valve Choices

All prosthetic valves fall into two broad groups: biologic and mechanical valves. Mechanical valves have the advantage of durability but the disadvantage of requiring lifelong anticoagulation. Bioprosthetic valves do not require anticoagulation; however, these are limited by a finite durability. Both the risk of embolism and the durability are determined, in part, by valve location. Biological aortic valve prostheses are more durable than the same valve in the mitral position, and mechanical valves in the aortic position have a lower risk of thromboembolism than in the mitral position.

Within each class of valve, mechanical and bioprosthetic, there are numerous types of prostheses; each type of valve is available in different forms (e.g., porcine vs. bovine pericardial or bileaflet vs. tilting disc).

Mechanical Valves

The original design mechanical valve was the ball-caged valve, which while durable has inefficient flow characteristics and requires higher levels of anticoagulation than the current generation of valves. The bileaflet mechanical valve is the most commonly used valve in the aortic position; while single leaflet tilting disc valves are available,

these are less frequently implanted. The risk of thromboembolism with anticoagulation is approximately 1% to 2% per year.

Bioprosthetic Valves

Stented and nonstented porcine valves are available, as well as stented valves fashioned from bovine pericardium. Like homografts, these valves do not require immunosuppression or anticoagulation. The risk of embolism for these types of valves is approximately 0.7% per year without anticoagulation; however, all the biological valves are prone to structural deterioration. The rate of deterioration is slower in older patients; consequently, the freedom from reoperation is 90% to 95% for patients who were older than 75 years at the time of implantation. Stentless valves do not have the valve mounting and are, therefore, more hemodynamically efficient for the same valve size; although initial data suggested regression of left ventricular hypertrophy, this has not been consistently noted in the literature, nor has the promise of improved survival, as a result of the reduction in ventricular hypertrophy, been realized.

Aortic Homografts

Cadaver valves that have been treated and cyropreserved unfortunately do not provide improved durability. Most data suggest either more rapid failure or at best comparable failure rates to other types of bioprosthetic valves. These valves can be more challenging to implant but are particularly useful in patients with endocarditis and tissue loss; additionally, the rate of thromboembolism is low, and, like the stentless porcine valves, these are very hemodynamically efficient especially at small sizes. Although there is no need for antirejection medications, the valve has a propensity to become heavily calcified, making replacement much more challenging.

Pulmonary Valve Autotransplants (Ross Procedure)

Mr. Donald Ross devised an operation to excise the patient's own pulmonary valve, which is used to replace the aortic valve, and then to replace the pulmonary valve with a homograft or bioprosthetic valve. Conceptually, the lower-pressure pulmonary circuit will allow for longer durability of the homograft or bioprosthetic valve in this circuit, and the aortic valve, which is now an autologous valve, would, therefore, also have increased durability. The operative morbidity and mortality for this procedure, especially in unfamiliar hands, are higher than bioprosthetic replacement. Although the ability of this procedure to accommodate growth makes it useful in pediatric patients, the increased procedural risk and limited benefit in the older patient rarely make it indicated in this population. A variation of this operation is also available for mitral replacement, but it is currently investigational and has the same limitations for use in the older patient.

Valve Repair

Repair of the aortic or mitral valves is the ideal. The ability to maintain ventricular geometry and to accommodate natural annular motion and durability makes mitral valve repair the best option for suitable patients; these advantages translate to lower operative mortality for mitral repair compared to replacement—1% to 2% versus 5.4% to 6.4%, respectively. Aortic valve repair for calcific disease is less durable and is rarely indicated; however, in the setting of normal leaflets, the aortic valve is repairable with excellent results (85% freedom from reoperation at 10 years).

The choice of replacement valve is sometimes determined by the contraindication to anticoagulation (which would necessitate the implantation of a bioprosthetic valve); otherwise, the choice resides with the patient. There are some data to suggest that the rate of bioprosthetic valve deteriorating slows down in older patients, prompting many surgeons to recommend bioprosthetic aortic valves for patients older than 65 years and bioprosthetic mitral valves for patients older than 70 years.

Other indirect factors may weigh the choice of valve in one direction or another: atrial fibrillation, multiple valve replacement, prior mechanical valve, prior cardiac surgery, annulus size—which might weigh the argument in favor of a mechanical valve rather than face the possibility of the third operation, etc. Essentially, the risk of the mechanical valve is the continuous low-level risk of anticoagulation and embolization, and the risk of the bioprosthetic valve is that of valve failure and reoperation. In the end, the choice of valve—unless there are contraindications to anticoagulation—belongs to the patient, since ultimately they must live with the perils of anticoagulation or the threat of reoperation.

Heart Failure

Michael W. Rich

Heart failure may be defined as an inability of the heart to pump sufficient blood to meet the metabolic needs of the body's tissues or the ability to do so only at the expense of elevated intracardiac pressures. Heart failure represents a clinical syndrome rather than a specific diagnosis, and, to a large extent, it is a geriatric syndrome in much the same way that dementia and incontinence are geriatric syndromes. Indeed, heart failure may be viewed as the quintessential disorder of cardiovascular aging since, as discussed later in this chapter, extensive age-related changes in cardiovascular structure and function, in conjunction with the rising prevalence of cardiovascular diseases with advancing age and the recent decline in premature cardiovascular deaths, all contribute to an exponential rise in the prevalence of heart failure with advancing age. Thus, although the clinical syndrome of heart failure has been recognized by physicians for more than 2000 years, it has only been within the past two decades that it has been identified as a major public health concern, a development that is largely attributable to the aging of the population.

EPIDEMIOLOGY AND ECONOMIC IMPACT

Despite progressive declines in age-adjusted mortality rates from coronary heart disease and hypertensive cardiovascular disease, both the incidence and the prevalence of heart failure are increasing, and it is projected that these trends will continue for the next several decades. As shown in Table 78-1, several factors have contributed to the progressive rise in heart failure. Foremost among these is the increasing number of older adults who, by virtue of advanced age and the high prevalence of hypertension, coronary heart disease, and cardiac valvular disorders in older individuals, are predisposed to the development of heart failure. In addition, advances in the treatment of other acute and chronic cardiac and noncardiac conditions, most notably atherosclerotic heart disease, hypertension, renal failure, cancer, and infectious diseases, have paradoxically contributed to the increasing burden of heart failure. Thus, individuals who 20

years ago might have died in middle age from acute myocardial infarction are now surviving to older age only to develop heart failure in their later years. Similarly, improved blood pressure control has led to a 60% decline in stroke mortality over the last 30 years, yet these same patients remain at risk of the subsequent development of heart failure as a complication of hypertension and left ventricular hypertrophy.

Heart failure affects approximately 5.2 million Americans, and 550,000 new cases are diagnosed each year. Moreover, both the incidence and the prevalence of heart failure are strikingly age dependent (Figures 78-1 and 78-2). Thus, heart failure is relatively uncommon in individuals younger than 40 years, but the prevalence doubles for each decade thereafter and exceeds 10% in adults older than 80 years. Similarly, heart failure mortality rates increase exponentially with advancing age in all major demographic subgroups of the U.S. population (Figure 78-3).

Heart failure is also a major source of chronic disability and impaired quality of life in older adults, and it is currently the leading indication for hospitalization in individuals older than 65 years. Moreover, the number of hospital discharges for heart failure increased by more than twofold from 1979 to 2004, primarily owing to the aging of the population (Figure 78-4). In 2004, there were 1.1 million hospital admissions in the United States with a primary diagnosis of heart failure (Table 78-2). Of these, 75% were in patients older than 65 years and more than 50% occurred in patients 75 years of age or older. The majority of heart failure patients younger than 65 years are males, but women comprise nearly 60% of heart failure admissions after the age of 65 years, and the proportion of females continues to rise with advancing age. The prevalence of heart failure in older Caucasians and African-Americans is similar, but hospital admission rates are lower in Hispanics and Asians. Whether this represents a true difference in population prevalence or a cultural difference in the likelihood that affected individuals will seek medical attention is unknown. Heart failure is also a common reason for outpatient physician office visits, with estimates ranging from

TABLE 78-1

Factors Contributing to the Rising Incidence and Prevalence of Heart Failure

Aging of the population
- Age-related cardiovascular changes
- High prevalence of cardiovascular disease

Improved therapy for coronary heart disease and hypertension
- Decline in coronary mortality
  - Thrombolytic therapy
  - Coronary angioplasty and bypass surgery
  - Aspirin, beta-blockers, and converting-enzyme inhibitors
  - Hypocholesterolemic agents
- Decline in stroke mortality
  - More widespread use of antihypertensive agents
  - Beneficial effects of treating diastolic and isolated systolic hypertension

Improved therapy for other disorders
- End-stage renal disease
- Cancer
- Pneumonia and other infections

3 to 12 million office visits annually. In this regard, heart failure ranks second only to hypertension among cardiovascular causes for outpatient physician visits.

As a result of its high prevalence and the need for intensive resource use in both the inpatient and the outpatient settings, it is not surprising that the economic burden of heart failure is staggering. Heart failure is currently the most costly diagnosis-related group in the United States, with estimated total annual expenditures in excess of $33 billion. Indeed, inpatient expenditures for heart failure exceed those for all cancers combined by a factor of 2.4 and for all myocardial infarctions combined by a factor of 1.7.

PATHOPHYSIOLOGY

Heart failure represents the prototypical disorder of cardiovascular aging in that age-related changes in the cardiovascular system in concert with an increasing prevalence of cardiovascular diseases at older age conspire to produce an exponential rise in heart failure prevalence with advancing age.

Aging is associated with extensive changes in cardiovascular structure and function (see Chapter 74). However, in the absence of coexistent cardiovascular disease, resting cardiac function is well pre-

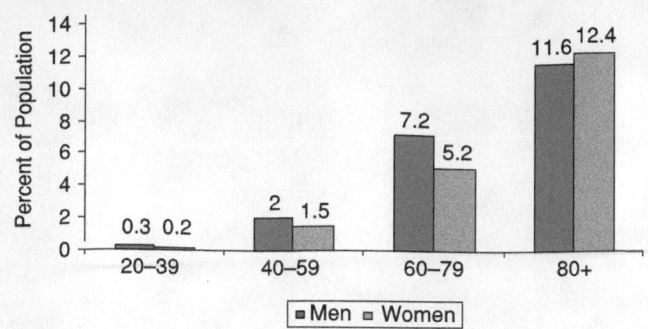

FIGURE 78-2. Prevalence of heart failure by age and sex in the United States. (*Source: National Health and Nutrition Examination Survey: 1999–2004.*)

served even at very elderly age. Thus, the resting left ventricular ejection fraction, an index of left ventricular systolic performance, is unaffected by age in healthy individuals. Similarly, most studies indicate that resting cardiac output is either maintained or declines minimally with normal aging.

From the clinical perspective, the changes associated with cardiovascular aging result in an impaired ability of the heart to respond to stress, whether that stress is physiologic (e.g., exercise) or pathologic (e.g., hypertension or myocardial ischemia). Four principal changes in the cardiovascular system contribute directly to the heart's attenuated capacity to augment cardiac output in response to stress. First, aging is associated with reduced responsiveness to β-adrenergic stimulation. The mechanism underlying this change has not been fully elucidated, but it is not caused by reduced circulating catecholamine levels, decreased β-receptor density on cardiac myocytes, or altered responsiveness to intracellular calcium. In any case, the diminished response to β-adrenergic stimulation limits the heart's capacity to maximally increase heart rate and contractility in response to stress, and β_2-mediated peripheral vasodilatation is also compromised.

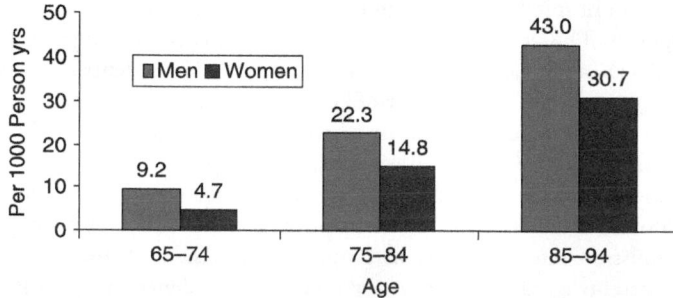

FIGURE 78-1. Incidence of heart failure in the United States by age and sex: 1980–2003. (*Source: Framingham Heart Study 1980–2003; National Heart, Lung, and Blood Institute.*)

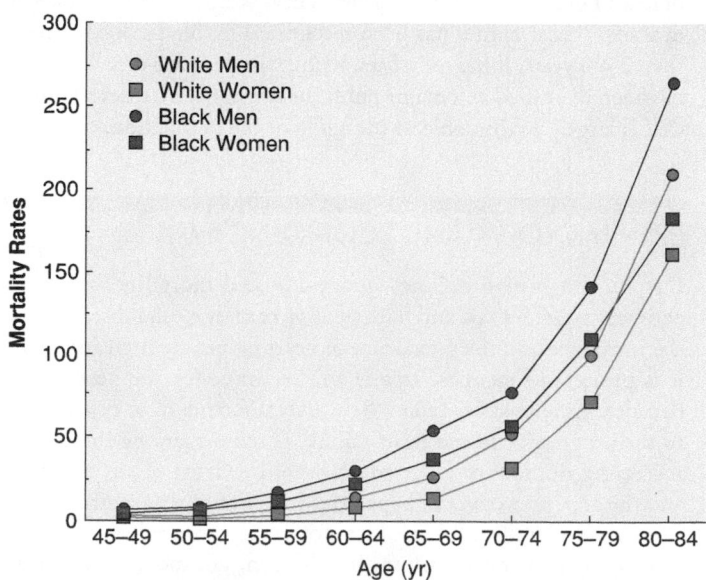

FIGURE 78-3. Mortality rates for congestive heart failure in the U.S. by age, sex, and race: 1990. (*Adapted with permission from Gillum RF. Epidemiology of heart failure in the United States. Am Heart J. 1993;126: 1042–1047.*)

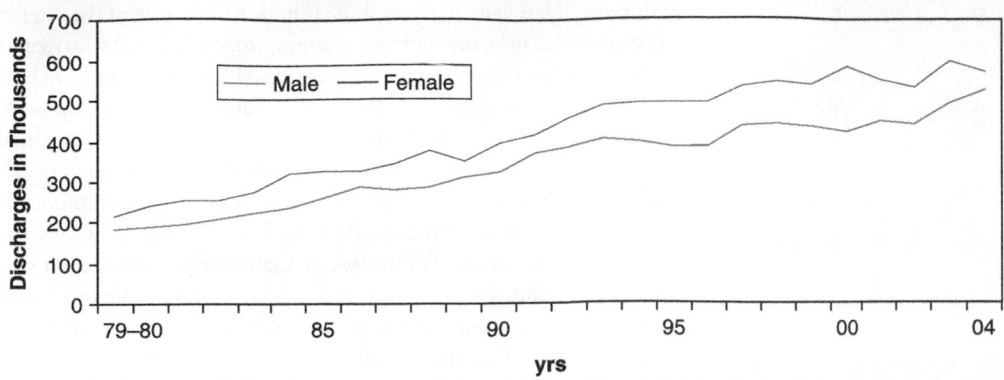

FIGURE 78-4. Hospital discharges for heart failure by sex: 1979–2004. *(Source: National Hospital Discharge Survey, National Center for Health Statistics.)*

A second major effect of aging is increased vascular stiffness, primarily because of increased collagen deposition and cross-linking and degeneration of elastin fibers in the media and adventitia of the large- and medium-sized arteries. Increased vascular stiffness results in increased impedance to left ventricular ejection (i.e., increased afterload), and it also contributes to the increased propensity of older individuals to develop isolated systolic hypertension.

A third major effect of aging is altered left ventricular diastolic filling. Diastole is characterized by four phases: isovolumic relaxation, early rapid filling, passive filling during mid-diastole, and late filling owing to atrial systole. The first two phases, isovolumic relaxation and early rapid filling, are largely dependent on myocardial relaxation, an active, energy-requiring process, whereas filling during the latter two phases is governed principally by intrinsic myocardial "stiffness," or compliance. Aging is associated with impaired calcium release from the contractile proteins and reuptake by the sarcoplasmic reticulum at the end of systole, leaving the heart in a state of "partial contraction" at the onset of diastole and inhibiting early diastolic relaxation. In addition, increased interstitial connective tissue content and collagen cross-linking reduce ventricular compliance. Compensatory myocyte hypertrophy in response to increased ventricular afterload and myocyte loss because of apoptosis further compromise left ventricular compliance. Thus, normal aging is associated with important changes that impair both relaxation and compliance, adversely impacting all four phases of diastole and substantially altering the pattern of left ventricular diastolic filling.

Age-related changes in diastolic filling and atrial function can be evaluated noninvasively using Doppler echocardiographic techniques to examine diastolic inflow across the mitral valve (Figure 78-5). In healthy young persons, the transmitral inflow pattern is characterized by a large E-wave, with a rapid upstroke representing rapid filling of the ventricle immediately following the opening of the mitral valve and corresponding to active ventricular relaxation (Figure 78-5A). This is followed by a period in which the rate of filling slows (the downslope of the E-wave), mid-diastolic diastasis (in which left atrial and left ventricular pressures are essentially equal), and a second burst of flow at the end of diastole corresponding to atrial contraction (the A-wave, or atrial "kick"). Importantly, the majority of ventricular filling occurs in the first half of diastole in young individuals, with a relatively small contribution from atrial contraction.

In older persons, alterations in cardiac relaxation and compliance result in characteristic changes in the pattern of diastolic filling (Figure 78-5B). Early filling is impaired, and the upstroke of the E-wave is delayed. Similarly, the downslope of the E-wave is less steep, as it takes a longer time to achieve diastasis. In order to compensate for increased resistance to emptying, the left atrium enlarges and hypertrophies. This results in a more forceful left atrial contraction

TABLE 78-2

Epidemiology of Heart Failure in the United States

POPULATION GROUP	PREVALENCE*	INCIDENCE	MORTALITY*	HOSPITAL DISCHARGES	COST†
Both sexes	5.2 million (2.5%)	550 000	57 700	1.099 million	$33.2
Men	2.6 million (2.8%)		22 501 (39%)	524 000	
Women	2.6 million (2.2%)		35 199 (61%)	575 000	
Race/ethnicity					
White men	2.8%		20 040		
White women	2.1%		31 785		
Black men	2.7%		2119		
Black women	3.3%		3017		
MA men	2.1%		NA		
MA women	1.9%		NA		

MA, Mexican American; NA, not available.
*Based on 2004 data.
†Estimated for 2007, in billions of dollars.
Rosamond W, et al. Heart disease and stroke statistics – 2007 update. A report from the American Heart Association Statistics Committee and Stroke Statistics Subcommittee. Circulation. 2007;115:e69–e171.

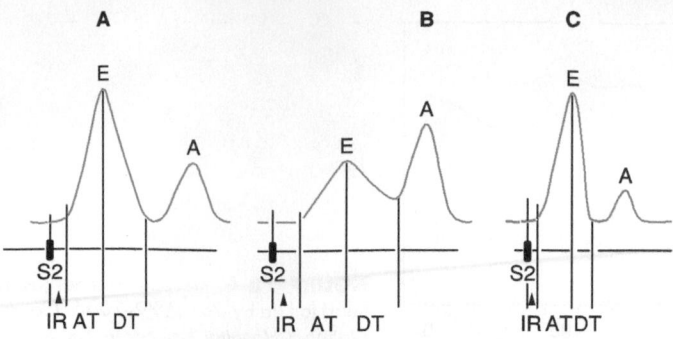

FIGURE 78-5. Schematic diagram of Doppler echocardiographic mitral valve inflow patterns. (A) Normal pattern. (B) Impaired filling pattern. (C) Restrictive pattern. AT, acceleration time; DT, deceleration time; IR, isovolumic relaxation; S2 aortic valve closure. *(Adapted with permission from Feigenbaum H. Echocardiography. 5th ed. Philadelphia: Lea & Febiger; 1994:152.)*

and an augmented A-wave. As a result of these changes, a greater proportion of filling occurs in the second half of diastole in older individuals, and as much as 30% to 40% of left ventricular end-diastolic volume may be attributable to atrial contraction. Thus, older individuals become increasingly reliant on the atrial "kick" to maximize left ventricular filling.

A third pattern of diastolic filling, referred to as the restrictive pattern, occurs when the left ventricle's ability to accept blood becomes severely compromised. In this situation (Figure 78-5C), very little flow occurs after the rapid filling phase in early diastole. This pattern is characterized by a tall, narrow E-wave with a rapid downslope, as diastasis is achieved early in diastole. Little additional flow occurs during mid-diastole, and the A-wave is typically small, with an amplitude that is less than 50% of the E-wave. A restrictive pattern generally indicates marked elevation of the left ventricular diastolic pressure, and it is generally associated with a poor prognosis, particularly in patients with concomitant systolic dysfunction. However, the restrictive pattern generally occurs in patients with advanced cardiac disease, and it rarely results from aging alone.

Age-related changes in diastolic filling have several important clinical implications. First, inability to distend the cardiac myocytes to an optimal fiber length results in a failure of the Frank–Starling mechanism, one of the cardinal adaptive responses (along with sympathetic activation) for acutely increasing cardiac output. Second, impaired diastolic filling results in a shift to the left in the normal ventricular pressure–volume relationship; i.e., a small increase in diastolic volume is associated with a greater increase in diastolic pressure in older compared to younger individuals. This increase in diastolic pressure is transmitted back to the left atrium, and left atrial myocytes become "stretched." This, in turn, increases the likelihood of atrial ectopic beats and atrial arrhythmias, especially atrial fibrillation. This accounts, in part, for the fact that atrial fibrillation, like heart failure, increases in prevalence with advancing age. In addition, atrial fibrillation itself is a common precipitant of heart failure in older adults for two reasons. First, the absence of a coordinated atrial contraction substantially compromises late diastolic filling as a result of loss of the atrial "kick." Second, the rapid, irregular ventricular rate associated with acute atrial fibrillation shortens the diastolic filling period, which further attenuates ventricular filling.

A third effect of altered diastolic filling is an increased propensity for older adults to develop diastolic heart failure (i.e., heart failure

with normal left ventricular systolic function). Because of the altered left ventricular pressure–volume relation, increases in left ventricular pressure owing to ischemia or uncontrolled hypertension may lead to pulmonary congestion and edema. Moreover, individuals with impaired diastolic function are often "volume sensitive"; i.e., small increments in intravascular volume, as may occur with a dietary salt load or intravenous fluid administration, are poorly accommodated by the noncompliant ventricle. As a result, intraventricular pressure rises abruptly and heart failure ensues. Conversely, intravascular volume contraction, which may arise from poor oral intake or overdiuresis, can cause a marked fall in intraventricular volume, which in turn leads to a fall in stroke volume and cardiac output.

The fourth major effect of cardiovascular aging is altered myocardial energy metabolism at the level of the mitochondria. Under resting conditions, older cardiac mitochondria are able to generate sufficient quantities of adenosine triphosphate to meet the heart's energy requirements. However, when stress causes an increase in adenosine triphosphate demands, the mitochondria are often unable to respond appropriately. Although the precise mechanism underlying this mitochondrial failure is unclear, the defect adds to the heart's inability to maintain normal metabolic function under stress.

To summarize, four major age-related changes in cardiovascular structure, function, and physiology combine to reduce cardiovascular reserve and greatly increase the risk of heart failure in older adults. Recalling that cardiac output is determined by four primary factors (heart rate, preload, afterload, and contractile state), and recognizing that each of these factors is adversely affected by one or more of the four major effects of aging on the heart, and that superimposed upon these changes is the high prevalence of cardiac disease in older adults, it is indeed not surprising that the incidence and prevalence of heart failure rise exponentially with advancing age.

It is also important to note that aging is associated with significant changes in other organ systems, which impact directly or indirectly on the development and/or management of heart failure. Aging is accompanied by a decline in glomerular filtration rate, and the aging kidney is less able to maintain intravascular volume and electrolyte homeostasis (see Chapter 85). The reduced capacity of the kidneys to respond to intravascular volume overload or dietary sodium excess further increases the risk of heart failure in older individuals. In addition, older patients are less responsive to diuretics and more likely to develop diuretic-induced electrolyte abnormalities than younger patients, factors that may complicate the management of heart failure in the older age group.

Aging is also associated with numerous changes in respiratory function, which serve to diminish respiratory reserve (see Chapter 82). Some of these effects, such as *V/Q* mismatching and sleep-related breathing disorders, may contribute directly to the development of heart failure by producing hypoxemia or pulmonary hypertension. Other changes reduce the capacity of the lungs to compensate for the failing heart by increasing tidal volume and minute ventilation, thereby contributing to the patient's sensation of dyspnea. In more severe cases of cardiac failure, such as pulmonary edema, acute respiratory failure may ensue, partly as a consequence of the inability of the lungs to maintain oxygenation and effective ventilation.

Age-related changes in nervous system function include an impaired thirst mechanism, which may contribute to dehydration and intravascular volume contraction in patients treated with diuretics, and reduced capacity of the central nervous system's autoregulatory mechanisms to maintain cerebral perfusion in the face of changes in systemic arterial blood pressure. The latter effect may contribute to subtle changes in mental function in older heart failure patients treated with vasodilators. Aging is also associated with widespread changes in reflex responsiveness. For example, impaired responsiveness of the carotid baroreceptors to acute changes in blood pressure may cause orthostatic hypotension or syncope, and these effects may further be aggravated by many of the drugs used to treat heart failure.

Finally, as is well recognized, aging is associated with significant changes in the pharmacokinetics and pharmacodynamics of almost all drugs. In addition, older patients tend to be at increased risk of both drug–drug and drug–disease interactions as a result of the high prevalence of comorbid conditions and the use of multiple pharmacological agents. These factors often lead to alterations in drug efficacy and an increased side-effect profile, and these effects must be taken into consideration when designing therapy for older heart failure patients (see Chapters 8 and 24).

ETIOLOGY AND PRECIPITATING FACTORS

In general, the etiology of heart failure is similar in older and younger patients (Table 78-3), but heart failure in older individuals is more often multifactorial. As in younger patients, hypertension and coronary heart disease are the most common causes of heart failure, accounting for more than 70% of cases. Hypertensive hypertrophic cardiomyopathy represents a more severe form of hypertensive heart disease most commonly seen in older women and often accom-

TABLE 78-3

Common Etiologies of Heart Failure in Older Adults

Coronary artery disease
- Acute myocardial infarction
- Ischemic cardiomyopathy

Hypertensive heart disease
- Hypertensive hypertrophic cardiomyopathy

Valvular heart disease
- Calcific aortic stenosis
- Mitral regurgitation
- Mitral stenosis
- Aortic insufficiency
- Prosthetic valve malfunction

Cardiomyopathy
- Dilated (nonischemic)
  - Alcohol
  - Anthracyclines
  - Idiopathic
- Hypertrophic
- Restrictive (especially amyloid)

Infective endocarditis

Myocarditis

Pericardial disease

High-output failure
- Chronic anemia
- Thiamine deficiency
- Hyperthyroidism
- Arteriovenous shunting

Age-related diastolic dysfunction

panied by calcification of the mitral valve annulus. These patients often manifest severe diastolic dysfunction and may exhibit dynamic left ventricular outflow tract obstruction indistinguishable from that seen in classical hypertrophic cardiomyopathy.

Valvular heart disease is an increasingly common cause of heart failure at older age. Calcific aortic stenosis is now the most common form of valvular heart disease requiring surgical intervention, and aortic valve replacement is the second most common open heart procedure performed in patients older than 70 years (after coronary bypass grafting). Mitral regurgitation in older individuals may be caused by myxomatous degeneration of the mitral valve leaflets and chordae tendineae (mitral valve prolapse), mitral annular calcification, valvular vegetations, ischemic papillary muscle dysfunction, or altered ventricular geometry owing to ischemic or nonischemic dilated cardiomyopathy. Importantly, mitral regurgitation may be acute (e.g., following acute myocardial infarction), subacute (e.g., endocarditis), or chronic (e.g., myxomatous degeneration), and the clinical manifestations may vary widely in each of these settings. In the United States, rheumatic mitral stenosis is a less common cause of heart failure in older adults, but it is still occasionally seen. Functional mitral stenosis owing to severe mitral valve annulus calcification with encroachment on the mitral valve orifice is an uncommon cause of heart failure, but it is associated with a poor prognosis. Aortic insufficiency may be either acute (e.g., because of endocarditis or type A aortic dissection) or chronic (e.g., annuloaortic ectasia or syphilitic aortitis), but it is a relatively infrequent cause of heart failure in older adults. Finally, prosthetic valve dysfunction should be considered as a potential cause of heart failure in any patient who has undergone previous valve repair or replacement.

Cardiomyopathies are classified into three categories: dilated, hypertrophic, and restrictive. In older adults, ischemic heart disease with one or more prior myocardial infarctions is the most common cause of dilated cardiomyopathy. Nonischemic dilated cardiomyopathy is less common in older than in younger individuals; when present, it is most often either idiopathic in origin or attributable to chronic ethanol abuse. Less frequently, dilated cardiomyopathy may be caused by cancer chemotherapy (e.g., anthracyclines and trastuzumab) or other causes. Classical hypertrophic cardiomyopathy, once thought to be rare in the geriatric age group, has been increasingly recognized in older adults since the advent of echocardiography. Similarly, restrictive cardiomyopathy, most commonly owing to amyloid deposition (so-called senile cardiac amyloid), is an occasional cause of heart failure. In one autopsy series, cardiac amyloid deposition was thought to be clinically important in approximately 10% of individuals 90 years of age or older.

Infective endocarditis is an uncommon but important cause of heart failure in older patients because it is one of the few etiologies for which curative pharmacological therapy is available. Endocarditis should be strongly suspected in any patient with persistent fever and either a prosthetic heart valve or a preexisting valvular lesion. It should also be considered in any patient with fever, recent dental work or other procedure, and a new or worsening heart murmur. It is important to recognize, however, that the clinical manifestations of endocarditis are often protean, and the absence of fever or a heart murmur does not exclude this diagnosis in older individuals.

Myocarditis is a relatively rare cause of heart failure in older adults. It may be infectious (e.g., postviral) or noninfectious (e.g., owing to sarcoid or collagen vascular disease). Pericardial effusions, for which there are numerous etiologies, occasionally present with heart failure symptomatology, including fatigue, exertional dyspnea, and edema. Constrictive pericarditis may be infectious (e.g., tuberculous) or noninfectious (e.g., postradiation), but it is a rare cause of heart failure in older patients.

High-output failure is an uncommon cause of heart failure in older adults, but when present the diagnosis is frequently overlooked. Potential causes of high-output failure include chronic anemia, hyperthyroidism, thiamine deficiency, and arteriovenous shunting (e.g., owing to a dialysis fistula or arteriovenous malformations).

Finally, in a small percentage of older heart failure patients, detailed investigation may fail to identify any primary cardiovascular pathology. In cases with normal left ventricular systolic function, heart failure may be attributed to age-related diastolic dysfunction.

Precipitating Factors

In addition to determining the etiology of heart failure, it is important to identify coexisting factors that may have contributed to the acute or subacute exacerbation (Table 78-4). The most common precipitant in patients with preexisting heart failure is noncompliance with medications and/or diet. Indeed, noncompliance may contribute to as many as two-thirds of heart failure exacerbations. In hospitalized patients, iatrogenic volume overload is also an important precipitant of heart failure.

Among cardiac factors, myocardial ischemia or infarction and new-onset atrial fibrillation or flutter are the most common causes of an acute episode of heart failure. Other cardiac causes include

TABLE 78-4

Common Precipitants of Heart Failure in Older Adults
Myocardial ischemia or infarction
Dietary sodium excess
Excess fluid intake
Medication noncompliance
Iatrogenic volume overload
Arrhythmias
• Atrial fibrillation or flutter
• Ventricular arrhythmias
• Bradyarrhythmias, especially sick sinus syndrome
Associated medical conditions
• Fever
• Infections, especially pneumonia or sepsis
• Hyperthyroidism or hypothyroidism
• Anemia
• Renal insufficiency
• Thiamine deficiency
• Pulmonary embolism
• Hypoxemia from chronic lung disease
• Uncontrolled hypertension
Drugs and medications
• Alcohol
• Beta-blockers (including ophthalmological agents)
• Calcium channel-blockers
• Antiarrhythmic agents
• Nonsteroidal anti-inflammatory drugs
• Corticosteroids
• Estrogen preparations
• Antihypertensive agents (e.g., clonidine and minoxodil)

ventricular arrhythmias, especially ventricular tachycardia, and bradyarrhythmias, such as marked sinus bradycardia or advanced atrioventricular block. Sick sinus syndrome, which is common in older adults, is a frequent cause of bradyarrhythmias in this population.

As previously discussed, older patients have limited cardiovascular reserve and they are less able to compensate in response to increased demands. As a result, heart failure in older adults is often precipitated by acute or worsening noncardiac conditions. Patients with acute respiratory disorders, such as pneumonia, pulmonary embolism, or an exacerbation of chronic obstructive lung disease, are particularly prone to exhibit deterioration in cardiac function. Other serious infections, such as sepsis or pyelonephritis, may also lead to heart failure exacerbations. In patients with hypertension, inadequate blood pressure control is a common cause of worsening heart failure. Thyroid disease, anemia (e.g., owing to gastrointestinal bleeding), and declining renal function may also contribute directly or indirectly to the development of heart failure.

Finally, numerous drugs and medications may contribute to heart failure exacerbations. Alcohol is a cardiac depressant, and it may also precipitate arrhythmias, especially atrial fibrillation. Beta-blockers (including ophthalmologic agents) and calcium antagonists are widely used in older individuals with cardiovascular disease, but both classes of agents are negatively inotropic and may exacerbate heart failure. Class Ia (e.g., quinidine, procainamide, and disopyramide) and Ic (e.g., flecainide and propafenone) antiarrhythmic agents have important myocardial depressant effects that may worsen cardiac function. Nonsteroidal anti-inflammatory drugs (NSAIDs), which are widely used by older adults, impair renal sodium and water excretion and may, therefore, contribute to intravascular volume overload. In addition, NSAIDs antagonize the effects of angiotensin-converting enzyme (ACE) inhibitors, thereby limiting the efficacy of these agents. Corticosteroids and estrogen preparations may cause fluid retention and an increase in total body water. Fluid retention is the most important side effect of the insulin-sensitizing thiazolidinediones (rosiglitazone and pioglitazone), and worsening heart failure may occur with these agents. The antihypertensive agent minoxodil also promotes fluid retention, and several other antihypertensive drugs (e.g., clonidine and guanethidine) may have unfavorable hemodynamic effects.

CLINICAL FEATURES

Symptoms

As in younger patients, the most common symptoms of heart failure in older adults are exertional shortness of breath, orthopnea, dependent edema, fatigue, and exercise intolerance. However, there is an increased prevalence of atypical symptomatology in older patients, particularly those older than 80 years (Table 78-5). As a result, heart failure in older adults is paradoxically both over- and underdiagnosed. Thus, shortness of breath and orthopnea in an older individual may be attributed to heart failure when the underlying cause is chronic lung disease, pneumonia, or pulmonary embolism. Similarly, fatigue and reduced exercise tolerance may be caused by anemia, hypothyroidism, depression, or poor physical conditioning. On the other hand, sedentary individuals and those limited by arthritis or neuromuscular conditions may not report exertional dyspnea

TABLE 78-5
Atypical Manifestations of Heart Failure in Older Persons

Nonspecific systemic complaints
- Malaise
- Lassitude
- Declining physical activity level

Neurological symptoms
- Confusion
- Irritability
- Sleep disturbances

Gastrointestinal disorders
- Anorexia
- Abdominal discomfort
- Nausea
- Diarrhea

or fatigue, and atypical symptoms such as those listed in Table 78-5 may be the first and only clinical manifestations of heart failure. In such cases, the physician must maintain a high index of suspicion, or the diagnosis of heart failure may be readily overlooked.

Signs

As with symptoms, the physical findings in older heart failure patients may be nonspecific or atypical. The classic signs of heart failure include moist pulmonary rales, an elevated jugular venous pressure, abdominojugular reflux, an S_3 gallop, and pitting edema of the lower extremities. However, pulmonary rales in older individuals may be due to chronic lung disease, pneumonia, or atelectasis, and peripheral edema may be caused by venous insufficiency, renal disease, or medication (e.g., calcium channel-blockers). Conversely, older patients may have an essentially normal physical examination despite markedly reduced cardiac performance. Alternatively, impaired sensorium or Cheyne–Stokes respirations may be the only findings to suggest the presence of heart failure.

Systolic versus Diastolic Heart Failure

The clinical manifestations of systolic and diastolic heart failure are similar, and no single clinical feature can reliably distinguish heart failure patients with intact left ventricular systolic function from those with impaired contractility. Nonetheless, certain features tend to favor one form or the other (Table 78-6). Based on the presence or absence of specific features, the probability of normal or reduced systolic function can be estimated, and there have been several attempts to develop algorithms for distinguishing these syndromes. Unfortunately, the predictive accuracy of these algorithms has been modest, and additional testing is essential in order to reliably differentiate systolic from diastolic heart failure.

DIAGNOSTIC EVALUATION

Heart failure may be difficult to diagnose in older patients with multiple comorbid conditions and either vague or nonspecific symptoms and signs. Thus, the first task facing the physician is to establish whether or not heart failure is present. This begins with a careful history and physical examination, giving due consideration to potential alternative etiologies for the patient's findings. As discussed in the previous section, physical signs may be unreliable in older patients. Nonetheless, certain findings, including pulsus alternans, an S_3 gallop, and the presence of jugular venous distension at rest or in response to the abdominojugular reflux maneuver, are highly specific signs of heart failure in older patients. In the absence of these findings, the diagnosis often remains in doubt, and additional laboratory studies are required.

To differentiate shortness of breath attributable to heart failure from that owing to other causes, the level of B-type natriuretic peptide (BNP—a 32 amino acid hormone released by the cardiac ventricles in response to increased wall tension) or its precursor N-terminal pro-BNP (NT-pro-BNP) is the single most useful test. However, BNP levels increase with age, especially in women (Figure 78-6), and with declining renal function. Therefore, the specificity

TABLE 78-6
Clinical Features of Systolic versus Diastolic Heart Failure

	Systolic Dysfunction	Diastolic Dysfunction
Demographics	Age <60 yr Male gender	Age >70 yr Female gender
Comorbid illnesses	Prior myocardial infarction Alcoholism Valvular insufficiency	Chronic hypertension Renal disease Obesity Aortic stenosis
Presentation	Progressive shortness of breath	Acute pulmonary edema Atrial fibrillation
Physical examination	Normotensive or hypotensive Jugular venous distention Displaced PMI S3 gallop Pitting edema	Hypertensive Absence of jugular venous distention Sustained PMI S4 gallop Absence of peripheral edema
Electrocardiogram	Q-waves and prior myocardial infarction	Left ventricular hypertrophy
Chest x-ray	Marked cardiomegaly	Normal or mildly increased heart size

PMI, point of maximum impulse.
Adapted with permission from Tresch DD, McGough MF. J Am Geriatr Soc. 1995;43:1035–1042.

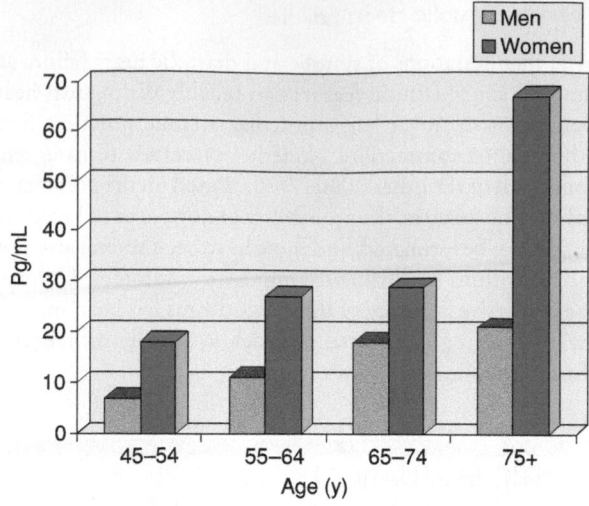

FIGURE 78-6. B-type natriuretic peptide levels by age and gender (mean values in healthy volunteers). *(Adapted with permission from Redfield MM, Rodeheffer RJ, Jacobsen SJ, et al. Plasma brain natriuretic peptide concentration: impact of age and gender. J Am Coll Cardiol. 2002;40:976–982.)*

of an elevated BNP level for clinical heart failure declines with age. BNP levels in excess of 500 pg/mL in the appropriate clinical context are highly suggestive of active heart failure, whereas a normal value (<100 pg/mL) in an older adult makes the diagnosis of heart failure much less likely. In addition to the BNP level, the chest radiograph remains useful for establishing the presence of active pulmonary congestion. In patients with moderate or severe heart failure, the chest film will usually demonstrate typical findings of cardiomegaly, pulmonary vascular engorgement, parenchymal edema, and pleural effusions. However, in patients with mild heart failure or coexisting pulmonary disease, the chest radiograph may be nondiagnostic.

Once the presence of heart failure has been established, the physician must address two crucial questions, the answers to which will serve as the basis for selecting appropriate therapy:

1. What is the underlying etiology and pathophysiology of heart failure (see Table 78-3)?
2. What additional factors, if any, contributed to or precipitated the development of heart failure (see Table 78-4)? Often, one or more precipitating factors can be identified, and alleviating these factors may significantly improve symptoms and reduce the likelihood of subsequent heart failure exacerbations.

In 2005, the American College of Cardiology and American Heart Association Task Force on Practice Guidelines published revised guidelines for the diagnosis and management of heart failure. Table 78-7 outlines an appropriate initial diagnostic assessment for patients with new-onset heart failure. Class I studies are defined as those that are indicated in most patients, Class II procedures are acceptable in some patients but are of unproven efficacy and may be controversial, and Class III studies are not routinely indicated and in some cases may be harmful. Briefly, basic laboratory studies, a thyroid function test, a chest radiograph, an electrocardiogram, and an echocardiogram with Doppler are recommended in all patients. Cardiac catheterization and coronary angiography are appropriate in patients with angina or significant ischemia on noninvasive testing, and in those who require surgical correction of a noncoronary car-

TABLE 78-7

Diagnostic Evaluation of Patients with Heart Failure

Class I (indicated in most patients)
- Complete blood count
- Blood chemistries: electrolytes, creatinine, blood urea nitrogen, fasting glucose, magnesium, calcium, liver function tests, and lipid profile
- Thyroid stimulating hormone (TSH)
- Urinalysis
- Chest radiograph and electrocardiogram (ECG)
- Echocardiogram: two-dimensional with Doppler
- Cardiac catheterization and coronary angiography in patients with angina or significant ischemia unless the patient is not eligible for revascularization

Class II (acceptable in selected patients; see text)
- Serum iron and ferritin
- Antinuclear antibody and rheumatoid factor
- If suspected, assessment for human immunodeficiency virus, amyloidosis, or pheochromocytoma
- Screening for sleep-disordered breathing
- Stress test to evaluate for ischemia in patients with unexplained heart failure who are potential candidates for revascularization
- Coronary angiography in all patients with possible or probable ischemia who are potential candidates for revascularization
- Endomyocardial biopsy when a specific diagnosis is suspected that would influence therapy

Class III (not routinely indicated, possibly harmful)
- Routine measurement of circulating neurohormone levels (e.g., norepinephrine)
- Routine signal-averaged electrocardiography
- Endomyocardial biopsy as a routine procedure in the evaluation of patients with heart failure

Data from Hunt SA, et al. ACC/AHA 2005 guideline update for the diagnosis and management of chronic heart failure in the adult – summary article. J Am Coll Cardiol. 2005;46:1116–1143.

diac lesion (e.g., aortic stenosis), unless the patient is not a suitable candidate for coronary revascularization.

The recommendations outlined in Table 78-7 are targeted toward a broad range of adult heart failure patients, and most are applicable in patients at an advanced age. Nonetheless, in older patients it is appropriate to consider the potential risks and benefits of each diagnostic procedure on an individualized basis, taking into account comorbid conditions, the extent of cardiac and noncardiac disability, and the wishes of the patient. For example, in a frail 85-year-old individual with diabetic nephropathy, the risk of precipitating dialysis-dependent end-stage renal disease as a complication of coronary angiography must be carefully weighed against the potential benefits to be derived from a successful revascularization procedure. Similarly, patient autonomy must be respected in all cases, and it is inappropriate to exert pressure on an older patient to undergo a procedure that the patient clearly does not desire. In this regard, it is imperative to discuss the therapeutic implications of specific procedures (especially invasive procedures) with respect to the patient's subsequent care (e.g., need for coronary bypass surgery) prior to performing the diagnostic assessment.

Systolic versus Diastolic Heart Failure

An important goal of the diagnostic evaluation, apart from determining the etiology of heart failure, is differentiating systolic from diastolic dysfunction, since the management of these two syndromes differs. As noted above, it is difficult to make this distinction on clinical grounds alone, and it is therefore essential to evaluate left ventricular function directly by echocardiography, radionuclide angiography, magnetic resonance imaging, or contrast ventriculography. In general, transthoracic echocardiography is the most useful technique because it is noninvasive, relatively inexpensive, and, in addition to providing information about systolic and diastolic function, it is helpful in evaluating chamber size, wall thickness and motion, valve function, and pericardial disease. Thus, transthoracic echocardiography is appropriate in virtually all older patients with newly diagnosed heart failure and in those with an unexplained change in symptom severity. The principal limitation of echocardiography is that adequate visualization of the heart may be unobtainable in a small percentage of patients, although the availability of echo-contrast agents has minimized this problem. Alternatively, radionuclide angiography can provide an accurate assessment of left ventricular function, as well as information about cavity size and regurgitant valvular lesions. Magnetic resonance imaging provides much the same information as echocardiography and radionuclide angiography but is less readily available and more expensive. For those patients who require cardiac catheterization, contrast left ventriculography is an excellent method for evaluating ventricular function.

Based on the results of echocardiography, radionuclide angiography, magnetic resonance imaging, or contrast ventriculography, heart failure may be classified as being primarily due to systolic dysfunction, as defined by a left ventricular ejection fraction of less than 40%; primarily due to diastolic dysfunction, as suggested by an ejection fraction of 50% or greater; or mixed, as indicated by an ejection fraction of 40% to 49%. However, it must be emphasized that systolic and diastolic dysfunction are not mutually exclusive. Indeed, almost all patients with significant systolic dysfunction also have concomitant diastolic dysfunction. Conversely, systolic dysfunction may play a role in the development of heart failure even when the ejection fraction under resting conditions is normal or near normal. Despite these limitations, the classification of heart failure as systolic or diastolic is useful in guiding therapy.

MANAGEMENT

The primary goals of heart failure therapy are to improve quality of life, reduce the frequency of heart failure exacerbations, and extend survival. Secondary goals include maximizing independence and exercise capacity, enhancing emotional well-being and reducing resource use and the associated costs of care.

To achieve these goals, optimal therapy in older patients comprises three principal components: correction of the underlying etiology whenever possible (e.g., aortic valve replacement for aortic stenosis or coronary revascularization for severe ischemia), attention to the nonpharmacological and rehabilitative aspects of treatment, and the judicious use of medications.

As discussed in the section on prognosis, the outlook for patients with established heart failure is poor. Therefore, the importance of effectively treating the primary etiology and all comorbid conditions predisposing to heart failure cannot be overemphasized. Since coronary heart disease and hypertension are the most common causes of heart failure in older adults, primary and secondary prevention of these conditions are critical if the development of heart failure is to be forestalled. Indeed, it has now been shown in multiple clinical trials

that effective treatment of both systolic and diastolic hypertension can reduce the incidence of heart failure by up to 50%. Similarly, appropriate management of other coronary risk factors, particularly hyperlipidemia and cigarette smoking, will undoubtedly further reduce the burden of heart failure through the primary prevention of coronary heart disease.

Nonpharmacological Therapy

Despite recent advances in the pharmacotherapy of heart failure, repetitive heart failure exacerbations are common and are more often precipitated by behavioral and social factors than by either new cardiac events (e.g., ischemia or an arrhythmia) or progressive deterioration in ventricular function. In one study, lack of adherence to prescribed medications and/or diet contributed to 64% of heart failure exacerbations among urban blacks, while emotional and environmental factors contributed to 26% of hospital readmissions. In another study involving 140 patients 70 years of age or older hospitalized with heart failure, 47% were readmitted at least once during a 90-day follow-up period. Behavioral and social factors contributing to readmission included medication and dietary noncompliance (15% and 18%, respectively), inadequate social support (21%), inadequate discharge planning (15%), inadequate follow-up (20%), and failure of the patient to seek medical attention promptly when symptoms recurred (20%). The findings suggest that interventions directed at behavioral and social factors could potentially reduce readmissions and improve quality of life in patients with heart failure, and this hypothesis has now been confirmed in numerous prospective randomized trials. In a recent meta-analytic review of 33 such trials, heart failure readmissions were reduced by 42%, all-cause readmissions were reduced by 24%, and mortality was reduced by 20% in patients with heart failure enrolled in a "disease management" program relative to conventional care.

Components of a comprehensive nonpharmacological treatment program are listed in Table 78-8. As with other aspects of geriatric care, it is important to structure the treatment program in order to accommodate the needs of each individual patient. Clearly, not every patient will require all of the components listed in the table. Similarly, the optimal intensity of any given component, e.g., patient education or follow-up care, will vary substantially. For these reasons, it is desirable to designate a single individual, such as a nurse case manager, to coordinate all aspects of the patient's care.

Physical Activity and Exercise

Traditionally, patients with heart failure have been advised to restrict physical activity on the grounds that rest is beneficial for the heart and that exercise could potentially worsen cardiac function or precipitate arrhythmias. However, it is now recognized that although some degree of activity restriction may be appropriate, excessive limitation of physical activity may contribute to a progressive decline in functional capacity as a result of cardiovascular and muscular deconditioning. In addition, several small studies have demonstrated that participation in an appropriately structured exercise program may result in significant improvements in functional capacity and quality of life in patients with heart failure. As a result, current guidelines recommend regular exercise for the majority of patients with heart failure.

Data from nine randomized trials on the effects of exercise training in patients with heart failure involving 801 patients have been

TABLE 78-8

Nonpharmacological Aspects of Heart Failure Management

Patient education
- Symptoms and signs of heart failure
- Detailed discussion of all medications
- Emphasize importance of compliance
- Specific information about when to contact nurse or physician for worsening symptoms
- Involve family/significant other as much as possible

Dietary consultation
- Individualized and consistent with needs/lifestyle
- Sodium restriction (1.5–2 g/d)
- Weight loss, if appropriate
- Low fat, low cholesterol, if appropriate
- Adequate caloric intake
- Emphasize compliance while allowing flexibility

Medication review
- Eliminate unnecessary medications
- Simplify regimen whenever possible
- Consolidate dosing schedule

Social services
- Assess social support structure
- Evaluate emotional and financial needs
- Intervene proactively when feasible

Daily weight chart
- Specific directions on when to contact nurse or physician for changes in weight
- Self-management of diuretic dosage based on daily weights in selected patients

Support stockings to reduce edema

Activity prescription (see text)

Vaccinations
- Annual influenza vaccine
- Pneumococcal vaccine

Intensive follow-up
- Telephone contacts
- Home visits
- Outpatient clinic

Contact information
- Names and phone numbers of nurse and physician
- 24-hour availability

TABLE 78-9

Contraindications to Exercise in Older Patients

Recent myocardial infarction or unstable angina (within 2 weeks)
Severe, decompensated heart failure (New York Heart Association Class IV)
Life-threatening arrhythmias not adequately treated
Severe aortic stenosis or hypertrophic cardiomyopathy
Any acute serious illness (e.g., pneumonia)
Any condition precluding safe participation in an exercise program

Association class, 6-minute walk distance, and quality of life, whereas control-group patients demonstrated no change from baseline in any of these parameters. In addition, patients receiving the intervention had significantly fewer hospital admissions relative to the control group. These data provide further support for a beneficial effect of exercise and cardiac rehabilitation in older patients with mild-to-moderate heart failure. Despite these findings, additional studies are needed to evaluate the safety and efficacy of regular exercise in older heart failure patients, especially those older than 75 years and patients with diastolic heart failure.

Exercise Prescription

A comprehensive exercise and conditioning program is appropriate for most older patients with mild-to-moderate heart failure symptoms and no contraindications to exercise (Table 78-9). Table 78-10 outlines the basic components of such a program. In general, patients should try to exercise every day. A typical session should include some gentle stretching exercises as well as strengthening exercises using elastic bands or light weights and targeting all of the major muscle groups. Suitable forms of aerobic exercise for older patients include walking, stationary cycling, and swimming. The choice of aerobic exercise should be tailored to the patient's wishes and abilities. When initiating an exercise program, the duration and intensity of the aerobic activity should be well within the patient's comfort range. The activity should be enjoyable, not stressful, and after completing the activity the patient should feel "positive" about the experience and not unduly fatigued. For many older patients with heart failure, this may mean starting with as little as 2 to 5 minutes of slow-paced walking. Once the patient feels comfortable exercising, the duration of exercise can be gradually increased over a period of several weeks. Weekly increases of 1 to 2 minutes per session are appropriate for most patients. Once the patient can exercise

summarized. Most of the studies excluded patients with preserved left ventricular systolic function, and none of the studies specifically targeted older patients. The average duration of training ranged from 8 to 60 weeks, with a mean follow-up of almost 2 years. The mode of exercise consisted primarily of walking and/or cycling. Exercise capacity consistently improved with training, primarily as a result of adaptations in the oxidative capacity of skeletal muscle without evidence for a beneficial effect on central cardiac hemodynamics. In addition, mortality was reduced by 35% and the combined end point of death or hospitalization was reduced by 28% in patients participating in an exercise program.

A more recent randomized trial of cardiac rehabilitation in 200 patients 60 to 89 years of age (mean 72 years, 66% male) with New York Heart Association Class II–III heart failure evaluated the effects of exercise prescription, education, occupational therapy, and psychosocial counseling. At 24 weeks follow-up, intervention group patients experienced significant improvements in New York Heart

TABLE 78-10

Exercise Prescription for Older Patients with Heart Failure

Components of conditioning program
- Flexibility exercises
- Strengthening exercises
- Aerobic conditioning

Frequency of exercise: daily, if possible
Duration of exercise: individualized; start low, go slow
Intensity of exercise: low to moderate (see text for details)
Rate of progression: gradual over weeks to months
Monitoring: heart rate, perceived exertion (see text)

continuously and comfortably for 20 to 30 minutes, the intensity of exercise may be increased, if desired. For example, if the patient is walking a half-mile in 30 minutes, he or she may gradually reduce the half-mile time to 20 minutes, while maintaining a total exercise duration of 30 minutes.

The two most common techniques for monitoring exercise intensity are the target heart rate method and the patient's subjective assessment of perceived exertion. For patients not taking medications that lower heart rate (e.g., beta-blockers), the maximum attainable heart rate in beats per minute (bpm) can be estimated from the following formula: 220 − age. The patient's resting heart rate is then subtracted from this figure to determine the *heart rate reserve*. A suitable target heart rate for low-intensity exercise can be calculated as the resting heart rate *plus* 30% to 50% of the heart rate reserve. For moderate-intensity exercise, the target range is the resting heart rate plus 50% to 70% of the heart rate reserve. For example, an 80-year-old individual has a predicted maximum heart rate of 220 − 80 = 140 bpm. If the resting heart rate is 80, the heart rate reserve is 60 (i.e., 140 − 80). For low-intensity exercise, 30% to 50% of the heart rate reserve would be 18 to 30 bpm. Adding this to the resting heart rate of 80 would yield a range for the target heart rate of 98 to 110 bpm.

For many older patients, calculating the target heart rate may be difficult. In addition, it may not be possible to accurately determine heart rate during exercise (unless a heart rate monitor is used). For these reasons, the patient's subjective assessment of perceived exertion is often the most practical method for monitoring exercise intensity. In addition, perceived exertion correlates reasonably well with exercise heart rate. A simple perceived exertion scale comprises five levels: very light, light, moderate, somewhat heavy, and heavy. Older patients with heart failure should begin with very light exercise, progressing to the light range as tolerated. After several weeks, some patients may wish to increase their perceived exertion level into the moderate range, but more strenuous exercise is not recommended for patients with heart failure.

Cessation of Exercise

All patients participating in an exercise program should be advised to discontinue exercise if they experience persistent chest discomfort, undue dyspnea or fatigue, dizziness, rapid or irregular heart beats, excessive sweating, or any other symptom suggesting that continuation of exercise may be unsafe. If the above symptoms do not resolve promptly with termination of exercise or if they occur repeatedly, the physician should be notified prior to continuing the exercise program.

Treatment of Systolic Heart Failure

From the therapeutic perspective, patients with heart failure and a left ventricular ejection fraction of less than 45% may be considered as having predominantly systolic heart failure, while those with an ejection fraction of 45% or greater may be considered as having predominantly diastolic heart failure. Although there is considerable overlap between these syndromes, their distinction is useful in designing therapy.

In general, the treatment of systolic heart failure in older patients does not differ substantially from that in younger patients. Table 78-11 lists currently available therapeutic options for systolic heart failure, and these are discussed in detail below.

TABLE 78-11

Treatment Options for Systolic Heart Failure

Angiotensin-converting enzyme inhibitors
Angiotensin II receptor blockers
Other vasodilators
Beta-adrenergic blocking agents
Diuretics • Aldosterone antagonists
Digoxin
Calcium channel-blockers
Antithrombotic agents • Aspirin • Warfarin

ACE Inhibitors

Numerous prospective randomized clinical trials using multiple different ACE inhibitors in a variety of clinical settings have conclusively demonstrated that these agents significantly reduce mortality and hospitalization rates and improve exercise tolerance and quality of life in patients with impaired left ventricular systolic function, even in the absence of clinical heart failure. Although none of these studies included patients older than 80 years, available evidence indicates that ACE inhibitors are as effective in older patients as in younger ones. Based on these findings, ACE inhibitors are now considered first-line therapy for all patients, regardless of age, with left ventricular systolic dysfunction with or without overt heart failure. However, despite these recommendations, ACE inhibitors remain underused, particularly in older patients.

ACE inhibitors approved for use in the United States for the treatment of heart failure include captopril, enalapril, lisinopril, ramipril, trandolapril, quinapril, and fosinopril. In older patients, therapy should be initiated with a low dose (e.g., captopril 6.25–12.5 mg tid–qid or enalapril 2.5–5 mg bid), and the dose should be gradually increased as tolerated. In hospitalized patients who are hemodynamically stable, the dose may be increased daily; in outpatients, the dose should be increased weekly or biweekly. Throughout the titration period, blood pressure, renal function, and serum potassium levels should be monitored.

For maintenance therapy, ACE inhibitor dosages should be commensurate with those used in the clinical trials. Recommended "target" doses for selected ACE inhibitors are as follows: captopril 50 mg tid, enalapril 10 to 20 mg bid, lisinopril 20 to 40 mg daily, ramipril 10 mg daily, trandolapril 4 mg daily, quinapril 40 mg bid, and fosinopril 40 mg daily. In patients unable to tolerate full therapeutic doses of ACE inhibitors, lower doses may be used; however, it must be recognized that clinical benefits may be attenuated. In addition, although captopril is an excellent agent for use during the titration phase, once the maintenance dose has been reached, it may be desirable to change to a once-daily ACE inhibitor at equivalent dosage for reasons of convenience, compliance, and cost.

The most common side effect from ACE inhibitors is a dry, hacking cough, which may be severe enough to require discontinuation of therapy in 5% to 10% of patients during long-term use. Less common but more serious side effects include hypotension, a decline in renal function, and hyperkalemia. These side effects tend to occur shortly after initiation of therapy and may be aggravated by intravascular volume contraction as a result of overdiuresis. Indications for downward titration or discontinuation of an ACE inhibitor include symptomatic hypotension, persistent increase in serum creatinine of 1 mg/dL or greater, or a rise in the serum potassium level above 5.5 meq/L. Note that asymptomatic low blood pressure does not mandate dosage reduction.

Although ACE inhibitors are generally well tolerated and can be taken safely in combination with most other medications, it is important to recognize that NSAIDs, which are widely used by older adults (both by prescription and over the counter), are potent ACE inhibitor antagonists. In addition, NSAIDs promote sodium and water retention and may adversely affect renal function. Therefore, NSAIDs should be avoided whenever possible in patients with heart failure. The use of aspirin in combination with an ACE inhibitor is controversial, as there is some evidence suggesting that aspirin may attenuate the effects of ACE inhibitors. However, recent studies indicate that aspirin does not adversely affect clinical outcomes in patients with heart failure treated with ACE inhibitors. Therefore, patients with a clear indication for aspirin therapy, such as coronary artery disease, peripheral arterial disease, cerebrovascular disease, or diabetes mellitus, should receive aspirin according to current treatment guidelines for these conditions. The value of prophylactic aspirin in older patients with heart failure without known vascular disease or diabetes is unknown, and additional study of this issue is needed.

Angiotensin II Receptor Blockers

Angiotensin II receptor blockers (ARBs) bind directly to angiotensin II receptors on the cell membrane. Unlike ACE inhibitors, ARBs do not inhibit the breakdown of bradykinins, thus eliminating bradykinin-mediated side effects, including cough.

The use of ARBs for the treatment of heart failure, either alone or in combination with an ACE inhibitor, has been evaluated in several studies. In the second Evaluation of Losartan in the Elderly trial (ELITE-II), losartan 50 mg once daily was compared to captopril 50 mg TID in 3152 patients 60 years of age or older (mean age 71 years) with moderate heart failure and an ejection fraction of 40% or less. After a mean follow-up of 18 months, there was no statistically significant difference in mortality between the two treatments, although there were 12% more deaths in the losartan group (280 vs. 250). As in the smaller ELITE-I trial, losartan was better tolerated than the ACE inhibitor captopril.

In the Valsartan Heart Failure trial (Val-HEFT), 5010 patients with heart failure and an ejection fraction of less than 40% were randomized to valsartan or placebo in addition to standard care, which included an ACE inhibitor in 93% of patients and a beta-blocker in 35%. During a 2-year follow-up period, mortality did not differ between patients treated with valsartan or placebo, but there was a significant 24% reduction in rehospitalizations for heart failure in the valsartan group, with similar effects in younger and older patients. However, patients receiving both an ACE inhibitor and a beta-blocker as background therapy experienced an unexplained increase in mortality when valsartan was added.

In the Valsartan in Acute Myocardial Infarction trial, 14 703 patients with clinical heart failure and/or an ejection fraction less than 35% within 10 days of experiencing an acute myocardial infarction were randomly assigned to receive valsartan, captopril, or both drugs. More than 70% of patients were also receiving beta-blockers. During a median follow-up of 24.7 months, there were no differences between groups with respect to all-cause mortality or the composite end point of fatal or nonfatal cardiovascular events. Median age was 65 years, and results were similar in older and younger patients. Hypotension and renal dysfunction were more common with valsartan, whereas cough, rash, and taste disturbances were more common with captopril. Limiting side effects were more common in patients receiving both drugs than in those receiving either drug alone.

The use of candesartan for the treatment of patients with heart failure and an ejection fraction of 40% or less has been evaluated in two large trials. In the Candesartan in Heart Failure: Assessment of Reduction in Mortality and Morbidity (CHARM)—Alternative study, 2028 patients intolerant to ACE inhibitors were randomized to candesartan or placebo and followed for a median of 33.7 months. Compared to patients in the placebo group, patients randomized to candesartan experienced a significant 30% reduction in the composite end point of cardiovascular death or hospitalization for heart failure. All-cause mortality was reduced by 17%, which was of borderline statistical significance. Hypotension, worsening renal function, and hyperkalemia, but not cough or angioedema, were more common in the candesartan group. The mean age of patients in the CHARM-Alternative study was approximately 66.5 years, and nearly one-fourth of patients were 75 years of age or older; however, subgroup analysis by age has not been reported.

In the CHARM-Added trial, 2548 symptomatic patients with heart failure and an ejection fraction of 40% or less who were receiving an ACE inhibitor were randomized to candesartan or placebo and followed for a median of 41 months. Compared to the placebo group, there was a significant 15% reduction in the composite end point of cardiovascular death or hospitalization for heart failure in patients randomized to candesartan. All-cause mortality was 11% lower in the candesartan group, but the difference was not significant. The mean age of patients in the CHARM-Added trial was 64 years, 19% of patients were 75 years of age or older, and similar results were reported in older and younger patients.

Based on these studies, ARBs are indicated for treatment of symptomatic heart failure in patients intolerant to ACE inhibitors and in patients with heart failure or left ventricular systolic dysfunction following acute myocardial infarction. In the United States, valsartan and candesartan are approved for the treatment of heart failure. The recommended starting dose of valsartan is 20 to 40 mg bid, and the dose should be titrated to 160 mg bid as tolerated. The starting dose of candesartan is 4 to 8 mg once daily, with titration to 32 mg once daily as tolerated. The major side effects of ARBs include hypotension, renal insufficiency, and hyperkalemia.

Other Vasodilators

In patients who are unable to tolerate an ACE inhibitor or ARB, the combination of hydralazine with oral or topical nitrates provides an acceptable alternative. In the first Veteran's Administration Heart Failure trial (V-HeFT-I), the hydralazine/nitrate combination was associated with a 36% mortality reduction compared to prazosin and placebo in patients with chronic heart failure and impaired systolic function. In a follow-up study (V-HeFT-II), patients with systolic heart failure were randomized to receive hydralazine/nitrates or enalapril. Although hydralazine/nitrates and enalapril had similar effects on exercise tolerance and quality of life, mortality was lower in the enalapril group.

More recently, the African-American Heart Failure trial (A-HeFT) randomized 1050 black patients with New York Heart Association Class III or IV heart failure to a fixed-dose combination of isosorbide dinitrate plus hydralazine or to placebo in addition to standard heart failure therapy. The study was stopped after an average follow-up of 10 months because of a significantly higher mortality rate in patients randomized to placebo. Heart failure hospitalizations were also lower and quality of life was improved in patients randomized to hydralazine-nitrates relative to placebo. Based on the results of A-HeFT, the fixed-dose combination of isosorbide dinitrate and hydralazine has been approved for treatment of heart failure in black patients in the United States. Although there was no upper-age restriction for the A-HeFT study, the average age of patients enrolled in the trial was only 57 years, so the efficacy of this therapy in elderly blacks remains unknown.

The dose of hydralazine used in the V-HeFT trials was 75 mg QID, and nitrates were administered as isosorbide dinitrate 40 mg QID. In A-HeFT, the total daily dose of hydralazine was 225 mg and of isosorbide dinitrate 120 mg. For older patients, treatment should begin with lower dosages (e.g., hydralazine 12.5–25 mg TID–QID; isosorbide dinitrate 10 mg TID–QID), followed by gradual upward titration to achieve the doses used in the trials. The most common side effects associated with hydralazine/nitrates in the V-HeFT and A-HeFT studies included headache and dizziness. A small percentage of patients in V-HeFT developed arthralgias or other symptoms suggestive of hydralazine-induced lupus.

Beta-Blockers

Traditionally, beta-adrenergic blocking agents have been considered contraindicated in patients with heart failure owing to their negative inotropic and chronotropic effects, both of which serve to diminish cardiac output. However, it is now recognized that persistent activation of the sympathetic nervous system is detrimental in patients with heart failure because it exacerbates ischemia, aids in arrhythmogenesis, promotes β-receptor down-regulation, and contributes to a progressive decline in ventricular function. These considerations led to the hypothesis that long-term treatment with β-blockers might be beneficial in patients with heart failure, and several large prospective randomized clinical trials have now confirmed that long-term beta-blockade improves left ventricular function and reduces both total mortality and sudden cardiac death in a broad range of patients with heart failure and impaired left ventricular systolic function.

These findings were recently confirmed in the Study of the Effects of Nebivolol Intervention on Outcomes and Rehospitalization in Seniors with Heart Failure trial, which randomized 2128 patients 70 years of age or older (mean age 76 years, 37% women) to nebivolol or placebo. During a mean follow-up of 21 months, the primary composite outcome of death or cardiovascular hospitalization was significantly lower in patients randomized to nebivolol, with similar results in younger and older patients, including those older than 85 years. Based on these studies, beta-blockers are now recommended as a standard therapy, along with ACE inhibitors, in almost all patients with symptomatic heart failure in the absence of contraindications.

In the United States, carvedilol and metoprolol have been approved for the treatment of heart failure. Starting dosages are carvedilol 3.125 mg bid and metoprolol 12.5 mg bid (or extended release metoprolol 25 mg once daily). The dose should be gradually increased at approximately 2 week intervals as tolerated, to achieve maintenance dosages of carvedilol 25 to 50 mg bid or metoprolol 100 to 200 mg daily.

Contraindications to the use of beta-blockers include severe decompensated heart failure, significant bronchospastic lung disease, marked bradycardia (resting heart rate less than 50/min), systolic blood pressure less than 90 to 100 mm Hg, advanced heart block (greater than first degree), and known intolerance to beta-blockade. In addition, as a result of the potential for significant adverse effects, it is important to monitor heart rate, blood pressure, clinical symptoms, and the cardiorespiratory examination during initiation and titration of therapy. Patients should be advised that they may experience a modest deterioration in heart failure symptoms during the first few weeks of beta-blocker therapy, but that in most cases these symptoms resolve and the long-term tolerability of beta-blockers is excellent. However, if severe adverse effects occur, dosage reduction or discontinuation of treatment may be necessary.

Diuretics

Diuretics are the most effective agents for relieving pulmonary congestion and edema, and for this reason they remain a key component of heart failure management. However, neither thiazide nor loop diuretics have been shown to alter the natural history of heart failure, and their beneficial effects are primarily palliative.

In patients with mild chronic heart failure, a thiazide diuretic (e.g., hydrochlorothiazide 12.5–50 mg daily) may be sufficient for relieving congestive symptoms and maintaining fluid homeostasis. However, most patients will require a more potent agent, and the "loop" diuretics, including furosemide, bumetanide, and torsemide, are the drugs most widely used. For optimal effectiveness, patients should be instructed to maintain a low sodium diet (1.5–2.0 g/d) and to avoid excessive fluid intake. Typical daily doses of "loop" diuretics range from 20 to 160 mg for furosemide, 0.5 to 5 mg for bumetanide, and 5 to 100 mg for torsemide. In patients hospitalized with an acute episode of heart failure, intravenous administration is more effective than the oral route in promoting diuresis, and continuous intravenous infusion is more effective than bolus dosing. In patients who fail to respond adequately to a loop diuretic, the addition of metolazone 2.5 to 10 mg daily often leads to a brisk diuresis.

The most common and important side effects of diuretics are electrolyte disturbances, including hypokalemia, hyponatremia, hypomagnesemia, and increased bicarbonate levels indicative of metabolic alkalosis. Owing to age-related changes in renal function as well as a higher prevalence of comorbid illnesses such as diabetes, older patients are at increased risk of serious diuretic-induced electrolyte abnormalities. For this reason, electrolytes should be monitored closely when diuretic therapy is being adjusted. This is particularly true when using metolazone, which can cause life-threatening hyponatremia after relatively short-term use.

Aldosterone Antagonists

The aldosterone antagonists spironolactone and eplerenone are relatively weak potassium-sparing diuretics that interfere with the effect of the neurohormone aldosterone. In the Randomized Aldactone Evaluation of Survival trial, spironolactone 12.5 to 50 mg once daily reduced mortality by 30% and heart failure hospitalizations by 35% in patients with New York Heart Association Class III or IV heart failure and a left ventricular ejection fraction ≤35%, despite therapy with an ACE inhibitor, digoxin, and loop diuretic. Moreover, the

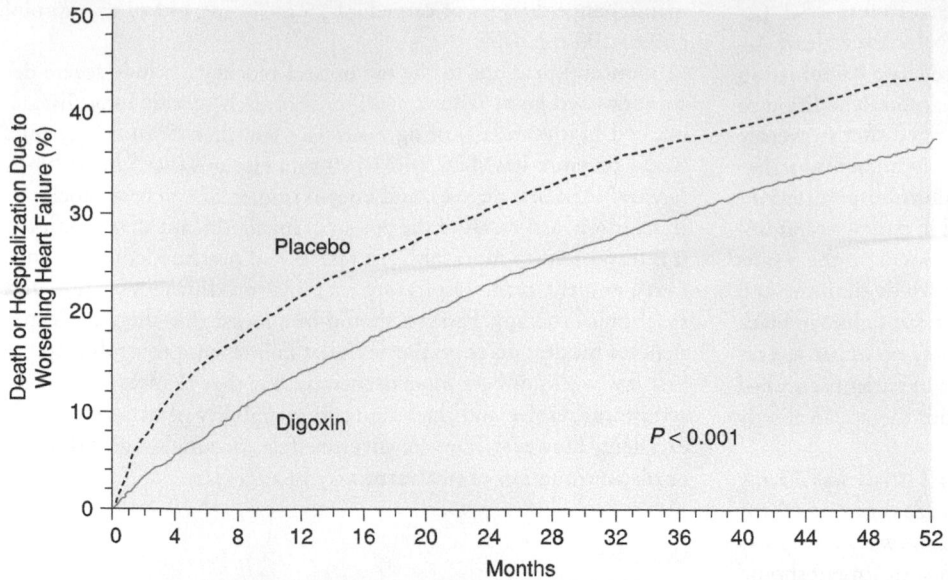

FIGURE 78-7. Incidence of death or hospitalization due to worsening heart failure in patients treated with digoxin versus placebo. The risk for the combined end point was 25% lower in the digoxin group. *(Adapted with permission from The Digitalis Investigation Group. The effect of digoxin on mortality and morbidity in patients with heart failure. N Engl J Med. 1997;336:525–533.)*

beneficial effects of spironolactone were at least as great in older as in younger patients. In the Eplerenone Post-Acute Myocardial Infarction Heart Failure Efficacy and Survival study, eplerenone 25 to 50 mg once daily significantly reduced mortality by 15% over a mean follow-up period of 16 months in patients with clinical evidence for heart failure and an ejection fraction of 40% or less within 3 to 16 days following acute myocardial infarction. Sudden death from cardiac causes and cardiovascular hospitalizations were also reduced in the eplerenone group. Compared to placebo, hyperkalemia occurred more commonly but hypokalemia occurred less frequently with eplerenone. The average age of patients in the Eplerenone Post-Acute Myocardial Infarction Heart Failure Efficacy and Survival study was 64 years, and although the relative benefit of eplerenone was somewhat less in older compared to younger patients, the difference was not statistically significant.

Based on the results of these studies, an aldosterone antagonist is recommended in patients with advanced heart failure symptoms and severe left ventricular systolic dysfunction, and in patients with heart failure and an ejection fraction of 40% or less following myocardial infarction. These agents are contraindicated in patients with significant renal dysfunction (creatinine ≥2.5 mg/dL) or preexisting hyperkalemia. Older patients may be at increased risk of adverse effects, and renal function as well as serum potassium levels should be monitored closely during initiation and titration of therapy. In addition, up to 10% of patients receiving long-term treatment with spironolactone may experience painful gynecomastia requiring discontinuation of the drug; this side effect occurs less frequently with eplerenone.

Digoxin

Digoxin inhibits the sodium–potassium exchange pump located within the myocyte membrane, producing a rise in intracellular sodium concentration. This facilitates sodium–calcium exchange, leading to an increase in intracellular calcium. Calcium binds with troponin C, which initiates the process of contraction by allowing myosin to bind with actin. By increasing calcium availability, digoxin induces a modest increase in the force of myocardial contraction (positive inotropic effect). This effect occurs whether or not heart failure is present, and it does not appear to be affected by advancing age.

In 1997, the Digitalis Investigation Group (DIG) reported the results of a prospective randomized trial involving 6800 patients with heart failure and ejection fractions less than 45%. Patients were randomized to receive digoxin or placebo in addition to diuretics and an ACE inhibitor, and the average duration of follow-up was 37 months. Overall mortality did not differ between digoxin and placebo (34.8% vs. 35.1%), but there were 28% fewer hospitalizations for heart failure in the digoxin group, and the combined end point of death or hospitalization for heart failure was significantly reduced (Figure 78-7). In addition, the beneficial effects of digoxin were similar in younger and older patients, including octogenarians. Subsequent analyses based on data from the DIG trial suggest that digoxin administered at low dosages to achieve serum concentrations in the range of 0.5 to 0.9 ng/mL may be associated with improved survival as well as a reduction in all-cause hospitalizations. These findings confirm that digoxin is beneficial in controlling heart failure symptoms and support the use of low-dose digoxin in patients who remain symptomatic despite appropriate dosages of an ACE inhibitor, beta-blocker, and diuretic.

Side effects from digoxin fall into three major categories: cardiac, neurological, and gastrointestinal. In the DIG study, side effects that occurred more frequently in patients receiving digoxin included nausea and vomiting, diarrhea, visual disturbances, supraventricular and ventricular arrhythmias, and advanced atrioventricular heart block. Although not reported in the DIG trial, older patients may be at increased risk of digoxin toxicity, especially cardiac toxicity, in part owing to a decreased volume of drug distribution. Patients with chronic lung disease, amyloid heart disease, and other conditions may also be at increased risk of digoxin toxicity.

In most older patients with relatively normal renal function, a digoxin dose of 0.125 mg daily is usually sufficient to achieve a therapeutic effect. Patients with renal impairment or small body habitus may require a lower dose. Serum digoxin concentration should be measured 2 to 4 weeks after initiating therapy, and periodically thereafter, to ensure that the level is in the therapeutic range of 0.5 to 0.9 ng/mL. It is also appropriate to measure the digoxin level whenever digitalis intoxication is suspected. In addition, since diuretic-induced hypokalemia and hypomagnesia potentiate digoxin's cardiotoxic effects, including proarrhythmia, it is important to maintain normal serum concentrations of these electrolytes in all patients receiving digoxin.

Calcium Channel-Blockers

First-generation short-acting calcium channel-blockers, including nifedipine, diltiazem, and verapamil, are contraindicated in patients with systolic heart failure because each of these agents has been associated with adverse clinical outcomes. In addition, although long-acting formulations of these agents may ultimately prove to be safe and effective, there is currently insufficient information to recommend their use.

The third-generation calcium channel-blockers amlodipine and felodipine have each been studied in prospective randomized trials involving heart failure patients with impaired systolic function. Although the initial Prospective Randomized Amlodipine Survival Evaluation (PRAISE) suggested that amlodipine might be beneficial in patients with nonischemic systolic heart failure, this was not confirmed in PRAISE-2. Similarly, the V-HeFT-3 trial failed to demonstrate a significant benefit in patients with heart failure treated with felodipine. In light of these findings, there are no currently approved indications for the use of calcium channel-blockers in patients with systolic heart failure, and their use in this condition is not recommended. However, in patients with heart failure and active anginal symptoms not controlled with beta-blockers and nitrates, the addition of amlodipine or felodipine is reasonable.

Antithrombotic Therapy

Patients with left ventricular systolic dysfunction are at increased risk of thromboembolic events, including stroke. However, in the absence of atrial fibrillation, rheumatic mitral valve disease, or a history of prior embolization, the value of antithrombotic treatment for the prevention of embolic events is unknown. In the Warfarin and Antiplatelet Therapy in Chronic Heart Failure trial, 1587 patients with New York Heart Association class II or III heart failure were randomized to receive aspirin 162 mg/day, clopidogrel 75 mg/day, or warfarin to maintain an international normalized ratio (INR) of 2.5 to 3.0. After a mean follow-up of 23 months, there were no differences between the three groups in the primary composite end point of death, myocardial infarction, or stroke. Hospitalizations for heart failure occurred more frequently in the aspirin group than with either clopidogrel or warfarin, whereas bleeding complications were more common with warfarin. The mean age of patients in the Warfarin and Antiplatelet Therapy in Chronic Heart Failure trial was 63 years; subgroup analysis by age has not been reported. Based on currently available data, anticoagulation with warfarin to achieve an INR of 2.0 to 3.0 is recommended in high-risk patients without major contraindications. Such patients include those with chronic or intermittent atrial fibrillation or atrial flutter, rheumatic mitral valve disease with left atrial enlargement, prior stroke or unexplained arterial embolus, a mobile left ventricular thrombus (as demonstrated by echocardiography or other imaging modality), or a left atrial appendage thrombus identified by transesophageal echocardiography. Routine use of warfarin in other circumstances is not recommended.

Aspirin is justified in patients with known coronary heart disease, particularly those with recent myocardial infarction, unstable angina, coronary angioplasty, or bypass surgery. Aspirin is also recommended for patients with peripheral arterial disease or diabetes. In addition, aspirin is appropriate in high-risk patients (as listed above) who are not suitable candidates for warfarin. As noted previously, additional study is needed to determine the value of aspirin in older patients with heart failure without established vascular disease or diabetes.

Statins

Statins have been shown to reduce mortality and nonfatal cardiovascular events in patients up to age 80 with coronary artery disease, peripheral arterial disease, or diabetes. In addition, several studies have suggested that statins may be beneficial in patients with heart failrue. However, the recently reported rosuvastatin in older patients with systolic heart failure trial, in which 5011 patients 60 years of age or older (mean age 73 years, 24% female) with ischemic cardiomyopathy and an ejection fraction of 40% or less were randomized to rosuvastatin or placebo and followed for an average of 33 months, failed to show a significant bebefit of rosuvastatin on either the primary outcome of death from cardiovascular causes, nonfatal myocardial infarction, or nonfatal stroke, or on total mortality. Hospitalizations for cardiovascular causes occurred less frequently in patients randomized to rosuvastatin. Based on these findings, rosuvastatin is not recommended for older patients with systolic heart failure. The role of other statins in this population requires further investigation.

Treatment of Diastolic Heart Failure

Despite the fact that approximately 50% of older patients with heart failure have preserved left ventricular systolic function, few large-scale clinical trials have evaluated specific pharmacologic agents for the treatment of this condition. As a result, therapy for diastolic heart failure remains largely empiric.

At least 70% to 80% of older persons with diastolic heart failure have hypertension, and coronary and valvular heart diseases are also highly prevalent in this population. Optimal therapy for diastolic heart failure begins with aggressive treatment of hypertension to target levels, as established by Joint National Committee guidelines. Myocardial ischemia should be treated with antianginal medications and/or coronary revascularization as indicated. Resting and exercise heart rate should be well controlled in patients with atrial fibrillation. Patients with severe valvular heart disease should be considered for valve repair or replacement, and less severe regurgitant valvular lesions should be treated with unloading agents, such as ACE inhibitors. As with systolic heart failure, nonpharmacologic aspects of therapy should be appropriately addressed.

Diuretics

Diuretics are an essential component of therapy for the relief of pulmonary and systemic venous congestion in patients with diastolic heart failure. However, such patients are often "volume sensitive." As a result, overly zealous diuresis can lead to a reduction in left ventricular diastolic volume, with a resultant decline in stroke volume and cardiac output, often manifested by increased fatigue, relative hypotension, and worsening prerenal azotemia. Thus, diuretics must be prescribed judiciously in order to relieve congestion while avoiding overdiuresis.

Beta-Blockers

Beta-blockers have little or no direct effect on diastolic function, but they may improve symptoms in patients with diastolic heart failure by slowing heart rate and lengthening the diastolic filling period. In patients with left ventricular hypertrophy, long-term beta-blockade and effective blood pressure control may aid in the regression of left ventricular hypertrophy, which in turn may be associated with improved diastolic function. In addition, in the Study of the Effects of Nebivolol Intervention on Outcomes and Rehospitalization in Seniors with Heart Failure trial, more than 20% of patients had relatively preserved left ventricular systolic function (ejection fraction ≥40%), and the benefits of nebivolol were similar in this group compared to those with ejection fractions <40%. These data support the use of beta-blocker therapy in all patients with heart failure, independent of whether left ventricular systolic function is preserved or impaired.

The goal of beta-blocker therapy in diastolic heart failure is to reduce the resting heart rate to less than 65 beats/min. The initial beta-blocker dose should be low and titration should be gradual. In the event that symptoms and exercise tolerance do not improve, alternative therapy should be considered.

ACE Inhibitors

ACE inhibitors may improve symptoms in diastolic heart failure both directly (by improving diastolic function) and indirectly (by promoting regression of left ventricular hypertrophy). The use of ACE inhibitors for the treatment of diastolic heart failure in patients of advanced age is supported by recently reported findings from the Perindopril in Elderly People with Chronic Heart Failure study, in which 850 patients ≥70 years of age (mean age 76 years, 55% women) with heart failure and relatively preserved left ventricular systolic function (estimated ejection fraction ≥40%) were randomized to perindopril 4 mg once daily or placebo and followed for an average of 2.1 years. Overall, there was no significant difference between groups with respect to the primary outcome of death or unplanned hospitalization for heart failure. However, heart failure hospitalizations were significantly reduced by 78% during the first 12 months of follow-up in patients randomized to perindopril. Relative to placebo, perindopril-treated patients also experienced significant improvements in New York Heart Association class and exercise tolerance during the first year of therapy. Perindopril is not currently approved for the treatment of heart failure in the United States, and the efficacy of other ACE inhibitors for the treatment of diastolic heart failure is unknown.

Angiotensin II Receptor Blockers

ARBs lower blood pressure and may have salutary effects on diastolic function similar to those observed with ACE inhibitors. In the CHARM-Preserved Trial, 3024 patients with New York Heart Association Class II–IV heart failure and an ejection fraction >40% were randomized to candesartan or placebo and followed for a median of 36.6 months. The mean age was 67 years, 27% were 75 years of age or older, and 40% were women. Mortality did not differ between groups, but patients randomized to candesartan experienced a significant 16% reduction in the risk of hospitalization for heart failure and 29% fewer total heart failure admissions. Subgroup analysis by age was not reported. Hypotension, hyperkalemia, and worsening renal function occurred more frequently in the candesartan group.

Taken together, the findings of Perindopril in Elderly People with Chronic Heart Failure and CHARM-Preserve indicate that ACE inhibitors and ARBs reduce hospitalizations and improve symptoms in patients with diastolic heart failure but have little or no effect on mortality. The ongoing Irbesartan in Heart Failure with Preserved Systolic Function (I-PRESERVE) trial, the largest study to date in patients with diastolic heart failure, should provide additional insight into the value of ARBs in the treatment of this condition. In the meantime, the favorable effects of ACE inhibitors and ARBs on quality of life and resource use imply that these agents should play an important role in the management of patients with diastolic heart failure, at least until more effective treatments have been established.

Aldosterone Antagonists

The aldosterone antagonists spironolactone and eplerenone reduce myocardial hypertrophy and fibrosis in laboratory animals and may have a favorable effect on left ventricular diastolic function. In addition, as discussed previously, both of these agents have been shown to improve mortality and other outcomes in patients with heart failure with reduced ejection fractions. Based on these considerations, the effects of spironolactone on clinical outcomes in patients with diastolic heart failure are now being evaluated in a large prospective randomized trial, sponsored by the National Heart, Lung, and Blood Institute.

Calcium Channel-Blockers

Calcium channel-blockers decrease intracellular calcium and may have a modest beneficial effect on diastolic function. Verapamil has also been shown to improve symptoms and exercise tolerance in selected patients with hypertrophic cardiomyopathy and normal systolic function. In addition, in 20 older patients with heart failure with an ejection fraction above 45%, it was found that, in comparison with placebo, verapamil at dosages of up to 120 mg tid improved symptoms, exercise capacity, and indices of diastolic function. On the other hand, some patients with diastolic heart failure may experience marked clinical deterioration when treated with verapamil. Moreover, the lack of benefit from calcium channel-blockers for the treatment of systolic heart failure tempers enthusiasm for their use in diastolic heart failure. There are also no ongoing clinical trials evaluating calcium channel-blockers for the treatment of diastolic heart failure. In light of these factors, calcium channel antagonists are not considered first-line agents for the treatment of this condition.

Nitrates

In addition to relieving ischemia, nitrates are effective venodilators and these lower pulmonary capillary wedge pressure. For these reasons, nitrates may serve as a useful adjunct to diuretics in relieving symptoms of pulmonary congestion, particularly orthopnea. However, nitrates have the potential for decreasing venous return to the heart, thereby reducing left ventricular diastolic volume and stroke volume. In addition, tolerance to the hemodynamic effects of nitrates occurs in the majority of patients. As a result, the value of nitrates in the long-term management of diastolic heart failure is uncertain.

Digoxin

Traditionally, digoxin has been considered contraindicated in patients with heart failure and normal systolic function. However, digoxin, as well as other inotropic agents, may exert a favorable effect on diastolic function by accelerating calcium reuptake by the sarcoplasmic reticulum at the onset of diastole. In the original DIG trial, 988 patients with heart failure and an ejection fraction of more than 45% were randomized to digoxin or placebo in an ancillary study. As in the main trial, digoxin had no effect on mortality. However, the combined end point of death or hospitalization for heart failure was reduced by 18% in patients receiving digoxin. In addition, all-cause mortality tended to be lower in patients with a serum digoxin concentration of 0.5 to 0.9 ng/mL. Although none of these differences were statistically significant, the findings suggest that digoxin may be beneficial in some patients with heart failure and preserved systolic function. Nonetheless, additional study is needed before digoxin can be recommended as routine therapy for patients with diastolic heart failure.

Summary

Studies published to date indicate that ACE inhibitors, ARBs, and beta-blockers have favorable effects on hospital admission rates and symptom severity in patients with diastolic heart failure, but none of these agents have been shown to reduce mortality and none are recommended as standard therapy in current practice guidelines. Management of diastolic heart failure should include aggressive treatment of the underlying cardiac disease, and a diuretic should be administered at low-to-moderate doses to relieve congestion and edema. The addition of an ACE inhibitor, ARB, or beta-blocker to improve symptoms and reduce the risk of hospitalization seems prudent. However, if the patient fails to respond to initial therapy, alternative treatment should be considered. Such therapy might include the use of nitrates, digoxin, a calcium channel blocker, or a combination of agents.

Refractory Heart Failure

Refractory heart failure may be defined as heart failure not amenable to primary corrective measures (e.g., valve replacement or revascularization) and not responsive to aggressive nonpharmacologic and pharmacologic therapy as described above. However, before designating heart failure as refractory, it is important to perform a careful search for potentially treatable causes, to carefully review the patient's medication regimen to ensure that therapy is optimal, and to discuss the patient's diet and medication habits in detail with the patient and family to ensure that an appropriate level of compliance is being maintained. The latter issue is of particular importance, since many cases of refractory heart failure can be traced to nonadherence to dietary restrictions, medications, or both.

In most cases, refractory heart failure simply represents the final common pathway of end-stage heart disease. Under these circumstances, the value of highly aggressive treatment is questionable, and decisions regarding the appropriateness of specific therapeutic interventions must be made on an individualized basis (see also Chapters 31 and 34).

Table 78-12 lists treatment options for refractory heart failure. In patients with systolic heart failure, intensifying the vasodilator regimen by using high doses of ACE inhibitors (e.g., up to 400 mg/day of captopril or 80 mg/day of enalapril), either alone or in combination with hydralazine/nitrates or an angiotensin II receptor blocker, may result in significant symptomatic improvement. This can often be accomplished in the outpatient setting, but titration must be very gradual, with frequent follow-up contacts to avoid adverse events. In patients who fail to respond to these measures,

TABLE 78-12

Treatment Options for Refractory Heart Failure

Systolic heart failure
Intensive vasodilator therapy
- High-dose ACE inhibitors
- Combination therapy
  - ACE inhibitor plus hydralazine/nitrates
  - ACE inhibitor plus angiotensin II receptor blocker
- Intravenous agents (e.g., nitroglycerin, nitroprusside, and niseritide)

Intensive diuretic therapy
- High-dose oral agents, especially in combination
- Continuous intravenous infusion

Chronic or intermittent inotropic therapy
- Dobutamine
- Milrinone

Pacemaker therapy

Dialysis
- Short-term or chronic dialysis
- Dry ultrafiltration

Investigational agents

Surgical options
- Myocardial resection
- Cardiomyoplasty
- Ventricular assist device

Diastolic heart failure
Intensive diuretic therapy (see above)
Empiric trial of inotropic therapy
Dialysis (see above)
A-V sequential pacemaker

ACE, angiotensin-converting enzyme.

intravenous vasodilator therapy with nitroglycerin, nitroprusside, or nesiritide (recombinant B-type natriuretic peptide, BNP) may lead to significant clinical and hemodynamic improvements.

In patients with persistent pulmonary congestion or peripheral edema, high-dose oral diuretics (e.g., furosemide 200 mg bid or bumetanide 10 mg daily), alone or in combination with metolazone, may be effective. Alternatively, a continuous intravenous infusion of furosemide 5 to 40 mg/h or bumetanide 0.5 to 1 mg/h will often facilitate diuresis.

The use of intravenous inotropic agents in the management of chronic heart failure is somewhat controversial, since these agents have not been shown to improve outcomes and they may increase the risk of life-threatening arrhythmias. Nonetheless, extensive clinical experience indicates that intermittent or continuous outpatient infusions of dobutamine or milrinone may significantly reduce symptoms and improve quality of life in selected patients with refractory heart failure.

Recently, biventricular pacing has been shown to improve symptoms, quality of life, and survival in patients with advanced heart failure and left bundle branch block or marked intraventricular conduction delay on the 12-lead electrocardiogram. This procedure should, therefore, be considered in appropriately selected patients with persistent Class III or IV heart failure symptoms.

If the above interventions fail, patients with significant renal dysfunction may benefit from short-term dialysis or dry ultrafiltration to remove excess fluid and stabilize electrolyte homeostasis. If the patient responds to short-term treatment, chronic dialysis may be considered. Finally, in highly selected patients, referral to a tertiary or quaternary facility for investigational medical or surgical treatment may be appropriate.

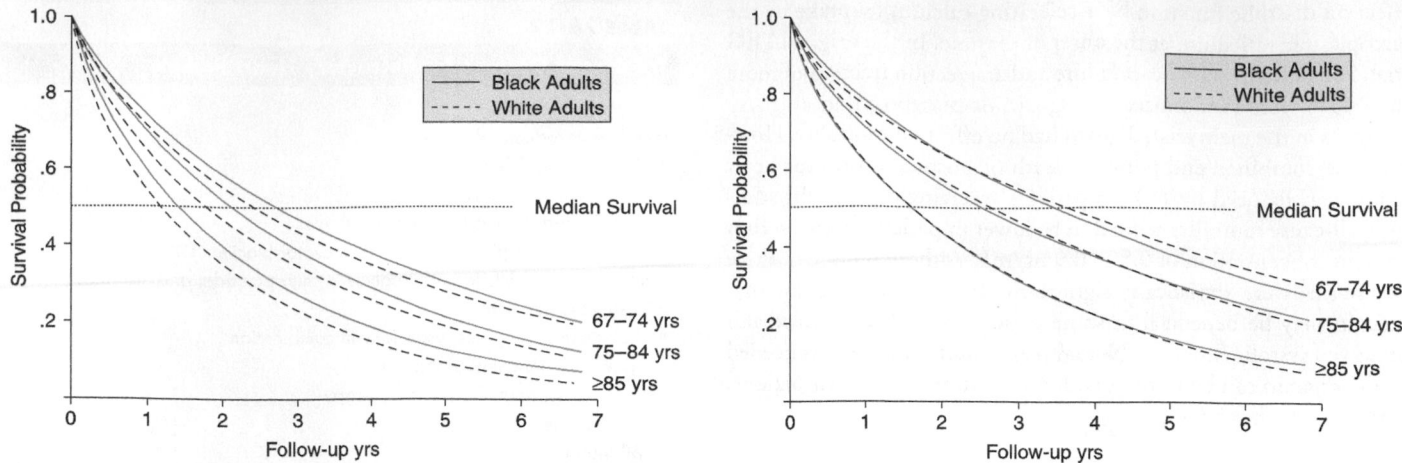

FIGURE 78-8. Probability of survival by age and race after first hospitalization for heart failure among older men (left panel) and women (right panel). (Adapted with permission from Croft JB, Giles WH, Pollard RA, et al. Heart failure survival among older adults in the United States: a poor prognosis for an emerging epidemic in the Medicare population. Arch Intern Med. 1999;159:505–510.)

For patients with refractory heart failure because of diastolic dysfunction, therapeutic options are limited (see Table 78-12). Intensive diuretic therapy may be attempted, but efficacy is often limited by the development of progressive prerenal azotemia. Similarly, a trial of inotropic therapy or dialysis may be considered, but the clinical response to these interventions is variable. Finally, although preliminary reports have suggested that some patients with diastolic heart failure may benefit from permanent dual-chamber pacing, this procedure remains investigational.

PROGNOSIS

The overall prognosis in patients with established heart failure is poor, and the 5-year survival rate is less than 50%. In elderly patients, the prognosis is even worse, and fewer than 20% of patients with heart failure older than 80 years survive more than 5 years (Figure 78-8). In general, the prognosis is worse in men than in women, in patients with systolic rather than diastolic dysfunction, and in patients with an ischemic rather than nonischemic etiology. Patients with more severe symptoms or exercise intolerance, as defined by the New York Heart Association functional class or as assessed by a 6-minute walk test, also have a less favorable outlook. Other markers of an adverse prognosis include elevated plasma norepinephrine, B-type natriuretic peptide, tumor necrosis factor-alpha, and endothelin-1 levels; low systolic blood pressure; hyponatremia; renal insufficiency; anemia; peripheral arterial disease; cognitive dysfunction; reduced heart rate variability; and the presence of atrial fibrillation or high-grade ventricular arrhythmias. In patients with chronic heart failure, 40% to 50% die from progressive heart failure, 40% die from arrhythmias, and 10% to 20% die from other causes (e.g., myocardial infarction or noncardiac conditions).

ETHICAL ISSUES AND END-OF-LIFE DECISIONS

As noted above, the prognosis for patients with heart failure is extremely poor, and 5-year survival rates are lower than for most forms of cancer. In addition, once heart failure symptoms have reached an advanced stage (e.g., New York Heart Association Class III or IV), quality of life is often severely compromised and therapeutic options are limited. Moreover, even patients with relatively mild or well-compensated heart failure are continually at risk of experiencing sudden cardiac arrest, and, if initial resuscitative efforts are successful, questions regarding life support and related issues may arise.

For these reasons, it is incumbent upon the physician to discuss the patient's wishes regarding the intensity of treatment and end-of-life care at a time when the patient is still capable of understanding the issues and making informed choices. In addition, since the patient's views may evolve over the course of illness, these issues should be readdressed at periodic intervals. The development of an advance directive and appointment of durable power of attorney should also be encouraged (see Chapter 51 and 34).

A related concern is the extent to which the physician should offer aggressive or investigational therapeutic options that are unlikely to substantially alter the natural history of disease or significantly improve quality of life. This concern applies not only to many of the treatment modalities discussed in the refractory heart failure section above, but also to such procedures as endotracheal intubation and intra-aortic balloon counterpulsation. In many cases, these interventions not only fail to modify the clinical course but actually contribute to the patient's pain and suffering in the terminal stages of disease. Moreover, the suggestion that a given intervention may help stabilize the patient and slow disease progression may create false hopes in the minds of the patient and family, and subsequent failure of the intervention may compound the emotional suffering that both the patient and the family are forced to endure. For these reasons, it is essential that the physician realistically appraise the potential benefits and attendant risks, both physical and emotional, prior to offering aggressive therapeutic options, which may provide little or no hope of improving the patient's quality of life over a clinically important period of time.

Finally, as the patient approaches the terminal stages of disease, there should be discussions with the patient and family regarding where the patient would like to spend his or her final days. For many patients, the idea of dying at home surrounded by close family is comforting, and this desire should be honored whenever possible. For some patients, a hospice that provides compassionate end-of-life

TABLE 78-13

Effect of Antihypertensive Therapy on Incident

	HEART FAILURE IN OLDER ADULTS			RISK REDUCTION FOR HEART FAILURE (%)
TRIAL	Year	N	Age (yr)	
EWPHE	1985	840	>60	22
Coope	1986	884	60–79	32
STOP-HTN	1991	1627	70–84	51
SHEP	1991	4736	≥60	55
STONE	1996	1632	60–79	68
Syst-Eur	1997	4695	≥60	36
Syst-China	2000	2394	≥60	38

EWPHE, European Working Party on Hypertension in the Elderly; SHEP, Systolic Hypertension in the Elderly Program; STONE, Shanghai Trial of Nifedipine in the Elderly; STOP-HTN, Swedish Trial in Old Patients with Hypertension; Syst-China, Systolic Hypertension in China Trial; Syst-Eur, Systolic Hypertension in Europe Trial.

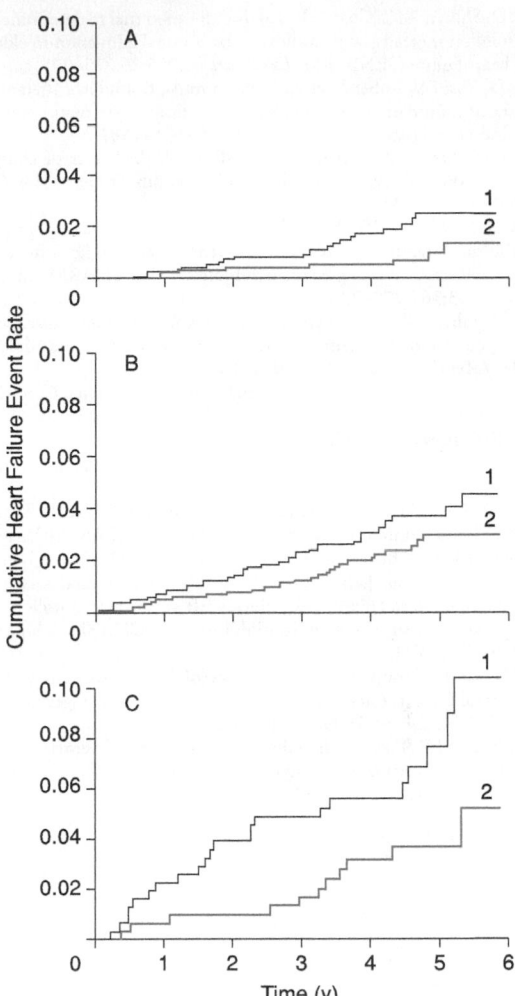

FIGURE 78-9. Effect of antihypertensive therapy on incident heart failure in patients with isolated systolic hypertension: the Systolic Hypertension in the Elderly Program (SHEP). Top panel: age 60 to 69 yrs; middle panel: age 70 to 79 yrs; lower panel: age ≥80 yrs. *(Adapted with permission from Kostis JB, Davis BR, Cutler J, et al. Prevention of heart failure by antihypertensive drug treatment in older persons with updated systolic hypertension. JAMA. 1997;278:212–216.)*

care may be a suitable alternative. For others, the hospital may be the most desirable environment, but an attempt should be made to secure a private room with open visitation hours. The intensive care unit, with its austere, "high-tech" facade, is the least desirable place to die, and this should be avoided whenever possible.

PREVENTION

In view of the exceptionally poor prognosis associated with established heart failure in older adults, it is essential to develop and implement preventive strategies. Appropriate treatment of hypertension has been repeatedly shown to reduce the incidence of heart failure by up to 50% (Table 78-13). Moreover, in the Systolic Hypertension in the Elderly Program, the greatest benefit was seen in patients older than 80 years (Figure 78-9). Treatment of hyperlipidemia has also been shown to reduce the incidence of heart failure, most likely through prevention of myocardial infarction and other ischemic events. Likewise, smoking cessation reduces the risk of myocardial infarction and stroke in older adults and likely has a similar effect on the development of heart failure. Unfortunately, despite abundant evidence that heart failure prevention is feasible through risk factor modification, such strategies are underused, especially in persons older than 80 years.

SUMMARY

Heart failure is an exceedingly common and important clinical problem in older adults, owing, in large part, to the complex interplay between age-related changes in the cardiovascular system, the high prevalence of cardiovascular and noncardiovascular diseases in the older population, and the widespread use of certain drugs and other therapies that may adversely affect cardiovascular physiology. As the population of the United States continues to age, heart failure will exact a progressively greater toll on our health-care delivery system. In addition, the impact of heart failure on quality of life and independence in the large number of older adults with this disorder is incalculable. Clearly, there is an urgent need to develop more effec-

tive strategies for the prevention and treatment of heart failure, with particular emphasis on the geriatric population.

FURTHER STUDIES

Ahmed A, Rich MW, Fleg JL, et al. Effects of digoxin on morbidity and mortality in diastolic heart failure: the ancillary Digitalis Investigation Group trial. *Circulation.* 2006;114:397–403.

Ahmed A, Rich MW, Love TE, et al. Digoxin and reduction in mortality and hospitalization in heart failure: a comprehensive post hoc analysis of the DIG trial. *Eur Heart J* 2006;27:178–186.

Austin J, Williams R, Ross, L, Moseley L, Hutchison S. Randomised controlled trial of cardiac rehabilitation in elderly patients with heart failure. *Eur J Heart Fail.* 2005;7:411–417.

Cleland JGF, Tendera M, Adamus J, Freemantle N, Polonski L, Taylor J. The perindopril in elderly people with chronic heart failure (PEP-CHF) study. *Eur Heart J.* 2006;27:2238–2245.

Cohn JN, Tognoni G; for the Valsartan Heart Failure Trial Investigators. A randomized trial of the angiotensin-receptor blocker valsartan in chronic heart failure. *N Engl J Med.* 2001;345:1667–1675.

Croft JB, Giles WH, Pollard RA, Keenan NL, Casper ML, Anda RF. Heart failure survival among older adults in the United States: a poor prognosis for an emerging epidemic in the Medicare population. *Arch Intern Med.* 1999;159:505–510.

Flather MD, Shibata MC, Coats AJ, et al. Randomized trial to determine the effect of nebivolol on mortality and cardiovascular hospital admission in elderly patients with heart failure (SENIORS). *Eur Heart J.* 2005;26:215–225.

Flather MD, Yusuf S, Kober L, et al. Long-term ACE-inhibitor therapy in patients with heart failure or left-ventricular dysfunction: a systematic overview of data from individual patients. *Lancet.* 2000;355:1575–1581.

Gottdiener JS, Arnold AM, Aurigemma GP, et al. Predictors of congestive heart failure in the elderly: the Cardiovascular Health Study. *J Am Coll Cardiol.* 2000;35:1628–1637.

Granger CB, McMurray JJV, Yusuf S, et al. Effects of candesartan in patients with chronic heart failure and reduced left-ventricular systolic function intolerant to angiotensin-converting-enzyme inhibitors: the CHARM-Alternative trial. *Lancet.* 2003;362:772–776.

Hunt SA, Abraham WT, Chin MH, et al. ACC/AHA 2005 guideline update for the diagnosis and management of chronic heart failure in the adult – summary article. *J Am Coll Cardiol.* 2005;46:1116–1143.

Kitzman DW. Heart failure with normal systolic function. *Clin Geriatr Med.* 2000;16:489–511.

Maisel A, Krishnaswamy P, Nowak RM, et al. Rapid measurement of B-type natriuretic peptide in the emergency diagnosis of heart failure. *N Engl J Med.* 2002;347:161–167.

McAlister FA, Ghali WA, Gong Y, Fang J, Armstrong PW, Tu JV. Aspirin use and outcomes in a community-based cohort of 7352 patients discharged after first hospitalization for heart failure. *Circulation.* 2006;113:2572–2578.

McMurray JJ, Ostergren J, Swedberg K, et al. Effects of candesartan in patients with chronic heart failure and reduced left-ventricular systolic function taking angiotensin-converting-enzyme inhibitors: the CHARM-Added trial. *Lancet.* 2003;362:767–771.

MERIT-HF Study Group. Effect of metoprolol CR/XL in chronic heart failure: Metoprolol CR/XL Randomised Intervention Trial in Congestive Heart Failure (MERIT-HF). *Lancet.* 1999;353:2001–2007.

Moser M, Hebert PR. Prevention of disease progression, left ventricular hypertrophy and congestive heart failure in hypertension treatment trials. *J Am Coll Cardiol.* 1996;27:1214–1218.

Packer M, Coats AJ, Fowler MB, et al. Effect of carvedilol on survival in severe chronic heart failure. *N Engl J Med.* 2001;344:1651–1658.

Packer M, Poole-Wilson PA, Armstrong PW, et al. Comparative effects of low and high doses of the angiotensin-converting enzyme inhibitor, lisinopril, on morbidity and mortality in chronic heart failure. ATLAS Study Group. *Circulation.* 1999;100:2312–2318.

Page J, Henry D. Consumption of NSAIDs and the development of congestive heart failure in elderly patients: an underrecognized public health problem. *Arch Intern Med.* 2000;160:777–784.

Pfeffer MA, McMurray JJV, Rouleau EJ, et al. Valsartan, captopril, or both in myocardial infarction complicated by heart failure, left ventricular dysfunction, or both. *N Engl J Med.* 2003;349:1893–1906.

Piepoli MF, Davos C, Francis DP, Coats AJS. Exercise training meta-analysis of trials in patients with chronic heart failure. *BMJ.* 2004;328:189.

Pitt B, Poole-Wilson PA, Segal R, et al. Effect of losartan compared with captopril on mortality in patients with symptomatic heart failure: randomised trial – the Losartan Heart Failure Survival Study ELITE II. *Lancet.* 2000;355:1582–1587.

Pitt B, Remme W, Zannard F, et al. Eplerenone, a selective aldosterone blocker, in patients with left ventricular dysfunction after myocardial infarction. *N Engl J Med.* 2003;348:1309–1321.

Pitt B, Zannad F, Remme WJ, et al. The effect of spironolactone on morbidity and mortality in patients with severe heart failure. Randomized Aldactone Evaluation Study Investigators. *N Engl J Med.* 1999;341:709–717.

Rich MW, McSherry F, Williford WO, Yusuf S; for the Digitalis Investigation Group. Effect of age on mortality, hospitalizations and response to digoxin in patients with heart failure: The DIG Study. *J Am Coll Cardiol.* 2001;38:806–813.

Roccaforte R, Demers C, Baldassarre F, Teo KK, Yusuf S. Effectiveness of comprehensive disease management programmes in improving clinical outcomes in heart failure patients. A meta-analysis. *Eur J Heart Fail.* 2005;7:1133–1144.

Taylor AL, Ziesche S, Yancy C, et al. Combination of isosorbide dinitrate and hydralazine in blacks with heart failure. *N Engl J Med.* 2004;351:2049–2057.

Yusuf S, Pfeffer MA, Swedberg K, et al. Effects of candesartan in patients with chronic heart failure and preserved left-ventricular ejection fraction: the CHARM-Preserved trial. *Lancet.* 2003;362:777–781.

Cardiac Arrhythmias

Xiao-Ke Liu ■ *Arshad Jahangir* ■ *Win-Kuang Shen*

OVERVIEW OF THE EFFECT OF AGING ON CARDIAC ELECTROPHYSIOLOGY AND EVALUATION OF ARRHYTHMIAS

Electrophysiology and Arrhythmias in the Elderly

In older patients without apparent cardiovascular disease, the number of cardiac myocytes declines, while residual myocytes enlarge. Concurrently, there is an increase in elastic and collagenous tissue in all parts of the interstitial matrix and conduction system with advancing age. Around the sinoatrial node, adipose tissue accumulates with age, producing a partial or complete separation of the sinoatrial node from the surrounding musculature. The number of pacemaker cells steadily decreases with age, such that by the age of 75 years, less than 10% of pacemaker cells remain functional. Calcification of the cardiac skeleton, which includes the aortic and mitral annuli, the central fibrous body, and the summit of the atrioventricular (AV) septum, also increases with age. Because of their proximity to these structures, the AV node (AVN), His-Purkinje bundle, and right and left bundle branches are frequently affected by aging. Prolongation of action potential duration and diminished autonomic response are also integral components of the aging process. Taken together, these changes provide the substrate for the age-related increase in propensity for chronotropic and dromotropic incompetence and for the development of atrial and ventricular arrhythmias.

The Baltimore Longitudinal Study on Aging demonstrated that basal heart rates in the supine position do not differ significantly among younger and older healthy subjects. Heart rate response to orthostatic challenge decreases slightly in older men and women. Heart rate variability during respiration diminishes with advancing age, reflecting changes in autonomic regulation. The PR interval increases slightly with aging, most likely owing to a delay in AVN conduction.

The prevalence of atrial premature beats on ambulatory monitoring increases with age, exceeding 80% in healthy volunteers and asymptomatic elderly subjects, particularly those older than 80 years. Brief salvos of supraventricular tachycardia occur in up to 50% of older subjects, and the prevalence doubles between the seventh and ninth decades of life. These arrhythmias have not been shown to have adverse prognostic significance. Atrial fibrillation (AF) and tachycardia–bradycardia syndrome are predominant conditions of the elderly.

Ventricular arrhythmias also increase with age. In longitudinal studies, the prevalence of ventricular arrhythmias on ambulatory monitoring is as high as 60% to 90% in asymptomatic elderly subjects. Complex forms such as pairs and triplets occur in up to 10% of such individuals. Exercise testing may induce ventricular arrhythmias in up to 60% of subjects in the ninth decade of life. The prognostic significance of these arrhythmias is dependent in large part on the presence of underlying cardiovascular disease. In patients with cardiovascular disease, frequent ventricular ectopy may adversely affect quality of life, may contribute to deterioration in myocardial function increasing susceptibility to heart failure, and may be a harbinger of symptomatic and sustained ventricular arrhythmias and cardiac arrest. Conversely, the prognostic impact of rest or exercise-induced ventricular arrhythmias is limited in the absence of cardiovascular disease. Reduced heart rate variability by fractal analysis has also been linked to the occurrence of sudden cardiac death (SCD) and non-sudden cardiac death in an unselected population of elderly subjects.

Clinical Testing

Several clinical tools are available for identification of patients at risk of cardiac arrhythmias or its consequences that may benefit from interventions to reduce morbidity and risk of sudden death. These include noninvasive tests, such as a standard 12 lead electrocardiogram

(ECG), exercise test or imaging to determine the severity of left ventricular systolic dysfunction, presence of late potentials on signal-average electrocardiography, severity of ventricular arrhythmias by ambulatory cardiac monitoring (Holter monitor or external or implantable event monitor), detection of repolarization instability by measurement of QT interval, QT dispersion and microvolt T-wave alternans, autonomic balance by heart rate variability or baroreflex sensitivity, or invasive tests to determine inducibility of sustained ventricular arrhythmias by programmed electrical stimulation. The effect of advanced age on predictability of these tests for risk stratification, however, has not been fully assessed.

A standard 12-lead ECG allows identification of underlying structural disease, such as conduction system abnormalities with heart block, bundle-branch block, ventricular hypertrophy, or prior infarction, as well as primary electrical disorders, such as the long-QT syndrome, short-QT syndrome, Brugada syndrome, or arrhythmogenic right ventricular cardiomyopathy. A prolonged QRS duration >120 milliseconds in patients with a severely depressed ventricular function or a prolonged QTc interval in the elderly predict higher risk of SCD. Absence of a slowly conducting zone, the electrophysiologic substrate for reentrant ventricular arrhythmias that is otherwise detected as late potentials on signal-average electrocardiography may be useful with its high negative predictive value to exclude a wide-complex tachycardia as a cause of unexplained syncope in the elderly patient with coronary artery disease.

The indications for ambulatory ECG recordings are similar between the younger and elderly populations. To detect a suspected arrhythmic event occurring frequently (e.g., greater than once every 48 hours or reproducible by outpatient activities), detect a precise count of ectopy, evaluate daily ventricular rate control in AF, or detect asymptomatic nonsustained ventricular tachycardia, a continuous ECG recorder such as a Holter is useful. Less frequent arrhythmias (e.g. ≥ 1 event per month but not occurring daily) can be investigated using an event recorder. A pre-event loop recorder is needed for patients with syncope or symptoms of brief duration. Even less frequent events or in patients who are unable to activate the event recorder, an implantable loop recorder such as the reveal device, which may record either automatically or by patient activation, can be very helpful in correlating symptoms to arrhythmias. Exercise ECG with or without cardiac imaging with echocardiogram or nuclear scan may also provide useful diagnostic and prognostic information in the evaluation of patients with known or suspected coronary artery disease or exercise-induced arrhythmias triggered by ischemia or catecholamine. Assessment of left ventricular systolic function and other structural and functional information about myocardial dimensions, wall thickness, and valvular and congenital heart disorders with imaging technique, such as echocardiogram, is an essential part of risk stratification of patients with ventricular arrhythmias at risk of SCD.

In most cases, the indications for invasive electrophysiologic study (EPS) in elderly patients are also the same as in younger patients (Table 79-1) and vary with the type and severity of heart disease. It is useful for arrhythmia assessment and risk stratification for SCD in elderly patients with ischemic heart disease and left ventricular dysfunction or syncope but plays only a minor role in the evaluation of patients with nonischemic cardiomyopathy or inherited arrhythmia syndromes, such as the long- or short-QT syndrome. It should be noted that Table 79-1 is based on the AHA/ACC guidelines from 1995, and there has been no recent update on indications for EPS. Some of the recommendations have changed as more data become available through multiple recent device trials, e.g., as discussed later in the chapter, EPS is no longer considered necessary for recommending device implantation in many patients with ischemic or nonischemic cardiomyopathy or in patients with documented out-of-hospital cardiac arrest. This section provides a brief overview of criteria for the selection of elderly patients for EPS, as well as a discussion of procedural risks.

Indications for EPS can be divided broadly into diagnostic and therapeutic purposes. In any patient, but especially in the elderly, the use of an intervention such as EPS, whether for diagnosis or therapy, should be determined from the clinical presentation and the specific goals of the study. Therefore, two key questions should be addressed before proceeding with EPS. First, is information obtained from the history and noninvasive evaluation sufficient to explain the clinical presentation, or is invasive EPS necessary to ensure an accurate diagnosis? Second, will the results of invasive EPS help guide therapy, or is catheter ablation being considered as a therapeutic option? Importantly, the decision to proceed with EPS remains a clinical judgment based on the history and physical findings, the probability of a cardiac cause of symptoms, and the likelihood that the results of EPS will substantially improve patient care and outcomes.

In general, procedural complications in the elderly are similar to those in younger patients. These include complications related to the procedure itself, such as (1) vascular damage, pneumothorax, or myocardial perforation leading to pericardial effusion and tamponade, and (2) exacerbation of preexisting medical conditions (e.g., chronic obstructive pulmonary disease and chronic heart failure). Exacerbation of preexisting conditions is most common with prolonged procedures, such as complicated ablation, and is rarely a problem during diagnostic EPS or straightforward catheter ablation. A widely held belief is that morbidity and mortality associated with invasive EPS are higher in elderly patients. Although this is not borne out by available data, which suggest similar rates of complications even in very elderly patients, one must be cognizant that patient selection bias is inevitably present in these observational studies. Thus, the potential risks and benefits of invasive EPS should be weighed on an individual basis and not merely by age.

BRADYARRHYTHMIA AND CARDIAC PACEMAKER THERAPY IN THE ELDERLY

Aging is associated with progressive fibrosis of the sinoatrial node and AV conduction system, resulting in bradycardia, which may be further exacerbated by disease and medications, resulting in symptoms requiring permanent pacemaker implantation. More than 80% of pacemaker recipients in the United States are older than 65 years, and the median age is 75 years. As the population ages, it is anticipated that the number of older persons requiring permanent pacemakers, as well as the associated costs, will continue to rise.

Standard Indications

Current guidelines for pacemaker implantation are updated regularly by the American College of Cardiology, American Heart Association, and North American Society of Pacing and Electrophysiology (now the Heart Rhythm Society). This section provides a synopsis of

TABLE 79-1

Indications for Invasive Electrophysiologic Study Based on AHA/ACC Guidelines (1995)

CLINICAL CONDITION OR INDICATION	CLASS I (APPROPRIATE)*	CLASS II (EQUIVOCAL)†	CLASS III (INAPPROPRIATE)‡
Recurrent syncope	Patients with recurrent syncope that remains unexplained after appropriate evaluation	Patients with recurrent unexplained syncope without structural heart disease and negative tilt	Patients with a known cause of syncope in whom treatment will not be guided by invasive EPS
Sinus node dysfunction	To establish association between symptoms and arrhythmia	Patients with documented sinus node dysfunction in whom other arrhythmias are suspected	Patients in whom an association has already been established or who are asymptomatic
Atrioventricular block	Symptomatic patients in whom atrioventricular block is suspected	Patients in whom knowledge of the site of block would help guide therapy	Patients in whom an association has already been established or who are asymptomatic or have pauses only during sleep
Intraventricular conduction delay	Symptomatic patients in whom the cause is unknown	Asymptomatic patients in whom pharmacologic therapy is planned	Symptomatic patients in whom an association has already been established or asymptomatic patients
Narrow complex tachycardia (QRS <120 ms)	Frequent or poorly tolerated tachycardia; patient preference	Intolerance of antiarrhythmic or atrioventricular nodal blocking drugs	Patients with few episodes of tachycardia or in whom ablation is not appropriate
Wide-complex tachycardia	Mechanism unclear or to help guide appropriate management	None	Patients in whom knowledge of the mechanism is clear from ECG or in whom knowledge is unnecessary
Out-of-hospital cardiac arrest	Survivors of cardiac arrest without obvious reversible cause	Cardiac arrest caused by documented bradycardia; patients in whom the results of EPS may be nondiagnostic or equivocal	Cardiac arrest within 48 h of AMI Cardiac arrest owing to clearly definable cause
Risk stratification for patients who may be candidates for implantable cardioverter defibrillator	Primary prevention in patients with MI, impaired LV function and nonsustained VT, or out-of-hospital cardiac arrest§	Patients with syncope and structural heart disease	Patients who are not candidates for implantable cardioverter defibrillator
Indications for catheter ablation procedures	Patients with symptomatic supraventricular arrhythmias owing to AVNRT or AVRT in whom ablation is preferred	Patients found to have a tachycardia substrate that is different from that suspected clinically	Patients with well-tolerated PSVT and who prefer conservative treatment to ablation
	Patients with symptomatic atrial tachyarrhythmias, such as typical atrial flutter, that may be amenable to catheter ablation therapy	Patients with atrial tachyarrhythmias in which catheter ablation may be successful in some cases	Patients with atrial tachyarrhythmias that are well tolerated or in whom catheter ablation is not preferred
	Patients with some forms of ventricular tachycardia that are amenable to catheter ablation therapy	Selected patients with VT because of reentry around a scar after (remote) myocardial infarction	Patients with well-tolerated ventricular arrhythmias or patients with multiple VT morphologic findings

AMI, acute myocardial infarction; AV, atrioventricular; AVNRT, atrioventricular nodal reentrant tachycardia; AVRT, atrioventricular reentrant tachycardia; ECG, electrocardiography; EPS, electrophysiologic study; LV, left ventricular; MI, myocardial infarction; PSVT, paroxysmal supraventricular tachycardia; VT, ventricular tachycardia.
*Class I: conditions for which there is general agreement that the form of therapy is appropriate.
†Class II: conditions for which there is divergence of opinion with respect to the necessity of the procedure.
‡Class III: conditions for which there is general agreement that the therapy is unnecessary or inappropriate.
§See text for comments.
From Brady PA, Shen WK. When is intracardiac electrophysiologic evaluation indicated in the older or very elderly patient? Complications rates and data. Clin Geriatr Med. 2002;18:339–360. By permission of Elsevier Science.

current indications for pacemaker implantation and outcomes from recent clinical trials relevant to pacemaker selection in older adults.

Acquired Advanced AV Block

Class I indications for permanent pacemaker implantation include third-degree AV block and advanced second-degree AV block in symptomatic patients. Pacing therapy is also recommended in patients with neuromuscular diseases and third-degree AV block

whether or not they are symptomatic, because progression of AV conduction slowing is not predictable in such patients.

AV Conduction Disease

Symptomatic patients (syncope and presyncope) with conduction system disease manifesting as bifascicular or trifascicular block on ECG in the absence of an alternative explanation for their symptoms are candidates for an EPS and/or permanent pacing. Prolongation of the HV interval beyond 80 milliseconds may be an index of potential high-degree AV block, and some clinicians recommend prophylactic permanent pacing in this setting. Other experts consider HV prolongation a marker of underlying heart disease and increased risk for sudden death but do not recommend pacemaker therapy unless the patient is symptomatic. According to the current guidelines, in the absence of syncope or presyncope, an HV interval of 100 milliseconds or more and/or nonphysiological infra-His block demonstrated during EPS are class IIa indications for pacemaker insertion.

Sinus Node Dysfunction

Pacemaker therapy is indicated in patients with symptomatic bradycardia (syncope, presyncope, dyspnea, and exercise intolerance) correlated to sinus node dysfunction (pauses, persistent bradycardia, or chronotropic incompetence). In elderly patients, sinus node dysfunction is often associated with atrial tachyarrhythmias, including AF. Because of the frequent association of sinus node dysfunction with AF, VVI and VVIR pacing were once considered the preferred pacing modes. Recent studies suggest that atrial-based pacing in patients with sinus node dysfunction is beneficial for preventing progression of AF. Current pacemaker technology allows mode switching from DDD to VVI or DDI in case of paroxysmal AF, thus avoiding ventricular tracking of fast atrial rates. These considerations have led to a progressive increase in the use of dual-chamber pacemakers in elderly patients. Some clinicians advocate AAI or AAIR pacing as the best pacing mode because these modes provide more physiological ventricular activation and are technically less complex. This approach has not been widely adopted in clinical practice because progression to AV block during long-term follow-up has been reported in up to 10% of elderly patients with sinus node dysfunction. Although maintaining AV synchrony during AV block and the availability of mode switch to reduce or eliminate inappropriate tracking during atrial tachyarrhythmia support the rationale for dual-chamber pacing in patients with sinus node dysfunction, recent data raised concerns whether excessive ventricular pacing from the right ventricular apex may cause increased incidence of heart failure and heart failure-mediated hospital admission. The clinical advantages of programmable features such as "AV delay hysteresis" or "managing ventricular pacing" to minimize ventricular pacing in the presence of AV conduction are currently under investigation.

Pacemaker Therapy

Prospective Trials of Ventricular (VVI) and Physiological (AAI or DDD) Pacing

In 1998, the results of the Pacemaker Selection in the Elderly trial were published. This randomized comparison of ventricular and dual-chamber pacing included 407 patients 65 years or older followed for 30 months. Patients with sinus node dysfunction, but not those with AV block, had a moderately better quality of life and cardiovascular functional status with dual-chamber pacing. One-fourth of all patients assigned to the VVI mode crossed over to dual-chamber operation because of symptoms suggesting "pacemaker syndrome." In the same year, Mattioli et al. reported a randomized trial involving 210 patients, which showed a higher incidence of AF and stroke in patients randomized to ventricular pacing.

Although the above trials were too small to assess the effect of pacemaker mode on mortality, three large mortality trials have now been completed (Table 79-2). The Canadian Trial of Physiologic Pacing enrolled 2568 patients who were scheduled for an initial implantation of a pacemaker to correct symptomatic bradycardia, did not have chronic AF, and were at least 18 years old. These patients were then randomized to ventricular pacing (VVIR) or a physiologic mode (AAIR or DDDR). At 4 years follow-up, there were no differences between the two groups in the primary study end point, the combination of cardiovascular death or stroke. In addition, all-cause mortality, stroke or arterial thromboembolism, hospitalization for heart failure, and performance on a 6-minute walk test did not differ between groups. Physiological pacing had a modest benefit in association with less new onset of AF, but there were also more perioperative complications, such as lead dislodgment or inadequate atrial pacing or sensing, in patients receiving physiological pacemakers.

The Mode Selection Trial randomized 2010 patients with sinus node dysfunction to single- or dual-chamber pacing. After a mean follow-up of 2.7 years, there was no difference between groups in the primary end point, death, or stroke. However, progression to chronic AF and heart failure symptoms were less frequent, and quality of life was better in the dual-chamber pacing arm.

In the prospective U.K. Pacing and Cardiovascular Events trial that enrolled 2021 patients older than 70 years with AV block,

TABLE 79-2

Randomized Clinical Trials of Pacemaker Mode Selection in Elderly Patients

TRIAL,* YEAR REPORTED	NO. ENROLLED	MEAN (Age yr)	GROUP	FOLLOW-UP (yr)	MODE OF PACING	RELATIVE RISK WITH VENTRICULAR VERSUS ATRIAL OR DUAL-CHAMBER PACING					
						Mortality	CHF	HF Hospitalization	AF	TE	QOL
PASE, 1998	407	76	SND or AVB	2.5	VVIR versus DDDR	NS	NS	NS	↑	NS	NS,† ↓ in SND
CTOPP, 2000	2568	73	SND or AVB	3	VVIR versus DDDR or AAIR	NS†	NS	NS	↑	NS†	Not stated
MOST, 2002	2010	74	SND	2.7	VVIR versus DDDR	NS†	↑	NS	↑	NS†	↓
UK-PACE, 2003	2021	80	AVB	4.6	VVI/VVIR versus DDD/DDDR	NS†	NS		NS	↑‡	Not stated

AF, atrial fibrillation; AVB, atrioventricular block; CHF, congestive heart failure; HF, heart failure; NS, no significant difference; QOL, quality of life; SND, sinus node dysfunction; TE, thromboembolism; ↑, increased; ↓, decreased.

*CTOPP, Canadian Trial of Physiologic Pacing; MOST, Mode Selection Trial; PASE, Pacemaker Selection in the Elderly; UK-PACE, U.K. Pacing and Cardiovascular Events.

†Designated primary end point of the trial.

‡Nonsignificant trend, VVI versus DDD.

Modified from Vliestra by permission of Le Jacq Communications, Inc.

morbidity and mortality were similar with VVI and DDD pacing, and there was also no difference in the incidence of AF between groups.

The main findings of these prospective randomized trials assessing the effect of pacing mode on long-term clinical outcomes are summarized in Table 79-2. The three largest trials conducted in three countries (United Kingdom, United States, and Canada), enrolling more than 6500 patients, did not find a beneficial effect of dual-chamber pacing for the prevention of stroke or improvement in survival when compared with ventricular pacing. However, the incidence and progression to chronic AF were reduced moderately in two of these studies. In addition, heart failure symptoms were reduced slightly and quality of life was better in patients receiving dual-chamber pacemakers for sinus node dysfunction, most likely because of the prevention of pacemaker syndrome.

SYNCOPE IN THE ELDERLY

Hypersensitive Carotid Sinus Syndrome

Carotid sinus hypersensitivity ($\geq$3-second pause or a decrease in systolic blood pressure $\geq$50 mm Hg during carotid sinus massage) predominantly affects elderly patients, although the prevalence in the general population has not been precisely defined. In elderly patients with recurrent syncope, carotid sinus hypersensitivity has been reported in up to 35% of cases. Permanent pacing in patients with carotid sinus syndrome (carotid sinus hypersensitivity associated with syncope) is indicated. Observational and randomized studies have shown that recurrent symptoms are significantly reduced after permanent pacemaker implantation in patients with carotid sinus syndrome. Dual-chamber pacing is considered the best choice for these patients, although data are lacking from randomized trials. Newer algorithms, such as the "rate-drop response" or "sudden-brady response," which accelerates the pacing rate when bradycardia is detected, are now available. However, the clinical utility of pacemakers with these newer algorithms compared with conventional pacemakers has not been determined in patients with carotid sinus syndrome.

Neurocardiogenic ("Vasovagal") Syncope

Vasovagal syncope is more common in younger patients but also should be considered in elderly patients with unexplained syncope. Although the triggering mechanisms are complex and may differ among young and elderly patients, the efferent responses generally can be categorized as cardioinhibitory (pauses of $\geq$3 seconds or heart rate <40 beats per minute for more than 10 seconds), vasodepressor (systolic blood pressure falls by 50 mm Hg or more without symptoms or 30 to 50 mm Hg with symptoms of syncope or presyncope, and the heart rate does not decrease by more than 10%), or mixed (heart rate decreases but the ventricular rate does not fall below 40 beats per minute for more than 10 seconds, and there are no pauses >3 seconds; blood pressure usually decreases before the heart rate drop). Of note, the vasodepressor component is frequently present in patients with vasovagal syncope, and pacing therapy does not necessarily eliminate or significantly reduce vasodepressor-mediated symptoms.

In three recent unblinded randomized trials (Vasovagal Pacemaker Study, Vasovagal International Study, and Syncope Diagnosis and Treatment) comparing pacing with conventional therapy (conservative or drug), recurrent symptoms were significantly reduced with pacemaker therapy. As a result, pacing for "significantly symptomatic and recurrent neurocardiogenic syncope associated with bradycardia documented spontaneously or at the time of tilt-table testing" is considered a class IIa indication for pacemaker implantation. However, following publication of these guidelines in 2002, the Vasovagal Pacemaker Study II trial, in which patients and investigators were blinded to pacing mode, failed to confirm a beneficial effect from pacing therapy in patients with vasovagal syncope.

In general, outcomes from pacing and drugs for treating vasovagal syncope reflect the heterogeneous patient population, complex underlying mechanisms, and sporadic nature of the neurocardiogenic reflex. On the basis of available evidence, it is reasonable to consider pacing as a class II indication in elderly patients who have recurrent syncope with documented bradycardia during a vasovagal response. Current data are insufficient to determine whether pacemakers with rate-drop or sudden-brady response features provide additional benefit.

Elderly Patients with Syncope of Uncertain Cause

Syncope is a common cause of falls, injuries, and hospitalizations in older adults. Normal age-related physiological changes often combine with pathological mechanisms to impair cerebral perfusion and induce syncope. Elderly community-dwelling patients have an average of 3.5 chronic illnesses, many of which predispose to syncope. In addition, elderly patients receive three times as many medications as the general population, further increasing their vulnerability to syncope. Numerous age-related autonomic and humoral changes also predispose older patients to syncope. Decreased heart rate responsiveness to postural changes and diminished baroreceptor sensitivity impair the ability to adapt to orthostatic stress. Reduced concentrations of plasma aldosterone, coupled with impaired thirst, place elderly patients at risk of volume depletion. These age-dependent changes, in combination with comorbid medical illnesses, increase the propensity for multiple potential etiologies of syncope in elderly patients. In turn, multiple-cause syncope is an independent predictor of poor clinical outcome.

The diagnostic approach to syncope is similar in older and younger patients and begins with a careful history and physical examination, recognizing that cardiogenic causes of syncope are more common in the elderly. Factors associated with an increased risk of cardiogenic syncope include a history of coronary artery disease, prior myocardial infarction, chronic heart failure, abrupt onset of symptoms (no prodrome), event occurring in the supine position, older age, abnormal cardiovascular examination (aortic stenosis murmur and S_3 gallop), abnormal ECG (Q waves, bundle branch block, or sinus bradycardia), and an abnormal echocardiogram (structural abnormality or reduced ejection fraction). Carotid sinus massage should be a routine part of examination in elderly patients presenting with syncope, unless there is a carotid bruit or prior history of stroke. In elderly patients with unexplained syncope and an increased risk of a cardiogenic cause, EPS should be considered. In patients at low risk of cardiogenic syncope, noninvasive cardiac monitoring or tilt-table testing may be appropriate. An implantable loop recorder should be considered in elderly patients with recurrent syncope of unknown cause, especially if structural heart disease is present. Once a cause of syncope has been established, treatment is similar in older and younger patients.

Despite advances in diagnostic technology for syncope evaluation, the cause of syncope remains undetermined in approximately 20% of patients after medical evaluation; many are elderly with an increased tendency for multiple etiologies. Current guidelines do not recommend "empirical" pacemaker therapy in elderly patients with recurrent syncope if carotid sinus massage, tilt-table testing, and EPS are all nondiagnostic. In such cases, an implantable loop recorder may be helpful in establishing a diagnosis. Data from implantable loop recorders for unexplained syncope have shown a predominance of bradycardic events among patients with recurrent symptoms during follow-up.

TACHYARRHYTHMIAS AND CARDIAC IMPLANTABLE DEFIBRILLATOR THERAPY IN THE ELDERLY

Atrial Fibrillation

Atrial Fibrillation affects approximately 2.3 million people in the United States and is the most common rhythm disorder among U.S. patients hospitalized with a primary diagnosis of an arrhythmia. The median age of AF patients is 75 years; 84% are older than 65 years. Pooled data from studies of chronic AF in North America, Britain, and Iceland suggest a prevalence of 0.5% to 1% in the general population. In two separate studies restricted to patients older than 60 years, the incidence was 5% to 9% after 5 to 15 years of follow-up. In the United States, hospitalization for AF has increased two- to threefold in the past 15 years and the size of the AF population is projected to triple by 2050. The genesis of this AF "epidemic" is strongly linked to the expanding elderly population.

AF has a substantial impact on both morbidity and mortality. It is a strong independent risk factor for stroke, responsible for an estimated 75 000 cerebrovascular accidents annually. AF is also associated with a more than twofold increase in all-cause mortality. Although AF frequently coexists with other medical conditions, especially cardiovascular and pulmonary disorders, mortality remains higher after adjusting for these and other conditions. (For a comprehensive review of AF, see: ACC/AHA/ESC Guidelines for the Management of Patients with Atrial Fibrillation; http://www.cardiosource.com/guidelines/guidelines/atrial_fib/pdfs/AF_final.pdf.)

Stroke Prevention in Atrial Fibrillation

Data supporting the use of anticoagulation for primary and secondary stroke prevention are more compelling than those for any other pharmacologic intervention in AF. The annual incidence of stroke in elderly patients with nonvalvular, chronic, or paroxysmal AF is approximately 5% in the absence of anticoagulation, compared with approximately 1% for comparable populations in sinus rhythm. Clinical risk factors for stroke in patients with AF include prior cerebrovascular accident, history of hypertension, diabetes mellitus, heart failure, and advanced age. Echocardiographic risk factors include increased left atrial size and decreased left ventricular systolic function.

Data from a pooled analysis of primary prevention studies indicate that the annual risk of stroke in patients with one or more clinical risk factors varies from 4% to 12% and that warfarin therapy reduces the risk by 60% to 70% (i.e., down to 1.2–4%). In patients older than 75 years, the beneficial effect of warfarin in embolic stroke prevention is offset by increased serious bleeding complications, especially in women. In the Stroke Prevention in Atrial Fibrillation (SPAF) II trial, combined embolic and hemorrhagic stroke rates were approximately 2% in patients less than 75 years of age and 5% in patients older than 75 years. From these data, current guidelines recommend maintaining the international normalized ratio (INR) near 2.0 in patients older than 75 years, particularly women.

Aspirin is substantially less effective than warfarin for preventing thromboembolic events, especially in elderly patients with risk factors for stroke, but aspirin is also associated with a lower risk of bleeding complications, including hemorrhagic stroke. In the Atrial Fibrillation, Aspirin, and Anticoagulation study, aspirin 75 mg daily was not significantly better than placebo for stroke prevention. However, aspirin 325 mg daily significantly decreased the risk of stroke in the SPAF trial, which enrolled younger patients than Atrial Fibrillation, Aspirin, and Anticoagulation study (mean age 67 vs. 75 years). Warfarin and aspirin were directly compared in the SPAF II trial, which failed to show a significant advantage of warfarin over aspirin in either of two age groups (60–75 years and >75 years). In SPAF II, patients 60 to 75 years old had a remarkably low event rate with either regimen, whereas in the older patients a reduction in the incidence of ischemic stroke was offset by a higher rate of intracranial bleeding in the warfarin arm. In contrast, the SPAF III study, which recruited patients with at least one risk factor for stroke in addition to AF, showed a clear advantage of warfarin adjusted to maintain an INR of 2 to 3 compared with a combination of aspirin 325 mg/day and a low, fixed-dose of warfarin (0.5–3.0 mg/day; INR, 1.2–1.5). Similarly, for secondary stroke prevention, the European Atrial Fibrillation trial demonstrated a 40% lower event rate with warfarin compared to aspirin.

The role of newer antiplatelet agents, such as clopidogrel, and antithrombotic agents, such as ximelagatran, for the prevention of thromboembolic events in elderly patients with AF is being determined. From the recent "clopidogrel plus aspirin versus oral anticoagulation for atrial fibrillation in Atrial fibrillation Clopidogrel Trial with Irbesartan for prevention of Vascular Events (ACTIVE W): a randomized controlled trial," the study was stopped early because warfarin was superior to clopidogrel plus aspirin for prevention of vascular events in patients (primarily elderly) with AF at higher risk of stroke. In the Stroke Prevention using an Oral Thrombin Inhibitor in Atrial Fibrillation III and V trials, ximelagatran, a new oral antithrombin, was not inferior to warfarin for the prevention of stroke in patients with AF. Major adverse effects, including bleeding, occurred less frequently in patients treated with ximelagatran than in those who received warfarin. Transient increases in liver enzymes were reported in approximately 6% of patients. Ximelagatran was not approved for clinical use primarily owing to the side effect of liver toxicity. Other oral antithrombin agents are currently under development and clinical investigation.

Current recommendations for stroke prevention in patients with AF are summarized in Table 79-3. More detailed discussion and models of stroke risk estimation including the CHADS2 score system are described in the 2006 AHA/ACC guidelines for management of AF. In elderly patients, the decision to initiate anticoagulation with warfarin must be balanced against the increased risk of intracerebral bleeding and bleeding related to injuries from falls.

TABLE 79-3

Risk-Based Approach to Antithrombotic Therapy in Patients with Atrial Fibrillation

PATIENT CHARACTERISTICS	ANTITHROMBOTIC THERAPY	GRADE OF RECOMMENDATION
Age <60 yr, no heart disease (lone AF)	Aspirin (81–325 mg/day) or no therapy	I
Age <60 yr, heart disease but no risk factors*	Aspirin (81–325 mg/day)	I
Age 60–74 yr, no risk factors*	Aspirin (81–325 mg/day)	I
Age 65–74 yr with DM or CAD	Oral anticoagulation (INR, 2.0–3.0)	I
Age ≥75 yr, women	Oral anticoagulation (INR, 2.0–3.0)	I
Age ≥ 75 yr, men, no other risk factors	Oral anticoagulation (INR, ≈2.0) or ASA (81–325 mg/day)	I
Age 65 yr or older, heart failure	Oral anticoagulation (INR, 2.0–3.0)	I
LV ejection fraction less than 35% or fractional shortening less than 25%, and hypertension	Oral anticoagulation (INR, 2.0–3.0)	I
Rheumatic heart disease (mitral stenosis)	Oral anticoagulation (INR, 2.0–3.0)	I
Prosthetic heart valves Prior thromboembolism	Oral anticoagulation (INR, 2.0–3.0 or higher)	I
Persistent atrial thrombus on TEE	Oral anticoagulation (INR, 2.0–3.0 or higher)	IIa

AF, atrial fibrillation; CAD, coronary artery disease; DM, diabetes mellitus; INR, international normalized ratio; LVEF, left ventricular ejection fraction; TEE, transesophageal echocardiography.

*Risk factors for thromboembolism include heart failure, left ventricular ejection fraction less than 35%, and history of hypertension.

From Fuster V, Rydén LE, Asinger RW, et al. ACC/AHA/ESC guidelines for the management of patients with atrial fibrillation: a report of the American College of Cardiology/American Heart Association Task Force on Practice Guidelines and the European Society of Cardiology Committee for Practice Guidelines and Policy Conferences (Committee to Develop Guidelines for the Management of Patients With Atrial Fibrillation). J Am Coll Cardiol. 2006;114:e257–e354. By permission of the American College of Cardiology, the American Heart Association, Inc, and the European Society of Cardiology.

Careful monitoring of warfarin dosing with frequent evaluation of the level of anticoagulation is warranted.

The risk of thromboembolism with acute cardioversion in patients with AF, which has been present for fewer than 48 hours, is low (0.8%). In patients with AF for longer than 48 hours or of unknown duration, warfarin therapy is recommended for 4 weeks before attempting cardioversion (either electrical or chemical). Recent data suggest that transesophageal echocardiography is effective for excluding atrial thrombi and allows earlier cardioversion in patients with AF of unknown duration. However, anticoagulation must be continued for at least 4 weeks after cardioversion because mechanical atrial stunning increases the risk of atrial thrombus formation.

Pharmacologic Therapy for Atrial Fibrillation

Rate Control Although urgent cardioversion is required for patients with AF associated with hemodynamic instability, persistent angina, or critical aortic stenosis, most acute-phase symptoms can be controlled by prompt reduction of the ventricular rate. Digitalis glycosides decrease ventricular rate in AF by augmenting cardiac vagal tone and increasing the level of block at the AVN. However, in both acute and chronic settings, digoxin is generally less effective at controlling rate than either β-adrenergic blockers or calcium channel-blockers (i.e., diltiazem or verapamil), especially during exercise or parasympathetic withdrawal. There are also no data to support the use of digoxin for chemical cardioversion or for the maintenance of sinus rhythm; in fact, digoxin theoretically may facilitate AF by shortening the atrial refractory period and increasing atrial automaticity.

β-Blockers and calcium channel-blockers reduce the ventricular rate in AF by slowing conduction through the AVN. The choice between these two groups of drugs primarily depends on the clinical context. For example, β-blockers are preferable for rate control of AF paroxysms precipitated by acute coronary ischemia, whereas calcium channel-blockers are chosen in the setting of asthma. Clonidine, a central α2-receptor agonist, can be moderately effective for reducing ventricular rate by decreasing central nervous system sympathetic outflow. In elderly patients, optimizing rate control with drugs may be difficult because of presence of comorbidities and susceptibility to adverse effects. Clinical conditions such as sinus node dysfunction, AV conduction delay, and ventricular dysfunction may result in significant bradyarrhythmia or worsening heart failure when rate-controlling agents are administered. In addition, rate control alone may be insufficient to alleviate symptoms in some patients, such as those with hypertrophic cardiomyopathy, in whom restoration of sinus rhythm may be beneficial.

Rhythm Control In the acute setting, rhythm control can be established by pharmacological or nonpharmacological cardioversion. The efficacy of intravenous and oral antiarrhythmic drugs for cardioversion of AF is highly variable, ranging from 30% to 75%. Efficacy also varies with the age of the patient, duration of the arrhythmia, presence of atrial flutter, underlying left ventricular function, and left atrial size. Ibutilide, a class III drug, is more effective in restoring sinus rhythm in atrial flutter than AF. Dofetilide, another class III agent, is effective for oral prophylaxis and safe in patients with left ventricular dysfunction. Single-dose oral propafenone has also been evaluated for AF cardioversion and has an excellent efficacy and safety profile. In general, higher cardioversion efficacy rates are reported for paroxysmal than for persistent AF. Elderly patients may be at increased risk of proarrhythmia with all of these agents, thus necessitating careful monitoring during and after cardioversion. The efficacy of intravenous amiodarone for termination of recent-onset AF is disputed. Although some studies suggest a high efficacy comparable to direct-current cardioversion, intravenous amiodarone was not more effective after 24 hours than placebo in a randomized trial of 100 patients with recent AF. This may be explained by the delayed onset of amiodarone's antiarrhythmic effects. Current data do not support the use of amiodarone for acute cardioversion.

TABLE 79-4

Atrial Fibrillation Clinical Trials: Rate versus Rhythm Control

TRIAL,* YEAR REPORTED	NO. ENROLLED	MEAN AGE (yr)	TYPE OF AF	PRIMARY END POINT	PRIMARY END POINT OUTCOME	COMMENTS		
						QOL	Hospi-talization	Stroke
PIAF, 2000	252	61	Persistent	Symptoms	NS	NS	↑	Not stated
AFFIRM, 2002	4060	70	Mostly persistent Paroxysmal <30%	All-cause mortality	NS (trend toward higher mortality in rhythm control)	NS	↑	(↑)
RACE, 2002	522	68	Persistent	Composite: cardiovascular death, hospitalized for heart failure, thromboembolic events, severe bleeding, drug side effects, and PM implantation	NS	NS	↑	(↑)
STAF, 2003	200	66	Mostly persistent	Composite: death, stroke, TIA, resuscitation from cardiac arrest, and peripheral emboli	Not stated	Not stated	↑	(↑)

AF, atrial fibrillation; NS, no significant difference; PM, pacemaker; QOL, quality of life; TIA, transient ischemic attack; ↑, significantly higher in rhythm control; (↑), higher, but not significantly, in rhythm control.

*AFFIRM, Atrial Fibrillation Follow-up Investigation of Rhythm Management; PIAF, Pharmacological Intervention in Atrial Fibrillation; RACE, Rate Control Versus Electrical Cardioversion for Persistent Atrial Fibrillation Study; STAF, Strategies of Treatment of Atrial Fibrillation.

External direct-current cardioversion can restore sinus rhythm in 75% to 90% of patients with AF. Catheter- or device-delivered internal cardioversion has a reported efficacy rate of close to 100%, even in patients in whom external cardioversion has failed. Internal cardioversion is indicated in patients who are refractory to external techniques and when restoration of sinus rhythm is deemed obligatory. Failure of external cardioversion is becoming uncommon because cardioverters with biphasic current waveforms, with improved efficacy in restoring sinus rhythm, are now used in routine clinical practice.

For maintenance of sinus rhythm in patients with recurrent AF, consideration is given to chronic antiarrhythmic therapy. Class Ia antiarrhythmic drugs such as quinidine, disopyramide, and procainamide; class Ic agents such as flecainide and propafenone; and class III agents such as sotalol, amiodarone, and dofetilide have all been used to prevent recurrent AF, with efficacy rates ranging from 30% to 80% during the first year of follow-up. Amiodarone is more efficacious and safer during short- and intermediate-term follow-up than class I agents, for which the risk of ventricular proarrhythmia must be carefully considered. The presence of structural heart disease, which is common in the elderly, increases the risk of proarrhythmia with class I agents. However, amiodarone is associated with considerable noncardiac side effects during long-term use, resulting in drug discontinuation rates of up to 20% at 1 year. In general, drugs with substantial negative inotropic effects, including procainamide, disopyramide, and flecainide, are contraindicated in patients with left ventricular systolic dysfunction. Class 1C drugs should not be used in patients with underlying coronary artery disease. Class Ia and III agents prolong ventricular repolarization and the QT interval owing to potassium channel blockade. Propafenone, sotalol, and amiodarone have a β-blocking effect that could be clinically significant in elderly patients with sinus node or AVN conduction disease. In patients with His-Purkinje disease (e.g., bifascicular or trifascicular block on electrocardiography), class I agents should be used with caution because of their potential to slow infranodal conduction.

Dofetilide, sotalol, and active metabolite of procainamide are predominantly excreted by the kidney and should be used with extreme caution in elderly patients with concomitant renal dysfunction.

Rate versus Rhythm Control Ideally, the goals of treating AF are to restore and maintain sinus rhythm, but all currently available therapeutic options are also associated with significant risks. Four randomized trials (Table 79-4) recently compared the effectiveness of rate control (i.e., controlling ventricular rate in AF) versus rhythm control (attempting to maintain sinus rhythm).

The largest of these studies was the Atrial Fibrillation Follow-up Investigation of Rhythm Management trial, which enrolled more than 4000 elderly patients with AF and at least one risk factor for stroke. After a mean follow-up of 3.5 years, there was a trend toward increased mortality in the rhythm control arm, but there was no difference between groups in a composite secondary end point that included stroke and other cardiovascular events. The Rate Control versus Electrical Cardioversion for Persistent Atrial Fibrillation study and the Strategies of Treatment of Atrial Fibrillation trial also found that rate control was not inferior to rhythm control for the prevention of death and cardiovascular morbidity. Functional outcomes were addressed in the Rhythm or Rate Control in Atrial Fibrillation—Pharmacological Intervention in Atrial Fibrillation study, in which patients were randomized to amiodarone for rhythm control or diltiazem for rate control. During a follow-up of 12 months, the proportion of patients who reported improvement in symptoms was similar in both groups. Exercise tolerance was better with rhythm control, although hospital admissions were significantly more frequent in the amiodarone-treated group.

Outcomes of the Atrial Fibrillation Follow-up Investigation of Rhythm Management, Rate Control versus Electrical Cardioversion for Persistent Atrial Fibrillation Study, Strategies of Treatment of Atrial Fibrillation, and Rhythm or Rate Control in Atrial Fibrillation—Pharmacological Intervention in Atrial Fibrillation trials suggest that medical therapy for rate control and chronic anticoagulation are the preferred approaches in asymptomatic or minimally symptomatic patients with persistent AF. These studies clearly show that an optimal drug therapy regimen for AF is not currently available; as a result, the most efficacious therapeutic strategy for the large population of patients with *symptomatic* AF, who are predominantly elderly (estimated to be at least 40% of the entire AF population), remains to be resolved.

Nonpharmacologic Therapy for Atrial Fibrillation

In the absence of a simple and effective drug-based treatment strategy, major efforts are being undertaken to develop and evaluate nonpharmacologic methods for treating recurrent AF. Before wide application of these approaches can be recommended in the elderly, clinically relevant end points, such as survival, stroke, major cardiovascular events, symptoms, and functional capacity, must be evaluated. General guidelines on catheter ablation, including ablation for AF, were updated in 2006: ACC/AHA/ESC 2006 guidelines for the management of patients with AF and 2007 (Heart Rhythm Society guidelines for AF ablation).

Rate Control In patients with severe symptoms and in whom drug therapy fails, ablation of the AVN and permanent pacing are effective for controlling ventricular rate. Although ablation of the AVN does not eliminate AF or the need for anticoagulation, it relieves symptoms and improves health-related quality of life, exercise tolerance, and left ventricular function. In addition, recent data from the Left Ventricular-Based Cardiac Stimulation Post AV Nodal Ablation Evaluation study suggest that biventricular pacing after AVN ablation is associated with improved 6-minute walk distance compared with conventional right ventricular apex pacing in patients with preexisting heart failure symptoms. Despite the efficacy of AVN ablation and pacemaker implantation for controlling symptoms in patients with AF, there is concern that the creation of complete AV block and the associated requirement for permanent pacing may have an adverse effect on long-term survival. However, in a large observational study, survival among patients who underwent ablation of the AVN to control ventricular rate for AF was similar to that among patients who received drug therapy.

Although ablation of the AVN plus pacemaker therapy seems to be a logical solution in the elderly with recurrent and symptomatic AF because the procedures are relatively straightforward with a high success rate (near 100%) and subsequent clinical improvement, most of the data accumulated thus far are from observational studies with a highly selected patient population. Large-scale randomized trials are needed to determine whether AVN ablation is beneficial to patients compared to pharmacologic rate control in the AF elderly population at large. In addition, large-scale randomized trials are needed to determine whether patients who have undergone AVN ablation should receive conventional pacemakers versus cardiac resynchronization therapy (CRT) pacemakers.

Rhythm Control Despite antiarrhythmic drug therapy, recurrent and refractory symptomatic AF is common in patients of all ages. Nonpharmacologic treatment options are increasingly being used to maintain sinus rhythm in these patients. However, the projected benefits must be weighed carefully against the potential risk of invasive procedures, especially in older patients with other comorbid conditions. The surgical maze procedure is highly effective in the treatment of refractory AF and has become an important adjunctive procedure for patients with AF undergoing cardiac surgery for other reasons. The long-term success rate has been reported to be as high as 90% during 4- to 5-year follow-up. The surgical experience has also provided impetus to develop catheter-based ablative techniques for the treatment of AF.

Currently, there are two general catheter approaches to target the arrhythmogenic AF substrate. Isolation of pulmonary veins, the first approach, is based on the premise that most AF is initiated or "triggered" from foci at the pulmonary vein and left atrial junction. This approach appears to be most suited for patients with paroxysmal AF and no significant preexisting heart disease; usually these patients are younger and likely to have a predominantly triggered mechanism initiating AF. The second approach is based on the concept that AF is usually sustained by a diffuse arrhythmogenic atrial substrate in patients with persistent AF and preexisting heart disease; usually these patients are older. The second approach requires a wider area of ablation involving the pulmonary vein orifices, the left atrium, and the right atrium. The success rate of catheter-based ablation for AF reported in the literature has been highly variable. Some explanations include, but not limited to, differences in patient selection, operator's experience, ablation techniques, procedural endpoints, follow-up, and definition of "success." In a recent survey from multiple centers around the globe, the success rate for catheter ablation has been estimated in the range of 60% to 70% in patients with paroxysmal AF and 40% to 60% in patients with persistent or permanent AF during an average follow-up of 2 years. One should also be aware that the mean age of patients undergoing primary AF ablation in most studies has been in the range of 50 to 65 years of age. Whether similar outcomes can be obtained in the majority of the AF patients, >80% older than 65 years, remain to be determined.

Major complications of AF ablation include death, stroke, tamponade, esophageal perforation or fistula, and pulmonary vein stenosis. The impact of AF ablation on stroke is also unknown; therefore, continuation of anticoagulation is recommended.

An alternative approach to the treatment of infrequent episodes of paroxysmal AF is the implantable atrial defibrillator. This device is safe and effective for terminating AF. However, its clinical application is limited because of discomfort experienced by conscious patients and the lack of evidence of a beneficial effect on long-term clinical outcomes.

Supraventricular Tachyarrhythmia

The principles of drug and nondrug management of supraventricular tachyarrhythmia (SVT) are similar to those outlined for AF. However, for most SVTs, the arrhythmogenic substrate is isolated and well defined. AV nodal reentrant tachycardia (localized to the region of AVN) and AV reentrant tachycardia (with use of an accessory pathway) are the two most common types of SVT. Atrial tachycardia can be reentrant or non-reentrant in mechanism, can be right or left atrial in origin, and can occur more frequently in the elderly population than in younger patients.

β-Blockers and calcium channel-blockers are effective for treating SVTs originating or using the sinoatrial node or AVN as a component of the tachycardia and for treating SVTs mediated by catecholamines. Class I and III antiarrhythmic agents are effective for treating SVTs involving conduction through an accessory pathway or atrial tissue. Ablative therapy is also highly effective for the treatment of SVTs (see Supraventricular Arrhythmias: ACC/AHA/ESC Guidelines for the Management of Patients with Supraventricular Tachyarrhythmias;

http://www.cardiosource.com/guidelines/guidelines/arrhythmias/sva_index.pdf).

Class I indications for catheter ablation are (1) symptomatic AV nodal reentrant tachycardia, (2) recurrent atrial flutter, (3) SVTs associated with preexcitation if the tachyarrhythmia is drug resistant or if the patient is drug intolerant or does not want long-term drug therapy, and (4) atrial tachyarrhythmias with rapid ventricular response as a result of conduction over an accessory pathway. Indications for catheter ablation in elderly and very elderly patients have not been separately defined and are the same as those for the general population. Success rates for catheter ablation of SVT range from 75% to more than 95%, depending primarily on the nature of the arrhythmia and the experience of the operator; notably, age is not predictive of procedural success.

The incidence of major complications associated with SVT ablation is approximately 3%, and the risk of minor complications is approximately 8%. Major complications include death, stroke, myocardial infarction, and complete heart block requiring permanent pacemaker implantation. The overall risk of thromboembolic complications is approximately 0.6%, but the risk is higher when ablation is performed in the left heart (1.8%–2%). Independent predictors of major complications include increasing age, the presence of heart disease, and multiple ablation targets.

Ventricular Tachyarrhythmia

Advancing age is associated with a progressive increase in the incidence of ventricular premature beats and nonsustained ventricular tachycardia in patients with or without manifest cardiac disease. These trends have been attributed to undetected cardiac disease, increased left ventricular mass, higher serum catecholamine levels, and intrinsic age-related changes in the cardiac myocyte and the extracellular matrix.

The management of ventricular arrhythmias in elderly patients is similar to that in the general population. In patients with asymptomatic nonsustained ventricular tachyarrhythmia, a careful evaluation for the presence of cardiac disease, including occult coronary artery disease, structural heart disease, and left ventricular dysfunction, is required. Premature ventricular contractions and nonsustained ventricular tachyarrhythmia are associated with a benign prognosis in the absence of any significant heart disease. The risk of SCD is increased in patients with compromised left ventricular ejection fraction, whether because of ischemic or nonischemic heart disease. Prevention of SCD entails optimization of therapy directed at the underlying disease and the use of implantable cardioverter-defibrillator (ICD) therapy in selected patients (ACC/AHA guidelines for implantation of cardiac pacemakers and antiarrhythmia devices). Note that although none of the indications for ICDs exclude or allude to special considerations in elderly patients, individual assessment and determination of primary therapeutic objectives are particularly pertinent in this population because comorbid medical illnesses are frequently present and life expectancy is shorter in the very elderly.

Secondary Prevention of Sudden Cardiac Death

Indications for implantation of a cardioverter defibrillator for secondary prevention of SCD include (1) cardiac arrest owing to ventricular tachycardia or ventricular fibrillation not related to a transient or reversible cause (e.g., acute myocardial infarction), (2) spontaneous sustained ventricular tachycardia in association with structural heart disease, and (3) syncope of undetermined origin with clinically relevant, hemodynamically significant sustained ventricular tachycardia or ventricular fibrillation induced at EPS when drug therapy is ineffective, not tolerated, or not preferred. Randomized, prospective clinical trials comparing antiarrhythmic drug therapy to ICD have demonstrated the usefulness of ICD in reducing the risk of SCD as a result of cardiac arrhythmias in those at risk of or resuscitated from cardiac arrest or life-threatening ventricular arrhythmias. However, none of these trials have focused specifically on the efficacy of ICD in the older-elderly. Overall, the average age of patients in the clinical trials of ICD has been in the sixties, ranging from the fifties into the high seventies. Data on octogenarian and nonagenarian patients are scant; however, using pooled data from the three major randomized ICD secondary prevention trials of SCD, a recent study by Healey et al. found no statistically significant reduction in all-cause mortality or arrhythmic death among patients aged 75 years, randomized to ICD therapy versus amiodarone. This highlights the importance of individualization when making decisions on ICD implantation in the older-elderly, taking into account the current guidelines, patient's preference, biological age, functional capacity, and underlying comorbidities.

Primary Prevention of Sudden Cardiac Death

Results from several recently completed trials have important implications for the primary prevention of SCD (Table 79-5). In patients with coronary artery disease, prior myocardial infarction, and ejection fraction of 30% or less, a survival benefit was found with prophylactic implantation of a cardioverter defibrillator compared with medical therapy (MADIT-II). In the MADIT-II trial, benefits in patients with preexisting left bundle branch block were more pronounced. In the Sudden Cardiac Death in Heart Failure Trial (SCD-HeFT), an ICD was associated with improved survival compared with amiodarone or medical therapy in patients with class II or III heart failure symptoms and an ejection fraction of 35% or less, and the benefit was evident in patients with or without ischemia (48%). Although not significant, the Defibrillators in Nonischemic Cardiomyopathy Treatment Evaluation trial also noted a trend toward improved survival in patients with nonischemic cardiomyopathy, nonsustained ventricular tachycardia, and an ejection fraction of 35% or less treated with an ICD compared with medical therapy.

Indications for the implantation of a cardioverter defibrillator for primary prevention of SCD were recently updated in 2006: ACC/AHA/ESC 2006 guidelines for management of patients with ventricular arrhythmias and prevention of sudden cardiac death (http://www.cardiosource.com/guidelines/guidelines/arrhythmias/va_scd.pdf). An ICD is currently approved by Medicare for use in patients with ischemic or nonischemic cardiomyopathy, ejection fraction of 35% or less, and class II or class III heart failure symptoms based on the MADIT-II and SCD-HeFT trial results. Patients who had history of MI (greater than 40 days after the event) and ejection fraction of 30% or less also qualify regardless of their functional status. In patients with ejection fractions between 35% and 40%, an ICD is indicated if a sustained ventricular tachyarrhythmia is inducible during EPS evaluation. As shown in Table 79-5, the mean age of patients in the primary prevention

TABLE 79-5

Primary Prevention of Sudden Cardiac Death: Major Trials of Implantable Cardioverter Defibrillators Since 2002*

TRIAL,[†] YEAR REPORTED	NO. ENROLLED	MEAN AGE (yr)	CONDITION	STUDY DESIGN	PRIMARY END POINT	PRIMARY END POINT OUTCOME	COMMENTS
CAT, 2002	104	52	Nonischemic EF ≤30% NYHA II, III	ICD versus medical therapy	Total mortality	NS	Low total mortality
MADIT-II, 2002	1232	64	CAD EF ≤30%	ICD versus medical therapy (control)	Total mortality	↓	Increased hospitalization for heart failure with ICD
AMIOVIRT, 2003	103	59	Nonischemic EF ≤35%	ICD versus amiodarone	Total mortality	NS	QOL not different Trend in favor of amiodarone in arrhythmia-free survival and cost
DEFINITE, 2004	558	58	Nonischemic EF ≤35% Nonsustained VT	ICD versus medical therapy	Total mortality	(↓) $P = 0.066$	Final numbers remain to be confirmed; pending publication
SCD-HeFT, 2005	1676	60	EF ≤35% NYHA II, III CAD = 52% Nonischemic = 48%	ICD versus medical versus amiodarone	Total mortality	↓	No difference between amiodarone and controls in mortality Survival benefit in CAD and non-CAD after ICD therapy
COMPANION, 2004	1520	67	EF ≤35% NYHA III, IV CAD = 55% Nonischemic = 45%	Medical versus CRT versus ICD/CRT	Mortality or hospitalization	↓	Survival benefit in CAD and non-CAD with ICD/CRT
DINAMIT, 2004	674	62	MI 6–40 d previously EF ≤35%	Medical versus ICD	Total mortality	No difference	Patients with recent MI do not benefit from prophylactic ICD

CAD, coronary artery disease; EF, ejection fraction; ICD, implantable cardioverter defibrillator; NS, no significant difference; NYHA, New York Heart Association; QOL, quality of life; ↓, significantly lower mortality in group that received an implantable cardioverter defibrillator.

*Excluding cardiac resynchronization treatment trials.

[†]AMIOVIRT, Amiodarone Versus Implantable Cardioverter-Defibrillator Trial; CAT, Cardiomyopathy Trial; DEFINITE, Defibrillators in Non-ischemic Cardiomyopathy Treatment Evaluation; MADIT-II, Multicenter Automatic Defibrillator Implantation Trial II; SCD-HeFT, Sudden Cardiac Death in Heart Failure Trials; COMPANION, Comparison of Medical Therapy, Pacing, and Defibrillation in Chronic Heart Failure.

Zipes DP, CA, Borggrefe M, et al. ACC/AHA/ESC 2006 guidelines for management of patients with ventricular arrhythmias and the prevention of sudden cardiac death: a report of the American College of Cardiology/American Heart Association Task Force and the European Society of Cardiology Committee for Practice Guidelines (Writing Committee to Develop Guidelines for Management of Patients With Ventricular Arrhythmias and the Prevention of Sudden Cardiac Death). J Am Coll Cardiol. 2006;48:e247–e346.

trials ranged from 52 to 64 years. Data for primary prevention of SCD in very elderly patients, octogenarians and older, are not available.

Cardiac Resynchronization Therapy and Implantable Cardioverter Defibrillator

CRT improves functional capacity and quality of life in patients with persistent class III and IV heart failure despite optimal medical therapy, and there is also evidence that CRT may reverse structural remodeling in selected patients. Although individual trials of CRT were underpowered to assess survival, a meta-analysis of outcomes from four randomized trials involving more than 800 patients found that CRT reduces mortality from heart failure. More recently, the Comparison of Medical Therapy, Pacing, and Defibrillation in Chronic Heart Failure trial found that CRT reduces hospitalizations and that CRT with an ICD reduces mortality in chronic heart failure. These benefits from CRT were further confirmed in the CARE-HF trial in which CRT was shown to significantly reduce all cause mortality. However, it must be recognized that very limited data are

available on the use of these devices in the very elderly. Therefore, recommendations for the use of CRT and ICDs in this age group must be individualized, taking into consideration the patient's life expectancy, concomitant medical illnesses, and therapeutic objectives.

AGING AND DRUG-INDUCED PROARRHYTHMIA

Changes in Pharmacokinetics Associated with Aging

There are several important changes in pharmacokinetics associated with aging that predispose the elderly to increased risk of drug-induced side effects including arrhythmia.

First, advanced age is accompanied by a decrease in overall body weight, total body water, lean body mass, and intravascular volume, resulting in a greater volume of distribution (V_d), which is defined by the drug dose divided by drug plasma concentration (V_d = dose/concentration). The reduced distribution volume will, therefore, lead to a higher drug concentration after a given dose in the elderly compared to the younger population. This effect will become more pronounced when elderly patients receive intravenous boluses of pharmacological agents, especially drugs that have a narrow therapeutic index.

The other significant change occurring in the elderly patients is decreased drug clearance secondary to either decreased hepatic metabolism or renal elimination. It is well known that liver and renal diseases are more common in the elderly, resulting in higher chances of drug-induced side effects. Even with normal aging, there is a trend toward decreased hepatic metabolizing capacity, which can affect the body's ability to clear therapeutic drugs and environmental chemicals. It was shown recently that the half-life of drugs processed by hepatic cytochrome P450 enzymes is typically 50% to 75% longer in those older than 65 years than in young adults. In addition to decreased hepatic clearance, renal clearance also decreased with age and is lower in women compared to men. It has been estimated that the glomerular filtration rate decreases by 10% per decade, which can result in significant increase in plasma concentration of these drugs eliminated by the kidneys.

Finally, polypharmacy in the elderly and the resulting potential drug interactions may also contribute significantly to their increased risk of adverse reactions. In a recently published survey conducted from 1998 to 1999 among ambulatory adults in the United States, it was found that women 65 years or older had the highest prevalence of medication use: 94% took at least one, 57% took five or more, and 12% took 10 or more. Men 65 years or older also reported a high prevalence of medication use, although not quite as high as among older women. As the number of medication used increases, the potential for drug interaction also increases exponentially.

Drug-Induced Arrhythmias

As discussed earlier in this chapter, there are intrinsic changes in the cardiac pacemaker cells and the cardiac conduction system associated with aging, which increase the propensity of the elderly population to develop chronotropic incompetence, conduction block, and bradycardia overall. Moreover, the already-at-risk elderly population is more likely to receive and is more sensitive to a variety of cardiovascular agents that may cause further bradycardia through suppression of the pacemaker activity or AV block.

In addition to bradyarrhythmias, the elderly are also at risk of drug-induced tachyarrhythmias. Acquired long-QT syndrome or drug-induced torsades de pointes is a form of ventricular tachyarrhythmia that can potentially degenerate into ventricular fibrillation and is an often overlooked cause of syncope and SCD. The underlying mechanism of drug-induced torsades de pointes has been attributed to the ability of multiple clinically used drugs to increase cardiac action potential duration and QT interval, leading to increased intracellular calcium loading and the generation of early afterdepolarization activity. Although data on the exact prevalence of drug-induced torsades de pointes in the elderly are lacking, the increased exposure of the elderly population to drugs that are capable of lengthening the QT interval, from reasons described above, may increase their likelihood of developing this life-threatening arrhythmia. Normal aging itself has also been reported to be associated with increased action potential duration as well as the propensity to develop calcium overload, which may lead to early afterdepolarization activities and, therefore, trigger torsades de pointes.

NOVEL, EMERGING THERAPIES FOR CARDIAC ARRHYTHMIAS

Biological Pacemakers for Bradyarrhythmias

Pacemaker implantation is the mainstay for treating bradyarrhythmias currently; however, this form of therapy does not cure the fundamental changes in cardiac electrophysiology that led to the arrhythmia and is associated with significant risks and complications. These include potential risk of bleeding, hematoma, pneumothorax, cardiac perforation, lead dislodgement, infection, need for battery replacement, inadequate rate response, and the potential to cause dyssynchrony and worsening heart failure.

In an effort to avoid the multiple potentially serious complications associated with pacemaker implantation, a number of innovative gene and cell therapy approaches have recently emerged as potential means to develop future biological alternatives of implantable electronic devices. These approaches are designed to reverse or modify the underlying electrophysiologic process accompanying aging and, therefore, may provide real "cure," rather than just palliative treatment using external pacemaker, for aging-related bradyarrhythmias.

The intrinsic cardiac pacemaker activity is based on spontaneous phase 4 depolarization of the cell membrane in the conduction system, as a result of the intricate balance of inward and outward currents that ultimately generates a net depolarization current triggering a new action potential. One of the key players in the generation of pacemaker activity is the inward pacemaker current called the "funny current," I_f, encoded by the hyperpolarization-activated cyclic-nucleotide-modulated (HCN) channel gene family. Any intervention that increases inward current such as the I_f or the calcium currents and/or decreases outward current such as potassium current will increase the pacemaker rate. Catecholamine binding to β-adrenergic receptors results in cyclic AMP generation, which in turn leads to faster membrane depolarization and increased rate by enhancing current through I_f and calcium channel.

One of the early genetic approaches in an attempt to develop alternative to extrinsic pacing involved enhancing the expression of β-2 adrenergic receptor in the atria of pigs through injection of plasmids encoding for the receptor. Injection of the β-2 adrenergic receptor construct significantly enhanced automaticity compared with control injections using saline. An increase in heart rate of $\geq 50\%$ was achieved. The problem with this approach was the potential arrhythmogenicity of β-adrenergic agonists. Another early approach that was tested was the use of adenoviral vector that harbors a genetic construct capable of suppressing one of the voltage-gated potassium channels, the inward rectifier, I_{K1}. When such viral vectors were injected into the guinea pig ventricles, these were able to "convert" normally quiescent ventricular myocytes into pacemaker cells with spontaneous, rhythmic activity. These transfected cells also responded to β-adrenergic stimulation (by isoproterenol) just as nodal cells do, by increasing their pacing rate. However, by prolonging cardiac repolarization, this approach may result in an increased risk of developing ventricular arrhythmia similar to the congenital long-QT syndrome. The third approach focused on the enhancement of the pacemaker current I_f, through viral vectors carrying potassium channel genes mutated to mimic certain characteristics of the HCN family. These are inserted via catheter injection into ventricles or atria of experimental animals to generate a variation on the pacemaker current I_f and, therefore, produce spontaneous pacemaker activity.

The methods described above all require use of a viral vector, typically an adenovirus. Although these vectors are deficient adenoviruses that have little infectious potential, there is always the possibility of only a transient improvement in pacemaker function and potential inflammatory responses. The use of retroviruses and other vectors carries a risk of carcinogenicity and infectivity that is unjustified, given the current success of electronic pacemakers. A possible alternative to the gene therapy that does not require the use of a viral vector is the use of cell therapy. Two major forms of this type of biological pacing strategy have been evaluated. The first form involves a combined cell and gene therapy approach in which cells can initially be modified ex vivo to express the required ionic channels and then injected into the myocardium. Proof of concept for this strategy was performed by using mesenchymal stem cells overexpressing the HCN-encoded pacemaker current (I_f). By means of electroporation, investigators were able to transfect the human mesenchymal stem cells with the HCN2 (mHCN2) gene. The HCN2 expressed in human mesenchymal stem cells was able to change the beating rate of cocultured neonatal rat ventricular myocytes and, when injected into the canine left ventricle, able to generate a spontaneous rhythm.

The second form of cell therapy involves the administration of fetal/neonatal cardiomyocytes or human embryonic stem cells developing into a cardiac lineage. The proof-of-concept experiment of using human embryonic stem cell has been successfully conducted recently. Investigators established an animal model of slow heart rate in pigs, mimicking the clinical scenario of patients having complete AV block, requiring the implantation of an electronic pacemaker. Following creation of AV block in these animals, spontaneously contracting embryonic bodies were injected into the posterolateral left ventricular wall and ECGs were monitored. Following cell grafting a few days later, episodes of a new ectopic ventricular rhythm could be observed and was confirmed to come from the transplanted cells.

Finally, in addition to the research to develop biological pacemaker for treatment of sick sinus syndrome, there has been other innovative, cell-based approaches designed to treat heart block. Recently, engineered tissue constructs in rat hearts harboring myoblasts were implanted into the AV groove and were shown to survive for the duration of the animal's natural life and there is evidence of permanent AV conduction through the implant in one-third of recipient animals using optical mapping and electrophysiological analyses.

Genetic and Cell Therapy for Tachyarrhythmias

The same genetic and cell approaches used for treatment of bradyarrhythmia can potentially be modified to treat tachyarrhythmias. Arrhythmogenesis typically results from increased automaticity, triggered activity, or reentry. Different genetic approaches can, therefore, be designed based on the individual mechanism.

For tachyarrhythmias caused by enhanced or abnormal automaticity, approaches opposite to that used for bradyarrhythmia for generating biological pacemaker may be used theoretically to reduce automaticity. Studies have demonstrated that overexpression of different potassium channels can be used to alter the action potential

properties in cardiomyocytes in vitro and even to suppress cardiac hyperexcitability in rabbit ventricular myocytes.

Arrhythmias secondary to early afterdepolarization and triggered activity can also be treated via genetic modification of the balance between inward and outward current, with an aim at reducing the action potential duration. Gene delivery of different potassium channels was suggested as a method to accelerate cardiac repolarization and abbreviate the QT interval for the treatment of the long-QT syndrome and was also proposed as a way to reverse the downregulation of potassium channels in cardiomyocytes isolated from failing hearts.

Finally, arrhythmias resulting from reentry could potentially be treated by genetic production of local conduction blocks to interrupt the reentry circuits. Genetically engineered fibroblasts, transfected to express the voltage-gated potassium channel Kv1.3, have been demonstrated to significantly alter the electrophysiological properties of the cardiomyocyte cultures. These changes were manifested by a significant reduction in the local extracellular signal amplitude and by the appearance of multiple local conduction blocks. The ability of these cells to cause conduction block may be used to facilitate ablations in the EP laboratory, reducing or even eliminating the need for cauterization and extensive tissue injury, thereby reducing procedure-related complications.

Modification of the AVN through gene or cell therapy is another innovative way to treat AF with rapid ventricular response. A study used viral gene transfer through catheter injection in the AV nodal artery to overexpress Gαi2 in swine AVN and was able to suppress baseline AV conduction and slow the heart rate during AF without producing complete heart block in the animals. This approach represents a novel strategy for ventricular rate control for AF, mimicking the effects of beta-adrenergic antagonists. Another study using direct injection of fibroblast into the slow and fast pathways of the AVN have been successfully shown to modify the electrophysiologic activities of the AVN. In this study, dogs injected with fibroblasts, especially those treated with TGF-β1, was able to significantly delay conduction over the AVN without causing AV block when compared to saline controls. This may suggest an alternative cell-based strategy to treat AF with rapid ventricular response.

SUMMARY

Guidelines on the treatment of cardiac arrhythmias continue to evolve and being updated regularly. Although many well-designed clinical trials have provided solid evidences for our clinical practice, the small number of very elderly patients (octogenarians and nonagenarians) participating in clinical trials poses significant limitations on a more specific practice recommendation in the elderly population. Live expectancy is finite; survival is expected to be less in the elderly. Clinical outcomes such as symptoms, quality of life, functional capacity, independent living, and hospitalization should be critically addressed when treating arrhythmias in this fastest growing segment of our population. Genetic and cell-based regenerative therapy for cardiac arrhythmia is evolving as experimental strategy for treatment of bradyarrhythmias through enhancement of pacemaker activity and facilitation of AV conduction or treatment of tachyarrhythmias through suppression of automaticity and/or creation of local conduction block. Multiple proof-of-concept experiments have been successfully conducted in several laboratories and have generated encouraging results. Although no human trials have been conducted to test the efficacy of these experimental therapies, safety and efficacy of cardiac cell therapy overall have already been evaluated in patients with heart failure and myocardial infarction in several clinical trials with overall promising results. Research in this area may provide ultimate cure for aging-associated arrhythmias through genetic reprogramming of the aging process or via cardiac regenerative therapy.

KEY POINTS

- Aging is associated with diffuse changes throughout the heart and conduction system, which predispose older individuals to the development of bradyarrhythmias, conduction disturbances, and supraventricular and ventricular tachyarrhythmias, all of which increase in incidence and prevalence with advancing age.

- The indications for invasive electrophysiological testing are generally similar in younger and older patients.

- The indications for permanent pacing for treatment of bradyarrhythmia are similar in older and younger patients, and more than 80% of permanent pacemakers are placed in patients 65 years of age or older, with sinoatrial dysfunction being the leading indication for pacemaker implantation in this age group.

- Compared with single-chamber ventricular pacing, dual-chamber pacing reduces the risk of AF but does not affect mortality or the risk of stroke.

- The median age for patients with AF is 75 years, and 84% of patients with AF are 65 years or older.

- Age of 75 years or older is a well-recognized risk factor for thromboembolism in patients with AF.

- In asymptomatic or minimally symptomatic patients with AF, a strategy of rate control and anticoagulation is associated with equivalent or better outcomes than a strategy of rhythm control during long-term follow-up.

- In patients with symptomatic AF refractory to pharmacological treatment, various catheter-based ablation procedures, as well as the surgical maze procedure, provide effective control of rate and/or arrhythmia in a high proportion of patients. Ablation of the AVN and permanent pacing for rate control are effective in reducing symptoms in selected elderly patients. Primary AF ablation for rhythm control has shown encouraging short-term outcomes predominantly in younger patients. Randomized trials with sufficient sample size for meaningful clinical outcomes comparing ablative therapy to the gold standard drug therapy are needed for the fast growing elderly population.

- The indications for ICDs and CRT are similar in older and younger patients, as are the benefits in terms of reducing mortality and improving symptoms; however, few data are available on the use of these devices in patients older than 80 years.

- Syncope is a common cause of falls and hospitalizations in older adults, and cardiovascular causes of syncope are more common in elderly than in younger patients; therefore, an evaluation for possible cardiovascular causes is warranted in older patients with unexplained syncope.

- Elderly patients are more prone to polypharmacy, drug interactions, and drug-induced brady- and tachyarrhythmias.

- Emerging research may provide novel gene- and cell-based therapies for arrhythmias in the elderly and ultimately lead to cardiac "rejuvenation."

FURTHER READING

Abraham WT, Fisher WG, Smith AL, et al.; for the Multicenter InSync Randomized Clinical Evaluation (MIRACLE) Study Group. Cardiac resynchronization in chronic heart failure. *N Engl J Med.* 2002;346:1845–1853.

Ammirati F, Colivicchi F, Santini M; for the Syncope Diagnosis and Treatment Study Investigators. Permanent cardiac pacing versus medical treatment for the prevention of recurrent vasovagal syncope: a multicenter, randomized, controlled trial. *Circulation.* 2001;104:52–57.

Bänsch D, Antz M, Boczor S, et al.; for the CAT Investigators. Primary prevention of sudden cardiac death in idiopathic dilated cardiomyopathy: the Cardiomyopathy Trial (CAT). *Circulation.* 2002;105:1453–1458.

Bardy GH, Lee KL, Mark DB, et al. Amiodarone or an implantable cardioverter-defibrillator for congestive heart failure. *N Engl J Med.* 2005;352:225–237.

Bradley DJ, Shen WK. Atrioventricular junction ablation combined with either right ventricular pacing or cardiac resynchronization therapy for atrial fibrillation: The need for large-scale randomized trials. *Heart Rhythm* 2007; 4:224–232.

Bradley DJ, Bradley EA, Baughman KL, et al. Cardiac resynchronization and death from progressive heart failure: a meta-analysis of randomized controlled trials. *JAMA.* 2003;289:730–740.

Brady PA, Shen WK. When is intracardiac electrophysiologic evaluation indicated in the older or very elderly patient? Complications rates and data. *Clin Geriatr Med.* 2002;18:339–360.

Brignole M, Alboni P, Benditt D, et al.; Task Force on Syncope, European Society of Cardiology. Guidelines on management (diagnosis and treatment) of syncope. *Eur Heart J.* 2001;22:1256–1306.

Brignole M, Alboni P, Benditt DG, et al.; Task Force on Syncope, European Society of Cardiology. Guidelines on management (diagnosis and treatment) of syncope – Update 2004. *Eur Heart J.* 2004;25:2054–2072.

Bristow MR, Saxon LA, Boehmer J, et al.; for the Comparison of Medical Therapy, Pacing, and Defibrillation in Heart Failure (COMPANION) Investigators. Cardiac-resynchronization therapy with or without an implantable defibrillator in advanced chronic heart failure. *N Engl J Med.* 2004;350:2140–2150.

Carlsson J, Miketic S, Windeler J, et al.; for the STAF Investigators. Randomized trial of rate-control versus rhythm-control in persistent atrial fibrillation: the Strategies of Treatment of Atrial Fibrillation (STAF) study. *J Am Coll Cardiol.* 2003;41:1690–1696.

Cazeau S, Leclercq C, Lavergne T, et al.; for The Multisite Stimulation in Cardiomyopathies (MUSTIC) Study Investigators. Effects of multisite biventricular pacing in patients with heart failure and intraventricular conduction delay. *N Engl J Med.* 2001;344:873–880.

Cheitlin MD, Gerstenblith G, Hazzard WR, et al. Database Conference January 27–30, 2000, Washington DC: do existing databases answer clinical questions about geriatric cardiovascular disease and stroke?. *Am J Geriatr Cardiol.* 2001;10:207–223.

Chen LY, Gersh BJ, Hodge DO, Wieling W, Hammill SC, Shen WK. Prevalence and clinical outcomes of patients with multiple potential causes of syncope. *Mayo Clin Proc.* 2003;78:414–420.

Connolly SJ, Sheldon R, Roberts RS, Gent M. The North American Vasovagal Pacemaker Study (VPS): a randomized trial of permanent cardiac pacing for the prevention of vasovagal syncope. *J Am Coll Cardiol.* 1999;33:16–20.

Connolly SJ, Sheldon R, Thorpe KE, et al.; for the VPS II Investigators. Pacemaker therapy for prevention of syncope in patients with recurrent severe vasovagal syncope: second vasovagal pacemaker study (VPS II): a randomized trial. *JAMA.* 2003;289:2224–2229.

Ginsberg G, Hattis D, Russ A, Sonawane B. Pharmacokinetic and pharmacodynamic factors that can affect sensitivity to neurotoxic sequelae in elderly individuals. *Environ Health Perspect.* 2005;113:1243–1249.

Hohnloser SH, Kuck K-H, Lilienthal J. Rhythm or rate control in atrial fibrillation: Pharmacological Intervention in Atrial Fibrillation (PIAF): a randomised trial. *Lancet.* 2000;356:1789–1794.

Jahangir A, Bradley DJ, Shen WK. ICDs for secondary prevention of sudden death in the older-elderly. *Eur Heart J.* 2007. doi:10.1093/eurheartj/ehl549.

Kadish A, Dyer A, Daubert JP, et al.; for the Defibrillators in Non-Ischemic Cardiomyopathy Treatment Evaluation (DEFINITE) Investigators. Prophylactic defibrillator implantation in patients with nonischemic dilated cardiomyopathy. *N Engl J Med.* 2004;350:2151–2158.

Lakatta EG. Age-associated cardiovascular changes in health: impact on cardiovascular disease in older persons. *Heart Failure Rev.* 2002;7(1):29–49.

Miake J, Marban E, Nuss HB. Gene therapy: biological pacemaker created by gene transfer. *Nature*. 2002;419:132–133.

Moss AJ, Zareba W, Hall WJ, et al.; for the Multicenter Automatic Defibrillator Implantation Trial II Investigators. Prophylactic implantation of a defibrillator in patients with myocardial infarction and reduced ejection fraction. *N Engl J Med*. 2002;346:877–883.

Ozcan C, Jahangir A, Friedman PA, et al. Long-term survival after ablation of the atrioventricular node and implantation of a permanent pacemaker in patients with atrial fibrillation. *N Engl J Med*. 2001;344:1043–1051.

Plotnikov AN, Shlapakova IN, Szabolcs MJ, et al. Adult human mesenchymal stem cells carrying HCN2 gene perform biological pacemaker function with no overt rejection for 6 weeks in canine heart. *Circulation*. 2005;112:II221.

Schwartz JB. Clinical pharmacology. In: Gerstenblith, ed. *Cardiovascular Disease in the Elderly*. Chapter 14. Totowa, NJ: Human Press. 2005;335–362.

Strickberger SA, Hummel JD, Bartlett TG, et al.; for the AMIOVIRT Investigators. Amiodarone versus implantable cardioverter-defibrillator: randomized trial in patients with nonischemic dilated cardiomyopathy and asymptomatic nonsustained ventricular tachycardia: AMIOVIRT. *J Am Coll Cardiol*. 2003;41:1707–1712.

Sutton R, Brignole M, Menozzi C, et al.; for the Vasovagal Syncope International Study (VASIS) Investigators. Dual-chamber pacing in the treatment of neurally mediated tilt-positive cardioinhibitory syncope: pacemaker versus no therapy: a multicenter randomized study. *Circulation*. 2000;102:294–299.

The ACTIVE Writing Group on behalf of the ACTIVE Investigators. Clopidogrel plus aspirin versus oral anticoagulation for atrial fibrillation in the Atrial fibrillation Clopidogrel Trial with Irbesartan for prevention of Vascular Events (ACTIVE W): a randomized controlled trial. *Lancet*. 2006;367:1903–1912.

The DAVID Trial Investigators. Dual-chamber pacing or ventricular backup pacing in patients with an implantable defibrillator: the Dual Chamber and VVI Implantable Defibrillator (DAVID) Trial. *JAMA*. 2002;288:3115–3123.

Van Gelder IC, Hagens VE, Bosker HA, et al.; for the Rate Control versus Electrical Cardioversion for Persistent Atrial Fibrillation Study Group. A comparison of rate control and rhythm control in patients with recurrent persistent atrial fibrillation. *N Engl J Med*. 2002;347:1834–1840.

Vliestra RE, Jahangir A, Shen WK. Choice of pacemakers in patients age 75 and older: VVI versus DDD. *Am J Geriatr Cardiol*. 2005;14:35–38.

Wyse DG, Waldo AL, DiMarco JP, et al.; for the Atrial Fibrillation Follow-up Investigation of Rhythm Management (AFFIRM) Investigators. A comparison of rate control and rhythm control in patients with atrial fibrillation. *N Engl J Med*. 2002;347:1825–1833.

Yankelson L, Gepstein L. From gene therapy and stem cells to clinical electrophysiology. *Pacing Clin Electrophysiol*. 2006;29:996–1005.

Peripheral Vascular Disease

Andrew W. Gardner ■ *John D. Sorkin* ■ *Azhar Afaq*

DEFINITION

Atherosclerotic cardiovascular disease is the most significant health problem in the United States, as heart and cerebrovascular diseases are leading causes of mortality and peripheral vascular disease is a leading cause of morbidity in elderly people. Peripheral arterial disease (PAD) is the most typical form of peripheral vascular disease. PAD is characterized by a partial or complete failure of the arterial system to deliver oxygenated blood to peripheral tissue. Atherosclerosis is, by far, the most common etiology of PAD. However, several other processes can lead to the clinical syndrome (Table 80-1). Although lesions (and symptoms) of PAD can occur in both the upper and the lower extremities, these are much more common in the lower extremity, which is the focus of this chapter.

EPIDEMIOLOGY

The ankle–brachial blood pressure index (ABI), defined as the systolic blood pressure measured at the ankle divided by the systolic blood pressure measured in the arm during supine rest, is the most widely used quantitative measure to identify subjects with PAD and to determine PAD severity. The ABI varies widely in the general population and is generally normally distributed with a long tail of low values (Figure 80-1). The prevalence of PAD is highly dependent on the exact ABI cutpoint used to detect inadequate peripheral circulation. The definition of an abnormal ABI has ranged between <0.80 and <0.97, with a value of ≤0.90 generally considered to be the best reference standard.

The prevalence of PAD is 16% in the general population older than 55 years of age when an ABI value of ≤0.90 and symptoms of intermittent claudication and rest pain are used as criteria of PAD. In the Edinburgh Artery Study, approximately 20% of the men and women aged 55 to 74 years were noted to have an ABI ≤0.90 and, thus, were diagnosed as having PAD. The prevalence of PAD increases with age and at all ages is higher in men than in women. At ages 65 to 69 years, the prevalence of PAD in men from the Cardiovascular Health Study was approximately 7%, and approximately 5% in women. In subjects aged 85 years and older, the prevalence was 23% in men and 21% in women.

PAD and coronary artery disease (CAD) share risk factors. In addition to age and male sex, risk factors for PAD include smoking, hypercholesterolemia, diabetes, hypertension, hyperhomocystinemia, elevated fibrinogen concentration, having a family history of premature atherosclerosis (suggesting that genetic factors may influence the development of PAD), and being nonwhite. Although PAD can be seen in the absence of clinical CAD, asymptomatic CAD is frequently present in patients with PAD. Every patient presenting with PAD should be considered to have CAD until proven otherwise. Evaluation and treatment for PAD should include evaluation and control of CAD risk factors.

PAD has important implications for function. PAD severity (assessed by ABI) is directly related to 6-minute walk distance, free-living energy expenditure, and steps taken per day. Of particular interest to geriatricians, patients with PAD are more likely to fall than are subjects without PAD.

PAD is not a static disease. Progression from intermittent claudication to rest pain or gangrene can occur in anywhere from 2% to 7% of patients per year. Furthermore, PAD is associated with increased risk for mortality, and this risk becomes greater as the severity of PAD increases (Figure 80-2).

Patients with PAD are at increased risk of coronary heart disease, coronary vascular disease, and all-cause mortality. This risk is independent of traditional risk factors, including age, sex, smoking, systolic blood pressure, plasma lipids, fasting glucose, body mass index, and preexisting clinical cardiovascular disease. Risk for mortality as a consequence of coronary heart disease and cardiovascular disease is three to six times higher in subjects with PAD than in subjects without PAD, even after accounting for traditional risk factors.

TABLE 80-1

Causes of Peripheral Arterial Disease

Atherosclerosis	Arterial entrapment
Thrombus	Adventitial cyst
Embolism	Fibromuscular dysplasia
Dissection	Trauma
Vasculitis	Vasospasm

PATHOPHYSIOLOGY

The atherosclerotic lesions that lead to PAD tend to form in a few well-defined locations in the vascular tree, and patients often will have lesions in more than one location. Thirty percent of the patients have lesions in the abdominal aorta, 80% to 90% have lesions in the femoral and popliteal arteries, and 40% to 50% have lesions in the tibial and peroneal arteries. The location of the arterial lesion will determine the clinical presentation. For example, aortoiliac disease (Leriche syndrome) leads to buttock, hip, and thigh pain along with erectile dysfunction; the more common femoral–popliteal disease leads to symptoms in the calf. The atherosclerotic process is similar to that in other major arteriostenoses and is discussed in Chapter 75.

PRESENTATION

Clinical PAD was recognized as early as 1831, when Jean-Francois Bouley Jeune observed a horse that, when pulling a cabriolet, limped with the hind legs. At autopsy, the horse was noted to have a partially thrombosed aneurysm of the abdominal aorta and occlusion of both femoral arteries.

Two schemes, both based on symptoms and clinical measures, are commonly used to classify the severity of PAD (Tables 80-2 and 80-3). In the early stages of PAD, the reduction in blood flow

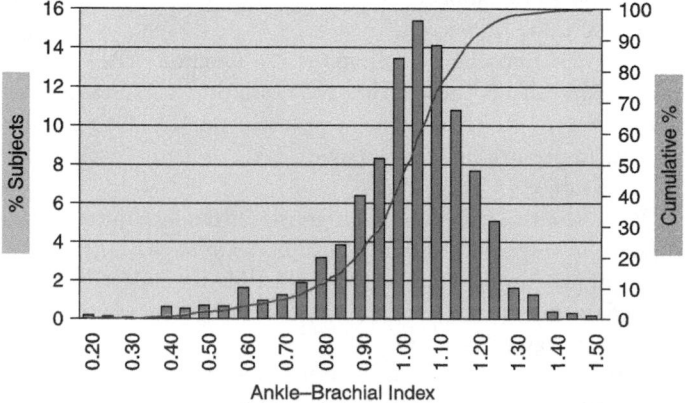

FIGURE 80-1. Ankle–brachial blood pressure index (ABI) in men and women in the Edinburgh Artery study. The bars and left-hand scale represent the percentage of subjects having a given ABI. The solid line and right-hand scale represent the cumulative percentage of subjects having an ABI at or below the ABIs listed on the abscissa. (Adapted from Fowkes FG. Epidemiological research on peripheral vascular disease. J Clin Epidemiol. 2001;54:863.)

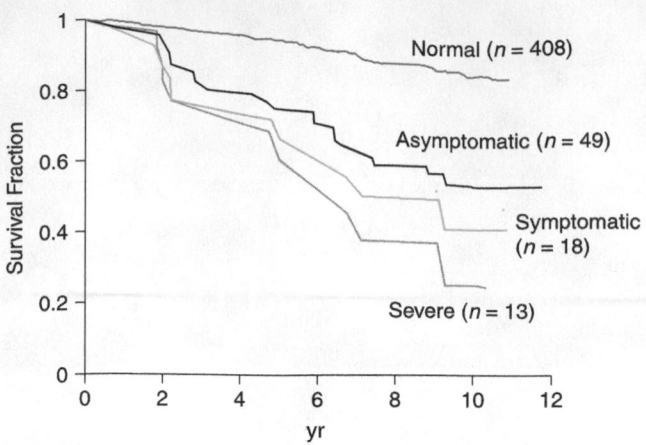

FIGURE 80-2. Relation of peripheral arterial disease (PAD) severity to mortality in subjects from Rancho Bernardo. (Adapted from Criqui MH, et al. Mortality over a period of 10 years in patients with peripheral arterial disease. N Engl J Med. 1992;326:381.)

and ABI does not result in any noticeable symptoms (asymptomatic PAD) and is defined as stage I according to the Fontaine classification system and grade I, category 0 according to the more widely accepted Rutherford classification system. As PAD progresses, ischemic pain in the leg musculature occurs when patients walk (intermittent claudication) and is classified as either Fontaine stage II-a or II-b, or Rutherford grade I, category 1, 2, or 3, depending on the walking distance and the change in ABI following walking. In more advanced stages of disease, ABI is reduced to such an extent that pain is experienced even while at rest, classified as either Fontaine stage III or Rutherford grade II, category 4. Further progression of the disease leads to ischemic ulcerations on the lower extremities, gangrene, and tissue loss, classified as either Fontaine stage IV or Rutherford grade II, category 5, or grade III, category 6. Patients in these categories have critical limb-threatening ischemia in which the ischemia endangers part or all of the lower extremity. These patients are candidates for aggressive limb salvage interventions such as percutaneous transluminal angioplasty or bypass surgery.

The presentation of PAD varies widely among patients. PAD can be present without any clinical signs, in which case diagnosis of PAD can only be made with laboratory tests. With mild disease, the peripheral pulses can be decreased. With more advanced disease, there may be an audible bruit or the distal pulses may be absent. The extremity may be pale or cyanotic at rest, upon raising the leg, or with exercise. The skin of the extremity can be cool, smooth and shiny with hair loss, and thickened nails. Dangling the legs following elevating the extremity can lead to delayed return of color to the skin (usual time approximately 10 seconds), delayed filling of the veins of the feet and ankles (normal approximately 15 seconds), and the development of a dusky rubor in the legs. Patients with the most severe disease will present with ulcers on their extremity or frank gangrene.

The patient may complain of a sensation of cold or numbness in the foot or toes. Patients with more severe disease will often complain of pain when the extremity is at rest. This pain will often occur at night and will be relieved by dangling the leg over the edge of the bed.

TABLE 80-2

Fontaine Classification of Peripheral Arterial Disease

STAGE	SYMPTOMS
I	Asymptomatic
II	Intermittent claudication
IIa	Pain free, claudication walking >200 m
IIb	Pain free, claudication walking <200 m
III	Rest/nocturnal pain
IV	Necrosis/gangrene

Adapted from Pentecost MJ, et al. Guidelines for peripheral percutaneous transluminal angioplasty of the abdominal aorta and lower extremity vessels. A statement for health professionals from a special writing group of the Councils on Cardiovascular Radiology, Arteriosclerosis, Cardio-Thoracic and Vascular Surgery, Clinical Cardiology, and Epidemiology and Prevention, The American Heart Association, Circulation 89(1):511–531, 1994.

EVALUATION

Pulse Palpation and San Diego Claudication Questionnaire

A number of noninvasive tests have been used to screen for and to evaluate the extent of a patient's PAD. The most basic clinical test is palpation and auscultation of the peripheral pulses. Little is known about the sensitivity of pulse palpation for the diagnosis of PAD. In situations in which direct examination of subjects is not feasible, such as epidemiological studies, the San Diego Claudication Questionnaire, which is a version of the Rose Questionnaire, is often used to screen subjects for PAD. Using these questionnaires, PAD is defined as leg pain associated with walking that goes away with rest. The sensitivity of the Rose Questionnaire has been reported as being anywhere from 10% to 50%.

Noninvasive Vascular Tests

The most common measure to assess the presence and severity of PAD is the ABI. PAD is typically defined by an ABI value ≤0.90. The sensitivity of using this cutpoint of ABI is >90%. Generally, a

TABLE 80-3

Rutherford Classification of Peripheral Arterial Disease

GRADE	CATEGORY	CLINICAL DESCRIPTION
I	0	Asymptomatic; not hemodynamically correct
	1	Mild claudication
	2	Moderate claudication
	3	Severe claudication
II	4	Ischemic rest pain
	5	Minor tissue loss; nonhealing ulcer, focal gangrene with diffuse pedal ischemia
III	6	Major tissue loss extending above transmetatarsal level; foot no longer salvageable

Adapted from Rutherford RB. Standards for evaluating results of interventional therapy for peripheral vascular disease. Circulation. 1991;83(suppl 2):16.

patient whose ABI is <0.8 will be symptomatic with intermittent claudication during exercise, and a patient whose ABI is <0.30 will generally complain of pain at rest. Very high ABIs, for example >1.3, are considered invalid because these do not reflect the true ankle blood pressure caused by arteries that have become calcified or noncompressible, termed calcific medial sclerosis, which is observed in patients with diabetes.

Segmental systolic blood pressure measures in the brachial, upper thigh, lower thigh, and ankle locations have been used to access the extent of PAD. Additional noninvasive tests for PAD include Doppler ultrasonography (i.e., measurement of blood flow velocity), plethysmography (pressure-wave tracing), and measurement of postocclusive reactive hyperemia. Postocclusive reactive hyperemia is performed by occluding arterial flow by inflating a blood pressure cuff above systolic pressure at the level of the upper thigh or knee for 3 minutes, followed by measurement of the systolic blood pressure at the ankle or calf blood flow 15 to 30 seconds after releasing the occlusion. When compared to patients without vascular disease, patients with PAD will demonstrate a lower postocclusive ABI and a delayed return to preocclusion pressures. The sensitivity of the postocclusive ABI is >95%. For individuals who present with classic claudication and who have ABI values in the borderline-to-normal range (0.91–1.30), or who have ABI values above normal (greater than 1.30), alternative diagnostic strategies should be used to confirm the diagnosis of lower extremity PAD. These alternative methods include the toe–brachial index, ABI after treadmill exercise, segmental systolic blood pressures, or duplex ultrasound.

Treadmill Testing

The main effect that PAD has on acute exercise is the development of claudication pain in the leg musculature as a result of insufficient blood flow. As a result, claudication and peripheral hemodynamic measurements obtained from a treadmill test are the primary criteria to assess the effectiveness of an exercise program. The specific claudication variables that are measured to assess the functional severity of PAD include the distances (or times) to onset and to maximal claudication pain. ABI measurements obtained before and after the treadmill test, in addition to claudication measurements, provide a more objective assessment of disease severity.

The primary objective of a treadmill test for patients with PAD is to obtain reliable measures of (1) the rate of claudication pain development, (2) the ABI response to exercise, and (3) the presence of coexisting coronary heart disease. The test should be a progressive test with gradual increments in grade. By having a test with small increases in exercise intensity, claudication distances of patients can be stratified according to disease severity. A highly reliable treadmill tests for patients with PAD uses a constant walking speed of 2 mph and gradual increases in grade of 2% every 2 minutes beginning at 0% grade. By using this treadmill protocol, typical distances to onset of pain and to maximal pain are approximately 170 m (3 minutes) and 360 m (6.5 minutes), respectively. Measurement of the ABI immediately after a treadmill exercise stress test can help diagnose PAD in difficult cases as well as determine the extent of impairment of the peripheral circulation. Exercise increases systemic blood pressure (i.e., the brachial pressure), while pressure distal to an arterial lesion in the lower extremity falls with exercise as a consequence of dilation of secondary arterioles. As a result, ABI typically drops from a resting value of 0.6 to approximately 0.2 immediately following the treadmill test. The sensitivity of ABI measured after treadmill walking is >95%.

Gas-exchange measures during the treadmill test show that PAD patients with intermittent claudication have peak oxygen consumption values in the range of 12 to 15 mL/kg/min, which is approximately 50% of age-matched controls. Favorable changes following a program of exercise rehabilitation should include greater walking distances covered before the occurrence of the onset and maximal claudication pain, an increase in peak oxygen consumption, and possibly a blunted drop in ABI and a faster rate of recovery in ABI to the resting baseline value.

Physical Function

Claudication distance and ABI are the most common measurements obtained in patients with claudication, because previous studies have been done from a vascular surgery perspective. However, a more gerontologic perspective would focus on the improvement in function of PAD, for example, in patients following exercise rehabilitation. Because the typical profile of a PAD patient is that of an elderly person with chronic ambulatory disability, the decline in physical functioning with aging may be accelerated in this population because of the extreme deconditioning brought about from the disease process. Consequently, performance on a 6-minute walk test, as well as measures of gait, walking economy (i.e., efficiency), balance, flexibility, lower extremity strength, and health-related quality of life, may be expected to be worse in PAD patients than in age-matched controls, but should improve after a program of exercise rehabilitation. However, little information is available on these measures in the PAD population.

MANAGEMENT

Risk Factor Modification

All patients with PAD need aggressive risk factor modification including cessation of cigarette smoking, control of diabetes, hypertension, and hypercholesterolemia along with dietary restrictions aimed at reducing cholesterol and obesity.

Smoking Cessation

Smoking is strongly associated with development of PAD. Smokers do worse in exercise performance compared to PAD patients who are nonsmokers. Similarly, walking distance has shown to be improved after smoking cessation. Smoking cessation slows the progression to more serious critical limb ischemia, reduces the need for revascularization, and improves graft patency in case of revascularization. As a result of these benefits, it is imperative that these patients should be referred to a smoking cessation program coupled with nicotine replacement therapy.

Hypercholesterolemia

Statins should be prescribed to all patients with PAD irrespective of whether CAD is also present or not. In a meta-analysis of more than 90,000 individuals, statin therapy reduced the 5-year incidence of major vascular events by approximately one-fifth per 1 mmol/L reduction in low-density lipoprotein concentration. This was irrespective of initial lipid profile or other characteristics, such as age, sex, or existing disease. Current PAD guidelines recommend target low-density lipoprotein concentration to be <100 mg/dL in all PAD patients, with an additional target of <70 mg/dL in patients with very high risk of ischemic events.

Hypertension

Control of hypertension is critical for prevention of stroke, myocardial infarction, and congestive heart failure. Antihypertensive therapy may decrease limb perfusion pressure and potentially exacerbate symptoms of claudication or chronic limb ischemia. However, most patients are able to tolerate therapy without worsening of symptoms. Furthermore, contrary to prior belief, β-blockers do not worsen intermittent claudication in PAD patients. Current PAD guidelines recommend using ACE inhibitors in symptomatic PAD patients based on the Heart Outcomes Prevention Evaluation study, where ramipril reduced the risk of myocardial infarction, stroke, or vascular death in patients with PAD by approximately 25%.

Diabetes

Diabetes is a strong risk factor for the development of PAD and is present in up to 20% of patients with PAD. Diabetic patients are prone to complications from severe PAD including critical limb ischemia, foot ulceration, and amputation. Thus, an annual comprehensive foot examination that includes palpation of pedal pulses and the use of a monofilament at specific sites to detect loss of sensation in the foot is recommended to identify risk factors predictive of ulcers and amputation. It is also recommended to control blood sugars with target HbA1C level <7% to reduce microvascular complications and potentially improve cardiovascular outcomes. Standard treatment in a diabetic patient who has PAD includes antithrombotic medication like aspirin, a statin, and an ACE inhibitor along with the usual oral hypoglycemic medications.

Antiplatelet and Anticoagulation Therapy

Aspirin is effective in preventing secondary events in patients with PAD, including delaying the rate of progression and decreasing the need of peripheral arterial procedures. Aspirin therapy does not improve walking distance or symptoms and, therefore, is not currently recommended for symptoms of patients with PAD. Clopidogrel is a useful alternative among patients intolerant of aspirin or can also be considered as the initial choice for patients with PAD. To date, there is no evidence to support the efficacy of combined aspirin and clopidogrel treatment versus a single antiplatelet agent in patients with lower extremity PAD. This combination is being used in patients who had endovascular intervention with a resultant stent placement in lower extremity vasculature.

Oral anticoagulation therapy with warfarin is not indicated to reduce the risk of adverse cardiovascular ischemic events in individuals with atherosclerotic lower extremity PAD.

Vasodilators

In addition to exercise rehabilitation, pharmacological intervention is another medical option to treat intermittent claudication. Pharmacological therapy for intermittent claudication in the United States is limited to pentoxifylline and cilostazol. Pentoxifylline, which has a hemorheologic effect by improving the flexibility of red blood cell membranes and by reducing platelet aggregation, was first studied in the United States in 1982. It was found to increase the distance to onset of claudication pain by 45% and the distance to maximal pain by 32% following 24 weeks of treatment, compared to 23% and 20% increases with placebo. Although this initial study demonstrated the efficacy of pentoxifylline, its usefulness in treating intermittent claudication has been questioned. Cilostazol is a newer medication with more potent vasodilatory and antiplatelet activity than aspirin. Cilostazol was found to increase the distances to onset and to maximal claudication pain by 40% and 42%, respectively, compared to 1% and -14% with placebo treatment. These studies suggest that pharmacological intervention may be used to treat intermittent claudication in some patients. However, exercise rehabilitation results in greater increases in walking distances in patients who are capable and motivated to walk on a regular basis.

Revascularization Therapy

Patients with lifestyle limiting claudication can be considered for revascularization with endovascular or surgical therapy. Endovascular intervention is recommended in case of failure of pharmacological or exercise therapy and or favorable risk–benefit ratio per 2005 ACC/AHA PAD guidelines. Endovascular interventions include percutaneous transluminal angioplasty, stenting, stent grafting, atherectomy, and cryotherapy. Initially percutaneous transluminal angioplasty and stenting were thought to be procedures of choice for shorter, more focal stenosis, whereas longer occlusions were thought to require surgical therapy. However, with improvement in endovascular techniques and experience, more complex procedures involving longer infrainguinal lesions are now being treated by endovascular intervention.

The indications for surgical treatment are the same as those for endovascular treatment. Comparable efficacy can often be achieved, with less risk imposed by endovascular intervention when both procedures are feasible. Choosing between endovascular versus surgical therapy depends on several factors including age, comorbidities, and type of the lesion (TransAtlantic Inter-Society Consensus [TASC] lesion classification). Surgery is usually reserved for individuals who have limb arterial anatomy that is favorable to obtaining a durable clinical result, and in whom the cardiovascular risk of surgical revascularization is low.

Effects of Exercise Rehabilitation

In contrast to either drug treatment or surgical procedures, the clinical management of intermittent claudication in patients with PAD can be significantly improved with little cost, morbidity, and mortality through physical conditioning. Significant improvements in claudication pain have occurred following exercise rehabilitation. For example, meta-analysis demonstrated that, in 21 exercise rehabilitation studies conducted between 1966 and 1993, the average distance walked on a treadmill to onset of claudication pain increased 179%, from a mean of 126 to 351 m following rehabilitation, and the average distance walked to maximal claudication pain increased 122%, from 326 to 723 m.

Numerous mechanisms have been proposed to explain the improvement in walking distances to the onset and to maximal claudication pain following exercise rehabilitation. The mechanisms primarily center on hemodynamic and enzymatic adaptations within the exercising musculature of the symptomatic leg(s). These mechanisms include an increase in blood flow to the exercising leg musculature, a more favorable redistribution of blood flow, greater use of oxygen because of a higher concentration of oxidative enzymes, improvement in hemorheologic properties of the blood, a decrease in the reliance upon anaerobic metabolism, and an improvement in the efficiency of walking. It is likely that a combination of changes in these factors contribute to the improved walking distances. Improvements in psychosocial attitude owing to accomplishments that are achieved during exercise rehabilitation may further enhance this effect.

Although substantial increases in the average distances to onset and to maximal claudication pain during treadmill walking have been noted following exercise, considerable variability among the studies exists; for example, the increased distance to onset of pain ranges between 73% and 746%, and the increased distance to maximal pain ranges between 61% and 765%. Differences in the components of exercise programs (e.g., intensity, duration, and frequency of exercise sessions) may largely account for these widely divergent responses.

To examine the contributions of the components of an exercise rehabilitation program, a meta-analysis was carried out. As displayed in Table 80-4, six components were examined: (1) duration of exercise (minutes per session), (2) frequency of exercise (sessions per week), (3) length of the program (weeks), (4) claudication pain end point used in the program (onset vs. near maximal pain), (5) mode of exercise (walking vs. a combination of exercises), and (6) level of supervision. All of the exercise rehabilitation components had a significant effect on the magnitude of change in the claudication distances except for the level of supervision. For example, programs that exercised patients to near-maximal claudication pain were more effective than programs that exercised patients to only the onset of pain. Additionally, programs consisting of higher exercise duration, higher frequency, greater program length, and walking as the only mode of exercise were more effective than programs consisting of lower exercise duration, lower frequency, and shorter program length, and having patients train by a variety of exercise modes. The addition of home exercise to supplement the amount of exercise performed in a supervised setting did not result in additional ambulatory benefit. Of the five components that had an effect on the change in the claudication distances, only three were found to have an independent effect through multivariate analyses. These components were the claudication pain end point used in the program, the length of the program, and the mode of exercise. The combination of these components explained nearly 90% of the variance in the increase in the walking distances following exercise rehabilitation.

Recommended Exercise Program for Treating Intermittent Claudication

Optimal improvements in claudication symptoms are elicited by having patients walk intermittently beyond the onset of pain for as long as they can safely tolerate and perform this exercise program for a minimum of 6 months. Although the duration and frequency of the exercise sessions are not independent predictors of the change in claudication pain times, patients should walk for at least 30 minutes per session and for at least three sessions per week, as these amounts

TABLE 80-4

The Effects of Exercise Program Components on Changes in Claudication Pain Distances from 21 Studies

COMPONENTS OF EXERCISE PROGRAMS	CHANGE IN THE DISTANCE TO ONSET OF PAIN (m)*	CHANGE IN THE DISTANCE TO MAXIMAL PAIN (m)*
Exercise duration		
≤30 minute/session (n = 8)	143 ± 163[†]	144 ± 419[‡]
>30 minute/session (n = 6)	314 ± 172[†]	653 ± 364[‡]
Exercise frequency		
<3 sessions/week (n = 7)	178 ± 130[†]	249 ± 349[†]
≥3 sessions/week (n = 11)	271 ± 221[†]	541 ± 263[†]
Length of program		
<26 weeks (n = 10)	132 ± 159[‡]	275 ± 228[‡]
≥26 weeks (n = 11)	346 ± 162[‡]	518 ± 409[‡]
Claudication pain end point used during training sessions		
Onset of pain (n = 15)	105 ± 91[‡]	195 ± 78[‡]
Near-maximal pain (n = 6)	350 ± 246[‡]	607 ± 427[‡]
Mode of exercise		
Walking (n = 6)	294 ± 290[†]	512 ± 483[†]
Combination of exercises (n = 15)	152 ± 158[†]	287 ± 127[†]
Level of supervision		
Supervised (n = 11)	238 ± 120	449 ± 292
Combination of home and supervised (n = 8)	208 ± 198	339 ± 472

*Values for each component are adjusted means ± standard deviations of the change in the distances to onset and to maximal claudication pain after statistically controlling for the other five exercise programs components.
[†]Significant difference between groups (P ≤ 0.05).
[‡]P ≤ 0.01.
Adapted from Gardner AW, Poehlman ET. Exercise rehabilitation programs for the treatment of claudication pain: a meta-analysis. JAMA. 1995;274:975.

are more beneficial than programs using a lower exercise duration and frequency. Table 80-5 summarizes recommendations for an exercise program for patients with PAD.

PREVENTION

Risk factors for PAD are typical of those for CAD, including cigarette smoking, race (nonwhite), diabetes, age, systolic blood pressure, body mass index, low-density lipoprotein cholesterol, total cholesterol, creatinine, and forced vital capacity. Thus, efforts at risk factor reduction make sense in trying to prevent PAD or its progression.

In addition, properties of blood rheology and coagulation also play a role in the development of arterial occlusive disease. Increased blood viscosity and red cell aggregation is associated with an increased risk of PAD. Fibrinogen is an independent risk factor for heart disease and stroke, and disorders of fibrinolysis such as increased plasminogen activator inhibitor are associated with ischemic heart disease. Consequently, fibrinogen and plasminogen activator inhibitor may be independent risk factors for PAD. An emerging body of evidence shows a beneficial effect of exercise training in reducing blood viscosity, red cell aggregation, fibrinogen, and increasing fibrinolytic activity both in healthy subjects and in PAD patients.

Thus, exercise training may improve the more traditionally accepted PAD risk factors (e.g., blood lipids, blood pressure, and obesity) as well as measures of blood rheology and coagulation. Finally, because physical activity level is associated with ABI, increasing the activity level may have a preventative role in the development of PAD.

TABLE 80-5

Recommended Exercise Program for Patients with Peripheral Arterial Disease

EXERCISE COMPONENT	COMMENT
Frequency	Three exercise sessions per week
Intensity	Initially, 50% of peak exercise capacity, with gradual progression to 80% by the end of the program
Duration	Initially 15 minute of exercise per session, with gradual progression to 40–50 minute by the end of the program
Mode	Weight bearing (e.g., walking and stair climbing); Non-weight-bearing tasks (e.g., bicycling) may be used for warming up and cooling down
Type of exercise	Intermittent walking to a claudication pain score of 3 using a four-point pain scale
Program length	Approximately 6 months

Data from Gardner AW. Guidelines for developing an exercise program for elderly patients with peripheral arterial occlusive disease. Clin Geriatr. 1995;3:41.

SUMMARY

PAD is a significant health concern in the elderly population, and it will continue to increase in future years. Conservative management of patients with asymptomatic PAD and patients with intermittent claudication is recommended to modify risk factors and improve ambulatory ability, while patients with more severe PAD typically require revascularization of the lower extremities. Exercise rehabilitation is a highly effective, conservative treatment to improve ambulation in patients with intermittent claudication. To date, the primary focus of attention on the benefits of exercise rehabilitation has centered on the increase in walking distances to onset and to maximal claudication pain during a treadmill test. Future research should focus on the improvement in other functional outcomes, which may be more representative of everyday activities such as submaximal exercise performance, walking economy, balance, flexibility, and lower extremity strength. Until these measures are obtained, the full benefit of exercise rehabilitation for PAD patients remains undefined.

FURTHER READING

Criqui MH, et al. Mortality over a period of 10 years in patients with peripheral arterial disease. *N Engl J Med.* 1992;326:381.

Fowkes FG. Epidemiological research on peripheral vascular disease. *J Clin Epidemiol.* 2001;54:863.

Gardner AW, Poehlman ET. Exercise rehabilitation programs for the treatment of claudication pain: a meta-analysis. *JAMA.* 1995;274:975.

Gardner AW, et al. Progressive versus single-stage treadmill tests for evaluation of claudication. *Med Sci Sports Exerc.* 1991;23:402.

Gardner AW, et al. Exercise rehabilitation improves functional outcomes and peripheral circulation in patients with intermittent claudication: a randomized controlled trial. *J Am Geriatr Soc.* 2001;49:755.

Hankey GJ, Norman PE, Eikelboom JW, et al. Medical treatment of peripheral arterial disease. *JAMA.* 2006;295:547.

Hiatt WR, et al. Benefit of exercise conditioning for patients with peripheral arterial disease. *Circulation.* 1990;81:602.

Hiatt WR, et al. Quality of the assessment of primary and secondary endpoints in claudication and critical leg ischemia trials. *Vasc Med.* 2005;10:207.

Hirsch AT, et al. Peripheral arterial disease detection, awareness, and treatment in primary care. *JAMA.* 2001;286:1317.

Hirsch AT, Haskal ZJ, Hertzer NR, et al. ACC/AHA 2005 Practice Guidelines for patients with peripheral arterial disease. *Circulation.* 2006;113(11):e463–e654.

McDermott MM, et al. Leg symptoms in peripheral arterial disease: associated clinical characteristics and functional impairment. *JAMA.* 2001;286:1599.

McKenna M, et al. The ratio of ankle and arm arterial pressure as an independent predictor of mortality. *Atherosclerosis.* 1991;87:119.

Montgomery PS, Gardner AW. The clinical utility of a 6-minute walk test in peripheral arterial occlusive disease patients. *J Am Geriatr Soc.* 1998;46:706.

Norgren L, et al. Inter-Society Consensus for the management of peripheral arterial disease (TASC II). *J Vasc Surg.* 2007;45:S5.

Pentecost MJ, et al. Guidelines for peripheral percutaneous transluminal angioplasty of the abdominal aorta and lower extremity vessels. *Circulation.* 1994;89:511.

Rutherford RB. Standards for evaluating results of interventional therapy for peripheral vascular disease. *Circulation* 1991;83(2 suppl):I6.

Stewart KJ, et al. Exercise training for claudication. *N Engl J Med.* 2002;347:1941.

Weitz JI, et al. Diagnosis and treatment of chronic arterial insufficiency of the lower extremities: a critical review. *Circulation.* 1996;94:3026.

Hypertension

Mark A. Supiano

INTRODUCTION

High blood pressure has the greatest impact on global attributable mortality of any other risk factor and accounts for the third leading cause of global burden of disease—64 million disability adjusted life years lost. The age-associated increase in blood pressure combined with the worldwide demographic increase in the aging population translates to an enormous emerging public health problem. In addition to the well-ascribed hypertension risk factors of cardiovascular disease and stroke, it is also a significant risk for chronic kidney disease, atrial fibrillation, congestive heart failure (CHF, including diastolic dysfunction), and cognitive impairment—each with a relative risk between 2.0 and 4.0. Lowering blood pressure by 10 mm Hg systolic and 5 mm Hg diastolic at age 65 years is associated with a reduction of up to 25% in myocardial infarction, 40% in stroke, 50% in CHF, and 10% to 20% overall decrease in mortality. Despite this knowledge, current rates of hypertension control are extremely low, especially among older women. In addition to illustrating the clinical importance of hypertension, these data are compelling in a call to improve both our knowledge concerning the mechanisms that underlie the age-associated increase in blood pressure to aid in its prevention as well as to make changes in the systems of care necessary to improve blood pressure control among those with hypertension.

EPIDEMIOLOGY

Although high blood pressure should not be construed to be a normal aspect of aging, there is clearly an age-associated increase in blood pressure and in the prevalence of hypertension. The National Health and Nutrition epidemiological surveys have documented that hypertension is a very prevalent condition among older Americans. Based on this study's definition of hypertension—the average of three readings ≥140 mm Hg systolic and/or ≥90 mm Hg diastolic or those receiving an antihypertensive medication—the overall prevalence for hypertension among those aged 65 years or older ranges between 50% and 75%. For women aged 75 years and older, the prevalence exceeds 75%. Of note, there is an age–gender interaction in hypertension prevalence across age. At younger ages, prevalence rates are higher among men while above the age of menopause, there is a crossover when the prevalence in women surpasses that of men.

Another viewpoint on epidemiology is to examine the lifetime risk of developing hypertension as has been done in participants in the Framingham Heart Study. This study identified that among men and women participants who had normal blood pressure readings at age 55 years, nearly 85% developed Stage 1 or higher hypertension over 20 to 25 years of follow-up, their residual lifetime risk.

CLASSIFICATION

The current scheme to classify various levels of hypertension published by the Joint National Committee on Prevention, Detection, Evaluation and Treatment of High Blood Pressure, JNC 7 makes no adjustment for age. This classification scheme incorporates recent evidence that the cardiovascular risks associated with high blood pressure are continuous beginning at a level of 115/75 mm Hg and includes a prehypertension category (systolic from 120 to 139 mm Hg or diastolic 80–89 mm Hg). A former category known as isolated systolic hypertension was deleted from the current classification system. Instead, the conjunction that links the systolic and diastolic blood pressure columns in the classification table that defines each stage of hypertension was changed from "and" to "or." Consequently, since isolated diastolic hypertension is so uncommon among older patients, one may correctly classify an older patient's hypertension based entirely on the level of their systolic blood pressure (i.e. Stage 1, between 140 and 159 mm Hg systolic, and Stage 2, ≥160 mm Hg systolic).

TABLE 81-1

Age-Related Physiological Changes that Contribute to Elevated Blood Pressure

- Arterial stiffness
- Decreased baroreceptor sensitivity
- Increased sympathetic nervous system activity
- Decreased alpha- and beta-adrenergic receptor responsiveness
- Endothelial dysfunction
- Decreased ability to excrete sodium load (sodium sensitivity)
- Low plasma renin activity
- Resistance to insulin's effect on carbohydrate metabolism
- Central adiposity

PATHOPHYSIOLOGICAL CHARACTERISTICS

A single factor is unlikely to explain the cause of essential hypertension regardless of its age of onset. However, a number of age-related changes in physiology have been identified and summarized in Table 81-1 that likely contribute to the age-associated increase in blood pressure and in the prevalence of hypertension. Lifestyle factors such as obesity, especially central adiposity, being sedentary, and eating a diet high in sodium content are also contributors commonly identified among older individuals.

Homeostatic regulation of blood pressure within its normal range while continuously maintaining adequate cerebral perfusion requires intricate and dynamic coordination of several complex interacting physiological systems. Under resting conditions, despite age-related physiological changes that occur in these systems, older individuals experience little difficulty maintaining their blood pressure and cerebral perfusion. However, when this balance is placed at risk by perturbations imposed by the intravascular volume shifts that occur with upright posture or following a meal, or the stimulus of exposure to one or more vasodilating medications, the older patient is less able to adapt and significant declines in blood pressure and inadequate cerebral perfusion may ensue.

Arterial stiffness, especially in the large arteries, is the pathophysiological characteristic that best exemplifies geriatric hypertension. It is directly related to the increase in peripheral vascular resistance, a pathognomonic characteristic of hypertension in the elderly population. In addition to age and body mass index, insulin resistance also appears to be independently related to increased arterial stiffness. The connection between arterial stiffness and the type of hypertension most commonly encountered in older patients, namely, systolic hypertension with high pulse pressure.

Beyond this structural change in the arteries, the regulation of vascular resistance is also affected by age-related changes in the autonomic nervous system and in the vascular endothelium. There is an age-associated decline in the sensitivity of the arterial baroreceptor. This effects the regulation of vascular resistance in two important ways. First, a larger change in blood pressure is required to stimulate the baroreceptor to invoke the appropriate compensatory response in heart rate. This also contributes to the age-related increase in blood pressure variability. Second, the decrease in baroreceptor sensitivity leads to relatively greater activation of sympathetic nervous system outflow for a given level of blood pressure. An age-associated increase in sympathetic nervous system activity has been demonstrated by higher plasma norepinephrine levels, rates of norepinephrine release derived from tracer kinetic studies, and muscle sympathetic nerve activity. If the increased activity of the sympathetic nervous system did not result in a corresponding decrease in adrenergic receptor responsiveness, one would expect a net increase in cardiovascular adrenergic responses. However, many studies have demonstrated age-associated declines in beta-adrenergic receptor chronotropic, inotropic, and vascular responses as well as alpha-adrenergic vasoconstrictor responses. Consequently, in normotensive older individuals, the increase in sympathetic nervous system activity does not lead to an overall increase in vascular tone and appears not to explain an age-related increase in blood pressure. In contrast, in older hypertensive subjects, arterial alpha-adrenergic receptor responsiveness has been shown to be elevated in relation to their high level of sympathetic nervous system activity possibly contributing to their higher blood pressure.

Regulation of vascular resistance by the vascular endothelium is also changed in relation to age. Endothelial dysfunction demonstrated by a decrease in the production of endothelial-derived nitric oxide has been identified to accompany aging as well as hypertension. Impaired nitric oxide–mediated vasodilation is a potential contributor to the age-related increase in peripheral vascular resistance.

Age-related changes in renal function and in particular in renal regulation of sodium balance may also contribute to an increase in blood pressure. Decreased renal blood flow and glomerular filtration rate impair the aging kidney's ability to excrete a sodium load. These renal changes in the regulation of sodium balance create a tendency for sodium retention. This likely plays a part in the finding that a high proportion of older hypertensive individuals, perhaps as high as two-thirds, are characterized as having salt sensitivity. Salt sensitivity is operationally defined as an increase in mean arterial blood pressure, commonly 5 mm Hg or more, during a high compared to a low dietary sodium intake.

Aging also alters the renin–angiotensin–aldosterone system in ways that may contribute both to elevated blood pressure as well as sodium sensitivity. In general, older hypertensive subjects are characterized by having low levels of plasma renin activity. The role of aldosterone as a contributor to elevated blood pressure, aside from overt primary hyperaldosteronism as a secondary cause of hypertension, in the age-related increase in blood pressure is being actively investigated. A direct relationship between plasma aldosterone levels within the physiologic range of normal and the future development of hypertension has been shown in normotensive individuals. Since higher levels of aldosterone have also been linked with central obesity, vascular stiffness, blunting of baroreceptor sensitivity, impaired endothelial function, insulin resistance, and sodium sensitivity, it seems very possible that aldosterone may prove to be a unifying factor that accounts for many of the age-related changes in these physiological features that also contribute to elevated blood pressure.

Abnormalities in glucose homeostasis and, in particular, resistance to insulin's effects on carbohydrate metabolism are evident with aging as well as in hypertension. Insulin resistance has been grouped together with a constellation of other characteristics—obesity, central adiposity (commonly measured as increased waist circumference), hyperlipidemia, and hypertension—referred to as the metabolic syndrome. Studies that have been careful to control for the confounding factors of obesity, central adiposity, physical inactivity, and hypertension demonstrate that age is not independently associated with insulin resistance. Therefore, although many older hypertensive individuals will be insulin resistant, and many may have impaired glucose tolerance if not meet criteria for type 2 diabetes, an isolated age-related change in insulin resistance appears not to directly contribute to elevated blood pressure in aging.

DIAGNOSTIC EVALUATION

Measurement Considerations

The first and most critical step in the diagnostic evaluation of hypertension among older individuals is the accurate measurement of blood pressure. In addition to the standard measurement instructions dictating cuff size and type of instrument, several factors regarding appropriate blood pressure measurement deserve emphasis. First, as a result of the observation that blood pressure is more variable in older people, the dictum that "hypertension should never be diagnosed on the basis of a single blood pressure measurement" is especially true. Studies have documented that there is considerable misdiagnosis of hypertension among older people. For example, up to one-third of subjects who were receiving antihypertensive therapy when they enrolled in the Systolic Hypertension in the Elderly Program failed to meet entry blood pressure criteria for the study after their medications had been withdrawn. The diagnosis of hypertension should be based on the average of a minimum of nine blood pressure readings that have been obtained on three separate visits.

Second, there is a strong association between arterial stiffness and the presence of an auscultatory gap. For this reason, if the blood pressure cuff is initially not inflated to a pressure above the true systolic pressure but falls within the range of the individual's auscultatory gap, the systolic pressure will be underestimated. One may palpate the systolic pressure by recording the pressure at which the radial artery pulse is first appreciated as the cuff is deflated to ensure that the true systolic pressure is obtained.

Third, while not directly related to the diagnostic classification of hypertension, another important factor in blood pressure measurement is to always obtain supine and upright standing readings to determine if there is evidence for an orthostatic or postural decrease in blood pressure. The commonly used definition of postural hypotension is a decrease in systolic blood pressure of 20 mm Hg or more from supine to upright positions within the first several minutes of standing. Elevated supine systolic blood pressure is one of the strongest predictors of postural hypotension. The presence of postural hypotension is an important risk factor for falls and may be exacerbated by almost all antihypertensive medications. Therefore, identifying those patients with postural hypotension at the outset and during therapy is of critical importance.

Fourth, some individuals may have in-office blood pressure readings that are markedly elevated compared with their in-home, self-taken readings, commonly referred to as white coat hypertension. For these individuals, it is worth considering further evaluation with carefully taken home readings using an appropriately calibrated instrument or obtaining 24-hour ambulatory monitoring. The 24-hour blood pressure monitor approach has an added advantage of defining both the daytime and the nocturnal as well as the overall average blood pressure values. The 24-hour average provides a good measure of the blood pressure load and correlates with indicators of target organ damage. The circadian blood pressure pattern may also

be informative in that individuals who fail to decrease their nocturnal blood pressure by at least 10% relative to their daytime blood pressure, referred to as nondippers, have been shown to have greater cardiovascular disease risk compared to those with the normal, dipper pattern.

A final point concerning blood pressure measurement is to emphasize the primacy of systolic over diastolic blood pressure as the pressure that confers the most significance with respect to cardiovascular risk. Moreover, the pulse pressure, the difference between systolic and diastolic pressure, appears to outweigh either systolic or diastolic blood pressure as a cardiovascular risk factor. Based on the pathophysiology of vascular stiffness discussed above, elevations in both systolic and pulse pressure are the expected correlates of increased vascular stiffness.

Evaluation

Similar to younger patients, more than 90% of older hypertensive patients have essential hypertension. A diagnostic evaluation for secondary and potentially reversible causes of hypertension should be completed following the standard guidelines that have been developed for younger patients. There are several factors that deserve special attention in an older patient population. First, since the majority of hypertension among this population is systolic hypertension, older patients who present with primarily diastolic hypertension merit a careful evaluation with a focus on a renovascular cause. This is especially true for those who present with relatively abrupt onset of diastolic hypertension. Second, older patients are apt to be receiving a number of medications, some of which could be contributing to elevated blood pressure. A complete medication review is warranted to search for medications that may be implicated, e.g., corticosteroids and nonsteriodal anti-inflammatory drugs including COX-2 inhibitors. Third, the prevalence of sleep apnea among older patients with hypertension is high and may be an important pathophysiological explanation for their elevated blood pressure. Fourth, although the incidence of pheochromocytoma is rare, there is a suggestion from an autopsy study that the incidence of this condition increases with increasing age.

Target Organ Damage and Risk Factor Assessment

The evaluation should also include a determination of target organ damage and a cardiovascular risk factor assessment and identification of comorbid conditions that may impact antihypertensive drug selection. Determining the extent of hypertension-related target organ damage may be complicated by the confounding effects of concurrent age- or disease-related changes. It is important to assess whether the patient has evidence of renal impairment, proteinuria, hypertensive retinopathy, electrocardiographic abnormalities or left ventricular hypertrophy. An assessment of overall cardiovascular risk—smoking history, alcohol intake, dietary salt and fat intake, and level of physical activity—should also be completed. Older patients presenting with hypertension are likely to have other conditions included among a group of abnormalities described collectively as the metabolic syndrome. Therefore, it is important to consider the coexistence of abdominal obesity; insulin resistance, impaired glucose tolerance, or overt type 2 diabetes mellitus; and hyperlipidemia and incorporate screening for these conditions into the diagnostic evaluation.

APPROACH TO TREATMENT

Treatment Effectiveness

Results from meta-analyses of numerous placebo-controlled randomized clinical trials that have been conducted in older hypertensive patients have confirmed that significant reductions in cardiovascular and cerebrovascular morbidity and mortality occur with antihypertensive therapy and that the treatments are also safe. Active treatment leads on average to a 12% to 25% decrease in the rate of death, a 35% reduction in stroke, and a 25% reduction in myocardial infarction in addition to significant decreases in the development of chronic kidney disease and congestive heart failure. Treatment may also be associated with a decreased rate in the development of dementia. Depending on the individual group's additional cardiovascular risk factors and assuming a 12 mm Hg decrease in systolic blood pressure for 10 years, between 9 (the highest risk group) and 81 (lowest risk group) patients would need to be treated to prevent one death. For these reasons, there is a clear consensus that treating hypertension in older patients is safe and effective.

Therapeutic Goals and Monitoring

In accordance with general geriatric principles, it is important to consider establishing individualized patient treatment goals. The general recommended target (for patients without diabetes or chronic kidney disease) is to decrease systolic blood pressure below 140 mm Hg and diastolic blood pressure below 90 mm Hg utilizing therapies that are least likely to produce adverse side effects or have a negative impact on quality of life. The goal for patients with diabetes or chronic kidney disease is a systolic blood pressure level below 130 mm Hg. Since the major risk factor, along with elevated pulse pressure, is the level of systolic pressure, lowering the systolic blood pressure to these goals without excessively lowering diastolic blood pressure (e.g., below 70 mm Hg) should be the primary therapeutic target.

The most common treatment-related adverse side effect, shared by all antihypertensive medications, is the development of postural hypotension. Patients may present with atypical symptoms such as generalized weakness or fatigue rather than noting postural lightheadedness or dizziness. For this reason, it is important not to treat blood pressure too aggressively and also to always determine supine and upright blood pressure measurements during monitoring of all older patients. If a patient's seated systolic blood pressure cannot be lowered to below 140 mm Hg without the development of postural hypotension, it is prudent to consider modifying that patient's target blood pressure goal to instead focus on their standing blood pressure. This may be more important from an overall perspective to minimize the patient's fall risk.

When patients present with markedly elevated blood pressures in the absence of a true hypertensive emergency (e.g., signs of target organ damage, hypertensive encephalopathy, intracranial hemorrhage, acute heart failure with pulmonary edema, dissecting aortic aneurysm, or unstable angina), it is not necessary and may in fact be harmful to reduce blood pressure to normal values too rapidly. Setting an intermediate treatment goal of 160 mm Hg may be appropriate for these patients. Dosage adjustments or additions of new therapies should be made gradually over time to avoid overtreatment. Similarly, once patients have reached their therapeutic target and have been maintained on stable therapy, their need for continued treatment should be periodically reassessed. Many patients will tolerate a dosage reduction or medication discontinuation, especially if they have been successful in making lifestyle modifications, achieved during a carefully monitored withdrawal period.

Lifestyle Modifications

Based on the physiological profile of the typical older hypertensive patient described in the preceding section—overweight, sedentary, and salt-sensitive—lifestyle modifications directed toward these characteristics would be predicted to be especially efficacious. Additional reasons to focus attention on lifestyle modification are that they will be adjunctive if medications are also needed, will lead to improvements in other cardiovascular risk factors (e.g., lipids), are associated with other salutary outcomes (notably exercise), and are associated with minimal adverse effects. For patients with Stage 1 hypertension (systolic levels between 140 and 160 mm Hg) who do not have diabetes mellitus, a 6-month treatment intervention with appropriate lifestyle modifications is the recommended first step in the treatment algorithm. Randomized controlled trials of multifactorial lifestyle interventions have been conducted and demonstrate the benefit in blood pressure reduction that is achieved as well as sustained in the intervention groups. A meta-analysis of 105 such trails (although few were directed solely to older subjects), demonstrated the overall benefits of weight reduction, aerobic exercise, and decreased intake of sodium and alcohol. Each of these modifications was associated on average with a 5 mm Hg reduction in systolic blood pressure, comparable to the level achieved with a single antihypertensive medication.

The Trial of Nonpharmacologic Intervention in the Elderly (TONE) targeted the effect of dietary sodium restriction and weight loss in older hypertensive patients. In this study, the intervention led to fairly modest declines in dietary sodium intake (average of 40 mmol/day) and body weight (average 4 kg), but there was a 30% decrease in the need to reinitiate antihypertensive therapy among the intervention group.

Pharmacological Therapies

Overview

Currently available evidence supports two general principles with respect to antihypertensive medication selection: one, that the level of blood pressure reduction achieved is more important than which drug is used, and two, that all classes of antihypertensive medications have been demonstrated to be efficacious in older patients. Following these principles, the initial antihypertensive drug selection should be based on patient-specific factors. For example, drug selection will depend on whether the patient's hypertension is simple or complicated by another coexisting condition. The presence of a coexisting condition will often dictate the optimal medication (e.g., an angiotensin converting enzyme [ACE] inhibitor for patients with type 2 diabetes or CHF). Beyond these factors, medications that are least likely to produce adverse effects should receive first priority. For this reason, as a general statement, centrally acting antihypertensive medications and direct vasodilators are best avoided in older

TABLE 81-2

General Treatment Recommendations for Stage 1 Hypertension

- Begin with nonpharmacological lifestyle modifications—weight loss, exercise, salt restriction for 6-month period.
- Focus treatment goal on systolic blood pressure reduction to below 140 mm Hg.
- If target blood pressure is not met, consider low dose thiazide-type diuretic as initial drug selection.
- Base alternative drug selection on individual patient characteristics.
- Consider combination of low doses of one or more agents if goal blood pressure not met with a single drug.
- When initiating drug therapy, begin at half of the usual dose, increase dose slowly, and continue nonpharmacological therapies.
- Aggressive therapy is not appropriate if adverse side effects (e.g., postural hypotension) cannot be avoided.

hypertensive patients due respectively to concerns regarding central nervous system sedating effects and association with marked postural hypotension. In addition, attention should be paid to selecting a once-daily medication to promote adherence and to avoiding any medication interactions with the patient's other medications.

An algorithmic approach to treating hypertension is provided in the JNC 7 report. As noted in the preceding discussion regarding hypertension classification, the category of prehypertension merits emphasis as this category calls attention to its importance as a risk factor and a determinant of future hypertension. Therapeutic recommendations are then stratified on the presence or absence of "compelling indications" such as diabetes, heart failure, and chronic kidney disease. In the absence of these conditions, there are some general recommendations for initial therapy based on the stage or severity of the patient's hypertension. For patients with Stage 1 hypertension in whom a 6-month lifestyle modification intervention strategy has failed to lower blood pressure to the goal level, a thiazide-type diuretic is the most commonly recommended initial medication. General treatment recommendations for Stage 1 hypertension are summarized in Table 81-2. Patients who present with Stage 2 hypertension will almost certainly require at least two drugs to control their blood pressure. Most often one of these two is a thiazide-type diuretic with the second agent selected either on compelling indications or on the basis of synergy with the initial agent (e.g. a thiazide diuretic combined with ACE inhibitor). It should be noted that regardless of the drug choice, the starting dose should be reduced and dosage titration be carried out gradually.

There are three additional general considerations to be made before a brief review of each of the major antihypertensive classes. (1) Beta-receptor antagonists are no longer recommended as an appropriate choice for the initial antihypertensive drug, especially among older patients. In part because of the age-related changes in sympathetic nervous system function discussed previously, older individuals are less responsive to beta-agonist stimulation. Beyond this physiological explanation, results from a meta-analysis concluded that unless there is a compelling indication for their use, beta-blockers should not be considered as a first-line antihypertensive agent in older (60 years and older) patients. Whereas beta-blockers were found to be equally efficacious in younger patient populations, this was not the case among the older population in whom compared with other agents, beta-blocker therapy was associated with an in-creased risk of a composite outcome of death, stroke, or myocardial infarction. (2) Although the algorithm provides overall recommendations, patient-specific factors that directly impact adherence also need to be taken into account. For example, thiazide diuretics are considered to be first-line agents, but persistence rates with their continued use are lower than with angiotensin receptor blockers. As with any prescription, cost, simplicity of the regimen, and absence of side effects are important factors impacting rates of adherence. (3) Especially for Stage 2 patients, currently available data are suggesting that prescribing a fixed and especially low-dose combination capsules may be associated with improved outcomes. Although the concept of a single multiple-medication capsule seems to contradict the general geriatric principle of avoiding polypharmacy, there appear to be benefits to this approach both with respect to improved efficacy and lower rates of side effects. For example, a fixed dose preparation of four antihypertensives (a thiazide diuretic, calcium antagonist, ACE inhibitor, and beta-blocker) each at one-quarter of their usual monotherapy starting dose was superior in blood pressure control to each of the agents administered individually when given at the usual monotherapy dosage. This evidence suggests that it may be preferable to add a second agent in lower dose rather than titrating up the dosage of the first medication if a patient is not at target blood pressure in response to the starting dose of the first agent.

Thiazide-type Diuretics

Table 81-3 summarizes the advantages and disadvantages for each of the major drug classes from the geriatric patient perspective. There are several reasons why thiazide-type diuretics have become the preferred initial antihypertensive agent for most older patients. The primary pathophysiological explanation is that diuretic therapy has been noted to reduce systolic blood pressure to a greater extent than diastolic blood pressure, and also achieves greater reductions in systolic pressure relative to other antihypertensive agents. Moreover, the majority of large-scale randomized controlled trials have utilized a thiazide-type diuretic in the treatment arm and there exist an abundance of outcome data demonstrating their therapeutic effectiveness in older hypertensive populations. Additional benefits include low cost, once daily dosing, and a favorable side effect profile. The most common adverse drug events are metabolic abnormalities, especially hypokalemia, as well as hyperuricemia and impaired glucose intolerance; and urinary frequency or incontinence. These side effects are quite uncommon at lower doses. Thus, 12.5 mg of hydrochlorothiazide or its equivalent is the recommended initial starting dose and since the blood pressure lowering effect plateaus at doses higher than 50 mg, 50 mg is considered to be the maximal dose. Finally, there is good synergy with most of the other commonly used medications, such that adding a second drug if needed to a thiazide-type diuretic is a reasonable approach.

Nonthiazide-type diuretics have been less well studied. Given that hypokalemia is a common side effect of thiazide-type diuretics, and that maintaining normal potassium levels aid in blood pressure control, combination drugs with a thiazide together with a potassium-sparing diuretic (e.g., amiloride or triamterene) have been developed. Owing to the similarities observed between the physiological effects of aldosterone and the age-related contributors to elevated blood pressure listed in Table 81-1, aldosterone receptor blockers (spironolactone or eplerenone) are other alternatives to consider.

TABLE 81-3

Advantages and Disadvantages of Antihypertensive Medication Classes Specific to Older Patients

ANTIHYPERTENSIVE CLASS	POTENTIAL ADVANTAGES	POTENTIAL DISADVANTAGES	CLINICAL SITUATIONS TO RECOMMEND USE	CLINICAL SITUATIONS TO RECOMMEND AGAINST USE, OR WHICH REQUIRE MONITORING
Thiazide-type diuretics	• Documented benefit in clinical trials • Produce greater reduction in systolic than diastolic blood pressure • Improve bone mineral density • Inexpensive	• Metabolic abnormalities (e.g., hypokalemia) • Urinary frequency	• Systolic hypertension	• Hyponatremia • Gout
ACE inhibitors and angiotensin receptor blockers	• Absence of CNS effects • Preservation of renal function • Decrease proteinuria	• Hyperkalemia, cough	• CHF, type 2 diabetes	• Renal insufficiency or renal artery stenosis
Calcium channel antagonists	• Benefit documented in clinical trials • Absence of CNS or metabolic effects	• Peripheral edema, constipation, heart block	• Systolic hypertension • Coronary artery disease	• Left ventricular dysfunction
Beta-adrenergic receptor antagonists	• None. Not recommended as monotherapy	• May increase peripheral vascular resistance • Metabolic abnormalities • CNS effects	• Postmyocardial infarction	• COPD, peripheral vascular disease, heart block, glucose intolerance, type 2 diabetes, hyperlipidemia, depression
Alpha-adrenergic receptor antagonists	• Improve urinary symptoms in BPH	• Increased rate of CHF hospitalizations as monotherapy relative to thiazide-type diuretics	• Prostatism	• Left ventricular dysfunction

ACE, angiotensin converting enzyme; COPD, chronic obstructive pulmonary disease; CHF, congestive heart failure; CNS, central nervous system; BPH, benign prostatic hypertrophy.

Angiotensin Converting Enzyme Inhibitors and Angiotensin Receptor Antagonists

ACE inhibitor agents and angiotensin receptor antagonists are good alternative choices for initial therapy or as second agents in combination with a thiazide-type diuretic. Their advantages include the absence of central nervous system or metabolic side effects and overall favorable side effect profile. They are also often used owing to the recommendations for their use in the setting of coexisting type 2 diabetes or systolic dysfunction. Another consideration favoring the use of these agents is the evidence that their use is associated with preservation of renal function and decreases in proteinuria in several clinical conditions.

Calcium Channel Antagonists

All three chemical classes of calcium channel antagonists have been shown to be effective in treating older hypertensive patients. Their mechanism of action—decreased peripheral vascular resistance—and lack of significant central nervous system or metabolic side effects provide a good match with the characteristics of the geriatric patient. Age-related changes in the pharmacokinetics of these drugs (decreased clearance and increased plasma levels) mean that lower doses need to be used in older patients. The longer acting agents in the dihydropyridine class of calcium channel antagonists have been the most widely studied in randomized controlled trials where their effectiveness in treating older patient populations has been demonstrated.

Adrenergic Receptor Antagonists

As discussed previously, beta-receptor antagonists are not an appropriate choice for monotherapy for older patients with uncomplicated hypertension. Beta-receptor antagonists should be reserved for patients with a compelling indication for their use, namely, as secondary prevention for those patients who have had prior myocardial infarction or in some patients with systolic dysfunction.

Several observations have limited the adoption of alpha$_1$-receptor antagonists as first-line treatment for older hypertensive patients. In addition to their predilection to produce postural hypotension, subjects who received an alpha$_1$-receptor antagonist as monotherapy in the Antihypertensive and Lipid Lowering Treatment to Prevent Heart Attack Trial (ALLHAT) were found to have a twofold higher risk of being hospitalized for CHF relative to the subjects randomized to the diuretic arm of the study. Based on these observations, alpha$_1$-receptor antagonist therapy should be considered for use as monotherapy, only in men in whom their use may be beneficial for symptoms related to benign prostatic hypertrophy, or in combination with another antihypertensive agent.

Barriers to Improving Blood Pressure Control

Since there is no cure for this chronic condition, effective treatment of hypertension requires a lifelong commitment to its management. For this reason, an approach that engages and sustains the patient's motivation and adherence over time is needed. Several methods may be recommended to promote the patient's efforts such as providing patient education materials, clear instructions for diet and exercise lifestyle recommendations, and prescribing once-daily medications to facilitate adherence. Some patients may benefit from the feedback and engagement that accompany home or self-taken blood pressure monitoring, although the effectiveness of this approach has not been proven. Another patient factor is the likelihood that the older hypertensive patient will have two or more additional chronic conditions. The complexity imposed by concurrently managing these comorbid conditions becomes extremely challenging. This is especially the case when treating a frail older individual when it is not clear how to best prioritize which of several guidelines should take precedence or for that matter if the guideline is still applicable to the patient's clinical situation.

In addition to these patient-specific factors, a number of barriers have been identified in the health care system that may impede progress in achieving better success in blood pressure control rates in the older population. The underdetection, undertreatment, and inadequate control of hypertension, especially among older patients, are well documented. Some of these system factors are limited access, lack of a team approach to care, constraints imposed by limited patient visit times, and the reimbursement system. Physician factors—the failure to modify treatment when the patient's target blood pressure goal has not been achieved—also contribute to this situation. Inadequate knowledge of the current guidelines and recommended goals outlined in the JNC 7 is one potential explanation for the failure of physicians to respond appropriately. Results from the TONE study demonstrated for example that there is systematic underutilization of the recommended thiazide-type diuretic among hypertensive patient populations. Moreover, many physicians overestimate their compliance with these standards as well as the proportion of their patient populations who have blood pressure levels below their target. However, solely providing education appears not to be an effective solution to changing physician behavior in this regard. The Assessing Care in the Older Vulnerable Elders (ACOVE) project has demonstrated that hypertension is one of many conditions for which quality indicators are not being met in this patient population. However, some quality improvement strategies have been demonstrated to be effective in improving hypertension management. The most effective strategies in this regard have involved a multidisciplinary team approach (assigning a nonphysician member of the team to assume responsibility for management), home blood pressure monitoring, and patient education. Thus, it appears that incorporating a geriatrics approach to hypertension management in the context of a quality improvement program is one effective way to eliminate some of the barriers to improving hypertension control in older patient populations.

UNANSWERED QUESTIONS AND FUTURE RESEARCH DIRECTIONS

Prior to the completion of the Hypertension in the Very Elderly Trial (HYVET) in 2007, very few subjects aged 80 years or older had been included in the controlled clinical trials of hypertension treatment. The HYVET study recruited 3,845 hypertensive individuals aged 80 years and older and randomized them to receive either active treatment (a diuretic plus an angiotensin-converting enzyme inhibitor if needed) or a placebo and followed outcomes (stroke and mortality rates were the primary outcomes) for 5 years. The HYVET study's Data Safety Monitoring Board ended the study early when an unexpected significant, 21%, reduction in overall mortality in

the active treatment group was identified. In the intention-to-treat analysis, the treatment group also had a 30% reduction in fatal and non-fatal stroke, and a 64% decrease in the rate of congestive heart failure. Moreover, active treatment was associated with fewer adverse events than placebo. While this trial's results clearly demonstrate the beneficial effects of antihypertensive therapy in patients 80 years of age and older, it is important to emphasize that its results cannot be generalized to frail older patients who would not have met the study's entry criteria. For example, the trial excluded those with dementia, who had an inability to walk or who had dementia.

Future research directions should increase our understanding of the mechanisms underlying the age-associated increase in blood pressure, with important implications for prevention and management. For example, it seems clear that understanding the predictors and modifiers of vascular stiffness is of critical importance in preventing the age-associated development of hypertension. Similarly, although none of the currently available antihypertensive agents specifically targets vascular stiffness, future advances in drug development aimed at preventing hypertension will likely address decreasing vascular stiffness as a mechanism of action.

Additional new approaches in antihypertensive therapy may derive from advances in understanding the genetic contributions to hypertension. In addition, improvements in the ability to genetically profile an individual patient based on the unique characteristics of their specific genes related to hypertension may be used in the future to better inform the selection of an appropriate antihypertensive medication. Pharmacogenetics or personalized medicine holds great promise for tailoring drug therapy to the individual patient and also may help to explain some of the racial/ethnic and perhaps age-related differences observed in response to therapy.

Research advances to define the physiological mechanisms for the nondipper effect, i.e., the absence of a nocturnal decrease in blood pressure, may help improve our understanding about this pattern, its implications, and how it may be treated. One intriguing prospect is the extent to which altered sleep patterns, especially sleep apnea, may be linked to the nondipper pattern of blood pressure.

Finally, additional investigation will aim to elucidate why hypertension is a significant risk factor for mixed dementia, the overlap of Alzheimer's and vascular dementia. Based on the results from several studies suggesting that antihypertensive therapy may help to prevent cognitive decline and decrease the incidence rate for dementia, controlling blood pressure may also confer beneficial effects in preserving cognitive function with aging. The interactions between elevated blood pressure, insulin resistance, and other aspects of the metabolic syndrome and cognitive function will be another area for productive future investigation.

SUMMARY

Key points for clinical practice highlighted in this chapter include:

1. Hypertension is not a normal aspect of aging, but its prevalence increases steadily with age. Hypertension is emerging as an extremely important global public health problem. The increasing prevalence of hypertension and its associated morbidity and mortality warrant increased attention to strategies to prevent the age-associated increase in blood pressure.

2. Older people primarily develop systolic hypertension most likely related to an age-related increase in arterial stiffness. Systolic

blood pressure and pulse pressure, both closely associated with arterial stiffness, confer the greatest significance as cardiovascular and cerebrovascular risk factors.

3. Age-related changes in systems that regulate blood pressure result in greater blood pressure variability. This dictates careful attention to accurate measurement and diagnosis of hypertension.

4. Older hypertensive individuals have physiological characteristics that are well suited to respond effectively to lifestyle modifications.

5. The focus of therapy should be on lowering the systolic blood pressure to the patient's target goal. Since the major antihypertensive drug classes have all been demonstrated to be effective in older patient populations, drug selection itself is less important and should take into consideration comorbidities and other patient-specific factors.

6. Thiazide-type diuretic drugs are preferred as the initial drug in most patients. Combination therapy with low doses of one or more agents should be considered if needed to control blood pressure below the target level.

7. Patients should be monitored for adverse drug events, especially postural hypotension, throughout treatment.

8. Current blood pressure control rates are inadequate, especially among the older patient population. Systems approaches that incorporate geriatric approaches to team care combined with quality improvement strategies need to be adopted to improve treatment outcomes.

FURTHER READING

Beckett NS, Peters R, Fletcher AE, et al. Treatment of hypertension in patients 80 years of age or older. *N Engl J Med.* 2008;358:1887–1898.

Chobanian AV, Bakris GL, Black HR, et al. The seventh report of the Joint National Committee on Prevention, Detection, Evaluation, and Treatment of High Blood Pressure: the JNC 7 report. *JAMA.* 2003;289:2560–2572.

Dickinson HO, Mason JM, Nicolson DJ, et al. Lifestyle interventions to reduce raised blood pressure: a systematic review of randomized controlled trials. *J Hypertens.* 2006;24:215–233.

Elliott WJ. Drug interactions and drugs that affect blood pressure. *J Clin Hypertens.* 2006;8:731–737.

Elmer PJ, Obarzanek E, Vollmer WM, et al. Effects of comprehensive lifestyle modification on diet, weight, physical fitness, and blood pressure control: 18-month results of a randomized trial. *Ann Intern Med.* 2006;144:485–495.

Ezzati M, Lopez AD, Rodgers A, et al. Selected major risk factors and global and regional burden of disease. *Lancet.* 2002;360:1347–1360.

Forette. F, Seux ML, Staessen JA, et al. Prevention of dementia in randomised double-blind placebo-controlled Systolic Hypertension in Europe (Syst-Eur) trial. *Lancet.* 1998;352:1347–1351.

Gueyffier F, Bulpitt C, Boissel J-P, et al. Antihypertensive drugs in very old people a subgroup meta-analysis of randomised controlled trials. *Lancet.* 1999;353:793–796.

Khan N, McAlister FA. Re-examining the efficacy of beta-blockers for the treatment of hypertension: a meta-analysis. *CMAJ.* 2006;174:1737–1742.

Langa KM, Foster NL, and Larson EB. Mixed dementia: emerging concepts and therapeutic implications. *JAMA.* 2004;292:2901–2908.

Lloyd-Jones DM, Evans JC, Larson MG, et al. Differential impact of systolic and diastolic blood pressure level on JNC-VI staging. *Hypertension.* 1999;34:381–385.

Lloyd-Jones DM, Evans JC, Levy D. Hypertension in adults across the age spectrum: current outcomes and control in the community. *JAMA.* 2005;294:466–472.

Mahmud A, Feely J. Low-dose quadruple antihypertensive combination: more efficacious than individual agents—a preliminary report. *Hypertension.* 2007;49:272–275.

Ostchega Y, Dillon CF, Hughes JP, et al. Trends in hypertension prevalence, awareness, treatment, and control in older U.S. adults: data from the National Health and Nutrition Examination Survey 1988 to 2004. *J Am Geriatr Soc.* 2007;55:1056–1065.

Sengstock DM, Vaitkevicius PV, Supiano MA. Arterial stiffness is related to insulin resistance in nondiabetic hypertensive older adults. *J Clin Endocrinol Metab.* 2005;90:2823–2827.

Staessen JA, Gasowski JG, Thijs L, et al. Risks of untreated and treated isolated systolic hypertension in the elderly: meta-analysis of outcome trials. *Lancet.* 2000;355:865–872.

Steinman MA, Fischer MA, Shlipak MG, et al. Clinician awareness of adherence to hypertension guidelines. *Am J Med.* 2004;117:747–754.

Supiano MA, Hogikyan RV, Sidani MA, et al. Sympathetic nervous system activity and alpha-adrenergic responsiveness in older hypertensive humans. *Am J Physiol.* 1999;276:E519–E528.

Vasan RS, Beiser A, Seshadri S, et al. Residual lifetime risk for developing hypertension in middle-aged women and men: the Framingham heart study. *JAMA.* 2002;287:1003–1010.

Vasan RS, Evans JC, Larson MG, et al. Serum aldosterone and the incidence of hypertension in nonhypertensive persons. *N Engl J Med.* 2004;351:33–41.

Walsh JM, McDonald KM, Shojania KG, et al. Quality improvement strategies for hypertension management: a systematic review. *Med Care.* 2006;44:646–657.

Whelton PK, Appel LJ, Espeland MA, et al. Sodium reduction and weight loss in the treatment of hypertension in older persons: a randomized controlled trial of nonpharmacologic interventions in the elderly (TONE). *JAMA.* 1998;279:839–846.

Aging of the Respiratory System

Paul L. Enright

INTRODUCTION

This chapter first reviews the changes in lung function with aging that are known to occur in healthy persons (normal, never smokers). Included are the major categories of pulmonary function tests: static lung volumes, maximal expiratory flow, lung mechanics, and gas exchange, plus bronchodilator (BD) response and nonspecific airway reactivity. Table 82-1 summarizes these changes. The chapter then adds a discussion of how lung function tests maybe used by a clinician to assist in the differential diagnosis of asthma and chronic obstructive pulmonary disease (COPD) in an elderly patient, and to objectively measure the efficacy of asthma and COPD therapy (see Chapter 83 for additional information on this topic).

LUNG VOLUMES

Total lung capacity (TLC) is the volume of air within the respiratory system when a subject makes a maximal voluntary inspiratory effort (and the air seen in the lungs on a chest x-ray). It is determined by the balance of forces between the maximally activated inspiratory muscles and the elastic recoil of the lung and chest wall. A decrease in TLC and other static lung volumes is called restriction.

The elastic recoil of lung tissue decreases with aging (just as the skin becomes less elastic), making the lungs easier to expand during a deep breath toward TLC. This reduction of elastic recoil tends to increase TLC; however, the chest wall (rib cage) becomes stiffer with aging, so that a maximal inspiratory effort is not able to achieve a higher lung volume even though the lungs themselves have become easier to expand. Thus, TLC normally remains stable throughout the aging process.

The volume of air remaining in the lungs when subjects have exhaled as much air as possible is called residual volume (RV). Because lung elastic recoil decreases as a consequence of normal aging, the RV and RV/TLC increase from young adulthood to older age. An abnormally high RV/TLC is called hyperinflation, can often be seen on a chest x-ray, and occurs with both asthma and COPD.

Vital capacity (VC) is the difference between the absolute lung volume at TLC and at RV, and the amount of air that a person can slowly exhale after inhaling maximally. Because TLC is relatively constant while RV increases with age, the VC decreases with age. Hutchinson coined the term vital capacity over 150 years ago because it predicted the vigor and length of life of his patients. Many modern epidemiologic studies have verified his observation.

MAXIMAL EXPIRATORY FLOW

Maximal expiratory flow, as seen during spirometry tests, varies as a function of lung volume because higher flows are possible at a higher lung volume. For forced exhalation beginning from a deep inhalation (the first phase of a spirometry maneuver), the initial (peak) flow (phase 2) is determined by the recoil of the lung and chest wall and the degree of effort expended by the patient, as well as by the speed with which the patient's respiratory muscles can generate positive pleural pressure. Once maximal flow is achieved, maximal flow throughout the remainder of the VC (phase 3) is determined by the intrinsic properties of the lung.

SPIROMETRY

Spirometry is the most common test of lung function, and is easily performed by 9 of 10 elderly patients. Modern office spirometers use a flow sensor, connected to a microprocessor that determines the forced expiratory volume in one second (FEV_1), forced vital capacity (FVC), and FEV_1/FVC from the best maneuver, as well as the predicted values. FEV_1 is the most important value, representing the volume of air (in liters) exhaled during the first second. Guidelines for spirometry methods and instrument accuracy are available from the American Thoracic Society.

TABLE 82-1

Effects of Aging on Lung Function

Lower maximal expiratory flows: FEV_1, FEV_1/FVC, FEF 75%
Increased FRC and RV, lower VC, but stable TLC
Lower diffusing capacity (oxygen uptake)
Lower PO_2 and SpO_2 as a consequence of V/Q mismatch (but no change in PCO_2)
Lower respiratory muscle strength and endurance
Stiffer chest wall (less compliant)
Increased lung tissue compliance (loss of lung recoil)
Reduced respiratory drive (for hypoxia, hypercarbia, and resistive loads)
Increased airway reactivity (but no change in bronchodilator responsiveness)

FEF, forced expiratory flow; FEV_1, forced expiratory volume in one second; FRC, functional residual capacity; FVC, forced vital capacity; PCO_2, partial pressure of carbon dioxide; PO_2, partial pressure of oxygen; RV, residual volume; S_pO_2, arterial oxyhemoglobin saturation; TLC, total lung capacity; VC, vital capacity; V/Q, ventilation/perfusion.

The presence of airways obstruction is determined by a low FEV_1/FVC ratio and visualized on the flow–volume ($F-V$) curve as concavity toward the volume axis or tail at the end of the maneuver (Figure 82-1). The descending limb of the $F-V$ curve of healthy young adults is a straight line of about 45 degrees until the end of the maneuver (shaped like a sail), corresponding to exponential emptying of the lungs. The shape of the $F-V$ curve becomes progressively more curvilinear as a healthy adult becomes older, corresponding to decreases in expiratory flows at low lung volumes. The reduced flow at low lung volumes, even in healthy elderly persons, is a result of a decrease in the mean diameter of small airways.

Adults normally experience a loss in FEV_1 of about one-third liter per decade (Figure 82-2). The decline in FEV_1 with aging is greater than the decline in FVC, so that the FEV_1/FVC also declines with age. Values below 0.65 usually indicate airway obstruction in patients aged 65 years and older.

Many nonpulmonary factors contribute to the decline in the FEV_1 in elderly persons (see Table 82-2 for a list). The strongest factors are cigarette smoking; a diagnosis of COPD or asthma; and wheezing symptoms—all of which are known to cause airway obstruction (a low FEV_1/FVC ratio). The inability to take a deep breath (restriction) also reduces the FEV_1, as with obesity, malnutrition, heart disease, and chest wall abnormalities. For a given height, gender, and age, the FVC and FEV_1 of healthy elderly African-Americans is approximately 12% lower than that of healthy elderly white persons, thus spirometry reference equations, which are race/ethnicity-specific (as from the NHANES III study), are used to calculate predicted values. Since spirometry tests require athletic-type breathing maneuvers, poorly trained technologists in outpatient settings often do not obtain maximal patient effort during one or more of the three phases of the maneuver, causing misclassification of the results.

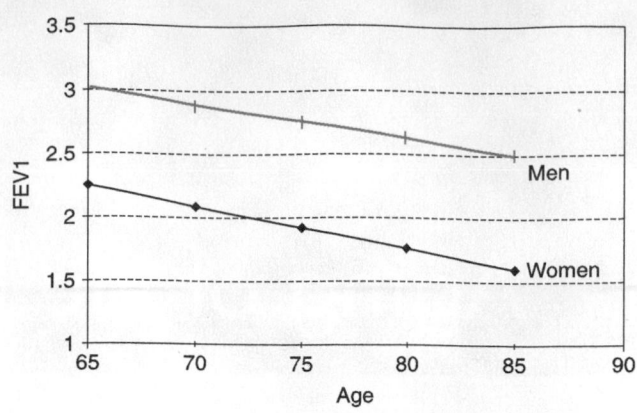

FIGURE 82-2. The FEV_1 normally declines about 30 mL per year with aging, even in healthy men and women without lung disease.

RESPIRATORY MUSCLE STRENGTH

Another vital component of respiratory function is respiratory muscle strength and endurance. Diaphragm strength is approximately 25% lower in healthy elderly persons as compared to young adults. The VC is reduced when the diaphragm is weak and when the expiratory muscles of the abdominal and thoracic wall cannot empty the

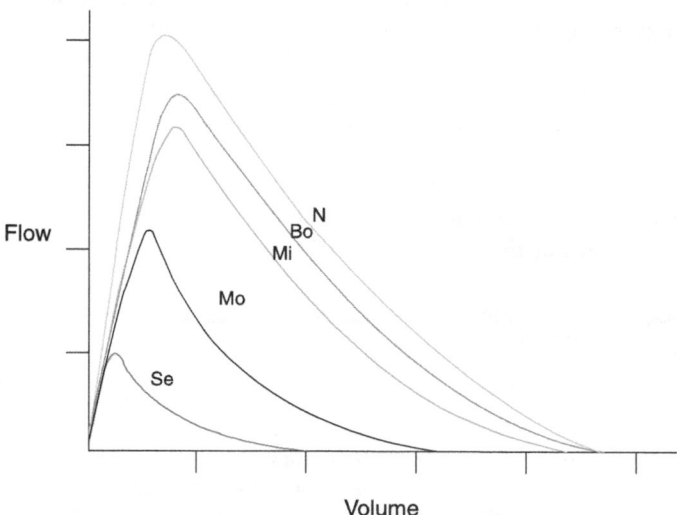

FIGURE 82-1. Flow–volume curves with increasing degrees of obstruction. Bo, borderline obstruction (85% predicted); Mi, mild obstruction (70% predicted); Mo, moderate obstruction (60% predicted); N, normal (100% predicted FEV_1); Se, severe obstruction (35% predicted).

TABLE 82-2

Factors Associated with a Lower FEV_1 in Elderly Individuals

Important factors associated with airway obstruction
Cigarette smoking (current, former, and pack-yrs)
Emphysema or chronic bronchitis (COPD)
A diagnosis of asthma at any time in the past
Wheezing (during or apart from colds, daytime or nighttime)
A history of workplace exposures to dust, fumes, smoke, or chemicals
Other factors associated with restriction of lung volumes
Dyspnea on exertion
Obesity or malnutrition
Hypertension or hypotension
Major ECG abnormality
Pitting ankle edema
Diabetes, on medication
Prior chest surgery

lungs below the resting respiratory position. The load on these respiratory muscles increases with aging, because chest wall compliance decreases.

Diaphragm strength maybe easily and inexpensively measured in the outpatient office. The patient exhales slowly, then makes a maximal attempt to inhale from a mouthpiece connected to a pressure gauge (−200 cm H_2O range, with a small leak) for 2 seconds. The largest pressure from five such maneuvers is reported as the Maximal Inspiratory Pressure (MIP). Respiratory muscle strength is stronger in men, but declines with aging in both sexes. The mean MIP for healthy 85-year-old men is approximately 30% lower than that for 65-year-old men (65 vs. 90 cm H_2O). A lower MIP is associated with many factors, including decreased handgrip strength, lower body mass index (malnutrition), and current smoking. A low MIP often causes a low FVC.

ARTERIAL BLOOD GASES

Acid–base balance is tightly controlled, and therefore, normal values for arterial pH and $PaCO_2$ (partial pressure of carbon dioxide in arterial gas) do not change throughout adult life in healthy persons. However, because of increased nonuniformity of ventilation with aging, mean arterial oxygen tension (PaO_2 [partial pressure arterial oxygen]) declines during middle life even in healthy never-smokers. Mean PaO_2 remains relatively constant at about 80 mm Hg from age 65 to 90 years in healthy elderly persons at sea level (Figure 82-3).

DIFFUSING CAPACITY

A test of the single-breath pulmonary diffusing capacity for carbon monoxide (DLCO) is available at hospital-based pulmonary function laboratories. The 15-minute noninvasive DLCO test is easier to perform than spirometry, yet clinically valuable for the differential diagnosis of both airway obstruction and restriction of lung volumes. DLCO is the amount of carbon monoxide (from a test gas containing 0.3% CO) that is absorbed into the blood during a 10-second breath-hold. The DLCO is an index of the ability of the lungs to take up oxygen from the environment and deliver it to red blood cells.

In smokers with airways obstruction, the DLCO is an excellent index of the degree of anatomic emphysema; a low DLCO correlates highly with a low mean lung tissue density on lung computed tomography (CT) scans and the degree of anatomic emphysema. Smokers with airways obstruction but normal DLCO values usually have chronic "obstructive" bronchitis but not emphysema, and non-smoking patients with asthma and borderline to moderate airways obstruction have normal or high (percent predicted) DLCO values.

In healthy persons, the absolute value of DLCO in adults varies with height, age, gender, and race. As with spirometry, reference values from the healthy subset of large population studies are used to obtain percent predicted values for individual patients. DLCO is higher in very obese persons and lower in patients with anemia. The DLCO declines about 5% per decade after age 40 years, even in healthy persons.

Differential Diagnosis of Asthma and COPD

The differential diagnosis of asthma and COPD in elderly persons is often more difficult than in younger adults because of the higher prevalence of comorbidity. The elderly are much more likely than middle-aged adults to have COPD and cardiovascular disease, both often a result of cigarette smoking, and both with symptoms that may mimic asthma, increasing the value of objective pulmonary function (PF) tests in the elderly patient.

Because intermittent airway obstruction is the primary physiologic manifestation of asthma, the first (and least expensive) PF test to perform is spirometry, especially if the patient is experiencing symptoms at the time of presentation (Figure 82-4). If the FEV_1/FVC ratio is below the lower limit of the normal range (assuming that appropriate reference equations for elderly patients are used and the quality of the test session was good), the patient has airway obstruction. The degree of severity of the obstruction is then determined by

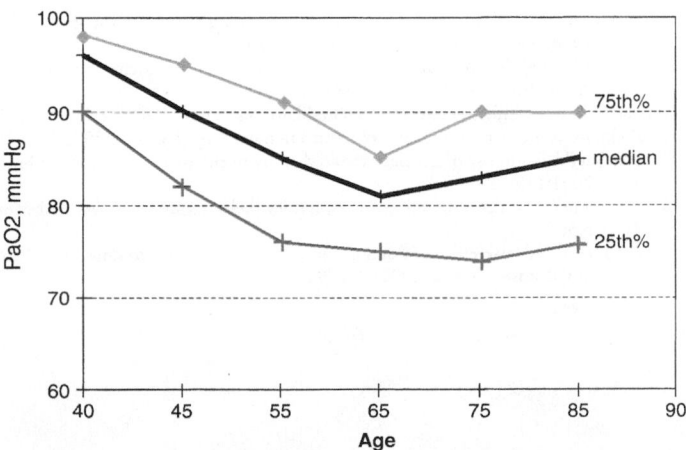

FIGURE 82-3. Arterial oxygen (PaO_2) decreases throughout middle age in healthy persons but stabilizes beyond age 65 years in healthy persons.

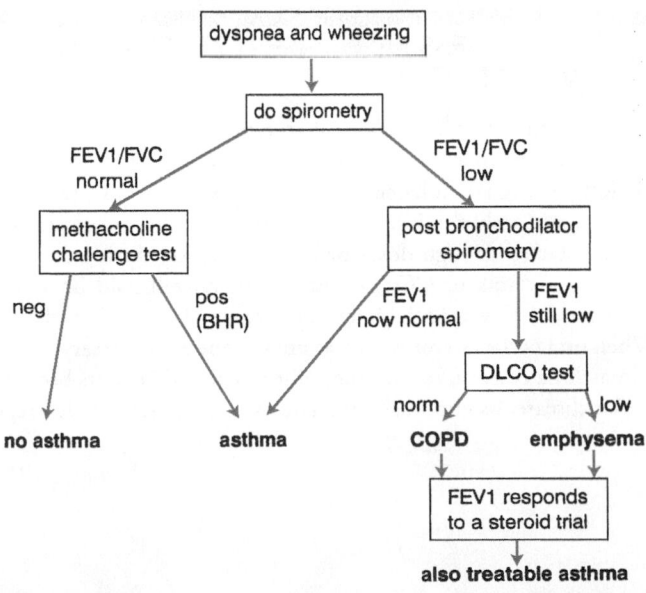

FIGURE 82-4. The role of PF tests in making a differential diagnosis of asthma versus COPD in a patient with chronic or intermittent dyspnea.

the percent predicted FEV$_1$. When compared to younger patients with asthma, one will often be surprised by more severe airway obstruction (an FEV$_1$ below 50% predicted) in elderly patients with asthma.

If the patient has airways obstruction, repeat spirometry approximately 45 minutes after administration of a combination of albuterol and ipratropium (post-BD) spirometry). A positive (significant) BD response is best defined as an increase of at least a 12% (and 0.20 L) improvement in percent predicted FEV$_1$ or FVC.

With good test quality, baseline airway obstruction followed by a BD response helps to confirm asthma in a patient with a history suggesting asthma. However, the lack of a positive BD response is of no help in making the diagnosis (does not rule out asthma), because chronic asthma often leads to airways inflammation that is not acutely reversible. Furthermore, many elderly patients with a history of smoking, current symptoms suggesting asthma, baseline airways obstruction, and a "positive" BD response, still have some "fixed" obstruction (a low FEV$_1$) following aggressive therapy for asthma. Some guidelines consider this pattern evidence for COPD.

Pre- and post-BD spirometry may be normal in patients with a history suggesting asthma. The patient maybe asked to return for retesting when symptoms occur; however, a methacholine challenge test (MCT) or measurement of exhaled nitric oxide (eNO) can quickly and safely detect the bronchial hyperresponsiveness (MCT) or the eosinophilic airway inflammation (eNO) characteristic of asthma. The MCT has optimal clinical utility when the pretest probability of asthma is intermediate. A high PC-20 (above 16 mg/mL) makes asthma highly unlikely, while a low PC-20 (below 4 mg/mL) in a patient with a history of asthma-like symptoms increases the pretest probability of asthma.

Measurement of the DLCO is quick, safe, and helps to distinguish between emphysema and other causes of chronic airway obstruction. Emphysema lowers the DLCO, obstructive chronic bronchitis does not affect the DLCO, and asthma frequently increases the DLCO. A lung CT scan may also differentiate asthma from emphysema in a cigarette smoker, although both diseases may coexist.

TESTS TO ASSESS RESPONSE TO THERAPY FOR ASTHMA AND COPD

The inhaled corticosteroids used to treat asthma and COPD frequently cause thrush (or other side-effects at high daily doses), while the long-acting BD inhalers may cause muscle cramps, tremors, insomnia, and arrhythmias. These asthma controller medications are usually started at high doses or in combination during an exacerbation of asthma or COPD, but this therapy should be adjusted downward a few months later after maximal control is obtained. When oral corticosteroids such as prednisone are necessary to maintain asthma control, serious morbidity frequently occurs because of ocular disease, osteoporosis, and glucose intolerance; therefore, ob-

jective measurements of the effectiveness of each newly prescribed asthma or COPD medication for each patient is highly desirable.

Two lung function tests are used as asthma therapy outcome measures in the outpatient clinic setting: the pre- or post-BD FEV$_1$ during a clinic visit, or peak expiratory flow (PEF) measured at home in the early morning. The FEV$_1$ is more accurate and more sensitive than peak flow for detecting narrow airways, and it is linearly related to the severity of asthma symptoms in groups of elderly patients. Pocket spirometers, which measure both FEV$_1$ and PEF, are now available for the same cost as a mechanical peak flow meter. Because many elderly patients become tolerant of severe, long-standing airway obstruction and consequently underreport respiratory symptoms, objective measurement of lung function is needed. FEV$_1$ improvement of more than 20% and 0.20 L is necessary to be confident that the change was not merely a result of measurement noise. The FEV$_1$ measured 10–30 minutes after albuterol is considered the best lung function that can be achieved on the day of the visit, and therefore, is a more stable measure in asthmatics than comparing visit-to-visit FEV$_1$ values without prior administration of albuterol. In the future, the availability of less expensive eNO analyzers for monitoring asthma in outpatient settings may complement or replace spirometry for this purpose.

FURTHER READING

American Thoracic Society. Standardization of Spirometry; Guidelines for Exercise and Methacholine Challenge Testing; Guidelines for the Six-Minute Walk; and Guidelines for the Measurement of Exhaled Nitric Oxide. These documents may be downloaded without charge from http://www.thoracic.org/sections/publications/statements/index.html. Accessed April 2007.

Barbee RA, Bloom JW. *Asthma in the Elderly.* New York, New York: Marcel Dekker; 1997.

Camhi SL, Enright PL. How to assess pulmonary function in older adults. *J Respir Dis.* 2000;21:395.

Celli B. The importance of spirometry in COPD and asthma: effect on approach to management. *Chest* 2000;117:15S.

Cerveri I, et al. Reference values of arterial oxygen tension in the middle-aged and elderly. *Am J Respir Crit Care Med.* 1995;152:934.

Enright PL, et al. Reduced vital capacity in elderly persons with hypertension, coronary heart disease, or left ventricular hypertrophy: The Cardiovascular Health Study. *Chest.* 1995;107:28.

Enright PL, et al. Correlates of respiratory muscle strength, and maximal respiratory pressure reference values in the elderly. *Am Rev Respir Dis.* 1994;149:430.

Enright PL, et al. ; for the Cardiovascular Health Study Research Group. Underdiagnosis and under-treatment of asthma in the elderly. *Chest.* 1999;116:603.

Goldstein MD, et al. Comparisons of peak diurnal expiratory flow variation, post-bronchodilator FEV$_1$ responses, and methacholine inhalation challenges in the evaluation of suspected asthma. *Chest.* 2001;119:1001.

Hankinson JL, et al. Spirometric reference values from a sample of the general US population. *Am J Respir Crit Care Med.* 1999;159:179.

Korenblat PE, et al. Effect of age on response to zafirlukast in patients with asthma. *Ann Allergy Asthma Immunol.* 2000;84:217.

Kradjan WA, et al. Effect of age on bronchodilator response. *Chest.* 1992;101:1545.

Quadrelli SA, Roncoroni A. Features of asthma in the elderly. *J Asthma.* 2001;38:377.

Sin DD, Tu JV. Underuse of inhaled steroid therapy in elderly patients with asthma. *Chest* 2001;119:720.

Tolep K, Kelsen SG. Effect of aging on respiratory skeletal muscles. *Clin Chest Med.* 1993;3:363.

Walsh LJ, et al. Adverse effects of oral corticosteroids in relation to dose in patients with lung disease. *Thorax.* 2001;56:279.

Chronic Obstructive Pulmonary Disease

Sachin Yende ■ *Anne B. Newman* ■ *Don Sin*

The smoking epidemic of the twentieth century has led to an increase in the incidence of chronic obstructive pulmonary disease (COPD), a largely preventable disease. The statistics concerning COPD have caused considerable alarm around the world. Globally, COPD is the fourth leading cause of mortality and the twelfth leading cause of disability. To address this growing problem, the World Health Organization partnered with the National Heart, Lung, and Blood Institute (NHLBI) to form a Global Initiative for Chronic Obstructive Lung Disease (GOLD). In 2001, they offered a global strategy to increase awareness of the disease and offer guidelines for disease prevention and treatment, referred to as the GOLD Guidelines. These guidelines and those created by leading medical societies are incorporated in this chapter.

Most patients are diagnosed with COPD in the sixth decade. Although it is an important chronic disease and a leading cause of disability in the elderly, it remains underrecognized. This chapter will focus on the early recognition and management of COPD, an important component of outpatient geriatric management.

DEFINITIONS

GOLD defines COPD as partially reversible or nonreversible airflow limitation, which is progressive, and cannot be reversed by current therapies. In contrast asthma is defined as a syndrome characterized by reversible airflow limitation. Although GOLD definitions did not include traditionally used terminologies, such as chronic bronchitis and emphysema, these definitions are important to understand the disease spectrum. Chronic bronchitis is defined clinically as cough with sputum production for 3 months of a year for 2 consecutive years. Emphysema is a pathological diagnosis defined as the destruction of alveolar walls with accompanying enlargement of air spaces distal to the terminal bronchiole.

Key differences between COPD and asthma are that, in COPD there is (i) a lack of complete reversibility of airflow obstruction; (ii) neutrophil predominance in the airways, especially in the lumen; (iii) significant smoking history (usually >10 pack years) or exposure to burning biomass fuel, such as wood and manure; (iv) chronic colonization of bacterial organisms in the airways, especially in patients with severe disease; and (v) emphysematous changes in the lung parenchyma often associated clinically with reduced diffusing capacity on a gas diffusion test.

It is important to recognize that some of these distinctions become blurred in the elderly. Firstly, many elderly asthmatics, even those who have never smoked, have evidence of poorly reversible airflow obstruction, similar to COPD. This is caused by permanent remodeling of the airways. Secondly, bronchial hyperresponsiveness, an exaggerated bronchoconstrictive response to a given stimulus, is seen in a majority of middle-aged smokers with COPD and is a strong predictor of progressive decline in lung function. Thirdly, adults with asthma, especially those with severe disease, often demonstrate neutrophilia in their airways. Lastly and perhaps most importantly, many adult patients with asthma are current or former smokers. It is likely that such patients have more than one pathological process and several pathways of inflammation. These patients are likely to have both COPD and asthma. This has raised a complexity of semantic issues that has not been resolved. One attempt has been to combine and describe such patients using the term asthmatic bronchitis (Figure 83-1).

An important limitation of current definitions of COPD is that they fail to identify a precise level of airflow limitation at which clinically relevant outcomes occur for each age group. This is an important issue in the elderly, in whom reduced elastic recoil of lung with aging maybe associated with increased incidence of airways obstruction. Using a commonly used criteria, such as forced expiratory volume in 1st second/forced vital capacity (FEV_1/FVC) ratio <70% may thus lead to over diagnosis. Using age-specific cutoffs of

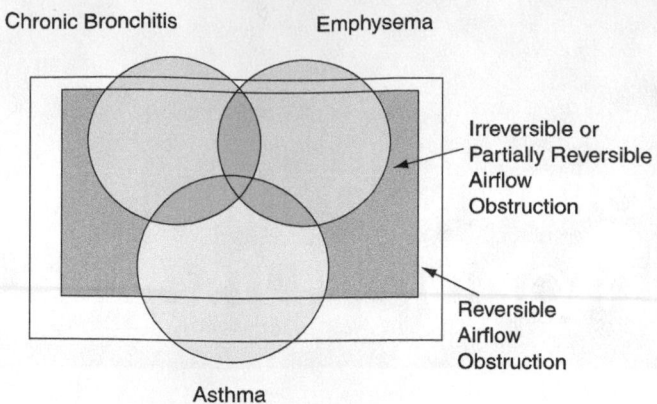

FIGURE 83-1. Subsets of COPD and asthma depicted by a Venn diagram. *(From Mannino DM. COPD: epidemiology, prevalence, morbidity and mortality, and disease heterogeneity [review]. Chest. 2002;121(5 Suppl):121S–126S.)*

FEV_1/FVC ratio to diagnose COPD is therefore important in the elderly.

EPIDEMIOLOGY

The different definitions of COPD, based on spirometry, clinical, or radiographic criteria, have important implications when estimating the global burden of disease. Using patient- or physician-reported diagnosis alone may underestimate the incidence of COPD. More than 50% of individuals with airway obstruction have never been diagnosed with COPD by a health care provider. Underdiagnosis is more common in the elderly because they fail to report symptoms or symptoms are attributed to other conditions.

Several recent studies used multiple approaches, including spirometry and clinical criteria, to estimate the prevalence of COPD. In the United States, the National Health and Nutrition Examination Survey (NHANES) III estimated prevalence of COPD from 1988 to 1994. In this survey, 14.3% of the adult population or 24.2 million individuals had airflow limitation by spirometry. Of these, 1.5% had moderate to severe disease, evidenced by FEV_1 <50%. However, only 2.9% or 4.8 million adults who met spirometry criteria report symptoms of chronic bronchitis or emphysema.

In the NHANES III survey, the prevalence of airflow obstruction increased with age and was highest among those 65 to 85 years of age. The prevalence of low lung function is higher with increasing age except in individuals 85 years or older, which maybe related to differential mortality or inability to do pulmonary function testing. This survey also underscored the difficulties in differentiating asthma and COPD. More than a fifth of the respondents reported that they had current asthma and current bronchitis or had current asthma and current emphysema.

Similar estimates have been obtained globally. For instance, a prevalence study in Japan estimated the prevalence of COPD in those 40 years or older to be 10.9% by spirometry criteria. In the Platino Study, which evaluated residents 40 years of age or older in five major Latin American cities (Sao Paulo, Santiago, Mexico City Montevideo, and Caracas), the prevalence estimates ranged from a low of 7.8% in Mexico City to a high of 19.7% in Montevideo. Similar estimates have been reported in European countries.

COPD is a leading cause of death worldwide. Globally, COPD is the fourth leading cause of mortality and the twelfth leading cause of disability. In 2004, chronic lower respiratory diseases, including chronic bronchitis and emphysema, were the fourth leading cause of death in United States and it is estimated that approximately 6% of deaths occur as a result of COPD. Patients with COPD often die as a result of influenza or pneumonia, the sixth leading cause of death in United States. These findings combined with the underdiagnosis of COPD suggests that current COPD mortality estimates maybe underestimated.

An alarming trend has been increasing mortality as a result of COPD over the past two decades. In United States, mortality caused by COPD has increased 44% from 1979 to 1993, and the highest increase in mortality has been experienced by women (Figure 83-2).

Rates per 100,000 Population

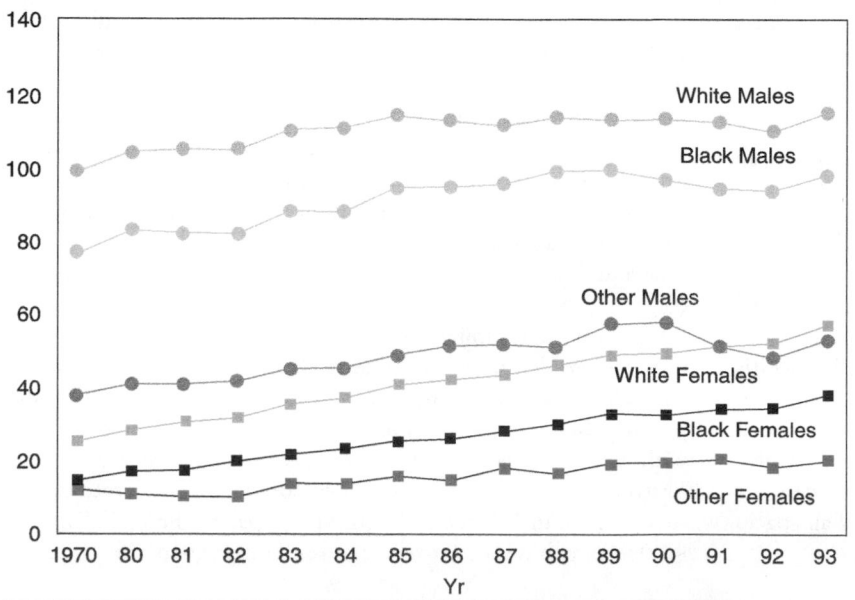

FIGURE 83-2. Trends in mortality as a result of COPD from 1979 to 1993 in the United States. *(From Mannino DM, et al. Obstructive lung disease deaths in the United States from 1979 through 1993. Am J Respir Crit Care Med 1997;156(3):814–818.)*

This is in sharp contrast to the declining mortality caused by cardiovascular disease and cancer. Worldwide it is estimated that by the year 2020, COPD will be the third leading cause of death and the fifth leading cause of disability.

Although accurate statistics regarding morbidity as a result of COPD are difficult to obtain, it represents an important cause of disability. The average number of days of restricted activities reported by patients with COPD is very high. In 1996, COPD was listed as the eighth leading cause of disability-adjusted life-years (DALYs) in men, and the seventh leading cause of DALYs among women. COPD is a leading cause of hospitalizations in United States. In 1998, nearly 2% of all hospitalizations were attributed to COPD and 7% had COPD as a contributing cause of hospitalization. More striking are COPD statistics regarding the elderly population. Nearly 20% of all hospitalizations in patients older than age 65 years had COPD as a primary or contributing cause. Owing to its impact on reduced physical activity, it is emerging as an important cause of reduced functional status and disability in older adults. The cost implications of treating COPD are huge and those with severe disease account for the highest cost.

PATHOPHYSIOLOGY

Risk Factors

Table 83-1 lists important risk factors for COPD. Exposure to inhalants, including tobacco, indoor and outdoor air pollution, are important environmental risk factors. Cigarette smoking is the most important risk factor for COPD. At least 15% of smokers develop COPD, though recent estimates suggest higher incidence among smokers. Both current and previous smokers are at increased risk of COPD. Pipe and cigar smokers and passive exposure to cigarette smoke also increases risk, though these individuals are at lower risk compared to cigarette smokers. In NHANES III survey, obstructive lung disease was present among 12.5% of current smokers, 9.4% of former smokers, and 3.1% of pipe or cigar smokers. Indoor pollution caused by cooking using biomass fuels is an important risk factor, especially for females in developing countries. The role of urban pollution in susceptibility to COPD is unclear.

The vast majority of individuals exposed to cigarette smoke do not develop symptomatic COPD. Thus host factors may explain differences in susceptibility. Genetics, especially gene–environment or gene–inhalant interaction, may play an important role. For instance, several studies in the 1970s observed higher rates of airflow obstruction in first-degree relatives of patients with COPD compared to control subjects. COPD also aggregates in families.

Severe alpha-1 antitrypsin deficiency is an important genetic risk factor and accounts for 1% of COPD patients. Alpha-1 antitrypsin, a serum protein, is synthesized in the liver. It inhibits proteolytic enzymes, such as trypsin, chymotrypsin, and neutrophil elastase. If neutrophil elastases are not inactivated by alpha-1 antitrypsin, these enzymes destroy lung connective tissue, particularly elastin, and cause emphysema. Understanding the role of alpha-1 antitrypsin in COPD has therefore provided a foundation for the protease–antiprotease hypothesis for the pathogenesis of COPD. The phenotype, also called Pi type, is determined by the independent expression of two independent alleles. More than 90% of severely deficient patients are homozygous for the Z allele. Such patients are designated Pi ZZ and have serum alpha-1 antitrypsin levels that are about 20% of the normal level. The phenotypic effects of having a single Z allele, heterozygote with Pi MZ genotype, are less clear. Individuals with alpha-1 antitrypsin deficiency develop COPD during the fourth or fifth decade.

Recent studies have also examined the role of other genes and their interaction with environmental factors to explain differences in susceptibility and outcomes of COPD. Candidate genes include tumor necrosis factor, microsomal epoxide hydrolase, glutathione S-transferases, heme oxygenase-1, and alpha-1-antichymotrypsin. Although preliminary studies suggest that these genetic variants may play an important role in COPD pathogenesis, results have not been consistent across studies.

Pathogenesis and Pathology

COPD is characterized by chronic inflammation in peripheral airways and alveoli. Macrophages, neutrophils, and CD8+ T lymphocytes are the predominant cells involved in inflammation. In contrast to asthma, eosinophils are not present in lung biopsy specimens. Important mediators include leukotriene B4, IL-8, and TNF-α. Cigarette smoking and other irritants activate resident macrophages to release chemotactic factors, which attract inflammatory cells from the circulation and release additional inflammatory mediators. The subsequent interaction between the molecular and cellular mediators is complex and poorly understood.

Two theories have been proposed to explain pathogenesis of COPD: protease–antiprotease imbalance theory and increased oxidative stress theory. These theories suggest that lung inflammation is amplified in the presence of excess proteases or oxidant stress. In the protease–antiprotease imbalance theory, proteases, such as elastase, proteinase 3, and matrix metalloproteinases, are induced by cigarette smoking and lead to alveolar wall destruction and mucus hypersecretion. These proteolytic enzymes are counteracted by antiproteases, particularly alpha-1 antitrypsin, and inhibitors of matrix metalloproteinases. The imbalance between proteases and antiproteases may lead to destruction of connective tissue and cause emphysema.

TABLE 83-1

Risk Factors for COPD

RISK FACTOR	COMMENT
Cigarette smoking	Most important risk factor and most cases of COPD are caused by smoking
Pipe and cigars	High risk, but lower than observed in cigarette smokers
Occupational exposure	Risk in coal miners, gold miners, grain handlers, cement and cotton workers
Environmental pollution	Indoor use of biomass fuels for cooking and heating in underdeveloped countries and particulate matter from urban pollution
Genetic factor	Alpha-1-antitrypsin deficiency known to cause early onset COPD. Other genetic risk factors may also increase risk
Socioeconomic	More common with low socioeconomic status
Childhood illnesses	Low birth weight, respiratory infections, and symptomatic childhood asthma may increase risk

The oxidative stress theory was proposed because of increase in markers of oxidative stress in exhaled breath and urine in COPD patients. Interestingly, the role of oxidative stress has also been implicated in aging. Oxidative stress is caused by the imbalance between reactive oxygen species and the body's ability to detoxify reactive oxygen species or the damage caused as a result. Excess oxidative stress has several consequences, including activation of inflammatory genes and inactivation of antiproteases, thereby leading to increased local inflammation.

The pathologic changes in COPD are found in the large and small airways and in the lung parenchyma. Structural changes in the airways include mucus hyperplasia, bronchiolar edema and smooth muscle hypertrophy, and peribronchiolar fibrosis. These changes result in narrowing of the small airways. Early pathophysiologic abnormalities in airways that are 2 mm and less in diameter have been referred to as "small-airway disease." Mucus hypersecretion occurs owing to increase in the size and number of the submucosal glands and an increase in the number of goblet cells on the surface epithelium.

Emphysema is a destructive process that occurs in the gas-exchanging airspaces, the respiratory bronchioles, alveolar ducts, and alveoli. It results in obliteration of airspace walls and coalescence of small distinct air spaces into larger ones. An important consequence of emphysema is loss of elastic recoil of the lungs and thereby increases airway obstruction. Emphysema also causes abnormal gas exchange.

In advanced stages, there are also changes in the pulmonary circulation, heart, and respiratory muscles. Alveolar hypoxia causes medial hypertrophy of vascular smooth muscle with extension of the muscularis layer into distal vessels that do not ordinarily contain smooth muscle. Intimal hyperplasia also occurs in advanced stages. These latter changes are associated with the development of pulmonary hypertension and its consequences, right ventricular hypertrophy. Loss of vascular bed also occurs with emphysema as a result of destruction of alveolar walls. In some patients with advanced COPD, there is atrophy of diaphragmatic muscle.

Changes in Respiratory Physiology in COPD

Pathologic processes affecting airways and lung parenchyma are accompanied by changes in respiratory physiology in COPD. The physiologic hallmark of COPD is the limitation of expiratory flow caused by airway narrowing and emphysematous changes in the lung. This is accompanied by a reduction in the FEV_1/FVC ratio. Early in the course of COPD, the expiratory flow–volume curve has a scooped out appearance in the expiratory limb as a result of reduced flow at low lung volumes (Figure 83-3). With disease progression, expiratory flow decreases at all lung volumes. Another important effect of decreased expiratory flow is nonuniform ventilation of the lungs, observed even in the earlier stages of COPD. Nonuniform ventilation can lead to ventilation–perfusion mismatches, which reduce arterial oxygen pressures.

Hypercapnia is usually observed in the end-stages of COPD, usually when FEV_1 is 1 L or lower. Pulmonary hyperinflation places the thoracic cage and diaphragm at a mechanical disadvantage and increases the work of breathing. Airflow obstruction also contributes to increased work of breathing. Finally, the destruction of lung parenchyma worsens ventilation perfusion mismatch and worsens both hypercapnia and hypoxemia.

Nonpulmonary Effects

There has been increased interest in understanding systemic consequences of COPD for several reasons. First, reduced exercise capacity observed in patient's with COPD patients is not limited by respiratory system abnormalities alone. Several studies suggest that cardiovascular and skeletal muscle changes also contribute to reduced exercise capacity. Second, most COPD patients die because

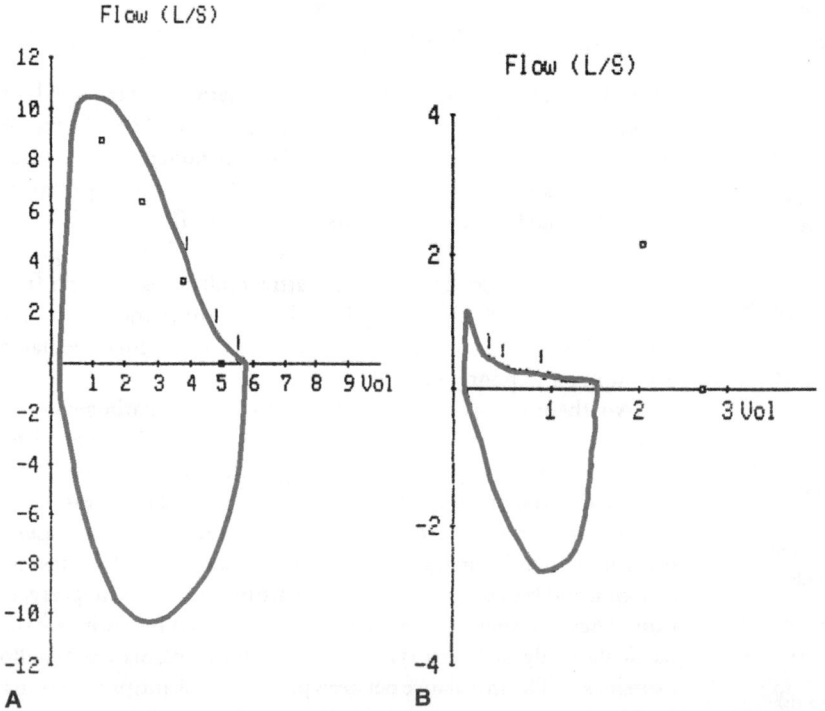

FIGURE 83-3. Flow–volume loop of a COPD patient compared to a normal individual. Notice the markedly diminished flow at all lung volumes.

A

B

of nonpulmonary causes, such as cardiovascular disease and cancer. Third, COPD patients have higher prevalence of reduced body mass index (BMI), osteoporosis, and increased systemic concentrations of inflammatory markers. These observations are underscored by a recently proposed multidimensional risk prediction score by Celli et al., in which survival prediction was improved by incorporating BMI, dyspnea scale, and exercise capacity in the traditional risk prediction model using FEV_1 alone. Although there is an improved understanding of the systemic consequences of COPD, the biologic mechanisms underlying these effects remain poorly understood.

COPD patients have reduced skeletal muscle strength. Upper extremity grip strength is usually well preserved in COPD, but the strength of the lower extremity quadriceps is reduced compared to age-matched controls. Respiratory muscle strength is also reduced, but it is more likely to occur because of hyperinflation of lung rather than intrinsic defect in the muscles. The decline in skeletal muscle strength in COPD patients is proportional to the reduction in FEV_1. During hospitalization for exacerbations, skeletal muscle strength is reduced further, but the long-term effect of an exacerbation on skeletal muscle strength is not known. Thigh muscle size and lower extremity lean body mass is also lower in COPD patients. Multiple factors may contribute to reduced skeletal muscle strength, including elevation of systemic inflammatory markers, particularly tumor necrosis factor or cachectin and IL-6, disuse atrophy, hypogonadism, poor nutrition, and hypoxemia.

COPD is also associated with changes in body composition. These patients have lower BMI and lean body mass. However, visceral fat appears to be similar to age-matched control population. Advanced COPD patients have higher risk of osteoporosis as a result of smoking, concomitant vitamin D deficiency, low BMI, hypogonadism, sedentary lifestyle, and use of glucocorticoids. The risk of osteoporosis is often underrecognized until the first fracture occurs.

There is a high prevalence of cognitive impairment in COPD. The most common disturbances are in verbal fluency, memory tasks, attention, and deductive thinking. Cognitive impairment in COPD has been related to age, educational background, depression, disability, exercise tolerance, and duration of respiratory failure. Although it is related to hypoxia, it does occur in nonhypoxemic COPD patients. Relationships between fatigue, depression, and cognitive function are poorly documented.

CLINICAL MANIFESTATIONS

Most clinical manifestations occur during the fifth and sixth decade of life. However, the onset of COPD symptoms maybe delayed to the seventh decade and beyond in smokers who stopped smoking in midlife. Dyspnea is the most common symptom of COPD and an important reason for reduced physical activity. Initially dyspnea is present only on exertion, but as lung function declines, patients experience dyspnea at rest too. Similar to dyspnea, chronic productive or nonproductive cough is intermittent initially and becomes persistent in severe disease. Chronic intermittent nonproductive cough can be present for several years prior to onset of dyspnea and maybe a subtle manifestation of mild COPD. Wheezing or chest tightness usually occurs with exertion.

An initial assessment of a COPD patient should include past medical history of asthma, detailed history of smoking and occupational exposures, family history of early onset COPD, and frequency of exacerbations or hospitalizations. Some symptoms may also be related to coexisting chronic health conditions, such as cardiovascular disease, which are common in these patients. Furthermore, COPD patients may develop secondary hypertension (*cor pulmonale*) that manifests as worsening dyspnea and lower extremity swelling. When patients develop rapid worsening of symptoms, alternative diagnoses should be considered, such as exacerbation of underlying disease, pneumothorax, or pulmonary thromboembolism.

Physical examination findings in the respiratory system are present in advanced disease and include barrel-shaped chest on inspection, prolonged expiration, distant heart sounds, and rhonchii on auscultation. Patients often use accessory muscles or pursed lips during breathing. Signs of *cor pulmonale* include pedal edema, a tender congested liver, loud pulmonary component of the second heart sound, and jugular venous distention. Careful attention should be paid to systemic manifestations, including cognitive deficits, reduced muscle strength, and recent weight loss.

Functional status assessment is important in COPD. Subjective and objective evaluations, based on activities of daily living and a 400-meter or a 6-minute walk test, is important to monitor disease progression and are independent predictors of mortality. Oxygen desaturation during an informal walk test in the office setting can identify patients who will benefit with supplemental oxygen.

DIAGNOSIS

Spirometry

Underdiagnosis or misdiagnosis of COPD is common in the elderly because symptoms of dyspnea and reduced functional status are often attributed to aging or coexisting disease. Therefore, spirometry, which includes an FEV_1 and FVC measurement with a flow volume loop, should be performed when COPD is suspected. A full pulmonary function test (PFT), which includes FEV_1, FVC, lung volumes, and diffusion capacity, can be performed in selected patients.

The peak expiratory flow (PEF) meter is often used to monitor disease in asthma. The PEF meter measures airflow obstruction in the larger airways. Since pathological changes occur predominantly in the smaller airways in COPD, the PEF meter underrepresents the severity of airflow obstruction in COPD, and therefore, should not be used for diagnosis or disease monitoring.

Challenges to perform spirometry in geriatric patients include difficulties in comprehension of instructions, dexterity problems, and reduced functional capacity. These problems often lead to poor quality results and are an important deterrent to performing spirometry in the elderly. Simple office-based spirometry tests using handheld spirometer are becoming more reliable and can be done in the outpatient office setting. These devices are easy to use and less demanding, and therefore, maybe particularly valuable in the diagnostic evaluation of older adults with suspected COPD.

A spirometer is a device that measures lung volumes through the forced expiration of air. Flow can also be assessed, by measuring the total volume of air that is expired in the first second of expiration. There are well-defined normal ranges that allow for the effects of age, race, sex, and height. Three measurements from the spirometer are commonly used in the diagnosis of COPD. FEV_1 measures the

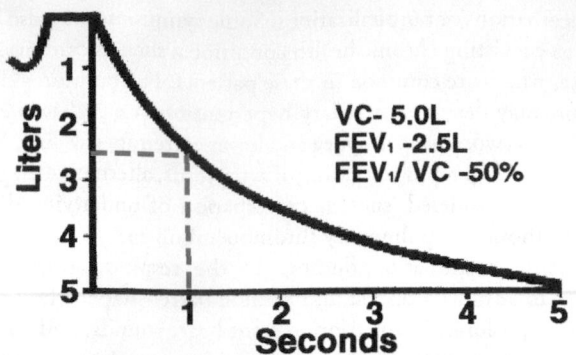

FIGURE 83-4. Forced vital capacity maneuver of patient with moderate COPD is shown on this spirogram. Both FEV$_1$ and FVC are reduced.

air exhaled in the first second of expiration. FVC is the maximum volume of air that can be forcibly expired. The ratio of FEV$_1$/FVC is expressed as a percentage and is the proportion of total volume of air that can be expired in the first second of expiration.

Spirometry results will only be of value if the tracings are performed satisfactorily and consistently. Two criteria should be met before results of spirometry are interpreted. First, the tracings should be reproducible, where at least two of the three FEV$_1$ measurements should be within 100 mL or 5% of each other. Second, the results should meet the acceptability criteria, where the measurements must continue until no more air can be exhaled. Exhalation is prolonged in COPD because of expiratory flow limitation and can take up to 15 seconds. Acceptability criteria can be assessed by examining the volume–time curve and at least 6 seconds of exhalation should be present or the exhalation should plateau for the last 2 seconds. Frequent coughing during spirometry may affect results.

COPD is diagnosed based on the FEV$_1$/FVC ratio less than 70% (Figures 83-3 and 83-4). However, in older adults, especially those over 70 years, this cutoff will overestimate disease. Therefore, age-adjusted ratios are preferred, though are cumbersome to use. However, for most older adults, a ratio below 60% is abnormal and suggestive of obstructive lung disease. Once obstruction is diagnosed, severity is graded based on the FEV$_1$ measurement (Table 83-2). The presence of reduced FEV$_1$, but a normal FEV$_1$/FVC ratio, is suggestive of restrictive lung disease, such as idiopathic pulmonary fibrosis. These findings should prompt referral for a full PFT and pulmonary consultation.

Improvement in FEV$_1$ in response to bronchodilators, termed bronchodilator reversibility, is based on increase in FEV$_1$ by 12% and 200 mL. Though bronchodilator reversibility suggests the diagnosis of asthma, many elderly subjects with asthma do not demonstrate response to bronchodilators. In individuals with an obstructive pattern on spirometry without evidence of airway reversibility, other clinical findings should be taken into account to differentiate asthma versus COPD. However, this distinction is often difficult in the elderly. It is important to emphasize that bronchodilator reversibility of findings on spirometry correlates poorly with clinical response to short or long-acting bronchodilators.

Bronchial or airway hyperresponsiveness is the exaggerated bronchoconstrictive response to nonspecific agonists, such as methacholine, hypertonic saline, adenosine, exercise, and hyperventilation. Although it is a hallmark of asthma, it can be present in several individuals with COPD and is associated with worse prognosis. Routine assessment of bronchial hyperresponsivess in elderly patients has limited value in clinical practice currently.

Other Tests

A chest x-ray is helpful during initial evaluation of the patient to rule out alternative diagnoses, such as congestive heart failure, or to identify a large bullous lesion, but is seldom helpful in the diagnosis of COPD. Findings suggestive of COPD on a chest radiograph include a low, flat diaphragm, an increased retrosternal airspace, and a teardrop-shaped heart (Figure 83-5). Pruning of the pulmonary arterial vessels and bullae are seen in emphysema. There is no benefit of obtaining routine yearly chest radiographs. A high-resolution CT scan of the chest maybe helpful when the diagnosis is doubtful or when lung reduction surgery is contemplated (Figure 83-6). Arterial blood gases are often recommended for patients with FEV$_1$ <50% predicted to identify hypercapnea. Other tests, such as complete blood count, echocardiogram, cardiopulmonary exercise tests, maybe necessary in special circumstances. For instance, a cardiopulmonary exercise will be useful in patients with concomitant

TABLE 83-2

Severity of COPD*		
	GLOBAL INITIATIVE FOR CHRONIC OBSTRUCTIVE DISEASE (GOLD)	**AMERICAN THORACIC SOCIETY (ATS)/ EUROPEAN RESPIRATORY SOCIETY (ERS)**
At risk	Risk factors and chronic symptoms but normal Spirometry	-
Mild	FEV$_1$/FVC<70% FEV$_1$≥80% predicted value	FEV$_1$≥70% predicted value
Moderate	FEV$_1$/FVC<70% 80%>FEV$_1$≥50% predicted value	70%>FEV$_1$≥60% predicted value 60%>FEV$_1$≥59% predicted value (moderately severe)
Severe	FEV$_1$/FVC<70% 50%>FEV$_1$≥30% predicted value	49%>FEV$_1$≥35% predicted value
Very severe	FEV$_1$/FVC<70% FEV$_1$≤30% predicted value	FEV$_1$<35% predicted value

*Although GOLD recommends using FEV$_1$/FVC cutoff of 70 to diagnose obstruction, using age-specific cutoffs is recommended by ATS and preferable in older adults.

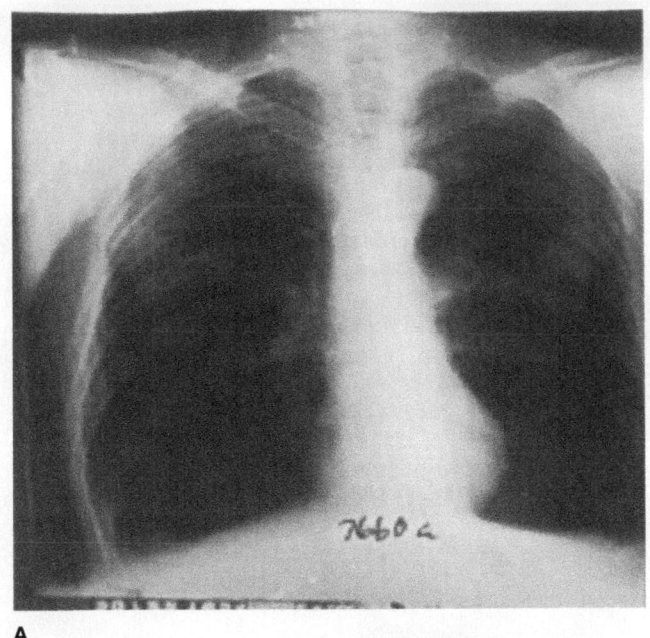

A

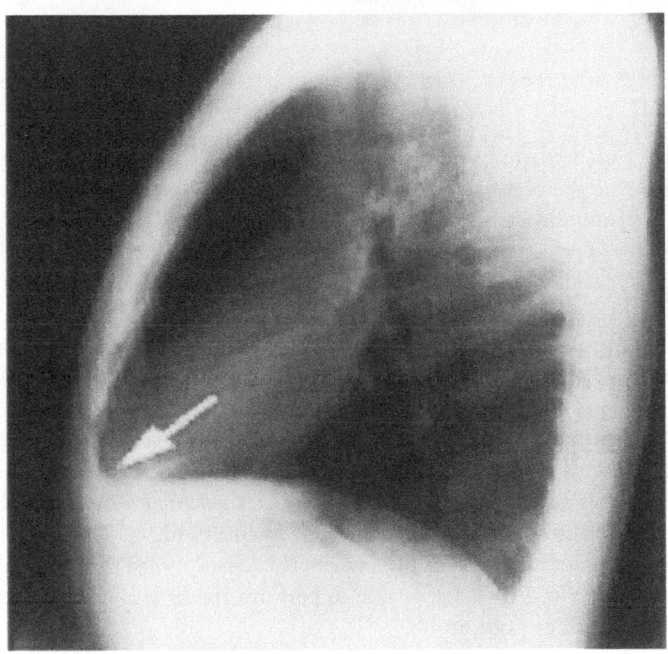

Normal

B

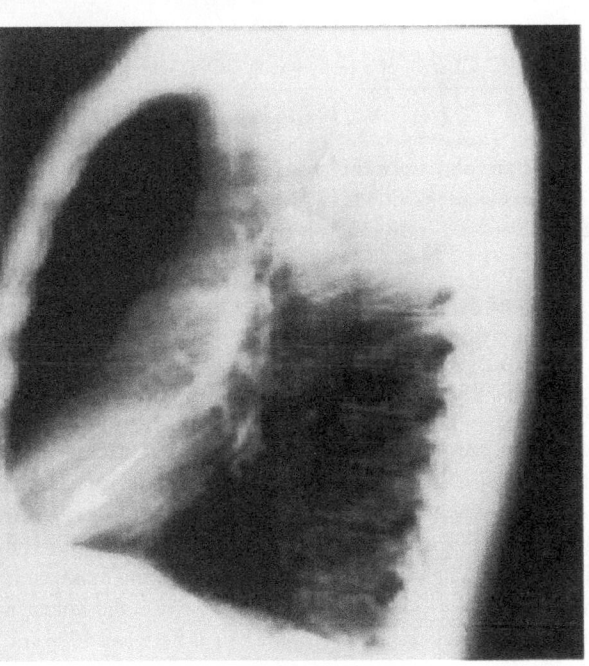

Hyperinflation

FIGURE 83-5. Chest radiograph of a patient with COPD. It shows flattened diaphragm and lung markings are reduced with hyperinflation. Heart is teardrop-shaped.

COPD and congestive heart failure to assess the contribution of each condition to the patients' symptoms.

SEVERITY OF COPD

Severity assessment is important for prognosis and to identify patients who are likely to benefit from specific therapies. Traditionally, severity of COPD was based on FEV_1 alone (Table 83-2). A reduction in FEV_1 was used to assess severity in most criteria because it is the most important predictor of mortality in COPD. FEV_1/FVC ratio is important to diagnose airflow limitation, but has limited value to assess disease severity.

As the systemic consequences of COPD are increasingly recognized, newer severity criteria have tried to incorporate nonpulmonary features of COPD. The BODE index by Celli et al. is the most extensively studied and validated. The BODE score is a 10-point scale and is based on body (B) mass index, obstruction (O) of airflow quantified by reduction in FEV_1, dyspnea (D) assessed by the modified Medical Research Council pulspnea scale, and exercise (E) capacity based on the 6-minute walk test. Higher scores correlate with higher mortality. The average age of subjects in the derivation

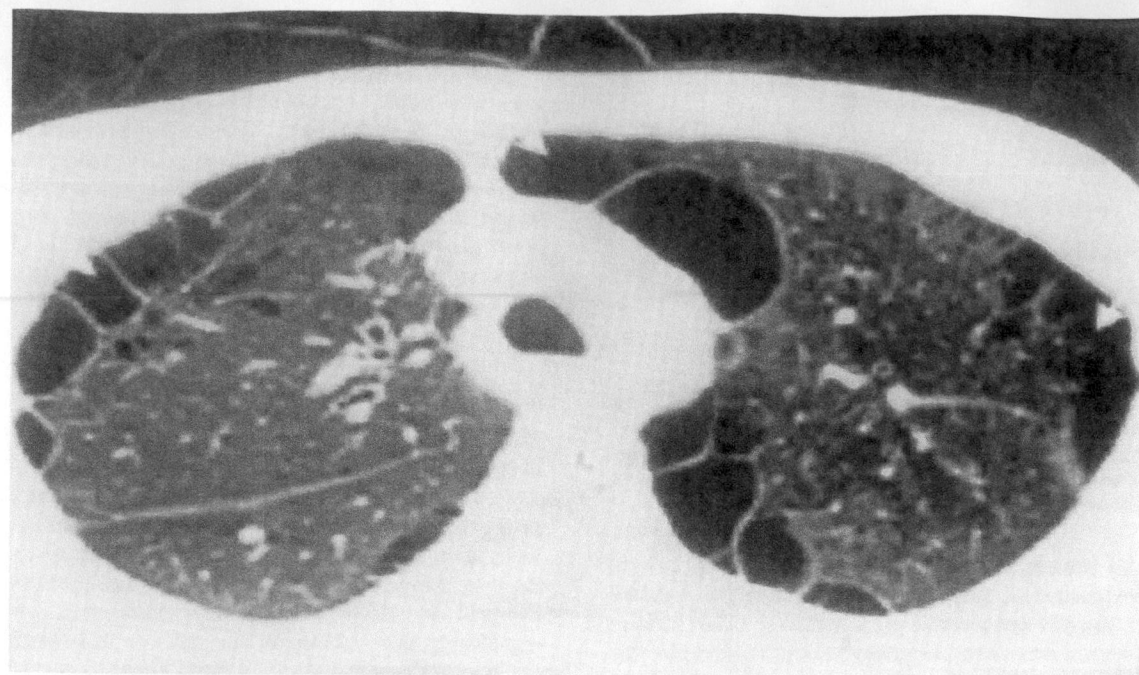

FIGURE 83-6. CT scan of a patient with COPD with bullous lesions.

and validation cohorts for this study was 66 years and few individuals over 80 years were included. Whether the BODE index can be generalized to very old individuals is not known.

NATURAL HISTORY OF COPD

After 25 years of age, FEV_1 declines continuously and smoothly over an individual's life (Figure 83-7). Nonsmokers without respiratory disease can expect to lose 25 to 30 mL per year after age 35 years. The rate of decline appears to accelerate with aging, but sudden large irreversible falls are very rare. Elderly current smokers experience a higher rate of decline compared to nonsmokers, approximately 48 mL per year. The rate of decline is higher among males compared to females and whites compared to blacks, with the lowest rate of decline among black females. When FEV_1 is between 40% and 59%

of predicted value, disability occurs. FEV_1 remains an important predictor of survival and when FEV_1 falls below 1 L, the 5-year mortality approaches 50%.

Few studies have examined the natural history of COPD, especially in the elderly. The Cardiovascular Health Study of 5888 subjects older than 65 years examined the effects of health behaviors and clinically diagnosed COPD on lung function. Spirometry was performed at baseline and at year 4 and 7. A diagnosis of COPD and smoking was associated with lower FEV_1 at baseline. However, current smoking was the only risk factor associated with accelerated FEV_1 decline. Former smokers had similar rate of decline in FEV_1 compared to nonsmokers. Paradoxically, a diagnosis of emphysema was associated with lower rate of decline in FEV_1. This is most likely because of survivor bias, where participants with the most rapid decline in FEV1 are unable to perform repeat spirometry because of death or poor health.

Smoking and Lung Function Decline

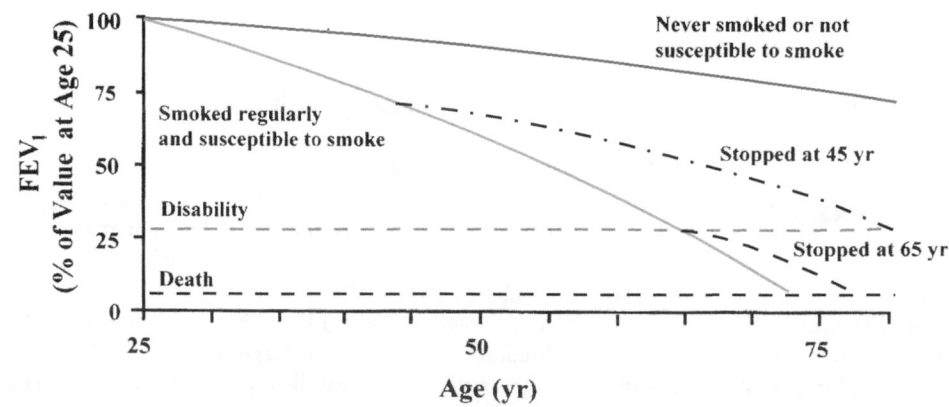

FIGURE 83-7. Natural history of COPD and effects of smoking cessation. (Adapted from Fletcher C, Peto R: BMJ. 1997;1:1645.)

The effect of smoking cessation on FEV_1 decline in susceptible smokers varies with age. When smoking cessation occurs early, before age 45 years, the rate of FEV_1 decline slows and approaches those seen among nonsmokers. A prospective multicenter longitudinal study, the Lung Health Study (LHS), examined effects of smoking cessation in patients identified with mild to moderate airflow obstruction. The LHS showed that smokers between 35 and 60 years old, who stopped with the help of an aggressive smoking intervention program, significantly reduced the decline in their FEV_1 over a 5-year study period when compared to those who continued to smoke. In contrast, smoking cessation in the elderly has a small effect on FEV_1 decline.

The slowly progressive course of COPD is often interrupted by acute respiratory illnesses or exacerbations, usually caused by viral or bacterial infections. Patients with milder stages of COPD will often develop one to two exacerbations per year; those with more severe disease are likely to have many more. Reduced FEV_1 is also the most important risk factor for community-acquired pneumonia. The risk of pneumonia is modest for mild or moderate reduction in FEV_1, but those with most severe reduction experience 3.6-fold higher risk. Patients with more frequent exacerbations have higher risk of decline in lung function.

Traditionally, it was believed that COPD survivors died largely as a result of respiratory failure. Recent studies suggest that death caused by cardiovascular disease and cancer is common among COPD patients. Although airway inflammation is a hallmark of COPD, it is increasingly recognized that these patients have higher systemic concentrations of inflammatory markers, including IL-6 and C-reactive protein (CRP). Increased systemic inflammation is associated with increased risk of atherosclerotic disease, including acute myocardial infarction and cerebrovascular accidents. These results suggest that COPD maybe associated with abnormalities of the immune system that predispose to increased risk of cardiovascular disease, repeat infections, and cancer. However, the exact biological mechanisms have not been elucidated. An important conclusion of these studies is that COPD is a systemic disease and reducing all-cause mortality may require novel and systemic approaches.

MANAGEMENT

Goals of Management of Stable Disease

Goals of management of stable COPD in the outpatient setting include slow disease progression, improvement of symptoms, particularly dyspnea and reduced exercise tolerance, prevent exacerbation, and reduce mortality. Smoking cessation and supplemental oxygen are the only interventions that have shown to reduce all-cause mortality. Current pharmacologic interventions neither reduce mortality nor influence the rate of decline of lung function. An overview of different therapies based on disease severity are shown in Fig. 83-8.

Smoking Cessation

Smoking cessation is difficult to achieve and more difficult to sustain in the general population. Physician-delivered smoking cessation interventions can significantly increase smoking abstinence rates. An empathetic, nonconfrontational interaction that maximizes patient participation is most effective. The essential elements of a smoking cessation program should include: (1) physician intervention (set a quit date) and appropriate follow-up; (2) group smoking cessation programs; and (3) pharmacologic therapy with nicotine replacement in highly dependent smokers. Such smokers can be identified as those who smoke a pack a day or more, require their first cigarette within 30 minutes of arising in the morning, and find it difficult refraining

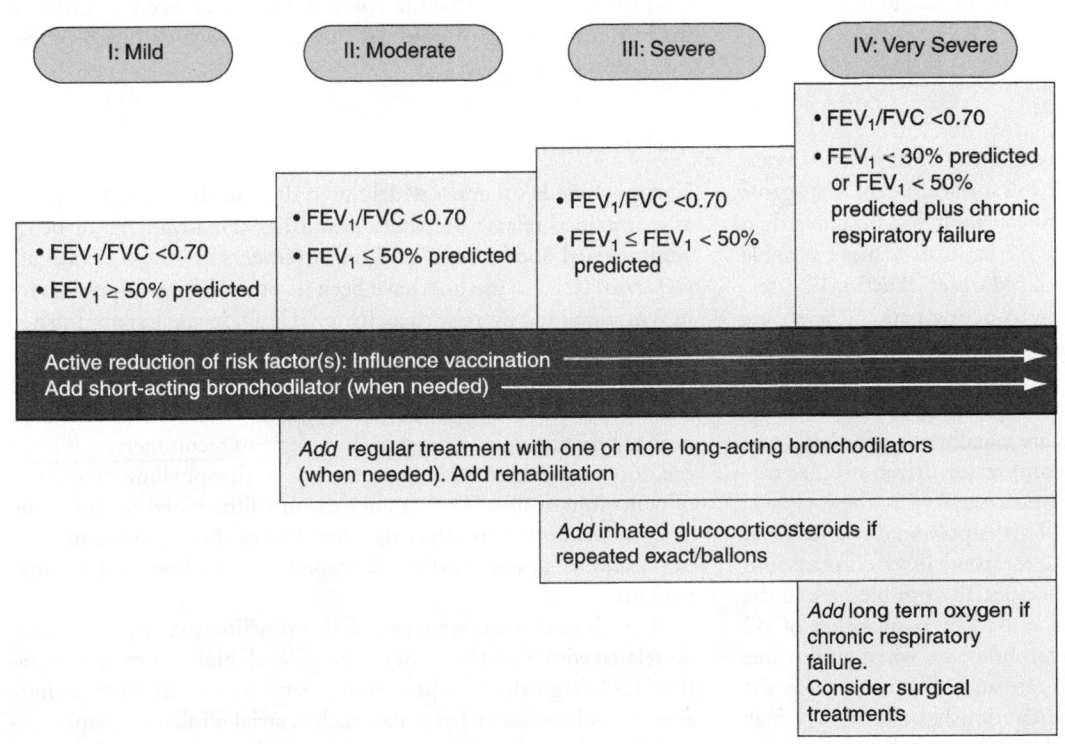

FIGURE 83-8. Overview of treatment for COPD by disease severity. (From GOLD. www.goldcopd.com)

from smoking in places where it is forbidden. Therapy with the antidepressants, such as bupropion hydrochloride and nortryptiline, are effective and when used with nicotine replacement can yield quit rates that approach 35%. The LHS showed that despite intensive antismoking efforts, middle-aged smokers with COPD are not likely to quit and only 22% were sustained quitters at 5 years.

Smoking cessation rates are similar in the elderly compared to younger individuals. For instance, the Wisconsin Tobacco Quit Line program, which targeted older smokers by providing free nicotine patches and phone counseling, showed that 43% of the senior participants had successfully quit at 9 months. A recent survey among adult smokers older than 60 years was conducted by the Center of Social Gerontology and revealed that a key motivation to quit smoking was to improve health. There were varying levels of awareness of smoking cessation aids among these participants. The lack of information from physicians recommending or educating them about smoking cessation aids was an important barrier to try these interventions. These observations underscore the need to educate smokers about the health benefits and the various aids to quit smoking. Older adults fear that they will fail to quit smoking and therefore, the elderly patient must be reminded that the average smoker who successfully quits has done so after five to six attempts. The clinician's responsibility is to remember that tobacco addiction is a chronic disease and treatment should be offered at every visit. Several hotlines are offered by the American Cancer Society and the National Cancer Institute to help quit smoking.

Pharmacologic Management

The goal of pharmacologic management is to provide symptomatic relief, improve exercise capacity, and prevent exacerbations. A step-wise approach is provided in Figure 83-8. The average age of subjects recruited in most clinical trials for COPD is 65 years and few subjects older than 85 years are recruited in these studies. Therefore, the efficacy and side-effect profile of these medications in the very old remains unclear.

Short- and Long-Acting Beta Agonist

These agents act by relaxing airway smooth muscle by a direct action on the β2-adrenergic receptors on the cell surface. While oral agents are available, their side effect profile makes them less desirable than the inhaled agents. The short-acting β2 agonists achieve variable degrees of bronchodilatation, with a rapid onset of action of a few minutes, and last for 4 to 6 hours. Short-acting beta2 agonists are used for symptom control. In contrast, long-acting beta2 agonist last for 12 hours and are useful for maintenance therapy. Both improve shortness of breath, cough, and in most patients, improve exercise capacity. Short-acting beta2 agonists are usually prescribed as a metered dose inhaler (MDI) or with a compressor-driven nebulizer.

Despite minimal systemic absorption seen with these agents, slight tachycardia may be observed. This is presumably a result of vasodilatation from stimulation of β2 receptors in vascular smooth muscle. Tremor may also occur and is especially troublesome in the geriatric patient. It is thought to be caused by stimulation of β2 receptors in skeletal muscle. In general, however, when given three or four times a day, β2 agonists are safe and effective even in the elderly. Higher doses should be used cautiously because they may cause hypokalemia, especially when the patient is taking a diuretic.

Salmeterol and formoterol are two long-acting beta2 agonists. In the recent TORCH trial, salmeterol alone reduced exacerbations compared to placebo and the combination of salmeterol and fluticose provided additional benefit. A similar benefit was seen with salmeterol on health-related quality of life. There is no evidence of tachyphylaxis with these agents. Though beta receptor function diminishes with age, the short- and long-acting β2 agonists should be used because of their proven track record.

Anticholinergic Agents

Ipratropium and tiotropium are two anticholinergic agents. These agents cause bronchodilatation and are capable of rapidly relieving symptoms. Muscarinic (M) receptors are present in the bronchial smooth muscles. M1 and M3 mediate bronchoconstriction, while M2 inhibits release of acetylcholine and thus results in feedback inhibition. Tiotropium has the advantage of prolonged action, lasting for 24 hours, and specifically inhibits M1 and M3 receptors, while it dissociates more quickly from M2 receptors. Ipratropium bromide has duration of action of 4 to 6 hours. Its onset of action is 30 minutes. This has made a single MDI of the combination of albuterol, a short-acting β2 agonist, and the anticholinergic, ipratropium bromide, very popular.

Tiotropium has a beneficial effect in reducing exacerbation rates compared to placebo or ipratropium bromide and improved health-related quality of life relative to placebo. An important beneficial effect of tiotropium is improvement in baseline FEV_1. Therefore, tiotropium is preferred over ipratropium in patients with severe COPD.

As these agents are poorly absorbed, the side effects are generally mild. Occasionally, patients complain of a dry mouth or metallic taste. Worsening symptoms of prostrate enlargement and acute glaucoma are rare. Plasma concentrations are higher in individuals with moderate or severe renal failure, and therefore should be used cautiously. Ophthalmic complications may occur because of inadvertent spraying of eyes and can easily be avoided with proper inhalation techniques.

Methylxanthines

Theophylline is the most widely used drug in this class. It is given as a sustained-release preparation and has the advantage of being administered once a day. Small improvements in lung function are seen with chronic use and have been associated with improvement in symptoms and exercise capacity in COPD. Its use has diminished over the past decade because of safety concerns, especially in the elderly. While there is in general a steady decline in drug metabolism from early to late adulthood, theophylline clearance does not appear to be sufficiently altered in the elderly to recommend reducing the dose. The narrow therapeutic range of theophylline, frequency of concomitant illnesses that alter theophylline kinetics, and many drug interactions that affect the clearance of theophylline, make it important to closely monitor the blood theophylline level in older patients.

The clinical manifestations of theophylline toxicity have been correlated with blood levels of the drug. With high serum concentrations ($>30\ \mu g/mL$), life-threatening events may occur. They include seizures and cardiac arrhythmias, such as atrial fibrillation, supraventricular tachycardia, ventricular ectopy, and ventricular tachycardia.

The most common cause for theophylline toxicity is a self-administered increase in medication. There is a stepwise increase in the frequency of life-threatening events caused by theophylline toxicity with advancing age. At comparable theophylline blood levels, patients older than age 75 years have a 16-fold greater risk of life-threatening events or death than do patients younger than age 25 years. The risk of theophylline toxicity can be minimized with careful patient monitoring, including checking blood levels and patient education. A range of 8 to 15 μg/mL is generally considered therapeutic and gives a margin of error that helps avoid toxicity.

Corticosteroids

Long-term oral corticosteroid treatment is not recommended for COPD. Some have advocated giving a short course of oral corticosteroids for 2 weeks to identify patients with asthma and bronchitis, but such a short-term response is not an effective predictor. Complications include cataracts, osteoporosis, secondary infection, diabetes, skin damage, and steroid myopathy, which contribute to respiratory muscle weakness, poor exercise tolerance, and respiratory failure.

Inhaled corticosteroids reduce exacerbation frequency, health-related quality of life, exercise capacity, and improve FEV_1. Although observational studies suggest that they may improve mortality, results of randomized clinical trials have failed to demonstrate improvement in all-cause mortality. Treatment with inhaled corticosteroids therefore has been recommended only for patients with moderate to advanced COPD. Two side effects, including bone loss and increased incidence of community-acquired pneumonia, can occur with chronic use, though the clinical relevance of pneumonia is uncertain. Different dosages of inhaled steroids have different potencies. In most clinical trials, 500 μg bid of fluticasone or 400 μg bid of budesonide has been used. Whether lower doses of inhaled corticosteroids can achieve similar efficacy is uncertain.

The combination of salmeterol and fluticasone has recently been shown to be better than individual medication in a randomized controlled trial of more than 6000 subjects. The average age of participants was 65 years. In this study, the combination of salmeterol and fluticasone reduced frequency of exacerbation, lung function decline, and improved health-related quality of life. Compared to placebo, the absolute reduction in all-cause mortality was 2.6% (relative reduction of 17.5%), but the results failed to reach statistical significance when adjusted for multiple interim analyses (adjusted p-value = 0.052 and unadjusted p-value = 0.04).

Inhalation Techniques

The inhaled route of therapy for COPD is preferred because it provides quicker action, fewer side effects, and greater bronchodilatation with smaller doses of medication. MDIs are the most commonly used methods for delivery of bronchodilators and corticosteroids. The great majority of the medication delivered by MDIs is deposited in the oropharynx, with only approximately 10% of the dose delivered to the lungs. Oropharyngeal deposition causes greater systemic absorption, more local irritation, and for corticosteroids, more likelihood of oropharyngeal candidiasis. Inadequate timing of actuation and inhalation is the most frequent error. Impaired mental function, weakened or deformed hands, and motor or musculoskeletal diseases are other reasons for inadequate MDI use. There are several solutions to this problem. One may deliver short-acting β agonists,

ipratropium, and corticosteroid, budesonide, as aerosolized solutions by pressurized handheld nebulizers. Alternatively, there is a breath-actuated pressurized MDI that obviates the need to synchronize activation with inhalation. The use of spacer devices fitted to the mouthpiece of the MDI can overcome most of the drawbacks of MDI therapy. Spacers are cheap, easy to carry, reduce oropharyngeal deposition, and increase intrapulmonary deposition. Lastly, newer dry-powder delivery devices that deliver inhaled corticosteroids and long-acting β agonists provide simple, easy-to-use preparations that do not require coordination or muscle strength.

Mucolytic Agents

Mixed results have been reported for the use of mucolytic agents, such as N-acetyl cysteine, and expectorants, such as Guaifenesin, as chronic maintenance therapy for COPD. Symptoms may improve in some patients with COPD, especially those with viscous sputum. However, overall the benefits are small and their widespread use is not recommended. Randomized controlled trials suggest that they are ineffective at shortening the course or improving outcomes of patients with acute exacerbations of COPD.

Phosphodiesterase (PDE)-4 Inhibitors

PDE-4 is a major regulator of cyclic adenosine monophosphate metabolism in smooth muscle and immune cells. Since cyclic adenosine monophosphate downregulates the activity of these cells, the inhibition of PDE-4 is an attractive target for COPD drug development. Early studies with a PDE-4 inhibitor, Cilomilast, suggest that it causes bronchodilatation and may improve quality of life. Further studies are necessary before this class of drugs can be recommended for routine use.

Adjunct Therapies

Treatment with calcium and vitamin D supplementation should be considered in older COPD patients with osteoporosis. Depression and anxiety are common in COPD patients and treatment may improve quality of life. Although pneumococcal and influenza vaccination have limited efficacy in the elderly, routine use is recommended in COPD patients because vaccination is associated with few side effects and these organisms are an important cause of acute exacerbations or community-acquired pneumonia.

Nonpharmacologic Interventions

Oxygen Therapy

Several controlled studies have been done regarding the efficacy of long-term oxygen. These have been summarized by Crockett et al. In addition to smoking cessation, it is the only intervention to improve survival in advanced COPD. The beneficial effect is related to the duration of oxygen use. For example, patients who receive oxygen for 19 hours or more a day are likely to survive longer than those who use it 12 or 15 hours a day. Patients who use chronic oxygen therapy are likely to have a significant fall in their pulmonary artery pressures and an increase in cardiac output. Table 83-3 provides recommendations for long-term oxygen use in COPD. Long-term oxygen therapy does not improve survival in patients with moderate

TABLE 83-3

Criteria for Home Oxygen in COPD

At rest
  Arterial partial pressure of oxygen (PaO_2) less than or equal to 55 mm Hg
  or arterial oxygen saturation (SaO_2) less than or equal to 88%
  PaO_2 levels between 56 and 59 or SaO_2 89% in the presence of
  pulmonary hypertension, *cor pulmonale*, edema secondary to right
  heart failure, or erythrocytosis with hematocrit greater than 55%

Following exercise (supplemental oxygen to be used during exercise only)
  Patients who desaturate to an SaO_2 less than or equal to 88% during
  exercise and who demonstrate improvement in both the hypoxia and
  dyspnea and/or exercise capacity when using oxygen

hypoxemia (PaO_2, 56 to 65 mm Hg) or in patients with nocturnal hypoxemia alone.

Pulmonary Rehabilitation

Pulmonary rehabilitation is a multidisciplinary program for patients with moderate to advanced COPD, especially those who have suffered deconditioning, significant weight loss, depression, and social isolation. The goals of a rehabilitation program are to improve exercise capacity, return the patient to more normal activities of daily living, and improve motivation, psychological well-being, and overall quality of life. With the use of lower-extremity exercise training and upper-extremity strength and endurance training, pulmonary rehabilitation improves dyspnea, endurance, and quality-of-life scores. Its effects on exacerbation are less clear and it does not influence survival. The benefits of pulmonary rehabilitation are short-lived and wane once the program is completed. Continuation of these exercises at home may have additional benefit. However, the benefit of repeat rehabilitation is less clear.

Weight Loss and Malnutrition

Weight loss, particularly skeletal muscle mass loss, is associated with a systemic inflammatory response in COPD. Resting energy expenditure is elevated and contributes to the negative energy balance. Nutritional supplements alone do not reverse the loss; results with anabolic steroids, growth hormone, and the progestational agent, megestrol acetate, show some effect on appetite and body weight. However, improved exercise tolerance and respiratory muscle function does not always follow, and side effects are often limiting.

Noninvasive Positive Pressure Ventilation

The chronic nocturnal use of noninvasive ventilation for COPD is controversial. There are theoretical advantages. Resting chronically fatigued muscles at night might improve daytime function. COPD patients have a high prevalence of nocturnal hypoxemia but the incidence of sleep apnea is similar. They have less rapid eye movement (REM) sleep and shorter sleep duration. Trials have examined the role of nocturnal noninvasive ventilation in COPD patients. These studies were small and have shown conflicting results. In general, nocturnal NIPPV for at least 3 months in hypercapnic patients with stable COPD had no consistent effect on lung function, gas exchange, respiratory muscle strength, sleep efficiency, or exercise tolerance.

Surgery for COPD

Lung volume reduction surgery (LVRS) has emerged as a treatment for far advanced COPD caused by emphysema. It involves resection of functionless areas of emphysematous lung in order to improve lung elastic recoil and lung and chest wall hyperinflation.

The National Emphysema Treatment Trial Research Group examined the role of LVRS in over 1200 subjects. The average age of participants in this study was 65 years. Overall mortality with the procedure ranges between 0% and 6% within 30 days of surgery and between 0% and 8% at 6-months although in patients with very severe degrees of airflow obstruction and/or hypercarbia, the rates are higher. The range of FEV_1 improvement pre- and post-surgery is approximately 250 to 350 mL and dyspnea scores and distance walked on the 6-minute walk test show improvement. Often patients no longer require oxygen following surgery. LVRS did not confer a survival advantage over medical therapy. It does yield a survival advantage for patients with both predominantly upper-lobe emphysema and low baseline exercise capacity. Currently, it is a modality that is being used in specialized centers for selected patients.

Resection of large bullae is occasionally necessary. The best results occur when the bullae occupy more than one-third of the hemithorax. Lung transplantation can be lifesaving in advanced cases, but is not offered to those of advanced age.

ACUTE EXACERBATION OF COPD

COPD exacerbation is an important cause of increased morbidity, health care costs, and mortality. Older adults are at higher risk of mortality following hospitalization for an exacerbation compared to younger patients. Exacerbations are also an important cause of disability in the elderly. Therefore, prevention and optimal management of exacerbations is important.

There are many definitions of acute exacerbation of COPD. The most widely quoted criteria, referred to as "the Winnipeg criteria," are based on worsening of dyspnea, an increase in sputum volume, and sputum purulence. Patients with type I exacerbations have all of the above symptoms. Patients with type II exacerbations have two of the three symptoms, while those with Type III exacerbations have at least one of these symptoms. Patients with COPD are accustomed to frequent symptom changes and thus new symptoms are underreported to physicians and patients often do not seek medical care. On an average, patients with COPD have three exacerbations every year, while those with more severe COPD have higher frequency of exacerbation.

Before the onset of an exacerbation of COPD, there is a prodromal period up to 1 week with symptoms of increased dyspnea, cough, sore throat, and rhinorrhea. This is not accompanied by a drop in lung function. On the day of the exacerbation, there is a small but significant drop in lung function, including peak flow rates, FEV_1, and FVC. Airway and systemic inflammatory marker concentrations also increase during an acute exacerbation. Peak flow rate recovery to baseline values is complete in 75% of patients by 1 month. Approximately 7% of patients with a COPD exacerbation do not return their peak flow rates to baseline by 3 months. This suggests that exacerbations of COPD may result in permanent loss of lung function.

The most frequent cause of an acute exacerbation of COPD is respiratory infection. The most common organisms isolated during an exacerbation are viruses, including rhinovirus, respiratory syncytial virus, coronavirus, influenza, and parainfluenza, and the pathogenic bacteria that colonize these patients. Pathogenic bacteria that colonize COPD patients include *Haemophilus influenzae, Streptococcus pneumoniae,* and *Moraxella catarrhalis.* Although these bacteria are often isolated during a COPD exacerbation, whether they play a causal role is unclear. Prior to an exacerbation, new strains of these bacteria are isolated in the lower respiratory tract. Airway inflammation is also higher in patients colonized with pathogenic bacteria. These results suggest that bacterial infection may play an important role in exacerbations. Clearly, environmental factors are also important. Hospital admissions for COPD appear to be high when air pollution levels in the ambient environment are high.

Irrespective of the cause of an acute exacerbation, it is clear that bronchial inflammation is enhanced during this event. Increased levels of myeloperoxidase have been found in the sputum indicating neutrophilic activity, and high levels of IL-8 and LTB4, well-known neutrophil chemoattractants, are also seen. During recovery, levels of sputum chemoattractants and inflammatory markers rapidly fall.

Diagnostic and Therapeutic Approaches

The diagnosis of COPD exacerbation is based on clinical criteria alone. The vast majority of patients with COPD exacerbations are managed in the outpatient setting. When patients present to a local emergency room or hospital with an acute exacerbation of COPD, it is useful to do a chest roentgenogram to rule out community-acquired pneumonia and congestive heart failure. Once a decision has been made to admit the patient, the best indicators for the need for mechanical ventilation include the blood gas values on admission. Significant predictors of hospital mortality include older age, lower BMI, poor functional status prior to admission, lower $PO_2:FIO_2$ (fraction of inspired oxygen) ratio, history of congestive heart failure, low serum albumin, and presence of *cor pulmonale.*

Spirometry has not been helpful in decision-making for patients with an acute exacerbation of COPD. There is poor correlation between arterial blood gases and the FEV_1 at the time of presentation. FEV_1 has also not been helpful in predicting need for hospital admission.

Most therapeutic interventions for the treatment of the acute exacerbation of COPD have been studied through randomized controlled trials. Beta2-agonists and anticholinergic agents appear to be equivalent in their usefulness and are superior to all parenterally administered medications including methylxanthines (Figure 83-8). The addition of a methylxanthine to inhaled bronchodilators does not improve outcomes. There appears to be only marginal improvement when two inhaled bronchodilators are used. The side effects of anticholinergic therapy are generally few and mild. The adverse effects of using repeated albuterol nebulized treatments in the acute setting include tremors, headache, and palpitations. Changes in heart rate, blood pressure, and electrocardiogram tracings are also possible. Chest physiotherapy and mechanical percussion of the chest are also ineffective and maybe potentially harmful.

Systemic steroids are indicated in the inpatient and outpatient setting for a COPD exacerbation. For patients admitted to the hospital, systemic steroids for 2 weeks improved combined end point of death, need for mechanical ventilation, intensification of pharmacologic regime, and readmission at 30 days, though these benefits were not observed at 6 months. Longer duration of steroid therapy did not demonstrate additional benefits. For patients treated in the outpatient setting, oral prednisone therapy for 10 days improved symptoms and heath-related quality of life. The most common adverse effect of steroids is hyperglycemia, which may require at least short-term treatment.

The use of antibiotics for COPD exacerbation is controversial. The beneficial effect of antibiotic therapy is seen patients with severe exacerbation (Type I exacerbation) and those with severe COPD. The choice of antibiotic is influenced by the age of the patient, the severity of underlying COPD, and the risk of antibiotic resistance. Commonly prescribed antibiotics include penicillin, such as amoxicillin with clavulanic acid, doxycycline, macrolides, such as azithromycin and clarithromycin, fluroquinolones, such as levofloxacin and moxifloxacin. Patients with severe underlying COPD have higher likelihood of being colonized with gram-negative organisms. Furthermore, there is an increasing prevalence of organisms that produce bacterial enzymes that inactivate traditional β-lactam antibiotics, especially with *H. influenzae* and *M. catarrhalis.* Therefore, many of the antibiotics traditionally used for bronchial infections may provide inadequate coverage. Yet, no studies have demonstrated improved outcomes with newer antibiotics. Newer antibiotics are more expensive and cost should be taken into consideration while prescribing antibiotics for the elderly. It is also important to consider local resistance patterns and patient compliance. All of these factors should be considered while prescribing antibiotics for the elderly patient with COPD exacerbation.

Noninvasive positive pressure ventilation (NPPV) is beneficial for patients who have a high likelihood of respiratory failure and thus may prevent need for invasive mechanical ventilation. Optimal NPPV for the COPD exacerbation requires close patient monitoring, usually in an intensive care setting.

SUMMARY

COPD is an important chronic disease and it is an important cause of disability in the elderly. Over the next decade, COPD will be the third leading cause of death worldwide. Yet, it is often under recognized. In the outpatient setting, spirometry should be performed in older adults with symptoms of persistent dyspnea, cough, or decreased exercise capacity. Prompt identification of cases allows initiation of pharmacological and nonpharmacological therapies. Smoking cessation remains the most important intervention and has shown to reduce all-cause mortality. Although current pharmacologic therapies do not improve mortality, they reduce frequency of exacerbations and improve exercise capacity and quality of life. Most pharmacological trials in COPD do not include individuals older than 80 years and efficacy of current therapies in this population is not known. There is increasing emphasis in understanding the systemic consequences of COPD rather than focusing on pulmonary impairments alone. Systemic approaches, using immunomodulatory agents, maybe necessary to effectively manage this disease in the future.

FURTHER READING

Aaron SD, Vandemheen KL, Hebert P, et al. Outpatient oral prednisone after emergency treatment of chronic obstructive pulmonary disease. *N Engl J Med.* 2003;348:2618–2625.

Anthonisen NR, Connett JE, Kiley JP, et al. Effects of smoking intervention and the use of an inhaled anticholinergic bronchodilator on the rate of decline of FEV1. The Lung Health Study. *JAMA.* 1994;272:1497–1505.

Anthonisen NR, Manfreda J, Warren CP, Hershfield ES, Harding GK, Nelson NA. Antibiotic therapy in exacerbations of chronic obstructive pulmonary disease. *Ann Intern Med.* 1987;106:196–204.

Barnes PJ. Theophylline: new perspectives for an old drug. *Am J Respir Crit Care Med.* 2003;167:813–818.

Bott J, Carroll MP, Conway JH, et al. Randomised controlled trial of nasal ventilation in acute ventilatory failure due to chronic obstructive airways disease. *Lancet.* 1993;341:1555–1557.

Calverley PMA, Anderson JA, Celli B, et al. Salmeterol and fluticasone propionate and survival in chronic obstructive pulmonary disease. *N Engl J Med.* 2007;356:775–789.

Casaburi R, Mahler DA, Jones PW, et al. A long-term evaluation of once-daily inhaled tiotropium in chronic obstructive pulmonary disease. *Eur Respir J.* 2002;19:217–224.

Celli BR, Cote CG, Marin JM, et al. The body–mass index, airflow obstruction, dyspnea, and exercise capacity index in chronic obstructive pulmonary disease. *N Engl J Med.* 2004;350:1005–1012.

Cole P, Rodu B. Declining cancer mortality in the United States. *Cancer.* 1996;78:2045–2048.

Crockett AJ, Cranston JM, Moss JR, Alpers JH. A review of long-term oxygen therapy for chronic obstructive pulmonary disease [review]. *Respir Med.* 2001;95(6):437–443.

Debigare R, Cote CH, Maltais F. Peripheral muscle wasting in chronic obstructive pulmonary disease. Clinical relevance and mechanisms. *Am J Respir Crit Care Med.* 2001;164:1712–1717.

Donaldson GC, Seemungal TAR, Bhowmik A, Wedzicha JA. Relationship between exacerbation frequency and lung function decline in chronic obstructive pulmonary disease. *Thorax.* 2002;57:847–852.

Fukuchi YF, Nishimura MF, Ichinose MF, et al. COPD in Japan: the Nippon COPD Epidemiology Study. *Respirology.* 2004;9(4):458–465.

Gan WQ, Man SF, Senthilselvan A, Sin DD. Association between chronic obstructive pulmonary disease and systemic inflammation: a systematic review and a meta-analysis. *Thorax.* 2004;59:574–580.

Global Initiative for Chronic Obstructive Lung Disease. www.goldcopd.com. Accessed Jan 31st 2008.

Griffith KA, Sherrill D, Siegel E, Manolio TA, Bonekat H, Enright PL. Predictors of loss of lung function in the elderly. The Cardiovascular Health Study. *Am J Respir Crit Care Med.* 2001;163:61–68.

Halbert RJ, Natoli JL, Gano AF, Badamgarav E, Buist AS, Mannino DM. Global burden of COPD: systematic review and meta-analysis. *Eur Respir J.* 2006;28(3):523–532.

Halbert RJ, Isonaka S, George D, Iqbal A. Interpreting COPD prevalence estimates: what is the true burden of disease?. *Chest.* 2003;123:1684–1692.

Hamilton AL, Killian KJ, Summers E, Jones NL. Muscle strength, symptom intensity, and exercise capacity in patients with cardiorespiratory disorders. *Am J Respir Crit Care Med.* 1995;152:2021–2031.

Heaton RK, Grant I, McSweeny AJ, Adams KM, Petty TL. Psychologic effects of continuous and nocturnal oxygen therapy in hypoxemic chronic obstructive pulmonary disease. *Ann Intern Med.* 1982;142:1470–1476.

Hu FB, Stampfer MJ, Manson JE, et al. Trends in the incidence of coronary heart disease and changes in diet and lifestyle in women. *N Engl J Med.* 2000;343:530–537.

Huan SL, Su CH, Chang S. Tumor necrosis factor-alpha gene polymorphism in chronic bronchitis. *Am J Respir Crit Care Med.* 1997;156:1436–1439.

Ishii T, Matsuse T, Teramoto S, et al. Glutathione S-transferase P1 (GSTP1) polymorphism in patients with chronic obstructive pulmonary disease. *Thorax.* 1999;54:693–696.

Jones PW, Bosh TK. Quality of life changes in COPD patients treated with salmeterol. *Am J Respir Crit Care Med.* 1997;155:1283–1289.

Jorgensen NR, Schwarz P, Holme I, Henriksen BM, Petersen LJ, Backer V. The prevalence of osteoporosis in patients with chronic obstructive pulmonary disease—a cross sectional study. *Respir Med.* 2007;101:177–185.

Kueppers F, Miller RD, Gordon H, Hepper NG, Offord K. Familial prevalence of chronic obstructive pulmonary disease in a matched pair study. *Am J Med.* 1977;63:336–342.

Lacasse YF, Brosseau LF, Milne S, et al. Pulmonary rehabilitation for chronic obstructive pulmonary disease. *Cochrane Database Syst Rev.* 2002;(3):CD003793; *Lancet.* 1996;748:1115–1119.

Lange P, Groth S, Nyboe GJ, et al. Effects of smoking and changes in smoking habits on the decline of FEV1. *Eur Respir J.* 1989;2:811–816.

Larson RK, Barman ML, Kueppers FF, Fudenberg HH. Genetic and environmental determinants of chronic obstructive pulmonary disease. *Ann Intern Med.* 1970;72(5):627–632.

Littner MR, Ilowite JS, Tashkin DP, et al. Long-acting bronchodilation with once-daily dosing of tiotropium (spiriva) in stable chronic obstructive pulmonary disease. *Am J Respir Crit Care Med.* 2000;161:1136–1142.

Lokke A, Lange P, Scharling H, Fabricius P, Vestbo J. Developing COPD: a 25 year follow up study of the general population. *Thorax.* 2006;61:935–939.

MacNee W. Right ventricular function in cor pulmonale [review]. *Cardiology.* 1988;75(Suppl 1):30–40.

Mannino DM, Brown C, Giovino GA. Obstructive lung disease deaths in the United States from 1979 through 1993. An analysis using multiple-cause mortality data. *Am J Respir Crit Care Med.* 1997;156:814–818.

Mannino DM, Gagnon RC, Petty TL, Lydick E. Obstructive lung disease and low lung function in adults in the United States: Data from the National Health and Nutrition Examination Survey, 1988–1994. *Arch Intern Med.* 2000;160:1683–1689.

Mannino DM, Sonia Buist A, Vollmer WM. Chronic obstructive pulmonary disease in the older adult: what defines abnormal lung function? *Thorax.* 2007;62:237–241.

Mannino DM. COPD: epidemiology, prevalence, morbidity and mortality, and disease heterogeneity [review]. *Chest.* 2002;121(5 Suppl):121S–126S.

Menezes AM, Perez-Padilla R, Jardim JB, et al. Chronic obstructive pulmonary disease in five Latin American cities (the PLATINO study): a prevalence study. *Lancet.* 2005;366:1875–1881.

Michaud CM, Murray CJL, Bloom BR. Burden of disease—implications for future research. *JAMA.* 2001;285:535–539.

Murray CJ, Lopez AD. Alternative projections of mortality and disability by cause 1990–2020: Global Burden of Disease Study. *Lancet.* 1997;349:1498–1504.

Murray CJ, Lopez AD. Global mortality, disability, and the contribution of risk factors: Global Burden of Disease Study. *Lancet.* 1997;349:1436–1442.

Murray CJ, Lopez AD. Mortality by cause for eight regions of the world: Global Burden of Disease Study. *Lancet.* 1997;349:1269–1276.

National Center for Health Statistics. www.cdc/nchs.gov. Accessed January 31, 2008.

National Emphysema Treatment Trial Research Group. A randomized trial comparing lung-volume-reduction surgery with medical therapy for severe emphysema. *N Engl J Med.* 2003;NEJMoa030287.

National Health Interview Survey. www.cdc.gov/nchs/about/major/nhanes/datalink.htm. Accessed Jan 31st 2008.

Niewoehner DE, Erbland ML, Deupree RH, et al. Effect of systemic glucocorticoids on exacerbations of chronic obstructive pulmonary disease. *N Engl J Med.* 1999;340:1941–1947.

Renwick DS, Connolly MJ. Do respiratory symptoms predict chronic airflow obstruction and bronchial hyperresponsiveness in older adults? *J Gerontol A Biol Sci Med Sci.* 1999;54(3):M136–M139.

Repine JE, Bast A, Lankhorst I. Oxidative stress in chronic obstructive pulmonary disease. Oxidative Stress Study Group. *Am J Resp Crit Car Med.* 1997;156:341–357.

Saint S, Bent S, Vittinghoff E, Grady D. Antibiotics in chronic obstructive pulmonary disease exacerbations. A meta-analysis. *JAMA.* 1995;273:957–960.

Schirnhofer L, Lamprecht B, Vollmer WM, et al. COPD prevalence in Salzburg, Austria: results from the Burden of Obstructive Lung Disease (BOLD) Study. *Chest.* 2007;131(1):29–36.

Seneff MG, Wagner DP, Wagner RP, Zimmerman JE, Knaus WA. Hospital and 1-year survival of patients admitted to intensive care units with acute exacerbation of chronic obstructive pulmonary disease. *JAMA.* 1995;274:1852–1857.

Sethi S, Evans N, Grant BJB, Murphy TF. New strains of bacteria and exacerbations of chronic obstructive pulmonary disease. *N Engl J Med.* 2002;347:465–471.

Sin DD, Anthonisen NR, Soriano JB, Agusti AG. Mortality in COPD: role of comorbidities. *Eur Resp J.* 2006;28:1245–1257.

Smith CA, Harrison DJ. Association between polymorphism in gene for microsomal epoxide hydrolase and susceptibility to emphysema. *Lancet.* 1997;350:630–633.

Soriano JB, Vestbo J, Pride NB, Kiri V, Maden C, Maier WC. Survival in COPD patients after regular use of fluticasone propionate and salmeterol in general practice. *Eur Resp J.* 2002;20(4):819–825.

Spruit MA, Gosselink R, Troosters T, et al. Muscle force during an acute exacerbation in hospitalised patients with COPD and its relationship with CXCL8 and IGF-I. *Thorax.* 2003;58:752–756.

Stockley RA. Neutrophils and protease/antiprotease imbalance. *Am J Respir Crit Care Med.* 1999;160:49S–52S.

Suissa S. Effectiveness of inhaled corticosteroids in chronic obstructive pulmonary disease: immortal time bias in observational studies. *Am J Respir Crit Care Med.* 2003;168:49–53.

Suki B, Lutchen KR, Ingenito EP. On the progressive nature of emphysema: roles of proteases, inflammation, and mechanical forces. *Am J Respir Crit Care Med.* 2003;168:516–521.

Tager IF, Tishler PV, Rosner BF, Speizer FE, Litt M. Studies of the familial aggregation of chronic bronchitis and obstructive airways disease. *Int J Epidemiol.* 1978;7(1):55–62.

Tzanakis N, Anagnostopoulou UF, Filaditaki VF, et al. Prevalence of COPD in Greece. Global burden of COPD: systematic review and meta-analysis. *Chest.* 2004;125(3):892–900.

Waterer GW, Wan JY, Kritchevsky SB, et al. Airflow limitation is underrecognized in well-functioning older people. *J Am Geriatr Soc.* 2001;49:1032–1038.

Wewers MD, Casolaro MA, Sellers SE, et al. Replacement therapy for alpha 1-antitrypsin deficiency associated with emphysema. *N Engl J Med.* 1987;316: 1055–1062.

Yamada N, Yamaya M, Okinaga S, et al. Microsatellite polymorphism in the heme oxygenase-1 gene promoter is associated with susceptibility to emphysema. *Am J Hum Genet.* 2000;66:187–195.

Yende S, Tuomanen EI, Wunderink RG, et al. Pre-infection systemic inflammatory markers and risk of hospitalization due to pneumonia. *Am J Respir Crit Care Med.* 2005;172:1440–1446.

Yende S, Waterer GW, Tolley EA, et al. Inflammatory markers are associated with ventilatory limitation and muscle dysfunction in obstructive lung disease in well functioning elderly subjects. *Thorax.* 2006;61:10–16.

Zielinski JF, MacNee WF, Wedzicha JF, et al. Causes of death in patients with COPD and chronic respiratory failure. *Monaldi Arch Chest Dis.* 1997;52(1):43–47.

Diffuse Parenchymal Lung Disease

Victor J. Thannickal ■ *Galen B. Toews*

INTRODUCTION

The lung brings the ambient air that we breathe into close proximity with the systemic circulation. This allows for its essential function in gas exchange. However, this also exposes the lung to a variety of potentially injurious infectious and noninfectious environmental agents. The normal host response to such insults is to eradicate the etiologic agent and to repair the injury caused either directly by the agent or indirectly by the associated inflammatory process. This complex but well orchestrated and tightly regulated host response leads to eventual resolution of injury and restoration of normal lung architecture and function in most cases. However, if the inflammatory and/or repair response is dysregulated, a chronic alveolar/interstitial remodeling process with varying degrees of inflammation and fibrosis ensues. Damage to the pulmonary vascular endothelium via the circulation (e.g., drugs, systemic rheumatic disorders) may produce similar inflammatory/fibrotic reactions in the lung. This results in the restrictive physiology and gas-exchange abnormalities characteristic of the diffuse parenchymal lung diseases (DPLDs). When all potential etiologic agents and associations are considered, the list of DPLDs includes over 150 different clinical entities (Table 84-1). Thus, DPLDs comprise a large and heterogeneous group of diseases that are grouped into a single category based on common features in their clinical, radiographic, and physiological presentations.

The most prevalent and devastating of all the DPLDs is idiopathic pulmonary fibrosis (IPF), a chronic fibrotic disease of unknown etiology. IPF is primarily a disease of elderly patients. Elderly patients maybe particularly susceptible to this disease because of inherent deficiencies in immune function and/or in their inability to mount an appropriate repair response. Alternatively, IPF may present in elderly patients as a result of accumulated insults or because early manifestations of the disease are difficult to recognize. In this chapter, we will focus on emerging new concepts regarding IPF pathogenesis and the challenges facing clinicians taking care of these patients.

We will also discuss other selected DPLDs that are relatively more common in the geriatric population.

EPIDEMIOLOGY

The prevalence of DPLD is estimated at about 20 to 40 per 100,000 in the United States DPLD accounts for 100,000 hospital admissions yearly. The increased use of pneumotoxic drugs to treat malignant and cardiovascular diseases in the elderly as well the rising median age of the U.S. population contribute to an increased incidence.

IPF has been reclassified into a group of diseases designated as the "idiopathic interstitial pneumonias" (IIPs) (Table 84-1). IIPs are rare in children, but increase with advancing age. IPF, the most common of the IIPs, has a prevalence of 6 to 14.6 per 100,000 persons in different series. In patients older than the age of 75 years, however, the prevalence may exceed 175 per 100,000. The median age of onset of IPF ranges from 50 to 70 years and the diagnosis is almost never made in a patient aged 40 years or younger. In contrast, other IIPs such as nonspecific interstitial pneumonia (NSIP) appear to occur in younger patients.

PROGNOSIS AND NATURAL HISTORY

DPLDs represent a group of clinical syndromes with varying histopathological patterns ranging from predominantly inflammatory to more fibrotic tissue reactions. This is well illustrated by the IIPs that comprise primarily inflammatory tissue reactions such as desquamative interstitial pneumonia (DIP) and NSIP, in contrast to fibrotic histopathological patterns such as usual interstitial pneumonia (UIP). The histopathological subtype has important clinical and prognostic significance. UIP, the histopathological correlate of IPF, carries the worst prognosis and is, in general, unresponsive

TABLE 84-1

Classification of Diffuse Parenchymal Lung Disease (DPLD)

Idiopathic Interstitial Pneumonias

Idiopathic pulmonary fibrosis (IPF)/Usual
  interstitial pneumonia (UIP)

Nonspecific interstitial pneumonia (NSIP)

Cryptogenic organizing pneumonia
  (COP; BOOP)

Acute interstitial pneumonia (AIP)

Respiratory bronchiolitis interstitial lung
  disease (RB-ILD)

Desquamative interstitial pneumonia (DIP)

Lymphoid interstitial pneumonia (LIP)

**Other DPLD (with Primary Lung
  Involvement)**

Sarcoidosis

Histiocytosis X

Lymphangioleiomyomatosis

**DPLD Associated with Systemic
  Rheumatic Disease**

Rheumatoid arthritis

Systemic lupus erythematosis

Scleroderma

Polymyositis-dermatomyositis

Sjogren's syndrome

Mixed connective tissue disease

Ankylosing spondylitis

**DPLD Associated with Drugs or
  Treatments**

Antibiotics

Anti-inflammatory agents

Cardiovascular drugs

Antineoplastic drugs

Illicit drugs

Dietary supplements

Oxygen

Radiation

Paraquat

**DPLD Associated with
  Environmental
  (Occupational) Exposures**

Organic dusts/hypersensitivity
  pneumonitis (> 40 known
  agents)

  Farmer's lung

  Air conditioner–humidifier
    lung

  Bird breeder's lung

  Baggasosis

Inorganic dusts

  Silicosis

  Asbestosis

  Coal worker's pneumoconiosis

  Berylliosis

Gases/fumes/vapors

  Oxides of nitrogen

  Sulfur dioxide

  Toluene diisocyanate

  Oxides of metals

  Hydrocarbons

  Thermosetting resins

**DPLD Associated with
  "Alveolar Filling"**

Diffuse alveolar hemorrhage

Goodpasture's syndrome

Idiopathic pulmonary
  hemosiderosis

Pulmonary alveolar proteinosis

Chronic eosinophilic pneumonia

Chronic aspiration syndrome

Lipoid pneumonia

**DPLD Associated with
  Pulmonary Vasculitis**

Wegener's granulomatosis

Churg–Strauss syndrome

Hypersensitivity vasculitis

Necrotizing sarcoid
  granulomatosis

Inherited DPLD

Familial idiopathic pulmonary
  fibrosis

Neurofibromatosis

Tuberous sclerosis

Gaucher's disease

Niemann–Pick disease

Hermansky–Pudlak syndrome

to anti-inflammatory and immune-modulating therapies. The finding of UIP on lung biopsy predicts a median survival of less than 5 years. Other baseline characteristics that predict a poor prognosis include a low DL_{CO}, increased $A–a$ gradient, desaturation during a 6-minute walk test (SaO_2 < 88%), pulmonary arterial hypertension (mPAP >25 mm Hg), and the finding of honeycombing on high-resolution computed tomography (HRCT). Dynamic predictors of poor prognosis include a decline in forced vital capacity (FVC)

≥ 10 (% predicted) over a 6-month period, decline in DLCO ≥ 15 (% predicted) over a 12-month period and serial changes in dyspnea score.

The precise relationships between different histopathological subtypes are not well defined. For example, it is not known if NSIP precedes UIP in the natural history of the disease or if they represent distinct tissue reaction patterns to an unknown injury in patients with varying host genetic/susceptibility factors (see section on "Pathogenesis"). With regard to the natural history of IPF, there is significant heterogeneity in the patient population. While the majority of patients experience a steady and inexorable decline in lung function, a significant proportion of patients with IPF succumb to acute exacerbations of the disease. The etiology and pathogenesis of these acute exacerbations are currently unknown.

PATHOGENESIS

The pathogenesis of the DPLDs is complex. Significant differences in pathogenesis likely exist among the histopathological subtypes of IIP. Since UIP is also the most common form of IIP and since UIP/IPF exhibits an age-dependent increase in prevalence, we will focus on the pathogenesis of this clinical syndrome. IPF is localized to the lung parenchyma. Early histopathological evidence of alveolar epithelial cell injury and apoptosis suggests an inhaled route of entry for a putative injurious agent and/or an intrinsic abnormality specific to the alveolar epithelial cell. The temporal and spatial heterogeneity of the fibrotic lesions in UIP suggests that the injury maybe recurrent and repetitive, occurring over many years. Although the identity of a specific extrinsic agent has not been identified, latent viral infections and environmental toxins, including cigarette smoke, have been implicated. Alternatively, or in concert, intrinsic defects in alveolar epithelial cell function and fate may drive the fibrogenic tissue response (Figure 84-1).

There is an increasing recognition that the aging process per se and the biology of cellular senescence influence tissue repair responses. Cellular senescence may affect the function and behavior of alveolar epithelial cells. Senescent epithelial cells with shortened telomeres are generally more susceptible to apoptosis. Genetic mutations in telomerase and surfactant protein-C have been shown to be associated with familial cases of IPF, suggesting a link to intrinsic defects in alveolar epithelial cell function. Familial pulmonary fibrosis appears to be inherited as an autosomal dominant trait with variable penetrance. No systematic assessment has been made of the heritability of IPF in the general population or the risk to relatives of affected individuals. Various forms of fibrotic lung disease have been associated with gene polymorphisms of interleukin-1-receptor antagonist, tumor necrosis-α, and major histocompatability complex loci. Transforming growth factor-β1 gene polymorphisms resulting in increased production of this cytokine have been associated with more rapid progression of the disease in patients with established IPF. Thus, aging and host genetic factors are likely to determine the susceptibility to fibrotic sequelae and, perhaps, in the type of pathologic repair that ensues in sporadic cases of fibrotic lung disease.

Complex disorders such as UIP/IPF are influenced by the actions of multiple genes and their interactions with each other and the environment. Environmental factors modulate the response of the lung to injury. Of these, the most intriguing is the role of cigarette smoke. There is a strong association with cigarette smoking in

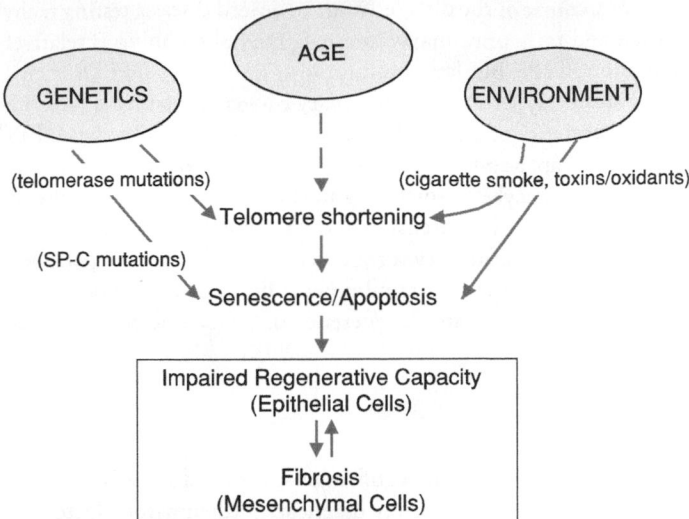

FIGURE 84-1. Host and environmental factors influence epithelial cell regenerative capacity. Mutations in the telomerase and surfactant protein-C (SP-C) genes have been linked to familial idiopathic pulmonary fibrosis; these telomerase and SP-C mutations induce cellular senescence and injury, respectively, leading to increased susceptibility of epithelial cells to apoptosis. Advancing age and extrinsic oxidative stress, including cigarette smoke, is also associated with telomere shortening and cellular senescence. Apoptosis of epithelial cells results in impaired re-epithelialization, loss of alveolar barrier function and activation of the underlying mesenchyme that culminates in fibrosis. The activated mesenchyme, in turn, may contribute to alveolar epithelial cell "dropout" by release of soluble mediators, further promoting epithelial dysrepair.

respiratory bronchiolitis-associated interstitial lung disease (RB-ILD) and DIP; cigarette smoke appears to play an etiologic role in the majority of these cases. Pulmonary histiocytosis X is diagnosed almost exclusively in active smokers. However, there is controversy regarding the role of cigarette smoke in IPF. Previous reports suggested that smoking was an independent risk factor for IPF. However, these studies may have included other cases of IIP, in addition to UIP. Some studies suggest a survival advantage in patients with IPF who

are cigarette smokers at the time of initial evaluation when compared with former smokers or never smokers. Interestingly, this presumed protection is associated with a histopathology that shows less interstitial cellularity and granulation/connective tissue formation but greater alveolar macrophage-predominant inflammation. The effect of cigarette smoke on the progression of IPF maybe as the result of factors that negatively regulate mesenchymal cell (myofibroblast) activation and/or promotes a specific type of inflammatory response.

The mesenchymal tissue response, in addition to the epithelium, may also be influenced by aging and cellular senescence. Age-related changes in extracellular matrix composition, expression of cell adhesion molecules, and altered cellular responses to growth factors have been reported in cells and tissues from various organ systems. For example, gene expression patterns in senescent fibroblasts have been shown to mimic chronic wound repair and, as such, senescent fibroblasts may contribute to ongoing fibrogenesis. Senescent fibroblasts may acquire an apoptosis-resistant phenotype. These observations support the establishment and perpetuation of an epithelial–mesenchymal paradox in which epithelial cells are in a continual state of disrepair and mesenchymal cells, in particular myofibroblasts, acquire resistance to apoptosis. Myofibroblasts in this context of lung injury-repair may derive from several sources, including the differentiation of lung-resident mesenchymal stem cells/fibroblasts, circulating fibrocytes or transdifferentiation from resident epithelial/endothelial cells (Figure 84-2) (Color Plate 12).

DIAGNOSTIC APPROACH

History

The most common presenting symptom is the insidious onset of exertional dyspnea that slowly progresses over many months and, in some cases, years. Initially, dyspnea is mild and the patient often does not seek medical attention. Dyspnea maybe attributed to other causes such as being "out-of-shape," normal aging, being overweight, or a viral infection. Patients may initially be misdiagnosed and

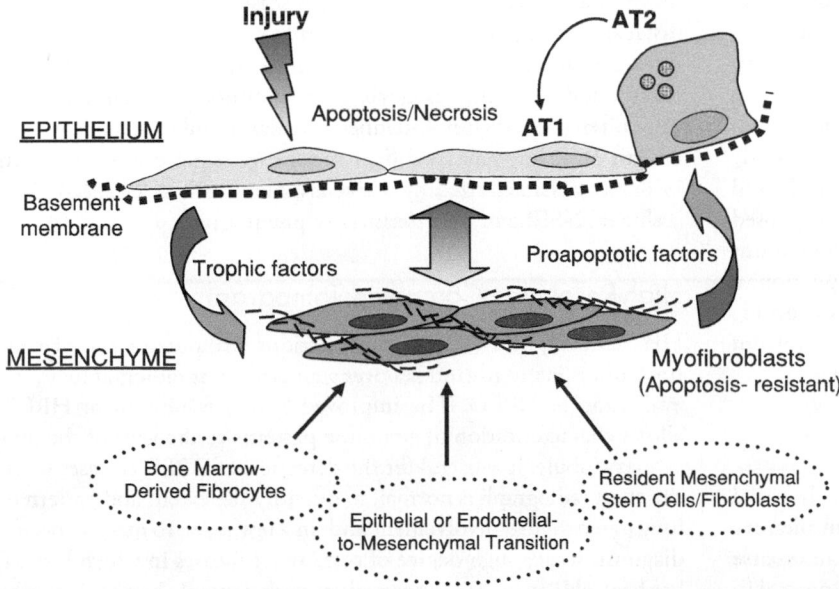

FIGURE 84-2. Epithelial–mesenchymal interactions in idiopathic pulmonary fibrosis (IPF). Current concepts on the pathogenesis of IPF suggest that repetitive alveolar epithelial injury result in aberrant or dysregulated repair responses with ensuing fibrosis. Alveolar type 1 (AT1) cells maybe more susceptible to injury/apoptosis, and alveolar type 2 (AT2) progenitor cells normally serve to reconstitute the alveolar epithelium by differentiating into AT1 cells. Recent studies suggest that AT2 cells in IPF may undergo epithelial–mesenchymal transition. Other potential sources of activated mesenchymal cells (myofibroblasts) include circulating fibrocytes and resident mesenchymal stem cells. Myofibroblasts, under the influence of trophic factors such as transforming growth factor-$\beta1$ acquire resistance to apoptosis. Additionally, activated myofibroblasts are capable of secreting soluble/diffusible factors such as angiotensin peptides, oxidants, and Fas ligand, which further contribute to impaired reepithelialization and unremitting fibrogenesis.

treated for other ailments (bronchitis, asthma, or heart failure). As the disease progresses, dyspnea occurs at rest. Nonproductive cough and fatigue are also prominent complaints. Cough is a frequent complaint in patients with cryptogenic organizing pneumonia (COP; also known as bronchiolitis obliterans organizing pneumonia, BOOP), eosinophilic pneumonia, RB-ILD, and IPF. Pleuritic chest pain may occur with DPLDs associated with systemic rheumatic disease and some drug-induced disorders. Pleuritic chest pain and sudden worsening of dyspnea should suggest a spontaneous pneumothorax, a characteristic finding in lymphangioleiomyomatosis, neurofibromatosis, tuberous sclerosis, and pulmonary histiocytosis X. Hemoptysis maybe the presenting complaint in patients with diffuse alveolar hemorrhage syndromes or lymphangioleiomyomatosis, but it is infrequent in other DPLDs. Hemoptysis should prompt a search for complications such as malignancy, superimposed infection, or pulmonary embolism.

The history often provides clues to a more specific diagnosis when a DPLD is associated with a systemic rheumatic disorder, an occupational or environmental exposure, or certain drug therapies. Most patients with DPLD associated with rheumatic diseases have an established diagnosis when pulmonary symptoms present or have extrapulmonary manifestations that provide clues to the underlying disorder. A careful history may also reveal an environmental or occupational exposure. A detailed, lifelong occupational history must be obtained because of the long latency periods between exposure and onset of symptoms or radiographic abnormalities for the majority of the occupational DPLDs. Exposure to agents that cause DPLD may also occur as a result of hobbies or recreational activities (bird breeder's lung, wood worker's lung, farmer's lung, sauna taker's disease). Accordingly, exposures outside the occupational setting should be explored. An increasing list of both prescribed and over-the-counter medications can cause DPLD. Chemotherapeutic drugs have variable latency periods ranging from a few weeks to many years; therefore, a history of both current and former drug therapies must be sought.

Other aspects of the history, although not indicative of a specific etiology, may aid in the diagnostic evaluation. A history of smoking has been strongly linked with histiocytosis X, RB-ILD, and pulmonary hemorrhage associated with Goodpasture's syndrome. In contrast, hypersensitivity pneumonitis and sarcoidosis occur less frequently in active smokers. The role of cigarette smoking in IPF is unclear. While it has been reported to be a risk factor for the development of IPF, cigarette smoking appears to have a negative influence on the rate of progression. Age and sex can be useful in initial evaluation. IPF is almost exclusively a disease of middle age and the elderly patient. Sarcoidosis, histiocytosis X, lymphangioleimyomatosis, and the inherited causes of DPLD (Table 84-1) are generally diagnosed before age of 40 years and, thus are uncommon initial presentations in the geriatric patient. Elderly patients are prone to aspiration; a history of gastroesophageal reflux suggests the possibility of chronic aspiration syndrome. The use of mineral oil nasal drops or petroleum products should raise the possibility of lipoid pneumonia.

Physical Examination

Patients with IPF and other UIP-associated DPLD typically reveal the characteristic bibasilar, crepitant ("Velcro-like") late-inspiratory rales (crackles) on lung auscultation. Wheezing, rhonchi, and coarse rales are occasionally heard. The lung examination can be normal in

the early course of the disease. With advanced disease, resting tachycardia and tachypnea maybe present. Digital clubbing is relatively common in IPF, but less common in certain other DPLDs such as sarcoidosis. Hypertrophic pulmonary osteoarthropathy is rare. The new appearance of digital clubbing in a patient with known DPLD should prompt a search for complicating lung malignancy. The heart examination maybe normal early in the disease. Later, with the onset of pulmonary hypertension and cor pulmonale, an accentuated P2, tricuspid insufficiency, a right ventricular heave, and peripheral edema maybe noted. Extrapulmonary findings involving the skin and joints may indicate the presence of a systemic rheumatologic disorder.

Laboratory Tests

Laboratory tests can either confirm or suggest a diagnosis in DPLD, but these studies are seldom diagnostic. Rheumatoid factor and antinuclear antibodies are occasionally present in patients with ILD, but their presence does not necessarily indicate an underlying collagen vascular disorder. Plasma immunoglobulin maybe elevated, but this finding is nonspecific. If hypersensitivity pneumonitis is suspected, serum-precipitating antibodies to a limited number of inhaled organic antigens maybe measured. Tests for antineutrophil cytoplasmic antibodies (ANCA) should be obtained if Wegener's granulomatosis is suspected. Tests for antibasement membrane antibodies should be obtained when Goodpasture's syndrome is suspected. The electrocardiogram (ECG) is usually normal in DPLD. With progressive loss of alveolar capillary units, the ECG may demonstrate a pattern of right atrial and ventricular strain.

Chest Radiography

The chest radiograph is a practical and useful screen for DPLD. The chest radiograph maybe normal in up to 10% of patients with DPLD detected by HRCT. When abnormal, a characteristic radiographic pattern in combination with the appropriate clinical history and physical examination findings may suggest or support a specific diagnosis. In DPLD, the chest radiograph typically reveals bilateral reticular opacities that are predominantly in the periphery and lower lung fields. With more severe disease, cystic dilatation of the distal air spaces ("honeycombing") and traction bronchiectasis with thickened and dilated airways are seen. In other DPLDs, nodular or reticulonodular infiltrates maybe more common. Alveolar filling diseases often present with ill-defined alveolar nodules (acinar rosettes) and air bronchograms. A diffuse ground glass pattern is often seen in diseases characterized by active alveolitis such as DIP, RB-ILD, "cellular" NSIP, and hypersensitivity pneumonitis.

High-Resolution Computed Tomography

HRCT, using thin (1 to 2 mm) sections without the use of contrast, offers many advantages over standard chest radiography in the evaluation of DPLD. The improved spatial resolution of HRCT allows characterization of anatomic patterns to the level of the pulmonary lobule. It is useful for the detection of DPLD in cases when the chest radiograph is normal, to quantify the extent and pattern of lung parenchymal involvement and, in a few cases, to make a specific diagnosis with a high degree of certainty. Diseases in which HRCT has been able to detect abnormalities with normal chest radiographs include asbestosis, silicosis, sarcoidosis, and scleroderma. Conversely, the HRCT maybe normal in some cases of biopsy-proven DPLD; therefore, HRCT cannot be used to exclude ILD with absolute certainty. In such cases, physiologic data such as gas exchange with exertion maybe more sensitive. HRCT is also valuable for following the response to therapy and in identifying a suitable site for transbronchial or open lung biopsy. Recent studies suggest that HRCT data when combined with the clinical information can result in a confident diagnosis of IPF when read by experienced pulmonologists or radiologists; this may obviate the need for a lung biopsy in certain patients.

Pulmonary Function Tests

Physiologic testing can identify the physiologic abnormalities associated with DPLD, determine the severity, and provide information on prognosis and response to treatment. The classic physiologic alterations in DPLD include reduced lung volumes (vital capacity, total lung capacity [TLC]), reduced diffusing capacity (DL_{co}), and a normal or supernormal ratio of forced expiratory volume in 1 second (FEV_1) to FVC. Static lung compliance is decreased (decreased lung volume for any given transpulmonary pressure) and maximal transpulmonary pressure is increased (a very high negative pressure must be generated to open fibrotic alveoli). Exceptions to this classic presentation are hisiocytosis X, lymphangioleiomyomatosis, neurofibromatosis, sarcoidosis, and tuberous sclerosis, in which airways disease can predominate, resulting in an increase in airflow limitation and increased TLC. A mixed restrictive and obstructive pattern is commonly seen in BOOP.

Arterial blood gas analysis typically shows mild hypoxemia. Carbon dioxide retention is rare. Most of the patients with DPLD have marked increases in minute ventilation both at rest and with exercise, resulting in reduced partial pressure of carbon dioxide (Pco_2) and compensated respiratory alkalosis. The increased minute ventilation is accomplished by increases in respiratory rate rather than in tidal volume. Hyperventilation is not caused by abnormalities in acid–base status or to hypoxemia, but rather to an increased stimulation of the respiratory center from neural signals arising from altered mechanoreceptors in the deranged lung parenchyma. Exercise tolerance in DPLD patients is markedly limited. With exercise, arterial partial pressure of oxygen (Po_2) falls and that of carbon dioxide (Pco_2) remain constant. Hypoxemia in patients with DPLD results primarily from abnormal ventilation–perfusion relationships and additionally from diffusion abnormalities with severe disease. The abnormalities in diffusion, which were originally believed to be the result of thickened alveolar walls, are now recognized to be caused by loss of capillary cross-sectional area and the passage of red blood cells through functioning pulmonary capillaries at a rate that is too rapid to permit full saturation of hemoglobin. Arterial pH is usually normal in DPLD but can fall with exercise as a result of anerobic metabolism in oxygen-deprived muscles.

Bronchoscopic Studies

Bronchoscopy should be performed when tissue abnormalities are distributed in the bronchovascular bundle, an alveolar filling disorder is present, or an infectious disease is suspected. The distinctive histopathologic abnormalities of sarcoidosis, lymphangitic carcinomatosis, and lymphangioleiomyomatosis are usually found in the bronchovascular bundle and transbronchial biopsy may demonstrate their characteristic lesions. Bronchoalveolar lavage (BAL) is diagnostic if an infectious agent or neoplastic cells are noted in the lavage specimen. BAL is also used to analyze the cellular constituents, cellular products, and proteins of the distal air spaces of the lung. A predominance of eosinophils in conjunction with appropriate clinical and radiographic picture can be diagnostic of eosinophilic pneumonia. In histiocytosis X, ultrastructural studies of BAL mononuclear cells reveal the typical Birbeck granule of the Langerhan's cell. Special stains for surfactant may suggest a diagnosis of alveolar proteinosis. However, BAL is usually nonspecific and it is not routinely indicated because of its limited ability to predict the underlying pathology (fibrosis vs. inflammation), to stage disease, or to predict response to therapy.

Lung Biopsy

The diagnosis of DPLDs, if not evident from the clinical, radiographic, and/or bronchoscopic findings, depends on histological studies of lung parenchyma obtained by surgical lung biopsy. Video-assisted thoracoscopic lung biopsy will secure a specific diagnosis in the majority of such cases. The mortality rate for open lung biopsy is less than 1% and the morbidity is less than 3%. The benefits of making a definitive diagnosis must be weighed carefully with potential risks, particularly in elderly patients with comorbid conditions. One must also consider the options for meaningful therapy once a diagnosis is made. Currently, for IPF, effective therapeutic options are limited.

THERAPEUTIC APPROACH

The principal aims of therapy are to remove exposure to injurious agents, to suppress any active inflammatory component, and to palliate or treat the complications of these diseases. Avoidance of the etiological agent, such as drugs and occupational exposures, should lead to resolution or stabilization. A short course of steroid therapy may also be indicated if the patient is symptomatic. In such cases, care must be taken to exclude infectious etiologies before embarking on empiric immunosuppressive therapy. Treatment of DPLDs associated with rheumatologic diseases is directed at suppressing the systemic immune response with prednisone with or without cyclophosphamide (Cytoxan). There are certain other DPLDs such as sarcoidosis and pulmonary vasculitides that are more responsive to such therapies.

The efficacy of anti-inflammatory agents in IIPs depends on the specific disease entity. In general, NSIP, COP, RB-ILD, DIP, and LIP are steroid-responsive whereas IPF/UIP and AIP are not. In cases where a lung biopsy cannot be obtained and a process other than IPF is suspected, a trial of anti-inflammatory therapy maybe initiated. When N-acteylcysteine (NAC) is added to a combination of prednisone and azathioprine, the rate of decline in FVC and DLCO is reduced. Immunosuppressive therapies are best limited to a 3- to 6-month period during which objective improvements in physiologic measures, radiographic findings, and clinical symptoms are assessed. Unfortunately, elderly patients tend to not respond well. In general, patients who respond to therapy are younger than 50 years of age, are likely to have coexistent NSIP, and are more likely to be females. In the absence of improvement, therapy with immunosuppressive agents must be discontinued. There appears to be no benefit to more potent anti-inflammatory therapy (such as cyclophosphamide) in steroid-unresponsive cases. In symptomatic scleroderma patients with evidence of active alveolitis (by BAL or HRCT), 1 year of oral cyclophosphamide appears to have a modest beneficial effect on lung function, dyspnea, thickening of the skin, and health-related quality of life.

Despite early promise, a Phase III clinical trial of interferon gamma-1b (Actimmune) for IPF was discontinued, as the overall survival result crossed a predefined stopping boundary for lack of benefit; among the 115 deaths in the 826 randomized patients, 14.5% were in the Actimmune group as compared to 12.7% in the placebo group. Other agents in Phase II/III clinical trials include pirfenidone (an orally active small molecule inhibitor of fibroblast activation and proliferation), bosentan (an endothelin receptor antagonist), and imatanib mesylate (a tyrosine kinase inhibitor). Several other agents are in Phase I or earlier stages of drug development. Currently, no FDA-approved drug therapies for IPF exist. Enrollment of such patients in clinical trials, including those sponsored by the National Institutes of Health, is strongly encouraged.

Early institution of oxygen therapy for patients with hypoxemia or desaturation (oxygen saturation $\leq 88\%$) at rest or with exercise is recommended; this is to prevent or delay complications related to pulmonary hypertension. Patients who develop pulmonary hypertension and *cor pulmonale* must be managed supportively with a combination of diuretics, inotropic agents, vasodilator therapy, and anticoagulation. Influenza and pneumococcal vaccines should be administered to all patients with chronic forms of DPLD.

Lung transplantation maybe an option for patients with end-stage DPLD refractory to medical therapy. Single lung transplantation is preferred for most patients. Most transplant centers currently do not list patients over the age of 65 years. Two-year survival ranges from 60% to 80%, with most deaths being caused by infections that complicate immunosuppressive therapy or to chronic allograft rejection. The 5-year survival is approximately 50% and is limited primarily by chronic allograft rejection.

FUTURE DIRECTIONS

The challenges facing clinicians who care for patients with DPLD, particularly those of the idiopathic variety (IIPs), include the ability to diagnose patients early in the disease course when the underlying inflammatory and repair processes may be more amenable to therapy and to accurately define the relative degree of inflammation versus fibrosis. In primarily fibrotic processes such as UIP/IPF, anti-inflammatory therapies are of no proven benefit. A number of "anti-fibrotic" strategies are now under investigation. Further understanding of the relationships between inflammation and fibrosis, and the molecular determinants that result in the varied manifestations of the IIPs may aid in the development of more targeted therapies. Evolving systems biology approaches that allow for more accurate genotyping/phenotyping of patients may aid in defining the underlying disease process and allow for more specific "personalized" therapies.

FURTHER READING

American Thoracic Society/European Respiratory Society International Multidisciplinary Consensus Classification of the Idiopathic Interstitial Pneumonias. This joint statement of the American Thoracic Society (ATS), and the European Respiratory Society (ERS) was adopted by the ATS board of directors, June 2001 and by the ERS Executive Committee, June 2001. *Am J Respir Crit Care Med.* 2002;165:277–304.

Collard HR, King TE, Jr., Bartelson BB, et al. Changes in clinical and physiologic variables predict survival in idiopathic pulmonary fibrosis. *Am J Respir Crit Care Med.* 2003;168:538–542.

Demedts M, Behr J, Buhl R, et al. High-dose acetylcysteine in idiopathic pulmonary fibrosis. *N Engl J Med.* 2005;353:2229–2242.

Flaherty KR, Travis WD, Colby TV, et al. Histopathologic variability in usual and nonspecific interstitial pneumonias. *Am J Respir Crit Care Med.* 2001;164:1722–1727.

Gross TJ, Hunninghake GW. Idiopathic pulmonary fibrosis. *N Engl J Med.* 2001;345:517–525.

Katzenstein AL, Myers JL. Idiopathic pulmonary fibrosis: clinical relevance of pathologic classification. *Am J Respir Crit Care Med.* 1998;157:1301–1315.

King TE, Jr., Schwarz MI, Brown K, et al. Idiopathic pulmonary fibrosis: relationship between histopathologic features and mortality. *Am J Respir Crit Care Med.* 2001; 164:1025–1032.

Lama VN, Flaherty KR, Toews GB, et al. Prognostic value of desaturation during a 6-minute walk test in idiopathic interstitial pneumonia. *Am J Respir Crit Care Med.* 2003;168:1084–1090.

Lama VN, Smith L, Badri L, et al. Evidence for tissue-resident mesenchymal stem cells in human adult lung from studies of transplanted allografts. *J Clin Invest.* 2007;117:989–996.

Raghu G, Brown KK, Bradford WZ, et al. A placebo-controlled trial of interferon gamma-1b in patients with idiopathic pulmonary fibrosis. *N Engl J Med.* 2004; 350:125–133.

Thannickal VJ, Toews GB, White ES, et al. Mechanisms of pulmonary fibrosis. *Annu Rev Med.* 2004;55:395–417.

Willis BC, Liebler JM, Luby-Phelps K, et al. Induction of epithelial-mesenchymal transition in alveolar epithelial cells by transforming growth factor-β1: potential role in idiopathic pulmonary fibrosis. *Am J Pathol.* 2005;166:1321–1332.

Changes in Kidney Function

Jocelyn Wiggins ■ *Sanjeevkumar R. Patel*

CLINICAL RELEVANCE

Kidney failure is a growing problem in the older population. Data on people reaching end-stage kidney disease (ESKD) is collected by the U.S. Renal Data System (USRDS). All dialysis units that receive funding from Medicare are required to file data with the USRDS, so that nationwide data are available on over 95% of people receiving renal replacement therapy. Information published in the 2006 USRDS annual data report shows that approximately 1.5 in 1000 persons aged 65 years or older are initiating treatment for ESKD each year—the highest rate of any age group. Over the last 10 years, the number of older people enrolling for treatment has increased by 41% in the group of people aged 75 years or older and by 48% in the 80+-year-old age group. Almost 4 in 1000 persons are currently maintained on renal replacement therapy, with the 75+-year-old age group growing at 10% per year. The peak incidence for ESKD is the 70- to 74-year-old age group, while the peak prevalence falls in the 65- to 69-year-old age group. In contrast, the incidence of ESKD in the 20- to 44-year-old age group has remained flat over the last 10 years, with only 6% growth in the 45- to 64-year-old group. Although some of the increase in renal replacement therapy for the older population indicates a greater willingness to offer treatment to older individuals, much of the increase is owing to people surviving to experience the chronic changes that occur with aging. The kidney undergoes significant age-related change. Other common diseases such as hypertension and diabetes accelerate these changes.

THE AGING PROCESS

Aging in the kidney is characterized by changes of both structure and function. It must be emphasized that many of the aging studies have been performed on laboratory animals, particularly rodents, that demonstrate quite different patterns of aging from humans. For example, kidney weight increases throughout life in rats while kidney mass and size in humans peaks in the fourth decade and declines thereafter. Care should be taken when reading the literature to keep in mind that changes seen in animal models may not be reflected by parallel changes in humans. Historical data from human postmortems describing changes in the kidney made no effort to exclude patients with kidney disease or significant comorbidities. More recently data on aging has been developed from longitudinal studies, such as the Baltimore Longitudinal Aging Study, in which the medical histories of the study volunteers are well documented. There are also data accumulating from the kidney transplant population. Older living donors are increasingly being used and are put thorough a rigorous medical workup for renal function and comorbid conditions before being accepted as donors. This has allowed acquisition of data on normal aging in the kidney, uncomplicated by the presence of medical comorbidities. Aging in the kidney is generally characterized by spontaneous progressive decline in renal function accompanied by thickening of the basement membrane, mesangial expansion, and focal glomerulosclerosis.

Functional Changes

Changes in renal function with age are well documented both in human and animal models. Although baseline homeostasis of fluids and electrolytes is maintained with normal aging, there is a progressive decline in renal reserve. This results in a compromise in the kidney's ability to respond to either a salt or water load or deficit. This manifests clinically in patients being vulnerable to superimposed renal complications during acute illnesses. Chronic conditions such as hypertension accelerate this age-related loss of renal reserve and increased vulnerability in these patients should be anticipated. Age-related changes in function will be considered by separate functional domain within the kidney.

Renal Blood Flow

Average renal blood flow decreases about 10% per decade, dropping from 600 mL per minute per 1.73 m² to 300 mL per minute per 1.73 m² by the ninth decade. This is accompanied by increasing resistance in both afferent and efferent arterioles. These changes occur independent of cardiac output or reductions in renal mass. This decline in renal blood flow is thought to contribute to the decline in efficiency with which the aging kidney responds to fluid and electrolyte load and loss.

Glomerular Filtration Rate

Newer data have shown a wide variation in the rate and extent of changes in the kidney within the older population. Approximately 30% of the population shows no measurable decline in renal function with normal aging. The bulk of the population loses about 10% of glomerular filtration rate (GFR) and 10% of renal plasma flow per decade after the fourth decade of life. Between 5% and 10% of the population shows accelerated loss, even in the absence of identifiable comorbidities. Since there is also a steady loss of muscle bulk with age, with concomitant reduction in creatinine production, serum creatinine should remain constant. Rises in serum creatinine should therefore be taken seriously and not dismissed as normal aging. As can be seen in Figure 85-1, serum creatinines at the upper limit of the "normal range" in an older individual represent significant functional decline, and thought should be given to renal dosing of medications. These curves were calculated using the Cockcroft Gault equation for a 70-kg man:

$$\text{Creatinine clearance} = \frac{(140 - \text{age})(\text{weight [kg]})}{72 \times \text{serum creatinine (mg/dL)}}$$

Results for women should be multiplied by 0.85, which shifts the curves downwards. In frail older women with very little residual muscle mass, this equation probably overestimates GFRs. This steady decline in renal function with age manifests itself clinically as impaired ability to excrete a salt or water load. Extra care should be taken when replacing fluids in an older individual to prevent extracellular fluid overload.

In 1999, an improved formula for estimating GFR was developed known as the MDRD formula (because it was developed as part of the Modification of Diet in Renal Disease study). Many routine laboratories now automatically calculate an MDRD glomerular filtration estimate when a basic or a comprehensive metabolic panel is ordered. In some institutions, it is necessary to order a "renal panel" for the calculation to be done. It is important to understand that this formula was based on data from community-dwelling volunteers aged 18 to 70 years. It has never been validated in an elderly or frail population. Several investigators have studied its performance in elderly patients and compared its efficacy with Cockroft Gault, creatinine clearances based on 24-hour urines or iothalamate clearances, or a combination of these methods. All of the studies have shown large discrepancies between these methods in patients with advanced age and at both extremes of the weight spectrum. These limitations should be kept in mind when using the formula in clinical geriatric practice. Although iothalamate clearance is the gold standard, it is expensive and impractical for routine use. The most reliable results come from calculating creatinine clearances based on 24-hour urine collection. This will always be an overestimate of the GFR, since some creatinine is actively excreted into the urine from the proximal tubule, not all of the urinary creatinine is filtered. It is however more reliable than the formula estimations in the very old and the frail.

Classification of Kidney Disease

The classification of kidney disorders has undergone a major revision over the past few years. A consensus committee, sponsored by the National Kidney Foundation, published new clinical practice guidelines in February 2002. The traditional chronic renal insufficiency (CRI) has become chronic kidney disease (CKD) and end-stage renal disease (ESRD) has become kidney failure. CKD is defined as either kidney damage or decreased kidney function for 3 or more months. Kidney failure is defined as a GFR of less than 15 mL/min or the need to start kidney replacement therapy. Along with renaming kidney disease, the committee also developed a system of staging,

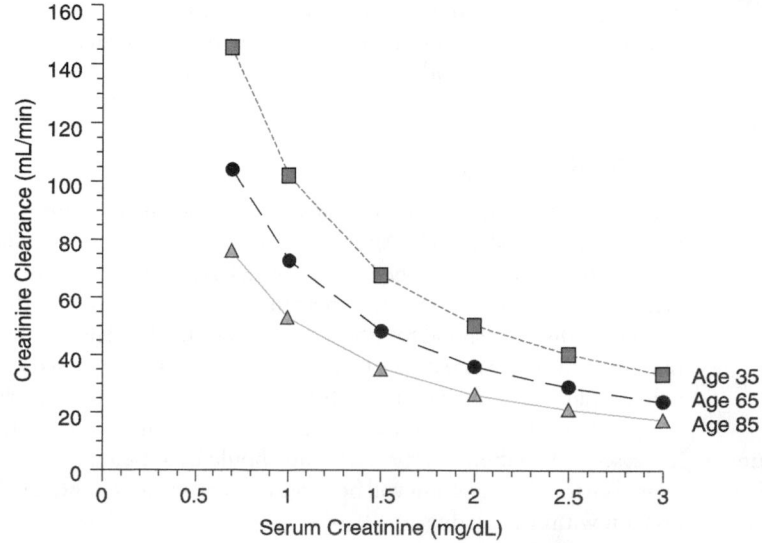

FIGURE 85-1. Relationship between serum creatinine and calculated creatinine clearance for men aged 35, 65, and 85 yrs. Calculations are based on a 70-kg man.

TABLE 85-1

TABLE 85-1

National Kidney Foundation Classification of Chronic Kidney Disease

STAGE	DESCRIPTION	GFR (mL/min/1.73 m²)
1	Kidney damage with normal or increased GFR	>90
2	Kidney damage with mild reduction in GFR	60–89
3	Moderate decrease in GFR	30–59
4	Severe decrease in GFR	15–29
5	Kidney Failure	<15 (or dialysis)

similar to the New York classification of congestive heart failure. It was felt that having a structure would help with standardizing diagnosis and opportunities for preventative management. CKD is now classified into five stages, regardless of underlying diagnosis. The classification defines stage 1 as kidney damage (primarily proteinuria) with preserved GFR and progresses to stage 5 kidney failure (Table 85-1). Declines in GFR are accompanied by a broad range of complications (Table 85-2). Early recognition of impaired kidney function allows the physician to screen for and manage these complications and thus prevent comorbidities and declines in quality of life. National Kidney Foundation Guidelines recommend referral to a nephrologist when a patient reaches stage 4 CKD for management of the complications of impaired function such as acidosis, phosphorus retention, and anemia. Preparation for kidney replacement therapy should also begin during stage 4.

Proteinuria

Despite the significant decline in GFR that occurs with aging, proteinuria is not a normal feature of the aging process. Proteinuria is always a pathological finding and requires a full workup. In contrast, in most rodent models, particularly in the rat, proteinuria is a normal feature of the aging kidney. This difference between humans and rodents should be kept in mind when reading the aging literature.

Tubular Function

Older individuals are well known to be more susceptible to acute renal failure. Much of the information on tubular function comes

TABLE 85-2

Complications of Chronic Kidney Disease

Hypertension
Anemia
Increased cardiovascular mortality and morbidity
Disorders of calcium and phosphorus metabolism
Compromised nutritional status
Metabolic bone disease
Neuropathy
Impaired functioning and well-being
Depression

from animal studies, particularly rat models. Rats spontaneously develop proteinuria with aging, and this protein load is believed to be toxic to the tubule. Since proteinuria is not a feature of normal aging in humans, these animal studies may not paint an accurate picture of changes in tubular function in humans. There are also large numbers of studies in experimental animals looking at vasoconstrictive and vasodilatory responses in the older kidney. Impaired response to ANP, acetylcholine, and blunted responses of cAMP to β-adrenergic stimulus have all been implicated. Virtually none of these findings have been confirmed in humans. Functional magnetic resonance imaging (MRI) in older volunteers has demonstrated decreased ability to modulate renal medullary oxygenation. Whether this is caused by fixed vascular changes or changes in renal autocrine systems such as prostaglandins, dopamine, nitric oxide (NO), naturetic peptides, or endothelin is not clear. The clinical result is increased sensitivity to acute ischemic renal failure.

Animal and human studies have shown impaired concentrating ability in the older kidney. Whether this is caused by intrinsic defects in the tubular epithelium or impaired response to ADH is not clear. Studies have also demonstrated impaired capacity to acidify urine manifested clinically as reduced excretion of an acid load. Whatever the underlying mechanism, older individuals are less likely to be able to maintain normal homeostasis when challenged. Although there is an age-related decline in tubular functions such as glucose and amino acid transport, these declines closely parallel the decline in GFR and are believed to correlate with the loss of nephrons rather than aging of the tubule. Age-related changes in sodium and potassium homeostasis, and water handling are discussed in Chapter 88.

Older individuals are also more sensitive to nephrotoxic injury. Careful thought should be given to the choice and dosing of antibiotics and other nephrotoxic drugs. Increased age is a risk factor for the development of radiocontrast nephropathy. Special care should be exercised before tests requiring radiocontrast are ordered.

Donor Organ Viability

Age also impacts on the viability of kidneys for transplantation. With the steady increase in living related and unrelated donations, more organs have become available for use in the older population. Although nationwide probably less than 5% of older individuals reaching ESKD are being considered for transplantation, many larger transplant programs are routinely offering transplantation to people in their late sixties and early seventies if they are otherwise in good health. Donated organs are commonly coming from a similar aged spouse or a family member. Age of the donated organ appears to be an independent risk factor for graft survival. This does not appear to be immune-mediated, as older recipients have lower risk of rejection. These organs typically show delayed graft function posttransplant, with chronic allograft nephropathy and result in higher baseline serum creatinines in the long term. It has been postulated that this is caused by impaired response to injury in the older kidney, but there is no real scientific evidence to support this at the current time.

Underlying Structural Changes

There is at least 100 years of meticulous research describing the anatomical changes that underlie the functional changes that we see in our patients as they age.

Gross Anatomy

Kidneys grow vigorously from birth through adolescence, reaching their maximum weight and volume during the third decade of life. In humans, although not in most laboratory animals, this weight starts to decline after the fourth decade and continues its decline throughout the remaining life span. Most of the decline in weight and volume appears to happen in the cortex, with relative sparing of the medulla.

Glomerulus

The young healthy human kidney contains roughly 1 million nephrons. There is no evidence for postnatal nephrogenesis. This underlies the hypothesis that low birth weight babies might have fewer initial nephrons and as a result are more susceptible to renal failure in later life. Although there is some observational data to support this hypothesis, no causal relationship has been proved. There is a steady decline in nephron number with age that starts around the fourth decade. This decline is believed to underlie the decline in GFR discussed above. Kidneys obtained at autopsy from patients with no known history of renal disease have been studied. Light microscopy showed the development of a focal sclerosing process, accompanied by thickening of the glomerular basement membrane. There was a steady progression with age in the percentage of glomeruli that were scared. By age 50 years, all subjects examined had some evidence of sclerosis, with the percentage of sclerotic glomeruli increasing steadily with age.

Age-Related Glomerulosclerosis

Sclerotic glomeruli typically first appear in the fourth decade of life. This starts as a segmental process with one part of a glomerulus becoming acellular and the normal architecture being replaced by extra cellular matrix. The glomerular tuft becomes adherent to Bowman's capsule (Figure 85-2) (Color Plate 13). Gradually an entire glomerulus becomes sclerosed and shrivels down with resultant loss of that nephron and its filtration capacity. It is not known what triggers this pattern of focal sclerosis, which is apparently randomly scattered throughout the cortex. The glomerular tuft increases in size with age. Concomitant with this expansion is an increase in endothelial and mesangial cells, such that the ratio of cells to glomerular area remains constant. Podocytes, the specialized cells that form the filtration barrier in the glomerulus, are postmitotic. They are not able to multiply in response to the increase in tuft volume, and become a progressively smaller percentage of the total cells making up the glomerular tuft. As the filtration area that they have to cover increases, it is believed that they may drop off the basement membrane, leaving a denuded area behind. It is this area of bare basement membrane that acts as the trigger for the sclerosing process. Many different experimental models of glomerulosclerosis have concluded that loss of the podocyte and its inability to be replaced is the sentinel event that triggers sclerosis. In our laboratory, we have developed a transgenic rat that expresses the diphtheria toxin receptor on the podocyte and allows us to deplete podocytes in a dose-dependent manner. We have shown that the loss of podocytes precedes the appearance of sclerosis, and podocytes markers can be detected in the urine prior to the development of global sclerosis.

Models of induced glomerular injury, of course, do not exist in humans. However, research has shown selective loss of podocytes in the kidneys of type I diabetics as diabetic nephropathy progresses. Podocyte number per glomerulus is the best predictor of progression of diabetic nephropathy in Pima Indians with type II diabetes. Thus, studies of the aging process in rat kidneys noted that a decline in podocyte counts accompanies by the appearance of glomerulosclerosis.

Some authors have suggested a role for the mesangial cell in initiating the sclerosis process. Certainly with aging, there is an increase in mesangial matrix and in mesangial cell numbers. However, this increase is just as marked in strains of rat that do not develop age-related glomerulosclerosis, as it is in strains that do. Several authors have looked at mesangial cell activation in rat models of

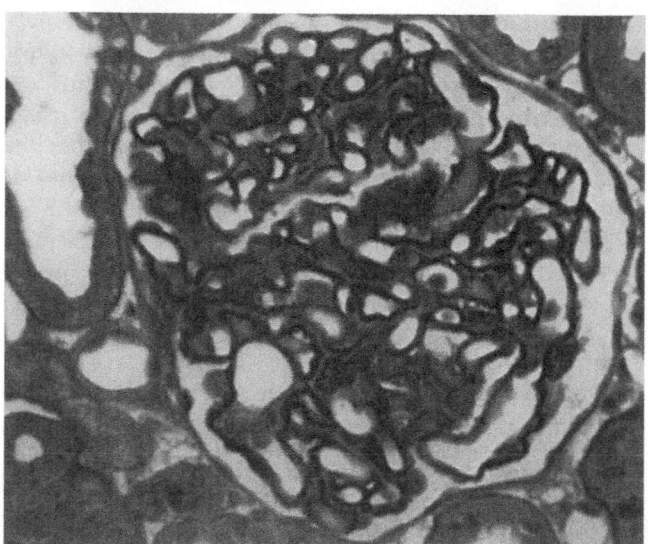 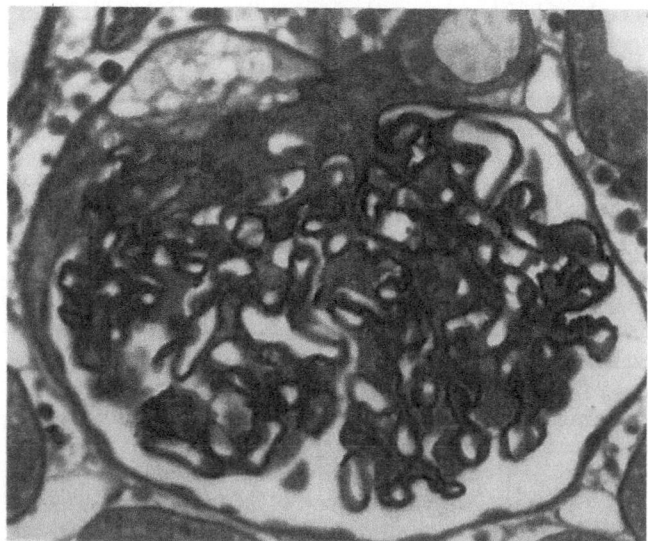

FIGURE 85-2. Renal glomeruli from a 24-month Fischer 344 rat stained with a podocyte marker, GLEPP1, and counterstained with PAS. Left panel: normal glomerulus showing normal architecture of the glomerular tuft. Right panel: age-related glomerulosclerosis showing normal cellular architecture replaced by extracellular matrix and adherence to Bowman's capsule.

glomerulosclerosis and found little or none. This suggests that mesangial expansion is a benign manifestation of the aging process rather than a pathological one.

Tubule

With the loss of the glomerulus, the tubular section of the nephron usually degenerates and is replaced by connective tissue. Tubular hypertrophy then occurs in the remaining nephrons, principally in the proximal convoluted tubule. This appears to result from both hypertrophy and hyperplasia. With thinning of the cortex, there is a decrease in tubule length and development of diverticuli in the distal convoluted tubule. As nephrons are lost, there is generalized tubular interstitial fibrosis. The structure of the distal tubule does not appear to change significantly with age.

Vasculature

Renal arteries undergo age-related thickening, similar to that seen throughout the circulation. Smaller arteries may become tortuous and show luminal irregularities. When a glomerulus becomes sclerosed, there is frequent formation of an arteriovenous shunt as the afferent and efferent arterioles develop a direct connection, as the glomerular capillary is lost. This shunt is very important in maintaining medullary blood flow. Physiological studies in both animals and humans have documented a decline in renal blood flow and an increase in vascular resistance with age. Studies of renal perfusion in healthy older individuals from a pool of potential kidney donors have shown steady declines in renal perfusion with age that exceeded the reduction in renal mass, suggesting that declines in blood flow were a significant factor in the changes seen in renal function with age. These changes contribute to the susceptibility of older individuals to acute renal failure, volume overload, and electrolyte abnormalities.

Infarcts may occur in the kidney, just as they do in other tissues of the body. Since one fifth of the circulating volume passes through the kidney each minute, the kidney is also particularly susceptible to embolization. If other signs of embolization are visible clinically, it is highly probable that the kidney is also undergoing embolization, and embolic disease should certainly be kept in mind in an older individual with widespread vascular disease who demonstrates accelerated loss of renal function.

MECHANISMS UNDERLYING THE DECLINE IN KIDNEY FUNCTION

There is no clear-cut consensus about what mechanisms may underlie the structural and functional changes occurring in the kidney in the older population. It is fairly clear however that there are both predisposing genetic and environmental factors that play a role.

Genetic Predisposition

There are as yet no genes known to cause age-related glomerulosclerosis. Accumulating evidence from animals studies, combined with evidence of genetic predisposition in humans, has led to a concerted effort to seek genes that may increase susceptibility to renal failure in individuals.

Animal Models

Rats are particularly susceptible to kidney failure and much of the work with models of renal disease has been carried out in laboratory rat strains. There are very marked strain differences in susceptibility to age-related glomerulosclerosis. Since these rats are maintained in pathogen-free environments and are fed uniform scientifically developed diets, this strongly suggests a genetic basis for the development of age-related glomerulosclerosis. The appearance of glomerulosclerosis has been reported as early as 5 months in the Milan normotensive rat, with extensive disease by 10 months of age. This occurs in the total absence of hypertension and is not ameliorated by administration of ACE inhibitors. Wistar rats were used as controls in this study and showed no significant disease during the same time period. In Sprague-Dawley rats, spontaneous age-related glomerulosclerosis first becomes apparent around 9 months of age, and disease became widespread by 18 months of age. In studies of aging in Fischer 344 rats, little glomerulosclerosis is seen until almost 2 years of age with fairly rapid progression thereafter. Other rat strains appear remarkably resistant to renal disease. Brown Norway rats show minimal sclerosis, even at 32 months of age, an advanced age in rat life span.

Human Studies

Clearly, these kinds of studies cannot be duplicated in humans. However, there is observational data that would support a similar variation in genetic susceptibility in humans. Cross-sectional studies, donor organ data, and longitudinal studies clearly show a wide variation in kidney function with age. Around 5% to 10% of the population show accelerated loss of kidney function with age even in the absence of accelerating factors such as hypertension, while 30% show no measurable decline. In the presence of predisposing comorbidities, there is also wide variation in the development of kidney disease. Some diabetics may never develop nephropathy, while others develop rapidly progressive kidney disease early in the course of their diabetes, suggesting an underlying genetic susceptibility. Within the African-American population rates of kidney disease are much higher than in the Caucasian population independent of the precipitating cause. Within an ethnic group, there are also distinct differences in vulnerability. An African-American who develops any predisposing disease, be it hypertension, diabetes, or lupus, who has a first degree relative on renal replacement therapy has a ninefold increased risk of developing kidney disease compared to another African-American with the same disease burden who has no family history of kidney disease. Similarly human immunodeficiency virus (HIV)-associated glomerulosclerosis occurs almost exclusively in the African-American population, while HIV-associated mesangial hyperplasia and immune-complex glomerular nephritis occur equally in all ethnic groups. Thus there is suggestive evidence for a genetic predisposition with respect to the development of glomerulosclerosis. Considerable effort and resources are currently being directed toward identifying genes that predispose to kidney disease, so we can expect to have greater understanding of this process soon.

Environmental Predisposing Factors

It has been well known for many years that several diseases predispose to kidney failure and will accelerate the progress of age-related glomerulosclerosis. By far the most frequent of these are hypertension and diabetes, both common disorders in the older population. There are however several other mechanisms that have been postulated to underlie the aging changes in the kidney.

Diet

One of the most striking aspects of rodent models of age-related nephropathy in the kidney is its complete reversal with calorie restriction. Both the anatomical and functional changes related to aging in the kidney are completely abolished in animals that are fed two-thirds of the calories given to their ad libitum-fed litter mates. Even though these animals live one third longer than their ad libitum-fed littermates, they do not develop age-related glomerulosclerosis. Several explanations have been proffered to account for this observation.

Free Radicals and Lipid Peroxides

One possible explanation for the profound effects of calorie restriction is a reduction in the generation of free radicals and lipid peroxides. There is a wide body of literature discussing the damaging effects of free radicals on cellular systems and the role that this plays in aging. It is not the scope of this chapter to review that literature. The main consequence of free radical production is lipid peroxidation, which results in damage to cellular proteins, lipids, and nucleic acids. Increased calorie intake is believed to fuel increased free radical production with accelerated aging damage. This hypothesis has generated interest in the role of antioxidants in slowing the aging process. The effects of supplementing the diets of Sprague-Dawley rats with vitamin E 50 IU/kg has been studied. Although they were able to measure reductions in markers of oxidative stress, and slowed the rate of decline in GFR, they were unable to prevent glomerulosclerosis. Studies in humans with vitamin E have also been disappointing.

Protein Restriction

The benefits of calorie restriction have been attributed to concomitant reductions in dietary protein. There is a large body of older literature on protein restriction in experimental animal models of kidney disease. In many of these studies, experimental and control animals were not fed isocaloric diets, and protein restriction also meant calorie restriction. Many of these studies have shown a slowing in the progression of established kidney disease, however the results were not corrected for total calorie content. Studies of spontaneous age-related glomerulosclerosis in Fischer 344 rats have shown that protein restriction was much less effective than calorie restriction in preventing age-related declines in kidney function. Modest benefits from protein restriction when rats were fed isocaloric diets have been demonstrated, as have some benefits when the type of protein in the diet was changed from casein to soy. In contrast, calorie-restricted animals had little or no decline in kidney function and they were not able to show significant glomerulosclerosis despite significantly increased longevity. Rats that were fed a high-protein diet, but restricted to 60% calorie intake compared to their ad libitum-fed litter mates, also showed dramatic reductions in age-related glomerulosclerosis. Clearly, protein restriction does have some benefit in the prevention of age-related nephropathy, but that advantage is small compared to those achieved with caloric restriction. Very few of the studies looked at changes in sodium, phosphate, and calcium content of the experimental diets. Many of the results of protein restriction can be duplicated by phosphate restriction. The relevance of these studies in humans remains unclear. An observational study that included individuals up to 80 years of age compared healthy vegetarians who consume an average of 30 g/day of protein with nonvegetarians who consume an average of 100 g/day showed no differences in kidney function between these groups. There is evidence to support protein restriction in patients with established renal disease to reduce symptoms of uremia, but none to support the role of protein restriction to prevent age-related changes in the human kidney.

Lipids

There is a well-established link between lipids and cardiovascular disease, and restriction of fat intake accompanied by treatment of hyperlipidemia has been shown to be efficacious in preventing or slowing the progress of cardiovascular disease. Certainly protecting the integrity and function of the vascular supply to the kidney is important to maintaining normal function. Evidence for benefits from the manipulation of lipids in kidney disease comes mainly from animal models of diabetes. Animal studies using high-fat diets have shown accelerated progress of kidney disease, but in most cases, diets were not corrected for total calorie intake. Lipogenic diets fed to Sprague-Dawley rats resulted in earlier appearance of widespread glomerulosclerosis, compared to standard fed animals. Use of lipid-lowering agents in a variety of animal models of glomerulosclerosis has shown reductions in the incidence of glomerular damage. Patients with established renal disease with or without diabetes have more rapid deterioration of kidney function in the presence of hyperlipidemia. The relevance of lipids to the age-related decline in kidney function remains to be established, but it would certainly be reasonable to recommend low-fat diet and lipid management in patients with declining renal function.

Hyperfiltration

The term hyperfitration is used to describe putative glomerular injury from long-term increases in intraglomerular pressure. Normal age-related loss of glomeruli causes intraglomerular hypertension with hypertrophy of remaining glomeruli. Persistent intraglomerular hypertension causes pressure-mediated renal injury. Most of the supporting evidence for this mechanism comes from animal models where one kidney and part of the remaining kidney are removed, leaving a partial kidney remnant. These animals develop a pattern of renal damage in the remnant indistinguishable from age-related glomerulosclerosis, but over an accelerated time course. Long-term follow-up in humans for over 20 years has not shown accelerated declines in renal function in people who have donated one of their kidneys for transplantation, even though the remaining kidney does undergo hypertrophy. Nutrition may also play a part in hyperfiltration. After a meal of protein, increases in both renal blood flow and GFR in animals as well as in humans have been demonstrated. Excessive intake, particularly of animal proteins, therefore could cause constant hyperperfusion in the kidney, leading to intraglomerular hypertension and accelerated glomerulosclerosis. This would certainly help to explain the benefits so clearly seen with calorie restriction in laboratory animals.

The efficacy of ACE inhibitors in preventing renal hyperperfusion damage early in the course of diabetes and hypertension would also lend support to the hyperfiltration hypothesis. Angiotensin II appears to be important in maintaining glomerular filtration pressure by vasoconstricting the efferent arteriole. ACE inhibition is believed to preserve renal function by blocking the vasoconstriction of the efferent arteriole and reducing intraglomerular pressure. Long-term ACE inhibition dramatically reduces the incidence of age-related glomerulosclerosis in Munich-Wistar rats. However, a sufficient dose of ACE inhibitor to significantly lower systolic blood pressure was administered in the treatment group as compared to the control animals. Whether low doses of ACE inhibitors would help to maintain normal renal function in humans, and prevent the appearance of age-related glomerulosclerosis is a matter for speculation. There is no doubt about their efficacy in preventing progressive decline in renal function when there is an underlying disease. It remains to be seen whether they have any role in modifying age-related changes.

CONSEQUENCES OF IMPAIRED KIDNEY FUNCTION

Patients who show signs of significantly diminished kidney function should be managed aggressively, regardless of their age. Individuals who reach dialysis have a mortality rate four to five times that of age-matched controls (Table 85-3) and are at 10 times the risk of a cardiovascular event. It costs more than $70 000 per annum to maintain someone on dialysis, without including the cost of treatment for any other health problems. Transplantation is also expensive and requires the patient to remain on toxic immunosuppressive regimes for the rest of their life. Patients who show signs of impaired kidney function should be managed with the idea of preventing them from reaching end-stage disease. Aggressive measures should be taken to reduce blood pressure with a goal of 125/75 if tolerated. A regimen should be used that includes an ACE inhibitor or an angiotensin receptor blocker. However, it should be kept in mind that neither of these classes of drug will confer significant renal protection in the absence of good blood pressure control. Lipids should also be aggressively managed, as should blood sugar and other potential accelerators of renal decline. Overweight patients should be encouraged to lose weight. Great care should be taken to avoid potential renal toxins, such as aminoglycoside antibiotics, nonsteriodal anti-inflammatory drugs (NSAIDs), and radiocontrast dyes.

Medications excreted by the kidney should be appropriately dosed in amount and frequency. Maintaining residual renal function confers on the patient a greatly superior prognosis when compared to those on renal replacement therapies. Hopefully the current emphasis on finding genes that predispose to declines in kidney function and the development of age-related glomerulosclerosis will help us to identify those at greatest risk before major losses of function have occurred. As with recent gains in the prevention of cardiovascular disease through control of risk factors, we anticipate that similar guidelines will be available for the prevention of age-related declines in kidney function.

In summary, kidney disease and failure are predominantly diseases of the older population. All older patients should have an estimate made of their GFR. If they have a deficit in their kidney function, they should be managed aggressively to prevent progression to kidney failure. As CKD progresses, special attention should be paid to choice of drugs and their dosing and to the use of contrast dyes for imaging.

FURTHER READING

Abrass CK. The nature of chronic progressive nephropathy in aging rats. *Adv Renal Replace Ther.* 2000;7(1):4–10.

Anderson S, Rennke HG, Zatz R. Glomerular adaptations with normal aging and with long-term converting enzyme inhibition in rats. *Am J Physiol.* 1994;36:F35–F43.

Blum M, Averbuch M, Wolman Y, Aviram A. Protein intake and kidney function in humans: its effect on "normal aging." *Arch Intern Med.* 1989;149(1):211–212.

Clark, B. Biology of renal aging in humans. *Adv Renal Replace Ther.* 2000;7(1):11–21.

Cockroft DW, Gault MH. Prediction of creatinine clearance from serum creatinine. *Nephron.* 1976;16:31–41.

Epstein M. Aging and the kidney. *J Am Soc Nephrol.* 1996;7:1106–1122.

Floege J, Hackman B, Kleim V, et al. Age-related glomerulosclerosis and interstitial fibrosis in Milan normotensive rats: a podocyte disease. *Kidney Int.* 1997;51:230–243.

Kaplan C, Pasternack B, Shah H, et al. Age-related incidence of sclerotic glomeruli in human kidneys. *Am J Pathol.* 1975;80:227–234.

Kriz W, Elger M, Nagata M, et al. The role of podocytes in the development of glomerular sclerosis. *Kidney Int.* 1994;45:S64–S72.

Kriz W, Gretz N, Lemley KV. Progression of glomerular diseases: is the podocyte the culprit? *Kidney Int.* 1998;54:687.

Levey AS, Bosch, JP, Lewis JB. *Ann Intern Med.* 1999;130(6):461–470.

Lindeman RD, Tobin J, Shock NW. Longitudinal studies on the rate of decline in renal function with age. *J Am Geriatric Soc.* 1985;33:278–285.

Luyckx VA, Brenner BM. Low birth weight, nephron number, and kidney disease. *Kidney Int Suppl.* 2005; 97:S68–S77.

Masoro EJ, Iwasaki K, Gleiser CA, McMahan CA, Seo E, Yu BP. Dietary modulation of the progression of nephropathy in aging rats: an evaluation of the importance of protein *Am J Clin Nutr.* 1989;49(6):1217–1227.

National Kidney Foundation. K/DOQI Clinical practice guidelines for chronic kidney disease: evaluation, classification and stratification. *Am J Kidney Dis.* 2002;39:S1–S246.

Pagtalunan ME, Miller PL, Jumping-Eagle S, et al. Podocyte loss and progressive injury in type II diabetes. *J Clin Invest.* 1997;99:342–348.

Porter LE, Hollenberg NK. Obesity, salt intake, and renal perfusion in healthy humans. *Hypertension.* 1998;32(1):144–148.

Reckelhoff JF, Kanji V, Racusen LC, et al. Vitamin E ameliorates enhanced renal lipid peroxidation and accumulation of F2-isoprostanes in aging kidneys. *Am J Physiol.* 1998;274(3 Pt 2):R767–R774.

Steffes MW, Schmidt D, McRery R, et al. Glomerular cell number in normal subjects and in type I diabetic patients. *Kidney Int.* 2001;59:2104–2113.

United States Renal Data System. 1999 Annual Data Report. Bethesda, MD: National Institutes of Health, National Institutes of Diabetes and Digestive and Kidney Diseases; April 1999.

Wharram B, Goyal M, Wiggins J, et al. Podocyte depletion causes glomerulosclerosis. Diphtheria toxin-induced podocyte depletion in rats expressing the human DTR transgene. *J Am Soc Nephrol.* 2005;16:2941–2952.

Wiggins J, Goyal M, Sanden S, et al. Podocyte hypertrophy, "adaptation" and "decompensation" associated with glomerular enlargement and glomerulosclerosis in the aging rat: prevention by calorie restriction. *J Am Soc Nephrol.* 2005;16:2953–2966.

TABLE 85-3

Life Expectancies for Selected Age Groups, Comparing Dialysis Patients with General Population Statistics		
AGE (yr)	DIALYSIS POPULATION	U.S. POPULATION
40–44	6.7–9.2	30.1–40.8
50–54	5.1–6.9	22.5–31.5
60–64	3.7–5.1	16.0–22.8
70–74	2.7–3.5	10.8–15.2
80–84	2.0–2.4	6.9–8.8

Numbers are shown as ranges to accommodate differences by gender and ethnic group.

Renal Disease

Lynn Schlanger ■ *Jeff M. Sands* ■ *James L. Bailey*

The normal aging process induces structural and functional changes in the kidney characterized by progressive development of glomerulosclerosis and interstitial fibrosis. The timing of these changes is highly variable and is not necessarily inevitable, and appears to hinge on associated comorbid factors. Nearly one-third of the elderly population will not demonstrate a decrement in glomerular filtration rate (GFR) with aging. Nevertheless, the average individual can expect to lose 0.8 mL/min/1.73 m²/year. Because the decline in GFR in individuals with aging is masked by a proportional decline in muscle mass, the serum creatinine generally remains constant. Failure to understand this fact can result in inappropriate dosing of medications with their associated morbidity. It can also result in underrecognition of renal pathology, for even subtle increases in serum creatinine in the elderly can represent a significant loss of renal function. This chapter reviews aspects of renal disease that are prevalent in the geriatric population.

EPIDEMIOLOGY

There has been an increase in the prevalence of renal disease with increasing age as a consequence of improved patient survival with comorbid conditions that result in renal dysfunction, such as congestive heart failure, hypertension, diabetes, and atherosclerotic vascular disease. Currently, more than 20% of individuals older than age 65 years who are living in the United States have some degree of renal impairment, and 60% of the patients with end-stage renal disease (ESRD) who are on chronic dialysis are older than age 65 years. Men and women are affected equally. This is surprising given the higher incidence of renal disease in young men; however, these statistics may reflect the higher survival rate for women in general.

The true incidence of acute renal failure (ARF) in the elderly population is unknown. Multicenter studies from Europe report a threefold increase in the prevalence of ARF in older people. In a recent prospective multicenter European study of ARF involving hos-

pitalized patients, more than 60% were older than age 60 years, with about one-third being older than age 70 years. The most frequent causes of ARF were acute tubular necrosis (ATN) (45%), prerenal azotemia (21%), acute on chronic renal failure (CRF) (13%), and obstructive uropathy (10%). Nearly half of the patients who later developed ARF had normal renal function on presentation to the hospital, and the mortality rate was 45%. The incidence of prerenal azotemia in the elderly population is probably much higher; data from a series of elderly patients in the United Kingdom and Spain show that of 571 patients with azotemia, approximately 40% had evidence of prerenal ARF.

The true incidence of glomerular disease cannot be determined in elderly patients because there are no population-based studies. Until recently, glomerulonephritis in geriatric patients received little attention because of fear of an increased risk of morbidity and mortality associated with renal biopsy, and to the more difficult interpretation of histopathological findings. The increased proportion of elderly people entering renal replacement therapy programs has prompted nephrologists to reconsider the actual prevalence of glomerulonephritis occurring in this population. Referral patterns suggest that proteinuria or renal dysfunction is the most common reason for renal biopsy. Of these cases, nearly one-third of the renal biopsies performed were for nephrotic syndrome, while another 50% were divided fairly equally between evaluation of acute and chronic renal insufficiency. Because of concerns for the safety and efficacy of the biopsy procedure in the past, older studies may not reflect the true incidence of disease. In fact, the Medical Research Council's glomerulonephritis registry in the United Kingdom shows that the percentage of elderly patients in this registry has increased from 6% in 1978 to 21% in 1990, suggesting that the number of geriatric patients undergoing a renal biopsy for the diagnosis of glomerular disease has also increased. As a result, the incidence of glomerulonephritis in the elderly population may be much higher than previously recognized and is probably higher than in younger groups less than 60 years of age. Idiopathic glomerulonephritis is

TABLE 86-1

Histology of Nephrotic Syndrome in Geriatric Patients

STUDY NO.	TOTAL (n)	NIL (%)	FSGS (%)	MEMB (%)	AMYLOID (%)	MCGN (%)	OTHER/PRO (%)	DIABETES (%)	OTHERS (%)
1	63	21	16	33	14	5	5	5	1
2	164	21	3	38	12	5	14	4	3
3	107	2	15	48	10	5	4	5	11
4	317	11	4	37	11	6	13	4	13
5	50	4	4	32	22	4	34	—	—
6	31	6	—	52	—	16	—	—	22
7	35	6	3	43	3	3	23	—	—
8	92	14	0	35	20	11	15	1	2
9	33	27	—	39	9	6	6	—	13
10	87	8	0	34	10	8	15	0	—
11	59	3	6	21	7	4	5	8	5
12	76	25	4	41	13	—	13	—	8
Total	1,114	11.2	7.4	37.7	11.1	6.6	13.3	3.7	9

NIL, minimal change; FSGS, focal segmental glomerulosclerosis; memb, membranous; amyloid, amyloidosis; MCGN, membranoproliferative or mesangiocapillary; Other/Pro, other proliferative glomerulonephritis; Diabetes, diabetic nephropathy; Others, nonproliferative glomerulonephritis.
Adapted from Cameron JS. Nephrotic syndrome in the elderly. Semin Nephrol. 1996;16:319.

the most common diagnosis, accounting for 65% to 70% of all reported cases. Whatever the histology, a renal biopsy from an elderly individual is more likely to show more than one pathological lesion as well as more evidence of senescence; there is more likely to be more glomerular scarring, interstitial fibrosis, and tubular dropout. Among the glomerulonephritides (Table 86-1), membranous appears to be most common (37.7%) while minimal change (11.2%), amyloidosis (11.1%), focal segmental (7.4%), membranoproliferative (mesangiocapillary) (6.6%), other proliferative (13.3%), and nonproliferative (9.0%) account for the bulk of the rest. Because most patients with diabetic nephropathy can be presumptively diagnosed based on certain clinical criteria, its true incidence is underreported. For patients presenting with ARF, crescentic glomerulonephritis (31%), acute interstitial nephritis (18.6%), ATN with nephrotic syndrome (7.5%), atheroemboli (7.1%), light-chain cast nephropathy (5.9%), and postinfectious (5.5%) are the most commonly reported lesions. Longitudinal studies from Italy depict a changing pattern of glomerulonephritis in the elderly population with a much higher incidence of crescentic glomerulonephritis. Elderly patients with chronic renal insufficiency are most likely to have hypertensive nephrosclerosis, focal segmental glomerulosclerosis, interstitial nephritis, or amyloidosis on renal biopsy.

There has been very limited information on the prevalence of renal disease in the very elderly (aged 80 years or older). Recently, a retrospective study reviewing renal biopsies from 2001 to 2003 compared the very elderly with other age groups. The most common indications for performing a renal biopsy in the very elderly group were ARF (23%), nephrotic syndrome (33%), and acute glomerulonephritis (20%). Other indications included: (1) rapidly progressing renal failure (6%), (2) chronic kidney failure (17%), and (3) asymptomatic urinary abnormalities (1%). Surprisingly, membranous nephropathy accounted for only a small percentage of idiopathic nephrotic syndrome (15%), while pauci-immune crescentic glomerulonephritis was the most common diagnosis (19%). At least

40% of the biopsies performed revealed pathological findings that would benefit from therapeutic intervention, suggesting that kidney biopsies can be beneficial in the very elderly.

Epidemiological surveys from England report that the prevalence and incidence of nephrotic syndrome in geriatric populations are similar if not higher than those in adult populations of all ages, with about 11 new cases per million people per year. Approximately 18% of newly diagnosed adults with nephrotic syndrome are aged 60 years or older. The incidence may be higher, but many geriatric patients are not referred for renal biopsy because of age and functional status. This is especially true for patients older than 80 years of age. Geriatric patients with type II diabetes mellitus are also generally underreported in renal biopsy registries because diabetic nephropathy may go unrecognized and because the diagnosis can often be made without the necessity of a renal biopsy. Yet, more than 40% of elderly patients with ESRD have underlying diabetic nephropathy as the etiology of their ESRD.

The frequency of renovascular disease in elderly patients is unknown. It may be an unexpected finding in patients investigated for nonrenal disease, but the prevalence of severe renal artery stenosis increases with age. Autopsy studies show that among those persons older than age 70 years at the time of death, 62% had severe renal artery disease. When present, renal artery stenosis was bilateral in 50% of cases.

A high incidence of renal artery stenosis among normotensive subjects also has been found in several patient cohort studies undergoing angiography. In one report of patients older than 50 years of age, 69% of patients with hypertension and 35% without hypertension had identifiable renal artery atherosclerotic disease. A prospective study from Duke University of 1302 patients undergoing elective diagnostic cardiac catheterization showed significant unilateral renal artery stenosis in 11% of patients and bilateral stenosis in 4%. Multivariate and univariate analyses identified several predictors of increased risk for significant renovascular disease, including older age, multivessel coronary artery disease, and congestive heart failure. Interestingly, a history of hypertension did not predict the presence of renal artery stenosis in this cohort. Other angiographic studies evaluating the prevalence of renal artery stenosis in patients with vascular disease have shown similar findings with a prevalence between 11% and 42%. The highest prevalence is found among patients with peripheral vascular and aorto-occlusive disease or aneurysms.

Renovascular disease may also occur in the setting of renal insufficiency. A recent report from Italy of a study that included elderly patients with renal insufficiency of unclear etiology and mild proteinuria (less than 1 g/d) showed a 56% prevalence of significant (>70%) stenosis at angiography. Other investigators have done angiographic screening of patients older than age 50 years entering renal replacement therapy programs and report finding renal artery stenosis in 11% to 16% of these patients.

ACUTE RENAL FAILURE

Definition

ARF is defined as a sudden deterioration in renal function, sufficient to cause retention of nitrogenous waste in the body. The anatomic and physiological changes occurring in the aging kidney, the presence of comorbid medical conditions, the use of excessive numbers of medications, and the higher prevalence of obstructive uropathy are all contributing factors that can cause ARF in the elderly.

Clinical Presentation

Prerenal azotemia, or functional ARF as a result of extracellular fluid contraction, is the main cause of ARF in the geriatric population (Table 86-2). The reduced renal blood flow and GFR associated with aging leads to a reversible state of ARF in the setting of superimposed volume contraction. Loss of fluids, internal fluid redistribution, decreased cardiac output, and medications are responsible for the majority of cases of prerenal ARF in older individuals. Common medications associated with ARF are nonsteroidal anti-inflammatory drugs (NSAIDs), angiotensin-converting enzyme inhibitors (ACEIs), and angiotensin II type 1 receptor antagonist blockers (ARBs). The development of ARF secondary to ACEIs or ARBs in patients with renal artery stenosis is well known; however, recent publications also report cases of ACEIs and ARB-related ARF in patients without renovascular disease. Furthermore, a study from France reported that 67.5% of ACEI-induced cases of ARF in elderly patients occurred in the absence of renal artery stenosis.

NSAID-induced ARF occurs more frequently in the elderly than in the general population, mainly because of the coexistence of conditions associated with decreased effective intravascular volume or true volume depletion. Under these conditions, the kidney is dependent on prostaglandins to maintain renal perfusion. Loss of this important autoregulatory mechanism results in ARF. Advanced age is an independent risk factor for developing ARF in patients taking NSAIDs, presumably because of the normal, aging-related decrease in GFR.

Parenchymal causes of ARF include ATN, acute interstitial nephritis, acute glomerulonephritis, and renovascular disease. The most common cause of biopsy-proven intrinsic renal failure in geriatric patients is rapidly progressive glomerulonephritis (RPGN). Vasculitis and idiopathic crescentic glomerulonephritis make up more than half of these cases.

ATN results from prolonged renal ischemia or from exposure to nephrotoxins. The causes of ATN are multifactorial; however, the most common cause in elderly patients is volume depletion associated with renal hypoperfusion and ischemia. Complications of major surgery including intraoperative hypotension, postoperative fluid loss, and arrhythmias account for approximately one-third of the cases of ATN in the elderly. Sepsis-induced ATN occurs just as commonly. Nephrotoxic drugs may also cause ATN. The former often results from a failure to consider age-related decreases in GFR while the latter is responsible for 10% of the cases or ARF. Aminoglycoside nephrotoxicity and radiocontrast-induced ARF are just two examples of drug-induced renal failure.

Cholesterol emboli are another important cause of ARF in the geriatric population. Cholesterol crystals can become dislodged from atherosclerotic plaques during intra-aortic procedures, or may even arise spontaneously, and cause ARF by obstructing small renal arteries. This entity is important to consider in any patient with ARF following cardiac catheterization or aortic angiography. Rhabdomyolysis, in the settings of acute immobilization, infectious disease, cerebrovascular accidents, crush injury, hyperosmolar conditions, hyponatremia, hypothermia, or falls is being recognized as a prevalent and underdiagnosed cause of ATN in the elderly.

Postrenal or obstructive renal failure is one of the most significant causes of ARF in the elderly and may occur in 5% of the cases presenting with ARF. Common causes of obstruction in the geriatric population include benign prostate hypertrophy; prostate carcinoma; retroperitoneal or pelvic neoplasms such as non-Hodgkin's lymphoma, carcinoma of the bladder, cervix, ovaries, or rectum; and neurogenic bladder caused by diabetes mellitus. Prompt diagnosis is extremely important because prognosis for recovery of renal function depends on the length of time that the kidney is obstructed. As such, it is considered a true urological emergency. Therefore, it is imperative to exclude the possibility of obstruction in any elderly patient presenting with ARF, especially in those situations of previous urological pathology or recent abdominal surgery.

Diagnosis

A complete history, with special attention to potential nephrotoxic drugs and clinical clues of obstruction, is fundamental in establishing the diagnosis of ARF. Physical findings may be very subtle in the elderly but postural hypotension is usually present in states of true volume depletion. The use of urinary sodium concentration or the fractional excretion of sodium as markers to differentiate between acute prerenal azotemia and established ATN are less reliable in the geriatric population than in the general population. Elderly individuals have a decreased ability to concentrate their urine or respond to sudden changes in sodium and water balance because of aging-related disturbances in the tubular handling of water and/or sodium reabsorption. Thus, in geriatric patients, the urinary indices may not be helpful in differentiating between prerenal and ATN as a result of the physiological changes associated with aging, and early nephrologic consultation is warranted in any patient with ARF. The most reliable indicator of prerenal azotemia is its reversal following

TABLE 86-2

Acute Renal Failure in the Elderly

Prerenal (acute reversible renal
  hypoperfusion) ARF
  Hypovolemia
    Fluid loss
      Gastrointestinal
        Diarrhea
        Fistulas
        Vomiting
      Renal
        Diuretic intake
      Salt wasting
      Redistribution of the extracellular
        volume
        Shock (septic, cardiogenic),
          hypoalbuminemia, nephrotic
          syndrome, liver diseases
  Malnutrition
  Hemorrhage
  Inappropriate fluid restriction
  Interference with renal autoregulatory
    mechanisms
    ACEIs
    Cyclosporine
    NSAIDs
  Cardiac failure
    Acute
      Acute myocardial infarction
      Arrhythmias
      Cardiac tamponade
      Malignant hypertension
  Chronic: ischemic and hypertensive
    cardiomyopathies
      Valvulopathies

Renal or intrinsic ARF
  Acute glomerulonephritis
    Mesangiocapillary
    Postinfectious
    Rapidly progressive
      Goodpasture's syndrome
      Idiopathic
      SLE
  Vasculitis
    Hypersensitivity angiitis
      Classic
      Hemolytic-uremic syndrome
      Henoch-Schönlein
      Mixed cryoglobulinemia
      Scleroderma
      Serum sickness
      Wegener's granulomatosis
    Polyarteritis nodosa
  Tubulointerstitial nephropathies
    Drugs
      ACEIs
      Allopurinol
      Ampicillin
      Analgesics (including NSAIDs)
      Cimetidine
      Diphenylhydantoin
      Methicillin
      Thiazides
    Infectious: acute pyelonephritis
    Infiltrative
      Leukemia
      Lymphoma
      Sarcoidosis
    Idiopathic
  Intratubular obstruction
    Myeloma proteins
    Myoglobin
    Sulfonamides
    Urates
  Hypercalcemia
  Hepatorenal syndrome
  Vascular obstruction
    Arterial
      Aneurysms
      Atheroembolic disease
      Venous: thrombosis of vena cava
  Tubule cell damage
    Nephrotoxin-related
      Antibiotics (aminoglycosides)
      Iodinated contrast media
      IV Immunoglobulin G
      Metals (Hg, Ag, Pt, Bi)
      Organic solvents

Obstructive ARF
  Ureteral and pelvic
    Intrinsic obstruction
      Blood clots
      Fungus balls
      Sloughed papillae
        Diabetics
        Analgesic abusers
      Stones
    Extrinsic obstruction
      Fecal impaction
      Malignancy
      Retroperitoneal fibrosis
  Bladder
    Bladder carcinoma
    Blood clots
    Neuropathic
    Prostatic hypertrophy
    Stones
  Urethra
    Phymosis
    Strictures

ACEI, angiotensin-converting enzyme inhibitor; ARF, acute renal failure; NSAID, nonsteroidal antiinflammatory drugs; SLE, systemic lupus erythematosis.
Modified from Macias-Nunez JF, et al. Acute renal failure in the aged. Semin Nephrol. 1996;16:333.

volume repletion, and a judicious volume challenge is indicated if the patient is not volume overloaded.

In the setting of ARF, ultrasonography is the imaging procedure of choice for the diagnosis of obstruction, kidney stones, or renal masses, and for the determination of renal size. Although there are a few case reports of urinary tract obstruction secondary to prior malignancy with minimal or no dilation of the collecting system on ultrasonography, these cases are rare, and duplex Doppler ultrasonography may prove to be a useful diagnostic tool in these instances. Computerized tomography (CT) scans often do not provide any further diagnostic information and should be reserved for the cases in which the kidneys are poorly visualized.

Indications for renal biopsy in elderly patients with ARF include the following: (1) prolonged oliguria (3 to 4 weeks); (2) ARF associated with systemic illnesses such as vasculitis; (3) RPGN; (4) acute tubulointerstitial nephritis; and (5) anuria in the absence of obstruction. Advanced age alone is not a contraindication for renal biopsy.

Treatment

The management of ARF in the elderly should follow the same principles as in the general population. Maintenance of adequate intravascular volume is paramount in maintaining renal blood flow. Hemodynamic monitoring in critically ill patients is preferable with right-heart catheterization as indicated to measure pulmonary capillary wedge pressure. The routine use of renal dose dopamine for ARF should be discouraged because of the lack of demonstrated efficacy in this setting. Fenoldopam, a dopamine-1 receptor agonist, has not been shown to have any benefit in the outcome of ATN. Moreover, combinations of α- and β-adrenergic agonists, or colloid and blood transfusions to increase cardiac output to supranormal levels are not helpful in the setting of established ATN. Medications should be adjusted for the degree of renal insufficiency and appropriate dietary sodium, potassium, and protein restrictions instituted. A Foley catheter should be placed to rule out and treat bladder outlet obstruction. A previously placed Foley catheter should always be replaced regardless of whether it flushes.

The indication for renal replacement therapy in ARF must be individualized for each patient and depends upon the volume status of the patient and the need for solute clearance. Timely renal consultation early in the course of ARF often obviates the need for dialysis intervention. For those patients with ARF requiring dialysis, the required dialysis dose has not been established and may hinge on volume status and catabolic state. Acute peritoneal dialysis (PD) and hemodialysis have been used in elderly patients with ARF with similar results and complications as in younger adult patients. Continuous renal replacement therapy (CRRT) offers the advantages of slow controlled ultrafiltration and efficient removal of small and middle molecules. The CRRT multicenter trials have shown mixed results in mortality compared with conventional dialysis but promising results with large volume hemofiltration CRRT. Biocompatible membranes are used routinely now because of improved outcomes in patients with ARF.

Nutritional considerations warrant special consideration for any elderly patient with renal disease. There are advantages in early appropriate restriction of sodium, potassium, phosphorus, and protein for the elderly patient with ARF. Restricting the dietary protein intake to 0.6 to 0.8 g/kg ideal body weight for those patients not yet on dialysis results in maintenance of nitrogen balance, control of metabolic acidosis, and control of elemental phosphorus normally excreted by the kidney. Potassium and sodium are restricted to 2 g per day based on nutritional requirements. For those patients on dialysis, the dietary protein restriction can be liberalized to 1 to 1.2 g/kg ideal body weight for hemodialysis patients and 1.2 to 1.4 g/kg ideal body weight for patients on PD.

Prognosis

The mortality rate for ARF remains high. For critically ill patients, mortality rates approach 60% with sepsis-induced ARF having a worse prognosis than nonseptic ARF. The influence of age on outcome of ARF is debated; however, the elderly patient generally has less renal reserve than a younger individual and is more prone to ARF. As a result, an elderly patient has a moderately worse prognosis than a corresponding younger patient. Nevertheless, age alone should not be used as a discriminating factor in therapeutic decisions concerning ARF.

GLOMERULAR DISEASES

There has been a change in the clinical approach toward patients with ARF or nephrotic syndrome in the geriatric population. Because of the routine use of ultrasonographic guidance for renal biopsies, as well as improvements in the size and accuracy of the biopsy needle, the success rate in obtaining a diagnostic renal biopsy that provides clinically useful information has improved to greater than 90%. This is important because ESRD caused by glomerulonephritis currently accounts for approximately 24% of patients requiring dialysis in Europe and a higher percentage in the United States. Recent reviews suggest that the clinical features, histopathologic classification, and clinical outcome of glomerulonephritis in elderly patients are comparable to those of younger adults. Based on these observations, a reliable diagnosis and an effective therapeutic plan have to be advocated in elderly patients similar to the approach taken in younger adult patients.

Clinical Presentation

Elderly patients with biopsy-proven glomerulonephritis usually present with the following major clinical syndromes (Table 86-3): (1) nephrotic syndrome (50% to 60% in some series), characterized by heavy proteinuria and a variable tendency toward edema, hypertension, renal failure, and hyperlipidemia; (2) acute glomerulonephritis or acute nephritic syndrome, characterized by the abrupt clinical onset of hematuria, proteinuria, decreased GFR, fluid and salt retention, hypertension, and occasionally, oliguria; (3) RPGN, whose clinical pattern includes a more insidious onset, progressive loss of renal function, and, frequently, oliguria; (4) chronic glomerulonephritis, characterized by CRF accompanied by various degrees of proteinuria, hematuria, and hypertension, and a clinical course that is usually progressive but which may be protracted over several years; and (5) urinary abnormalities with few or no symptoms. Although an asymptomatic urinary abnormality is the single most common clinical presentation in younger patients, it is rarely found

TABLE 86-3

Comparison of Mode of Presentation Between Patients Aged Older Than 65 Yrs and Those Aged 20 to 65 Yrs at the Time of Biopsy and Reported as Having Idiopathic Glomerulonephritis

MODE OF PRESENTATION	AGE			
	>65 Yrs		20–65 Yrs	
	(n)	(%)	(n)	(%)
Acute renal failure	37	14	240	11
Asymptomatic urinary abnormality	17	6	841	38
Chronic renal failure	54	20	168	7
Hypertension	4	1	40	2
Nephrotic syndrome	140	52	715	32
Unknown	19	7	226	10
Total number	271	100	2230	100

Modified from Davison AM, Johnston PA. Idiopathic glomerulonephritis in the elderly. Contrib Nephrol. 1993;105:41.

TABLE 86-4

Classification of Rapidly Progressive Glomerulonephritis

Primary diffuse crescentic glomerulonephritis
  Type I: anti-GBM-mediated disease without pulmonary hemorrhage (with anti-GBM)
  Type II: immune complex-associated disease (without anti-GMB or ANCA)
  Type III: pauci-immune (with ANCA)
  Type IV: mixed pattern (with anti-GBM and ANCA)
  Type V: pauci-immune (without ANCA or anti-GBM)
  Fibrillary and immunotactoid glomerulonephritis
  Focal sclerosis (rare)
  IgA nephropathy
  Mesangiocapillary glomerulonephritis (especially type II)
  Membranous glomerulonephritis (with or without anti-GBM)
  Superimposed on another primary glomerular disease

Associated with infectious disease
  Hepatitis B and C
  Histoplasmosis
  Infective endocarditis
  Influenza (?)
  Mycoplasma infection
  Poststreptococcal glomerulonephritis
  Visceral abscesses

Associated with multisystem disease
  Carcinoma (lung, bladder, prostate)
  Goodpasture disease (anti-GBM with pulmonary hemorrhage)
  Lymphoma
  Mixed (IgG/IgM) cryoimmunoglobulinemia (hepatitis C)
  Relapsing polychondritis
  Henoch–Schönlein purpura
  Systemic lupus erythematosus
  Systemic polyangiitis
    Churg–Strauss syndrome
    Microscopic polyangiitis (with ANCA)
    Wegener granulomatosis (with ANCA)
    Other variants

Associated with medications
  Allopurinol
  Bucillamine
  D-Penicillamine
  Hydralazine
  Rifampin

ANCA, antineutrophil cytoplasmic antibodies; GBM, glomerular basement membrane.
Modified from Glassock RJ. Syndromes of glomerular diseases. In: Massry SG, Glassock RJ, eds. Textbook of Nephrology. 4th ed. Baltimore: Williams and Wilkins; 2000:650.

in geriatric populations (age ≥60 years). The reason for this difference may be the aging-related reduction in renal function, or the lack of routine urine testing in elderly patients even though they are more likely to be seeking advice for medical complaints.

Acute Glomerulonephritis and Rapidly Progressive Glomerulonephritis

These two clinical syndromes often present as ARF in the elderly. The glomerular findings are similar to younger adults presenting with crescentic glomerulonephritis. Indeed, crescentic glomerulonephritis is the most common lesion found on renal biopsy in this group of geriatric patients. With aging, the glomerular basement membrane (GBM) becomes thickened and the glomerular surface area decreases. These changes tend to render the glomerulus more liable to immune complex-mediated damage. In addition, the increased prevalence of autoantibody and immune complexes in the elderly increase the risk of immunological-mediated glomerular injury, but these factors may be offset by the reduced renal plasma flow and the aging-associated impairment of cell-mediated immunity. This leads some investigators to believe that there may be other, currently unrecognized factors that increase the risk of developing glomerulonephritis in geriatric patients.

Postinfectious glomerulonephritis is present in approximately 6% to 8% of biopsy series of geriatric patients presenting with ARF. The clinical features are similar to those found in younger adults, but the clinical course is associated with a higher incidence of hypertension, azotemia, and ESRD. Underrecognized is postinfectious glomerulonephritis associated with aortofemoral bypass graft infections, especially those caused by *Salmonella*, which result in increased risk for morbidity and mortality.

Renal biopsies from patients with RPGN demonstrate extensive accumulation of cells in Bowman's space (crescents). Although the disorders associated with RPGN can be classified as either primary glomerular disorders or secondary forms associated with infectious processes, multisystem disorders, or drug reactions (Table 86-4), three disorders deserve special attention in the elderly: antineutrophil

cytoplasmic antibody (ANCA)-associated renal disease, hepatitis C-associated cryoglobulinemia, and Henoch–Schönlein purpura.

ANCA-associated renal disease presents as a small-vessel systemic vasculitis or as an isolated primary pauci-immune necrotizing and crescentic glomerulonephritis. The clinical manifestations depend on the severity and stage of the underlying renal injury. The light microscopy morphologic findings range from focal sclerosing glomerulonephritis associated with hematuria and/or proteinuria, to more aggressive patterns including necrosis with a few crescents to overt cellular crescentic changes associated with acute nephritis and a rapid loss of renal function. In addition, a few biopsy specimens will depict changes compatible with chronic glomerulonephritis and global glomerular sclerosis associated with slowly progressive nephritis and CRF.

The most common finding in elderly patients undergoing renal biopsy for the clinical syndrome of RPGN is isolated primary pauci-immune glomerulonephritis. The ANCA is positive in approximately 45% to 55% of these cases. Another 20% to 25% of patients present with identical histological findings associated with small vessel vasculitis in an extrarenal location. This group of patients has been classified as microscopic polyangiitis (MPA) according to the Chapel Hill Consensus Conference on the Nomenclature of Systemic Vasculitis. In addition to the renal histological pattern described above, another 12% to 15% of patients present with granulomatous inflammation involving the respiratory tract and will be diagnosed with Wegener's granulomatosis.

The two known staining patterns of ANCA are perinuclear and cytoplasmic. The perinuclear pattern (P-ANCA) is usually associated with specific reactivity against myeloperoxidase and is associated with MPA in approximately 40% to 55% of cases. This pattern is strongly associated with primary pauci-immune crescentic glomerulonephritis in 60% to 70% of cases. Finally, approximately 15% to 25% of patients with Wegener's granulomatosis present with reactivity to perinuclear ANCA.

The cytoplasmic ANCA (C-ANCA) pattern is associated with reactivity against a serine proteinase (proteinase 3, PR3), and is found in 65% to 75% of patients classified as Wegener's granulomatosis, 35% to 45% of patients with MPA, and 30% to 40% of patients with primary pauci-immune glomerulonephritis. Patients with one of these three diagnoses are ANCA-negative in 10% to 20% of the cases. The treatment of this group of disorders has only been reported in uncontrolled studies.

In addition to testing patients presenting with vasculitis for ANCA, it is important to test for antiglomerular basement membrane (anti-GBM) disease and for systemic lupus erythematosus, because the treatment options for these two diseases are quite different. Referral to a nephrologist is essential for proper diagnosis and therapy.

Most patients with MPA or primary necrotizing and crescentic glomerulonephritis achieve remission with therapeutic regimens based on corticosteroids in combination with either intravenous or oral cyclophosphamide. Recent reviews report a long-term remission rate of 60% to 85% in patients with these disorders, but relapse occurs in up to 40% of patients within 18 months. For those patients with systemic vasculitis such as Wegener's granulomatosis, long-term remission is not possible without the use of cyclophosphamide. The 5-year survival rates cited for patients older than 60 years of age at the time of diagnosis (31%) compared with those subjects younger than 60 years of age (83%), is partly a result of the reluctance of clinicians to use cyclophosphamide in the elderly patient. Although the toxicity and side effects of steroids and cytotoxic drugs increases with age, these medications should not be necessarily withheld in the elderly patient. Careful examination of the renal biopsy, clinical presentation, and the ANCA reactivity are needed to design an appropriate treatment strategy with the benefits and risks of therapy individualized for each patient. The reader is referred to reference sources listed at the end of this chapter for details about specific therapeutic protocols.

Hepatitis C-associated cryoglobulinemia associated with vasculitis and hepatitis can also present with RPGN. Associated findings include purpuric and necrotizing skin lesions in exposed areas, fever, acroparesthesia, Raynaud's phenomenon, urticaria, neuritis, arthralgia, and hepatosplenomegaly. Some series from Italy report hepatitis C as the second most common cause of secondary glomerulonephritis in the elderly population; amyloidosis is the most common cause. Warm serum immunoelectrophoresis shows abnormal circulating immunoglobulins that precipitate in the cold with a polyclonal immunoglobulin (Ig) G component and a monoclonal IgM or IgA with rheumatoid factor activity (type II cryoglobulinemia). Light microscopic examination of renal biopsies reveals diffuse endocapillary proliferation with a few crescents. Electron microscopic findings of typical intracapillary deposits and subendothelial electron-dense deposits, with a crystalline substructure, confirm the diagnosis.

In the past, immunosuppressive therapy was used for cryoglobulinemia-related vasculitis, but the effect of immunosuppression on chronic hepatitis C infection has not been well defined and could potentially accelerate viral replication. Reduction in the level of cryoglobulins by intensive plasma exchange may be associated with clinical remission, while the administration of interferon-α and ribavirin have the potential to revolutionize therapy for this disease but await future controlled trials.

Henoch–Schönlein purpura presents as a small-vessel vasculitis with IgA-dominant immune deposits, typically involving the skin, gut, and glomeruli, and is frequently associated with arthralgias or arthritis. Potential precipitating conditions in the elderly include alcohol abuse, malignancies, and some medications. This pattern of etiologic agents contrasts with the pattern in younger patients in whom infections are the most common etiologic agent. In general, Henoch–Schönlein purpura is a benign, self-limited disorder, but the renal dysfunction is significantly worse in geriatric patients than in younger adults. Elderly patients present with a higher prevalence of hypertension, azotemia requiring renal replacement therapy, and histopathological features of IgA mesangial deposits and proliferation with crescentic glomerulonephritis. Improvement in renal function has been noted in some patients after plasma exchange and immunosuppressive therapy, but the small number of cases reported and the lack of a controlled study prevent any firm therapeutic recommendations.

NEPHROTIC SYNDROME

Definition

The nephrotic syndrome consists of urinary protein losses in excess of 3.5 g per 1.73 m^2 body surface area per day in association with hypoalbuminemia, hypercholesterolemia, and peripheral edema. The onset is usually insidious but it can be explosive. As the major clinical manifestation of nephrotic syndrome is generalized edema, many geriatric patients are often misdiagnosed as having congestive heart failure. The etiologies of nephrotic syndrome include the primary glomerular diseases (minimal change disease, focal and segmental glomerulosclerosis, membranous glomerulonephropathy, membranoproliferative glomerulonephropathy), and glomerulonephritis secondary to systemic infiltrative diseases, neoplasms, chronic infectious diseases, atheroembolic disease, or medications.

Pathophysiology

The glomerular capillary wall consists of three components: the endothelial cells, basement membrane, and the podocytes. The membrane component or components responsible for the loss of the filtration barrier have been debated. Over the past decade, the podocytes' molecular structure has been found to play a major role in maintaining the integrity of the basement membrane. The molecules in the slit diaphragm allow for interdigitation of adjacent podocytes, maintenance of distance between the slits (35 to 45 nm), and the polarity of the podocytes. Loss of the function of certain podocytes molecules, podocin, nephrin, CD2AP, and α-4 actinin, are responsible for congential nephrotic syndrome. Immunohistochemical studies in rats and human with nephrotic syndrome have shown redistribution of the nephrin in the podocytes. The function of these various molecules in the podocytes may have a major effect on the course of treatment in adult nephrotic syndrome.

Clinical Manifestations

The nephrotic syndrome often goes unrecognized in geriatric individuals since it frequently presents in an atypical manner. Because many geriatric patients have poor tissue turgor, edema frequently develops only in dependent portions of the body. Moreover, many geriatric patients with nephrotic syndrome will develop edema at higher plasma albumin concentrations than younger adults, who, in turn, develop edema at higher albumin levels than children. Hypercoagulability is a frequent complication of nephrotic syndrome and is particularly concerning in a geriatric patient who is bedridden. In some series, the proportion of patients who present with a significant complication such as deep venous thrombosis (DVT) or pulmonary embolus (PE) approaches 50%. Compared to younger adults, geriatric patients with nephrotic syndrome have a higher incidence of hypertension, hypercholesterolemia, and nonselective proteinuria, a lower value of GFR, and often present with microscopic hematuria. Microscopic hematuria is particularly common in geriatric patients with minimal change disease or hypertensive glomerulosclerosis. Geriatric age individuals with biopsy-proven minimal change disease present with persistent hematuria in 30% of cases and with hypertension in 44% of cases.

The pathogenesis of coincident nephrotic syndrome and ARF remains obscure. Some investigators suggest that ARF results from an increase in intrarenal pressure and the presence of proteinaceous casts, which obstruct tubule lumens. This pathogenetic mechanism suggests that a renal biopsy should be obtained to aid in the management of the nephrotic syndrome in the elderly.

Approximately 5% of geriatric patients who present with nephrotic syndrome will have an underlying malignancy or develop one within 1 year. Of these patients, 33% will be diagnosed with membranous glomerulonephritis. In older series, 10% to 33% of geriatric individuals with nephrotic syndrome caused by membranous glomerulonephritis were found to have a malignancy, but recent studies suggest that patients with nephrotic syndrome do not have a higher incidence of malignant disease when compared to age-matched individuals without nephrotic syndrome. Currently, most investigators recommend that the only test that should be performed in all patients presenting with nephrotic syndrome is a chest x-ray, because carcinoma of the lung is the most common malignancy associated with membranous glomerulonephritis, and a stool guaiac, because carcinoma of the colon is the next most common location for an unsuspected malignancy. If no evidence for a malignancy is found on physical examination, chest x-ray, or by occult blood testing, the patient should be carefully followed for the next 15 months for the appearance of a malignancy, and receive routine care thereafter.

The clinical presentation of nephrotic syndrome secondary to another systemic illness does not differ substantially between geriatric and younger adult patients. All patients presenting with nephrotic syndrome should be evaluated for amyloidosis, plasma cell dyscrasias, diabetes mellitus, hepatitis, syphilis, human immunodeficiency virus (HIV), collagen vascular disorders, and cryoglobulins.

Histopathology Findings

The interpretation of the histologic appearance of renal biopsy specimens from geriatric individuals with nephrotic syndrome represents a challenge to the nephropathologist because of the normal aging-related changes that occur in the kidney. Glomerulosclerosis (which can occur in up to 40% of remaining glomeruli), vascular changes (especially hypertension-induced changes), and interstitial fibrosis are common findings in normal kidneys from geriatric individuals and must be considered in evaluating renal pathology. However, minimal change disease and membranous glomerulopathy retain their typical histological appearance and can be diagnosed by an experienced nephropathologist.

Secondary amyloidosis should be distinguished from primary amyloidosis because its prognosis is better and specific therapy aimed at the underlying disease may be available. Special stains including immunofluorescent antibodies against amyloid A protein are useful in diagnosing cases of secondary amyloidosis. Amyloid may be found infiltrating the glomerulus and may also be found infiltrating blood vessels and, occasionally, peritubular spaces. Light-chain glomerulopathy is characterized by the deposition of immunoglobulin light chains in a nodular or diffuse fashion along the basement membranes within the kidney. Kappa light chains are found more frequently than lambda light chains.

Occasional patients will show histological findings compatible with nonamyloid fibrillary glomerulopathies. Two categories are recognized on the basis of their ultrastructural appearance: fibrillary glomerulonephritis with extracellular deposits randomly oriented (10 to 30 nm diameter fibrils) and immunotactoid glomerulonephritis characterized by microtubular structures in a parallel array (25 to 45 nm diameter). Because these entities are fairly uncommon, the prognosis and therapeutic interventions remain obscure.

Focal segmental glomerulosclerosis was recently associated with atheroembolic renal disease. The pathologic changes produced by cholesterol atheroemboli show distinctive pathological findings including glomerular collapse, foot process fusion, podocyte hypertrophy, and frequently, acute tubular injury. Very few elderly patients present with IgA nephropathy with nephrotic range proteinuria.

Diagnosis

Nephrotic syndrome is often masked by other comorbid conditions in geriatric individuals. The patient evaluation should include microscopic examination of the urine by a nephrologist; serum creatinine; blood urea nitrogen (BUN); albumin; and cholesterol; 24-hour urine collection to quantitatively measure proteinuria and creatinine clearance; serum protein electrophoresis and immunoelectrophoresis; urine protein electrophoresis and immunoelectrophoresis; antinuclear antibody (ANA); antideoxyribonucleic acid (anti-DNA) antibody titer; hepatitis B and C serologies; syphilis serology; complement profile; cryoglobulins; lipoprotein profile; HIV; chest x-ray; and stool guaiac. Renal biopsy is essential for establishing the definitive histopathological diagnosis.

Treatment and Prognosis

Definitive treatment for the nephrotic syndrome depends upon the histologic type. Regardless of the histology, some generalizations about therapy can be made. Every effort should be made to control blood pressure. ACEIs and ARBs are rapidly becoming mainstays in treatment because of their efficacy in reducing proteinuria and numerous studies suggesting that they may slow progression of renal disease. If these agents are not tolerated, other agents can be substituted with a goal of maintaining the blood pressure at around 125/75 mm Hg. Low-protein diets also have their utility, especially for those patients with heavy proteinuria and dietary counseling, which is reimbursed by Medicare, can prove to be invaluable. The value of hydroxymethylglutaryl coenzyme A (HMG-CoA) reductase inhibitors remains unproven in patients older than age 75 years, but should be considered for younger patients. Any discussion of therapy should take into consideration the patient's financial status, as some medications may prove to be prohibitively expensive.

The treatment of membranous nephropathy remains controversial because the natural history of the disease includes spontaneous remissions and exacerbations. In general, one third of patients will be expected to improve; another third will follow an indolent course, while the final third will progress to ESRD. Risk factors for progression include male sex, poorly controlled hypertension, renal insufficiency, and heavy proteinuria. Recent reevaluation of data from multiple trials suggests that targeted therapy to those individuals most likely to progress is beneficial. ACEIs and/or ARBs should be considered for control of both hypertension and proteinuria. Likewise, for those individuals likely to progress, a combination of steroids with cytotoxic agents or cyclosporine A should be considered with careful consideration of dose, duration, and other comorbid factors, but treatment with steroids alone is not beneficial. In most instances, it may be more prudent to carefully observe the patient and watch for signs of progression before embarking on a course of steroids and immunosuppressive therapy. Because therapy continues to evolve, nephrology consultation is appropriate.

Geriatric patients with minimal change disease tend to have as favorable a prognosis as younger cohorts and respond equally well to corticosteroid therapy. Moreover, relapses following cessation of prednisone therapy are relatively infrequent. For some individuals, stopping NSAID therapy is the only intervention necessary. Otherwise, patients with minimal change disease should be treated with prednisone for 2 to 4 months before they are diagnosed as corticosteroid-resistant. If a relapse does occur, these patients should be treated in the same way as younger adults. In steroid-resistant geriatric patients, cyclophosphamide can be used, but the normal age-associated decrease in GFR should be taken into account in determining the appropriate dose. In most instances, a dose of 1 to 2 mg/kg body weight per day that is commonly used in younger patients must be reduced, and the white blood cell count monitored carefully. Other treatment options include calcineurin inhibitors or mycophenolate.

The management of renal amyloidosis is supportive and specific treatment depends on the type: primary versus secondary. For primary amyloidosis, there is no specific therapy but selective cases may benefit from chemotherapy and autologous or allogeneic hematopoietic cell transplantation. The role of this therapeutic approach is difficult to define in geriatric populations since many patients die before any benefit can be seen. For secondary amyloidosis, further amyloid deposition can be prevented if the underlying disease process can be treated. No therapy is available that effects the resolution of amyloid deposits, but treatment that reduces the supply of amyloid fibril precursor proteins can improve survival and preserve renal function.

Patients presenting with histologic features of light chain glomerulopathy have a 5-year renal survival of 40%. These patients should undergo bone marrow examination to test for the presence of multiple myeloma. Treatment with cytotoxic drugs (melphalan and prednisone) may diminish proteinuria and preserve renal function. However, cytotoxic therapy in the absence of multiple myeloma is controversial. Plasmapheresis, in addition to cytotoxic therapy, should be considered for patients with ARF caused by multiple myeloma, but the likelihood of success of this intervention hinges on the blood paraprotein level.

RENOVASCULAR DISEASE

Definition

Renovascular disease is an important cause of secondary hypertension and progressive renal insufficiency in the elderly population. The spectrum of diseases that can cause anatomic narrowing of a main renal artery or its branches include many different disease entities (Table 86-5). The two main types of renal arterial lesions are atherosclerosis and fibrous dysplasia, but atherosclerosis accounts for almost 90% of cases in the elderly population.

TABLE 86-5

Categories of Renal Artery Disease
Aneurysms
Arteriovenous malformations
Atherosclerosis
Dissection of the aorta
Embolic disease
Fibrous dysplasia
Kawasaki disease
Neurofibromatosis
Other systemic necrotizing vasculitides
Polyarteritis nodosa
Takayasu arteritis
Thromboangiitis obliterans
Thrombotic diseases
Trauma
Vasculitis involving the renal artery

Modified from Greco BA, Breyer JA. Natural history of renal artery stenosis. Semin Nephrol. 1996;16:3.

TABLE 86-6

Prevalence of Unsuspected Renal Artery Stenosis (RAS): Angiographic Studies

STUDY NO.	YEAR	NO. OF PATIENTS	INDICATIONS	% OF PATIENTS WITH >50% RAS
1	1975	190	AAA	22
2	1990	100	PVD	42
3	1992	1302	Cardiac catheterization	11
4	1995	196	Cardiac catheterization	18
5	1994	127	PVD	16
6	1990	395	Aortic/PVD	33–39
7	1990	374	PVD	14
8	1992	450	PVD	23
9	1993	346	AAA/AOD	28
10	1989	118	Cardiac catheterization	23
11	1996	100	PVD	11
12	1990	100	PVD	22

AAA, abdominal aortic aneurysm; AOD, atherosclerotic disease; PVD, peripheral vascular disease; RAS, renal artery stenosis.
Modified from Greco BA, Breyer JA. Natural history of renal artery stenosis. Semin Nephrol. 1996;16:5.

Clinical Features

As mentioned above, the clinical presentation of renal artery stenosis ranges widely from asymptomatic forms to the two well-known clinical syndromes: renovascular hypertension and ischemic nephropathy (Table 86-6). Renovascular hypertension is defined as the secondary elevation of blood pressure produced by any of a variety of conditions that interfere with the kidney's arterial circulation and cause renal hypoperfusion. With the exception of oral contraceptive use (not common in the elderly) and alcohol ingestion, renovascular hypertension is the most common cause of potentially remediable secondary hypertension. Renovascular hypertension has an estimated prevalence of 2% to 3% in the general hypertensive population. It is important to differentiate between renal artery stenosis and renovascular hypertension because the diagnosis of the latter requires verification that sufficient stenosis (>75% to 80%) is present to produce renal tissue ischemia and to initiate the sequence of events leading to hypertension. Clinical clues that might prompt the clinician to diagnose renal artery stenosis in elderly patients are onset of hypertension after the age of 50 years; accelerated or difficult to control hypertension; coexisting diffuse atherosclerotic vascular disease; acute or subacute renal insufficiency after initiation of therapy with ACEIs or ARBs; recurrent pulmonary edema; grades III to IV hypertensive retinopathy; abdominal or flank bruit; hypokalemia in the absence of diuretic use; erythrocytosis; microangiopathic hemolytic anemia; and hyperuricemia. Although renovascular hypertension is thought to occur primarily in white patients, recent cohort studies report a similar prevalence in selected African-American and white patients. Whether these racial variations are a result of differences in screening and referral patterns or true differences in the prevalence of renovascular hypertension remains to be determined.

Ischemic nephropathy can be defined as a clinically significant reduction in the GFR resulting from a partial or complete luminal obstruction of the preglomerular renal arteries of any caliber. It occurs in patients with hemodynamically significant stenosis in the renal artery of a solitary kidney or in both renal arteries if two kidneys are present.

Patients with atheromatous renovascular disease may present with different clinical courses. ARF can be precipitated by treatment of hypertension with ACEIs or ARBs during a period of days to weeks after initiating therapy. This form of ARF may be associated with hypoperfusion of the kidneys caused by inhibition of angiotensin II–dependent autoregulatory pathways in the glomerulus. Nevertheless, many patients with renovascular disease tolerate these agents and are usually not referred for additional noninvasive studies. Thus, the sensitivity of using the response to ACEIs or ARBs as a screening test for the presence of renovascular disease is unknown. Currently available clinical data estimate that 6% to 38% of patients with significant renal vascular disease will develop ARF following ACEI or ARB therapy. Other antihypertensive agents have been reported to cause reversible ARF in the setting of ischemic nephropathy. These cases should be distinguished from those hypertensive patients without ischemic nephropathy who develop ARF in the setting of renin-dependent decreases in renal perfusion such as intravascular volume depletion or low effective circulating volume states such as congestive heart failure or cirrhosis.

Renovascular disease may also present as progressive azotemia in a patient with suspected or documented renovascular hypertension (Table 86-7) or as recurrent pulmonary edema associated with poorly controlled hypertension and renal insufficiency (23% prevalence in some series). Postulated mechanisms include angiotensin II-induced myocardial dysfunction, diastolic dysfunction secondary to left ventricular hypertrophy, and reduced pressure natriuresis in conjunction with subsequent volume expansion. Azotemia in an elderly patient, in the absence of clinical and laboratory signs, that is suggestive of another renal disease, or of unexplained azotemia requiring initiation of renal replacement therapy, should prompt an evaluation for renovascular disease. Because the age of patients with ESRD is increasing, there is a significant proportion of patients on dialysis with renovascular disease.

Atheroembolic renal disease falls into the category of renal insufficiency induced by preglomerular ischemia. This entity has been usually described in patients with clinical evidence of atheromatous occlusive disease following invasive intra-aortic diagnostic or

TABLE 86-7

Natural History of Atheromatous Renovascular Disease					
STUDY NO.	YEAR	NO. OF PATIENTS	MEAN FOLLOW-UP	PROGRESSIVE NARROWING OF RENAL ARTERY (%)*	RENAL FUNCTION DETERIORATION (%)
1	1981	41	36	(?)	37
2	1968	39	27 (?)	36	(?)
3	1984	85	87	44	38
4	1991	48	97	1	(?)
5	1968	30	28	60	19
6	1987	36	48	40	44.4

*On serial angiography.

Data from Zucchelli P, Zuccala A. Ischemic nephropathy in the elderly. Contrib Nephrol. 105:13, 17.

therapeutic procedures, although spontaneous embolic episodes have been described. Important clinical clues associated with this disease are the presence of unexplained eosinophilia, purpuric-ischemic skin lesions, and the presence of heavy proteinuria, which can be in the nephrotic range.

Diagnostic Approach

There are three basic steps in making the diagnosis of renovascular hypertension: (1) renal artery stenosis must be demonstrated by angiography; (2) the stenotic lesion must be pathophysiologically significant; and (3) the hypertension is corrected by intervention to relieve the stenosis. In practice, the diagnosis of ischemic nephropathy is almost always made in the context of coexisting hypertension.

In the appropriate clinical setting such as those just described (worsening renal failure, bland urinary sediment, proteinuria <1 g/day, hypertension, and evidence of peripheral vascular disease), the clinician should develop a high index of suspicion for the disease. According to the triage approach proposed by Mann and Pickering, the patient may be classified as having a low (less than 1% prevalence), moderate (5 to 15% prevalence), or high (>25% prevalence) pretest probability for renovascular disease. Patients classified in the low-risk group should not undergo further workup. The presence of azotemia in the high-risk group may impair the reliability of the noninvasive tests and may justify performing renal angiography regardless of the results of noninvasive tests. In patients with intermediate probability, noninvasive testing has the most important diagnostic role.

ACEI radionuclide scintirenography is currently the most thoroughly evaluated noninvasive test for the diagnosis of renovascular hypertension. This study should be preceded by measurement of a random morning plasma renin activity (PRA). Evaluation of ACEI renography by using technetium-99m diethylenetriamine pentaacetic acid (^{99m}Tc-DTPA) has shown high sensitivity and specificity (91% to 94%) for renovascular hypertension. Currently, renal scintigraphy with Hippuran or Mag3 (renal plasma flow tracers) before and after ACEIs is the functional test of choice to diagnose ischemic nephropathy. Two limitations should be kept in mind: (1) these tests have not been evaluated in patients with azotemia and (2) while a positive test predicts an improvement in blood pressure, it is not known whether it also predicts an improvement in renal function.

Duplex ultrasound scanning of the renal arteries is a screening tool with promising early results. Duplex ultrasound scanning also allows measurement of kidney size and is not affected by medications or the level of GFR. The reported sensitivity and specificity values are in the low to mid-90% range. The main disadvantage of this test is that it is technically demanding and has a steep learning curve for each center that performs this test. Another caveat is that accessory renal arteries are difficult to detect and study.

The magnetic resonance angiography (MRA) has been effective in screening for the presence of renal artery stenosis with the advantage of being less exposure to contrast media and less invasive than the arteriogram. A publication from Italy reports overall accuracy of 97% for correct depiction of severe renal artery stenosis when compared head-to-head to conventional angiography. However, there have been recent case reports of patients with chronic kidney disease (CKD) developing nephrogenic systemic fibrosis (NSF)/nephrogenic fibrosing dermopathy (NFD) thought to be secondary to gadolinium exposure. Therefore, the future use of MRA for defining renal artery stenosis in patients with kidney disease needs to be redefined. Another highly accurate noninvasive study for screening for renal artery stenosis is the spiral (helical) CT scan with CT angiography, but there is a risk of contrast nephropathy with the spiral CT scan in patients with CKD.

The gold standard for diagnosing renal artery stenosis is selective renal angiography. Intra-arterial digital subtraction angiography (IA-DSA) or a CO_2 angiogram also provides excellent anatomic detail and requires less contrast than conventional angiography. The technique of intravenous DSA, although less invasive, does not provide comparable resolution to the aforementioned tests because of the high degree of bowel gas and motility artifacts, and usually requires a significantly larger amount of nephrotoxic contrast material.

The second step in making the diagnosis of renovascular hypertension is to determine the pathophysiological significance of the lesion. Some of the diagnostic tests already mentioned are also used to assess this issue. Selective renal vein renin measurement is the gold standard for establishing the functional nature of the stenotic lesion and helps predict the blood pressure response to revascularization. In general, a renal vein renin ratio of ≥ 1.5 between the two renal veins is predictive of a beneficial blood pressure response following surgery or angioplasty, but failure to lateralize does not predict a negative response. Overall, the blood pressure response to revascularization cannot be determined with confidence by using renal vein renin measurements. A positive captopril renogram with ^{99m}Tc-DTPA has been reported to accurately predict the blood pressure response to revascularization. The predictive value of all of these

TABLE 86-8

Results of Surgical Revascularization for Atherosclerotic Ischemic Nephropathy

Study No.	Year	No. of Patients	No. (%) Improved	No. (%) Stable	No. (%) Deteriorated
1	1992	40	22 (55%)	10 (25%)	8 (20%)
2	1987	91	20 (22%)	48 (53%)	23 (25%)
3	1992	70	34 (49%)	25 (36%)	11 (15%)
4	1992	91	45 (49%)	31 (35%)	15 (16%)
5	1987	161	93 (58%)	50 (31%)	18 (11%)
6	1993	13	9 (69%)	3 (23%)	7 (8%)

Data from Pohl MA. Ischemic nephropathy. American Society of Nephrology's Board Review Course Syllabus, 1996;14.

tests in terms of the renal function outcome after revascularization is largely unknown and awaits further study.

Treatment

Several studies clearly demonstrate that renovascular disease is a progressive disease. Of patients with the disease, 50% can expect their stenosis to worsen, with reported rates varying between 1.5% and 5% per year. In general, the rate of progression of renal insufficiency and the likelihood of deterioration of renal function correlates positively with the extent of stenosis at the time of diagnosis. This implies that correction of renal artery stenosis might be worthwhile in preventing renal failure or to improve renal function. This is important because elderly patients with progressive atherosclerotic renal artery obstruction leading to ESRD do not respond well to renal replacement therapy. Of all geriatric patients with ESRD, these patients have the poorest overall survival, with a 27-month median survival rate and only a 12% 5-year survival rate.

There is no universally accepted treatment in patients with renovascular disease. Therapy must be individualized and based upon the general status of the patient, the presence of any concomitant disease, and the local surgical or angiographic experience of the center. The role of surgical revascularization in the management of renovascular hypertension was first established by the U.S. Cooperative study 20 years ago. Increasingly good results have been reported (Table 86-8). The combined cured and improved rate is reported to be approximately 82% with a mortality rate of approximately 1% when one includes patients of all ages. The results are less favorable in elderly patients with atherosclerotic renal artery stenosis because their prognosis is determined by the extent of atherosclerosis elsewhere and the potential risk of cholesterol embolization during the operation.

Recovery of renal function after surgical revascularization depends upon whether the patient has unilateral or bilateral atherosclerotic renal disease, or a solitary kidney. With regard to unilateral stenosis, revascularization has only a modest beneficial effect on renal function. This occurs mainly because any increase in GFR in the revascularized, poststenotic kidney, is often offset by a decrease in the GFR of the contralateral kidney. Furthermore, when severe azotemia is present in a patient with unilateral stenosis, it is usually a result of severe bilateral nephrosclerosis, that is, bilateral renal parenchymal damage, which will not be improved by revascularization.

In bilateral stenosis, there are two possible clinical presentations. The first is bilateral occlusion of the renal arteries. This situation does not necessarily imply irreversible damage because the viability of the kidneys may be maintained by a collateral blood supply. This is particularly true in patients who have a gradual onset of arterial occlusion. Clinical clues suggesting parenchymal salvageability include the following: angiographic demonstration of retrograde filling of the distal renal arterial system by collateral vessels; renal biopsy showing preserved glomerular architecture; kidney size >9 cm by ultrasound; and function of the involved kidney on renal scintigraphy. Some centers perform kidney biopsies in surgical candidates if their serum creatinine is higher than 4 mg/dL. In patients with serum creatinine less than 3 mg/dL, improved renal function (defined as a reduction in serum creatinine of >20% from the baseline value) postrevascularization can be expected in nearly half of patients undergoing this procedure.

The second scenario is bilateral stenosis without total occlusion or stenosis in a solitary kidney. Improvement in renal function is frequently seen after reconstructive surgery in 75% to 89% of these patients. Unlike cases with total renal occlusion, revascularization to preserve renal function is not worthwhile in patients with severe renal insufficiency (serum creatinine >4 mg/dL) because they usually have advanced underlying renal parenchymal disease (nephrosclerosis and/or atheroembolic disease), which is not improved by revascularization. In older patients, severe atherosclerosis of the abdominal aorta may render an aortorenal bypass technically impossible. In such cases, alternate bypass techniques have been used, such as splenorenal bypass for left-kidney revascularization and hepatorenal bypass for right-kidney revascularization. Considering the significant risks of progressive renal occlusive disease and renal failure that are associated with medical management of this condition in elderly patients, the surgical results showing a favorable influence of revascularization on the natural history of untreated atherosclerotic renal artery disease are of interest and merit further study.

Initially percutaneous transluminal renal angioplasty (PTRA) had a limited role in elderly patients because of the concomitant presence of aortic atherosclerotic disease, making any endovascular procedure hazardous and technically difficult. Restenosis following dilatation of atheromatous lesions was quite common and a significant number of elderly patients present with ostial lesions, which are not amenable to PTRA. PTRA with the use of endovascular stenting devices have come into vogue with improved outcome of the revascularization of these ostial lesions. Surgical intervention is presently recommended for more complicated lesions, or angioplasty failures. One advantage of angioplasty over surgery is that it can be undertaken in patients who have prohibitively high surgical risks that are related to systemic atherosclerosis.

TUBULOINTERSTITIAL NEPHRITIS

Tubulointerstitial nephritis involves a heterogeneous group of disorders that primarily affect the renal interstitium and tubules and only secondarily involve the other structures of the kidney. The etiology of these diseases includes medications, infectious agents, physical, chemical, immunological, hereditary, and unknown causes. Elderly patients are predisposed to the development of this entity because of the high prevalence of polypharmacy, comorbid diseases, and impaired immunological mechanisms to control infections. Interstitial disease in the geriatric patient should be thoroughly investigated. Aging-related interstitial changes may precipitate clinical features compatible with tubulointerstitial nephritis but should be considered as a diagnosis of exclusion after other possible underlying conditions are ruled out.

Functional Defects

The pattern of tubular dysfunction will vary depending on the major site of injury. Salt retention, hypertension, edema, and heavy proteinuria are absent in the early phases of the disease. The tubulointerstitial lesions are localized either to the cortex or to the medulla. Cortical lesions can affect either the proximal or distal tubule. Proximal lesions are characterized by Fanconi's syndrome (bicarbonaturia, glucosuria, hyperuricosuria, hyperphosphaturia, and aminoaciduria). Distal lesions are associated with impaired ability to secrete protons (distal tubular acidosis) and potassium, and decreased reabsorption of sodium. Medullary lesions that involve the papilla manifest by sodium wasting and an impaired ability to concentrate the urine maximally.

In addition to abnormalities associated with tubular defects, other clinical features are also suggestive of tubulointerstitial nephritis. Anemia that is out of proportion to azotemia may signify the early failure of erythropoietin synthesis. High levels of parathyroid hormone (PTH) with mild azotemia may be secondary to reduced tubular generation of the biologically active form of vitamin D, 1,25-$(OH)_2D_3$. Microscopic examination of the urine sediment typically shows leukocytes and white cell casts, but may be surprisingly bland as well. Eosinophiluria, detected by Hansel's stain, may be seen in the setting of drug-induced tubulointerstitial nephritis, especially when it is secondary to β-lactam antibiotics. Despite the number of typical clinical manifestations, early renal consultation should be obtained because the diagnosis of tubulointerstitial disease can only be established by renal biopsy.

Acute Tubulointerstitial Nephritis

Tubulointerstitial nephritis can be divided into acute and chronic forms. Of the etiologies associated with acute tubulointerstitial nephritis, two entities deserve special attention in geriatric populations: acute bacterial pyelonephritis and acute drug-induced hypersensitivity reactions.

Acute Bacterial Pyelonephritis

For most, but not all, elderly individuals, the presentation and course of infection involving the urinary tract is no different from that found in younger patients. Bacterial pyelonephritis occurs equally in both sexes and is the most common form of renal disease in the elderly. Prostatic hypertrophy and the decreased antimicrobial properties of prostatic fluid may be the cause of increased incidence in elderly men. In geriatric-aged women, the vaginal pH changes as the epithelium atrophies, resulting in replacement of the usual microbial flora by gram-negative organisms. These changes predispose the patient to infection. Urinary tract infection is strongly correlated with dementia, which may be caused by fecal incontinence and perineal soiling in women, although the reason in men is unknown.

In those patients with an atypical presentation, the disease is a diagnostic challenge. Costovertebral angle tenderness and urinary symptoms may be absent, whereas bacteremia (>50%), central nervous system changes, tachypnea, and hypotension are common. There are even case reports of asymptomatic acute pyelonephritis presenting as ARF.

Therapy includes hemodynamic support and eradication of the infection. Uncomplicated pyelonephritis improves within 48 to 72 hours after initiation of adequate antimicrobial agents. Ultrasonographic surveillance is indicated if no improvement is noted in this time frame to exclude obstructive lesions or perinephric abscess.

Drug Hypersensitivity

Drug-induced acute interstitial nephritis has been reported with most medications. The classic description is the one associated with methicillin (and other β-lactam antibiotics). The sulfonamides were the first antibiotics reported to cause acute interstitial nephritis and were followed by the penicillins in the 1950s. Methicillin was implicated in numerous, well-documented, biopsy-proven cases and became the prototype for drug-induced acute interstitial nephritis. Subsequent reports included a vast number of antibiotics as the cause of this syndrome. Unfortunately, many of the anecdotal reports lack large numbers of cases and do not include biopsy findings, thereby bringing into question the validity of the causal association. A high index of suspicion of acute interstitial nephritis in the clinical setting of acutely deteriorating renal function is the key to diagnosis.

The clinical presentation is characterized by the tetrad of rash, arthralgia, fever, and ARF, which are present in only 10% of cases. The urine sediment shows nonephrotic range proteinuria, white cell casts, and eosinophiluria in 40% of the cases.

The other significant group of drugs causing acute interstitial nephritis in the elderly population are the NSAIDs. All classes of NSAIDs induce this syndrome, with or without minimal change nephropathy. Acute interstitial nephritis has been reported after 2 to 18 months of NSAID therapy and may be sufficiently severe as to require renal replacement therapy. Most cases are reversible after the drug is stopped. Unlike antimicrobial-induced interstitial nephritis, signs of hypersensitivity (fever, rash, eosinophilia, eosinophiluria) are usually absent. Some cases are associated with nephrotic range proteinuria and glomerular lesions similar to minimal change or membranous nephropathy. The most culpable NSAID appears to be fenoprofen, although all NSAIDs induce this pathology.

The best therapeutic option for treating drug-induced acute interstitial nephritis is to identify and withdraw the offending agent, although this may not be obvious in a hospitalized patient on multiple medications. Although there are anecdotal reports of using corticosteroids for treatment, there are no controlled trials showing that their use alters the rate or extent of renal recovery.

Chronic Tubulointerstitial Nephritis

The clinical course of tubulointerstitial disease depends on the primary cause and the magnitude of the renal insult. Sporadic exposure to nephrotoxic materials results in a more indolent clinical course and progressive loss of renal function. Chronic tubulointerstitial nephritis is associated with tubular atrophy and interstitial polymorphonuclear and mononuclear cell infiltrates. The etiological factors and the pathogenetic mechanisms are essentially the same as in the acute forms of interstitial nephritis. Special considerations in elderly populations are the chronic forms associated with analgesic abuse, neoplasms, and aging-associated interstitial disease.

Analgesic Nephropathy

There are no scientifically acceptable data documenting the safety of NSAIDs on renal structure and function when taken chronically. Epidemiologic data show a ninefold increased relative risk of ESRD in subjects ingesting 5000 or more doses of NSAIDs when compared with age-matched control subjects; however, it has been difficult to demonstrate a cause-and-effect relationship between analgesic use and CRF or ESRD. In an intriguing study from Sweden, regular use of acetaminophen and aspirin as analgesics was associated with an increased risk of CRF. In fact, subjects who chronically took more than 1.4 g of acetaminophen per day had a fivefold increased risk for CRF. The risk was higher in those patients with preexisting CRF. This is particularly germane to the elderly population, which has a high incidence of CRF. Although the incidence of analgesic nephropathy in the ESRD population has declined in those countries where analgesic combinations containing phenacetin were removed from the market, the incidence of this condition appears to be increasing in the elderly population in some countries outside of the United States. The frequency of renal papillary necrosis, the hallmark lesion of analgesic associated nephropathy, as a primary cause or contributing cause of ESRD is unknown because of the infrequent radiographic proof of this diagnosis.

A review of the literature that included studies from Europe, Australia, and North America concluded that the use of NSAIDs in the general population is safe and effective when used in therapeutic dosages for a limited period of time. There are no acceptable epidemiologic or clinical data regarding the risk of NSAIDs for CRF, renal papillary necrosis, or ESRD. There are also no experimental or clinical data on whether NSAIDs affect the rate of progression of renal disease. Consequently, the National Kidney Foundation recommends the design and implementation of controlled studies on the renal and cardiovascular safety of chronic NSAIDs by themselves, or in the presence of another known cause of renal disease, and the prospective evaluation of combinations of NSAIDs and other analgesics prior to their release onto the market.

Neoplastic Diseases Associated with Interstitial Nephritis

Many neoplastic diseases infiltrate the interstitium of the kidney with variable clinical implications. Leukemias and lymphomas are the most common malignancies associated with direct invasion of the renal parenchyma. Multiple myeloma may affect the kidney by several different mechanisms. One is involvement of the tubulointerstitial structures resulting from the filtration of toxic light chains and the formation of intratubular casts from aggregates of light chains

and Tamm–Horsfall mucoprotein. This clinical entity is known as myeloma kidney and may present as an indolent, chronic form of renal failure, or as isolated tubular dysfunction with well-preserved GFR. The clinical manifestations of the tubular involvement include the Fanconi's syndrome, renal tubular acidosis types I or II, and hyperphosphaturia.

The diagnosis of myeloma kidney should be confirmed by kidney biopsy when the clinical picture suggests tubulointerstitial involvement. The presence of tubular involvement has important therapeutic implications. Even though plasmapheresis has been used with rewarding results in the settings of acute myeloma kidney, the role of plasma exchange in chronic tubulointerstitial nephritis secondary to light chain cast nephropathy awaits further investigation and definition. The addition of high-intensity chemotherapy has improved survival rates in cases associated with ARF but optimal therapy for chronic tubulointerstitial nephritis is less certain. Prevention is the most effective therapy for myeloma kidney. Institution of effective chemotherapy and prevention of tubular obstruction are fundamental. The role of colchicine to inhibit the intratubular cast formation is still experimental and should be used only in controlled studies.

Aging-Associated Interstitial Disease

Tubulointerstitial nephropathy of the elderly is defined as the decreased renal tubular function associated with aging, including decreased ability to concentrate urine; decreased renin and aldosterone production; and histologic changes, including interstitial fibrosis and mononuclear cell infiltrates. The clinical presentation is essentially identical to any other form of interstitial nephritis. This entity should be considered only as a diagnosis of exclusion.

CHRONIC KIDNEY DISEASE

The clinical presentation of CDK as a result of irreversible damage to renal parenchyma in elderly patients includes essentially the same constellation of symptoms and signs as in the general population. Medical management directed to potassium homeostasis, sodium and water balance, acid–base status, calcium and phosphate metabolism, hypertension, cholesterol, anemia, and nutritional support, follow the same guidelines and parameters as described for the general population. The reader is referred to a general nephrology textbook for details.

Recently, CDK has been divided into various stages ranging from CKD stage 1 to 5 depending on the estimated glomerular filtration rate (eGFR) (Table 86-9). Levey's formula for eGFR was derived from data obtained from the Modification of Diet in Renal Disease (MDRD) Study and takes into account various variables including age, gender, race, serum creatinine, serum albumin, and serum urea. The eGFR was initially established primarily in Caucasians with moderate renal insufficiency, but was later validated in African-Americans, diabetic and renal transplant recipients. However, the equation has not been validated in the elderly (older than 70 years). Another limitation of the eGFR is that the assay used for measurement of the serum creatinine has not been standardized, making it difficult to interpret between different institutions. Although there are limitations with the eGFR, it is recommended for clinical use by established organizations with some exceptions, including muscle

TABLE 86-9

Ischemic Renal Disease: Outcome of Angioplasty						
STUDY NO.	YEAR	NO. OF PATIENTS	ANGIOPLASTY OUTCOME			
			No. (%) Improved	No. (%) Stable	No. (%) Worse*	No. (%) Death
1	198	20	7 (35)	10 (50)	3 (15)	0 (0)
2	1983	12	3 (25)	5 (42)	4 (33)	0 (0)
3	1992	17	9 (53)	2 (12)	6 (35)	5 (29)
4	1986	55	26 (47)	19 (35)	10 (18)	NA
5	1993	21	10	38	3	
Total		104	45 (43)	36 (35)	23 (22)	5 (5)

*Includes all deaths; NA, not available.
Data from Pohl MA. Ischemic nephropathy. American Society of Nephrology's Board Review Course Syllabus, 1996;14.

wasting states, ARF, pregnancy, paraplegic, vegetarian, and extreme weights.

In the NHANES III, the prevalence of CKD in the United States was 11% (19.2 million). A large percentage had CDK stage 3 (7.6 million) with a smaller percentage had CKD stage 4 (400 000). The elderly account for approximately 60% to 80% of those with eGFR less than 60 mL/min/1.73 m². The rate of progression in elderly is similar to the general population in those with diabetes and severe CDK.

CDK has been associated with an increase in cardiovascular risk and metabolic derangements. Fried et al. demonstrated that there is an increased association in both morbidity and mortality in the elderly with CKD stage 3. Cardiovascular morbidity and mortality increased with worsening renal function compared with those with normal renal function. The high incidence of cardiovascular disease in the elderly is probably secondary to both traditional and non-traditional risk factors (elevated homocysteine, C-reactive protein, albuminuria, uremic toxins, anemia, and renal bone disease). Interestingly, elderly patients with mild decrease in eGFR (50 to 59 mL/min/1.73 m²) have been shown to have less increase in mortality than their younger cohorts. But when the eGFR decreases further, there is an increase in mortality similar to the younger cohorts, suggesting that mortality stratification may differ in different age groups at certain CKD stages.

The renal osteodystrophy from secondary hyperparathyroidism begins at CKD stage 3. The interplay between the decreased production of 1,25-(OH)$_2$ vitamin D$_3$, an increased serum phosphate, and a low serum calcium results in hyperplasia of the parathyroid gland and increase production of the PTH. In the elderly, there is less exposure to ultraviolet rays, resulting in a decreased synthesis of vitamin D 3, cholecalciferol, which is the substrate for 25-hydroxylase in the liver. Because of the low level of 25-(OH) vitamin D$_3$, there is less conversion to the active form, 1,25-(OH)$_2$ vitamin D$_3$ Both the decreased sun exposure and the gradual loss of renal function contribute to the low level of 1,25-(OH)$_2$ vitamin D$_3$. Acceptable intact PTH levels for CKD stages 3, 4, and 5, are 35 to 70, 70 to 110, and 150 to 300 pg/mL, respectively. For values over these limits, the patient is considered to have secondary hyperparathyroidism. Both the 25-(OH) vitamin D$_3$ and PTH level should be measured. If the intact PTH level is elevated, 25-(OH) vitamin D$_3$ should be replaced for CKD stages 3 and 4 according to Tables 86-10 and 86-11. For CKD stage 5, the active form of vitamin D, 1,25-(OH)$_2$ vitamin D$_3$

should be prescribed to maintain the intact PTH level between 150 and 300 pg/mL. The complications from renal osteodystrophy can have a significant morbidity in the elderly, with an increased incidence of bone fracture, height loss, soft tissue deposition of calcium, and cardiovascular disease. The early detection of secondary hyperparathyroidism lessens the likelihood of parathyroid hyperplasia and associated morbidities.

Anemia is a common finding in the elderly and has been linked to an increased morbidity and mortality associated with left ventricular hypertrophy, worsening congestive heart failure and myocardial ischemia. The NHANES III study found that CDK accounted for 12% of all causes of anemia in the elderly. As kidney disease advances, the production of erythropoietin is decreased and accounts for the anemia; however, other causes for anemia need to be excluded. For CKD stages 3, 4, and 5, the goal for anemia management is a hemoglobin between 11 and 12 mg/dL. Higher hemoglobin valves have not been found to decrease cardiovascular events.

Renal replacement modalities are initiated at CKD stage 5 and have become commonplace for the elderly within the last decade. The U.S. Renal Data System (USRDS) from 2006 show that approximately 48% of the incident patients receiving some form of renal replacement therapy are older than 65 years of age and 25% are older than 75 years of age. Those patients older than 75 years of age constitute the fastest growing segment on dialysis, with their numbers tripling in the last decade. Moreover, it is estimated that 60% of all ESRD patients are older than age 65 years. These statistics should not be surprising given the high incidence of hypertension and diabetes mellitus in the elderly, accounting for 40% to 60% of the new cases of ESRD. Tubulointerstitial disorders (13.5%),

TABLE 86-10

Stages of Chronic Kidney Disease
CKD stage GFR (mL/min/1.73m²) description
Stage 1 >90 kidney damage
Stage 2 60–89 kidney damage mild dec GFR
Stage 3 30–59 kidney damage mod dec GFR
Stage 4 15–29 kidney damage sever dec GFR
Stage 5 < 15 end stage (dialysis)

Modified from K/DOQI clinical practice guidelines from chronic kidney disease. Am J Kidney Dis. 2002;39:1.

TABLE 86-11

Vitamin D Supplement Therapy for CKD Stages 3 and 4

25(OH)VIT D	ERGOCALCIFEROL DOSE (VIT D2)	DURATION
<5 mg/dL recheck 25 (OH) vit D	50,000 IU/wk orally × 12 weeks then monthly or 500,000 IU IM	6 months
5–15 mg/dL recheck 25 (OH) vit D	50,000 IU/wk orally × 4 weeks then 50,000 IU/ month	6 months
16–30 mg/dL	50,000 IU orally every month	6 months

obstructive uropathy (11%), glomerular disease (10.5%), and poly-cystic kidney disease (2%) account for other causes of ESRD.

The selection of the type of renal replacement therapy for a geriatric patient must be individualized and requires a comprehensive evaluation that takes into account the medical and psychosocial problems that affect each individual patient. The fact that life expectancy is limited for the aged population does not justify depriving them of treatment. In fact, the first year survival on hemodialysis for octogenarians and nonagenarians can be greater than 50% and in a selective population of octogenarians 2-year survival rate can exceed 75%. Elderly patients with ESRD have multiple therapeutic options available, including center or home hemodialysis, PD, renal transplantation, and acceptance of death from uremia. Consultation with a nephrologist is essential for counseling the patient on the advantages and disadvantages of the various types of renal replacement therapy; planning for the start of renal replacement therapy, for provision of renal replacement therapy, and for formulating advance directives regarding cessation of renal placement therapy.

HEMODIALYSIS

The primary treatment modality for geriatric patients with ESRD is in-center hemodialysis (78%). Despite their complex medical and psychosocial conditions, survival rates and rehabilitation rates are acceptable in elderly patients undergoing dialysis. In addition, these patients tend to be more compliant. The risk of death in patients undergoing dialysis increases with age and with coexisting diseases. Several studies report that age, diabetes, and cardiovascular disease are associated with a shorter survival. Survival for at least 5 years was 15% lower for patients older than 65 years of age at the initiation of hemodialysis than for younger adults in Europe. Early mortality (within the first 90 days after starting hemodialysis) is mainly secondary to comorbid conditions. The principal reported causes of death are acute myocardial infarction, cardiac arrest, sepsis, and malignancies. There are no significant differences in the percentage of deaths as a result of these various causes between geriatric patients and those younger than 65 years of age with the exception of cachexia, which accounts for 10% of the deaths in patients younger than age 65 years and increases to 36% in geriatric patients. Withdrawal from dialysis has been reported as the leading cause of death in dialysis patients older than 70 years of age. Other important factors associated with the decision to withdraw from dialysis are malnutrition, cancer, and dissatisfaction with the quality of life.

The success rate for vascular access for chronic hemodialysis in the elderly is similar to the rate in younger patients. The USRDS 2006 annual report indicated that the types of access for patients older than 65 years of age were catheters, arteriovenous fistulas, and polytetrafluoroethylene grafts. There has been a noticeable change in the type of access placed with a decrease in the grafts, doubling of the catheters and no significant change in ateriovenous fistulas. The elderly experienced more access-related hospital stays than younger patients. Many investigators report a greater number of hospitalization days per year for the elderly patient on hemodialysis. This higher morbidity rate in geriatric patients on hemodialysis is the result of complications secondary to hypertension, cardiovascular disease, coronary or cardiac insufficiency, or left ventricular hypertrophy. Nevertheless, multiple surveys on geriatric patients with ESRD report a more positive overall satisfaction with life when compared to younger dialysis patients. Other investigators have reported that age has no value as a predictor of quality of life in patients with ESRD.

It is important to note that the quality of hemodialysis has improved markedly during the past decade facilitated by both new technology and new medications. Thus, historical data on hemodialysis may not be applicable to the way hemodialysis is performed currently in state-of-the-art hemodialysis centers. Technologic improvements include the development of high-flux hemodialysis, improved biocompatible membranes, bicarbonate dialysis, computer-controlled hemodialysis machines, and improved vascular accesses that can produce the high blood flows needed for high-flux hemodialysis. Major medical improvements include the availability of erythropoietin and intravenous iron for treating the anemia of ESRD, and intravenous vitamin D or its analogs and calcimimetic agent for preventing and treating secondary hyperparathyroidism. These advances have resulted in improved hemodialysis with shorter treatment times, less cardiovascular stress during hemodialysis, and an improved quality of life for hemodialysis patients of all ages.

PERITONEAL DIALYSIS

Peritoneal dialysis has undergone dramatic changes within the last decade with the development and introduction of smaller, portable cycling dialysis machines that introduce and remove dialysis fluid in a timely, programmed manner. This has resulted in alterations in the dialysis prescription such that in most cases, the bulk of the dialysis exchanges can be done mechanically at night, limiting manual exchanges to one a day. The percentage of elderly patients treated with PD varies from country to country; in the United Kingdom 50% of elderly ESRD patients are treated with this modality, while in the United States, fewer than 10% of the geriatric patients with ESRD are on PD.

For the elderly patient, PD has important advantages, including decreased cardiovascular instability and arrhythmias, better maintenance of residual renal function, good control of hypertension, no need for vascular access surgery, efficacy of intraperitoneal insulin therapy (for diabetics), and better clearance of middle molecules. Despite its many advantages, many elderly patients do not choose this mode for psychosocial reasons such as inadequate family support, poor eyesight, and physical and mental impairment. Unlike in center hemodialysis, PD must be done daily and does require manual strength to lift 5-kg bags if a cycling dialysis machine is used.

The rate of infectious complications in elderly patients on PD is similar to that of younger patients, but elderly patients tend to have a more protracted course with increased morbidity and longer hospital stays. Unfortunately, the incidence of peritonitis is still unacceptably high and varies from 0.5 to 3 episodes per patient per year. Moreover, more frequent episodes of peritonitis are associated with catheter loss.

As in hemodialysis patients, the incidence of malnutrition is increased in the elderly patient. The causes of malnutrition include comorbid conditions, as well as protein losses of 7 to 15 g/day with the dialysis procedure.

The choice of dialysis modality ultimately hinges on patient preference. Each modality has its own advantages and disadvantages and optimal rates of survival can be garnered through careful and planned counseling of the pre-ESRD patient.

RENAL TRANSPLANTATION

Despite the high incidence of ESRD in the aged population, the USRDS indicates that fewer than 5% of geriatric ESRD patients have a working renal allograft as renal replacement therapy. Previous studies reported a higher mortality rate in older patients receiving a renal transplant. One-year patient and graft survival for patients older than 60 years of age averaged 62% and 57%, respectively, before the introduction of cyclosporine A. Improved pre- and postoperative management and better immunosuppressive therapy have improved survival to rates equivalent to those obtained in younger transplant populations. The reluctance for renal transplant in the elderly patients with ESRD is a result of their limited life expectancy. The probability of 10-year patient survival for deceased donor transplant recipients aged 65 to 69 years in the United States is 8%, contrasting with 50% to 85% 10-year survival rates in patients younger than 44 years of age.

Current data on elderly patients receiving transplant of deceased donor renal transplant report a 1-year patient survival rate ranging between 80% and 91% and 5-year survival exceeding 55%. Graft survival has increased to 80% at 1 year and 55 to 60% at 5 years. Patients dying with functioning renal allografts account for the majority of graft loss in older recipients (50%). Review of the USRDS database shows a lower incidence of rejection (accounting for 11% to 28% of graft loss at 1 year) when compared with younger renal allograft recipients. This difference may be explained by age-related "tolerance." Living-related transplantation offers improved patient and graft survival, and should be investigated in elderly patients with ESRD who are suitable candidates for transplantation. Another option for the elderly recipients is to be placed on the kidney transplant list for extended criteria donors (ECD). The ECD kidneys are marginal but allow for a larger donor pool and a decrease in waiting time for the elderly patients.

The leading causes of death in elderly patients receiving transplant are cardiovascular and infection. The majority of infections occur in the first 6 months posttransplant and are related to the degree of immunosuppression. Other series report cardiovascular events as the major cause of death in older transplant patients. Underlying cardiovascular disease may be a natural consequence of older age that is exacerbated by transplant-related complications such as posttransplant hypertension and steroid-induced diabetes. Other important causes of death include malignancy (13% to 16%) and gastrointestinal hemorrhage (16%).

The selection of transplant recipients in the elderly should follow the same clinical practice guidelines dictated for younger patients. In addition, a routine voiding cystourethrogram is recommended for this age group. Careful attention should be given to the effect of transplantation on the quality of life and should ensure that patient's expectations as to benefits of transplantation are realistic.

Attenuated immune responsiveness in elderly patients undergoing transplant decreases the likelihood of immunologic rejection, but it is offset by a potentially increased risk of infection. The goal of any immunosuppression protocol in an elderly patient should be to decrease the risk of infection without causing rejection. Acute rejection requires the use of high doses of immunosuppression to prevent graft loss. The optimal immunosuppression regimen, involving cyclosporine A, prednisone, rapamycin, mycophenolate mofetil, tacrolimus, and azathioprine for long-term immunosuppression has not yet been addressed in prospective studies of elderly recipients undergoing renal transplant. In addition, new immunosuppressive agents, such as monoclonal antibodies, may confer a greater potential for reducing steroid and other immunosuppressive dosages while retaining excellent graft and patient survival.

FURTHER READING

Appel RG, et al. Renovascular disease in older patients beginning renal replacement therapy. *Kidney Int.* 1995;48:171.

Baraldi A, et al. Acute renal failure of medical type in an elderly population. *Nephrol Dial Transplant.* 1998;13:25.

Becker BN, et al. Renal transplantation in the older end stage renal disease patient. *Semin Nephrol.* 1996;16:353.

Cameron JS. Nephrotic syndrome in the elderly. *Semin Nephrol.* 1996;16:319.

Collins AJ, et al. Excerpts from the United States Renal Data System 2006 annual data report. *Am J Kidney Dis.* 2007;49:S1.

Cozzolino M, et al. Vitamin D retains an important role in pathogenesis and management of secondary hyperparathyroidism in chronic renal failure. *J Nephrol.* 2006;19:566.

Coresh J, et al. Prevalence of chronic kidney disease and decreased kidney function in the adult US population: Third National Health and Nutrition Examination Survey. *Am J Kidney Dis.* 2003;41:1.

Davison AM, Johnston PA. Idiopathic glomerulonephritis in the elderly. *Contrib Nephrol.* 1993;105:38.

Donadio JV Jr. Treatment and clinical outcome of glomerulonephritis in the elderly. *Contrib Nephrol.* 1993;105:49.

Doublier S, et al. Nephrin redistribution on podocytes is a potential mechanism for proteinuria inpatients with primary acquired nephrotic syndrome. *Am J Pathol.* 2001;158:1723.

Drueke TB, et al. Normalization of hemoglobin level in patients with chronic kidney disease. *New Engl J Med.* 2006;355:2071.

DuBose TD, et al. Acute renal in the 21st century: Recommendations for management and outcomes assessment. *Am J Kidney Dis.* 1997;29:793.

Fored CM, et al. Acetaminophen, aspirin and chronic renal failure. *N Engl J Med.* 2001;345:1801.

Fried LF, et al. Renal insufficiency as a predictor of cardiovascular outcomes and mortality in the elderly individuals. *J Am Coll Cardiol.* 2003;41:1364.

Glassock RJ. Syndromes of glomerular diseases. In: Massry SG, Glassock RJ, eds. *Textbook of Nephrology.* 3rd ed. Baltimore: Williams and Wilkins; 1995:681.

Grapsa I, Oreopoulos DG. Practical ethical issues of dialysis in the elderly. *Semin Nephrol.* 1996;16:339.

Greco BA, Breyer JA. Natural history of renal artery stenosis. *Semin Nephrol.* 1996;16:2.

Haas M, et al. Etiologies and outcome of acute renal insufficiency in older adults: a renal biopsy study of 259 cases. *Am J Kidney Dis.* 2000;35:433.

Hemmelgarn BR, et al. Progression of kidney dysfunction in the community-dwelling elderly. *Kidney Int.* 2006;69:2155.

Johnston PA, et al. Renal biopsy findings in patients older than 65 years of age presenting with the nephrotic syndrome. A report from the MRC glomerulonephritis registry. *Contrib Nephrol.* 1993;105:127.

Johnson JM II, et al. A prospective evaluation of the glomerular filtration rate in older adults with frequent night time urination. *J Urol.* 2002;107:146.

K/DOQI. National Kidney Foundation. K/DOQI clinical practice guidelines for bone metabolism and disease in chronic kidney disease. *Am J Kid Dis.* 2003;42:S1.

K/DOQI. National Kidney Foundation. K/DOQI Clinical practice guidelines and clinical practice recommendations for anemia in chronic kidney disease. *Am J Kidney Dis.* 2006;47:S11.

K/DOQI. National Kidney Foundation K/DOQI Clinical practice guidelines for chronic kidney disease: evaluation, classification, and stratification. *Am J Kidney Dis.* 2002;39:S1.

Macias-Nunez JF, et al. Acute renal failure in the aged. *Semin Nephrol.* 1996;16:330.

Mandal AK, et al. Management of acute renal failure in the elderly. Treatment options. *Drugs Aging.* 1996; 9:226.

Moran D, et al. Is renal biopsy justified for the diagnosis and management of the nephrotic syndrome in the elderly?. *Gerontology.* 1993;39:49.

Naire R, et al. Renal biopsy in patients aged 80 years and older. *Am J Kidney Dis.* 2004;44:618.

O'Hare AN, et al. Mortality risk stratification in chronic kidney disease: one size for all ages?. *Am Soc Nephrol.* 2006;17:846.

Pascual J, et al. The elderly patient with acute renal failure. *J Am Soc Nephrol.* 1995;6:144.

Ponticelli C, et al. Primary nephrotic syndrome in the elderly. *Contrib Nephrol.* 1993;105:33.

Safian RD, Textor SC, et al. Renal artery stenosis. *N Engl J Med.* 2001;344:431.

Stevens LA, Levey AS, et al. Measurement of kidney function. *Med Clin N Am.* 2005;89:457.

Woodman R, et al. Anemia in older adults. *Curr Opin Hematol.* 2005;12:123.

Zent R, et al. Idiopathic membranous nephropathy in the elderly: a comparative study. *Am J Kidney Dis.* 1997;29:200.

Zucchelli P, Zuccala A. Ischemic nephropathy in the elderly. *Contrib Nephrol.* 1993;105:13.

End-Stage Renal Disease

Mark L. Unruh

DEFINITION

End-stage renal disease (ESRD) or kidney failure has been defined as having kidney function less than 15 mL/min/1.73 m^2. Kidney failure may be caused by progression of a chronic nephropathy or by acute kidney injury (AKI). Kidney failure is associated with the inability to excrete waste products, control serum electrolytes, handle the daily dietary and metabolic acid load, and maintain fluid balance. In addition, kidney failure causes inadequate production of erythropoietin, deranged calcium and phosphorous metabolism, high blood pressure, and accelerated progression of cardiovascular disease. Uremia is the term used to describe the symptoms or symptom complex attributable to advanced kidney failure or ESRD. Most chronic nephropathies demonstrate inexorable progression to kidney failure. In general, there is a straight line relationship between the decrement in kidney function over time when the kidney function is plotted longitudinally. The rates of decline in kidney function vary by underlying nephropathy, by severity of hypertension and proteinuria, by modifying factors, and between individuals. Historically, the rate of decline could be estimated as 7 to 10 mL/min/year in those with untreated chronic nephropathies such as diabetic nephropathy. However, chronic nephropathies have similar effects on electrolyte homeostasis, causes of progressive decline in function, and manifestations of kidney failure so that classification by severity permits a better understanding of underlying routes to progression, symptoms, and hopefully, treatments of chronic kidney disease (CKD). In parts of the world with access to dialysis and kidney transplantation, renal replacement therapy (RRT) has been thought to be necessary when the glomerular filtration rate (GFR) decreases to less than 15 mL/min. "Kidney damage" has been defined as structural or functional abnormalities of the kidney, initially without decreased GFR, which over time can lead to decreased GFR. Markers of kidney damage include abnormalities in the composition of the blood or urine, or abnormalities in imaging tests. Proteinuria as a marker of kidney damage has been studied most thoroughly. CKD is the term used to describe patients with a chronic decrease in GFR. There are different levels of CKD, and these levels have underpinned an international classification system (Table 87-1). It has been proposed that advanced CKD (GFR estimated <15mL/min/1.73m^2) be classified as CKD Stage 5 with a suffix to classify the treatment modality. For example, a person treated by hemodialysis would be characterized as CKD Stage 5-D.

EPIDEMIOLOGY

The prevalence of kidney failure is increasing rapidly worldwide; the projections are that the number of patients with kidney failure will double in the next 10 to 15 years. However, this is just the tip of the iceberg. Estimates are that there are 30 times as many people with CKD as compared to kidney failure. Approximately 14.7% of the U.S. adult population is thought to have some form of CKD. The majority of those with CKD Stage 1 and Stage 2 may not even be aware of their kidney disease. Nonmodifiable risk factors are important for risk stratification and for understanding the pathophysiology of CKD progression (Table 87-2). African-American patients with diabetes have a two- to threefold higher risk of developing kidney failure compared to white patients. Modifiable risk factors are important for both understanding disease progression and as a possible option for prevention or therapy. For example, the heavy consumption of analgesics has been associated with the development of kidney failure. The number of patients who develop kidney disease and at risk for developing kidney disease will increase with the increasing prevalence of diabetes and the aging of the population.

The burgeoning number of elderly with kidney failure has been caused by an increased incidence of kidney failure, greater access to RRT, and improved survival of both dialysis patients and kidney transplant recipients. The majority of patients in the United

TABLE 87-1

Classification of Chronic Kidney Disease

STAGE	DESCRIPTION	GFR mL/min/ 1.73 m²	RELATED TERMS	CLASSIFICATION BY TREATMENT
1	Kidney damage with normal or ↑ GFR	≥90	Albuminuria, proteinuria, hematuria	
2	Kidney damage with mild ↓GFR	60–89	Albuminuria, proteinuria, hematuria	
3	Moderate ↓GFR	30–59	Chronic renal insufficiency	
4	Severe ↓GFR	15–29	Chronic renal insufficiency, pre-ESRD	
5	Kidney Failure	<15 (or dialysis)	Renal failure, uremia, end-stage renal disease	D if dialysis T if kidney transplant recipient

Adapted from KDIGO definition and classification of chronic kidney disease: a position statement from Kidney Disease: Improving Global Outcomes (www.kdigo.org).

States receiving hemodialysis are aged 65 years and older and the proportion of older patients undergoing hemodialysis is rapidly increasing (Figure 87-1). Hence, the growth of the ESRD population has been driven by those patients older than 65 years. This has been a worldwide phenomenon with a sevenfold increase in the rate of incident dialysis patients older than 75 years over the past two decades in Canada. Similar rates of increase of kidney failure in the elderly have been noted in Europe and Japan with a 10-fold increase in octogenarian hemodialysis patients in Japan. Indeed, the very recent marked increase in incidence of end-stage kidney failure documented by renal registries suggests that this spike of disease has been driven by the increased access to RRT. Older and sicker patients have been referred for hemodialysis in Asia, Australia, Europe, and North America as a result of perceived improvements in quality of life on dialysis, as well as economic and cultural factors. Once referred for kidney failure, older patients have been surviving longer with RRT as dialysis adequacy has increased and kidney transplant outcomes have improved. As a result of improvements in technology and greater access to dialysis, the increased prevalence of older adults undergoing RRT generally mirrors the aging trend of the general population.

Acute Kidney Injury in the Elderly

AKI has been defined as an abrupt decrease in kidney function. This decrement in kidney function is reflected by an increase of serum creatinine from baseline of at least 50% often in the setting of reduced urine output. More than 50% of patients with AKI are older than 60 years of age. The elderly are thought to be predisposed to AKI owing to a reduced GFR, comorbid illness, and use of medications such as nonsteroidal anti-inflammatories and angiotensin-converting enzyme inhibitors. AKI may occur in elderly patients both in the outpatient or inpatient setting. Obstruction from prostatic hypertrophy, volume depletion, and medications are prominent causes of AKI among the community-dwelling elderly. In the hospital setting, AKI may occur in up to 25% of critically ill patients and has been associated with a marked increase in mortality. Among hospitalized patients, AKI often arises from acute tubular necrosis or acute interstitial nephritis, although AKI merits a thorough evaluation for reversible causes. At present, the care of patients with AKI has been supportive care with acute dialysis and avoidance of further kidney injury from nephrotoxins. The indications for initiation of emergent or acute dialysis therapy in the elderly population vary little from younger patients (Table 87-3). The prognosis for survivors of AKI depends on severity of illness, chronic health conditions, length of time requiring dialysis, and preexisting kidney disease. A majority of patients who survive the initial insult of acute renal failure caused by acute tubular necrosis requiring dialysis will recover renal function and have adequate long-term kidney function. A large randomized trial of AKI in the hospitalized patient will determine the optimal frequency and intensity of dialysis following kidney failure caused by AKI in both young and old critically ill patients.

PRESENTATION

Etiology of End Stage Renal Disease in the Elderly Population

The most common reported causes of ESRD in the elderly population have been shown to diabetes and hypertension in the United States and worldwide (Figure 87-2). The high proportion of kidney failure diagnosed as nephropathy as a result of diabetes and hypertension maybe in part because of a hesitance to perform a kidney biopsy in elderly patients in the face of usual indications such as nephrotic range proteinuria or unexplained renal failure. It may also be that age-related changes seen in many kidneys contribute to the disease-related changes of diabetes and hypertension to cause kidney failure in the elderly. However, several disease processes including primary kidney and vascular diseases present in older patients with kidney failure. Minimal change disease, usually more associated with a pediatric population, has a second peak in incidence during the sixth decade of life. The declining immunity associated with aging may also play a role in the second peak in incidence of poststreptococcal glomerulonephritis seen in the elderly. Pauci-immune necrotizing glomerulonephritis is also more common among those

TABLE 87-2

Chronic Kidney Disease Risk Factors

NONMODIFIABLE RISK FACTORS	MODIFIABLE RISK FACTORS
Older age	Hypertension
Male gender	Obesity
Black race	Proteinuria
Genotype	Dyslipidemia
	Hyperuricemia
	Smoking

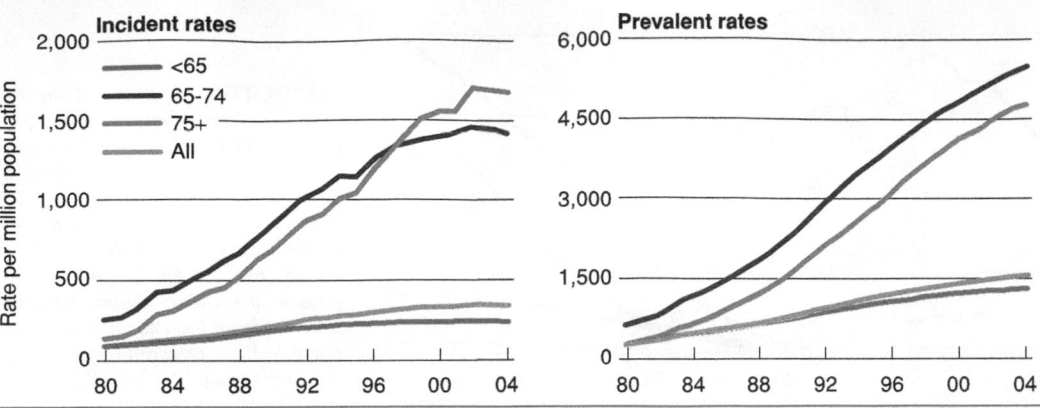

FIGURE 87-1. Incident and prevalence rates for ESRD patients aged 75 yrs and older from 1980 to 2004. Rates adjusted for gender and race. *(2006 Annual Data Report: Atlas of End-Stage Renal Disease in the United States. Bethesda, MD: National Institutes of Health, National Institute of Diabetes and Digestive and Kidney Diseases; 2006.)*

older than 65 years. In addition to immune-mediated kidney disease, renovascular disease, a term used to describe arterial sclerosis in the kidney, is more common in older individuals. The presence of a clinically significant narrowing of the renal artery may lead to marked hypertension and kidney failure. Diagnosis involves magnetic resonance angiography, renal ultrasounds with Doppler, or a captopril renogram. The treatment of renal artery stenosis depends on the severity of the lesion and the clinical presentation. Options for treatment include renal angioplasty and stenting, renal bypass surgery, or medical management. The best treatment of renal artery stenosis among the elderly remains controversial with the current literature supporting conservative medical management. When older patients with CKD present with an acute increase in creatinine, they should be evaluated for reversible causes of their kidney failure such as obstruction or volume depletion.

REFERRAL OF PATIENTS TO NEPHROLOGY

The geriatrician can influence the outcome of kidney failure with the timing of referral. In the past, physicians would limit access to dialysis and transplantation simply by not sending a patient to a nephrologist. While this still happens widely and is common in certain practices and in parts of the world with more limited health care, many patients should be referred for kidney-targeted therapy. Older patients with kidney failure maybe referred late to nephrologists with resulting poor outcomes. These patients may lose the opportunity to consider conservative therapy and require dialysis. The National Kidney Foundation Kidney Disease Outcomes Quality Initiative ("K/DOQI") CKD Guidelines advises referral to a nephrologist after diagnosis under the following circumstances: a clinical action plan

TABLE 87-3

Indications for Urgent Hemodialysis

Refractory
   Progressive fluid overload
   Hyperkalemia
   Metabolic acidosis

Uremia
   Nausea, vomiting, poor appetite
   Altered mental status (encephalopathy)
   Bleeding diathesis (uremic platelet dysfunction)
   Pericarditis

cannot be prepared based on the stage of the disease, the prescribed evaluation of the patient cannot be carried out, or the recommended treatment cannot be carried out. In general, patients with GFR <30 mL/min/1.73 m^2 (CKD Stages 4 and 5) should be referred to a nephrologist. It is difficult to estimate the proportion of late referrals that have been caused by the failure to recognize kidney failure in the elderly.

While most geriatricians may feel comfortable managing CKD and the concomitant metabolic and endocrine derangements, it is important to have nephrology involvement for patient education and preparation for dialysis. As outlined below, older patients with worsening CKD have a wide spectrum of choices for the treatment of kidney failure. It may take some time for the older patient to be educated and accept another chronic illness in the form of CKD, and then time to select a therapeutic approach to the kidney failure. Once therapy has been selected, some of the treatments require lead time prior to the development of an urgent indication for dialysis. For example, the placement of a vascular access may require a referral to a vascular surgeon, vein mapping, and months for fistula maturation and monitoring. A large European Study has demonstrated that late referral was associated with poor outcomes and that outcomes among older patients referred late were significantly worse than younger patients referred late. In many studies of referral timeliness, the cutpoint has been arbitrarily set at 3 to 4 months; however, it is likely that this is still too short of a time to optimize the care of the older patient with kidney failure.

Chronic Kidney Disease and Management of Chronic Health Conditions

Since the access to dialysis and kidney transplantation has been liberalized, there has been a steady shift of the population to not only older patients, but also to those burdened with comorbid disease. In one cohort of adult patients treated with maintenance hemodialysis in the United Kingdom, 90% of patients older than 65 years of age had two or more chronic health conditions. These findings are underscored by data from the 2006 United States Renal Data System, which demonstrate that patients 65 to 74 years of age have the multiple chronic health conditions and that the number of comorbid illnesses has been steady or increased in this population (Figure 87-3). Cardiovascular, musculoskeletal, and neurological problems predominate and adversely affected morbidity, hospitalizations mortality, and quality of life. Given the complexity of managing older patients with a high burden of comorbid disease, the geriatric team has the opportunity to play a crucial role in the care of these patients.

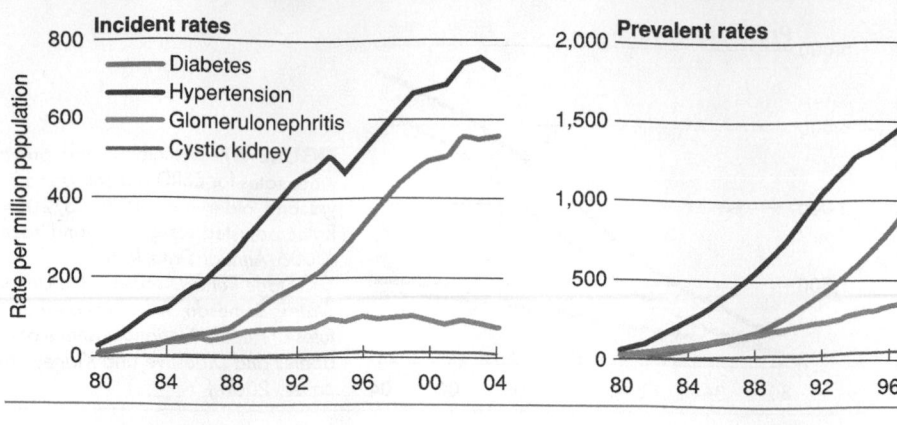

FIGURE 87-2. Incident and prevalent rates, by primary diagnosis from 1980 to 2004 for patients aged 75 yrs and older at initiation, and December 31 point prevalent ESRD patients, aged 75 yrs and older. Rates adjusted for age, gender, and race. (2006 Annual Data Report: Atlas of End-Stage Renal Disease in the United States. Bethesda, MD: National Institutes of Health, National Institute of Diabetes and Digestive and Kidney Diseases; 2006.)

The role of the primary care provider for older patient on dialysis or following kidney transplantation varies by local practice patterns and resources. At times, the nephrologist may subsume the role of the geriatric team given the frequent interaction with the patient at the dialysis units or the complexities of immunosuppressant following kidney transplantation. In other instances, geriatricians retain the primary role and nephrologists administer the dialysis in more of a consulting role. Those with advanced CKD have been shown to have gaps in their primary care, diabetes care, and cardiovascular disease care. This has been illustrated by The U.S. Renal Data System (USRDS) data demonstrating worse diabetes care among CKD Stage 4 to 5 patients compared to the general Medicare population as assessed by the performance of screening tests (Figure 87-4). It may be that nephrologists would benefit from targeted geriatric training, or as some propose, that there should be special geriatric dialysis units in order to address these gaps in care.

INDICATIONS FOR INITIATION OF DIALYSIS

The most common symptoms present before initiation of maintenance dialysis in older patients tend to be anorexia, weight loss, fatigue, nausea, and vomiting. The recognition of uremia in the elderly patient, however, may prove more difficult than in the younger patient. Behavioral changes, unexplained dementia, "adult failure to thrive," unexplained worsening of congestive heart failure, or a change in sense of well-being may represent uremia in the geriatric patient.

The trend has been for earlier initiation of dialysis in older patients, perhaps because of the increased burden of comorbid dis-

ease (Figure 87-5). The Center for Medicare and Medicaid Services (CMS) bases reimbursement for chronic hemodialysis upon a creatinine clearance below 10 mL/min for patients not having diabetes and less than 15 mL/min for patients with diabetes. Creatinine clearance can be calculated by using one of the formulas illustrated in Chapter 44 or with a 24-hour urine collection.

Timely initiation of RRT (Table 87-4) not only avoids the need for urgent dialysis, but also is associated with decreased mortality. A strong correlation between "baseline" serum albumin just prior to initiation of dialysis and patient survival has been demonstrated. Although hypoalbuminemia itself does not necessarily indicate protein-energy malnutrition, it is believed to be a major contributing factor. Analysis of the Modification of Diet in Renal Disease (MDRD) study showed that patients tend to adapt to their declining GFR and associated uremic symptoms by reducing their protein intake. Nevertheless, approximately 60% of American ESRD patients experience nausea and vomiting at the time dialysis is initiated. NKF-K/DOQI guidelines (Table 87-5) recommend evaluating renal function by monitoring weekly urea clearance ($K_t t/V_{urea}$). Once the $K_t t/V_{urea}$ falls below 2.0 (equivalent to a creatinine clearance of 9 to14 mL/min/1.73 m^2), there is increased risk for development of uremic anorexia leading to malnutrition, and RRT should be considered.

Contraindications to Renal Replacement Therapy

There are few absolute medical contraindications to RRT. Some authors propose that advanced dementia, metastatic cancer, and advanced liver disease are reasons for withholding RRT. However, progressive dementia can be confused with uremia-induced delirium in

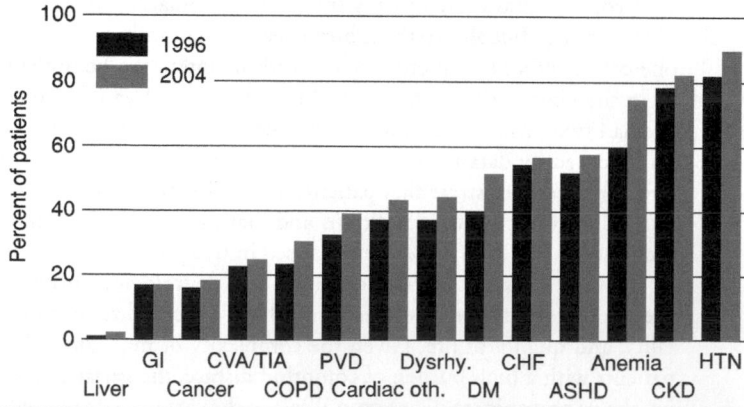

FIGURE 87-3. Comorbid conditions developed in the 2 yrs prior to ESRD initiation. Mean glomerular filtration rate (GFR) at initiation of hemodyalisis by age for incident patients in 1999. (2006 Annual Data Report: Atlas of End-Stage Renal Disease in the United States. Bethesda, MD: National Institutes of Health, National Institute of Diabetes and Digestive and Kidney Diseases; 2006.)

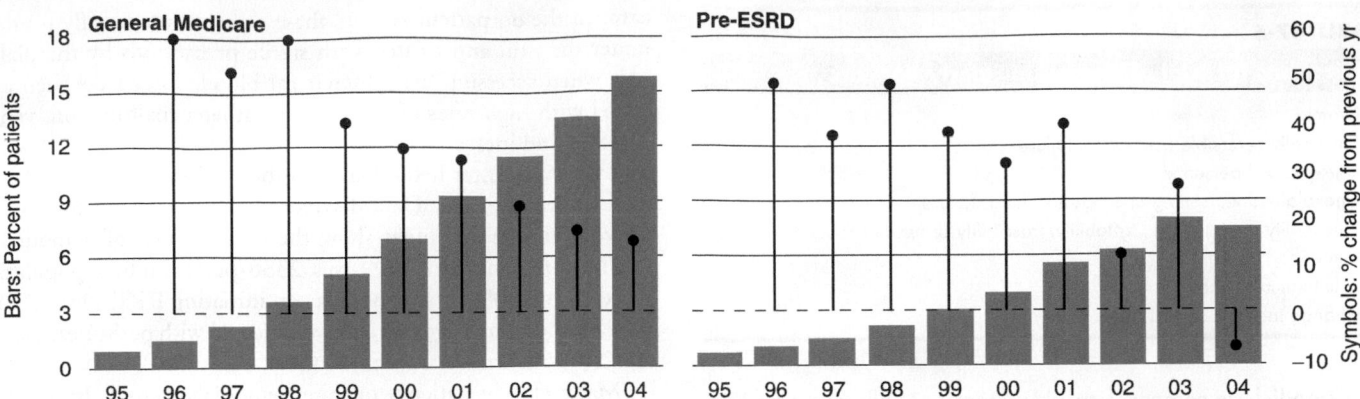

FIGURE 87-4. Percent of diabetic patients receiving all four diabetic preventive care tests. General Medicare: patients diagnosed with diabetes in each year, aged 67 yrs and older on December 31 of the diagnosis year, and continuously enrolled in Medicare during the diagnosis year and the previous year. Claims from diagnosis year and the previous year searched for eye examination codes; claims from diagnosis year searched for lipid, HbA1c, and microalbuminuria testing codes. Pre-ESRD: incident patients aged 67 yrs and older at initiation, and with diabetes 1 yr prior to start of ESRD. Eye examinations tracked 2 yrs prior to start of ESRD; lipid, HbA1c, and microalbuminuria testing tracked 1 yr prior to start of ESRD. (*2006 Annual Data Report: Atlas of End-Stage Renal Disease in the United States. Bethesda, MD: National Institutes of Health, National Institute of Diabetes and Digestive and Kidney Diseases, 2006.*)

a patient with advanced kidney dysfunction, and a "trial" of dialysis is often justified. It may take as long as 3 to 4 weeks to clear uremic symptoms with dialysis. The patient's family should be aware that if the patient's mental status fails to improve, RRT may be inappropriate. Similarly, providing dialysis for a patient with metastatic cancer or end-stage liver disease may allow the patient to get their affairs in order and spend some quality time with friends and family. Cognitive and behavioral contraindications may play an even larger role in the elderly than medical contraindications. Dialysis units are communities where a patient with inappropriate, unsafe, or violent behavior adversely impacts care provided to others at that unit. For example, most nephrologists would discourage the use of dialysis in a patient who is severely cognitively impaired and unable to understand the requirements for safe dialysis treatment.

Health-Related Quality of Life

Maintaining health-related quality of life (HRQOL) may be the most important role of health care in elderly patients with chronic illness. Studies of older patients undergoing dialysis have shown markedly lower functional status compared to older community-dwelling adults. However, hemodialysis has improved since these early studies and there have been advances in technology, treatment of comorbidities such as anemia and hyperparathyroidism, and quality improvement initiatives that have improved the HRQOL of patients on dialysis. While HRQOL was impaired in the hemodialysis population, the HRQOL scores at baseline reflect a preserved multidimensional quality of life among respondents in the HEMO Study >70 years compared to younger hemodialysis patients. A large study in the Netherlands demonstrated decline in scores on physical domains over time in the age groups >55 years. Stability of mental domains is consistent with a previous study of incident patients remaining on hemodialysis over 18 months. These authors also suggest that comorbid disease burden rather than age was associated with a composite outcome of hospitalization, decline in albumin, and a quality of life score of 2 standard deviations below the general population mean score. These longitudinal HRQOL data are also consistent with the North-of-Thames Study findings showing rather moderate use of resources and cross-sectional differences in quality of life among hemodialysis patients older than 65 years. In cross-sectional studies of HRQOL in the ESRD population, there have been larger differences in HRQOL for younger patients on hemodialysis compared to younger norms than for older patients

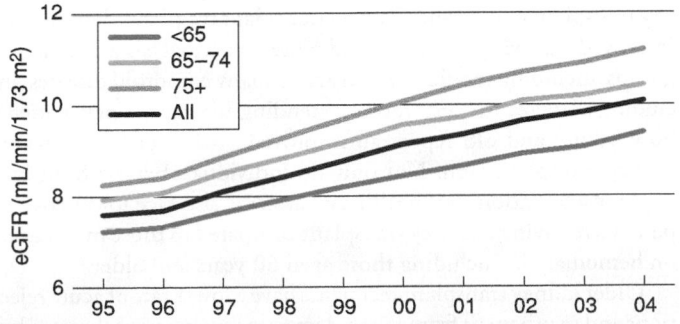

FIGURE 87-5. Estimated glomerular filtration rate, by age. (*2006 Annual Data Report: Atlas of End-Stage Renal Disease in the United States. Bethesda, MD: National Institutes of Health, National Institute of Diabetes and Digestive and Kidney Diseases; 2006.*)

TABLE 87-4

Timely Initiation of Renal Replacement Therapy
RRT should be initiated when:
GFR of approximately 10 mL/min/1.73 m²
Protein-energy malnutrition develops or persists because of decreased nutrient intake without apparent cause for malnutrition
Unless there is:
Stable or increased edema-free body weight
Complete absence of clinical signs or symptoms of uremia
Serum albumin within normal range and stable or increasing

Data from The National Kidney Foundation Kidney Disease Outcomes Quality Initiative (KDOQI) Clinical Practice Guideline on Peritoneal Dialysis Adequacy, 1997 and modified using KDOQI Dialysis Adequacy 2006.

TABLE 87-5

Indications for Trial of Dialysis in Elderly Patients

- Uremia
- Potentially reversible acute renal failure
- Unexplained dementia
- Unexplained worsening of congestive heart failure
- Personality change (e.g., irritability/irascibility or newly subdued demeanor)
- Adult failure to thrive
- Change in sense of well-being

on hemodialysis compared to older norms. While these findings may be informative to older patients and health care providers, they also underline the need to improve HRQOL among all patients undergoing dialysis. Interventions aimed at preserving residual renal function, monitoring HRQOL, treatment of anemia, engaging the patient in physical therapy and rehabilitation, applying palliative care principles, and perhaps more frequent and longer hemodialysis treatments may preserve HRQOL among elderly patients undergoing hemodialysis.

Management

Choice of Renal Replacement Modality

When faced with kidney failure, the elderly patient has a number of choices to make regarding therapy consistent with their level of care and plans for the future. The most common form of RRT are three times weekly outpatient hemodialysis, peritoneal dialysis, and renal transplantation. There has been a proliferation of home therapies and therapies tailored to the elderly such as nursing home–based dialysis units. The elderly patient may also choose conservative management and thereby avoid dialysis. The patients should have time to develop a relationship with the nephrologist and team in order to have discussions of goals for care and how RRT may be tailored to meet those goals.

Hemodialysis Hemodialysis removes excess fluids and solutes from the blood in order to maintain euvolemia and homeostasis. The conventional hemodialysis schedule requires three treatments for 1 per week for approximately 4 hours per treatment. In order to perform hemodialysis, the patient must have an access placed to circulate the blood through the hemodialysis filter. The three options for hemodialysis access include arteriovenous (AV) fistula, AV graft, and temporary hemodialysis catheters. Permanent hemodialysis access requires minor surgery in the arm or leg. The AV fistula, which creates a connection between the native artery and then the AV fistula vein, matures and thickens to handle the higher blood flow rates and permit the use of a needle for access after approximately 3 months. The use of an AV fistula has been associated with better access survival, fewer infections, fewer hospitalizations, and longer patient survival. The AV Graft uses a synthetic bridge between the artery and the vein. The graft has been used in a broader population than the AV fistula but has the major limitations of shorter access survival as well as more infections and hospitalizations. For elderly patients who have been referred late or who have acute kidney failure, hemodialysis is performed using a dialysis catheter. This is a large bore catheter placed in a major vessel such as the superior vena

cava. In the outpatient setting, these catheters are usually tunneled under the skin and treated with sterile precautions by the dialysis unit when accessing the catheters for blood. They have been associated with high rates of bacteremia, catheter malfunction, venous stenosis, and increased costs.

By far, in-center hemodialysis is the predominant form of RRT in the United States. Data derived from the USRDS for patients 65 years of age and older show the incident rate of hemodialysis (by first modality) in 1999 was 2336 per 1 million population, representing 50% of that population initiating RRT. Only 10% of patients older than age 65 years were treated with peritoneal dialysis, and 5% with renal transplantation.

Many elderly patients tolerate hemodialysis well. In addition, some studies demonstrate that older dialysis patients seem to enjoy the scheduled social interaction that in-center dialysis provides them. While most patients maintain a certain quality of life on hemodialysis, the drawbacks to in-center hemodialysis therapy include pain, fatigue, depression, loss of freedom, dietary restrictions, and concern about burden to caregivers.

Peritoneal Dialysis Peritoneal dialysis (PD) permits elderly patients to maintain more control over their schedule and play a larger role in the management of their kidney failure. PD uses the peritoneal membrane as a dialysis membrane by drawing excess fluid and toxins from the blood and into the peritoneal cavity where the fluid will then be drained through a plastic catheter that has been placed into the abdomen. Depending on the dialysis prescription, the peritoneal cavity is filled with fluid and drained a number of times over the course of the day or night. The advantages to using PD include a less-restrictive diet and avoiding the need to travel to a dialysis unit for treatment. However, the disadvantages include back pain, peritonitis, hyperglycemia, obesity, and hernia formation. PD has been successfully used in elderly patients, but its use in patients with poor functional status depends on a caregiver willing to commit to performing the daily therapy. PD can also be performed safely and effectively in a long-term care facility by staff with specialized training. The preferred mode of peritoneal dialysis in this setting is continuous cyclic peritoneal dialysis or nocturnal peritoneal dialysis, which requires less nursing time, allows patients to be more fully integrated into social activities, and allows interruption-free intensive rehabilitation.

Kidney Transplantation Kidney transplantation represents the optimal therapy for those with kidney failure and access to kidney transplant has increased among elderly patients. Elderly patients, in fact, currently make up the fastest growing segment of the kidney transplant population. Kidney transplant recipients demonstrate improved survival over wait-listed patients on dialysis across all age groups, including the elderly, and across many comorbid diseases, including diabetes. In addition to extending life expectancy, patients both young and old report an improved quality of life following kidney transplantation. Not only do individuals benefit from kidney transplantation, but health care systems also face lower costs in patients receiving a kidney transplant compared to those maintained on hemodialysis, including those aged 60 years and older.

Older kidney transplant recipients have a lower rate of acute rejections and may benefit from tailored immunosuppressant therapy, but have a higher risk of infection, cardiovascular events, and malignancy after kidney transplantation compared to younger patients. Furthermore, older patients may experience more drug toxicity and more drug side effects compared to their younger counterparts. Many older kidney transplant recipients face not only immunological risk but also significant nonimmunological risk of baseline medical comorbidity that may increase their vulnerability to morbidity and mortality associated with delayed or suboptimal graft function.

Because the deceased donor kidney remains a scarce resource, the pursuit of an allocation policy that maximizes the life-year benefit of donor organs has generated strategies, which include matching kidneys with lower expected graft survival time to older patients with lower expected longevity. The elderly are more often offered and more likely to accept expanded criteria donor (ECD) kidneys. ECD kidneys are obtained from donors aged 60 years and older or from donors between the age of 50 and 59 years with at least two of the following risk factors: death from cerebrovascular accident, serum creatinine greater than 1.5mg/dL, or history of hypertension, which carry a higher relative risk of graft failure compared to a reference group of donors aged 10 to 39 years without any of these three conditions. However, older patients may be at increased risk of morbidity and mortality following transplantation with ECD kidneys because of increased baseline comorbidity and decreased physical reserve. Recent discussions focusing on the development of kidney allocation systems to maximize the life-year benefit of donor kidneys has involved "old kidney-for-old recipient" strategies. A potential increase in overall graft survival, with significant associated cost savings to society might be realized by allocating younger kidneys to younger recipients. However, it is important to assess the perception of fairness of such a potentially age-ist allocation schema. In the United States, transplant centers rarely discourage elderly patients from seeking kidney transplantation. Some physicians may be reluctant to encourage elderly transplant candidates to accept kidneys presumed to be of lower quality for the objective of maximizing social justice. Others will be willing to accept such kidneys, using the argument of medical efficacy, while providing subtle or even overt encouragement to the elderly to accept ECD kidneys by framing the option as a means to decrease time on the waiting list. This may in part explain why the odds ratio for willingness to accept an ECD kidney increases significantly with age. In an attempt to ensure good outcome of their grafts in elderly recipients, strict rules have been imposed to limit ischemic damage in the donor and immunological risk by the Eurotransplant Senior Program. Preliminary reports from this program have been positive and this may serve as a model for maximizing kidney resources while offering older patients an opportunity for kidney transplantation.

The degree to which comorbidity influences graft and patient outcomes is significantly less in recipients of living donor kidneys compared to recipients of deceased donor kidneys. A living donor kidney may offset some of the risk of increased comorbidity in the elderly recipient and highlights living donor kidney transplantation as an important opportunity for elderly patients with kidney failure to receive optimal treatment. If the allocation of deceased donor kidneys in the future increasingly favors younger patients over older patients in the distribution of this scarce resource, living donor kidney transplantation may become the only realistic chance at successful kidney transplantation for older patients.

Time-Limited Trial of Dialysis

When the patient, family, or physician is unsure about the prognosis or the impact that dialysis will have upon the patient's quality of life,

it is reasonable to offer a time-limited trial of dialysis. If a trial of dialysis is to be conducted, it is important to predetermine a time period (usually 4 to 6 weeks) and to inform all the members of the dialysis team. Such measures will ease the appropriate withdrawal from dialysis.

Conservative Management

It is difficult to assess the frequency of conservative palliative therapy, but it is likely that the geriatrician plays a primary role in the decision-making process and management of these patients. In a study from the UK, 84% of patients with CKD Stages 3 to 5 were not referred to nephrology. The proportion of referred patients declined dramatically with older age, with a maximum referral rate of 68% for those 40 to 49 years of age, and 4% of those older than 80 years of age. Another study presented 19% with palliative care as a recommended option based on age and comorbid disease burden; 76% of those recommended for palliative care followed through with management of kidney failure without dialysis. While it was somewhat difficult to provide accurate comparisons of survival times, these investigators reported no substantial difference in expected survival time for those undergoing palliative care compared to hemodialysis. Significantly fewer palliative care deaths (27%) took place in the hospital compared to the proportion of deaths among those patients undergoing hemodialysis (67%). In a study of octogenarians in a single-center where older patients were advised not to undergo dialysis, 25% were conservatively managed. In this report, the median survival of those undergoing conservative management was 8.9 months compared to 28.9 months among those undergoing dialysis. In addition, the cause of death of those managed without dialysis was uremia or pulmonary edema in approximately 60%.

Conservative management should aim to maintain quality of life while keeping in mind the shared decision to avoid dialysis therapy. In addition to continuing to manage fluid status, anemia, electrolytes, and bone metabolism, symptoms should be addressed by the geriatric, nephrology, and palliative care teams. Among both groups of patients undergoing dialysis and receiving palliative care, symptoms should be treated since pain, dry itchy skin, poor sleep, and fatigue impact mood and quality of life. A study has recently shown improvement in pain among ESRD patients managed using the World Health Organization (WHO) three-step analgesic ladder. A nutritional approach to avoiding dialysis therapy was assessed in nondiabetic patients older than 70 years. In this randomized study, patients with kidney failure were assigned a supplemented very low protein diet compared to usual care with dialysis. This study found that those patients assigned the dietary intervention spent an additional 10.7 months off dialysis without substantial differences in survival between groups. These findings suggest that nutrition may play an important role in managing patients who elect to avoid dialysis.

Management of End Stage Renal Disease on Dialysis

Anemia

Anemia is a common problem with CKD and kidney failure. The fall in hematocrit correlates roughly with the severity of the renal disease, although individual variation is considerable. In general, anemia presents when the GFR is around 35 mL/min. The bone marrow is hypoproliferative while peripheral blood (red cell) indices are normal unless there is superimposed deficiency of iron or folic acid. Thus, the anemia seen with kidney failure is typically a normochromic, normocytic anemia. The lack of erythropoietin production, which occurs with CKD, is the primary cause of anemia with kidney failure. Since erythropoietin production occurs primarily in the kidney, erythropoietin levels are inadequate with CKD, thus depriving the bone marrow of the stimulus necessary for production of red blood cells. The isolation of human erythropoietin and subsequent production of recombinant erythropoietin has been a major advance in the care of those with CKD. Beginning in 1989, synthetic erythropoietin has been available and effectively treats the anemia of CRF. Recently another recombinant form, darbepoetin, has become available and permitted less frequent dosing regimens. Correction of anemia has improved quality of life, reduced the need for transfusions, improved cognitive performance, and decreased left ventricular hypertrophy. There are adverse effects of using erythropoietin in the patient with CKD, including iron deficiency (the stimulation of red blood cell production outstrips iron stores), hypertension, and vascular thrombosis.

The optimal hemoglobin target for patients with anemia caused by chronic kidney failure remains somewhat unclear. Recent data in the CKD population suggest untoward cardiovascular outcomes at higher hemoglobin levels. The current conservative target is a hemoglobin count between 11 and 12 mg/dL. In addition to close attention to erythropoietin dosing and hemoglobin levels, adequate anemia management requires routine analysis and treatment of iron deficiency. Iron levels tend to drop in patients on erythropoietin therapy because of increased iron utilization. All patients, however, should receive routine screening of stool for occult blood and periodic screening colonoscopy. Iron-deficient ESRD patients usually receive intravenous replacement iron at the end of their dialysis treatments, either as dextran, gluconate, or sucrate solution. Because they absorb oral iron poorly, ESRD patients have "functional" iron deficiency when their transferrin falls below 100 ng/mL or their iron saturation is less than 20%.

Cardiovascular Disease

Many more patients have CKD compared to the numbers receiving RRT. The disparity between the number receiving RRT and the number with CKD is explained by the high mortality from cardiovascular disease prior to needing dialysis in the CKD population. Even on dialysis, the risk of death from cardiovascular disease remains 10 to 100 times higher than the risk of a person from the general population. While traditional risk factors account for only a portion of the increased risk associated with kidney disease, the etiology of the increased cardiovascular risk is unclear. There are a number of potential factors that represent classical risk factors shared between atherosclerosis and kidney disease such as age, hypercholesterolemia, hypertension, smoking, and obesity. In addition, there are a number of factors specific to kidney failure such as anemia, hyperhomocysteinemia, hypervolemia, and hyperparathyroidism. These factors can act to promote both cardiomyopathy and ischemic heart disease. The current treatment recommendations focus on optimizing management of known cardiovascular risk factors and on recognizing harbingers of active cardiovascular disease. Those caring for patients with CKD should consider the cardiovascular disease management as an important part of their care.

Calcium, Phosphorous, Hyperparathyroidism, and Bone Disorders

Kidney failure is associated with abnormalities of divalent ions (Ca^{2+}, P) and of the hormones that regulate the concentration of these minerals in body fluids. One of the earliest detectable abnormalities in kidney failure is a rise in parathyroid hormone (PTH), which can occur at a GFR of 40 mL/min. Secondary hyperparathyroidism is a major cause of bone disease in patients with kidney failure. Two inhibitors of parathyroid hormone are ionized calcium (the active form of calcium) and $1,25\text{-}(OH)_2D_3$, which has an independent inhibitory effect on parathyroid hormone release. No difference has been found in hyperphosphatemia or severity of renal osteodystrophy in elderly dialysis patients as compared with younger dialysis patients, and there is no correlation between plasma 1,25-dihydroxyvitamin D_3 levels and age in patients with kidney failure. Elderly female dialysis patients have significantly lower bone mineral content and bone width when compared with younger dialysis patients matched for duration of dialysis. There is a higher incidence of pathologic fracture, vascular or metastatic calcification, and bone pain in elderly patients on dialysis than in younger patients. The overall result of these disturbances is that patients with ESRD may develop a complex form of bone disease (renal osteodystrophy). Furthermore, there has been a strong association of disordered bone and mineral metabolism and risk of cardiovascular disease. This association between calcium and phosphate metabolism has been most striking when images of the heart demonstrating extensive calcification have been related to levels of both calcium and phosphate.

Treatment of renal osteodystrophy and secondary hyperparathyroidism in the geriatric renal patient is similar to the younger patient. However, the optimal management of patients has been controversial. Hyperphosphatemia is treated with a low phosphate diet and with various phosphate binders. Recent recommendations advise that daily calcium in the phosphate binder should be less than 2 g. Hypocalcemia can be treated with oral calcium, oral or intravenous calcitriol, or other Vitamin D analog, or higher dialysate calcium. Refractory hyperparathyroidism can be treated with parathyroidectomy or with a trial of a calcimimetic. While the agents used to regulate calcium and phosphate levels remain controversial, the goals of normalizing calcium and phosphate levels and improving bone health are widely accepted as important in the management of CKD patients.

Metabolic Acidosis

The acidosis associated with renal disease is not more severe in the elderly patient despite the decreased ability to handle an acid load seen with normal aging. Acidemia caused by metabolic acidosis is associated with increased oxidation of branched chain amino acids, increased protein degradation, and decreased albumin synthesis. Because of the adverse metabolic effects of chronic acidosis, such as accelerated bone loss and muscle wasting, goals of therapy should be directed at achieving predialysis serum bicarbonate levels of at least 22 mmol/L. If predialysis levels routinely fall below 22 mmol/L, acidemia may be treated by increasing the dialysis bicarbonate in those undergoing hemodialysis, or supplementation with oral sodium bicarbonate tablets.

Malnutrition

Nutrition plays an important role in the health and well-being of patients with kidney failure. Patients with kidney failure are thought to benefit from intensive monitoring of nutritional status. The recommended assessments include body weight, dietary interviews and diaries, serum albumin, and total nitrogen appearance. A renal dietician may offer alternative foods and recommendations to patients that feel limited by fluid, sodium, potassium, and phosphate restrictions. Weight loss and inability to maintain nutritional status are indications for initiating hemodialysis and adequacy of dialysis therapy should be evaluated to avoid anorexia and nausea. Dietary supplements and vitamin and mineral supplements, such as zinc or oral pyridoxine (50 mg/day), might be helpful. It is unclear whether intradialytic parenteral nutrition offers real benefit. There are no controlled studies available, and are very expensive to conduct. Dietary restrictions in the elderly patient undergoing dialysis should be minimal. Patients with inadequate intake rarely need food restrictions.

Pruritus

Itching in patients with kidney failure can adversely affect sleep and quality of life. The causes of itching in elderly patients with kidney failure would include xerosis, uremic itching, medication sensitivity, and other chronic health conditions such as diabetes. Pruritus is common in the elderly dialysis patient, possibly because of skin changes seen with aging. As a part of an approach to managing uremic itching, it has been recommended to optimize dialysis treatment by increasing dialysis dose, treating anemia and iron deficiency, and maintaining a low serum phosphate. Treatment of itching caused by xerosis or uremia has been largely symptomatic local treatment consisting of keeping the skin moist with emollients, bathing less frequently and with tepid rather than hot water, and increasing ambient humidity with vaporizers or humidifiers. Capsaicin cream may also be effective. A promising new approach has been tested in two randomized trials of nalfurafine, a k-opioid receptor agonist. These studies of patients with severe uremic itching demonstrated improvement in itching intensity and sleep disturbances compared to placebo. Antihistamines such as diphenhydramine or hydroxyzine may be used, but may cause sedation and cognitive impairment in elderly patients.

SPECIAL ISSUES

Prognosis and Survival

Kidney failure is associated with a decrease in life expectancy for all age groups when compared to age-matched patients. The need for dialysis impacts the risk of death in the patient older than age 75 years to a lesser degree than it impacts patients 45 years of age, with a threefold versus 20-fold increased risk as compared to nondialysis patients, respectively. The survival of older patients undergoing dialysis has been recently assessed in the USRDS. The number of patients older than 80 years of age roughly doubled from 1996 to 2003. Overall, the 1-year survival rate for octogenarians and nonagenarians after dialysis initiation was 54%. The characteristics strongly associated with death were older age, nonambulatory status, and

more comorbid conditions (Figure 87-6). In addition to survival, it is important to convey the impact of dialysis on HRQOL. In the HEMO Study, a randomized clinical trial of dialysis dose and membrane flux, patients were assessed for HRQOL at baseline and annually. Among those with HRQOL data at the first three annual assessments, there were no substantial mean declines in physical or mental well-being over the 3-year period. However, there were high rates of adverse HRQOL events in all age groups and significantly higher adverse event rates of either death or clinically significant decline in HRQOL over 3 years among those older than 70 years. The composite outcomes of clinically significant decline in HRQOL or death of those older than 70 years over 3 years was approximately 70%. These findings underline the importance of conveying the limited life expectancy of those patients who are not transplant candidates, and particularly those with limited functional status and comorbidity. While life span is limited, it remains up to the individual whether to pursue dialysis or palliative therapy.

Withdrawal from Dialysis

Stopping dialysis has been a common reason for death in the dialysis population, especially for older patients. Up to one-third of patients are withdrawn or voluntarily withdraw from dialysis therapy annually. The factors associated with dialysis discontinuation in the United States include white race, diabetes, female sex, symptoms, and older age. While dialysis patients should understand that they have the right to stop treatment, the health care team should ensure that the patient is not withdrawing because of "burdens" that can be ameliorated. One prospective observational study of 131 adult (average age 70 years) maintenance dialysis patients examined the quality of dying following dialysis termination. Quality of death was evaluated by the use of a quality-of-dying tool that quantified the duration (length of time it took to die), pain and suffering, and psychosocial factors. Death occurred on average 8 days after the last dialysis treatment. Thirty-eight percent of the patients on dialysis had a "very good" death, 47% had "good" deaths, and only 15% had "bad" deaths. However, during the last day of life, 42% of the patients had some pain (5% severe) reiterating the importance end-of-life palliation once the decision to withdraw therapy is made. While the end-of-life issues in renal failure have received increasing attention, there remain many barriers to management of these issues, as underscored by the fivefold lower use of hospice among patients undergoing hemodialysis compared to those older patients not using dialysis. In order to overcome the barriers to a good death for those on dialysis, it is important to have a multidisciplinary approach and an awareness of local hospice services.

Advance Directives

A complete review of treatment options, prognosis, and quality of life should be included when discussing advanced directives of a patient with CKD Stages 4 and 5. Having the patients wishes expressed prior to starting dialysis makes the burden of decision-making much easier for the families and physicians should the patient become critically ill. It is crucial to involve the family and surrogates in the advanced directives process and to fully document the directives in order to avoid a change in direction with an unplanned hospitalization. Patients who decide not to undergo dialysis should have clear documentation

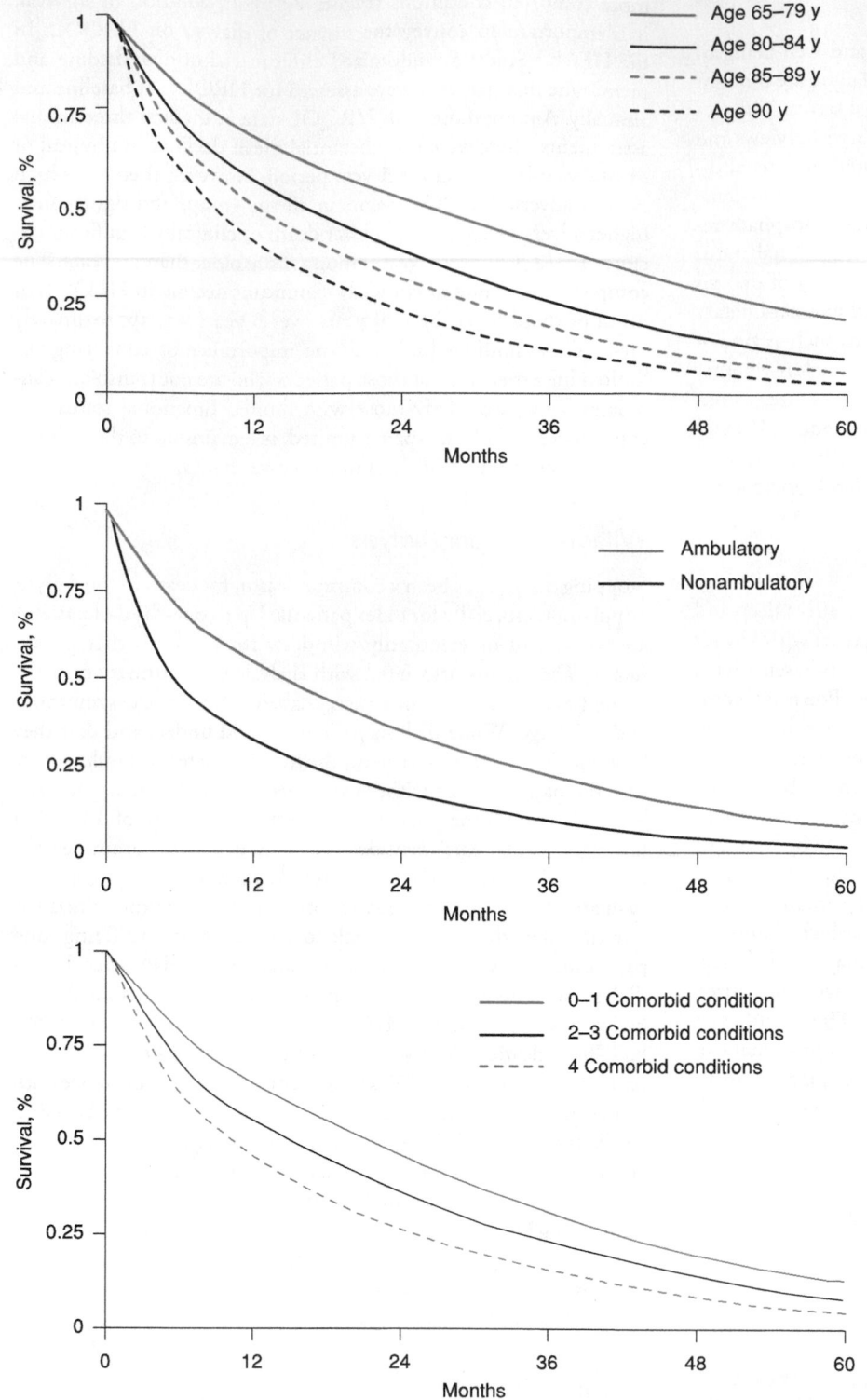

FIGURE 87-6. Survival of octogenarians and nonagenarians at dialysis initiation by age group (top), ambulatory status (middle), and number of comorbid conditions (bottom). *(Kurella M, Covinsky KE, Collins AJ, et al. Octogenarians and nonagenarians starting dialysis in the United States. Ann Intern Med. 146:177–183, 2007.)*

in their medical records. There should be similar documentation of do-not-resuscitate orders, wishes regarding artificial nutrition and other measures, and identification of their health care surrogate.

SUMMARY

As the population ages, there will be increasing numbers of older patients with advanced CKD and kidney failure. The elderly patient

with kidney failure now has a multitude of choices for RRT including hemodialysis, peritoneal dialysis, conservative management, and kidney transplantation. Primary care physicians and geriatricians should identify CKD in older patients who have risk factors and refer them kidney disease management. After referral, the geriatric team may remain in the key role of addressing advanced directives and planning long-term care, since they may have a long-standing relationship with the patient and have the best insight into the patient's goals and values. In addition, the geriatric team may choose to continue managing other health issues in the kidney failure patient so that it remains clear who will manage comorbid illnesses. Elderly patients with CKD will remain an economic and medical challenge, but a multidisciplinary approach to care of these patients will provide the best long-term outcomes.

FURTHER READING

Bellomo R, Ronco C, Kellum JA, et al. Acute renal failure—definition, outcome measures, animal models, fluid therapy and information technology needs: the Second International Consensus Conference of the Acute Dialysis Quality Initiative (ADQI) Group. *Crit Care.* 2004;8:R204–R212.

Brown WW. Hemodialysis in elderly patients. *Int Urol Nephrol.* 2000;32:127–135.

Brunori G, Viola BF, Parrinello G, et al. Efficacy and safety of a very-low-protein diet when postponing dialysis in the elderly: a prospective randomized multicenter controlled study. *Am J Kidney Dis.* 2007;49:569–580.

Coresh J, Astor BC, Greene T, et al. Prevalence of chronic kidney disease and decreased kidney function in the adult US population: Third National Health and Nutrition Examination Survey. *Am J Kidney Dis.* 2003;41:1–12.

Fabrizii V, Winkelmayer WC, Klauser R, et al. Patient and graft survival in older kidney transplant recipients: does age matter? *J Am Soc Nephrol.* 2004;15:1052–1060.

Galla JH. Clinical practice guideline on shared decision-making in the appropriate initiation of and withdrawal from dialysis. The Renal Physicians Association and the American Society of Nephrology. *J Am Soc Nephrol.* 2000;11:1340–1342.

Germain MJ, Cohen LM, Davison SN. Withholding and withdrawal from dialysis: what we know about how our patients die. *Semin Dial.* 2007;20:195–199.

Jassal SV, Krahn MD, Naglie G, et al. Kidney transplantation in the elderly: a decision analysis. *J Am Soc Nephrol.* 2003;14:187–196.

John R, Webb M, Young A, et al. Unreferred chronic kidney disease: a longitudinal study. *Am J Kidney Dis.* 2004;43:825–835.

Johnson DW, Herzig K, Purdie D, et al. A comparison of the effects of dialysis and renal transplantation on the survival of older uremic patients. *Transplantation.* 2000;69:794–799.

Joly D, Anglicheau D, Alberti C, et al. Octogenarians reaching end-stage renal disease: cohort study of decision-making and clinical outcomes. *J Am Soc Nephrol.* 2003;14:1012–1021.

Kauffman HM, McBride MA, Cors CS, et al. Early mortality rates in older kidney recipients with comorbid risk factors. *Transplantation.* 2007;83:404–410.

Keithi-Reddy SR, Patel TV, Armstrong AW, et al. Uremic pruritus. *Kidney Int.* 2007;72(3):373–377.

Kurella M, Covinsky KE, Collins AJ, et al. Octogenarians and nonagenarians starting dialysis in the United States. *Ann Intern Med.* 2007;146:177–183.

Kutner NG, Brogan D, Hall WD, et al. Functional impairment, depression, and life satisfaction among older hemodialysis patients and age-matched controls: a prospective study. *Arch Phys Med Rehabil.* 2000;81:453–459.

Levey AS, Eckardt KU, Tsukamoto Y, et al. Definition and classification of chronic kidney disease: a position statement from Kidney Disease: Improving Global Outcomes (KDIGO). *Kidney Int.* 2005;67:2089–2100.

Oniscu GC, Brown H, Forsythe JL: How great is the survival advantage of transplantation over dialysis in elderly patients? *Nephrol Dial Transplant.* 2004;19:945–951.

Oniscu GC, Brown H, Forsythe JL. How old is old for transplantation? *Am J Transplant.* 2004;4:2067–2074.

Rebollo P, Ortega F, Baltar JM, et al. Is the loss of health-related quality of life during renal replacement therapy lower in elderly patients than in younger patients?. *Nephrol Dial Transplant.* 2001;16:1675–1680.

Schwenger V, Morath C, Hofmann A, et al. Late referral—a major cause of poor outcome in the very elderly dialysis patient. *Nephrol Dial Transplant.* 2006;21:962–967.

Shapiro R. Kidney allocation and the perception of fairness. *Am J Transplant.* 2007;7:1041–1042.

Disorders of Fluid Balance

Myron Miller

Characteristic of the normal aging process is a decline in physiologic reserve in many body regulatory systems, including those involved in the maintenance of fluid balance. The confluence of normal aging changes, common diseases, and the administration of many classes of drugs can readily lead to clinically evident disturbances of fluid balance, such as water retention or loss and to hyponatremia or hypernatremia with resultant symptomatic consequences. In some individuals, an impaired ability to conserve water may underlie the development of nocturnal urinary frequency as well as urinary incontinence.

The normal regulation of water and electrolyte balance involves the interplay of many homeostatic systems that operate to maintain the composition of fluid and electrolyte compartments within a narrow range. Because of alterations in the normal aging process, these homeostatic systems maybe compromised. The key regulatory components of fluid balance include (1) thirst perception, which governs fluid intake, (2) the kidney, which is governed by hemodynamic forces, and (3) hormonal influences of arginine vasopressin (AVP) or antidiuretic hormone (ADH), atrial natriuretic hormone (ANH), and the renin–angiotensin–aldosterone system, which control renal water and electrolyte excretion. Clinicians who are involved in the care of the elderly recognize that disturbances of water and electrolyte balance are common in this age group, especially when older persons are challenged by disease, drugs, or extrinsic factors such as access to fluids or control of diet composition.

EFFECTS OF NORMAL AGING ON FLUID REGULATORY SYSTEMS (Table 88-1)

Body Composition

Aging effects on body composition have the potential to contribute to derangements in fluid balance. Normal aging is accompanied by a decrease in lean body mass, an increase in fat mass, and a decrease in total body water. Thus, total body water declines from the approximate values of 60% of body weight in young men and 52% in young women to 54% and 46%, respectively, in individuals older than age 65 years, primarily through a decrease in the intracellular fluid compartment. The decrease in total body water may place the elderly patient at increased risk for dehydration and/or hyponatremia when challenged by fluid loss or decreased fluid intake and at increased risk for fluid overload and hyponatremia when exposed to excessive oral or parenteral fluid intake.

Thirst and Fluid Intake

The ability to ingest a sufficient volume of fluid to meet body needs requires that thirst perception be present, that a suitable source of fluid be available, and that the individual be physically capable of obtaining and consuming the fluid. Under normal conditions, the requirement for daily fluid intake is approximately 30 mL/kg body weight. This requirement is further increased when there is high environmental temperature, fever, increased gastrointestinal, urinary, or respiratory fluid loss. Urine production typically ranges from 1.0 to 2.5 L per 24 hours and is modestly higher in men older than the age of 60 years. Older persons maybe challenged by increased amounts of fluid by either oral or parenteral routes, especially when they are in institutional acute care or long-term care settings and not in control of their fluid intake. In this circumstance, there is risk of volume overload and hyponatremia.

In healthy individuals, fluid intake is largely controlled by thirst sensation, which is regulated by both extracellular fluid volume and blood tonicity. Blood osmolality is the most important factor in the day to day perception of thirst. Thirst is usually stimulated when plasma osmolality rises to values greater than 292 mOsm/kg. Healthy persons older than age 65 years have shown evidence of an age-associated impairment in thirst perception so that when they were subjected to water deprivation sufficient to raise plasma osmolality to greater than 296 mOsm/kg, they exhibited diminished subjective

TABLE 88-1

Aging Effects on Water and Sodium Regulatory Systems

Body composition
  Decreased total body water
  Decreased intracellular fluid compartment

Fluid intake
  Decreased thirst perception

Renal function
  Decreased kidney mass
  Decline in renal blood flow
  Decline in glomerular filtration rate
  Impaired distal renal tubular diluting capacity
  Impaired renal concentrating capacity
  Impaired sodium conservation
  Impaired renal response to vasopressin

Hormonal systems
  Vasopressin
    Normal or increased basal secretion
    Increased response to osmotic stimulation
    Decreased nocturnal secretion
  Atrial natriuretic hormone
    Increased basal secretion
    Increased response to stimulation
  Decreased plasma renin activity
  Decreased aldosterone production

awareness of thirst and consumed significantly less water than young subjects who were similarly water deprived and whose plasma osmolality rose to a lesser level (mean, 290 mOsm/kg). Other studies of elderly patients with cerebrovascular accidents have similarly documented impaired thirst perception in the face of volume depletion and hyperosmolality, both normally being potent stimuli for thirst. Elderly patients with Alzheimer's disease fail to drink adequately when exposed to water deprivation in spite of the accompanying elevation of blood osmolality to levels above the usual thirst threshold. Further confounding the ability of the elderly person to ingest adequate amounts of fluid is the frequent presence of physical disability (e.g., blindness, arthritis, stroke) and impaired mobility, thus limiting the capacity of the patient to gain access to fluids.

Renal Changes of Normal Aging (Also See Chapter 85)

Structural and Functional Changes

Normal aging is accompanied by changes in renal anatomy and in renal function. Kidney mass undergoes progressive decline from a normal combined weight of approximately 250 to 280 g in young adults to between 180 and 200 g by age 80 to 90 years, with corresponding decrease in length and volume. Histologically, the number of glomeruli decline by 30% to 40% with increasing age and the percent of glomeruli that are hyalinized or sclerotic, increase to 10% to 30%. This process accelerates after the age of 40 years, and the residual glomeruli also undergo changes with age. Thus, there is a decrease in effective filtering surface, and an increase in the number of mesangial cells, a decrease in number of epithelial cells, and thickening of the glomerular basement membrane.

As part of the normal aging process, there are changes in the renal vasculature that lead to obliteration of the arteriolar lumen and loss of the glomerular capillary tuft. These changes take place primarily in the cortical glomeruli. In the juxtamedullary area, glomerular sclerosis may lead to anastomosis between afferent and efferent arterioles with direct shunting of blood between these vessels. Blood flow to the medulla, through the arteria rectae, is maintained in old age.

The anatomic changes of the aging kidney are paralleled by alterations in renal function although a direct relationship between anatomic and functional changes is not firmly established. Renal blood flow declines during the course of normal aging by approximately 10% per decade after young adulthood so that by the age of 90 years, the renal plasma flow is approximately 300 mL/min—a reduction of 50% of the value found at 30 years of age. The decrease in renal perfusion is most extensive in the outer cortex with lesser impairment of inner cortex and minimal effect on the medulla.

Glomerular filtration rate (GFR) remains relatively stable until age 40 years, after which it undergoes decline at an annual rate of approximately 0.8 mL/min/1.73 m^2. Because there is much individual variability within the elderly population, longitudinal studies show that not all aging persons will undergo a decline in GFR. The Cockcroft–Gault formula for creatinine clearance has been used to estimate GFR. A more accurate estimate of GFR is now recommended using the abbreviated version of the Modification of Diet in Renal Disease (MDRD) formula, which is based on serum creatinine, age, gender, and race. The calculation can easily be made by use of a downloadable Web-based calculator (http://www.nkdep.nih.gov/GFR-cal-adult-htm). In persons older than the age of 70 years, approximately 26% will have estimated GFR less than 60 mL/min/1.73 m^2.

Water Regulatory Capacity

Renal Water Retention The aging kidney exhibits a modest age-related impairment in the ability to dilute the urine and excrete a water load. The ability to generate free water is dependent on several factors, including adequate delivery of solute to the diluting region (sufficient renal perfusion and GFR), a functional intact distal diluting site (ascending limb of Henle's loop and the distal tubule), and suppression of ADH in order to escape water reabsorption in the collecting duct. The age-related decline in GFR is the most important factor in the aged kidney's diluting capacity. The presence of an age-related diluting defect that is independent of changes in GFR remains controversial.

The diluting capacity of the aging kidney has been evaluated in men by determining the urine osmolality and free water clearance response to acute water loading. In young men (mean age 31 years), minimum urine osmolality was 52 mOsm/kg, whereas in middle-aged men (mean age 60 years), minimum urine osmolality was 74 mOsm/kg, and in the older men (mean age 84 years), it was 92 mOsm/kg. The free water clearance was lowest in the older group. However, when these results were expressed as free water clearance per mL of GFR, the values were not different, suggesting that the defect in diluting capacity was a consequence of an age-related reduction in GFR. In a similar study in which healthy elderly subjects aged 63 to 80 years (mean, 72 years) and healthy young subjects aged 21 to 26 years (mean, 22 years) were administered a water load, the peak free water clearance was 5.7 mL/min in the older group and

8.4 mL/min in the younger group. However, when adjustments were made for changes in creatinine clearance, the difference in these indices was not statistically significant.

Other studies suggest that age-related free water clearance defects persist following correction for a lower GFR. A significantly lower free water clearance/creatinine ratio was found in elderly nursing home residents as compared to healthy younger subjects. The maximal urinary dilution (urinary/plasma osmolality) declined from 0.247 in younger subjects to 0.418 in elderly subjects.

In addition to impaired diluting capacity, the age-related decrease in renal plasma flow and GFR can lead to passive reabsorption of fluid, thereby increasing the risk of water overload and hyponatremia. This effect is clinically evident in elderly patients who have congestive heart failure, extracellular volume depletion, and hypoalbuminemia.

Diuretics, especially thiazides, can decrease renal diluting capacity. In the elderly, this effect becomes especially important when it is superimposed on the already diminished diluting capacity of the aged kidney, thus increasing the risk of developing water intoxication by impairing the ability to excrete excess water promptly.

Renal Water Loss It has been known for many years that there is an age-related change in renal concentrating capacity. In a study of healthy men aged 40 to 101 years who underwent 24 hours of water deprivation, maximum attainable urine specific gravity declined from 1.030 at 40 years to 1.023 at 89 years. Hospitalized men aged 23 to 72 years who underwent 24 hours of dehydration demonstrated a progressive decline in maximum urine osmolality with increasing age. In healthy, active community-dwelling participants in the Baltimore Longitudinal Study of Aging, young subjects responded to 12 hours of water deprivation with a marked decrease in urine flow (1.02 ± 0.10 to 0.49 ± 0.03 mL/min) and a moderate increase in urine osmolality (969 ± 41 to 1109 ± 22 mOsm/kg), whereas elderly subjects were unable to significantly alter urine flow (1.05 ± 0.15 to 1.03 ± 0.13 mL/min) or osmolality (852 ± 64 to 882 ± 49 mOsm/kg). This age-related decline in urine concentrating ability persisted after correction for the age-related decrease in GFR.

The effect of age on renal tubular response to vasopressin has been assessed by measuring the urine-to-plasma inulin concentration ratio in men who ranged in age from 26 to 86 years and who were free of clinically demonstrable cardiovascular and renal disease. The ratio fell from 118 in young men (mean age 35 years) to 77 in the middle-aged group (mean age 55 years) and to 45 in the older men (mean age 73 years). The decreased renal sensitivity to vasopressin with age maybe a result of an age-related increase in vasopressin secretion. Animal studies demonstrate that chronic exposure of the kidney to increased vasopressin results in diminished renal responsiveness to the hormone. Thus, an age-related increase in vasopressin secretion may result in down-regulation of renal AVP receptors and be the basis for decreased renal concentrating capacity in the elderly.

Sodium Regulatory Capacity

Renal Sodium Retention Several situations may lead to sodium retention and accompanying water overload in the elderly. The previously described age-related decrease in renal blood flow and GFR favors enhanced conservation of sodium. Disease states resulting in secondary hyperaldosteronism, such as congestive heart failure,

cirrhosis, or nephrotic syndrome, are common in the elderly. In addition, drugs such as nonsteroidal anti-inflammatory agents, which are frequently used in the elderly, may promote sodium retention.

Renal Sodium Loss Elderly individuals are more likely to have exaggerated natriuresis after a water load than are younger subjects. Patients with benign hypertension have an excess of sodium excretion in association with increased age. The aged kidney's response to salt restriction is sluggish so that restriction in sodium intake to 10 mEq/d was followed by a half-time for reduction of urinary sodium excretion of 17.6 hours in young individuals and 30.9 hours in old individuals. These data suggest that the aging kidney is more prone to sodium wasting. Mechanisms underlying this tendency maybe multifactorial and are related to the effects of age on ANH, the renin–angiotensin–aldosterone system, and renal tubular function.

Vasopressin System in Normal Aging (Table 88-2)

Neurohypophyseal System

The magnocellular neurons of the hypothalamus where AVP is synthesized do not appear to undergo age-related degenerative changes. There is no evidence of the cell destruction, neuronal dropout, or loss of dendritic arborization found in other segments of the aged brain. Moreover, neurosecretory material in supraoptic nuclei (SON) and paraventricular nuclei (PVN) in elderly persons does not appear to differ in amount from that in younger subjects.

Morphologic data provide evidence that these nuclei, in fact, become more active with age. In the human hypothalamic neurohypophyseal system of subjects ranging from 10 to 93 years of age, a gradual increase in the size of the SON and PVN was observed after 60 years of age, suggesting that AVP production increases in senescence. Similar changes have been observed in the nuclear size of AVP neurons. Possibly contributing to the maintenance of normal or increased amounts of AVP in the magnocellular neurons is the observation of a 25% reduction in the rate of axonal transport of AVP and its associated neurophysin with advancing age. Thus, it appears that neurosecretory activity of hypothalamic AVP neurons

TABLE 88-2

Aging Effects on the Vasopressin System*
Morphology of the neurohypophyseal system
Normal or increased supraoptic nucleus cell number/AVP content
Normal or increased paraventricular nucleus cell number/AVP content
Decreased suprachiasmatic nucleus cell number/AVP content
Normal extrahypothalamic nuclei cell number/AVP content
Hypothalamic vasopressin content
Normal or increased
Cerebrospinal fluid vasopressin concentration
Normal
Blood vasopressin concentration
Normal or increased basal
Increased after osmotic and pharmacologic stimulation
Decreased response to volume/pressure stimulation
Decreased nocturnal secretion
Renal response to vasopressin
Decreased

*Changes are in comparison to values observed in the young.

does not decrease but, in fact, remains constant or is elevated with age.

Basal Plasma Vasopressin Levels

There are conflicting data regarding basal concentration of AVP in the blood during normal aging. In young normal individuals, there is a diurnal rhythm of vasopressin secretion, with greatest AVP secretion occurring at night. This rhythm appears to be linked to the wake–sleep cycle rather than to time of day. The sleep-associated peak is absent in the majority of healthy elderly persons. Low AVP levels and the lack of definite diurnal rhythm may, to some extent, explain increased diuresis during the night in some elderly individuals.

Healthy elderly subjects have been found to have basal plasma AVP levels that were significantly lower than in young subjects. In association with the reduced AVP concentration, plasma osmolality was elevated, suggesting that the elderly subjects had a water-losing state similar to partial diabetes insipidus.

Other studies indicate that basal plasma levels of AVP did not differ among young, middle-aged, and elderly healthy individuals who were studied under both supine and ambulatory conditions. Furthermore, there were no differences in plasma osmolality between the groups.

In contrast to the above are reports of elevated basal vasopressin levels in healthy elderly persons as compared with younger individuals. Healthy human subjects aged 20 to 80 years have been observed to exhibit a progressive rise in plasma AVP concentration with age, which become most evident in subjects older than age 60 years. Baseline plasma AVP correlates with serum osmolality in younger adults but not in elderly subjects.

Debate exists regarding a sex-related difference in plasma AVP levels in the elderly population. There are reports of a twofold higher plasma AVP concentration in elderly men as compared to women, while other studies fail to identify a gender effect on basal plasma AVP.

A rise in basal plasma AVP with age cannot be attributed to age-related changes in vasopressin metabolism. No differences were found between young and old subjects in vasopressin half-life, volume of distribution, or clearance. Thus, evidence of increased basal plasma vasopressin most likely reflects age-related changes in central control systems for vasopressin release.

Vasopressin Stimulation

Secretion of AVP normally varies in response to changes in blood tonicity, blood volume, and blood pressure. Hormone release is also affected by other variables such as nausea, pain, emotional stress, a variety of drugs, cigarette smoking, and glucopenia. In recent years, a growing body of information suggests that normal aging affects the way these stimuli act and interact to influence AVP release.

The major physiologic stimulus for vasopressin secretion in humans, plasma osmolality, is regulated by hypothalamic osmoreceptors. Osmoreceptor sensitivity in the elderly population has been assessed by comparing the AVP response to hypertonic saline infusion in healthy elderly persons (age 54–92 years) to the response in younger individuals (age 21–49 years). Hypertonic saline raised plasma osmolality with a consequent increase in plasma AVP in both groups, but the hormone concentrations in the older subjects were almost double those in the younger subjects. Thus, for any given level

of osmotic stimulus, there was a greater release of AVP in the elderly, suggesting that aging resulted in osmoreceptor hypersensitivity.

Use of water deprivation as a stimulus for vasopressin secretion has supported the concept of an age-related enhancement in vasopressin secretion. Water deprivation for 24 hours in young healthy individuals (age 20–31 years) and healthy elderly men (age 67–75 years) demonstrated that the older persons responded with higher serum concentrations of AVP than the younger individuals.

The sensitivity of the hypothalamic–neurohypophyseal axis to volume/pressure stimuli has been studied. In response to acute upright posture after overnight water deprivation, older subjects (age 62–80 years) demonstrated the expected changes in pulse and blood pressure but only 8 of 15 older individuals experienced increased plasma vasopressin in contrast to a rise in plasma vasopressin in all young subjects (age 19–31 years). This and other studies suggest the presence of an aged-related impairment of volume-/pressure-mediated vasopressin release.

The ability of intravenous ethanol infusion to inhibit AVP secretion has been evaluated in young (age 21–49 years) and old (age 54–92 years) subjects. Younger subjects demonstrated a sustained inhibition of AVP secretion during the infusion of ethanol, whereas there was a paradoxical response in the older group with initial AVP inhibition followed by breakthrough secretion and rebound to twice basal levels. Not only was ethanol less effective in inhibiting AVP release in the elderly, but it eventually lost its suppressive effect entirely as a result of the introduction of a hyperosmotic stimulus resulting from the ethanol-induced constriction in plasma volume.

Metoclopramide can stimulate vasopressin secretion in humans through cholinergic mechanisms. Intravenous metoclopramide administration to normal elderly subjects aged 65 to 80 years and to normal young subjects aged 16 to 35 years produced significantly higher plasma AVP concentrations in the older group with no significant changes in plasma osmolality, blood pressure, or heart rate. Response of AVP to cigarette smoking and insulin-induced hypoglycemia, as well as to metoclopramide, has been evaluated in male subjects aged 22 to 81 years. The AVP response to metoclopramide and to smoking was significantly higher in the older group as compared to two younger groups. In contrast, the AVP response during the insulin hypoglycemia test was identical in pattern and magnitude in all age groups.

The stimulation studies indicate that, in aging, AVP response to osmotic stimuli is increased because of a hyperresponsive osmoreceptor, whereas AVP response to upright posture is reduced because of impaired baroreceptor function. Input from the baroreceptor to the osmoreceptor is usually inhibitory, so that a defect in this reflex arc would result in lesser dampening and consequent heightening of osmotically stimulated ADH release. When coupled with the many alterations in renal function that occur with aging, these changes can increase the risk of elderly persons for hyponatremia by impairing their ability to excrete excess water promptly.

Age-Related Changes in Atrial Natriuretic Hormone Secretion, Regulation, and Action

ANH is synthesized, stored, and released in the atria of the heart. Through its action on the kidney, ANH produces a pronounced natriuresis and diuresis; through its action on blood vessels, it produces vasodilation and decreases blood pressure in both normal and hypertensive individuals. As an important regulator of sodium excretion, ANH maybe a significant factor in mediating the altered renal sodium handling of age.

In a comparison of young normal men with elderly male nursing home residents, a fivefold increase in mean basal ANH levels and an exaggerated ANH response to the stimulus of saline infusion has been observed in the elderly group. In response to the stimulus of head-out water immersion, ANH levels in healthy old individuals (age 62–73 years), which were twice as high at baseline than in young subjects (age 21–28 years), rose to a greater extent than in the young. Healthy male and female subjects aged 22 to 64 years have been studied to determine the influence of age on circulating levels of ANH, both under basal conditions and after the physiologic stimulation of ANH release by controlled exercise using a bicycle ergometer to increase heart rate to 80% of maximum predicted rate. Subjects older than 50 years of age had higher baseline levels and a greater response to exercise when compared to subjects younger than age 50 years. Thus, increasing age results in increased ANH basal levels and an increased ANH response to both physiologic and pharmacologic stimuli, perhaps as a consequence of age-related decrease in cardiac muscle compliance.

The renal effects of ANH maybe exaggerated in elderly versus young individuals. The natriuretic response to a bolus injection of ANH was higher in older individuals (mean age 52.3 years) as compared with younger subjects (mean age 26 years). No change with age was noted in the blood pressure response to ANH intravenous infusion after correction for higher ANH levels in the elderly.

ANH is known to interact with the renin–angiotensin–aldosterone system. Increases of ANH result in suppression of renal renin secretion, plasma renin activity, plasma angiotensin II, and aldosterone levels, suggesting indirect inhibition of aldosterone secretion by ANH. Minimal increases in ANH within physiologic levels produced by slow-rate ANH infusion can inhibit angiotensin II-induced aldosterone secretion in normal men, suggesting a direct inhibitory effect of ANH on aldosterone release. Thus, ANH may promote renal sodium loss both through inhibition of aldosterone release and through a direct natriuretic action.

ANH maybe an important mediator of age-related renal sodium loss. This effect maybe the consequence of increased basal ANH levels, increased ANH response to stimuli, increased renal sensitivity to ANH, and ANH-induced suppression of adrenal sodium-retaining hormones.

Renin–Angiotensin–Aldosterone

A substantial body of evidence indicates that the normal aging process affects the renin–angiotensin–aldosterone system. Healthy older individuals (age 62–70 years) with normal dietary sodium intake have lower plasma renin activity and aldosterone concentration while in the supine position than do young healthy persons (age 20–30 years). Under the stimuli of upright posture and sodium depletion, significant increases in circulating renin and aldosterone occurred in both age groups, but mean values achieved were always significantly lower in the elderly group. The decrease in plasma renin activity in the elderly population is not a result of changes in plasma renin substrate concentration; rather, it is a result of a decrease in active renin concentration, perhaps caused by decreased conversion of inactive to active renin. The decrease in plasma renin activity may also be related to the inhibitory effect of increased amounts of ANH on renin secretion (see above). Decreased aldosterone concentration

with age appears to be a direct result of age-related decrease of plasma renin activity and not to aging changes in the adrenal gland because aldosterone and cortisol responses to corticotropin infusion are not altered in the elderly person. It is likely that the age-related decrease in aldosterone concentration is a predisposing factor to renal salt wasting in the elderly person.

Intrinsic renal tubular changes may also play a role in sodium wasting. An impaired capacity to reabsorb sodium has been described along with decreased tubular responsiveness to aldosterone administration. However, a subsequent study failed to find an effect of age on renal tubular sensitivity to aldosterone.

The age-associated decline in the renin–angiotensin–aldosterone system maybe linked to alterations in potassium regulation. Hyporeninemic hypoaldosteronism occurs most commonly in elderly persons, especially those with diabetes mellitus. The hyperkalemia characteristic of the disorder responds to treatment with mineralocorticoid and maybe the consequence of interaction of chronic renal disease with the hormonal changes of normal aging. The risk of angiotensin-converting enzyme (ACE) inhibitors in producing hyperkalemia is especially high in elderly persons, and may also be related to the interplay between drug action and physiologic alterations caused by aging.

DISORDERS OF FLUID REGULATION

Hyponatremia

Despite wide ranges in intake of sodium and water in normal persons, serum sodium concentration is tightly maintained within the range of 136–144 mEq/L. Hyponatremia is usually defined as a serum sodium concentration of ≤135 mEq/L. It appears when there is an excess of water relative to sodium in the extracellular body fluid compartment and can be the consequence of either a decrease in extracellular sodium content (i.e., sodium depletion) or an increase in extracellular water (i.e., dilutional hyponatremia). In the elderly person, dilutional hyponatremia is the more common mechanism and most frequently is caused by the syndrome of inappropriate antidiuretic hormone secretion (SIADH).

The altered relationship of sodium to water can occur in the setting of decreased (hypovolemic), normal (euvolemic), or increased (hypervolemic) intravascular volume. Hypovolemic hyponatremia can result from increased sodium loss from the gastrointestinal tract, from increased urinary loss, and from sweat. Euvolemic hyponatremia is characteristic of SIADH. Hypervolemic hyponatremia is seen in edematous states such as congestive heart failure, cirrhosis with ascites and nephrotic syndrome.

Dilutional versus Depletional Hyponatremia

A key determination in the patient with hyponatremia is whether hyponatremia is of dilutional, depletional, or mixed origin and can generally be made by history and physical examination and by commonly available laboratory measurements (Table 88-3). The characteristic features of dilutional hyponatremia and SIADH are hyponatremia and serum hypoosmolality with clinical euvolemia and absence of edema, failure of the urine to be appropriately dilute, excretion of sodium in the urine at a concentration of >20 mEq/L, and

TABLE 88-3

Clinical Features of Depletional versus Dilutional Hyponatremia

Feature	Depletional	Dilutional
History	Low dietary Na intake Na loss 　Vomiting 　Diarrhea 　Nasogastric suction Use of diuretics Diseases 　Renal 　Adrenal	Increased fluid intake (oral, IV) Drugs Diseases 　CNS 　Pulmonary 　Malignancy
Physical examination	Dry mucous membranes Decreased skin turgor Hypotension, tachycardia, orthostatic changes	Euvolemia or edema Evidence of CNS, pulmonary disease, malignancy
Laboratory evaluation	Increased hematocrit, BUN, creatinine Urinary Na excretion <20 mEq/L	Normal or decreased BUN, creatinine, uric acid, albumin Urinary Na excretion >20 mEq/L

BUN, blood urea nitrogen; CNS, central nervous system; NA, sodium.
Reproduced with permission from Miller M. Hyponatremia: age-related risk factors and therapy decisions. Geriatrics. 1998;53:32.

the absence of other hyponatremia-producing disease states such as hypothyroidism, adrenal insufficiency, congestive heart failure, cirrhosis, or renal disease.

Depletional hyponatremia typically results from a prolonged period of inadequate sodium intake and/or from increased gastrointestinal tract or urinary sodium loss. Extracellular fluid volume depletion is often present with physical findings and laboratory values related to hypovolemia.

Epidemiology

Hyponatremia is a common finding in elderly persons. Analysis of plasma sodium values in healthy individuals has shown an age-related decrease of approximately 1 mEq/L per decade from a mean value of 141 ± 4 mEq/L in young subjects. In a population of individuals older than age 65 years who were living at home and who were without acute illness, a 7% incidence of serum sodium concentration of 137 mEq/L or less was observed. Similarly, there was a 11% incidence of hyponatremia in the population of a geriatric medicine outpatient practice. In hospitalized patients, hyponatremia is even more common with an incidence of about 1% and a prevalence of 3% to 4%, increasing to as high as 30% in intensive care unit patients. An analysis of 5000 consecutive sets of plasma electrolytes from a hospital population with a mean age of 54 years revealed a mean serum sodium of 134 ± 6 mEq/L, with the values skewed toward the hyponatremic end of the distribution curve. A high prevalence of hyponatremia has been found in patients hospitalized for a variety of acute illnesses, with the risk being greater with increasing age of the patient.

Elderly residents of long-term care institutions appear to be especially prone to hyponatremia. In a study of patients with a mean age of 72 years who resided in a chronic disease hospital, 22.5%

had repeated serum sodium determinations of less than 135 mEq/L. Of patients admitted to an acute geriatric unit, 11.3% were found to have serum sodium concentrations of ≤130 mEq/L. A survey of nursing home residents aged >60 years revealed a prevalence of 18% with serum sodium less than 136 mEq/L. When this population was observed on a longitudinal basis over a 12-month period, 53% were observed to experience one or more episodes of hyponatremia. Persons with central nervous system (CNS) and spinal cord disease were at highest risk, and water-load testing indicated that most hyponatremic patients had features consistent with SIADH.

Risk Factors (Table 88-4)

A major risk for the development or worsening of hyponatremia is the administration of hypotonic fluid, either as an increase in oral water intake or as intravenous 0.45% saline solution or 5% glucose in water, a finding in 78% of nursing home residents with hyponatremia. Low sodium intake coupled with age-associated impaired renal sodium-conserving ability can, over time, lead to sodium depletion with hyponatremia. Many patients whose nutritional support is primarily or entirely provided by tube feeding develop either intermittent or persistent hyponatremia. The underlying cause appears to be sodium depletion because of the low sodium content of most tube-feeding diets. The hyponatremia usually resolves in response to increasing the dietary sodium intake.

TABLE 88-4

Risk Factors for Hyponatremia in the Elderly Person

Physiologic changes of normal aging
　Decreased renal sodium-conserving ability
　　Altered renal tubular function
　　Increased atrial natriuretic hormone secretion
　　Decreased renin–angiotensin–aldosterone secretion
　Decreased renal water-excretion ability
　　Decreased renal blood flow and glomerular filtration rate
　　Decreased distal renal tubular diluting capacity
　　Increased renal passive reabsorption of water
　　Increased vasopressin secretion

Diseases accompanied by SIADH (see Table 88-5)

Drugs accompanied by sodium loss or SIADH (see Table 88-6)

Increased water intake
　Oral fluids
　Intravenous hypotonic fluids

Decreased sodium intake
　Low-sodium diet
　Tube feeding

Increased sodium loss
　Renal disease
　Gastrointestinal tract
　　Vomiting
　　Diarrhea
　　Gastric suctioning
　Cerebral salt wasting

Idiopathic SIADH of the elderly person
　Age >80 yr
　Race other than African-American

SIADH, syndrome of inappropriate antidiuretic hormone secretion.
Reproduced with permission from Miller M. Hyponatremia: age-related risk factors and therapy decisions. Geriatrics. 1998;53:32.

Advanced age itself may be a risk factor for hyponatremia. SIADH has been described in elderly individuals, generally older than age 80 years, in whom no identifiable cause for hyponatremia could be found, suggesting that there is an idiopathic form of SIADH that may represent the clinical expression of physiologic changes that take place in the regulation of water balance during aging. Race may play a role because African-Americans appear to be at lower risk than whites or Hispanics.

Hyponatremia often is a marker for severe underlying disease with poor prognosis and high mortality. The presence of hyponatremia in patients with congestive heart failure is an independent risk factor for death. Hyponatremia is common in patients with liver cirrhosis, in whom it is associated with a significantly worse prognosis. It is unclear whether hyponatremia is the direct cause of death in these patients, but its prompt diagnosis and effective treatment are important in improving patient outcomes.

Syndrome of Inappropriate Antidiuretic Hormone Secretion

Diseases Many diseases that are common in the elderly population can cause SIADH (Table 88-5). Almost all CNS disorders can lead to dysfunction of the hypothalamic system involved in the normal regulation of AVP secretion with resultant increased secretion of the hormone and consequent risk for water retention and hyponatremia. Such CNS disorders include vascular injury (thrombosis, embolism, hemorrhage), trauma with subdural hematoma, vasculitis, tumor, and infection. Malignancies can cause SIADH as a result of autonomous release of AVP from cancer tissue where it is synthesized, stored, and discharged in the absence of known stimuli. The malignancy most commonly associated with SIADH in the elderly population is small-cell carcinoma of the lung, in which as many as 68% of patients have been found to have evidence of impaired water excretion and elevated blood AVP concentration. Other malignancies include pancreatic carcinoma, thymoma, pharyngeal carcinoma, lymphosarcoma, and Hodgkin's disease. Inflammatory lung diseases can also cause SIADH, perhaps as a result of AVP production by diseased pulmonary tissue, and include such entities as bronchiectasis, pneumonia, lung abscess, and tuberculosis.

Drugs Numerous drugs taken by elderly persons can affect water balance by direct action on the kidney or by altering AVP release from the neurohypophyseal system or its action on the kidney (Table 88-6). In particular, many drugs increase the risk for SIADH.

Hyponatremia with the characteristics of SIADH is recognized as a side effect of several older antipsychotic agents, such as fluphenazine, thiothixene, and phenothiazine, and the tricyclic antidepressants. There is evidence that the selective serotonin reuptake inhibitors (SSRIs) antidepressants can also induce SIADH, with a reported incidence of 3.5 to 6.3 per 1000 people treated per year. Although fluoxetine is the SSRI most commonly reported to produce hyponatremia, other SSRIs, including paroxetine, sertraline, fluvoxamine, citalopram and escitalopram, have also been involved. Individuals at highest risk for SSRI-induced hyponatremia are those older than age 65 years in whom the onset of hyponatremia typically occurs within 2 weeks after initiation of drug therapy. More recently, there is evidence that drugs with combined SSRI/norepinephrine reuptake inhibitor (SNRIs) activity, such as venlafaxine and duloxetine, are also capable of producing SIADH-type hyponatremia.

TABLE 88-5

Diseases/Disorders Associated with Hyponatremia in the Elderly Population

Central nervous system disorders
   Vascular diseases (thrombosis, embolism, hemorrhage, vasculitis)
   Trauma (subdural hematoma, intracranial hemorrhage)
   Tumor
   Infectious disease (meningitis, encephalitis, brain abscess)

Malignancy with ectopic AVP production
   Pulmonary (small-cell carcinoma)
   Pancreatic carcinoma
   Pharyngeal carcinoma
   Thymoma
   Lymphosarcoma, reticulum cell sarcoma, Hodgkin's disease

Pulmonary disease
   Pneumonia
   Tuberculosis
   Lung abscess
   Bronchiectasis

Endocrine disease
   Hypothyroidism
   Diabetes mellitus with hyperglycemia
   Adrenal insufficiency

Other
   Acquired immunodeficiency syndrome (AIDS)
   Idiopathic SIADH of the elderly person

Modified with permission from Miller M. Hyponatremia: age-related risk factors and therapy decisions. Geriatrics. 1998;53:32.

TABLE 88-6

Drug-Induced Changes in Sodium and Water Regulation

Sodium retention
   Nonsteroidal antiinflamatory agents

Sodium loss
   Thiazide and loop diuretics

Impaired diluting capacity
   Thiazide diuretics

Impaired concentrating capacity
   Lithium
   Demeclocycline
   Potassium-losing diuretics

Syndrome of inappropriate antidiuretic hormone secretion
   Central nervous system agents
     Tricyclic antidepressants
     SSRI and SNRI antidepressants
     Phenothiazine antipsychotics
     Carbamazepine anticonvulsant
   ACE inhibitors
   Antineoplastic drugs
     Vincristine
     Vinblastine
     Cyclophosphamide
   Chlorpropamide
   Clofibrate
   Narcotics

Reproduced by permission from Miller M. Hyponatremia: age-related risk factors and therapy decisions. Geriatrics 1998;53:32.

ACE inhibitor use in the elderly population is associated with the development of hyponatremia. In most of the cases, the level of hyponatremia has been clinically significant with serum sodium concentrations as low as 101 mEq/L and with symptoms ranging from confusion to seizures and coma. Although initial reports indicated that the risk was greatest when ACE inhibitors were used in combination with thiazide diuretics, it now appears that the ACE inhibitors alone can precipitate hyponatremia. The hyponatremia appears to be dilutional with features of SIADH and maybe mediated by potentiation of plasma renin activity with subsequent increase in brain angiotensin levels, which, in turn, stimulate both release of AVP from the hypothalamus and an increase in thirst. Discontinuing the ACE inhibitor is associated with rapid resolution of the hyponatremia.

Diuretics, both of the loop and thiazide types, can produce hyponatremia. Loop diuretics appear to have a greater natriuretic effect in older persons than in younger persons. Hyponatremia can occur when diuretic-induced sodium and water loss are replaced by hypotonic fluids, resulting in a combined depletional and dilutional hyponatremia. With thiazide diuretics, the induced sodium loss is often accompanied by loss of total body potassium with consequent decrease in intracellular solute content and decreased cell volume. This circumstance can activate hypothalamic pathways, leading to increased AVP discharge, water retention, and SIADH. This form of thiazide-induced hyponatremia occurs almost entirely in the elderly population and can be reversed by correcting the underlying potassium depletion.

Other drugs associated with development of hyponatremia in the elderly population include the sulfonylurea chlorpropamide, the anticonvulsant carbamazepine, and the antineoplastic agents vincristine, vinblastine, and cyclophosphamide. Analgesics, particularly the narcotics, maybe responsible for the occurrence of hyponatremia in the elderly postoperative patient.

Cerebral Salt Wasting   Renal sodium excretion from the excessive release of natriuretic factor in the brain can lead to cerebral salt wasting (CSW). CSW and SIADH are both syndromes of hypoosmotic serum and increased urine sodium excretion. Patients with CSW, however, have a low effective intravascular blood volume as a consequence of marked natriuresis and secondary osmotic diuresis. In contrast, patients with SIADH are usually euvolemic or have mildly increased extracellular fluid volume. CSW can be diagnosed by the clinical and laboratory findings that define diminished extracellular fluid volume, including orthostatic hypotension, tachycardia, and elevated hematocrit, blood urea nitrogen (BUN), and creatinine levels.

Clinical Presentation

Mild chronic hyponatremia may appear to be asymptomatic. However, recent evidence from a case–control study suggests that mild chronic hyponatremia may have serious consequences in the elderly, even when symptoms appear to be absent. This study examined the frequency of falls in 122 patients (mean age 72 years) with chronic hyponatremia (serum sodium 115–132 mEq/L) admitted to a medical emergency department. The frequency of reported falls was significantly greater among patients with hyponatremia (21.3%) than among control subjects (5.3%) and was unrelated to the level of serum sodium. Alterations in gait and attention were detected in patients with hyponatremia and suggest that these impairments may have contributed to the higher incidence of falls in this group. The data suggest that prompt recognition of even apparently asymptomatic hyponatremia and early initiation of appropriate treatment maybe important for preventing hyponatremia-related consequences.

The clinical severity of hyponatremia is dependent on both the magnitude of the hyponatremia and the rate at which the serum sodium level has declined. There is often a poor correlation between serum sodium concentration and severity of symptoms. Serum sodium levels <125 mEq/L maybe accompanied by lethargy, fatigue, anorexia, nausea, and muscle cramps. With worsening hyponatremia, CNS symptoms predominate and range from confusion to coma to seizures. There is substantial risk of death in severely symptomatic patients with serum sodium <110 mEq/L who also have underlying disease with cachexia.

Management (Table 88-7)

Treatment of hyponatremia is based on the absence or presence of symptoms and their severity, whether the onset is acute or chronic, and if acute, the rapidity of onset. Hyponatremia caused by sodium depletion is often accompanied by extracellular fluid volume depletion and treatment is directed at correcting the volume deficit with intravenous 0.9% saline. Milder depletional hyponatremia, such as that occurring in persons whose nutrition is predominantly from enteral feedings, can be corrected by adding saline solution or crushed sodium chloride tablets to the enteral feedings.

For patients thought to be asymptomatic, conservative management is appropriate with fluid restriction and an attempt to identify and correct the underlying cause, if possible. Mildly symptomatic patients with serum sodium >125 mEq/L can be treated with fluid

TABLE 88-7

Treatment of Dilutional Hyponatremia		
Presentation	**Treatment Modality**	**Potential Adverse Outcomes**
Acute	IV 3% saline, 300–500 mL over 4–6 h, followed by 100 mL/h until serum Na reaches ~125 mEq/L at rate of increase of 0.5–1 mEq/L/h (maximum increase 12 mEq/L over 24 h)	Central pontine myelinolysis, congestive heart failure
	IV furosemide 1 mg/kg body weight	Hypokalemia, hypomagnesemia
Chronic	Correction of underlying cause	
	Fluid restriction to 800–1000 mL per 24 h	Thirst stimulation, dehydration
	Demeclocycline 600–1200 mg per 24 h	Photosensitivity, azotemia, nephrotoxicity in patients with hepatic disease or congestive heart failure

Reproduced by permission from Miller M. Hyponatremia: Age-related risk factors and therapy decisions. Geriatrics 1998;53:32.

restriction to a level of 800 to 1000 mL/24 hours. The patient with acute onset of symptomatic dilutional hyponatremia requires prompt intervention and is best managed in an intensive care unit setting and treated with intravenous 3% saline infusion at a rate sufficient to raise serum sodium by 0.5 to 1 mEq/L/h. The goal is a maximum increase in serum sodium of no more than 12 mEq/L in the first 24 hours, and to a value no higher than 125 mEq/L, in order to avoid central pontine myelinolysis. Occasionally, patients either with fluid overload and pulmonary edema or with symptoms of coma or seizures who have very low serum sodium levels may require initial treatment with intravenous furosemide in a dose 1 mg/kg body weight along with the 3% saline. In this circumstance, attention will need to be given to possible diuretic-induced potassium and magnesium depletion.

Strategies currently used for the treatment of stable, asymptomatic or mildly symptomatic chronic hyponatremia include mainly fluid restriction and occasionally demeclocycline. Demeclocycline in doses of 600 to 1200 mg daily blocks AVP effect on the renal distal and collecting tubules with production of a mild state of nephrogenic diabetes insipidus, thus promoting an increase in urine production and a corresponding increase in serum sodium. Both chronic fluid restriction and demeclocycline administration are limited by poor compliance, inconsistent or delayed response and, in the case of demeclocycline, renal and hepatotoxicity.

Role of Aquaretics in the Treatment of Hyponatremia

AVP receptor antagonists, a new class of drugs called "aquaretics," which promote electrolyte-free excretion of water, may provide a more reliable approach to the treatment of both acute and chronic hyponatremia. AVP promotes renal water reabsorption by increasing the water permeability of epithelial cells in the renal-collecting ducts. This and other biological effects of AVP are mediated by the interaction of the hormone with various receptors: V_{1A}, V_{1B}, and V_2. It is the binding of AVP to V_2 receptors in renal collecting duct cells that promotes renal reabsorption of water. Interaction of AVP with these receptors initiates a series of events culminating in the insertion of aquaporin-2 water channels in the apical plasma membrane. The interaction of AVP with V_{1A} receptors in vascular smooth muscle cells, hepatocytes, and platelets mediates vasoconstriction, glycogenolysis, and platelet aggregation. Corticotropin release is regulated via V_{1B} receptors located predominantly in the anterior pituitary.

Excess or inappropriate secretion of AVP acting on renal V_2 receptors causes the retention of water and can lead to dilutional hyponatremia. The blockade of these AVP V_2 receptors thus represents a rational approach to the treatment of hyponatremia. The development of AVP receptor antagonists began several decades ago with the synthesis of peptide AVP analogs capable of antagonizing the water-reabsorbing effect of AVP in a number of animal species. A major advance in the early 1990s was the development of nonpeptide molecules, which were able to bind to AVP receptors and function as V_1 and/or V_2 receptor antagonists. The nonpeptide AVP receptor antagonists subsequently created—tolvaptan, lixivaptan, sativaptan, and conivaptan—exhibit a long half-life and no agonist activity.

At the present time, conivaptan is the only agent in this class to be approved by the Food and Drug Administration and is limited to its intravenous form for the treatment of euvolemic hyponatremia in hospitalized patients. Conivaptan blocks the action of AVP at both the V_2 receptor that mediates renal excretion of water and the

TABLE 88-8

Aquaretic Agents

Drug	Route of Administration	Hyponatremic Population Studied
Conivaptam*	i.v.	SIADH
Lixivaptam	Oral	Cirrhosis with ascites, CHF, SIADH
Satavaptam	Oral	SIADH
Tolvaptam	Oral	Cirrhosis with ascites, CHF, SIADH

SIADH, syndrome of inappropriate antidiuretic hormone secretion; CHF, congestive heart failure.
*Only drug listed approved by the U.S. Food and Drug Administration.

V_{1A} receptor that mediates systemic vasoconstriction. Several of the other aquaretic agents have been studied extensively in normal human subjects and in clinical trials in patients with hyponatremia. Tolvaptan, lixivaptan, and sativaptan are effective by oral administration and bind to V_2 receptors in the renal tubules to block the action of AVP. In clinical trials, these three drugs have been demonstrated to promote acute aquaresis in patients with SIADH and in patients with hyponatremia caused by congestive heart failure and also to maintain improvement in serum sodium for up to 12 months of chronic treatment (Table 88-8).

The AVP receptor antagonists may provide a more direct approach to the treatment of both acute and chronic euvolemic and hypervolemic hyponatremia than currently available therapies. Preliminary experience with the AVP receptor antagonists suggests that these agents are effective and well tolerated both acutely and following prolonged administration. Continued investigation should further define the role of AVP receptor antagonists in the treatment of acute and chronic hyponatremia in the elderly. The ability of the drugs to normalize serum sodium in patients who have chronic and apparently asymptomatic hyponatremia will help determine the clinical significance of this common electrolyte disturbance.

Hypernatremia and Dehydration

Hypernatremia, generally defined as a serum sodium of ≥ 148 mEq/L, most commonly occurs when there is excessive loss of body water relative to loss of sodium in association with inadequate fluid intake. In this circumstance, hypernatremia is accompanied by dehydration. When fluid loss is accompanied by sodium loss, dehydration can occur without associated hypernatremia. In rare circumstances, hypernatremia can be caused by excessive sodium intake without corresponding increased fluid intake and thus be associated with euvolemic or hypervolemic volume status.

Epidemiology

In a study of 15,187 hospitalized patients older than age 60 years, a 1% incidence of hypernatremia was reported, with a mean serum sodium concentration of 154 mEq/L. Similarly, a study of elderly residents in a long-term care institution revealed a 1% incidence of hypernatremia, which increased to 18% over a 12-month observation period. Of 264 nursing home residents in whom acute illness developed requiring hospitalization, 34% became markedly hypernatremic with serum sodium concentration greater than 150 mEq/L.

TABLE 88-9

Risk Factors for Hypernatremia in the Elderly Population

Increased water loss
  Renal
    Age-associated impaired concentrating capacity
    Resistance to vasopressin action
      Age-associated
      Acquired (drugs, hypokalemia, hypercalcemia)
    Osmotic diuresis (glycosuria, diuretic-induced natriuresis)
    Renal tubular disease
  Gastrointestinal tract
    Vomiting
    Diarrhea
  Skin (sweating)
  Lung (tachypnea)

Decreased water intake
  Impaired thirst perception
  Impaired cognition (delerium, dementia)
  Impaired access to fluids

Risk Factors

The renal and hormonal alterations of aging described above are physiologic factors associated with an increased risk for hypernatremia (Table 88-9). Frequent pathologic factors are febrile illness with increased insensible fluid loss, tachypnea with increased water loss from the lungs, vomiting or diarrhea, and osmotic-induced polyuria from poorly controlled diabetes mellitus or use of loop diuretics. There is a high morbidity and mortality in elderly patients who develop serum sodium concentrations above 148 mEq/L and such elevations of serum sodium are often a consequence of a severe underlying disease process.

CSW, described above, can lead to marked intravascular volume depletion and hypotonic dehydration. Typical clinical features are related to the volume depletion and include orthostatic hypotension, tachycardia, and increases in blood hemoglobin, hematocrit, urea nitrogen, and creatinine.

Clinical Presentation

The symptoms of both moderate hypernatremia and dehydration maybe nonspecific and commonly include weakness and lethargy. More severe hypernatremia, often with serum sodium concentration >152 mEq/L, maybe accompanied by obtundation, stupor, coma, and seizures. The clinical signs are those of volume depletion and dehydration with weight loss, decreased skin turgor, dry mucous membranes, tachycardia, and orthostatic hypotension. In addition to the elevated serum sodium, laboratory findings are those of hemoconcentration with increased hematocrit, BUN, creatinine, and serum osmolality. Urine osmolality may not be greatly increased because of age-related impairment in renal concentrating capacity.

Management

The correction of hypernatremia requires replacement of body water deficits, which maybe as large as 11 L or 30% of total body water. When hypernatremia is caused almost entirely by water loss

alone, the water deficit can be estimated by means of the following calculation:

$$\text{Current total body fluid volume (L)} = \frac{140 \text{ mEq/L} \times \text{basel body weight (kg)} \times 0.45}{\text{current serum Na (mEq/L)}}$$

where 0.45 represents the approximate proportion of body weight that is water. Total body water is subtracted from estimated normal total body water of 0.45 × body weight to give an approximate value for the water deficit.

Modest fluid deficits of 1 to 2 L can be corrected by oral fluid intake. More significant volume deficits require intravenous fluid therapy, preferably starting with 0.9% saline given at a rate sufficient to resolve orthostatic hypotension and tachycardia and to replace approximately 50% of the estimated fluid deficit in the first 24 hours and to reduce serum sodium by no more than 2 mEq/L/h. Excessively rapid correction can lead to cerebral edema with consequent brain damage or death. The goal is then to correct remaining volume depletion and hypernatremia over 48 to 72 hours by using 0.45% saline.

Treatment of dehydration without hypernatremia is directed at correction of intravascular volume depletion and involves fluid replacement with intravenous 0.9% saline. Clinical indicators of effectiveness of therapy are correction of orthostatic hypotension and tachycardia and reduction in BUN and serum creatinine concentrations.

Nocturnal Polyuria

In normal young persons, there is a diurnal pattern of vasopressin secretion with highest levels occurring during sleep. This is reflected by a lower rate of urine flow at night (40–60 mL per hour) than during the daytime (60–80 mL per hour) so that nighttime urine volume is approximately 25% or less of total 24-hour urine volume. In many older persons, there is loss of nocturnal vasopressin secretion and an accompanying reversal of day/night urine production so that nighttime urine flow rate exceeds the daytime flow rate. This alteration in renal function leads to a diabetes insipidus-like nocturnal polyuria. Nocturnal polyuria is considered to be present when any of the following criteria are met: urine production during 8 hours of sleep is ≥33% of 24-hour urine production; nighttime urine production rate is ≥0.9 mL/min; 7 P.M. to 7 A.M. urine volume is ≥50% of total 24-hour volume (Table 88-10). Nocturnal

TABLE 88-10

Nocturnal Polyuria

Definitions
  Urine production during 8 h of sleep ≥33% of 24-h urine production
  Nighttime urine production rate >0.9 mL/min
  7 P.M. to 7 A.M. urine volume ≥50% of total 24-h volume

Causes
  Normal aging
  Multiple system atrophy
  Alzheimer's disease
  Spinal cord injury

polyuria is a common finding in community-residing elderly persons with nocturia. The prevalence can be as high as 50% in nursing home residents, particularly those with Alzheimer's disease. It is also often seen in patients with central autonomic insufficiency (Shy-Drager syndrome/multiple system atrophy) or spinal cord injury (Table 88-10).

Both reduced bladder capacity and detrusor instability are commonly present in elderly persons, with prevalence in both men and women increased with increasing age. High nighttime urine production in persons with nocturnal polyuria coupled with these bladder alterations maybe a contributing factor to the nocturnal urinary frequency seen so commonly in older persons.

Evaluation

Individuals with nocturia can be evaluated for the presence of nocturnal polyuria by means of a voiding diary in which the time and volume of each void is recorded for a 72-hour period. In addition, urine production during 8 hours of sleep can be measured in a timed urine collection and compared with urine production during the remainder of a 24-hour period. Both approaches allow demonstration of increased nocturnal urine production meeting the above cited criteria.

Management

The vasopressin analog DDAVP (deamino-8-D-arginine vasopressin) may be helpful in treating both nocturnal frequency and nocturnal urinary incontinence among patients without other treatable causes of these symptoms. DDAVP can be given either intranasally in a dose of 5 to 20 μg or orally in a dose of 200 to 400 mg taken in the evening. Because DDAVP has a duration of action of 12 to 24 hours, care must be taken to monitor serum sodium to avoid the possible development of dilutional hyponatremia. A meta-analysis of published reports on the use of either intranasal or oral DDAVP in treatment of nocturia in older adults has identified hyponatremia as a common occurrence with a pooled incidence of 7.6%. In the authors' experience, hyponatremia has been observed in as many as 20% of older persons treated with oral DDAVP. Patients treated with DDAVP should therefore have serum sodium monitored within 3 to 7 days of initiating therapy, and periodically thereafter.

Water Balance in Alzheimer's Disease

Persons with Alzheimer's disease are at increased risk for disturbed water regulation (Table 88-11). The secretion of vasopressin maybe lower in those with Alzheimer's disease than in comparably aged persons with normal cognitive function and there is absence of the nocturnal rise in hormone secretion. Following dehydration, individuals with Alzheimer's disease show a lesser rise in plasma vasopressin than do age-matched normal subjects. Similarly, pharmacologic stimulation with metoclopramide or physostigmine is accompanied by marked blunting of plasma vasopressin response. These changes contribute to a high prevalence of nocturnal polyuria and nocturia in patients with Alzheimer's disease. In patients with Alzheimer's disease, the cognitive impairment can cause the nighttime polyuria to be clinically expressed as urinary incontinence.

TABLE 88-11

Alzheimer's Disease and Disordered Water Regulation

Alterations in water regulation
    Impaired thirst perception
    Decreased vasopressin secretion
        Basal
        Response to stimulation
        Diurnal pattern
Clinical consequences
    Increased risk of dehydration
    Hypertonicity (increased serum sodium and osmolality)
    Reversal of day/night urine flow rate
    Nocturnal polyuria and incontinence

Clinically, the combination of impaired water conservation along with an impairment of thirst perception puts patients with Alzheimer's disease at increased risk for dehydration. In studies of patients with Alzheimer's disease, overnight fluid restriction results in greater rise in plasma osmolality, greater water loss, and, in spite of these stimuli for thirst, marked reduction in spontaneous water intake. A direct correlation has been demonstrated between mini mental status examination score and impairment of water intake.

SUMMARY

Normal aging is accompanied by many changes in the various regulatory systems involved in the control of sodium and water balance. As a consequence of these alterations, the elderly person has a diminished capacity to withstand the challenges of illness, drugs, and physiologic stresses, and, thus, has an increased risk for the development of clinically significant alterations in sodium and water balance, which may have adverse effects on functional status and mortality. Awareness of the limitations of homeostatic ability can allow the physician to anticipate the impact of illnesses and drugs on volume and electrolyte status of the elderly patient and lead to a more rational approach to therapeutic intervention and management.

The recent availability of AVP antagonists should make it possible to normalize serum sodium in persons with chronic hyponatremia and, in so doing, allow the impact of hyponatremia on many areas of function to be clarified, especially the role of hyponatremia on worsening cognitive function in persons who already have underlying disorders of cognition. The potential ability of long-term treatment with AVP antagonists to alter diminished quality of life and mortality of persons with hypervolemic hyponatremia, such as occurring in congestive heart failure and in cirrhosis with ascites, remains an area for future investigation.

FURTHER READING

Anderson RJ, Chung H, Kluge R, et al. Hyponatremia: A prospective analysis of its epidemiology and the pathogenetic role of vasopressin. *Ann Intern Med.* 1985;102:164.

Asplund R, Aberg H. Diurnal variation in the levels of antidiuretic hormone in the elderly. *J Intern Med.* 1991;299:131.

Bauer JH. Age-related changes in the renin–aldosterone system: physiological effects and clinical implications. *Drugs Ageing.* 1993;3:238.

Espiner EA, Richard AM, Yandle TG, et al. Natriuretic hormones. *Endocrinol Metab Clinics North Am.* 1995;24:481.

Helderman JH, Vestal RE, Rowe JW, et al. The response of arginine vasopressin to intravenous ethanol and hypertonic saline in man. The impact of aging. *J Gerontol.* 1978;33:39.

Johnson AG, Crawford GA, Kelly D, et al. Arginine vasopressin and osmolality in the elderly. *J Am Geriatr Soc.* 1994;42:399.

Lindeman RD, Tobin JD, Shock NW, et al. Longitudinal studies on the rate of decline in renal function with age. *J Am Geriatr Soc.* 1985;33:278.

Miller M. Nocturnal polyuria in older people: Pathophysiology and clinical implications. *J Am Geriatr Soc.* 2000;48:1321.

Miller M. Hyponatremia and arginine vasopressin dysregulaton: mechanisms, clinical consequences, and management. *J Am Geriatr Soc.* 2006;54:345.

Miller M, Hecker MS, Friedlander DA, et al. Apparent idiopathic hyponatremia in an ambulatory geriatric population. *J Am Geriatr Soc.* 1996;44:404.

Miller M, Morley JE, Rubenstein LZ, et al. Hyponatremia in a nursing home population. *J Am Geriatr Soc.* 1995;43:1410.

Miller M, Gold GC, Friedlander DA, et al. Physiological changes of aging affecting salt and water balance. *Rev Clin Gerontol.* 1991;1:215.

Ouslander J, Schnelle J, Simmons S, et al. The dark side of incontinence: Nighttime incontinence in nursing home residents. *J Am Geriatr Soc.* 1993;41:371.

Palevsky PM, Bhagrath R, Greenberg A, et al. Hypernatremia in hospitalized patients. *Ann Intern Med.* 1996;124:197.

Palm C, Pistrosch F, Herbrig K, et al. Vasopressin antagonists as aquaretic agents for the treatment of hyponatremia. *Am J Med.* 2006;119 (Suppl 7A):S87.

Phillips PA, Rolls BJ, Ledingham JGG, et al. Reduced thirst after water deprivation in healthy elderly men. *N Engl J Med.* 1984;311:753.

Raman A, Schoeller DA, Subar AF, et al. Water turnover in 458 American adults 40–79 yr of age. *Am J Physiol Renal Physiol.* 2004;286:F394.

Renneboog B, Musch W, Vandermergel X, et al. Mild chronic hyponatremia is associated with falls, unsteadiness, and attention deficits. *Am J Med.* 2006;119:71;e1.

Rowe JW, Andres RA, Tobin JD, et al. The effect of age on creatinine clearance in man: a cross-sectional and longitudinal study. *J Gerontol.* 1976;311:155.

Snyder NA, Feigel DW, Arieff AI, et al. Hypernatremia in elderly patients. A heterogeneous, morbid, and iatrogenic entity. *Ann Intern Med.* 1987;107:309.

Tsunoda K, Abe K, Goto T, et al. Effect of age on the renin–angiotensin–aldosterone system in normal subjects: simultaneous measurement of active and inactive renin, renin substrate, and aldosterone in plasma. *J Clin Endocrinol Metab.* 1986;62:384.

Verbalis JG. Adaptation to acute and chronic hyponatremia: implications for symptomatology, diagnosis, and therapy. *Semin Nephrol.* 1998;18:3.

Wilkinson TJ, Begg EJ, Winter AC, et al. Incidence and risk factors for hyponatremia following treatment with fluoxetine or paroxetine in elderly people. *Br J Clin Pharmacol.* 1999;47:211.

Effect of Aging on Gastrointestinal Function

Karen E. Hall

The aging process has clinically significant effects on oropharyngeal and upper esophageal motility, colonic function, gastrointestinal (GI) immunity, and GI drug metabolism (Figure 89-1). On the other hand, because the GI tract exhibits considerable reserve capacity, many essential aspects of GI function, such as intestinal secretion, are preserved with aging. Despite such adaptation, superimposed effects of chronic diseases and environmental/lifestyle exposures (medications, alcohol, tobacco) can further impair GI function in older patients. A modest decline in gastric mucosal cytoprotection or esophageal acid clearance may become significant when superimposed side effects of certain medications or concurrent disease are also present. Certain age-related changes in GI function, such as constipation, are viewed as dysfunctional by patients and health care providers. Research areas that have been identified as important in aging include the pathophysiology of swallowing disorders, esophageal reflux, dysmotility syndromes, GI immunobiology, and the cellular mechanisms of neoplasia in the GI tract. Animal studies provide important insights into the cellular physiology of aging, despite the issue of species variation.

OROPHARYNGEAL FUNCTION

The increasing likelihood of dental decay and tooth loss with aging affects the efficiency and completeness of mastication (also see Chapter 42). Chewing and swallowing are impaired by xerostomia, which affects roughly 25% of older patients, while as many as 50% have subjective complaints of dry mouth. Medication side effects are a common cause of xerostomia, while a minority is caused by specific diseases affecting the salivary glands, such as Sjogren's syndrome. A mild loss of saliva production appears to occur with normal aging.

After food is broken up in the mouth by mastication, the act of swallowing moves the food bolus from the oral cavity into the pharynx and esophagus (also see Chapter 41). The oral and pharyngeal stages of swallowing are regulated by cortical input to medullary swallowing centers, which innervate skeletal muscle groups in the pharynx. The proximal esophagus contains skeletal muscle controlled by nerves from the medullary swallowing centers, whereas the mid- and distal esophagus consists of smooth muscle regulated by intrinsic enteric innervation and extrinsic innervation by the vagus nerve.

Oropharyngeal swallowing disorders are most commonly observed in patients with cognitive and/or perceptual dysfunction secondary to stroke or dementia, or chronic neurodegenerative diseases that affect the brainstem or motor neurons, such as Parkinson's disease, myasthenia gravis, or amyotrophic lateral sclerosis. Normal aging, however, is associated with alterations that predispose older individuals to dysphagia. Video fluoroscopy demonstrates abnormal transfer of a food bolus from the oral cavity to the pharynx in up to 60% of elderly patients without dysphagia. Other anatomic changes in esophageal neuromuscular anatomy occur in the aged orpharynx, such as cricopharyngeal bars caused by osteoarthritic spine disease. The pathophysiological significance of these are not clear, however, as they are seen in older patients with normal deglutition. Upper esophageal sphincter pressure gradually decreases with age, and is associated with a delay in relaxation after deglutition. Aspiration risk is increased in older subjects by delayed elevation of the larynx and decreased ability to clear food from the pharynx compared to younger subjects. However, clinically significant aspiration usually does not occur unless there are superimposed risk factors such as neurodegenerative diseases (e.g., Parkinson's disease) or medications that affect neuromuscular function. Figure 89-2 illustrates how various risk factors may interact with aging effects to lead to clinical swallowing problems, and is a model that may apply to how aging contributes to other GI tract disorders as well.

ESOPHAGEAL FUNCTION

Age-associated changes in the anatomy of the esophageal body appear to be minimal. Thickness of esophageal smooth muscle and

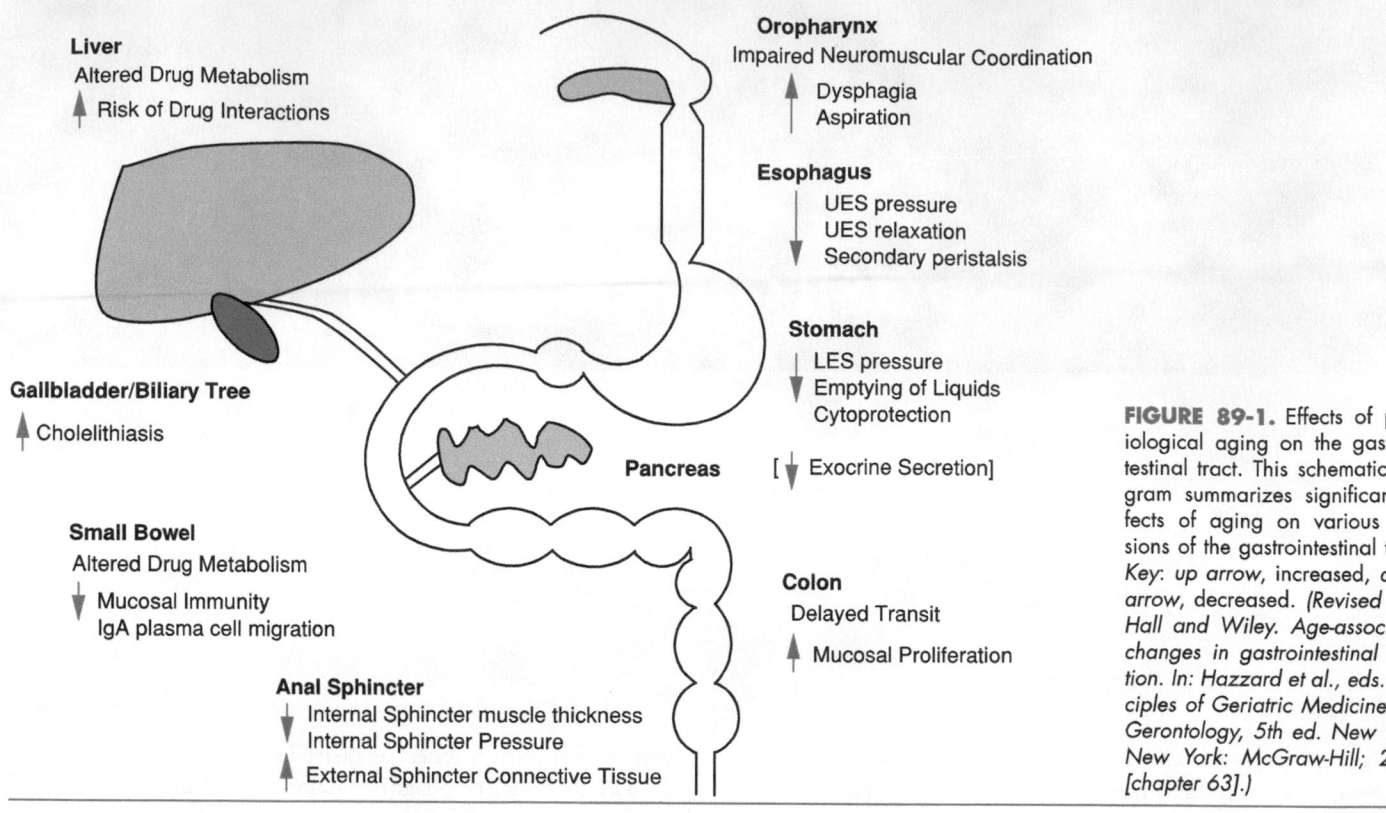

Liver
Altered Drug Metabolism
↑ Risk of Drug Interactions

Oropharynx
Impaired Neuromuscular Coordination
↑ Dysphagia
   Aspiration

Esophagus
↓ UES pressure
↓ UES relaxation
   Secondary peristalsis

Stomach
↓ LES pressure
↓ Emptying of Liquids
   Cytoprotection

Gallbladder/Biliary Tree
↑ Cholelithiasis

Pancreas   [↓ Exocrine Secretion]

Small Bowel
Altered Drug Metabolism
↓ Mucosal Immunity
   IgA plasma cell migration

Colon
Delayed Transit
↑ Mucosal Proliferation

Anal Sphincter
↓ Internal Sphincter muscle thickness
↓ Internal Sphincter Pressure
↑ External Sphincter Connective Tissue

FIGURE 89-1. Effects of physiological aging on the gastrointestinal tract. This schematic diagram summarizes significant effects of aging on various divisions of the gastrointestinal tract. Key: up arrow, increased, down arrow, decreased. (Revised from Hall and Wiley. Age-associated changes in gastrointestinal function. In: Hazzard et al., eds. Principles of Geriatric Medicine and Gerontology, 5th ed. New York, New York: McGraw-Hill; 2003 [chapter 63].)

amplitude of peristaltic contractions appear unaffected by aging. Although the number of myenteric neurons in the esophagus decreases with age, the functional significance is unclear. While some studies have reported impaired relaxation or decreased contractions of the lower esophageal sphincter (LES) with aging, more recent reports suggest that concomitant disease accounts for altered resting pressure of the aged LES.

Complaints of dysphagia, regurgitation, chest pain, and heartburn are fairly common in the geriatric population, with a prevalence of 35% reported in the general population aged 50 to 79 years (see Chapter 91). However, it is difficult to demonstrate a consistent relationship between symptoms and underlying pathophysiology, as demonstrable esophageal abnormalities are found in only 20% to 30% of symptomatic patients. A particular concern in an elderly patient is that symptoms of dysphagia are more likely to have a serious underlying etiology, such as malignancy. Elderly patients also appear to be more susceptible to complications of inadequately treated chronic esophageal disease, such as aspiration, malnutrition, and Barrett's metaplasia. Attempts at symptom analysis to identify subgroups at risk for serious underlying disease have met with mixed success.

The term "presbyesophagus" was coined to describe age-related changes in esophageal function, including decreased contractile amplitude, polyphasic waves in the esophageal body, incomplete relaxation of the lower esophageal sphincter, and esophageal dilation. The most common alteration in motility observed in older subjects was an increase in rapidity of propagation of the peristaltic wave, together with increased simultaneous contractions. Esophageal dysmotility in older patients is more often a result of diabetes mellitus and neurological disorders, or the side effects of medications, rather than aging per se.

Symptoms related to gastroesophageal reflux disease (GERD) are a frequent complaint of elderly patients (see Chapter 91). Risk factors for reflux-induced esophageal damage include decreased esophageal clearance, gastric factors such as decreased emptying or increased gastric pressure, decreased LES pressure, inappropriate LES relaxation, or the presence of a hiatal hernia, and increased gastric acid secretion. Older patients appear to have an increase in esophageal acid exposure and longer duration of reflux episodes. This maybe caused by decreased occurrence of secondary esophageal peristalsis, an important clearance mechanism for refluxed acid. Other factors, such as gastric emptying and frequency of LES relaxation, are relatively unchanged with aging. Concurrent disease and side effects of medications may play an important role in the pathophysiology of GERD in older patients.

GASTRIC FUNCTION

Decreased clearance of liquids from the stomach has been documented in older patients, and can be exacerbated by anticholinergic medications. Aging is also associated with decreased perception of gastric distension as measured by subjective fullness during inflation of a gastric barostat balloon. Delayed emptying may prolong the gastric contact time of noxious agents, such as nonsteroidal anti-inflammatory drugs (NSAIDs). This may have serious consequences, as significant age-related changes do occur in gastric mucosal defense mechanisms. These may predispose aged people to gastric mucosal injury and subsequent complications of ulceration. Increased risk of gastric injury does not appear to be to the result of excessive secretion of agents that promote mucosal injury, as most healthy older individuals have decreased, not increased, acid and pepsin output.

A   Relationship of Risk Factors and Aging on Swallowing

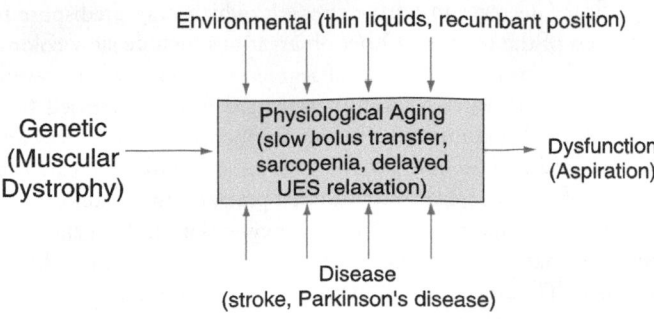

B   Oropharyngeal Dyskinesia and Aspiration Risk

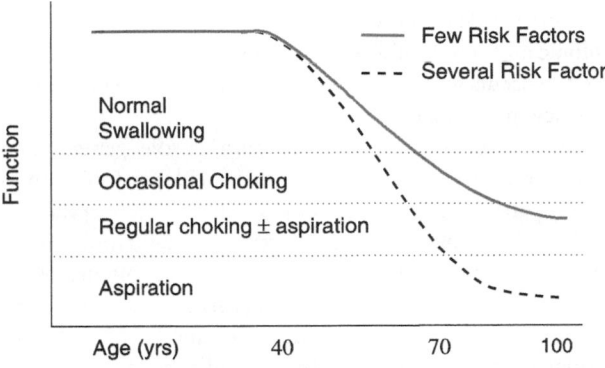

FIGURE 89-2. (A) Physiological aging maybe thought of as a baseline state upon which can be superimposed the effects of risk factors such as genetic predisposition, environmental exposure, and superimposed disease. The net result is symptomatic dysfunction in senescence that results in impairment. An example of this kind of synergy is dysphagia, which can manifest as a result of a combination of superimposed risks such as neurodegenerative disease and drug-induced damage on age-related oropharyngeal dyskinesia. UES, upper esophageal sphincter. (B) Graph illustrating how risk factors may affect swallowing function at various ages. Horizontal solid lines indicate three theoretical thresholds for clinically significant dysphagia (mild, moderate, severe symptom). Physiological aging of the gastrointestinal tract in individuals with few risk factors for dysphagia (solid blue line) results in minimal alterations in swallowing in middle age through the sixth decade. Superimposed risk factors such as neuromuscular disease (dashed line) can lead to earlier onset of dysphagia, and increased risk of moderate or severe dysphagia.

A small minority has severe acid hyposecretion (achlorhydria) associated with atrophic gastritis. Animal studies have shown a small age-related reduction in gastric acid secretion. Gastrin levels tend to rise with age in humans, possibly as a compensatory response to decreased acid production as a result of increased gastric autoantibodies and *Helicobacter pylori* colonization. The increased prevalence of *H. pylori* carriage in the elderly population does not appear to result in increased rates of duodenal ulceration, but is associated with increased risk of pernicious anemia and gastric lymphoma.

Increased susceptibility to gastric mucosal injury from NSAIDs in elderly people appears to be caused by a reduction in gastric mucosal cytoprotective factors such as mucosal prostaglandins. Human and animal aging is associated with a significant decrease in gastric bicarbonate, sodium ion and nonparietal fluid secretion, and thinning of the mucus gel layer, particularly in *H. pylori*-positive individuals. Aging is also associated with a decrease in the basal and

injury-induced rate of proliferation of stem cells in the neck of gastric glands in rats. In vivo expression and activity of several intestinal growth factors, such as transforming growth factor alpha (TGFα) and epithelial growth factor (EGF), is decreased in animal models of aging, However, activation of EGFR by membrane-bound TGF-alpha in vitro is actually increased in gastric and colonic mucosa of aged rats, suggesting that the relative lack of activity may not be caused by intrinsic inactivation.

Mucosal blood flow plays an essential role in maintaining gastric mucosal integrity. In rats, aging is associated with a decrease in basal gastric blood flow associated with impaired healing of acid-induced mucosal lesions. Impaired healing of gastric ulcers has also been associated with underlying impairment in sensory neuron function in several aging models.

Gastric secretion of intrinsic factor is necessary for vitamin B-12 absorption in the small bowel. Decreased secretion of intrinsic factor in aging is invariably caused by atrophic gastritis, not aging per se.

SMALL INTESTINAL FUNCTION

The small intestine has a large functional reserve capacity, because of the substantial mucosal surface area available for secretion and absorption. Intestinal surface area does not change after 6 weeks of age in rats. It is unclear whether the specific activity of intestinal disaccharidases and amino-peptidases is affected by aging, as both higher and lower activity has been reported in aged animals compared to youthful controls. Delayed maturation and expression of brush-border enzymes in small intestinal villous epithelial cells during crypt-to-villous migration appears to be the underlying cause. However, absorption of lactose, mannitol, and lipid in individuals greater than 60 years of age is unaffected. Vitamin D absorption and sensitivity is significantly impaired in aged rats. This is also a concern in human studies, which have documented decreased uptake of vitamin D, folic acid, vitamin B-12, calcium, copper, zinc, fatty acids, and cholesterol in aged subjects. Current recommendations by the U.S. Department of Agriculture to increase calcium, B-12, and Vitamin D supplementation in persons older than 70 years of age reflect this new information. Iron is one nutrient that is usually present in overabundance in the diet for older individuals. Older patients maybe at risk of diseases such as hepatic iron overload (particularly in individuals who are monozygotic for hemochromatosis), and iron overload has been implicated in some models of oxidative stress. Older men and postmenopausal women do not require additional iron unless there is superimposed blood loss or bone marrow impairment.

There is little evidence that older individuals are at risk for impaired absorption of most macronutrients in the absence of superimposed disease or surgical resection of small bowel. Limited data suggests that absorption of raw and heat-treated soybeans is impaired in old rats compared to youthful animals, while casein, skim milk powder, and autoclaved soybean powder were absorbed equally well. This may have implications for older individuals who follow a macrobiotic diet. Studies of protein turnover indicate that rapidly absorbed proteins such as whey protein resulted in greater net protein gain in older subjects compared to younger individuals, although the effect disappeared if fat and carbohydrate were added to the test meal. It is not clear whether this indicates a true impairment in protein absorption, or effects of fat and carbohydrate on small bowel motility.

Aging may alter visceral chemosensitivity or hormone responsiveness, as an enhanced satiating effect of carbohydrates delivered into the small intestine by infusion has been reported in older men. Mucosal regeneration is actually increased in aging. Crypt cell proliferation rates in all segments of the small intestine were found to be greater in aged rats compared to their youthful counterparts. These studies suggest that aged animals have increased cell production as a result of greater number of crypt cells undergoing cell division.

Minor effects of aging on small bowel motility have been described despite reports that several neuronal subtypes (substance P-, VIP-, somatostatin-, and nitric oxide-containing) are decreased in aged animals models. Studies in cats do not demonstrate significant effects of age on small bowel transit of radiolabeled lipids. In human studies, small bowel transit time measured by breath hydrogen was shorter in elderly males, but not women. Caloric restriction to 70% of normal intake prevents ileal myenteric neuronal loss in Sprague-Dawley rats up to 30 months of age, similar to beneficial effects of calorie restriction on other changes in aging.

COLONIC FUNCTION

Aging is associated with diverse effects on the large intestine including alterations in mucosal cell growth, differentiation, metabolism, and immunity. Disorders commonly observed in elderly patients include colon cancer, diverticulosis, and altered bowel habits, leading to constipation or diarrhea (see Chapters 92 and 93). While constipation is a common complaint in elderly people, age-associated alterations in colonic motility have been difficult to demonstrate. Some studies indicate that colonic transit slows with aging, particularly in women, while others found no significant difference in transit between young and elderly subjects. Inclusion of chronic laxative users in investigations of colonic function in aging should be interpreted cautiously, as chronic use of phenolphthalein results in loss of interneurons. Other cathartic laxatives, such as senna, do not cause significant anatomic damage in animal studies when used for up to 5 months.

Age-associated reduction in the nitric oxide–containing neurons in the myenteric plexus involved in receptive relaxation has been reported. The remaining myenteric neurons maybe functionally impaired. Release of the excitatory neurotransmitter acetylcholine was diminished in the colon of aged rats, an effect that appeared to be caused by decreased calcium influx. Neurotransmitter release from myenteric neurons in the aged colon could be restored to youthful levels by use of calcium ionophores that bypass membrane calcium channels. Similar impairment of calcium signaling with aging has also been demonstrated in peripheral sensory neurons and muscle.

Diverticulosis is an abnormality commonly described in the aging colon, and predisposes to the subsequent development of diverticulitis. By 50 years of age, one-third of Americans will have diverticulosis coli, and by 80 years of age, approximately two thirds. Most are asymptomatic, with 10% to 20% developing complications such as diverticulitis or hemorrhage. Diverticulosis is an abnormality commonly described in the aging colon and predisposes to the subsequent development of diverticulitis. Diverticulosis is observed in otherwise healthy individuals, suggesting that some effect of aging on colonic neuromuscular anatomy or function maybe responsible. Decreased tensile strength of the muscle wall and increased intra-abdominal pressures required for evacuation have been implicated in the development of diverticuli. Human aging is associated with an increase in collagen in the colon wall that is accompanied by a significant decrease in tensile strength, which may predispose to herniation of the mucosa. Other observations include slow colonic transit and increased frequency of segmenting contractions, resulting in increased water resorbtion and hard feces. Decreased fiber intake likely also contributes to the production of hard feces and excessive straining, as both animal and human studies indicate that addition of fiber decreases intraluminal pressures in the colon.

Elderly patients may present with new-onset fecal urgency and frequency that is similar to diarrhea-predominant irritable bowel syndrome. The onset may coincide with an acute diarrheal illness caused by viral or bacterial infection. However, many patients continue to have distressing urgency, resulting in considerable lifestyle impairment. Many curtail their travel and social activities outside the home for fear of fecal incontinence. The etiology is often multifactorial. Side effects of medications that increase small bowel and colonic motility should always be considered. Decreased rectal compliance occurs with aging, and may contribute to sensations of fecal urgency in these patients.

Fecal incontinence is uncommon in the general population (2.2%) but has a significantly higher incidence (10%) in older patients, particularly nursing home residents and hospitalized elderly patients. Fecal incontinence can result from fecal impaction and subsequent overflow, internal anal sphincter incompetence, decreased rectal or anal sensation, or from other structural impairments in the pelvic floor or anorectal neuromuscular function caused by trauma or iatrogenic damage from surgery or irradiation. In younger patients, fecal incontinence and fecal impaction are most commonly seen in the setting of structural or neuromuscular disease. In older patients, the added risks of immobility and use of anticholinergic drugs can dramatically increase the risk of constipation and subsequent fecal impaction. Aging maybe associated with a reduction in anal function in women. Healthy elderly women demonstrated thinning of the internal anal sphincter, resulting in decreased resting and maximum squeeze pressures in the anal canal. Although thickening of the external sphincter is also observed, it does not correlate with increased ability to maintain continence. In the absence of disease, the effects of aging on male anal sphincter function appear minimal. Other pathological factors that contribute to fecal incontinence in elderly people are the presence of neurological disorders that may predispose to impairment in the ability to interpret the need to defecate (dementia) or in the ability to coordinate defecation (myasthenia gravis or stroke).

COLONIC NEOPLASIA

Colon cancer is a common disorder in older patients, primarily because most colon cancers occur sporadically and are associated with polyp formation. The observation that crypt cell production rate is significantly higher in colonic tissue from aged rats raises the question of whether normal aging predisposes the colon to malignant transformation. The aged colon maybe more sensitive to the oncogenic effects of growth factors and carcinogens. Methylazoxymethanol, the active metabolite of the colonic carcinogen azoxymethane, induces a greater stimulation of ornithine decarboxylase activity and tyrosine kinase activity in aged rats compared to their younger counterparts. Similar results have been reported with TGFα and insulin-like growth factor-1 (IGF-1), both potent mitogens for a variety of tissues in the GI tract including the colon. It is not yet clear whether changes in the expression and/or affinity of TGFα receptors or altered postreceptor events contribute to this process.

HEPATIC AND BILIARY FUNCTION

There is no effect of age on conventional liver function tests, such as serum concentrations of aminotransferases, hepatic alkaline phosphatase, and bilirubin. However, dynamic assessments of liver function do show a decrease with aging. In healthy subjects, liver size, blood flow, and perfusion decrease by 30% to 40% between the third and tenth decade. Aminopyrine demethylation, galactose elimination, and caffeine clearance decrease in parallel with the reduction in liver volume and blood flow. Studies in isolated perfused livers from young adult and senescent Sprague-Dawley rats indicated age-associated reductions of approximately 50% in bile acid-dependent and -independent bile flow as well as hepatocellular uptake of taurocholate and rates of bile acid secretion. Tight junction permeability and transcellular transport were decreased modestly in senescent rats. Based on studies of hepatic impairment, including subtotal resection and diseases such as hepatitis or cirrhosis, it is likely that a decrease of greater than 70% of the total functional hepatic reserve would result in clinically relevant impairment of hepatic function in aging. In general, physiologic aging does not result in this degree of diminution in hepatic function.

However, the senescent liver maybe more susceptible to stress insult from diet, alcohol consumption, tobacco use, nutritional status, coexistent diseases, and genetic factors. Liver injury is associated with a regenerative response characterized by increased hepatocyte mitogen activated protein (MAP) kinase activity. Aged animals have an age-associated decline in MAP kinase activity and epidermal growth factor–stimulated hepatocytes. Specific impairment of intracellular transcription factors that are involved in transducuction of growth hormone receptor activation has been reported in senescent mice. Mitogenic stimulation of these pathways in aged mice results in hepatic regeneration following partial hepatectomy that is equivalent to that seen in younger animals. This has potential implications for management of hepatic resection in older patients, such as that used in treatment of solitary hepatoma. Animal studies suggest that hepatic damage may also be related to accumulation of oxidative metabolites with age.

The prevalence of cholelithiasis increases with age (see Chapter 90). Bile appears to become increasingly lithogenic as a function of aging, with precipitation of supersaturated bile and concomitant crystallization of cholesterol or calcium bilirubinate. Much of the available human data has been obtained from subjects aged younger than 65 years, therefore it is unclear whether gallbladder function is altered in old age. Some studies have demonstrated impaired gallbladder function in older subjects. Fasting and postprandial gallbladder volumes are increased in subjects older than 35 years of age, with less complete emptying following a meal observed in older individuals. Increased gallbladder volumes correlate with cholelithiasis, however no difference in fat-induced gallbladder emptying is observed in either male or female subjects older than 50 years of age, compared to younger individuals. As in younger age groups, aged females maybe more susceptible to impaired gallbladder contractility, with decreased contractile response to acetylcholine in post-

menopausal females compared to aged males. Animal studies in aged guinea pigs suggest that deceased density of receptors for hormones such as cholecystokinin (CCK) and galanin may underlie the decreased gallbladder contractility and increased gallstone formation in this model. Impairment in intracellular calcium mobilization and decreased muscle compliance correlate with decreased CCK responsiveness. The functional significance of these animal studies to humans is unclear, as decreased CCK responsiveness in older human subjects maybe compensated by increased CCK release, with no net change in gallbladder kinetics in aging.

PANCREATIC STRUCTURE AND FUNCTION

The exocrine pancreas possesses adequate reserve to maintain normal digestive capacity with aging. While there are some contradictory reports, there is little evidence for clinically significant decreases in pancreatic exocrine function in the elderly human. Age-related changes in pancreatic anatomy and histology include decreased pancreatic weight after the seventh decade in humans, with ductal epithelial hyperplasia, interlobular fibrosis, and acinar cell degranulation. A modest decrease in bicarbonate and enzyme output in response to secretin and caerulin in elderly subjects compared to their younger counterparts has been reported. However, secretin and caerulin (CCK receptor agonist)-mediated stimulation of sphincter of Oddi motor function, pancreatic bicarbonate, enzyme and volume output are not significantly changed in individuals older than 60 years of age. In contradistinction to human studies, animal models of pancreatic function do show significant effects of aging on trophic response to hormonal stimulation. Caerulin and secretin administration increased pancreatic weight, protein content, mRNA expression, enzyme, and polyamine concentrations in young and aged rats, but the magnitude of the responses were greater in young rats. The pancreas of aged animals demonstrates a diminished capacity to increase pancreatic lipase and amylase content in response to a high fat or high carbohydrate diet. Given the significant reserve capacity of the exocrine pancreas, the clinical significance of these observations to healthy aged individuals is questionable.

GASTROINTESTINAL IMMUNITY

The GI tract is the largest immunological system in mammals. Elderly people are relatively susceptible to infections that enter the body via the GI tract. This observation suggests that aging may impair mucosal immunity. The GI mucosal immune response in the small intestine is a complex process that involves a series of events: antigen uptake and presentation of antigen at the mucosal surface by specialized epithelial cells (M cells) overlying Peyer's patches in the small intestine; differentiation and migration of immunologically competent lymphocytes to the lamina propria; regulation of local antibody production in the intestinal wall; and mucosal epithelial cell receptor–mediated transport of antibodies to the intestinal lumen. The effect of aging on the first two steps, antigen uptake and presentation in animal studies is unclear. In rats, there was no change in the number of Peyer's patches or the yield of lymphocytes per patch in the small bowel. Increased T suppressor/cytotoxic lymphocytes could explain the observed decrease in lamina propria IgA plasma cells because of decreased cytokine-mediated differentiation

gallstones with ursodiol. Ursodiol is a naturally occurring bile salt that inhibits 3-hydroxy 3-methylglutaryl coenzyme A reductase, the rate-limiting enzyme in cholesterol synthesis. It also acts by dissolving cholesterol from the stone surface. Therefore, this medication is only useful in the setting of cholesterol gallstones. A meta-analysis of randomized trials using ursodiol for treatment of gallstones found a dissolution rate of 37% after 6 months with doses of at least 7 mg/kg or greater than 500 mg/day. However, at least 50% of patients treated with ursodiol for gallstones will have recurrent stone formation.

Carcinoma

Gallbladder Cancer

Cancer of the gallbladder is uncommon in the United States and carries a poor prognosis. Often, this diagnosis is not made until late in its course. The 5-year survival for local disease is 42%, but drops to 0.7% with distant spread of disease. SEER data show that gallbladder cancer occurs primarily in the elderly. Approximately 75% of cases occur in patients older than 65 years. Ninety percent of all gallbladder cancers are carcinomas and occur in approximately 3:1 female to male ratio. Ethnic background and geographic distribution appear to influence the development of gallbladder cancer, as the highest incidence rates are found in those of native North American and Mexican descent and those living in the region of the Andes. It has been noted that 80% of patients with gallbladder cancer have a history of cholelithiasis. Chronic inflammation from gallstones is thought to induce metaplasia of the gallbladder. Size and duration of gallstones appear to be important in carcinogenesis. Prophylactic cholecystectomy in certain higher risk groups is controversial. Among those who may benefit from this procedure include patients with a porcelain gallbladder and patients with a congenital defect in the junction of the pancreato–biliary duct.

Cancer of the Extra-Hepatic Bile Ducts

Primary bile duct cancers account of less than 3% of all cancers diagnosed in the United States. Cancer of the extrahepatic bile ducts is more common in the elderly, as 65% of cases are found in those older than 65 years and 69 is the median age. Ninety-nine percent of these are carcinomas. The 5-year survival rate ranges from 26.5% with localized disease to 1.3% with distant spread. The incidence is 1.2 per 100 000 in males and 0.8 per 100 000 in females. The tumors tend to infiltrate along the wall of the bile duct and may be difficult to differentiate from benign strictures. Patients present with signs and symptoms of biliary obstruction with jaundice, pruritus, and weight loss. Treatment is primarily surgical, most commonly with a Whipple procedure. For those who are not surgical candidates, biliary decompression by stent placement is a reasonable option for palliation to maintain patency of biliary drainage.

PANCREATIC DISEASE

Anatomy

See Figure 90-1 for the gross anatomy of the pancreas. The pancreas can be broken into the endocrine and the exocrine pancreas. Four different types of islet cells comprising the endocrine pancreas produce hormones such as insulin, glucagon, pancreatic polypeptide, and somatostatin. The exocrine pancreas is the focus of this chapter. The exocrine pancreas is composed primarily of acinar cells and duct cells. The acinar cells produce the digestive enzymes. The key enzyme is trypsinogen. The duct cells produce the bicarbonate-rich fluid for secretion.

Physiology

The exocrine pancreas has proteases, lipases, glycosidases (amylase), and nucleases. The proteases and the nucleases are stored in an inactive form. The proteases constitute greater than 75% of the pancreas by weight. Trypsinogen is the primary protease. Trypsinogen is activated to trypsin in the duodenum by enterokinase—the only physiological function of this enzyme. Trypsin subsequently activates the other digestive enzymes and in the presence of calcium activates trypsinogen to trypsin. In the absence of calcium, trypsin has negative feedback by degrading other trypsin molecules. Trypsin's primary site of action is on arginine and lysine amino acids. The most common defect in hereditary pancreatitis is R122 H or

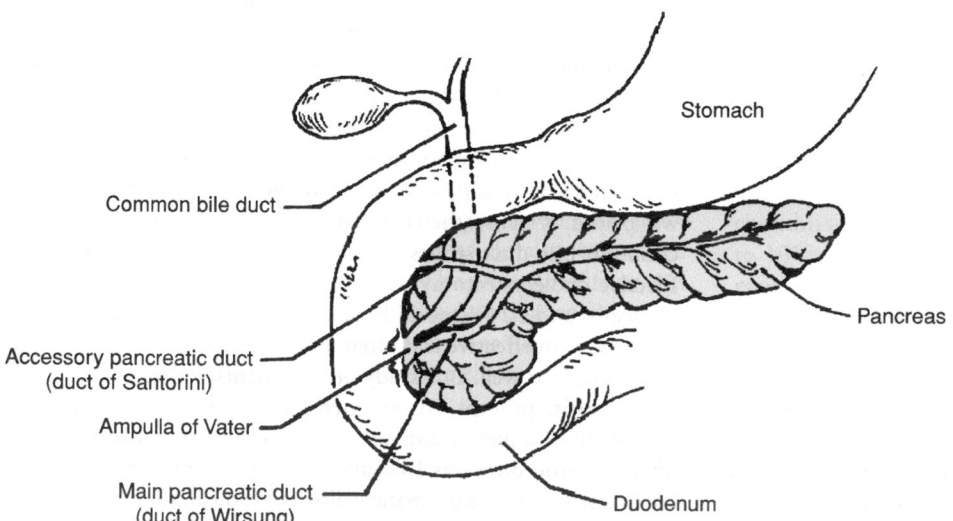

FIGURE 90-1. Normal anatomy of the pancreas. (From Steinberg W, Tenner S. Acute pancreatitis. N Engl J Med. 1994;330:1198.)

Stomach

Common bile duct

Pancreas

Accessory pancreatic duct (duct of Santorini)

Ampulla of Vater

Main pancreatic duct (duct of Wirsung)

Duodenum

arginine being replaced at position 122 (important regulatory site) by histidine. This defect negates the negative feedback safety mechanism for trypsin regulation.

There are two additional important mechanisms regulating pancreatic function. First, acid in the duodenum stimulates secretion of the hormone secretin and through vagal mediation leads to the duct cells of the pancreas to secrete bicarbonate. The second regulatory mechanism involves the cholecystokinin (CCK) feedback loop. Human pancreatic acini lack CCK receptors. The presence of protein in the duodenum effectively increases cholecystokinin releasing factor (CCK RF), which stimulates CCK release. The elevated CCK level is recognized by the brain leading to vagal stimulation of the acinar cells of the pancreas to secrete more digestive enzymes.

Aging and the Pancreas

Table 90-5 outlines the age-related changes of the pancreas. The maximal pancreatic volume excreted in response to secretin and CCK stimulation increases until the fifth decade and thereafter decreases steadily. Bicarbonate decreases steadily after the fourth decade of life. Also, in ERCP studies, a slight increase in size of the pancreatic duct in the head and body but not the tail has been noted with aging. Despite these anatomic and physiologic changes, only rare cases of pancreatic exocrine deficiency are clinically apparent in the healthy elderly.

Over and above the normal changes of aging, advanced age poses other threats to pancreatic structure and function. Pancreatitis secondary to alcohol tends to be a disease of the middle age, while gallstone disease continues to have a relatively high incidence in older cohorts. The biggest risk to the elderly pancreas is an increased incidence of malignancy, particularly adenocarcinoma. In addition, during imaging studies of the abdomen, incidental small cystic and solid lesions of the pancreas are now frequently found.

Acute Pancreatitis

Acute pancreatitis has a variety of etiologies, but all eventually lead to activation of the digestive enzymes particularly trypsin in the pancreatic acinar cells. The most common etiologies for acute pancreatitis are gallstones and alcohol. However, in an elderly patient without gallstones or a history of chronic excessive use of alcohol, the suspicion for underlying malignancy needs to be especially high. Inherited defects in the trypsinogen to trypsin pathway may lead to rare forms of acute pancreatitis, termed "hereditary pancreatitis." Obstruction of the pancreatic duct by a gallstone is an important mechanism of initiating pancreatic injury. Alcohol, on the other

TABLE 90-5

Aging and the Pancreas
Fat, fibrosis, and reduced weight after seventh decade
Bicarbonate decreases steadily after the fourth decade of life
Pancreatic exocrine deficiency: rare in the elderly without underlying pathology
Alcoholic pancreatitis: a disease of the middle age
Gallstone prevalence, and therefore gallstone pancreatitis, increases with age
Increased incidence of malignancy, particularly adenocarcinoma

TABLE 90-6

Etiologies for Pancreatitis
Gallstones
Alcohol
Hypertriglyceridemia
Medications/toxins
Hereditary pancreatitis
Cystic fibrosis gene mutation
Autoimmune pancreatitis
Pancreatic divisum
Trauma
Post-ERCP
Tumors
Elevated calcium
Idiopathic

hand, causes mitochondrial dysfunction, which allows for increased levels of intracellular calcium and subsequent activation of trypsin. Hypertriglyceridemia is often overlooked as a cause of acute pancreatitis. Triglycerides should be measured on admission to hospital because levels will often quickly decrease with bowel rest and fluids. Many medications may cause acute pancreatitis or elevate levels of triglycerides. See Table 90-6 for etiologies of acute pancreatitis.

The predominant symptom of acute pancreatitis is epigastric pain, commonly with radiation into the back. Nausea and vomiting are also frequently present. The diagnosis is a clinical diagnosis with support from elevated serum amylase and lipase. Levels at least 3 times the upper limit of normal are typical of acute pancreatitis. Many other conditions cause minor elevations in amylase or lipase. Radiographic studies have little role in diagnosis, but do play important roles in evaluating etiology (gallstones, neoplasia, pancreatic calcification indicating chronic pancreatitis) and complications such as necrosis, and pseudocysts. Care needs to be taken in the acute setting not to add intravenous contrast load to a patient that is extremely intravascularly depleted already. Acute pancreatitis can be divided into mild and severe pancreatitis. The range of disease is from self-limited disease to multiorgan failure and death. A variety of grading systems including Ranson criteria, Apache score, Glasgow score, and the Baltazar CT grade +/− necrosis do correlate with morbidity and mortality.

Treatment of mild pancreatitis is accomplished with bowel rest, +/− parenteral feeding, intravenous fluids, and pain control. Gallstone pancreatitis is treated with ERCP, sphincterotomy, and stone extraction if cholangitis or evidence of biliary obstruction is present. Severe pancreatitis often becomes management of multiorgan failure. Placement of nasojejunal tubes with subsequent enteral feedings has become the standard of care at the University of Wisconsin Hospital. Evidence of necrosis on CT scan warrants intravenous antibiotics with good pancreatic penetration such as imipenem. Pancreatic necrosis should be surveyed by radiology by biopsy and culture. Evidence of infection may require surgical debridement.

Pseudocyst formation is an important complication of acute pancreatitis. Approximately 10% of patients with acute pancreatitis proceed to formation of these fluid collections. Most pseudocysts resolve with time; however, if symptoms are present (early satiety, pain, infection, bleeding) then drainage may be necessary.

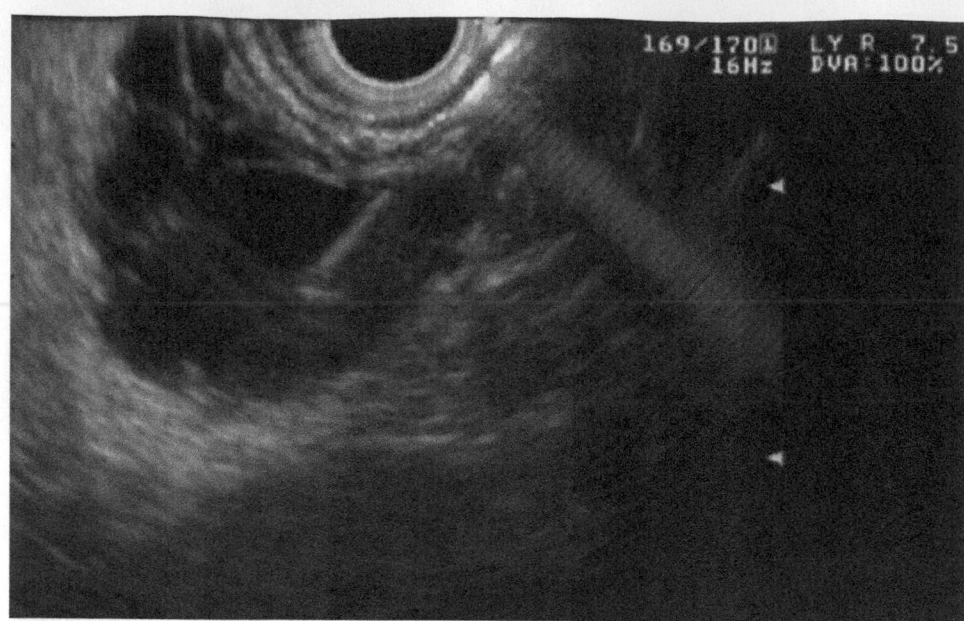

FIGURE 90-2. Endoscopic ultrasound with FNA needle in pancreatic cyst. This cyst proved to be a serous cystadenoma. *(Image courtesy of Deepak Gopal, MD, University of Wisconsin, Madison, WI.)*

Chronic Pancreatitis

Alcohol abuse accounts for approximately 70% of chronic pancreatitis. Idiopathic causes are the second most common cause of chronic pancreatitis. Cystic fibrosis gene mutations are now frequently being identified as an etiology in approximately a third of idiopathic pancreatitis diagnosis. Hereditary pancreatitis frequently leads to chronic pancreatitis at a young age. In the elderly, it is important to evaluate for tumors compressing the pancreatic duct as the etiology.

The diagnosis of chronic pancreatitis can be a challenging diagnosis to make. Amylase and lipase can be mildly elevated or normal. Evidence of calcifications by x-ray or by CT scan is found in 30% to 40% of cases and can give a diagnosis. Often, more advanced imaging studies such as ERCP, MRCP, or endoscopic ultrasound (EUS) are used to evaluate the anatomy of the pancreas and give a diagnosis. The major features of chronic pancreatitis include pain, malabsorption, and frequently diabetes.

Treatment is based on resolving malabsorption with pancreatic enzyme replacement, which also down regulates the CCK feedback loop decreasing pancreatic stimulation. Narcotic pain medication is often needed. If a dilated main pancreatic duct is present, a pancreaticojejunostomy (Puestow procedure) can be helpful. In some cases, near total pancreatectomy is needed with or without islet cell transplantation.

Pancreatic Cancer

Approximately 33,700 new cases of pancreatic cancer will be diagnosed, and 32,600 patients will die secondary to pancreatic cancer in 2007. Approximately 87% of patients will be older than age 55 at diagnosis with the median age being 72. The overall 5-year survival is 5%. Unfortunately, little progress has been made to change the mortality from this disease over the last several decades. The genetics have now been further elucidated showing that 85% of adenocarcinomas of the pancreas have an activating point mutation in the K-ras oncogene. In addition, 95% have an inactivated p16 tumor-suppressor gene. Genetic changes and new knowledge about the cytokine milieu are current areas of active research.

More than 70% of adenocarcinomas arise in the head of the pancreas, which leads to common presentations including jaundice, gastric outlet obstruction, and pain. Approximately 15% of lesions do not have vasculature invasion or metastatic disease on presentation making surgical resection possible, with curative intent. The 5-year survival in this population is approximately 20%. Staging with CT scans and EUS to evaluate for metastatic disease and vascular invasion is thus important. In addition, tissue diagnosis can be made with EUS and fine needle aspiration (FNA). Autoimmune pancreatitis (sclerosing pancreatitis) can present as a pancreatic head mass and obstructive jaundice making this diagnosis important to consider prior to surgical or medical therapy for presumed pancreatic cancer. Autoimmune pancreatitis has elevated ANA as well as IgG4 autoantibodies in the majority of cases and responds to prednisone.

Other tumors exist in the pancreas including neuroendocrine tumors and many types of cystic lesions of the pancreas. Neuroendocrine tumors of the pancreas are typically solid tumors. Evaluation by EUS +/− FNA and surgical resection are often performed except in multiple endocrine neoplasia (MEN) 1 where the pancreatic lesions are often multifocal in nature. Cystic lesions of the pancreas are becoming increasingly recognized because of more widespread abdominal imaging. These lesions can vary from congenital cysts to pseudocysts to benign cysts to premalignant and malignant lesions. According to the ASGE guidelines, cystic lesions of the pancreas, even when found incidentally, may represent malignant or premalignant neoplasms and require diagnostic evaluation regardless of size. EUS with FNA can obtain fluid for cytologic evaluation and for tumor markers and amylase. See Figure 90-2.

FURTHER READING

Aithal GP, Breslin NP, Gumustop B. High serum IgG4 concentrations in patients with sclerosing pancreatitis. *N Engl J Med.* 2001;345(2):147–148.

Anand BS, Vij JC, Mac HS, et al. Effect of aging on the pancreatic ducts: a study based on endoscopic retrograde pancreatography. *Gastrointest Endosc.* 1989;35(3):210–213.

Carriaga MT, Henson DE. Liver, gallbladder, extrahepatic bile ducts, and pancreas. *Cancer.* 1995;75:171–190.

Cohn JA, Friedman KJ, Noone PG, et al. Relation between mutations of the cystic fibrosis gene and idiopathic pancreatitis. *N Engl J Med.* 1998;339(10):653–658.

Fritz E, Kirchgatterer A, Hubner D, et al. ERCP is safe and effective in patients 80 years of age and older compared with younger patients. *Gastrointest Endosc.* 2006;64(6):899–905.

Grace WA, Ransohoff DF. The natural history of silent gallstones: the innocent gallstone is not a myth. *NEJM.* 1982;307(13):798–800.

Henson DE, Abores-Saavedra J, Corle D. Carcinoma of the gallbladder: histologic types, stage of disease, grade and survival rates. *Cancer.* 1992;70:1493–1497.

Jacobson BC, Baron TH, Adler DG, et al. ASGE guideline: the role of endoscopy in the diagnosis and the management of cystic lesions and inflammatory fluid collections of the pancreas. *Gastrointest Endosc.* 2005;61(3):363–370.

Katsinelos P, Paroutoglou G, Kountouras J, et al. Efficacy and safety of therapeutic ERCP in patients 90 years of age and older. *Gastrointest Endosc.* 2006;63(3):417–423.

Keswani RN, Ahmed A, Keeffe EB. Older age and liver transplantation: a review. *Liver Transpl.* 2004;10(8):957–967.

Laugier R, Bernard JP, Berthezene P, Dupuy P. Changes in pancreatic exocrine secretion with age: pancreatic exocrine secretion does decrease in the elderly. *Digestion.* 1991;50(3-4):202–211.

Li D, Xie K, Wolff R, Abbruzzese JL. Pancreatic cancer. *Lancet.* 2004;363(9414):1049–1057.

Marcus EL, Tur-Kaspa R. Viral hepatitis in older adults. *J Am Geriatr Soc.* 1997;45(6):755–763.

May GR, Sutherland LR, Shaffer EA. Efficacy of bile acid therapy for gallstone dissolution: a meta-analysis of randomized trials. *Aliment Pharmacol Ther.* 1993;7:139–148.

Morrow DJ, Thompson J, Wilson SE. Acute cholecystitis in the elderly: a surgical emergency. *Arch Surgery.* 1978;113(10):1149–1152.

Newton JL, Burt AD, Park JB, et al. Autoimmune hepatitis in older patients. *Age Ageing.* 1997;26(6):441–444.

Regev A, Schiff ER. Liver disease in the elderly. *Gastroenterol Clin North Am.* 2001;30(2):547–563.

Schmucker DL. Age-related changes in liver structure and function: implications for disease? *Exp Gerontol.* 2005;40(8-9):650–659.

Van Dam J, Zeldis JB. Hepatic diseases in the elderly. *Gastroenterol Clin North Am.* 1990;19(2):459–472.

Zeeh J, Platt D. The aging liver: structural and functional changes and their consequences for drug treatment in old age. *Gerontology.* 2002;48(3):121–127.

Upper Gastrointestinal Disorders

Alberto Pilotto ■ *Marilisa Franceschi*

GASTROESOPHAGEAL REFLUX DISEASE IN THE ELDERLY

Definition

Gastroesophageal reflux disease (GERD) is defined by symptoms and/or histopathological alterations (esophagitis) caused by reflux of gastric contents into the esophagus. Manifestations of GERD range from mild episodes of heartburn and acid regurgitation, without esophagitis, to chronic mucosal inflammation with erosive esophagitis and ulceration, complicated in severe cases by stricture and bleeding. While it is still unclear whether the incidence and prevalence of GERD symptoms increase with aging, several studies suggest that frequency of esophagitis is significantly higher in the elderly than in adult or young subjects. Indeed, older age was found to be a significant risk factor in the development of severe forms of GERD in both epidemiological and clinical studies from the United States, Japan, and Europe.

Pathophysiology

Pathophysiological changes in esophageal functions that occur with aging may be responsible, at least in part, for the high prevalence of GERD in old age. These include (1) a shorter intra-abdominal segment of the lower esophageal sphincter (LES), (2) a reduction of secondary peristalsis, (3) an increase in the prevalence of tertiary contractions, (4) alterations in salivary secretion, (5) a reduction in gastric emptying, (6) a decreased esophageal mucosal resistance resulting from impaired epithelial cell regeneration, and (7) duodenogastroesophageal reflux of bile salts (Table 91-1). Elderly subjects have a high prevalence of other risk factors that predispose the aging esophagus to lesions (Table 91-1): (1) difficulty in maintaining an upright position after meals; (2) hiatus hernia associated with both repeated episodes of acid reflux and with more severe diseases sucs as Barrett esophagus; (3) increased drug use, including those that may have a directly damaging effect on esophageal mucosa or an indirect effect on reducing LES pressure; and (4) delayed esophageal transit time of many drugs, creating a potentially dangerous situation when it coexists with acid reflux, as reported for alendronate and nonsteroidal anti-inflammatory drugs (NSAIDs) (Table 91-2).

Symptomatology

Particular attention has been given to the clinical presentation of GERD in the elderly since important differences between young and adult patients have been reported. Indeed, with advancing age, a significantly lower prevalence of typical symptoms, i.e., heartburn, acid regurgitation, and epigastric pain was reported by patients (Figure 91-1). Atypical symptoms also are relatively rare in the elderly (Table 91-3). In contrast, the prevalence of nonspecific symptoms, i.e., vomiting, anorexia, weight loss, and anemia significantly increased with age (Figure 91-2). Reflux esophagitis in the elderly may thus be missed, and a substantial number of patients may suffer subclinical relapses of the disease. The cause of such a different clinical expression of the disease in the elderly is not clear, but a diminished sensitivity to visceral pain has been documented in the elderly. Moreover, 24-hour esophageal pH monitoring and endoscopy examinations demonstrated an age-related reduction in acid chemosensitivity and a reduced symptom severity despite a tendency toward increased severity of esophageal mucosal injury.

Diagnosis

Since the presentation of GERD is often with nonspecific symptoms in the elderly, *endoscopy* should be undertaken early as the initial diagnostic test in all elderly patients suspected of having GERD. Early endoscopy is very useful in diagnosing the presence and the grade

TABLE 91-1

Pathophysiological Changes in Esophageal Functions That Occur with Aging	
FUNCTIONAL CAUSES	**ANATOMICAL CAUSES**
Impaired motility of the esophagus	Hiatus hernia
Reduced LES pressure and length	Difficulty in maintaining an
Normal gastric acid secretion	upright position
Delayed gastric emptying transit time	
Reduced salivary secretion	
Decreased tissue resistance as a result of impaired epithelial cell regeneration	
Duodenogastroesophageal reflux of bile salts	

TABLE 91-2

Drugs That May Increase the Risk of Severe GERD	
DIRECT EFFECT ON ESOPHAGEAL MUCOSA	**REDUCTION IN LES PRESSURE**
Aspirin	Theophylline
NSAIDs	Nitroderivates
Potassium salts	Calcium channel-blockers
Ferrous sulfate	Benzodiazepines
Corticosteroids	Dopaminergics
Alendronate	Tricyclic antidepressants
	Anticholinergics

of severity of esophagitis (Table 91-4) and/or hiatus hernia, which are important prognostic factors to be considered in the long-term treatment of patients. Endoscopy will also identify GERD complications, especially esophageal stricture and Barrett esophagus, and concomitant gastroduodenal diseases, that is, gastric or duodenal ulcers and/or *Helicobacter pylori* (*H pylori*) infection. *Barium radiography* of the esophagus is a useful test to establish the presence of a hiatus hernia and is indicated as part of the evaluation of the patient with suspected motility abnormalities or peptic stricture. A barium study may also identify rings and webs or other obstructive lesions. The barium swallow test is also a key test in studying elderly patients with dysphagia, and it should be performed in conjunction with endoscopy in all elderly patients with this symptomatology. Barium studies are widely available and usually well tolerated by older people. *Esophageal 24-hour pH testing* is helpful before antireflux surgery and in those patients not responsive to medical treatment. In the endoscopy-negative patient, an abnormal esophageal pH test may suggest the need for more aggressive drug therapy, whereas a normal test may indicate the presence of a functional disorder. In the patient with persistent esophagitis, a normal test could differentiate

pathophysiological mechanisms, that is, a drug-induced esophagitis from acid reflux disease. *Esophageal manometry* is useful in identifying abnormalities of LES pressure or esophageal motility. In elderly patients, its major use is reserved for the localization of LES before pH testing and for obtaining preoperative information on esophageal peristalsis.

A therapeutic trial with proton pump inhibitors (*PPI-test*) has been suggested as a useful diagnostic test in patients with GERD. Meta-analyses of clinical studies demonstrated that the PPI test has 78% sensitivity and 54% specificity in confirming the diagnosis of GERD when compared with endoscopy or 24-hour esophageal pH monitoring. In patients with noncardiac chest pain, sensitivity and specificity are reported to be 80% and 74%, respectively. Since typical (heartburn, acid regurgitation) and extraesophageal symptoms (asthma, chronic cough, noncardiac chest pain) of GERD are often absent in elderly patients, the patient's history is less reliable and high prevalences of severe esophagitis are common despite mild symptoms, a trial with PPIs should be used with great caution in older patients, possibly only after endoscopy as a first diagnostic test.

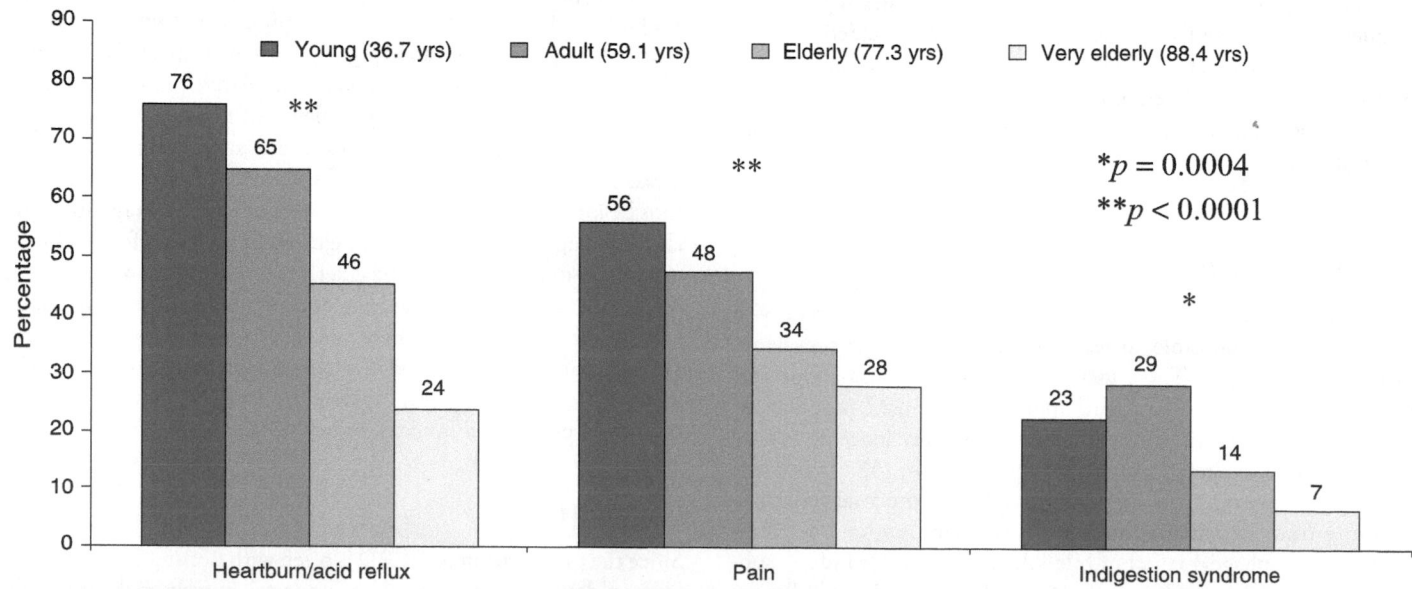

FIGURE 91-1. Prevalence of typical symptoms in 840 subjects with reflux esophagitis divided according to age. (*Adapted from Pilotto A, Franceschi M, Leandro G, et al. Clinical features of reflux esophagitis in older people: a study of 840 consecutive patients. J Am Geriatr Soc. 2006;54:1537–1542.*)

TABLE 91-3

Typical and Atypical Symptoms of Gastroesophageal Reflux Disease

TYPICAL SYMPTOMS	ATYPICAL SYMPTOMS
Heartburn	Pulmonary symptoms:
Acid regurgitation	Bronchial asthma
Epigastric pain	Bronchiectasis
	Chronic bronchitis
	Chronic cough
	Otorhinolaryngeal symptoms:
	Hoarseness
	Chronic laryngitis
	Odynophagia
	Noncardiac chest pain

TABLE 91-4

Endoscopic Classification of Esophagitis (According to the Los Angeles Classification)

GRADE	DESCRIPTION	
Grade A	One or more mucosal breaks no longer than 5 mm, none of which extends between the tops of the mucosal folds	
Grade B	One or more mucosal breaks more than 5 mm long, none of which extends between the tops of two mucosal folds	
Grade C	Mucosal breaks that extend between the tops of two or more mucosal folds, but which involve less than 75% of the esophageal circumference	
Grade D	Mucosal breaks that involve at least 75% of the esophageal circumference	

Lundell LR, Dent J, Bennett JR, et al. Endoscopic assessment of oesophagitis: clinical and functional correlates and further validation of the Los Angeles classification. Gut. 1999;45:172–80.

Treatment

The objectives of GERD treatment are (1) relief of symptoms, (2) healing of the esophagitis, (3) prevention of the relapses of the disease, and (4) prevention of the complications.

Lifestyle and Dietary Modifications

Recommendations for lifestyle modifications are based on the presumption that certain foods, body position, tobacco, alcohol, and obesity contribute to a dysfunction in the body's antireflux defense system. Although there is clinical and physiologic evidence that smoking, alcohol, chocolate, peppermint, coffee, fatty or citrus intake may adversely affect symptoms or esophageal pH, there is little evidence that cessation of these agents will improve GERD variables. Elevation of the head of the bed and weight loss, however, have been associated with improvement in GERD variables in case–control studies. Medications that decrease LES pressure and promote gastroesophageal reflux as well as drugs that may cause direct esophageal injury (Table 91-2) should be avoided when possible or used with caution in older patients with GERD. In any case, these drugs must be taken while maintaining an upright position and with a full glass of water.

Pharmacological Treatment: Short-Term Therapy

Antacids and alginic acid provide symptomatic relief in mild nonerosive esophagitis. Prokinetic drugs, either alone or in combination with antisecretory drugs, are only moderately effective in GERD. Possible side effects of antacids include salt overload, constipation, hypercalcemia, and interference with absorption of other drugs, particularly antibiotics such as tetracycline, azithromycin, and quinolones. Currently, prokinetic drugs include metoclopramide,

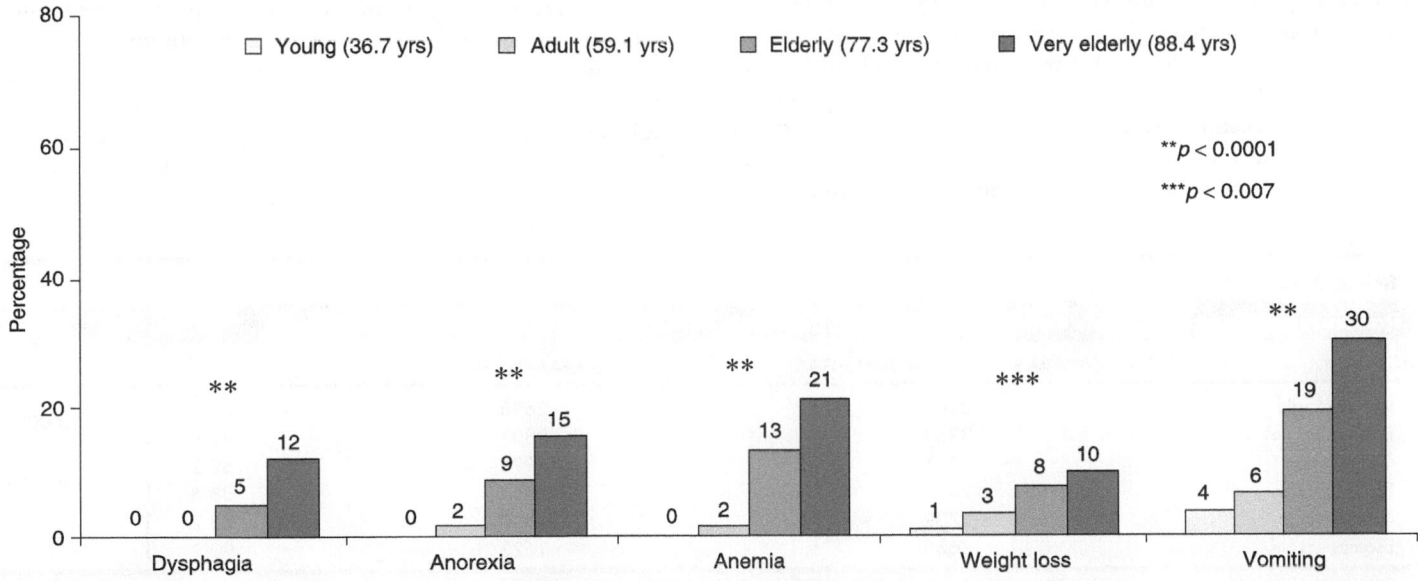

FIGURE 91-2. Prevalence of nonspecific symptoms in 840 subjects with reflux esophagitis divided according to age. (Adapted from Pilotto A, Franceschi M, Leandro G, et al. Clinical features of reflux esophagitis in older people: a study of 840 consecutive patients. J Am Geriatr Soc. 2006;54:1537–1542.)

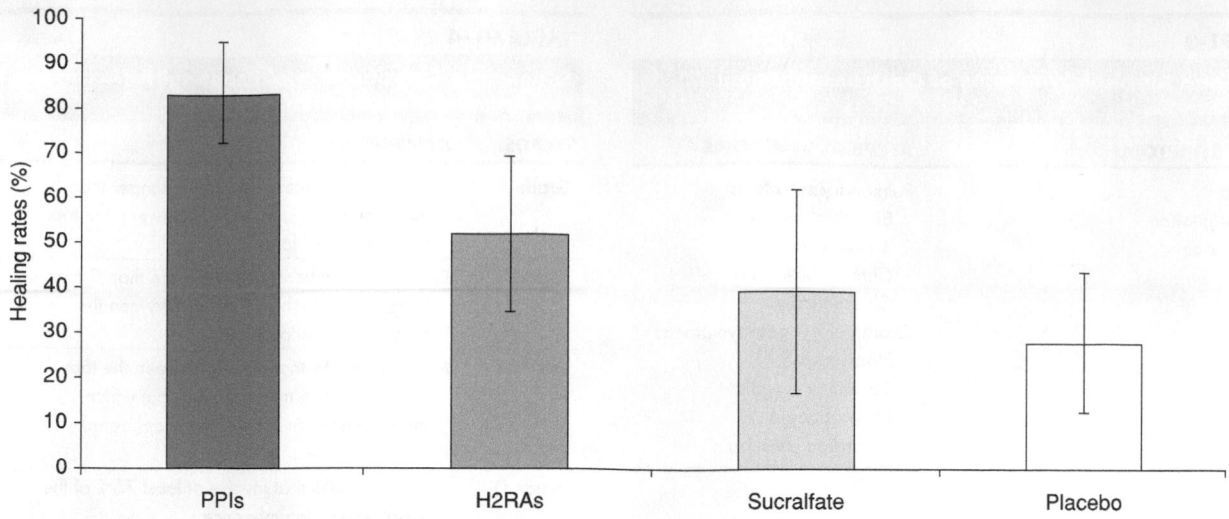

FIGURE 91-3. Percentage of patients that experience complete healing after treatment for grade II to IV reflux esophagitis with the indicated therapies. PPIs, proton pump inhibitors; H2RAs, histamine type 2 receptor antagonists. *(Adapted from Chiba N, De Gara CJ, Wilkinson JM, et al. Speed of healing and symptom relief in grade II to IV gastroesophageal reflux disease: a meta-analysis. Gastroenterology. 1997;112:1798–1810.)*

clebopride, domperidone, and partially levosulpiride. Unfortunately, no controlled clinical trials have evaluated the role of these drugs in the treatment of GERD in the elderly. Antireflux therapy is focused largely on suppressing gastric acid secretion with H2-blockers and proton pump inhibitors (PPI). Meta-analysis of 43 articles including more than 7600 patients aged 18 to 89 years with grade II to IV esophagitis treated for ≤12 weeks reported higher healing rates with PPIs (83.6% ± 11.4) than H2-blockers (51.9% ± 17.1), sucralfate (39.2% ± 22.4), or placebo (28.2% ± 15.6). Moreover, PPIs provided faster and more complete heartburn relief than H2-blockers (Figure 91-3). Currently, five PPIs are available: omeprazole, lansoprazole, rabeprazole, pantoprazole, and esomeprazole. Some age-associated differences in pharmacokinetics and pharmacodynamics of the PPIs have been reported. However, it is unknown if these differences are associated with different clinical effects, particularly in older patients. Indeed, a series of meta-analyses evaluating acute therapy of esophagitis reported that the PPIs were superior to ranitidine and placebo in healing erosive esophagitis, without significant differences in efficacy between omeprazole 20 mg daily and lansoprazole 30 mg daily or pantoprazole 40 mg daily or rabeprazole 20 mg daily. Recently, a systematic review of randomized controlled trials comparing standard dose PPIs reported a lower 8-week healing rate of esophagitis with omeprazole 20 mg or lansoprazole 30 mg

daily, but not with pantoprazole 40 mg daily, compared to esomeprazole 40 mg daily (Table 91-5). The recent finding that omeprazole has considerable potential for drug interactions, since it has higher affinity for the cytochrome CYP2C19 than other PPIs, may explain these differences in efficacy, especially in elderly patients who are treated with concomitant therapies.

Long-Term Maintenance Therapy

GERD is a chronic disease with a 70% to 90% annual relapse rate after the interruption of an effective antisecretory therapy. Risk factors for relapse of the disease are shown in Table 91-6. Maintenance therapy with antisecretory drugs is a significant protective factor in reducing the occurrence of relapse of GERD in elderly patients. Several studies have shown higher efficacy of PPIs over H2-blockers and prokinetics in maintaining a healed esophagitis. There are two main approaches to drug therapy for GERD: step-up and step-down. In the step-up approach, therapy is initiated with weak inhibition of gastric acid (e.g., an H2-blocker or half dosage of a PPI), and progresses to a higher degree of acid inhibition (standard and then escalating doses of PPI), until adequate symptom control is obtained. The step-down approach involves starting with the most effective regimen (full dosage of a PPI) and switching to lower doses of PPI

TABLE 91-5

Randomized Controlled Trials Comparing Standard Dose PPIs in the Healing of Esophagitis at 8 Weeks

	TOTAL NUMBER OF PATIENTS	ESOPHAGITIS HEALED	%	*p*
Lansoprazole	3262	2698	82.7	0.0001
Esomeprazole	3264	2807	85.9	
Omeprazole	2431	1998	82.2	0.0001
Esomeprazole	2446	2167	88.6	
Pantoprazole	1709	1507	88.2	ns
Esomeprazole	1688	1523	90.2	

(Data from Edwards SJ, Lind T, Lundell L. Systematic review: proton pump inhibitors (PPIs) for the healing of reflux oesophagitis-a comparison of esomeprazole with other PPIs. Aliment Pharmacol Ther. 2006;24:743–750.)

TABLE 91-6

Risk Factors for Relapse of Esophagitis

RISK FACTORS

Patient's characteristics
  Old age
  High body mass index (BMI)

Clinical features
  Long history of reflux symptoms
  Latency prolonged between appearance of symptoms and therapy
  Persistence of symptoms after the healing of esophagitis

Endoscopic characteristics
  Severity of the esophagitis at baseline
  Presence of a large hiatus hernia

Pathophysiology features
  Reduced pressure of the lower esophageal sphincter (manometry)
  Modified curve at the 24-h pH-metry

for maintenance therapy once symptoms are under control. This latter approach is perhaps more rational, based on evidence showing superior efficacy of PPIs over H2-antagonists across all grades of severity of GERD. Withdrawal of maintenance therapy with PPI after 6 months significantly reduces the percentage of remission of esophagitis at 1 year from 95% to 33% in patients older than 65 years (Figure 91-4). Presently, no comparative studies have been carried out to evaluate which strategy (step-down vs. step-up) is more cost-effective in older subjects.

Safety of Long-Term Antisecretory Treatment

A study explored the long-term safety of omeprazole for up to 11 years in patients (including some elderly) with refractory reflux esophagitis. Annual incidence of gastric corpus mucosal atrophy was 4.7% in *H pylori*-positive individuals and 0.7% in *H pylori*-negative patients. Moreover, mucosal atrophy was mainly observed in elderly patients who had moderate or severe gastritis at entry into the study. Corpus intestinal metaplasia was rare and no dysplasia or neoplasms were observed. Long-term therapy with a PPI does not appear to

have marked effects on protein and carbohydrate digestion. Antisecretory drugs, however, may interfere with calcium absorption through induction of hypochlorydria; PPIs, moreover, may reduce bone resorption through inhibition of the osteoclastic vacuolar proton pump. Indeed, a long-term PPI therapy has been associated with an increased risk of hip fractures. Inhibition of acid secretion may induce an increase of the bacterial flora at the gastrointestinal level with potential to increase the incidence of systemic infections particularly in immunodepressed elderly subjects. Indeed, the use of antisecretory drugs has been associated with an increased risk of infections of the lower gastrointestinal tract, mainly because of *Salmonella* spp. and *Clostridium difficile*. Recent studies, moreover, reported that the use of PPIs may be associated with an increased risk of community-acquired pneumonia.

Since PPIs are mainly metabolized by the cytochrome P450 (CYP), particularly the subfamily CYP2C19, clinically relevant drug interactions may occur in case of concomitant administrations of CYP-2C19-metabolized drugs. For these reasons a thorough surveillance of the long-term antisecretory therapy is suggested in elderly patients who frequently present with infections, malabsorption and/or diarrhea, osteoporosis, and/or are treated with CYP450-metabolized medications.

The Role of Surgery

The role of surgery in the treatment of GERD is controversial. Laparoscopic fundoplication has greatly reduced the morbidity and mortality of antireflux surgery, also in the elderly. Thus, the indications for surgery seem to be evolving. At present, evidence suggests that surgery may be indicated in elderly patients who (1) are medical treatment failures; (2) have severe complications, i.e., strictures not treatable by endoscopy; (3) have severe dysphagia, aspiration, or atypical symptoms associated with a large hiatal hernia; and/or (4) have preneoplastic lesions, that is, Barrett esophagus with high-grade dysplasia. Randomized clinical studies are needed to compare the outcome of antireflux surgery with that of medical therapy in the elderly. Furthermore, surgery for GERD should be centralized to units specialized in these techniques to reduce surgical complications and improve successful clinical outcomes.

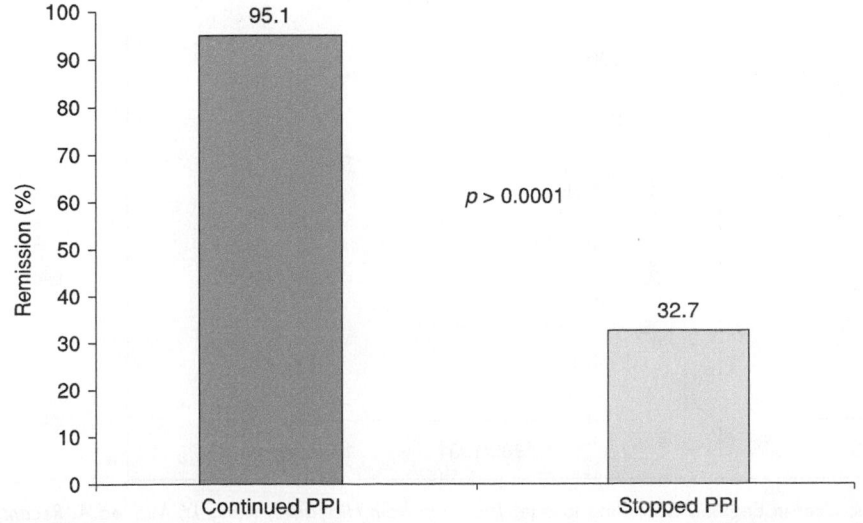

FIGURE 91-4. Remission at 12 months in elderly patients with esophagitis who continued versus stopped PPI maintenance treatment after 6 months. (Data from Pilotto A, Leandro G, Franceschi M, et al. Short- and long-term therapy for reflux oesophagitis in the elderly: a multi-centre, placebo-controlled study with pantoprazole. Aliment Pharmacol Ther. 2003;17:1399–1406.)

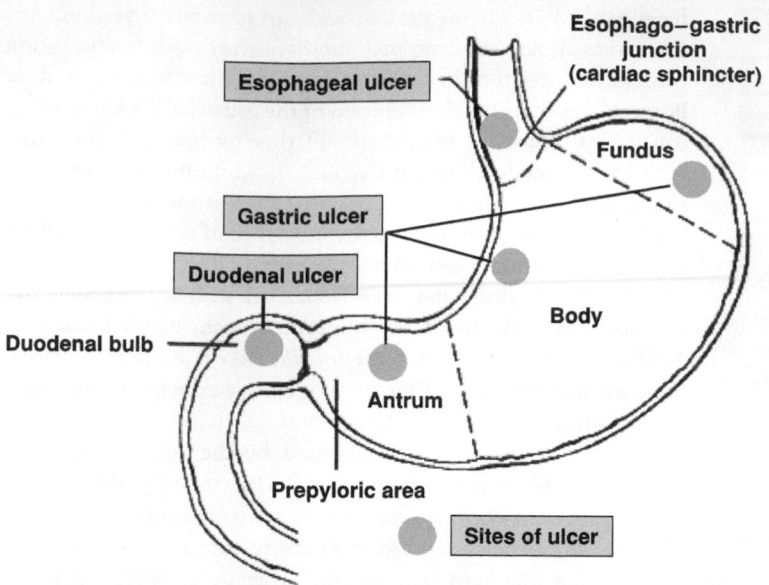

FIGURE 91-5. Anatomical location of peptic ulcers.

PEPTIC ULCER DISEASE

Definition

Peptic ulcer is a break of the mucosa lining the stomach or the duodenum. According to their anatomical location, peptic ulcers are divided into *gastric ulcers*, i.e., peptic ulcers of the gastric fundus, body or antrum, *prepyloric and pylori ulcers*, i.e., located within 3 cm from the pyloric ring and in the pyloric ring respectively, and *duodenal ulcers*, i.e., located into the bulb or in the second portion of the duodenum (Figure 91-5).

Epidemiology

The worldwide peptic ulcer prevalence differs, with duodenal ulcers dominating in western populations and gastric ulcers being more frequent in Asia. Although the incidence of peptic ulcer disease in western countries has declined over the past 100 years, almost 1 in 10 Americans is still affected. Even if the most recent epidemiological studies indicate that the prevalence and the incidence of the peptic ulcer show a constant decline in the general population, the incidence of complicated gastric and duodenal ulcer hospitalization (Figure 91-6) and mortality (Figure 91-7) remain very high in older patients.

Pathophysiology

Two main factors that might explain the observed increase in the incidence of peptic ulcer in elderly patients are the high prevalence of *H pylori* infection and the increasing use of damaging drugs, i.e., NSAIDs and/or aspirin. Nevertheless, in elderly subjects, around 20% of all the peptic ulcers are not associated with the use of damaging drugs or with an *H pylori* infection (Figure 91-8). Pathophysiology of these "idiopathic" non-NSAID, non-*H pylori* peptic ulcers

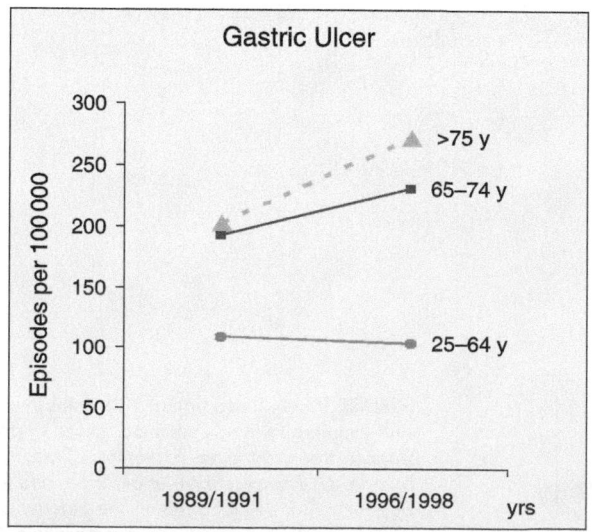

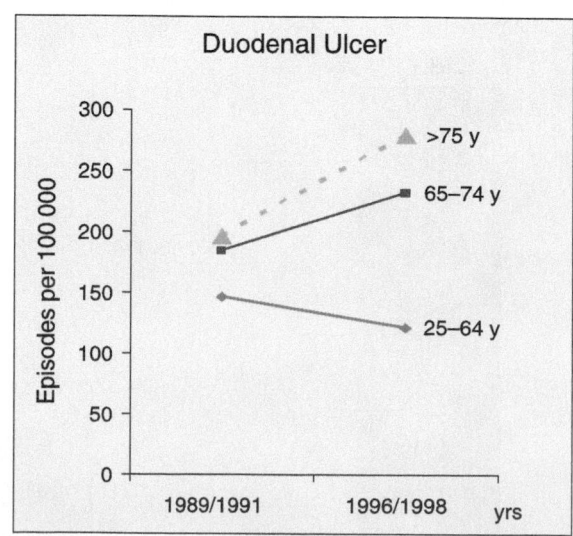

FIGURE 91-6. Trends in hospital admission owing to peptic ulcer in England according to age. (*Adapted from Higham J, Kang JY, Majeed A. Recent trends in admissions and mortality due to peptic ulcer in England: increasing frequency of haemorrhage among older subjects. Gut. 2002;50:460–464.*)

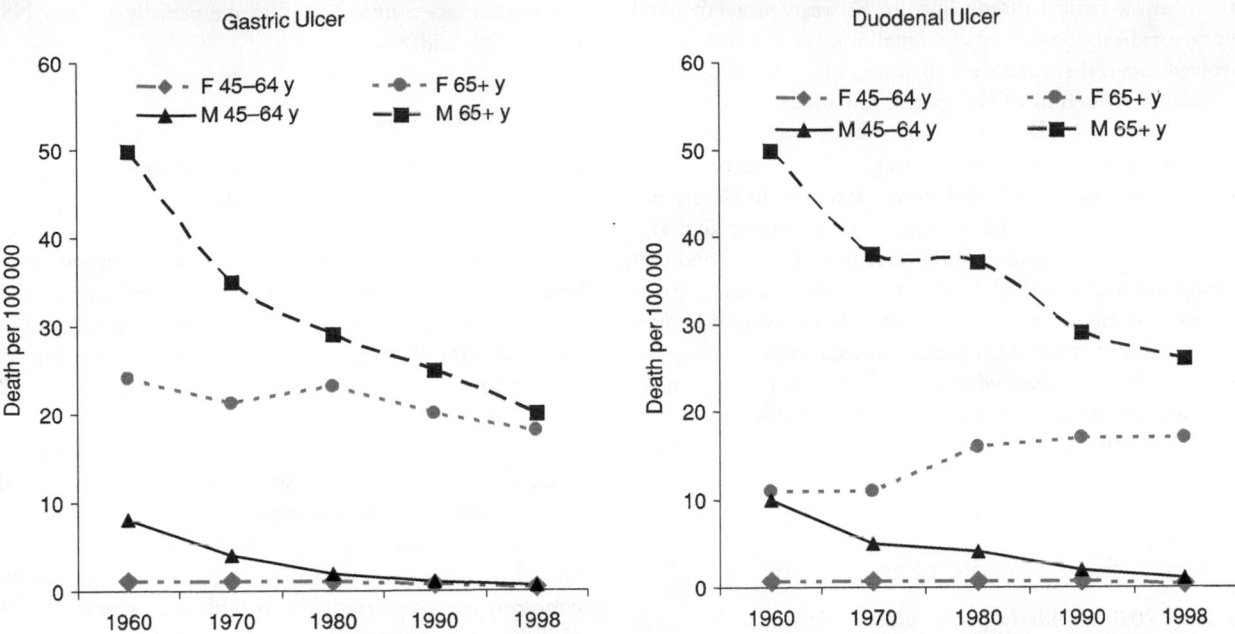

FIGURE 91-7. Age specific mortality rates for males (M) and females (F) for gastric and duodenal ulcer in England. *(Adapted from Higham J, Kang JY, Majeed A. Recent trends in admissions and mortality due to peptic ulcer in England: increasing frequency of haemorrhage among older subjects. Gut. 2002;50:460–464.)*

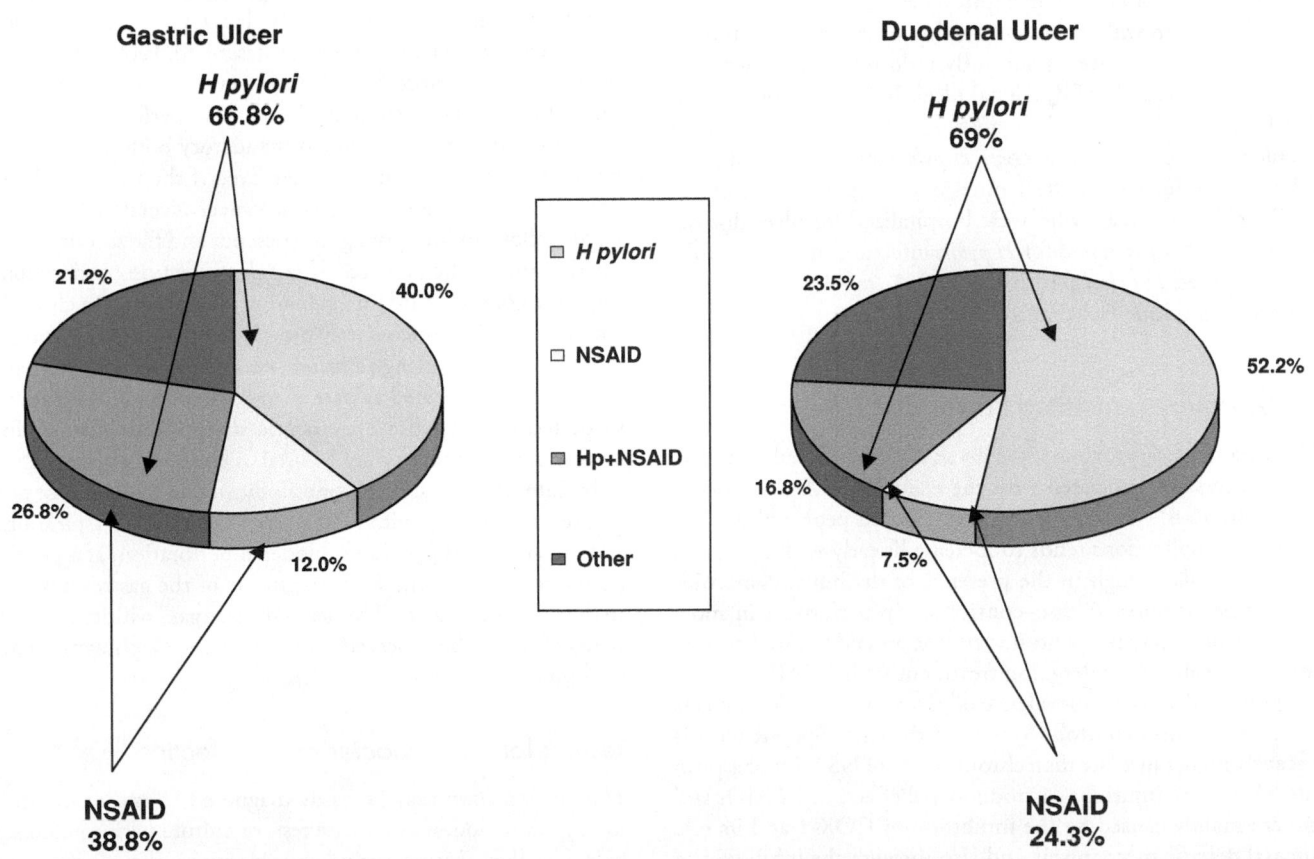

FIGURE 91-8. Prevalence of gastric and duodenal ulcer in elderly patients divided according to the presence of *H pylori* infection and/or NSAID use. *(Adapted from Pilotto. Aging and upper gastrointestinal disorders. Best Pract Res Clin Gastroenterol. 2004;18:73–81.)*

is still uncertain; a critical disequilibrium between protective and aggressive factors in the gastric or duodenal mucosa, however, seems to be involved. Several studies demonstrated that advancing age is associated with a reduction of the gastric mucosal barrier, i.e., the capacity to resist external damage owing to secretion of gastric mucus, bicarbonate secretion, mucosal prostaglandins, gastric mucosal proliferation and/or mucosal blood flow. Moreover, in elderly patients with peptic ulcer, normal or high levels of gastric acid and pepsin secretions have been observed. Previous studies reported that advancing age was independently related to chronic atrophic gastritis and a functional status of hypo/achlorhydria. More recent data suggested that atrophic changes of the gastric mucosa are associated with *H pylori* infection rather than with aging. Emotional stress, smoking tobacco and/or alcohol use are even potential risk factors that may contribute to the development of peptic ulcer in predisposed subjects.

Helicobacter pylori-Associated Peptic Ulcer

Approximately 70% of elderly peptic ulcer patients are *H pylori*-positive (Figure 91-8). Controlled studies, performed on elderly patients, reported that the treatment of *H pylori* infection healed ulcers in more than 95% of patients and improved symptoms in more than 85% of patients. Moreover, long-term studies performed in elderly patients with peptic ulcer demonstrated that the eradication of *H pylori* infection significantly improved clinical outcome, reducing ulcer recurrences and symptoms. Significant reduction of ulcer relapses after *H pylori* eradication is the main factor that demonstrated the pathogenic role of *H pylori* in peptic ulcer disease. Indeed, health programs leading to widespread eradication of *H pylori* infection in symptomatic patients have significantly reduced the prevalence of peptic ulcer, particularly of duodenal ulcer, both in Europe and in the Far East. Unfortunately, the percentage of elderly patients with peptic ulcer who are treated for their *H pylori* infection is still quite low. A study performed in the United States reported that of patients older than 65 years who were hospitalized for ulcer disease, only 40% to 56% were tested for *H pylori* infection; among the subjects who resulted *H pylori*-positive, only 50% to 73% were treated with specific antibiotic-based anti-*H pylori* therapy.

NSAID/Aspirin-Associated Peptic Ulcer

In elderly patients, approximately 25% of duodenal ulcers and 40% of gastric ulcers are associated with the use of NSAIDs and/or aspirin (Figure 91-8). The risk of NSAID-related peptic ulcers and their severe complications tends to increase linearly with aging and becomes particularly high in the presence of disability, comorbidity, and comedications. A case–control study performed in more than 3000 elderly patients who underwent an endoscopy has documented that subjects undergoing treatment with NSAIDs and/or aspirin presented a higher prevalence of gastric and duodenal ulcers compared to nonuser controls. Moreover, the risk of peptic ulcer is significantly higher in acute than chronic users of NSAIDs or aspirin (Figure 91-9). The injurious gastroduodenal effects of NSAIDs and aspirin are mainly caused by the inhibition of COX-1 and its role in mucosal defense mechanisms and also through the inhibition of thromboxane A2, which reduces platelet functions, resulting in a higher risk of bleeding. However, a direct effect on gastroduodenal mucosal surface cannot be excluded especially by those NSAIDs that have a high acid/base pK ratio.

Clinical Features

In the elderly, peptic ulcer is often difficult to diagnose. Indeed, symptoms of peptic ulcer may be atypical in old age. The patient's concomitant diseases and treatments may cause symptoms that mask those of the ulcer. A study reported that in patients older than 60 years, only one-third suffered from typical epigastric pain, and two-thirds experienced vague abdominal pain as a main symptom. Moreover, the intensity of pain may be less severe in older subjects and therefore may not receive the full attention of the physician or may not be taken seriously by the patient him/herself. Frequently, symptomatology includes nausea, vomiting, weight loss, and/or anorexia as the first, or even the only, symptom of peptic ulcer in the elderly. Unfortunately, it is not rare that the first symptom might be owing to a severe complication, especially bleeding or stenosis. In a study carried out in patients aged 80 years or more, the most common symptom was epigastric pain in both gastric and duodenal ulcers, while anemia and vomiting were most common among the patients suffering from duodenal ulcers. Because of the insidious clinical presentation of the disease in elderly patients, the consequences of peptic ulcer disease are more serious than those in younger subjects.

Diagnostic Tests

Upper GI *endoscopy* is always indicated for elderly subjects with new abdominal symptoms because of the high prevalence of serious gastric diseases in this age group. By direct visual identification, the location and size of an ulcer can be described. Peptic ulcer is a round to oval mucosal defect, from 5 mm to even 4 cm in diameter, with a smooth base and perpendicular borders. To perform a series of biopsies for excluding malignancy is mandatory both in the center and on the borders of the gastric ulcer, even if they are not elevated or irregular as in the advanced gastric cancer-ulcerative forms. Gastric *biopsies* allow for identifying the presence and the severity of chronic gastritis and/or the presence of *H pylori* infection. Endoscopic healing is the gold standard for evaluating ulcer healing in clinical trials. The surrounding mucosa may present radial folds, as a consequence of the parietal scarring. *Barium radiography* of the stomach and duodenum is indicated as part of the evaluation of the patient with suspected motility disorders, peptic strictures, or fistulas. In these last cases, gastrograffin may be used as contrast medium alternative to barium. Radiography is contraindicated in the presence of bleeding, severe vomiting with a high risk of pulmonary aspiration, or in cases of suspected gastric or duodenal perforation. If a peptic ulcer perforates, air will leak from the inside of the gastrointestinal tract to the peritoneal cavity. This leads to "free gas" within the peritoneal cavity that may be observed underneath the diaphragm on an erect or supine lateral *abdominal x-ray*.

Testing for Helicobacter pylori Infection

H pylori infection may be easily diagnosed by means of either histology evaluation, rapid urease test, or culture performed on gastric biopsies taken during endoscopy. However, the biopsy site needs to be selected with care, since *H pylori* may only be found in the fundus or body and not in the antral mucosa of elderly patients who

	NSAID Acute Users		NSAID Chronic Users	
	OR	95% CI	OR	95% CI
Gastric ulcer	4.47	3.19–6.26	2.80	1.97–3.99
Duodenal ulcer	2.39	1.73–3.31	1.68	1.22–2.33

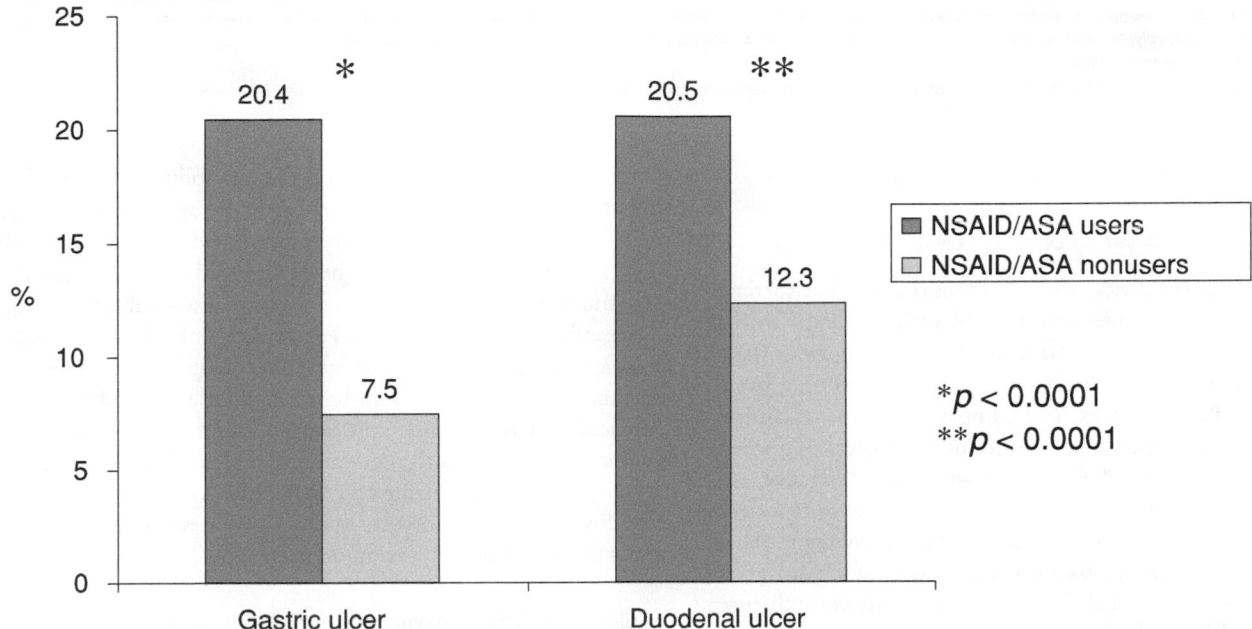

FIGURE 91-9. Prevalence of gastric ulcer and duodenal ulcer in NSAID users and NSAID nonusers. *(Data from Pilotto A, Franceschi M, Leandro G, et al. Proton-pump inhibitors reduce the risk of uncomplicated peptic ulcer in elderly either acute or chronic users of aspirin/non-steroidal anti-inflammatory drugs. Aliment Pharmacol Ther. 2004;20:1091–1097.)*

are taking antisecretory drugs. Moreover, the presence of chronic atrophic gastritis as a result of a past colonization of *H pylori* may be associated with a lower prevalence of the bacterium in the gastric biopsy specimens in the elderly than in adult or young patients. For the same reasons, the rapid urease test performed on gastric biopsies has lower sensitivity in subjects 60 years and older compared with younger patients. These findings suggest that in the elderly (1) it is advisable to perform gastric biopsies from both the antrum and the body of the stomach; and (2) a second test for *H pylori* should be performed in this age group if a urease-based or histological test is negative.

Posttreatment *Helicobacter pylori* Evaluation

Successful eradication should always be confirmed by a noninvasive or an invasive test if endoscopy is clinically indicated. Elderly patients with a diagnosis of peptic ulcer (especially gastric ulcer), gastric mucosa-associated lymphoid tissue, lymphoma, or severe gastritis should be evaluated by endoscopy and gastric mucosal histology after completion of anti-*H pylori* therapy. Most experts agree that this evaluation must be carried out at least 1 month after completion of therapy in order to minimize false-negative results. Elderly patients with mild or moderate forms of chronic gastritis may be evaluated after therapy by a noninvasive test. The ^{13}C-urea breath

test demonstrated significantly higher sensitivity, specificity, and diagnostic accuracy than serology (IgG anti-*H pylori* antibodies) in elderly subjects. An *H pylori* stool antigen (HpSA) test for the detection of *H pylori* was suggested as a valuable option with a high-potential role in the diagnosis after eradication therapy. The HpSA test is an easy and quick procedure that does not require expensive equipment. In hospitalized frail older patients, the HpSA was significantly less accurate than the ^{13}C-urea breath test, while antibiotic therapy and corpus atrophy decreased the positivity rate. Another study of geriatric subjects reported that HpSA test had a posttreatment diagnostic accuracy comparable to the ^{13}C-urea breath test (91% vs. 92%) without influence by cognitive status, disability, concomitant diseases, and cotreatments.

Other Noninvasive Tests

Serum pepsinogen I and II levels (sPGI, sPGII) are known to increase in the presence of *H pylori*-related nonatrophic gastritis. sPGII levels are higher in subjects with both gastric and duodenal ulcer, and levels correlate with the severity of inflammation. A study in older people reported that sPGII levels decreased significantly after a successful *H pylori* cure. The clinical usefulness of serum pepsinogens for monitoring elderly peptic ulcer patients remains to be established.

TABLE 91-7

Cumulative Results of Clinical Trials Evaluating 1-Week PPI-Based Triple Therapies Against *Helicobacter pylori* Infection in Elderly Patients

TRIPLE THERAPY	PATIENTS (n)	ERADICATION		DROP OUTS (%)	SIDE EFFECTS (%)
		ITT (%)	PP (%)		
PPI + C + M or T	296	88.2	90.9	3.0	3.4
PPI + A* + C	253	84.2	89.1	5.5	7.1
PPI + A* + M	154	79.8	83.7	4.5	7.1

ITT, intention-to-treat analysis; PP, per-protocol analysis; PPI, proton pump inhibitors, i.e., omeprazole 20 mg daily or twice daily, lansoprazole 30 mg twice daily, or pantoprazole 40 mg daily; C, clarithromycin 250 mg twice daily; M, metronidazole 250 mg four times a day or 500 mg twice daily; T, tinidazole 500 mg twice daily; A, amoxicillin.

*1 g twice daily or 500 mg three times a day.

Modified from Pilotto A, Franceschi M, Perri F, et al. Treatment options for Helicobacter pylori infection in the elderly. Aging Health. 2006;2:661–668.

Treatment Options for Peptic Ulcer Disease

Eradication of *Helicobacter pylori* Infection

There is currently a worldwide consensus that the first-line therapy for eradication of *H pylori* infection should be triple therapy with a PPI twice daily combined with clarithromycin 500 mg twice daily and amoxicillin 1 g twice daily or a nitroimidazole 500 mg twice daily for a minimum of 7 days. The cumulative results of clinical trials evaluating anti-*H pylori* therapies in elderly subjects confirmed that PPI-based triple therapies for 1 week were highly effective and well tolerated. Adverse event rates of less than 13% were reported, with less than 6% of patients discontinuing therapy owing to these effects (Table 91-7). In elderly patients, a reduction of the dosage of the PPI from a twice to once daily standard dose did not influence cure rates of the PPI-triple therapies. Since aging may modify the pharmacokinetic distribution of clarithromycin, independent of renal function, clinical trials evaluated the efficacy of PPI-based triple therapies including clarithromycin at a low dose of 250 mg twice daily in combination with a PPI and amoxicillin (at the standard dosage of 1 g twice daily) or metronidazole (at the dosage of 400 mg or 500 mg twice daily) in older patients. Results demonstrated no significant differences in cure rates and tolerability between clarithromycin 250 mg versus 500 mg twice daily. All these findings suggest that in elderly patients, 1-week PPI-based triple therapies should include low doses of both PPIs and clarithromycin, in combination with standard doses of either amoxicillin or a nitroimidazole to obtain excellent cure rates and tolerability. Increasing the duration of treatment from 7 days to 14 days is associated with higher eradication rates. At present, however, no studies have evaluated the clinical usefulness of these 2-week triple therapy regimens specifically in elderly patients. Low compliance and antibiotic resistance are the two major reasons for treatment failure. Primary resistance to amoxicillin remains uncommon, but the frequency of clarithromycin resistance is now around 10% in most European countries and the United States. Metronidazole resistance ranges between 20% and 30% and is more frequent among women and in developing countries. Consensus exists in using clarithromycin and metronidazole for *H pylori* eradication therapies when prevalences of antibiotic resistance are lower than 15% and 40%, respectively. A multicenter study from north-eastern Italy, carried out in subjects 25 to 90 years old, documented that primary resistance to metronidazole was 15% and to clarithromycin 1.8%, without significant differences in patients of different ages. Because failure of therapy is often associated with secondary antibiotic resistance, re-treatment should ideally be guided by data on susceptibility. Since, such information is often unavailable, quadruple therapies, in which a PPI or an H2-blocker is added to a bismuth-based triple regimen with high-dose metronidazole, have been proposed as second-line therapy. Another retreatment approach without susceptibility testing is to prescribe a second course of PPI–based triple therapy, avoiding antimicrobial agents against which prior therapy may have induced resistance. If a clarithromycin-based regimen was used first, PPI–amoxicillin or tetracycline and metronidazole regimens should be recommended if bismuth is not available. Unfortunately, no data in elderly patients are available on possible alternative rescue therapies including rifabutin or the new fluoroquinolones as well as probiotic agents as part of an eradication regimen.

Treatment and Prevention of NSAID-Related Peptic Ulcer

NSAID- or aspirin-associated peptic ulcers usually heal after 4 to 8 weeks of treatment with a PPI. Healing rates are higher if NSAID or aspirin treatments are stopped. Presently, no consensus exists on the clinical usefulness of a maintenance therapy with antisecretory drugs in patients who stopped NSAID or aspirin treatment after healing an NSAID-related peptic ulcer. The following strategies have been suggested to prevent NSAID- or aspirin-related gastroduodenal peptic ulcer in the elderly (Table 91-8).

Identify the High-Risk Patient. Current strategies to reduce ulcer relapse and/or complications are considered cost-effective in

TABLE 91-8

Strategies for the Prevention of NSAID- or Aspirin-Related Gastroduodenal Peptic Ulcer in the Elderly

STRATEGIES

1. Identify the high-risk patient
   History of upper GI symptoms
   History of peptic ulcer and bleeding
   Old age
   Disability
   Comorbidity
   Comedications (oral steroids, antiplatelet drugs, warfarin)
2. Reduce dosage and use less damaging NSAIDs
3. Use of coxibs
4. Cotreatment with gastroprotective drugs
5. Eradication of H pylori infection
6. Educational programs

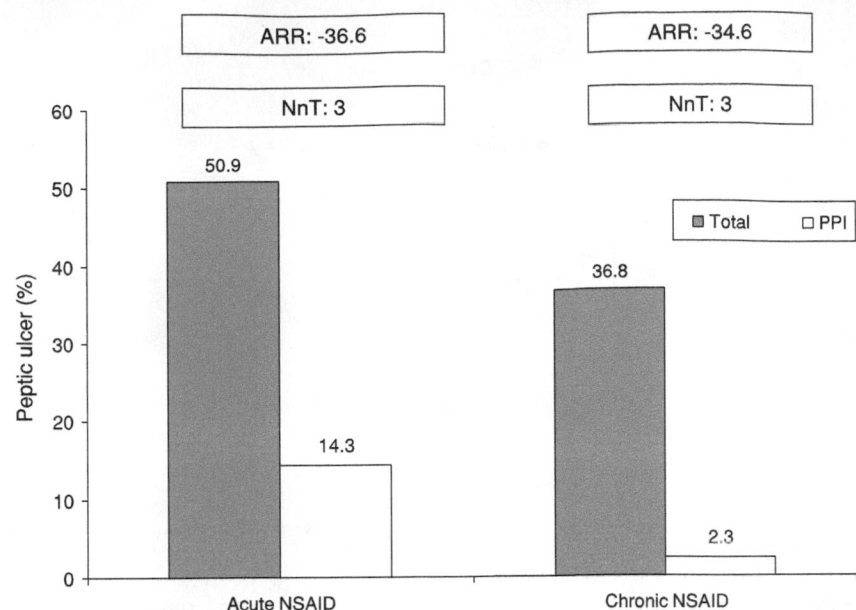

FIGURE 91-10. Absolute risk reduction (ARR) of peptic ulcer and the number needed to treat (NnT) in elderly acute and chronic users of nonsteroidal anti-inflammatory drugs (NSAID) and/or aspirin concomitantly treated with proton pump inhibitors (PPIs). *(Data from Pilotto A, Franceschi M, Leandro G, et al. Proton-pump inhibitors reduce the risk of uncomplicated peptic ulcer in elderly either acute or chronic users of aspirin/non-steroidal anti-inflammatory drugs. Aliment Pharmacol Ther. 2004;20:1091–1097.)*

high-risk patients. Great importance is placed, therefore, on defining those patients who are at high risk for peptic ulcer when treated with NSAIDs or aspirin. A history of upper GI symptoms, peptic ulcer and/or bleeding; old age; the presence of disability, comorbidity; and concomitant medications, particularly oral steroids, antiplatelet drugs, and warfarin increase the risk of NSAID-related peptic ulcer and/or its complications. Thus, a comprehensive geriatric assessment may be useful in the evaluation of the multidimensional risk of elderly patient.

Reduce Dosage and Use Less Damaging NSAIDs. The risk of peptic ulcer and its complications appears to be directly related to dose of the given NSAID and coxib. Lower risk of upper GI damage has been reported with NSAIDs with a short plasma half-life versus those with a prolonged plasma half-time. Independent of this, however, slow release formulations present an augmented risk of ulcer complications.

Use of Selective Inhibitors of Cyclo-Oxygenase-2 (Coxibs). The selective inhibitors of cyclo-oxygenase (COX)-2 are claimed to be as effective in relieving pain and inflammation in osteoarthritis patients as traditional NSAIDs. Postmarketing observational studies indicate a lower ulcer complications in elderly patients treated with coxibs versus conventional NSAIDs. Concomitant use of aspirin, however, negates their superior gastrointestinal safety over NSAIDs. In high-risk patients, that is, elderly patients with a previous history of NSAID-related ulcer or bleeding, who need anti-inflammatory treatments, the use of celecoxib is not safer than a combination of the NSAID diclofenac and the PPI omeprazole. Moreover, combination treatment with a celecoxib plus a PPI is more effective than coxib alone in preventing peptic ulcer and its complication. Since selective inhibition of COX-2 may induce both cardiovascular and renal adverse events as do traditional NSAIDs, a very careful evaluation of the elderly patient is recommended before prescribing these medications.

Cotreatment with Gastroprotective Drugs. Several meta-analyses of controlled trials on gastroprotective drug treatments reported that misoprostol and PPIs are more effective than H2-blockers in preventing both gastric and duodenal severe damage. Indeed, misoprostol administered at effective doses of 200 μg four times daily induced significantly higher adverse effects, particularly diarrhea, than PPIs and placebo. PPIs were very effective in preventing gastroduodenal injuries in both acute and chronic elderly users of NSAIDs (Figure 91-10). Similarly, significant efficacy of PPIs for the prevention of peptic ulcer and its complications has been reported in elderly patients treated with low-dose aspirin as antiplatelet therapy, independent of the presence of *H pylori* infection.

Eradication of *Helicobacter pylori* Infection. NSAID-use and *H pylori* infection are independent risk factors for peptic ulcer and gastroduodenal bleeding in elderly subjects. In *H pylori*-positive patients who are starting long-term treatment with NSAIDs, the cure of *H pylori* infection significantly reduces the 6-month risk of peptic ulcer. In elderly high-risk patients, however, the use of PPIs concomitantly with the NSAID reduces the occurrence of both acute and chronic NSAID-related gastroduodenal damage more effectively than the eradication of *H pylori* infection. Moreover, after the eradication of *H pylori*, maintenance treatment with a PPI is more effective than placebo in the prevention of ulcer bleeding in elderly patients. All these findings suggest that *H pylori* eradication may be a useful strategy, but it is not sufficient for the prevention of severe gastroduodenal damage in elderly *H pylori*-positive NSAID and aspirin users.

Educational Programs. A crucial strategy in the prevention of NSAID-related adverse events is the discontinuation of NSAID therapy. Indeed, a study from Canada reported an estimated 37% of unnecessary NSAID prescriptions in elderly patients with osteoarthritis. Similarly, a study from the United States reported that almost 50% of NSAID prescriptions in elderly patients were inappropriate. Active interventions to improve appropriateness of drug prescription, particularly in the elderly, demonstrated a reduction in NSAID prescriptions. A significant reduction in NSAID use was observed by a nurse-delivered advice intervention on NSAID use involving patients in general practice. A significant reduction in

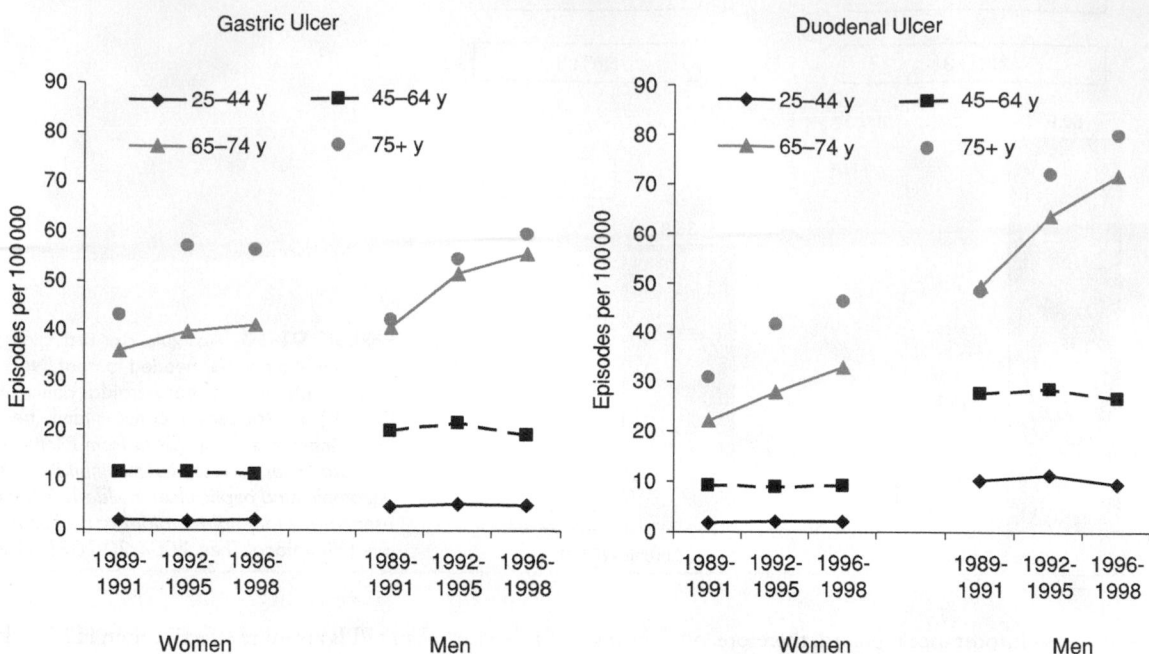

FIGURE 91-11. Average annual age-standardized rate for peptic ulcer hemorrhage in England from 1989 to 1998. (*Adapted from Higham J, Kang JY, Majeed A. Recent trends in admissions and mortality due to peptic ulcer in England: increasing frequency of haemorrhage among older subjects. Gut. 2002;50:460–464.*)

re-hospitalization rates for peptic ulcer as well as mortality rates within 1-year was observed in elderly subjects who participated in a quality improvement project in the United States that involved counseling of patients and their caregivers about NSAID toxicity.

Non-NSAID, Non-*Helicobacter pylori* Ulcers

Antisecretory therapy remains the cornerstone of treatment to promote ulcer healing. Standard doses of PPIs should be prescribed at least for 4 weeks in patients with duodenal ulcers and for 8 weeks in patients with gastric ulcers. Generally, patients respond well to these therapies, and no established evidence supports the need for a longer duration or higher dose of antisecretory therapy in uncomplicated idiopathic ulcer. Elderly nonresponders should be investigated for any possible underlying pathophysiology, including compliance, acid hypersecretory state, or use of damaging drugs.

Bleeding Peptic Ulcer

Epidemiological studies reported that the prevalence of bleeding complications of peptic ulcer has increased during the last 10 to 15 years in patients who are older than 65 (Figure 91-11). A study performed in elderly residents in the United States has confirmed that the risk of hospitalization for bleeding was significantly associated with an age above 80 years, a limitation in the instrumental activities of daily living, comorbidity, and multiple drugs used. Recent meta-analyses indicate that best management of acute bleeding ulcer includes a combination treatment with endoscopy (heater probe or laser coagulation and/or injection of vasoactive drugs) and PPIs. These treatments might reduce the rates of re-bleeding and surgery interventions; unfortunately, no modification of short- and long-term mortality rates has been observed with all these strategies (Table 91-9). In elderly patients with bleeding, however, a comprehensive geriatric assessment demonstrates a very high prognostic value

TABLE 91-9

PPI Therapy and Outcome of Endoscopic Hemostasis in Bleeding Peptic Ulcer			
	RE-BLEEDING	**SURGERY**	**MORTALITY**
EndoTx + PPI vs. PPI alone	0.2 (0.09–0.4)	0.17 (0.06–0.4)	NS
EndoTx + PPI vs. EndoTx alone	0.5 (0.37–0.7)	NS	NS
EndoTx + PPI bolus vs. infusion	NS	NS	NS
PPI after EndoTx vs. EndoTx alone	0.52 (0.4–0.7)	0.53 (0.35–0.8)	NS
Oral PPI	0.32 (0.2–0.5)	0.38 (0.2–0.6)	NS
Intravenous PPI	0.57 (0.4–0.7)	0.67 (0.5–0.9)	NS

Data from Andriulli A, Annese V, Caruso N, et al. Proton-pump inhibitors and outcome of endoscopic hemostasis in bleeding peptic ulcers: a series of meta-analyses. Am J Gastroenterol. 2005;100:207–219 and Leontiadis GI, Sharma VK, Howden CW. Systematic review and meta-analysis of proton pump inhibitor therapy in peptic ulcer bleeding. BMJ. 2005;330:568–570.

for mortality. This finding suggests that general conditions and the severity of multidimensional impairments of elderly patients are crucial points in evaluating the outcome of this severe clinical condition.

NEOPLASM OF THE ESOPHAGUS

Esophageal Cancer

Two major histologic types of esophageal cancer are described: squamous cell carcinoma and adenocarcinoma. Although the incidence of squamous cell carcinoma has remained relatively static during the last decades, the incidence of esophageal adenocarcinoma has increased dramatically.

Squamous Cell Carcinoma

Esophageal squamous cell cancer accounts for 5% to 7% of all gastrointestinal malignancies. The annual incidence in the United States is 3 to 4 cases per 100 000 persons. The incidence increases with age, being most common in men in their sixth and seventh decades of life. Risk factors (Table 91-10) for squamous cell cancer include alcohol and tobacco use, caustic esophageal injury, chronic strictures, achalasia, squamous carcinoma of the nasopharynx, partial gastrectomy, and human papilloma virus. The incidence and mortality rates are much higher in elderly black men when compared to other group populations. Symptoms of esophageal cancer generally develop only when the tumor has grown to the extent that it has narrowed the lumen of the esophagus substantially, has invaded local structures, or has metastasized. Dysphagia is the most common symptom; other manifestations include coughing and/or choking (because of invasion of the tumor into of the tracheobronchial tree), hoarseness (because of invasion of a recurrent laryngeal nerve), or hematemesis (because of tumor invasion of aorta or the presence of an aorto-esophageal fistula). Ulcerated tumors can cause odynophagia. Since anorexia and weight loss usually precede the onset of dysphagia, the physical examination of these patients at the time of the diagnosis

TABLE 91-10

Common Risk Factors for Esophageal Cancers	
SQUAMOUS CELL CARCINOMA	**ADENOCARCINOMA**
60–70 yrs of age	50–60 yrs of age
Achalasia	Barrett esophagus
Alcohol abuse	Gastroesophageal reflux disease
Black populations	Caucasian populations
Male sex	Male sex
High-starch diet without fruits and vegetables	
Lye ingestion	
Plummer–Vinson syndrome	
Previous head and neck squamous cell carcinoma	
Radiation therapy	
Smoking	

often reveals malnutrition and dehydration. Metastatic disease may be responsible for bone pain.

Adenocarcinoma

Adenocarcinoma of the esophagus has been increasing in frequency at an alarming rate over the past few decades, now accounting for more than 50% of the newly diagnosed esophageal cancers. The annual incidence of adenocarcinoma of the esophagus and gastric cardias is 5.1 cases per 100,000 persons. Unlike squamous cell carcinoma, adenocarcinoma typically affects elderly white males. Barrett esophagus secondary to long-standing reflux disease is the single most important risk factor for adenocarcinoma (Table 91-10). Patients with Barrett esophagus are 30 to 125 times more likely to have adenocarcinoma of the esophagus than the general population. The estimated incidence of adenocarcinoma in patients with Barrett esophagus is 0.2% to 2.1% per year.

The clinical presentation is similar to that of squamous cell carcinoma, but malnutrition, fistulas, and recurrent laryngeal nerve involvement are less common and extension into the stomach, diaphragm, and the liver are more frequent. More than 80% of the tumors are in the distal esophagus. The diagnostic evaluation, treatment modalities, and prognosis are similar to those for squamous cell carcinoma. However, with increased use of endoscopic surveillance, adenocarcinoma can be diagnosed at an earlier stage than squamous cell carcinoma.

Diagnosis

Endoscopy with biopsies and cytology is the best way to establish the diagnosis. The mid-esophagus and/or the distal esophagus are the most common sites affected. The majority of symptomatic lesions are ulcerated in the center with heaped up margins and encroachment on the lumen. However, early lesions may be subtle and almost normal in appearance. In vivo staining with Lugol iodine or toluidine blue may be helpful for discovering the abnormal mucosa. *Barium esophagogram* may show tumors, but has low sensitivity in the detection of early tumors. Usually *computed tomography* of the chest and abdomen is recommended to assess the extent of disease within the chest and to look for metastases. However, the sensitivity and specificity of CT for determining the depth of esophageal tumor penetration (the T status) and the presence of regional lymph node metastases (the N status) are poor. *Endoscopic ultrasonography* is superior to CT in this regard, accurately predicting the T and N status in 70% to 80% of patients.

Treatment

Cancer of the esophagus usually is disseminated at the time of diagnosis and because there is no treatment that reliably eradicates metastatic disease, cure is not possible in most cases. Initial treatment usually involves a choice between surgery, radiation therapy, chemotherapy, and some combination of these three modalities. Squamous cell cancer and adenocarcinoma are treated similarly, with similarly poor survival rates. Overall cure rates for cancer of the esophagus remain below 10%. Treatment and survival, therefore, depends on the stage of the disease. Elderly patients, especially white men, should be screened for Barrett esophagus, and if identified, patients should be placed in endoscopic *surveillance programs* and on aggressive antireflux therapy with PPIs. However, PPIs as

TABLE 91-11

Endoscopic Surveillance of Barrett Esophagus

DYSPLASIA	ENDOSCOPY
Absent	Every 2–3 yr after at least two endoscopies negative for dysplasia
Low grade	At 6–12 mo, every yr (in absence of progression)
High grade	Histological confirmation Focal: every 3 mo Focal multiple: esophageal resection or endoscopic ablation

Modified from Sampliner RE. Practice guidelines on the diagnosis, surveillance, and therapy of Barrett's esophagus. The Practice Parameters Committee of the American College of Gastroenterology. Am J Gastroenterol. 1998;93:1028–32.

well as antireflux surgery have not been shown to consistently cause regression of the Barrett epithelium or prevention of esophageal cancer. Surveillance involves obtaining four-quadrant biopsies at 2-cm intervals in the Barrett segment using a jumbo biopsy forceps as well as biopsies of any other mucosal abnormalities such as nodules or ulcers. If the biopsies are negative for dysplasia, endoscopy should be repeated within 1 year, followed by endoscopy every 2 to 3 years. If low-grade or indefinite dysplasia is identified, the surveillance interval is shortened to every 6 months for 1 year, followed by annual surveillance. If high-grade dysplasia is found, endoscopy is repeated at 1 month. If high-grade dysplasia is confirmed by two independent pathologists, options include esophagectomy or continued surveillance every 3 months. Ablative endoscopic therapies such as photodynamic therapy, laser, argon plasma coagulation, and multipolar electrocoagulation appear to be very promising especially in patients who are poor surgical candidates (Table 91-11).

Early cancers, that is, limited to the mucosa and the submucosa, can be cured by esophagectomy, but cure is not always possible because of presentation of cancers at a late stage. In patients with *superficial cancers* limited to the mucosa who are poor candidates for surgery, options include endoscopic mucosal resection or ablation with electrocautery, argon plasma coagulation, laser or photodynamic therapy. In locally *advanced cancer*, a multimodality approach involving surgery, radiation, and chemotherapy provides the best chance for survival. Squamous cell cancer, unlike adenocarcinoma, is radiosensitive. Majority of patients have some response to radiation therapy, but the response is brief, averaging approximately 3 months. The most widely used combination for chemotherapy, cisplatin and 5-fluorouracil, has shown a response in 20% to 40% of cases, but has no impact on survival.

Palliative Therapy

In patients with metastatic disease, treatment is mainly palliative. Palliative measures for dysphagia include esophageal dilation, stent placement, or endoscopic tumor ablation. The 5-year survival rates for TNM stage I, II, III, and IV cancers are 60%, 31%, 20%, and 4.1%, respectively.

Benign Tumors

Benign tumors are a rare entity representing less than 1% of all the esophageal neoplasms. Leiomyoma is the most common benign esophageal tumor. Esophageal leiomyomas may produce dysphagia and retrosternal chest pain, but in most cases are asymptomatic. If leiomyomas are symptomatic, surgical enucleation is indicated. Others benign tumors are squamous cell papillomas, fibrovascular polyps, and granular cell tumors.

GASTRIC CANCER

Epidemiology

Gastric cancer is an important disease in elderly patients with an estimated 21 700 new diagnoses in the United States in 2001. On a global scale, gastric cancer remains the world's second most common malignancy after lung cancer. The incidence of gastric cancer shows marked worldwide variation; while in industrialized countries, the incidence of gastric cancer is decreasing, in less developed countries gastric cancer is extremely common and often affects younger people. While distal gastric adenocarcinoma is more common in Afro-Asian populations, carcinoma of the cardia and fundus are more common in Caucasians, and their incidence is rising at an alarming rate. Adenocarcinoma makes up 90% of malignant gastric tumors with lymphoma accounting for a further 5%. The Lauren classification is traditionally used to divide adenocarcinoma into (1) an intestinal form, where the malignant cells form a glandular like structure; and (2) a diffuse form, where the cells infiltrate through the wall of the stomach with relatively little disturbance of the mucosa itself, making endoscopic diagnosis more difficult. Despite significant advances in the understanding of its etiology and pathogenesis, the mortality rate remains high and no more than 10% of patients will be alive 5 years from diagnosis. The risk of gastric cancer is strongly related to age. The median age of patients presenting with this cancer is around 72 years, and from the early 1990s, one-quarter of newly diagnosed gastric cancer patients are older than 80 years.

Etiology and Risk Factors

Pernicious anemia with its hallmark of atrophic gastritis has long been known to confer an increased risk of gastric cancer. Similarly, it is well established that benign ulcer surgery, such as partial gastrectomy, is associated with gastric cancer with a lead in time of 15 to 30 years. Following gastric surgery, inflammation of the gastric remnant is common and usually associated with the reflux of bile. Although the histological appearances are different, both pernicious anemia and the surgical stomach share a common pathophysiological abnormality—hypochlorhydria. Gastric cancer and gastric MALT lymphoma (lymphoma of the mucosa-associated lymphoid tissue) have been associated with *H pylori* infection, and the bacterium has been categorized as a group I carcinogen by the International Agency for Research on Cancer (IARC). *H pylori* infection induces, in genetically predisposed hosts, a cascade of events that could ultimately lead to gastric neoplasia. Several studies reported that the increased proliferation induced by inflammation creates a genetically unstable gastric mucosa, which is further compromised by the presence of genotoxic substances generated by inflammatory and bacterial products. The key pathophysiological events include the onset of gastric atrophy and hypochlorhydria. Hypochlorhydria itself contributes to bacterial overgrowth, which further exacerbates the inflammation and leads to generation of carcinogenic nitrogenous products. Diets that are high in salt content and lacking in

TABLE 91-12

Risk Factors for Stomach Cancer

RISK FACTORS

Male sex
Old age
H pylori infection
Foods that contain nitrites and nitrates
Tobacco use
Previous gastric surgery
Adenomatous polyps larger than 1 centimeter in diameter
Familial adenomatous polyposis (mutations in the BRCA1 and BRCA2 genes)
Hereditary diffuse gastric cancer
Atrophic gastritis
Type A blood group
Environmental cold dust, asbestos, and nickel exposure
Obesity

fresh fruits and vegetables are likely to contribute to the malignant transformation (Table 91-12). The role of time, that is, a long lasting infection with *H pylori*, is probably important in the development of all these mechanisms. Indeed, chronic atrophic gastritis and *H pylori* infection are commonly found in the same elderly subject. Most of the studies suggested that atrophic changes of the gastric mucosa are associated with *H pylori* infection rather than with aging itself. A prospective study was carried out in a group of elderly men with *H pylori* infection and atrophic corpus gastritis. During a 7.5-year period prior to eradication therapy, no significant changes were observed in the mean atrophy and intestinal metaplasia scores. However, after *H pylori* eradication, a significant improvement occurred in the mean histological score of inflammation, atrophy, and intestinal metaplasia. These findings suggest that advanced atrophic gastritis may improve after *H pylori* eradication also in elderly subjects.

Clinical Features

A symptomatic presentation is very often indicative of advanced stage. In western countries, the most common presenting symptoms are weight loss followed by abdominal pain, nausea and vomiting, anorexia, and dysphagia. Most of these symptoms are nonspecific and are very common in elderly patients for other reasons. In some studies, 40% of patients had symptoms for less than 3 months, but 60% were symptomatic for 3 months or longer and up to 20% for over 1 year. The late presentation of the disease probably explains why its prognosis remains so severe with only 10% of patients alive at 5 years. The clinical manifestations also depend critically on the anatomical location of the tumor. Large tumors in the fundus and body may simply manifest with occult blood loss. In contrast, tumors of the antrum will delay gastric emptying and lead to early satiety, anorexia, and eventually the features of gastric outlet obstruction. Tumors of the proximal stomach may involve the distal esophagus and present with dysphagia.

Diagnosis

The diagnosis of gastric cancer is easy in advanced cases, but may require a high index of suspicion: a careful history and examination are essential. Physical examination is frequently unrewarding even in advanced gastric cancer. A hypochromic, microcytic anemia is a common finding and the fecal occult blood test may be positive, although this does not localize the source of blood loss and as such it is not a helpful diagnostic tool in old age. *Upper GI endoscopy* has been shown to be more accurate than *barium radiology* in the diagnosis of gastric cancer. Endoscopy allows a close inspection of the mucosa, which is generally the only circumstance under which early gastric carcinoma is found. *Histological examination* of multiple biopsies is essential for diagnosis. As mentioned previously, gastric atrophy and intestinal metaplasia are common findings in elderly patients. The presence of dysplasia, however, should always be regarded as significant because it may indicate a high risk of malignant transformation, or it may reflect the presence of adjacent malignancy. Currently the diagnostic usefulness of the barium meal is limited in defining the extent of a tumor or in identifying eventual gastroenteric fistulas. *Ultrasonography* of the abdomen is useful for assessing the spread of gastric carcinoma. It may detect evidence of lymphadenopathy but can be particularly valuable in detecting metastases within the liver. A number of studies suggest that *endoscopic ultrasound* has an accuracy of 90% in defining the depth of invasion within the stomach itself. It is also sensitive to wall thickening and will pick up diffuse carcinomas, and it may allow for the identification of regional lymph nodes.

Treatment of Gastric Cancer

Age in itself is not a contraindication to aggressive treatment including curative surgery. Nevertheless, the operative risk must be well defined by a comprehensive geriatric assessment.

Surgery and Endoscopic Procedures

Surgical resection remains the only proven method of providing long-term survival in patients with gastric cancer, but it is effective only if a complete macro- and microscopic clearance of the tumor is possible (R_0 resection). In patients with very early tumors, alternatives to resection have been proposed including laser ablation, photodynamic therapy, and endoscopic mucosal resection. Clearly, such treatments avoid both the immediate and long-term morbidity associated with surgery, but can only be recommended for tumors limited to the gastric mucosa in which the incidence of lymphatic spread is minimal. In patients with mucosal disease, a policy of regular endoscopic surveillance combined with ablation of the surrounding mucosa is mandatory. As tumor invades into the submucosa, the incidence of lymphatic spread increases, and mucosal ablative techniques are unlikely to achieve clearance of the disease. If there is evidence of submucosal invasion, a formal resection is performed. Lesions that are ulcerated pose particular problems with infiltration and may also be difficult for the pathologist to interpret. Furthermore, some reports have indicated that such lesions may metastasize early to regional lymph nodes, and accordingly endoscopic mucosal resection is not recommended for these tumors.

Chemotherapy

The low survival associated with gastric cancer has prompted investigation into postoperative (adjuvant) chemotherapy, and preoperative treatment (neoadjuvant). In patients with gastric cancer, there is no evidence that either adjuvant or neoadjuvant chemotherapy is of value in patients in whom a complete surgical resection is possible. The elderly are more likely to have cardiac and renal impairments and therefore less likely to tolerate chemotherapy well and have a greater risk of side effects. A comprehensive geriatric assessment that exactly defines the multidimensional impairments of elderly patients is crucial in evaluating the role of adjuvant chemotherapy. This treatment must offer significant survival benefits weighed against the toxic effects and eventual hospitalizations and complications, particularly in very old subjects.

Palliative Therapy

The majority of elderly patients present with late gastric cancer at an advanced stage. Most will not be amenable to curative surgical resection, and the issue of palliation is therefore very important. Distal tumors involving the antrum frequently progress to *obstruction*. In some patients, this will be owing to physical stenosis of the pylorus, while in others gradual infiltration of the antrum leads to loss of functionality and a failure in gastric emptying. Medical treatment of outlet obstruction with prokinetics is usually unhelpful. The symptoms are usually unpleasant with vomiting, regurgitation and reflux, and rapid nutritional failure. Because of this, palliative surgical therapy is often justified and options include antrectomy or, more commonly, the formation of a gastroenterostomy to relieve obstruction. Alternative approaches may include laser to more localized lesions. If the distal esophagus is involved, patients with large tumors may also develop dysphagia. This complication is usually managed with stenting or sometimes with laser therapy. Large tumors frequently bleed and result in *chronic blood loss*. This may on occasion warrant consideration of surgery, although the difficulties of performing this on frail elderly patients should not be underestimated. Another alternative is to try to shrink the tumor using a neodymium YAG laser, but results on this technique for treating chronic blood loss are conflicting. Most patients with advanced gastric cancer develop *nutritional problems*, and weight loss is almost invariable. Extensive infiltration alters the compliance of the stomach and frequently leads to sensations of early satiety and loss of appetite. In addition, advanced gastric cancer frequently leads to profound metabolic effects such as cachexia and loss of muscle bulk. Some patients may benefit from radiotherapy, but adenocarcinoma is frequently not radiosensitive. The role of hospice and organized palliative care and pain teams is extremely important in improving the comfort of patients.

FURTHER READING

Andriulli A, Annese V, Caruso N, et al. Proton-pump inhibitors and outcome of endoscopic hemostasis in bleeding peptic ulcers: a series of meta-analyses. *Am J Gastroenterol.* 2005;100:207–219.

Barkun A, Bardou M, Marshall JK; Nonvariceal Upper GI Bleeding Consensus Conference Group. Consensus recommendations for managing patients with nonvariceal upper gastrointestinal bleeding. *Ann Intern Med.* 2003;139:843–857.

Dicken BJ, Bigam DL, Cass C, et al. Gastric adenocarcinoma: review and considerations for future directions. *Ann Surg.* 2005;241:27–39.

Garcia Rodriguez LA, Barreales Tolosa L. Risk of upper gastrointestinal complications among users of traditional NSAIDs and COXIBs in the general population. *Gastroenterology.* 2007;132:498–506.

Gee DW, Rattner DW. Management of gastroesophageal tumors. *Oncologist.* 2007;12:175–185.

Lanas A, Ferrandez A. Inappropriate prevention of NSAID-induced gastrointestinal events among long-term users in the elderly. *Drugs Aging.* 2007;24:121–131.

Leontiadis GI, Sharma VK, Howden CW. Proton pump inhibitor therapy for peptic ulcer bleeding: Cochrane collaboration meta-analysis of randomized controlled trials. *Mayo Clin Proc.* 2007;82:286–296.

Malfertheiner P, Megraud F, O'Morain C, et al. Current concepts in the management of *Helicobacter pylori* infection: the Maastricht III Consensus Report. *Gut.* 2007;56:772–781.

Pilotto A, Ferrucci L, Scarcelli C, et al. Usefulness of the comprehensive geriatric assessment in older patients with upper gastrointestinal bleeding: a two-year follow-up study. *Dig Dis.* 2007;25:124–128.

Pilotto A, Franceschi M, Leandro G, et al. Clinical features of reflux esophagitis in older people: a study of 840 consecutive patients. *J Am Geriatr Soc.* 2006;54:1537–1542.

Pilotto A, Franceschi M, Perri F, et al. Treatment options for *Helicobacter pylori* infection in the elderly. *Aging Health.* 2006;2:661–668.

Pilotto A, Malfertheiner P, Holt PR, editors. Aging and the gastrointestinal tract. *Interdisciplinary Topics in Gerontology.* Karger AG Press, Basel, Switzerland: 2003;32:1–218.

Richter JE. Gastroesophageal reflux disease in the older patient: presentation, treatment, and complications. *Am J Gastroenterol.* 2000;95:368–373.

Yuan Y, Padol IT, Hunt RH. Peptic ulcer disease today. *Nature Clin Pract Gastroenterol Hepatol.* 2006;3:80–89.

Common Large Intestinal Disorders

Leon S. Maratchi ■ *David A. Greenwald*

In the elderly, gastrointestinal (GI) disorders, especially those of the large intestine, account for a significant portion of physician visits, inpatient hospitalizations, and health care expenditure in the United States. Not only are large intestinal disorders common, but in the elderly their presentations, complications, and treatment may be different than in the young. This chapter focuses on diagnosis and treatment of a variety of diseases of the large intestine, including diverticular disease, *Clostridium difficile*-associated diarrhea, microscopic colitis, inflammatory bowel disease, colonic ischemia, colonic obstruction, and lower GI bleeding.

Diagnosis of GI disorders in an elderly patient poses several additional challenges to the physician on top of those present for all patients. First, comorbid illnesses are frequent and often numerous, and some such as dementia and depression may impair adequate communication between patient and caregiver. Second, medications and their side effects may cloud the clinical picture; polypharmacy is common in the elderly. Lastly, symptoms attributable to the large intestine may be manifestations of different diseases in the elderly than they would in the young. The astute geriatrician must take these factors into consideration when treating all patients.

DIAGNOSTIC TESTING

Symptoms of digestive diseases may be misinterpreted or atypical in the aged. For example, constipation may be a symptom of irritable bowel syndrome in a young patient, whereas it might herald an obstructing lesion in an older patient. Rectal bleeding in a young person is most commonly from hemorrhoids or inflammatory bowel disease. In the elderly, diverticulosis or colon cancer more commonly cause rectal bleeding. A complete and thorough history is imperative in patients, especially the elderly. Subtle clues to the diagnosis are sometimes dismissed as physiologic aspects of aging. Physical examination and some laboratory tests including tests of liver function

are unaffected by aging, and any abnormality should be evaluated for the presence of a disease state and not dismissed as an age-related change (Table 92-1).

Endoscopic Procedures

Colonoscopy

Colonoscopy in the elderly is safe and well tolerated. Several studies of indications and outcomes of patients older than 80 years having elective and emergency endoscopic procedures found those tests to be safe; advanced age is not a contraindication to endoscopy. Moreover, the yield for diagnostic testing with colonoscopy in the elderly is relatively high.

Adequate bowel preparation is critical to a successful colonoscopic examination. Bowel cleansing in the elderly should be performed with care. Preparation with standard doses of polyethylene glycol based lavage solutions (PEG-ELS) in the elderly is well tolerated and produces satisfactory bowel cleansing in more than 95% of all cases. Sodium phosphate osmotic laxative preparation may also be used for bowel preparation, but causes significant fluid shifts and may cause electrolyte abnormalities or renal failure in this subset of patients. Sodium phosphate laxatives should be used with caution in the elderly and those with kidney or heart disease.

Most colonoscopies are performed under conscious sedation. Sedation for colonoscopy usually includes a combination of a benzodiazepine (midazolam or diazepam) and a narcotic (meperidine or fentanyl), or may include a short-acting anesthetic agent such as propofol. The elderly may be more sensitive to the agents used for sedation in GI endoscopy; small incremental doses should be given and the patient monitored closely for signs of cardiopulmonary compromise. Nevertheless, age alone is not a major determinant of morbidity; rapid or excessive dosing contributes more to complications from sedation than does age itself.

TABLE 92-1

Influence of Age on Likely Diagnosis of Lower Gastrointestinal Symptoms

SYMPTOM	YOUNG PATIENT	ELDERLY PATIENT
Rectal bleeding	Hemorrhoids	Diverticulosis
	Inflammatory bowel disease	Vascular ectasia
	Colonic polyp	Colon cancer
Constipation	Irritable bowel syndrome	Obstructing lesion
Anal stricture	Inflammatory bowel disease	Neoplasm
		Radiation-induced injury

Endoscopic Ultrasound

Endoscopic ultrasound (EUS) can be used to diagnose and manage disease of the anorectum. EUS utilizes high frequency ultrasound waves emitted from a probe attached to an endoscope to delineate the layers of the rectal wall, the internal and external anal sphincters, and the pelvic floor muscles. EUS may be helpful in evaluating these structures in patients with fecal incontinence. EUS also is frequently used to stage rectal malignancy, providing information about the depth of tumor invasion and the status of regional lymph nodes. Direct tissue sampling is available through fine needle aspiration at the time of the EUS.

Radiology

Contrast Studies

Contrast studies of the large intestine involve coating the colonic mucosa with a contrast medium, usually barium sulfate, following thorough colonic preparation. Barium enemas may be performed by either single- or double-contrast method; in the latter, air is insufflated as well as barium. The single-contrast technique often is used to diagnose colonic strictures, fistula, obstruction, or diverticulitis. Double-contrast barium enema more commonly is used to detect polyps or mucosal abnormalities.

There exists some controversy concerning whether double-contrast barium enema is effective as a screening tool for colon cancer. Many experts consider colonoscopy to be the gold standard screening test. Colonoscopy is safe in the elderly and is widely available. However, contrast studies may be reasonable as a first-line test when colonic strictures are suspected or the presence of likely or known obstruction might make colonoscopy unsafe.

CT Colonography

CT colonography (virtual colonoscopy) is a radiographic technique that combines helical CT and graphics software to create a three-dimensional view of the colonic lumen. This technology was developed to detect colonic polyps. In preliminary trials of CT colonography, detection rates for polyps greater than 5 mm were similar to those for optical colonoscopy. Debate remains about the significance of finding polyps of different sizes; comparisons of CT colonography with optical colonoscopy rest on what the investigators deem to be a "significant" polyp, with much disagreement about the significance of polyps less than 5 mm. Nonetheless, CT colonography will likely play an increasingly important role in colon cancer screening in the coming years.

There are several limitations of CT colonography. First, the procedure requires formal bowel preparation, similar to that required for optical colonoscopy. Moreover, polyps and other abnormalities found at CT colonography, detected in 10% to 30% of all examinations, require conventional colonoscopy for removal. Lastly, in addition to colonic lesions, incidental extracolonic findings on CT colonography such as gall bladder, liver, and renal/adrenal abnormalities may require evaluation and possibly further invasive testing.

DIVERTICULAR DISEASE

Colonic diverticula are herniations of colonic mucosa through the smooth muscle layers of the colon. Strictly speaking, because colonic diverticula do not involve the muscle layer but rather are herniations of the mucosa and submucosa, they are actually pseudodiverticula. Diverticulosis has been increasingly recognized in western society and is thought to be a disorder of older individuals. Diverticula are present in approximately one-third of persons by age 50 and in approximately two-thirds by age 80. In western society, the predominance of diverticula occurs on the left side of the colon, specifically the sigmoid colon, although diverticula can occur anywhere in the colon.

Pathophysiology

There are three factors implicated in the pathogenesis of colonic diverticulosis. First, altered colonic motility results in increased luminal pressure along segments of the colon, and the resulting high-pressure areas cause out-pouchings at areas of weakness. Second, low intake of dietary fiber predisposes to diverticular disease, because low stool weights and slower stool transit times allow for relative increases in colonic intraluminal pressure. Third, with age the structural integrity of the colonic muscular wall decreases, and diverticula are more likely to form as a result.

Asymptomatic Diverticulosis

Diverticulosis is usually an incidental finding in patients undergoing radiographic studies or colonoscopy for other reasons. There is no clear indication for therapy or follow-up in such patients. Large cohort studies suggest that complications of diverticular disease may be prevented by intake of a high-fiber diet. Although prospective, randomized studies are lacking, a diet high in fiber and low in fat appears to be reasonable, and one that likely provides other health benefits as well as potentially decreasing the risk of complications from diverticulosis.

Painful Diverticular Disease

Some patients with diverticulosis have left lower quadrant pain, and when examined, do not have evidence of inflammation. These patients may have painful diverticular disease. Pain often is described as crampy, located in the left lower abdomen, and may be associated with diarrhea or constipation as well as tenderness over the affected area. The pain is often exacerbated by eating and diminished by defecation or the passage of flatus. The symptoms of painful diverticular disease often overlap with those of irritable bowel syndrome, and therefore painful diverticular disease is considered part of the spectrum of functional bowel disorders. It is important to consider other causes of left lower quadrant pain such as diverticulitis, colonic obstruction, and incarcerated hernias in such patients.

Diverticulitis

Diverticulitis, defined as having diverticulosis in association with inflammation, infection, or both, is probably the most common clinical manifestation of diverticular disease. Diverticulitis develops in approximately 10% to 25% of individuals with diverticulosis who are followed for 10 years or more; however, less than 20% of these patients require hospitalization.

The process by which a diverticulum becomes inflamed has been compared to appendicitis, in which the diverticulum becomes obstructed by stool in its neck. The resulting obstruction eventually leads to micro- or macroperforation of the diverticulum. Fever, leukocytosis, and rebound tenderness often ensue. In an elderly patient, absence of these findings unfortunately does not rule out diverticulitis, and an aggressive evaluation is indicated if this diagnosis is suspected.

An abdominal and pelvic CT scan often confirms the diagnosis when the clinical suspicion is for diverticulitis, and the radiographic finding may or may not include evidence of a pericolic abscess. Colonoscopy or barium enema should be delayed until inflammation has improved because of an increased risk of colonic perforation with these studies. Patients with severe pain, nausea, and vomiting often require hospitalization and benefit from intravenous antibiotics. Most patients with diverticulitis will improve within 48 to 72 hours, and then a 5 to 7 day course of oral antibiotics with gradual introduction of oral intake is adequate therapy. Selected patients with relatively mild symptoms and who are able to tolerate oral intake may be managed with close outpatient monitoring including oral antibiotics and bowel rest. Given the high incidence of complicated disease, there should be a low threshold for hospitalization in elderly patients with diverticulitis.

Patients with complicated disease including those with abscesses may need drainage by surgery or interventional radiology. Surgery is recommended for patients with diverticulitis who fail to respond to medical therapy within 72 hours, those with two or more attacks, and those with one attack complicated by abscess, obstruction, or when the inflammatory process involves the bladder. The operation can usually be done in one stage with a primary bowel anastomosis. Sometimes, however, a two-stage procedure with a temporary colostomy may be necessary.

Diverticular Hemorrhage

Three to five percent of patients with diverticulosis have hemorrhage from a diverticulum. Diverticular hemorrhage is the most common identifiable cause of significant lower GI bleeding, accounting for 30% to 40% of cases with confirmed sources.

Bleeding associated with diverticula is typically brisk, and painless. While the majority of diverticula are located in the left colon, bleeding from diverticular disease usually arises from the right colon. Bleeding is said to arise from arterial rupture of the vasa recta as it courses over the dome of a diverticulum. Bleeding ceases spontaneously in 70% to 80% of patients, and re-bleeding rates range from 22% to 38%. Re-bleeding is more likely when the initial bleed is severe.

The initial step in the management of patients with hemodynamically significant bleeding from diverticulosis is stabilization with intravenous fluid and blood products as necessary. Stable patients with suspected diverticular hemorrhage may undergo colonoscopy following rapid colonic purge. Colonoscopy in this setting allows for the ability to identify a diverticular source, to exclude alternative diagnoses, and to provide therapy of actively bleeding lesions.

In patients with recurrent bleeding, nuclear tagged red blood cell scans (scintigraphy) may localize the bleeding site. A positive bleeding scan may lead to angiography, which may allow for nonsurgical management of diverticular hemorrhage. Patients who require more than three units of packed red cell transfusions over 24 hours, have bleeding refractory to treatment, or are hemodynamically unstable may require surgical management. Preoperative nuclear red blood cell scans or angiography often help localize the diseased segment and allow for limited bowel resections. Blind total colectomy is rarely indicated.

CLOSTRIDIUM DIFFICILE COLITIS

Clostridium difficile, an anaerobic gram-positive, spore forming toxigenic bacillus was first isolated in 1935. It was not until 1978 when the association between the toxin elaborated by this bacteria and antibiotic-associated pseudomembranous colitis was made. The organism is now recognized as the single most important cause of nosocomial infectious diarrhea in the United States.

Pathogenesis

The pathogenesis of *C. difficile* colitis involves several steps. Patients must first be exposed to antibiotics. While the most common antibiotics associated with *C. difficile* colitis are ampicillin, amoxicillin, cephalosporins, and clindamycin, virtually all antibiotics (including those used to treat *C. difficile* colitis) have been implicated in causing disease (Table 92-2).

Next, exposure to antibiotics leads to altered colonic microflora, which in turn changes the protective barrier typically present in the colon against *C difficile*. Colonization of the organism in the colon is then possible. *C difficile* infection may result in an asymptomatic carrier state, or patients may develop diarrhea and colitis. Patients with intact immune systems and an ability to mount an early antibody response to *C difficile* toxin usually become asymptomatic carriers of the organism. On the other hand, patients lacking sufficient

TABLE 92-2

Antibiotics Associated with *Clostridium difficile* Colitis	
COMMON	**LESS COMMON**
Ampicillin and Amoxicillin	Chloramphenicol
Cephalosporins	Macrolides
Clindamycin	Sulfonamides
Fluoroquinolones	Tetracyclines
	Trimethoprim

TABLE 92-3

Risk Factors for *Clostridium difficile* Infection

Antimicrobial therapy

Older Age

Use of nasogastric tube

Gastrointestinal procedures

Acid antisecretory medications

Intensive care unit stay

Length of hospitalization

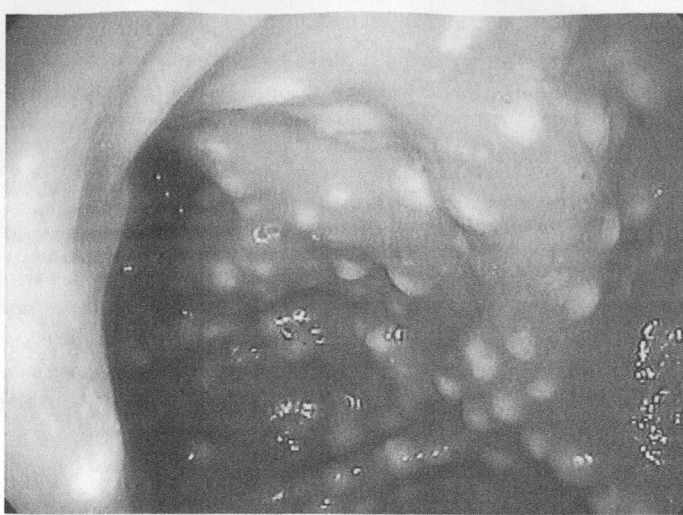

FIGURE 92-2. Pseudomembranes.

ability to mount an adequate immune response develop diarrhea and colitis.

Risk factors for the development of *C difficile* colitis include advanced age, multiple comorbid illnesses, intensive care unit stay, use of a nasogastric tube, acid antisecretory medications, and length of hospital stay (Table 92-3).

Clinical Manifestations

Clinical manifestations of *C difficile* infection range from asymptomatic carriage to mild to moderate diarrhea to life-threatening pseudomembranous colitis (Figure 92-1). Asymptomatic carriage of *C difficile* is common in hospitalized patients, and in fact, studies have shown that 10% to 16% of hospitalized patients receiving antibiotics are carriers of *C difficile*. Asymptomatic carriers should not be treated. In patients who develop diarrhea with *C difficile*, symptoms often develop soon after colonization. Fever, abdominal pain, and leukocytosis accompany the watery, nonbloody diarrhea. Mucus or occult blood may be present, but hematochezia should prompt an evaluation for other disease states. Patients with more severe disease may develop colonic ileus or toxic dilation without diarrhea. Abdominal radiographs will often reveal the colonic dilation.

Diagnostic Tests

There are several tests for diagnosing *C difficile* colitis. The most widely used is an enzyme linked immunoassay. This assay detects either one of the two *C difficile* toxins. While the main advantages

are speed, cost, ease of testing, and high specificity, this immunoassay has relatively low sensitivity. Other diagnostic tests including *C difficile* culture, tissue culture cytotoxic assay, and PCR for detection of toxin genes are rarely used because of their high cost, need for specialized laboratory techniques, and length of time to make the diagnosis.

Colonoscopy, or more often flexible sigmoidoscopy, may be helpful in making the diagnosis of *C difficile* colitis but is not necessary. Endoscopy is most useful when the diagnosis is in doubt or when disease severity demands rapid diagnosis. The finding of colonic pseudomembranes in a patient with antibiotic-associated diarrhea is almost pathognomonic for *C difficile* colitis (Figure 92-2).

Treatment

Therapy for *C difficile* colitis begins with withdrawal of the precipitating antibiotics if possible. Metronidazole and vancomycin are both effective in the treatment of *C difficile*-associated disease. (Note that the only FDA-approved drug for treating *C difficile* colitis in the United States is vancomycin). Metronidazole is by far less expensive, and the use of vancomycin carries with it a concern for the induction of vancomycin-resistant enterococci; therefore, the usual initial therapy is with a 10 to 14 day course of oral metronidazole. This is effective in treating the majority of patients. In patients who are too ill or cannot take oral medication, IV metronidazole can be substituted. Patients who do not respond to metronidazole can be switched to oral vancomycin. Because intravenous vancomycin does not penetrate the colonic lumen, this formulation is not effective in treating *C difficile* colitis. Probiotic agents such as *Lactobacillus* GG and *Saccharomyces boulardii* have been used to reconstitute the colonic microflora, and are occasionally added to metronidazole or vancomycin to treat *C difficile* colitis, but their effectiveness has not been demonstrated in well-designed trials.

Unfortunately, recurrent *C difficile* infection is a common problem and particularly prevalent in older adults. Symptomatic recurrence may result from reinfection with either the same or a different strain of *C difficile*. Resistance to metronidazole or vancomycin is seldom if ever an important factor in recurrence. Therefore,

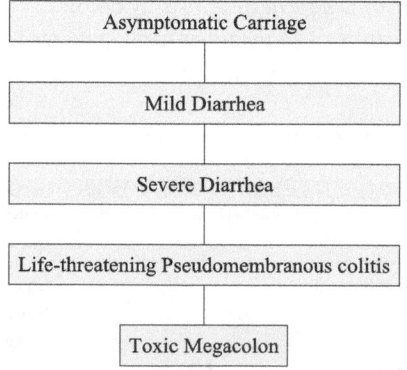

| Asymptomatic Carriage |
| Mild Diarrhea |
| Severe Diarrhea |
| Life-threatening Pseudomembranous colitis |
| Toxic Megacolon |

FIGURE 92-1. Clinical Manifestations of *Clostridium difficile* infection.

TABLE 92-4

Vancomycin Taper for Second Relapse of *Clostridium difficile* Colitis
Vancomycin 125 mg po qid for 7 days
Vancomycin 125 mg po bid for 7 days
Vancomycin 125 mg po qd for 7 days
Vancomycin 125 mg po qod for 7 days
Vancomycin 125 mg po q 3 days for 7 days

patients with recurrent *C difficile* colitis generally are given another trial with the antibiotic used to treat the initial infection. In some patients, a prolonged taper of vancomycin as well as the addition of cholestyramine over many months may be needed to prevent further recurrence (Table 92-4). A variety of other strategies, including the use of some nonabsorbable antibiotics and fecal transplantation, have been used in the treatment of recurrent *C difficile* infection.

MICROSCOPIC COLITIS

The term "microscopic colitis" refers to two distinct but similar clinical entities, lymphocytic and collagenous colitis. Combined, they are characterized by chronic watery diarrhea and feature histologic evidence of chronic mucosal inflammation in the absence of endoscopic or radiological abnormalities of the large intestine. They differ principally by the presence or absence of a thickened collagenous band, which when present in collagenous colitis is located in the colonic subepithelium.

Both lymphocytic and collagenous colitis occur most commonly in people in their sixth to eighth decade. There is a strong female predominance. Most patients present with chronic watery stools for months to years. The pattern of symptoms in patients with microscopic colitis fluctuates and consists of exacerbations and remissions over years. Crampy abdominal pain is common, and symptoms often improve with fasting. Physical examination in patients with microscopic colitis is usually unremarkable, and occult blood in the stool is uncommon. Colonoscopic examinations are usually normal. It is important to exclude infectious causes of diarrhea by testing the stool for ova and parasites, bacterial pathogens, and *C. difficile* toxin prior to making the diagnosis of microscopic colitis. The diagnosis relies on histopathologic evaluation of biopsied material from the diseased colon.

Pathology

Microscopic colitis is characterized by increased mononuclear cells in the lamina propria and between crypt epithelial cells, while collagenous colitis features a thickened subepithelial collagen layer. Contrasted to the normal colon where the collagen layer typically is 4 to 5 micrometers thick, in collagenous colitis the collagen layer is greater than 10 micrometers thick and averages 20 to 60 micrometers. The thickened layer is predominantly made up of type VI collagen, and it is this thickened collagen band that distinguishes collagenous colitis from lymphocytic colitis. Although inflammatory changes may be found diffusely throughout the colon in microscopic colitis,

multiple biopsies of the left colon proximal to the rectosigmoid usually are sufficient to make the diagnosis.

Treatment

There have been few controlled trials regarding treatment for microscopic colitis, and therapy is largely empiric. Most reports suggest that no single agent works. The pattern of the diarrhea in microscopic colitis often is relapsing; patients sometimes find relief with one agent, but unfortunately symptom improvement may not be permanent. Almost one-third of patients respond to antidiarrheal agents like loperamide as well as stool bulking agents like psyllium or methylcellulose; however, these agents do not improve the subepithelial inflammation or reduce the thickness of the collagen band.

Other treatment trials in microscopic colitis have examined the effect of aminosalicylates, corticosteroids, and bile acid absorbing resins. Alone or in combination, these agents reduce subepithelial inflammation and collagen thickness. Budesonide, an orally administered, topically active synthetic corticosteroid with significant first-pass metabolism has shown considerable promise in the treatment of microscopic colitis. Budesonide is an attractive agent here because of limited systemic side-effects and improvement of symptoms with once daily dosing, but unfortunately relapse after stopping the drug is common. In severe refractory cases, diverting ileostomy or proctocolectomy is a treatment of last resort.

INFLAMMATORY BOWEL DISEASE

Crohn's disease and ulcerative colitis comprise the vast majority of inflammatory bowel disease (IBD) (Table 92-5). They are characterized by a tendency for immune activation and inflammation within the GI tract. IBD commonly has its onset in the young adult population, but is found with increasing frequency in the elderly as well.

The age of diagnosis may range from early childhood through the entire lifespan. Epidemiological studies suggest there is a bimodal distribution of the age of onset, with the peak incidence of IBD occurring in the second and third decades, and a second smaller peak in the elderly between the ages of 60 and 70 years. "Late-onset" IBD accounts for approximately 12% cases of ulcerative colitis and 16% cases of Crohn's disease. However, in the elderly, presenting

TABLE 92-5

Differentiating Crohn's Disease and Ulcerative Colitis		
	CROHN'S DISEASE	**ULCERATIVE COLITIS**
Distribution	Throughout the GI tract, with skipped segments	Continuous disease from the rectum involving only the colon
Rectum	Relatively spared	Typically involved
Mucosal lesions	Aphthous ulcers, cobblestoning	Micro ulcers, linear ulcers
Rectal bleeding	Uncommon	Common
Depth of inflammation	Transmural	Mucosal
Fistulas	Present	Not present

symptoms of IBD often are presumed to be attributable to another cause, and initially the correct diagnosis is sometimes overlooked. On the other hand, many experts believe that much of what was previously considered to be IBD in the elderly is actually attributable to other causes, and in particular, to ischemic colitis.

Crohn's Disease

Crohn's disease is a chronic inflammatory process of unknown etiology, which most often affects the distal ileum, but can affect any segment of the GI tract including the colon. It is characterized by transmural inflammation of the bowel wall, the presence of apthae and ulcers, and the interspersing of segments of involved bowel with uninvolved bowel, i.e. skip lesions. Fissures, fistulas, and strictures are common in Crohn's disease. According to most published series, Crohn's disease of the colon, also known as Crohn's colitis, is more common in the elderly than in the young.

Symptoms and Signs

The presentation of Crohn's disease may be subtle and varies considerably. The clinical picture of Crohn's disease in the elderly as compared to the young has its roots in the propensity for Crohn's disease in the elderly to involve the colon. Consequently, intestinal obstruction, perforation, and fistula—features often associated with small bowel disease are less common. The majority of elderly patients with Crohn's disease manifest their disease with abdominal pain, weight loss, fever, and diarrhea. The diarrhea, typically watery in Crohn's disease can be bloody when the colon is involved.

Common laboratory abnormalities such as anemia, leukocytosis, thrombocytosis, hypoalbuminemia, and elevated erythrocyte sedimentation rate, as well as C-reactive protein levels vary with the severity of the illness. Interestingly, anemia in Crohn's disease can be because of either iron deficiency from chronic GI blood loss or from vitamin B-12 deficiency if the Crohn's disease involves a large enough segment of the distal ileum, the site for B-12 absorption in the small bowel.

Unfortunately, no single symptom, sign, or diagnostic test definitively establishes the diagnosis of Crohn's disease, and prolonged delays in diagnosis probably occur more frequently in elderly patients. Ultimately, a constellation of suggestive symptoms and laboratory abnormalities should prompt further evaluation. Common intestinal infections should be excluded, and tests may include stool cultures, stool examination for ova and parasites, and assays for *C. difficile* toxin.

Ultimately, the diagnosis of Crohn's disease is confirmed by findings on barium studies, colonoscopy, and histopathology. Colonoscopy and barium studies can identify the characteristic linear ulcers, skip lesions, and mucosal edema in Crohn's disease. Barium studies are superior for finding fistulas and defining the anatomic location of disease. CT and MR enterography may play an increasing role in the diagnosis of Crohn's disease. Because of its ability to see the mucosa directly and sample it for histopathologic examination, colonoscopy complements radiologic studies in making the diagnosis of Crohn's disease.

Computed tomography studies provide superior definition of the colon wall, can identify pyogenic complications like abscesses and perforations, and also can detect other intra-abdominal pathology that might mimic the presentation of Crohn's disease, such as appendicitis or nephrolithiasis. On the other hand, CT does not demonstrate fine mucosal detail and often appears normal early in the course of disease.

Management

The principles of IBD management are the same regardless of the age of the patient. Nonetheless, there are several important considerations when treating elderly patients with IBD. The most commonly used medications in the treatment of Crohn's disease include sulfasalazine, mesalamine (5-aminosalicylic acid), and corticosteroids; all of these are well tolerated in the elderly population. However, corticosteroid use confers a higher risk of complications in the elderly, including accelerated bone loss and fractures, hypertension, and glucose intolerance (Table 92-6).

Immunomodulators like azathioprine, 6-mercaptopurine, and methotrexate are used effectively in the young to maintain remission of Crohn's disease. These agents are usually well tolerated in the elderly as well; however, some authorities argue against their use in older patients on the theoretical grounds that they may further impair the immune dysfunction associated with aging and result in increased risk of infection or possibly malignancy.

Finally, some antibiotics such as metronidazole and ciprofloxacin have been shown to be effective in inducing and maintaining remission, as well as healing perineal fistulas, in patients with Crohn's disease. The long-term use of antibiotics typically is limited by the occurrence of significant side effects. Specifically, irreversible peripheral neuropathy can occur with the use of metronidazole, while antibiotic-associated diarrhea may be a complication of prolonged ciprofloxacin use.

TABLE 92-6

Doses and Adverse Reactions with Commonly Used Medications to Treat Inflammatory Bowel Disease

MEDICATION	DOSE	ADVERSE REACTIONS
Sulfasalazine	4–6 g/d	Nausea, folate deficiency, hemolytic anemia with glucose-6-phosphatase dehydrogenase deficiency
Mesalamine	Up to 4.8 g/d	Headaches
Prednisone	Up to 60 mg/day	Cushingoid appearance, glucose intolerance, osteoporosis, avascular necrosis, proximal myopathy, irritability, hypertension, cataract, glaucoma
6-Mercaptopurine, azathioprine	6-MP 1.5 mg/kg AZA 3 mg/kg	Pancreatitis, pancytopenia, hepatitis
Metronidazole	Up to 1 g/d	Anorexia, nausea/vomiting, disulfiram-like effect, peripheral neuropathy
Ciprofloxacin	Up to 1 g/d	Nausea/vomiting, rash, hepatitis, spontaneous tendon rupture

Elderly patients with ileal or ileal–colonic Crohn's disease occasionally require intestinal resection, but generally tolerate surgery well and appear to have low rates of postoperative recurrence. Proctocolectomy with ileostomy is a common surgical option for patients with extensive Crohn's colitis. In elderly patients who are debilitated or malnourished, an initial subtotal colectomy with ileostomy is less debilitating and permits weight gain and improved physical well-being. If proctocolectomy is subsequently required, it can be done with a low complication rate, but may not be necessary at all if rectal disease is absent. A conventional ileostomy is generally favored in elderly patients following colectomy, because anal sphincter sparing surgical procedures, such as an ileal pouch–anal anastomosis, often have poor functional results in older patients.

Ulcerative Colitis

Ulcerative colitis (UC) is a chronic inflammatory disorder of the GI tract of unknown etiology that affects the mucosa and submucosa of the large intestine in a continuous fashion. The inflammatory process invariably involves the rectum and extends proximally to variable distances, but does not involve the GI tract proximal to the colon. For many elderly patients, UC is a relatively mild illness, because colonic inflammation often is limited to the rectum or sigmoid colon. This distribution of disease is generally associated with less systemic manifestations, better response to medical therapy, and less need for surgery than more extensive UC.

Symptoms and Signs

The severity of UC may be subjectively classified as mild, moderate, or severe and is generally proportional to the extent of colonic inflammation. Symptoms in elderly patients are similar to those seen in young patients, and include bloody diarrhea, rectal pain, tenesmus, urgency, and abdominal pain. In comparison to Crohn's disease, the diarrhea in UC almost always is bloody. Fecal urgency, a sensation of incomplete evacuation, and fecal incontinence also are common. Unfortunately, older patients appear to be more likely than younger patients to present with a severe initial attack, and that first severe manifestation is associated with a relatively high fatality rate.

Laboratory findings in UC are nonspecific and reflect the severity of the underlying disease. In patients with limited distal disease, laboratory abnormalities may be absent except perhaps for mild anemia. In patients with extensive disease, severe iron deficiency anemia, hypoalbuminemia, leukocytosis, and thrombocytosis are common.

Toxic megacolon is a feared complication of UC, and it occurs more frequently in older patients. One should be suspicious of toxic megacolon in a patient whose diarrhea improves but whose abdomen is distended and tympanic. Other markers of worsening systemic inflammation, such as fever and leukocytosis, will also be present. The diagnosis is usually made by abdominal radiography. Colonoscopy should not be attempted when there is a suspicion for toxic megacolon, as perforation may ensue.

Similar to the situation in Crohn's disease, there is no single test that can definitively diagnose UC with acceptable sensitivity and specificity. In elderly people, it is important to exclude other diseases that may mimic UC, like ischemic colitis, radiation proctocolitis, diverticulitis, malignancy, and infectious colitis.

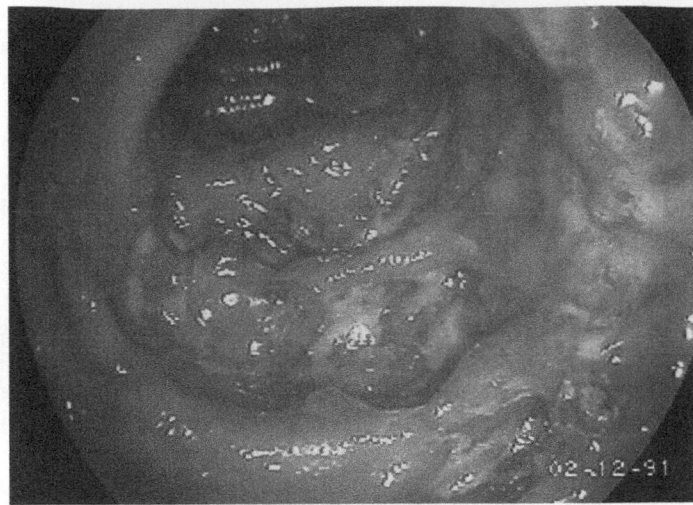

FIGURE 92-3. Ulcerative colitis as seen on colonoscopy.

Again, the constellation of characteristic signs and symptoms often prompts an endoscopic examination, which may show the classic findings of diffuse erythema, mucosal edema, granular mucosa, and ulcerations starting in the rectum without intervening areas of normal mucosa (Figure 92-3). In the proper clinical setting, flexible sigmoidoscopy with biopsy is usually sufficient to establish a diagnosis of UC. Complete colonoscopy with ileoscopy is necessary to determine the extent of disease and to exclude Crohn's disease. However, complete colonoscopy is not recommended in patients with active UC for fear of perforation; the procedure can be safely performed once active disease has been controlled.

Management

Most elderly patients with UC respond favorably to medical management. Once in remission, relapse occurs less frequently in the elderly regardless of the severity of the initial attack. A range of agents is available for medical therapy of UC, and these may be administered orally, rectally, or parenterally depending on the site and severity of disease. Pharmacologic agents used to treat UC in the elderly are similar to the ones used to treat Crohn's disease and include sulfasalazine, mesalamine, corticosteroids, and immunomodulators.

The mainstays of treatment for UC are aminosalicylates, and they may be administered orally or rectally. Formulations designed either for enema or suppositories are reasonable choices when treating distal disease. Unfortunately, distal disease in elderly patients is more refractory to topical therapy than in the young, and so often elderly subjects with distal disease will require oral formulations of aminosalicylates to achieve and maintain remission.

In addition to aminosalicylates, corticosteroids are effective in achieving remission, but steroid use is associated with frequent side effects. Therefore, corticosteroids should only be used temporarily in UC as a means to induce remission. They should not be used long-term as they have not been shown to be effective at preventing relapses, and their side effect profile makes prolonged use unsatisfactory.

In patients who do not respond to aminosalicylates, immunomodulators such as azathioprine or 6-mercaptopurine can be introduced. These drugs are purine analogues, interfere with nucleic acid metabolism and cell growth, and exert their cytotoxic effects on lymphoid cells. Azathioprine and 6-mercaptopurine use is subject to a delayed response; patients may require up to 6 to 12 weeks to see an effect from these agents. Fortunately, they are effective at maintaining remission, once a response is achieved.

Surgery for UC is indicated in patients who fail medical therapy, have acute fulminant disease, are steroid dependent, or develop a dysplastic lesion or cancer. UC is cured following total proctocolectomy. In the elderly, total proctocolectomy with ileostomy remains a popular choice, because restorative procedures like ileo–anal anastomosis are limited by functional morbidity. An alternative surgical procedure is a subtotal colectomy. In patients who have a subcolectomy, a rectal stump is left that provides the patient with an improved chance for fecal continence. Such patients, however, continue to have colonic mucosa, as such have an ongoing increased risk for colon cancer to develop in the diseased segment, and require periodic surveillance of the retained rectum.

Colon Cancer in IBD

The risk of colon cancer in patients with long-standing IBD is a significant complication of the disease. Colon cancer rates generally are higher in patients with UC than those with Crohn's disease; it appears to be the degree of ongoing inflammation in the colon that confers an increased risk of colon cancer. As such, patients with Crohn's colitis are believed to have an equally high risk of developing colon cancer as their UC peers. In patients with long-standing UC, surveillance for colon cancer includes annual colonoscopy with random mucosal biopsies of the entire colon looking for evidence of early or advanced dysplasia. Areas that appear suspicious are also targeted. The risk of colon cancer increases substantially after 8 to 10 years of disease, and after many years approaches nine times the risk of the general population in patients of the same age group. During surveillance, patients found to have low- or high-grade dysplasia or carcinoma generally are offered proctocolectomy.

COLON ISCHEMIA

Colon ischemia (CI) is the most common intestinal vascular disorder in the elderly. Until the 1950s, the only well-described form of CI was gangrene. During the 1950s, however, a variety of ischemic manifestations other than gangrene were noted after ligation of the inferior mesenteric artery during abdominal surgery. Careful review of these cases revealed a spectrum of diseases in addition to infarction that included healed ulcers, strictures, pseudotumors, and ischemic UC.

Pathophysiology

The colon receives its blood supply from branches of the superior mesenteric artery and inferior mesenteric artery. The colon is protected from ischemia by an abundant collateral circulation formed by the marginal arterial complex of Drummond, central anastomotic artery, and arc of Riolan. Occlusion of a major vessel results in opening of collateral pathways in response to arterial

TABLE 92-7

Causes of Colonic Ischemia	
Inferior mesenteric artery thrombosis	Volvulus
Arterial embolus	Strangulated hernia
Cholesterol emboli	Vasculitis
Cardiac arrhythmia	Inherited and/or acquired hypercoagulable states
Shock	Medications

hypotension distal to the occlusion. Increased blood flow through collateral pathways maintains adequate perfusion for a variable but brief period of time. If blood flow is diminished for a prolonged period, vasoconstriction develops in the affected bed and may persist after the primary cause of the mesenteric ischemia is reversed.

In most cases, the cause of an episode of CI cannot be established with certainty, and no vascular occlusion can be identified. The causes of CI are vast and include thrombosis, embolus, shock, volvulus, hematologic disorders, infections, trauma, surgery, and medications (Table 92-7). The colon is particularly susceptible to ischemia, perhaps owing to its relatively low blood flow during periods of functional activity, and its sensitivity to autonomic stimulation. What triggers a specific episode of CI, however, usually is not known.

CI encompasses a spectrum of injury. The specific conditions resulting from ischemic injury to the colon are classified as reversible or irreversible, and then can be characterized further as reversible ischemic colonopathy, reversible or transient ischemic colitis, chronic ulcerative ischemic colitis, ischemic colonic stricture, colonic gangrene, and fulminant universal ischemic colitis.

Clinical Features

Despite a growing understanding of the pathophysiology of CI and its disparate clinical presentations, many cases of transient or reversible ischemia still are missed because diagnostic studies are not performed early enough in the course of disease. This is because patients may not seek medical advice for a disease that is self-limited or the initial symptoms may be confused with other conditions such as IBD.

Approximately 90% of persons with CI are older than age 60 and have widespread evidence of atherosclerosis. Up to 10% of patients may have a potentially obstructing lesion of the colon, including carcinoma, benign stricture, and diverticulitis. Patients with CI usually are not critically ill at the time of diagnosis, and their abdominal pain typically is mild. Mesenteric angiography plays little role in the diagnosis and management of this condition; since colonic blood flow usually has normalized by the time of presentation, the prognosis is excellent.

Typically, CI presents with the sudden onset of mild crampy left lower quadrant abdominal pain. The pain frequently is accompanied, or followed within 24 hours, by bloody diarrhea or bright red blood per rectum. In most cases, blood loss is minimal; hemodynamically significant bleeding should prompt consideration of other diagnoses, such as diverticular bleeding. Severe pain is unusual and may indicate irreversible transmural necrosis.

TABLE 92-8

Medications Associated with Colon Ischemia

Digitalis	Vasopressin
Gold	Pseudoephedrine
Sumatriptan	Cocaine
Methamphetamine	Nonsteroidal anti-inflammatory drugs
Imipramine	Saline laxatives
Estrogens	Psychotropic drugs

The differential diagnosis of CI includes infectious colitis, IBD, pseudomembranous colitis, diverticulitis, and colon carcinoma. In all patients suspected of having colonic ischemia, infection with organisms such as *Salmonella, Shigella, Campylobacter, and E. coli* O157:H7 should be excluded. In fact, *E. coli* O157:H7 infection induces a colitis that mimics or may even cause CI. Many commonly used medications are associated with CI, and include digitalis, nonsteroidal anti-inflammatory drugs, imipramine, danazol, and sumatriptan (Table 92-8).

An elderly patient who presents with the sudden onset of abdominal pain and rectal bleeding or bloody diarrhea may benefit from a gentle barium enema or colonoscopy within 48 hours, once other more serious life threatening diagnoses are excluded. Colonoscopy is preferable because it is more sensitive in demonstrating mucosal abnormalities and permits histopathologic evaluation of the colon mucosa. Conventional sigmoidoscopy is of value only if the segment of involved bowel is within reach of the sigmoidoscope; CI involves the sigmoid in 50% to 60% of patients and the rectum in less than 10% of cases. Findings vary greatly depending on the stage at which sigmoidoscopy or colonoscopy is performed. At the outset, purplish blebs representing mucosal and submucosal hemorrhage may be seen. As hemorrhage is absorbed, varying degrees of necrosis, inflammation, ulceration, and mucosal sloughing occur, resembling UC or Crohn's disease.

Thumbprinting is the major radiologic finding in the acute presentation of CI. Thumbprints represent submucosal hemorrhage and edema. A barium enema repeated 1 week after an initial study should reflect evolution of the injury; either the areas of hemorrhage resorb and the study returns to normal or the thumbprints are replaced by a segmental pattern of colitis as the mucosa ulcerates.

Management

The treatment of CI is based on early diagnosis and continued monitoring, with special attention to the radiologic or colonoscopic appearance of the colon. This form of surveillance is essential in that it establishes the diagnosis and verifies its reversibility or shows progression to chronic ischemic colitis or stricture. Management includes stabilization of the patient, optimization of cardiac function, and bowel rest. Systemic antibiotics are administered routinely in most cases. Systemic glucocorticoids are of no proven value and increase the risk of perforation. If abdominal examination, fever, and leukocytosis suggest deterioration or if the patient experiences diarrhea or bleeding for more than 2 weeks, irreversible damage is likely, and surgical resection is usually indicated.

COLONIC OBSTRUCTION

Colonic obstruction results in dilation of the colon, abdominal distention and in some cases, colonic perforation. The majority of colonic obstructions are the result of mechanical obstruction from cancer, volvulus, stricture, impacted stool, surgical adhesion, or bowel intussusception. Patients with acute colonic obstruction can develop megacolon, the diagnosis of which is based on a cecal diameter of 12 centimeters or greater. Cecal distension is critical, because the cecum is the part of the colon that is most susceptible to ischemia and perforation based on LaPlace's law:

$$T = P \times R,$$

where T is wall tension, P is pressure, and R is the radius. With obstruction, as fluid and gas accumulate in the colon and intraluminal pressure increases, the radius of the colon increases. Wall tension is the greatest, and hence the risk for perforation most acute, at the area of greatest radius, which is generally in the cecum.

Acute Colonic Pseudo-obstruction

Acute colonic pseudo-obstruction, also known as Ogilve syndrome, usually presents as intestinal ileus with massive bowel dilation postoperatively or in the setting of a severe intercurrent illness.

Pathophysiology

The colon is innervated extrinsically via the sympathetic and parasympathetic nervous systems and locally via the enteric neurons. The sympathetic nervous system, by inhibition of acetylcholine release, inhibits colonic motility. On the other hand, the parasympathetic nervous system, via acetylcholine release from the vagus and sacral nerves, stimulates colonic motility. An imbalance of these two systems favoring colonic inhibitory motor input results in colonic ileus and acute colonic pseudo-obstruction.

Clinical Features

Acute colonic pseudo-obstruction usually presents in patients with severe underlying illness like stroke, myocardial infarction, or sepsis, or after surgical procedures. It is most common after orthopedic procedures of the pelvis, hips or knees, abdominal surgery, or obstetric procedures.

The presentation of acute colonic pseudo-obstruction may be subtle and variable, although the most characteristic clinical feature is severe abdominal distention and failure to pass flatus or stool. Some patients report only mild distention and minimal pain. Indeed, a high level of suspicion is necessary to make the diagnosis, because patients often present after surgery with perioperative bowel cleansing and so early passage of stool is not expected.

The hallmark of the disease is colonic dilation on standard abdominal radiography. The entire colon can be affected, although in some cases just the right sided segments can be dilated. The presence of air in the rectum implies that there is no mechanical obstruction, and is therefore important to note before making a diagnosis of acute colonic pseudo-obstruction.

TABLE 92-9

Contraindications to Use of Neostigmine

ABSOLUTE	RELATIVE
Hypersensitivity to neostigmine	Recent myocardial infarction
Mechanical urinary or intestinal obstruction	Acidosis
	Asthma
	Bradycardia
	Peptic ulcer disease
	Therapy with beta-blockers

Management

Initial management of acute colonic pseudo-obstruction involves correcting reversible causes of colonic ileus such as electrolyte imbalances, hypoxemia, hypovolemia, and removal of medications that can exacerbate the problem. The vast majority of patients are successfully treated with these relatively simple measures. Bowel rest and intravenous hydration is imperative. Colonoscopic decompression, with or without placement of a decompression tube, is an option in patients with prolonged pseudo-obstruction. In fact, through the 1990s, the primary therapeutic approach for patients with acute colonic pseudo-obstruction who had not responded to conservative measures was endoscopic decompression of the colon.

Recently, a placebo-controlled study confirmed the efficacy of the cholinesterase inhibitor neostigmine (1–2 mg IV or SQ) in patients with acute colonic pseudo-obstruction. Relative contraindications to the use of neostigmine include a heart rate <50 beats per minute or systolic blood pressure <90 mm Hg; sick sinus syndrome or history of second- or third-degree arteriovenous block without a pacemaker; serum creatinine greater than 3 mg/dL; or active bronchospasm requiring medication (Table 92-9). Following neostigmine administration, patients should be monitored closely. A second administration of neostigmine can be attempted if there is partial or no response to the first trial.

In selected patients who fail conservative and medical management, colonoscopic decompression of the unprepped bowel can be attempted. However, care is required since during colonoscopy air is insufflated into an already dilated colon. Recalling the principles of LaPlace's law, by increasing intraluminal pressure, wall tension increases in proportion to the radius of the colon, and therefore additional air insufflation carries with it an increased risk of colonic perforation. Surgical decompression, sometimes via placement of a cecostomy tube, remains another option for patients who do not respond to medical and endoscopic interventions.

The overall prognosis of patients with acute colonic pseudo-obstruction is poor, with an in-hospital mortality approaching 30%, attributable primarily to the severity of the underlying illness. The most significant complication of acute dilatation is colonic perforation, which occurred in 3% of cases in one retrospective series.

LOWER GASTROINTESTINAL BLEEDING

Lower GI bleeding is defined as that which arises distal to the ligament of Treitz. Lower GI bleeding occurs less frequently and is less severe than upper GI bleeding.

TABLE 92-10

Causes of Lower GI Hemorrhage

Diverticulosis
Ischemic colitis
Vascular ectasia
Hemorrhoids
Neoplasm
Postpolypectomy
Inflammatory bowel disease
Infectious colitis
NSAID-induced colopathy
Radiation colopathy
Dieulafoy lesion
Colonic ulcerations
Meckel diverticulum
Rectal varices
Aortoenteric fistula
Small-bowel sources

The incidence of lower GI bleeding increases significantly with age. The majority of lower GI bleeding in the elderly is the result of diverticula, vascular ectasias, and CI (Table 92-10). This section will focus on the approach to the patient with lower GI bleeding and bleeding from vascular ectasias. Diverticular hemorrhage and CI were discussed previously.

Acute lower GI bleeding presents with bright red blood per rectum, hematochezia, or melena depending on the location of the bleeding. Bright red blood per rectum usually indicates a distal colonic source or rapidly bleeding upper source. Melena usually indicates a right sided colonic lesion or upper source.

The first goal in the management of a patient with lower GI bleeding is resuscitation and hemodynamic stabilization. This may include administration of crystalloid intravenous fluids and blood products. Initial testing usually includes complete blood count, blood chemistry, coagulation profile, and blood type and cross-match, and the results help guide further management. For example, a low mean corpuscle volume often is a sign of chronic blood loss; a BUN-to-creatinine ratio of greater than 20:1 usually indicates an upper GI source; an elevated INR requires consideration of reversal in the face of hemodynamically significant bleeding.

Approximately 12% of patients thought to have lower GI bleeding have an upper GI bleeding source. It is important to exclude upper GI bleeding in patients with presumed lower GI bleeding, and often this can be accomplished with passage of a nasogastric tube and analysis of the gastric aspirate. Bilious fluid without blood in the nasogastric tube aspirate usually confirms the suspicion of lower GI bleeding. If an upper GI source is still in question, urgent upper endoscopy may be performed.

Although urgent upper endoscopy for the diagnosis and treatment of upper GI bleeding is predicated on sound data, urgent colonoscopy in lower GI bleeding has been practiced less consistently. Colonoscopy has the advantage of allowing for the diagnosis and immediate treatment of actively bleeding lesions. A number of reports have shown that "urgent colonoscopy" is safe and yields a

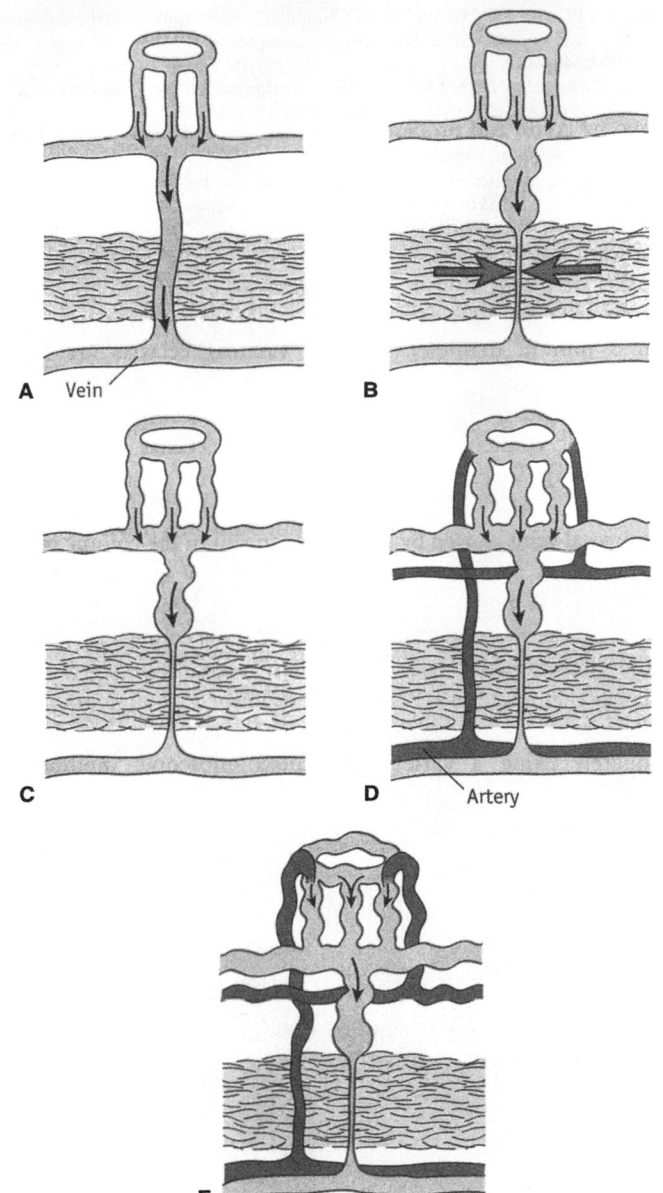

FIGURE 92-4. Proposed concept of the development of cecal vascular ectasias. **A,** Normal state of vein perforating muscular layers. **B,** With muscle contraction or increased intraluminal pressure, the vein is partially obstructed. **C,** After repeated episodes over many years, the submucosal vein becomes dilated and tortuous. **D,** Later, the veins and venules draining into the abnormal submucosal vein become similarly dilated and tortuous. **E,** Ultimately, the capillary ring becomes dilated, the precapillary sphincter becomes incompetent, and a small arteriovenous communication is present through the ectasia.

have positive red blood cell scintigraphy. Tagged red blood cell scans can detect bleeding at a rate greater than 0.1 mL/min and are useful to localize the site of bleeding, but unfortunately offer no option for therapy. If a patient has a positive bleeding scan, angiography with selective embolization can be performed to attempt to stop the bleeding. In order to detect active bleeding, angiography requires a higher rate of bleeding than scintigraphy, 0.5 mL/min compared to 0.1 mL/min. Transcatheter embolization of a lower GI bleeding source is usually effective in 70% to 90% of patients. If bleeding cannot be stopped with angiography, surgery to remove the bleeding colonic segment may be necessary. If a specific bleeding site can be localized with the above studies, a limited surgical resection can be performed rather than a subtotal colectomy.

Vascular Ectasias

Vascular ectasias, which arise from an age-related degeneration of previously normal blood vessels, typically occur in the cecum and proximal ascending colon. Along with diverticular bleeding, they are responsible for the majority of significant lower GI bleeding episodes in the elderly. Ectasias are found in up to 25% of persons older than 60 years who do not have symptoms; they typically are multiple and less than 5 mm in diameter. Despite a long standing belief to the contrary, there is no etiologic connection between vascular ectasias and aortic stenosis. Vascular ectasias probably arise as a result of repeated episodes of incomplete, low-grade obstruction of submucosal veins caused by increased tension in the colonic wall. The ultimate result is tortuosity and dilation of the venules and the arteriolar–capillary unit that feeds it, resulting in a small arteriovenous communication (Figure 92-4).

Lower GI bleeding caused by a vascular ectasia may be clinically indistinguishable from diverticular bleeding and is characterized by painless hematochezia. Bleeding from vascular ectasias may be hemodynamically significant, and a variety of treatment options exists including electrocoagulation, injection therapy, heater probe application, or argon plasma coagulation.

SUMMARY

Diseases of the large intestine that occur in the elderly are a heterogeneous group of disorders, which are a major cause of morbidity and mortality in this population. The fundamental principle of thorough history and physical examination skills will aid the clinician at arriving at these diagnoses. With the help of modern therapeutic modalities, we can alleviate the pain and suffering associated with many of these diseases.

FURTHER READING

Brandt LJ, Boley SJ. Colon ischemia. *Surg Clin N Am.* 1992;72:203.

Brandt LJ, Greenwald DA. Gastrointestinal diseases in the elderly. In: Brandt LJ, Daum F, eds. *Clinical Practice of Gastroenterology.* New York, New York: Churchill Livingstone; 1998:1582–1583.

Farrell JJ, Friedman LS. Colitis in the elderly. In: Bayless TM, Hanauer SB, eds. *Advanced Therapy of Inflammatory Bowel Disease.* London: BC Decker; 2001: 619–624.

Greenwald DA, Brandt LJ, Reinus JF. Ischemic bowel disease in the elderly. *Gastroenterol Clin.* 2001;30:2.

Hurley BW, Nguyen CC. The spectrum of pseudomembranous enterocolitis and antibiotic associated diarrhea. *Arch Intern Med.* 2002;162:19.

specific diagnosis in a high proportion of elderly patients with lower GI bleeding. On the basis of a high diagnostic yield, low rate of complications, and theoretical therapeutic potential, urgent colonoscopy following a rapid colonic purge has been recommended as the diagnostic procedure of choice in most patients with hemodynamically significant lower GI bleeding.

Other diagnostic tests in patients with active lower GI bleeding include scintigraphy (nuclear tagged red blood cell scans) and angiography. Approximately 45% of patients with lower GI bleeding

Jensen DM, Machicado GA, Jutabha R, et al. Urgent colonoscopy for the diagnosis and treatment of severe diverticular hemorrhage. *N Engl J Med.* 2000;342:78.

Kang JY, Melville D, Maxwell JD. Epidemiology and management of diverticular disease of the colon. *Drugs Aging.* 2004;21:4.

Katz JA. Advances in the medical therapy of inflammatory bowel disease. *Curr Opin Gastroenterol.* 2002;18:4.

Loftus EV, Silverstein MD, Sandborn WJ, et al. Crohn's disease in Olmsted County, Minnesota, 1940–1993: incidence, prevalence, and survival. *Gastroenterol.* 1998;114:6.

Pardi DS, Smyrk TC, Tremaine WJ, et al. Microscopic colitis: a review. *Am J Gastroenterol.* 2002;97:4.

Pickhardt PJ, Choi JR, Hwang I, et al. Computed tomographic virtual colonoscopy to screen for colorectal neoplasia in asymptomatic adults. *N Engl J Med.* 2003;349:24.

Ponec RJ, Saunders MD, Kimmey MB. Neostigmine for the treatment of acute colonic pseudo-obstruction. *N Engl J Med.* 1999;341:137.

Ure T, Dehghan K, Vernava AM, et al. Colonoscopy in the elderly: low risk, high yield. *Surg Endos.* 1995;9:5.

Wald A. Other diseases of the colon and rectum. In: Feldman M, Friedman LS, Brandt LJ, eds. *Sleisenger and Fordtran's Gastrointestinal and Liver Disease.* 8th ed. Philadelphia, PA: Saunders; 2006:2811–2814.

Constipation

Danielle Harari

INTRODUCTION

Constipation is a frequent health concern for older people in every health care setting. Primary care visits for constipation increase markedly in people older than 60 years, as does regular use of laxatives. Self-reported constipation in older people is associated with anxiety, depression, and poor health perception, while clinical constipation in vulnerable individuals may lead to complications such as fecal impaction, overflow incontinence, sigmoid volvulus, and urinary retention. Constipation is an expensive condition, with high costs ranging from laxative expenditure to nursing time. For instance, it is estimated that 80% of community nurses working with older people in the United Kingdom are managing constipation (particularly fecal impaction) as part of their case-load. An Australian study used in-depth, semistructured interviews to explore older individuals' experiences with constipation, and their findings largely summed up feelings and problems, no doubt, shared by many older people across the developed world:

- They feel "not right" in themselves when they are constipated.

- Physicians can have a dismissive attitude about constipation and do not consider the problem seriously.

- Patients are keen to find a solution, but feel useful and empathic advice and information are generally unavailable.

- At the same time, they have a strong imperative for self-management including use of over-the-counter laxatives.

- There are some barriers to lifestyle approaches, for example, expense of fruit and vegetables, fear of urinary incontinence with increased fluid intake, reluctance to walk out alone.

- One-quarter still need to do self-manual removal despite measures taken.

This chapter will describe the epidemiology, risk factors, clinical presentation, assessment, and treatment of constipation in older adults. Data sources were a computer search of the English language literature (1966 to 2006), systematic review Web sites including the Cochrane database, reference lists from recent systematic reviews and book chapters, and expert committee reports and opinion. Levels of evidence are as used by the U.S. Preventive Task Force:

- Good evidence Level [1]: consistent results from well-designed, well-conducted studies

- Fair evidence Level [2]: results show benefit, but strength limited by number, quality, or consistency of studies

- Poor evidence Level [3]: insufficient because of limited number, power, or quality of studies

DEFINITIONS

Definitions of constipation in older people in medical and nursing literature have been inconsistent. Studies of older people have tended to define constipation

- subjectively by self-report,

- according to specific bowel-related symptoms, or

- by daily laxative usage.

Few use objective assessment–based definitions (e.g., fecal loading). The feeling of being constipated frequently means different things to different individuals. While the nonspecific self-reporting of constipation ("I suffer from constipation") provides insight into how individuals perceive their bowel habit, standardized definitions based on specific symptoms (Rome II criteria) are now widely used in both clinical practice and research (Table 93-1). A recent systematic review reported that approximately 63 million people in North America meet the Rome II criteria for constipation with a disproportionate number being older than 65. An important subtype of constipation in older people is rectal outlet delay, which affects 21% of community dwellers aged 65+. The Rome II definitions for constipation and rectal outlet delay are symptom-based;

TABLE 93-1

Definitions of Constipation

Constipation (Rome II Criteria)

Two or more of the following symptoms present on more than 25% of
  occasions for at least 12 weeks in the last 12 months:

  Two or less bowel movements per week

  Straining at stool

  Hard stools

  Feeling of incomplete evacuation

Rectal Outlet Delay (Rome II Criteria)

Feeling of anal blockage at least a quarter of the time *and*

Prolonged defecation (>10 min to complete bowel movement); *or*

Need for self-digitation (pressing in or around the anus to aid evacuation) on
  any occasion

Clinical Constipation

Large amount of feces (hard or soft) in rectum on digital examination *and/or*

Colonic fecal loading on abdominal radiograph

objectively, however, the clinical definition of constipation relies on
finding fecal loading in the rectum and/or colon. Such objective
assessment is particularly important in frail older people owing to
factors listed in Table 93-2.

PREVALENCE OF CONSTIPATION AND CONSTIPATION-RELATED SYMPTOMS

Table 93-3 provides practice guidance based on evidence from epidemiological studies (prevalence, symptomatology, and risk factors)
of constipation in older people.

Self-Reported Constipation

One older community-based study of 3166 persons aged 65 years
and older asked the question, "Do you have recurrent constipation?"
and found a prevalence of 26% in women and 16% in men; in the
84+ years age group, prevalence was 34% and 26%, respectively. Age
was a strong independent risk factor for self-reported constipation.
Other community studies support this relationship with age and
show prevalence rates of up to 34% of women and 30% of men
older than age 65 years. The preponderance of women over men
reporting constipation tends to equalize after the age of 80 years.

TABLE 93-2

**Factors Potentially Leading to Underestimation of
Constipation in Frail Older People**

Frail older people may

- be unable to report bowel-related symptoms owing to communication or
  cognitive difficulties;
- have regular bowel movements despite have rectal or colonic fecal
  impaction;
- have impaired rectal sensation and inhibited urge to go and so be
  unaware of rectal stool impaction;
- have nonspecific symptoms associated with colonic fecal impaction
  (e.g., delirium, anorexia, functional decline).

TABLE 93-3

Practice Guidance Based on Epidemiological Evidence

Screening

Constipation symptoms should be routinely asked about in patients aged
  65+ in view of the high prevalence of the condition in this population [2]

Men and women in their eighth decade and beyond should be regularly
  screened for constipation symptoms, as prevalence increases with
  advancing age [2]

Periodic objective assessment for constipation in elderly nursing home
  residents should be incorporated into routine nursing and medical care
  [2]. Patients unable to report symptoms owing to cognitive or
  communication difficulties should be especially targeted [3]. Such an
  assessment should occur at minimum every 3 months (3 monthly
  incidence rate of new-onset constipation is 7% in nursing home
  residents), and optimally monthly [3].

Identifying Risk Factors

The identification of risk factors for constipation in older people is critical to
  effectively managing the condition [2]

Systematic identification of multiple risk factors in vulnerable older people
  with constipation should be incorporated into good practice guidelines in
  all health care settings [3]

Patients at increased risk of constipation from recognized comorbidities
  (e.g., Parkinson disease, diabetes) should be regularly assessed for the
  condition [2]

Assessment

Identifying specific bowel symptoms in older individuals reporting
  constipation is important to guide appropriate management of this
  common complaint [2]

Reduced bowel movement frequency is not a sensitive clinical indicator for
  constipation in older people [2], though it is specific [3]

Difficulty with evacuation and rectal outlet delay are primary symptoms in
  older individuals [2]

An objective assessment should be undertaken in frail older people with
  constipation as these patients are at increased risk of developing
  complications [2]

Older patients being prescribed laxatives on a daily basis should be
  regularly reviewed for symptoms of constipation and the appropriateness
  of long-term laxative therapy [3]

Level [1] indicates good evidence, i.e., consistent results from well-designed, well-conducted
studies.
Level [2] indicates fair evidence, i.e., results show benefit, but strength limited by number,
quality, or consistency of studies.
Level [3] indicates poor evidence, i.e., insufficient because of limited number, power, or quality
of studies.

Infrequent Bowel Movements

Two or fewer bowel movements per week are below normal range
and tend to signify slow transit constipation. Weekly frequency of
bowel movements does not, however, alter with age alone, in contrast
to self-reporting of constipation. In community-based studies, it has
been found that

- only 1% to 7% of both younger and older community-dwelling
  individuals report two or fewer bowel movements a week;
- this consistent bowel pattern across age groups persists even after
  statistical adjustment for the greater amount of laxatives used by
  older people;
- among older people complaining of constipation, less than 10%
  report two or fewer weekly bowel movements, and more than
  50% move their bowels daily.

TABLE 93-4

Complications of Constipation in Older People
Fecal incontinence [1]
Fecal impaction [1]
Stercoral perforation [3]
Urinary retention [2]
Sigmoid volvulus [2]
Acquired megacolon [2]
Rectal prolapse [3]
Diverticular disease [2]
Impaired quality of life [3]
Agitation in patients with dementia [3]

Level [1] indicates good evidence, i.e., consistent results from well-designed, well-conducted studies.

Level [2] indicates fair evidence, i.e., results show benefit, but strength limited by number, quality, or consistency of studies.

Level [3] indicates poor evidence, i.e., insufficient because of limited number, power, or quality of studies.

Difficult Evacuation

So, what are the symptoms other than infrequent bowel movements that drive self-reporting of constipation in older people? Theses symptoms are predominantly straining and passage of hard stools. Of older people reporting constipation in a U.S. community study, 65% had persistent straining and 39% had passage of hard bowel movements. Difficult rectal evacuation is a primary cause of constipation in older people. Twenty-one percent of community-dwelling people aged 65+ had rectal outlet delay (according to Rome II criteria), and many describe the need to self-evacuate. Among frailer individuals, difficult evacuation can lead to rectal impaction and fecal soiling.

Constipation Symptoms in the Long-Term Care Setting

Long-term care residents are at increased risk of developing complications of constipation (Table 93-4) that may precipitate acute hospital admissions. Physical frailty in older persons does increase the prevalence of infrequent bowel movements, with 17% of nursing home residents and 14% of geriatric day-hospital attendees reporting two or fewer bowel movements a week. Among long-term care residents self-reporting constipation, 33% have two or fewer bowel movements a week. A Finnish study showed the prevalence of chronic constipation and/or rectal outlet delay to be 57% in women and 64% in men living in residential homes, and 79% and 81% respectively in the nursing home setting. A U.K. study found that 64% of nursing home residents taking laxatives still reported straining on more than 1 in 4 occasions. This and the fact that 50% to 74% of long-term care residents use daily laxatives suggest that rectal evacuation difficulties are not being well managed in this population.

PATHOPHYSIOLOGY

Physiological studies suggest that changes in the lower bowel predisposing toward constipation in older people are not primarily age-related. This is compatible with the epidemiology showing that (1) bowel movement frequency does alter with aging, and (2) constipa-

tion symptoms are more prevalent in older people with comorbidities. Extrinsic causes such as reduced mobility, fluid intake, dietary fiber, comorbidities, and medication all impact colonic motility and transit, and influence the pathophysiology of constipation.

Colonic Function

Colonic motility depends on the integrity of the central and autonomic nervous systems, gut wall innervation and receptors, circular smooth muscle, and gastrointestinal hormones. Propagating motor complexes in the colon are stimulated by increased intraluminal pressure generated by bulky fecal content. Studies of total gut transit time (passage of radiopaque markers from mouth to anus, normally 80% passed within 5 days), colonic motor activity, and postprandial gastrocolic reflex show no differences between healthy older and younger people. Older people with chronic constipation do, however, tend to have a prolonged total gut transit time, ranging from 4 to 9 days. Radiologic markers pass especially slowly through the left colon with striking delay in the rectosigmoid, suggesting that total transit time is prolonged because of segmental dysmotility in the "hindgut." The prolongation in transit time is even greater in institutionalized or bedridden patients with constipation, with total gut transit time ranging from 6 to more than 14 days. Slow transit results in a cycle of worsening colonic dysfunction by reducing water content of stool (normally 75%) and shrinking fecal bulk, which then diminishes the intraluminal pressures, and hence the generation of propagating motor complexes and propulsive activity.

Intrinsic Mechanisms for Colonic Dysfunction in Older People with Constipation

Certain intrinsic mechanisms for altered colonic function in older persons with constipation have been postulated from physiologic studies (Table 93-5). Overall collagen deposition in the left side of the colon increases with aging, and this could alter colonic compliance and motility. Direct electrophysiologic measurement of colonic motor activity in elderly subjects has shown that the sigmoid motor response to intraluminal Bisacodyl (a direct stimulant of the myenteric

TABLE 93-5

Pathophysiological Mechanisms for Constipation in Older People
Chronic Constipation
Intrinsic myenteric plexus dysfunction
Increased collagen deposit in colon (age-related)
Reduced inhibitory nerve input to circular muscle (age-related)
Increased binding of plasma endorphins to gut receptors (age-related)
Prolonged transit owing to extrinsic factors (immobility, diet, drugs, comorbidity)
Rectal Outlet Delay
Rectal dyschezia secondary to suppression or disregard of urge to pass stool
Sacral cord dysfunction
Pelvic floor descent
Pelvic floor dyssynergia (paradoxical contraction of pelvic floor muscles and external sphincter)
Irritable bowel disease
Weak abdominal musculature

plexus) is diminished in patients who are constipated, implying a deficit in intrinsic innervation. Myenteric plexus dysfunction may partially account for impaired gut motility in elderly persons with constipation. The total number of neurons in the myenteric plexus is decreased, and this neuronal loss bears no relation to the presence of pseudomelanosis coli cells, implying that use of anthraquinone laxatives is not the primary cause.

Another possible intrinsic factor is age-related deficit in the density of inhibitory nerves, or in the binding sites on smooth muscle for inhibitory gut neuropeptides. In vitro studies of colons across age groups showed an age-related reduction in the amplitude of inhibitory junction potentials, but no decrease in the levels of inhibitory gut neuropeptides. This age-related decline occurs earlier in women as compared with men. Such a decrease in inhibitory nerve input to the circular smooth muscle could result in segmental motor incoordination, which may lengthen transit time and promote constipation in older persons with other predisposing risk factors. Individuals older than age 60 years have higher plasma concentrations of *beta*-endorphin with increased binding to opiate receptors in the gut wall and myenteric plexus. Higher opiate binding has the effect of relaxing colonic tone, reducing motility, and inhibiting the gastrocolic reflex.

Finally, it is interesting to note that constipation is more prevalent in patients with nonulcer dyspepsia, the two clinical conditions being linked by gastrointestinal hypomotility.

Anorectal Function

In normal defecation, colonic activity propels stool into the rectal ampulla causing distension and intrinsically mediated relaxation of the smooth muscle of the internal anal sphincter (or anal canal). This is followed promptly by reflex contraction of the external anal sphincter and pelvic floor muscles, which are skeletal muscles innervated by the pudendal nerve. The brain registers a desire to defecate, the external sphincter is voluntarily relaxed, and the rectum is evacuated with assistance from abdominal wall muscle contraction.

Age-Related Changes in Anorectal Function

There is a tendency toward an age-related decline in internal sphincter tone, particularly in the eighth decade onward. Clinically, this predisposes older individuals to fecal incontinence, particularly with loose stools. There is a more definite age-related decline (greater in women than men) in external anal sphincter and pelvic muscle strength, which can contribute toward evacuation difficulties. Failure of the anorectal angle to open and excessive perineal descent in older women can lead to constipation. In simulated defecation studies, 37% of nonconstipated older subjects were unable to evacuate a small solid sphere. Consequent prolonged straining may compress the pudendal nerve, further exacerbating any preexisting weakness. There appears to be a reduction in rectal motility with normal aging, again in older old age. Rectal sensation does not alter with normal aging.

Anorectal Dysfunction in Older Persons

There are three types of anorectal dysfunction that predispose older people to rectal outlet delay.

The most common is *rectal dysmotility* characterized by reduced rectal motility, increased rectal compliance with a variable degree of rectal dilatation, and impaired rectal sensation such that the urge to pass stool is blunted. Over time, an increasing degree of rectal distension is required to reflexly trigger the defecation mechanism. These patients have rectal retention of hard or soft stool on digital examination of which they may be unaware. The resulting rectal distension leads to relaxation of the internal sphincter and hence to fecal soiling. One study showed that rectal contractions could be elicited in only 14% of older people with a history of rectal impaction. One postulated cause for rectal dysmotility is diminished parasympathetic outflow as a result of impaired sacral cord function, for example, from ischemia or spinal stenosis (Table 93-5). In a significant number of older people, rectal dysmotility can develop through a persistent disregard or suppression of the urge to defecate as a result of dementia, depression, immobility, or painful anorectal conditions. Voluntary increase in intra-abdominal pressure during defecation could overcome rectal dysmotility to produce enough of an increase in rectal pressure for evacuation to occur, but older people often have weakened abdominal musculature, limiting their ability to compensate in this way.

Pelvic floor dyssynergia, though more common in younger women, can cause rectal outlet delay in older people. This is caused by paradoxical contraction or failure to relax the pelvic floor and external anal sphincter muscles during defecation, and manometric studies show paradoxical increases in anal canal pressure on straining. This abnormal expulsion pattern may be seen in individuals with severe and long-standing symptoms of rectal outlet delay, and in patients with Parkinson disease.

Another type of anorectal dysfunction is *irritable bowel syndrome* (IBS) characterized by increased rectal tone and reduced compliance. Sensation of pain on distending the rectum during anorectal function tests has been shown to be greater in patients with IBS than controls. IBS is usually constipation-predominant in older people. These patients are likely to have a many year history of difficult passage of small fecal pellets and other IBS symptoms such as passing mucus, abdominal distension, and pain.

RISK FACTORS FOR CONSTIPATION IN OLDER PEOPLE

Both the epidemiology and pathophysiology of constipation in older people point to the enormous importance of identifying predisposing causes for the condition in each affected individual. One prospective study examined baseline characteristics predictive of new-onset constipation in elderly nursing home patients, using the U.S. Minimum Data Set instrument. Seven percent ($n = 1291$) developed constipation over a 3-month period. Independent predictors were white race, poor consumption of fluids, pneumonia, Parkinson disease, allergies, decreased bed mobility, arthritis, greater than five medications, dementia, hypothyroidism, and hypertension. The authors postulated that allergies, arthritis, and hypertension were associated primarily because of the constipating effect of drugs used to treat these conditions. Other studies have shown that institutionalization itself is an independent risk factor for symptom-based constipation in older people. Table 93-6 summarizes evidence-based risk factors of constipation in the elderly population.

TABLE 93-6

Risk Factors for Constipation in Older People

Medications
  Polypharmacy (≥5 medications) [2]
  Anticholinergic drugs (tricyclics, antipsychotics, antihistamines,
    antiemetics, drugs for detrusor hyperactivity) [1]
  Opiates [2]
  Iron supplements [3]
  Calcium channel antagonists (nifedipine and verapamil) [2]
  Calcium supplements [2]
  Nonsteroidal anti-inflammatory drugs [2]

Impaired mobility [2]

Nursing home residency [2]

Neurological conditions
  Dementia [2]
  Parkinson disease [1]
  Diabetes mellitus [1]
  Autonomic neuropathy [2]
  Stroke [3]
  Spinal cord injury or disease [1]

Depression [3]

Dehydration [2]

Low dietary fiber [3]

Metabolic disturbances
  Hypothyroidism
  Hypercalcemia
  Hypokalemia
  Uremia
  Patients receiving renal dialysis [3]

Mechanical obstruction (e.g., tumor, rectocele)

Lack of privacy or comfort

Poor toilet access [3]

Level [1] indicates good evidence, i.e., consistent results from well-designed, well-conducted studies.
Level [2] indicates fair evidence, i.e., results show benefit, but strength limited by number, quality, or consistency of studies.
Level [3] indicates poor evidence, i.e., insufficient because of limited number, power, or quality of studies.

Reduced Mobility

Impaired mobility is a common risk factor for constipation in older people. Greater physical activity (including regular walking) is associated with less self-reported and symptom-specific constipation in older people living both at home and in long-term care. Reduced mobility was found to be the strongest independent correlate of heavy laxative use among nursing home residents, following adjustment for age, comorbidity, and other relevant clinical factors. Gut transit time in elderly subjects was measured independently as 3 days in ambulant, and 3 weeks in bedridden patients, although comorbid factors were likely to be contributory. A study of healthy young male volunteers showed that after only 1 week of bed rest, both transit through the sigmoid colon and stool frequency were reduced. It is well documented that exercise increases colonic propulsive activity ("joggers diarrhea"), especially when measured postprandially. In a population survey of younger women (36–61 years), daily physical activity was associated with less constipation (defined as two or fewer bowel movements per week), and the association strengthened

with increased frequency of physical activity. This leads to speculation that increasing physical activity in adulthood may reduce the likelihood of constipation problems in older age.

Polypharmacy/Drug Side Effects

Polypharmacy itself increases the risk of constipation in older patients, particularly in nursing homes where each individual takes an average of six prescribed medications per day.

Anticholinergic medications reduce contractility of the smooth muscle of the gut via an antimuscarinic effect at acetylcholine receptor sites, and in some cases (e.g., patients with schizophrenia taking neuroleptics), long-term use may result in chronic megacolon. In two cross-sectional studies of nursing home residents, anticholinergic antidepressants were independently associated with daily laxative use following adjustment for age, gender, function, and cognition. Anticholinergic neuroleptics and antihistamines were also independently associated in one of the studies; nonanticholinergic sedatives, however, were not found to be constipating. A recent study of 532 community-dwelling older U.S. veterans found that among the 27% using anticholinergic drugs, the rate of constipation (42%) was significantly greater than those not using the drugs.

While older people are very susceptible to the constipating effects of *opiate analgesia*, a recent U.S. study of nursing home residents with persistent nonmalignant pain found that there was no increased rate of constipation in chronic opiate users over a 6 month period compared to those not taking opiates. They also observed a general improvement in functional status and social engagement. Constipation in chronic opiate users can be effectively managed (by laxative or suppository coprescription where needed)—an important finding as chronic pain is often undertreated in frailer older people perhaps owing to fear of the adverse effects of analgesic drugs. In terms of different preparations, community-based studies of adults receiving opiates for chronic pain have shown equal constipation risk for all sustained-release oral preparations. Transdermal patches (e.g., fentanyl), however, are associated with lower risk of constipation than oral preparations.

All types of *iron supplements* (sulphate, fumarate, and gluconate) cause constipation in adults, the constipating factor being the amount of elemental iron absorbed. Slow-release preparations have a lesser impact on the large bowel, but this is because they tend to carry the iron past the first part of the duodenum into an area of the gut where elemental iron absorption is poorer. Administration of iron sulfate in doses greater than 325 mg per day does not substantially increase iron absorption in elderly persons and may significantly increase gastrointestinal side effects. Intravenous iron does not cause constipation and may be an alternative in patients with chronic anemia (e.g., chronic kidney disease) who have symptomatic constipation on oral iron.

In a recent 5-year study of *calcium supplementation* in older women, the only side effect was constipation (treatment 13.4% vs. placebo 9.1%). The study showed that calcium supplementation reduced bone loss and turnover and fracture rates in older women who took it, but long-term compliance was poor, and constipation may have contributed to this.

Calcium channel antagonists impair lower gut motility, particularly in the rectosigmoid, by inhibiting calcium uptake into smooth muscle cells and altering intraluminal electrolyte and water transportation. Severe constipation has been reported in older patients taking calcium channel antagonists, with nifedipine and verapamil being the most potent inhibitors of gut motility in this class of drugs.

Nonsteroidal anti-inflammatory drugs (NSAIDs) increase the risk of constipation in older people, most likely through prostaglandin inhibition. In a large case-controlled primary care study, constipation and straining was a more common reason for stopping NSAIDs than dyspepsia. NSAIDs have also been implicated in causing stercoral perforation in patients with chronic constipation. Using 15 or more aspirin tablets a week has been linked to constipation in a middle-aged cohort of women.

Aluminium antacids have been associated with constipation in older people living in both nursing homes and in the community.

Dietary Factors

Fiber

Low consumption of wheat bran, fiber, vegetables, fruit, rice, and calories can all predispose toward constipation. A U.K. survey showed that consumption of fruit, vegetables, and bread decreases with advancing age. It has been suggested that the prevalence of constipation is rising because modern food processing produces refined food with low roughage. Community studies of older Europeans who eat a Mediterranean diet rich in fruit, vegetables, and olive oil show a low prevalence of constipation (4.4% in people aged 50+). Conversely, a German questionnaire survey of adults with and without constipation reported that chocolate, white bread, and bananas were the foodstuffs most strongly perceived to harden stools.

Calories

Low calorie intake in older people (adjusted for fiber intake) has been linked to constipation. One study looked at nutritional factors across all nursing homes in Finland and found that malnutrition and constipation were associated. This may be a two-way association in that marked constipation or fecal impaction can cause anorexia, while low calorie intake can promote constipation.

Enteral Nutrition

Constipation is a recognized problem in patients receiving enteral nutrition. A prospective survey from Spain of hospitalized patients (mean age 76) receiving nasogastric tube feeding identified constipation as a complication of treatment in 30%. Enteric feeding products containing fiber are available, though there are no data on whether constipation is any less of a problem with their use.

Fluid Intake

Amount

Low fluid intake in older adults has been related to symptomatic constipation in epidemiologic surveys and (in an unadjusted analysis) to slow colonic transit. In patients with Parkinson disease, low water intake correlated with severity of constipation. Withholding fluids over a 1-week period in young male volunteers significantly reduced stool output. Elderly people are at greater risk of dehydration because of

- impaired thirst sensation,
- less effective hormonal responses to hypertonicity,
- limited access to drinks because of coexisting physical or cognitive impairments,
- voluntary fluid restriction in an attempt to control urinary incontinence.

Alcohol and Coffee

A large Japanese survey of constipation symptoms found that alcohol consumption was a preventive factor in men. A population survey of middle-aged women in the United States showed that daily alcohol consumption (exceeding 12 g/d) and low-moderate caffeine intake were independently inversely related to infrequent bowel movements. Black coffee has been shown to increase colonic motility specifically in the rectosigmoid within 4 minutes of ingestion in young healthy volunteers (a reaction not observed with ingestion of hot water), implying that caffeine triggers the gastrocolic reflex.

Parkinson Disease

Patients with Parkinson disease suffer from three primary pathologies that lead to constipation:

- Primary degeneration of dopaminergic neurons in the myenteric plexus resulting in prolonged colorectal transit
- Pelvic dyssynergia causing rectal outlet delay and prolonged straining
- Small increases in intra-abdominal pressures on straining (compared with age-matched controls)

Constipation can become prominent early in the course of the disease, even 10 to 20 years prior to motor symptoms. In a 24-year longitudinal study (Honolulu), less than one bowel movement a day was associated with a threefold elevated risk of future Parkinson disease in men. A recent study of patients at a Parkinson disease clinic found that 59% were constipated according to the Rome criteria (vs. 21% in age-matched control group without neurological disease), and 33% were very concerned by their bowel problem. Antiparkinsonian drugs can further exacerbate constipation. Pelvic dyssynergia affects 60% of people with Parkinson disease and may be hard to treat. Botulinum toxin injected into the puborectalis muscle has been used to improve rectal emptying in Parkinson disease patients with good effect, though repeat injections every 3 months are required to maintain clinical benefit.

Diabetes Mellitus

A Turkish study of outpatients with type 2 diabetes showed that 56% complained of constipation (vs. 30% of controls). Neuropathy symptom scores correlated with laxative usage and straining. Diabetic patients with autonomic neuropathy are more likely to be constipated because of markedly slowed transit throughout the colon and impairment of the gastrocolic reflex. However, one-third of diabetic patients with constipation do not have neuropathic symptoms, so additional potentially reversible factors should be considered particularly in older people (e.g., drugs, mobility, fluids). Indeed, a U.S. community study found that constipation and/or laxative use was increased in type 1 versus type 2 diabetic men, but this difference was associated with use of calcium channel-blockers rather than with neuropathy symptoms. Acute hyperglycemia inhibits the gastrocolic reflex and colonic peristalsis, so glycemic control is important. Colonic transit time in frail and immobile older people with diabetes is extremely prolonged at 200 ± 144 hours. An Israeli study showed that this very long transit time in long-term care residents with diabetes can be significantly reduced by administering acarbose, an alpha-glucosidase inhibitor with a potential adverse effect of causing diarrhea. Overall, gut dysmotility can lead to bacterial overgrowth and the clinical problem of explosive diarrhea; treatment with erythromycin and long-term motility agents such as metoclopramide should be considered in these individuals.

Dementia

Dementia predisposes individuals to rectal dysmotility, partly through ignoring the urge to defecate. A study in which young men deliberately suppressed defecation resulted in prolonged transit through the rectosigmoid with a marked reduction in frequency of bowel movements. Epidemiological studies show a significant association between cognitive impairment and nurse-documented constipation in nursing home residents. Patients with non-Alzheimer dementias (Parkinson disease, Lewy body, vascular dementia) compared to those with Alzheimer dementia are more likely to suffer from autonomic symptoms, including constipation.

Mood-Related Disorders

Depression, psychological distress, and anxiety are all associated with increased self-reporting of constipation in older persons. In certain cases, the symptom of constipation is a somatic manifestation of psychiatric illness. A careful assessment is required to differentiate subjective complaints from clinical constipation in depressed or anxious patients.

Stroke

Constipation affects 60% of those recovering from stroke on rehabilitation wards, and a high number of these have combined rectal outlet delay and slow transit constipation. For stroke survivors living in the community, problems relating to bowel evacuation are greatly worsened by difficulties accessing the toilet owing to functional impairment. Fecal incontinence in stroke survivors has been shown to relate more to modifiable disability-related factors such as toilet access and anticholinergic medication use than to stroke-related factors (such as severity and lesion location). Weakness of abdominal and pelvic muscles following stroke also contribute to problems with evacuation.

Spinal Cord Injury/Disease

Constipation affects the majority of people with spinal cord disease or injury. Age and duration of injury interact to promote complications of chronic constipation such as acquired megacolon, which affects more than half of patients with spinal cord injury. Lumbar stenosis in older people caused by degenerative joint disease may lead to cauda equina problems with severe rectal outlet delay. One study in younger people showed that an average of 27% (range 0–44%) of rectosigmoid emptying was achieved with each defecation in patients with cauda equina syndromes, versus 81% (range 53–100%) in healthy controls.

Metabolic Disorders

Hypokalemia produces neuronal dysfunction that minimizes acetylcholine stimulation of gut smooth muscle and so prolongs transit through the gut. It should be excluded in cases of colonic psuedoobstruction and sigmoid volvulus. *Hypercalcemia* causes conduction delay within the extrinsic and intrinsic innervation of the gut. Surgical treatment of hyperparathyroidism reverses the neuromuscular bowel dysfunction seen with this condition. Patients with *myxedema* have been observed to have edema of the gut wall with mucopolysaccharide deposition, although whether this contributes to the colonic hypomotility seen commonly in *clinical hypothyroidism* is uncertain. Patients on *long-term renal dialysis* have prolonged age-adjusted transit time, more so in hemo- than peritoneal dialysis. In a questionnaire study from Japan, 63% of hemodialysis patients complained of constipation. Important contributors to this problem were thought to be high (49%) use of resin to avoid hyperkalemia, suppression of the defecation urge while undergoing dialysis, and low fiber intake. Resin administration also places elderly inpatients at risk of fecal impaction.

Colorectal Cancer

Colorectal cancer has been linked with both constipation and use of laxatives, although this risk association is likely to be confounded by the influence of underlying habits. One study, adjusted for age and potential confounders, found that having fewer than three reported bowel movements a week was associated with a greater than twofold risk of colon cancer, with the association being most strong in black women. As the prevalence of colorectal cancer increases with age, index of suspicion should be higher in older adults. Constipation alone, however, is not an indication for proceeding to colonoscopy (see below).

Rectocele

Posterior vaginal wall prolapse and rectocele is not uncommonly seen in older multiparous women. These individuals have an increased risk of rectal outlet delay, particularly incomplete emptying and need for digital evacuation. This is presumably caused by mechanical obstruction, as this association is not seen in women with anterior pelvic prolapse.

PRESENTATION

Table 93-7 lists the important aspects of the bowel history that should be elicited from an elderly person who complains of constipation. It is essential to identify rectal evacuation difficulties where present in order to manage the patient effectively. Table 93-2 lists reasons why constipation may be underestimated in frail elderly patients. Conversely, studies have shown that adults complaining of constipation frequently underestimate the number of bowel movements per week,

TABLE 93-7

Diagnosis of Constipation in Older People

Bowel History
Number of bowel movements per week
Stool consistency
Straining/symptoms of rectal outlet delay
Duration of constipation
Fecal incontinence/soiling
Irritable bowel syndrome symptoms (abdominal pain, bloating, passage of
    mucus)
Rectal pain or bleeding
Laxative use, prior and current
Psychological and quality of life impact of bowel problem
Urinary incontinence/lower urinary tract symptoms

General History
Mood/cognition
Symptoms of systemic illness (weight loss, anemia)
Relevant comorbidities (e.g., diabetes, neurological disease)
Mobility
Diet
Medications
Toilet access (location of bathroom, manual dexterity, vision)

Specific Physical Examination
Digital rectal examination including external and internal sphincter tone
Perianal sensation/cutaneous anal reflex
Rectal prolapse/hemorrhoids
Pelvic floor descent/rectocele
Abdominal palpation, auscultation
Neurological, cognitive, and functional examination

Tests
Indications for plain abdominal radiograph
    Empty rectum with clinical suspicion of constipation
    Evaluation for fecal impaction
    Persistent fecal incontinence despite clearing of any rectal impaction
    Evaluation of abdominal distension, pain, or acute discomfort
    Persisting complaints of constipation with increasing laxative usage
Indications for colonoscopy
    Systemic illness (weight loss, anemia etc.)
    Bleeding per rectum
    Recent change in bowel habit without obvious risk factors
Indications for anorectal function tests
    Severe or persistent symptoms of rectal outlet delay
    Persistent fecal incontinence with clinical evidence of anal sphincter
        weakness

so it is helpful to have them keep a stool chart for 1 week to document frequency and characteristics of their bowel movements and associated symptoms. A recent history of altered bowel habit should prompt an exploration of precipitants (e.g., medications, stroke), and where unexplained, an evaluation for colorectal cancer. Abdominal pain, rectal bleeding, and certainly any systemic features such as weight loss and anemia should prompt further investigations for underlying neoplasm.

Perianal fecal soiling should be asked about and looked for; it is a common and embarrassing symptom that patients are reluctant to volunteer. In one large nursing home study, 38% of elderly individuals who complained of constipation reported fecal soiling of undergarments. Overflow fecal incontinence typically presents as frequent passive leakage of watery stool, sometimes confusing patients and carers (and occasionally health care providers) into thinking they

have "diarrhea" rather than constipation. Impaction must be ruled out in the presence of fecal soiling or incontinence. The other important diagnoses to consider in older people are loose stools caused by inappropriate laxative use, other drug side effects, or undiagnosed bowel disease. Bowel diseases that are especially prevalent in older people include *Clostridium difficile* colitis, lactose intolerance (more common in people aged 60–79 than in those aged 40–59 years), late-onset Crohn, and tumor.

IBS should be a diagnosis of exclusion in older people, and only made in those with a many year history of intermittent IBS symptoms such as abdominal distension or pain relieved by defecation, passage of mucus, and feeling of incomplete emptying (Rome criteria). Rectal pain associated with defecation should alert the physician to rectal ischemia as well as to other more common anorectal conditions. Rectal bleeding should prompt further evaluation for underlying tumor disease, unless examination clearly reveals bright red blood from anal fissure or hemorrhoids. Lower urinary tract symptoms may be exacerbated by constipation and should be documented.

A person's attitude to their bowel problem (positive, acceptance, denial, distress, apathy) and the impact on their quality of life (changes in usual family, social, physical, and work-related activities) should be included when taking a history. Some health care providers share the generally held belief that constipation is an inevitable consequence of aging, and qualitative work has shown that patients can feel that their problem is not being taken seriously. A thorough clinical history and assessment is an important first step in developing a sound patient–physician partnership, which enhances successful outcomes in managing what is usually a chronic condition.

CLINICAL EVALUATION

Digital Rectal Examination

Digital rectal examination is required in all patients who report constipation to reveal rectal impaction, rectal dilatation, hemorrhoids, anorectal disease, and perianal fecal soiling. Retained stool in rectal impaction does not have to be hard; loading with soft stool is commonly seen in older people taking laxatives who have problems with rectal outlet delay. Absence of stool on rectal examination does not exclude the diagnosis of constipation. A dilated rectum with diminished sensation and retained stool suggests rectal dysmotility. External sphincter tone is assessed by asking the patient to "squeeze and pull up" around the examining finger. Indicators of reduced internal anal tone are easy insertion of the finger into the anal canal and gaping of the anus on applying gentle traction to the anal margin. Anal sphincter weakness should prompt (1) careful prescribing to avoid causing fecal leakage though excessive laxative-induced softness of stool, and (2) instruction in anal sphincter strengthening exercises (Table 93-8). Absent cutaneous-anal reflex (gentle scratching of the anal margin should normally induce a visible contraction of the external sphincter) and, in particular, perianal anesthesia points to significant sacral cord dysfunction with associated rectal dysmotility. Proctoscopy is a simple, quick, and useful test for diagnosing internal hemorrhoids, and abnormalities of the rectal wall. Where rectal impaction or outlet delay is identified, a postvoid residual volume should be measured as urinary retention may coexist.

TABLE 93-8

Patient Education

Toilet Habits and Positioning

Do not delay having a bowel movement when you feel the urge.

Put aside a particular time each day (we would advise after breakfast) when you can sit on the toilet without being in a hurry.

A relaxed attitude to bowel evacuation will especially help if you have problems with straining or a feeling of anal blockage.

If straining is a problem, it is helpful to have a footstool under your feet while sitting on the toilet as this increases the ability of your abdominal muscles to help evacuation of stool.

Abdominal Massage

Lie on the bed with pillows under your head and shoulders.

Your knees should be bent up with a pillow underneath them for support.

Cover your abdomen with a light sheet.

Massage your abdomen with firm but gentle circular movements starting at the right side and working across to the left side.

Continue the massage for approximately 10 minutes.

This massage should be a pleasant experience—if you feel any discomfort then stop.

Diet

To help prevent constipation you should eat more of the foods from List A and less of the foods from List B. Foods in list A tend to make the stool softer and easier to pass, because they are high in fiber. Foods in List B tend to make the stool harder, because they bind together the contents of the bowel.

List A: Fresh fruit, prunes and other dried fruit, whole meal bread, bran cereals and porridge, salad, cooked vegetables (with skin where possible), beans, lentils.

List B: Milk, hard cheese, yogurt, white bread or crackers, refined cereals, cakes, pancakes, noodles, white rice, chocolate, creamed soups.

You should increase your fiber intake gradually because sudden change in fiber content may cause temporary bloating and irregularity. It is important to eat the foods that contain fiber all through the day and not just at one meal such as breakfast.

Increase the amount of fluid that you drink gradually up to 8 to 10 glasses a day. Try to drink more water, fruit juices, and fizzy drinks.

Sphincter Strengthening

Learning to do your exercises

Sit in a comfortable position with your knees slightly apart. Now imagine that you are trying to stop yourself passing wind from the bowel. To do this you must squeeze the muscle around the back passage. Try squeezing and lifting that muscle as tightly as you can. You should be able to feel the muscle move.

Your buttocks, abdomen, and legs should not move at all. You should be aware of the skin around the back passage tightening and being pulled up and away from your chair. Really try to feel this. You are now exercising your anal sphincter muscles. (You do not need to hold your breath when you tighten the muscles!)

Practicing your exercises

Tighten and pull up the anal sphincter muscles as tightly as you can. Hold tightened for at least 5 seconds, then relax for at least 10 seconds.

Repeat this exercise at least 5 times. This will work on the strength of your muscles.

Next, pull the muscles to approximately half of their maximum squeeze. See how long you can hold this for. Then relax for at least 10 seconds.

Repeat at least 5 times. This will work on the endurance or staying power of your muscles.

Pull up the muscles as quickly and tightly as you can and then relax and then pull up again, and see how many times you can do this before you get tired. Try for at least 5 quick pull-ups. Try this quick pull-up exercise at least 10 times each day.

Do all these exercises as hard as you can and at least 5 times a day. As the muscles get stronger, you will find that you can do more pull-ups each time without the muscle getting tired.

It takes time for exercises to make muscle stronger. You may need to exercise regularly for several months before the muscles gain their full strength.

Instructions for Using Suppositories

These may be inserted into your rectum (back passage) by your nurse or carer or yourself if you are physically able to do it.

If necessary go to the toilet and empty your bowels if you can.

Wash your hands.

Remove any foil or wrapping from the suppository.

Either lie on your side with your lower leg straight and your upper leg bent towards your waist or squat.

Gently but firmly insert the suppository, narrow end first, into the rectum using a finger. Push far enough (approximately one inch) so that it does not come out again.

You may find your body wanting to push out the suppository. Close your legs and keep still for a few minutes.

Try not to empty your bowels for at least 10 to 20 minutes.

Pelvic Floor/Rectal Prolapse

Excessive perineal descent is observed by asking the patient to "bear down" while lying in the lateral position. Normal perineal descent is less than 4 cms (can be eye-balled by drawing an imaginary line between that ischeal prominences). Rectal prolapse may also be observed in this manner, though lesser degrees of prolapse may only be identified by having the patient strain while sitting on a toilet or commode. An examination for posterior vaginal prolapse (bearing down in the gynecological position) is appropriate in all women with constipation, especially those reporting incomplete rectal emptying and the need to manually evacuate.

General Assessment

A broad assessment should be undertaken in older patients with constipation, focusing on predisposing causes. History should include over-the-counter medications, diet, and fluid intake. Examination should include cognition, mood, and function. Appropriate laboratory tests include complete blood count; plasma electrolytes; glucose; and bone, liver, and thyroid profiles.

Plain Abdominal X-Ray

Clinical diagnosis can usually be made on the basis of a thorough history and examination. However, a plain abdominal radiograph is useful in patients without rectal impaction in whom colonic loading is suspected because of a high-risk profile, constipation-related symptoms, or fecal incontinence. In those patients who continue to report troublesome constipation-related symptoms despite regular laxative use it can guide management by showing the following:

- No stool—patient may require education about what constitutes a normal bowel habit and no increase and possibly a reduction in laxative usage.
- Colonic fecal loading—patient requires education on lifestyle measures and a change in type or increased dose of laxative.
- Rectal loading with a clear colon—patient requires suppositories or enemas, and no increase and possibly a reduction in laxatives.

Marked fecal loading in the descending and sigmoid colon correlates well with prolonged transit time, as does the presence of feces rather than air in the cecum (Figure 93-1). Dilatation of the colon (>6.5 cm maximum diameter) in the absence of acute obstruction points to a neurogenic component to bowel dysfunction, and thus identifies patients at risk of recurrent colonic impaction. Rectal dilatation (>4 cm) implies dysmotility and evacuation problems. Finally, in patients with abdominal distension and/or pain, an abdominal radiograph has to be done to rule out acute problems such as sigmoid volvulus and small bowel obstruction secondary to severe impaction.

Colonoscopy/Bowel Preparation

Chronic constipation alone is not an appropriate indication for colonoscopy; the range of neoplasia found is similar to that in asymptomatic patients undergoing primary colorectal cancer screening. Further investigation is of course warranted in the context of systemic illness or laboratory abnormalities. Barium enema has now largely

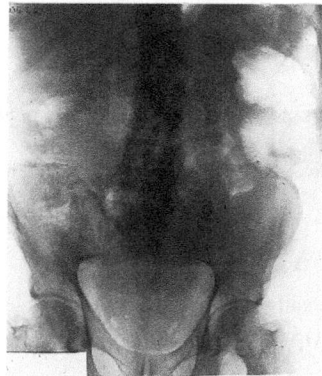

FIGURE 93-1. Abdominal radiograph of an 83-yr-old man with Parkinson disease and long-standing symptoms of continuous fecal leakage. As his caregiver at home, his wife was changing his clothing up to six times a day. The rectosigmoid colon is completely impacted, and the dilated bowel loop implies obstruction. He was briefly hospitalized for disimpaction with enemas and laxatives, resulting in complete resolution of incontinence. He and his wife were educated in regular use of laxatives and suppositories, as well as in lifestyle measures.

TABLE 93-9
Bowel Preparation in Older People

Give regular laxatives (e.g., Movicol 2 sachets daily) and enemas or suppositories for at least 1 week before the procedure, with a longer run up period in patients known to have constipation, or with comorbidities such as diabetes
Individualize the cathartic regimen (e.g., 1–2 L of GoLYTELY daily over 2 to 3 days in those unable to drink 4 L, or use of alternative preparations such as sodium picosulfate)
Identify potential nonadherence ("Can the patient drink 4 L of GoLYTELY in 24 h?")
Preempt unpleasant side effects ("Will the patient be able to reach the toilet in time to avoid fecal leakage?")
Use oral phosphosoda with caution as administration in older people increases in serum phosphate, even in patients with normal creatinine clearance
Consider preprocedure plain abdominal x-ray for evaluation of persisting fecal loading
Where possible, give clear fluid diet prior to administration of bowel preparation

been superceded by colonoscopy in older patients—colonoscopy causes significantly less discomfort than barium enema as well as is diagnostically more sensitive. A review of 400 colonoscopies in octagenarians and upwards showed a good safety profile but low cancer detection rate for symptoms (e.g., constipation, abdominal pain) other than bleeding (2% vs. 12%).

Inadequate colonoscopies are common in older people because of poor bowel preparation. Older age, constipation, reported laxative use, tricyclic antidepressants, stroke, and dementia have been associated with inadequate preparation and thus taking longer to instrument the cecum. A study of 101 inpatients showed that even in those who took 75% to 100% of their prescribed treatment, bowel preparation was satisfactory in only 50%. Table 93-9 lists issues relevant to bowel preparation in older people.

Anorectal Function Tests

Anorectal function tests are rarely required in assessment of constipation in older people. They may be indicated in patients with severe and persistent rectal outlet delay, in order to diagnose pelvic dyssynergia, which is more effectively treated by biofeedback than laxatives. Another indication is fecal incontinence of formed stool that persists despite clearing of fecal impaction. Anorectal tests (including endoanal ultrasound) can measure the integrity of the anal sphincters and thus guide management of incontinence toward conservative treatment (sphincter strengthening exercises and biofeedback therapy), or surgical intervention (sphincter reconstruction).

COMPLICATIONS OF CONSTIPATION IN THE ELDERLY

Fecal Incontinence

Constipation is a common, treatable, preventable, and often overlooked cause of fecal incontinence in older people (Table 93-4). Few medical symptoms are as distressing and social isolating for older people as fecal incontinence, a condition that places them at greater risk of morbidity, mortality, dependency, and nursing home placement. All too often, untreated overflow leads to hospitalization of vulnerable older patients. Many older individuals in the community with fecal incontinence will not volunteer the problem to their general practitioner and, regrettably, physicians and nurses do not routinely inquire about the symptom. This "hidden problem" therefore leads to social isolation and a downward spiral of psychological distress, dependency, and poor health. Even when older people are noted by health care professionals to have fecal incontinence, the condition is often poorly assessed and passively managed, especially in the long-term care setting where it is most prevalent.

Overflow (continuous fecal soiling and fecal impaction on rectal examination) was identified as the underlying problem in 52% of frail nursing home residents with long-standing fecal incontinence in one study. A therapeutic intervention consisting of enemas until no further response followed by lactulose achieved complete resolution of incontinence in 94% of those in whom full treatment compliance could be obtained. Notably, this study showed that only 4% of nursing home residents with long-standing fecal incontinence had been referred to their primary care physician for further assessment, reflecting a tendency toward unnecessarily conservative nursing management (e.g., use of pads and pants only). Another nursing home study found that daily lactulose and suppositories plus weekly enemas only effectively resolved overflow incontinence when complete rectal emptying was consistently achieved over a period of 2 months. An effective therapeutic program for overflow incontinence depends on the following:

- Regular toileting (ideally 2 hourly, which also promotes mobility)
- Monitoring of treatment effect by rectal examination and bowel chart
- Responsive stepwise drug and dosage changes
- Prolonged treatment (at least 2 weeks)
- Subsequent maintenance regimen to prevent recurrences

Fecal Impaction

Fecal impaction is an important cause of comorbidity in older patients, increasing the risk of hospitalization and of potentially fatal complications. A survey of patients admitted to acute geriatric units in the United Kingdom over 1 year reported that fecal impaction was a primary reason for hospitalization in 27%. In frail patients, fecal impaction may present as a nonspecific clinical deterioration; more specific symptoms are anorexia, vomiting, and abdominal pain. Findings on physical examination may include fever, delirium, abdominal distension, reduced bowel sounds, arrhythmias, and tachypnea secondary to splinting of the diaphragm. The mechanism for the fever and leucocytosis response is thought to be microscopic stercoral ulcerations of the colon. A plain abdominal radiograph will show colonic or rectal fecal retention associated with lower bowel dilatation (Figure 93-2). Presence of fluid levels in the large or small bowel suggests advanced obstruction; the closer the fecal impaction is to the ileocecal valve, the greater the number of fluid levels seen in the small bowel.

Urinary Retention/Lower Urinary Tract Symptoms

Rectosigmoid fecal loading may impinge on the bladder neck causing some degree of urinary retention. At a population level, two

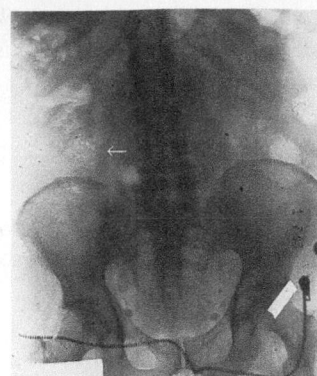

FIGURE 93-2. Abdominal radiograph of a 73-yr-old man with chronic schizophrenia who has taken anticholinergic neuroleptics for many years. This was his third hospital admission for colonic impaction. The arrow points to the cecum, which is full of stool, indicative of slow transit. Fecaliths are visible in the pelvic region.

recent Finnish studies of older women and men showed an independent association between constipation and lower urinary tract symptoms (LUTS) in both genders. A case–control study from Singapore looked at risk factors for urinary retention (defined as postvoid residual volume [PVRV] >100 mL by portable bladder scan) in hospitalized women aged 65+ and found that after adjustment for relevant confounders, constipation was the primary predictor, increasing the risk of retention fourfold (other predictors were urinary tract infection and previous urinary retention). Urinary symptoms of difficult voiding were unreliable in diagnosing retention in this study, suggesting that it is good practice to do screening PVRVs in hospitalized older women with constipation, particularly in the context of coexisting urinary tract infection. A prospective cohort study from Israel examined the impact of treating chronic constipation on coexistent LUTS in older people (mean age 72). After 4 months, there was a significant improvement in constipation symptoms, LUTS (including urgency, frequency, and voiding), mean PVRV (reduced from 85–30 mL), and fewer urinary tract infections. There are case reports in frail older people, of bilateral hydronephrosis associated with renal failure that resolved following fecal disimpaction.

Stercoral Perforation/Colon Ischemia

Fecal impaction increases the risk of stercoral perforation of the wall of the colon (usually sigmoid) secondary to ischemic necrosis. Stercoral perforation can also occur in chronically constipated persons where pressure from a hard fecaloma produces an ulcer with characteristically necrotic and inflammatory edges; these individuals tend to present with sudden onset of acute abdominal pain. Prompt surgical intervention and rigorous treatment of peritonitis are needed to prevent the high mortality rate associated with this condition. A case–control study found that the most prevalent risk factor for colon ischemia in 700 cases was the use of drugs that cause constipation (one in three cases compared to only one in nine controls).

Sigmoid Volvulus

Chronic constipation in frail older people is the leading cause of sigmoid volvulus in the developed world. Volvulus is

- the third commonest cause of large bowel obstruction in the United States;

- more likely in constipated patients with Parkinson disease and neuropathic colon (e.g., from spinal cord disease or long-term neuroleptic treatment);
- associated with hypokalemia;
- treated in the first instance by sigmoidoscopic detorsion (high recurrence rate);
- managed surgically, usually by partial colectomy, when sigmoidoscopic deflation fails (in approximately two-thirds of cases).

Colonic Pseudo-obstruction

Acute colonic pseudo-obstruction (Ogilvie syndrome) is most likely to occur in hospitalized frail older people with a history of chronic constipation who are acutely medically ill, or in postoperative phase. It presents with abdominal distension and colonic dilatation on x-ray, with a cecal diameter of 10 cm or more. Nil by mouth, flatus tube, and correction of electrolyte imbalances (particularly potassium and magnesium) are initial treatments, progressing to neostigmine (if no cardiac contraindications), and then endoscopic decompression if dilatation persists. Administration of polyethylene glycol (PEG) after initial resolution of colonic dilatation has been shown to reduce the likelihood of recurrence requiring escalation of therapy.

Rectal Prolapse

Prolonged straining at stool in constipated patients can result in rectal prolapse of varying degrees, and older people are more at risk from developing fecal soiling as a result. Surgery should be considered for full thickness prolapses, and laparoscopic versus transabdominal repair is now an effective treatment (including improving bowel-related symptoms) with a low recurrence rate.

Diverticular Disease

Left-sided diverticulosis coli affects 30% to 60% of people older than 60 in developed countries. Etiology has been attributed to high intraluminal pressures while straining at stool in people who have a low fiber diet. A case–control study of patients (mean age 68) with acute uncomplicated diverticulitis showed 74% to have prolonged transit (longest in those with constipation symptoms), and 59% small intestinal bacterial overgrowth. New approaches to preventing recurrence of symptomatic flare-ups of diverticular disease are use of mesalazine and *Lactobacillus casei*, separately or in combination.

Psychological Impact/Quality of Life

Quality of life and daily living are affected by functional bowel symptoms in older people, even following adjustment for other chronic illnesses. Patients with constipation generally have an impaired quality of life compared with the general population, though few studies have looked at this specifically in older people. A Hong Kong study of community-living people aged 70+ showed an independent association between constipation and low morale as measured by the *Philadelphia Geriatric Morale Scale*. One large Canadian study of the general population found association between constipation and a low *SF-36* score, with the rate of physician visits for constipation being strongly predicted by the physical component of the *SF-36*.

The *Patient Assessment of Constipation Quality of Life* questionnaire is a validated tool for assessing quality of life over time that has been used in older adults in long-term care; scores correlate with abdominal pain and constipation severity. Patients whose constipation is associated with abdominal pain or IBS symptoms score even lower on quality of life measures, plus have poor general health perception. For patients with spinal cord injury, a *neurogenic bowel dysfunction score* has been constructed and validated that correlates to quality of life score. Fecal incontinence has a demonstrable negative impact on quality of life in community surveys, correlating with self-reported symptom severity.

Constipation in long-term care residents unable to communicate because of dementia has been linked to physically aggressive behavior by independent association. A U.S. study of almost 9000 care home residents looked at independent characteristics associated with the development of wandering behavior over a 1-year period and found that constipation increased the risk almost twofold. The authors postulate that residents with dementia may wander to alleviate constipation-related discomfort, and care home providers should be alert to this.

NONPHARMACOLOGICAL TREATMENT

More often than not, the consultation between a general practitioner and an older person reporting constipation will result in a laxative being prescribed. Among frailer older people, nursing home studies show high rates of self-reported constipation, despite very substantial levels of laxative prescribing. These observations have led to speculation that nonpharmacological treatments for constipation are underused as first-line treatment in nonsevere constipation, and as adjunctive treatment even when laxatives are deemed necessary. Symptoms of difficult evacuation may be particularly amenable to nonpharmacological approaches such as stool softening and bulking through increasing fiber and fluid intake, pelvic muscle strengthening exercises, and footstool elevation of the legs during evacuation (see below). A systematic review examining nonpharmacological treatment of chronic constipation in older people in 1997 found no studies evaluating the effect of exercise therapy and only a few nonrandomized trials examining fiber and fluid supplementation, and there has been little further research in this area since then. Available data, expert opinion, and practical recommendations are summarized below.

Education

Educating patients as to what constitutes normal bowel habit should be one of the first steps in managing self-reported constipation. Patients with no or mild symptoms of constipation should be encouraged to discontinue chronic laxative therapy. Withdrawal may be easier to achieve in the more controlled environment of a nursing home, than in the community where over-the-counter medications are so readily available. Patients who require laxative treatment for constipation should be told to aim for regular, comfortable evacuation rather than daily evacuation, which is often their preconceived norm.

Educational interventions promoting lifestyle changes for patients with chronic constipation should focus on exercise and diet, and ideally be based on the cognitive Theory of Planned Behavior.

In order to persuade older people with constipation to change their lifestyle, they need to be convinced that

- their current behaviors are "bad for their bowels";
- bowel-related and general health improvements associated with recommended measures are worth the trouble and expense of changing;
- it is they who are responsible for what they eat, how much exercise they take, and so on (internal locus of control);
- they have the skills and knowledge to modify their own lifestyle to improve their constipation, if they choose to do so (self-efficacy).

It is important to provide people with clearly written educational materials. An RCT in stroke survivors with constipation evaluated the impact of a one-off nurse-led assessment (with feedback to primary care physician) and educational session including provision of booklet. At 6 months, postintervention subjects reported improved bowel function in terms of number and normality of bowel movements; at 1 year, they were more likely to still be altering their diet and fluid intake to control their bowel problem. Table 93-8 illustrates some of the patient-centered instructions from this study booklet, which are relevant to all older people with constipation.

Other RCTs have sought to influence fiber intake at a population level. Nutrition newsletters sent to older Americans in their homes significantly improved their dietary fiber intake. Another community intervention used media and social marketing in educational targeting of small retirement communities under the theme "Bread: It's a Great Way to Go," and reported a result of a 49% decrease in laxative sales and 58% increase in sales of whole meal and whole grain bread.

Educating home carers on maintaining fecal continence in patients with dementia (with focus on constipation and other contributing factors) increased knowledge levels significantly. Home carer involvement in bowel care plans is also crucial in patients with chronic neurological diseases other than dementia such as Parkinson disease, stroke, and neuropathic bowel.

Diet

A meta-analysis of 20 nonrandomized studies in younger adults with constipation associated additional wheat bran with increased stool weight and decreased transit time. Evidence for the effectiveness of fiber in treatment of constipation in elderly people is more equivocal. In one community study, higher fiber intake was associated with lower laxative use among older women, but in another study, higher intake of bran was associated with no reduction in constipation symptoms and greater fecal loading in the colon on abdominal radiography. In older hospitalized patients, daily bran supplementation increased weekly bowel movement frequency and improved overall symptoms as compared with placebo. There have been several "before and after" studies in nursing home residents reporting that addition of dietary fiber (ranging from bran to processed pea hull) or fruit mixtures (apple puree to fruit porridge) to the daily diet improved bowel movement frequency and consistency, and reduced laxative intake and the need for nursing intervention. Bias cannot be excluded from these nursing home studies, including that of concomitant increased fluid intake contributing to these positive results. But despite these reservations, these observational studies emphasize the usefulness of increasing dietary fiber, fluid, and fruit in older

people at high risk of constipation. Additional benefits should not be discounted; for instance, adding oat bran to the diet in one study reduced cholesterol levels more markedly in older versus younger women.

In practical terms, at least 10 g of fiber with additional fluids should be recommended to patients. While coarse bran rather than more refined fiber is more effective in increasing stool fluid weight, it is far less palatable, and is more likely to cause initial symptoms of increased bloating, flatulence, and irregular bowel movements. Fiber should therefore be recommended to older individuals in the form of foods such as whole meal or whole grain bread, porridge, fresh fruit (preferably unpeeled), seeded berries, raw or cooked vegetables, beans, and lentils. A crossover trial in subjects aged 60+ that entailed taking a daily kiwi fruit resulted in bulkier and softer stools and increased bowel movement frequency. Fiber supplementation should also be culturally appropriate. Chinese food is typically low-fiber, and dietary additives such as konjac glucomannan can serve as "natural laxatives." Other examples of natural laxatives are aloe vera and rhubarb, both of which contain stimulant anthraquinone derivatives like senna.

Fluids

An Italian RCT in adults aged 18 to 50 with chronic constipation showed that the beneficial effect of increased dietary fiber was significantly enhanced by increasing fluid intake to 1.5 to 2 L daily. Upping fluid intake by two 8-ounce beverages a day for 5 weeks in dependent nursing home residents significantly increased bowel movement frequency and reduced laxative use. This "hydration program" used a colorful beverage cart and four beverage choices to stimulate residents' interest in drinking. Regarding type of fluids, a RCT comparing the effect of drinking carbonated versus tap water found that the former significantly improved constipation scores, as well as functional dyspepsia and gallbladder emptying. Caffeine is known to increase both bowel and bladder smooth muscle activity, though its impact on constipation in older people is not documented. Subjects randomized to receive juice containing probiotics (*Lactobacillus rhamnosus* and *Propionibacterium freudenreichii*) for 4 weeks had a 24% increase in defecation frequency compared to those receiving unsupplemented juice.

Physical Activity

An RCT in middle-aged inactive patients with chronic constipation showed that regular physical activity (30-min brisk walk and 11-min home exercises a day) decreased colonic and rectosigmoid transit time and improved defecation pattern according to Rome II criteria. A review of physical activity interventions in older adults concluded that incorporating exercise naturally into a person's day tends to provide the most effective means for increasing activity levels. Studies conducted in older nursing home patients showed the following outcome:

- Six months of moderate intensity exercise training had no impact on constipation symptoms or habitual physical activity (RCT).
- Six months of 2 hourly prompted toileting improved measures of daily physical activity and functional performance, but did not alter bowel movement frequency (RCT).

- Daily exercise in bed and the use of abdominal massage reduced laxative and enema use in chair-fast patients, although transit time was unaffected (non-RCT).

Existing evidence would tend to support exercise programs to influence constipation in nursing home residents within the context of addressing other risk factors also. Daily exercise for immobile elderly patients, including positioning out of bed into a chair for up to 60-minute periods with chair-lifts at 15-minute intervals, may also have benefits.

Abdominal Massage

Abdominal massage added to the standard bowel regimen in spinal cord patients has been shown to shorten colonic transit time and increase weekly bowel movement frequency. A vibrating device that applied kneading force to the abdomen once a day for 20 minutes was evaluated in elderly constipated nursing home residents in Greece, and after 12 weeks resulted in softening of stool, increased bowel movement frequency, and a 47% reduction in transit time. Case reports show that physiotherapists can incorporate daily 10 minute abdominal massage into home activity programs for community-dwelling people suffering from constipation with good effect.

Pelvic Floor and Sphincter Strengthening Exercises

Where rectal outlet delay and/or persistent straining is associated with excessive pelvic floor descent, pelvic strengthening exercises should be taught. In women, it is helpful to do the teaching while undertaking a pelvic examination (with the examining hand resting on the posterior vaginal wall), so that positive verbal feedback can be given when the patient correctly contracts the pelvic floor. Pelvic floor retraining can help rectal outlet symptoms, but a greater degree of perineal descent is predictive of poorer treatment responses. Sphincter strengthening exercises (Table 93-8) should be taught to patients with fecal soiling and/or weak external sphincter.

Toileting Habits

Small nonrandomized studies show that regular toileting habits (scheduled evacuation) restores comfortable evacuation in stroke survivors (with the assistance of digital stimulation) and in older postoperative inpatients. The preservation of the gastrocolic reflex with aging supports the rationale for postprandial toilet visits. Care should be given to treating hemorrhoids and any other anorectal condition in these patients. Expert opinion supports the use of footstools during evacuation in individuals with weakened abdominal and pelvic muscles to optimize the Valsalva maneuver.

Toileting Access—Privacy and Dignity

Toilet access should be assessed and facilitated particularly in patients with mobility, visual, or dexterity impairments. Bathroom comfort and privacy must be considered, particularly for individuals in institutional settings. Reluctance to use the toilet in institutional settings has been linked to residents developing fecal impaction in case reports. Table 93-10 summarizes basic but important recommendations relating to toileting and maintaining privacy and dignity.

TABLE 93-10

Toilets and Toileting—Maintaining Privacy and Dignity

A multidisciplinary assessment should be made of older person's ability to access and use the toilet [3]

Commodes/sani-chairs/shower chairs
- should be available to residents in institutional settings [3];
- should provide a safe seated position for prolonged use by older people with skin vulnerability and trunk support problems (e.g., padded seat, footstool if feet are unsupported, back and arm support, grab rails etc.) [3].

Older people should be given the opportunity to use the toilet (either directly or by using a sani-chair or shower chair) rather than a bedside commode [3]

Bedpans should be avoided for defecation purposes

Transportation to the toilet and use of the toilet or commode should be carried out with due regard to privacy and dignity

A direct method of calling for assistance should be provided when an older person is left on the toilet/commode

When using a commode
- methods to reduce noise and odor should be offered;
- methods to facilitate bottom wiping should be available;
- in living area and cannot be emptied immediately, a chemical toilet should be offered instead [3].

Level [1] indicates good evidence, i.e., consistent results from well-designed, well-conducted studies.
Level [2] indicates fair evidence, i.e., results show benefit, but strength limited by number, quality, or consistency of studies.
Level [3] indicates poor evidence, i.e., insufficient because of limited number, power, or quality of studies.
Adapted from Potter et al. Bowel Care in Older People.

Medication Review

A careful review of the medication regimen is necessary to eliminate, reduce the dosage, or substitute other medications for those that predispose to constipation. As an example, a selective serotonin reuptake inhibitor may provide an effective alternative to tricyclic therapy for elderly patients with depression and persistent constipation. Newer antipsychotic agents (e.g., quetiapine) are less likely to cause severe constipation in older people than older agents.

PHARMACOLOGICAL TREATMENT

Laxative and Enema Use and Abuse in Older People

A Food and Drug Administration (FDA) Advisory Panel has registered concern over the widespread overuse of over-the-counter (OTC) laxatives; laxatives are second only to analgesics as the most commonly used OTC medications by older people. OTC laxative use is common in the United States and Europe, and is encouraged by advertising and popular ignorance of adverse effects. Only 38% of OTC laxative users in Italy were guided in their choice of laxative by a physician; the remainder were influenced by pharmacists (21%), relatives or friends (16%), and advertisements (12%). Six percent of users reported adverse effects.

Several researchers have documented an enormous increase in the use of laxatives in older people in the community with little relation to either frequency of bowel movements or the need to strain. One-fifth to one-third of regular laxative users do not consider themselves to be constipated, and many people take them through a misguided belief in the benefits of regular purgation. One study showed that 78% of elderly persons who used laxatives regularly had never gone for more than 3 days without a bowel movement. Habitual rather than surreptitious abuse is more likely in older individuals; repeated purging empties the colon of stool that would normally descend into and distend the rectal ampulla, thereby removing the urge to defecate, and prompting the patient to take further laxatives. This habitual profile of overuse means that older people are less likely to have the electrolyte imbalances that have been documented in younger people who abuse laxatives. However, chronic laxative use in patients aged 80+ has been associated with increased plasma homocysteine, independently of other relevant factors such as institutionalization and dementia. This may be caused by impaired absorption of folate; low folate levels have also been associated with long-term laxative use in older people.

Although patients in hospitals and nursing homes are at higher risk for clinical constipation, this does not entirely justify the very high levels of cathartic prescribing in these settings. Seventy-six percent of hospitalized elderly are prescribed at least one type of laxative. A prospective study of 2355 nursing home residents in the Netherlands showed that over the course of 2 years, 47% were started on laxatives, with 79% of these continuing with the treatment long-term. Prescribing rates in U.S. nursing homes are high at 54% to 74%, with almost half of these users being prescribed more than one agent. Most commonly prescribed agents are stool softeners (26%), magnesium salts (18%), and stimulants (16%). Two contributing factors may lead to over-prescribing of laxatives to older patients:

- Lack of objective confirmation of the diagnosis by the prescribing physician or nurse
- Prescribing patterns of laxatives that are clinically ineffective

For instance, in U.S. nursing homes, docusate (a fecal softener with little or no laxative effect) is the predominantly prescribed agent.

Evidence-Based Summary of Laxative, Suppository, and Enema Treatment in Older Persons

Many reported trials of laxative and enema treatment in older people are low quality, limited by unclear definitions for constipation, inconsistent outcome measurement, and underreporting of potential confounding factors during the trial period (e.g., fiber intake). The absence of good level evidence may in part underlie the somewhat empirical way in which laxatives are prescribed to older people. A 1997 systematic review of effective laxative treatment in elderly persons found that the few published randomized controlled trials were potentially flawed owing to small numbers and other methodologic concerns. In the 10 years since that review, there has been little rigorous research specific to the older population. The following conclusions are drawn from meta-analytical reviews (1997, 2001, 2002, 2004) of efficacy of laxatives in treating chronic constipation in adults:

- Availability of published evidence is poor for many commonly used agents including senna, magnesium hydroxide, Bisacodyl, and stool softeners.

- In trials conducted in older people, significant improvements in bowel movement frequency were observed with a stimulant laxative (cascara) [3] and with lactulose [2], while psyllium [2] and lactulose [2] were individually reported to improve stool consistency and related symptoms in placebo-controlled trials.
- Level [1] evidence supports the use of PEG in adults.
- Level [2] evidence supports the use of lactulose and psyllium in adults.
- None of the currently available trials include quality of life outcomes.
- In trials conducted in older adults (>55 years), there is little evidence of differences in effectiveness between categories of laxatives.
- A stepped approach to laxative treatment in older people is justified, starting with cheaper laxatives before proceeding to more expensive alternatives.

Table 93-11 summarizes the onset of action, mechanisms of action, potential side effects, and benefits of selected laxatives in current usage, and the following discussion describes efficacy and safety.

Stimulant Laxatives

Senna is a cheap and safe agent for use in elderly people with functional constipation. A trial of cascara (a similar plant-derived stimulant laxative) in older hospitalized patients increased bowel movement frequency by an average of 2.6 bowel movements per week as compared to placebo. Administration of 20 mg of senna daily for 6 months to patients older than 80 did not cause any significant losses of intestinal protein or electrolytes, and repeated studies in mice show no evidence of myenteric nerve damage resulting from its use. Senna generally induces evacuation 8 to 12 hours following administration, and should therefore be taken at bedtime. Frail elderly patients may have even slower response times, and may also require several weeks of daily use before achieving regular bowel habit. Maintenance therapy with senna is appropriate in patients with chronic constipation, and it can be used in higher doses for short-term treatment of fecal impaction. In patients with weak anal sphincters, the senna alone may be sufficient to treat constipation without causing or exacerbating fecal incontinence through excess stool softening.

Bisacodyl is a useful alternative stimulant laxative to senna. A recent treatment (Bisacodyl 10 mg daily) versus placebo RCT in primary care patients (mean age 62) with chronic constipation showed improved stool frequency and consistency without side effects.

Phenolphthalein and castor oil should not be used in older people because of a high risk of side effects including malabsorption, dehydration, lipoid pneumonia, and, with heavy prolonged use, cathartic colon.

Bulk Laxatives

Bulk laxatives are generally underprescribed to older people, despite evidence that they increase bowel movement frequency (by a mean of 1.4 bowel movements per week as compared to placebo), and improve consistency and ease of evacuation. This may partly be because of intolerance in the form of bloating and unpredictable bowel habit in the first weeks of taking them, and also of caution

TABLE 93-11

Laxative and Enemas Used in Older People with Constipation

AGENT AND TYPE	ONSET	MECHANISMS OF ACTION, SIDE EFFECTS, AND BENEFITS
Senna/cascara/Bisacodyl *Stimulant*	8–12 h	Direct stimulation of myenteric plexus, alteration of salt and water transportation, prostaglandin E-like effect. May cause dose-dependent cramps and diarrhea, so titrate dosage. Long-term use associated with melanosis coli, but does not cause 'cathartic colon'. May cause false-positive urine test for urobilinogen. Improves propulsive action, softens stool, shortens transit time. Suitable for long-term use.
Psyllium Methyl cellulose Calcium polycarbophil *Bulk*	12–72 h	Hydrophilic fibers, resistant to bacterial degradation, leads to bulkier and softer stool and peristaltic stimulation. May cause transient bloating, flatulence. Good fluid intake needed. Avoid use in bedridden or dehydrated patients. Causes more frequent passage of well-formed stools, reduces evacuation discomfort caused by hard stools. Suitable for long-term use.
Magnesium hydroxide (milk of magnesia) *Magnesium salt*	0.5–3 h	Stimulates release of cholecystokinin, increases secretion of electrolytes and water into gut lumen. Rapid action may cause watery stool, dehydration, fecal incontinence. Hypermagnesemia in renal insufficiency. Avoid magnesium citrate. Unsuitable for long-term use.
Lactulose/sorbitol *Hyperosmolar*	24–48 h	Nonabsorbable disaccharides degraded into low-molecular-weight acids, which osmotically draw water into the colon causing reflex prolonged tonic gut contractions. May cause abdominal cramps and flatulence, especially if taken with large amount of fruit. Increases transit, softens stool. Safe for use in diabetic patients and renal failure. Suitable for long-term use.
Polyethylene glycol *Hyperosmolar*	30–60 mins	Potent hyperosmotic action, shortens transit time. May cause nausea, abdominal cramps, incontinence, and loose stool, dose should be titrated against effect. Useful in treatment of fecal impaction, bowel preparation. Long-term use in patients with hypotonic colon or resistant constipation.
Docusate sodium *Softener*	24–72 h	Stimulates cyclic-AMP increasing fluid secretions, reduces surface tension, and promotes penetration of water into stool. Ineffective in treatment of constipation. Risk of fecal soiling in older women. Long-term use alters morphology of gut mucosa. Unsuitable for long-term use.
Phosphate (Fleets) Sodium citrate Arachis oil Tap water *Enemas*	2–15 min	Contractile response to gut dilatation, lavage effect. Phosphate: hyperphosphatemia, tetany, fluid retention, avoid use in renal failure. Mineral oil: useful for acute disimpaction. Tap water: useful for disimpaction. Can be used long-term in patients with recurrent impactions.
Bisacodyl/glycerine *Suppositories*	10–45 min	Rectal contractile response to increased volume Daily Bisacodyl use may cause rectal burning and cramps. Suppositories helpful for rectal outlet delay, persistent straining, prevention of recurrent rectal impactions. Suitable for long-term use.

on the part of prescribers because of the documented risk of impaction with these agents in frailer patients with poor fluid intake. Psyllium has been associated with increased stool frequency in people with Parkinson disease, but was not shown to alter transit time. Bulking agents are generally useful in older individuals with mild to moderate constipation who are able to tolerate them and who drink sufficient fluids. They have the additional benefit of reducing abdominal pain in patients with irritable bowel syndrome, limiting flare-ups of diverticulitis, and facilitating painful defecation associated with hemorrhoids. Furthermore, psyllium significantly lowers serum cholesterol by binding bile acids in the intestine. Available preparations are natural nonwheat fibers such as psyllium and ispaghula husk, and synthetic compounds such as calcium polycarbophil and methylcellulose. The synthetic compounds tend to be cheaper and are available in more easily administrated tablet forms, as compared to reconstituted powder, which can be hard for older patients to swallow. The synthetic bulking agents and the natural fibers are equally effective in increasing stool frequency and volume. It should be noted that bran in tablet form is considerably cheaper than bulk laxatives, but the former may cause even more bloating and unpredictability of bowel habit, and may also, unlike bulking agents, predispose to malabsorption of iron or calcium in elderly people.

Magnesium Salts

Magnesium salts are the most commonly prescribed type to elderly in hospital, and magnesium hydroxide is popular in OTC laxative sales. There is only one published study evaluating magnesium hydroxide in elderly people, a small trial in nursing home residents, which suggested that this laxative was more effective than a bulking agent in increasing bowel movement frequency and softening stool. Magnesium salts may be favored by physician and patient alike because of their rapid action, but in general, a gradual catharsis is preferable to restore regular bowel habit in older persons. Their potent catharsis increases the risk of fluid and electrolyte losses, and of fecal incontinence in less-mobile people, or in those with weak sphincters. Furthermore, magnesium levels should be monitored in all elderly people who are using magnesium hydroxide on a regular basis, as hypermagnesemia can occur even with normal serum creatinine levels.

Long-term use of magnesium hydroxide is contraindicated in chronic kidney disease. The more potent salt magnesium citrate carries an even greater risk of side effects, including promoting colonic pseudo-obstruction in frailer patients, and is therefore not recommended for use in the elderly population. Based on evidence and known side effects, there is no clear role for using magnesium salts in treatment of chronic constipation in older people.

Hyperosmolar Laxatives

Hyperosmolar laxatives are the most rigorously studied laxative group in the current literature. The following summarizes findings from nursing home studies:

- Lactulose (or the related agent lactitol) versus placebo shortened transit time, increased bowel movement frequency (by an average of 1.9 bowel movements per week), and improved stool consistency.

- In a comparison study with a bulking/stimulant combination agent, lactulose was a little less effective in influencing bowel pattern and consistency.

- Lactulose and sorbitol were equally effective in mostly eliminating the use of other laxatives and enemas in residents with dementia and chronic constipation, with sorbitol being considerably cheaper.

In the community, a well-designed trial of ambulatory older veterans with severe constipation also showed lactulose and sorbitol to be equally efficacious. Lactulose and sorbitol are effective agents in treating chronic constipation in older people in all health care settings, with sorbitol being the cheaper option.

Polyethylene glycol (PEG, GoLYTELY, Movicol) is a more potent hyperosmolar laxative than lactulose as demonstrated by its impact on transit time in normal subjects. In an RCT of hospitalized patients (mean age 55 years), in comparison to lactulose, PEG produced a greater increase in bowel movement frequency and a greater reduction in straining, but at the expense of a higher mean number of liquid stools. A similar efficacy and side-effect profile plus a reduction in laxative expenditure were shown with use in long-stay residents of a mental health institute with constipation. Its use in treatment of fecal impaction (in combination with daily enemas) in elderly nursing home residents showed greater efficacy than lactulose, without the dehydration or hemodynamic side effects. Another RCT of adults (aged 17–88) with fecal loading on x-ray or rectal examination, and bowels not open for 3 to 5 days showed that 1L (or 8 sachets) a day of PEG plus electrolytes for 3 days resolved impaction in 89% of patients, with few adverse effects. The current evidence base suggests that the role of PEG in older people is for acute disimpaction (ensuring that easy toilet access is guaranteed) and for regular use as a laxative only in high-risk people whose constipation has proved resistant to milder and cheaper alternatives.

Fecal Softeners

Docusate sodium has been shown experimentally to have no effect on colonic motility, and little or no laxative action, even at doses of 300 mg/day. In an RCT of adults with severe constipation comparing docusate with psyllium, docusate proved significantly inferior for both softening stools and increasing bowel movement frequency. A systematic review of prospective controlled trials evaluating oral docusate in chronically ill people (though hampered by poor data) showed only a small trend toward increased stool frequency, and concluded that there was insufficient evidence to support its use in this population. Nevertheless, docusate is frequently recommended and used in older people as a laxative as well as fecal softener. This is of particular concern in the nursing home and hospital settings, where constipation may as a result be undertreated with an increased risk of fecal impaction. Furthermore, docusate (in combination with the stimulant danthron) increases the risk of fecal incontinence in nursing home residents. Current evidence suggests that docusate is unhelpful in the treatment of constipation or rectal outlet delay in frail older people.

Enemas

Enemas have a role in both acute disimpaction and in preventing recurrent impactions in susceptible patients. They induce evacuation as a response to colonic distension, as well as by plain lavage; the commonest reason for a poor result from an enema is inadequate administration. In one study of nursing home residents with overflow incontinence associated with fecal impaction on rectal examination, daily phosphate enemas continued until no further results was effective in completely resolving incontinence in 94% of patients. Some frail elderly patients with poor mobility and some individuals with neurogenic bowel dysfunction may have recurrent stool impactions despite regular laxative and suppository use, and they will benefit from weekly enemas.

Regular use of phosphate enemas should be avoided in patients with renal impairment as dangerous hyperphosphatemia has been reported. Tap water enemas are the safest type for regular use, although they take more nursing administration time than phosphate enemas, and are not available in certain countries. Soapsuds enemas should never be administered to older patients. Arachis oil retention enemas are particularly useful in loosening colonic impactions. In patients who have a firm and large rectal impaction, manual evacuation should be performed before inserting enemas or suppositories, using local anesthetic gel if needed to reduce discomfort.

Suppositories

The predominance of rectal outlet delay (including manual evacuation) in older people, many of whom take regular laxatives, is likely to be linked to underuse of suppositories in these patients. Although research data are lacking, clinically suppositories are very useful in treatment of rectal outlet delay, or where symptoms of prolonged straining predominate. Regular suppository administration (usually three times a week, and ideally after breakfast) can effectively control symptoms in these patients. A study of frail nursing home patients with overflow incontinence found that a regimen of daily lactulose and suppositories plus weekly enemas was only effective in restoring continence when long-lasting and complete rectal emptying was achieved. Regular use of suppositories is indicated in older patients with rectal motility and/or recurrent rectal impactions. With appropriate education, many older people can themselves use suppositories; they are easier to insert and more effective if used blunt end first (Table 93-8), and people with impaired dexterity can be helped with suppository inserters designed for spinal cord conjured patients. First-line suppository use is with glycerin, a hyperosmolar laxative used solely in suppository form. If ineffective, Bisacodyl suppositories (in

TABLE 93-12

Pharmacological Treatment of Constipation in Older People—Stepwise Approach

Chronic Constipation

In ambulant older people

Bulk laxative (psyllium) 1–3 times daily with fluids as required

If symptoms persist add senna 1–3 tablets at bedtime

In individuals with questionable fluid intake or those intolerant of bulk laxatives, start with senna 1–2 tablets at bedtime

If symptoms persist, add sorbitol or lactulose 15 mL daily as needed, titrating the dose to achieve regular (≥3 times a week) and comfortable evacuation

In high-risk patients (bedridden individuals, patients with neurological disease, and patients with history of fecal impaction)

Senna 2–3 tablets at bedtime and sorbitol or lactulose 30 mL daily, titrating upwards as needed

If symptoms persist, give PEG (half to two sachets of Movicol daily)

Colonic Fecal Impaction

Clinical or radiological obstruction

Daily retention enemas (e.g., arachis oil) until obstruction resolves, before starting oral laxatives

Colonic disimpaction

Daily enemas (preferably tap water) until no further washout result

PEG (0.5–2 L daily or 2–3 sachets of Movicol) with fluids

Ensure that patient has easy access to toilet to avoid fecal incontinence

When impaction resolves, give laxative regimen for chronic constipation in high-risk patients for long-term to avoid recurrence

Rectal Outlet Delay

Rectal disimpaction

Manual disimpaction where necessary, followed by phosphate enema(s) for initial complete clearance of rectal impaction

Regular treatment

Glycerine suppositories at least once a week and as required to relieve symptoms

For persistent symptoms, use Bisacodyl suppositories instead of glycerine suppositories

In patients at high risk of rectal impaction (rectal dysmotility, neurological disease) give regular enemas (usually once weekly) and daily suppositories

If stool is hard or infrequent, add daily laxative as for chronic constipation

TABLE 93-13

What We Do Not Know—Research Ideas

Can constipation be prevented in older people? For example, prevention of postoperative constipation in older people with normal preoperative bowel habit undergoing elective orthopedic or cardiac surgery.   [RCT]

What are the different characteristics between constipation sufferers who seek help and those who do not?   [Case–Control Study]

What drives constipation sufferers to seek help?   [Qualitative Research]

How can standardized "constipation protocols" for case-finding and risk assessment be implemented across community and institutional health care setting where frail older patients are cared for?   [Action Research, Quality Improvement Study]

Why is the prevalence of constipation in nursing homes so high despite heavy laxative use? Is it
ineffective laxative prescribing?
substandard assessment of patients?
underuse of nonpharmacological treatments?   [Observational]

What is the impact of nonpharmacological interventions targeting constipation risk factors on bowel and health-related outcomes in frail older people?   [RCT]

What are the barriers to older people adopting bowel-related lifestyle measures?   [Qualitative Research]

What are the psychosocial and quality of life effects of chronic constipation on older individuals and carers?   [Questionnaire Population Studies, Qualitative Research]

What is the effectiveness of enemas and suppositories in treating constipation and rectal outlet delay in older people?   [RCT]

Is biofeedback an effective treatment for pelvic dyssynergia in older people with rectal outlet delay?   [RCT]

How common is manual self-evacuation in older people, and does prolonged use affect anal sphincter function?   [Questionnaire Survey, Anorectal Function Study]

What is the cost-effectiveness of a stepwise approach to laxative treatment in older people with constipation in different health care settings (community, hospital, long-term care)?   [RCT]

How effective and safe are new enterokinetic agents (serotonin agonists) in treatment of chronic constipation in older people, including frail individuals?   [RCT]

Data from Potter et al. Bowel Care in Older People.

PEG base) should be used, although daily use can sometimes causes symptoms of rectal discomfort or burning. Bisacodyl suppositories have been shown to be effective in treating severe constipation in patients with spinal cord injuries. The onset of action of suppositories varies by individual from 5 to 45 minutes (most likely influenced by the neurogenicity of the rectum), and so patients should be advised to set a quiet time aside for effective evacuation.

Enterokinetic Agents

Altered serotonin (5-HT) signaling may predispose to chronic constipation, and 5-HT4 agonists (e.g., tegaserod) have been shown to stimulate gastrointestinal motility and increase stool water content. The efficacy and safety of tegaserod in treating chronic constipation were evaluated in an RCT where 13% of participants were aged 65 years and above, but no subgroup analysis was undertaken to look at the specific effects in these older subjects. Tegaserod improves symptoms of constipation in younger people, particularly women with irritable bowel syndrome, but its side-effect profile includes headaches and diarrhea, and there have been postmarketing reports of ischemic colitis. Serotonin-receptor modulators are also emerging as useful agents in treatment of nonulcer dyspepsia, a motility disorder linked to constipation. The enterokinetic drug prucalopride proved disappointing in treating constipation in people with Parkinson disease. Presently, these agents are not recommended for routine use in older people.

TREATMENT GUIDANCE

The 1997 systemic review from the United Kingdom concluded that based on the somewhat limited current evidence, older patients should first be prescribed the cheapest laxative, with alternatives given if this treatment fails. Table 93-12 represents a combination of

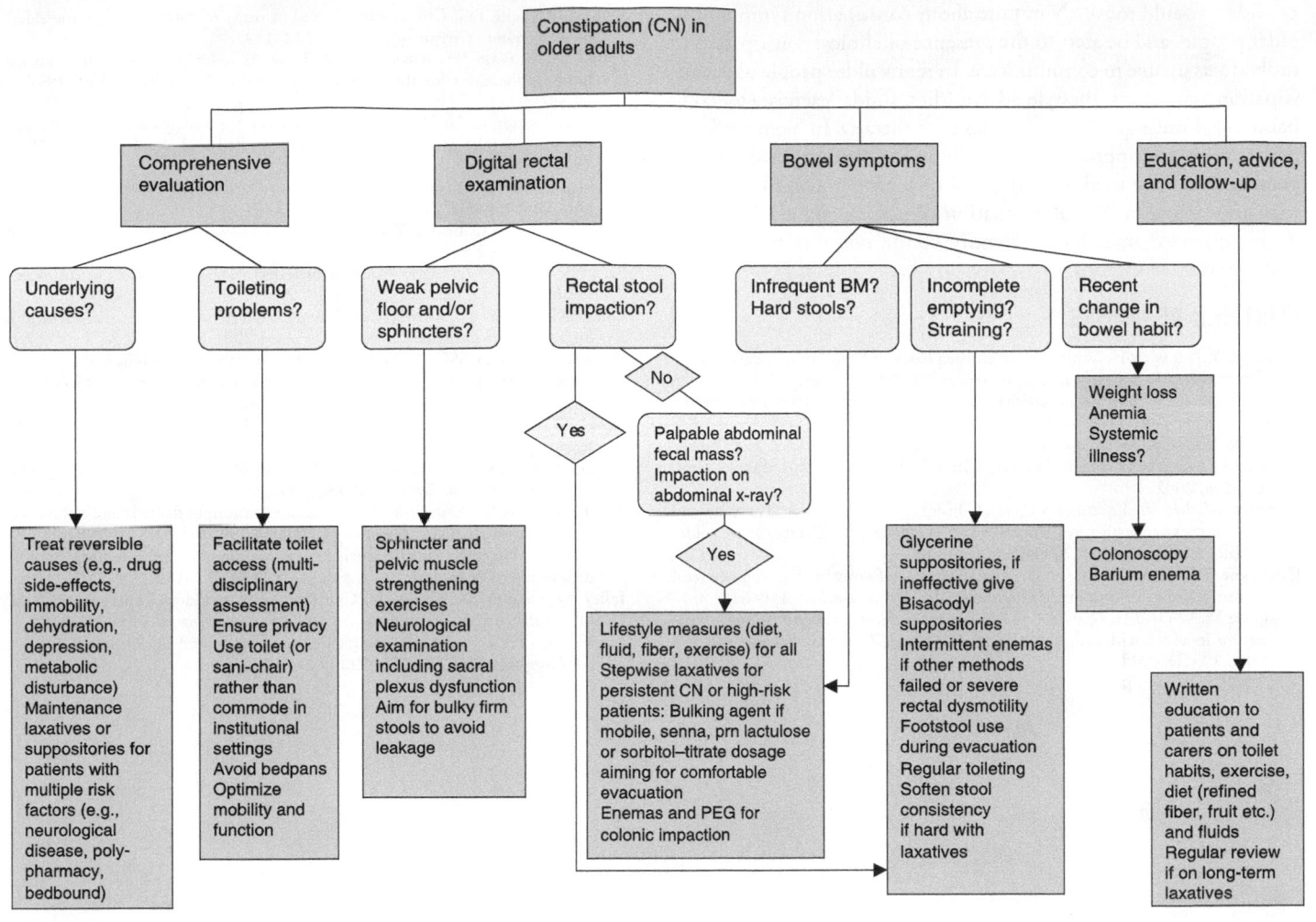

FIGURE 93-3. A practical approach to assessment and treatment of constipation in older people.

evidence-based and expert opinion in providing treatment guidance, which can be summarized as follows:

- In ambulant elderly with functional constipation, a daily bulk laxative is appropriate for both rectal outlet delay and slow-transit constipation.

- If the bulking agent is not tolerated, or proves ineffective, then senna may be substituted (1–3 tablets at night) with prn sorbitol (or lactulose) if needed to achieve patient-centered goals of comfortable regular evacuations.

- In frailer, less-mobile elderly people at higher risk of impaction, a combination of regular senna and sorbitol (or lactulose) should be used with dosage titration.

- In patients with colonic impaction, oil retention enemas should be administered daily until there are no clinical or radiologic signs of obstruction, and then tap water enemas continued regularly until they produce no further result.

- Where the patient has easy access to a toilet, PEG 0.5 to 2 L daily (or 1–2 sachets of Movicol) should be given as long as is needed to clear the impaction, followed by a regular maintenance laxative regimen of senna and lactulose to avoid recurrence of fecal impaction.

- In cases where toilet access is not so easy (e.g., at home with stairs), a more gradual clear-out using higher-dose senna and lactulose is appropriate to limit problems with incontinence.

- For rectal outlet delay or a predominant complaint of straining, the first-line approach should be regular use of suppositories, and laxatives should only be given for coexisting symptoms of hard or infrequent bowel movements.

FURTHER RESEARCH

Table 93-13 lists what we do not know about constipation in older people, and ideas for further research. The overall aim in both clinical practice and research should be to develop common evidence-based policies, procedures, guidelines, and targets to promote integrated bowel care for older people within all health care settings.

CONCLUSIONS

Figure 93-3 illustrates a practical algorithmic approach to assessment and treatment of constipation in older people. Health care providers should routinely inquire about constipation symptoms in older people, and be alert to the presence of clinical constipation in individuals unable to communicate. In many older people with constipation symptoms, lifestyle advice (diet, fluids, exercise, toileting habits) will preempt the need for laxative therapy. In higher-risk patients, a stepwise approach to prescribing laxatives, suppositories, or enemas should be used, with the goal of achieving comfortable and regular evacuation. Rectal evacuation difficulties should be specifically addressed in order to identify conditions that may require additional interventions.

FURTHER READING

Abbott RD, Petrovich H, White LR, et al. Frequency of bowel movements and the future risk of Parkinson's disease. *Neurology.* 2001;57:456–462.

Annells M, Koch T. Older people seeking solutions to constipation: the laxative mire. *J Clin Nurs.* 2002;11:603–612.

Potter, Norton, Cottenden, eds. *Bowel Care in Older People. Research and Practice.* Royal College of Physicians London, Clinical Effectiveness & Evaluation Unit, London, 2002.

Camilleri M, Lee JS, Viramontes B, et al. Insights into the pathophysiology and mechanisms of constipation, irritable bowel syndrome, and diverticulosis in older people. *J Am Geriatr Soc.* 2000;48:1142–1150.

Chassagne P, Jego A, Gloc P, et al. Does treatment of constipation improve fecal incontinence in institutionalized patients. *Age Ageing.* 2000;29:159–64.

Coggrave M, Wiesel PH, Norton C. Management of fecal incontinence and constipation in adults with central neurological diseases. *Cochrane Database Syst Rev.* 2006;19:CD002115.

Donald IP, Smith RG, Cruikshank JE, et al. A study of constipation in the elderly living at home. *Gerontology.* 1985;31:112–118.

Harari D, Gurwitz JH, Avoru J, et al. How do older persons define constipation? Implications for therapeutic management. *J Gen Intern Med.* 1997;12: 63–66.

Harari D, Norton C, LockWood L, et al. Treatment of constipation and fecal incontinence in stroke patients: randomized controlled trial. *Stroke.* 2004;35:2549–2555.

Kinnunen O. Study of constipation in a geriatric hospital, day hospital, old people's home and at home. *Aging.* 1991;31:161–170.

Petticrew M, Sheldon T. Effectiveness of laxatives in adults. *Qual Health Care.* 2001;10:268–273.

Petticrew M et al. Systematic review of the effectiveness of laxatives in the elderly. *Health Technol Assess.* 1997;1(13):i, 1–52.

Phillips C, Polakof FD, Mave JK, et al. Assessment of constipation management in long-term care patients. *J Am Med Dir Assoc.* 2001;2:149–154.

Ramkumar D, Rao SSC. Efficacy and safety of traditional medical therapies for chronic constipation: systematic review. *Am J Gastroenterol.* 2005;100:936–971.

Read NW, Abouzerry L, Read MG, et al. Anorectal function in elderly patients with fecal impaction. *Gastroenterology.* 1985;89:959–966.

Robson KM, kiely DK, Lembo T. Development of constipation in nursing home residents. *Dis Colon Rectum.* 2000;43:940–943.

Ron Y, Leibovitz A, Monastirski N, et al. Colonic transit in diabetic and nondiabetic long-term care patients. *Gerontology.* 2002;48:250–253.

Sardinha TC, Nogveras JJ, Ehrenpreis ED, et al. Colonoscopy in octogenarians: a review of 428 cases. *Int J Colorectal Dis.* 1999;14:172–176.

Talley NJ, Fleming KC, Evans JM. Constipation in an elderly community: a study of prevalence and potential risk factors. *Am J Gastroenterol.* 1996;91:19–25.

Tan TL, Lieu PK, Ding YY, Urinary retention in hospitalised older women. *Ann Acad Med Singapore.* 2001;30:588–592.

Oncology and Aging: General Principles

Arati V. Rao ■ *Harvey Jay Cohen*

This chapter discusses many of the general relationships of oncology and aging. It focuses on the epidemiological, basic etiological, and biological relationships between the processes of aging and neoplasia, and on the generalizable aspects of management of malignant disease in the elderly patient. This chapter discusses clinical management of individual malignancies only as an example of general principles. The approach to specific malignancies is covered in subsequent chapters related to the appropriate organ system.

It is now well recognized that cancer is a major problem for elderly individuals. It is the second leading cause of death after heart disease in the United States, and age is the single most important risk factor for developing cancer. Approximately 60% of all newly diagnosed malignant tumors and 70% of all cancer deaths occur in persons 65 years or older according to the NCI Surveillance. As illustrated in Figure 94-1, the total cancer incidence rises progressively through the middle years and then falls off in the later years. However, the age-specific cancer incidence rises progressively throughout the age range. Thus, while the rate of increase diminishes somewhat in the oldest age groups, and the rate actually falls slightly in the very oldest (perhaps a survivor effect), the overall risk for developing cancer is certainly greatest in the later years. Because the number of people in this country older than age 65 years is rising rapidly and the oldest of the old, that is, those older than age 85 years, are increasing at the greatest rate, geriatricians, generalists, and internists will be encountering increasing numbers of elderly individuals with cancer in their practices.

The median age range for diagnosis for most major tumors, common to both men and women, is 68 to 74 years; the median age range at death is 70 to 79 years. The overall pattern for the incidence of age-specific cancer shows a rise with age; overall, 60% of cancers occur in those age 65 years or older (Table 94-1). This is not uniform for individual cancers and in some malignancies, there is an apparent decrease in incidence in people older than age 80 years. This may be a result of a number of factors, including underreporting or natural selection, which would allow the less-cancer-prone

population to survive. However, cohort effects may have the most significant impact. For example, age-specific annual cancer incidence rates from the SEER Program indicate a fall in incidence in the oldest age groups for both prostate and lung cancer. This changes when the data are corrected for certain known risk factors. For prostate cancer, when only men are considered in the base population at risk, the incidence continues to rise into the oldest age groups. For lung cancer, an apparent decrease in lung cancer incidence in the older age groups might be explained by a smaller high-risk population because of decreased prevalence of smoking in the older age groups. When data derived from the Lung Cancer Early Detection Project for annual cancer incidence in male smokers older than the age of 45 are used, one notes a continuing increase into advanced age. There is little change in the case of colorectal cancer, because the entire population appears to be at risk. For women with breast cancer, data indicate an incidence that continues to rise slowly into advanced age. It has been suggested that data from the most recent survey showing a decrease in breast cancer risk at older ages (>75 years) may be an artifact of recent increases in breast cancer screening in the United States. For other gynecologic malignancies, there does appear to be a decrease, perhaps because of different interactions of hormonal status and neoplasia in hormonally responsive target organs.

Other types of patterns in age-specific incidence may also be seen. For example, Hodgkin's disease has a distinct bimodal distribution in incidence with a peak in the early years and another peak after late middle age. This has led to the suggestion that there actually may be two different diseases involved, one in the young individual and one in the older one, but that they assume similar morphologic features, and so with current technologies we are unable to tell them apart. This impression is further substantiated by the markedly different response to treatment in younger and older groups of individuals with this disease. On the other hand, the most common leukemias and lymphomas in elderly patients are those derived from the B-lymphocyte arm of the immune system. These, including chronic lymphocytic leukemia and multiple myeloma,

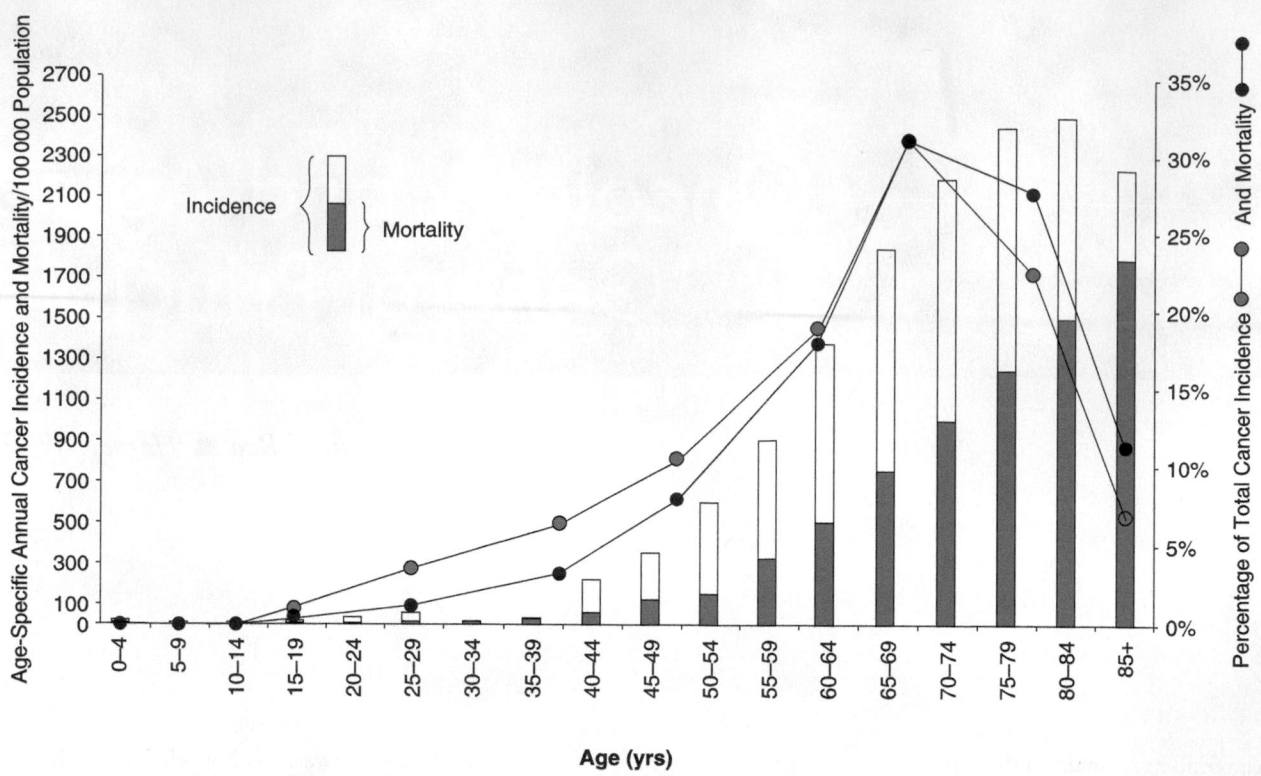

FIGURE 94-1. Comparison of the percentage of total cancer incidence and mortality by age with age-specific incidence and mortality. *(Data from SEER Cancer Statistics Review: 1973–1994. Bethesda, MD: National Cancer Institute, 1997.)*

rise dramatically in incidence throughout life, with the real majority of these disorders found in elderly individuals. Whether this dramatic relationship is caused by an enhanced susceptibility of the B-lymphocyte to neoplastic transformation in older individuals is a question relevant to the entire issue of the relationship between the

aging process and the neoplastic process, a subject that is considered next.

Not only does cancer occur at an increased rate in older individuals, but it makes a significant impact on such people's lives, from the standpoint of both increasing morbidity and mortality. As Figure 94-1 also demonstrates, the age-specific cancer mortality continues to rise as a function of age, as does incidence. In support of this observation is the report from the SEER Program that 5-year survivals for most types of cancer decrease with advancing age.

TABLE 94-1

Cancer Incidence in U.S. Patients Age 65+ Years of All Races and Both Sexes

CANCER	% 65+
Prostate	63.8
Colon	70.2
Pancreas	69.2
Urinary bladder	72.2
Stomach	65.5
Rectum	57.0
Lung and bronchus	67.8
Leukemias	54.3
Corpus uteri	45.3
Non-Hodgkin's lymphoma	54.3
Breast	42.3
Ovary	47.0
All Cancers Combined	**55.8**

Note: For breast cancer, cancer of the ovary, and corpus uteri only female patients included, and for prostate cancer only male patients included.
Data from SEER Cancer Statistics Review: 1975–2004. Bethesda, MD: National Cancer Institute; 2004.

RELATIONSHIP OF AGING AND NEOPLASIA

It is difficult to discuss a relationship between two processes—aging (senescence) and neoplastic transformation—both of which are still incompletely understood at this time. To explore the relationship, however, we must first briefly describe the current understanding of the multistep process of carcinogenesis. The first stage of cancer development is known as initiation. In this process, chemical or physical carcinogens, or certain viruses, cause a change in the cell that predisposes it to a subsequent malignant transformation. This change appears to be an irreversible lesion in the genomic deoxyribonucleic acid (DNA) of a stem cell; the lesion may remain stable for a long period. It is not clear whether such an initiated cell can be recognized clinically, but certain disorders such as myelodysplasia or carcinoma in situ, may be a manifestation of this phenomenon.

The next stage of carcinogenesis is called promotion and involves a proliferative phase. Promoters are agents that can induce mitogenesis, or cell division, in an initiated cell. This phenomenon includes the activation of a number of growth factors and transcription factors, which promote cell proliferation, and which may arise through the events related to changes in oncogenes or tumor suppressor genes noted later. While it appears that a single initiating event is sufficient to begin the process, promotion appears to be most successful when it is repetitive. This may occur shortly after initiation or after a delay and appears to be dose-dependent as well as reversible. For this reason, researchers believe that cessation of cigarette smoking (containing both initiators and promoters) reduces the cancer incidence of former smokers when compared with those who continue to smoke.

The final stage of cancer development in this model is progression. This is actually multiphasic itself and involves the transformation of a cell from a premalignant to a malignant state, the potential clonal evolution of a subset of such cells, and the potential development of metastasis. The latter two phenomena are quite important and have led to the concept of tumor cell heterogeneity. Although we believe that tumors arise from a single "clone of cells," tumor cells are genetically more unstable than normal cells, yielding progeny with variable proliferative and metastatic potential. Thus, not all cells within a given tumor are the same. Clinically, this may explain such diversity as variable chemosensitivity of tumor cells, the selection of resistant cells, the differential behavior of different metastatic lesions compared with the original tumor and with other metastatic lesions, and sometimes the unpredictable behavior of a particular cancer. Other factors relating to the tumor's impact on host tissue may also play an important role at this stage. These include the ability to disrupt stromal elements such as the basement membrane and the ability to promote angiogenesis, which supports further tumor growth.

It is clear that alterations in growth regulatory gene function play a critical role in the development of neoplasia. There are two major classes of such genes—oncogenes and tumor-suppressor genes. Oncogenes, or cancer genes, were initially described as viral genes capable of transforming normal cells to malignant ones. Of the various genes, approximately 100 to 200 have been shown to be targets for oncogenic disruption of their DNA structure. Oncogene activation can result in one of two pathways: First, the decision of a cell to divide or undergo senescence and apoptosis (programmed cell death) is altered such that the balance is shifted away from cell death and toward cell survival and proliferation. Second, the oncogene mutations might affect DNA repair, thus predisposing cells to additional DNA damage and activation of additional oncogenes. Oncogenes can be either dominant or recessive. Dominant oncogenes are those for which a functional alteration in one allele contributes to the malignant phenotype despite the persistence of the normal contralateral allele. Recessive oncogenes are called tumor suppressor genes, which normally limit cell growth, enhance apoptosis, and control differentiation and require both alleles to be disrupted to contribute to the cancer process.

A large number of oncogenes have been described. They appear to have the potential for growth-enhancing activity at a series of steps along the mitogenic pathway, including activating signal transduction at the cell surface, producing endogenous growth factors at the cytoplasmic level (e.g., ras-like), and increasing the sensitivity of the cell to exogenous (or endogenous) growth factors at the nuclear level (e.g., myc-like). Another oncogene, bcl-2, codes for an inner mitochondrial protein that blocks apoptosis, or programmed cell death. This mechanism may be of particular interest in the context of senescence, as it may operate by increasing cell longevity rather than proliferation. Increased cellular oncogenic expression has been noted in many tumors and can be mimicked experimentally by altering the DNA encoding for the oncogene, usually at or near the promoter. Thus, it is possible that the chromosomal damage noted in neoplasia during the initiation and promotion phases, if it occurred near the region of an oncogene, could result in transformation and clonal evolution of the cancer. The evolutions noted in Burkitt lymphoma and chronic granulocytic leukemia may be examples of this process. The expression of more than one oncogene is necessary to cause transformation.

A number of tumor-suppressor genes have been described, and mutations in such genes as Rb and p53 have been described in many human tumors. The normal function of such genes appears to prevent uncontrolled growth as a result of the action of various growth-promoting factors. It has even been suggested that senescence may act as a form of tumor suppression. In fact, the two tumor-suppressor genes just noted, p53 and Rb, are essential for maintaining the senescent phenotype of cells in culture. Inactivation of either gene extends the replicative life span of such cells, and mutations of Rb have been linked to both cancer incidence and longevity in mice. This phenomenon would appear to enhance the likelihood of acquiring further mutations, leading to the ultimate development of malignancy. Indeed deletions of p53, Rb, or both, are frequently found in common solid tumors, such as lung, breast, and colon. Although the inactivation of tumor suppressor genes is important in the development of neoplasia, it is likely that alterations in both oncogenes and tumor-suppressor genes are necessary in many cases to achieve full malignant potential.

It is also important to understand the theory of the "two-hit hypothesis." As described above, certain tumor suppressor genes are responsible for suppressing the malignant phenotype. In normal individuals, both alleles of such genes would need to be eliminated by random or environmentally induced errors thus requiring "two-hits." In contrast, families with certain genetic mutations that make them susceptible to cancer already have one abnormal allele of the tumor suppressor gene. Thus, the "first-hit" preexists making them substantially more susceptible to carcinogenic action of the "second random hit."

How then might the aging process influence the process of neoplastic transformation to result in the markedly increased rates of cancer in older people? General aspects of the aging process were discussed in Chapter 1, and only certain specific aspects relevant to the process under discussion will be reiterated here. Table 94-2 lists the types of theories that appear relevant to an explanation of the striking epidemiologic relationship.

TABLE 94-2

Theories for Cancer Increase with Age

Longer duration of carcinogenic exposure
Increased susceptibility of cells to carcinogens
Decreased ability to repair DNA
Oncogene activation or amplification
Decrease in tumor suppression gene activity
Telomere shortening and genetic instability
Microenvironment alterations
Decreased immune surveillance

1. Longer duration of carcinogenic exposure: It is possible that aging simply allows the time necessary for the accumulation of cellular events to develop into a clinical neoplasm. There is evidence for age-related accumulation and expression of genetic damage. Somatic mutations are believed to occur at the rate of approximately 1 in 10 cell divisions, with approximately 10 cell divisions occurring in a lifetime of a human being. Certainly, the complex set of events required in the multistep process of carcinogenesis, for example, as described for colon cancer in humans, does occur over time. The passage of time alone, however, is not likely to explain the phenomenon, as the time for a mutated cell to become a malignant cell and then subsequently to become a detectable tumor has been estimated to be approximately 10% to 30% of the maximum life span for a given animal species, which may vary from just a few years to more than 100 years.

2. Altered susceptibility of aging cells to carcinogens: Data in this area are somewhat contradictory. In some cases, the incidence of skin tumors in mice produced with benzopyrene has been more related to dose than to age, whereas in other models, accelerated carcinogenesis as a function of age has been demonstrated, as, for example, when dimethyl benzanthracene (DMA) was applied to skin grafts of young and old mice. In addition, an age-related increase in the sensitivity of lymphocytes to cell-cycle arrest and chromosome damage after radiation has been demonstrated. It is also possible that there are alterations in carcinogen metabolism with age, but the findings from such studies have also been contradictory.

3. Decreased ability to repair DNA: It is possible that damage, once initiated, is more difficult to repair in older cells. A number of studies demonstrate decreased DNA repair as a function of age following damage by carcinogens as well as radiation. Such repair failures may also be reflected in increased karyotype abnormalities in aged normal cells as well as in older patients with neoplastic disease.

4. Oncogene activation or amplification or decrease in tumor suppressor gene activity: These processes might be increased in the older host, resulting either in increased action or promotion or in differential clonal evolution. Although evidence is currently limited, there have been observations of increased amplification of proto-oncogenes and their products in aging fibroblasts in vitro as well as evidence for increased c-myc transcript levels in the livers of aging mice. Alternatively, such factors as genetic alterations or DNA damage could lead to inactivation of cancer-suppressor genes. Given that age-related mutations frequently appear to result in the loss of function, alterations in tumor-suppressor genes may prove to be an important mechanism.

5. Telomere shortening and genetic instability: The function of telomeres and the enzyme telomerase appears to be intimately involved in both the senescence and neoplasia processes. Telomeres, the terminal end of all chromosomes, shorten progressively as cells age. This functional decline begins at age 30 and continues at a loss of approximately 1% per year. This shortening appears to be causally related to controlled cell proliferation and limitation of population doubling. It is thought that each time a cell divides, 30 to 200 base pairs are lost from the end of that cell's telomeres. Because the major function of telomeres is to protect the stability of the more internal coding sequences (i.e., allow cells to divide without losing genes), the loss of this function may lead to genetic instability, which may promote mutations in oncogenic or tumor-suppressor gene sequences. Without telomeres, chromosome ends could fuse together and degrade the cell's genetic blueprint, making the cell malfunction, become cancerous, or even die. Telomere length is a predictor of mortality in people aged 60 or older.

The enzyme telomerase is responsible for adding back telomeric repeats to the ends of chromosomes, that is, regenerate the telomeres. This enzyme is generally not expressed in normal cells, but it is activated in malignant cells. While telomerase can reverse replicative cell senescence, the indiscriminate expression of this enzyme might increase the likelihood of tumor formation. It is also possible that p53 or Rb inactivation that occurs in senescent cells, or the inactivation of other tumor-suppressor genes, may allow the activation of the telomerase gene and promote cell immortalization and ultimately malignancy.

6. Microenvironment alterations: Older people accumulate senescent cells as shown by β-galactosidase staining. They also have higher levels of IL-6, which is one of the causes of frailty. A number of factors in the tumor microenvironment are critical for the development of the malignant phenotype, especially invasion and metastasis. Senescent cells can compromise tissue renewal capacity, and secrete multiple factors that alter tissue homeostasis. These factors include inflammatory cytokines like IL-1 and epithelial growth factors (e.g., heregulin, and matrix metalloproteinases like MMP-3) and can disrupt the architecture and function of the surrounding tissue and stimulate or inhibit the proliferation of neighboring cells.

Senescent fibroblasts disrupt epithelial alveolar morphogenesis, functional differentiation, and branching morphogenesis. Senescent human and mouse fibroblasts also increase vascular endothelial growth factor expression, and hypoxia further induces endothelial growth factor in senescent cells. Thus, senescent cells can create a tissue environment that synergizes with mutation accumulation to facilitate the progression of malignancies.

7. Decreased immune surveillance: A decrease in immune surveillance, or immunosenescence, could contribute to the increased incidence of malignancies. With respect to tumor-related immunity, however, there is a considerable amount of evidence in animal models for a loss of tumor-specific immunity with progressive age. This includes the altered capacity of old mice to reject transplanted tumors, the close relationship between susceptibility to malignant melanomas and the rate of age-related T-cell-dependent immune function decline, and the ability by immunopharmacologic manipulation to increase age-depressed tumoricidal immune function and to decrease the incidence of spontaneous tumors. The evidence linking such data to age-associated immune deficiency and the rise of cancer incidence in humans, however, is mainly circumstantial and not likely to be fully explanatory, as the types of tumors seen in the most striking examples of immune deficiency are very different from those seen in the usual aging human.

Figure 94-2 summarizes in a schematic fashion the potential interaction of these many factors that may be of importance in the increase of cancer with age. It indicates the interface of time and age-related events, such as free radical and other carcinogenic exposure, resulting in initiation, then cumulative promoting events, including mutations and other alterations in critical genes, which

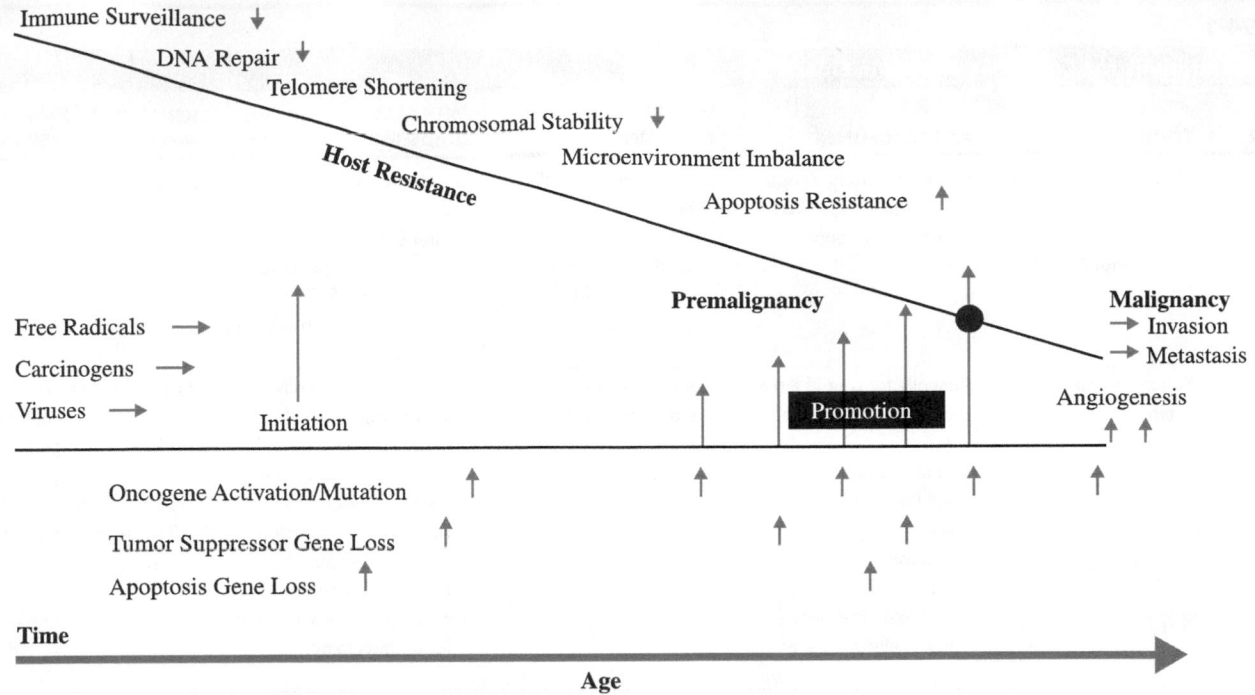

FIGURE 94-2. Age and cancer susceptibility. This figure presents a model incorporating the various factors that may play a role in the increased incidence of cancer with age.

alternately exceed a threshold of host resistance factors, which have been progressively reduced during the aging process.

Cellular senescence suppresses cancer by arresting cells at risk of malignant transformation. However, senescent cells also secrete molecules that can stimulate premalignant cells to proliferate and form tumors, suggesting that the senescence response is antagonistically pleiotropic. Thus, cellular senescence-induced suppression of malignant transformation, a function important for the organism in early life (through the reproductive period), may be selected for, despite the fact that cellular senescence may be quite injurious in later life. In this case, senescence could be viewed as the price we pay in later life for the rigorous attempt to control proliferation to avoid neoplasia early on. The progressive, and no doubt multifactorial, loss of the controls with aging ultimately results in an increase in neoplasia in advanced age despite the early control. From the standpoint of natural selection, both of these outcomes would be acceptable, as they tend to occur long after the reproductive life span. It is likely that through research at the basic level concerning the interactions of aging and neoplasia, we will learn a great deal about the fundamental basis of each. It is hoped that such information will enhance our ability to engage in prevention at the primary and secondary levels.

A large proportion of cancers are potentially preventable. The most obviously available modalities in this regard are avoidance of known and suspected carcinogenic exposures such as tobacco smoke, occupational and environmental chemicals, excessive sunlight, and dietary factors such as excessive fat and smoked, salted, and pickled foods. Although older individuals have potentially acquired a lifetime exposure to such carcinogens, they should still accrue benefits from modifying these behaviors as well as from engaging in positive ones such as the suggested intake of fiber,

vitamins, and fresh vegetables. In recent years, there has been increased interest in cancer prevention through chemopreventive intervention approaches. However, results are inconsistent and some have shown adverse effects. The evidence for tamoxifen as a preventive agent for breast cancer is the strongest, but the agent appears to be less effective in elderly women.

In 2006 the Food and Drug Administration (FDA) approved the use of a human papillomavirus-16 (HPV-16) live particle vaccine to prevent cervical cancer, precancerous genital lesions, and genital warts caused by HPV types 6, 11, 16, and 18. The vaccine is approved for use in females 9 to 26 years of age and has not been studied in elderly patients. The Selenium and Vitamin E Cancer Prevention Trial (SELECT) is an ongoing randomized, prospective, double-blind study designed to determine whether selenium and vitamin E alone and in combination can reduce the risk of prostate cancer among healthy men. The final results from this study are anticipated in the year 2013. Thus, currently there is no compelling evidence for the efficacy of the use of chemopreventive agents among the elderly population, and it still must be considered experimental.

CLINICAL PRESENTATIONS AND DISEASE BEHAVIOR

Screening in Asymptomatic Individuals

Elderly patients continue to be underscreened and thus underdiagnosed with cancer. Screening examination for oral and skin cancers is reasonable for high-risk older people as part of an office examination. It is well known that mammography and Papanicolaou (Pap) tests are underutilized in certain older racial and ethnic minority

TABLE 94-3

Recommendations for Cancer Screening in Elderly People

CANCER	TEST(S)	ACS GUIDELINES	USPSTF GUIDELINES	MEDICARE GUIDELINES	REIMBURSEMENT/ MEDICARE COVERAGE
Breast	Mammography (with or without clinical breast examination)	Annually starting at age 40 yr for as long as patient is in good health	Annually or biennially between ages 50 and 69 yr; consider continuing if patient has reasonable life expectancy	Start biennial screening at age 50 yr, continue to offer between 70 and 80 yr if life expectancy greater than 5–7 yr; explain risks, explore barriers	Annual mammography will be reimbursed for women older than age 40
Cervical	Papanicolaou (Pap) test	Annually for 3 yr. If three or more consecutive satisfactory normal annual examinations, the Pap test may be performed less frequently at the discretion of her physician then less frequently, no upper age limit	Biennially or triennially, may stop at age 65 yr if has had regular, normal smears	Biennially or triennially, stop at age 65 yr if patient has had regular, normal smears; obtain history of prior Pap smears and risk factors; perform speculum examination before excluding from screening for hysterectomy	Pap and pelvic every 3 yr. Yearly screening for women who are at high risk for cervical or vaginal cancer or who have had an abnormal Pap smear in the preceding 3 yr
Colorectal	FOBT; flexible sigmoidoscopy; colonoscopy; ACBE	At age 50 yr, offer: annual FOBT, flexible sigmoidoscopy every 5 yr, annual FOBT and flexible sigmoidoscopy every 5 yr, colonoscopy every 10 yr, or ACBE every 5–10 yr	At age 50 yr, offer annual FOBT; flexible sigmoidoscopy every 5 yr; or annual FOBT and flexible sigmoidoscopy every 5 yr	At age 50 yr, offer annual FOBT with or without flexible sigmoidoscopy every 5 yr; consider one-time colonoscopy or combined flexible sigmoidoscopy and ACBE	For individuals older than 50 yr, screening FOBT reimbursed once a year, flexible sigmoidoscopy once every 4 yr or once every 2 yr if patient is high risk. Colonoscopy reimbursed every 2 yr for high-risk patients
Prostate	Digital rectal examination; PSA assay	Both tests annually, starting at age 50 yr	Neither test recommended for the general population	Neither test recommended except in high-risk patients (e.g., family history of disease, African-American)	Annual digital rectal examination and PSA will be reimbursed in men older than age 50
Lung	Chest x-ray; sputum cytology; spiral CT scan; fluorescence bronchoscopy	None of these tests are yet recommended	None of these tests recommended for the general population	None of these tests recommended	No reimbursement
Ovary	Pelvic examination; CA-125 assay; transvaginal ultrasound	None of these tests are recommended	None of these tests recommended	None of these tests recommended	No reimbursement

ACBE, air-contrast barium enema; ACS, American Cancer Society; CT, computed tomography; FOBT, fecal occult blood test; PSA, prostate-specific antigen; USPSTF, United States Preventive Services Task Force.

groups and in those who have less than high school education or live below the poverty level. Only 17% of American Indian/Alaska Native women who are 60 years or older have ever had a mammogram, compared to 38% among all U.S. women of that age. The situations in which periodic routine screening is recommended for all individuals regardless of age are relatively few. A number of organizations have made recommendations, and there is some variation among them. It should be recognized that when applied to elderly persons, especially those older than age 75 years, such information is largely empirically derived. These recommendations are directed at mass screening of populations. When applied to individuals within a physician's office or other practice, they serve only as general guide-

lines for decisions that may be, and often should be, modified by many other factors. Table 94-3 shows the current guidelines of the American Cancer Society relevant to the older adult, those of the U.S. Preventive Health Task Force, a synthesized recommendation by the authors, and Medicare reimbursement. Most of these recommendations do not directly address alterations in strategy for people at more advanced ages. Moreover, there is obvious variability in the recommendations. In general, for malignancies for which screening modalities are potentially useful, in the absence of upper age limits, the expectation of 5 to 10 years of life would appear reasonable as a cut-point. The problem is that assessment of remaining life expectancy for an individual patient may be difficult.

Breast Cancer

Arriving at a specific recommendation for breast cancer screening in older women has been complicated by several factors. In addition to the lack of specific outcome data for women older than 75 years of age, factors such as increased mammographic detectability of cancers in older women because of the increase in fatty tissue of the breast with age, contrasted with the increased prevalence of co-morbid disease, make decision making difficult. The United States Preventive Services Task Force (USPSTF) does not recommend continued screening in elderly women, because most studies of breast cancer efficacy included inadequate numbers of these women. Few, if any, studies have yielded evidence that screening is ineffective in women 70 and older. Given the higher breast cancer incidence and mortality seen in elderly women, as well as the increased life expectancy with little or no activity limitation seen among today's elderly, consideration should be given to including elderly women in the recommendation to receive timely breast cancer screening. Since surgical and adjuvant therapy for breast cancer in older women can often be accomplished without major complications, the cost–benefit ratio for breast cancer screening in this age group may prove to be promising. Thus, breast cancer screening should be a lifelong activity, although cessation has been suggested if remaining life expectancy is less than 5 years. While there are no specific outcome data to support breast self-examination in older women, if it is practiced, it should be made clear that it is not a substitute for mammography and clinical examination.

Cervical Cancer

In the past, recommendations concerning cervical cancer and the Pap test have been controversial. The effectiveness of this screening modality is widely accepted. Controversy has been centered more around the frequency of testing required and whether testing could be suspended either at a certain age or after a certain number of negative tests. The current American Cancer Society guideline for detection of cervical cancer in asymptomatic women appears to be a consensus position that should adequately address the issue. The guideline states, "All women who are, or who have been, sexually active, or have reached age 18 years, [should] have an annual Pap test and pelvic examination. After a women has three or more consecutive satisfactory normal annual examinations, the Pap test may be performed less frequently at the discretion of her physician." This recommendation has no specific upper-age limitation, and the discussion of these recommendations contains a reminder that "mature women, those older than 65, also require testing." This is considered to be critical if such women have not had a history of regular Pap testing in their younger years. Thus, we recommend that for the older patient whose history of previous screening is not clear, Pap testing be done until the recommendations have been fulfilled. In addition, in 2003, the FDA approved the HPV DNA test to be used simultaneously with the Pap test to screen for cervical cancer in women age 30 and older. If both the Pap and the HPV DNA test results are negative, a woman's physician may advise her to wait for 3 years before being retested, according to guidelines from the American College of Obstetricians and Gynecologists (ACOG). But more frequent testing is recommended if other high-risk factors are present, such as a weakened immune system or a history of cervical cancer. If only one of the tests is negative, the physician may advise the woman to return for retesting in 6 to 12 months. For ovarian cancer, acceptable screening methods have not yet been shown to have an impact on tumor-related outcomes.

Colon Cancer

Recommendations for colon cancer screening center on general agreement over the use of fecal occult blood testing and sigmoidoscopy, with the use of colonoscopy and double-contrast barium enema being more questionable. Prostate cancer screening remains controversial. While some agencies recommend prostrate-specific antigen (PSA) screening, this has been done on the basis only of a demonstration of increased ascertainment. There are yet no data on impact on mortality or even quality of life over long periods. Given the large number of false-positives requiring considerable work-up and the high incidence of very indolent disease in older men, the USPSTF decision not to recommend such screening appears reasonable. In any event, if screening is to be considered, a thorough discussion of the risks as well as benefits should first ensue. In such consideration, it would appear that at least a 10-year life expectancy would be required before there is any chance of seeing a positive benefit overall.

Lung Cancer

For lung cancer, one of the most common malignancies in both genders, specific mass screening is not yet recommended. This is based on a lack of demonstrated cost–benefit efficacy, even in high-risk smoking groups. However, the International Early Lung Cancer Action Project (I-ELCAP) used low-dose spiral CT screening to diagnose lung cancer in 484 of approximately 30 000 participants. Of these 484 patient's, 412 (85%) had clinical stage I lung cancer, and the estimated 10-year survival rate was 88% in this subgroup. Thus, spiral CT screening may detect lung cancer that is curable. Of note, ~55% of patients in this study were 60 years or older (predominantly previous or current smokers). Formal recommendations regarding the use of spiral CT scans to screen for lung cancer have not been made.

Despite these widely disseminated recommendations, many individuals do not follow them. This appears to relate to both physician- and patient-derived factors. Despite the increased risk of cancer in the older age group, such individuals appear to avail themselves of routine screening even less frequently than their younger counterparts. The physician and other health care professionals should ensure that the older individual is aware of the importance of screening, that the opportunity for such examinations is provided, and that fears and anxieties about these tests are allayed to as great an extent as possible. Screening education materials, made user friendly for the older person, have been developed and should be used.

Initial Presentation

As an extension of the screening concept, the goal for initial cancer detection is to make the diagnosis as early as possible, with the hope that treatment at the earliest stages of disease would yield the best survival rates. It is, therefore, of great importance that both patient and physician pay attention to symptoms that may herald the onset of the neoplastic process. Although information on "warning signs of cancer" has been widely disseminated by the American Cancer

TABLE 94-4

Cancer Symptom Confusion

SYMPTOM OR SIGN	POSSIBLE MALIGNANCY	AGING "EXPLANATION"
Increase in skin pigment	Melanoma, squamous cell	"Age spots"
Rectal bleeding	Colon or rectum	Hemorrhoids
Constipation	Rectal	"Old age"
Dyspnea	Lung	Getting old, out of shape
Decrease in urinary stream	Prostate	"Dribbling"—benign prostatic hypertrophy (BPH)
Breast contour change	Breast	"Normal" atrophy, fibrosis
Fatigue	Metastatic or other	Loss of energy owing to "aging"
Bone pain	Metastatic or other	Arthritis: "aches and pains of aging"

Society and others, it is often ignored. This is due in part to a lack of knowledge of the implications of such warning signs. Indeed, some have indicated that elderly persons know less about potential cancer symptoms and their significance than do young individuals, which might lead to a delay in presentation. Another factor that might interfere with early diagnosis is what might be called "cancer symptom confusion," that is, a tendency to write off the symptom as simply another change caused by the aging process. Table 94-4 lists examples of such possibilities. Physicians and patients alike may be prone to such assumptions and should be alerted to the fact that a new symptom or a change in symptoms should be appropriately pursued in the elderly individual.

Once having noticed a symptom that appears to be related to cancer, most older individuals do not delay appreciably in seeking medical help. However, in one study from New Mexico of 800 patients older than 65 years, 19.2% of the subjects delayed seeking care for at least 12 weeks and 7.4% delayed at least 1 year. In another study from Finland, women older than 80 years had a longer interval between first symptom and first medical examination for the diagnosis of colorectal cancer when compared to their younger counterparts. Older women, who are at greater risk of developing breast cancer, are also more likely to delay their presentation. Factors associated with delayed presentation include having a nonlump symptom, reservations about seeing a general practitioner, and fear of the consequences of cancer.

Physicians may also be guilty of delaying further diagnostic pursuits in elderly patients. Part of the problem may lie in a failure to recognize new signs and symptoms in patients with multiple disease processes. It is easy to attribute such symptoms as anorexia, weight loss, or decrease in performance status to chronic diseases and to social or psychological changes. The increasing prevalence of findings such as anemia in elderly patients may lower the index of suspicion for attributing the factor to a new specific neoplastic process. The remarkable age-related increase in cancer incidence described earlier in this chapter should be sufficient to promote the maintenance of vigilance in this regard, although it must be balanced by judgment concerning the risk–benefit ratio for diagnostic evaluations in

individual patients depending on their other medical status. Thus, the initial discovery of a new symptom in a previously totally well, active 80-year-old may be pursued rather differently than a similar discovery in a severely demented, bed-bound individual with severe congestive heart failure, diabetes, and pulmonary failure.

Biological Behavior of Tumors in the Elderly Host

The effect of the aging process on the clinical course of cancer, or to put it another way, whether cancer behaves differently in the older individual—is not clear. Although the SEER data noted previously suggested that in many cancers the 5-year survival rate is lower for older people, it is possible that this is related more to comorbid disease and other factors rather than simply to aging per se. On the other hand, there is a widespread belief that cancers may behave more indolently in elderly patients. These are important issues because they may, to a considerable degree, affect decisions regarding treatment. Both clinical and experimental evidence support both sides of this issue, and it is likely that there is a spectrum of responses dependent on initial tumor types as well as individual host status. One indicator of the phenomenon is the extent of disease at presentation. For most cancers examined, there has been no consistent difference in the stage of disease or presentation for different age groups. For those that have been determined, the directions are not always the same. For malignant melanoma, older patients have been consistently found to have more advanced-stage local disease with deeper penetrating lesions at presentation. For breast cancer, some studies show a greater proportion of older patients with distant metastatic spread at presentation, whereas for lung cancer the opposite has been found, and older patients have been noted to present with localized disease in a greater proportion of cases. Uterine and cervical cancers have in some cases been noted to be later in the course of disease at presentation in older individuals. Of course, even these differences might be related to such phenomena as delay in the patient's presenting for diagnosis (which does not appear to be the case), delay in pursuing the diagnosis, intensity of diagnostic endeavors, or a combination of these factors, or, on the other hand, a greater chance for a serendipitous finding because of more frequent visits to physicians.

Another biologic factor that may influence neoplastic behavior in differently aged hosts is the histologic subtype of the tumor. Thus, while thyroid cancer overall appears to behave more aggressively in the older host, it is also true that a larger proportion of thyroid neoplasia in elderly patients is made up by anaplastic carcinoma, which at any age has more aggressive behavior. However, there is a poorer overall prognosis for older individuals with thyroid cancer, independent of histologic type when compared to their younger counterparts. Similarly, for malignant melanoma, although there is an increased proportion of older people who have melanomas of poor prognostic histologic type and location at presentation, older individuals have a poorer prognosis for survival than do younger ones independent of this phenomenon even for localized disease. Similarly, for lung cancer, the increased proportion of elderly patients with squamous carcinoma of the lung—which is the histologic subset most likely to present as localized disease—partially, but not completely, explains some of the findings just noted. Such biologic differences may be manifested in other ways, as in the case of breast cancer, in which older women have an increased frequency of estrogen receptor–positive breast cancer, probably related to hormonal influences of the postmenopausal state. An additional factor is the longer tumor doubling time seen in breast cancer cells from older women. Because estrogen-receptor positivity and longer doubling times are associated with better prognosis, with more slow-growing tumors and with longer disease-free survivals, these phenomena—rather than age per se—might provide the reason why this cancer appears to behave more indolently in an older individual. Despite this, overall cancer-related survival is lower in older women, emphasizing the complex interactions of tumor and host that must be considered.

Acute myelogenous leukemia (AML) has a much poorer prognosis in older patients. The biology underlying the poor prognosis and poor treatment outcome of AML in elderly patients has been extensively studied. Among the findings to date are a high incidence of poor-prognosis karyotypes (5q-, 7q-), high frequency of preceding myelodysplastic syndromes, and an increased expression of proteins involved in intrinsic resistance to chemotherapeutic agents. Compared to younger patients, leukemic blasts from elderly patients with AML have a lower propensity to apoptosis following traditional remission-induction treatment with ara-C and daunorubicin. These findings suggest that leukemia in the elderly patient may arise from an earlier stem cell; thus, such a patient may have an impaired capacity for hematopoietic recovery after chemotherapy.

Experimental data in animal models likewise show this spectrum in rate of tumor growth and progression as a function of age. In these studies, the ability to contain tumor growth depends on the particular host tumor system used, thus mimicking the clinical situation to some extent. A proposed explanation for the situation in which the older host more effectively controls the rate of tumor is a paradoxical effect of decreasing immune function with age, that is, decreased activity of those cells in the old host's immune system, which—under the stimulation of the neoplastic process—produce tumor-enhancing factors such as angiogenesis factor. When this occurs, tumor growth might be expected to be diminished. To what extent these various factors play a role in the biological behavior of neoplasia in the aging human host remains a fascinating puzzle to be unraveled.

MANAGEMENT

This section examines the utility of the major modalities of cancer treatment in the elderly individual. The use of such modalities is heavily conditioned by the initial decision-making process, that is, whether to screen, whether to pursue diagnostic work-ups, whether to treat at all, and how intensively to treat. In such decisions, the physician is often placed in the position of weighing benefits versus risks of diagnostic and therapeutic interventions. This is as it should be, and the physician should take into account the various biologic, psychological, and social factors involved in the patient's well-being. Of great importance in this regard is the patient's own assessment of the value of both quantity and quality of potential survival during and after the treatment for malignancy. In this process, there is a clear need to individualize such decisions, and a decision made for a well elderly patient may be appropriately different than that for a frail elderly patient.

Unfortunately, age bias in diagnostic and treatment decisions for older patients with cancer does exist, and elderly patients are continually underrepresented in clinical trials. Analysis of data on ~60 000 patients treated in phase II and III trials sponsored by the National Cancer Institute between 1997 and 2000 found that only 32% of the participants were aged 65 years or older, despite the fact that this age group accounted for 61% of patients with cancer. Thus, while differences in decisions may be entirely appropriate in certain situations, these must be based on specific individualized patient information and not on categorical decisions made purely on the basis of chronologic age.

We proposed one framework in which the general aspects of such decision making can be considered for the individual patient. This is shown in Figure 94-3 and is called the Comprehensive Geriatric Model. It graphically presents a number of the concepts critical to the care of the elderly patient, that is, that there is a decreased functional reserve and that, as an extension of Engel's Bio-Psycho-Social Model, all of these various aspects of the individual's background must be taken into account when making decisions about the new process, that is, the cancer. Each of these levels, for example, biologic or psychological, can create interactions that influence both the cancer and the host, and, likewise, any intervention directed at the cancer may influence both the cancer and each of these levels of the host's function. Conversely, each of these levels of function, when compromised by the aging process or other comorbid diseases, may influence the ability to deliver these various interventions. Thus, in a sense, a conceptual checklist is presented in which a four-way interaction of various factors can be systematically considered when making decisions. Examples of ways in which physiologic changes occurring with age can impact on cancer treatment are shown in Table 94-5.

The implementation of this concept is through the application of geriatric assessment (as described in detail in Chapter 11) to the elderly cancer patient so that the domains of physiological status, comorbidity, geriatric syndromes, and functional and cognitive status can be assessed and define levels of frailty. One feasibility study to evaluate cancer-specific geriatric assessment included validated measures of geriatric assessment in the following domains: functional status, comorbidity, cognition, psychological status, social functioning and support, and nutritional status. The assessment was administered to 43 patients with breast, lung, and colorectal cancers or lymphoma who were receiving chemotherapy. The average age of these patients was 74 years, and the majority of patients had stage IV disease. The mean time to complete the assessment was 27 minutes, 78% patients were able to complete the self-administered portion of the assessment without assistance, and 90% of patients were satisfied with the questionnaire length. Another report has suggested that care of elderly cancer patients in geriatric evaluation and management units has a positive and sustained effect on their quality of life, including emotional limitation, mental health, and bodily pain. Thus, oncogeriatricians now feel that this information, rather than age per se, should weigh more heavily on subsequent management decisions for use of diagnostic as well as therapeutic technologies for the elderly patient with cancer. The optimal mechanism for practically implementing this approach (e.g., clinic team, inpatient unit, consultation) remains to be determined.

MAJOR THERAPEUTIC MODALITIES

Surgery

Surgery and other invasive procedures are frequently involved in initial diagnostic as well as in therapeutic approaches to the elderly

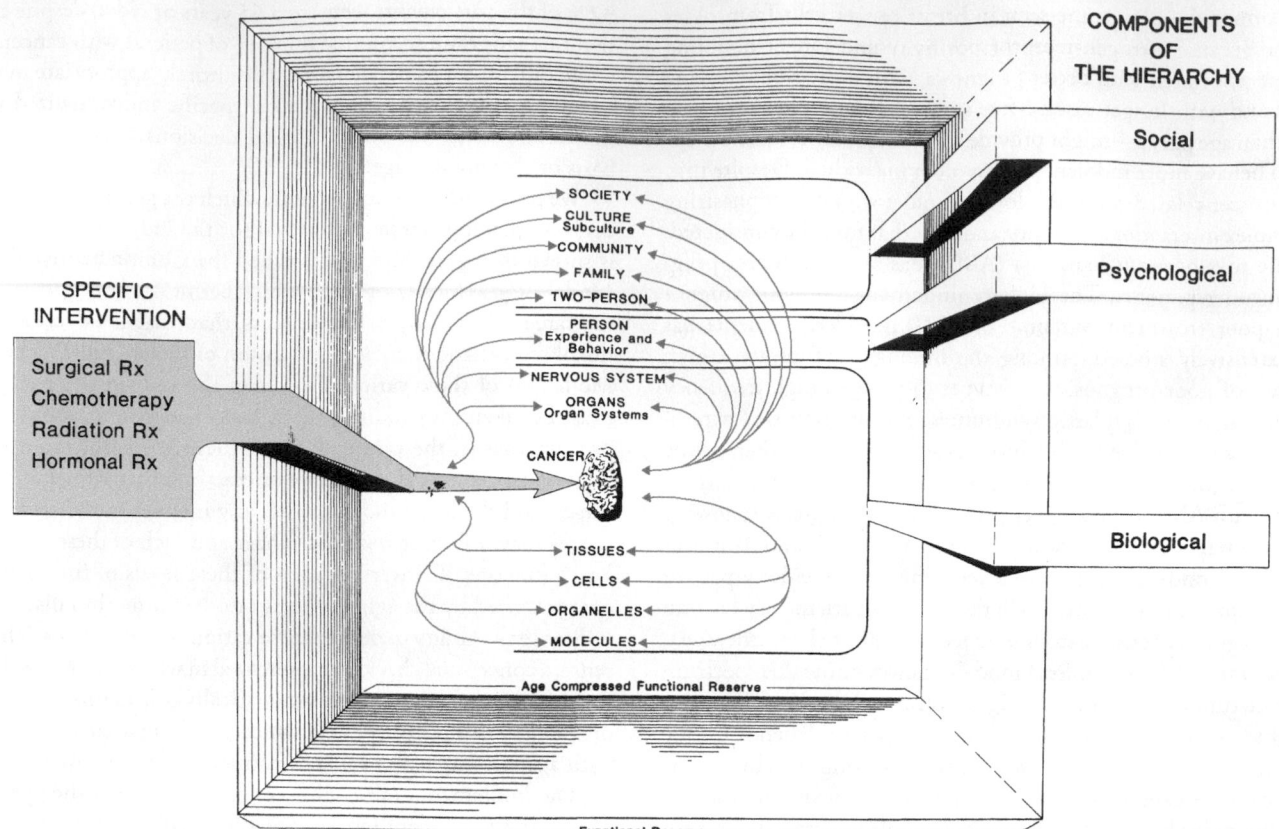

FIGURE 94-3. The Comprehensive Geriatric Model. *(Reproduced with permission from Cohen HJ, DeMaria L: In: Lazlo J, ed. Physician's Guide to Cancer Care Complications. New York, New York: Dekker; 1986:240.)*

patient with cancer. The general aspects of surgery in the elderly patient are discussed thoroughly in Chapter 37. Cancer surgery may be accomplished in elderly patients with mortality and morbidity rates that are often similar to those for younger patients and appear to be conditioned more by the extent of comorbid disease and declines in measurable physiologic functions than by chronologic age. In com-

paring potential alternative modalities, it is well to remember that the acute and time-limited stress of surgery may be preferable to many older patients than the more chronic or protracted courses of therapy frequently involved in radiation therapy and/or chemotherapy.

Radiation Therapy

Radiation therapy is used in the treatment of malignancies with both curative and palliative intent. In an attempt to cure local or regional disease, given that both radiation therapy and surgery might be considered, one must consider whether the cure rate is equivalent and whether there are differences in morbidity or mortality between the procedures that would favor one over the other. Radiation therapy is generally not contraindicated by associated medical conditions, and it may allow maintenance of function of the organ in which the tumor arises. For example, for an elderly person, radiating laryngeal carcinoma and maintaining speech, rather than requiring the learning of laryngeal speech postoperatively, may be of considerable advantage. On the other hand, radiation treatment frequently involves a protracted course of therapy and can cause significant fatigue.

Radiation therapy is also used as an effective adjunct to surgery or chemotherapy or both. For those surgical procedures with high operative mortality, using adjunct radiation therapy to reduce the degree of surgery required may be especially attractive to an elderly patient. The results for adjunct radiation therapy and approaches such as quadrantectomy in breast cancer or lymph node excision in head or neck cancer have been demonstrated to be equivalent

TABLE 94-5

Aging Physiology and Cancer	
AGING PHYSIOLOGY	**CANCER RELEVANCE**
Cardiopulmonary	
↓ Max CO, VO₂ Max	Surgery
↓ Elasticity	C/P toxic drugs
Skin—↓ wound healing	Surgery
CNS—↓ brain weight, cerebral blood flow	Patient interactions CNS toxic drugs
Special senses—↓ taste, smell, salivary flow	Nutrition radiation therapy
Hematopoiesis—↓ response under stress	Chemotherapy and radiation therapy
Immune system—↓ response	Infection
Body composition—↓ lean, ↓ fat	Drug distribution
Liver—↓ mass and flow	Hepatic drug metabolism
Kidney—↓ GFR	Renal drug excretion

CNS, central nervous system; C/P, cardiopulmonary; GFR, glomerular filtration rate.

to more extensive surgical procedures. Radiation is also used in a "neoadjuvant" setting, that is, prior to surgery in an attempt to reduce tumor mass and allow greater operability. Palliative, radiation therapy can be extremely effective in providing relief from pain from bone metastases, the effects of brain metastases, control of local obstructive symptoms, and spinal cord compromise. Such treatments can frequently be delivered in courses of 1 to 2 weeks' duration rather than the longer courses of therapy that may be more difficult to tolerate. However, short courses of high-dose radiation may be associated with a higher incidence of acute side effects. The results of treatment, as well as the incidence of complications, greatly depend on the technology available and its correct application.

The side effects of therapy may create problems for the older patient. The radiation effect on normal tissue is said to be enhanced approximately 10% to 15% in the elderly patient. Logically, those organs with more marked physiological decline would be at greatest risk. Radiation to the oral pharynx and oral cavity can produce a loss of taste, dryness of mucous membranes, and involution of salivary glands, which when combined with a precarious nutritional intake in a frail and elderly individual might be lethal, or certainly contribute a considerable amount of morbidity, if not recognized. Moreover, if daily treatment is tolerated poorly owing to nausea or weakness, treatment may be compromised because of the decreased daily doses, the patient's unscheduled absences, or decrease in the total planned dose. Because radiation therapy is frequently used in the treatment of lung cancer, pulmonary complications may be of particular importance. In one study, severe radiation pneumonitis was noted more frequently in elderly individuals than in younger ones, regardless of field size and other therapies. Alterations in schedule can be made and still deliver potentially curative radiation therapy to older individuals. This must be done with care, however; although decreasing the daily fraction has not been shown to be detrimental to local control of neck and head cancer, split-dose schedules are associated with significantly lower control rates for some tumor sites.

Chemotherapy and Hormonal Therapy

Thorough discussions of the principles of pharmacology and of medication use in elderly persons can be found in Chapters 8 and 24. Although still understudied, there are a growing number of direct studies of the effect of age on the pharmacokinetics of orally or parenterally administered chemotherapeutic agents. The declining ability of senescent cells to repair DNA damage may prolong toxicity. Increased destruction of and lower numbers of rapidly renewing mucosal stem cells increase susceptibility to mucositis. Also, reduced hematopoietic stem cell reserve may slow recovery of cytopenias after chemotherapy in older persons. In general, absorption of drugs appears to be affected relatively little as a consequence of age, but may become more relevant as newer oral agents (e.g., fluorinated pyrimidines) become more widely used. Decreased gastric motility and gastric secretions can also add to increased toxicity from these agents. Higher proportions of body fat may increase the volume of distribution of lipid-soluble drugs, such as nitrosoureas. In people with reduced albumin, volume of distribution for drugs bound to albumin, such as etoposide, is increased. Also, drugs like taxanes and anthracyclines that are highly bound to red blood cells are affected when anemia is present. Drug metabolism is also affected by lower hepatic mass and decreased activity of cytochrome P-450 enzymes in elderly patients. Renally excreted drugs are affected by decreased nephron mass in elderly patients.

The potential for response and degree of toxicity for various regimens in elderly patients appear to constitute a spectrum depending predominantly on the aggressiveness of the therapeutic regimen. The major limiting factor for most drugs is bone marrow reserve. Decreased reserve capacity has been demonstrated in both experimental animals and humans, but clinical toxicity depends on the degree to which bone marrow reserve is stressed. Age is an independent risk factor for neutropenia in elderly patients with lymphomas and leukemias. Other toxicities, such as the pulmonary toxicity of bleomycin, the cardiotoxicity of doxorubicin, and the peripheral nerve toxicity of vincristine, also appear to be increased somewhat, although, again, depending on the aggressiveness of the regimen. Comorbidity has a negative effect on survival in patients with cancer, and one study found that hospitalization for chemotherapy-induced toxicity in older patients increased significantly with their comorbidity score. Patients with stage II and III colon cancer treated with adjuvant therapy had a higher rate of cancer recurrence and mortality and grade 3 or 4 diarrhea if they also had concurrent diabetes mellitus.

Despite these risks in older people, a number of studies of adjuvant chemotherapy indicate similar benefits and toxicities in equivalently selected younger and older patients. Yet, older age is associated with less use of adjuvant chemotherapy in elderly patients with breast cancer independent of comorbidities. The phenomenon of "risk aversion" is underdosing in an attempt to avoid toxicities, but it effectively abrogates chances of a positive therapeutic response. This occurred in trials of adjuvant chemotherapy for breast cancer wherein poor results were seen in those elderly women who had lower than the prescribed dosage of adjuvant therapy, presumably in an attempt to avoid toxicities. In contrast, in those older women who had received doses of therapy equivalent to those of younger women, an equal effect was noted. The use of adjuvant hormonal therapy as with tamoxifen increases after the age of 65 years, peaking at 68% in women 70 to 79 years of age. Still, in patients who are 85 years or older, there is undertreatment with tamoxifen, placing these patients at risk for recurrence of their primary cancer.

When one considers somewhat more aggressive combination chemotherapy, such as for small-cell carcinoma of the lung, equivalent response rates have been obtained for older individuals, but this has come at the cost of increased marrow toxicity. However, 78% of patients younger than 65 years are actively treated for their lung cancer compared to only 49% of those older than 75 years. Similarly in a study of ~2000 patients with colorectal cancer, 88% of patients younger than 55 years were treated with chemotherapy compared to only 11% of those 85 years or older. Comorbidities and advanced age seem to be more common reasons for not using therapy in patients 75 years or older than was patient refusal.

Likewise, elderly patients with non-Hodgkin's lymphoma are more likely to be treated with lower chemotherapy doses and with less aggressive regimens than those given to younger patients. This is despite the evidence that responses and survival in older patients are better with more aggressive multi-agent chemotherapy regimens. The addition of rituximab, a monoclonal antibody against the CD-20 antigen, to routine chemotherapy has significantly increased the complete response rates and overall survival in patients between 60 and 80 years without a clinically significant increase in toxicity.

Also, in elderly patients, AML, attenuated chemotherapy, or palliative chemotherapy leads to worse response rates and survival when compared to patients who receive traditional remission-induction chemotherapy. However, early treatment-related toxicity especially as a result of myelosuppression is significant. A monoclonal antibody against the CD-33 antigen has now been approved for use for AML relapse in patients who are 60 years or older.

When approaching decisions about chemotherapy in treating the elderly patient, the clinician should use those modalities that in the prescribed dosages have acceptable responses with acceptable levels of toxicity. In those tumor types that require extremely aggressive therapy, the physician may need to seek modifications and new approaches in order to achieve lower levels of toxicity. Such situations may be amenable to clinical trials (but in which elderly subjects are currently underrepresented) so that the best approaches to therapy can be delineated.

Supportive Care

The effects of cancer and its treatment may be devastating to elderly patients and may require substantial supportive care. The goal of such therapy is to maximize the ability of patients to tolerate the treatment as well as the disease. Underlying problems requiring symptomatic relief need to be actively sought by the physician, because elderly patients more frequently underreport their symptoms. Many of the specific aspects of supportive care are covered in other chapters and are only mentioned here to stress their importance for the management of the elderly cancer patient. These include the extreme importance of effective pain management (see Chapter 30); maintenance of appropriate nutritional support (see Chapter 40); the supportive role of nursing and team care (see Chapter 26); the importance of patient, physician, and family discussions concerning decisions regarding terminal care and other issues (see Chapters 31–34); and the utility of hospice care (see Chapter 31).

One complication frequently seen in treatment of the elderly patient with cancer is nausea and vomiting. These side effects can seriously compromise the ability to deliver effective chemotherapy, and they create a considerable degree of morbidity. General guidelines to prevent morbidity from nausea and vomiting include (1) all elderly patients on chemotherapy should be well hydrated; (2) eliminate environmental factors, such as food and other odors, that may trigger vomiting; (3) if oral feeding is attempted, patients should use dry bland foods that are generally well tolerated; and (4) avoid high-protein diets. The importance of the prophylactic administration of antiemetics is recognized by various evidenced-based U.S. guidelines. All these guidelines recommend antiemetic prophylaxis with a 5-HT$_3$-receptor antagonist in combination with a steroid in patients receiving moderately to highly emetogenic chemotherapy or radiotherapy. In all patients receiving cisplatin, a corticosteroid plus a 5-HT$_3$-receptor antagonist is recommended for the prevention of delayed and anticipatory chemotherapy-induced nausea and vomiting. In patients receiving high-risk, noncisplatin regimens, a prophylactic corticosteroid with or without either a 5-HT$_3$-receptor antagonist or metoclopramide is suggested. Overall, the prophylactic use of the most effective antiemetic regimen appropriate to the chemotherapy employed is suggested to prevent acute, delayed, and anticipatory nausea and vomiting. Such regimens must be used with the initial chemotherapy in order to prevent the occurrence of symptoms, rather than waiting to assess the patient's emetic response with less effective treatment. These general guidelines can also be applied to elderly cancer patients.

Other side effects from chemotherapeutic agents that elderly patients are predisposed to include constipation from vincristine, and neuropathy from platinum analogues and taxanes.

Another significant problem as a result of the cancer itself or therapy for cancer is the occurrence of fatigue in elderly patients. This is one of the most common symptoms and significantly affects a patient's quality of life. In one systematic review, the prevalence of fatigue was 40% to 90% during treatment and 19% to 80% after completion of treatment. The etiology of fatigue is multifold ranging from immobility and deconditioning to anemia, depression, pain, poor nutrition, drugs, and metabolic causes. Treatment of fatigue is to usually treat the underlying causes, e.g., treat anemia with hematinics, iron, B-12, folate. Exercise programs can play a very positive role in the treatment of cancer-related fatigue. Drugs like methylphenidate and modafinil have been used to treat cancer-related fatigue, but have yet to be studied in older cancer patients.

Cytopenias resulting from the bone marrow suppressive effects of chemotherapeutic agents should be appropriately treated with transfusion of blood products or use of growth stimulating factors. The American Society of Clinical Oncology 2006 guidelines recommend preventive use of white blood cell growth factors for patients whose risk of febrile neutropenia is 20% or higher. The indications include elderly patients with diffuse aggressive lymphomas treated with curative intent and patients with AML older than 55 during induction and consolidation chemotherapy. Different types of white cell growth factors somewhat reduce the incidence of infections during aggressive chemotherapy in elderly patients, but they have had little impact on treatment outcomes and on survival. The cost–benefit ratios of these therapies must be weighed carefully.

Finally, the all important area of psychological support for elderly patients with cancer and their caregivers must be considered. This begins with effective physician–patient communication and acknowledgment of the patient's views and values at every stage of the disease. When appropriate, caregiver involvement can be critical. An assessment of the patient's coping skills and strategies will be very helpful. Acknowledgment and support of those who appear to work best for the patient are important. The patient's spiritual state and use of religious coping strategies are also important to assess and support. It is ironic that despite the increase in physical frailty and other decrements in function with age, older cancer patients appear to cope better with the psychological stress of the illness than do younger patients. This may be a result of the development of effective coping strategies from dealing with many other stressors over the years.

CONCLUSION

Cancer occurs with great frequency in elderly patients. The relationship of cancer to aging poses a challenge to our scientific understanding of these processes as well as to our clinical approach to the elderly patient. Further research is required to resolve the former, but a systematic, logically developed diagnostic and treatment plan can produce effective and gratifying results in the latter.

FURTHER READING

Albin RL. Antagonistic pleiotropy, mutation accumulation, and human genetic disease. *Genetica.* 1993;91(1–3):279–286.

Audisio RA, Bozzetti F, Gennari R, et al. The surgical management of elderly cancer patients; recommendations of the SIOG surgical task force. *Eu J Cancer.* 2004;40(7):926–938.

Balducci L, Hardy CL, Lyman GH. Hemopoietic reserve in the older cancer patient: clinical and economic considerations. *Cancer Control.* 2000;7(6):539–547.

Campisi J. Aging and cancer: the double-edged sword of replicative senescence. *J Am Geriatr Soc.* 1997;45(4):482–488.

Cohen HJ. Biology of aging as related to cancer. *Cancer.* 1994;74(7 Suppl):2092–2100.

Crivellari D, Aapro M, Leonard R, et al. Breast cancer in the elderly. *J Clin Oncol.* 2007;25(14):1882–1890.

Dale DC. Poor prognosis in elderly patients with cancer: the role of bias and undertreatment. *J Support Oncol.* 2003;1(4 Suppl 2):11–17.

Ershler WB, Keller ET. Age-associated increased interleukin-6 gene expression, late-life diseases, and frailty. *Annu Rev Med.* 2000;51:245–270.

Gridelli C, Langer C, Maione P, Rossi A, Schild SE. Lung cancer in the elderly. *J Clin Oncol.* 2007;25(14):1898–1907.

Hanahan D, Weinberg RA. The hallmarks of cancer. *Cell.* 2000;100(1):57–70.

Heflin MT, Cohen HJ. Cancer screening in the elderly. *Hosp Pract (Minneap).* 2001;36(3):61–69.

Hurria A, Gupta S, Zauderer M, et al. Developing a cancer-specific geriatric assessment: a feasibility study. *Cancer.* 2005;104(9):1998–2005.

Kaesberg PR, Ershler WB. The change in tumor aggressiveness with age: lessons from experimental animals. *Semin Oncol.* 1989;16(1):28–33.

Lewis JH, Kilgore ML, Goldman DP, et al. Participation of patients 65 years of age or older in cancer clinical trials. *J Clin Oncol.* 2003;21(7):1383–1389.

Lichtman SM, Villani G. Chemotherapy in the elderly: pharmacologic considerations. *Cancer Control.* 2000;7(6):548–556.

Rao AV, Hsieh F, Feussner JR, Cohen HJ. Geriatric evaluation and management units in the care of the frail elderly cancer patient. *J Gerontol Ser Biol Sci Med Sci.* 2005;60(6):798–803.

Smith TJ, Khatcheressian J, Lyman GH, et al. 2006 update of recommendations for the use of white blood cell growth factors: an evidence-based clinical practice guideline. *J Clin Oncol.* 2006;24(19):3187–3205.

Wright WE, Shay JW. Telomere biology in aging and cancer. *J Am Geriatr Soc.* 2005;53(9 Suppl):S292–S294.

Yancik R, Ries LA. Aging and cancer in America. Demographic and epidemiologic perspectives. *Hematol Oncol Clin North Am.* 2000;14(1):17–23.

Zachariah B, Balducci L. Radiation therapy of the older patient. *Hematol Oncol Clin North Am.* 2000;14(1):131–167.

Breast Disease

Gretchen G. Kimmick ■ *Hyman B. Muss*

The breast, or mammary gland, is a fibrofatty organ that produces all the necessary nutrients for a newborn. In women of childbearing age, the breast responds to cyclic hormone production and contains an abundance of epithelial structures and stroma that enable the production of milk. In postmenopausal women, declining ovarian function in late menopause leads to regression of these structures. The postmenopausal breast contains a ductal system, but the lobules shrink and collapse, leaving an organ that is composed primarily of fat. While a breast lump in a premenopausal woman is likely to be a benign problem related to cyclic hormonal changes, in a postmenopausal woman, this is not the case and the most important breast disease is cancer.

Cancer is the leading cause of death in women aged 55 to 74 years and is second to heart disease in women aged 75 and older. The incidence of cancer increases dramatically with age. In particular, breast cancer—the most common cancer in American women—is a major health concern. According to 2007 American Cancer Society estimates, breast cancer is the most common cancer in women, accounting for 31% of all newly diagnosed malignancies (178,480 new cases) and the second leading cause of cancer-related death (40,460 deaths). Moreover, U.S. incidence and mortality data from the 1980s suggest that 12% of all women will be diagnosed with breast cancer during their lifetime and that 3.5% will die from it.

Approximately half of the cases of breast cancer occur in women older than age 65 years. In addition, 1999 National Vital Statistics indicate that the incidence increases dramatically with age (Figure 95-1) from an invasive breast cancer rate of 15 per 1000 in women aged 40 to 50 years to a rate of 43 per 1000 in women aged 70 to 80 years. Older age has also been associated with a lower breast cancer specific survival rate (Figure 95-1).

Breast cancer is a major health concern and will become of even greater importance as the size of the older population grows. Although breast cancer is more common in older women, they are also less likely to be appropriately screened, more likely to present for care at a more advanced stage and to receive inferior surgical and postoperative management, and are less likely to be entered into clinical trials.

RISK FACTORS AND BIOLOGY

The specific cause of breast cancer is unknown. Many factors associated with increased risk have been identified. These include the following: increasing age, white race, family history of breast cancer (especially in a first-degree relative), early menarche, late age at birth of first child (older than 30 years), late menopause, history of benign breast disease (hyperplasia or atypical hyperplasia), heavy radiation exposure, obesity, increasing height, postmenopausal estrogen replacement therapy, and moderate to excessive alcohol use. Most of these factors are associated with relative risks in the range of 1.4 to 2 times the risk in the general population. There is a breast cancer risk assessment tool, based on the Gail Model, available. This tool calculates the 5-year risk of breast cancer, using risk factors of age, age at first menses, age at first live birth, presence of first-degree relatives with breast cancer, number of past breast biopsies and whether or not atypical hyperplasia was found, and race/ethnicity. There is also geographic, economic, and racial variability in breast cancer incidence, with the highest incidence being found in affluent white populations. The reason for these differences is probably related to risk factor distribution, as well as genetic and environmental factors. Although breast cancer incidence differs among racial groups, such differences are minimized or lost when racial groups that are at low risk migrate to a high-risk environment.

A family history of breast cancer, implying a genetic defect, may be important in 5% to 20% of all cases of breast cancer. Genetic predisposition is particularly important in early-onset breast cancer (diagnosed before age 50 years), but is probably not a major factor in the geriatric population. BRCA1 accounts for approximately 45% of familial breast cancers. Another gene, BRCA2, is responsible for approximately 35% of genetic abnormalities in high-risk families.

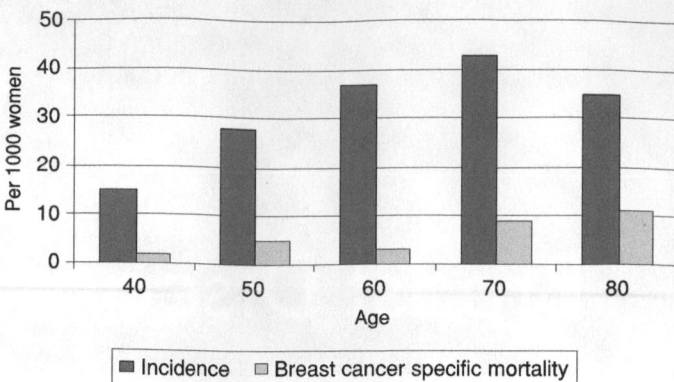

FIGURE 95-1. Breast cancer incidence and mortality by age.

Both BRCA1 and BRCA2 portend increased risks for breast cancer and ovarian cancer, ranging from 36% to 85% for breast cancer and 16% to 60% for ovarian cancer. There are many modifying factors, including genetic, hormonal, and environmental, that determine whether a genetic mutation will lead to cancer.

Most breast cancers originate from ductal epithelium. Comparisons of older and younger patients with breast cancer reveal that infiltrating ductal carcinoma is the most common histological type in both groups, accounting for 75% to 80% of cases, with lobular carcinoma accounting for approximately 5% to 10%. Mucinous carcinoma and papillary carcinoma, histological types that are associated with a somewhat lower risk of recurrence, are more common in older patients, while inflammatory carcinoma, an aggressive lesion with a poor prognosis, is extremely uncommon in such persons. Cancers in older patients are more likely to be well-differentiated and moderately differentiated, be estrogen and progesterone receptor positive (60–70% of patients), have lower rates of tumor proliferation (the number of cells synthesizing deoxyribonucleic acid [DNA]), and less frequently express the HER2 oncogene, when compared with cancers in younger patients. These data suggest that breast cancer in older patients is biologically less aggressive than it is in younger women. Mortality from breast cancer, however, is not lower in older women, leading us to explore issues associated with treatment choice and other patient- and tumor-related factors that might affect disease specific survival.

DIAGNOSIS

Primary Prevention, Screening, and Diagnosis

Primary Prevention

Except for draconian measures such as prophylactic mastectomy, which is not 100% effective, there is no known effective means of preventing breast cancer. As the pathogenesis of breast cancer is likely to be related to interactions of estrogens, other hormones, and breast tissue, current research efforts toward prevention focus on the use of agents that lower breast tissue estrogen exposure, such as selective estrogen receptor modulators (SERMs) and aromatase inhibitors.

The SERMs, tamoxifen and raloxifene, decrease incidence of hormone receptor–positive breast cancer. Data from the Early

Breast Cancer Trialists' Collaborative Group meta-analysis involving 75 000 patients with early-stage breast cancer suggest that the use of tamoxifen decreases contralateral breast cancer risk by 40% to 50% in postmenopausal women. A national trial (National Surgical Adjuvant Breast Project [NSABP] P1) comparing tamoxifen with placebo as a means of prevention in women at high risk for breast cancer (a risk of 1.66% of invasive breast cancer over 5 years) showed that tamoxifen decreased the incidence of noninvasive and invasive breast cancer by approximately 40%, with the majority of the benefit in decreasing the risk of hormone receptor–positive breast cancer and no decrease in risk of hormone receptor–negative breast cancer. Thirty percent of women in this trial were older than 60 years and 6% were older than 70 years; similar risk reductions were seen in all age groups. A second, large randomized trial proved that raloxifene was as effective as tamoxifen in decreasing the incidence of hormone receptor–positive breast cancer. The SERMs, however, are also weakly estrogenic and increase the risk of thromboembolism. Further, tamoxifen, but not raloxifene, increases the risk of endometrial cancer. In clinical practice, the benefit of SERM treatment must be weighed against risk and can be estimated from a model developed from Gail and colleagues. At present there are large trials studying the use of aromatase inhibitors, which do not increase thromboembolic risk, compared to SERMs, to decrease the risk of breast cancer in postmenopausal women; older patients should be encouraged to participate in these trials. Maintaining an ideal body mass and exercise should also be encouraged.

Screening

Breast cancer screening in a postmenopausal woman includes mammography and a physical examination. After menopause, as estrogen levels diminish, breast glandular tissue and ductal tissue decrease and fat tissue increases. In addition, postmenopausal patients have fewer cysts and fibroadenomas. These age-related biological changes in breast tissue, especially the increased percentage of fat tissue, allow for improved contrast between small foci of malignancy and the surrounding breast tissue, resulting in fewer false-negative mammographic examinations. Several studies show that the routine use of screening mammography in women aged 50 through 70 years improves survival by detecting breast carcinoma at an earlier stage and before metastatic dissemination.

It is estimated that a 25% to 30% reduction in 5-year breast cancer mortality could be achieved if all women aged 50 to 70 years received appropriate screening with mammography. Controversy persists, however, because data are sparse in women older than 70 years. An overview analysis did suggest that mammography will be of benefit in this group. The average life expectancy of a healthy older woman who is 75 years old is 10 more years, and for a healthy woman aged 85 years, it is 7 more years, making it important to decrease cancer-related morbidity. When the estimated life expectancy exceeds 5 years, it is prudent to offer yearly screening mammogram.

Ten to twenty percent of all breast cancers are not visualized on a mammogram. Physical examination by health professionals and breast self-examination, therefore, remain essential and complementary adjuncts to mammographic screening. The patient–physician interaction is also important because, as several studies show, the most important factor for the physician to inducing an older patient to have a screening mammogram is to personally recommend it to the patient. Medicare law provides for payment for screening

TABLE 95-1

Screening Guidelines for Breast Cancer in Women Older Than 70 Yrs		
	FREQUENCY	**COMMENT**
Breast self-examination	Monthly	Value uncertain, but many breast cancers are still detected by the patient
Physical examination	Yearly	By physician or other health professional; detects 15% of cancers *not* discovered on screening mammogram
Mammography	Every 1–2 yr	Value in improving survival in women older than 75 yr is unproven, but extrapolation of data from studies in postmenopausal patients suggests benefit if life expectancy is 5 yr or more

mammography on an annual basis. Table 95-1 presents our recommendations for the screening of older women.

Diagnosis

Breast cancer usually presents either as a breast mass or as a suspicious finding on a mammogram. The discovery of a breast mass in a postmenopausal woman requires prompt attention, as the majority of palpable masses in this age group are malignant. All breast masses require biopsy in this patient population. Although it is not essential to the diagnosis in a woman who presents with a mass, mammography helps to define the nature of a mass and finds other nonpalpable lesions; it is, therefore, indicated when a breast mass is found. New mammographic findings also prompt evaluation. Typically, a step-wise process of diagnosis and definitive surgery is followed, as depicted in Figure 95-2. This allows pathological confirmation of cancer and time to contemplate surgical treatment choice.

For palpable lesions, core-needle biopsy is preferable to fine-needle aspiration biopsy, because core biopsy can distinguish invasive from in situ lesions in most patients. Although concerns have been expressed that needle biopsy may be associated with tracking of malignant cells and a higher risk of local recurrence, such fears are unfounded. If the core biopsy or fine-needle aspiration is negative or inconclusive, unless the mass proves to be a cyst and resolves after aspiration, further biopsy, preferably excision, is necessary. For patients who have a mass that is characteristic of malignancy on physical examination or mammography, initial excision of the lesion or intraoperative biopsy to confirm invasive cancer and then lumpectomy or mastectomy, with or without sentinel lymph node biopsy or axillary dissection, may be preferable to a two-stage procedure involving a needle, core, or excisional biopsy.

For nonpalpable lesions that are found mammographically, ultrasound is recommended for further evaluation. If ultrasound finds a solid, suspicious lesion, ultrasound-guided biopsy can be done. If not visible by ultrasound, either stereotactic biopsy or needle-localized

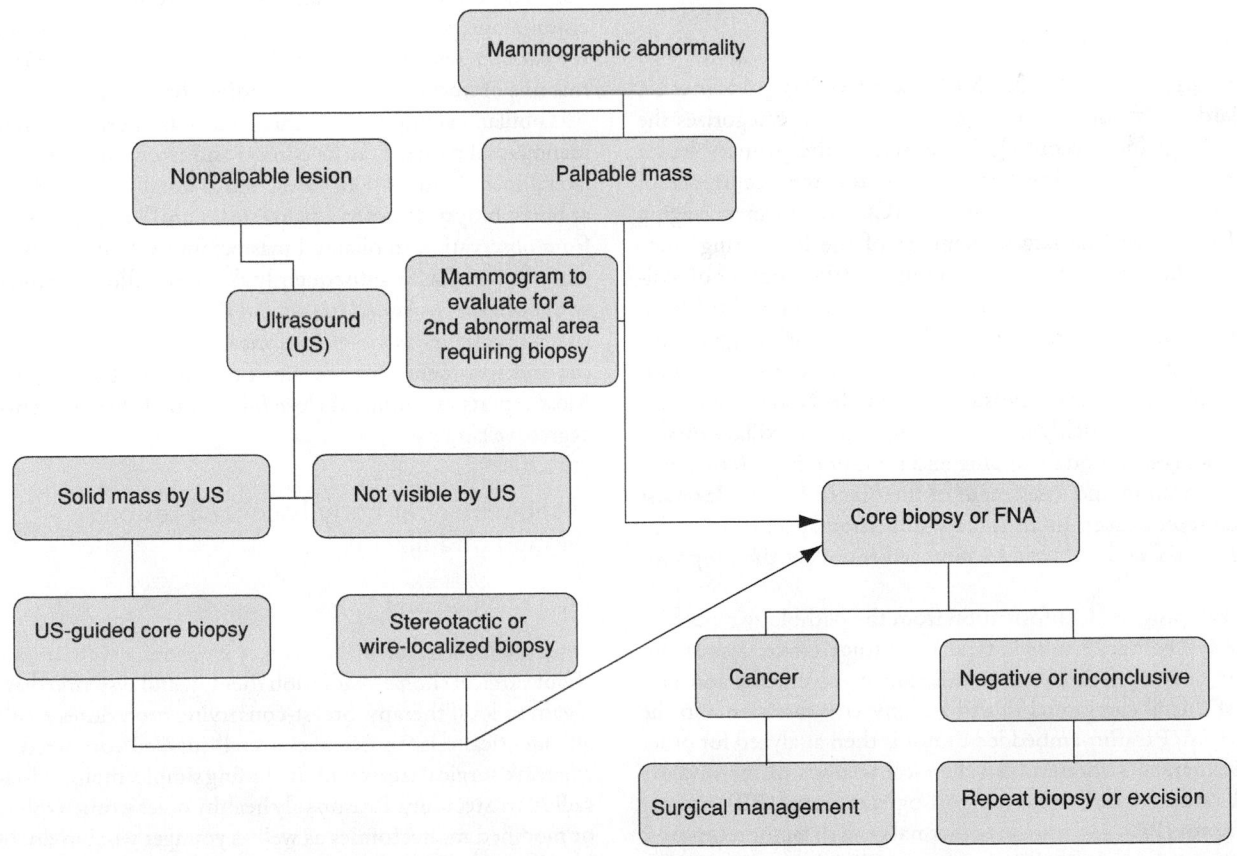

FIGURE 95-2. Approach to a suspicious breast lesion in an older woman.

biopsy will be necessary. Stereotactic biopsy uses mammographic guidance to obtain a core biopsy specimen and is preferred because it allows pathologic diagnosis without anesthesia. The prone position required for the stereotactic procedure, however, may be difficult for some older patients. Needle-localized biopsy uses mammographic guidance to place a needle within the area of suspicion, after which the area is surgically excised, a procedure that typically involves anesthesia. If atypical hyperplasia is found on core biopsy, excisional biopsy is required, because a small proportion of suspicious lesions for which core biopsy finds only atypical hyperplasia will also contain in situ or invasive cancer when excised.

When biopsy is diagnostic of malignancy or definitive surgery is scheduled, preoperative evaluation includes a complete history and physical examination, a complete blood count and chemistry profile, and a chest x-ray. MRI of the breasts may also be helpful in management of older women, but is not recommended for routine screening. These studies are generally more helpful in determining the presence of comorbid illness than they are in finding metastases. Bone, computerized tomographic, or magnetic resonance imaging scans should be done to investigate signs or symptoms suggestive of metastasis, but are not necessary in asymptomatic patients. Bilateral mammography should be performed on all these patients to evaluate both the ipsilateral breast and the contralateral breast for other nonpalpable lesions.

It is important to remember that mammography is normal in 20% of patients with cancer. A palpable lesion in a postmenopausal woman always requires biopsy; mammography is of value mainly for detecting nonpalpable lesions in either the involved or the contralateral breast.

Staging

The American Joint Committee for Cancer (AJCC) guidelines set the standard for breast cancer staging. This system categorizes the extent of malignancy according to the size of the primary lesion (T), the extent of nodal involvement (N), and the occurrence of metastasis (M). Table 95-2 presents the AJCC breast cancer staging criteria. Tumor size (the largest diameter of the infiltrating component) and the extent of nodal involvement (the number of axillary nodes removed and the number positive) are determined from pathologic examination and are included in the pathology report. Less than 5% of the time, breast cancer presents as a diffuse infiltrating lesion and cannot be measured accurately. Nodal assessment is done either by sentinel lymph node biopsy or by axillary dissection. Sentinel lymph node mapping and sampling is preferred as it allows identification and assessment of the one to four nodes most likely to contain cancer. In an axillary dissection specimen, a sample of at least six nodes should be removed to reflect the prognosis accurately.

Other key prognostic information from the pathology report includes the following: histologic type and tumor grade, assessment of vascular or lymphatic invasion and skin involvement, and percentages of ductal carcinoma in situ and invasive carcinoma in the primary lesion. Paraffin-embedded tumor is then analyzed for other prognostic markers. Immunohistochemical analysis of the invasive cancer cells is also done to determine estrogen receptor (ER), progesterone receptor (PR), and human epidermal growth factor receptor-2 (HER2) status. An intermediate result for HER2 by immunohistochemistry necessitates analysis by fluorescent in situ hybridization

("FISH"). Other markers, such as epidermal growth factor receptor and proliferative indices, are not of consistent benefit and are not needed on a routine basis.

After definitive surgical management, asymptomatic patients who have had an unremarkable preoperative evaluation, including history and physical examination, mammography, chest x-ray, complete blood count, and serum chemistries (with liver function tests and calcium), require no further staging procedures. The use of tumor markers, such as the carcinoembryonic antigen and mucin antigens (CA27.29 and CA15.3), in patient management is controversial and is not recommended on a routine basis.

TREATMENT OF BREAST CANCER

Carcinoma In Situ

The more widespread use of screening mammography has led to a major increase in the diagnosis of ductal carcinoma in situ (DCIS). Before the common use of screening mammograms, DCIS was uncommon, usually detected on physical examination, was large in size and the cure rate exceeded 95% with mastectomy. In a screened population, most DCIS lesions are nonpalpable and small and are suggested by microcalcifications found on screening mammography. Mastectomy cures almost all patients, but breast conserving procedures followed by breast irradiation are as effective for patients with smaller lesions.

Axillary dissection or sentinel node biopsy finds metastases in less than 1% of patients and is generally not recommended. Excision alone, without local radiation therapy, may be appropriate for patients with lesions less than 2.5 cm with generous (>1 cm) margins of normal tissue surrounding the in situ component.

Lobular carcinoma in situ (LCIS) is more common in premenopausal patients, lacks clinical and mammographic signs, is bilateral in 25% to 35% of cases, and is usually an incidental finding at breast biopsy. It is not a palpable lesion. Treatment options range from observation to bilateral mastectomy. Of note, 20% to 40% of patients with LCIS subsequently develop infiltrating ductal cancer, with both the ipsilateral breast and the contralateral breast at similar risk. LCIS serves as a high-risk marker for subsequent invasive cancer, and treatment selection must rest on the desires of the patient. Most experts recommend close follow-up of these patients, without aggressive surgery.

Management of Early Localized Lesions (Stage I and II)

Local Management

Once a diagnosis of breast cancer is made, a woman is counseled about surgical choices, radiation therapy, and systemic therapy. With regard to local therapy, breast-conserving procedures result in virtually identical relapse-free and overall survival compared with more extensive surgical treatment, including simple, modified-radical, and radical mastectomy. Reasonably healthy older women tolerate simple or modified mastectomies as well as younger women do, but should be offered the option of breast-conserving surgical procedures when clinically appropriate.

TABLE 95-2

AJCC Staging Criteria for Breast Cancer (Sixth Edition, 2002)

SYMBOL TNM SYSTEM	MEANING
Primary tumor (T)	
TX	Primary tumor cannot be assessed
T0	No evidence of primary tumor
Tis	Carcinoma in situ; intraductal carcinoma, lobular carcinoma in situ, or Paget disease of the nipple with no tumor
T1	Tumor $\leq$ 2 cm in greatest dimension
	T1a $\leq$ 0.5 cm in greatest dimension
	T1b > 0.5 cm but not > 1 cm in greatest dimension
	T1c > 1 cm but not > 2 cm in greatest dimension
T2	Tumor > 2 cm but not > 5 cm in greatest dimension
T3	Tumor > 5 cm in greatest dimension
T4	Tumor of any size with direct extension to chest wall or skin (includes inflammatory carcinoma)
Regional lymph nodes (N)	
NX	Regional lymph nodes cannot be assessed (e.g., previously removed)
N0	No regional lymph-node metastasis; no additional examination for isolated tumor cells (ITCs, defined as single tumor cells or small clusters not greater than 0.2 mm, usually detected only by immunohistochemical or molecular methods but which may be verified on hematoxylin and eosin [H & E] stains). ITCs do not usually show evidence of malignant activity (e.g., proliferation or stromal reaction) • pN0 (i –): No histologic nodal metastasis, and negative by immunohistochemistry (IHC) • pN0 (i +): No histologic nodal metastasis but positive by IHC, with no cluster greater than 0.2 mm in diameter • pN0 (mol –): No histologic nodal metastasis and negative molecular findings (by reverse transcriptase polymerase chain reaction, RT-PCR) • pN0 (mol +): No histologic nodal metastasis but positive molecular findings (by RT-PCR)
N1	Metastasis in 1–3 ipsilateral axillary lymph node(s) and/or in internal mammary nodes with microscopic disease detected by SLND but not clinically apparent • pN1mi: Micrometastasis (greater than 0.2 mm, none greater than 2.0 mm) • pN1a: Metastasis in 1–3 axillary lymph nodes • pN1b: Metastasis to internal mammary lymph nodes with microscopic disease detected by SLND but not clinically apparent • pN1c: Metastasis in 1–3 ipsilateral axillary lymph node(s) and in internal mammary nodes with microscopic disease detected by SLND but not clinically apparent. If associated with more than 3 positive axillary nodes, the internal mammary nodes are classified as N3b to reflect increased tumor burden.
N2	Metastasis in 4–9 axillary lymph nodes or in clinically apparent internal mammary lymph nodes in the absence of axillary lymph nodes • pN2a: Metastasis in 4–9 axillary lymph nodes (at least one tumor deposit >2 mm) • pN2b: Metastasis in clinically apparent internal mammary lymph nodes in the absence of axillary lymph nodes
N3	Metastasis in 10 or more axillary lymph nodes, or in infraclavicular lymph nodes, or in clinically apparent ipsilateral internal mammary lymph nodes in the presence of one or more positive axillary nodes; or in more than three axillary lymph nodes with clinically negative microscopic metastasis in internal mammary lymph nodes; or in ipsilateral supraclavicular lymph node(s) • pN3a: Metastasis in 10 or more axillary lymph nodes (at least one tumor deposit greater than 2.0 mm), or metastasis to the infraclavicular lymph nodes • pN3b: Metastasis in clinically apparent ipsilateral internal mammary lymph nodes in the presence of one or more positive axillary nodes; or in more than three axillary lymph nodes with microscopic metastasis in internal mammary lymph nodes detected by SLND but not clinically apparent • pN3c: Metastasis in ipsilateral supraclavicular lymph node(s)
Distant metastasis (M)	
MX	Presence of distant metastasis cannot be assessed
M0	No evidence of distant metastasis
M1	Distant metastasis (including metastasis to ipsilateral supraclavicular lymph nodes)
Clinical stage	
0	Tis, N0, M0
1	T1, N0, M0
IIA	T0, N1, M0
	T1, N1, M0
	T2, N0, M0
IIB	T2, N1, M0
	T3, N0, M0
IIIA	T0 or T1, N2, M0
	T2, N2, M0
	T3, N1 or N2, M0
IIIB	T4, any N, M0
	Any T, N3, M0
IV	Any T, any N, M1

Adapted from Singletary SE, Allred C, et al. Revision of the American Joint Committee on Cancer staging system for breast cancer. J Clin Oncol. 2002;20(17):3628–3636.

Management of the Breast. The breast-conserving approach to breast cancer management involves removing the tumor mass with a clear margin of several millimeters of surrounding normal breast tissue (lumpectomy, tylectomy, quadrantectomy, etc.), assessing axillary lymph nodes, and delivering local breast irradiation after surgery. Ipsilateral axillary node assessment is recommended by most medical, surgical, and radiation oncologists to provide important prognostic data. Breast-conserving procedures require close cooperation among the radiologist, surgeon, pathologist, and radiation oncologist in order to locate and remove the area of concern, assure negative margins, and provide the best cosmetic result with lowest risk of local recurrence. Breast irradiation after removal of tumor mass reduces the likelihood of recurrence in the affected breast from 40% to less than 10% and may improve survival. Most breast relapses occur in or in close proximity to the previously resected lesion. Other techniques, such as brachytherapy (localized radiation therapy [RT] may prove to be as effective as whole-breast RT and can be completed over a period of several days. Two trials have shown that lumpectomy and tamoxifen confers the same short-term survival benefit as lumpectomy, tamoxifen, and breast RT, but that breast RT is better than tamoxifen in preventing in-breast recurrence. For healthy older patients at high risk for in-breast recurrence and reasonable life expectancy, breast radiation is recommended.

Contraindications to breast-conserving surgery include two or more gross tumors in separate quadrants of the breast, diffuse indeterminate or malignant-appearing microcalcifications, and a history of therapeutic irradiation of the breast region. Relative contraindications to breast-conserving surgery include the following: large tumor/breast size ratio (mass more than 5 cm in size), which interferes with cosmesis; large breast size, which makes radiation delivery difficult and interferes with cosmesis; and a history of collagen vascular disease, which has been reported anecdotally to increase the likelihood of fibrosis associated with radiation. It is important, however, not to underestimate the value to a patient of preserving her own breast, with sensation intact, even if the cosmetic appearance is not perfect. It is now well established that preoperative ("neoadjuvant") chemotherapy or endocrine therapy (for women with ER- or PR-positive breast cancer) can shrink large breast cancers, allowing breast conservation for many patients without sacrificing distant recurrence or survival outcomes and without the need for preoperative chemotherapy.

Breast-conservation is more costly than mastectomy because of the time, inconvenience, and monetary expense of postoperative RT. Nevertheless, such treatment is preferred by many women, irrespective of age. The option for breast-conserving surgery provides motivation for detecting early-stage lesions through screening. Patients who have had breast-conserving procedures also have higher self-appraisals of body image and sexuality than do women who have had more extensive surgical intervention.

Breast Reconstruction. For older women who have had a mastectomy, breast reconstruction represents another option for restoring body image. Many physicians, because of personal bias, are unlikely to discuss reconstruction with older patients. This procedure can be done safely in an older patient and should be discussed, with subsequent surgical consultation if desired.

Radiation After Mastectomy. The likelihood of local recurrence is directly proportional to both the size of the primary lesion and the number of involved axillary nodes. Postoperative adjuvant irradiation, therefore, is recommended for patients with large primary lesions (greater than 5 cm) or with four or more positive nodes. It is also considered reasonable for any woman with breast cancer that involves lymph nodes to receive postmastectomy "adjuvant" irradiation therapy to the chest wall and the contiguous regional lymph nodes (internal mammary, supraclavicular, and upper axilla), because it reduces the likelihood of local recurrence (recurrence in the mastectomy site or contiguous nodal areas) by 70% and improves overall breast cancer–specific survival rates by several percent. Delaying postoperative irradiation for 4 to 6 months to allow the completion of adjuvant chemotherapy is feasible and does not increase the risk of subsequent local recurrence.

Axillary Assessment. Tumor size and axillary nodal status are the most consistent predictors of the risk of recurrence and, therefore, key in making decisions about the risk/benefit ratio of adjuvant systemic treatment. Node involvement is found in 5% to 37% of women with very small tumors (less than 1 cm), and physical examination is only of modest benefit in predicting nodal involvement, with false-negative and false-positive rates of 35% and 25%, respectively. Because arm problems, such as swelling (lymphedema), pain, numbness, weakness, and impaired shoulder mobility, may complicate axillary dissection, the argument has been made that its prognostic benefit is not worth the risk of side effects in women with primary tumors less than 1 cm in size. Sentinel lymph node mapping and sampling, with its lower risk of arm morbidity, is the procedure of choice, if axillary assessment is deemed necessary.

In older women, the role of assessing axillary nodes is quite controversial because of the risk of arm morbidity. If adjuvant chemotherapy is not a consideration because of physician or patient choice, the risk of axillary dissection is not worth its prognostic yield, regardless of the primary tumor size. It is generally acceptable to omit axillary assessment in older women with small (2 cm or less), clinically node-negative, ER-positive breast cancer, who will take adjuvant hormonal therapy for at least 5 years.

Lymphatic mapping with sentinel node biopsy is associated with less arm morbidity and is the standard method to assess axillary lymph nodes in women who have breast cancer and in whom there are no clinically evident ipsilateral axillary nodes. This procedure allows identification and sampling of the first nodes in the lymphatic basin to receive lymphatic flow, that is, presumptive removal of the initial site of metastatic nodal involvement. When the sentinel lymph node(s) is positive, the likelihood of finding further positive nodes after a more complete axillary dissection is approximately 50% and, therefore, a standard level I and II node dissection is indicated. Standard axillary dissection should be performed in any woman with breast cancer who has clinically palpable axillary lymph nodes.

Adjuvant Systemic Therapy

Adjuvant systemic therapy involves preoperative, perioperative, or postoperative administration of endocrine therapy and/or chemotherapy to patients with localized breast cancer for the purpose of reducing risk of and delaying relapse and improving survival. Such treatment is aimed at eradicating occult, clinically undetectable metastasis.

Figure 95-3 shows 8-year breast cancer survival by age and stage and Table 95-3 describes 10- and 15-year overall survival according

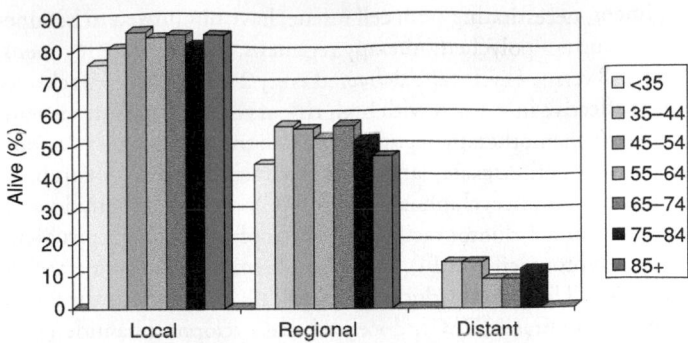

FIGURE 95-3. Eight-year breast cancer survival by age and stage.

to current breast cancer staging criteria. Adjuvant therapy is chosen on the basis of the risk:benefit ratio. The anticipated risk reduction for metastatic disease is weighed against the risk of toxicity from adjuvant therapy. Estimated improvements in relapse-free and overall survival for adjuvant systemic therapy are provided by the Early Breast Cancer Trialists' Collaborative Group (EBCTCG) (Table 95-4). This group provides collaborative meta-analyses of 194 randomized trials studying adjuvant chemotherapy and hormonal therapy every 5 years and was last updated in 2005, with the ability to show 15-year effects. These data clearly confirm the benefits of adjuvant endocrine therapy and chemotherapy in significantly reducing the risk of recurrence and death in women with early breast cancer. Table 95-5 summarizes the overview of results of adjuvant therapy for postmenopausal patients by age. Table 95-5 depicts the benefits of adjuvant therapies by age group.

In postmenopausal women, the majority of trials using adjuvant endocrine therapy compared tamoxifen with either no treatment or with chemotherapy and tamoxifen. In women older than 70 years, there was a significant decrease in the annual recurrence rate (51%) and deaths (37%) among those treated with approximately 5 years of tamoxifen versus not. Patients with positive ER or PR derived greatest benefit from tamoxifen. In addition, tamoxifen significantly decreased the annual odds of developing contralateral breast cancer by approximately 40%. Several studies have confirmed that tamoxifen decreases cardiovascular morbidity, lowers cholesterol and low-density lipoprotein levels, and increases or preserves vertebral bone density in postmenopausal women, but there is a small increased risk of thrombotic events and of endometrial cancer. Based on this information, adjuvant hormonal therapy for 5 years is recommended

TABLE 95-3

Ten- and Fifteen-Year Overall Survival (OS) in Current TNM Staging System

	10-YR OS (%)	15-YR OS (%)
II	76	62
IIa	81	72
IIb	70	52
III	50	40
IIIa	59	49
IIIb	36	18
IIIc	36	28

TABLE 95-4

Risk Reduction for Adjuvant Systemic Therapy in Women Aged 50–69 Yrs

	ANNUAL EVENT RATIO* % (SE)	
	Recurrence	**Breast Cancer Specific Death**
Chemotherapy type (vs. nil)		
CMF-based	0.81 (0.03)	0.90 (0.03)
Anthracycline-based	0.79 (0.04)	0.83 (0.05)
Other polychemotherapy	0.89 (0.06)	0.93 (0.07)
Presence or absence of tamoxifen		
Chemo + tam vs. tam alone	0.84 (0.03)	0.90 (0.03)
Chemo then tam vs. tam alone	0.77 (0.08)	0.80 (0.10)
Chemo alone vs. nil	0.78 (0.04)	0.87 (0.04)
ER status and tamoxifen		
Polychemotherapy alone vs. nil	0.67 (0.07)	
ER-poor	0.84 (0.07)	
ER-positive	0.81 (0.06)	0.74 (0.08)
Unknown		0.95 (0.08)
Polychemotherapy + tamoxifen vs.	0.75 (0.06)	0.88 (0.06)
tamoxifen only	0.85 (0.04)	
ER-poor	0.86 (0.07)	0.86 (0.07)
ER-positive		0.89 (0.04)
Unknown		0.88 (0.08)
Nodal status		
Node-negative	0.77 (0.05)	0.77 (0.06)
Node-positive	0.83 (0.03)	0.90 (0.03)
Period of follow-up		
Yrs 0–1	0.64 (0.03)	0.82 (0.06)
Yrs 2–4	0.92 (0.04)	0.87 (0.04)
Yrs 5–9	0.99 (0.05)	0.91 (0.05)
Yrs ≥ 10	0.84 (0.10)	0.90 (0.08)

CMF = cyclophosphamide, methotrexate, and fluorouracil.
*Annual Event Ratio for treatment versus control.

for most women with estrogen and/or progesterone-receptor node-negative and node-positive early breast cancer.

Newer data, not included in the EBCTCG meta-analysis, show that the aromatase inhibitors (anastrozole, letrozole, and exemestane), compounds that inhibit the enzyme involved in estrogen production, are more effective and less toxic alternatives to tamoxifen as adjuvant treatment for hormone receptor–positive breast cancers in postmenopausal women. Use of the aromatase inhibitors (AIs) is not associated with increased blood clot risk or endometrial cancer and, overall, studies show that AIs have fewer side effects than tamoxifen. Based on results from clinical trials, AIs are acceptable and, in most cases, preferable agents to tamoxifen in the adjuvant setting, unless there is another reason to prefer tamoxifen, such as the presence of osteoporosis. Side effects of AIs include menopausal symptoms, musculoskeletal aches and pains, and accelerated osteoporosis. In women who have osteopenia or osteoporosis, bone density is monitored carefully during treatment with AIs. There are three options for use of AIs in the adjuvant setting: (1) 2 to 3 years of tamoxifen followed by 2 to 3 years of an AI to complete a 5-year course of adjuvant hormonal therapy, (2) 5 years of an AI, or (3) 5 years of tamoxifen followed by an AI for 2–5 years. The optimal duration of

TABLE 95-5

Risk Reduction in Recurrence and Mortality for Adjuvant Systemic Therapy by Age Group (Years)

	ANNUAL EVENT RATIO* % (SE)	
	Recurrence	Breast Cancer Specific Death
Single-agent		
Age <40	0.72 (0.15)	0.86 (0.16)
Age 40–49	0.82 (0.09)	0.91 (0.09)
Age 50–59	0.87 (0.08)	0.94 (0.08)
Age 60–69	0.94 (0.09)	1.06 (0.10)
Age ≥ 70	0.75 (0.20)	NS
Polychemotherapy		
Age <40	0.60 (0.06)	0.71 (0.07)
Age 40–49	0.64 (0.04)	0.70 (0.05)
Age 50–59	0.77 (0.03)	0.85 (0.04)
Age 60–69	0.87 (0.03)	0.91 (0.04)
Age ≥ 70	0.88 (0.11)	0.87 (0.12)
Anthracycline-based regimen vs. CMF		
Age <50	0.90 (0.04)	0.90 (0.03)
Age 50–69	0.87 (0.05)	0.83 (0.05)
Age ≥ 70	NS	NS
Approximately 5 yr of tamoxifen vs. not in ER-positive (or unknown)		
Age <40	0.56 (0.10)	0.61 (0.12)
Age 40–49	0.71 (0.07)	0.76 (0.09)
Age 50–59	0.66 (0.05)	0.76 (0.07)
Age 60–69	0.55 (0.05)	0.65 (0.06)
Age ≥ 70	0.49 (0.12)	0.63 (0.15)

CMF = cyclophosphamide, methotrexate, and fluorouracil; NS = not specified and not significant.

*Annual Event Ratio for treatment versus control.

adjuvant hormonal therapy with AIs is not yet defined and may be longer than 5 years.

The overview found a significant decrease in the annual odds of recurrence and death for both node-negative and node-positive tumors in women aged 50 to 70 years who were treated with combination chemotherapy (polychemotherapy); unfortunately, not enough data were available to see a statistically significant benefit of chemotherapy in patients older than 70 years. In postmenopausal women in general, however, the combination of tamoxifen and chemotherapy was superior to tamoxifen alone in prolonging relapse-free and overall survival. Chemotherapy programs using anthracycline-containing combinations were superior to nonanthracycline regimens in improving both relapse-free and overall survival. Current controversies revolve around the optimal duration and intensity of adjuvant chemotherapy and the choice of adjuvant therapy based on the breast cancer cell type.

With regard to the optimal duration of adjuvant chemotherapy, short treatment courses of 3 to 6 months appear to be as effective as treatment of longer duration. With regard to the optimal dose intensity of adjuvant chemotherapy (the dose administered during a specific time period), more intense regimens are more effective, even in older patients. Adjuvant chemotherapy regimens that have shown a survival benefit for women aged 50 to 70 years are also well tolerated in healthy women older than 70 years. Although high-dose

regimens, necessitating stem cell rescue, have not proven to be superior to current polychemotherapy regimens, more intense regimens, such as 8 versus 4 cycles and delivered every 2 versus every 3 weeks, are more effective in women with high risk of recurrence. Current standard polychemotherapy regimens include the following: cyclophosphamide, methotrexate, and 5-fluorouracil (CMF); doxorubicin (Adriamycin) and cyclophosphamide (AC); cyclophosphamide, doxorubicin, and 5-fluorouracil (CAF); cyclophosphamide, epirubicin, and 5-fluorouracil (CEF); cyclophosphamide, epirubicin, and 5-fluorouracil followed by docetaxel (CEF-T); docetaxel, doxorubicin, and 5-fluorouracil (TAC); docetaxel and cyclophosphamide (TC); and AC plus a taxane (paclitaxel and docetaxel) (AC-T). Unlike tamoxifen, however, chemotherapy had little effect on the risk of developing contralateral breast cancer in the overview analysis.

With regard to tumor type, molecular strategies have defined three categories of breast cancer—hormone receptor positive, HER2 positive, and hormone receptor/HER2 negative (triple negative)—and future research may further classify subtypes and define sensitivity to adjuvant treatments. Benefit of adjuvant therapy for women who have hormone receptor–positive breast cancer is derived primarily from hormonal agents, and the additional benefit of chemotherapy is questionable. Techniques to define risk—based on the molecular profile of these tumors, especially those that are node-negative—are increasingly used in practice to help decide which patients are at high enough risk to justify the addition of chemotherapy to hormonal adjuvant therapy. The addition of trastuzumab (Herceptin™), a humanized monoclonal antibody targeted against the HER2 gene product, to adjuvant chemotherapy for HER2-positive tumors further decreases the risk of recurrence by 50% and the risk of death by 30%, according to randomized trials with 3 years of follow-up. Cardiac monitoring, with echocardiogram or MUGA scan to evaluate cardiac ejection fraction at least every 3 months, is recommended during treatment, as trastuzumab may cause reversible decline in cardiac function. Up to one-fifth of the women will not complete the entire year of therapy owing to asymptomatic decline in ejection fraction (15%), development of congestive heart failure or other cardiac event (5%). For patients with hormone receptor– and HER2-negative tumors, more intense chemotherapy regimens are generally utilized.

As a result of the paucity of data, the role of adjuvant chemotherapy in the management of older patients remains unclear to most oncologists. More carefully designed trials of chemotherapy for older women are needed and should include drug combinations that provide dose intensity similar to that of other currently effective therapies. One such trial, comparing standard chemotherapy with an oral chemotherapeutic agent (capecitabine) (Cancer and Leukemia Group B trial 49907; www.calgb.org), completed accrual and showed a significant benefit for standard chemotherapy in improving both relapse-free and overall survival.

Follow-up for Women with Early Breast Cancer

There is good evidence that close follow-up after diagnosis or adjuvant therapy does not result in improved overall survival, but that detection of early skin or lymph node (soft tissue) recurrence may result in more effective palliation. Mammography is an exception and should be performed yearly to detect new primary lesions. Because a history of breast cancer is a risk factor for another breast cancer, follow-up visits do provide an opportunity for patients to

TABLE 95-6

Follow-up of Early Breast Cancer After Diagnosis and Initial Treatment

	FREQUENCY OF EXAMINATION		
	1–3 YR	3–5 YR	5+ YR
History and physical examination	Every 3–6 mo	Every 6–12 mo	Yearly
Breast self-examination	Monthly	Monthly	Monthly
Mammogram*	Yearly	Yearly	Yearly
Gynecologic examination†	Yearly	Yearly	Yearly
Other‡	PRN	PRN	PRN

*In patients treated with lumpectomy and breast irradiation, more frequent mammograms of the radiation-treated breast (every 6 months) may be recommended for the first 3 yrs. Breast MRI are not recommended as part of routine screening.

†Yearly gynecologic examinations are recommended; they are required for women on tamoxifen who have an intact uterus.

‡Tumor marker studies, complete blood count, and automated chemistry studies, chest and skeletal x-rays, ultrasound, and radionuclide, computer tomographic, and positron emission tomographic scans are not necessary in asymptomatic patients. Appropriate studies should be obtained for patients with signs or symptoms of recurrence.

Data from Recommended Breast Cancer Surveillance Guidelines. American Society of Clinical Oncology, 2006.

express concerns and for physicians to give them reassurance. Extensive laboratory and radiologic procedures are now available for the detection of metastatic disease, but trials have indicated that a brief, focused history and a limited physical examination (skin, chest, breast, and abdominal examination) detect more than 75% of metastases. Because of the growing concern over health care costs, many organizations are formulating guidelines for follow-up.

Table 95-6 presents guidelines developed by the American Society of Clinical Oncology. In addition to mammograms and follow-up visits with the oncologist and gynecologist, patients should be educated about the symptoms of breast cancer recurrence so that those symptoms are reported and evaluated promptly.

Treatment of Metastatic Disease

Patients with metastatic breast cancer are currently incurable and have a median survival of approximately 2 to 7 years after the discovery of recurrence, depending on what series is considered. Nevertheless, patients may derive considerable palliative benefit from judiciously chosen therapy. Bone, soft-tissue (skin and lymph nodes), pleural, and pulmonary metastases are the most common sites of breast cancer recurrence. Women with localized symptomatic lesions in brain, skin, lymph nodes, and bone should be considered for palliative radiation therapy, which relieves symptoms in the majority of patients.

Patients with disseminated metastases should be considered for palliative systemic treatment. Table 95-7 describes endocrine and cytotoxic agents used in the treatment of breast cancer and their common and major side effects. Endocrine therapy usually is associated with minimal toxicity, while the toxicity associated with chemotherapy is frequently substantial and, in a small percent of patients, may be life threatening. Provided that metastases are not rapidly progressive or life threatening, all women with metastatic breast cancer should have a trial of endocrine therapy, irrespective of the ER and PR status of the tumor. Even in receptor-negative patients, endocrine therapy results in complete and partial response (greater than 50% shrinkage of the tumor mass) in 10% to 20% of those treated. Chemotherapy should be considered when metastases become refractory to endocrine treatment; such a strategy has been shown to be safe and most likely maintains the highest quality of life for the longest time period.

The choice of initial hormone agent for therapy of metastatic breast cancer is dependent on which agent was used in the adjuvant setting and if the patient is still taking that agent. If relapse occurs soon after starting adjuvant hormonal therapy, it is reasonable to try on more, noncross-resistant hormonal agent. If the tumor progresses soon after changing to the second hormonal agent, it is generally deemed hormone refractory and chemotherapy is used. If relapse occurs 6 months or more after starting adjuvant hormonal therapy, another hormonal agent is generally tried. Historically, the most experience is with tamoxifen and response rates of approximately 30% are seen in unselected patients. As first-line treatment for metastatic disease, AIs (agents that block the synthesis of estrogens in postmenopausal women) are as effective as or more effective than tamoxifen. Responses to endocrine treatment generally last an average of 1 year, but in a small percentage of patients, response may last many years. Patients with receptor-positive tumors, time intervals greater than 2 years from initial diagnosis to recurrence, soft-tissue or bone metastases, or a prior response to endocrine therapy are the most likely to respond. For patients who have responded to one agent or who have prolonged periods where the tumor does not grow (stable disease), other hormonal agents should be used in succession, until it is clear that the metastases are refractory to endocrine therapy. Patients who respond to one endocrine agent are likely to respond to another at the time of progression; the use of successive endocrine agents in patients with minimally symptomatic metastases is an excellent treatment strategy. In addition to tamoxifen and AIs, pure anti-estrogens, progestins and estrogens may be effective; moreover, patients who have previously responded or had prolonged stable disease and then had tumor progression may respond to the same agent after being treated with other therapy.

Once breast cancer is deemed refractory to hormonal therapy, chemotherapy is the treatment of choice. Older patients with metastatic disease, whose general health is otherwise satisfactory, display response and toxicity profiles to chemotherapy similar to those of their younger counterparts. Most cytotoxic drugs are metabolized in the liver with only a select few dependent on renal excretion (methotrexate, carboplatin, and cisplatin); major liver dysfunction probably is required to alter drug metabolism significantly. Chemotherapy-related myelosuppression is more common in older patients as a result of diminished bone marrow reserve with aging; nausea and vomiting are seen less frequently than they are in younger

TABLE 95-7

Endocrine and Cytotoxic Agents Used in the Treatment of Breast Cancer

CLASS	COMMON AND MAJOR TOXICITIES
Endocrine therapy	
Selective estrogen receptor modulators (SERMs)	Hot flashes, nausea, thrombosis, endometrial hyperplasia/ carcinoma
Tamoxifen	
Toremifene	
Aromatase inhibitors	
Anastrozole	Nausea
Letrozole	
Exemestane	
Pure Anti-estrogen	
Fulvestrant	Hot flashes, malaise
Progestin	
Megace	
Estrogen	
Stilbestrol	Weight gain
Androgen	Nausea and vomiting (N+V), edema, fluid retention
Fluoxymestrone	N+V, fluid retention, masculinization
Cytotoxic agents	
Alkylating agents	
Melphalan (L-PAM)	Myelosuppression (M)
Chlorambucil	M
Cyclophosphamide	M, N+V, cystitis
Carboplatin	M, N+V (mild)
Antitumor antibiotics	
Doxorubicin, epirubicin, liposomal doxorubicin	M, N+V, mucositis (MS), alopecia, cardiomyopathy, vesication
Mitoxantrone	M, N+V, mild alopecia, cardiomyopathy
Mitomycin	M, N+V, MS, alopecia, vesication
Antimetabolites	
Methotrexate	M (uncommon), nephrotoxicity, MS
Fluorouracil	M (uncommon), N+V (uncommon), rash (rare)
Capecitabine	Diarrhea, "hand–foot" syndrome
Gemcitabine	M, N+V (mild)
Taxanes	
Paclitaxel	M, hypersensitivity reactions (HR), neuropathy, MS, arthralgia/myalgia, alopecia, MS (rare)
Docetaxel	M, HR (rare), neuropathy, fluid retention, rash, alopecia
Nanoparticle albumin-bound paclitaxel	M, neuropathy, arthralgia/myalgia, alopecia
Ixabepilone	
Vincas	Peripheral neuropathy, alopecia, M (rare), vesication
Vincristine	M, neuropathy (uncommon), vesication
Vinblastine	M, neuropathy, vesication
Vinorelbine	
Immunotherapy	
ErbB-2 (Her2/neu) tyrosine kinase inhibitor	Cardiomyopathy, infusion reactions (rarely fatal)
Trastuzumab	
Epidermal growth factor receptor	
(EGFR) and ErbB-2 (Her2/neu) dual tyrosine kinase inhibitor	Diarrhea, rash, decrease in left ventricular function
Lapatinib	
Anti-angiogenesis (anti-VEGF antibody)	Slow or incomplete wound healing, thrombosis, hypertension, reversible posterior
Bevacizumab	leukoencephalopathy syndrome, nephrotic syndrome, M, N+V, congestive heart failure

patients. Of importance, psychosocial adjustments to chemotherapy appear to be better for older than for younger patients. Complete and partial responses to most single chemotherapy agents range from 20% to 30%, while responses to combination chemotherapy average 50% to 70%. The use of sequential single agents to maximize quality of life, yet maintain tumor control, is as effective as treatment with several agents in combination, and is a less toxic strategy. Responses generally last an average of 6 to 12 months; response rates to subsequent "salvage" regimens are generally low and last only several months.

Biologically engineered monoclonal antibodies with antitumor activity are showing efficacy in treatment of cancer. For breast cancer, the following have been shown to be beneficial for use in combination with chemotherapy agents: trastuzumab (Herceptin™), the

TABLE 95-8

Essential Information for the Management of Breast Cancer

Patient characteristics
Significant comorbidities
Complete blood count
Chemistry profile, including liver and renal function
Chest x-ray
Bilateral mammography

Type of initial treatment
Mastectomy or lumpectomy
Radiation therapy – type
Axillary lymph node dissection or sentinel lymph node biopsy

Pathology
Histologic type
Tumor grade
Presence of vascular or lymphatic involvement
Percent of invasive and intraductal cancer
Tumor size (maximum diameter of invasive component)
Number of axillary nodes removed
Number of axillary nodes involved
Estrogen and progesterone receptors
Human epidermal growth factor receptor-2 (HER2)

Social environment
Physical and mental function
Access to clinic (transportation)
Family and social support
Financial resources (coinsurance)

humanized-monoclonal antibody that inhibits erbB-2 (Her2/neu) tyrosine kinase; lapatinib (Tykerb™), an epidermal growth factor receptor (EGFR) and ErbB-2 (Her2/neu) dual tyrosine kinase inhibitor; and bevacizumab (Avastin™), an anti-angiogenesis, anti-VEGF antibody. Trastuzumab is approved for use in women with metastatic breast cancer whose tumors over-express the HER2 gene. It is well tolerated and associated with tumor response rates of approximately 25% when used as a single agent. Concomitant use of trastuzumab and chemotherapy improves in response rates when compared to chemotherapy alone. Lapatinib is approved for use in combination with capecitabine for treatment of HER2-overexpressing advanced or metastatic breast cancer that has been previously treated with an anthracycline, a taxane, and trastuzumab. Bevacizumab is approved for first-line use in breast cancer patients in combination with paclitaxel. Compared to younger patients, older patients have higher risks of thrombosis and bleeding events with bevacizumab.

SPECIAL CONSIDERATIONS

Endocrine Therapy as Initial Treatment

For many older patients, especially those with advanced but localized lesions (T3 and T4) and those with significant comorbidity or frailty, initial treatment with hormonal therapy is appropriate. Tumor shrinkage occurs in 40% to 70% of patients. Although surgery is more likely to be effective (and potentially curative) in patients with small lesions, several randomized trials comparing surgery with hor-

monal treatment for initial therapy suggest that long-term survival is not changed by using hormonal therapy as the initial treatment and reserving surgical management for patients with tumor progression. Radiation therapy also can be used as "salvage" treatment after hormonal therapy fails, but large tumor masses, especially those greater than 3 cm and those with extensive skin involvement, frequently respond only partially. For patients treated with hormonal therapy because comorbidity precludes surgical therapy, radiation therapy should be considered when tumor shrinkage is maximal to try to prolong the duration of local tumor control. In the authors' opinion, older women with localized breast cancer should be offered the same initial treatment options as offered to younger patients in most cases. The majority of patients treated initially with hormonal therapy do not achieve complete tumor regression and, over time, probably will need surgery or other treatments to control the primary lesion.

Male Breast Cancer

Male breast cancer is uncommon and accounts for less than 1% of all breast cancer incidence. The natural history of male and female breast cancer is similar, but males usually present at a later stage, probably because of a delay in diagnosis. Almost all cases are sporadic, except for males with Klinefelter syndrome (sex chromosomes XXY)—in which the prevalence of breast cancer ranges from 3% to 6%—or men with the BRCA-2 gene, which is associated with a 5% to 10% risk of male breast cancer. A careful family history is mandatory in all males with breast cancer. Mastectomy with axillary dissection is the standard approach to treatment but breast conserving surgery and irradiation is appropriate for males with small tumors. Histologically, most lesions are infiltrating ductal carcinomas, and the frequency of estrogen receptor–positive lesions is 70% to 80%. Because of the rarity of male breast cancer, there are few data on the role of adjuvant systemic therapy, and it is unlikely that large randomized trials will be undertaken. Many oncologists use the same guidelines for adjuvant therapy in men that are used in women with a similar stage and receptor status. Uncontrolled trials suggest that such treatment is similar in efficacy in men to that in women.

Males with metastatic breast cancer are incurable but frequently respond to endocrine therapy, including tamoxifen and orchiectomy. There is little experience with AIs in men with breast cancer. The results with systemic chemotherapy are similar to those in females.

CONCLUSIONS

Breast cancer is a major gerontologic problem. Both physician education and patient education concerning screening, early diagnosis, and management of breast cancer in this age group are required. Available data indicate that optimal treatment of breast cancer in older women results in outcomes similar to those from treatment of younger women. Although significant comorbid illness is encountered more frequently in older patients and may complicate breast cancer treatment, most patients can be managed with judicious "state-of-the-art" therapy. Barriers to the treatment of breast cancer in older women are generic to the treatment of all illnesses in this age group and include access to care, transportation, adequate family and social support, physician bias, and treatment costs.

Changes in health care policy, as well as focused research related to cancer in the geriatric population, will be needed to overcome these obstacles.

FURTHER READING

Abe O, Abe R, Enomoto K, et al. Effects of chemotherapy and hormonal therapy for early breast cancer on recurrence and 15-year survival: an overview of the randomised trials. *Lancet.* 2005;365(9472):1687–1717.

Eifel P, Axelson JA, Costa J, et al. National institutes of health consensus development conference statement: adjuvant therapy for breast cancer, November 1–3, 2000. *J Natl Cancer Inst.* 2001;93(13):979–989.

Extermann M, Balducci L, Lyman GH. What threshold for adjuvant therapy in older breast cancer patients? *J Clin Oncol.* 2000;18(8):1709–1717.

Gail MH, Costantino JP, Bryant J, et al. Weighing the risks and benefits of tamoxifen treatment for preventing breast cancer [Review]. *J Natl Cancer Inst.* 1999;91(21):1829–1846.

Harris JR, Lippman ME, Morrow M, Osborne CK. *Diseases of the Breast.* 3rd ed. Philadelphia, PA: Lippincott, Williams, and WIlkins; 2004.

Havlik RJ, Yancik R, Long S, et al. The National Institute on Aging and the National Cancer Institute SEER collaborative study on comorbidity and early diagnosis of cancer in the elderly. *Cancer.* 1994;74:2101–2106.

Khatcheressian JL, Wolff AC, Smith TJ, et al. American society of clinical oncology 2006 update of the breast cancer follow-up and management guidelines in the adjuvant setting. *J Clin Oncol.* 2006;24(31):5091–5097.

Kimmick G, Kornblith A, Mandelblatt J, et al. A randomized controlled trial of an educational program to improve accrual of older persons to cancer treatment protocols: CALGB 360001. *J Clin Oncol.* 2005;23(10):2201–2207.

Lichtman SM, Skirvin JA. Pharmacology of antineoplastic agents in older cancer patients. *Oncology (Williston Park).* 2000;14(12):1743–1755; discussion 1755, passim.

Lyman GH, Giuliano AE, Somerfield MR, et al. American Society of Clinical Oncology guideline recommendations for sentinel lymph node biopsy in early-stage breast cancer. *J Clin Oncol.* 2005;23(30):7703–7720.

Mandelblatt JS, Wheat ME, Monane M, et al. Breast cancer screening for elderly women with and without comorbid conditions. A decision analysis model. *Ann Intern Med.* 1992;116:722–730.

Muss HB, Woolf S, Berry D, et al. Adjuvant chemotherapy in older and younger women with lymph node-positive breast cancer. *JAMA.* 2005;293(9):1073–1081.

Singletary SE, Allred C, Ashley P, et al. Revision of the American Joint Committee on Cancer staging system for breast cancer. *J Clin Oncol.* 2002;20(17):3628–3636.

Smith TJ. The American society of clinical oncology recommended breast cancer surveillance guidelines can be done in a routine office visit. *J Clin Oncol.* 2005;23(27):6807.

Vogel VG, Costantino JP, Wickerham DL, et al. Effects of tamoxifen vs raloxifene on the risk of developing invasive breast cancer and other disease outcomes: the NSABP Study of Tamoxifen and Raloxifene (STAR) P-2 trial. *JAMA.* 2006;295(23):2727–2741.

Welch HG, Albertsen PC, Nease RF, et al. Estimating treatment benefits for the elderly: the effect of competing risks. *Ann Intern Med.* 1996;124:577–584.

Woodward WA, Strom EA, Tucker SL, et al. Changes in the 2003 American Joint Committee on Cancer staging for breast cancer dramatically affect stage-specific survival. *J Clin Oncol.* 2003;21(17):3244–3248.

Yancik R, Wesley MN, Varicchio CG, et al. Effect of age and comorbidity in postmenopausal breast cancer patients aged 55 years and older. *JAMA.* 2001;285(7):885–892.

Prostate Cancer

Kenneth J. Pienta

EPIDEMIOLOGY AND RISK FACTORS

Prostate cancer remains the most common noncutaneous malignancy diagnosed in American men and is the second leading cause of cancer-related deaths in that group. In the year 2008, almost 187,000 will be diagnosed with prostate cancer and an estimated 29,000 men will die of the disease.

The only undisputed risk factors for prostate cancer are older age, African-American race, and positive family history. Prostate cancer is generally a disease of elderly men; risk increases exponentially with age, with a median age at presentation of 68 years. Eighty percent of prostate cancer diagnoses and 90% of prostate cancer deaths occur in men older than 65. The incidence rates of the disease among African-American men are higher than rates for men in *any* other racial or ethnic background. African-American men are more likely to be diagnosed with prostate cancer and to die from it than their Caucasian counterparts. The estimated lifetime risk of prostate cancer is 17.6% and 20.6% respectively for Caucasians and African-Americans, while the estimated lifetime risk of death is 2.8% and 4.7%. Studies suggest that early onset prostate cancer may be inherited in an autosomal dominant fashion, and it is estimated that approximately 10% of all prostate cancer cases are hereditary. A large twin study suggests that genetic factors may account for as much as 42% of prostate cancer risk, although the absence of clear, highly penetrant markers suggests that in the majority of men, prostate cancer risk involves a complex interaction of multiple genetic and environmental factors.

Additional factors such as diet, obesity, hormones, inflammation and sexually transmitted diseases, and occupational exposure have all been implicated in prostate carcinogenesis, but without consistent results. Dietary fat may be a risk factor for prostate cancer. Multiple epidemiological, case–control, and cohort studies have suggested a moderate to strong increased risk of developing prostate cancer, particularly advanced disease, associated with total dietary fat, saturated fat, alpha linolenic fatty acid, and cooked red meat.

Two large prospective studies and a smaller case–control study suggest that fish intake may be protective, possibly owing to marine omega-3 fatty acids—known antagonists of arachidonic acid, which suppress the production of proinflammatory cytokines. Evidence for the association with dietary fat is further correlated with worldwide incidence patterns; prostate cancer is more common in the United States and northern European countries and is relatively rare in Asia and Africa. When Asian men migrate to the West and change from a low-fat to a high-fat diet, their risk of prostate cancer increases. These studies, however, are complicated by the fact that many of the men migrating from low-fat diet areas also consume green tea and soy products, which contain isoflavones and estrogen that may act as antioxidants and chemoprotectants against prostate-specific carcinogenesis. Several epidemiologic studies have suggested an inverse relationship between soy intake and prostate cancer risk.

Most studies have not demonstrated an association between obesity and prostate cancer incidence, but there is growing evidence to support an association between obesity and aggressive prostate cancer, recurrence after primary therapy, and death from prostate cancer. Data from the Prostate Cancer Prevention Trial (PCPT) suggest that obesity increases the risk of higher-grade cancers, but decreases the risk of low-grade prostate cancer. While BMI ≥ 30 was associated with an 18% decrease in low-grade cancers (Gleason grade < 7) there was a 29% increase in Gleason grade of 7 and above and a 78% increase in high-grade cancers (Gleason 8–10). These data suggest that obesity may differentially affect the development of aggressive and nonaggressive prostate cancer and may somehow play a role in the progression from latent to clinically significant prostate cancer. Although the specific role obesity plays in prostate cancer risk is unclear, it may be linked to other risk factors such as dietary fat and meat intake, hormone metabolism, and insulin metabolism. The prevalence of obesity also correlates with prostate cancer risk across populations and may provide a link between the increased risk of prostate cancer with westernization.

Although a diet rich in fruits and vegetables is associated with reduced risk in several cancers, their effect on prostate cancer risk is still unclear. Several studies have shown an inverse association with tomatoes and tomato products, presumably owing to the effects of lycopene, the most common carotenoid in the human body and one of the most potent carotenoid antioxidants. Data from the large Health Professionals Follow-Up Study (HPFS) suggest that frequent consumption of tomato products is associated with a decreased risk of prostate cancer, and in a meta-analysis of 21 case–control and cohort studies, a statistically significant 10% to 20% risk reduction was associated with high versus low intake of tomatoes. The majority of these studies also show a stronger effect for cooked versus raw tomatoes.

Although it seems intuitive that testosterone levels may influence the incidence of prostate cancer, no evidence exists to confirm this association. Dihydrotestosterone, the active hormone produced from the conversion of testosterone by the enzyme 5α-reductase, is associated in some studies with increased risk. A prospective, population-based study of 1156 men showed no correlation between 17 different hormones and prostate cancer development, with the possible exception of androstanediol glucuronide. Importantly, no dose–response relationships were seen, suggesting that serum hormonal levels may not be useful even in risk stratification.

There is some evidence that chronic inflammation may increase prostate cancer risk. One meta-analysis of 11 studies on prostatitis and prostate cancer showed an overall relative risk of 1.6, while another meta-analysis of aspirin and cancer showed that regular aspirin use was associated with an approximately 15% decrease in prostate cancer risk. Population based studies have suggested an increased risk of prostate cancer in patients with STDs, including syphilis, recurrent gonorrhea, HPV, and HIV. A meta-analysis of 17 studies of prostate cancer and sexual patterns suggested that an increased number of sexual partners was associated with an increased prostate cancer risk, possibly through an increased exposure to STDs. There are currently no strong data to suggest a link between benign prostate hypertrophy (BPH) and prostate cancer risk.

PREVENTION

Chemoprevention is an area of ongoing research, and in many ways, prostate cancer is an ideal disease for this approach—relatively slow growing, centered in the elderly population, yet with devastating effects and difficult management after the onset of metastasis.

Finasteride

Finasteride is a drug that blocks the actions of 5α-reductase, the enzyme that converts testosterone to dihydrotestosterone. The PCPT enrolled 18,000 men between January 1994 and May 1997 to study the efficacy of finasteride for decreasing the period prevalence of prostate cancer. The trial was based on two observations: androgens are required for prostate cancer development and men with congenital 5α-reductase deficiency develop neither BPH nor prostate cancer. This randomized, double-blind, placebo-controlled trial was closed early because of a perceived risk reduction with finasteride. After 7 years of treatment, prostate cancer was diagnosed in 18.4% of the men on finasteride and 24.4% of the men on placebo, a 6% absolute risk reduction and 24.8% relative risk reduction. The

risk reduction associated with finasteride was apparent across all risk groups defined by age, family history, race, and PSA. Finasteride use was also associated with increased sexual dysfunction, but decreased lower urinary tract symptoms.

Results from the trial, however, were tempered by an apparent increase in high-risk cancers in the finasteride group; 6.4% of the cancers in the finasteride group were Gleason grade 8 to 10 versus 5.1% in the controls. This represented a statistically significant 1.3% absolute increase in the risk of high-grade cancer associated with finasteride. Since high-grade cancers are associated with a poorer prognosis after definitive therapy, the role of finasteride in the prevention of prostate cancer remains controversial at this time. Several experts, however, have questioned whether the increase in high-grade cancers associated with finasteride in the PCPT is real or artifact. If finasteride induced higher-grade tumors, the incidence of prostate cancer in the finasteride arm should increase at a greater rate, particularly as the trial progressed and the duration of prostate exposure to finasteride increased. This was not the case however. Furthermore, ultrasound evaluation showed a 24.1% decrease in prostate volume in the treatment arm (median volume 25.5 cm^3 versus 33.6 cm^3). There is evidence to suggest that the risk of missing high-grade cancers increases as prostatic volume increases; with a smaller volume, a larger proportion of the gland is biopsied and evaluated, increasing the chance of detecting cancer. Thus, some experts claim that the increased risk of high-grade cancer in the finasteride group could be because of increased sampling rather than a medication effect. Finally, there is new evidence to suggest that finasteride enhances the sensitivity of PSA for prostate cancer, by decreasing BPH and thus its effect on PSA levels.

Further evaluation of the role of 5α-reductase inhibitors in prostate cancer prevention will occur with The Reduction by Dutasteride of Prostate Cancer Events (REDUCE), a randomized, double-blind, placebo-controlled trial currently enrolling patients in Europe and the United States, randomizing men to Avodart, a new 5α-reductase inhibitor, versus placebo. Until these results are available, widespread use of finasteride for chemoprevention is currently not being advocated by most experts in the field. It remains, however, an effective treatment for BPH.

Vitamin E and Selenium

In recent years, the role of oxidative stress in the development of prostate cancer has been investigated. The damage caused by reactive oxygen species is not limited to deoxyribonucleic acid (DNA); it can encompass lipids and proteins as well. The association of prostate cancer and a high-fat diet may be secondary to the generation of increased fatty acids, which can cause lipid peroxidation. The two most exciting agents in the area of chemoprevention are selenium and vitamin E.

Selenium is an essential trace nutrient, which enters the food chain via consumption of plants and plant eating animals. Since there is marked geographic variability in foods, linked to local soil content, selenium intake cannot be easily linked to dietary sources. Selenium was initially investigated in the prevention of recurrent basal and squamous cell skin cancers, and although it did not affect the incidence of recurrent skin cancer, an unexpected finding was a decrease in the risk of prostate, colorectal, and lung cancer. Remarkably, the incidence of prostate cancer decreased by 65%. Subsequently, both case–control and randomized placebo-controlled trials have demonstrated a decrease in the risk of developing prostate cancer associated with selenium supplementation.

Alpha tocopherol is the most active and abundant source of vitamin E, and its antioxidant properties have been studied extensively in a variety of prostate cell lines and animal models. Results from human studies are conflicting. In one prospective study, there was no protective association between increased serum levels of vitamin E and the risk of prostate cancer, while other studies have shown a statistically significant positive effect. The Alpha-Tocopherol, Beta-Carotene Cancer Prevention Trial (ATBC) randomized 29,133 male smokers to either α-tocopherol (50 mg daily), beta carotene (20 mg daily), both or placebo. Although the primary endpoint was lung cancer incidence and mortality, the trial demonstrated a statistically significant 32% decrease in prostate cancer incidence and a 41% decrease in prostate cancer mortality in the groups taking α-tocopherol supplements. A recent meta-analysis of 19 randomized clinic trials, however, suggested that long-term supplemental vitamin E ≥ 400 IU daily was associated with an increase in mortality from all causes. This has caused many to question the long-term use of this supplement as a chemoprotectant in the absence of data demonstrating clear benefit.

SELECT (Selenium and Vitamin E Cancer Prevention Trial) is an NCI sponsored, randomized, prospective, double-blind trial designed to determine whether selenium and vitamin E decrease the risk of prostate cancer in healthy men. It will enroll 32,400 healthy men with a normal digital rectal examination and a prostate-specific antigen (PSA) ≤ 4 ng/mL. The 2×2 factorial design includes four study arms: vitamin E + placebo, selenium + placebo, vitamin E + selenium, and placebo + placebo. The primary end point of the trial is the clinical incidence of prostate cancer; secondary endpoints include prostate cancer-free survival, mortality from any cause, and the incidence and mortality of other cancers or diseases affected by chronic supplementation with vitamin E and/or selenium. The planned duration of the study is 12 years with a minimum 7 years of treatment, and final results are expected by 2013. As prostate cancer incidence increases with age, it is important to enroll as many geriatric patients as possible, as the greatest risk reduction may be possible in this group.

PRESENTATION

Most men who present with prostate cancer are asymptomatic, particularly in the era of PSA testing, which detects many cancers long before they are clinically apparent. Patients rarely have urinary symptoms, as the majority of cancers arise in the posterior aspect of the prostate. Most men undergo evaluation after routine screening reveals either an elevated PSA or abnormal digital rectal examination (DRE). Since the advent of PSA testing and regular screening, there has been a demonstrated risk migration, and presently in the United States, the majority of patients have clinically localized, intermediate-risk prostate cancer at diagnosis. A minority of patients are diagnosed when they present with symptomatic metastatic disease, usually manifested as bony pain; CapSure data demonstrate that while in 1988, 14% of new prostate cancer patients presented with metastatic disease, that number had fallen to 3.3% by 1998. Although screening has strongly influenced this downward stage migration, there are no data to suggest that it has significantly decreased prostate cancer–specific mortality; there is some concern that

screening may detect a significant number of clinically insignificant cancers. The wide discrepancy between incidence and mortality attributed to prostate cancer demonstrates that some slow growing cancers may never be life threatening. Published guidelines do exist, notably from the NCCN (National Comprehensive Cancer Network). Currently, there are two large scale, long-term, randomized clinical trials ongoing in the United States and Europe evaluating whether screening decreases mortality; these trials may ultimately provide evidence for the validity of wide-based screening.

A difficult task for primary physicians is thus deciding which patients should undergo screening for prostate cancer. In the absence of definitive data, a reasonable approach to screening should involve an active discussion between the physician and patient, taking into consideration the patient's overall health and treatment preferences. Men with a life expectancy of 10 to 15 years (owing to age or comorbidities) should be informed that screening may not be beneficial. Younger men with a family history of prostate cancer and African-American men should be encouraged to undergo screening, as the disease prevalence is high in these groups. Any patient with symptoms that may be referable to prostate cancer (bone pain, hypercalcemia, symptomatic pelvic lymphadenopathy) warrants a PSA evaluation as a part of his initial evaluation, since symptomatic patients can enjoy significant improvement with the institution of hormonal therapy. An ongoing challenge for the geriatrician is the need to remain current on the development of new treatments. In the future, as more targeted and less toxic therapies are identified, PSA screening may become a routine part of health maintenance for all men.

EVALUATION

The appropriate screening examinations for prostate cancer include a serum PSA and DRE. PSA is a protein produced and secreted by both normal prostate and prostate cancer cells. It provides a sensitive but not highly specific screening test, as it is also elevated with BPH, inflammation, and infection of the prostate. The proposed cutoff is 4.0 ng/mL, but studies have shown that 15% of men with normal PSA levels will have prostate cancer and 2% will have high-grade prostate cancer. PSA is, however, more sensitive than DRE, detecting more cancers and earlier stage and smaller sized cancers than rectal examination alone. PSA-doubling time is also a significant factor in prostate assessment, and any patient with a rapid PSA-doubling time should be sent for further evaluation, even if the absolute value of the PSA is below the normal cutoff level. DRE yield alone is low; estimates are that only 3% to 6% of examinations yield suspicious results. On the basis of an elevated PSA or an abnormal DRE, the patient should be referred for a transrectal ultrasound-guided prostate biopsy. In general, six to twelve cores are taken for evaluation; areas that are abnormal on DRE may receive more biopsy attempts.

If the biopsy is positive, a Gleason score is assigned. This score is one of the most important determinants of prognosis. The pathologist assigns a numerical value (on a scale of 1 to 5) to the most prevalent and the second most prevalent grades of cancer seen in the specimens. The score is then reported on a scale of 2 to 10, with 10 being the most aggressive cancer. Gleason scores should be reported separately, for example, $3 + 4 = 7$, as the primary pathology has prognostic implications.

Risk stratification plays an important role in both the selection and timing of treatment and is an important part of the initial evaluation. After diagnosis, the natural course of prostate cancer can be estimated from tumor volume, aggressiveness, PSA level, and extent of disease. Tumor volume assessment includes local stage, the number of positive biopsy cores, and the extent of cancer in affected cores. Gleason score is currently the standard measurement of aggressiveness with Gleason 5 to 6 cancers considered low grade, Gleason 7 intermediate grade, and Gleason 8 to 10 high grade. Taking all of these prognostic factors into effect, newly diagnosed patients are classified as having low-, intermediate-, or high-risk disease. In addition to these broad risk groups, multiple nomograms are available to help clinicians estimate an individual patient's probability of localized disease, risk of progression without intervention, and risk of recurrence after definitive therapy. Several of these tools are available online, and they can sometimes be more helpful than the broad categories in assessing an individual's risk, as they allow integration of discordant factors (e.g., high PSA with low Gleason score). PSA velocity prior to diagnosis may also provide valuable information in risk assessment; a PSA velocity ≥2.0 ng/mL in the year prior to radical prostatectomy is predictive of greater risk of biochemical recurrence, cancer-specific mortality, and overall mortality.

The staging evaluation for men with known prostate cancer or symptoms that could be attributable to metastatic prostate cancer includes serum chemistries, PSA, bone scan, and computed tomography (CT) scan of the abdomen and pelvis. These initial tests provide evaluation of the most likely sites of metastatic disease to avoid inappropriate surgical intervention or radiation therapy. The extent of evaluation for metastatic disease relates to the likelihood of finding disease. A recent prospective survey of 3690 men described the positive yield of bone scan, and CT was <5% and 12%, respectively, for men with a PSA of 4 to 20 ng/mL. The yield decreased to 2% and 9% for those who also had a Gleason score of ≤6. Only the combination of a Gleason score of 8 to 10 and a PSA >20, or a PSA >50 alone, identified a group of men who had a >10% yield on bone scan and a 20% yield on CT scan. To stage in an appropriate and cost-effective manner, patients with low PSAs and low to intermediate Gleason scores do not require evaluation. More risk factors increase the degree of preoperative evaluation. Table 96-1 provides guidelines for preoperative staging. These studies also provide a baseline for follow-up. Figure 96-1 illustrates a stepwise approach to evaluation, monitoring, and treatment.

MANAGEMENT

After an initial diagnosis of prostate cancer, treatment decisions should take into consideration a number of factors including the individual patient's remaining life expectancy (which can be estimated using social security tables), comorbidities, baseline quality of life, treatment preferences, and disease characteristics/risk factors.

Observation

The concept of observation or watchful waiting involves deferring treatment until patients develop symptomatic disease. It was first proposed in the 1970s after the results of the Veterans Administration Cooperative Urological Research Group (VACURG) trial suggested that delaying therapy until the onset of symptoms did not increase prostate cancer-specific mortality in patients with locally advanced or metastatic disease. To evaluate watchful waiting in the modern era, from 1985 until 1993 the Medical Research Council Trial randomized 938 men with locally advanced or asymptomatic metastatic prostate cancer to either immediate or deferred treatment with hormonal therapy. In this study, 67% of patients died secondary to prostate cancer, a substantial increase from the findings of the VACURG trial. Overall survival was significantly longer in the patients treated immediately, with the most pronounced difference in men who initially had no evidence of metastatic disease. The rate of complications, such as bone pain, pathological fractures, spinal cord compression, and ureteral obstruction was higher in the deferred group. Because PSA testing allows detection of cancers some 5 to 15 years earlier than DRE, men with T1c (PSA detected) tumors treated with watchful waiting may have better than 20-year disease-specific survival. Thus, watchful waiting, either at the time of initial diagnosis or at the time of progression, may still be applicable in a subset of elderly men without metastatic disease. However, if the patient is not a candidate for treatment and has no symptoms attributable to the disease, both the patient and the physician should reflect on why screening was undertaken.

Active Surveillance

Active surveillance or expectant management differs from watchful waiting in the intensity of monitoring and the expectation of delayed but successful definitive, potentially curative therapy. This strategy is based on the observation that there is tremendous heterogeneity

TABLE 96-1

Guidelines for Staging Evaluation			
PARAMETERS	**RISK**	**METASTATIC EVALUATION**	**REFERENCES**
PSA < 15, Gleason 2–7, clinical stage ≤ T2b	Low	No screening	All 237 patients had negative bone scan and all 244 patients had negative CT scans in this category
PSA 15–50, Gleason 2–7, clinical stage ≤ T2b	Intermediate	Consider bone scan and perform CT scan of abdomen/pelvis	3 of 308 patients had positive bone scan and 8 of 174 patients had positive CT scan in this category
PSA > 50, Gleason 8–10, clinical stage ≥ T2c	High	Perform bone scan and CT scan of abdomen/pelvis	OR for positive CT scan 6.17 for Gleason 8–10 vs. 2–6
Symptoms		Appropriate evaluation for symptoms noted	

CT, computed tomography; OR, odds ratio; PSA, prostate-specific antigen.

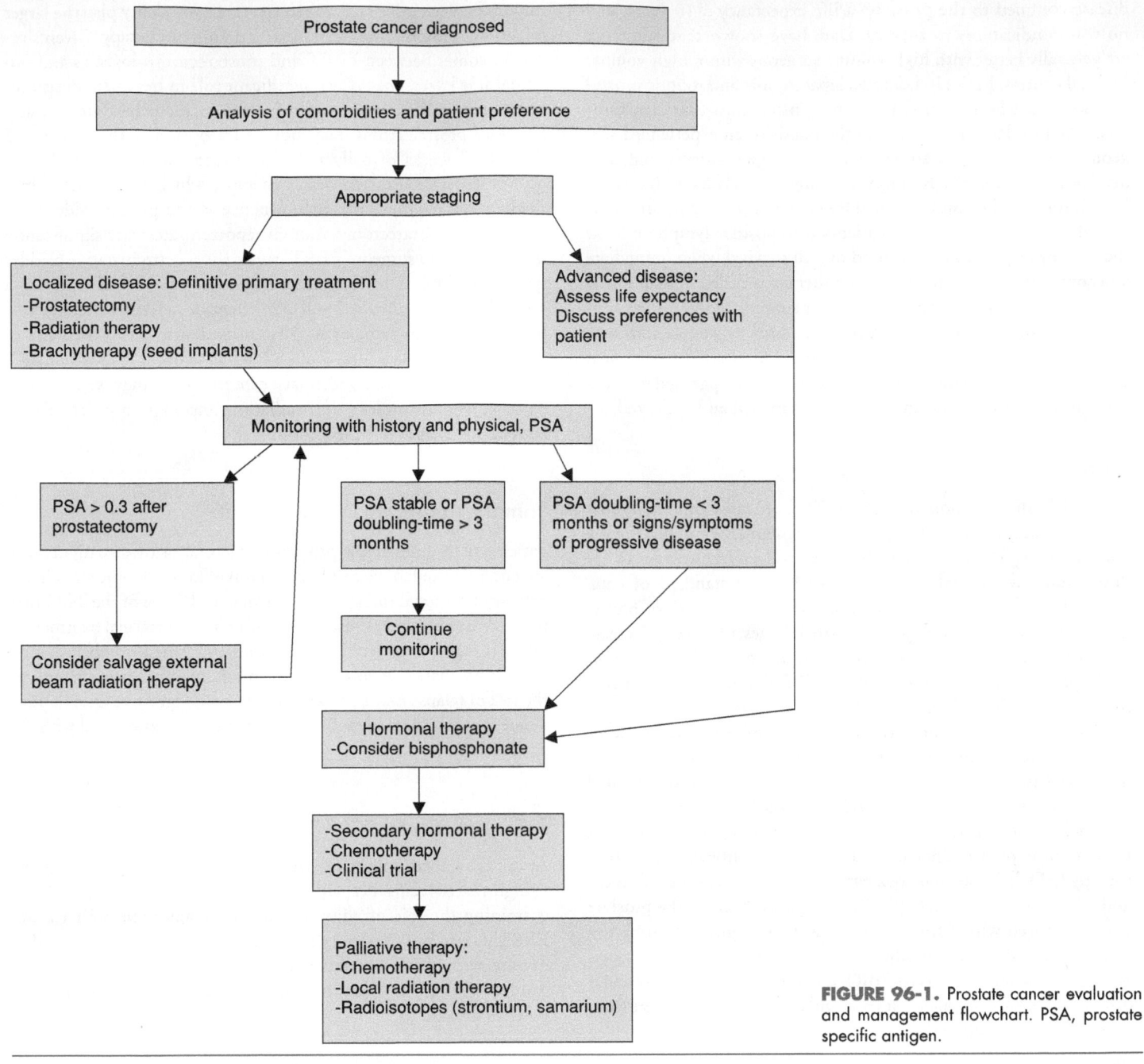

FIGURE 96-1. Prostate cancer evaluation and management flowchart. PSA, prostate specific antigen.

in the natural history of prostate cancer, and a significant number of men may be "overdiagnosed" in the sense that diagnosis and treatment may not improve either quality of life or survival. Active surveillance involves regular monitoring with PSA every 3 months, clinical examination with DRE every 6 months, and repeat biopsies as warranted by PSA and DRE (which can occur as frequently as once a year). An increase in PSA velocity (doubling time <3 years), primary Gleason pattern of 4 or 5 on repeat biopsy, or an increased number or extent of positive biopsy cores suggests progression of disease, and intervention with appropriately selected therapy should be initiated. Many experts feel that this is a reasonable approach for men with low-risk disease and may represent a practical compromise between radical treatment for all patients and watchful waiting with palliative treatment only (a strategy that undertreats aggressive disease). Although active surveillance may avoid overtreatment and

allow patients to maintain their baseline quality of life, the strategy carries with it a risk of local or metastatic progression before active treatment is initiated. It is important, therefore, that patients are made aware that even the most careful monitoring may miss the window for administering curative therapy.

Local Therapy: Surgery, Radiation, or Brachytherapy

Surgery, radiation, or brachytherapy for early-stage disease is performed with curative intent.

Radical Prostatectomy

Radical prostatectomy (RP) involves removal of the prostate and seminal vesicles, and is an appropriate therapy for any patient with disease confined to the prostate, a life expectancy >10 years, and no contraindications to surgery. Data have shown that outcomes are generally better with high-volume surgeons within high-volume medical centers. In the last decade, laparoscopic and robotic prostatectomies have been refined and moved into mainstream care. Outcome data to date suggest that in the hands of an experienced surgeon, these approaches are comparable to open surgery and may involve less morbidity. Randomized clinical trials have shown no benefit for neoadjuvant hormonal therapy with RP. There are, however, data demonstrating that patients with positive lymph nodes at the time of surgery have improved overall survival when immediate and continued androgen deprivation therapy is added to their initial treatment. Pathologic examination after surgery allows for verification of organ confinement and margin status as well as complete histological examination; several studies have reported that almost 50% of patients with biopsy Gleason 6 disease are upgraded to Gleason 7 or higher, once the entire gland is removed and evaluated.

External Beam Radiation Therapy

External beam radiation therapy (EBRT) in most centers is now delivered using advanced CT planning or intensity-modulated radiation therapy. These newer techniques, collectively known as "3-dimensional conformal therapy," have become standard of care. They allow for increased accuracy and thus the delivery of higher doses to the prostate while sparing normal tissues, ultimately decreasing both acute and delayed side effects. Often gold fiducial markers are implanted in the prostate prior to EBRT to provide landmarks for accurate daily dosing.

Radiation dosing is currently based on risk of recurrence. Patients with low-risk prostate cancer are generally treated with 70 to 75 Gy in 35 to 41 fractions. Higher doses of 75 to 80 Gy are recommended for patients with intermediate- and high-risk features. In addition, studies have shown that intermediate-risk patients benefit from 4 to 6 months of neoadjuvant and adjuvant androgen deprivation therapy (ADT), while high-risk patients should receive neoadjuvant and adjuvant ADT for a total of 2 to 3 years. Because the prostate is not removed with EBRT, there is no pathological confirmation of the extent of disease or adjustment of the biopsy Gleason score. Relative contraindications to EBRT include active collagen vascular disease, inflammatory bowel disease, and microvascular damage from hypertension or diabetes.

Brachytherapy

Brachytherapy involves radioactive iodine (^{125}I) or palladium (^{103}Pd) implants, which are placed in the prostate under general anesthesia. They emit short-range radiation within the prostate, generally avoiding the bladder and rectum, and lose their radioactivity gradually. Prostate brachytherapy as monotherapy is indicated for patients with low-risk disease and small prostate volume (<60 g). For intermediate-risk patients, brachytherapy is frequently combined with external beam radiation (40–50 Gy). High-risk patients are generally considered poor candidates for this treatment modality.

Although there are no good randomized data comparing local treatment modalities, a review of 2991 patients treated at the Cleveland Clinic and Memorial Sloan-Kettering Cancer Center showed similar 5-year biochemical relapse-free survival rates for RP, EBRT, and brachytherapy, leading the authors to conclude that intrinsic tumor characteristics rather than treatment modality play the larger role in determining progression after definitive therapy. Given similar outcomes between EBRT and prostatectomy, logistics and potential side effects may play a significant role in treatment decisions. Some men may not be candidates for major pelvic surgery, and therefore prostatectomy may not be an option. Others may find the 8 to 9 weeks of daily radiation treatments unacceptable and opt for prostatectomy or brachytherapy, which is completed in a single surgical procedure. Incontinence is the primary side effect noted after prostatectomy, though reported rates vary significantly from surgeon to surgeon. EBRT causes short-term irritative bladder symptoms; long-term incontinence is rare. Bowel dysfunction is a potential short and/or delayed side effect of radiation therapy. Impotence occurs in as many as 50% of patients treated with any of the three local approaches, though it tends to occur later with EBRT than with prostatectomy. Primary care providers may want to refer patients to both urology and radiation oncology in order to fully educate patients about their choices.

Primary Androgen Deprivation

Patients with unfavorable prognostic factors, or those patients who are not interested in the risk:benefit ratio of local therapy, may choose primary hormonal therapy. Approximately 12.5% of the 3486 men in the Prostate Cancer Outcomes Study chose hormonal treatment as initial therapy, considered to be a surprisingly high number. Clearly, there is no chance of cure with this modality, but for some patients the risk of relapse may be too high to pursue aggressive local therapy. There is also scant evidence about the outcomes associated with this approach.

Adjuvant Therapy

At this time, there is no standard adjuvant chemotherapy for patients at high-risk of recurrence, although there are several intergroup trials examining the role of adjuvant chemotherapy with both RP and EBRT. Adjuvant hormonal therapy, as noted above, is now standard of care with EBRT in patients with intermediate- and high-risk disease; after RP, it is recommended only for patients with node-positive disease.

POSTTREATMENT SURVEILLANCE

The scheduled follow-up after definitive local therapy depends upon the risk of recurrence and the potential for curative salvage therapy. Patients at high risk of recurrence who would be good candidates for further intervention should have regular PSA testing (every 1–3 months) and DRE at least annually. Patients at low risk of recurrence or poor intervention candidates are more appropriately followed with evaluations every 4 to 6 months for the first 5 years and annually thereafter. Pound and colleagues found that 45% of patients who recur after prostatectomy do so within 2 years. Seventy-seven percent of recurrences occur within the first 5 years after prostatectomy and 96% within 9 years. Any patient with symptoms referable to local or systemic relapse (particularly new bone pain) should be evaluated with repeat serum and radiologic tests.

Biochemical Recurrence

Biochemical recurrence after RP is defined as a PSA level greater than 0.3 ng/mL and rising on two or more determinations. Recurrence after EBRT has recently been redefined by ASTRO consensus as nadir PSA plus 2. The pattern of local recurrence is usually 1 to 3 years after primary therapy, with a slowly rising PSA or new finding on DRE; these patients should be followed closely and referred for local salvage therapy, if appropriate. The need for biopsy of radiologically proven disease in this setting is controversial. Patients who relapse quickly after local therapy (<6 months) are more likely to have metastatic disease that was not discovered prior to definitive local therapy and are therefore unlikely to respond to local salvage therapy.

Patients with a rising PSA and no clinical, symptomatic, or radiographic evidence of disease present a therapeutic dilemma, as there is no clear consensus as to the timing of further therapy. Some men with biochemical recurrence will eventually die of prostate cancer, while others will have indolent disease and ultimately die of other causes. Prognosis is best estimated by considering initial stage, Gleason grade, and PSA in addition to the absolute value of the PSA at the time of recurrence and the PSA-doubling time. PSA-doubling time has been shown to be a useful parameter for monitoring patients and deciding when to initiate treatment after biochemical recurrence. One analysis of 587 men who had undergone an RP for clinically localized disease analyzed the significance of PSA-doubling time as a predictor of clinical progression after biochemical (PSA) failure. In a multivariate model, PSA-doubling time was a significant risk factor ($p < 0.001$) for both metastatic progression and local recurrence. The mean 5-year progression-free survival was 99% with a PSA-doubling time of > 10 years, 95% with a PSA-doubling time of 1 to 9.9 years, 93% with a PSA-doubling time of 6 to 11 months, and 64% with a PSA-doubling time of less than 6 months. As expected, patients with a PSA-doubling time of less than 6 months were far more likely to have metastatic disease than local recurrence. PSA-doubling time of ≤3 months has been shown in multiple studies to predict cancer-specific mortality among patients with biochemical recurrence after either RP or EBRT.

Salvage Local Therapy

Patients whose PSA levels do not fall to an undetectable level after surgery should be evaluated for adjuvant or salvage therapy, including EBRT with or without ADT, or ADT alone. Approximately 20% to 25% of men with local recurrence postprostatectomy can be cured with early salvage EBRT. Several factors have been demonstrated to predict long-term response to salvage ERBT: Gleason score ≤7,

positive surgical margins at RP, negative nodal or seminal vesicle involvement, and post-RP PSA kinetics consistent with local failure (>3 year interval from RP to biochemical failure, PSA-doubling time >10 to 12 months, and an absolute PSA at salvage of ≤1.0). Patients who recur immediately after definitive radiation therapy are candidates for ADT, observation, or, in selected cases, salvage prostatectomy.

ADVANCED DISEASE

A positive bone scan and pain in a weight-bearing area correlating to the scan should prompt an x-ray to assess for impending pathologic fractures. Patients should be made non-weight-bearing and immediately referred for both surgical and radiation consultation. The possibility of cord compression should be suspected in any man with a history of prostate cancer and new onset back pain. Pain from spinal cord compression is often severe and generally predates neurologic symptoms. A negative neurologic examination should not delay a definitive radiologic study (preferably magnetic resonance imaging [MRI] or CT myelogram), and patients with suspected cord compression should be initiated and maintained on steroids until compression is ruled out.

Hormonal Therapy

First-Line Hormonal Therapy

Patients with advanced disease at presentation, or patients who relapse after definitive local therapy are initially treated with some form of ADT. Timing of hormonal therapy should take into consideration the aggressiveness of the cancer as well as patient preferences. There is some evidence to suggest that starting ADT earlier rather than later improves outcomes, but the impact of early treatment on survival has yet to be defined.

The goal of ADT is to decrease the level of testosterone available to potentiate growth of the prostate cancer cells. A variety of treatments can achieve this goal; Table 96-2 outlines the spectrum of drugs, which either alone or in combination are used as first-line hormonal therapy. Currently, the majority of men on ADT are treated with LHRH agonists alone (monotherapy) or in combination with an antiandrogen (combined androgen blockade). Although some physicians routinely use combination therapy, others prefer LHRH monotherapy, and there are no clear data showing benefit of one strategy over the other. Patients with known metastatic disease, however, need to be on an antiandrogen for at least 30 days, starting 7

TABLE 96-2

Commonly Used First-Line Hormonal Therapy Options			
TREATMENT	MECHANISM	EXAMPLE	ADMINISTRATION
Orchiectomy	Removal of major source of testosterone		Surgical
LHRH agonist	Stops the pulsatile secretion of LHRH from the pituitary and production of testosterone by the testes	Zoladex, Lupron	By depot injection, every 3–4 months
Antiandrogen	Androgen-receptor antagonist	Casodex, Eulexin, Nilandron	Daily pill

to 10 days prior to initiation of LHRH agonist therapy to avoid the initial testosterone flare associated with LHRH therapy.

Orchiectomy (surgical castration) may be an underused and underappreciated form of hormonal treatment. Clearly, with advances in surgical techniques, the morbidity associated with the procedure is minimal and barring unforeseen complications, it is an outpatient procedure. Data from the Prostate Cancer Outcomes Study provided an update on quality-of-life issues for patients receiving hormonal therapy. Men who chose LHRH agonist therapy reported greater problems than orchiectomy patients did with their overall sexual functioning, despite both groups having similar levels of function prior to beginning treatment. LHRH patients were also less likely to perceive themselves as free of cancer, likely because of the need for ongoing injections.

The duration of response to first-line ADT is typically 18 to 24 months, although patients who initiate therapy for biochemical relapse alone may show PSA responses for much longer. The continuation of ADT in the setting of hormone refractory disease is a subject of some controversy. A retrospective analysis by the Southwest Oncology Group (SWOG) showed no improvement in survival for patients remaining on LHRH therapy, while an Eastern Cooperative Oncology Group (ECOG) analysis showed a slight survival benefit. Given the potential for improved survival for patients remaining on testicular androgen suppression, many physicians continue to administer LHRH agonists for the duration of treatment with secondary hormonal therapies and chemotherapy.

Side effects from hormonal therapies include hot flashes, insomnia, decreased libido, erectile dysfunction, weight gain/fluid retention, diabetes, increased risk of cardiovascular events, and breast enlargement/nipple tenderness. Breast enlargement can be curtailed, although not reversed, by a few treatments of electron beam radiation directly to the breast stem cells underneath the areola. This low-risk treatment can provide significant physical and psychological benefit. Antiandrogen treatment can lead to hepatic dysfunction, requiring monitoring of liver function tests after the initial month of therapy, and every 3 months thereafter. Antiandrogens are also associated with gastrointestinal effects, including nausea, diarrhea, and constipation. Estrogens can predispose patients to thromboembolic complications, including deep vein thrombosis, pulmonary embolism, and myocardial infarction.

Patients with decreased testosterone caused by orchiectomy or ADT also have a significantly increased risk of bone loss. Most studies have demonstrated a 2% to 3% decrease per year in bone mineral density (BMD) of the hip and spine during initial testosterone suppressing therapy and BMD continues to decline during long-term therapy. Fracture rates are also higher in patients on ADT. Three large, claims-based studies have shown that LHRH treatment is independently associated with fracture risk. Patients on testosterone suppressing therapy should, therefore, be encouraged to take daily calcium (500 mg) and vitamin D (400 IU) supplements to prevent bone loss. In addition, patients may benefit from BMD testing to evaluate overall bone health. Men with osteopenia or osteoporosis should be considered for treatment with oral bisphosphonates (see section on "Supportive Care").

Intermittent Androgen Deprivation

Intermittent androgen blockade has been advocated as a way to decrease side effects from ADT, and also to, potentially, increase the time to androgen independence. With this strategy, patients are cycled on and off hormonal therapy based on PSA response. Once patients achieve an undetectable PSA in response to ADT, they are taken off therapy and monitored; treatment is reinitiated based on absolute PSA value and/or PSA-doubling time. Although intermittent ADT is now widely used and in most cases decreases the side effects attributable to ADT, its long-term efficacy is as yet unproven. A large intergroup trial is currently evaluating this strategy, randomizing patients to intermittent versus continuous ADT; primary endpoints are survival and quality of life.

Second-Line Hormonal Therapy

There are several potential second- (and third-) line hormonal treatments for patients who fail first-line therapy. If the patient is receiving combined androgen blockade, the first treatment modality is antiandrogen withdrawal. The maximum duration of response is approximately 5 months. To date, there have been no identified predictors of androgen withdrawal response, although a longer duration of treatment with flutamide has been associated with response in two larger trials.

After withdrawal of one antiandrogen, some patients can derive benefit from the addition of a different antiandrogen, such as high-dose bicalutamide (150 mg daily). Ketoconazole, which decreases the production of adrenal androgens, has also been widely studied and has demonstrated transient response rates in patients with progression after ADT. Most ketoconazole trials, however, are confounded by the concomitant use of hydrocortisone (to prevent adrenal insufficiency); an evolving body of evidence suggests that steroids alone could be responsible for the PSA decline and improvement in quality of life. The first reported study of low-dose prednisone showed that 40% of patients had improved quality of life at 1 month, which was sustained for a median of 4 months in 20% of patients.

Estrogens, such as diethylstilbestrol, show promise both singly and in combination, although estrogen therapy is associated with side effects such as edema and increased incidence of thromboembolic complications. Judicious use of prophylactic agents, such as warfarin or low-dose aspirin, have been used in these trials, but not studied prospectively.

The decision to pursue secondary hormonal manipulations will likely depend on several factors. Available data suggest that patients with a significant and prolonged response to initial hormonal therapy, or a significant antiandrogen withdrawal response, may be good candidates for a trial of secondary hormonal therapy. Poor performance status and the presence of other medical problems may render attempts at further hormonal manipulation an attractive option as these patients are often intolerant of the side effects associated with chemotherapy. Patients with rapid PSA-doubling times are likely to have more aggressive disease and may receive more benefit from chemotherapy or a clinical trial with a novel agent.

Chemotherapy

The use of chemotherapy in androgen-independent prostate cancer has undergone a revolution in the past decade. Although androgen-independent prostate cancer was once labeled "chemotherapy resistant," new agents show great promise in both palliative and response end points. Docetaxel is the first chemotherapeutic agent with demonstrated survival benefit in prostate cancer and has become standard of care for first-line therapy in hormone refractory disease. In phase II and III clinical trials, docetaxel in combination with prednisone showed an increased median survival, PSA response, and quality of life compared with mitoxantrone. Mitoxantrone with prednisone has demonstrated palliative benefits in patients with bone metastases and is generally well tolerated; it may be used as a second-line option for symptomatic patients or as first-line for frailer patients who are poor candidates for docetaxel.

SUPPORTIVE CARE

Bisphosphonates

Bisphosphonates are synthetic analogues of inorganic pyrophosphates with high avidity for calcium and areas of bone mineralization. These compounds have been used for many years to treat disorders associated with bone resorption such as osteoporosis, Paget disease, and metastatic bone disease. Although various bisphosphonates have been tested in multiple clinical trials in the setting of advanced prostate cancer, only zoledronic acid—a potent, intravenous bisphosphonate—has a demonstrated effect on bone metastases in this population. In two placebo-controlled, randomized clinical trials, zoledronic acid decreased the incidence of skeletal events by 25% compared with placebo. Intravenous bisphosphonates are generally well tolerated, though patients should have regular creatinine assessment as renal toxicity is a known, but relatively uncommon, side effect. In addition, recent evidence has linked bisphosphonate use with osteonecrosis of the jaw—a rare but potentially devastating complication, which appears to be most prevalent in patients who have received these drugs over a period of several years. It may be prudent, therefore, for patients to have a dental examination prior to initiating therapy, and clinicians should ask patients regularly about their dental health.

As both increasing age and androgen ablation place men at higher risk of osteoporosis, bisphosphonates may also be useful in prevention of secondary fractures in this population. Even in a study of intermittent androgen blockade, evaluation of BMD in the lumbar spine revealed osteopenia in 46% and osteoporosis in 20% of patients, with similar values seen for the hip. A similar study found that 50% of men on androgen blockade for at least 12 months had asymptomatic vertebral fractures. A recent study of 47 men with hormone-sensitive prostate cancer compared BMD in men receiving the LHRH agonist leuprolide alone to BMD in men receiving the combination of pamidronate and leuprolide. Pamidronate showed significant protection of BMD in the lumbar spine, greater trochanter, and total hip. Although the study was only of 48 weeks duration, it underscored the startling amount of bone loss in patients on LHRH monotherapy for this period: 3.3% in the lumbar spine, 2.1% in the trochanter, and 1.8% in the total hip. As bone is a ready target for prostate cancer metastases as well, bone protection should be paramount, especially in the early stages of the disease. At this time, however, only oral bisphosphonates are FDA approved for the prevention and treatment of osteoporosis.

Pain Control

The majority of men with advanced prostate cancer have bone metastases, which are frequently very painful. Pain control is thus a critical

issue in these patients and needs to be frequently monitored. Bone pain generally responds well to treatment with both nonsteroidal anti-inflammatory drugs and opioids, used alone or in combination. Although some elderly patients are very tolerant of narcotic analgesics, as a rule they should be started on low doses with careful dose titration and individualized treatment plans to achieve maximal analgesia and maintain quality of life. Constipation, the most common side effect of pain medications, should be aggressively addressed, but is generally well controlled with laxatives.

Palliative Radiation and Systemic Radioisotopes

Palliative radiation therapy can provide significant pain relief for symptomatic bony metastases and is also used to prevent impending pathologic fracture, particularly in the femora. Thus, patients with one or two areas of severe bone pain, which is either inadequately controlled with narcotics or which requires unacceptably high doses of narcotics, should be referred to radiation oncology for consultation. Most palliative radiation is given in one to 10 dose fractions, and 80% to 90% of prostate cancer patients who receive palliative radiation for bone metastases experience significant and durable pain relief. The onset of pain relief may be as soon as 48 hours after the initiation of therapy, although some patients will not experience maximal relief for up to 2 weeks after therapy is complete. Systemic radioisotopes such as strontium-89 and samarium-153 deliver high-dose radiation to bone lesions without significantly affecting normal bone and can provide palliative benefit to patients with widespread, painful bone metastases, which are refractory to palliative chemotherapy or narcotic analgesia. These agents generally provide significant pain relief and can be re-administered if needed. They do, however, have the potential to cause significant myelosuppression and thrombocytopenia and should be used cautiously in patients with low baseline blood counts or patients receiving concomitant chemotherapy.

FURTHER READING

Albertson PC et al. The positive yield of imaging studies in the evaluation of men with newly diagnosed prostate cancer: a population-based analysis. *J Urol.* 2000;163:1138.

Albertsen PC, Hanley JA, Fine J. 20-year outcomes following conservative management of clinically localized prostate cancer. *JAMA.* 2005;293(17):2095.

Aus G, Robinson D, Rosell J, et al. South-East Region Prostate Cancer Group. Survival in prostate carcinoma—outcomes from a prospective, population-based cohort of 8887 men with up to 15 years of follow-up: results from three countries in the population-based National Prostate Cancer Registry of Sweden. *Cancer.* 2005;103(5):943.

Carter HB, Ferrucci L, Kettermann A, et al. Detection of life-threatening prostate cancer with prostate-specific antigen velocity during a window of curability. *J Natl Cancer Inst.* 2006;98(21):1521.

Clark L et al. Effects of selenium supplementation for cancer prevention in patients with carcinoma of the skin: a randomized controlled trial. *JAMA.* 1996;276:1957.

Goodman PJ, Thompson IM, Jr, Tangen CM, et al. The prostate cancer prevention trial: design, biases and interpretation of study results. *J Urol.* 2006;175(6):2234.

Hussain M et al. Effects of continued androgen-deprivation therapy and other prognostic factors on response and survival in phase II chemotherapy trials for hormone-refractory prostate cancer: a Southwest Oncology Group report. *J Clin Oncol.* 1994;12:1868.

Keating NL, O'Malley AJ, Smith MR. Diabetes and cardiovascular disease during androgen deprivation therapy for prostate cancer. *J Clin Oncol.* 2006;24(27):4448.

Kirk D. The Medical Research Council Prostate Cancer Working Party Investigators Group. Intermediate versus deferred treatment for advanced prostatic cancer: initial results of the Medical Research Council trial. *Br J Urol.* 1997;79:235.

Lawton CA et al. Updated results of phase III Radiation Therapy Oncology Group (RTOG) trial 85–31 evaluating the potential benefit of androgen suppression following standard radiation therapy for unfavorable prognosis carcinoma of the prostate. *Int J Radiat Oncol Biol Phys.* 2001;49:937.

Lee N et al. Which patients with newly diagnosed prostate cancer need a computed tomography scan of the abdomen and pelvis? An analysis based on 588 patients. *Urology.* 1999;54:490.

Leventis AK et al. Prediction of response to salvage radiation therapy in patients with prostate cancer recurrence after radical prostatectomy. *J Clin Oncol.* 2001;19:1030.

Lippman SM, Goodman PJ, Klein EA, et al. Designing the Selenium and Vitamin E Cancer Prevention Trial (SELECT). *J Natl Cancer Inst.* 2005;97(2):94.

Loberg RD, Logothetis CJ, Keller ET, Pienta KJ. Pathogenesis and treatment of prostate cancer bone metastasis: targeting the lethal phenotype. *J Clin Oncol.* 2005;23(32):8232.

Mohr BA et al. Are serum hormones associated with the risk of prostate cancer? Prospective results from the Massachusetts Male Aging Study. *Urology.* 2001;57:930.

Oesterling JE et al. Serum prostate-specific antigen in a community-based population of healthy men. Establishment of age-specific reference ranges. *JAMA.* 1993;270:860.

Palapattu GS, Sutcliffe S, Bastian PJ, et al. Prostate carcinogenesis and inflammation: emerging insights. *Carcinogenesis.* 2004;26:1170.

Pienta K, Bradley D. Mechanisms underlying the development of androgen-independent prostate cancer. *Clin Cancer Res.* 2006;12(6):1665.

Potosky AL et al. Quality-of-life outcomes after primary androgen deprivation therapy: results from the prostate cancer outcomes study. *J Clin Oncol.* 2001;17:3750.

Saad F, Gleason DM, Murray R, et al. Long-term efficacy of zoledronic acid for the prevention of skeletal complications in patients with metastatic hormone-refractory prostate cancer. Zoledronic Acid Prostate Cancer Study Group. *J Clin Oncol.* 2004;96:1480.

Smith MR et al. Pamidronate to prevent bone loss during androgen deprivation therapy for prostate cancer. *N Engl J Med.* 2001;345:949.

Stanford JL et al. Urinary and sexual function after radical prostatectomy for clinically localized prostate cancer: the Prostate Cancer Outcomes Study. *JAMA.* 2000;283:354.

Tannock IF, de Wit R, Berry WR, et al. Docetaxel plus prednisone or mitoxantrone plus prednisone for advanced prostate cancer. *N Engl J Med.* 2004;351:1502.

Zhou P, Chen MH, McLeod D, et al. Predictors of prostate cancer-specific mortality after radical prostatectomy or radiation therapy. *J Clin Oncol.* 2005;23(28):6992.

Lung Cancer

Daniel Morgensztern ■ *Ramaswamy Govindan* ■ *Michael C. Perry*

EPIDEMIOLOGY

According to American Cancer Society statistics, there will be 232,270 new cases of lung cancer in 2008, accounting for approximately 15% of cancer diagnoses. The likelihood of developing lung cancer is 1 in 2500 in men younger than 39 years of age and 1 in 15 in men between the ages of 60 and 79 years.

The vast majority of patients with lung cancer will still die of the disease. It is estimated that 166,280 patients will die of lung cancer in 2008, accounting for 31% of all cancer deaths in men and 26% of cancer deaths in women. Among women, the rate of deaths from lung cancer remains high. Since 1987, more women have died from lung cancer than from breast cancer. Despite an enormous effort to find effective therapies for lung cancer, the overall 5-year survival remains only 15%. The high mortality rate and low 5-year survival rate are largely the result of an inability to diagnose lung cancer at an early stage, when it is still potentially curable. Only 15% of lung cancers are diagnosed at this early stage. The uniformly poor results obtained with current therapies are a strong argument for the inclusion of all possible patients into clinical trials.

ETIOLOGY

Risk Factors

Tobacco Smoking

Smoking is by far the most common cause of lung cancer. Approximately 85% to 90% of lung cancer cases can be attributed directly to tobacco smoking. The risk of lung cancer is directly related to the length of time a person smokes, the number of cigarettes smoked per day, the age at which a person starts smoking, and the amount of tar contained in the cigarettes. The risk of developing lung cancer is 9- to 10-fold higher in an average smoker and up to 25-fold higher for a heavy smoker. However, not all tobacco smokers develop lung cancer. This may be attributable to differences in an individual's inherited predisposition to cancer development. There is also evidence that nonsmokers exposed to tobacco smoke (passive smokers) have an increased risk of developing lung cancer. It has been estimated that up to 25% of lung cancers in nonsmokers are caused by passive smoking. The risk of lung cancer declines steadily once a person stops smoking, but it takes up to 15 to 20 years for the risk to return to the level of nonsmokers. However, it never reaches this level if they had smoked two packs per day or more.

Other Risk Factors

Other factors reported to cause lung cancer include occupational exposure to arsenic, asbestos, nickel, uranium, chromium, silica, beryllium, and diesel exhaust. Dietary deficiency of vitamins A, C, and E, retinoids, carotenoids, and selenium, and air pollution, lung scars, and oncogenes have all been implicated in the causation of lung cancer. Asbestos is the most common occupational cause of lung cancer and increases the risk of lung cancer fivefold. Tobacco smoking and asbestos exposure act synergistically, and the risk of lung cancer in smokers who have been exposed to asbestos becomes as high as 80-fold to 90-fold higher than the risk in nonsmokers. Radon, produced by the decay of uranium, has a well-established association with lung cancer in underground miners. However, the association between lung cancer and residential exposure to radon is less well established.

SCREENING

Most patients with lung cancer present with advanced-stage disease, when the outcome is dismal. Therefore, there has been an interest in screening high-risk people to detect lung cancers when they are smaller and presumably at earlier and more curable stages. Earlier trials using chest radiography, cytologic examination of the sputum, or both, however, failed to decrease the disease-specific mortality. These trials have been criticized for their study design, statistical analysis, contamination, and older forms of technology. With the development of newer imaging technology, specifically low-dose spiral CT scans, there has been a new interest in screening for lung cancer. The International Early Lung Cancer Action Program screened 31,567 asymptomatic patients, with 27,456 repeat screenings and found lung cancer in 484 participants. Of these, 85% had stage I disease with an estimated 10-year survival rate of 88%. Although intriguing, this study has been criticized on methodological grounds. Another longitudinal study of 3246 asymptomatic patients from three centers found 144 lung cancers, compared to 44.5 expected cases. There was no evidence of a decline in the number of diagnoses of advanced lung cancers.

In addition to the overdiagnosis of small tumors detected during screening, which could otherwise remain silent until the patient dies from other causes, screening for lung cancer with spiral CT scan could potentially cause harm secondary to morbidity and mortality associated with thoracotomy, since lung tumors appear as noncalcified nodules and only a small fraction of those nodules actually represent lung cancer. The ongoing National Lung Cancer Screening Trial is carefully studying the role of CT scans in the screening of lung cancer in patients with a strong history of tobacco smoking. The issues of lead-time bias and additional morbidity and mortality are particularly relevant in the population of older adults in whom competing causes of death and multiple comorbidities are frequently encountered. At the present time, we do not believe there is enough evidence to recommend CT screening for lung cancer outside the context of clinical trial.

With better understanding of the molecular pathology of lung cancer, an interesting area of research is to examine the utility of molecular and genetic biomarkers in screening high-risk people. Because cancer is a multistep process, identification of these biomarkers in the sputum of high-risk individuals may help to identify the early clonal phase of progression of lung cancer. If this becomes reality, then it may enable detection of cancers earlier than with spiral CT. It could also be complementary to spiral CT screening.

PATHOLOGY

Based on the light microscopic features, lung cancers are divided into two major groups: small-cell lung cancer (SCLC) and non–small-cell lung cancer (NSCLC). The later include squamous cell carcinoma, adenocarcinoma, and large-cell carcinoma (Table 97-1).

TABLE 97-1

Most Common Histological Subtypes of Lung Cancer
Small-cell carcinoma
Adenocarcinoma
Squamous cell carcinoma
Large-cell carcinoma
Adenosquamous carcinoma
Undifferentiated carcinoma

Bronchoalveolar carcinoma is subclassified under adenocarcinoma. The distinction between small- and non–small-cell histology is important clinically, because small-cell histology is more aggressive and more responsive to chemotherapy and radiation.

In the past, the most common histology was squamous cell carcinoma, which accounted for 40% of lung cancers. However, now in the United States only 20% to 25% of lung cancers are squamous cell cancers. Squamous cell carcinoma is the classic lung cancer—central in location, endobronchial in nature, sometimes with central cavitation, and commonly associated with lobar collapse, obstructive pneumonia, or hemoptysis, with late development of distant metastases. On the other hand, adenocarcinomas, which in earlier times constituted 20% to 25% of all lung cancers, are now the most prevalent histology, accounting for almost 40% of all lung cancers. This increase in prevalence has been greater in North America than in Europe, where squamous cell cancer is still the most common type. Changes in smoking habits and other environmental factors are thought to account for this shift in histology.

Adenocarcinoma is not as strongly associated with smoking as other types of carcinomas and is the most common type in nonsmokers. It is characterized by the early development of metastases, even when tumor still appears to be a solitary lesion. Adenocarcinoma is most frequently a peripheral lung lesion and is commonly accompanied by a malignant pleural effusion.

The incidence of squamous cell carcinoma rises with increasing age, while that of adenocarcinoma falls. This, in combination with the fact that elderly patients seem to have more localized disease at presentation, correlates with a greater likelihood that older patients will have resectable and thus potentially curable disease.

Bronchoalveolar carcinomas and large-cell carcinomas are less common. The former is either unifocal or multifocal, which can mimic pneumonia. It may be detected in the setting of prior fibrotic lung disease, such as idiopathic pulmonary fibrosis, scleroderma, or asbestosis. Large-cell carcinomas account for approximately 10% of all lung cancers. The lesions are usually peripheral and sometime cavitate because of necrosis. Small-cell carcinomas account for approximately 20% of all lung cancers. Among all the lung cancer types, they have the strongest association with smoking. These commonly form central masses and grow rapidly, with a tendency to early metastasis. Rarely, tumors contain two histologies.

CLINICAL PRESENTATION

The initial clinical presentation of lung cancer patients is variable. Patients may seek medical attention for symptoms related to the primary tumor, mediastinal disease, distant metastases, or paraneoplastic syndromes (Table 97-2). In advanced cases, patients may present with systemic signs of anorexia, weight loss, fatigue, and weakness. Symptoms related to the primary tumor depend upon the location of the tumor: central or peripheral. Central tumors produce cough, dyspnea, hoarseness, stridor, hemoptysis, and postobstructive pneumonia. Superior sulcus tumors may produce shoulder pain, arm pain, or brachial plexopathy, or Horner syndrome. Peripheral lesions may cause pleuritic chest pain suggesting pleural involvement. Symptoms related to mediastinal disease include hoarseness caused by the involvement of left recurrent laryngeal nerve with left-sided tumors and obstruction of the superior vena cava with right-sided tumors

TABLE 97-2

Clinical Presentation of Lung Cancer

LOCAL	INTRATHORACIC SPREAD	EXTRATHORACIC SPREAD	PARANEOPLASTIC
Cough	Chest wall pain	Abdominal pain	Clubbing
Chest pain	Dysphagia	Bone pain	Cushing syndrome
Dyspnea	Hoarseness	Headaches	Hypercalcemia
Hemoptysis	Pleural effusion	Jaundice	Hypertrophic osteoarthropathy
	SVC obstruction	Lymphadenopathy	Lambert–Eaton syndrome
		Paralysis	SIADH
		Seizures	

or associated lymphadenopathy. Less common features include dysphagia caused by esophageal obstruction and hypotension caused by pericardial tamponade. Direct involvement of the myocardium is rare, although pericardial effusions are sometimes seen and may produce severe dyspnea and refractory hypotension. Phrenic nerve involvement leads to paralysis of the ipsilateral diaphragm, most commonly seen as elevation of the affected diaphragm on a plain chest radiograph.

Metastases from lung cancer are common. Sites of spread include the brain, pleural cavity, bone, liver, adrenal glands, and contralateral lung. Because more than half of patients have metastases at presentation, initial symptoms related to a metastatic site are frequent, particularly in patients with adenocarcinoma or small-cell carcinoma.

PARANEOPLASTIC SYNDROMES

Although lung cancer is associated with a variety of paraneoplastic syndromes, presentation with symptoms related to a paraneoplastic syndrome is uncommon. Apart from hypercalcemia and hypertrophic pulmonary osteoarthropathy that are associated with squamous cell carcinoma, all others are linked to SCLCs. These include the syndrome of inappropriate secretion of antidiuretic hormone (SIADH), Cushing syndrome, and various neurological syndromes such as Eaton–Lambert reverse myasthenia syndrome, encephalitis, subacute sensory neuropathy, opsoclonus and myoclonus, cerebellar degeneration, and limbic degeneration. Hypercoagulability resulting in deep venous thrombosis is common in advanced lung cancers, particularly adenocarcinoma. Occasionally, lung cancers are diagnosed during work-up of patients with dermatomyositis or membranous glomerulonephritis.

DIAGNOSIS

An accurate diagnosis with proper distinction between SCLC and the various non-small-cell types is essential before any further staging work-up can be performed. A change in the usual symptoms of cough and dyspnea in a chronic smoker is often an indication for a chest x-ray, which if abnormal, leads to further evaluation. Because benign and other malignant conditions can mimic lung cancer on radiologic studies, histological confirmation of the diagnosis is essential. Depending on the location of the tumor, this can be achieved through examination of sputum cytology, fiberoptic bronchoscopy, or transthoracic biopsy.

Sputum cytology is a cost-effective and easy way of reaching a diagnosis. The yield is high for endobronchial lesions such as small-cell tumors and squamous cell carcinomas, but it is low for peripheral lesions of adenocarcinoma and large-cell carcinoma. The false-positive rate for cytology is less than 1%, but the false-negative rate is 41% to 43%. A cytological specimen that is positive for malignancy is accurate in approximately 90% of cases, but the distinction between individual histologic types is not as accurate, and discordant results are often seen between cytology and histology bronchoscopy and needle-biopsy specimens.

In contrast, fiberoptic bronchoscopy provides direct visualization of the bronchial tree, and diagnostic material can be obtained with bronchial brushings, washings, and biopsy of the directly visualized tumor, or with a transbronchial biopsy. Fiberoptic bronchoscopy is well tolerated by elderly patients, and age alone should not exclude an appropriate diagnostic evaluation. For tumors not visualized, the yield for washing and brushing is approximately 75% in central lesions and 55% in peripheral lesions. Therefore, the yield in small-cell and squamous cell carcinomas is higher than in adenocarcinomas and large-cell carcinomas.

Percutaneous fine-needle aspiration of a lung lesion gives a high yield (more than 85%), with a high accuracy for histological subtype. This technique is very useful to establish a diagnosis for peripheral lesions and in patients who are not surgical candidates for an open thoracotomy. One deterrent for performing percutaneous fine-needle aspiration is the risk of inducing iatrogenic pneumothorax; however, chest tube placement is required only in approximately 5% of patients. The same technique is used in obtaining tissue from metastatic sites such as supraclavicular lymph nodes, adrenal glands, and liver. In patients with a classic solitary lesion that is surgically resectable, many times a diagnosis is made after a thoracotomy. This is because the management of the lesion is unlikely to be changed if a percutaneous biopsy is performed first. In patients with a pleural effusion, either cytological examination of the pleural fluid or, if that is inconclusive, thoracoscopic biopsy of pleural lesions is the method of obtaining a biopsy material. An additional method of obtaining a tissue is mediastinoscopy.

Staging

Following the diagnosis of lung cancer, patients should be evaluated for the presence of spreading to regional lymph nodes or distant organs. Adequate staging of lung cancer provides important prognostic information and is one of the most important determinants of the optimal treatment for each individual patient. The staging system for patients with NSCLC is the TNM staging, which takes into account the degree of involvement by the primary tumor (T), the extent of lymph node involvement (N), and the presence or absence of distant spread (metastasis, M). Although the TNM system can be used to stage SCLC, the high propensity for early metastasis led to the development of a more practical staging system, which divides these tumors into limited disease or extensive disease. Limited disease is defined as a tumor that can be encompassed within a single and tolerable radiation port and any spreading to sites beyond the definition of limited-stage disease is classified as extensive disease.

In the assessment of metastatic spread, the history and physical examination are the most helpful tests, supplemented by liver function tests. Chest CT provides information about the primary tumor as well as about the lymph node status of the mediastinum. The abdominal CT is used to examine the liver and adrenal glands. Magnetic resonance imaging (MRI) of the chest and abdomen does not appear to improve the accuracy of staging. Brain CT or MRI scan is indicated in all patients with SCLC and selected patients with NSCLC, including patients with stage III disease planned to receive chemoradiotherapy and those with neurological symptoms. Likewise, radionuclide bone scanning is only recommended in patients with symptoms of bone metastases, elevated alkaline phosphatase, or hypercalcemia. The yield of bone scans in asymptomatic patients is very low. Other invasive staging procedures employed in the staging of lung cancer include mediastinotomy and video-assisted thoracoscopy.

Metabolic Staging

Noninvasive staging with CT scan is not very accurate in predicting the presence and absence of metastatic disease. This anatomic staging is dependent on the size of the underlying lymph nodes, which, when enlarged, could be reactive in pathology. On the other hand, CT scans can miss metastatic disease in a normal-sized lymph node. In a series of 102 patients, it was reported that CT scan has a sensitivity of 75% and a specificity of 66% for mediastinal staging for nodal disease. In a large meta-analysis, the overall sensitivity and specificity of CT scan were 60% and 77%, respectively. In these situations, the gold standard is to subject all potentially resectable patients to invasive procedures such as mediastinoscopy, mediastinotomy, and video-assisted thoracoscopy. With the advent of positron emission tomogram (PET) scanning, it is now possible to use metabolic staging whenever there is suspicion of occult metastases in the mediastinum or elsewhere. PET uses fluorodeoxyglucose (FDG) as a tracer with the underlying knowledge that there is increased glucose metabolism in tumor cells. FDG, a glucose analogue labeled with a positron emitter, concentrates in the tumor cells and is trapped because it does not proceed along the usual metabolic pathways. A PET scanner then picks up the tissue distribution. A higher concentration in the tumor could be easily observed on a computer-generated image. Despite some limitations, PET scan is more sensitive (91%) and specific (86%) than a CT scan.

The American Society of Clinical Oncology (ASCO) currently recommends the use of FDG-PET scan in patients without evidence of metastatic disease in the chest CT. Furthermore, owing to the high negative predictive value of FDG-PET scan, which is typically above 90%, patients without enlarged mediastinal lymph nodes in the CT scan and no increased uptake by FDG-PET may not require staging mediastinoscopy.

Sixty to seventy percent of patients with SCLC have extensive-stage disease at presentation.

PROGNOSTIC FACTORS

For all lung cancers, the most consistent prognostic factor is the extent (stage) of disease and the performance status, measured by either the Zubrod or the Karnofsky scale. Simply stated, ambulatory patients (Zubrod scores of 0, 1, and 2, or Karnofsky scores of 70% or higher) survive longer than do nonambulatory patients. For patients with NSCLC, advanced disease stage and unintentional weight loss greater than 10% in the last 6 months are adverse prognostic indicators. For SCLC patients, extensive stage, male sex, increased age, elevated serum lactic acid dehydrogenase, elevated serum alkaline phosphatase, and hyponatremia are significant adverse prognostic indicators.

TREATMENT OF NON–SMALL-CELL LUNG CANCER

Stage I (T1N0, T2N0)

Stage I patients are best treated by surgical resection with the aim of cure. The standard surgical procedure in fit patients consists of at least lobectomy. Despite undergoing surgery with curative intent, the 5-year overall survival is approximately 60% for clinical stage IA and 38% for stage IB. Current data do not support the use of chemotherapy in patients with resected stage I NSCLC.

In patients who are medically unfit for curative resection, primary radiotherapy offers a cure rate of approximately 25%. This option is commonly used in elderly patients who may have comorbid conditions making them high risk for surgery. In a single report of patients older than 70 years who had resectable lesions smaller than 4 cm but who were medically inoperable or who refused surgery, survival at 5 years following radiation therapy with curative intent was comparable to a historical control group of patients of similar age resected with curative intent. In the two largest retrospective radiation therapy series, patients with inoperable disease treated with definitive radiation therapy achieved 5-year survival rates of 10% and 27%. Both series found that patients with T1N0 tumors had better outcomes, with 5-year survival rates of 60% and 32% in this subgroup. Primary radiation therapy should consist of approximately 6000 cGy. Careful treatment planning with precise definition of target volume and avoidance of critical normal structures to the extent possible is needed for optimal results and requires the use of a simulator. Stereotactic radiosurgery is becoming increasingly popular for the treatment of appropriately located small lesions in patients who are not candidates for surgery owing to comorbid conditions. Another option for patients who cannot undergo proper cancer surgery is wedge resection; however, despite achieving negative margins, the local failure rate is very high.

Stage II (T1N1, T2N1, T3N0)

These patients are also treated by surgical resection with a curative intent. The types of surgical procedures considered standard care are lobectomy or pneumonectomy. However, the 5-year survival rate is worse than stage I with 5-year survival ranging from 39% to 55%. Various attempts have been made to improve the cure rate with the use of postoperative radiation therapy or chemotherapy. In a large randomized trial of adjuvant radiation therapy in early-stage lung cancer, despite a decrease in local recurrence, there was no effect on the overall survival of the patients. A large meta-analysis of randomized clinical trials found that adjuvant radiation after curative resection was detrimental to patient survival. Cisplatin-based adjuvant chemotherapy improves survival in patients with resected stage II NSCLC.

Patients with inoperable stage II disease but with sufficient pulmonary reserve may be considered for radiation therapy with curative intent. Among patients with excellent performance status, up to a 20% 3-year survival rate may be expected if a course of radiation therapy with curative intent can be completed. In the largest retrospective series reported to date, 152 patients with medically inoperable NSCLC treated with definitive radiation therapy achieved a 5-year overall survival rate of 10%; however, the 44 patients with T1 tumors achieved an actuarial disease-free survival rate of 60%. This retrospective study also suggested that improved disease-free survival was obtained with radiation therapy doses greater than 6000 cGy.

Stage IIIA (T3N1, T1–3N2)

Stage IIIA is a heterogeneous group of tumors that can be broadly classified into three distinct subgroups; incidental IIIA, potentially resectable IIIA, and bulky or unresectable IIIA. Patients with incidentally diagnosed stage IIIA at the time of thoracotomy should receive adjuvant chemotherapy. The role of adjuvant radiation in this setting is not clearly defined. A large intergroup study conducted in North America did not find any improvement in survival with the addition of surgery following chemotherapy and radiation in patients with resectable stage III NSCLC. However, patients with limited mediastinal lymph node involvement and excellent lung function who are likely to need only lobectomy (and not pneumonectomy) may be considered for neoadjuvant chemoradiotherapy followed by surgical resection. For those with bulky mediastinal adenopathy, the recommended treatment is the combination of chemotherapy and radiation, preferably given concurrently. Patients with poor performance status may be treated with sequential chemotherapy and radiotherapy or either modality alone.

Stage IIIB (T4N0, any TN3)

While selected patients with stage IIIB because of T4 extension other than malignant pleural effusion may be treated surgically with curative intent, patients with contralateral mediastinal or supraclavicular involvement are not surgical candidates and should be treated with chemotherapy and radiation. Patients with stage IIIB NSCLC and malignant pleural effusion are incurable and should be treated as stage IV, with chemotherapy alone for palliation.

Stage IV (any T, any N, M1)

Patients with stage IV NSCLC are treated with chemotherapy (Table 97-3), which improves survival compared with best supportive care. Typical results from randomized clinical trials of combination chemotherapy in this setting include response rates of approx-

TABLE 97-3

Chemotherapy Agents Commonly Used in Non–Small-Cell Lung Cancer

FIRST-LINE	SECOND-LINE
Platinum agent	Docetaxel
Cisplatin	Pemetrexed
Carboplatin	Erlotinib
Taxane	
Docetaxel	
Paclitaxel	
Gemcitabine	
Vinorelbine	

imately 30%, median survival times of 8 to 9 months, and 1-year survivals of 35%. Bevacizumab, a vascular endothelium growth factor inhibitor, recently demonstrated survival benefit when combined with standard chemotherapy in a randomized trial, with a median survival of greater than 12 months. Early studies, however, showed increased risk of fatal hemoptysis in patients with centrally located tumors, squamous cell carcinoma histology, and previous history of hemoptysis. Therefore, the addition of bevacizumab to chemotherapy represents the new standard of care in stage IV NSCLC in the patients without these risk factors. Since the disease is incurable, virtually every patient with metastatic NSCLC will develop progressive disease. Several randomized studies have already shown survival benefit from second-line therapy. Several molecularly targeted therapies are being studied in NSCLC. Epidermal growth factor receptor tyrosine kinase inhibitors such as gefitinib and erlotinib have been associated with striking response in patients who are lifelong never smokers with NSCLC. In a randomized study, erlotinib improved survival over best supportive care in unselected group of patients (smokers and nonsmokers) with advanced NSCLC who had progressive disease following initial therapy. Approved therapies in this setting include docetaxel, pemetrexed, and erlotinib.

Patients with solitary metastasis to the brain or adrenal gland may be candidates for curative resection.

Radiation therapy may be effective in palliating symptomatic local involvement from NSCLC such as tracheal, esophageal, or bronchial compression, bone or brain metastases, pain, vocal cord paralysis, or hemoptysis. In some cases, endobronchial laser therapy and/or brachytherapy have been used to alleviate proximal obstructing lesions. Such therapeutic intervention is important in maintaining the quality of life of the patient. In the rare patient with synchronous presentation of a resectable primary tumor in the lung and a single brain metastasis, surgical resection of the solitary brain lesion is indicated with resection of the primary tumor and appropriate postoperative chemotherapy and/or irradiation of the primary tumor site and with postoperative whole-brain irradiation delivered in daily fractions of 180 cGy to 200 cGy to avoid long-term toxic effects to normal brain tissue.

Aging is usually associated with decreased marrow reserve and renal function as well as the development of accumulative comorbidities. Consequently, elderly patients frequently undergo less aggressive therapy and are commonly excluded from clinical trials. Several retrospective studies, however, demonstrated benefit from chemotherapy over best supportive care in this patient population. Recent studies have demonstrated that age by itself should not be a determinant to guide the therapeutic decision in patients with lung cancer. Elderly patients with good performance status and no significant comorbidities should be considered for aggressive therapy including surgical resection, chemoradiotherapy, and combination chemotherapy when appropriate.

SMALL-CELL LUNG CANCER

SCLC is the most aggressive type of lung cancer, and without therapy, the median survival is only 6 to 12 weeks. Though initially very sensitive to chemotherapy and radiation, relapse of the disease is very common (Table 97-4). The combination of platinum and etoposide continues to be the standard therapy for now nearly three decades.

Patients with limited disease are typically treated with cisplatin, etoposide, and concurrent thoracic radiation. Because radiation is very effective in small-cell lung patients, earlier investigators wondered whether thoracic radiation could be combined with systemic chemotherapy. Randomized trials have shown improved survival with addition of radiation to chemotherapy in patients with limited-stage without the development of unacceptable toxicity. This benefit is usually greater, if the radiation is administered during the first several cycles of therapy. A meta-analysis of trials comparing chemotherapy alone with combined chemotherapy and thoracic radiotherapy found that combined treatment improved survival among patients with limited-stage SCLC. Cisplatin and etoposide have largely supplanted the older regimens of cyclophosphamide, doxorubicin, and vincristine because of the absence of toxic side effects on intrathoracic organs and the ability to use concurrent thoracic radiation. Surgery in limited-stage SCLC is only performed when a peripheral lung nodule is surgically resected for presumed NSCLC. Even these patients are further treated with systemic chemotherapy with or without thoracic radiation. On the other hand, patients with extensive-stage disease are usually treated with four cycles of etoposide with either cisplatin or carboplatin.

The response rates to combination chemotherapy are high, up to 75% to 80% in extensive-stage disease and 85% to 95% in limited-stage disease, with complete responses in 20% to 25% and 50% to 60%, respectively. The duration of chemotherapy treatment is typically four to six cycles. The median survival is 7 to 10 months in extensive-stage and 14 to 20 months for limited-stage patients. Patients with limited-stage disease have a 2-year survival of 20% to 30% and those with extensive-stage have 2-year survival rates of 5% to 10%.

SCLC has a high propensity for brain metastases. The actuarial risk of developing brain metastases in patients with limited-stage lung cancer whose disease is controlled with combination therapy is 60% in the next 2 to 3 years. Many times the brain is the only site of metastases. Prophylactic cranial irradiation (PCI) decreases the risk of clinically apparent lesions in the brain by more than 50% with doses of 2400 cGy. A meta-analysis of seven randomized trials evaluating the value of PCI in patients in complete remission reported improvement in brain recurrence, disease-free survival, and overall survival with the addition of PCI. The 3-year overall survival was improved from 15% to 21% with PCI. PCI is now the standard therapy in patients with limited-stage disease who have a complete response to thoracic radiation and systemic chemotherapy. A European study recently demonstrated a near twofold increase in 1-year survival with the addition of PCI following chemotherapy in patients with extensive-stage disease who achieve a good response or stable disease.

The standard second-line therapy is topotecan, which was found to be as effective as CAV but with less toxicity. Patients with progression-free interval greater than 3 months are called chemotherapy sensitive and have better probability of response to second-line therapy. Patients with no initial response or progression within 3 months from the last cycle of first-line therapy are called chemotherapy refractory and have poor response to available chemotherapy agents.

Fear of increased toxicity from chemotherapy in elderly patients led some physicians to avoid combination therapy in these patients. Until recently, oral etoposide as a single agent was considered to be both well tolerated and effective in SCLC, with an overall response rate of 79% and a complete response rate of 17%. However, studies by the Medical Research Council Lung Cancer Working Party and the London Lung Cancer Study group compared single-agent etoposide with standard combination chemotherapy. Both trials found that oral etoposide was inferior to standard intravenous combination chemotherapy with fewer responses, a worse quality of life, and worse survival.

SPECIAL PROBLEMS

Pancoast (Superior Sulcus) Tumors

Pancoast tumors are carcinomas that develop peripherally in the apex of the lungs and invade the superior sulcus. They are a unique category of tumors that are locally invasive with a reduced tendency for distant metastases. Typically they cause symptoms of pain in the shoulder and along the vertebral border of the scapula and down the arm. As they extend into the thoracic inlet, they invade the sympathetic chain and stellate ganglion, causing Horner syndrome. If the tumor is relatively confined and there is no evidence of distant spread, the treatment is local with curative potential, especially for T3N0 disease. Radiation therapy alone, radiation therapy preceded or followed by surgery, or surgery alone (in highly selected cases) may be curative in some patients, with a 5-year survival rate of 20% or more in some studies. The best results have been achieved with a combination of chemotherapy and concurrent radiation therapy. Patients with more invasive tumors of this area, or true Pancoast tumors, have a worse prognosis and generally do not benefit from primary surgical management. Follow-up surgery may be used to

---

TABLE 97-4

Chemotherapy of Small-Cell Lung Cancer

FIRST-LINE	SECOND-LINE
Cisplatin and etoposide	Topotecan
Carboplatin and etoposide	Irinotecan
Cisplatin and irinotecan	Gemcitabine
Cyclophosphamide, doxorubicin,	Oral etoposide
and vincristine (CAV)	CAV

verify complete response in the radiation therapy field and to resect necrotic tissue.

Chest Wall Tumors

Selected patients with bulky primary tumors that directly invade the chest wall can obtain long-term survival with surgical management provided that their tumor is completely resected. Standard treatment options include surgery, radiation, surgery and radiation, and chemotherapy combined with other modalities.

Superior Vena Cava Syndrome

Approximately 80% of cases of the superior vena cava syndrome are caused by malignancy and carcinoma of the lung, particularly small-cell carcinoma, which accounts for the majority of these cases. The syndrome consists of edema of the face and neck with dilated veins in the neck and upper torso. Although considered by some to be a medical emergency, this is, in fact, only an urgency. If the patient's condition permits, a rapid search for histologic confirmation of the diagnosis should be sought (as above), followed by appropriate treatment. If the patient is clearly deteriorating, urgent radiation therapy is appropriate, followed by diagnostic evaluation at a subsequent time.

Solitary Brain Metastases

Patients who present with a solitary cerebral metastasis after resection of a primary NSCLC lesion and who have no evidence of extracranial tumor can achieve prolonged disease-free survival with surgical excision of the brain metastasis and postoperative whole-brain irradiation. Unresectable brain metastases in this setting may be treated with radiosurgery. Because of the small potential for long-term survival, radiation therapy should be delivered by conventional methods in daily doses of 180 to 200 cGy, while higher daily doses over a shorter period of time (hypofractionated schemes) should be avoided because of the high risk of toxic effects observed with such treatments. Patients, including elderly ones, who are not suitable for surgical resection should receive conventional whole-brain radiation therapy. Selected patients with good performance status and small metastases can be considered for stereotactic radiosurgery. Approximately one-half of patients treated with resection and postoperative radiation therapy will develop recurrence in the brain; some of these patients will be suitable for additional treatment. In those selected patients with good performance status and without progressive metastases outside of the brain, treatment options include reoperation or stereotactic radiosurgery. For most patients, additional radiation therapy can be considered; however, the palliative benefit of this treatment is limited.

SUPPORTIVE CARE

All lung cancer treatments produce some degree of adverse effects in every patient; therefore, supportive care has become an important aspect of cancer management. Irrespective of whether patients undergo surgery, radiation, or chemotherapy, they all will experience a decline in their nutritional status. This is more pronounced in patients who are elderly and those who are treated with combined modality therapy. It is therefore imperative that all such patients receive proper nutritional support. There should be a low threshold for involving clinical dietitians in cancer management. Many patients have anorexia and weight loss because of their advanced cancer. These patients should be offered medroxyprogesterone or prednisone, which are beneficial in such circumstances.

Two of the major side effects of systemic chemotherapy are nausea and vomiting. Cisplatin, the most commonly used chemotherapeutic drug in lung cancer, is highly emetogenic. However, with prophylactic doses of dexamethasone and $5HT_3$ antagonists (ondansetron and granisetron), severe nausea and vomiting are now seldom seen. Even delayed nausea and vomiting are now controlled with dexamethasone and lorazepam. All patients should be kept well hydrated while nausea and vomiting are being treated. Mucositis is frequently seen in patients receiving thoracic radiation with or without systemic chemotherapy. Amifostine is now used as an adjunctive drug in these situations, but it may not influence esophagitis.

Infections caused by the disease itself or by myelosuppression from chemotherapy should be treated aggressively with appropriate antibiotics. The use of colony-stimulating factors in selected patients may decrease the severity and shorten the duration of neutropenia. The American Society of Clinical Oncology now supports the use of colony stimulating factors in elderly patients who are high risk for the development of neutropenic fever.

Anemia is a major issue in patients on systemic chemotherapy. Those who receive radiation concurrently are at higher risk for developing symptomatic anemia. A number of studies have demonstrated that weakness and fatigue associated with chemotherapy negatively affect the quality of life and that such symptoms may improve with correction of anemia. Recombinant erythropoietin is now commonly used in this subset of patients and has made a significant impact on patients' well being.

Pain control is probably the most important aspect of supportive care in cancer patients (see Chapter 53). All patients experiencing pain should be on appropriate pain medications. The judicious use of long-acting narcotic analgesics with short-acting agents for breakthrough pain and adjuvant drugs such as nonsteroidal anti-inflammatory drugs and amitriptyline goes a long way toward promoting a sense of well being and improving performance status.

A cancer diagnosis has a major impact of the psychological state of patient and their family. Psychosocial issues, financial concerns, and family stress are all best managed by physicians, nurses, social workers, and dietitians working as a team. Thus, cancer is now a multidisciplinary disease, and coordination and communication between all members of the team are essential.

FURTHER READING

Bach PB, Jett JR, Pastorino U, Tockman MS, Swensen SJ, Begg CB. Computed tomography screening and lung cancer outcomes. *JAMA*. 2007;297:953–961.

Beckels M, Spiro SG, Colice GL, et al. The physiological evaluation of patients with lung cancer being evaluated for resectional surgery. *Chest*. 2003;123:105S–114S.

Berlangeri SU, Scott AM. Metabolic staging of lung cancer. *N Engl J Med*. 2000;343:290.

Dosoretz D, Katin MJ, Blitzer PH, Dosoretz D, et al. Radiation therapy in the management of medically inoperable carcinoma of the lung: results and implications for future treatment strategies. *Int J Radiat Oncol Biol Phys*. 1992;24(1):3.

Furuta M, Hayakawa K, Katano S, et al. Radiation therapy for stage I–II non–small-cell lung cancer in patients aged 75 years and older. *Jpn J Clin Oncol*. 1996;26(2):95.

Gridelli C. Lung cancer in the elderly. *J Clin Oncol*. 2007;25:1898–1907.

Hoffman PC, Mauer AM, Vokes EE. Lung cancer. *Lancet*. 2000;355:479–485.

International Early Lung Cancer Action Program Investigators. Survival of patients with stage I lung cancer detected on CT screening. *N Engl J Med.* 2006;355: 1763–1761.

Jemal A, Siegel R, Ward E, Murray T, Xu J, Thun MJ. Cancer statistics, 2007. *CA Cancer J Clin.* 2007;57:43–66.

Johnson DH. Small-cell lung cancer in the elderly patient. *Semin Oncol.* 1997;24: 484.

Lally BE, Urbanic JJ, Blackstock AW, et al. Small cell lung cancer: have we learned anything in the last 25 years? *Oncologist.* 2007;12(9):1096–104.

Lee-Chiong TL, Jr, Matthay RA. Lung cancer in the elderly patient. *Clin Chest Med.* 1993;14(3):453.

Makrantonakis PD. Non-small cell lung cancer in the elderly. *Oncologist.* 2004;9:556–560.

Mountain CF. Revisions in the international system for staging lung cancer. *Chest.* 1997;111(6):1711.

Mulshine JL, Sullivan DC. Lung cancer screening. *N Engl J Med.* 2005;352:2714–2720.

Noda K, Nishiwaki Y, Kawahara M, et al. Irinotecan plus cisplatin compared with etoposide plus cisplatin for extensive small cell-lung cancer. *N Engl J Med.* 2002;346:85–91.

Perry MC, Eaton WL, Propert KJ, et al. Chemotherapy with or without radiation therapy in limited small-cell carcinoma of the lung. *N Engl J Med.* 1987;316(15):912–918.

Pfister DG et al. American Society of Clinical Oncology treatment of unresectable non-small cell lung cancer guideline: update 2003. *J Clin Oncol.* 2004;22:330–353.

Pisters KM, Le Chevalier T. Adjuvant chemotherapy in completely resected non-small-cell lung cancer. *J Clin Oncol.* 2005;23:3270–3278.

Robinson LA et al. Treatment of stage IIIA non-small cell lung cancer. *Chest.* 2003;123:202S–220S.

Sandler A, Gray R, Perry MC, et al. Paclitaxel-carboplatin alone or with bevacizumab for non-small-cell lung cancer. *N Engl J Med.* 2006;55:2542–2550.

Shepherd FA, Amdemichael E, Evans WK, et al. Treatment of small-cell lung cancer in the elderly. *J Am Geriatr Soc.* 1994;42(1):64–70.

Shepherd FA, Rodrigues Pereira J, Cluleanu T, et al. Erlotinib in previously treated non-small cell lung cancer. *N Engl J Med.* 2005;353:123–132.

Sone S, Takashima S, Li F, Yang Z, et al. Mass screening for lung cancer with mobile spiral computed tomography scanner. *Lancet.* 1998;351:1242–1245.

Spira A, Ettinger DS. Multidisciplinary management of lung cancer. *New Engl J Med.* 2004;350:379–392.

Gastrointestinal Malignancies

Nadine A. Jackson ■ *Peter C. Enzinger*

INTRODUCTION

Gastrointestinal cancers are primarily diseases of persons in their sixth, seventh, and eighth decade of life. Both incidence and mortality of gastrointestinal cancers increase with advancing age (Figures 98-1 and 98-2). Many elderly persons, however, have additional medical problems that almost certainly contribute to this inferior outcome. This chapter will explore the epidemiology, presentation, treatment options, and disparities in the care of older persons with gastrointestinal malignances.

In general, the symptoms and presentation of gastrointestinal cancers in older individuals appear similar to those of persons of younger age. Although treatments for these cancers have been developed primarily in younger patients, greater expertise over time has permitted similarly safe and efficacious therapy to be extended to older age groups. Since the greatest percentage of gastrointestinal cancers are located in the colon and rectum, most of the information regarding older persons focuses on colorectal cancer. Unfortunately, there is a paucity of information concerning the treatment of elderly patients with other gastrointestinal malignancies. In this chapter, gastrointestinal malignancies are ordered by incidence in the U.S. population.

COLORECTAL CANCER

Colorectal cancer accounts for approximately 10% of all new cancer cases and 10% of all cancer-related deaths in the United States. In fact, colorectal cancer causes more deaths than prostate cancer in men 60 to 79 years of age and more deaths than breast cancer in women 80 years or older. In 2008, 108,070 new cases of colon cancer and 40,740 new cases of rectal cancer will be diagnosed. The probability of developing colorectal cancer increases from 0.07% in the first four decades of life to 4.3% for females and to 4.8% for males in the

seventh decade of life. Although the 5-year relative survival (66%) with this cancer is identical for persons younger than 65 and for persons 65 to 74 years, it declines to 60% for individuals 75 years or older (Figure 98-3 and Figure 98-4).

Six out of seven studies suggest that elderly patients present at the time of diagnosis with the same probabilities of having localized and advanced colon cancer as younger patients. In randomized studies, elderly patients are reported to have the same performance status and incidence of tumor-related symptoms as younger patients, but tend to have more disease-related weight loss. Older patients also appear to have a greater incidence of right-sided (proximal) tumors and higher rates of obstruction and perforation. This in turn results in a greater likelihood of acute presentations, leading to a higher perioperative mortality rate in this older age group.

While some investigators have noted that overall survival is shorter in elderly patients, this difference is not significant if non-cancer deaths are excluded. In fact, comorbid illnesses account for a substantial number of deaths among older patients with colorectal cancer. In one study of 29,733 patients 67 years and older with localized colorectal cancer in the Surveillance, Epidemiology and End Results (SEER)/Medicare database, congestive heart failure, chronic obstructive pulmonary disease, and diabetes mellitus accounted for 9.4%, 5.3%, and 3.9% of deaths, respectively.

Risk Factors of Colorectal Cancer

As in younger individuals, most older persons have no clearly defined risk factors for the development of their colorectal cancer. Hereditary syndromes, such as familial adenomatosis polyposis or hereditary nonpolyposis colorectal cancer, have less impact in this older age group, since the majority of cases are diagnosed before the age of 65 years. There is one risk factor specific to men who were curatively treated with radiation for localized prostate cancer. These men have a 70% increased risk of developing cancer in previously

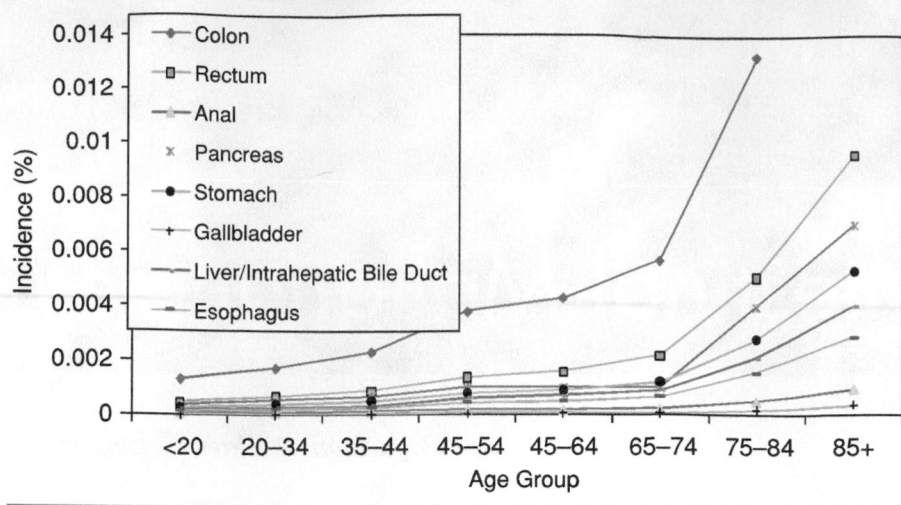

FIGURE 98-1. Percentage of incident cases by age group for GI malignancies (2000–2003), adjusted for 2003 U.S. census.

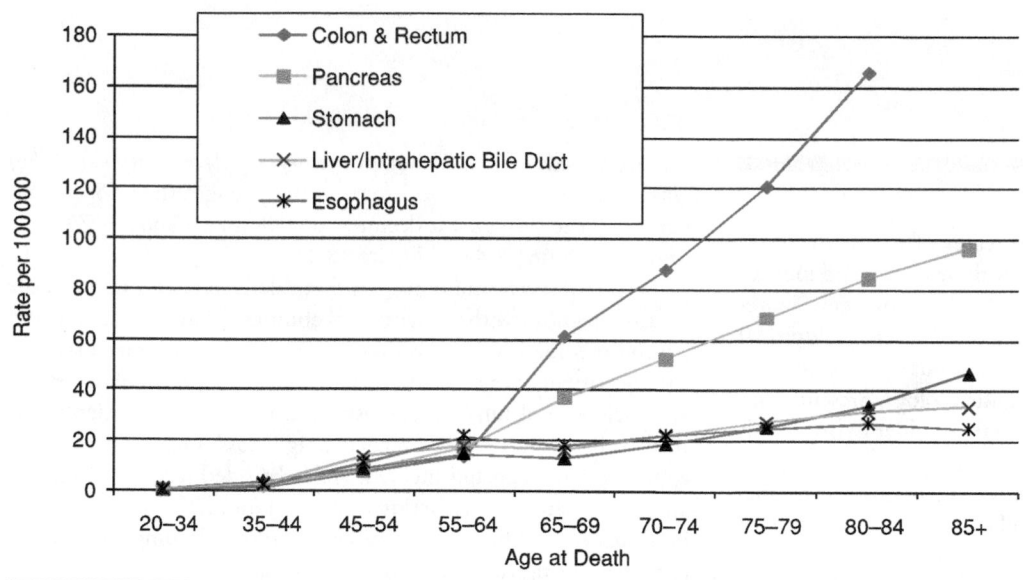

FIGURE 98-2. Mortality rates for GI malignancies (2000–2003) by age at death.

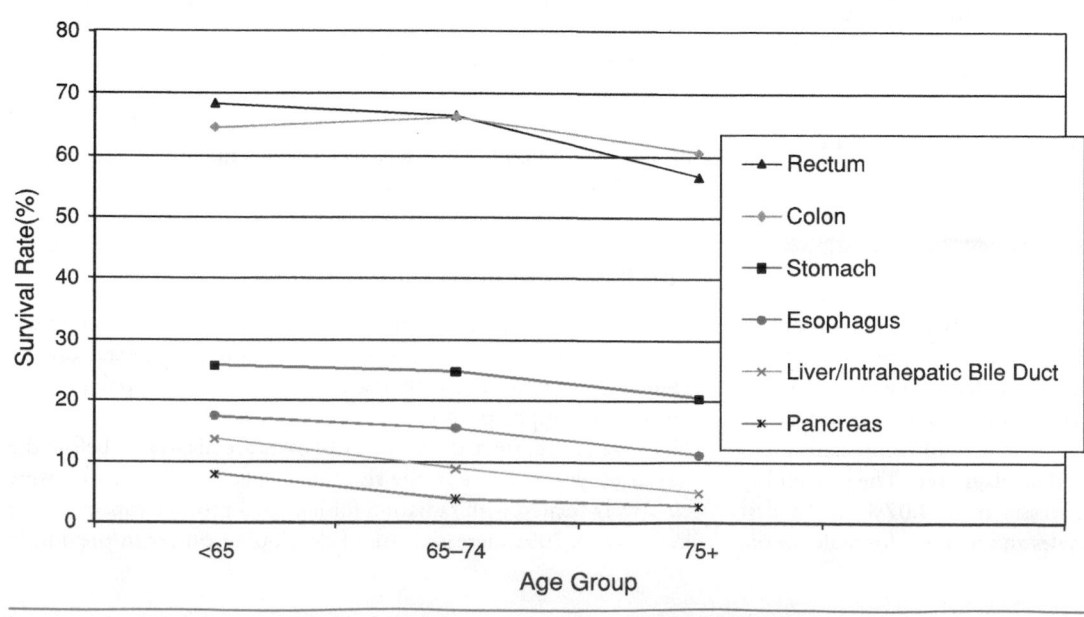

FIGURE 98-3. Five-year survival rates for GI malignancies by age group.

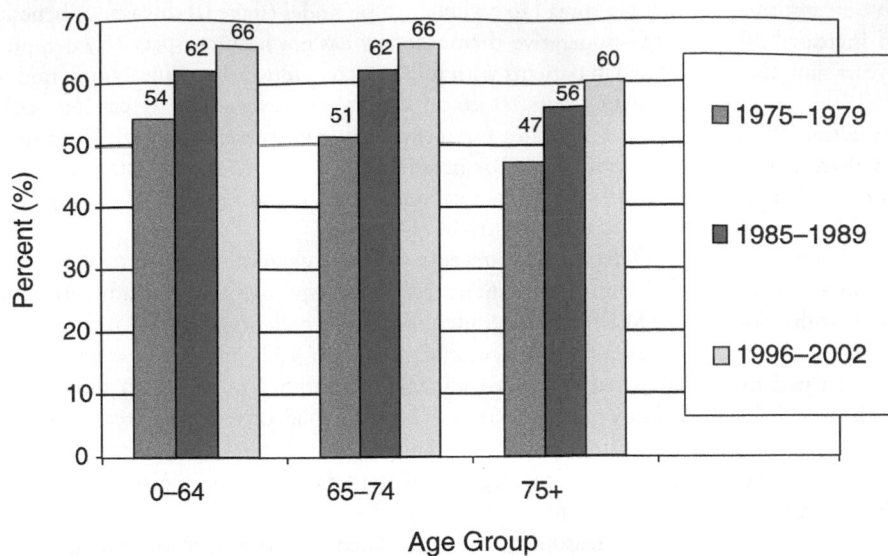

FIGURE 98-4. All-stage 5-yr survival by age group for colon and rectal cancer.

irradiated portions of the bowel and could potentially benefit from more frequent colorectal cancer screening.

Chemoprevention of Colorectal Cancer

Various dietary supplements and drugs have been proposed as chemopreventive agents for colorectal neoplasia. Of these, aspirin has been the most widely studied; the regular use of this drug appears to confer a significant risk reduction (relative risk 0.56–0.68).

In at least two prospective cohort studies, the use of post-menopausal estrogens has been shown to reduce the risk of colorectal cancer by approximately 30%. Estrogen supplementation, however, has been associated with an increased risk for coronary heart disease, breast cancer, thromboembolic events, and early mortality in at least one large randomized study of postmenopausal women, thereby limiting its use as a chemopreventive agent in older women.

Most recently, it has been reported that cholesterol-lowering "statins" can significantly reduce the risk of colorectal cancer. As compared to individuals who did not use statins, individuals who used these agents for at least 5 years were able to reduce their relative risk of colorectal cancer by one-half.

Screening of Colorectal Cancer

Approximately one in two persons will have an adenomatous polyp in their colon by the age of 70 years. The risk of sporadic colorectal cancer can be reduced by 50% to 90%, if adenomatous polyps are implicated by fecal occult blood testing or are visualized by barium enema, sigmoidoscopy, or colonoscopy and are then removed before they transform into a malignancy over a 5 to 10 year period. Three randomized trials have demonstrated that routine fecal occult blood testing can diminish colon cancer mortality by 15% to 20% during an 8 to 18 year follow-up period. The mortality benefit for older patients was slightly lower (10%–16%) than for younger patients (19%–23%).

Case–control studies suggest that lower endoscopy and removal of polyps may decrease the incidence and mortality of colorectal carcinoma by 50% to 80%. However, screening extends life to a lesser degree with advancing age. Although colonoscopy appears to be particularly beneficial in older patients who have a higher incidence of proximal neoplasms, which are beyond the view of a flexible sigmoidoscopy, the risk of perforation from colonoscopy is higher than from sigmoidoscopy (OR 1.8). This risk increases with advancing age and number of comorbidities. Therefore, screening decisions must be individualized for every elderly patient.

Since only a small percentage of persons at risk for colorectal neoplasia undergo routine screening in the United States, Medicare now provides reimbursement for surveillance fecal occult blood testing plus sigmoidoscopy or barium enema or colonoscopy for all beneficiaries. This has increased the prevalence of "screening within 1 year" for fecal occult blood testing from 20% in persons younger than 65 years to 26% in persons 65 years and older and the prevalence of "endoscopy within 5 years" from 37% in persons younger than 65 years to 48% in persons 65 years or older.

Most older persons have a stated preference to continue colorectal cancer screening, feeling that their own life expectancy does not factor into this decision. Since the risk of advanced neoplasia and colorectal cancer is highest in the oldest individuals, it seems doubtful that screening should be arbitrarily discontinued after a certain age. In the United States, an individual who reaches the age of 80 years has an average life expectancy of an additional 8.6 years for women and 6.7 years for men. At age 85 years, average survival is 6.7 years for women and 4.7 years for men. This estimate must be adjusted for the number and severity of chronic diseases affecting the individual, as well as his or her functional status. It may be reasonable to discontinue screening when life expectancy is shorter than the time a polyp progresses to a cancer, that is, 5 to 10 years.

Localized Colorectal Cancer

Surgery—Localized Colon Cancer

Cancers of the colon are typically resected with a hemicolectomy. Whether older age is an adverse prognostic factor in resection of localized colon cancer is controversial. Data on 20,862 patients undergoing surgery in 1997 for colon cancer from the Nationwide Inpatient Sample, a claims-based database, suggest that perioperative mortality increases gradually with advancing age until the age of 80 years, after which a substantial increase in mortality is seen (6.9% for patients older than 80 years). In Australia, patients 70 years and older had a worse prognosis for early-stage colon cancer treated with surgery alone. A European study also showed increased 30-day morbidity and mortality rates for patients 80 years and older compared to their younger counterparts.

Older patients in the Nationwide Inpatient Sample from 1997 had lower mortality rates at high-volume hospitals than at low-volume institutions: 3.1% versus 4.5% for patients older than 65 years (p = 0.03). This effect was even more pronounced for patients older than 80 years, where 4.6% of patients died at high-volume centers compared to 7.3% at smaller institutions (p = 0.04). Therefore, it may be preferable to send the very oldest patients with colon cancer to high-volume hospitals for their resections.

A tendency to perform less aggressive surgery in older patients may be evident from a recent analysis of 116 995 adults with localized colorectal cancer in the SEER database (1988–2001). This retrospective study revealed that patients 71 years or older were half as likely to receive adequate lymph node evaluation (examination of at least 12 lymph nodes) as younger patients. Multiple studies have now demonstrated that inadequate lymph node evaluation correlates with inferior survival. These data would suggest that less aggressive surgical intervention predisposes elderly patients to a higher risk of recurrence and cancer-related death.

Increasingly, laparoscopy-assisted colectomies are being performed in the United States and elsewhere. Randomized studies indicate that patients undergoing this procedure have a similar outcome to patients undergoing an "open" colectomy, with slightly less postoperative pain and a one-day shorter hospital stay. Persons 75 years or older tolerate laparoscopic-assisted colectomy equally well as younger individuals. One study compared 51 patients 70 years or older who underwent laparoscopic colectomy to 102 age-matched patients who underwent open colectomy. Older patients had less overall morbidity with laparoscopic colectomy (17.6%) than with open surgery (37.3%), suggesting that laparoscopic surgery may lessen surgical morbidity for frail, elderly individuals (p = 0.01).

Surgery—Localized Rectal Cancer

A radical resection with anastomosis or ostomy is the standard surgical procedure for cancers of the rectum. A Veteran's Administration study of 7243 patients who underwent surgery for their rectal cancer during the period of 1990 to 2000 revealed that 30-day mortality following resection for rectal cancer was 2.1% for patients younger than 65 years compared with 4.9% for patients 65 years or older (*p* < 0.0001). Five-year survival was 60% versus 48%, respectively (*p* < 0.0001). French investigators reviewed the records of 92 surgical patients who were 80 years or older and matched these to records of 276 younger patients who underwent resection during the same time interval. Although not statistically significant, older patients had a higher operative mortality than younger patients (8% vs. 4%, respectively). Among elective surgeries, the operative mortality was nearly identical (3%–4%). Although 5-year overall survival was greater for younger patients, 5-year cancer-specific survival was comparable for the two groups.

Adjuvant Therapy—Localized Colon Cancer

Since the publication of a National Institutes of Health (NIH) consensus statement in 1990, 5-fluorouracil (5-FU)-based adjuvant therapy has represented the standard of care for patients in the United States following the complete resection of colon cancer

that has spread to regional lymph nodes (stage III disease). A benefit for postoperative chemotherapy has not been prospectively demonstrated in patients with fully resected, muscle-invasive, lymph node-negative (stage II) colon cancer. However, stage II cancers with high-risk features for recurrence (e.g., presentation with obstruction, perforation, or invasion into adjacent organs—stage IIb) are often treated by medical oncologists and are included in many randomized adjuvant trials.

Older patients receive adjuvant chemotherapy less often than their younger counterparts. A retrospective cohort study, utilizing the SEER database, identified 6262 patients 65 years or older with resected stage III colon cancer from 1991 to 1996. Overall, 55% of patients received adjuvant chemotherapy within 3 months of colon cancer resection. The likelihood of receiving treatment declined steeply with increasing age (Table 98-1). Similar results were noted in an Italian study of 1014 patients with resected stage II/III colon cancer.

The reason for this age-related disparity in management is not entirely clear. In one study utilizing the California Cancer Registry, oncologists cited patient refusal, comorbid illness, or advanced age as the most common reasons for not providing chemotherapy to elderly patients with resected colon cancer. Financial considerations and logistical problems may also prevent some elderly from seeking care. Additionally, treatment for older patients is more frequently discontinued, suggesting reluctance by physicians to treat older patients who have experienced some degree of side effects to chemotherapy.

A pooled analysis of 3351 patients in the United States, stratified by decade of life, from seven randomized trials evaluated the benefit of adjuvant chemotherapy in elderly persons with stage II or III colon cancer. The primary conclusion of this pooled analysis was that elderly patients derive the same clinical benefit from postoperative chemotherapy as younger patients. Treatment-related toxicity was somewhat higher for older patients, yet not statistically significant. Another U.S. study, however, could not extend this observation to patients 75 years and older, given limitations in the data.

Adjuvant chemotherapy also appeared to be slightly more toxic for elderly patients in a SEER-derived retrospective cohort study (Table 98-2). Hospitalization for various chemotherapy-related toxicities increased steadily with advancing age. Prospective data from the Royal Marsden Hospital in London confirmed this trend toward higher rates of severe toxicity in patients 70 years or older.

In conclusion, it appears that postoperative chemotherapy in stage III colon cancer is as beneficial in elderly patients, as it is in younger individuals. A slight increase in toxicity should not prevent the clinician from treating these older patients, although increased vigilance during chemotherapy is warranted.

Adjuvant Therapy—Localized Rectal Cancer

Chemoradiation before or after surgery reduces the local recurrence rate and increases disease-free survival in patients with deeply invasive (T3–4) or lymph node–positive rectal cancer. Although there are few data to suggest that elderly patients respond any differently to chemoradiotherapy than younger patients, they are less frequently referred to oncologists for this treatment. Analysis of the SEER database identified patients 65 years or older with stage II or III rectal cancer who underwent surgical resection between 1992 and 1996. Increasing age corresponded inversely with the percentage of patients who received adjuvant therapy (Table 98-1). Overall,

TABLE 98-1

Use of Chemotherapy for Colorectal Cancer by Age

	AGE	TOTAL NUMBER OF PATIENTS	PERCENTAGE OF PATIENTS TREATED	HOSPITALIZATIONS FOR CHEMOTHERAPY-RELATED TOXICITY
Stage III colon cancer	65–69	1261	78%	7%
Schrag 2001	70–74	1552	74%	8%
	75–79	1492	58%	9%
	80–84	1100	34%	12%
	85–89	604	11%	13%
Stage II/III rectal cancer	65–69	367	60%*	
Schrag 2001	70–74	392	52%*	
	75–79	301	36%*	
	80–84	231	23%*	
	85+	120	12%*	
Stage IV colorectal cancer	65–69	377	45%	
Sundararajan 1999	70–74	411	41%	
	75–79	366	27%	
	80–84	262	18%	
	85+	214	5%	

*Chemotherapy and radiation therapy.

chemoradiation therapy was associated with a 17% reduced risk of death among all cases, with a 29% reduced risk of death in stage III patients, but no statistically significant improvement in stage II cases, similar to the results reported in younger patients.

Postoperative Surveillance—Localized Colorectal Cancer

There is general agreement that all patients with resected colorectal cancer should undergo regular surveillance screening with colonoscopy, CEA testing, and possibly an annual CT scan. Analysis of 52,283 Medicare beneficiaries treated for locoregional colorectal cancer between 1986 and 1996 suggests that younger patients are more likely to undergo periodic surveillance endoscopies, and that the median time to first follow-up endoscopy is significantly shorter ($p < 0.0001$) for patients at younger ages.

Advanced Colorectal Cancer

Surgery—Advanced Colorectal Cancer

Removal of the primary cancer is indicated in patients who have an (impending) obstruction, uncontrollable bleeding, or oligometastatic disease that may potentially be cured with aggressive therapy. In spite of these restrictive criteria, a recent pattern of care study, utilizing the SEER database, revealed that the majority of patients 65 years or older with stage IV colorectal cancer undergo resection of their primary tumor. Overall, 72% of patients underwent this primary-cancer-directed surgery. The percentage of patients undergoing surgery declined gradually from 76% in patients 65 to 69 years old, to 70% in patients 80 to 84 years old, and then dropped to 62% in patients 85 years or older.

In this pattern of care study, the 30-day mortality was 10% for all patients. However, higher perioperative mortality rates for elderly patients with advanced colorectal cancer have been reported elsewhere; in patients 70 to 79 years of age, the mortality may be as high as 21% and in octogenarians it may reach 38%. Overall, improvements in surgical technique and postoperative care have led to a decrease in operative mortality particularly in older patients, so that current operative survival figures for elderly patients now approach those reported for younger patients a decade ago.

Elderly patients with oligometastatic disease or isolated recurrences of their colorectal cancer may be candidates for a "curative-intent" resection. In a series from the Memorial Sloan-Kettering

TABLE 98-2

Severe Toxicity to 5-Fluorouracil-Based Therapy by Age in a Pooled Analysis of 1748 Patients with Advanced Colorectal Cancer Treated by the North Central Cancer Treatment Group

SEVERE TOXICITY (NCI CTC GRADE $\geq$3)	AGE			P VALUE*
	<66 YR	66–70 YR	>70 YR	
Any	46%	53%	53%	0.01
Diarrhea	16%	23%	21%	0.01
Leukopenia	14%	18%	17%	0.23
Nausea/vomiting	9%	9%	9%	0.95
Stomatitis	13%	18%	17%	0.03
Infection	2%	5%	4%	0.02

*The P value compares the rate of toxicity for the three age groups using χ^2 test with 2 degrees of freedom.

Cancer Center, 128 patients 70 years or older underwent liver resection for metastatic colorectal cancer between 1985 and 1994. While these patients experienced a 4% perioperative mortality rate and a 42% complication rate, their median survival was 40 months and 5-year survival rate was 35%. These older patients had a similar outcome to 449 patients younger than 70 years who underwent comparable liver resections during the same time period. In a retrospective analysis of patients 65 years and older in the SEER database, only 6.1% of the 13,599 patients identified with colorectal metastases limited to the liver underwent hepatic resection. The 30-day mortality rate was 4.3%. Five-year survival for resected patients was superior to those who did not undergo resection (32.8% vs. 10.5%; p < 0.0001). Additionally, investigators have reported that appropriately selected elderly patients can tolerate resection of colorectal lung metastases with similar outcome as younger patients, with acceptable morbidity and mortality.

Chemotherapy—Advanced Colorectal Cancer

5-Fluorouracil. Until the early 1990s, the only active treatment for advanced colorectal cancer was 5-FU, a thymidylate synthase inhibitor. Multiple studies have now demonstrated that this agent, given as a bolus with leucovorin or as an infusion with or without leucovorin, is effective and well tolerated in the elderly population, with similar response rates and overall survival compared to younger cohorts.

Folprecht and colleagues carried out a pooled analysis of 22 randomized European trials in which patients received palliative 5-FU-based therapy. In this retrospective analysis, overall survival (10.8 months for younger patients vs. 11.3 months for older patients, $p = 0.31$) and response rate (20.8% for younger patients vs. 17.6% for older patients, $p = 0.14$) were nearly identical in younger and older patients. Infusional 5-FU proved to be superior to bolus 5-FU in all age groups. Similar results were obtained in a meta-analysis of four large trials of 5-FU-based therapy to examine the efficacy and toxicity of 5-FU in patients 70 years and older ($n = 303$) compared to younger individuals ($n = 1181$). While severe neutropenia (40.4% vs. 33.6%) and stomatitis (10% vs. 4.6%) were significantly increased in older patients, overall response rate (39.5% vs. 33.1%) and overall survival (15.9 vs. 15.4 months) were similar to that of younger patients.

The North Central Cancer Treatment Group (NCCTG) conducted another pooled analysis of 1748 patients with advanced colorectal cancer treated with 5-FU-based therapy. No significant differences in response rate ($p = 0.90$) or overall survival ($p = 0.42$) were observed between patients younger than 56 years and older than 70 years. Patients 65 years or older had more overall severe toxicity than their younger counterparts (53% vs. 46%, $p = 0.01$). Statistically significant differences in severe diarrhea and stomatitis were reported. Other studies have also noted higher rates of 5-FU-related palmar–plantar erythrodysthesia in older patients.

Capecitabine. The oral 5-FU prodrug, capecitabine, has similar efficacy to monthly intravenous 5-FU and leucovorin (Mayo Clinic Regimen) in the metastatic and adjuvant setting. In patients 70 years or older with metastatic colorectal cancer, the overall response rate with capecitabine was 24% and the overall survival time was 11 months. In patients 70 years and older with resected colon cancer, capecitabine offered the same disease-free survival advantage as standard 5-FU and leucovorin. In this adjuvant trial, severe capecitabine-related toxicity was noted in only 12% of patients. Overall, the results with capecitabine in older patients appear similar to those seen in younger individuals.

Irinotecan. Irinotecan, a topoisomerase I inhibitor, is another active drug in metastatic colorectal cancer. A multi-institutional phase II study found similar rates of severe toxicity in patients 65 years or older and those younger than 65 years receiving a weekly schedule of this agent. In a trial comparing the weekly and the tri-weekly dosing regimens of this drug as second-line therapy for metastatic disease, more than one-third of 291 patients were at least 70 years of age. Age greater than 70 years did not affect survival or time to progression, but was associated with an increased risk of severe neutropenia and diarrhea compared to patients younger than 70 years of age.

Various trials have evaluated irinotecan-based chemotherapies in elderly patients with metastatic colorectal cancer. These have included combinations of irinotecan, bolus 5-FU, and leucovorin; irinotecan, infusional 5-FU, and leucovorin; irinotecan and capecitabine; and irinotecan and oxaliplatin. These trials uniformly revealed that response to chemotherapy, median survival times, and degree of toxicity in these elderly patients appear to be similar to those observed in younger patients.

Oxaliplatin. Oxaliplatin is a third-generation platinum analogue, which induces platinum-DNA adducts, inhibiting the replication of DNA. Although it has limited activity as a single agent in colorectal cancer, oxaliplatin has notable synergy with 5-FU and leucovorin (FOLFOX). In metastatic colorectal cancer, the toxicity following treatment with FOLFOX was evaluated for patients 70 years and older in a pooled analysis of four randomized clinical trials. Although severe hematologic toxicity was increased in older patients, there was no difference in other severe toxicities or 60-day mortality.

For patients with resected colon cancer, a randomized adjuvant trial, in which 35% of patients were 65 years or older, has suggested that disease-free survival can be enhanced if oxaliplatin is added to 5-FU and leucovorin. Subgroup analysis suggested a similar benefit for elderly patients as for the group as a whole. For those older patients with resectable liver metastases, preoperative FOLFOX therapy may be superior to 5-FU therapy. In this study, 2-year overall survival was prolonged in the "FOLFOX group" compared to the "5-FU group" or to the "no chemotherapy group" (84% vs. 60% vs. 23%).

The combination of capecitabine and oxaliplatin (CAPOX) has been evaluated in 76 patients 70 years and older with metastatic colorectal cancer. Overall response was 41%, median progression-free survival was 8.5 months and median overall survival was 14.4 months with little severe toxicity (3% peripheral neuropathy and 13% palmar–plantar erythrodysthesia). A recent randomized study has suggested that the FOLFOX and CAPOX regimens have similar efficacy and rates of toxicity.

Bevacizumab. The humanized monoclonal antibody, bevacizumab, binds to the vascular epidermal growth factor, reducing the vascularity of tumors, leading to hypoxia and necrosis. It also appears to lower interstitial fluid pressure in cancer nodules, promoting diffusion of other chemotherapeutic agents into these tumors. Three pivotal studies in patients with advanced colorectal cancer have established that this agent consistently enhances the efficacy of 5-FU-based therapy with either irinotecan or oxaliplatin for patients of all age groups. A fourth study compared bolus 5-FU and leucovorin alone or in combination with bevacizumab in patients 65 years and older or in patients of poor performance status. This study demonstrated that bevacizumab could significantly improve survival by 4 months in "suboptimal" patients without significantly increasing toxicity.

Bevacizumab may increase the risk of arterial thrombosis, i.e., myocardial infarction, stroke, or peripheral arterial thrombotic event. In a multivariate analysis, persons 65 years or older increased their risk of arterial thrombosis from 2.3% with chemotherapy alone to 7.1% with chemotherapy plus bevacizumab. This risk increased further to 17.9%, if the patient had a history of prior arterial thrombosis. However, progression-free and overall survival was better for those receiving the bevacizumab combination than for those receiving chemotherapy alone. Therefore, bevacizumab can still provide a benefit in carefully selected elderly patients with a history of atherosclerosis-related disease.

Cetuximab/Panitumumab. Cetuximab and panitumumab are monoclonal antibodies to the epidermal growth factor receptor. Blockade of this receptor in colorectal cancer cells induces apoptosis and cell death. In individuals with extensively treated metastatic colorectal cancer, these agents can induce significant tumor regressions in 8% to 11% of patients; cetuximab in combination with irinotecan has a response rate of 23%. The most common severe toxicities of these agents include dyspnea, asthenia, and an acneiform rash. Cetuximab may also cause a hypersensitivity reaction. In one phase II study of 114 patients 65 years and older with metastatic colorectal cancer refractory to irinotecan, oxaliplatin, and 5-FU, cetuximab achieved a response rate of 9.6% compared to a 12.5% response rate in 232 patients younger than 65 years (p = nonsignificant). In a randomized trial for patients with chemotherapy-refractory metastatic colorectal cancer, panitumumab resulted in partial response rate of 8% and a 46% reduction in risk of tumor progression compared to best supportive care. Similar to cetuximab, rash is the predominant adverse effect of panitumumab therapy. A severe rash early in the treatment course is predictive of enhanced response and survival with either agent.

PANCREATIC CANCER

In the United States, the number of expected new cases and the number of anticipated deaths for pancreas cancer in 2008 are almost identical (37,680 and 34,290, respectively). Overall, the probability of 5-year survival for this cancer is less than 5%. The median age at presentation is 72 years, and thus a significant proportion of patients are elderly. A tissue confirmation of pancreas cancer is established less frequently in older individuals. Thus, a disproportionate number of elderly patients may be misdiagnosed with this malignancy and may be incorrectly given a poor prognosis in an attempt to spare them the discomfort of an accurate pathological diagnosis.

Treatment—Localized Pancreas Cancer

Older patients are more likely than younger patients to present with early-stage pancreas cancer. Pancreaticoduodenectomy, the Whipple procedure, is the only potentially curative therapy for this malig-

nancy. There is ample evidence that this procedure can be performed safely in geriatric patients. For example, in 206 patients older than 70 years who underwent surgery at the Mayo Clinic between 1982 and 1987, operative morbidity and mortality rates were 28% and 9%, respectively. Overall median survival was 19 months and 5-year survival was 4%. Similarly, the operative mortality in 138 patients older than 70 years who underwent pancreatic resection at Memorial Sloan-Kettering Cancer Center was 6%, and the major complication rate was 45%. These results are virtually identical to those of younger patients. However, the probability of 5-year survival was slightly lower in this group of older patients (21% vs. 29%, p = 0.03), possibly because of an enhanced risk from comorbid diseases.

Patients with grossly resected pancreas cancer or locally unresectable pancreas cancer may benefit from chemoradiation therapy. Alternatively, a recent prospective study evaluating the benefit of gemcitabine, a nucleoside analogue, after complete resection of pancreatic cancer demonstrated a disease-free but not an overall survival benefit in comparison to the observation arm. Although patients up to 82 years were included in this study, there was no specific evaluation of the effect of adjuvant gemcitabine in older patients.

Treatment—Advanced Pancreas Cancer

Gemcitabine is considered the standard initial therapy for patients with metastatic pancreas cancer. Patients treated with gemcitabine have a median survival time of 5 to 7 months and a 1-year survival rate of 20%. In the pivotal trial of this agent, median age was 62 years and individuals as old as 79 years of age were enrolled, indicating tolerance of such treatment in the elderly. Although the addition of erlotinib, an epidermal growth factor receptor inhibitor, to gemcitabine demonstrated a small survival benefit in younger patients, no such advantage was demonstrated in the 268 patients 65 years or older.

GASTRIC CANCER

Gastric cancer is the second leading cause of cancer death (after lung cancer) in the world. In the United States, the predicted number of new cases for 2008 is 21,500, with 10,880 deaths expected. The results of a German study have suggested that cancers with diffuse histology are more common in younger patients than in patients 70 years or older. In Japan, patients 80 years or older are found to have more advanced disease than younger patients, perhaps because of a later time to diagnosis.

Treatment—Localized Gastric Cancer

Gastrectomy is the only curative treatment for gastric cancer. In patients who undergo the resection of all macroscopic and microscopic disease, the long-term survival is approximately 35%. A prospective review of 310 elderly patients with gastric cancer found that surgery in this group was reasonably well-tolerated and led to survival duration comparable to the results obtained in younger patients. Most, but not all, studies suggest a similar perioperative morbidity and mortality risk for gastrectomy in older and younger patients. For instance, a British multicenter prospective cohort study showed that surgical morbidity and mortality did not differ significantly by age. Of the 955 patients who underwent esophagectomy or gastrectomy, morbidity for patients younger than 70 years and older than 70 years was 50% and 48%, respectively. Mortality was also similar at 10% and 14% for those two age groups. In Italy, age was found to be an independent predictor of recurrence in 536 patients following gastric cancer resection.

Although data specific to elderly patients are not currently available, it is generally recommended that patients with localized gastric cancer be considered for perioperative chemotherapy or postoperative chemoradiation. In a randomized controlled trial of perioperative chemotherapy for resectable esophageal, gastroesophageal junction, and gastric cancers, two cycles of combination chemotherapy administered before and after surgical resection provided a 4 month improvement in median survival compared with surgical resection alone. In another study of 556 patients with resected gastric or gastroesophageal junction cancer, individuals who received adjuvant chemoradiotherapy had a 9-month increase in overall survival compared to those who underwent surgery alone. It is currently uncertain which one of these two approaches is better tolerated and offers a superior survival advantage.

Treatment—Advanced Gastric Cancer

The efficacy of chemotherapy programs for gastric cancer has not been specifically analyzed by patient age. Single-agent therapy generally results in less toxicity than is observed with platinum-based combinations and may be better suited for older individuals. Platinum analogues must be carefully dosed, since renal platinum clearance declines with increasing age. Single agents commonly used in gastric cancer include 5-fluorouracil, capecitabine, the taxanes, and irinotecan. Recent trials, including combinations of 5-FU, leucovorin, and oxaliplatin; capecitabine and oxaliplatin; irinotecan and cisplatin; 5-FU, leucovorin, and irinotecan, have included patients 65 years or older. However, subgroup analyses evaluating response and toxicity in these older patients have not been performed. Thus, it is unclear how older patients fare with more aggressive regimens. Small, single-institution trials have shown a benefit for combination therapy in selected, fit elderly patients. One such study of cisplatin, leucovorin, and fluorouracil in 58 patients 65 years and older with metastatic gastric cancer noted significant responses in 43% of patients. Investigators noted that the therapy was well tolerated.

PRIMARY LIVER CANCER

Primary liver cancer—hepatocellular carcinoma (HCC) and intrahepatic cholangiocarcinoma—is the fourth most common cause of cancer death in the world, leading to almost half a million deaths annually. In contrast, the annual incidence in the United States has been relatively low, with 21 370 new cases and 18 410 deaths expected in 2008. In the United States, the incidence of HCC levels off at older age in males (70 years for Caucasian males and 55 years for African-American males), whereas the incidence of intrahepatic cholangiocarcinoma continues to climb with increasing age for both genders. The risk factors for primary liver cancer do not vary by age, but Japanese investigators suggest that the presence of portal vein thrombosis is a more important prognostic factor than tumor size or the number of tumors for patients 80 years and older.

Treatment—Primary Liver Cancer

Treatment options for elderly patients with HCC restricted to the liver include operative resection, transarterial hepatic chemoem-

bolization, or nonsurgical tumor ablation. Surgery and chemoembolization in the geriatric population have been found to be tolerable in some but not all experiences. In one Italian study, the operative mortality was 8% in patients 65 years or older, with 1-year, 3-year, and 5-year survival probabilities of 89%, 61%, and 45%, respectively. These percentages were nearly identical to those of patients younger than 65 years of age. Localized tumor ablation with ethanol, cryotherapy, or radiofrequency has been increasingly utilized to eradicate small tumors and may be particularly appropriate for older patients, who are frequently considered poor candidates for surgery.

In a recent review of the 2696 Medicare patients with HCC between 1992 and 1999, 13% had procedures with curative intent (0.9% transplant, 8.2% resection, 4.1% local ablation), 4% underwent transarterial chemoembolization, 57% received palliative therapy, and 26% did not get treatment. Only 34% of patients with solitary lesions or lesions less than 3 cm in diameter received therapy with curative intent, suggesting underutilization of curative interventions in eligible elderly patients. Three-year survival for transarterial chemoembolization or local ablation was less than 10%.

Surgical resection of liver tumors is well tolerated in older patients. In a recent European study, cirrhotic patients with HCC aged 70 years and older were compared to patients younger than 70 years. The operative morbidity and liver failure rates were lower in the subset of older patients (23.4% vs. 42.4% and 1.6% vs. 12.9%, respectively). Operative mortality and 5-year survival rates were not significantly different between the two groups. Although smaller tumor size was predictive of better outcome for younger patients, this was not noted for older patients. Similar findings were reported by investigators in Taiwan.

ESOPHAGEAL CANCER

Squamous cell carcinomas and adenocarcinomas of the esophagus are the sixth leading cause of cancer death worldwide. In the United States, esophageal cancer is less common, with 16 470 new cases and 14 280 deaths anticipated in 2008. Between 1974 and 1994, the appearance of adenocarcinomas of the esophagus has increased substantially, particularly in white men between 65 and 74 years of age, while the incidence of squamous cell carcinomas has declined slightly. The epidemiologic pattern of esophageal carcinoma does not appear different in elderly patients. Most studies report similar clinical symptoms at the time of presentation, as well as similar distribution of histology, stage, and location of tumors for patients older and younger than 70 years of age. In these series, approximately 50% to 75% of the older patients were found to have adenocarcinoma and 25% to 50% had squamous cell carcinoma.

It is unclear if the incidence of Barrett's associated adenocarcinoma increases with advanced age. Although one study has suggested a higher incidence in older patients, another study suggested this incidence is not age dependent. The location of tumors in the esophagus does not differ between older and younger patients—distal esophageal tumors predominate in all groups. A similar distribution in early- and late-stage cancers has also been reported.

Treatment—Localized Esophageal Cancer

Most but not all studies suggest that age is not a limiting factor in surgery of the esophagus. Although elderly patients tend to have a higher incidence of respiratory and cardiovascular complications than younger patients, this does not appear to have a significant effect on operative mortality or survival. In one series, 50 patients older than 70 years were compared to 89 patients younger than 70 years; postoperative complications and inhospital mortality occurred in 38% and 3% of younger patients and in 44% and 0% of older patients. The mean duration of hospitalization was 17.9 days for younger patients and 18.6 days for older patients. The severity of postoperative dysphagia and weight loss were similar for both groups. The likelihood of survival after 8 years was identical at 20%.

In a second study of 60 patients 70 years and older, no difference was observed in the rate of resection with curative intent, surgical complications, or hospital mortality rate in comparison to a younger population. This was confirmed in another study, demonstrating equivalent surgical morbidity and mortality for older patients stratified by performance status and overall fitness in comparison to younger patients. A contradictory study suggested that age was predictive of morbidity and mortality following esophagectomy in multivariate analysis ($p = 0.002$). Age and comorbidity were also noted to be significant predictors of outcome in a simple risk score developed to predict surgical mortality for esophageal cancer.

Although the rate of surgical complications may not be significantly increased in the elderly, the presence of such complications significantly worsens survival. This was the conclusion in a review of 510 patients who underwent resection of esophageal or gastroesophageal junction carcinoma at the Memorial Sloan-Kettering Cancer Center from 1996 to 2001. Surgical complications occurred in 31.8% of the 173 patients 65 to 74 years old and in 34.8% of the 66 patients 75 years and older. Although survival at 30 days did not differ significantly between patient groups who did and did not experience surgical complications, there was a notable decline in 1-year survival for patients 65 years and older who had suffered a perioperative complication. In a separate study at the same institution, octogenarians were noted to have more than a threefold higher mortality rate than patients 50 to 79 years old, although they experienced similar rates of operative complications (blood loss, cardiopulmonary complications, infection, and anastomotic leak).

A review of 945 patients in the Veteran's Administration National Surgical Quality Improvement Program found no difference in 30-day surgical mortality and morbidity between transthoracic and transhiatal esophagectomies. Age did significantly impact the overall mortality rate for both surgical techniques, with increasing age associated with an increased risk of surgical mortality. The same age-related surgical mortality risk was also noted in a French study of gastroesophageal junction adenocarcinomas.

Although age may not be a significant factor in the rate of curative resection, curative surgery is still underutilized in older racial minority patients. African-American patients 65 years and older were noted to have a lower rate of surgical consultation and half the rate of curative surgery as their elderly Caucasian counterparts (70% vs. 78%, $p < 0.001$ and 25% vs. 46%, $p < 0.001$, respectively).

Chemoradiation therapy appears equally effective in patients 70 years of age and older as in younger individuals. Furthermore, there appears to be no association between age and toxicity in patients of good performance status. At Memorial Sloan-Kettering Cancer Center, 24 elderly patients (median age 77 years) with locally advanced esophageal cancer were treated with 5040 cGy of radiation and infusional 5-fluorouracil plus mitomycin C over a 6-week period of time. Nine of these individuals (38%) required hospitalization for toxicity and three required dose reductions. Sixteen patients achieved a clinical remission and 10 remained without evidence of disease after a median follow-up of 1.2 years, suggesting that selected chemoradiation therapy is a feasible and well-tolerated alternative to esophagectomy in elderly patients.

Treatment—Advanced Esophageal Cancer

Single agents, such as the taxanes, irinotecan, 5-fluorouracil, capecitabine, and vinorelbine, have some efficacy in palliating metastatic esophageal cancer and represent management options for elderly patients, particularly for those with lower performance status or significant comorbidities. Combination chemotherapy regimens tend to have more side effects and have not been systematically evaluated in older patients with esophageal cancer. Preliminary results of one study in patients 70 years or older suggested that the combination of weekly docetaxel and infusional 5-FU is well tolerated in this age group. Toxicities were primarily neutropenia and mucositis.

GALLBLADDER CANCER

Cancers of the gallbladder occur infrequently in the United States. The incidence increases with age and reaches its peak in the seventh decade of life. In 2008, 9520 new cases and 3340 deaths are expected. The presentation and clinical features of this cancer do not appear to differ appreciably between older and younger patients. Endoscopic retrograde cholangiopancreatography (ERCP) is often used in the diagnosis of gallbladder cancer and is well tolerated in older patients—even the very old. In a study of 126 patients 90 years and older who underwent a total of 147 ERCP procedures, 9.5% were noted to have malignant stenosis. The overall morbidity and mortality rates were low at 2.5% and 0.7%, respectively.

Treatment—Gallbladder Cancer

Surgery is the only potentially curative treatment for this disease. A retrospective single institution study from Japan reviewed the cases of 54 patients who were 75 years or older and compared them to 152 patients less than 75 years of age. Approximately 58% of patients in both age groups underwent a radical resection (rather than a simple cholecystectomy). Operative mortality and survival rates were similar between the two age groups. The investigators noted that the likelihood of 5-year survival was better for those elderly patients who had undergone a radical resection, compared to those who had undergone a simple cholecystectomy (61% vs. 14%, $p = 0.01$). These uncontrolled results have not been validated through a randomized trial.

Although advanced gallbladder cancer is highly resistant to chemotherapy, single agents such as gemcitabine, 5-FU, and capecitabine are generally well tolerated in elderly patients and may offer some palliation in this disease. In a small study of advanced biliary tract cancers and gallbladder cancer, treated with the combination of gemcitabine and cisplatin, no difference in response rate was noted between 10 patients 60 years and older and 30 younger patients, although the older patients had higher rates of hematologic toxicity.

ANAL CANCER

Squamous cell carcinoma of the anal canal is the least common but most treatable of the gastrointestinal malignancies. In 2008, 5070 new cases but only 680 deaths are expected for this malignancy. The risk factors for anal cancer and genital malignancies are similar. The risk of HPV-related anal cancer in men who have sex with men increases with age. Older age at first receptive intercourse was associated with increased prevalence of both low- and high-grade squamous dysplasia, the precursor lesions to anal cancer. The higher incidence of anal cancer is more pronounced in patients 65 years and older than in younger age groups. Five-year survival does not differ significantly by gender or age.

Treatment—Anal Cancer

Since the 1970s, the standard treatment for anal cancer has been the combination of 5-FU, mitomycin, and radiation therapy. With this technique, 60% to 73% of patients will remain free of disease recurrence and a colostomy at 4 years. A small study evaluating this nonsurgical strategy in patients 75 years or older demonstrated similar complication rates to those seen in younger patients, suggesting that sphincter-conserving treatment is feasible in older patients with anal carcinoma. In an Australian study of 62 patients, treated with chemoradiation (mitomycin C and 5-FU) and anal sphincter preservation surgery, the local control rate was 86% and the colostomy-free survival at 2 years was 83%. This study included 38 patients 60 years and older.

Radiation used in the treatment of anal cancer in women 65 years or older can lead to a threefold increased risk of pelvic fracture. These women are at greater risk for fracture than women treated with radiation therapy for cervical or rectal cancer. Therefore, older women treated with chemotherapy and radiation therapy for anal cancer should undergo regular bone densitometry screening and bisphosphonate therapy.

CLINICAL TRIALS

While 70% to 75% of colorectal cancers are diagnosed in patients older than 65 years, only 40% to 48% of patients enrolled in NCI-sponsored or cooperative group trials are drawn from this age group. This underrepresentation of elderly patients with colorectal cancer has not improved in the past several years. During the 2000 to 2002 time period, only 2% of colorectal cancer patients 65 to 74 years old and 0.5% of colorectal cancer patients 75 years or older enrolled in NCI-sponsored trials, substantially less than the 4% enrollment recorded for patients 30 to 64 years old. Similar data are not available for the less common gastrointestinal malignancies.

A possible explanation for this discrepancy may be financial, although a similarly low rate of enrollment for older patients has been documented in Canada, where the national health care program provides reimbursement for all health care costs. More plausible explanations for the lack of participation of elderly patients in clinical trials may include lack of social and home care support, physician reluctance to offer research protocols to older individuals, difficulties with access to clinics and hospitals, potential noncoverage of investigational treatments by Medicare, patient re-fusal, increasing concomitant medication usage and co-morbidities with advancing age, and fewer trials specifically aimed at elderly patients.

FURTHER READING

Ayanian JZ, Zaslavsky AM, Fuchs CS, et al. Use of adjuvant chemotherapy and radiation therapy for colorectal cancer in a population-based cohort. *J Clin Oncol.* 2003;21(7):1293–1300.

Colorectal Cancer Collaborative Group. Palliative chemotherapy for advanced colorectal cancer: systematic review and meta-analysis. *Br Med J.* 2000;321:531–535.

Cunningham D, Allum WH, Stenning SP, et al. ; for the MAGIC Trial Participants. Perioperative chemotherapy versus surgery alone for resectable gastroesophageal cancer. *N Engl J Med.* 2006;355(1):11–20.

Dobie SA, Baldwin LM, Dominitz JA, Matthews B, Billingsley K, Barlow W. Completion of therapy by medicare patients with stage III colon cancer. *J Natl Canc Inst.* 2006;98(9):610–619.

El-Serag HB, Siegel AB, Davila JA, et al. Treatment and outcomes of treating of hepatocellular carcinoma among medicare recipients in the United States: a population-based study. *J Hepatol.* 2006;44(1):158–166.

Goldberg RM, Rabah-Fisch I, Bleiberg H, et al. Pooled analysis of safety and efficacy of oxaliplatin plus fluorouracil/leucovorin administered bimonthly in elderly patient with colorectal cancer. *J Clin Oncol.* 2006;24(25):4085–4091.

Gross CP, Andersen MS, Krumholz HM, McAvay GJ, Proctor D, Tinetti ME. Relation between medicare screening reimbursement and stage at diagnosis for older patients with colon cancer. *J Am Med Assoc.* 2006;292(23):2815–2822.

Gross CP, Guo Z, McAvay GJ, Allore HG, Young M, Tinetti ME. Multimorbidity and survival in older persons with colorectal cancer. *J Am Geriatr Soc.* 2006;54:1898–1904.

Gross CP, McAvay GJ, Krumholz HM, Paltiel D, Bhasin D, Tinetti ME. The effect of age and chronic illness on life expectancy after a diagnosis of colorectal cancer: implications for screening. *Ann Intern Med.* 2006;145:646–653.

Iwashyna TJ, Lamont EB. Effectiveness of adjuvant fluorouracil in clinical practice: a population-based cohort study of elderly patients with stage III colon cancer. *J Clin Oncol.* 2002;20(19):3992–3998.

Lichtman SM. Management of advanced colorectal cancer in older patients. *Oncology.* 2005;19(5):597–602.

Lin OS, Kozarek RA, Schembre DB, et al. Screening colonoscopy in very elderly patients. *J Am Med Assoc.* 2006;295:2357–2365.

Ma JY, Wu Z, Wang Y, et al. Clinicopathologic characteristics of esophagectomy for esophageal carcinoma in elderly patients. *World J Gastroenterol.* 2006;12(8):1296–1299.

Makary MA, Winter JM, Cameron JL, et al. Pancreaticoduodenectomy in the very elderly. *J Gastrointest Surg.* 2006;10:347–356.

McCulloch P, Ward J, Tekkis PP. Mortality and morbidity in gastro-oesophageal cancer surgery: initial results of ASCOT multicenter prospective cohort study. *Br Med J.* 2003;327:1192–1197.

Neugut AI, Fleischauer AT, Sundararajan V, et al. Use of adjuvant chemotherapy and radiation therapy for rectal cancer among the elderly: a population-based study. *J Clin Oncol.* 2002;20(11):2643–2650.

Neugut AI, Matasar M, Wang X, et al. Duration of adjuvant chemotherapy for colon cancer and survival among the elderly. *J Clin Oncol.* 2006;24:2368–2375.

Potosky AL, Harlan LC, Kaplan RS, Johnson KA, Lynch CF. Age, sex, and racial differences in the use of standard adjuvant therapy for colorectal cancer. *J Clin Oncol.* 2002;20(5):1192–1202.

Sargent DJ, Goldberg RM, Jacobson SD, et al. A pooled analysis of adjuvant chemotherapy for resected colon cancer in elderly patients. *N Engl J Med.* 2001;345(15):1091–1097.

Schrag D, Cramer LD, Bach PB, Begg CB. Age and adjuvant chemotherapy use after surgery for stage III colon cancer. *J Natl Canc Inst.* 2001;93(11):850–857.

Shore S, Vimalachandran D, Raraty MGT, Ghaneh P. Cancer in the elderly: pancreatic cancer. *Surg Oncol.* 2004;13:201–210.

Sundararajan V, Grann V, Neugut A. Population based variation in the use of chemotherapy for colorectal cancer in the elderly. *Proc Am Soc Clin Oncol.* 1999;18:A1598.

Trumper M, Ross PJ, Cunningham D, et al. Efficacy and tolerability of chemotherapy in elderly patients with advanced oesophago-gastric cancer: a pooled analysis of three clinical trials. *Eur J Cancer.* 2006;42:827–834.

Intracranial Neoplasms

Noelle K. LoConte ■ *Julie E. Chang* ■ *H. Ian Robins*

Older patients with central nervous system (CNS) disease present a unique set of problems for the health care provider. Often their presentation can be atypical, potentially confounding or delaying the correct diagnosis. For example, older patients often present with cognitive dysfunction suggesting dementia, or personality changes suggesting depression rather than more typical symptoms such as headache. This population also has various comorbidities, which often complicate the potential for neurosurgery. Additionally, this group of patients may have a tendency to tolerate radiation, chemotherapy, or supportive agents (such as steroids or antiepileptics) poorly. Also, CNS tumors in general carry with them a significant risk of morbidity and mortality, independent of the patient's age, which may only further complicate the decision making process in the older adult patient. In this chapter, various intracranial neoplastic disease processes and their management in the older adult are considered.

GLIOMAS

Low-Grade Gliomas

Low-grade gliomas (i.e., astrocytomas and oligodendrogliomas) are relatively uncommon in patients older than 65 years. Therapy usually involves maximally feasible resection. Radiation therapy (RT) may be reserved for symptomatic patients, or patients with recurrent disease. In a randomized European trial, RT did not improve overall survival, but did improve progression free survival. Another indication for RT relates to a patient for whom minimal disease progression might result in significant neurological deterioration. It should be noted that low-grade oligodendrogliomas with chromosomal deletions in the 1p and 19q loci are very sensitive to both radiation and chemotherapy. This enhanced sensitivity to therapy is also true for anaplastic oligodendroglioma (discussed below).

Anaplastic Gliomas

Grade 3 astrocytomas, as well as anaplastic oligodendroglioma, are also less common in older patients with a peak incidence in adults during the third decade of life. The mainstay of therapy is surgery and RT. The definitive role for chemotherapy is yet to be defined in these diseases. By extrapolation from the success of temozolomide chemotherapy (TMZ) in the treatment of newly diagnosed grade 4 astrocytoma (i.e., glioblastoma multiforme [GBM, discussed below]), some oncologists feel there is a role for TMZ chemotherapy in treating these patients at the time of diagnosis. There are, however, no level one data to support this therapeutic approach currently.

Glioblastoma Multiforme

Background

Geriatric patients have an increasing incidence of GBM. This diagnosis in a geriatric patient population is typically associated with shorter survivals (than comparable patients who are younger) and may not be treated as aggressively (Table 99-2). Reasons for this may include the "biology" of primary GBM in these patients, comorbidities, and the inability to tolerate toxic therapies. Elderly patients with GBM appear to be less responsive to chemotherapy, and age appears to have a negative correlation with the tumor's response to treatment and time to disease progression, but a positive correlation with toxicity for patients older than 60 years (Table 99-1). Several studies have demonstrated that overall survival declines with increasing age and decreasing performance status, as measured by Karnofsky performance status (KPS).

Many studies have been performed in elderly patients in an attempt to determine the optimal management; the majority of these studies have used a "less is better" approach to treatment. This literature is summarized under two main points: what constitutes "elderly" is not well defined, and may be as low as 60 years of age, and studies have used different parameters for "good" versus "poor" performance status, (e.g., KPS). Both of these factors impact outcome. Another confounder to interpreting outcome data in GBM is extent of surgery. Gross total resection surgery appears to have a modest benefit on survival, particularly in patients with good performance status. This is a surgery that removes all tumor visible to the naked eye. Relative to this, many older patients simply undergo a biopsy or partial resection, resulting in an incomplete surgical removal of tumor.

Radiation Therapy

Most radiation studies in the geriatric patient population have focused on abbreviated courses of RT. Survivals obtained are similar or slightly less than the standard 6-week course, but require less time for treatment. The benefits of RT decrease with increasing age and are affected to some degree by extent of surgical resection. Villa et al. (1998) treated patients (median age 70) with 54 to 66 gray (Gy) of external beam radiation with a median survival of 18.1 weeks for all patients and 45 weeks for those who started RT. The median survival of patients younger than 70 years was 55 weeks, compared to 34 weeks for patients older than 70 years. Pierga et al. (1999) treated 30 patients (median age 73 and KPS 60–70) with 45 Gy for more than 5 weeks after maximal resection and found a median survival of 36 weeks. Philips et al. (2003) found that non-significant survival advantage for patients treated with 60 Gy (median survival of 41 weeks) versus 35 Gy (35 weeks). McAleese et al. (2003) compared patients treated with 30 Gy to a case matched control group of patients treated with 60 Gy and found an increase in survival of 2.5 to 4.5 months longer; the authors questioned whether the lesser survival was outweighed by an improved quality of life. Chang et al. (2003) treated 59 patients (median age 65) with 50 Gy in 4 weeks and found a median survival of 28 weeks, which was comparable to the Radiation Therapy Oncology Group (RTOG) database. Roa et al. (2004) randomized patients >60 (median was 72 years) to 60 Gy in 6 weeks or 40 Gy in 3 weeks. Median survival was similar at 20 weeks and 21 weeks with fewer patients in the lower dose group requiring an increase in steroids.

Chemotherapy

The first glimpse of a therapeutic breakthrough in the treatment of GBM occurred in 2002 when Stupp and coworkers reported results

TABLE 99-1

Median Survival of Various Gliomas as a Function of Histology

GLIOMA TYPE	MEDIAN SURVIVAL (yr)	CHROMOSOMAL ABNORMALITY
Low-grade oligodendroglioma	4–10	
Low-grade astrocytoma	5	P53 gene, chromosome 22q
Anaplastic oligodendroglioma	3–5	Chromosomes 9p, 13q, 19q
Anaplastic astrocytoma	3	
Glioblastoma multiforme	~1	Chromosome 10

TABLE 99-2

General Characteristics of High-Grade Gliomas

CHARACTERISTIC	ANAPLASTIC ASTROCYTOMA	GLIOBLASTOMA MULTIFORME
Grade	3	4
Mean age of onset	40–50 yr	65 yr
Median survival	3–4 yr	12–14 mo with surgery and chemotherapy
Recurrence pattern	Often as grade 4	Rapid tumor growth and recurrence
Clinical challenge	Achieving gross total surgical resection	

of the use of daily TMZ (75 mg orally per square meter body surface area) during radiation (approximately 6–7 weeks), followed by 6 months of adjuvant therapy at 150 to 200 po mg/m^2 on days 1 through 5 of a 28-day cycle. The median survival in this phase II study was 16 months. The rationale for this approach included the possibility of radiosensitization. The concept of daily dosing was an attempt to overcome TMZ drug resistance. The background for this related to observations demonstrating that the repeated administration of TMZ depletes the DNA-repair enzyme 0^6-methylquanine-DNA methyltransferase (MGMT). MGMT is a resistance mechanism for TMZ. Thus, it is termed a "suicide enzyme." After MGMT removes a methyl group from DNA (deposited by TMZ), it is no longer active. The use of adjuvant TMZ starting 1 month postradiotherapy was predicated on the inherent antitumor activity of the drug. As the study by Stupp et al. demonstrated a promising 2-year survival rate of 31%, the European Organization for Research and Treatment of Cancer (EORTC) and the National Cancer Institute of Canada (NCIC) launched a phase III trial comparing this phase II regimen to radiotherapy alone. Recently, data presented from Stupp et al. in a randomized phase 3 study (2005) demonstrated that the combination of RT and TMZ followed by 6 months of TMZ was better than RT alone in terms of overall survival and disease control. This has become the new standard of care for GBM. Patients treated with chemotherapy and radiation had a progression free survival of 6.9 months compared to 5 months, a median survival of 14.6 months compared to 12.1 months, and a 2-year survival of 27% compared to 10%; all values were statistically significant. Importantly, in that study, patients older than 70 years were not eligible so the benefit in this group remains undefined. It is notable that the American Radiation Therapy Oncology Group (RTOG) in cooperation with the EORTC and the NCIC has launched a new phase 3 trial (RTOG 0525): one arm is the aforementioned Stupp regimen; the other is a dose dense TMZ treatment (75 mg/m^2 for 21 days on a 28-day schedule) postradiation (in an attempt to overcome resistance). This study will have no age limitation, and therefore should provide important new data.

Despite the data available, the best approach for the elderly patient is not known with a variable approach depending on the biases of individual practitioners. For patients with a good performance status and no significant comorbidities, maximal resection followed by RT (60 Gy) + TMZ followed by TMZ for 6 months should probably be the approach to use. It has become a convention in the United States to treat patients with TMZ for 1 year post-RT, but there is no level one data to support this practice.

A geriatric patient population with newly diagnosed GBM is the ideal one for further study. One possible aim is the evaluation of the potential benefits of adjuvant TMZ. In a nongeriatric patient population, the benefit of concurrent and adjuvant chemotherapy as an overall treatment has been demonstrated, but the benefits of adjuvant chemotherapy (i.e., TMZ post-RT) as a portion of that approach has not been assessed. In a phase II ($n = 55$) study done in Germany with a somewhat older patient population, TMZ was given with RT at a dose of only 50 mg/m^2 rather than the 75 mg/m^2 as in the Stupp study; no TMZ was given post-RT. The overall survival in this study approximated the Stupp trial. As many patients fail to complete the adjuvant treatment, it is possible that the concurrent therapy (TMZ/RT) is most important. In older patients, the decision to offer a trial comparing these options is justified by the greater uncertainty about the benefits of the overall treatment program with TMZ, as well as, the greater risk of toxicity of these regimens in older patients, and the poorer overall survival. The issue of survival is relevant as adjuvant therapy may occupy a period of time greater than the predicted median survival for the population.

A few studies have looked at the role of TMZ chemotherapy in the elderly post-RT only, or as sole treatment without RT. A small series of 23 GBM patients (mean age 68, all with good performance status) treated with surgery, TMZ and RT, with a median survival time of 15.38 months. Notable in this series was the development of leukoencephalopathy in 2 patients older than 70 years old. TMZ alone has been retrospectively compared to survival for RT alone, with no statistical difference between the two groups. Consistently, performance status was a predicator of survival. In prospective studies of TMG alone, neurologic improvement has been reported in 50% of patients with an overall survival of 6.4 months, and a median progression free survival of 5 months.

In spite of the advances described above, the overall prognosis for patients with GBM (in general, and particularly for the elderly) remains poor. Interestingly, the marked genetic heterogeneity of GBM may provide another opportunity for directed therapy. Recent elucidation of signaling pathways and evaluation of targeted agents has been an exciting approach in the treatment of cancer patients in general. For GBM, there are several promising targets. For example, GBM tends to overexpress epidermal growth factor receptor (EGFR). Additionally, research suggests that the status of the PTEN gene involved in the activity of the Akt signal transduction pathway (which is involved in resistance to apoptosis and acceleration of cell proliferation) may have implications for prognosis as well as response to EGFR tyrosine-kinase inhibitors for GBM. In a retrospective study, Mellinghoff et al. found that activated EGFR, (i.e., EGFR vIII) in combination with wild-type PTEN was associated with a very high response rate to the EGFR tyrosine kinase inhibitors erlotinib and gefitinib. Similarly, another group reported that EGFR amplification and low levels of protein kinase B/Akt phosphorylation was associated with response.

Taken collectively, such studies point the way for prospective trials, allowing for selection of patients based on the molecular characteristics of their tumors. In the now active RTOG study 0525, discussed above, such data will be collected prospectively, so that at the time of relapse such concepts can be clinically tested in specific cohorts of patients.

In conclusion, it is noteworthy that cooperative groups throughout the world have increasingly focused on age as a determinant in the outcome of geriatric GBM patients. This has resulted in recent design of studies targeting geriatric studies, as well as open studies without age restrictions but with stratification for age. This awareness coupled with the increasing propagation of new agents, and biologic markers to allow for directed therapy will hopefully result in a significant improvement in outcome for these older patients.

PRIMARY NERVOUS SYSTEM LYMPHOMAS

Primary central nervous system lymphoma (PCNSL) is a rare type of intracranial neoplasm, representing only 1% to 4% of all primary brain tumors. PCNSL is a subtype of extranodal non-Hodgkin's lymphoma that is confined to the brain, spinal cord, meninges, and eye. Patients may present with symptoms related to increased intracranial pressure, local mass effect, ocular involvement, or from focal involvement at cranial or spinal nerve roots. Diagnostic imaging of PCNSL is best achieved with magnetic resonance imaging (MRI), with PCNSL having the characteristic appearance of a periventricular homogenous, hypointense mass with indistinct borders.

Consideration of PCNSL in the differential diagnosis of an intracranial mass is important given the divergence in treatment modalities employed for PCNSL compared with other primary or metastatic brain tumors. In particular, PCNSL is frequently exquisitely sensitive to steroids, and initiation of high-dose steroids in cases of PCNSL may result in significant or complete regression of the mass prior to a diagnostic biopsy. Surgical resection should be avoided in cases where PCNSL is considered until a definitive tissue diagnosis is made, given the results of multiple retrospective series showing that gross total resection of PCNSL only results in increased morbidity without improving outcome. This is somewhat surprising given the important role of surgical resection in improving outcomes in other primary brain tumors and some metastatic brain tumors. Lastly, proper histologic diagnosis of PCNSL is important in order to adequately assess for other common sites of disease, including the eyes and leptomeninges. Failure to do so will result in inadequate treatment for occult or subclinical disease sites.

PCNSL may occur in immunocompromised or immunocompetent patients, although a discussion of treatment will be limited to the setting of immunocompetent patients. Whole-brain radiation therapy (WBRT) has been the mainstay of PCNSL treatment for more than a decade, with reported median survivals of 12 to 18 months. Ongoing efforts are underway to improve outcomes with the incorporation of chemotherapy. In contrast to other subtypes of non-Hodgkin's lymphoma, the most active agent in treatment of PCNSL is methotrexate, given at doses high enough to penetrate the blood-brain barrier (doses ≥ 1 g/m^2). Previously, it has been reported that the best outcomes are observed with doses of methotrexate ≥ 3.5 g/m^2. Combined modality therapy with methotrexate-based regimens and consolidation WBRT have been associated with improved median survival, but with high rates of neurotoxicity related to leukoencephalopathy. In patients older than age 60, the rates of severe neurocognitive dysfunction have approached as high as 60% to 80% in patients treated with high-dose methotrexate and WBRT. Recently, the long-term retrospective experience at Memorial Sloan-Kettering Cancer Center has suggested improved median survival in older patients treated with chemotherapy alone. In this series of patients with PCNSL treated with a methotrexate-based regimen with or without WBRT, age again emerged as an important prognostic variable in terms of overall survival and risk for neurotoxicity.

A median survival of 29 months was observed in the patients aging 60 years or older, which is significantly improved in comparison with historical data in older patients receiving WBRT alone (median survival 7–12 months).

Neurotoxicity was a significant problem in older patients receiving chemotherapy and WBRT, with rates of neurotoxicity of 75% compared with 12% in older patients treated with chemotherapy alone. Similarly, Abrey et al recently reported a prognostic scoring system in PCNSL in which age and KPS are significant predictors of outcome in terms of overall and failure-free survival in PCNSL.

Ongoing trials are investigating novel methotrexate-based regimens with the incorporation of agents known to cross the blood-brain barrier (e.g., temozolomide, procarbazine, cytarabine) as well as newer agents that have established activity in lymphoma (e.g., rituximab). Clearly, better means of assessing and detecting neurocognitive changes are needed as part of ongoing treatment of PCNSL, especially in older patients who are at highest risk for these complications. The recent description of a prognostic model based on age and performance status in PCNSL will aid in identifying patients who are candidates for more aggressive treatment strategies and will also serve as an important tool in clinical trial development. In older patients with a poor performance status at diagnosis, palliative WBRT remains a reasonable and effective treatment option.

BRAIN METASTASES

Brain metastases represent the most common intracranial neoplasm in adults. Brain metastases may carry with them devastating functional impairments as well as generally carrying a poor prognosis. Several common solid tumors have a particular predilection to metastasize to the brain, including breast and lung cancer, as well as melanoma. The presenting signs and symptoms for a patient with brain metastases are similar to those with primary brain tumors; seizures, headaches, and focal neurological deficits tend to dominate the presentation. Conventional whole-brain RT remains the mainstay of treatment for brain metastases among patients of all ages. There is an emerging role for surgery, novel ways of delivering RT and chemotherapy.

Radiation Therapy

The treatment typically given for intracranial metastases is whole-brain radiotherapy (treating the entire brain with equal amounts of radiation). The dose given ranges from 30 to 37.5 Gy of radiation, usually divided in 2 to 3 Gy fractions. A higher total dose is no more effective in increasing median survival, nor is shortening the duration of treatment to as little as one high-dose fraction. For patients whose overall survival is expected to be longer than 6 months, pursuing low per-fraction doses (i.e., 2 Gy per fraction) may reduce long-term complications of RT.

Reirradiation is generally not considered useful, except in usual circumstances, such as if a patient were to have a long disease-free period between initial radiation and reradiation. Of note, the risk of neurotoxicity and worsened cognitive function is higher with repeat radiation treatments.

Age and performance status do predict outcome. That is, the older or poorer the performance status, the worse the overall survival (2.3 vs. 7.1 months). Controlling the primary disease outside of the brain is also an important consideration.

Newer techniques for delivering radiation, including stereotactic radiosurgery, have a role in the management of brain metastases as well. Stereotactic radiosurgery delivers one to a few fractions of high-dose radiation to a well-circumscribed area. This treatment is more targeted than whole-brain RT, involves less fractions of treatment, and is typically delivered as an outpatient. This modality can be particularly useful for patients who, for whatever reason, cannot have surgical resection, and in patients with up to 3 metastatic deposits of disease without mass effect. There have been no randomized trials comparing radiosurgery versus conventional resection.

Surgery

The role of surgery is largely in patients with oligometastatic disease, normally with only one or two metastatic deposit in the brain, and in whom their systemic disease is either resolved or well controlled. Surgery to remove the tumors, given in conjunction with postoperative whole-brain RT, improves local control as well as median survival when compared to surgery alone. Notably RT was started within 14 days of surgery, and the majority of the studies included patients with only one metastasis. A retrospective review, however, suggested that there is also a benefit for patients with multiple metastases if all sites of disease can be removed.

Prognosis

Prognosis is best for patients with a solitary brain metastasis, excellent performance status, and little or no disease outside of the brain. Even in this good prognosis category, median survival is still only approximately 12 months. In patients with a low performance status and a high extracranial burden of disease, survival is only weeks to months and consideration should be given to palliative care alone.

MENINGIOMAS

Meningiomas are normally benign, slowly growing intracranial neoplasms, though they can rarely be found to be malignant. The management of benign meningiomas is discussed below. These tumors are normally seen attached to the dura mater, and are a common incidental finding on imaging pursued for other reasons than a suspected intracranial neoplasm. On neuroimaging, meningiomas are frequently calcified and extraxial in location, and may be accompanied by edema, occasionally in significant amounts. The histologic variant of a meningioma is generally not helpful in defining prognosis or optimal treatment. The peak age for meningiomas to be diagnosed is in mid-40s, and there is a female to male predominance. Meningiomas are also more common in African-Americans than whites. Surgical resection is the treatment of choice, though radiosurgery may also be a reasonable option. Importantly, if a meningioma is discovered incidentally, observation or a plan for expectant reimaging may also be a reasonable consideration, particularly if the patient has no symptoms or has other life-limiting comorbidities. Surgery in the older adult should be approached cautiously, as older age is associated with worse outcomes, including higher in-hospital mortality, longer mean hospital stay, and higher likelihood of discharge to a nursing facility. In the event of a positive margin or a recurrence in the bed of a prior resection, radiation may be used as a salvage therapy. The prognosis for meningiomas is excellent with a 5 years survival of more than 90%; the issue of greatest concern is the neurological deficit that remains after resection. Meningiomas also can recur as late as 20 years after the original resection, so a long period of follow-up may be necessary, as appropriate.

NEUROMAS

The most common neuromas in the older adult patient are acoustic neuromas, which are benign schwannomas of the vestibular nerve. These represent only 5% to 7% of intracranial neoplasms. They are slightly more common in women, and are also seen in association with neurofibromatosis type 2. These tumors arise from a mutation in the *NF2* gene, resulting in lack of production of the merlin protein. There are several approaches to this tumor depending on symptoms and patient's health condition. Although they are benign tumors, they may cause many symptoms depending on their location and proximity to the cranial nerves and brainstem. Presenting symptoms may include hearing loss, ringing in the ears and balance difficulties. Treatment options include surgery, expectant observation, or radiosurgery. The treatment plan for most acoustic neuromas is made by a multidisciplinary team of practitioners, as all approaches bring with them potential serious morbidity given the tumor's location.

GENERAL CONSIDERATIONS

Clinical Presentation

The older adult can present in different way clinically than the younger patient, perhaps owing to brain changes with age, which allow tumors to grow without much in the way of mass effect or elevated intracranial pressure, such as headaches, seizures, or papilledema. Conversely, older adults are more likely to present with mental status changes, memory problems, and confusion. On examination, a focal neurologic finding should be strongly suggestive of a possible brain tumor. Importantly, frontal brain tumors are more likely to present without focal findings, but instead personality change. Slowly growing tumors, such as meningiomas may present with a long history of symptoms.

Diagnostic Evaluation and Imaging

Where possible, initial imaging for an intracranial neoplasm should include MRI with and without gadolinium contrast, as this provides a superior sensitivity for tumors when compared to computed tomography (CT), and also provides multiplanar imaging, useful in treatment planning. CT has a role in defining extent of bony invasion, or for a rapid clinical deterioration where the delay in acquiring an MRI may be too long. Positron emission tomography (PET) can be used to differentiate residual or recurrent tumor from necrosis after treatment, particularly RT. A brain biopsy may be useful in determining the World Health Association grade of a tumor (Table 99-3).

Non-Chemotherapy Medication Considerations

Corticosteroids (most commonly dexamethasone) are commonly used in the setting of CNS neoplasms to reduce or prevent edema.

TABLE 99-3

WHO Classification of Common Brain Tumors

TUMOR TYPE	WHO PATHOLOGICAL GRADE
Glioblastoma multiforme	4
Anaplastic astrocytoma	3
Meningioma	1
Primary CNS lymphoma	3–4
Astrocytoma	1–2
Atypical meningioma	2–3

The dose of steroid may be tapered after several weeks of treatment if symptoms have stabilized. The lowest possible dose to control symptoms should be used. Common or serious side effects with this medication include oral thrush, hyperglycemia and steroid induced diabetes mellitus, insomnia, weight gain, agitation and delirium, all of which may complicate use in the older patient. It is our practice to start empiric antithrush prophylaxis at the time of starting corticosteroids. We also check blood glucoses while on higher doses of steroids. Patients and their caregivers should be counseled about the side effects of corticosteroids prior to administration.

Antiepileptics are commonly used to treat seizures associated with brain tumors or the accompanying edema. They are not required without a history of seizures except perhaps for prophylaxis around the time of surgery. The provider should recall that most antiepileptics agents interact with many medications by hepatic interactions, including dexamethasone, some chemotherapies, and anticoagulants, such as warfarin. There are a few antiepileptics (such as gabapentin and levetiracetam) that are not hepatically processed, and so may have fewer of these drug interactions. Antiepileptic drugs also carry the risk of the serious dermatological side effect of Stevens-Johnson syndrome. Any rash that develops in a patient with a brain tumor and concurrent antiepileptic use must be watched carefully.

The majority of patients with CNS neoplasms have some degree of a reactive depression, which should be treated in all but the minority of cases. This depression appears to be more severe in the older patients. Although the discussion regarding which antidepressant should be used is beyond the scope of this chapter, it is notable that the tricyclic and monoamine oxidase inhibitors should be avoided in patients on procarbazine chemotherapy.

CONCLUSIONS

Taken collectively, CNS disease in the older adult patient presents unique therapeutic challenges. Continued laboratory and clinical investigation should provide development of new less toxic and more efficacious approaches to therapy. Relative to this, the continued elucidation of resistance mechanisms, which may be modified by specific clinical strategies, should prove beneficial. Further, in the past year, laboratory correlative studies have opened the potential for the therapeutic application of signal transduction modifiers. Finally, the continued exploration of approaches to minimize toxicity in this fragile patient population is an ongoing research aim, which is now receiving significant interest by various acknowledged investigative groups.

FURTHER READING

Abrey LE, Ben-Porat L, Panageas KS, et al. Primary central nervous system lymphoma: the Memorial Sloan-Kettering Cancer Center prognostic model. *J Clin Oncol.* 2006;24:5711–5715.

Barker FG, Chang SM, Larson DA, et al. Age and radiation response in glioblastoma multiforme. *Neurosurgery.* 2001;49(6):1288–1298.

Bateman BT, Pile-Spellman J, Gutin PH, et al. Meningioma resection in the elderly: nationwide inpatient sample, 1998–2002. *Neurosurgery.* 2005;57(5):866–872.

Bindahl RK, Sawaya R, Leavens ME, et al. Surgical treatment of multiple brain metastases. *J Neurosurg.* 1993;79:210–216.

Brandes AA, Vastola F, Basso U, et al. Temozolomide in glioblastoma multiforme of the elderly. *Tumori.* 2002;88(1):S69-S70.

Chatani M, Matayoshi Y, Masaki N, et al. Prognostic factors in patients with brain metastases from lung carcinoma. *Strahlenther Onkol.* 1994;170:155–161.

Chinot OL, Barrie M, Frauger E, et al. Phase II study of temozolomide without radiotherapy in newly diagnosed glioblastoma multiforme in an elderly populations. *Cancer.* 2004;100(10):2208–2214.

DeAngelis LM, Hormigo A. Treatment of primary central nervous system lymphoma. *Semin Oncol.* 2004;31:684–692.

Gaspar LE, Scott C, Rotman M, et al. Recursive partitioning analysis (RPA) of prognostic factors in three radiation therapy oncology group brain metastases trials. *Int J Radiat Oncol Biol Phys.* 1997;37:745–751.

Gavrilovic IT, Hormigo A, Yahalom J, et al. Long-term follow-up of high-dose methotrexate-based therapy with or without WBRT for newly-diagnosed PCNSL. *J Clin Oncol.* 2006;24:4570–4574.

Grant R, Liang BC, Page MA, Crane DL, Greenberg HS, Junck L. Age influences chemotherapy response in astrocytomas. *Neurology.* 1995;45(5):929–933.

McAleese JJ, Stenning SP, Ashley S, et al. Hypofractionated radiotherapy for poor prognosis malignant glioma: matched pair survival analysis with MRC controls. *Radiother Oncol.* 2003;67:177–182.

Mellinghoff IK, Wang MY, Vivanco I, et al. Molecular determinants of the response of glioblastomas to EGFR kinase inhibitors. *N Engl J Med.* 2005;353:2012–2024.

Mohan DS, Suh JH, Phan JL, Kupelian PA, Cohen BH, Barnett GH. Outcome in elderly patients undergoing definitive surgery and radiation therapy for supratentorial glioblastoma multiforme at a tertiary care institution. *Int J Radiat Oncol Biol Phys.* 1998;42(5):981–987.

Murray KJ, Scott C, Greenberg HM, et al. A randomized phase III study of accelerated hyperfractionation versus standard in patients with unresected brain metastases: a report of the radiation therapy oncology group (RTOG) 9104. *Int J Radiat Oncol Biol Phys.* 1997;39:571–574.

Nelson DF. Radiotherapy in the treatment of primary central nervous system lymphoma (PCNSL). *J Neurooncol.* 1999;43:241–247.

Patchell RA, Tibbs PA, Regine WF, et al. Postoperative radiotherapy in the treatment of single metastases to the brain: a randomized trial. *JAMA.* 1998;280:1485–1489.

Philips C, Guiney M, Smith S, Hughes P, Narayan K, Quong G. A randomized trial comparing 35 Gy in ten fractions with 60 Gy in 30 fractions of cerebral irradiation for glioblastoma multiforme and older patients with anaplastic astrocytoma. *Radiother Oncol.* 2003;68:23–26.

Reni M, Ferreri AJM, Guha-Thakurta N, et al. Clinical relevance of consolidation radiotherapy and other main therapeutic issues in primary central nervous system lymphomas treated with upfront high-dose methotrexate. *Int J Radiat Oncol Biol Phys.* 2001;51:419–425.

Roa W, Brasher PMA, Bauman G, et al. Abbreviated course of radiation therapy in older patients with glioblastoma multiforme: a prospective randomized clinical trial. *J Clin Oncol.* 2004;22(9):1583–1588.

Stupp R, Mason WP, van den Bent MJ, et al. Radiotherapy plus concomitant and adjuvant temozolomide for glioblastoma. *N Engl J Med.* 2005;352:987–996.

Villa S, Vinolas N, Verger E, et al. Efficacy of radiotherapy for malignant gliomas in elderly patients. *Int J Radiat Oncol Biol Phys.* 1998;42(5):977–980.

Skin Cancer

Mathew W. Ludgate ■ *Timothy M. Johnson* ■ *Timothy S. Wang*

INTRODUCTION

Nearly 1.5 million new skin cancers are diagnosed in the United States each year, which represents more than half of all new U.S. cancer diagnoses. Approximately 10 000 people die annually of skin cancer in the United States; one an hour from melanoma and one every 4 hours from nonmelanoma skin cancer. There are three main types of skin cancer: basal cell carcinoma (79% of skin cancers), squamous cell carcinoma (14%), and melanoma (5%). Other skin cancer types comprise the remaining 2%. While melanoma accounts for only 5% of skin cancer diagnoses, it accounts for 75% of skin cancer deaths. Basal and squamous cell carcinomas are considerably less lethal, but these tumors are associated with significant morbidity. As with most malignancies, the incidence of skin cancer increases with age. Owing to their sheer numbers, the public health burden from skin cancer is great.

One in five people in the United States and one in three Caucasians will develop skin cancer during their lifetime. Since 1960, the incidence of skin cancer has risen by 4% to 8% per year. It continues to rise faster than any other cancer, and skin cancer has been labeled as "today's epidemic" in the lay press. It is likely that much of the data on the incidence and prevalence of skin cancer are an underestimation, as many biopsies of nonmelanoma skin cancer are interpreted in physicians' offices, and thus go unreported to hospital-based registries.

ETIOLOGY

Both genetic and environmental risk factors are implicated in the development of skin cancer. The most common known environmental risk factor is chronic and/or acute intense intermittent ultraviolet light exposure in the form of sunlight, artificial tanning devices (tanning booths), and sunburns. The Centers for Disease Control

Behavior Risk Factor Surveillance System data report that nearly 32% of all adults (57% of those aged 18–29) and more than 40% of children in the United States develop at least one sunburn annually. Ultraviolet B (UVB), at wavelengths between 290 to 320 nm, causes most of what we see as sun tanning and sun burns and is responsible for much of the actinic skin damage caused by sunlight. Ultraviolet A (UVA), 320 to 400 nm penetrates more deeply into the skin and is also an important factor in photoaging and skin cancers. UVB radiation induces skin cancer by a variety of mechanisms including direct DNA damage, damage to DNA repair systems, and alteration of the local cutaneous immune system. Some of the strongest evidence that implicates ultraviolet light as being important in the etiology of skin cancer comes from epidemiologic and experimental data correlating the incidence of tumors with the degree of pigmentary protection. Fair-skinned individuals with blue or green eyes and red, blonde, or light brown hair are at highest risk. These patients also typically tan poorly and sunburn and freckle easily. The risk of skin cancer varies with race and ethnic group with Caucasians of Celtic ancestry having the highest incidence rates. Skin cancer is less common in African-Americans, Asians, and Hispanics, but a rise in the Hispanic and Asian population is occurring. Other strong epidemiologic data correlate an increased incidence of skin cancer with residence at lower latitudes where there are higher levels of ambient UVB radiation.

The changes that most persons equate with aging of the skin are a result of chronic solar damage. Prolonged exposure to ultraviolet light leads to cutaneous atrophy, alterations in pigmentation, wrinkling, dryness, telangiectasia, and solar elastosis. Ultraviolet light from the sun or artificial tanning devices is believed to be the most common cause of nonmelanoma skin cancer (NMSC) and may account for some melanomas. Most NMSCs occur on sun-exposed sites such as the face, head, neck, or extensor arms and hands. Understandably, skin cancer is a significant occupational hazard for people who work outdoors. Although NMSCs usually occur on sun-exposed sites, they also rarely occur in sun-protected sites such as the anogenital area, mucous membranes, palms, and soles.

Other environmental/exposure factors associated primarily with squamous cell carcinoma (SCC) include chronic exposure to chemicals such as hydrocarbons (coal tars, soot, cutting oils, and asphalt). Chronic exposure to arsenic is associated with NMSC on both sun-exposed and sun-protected sites. PUVA (psoralen in combination with UVA) used in the treatment of psoriasis and other inflammatory dermatoses produces a dose-dependent increase in SCC and melanoma. Cigarette smoking is linked to SCC of the lip and mouth. The human papilloma virus has been associated with cutaneous SCC in the genital and acral/periungual areas. The carcinogenic effect of ionizing radiation inducing NMSC is documented in human and animal models. Other conditions associated with NMSC include burn and vaccination scars, chronic inflammatory processes and ulcers, and immunosuppression.

A number of genetic syndromes are associated with an increased risk of developing NMSC. Nevoid basal cell carcinoma syndrome (Gorlin syndrome) is an autosomal dominant or mosaic disorder associated with the occurrence of hundreds to thousands of lifetime basal cell carcinomas beginning in childhood or young adulthood. Jaw cysts, palmoplantar pits, abnormal ribs and vertebrae, frontal bossing, and hypertelorism are also found. Albinism, which can occur owing to one of several causal genetic defects, is associated with an increased risk of all skin cancer types. It is characterized by partial or complete failure to produce or distribute ocular, hair, and/or cutaneous UV protective melanin pigment. Xeroderma pigmentosum is a rare autosomal recessive disorder that results in the inability to repair UV-induced DNA damage. It is characterized by hypersensitivity to UV light and the relentless development of skin cancer, especially SCC and melanoma. Individuals with xeroderma pigmentosum are usually diagnosed with their first cancer prior to the age of 10.

A genetic component is also implicated in the pathogenesis of melanoma. Currently, a small percentage of melanomas are known to be associated with chromosomal mutations in CDKN2 A (p16), MC1R, or BRAF. The hereditary nature of melanoma is also noted in families with >100 normal nevi or any number of atypical appearing (dysplastic) nevi. Atypical nevi are not "premelanoma" *per se* but represent a phenotypic marker for an increased risk of melanoma. A positive family history of melanoma is present in 5% to 15% of melanoma patients. Five to ten percent of individuals with a prior melanoma develop a second melanoma. The genetic etiology of melanoma represents an area of future discovery.

Congenital nevi (CN) are present at birth or appear within the first 6 months of life. The risk of melanoma developing in CN <20 cm in diameter is similar to that of any other area of skin. Melanoma in CN usually occurs after childhood and arises at the dermoepidermal junction making early detection possible. Thus, in the absence of warning signs or symptoms, routine prophylactic removal of CN <20 cm in diameter is rarely indicated. Large (≥20 cm) CN are at increased risk for developing melanoma (5% to 20%), tend to progress to melanoma prior to age 10 (70%), and may originate deep in the lesion resulting in later detection.

NONMELANOMA SKIN CANCER

Basal Cell Carcinoma

Basal cell carcinoma (BCC) is the most common type of skin cancer and has no known precursor lesion. Approximately 80% of BCCs occur on the head and neck. BCCs are classified by clinical appearance and histologic pattern and include nodular, superficial, aggressive growth, and pigmented subtypes. BCCs rarely metastasize and grow slowly for years prior to sometimes developing a more rapid growth rate. Although they can appear quite indolent, BCCs grow relentlessly and if left untreated can cause extensive local destruction. Occult local invasion can also occur and may be deep and asymmetric with root-like extensions sometimes several centimeters beyond their apparent borders. Metastatic BCC is a rare event (0.03% of all BCCs), most often spreading to the regional lymph nodes followed by the lungs, bones, and skin. The 5-year survival rate for patients with metastatic BCC is poor and patients with distant disease have a median survival of only 10 and 14 months.

The most common BCC subtype is the well circumscribed nodular or noduloulcerative variant. This typically begins as a small, translucent or waxy flesh-colored or pink, pearly papule or nodule with small telangiectasias on the surface and a translucent, rolled border (Figure 100-1) (Color Plate 14). They may be pruritic or bleed. With time, the nodule increases in size and undergoes central ulceration. Most nodular BCCs present as small (< 1 cm) papules, however, patients still occasionally present with large, disfiguring lesions that have been neglected for many years. Classic histologic features of the nodular BCC include the presence of well circumscribed, basaloid tumor lobules of various sizes in the dermis. The basal cells at the tumor periphery appear to line up, a phenomenon known as peripheral palisading. Areas of separation or retraction artifact between tumor nodules and the adjacent connective tissue embedded in a pale mucinous stroma are also seen.

Superficial BCCs occur predominantly on the trunk and usually present as a pink to red, flat scaly lesion, sometimes with a fine, thread-like translucent border with central areas of hypopigmentation or atrophy (Figure 100-2) (Color Plate 15). They are sometimes confused with scaly skin conditions such as psoriasis or other eczematous dermatoses, and may closely resemble actinic keratosis or Bowen disease. Significant and sometimes extensive superficial subclinical involvement is common as they grow by peripheral extension. Histological features of the superficial BCC include numerous, multifocal small buds of basaloid tumor cells that arise in the epidermis and extend into the superficial dermis and down and around hair follicles.

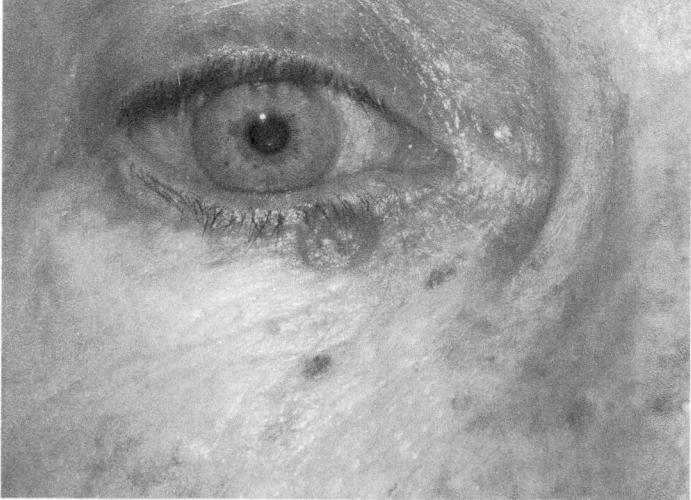

FIGURE 100-1. Nodular BCC on the lower eyelid. Small pearly papule with telangiectatic blood vessel visible at superior aspect of lesion.

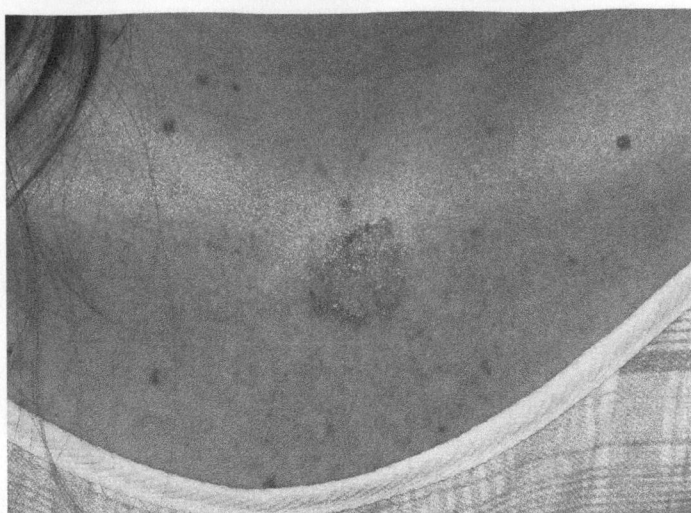

FIGURE 100-2. Superficial BCC occurring on the chest. Pink, flat lesion with slightly raised scaly borders.

The aggressive BCC subtype usually presents as a flat, firm, indurated, pale, white-to-yellow papule or plaque with harder to detect clinical borders and a "scar like" appearance. This subtype is also known as infiltrating, morpheaform, sclerosing, sclerotic, and fibrotic BCC. Clinically, aggressive BCCs can exhibit subclinical extension widely beyond (>1 cm) their apparent borders, and can also ulcerate (Figure 100-3) (Color Plate 16). They have a higher rate of recurrence following standard treatment modalities because of distant, small finger-like projections of tumor cells that may deeply invade into the dermis, subcutis, and muscle and skate along fascial planes, cartilage, and bone. These small, finger-like islands are often missed with standard histologic margin control. Histological features of aggressive-growth BCC include small islands and spiky finger-like linear strands and cords of basaloid tumor cells embedded in a dense, fibrous sometimes sclerotic connective tissue stroma. Peripheral palisading and stromal retraction is often subtle or absent and perineural invasion is more common. Micronodular BCC similar to aggressive

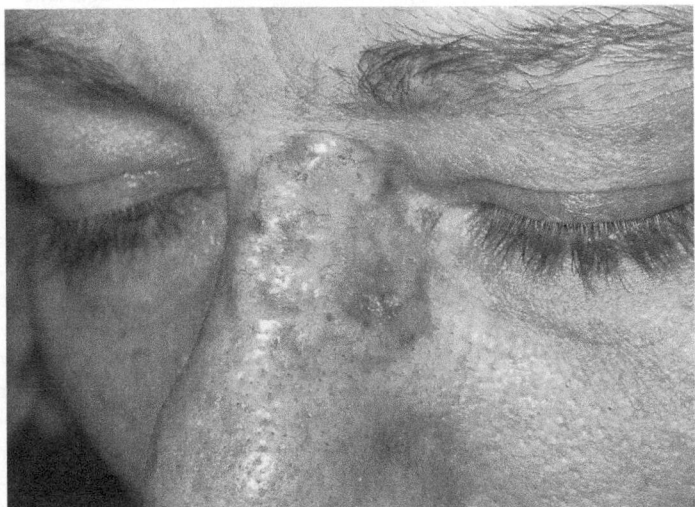

FIGURE 100-3. Aggressive BCC. Note the very subtle clinical features with an indurated plaque with telangiectasia present. This lesion is likely to have wide subclinical extension present.

BCC often has significant subclinical extension through the dermis or subcutis. Histologically, smaller tumor islands similar in size to hair bulbs, characterize micronodular BCC. In some cases, a BCC has histologic features of squamous metaplasia and keratinization. These tumors have basosquamous differentiation and may become more aggressive and develop regional lymphatic spread. It is important for the pathologist to convey the BCC histologic subtype pattern to the clinician, especially for aggressive-growth BCC. Multiple histologic patterns may be present in up to 35% to 50% of BCC with the most aggressive pattern correlating with biologic behavior.

Pigmentation from melanin can be seen in all BCC subtypes, but is most commonly seen in nodular BCCs. Some lesions categorized as pigmented BCC are heavily pigmented and can bear a striking resemblance to melanoma or pigmented seborrheic keratoses.

BCC is thought to originate from immature pluripotential epidermal cells. The cytokeratin pattern in BCC resembles that found in the outer root sheath of the hair follicle below the isthmus in the bulge area rather than that of the epidermis, supporting a follicular origin for the tumor. These cells can mature and differentiate in a pattern resembling any of the epithelial structures. BCC can develop in both a hereditary and sporadic fashion. Mutations in the patched (PTCH) gene have been identified in nevoid BCC syndrome and in sporadic BCC. PTCH is a cell membrane receptor for a family of proteins called hedgehog (Hh). The PTCH protein binds and inhibits a transmembrane protein known as smoothened (SMO). Mutations in either PTCH or SMO lead to increased SMO signaling and growth promotion with subsequent cancer formation. The activation of the SMO pathway leads to induction of a number of proteins via the Gli1 transcription factor, including transforming growth factor (TGF-β), platelet-derived growth factor receptor-α, PTCH, and Gli1 and are relevant to cancer development. Mutations that inactivate the tumor suppressor gene p53 have also been identified in more than half of BCCs, but a causal role for p53 mutations in BCC development or progression has not been demonstrated. Patients with Li–Fraumeni syndrome, characterized by an inherited mutation in the p53 gene, have an increased incidence of a number of malignancies, but an increase in NMSC has not been reported.

Squamous Cell Carcinoma

SCC is the second most common skin cancer type. It possesses the potential to metastasize, the risk of which depends on various risk factors. The most common site of metastasis is the regional lymph nodes, which occurs in 85% of metastatic cases. Approximately 15% of metastases involve distant sites such as the lungs, liver, brain, bone, and skin. The prognosis for patients with metastatic SCC is poor with 10-year survival rates of <20% for patients with advanced regional lymph node involvement and <10% for patients with distant metastases. Fortunately, the majority of cutaneous SCCs are low-risk lesions that are treated with high cure rates.

SCC has a precursor "premalignant" lesion termed actinic keratosis (AK). AKs are extremely common in fair-skinned elderly Caucasian individuals who have had significant chronic sun exposure. AKs usually occur in areas damaged by sun exposure, such as the bald scalp, face, and extensor forearms/hands. AKs occur as well-demarcated, scaly, rough patches or plaques on chronic sun-exposed skin surfaces. Their color can vary from skin colored, erythematous, pink, or to brown, and they are often more easily palpated than seen. The majority of cutaneous SCCs arise in AKs. However, the incidence of progression of an individual lesion from AK to SCC in situ (Bowen disease) and then to invasive SCC remains low, ranging from 0.025% to 20% and occurs slowly over years in immunocompetent individuals. The cumulative risk depends on the number of lesions and the length of time they persist. AKs are easily treatable with cryotherapy or topical agents such as 5-fluorouracil for more numerous lesions. Other conditions predisposing to SCC include radiation exposure; scarring from a previous injury such as a burn, chronic inflammatory processes such as chronic wounds or ulcers, osteomyelitis, sinuses, or discoid lupus; human papilloma virus particularly in acral and genital sites; and chronic arsenic or hydrocarbon exposure.

Patients who are immunosuppressed following organ transplant deserve special consideration and attention. SCC is the most common skin cancer in immunosuppressed organ transplant recipients, occurring 65 to 250 times more frequently than in the general population. Large numbers of premalignant AKs can rapidly develop and progress in fair-skinned, immunosuppressed individuals with a history of significant sun exposure. Moreover, these AKs behave more aggressively and tend to transform into invasive, rapidly growing SCCs with a more aggressive behavior and increased risk of metastasis. Frequent clinical surveillance and early intervention and prevention are thus essential in these patients. Almost half of the malignancies that arise in patients with impaired immune surveillance occur in the skin. The great majority of these are squamous cell cancers, occur in sun-exposed areas, and almost 50% of patients have multiple tumors.

Ultraviolet-induced mutations of the p53 tumor-suppressor gene interfere with apoptosis of the damaged cells, permitting damaged cells to proliferate. More than half of cutaneous SCCs and AKs have p53 gene mutations. Nucleotide sequence analysis demonstrates that these mutations are specifically associated with exposure to UVB light.

Clinically, cutaneous SCCs most commonly develop (80%) on chronically sun-exposed areas on the head and neck and extremities, followed by the trunk. Clinical presentation varies, but most commonly occurs as a 0.5 to 1.5 cm firm, sometimes tender, hyperkeratotic pink to red papule, nodule, or plaque (Figures 100-4 and 100-5) (Color Plates 17 and 18). Ulceration and easy bleed-

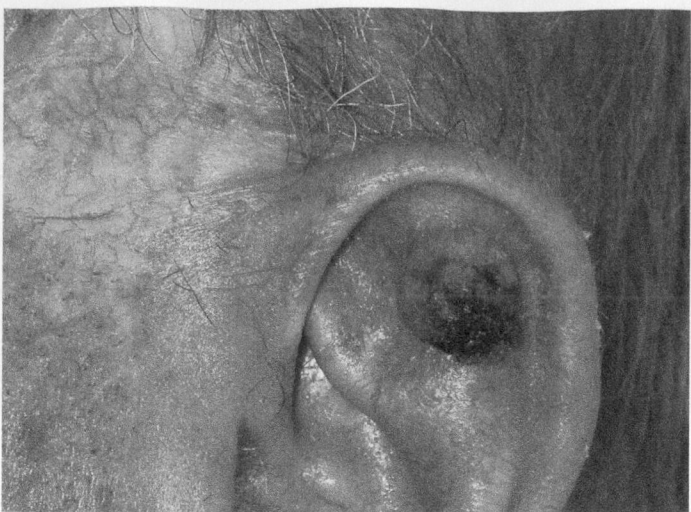

FIGURE 100-5. Invasive SCC on the ear. Ulcerated crusted lesion on the ear associated with a high risk of regional metastasis.

ing is a relatively common finding. Rapid and deep local invasion may occur. In darker skinned patients, SCC may present in non sun-exposed areas and is most commonly associated with chronic inflammatory or scarring processes.

Histologically, several subtypes of SCC exist, but the conventional subtype is the most common. Other subtypes include adenoid/ acantholytic, bowenoid, spindle/pleomorphic, small cell, verrucous, and keratoacanthoma. The conventional subtype is associated with irregular masses of epidermal cells proliferating downward and invading the dermis. The invading tumor masses are composed of varying proportions of normal squamous cells and atypical cells. These atypical cells demonstrate variations in the size and shape of the cells, hyperchromasia and hyperplasia of the nuclei, absence of intracellular bridges, keratinization of individual cells, and the presence of atypical mitotic figures. In SCC, differentiation is toward keratinization. Horn pearls, which are concentric layers of squamous cells with gradually increasing keratinization toward the center, can also be seen. The dermis often shows a marked inflammatory reaction. Histologic grading of SCC depends on the percentage of keratinizing cells, percentage of atypical cells, number of mitotic figures, and depth of invasion. The Broders classification system is based on the degree of de-differentiation of the cells: in grade 1, <25%; in grade 2, <50%; in grade 3, <75%; and in grade 4, >75% of the cells are undifferentiated (poorly differentiated).

Treatment for BCC and SCC

Prior to any treatment, a biopsy confirming the diagnosis is mandatory. Numerous surgical and nonsurgical modalities are effective in treating BCC and SCC. Despite the enormous amount of literature pertaining to the treatment of BCC and SCC, there is relatively little high-level evidence–based research on the efficacy of the treatment modalities used. Most of the reported literature is retrospective, not randomized, and suffers from selection bias, such as allowing treatment modality to be influenced by whether the lesion is low- or high-risk. Based on the best available cumulative evidence, the selection of therapy is based upon several clinical and histologic risk factors noted in Table 100-1. The majority of lesions are relatively low risk and can be treated effectively with standard techniques such

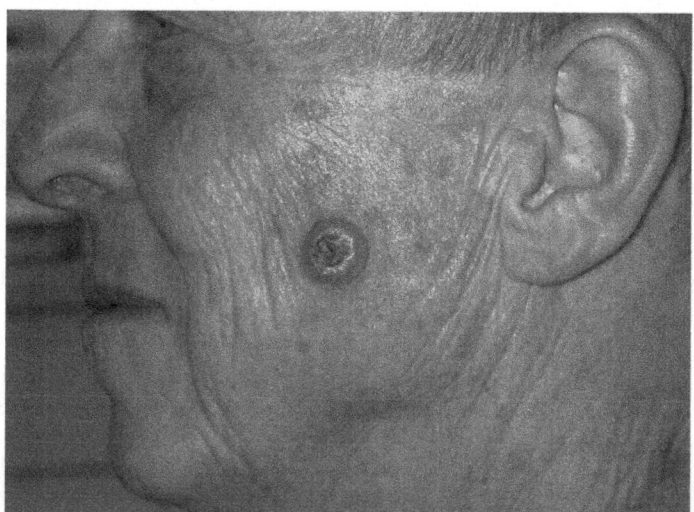

FIGURE 100-4. Invasive SCC on the cheek. Large ulcerated nodule with central core filled with hyperkeratotic material.

TABLE 100-1

Basal Cell Carcinoma (BCC) and Squamous Cell Carcinoma (SCC) Risk Factors for Occult Subclinical Invasion and Recurrence

Recurrent tumor

Location
  High-risk: mask areas of face (eyelid, eyebrow, periorbital, nose, lip, chin, mandible, temple, ear, in front or behind the ear), genitalia, hands, and feet
  Medium-risk: cheeks, forehead, scalp, and neck
  Low-risk: trunk, extremities

Size
  Lesions > 5 mm on high-risk area: mask areas of face, genitalia, hands, and feet
  Lesions > 9 mm on medium-risk area: cheeks, forehead, scalp, and neck
  Lesions > 19 mm on low-risk area: trunk and extremities

Histology
  BCC: aggressive growth (morpheaform, fibrosing, sclerosing, infiltrating, micronodular)
  SCC: poorly differentiated, invades deep reticular dermis or adipose

Ill-defined clinical borders

Perineural invasion

Immunosuppression

Etiology: development in site of prior radiation, scar, chronic inflammatory process

SCC-depth of invasion

SCC-rapid growth

---

as electrodessication and curettage, curettage alone, standard surgical excision, radiation, or ablative cryosurgery with 92% to 98% local control rates for low-risk tumors. As the lesions develop additional risk factors noted in Table 100-1, the control (cure) rate begins to drop precipitously. For higher risk lesions, Mohs surgery or surgical excision with comprehensive margin control or wide margins still results in 95% to 99% local control rates in the majority of cases.

Electrodessication and Curettage

Electrodessication and curettage (ED&C) is a common, effective, operator-dependent treatment option. ED&C causes local tissue destruction and is quickly performed with local anesthesia in the office. First, a curette is used to remove the gross tumor, which is soft and friable. This is followed by electrodessication of the periphery and base of the wound to destroy residual tumor cells. This process is repeated with both a large and small curettes and electrodessicated for 2 to 4 cycles depending upon the size and feel of the lesion. The experienced operator can provide similar high cure rates with curettage alone, omitting electrodessication. The resulting wound heals by granulation with a hypopigmented, atrophic, and sometimes a depressed scar. If the curette extends into the subcutis or a sclerotic "feel" is noted, ED&C should be discontinued and excision of the site should be performed. The major disadvantage of ED&C is the lack of a surgical specimen to examine for margin control.

Cryosurgery

Ablative cryosurgery is another treatment option, but less frequently used. It is also quickly performed using local anesthesia in the office.

Liquid nitrogen is delivered to the tumor and a margin of normal appearing skin, which causes deep-freezing to −50° to −60°C and significant local destruction and tissue necrosis. Common side effects include edema, pain, extensive blister formation, and erythema. Chondritis and cartilage necrosis may occur for auricular lesions. The drawbacks of poorer cosmetic result, time to heal, and lack of a tissue specimen are similar to those seen with ED&C. Cryosurgery is an effective treatment for low-risk BCCs as well as for some SCCs.

Topical Chemotherapy

Topical chemotherapy can be an effective treatment modality for AKs and has been used for select low-risk BCC. The two main agents available are topical 5-fluorouracil (5-FU) and the imidazoquinoline, imiquimod. Topical 5-FU is usually used in a 5% cream formulation, applied twice daily for 2 to 4 weeks. Topical 5-FU is particularly useful for treating larger areas of AKs, when more localized treatment such as cryosurgery becomes impractical. It has also been used for low-risk superficial BCC. Local inflammation and irritation are the main complications of therapy. Topical imiquimod 5% cream is also an effective treatment for AKs and is also used for select low-risk superficial BCC. Imiquimod is an immune response modifier and exerts its effect via toll-like receptors to increase inflammatory cytokine production. Similar to topical 5-FU, local inflammatory reactions are common, and some patients can also develop systemic flu-like symptoms.

Radiotherapy

Fractionated radiation therapy (RT), usually performed in 15 to 25 daily treatments over 3 to 5 weeks, is an effective therapy for lower risk NMSC especially in patients who are poor surgical candidates. Experience and a clinical understanding of NMSC are vitally important to achieve good results. While early cosmetic results are better than destructive techniques, long-term results are not. Contraindications for RT include genodermatoses predisposing to skin cancer (nevoid BCC syndrome and xeroderma pigmentosum) and connective tissue disease (lupus and scleroderma). Local recurrences following RT are more aggressive and as with destructive techniques, a surgical specimen to examine for margins is lacking.

Surgical Excision

Surgical excision is an effective treatment modality for all types of NMSC and possesses the advantage of a tissue specimen for histologic assessment of margins. Excisions heal more rapidly often with superior cosmetic results when compared with destructive techniques. Recommended margins for excision of NMSC generally range from 4 to 10 mm. Surgical excision is more invasive, more expensive for low-risk lesions, and requires training and experience. Many cases can be performed in a treatment room with local anesthesia, but larger cases may require general anesthesia or intravenous sedation in the operating room. High-risk lesions require more comprehensive histological processing and evaluation or widely clear margins with standard tissue processing to achieve high control rates. Standard histopathologic (bread loaf) processing of standard surgical excision specimens examines <1% of the true surgical margin. This may be problematic for higher risk NMSC such as those with greater subclinical extension. Following an incompletely excised NMSC by observation is not appropriate therapy. Rather, re-excision by either Mohs surgery, or additional therapeutic intervention should be performed. The cure rate of low-risk lesions by excisional surgery is similar to those of destructive techniques and RT.

Mohs Micrographic Surgery

Mohs surgery is a highly effective treatment for NMSC when done by experienced, appropriately trained Mohs surgeons and results in the highest local control (cure) rates with maximal sparing of normal tissue. Mohs surgery avoids many of the problems associated with the aforementioned treatments for skin cancer. Originally developed in the 1930s using a zinc chloride chemical paste to fix the tissue in vivo, the procedure is named after its inventor Dr. Frederic E. Mohs. The technique was refined in the 1970s to its current "fresh tissue" technique, which essentially involves serially excising cancerous tissue with 1 to 3 mm margins per stage, and examining the entire undersurface and edges of the specimen. When done properly, nearly total (theoretical 100%) margin control can be obtained. Of all NMSC treatments, Mohs surgery offers the highest cure rate (often >99%), lowest likelihood of recurrence, potential for minimal scarring and disfigurement, and unmatched precision. By definition, the Mohs surgeon performs a dual role as both surgeon and pathologist, and through advanced 1 to 2 year postgraduate fellowship training, the Mohs surgeon is adept at microscopic interpretation of horizontally cut frozen sections as well as local flap and graft soft tissue reconstruction techniques to repair the resulting wounds.

Mohs surgery is performed under local anesthesia in an office-based setting. Briefly, the visible portion of the tumor is outlined and anesthetized, then all gross tumor is removed by curettage. With the scalpel blade held at a 45-degree angle to the skin to facilitate tissue processing of the deep and peripheral margins, the surgeon excises a layer of tissue in the shape of a saucer with 1 to 3 mm deep and peripheral margins around and under the curettage defect. The specimen is divided into sections, color coded with dyes, and a schematic map is made for precise anatomic orientation. The specimen is then turned over and flattened into one plane so that the beveled skin edge is placed in the same horizontal plane as the deep margin. The Mohs histotechnician processes horizontal frozen sections that incorporate the entire deep and peripheral margin for interpretation.

The undersurface and edges of each section are examined by the Mohs surgeon under the microscope for evidence of remaining cancer. If cancer cells are noted, the surgeon marks their precise location on the map and returns to the patient to remove another layer of skin at the corresponding site of residual tumor. This layer is again examined microscopically for additional cancer cells. The process continues layer by layer in stages until no detectable cancer cells remain. Maximal normal tissue conservation is preserved, and nearly 100% of the margin is examined resulting in exceedingly high local control rates. Reconstruction is performed without delay after margins are free. In cases involving extensive defects or very large or complex tumors, a collaborative multidisciplinary team approach is important. Adjunctive RT may be indicated in cases of extensive perineural spread and in cases of SCC with a significant risk of lymphatic spread.

Mohs surgery is a labor-intensive technique and requires an experienced team. Surgical training is often highly variable with practice ranging from no postgraduate training; weekend courses to postgraduate Mohs College approved fellowship training, and ACGME approved postgraduate training. To achieve high cure rates, the Mohs surgeon must be provided high quality Mohs frozen section slides. This requires specialized histotechnician training and experience. Mohs surgery is considered the "gold standard" for removal of higher risk NMSC. However, for small lower risk lesions, the cure rates for the treatment of NMSC with Mohs versus standard therapies are comparable.

MELANOMA

Melanoma results from the malignant transformation of melanocytes usually located at the dermal–epidermal junction. Melanoma confined to the epidermis is termed melanoma in situ, which is theoretically 100% curable. With time, the melanoma invades vertically into the dermis where it can metastasize to the regional lymph nodes and/or other distant visceral organ systems via the lymphatic or vascular systems. The deeper melanoma invades, the greater the risk for metastasis and advanced systemic disease, which is by and large fatal.

Melanoma occurs in a younger age group than many cancers with approximately 25% occurring in patients <45 years of age, including children. Melanoma is one of the leading cancer types in terms of average years of potential life lost because of cancer-related death. In the United States, melanoma is the most common cancer type in Caucasian women aged 25 to 29, is second only to breast cancer in women 30 to 34 years of age, and is the most common type of cancer in Caucasian men in Michigan aged 25 to 44. The incidence in Caucasians has more than tripled since 1980. Encouragingly, the 5-year survival rate has increased from 50% in 1954 to 85% to 90% in 2006. This is largely a reflection of earlier detection. The annual direct cost of treating melanoma in 1997 was estimated at $563 million with projections exceeding $5 billion by 2010 for Medicare alone. Approximately 90% of this cost is attributable to the less than 20% of patients with more advanced disease, highlighting the importance of early detection, diagnosis, and treatment.

Primary care practitioners are often the patient's first contact with the health care system, and therefore they play a vital role in the early detection of melanoma. Primary care practitioners knowledgeable about persons at risk and who have a heightened awareness of melanoma have a "golden" opportunity for early melanoma detection and education. Lives can be saved and health care costs reduced by early detection of this potentially fatal skin cancer. Although fewer than 20% of melanomas are detected by physicians and health care providers, provider-detected melanomas are significantly thinner, resulting in a better prognosis and lowered costs for treatment. Patients taught to examine their skin and the importance of bringing suspicious skin lesions to the attention of their providers also detect earlier lesions.

Melanoma can arise anywhere on the skin surface. One-third occur within a preexisting pigmented lesion and two-thirds occur with no precursor lesion or nevus on clinically normal appearing skin. The most frequent site for melanoma in men is the trunk, particularly upper back and shoulders. The most frequent sites for melanoma in women are the legs followed by the trunk. Melanoma can also rarely occur in mucosal, genital, nail bed, and ocular sites. In the African-American population, the hands and feet are common sites for melanoma. Risk factors for the development of melanoma include blue or green eyes, blonde or red hair, fair complexion with a tendency to freckle, sunburn and to tan poorly, the presence of dysplastic nevi or >100 normal appearing nevi, a personal or family history of melanoma, and a history of significant UV exposure or sunburns.

The earliest clinical features of melanoma include a change in the size, shape, or color and occasionally persistent itching in a lesion. Later features include ulceration, bleeding, and/or tenderness. Classically an ABCD rule has been used to help recognize lesions suspicious for melanoma. "A" stands for asymmetry—one half of the lesion does not match the other half as a mirror image when drawing an imaginary line through the center of the lesion. "B" stands for irregularity of the borders—the edges of the lesion are ragged, notched, jagged, scalloped, or fuzzy. "C" stands for color—the color is not homogeneous throughout the lesion. Varying and mottled shades of tan, dark brown to jet-black, or shades of red, white, and/or blue may be present. Historically, "D" stands for diameter >6 mm, which has proven to be relatively insensitive as an independent factor. At our melanoma center and in many in the United States, "D" now stands for difference whose meaning is two-fold. The first application of "difference" describes any change or difference in an individual lesion, especially with respect to size, shape, color, or persistent itching. The second applies more to the evaluation of multiple nevi. In patients with multiple normal or slightly abnormal appearing nevi, those nevi when viewed as a group should grossly appear similar to one another. That is that they should have a "family" resemblance. Any members of the family that look "different", like they do not belong to the family, should be examined. This has also been called the "ugly duckling" sign. The presence of atypical nevi represents a risk factor for the development of melanoma anywhere on the skin. The ABCD rule and other diagnostic aids enhance early detection, but do not provide the ability to differentiate between benign and malignant in every setting. Some advocate adding an "E" to denote evolution and change.

Early melanomas often lack all of these classic ABCD features. Therefore, any changing pigmented lesion or new atypical lesion should be evaluated and considered for biopsy especially in a patient with risk factors for melanoma. Melanomas can completely lack pigmentation (amelanotic melanoma) in 3% to 4% of cases. Understandably, these are often associated with later detection. As previously mentioned, melanoma arises within a preexisting nevus in only 33% of cases, and therefore it occurs *de novo* on clinically normal appearing skin in 66% of cases. Although one's threshold for biopsy should be low and suspicion for melanoma high, prophylactic removal of preexisting nevi is therefore rarely indicated.

Historically, melanomas are classified by histological patterns and clinical characteristics into four major subtypes: superficial spreading melanoma, lentigo maligna melanoma, nodular melanoma, and acral lentiginous melanoma. These classifications are of little prognostic value as the biological behavior and risk of metastasis today are based mainly on the thickness of the primary tumor (Breslow depth).

Superficial spreading melanoma comprises approximately 60% to 70% of melanomas and represents the most common melanoma subtype. They often arise in a preexisting nevus and typically develop as a spreading pigmented plaque with irregular borders and variation in color and surface contour. They often exhibit the classic clinical features of melanoma (Figures 100-6 to 100-8) (Color Plates 19, 20, 21). Areas of regression may result in pink to white areas within the black or brown tumor. They may progress to a vertical growth phase faster than lentigo maligna.

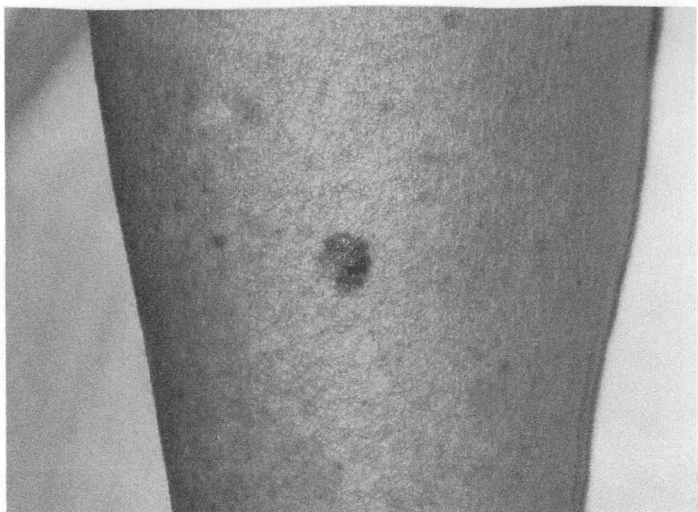

FIGURE 100-6. Early superficial spreading melanoma. Note asymmetry and irregular border.

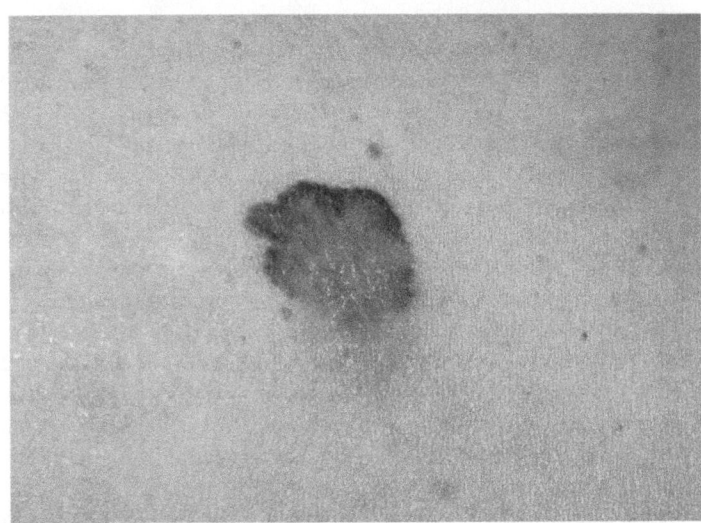

FIGURE 100-7. Superficial spreading melanoma showing all of the ABCD features. Breslow depth 3.5 mm.

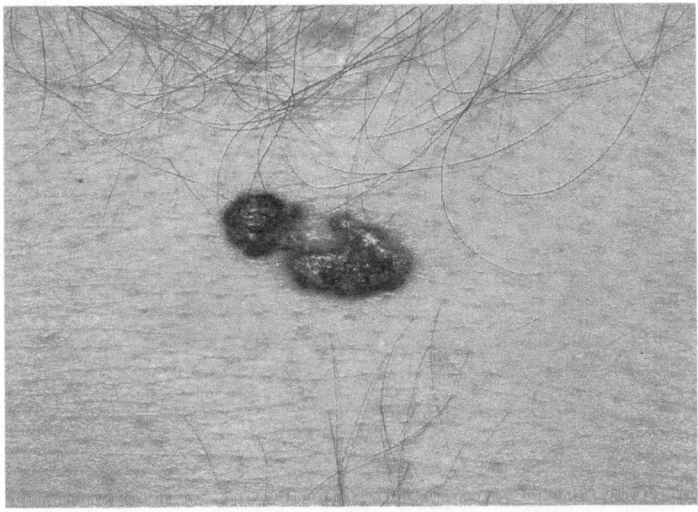

FIGURE 100-8. Superficial spreading melanoma. Breslow depth 1.1 mm.

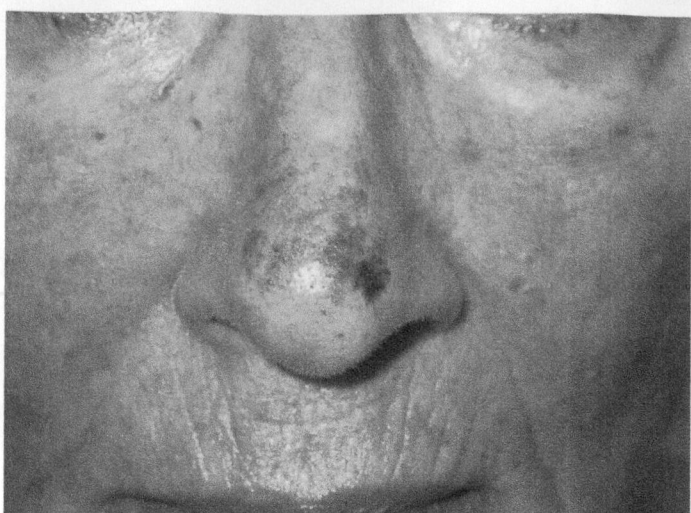

FIGURE 100-9. Lentigo melanoma (melanoma in situ) on the dorsum of the nose. Irregularly pigmented flat macule that had been slowly enlarging over a number of years.

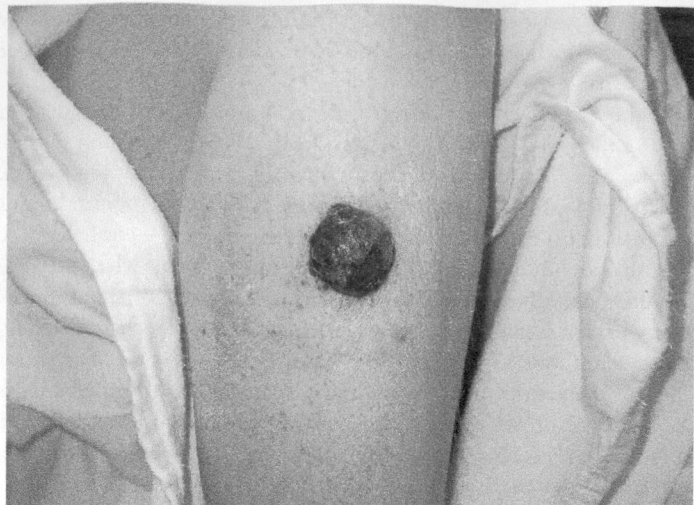

FIGURE 100-10. Large nodular melanoma. Breslow depth 11.5 mm with ulceration associated with 45% 5-yr survival (stage IIc).

The lentigo maligna melanoma subtype comprises approximately 10% to 15% of all melanomas and usually begins as a pigmented macular lesion with variation in black and brown color (Figure 100-9) (Color Plate 22). They are most common on the chronically sun-exposed areas of the head and neck, most often in older individuals. Lentigo maligna represents the in situ phase and with time, progresses to the invasive phase then termed lentigo maligna melanoma. These lesions have irregular outlines and may slowly enlarge over many years with progression to black and development of other classic melanoma features. The malignant cells may extend asymmetrically several centimeters beyond the clinical lesion and extend down hair follicles and other skin appendages. These characteristics can make lentigo maligna and lentigo maligna melanoma difficult to cure by superficial treatments and result in higher recurrence rates with standard surgical margins. Amelanotic and desmoplastic melanoma with neurotropism may occur more frequently in the setting of lentigo maligna melanoma.

Nodular melanoma often arises without evidence of a preexisting lesion. They constitute approximately 15% to 30% of melanomas and have a minimal radial–lateral growth phase. These tumors are more aggressive because they are often thicker when detected, stressing the importance of lesion change and difference for early detection. Nodular melanomas usually appear as a raised, nodular, or polypoid lesion with more uniform color and regular borders. They often present as <6 mm, may become ulcerated with rapid growth, and can lack the classic melanoma features (Figure 100-10) (Color Plate 23).

Acral lentiginous melanoma represents approximately 2% to 8% of melanomas in Caucasians, but 35% to 60% in people of color. They usually occur on acral sites, i.e., the hands, feet, fingers, toes, and under the nails. Subungual melanomas can present as an irregular, tan-brown longitudinal streak in the nail. Approximately 75% of subungual melanomas involve the great toe or thumb and are often confused with subungual hematoma.

Staging and Prognosis

Accurate staging is necessary for counseling, treatment recommendations, and survival. Additionally, stage grouping better defines homogeneous populations for clinical trials. The guidelines for management of melanoma continue to rapidly evolve owing to a wealth of new knowledge and research. Tumor thickness as measured in millimeters is termed the Breslow depth and is the single most important independent factor of the primary lesion that determines treatment, follow-up, and prognosis. The presence or absence of ulceration in the primary lesion is also an independent prognostic and staging factor. The American Joint Committee on Cancer (AJCC) uses a five-stage system that is based on classifying melanoma according to tumor thickness (T), nodal status (N), and metastatic disease (M). Five stages exist, which correlate with prognosis: stage 0 (in situ melanoma), stage I (local disease), stage II (local disease), stage III (regional nodal disease, satellitosis or in-transit metastases), and stage IV (distant metastases). Distant metastasis portends a poorer prognosis. Melanoma metastasizes most frequently to the skin, subcutaneous tissue, and lymph nodes. Visceral metastases manifest most commonly in the lungs, liver, brain, bone, and intestines but may occur in any organ. A thorough description of the current TNM classification and melanoma staging system is found in a seminal article referenced: Balch M, Buzaid AC, Soong SJ, et al. Final version of the American Joint Committee on Cancer Staging System for Cutaneous Melanoma. *J Clin Oncol.* 2001;19:3635–3648.

Microstaging

The most important histologic prognostic factor of melanoma is the Breslow depth of the primary tumor. Breslow depth is the measured thickness (in millimeters) of the primary tumor from the top of the granular layer (the uppermost layer of the epidermis) to the base of the tumor. As above, the presence of ulceration is also an independent prognostic factor. Breslow depth and the presence or absence of ulceration often determines work-up, treatment, and prognosis. Poorer prognosis generally correlates with deeper Breslow depth and the presence of ulceration. Five-year survival rate range from greater than 95% for those diagnosed with melanoma less than 1.00 mm thick with no ulceration to 45% for those with melanoma greater than 4.00 mm thick with ulceration.

The status of the regional lymph node basin is the most powerful predictor of overall survival. For those with nodal metastasis, the tumor burden (both microscopic vs. macroscopic disease and the number of involved lymph nodes) has an inverse correlation with survival. The 5-year survival rate for patients with involved lymph nodes ranges from 25% to 70% based primarily on tumor burden and ulceration status of the primary lesion. The use of sentinel lymph node biopsy (SLNB) for melanoma deeper than 1.0 mm in Breslow depth or 0.75 to 1.0 mm with other adverse features can identify patients with micrometastatic nodal disease who have a favorable prognosis compared to those with macroscopic nodal involvement. The lymph node status and tumor burden based on SLNB is incorporated into the current AJCC staging system. A thorough description of prognosis based on Breslow depth and other prognostic factors is found in a seminal article referenced: Balch M, Soong SJ, Gershenwald JE, et al. Prognostic factors analysis of 17600 melanoma patients: validation of the American Joint Committee on Cancer Melanoma Staging System. *J Clin Oncol.* 2001;19:3622–3634.

Treatment of Melanoma

Biopsy

The primary lesion of melanoma can vary in depth, and prognosis is based on the deepest measured area of invasion. Therefore, a full-thickness excision with narrow margins oriented parallel to the lines of lymphatic drainage is the preferred method to evaluate a suspicious pigmented lesion with the goal being to provide the pathologist a complete specimen for histologic interpretation and accurate microstaging. A superficial shave biopsy is never recommended for a lesion suspicious for melanoma, because if the melanoma is transected, the ability to obtain an accurate measurement of tumor thickness may be lost. Performing a wide excision with 0.5 cm margins or greater as the initial step is similarly discouraged as it may result in the inability to accurately perform a subsequent SLNB. For suspicious lesions too large for complete excision, a full-thickness incisional biopsy deep enough to avoid transecting the lesion at the deep margin may be performed using an ellipse, deep saucerization shave, or punch. Incisional biopsies of melanoma do not increase the risk of metastasis. Formalin-fixed, paraffin-embedded, permanent sections are required for accurate microstaging and diagnosis of the primary lesion. The biopsy should be interpreted by a dermatopathologist with experience in melanocytic lesions. Frozen sections and fine-needle aspiration have no role in the diagnosis of primary cutaneous melanoma, but can be useful in the diagnosis of metastatic disease in palpable nodules found in the nodal basin or soft tissues.

In the case of recently diagnosed melanoma and in the presence of an unremarkable history and physical examination, the National Comprehensive Cancer Network (http://www.nccn.org/) in 2007 recommends (1) no routine tests for local disease <1 mm Breslow depth, (2) no routine tests versus optional CXR and serum LDH plus SLNB (if indicated to follow) for local disease ≥1 mm, and (3) CXR, LDH, pelvic CT if groin nodes involved versus CT chest/abdomen/pelvis and MRI head for regional disease. Work-up for stage IV disseminated melanoma is often dictated by clinical trial protocols. Significant emotional distress of many patients with melanoma occurs, regardless of disease stage. Thus, access to psychooncology services is an important aspect of the overall management in the patient with melanoma.

Surgical Excision of the Primary Tumor

Surgical excision of the primary tumor is the standard therapy for melanoma to prevent local recurrence caused by persistent disease.

For melanoma in situ, excision margins of 0.5 to 1 cm are indicated. For invasive melanoma, excision with margins of 1 cm for melanoma ≤1 mm thick, 1 to 2 cm for those 1 to 2 mm thick, and 2 cm for those >2 mm thick is indicated for local control. For the clinically ill-defined lentigo maligna melanoma, these standard margin recommendations may be inadequate because of potentially extensive (up to several centimeters) subclinical extension. Histological confirmation of negative margins is necessary for complete surgical resection of lentigo maligna melanoma, preferably using permanent section processing.

Regional Node Management

Sentinel Lymph Node Biopsy.
The concept of SLNB is based on the hypothesis that in some patients melanoma involvement of a nodal basin develops in an orderly fashion with metastasis to the SLN as the first step in the metastatic process. With the intradermal injection of lymphatic tracers such as blue dye (Lymphazurin) and/or a radiolabeled colloid solution, the first draining node from the primary lesion site, the sentinel lymph node, can be identified and used to accurately stage the entire nodal basin. The technique of SLNB is most often performed in conjunction with the wide excision of the primary tumor and is routinely performed as an outpatient procedure. If the SLN is negative for melanoma, the remaining lymph nodes are free of involvement in >96% of cases, the prognosis is more favorable and observation is indicated. If the SLNB is positive for melanoma, regional therapeutic lymphadenectomy is indicated based on potential survival and clinical benefit.

Patients without clinical evidence of metastasis with primary melanoma ≥1 mm in thickness should be counselled for SLNB. For some subgroups with melanoma Breslow depth 0.75 to 1.0 mm including young patients, evidence of ulceration, extensive dermal regression to 1.0 mm, or ≥ 1.0 mitosis/mm^2 in young patients, SLNB may also be considered. The rate of SLNB positivity in patients with melanoma >1 mm is approximately 15% with the rate positivity increasing with Breslow depth. Reasons not to perform SLNB include a low risk of regional nodal metastasis, significant medical comorbidities, wide excision already performed in ambiguous draining areas, or the patient does not desire SLNB after an informed discussion.

SLN status is the most powerful independent factor predicting survival and provides the highest sensitivity and specificity of any nodal staging test available in 2007. Additionally, SLNB followed by immediate complete lymphadenectomy may result in improved regional control compared to delayed complete lymphadenectomy after clinical evidence of nodal disease occurs. No definitive evidence exists that a positive SLNB followed by immediate complete lymph node dissection improves overall survival in patients with melanoma. However, interim evidence suggests a potential subset survival benefit of approximately 20% at 7 years. This interim evidence suggests that in a subset of patients with occult SLN metastasis, immediate complete lymphadenectomy prolongs disease-free survival compared with delayed complete lymphadenectomy when nodal metastasis becomes clinically evident.

Lymphadenectomy Indications.
Therapuetic complete lymphadenectomy of metastases to regional lymph nodes is potentially curative. The 5-year survival rate for patients who undergo therapuetic lymphadenectomy for nodal disease ranges from 25% to 70% and correlates with tumor burden. In addition, for those patients

not cured by lymphadenectomy, complete lymphadenectomy can still be beneficial by preventing potential painful uncontrolled nodal disease. After surgical resection of regional nodal disease in the absence of known distant metastasis, high-dose protocol interferon-α2b (IFN-α) is the only adjuvant treatment that has demonstrated a modest benefit in disease-free survival. IFN-α is associated with significant side effects, and many patients are thus not good candidates. Clinical trials involving investigational drugs, often versus IFN-α are available.

Treatment of Disseminated Melanoma (Stage IV)

Cure for Stage IV melanoma is rare. Dacarbazine is the main, single-agent chemotherapeutic drug for treatment of disseminated melanoma with response rates in the range of 10% to 20%. Complete responses are rare and usually brief, often less than 6 months. Combination chemotherapy with multiple agents has been used, but unfortunately with results not significantly better than single-agent dacarbazine. Systemic interleukin-2 (IL-2) may result in a 15% to 20% response rate, but is associated with high toxicity and is thus often used in otherwise relatively young and healthy patients with advanced melanoma. Approximately 5% of patients have a complete response, which may be durable for a prolonged period of time. Several immunotherapeutic trials exist for disseminated metastatic melanoma in select patients. Trials with adoptive immunotherapy, dendritic cells, and vaccines with and without the concomitant use of IL-2 and chemotherapeutic agents, gene therapy, and combinations of IL-2 and/or IFN-α with chemotherapy (biochemotherapy) are ongoing. RT may be used for palliation of bone pain secondary to metastatic disease or brain metastasis but has little role in the treatment of primary melanoma. Surgical resection of metastatic melanoma may be useful for palliation in patients with isolated recurrences in the skin, brain, lung, and gastrointestinal tract. Isolated hyperthermic limb perfusion of chemotherapeutic agents may be considered in a small subgroup of patients with nonresectable subcutaneous or skin metastases confined to a lower limb.

OTHER CUTANEOUS TUMORS

There are a number of less-common cutaneous tumors that are beyond the scope of this chapter. The reader is referred to a standard dermatology text for discussion of the following:

- Merkel cell carcinoma
- Cutaneous T-cell and B-cell lymphoma
- Histiocytic tumors
- Mast cell tumors
- Malignant adnexal tumors (hair follicle origin—malignant proliferating tricholemmal tumor, tricholemmoma carcinoma, malignant pilomatrixoma; eccrine gland origin—malignant eccrine poroma, hidradenocarcinoma, malignant chondroid syringoma, malignant spiradenoma, malignant cylindroma, eccrine ductal carcinoma, mucoepidermoid carcinoma, microcystic adnexal carcinoma, eccrine epithelioma, adenoid cystic carcinoma, mucinous carcinoma, aggressive digital papillary adenocarcinoma; apocrine gland origin—extramammary Paget disease, apocrine adenocarcinoma; sebaceous gland origin—sebaceous epithelioma, sebaceous carcinoma)
- Cutaneous sarcoma—fibrosarcoma, malignant fibrous histiocytoma, dermatofibrosarcoma protuberans, liposarcoma, synovial sarcoma, leiomyosarcoma, rhabdomyosarcoma, malignant nerve sheath tumor, angiosarcoma, lymphangiosarcoma, malignant hemangiopericytoma, Kaposi sarcoma, alveolar soft part sarcoma, epithelioid sarcoma of Enzinger, clear cell sarcoma of tendons and aponeuroses, extraskeletal osteosarcoma, extraskeletal chondrosarcoma
- Metastatic cancer to the skin

FURTHER READING

Alam M, Ratner D. Cutaneous squamous-cell carcinoma. *N Engl J Med.* 2001; 344:975–83.

Albert MR, Weinstock MA. Keratinocyte carcinoma. *CA Cancer J Clin.* 2003;53:292–302.

Armstrong BK, Kricker A. The epidemiology of UV induced skin cancer. *J Photochem Photobiol B.* 2001;63:8–18.

Balch M, Buzaid AC, Soong SJ, et al. Final version of the American Joint Committee on Cancer Staging System for Cutaneous Melanoma. *J Clin Oncol.* 2001;19:3635–48.

Balch M, Soong SJ, Gershenwald JE, et al. Prognostic factors analysis of 17600 melanoma patients: validation of the American Joint Committee on Cancer Melanoma Staging System. *J Clin Oncol.* 2001;19:3622–34.

Berg D, Otley CC. Skin cancer in organ transplant recipients: epidemiology, pathogenesis, and management. *J Am Acad Dermatol.* 2002;47:1–17.

Berwick M, Wiggins C. The current epidemiology of cutaneous malignant melanoma. *Front Biosci.* 2006;11:1244–54.

Christenson LJ, Borrowman TA, Vachon CM, et al. Incidence of basal cell and squamous cell carcinomas in a population younger than 40 years. *JAMA.* 2005;294:681–90.

Housman T, Feldman S, Willford P, et al. Skin cancer is among the most costly of all cancers to treat for the Medicare population. *J Am Acad Dermatol.* 2003;48:425–9.

Johnson T, Rowe DM, Nelson BR, et al. Squamous cell carcinoma (excluding lip and oral mucosa). *J Am Acad Dermatol.* 1992;26:467–84.

Johnson TM, Bradford CR, Gruber SB, et al. Staging workup, sentinel node biopsy, and follow-up tests for melanoma: update of current concepts. *Arch Dermatol.* 2004;40:107–13.

Johnson TM, Chang A, Redman B, et al. Management of melanoma with a multidisciplinary melanoma clinic model. *J Am Acad Dermatol.* 2000;42:820–6.

Johnson TM, Sondak VK, Bichakjian CK, et al. The role of sentinel lymph node biopsy for melanoma: evidence assessment. *J Am Acad Dermatol.* 2006;54:19–27.

Morton DL, Thompson JF, Cochran AJ, et al. Sentinel-node biopsy or nodal observation in melanoma. *N Engl J Med.* 2006;355:1307–17.

National Comprehensive Cancer Network. http://www.nccn.org/. Accessed March 2007.

Paek SC, Griffith KA, Johnson TM, et al. The impact of factors beyond Breslow depth on predicting sentinel lymph node positivity in melanoma. *Cancer.* 2007;109:100–8.

Rowe D, Carroll R, Day CJ. Long-term recurrence rates in previously untreated (primary) basal cell carcinoma: implications for patient follow-up. *J Dermatol Surg Oncol.* 1989;15:315–28.

Rubin AI, Chen EH, Ratner D. Basal-cell carcinoma. *N Engl J Med.* 2005;353:2262–9.

Stasko T, Brown MD, Carucci JA, et al. Guidelines for the management of squamous cell carcinoma in organ transplant recipients. *Dermatol Surg.* 2004;30:642–50.

Tsao H, Atkins MB, Sober AJ. Management of cutaneous melanoma. *N Engl J Med.* 2004;351:998–1012.

Aging of the Hematopoietic System

Gurkamal S. Chatta ■ *David A. Lipschitz*

INTRODUCTION

Aging of the lymphohematopoietic system often manifests as a blunted response to hematopoietic stress and is thought to be associated with an increased incidence of neoplasia, autoimmune diseases, and infections in elderly people. Although the physiological basis of this suboptimal response remains unclear, our understanding of human hematopoiesis has increased exponentially over the last two decades. However, most of the initial breakthroughs, as well as the seminal findings in the biology of hematopoiesis, have occurred in murine models. This review will discuss (1) the biology of hematopoiesis, (2) age-related changes in lymphohematopoiesis, and (3) indications for the use of hematopoietic growth factors in elderly patients.

BIOLOGY OF HEMATOPOIESIS

The hematopoietic system derives from a small pool of hematopoietic stem cells (HSCs), which can either self-renew or differentiate along one of several lineages to form mature leukocytes, erythrocytes, or platelets. HSCs differentiate into mature cells through an intermediate set of committed progenitors and precursors, each with decreasing self-renewal potential and increasing lineage commitment. Hematopoiesis is tightly regulated by a complex series of interactions between HSCs, their stromal microenvironment, and diffusible regulatory molecules (hematopoietic growth factors) that effect cellular proliferation. The orderly development of the hematopoietic system in vivo and the maintenance of homeostasis require that a strict balance be maintained between self-renewal, differentiation, maturation, and cell loss.

Murine Hematopoiesis

HSCs cannot be directly observed, but are defined and identified by their ability to reconstitute and maintain hematopoiesis. The earliest morphologically recognizable cells of the myeloid and erythroid series are the myeloblasts and proerythroblasts (Figure 101-1). These cells are derived from morphologically unrecognizable progenitors that were first identified by in vitro culture techniques. There are two forms of erythroid progenitors: a more primitive precursor referred to as a burst-forming unit–erythroid (BFU-E), and a more mature progenitor referred to as the colony-forming unit–erythroid (CFU-E). A committed myeloid progenitor, also known as colony-forming unit–granulocyte/macrophage (CFU-GM), is the immediate precursor of the myeloblast. The committed progenitor cell compartments are supplied, in turn, by a common pluripotent stem cell, which has the capacity to differentiate into either hematopoietic or lymphoid cells. Figure 101-1 shows the hierarchy of cellular proliferation and differentiation in this pathway. The pluripotent HSC is called a colony-forming unit–spleen (CFU-S) by virtue of its ability (1) to produce colonies in spleens of lethally irradiated mice and (2) to repopulate the marrow of lethally irradiated recipients. There is evidence that the number of CFU-S in cell cycle is minimal, but that cycling can be greatly increased if demands for regeneration are increased. The CFU-S has a heterogeneous self-renewal capacity whereby an uncommitted CFU-S with high self-renewal capacity produces more committed CFU-S with decreasing self-renewal capacity and increasing differentiation potential.

Modern multichannel flow cytometry together with the availability of antibodies for different progenitor cell surface markers has validated the above findings, by allowing the identification of distinct progenitor cell populations with variable potential for hematopoietic reconstitution in lethally irradiated recipients. All HSC activity

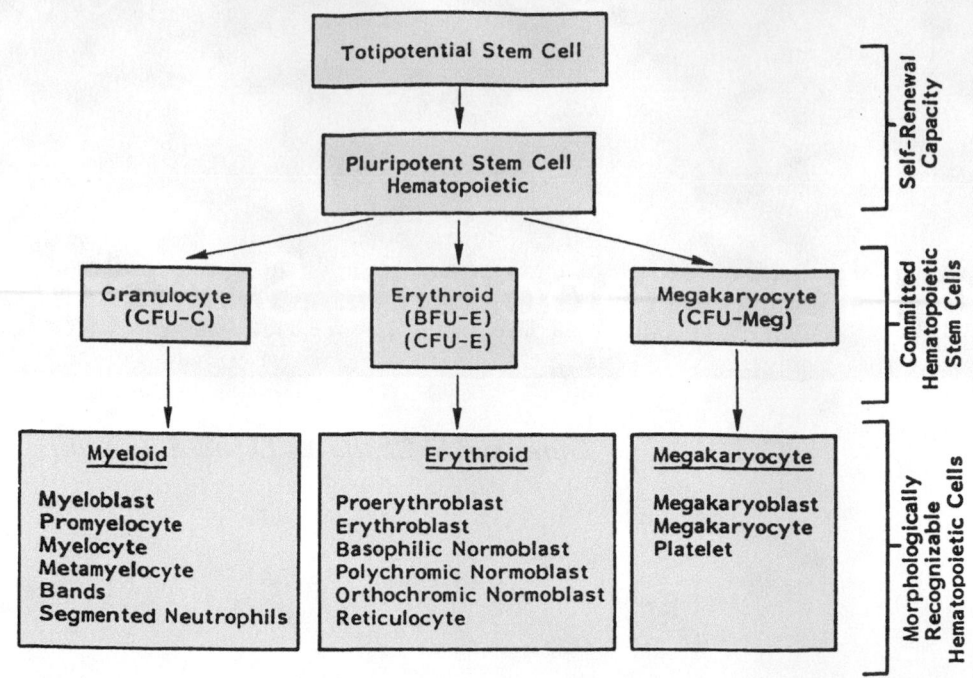

FIGURE 101-1. The hierarchy and production of hematoietic precursors from primitive pluripotent stem cells.

in many strains of mice is contained within a minor bone marrow population with a cell surface phenotype of c-<u>k</u>it positive (K), lineage negative (L), and Sca-1 positive (S), also known as the KLS cell fraction. However, only 1 in 30 KLS cells have true stem cell function. Two additional murine bone marrow markers, flk 2 and murine CD34, have also been identified. Thus, the KLS, flk2−, CD34− cells are the only cells within the KLS fraction, which possess long-term multilineage reconstituting HSC ability and are also known as the long-term repopulating stem cells or the LT-HSC. The KLS, flk2+, CD34+ cell fraction has limited repopulation potential and is known as the ST-HSC.

Effect of Age on CFU-S and LT-HSC

A major question with regard to the aging hematopoietic system is whether or not the pluripotent HSC has a finite replicative capacity. Studies of long-term bone marrow culture show that maintenance of hematopoiesis varies inversely with the age of the donor from which the culture was initiated. Additional studies using serial transplantation, whereby HSCs are subjected to in vivo serial transfer into recipient animals in which hematopoiesis has been ablated, also reveal a gradual loss in the ability to self-replicate. Thus, CFU-S from young donors is better able to repopulate the marrow of irradiated mice than CFU-S from old donors. A finite replicative capacity of the HSC was also found in an in vivo mouse model. Although finite, the lifespan of HSCs is thought to be well in excess of the potential lifespan of a species.

With the ability to detect stage-specific membrane markers, it is now possible to distinguish between long-term (LT) and short-term (ST) HSCs, and thus more accurately dissect the changes in the subtypes of CFU-S with age. Isolated bone marrow cells bearing the phenotype of LT-HSC and ST-HSC demonstrate a fivefold increase in the frequency of cells orwith stem cell phenotype from older mice. However, their functional capacity was only a quarter of that seen with these cells from younger mice. The impact of aging on the

lineage potential of stem cells has now been studied by transplanting limited numbers of purified LT-HSC from young and old mice into young congenic recipients, followed by analysis of donor cell contribution to B-cell, T-cell, and myeloid cell lineages at multiple time points posttransplant. These studies demonstrated that total donor reconstitution was consistently diminished in mice transplanted with old HSC. Furthermore, it was also noted that LT-HSCs from old mice had an increased propensity for myeloid differentiation and were deficient in generating mature lymphocytes. This skewed pattern of myeloid–lymphoid differentiation was not influenced by the aging marrow microenvironment, and was primarily thought to be an inherent attribute of the aging LT-HSC. Furthermore, in a murine model of chronic myeloid leukemia (CML), older animals with CML primarily developed a myeloid disorder with rare lymphoid involvement, as opposed to involvement of both myeloid and lymphoid lineages in younger animals with CML. Thus, it has been postulated that the myeloid dominance of adult leukemia may in part be driven by age-related deficient lymphopoiesis. Gene expression analysis of aging LT-HSCs supports this hypothesis by revealing (1) a 2- to 12-fold down-regulation of lymphoid lineage genes, (2) a two- to sixfold up-regulation of myeloid genes, and (3) a two- to fivefold up-regulation of leukemic proto-oncogenes like Aml 1, Pml, and Eto. In all, more than 700 genes were found to be differentially regulated with aging in the LT-HSCs, with genes involved in inflammatory and stress responses being up-regulated, and genes regulating chromatin remodelling and DNA repair being down-regulated.

Effect of Aging on Bone Marrow Function

The effect of age on committed HSC number and on the number of differentiated hematopoietic bone marrow cells has also been examined. In mice, no age-related reduction in the number of erythroid (BFU-E, CFU-E) or myeloid/macrophage (CFU-GM) progenitor cells occurs. Red blood cell survival is unchanged with aging, the plasma iron turnover and erythron iron turnover are unchanged, and the red blood cell mass is normal. The apparent anemia frequently observed in aged mice appears to be caused by an expansion of plasma volume. These findings and those of others indicate that no change in basal hematopoiesis occurs with aging. However, the ability of the aged hematopoietic system to respond to increased demands appears to be compromised. For example, older mice recover their hemoglobin values more slowly after phlebotomy than do young mice. Furthermore, when aged animals are placed in a high-altitude chamber, the expected increase in hemoglobin level is more variable and tends to be lower in older, as compared with younger, animals. Similar observations have also been made for the myeloid lineage, whereby bacterially challenged older mice undergo myeloid exhaustion earlier than younger mice.

The fragility of the aged hematopoietic system is further highlighted by studies on mice approaching their maximal life expectancy. When 48-month-old C57 BL/6 mice were housed in individual cages (one animal per cage), no change in hematopoiesis was seen. If, however, they were housed in groups of five animals per cage, the animals became more anemic and the number of stem cells in their bone marrow decreased. Thus, a suboptimal response in the face of stimulus-driven hematopoiesis and a failure to maintain homeostasis is a central characteristic of the aging hematopoietic system.

The mechanism/s responsible for the decline in HSC function remain unclear. Recently, accumulated DNA damage has been proposed as the principal and unifying mechanism underlying age-dependent HSC decline. HSC reserves and function with age in mice deficient in several genomic maintenance pathways including nucleotide excision repair (XPD^{TTD} mice), telomere maintenance ($mTR^{-/-}$ mice) and nonhomologous end-joining ($Ku80^{-/-}$ mice) have been studied. None of the knock-out mice had a diminution either in HSC number or stem cell frequency. However, HSC functional capacity was severely affected under conditions of stress, leading to loss of reconstitution and proliferative potential, diminished self-renewal, increased apoptosis and, ultimately, functional exhaustion. Furthermore, endogenous DNA damage was noted to accumulate with age in wild-type HSCs. These data were thought to be consistent with DNA damage accrual being a physiological mechanism of stem cell aging that may contribute to the diminished capacity of aged tissues to return to homeostasis after exposure to acute stress or injury. Efforts are also underway to dissect the molecular mechanisms of HSC senescence. Analyses of cell cycle genes have implicated reciprocal roles for the cycle-dependent kinase inhibitors p21 and p18 in HSC function, with a deletion of p21 accelerating hematopoietic exhaustion and a deletion of p18 improving the engraftment potential of LT-HSC in serial transplantation experiments in mice.

THE EFFECT OF AGE ON HEMATOPOIESIS IN HUMANS

Normal Hematopoiesis

The human hematopoietic system derives from a small pool of stem cells that can either self-renew or differentiate along one of several lineages to form mature leukocytes, erythrocytes, or platelets. Marrow progenitors can be enriched on the basis of surface markers expressed at sequential stages of maturation. With respect to the myeloid lin-

eage, the relevant surface markers are CD33 and CD34. CD33 is found on most cells of the myeloid lineage in the marrow, and CD34 is expressed only by more primitive progenitors (1% to 4% of the marrow cells). Thus, precursors of myeloid colony-forming cells (pre-CFC) express CD34 and lack expression of CD33 and other antigens expressed by mature lymphoid and myeloid cells. Since CD34+ marrow cells can engraft and reconstitute hematopoiesis in lethally irradiated baboons and humans, surface expression of CD34 on marrow and circulating cells serves as a surrogate for stem cell function.

Proliferation and differentiation of progenitor cells to become mature blood cells requires intimate contact between stem cells, stromal cells, and the extracellular matrix, and is thought to be mediated by the hematopoietic growth factors (HGFs). The HGFs are produced by multiple cell types and, on the basis of their actions, are characterized either as multilineage hematopoietins, e.g., stem cell factor (SCF), or mast cell growth factor (MGF), interleukin-3 (IL-3), and granulocyte-macrophage colony-stimulating factor (GM-CSF); or as lineage restricted hematopoietins, for example, granulocyte colony-stimulating factor (G-CSF), macrophage colony-stimulating factor (M-CSF), erythropoietin (EPO), thrombopoietin (TPO), and T-cell growth factor (IL-2). In addition to the above growth factors, lymphohematopoiesis is also modulated by an ever-expanding list of other cytokines (Table 101-1). These are produced by diverse cell types, have wide-ranging biological effects, and participate in a variety of cellular responses. Currently, G-CSF, GM-CSF, EPO, and IL-2 are in common clinical use.

G-CSF is a 24kD glycoprotein promoting the growth and maturation of myeloid cells and in particular, the proliferation and differentiation of neutrophil progenitors both in vitro and in vivo. There are two recombinant forms of G-CSF currently available.

TABLE 101-1

Cytokines Modulating Hematopoiesis	
LYMPHOKINE	**MAJOR BIOLOGICAL PROPERTIES**
IL-1	Activates resting T-cells; induces fever; activates endothelial cells and macrophages
IL-2	Growth factor for activated T-cells; synthesis of other lymphokines
IL-3	Supports growth of multilineage bone marrow stem cells
IL-6	B-cell growth factor
IL-7	B-cell and T-cell growth factor
IL-12	Differentiation of naive CD4 T cells to the Th1 subset
Stem cell factor (SCF)	Promotes proliferation of primitive progenitors
Granulocyte-macrophage colony-stimulating factor (GM-CSF)	Promotes growth of neutrophilic, eosinophilic and macrophage cell lineages
Granulocyte CSF (G-CSF)	Promotes growth of neutrophilic cells
Macrophage CSF (M-CSF)	Promotes growth of monocytes and macrophage
Erythropoietin (EPO)	Promotes growth of erythroid cells
Thrombopoietin (TPO)	Stimulates megakaryocyte and platelet production

CSF, colony-stimulating factor; IL, interleukin.

Filgrastim (Neupogen®) is a nonglycosylated, smaller molecule than its endogenous counterpart, but has the same biological activity. Pegfilgrastim (Neulasta®) is pegylated formulation of G-CSF, allowing for an increased plasma half-life permitting once a chemotherapy cycle (every 14 to 21 days) administration as opposed to daily administration with nonpegylated G-CSF. Pegfilgrastim has shown a comparable safety and efficacy profile to filgrastim in three randomized clinical trials. Phase III studies established the safety and efficacy of recombinant human (rh) G-CSF in ameliorating chemotherapy-related neutropenia in cancer patients and for the treatment of severe chronic neutropenia. G-CSF is also routinely used for the purposes of mobilizing peripheral blood stem cells (PBSCs). Its role in the treatment of acute leukemia and myelodysplasia is controversial. It is usually administered subcutaneously, is well tolerated, and other than medullary bone pain and a skin rash at the site of injection, no significant side effects have been reported.

GM-CSF is a glycosylated 22-kDa peptide that has a broader range of cellular targets than G-CSF. The two forms of recombinant human GM-CSF currently in use are sargramostim (Leukine®), and molgramostim (nonglycosylated or *E coli*–derived). The effects of GM-CSF both in causing neutrophilia and in mobilizing PBSC are very similar to those of G-CSF. GM-CSF was first reported to enhance marrow recovery in the setting of autologous marrow transplantation for lymphoid malignancies. Currently, GM-CSF is approved for use in AML in elderly patients. The use of GM-CSF as a vaccine adjuvant, in particular its ability to recruit dendritic cells to the site of injection, is under investigation. Because of its wider spectrum of biological effects, GM-CSF has more systemic toxicity and at high dosage levels, the capillary leak syndrome is a particular concern.

EPO is a 34- to 39-kDa glycoprotein that selectively acts on the erythroid lineage. EPO has been in clinical use since 1985 for pa-tients with end-stage renal disease. Erythropoiesis can be stimulated by the exogenous administration of two FDA approved agents: the recombinant human erythropoietin (Epogen® or Procrit®), and dar-bepoetin alfa (Aranesp®). The latter is more heavily glycosylated and longer acting than the former. EPO is also widely used for the treatment of cancer-related anemia. The target hemoglobin is typically 11 g%, with there being continued controversy as to whether higher levels are desirable or detrimental. EPO is well tolerated and most of its side effects, that is, thromboembolic phenomena, have been described in the setting of dialysis.

Age-Related Changes in Lymphohematopoiesis

The evaluation of hematopoiesis in older humans is made exceedingly difficult by the complex interaction of environmental variables with the host over extended periods of time. Figure 101-2 illustrates the large number of factors that may modulate erythropoietic function in elderly subjects.

An extensive study performed on a group of carefully selected, hematologically normal (Table 101-2) healthy young and elderly subjects revealed no significant differences in peripheral blood or ferrokinetic data. Furthermore, quantitation of marrow progenitors and differentiated precursors demonstrated no significant differences between the young and the elderly group. A series of longitudinal studies of hematological parameters on a group of affluent subjects in New Mexico also demonstrated no obvious hematologic problem, and no abnormalities developed during a 3-year follow-up. Based upon these observations and the animal studies described above, the aging process is thought to primarily affect stimulus-driven hematopoiesis, with little or no impact on the basal state. The blunted hematopoietic response to stress has been ascribed to age-related deficits in marrow progenitor cell numbers, changes in

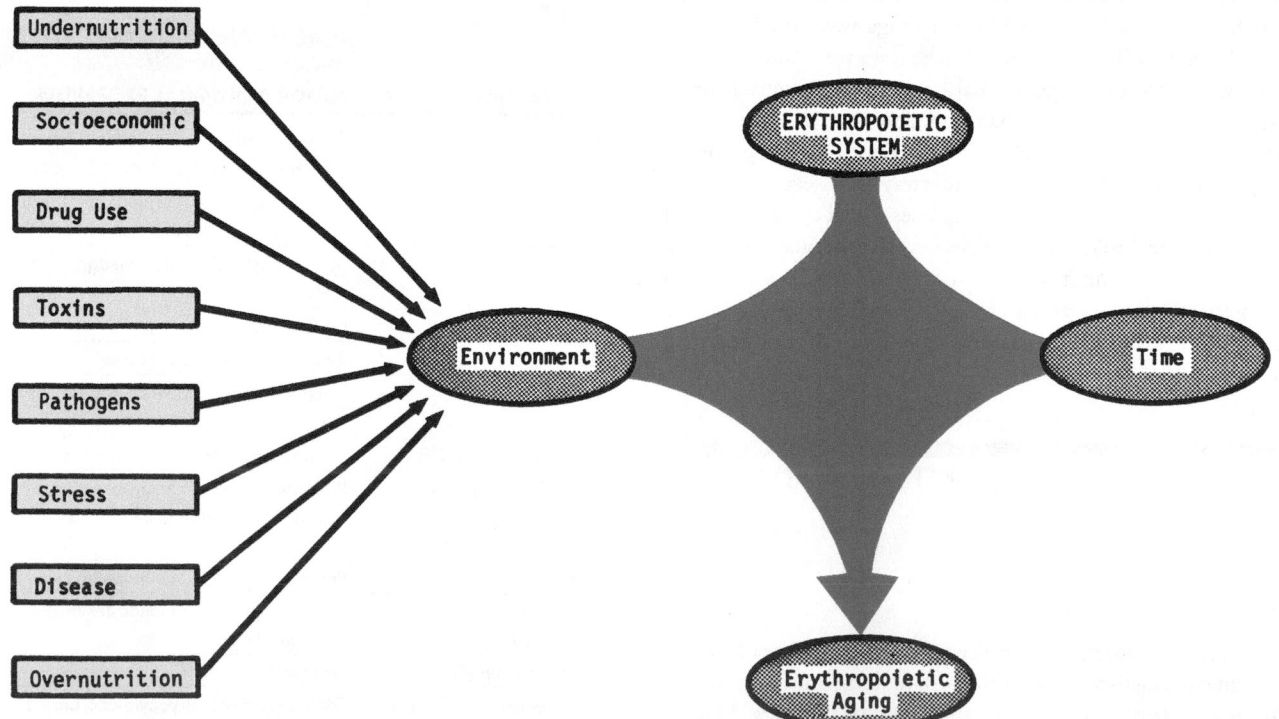

FIGURE 101-2. External variables likely to modify age-related decrements in erythropoiesis.

TABLE 101-2

Hematological Profile in Young and Elderly Hematologically Normal Subjects

	YOUNG	ELDERLY
Age (yrs)	34 ± 2.0*	78 ± 2.0
Hemoglobin (g/dL)	15 ± 0.3	15 ± 0.2
Mean corpuscular volume (fl)	89 ± 0.9	91 ± 1.8
Serum iron (μg/dL)	107 ± 8.1	93 ± 5.0
TIBC (μg/dL)	297 ± 10	307 ± 13
Saturation (%)	36 ± 3.0	30 ± 2.2
Serum ferritin (ng/mL)	126 ± 17	219 ± 26
Proto:heme (μmol/mol)	24 ± 1.4	22 ± 1.8
Vitamin B-12 (μg/mL)	476 ± 34	451 ± 34
Serum folate (ng/mL)	5.6 ± 0.8	4.8 ± 0.5
Retic index	1.1 ± 0.3	1.0 ± 0.2
Leukocyte ($\times 10^3$/μL)	8.8 ± 0.4	7.6 ± 0.5
Neutrophils ($\times 10^3$/μL)	5.9 ± 0.3	4.5 ± 0.6
Lymphocyte ($\times 10^3$/μL)	1.9 ± 0.8	1.9 ± 0.3
Platelet ($\times 10^3$/μL)	361 ± 38	277 ± 2.1
EIT†	0.5 ± 0.1	0.5 ± 0.1
Total myeloid precursors ($\times 10^9$ cells/kg)	38 ± 16	40 ± 15
CFU-C (–10^6/kg)	0.9 ± 0.3	0.7 ± 0.2

*Mean ± SE.
†Erythron iron turnover (mg/dL whole blood per day).
Data from Lipschitz DA, Nutrition, aging, and the immunohematopoietic system. Clin Geriatr Med. 1987;3(2):p319–28.

the marrow microenvironment, decreased production of regulatory growth factors, or a combination of these mechanisms. However, in a number of areas, the data are conflicting. This is partly a result of the tremendous heterogeneity of the aging process and partly a result of the difficulty in separating the effects of age per se from the effects of occult diseases. The effects of age on lymphohematopoiesis are summarized in the following sections.

Myeloid Lineage

Hematopoietic Progenitors

Studies on marrow hematopoietic progenitors report increased, decreased, and no change in colony numbers in aging humans. When isolated marrow CD34+ cells from the young and elderly persons were assayed in culture, similar proportions of committed marrow progenitors, that is, CD34+ marrow cells, were found in the two groups. However, "in vitro" colony formation by marrow CD34+ cells from elderly individuals required a twofold higher concentration of G-CSF to induce equivalent levels of colony formation as cells from young people. The number of subjects evaluated in all these studies was relatively small, and at present, in humans there are no reports on the effects of age on the very primitive marrow progenitors, that is, CD34+Lin− cells. There is also little information on circulating progenitors in human aging. However, it has been reported that at least in response to G-CSF, the ability of elderly persons to mobilize peripheral blood colony-forming cells is reduced. This is of potential clinical significance, given the increasing use

of cytokine-mobilized PBSC as a part of high-dose chemotherapy protocols.

Telomere length, which is known to correlate with the replication history of somatic cells, has also been investigated in hematopoietic cells: adult CD34+ CD38^{lo} stem cells have shorter telomeres than their counterparts from fetal liver and umbilical cord blood; blood cell telomeres of marrow transplant recipients were on average 0.4 kilobase (kb) shorter than those of their respective donors, equivalent to that seen with around 15 years of aging. This suggests that stem cells in humans probably have a finite replicative capacity, which is further attenuated in the presence of replicative stress.

Polymorphonuclear Neutrophils. Polymorphonuclear neutrophils (PMNs) phagocytose and kill bacteria by the generation of a series of toxic radicals and by the release of enzymes located in neutrophil granules. The process of bacterial killing is associated with a 100-fold increase in neutrophil metabolism and oxygen uptake in a reaction referred to as the respiratory burst. Thus, PMN function can be assessed by exposing PMNs to a series of chemotactic peptides or other reagents, which stimulate the respiratory burst, and evaluating oxygen metabolism in the cells. The respiratory burst activity of neutrophils from elderly individuals has been found to be decreased and the level of various neutrophil enzymes secreted during degranulation reduced. The prime defect with age appears to be a decline in the concentration of the metabolically active phosphoinositide precursors of inositol triphosphate and diacylglycerol. This defect in PMN function is not large enough to interfere with the ability of neutrophils from elderly people to phagocytose or to kill bacteria. However, this diminution in PMN reserve capacity may have clinical relevance when patients are protein-deficient. This observation maybe a partial explanation for the high prevalence of serious bacterial infections in hospitalized older individuals who are also frequently malnourished. Other studies evaluating different aspects of PMN function in aging, such as adherence, chemotaxis, phagocytosis, microbicidal capability, and response to cytokines, report that neither PMN counts nor PMN function at the level of the individual cell are altered with aging. Thus, at least in healthy elderly people, both neutrophil production and function can be upregulated to levels comparable to young adults with the exogenous administration of G-CSF.

Monocytes and Macrophages. Circulating monocytes are transformed into tissue macrophages and are the principal cells for processing antigens. Their number and function are not affected by the aging process. There is little information on age-related changes (if any) in the ability of dendritic cells to process and present antigens.

Red Cells. Although unexplained anemia is often seen in healthy elderly people, it is unclear whether baseline counts are affected with aging. However, the erythroid response to hematopoietic stress is known to be blunted in aged animals and thought to be suboptimal in elderly persons.

Hematopoietic Growth Factors

The blunted hematopoietic response to stress has been attributed to age-related decrements in growth factor secretion, particularly by marrow stromal cells. However, in humans, available data indicate that at least with severe infections, G-CSF levels can rise to a comparable degree in young and elderly patients. Erythropoietin levels in the anemic elderly patient are also not significantly different from young controls, but altered responsiveness of erythroid precursors has been invoked as a possible cause for the unexplained anemia in healthy elderly people. Animal data are more compelling for age-associated defects in stimulus-driven hematopoiesis—bacterially challenged, aged mice had blunted myelopoiesis when compared to younger animals challenged in a similar fashion. The production of the growth factor IL-6 has also been reported to go up with the aging process. Hence, according to one view, aging is associated with inappropriate underproduction and overproduction of different cytokines leading to a dysregulated hematopoietic state.

Lymphoid Lineage

Most components of the immune system undergo age-related restructuring, leading to both enhanced as well as reduced function in different components. The effect of aging on cell-mediated and humoral immunity is reviewed in detail in Chapter 3 and is not included in this chapter.

HEMATOPOIETIC GROWTH FACTORS IN ELDERLY PERSONS

There is emerging consensus that aging per se has no appreciable effect on steady state hematopoiesis. Age-related deficits tend to be subtle and are of clinical import either when present cumulatively or under conditions of hematopoietic stress. Relatively few studies have specifically addressed the use of growth factors in the elderly population. The effects of administration of growth factors in the context of cancer chemotherapy, aplastic anemia, myelodysplasia, chronic neutropenia, and anemia, and involving the use of either recombinant GM-CSF, G-CSF, or erythropoietin have been studied. When the hemoglobin level and the total neutrophil count were the end points, there was no age-related difference either in the mean time to response or in the level of absolute hematopoietic response at different doses of the growth factors.

In one prospective randomized study, the effects of rhG-CSF on the blood and marrow were evaluated in 19 young and 19 healthy elderly volunteers. When rhG-CSF was administered subcutaneously to young and healthy elderly volunteers over a 2-week period, rhG-CSF was well tolerated in both age groups, with an equivalent increase in PMN response in both groups. The increase in PMNs in blood was dose dependent, being fivefold at 30 μg and 15-fold at 300 μg. No age-related compromise, either in the magnitude or in the timing of the PMN response to rhG-CSF, was found. In the marrow, rhG-CSF caused expansion of the mitotic pool primarily at the promyelocyte and myelocyte stage, with no significant change in marrow myeloblasts. This finding suggests that G-CSF expands the marrow myeloid pool at or distal to the CFU-GM stage and that this portion of the myeloid pathway is well preserved in healthy elderly people. The only age-related change observed was the reduced ability of elderly people to mobilize peripheral blood CFU-GM in response to rhG-CSF. The doses of G-CSF used in this study were relatively modest (5 μg/kg). Hence, it is unclear whether routinely used mobilization dosages of G-CSF, that is, 10 to 30 μg/kg/d would further accentuate or blunt differences between young and the elderly people.

TABLE 101-3

Use of Growth Factors in Elderly Patients

GROWTH FACTOR	MOLECULAR WEIGHT	INDICATIONS
Granulocyte colony-stimulating factor	24 kD	Chemotherapy-related neutropenia Chronic and drug-induced neutropenia Peripheral blood stem cell transplantation ?Myelodysplasia
Erythropoietin	34–39 kD	Renal disease with anemia Anemia in cancer patients ?Myelodysplasia
Granulocyte-macrophage colony-stimulating factor	22 kD	As for G-CSF

Thus, on the basis of the available data, the indications for the use of hematopoietic growth factors in the elderly population are no different from the general population. Table 101-3 summarizes the growth factors that have special relevance for use in elderly people. Given the increased susceptibility of the elderly cancer patients to treatment-related morbidity and mortality, there may be even more compelling reason for the use of growth factors to obviate complications like bleeding and infections.

SUMMARY

Evaluation of the effect of age on hematopoiesis at the organ or cellular level demonstrates evidence of a diminished reserve capacity. In addition to being lower, the aged response tends to be more variable. Given a comparable stress, hematological abnormalities are likely to occur earlier and to be of greater severity in elderly people as compared to the young. Age-related changes in the early stages of hematopoiesis in humans remain to be elucidated, with most of the breakthroughs in HSC biology coming from murine models. Given the inability to conduct gene knockouts or do serial transplantation experiments in larger animals, much effort has been expended on alternate experimental strategies. HSC kinetics and replication rates have been studied in small and large animals using the tracking of transgene expression after retroviral-mediated gene transfer and quantitation of the average telomere length of granulocytes. This work suggests that baboon and macaque HSCs replicate more slowly than both cat and mouse HSCs. However, the mean number of times that an HSC will replicate during a mammal's lifespan is reasonably constant across species.

There is increasing recognition that genomic instability, impaired DNA repair, and consequent genetic and epigenetic changes impact many aspects of the aging hematopoietic system. This is further underscored by the link between premature aging syndromes, defective DNA repair, and impaired HSC function. Thus, accumulated DNA damage may be a common unifying mechanism responsible for age-related declines. The availability of several new animal models of the different DNA repair pathways provides the opportunity for linking specific DNA repair pathways with either preserving or impairing stem cell function. Dissection of these pathways may also provide targets for manipulating stem cell function to reverse age-related hematopoietic decline.

FURTHER READING

Balducci L, Hardy CL, Lyman GH. Hematopoietic growth factors in the older cancer patient. *Curr Opin Hematol.* 2001;8(3):170–187.

Chambers SM et al. Aging hematopoietic stem cells decline in function and exhibit epigenetic dysregulation. *PLoS Biol.* 2007;5(8):e201.

Chatta GS, Dale DC. Aging and haemopoiesis. Implications for treatment with haemopoietic growth factors. *Drugs Aging.* 1996;9(1):37–47.

Chatta GS et al. Effects of in vivo recombinant methionyl human granulocyte colony-stimulating factor on the neutrophil response and peripheral blood colony-forming cells in healthy young and elderly adult volunteers. *Blood.* 1994;84(9):2923–2929.

Chatta GS et al. Hematopoietic progenitors and aging: alterations in granulocytic precursors and responsiveness to recombinant human G-CSF, GM-CSF, and IL-3. *J Gerontol.* 1993;48(5):M207–M212.

Globerson A. Hematopoietic stem cells and aging. *Exp Gerontol.* 1999;34(2):137–146.

Kamminga LM et al. The Polycomb group gene Ezh2 prevents hematopoietic stem cell exhaustion. *Blood.* 2006;107(5):2170–2179.

Lichtin A. The ASH/ASCO clinical guidelines on the use of erythropoietin. *Best Pract Res Clin Haematol.* 2005;18(3):433–438.

May G, Enver T. The lineage commitment and self-renewal of blood stem cells. In: Zon LI, ed. *Hematopoiesis: A Developmental Approach.* New York, New York: Oxford University Press; 2001.

Metcalf D. On hematopoietic stem cell fate. *Immunity.* 2007;26(6):669–673.

Morrison SJ et al. The aging of hematopoietic stem cells. *Nat Med.* 1996;2(9):1011–1016.

Nijnik A et al. DNA repair is limiting for haematopoietic stem cells during ageing. *Nature.* 2007;447(7145):686–690.

Park Y, Gerson SL. DNA repair defects in stem cell function and aging. *Annu Rev Med.* 2005;56:495–508.

Rossi DJ, Bryder D, Weissman IL. Hematopoietic stem cell aging: mechanism and consequence. *Exp Gerontol.* 2007;42(5):385–390.

Rossi DJ et al. Deficiencies in DNA damage repair limit the function of haematopoietic stem cells with age. *Nature.* 2007;447(7145):725–729.

Rowe JM et al. A randomized placebo-controlled phase III study of granulocyte-macrophage colony-stimulating factor in adult patients (> 55 to 70 years of age) with acute myelogenous leukemia: a study of the Eastern Cooperative Oncology Group (E1490). *Blood.* 1995;86(2):457–462.

Smith TJ et al. 2006 update of recommendations for the use of white blood cell growth factors: an evidence-based clinical practice guideline. *J Clin Oncol.* 2006;24(19):3187–3205.

Stone RM et al. Granulocyte-macrophage colony-stimulating factor after initial chemotherapy for elderly patients with primary acute myelogenous leukemia. Cancer and Leukemia Group B. *N Engl J Med.* 1995;332(25):1671–1677.

Van Zant G, Liang Y. The role of stem cells in aging. *Exp Hematol.* 2003;31(8):659–672.

Yu H et al. Hematopoietic stem cell exhaustion impacted by p18 INK4 C and p21 Cip1/Waf1 in opposite manners. *Blood.* 2006;107(3):1200–1206.

Anemia

Paulo H. M. Chaves

Anemia, a common clinical syndrome in older adults, has been the focus of renewed attention over the last decade, as attested by the increasing number of publications addressing its clinical epidemiology. Anemia in older persons tends to be multifactorial in origin, and is often associated with a combination of chronic medical conditions. The clinical presentation of anemia in older adults is complex, and symptoms are often insidious and nonspecific. Unless severe, anemia it is often perceived as a relatively benign condition that is either a normal accompaniment to aging and/or merely a marker of prevalent chronic diseases. However, data gathered to date have established that this maybe an incorrect perception. Consistently, several studies have shown that anemia, even if mild, is a strong, independent, risk factor for major adverse outcomes in older adults, including decline in physical and cognitive function, frailty, disability, and mortality. Aside from its prognostic implication, it has been hypothesized that even nonsevere anemia could causally contribute to the occurrence of these adverse outcomes, and that anemia correction could potentially lead to improved outcomes in older adults. These hypotheses remain to be proven. Future studies, including large randomized clinical trials (RCTs), are expected to contribute key insight as to whether correction of anemia that is nonsevere in the broad older population could prevent additional morbidity and/or mortality. In this context, aiming to summarize valuable information for the health professional involved with the care of older adults, this chapter presents basic information on a number of relevant issues related to the topic of anemia in older adults, including insight regarding prevalence, associations with major adverse clinical outcomes, and potential intervention opportunities.

DEFINITION OF ANEMIA IN OLDER ADULTS

Conceptually, anemia is a clinical syndrome caused by a reduced mass of circulating red blood cells (RBCs). In practice, anemia is often operationally defined as a decreased level in any of the following parameters: the concentration of hemoglobin (Hb) in the whole blood; the proportion occupied by RBCs in a sample of whole blood—that is, hematocrit (Hct); and/or the number of RBCs in a standardized volume of whole blood. Often, Hb is expressed as g/dL, Hct as %, and RBC count as the number of RBCs in millions per microliter. Consistent with the literature, we will use Hb as the key parameter to define anemia in this chapter.

A widely used standard to define anemia in older adults is the one usually referred to as the World Health Organization (WHO) criteria, published in the 1968 WHO report on nutritional anemias. According to this criteria, anemia is defined as a Hb less than 12 g/dL in older women, and less than 13 g/dL in older men. This gender difference is primarily because of the differences in the distributions of Hb in older men and women. These criteria are the same as proposed earlier (1933) by Wintrobe. Lower Hb cutoffs have also been proposed for anemia definition in older adults, under the nonempirical argument that the concentration of Hb is "normally" lower in older populations. Important limitations of the methods used to define anemia in older adults should be acknowledged, however. Current criteria used to select the Hb cutoff for anemia have been derived primarily on the basis of statistical distribution considerations; i.e., the Hb cutoff used to separate subjects with and without anemia being the one corresponding to minus 2 standard deviations (–2 SD) below the mean calculated in an apparently healthy, standard population. Although this constitutes a useful and traditional method for defining the lower limit of the "normal range" of a biological parameter in general, it has limitations. Apparently healthy older populations, which are often defined in terms of self-reported clinical diseases, are likely to include older adults with subclinical diseases and health status changes (e.g., inflammation, decline in kidney function, etc.). These subclinical factors may shift the Hb distribution in the whole older population to the left (toward lower values). Thus, the use of –2 SD as the key criterion may result in biased, lower-than-optimal Hb cutoffs for a definition. Additionally, this statistical distribution method, which assumes a meaningful threshold difference between

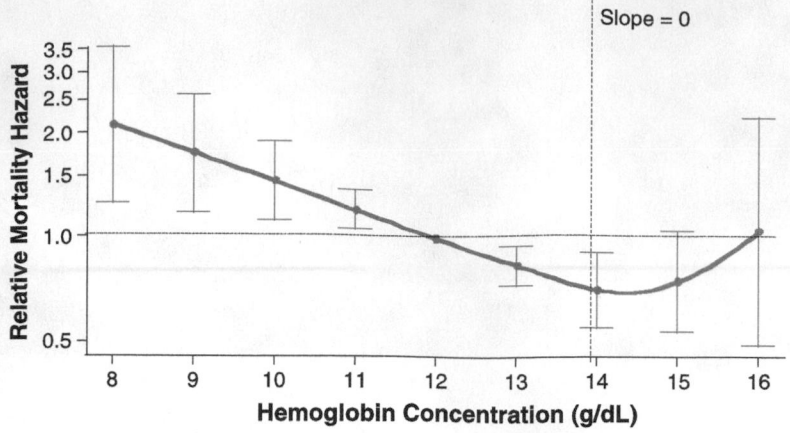

FIGURE 102-1. Relationship between hemoglobin (Hb) concentration and 5-yr all-cause mortality in community-dwelling disabled older women (Women's Health and Aging Study I, 1992–2000). The figure shows a graphical display of relative risk estimates for the mortality linked to specific Hb concentrations compared with the risk linked to Hb of 12 g/dL. The curve represents smoothed relative mortality hazards across Hb concentrations, and the bars indicate their 95% confidence intervals. Also indicated is the 13.9 g/dL Hb threshold at which the slope of mortality risk decline was no longer statistically significant (i.e., the 95% confidence interval for the slope of the tangent included 0). The y-axis was transformed so that, for example, the graphical display of an increase in risk of the magnitude of two (hazard ratio (HR) = 2) would be equivalent to that of a decrease in risk of the same magnitude (HR = 0.5) in terms of scale size. Risk estimates are adjusted for age, race, congestive heart failure, coronary heart disease, peripheral artery disease, stroke, pulmonary disease, cancer, estimated creatinine clearance, ankle–arm index, depression, body mass index, smoking status, education, disability performing basic activities of daily living, and number of domains with difficulty. *(Chaves PHM, Xue Q-L, Guralnik JM, et al. What does constitute normal hemoglobin concentration in community-dwelling disable older women? J Am Geriatr Soc. 2004;52(11):1811–1816. Modified, reprinted with permission.)*

subjects with Hb levels below –2 SD (abnormally low) versus those with Hb levels between –2 SD and +2 SD ("normal" range), does not take into account the direct relationship between Hb and the risk of clinically relevant outcomes. In fact, recent observational epidemiologic studies have demonstrated that Hb is related to the risk of major adverse clinical outcomes in a rather continuous, curvilinear pattern (see "Outcomes Associated with Anemia"). The observed pattern was marked by an association of highest risk of outcomes with lowest Hb levels, and a monotonically risk decrement with increasing Hb levels up to mid-normal Hb levels (Figure 102-1). Even within the "normal range," a risk gradient was observed, with Hb levels considered per current standards as low-normal being associated with a higher risk of outcomes such as frailty, disability, and mortality, as compared to levels currently perceived as mid-normal Hb. Consistently, analysis of the relationship between Hb and serum erythropoietin in older women revealed that that serum erythropoietin levels were significantly higher at low-normal Hb, as compared to mid-normal Hb, where serum erythropoietin levels were lowest (Figure 102-2). Collectively, current evidence suggests that while the WHO criteria constitute a valid approach to define data in older adults, it may not be optimal, at least from the risk prediction perspective.

Arguments have been made in favor of the use race-specific criteria for anemia definition. This perspective is supported by a recent observational study conducted in the Health, Aging, and Body Composition Study. In that study, although concerns with residual confounding by comorbidity burden as well as with selection bias at least partially explaining study findings cannot be discarded, race was shown to be an effect modifier of the associations of WHO-defined anemia with all-cause mortality (over 6 years) as well as incident mobility disability (over 4 years); that is, anemia was associated with an increased risk of mortality and disability in white, but not in black older adults.

Finally, it should be acknowledged that what may constitute best naturally occurring levels of Hb in observational studies of older adults from a risk prediction perspective does necessarily constitute optimal levels from other clinical decision-making perspectives. In fact, major discrepancies have been reported between Hb levels linked to lowest risk of adverse outcomes in older adults in observational studies with "optimal" target Hb of recombinant erythropoietin in RCTs (see "Therapeutic Considerations").

PREVALENCE AND TYPES OF ANEMIA

Prevalence

The prevalence of anemia in older adults varies according to the setting in which it is estimated. Higher prevalence estimates have been reported in long-term care facilities such as nursing homes than in the general community-dwelling older population. This difference maybe explained by the fact that, in general, anemia is associated with poorer health status. Differences in prevalence estimates within similar settings have also been reported, and maybe primarily attributed to methodological differences, such as variations in background characteristics of targeted populations, response rates, and the way anemia was defined.

A recent study reported on the prevalence of anemia in the large U.S.-representative sample of noninstitutionalized older adults who participated in the Third National Health and Nutrition Examination Survey (NHANES III, 1988–1994). In that study, the prevalence of anemia was 11% in older men and 10.2% in older women. Overall, the prevalence in the population of community-dwelling subjects 65 years and older was 10.6%. There were, nonetheless, significant differences according to age groups (Figure 102-3). In both men and women 65 years and older, the prevalence of anemia steadily increased with advancing age, being highest in the 85+-year age group. In subjects who were 65 to 74 years old, the prevalence

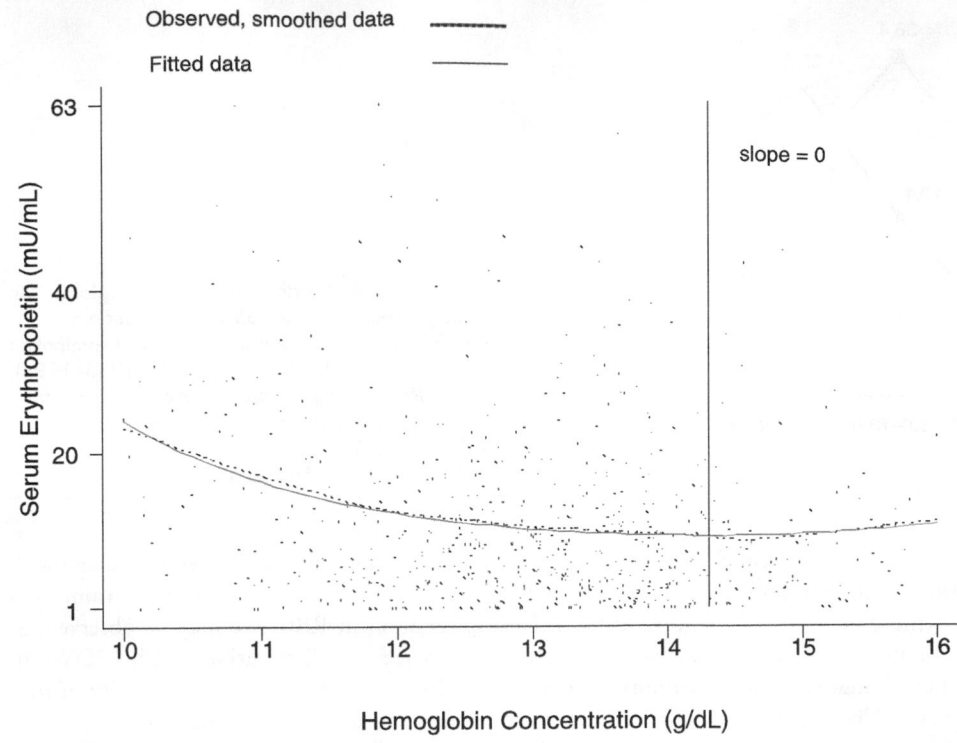

FIGURE 102-2. Graphical display of the curvilinear relationship between serum erythropoietin and hemoglobin (Hb) concentration in community-dwelling disabled older women (Women's Health and Aging Study I, 1992–1995). The slope of the tangent line to the EPO versus the Hb curve was equal to zero at the Hb threshold point of 14.3 (95% CI = 13.2–15.4). EPO at a Hb concentration of 12 g/dL was 28% greater than EPO at a Hb concentration of 13.9 g/dL (95% CI = 15–44%). Adjustment for age, race, and creatinine clearance did not change this difference estimate. Similarity between observed (smoothed) and fitted curves indicated proper model fit. (Chaves PHM, Xue Q-L, Guralnik JM, et al. What does constitute normal hemoglobin concentration in community-dwelling disable older women? J Am Geriatr Soc. 2004;52(11):1811–1816. Modified, reprinted with permission.)

of anemia was slightly higher in women than in men; however, in the age groups 75 to 84 years and 85+ years old, the prevalence of anemia was substantially higher in men than in women.

As compared to the distribution of Hb in older men, anemia in older women was shifted to the left; that is, toward lower values (Figure 102-4). Only a very small minority of anemia in community-dwelling older adults is severe, with less than 1% of the total sample having Hb levels lower than 10 g/dL (see Figure 102-4). Additionally, in that study, significant differences in the prevalence of anemia according to race and ethnicity were reported (Figure 102-5). The prevalence of anemia was lowest in non-Hispanic whites, and highest in non-Hispanic blacks. Anemia prevalence in Mexican Americans was only slightly higher than that of non-Hispanic whites.

Types of Anemia

Anemia maybe classified in a number of different ways. A practical scheme used in the geriatrics literature involves the classification of

anemia in the following major categories: (a) nutrient deficiency, (b) anemia of chronic kidney disease (CKD), (c) anemia of chronic inflammation (ACI; previously referred to as anemia of chronic disease), and (d) unclassified (also called "unexplained" anemia). These broad categories should not be seen as exclusive, as more than one type of anemia maybe present. For example, in patients with anemia of CKD, nutrient absolute or functional nutrient deficiency, and/or chronic inflammation may also contribute to impaired erythropoiesis and anemia. Other schemes for classification of anemia exist, including ones appropriately more refined for the investigation of causes of anemia in the clinical setting (see below).

Nutrient-deficiency Anemia

Anemia with nutrient deficiency is common. In a recent study that analyzed NHANES III data from community-dwelling adults 65 years and older, approximately one third of all causes of anemia met the study criteria for iron, folate, and/or vitamin B-12 deficiency.

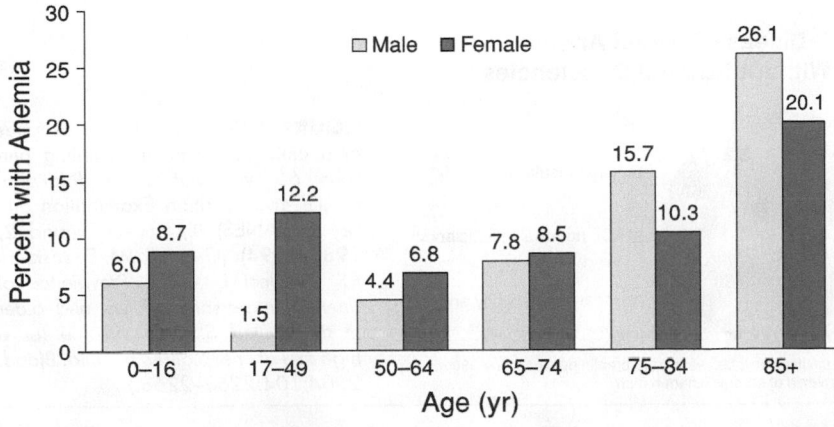

FIGURE 102-3. Percentage of persons with anemia according to age and sex (National Health and Nutrition Examination Survey (NHANES) III, phases 1 and 2, 1988–1994). (Guralnik IM, Eisenstaedt RS, Ferrucci L, et al. Prevalence of anemia in persons 65 yrs and older in the United States: evidence for a high rate of unexplained anemia. Blood. 2004;104:2263–2268.)

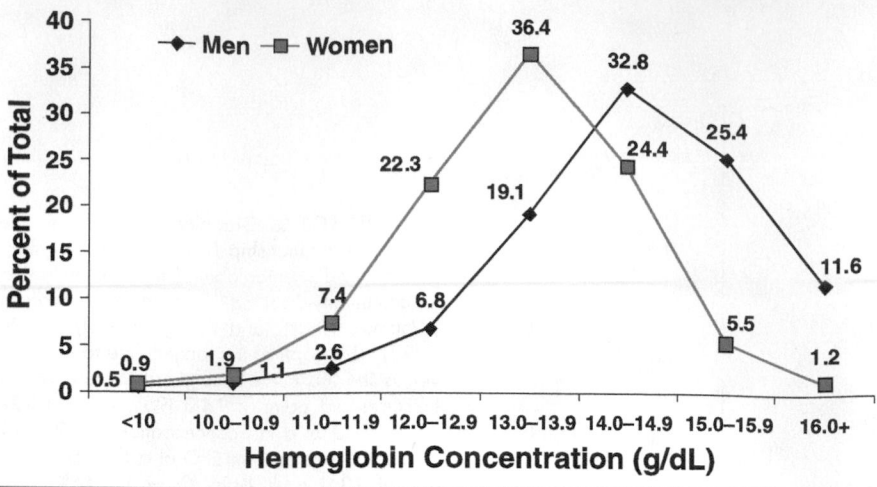

FIGURE 102-4. Distribution of hemoglobin in community-dwelling persons 65 yrs and older according to sex (National Health and Nutrition Examination Survey (NHANES) III, phases 1 and 2, 1988–1994). (Guralnik JM, Eisenstaedt RS, Ferrucci L, et al. Prevalence of anemia in persons 65 yrs and older in the United States: evidence for a high rate of unexplained anemia. Blood. 2004;104:2263–2268.)

Anemia with Iron Deficiency Iron deficiency is by far the most common cause of nutrient-deficient anemia. Along with protoporphyrin IX, iron is a key component of the heme complex, the nonprotein pigment of the hemoglobin molecule in RBCs that is directly involved with oxygen binding and transport. Reduced availability of iron may cause anemia through impaired Hb synthesis. Iron-deficiency anemia is usually the endpoint of a negative overall iron balance disorder that gradually progresses over time. While decreased oral iron intake as well as reduced absorption maybe important contributing factors, it is believed that iron-deficiency anemia in older adults is primarily caused by chronic blood loss, in particular from the gastrointestinal (GI) tract. Iron-deficiency anemia constitutes an advanced stage of iron deficiency. The earlier stages of iron deficiency are marked by progressive depletion of iron stores. With exhaustion of iron stores, Hb synthesis becomes compromised, and results in erythropoiesis impairment. Eventu-

ally, Hb drops below specific thresholds, and anemia is diagnosed. Early in iron-deficiency anemia, anemia maybe normochromic and normocytic. Increased variation in RBC size may be observed, as assessed by an increase in red cell distribution width (RDW) in automated analysis of RBCs. As the duration and severity of iron deficiency increases, overt iron-deficiency anemia ensues. At this more advanced stage, the production of microcytic (small-sized), hypochromic (with decreased Hb content) erythrocytes is characteristic. Other typical laboratory abnormalities of advanced, overt iron-deficiency anemia include low serum ferritin concentration, low serum iron concentration, increased total iron-binding capacity (TIBC), low transferrin saturation ratio (serum iron divided by TIBC), and increased levels of soluble transferrin receptor (sTfR) (see below). Complementary laboratory tests maybe useful to further characterize the different stages of iron deficiency and iron-deficiency anemia.

All Anemia Cases

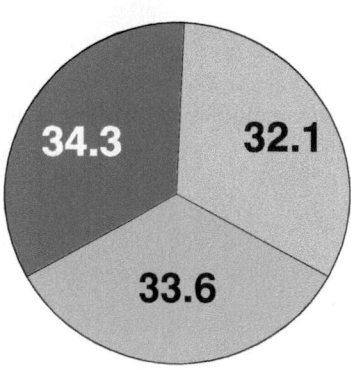

- With nutrient deficiency
- Disease-related, without nutrient deficiencies
- Unexplained, without nutrient deficiencies

Anemia with Nutrient Deficiency

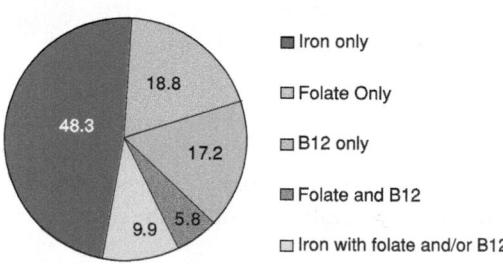

- Iron only
- Folate Only
- B12 only
- Folate and B12
- Iron with folate and/or B12

Disease-Related Anemia, Without Nutrient Deficiencies

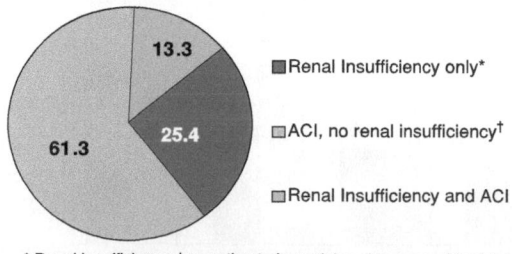

- Renal Insufficiency only*
- ACI, no renal insufficiency†
- Renal Insufficiency and ACI

* Renal insufficiency; i.e., estimated creatinine clearance <30 mL/min
† ACI, anemia of chronic inflammation

FIGURE 102-5. Distribution of types of anemia in community-dwelling persons 65 yrs and older (National Health and Nutrition Examination Survey (NHANES) III, phases 1 and 2, 1988–1994). (Guralnik JM, Eisenstaedt RS, Ferrucci L, et al. Prevalence of anemia in persons 65 yrs and older in the United States: evidence for a high rate of unexplained anemia. Blood. 2004;104:2263–2268.)

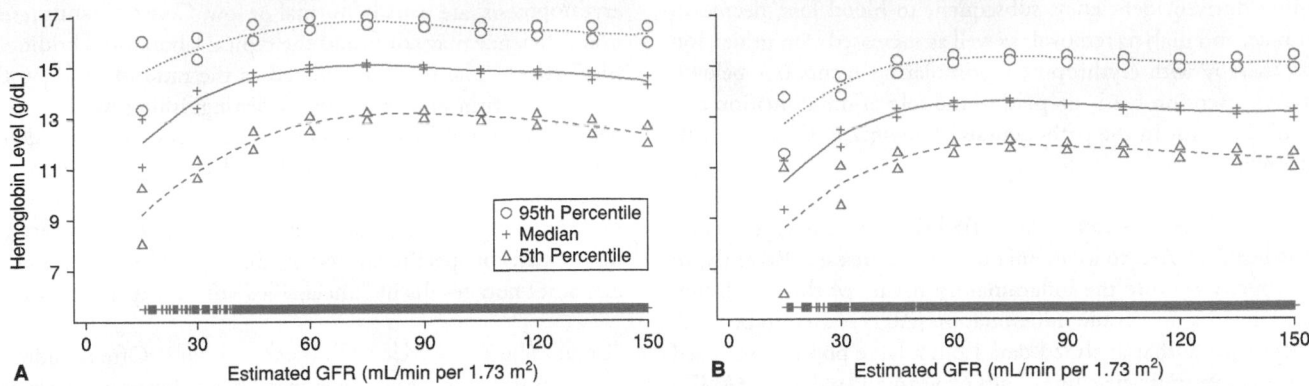

FIGURE 102-6. Median and 5th and 95th percentiles of hemoglobin levels among men (A) and women (B) 20 yrs and older who participated in the Third National Health and Nutrition Examination Survey (1988–1994). All values are adjusted to the age of 60 yrs. Estimates and 95% confidence intervals are demarcated at selected levels of estimated glomerular filtration rate (GFR). Marks near the abscissa indicate the estimated GFRs of individual data points. (Astor BC, Muntner P, Levin A, et al. Association of kidney function with anemia: the Third National Health and Nutrition Examination Survey (1988–1994). Arch Intern Med. 2002;162(12):1401–1408, reprinted with permission.)

Anemia with Vitamin B-12 (Cobalamin) and/or Folate Deficiency

The remaining cases of nutrient-deficiency anemia are largely caused by deficiency of folate and/or vitamin B-12. These deficiencies may impair erythrocyte maturation and proliferation through their adverse effect on DNA synthesis and result in macrocytic anemia, i.e., anemia with oversized RBCs, usually quantified as a mean corpuscular volume (MCV) greater than 100 femtoliters (fL). Analogously to iron deficiency, vitamin B-12 deficiency usually progresses across stages of severity. In its earlier stages, one is able to maintain erythropoiesis using vitamin B-12 from body stores. After, stores become depleted, erythropoiesis becomes impaired, and megalobastic anemia ensues. Often, vitamin B-12 deficiency, as assessed by low serum vitamin B-12 levels, as well as macrocytic changes maybe noted before the drop of Hb below the level in which anemia is diagnosed. Typically, other laboratory abnormalities that accompany the macrocytic anemia of vitamin B-12 deficiency include the presence of hypersegmented granulocytes on blood smears; giant platelets may also be observed. Thrombocytopenia, as well as leucopenia may also occur. Presence of iron deficiency concomitant to vitamin B-12 deficiency anemia may mask typical abnormalities of the latter. Often, vitamin B-12 deficiency anemia is caused by gastric and intestinal disorders that prevent the proper digestion of vitamin B-12, involving either impaired release of cobalamin from the ingested food and/or the absorption of free cobalamin in the GI tract. Examples of these disorders include hypochlorhydria, surgical procedures involving the stomach, atrophic gastritis (involving a deficiency in the production of intrinsic factor by parietal cells of the gastric mucosa), pancreatic insufficiency, and small bowel bacterial overgrowth. Vitamin B-12 deficiency, resulting from dietary deficiency is not common, but may occur in subjects with severe long-term avoidance to meat products, as maybe found in strict vegetarians. Folate deficiency, on the other hand, is often caused by poor nutritional intake. GI disorders result in decreased absorption of folate (e.g., hypochlorhydria associated with atrophic gastritis or acid-suppressive therapy, celiac disease) and adverse effects of drugs (e.g., alcohol, methotrexate, anticonvulsants). Like vitamin B-12 deficiency, folate deficiency typically presents as a macrocytic anemia. Laboratory tests are useful to distinguish folate- versus vitamin B-12 deficiency. The distinction is important vis-à-vis therapeutic implications (see below). Other vitamins and trace minerals have also been hypothesized to impair erythropoiesis, and potentially contribute to the development of anemia, when other mechanisms are also present, including deficiencies in vitamins A, C, E, and pyridoxine and riboflavin (vitamin B group), as well as copper, selenium, and zinc.

Anemia of CKD With increasing age, the prevalence of CKD increases, kidney function declines, and the prevalence of anemia—a common complication of CKD, particularly when the latter is advanced—increases. Figure 102-6 displays data on the age-adjusted, cross-sectional relationship between renal function, as assessed by estimated glomerular filtration rate (eGFR) levels, and the continuous distribution of Hb observed in a nationally representative sample of 15 625 noninstitutionalized Americans 20 years and older. Stable Hb levels were observed across eGFR levels greater than 60 mL/min per 1.73 m^2; below this threshold, lower eGFR levels were associated with progressively lower Hb levels. In another study that analyzed NHANES III data and used a strict definition for anemia of CKD, 8.2% of all cases of anemia were attributed to anemia of CKD only, and an additional 4.3% to anemia of CKD in combination with ACI (see below). The definition of anemia of CKD in that study was the following: Hb <12 g/dL in women and <13 g/dL in men, an eGFR less than 30 mL/min per 1.73 m^2 and no evidence of iron, folate, or vitamin B-12 deficiency. Had more sensitive eGFR cutoffs (e.g., eGFR <45 or <60 mL/min per 1.73 m^2) been used to define anemia of CKD, higher prevalence estimates of this type of anemia would have been yielded. Typically, anemia of CKD is normocytic and normochromic. The primary mechanism through which CKD causes anemia is a deficiency in the production of erythropoietin, a naturally occurring erythropoiesis-stimulating hormone mainly produced by the kidneys in adults, which is secreted in response to hypoxia. The diminished renal production of erythropoietin is most noticeable in the most advanced stages of renal failure. In the failing kidney, in addition to the absolute deficiency in erythropoietin, the decline in the renal excretory function also plays a part in the pathogenesis of anemia, as it may contribute to a shortened life span of RBCs and bone marrow suppression. Other concomitant factors may also inhibit erythropoiesis in anemic subjects with CKD, including nutrient deficiency, subsequent to blood loss, decreased oral intake, and dialysis removal, as well as increased iron utilization during therapy with erythropoiesis stimulating agents (see below). Increasing attention has been paid to the role of inflammation as a mechanistic factor in the pathogenesis of anemia in CKD patients (see below).

Anemia of Chronic Inflammation Traditionally, this type of anemia has been referred to as anemia of chronic disease. Recently, to more properly capture the inflammatory nature of this condition, the term anemia of chronic inflammation (ACI) started to be used. In a recent study that analyzed data from a large population-based sample of community-dwelling adults 65 years and older (NHANES III), more than 20% of all cases of anemia met the criteria for ACI. In that study, the overall prevalence of ACI (24%) was slightly higher than that attributed to anemia with iron deficiency (20%). ACI is associated with a wide variety of inflammatory conditions, including chronic infection, cancer, diabetes, rheumatoid arthritis, and congestive heart failure, and trauma. It is said that the severity of ACI and that of the underlying disease(s) are positively correlated.

Several mechanisms mediated by inflammatory cytokines have been proposed to explain ACI. The key one involves unavailability of iron for erythropoiesis despite adequate, if not elevated total iron stores, mediated by inflammation. This dysregulation of iron homeostasis results from sequestration of iron in the cells of the reticuloendothelial system, with consequent inadequate availability of iron for erythropoiesis. Interleukin-6 (IL-6), a proinflammatory cytokine, has been shown to stimulate the hepatic production of hepcidin, a polypeptide that is a major regulator of iron homeostasis. Hepcidin inhibits the release of iron from the reticuloendothelial and macrophage systems, as well as iron intestinal absorption. High levels of IL-6 have been shown to induce an increased production of hepcidin, which in turn can lead to sequestration of iron by reticuloendothelial cells, reduced amount of iron available for erythropoiesis, and, ultimately anemia. Additional mechanisms maybe involved in the pathogenesis of ACI, including the inhibition of the proliferation and differentiation of erythroid progenitor cells, which may result from inflammation-mediated induction of apoptosis of progenitor cells, and/or through a direct toxic effect of inflammation on progenitor cells. Another mechanism involves a blunted erythropoietin response, i.e., an attenuated compensatory response in erythropoietin production in relation to the degree of anemia, resulting in a relative erythropoietin deficiency. Support for this explanation include in vitro evidence of inhibition of erythropoietin production by proinflammatory cytokines, such as tumor necrosis factor alpha (TNF-α) and interleukin-1, as well as evidence of lower levels of serum erythropoietin in patients with ACI as compared to patients with iron-deficiency anemia for the same level of anemia. Controversy exists though as to whether the iron-deficiency group is a proper control group, given its exacerbating impact on hypoxia homeostatic mechanisms. Shortened RBC life span may also contribute to the pathogenesis of ACI.

Characteristically, laboratory evaluation of ACI reveals a normochromic, normocytic anemia. As ACI progresses over time, anemia may become macrocytic. Reflecting its pathogenesis, the hallmark ACI is the presence of low serum iron along with evidence of adequate iron stores, as indicated by normal or increased levels of serum ferritin. Typically, serum transferrin levels are low, and so is the TBIC. Serum levels of sTfR, which reflects bone marrow

erythropoiesis, are usually normal or low. Concomitant presence of iron deficiency may confound the typical laboratorial findings identified above. The index calculated as the ratio of sTfR by the log of serum ferritin maybe useful for distinguishing ACI without iron deficiency, from ACI with iron deficiency, as well as iron-deficiency anemia without ACI (see below). Reflecting an improved knowledge about the pathogenesis and measurement of ACI, diagnosis of ACI is no longer a diagnosis of exclusion, but rather it is established on the basis of specific laboratory findings. The exclusion of other diagnoses now results in "unclassified" or "unexplained" anemia.

"Unclassified" or "Unexplained" Anemia Often, older adults have anemia that does not meet specific classification criteria. In these cases, anemia is said to be unclassified or unexplained. This occurs commonly in community-dwelling subjects. Investigators analyzing NHANES III data reported that, after excluding other possible causes of anemia according to study criteria (which used laboratory tests for classification of the type of anemia consistent with that commonly used in the clinical setting by geriatricians), about one third of all cases of anemia in community-dwelling men and women 65 years and older were "unclassified." It is possible that a more comprehensive and repeated assessment, particularly in the case of long-duration and more severe anemia, may increase the likelihood of detection of a specific etiology. The "unclassified" group of anemia is likely a heterogeneous one; reflecting this, it has been speculated that all mechanisms listed above could play a role in the pathogenesis of "unclassified" anemia. More recently, it has been demonstrated that, as a group, unclassified anemia is marked by low levels of serum erythropoietin, and low levels of circulating proinflammatory markers.

OUTCOMES ASSOCIATED WITH ANEMIA

Observational findings from epidemiological studies have documented that anemia is a strong and independent risk factor for major adverse clinical and public health outcomes in older adults, including mortality, frailty, decline in physical function, disability, and cognitive impairment (Figure 102-7). Additionally, studies have

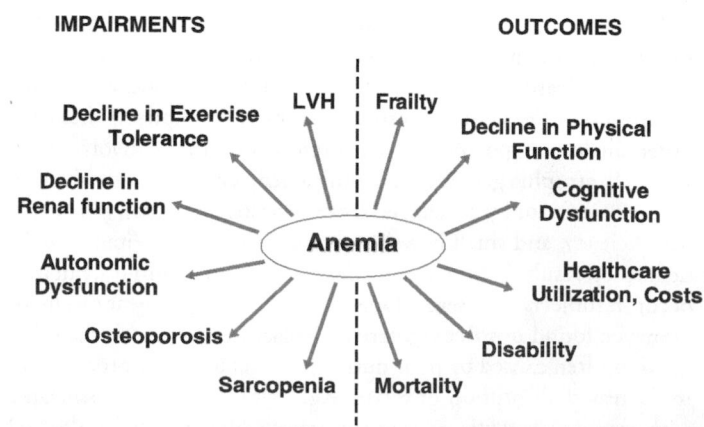

FIGURE 102-7. Anemia, physiological impairments, and clinical outcomes. Anemia has been linked to a number of physiological impairments and clinical outcomes in community-dwelling older populations, including the ones highlighted.

shown that presence of both anemia and prevalent comorbidities are associated with a synergistically increased risk of adverse outcomes. These findings have been consistently replicated in different settings, including population- and patient-based studies involving older adults with specific diseases (e.g., CKD, cardiovascular disease, and diabetes), as well as subjects representative of the broad population of older adults living in the community. In this section, we review data on selected outcomes and discuss the nature of the documented associations.

Mortality

The association between prevalent anemia and increased risk of mortality has been well documented by a number of large epidemiological studies of noninstitutionalized older adults. For example, in a large ($n = 755$) community-based study of adults aged 85 years and older in Leiden the Netherlands, it was estimated that 5-year all-cause mortality risk was 1.84 (95% confidence interval [CI]: 1.50–2.25) times higher in those with prevalent anemia (as defined according to the WHO criteria; that is, Hb <12 g/dL in women and Hb <13 g/dL in men) as compared to those without it, after adjustment for age and gender. Additional insight was provided by a subsequent study that examined the relationship between the continuous Hb distribution and all-cause mortality risk over a median follow-up period of 5 years in 686 community-dwelling women 65 years and older with moderate-to-severe physical disability (see Figure 102-1). In the latter study, there was evidence of a reversed J-shape curve characterized by highest mortality risk at lowest Hb levels, and lowest mortality risk at mid-normal Hb levels around 13.9 g/dL; above this Hb threshold, mortality risk increased with higher Hb levels. The highest mortality risk associated with mild anemia persisted even after comprehensive adjustment for major confounders, such as demographics, comorbidity, and disease severity indicators; e.g., as compared to a Hb level of 12 g/dL, a Hb of 11 g/dL was associated with a 20% (95%CI: 10–40%) higher mortality risk in adjusted analysis. Additionally, this study also showed that a Hb of 12 g/dL, a level that is considered low-normal by WHO and current clinical practice standards, is independently associated with a significantly higher mortality risk, as well as increased serum

erythropoietin levels, as compared to mid-normal Hb levels such as 14 g/dL. Collectively, recently published data have consistently demonstrated that, in community-dwelling older adults, (a) WHO-defined anemia, which primarily corresponds to mild anemia, is an independent risk factor for 5-year all-cause mortality; (b) there is a dose–response in mortality risk associated with increasing anemia severity; and (c) there is a meaningful mortality risk gradient even within the Hb range currently perceived as normal. Also relevant were findings of interactions of anemia with other comorbidities—including CKD, left ventricular hypertrophy (LVH), and CVD—in regard to increased mortality risk in older patients.

Decline in Physical Function

Aside from mortality, anemia has also been related to decline in physical function, as well as physical disability. A recent cross-sectional study evaluated the association of prevalent anemia with self-reported and objectively measured mobility function in 633 community-dwelling women aged 70 to 80 years with Hb higher than 10 g/dL (mean ±) participating in the Women's Health and Aging Studies (WHAS) I and II. As compared to mid-normal Hb levels such as 14 g/dL, where the likelihood of mobility disability was lowest and mobility performance was best, Hb levels corresponding to mild anemia and even low-normal Hb were associated with increased likelihood of mobility disability (defined as difficulty in walking one-quarter mile or climbing 10 steps) (Figure 102-8) and worse mobility performance (objectively assessed by the Short Physical Performance Battery (SPPB) scores, based on tests that the assessed ability to hold balance on different standing positions, the time to walk a few meters at usual pace, and the time to raise from a chair as quickly as possible five times), even after adjustment for demographics, disease, and other major health indicators. Subsequently, a prospective study conducted in 1146 older subjects (mean age 77 ± 5 years; 70% female) participating in the Established Populations for Epidemiologic Study of the Elderly (EPESE) provided further insight by documenting an independent association of WHO-defined anemia with subsequent, meaningful decline in objectively measured mobility performance (as assessed by SPPB scores) over a 4 year-period both in women as well as in men

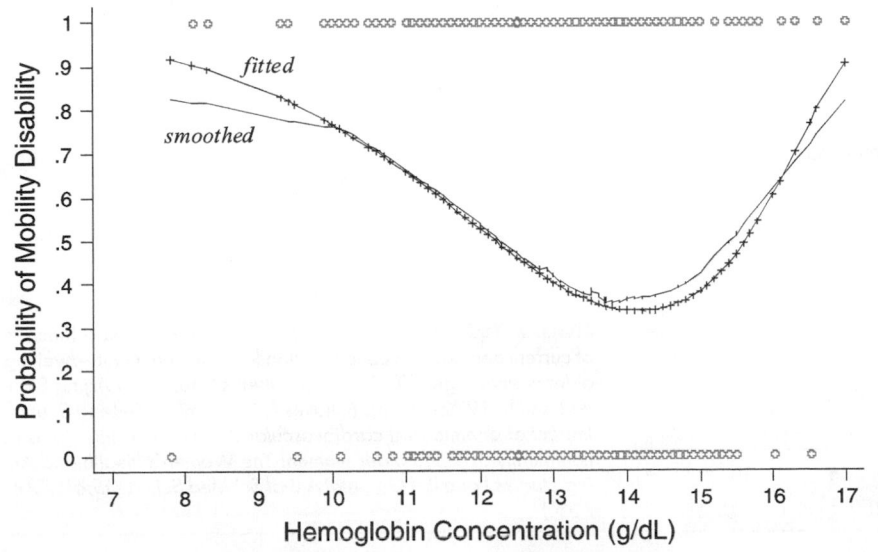

FIGURE 102-8. Relationship between mobility disability and hemoglobin concentration (Women's Health and Aging Studies I and II, 1992–1996). The figure shows graphical display of the probability of having mobility disability (difficulty walking one-quarter mile or climbing up 10 steps) as a function of hemoglobin concentration levels. Shown are observed, smoothed (straight line) and fitted curves (line with "+" signs). A nonlinear relationship pattern was documented, with the probability of mobility difficulty being lowest at mid-normal Hb levels around 14.0 g/dL, and highest at Hb extremes. Hypothesis testing confirmed that the likelihood of mobility difficulty was not constant between 12.0 and 16.0 g/dL of Hb ($p < .01$). (Chaves PHM, Ashar B, Guralnik JM, Fried LP. Looking at the relationship between hemoglobin concentration and prevalent mobility difficulty in older women. Should the criteria currently used to define anemia in older people be reevaluated? J Am Geriatr Soc. 2002;50:1257–1264. Modified, reprinted with permission.)

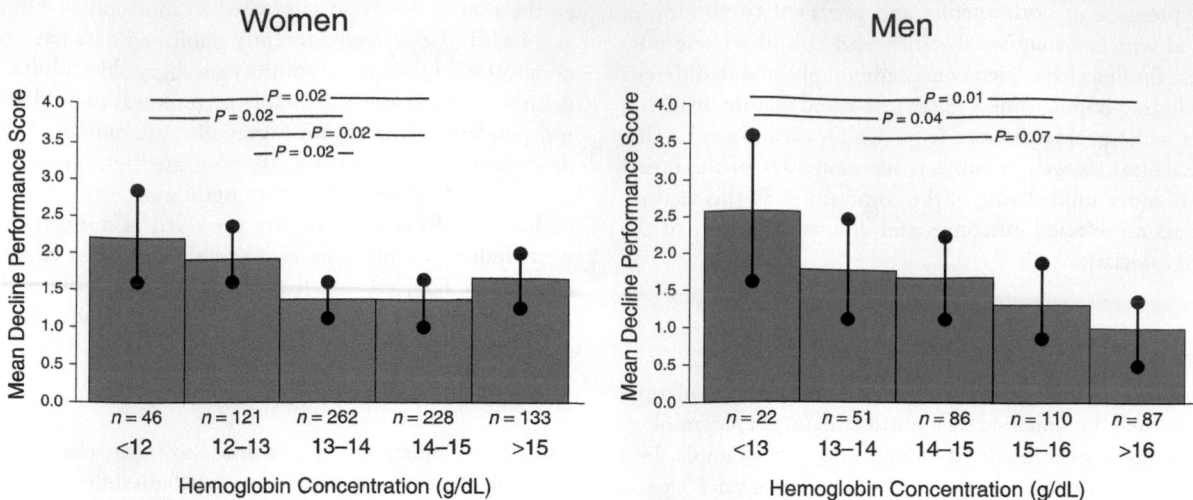

FIGURE 102-9. Adjusted mean decline in mobility performance, as assessed by Short Physical Performance Battery (SPBB) scores, as a function of hemoglobin concentration in community-dwelling older women and men (Established Populations for Epidemiologic Study of the Elderly, 1988–1992). Decline in performance corresponds to a negative change in score. Decline is adjusted for baseline performance score, age, education, smoking, blood pressure, body mass index, coronary heart disease, heart failure, stroke, diabetes, cancer, lung disease, infectious disease, and renal disease. *P* values indicate significant differences between categories. *(Penninx BW, Guralnik JM, Onder G, et al. Anemia and decline in physical performance among older adults. Am J Med. 2003;115:105–110.)*

(Figure 102-9). Consistently, several studies have reported associations of anemia with a number of intermediate endpoints—for example, reduced aerobic capacity, exercise tolerance symptoms such as fatigue, and decreased muscle strength—and distal outcomes of the disablement process, such as difficulty and dependency carrying out basic activities of daily living (ADLs), a more severe types of physical disability than mobility disability.

Frailty Status

Frailty has been conceptualized as a clinical syndrome whose hallmark is increased clinical vulnerability to stressors caused by loss of physiological reserve. While related to aging and disability, frailty has been conceptually regarded as being a separate entity. In fact, many have proposed frailty as a risk factor for disability in older adults (see

Chapter 52). The relationship between anemia and frailty status was examined in a study that analyzed data from WHAS I and II. In that study, frailty was defined according to a validated set of criteria as the presence of at least three out of the following five manifestations: shrinkage, slowness, weakness, exhaustion, and low energy expenditure. The relationship between frailty and anemia was best described by a reversed J-shaped curve that was consistent with that reported for mortality and physical disability (Figure 102-10). As compared to mid-normal Hb levels such as 13.5 g/dL, the likelihood of being classified as frail was significantly higher for lowest and highest Hb levels, even after adjustment for major confounders. Another major finding of that study was evidence of a synergistic interaction between anemia and cardiovascular disease in regard to the likelihood of frailty. Clinically, such an interaction could be thought of as follows. In older adults, the likelihood of frailty might be minimized

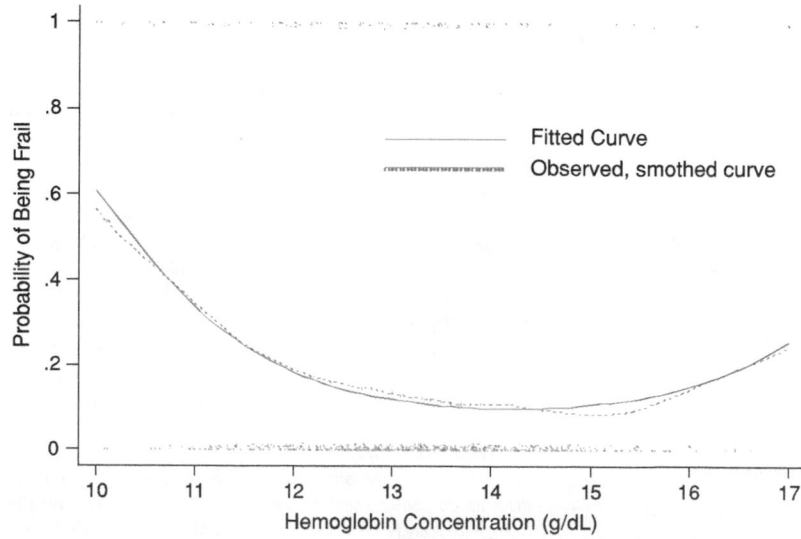

FIGURE 102-10. Probability of prevalent frailty as a function of current hemoglobin concentration levels in community-dwelling older women aged 70–80 yrs (Women's Health and Aging Studies I and II, 1992–1996). *(Chaves PHM, Semba RD, Leng S, et al. Impact of anemia and cardiovascular disease on frailty status of community-dwelling older women: The Women's Health and Aging Studies I and II. J Gerontol A Biol Sci Med Sci. 2005;60:729–735.)*

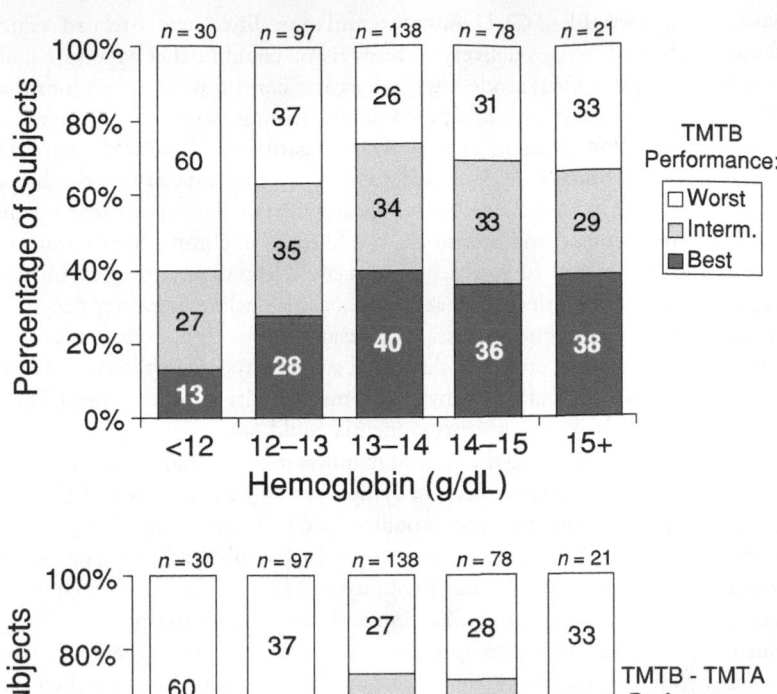

FIGURE 102-11. Performance in cognitive tests that reflect executive function according to hemoglobin levels in high physically functioning women 70–80 yrs of age free of dementia (Women's Health and Aging Studies II, 1994–1996). Shown are distributions of performance as assessed by two measures: (A) time to complete the Trail Making Test Part B (TMT-B) and (B) time to complete TMT-B minus the time to complete the Trail Making Test Part A (TMT-A) stratified by hemoglobin categories. Anemia was associated with worst performance. The sum of percentages in each column may not add exactly to 100% because of rounding. (Chaves PHM, Carlson M, Ferrucci L, et al. Association of mild anemia with executive function impairment in community-dwelling older women: The Women's Health and Aging Study II. J Am Geriatr Soc. 2006;54:1429–1435. Modified, reprinted with permission.)

in subjects without anemia or CVD, and increased, to a certain extent, when CVD is present. If anemia is present, but key physiologic cardiovascular system-mediated compensatory capacity is compromised because of prevalent CVD, the likelihood of frailty or clinical vulnerability to adverse events might be substantially increased. Such an enhancement in the risk of adverse outcomes in older adults with prevalent comorbidities in the presence of anemia, which has been documented for other outcomes in a number of studies, highlights the clinical importance underlying interactions across comorbidities in older adults and is of particular relevance for professionals caring for the health of older adults.

Cognitive Function

The relationship between anemia and cognitive function, which has been less studied than the relationships of anemia with mortality or physical disability, has been the focus of recent observational studies. In a study of 364 high-functioning women aged 70 to 80 years who had Mini-Mental Status Examination (MMSE) scores ≥ 24 and were living in the community, subjects with mild anemia (Hb between 10 and 12 g/dL) were four to five times more likely to perform worst on tests reflective of executive function (Trail Making Test Parts A and B) compared with those without anemia, even after

controlling for age, education, race, prevalent diseases, and relevant physiological and functional parameters (Figure 102-11). Executive function refers to a set of high-order cognitive abilities including planning, monitoring, and problem solving of goal-oriented tasks. Executive function impairment, which occurs commonly even in nondemented older adults, has been linked to subsequent functional decline and disability in instrumental activities of daily living. Associations of mild anemia with prevalent impaired cognition, assessed by a MMSE <24, as well as with incident dementia have also been documented in community-dwelling older adults. Consistently, associations of severe anemia with cognitive impairment in patients with CKD, as well as cancer have also been reported.

Other Selected Outcomes

Anemia is a well-recognized independent risk factor for LVH, an intermediate CVD endpoint, as well as incident CVD outcomes such as coronary heart disease events. This has been well documented in studies involving middle-aged subjects and/or subjects with CKD (including both middle-aged and older adults). Presence of anemia has also been associated with accelerated CKD progression. Additionally, it has been demonstrated that, in subjects with CKD or LVH, the risk of CVD-related outcomes is synergistically increased in the presence of anemia. Not surprisingly, given the strong association of anemia with increased comorbidity and disability, studies have consistently documented associations of anemia with increased hospitalization, health care utilization, and health care costs.

Nature of Associations: Anemia as a Causal or Noncausal (Marker) Risk Factor?

A clear understanding about the nature of the associations of anemia with adverse outcomes described above is critical for clinical decision-making. Both causal and noncausal associations maybe useful for prognostic screening. However, only causal associations may offer a potential opportunity for direct therapeutic intervention. To make inferences about causality, a number of considerations are evaluated.

Biological plausibility refers to whether the observed association maybe potentially explained in light of current biological and physiological knowledge. In this regard, several hypotheses in support of the notion that associations of anemia with clinical adverse outcomes might be biological plausible have been proposed. Chronic anemia, particularly if severe, promote a series of hemodynamic adaptations—including, for example, increase in cardiac preload, and decrease in cardiac afterload—that may lead to increased cardiac output, and ultimately to LVH, which in turn has been linked to in-

creased risk of CVD outcomes and mortality. Anemia-related reduction of oxygen delivery to heart tissue could further aggravate maladaptive LV remodeling changes and contribute to subendocardial ischemia, which could potentially explain, at least partly, observed interactions of anemia with CKD in regard to CVD-related outcomes.

Secondary to decreased oxygen-carrying capacity of the blood linked to anemia, it has also been hypothesized that persistent anemia over time, even if nonsevere, could result in chronic hypoxemia in a number of tissues, which in turn could lead to physiological impairments (e.g., decreased aerobic capacity, decline in kidney function, sarcopenia, osteoporosis, cardiac autonomic dysfunction, executive dysfunction, etc.), and decreased overall physiologic reserve. The latter is a key feature of the syndrome of frailty in older adults (Figure 102-12). In this scenario, anemia could potentially contribute in a causal manner to the clinical manifestations of frailty, such as occurrence of exercise-tolerance symptoms, as well as decreased physical activity, strength, and mobility speed. Anemia may also promote further physical deconditioning, which could lead to the onset and progression of physical disability and its complications, such as increased health care utilization and costs and mortality.

It has also been speculated that anemia could potentially have an adverse effect on cognitive function. Potential mechanisms might involve chronic reduction of cerebral oxygenation; physical

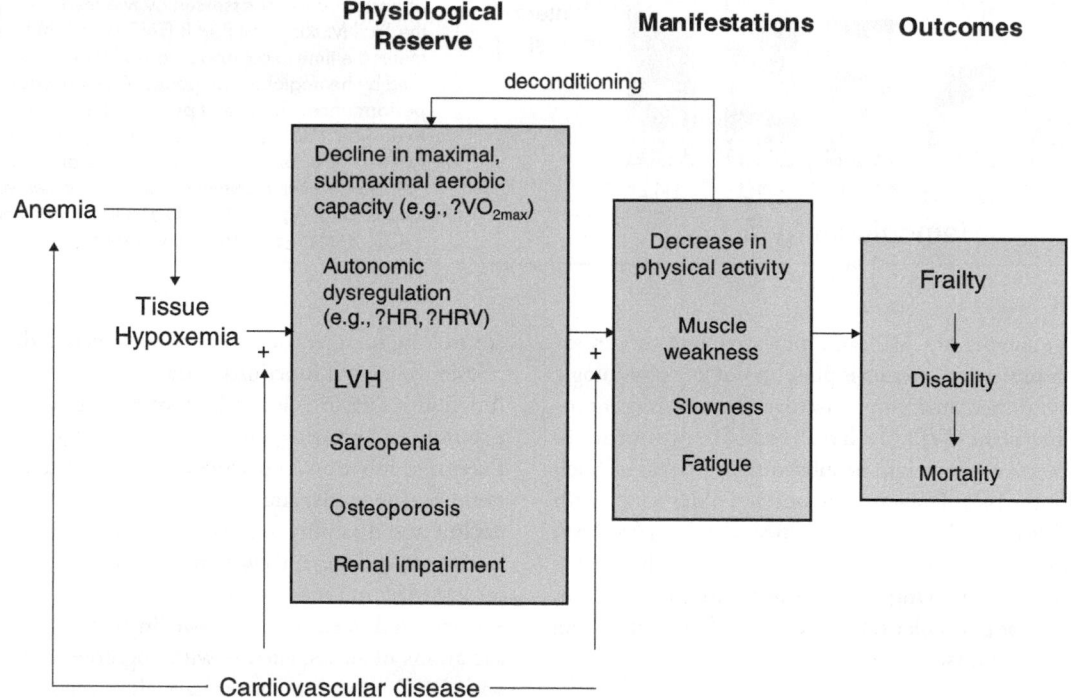

FIGURE 102-12. Proposed mechanisms through which anemia could contribute to the development of frailty. Anemia, particularly when severe, decreases the oxygen-carrying capacity of the blood, and thus may lead to tissue hypoxemia. It has been hypothesized that milder forms of anemia could also promote physiologically relevant chronic tissue hypoxemia, which would result in a number of impairments, including reduction in maximal and submaximal aerobic capacity, sarcopenia, osteoporosis, and progression of renal impairment. Chronic anemia also promotes a series of hemodynamic adaptations, which may result in autonomic dysregulation and left ventricular hypertrophy (LVH). Cardiovascular disease (CVD), an outcome that has been linked to anemia-related physiological impairments, including decreased physical activity, LVH, and autonomic dysregulation, might synergistically enhance the adverse impact of anemia on tissue oxygenation through perfusion impairment. Anemia-related physiological impairments may lead to a number of manifestations typical of frailty that reflect limitation in exercise tolerance, including decreased physical activity and/or fatigue, as well as muscle weakness, and slowness. Behavioral modifications such as excessive reduction in physical activity may in turn promote further physical deconditioning, which can contribute to further physiological decline. Presence of chronic diseases such as CVD or pulmonary diseases precluding optimal cardiorespiratory physiologic adaptive responses to anemia may contribute to the development of frailty-related manifestations. Reduction in physiologic reserve beyond a certain threshold may compromise physiologic resilience, thus increasing vulnerability to stressors—the clinical hallmark of frailty—and ultimately contributing to major frailty outcomes, including disability and mortality. HR, heart rate; HRV, heart rate variability; LVH, left ventricular hypertrophy.

deconditioning, leading to a decrease in brain-derived neurotrophin factor or a parasympathetic-related efficiency of prefrontal neural function; autonomic dysfunction; and incident CVD outcomes.

Other considerations for inferences about causality include temporal relationship, strength of association, dose–response relationship, and replication. In this regard, review of the literature reveals a clear, consistent documentation of coherent, independent, strong, dose–response associations of anemia with a number of clinical adverse outcomes in older adults by observational studies in different settings. While promising, current evidence is *not* conclusive that anemia is, in fact, a causal risk factor for these outcomes. This is a reflection of a number of important limitations inherent to observational studies of anemia in older adults. One major limitation has to do with the possibility of residual confounding by chronic disease burden, of which anemia is a well-established marker. Chronic disease burden is a causal risk factor for outcomes including physical disability, frailty, cognitive impairment, and mortality. Thus, it is theoretically possible that associations of anemia with outcomes such as the ones listed above could be not be a direct consequence of anemia, but rather indirectly, as a consequence of the fact that anemia is a marker of prevalent chronic disease burden. While epidemiologic design approaches and statistical techniques used in the analysis of observational studies (e.g., adjustment by regression models) may help minimizing confounding effects, they may not eliminate it.

Another important causality criterion refers to the documentation of change, i.e., reduction, in the risk of outcome resulting from correction of the risk factor hypothesized to be causal. In this context, intervention studies are pivotal. Observational studies unfortunately do not constitute an adequate setting for assessment of the ability of anemia correction in improving major clinical outcomes in the broad population of older adults, as treatment is currently available for only the minority of anemia cases (see below) and because of potential selection biases. Preliminary clinical trials examining the potential efficacy of therapy with erythropoiesis-stimulating agents (ESAs) in improving outcomes of anemia, including LVH, kidney function decline, and mortality in CKD patients with severe anemia did show initial promising evidence. However, generalization of these findings to milder and/or other types of anemia that are often present in the population of older adults at large should not be made automatically. Additionally, larger RCTs more recently completed have failed to document improvement in key outcomes associated with correction of milder anemia in CKD patients (see below). In summary, future large RCTs are expected to provide key insight into the causality, as well as potential clinical impact, of observed association of anemia with major adverse outcomes.

DIAGNOSTIC CONSIDERATIONS

Current published evidence supports the notion that anemia is not a "normal," clinically appropriate finding in older adults, whether in community or institutionalized settings. As outlined above, the presence of anemia is associated with a variety of adverse outcomes, but is should also be recognized that anemia may be a manifestation of major underlying disorders such as occult malignancy. A long-time clinical axiom is that anemia is often, If not always, secondary to an underlying disorder. In this context, evaluation of anemia is warranted, and may help clinicians in understanding potential opportunities for anemia treatment, as well as in diagnosing major potentially treatable underlying diseases.

An initial important consideration is that the clinical presentation of anemia in older adults may differ from that in other age groups. Clinical symptoms of anemia depend on the severity and onset of anemia. Mild, chronic, and gradually developing anemia occurs commonly in older adults. Additionally, the number of prevalent comorbidities is significant in this segment of the population, which may confound the presentation of anemia. These factors, along with possible physiologic changes secondary to age- and/or disease-related changes, and behavioral modifications (e.g., older subjects may have cut down on the frequency and/or intensity of task performance to avoid exercise tolerance symptoms) may contribute to the fact that anemia symptoms are often nonspecific, insidious in older adults. This is analogous to the increased occurrence of subclinical presentation of diseases (e.g., CVD) in this segment of the population.

The clinical investigation of anemia in older adults involves the determination of its presence, classification, as well as identification of its underlying causes. While the overall classification scheme discussed earlier in this chapter is useful for the classification of anemia in the research setting, other more refined approaches are used in the clinical setting in clinical decision-making. These approaches are based on comprehensive evaluation of the patient's medical history—including detailed assessment of prevalent comorbidities and use of medications, which are often overlooked—and physical examination as well as laboratory tests. This information serves as the basis for the classification of anemia according to kinetic and/or morphologic considerations. Kinetic considerations involve the classification of anemia in three overall mechanistic groups that are primarily marked by (a) decreased production, (b) increased destruction, or (c) loss of RBCs. Each group has further subdivisions. Morphological considerations refer to the classification of anemia on the basis of the size of RBC, as usually determined by the RBC MCV index, in combination with the reticulocyte count. Based on the MCV index, anemia can be classified as microcytic, macrocytic, or normocytic. Both MCV and reticulocyte count can be obtained by automated cell counting methods. Review of peripheral blood smear may contribute to the evaluation of anemia by allowing direct evaluation of morphological features of blood cells.

Several clinical algorithms have been developed to assist in the clinical investigation of anemia. They are readily accessible elsewhere. Results from a number of laboratory tests are incorporated in these algorithms. Tests that are commonly used in the preliminary steps of the evaluation of anemia include assessment of a complete blood count (CBC), which quantitatively estimates (either directly measured or calculated from measured parameters) a number of key parameters, including RBC count; white blood cell (WBC) count, including total and differential WBC; hemoglobin concentration (Hb); hematocrit (Hct); RBC indices, including MCV, mean corpuscular hemoglobin (MCH), mean corpuscular hemoglobin concentration (MCHC), RDW; and platelet count. Absolute reticulocyte count and the reticulocyte production index are routinely assessed. The peripheral blood smear is often reviewed.

Additional tests that are always useful in the evaluation of anemia include the following:

(a) Tests to assess iron deficiency, including serum iron, TIBC, serum ferritin, transferrin saturation, and serum sTfR. The latter reflects the product of proteolytic cleavage of transferrin receptors that are predominantly expressed on the surface of cells with high iron requirements, such as erythroid progenitor cells. In situations of iron deficiency, there is increased expression of transferrin receptors on the cellular membrane, and, concomitantly, increased sTfR levels. Serum levels of sTfR are positively correlated with bone marrow erythropoietic activity and negatively with the amount of iron stores. Serum levels of sTfR, and in particular, the index calculated as the ratio between sTfR serum transferrin receptor and the log of serum ferritin have been proposed as a particularly useful, sensitive method for differential diagnosis between iron-deficiency anemia and ACI with and without iron deficiency. Increased serum levels of sTfR and the ratio of sTfR by the log of serum ferritin are found in iron-deficiency anemia, but not in ACI. Whether measurement of sTfR levels could help improving current approaches used for monitoring of functional iron deficiency during therapy with ESAs remains to be established.

(b) Tests to assess vitamin B-12 deficiency, including serum vitamin B-12, serum methylmalonic acid (MMA), and serum total homocysteine. Measurements of serum MMA and/or total homocysteine provide a more sensitive approach to assess tissue vitamin B-12 deficiency than measurement of serum vitamin B-12 levels. This is because elevation of serum MMA and homocysteine levels tends to occur before serum vitamin B-12 falls below normal levels.

(c) Tests to assess folate deficiency, including serum folate, and RBC folate

(d) Tests to assess renal function, aiming at calculation of eGFR

(e) Tests of liver function

(f) Tests for evaluation of hemolysis, including serum lactate dehydrogenase (LDH), indirect bilirubin concentrations, and serum haptoglobin concentration

(g) Tests to evaluate occult GI bleeding, including fecal occult blood detection and endoscopy

(h) Tests to directly evaluate bone marrow, including aspiration and biopsy

(i) Tests to evaluate selected endocrine disorders, including thyroid dysfunction, and hypogonadism. Assessment of testosterone-related measures, for example, are currently recommended only if male hypogonadism is suspected, and not specifically for anemia evaluation.

There are also a number of additional measurements that, while not systematically used in the current evaluation of anemia in older adults, may eventually become part of anemia algorithms. Further clinical epidemiologic characterization of theses measurements are warranted. They include serum erythropoietin, proinflammatory markers, and hepcidin. Serum erythropoietin increases as severity of anemia increases. The increase in serum erythropoietin, a key stimulator of erythropoiesis, reflects a compensatory physiologic response to tissue hypoxemia promoted by complex hypoxia-sensing homeostatic mechanisms. However, serum erythropoietin levels are not presently measured routinely in patients with anemia because the level is abnormally increased only when severe anemia is present. Another contributing factor is that serum erythropoietin levels maybe inaccurately low for the degree of anemia as a result of the blunted erythropoietin response discussed above (Figure 102-13). Recent

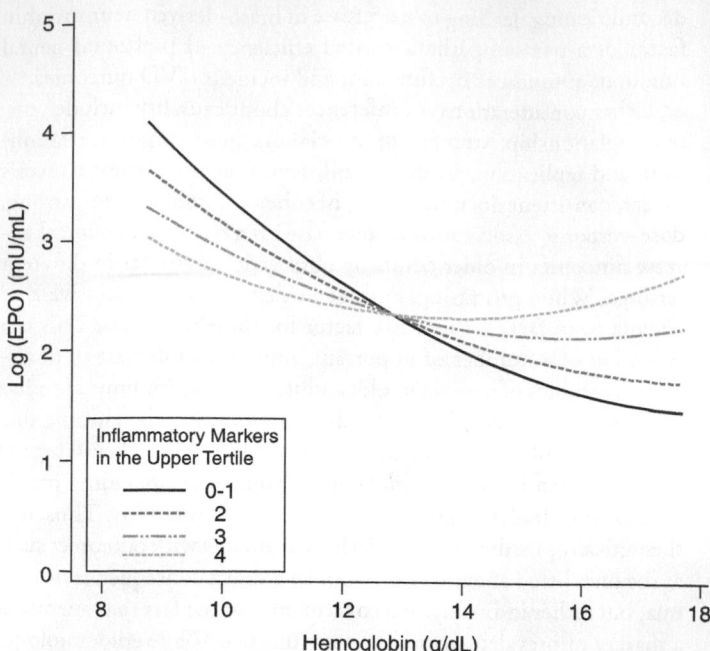

FIGURE 102-13. Scatterplot of the relationship between hemoglobin and log(erythropoietin), according to level of inflammation expressed by the number of proinflammatory markers (C-reactive protein, IL-6, IL-1β, TNF-α) in the upper tertile. The lines were obtained from a linear regression model predicting log(erythropoietin) including age, sex, hemoglobin, squared hemoglobin, inflammatory index (dummy variables), and appropriate terms for the interactions of the inflammatory index with hemoglobin and squared hemoglobin. *(Ferrucci L, Guralnik JM, Woodman RC, et al. Proinflammatory state and circulating erythropoietin in persons with and without anemia. Am J Med. 2005;118(11):1288.)*

data have suggested, nonetheless, that even within its normal range, serum erythropoietin levels may reflect significant differences across Hb levels in the mid-normal to moderately reduced range (see Figure 102-2). High-sensitivity C-reactive protein, high-sensitivity IL-6, and TNF-α, among others, are well established proinflammatory markers. Given the role of inflammation on the pathogenesis of anemia, particularly of ACI, one may expect that measurement of proinflammatory markers may become useful in the evaluation of anemia in older adults the future. Major methodological progress has been recently made in regard to the measurement of hepcidin in the blood and the urine. Given that hepcidin is an important modulator of iron metabolism and may play a major role in the pathogenesis of ACI, it may be that measurement of hepcidin will prove useful in anemia-related clinical decision-making in the future.

THERAPEUTIC CONSIDERATIONS

Nutrient-deficiency Anemia

Intervention involves two critical components: replacement of the nutrient that is deficient and treatment of the underlying disorder that is causing the deficiency. Available interventions for this type of anemia are effective, safe, and relatively inexpensive. Iron-deficiency anemia is traditionally treated with oral iron replacement. This is usually accomplished through the use of oral iron supplements, though recommendation of ingestion for high-iron-content foods should not be forgotten. Usually, initial hematological response is rapid, as assessed by a marked increase in the number of reticulocytes within 7 to 10 days of therapy. Continued iron replacement, however, is important for repletion of total body iron stores. Often, adverse GI symptoms may occur, threatening treatment compliance and requiring adjustments. If the underlying condition has not been corrected (e.g., blood loss), effectiveness of treatment maybe delayed or even precluded. In community-dwelling older adults with mild-to-moderate anemia, parenteral iron replacement is rarely pursued. Several studies have shown that IV iron therapy maybe particularly useful in patients with cancer or CKD undergoing treatment with ESAs.

Folate deficiency is primarily treated with oral folate replacement. Vitamin B-12 typically is replaced through parenteral therapy, for example, intramuscular, monthly doses of vitamin B-12. Alternative routes of administration, including oral vitamin B-12 therapy, have also been proposed. In patients lacking intrinsic factor, high oral doses of vitamin B-12 maybe considered. In patients with deficient food digestion resulting in impaired release of vitamin B-12 from ingested foods leading to poor absorption of free vitamin B-12, oral doses of vitamin B-12 not as high as that for patients with pernicious anemia maybe effective. Initial hematopoietic response to vitamin B-12 replacement in vitamin B-12-deficiency and to folate in folate-deficiency anemia is also rapidly observed, as assessed by a substantial increase in the reticulocyte count within 1 week of therapy. Folate replacement may produce a transient, suboptimal hematological improvement in anemia as a result of vitamin B-12 deficiency; however, vitamin B-12 neurologic complications may appear and progress without vitamin B-12 replacement.

Anemia of CKD

The use of ESAs is the keystone of management of anemia in older adults with CKD. Several studies have been shown that ESA therapy constitutes an effective, safe therapy to treat anemia and lead to improvement in quality of life parameters in CKD patients. At the time this chapter is being written, there are two ESAs licensed for the treatment of anemia of CKD in the Unites States: epoetin alfa and darbopoetin alfa. Both are glycoproteins that are manufactured using recombinant DNA technology. They stimulate erythropoiesis through the same mechanism of action as endogenous erythropoietin. Epoetin alfa is a recombinant human erythropoietin (rHuEPO) that has the same amino acid sequence of naturally occurring erythropoietin. It was originally licensed in 1989 for the treatment of anemia in patients with anemia of CKD. Subsequently, epoetin alfa therapy was approved for additional indications, including the treatment of anemia in cancer patients on chemotherapy, and anemia in zidovudine-treated patients infected with the human immunodeficiency virus (HIV). Darbopoetin alfa is a rHuEPO analog that contains extra carbohydrate chains, which increases the molecular weight of the glycoprotein. As compared to epoetin alfa, darbopoetin alfa has a longer half-life. Additional ESAs are currently being investigated.

Detailed guidelines exist to guide ESA therapy in patients with CKD. Varying administration schemes provide therapy flexibility. Traditional outpatient regimens involve the subcutaneous administration of ESA once per week or every 2 weeks. More recently, extended-dosing regimens involving ESA administration every

3 weeks and even once monthly have been proposed. To avoid impaired erythropoiesis caused by true iron deficiency or functional iron deficiency, iron stores should be fully replenished before and during ESA therapy. This may initially be attempted through oral iron replacement, though often IV iron therapy is required. ESA therapy is considered safe. However, major adverse effects should be acknowledged, including an increased risk of death, thromboembolic complications, stroke, heart attack, aplastic anemia, tumor progression, and others. To minimize risks of these adverse events, careful monitoring of hemoglobin levels, along with adjustment of ESA dosing, to maintain the lowest hemoglobin level clinically needed is recommended. The target Hb level that should be pursued in patients with anemia of CKD remains a subject of controversy (see below). Current clinical recommendations at the time this chapter is being written suggest a target Hb range between 11 and 12 g/dL.

Before the advent of recombinant erythropoietin, androgens were regularly used for treatment of anemia in patients with end-stage CKD. Hypothesized mechanisms included stimulation of erythropoietin production, a direct effect on the bone marrow enhancing the response of erythroid progenitors to erythropoietin, and increase in RBC survival. However, adverse effects of androgen therapy, along with availability of recombinant erythropoietin, obviate the use of androgen therapy for anemia of CKD. Current guidelines recommend against use of androgens as adjuvant therapy to ESA treatment.

Anemia of Chronic Inflammation

Treatment of underlying chronic inflammatory diseases constitutes the cornerstone therapy for ACI. This axiom remains valid to this date. Cases exist though of refractory ACI despite proper treatment for underlying diseases, including, for example, rheumatoid arthritis, inflammatory bowel disease, and congestive heart failure. At this time, there is no approved specific treatment for ACI. Preliminary small pilot studies of short duration have suggested that the use of ESAs along with iron replacement may result in hematological response and anemia correction. Further large RCT studies will be necessary to establish whether pharmacologic correction of anemia with ESAs could ultimately lead to improved hard outcomes, for example, increased survival, in older adults with specific diseases survival and/or in the broad older population.

"Unclassified" or "Unexplained" Anemia

Reflecting the limited knowledge about pathogenic mechanisms involved with this heterogeneous anemia group, no specific anemia treatment is currently recommended. Considering the axiom that anemia is always secondary to a specific cause, i.e., not simply caused by aging per se, it is possible that a specific etiology may eventually become apparent as a consequence of continued clinical investigation over time.

Impact of Anemia Correction with Recombinant Erythropoietin on Clinical Outcomes

Over the last decade, data from several intervention studies that included older adults in different settings helped establishing the efficacy of recombinant erythropoietin therapy in safely increasing Hb levels in older adults. More important, increasing Hb levels through recombinant erythropoietin therapy has been consistently shown to improve health-related quality of life in patients with severe and/or moderate anemia and specific diseases, including CKD and cancer. However, discrepancy of evidence from observational studies and small preliminary trials with that from recent major RCTs have been documented in regard to the ability to improve hard outcomes, as a result of anemia correction via ESA therapy. For example, recent RCTs conducted in CKD patients have shown that recombinant erythropoietin targeting Hb levels currently considered in the "normal" range ("full correction of anemia") as opposed to below "normal" levels ("partial anemia correction") did not show hypothesized results in terms of improving mortality, left ventricular mass changes, CVD events, and slowing of renal function decline. In fact, recent RCT data have, in fact, raised concerns that increase in Hb levels with recombinant erythropoietin up to levels until recently thought of as normal may in fact increase the risk of serious adverse events. These concerns even have motivated the United States Food and Drug Administration's (FDA) to recently (March 2007) issue a warning to health care professionals in regard to the in regard to the risk of these serious adverse complications associated with ESA therapy complications.

CONCLUSION

Anemia is a major clinical syndrome in older adults. Recent advances have been made in the characterization of important mechanisms underlying the pathogenesis of this syndrome and of the relationship of anemia with major outcomes in older populations. Treatment data that have become recently available have contributed novel insight not only on the ability to correct anemia with ESA therapy, but more importantly, on the potential impact of this therapy on major clinical outcomes. Despite these advances, many questions remain to be answered at this time, including the selected topics regarding the clinical epidemiology of anemia in older adults identified below:

(a) In older adults with anemia and specific diseases for which ESA therapy is currently approved, can anemia correction with ESA therapy slow declines in physical and cognitive function, prevent frailty and disability, and/or improve survival? If so, what should the target Hb be to optimally improve clinical outcomes?

(b) Can correction of mild ACI with ESA therapy improve major outcomes such as the ones listed in (a) in the broad population of community-dwelling older adults?

(c) How should health status heterogeneity impact anemia-related clinical decision-making in older adults? For example, how should screening and treatment considerations differ for community-dwelling older adults without advanced disability versus nursing home residents?

(d) In regard to the definition of anemia in older adults, should criteria differ according to race?

(e) What are the major mechanisms underlying unclassified/ unexplained anemia? Does ESA therapy constitute a therapeutic approach in this type of anemia?

FURTHER READING

Astor BC, Muntner P, Levin A, et al. Association of kidney function with anemia: the Third National Health and Nutrition Examination Survey (1988–1994). *Arch Intern Med.* 2002;162(12):1401–1408.

Balducci L. Epidemiology of anemia in the elderly: information on diagnostic evaluation. *J Am Geriatr Soc.* 2003;51(3 Suppl):S2–S9.

Besarab A, Bolton WK, Browne JK, et al. The effects of normal as compared with low hematocrit values in patients with cardiac disease who are receiving hemodialysis and epoetin. *N Engl J Med.* 1998;339(9):584–590.

Chaves PHM, Xue Q-L, Guralnik JM, et al. What does constitute normal hemoglobin concentration in community-dwelling disable older women? *J Am Geriatr Soc.* 2004;52:1811–1816.

Chaves PHM, Ashar B, Guralnik JM, Fried LP. Looking at the relationship between hemoglobin concentration and prevalent mobility difficulty in older women. Should the criteria currently used to define anemia in older people be reevaluated? *J Am Geriatr Soc.* 2002;50:1257–1264.

Chaves PHM, Semba RD, Leng S, et al. Impact of anemia and cardiovascular disease on frailty status of community-dwelling older women: The Women's Health and Aging Studies I and II. *J Gerontol A Biol Sci Med Sci.* 2005;60:729–735.

Chaves PHM, Carlson M, Ferrucci L, et al. Association of mild anemia with executive function impairment in community-dwelling older women: The Women's Health and Aging Study II. *J Am Geriatr Soc.* 2006;54:1429–1435.

Colcombe S, Kramer AF. Fitness effects on the cognitive function of older adults: a meta-analytic study. *Psychol Sci.* 2003;14:125–735.

Drueke TB, Locatelli F, Clyne N, et al. Normalization of hemoglobin in patients with chronic kidney disease, *N Engl J Med.* 2006;355;2071–2084.

Ferrucci L, Guralnik JM, Bandinelli S, et al. Unexplained anaemia in older persons is characterized by low erythropoietin and low levels of pro-inflammatory markers. *Br J Haematol.* 2007;136(6):849–855.

Ferrucci L, Guralnik JM, Woodman RC, et al. Proinflammatory state and circulating erythropoietin in persons with and without anemia. *Am J Med.* 2005;118(11):1288.

Ganz T. Molecular control of iron transport. *J Am Soc Nephrol.* 2007;18(2):394–400.

Guralnik JM, Eisenstaedt RS, Ferrucci L, et al. Prevalence of anemia in persons 65 years and older in the United States: evidence for a high rate of unexplained anemia. *Blood.* 2004;104:2263–2268.

Izaks GJ, Westendorp RG, Knook DL. The definition of anemia in older persons. *JAMA.* 1999;281:1714–1717.

National Kidney Foundation. KDOQI Clinical Practice Guidelines and Clinical Practice Recommendations for Anemia in Chronic Kidney Disease. *Am J Kidney Dis.* 2006;47 (suppl 3):S1–S146.

Patel KV, Harris TB, Faulhaber M, et al. Racial variation in the relationship of anemia with mortality and mobility disability among older adults. *Blood.* 2007;109(11):4663–4670.

Penninx BW, Guralnik JM, Onder G, et al. Anemia and decline in physical performance among older adults. *Am J Med.* 2003;115:105–110.

Roger SD, Levin A. Epoetin trials: randomised controlled trials don't always mimic observational data. *Nephrol Dial Transplant.* 2007;22(3):684–686.

Singh AK, Szczech L, Tang KL, et al. Correction of anemia with epoetin alfa in chronic kidney disease. *N Engl J Med.* 2006;355:2085–2098.

Spivak JL. Anemia in the elderly: time for new blood in old vessels? *Arch Intern Med.* 2005;165(19):2187–2189.

Weiss G, Goodnough LT. Anemia of chronic disease. *N Engl J Med.* 2005;352(10):1011–1023.

White Cell Disorders

Heidi D. Klepin ■ *Bayard L. Powell*

White blood cells (WBC) provide major host defense mechanisms against invading pathogens through phagocytosis and the immune response. In addition, lymphocytes provide immune surveillance against the development of cancer and are important mediators of disorders of the immune system. White cell disorders are usually the result of overproduction or underproduction of one or more of the WBC series, which include the granulocytes—neutrophils, basophils, and eosinophils—and/or mononuclear cells—lymphocytes and monocytes. Less frequently, WBC disorders result from WBC dysfunction despite normal number of cells. The acuity and severity of these disorders are related to the number of white cells, the subset(s) of WBC involved, their degree of maturity, and their functional capacity.

Initial clinical manifestations of WBC disorders can vary widely but often include signs and symptoms of infection. Disorders of WBC, benign or malignant, frequently also involve abnormalities of the red blood cells (RBCs) and platelets. In these situations, the signs and symptoms of disease at presentation may include those related to anemia (i.e., weakness and easy fatigability) and/or thrombocytopenia (i.e., easy bruisability, mucosal or gastrointestinal bleeding, and hematuria). A careful history and physical examination with evaluation of the peripheral blood, and bone marrow when needed, will establish a diagnosis in many cases.

Aging is not associated with significant changes in the peripheral WBC count or WBC differential (Table 103-1). Therefore, abnormalities in white cell numbers should be evaluated as a probable sign of an active disease process. Most white cell disorders are more common with increased age and the most common WBC disorders in the elderly are neoplastic diseases. Table 103-2 lists the spectrum of white cell disorders encountered in clinical practice. Full descriptions of these processes are available in textbooks of hematology and oncology. This chapter focuses on these disorders as related to geriatric medicine.

The most common assessment of white cells is quantitative evaluation of their numbers. Careful attention should also be paid to the distribution of the different types of white cells (WBC differential). Equally important is the microscopic examination of the peripheral blood smear (and bone marrow when needed) for morphologic changes in the WBC as well as the red cells and platelets. Specific quantitation of WBC subsets by immunophenotyping techniques can aid in the diagnosis of many neoplastic WBC disorders. Qualitative or functional defects are more difficult to establish with laboratory techniques and are usually strongly suggested by the medical history.

DECREASED WHITE BLOOD CELLS

Leukopenia may occur with a broad array of medical problems. Leukopenia can range from a mild suppression of the WBC to clinically significant neutropenia (Table 103-3). Most intrinsic (hereditary/familial) disorders and syndromes are detected during infancy or childhood. Leukopenia in older adults is generally the result of acquired or secondary disorders, either reactive (drugs, nutritional, infections, immune) or malignant. Table 103-4 presents key components in the clinical workup of neutropenia.

Drug/Toxin Effects

Elderly patients commonly consume many prescribed and over-the-counter medications and are at higher risk for developing drug-related neutropenia or pancytopenia. The bone marrow is one of the more rapidly proliferating organs of the body; therefore, it is not surprising that exposure to noxious agents may temporarily or permanently inhibit production of one or more elements of the blood. The list of possible offenders is extensive and constantly evolving with new drug development. Table 103-5 lists some of the more commonly reported offenders. In a situation of neutropenia, leukopenia, or pancytopenia, the physician should thoroughly review the patient's medications and the duration of the medication

TABLE 103-1

Normal WBC Counts for Adults

TEST	RANGE ($\times 10^3/\mu L$)
WBC	4.5–11.0
Segmental neutrophils	1.6–7.3
Band neutrophils	0.0–0.2
Lymphocytes	1.0–5.1
Monocytes	0.1–0.9
Eosinophils	0.0–0.5
Basophils	0.0–0.5

TABLE 103-3

Neutropenia

ANC*	INFECTION RISK
≥1000	Essentially normal
500–1000	Slight ↑ risk
<500	"Significant" risk
<100	Severe risk

*Absolute neutrophil count (ANC) = WBC ×%(seg + bands).

exposure. In the absence of alternative explanations, medications administered within 4 weeks of onset of neutropenia should be evaluated. Short duration of exposure does not remove the possibility of a drug-induced cytopenia; it could be an idiosyncratic reaction. Diagnosis involves identification of a possible offending agent and exclusion of alternative etiologies for the leukopenia. A bone marrow

biopsy is often indicated as part of the workup if the leukopenia is severe.

Drug effects on the bone marrow range from mild neutropenias (more common) to agranulocytosis; lymphocytopenia occurs less frequently. The RBC and platelets may or may not be affected. Drug-induced reduction of the granulocytic series may be a direct toxic effect, as with many cancer chemotherapeutic drugs or may be the result of an immunologic phenomenon wherein a drug–antibody complex reacts with mature neutrophils and/or their precursors in the peripheral blood or bone marrow. Treatment usually consists of supportive care, with administration of antibiotics for febrile patients. Upon withdrawal of the offending agent, there may be a relatively brisk marrow recovery within 14 to 21 days. A bone marrow examination during this recovery period may reveal an increased number of immature elements, which can be confused with a malignant process such as an acute leukemia or myelodysplasia. If this is a possibility, close follow-up for an additional 2 to 3 weeks will usually provide the answer. The recovering marrow will go on to differentiate, but the malignant marrow will either stay the same

TABLE 103-2

Disorders of White Blood Cells

I. Lack of production
  A. Drug or toxin suppression, which may be temporary or permanent
  B. Ineffective myelopoiesis secondary to B-12 or folate deficiency
  C. Bone marrow failure (aplastic anemia)
  D. Neoplastic causes of decreased WBC (e.g., MDS, acute leukemia, LGL leukemia)
II. Increased destruction
  Immune neutropenia secondary to rheumatologic disorders, Felty's syndrome, and lymphoproliferative malignancies
III. Increased splenic sequestration
  Congestive splenomegaly with cirrhosis, Gaucher's disease, etc.
IV. Nonneoplastic increases in WBC
  A. Response to stress (e.g., infection)
  B. Response to drug (e.g., corticosteroids, granulocyte colony-stimulating factor)
  C. Other reactive increases (e.g., inflammation)
V. Neoplastic diseases
  A. Primary hematologic
    1. Myelodysplastic syndromes (MDS)
    2. Acute leukemias
      a. Acute myelogenous leukemia (AML)
      b. Acute lymphocytic leukemia (ALL)
    3. Chronic leukemias
      a. Chronic lymphocytic leukemia (CLL)
      b. Chronic myelogenous leukemia (CML)
      c. Hairy-cell leukemia
      d. Large Granular Lymphocytic Leukemia (LGL leukemia)
    4. Other myeloproliferative diseases
    5. Non-Hodgkin's lymphoma (with circulating lymphoma cells)
  B. Cancers metastatic to bone marrow
  Most commonly breast, lung, prostate, and lymphomas
VI. Normal count with impaired function
  A. Diabetes mellitus: impaired polymorphonuclear neutrophil function
  B. Chronic renal failure: Impaired polymorphonuclear neutrophil and lymphocyte function
  C. Drugs (e.g., corticosteroids)

TABLE 103-4

Key Components in the Evaluation of Neutropenia

1. Clinical history	Duration (acute vs. chronic)
	History of infection
	History of bleeding/bruising/fatigue
	Medication history
	Presence of comorbidities (rheumatologic disease, cirrhosis, malabsorption)
2. Examination	Evaluate for signs of infection including careful skin and mucosal examination
	Evidence of bleeding/bruising
	Splenomegaly
3. Complete blood count	Severity of neutropenia
	Presence of anemia or thrombocytopenia
	Macrocytosis
	Immature granulocytes on differential
4. Peripheral smear	Toxic granulation/vacuolation of neutrophils
	Presence of dysplastic features
	Immature granulocytes
	Nucleated red cells
	Megaloblastic changes (hypersegmentation of neutrophils)
5. Bone marrow biopsy	Indicated for severe neutropenia, pancytopenia, evidence of dysplasia or granulocytic immaturity on peripheral smear

TABLE 103-5

Drugs Associated with Agranulocytosis/Neutropenia

1. Cancer chemotherapeutic agents
2. Psychotropic drugs:
   Clozapine
   Risperidone
   Olanzapine
   Haloperidol
   Phenothiazine
   Tricyclic antidepressants
   Meprobamate
3. Anti-inflammatory/antiarthritic drugs:
   Sulfasalazine
   Nonsteroidal anti-inflammatory agents
   Colchicine
   Immunosuppressive agents
   Penicillamine
   Gold salts
   Allopurinol
   Immunosuppressants
4. Thyroid suppressants:
   Propylthiouracil
5. Cardiovascular drugs:
   Antiarrhythmic agents (procainamide, quinidine, amiodarone)
   ACE inhibitors (captopril, enalapril)
   Nifedipine
   Hydralazine
   Propranolol
   Methyldopa
   Ticlopidine
   Dipyridamole
   Digoxin
6. Antibiotics:
   Sulfa drugs
   Semisynthetic penicillins
   Cephalosporins
   Macrolides
   Vancomycin
   Rifampin
   Clindamycin
   Gentamicin
   Linezolid
7. Anticonvulsants:
   Phenytoin and derivatives
   Carbamazepine
8. Thiazide diuretics
9. Antihistamines- H_2 blockers
10. Oral hypoglycemia drugs

or worsen. Other marrow toxins include a variety of household and industrial chemicals, especially organic solvents, naphthalenes, insecticides, and herbicides. Inquiries about chemical exposure from hobbies or occupations must therefore be part of history taking. While the hematologic effects of drug and chemical exposure are frequently reversible, some may result in myelodysplastic syndromes (MDS) or aplastic anemia which, in turn, may evolve into acute myelogenous leukemia (AML).

Nutritional Deficiency

Mild neutropenia may be associated with nutritional anemias secondary to folate or B-12 deficiency. Older individuals, especially those living alone, may not be attentive to their diet for various socioeconomic, psychological, or medical reasons. The main sources of folates are fresh green vegetables, many fruits, and beans. Cooking and canning destroys folates. The body's folate stores can be depleted after 4 to 5 months of poor dietary intake. Thus, a dietary history may provide an important clue to the diagnosis of the hematologic problem. Dietary folate deficiency may be aggravated by alcoholism and chronic hemolysis. Additional hematologic findings of folate deficiency include macrocytic anemia and hypersegmented neutrophils. Potential folate deficiency is best evaluated by measuring RBC folate.

In contrast, body stores of vitamin B-12 are not readily depleted by poor dietary habits alone. It takes 3 to 5 years to deplete the body stores of vitamin B-12. However, gastric atrophy is more common with increasing age, and this may lead to failure of gastric secretion of intrinsic factor, which binds to dietary cobalamin—a necessary step in the absorption of vitamin B-12 in the ileum. Other conditions that cause a B-12 deficiency include gastrectomy or subtotal small-bowel (ileal) resection. It should be noted that neurologic signs and symptoms of B-12 deficiency may be confused with other neurologic problems in the elderly patient. These include peripheral paresthesias (peripheral neuritis), loss of balance (posterior column damage), spasticity (lateral column damage), and impaired cognitive function. Any of these neurological signs and symptoms may be mistakenly attributed to "old age," but if caused by B-12 deficiency may be corrected with vitamin B-12 replacement therapy. Low serum cobalamin levels (<200 ng/L) are diagnostic of deficiency and will be found in the majority of patients who are symptomatic. Subclinical cobalamin deficiency can be detected by measuring serum methylmalonic acid. Subclinical cobalamin deficiency is characterized by low normal serum cobalamin level (200–350 ng/L) and an elevated methylmalonic acid level. It should be noted that homocysteine will be elevated in both folate and cobalamin deficiency.

Copper deficiency is a more recently reported but uncommon cause of neutropenia. Neutropenia is typically associated with anemia and may be confused with early MDS, particularly in an older adult. Copper deficiency is most commonly associated with malabsorption, malnutrition, use of total parenteral nutrition, or excess oral zinc supplementation. The diagnosis is suggested by the appropriate clinical setting and a low serum copper level. Hematological changes are potentially reversible with oral copper supplementation.

Infections

A number of infections can be associated with neutropenia and/or leukopenia in older adults. These infections include viral (e.g., influenza, varicella, hepatitis A, B, or C, cytomegalovirus, human immunodeficiency virus, parvovirus B19), and bacterial (e.g., *Staphylococcus aureus*, brucellosis, tularemia, rickettsia, and tuberculosis). Neutropenia associated with most viral illnesses is self-limited and of minimal clinical consequence. A few viruses (hepatitis B, Epstein–Barr, and human immunodeficiency virus) can cause protracted, clinically significant neutropenia. Bacterial septicemia, particularly with Gram-negative organisms, is a serious cause of acquired neutropenia and confers a poor prognosis. The mechanism of leukopenia is usually bone marrow suppression, but in the case of overwhelming bacterial sepsis, can result from exhaustion of bone marrow reserves. Treatment focuses on supportive care including use of antibiotics for infection; the role of myeloid growth factors in this setting is unproven.

Bone Marrow Failure

Severe and prolonged bone marrow failure may occur in association with drugs, toxins, or infections, but is frequently idiopathic. Aplastic anemia is characterized by severe pancytopenia and bone marrow hypoplasia. Clinical signs and symptoms reflect the cytopenias: infection, bleeding, and/or the signs/symptoms of anemia. Pure white cell aplasia occurs rarely. Treatments for this life-threatening disease include supportive care (transfusion, antibiotics), immunosuppression (antithymocyte globulin, cyclosporine, steroids), and stem cell transplant (limited application in the elderly population).

Increased Destruction

Immune neutropenia may be associated with various rheumatologic conditions such as systemic lupus erythematosus, rheumatoid arthritis, polyserositis, and lymphoproliferative malignancies. In these situations, neutropenia is caused by the elimination of immunoglobulin-coated granulocytes by the reticuloendothelial system. Immune-mediated neutropenia is often clinically significant with absolute neutrophil count (ANC) <500 cells/mm^3, predisposing to increased infection risk. In general, the bone marrow is hypercellular or normocellular and lacking in mature neutrophils. Neutropenia of Felty's syndrome (rheumatoid arthritis, splenomegaly, and neutropenia) has a complex etiology that includes immune destruction and suppression as well as splenic sequestration. These neutropenias frequently respond to granulocyte colony-stimulating factors (G-CSF) or granulocyte-macrophage colony-stimulating factors (GM-CSF).

Splenic Sequestration

Any condition causing splenomegaly (e.g., hepatic cirrhosis) may lead to sequestration of sufficient neutrophils to cause mild-to-moderate neutropenia as a component of the pancytopenia of hypersplenism. The mild-to-moderate neutropenia usually does not predispose to increased infections and often occurs in association with anemia and/or thrombocytopenia.

Neoplastic Causes of Decreased WBC

Malignancies (hematological and nonhematological) can present with neutropenia and need to be considered in the evaluation of this finding. Details of the presentation and workup of many of these disorders will be presented later in this chapter.

INCREASED WBC

Benign Causes of Leukocytosis

The most common causes of sustained increases in WBC are neoplastic diseases. However, there are a number of nonneoplastic etiologies for increases in one or more white cell forms. The most common among these is a leukocytosis, specifically neutrophilia, in response to infection. This is associated with a "left shift" in the differential, with increases in bands and other less-mature granulocytes, including metamyelocytes and myelocytes. Such a normal granulocytosis can also be seen in response to an exogenous steroid. Increases in specific subsets of white cells (e.g., eosinophils or basophils) can occur in response to a number of exposures or illnesses. Hereditary and familial (e.g., Down syndrome) causes of leukocytosis are rare and usually detected early in life.

Infection

Infection stimulates the acute release of neutrophils from the marginated storage pools of the bone marrow. Neutrophilia commonly occurs with acute bacterial infections, and is less predictably seen with viruses. An increase in band neutrophils and metamyelocytes is most common. Toxic granules in those cells are frequently present on review of the peripheral blood smear. A dramatic "leukemoid reaction," characterized by a WBC >50,000/μL, a marked left shift with increased immature granulocytes including myelocytes, promyelocytes, and even blasts, may be confused with malignant disorders, especially chronic myelogenous leukemia (CML). Leukemoid reactions are characterized by a high-leukocyte alkaline phosphatase (LAP [low in CML]) and absence of the Philadelphia chromosome. Leukemoid reactions are uncommon and the probability of an underlying bone marrow disorder should always be suspected in this setting.

Drug-Induced Leukocytosis

Corticosteroids are the most common medications associated with increases in WBC, primarily neutrophilia. The mechanism includes reduced neutrophil adhesion and release from marrow stores. The hematopoietic colony-stimulating factors (e.g., G-CSF, GM-CSF) are designed to stimulate neutrophilia, and lithium can induce neutrophilia through similar CSF pathways. Beta-adrenergic agonists also frequently stimulate acute release of neutrophils from marginated pools.

Other Reactive Leukocytosis

Mild neutrophilia (WBC 12,000–20,000/μL) can occur after a stress, resulting from release of neutrophils from marginated pools into the bloodstream. Stressful stimuli include exercise, seizures, anesthesia, and surgery. Acute inflammation and tissue necrosis are also associated with neutrophilia. Examples include burns, electric shock, trauma, and infarction. Asplenia can be associated with moderate leukocytosis. Chronic inflammatory conditions such as colitis, rheumatoid arthritis, and vasculitis may stimulate a modest increase in bone marrow production and release of neutrophils. Mild to moderate leukocytosis (WBC <30,000/μL) may also occur in association with a variety of malignancies without bone marrow involvement.

Isolated increases in WBC subsets occur with or without increase in total WBC. Monocytosis may be associated with inflammatory diseases, specifically infections, autoimmune and granulomatous diseases, and numerous malignancies. Eosinophilia (>600/μL) usually represents a reaction to drugs, infection (e.g., fungi, parasites), allergic disorders, vasculitis, or malignancies. Lymphocytosis, though frequently representing malignancy, may occur in response to infection.

MALIGNANT DISEASE OF THE HEMATOPOIETIC SYSTEM

Hematologic malignancies, although most frequently characterized by elevated WBC, can be associated with low, normal, or high WBC. The WBC differential, as well as the red cell and platelet counts, are usually abnormal.

Malignant diseases of the WBCs include the four major subtypes of leukemia—AML, acute lymphocytic leukemia (ALL), CML, and chronic lymphocytic leukemia (CLL); as well as the MDS (preleukemias); the myeloproliferative disorders other than CML; hairy cell leukemia; large granular lymphocytic leukemia; metastatic cancers to the bone marrow; and circulating non-Hodgkin's lymphoma cells. Older adults make up a large proportion of incident and prevalent cases of these diseases. In fact, the age-specific incidence rates of all leukemias increase in the elderly population (Figure 103-1). As the population ages, the burden of these diseases is nearly certain to rise, with the elderly population being most affected.

The effectiveness of treatments has improved substantially over recent decades for most hematologic malignancies. Unfortunately, the response rates and cure rates in elderly patients have lagged behind for a number of reasons, including the more common occurrence of chronic leukemias, MDS, and myeloproliferative disease in the elderly person, limited ability of the elderly person to tolerate the more aggressive curative approaches for acute leukemia, underrepresentation of older adults in clinical trials, and the more common occurrence of multiple poor prognostic factors in elderly patients. With the increased focus on elderly specific clinical trials and the ongoing development of less toxic, targeted therapies, opportunities for effective treatment of older adults with malignant WBC disorders should improve.

Myelodysplastic (Preleukemia) Syndromes

The myelodysplastic syndromes, frequently referred to as preleukemia, encompass a heterogenous group of clonal hematopoietic disorders characterized by ineffective hematopoiesis, peripheral blood cytopenias, and hypercellularity of the bone marrow. In these diseases, cells of the affected lineage are unable to undergo maturation and differentiation, resulting in cytopenias. The major clinical significance of these disorders is the morbidity associated with profound cytopenias and the potential to evolve into AML.

The true incidence of myelodysplastic syndromes is not known, but currently estimated at 15,000 to 20,000 new cases per year in the United States. About two thirds of patients with MDS are elderly males. MDS are clearly diseases of aging patients, with a median age at diagnosis of 65 to 70 years. The nomenclature associated with myelodysplastic syndromes is confusing. Terms found in the literature include odoleukemia (threshold of leukemia), subacute myeloid leukemia, smoldering leukemia, dysmyelopoietic syndrome, and preleukemia.

Diagnosis of MDS relies mainly on peripheral blood and bone marrow findings. The diagnosis should be suspected in individuals presenting with cytopenia. In clinical studies, the majority of patients have a hemoglobin of less than 11, platelet count <100,000, and an ANC <1000 at the time of diagnosis. However, careful attention should be paid to consistent decreases in blood counts over time in an older adult, which may signify early developing MDS. Many patients are asymptomatic at the time of diagnosis. However, careful history taking should include questions regarding recurrent infections, bruising, and bleeding. The differential diagnosis for suspected MDS includes AML, aplastic anemia, megaloblastic anemia (B-12 and folate deficiency), copper deficiency, viral infections (HIV), large granular lymphocytic leukemia, and heavy metal poisoning.

The initial serologic workup includes a complete blood count (CBC) with differential, reticulocyte count, RBC folate, serum B-12, iron studies, and review of the peripheral smear. Classic peripheral blood findings associated with MDS include macrocytosis and hypogranular, hypolobated (dysplastic) neutrophils. A bone marrow biopsy with cytogenetic analysis is required to confirm the diagnosis. The bone marrow is typically hypercellular and demonstrates evidence of dysplasia. Cytogenetic abnormalities play a critical role in the diagnosis and natural history of MDS. Common cytogenetic abnormalities involve chromosomes 5, 7, 8, 17, or 20.

The classification of MDS has evolved over the past 10 years. In 1982, the French-American-British (FAB) Cooperative Group established a classification system with five diagnostic categories based on peripheral blood and bone marrow characteristics. These include refractory anemia (RA), RA with ring sideroblasts (RARS), RA with excess blasts (RAEB), RAEB in transformation (RAEBT), and chronic myelomonocytic leukemia (CMML). Details of this classification system are presented in Table 103-6.

A more recent classification scheme was proposed by the World Health Organization (WHO), which incorporates evolving knowledge of the biology of disease including the significance of cytogenetic abnormalities. This classification scheme is presented in Table 103-7 and better reflects the heterogeneity of MDS. There are several important differences between the FAB and WHO classifications. The WHO classification defines ≥20% blasts (RAEBT) as AML; defines CMML as a myelodysplastic/myeloproliferative disease; and adds new categories of MDS such as the 5q-syndrome.

The natural history of patients with MDS syndromes is quite variable and can range from a chronic relatively indolent disease to an acute fulminant and progressive process. It is well established that mutagen-induced MDS is associated with a poor prognosis and that increased age is also a negative prognostic factor. However, the heterogeneity of this disease has complicated accurate prognostication in de novo MDS. The International Prognostic Scoring System (IPSS) (Table 103-8) was developed to risk stratify patients at the time of diagnosis based on cytogenetic, morphologic, and clinical data. The IPSS for MDS was developed based on an analysis of 816 patients, which demonstrated that specific cytogenetic abnormalities, the percentage of marrow blasts in the bone marrow, and the number of hematopoietic lineages involved in the cytopenia were the most important variables in disease outcome. Risk scores are determined based on these variables, and a categorization of low risk, intermediate-1, intermediate-2, and high risk is assigned (Table 103-9). The IPSS has demonstrated improved prognostic discrimination over earlier classification schemes and has been incorporated into clinical practice and subsequent trial design.

There are few effective therapies for MDS. However, treatment strategies have been evolving in recent years to target higher risk MDS and subgroups defined by specific cytogenetic abnormalities. Current treatment recommendations involve a risk-adapted therapeutic approach. In general, the National Comprehensive Cancer Center guidelines recommend classifying patients into relatively low risk (IPSS Low or Intermediate-1 categories) and higher risk (IPSS Intermediate-2 and High categories). Supportive care aimed

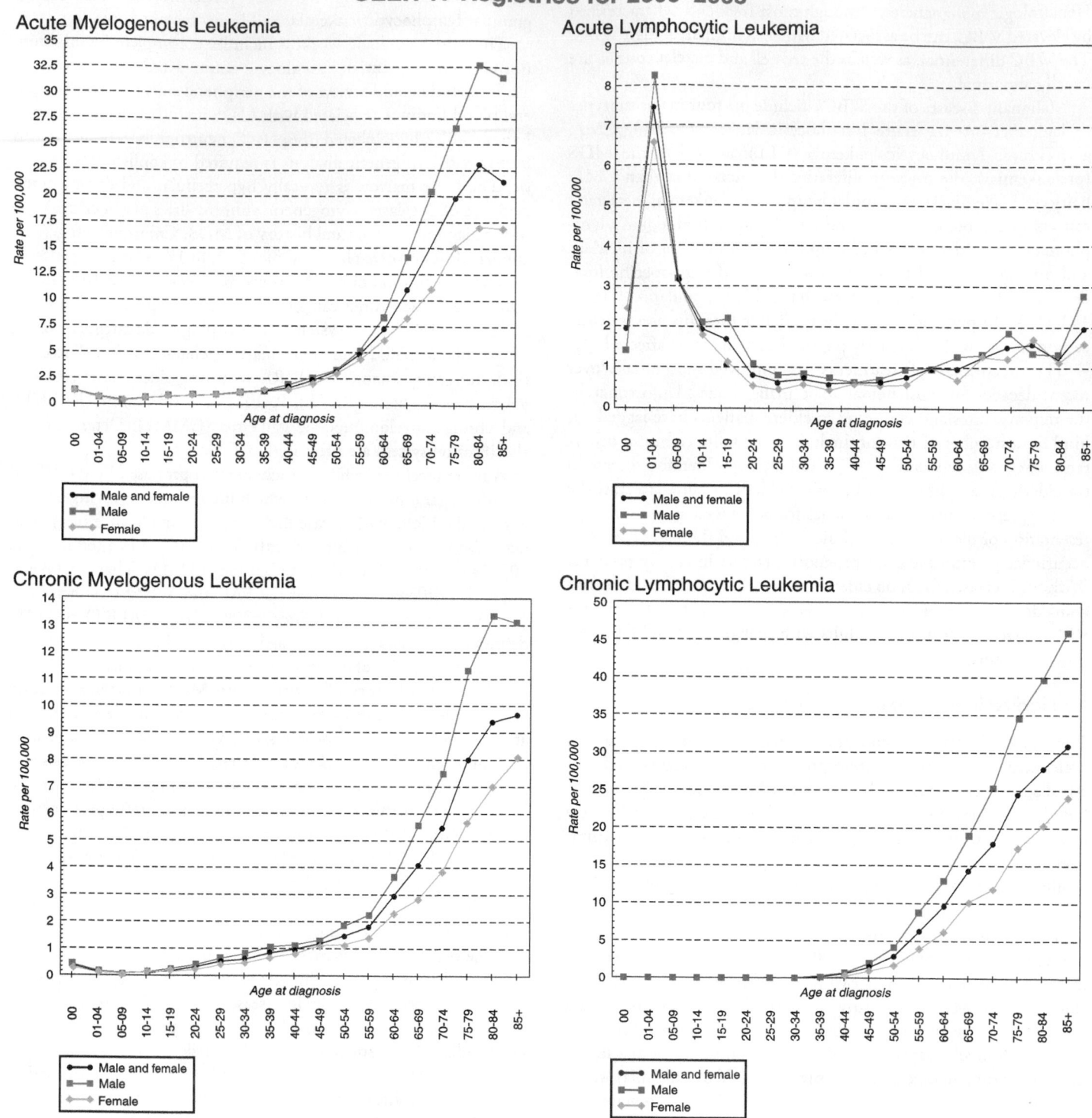

FIGURE 103-1. Age-specific incidence rates for leukemia. (*From http://seer.cancer.gov.*)

at controlling symptoms related to cytopenias is the mainstay of treatment for lower risk patients. Supportive care with red cell and platelet transfusions and antibiotics for infection has long been considered standard therapy for most patients with MDS. Hematopoietic growth factors such as erythropoietin are used to try to minimize transfusion requirements in responding patients. Over time, most patients become transfusion-dependent, increasing the risk of iron overload. Iron chelation therapy should be initiated after 20 to 30 units of red cells have been transfused or the serum ferritin is >2500 mcg/L. Supportive care is also recommended for adults with higher risk disease who have poor performance status and are more likely to suffer complications from aggressive therapies.

TABLE 103-6

Characteristics and Prognosis of Myelodysplastic Syndromes

FAB SUBGROUP	PERIPHERAL BLOOD BLASTS (%)	BONE MARROW BLASTS (%)	PROGRESSION TO AML (%)	MEDIAN SURVIVAL (MONTHS)
Refractory anemia	<1	<5	10	70
Refractory anemia with ring sideroblasts	<1	<5	15	65
Chronic myelomonocytic leukemia	<5	≤20	30	10
Refractory anemia with excess blasts	<5	5–20	40	10
Refractory anemia with excess blasts in transformation	≥5	21–30	60	5

Patients in the higher risk IPSS categories are more likely to experience morbidity related to cytopenias and to progress to acute leukemia in a shorter time interval from diagnosis. Publications by Silverman and Kornblith described improvements in survival, quality of life, and a longer time to progression to acute leukemia, in patients with MDS who received 5-azacytidine (vs. observation) in a randomized trial of the national cooperative group Cancer and Leukemia Group B (CALGB). The strongly positive results of this large randomized study support 5-azacytidine as a standard of care for treatment of MDS. The FDA also recently approved decitabine, a second pyrimidine nucleoside analog of cytidine, which inhibits DNA methylation for the treatment of higher risk MDS. While these medications are associated with toxicity, they represent the mainstay of treatment for good performance status older adults with higher risk MDS. Higher intensity therapy such as allogeneic transplantation, to date the only curative therapy for MDS, is restricted to younger adults with acceptable donors because of the high morbidity and mortality associated with the therapy itself.

Treatment options have expanded for patients with the 5q-syndrome. This subset of MDS is defined by a deletion of the long arm of chromosome 5 as the sole abnormality. The 5q-syndrome typically manifests as refractory anemia and is considered a more

TABLE 103-7

WHO Classification of Peripheral Blood and Bone Marrow Findings in Myelodysplastic Syndromes

DISEASE	BLOOD FINDINGS	BONE MARROW FINDINGS
Refractory anemia	Anemia No or rare blasts	Erythroid dysplasia only <5% blasts <15% ringed sideroblasts
Refractory anemia with ringed sideroblasts	Anemia No blasts	≥15% ringed sideroblasts Erythroid dysplasia only <5% blasts
Refractory cytopenia with multilineage dysplasia (RCMD)	Cytopenias (bicytopenia or pancytopenia) No or rare blasts No Auer rods <1 × 10^9/L monocytes	Dysplasia in ≥10% of the cells of two or more myeloid cell lines <5% blasts in marrow No Auer rods <15% ringed sideroblasts
Refractory cytopenia with multilineage dysplasia and ringed sideroblasts (RCMD-RS)	Cytopenias (bicytopenia or pancytopenia) No or rare blasts No Auer rods <1 × 10^9/L monocytes	Dysplasia in ≥10% of the cells in two or more myeloid cell lines ≥15% ringed sideroblasts <5% blasts No Auer rods
Refractory anemia with excess blasts-1 (RAEB-1)	Cytopenias <5% blasts No Auer rods <1 × 10^9/L monocytes	Unilineage or multilineage dysplasia 5–9% blasts No Auer rods
Refractory anemia with excess blasts-2 (RAEB-2)	Cytopenias 5–19% blasts Auer rods ± <1 × 10^9/L monocytes	Unilineage or multilineage dysplasia 10–19% blasts Auer rods ±
Myelodysplastic syndrome-unclassified (MDS-U)	Cytopenias No or rare blasts No Auer rods	Unilineage dysplasia: one myeloid cell line <5% blasts No Auer rods
MDS associated with isolated del (5q)	Anemia Usually normal or increased platelet count <5% blasts	Normal to increased megakaryocytes with hypolobated nuclei <5% blasts Isolated del(5q) cytogenetic abnormality No Auer rods

From Brunning R, et al. Tumors of Hematopoietic and Lymphoid Tissues. Geneva:World Health Organization; 2001.

TABLE 103-8

International Prognostic Scoring System (IPSS) for MDS

	SCORE VALUE				
Prognostic variable	0	0.5	1.0	1.5	2.0
Bone marrow blasts (%)	<5	5–10	–	11–20	21–30
Karyotype*	Good	Intermediate	Poor	–	–
Cytopenias	0/1	2/3	–	–	–

*Karyotype definitions:
Good risk: Normal; -Y, del(5q), del (20q). Poor risk: ≥3 abnormalities; abnormal chromosome 7. Intermediate risk: All other abnormalities.
Data from Greenberg P, et al. International scoring system for evaluating prognosis in myelodysplastic syndrome. Blood. 89:2079, 1997.

favorable MDS subset because a large percentage of patients do not progress to acute leukemia. In a recent clinical study, lenalidomide, an oral immunomodulatory drug, significantly decreased transfusion requirements and demonstrated reversal of cytogenetic abnormalities in patients with 5q-syndrome. This drug has become the standard of care for treatment of transfusion-dependent, lower risk patients with 5q-syndrome and reinforces the clinical and therapeutic importance of cytogenetic evaluation in MDS.

Acute Myelogenous Leukemia

AML refers to a group of clonal hematopoietic disorders that are characterized by proliferation of immature myeloid cells in the bone marrow. Accumulation of leukemic cells impairs the normal hematopoietic function of the bone marrow, resulting in cytopenias with or without leukocytosis.

AML is a disease of older adults, with a median age at diagnosis of 67 years. The American Cancer Society estimated that 11 930 patients would be diagnosed with AML in 2006 with an anticipated 9040 dying of disease. The incidence increases with age (see Figure 103-1). According to the Surveillance Epidemiologic and End Results (SEER) statistics from 2000 to 2003, over 55% of incident cases of AML were diagnosed in adults aged 65 years and older.

Risk factors for the development of AML include a history of preceding MDS, exposure to certain chemotherapy drugs (alkylating agents, topoisomerase 2 inhibitors, and nitrosoureas), radiation or benzene exposure, and a history of Down's syndrome. The majority of diagnosed cases of AML, however, are not linked to any known risk factor.

The clinical signs and symptoms of AML can be varied and non-specific. Patients usually present with evidence of bone marrow failure: anemia, thrombocytopenia, granulocytopenia. Fatigue, dyspnea, bleeding, fever, and infection are common upon presentation. Leukemic infiltration of tissues outside the bone marrow such as liver, spleen, skin, lymph nodes, and central nervous system (CNS) can produce a variety of other symptoms specific to the site of involvement. Some patients present with severe leukocytosis, which can produce symptoms of leukostasis as a result of a large blast fraction in the peripheral blood. Peripheral blood findings range from pancytopenia with or without circulating blasts cells to severe leukocytosis with circulating blasts typically with anemia and thrombocytopenia.

The diagnosis of AML depends primarily upon detection of leukemic blasts of myeloid lineage (≥20%) in the bone marrow. Morphologic evaluation can be aided by immunohistochemical and flow cytometry techniques to confirm myeloid versus lymphoid origin. The traditional international classification system (FAB) details subtypes of AML (M1 through M7) based on morphology, histochemical characteristics, and immunophenotyping. The more recently proposed WHO classification of AML (Table 103-10)

TABLE 103-9

Median Survival by IPSS Score Category for MDS

IPSS RISK CATEGORY	OVERALL SCORE	MEDIAN SURVIVAL (yr)
Low	0	5.7
Intermediate-1	0.5–1.0	3.5
Intermediate -2	1.5–2.0	1.2
High	≥2.5	0.4

Adapted from Greenberg P, et al. International scoring system for evaluating prognosis in myelodysplastic syndrome. Blood. 89: 2079, 1997.

TABLE 103-10

Classification of Acute Myeloid Leukemia

Acute myeloid leukemia with recurrent genetic abnormalities
    Acute myeloid leukemia with t(8;21)(q22;q22); (AML1/ETO)
    Acute myeloid leukemia with abnormal bone marrow eosinophils
        inv(16)(p13q22) or t(16;16)(p13;q22); (CBFβ/MYH11)
    Acute promyelocytic leukemia (AML with t[15;17][q22;q12] [PML/RARα] and variants)
    Acute myeloid leukemia with 11q23 (MLL) abnormalities

Acute myeloid leukemia with multilineage dysplasia
    Following a myelodysplastic syndrome or myelodysplastic syndrome/myeloproliferative disorder
    Without antecedent myelodysplastic syndrome

Acute myeloid leukemia and myelodysplastic syndromes, therapy-related
    Alkylating agent-related
    Topoisomerase type II inhibitor-related (some may be lymphoid)
    Other types

Acute myeloid leukemia not otherwise categorized
    Acute myeloid leukemia minimally differentiated
    Acute myeloid leukemia without maturation
    Acute myeloid leukemia with maturation
    Acute myelomonocytic leukemia
    Acute monoblastic and monocytic leukemia
    Acute erythroid leukemia
    Acute megakaryoblastic leukemia
    Acute basophilic leukemia
    Acute panmyelosis with myelofibrosis
    Myeloid sarcoma

From Brunning R, et al. Tumors of Hematopoietic and Lymphoid Tissues. Geneva: World Health Organization; 2001.

incorporates morphologic, immunophenotypic, genetic, and clinical features. There are four major categories, each with two or more subtypes described by Brunning et al. The WHO classification highlights the importance of a cytogenetic classification for prognosis and treatment. In recent years, subsets of AML defined by specific cytogenetic abnormalities have been shown to be associated with improved prognosis such as the core binding factor leukemias (inv 16, t(8;21), t(16;16)), and acute promyelocytic leukemia (t(15;17)). Risk-adapted treatment strategies have been developed to maximize clinical outcomes and minimize toxicity based upon cytogenetic classification.

If untreated or unresponsive to chemotherapy, AML may be rapidly fatal (median survival < 2 months). The major causes of death are overwhelming infection and hemorrhage related to the disease-associated cytopenias.

Standard induction therapy for AML is combination chemotherapy that includes cytosine arabinoside (ara-C) and an anthracycline such as daunorubicin. These drugs yield complete remissions (CRs) in 50% to 80% of patients, depending upon various prognostic factors. Increased age is an important negative prognostic factor. The poorer prognosis associated with increased age is related to both a higher frequency of fatal infections and hemorrhage during the period of disease and treatment-related marrow hypoplasia (induction deaths) and to chemotherapy failure (residual or resistant leukemia). While CR rates have usually been 60% to 80% in younger patients with AML, the CR rate in patients aged 60 years and older has generally been ≤50% (with induction death rates of 20% to 40%).

Tumor biology contributes to worse prognosis in older adults with AML. As a group, older patients with AML have a higher percentage of unfavorable cytogenetic abnormalities and a lower percentage of favorable cytogenetic abnormalities compared to younger patients. Unfavorable cytogenetic abnormalities are associated with decreased rates of remission and shortened overall survival. Expression of MDR1, which confers resistance to chemotherapeutic agents, is more common in older AML patients. Older patients are more likely to have a secondary AML arising from underlying myelodysplastic syndrome, which is less responsive to standard therapy. Clinical characteristics including increased comorbidity, age-associated physiologic changes, polypharmacy, and functional and cognitive impairment complicate therapy in older adults and likely also contribute to outcome disparities.

To date, the optimal treatment strategy for older adults remains controversial with recommendations ranging from supportive care alone to standard aggressive therapies. A landmark randomized study by Lowenberg et al. demonstrated improved survival in selected patients aged 65 years and older treated with induction chemotherapy versus supportive care alone. This study demonstrated a potential benefit to aggressive treatment for selected older adults. However, outcomes remain suboptimal in this population. Attempts to improve response rates in older patients with AML have included attenuated doses of standard therapy; these treatments have resulted in decreased induction death rates but without improved CR rates. The roles of gemtuzumab ozogamicin (Mylotarg), a monoclonal antibody directed at CD33, and other directed therapies are yet to be determined. Patients in the subgroup with acute promyelocyte leukemia (APL; AML-M3) are now treated very effectively with oral all-*trans*-retinoic acid (ATRA) plus chemotherapy; AML-M3, however, occurs uncommonly in older patients. The role of more aggressive therapies, including stem cell transplantation (high-dose therapy with stem cell rescue), has been limited in elderly patients by the high rates of complications and prohibitive toxicity. However, improvements in supportive care have allowed for increased investigation of dose-intensive therapies in older patients.

The median duration of CR is approximately 1 year, and a small percentage (≤15%) of older (60 years of age and older) patients will be cured of their leukemia. Patients who achieve CRs should be considered for therapy after remission in an attempt to prevent or delay relapse. However, the exact role and optimal type of such postremission therapy in older patients remain poorly defined.

Treatment decisions for older adults with AML should be individualized. Decisions should include risk stratification based on tumor biology (cytogenetic risk groups) and an estimate of physiologic reserve based on clinical characteristics such as comorbidity and functional status. Older adults with favorable cytogenetics and good functional status should be considered for aggressive curative treatment. Poor-risk patients based on tumor biology or clinical characteristics could be considered for novel treatments on clinical trials or supportive care in an effort to maximize quality of life.

Acute Lymphoblastic Leukemia

ALL is primarily a disease of children, but in adults, age-adjusted incidence increases in the elderly. There are approximately 3900 new cases of adult ALL in the United States annually, with a slight male predominance (1.2:1). With available therapy today, childhood ALL is curable in the majority of patients. ALL in adults is not the same as the childhood disease. First, the frequency of complete response is lower—70% to 75% in adults as opposed to more than 90% in children. Second, the remission duration and curability using the same therapy is considerably less. Important prognostic features for outcome in the treatment of ALL include age, cytogenetics, and immunophenotype. Poor prognosis is especially associated with the presence of chromosomal translocations such as Philadelphia (Ph) chromosome t(9;22), t(4;11), t(8;14), t(2;8), or t(8;22), and with a phenotype indicating mixed lymphoid–myeloid leukemia (also called biphenotypic leukemia).

The initial goal of therapy for adult ALL is to correct problems secondary to bone marrow failure; that is, to treat anemia with blood transfusions, treat documented or suspected infection, and control bleeding. Specific antileukemia treatment is then directed toward the achievement of a CR. Induction chemotherapy therapy for ALL, very different from that for AML, usually includes the use of prednisone, vincristine, daunorubicin, and asparaginase. While these drugs are well-tolerated in children, increasing age is associated with poorer drug tolerance. Mortality, usually from infection and/or bleeding during the induction process, may occur in 10% to 20% of elderly patients.

In contrast to the treatment of AML, it is widely accepted that patients with ALL require therapy after CR. These phases of treatment once the patient is in CR have been referred to as intensification therapy and maintenance therapy. The optimal therapy after remission and the duration of such therapy in older patients are not clearly defined. Most programs use multiple drugs administered in a cyclic fashion over a 2-year period; the more intensive therapy is given over about 6 months after CR is achieved (intensification or consolidation), followed by a less-intensive outpatient maintenance regimen for approximately 18 months.

Directed treatment to the craniospinal axis (CNS prophylaxis) is standard practice in the treatment of childhood ALL. While the incidence of CNS leukemia is lower in adults than in children,

TABLE 103-11

Immunophenotype of Mature B-cell Neoplasms

DIAGNOSIS	SIg*	CD5	CD10	CD23	CD43	CD103
B-CLL	+/−	+	−	+	+	−
Mantle cell lymphoma	+	+	−	−	+	−
B-cell prolymphocytic leukemia	++	+/−	−	−	−	−
Splenic marginal zone lymphoma	+	−	−	−	−	−
Hairy-Cell leukemia	+	−	−	−	−	++

*Surface immunoglobulin.

treatment to the CNS is also part of ALL therapy in adults. This usually consists of intrathecal methotrexate in conjunction with high-dose systemic therapy such as high-dose methotrexate and ara-C, or cranial radiation.

With the above intensive treatment plan, the median duration of remission is approximately 2 years, with 35% to 45% of adult patients disease-free at 5 years; however, prognosis is poorer for older adults. One contributing feature to this poorer response duration in adults as opposed to children is the inability to deliver optimal chemotherapy at maximal doses caused by comorbid diseases and increased susceptibility to toxicity.

Chronic Lymphocytic Leukemia

CLL is the most common leukemia in the western hemisphere and may be commonly encountered in a geriatric practice. CLL is a disorder of clonal proliferation of mature lymphoid cells in the peripheral blood, bone marrow, and lymphoid organs. CLL occurs predominantly in older adults, with median age at diagnosis of approximately 70 years. The reported incidence of 3.8 per 100,000 population in western countries (about 10,000 new cases per year in the United States) may be an underestimate because many patients are asymptomatic for years; incidence in persons older than age 60 years is about 20 per 100,000 population. There is no racial difference in the United States between blacks and whites, but there are very few cases in the Far East and among persons of Oriental descent; the male:female ratio is approximately 2:1. Current diagnostic studies, especially immunophenotyping, allow for differentiation of the chronic lymphoid malignancies: B-cell CLL, T-cell CLL, prolymphocytic, circulating non-Hodgkin's lymphomas, and hairy cell leukemia.

B-cell CLL

B-cell CLL accounts for over 95% of all CLL. Twenty-five percent of such patients are identified with asymptomatic lymphocytosis during evaluation for other medical problems. Symptomatic patients may present with weight loss, fatigue, recurrent infections, fevers, or pain associated with hepatosplenomegaly or bulky lymphadenopathy. In most patients, the disease has a gradual progression spanning several years and the extent of the lymphoid burden at diagnosis correlates well with length of preexisting disease. In some patients, the disease has a more aggressive course and progression to advanced clinical stages may occur within a few months of diagnosis. Identification of molecular and protein markers are beginning to explain the heterogenous natural history observed in this disease.

The diagnosis of CLL is based on peripheral blood lymphocytosis >10,000 lymphocytes/μL and a specific immunophenotyping pattern (coexpression of CD5 and CD20/23 with weak expression of surface immunoglobulin) showing a clonal proliferation of lymphocytes. Diagnosis and staging of CLL can usually be established by history, physical examination (careful evaluation for lymphadenopathy and splenomegaly), CBC with review of the blood smear, and immunophenotyping of the peripheral blood using flow cytometry. Classic findings on the peripheral smear include increased mature appearing lymphocytes and smudge cells (peripheral smear artifact reflecting the fragility of the B-CLL cells to mechanical manipulation). Bone marrow studies are usually not needed for diagnosis.

The differential diagnosis for B-CLL includes other mature B-lymphoproliferative disorders such as mantle cell lymphoma, prolymphocytic leukemia, hairy cell leukemia, and splenic lymphoma with villous lymphocytes. The clinical course and treatments differ widely for these disorders, particularly mantle cell lymphoma. Evaluation of clinical presentation, morphology, and immunophenotype are necessary to arrive at the correct diagnosis (Table 103-11).

The original Rai classification (Table 103-12) implied an orderly progression from lymphocytosis alone to the successive development of adenopathy, organomegaly, and, eventually, anemia and thrombocytopenia. The prognostic importance of these variables has been confirmed. Specific cytogenetic abnormalities correlate with

TABLE 103-12

CLL Rai Clinical Classification

STAGE	RISK*	CLINICAL FINDINGS	SURVIVAL (yr)
0	Low	Lymphocytosis only	≥12
1	Intermediate	↑ Lymphs plus ↑ nodes	7–10
2	Intermediate	↑ Lymphs plus ↑ spleen and/or liver ± ↑ Nodes	4–9
3	High	↑ Lymphs plus ↓ Hgb (<11 g/dl) ± ↑ Nodes, ↑ liver, ↑ spleen	1.5–2
4	High	↑ Lymphs plus ↓ platelets (<100, 000/ul) ± ↑ Nodes, ↑ liver, ↑ spleen, ↓ Hgb	1.5–2

*Data from Rai classification.

prognosis. A 13q deletion is associated with a better prognosis, compared to deletions of 11q and 17p, which confer a worse prognosis. Additional molecular markers of prognostic significance include presence of CD38 and ZAP-70.

Therapy for B-cell CLL has been considered palliative and therefore has been reserved for patients who are symptomatic or who progress to develop cytopenias (Rai stages 3 or 4). The mainstay of therapy has been oral alkylating agents (chlorambucil or cyclophosphamide) for control of lymphoid proliferation and steroids for autoimmune complications. Leukocytosis alone (stage 0) does not require therapy, because the prognosis of these patients is excellent in the absence of the other poor prognostic factors. The rate of increase of leukocytosis is a better indicator of disease activity than the absolute count. Leukostasis associated with high circulating blast counts in acute leukemias does not generally occur in this condition because most of the lymphocytes are mature, small cells.

Treatment with chemotherapy or local radiation can be used to control symptoms in patients with stage I or II disease; however, symptomatic improvement does not appear to prolong survival. In contrast, when treated with combination chemotherapy, patients with stage III or IV CLL have an improved median survival, which ranges from 1.5 years to more than 4 years. The development of more effective initial therapies for CLL such as nucleoside analogs (e.g., fludarabine) have resulted in an increased number of patients achieving CR. It is not yet clear that these remissions result in prolonged survival, although data from recent clinical trials are encouraging. These promising results have encouraged many hematologists and oncologists to institute therapy at an earlier stage. A monoclonal antibody against CD-52, altuzemab, has been approved as second line therapy for patients previously treated with alkylating agents and fludarabine. The best way to integrate newer agents such as fludarabine and monoclonal antibodies (e.g., rituximab and alemtuzumab) with each other and/or with more traditional therapies (alkylators and steroids) are not yet well-defined. There are multiple clinical trials currently evaluating different combinations of these medications (concurrent or sequential). Unfortunately, each of these agents has been associated with increased risk of opportunistic infections, particularly in the older adult.

Autoimmune manifestations of CLL are common and include development of antibodies to platelets and red cells (IgG and C3 on direct antiglobulin test) and to erythroid precursors, resulting in red cell aplasia. For anemic patients, reticulocyte counts and direct Coomb's testing should be obtained to help differentiate hemolysis from decreased bone marrow production. All of the autoimmune complications are indications for therapy with steroids or intravenous gamma globulin for refractory cases of red cell aplasia.

Recurrent infections are the most common complications leading to death in CLL. Patients with stage 0 CLL have minimal increased risk of infection. In anticipation of gradual deterioration in immune response, however, pneumococcal vaccine and boosters should be administered while the potential for response is still intact. All other patients have higher risks for infection. As the disease advances clinically, immune function becomes progressively compromised, with increased susceptibility to viral, bacterial, and fungal infection. Patients should avoid direct contact with the body fluids of children who have received live-virus vaccines (oral polio, measles-mumps-rubella) for the duration of viral shedding. The subset of patients presenting with recurrent bacterial infections may benefit from administration of intravenous gamma globulin.

B-Cell Prolymphocytic Leukemia

This rare subtype of lymphoid leukemia is characterized by marked lymphocytosis (often >100,000 lymphocytes/μL), extensive bone marrow infiltration, massive splenomegaly, and minimal to absent adenopathy. Prolymphocytes comprise the majority of circulating WBC (>55%; often >90%). The prolymphocyte is about twice the size of a normal lymphocyte, with a characteristic dense border outlining a prominent nucleolus. B-cell prolymphocytic leukemia (B-PLL) cells usually express CD19, CD20, CD22, CD79a, FMC7, and strong surface IgM; CD23 is usually negative.

Most patients with B-PLL have advanced clinical disease at presentation, with a prognosis similar to that of patients with stage III and IV B-cell CLL. Therapy for these patients has included multi-agent chemotherapy to control the splenomegaly and leukocytosis, and radiation therapy to palliate splenic engorgement. Patients become increasingly refractory to therapy, with an expected survival of 1.5 years and death caused by uncontrolled disease. Recent data suggest that more aggressive newer agents such as alemtuzumab (CAMPATH-1H) are more effective than previous therapies for PLL, with improved response rates and survival.

T-Cell PLL/CLL

T-cell PLL/CLL is a rare subtype that accounts for 2% to 3% of all small lymphocytic leukemia ("CLL") cases. Clinical manifestations include lymphocytosis, hepatosplenomegaly, generalized lymphadenopathy, skin infiltration (20%), and bone marrow involvement. Immunophenotyping in the peripheral blood shows a clonal proliferation of the malignant T cells—CD2, CD3, CD7 positive with weak CD3; in approximately 60% of patients, the cells are CD4+/CD8−, 25% are CD4+/CD8+, and 15% are CD4−/CD8+. Prognosis is generally poor, with limited responsiveness to therapy though newer agents (e.g., alemtuzumab) appear to be active.

Hairy Cell Leukemia

Hairy cell leukemia is rare and almost exclusively seen in men older than age 60 years. The clinical features include massive splenomegaly, absence of adenopathy, and peripheral pancytopenia. The diagnosis is made by the morphologic characteristics of the circulating lymphocytes, which are small and have cytoplasmic projections ("hairs"). Diagnosis, previously made histochemically with the tartrate-resistant acid phosphatase (TRAP) stain, is now made with immunophenotyping that shows positive sIgM, CD19, CD20, CD22, CD79a, CD11c, CD25, and CD103; negative CD5, CD10, and CD23. Bone marrow aspiration usually yields little material (dry tap) and bone marrow biopsy shows increased cellularity with diffuse infiltration by the hairy cells. The spleen is infiltrated with the same clone of cells. Infections with Gram-negative and staphylococcal species is the predominant complication.

Splenectomy was the treatment of choice in the past with improvement of neutropenia in about 50% of patients for 8 to 10 years. Interferon (IFN)-α produced partial and CRs in more than 50% of patients, sparing many patients a surgical procedure and the effects of the splenectomy on the immune system. Interferon has now been replaced by the nucleoside analogs, especially cladribine (2-CdA), which is very well tolerated. This 5-day treatment yields high remission rates, frequently after only one course of therapy.

T-cell Large Granular Lymphocytic Leukemia

T-cell large granular lymphocytic (T-LGL) leukemia is a rare clonal disorder of cytotoxic T lymphocytes, which typically presents with chronic neutropenia. T-LGL leukemia represents approximately 4% of lymphoproliferative disorders. Patients tend to be older, with a median age of 60 years. Many patients are asymptomatic and will have chronic neutropenia, mild lymphocytosis with or without anemia. Symptoms are typically related to recurrent infections particularly of the skin, oropharynx, and perirectal regions. Splenomegaly is common but lymphadenopathy is uncharacteristic. The peripheral blood demonstrates a proliferation of large granular lymphocytes. These can also be seen in reactive disorders such as viral infections. The diagnosis depends upon establishing a clonal T-cell receptor gene rearrangement within the population of large granular lymphocytes using polymerase chain reaction (PCR) or flow cytometry techniques on the peripheral blood. The diagnosis is supported by the characteristic immunophenotype of CD3+, CD8+, CD16+, and CD57+. T-LGL leukemia is a relatively indolent disease with median survival >10 years. Indications for treatment include severe neutropenia (ANC < 500), recurrent infections, and transfusion-dependent anemia. Treatment involves immunosuppression with agents such as methotrexate, cyclosporine, or steroids.

Chronic Myelogenous Leukemia

CML is a myeloproliferative disorder characterized by excess production of mature granulocytes that eventually progresses to a clinical picture similar to acute leukemia with an overgrowth of immature cells (blast crisis). It accounts for 15% to 20% of all leukemias, with an age-adjusted incidence rate of 1.5 per 100,000 population without geographic, sex, or racial differences. The incidence increases with age and the median age at diagnosis is 67 years.

Diagnosis is suspected by the demonstration of granulocytosis in the peripheral blood with a predominance of segmented neutrophils and myelocytes, increased basophils and eosinophils, increased bone marrow cellularity, a low LAP score. The presence of the Philadelphia chromosome t(9;22) and or its products (*BCR/ABL* fusion mRNA, *Bcr/Abl* protein) are required to confirm the diagnosis. Diagnosis can be made on peripheral blood using PCR or fluorescence in-situ hybridization (FISH) techniques. Bone marrow biopsy is still required for complete cytogenetic evaluation.

The disease characteristically proceeds through three phases: chronic, accelerated, and terminal (blastic) phase (Table 103-13). The length of the chronic phase is highly variable, from 1.5 years to 14 years (median duration of 3 years). In the chronic phase, the disease is easily controlled without aggressive therapy. The accelerated phase begins with gradual increases in white cells, platelets, and spleen size. Initially good maturation persists, but eventually more blasts are seen in the peripheral blood, and higher doses of medication are required to maintain control. This phase generally lasts a few months but may extend over 1 year. The terminal phase of the disease is indistinguishable from acute leukemia. The blasts have myeloid surface markers in 85% of the patients and lymphoid markers in the remaining 15%.

Treatment for CML has changed dramatically in recent years, altering the natural history of this disease. IFN-α was the first drug to change the natural history of CML, decreasing the percentage of cells exhibiting the Ph chromosome and prolonging the chronic

TABLE 103-13

CML Classification

CHRONIC PHASE	ACCELERATED PHASE	BLAST PHASE
<10% blasts	Any of the following: 10–19% blasts Thrombocytopenia <100,000/cmm Peripheral basophilia >20% Appearance of additional cytogenetic abnormality Increasing spleen size or WBC on therapy	Any of the following: >20% blasts Extramedullary blasts

From Brunning R, et al. Tumors of Hematopoietic and Lymphoid Tissues. Geneva: World Health Organization; 2001.

phase by 1 to 2 years. Imatinib mesylate (Gleevec; STI-571), a targeted tyrosine kinase inhibitor designed specifically for the treatment of CML (in oral formulation), proved to have significant activity in the blast phase and accelerated phase of CML. In chronic phase CML, imatinib mesylate yielded marked improvements in clinical and cytogenetic responses, rates of disease progression, and treatment related toxicity compared to IFN-α plus low-dose ara-C in a randomized clinical trial. Based on these results, imatinib mesylate has replaced interferon regimens as the standard of care for patients with chronic phase CML. Imatinib is very well tolerated, which is particularly relevant for the elderly population. Many patients who would not have been good candidates for cytotoxic therapy or interferon can be effectively treated with imatinib. It is too early to determine the duration of remissions for elderly patients treated with this medication. However, second line therapy with newer tyrosine kinase inhibitors (dasatinib, nilotinib) have demonstrated activity in patients who have progressed on imatinib providing additional treatment options for older adults.

Allogeneic stem cell transplantation in the chronic phase, a promising intervention in younger patients, has limited benefit in the elderly patient because of the morbidity and mortality of this treatment. Imatinib mesylate should be the initial treatment for both the accelerated and blastic phases of CML if not already used during the chronic phase of the disease. Treatment of the blastic transformation (after imatinib) depends on the cell origin of the blasts. Myeloid blastic states respond poorly to standard AML therapies, and no standard therapy is available. Lymphoid blastic states can be controlled for 6 to 12 months, with standard combination regimens as used for de novo ALL.

Myeloproliferative Diseases

Myeloproliferative diseases include CML (described above), polycythemia vera, myelofibrosis, and essential thrombocytosis. Both polycythemia vera and myelofibrosis can be associated with increased WBC. Polycythemia vera is usually associated with mild increases in white count with a relatively normal differential, while myelofibrosis is frequently associated with immature WBCs in addition to nucleated RBCs. The leukocytosis associated with polycythemia vera is usually of little consequence and treatment is directed towards the control of the increased red cells. Myelofibrosis can be associated with variable abnormalities in WBC numbers, either increased WBC with circulating immature precursors or decreased WBCs, especially in the present of massive splenomegaly.

Cancers Metastatic to Bone Marrow

Many of the common malignancies have a propensity for metastasis to the bone and bone marrow. These include carcinomas of the breast, lung, prostate, and the lymphomas. Space-occupying lesions in the bone marrow, which crowd out normal hematopoietic elements, are termed myelophthisis. Manifestations of myelophthisis in the peripheral blood include pancytopenia and leukoerythroblastosis. Pancytopenias may be aggravated by nutritional deficiencies, especially folate deficiency.

FURTHER READING

Appelbaum F, Gundacker H, Head DR, et al. Age and acute myeloid leukemia. *Blood.* 2006;107(9):3481.

Brunning R, et al. *Tumors of Hematopoietic and Lymphoid Tissues.* Geneva: World Health Organization; 2001.

DeVita VT, Hellman S, Rosenberg SA, et al. *Cancer: Principles and Practice of Oncology.* Philadelphia: Lippincott Williams and Wilkins; 2001.

Druker BJ, Guilhot F, O'Brien SG, et al. Five year follow-up of patients receiving imatinib for chronic myeloid leukemia. *N Engl J Med.* 2006;355:2408.

Greer J, et al., eds. *Wintrobe's Clinical Hematology,* 11th edition. Philadelphia: Lippincott Williams and Wilkins; 2004.

Greenberg P, Cox C, LeBeau MM, et al. International scoring system for evaluating prognosis in myelodysplastic syndrome. *Blood.* 1997;89:2079.

Huff JD, Keung YK, Thakuri M, et al. Copper deficiency causes reversible myelodysplasia. *Am J Hematol.* 2007;82:625–30.

Jaffe ES, et al., eds. *World Health Organization Classification of Tumours. Pathology and Genetics of Tumours of Haematopoietic and Lymphoid Tissues.* Lyon: IARC Press; 2001.

Kantarjian H, O'brien S, Cortes J, et al. Results of intensive chemotherapy in 998 patients age 65 years or older with acute myeloid leukemia or high risk myelodysplastic syndrome. *Cancer.* 2006;106:1090.

Kornblith AB, Herndon JE, Silverman LR, et al. Impact of azacytidine on the quality of life of patients with myelodysplastic syndrome treated in a randomized phase III trial: A Cancer and Leukemia Group B study. *J Clin Oncol.* 2002;20:2441.

Lenhard RE, et al., eds. *The American Cancer Society's Clinical Oncology.* Atlanta, GA: American Cancer Society, 2001.

Lichtman M, et al., eds. *Williams Hematology,* 7th ed. New York, New York: McGraw-Hill; 2006.

List A, Dewald G, Bannett J, et al. Lenalidomide in the myelodysplastic syndrome with chromosome 5q deletion. *N Engl J Med.* 2006;355:1456.

Lowenberg B, Zittoun R, Kerkhofs H, et al. On the value of intensive remission–induction chemotherapy in elderly patients of 65+ years with acute myeloid leukemia: A randomized phase 3 study of the European Organization for Research and Treatment of Cancer Leukemia Group. *J Clin Oncol.* 1989;7:1268.

Lowenberg B, Downing JR, Burnett A, et al. Acute myeloid leukemia. *N Engl J Med.* 1999;341:1051.

Lubran MM. Hematologic side effects of drugs. *Ann Clin Lab Sci.* 1989;19:114.

Silverman LR, Demakos EP, Peterson BL, et al. Randomized controlled trial of azacitidine in patients with the myelodysplastic syndrome: A study of the Cancer and Leukemia Group B. *J Clin Oncol.* 2002;20:2429.

Surveillance, Epidemiology, and End Results (SEER) Program (www.seer.cancer.gov) SEER*Stat Database: Incidence—SEER 17 Regs Public-Use, Nov 2005 Sub (2000–2003), National Cancer Institute, DCCPS, Surveillance Research Program, Cancer Statistics Branch, released April 2006, based on the November 2005 submission.

Non-Hodgkin's and Hodgkin's Lymphomas and Myeloma

William B. Ershler ■ *Dan L. Longo*

Lymphoid malignancies include nearly 40 named entities; however, they can be divided into roughly five large categories based on the clinical syndrome they cause: acute lymphoid leukemias, chronic lymphoid leukemias, non-Hodgkin's lymphomas, Hodgkin's disease, and plasma cell disorders (chiefly multiple myeloma). In 2007, 111,820 people were diagnosed with a lymphoid malignancy and 36,440 patients died from a lymphoid malignancy. Figure 104-1 shows a distribution of the annual incidence in a pie chart. Acute and chronic lymphoid leukemias are covered in a separate chapter. We shall discuss non-Hodgkin's lymphomas, Hodgkin's disease, and plasma cell disorders in this chapter.

NON-HODGKIN'S LYMPHOMA

The non-Hodgkin's lymphomas (NHLs), the most common lymphoid malignancies, are a heterogeneous group of cancers that have in common the clonal expansion of cells of lymphoid origin. The heterogeneity stems from the very large number of distinct lymphocyte subsets and diverse molecular and genetic pathways to neoplasia. Mutations, chromosome translocations, or other alterations in certain genes (e.g., *BCL2, c-MYC, FAS, BCL6*) contribute to the pathogenesis in many cases and gene expression profiling has identified subsets of NHL with varying aggressiveness and response to chemotherapy. About 88% of all NHLs are derived from B cells. Despite insights into the alterations associated with specific NHL types, the mainstay of current therapy remains empiric and typically includes cytotoxic chemotherapy combined with monoclonal antibody directed at the CD20 molecule, which is expressed on nearly all B cells. Clinical trials suggest that elderly patients may safely receive these agents with expectations similar to their younger counterparts.

Epidemiology

In 2007, 63,190 new cases of NHL were diagnosed and about half occurred in persons aged 60 years or older. National Cancer Institute data indicates an approximate 25% increase in NHL incidence since 1950, although there is some evidence that the rate of rise has declined somewhat since 1990. Although some of the increase can be related to the acquired immunodeficiency syndrome (AIDS) epidemic, particularly in young and middle-aged persons, the bulk of the cause of the increase is undefined, particularly in the aged population. With more effective human immunodeficiency virus (HIV) treatment, HIV-associated lymphoma is becoming less frequent. However, NHL affects older patients (one third are 70 years or older) and is the fifth leading cause of cancer deaths in women aged 80 years and older. Furthermore, current cancer surveillance statistics indicate that despite the fact that incidence is declining for the population as a whole, for those aged older than 65 years, there is a net increase of 1.3% compared to a rate of −1.5% for the younger population.

Classification

Lymphoma classification was a contentious field until 1999 when the World Health Organization Classification was developed by an international panel of hematopathologists and clinicians based on consensus criteria including histology, immunology, genetics, and clinical features of diseases (Table 104-1). The classification includes nearly 40 named entities; however, the 10 most frequent diagnoses are printed in bold type. Fortunately, about 75% of patients have one of two histological types, diffuse large B-cell lymphoma (DLBL) (~40% to 45% of lymphomas in the United States) and follicular lymphoma (FL) (~30% of lymphomas in the United States). These two prototypical forms of lymphoma highlight an intriguing paradox. In general, FLs, which have a more indolent natural history, frequently present with few symptoms but with widespread disease and are generally considered incurable with the current modalities. The more aggressive DLBLs present with more constitutional symptoms and more often at earlier stages and are in most cases curable, even at an advanced stage. The challenge for those treating lymphomas in elderly patients is to balance the likelihood of a meaningful treatment response against the potentially enhanced rate and severity of

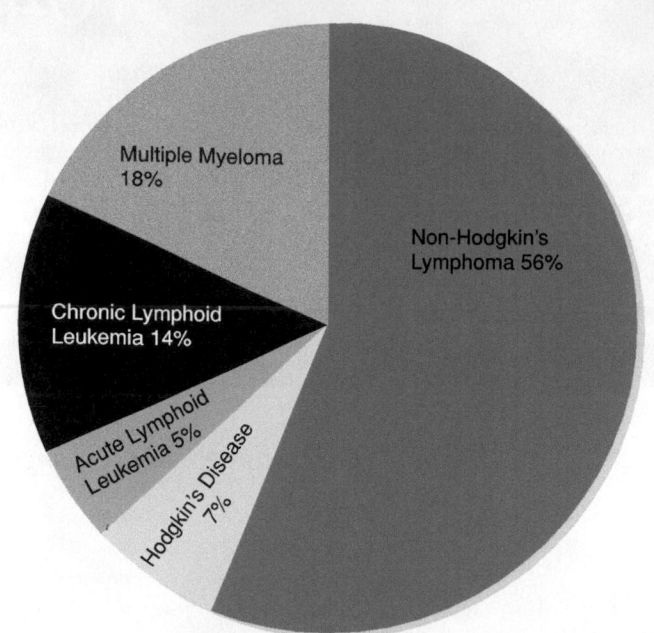

FIGURE 104-1. Distribution of lymphoid malignancies in the United States.

Less detailed discussion will be provided for a handful of more unusual lymphomas. The approach to the patient with lymphoma is similar regardless of the specific diagnosis. One first seeks to establish the extent of the disease and establish the clinical stage (see later). A variety of specialized tools have been applied to the diagnosis of lymphomas including cytogenetics and flow cytometry to define the expression of certain cell surface markers, and immunohistochemistry and molecular biology techniques. These tests can sometimes be helpful in making a difficult diagnosis, but often the results are not available in a clinically useful time frame. Similarly, the development of microarray technology and the demonstration that various patterns of gene expression correlate with clinical outcomes is of interest; however, it is not clear that these techniques are suitable for clinical application to a particular patient.

Etiology

For most lymphomas, the cause is unknown. Lymphomas are increased in the setting of primary and secondary immunodeficiency disease and certain autoimmune diseases (Sjogren's syndrome, celiac disease, rheumatoid arthritis, systemic lupus erythematosus). A number of lymphoma types are associated with infectious agents. For example, gastric mucosa-associated lymphatic tissue (MALT) lymphoma is associated with *Helicobacter pylori* infection. Exposure to agricultural chemicals seems to be associated with an increased risk of lymphoma. However, the factors that produced an increasing incidence between 1950 and 1990, which has leveled off in recent years, is unexplained. Many types of lymphomas have characteristic

treatment toxicity in the setting of an individualized assessment of the patient's functional status and projected longevity.

Given that most lymphomas are either follicular or DLBL, most of the discussion will deal with management of these two entities.

TABLE 104-1

WHO Classification of Lymphoid Malignancies		
B CELL	**T CELL**	**HODGKIN'S DISEASE**
Precursor B cell neoplasm	**Precursor T cell neoplasm**	Nodular lymphocyte-predominant Hodgkin's disease
Precursor B lymphoblastic leukemia/lymphoma (precursor B cell acute lymphoblastic leukemia)	Precursor T cell lymphoblastic lymphoma/leukemia (precursor T cell acute lymphoblastic leukemia)	
Mature (peripheral) B cell neoplasms	**Mature (peripheral) T cell neoplasms**	Classic Hodgkin's disease
B cell chronic lymphocytic leukemia/small lymphocytic lymphoma	T cell prolymphocytic leukemia	Nodular sclerosis Hodgkin's disease
B cell prolymphocytic leukemia	T cell granular lymphocytic leukemia	Lymphocyte-rich classic Hodgkin's disease
Lymphoplasmacytic lymphoma	Aggressive NK cell leukemia	Mixed-cellularity Hodgkin's disease
Splenic marginal zone B cell lymphoma (± villous lymphocytes)	Adult T cell lymphoma/ leukemia (HTLV-I +)	Lymphocyte-depletion Hodgkin's disease
Hairy cell leukemia	Extranodal NK/T cell lymphoma, nasal type	
Plasma cell myeloma/plasmacytoma	Enteropathy-type T cell lymphoma	
Extranodal marginal zone B cell lymphoma of MALT type	Hepatosplenic $\gamma\delta$ T cell lymphoma	
Mantle cell lymphoma	Subcutaneous panniculitis-like T cell lymphoma	
Follicular lymphoma	**Mycosis fungoides/Sézary syndrome**	
Nodal marginal zone B cell lymphoma (± monocytoid B cells)	Anaplastic large cell lymphoma, primary cutaneous type	
Diffuse large B cell lymphoma	**Peripheral T cell lymphoma, not otherwise specified (NOS)**	
Burkitt's lymphoma/Burkitt cell leukemia	Angioimmunoblastic T cell lymphoma	
	Anaplastic large cell lymphoma, primary systemic type	

HTLV, human T cell lymphotropic virus; MALT, mucosa-associated lymphoid tissue; NK, natural killer; WHO, World Health Organization.
Adapted from Harris NL, Jaffe ES, Diebold J, et al. World Health Organization classification of neoplastic diseases of the hematopoietic and lymphoid tissues: report of the Clinical Advisory Committee meeting—Airlie House, Virginia, November 1997. J Clin Oncol. 1999;17:3835–3849.

TABLE 104-2

Staging for Lymphoma—Ann Arbor Classification, Cotswolds Modifications

I	Involvement of a single lymph node region or lymphoid structure (e.g., spleen, thymus, Waldeyer's ring)
II	Involvement of two or more lymph node regions on the same side of the diaphragm (the mediastinum is a single site; hilar lymph nodes should be considered "lateralized" and, when involved on both sides, constitute stage II disease)
III	Involvement of lymph node regions or lymphoid structures on both sides of the diaphragm
III1	Subdiaphragmatic involvement limited to spleen, splenic hilar nodes, celiac nodes, or portal nodes
III2	Subdiaphragmatic involvement includes paraaortic, iliac or mesenteric nodes plus structures in III1
IV	Involvement of extranodal sites(s) beyond that designated as "E"; more than one extranodal deposit at any location; any involvement of liver or bone marrow
A	No symptoms
B	Unexplained weight loss of >10% of body weight during the 6 months before staging
	Unexplained, persistent, or recurrent fever (T>38 degrees C) in the previous month
	Recurrent drenching night sweats in the previous month
E	Localized, solitary involvement of extralymphatic tissue, excluding liver and bone marrow

chromosomal translocations that are thought to play a role in their origin. However, lymphomagenesis remains largely undefined. Only the *c-myc* translocations in Burkitt's lymphoma are sufficient to produce the lymphoma they are associated with. Other characteristic translocations seem to be one of several molecular alterations required to produce disease.

Evaluation and Staging

The Ann Arbor staging system that was developed for Hodgkin's disease is also applied to patients with NHL, but often the system applies to NHL patients poorly. With the widespread use of systemic therapy to treat all stages of NHL and Hodgkin's disease (see later), precise pathological staging (Table 104-2) is less critical than it was when eligible patients were treated with localized therapies (e.g., radiation therapy). For example, in the low-grade lymphomas, the disease may be stage IV without much change in prognosis compared with earlier stages, and in the higher-grade aggressive lymphomas, systemic treatment is necessary even when disease is confined to one anatomical region. A patient with stage II DLBL could have small-volume disease involving two lymph node groups and an outstanding prognosis with a shortened course of chemotherapy or could instead have a football size mass in the abdomen with a poorer prognosis. Because anatomical staging does not define prognosis well in NHL, other supplementary systems have been developed. The International Prognostic Index (IPI) was developed for DLBL based on outcome of treating patients with CHOP (cyclophosphamide, hydroxydaunarubicin [doxorubicin], vincristine, prednisone) or CHOP-like regimens. The addition of rituximab to CHOP improved prognosis substantially and altered the prognostic significance of the IPI factors; these alterations have been incorporated into a new revised IPI (Table 104-3). A similar prognostic index has been developed for FL

TABLE 104-3

Revised International Prognostic Index (IPI) for Diffuse Large B-Cell Lymphoma Treated with R-CHOP

Five clinical prognostic factors:
1. Age $\geq$ 60 yrs
2. Serum lactate dehydrogenase levels elevated
3. Performance status $\geq$ 2 (ECOG) or $\leq$ 70 (Karnofsky)
4. Ann Arbor stage III or IV
5. More than one site of extranodal involvement

0 factors = very good risk, 10% of patients, 94% 4-yr survival.
1,2 factors = good risk, 45% of patients, 79% 4-yr survival.
3,4, to 5 factors = poor risk, 45% of patients, 55% 4-yr survival.

in which hemoglobin level and number of sites of nodal involvement replace Ann Arbor stage III or IV and > 1 extranodal site of disease in the IPI (Table 104-4). The staging workup for lymphomas (NHL and Hodgkin's) is shown in Table 104-5. Aggressive histology lymphomas, such as diffuse large B cell, Burkitt's and lymphoblastic, may require evaluation of the central nervous system (CNS) with a head computed tomogram (CT) and lumbar puncture, especially in patients with diffuse histology, bulky abdominal lymphadenopathy, or bone or bone marrow involvement. Keep in mind that older patients are more likely to present with more advanced disease. This may reflect a delay in diagnosis, as has been demonstrated for older people with solid tumors.

Overall, it does not appear that lymphomas in older patients have distinct clinical or pathological features from those same lymphomas occurring in younger people, though the confidence in that conclusion is undermined by the general underrepresentation of older patients on clinical trials. However, in certain series, it has been reported that older patients are more likely to have diffuse histology and present with extranodal disease involving gastric or bone marrow sites.

Clinical Features and Therapy

Diffuse Large B-Cell Lymphoma

DLBL is the most common form of lymphoma in the United States accounting for 40% to 45% of cases. DLBL often presents with diffuse adenopathy or an abdominal mass, and extranodal sites are involved in about 45% of cases. Factors influencing prognosis have been incorporated into a prognostic index (Table 104-3). The median age is about 64 years. The male-to-female ratio is 55:45. About one third of patients have B symptoms and about 50% present

TABLE 104-4

International Prognostic Index for Follicular Lymphoma (FLIPI)

Five clinical prognostic factors:
1. Age $\geq$ 60 yrs
2. Serum lactate dehydrogenase levels elevated
3. Performance status $\geq$ 2 (ECOG) or $\leq$ 70 (Karnofsky)
4. Hemoglobin level < 12 g/dL
5. Number of nodal groups involved > 4

0,1 factor = low risk, 36% of patients, 83% 8-yr survival.
2 factors = intermediate risk, 37% of patients, 62% 8-yr survival.
$\geq$ 3 factors = poor risk, 27% of patients, 51% 8-yr survival.

TABLE 104-5

Staging Recommendations for Lymphoma

History, with special attention to "B" symptoms, including fevers, night sweats, and >10% loss in body weight

Physical examination with special attention to node-bearing areas, liver, and spleen

Initial blood work to include a complete blood count with white cell differential and platelet count, serum chemistries including liver function tests, creatinine, albumin, total protein, and erythrocyte sedimentation rate

Radiologic studies to include chest x-ray, positron emission tomography (PET), superimposed upon chest, abdomen and pelvis CT

Bilateral iliac crest bone marrow biopsies

(Selected cases) Bipedal lymhangiogram

(Selected cases) Laparotomy with exploration of lymph node–bearing areas, liver biopsies, and splenectomy; if laparotomy is not to be performed, consider percutaneous or laparoscopic-guided liver biopsies

---

with advanced stage disease. A small subset of patients has disease restricted largely to the mediastinum and the tumor is encased in dense fibrotic tissue. This mediastinal DLBL predominantly affects younger patients (median age 37 years) and women are affected twice as commonly as men. The approach to the patient is not influenced by the differences in presentation.

Most DLBL occurs de novo in the absence of known underlying disease. However, DLBL can also occur in the setting of immunosuppression, either from primary immunodeficiency diseases or AIDS or from iatrogenic immunosuppression in the setting of organ transplant. Often the Epstein–Barr virus (EBV) is an etiological agent of lymphomas occurring in immunosuppressed patients. EBV is also associated with primary CNS lymphoma and some cases of Hodgkin's disease, particularly cases of mixed cellularity histology. DLBL frequently manifest mutations in p53 and alterations in the Bcl-6 gene on chromosome 3q27. Distinct subsets have been defined by gene expression profiling, but such data are not usually relevant to the management of patients.

The treatment of choice for DLBL is a five-drug regimen called CHOP-R (cyclophosphamide, doxorubicin, vincristine, prednisone and rituximab). Patients with early stage disease may receive four to six cycles and those with advanced disease six to eight cycles. Overall survival at 4 years ranges from 94% for those with no poor prognostic factors to 55% for those with three or more poor prognostic factors. Patients who do not relapse within the first 2 years of achieving a complete response are very unlikely to do so. Overall, complete response rates are 70% to 100% with less than one third of complete responders relapsing. Untreated patients survive only 4 to 6 months. About 40% of patients who relapse are curable with high-dose therapy and autologous hematopoietic stem cell transplantation. Overall, more than two thirds of patients with DLBL are cured.

The curability of the disease makes it essential that the treating physician carefully inform the patient of the options available to them. CHOP-R is generally well-tolerated with predictable dose-related toxicities. Even very old patients can be successfully treated. In addition, infusional regimens like R-EPOCH (rituximab, etoposide, prednisone, vincristine, cyclophosphamide, doxorubicin) are also safe and highly effective in older patients.

The new standard treatment represents a true advance in therapy. In an earlier study, the Nebraska Lymphoma Study Group used the CAP/BOP regimen (cyclophosphamide, doxorubicin, procarbazine, bleomycin, vincristine, and prednisone) to treat all patients with DLBL. They found a similar overall complete remission (CR) rate of 65% in patients older and younger than 60 years of age; however, patients younger than 60 years had a 62% 5-year survival, whereas those older than 60 years had a 35% 5-year survival. They found that treatment toxicity was similar and that deaths from apparently unrelated causes accounted for most of the survival difference. However, as therapy has improved, the contribution of age to prognosis has decreased.

Follicular Lymphoma

FL is the second most common form of lymphoma in the United States accounting for about 33% of cases. Thus, FL and DLBL together account for about 75% of lymphomas. FL is predominantly a disease of lymph nodes. New painless adenopathy is the predominant presenting symptom. Some patients give a history of adenopathy that has waxed and waned in the past. B symptoms occur in less than 25% of patients and the disease is often widely disseminated at presentation with involvement of bone marrow noted in over 40%. Females are affected slightly more commonly than males and the median age is 59 years.

FL is associated with a characteristic genetic lesion, a t(14;18) that results in the expression of bcl-2, an antiapoptotic protein. How bcl-2 expression is related to lymphomagenesis is undefined. An important biologic feature of FL is its genetic instability. Normal follicle center B cells undergo extensive somatic hypermutation to increase the ability of the antibody it produces to bind to antigens. In neoplastic follicular center cells, the mutation process is not restricted to the immunoglobulin genes. As mutations in other genes accumulate, the disease has a tendency to undergo transformation to DLBL with an acceleration in natural history and often an increased resistance to therapy. Histologic progression occurs at a rate of 5% to 7% per year and is not increased by therapy. The vast majority of patients with FL who die have DLBL as the cause of death. Median survival appears to have been increasing in the last 20 years from a median of 8 years to a median of 13 years. The basis for the improvement is not defined.

Patients in whom FL is restricted to lymph nodes may be cured by involved-field radiation therapy. Early studies of radiation therapy in early stage disease documented long-term disease-free survival in 90% of patients. The relegation of a patient to a watch-and-wait approach without staging the disease is indefensible. Many patients with localized disease have experienced disease progression while under "observation" and are thereby denied the potential for cure of early stage disease.

Management of patients with advanced stage disease is controversial. Because of the indolent course of disease, an initial period of "watchful waiting" is very appealing, especially in the elderly. In prospective trials, no overall survival difference has been demonstrated between observation and early chemotherapy. However, it should be noted that the CR rates and duration of the remissions are longer in the group treated initially compared with the observation groups. If one withholds treatment until a clinical indication emerges, the median time to initiation of chemotherapy is between 2 and 3 years. In one study, about one-fifth of the patients in the observation protocol remained free from an indication to begin chemotherapy at 10 years. In a large prospective British trial, which had a 19-year follow-up, the actuarial survival without needing treatment in elderly patients was 40% (out of 51 patients). If one is to choose the watchful waiting approach, careful patient selection is essential. The presence of B symptoms, peripheral blood cytopenia, kidney or liver involvement, and any life-endangering organ involvement suggest a more aggressive disease requiring immediate treatment.

A single agent oral alkylating agent like chlorambucil or cyclophosphamide may be an attractive choice in the elderly because of ease of administration and relatively low toxicity. When used alone, this therapy results in response rates of 60% to 80% with about half of all patients achieving a complete response. Combination chemotherapy with cyclophosphamide, vincristine, and prednisone (CVP) is also effective and may result in slightly higher CR of 60% to 70%. Fludarabine, a purine nucleotide analog, is also an active agent used in the treatment of indolent lymphoma. Used alone, it can induce remissions in about 60% to 80% of all treatment naive patients.

The use of interferon for treatment of indolent lymphoma remains controversial. A meta-analysis demonstrated usefulness as a maintenance therapy in patients treated with aggressive combination chemotherapy who had responded to the therapy. It was shown that the DFS was increased with addition of interferon alfa as a maintenance agent. However, many patients on interferon have symptoms of fatigue and depression that affect their quality of life.

When used as a single agent in previously untreated patients, rituximab produces response in 47% to 73% of patients with up to 37% achieving a CR. Moreover, when combined with combination chemotherapy such as CHOP, rituximab has shown an excellent overall response rate (100%) and CR (87%). When combined with CVP (cyclophosphamide, vincristine, prednisone), R-CVP yields better overall survival (81% vs. 50%), CR (57% vs. 10%), and time to progression (median 27 months vs. 7 months) than CVP alone.

Patients with advanced stage disease including involvement of extranodal sites should be informed that recent advances in treatment appear to be associated with longer remissions and longer survival, but definitive evidence of disease curability is still scarce. Formerly, CRs could be achieved with a wide range of interventions including radiation therapy, single agent and combination chemotherapy, antibodies, interferon, and various combinations. However, the CRs tended to be short-lived, with a median duration of 2 years. More active regimens and agents are changing this picture. Combination chemotherapy programs including CHOP (see earlier in the chapter) or fludarabine with rituximab produce complete responses in 90% or more of patients with median durations of complete responses exceeding 8 years. Because patients with FL can survive for many years with lymphoma, treatment-induced improvement in overall survival has been more difficult to demonstrate. However, some evidence of treatment benefit is beginning to emerge from studies that use effective drugs with rituximab during induction therapy and some sort of maintenance therapy (either rituximab or interferon). It is not clear if maintenance therapy is merely keeping disease at a subclinical level or is eradicating disease. Another benefit from aggressive treatment approaches seems to be a reduction in the rate of histologic progression.

Once a relapse occurs, the disease is likely to respond to treatment again, but the response rates and duration decrease with each relapse. Some data support the use of high-dose therapy with autologous stem cell transplant in selected (usually younger) patients. Two radionuclides have been approved by the FDA in the treatment of rituximab refractory indolent NHL. Yttrium-90-conjugated ibritumomab tiuxetan and iodine-131-conjugated tositumomab produce responses in two-thirds to three-fourths of rituximab-resistant patients. [131]I tositumomab is also effective as a single agent in previously untreated patients with over 90% OR and 75% CR. However, use of these agents as a primary therapy requires further randomized studies.

The confusion in the field is evident when expert recommendations range from watch and wait to high-dose therapy with transplant. However, a reasonable approach is to treat all patients with stage I or II disease with curative intent with radiation therapy. Patients with advanced disease should be assessed for intercurrent illness and life expectancy. Patients whose life expectancy is greater than 10 years may be candidates for an initial attempt at inducing durable remission with R-CHOP. Those with a shorter life expectancy with intercurrent illness can be observed and treated palliatively with single agent oral chlorambucil with or without prednisone when needed to control symptoms.

Small Lymphocytic Lymphoma/Chronic Lymphocytic Leukemia

Small lymphocytic lymphoma (SLL) is the tissue counterpart of chronic lymphocytic leukemia (CLL) and occurs in patients with a median age of 65 years. CLL is the most common form of leukemia in the United States (Figure 104-1; ~15 500 cases/year) while SLL accounts for only 6% to 7% of lymphomas (~4160 new cases/year). Initially, there are few symptoms of SLL/CLL and many patients are diagnosed incidentally based on abnormal lymphocytes on the peripheral blood smear. Fevers, sweats, and weight loss (the typical "B" symptoms) are uncommon and should prompt evaluation for other potential causes, such as infection, histologic conversion (see later), or second malignancy. The disease is nearly always in advanced stage at diagnosis.

The malignant cell in SLL/CLL is a CD5+ B cell. The difference between SLL and CLL is thought to depend on the expression of adhesion molecules that either favor lymph node-based growth or not.

Immunologic abnormalities are not demonstrable in most histologic types of lymphoma except SLL, which is similar in nature to CLL. In this disorder, hypogammaglobulinemia is common and is associated with a propensity to infection, primarily with encapsulated bacterial organisms but also with common viruses. Monoclonal gammopathy may be noted, particularly if examined by sensitive techniques. Circulating tumor cells can be detected by immunoglobulin gene-rearrangement studies even when peripheral lymphocyte counts are not elevated. Hemolytic anemias, especially cold-agglutinin disease (1.7%), and immune thrombocytopenia (0.4%) are uncommon but well-known complications.

Occasionally (in ~5% of patients), and less commonly than FL, SLL/CLL may convert to a more aggressive large cell lymphoma after 5 to 8 years of clinically indolent disease (Richter's conversion). These aggressive tumors demonstrate more rapid growth, are more resistant to treatment, and are associated with a median survival of less than 6 months. Suspicion for such a conversion is raised when a single node or group of nodes is found to be growing disproportionately to nodes at other sites, and biopsy reveals the large cell lymphoma, with SLL still being present in other nodes or in the bone marrow.

Treatment for SLL/CLL is generally based on fludarabine-containing combination chemotherapy. Cyclophosphamide plus fludarabine plus rituximab is an active regimen that obtains excellent responses in the majority of treated patients. When used in CLL, 70% of patients have complete responses that may last many years. Large series of SLL have not been reported, but the disease generally responds identically to CLL. Even though nodal masses predominate in SLL, 80% of patients have marrow involvement and it is marrow compromise that is the main life-threatening feature of the disease. In the face of progressive anemia or thrombocytopenia, it is important to assess whether the cause is immune destruction or marrow replacement. Immune destruction can be managed with prednisone while marrow replacement requires antitumor therapy.

Marginal Zone Lymphoma

The marginal zone lymphomas (MZL) are considered indolent in natural history. Various subtypes of MZL exist, including nodal MZL, splenic MZL, and extranodal MZL. Extranodal MZL, which may involve mucosa-associated lymphoid tissue (MALT), is the most common form. The nodal MZL behaves very similar to FL. Splenic MZL is rare and is managed successfully by splenectomy. Extranodal MZL of the MALT type appears to begin as a consequence of chronic antigenic stimulation and where it is possible, removing the stimulus may cause tumor regression.

MALT lymphoma accounts for about 7.6% of lymphomas in the United States. Median age is 60 years. It commonly presents in the stomach, although it may involve other extranodal sites including orbit, intestine, thyroid, lung, breast, salivary gland, urinary bladder, kidney, and CNS. Gastric MALT lymphoma is a consequence of infection by *Helicobacter pylori*. Thyroid lymphomas of MALT type are usually associated with Hashimoto's thyroiditis. MALT lymphomas of the salivary glands are usually associated with Sjogren's syndrome. Orbital MALT lymphomas have been linked to *Chlamydia psittaci* infection. Gastric MALT lymphoma is the most common form of extranodal MZL. The disease often presents with symptoms of ulcer and is discovered at the time of upper endoscopy. Treatment of *H. pylori* may result in gradual tumor regression and even CR. If the tumor does not regress completely within a year of eradicating the bacterium, chemotherapy is usually required. Two distinct genetic forms of gastric MALT lymphoma have been defined: about half the cases have t(11;18), which creates an API/MALT1 fusion product and is genetically stable; the other form is characterized by genetic instability and may show trisomies of chromosomes 3, 7, 12, or 18. The latter form has the propensity to evolve into DLBL of the stomach and requires R-CHOP therapy. The patients who achieve CR with just antibiotics (~50% of patients) almost always have a very superficial form of the disease. For those not responding completely to antibiotics, chemotherapy or radiation therapy is generally required. Treatment with combination chemotherapy using CVP (cyclophosphamide, vincristine, prednisone) with or without involved field radiation leads to cure in most patients. Five-year survival is 72%.

Splenic MZL is responsible for about one fourth of low-grade B cell tumors affecting the spleen. Hepatitis C infection may be associated with this lymphoma. Splenectomy is effective therapy as is treatment of the underlying hepatitis C infection. However, a poor response to alkylating agents is often seen with this subgroup. Both nodal MZL and splenic MZL can transform to aggressive DLBL, conferring a poor prognosis.

Mantle Cell Lymphoma

Mantle cell lymphoma (MCL), first described as an independent entity in 1992, is a lymphoid malignancy in which the malignant cells are usually CD5+ and overexpress cyclin D1, usually as a result of a t(11:14) chromosomal translocation. It comprises ~6% of all lymphomas and with a median age of 63 years. It is commonly seen in the elderly. The male-to-female ratio is 3:1. MCL commonly involves lymph nodes, spleen, bone marrow, Waldeyer's ring, and gastrointestinal tract and has been associated with lymphomatous polyposis. It tends to be clinically aggressive though a wide range of natural histories have been seen. Five-year survival is only 27%. Aggressive chemotherapy regimens such as Hyper C-VAD plus rituximab are improving complete response rates and remission durations, but convincing evidence for improved overall survival has not yet been generated. Bortezomib, a proteasome inhibitor, also has some antitumor activity.

Highly Aggressive Lymphomas

The highly aggressive lymphomas are the precursor B and T cell malignancies and Burkitt's lymphoma. These entities can either cause a leukemia clinical picture or have a dominant pattern of tissue involvement that spares the peripheral blood and looks like a lymphoma. However, their rapid natural history usually manifests in a short prodrome (less than 2 weeks between symptoms appearing and diagnosis) and an untreated natural history of a few weeks. When the precursor B and T cell malignancies produce lymphoma, they are generally called lymphoblastic lymphoma. Since lymphoblastic lymphoma is almost completely a disease of adolescence and young adulthood, it will not be discussed here except to note that, unlike other lymphomas, lymphoblastic lymphomas are most commonly of T cell origin. Burkitt's lymphoma too has a median age of onset of 31 years, but rare older persons may have this disease and it may occur in people with AIDS.

In the United States, the Burkitt lymphomas usually present with rapidly expanding abdominal masses, high LDH and uric acid levels, and systemic symptoms. The growth fraction of the tumor is nearly 100%; thus, the evaluation and workup of patients with Burkitt's lymphoma should be geared toward the rapid institution of combination chemotherapy with appropriate prophylaxis for tumor lysis syndrome. Although Epstein–Barr virus is associated with the endemic (African) form, its role in the pathogenesis of sporadic Burkitt's lymphoma in the United States is unclear. These tumors arise from mature B cells of follicular center phenotype, as evidenced by the expression of surface immunoglobulin (SIg), CD19, CD20, and CD22, and the presence of mutated immunoglobulin genes. The tumor can be identified karyotypically by one of three characteristic chromosomal translocations [t(8;14), t(8;22), and t(2;8)], all of which result in juxtaposition of the *c-myc* proto-oncogene (chromosome 8) to one of the three immunoglobulin genes, heavy chain on chromosome 14, or lambda or kappa light chain genes on chromosomes 8 and 22, respectively.

The prognosis is poor in older patients because of the need for extremely aggressive and specialized leukemia-like treatment. Often the bone marrow is involved. Treatment requires prophylaxis against tumor lysis syndrome (intravenous fluids, alkalinization of the urine, and allopurinol), intensive doses of chemotherapy for several months, and CNS prophylaxis with intrathecal chemotherapy and whole brain irradiation.

HODGKIN'S LYMPHOMA

Hodgkin's lymphoma (HL) in the United States has a bimodal age incidence. The early peak occurs between the ages of 20 and 30 years, and the later peak occurs between ages 70 and 80 years, with the incidence starting to increase around the age of 50 years. Men far outnumber women in the later peak. HL is one cancer in which the disease may differ in older patients. Age >50 years is a prognostic factor and a decreasing ability to tolerate treatment does not appear to influence outcome. HL was diagnosed in 8190 people in the United States in 2007; its incidence has been stable for many years. Only 1070 people died from the disease, indicating the widespread implementation of effective treatment programs.

There has been a curious association of Epstein–Barr virus and HL. The risk of HL is increased in patients with a history of infectious mononucleosis, and the Epstein–Barr virus has been demonstrated directly in some cases. However, this association is not found in HL developing in older patients. The contribution of age-associated immune dysregulation to the pathogenesis in late-life HL has theoretical appeal, but there are no supporting data.

Presentation

Adenopathy, usually in the neck, is the most common presenting sign of HL in all age groups. However, as a presenting complaint, adenopathy is less frequent and systemic symptoms (fever, night sweats, weight loss) are more frequent in older patients. Abdominal disease is also more common in older patients. In a study from Stanford University, unexplained adenopathy was still the most common presentation in patients aged older than 60 years (65%) and "B" symptoms were the presenting complaint in 29%. Because nearly every patient (except those with peripheral IA disease) receive combination chemotherapy as a component of their treatment, pathological staging with staging laparotomy is only rarely performed and is restricted to patients in whom it will influence choice of treatment (radiation therapy vs. chemotherapy). The staging schema is shown in Table 104-2.

Histologies

The diagnosis of HL depends on detecting the characteristic malignant cell, the Reed-Sternberg (RS) cell, in a setting of a pleiomorphic inflammatory infiltrate that includes lymphocytes, macrophages, and eosinophils with a variable degree of fibrosis. The infiltrate effaces the nodal architecture. The RS cell is a large binucleated cell with at least two prominent nucleoli. The cell is often said to display an "owl's eyes" appearance, particularly in mixed cellularity HL. In nodular sclerosis HL, it takes the form of a so-called "lacunar cell" because of cytoplasmic retraction during fixation and in lymphocyte predominant HL, it may have a convoluted nucleus that looks like popcorn and is called a "popcorn cell." Although there has been controversy on the cell of origin of HL for many years and at least some heterogeneity exists, the vast majority of cases originate from a B cell of follicular center phenotype that have rearranged and mutated their immunoglobulin genes but do not transcribe them.

HL is divided into two categories in the WHO classification (Table 104-1): classical Hodgkin's disease accounts for 95% of HL and nodular lymphocyte predominant Hodgkin's disease accounts for about 5%. Classical Hodgkin's disease has four histologic subsets: lymphocyte-predominant, nodular sclerosis, mixed cellularity, and lymphocyte-depleted. Of these types, nodular sclerosis is by far the most common in the United States accounting for 65% to 75%. Mixed cellularity is next most common (20%) and most of the rest are lymphocyte-predominant. Lymphocyte-depleted histology is rare and can be confused with DLBL. Mixed cellularity is more common in South American and in HIV-infected patients. In addition, mixed cellularity appears to increase in frequency with age (Table 104-6).

The Finsen Institute study involved 506 unselected patients who were studied for the age distribution of histology. In the younger groups, nodular sclerosis was the most common histological type and this type was also most common in patients older than 60 years, but to a lesser extent. Mixed cellularity histology, uncommon in the younger groups, appeared almost as frequently as nodular sclerosis in the older group. Lymphocyte-predominant and lymphocyte-depleted histologies were notably uncommon in the elderly.

Staging

Anatomical staging has been an important factor in HL management. The disease tends to originate in nodes (particularly the cervical nodes) and march to adjacent nodal groups in a stepwise fashion. The first site of intraabdominal involvement is often the spleen and the liver, though rarely involved, is never involved unless the spleen is involved. A suggested staging workup is found in Table 104-5. A careful medical history and thorough physical examination are essential. Clinical staging also includes CT of the chest, abdomen and pelvis, and positron emission tomography (PET). The

TABLE 104-6

Influence of Age on Histological Patterns of Hodgkin's Lymphoma					
	SPECHT AND NISSEN		PETERSON ET AL.		WEDELIN ET AL.
Histology	Age <40 (%)	Age >60 (%)	Age <40 (%)	Age >60 (%)	Age <50 (%)	Age >50 (%)
Lymphocyte predominant	12	12	7	11	12	17
Nodular sclerosing	61	44	30	7	49	21
Mixed cellularity	25	37	42	52	29	46
Lymphocyte depleted	<1	2	14	20	7	13
Unclassified	2	4	7	11	4	4

lymphangiogram provides unique information about the involvement of paraaortic nodes and can also allow the physician to follow the response monthly with a plain abdominal film as involved nodes shrink under therapy, but the expertise to conduct this test is vanishing and it is rarely employed today. Bilateral bone marrow biopsies will indicate the presence of marrow involvement in a subset of patients (perhaps 10%) for whom staging to that point did not indicate any suspicion of extranodal disease. In older individuals, the marrow cellularity and evidence for adequate hematopoiesis are of additional value for planning therapy.

In general, management of all stages of HL involves combination chemotherapy plus or minus radiation therapy. Therefore, most patients do not require a staging laparotomy. However, for patients who have clinical early stage disease and who have intercurrent illness that would make the use of combination chemotherapy particularly hazardous, a staging laparotomy should be considered. This involves careful abdominal exploration with routine biopsies of paraaortic, celiac, splenic hilar, mesenteric, portal, and iliac nodes; wedge and core biopsies of the liver; and splenectomy. Staging laparotomy will demonstrate more advanced disease (upstage) about 35% of the time, but in some cases (10% to 15%) radiographically suspicious lesions are shown to be not Hodgkin's and downstaging is the result. An enlarged spleen on CT scan is involved with Hodgkin's disease only two thirds of the time. If the staging laparotomy is negative, one could consider the use of radiation therapy alone to treat a patient too ill to receive systemic therapy. Before taking a patient to splenectomy, pneumococcal vaccine should be given, preferably at least 2 weeks in advance of splenectomy.

A staging laparotomy is a major surgery and may not be well tolerated in elderly patients. The benefits of more accurate assessment and more precise therapy have to be weighed against the operative risks. Alternative staging approaches, including new visualizing techniques, are being explored. However, for patients in whom radiation therapy alone is being considered, staging laparotomy remains the standard evaluative approach.

Therapy

The therapy for HL has become better defined as a result of clinical trials (Table 104-7). The main debate centers on whether to add radiation therapy to chemotherapy versus relying on chemotherapy alone. Nearly every patient received chemotherapy. The source of the controversy is the very high rate of late, fatal complications from the use of radiation therapy. Long-term follow-up studies demonstrate a threefold increased rate of *fatal* myocardial infarctions in patients who received mantle-field radiation therapy. In addition, the risk of strokes is increased. Furthermore, patients who received radiation therapy begin developing second malignancies about 5 to 7 years after completing treatment and by 25 years after treatment, 25% to 30% of patients have a second cancer. These cancers are mainly in or adjacent to treatment fields and include lung cancer, breast cancer, head and neck cancer, melanoma, and sarcomas. Chemotherapy-treated patients have not demonstrated this increased risk of second cancers, heart disease, or stroke.

In older patients, the intervention should be based on the life expectancy in the absence of HL. If a patient with HL is expected to live more than 20 years if the HL is cured, it would be best to avoid radiation therapy as a component of treatment. On the other hand, older patients with intercurrent illnesses and a life expectancy independent of HL of less than 10 years could be treated with radiation therapy alone to avoid the acute and chronic toxicities of combination chemotherapy. The main acute side effect of the active chemotherapy programs is myelosuppression. ABVD (doxorubicin, bleomycin, vinblastine, dacarbazine) is the most widely used regimen and involves intravenous therapy every 2 weeks for 24 weeks. Doxorubicin can compromise cardiac function in a patient with preexisting heart failure, while more cardiac-sparing anthracyclines can be substituted (e.g., mitoxantrone, liposomal doxorubicin), an alkylating agent-based regimen may be preferable. Bleomycin can induce pulmonary fibrosis and should not be given to patients with preexisting compromise of their diffusing capacity.

MOPP (nitrogen mustard, vincristine, procarbazine, prednisone) and ChlVPP (chlorambucil, vinblastine, procarbazine, prednisone) are effective alternatives to ABVD in those with contraindications. They are myelotoxic acutely in a dose-related fashion. The main late toxicity is infertility, which is rarely a consideration in the elderly. When combined with radiation therapy, the alkylating agent-based regimens produce acute leukemia in about 3% of treated patients and older patients may be more susceptible to this late effect. However, the window of risk seems to be 3 to 10 years following treatment, after which the risk declines sharply. If given without radiation therapy, the leukemia risk is decreased about 90%.

Other regimens used to treat HL include Stanford V and BEACOPP. Stanford V uses a short course of chemotherapy together with radiation therapy in every patient. It has been hoped that the use of a lower total dose of radiation therapy will reduce the incidence of late fatal complications but this hope has not yet been validated by actual data. BEACOPP employs higher doses and more agents than either ABVD or MOPP and is more difficult to administer to older patients. It is not clearly superior to six cycles of ABVD. Studies combining MOPP and ABVD have not shown an improvement over ABVD alone.

In light of the controversies, consensus treatment recommendations have not been developed. However, it is rational to assess every patient and make individualized treatment programs. For most patients, clinical staging followed by six cycles of ABVD chemotherapy will be an effective approach to patients of all stages. In those with cardiac or pulmonary problems, MOPP or ChlVPP are equally active alternatives to ABVD. For patients with localized (stage I or II) disease in whom chemotherapy is attempted, but toxicities prevent

TABLE 104-7

Recommended Therapy for Hodgkin's Lymphoma	
STAGE	**THERAPY**
I, II (A or B, negative laparotomy)	Subtotal lymphoid irradiation or combination chemotherapy
Clinical stage I, II (no laparotomy)	Combination chemotherapy
I, II (A or B with mediastinal mass >1/3 diameter of chest wall)	Combination chemotherapy followed by irradiation to involved field
IIA$_1$ (minimal abdominal disease)	Combination chemotherapy
IIIA$_2$ (extensive abdominal disease)	Combination chemotherapy alone or with irradiation to persistent PET-positive sites
IIIB	Combination chemotherapy
IV (A or B)	Combination chemotherapy

the administration of more than 50% of the doses or lead to treatment delays, it is reasonable to use radiation therapy. Involved-field radiation therapy may eradicate the disease.

Radiation therapy is appropriate in two other settings. In patients who respond well to chemotherapy but still have PET positive sites after four or six cycles of chemotherapy, radiation therapy to the positive site can convert many patients into durable complete responders. Often the residual positivity is in the mediastinum. In addition, patients who have massive mediastinal disease at presentation may benefit from involved-field radiation therapy after chemotherapy.

Toxicity from both radiotherapy and chemotherapy increases with age. The typical side effects of radiation therapy for HL include acute and transient anorexia with occasional nausea, vomiting, diarrhea, transient and occasionally permanent drying of salivary secretions, transient pharyngitis and esophagitis, fatigue, and cytopenias. The long-term side effects include hypothyroidism (common), pneumonitis, constrictive pericarditis, rare endocardial or myocardial fibrosis, skin pigmentation and breakdown, and second malignancies. Long-term follow-up of patients who have received radiation therapy to upper mantle areas should include periodic thyroid evaluations.

The side effects of chemotherapy are also enhanced in older patients and certain drugs are particularly difficult for the older patient. Those used commonly in the treatment of HL include vinblastine and doxorubicin. Liver metabolism of other drugs is probably slowed in older persons.

Although there is an increased risk for toxicity, older HL patients may still be treated safely and with curative intent. Even for those in whom curative treatment is not indicated or who relapse from CR, significant palliation and prolongation of life can be achieved with localized radiation and single-agent or multiagent chemotherapy.

Response to Treatment and Survival

Many published series have demonstrated poorer survival in older patients with HL, but these series have been difficult to interpret because modern staging and treatment were not applied consistently, and it is now understood that age bias may influence cancer therapy outcomes.

The ECOG study cited earlier reported decreasing freedom from relapse with increasing age in patients treated from 1968 to 1981. The 5-year freedom-from-relapse rate was 81% for those younger than age 17 years, 70% for those aged 17 to 49 years, 63% for those aged 50 to 59 years, and 38% for those aged 60 years and older. Multivariate analysis revealed that age was the most important factor in determining freedom from relapse. Older patients with HL have not been a focus of clinical research as yet and it seems likely that improvements in outcome are at hand.

Multiple Myeloma and Related Plasma Cell Dyscrasias

Malignant plasma cells typically remain in the bone marrow and grow as either a solitary mass (solitary myeloma of bone [SMB]) or as nests of cells distributed throughout the bone marrow (multiple myeloma [MM]). Occasionally, plasma cell tumors will arise outside of the marrow, particularly within the aerodigestive tract (extramedullary plasmacytoma [EMP]). Whereas SMB and EMP are relatively uncommon, MM accounts for approximately 17.8% of lymphoid malignancies (Figure 104-1) or 19 900 cases in 2007. MM is a disease characterized by destructive bone disease and circulating monoclonal protein that can increase serum viscosity and infiltrate and damage organs.

Epidemiology

In the United States, there are approximately 4 new cases per 100 000 population per year. Myeloma accounts for 1% of all malignancies. Although the age range is wide, it is considered a disease of older adults. The median age is 68 years. Cases are rare before 30 years of age. Males are affected slightly more frequently than females, and myeloma is nearly twice as common in African-Americans as in other races.

Etiology

The cause of myeloma is not known. Radiation or other carcinogen exposure is involved in the cause of this disease. Japanese atomic bomb survivors have had a fivefold increase in risk. A number of chromosome alterations have been noted including 13q14 deletions, 17p13 deletions, and 11q abnormalities. The most common translocation is t(11;14) and many tumors show changes suggesting errors in heavy chain gene switch recombination, the process that occurs when cells change from producing IgM to another heavy chain isotype. Cytokine [particularly interleukin-6 (IL-6)] dysregulation is also an important feature of MM. IL-6 triggers proliferation through the Ras, Raf, MEK, mitogen-activated protein kinase cascade, and promotes cell survival by upregulation of antiapoptotic molecules. Serum levels of IL-6 are very high and correlate with tumor mass, the extent of bone destruction, and survival. Furthermore, in murine models of myeloma, plasma cell tumors did not develop in mice that were genetically engineered to be IL-6-deficient (IL-6 "knockouts"). Interactions between myeloma cells and bone marrow stromal cells and the extracellular matrix are critical to myeloma cell growth and survival. In addition to IL-6, insulin-like growth factor, vascular endothelial growth factor (VEGF), and the chemokine, stromal cell derived (SDF) 1-alpha play a role.

The frequency of particular heavy chain classes in myeloma roughly corresponds to the relative frequency of the different isotypes in the serum (Table 104-8).

Clinical Manifestations of Disease and Their Pathogenesis

Many of the features of myeloma are caused by the effect of the paraprotein and other tumor products.

TABLE 104-8

Plasma Cell Disorders			
DISEASE		FREQUENCY (%)	PROGNOSIS (MONTHS)
Multiple myeloma	IgG	52	29–35
	IgA	21	19–22
	IgD	2	9
	IgE	<0.01%	—
	Light chains only Non-secretor	11	10–28
Waldenström's macroglobulinemia	IgM	12	50

Bone Pain

Bone pain is the most common symptom in patients with myeloma (70%). Pain usually involves the back and ribs and is made worse by movement. X-rays reveal either localized "punched-out" lytic lesions or diffuse osteoporosis, usually in bones with active hematopoietic tissue. The discrete lytic lesions are characterized by numerous osteoclasts on the bone-reabsorbing surface without osteoblastic activity. Thus, bone scans are not useful in diagnosis as they detect new bone formation. The osteoclasts are activated by osteoclast-activating factors (OAF) made by the tumor including IL1, lymphotoxin, IL6, vascular endothelial growth factor (VEGF), receptor activator of NF-kB (RANK) ligand, and others. Localized bone lesions may expand to the point where they produce soft tissue masses and collapsed vertebrae can lead to cord compression.

With bone demineralization caused by osteoclast activation and with decreased activity because of pain, hypercalcemia may be expected. The symptoms of hypercalcemia (drowsiness, confusion, nausea, and thirst) are nonspecific, but their occurrence should alert the physician to investigate this possibility. Cardiac arrhythmias, renal insufficiency, and profound CNS depression can develop as hypercalcemia progresses.

Infection

Susceptibility to bacterial infections is also a serious clinical problem in patients with myeloma. The most common sites of infection are the lungs and kidneys and the most common causative agents are *Streptococcus pneumoniae*, *Staphylococcus aureus*, and *Klebsiella pneumoniae* in the lungs and *Escherichia coli* and other Gram-negative organisms in the urinary tract. Recurrent infection is the presenting symptom in 25% of patients and >75% will have a serious infection at some time in the course of the disease. Several factors contribute to the susceptibility. If one discounts the paraprotein, most patients with myeloma have hypogammaglobulinemia related to both decreased production and increased catabolism of normal antibodies. In addition, granulocyte lysozyme levels and migration are impaired by products of the tumor. Complement functions are also abnormal. Furthermore, some therapeutic interventions also increase the risk of infection.

Renal Failure

Renal failure occurs in about one-fourth of myeloma patients and some renal pathology is seen in over half. Its causes are many (Table 104-9). Hypercalcemia is the most common cause. In addition, glomerular deposits of amyloid, hyperuricemia, recurrent infections,

TABLE 104-9

Causes of Renal Failure in Myeloma

Light-chain deposition in tubules ("myeloma kidney")
Hyperviscosity
Hypercalcemia
Hyperuricemia
Infection
Dehydration (especially after an intravenous pyelogram)
Associated amyloidosis

use of nonsteroidal anti-inflammatory agents, radiographic contrast material, bisphosphonate use, and occasional myeloma cell infiltration of the kidney can all contribute to the renal dysfunction. Renal tubular dysfunction is very common as a result of damage to the tubules by light chains. This tubular damage is often reflected in a type 2 proximal renal tubular acidosis with loss of glucose and amino acids and problems concentrating and acidifying the urine. Monoclonal lambda light chains are more likely to produce tubular injury than are kappa chains.

Anemia and Bleeding

Anemia is seen in 80% of patients. It is generally related to the inhibition of hematopoiesis by products of the tumor cells, but in late stages of disease can be caused by crowding of normal hematopoietic cells in the marrow. The anemia is usually normocytic and normochromic. The high concentrations of serum protein interact with erythrocyte membranes and cause a coin-like stacking of red cells known as rouleaux formation. Mild hemolysis may be present and other causes of anemia (such as vitamin B-12 deficiency) may coexist. Coating of platelets results in diminished aggregation and purpura. The high protein level also may interfere with coagulation factors by inhibiting fibrin polymerization, and bleeding may result.

Hyperviscosity

Hyperviscosity may occur at different levels of paraprotein based on its physical characteristics. Normal serum is about 1.8 times as viscous as water and symptoms of hyperviscosity (decreased cerebral blood flow, producing headache, nausea, visual impairment, and mental clouding) occur when the serum becomes five to six times more viscous than water. This level is generally reached at paraprotein levels of 4 g/dL for IgM, 5 g/dL for IgG3, and 7 g/dL for IgA. Decreased renal blood flow may contribute to the renal failure that is so common in MM. Total blood volume expands and may predispose to congestive heart failure.

Neurological Symptoms

A minority of patients may experience neurologic signs or symptoms. Hypercalcemia may produce lethargy, fatigue, depression, and confusion. Hyperviscosity compromises CNS function and causes visual disturbances. Cord compression can result from bony destruction. Infiltration of peripheral nerves with amyloid or a paraprotein with antigen specificity for a nerve component can produce sensorimotor mono- and polyneuropathies.

Diagnosis and Staging

The classic triad of myeloma is marrow plasmacytosis of 10% or greater, lytic bone lesions, and a serum and/or urine paraprotein. Bone marrow plasma cells are monoclonal and express CD138. A number of diseases may produce a monoclonal gammopathy including other lymphoid malignancies, other solid tumors (breast cancer, colon cancer), cirrhosis, sarcoidosis, parasitic diseases, Gaucher disease, and a number of autoimmune disorders including rheumatoid arthritis, myasthenia gravis, and cold agglutinin disease. However, the most common differential diagnosis is between myeloma and monoclonal gammopathy of uncertain significance (MGUS). Patients with myeloma typically have paraprotein levels >3 g/dL and some stigmata of end-organ damage such as lytic bone lesions, hypercalcemia, renal dysfunction, recurrent bacterial infections, or anemia.

Monoclonal Gammopathy of Uncertain Significance

MGUS is an elevation of a clonal immunoglobulin molecule in the serum generally present at <3 g/dL. It occurs in about 1% of people aged older than 50 years and up to 10% of people aged older than 75 years. It is an indicator of dysregulated B-cell clonal expansion, but it is not considered to be the antecedent of MM. Patients with MGUS have fewer than 10% plasma cells in the bone marrow, have no lytic bone lesions, and are normocalcemic. Although not a malignant process itself, patients with MGUS have a 2-year decline in life expectancy compared with age-matched unaffected controls. About 15% of people with MGUS progress to overt myeloma after periods of up to 30 years and generally these individuals had higher levels of paraprotein at MGUS diagnosis. Typically, MGUS is distinguished from myeloma through examination of bone marrow, skeletal x-rays, renal function, and serum $\beta2$ microglobulin levels (Table 104-10). Early myeloma will show signs of disease progression over time and an increase in myeloma-related organ and tissue impairment, whereas MGUS will have stable protein readings, no bone disease, and a marrow that may or may not show a mild-to-moderate plasmacytosis but without dysplastic appearing plasma cells. It is important to make this distinction because MGUS is so much more common than myeloma and does not require therapy.

Smoldering Myeloma

A small subset of patients who make diagnostic criteria for myeloma have a very slow progression of disease. It differs from MGUS in having 10% of greater plasmacytosis in the bone marrow and at least 3 g/dL of paraprotein. However, like MGUS, it is not associated with the usual myeloma-associated tissue or organ impairment (hypercalcemia, lytic bone lesions, renal dysfunction, infections). The rate of progression to overt myeloma is higher than MGUS; actuarial risk is 73% over 15 years. However, it is not clear that early treatment is beneficial and most authorities recommend that patients be observed until disease progression to organ impairment before treatment is begun.

Myeloma Staging

A number of staging schemes have been developed. However, the international staging system is now the most widely used. The staging system is based on serum albumin levels and serum beta-2-microglobulin levels. If the beta-2-microglobulin levels are less than 3.5 μg/mL and the serum albumin is equal to or greater than 3.5 g/dL, patients are said to be stage I. This accounts for about 28% of all patients and is associated with a median survival of about 5 years. In stage II, the beta-2-microglobulin level is less than 3.5 μg/mL and the albumin level is less than 3.5 μg/mL or beta-2-microglobulin levels are 3.5 to 5.5 μg/mL. Thirty-nine percent of patients are stage II and their median survival is about 4 years. Stage III patients are those with any albumin level and beta-2-microglobulin levels > 5.5 μg/mL. This accounts for 33% of patients and is associated with a median survival of 29 months.

Therapy

Effective treatment for myeloma patients includes chemotherapy, radiation therapy, and the use of several supportive care measures.

Three regimens are commonly used in newly diagnosed myeloma: intermittent oral melphalan (phenylalanine mustard) and prednisone with response rates of about 50% to 60%; melphalan plus prednisone with daily thalidomide added with response rates of 70% to 75%; and thalidomide plus dexamethasone with response rates around 65%. Younger patients are often managed with tandem autologous bone marrow transplants with the result that a substantial fraction experience long-term disease-free survival. Lenalidomide, a thalidomide analog, is being evaluated in first-line therapy as it has the advantage of being a more potent inhibitor of inflammatory cytokine production as well as being less sedating and with much diminished associated neuropathy. When used with dexamethasone response rates have been reported to be 70% to 90% with progression-free survival of greater than 1 year. Curiously, lenalidomide with dexamethasone is associated with an increased risk of deep vein thrombosis, but this does has not been observed when lenalidomide is used alone. Boretezomib is an antineoplastic agent that inhibits proteolytic activity of the proteosome. Bortezomib either alone or with dexamethasone, has shown excellent response rates; it is especially useful in the salvage setting. Secondary analyses of both lenalidomide and bortezomib studies reveal both to be well-tolerated in older patients. The current trend in therapy is to use lenalidomide and dexamethasone initially and to use bortezomib at the time of relapse.

Localized radiation therapy is used for pain relief and to decrease the risk of fractures. Measures designed to maintain activity and hydration are also important. Analgesics, orthopedic surgery, and orthotic supports facilitate mobilization. With adequate mobilization and fluid intake, the symptom complex of hypercalcemia, dehydration, and renal failure can usually be avoided. Bisphosphonates such as pamidronate or zoledronate have proven useful in both the prevention and treatment of myeloma-associated hypercalcemia and the American Society of Clinical Oncology recommends administration of either drug at monthly intervals for myeloma patients with lytic bone disease and without overt renal failure.

TABLE 104-10

Myeloma versus Monoclonal Gammopathy of Uncertain Significance (MGUS)		
	MYELOMA	**MGUS**
Pathogenesis	Neoplastic plasma cell disorder (malignant)	Disordered immunoregulation
Bone marrow	Frequently >10% plasma cells	Usually less than 10% plasma cells, and these appear normal
Bone	Majority will have bone erosions or diffuse osteoporosis (even early)	No bone disease
Symptoms	Bone pain, fatigue, weight loss, or those associated with kidney failure	Usually no symptoms
Serum spike	Progressively rising	Stable level IgG <3 g/dL IgA <2 g/dL BJ <1 g/24 h (urine)

Other Plasma Cell Dyscrasias Seen in Geriatric Populations

Waldenström's Macroglobulinemia

This disorder is caused by a proliferation of a neoplastic clone of IgM-producing cells called lymphocytoid plasma cells. Bone destruction is not a feature of the disease. In many respects, macroglobulinemia resembles a SLL with infiltration of the marrow by lymphocytes or lymphocytoid plasma cells, lymphadenopathy, and splenomegaly.

The circulating monoclonal IgM (macroglobulin) appears to explain much of the pathophysiology. The macroglobulin coats platelets and interferes with clotting. The oncotic expansion of the plasma volume leads to spurious anemia and may result in congestive heart failure. The hyperviscosity syndrome is common.

Therapy is directed at both the proliferating malignant clone of cells and the abnormal circulating protein. Alkylating agents such as chlorambucil or cyclophosphamide or purine analog such as fludarabine have proven to be effective in prolonging survival. Rituximab has been used with moderate success and may be of particular value for those patients with Waldenstrom's associated polyneuropathy. Plasmapheresis is indicated for the acute management of patients with symptoms of hyperviscosity as 80% of IgM remains intravascular. Plasmapheresis removes a substantial fraction of the body's IgM paraprotein.

Heavy-Chain Disease

These rare malignancies are characterized by the proliferation of plasma cells that produce an abnormal monoclonal heavy chain without associated light-chain synthesis. Like macroglobulinemia, these disorders resemble lymphoma more than they do myeloma. Bone disease does not occur, but lymphadenopathy and hepatosplenomegaly are common. Gamma, alpha, and mu heavy-chain diseases have been described. Alpha chain disease usually is associated with lymphoma involving the gastrointestinal tract and with malabsorption, whereas the mu heavy-chain disease is associated with long-standing CLL. Gamma heavy-chain disease can present as a lymphoma that histologically resembles HL.

Amyloidosis

Amyloidosis is a heterogeneous group of disorders characterized by the deposition of insoluble proteins in tissues, with eventual compromise in the function of the involved organs. Several different proteins have been identified in deposits, but two are common. In type I amyloid, the principal protein is immunoglobulin light chains, whereas in type II, a nonimmunoglobulin protein (protein A) is found. In both types, the proteins form noncovalent polymers in a fibrillar pattern, which can be recognized on electron microscopy. Different patterns of tissue distribution are associated with the different types of protein deposited.

When amyloidosis is associated with plasma cell dyscrasia (type I), amyloid deposits are found primarily in the muscles (including the heart and tongue), gastrointestinal tract, and skin. In conditions associated with protein A deposition (such as chronic infections and familial Mediterranean fever), amyloid deposition occurs in the kidney, spleen, liver, and adrenals. Mixed patterns, however, are common, and the presenting site of involvement is not sufficient to classify the type of amyloid involved.

TABLE 104-11

Summary Points for the Practicing Geriatrician

General

Older patients will present with more advanced disease.

Published cooperative trials on which standard therapy is based include disproportionately few elderly patients.

Older patients are not a priori more resistant to chemotherapy. However, end organ toxicity, especially heart, lung, and bone marrow, may be greater.

Do not risk letting your patient die from a curable tumor out of a fear of toxicity. Many older patients have less toxicity than expected.

Non-Hodgkin's lymphoma

Increases in frequency with advancing age.

DLBL (the most common lymphoma) is curable and must be treated aggressively or survival will be short.

Hodgkin's lymphoma

Older patients have relatively more "unfavorable" histologies (i.e., mixed cellularity or lymphocyte-depleted).

Chemotherapy has been less successful in achieving cures in older patients, perhaps because of comorbidity.

Multiple myeloma

It is important to differentiate myeloma from benign monoclonal gammopathy (see Table 104-10).

Myeloma should be a consideration for all older patients with persistent bone (especially low back) pain. The average delay in diagnosis from first seeking medical attention is 6 mo or more.

TAKE HOME POINTS FOR THE GERIATRICIAN

Older patients with lymphoid malignancies should not be assumed to be incurable. Patients can be cured sometimes, have their lives extended often, and made more comfortable always. It should not be assumed that a patient will experience more treatment-related toxicity on the basis of chronological age alone. Nearly always any toxicity encountered in an individual patient will permit rational modifications of dose (and sometimes schedule) to permit delivery of effective treatment. The time for failing to treat a treatable illness in the name of "doing no harm" has passed. Any older patient with a lymphoid malignancy should be evaluated by a specialist before it is assumed that the treatment is worse than the disease. Table 104-11 summarizes some important points about NHLs, Hodgkin's disease, and myeloma.

FURTHER READING

Ardeshna KM, Smith P, Norton A, et al. Long-term effect of a watch and wait policy versus immediate systemic treatment for asymptomatic advanced-stage non-Hodgkin's lymphoma: a randomised controlled trial. *Lancet.* 2003;362:516–522.

Begg CB, Carbone PP. Clinical trials and drug toxicity in the elderly. The experience of the Eastern Cooperative Oncology Group. *Cancer.* 1983;52:1986–1992.

Coiffier B, Lepage E, Briere J, et al. CHOP chemotherapy plus rituximab compared with CHOP alone in elderly patients with diffuse large B-cell lymphoma. *N Engl J Med.* 2002;346:235–242.

Czuczman MS, Weaver R, Alkuzweny B, Berlfein J, Grillo-Lopez AJ. Prolonged clinical and molecular remission in patients with low-grade or follicular non-Hodgkin's lymphoma treated with rituximab plus CHOP chemotherapy: 9-year follow-up. *J Clin Oncol.* 2004;22:4711–4716.

Dispenzieri A, Kyle RA. Multiple myeloma: clinical features and indications for therapy. *Best Pract Res Clin Haematol.* 2005;18:553–568.

Harris NL, Jaffe ES, Diebold J, et al. World Health Organization classification of neoplastic diseases of the hematopoietic and lymphoid tissues: report of the Clinical Advisory Committee meeting—Airlie House, Virginia, November 1997. *J Clin Oncol.* 1999;17:3835–3849.

Herold M, Haas A, Srock S, et al. Rituximab added to first-line mitoxantrone, chlorambucil, and prednisolone chemotherapy followed by interferon maintenance prolongs survival in patients with advanced follicular lymphoma: and East German Study Group Hematology and Oncology Study. *J Clin Oncol.* 2007;25:1986–1992.

Jemal A, Sigel R, Wood E, et al. Cancer statistics, 2007. *CA Cancer J Clin.* 2007;57:43–66.

Keating MJ, O'Brien S, Albitar M, et al. Early results of a chemoimmunotherapy regimen of fludarabine, cyclophosphamide, and rituximab as initial therapy for chronic lymphocytic leukemia. *J Clin Oncol.* 2005;23:4079–4088.

Kuppers R, Rajewsky K, Zhao M, et al. Hodgkin's disease: Hodgkin's and Reed-Sternberg cells picked from histological sections show clonal immunoglobulin gene rearrangements and appear to be derived from B cells at various stages of development. *Proc Natl Acad Sci U S A.* 1994;91:10962–10966.

Lichtman SM, Villani G. Chemotherapy in the elderly: pharmacologic considerations. *Cancer Control.* 2000;7:548–556.

Lokich JJ, Pinkus GS, Moloney WC. Hodgkin's disease in the elderly. *Oncology.* 1974;29:484–500.

Marcus R, Imrie K, Belch A, et al. CVP chemotherapy plus rituximab compared with CVP as first-line treatment for advanced follicular lymphoma. *Blood.* 2005;105:1417–1423.

Peterson BA, Pajak TF, Cooper MR, et al. Effect of age on therapeutic response and survival in advanced Hodgkin's disease. *Cancer Treat Rep.* 1982;66:889–735.

Sehn LH, Berry B, Chhanabhai M, et al. The revised International Prognostic Index (R-IPI) is a better predictor of outcome than the standard IPI for patients with diffuse large B-cell lymphoma. *Blood.* 2007;109:1857–1861.

Solal-Celigny P, Roy P, Colombat P, et al. Follicular lymphoma international prognostic index. *Blood.* 2004;104:1258–1265.

Specht L, Nissen NI. Hodgkin's disease and age. *Eur J Haematol.* 1989;43:127–135.

Vijay A, Gertz MA. Waldenstrom macroglobulinemia. *Blood.* 2007;109:5096–5103.

Vose JM, Armitage JO, Weisenburger DD, et al. The importance of age in survival of patients treated with chemotherapy for aggressive non-Hodgkin's lymphoma. *J Clin Oncol.* 1988;6:1838–1844.

Thrombosis

Martin O'Donnell ■ *Jeffrey S. Ginsberg* ■ *Clive Kearon*

Venous thromboembolism (VTE), which includes deep venous thrombosis (DVT) and pulmonary embolism (PE), affects about 1 in 1000 persons annually. The incidence and case-fatality of venous and arterial thromboembolic events increase with age. The increased risk of VTE in elderly patients reflects the increased prevalence of risk factors (temporary and permanent), prothrombotic changes in coagulation with advanced age, and an independent contribution of advancing age.

The diagnosis of VTE is more challenging in the elderly patient, as clinical presentations are more often atypical than in younger patients and the diagnostic properties of some tests appear to be influenced by advancing age. However, the general approach to diagnosis of VTE in the elderly is much the same as in younger patients.

While anticoagulant therapies have comparable relative risk reductions for prevention of VTE in older compared to younger patients, elderly patients are at increased risk of major bleeding and particularly intracranial bleeding. Therefore, decisions regarding optimal duration of anticoagulant therapy for VTE are influenced by the patient's age.

In this chapter, we review the epidemiology, pathophysiology, natural history, diagnosis, and treatment of VTE in the elderly patient.

EPIDEMIOLOGY

Incidence of VTE

The incidence of VTE increases exponentially with advancing age (i.e., approximately twofold increase with each decade) rising from an annual incidence of 0.03% at age 40 years, to 0.09% at 60 years, and 0.26% at age 80 years.

Risk Factors

Most patients with VTE have one or more clinical risk factors for venous thrombosis. The most common risk factors in hospitalized elderly patients are recent surgery, previous VTE, trauma, and immobility, as well as serious illness, including malignancy, chronic heart failure, stroke, chronic lung disease, acute infections, and inflammatory bowel disease. A particularly important major risk factor for VTE in elderly patients is major orthopedic surgery, both elective and after hip fracture, where fatal PE is a leading cause of in-hospital death. Common risk factors in outpatients include hospital admission within the past 3 months, malignancy, previous VTE, cancer chemotherapy, estrogen therapy, presence of an antiphospholipid antibody, and familial thrombophilia. Less common risk factors are paroxysmal nocturnal hemoglobinuria, nephrotic syndrome, and polycythemia vera. A recent study of elderly patients has reported frailty to be a risk factor for VTE.

Age is thought to have at least an additive influence on the risk of VTE when combined with other risk factors for VTE and the prevalence of many risk factors is greater in the elderly. Consequently, the risk of VTE in high-risk situations, such as following surgery, is greater in older than younger persons.

The risk of thrombosis is about 50-fold higher in persons with a previous VTE than in the general population, and recurrent thrombosis accounts for about one quarter of all acute episodes of VTE. When anticoagulant therapy is stopped after 3 or more months of treatment, the subsequent risk of recurrent VTE in the first year varies from about 2% in patients who had VTE provoked by a transient risk factor, to about 10% in those with an unprovoked VTE or a continuing risk factor for thrombosis. There is some evidence that older age may be associated with a higher risk of recurrent VTE after anticoagulants are stopped, but this is uncertain and poorly quantified.

PATHOPHYSIOLOGY

Venous stasis and damage to the vessel wall predispose to thrombosis. Venous stasis is produced by immobility, obstruction or dilatation of veins, increased venous pressure, and increased blood viscosity. The critical role of stasis in the pathogenesis of venous thrombosis is illustrated by the observation that thrombosis occurs with equal frequency in the two legs of paraplegic patients but occurs with much greater frequency in the paralyzed limb than in the nonparalyzed limb in stroke patients.

Venous thrombi usually arise at sites of vessel damage, or in the large venous sinuses of the calves, or the valve cusp pockets of the deep veins of the calves, and are composed predominantly of fibrin and red blood cells. Thrombosis occurs when blood coagulation overwhelms the natural anticoagulant and fibrinolytic systems. Coagulation is usually triggered by exposure of blood to tissue factor on the surface of activated monocytes that are attracted to sites of tissue damage or vascular trauma. Clinical risk factors that activate blood coagulation include extensive surgery, trauma, burns, malignant disease, myocardial infarction, cancer chemotherapy, and local hypoxia produced by venous stasis.

Tissue damage also results in impaired fibrinolysis, which occurs through the release of inflammatory cytokines in response to the damage. These cytokines induce endothelial cell synthesis of plasminogen activator inhibitor-1 (PAI-1) and reduce the protective effect of the vascular endothelium by downregulating the endothelial-bound anticoagulant thrombomodulin.

Stasis resulting from venous dilatation occurs in elderly patients, in patients with varicose veins, and in women who are pregnant or using supplemental estrogen. Venous obstruction contributes to the risk of venous thrombosis in patients with pelvic tumors. Increased blood viscosity, which also causes stasis, may explain the risk of thrombosis in patients with polycythemia vera, hypergammaglobulinemia, or chronic inflammatory disorders. Direct venous damage may lead to venous thrombosis in patients undergoing hip surgery, knee surgery, or varicose vein stripping and in patients with severe burns or trauma to the lower extremities.

Blood coagulation is modulated by circulating, or by endothelial cell-bound, inhibitors of thrombosis. The most important circulating inhibitors of coagulation are antithrombin, protein C, and protein S. An inherited deficiency of one of these three proteins is found in about 20% of patients who have a family history of VTE and whose first episode of VTE occurs before 41 years of age. Some types of congenital dysfibrinogenemias can also predispose patients to thrombosis, as can a congenital deficiency of plasminogen. However, these are rare causes of venous thrombosis in the elderly presenting with first VTE episode. An inherited thrombophilic defect known as activated protein C (APC) resistance, or factor V Leiden, is the most common cause of inherited thrombophilia, occurring in about 5% of whites who do not have a family history of VTE and in about 20% of patients with a first episode of VTE. One case–control study reported that factor V Leiden was not a risk factor for VTE in patients older than 70 years but associated with threefold increase in younger patients. The second most common thrombophilic defect is a mutation (G20210A) in the 3'-untranslated region of the prothrombin gene that results in about a 25% increase in prothrombin levels. This mutation is found in about 2% of whites with no family history of VTE and in about 5% of patients with a first episode

of VTE. Elevated levels of clotting factors VIII and XI also predispose patients to thrombosis. Randomized trials have shown that the administration of estrogens in the doses used for postmenopausal hormone replacement therapy increase the risk of a first or recurrent thromboembolism about threefold, with highest risk being within the first 6 months of starting therapy.

NATURAL HISTORY

Most venous thrombi produce no symptoms and are confined to the intramuscular and deep veins of the calf. Many calf vein thrombi undergo spontaneous lysis, but some extend into the popliteal and more proximal veins. Complete lysis of proximal vein thrombosis is less common. Most symptomatic pulmonary emboli and virtually all fatal emboli arise from thrombi in the proximal veins of the legs.

Although venous thrombosis can occur in any vein in the body, it usually involves superficial or deep veins of the legs. Thrombosis in a superficial vein of the leg is generally benign and self-limiting but can be serious if it extends from the long saphenous vein into the common femoral vein. Superficial thrombophlebitis is easily recognized by the presence of a tender vein surrounded by an area of erythema, heat, and edema. A thrombus can often be palpated in the affected vein. Thrombosis involving the deep veins of the leg maybe confined to calf veins or may extend into the popliteal or more proximal veins. Thrombi confined to calf veins are usually small, often asymptomatic, and are rarely associated with PE. About 20% of calf vein thrombi, however, extend into the popliteal vein and beyond, where they can cause serious complications. In most cases, extension of calf vein thrombosis occurs within a week. About 50% of patients with symptomatic proximal vein thrombosis also have clinically silent PE, and about 70% of patients with symptomatic PE have DVT, which is usually clinically silent. Untreated or inadequately treated VTE is associated with a high rate of complications, with about 50% of untreated proximal vein thrombi undergoing symptomatic extension or embolization (see "Treatment").

Acute Consequences of Venous Thromboembolism

In general, one-third to one-half of first episodes of VTE present as PE, the remainder presenting as DVT. It is estimated that about 10% of symptomatic PE are rapidly fatal and that about 5% of patients that are treated for PE die of a recurrence (mostly within the first 3 months). There is evidence that in the elderly, a larger proportion of episodes of VTE presents as PE and, when PE occurs, it is more likely to be fatal (i.e., four times higher than in patients 45 years of age or younger). In patients who are being closely monitored (e.g., in clinical trials), about 5% of recurrent episodes of VTE that occur after anticoagulants have been stopped are fatal. If the initial episode of VTE is a PE, recurrent episodes are also more likely to be a PE than DVT and, therefore, are more likely to be fatal. As with a first episode of VTE, the case-fatality of recurrent episodes of thrombosis may be higher in the elderly although this is uncertain.

Chronic Complications of Venous Thromboembolism

While PE is the most serious and most feared complication of venous thrombosis, important chronic conditions may also occur after acute VTE. Postthrombotic syndrome is the most frequent chronic complication of DVT of the leg. Characterized by pain and swelling, it is responsible for considerable personal disability, reduced quality of life, and substantial health care costs (estimated at $250 million per year in North America). The postthrombotic syndrome occurs as a long-term complication in about 25% (and is severe in about 10%) of patients with symptomatic proximal vein thrombosis in the 8 years after the acute event, with most cases developing within 2 years. The postthrombotic syndrome typically presents as chronic leg pain and swelling, which is worse at the end of the day. Some patients also have stasis pigmentation, induration, and skin ulceration. In a minority of patients, there is venous claudication on walking, caused by persistent obstruction in the iliac veins. Chronic pulmonary hypertension is a more serious complication that occurs in about 4% of patients within 2 years of treated PE.

DIAGNOSIS

Deep Vein Thrombosis (Tables 105-1 and 105-2)

Clinical Features

The clinical features of DVT include localized swelling, redness, tenderness, and distal edema. As these symptoms are nonspecific, the diagnosis should always be confirmed by objective investigations. However, clinical assessment does allow division of patients into low, moderate, and high probabilities of DVT, corresponding to prevalence of 15%, 25%, and 60%, respectively. Clinical prediction rules, such as the Well's Score, are based on four factors; (1)

TABLE 105-1

Model for Determining Clinical Suspicion of Deep Vein Thrombosis

VARIABLES	POINTS*
Active cancer (treatment ongoing or within previous 6 mo or palliative)	1
Paralysis, paresis, or recent plaster immobilization of the lower extremities	1
Recently bedridden for more than 3 d, or major surgery within the past 4 wk	1
Localized tenderness along the distribution of the deep venous system	1
Entire leg swollen	1
Affected calf 3 cm greater than asymptomatic calf (measured 10 cm below tibial tuberosity)	1
Pitting edema confined to the symptomatic leg	1
Dilated superficial veins (nonvaricose)	1
Alternative diagnosis is at least as likely as that of deep vein thrombosis	–2
Total points	

*Pretest probability is calculated as follows: total points, ≤0, low probability; 1 to 2, moderate probability; ≥ 3, high probability.

the presence or absence of risk factors (e.g., recent immobilization, hospitalization within the past month, or malignancy), (2) symptoms and signs at presentation are considered typical or atypical, and their severity, (3) severity of symptoms and signs, and (4) whether there is an alternative explanation for the symptoms and signs considered at least as likely as DVT (Table 105-1). The conditions

TABLE 105-2

Test Results That Effectively Confirm or Exclude Deep Vein Thrombosis

PURPOSE	TEST	SIGNIFICANT RESULT
Diagnostic for first DVT	Venography	Intraluminal filling defect
	Venous ultrasonography	Noncompressible proximal veins at two or more of the common femoral, popliteal, and calf trifurcation sites*
Excludes first DVT	Venography	All deep veins seen, and no intraluminal filling defects
	D-dimer	Negative result on a test that has at least a moderately high sensitivity (≥85%) and specificity (≥70%) and (1) normal results on venous ultrasonography of the proximal veins or (2) low clinical suspicion of DVT at presentation
		Negative result on a test that has a high sensitivity (≥98%)
	Venous ultrasonography	Normal proximal veins and (1) low clinical suspicion for DVT at presentation, or (2) normal D-dimer test at presentation, or (3) normal second test after 7 d
		Normal proximal and distal veins*
Diagnostic for recurrent DVT	Venography	Intraluminal filling defect
	Venous ultrasonography	(1) A new noncompressible common femoral or popliteal vein segment or (2) a ≥ 4.0 mm increase in diameter of the common or popliteal vein since a previous test†
Excludes recurrent DVT	Venography	All deep veins seen and no intraluminal filling defects
	Venous ultrasonography	Normal or ≤ 1 mm increase in diameter of the common femoral or popliteal veins on venous ultrasound since a previous test and continuing normal results (no progression of venous ultrasound) at 2 and 7 d
	D-dimer	Results as described as for a first episode of DVT; however, these criteria are less well evaluated for diagnosis of recurrence

*The accuracy of, and need to treat, isolated distal vein abnormalities on ultrasound are uncertain. For this reason, and because examination of the calf veins is difficult to perform, many centers confine the examination to the proximal veins.
†If other evidence is not consistent with recurrent DVT (e.g., clinical assessment, or D-dimer), venography should be considered.

that are most likely to simulate DVT are ruptured Baker cyst, cellulitis, muscle tear, muscle cramp, muscle hematoma, external venous compression, superficial thrombophlebitis, and the postthrombotic syndrome. The prevalence of VTE is higher in the elderly who are investigated, compared to younger patients.

Diagnostic Testing

Four objective tests—venography, impedance plethysmography, and venous ultrasonography, and D-dimer testing—have been rigorously evaluated for the diagnosis of DVT. Impedence plethysmography is now used infrequently, and will not be considered in the following review. Magnetic resonance venography and computed tomography (CT) venography appear to be promising new modalities but are less well evaluated.

Venography
Venography provides the reference standard for diagnosis of DVT. It involves the injection of a radiocontrast agent into a distal vein. Venography detects both proximal vein thrombosis and calf vein thrombosis. However, it is technically difficult, expensive, requires injection of contrast dye and can be painful. Since contrast dye can cause allergic reactions or exacerbate renal impairment, venography is usually reserved to resolve discrepancies between findings on venous ultrasonography and clinical assessment of probability of DVT, or when venous ultrasonography is nondiagnostic (often in patients with previous DVT). The increased prevalence of renal impairment makes venography an even less attractive investigation option in the elderly.

Venous Ultrasonography
Venous ultrasonography is the noninvasive imaging method of choice for diagnosing DVT. It is not painful and it is easier to perform than venography. The common femoral vein, femoral vein, popliteal vein, and calf vein trifurcation (i.e., very proximal deep calf veins) are imaged in real time and compressed with the transducer probe. Inability to fully compress or obliterate the vein is diagnostic of DVT. Duplex ultrasonography, which combines real-time imaging with pulsed Doppler and color-coded Doppler technology, facilitates imaging of the deep veins of the calf.

Venous ultrasonography is highly accurate for the detection of proximal vein thrombosis in symptomatic patients, with reported sensitivity and specificity approaching 95%. The sensitivity for symptomatic calf vein thrombosis is considerably lower and appears to be operator dependent. For this reason, many centers do not examine the deep veins of the calf with ultrasonography. Instead, if the initial test excludes proximal DVT, anticoagulants are withheld and the test is repeated in 7 days to exclude progression of a calf vein thrombosis not identified at the initial presentation. If the test remains negative after 7 days, the risk that thrombus is present and will subsequently extend to the proximal veins is negligible, and it is safe to continue withholding treatment.

While ultrasonography is an accurate test, if the results are inconsistent with the pretest probability, further investigations maybe warranted. For example, if the pretest clinical suspicion for DVT is low and the ultrasound shows a localized abnormality (i.e., less convincing findings), or if clinical suspicion is high and the ultrasound is normal, venography should be considered. In about one quarter of such cases, the results of venography differ from those of the ultrasound. Because the prevalence of DVT is only about 2% (most of which is distal), a follow-up test is not necessary when the clinical suspicion of thrombosis is low and the result of an initial proximal venous ultrasound is normal.

D-dimer Blood Testing
D-dimer is formed when cross-linked fibrin in thrombi is broken down by plasmin; thus, elevated levels of D-dimer can be used to detect DVT and PE. A variety of D-dimer assays are available, and they vary markedly in their accuracy as diagnostic tests for VTE.

All D-dimer assays have a low specificity for DVT and, therefore, an abnormal result is associated with a low positive predictive value and cannot be used to diagnose DVT. D-dimer assays that are used for diagnosis of VTE can be divided into two groups based on their sensitivity and specificity. Very highly sensitive D-dimer assays (e.g., sensitivity $\geq$ 98%; specificity ~40%) have a sufficiently high negative predictive value ($\geq$98%) that a normal result can be used to exclude VTE without the need to perform additional diagnostic testing. Moderate to highly sensitive D-dimer assays (sensitivity 85% to 97%; specificity 50% to 70%) need to have a negative result combined with another assessment that identifies patients as having a lower prevalence of VTE in order to exclude DVT or PE. Management studies have shown that it is safe to withhold anticoagulant therapy in patients who have a normal result on a moderately sensitive D-dimer test in combination with (1) a low clinical suspicion for DVT or (2) a normal result on venous ultrasonography of the proximal veins. Baseline D-dimer levels are known to increase with age. Therefore, D-dimer testing are much less specific and, therefore, of less clinical utility (fewer negative tests among those without venous thrombosis) in the elderly. Also, D-dimer testing has less clinical utility among patients with a high clinical suspicion of VTE as negative results are rarely obtained, and the predictive value of a negative test is lower in this group, because of a higher prevalence of disease.

Recurrent Deep Vein Thrombosis

The diagnosis of acute recurrent DVT can be difficult. A negative D-dimer test can exclude recurrent DVT, although the safety of this approach has been less well evaluated than for first episodes of DVT, and D-dimer test is less often negative compared with patients without a history of venous thrombosis. If D-dimer testing is positive, or has not been performed, venous ultrasonography is performed. If the result is normal, the test should be repeated twice over the next 7 to 10 days. If the result is positive in the popliteal or common femoral vein segments, and the result of the previous test was negative at the same site, a recurrence is diagnosed. This diagnosis can also be made if venous ultrasonography shows other convincing evidence of more extensive thrombosis than was seen on a previous examination (e.g., an increase in thrombus diameter of $\geq$4 mm at the inguinal ligament or the mid-popliteal fossa; unequivocal extension within the femoral vein of the thigh). If findings on venous ultrasonography are equivocal, as compared with a previous scan, or a previous scan is not available for comparison, venography should be performed or the test can be repeated twice over the next 7 to 10 days to detect extension of thrombosis. If the venogram shows a new intraluminal filling defect or evidence of thrombus extension since a previous venogram, recurrent DVT is diagnosed. If the venogram outlines all of the deep veins and does not show an intraluminal filling defect, recurrent DVT is excluded. If the venogram is nondiagnostic (i.e., nonfilling of segments of the deep veins), the patient

TABLE 105-3

Model for Determining a Clinical Suspicion of Pulmonary Embolism

VARIABLES	POINTS*
Clinical signs and symptoms of deep vein thrombosis (minimum leg swelling and pain with palpation of the deep veins)	3.0
An alternative diagnosis is less likely than pulmonary embolism	3.0
Heart rate > 100 beats/min	1.5
Immobilization or surgery in the previous 4 wk	1.5
Previous deep vein thrombosis/pulmonary embolism	1.5
Hemoptysis	1.0
Malignancy (treatment ongoing or within previous 6 mo or palliative)	1.0
Total points	

*Pretest probability is calculated as follows: a total score of ≤ 4 indicates a low probability (also termed "unlikely"); a score of 4.5 to 6 indicates moderate probability; and a score of > 6 indicates high probability.

can be followed with repeat venous ultrasonography (as described above) or recurrent DVT can be diagnosed based on the results of all assessments, including clinical features.

Pulmonary Embolism (Tables 105-3 and 105-4)

Clinical Features

Dyspnea is the most common symptom of PE. Chest pain is also common; it is usually pleuritic but can be substernal and compressive. Tachycardia is relatively common and hemoptysis is less frequent. Although most patients with PE also have DVT, fewer than 25% have associated clinical features. However, the clinical features of PE, like those of DVT, are nonspecific, and in only about one quarter of patients suspected with PE is the diagnosis confirmed by objective tests. Furthermore, elderly patients are more likely to

present with atypical symptoms and signs such as fatigue, dizziness, and syncope.

In the past, clinical assessment of the probability of PE was not standardized; physicians made the assessment informally on the basis of their experience and the results of initial routine tests (e.g., chest x-ray and electrocardiogram). Two groups have published explicit criteria for determining the clinical probability of PE. The model created by Wells and colleagues incorporates an assessment of symptoms and signs, the presence of an alternative diagnosis to account for the patient's condition, and the presence of risk factors for VTE. With this model, a patient's clinical probability of PE can be categorized as low or unlikely (prevalence of PE <10%), moderate (prevalence ~ 25%), or high (prevalence of 60%) (Table 105-2).

Diagnostic Tests

Chest Radiography and Electrocardiography In patients with PE, chest x-rays show either normal or nonspecific findings. Chest radiography, however, is useful for exclusion of pneumothorax and other conditions that can simulate PE. The electrocardiogram also frequently shows normal or nonspecific findings, but it is valuable for excluding acute cardiac conditions (e.g., myocardial infarction, acute pericarditis). In the appropriate clinical setting, electrocardiographic (ECG) evidence of right ventricular strain suggests PE.

Pulmonary Angiography Pulmonary angiography is considered the reference standard for PE, however, it is now rarely performed as it is invasive and can usually be replaced by computed tomographic pulmonary angiography (CTPA). Pulmonary angiography can be complicated by arrhythmias, cardiac perforation, cardiac arrest, and hypersensitivity to the contrast medium. Complications occur in 3% to 4% of patients undergoing pulmonary angiography.

Ventilation–Perfusion Lung Scanning In the past, ventilation–perfusion lung scanning was the most important test for diagnosing PE. More recently, CTPA has supplanted lung scanning, although

TABLE 105-4

Test Results that Effectively Confirm or Exclude Pulmonary Embolism

CONCLUSION	TEST	RESULT
Diagnostic for PE	Pulmonary angiography	Intraluminal filling defect
	CT pulmonary angiography (CTPA)	Intraluminal filling defect in a main or lobar or segmental pulmonary artery and moderate/high clinical probability
	Ventilation–perfusion scan	High-probability scan and moderate/high clinical probability
	Tests for DVT*	Evidence of acute DVT with nondiagnostic ventilation-perfusion scan or CTPA
Excludes PE	Pulmonary angiography	Normal
	CT pulmonary angiography	Negative†
	Lung perfusion scan	Normal
	High-sensitivity D-dimer test‡	Negative
	Moderate-sensitivity D-dimer test§	Negative, plus (1) low clinical suspicion of PE or (2) normal alveolar dead space fraction or (3) nondiagnostic lung scan and negative ultrasonography of proximal leg veins
	Combination of clinical assessment, ventilation-perfusion scan, ultrasonography of proximal leg vein	Low clinical suspicion, nondiagnostic scan, and negative ultrasonography

DVT, deep vein thrombosis; PE, pulmonary embolism.
*See Table 105-3.
†If high clinical suspicion, supplemental bilateral ultrasonography of the proximal leg veins is recommended.
‡D-dimer assay with very high sensitivity (i.e., 98%) and at least moderate specificity (i.e., 40%).
§ D-dimer assay with at least moderately high sensitivity (i.e., 85%) and specificity (i.e., 70%).

lung scanning is still used, particularly when CTPA is contraindicated because of renal failure or associated radiation exposure to the chest (e.g., in young women). A normal perfusion scan excludes a diagnosis of PE, however, a normal result is only obtained in about 25% of consecutive patients with suspected PE and an even smaller proportion of elderly patients. An abnormal perfusion scan is nonspecific. Ventilation imaging improves the specificity of perfusion scanning for the diagnosis of PE; when the ventilation scan is normal at the site of a segmental or larger perfusion defect, the prevalence of PE is 85% or higher (termed a "high probability" lung scan, which justifies anticoagulant therapy). About half of patients who have PE have a "high probability" lung scan. Therefore, among consecutive patients who are investigated for PE, about 25% have a normal perfusion scan and can have the diagnosis excluded, about 15% have a "high probability scan" and can (provided clinical probability is not low) have PE diagnosed, and about 60% have an abnormal but nondiagnostic lung scan that requires further diagnostic testing.

Computed Tomographic Pulmonary Angiography

CTPA, performed using helical CT (also known as spiral or continuous volume CT), is able to directly visualize the pulmonary arteries. Helical CT technology has rapidly advanced from use of single detector scanners to use of progressively larger numbers of detectors (termed multidetector CT) and enables more detailed examination of the pulmonary arteries.

Current evidence from the PIOPED II study suggests that CTPA is nondiagnostic in 6% of patients, and that among adequate examinations, sensitivity is 83%, specificity is 96%, positive predictive value is 86%, and negative predictive value is 95%. Accuracy varies according to the size of the largest pulmonary artery involved: positive predictive value was 97% for abnormalities in the main or lobar artery, 68% for those in segmental arteries, and 25% for subsegmental abnormalities (4% of pulmonary emboli in this study). Predictive values were also influenced by clinical assessment of PE probability; positive predictive value was 96% with high, 92% with intermediate, and 58% with low clinical probability (8% of patients); negative predictive value was 96% with low, 89% with intermediate, and 60% with high clinical probability (3% of patients).

The ability of CTPA to exclude PE has also been evaluated in management studies in which anticoagulant therapy was withheld in patients with negative CTPA. More recent studies suggest that less than 2% of patients with a negative CTPA for PE will return with symptomatic VTE during follow-up.

Magnetic resonance imaging (MRI) is less well evaluated than helical CT for the diagnosis of PE and is expected to be less accurate. Both helical CT and MRI have the advantage of being able to identify alternative pulmonary diagnoses. MRI does not expose the patient to radiation. Both MRI and helical CT can be extended to look for concomitant DVT.

D-dimer Blood Testing

As was discussed for evaluation of suspected DVT, D-dimer testing is also a valuable test for the exclusion of PE, either used alone (very sensitive D-dimer assay) or in combination with other assessments that are associated with a reduced prevalence of PE (e.g., low clinical probability for PE; nondiagnostic ventilation–perfusion scan in combination with a negative ultrasound of proximal lower limb veins [see below]).

Compression Ultrasonography

Compression ultrasonography, usually evaluating the proximal deep veins of the legs, can aid in the diagnosis of PE. Demonstration of DVT, which occurs in about 5% of patients with nondiagnostic ventilation–perfusion lung scans, can serve as indirect evidence of PE. Exclusion of proximal DVT does not rule out PE in a patient with a nondiagnostic ventilation–perfusion scan, although it does reduce that probability somewhat. However, if there are no proximal DVT on the day of presentation, and if no proximal DVT are detected on two subsequent examination 1 and 2 weeks later (DVT is diagnosed during serial testing in ~2% of patients), anticoagulant therapy can be withheld with a very low risk that patients will return with VTE (less than 2% during 3 months of follow-up). Earlier studies that evaluated CTPA suggested that a negative result did not exclude PE and, therefore, should be followed by bilateral ultrasonography of the proximal veins. However, more recent studies of CTPA, which used mostly multidector scanners, do not support the need for routine ultrasonography of the proximal deep veins in patients with a negative CTPA. Instead, it appears to be reasonable to only perform ultrasonography of the proximal deep veins in patients with a negative CTPA if clinical suspicion for PE is high. As for patients who have nondiagnostic ventilation–perfusion lung scans, withholding of anticoagulant therapy and performance of serial ultrasonography is a reasonable approach to management of patients who have a CTPA that is suspicious for isolated subsegmental PE.

Uncommon Thromboembolic Disorders

Subclavian or Axillary Veins

Thrombosis of the subclavian or axillary veins may be idiopathic or may occur as a complication of local vascular damage. It is now most frequently seen as a complication of chronic indwelling catheter use, but it also occurs as a complication after mastectomy and local radiotherapy for breast cancer. Idiopathic subclavian or axillary vein thrombosis may occur in young muscular individuals and maybe preceded by repetitive, strenuous activity involving the affected arm. Some of these persons have a fixed stenosis of the subclavian vein that is thought to be caused by compression of the vein between the first rib and the clavicle. Thrombosis of the subclavian vein or the superior vena cava is a rare complication of a transvenous cardiac pacemaker.

Subclavian or axillary thrombosis causes pain, edema, and cyanosis of the arm. In rare cases, the thrombosis extends into the superior vena cava and causes edema and cyanosis of the face and neck.

Definitive diagnosis is made by venography, venous ultrasonography, or CT angiography. Subclavian or axillary vein thrombosis is treated with anticoagulants using a similar approach for lower limb DVT and PE (see "Treatment"). Regional or systemic thrombolytic therapy is usually reserved for select young patients without contraindications.

Mesenteric Vein

An uncommon disorder, mesenteric vein thrombosis usually occurs in the sixth or seventh decade of life. It generally involves segments of the small bowel, leading to hemorrhagic infarction. Affected patients often have associated disorders, such as inflammatory bowel disease, malignancy, portal hypertension, familial thrombophilia, or polycythemia vera, or they may have a history of recent abdominal surgery. In about 20% of cases, no underlying cause is found.

The clinical manifestations of mesenteric vein thrombosis include intermittent abdominal pain, abdominal distention, vomiting, diarrhea, and melena. Blunt, semiopaque indentations of the bowel lumen ("thumbprinting") caused by mucosal edema, or gas in the wall of the bowel or the portal vein, or free peritoneal air may occur secondary to bowel infarction. CT, which shows an intraluminal filling defect in the mesenteric vein, is the diagnostic test of choice, and both Doppler ultrasonography and MRI are also helpful. Management includes acute and long-term anticoagulation, supportive care and surgery if bowel resection is being considered, followed by anticoagulant therapy. Mortality is about 30%, and up to 30% of patients experience recurrence.

Renal Vein Thrombosis

Renal vein thrombosis can be idiopathic or a complication of the nephrotic syndrome. Patients maybe asymptomatic or may present with abdominal, back, or flank pain and tenderness. PE is a relatively common complication of renal vein thrombosis. Anticoagulant therapy results in a gradual improvement in renal function, but patients may have long-standing proteinuria. Thrombolytic agents have been used, but the data are inadequate for critical appraisal of this form of treatment.

TREATMENT OF VENOUS THROMBOEMBOLISM

A detailed review of anticoagulants is provided in Chapter 106.

Management of Acute Venous Thromboembolism

Overview

The objectives of treating patients with VTE are to prevent PE, the postthrombotic syndrome, thromboembolic pulmonary hypertension, recurrent VTE and to alleviate the discomfort of the acute event.

Superficial venous thrombosis usually can be treated conservatively with anti-inflammatory drugs. If superficial phlebitis is extensive or very symptomatic, a 2- to 4-week course of heparin or low-molecular-weight heparin (LMWH) therapy can be used. In patients with DVT or PE, anticoagulants reduce morbidity and mortality from recurrent DVT and PE. Vena caval interruption is generally used only if anticoagulant therapy has failed or is contraindicated because of the risk of serious hemorrhage. Retrievable inferior caval filters are an option in patients with an expected temporary contraindication to anticoagulants (e.g., acute VTE less than 2 weeks before major surgery).

Thrombolytic therapy is more effective than heparin in achieving early lysis of VTE and can reduce mortality in patients with massive PE associated with shock. A regimen of 100 mg of rt-PA administered over 2 hours is generally recommended. The role of thrombolytic therapy in the treatment of DVT is uncertain. Systemic thrombolytic therapy increases lysis of DVT, and may reduce the risk of developing the postthrombotic syndrome, however, it increases the frequency of major bleeding, including intracranial hemorrhage. Thromboendarterectomy is effective in selected cases of

chronic thromboembolic pulmonary hypertension caused by proximal pulmonary arterial obstruction. Routine early use of graduated compression stockings for 2 years has been reported to reduce the incidence of the postthrombotic syndrome by about 50%.

Anticoagulant Therapy

Anticoagulants are the mainstay of treatment for most patients with VTE. In the past, the initial treatment of choice was heparin administered by continuous intravenous infusion or subcutaneous injection in doses sufficient to produce an adequate anticoagulant response. Current evidence indicates that LMWH administered by subcutaneous injection without laboratory monitoring is at least as effective and safe as heparin given intravenously.

Heparin therapy is usually monitored by the activated Partial Thromboplastin time (aPTT) and less frequently by heparin assays, which measure the ability of heparin to accelerate the inactivation of factor Xa or thrombin by antithrombin. The starting dose of intravenous heparin is a bolus of 80 U/kg (or a set dose of 5000 U) followed by an initial infusion of 18 U/kg/h (or a set dose of about 1300 U/h). The anticoagulant effect should be monitored every 6 hours until the aPTT is in the therapeutic range, and then daily. The therapeutic range of aPTT is equivalent to a heparin level between 0.35 and 7.0 U/mL as measured by an antifactor Xa assay. For many aPTT reagents, this range is an aPTT ratio of 1.8 to 2.5 times the mean of the normal laboratory control value. A recent study showed that acute VTE can be treated with subcutaneous, weight-adjusted, heparin without dose-adjustment and laboratory monitoring (initial dose of 333 U/kg followed by 250 U/kg every 12 hours).

LMWH is administered subcutaneously on a weight-adjusted basis at a dosage of about 100 anti-Xa U/kg every 12 hours or 150 to 200 anti-Xa units once daily. Monitoring is not required in the absence of marked renal impairment.

Treatment with heparin or LMWH is recommended for 5 to 6 days; warfarin therapy is started on the first or second day, overlapping the heparin therapy for 4 or 5 days, and is continued until an International Normalized Ratio (INR) of 2.0 is maintained for at least 24 hours. A 4- to 5-day period of overlap is necessary because the antithrombotic effects of oral anticoagulants are delayed. The initial course of heparin should be followed by warfarin for at least 3 months. Extended treatment with low-intensity warfarin (INR 1.5–2.0) is less effective than standard intensity (INR 2.0–3.0) and has not been shown to reduce bleeding. However, low-intensity warfarin has been used with less frequent INR monitoring (i.e., about every 2 months). Full to intermediate-dose LMWH can also be used in place of warfarin for long-term treatment and has been shown to be preferable to warfarin in patients with VTE and active cancer.

Duration of Anticoagulant Therapy During the past decade, a series of well-designed studies has helped to define the optimal duration of anticoagulation. The findings of these studies are summarized in Table 105-5. Whether anticoagulant therapy (INR = 2.0–3.0) for proximal DVT or PE is recommended for 3 months, or an indefinite period (with annual review), depends primarily on the presence of a provoking risk factor for VTE (i.e., transient risk factor, no risk factor, or cancer), risk factors for bleeding, and patient preference (i.e., burden associated with treatment). Secondary factors that support indefinite therapy for unprovoked VTE include a second episode of VTE and presentation with PE rather than DVT. A

TABLE 105-4

Findings from Randomized Controlled Trials and Observational Studies that Influence Optimal Duration of Oral Anticoagulant Therapy

- Shortening the duration of anticoagulation from 3 or 6 mo to 4 or 6 wk results in a doubling of the frequency of recurrent VTE during 1–2 yr of follow-up.
- Patients with VTE provoked by a transient risk factor have a lower (about one third) risk of recurrence than those with an unprovoked VTE or a persistent risk factor.
- Three months of anticoagulation is adequate treatment for VTE provoked by a transient risk factor; subsequent risk of recurrence is about 3% in the first year of follow-up.
- After about 3 mo of anticoagulation, recurrent DVT is as likely to involve the contralateral leg; this suggests that systemic rather than local (including inadequate treatment) factors are responsible for recurrences after 3 mo of treatment.
- There is a persistently elevated risk of recurrent VTE after a first episode of VTE; this appears to be about 10% in the first year, and about 30% in the first 5 yr, after 6 or more mo of treatment for an unprovoked proximal DVT or pulmonary embolism.
- Extending duration of anticoagulation beyond 3–6 or 12 mo may delay, but ultimately not reduce, the risk of recurrence if therapy is then stopped.
- After 3 mo of initial treatment of unprovoked VTE with oral anticoagulants targeted at an INR of 2.5 (INR range 2.0–3.0), continuing treatment with:
  —oral anticoagulants targeted at an INR of ~2.5 reduces the risk of recurrent VTE by over 90%;
  —oral anticoagulants targeted at an INR of ~1.75 reduces the risk of recurrent VTE by about 75%;
  —oral anticoagulants targeted to an INR of ~2.5 are more effective than using an INR target of ~1.75, without evidence of increased bleeding.
- A second episode of VTE predicts a higher risk of recurrence and favors indefinite anticoagulation after unprovoked VTE.
- Risk of recurrence is lower (about half) following an isolated calf (distal) DVT than after proximal DVT or PE; this favors a shorter duration of treatment.
- Risk of recurrence off treatment is similar after an episode of proximal DVT or PE.
- About 5% of recurrent episodes of VTE are expected to be fatal.
- Recurrent VTE is usually (about 60% of episodes) a PE after an initial PE, and usually (about 80% of episodes) a DVT after an initial DVT; this effect is expected to increase mortality from recurrent VTE by two- to threefold after a PE compared to after a DVT.
- Risk of recurrence is about threefold higher in patients with active cancer.
- Long-term treatment with low-molecular-weight heparin is more effective than warfarin in patients with VTE associated with cancer, and is a preferred option for such patients for at least 3 mo.
- Estrogen therapy is an important risk factor for first and recurrent episodes of VTE; consequently, if VTE occurred while on estrogen therapy, the risk of recurrent VTE is expected to be lowered by stopping estrogens.
- Risk of recurrence appears to be somewhat higher with antiphospholipid antibodies (anticardiolipin antibodies and/or lupus anticoagulants) and inherited thrombophilias.
- Males appear to have about a 50% higher risk of recurrent VTE than females.
- Other risk factors for recurrences may include: advanced age; elevated levels of clotting factors VIII, IX, XI and homocysteine; elevated D-dimer levels after stopping anticoagulant therapy; venal caval filters; and residual deep vein thrombosis on ultrasound; currently, these factors do not have clear implications for duration of treatment.
- The risk of anticoagulant-induced bleeding is highest during the first 3 mo of treatment and stabilizes after the first year.
- Risk of bleeding differs markedly among patients depending on the prevalence of risk factors (e.g., advanced age; previous bleeding or stroke; renal failure; anaemia; antiplatelet therapy; malignancy; poor anticoagulant control).
- About 10% of episodes of major bleeding are fatal.
- The risk of major bleeding in younger patients (e.g., younger than 60 yr) that do not have risk factors for bleeding and have good anticoagulant control (target INR 2–3) is about 1% per year. The risk of major bleeding is expected to be at least 10-fold higher in patients with multiple risk factors for bleeding.

key consideration in elderly patients is assessment of risk for major bleeding and we generally do not recommend indefinite anticoagulant therapy for a first unprovoked proximal DVT or PE in patients older than 75 years of age because of their increase risk of bleeding (see below).

Primary Prevention of Venous Thromboembolism

Overview

The most effective way of reducing the mortality associated with PE and the morbidity associated with the postthrombotic syndrome is to use primary prophylaxis in patients at high risk for VTE. Prophylaxis is achieved either by reducing blood coagulability or by preventing venous stasis using the following approaches: (1) low-dose subcutaneous heparin, (2) LMWHs, (3) fondaparinux, (4) coumarin anticoagulants, (5) graduated compression stockings, or (6) intermittent pneumatic compression of the legs. Antiplatelet agents, such as aspirin, are not recommended as sole therapy as they are less effective than the previously noted methods.

On the basis of well-defined clinical criteria, patients can be classified as being at low, moderate, or high risk for VTE, and the choice of prophylaxis should be tailored to the patient's risk of VTE and of bleeding (Table 105-6). In the absence of prophylaxis, the frequency of fatal postoperative PE ranges from 0.1% to 0.4% in patients undergoing elective general surgery and from 1% to 5% in patients undergoing elective hip or knee surgery, emergency hip surgery, major trauma, or spinal cord injury. Prophylaxis is cost-effective for most moderate and high-risk groups. Despite the merits of venous thromboprophylaxis, adherence with current guidelines for hospitalized patients is often poor, particularly in elderly patients.

Therapies

Low-dose heparin is given subcutaneously at a dose of 5000 units 2 hours before surgery and 5000 U every 8 or 12 hours after surgery. In patients undergoing major orthopedic surgical procedures, low-dose heparin is less effective than warfarin, LMWH, or fondaparinux and is not recommended. Intermittent pneumatic compression of the legs enhances blood flow in the deep veins and may increase

TABLE 105-5

Risk Categories for Venous Thromboembolism and Recommendations for Prophylaxis

	HIGH RISK	MODERATE RISK
Calf vein thrombosis	20%–50%	10%–20%
Proximal vein thrombosis	5%–20%	0.4%–5%
Fatal pulmonary embolism	2%–5%	0.1%–0.4%
Recommended prophylaxis	Low-molecular-weight heparin, oral anticoagulants, or fondaparinux (can be combined with graduated compression stockings or pneumatic compression)	Low-dose heparin, external pneumatic compression, or graduated compression stockings

*Usually asymptomatic and detected by screening venography about 10 days after surgery.

blood fibrinolytic activity. This method of prophylaxis is particularly useful in patients who have a high risk of serious bleeding. It is the method of choice for preventing venous thrombosis in patients undergoing neurosurgery, is effective in patients undergoing major knee surgery, and is as effective as low-dose heparin in patients undergoing abdominal surgery.

Graduated compression stockings reduce venous stasis and prevent postoperative venous thrombosis in general surgical patients and in medical or surgical patients with neurologic disorders, including paralysis of the lower limbs. In surgical patients, the combined use of graduated compression stockings and low-dose heparin is more effective than use of low-dose heparin alone.

Standard-dose warfarin (INR = 2.0–3.0) is effective for preventing postoperative VTE and is started at the time of surgery, or in the early postoperative period. Because it is complex to use, warfarin is generally reserved for patients at very high risk, including patients with hip fractures and those who undergo joint replacement.

LMWH is a safe and effective form of prophylaxis in high-risk patients undergoing elective hip surgery, major general surgery, or major knee surgery, as well as in patients who have experienced hip fracture, spinal injury, or acute medical illness. LMWH is more effective than low-dose heparin in high-risk patients.

In patients who undergo hip or major knee surgery, LMWH is more effective than warfarin while patients are in hospital but is associated with more frequent bleeding; both of these differences may be caused by a more rapid onset of anticoagulation with LMWH. Fondaparinux reduces the frequency of venographically detected DVT (about 10 days after surgery) by 50% compared to LMWH but causes a small increase in bleeding.

Indications for Venous Thromboembolism Prophylaxis

General Surgery and Medicine

Low-dose heparin or LMWH prophylaxis is the method of choice for moderate-risk general surgical and medical patients. It reduces the risk of VTE by 50% to 70% and is simple, inexpensive, convenient, and safe. Heparin-induced thrombocytopenia may occur, particularly in surgical patients who receive heparin for more than 5 days. If anticoagulants are contraindicated because of an unusually high risk of bleeding, graduated compression stockings, intermittent pneumatic compression of the legs, or both, should be used.

Major Orthopedic Surgery LMWH, fondaparinux, or oral anticoagulants provide effective prophylaxis for VTE in patients who have undergone hip surgery. LMWH, warfarin, fondaparinux, and intermittent pneumatic compression are effective in preventing VTE in patients undergoing major knee surgery.

Extended prophylaxis with LWMH, fondaparinux, or warfarin for an additional 3 weeks after hospital discharge should be considered after major orthopedic surgery and is strongly recommended for high-risk patients (e.g., those with previous VTE or active cancer). If extended prophylaxis with LMWH or fondaparinux is not used, there is indirect evidence supporting use of aspirin for 1 month after stopping anticoagulant therapy.

Genitourinary Surgery, Neurosurgery, and Ocular Surgery Intermittent pneumatic compression, with or without graduated compression stockings, is effective prophylaxis for VTE and does not increase the risk of bleeding.

Complications of Antithrombotic Agents

Risks of Major Bleeding

Bleeding is the main complication of antithrombotic therapy. "Major bleeding" is usually defined as clinically overt bleeding that results in a 2 gm/dL drop in hemoglobin, the need for transfusion or hospitalization, or serious residual consequences. With all antithrombotic agents, the risk of bleeding is influenced by the dose and by patient-related factors, the most important being recent surgery or trauma. Other patient characteristics that increase the risk of bleeding are older age, recent stroke, generalized hemostatic defect, a history of gastrointestinal hemorrhage, renal failure, and other serious comorbid conditions.

With heparin, the incidence of bleeding is influenced by dosage; independently of dosage, there is no clear relationship between bleeding and the aPTT. Bleeding rates appear to be lower with LMWH than with intravenous heparin.

Bleeding associated with coumarin anticoagulants is influenced by the intensity of anticoagulant therapy, particularly with progressive increases of the INR above 3.0. A study that compared long-term treatment of VTE with warfarin targeted to an INR of 1.75 compared with an INR of 2.5 found no difference in the rates of bleeding, suggesting that differences in the INR between 1.5 and 3.0 are not associated with clinically important difference in bleeding risk. Both heparin-induced bleeding and warfarin-induced bleeding are increased by concomitant use of aspirin, which impairs platelet function and produces gastric erosions. When the INR is less than 3.0, coumarin-associated bleeding frequently has an obvious underlying cause or is from an occult gastrointestinal or renal lesion.

Long-term anticoagulant therapy is associated with an average annual risk of major bleeding of about 1% to 3%. Advanced age is an independent risk factor for anticoagulant-induced major bleeding with patients greater than 65 years of age having a twofold or greater risk of bleeding than younger patients.

Intensity of anticoagulation is the strongest predictor of major bleeding and avoiding INR values above 3.0 appears to be particularly important in the elderly. This was most clearly shown in the Stroke Prevention in Atrial Fibrillation II (SPAF II) study that compared oral anitcoagulation (INR 2.0–4.5) with aspirin. In the subgroup of patients older than 75 years of age, much of the benefit of anticoagulant therapy was lost because of a high frequency of intracranial bleeding that was attributable to the high intensity of anticoagulation. Additional risk factors for bleeding include (1) previous history of bleeding (e.g., gastrointestinal or intracerebral), (2) previous noncardioembolic stroke, (3) renal failure, (4) anemia, (5) erratic control of anticoagulant therapy, (6) malignancy, and (7) concomitant use of antiplatelet therapy. The risk of anticoagulant-induced bleeding differs markedly among patients. Patients less than 65 years of age without risk factors for bleeding have an annual risk of major bleeding of about 1%. This risk maybe 10%/year or higher in patients with multiple risk factors. Careful control of anticoagulant therapy, with use of an expert clinical service and patient education, has been shown to reduce the risk of bleeding in the elderly.

Consequences of Bleeding in Elderly

On average, about 10% of major bleeds that occur in anticoagulated patients are fatal. The most feared type of bleed is intracranial hemorrhage that is fatal in about 70% of cases. The risk of life-threatening bleeds is three to four times higher in patients aged 80 years or older compared with patients 50 years of age or younger. This reflects both a higher frequency of bleeding and a higher incidence of intracranial hemorrhage in older patients (relative risk of 3.2 for age 75 years or older when compared with younger patients).

FURTHER READING

Beyth RJ, Quinn LM, Landefeld S. Prospective evaluation of an index for predicting the risk of major bleeding in outpatients treated with warfarin. *Am J Med.* 1998;105:91–99.

Bates SM, Ginsberg JS. Clinical practice. Treatment of deep-vein thrombosis. *N Engl J Med.* 2004;351(3):268–277.

Douketis JD, Kearon C, Bates S, Duku EK, Ginsberg JS. Risk of fatal pulmonary embolism in patients with treated venous thromboembolism. *JAMA.* 1998;279:458–462.

Lee AYY, Levine MN, Baker RI, et al.; for the Randomized Comparison of Low-Molecular-Weight Heparin versus Oral Anticoagulant Therapy for the Prevention of Recurrent Venous Thromboembolism in Patients with Cancer (CLOT) Investigators. Low-molecular-weight heparin versus a coumarin for the prevention of recurrent venous thromboembolism in patients with cancer. *N Engl J Med.* 2003;349:146–153.

Linkins L, Choi PT, Douketis JD. Clinical impact of bleeding in patients taking oral anticoagulant therapy for venous thromboembolism: a meta-analysis. *Ann Intern Med.* 2003;139:893–900.

Hirsh J, O'Donnell M, Weitz JI. New Anticoagulants. *Blood.* 2005;105(2):453–463.

Kearon C. Hirsh J. Venous thromboembolism. In: Dale DC, Federman DD, eds. *Scientific American Medicine. ACP Medicine Online.* New York, New York: WebMed Inc.; 2006. http://acpmedicine.com. [Chapter XVIII]. Accessed June 10. 2007.

Kearon C. Natural history of venous thromboembolism. *Circulation.* 2003;107(23, Suppl 1):I22–I30.

Kearon C. Diagnosis of pulmonary embolism. *CMAJ.* 2003;168(2):183–194.

Kearon C. Long-term management of patients after venous thromboembolism. *Circulation.* 2004;110(Suppl I):I-10–I-18.

McRae S, Ginsberg JS. Initial treatment of venous thromboembolism. *Circulation.* 2004;110(9, Suppl 1):I3–I9.

Rosenthaal FR, Van Hylckama A, Doggen CJM. Venous thrombosis in the elderly. *J Thromb Haemost.* 2007;5 (Suppl 1):310–317.

Wan S, Quinlan DJ, Agnelli G, Eikelboom JW. Thrombolysis compared with heparin for the initial treatment of pulmonary embolism: a meta-analysis of the randomized controlled trials. *Circulation.* 2004;110(6):744–749.

Wells PS. Integrated strategies for the diagnosis of venous thromboembolism. *J Thromb Haemost.* 2007;5(Suppl 1):41–50.

Wells PS, Anderson DR, Rodger M, et al. Evaluation of D-dimer in the diagnosis of suspected deep-vein thrombosis. *N Eng J Med.* 2003;349:1227–1235.

Hemorrhagic Disorders

Julia A. M. Anderson ■ *Agnes Y. Y. Lee*

Although hemorrhage caused by intracranial, aneurysmal, and gastrointestinal pathologies account for a significant proportion of all deaths in the older-than-60-year age group, fatal bleeding caused by primary defects in coagulation and platelets are less common. Nevertheless, the development of a bleeding diathesis in an elderly patient presents clinical challenges that form the focus of this chapter.

Hemostasis is a highly regulated process involving a dynamic balance between coagulation and fibrinolytic proteins and their inhibitors, platelets, and the vascular endothelium. The overall aim of the coagulation system is to rapidly generate a hemostatic plug at sites of vascular injury to prevent catastrophic blood loss from severed vessels. Congenital or acquired disturbances of the delicate balance between coagulation and fibrinolysis may result in thrombotic or hemorrhagic clinical manifestations.

Elderly patients more commonly present with acquired bleeding disorders, but occasionally a mild congenital bleeding diathesis may remain hidden until later years when surgical procedures become common, when comorbid disease develops (such as renal or hepatic dysfunction), or when an additional acquired condition creates an additive challenge to the hemostatic system, such as the introduction of antiplatelet agents or anticoagulant therapy. Focusing on bleeding in the elderly, this chapter (a) provides a brief overview of hemostatic mechanisms, (b) discusses the clinical assessment of an elderly patient with a history of bleeding, (c) details the main inherited and acquired hemorrhagic conditions and their presentation in an elderly population, and (d) outlines the treatment of elderly patients with hemorrhagic states.

OVERVIEW OF HEMOSTASIS

Following damage to the endothelium, blood is exposed to subendothelial components, such as von Willebrand factor (vWF) and collagen. Platelets adhere to the subendothelium and are activated, releasing substances that further recruit and activate platelets inducing platelet aggregation. A platelet plug is formed at the site of injury providing initial arrest of bleeding, in a process known as "primary hemostasis". A process referred to as "secondary hemostasis" follows to ensure stabilization of the platelet plug.

Vascular injury also exposes tissue factor (TF), a membrane-bound procoagulant factor that triggers the coagulation cascade. The coagulation cascade is a highly regulated series of enzymatic reactions involving the sequential conversion of proenzymes into their active forms. Activated platelets provide a phospholipid surface membrane on which coagulation enzymes localize and assemble into complexes that accelerate the serial enzymatic reactions. Such amplification processes translate a small initiating signal into an explosion of thrombin generation, thereby resulting in rapid fibrin formation. The polymerization of fibrin stabilizes the platelet plug and results in secondary hemostasis.

Removal of the fibrin clot takes place by activation of the fibrinolytic system. Plasminogen, a zymogen, is converted into plasmin, an enzyme that degrades the fibrin matrix of the clot into soluble fragments. Hemostatic mechanisms rely on dynamic interactions between platelets, the coagulation cascade, the fibrinolytic system, and the endothelium (see Figure 106-1). Disturbances of the equilibrium, caused by acquired or congenital factors, may result in unexpected or excessive bleeding or thrombosis.

Age-Related Effects on the Hemostatic System

Two large epidemiological studies of men and women aged 25 to 74 years (the MONICA Project), and 60 to 79 years, demonstrate a significant effect of the ageing process on coagulation factors, inhibitors, and activation markers. However, these age-related changes do not cause an increased tendency to hemorrhage; instead, increases in fibrinogen and coagulation factors VII (fVII), VIII (fVIII), IX (fIX), and vWF are greater than increases in the coagulation inhibitors, antithrombin (AT), protein C, and protein S, resulting in a tendency toward thrombosis. This net procoagulant

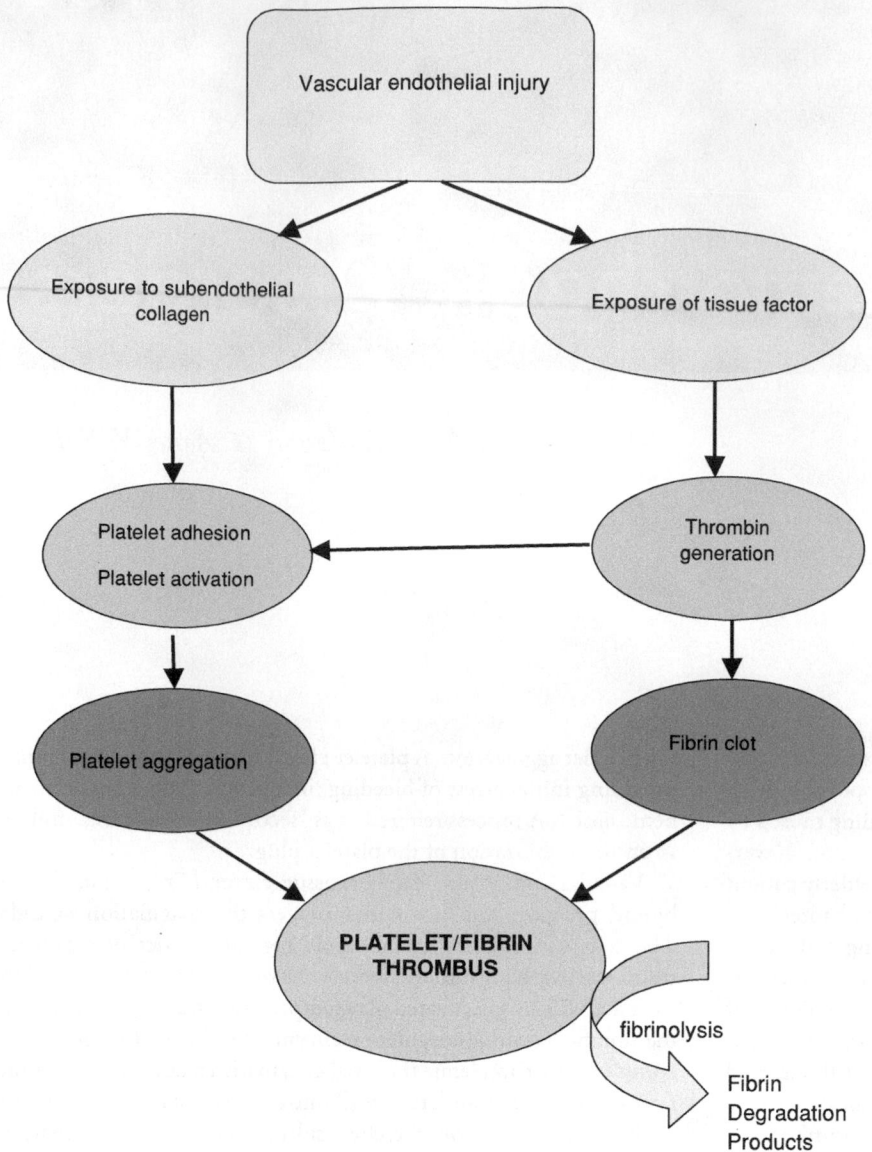

FIGURE 106-1. The hemostatic mechanism involves a dynamic relationship between the vascular endothelium, platelets, coagulation cascade, and fibrinolysis. Abnormalities of any parts of the system can cause a bleeding diathesis. (Modified with permission from Liaw PC, Weitz JI. Coagulation overview. Section 8. Hematologic problems. In Albert RK, Slutsky A, Ranieri M, Takala J, Torres A, eds. Clinical Critical Care Medicine. Philadelphia: Elsevier; 2006:543–553).

effect appears to be more pronounced in men than women, and is reflected by an increase in thrombin–AT complexes, high plasma levels of activation peptides cleaved from prothrombin, fIX, and factor X (fX), and minor changes in thromboelastograph variables. Levels of plasminogen activator inhibitor-1 (PAI-1), an inhibitor of the tissue plasminogen activator (tPA), also increase in an age-dependent manner, adding to the relative prothrombotic state with ageing.

Megakaryopoiesis does not appear to alter with the aging process. Platelets are present in similar numbers with only a normal or moderate reduction in life span compared with platelets in younger individuals.

CLINICAL APPROACH TO BLEEDING IN THE ELDERLY PATIENT

A patient may present for evaluation of new symptoms of bleeding or bruising, or may be referred postoperatively or postprocedurally following difficulty securing hemostasis. The immediate assessment

of a patient who has been bleeding intraoperatively can be particularly challenging from a laboratory viewpoint, and reassessment may be necessary several weeks later once the hemostatic system has had time to rebalance. Accurate historical details are essential in the overall evaluation process (see Table 106-1). Accompanying caregivers are often helpful in providing extra details about patients who cannot provide a reliable history.

Age of Onset of Symptoms

Bleeding issues that are lifelong are likely to hold a congenital basis, rather than a recently acquired etiology. An assessment of previous hemostatic challenges should be made, such as dental surgery, trauma, and operations, including operations commonly performed in childhood such as tonsillectomy and adenoidectomy. Bleeding around the time of childbirth may be more difficult to interpret, but the need for blood transfusion is valuable information that may point to the severity of hemorrhage. Congenital causes may manifest late in life if they are mild and the patient has not experienced any previous hemostatic challenges.

TABLE 106-1

Evaluation of Bleeding in the Elderly: Points of Historical Relevance

HISTORICAL DETAILS	POINTS TO ELICIT
When did the bleeding start?	Duration of symptoms Lifelong or recent onset?
Nature of the bleeding?	Spontaneous or post trauma/procedure? Epistaxis, gingival bleeding Previous history of menorrhagia Joint bleeds, muscle bleeds
How long did the bleeding persist?	
Was the bleeding immediate or delayed?	
Any other associated forms of bleeding?	Gastrointestinal, hematuria
Response to past operative or dental challenges Medications Diet	Dental extraction is a hemostatic challenge Include all recent medications Include herbal remedies Any history of malabsorption? Recent administration of antibiotics? Balanced diet?
Family history	Are male and female members of the family equally affected?
Other questions	Any comorbidity to exacerbate a bleeding tendency? Does the bleeding require urgent attention or is this an evaluation to assess the potential to bleed during future operations?

Bleeding Symptoms

The nature of bleeding symptoms may determine the etiology of the hemostatic defect: mucosal bleeding, epistaxis, and menorrhagia highlight defects in platelets or their interaction with the vascular wall; delayed bleeding, spontaneous hemarthroses, and muscle bleeds are consistent with coagulation factor deficiencies such as hemophilia. The significance of symptoms such as bruising, epistaxis, and menorrhagia may be challenging to define as there is a strong subjective component to each, and they are common symptoms. Sometimes it is useful to assess for any temporal changes in severity of these events. The clinician should also determine whether bleeding occurs spontaneously, or secondary to trauma or surgery.

Bruising, Purpura, Petechiae, and Ecchymoses

The term "purpura" refers to a spontaneous extravasation of blood from the capillaries into the skin. "Petechiae" are purpuric lesions of pin-head size and ecchymoses are larger lesions.

The location and extent of bruising may be indicative of an underlying bleeding disorder. For example, large ecchymoses, presenting on the trunk without known trauma, may suggest an underlying bleeding disorder, whereas minor bruising on extremities are more likely benign. In an older person with no prior history of bleeding, extensive or truncal ecchymoses may suggest the development of

an acquired coagulation disorder such as liver disease, disseminated intravascular coagulation (DIC), or acquired hemophilia.

Oral Mucosal Bleeding

Tonsillectomy, adenoidectomy, and dental extraction of the molar teeth create a significant hemostatic challenge, and the patient's response to the challenge is of historical importance; bleeding that required resuturing or excessive packing, or that continued for several hours to days is suggestive of an underlying hemostatic disorder.

Menorrhagia

This complaint is highly subjective and poorly correlates to actual blood loss; description of the passage of clots, a history of past iron-deficiency anemia, the requirement for blood transfusion or for hysterectomy at a young age may all highlight an underlying bleeding diathesis.

Gastrointestinal Bleeding, Hemoptysis, and Hematuria

These symptoms are usually caused by localized blood loss from underlying pathology; an acquired or congenital bleeding disorder may unmask the symptoms and make them more florid. In an older person, such bleeding should prompt urgent investigations for the underlying cause as bleeding from such sites could be potentially life-threatening and may be a harbinger of malignancy or other serious conditions.

Family History of Bleeding

A patient's first hemostatic challenge may occur in older age, leading to the presentation of a hidden mild congenital disorder. A careful family history should record any hemorrhagic events affecting family members, including immediate and more distant relatives. However, one-third of cases of hemophilia A and B arise as a result of *de novo* mutations in whom there may be no family history. Female carriers of factor VIII (fVIII) or factor IX (fIX) deficiency, or male patients with mild hemophilia may have no bleeding history if coagulation factor levels are greater than 30% to 50%; lower baseline factor levels may cause bleeding problems after surgical or dental challenge.

Medications

A careful history should be taken of all medications and herbal remedies (see Table 106-2) being administered. Aspirin, a cyclo-oxygenase-1 inhibitor, and ADP-receptor antagonists such as clopidogrel and ticlopidine cause platelet dysfunction; quinine, carbimazole, and penicillins may cause drug-induced immune thrombocytopenia (d-ITP) and anticoagulants including heparin, low-molecular-weight heparin, and warfarin may all cause hemorrhagic complications in elderly patients. The chronic administration of steroids may thin the skin increasing the likelihood of purpura (steroid-induced purpura). It may be difficult to solicit an accurate history of all medications used, so patients should be encouraged to bring all medications and dietary supplements with them to their consultation. It is also important to review the doses and frequency of administration.

TABLE 106-2

Commonly Used Herbal Medicines That May Alter Hemostasis

MEDICINE	ACTION	COMMENTS
Garlic	Inhibition of platelet aggregation; increased fibrinolysis	May increase bleeding when combined with other antiplatelet drugs
Gingko	Inhibition of platelet activation	May increase bleeding when combined with other antiplatelet drugs
Ginseng	Increases PT and aPTT	May increase bleeding risk; also reduces anticoagulant effect of warfarin
St John's Wort	Induction of cyt P450 enzymes	Interacts with warfarin

Data from, Ang-Lee MK, Moss J, Chiu-Su Y, et al. JAMA. 2001;286(2):208–216. © American Medical Association.

Diet

In an elderly patient presenting with new onset bleeding, an assessment of nutritional status is important. The most common dietary deficiencies that contribute to bleeding or a coagulopathy are those of vitamin B-12, folate, vitamin K, and vitamin C.

Vitamin B-12 and folate are essential for normal hematopoiesis because of their roles in DNA synthesis. Although vitamin B-12 or folate deficiency may cause megaloblastosis and pancytopenia, including thrombocytopenia, these conditions alone are unlikely to present with a bleeding diathesis unless the patient is taking concurrent anticoagulants or antiplatelet medications, or other comorbidity is present. Nevertheless, it is important to exclude vitamin B-12 and folate deficiency in patients presenting with thrombocytopenia or other cytopenias as it is easily correctable.

Acute folate deficiency can develop quite rapidly, within a 3-week period; this may be found in up to one-third of hospitalized patients. Risk factors include anorexia, acute alcohol ingestion, and in patients receiving anticonvulsants. Rich sources of dietary folate include green leafy vegetables, fresh and minimally cooked, as folate is thermolabile and is destroyed following prolonged cooking.

Vitamin B-12, a cobalamin, is synthesized by microorganisms, and must be solely obtained from the diet; foods rich in vitamin B-12 include meat, fish, milk, and eggs. The normal body store is 2 to 5 mg in adults, and it usually takes 3 to 4 years to deplete if there is inadequate dietary intake. Vegetarian and vegans often have inadequate dietary intake of cobalamin and may develop low body stores. Other causes of vitamin B-12 deficiency include atrophic gastritis, total or partial gastrectomy, pernicious anemia, and malabsorption in the small bowel secondary to inadequate pancreatic protease and reduction of intrinsic factor-cobalamin receptors in the ileum.

Vitamin K is the cofactor required for gamma-carboxylation of glutamic acid residues on prothrombin, factors VII, IX, X, protein C, and protein S. Vitamin K deficiency occurs as a result of poor nutrition, malabsorption of fat-soluble vitamins, or intrahepatic cholestasis and may be present in any hospitalised or ill patient; patients with inadequate dietary intake are unlikely to develop severe vitamin K deficiency unless concurrently taking antibiotics, when the intestinal source of vitamin K_2 is eliminated.

Vitamin C is necessary for the conversion of hydroxyproline to proline, vital for collagen turnover. Inadequate vitamin C intake over a 2- to 3-month period may cause the clinical condition of scurvy manifested by bruising, ecchymoses, and perifollicular hemorrhage.

Physical Examination

General Examination

Clinical signs of chronic liver disease or renal impairment, abdominal masses, splenomegaly, and lymphadenopathy (indicative of bone marrow pathology such as leukemia, lymphoma, or myeloproliferative diseases), bone tenderness (paraproteinemia), and joint swelling (rheumatoid arthritis, connective tissue diseases) may all provide diagnostic information. An assessment should be made of skin elasticity and joint hypermobility, such as found in Ehlers Danlos or pseudoxanthoma elasticum, conditions that may present with microvascular hemorrhage. Infectious causes of purpura include infective endocarditis (clinical signs may include the presence of a new heart murmer, Osler's nodes, finger clubbing, and splinter hemorrhages) and meningococcal septicemia because of their associated DIC.

Purpura

Evidence of skin bruising, its site, and extent should be recorded: this includes the presence of petechiae, ecchymoses, and subcutaneous hematoma. The site of purpura may provide diagnostic information: petechiae found on the distal limbs is suggestive of thrombocytopenia, on the face and periorbital area may be suggestive of amyloid and purpura sited on the extensor surfaces of legs, arms, and buttocks is a feature of vasculitic conditions. The presence of spongy-looking bleeding gums, purpura, and corkscrew hairs is suggestive of scurvy. Telangiectasia may appear to look purpuric, but classically these lesions are blanchable. Telangiectasiae affecting the face, mouth, tongue, and lips is diagnostic of hereditary hemorrhagic telangiectasia (HHT), a condition that may cause epistaxis and gastrointestinal bleeding throughout the patient's life, resulting in severe chronic iron-deficiency anemia. Telangiectasia is also associated with scleroderma, CREST (calcinosis, Raynaud's phenomenon, esophageal dysmotility, sclerodactyly and telangiectasia) syndrome, and may be evident in patients who have received radiotherapy or solar damage.

Importance of Correlation of Clinical and Laboratory Findings

Information from the history and physical examination must be carefully correlated with laboratory findings. A patient may be referred for laboratory evaluation of a hemostatic abnormality either as a result of a clinical history of bleeding, or to further assess abnormal blood tests found coincidentally or following routine screening. Screening tests are performed, with a view to focus on more specific tests of platelet, coagulation, and fibrinogen components of the hemostatic system if suggested by historical details, or if any laboratory screening defects are detected (see Table 106-3). No single global assay exists to predict the risk of either bleeding or thrombosis. Several assessments over a period of time may need to be performed to arrive at a diagnosis or an assessment of bleeding risk.

TABLE 106-3

Screening Tests of Hemostasis	
LABORATORY TEST	**DETAILS**
Complete blood count	
Blood film examination	
Coagulation screen	Prothrombin time (PT)
	Activated partial thromboplastin time (aPTT)
	Thrombin time
	Fibrinogen
	D-dimer or fibrinogen degradation products (FDPs)
Tests of thyroid function	TSH, T_4, T_3
Tests of renal function	Urea, creatinine
Tests of liver function	Albumin, bilirubin, transaminases

TABLE 106-4

Causes of Acquired Thrombocytopenia in the Elderly	
Immune	**Non-immune**
Immune thrombocytopenia	*Decreased production*
Primary	Megaloblastic anemia; B-12 and
Secondary: SLE	folate deficiency
Posttransfusion purpura	Primary bone marrow disorders:
Drug-induced: vancomycin,	leukemia, lymphoma, myeloma
quinine, heparin	Aplastic anemia
	Infiltration by solid tumor, TB,
	sarcoidosis
	Drugs: chemotherapy
	Alcohol
	Sequestration: hypersplenism

QUANTITATIVE DISORDERS OF PLATELETS

Isolated Thrombocytopenia

There are numerous causes of isolated thrombocytopenia in the elderly and many are listed in Table 106-4. The most common and relevant causes of thrombocytopenia are discussed here.

Pseudothrombocytopenia

Pseudothrombocytopenia is a relatively common phenomenon (found in approximately 0.1% of adults) caused by platelet clumping in the presence of the anticoagulant ethylenediaminetetraacetic acid (EDTA), which is used in vaccutainer tubes for drawing complete blood counts. It should be excluded in any patient with an unexpected low platelet count by examination of the blood film (see Figure 106-2). An accurate platelet count can be estimated by prompt analysis of a fresh blood sample in an alternative anticoagulant such as citrate buffer. Abciximab, a glycoprotein (GP) IIb/IIIa antibody, commonly used in patients with acute coronary syndromes, can cause pseudothrombocytopenia as well as a true drug-induced thrombocytopenia.

Immune Thrombocytopenia

Immune thrombocytopenia (ITP) is an autoimmune disorder characterized by a persistently low platelet count ($<150 \times 10^9$/L). It is caused by autoantibodies binding to platelet antigen(s) and the resultant premature destruction of the platelets by the reticuloendothelial system, especially the spleen. The diagnosis is made by the exclusion of pseudothrombocytopenia and other causes of true thrombocytopenia. Differentiating between hereditary and acquired thrombocytopenia, especially ITP, is of clinical importance to ensure

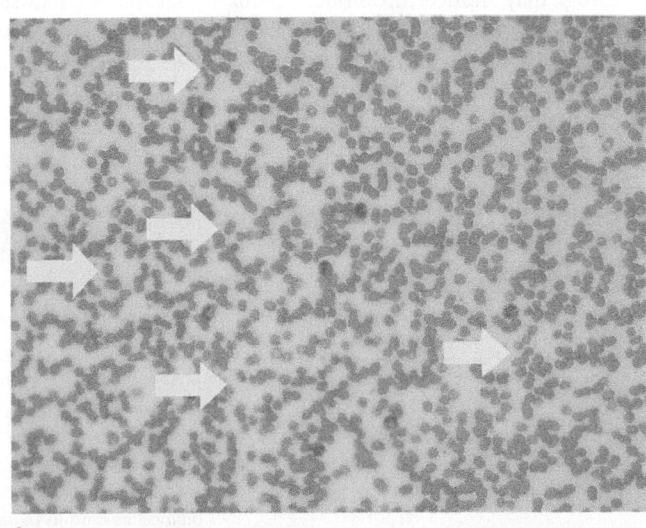

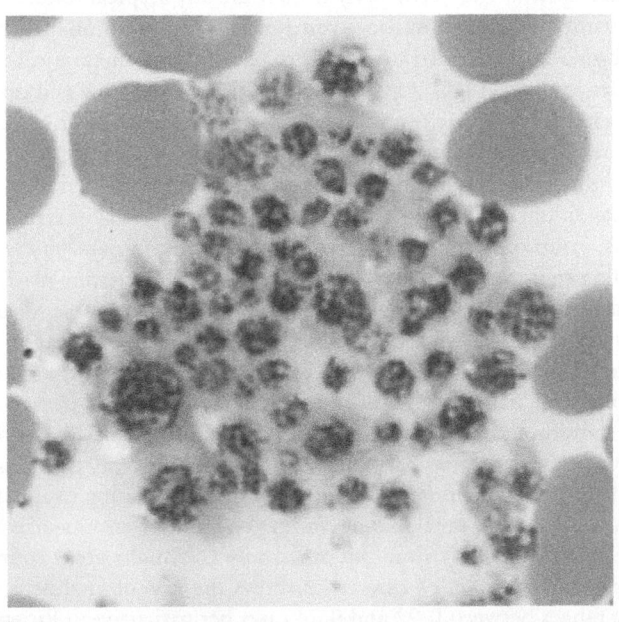

A   **B**

FIGURE 106-2. Blood film. (A) low power magnification demonstrating platelet clumping, a cause of pseudothrombocytopenia; (B) high power view. *(With permission from Dr M Crowther, Hematology Regional Laboratory Medicine Program, Hamilton Health Sciences, Hamilton, Ontario).*

TABLE 106-5

Differentiating Congenital and Acquired Thrombocytopenia from the History

Clinical Details	Hereditary Thrombo-cytopenia	Immune Thrombo-cytopenia
Duration of thrombocytopenia	Lifelong	Recent
History of bleeding after previous procedures	Yes/No	No
Positive family history of thrombocytopenia or of bleeding	Yes	No
Prior normal platelet count?	Never	Yes
Response to treatment with steroids, ivIgG, anti-D?	None/small effect	Increases platelet count
Response to platelet transfusion?	Normal increment	Poor response

Modified with permission from Drachman JG. Blood. 2004;103:390–398.

the patient is not subjected to potentially harmful therapies or procedures (see Table 106-5).

The incidence of adult chronic ITP in United States is approximately 60 new cases per 1 million population per year. The majority of cases are idiopathic. In contrast, childhood ITP has a higher incidence and often presents abruptly following a viral illness or immunization. Secondary ITPs occur in patients with systemic lupus erythematosus or malignant disease, such as chronic lymphocytic leukemia (CLL).

In ITP, the blood film shows no abnormalities excepting a low platelet count. Bone marrow morphology appears normal with increased numbers of megakaryocytes, in addition to normal myelopoiesis and erythropoiesis. Bone marrow examination is not necessary in childhood or young adults, but may be appropriate in older patients to exclude underlying marrow pathology such as myelodysplasia, and particularly if there are any atypical features to the history, examination, or investigations. An autoimmune profile should be performed to exclude other autoimmune diseases. As platelet-associated IgG may be elevated in both immune and non-ITP, assays of antiplatelet antibodies are not informative and are not routinely used in the management of patients with ITP.

Adult ITP differs from the acute disorder in childhood: it usually has an unclear date of onset with no preceding viral or systemic illness; symptoms and signs vary from mild bruising and mucosal bleeding to frank hemorrhage dependent on the presenting platelet count, the presence of comorbidities and if the patient is taking antiplatelet drugs. Overall, bleeding is uncommon unless the ITP is severe (platelet count $< 30 \times 10^9$/L). At any age, there can be spontaneous remission, but one-third of patients may require treatment with steroids and/or splenectomy. In young adults, the 5-year mortality rate is around 5% and it is unclear if this rate increases with age.

There are few randomized controlled trials addressing treatment so an individual approach is necessary. The aim of treatment is to achieve a safe platelet count, not necessarily a normal platelet count. Review of data from 17 case series shows the rate of fatal hemorrhage ranges between 0.02 and 0.04 cases per patient-year. Patients with persistent platelet counts of more than 30×10^9/L need to be followed but interventions are usually not needed. However, such patients should be referred to a hematologist if invasive procedures are needed.

For patients with platelet counts of less than 30×10^9/L or those who experience bleeding, first-line therapy includes corticosteroids and intravenous immunoglobulin G (ivIgG) with a view to splenectomy if medical therapies fail. Anti-D may also have a role in selected patients. About 11% to 35% of patients will fail to respond to corticosteroids, ivIgG, or splenectomy, and can be problematic to manage. Commonly considered second-line therapies include danazol, dapsone, and intensive immunosuppressive regimens, including the combination of cyclophosphamide, vincristine, and methylprednisolone. Rituximab, a selective immunosuppressive agent (anti-CD20 monoclonal antibody) developed for patients with low-grade B-cell lymphoma, has been used with some success to treat refractory ITP.

Posttransfusion Purpura

Posttransfusion purpura (PTP) is a rare bleeding disorder characterized by severe and sudden thrombocytopenia (usually $<10 \times 10^9$/L) within 3 to 12 days following a transfusion. It is caused by preformed antibodies directed against common human platelet alloantigens (HPA), especially HPA-1a. The majority of the affected patients are multiparous women who have been sensitized during a previous pregnancy. Thrombocytopenia usually resolves spontaneously within several weeks, but patients may develop severe or fatal bleeding during the course of the disease. Ecchymoses, bleeding from mucosal surfaces, and postoperative wounds are common presenting features. Bone marrow examination reveals normal numbers of megakaryocytes, and a coagulation screen reveals no abnormalities. The diagnosis is confirmed by the finding of antibodies to platelet-specific antigens, and the active exclusion of disseminated intravascular coagulation (DIC) and heparin-induced thrombocytopenia. Management includes ivIgG, corticosteroids, and plasmapheresis. Platelet transfusion is ineffective and may worsen the clinical condition. The recurrence of PTP is minimized by using blood products from a platelet-compatible donor.

Drug-Induced Thrombocytopenias

Drugs may induce thrombocytopenia by several mechanisms (see Table 106-6), including generalized or selective suppression of megakaryopoiesis and increased platelet destruction by immune and nonimmune mechanisms. Drug-induced thrombocytopenias may

TABLE 106-6

Mechanisms of Drug-Induced Thrombocytopenia

Mechanism	Example	Further Details
Myelosuppression	Chemotherapeutic agents	Dose-dependent, predictable
Immune mediated	Gold	Autoantibody-induced immune thrombocytopenia
	Quinine	Drug-dependent antibodies against drug/platelet glycoprotein complexes
	Heparin	IgG antibodies bind to platelet factor 4 and heparin causing platelet activation and generation of platelet-derived microparticles

present with clinical features of bleeding, bruising, and petechiae or may be asymptomatic. Heparin-induced thrombocytopenia can cause severe and rapid drops in the platelet count but is associated paradoxically with thrombosis, not bleeding.

The management of drug-induced thrombocytopenia involves immediate cessation of the drug, plus supportive measures to increase the platelet count, such as ivIgG.

QUALITATIVE DISORDERS OF PLATELETS

In the elderly, a number of disorders may cause acquired platelet dysfunction (see Table 106-7).

Antiplatelet Agents

The most common cause of acquired platelet dysfunction is the use of antiplatelet agents. Five classes of drugs are administered therapeutically to specifically inhibit platelet function (see Figure 106-3). These include the cyclo-oxygenase inhibitors, such as aspirin and nonsteroidal anti-inflammatory agents, ADP receptor antagonists, such as ticlopidine and clopidogrel, GP IIb/IIIa antagonists, such as abciximab, tirofiban, and eptifibatide, and drugs that increase cyclic AMP or cyclic GMP, such as phosphodiesterase inhibitors, including dipyridamole. Many other drugs also adversely affect platelet function, including antimicrobials such as penicillins and cephalosporins, tricyclic antidepressants, and phenothiazines. The administration of these drugs should be avoided, if possible, in patients with moderate and severe thrombocytopenia to prevent hemorrhagic issues.

Myeloproliferative Disorders

Myeloproliferative disorders are clonal stem cell disorders and include polycythemia rubra vera (PRV), essential thrombocythemia (ET), and myelofibrosis; all three conditions show features of bone marrow hypercellularity, varying degrees of leukocytosis and thrombocytosis, and elevated hematocrit.

Platelet dysfunction is usually encountered when the absolute platelet count increases over $1500 \times 10^9/L$ and may be caused by a reduction in platelet survival, loss of high-molecular-weight vWF, and decreased platelet aggregation responses. Treatment of the underlying myeloproliferative disorder is required to control any bleeding diathesis.

TABLE 106-7

Causes of Acquired Disorders of Platelet Function in the Elderly

Primary bone marrow disorders
  Myeloproliferative disorders: PRV, ET, MF

Medications
  Inhibition of cyclo-oxygenase: ASA, nonsteroidal anti-inflammatory drugs
  Inhibition of ADP receptors: clopidogrel, ticlopidine
  Inhibition of GPIIb/IIIa: abciximab, eptifibatide

Chronic renal failure

Cardiopulmonary bypass

Paraproteinemias

See text for abbreviations.

Uremia/Chronic Renal Failure

Chronic renal failure creates a complex coagulopathy of unclear clinical significance. The primary hemostatic abnormality is partly caused by platelet dysfunction. Hence laboratory findings of a prolonged bleeding time and abnormal platelet aggregation are common. However, these parameters are poor predictors of the risk of bleeding, fail to correlate with the degree of renal dysfunction, and do not constitute an indication for therapeutic intervention. In addition, anemia of chronic renal failure is associated with an increased bleeding time as a result of the diminished displacement of platelets to the periphery of the blood vessel, causing a reduced platelet–endothelial interaction. Anemia is an independent cause of a prolonged bleeding time and the relationship of the hematocrit to the bleeding time is well recognized and corrected by transfusion of packed red blood cells and administration of erythropoietin.

L-Deamino-8-o-arginine vasopressin (DDAVP, desmopressin) has been used in the management of bleeding in uremia. The effect is transient, lasting 1 to 4 hours, and correlates to increases in vWF functional activity. Its mode of action is by the stimulation of release of vWF from Weibel–Palade bodies in the endothelium. Side effects include facial flushing, tachycardia, water retention and hyponatremia of sufficient severity to cause cerebral edema, coma, and seizures. Conjugated estrogens have been reported to shorten bleeding times in rat models of uremia, and remain an option in problematic cases. Both peritoneal dialysis and hemodialysis improve platelet function and normalize the bleeding time, reducing the risk of bleeding. Should bleeding remain problematic, the patient should be investigated as in any other patient.

COAGULATION DISORDERS

Congenital Coagulation Disorders in Elderly Patients

It is unusual for classic hemophilias and severe von Willebrand's disease to present late in life but many patients with congenital coagulation disorders are living longer and will require ongoing specialized support. Referral of such patients to comprehensive hemophilia centres or specialists with expertise in their management is mandatory.

Acquired Coagulation Factor Inhibitors

Acquired Hemophilia (Inhibitors to Factor VIII (fVIII)

The spontaneous development of an inhibitor to fVIII in an individual with previously normal hemostatic function and no clinically significant personal or family history of bleeding episodes is known as acquired hemophilia.

Although rare, with an incidence of 0.2 to 1.0 cases per 1 million persons per year, acquired hemophilia mainly affects individuals older than of 60 years of age, and may present with spontaneous life- and limb-threatening bleeding manifestations (see Figure 106-4). It commonly presents with bleeding into soft tissues, mucous membranes, and skin, as well as the retroperitoneal and retropharyngeal spaces. This is distinctly different from the pattern of bleeding encountered in congenital hemophilia, where intramuscular and intra-articular bleeds are more common (see Table 106-8).

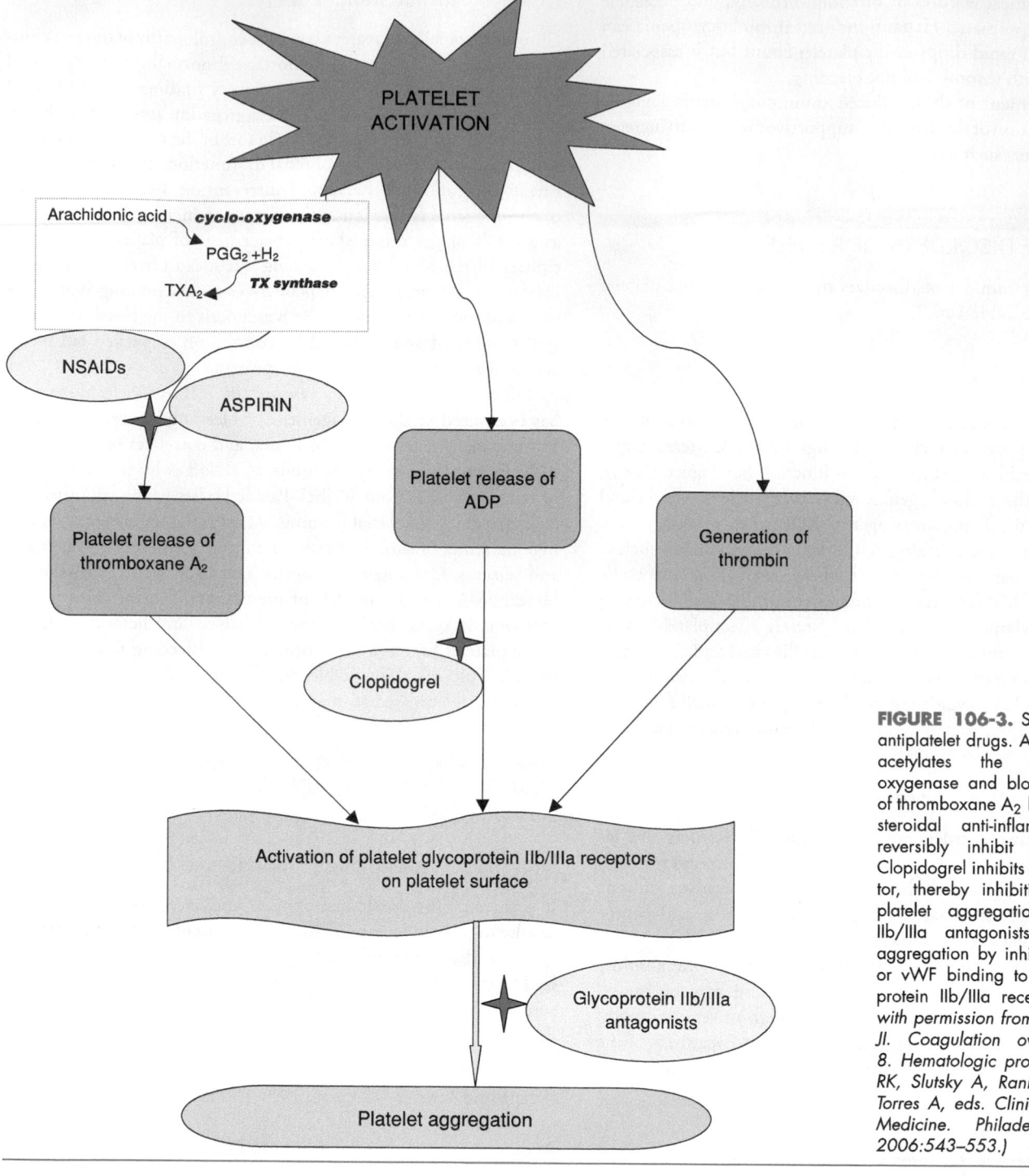

FIGURE 106-3. Sites of action of antiplatelet drugs. Aspirin irreversibly acetylates the enzyme cyclo-oxygenase and blocks the synthesis of thromboxane A_2 by platelets. Nonsteroidal anti-inflammatory agents reversibly inhibit cyclo-oxygenase. Clopidogrel inhibits a key ADP receptor, thereby inhibiting ADP-induced platelet aggregation. Glycoprotein IIb/IIIa antagonists block platelet aggregation by inhibiting fibrinogen or vWF binding to activated glycoprotein IIb/IIIa receptors. (Modified with permission from Liaw PC, Weitz JI. Coagulation overview. Section 8. Hematologic problems. In: Albert RK, Slutsky A, Ranieri M, Takala J, Torres A, eds. Clinical Critical Care Medicine. Philadelphia: Elsevier; 2006:543–553.)

TABLE 106-8

Bleeding Symptoms in Acquired and Congenital Hemophilia

CONGENITAL	ACQUIRED
Hemarthroses	Subcutaneous hematoma
Muscle bleeds	Frank hematuria
Soft tissue bleeds	Retropharyngeal hematoma
	Retroperitoneal hematoma
	Cerebral hemorrhage
	Compartment syndrome

Acquired hemophilia has been reported in association with autoimmune disorders, systemic lupus erythematosus, rheumatoid arthritis, and solid and hematologic malignancies (see Table 106-9) but in 50% of cases, there may be no obvious associated disease state. Drugs such as sulphonamides, penicillin, and phenothiazines have also been reported as causes. One-third of cases resolve spontaneously. Autoantibody inhibitors are usually of IgG_1 and IgG_4, subclasses that appear to disrupt assembled coagulation factors on the surface of the phospholipid membrane that are integral to the production of activated coagulation factors.

If acquired hemophilia is suspected, an urgent hematology (hemostasis) consultation is recommended. The diagnosis is made by

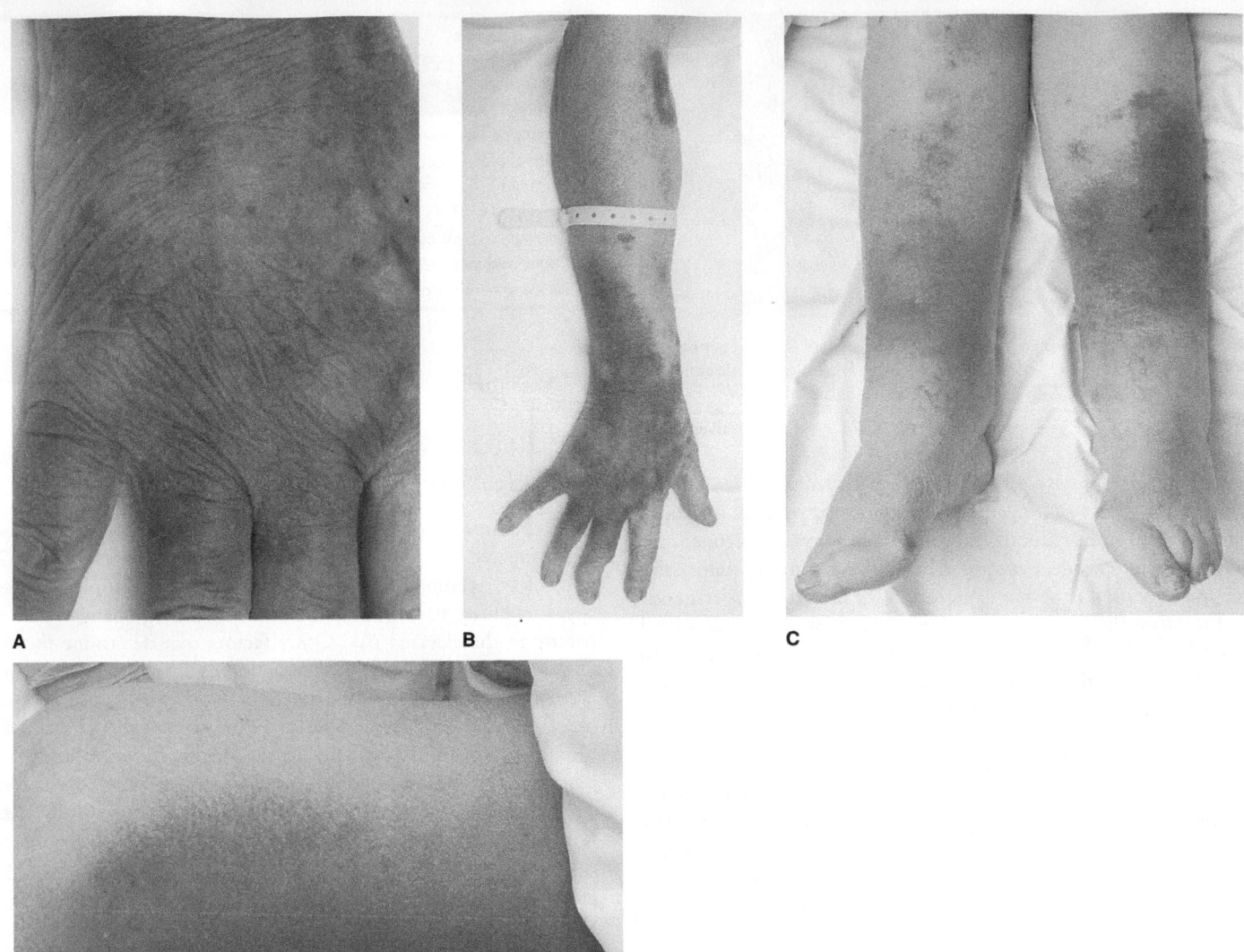

FIGURE 106-4. Severe bleeding diathesis in a patient with an acquired inhibitor to factor VIII (acquired hemophilia). (A) Close-up view of right hand; (B) right arm; (C) lower limbs; (D) hematoma in medial aspect of right thigh. *(With permission from Dr. E Horn, Edinburgh Royal Infirmary.)*

the demonstration of a solitary prolonged activated partial thromboplastin time (aPTT) that fails to correct on mixing with equal volumes of normal plasma (50:50 mix). The prothrombin time (PT), thrombin time (TT), and fibrinogen activity are all normal. The presence of lupus anticoagulant must be excluded.

The diagnosis of an inhibitor to fVIII is confirmed by specific assays of the factor and quantification of the inhibitor by a Bethesda assay.

TABLE 106-9

Etiology of Acquired Inhibitors to Factor VIII

- Elderly with no apparent underlying disease
- Postpartum (rarely during pregnancy)
- Underlying disorders
  - Autoimmune disorders e.g., SLE, rheumatoid arthritis
  - Adverse drug reactions (especially penicillins; phenothiazines)
  - Malignancy (solid, lymphoproliferative)
  - Monoclonal gammopathies

The management of acquired hemophilia depends on the underlying disease state, the extent and severity of the hemorrhagic complications, and the magnitude of the Bethesda titer. Prevention of further bleeds by careful nursing and the avoidance of frequent venepunctures are simple practical measures. Antiplatelet drugs, heparin, and anticoagulants must not be administered and intramuscular injections are contraindicated. Invasive diagnostic procedures should be avoided as hemostasis is often difficult to secure.

With a low-inhibitor titer (<5 Bethesda Unit/mL), patients can be treated with human factor VIII concentrates given at sufficiently high dose to overcome the inhibitor effect. Desmopressin may be used in patients with low titer inhibitors for minor bleeds, but may have side effects of hyponatremia and hypotension, limiting its use. With higher inhibitor titers (>5 Bethesda Unit/mL), fVIII concentrates and DDAVP are not effective and more aggressive therapy is needed. Bypassing agents, so called because they bypass critical steps in the coagulation pathway requiring fVIII, are plasma-derived factor concentrates that contain activated vitamin K-dependent coagulation factors, and may be used to treat hemorrhage. By generating thrombin, these agents have potential side effects of

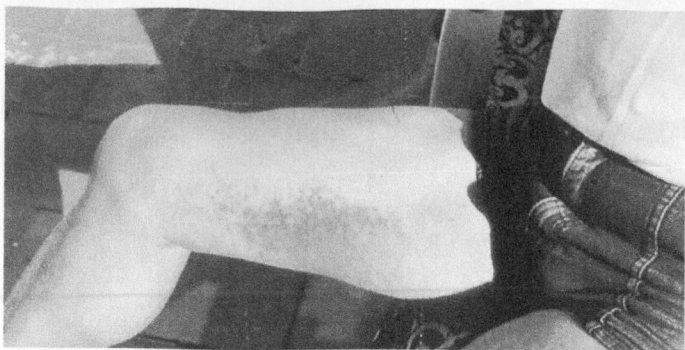

FIGURE 106-5. Extensive ecchymosis in a patient with acquired von Willebrand's Syndrome. *(With permission from Professor C.A. Ludlam, Edinburgh University.)*

TABLE 106-11

Laboratory Evaluation of Acquired von Willebrand's Syndrome

- Prolonged bleeding time
- Normal platelet count
- Normal PT
- Prolonged aPTT
- Decreased levels of von Willebrand factor antigen and functional activity
- Decreased factor VIII levels
- Absence of inhibitor to factor VIII

thromboembolism. Recombinant-activated factor VIIa (rfVIIa) (Novoseven, Niastase), a genetically engineered product, has been demonstrated to be clinically safe and efficacious as a treatment for acute bleeding episodes in acquired hemophilia. Immunosuppressive therapies are used in severe cases to inhibit the cell clone responsible for the synthesis of the autoantibody. Cyclophosphamide is used as a sole agent, or in combination with corticosteroids, for a 3- to 6-week period and the doses adjusted to the therapeutic response. The blood count must be monitored carefully in view of potential neutropenia and myelosuppression.

High-dose ivIgG has been shown to be effective in reducing the inhibitor titer in certain individuals and can be considered as a therapy in patients who do not respond, or are intolerant of, other immunosuppressive regimens. Cyclosporine, 2-chlorodeoxyadenosine (2-CDA), and interferon alpha have also been successfully used. Rituximab has been used with success; however, the optimal dose, its mechanism of action and long-term side effects are unclear.

Acquired von Willebrand's Syndrome

Acquired von Willebrand's Syndrome (AVWS) is a rare, adult-onset bleeding diathesis, mainly presenting with mucocutaneous and skin bleeding (see Figure 106-5 and Table 106-10). AVWS is most commonly associated with underlying low-grade hematological malignancies, in addition to solid tumors and autoimmune disease (see Table 106-11).

Desmopressin and plasma-derived vWF-rich concentrates can be used to treat hemorrhagic episodes, but are limited by their extremely short duration of action. Long-term disease modification of

TABLE 106-10

Etiology of Acquired von Willebrand's Syndrome

- Hematological disorders
  - Myeloproliferative disorders
  - Lymphoproliferative disorders
  - Monoclonal gammopathy of undetermined significance
  - Autoimmune disorders
  - Solid tumors
  - Hypothyroidism
  - Loss of high-molecular-weight multimers: aortic stenosis, angiodysplasia

the AVWS can be achieved by high-dose ivIgG and usually induces a transient correction of vWF parameters for 1 to 3 weeks.

Anticoagulants

Older persons have a higher risk for anticoagulant-related bleeding compared with younger persons. In particular, older than 75 years of age, comorbid disease, concurrent use of antiplatelet therapy, propensity to falls, and the need for dosing changes all contribute to the elevated risk. Other factors that determine the risk of anticoagulant-related bleeding, including intensity of anticoagulation, duration of exposure, genetic polymorphism, also apply to older persons. The most important comorbidities associated with bleeding during anticoagulant therapy include uncontrolled hypertension, cerebrovascular disease, ischemic stroke, history of gastrointestinal bleeding, malignancy, liver disease, and renal insufficiency. Older patients may also tolerate the consequences of bleeding and the necessary interventions, such as surgery, less well than younger patients.

For warfarin, it is clearly established that the risk of bleeding, in particular intracranial hemorrhage, is strongly determined by the intensity of the anticoagulant effect. The risk increases dramatically with an international normalized ratio (INR) greater than 4.0. Therefore, because of warfarin's narrow therapeutic effect, its unpredictable interpatient and intrapatient variability in the dose response and the borderline nutritional status in many older persons, frequent laboratory monitoring of the INR is important. This can be a burden to patients who do not have reliable means of transportation or have difficulty understanding the needs for dose adjustment. Older persons often require lower doses than younger patients. One study showed that a starting dose of 5 mg per day led to overanticoagulation in an estimated 82% of female patients and 65% of male patients older than 70 years of age. Interaction with other drugs is another limitation with warfarin. Concurrent use of drugs that may interact with warfarin is associated with a 3- to 4.5-fold increased risk of serious bleeding in long-term warfarin users. This is a real and challenging concern in elderly patients who are often subjected to polypharmacy. Computer-based surveillance systems in long-term care facilities, and drug-alerts systems within hospitals and community pharmacy settings, have been demonstrated to reduce the potential for serious drug interactions between warfarin and other medications.

Anticoagulation with unfractionated heparin, low-molecular-weight heparin, or fondaparinux is also associated with a high bleeding risk. As these agents are excreted by the renal route, an assessment of renal function is essential when they are prescribed. Body weight is also important for guiding the doses of these agents. Weight-based nomograms are available for heparin infusions and should be used to facilitate rapid achievement of a therapeutic anticoagulant effect and reduce the risk of overdose.

Management of patients with anticoagulant-related bleeding is similar to other bleeding situations. The drug should be discontinued and supportive blood products given if necessary. The anticoagulant effect of warfarin should be reversed with vitamin K, given either orally or parentally. However, it will take a minimum of 6 to 8 hours before functional coagulation factors are produced by the liver so the INR correction will be delayed. Fresh frozen plasma should be given in the interim if the patient has active bleeding. Protamine sulfate can be used for reversing the anticoagulant effects of heparin and low-molecular-weight heparin. Repeat boluses or continuous intravenous infusions of protamine sulfate are required to provide adequate neutralization of the anticoagulant effects. A specific antidote for fondaparinux is not available but recombinant activated factor VII will reverse abnormal laboratory parameters and is likely effective in stopping active hemorrhage. Because spontaneous bleeding does not occur with therapeutic doses of anticoagulants, aggressive measures should be undertaken in such circumstances to identify and eliminate, if possible, the bleeding source. Following an episode of serious bleeding, reintroduction of anticoagulant therapy should be considered only if the source of bleeding is identified, reversed, and the overall risk–benefit ratio continues to favor anticoagulation.

COMBINED HEMOSTATIC DEFECTS

Disseminated Intravascular Coagulation

Disseminated intravascular coagulation (DIC) is a clinicopathologic syndrome characterized by the systemic activation of coagulation. The mainstay of the syndrome involves the dysregulated and excessive generation of thrombin and a reactive fibrinolytic response. This leads to the widespread deposition of fibrin in the circulation contributing to microvascular thrombosis and multiorgan failure. Further activation of the coagulation system depletes platelets and coagulation factors, and may precipitate bleeding manifestations. Clinical manifestations are diverse, forming a spectrum from asymptomatic laboratory abnormalities to hemorrhagic and thrombotic complications.

The presence of DIC is clinically important as the syndrome increases the risk of mortality beyond that associated with the primary disease. No single test exists with sufficient diagnostic accuracy to confirm the diagnosis of DIC; the diagnosis rests on the correlation of clinical features, taking into account the relevant causative factor (see Table 106-12), and laboratory findings (Table 106-13). Monitoring the trend in serial tests is often more important than the absolute results. Screening for the presence of overt DIC can be made by a combination of simple, reliable, readily available laboratory tests, and forms the basis of a clinical scoring system. A scoring system is also being developed for the diagnosis of nonovert stages of DIC.

The management of DIC involves an individual approach, with prompt recognition and removal of the precipitating cause (Table 106-14). The efficacy of treatment with plasma, fibrinogen, cryoprecipitate or platelets lacks clinical trial evidence, but is widely accepted

TABLE 106-12

Clinical Conditions Associated with Overt DIC

Diagnosis	Causes
Sepsis, severe infection	Gram-negative and gram-positive bacterial infections Viral infections Fungal infections Parasitic infections
Trauma	Shock, hypoxia, brain injury, burns, heat stroke
Malignancy	Solid tumors, including mucin-producing adenocarcinoma; Hematological malignancies, especially acute promyelocytic leukemia
Obstetric emergencies	Amniotic fluid embolism, abruptio placentae, retained dead fetus, eclampsia
Vascular abnormalities	Large vessel aneurysm, giant hemangioma including Kasabach-Merrit syndrome
Toxic	Drugs (recreational) Venoms—snake and spider bites
Immunological	Drugs (therapeutic)—heparin-induced thrombocytopenia ABO incompatible transfusion
Advanced liver disease	LeVeen shunt

as supportive and aimed at replacing depleted coagulation factors. Plasma and blood product therapies should not be administered on the basis of laboratory results alone but are given only in a patient with active bleeding or someone with a high bleeding risk who must undergo invasive procedures. The use of coagulation factor concentrates, such as prothrombin complex concentrates (PCCs), are not usually appropriate as they contain only single or a small combination of factors; minute traces of activated coagulation factors may precipitate thromboembolism or worsen the coagulopathy.

The successful use of heparin and low-molecular-weight heparin have been anecdotally reported in specific settings such as chronic DIC associated with solid tumors, and in overt cases of thromboembolism or situations involving extensive fibrin deposition, such as purpura fulminans and acral necrosis. A beneficial effect of heparin on clinically important outcome events in patients with DIC has never been demonstrated in clinical trials.

Fibrinolytic inhibitors act by blocking secondary fibrinogenolysis, and in the setting of DIC may have adverse consequences such as

TABLE 106-13

Screening Tests for Overt DIC

Blood count and blood film: Decreasing trend in the platelet count is a sensitive marker of DIC; blood film may show red cell fragmentation; also may highlight cause of DIC, e.g., blasts in acute leukemia; toxic granulation in sepsis

Global assays of hemostasis: Prolongation of PT, aPTT, TCT; reflective of factor consumption and reduced factor synthesis

Fibrinogen: As an acute phase reactant may remain normal before falling; hypofibrinogenemia is found in acute head injury, prostatic adenocarcinoma and obstetric calamities

Fibrinogen degradation products

TABLE 106-14

Management of DIC

- Removal of precipitating cause
- Supportive care
  Maintain oxygenation
  Prevent acidosis and hypothermia
  Replace folate
  Replace vitamin K
- Plasma and blood products
  If active bleeding
  At high risk of bleeding
  Undergoing invasive procedures
- Anticoagulant therapy
  Chronic DIC in the setting of hyperfibrinolysis
- Fibrinolytic inhibitors
  Used on occasion in fibrinogenolysis, such as vascular malformations
- Activated protein C concentrate
  Efficacy demonstrated in randomized clinical trials of DIC in sepsis

the prevention of tissue perfusion. Consideration may be warranted in situations of intense fibrinogenolysis such as the Kasabach-Merrit syndrome, vascular malformations, and in coagulopathies secondary to metastatic prostate cancer and acute promyelocytic leukemia.

Phase III clinical trials have been performed with three natural anticoagulants—AT, activated protein C (aPC), and TF pathway inhibitor (TFPI)—in the setting of patients with severe sepsis. To date, only a beneficial effect of recombinant human aPC (rhaPC) has been demonstrated. Recombinant human aPC is licensed for the treatment of patients with severe sepsis and two or more organ failures. It is administered as a 96-hour intravenous infusion, but caution is required in patients with thrombocytopenia ($<30 \times 10^9$/L) to avoid the risk of intracranial hemorrhage. In situations where protein C is not available, the strategy to replace protein C by plasma exchange has proven successful in a small case series.

Liver Disease

Acute hepatic failure and end-stage liver disease (ESLD) cause many hemostatic defects (Table 106-15). The management of coagulation issues in elderly patients with severe liver disease requires an individual approach with attention to the nature, site, and extent of bleeding. Surgical, endovascular, and pharmacologic interventions may be necessary to reduce the portal pressure. Administration of

TABLE 106-15

Underlying Hemostatic Defects in End-Stage Liver Disease

- Reduced synthesis of coagulation factors
- Vitamin K deficiency: Causing deficiencies of procoagulant and anticoagulant systems
- Thrombocytopenia: Secondary to hypersplenism and portal hypertension
- Platelet dysfunction
- Impaired synthesis of fibrinolytic proteins
- Impaired clearance of activated coagulation factors
- Acquired dysfibrinogenemia
- Hyperfibrinolysis

vitamin K slowly by the intravenous route for a few days is advisable to correct any underlying deficiency of vitamin K.

Fresh frozen plasma (FFP) contains all the coagulation factors and inhibitors except vWF present in circulating blood. It may be given to correct hemostatic defects prior to invasive procedures and to control active bleeding. Effective replacement may be difficult as large amounts of plasma are necessary to correct a prolonged PT as a result of the short half-life of factor VII, and infusions of FFP every 6 to 12 hours may be necessary. Fibrinogen can be replaced using cryoprecipitate.

Platelet transfusions may be helpful in patients with severe thrombocytopenia and bleeding, although the platelet increment may be less than anticipated as a result of sequestration within an enlarged spleen. PCCs are pooled plasma-derived factor concentrates that contain fIX and variable concentrations of factors X, VII, and II and protein C. PCCs may transiently correct deficiencies of vitamin K-dependent factors but also contain variable amounts of activated coagulation factors that may give rise to thromboembolic complications including venous thromboembolism and DIC, particularly in liver failure where clearance of activated coagulation factors may be impaired.

Clinical trials of recombinant fVIIa (rfVIIa) in patients with liver cirrhosis with active bleeding, and in patients undergoing orthotopic liver transplantation, have failed to demonstrate any significant benefit with this agent to date. Fibrinolytic inhibitors, such as ε-aminocaproic acid (EACA) and tranexamic acid, can be considered in the setting of hyperfibrinolysis and may be useful in patients with diffuse mucosal, subcutaneous, or gastrointestinal bleeding, but prospective controlled studies to demonstrate efficacy are lacking.

VASCULAR PURPURA

Elderly patients with normal hemostatic parameters may present with purpura secondary to vascular abnormalities (see Table 106-16).

Senile Purpura

With the aging process, the turnover of collagen and elastin are altered, and along with chronic solar damage, skin thins causing a characteristic pattern of purpura on the forearms and hands. In this benign condition, vitamin C administration is not effective.

TABLE 106-16

Causes of Purpura in Elderly Patients with Normal Coagulation Parameters

Senile purpura
Vasculitis Polyarteritis nodosa, Wegener's granulomatosis,
Steroid excess: Cushing's syndrome, exogenous steroids
Vitamin C deficiency
Abnormal connective tissue disorder: Ehler Danlos, Pseudoxanthoma elasticum
Amyloid infiltration of blood vessels
Infections: Bacterial, fungal

Scurvy

Vitamin C stores are readily depleted after 1 month on a vitamin C-free diet. Initial symptoms include fatigue, depression, and lethargy. Scurvy is primarily found in persons addicted to alcohol with poor nutritional intake, persons who have a liking for food fads, and in individuals eating highly refined or purified diets. The last group of individuals includes elderly patients with swallowing difficulties, or who may be edentulous, often in long-term institutional care. The most common presenting symptoms are bruising, arthralgia, or joint swelling. Hemorrhagic manifestations occur late in the disease and include perifollicular hemorrhages with corkscrew hairs affecting the arms, legs, back, and buttocks, "plate-like ecchymoses" affecting the legs or trunk; spongy friable gums and loosening of teeth. The finding of a serum ascorbic acid level lower than 2.5 mg/L confirms the diagnosis; the administration of vitamin C resolves the symptoms and signs promptly.

Hereditary Hemorrhagic Telangiectasia (Osler-Weber-Rendu Syndrome)

HHT is an uncommon, often under-recognised condition that presents with characteristic mucocutaneous telangiectasia (not purpura) affecting the buccal area, lips, and finger tips. Epidemiological studies in Europe and Japan point to an incidence of 1:5000–10,000. Diagnostic criteria were established in 2000, and the clinical diagnosis is based on the presence of at least three of the following features: recurrent epistaxis, mucocutaneous telangiectases, evidence of autosomal dominant inheritance and visceral arteriovenous malformations. Telangiectasia consists of localized collections of noncontractile capillaries that bleed for a prolonged time following rupture. The manifestations are often not present at birth, but develop with age, and presentation is with persistent nasal, oropharyngeal bleeding, and gastrointestinal bleeding, leading to chronic iron deficiency. The management involves the aggressive replacement of depleted iron stores with intravenous iron.

Methods to arrest bleeding include packing, electrocautery, cryosurgery, arterial embolization, arterial ligation, and hormonal manipulation (estrogens), in addition to the use of lasers. An evidence base is accumulating, but at present no single method to arrest bleeding has been demonstrated to be superior to others.

CONCLUSIONS

The correct and timely diagnosis of a bleeding diathesis in an elderly patient involves attention to meticulous history taking, careful general examination, and focused investigation. The ageing process itself does not cause a tendency to bleed. However, polypharmacy, increased comorbidities, and other acquired risk factors for bleeding may unmask underlying mild congenital disorders or other primary pathologies. The rare disorders of acquired hemophilia and PTP predominantly affect elderly patients and must be quickly recognized and referred on to a hematologist.

FURTHER READING

Ang-Lee MK, Moss J, Chun-Su Y. Herbal medicines and perioperative care. *JAMA*, 2001;286(2):208–216.

Begbie ME, Wallace GMF, Shovlin CL. Hereditary haemorrhagic telangiectasia (Osler-Weber-Rendu syndrome). *Postgrad Med J.* 2003;79:18.

Bernard GR, Ely EW, Wright TJ. Safety and dose relationship of recombinant human activated protein C for coagulopathy in severe sepsis. *Crit Care Med.* 2001;29:2051–2059

Bernard GR, Vincent AL, Laterre PF, LaRosa S. Efficacy and safety of recombinant human activated protein C for severe sepsis. *N Engl J Med.* 2001;344:699–709.

British Committee for Standards in Haematology. Guidelines for the investigation and management of idiopathic thrombocytopenic purpura in adults, children and pregnancy. *Br J Haematol.* 2003;120:574–596.

Cohen AJ, Kessler CM. Acquired inhibitors. *Ballieres Clin Hematol.* 1996;9:331–354.

Copplestone JA. Bleeding and coagulation disorders in the elderly. *Ballieres Clin Haematol.* 1987;1(2):559–580

Drachman JG. Inherited thrombocytopenia: when a low platelet count does not mean ITP. *Blood.* 2004;103:390–398

Franchini M. Acquired hemophilia A. *Hematology.* 2006;11[2]:119–125.

Hamilton PJ, Allardyce M, Ogston D, Dawson AA, Dawson AS. The effect of age on the coagulation system. *J Clin Path.* 1974;27:980–982.

Hay CRM, Baglin TTP, Collins PW, Hill FGH, Keeling DM. The diagnosis and management of factor VIII and factor IX inhibitors: a guideline from the UK Haemophilia Centre Doctors' Organization (UKHCDO). *Br J Haematol.* 2000;111:78–90.

Kujovich J. Hemostatic defects in end stage liver disease. *Crit Care Clin.* 2005;21:563–587.

Levi M. Current understanding of disseminated intravascular coagulation. *Br J Haematol.* 2004;124:567–576.

Liaw PC, Weitz JI. Coagulation overview. Section 8. Hematologic problems. In: Albert RK, Slutsky A, Ranieri M, Takala J, Torres A, eds. *Clinical Critical Care Medicine.* Philadelphia: Elsevier; 2006:543–553

Lowe GD, Rumley A, Woodward M, et al. Epidemiology of coagulation factors, inhibitors and activation markers: The Third Glasgow MONICA Survey I. Illustrative reference ranges by age, sex and hormone use. *Br J Haematol.* 1997;97:775–784.

Mannucci PM. Hemophilia: treatment options in the twenty-first century. *J Thrombosis Haemostasis.* 2007;1:1349–1355

Mapp SJ, Coughlin PB. Scurvy in an otherwise well young man. *Med J Aust.* 2006;185[6]:331–332.

Mari D, Mannucci PM, Coppola R, Bottasso B, Bauer KA, Rosenberg RD. Hypercoagulability in centenarians: the paradox of successful aging. *Blood.* 1995;85[11]:3144–3149.

Michiels JJ, Budde U, van der Planken M, van Vliet HH, Shroyens W, Berneman Z. Acquired von Willebrand's syndrome: clinical features, aetiology, pathophysiology, classification and management. *Best Pract Res Clin Haematol.* 2001;14:401–436.

Olmedo JM, Yiannias JA, Windgassen EB, Gornet MK. Scurvy: a disease almost forgotten. *Int J Dermatol.* 2006;45(8):909–913.

Rumley A, Emberson JR, Wannamethee SG, Lennon L, Whincup PH, Lowe GDO. Effects of older age on fibrin D-dimer, C-reactive protein, and other hemostatic and inflammatory variables in men aged 60–79 years. *J Thromb Haemost.* 2006;4:982–987.

Sie P, Montague J, Blanc M, et al. Evaluation of some platelet parameters in a group of elderly people. *Thromb Haemost.* 1981;45:197–199.

Street A, Hill K, Sussex B, Warner M, Scully M-F. Haemophilia and ageing. *Haemophilia.* 2006;12[Suppl 3]:8–12.

Taylor FB, Toh CH, Hoots WK, Wada H, Levi M. Towards definition, clinical and laboratory criteria and a scoring system for disseminated intravascular coagulation. *Thromb Haemost.* 2001;86:1327–1330.

Toh CH, Dennis M. Disseminated intravascular coagulation: old disease, new hope. *BMJ.* 2005;327:974–977.

van Genderen PJ, Michiels JJ. Acquired von Willebrand disease. *Ballieres Clin Haematol.* 1998;11[2]:319–320.

Warkentin TE. Heparin-induced thrombocytopenia: pathogenesis and management. *Br J Haematol.* 2003;121:535–555.

Warkentin TE. Drug-induced immune-mediated thrombocytopenia—from purpura to thrombosis. *N Eng J Med.* 2007;356:891–893.

Waters AH. Post-transfusion purpura. *Blood Rev.* 1989;3:83–87.

Aging of the Endocrine System and Selected Endocrine Disorders

David A. Gruenewald ■ *Alvin M. Matsumoto*

PRINCIPLES OF GERIATRIC ENDOCRINOLOGY

Impaired Homeostatic Regulation

As in other organ systems, the normal aging of the endocrine system is characterized by a progressive loss of reserve capacity, resulting in a decreased ability to adapt to changing environmental demands. This loss of homeostatic regulation reflects important alterations in hormonal synthesis, metabolism, and action, but these changes may not be clinically apparent under baseline conditions. In fact, basal plasma concentrations of many hormones and metabolic fuels are essentially unchanged with normal aging. This is illustrated by fasting plasma glucose levels that exhibit little change with normal aging, but after a glucose challenge, glucose levels increase much more in healthy older persons as compared to young adults. In some instances, the function of aging endocrine systems is maintained by compensatory changes in secretion of one hormone to offset the loss of function of another hormone in a feedback system, or to compensate for alterations in metabolic clearance. For example, in many older men with testosterone levels in the normal range, pituitary luteinizing hormone (LH) secretion and serum LH levels are increased (although levels usually remain within the normal range), partially offsetting a reduction in testicular testosterone secretion. However, in other cases, these compensatory mechanisms are inadequate to maintain normal function with aging even under basal conditions. For example, unlike cortisol, adrenal production of aldosterone and dehydroepiandrosterone (DHEA) declines disproportionately to clearance rates with aging, leading to age-related decreases in plasma levels of these hormones even under baseline conditions.

Altered Presentation of Endocrine Diseases

The presenting manifestations of endocrine disorders in older adults are often nonspecific, muted, or atypical. For example, hypothyroidism and hyperthyroidism may present similarly with nonspecific symptoms in older people, such as weight loss, fatigue, weakness, constipation, and depression. Endocrine diseases may also present with signs and symptoms that are classic for older patients yet atypical compared to those commonly observed in younger patients. As illustrations, thyrotoxic older patients may exhibit apathy and depression with psychomotor retardation ("apathetic hyperthyroidism"), and diabetes mellitus may present with hyperosmolar nonketotic state, a classic presentation rarely seen in individuals younger than age 50 years (see Chapters 108 and 109). In addition, with aging, it is increasingly common for illnesses to present without any appreciable symptoms, such as hypothyroidism or hypercalcemia secondary to hyperparathyroidism. Finally, the manifestations of endocrine disease may be altered or masked by coexisting illnesses and medications used to treat comorbidities that commonly occur in older people. For example, exacerbations of congestive heart failure or angina may be precipitated by hyperthyroidism in older patients with preexisting cardiac disease, but practitioners may mistakenly attribute the symptoms to worsening primary cardiac disease rather than to thyrotoxicosis in such patients.

Changes in Diagnostic and Therapeutic Approach

Based on the above discussion, it is clear that a high index of suspicion for endocrine (and other) diseases is required in older patients with nonspecific signs and symptoms or functional decline. Indeed, the presence of these diseases may be appreciated only upon routine laboratory screening. However, there is no firm consensus on appropriate screening practices for endocrine disorders in asymptomatic older adults. Furthermore, even with normal aging, alterations in endocrine system function may have an important impact on the diagnostic evaluation of the older patient. For example, several factors contribute to an age-related decrease in intestinal calcium absorption, including decreased renal production of 1,25-dihydroxyvitamin D ($1,25(OH)_2D$) and reduced intestinal responsiveness to 1,25(OH)$_2$D. In turn, these alterations in vitamin D metabolism and action cause an increase in parathyroid hormone (PTH) levels to maintain calcium homeostasis, and ultimately a reduction in bone mass. As a result of these changes, together with the effects of sex hormone deficiency (a common problem in both older women and men), many asymptomatic older people require evaluation for osteoporosis (see Chapter 117). In addition, the presence of concomitant medical problems, medications, and changes in nutritional status and body composition may lead to a mistaken impression of endocrine disease in older as well as in younger people. For example, decreased serum triiodothyronine and thyroxine levels may occur in patients who are systemically ill but euthyroid ("euthyroid sick" syndromes), or thyroxine levels may be increased in others receiving certain medications such as estrogen supplements, falsely giving the impression of an endocrine abnormality (see Chapter 108).

Another factor complicating the evaluation of the older patient is the lack of age-adjusted normal ranges for most endocrine laboratory tests. Normal values for these tests are usually determined in healthy young subjects, or young to middle-aged blood donors, which may or may not reflect normal values in healthy older adults. Furthermore, most studies of aging and endocrine function are cross-sectional rather than longitudinal. Because interindividual variability and heterogeneity are important concomitants of aging, the usefulness of cross-sectional studies in predicting age-related changes within an individual is limited. Finally, normative studies in older populations are often confounded by the inclusion of subjects with age-associated diseases.

Alterations in the therapeutic approach for geriatric patients with endocrine disease are similar to those required in older people with illnesses involving other body systems. First, treatment plans must take into account coexisting medical illnesses, medications, alterations in clearance rate of hormones and medications, and changes in target organ sensitivity and effects. As a result of these factors, interventions such as hormone replacement may have different outcomes in older than in young persons. For example, data from the Women's Health Initiative suggest that postmenopausal estrogen replacement therapy has a favorable benefit/risk ratio in many newly postmenopausal women, whereas in older women the risk of adverse effects such as coronary heart disease events tends to outweigh the benefits. Second, to minimize the risk of drug toxicity and polypharmacy, dosage levels for hormone replacement and medications must be adjusted for changes in clearance rate with aging, and patients should receive the lowest dose of medication needed to achieve the therapeutic effect. Third, new medications should be initiated at low doses and increased very gradually if needed. Fourth, the medication regimen should be reviewed periodically and medications should be discontinued if no longer needed. Finally, approaches that improve physical or cognitive function are of paramount importance for older people.

NEUROENDOCRINE REGULATION

Neurotransmitters and Neuropeptides

Studies directly assessing parameters of hypothalamic neuroendocrine function have not been performed in vivo in humans. However, age-related effects on hypothalamic function may be studied indirectly by examining alterations in pulsatile secretion of pituitary hormones, which reflect changes in pulsatile secretion of hypothalamic releasing and/or inhibiting hormones. Other indices of the effects of aging on hypothalamic function in humans include pituitary hormonal responses to administration of (1) hypothalamic releasing hormones, (2) agents that block end-organ feedback (e.g., clomiphene and metyrapone), and (3) agents that stimulate hypothalamic/pituitary hormonal secretion (e.g., the use of hypertonic saline to stimulate antidiuretic hormone [ADH] secretion, or arginine to stimulate growth hormone [GH] secretion).

A number of neurotransmitters and neuropeptides within the central nervous system (CNS) have been found to affect the secretion of hypothalamic and pituitary hormones. Changes in activity of these neurotransmitters and neuropeptides are responsible for many age-related alterations in the function of the endocrine system.

Dopamine

Dopamine released by hypothalamic neurons inhibits pituitary prolactin secretion. In turn, prolactin stimulates hypothalamic dopaminergic neurons, forming a short feedback loop. In humans, to a greater extent than some of the other hypothalamic neurotransmitters, changes in dopamine secretion are indirectly observable with commonly available methods. This is because dopamine is the major regulator of prolactin secretion, and changes in hypothalamic dopamine activity can be inferred through observation of changes in pulsatile prolactin secretion. The frequency of pulsatile prolactin secretion is unchanged with aging, suggesting an intact pulse generator. However, humans become relatively hypoprolactinemic with normal aging. Furthermore, the circadian rhythm of prolactin secretion is altered in older men, with a blunted or absent nocturnal rise in prolactin and reduced amplitude of prolactin pulses, as compared to young controls. Metoclopramide, a dopamine antagonist, increases nocturnal prolactin secretion to a greater degree in older people than in young subjects, suggesting that this blunted nocturnal elevation in prolactin in older men may be caused by an increase in dopaminergic tone with aging. In turn, these age-related alterations in dopaminergic activity may contribute to alterations in secretion of other anterior pituitary hormones. For example, after administration of the dopamine precursor L-dopa, plasma gonadotropins increase and thyroid-stimulating hormone (TSH) levels decrease in old but not in young male subjects, implying altered dopaminergic regulation of these hormones with aging.

Norepinephrine

Studies of postmortem brain tissue in normal older persons demonstrate a modest decrease in the number of noradrenergic neurons in the locus coeruleus, the primary source of noradrenergic innervation within the CNS. However, levels of norepinephrine (NE) in the cerebrospinal fluid (CSF) of normal older subjects are increased as compared to young adults, both in the basal state and in response to yohimbine, a stimulator of central noradrenergic activity. CSF NE is thought to be produced by noradrenergic neurons within the CNS rather than the peripheral sympathetic nervous system. Taken together with the observation that NE clearance from the CNS is unchanged in older adults, these findings suggest that central noradrenergic neuronal activity is increased with aging.

The noradrenergic neuronal system is thought to exert an important influence on pituitary secretion of a number of hormones, including GH, TSH and LH; therefore, an age-associated increase in central noradrenergic tone may be an important factor underlying age-related changes in the secretion of these hormones.

Opioid Peptides

Endogenous opioid peptides are believed to be important regulators of neuroendocrine systems. The products of proopiomelanocortin metabolism are the most extensively studied of these peptides, including adrenocorticotropic hormone (ACTH), β-endorphin, β-lipotropin, and α-melanocyte-stimulating hormone. β-Endorphin, for example, is thought to exert a tonic inhibitory influence on gonadotropin-releasing hormone (GnRH) secretion and to be an important regulator of reproductive function. In older men, administration of the opioid receptor antagonist naltrexone causes a smaller increase in LH levels than it causes in young men, and unlike in young men, there is no increase in LH pulse frequency. Taken together, these observations suggest a decrease in central opioid tone with aging. However, in the periphery, basal plasma levels of β-endorphin are unaffected, and basal ACTH levels are unchanged or increased with normal aging. Furthermore, plasma ACTH, cortisol and β-endorphin responses to physostigmine, a drug that increases CNS cholinergic activity, and ACTH and cortisol responses to administration of corticotropin-releasing hormone (CRH), are increased in older compared to younger adults. Increased responsiveness of β-endorphin and the hypothalamic–pituitary–adrenal (HPA) axis with aging may alter the function of other endocrine systems.

Melatonin

Melatonin is a hormone produced in the pineal gland that is involved in the organization of circadian and seasonal biorhythms. Its synthesis and release are stimulated by darkness and inhibited by light. Therefore, the diurnal rhythm of melatonin secretion mirrors the day–night cycle. This circadian rhythm of melatonin production is controlled by a "pacemaker" in the suprachiasmatic nucleus of the brain, but changes in environmental lighting can alter the timing of this rhythm. For example, light exposure inhibits melatonin release in a dose-dependent fashion and it is possible to reverse the diurnal melatonin rhythm within a few days by reversing the diurnal pattern of light exposure. Melatonin affects reproductive function in a variety of species, with antigonadotropic effects that are more pronounced in species with marked seasonal variation in reproductive function and breeding patterns. However, even in humans dwelling in the Arctic, conception rates and pituitary–gonadal function are reduced during the winter as compared to the summer. Melatonin levels are increased in women with hypothalamic amenorrhea, and there has been some interest in very-high-dose melatonin (75–300 mg) as a potential contraceptive agent, used in combination with a progestin.

During development and aging, melatonin production is negligible in young infants, but rises markedly between 3 months and 1 to 3 years of age, when nighttime levels are at their highest. After early childhood, melatonin secretion appears to gradually decrease, with a progressive decline in melatonin secretion by the age of 30 years. Nocturnal and 24-hour melatonin secretion appears to be similar in healthy older men and women free of confounding conditions and medications, as compared to healthy young men. Additionally, MT1 melatonin receptor expression is reduced in suprachiasmatic nucleus neurons of aged subjects and to a greater extent in persons with Alzheimer's disease, compared to young adult subjects.

Melatonin has long been known to have sedative effects, suggesting a role in sleep production. A meta-analysis of 17 studies of the effects of exogenous melatonin on sleep in subjects of various ages showed improvement in several parameters of sleep quality. In older people with insomnia, serum melatonin levels were lower than in age-matched controls without insomnia, suggesting that insomnia in older adults is caused, at least in part, by melatonin deficiency. Older adults are often exposed to significantly less environmental light than younger adults, a factor that is associated with diminished nocturnal melatonin secretion. Supplementary exposure to bright light during midday increased melatonin secretion in older adults, and tended to improve sleep disturbances in older insomniacs. In older insomniacs, short-term administration of melatonin in doses of 0.1 to 6 mg per day improved some measures of sleep quality. In older people without sleep complaints, melatonin improved sleep quality in some studies but not others. No long-term studies of melatonin supplementation have been performed in older subjects. Ramelteon, an MT1/MT2 melatonin receptor agonist, improved some measures of sleep quality in older people with chronic primary insomnia, and is approved by the U.S. Food and Drug Administration for improving sleep in individuals with difficulty falling asleep and has not been associated with dependence.

Melatonin is a potent free radical scavenger and it has been proposed that if the age-related decline in melatonin were prevented, then potentially the degenerative changes of aging could also be delayed. However, others have noted that the reported antioxidant effects of melatonin probably occur only at pharmacologic concentrations. In humans, high-affinity melatonin receptors are present on CD4 T lymphocytes and mononuclear cells in peripheral blood synthesize melatonin. Moreover, inhibition of serotonin-N-acetyltransferase, the enzyme catalyzing melatonin synthesis, was reported to cause a significant decrease in interleukin-2 (IL-2) secretion that was restored by melatonin administration. It has been proposed that melatonin may be an intracrine and paracrine regulator of immune function.

Based in part on the assumption that a decline in endogenous hormone levels constitutes a deficiency needing replacement, there has been considerable enthusiasm in the lay community for supplementation of certain hormones, including melatonin. Melatonin is readily available without a prescription in the United States, and many older people take melatonin without physician consultation. It is noteworthy that melatonin dosages of 1 to 5 mg contained in preparations commonly available over-the-counter boost nighttime levels 10 to 100 times higher than the usual maximum within an hour after administration, and only very low doses (0.1–0.3 mg) achieve peak serum levels within the normal nighttime range. Thus far, no serious side effects have been reported in humans after melatonin ingestion (aside from sleepiness after the dose), even with pharmacologic melatonin doses. However, large, long-term studies of melatonin use are still lacking, and the long-term risks and benefits of melatonin supplementation remain to be determined. Until this information is available, it is premature to advocate its use.

Hormonal Changes in Alzheimer's Disease

Alzheimer's disease is characterized by a profound impairment of cholinergic neuronal function within the CNS, but changes in the function of many other neurotransmitter and neuropeptide systems have also been described. In turn, these CNS alterations are associated with changes in pituitary and peripheral hormone levels. One important endocrine system abnormality observed in patients with Alzheimer's disease is an increase in HPA axis activity with elevated plasma ACTH and cortisol levels, and lack of suppression of cortisol levels by dexamethasone, suggesting decreased glucocorticoid feedback inhibition. In addition, ACTH responses to exogenous administration of CRH are blunted, which may be a result of down-regulation of pituitary responsiveness to CRH secondary to chronically increased hypothalamic CRH stimulation. Elevated cortisol levels are associated with memory impairment in older nondemented people, and appear to predict subsequent decline in memory function. Finally, cortisol and ACTH responsiveness to physostigmine, which increases central cholinergic activity, is markedly increased in patients with Alzheimer's disease and normal older persons, as compared to young subjects.

This elevated glucocorticoid milieu may play a role in the pathogenesis of Alzheimer's disease. It has been hypothesized that chronically increased glucocorticoid stimulation damages the hippocampal neurons that mediate glucocorticoid feedback inhibition of the HPA axis, leading, in turn, to a "glucocorticoid cascade" of neurodegeneration in Alzheimer's disease (and to a lesser extent in the aging brain). While controversial, this hypothesis remains under active study to determine whether glucocorticoid levels are a potentially modifiable risk factor for Alzheimer's disease.

Numerous epidemiological studies indicate a link between type 2 diabetes mellitus and increased risk of Alzheimer's disease. In normal physiology, and when exogenous insulin is administered at optimal doses, insulin appears to enhance some aspects of memory. However, the presence of insulin resistance as in the metabolic syndrome and type 2 diabetes mellitus is associated with an increased risk of cognitive dysfunction and possibly of Alzheimer's disease. Insulin might play a role in the pathophysiology of Alzheimer's disease through a number of mechanisms. For example, insulin may increase levels of beta-amyloid, the primary component of senile plaques, by competing with beta-amyloid for insulin-degrading enzyme, which catalyzes the breakdown of both peptides within the CNS. Insulin-degrading enzyme has a high affinity for insulin, so under conditions of high insulin availability in the brain insulin degradation is favored over degradation of beta-amyloid, thereby potentially promoting plaque formation. Additionally, increased insulin may promote cerebral inflammation, which is thought to be part of the pathophysiology of Alzheimer's disease. Inflammatory markers such as C-reactive peptide and interleukin-6 are elevated in older people with insulin resistance, and peripheral administration of high doses of insulin under hyperinsulinemic-euglycemic clamp conditions increases levels of proinflammatory cytokines within the CNS.

Many other alterations in hormone, hormone receptor, neuropeptide, and neurotransmitter levels have been reported in plasma, CSF, and postmortem brain tissue specimens in Alzheimer's disease. However, such changes have not generally controlled for the effects of nutritional status, medications, or coexisting medical illnesses and depression. NE levels in CSF are increased both in individuals with Alzheimer's disease and in normal older people. This increase is apparently caused by an increase in NE biosynthesis without a change in NE clearance. Because there is a marked loss of noradrenergic neurons in the locus coeruleus of the brain in patients with Alzheimer's disease, these findings suggest compensatory activation of the remaining noradrenergic neurons in these patients.

Anterior Pituitary

Prolactin

Healthy aging is associated with a decrease in prolactin secretion in both men and postmenopausal women, reflecting a decrease in both basal prolactin secretion and the amplitude of pulsatile prolactin release. However, serum prolactin levels may vary considerably as they can increase in many situations including stress, exercise, and sleep. Mild hyperprolactinemia observed in some older adults may result from any of several underlying causes (Table 107-1), including hypothalamic diseases that interfere with the production of dopamine (prolactin-inhibitory factor). A number of medications commonly used by older adults inhibit dopaminergic activity and increase prolactin levels, and primary hypothyroidism increases thyrotropin-releasing hormone (TRH), which stimulates prolactin secretion.

The clinical manifestations of hyperprolactinemia are typically subtle and often unrecognized. Hyperprolactinemia causes secondary hypogonadism and may exacerbate sexual dysfunction and cause gynecomastia. Rarely, galactorrhea may occur. In addition, hyperprolactinemia can accelerate age-related bone loss primarily because of the antigonadotropic effects of prolactin and resulting hypogonadism. Thus, measurement of prolactin is important in the

TABLE 107-1

Causes of Hyperprolactinemia in Older Adults

Hypothalamic diseases
  Tumors
    Metastatic disease
    Meningioma
    Glioma
  Granulomatous diseases
    Sarcoidosis
    Tuberculosis
  Irradiation
Primary hypothyroidism
Pituitary stalk section
  Suprasellar extension of pituitary adenoma
  Trauma
Pituitary prolactinoma
Chronic renal failure
Chronic liver disease
Chest wall lesions
  Herpes zoster
  Surgery
Drugs
  Phenothiazines
  Cimetidine
  Opiates
  Metoclopramide
  Estrogens

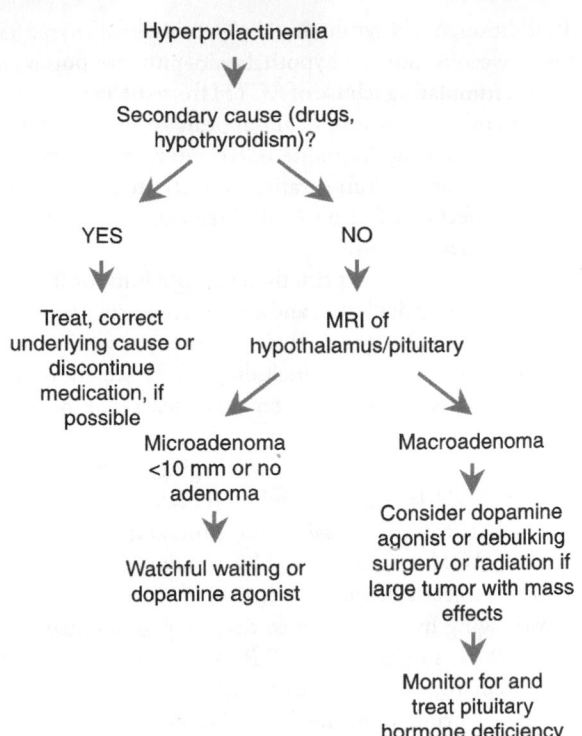

Hyperprolactinemia

↓

Secondary cause (drugs, hypothyroidism)?

YES → NO

YES:
Treat, correct underlying cause or discontinue medication, if possible

NO:
MRI of hypothalamus/pituitary

↓

Microadenoma <10 mm or no adenoma → Watchful waiting or dopamine agonist

Macroadenoma → Consider dopamine agonist or debulking surgery or radiation if large tumor with mass effects → Monitor for and treat pituitary hormone deficiency

FIGURE 107-1. Diagnostic approach for older adults with hyperprolactinemia.

evaluation of secondary causes of osteoporosis, especially when hypogonadism is present. The diagnostic approach for older adults with hyperprolactinemia is summarized in Figure 107-1. If drugs and hypothyroidism have been ruled out as causes of hyperprolactinemia, it is appropriate to obtain magnetic resonance imaging (MRI) to rule out the presence of a pituitary tumor or hypothalamic lesion (computerized tomography is much less sensitive.). Dynamic pituitary testing, such as a TRH test, is of no value in the diagnosis of this disorder.

If the hyperprolactinemia is secondary to another disorder such as hypothyroidism or a medication, the underlying cause should be corrected or the offending medication should be discontinued if possible, which often results in normalization of prolactin levels. However, if the etiology is a microadenoma (defined as a pituitary tumor <10 mm in size) or idiopathic hyperprolactinemia, options include watchful waiting or dopamine agonist medications. The natural history of microadenomas is incompletely understood, especially in older adults, but most prolactin-producing microadenomas are stable or involute with time. Accordingly, observation is the most appropriate strategy in many patients although treatment may be indicated if sexual dysfunction or additional risk factors for osteoporosis are present. Dopamine agonists such as bromocriptine or cabergoline are effective in reducing prolactin levels and normalizing reproductive axis function in most patients, but gastrointestinal, behavioral, and other side effects such as hallucinations are common in older patients. These side effects can be minimized by following a "start low, go slow" approach when beginning these medications. Of note, high doses of cabergoline may be associated with an increased risk of valvular heart disease. Surgery is rarely indicated, but may be necessary in those with macroadenomas (>10 mm) and persistent visual field defects or inability to tolerate dopamine agonists.

Alternatively, radiation therapy may be an option for patients with large tumors who are unable to tolerate medical therapy and are not surgical candidates. However, the clinical response to radiation is often delayed for months to years, and anterior pituitary insufficiency eventually occurs in many, if not most, of these patients.

Age-associated alterations in secretion of other anterior pituitary hormones are discussed below, under the individual hormonal systems, and in Chapter 108 (Thyroid Disorders) and Chapter 46 (Menopause and Midlife Health Changes).

Pituitary Adenomas

Although the incidence of pituitary tumors increases with aging, symptomatic pituitary tumors are uncommon even in people of advanced age. However, the prevalence of pituitary tumors at autopsy ranges from 8.5% to 27%, indicating that the vast majority of these tumors are clinically "silent." In case series of pituitary tumors in older adults, the majority of lesions are apparently nonfunctioning adenomas, whereas 9% to 17% are GH-secreting tumors and 4.5% to 10% are prolactinomas. However, many, if not most, apparently nonfunctioning adenomas actually produce quantities of gonadotropins or the α-subunit of these glycoprotein hormones.

Nonsecreting tumors and tumors that secrete LH, follicle-stimulating hormone (FSH), or α-subunit are usually large at the time of diagnosis, because there are few or no symptoms of hormone overproduction. Gonadotropin hypersecretion from such tumors usually does not result in excessive gonadal hormone secretion although LH hypersecretion occasionally results in elevated testosterone levels. Clinical manifestations of these tumors are usually a result of a mass effect, including visual field abnormalities caused by compression of the optic chiasm, headaches, and panhypopituitarism. Gonadotropin-secreting pituitary tumors are particularly difficult to diagnose in postmenopausal women in whom gonadotropin levels are elevated as a result of ovarian failure. For these women, exaggerated α, LH-β, and FSH-β subunit responses, and/or intact gonadotropin responses to TRH are useful in diagnosing these tumors. However, pituitary "incidentalomas" are being increasingly identified during neuroimaging evaluations for comorbid conditions, accounting for 5% to 15% of pituitary tumors identified in older adults. Most of these are asymptomatic though endocrine and visual disturbances should be sought in these patients. Diagnosis of pituitary tumors depends on neuroimaging (especially magnetic resonance imaging). Management of large pituitary tumors usually involves transsphenoidal decompression and debulking, along with assessment of anterior pituitary hormone function and replacement of hormone deficiencies. Macroprolactinomas may be managed with dopamine agonists in many cases even when large or associated with visual field changes although these agents may be less effective in older than in young adults (Figure 107-1). Pituitary function should be reassessed in patients started on dopamine agonists for a prolactinoma because recovery of pituitary function occurs in some individuals treated with these medications.

Hypopituitarism and the Empty Sella Syndrome

As a pituitary macroadenoma grows, destruction of normal surrounding pituitary tissue occurs, leading ultimately to a predictable

TABLE 107-2

Causes of Hypopituitarism in Older Persons

Pituitary adenomas

Sequelae of irradiation or surgery for pituitary tumors

Peripituitary tumors (e.g., meningioma, glioma, metastatic cancer)

Vascular conditions (e.g., pituitary infarction, carotid artery aneurysm, subarachnoid hemorrhage)

Traumatic brain injury (e.g., stalk section)

Infiltrative or granulomatous diseases (e.g., lymphocytic hypophysitis, hemochromatosis, histiocytosis X, sarcoidosis)

Infections (e.g., tuberculosis, mycoses, abscesses)

loss of gonadotropins and GH followed by TSH and eventually ACTH secretion. The resulting panhypopituitarism may present clinically as a constellation of symptoms including supine and/or postural hypotension, fatigue, loss of libido, weight loss, hypogonadism, hyponatremia, and hypoglycemia. Many of these symptoms are nonspecific and common in older patients without panhypopituitarism, so a high index of suspicion is required to make the diagnosis. Causes of hypopituitarism in adults are summarized in Table 107-2.

Initially, measurements of basal serum levels of morning cortisol and ACTH; total or free testosterone (in men) and gonadotropins; free thyroxine and TSH; IGF-1; and prolactin may be sufficient to confirm panhypopituitarism. Measurement of both the pituitary hormone and the target hormone concentration allows assessment of the appropriateness of both levels together. Dynamic ACTH (cortrosyn) stimulation testing is indicated to confirm the diagnosis of secondary hypoadrenalism. ACTH and other dynamic tests of adrenal function are discussed below under "Laboratory Testing of HPA Axis Function" (also see Chapter 108).

As computed tomography (CT) and MRI have come into widespread use, it is increasingly common to discover incidentally the presence of both pituitary masses and empty sella syndrome. MRI studies of healthy young and older subjects found that pituitary height and volume tend to decrease with aging, with empty sella occurring in 19% of subjects. No relationship was found between pituitary volume and anterior pituitary hormone levels. Most cases of primary empty sella syndrome (i.e., not associated with prior pituitary tumor, surgery or irradiation) occur in obese, hypertensive middle-aged women. Clinically apparent pituitary dysfunction is uncommon, although up to 15% of subjects may manifest endocrine dysfunction including hyperprolactinemia, hypogonadism, or panhypopituitarism. However, the functional significance of an empty sella as an incidental finding on imaging studies in apparently healthy older patients is unclear. In such patients, conservative management is appropriate, including visual field testing and serum hormone testing to rule out subclinical pituitary dysfunction and suprasellar involvement.

Posterior Pituitary

Antidiuretic hormone (ADH), or arginine vasopressin (AVP), is synthesized in "magnocellular" neurons of the hypothalamus and released into the systemic circulation from nerve terminals in the posterior pituitary gland in response to increased plasma osmolality, decreased arterial pressure, and reductions in circulating blood vol-

ume. In addition, ADH synthesized in "parvocellular" hypothalamic neurons is released into the hypothalamic–pituitary portal circulation, in turn stimulating release of ACTH from the anterior pituitary into the systemic circulation. ADH appears to be colocalized with corticotrophin-releasing hormone (CRH) in parvocellular neurons of the hypothalamus. Administration of ADH together with CRH amplifies the effect of CRH on ACTH release, suggesting a role for ADH in responses to stress.

Older people are at higher risk than young adults for the development of both volume depletion and excess free water states. This is a result of age-related changes occurring in the systems that maintain volume status and osmolality, including ADH secretion, osmoreceptor and baroreceptor systems, renal concentration of urine and hormone responsiveness, and thirst mechanisms. There is evidence for a state of relative ADH excess with aging, with normal to increased basal ADH levels, increased ADH release after an osmotic stimulus such as hypertonic saline infusion, and impaired ethanol inhibition of ADH secretion in older persons, as compared with young adult subjects. Furthermore, renal free water clearance decreases with aging in proportion to declining glomerular filtration rate (GFR). With a reduction in GFR, proximal renal tubular fluid absorption is increased, leading to a decrease in fluid delivery to the distal diluting portions of the nephron. The net result is a decrease in the diluting capacity of the kidney and a decreased ability to excrete a free water load. This age-related reduction in free water clearance, together with relative ADH excess and the increased prevalence of conditions such as congestive heart failure, hypothyroidism, and the use of sulfonylurea and diuretic medication all contribute to the common occurrence of free water excess and hyponatremia in older people. When present, hyponatremia in frail older adults is usually mild and asymptomatic, but these individuals may develop more marked symptomatic hyponatremia in the setting of acute illness.

In contrast to the increased osmoreceptor sensitivity to ADH, baroreceptor regulation of ADH is decreased with aging, resulting in decreased ADH release in response to hypotension or hypovolemia and increased risk of volume depletion. Furthermore, renal responsiveness to ADH is diminished with aging, possibly because of chronic exposure to elevated ADH levels, leading to a decrease in maximal urine concentrating ability. Decreased aldosterone and increased atrial natriuretic hormone activity with aging contribute to the potential for volume depletion by decreasing the capacity of the kidneys to conserve sodium under conditions of fluid deprivation (see "Renin–Angiotensin–Aldosterone System" later in this chapter). Finally, healthy older adults exhibit decreased thirst and reduced fluid intake in response to fluid deprivation, hyperosmotic stimuli, and hypovolemia, further contributing to the risk of dehydration with aging. Older patients with immobility or dementia, such as nursing home residents, are at particularly high risk for severe dehydration and hypernatremia.

A number of factors predispose older people to nocturnal polyuria. These include age-related blunting of the circadian rhythm of circulating ADH, with loss of the nocturnal increase in ADH levels, and an increase in nighttime plasma atrial natriuretic hormone levels. Patients with Alzheimer's disease have lower circulating ADH levels than cognitively intact people of the same age, and appear to be particularly prone to nocturnal polyuria. Superimposed on age-related changes in bladder function and mobility, altered ADH regulation can contribute to urinary incontinence. Older patients with nocturnal polyuria may benefit from administration of the ADH

TABLE 107-3

Alterations in Hypothalamic–Pituitary–Glucocorticoid Axis Function with Aging

ACTH levels	↔
ACTH response to CRH stimulation	↔
Cortisol production	↓
Cortisol clearance from plasma	↓
Plasma cortisol levels	↔
Cortisol response to stimulation	
ACTH	↔
Metyrapone, hypoglycemia	↔/↑
Surgical stress	↑
HPA axis sensitivity to glucocorticoid feedback	↓

↓, decreased; ↔, unchanged; ↑, increased; ACTH, adrenocorticotropic hormone; CRH, corticotropin-releasing hormone; HPA, hypothalamic–pituitary–adrenal.

analog desmopressin (DDAVP), in addition to other interventions such as detrusor muscle relaxants and behavioral interventions.

See Chapter 88 for additional information on effects of aging on salt and water regulation.

HYPOTHALAMIC–PITUITARY–ADRENAL AXIS

Physiology

Compared to the other hypothalamic–pituitary–end-organ axes, hypothalamic–pituitary–glucocorticoid function is relatively intact with aging in humans (Table 107-3). The cortisol secretion rate is decreased with aging, but this is matched by a decrease in the cortisol metabolic clearance rate. As a result, basal plasma concentrations of cortisol are unchanged with aging even in very old subjects. Consistent with intact cortisol secretion, basal ACTH levels are also unaffected by aging. Furthermore, glucocorticoid responsiveness of the HPA axis to stimulation is well-maintained in older adults, with intact cortisol responses to exogenous ACTH stimulation (except at very low doses of ACTH [0.06 μg]) and normal or slightly prolonged cortisol and ACTH responses to metyrapone, ovine CRH,

and insulin-induced hypoglycemia. ACTH pulse frequency appears to be maintained in older men, suggesting intact hypothalamic regulation of glucocorticoid function. Moreover, the circadian rhythm of ACTH and cortisol secretion is intact in healthy older subjects although the amplitude of the cortisol rhythm is reduced and the nighttime cortisol nadir is increased in older compared to young adults. In addition, a phase advance of the cortisol rhythm occurs in older people, with earlier nadir and peak secretion, as compared to young adults. This phase advance has been attributed to behavioral changes, possibly reflecting an earlier bedtime in older adults.

Although still controversial, many studies have reported age-related alterations in the cortisol response to stress. After a stressful stimulus such as surgery, peak cortisol levels are higher and remain elevated longer in older compared to young adult subjects. Furthermore, dexamethasone is less effective in suppressing cortisol levels in older subjects, and in studies using metyrapone to remove endogenous cortisol feedback inhibition, the decline in ACTH levels after exogenous cortisol infusion was blunted and delayed in older compared to young adult subjects. Taken together, these studies indicate that the sensitivity of the HPA axis to glucocorticoid negative feedback is decreased with aging. The clinical implications of this decreased responsiveness to glucocorticoid feedback inhibition are unclear. However, it has been proposed that the resulting chronic increase in glucocorticoid exposure may damage hippocampal neurons regulating glucocorticoid secretion and important to cognitive function, leading to a vicious cycle of further glucocorticoid hypersecretion and damage to mechanisms regulating HPA feedback inhibition.

Laboratory Testing of HPA Axis Function

Although glucocorticoid function is well-preserved with aging, certain factors may interfere with testing of HPA axis function in older patients (Table 107-4). For example, excretion of steroids commonly measured in urine is decreased with renal impairment, and measurements are unreliable in people with a creatinine clearance of less than 50 mL/min. Moreover, because the acute cortisol stress response may be higher and prolonged in older patients, testing for Cushing's syndrome should be delayed for at least 48 hours after major stresses such as high fever, trauma; or surgery.

TABLE 107-4

Potential Pitfalls in Laboratory Diagnosis of Cushing's Syndrome in Older Adults

TEST	POTENTIALLY CONFOUNDING FACTORS	TEST ALTERATION	COMMENTS
24-hour urine cortisol	Renal impairment, undercollection Overcollection, severe malnutrition, stress, chronic anxiety, alcoholism, depression	False-negative urine cortisol False-positive urine cortisol	Normal level excludes Cushing's syndrome
DST	Obesity, estrogens, anticonvulsant medications, depression, alcoholism, acute illness	False-positive DST (Pseudo-Cushing's)	Cortisol nonsuppression common in older adults (high sensitivity but low specificity)
Late-night salivary cortisol	Hypertension, advanced age, psychiatric diagnoses	False-positive (increased) salivary cortisol	Repeat testing often normal in false-positive situations
Urine 17-hydroxycorticosteroid levels	Medications (e.g., phenytoin, phenobarbital)	Falsely decreased urine 17-hydroxycorticosteroid levels (false-negative test for hypercortisolism)	

DST, dexamethasone suppression test.

The ACTH stimulation test is used to screen for both primary and chronic secondary (central) adrenal insufficiency. Expected cortisol responses to the standard dose of 250 μg of ACTH (absolute serum cortisol level of > 20 μg/dL at 30 or 60 minutes after an IV bolus of ACTH or cortrosyn) do not change with aging. The rationale for its use in assessing pituitary function is that in patients with chronic pituitary disease, the absence of sufficient stimulation of the adrenal glands by endogenous ACTH leads to adrenal atrophy and hyporesponsiveness to exogenous ACTH. Thus, a serum cortisol > 20 μg/dL either at baseline or after ACTH rules out adrenal insufficiency. However, the standard ACTH stimulation test lacks sensitivity for mild secondary adrenal insufficiency. The low-dose ACTH stimulation test, performed with 1 μg of ACTH and measurement of cortisol 30 minutes after injection, has been proposed as a more sensitive test, but a meta-analysis demonstrated similar diagnostic utility for the low-dose and standard-dose ACTH tests. In patients with a positive ACTH stimulation test, a plasma ACTH level obtained at 8:00 A.M. may help to distinguish primary from secondary adrenal insufficiency with a high plasma ACTH, indicating primary adrenal insufficiency and normal or low ACTH indicating secondary adrenal insufficiency. However, additional dynamic testing of adrenal axis function may be indicated for borderline abnormal ACTH stimulation test results. Furthermore, the ACTH stimulation test should never be used in cases of suspected acute or recent onset of hypopituitarism, because the adrenal glands may still be able to respond normally to any ACTH challenge. In patients with septic shock, a reduced increment between basal and post-ACTH cortisol level (< 9 μg/dL) may be a more useful indicator of "relative adrenal insufficiency" that is associated with improved pressor responsiveness and mortality in response to glucocorticoid treatment.

The cortisol response to insulin-induced hypoglycemia is a reliable test for primary or secondary adrenal insufficiency, but may be inappropriate in frail older patients because of the potential risks associated with severe hypoglycemia. In patients with a normal response to ACTH stimulation, the metyrapone test can be used to confirm suspected secondary adrenal insufficiency. Metyrapone inhibits 11β-hydroxylase, the final step in cortisol synthesis, and in normal individuals, ACTH secretion increases, stimulating adrenal secretion of 11-deoxycortisol. However, oral metyrapone may cause dizziness, nausea, and vomiting in some older patients, and it has been suggested that intravenous metyrapone infusion is safer and better tolerated in older people.

Hyperadrenocorticism

Cushing's syndrome is an eponym for the constellation of signs and symptoms of chronic corticosteroid excess, including central obesity; catabolic effects on muscle, skin, and bone; glucose intolerance; hypertension; hypogonadism; and hirsutism and acne (in women).

Glucocorticoid Therapy

The most common cause of Cushing's syndrome in older adults, as in other age groups, is the pharmacological administration of glucocorticoids. The undesirable effects of glucocorticoid treatment are similar in older and younger patients, but in older people glucocorticoids may cause major adverse effects upon function (Table 107-5). When it is necessary to use pharmacologic doses of glucocorticoids, older patients should receive the minimum necessary dosage for the shortest possible period of time, and the dosage requirement should

TABLE 107-5

Adverse Effects of Glucocorticoids in Older Patients

Central nervous system
  Impaired cognition
  Emotional lability
  Depression
  Psychosis
Bone
  Osteoporosis
  Fractures
Muscle
  Proximal muscle wasting
  Weakness
Fluid and electrolytes
  Sodium retention, edema
  Hypokalemia
Metabolic
  Central obesity
  Hyperglycemia
  Hypertriglyceridemia
Cardiac
  Congestive heart failure
  Hypertension
Gastrointestinal
  Peptic ulcer disease
Skin
  Fragility
  Impaired wound healing
Vision
  Cataracts
  Glaucoma
Immune system
  Decreased cell-mediated immunity
  Increased risk of infections
Functional
  Impaired ambulation and transfers
  Falls
  Loss of independence

be reviewed at frequent intervals. Bone densitometry measurements using dual-energy x-ray absorptiometry (DXA) should be performed prior to initiating long-term corticosteroid therapy and after 6 to 12 months of therapy (Figure 107-2). As for the evaluation of osteoporosis not associated with corticosteroid use, all patients should be assessed for modifiable osteoporosis risk factors, secondary causes of osteoporosis, primary hyperparathyroidism, and vitamin D deficiency.

Some of the adverse effects of corticosteroid use in older people can be minimized with other interventions (Figure 107-2). For example, because corticosteroids decrease intestinal calcium absorption and increase urinary calcium losses, ensuring an intake of at least 1500 mg elemental calcium per day together with at least 800 to 1000 IU/day of vitamin D helps to minimize bone loss. In individuals with low 25-hydroxyvitamin D levels (< 32 ng/mL), high-dose vitamin D (e.g., ergocalciferol 50 000 IU should be given weekly for 12 weeks after which a repeat 25-OH vitamin D level should be performed; the goal is to normalize the 25-OH vitamin D level). Occasionally, high-dose vitamin D (ergocalciferol 50 000 IU weekly or twice weekly) or calcitriol (0.25 or 0.50 μg/day) may be needed to maintain vitamin D sufficiency, but follow-up of both serum and

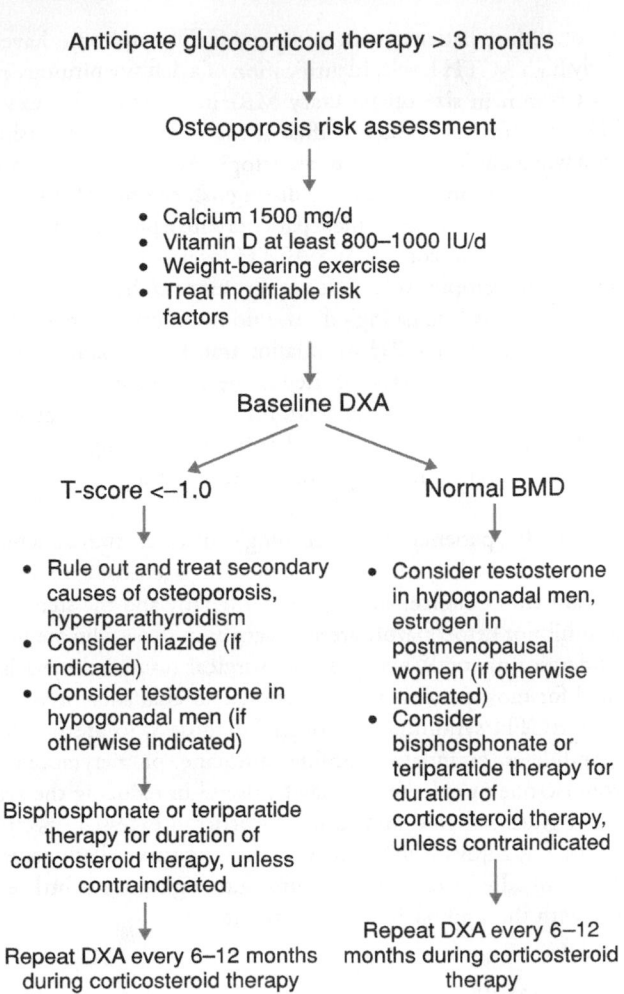

FIGURE 107-2. Prevention and management of glucocorticoid-induced osteoporosis. DXA, dual-energy x-ray absorptiometry; BMD, bone mineral density.

urine calcium levels is required. Furthermore, dietary sodium restriction (2–3 g/d) and thiazide diuretics (e.g., hydrochlorothiazide, 25 mg/day) are useful to reduce hypercalciuria associated with corticosteroid use, although their effects on bone density have not been adequately determined in patients receiving corticosteroids.

Hormone replacement therapy can be considered to counteract corticosteroid-induced suppression of sex hormones. Estrogen supplementation (e.g., conjugated estrogens 0.625 mg/day with medroxyprogesterone acetate 2.5–5.0 mg daily for women with an intact uterus) may help postmenopausal women taking corticosteroids, but its use is controversial. Men with corticosteroid-induced and/or other causes of hypogonadism should receive androgen-replacement therapy (e.g., testosterone enanthate or cypionate, 100–200 mg IM every 2 weeks, or daily transdermal application of a testosterone patch or gel). Although testosterone therapy in hypogonadal men has not been demonstrated to reduce fracture risk, it has been shown to improve bone mineral density and to ameliorate other manifestations of androgen deficiency. Bisphosphonates should be considered as first-line therapy for patients who will be taking the equivalent of prednisone 7.5 mg per day or more for at least 3 months, because clinically significant bone loss may occur with this dose and duration of therapy. Bisphosphonates used for prevention and treatment of corticosteroid-induced osteoporosis increase bone mineral density at the lumbar spine and hip, and reduce the risk of

fractures of the vertebral spine. However, the cost effectiveness of bisphosphonates in the treatment of glucocorticoid-induced osteoporosis is best established in individuals of more advanced age and with lower (more abnormal) T-scores for bone mineral density. Options include alendronate 70 mg weekly (or 10 mg daily), risedronate 35 mg weekly (or 5 mg daily), or ibandronate 150 mg monthly. For patients who cannot tolerate oral bisphosphonates, intravenous bisphosphonates (e.g. zolendronic acid 5 mg iv once yearly) may be considered, although its efficacy in glucocorticoid-induced osteoporosis has not been established. As an alternative to bisphosphonates in persons with severe glucocorticoid-induced osteoporosis, teriparatide (recombinant human PTH 1–34) 20 μg sc daily may be used. However, expense and daily subcutaneous injections from cartridges requiring refrigeration may make teriparatide therapy less desirable for older persons. Calcitonin (e.g., 200 IU intranasally per day) preserves bone mass at the lumbar spine but not at the femoral neck in patients taking glucocorticoids. However, it is a weak antiresorptive agent that has significant tachyphylaxis and its efficacy in fracture prevention in these patients has not been established.

Corticosteroid-induced myopathy is characterized by weakness and atrophy of the muscles of the hip, thigh, and proximal upper extremities, which may result in an increased risk of falls in older people with age-related loss of muscle mass. The best approach for this difficult problem is to minimize the dose of corticosteroid or to eliminate it altogether if possible. For those who require ongoing corticosteroid therapy and cannot be tapered off these drugs, resistance and endurance exercise, and androgen-replacement therapy in men, may help to prevent glucocorticoid-induced muscle atrophy. However, the effectiveness of these approaches in preventing functional decline in older patients has not been determined.

Hypercortisolism

Cushing's disease, or hypercortisolism caused by excessive pituitary ACTH secretion, is most common in persons between 20 and 40 years of age. Accounting for approximately two-thirds of cases of endogenous hypercortisolism in younger adults, Cushing's disease is a much-less-common cause of cortisol excess in older people, although its exact prevalence in older adults is unclear. In contrast, the ectopic ACTH syndrome is more common in older people, most of whom have obvious neoplasms such as small cell lung cancer although other tumors may be clinically undetectable as in the case of some bronchial carcinoid tumors. Patients with the ectopic ACTH syndrome caused by small-cell lung cancer or other rapidly growing tumors typically present with cachexia rather than central obesity, hypertension, and metabolic disturbances including hypokalemia, metabolic alkalosis, and hyperglycemia. Cortisol-producing adrenal carcinomas are more common in older people than in young adults, with a bimodal peak incidence in children and in people older than age 60 years. These tumors may produce severe Cushing's syndrome with virilization in women and mineralocorticoid excess, although many of these tumors are nonfunctioning and do not cause symptoms of Cushing's syndrome. Adrenocortical carcinomas are typically large (>100 g) and palpable unlike benign adrenal adenomas which are usually 10 to 20 g (size 1–6 cm) at presentation.

Diagnostic Testing If there is a clinical suspicion of Cushing's syndrome, diagnostic options include a 24-hour urinary free cortisol, a

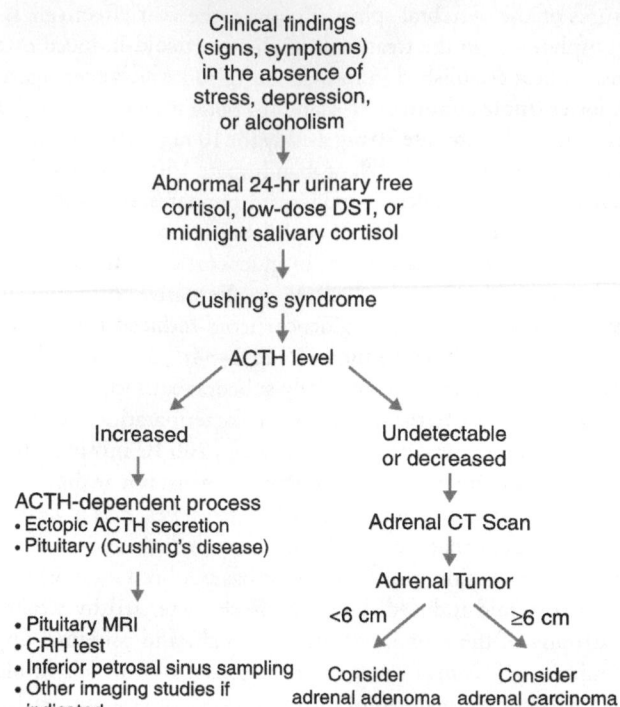

FIGURE 107-3. Diagnostic evaluation for suspected Cushing's syndrome. ACTH, adrenocorticotropic hormone; CRH, corticotropin-releasing hormone; DST, dexamethasone suppression test.

low-dose dexamethasone suppression test (DST), or a midnight salivary cortisol level (Figure 107-3). False-positive results are common with the low-dose DST in older people, even in apparently normal individuals, and the urinary-free cortisol test may be confounded by inadequate urine collections or the presence of renal insufficiency. Additionally, one or both tests may be confounded by other conditions commonly encountered in older adults including obesity, medications such as phenytoin, depression, active alcoholism, or other coexisting stressful illnesses (Table 107-4). In these instances of "pseudo-Cushing's syndrome," patients retain normal circadian variation in serum cortisol levels despite increased cortisol secretion, whereas circadian rhythmicity is lost in patients with bona fide Cushing's syndrome. A midnight salivary cortisol level distinguishes patients with Cushing's syndrome from those with pseudo-Cushing's syndrome with a high degree of specificity and sensitivity in young and middle-aged adults. However, elevated late-night salivary cortisol levels are common in older adults and individuals with type 2 diabetes mellitus without Cushing's syndrome, suggesting a need to increase the diagnostic threshold of the test in these populations. Cortisol secretion usually normalizes in patients with pseudo-Cushing's syndrome with remission of the underlying condition.

After the diagnosis of Cushing's syndrome is established, simultaneous plasma ACTH and cortisol levels are obtained to determine whether the cortisol excess is ACTH-dependent or ACTH-independent. If ACTH levels are undetectable or low and cortisol levels are high, then an ACTH-independent process is present, suggesting an adrenal tumor. In this case, CT scanning of the adrenals is indicated to confirm the diagnosis. If ACTH and cortisol levels are increased, then hypercortisolism is ACTH-dependent, usually reflecting a pituitary adenoma (Cushing's disease) or ectopic ACTH

secretion. Most patients with ectopic ACTH syndrome have extremely high ACTH levels. Identification of a definite pituitary mass at least 6 mm in size on pituitary MRI in patients with elevated ACTH and cortisol levels is sufficient for a diagnosis of Cushing's disease when clinical features of an ectopic ACTH secreting tumor are absent. Infusion of CRH can distinguish ectopic ACTH secretion from Cushing's disease; most patients with a pituitary tumor will show an increase in cortisol and ACTH levels after CRH, whereas patients with ectopic ACTH-secreting tumors will not. However, many patients with Cushing's disease do not meet the stringent response criteria for the CRH stimulation test. Venous sampling from the inferior petrosal sinus is required in these cases, and referral to an endocrinologist is usually indicated. Imaging to search for an occult ACTH secreting tumor is indicated only after Cushing's disease has been ruled out with inferior petrosal sinus sampling.

Treatment In patients with Cushing's disease, transsphenoidal surgery performed by a neurosurgeon with extensive experience is the treatment of choice, although radiotherapy and the steroidogenesis inhibitor ketoconazole are alternatives in those who are unable to undergo surgery. When possible, surgical tumor removal is indicated for most patients with functional adrenal adenomas or the ectopic ACTH syndrome, although for those who are not surgical candidates, aminoglutethimide, mitotane, or metyrapone and spironolactone or eplerenone may be useful in reducing the symptoms of glucocorticoid and mineralocorticoid excess, respectively. Additionally, adjuvant mitotane may prolong survival after surgical resection of adrenocortical carcinoma, although there is little experience with this approach in older patients.

Adrenal Insufficiency

Primary adrenal insufficiency is less common in older persons than in young adults; less than 10% of patients with adrenocortical failure are older than age 60 years at initial presentation. As in younger patients, most cases of adrenal insufficiency in older people are a result of acute stress or rapid withdrawal of glucocorticoids in patients with suppressed adrenal function caused by chronic glucocorticoid administration. Autoimmune adrenocortical insufficiency is rare in older patients, but other causes of adrenal insufficiency, including tuberculosis, adrenal hemorrhage, and metastatic disease, are much more common in older persons than in young adults. Tuberculous involvement of the adrenals is nearly always associated with evidence of past or current tuberculosis infection elsewhere in the body, and may manifest with large calcified adrenal glands on plain x-rays or CT scans. Adrenal hemorrhage typically presents acutely in anticoagulated patients with symptoms such as nausea, vomiting, hypotension, and tachycardia, and is likely to be the cause if bilateral adrenal enlargement is demonstrated on CT scan. Metastatic disease involving the adrenals occurs most commonly with lymphomas and carcinomas of the lung, colon, and prostate, although even when metastases are present, it is unusual for cortisol secretion to be impaired.

The presentation of chronic adrenal insufficiency is usually vague and nonspecific in older patients, with symptoms of "failure to thrive" including weight loss, anorexia, confusion, weakness, and decreased functional status. Examination findings may include orthostatic hypotension, supine hypotension, cachexia, and hyperpigmentation, and laboratory testing may reveal hyponatremia, hyperkalemia, azotemia, and hypoglycemia. However, one-third of older patients with primary adrenal insufficiency are not hyperkalemic at initial presentation, and hyperpigmentation, hyperkalemia, and orthostatic hypotension are not present in patients with secondary adrenal insufficiency. These signs and symptoms are nonspecific and common in older people and are, therefore, easily attributable to another condition. Consequently, it is important to suspect this diagnosis in older patients with worsening functional status and vague symptoms. Unfortunately, adrenal insufficiency has historically been more commonly fatal in older people and more likely to be diagnosed only at autopsy, as compared to younger patients.

Once the diagnosis is suspected, the evaluation is the same as for younger patients: the ACTH stimulation test establishes the diagnosis. Treatment is also the same as in young adults. In patients with primary adrenal insufficiency and less-severe mineralocorticoid deficiency, replacement doses of hydrocortisone may provide sufficient mineralocorticoid activity. However, those with absent mineralocorticoid function (manifested by orthostatic hypotension and electrolyte abnormalities such as hyperkalemia and hyponatremia) also require fludrocortisone, titrated to normalize electrolyte abnormalities. These patients should be monitored closely to avoid volume overload and hypertension. During minor illnesses or other stresses, maintenance glucocorticoid doses should be doubled for 2 to 3 days, whereas for major surgery or trauma, much higher doses of hydrocortisone (e.g., 50 to 100 mg intravenously every 8 hours) are usually administered initially. Patients with adrenal insufficiency should be given a parenteral glucocorticoid to be used if nausea and vomiting prevent ingestion of oral glucocorticoid replacement, and they should also have a bracelet or necklace identifying them as being adrenally insufficient.

Women with adrenal insufficiency and impaired mood and health-related quality of life may benefit from replacement of the adrenal androgen DHEA (25–50 mg per day), which has been shown to improve mood, fatigability, sexuality, and sense of well-being in these patients. Of note, high-density lipoprotein cholesterol levels decreased in one study of DHEA replacement in women with adrenal insufficiency. The long-term safety of DHEA replacement in people with adrenal insufficiency has not yet been established, including the possible risk of sex steroid-dependent tumor growth (see Adrenal Androgens and Aging).

Chronic glucocorticoid therapy suppresses HPA axis function and results in adrenal atrophy because of the loss of ACTH stimulation. As a result, cessation of corticosteroids may be associated with a prolonged period of decreased pituitary ACTH secretion and adrenal responsiveness to ACTH. Recovery of HPA axis responsiveness is variable and may not occur for months in some individuals. Older people may be particularly at risk to develop adrenal insufficiency as a consequence of withdrawal of steroid therapy for several reasons. For example, older adults may forget medicines or become confused about their medicines because of a complicated regimen or associated cognitive impairment. Other patients may discontinue medicines abruptly without consulting their physician because of expense or unacceptable side effects. The clinical features of adrenocortical insufficiency secondary to withdrawal of glucocorticoids (or hypopituitarism) are nonspecific and similar to those of primary adrenal insufficiency, although findings suggesting mineralocorticoid insufficiency (orthostatic hypotension and hyperkalemia) and hyperpigmentation (associated with high ACTH production) are

usually absent. Based on the foregoing, a high index of suspicion is necessary to detect adrenocortical insufficiency in older people caused by cessation of chronic glucocorticoid therapy. It is appropriate to perform the ACTH stimulation test in such patients, and those with persistent adrenocortical insufficiency should receive glucocorticoid coverage for major surgery or other stresses until HPA axis function has normalized.

Adrenal Androgens and Aging

The adrenal steroids DHEA and its sulfated form (DHEAS) are the most abundant steroids in the human circulation. DHEA and DHEAS are precursors of both male and female sex steroids including testosterone, estradiol, and progesterone, as well as the glucocorticoid corticosterone. Neither DHEA nor androstenedione bind to or activate the androgen receptor to a significant degree, so they are considered to be very weak androgens that act mostly as prohormones. However, these prohormones may exert physiological actions indirectly via tissue-specific conversion to active androgens or estrogens.

In men, 5% to 30% of DHEA is of testicular origin, with the remainder synthesized in the zona reticularis of the adrenal cortex. In women, DHEA is produced almost exclusively by the adrenal cortex, whereas androstenedione and testosterone are secreted by both the adrenal glands and the ovaries. Total circulating androgens decline with aging as a result of both ovarian failure and a decrease in adrenal production of androgens and androgen precursors. However, in contrast to estrogen deficiency, ovarian androgen secretion may persist after menopause and the decline in androgens is more gradual, typically beginning at least a decade before menopause.

The Princeton Consensus Statement proposed a definition of "female androgen deficiency syndrome" consisting of symptoms of impaired libido and well-being in the setting of low testosterone levels and adequate estrogenization either through normal ovarian function or estrogen replacement therapy. This definition has been criticized on several grounds. First, impairment of libido is typically multifactorial in origin and is not a specific indicator of androgen deficiency. Additionally, clinical studies in women across the life span have not found a correlation between testosterone levels and sexual function although interpretation of such studies is confounded by the lack of testosterone assays with sufficient sensitivity and accuracy at the very low concentrations of testosterone present in women, the lack of consensus on the most appropriate measures to assess sexual function, and other issues. Furthermore, the risks and feasibility of offering androgen replacement to all women with self-rated impaired well-being and low circulating androgen levels has been questioned.

Women who have undergone bilateral oophorectomy or who develop adrenal insufficiency develop severe androgen deficiency and may present with symptoms of decreased libido, energy, and well-being. Androgen replacement therapy may be justifiable in these women to treat severe, symptomatic androgen deficiency. On the other hand, a recent Endocrine Society guideline recommended against attempts to diagnose androgen deficiency in women at present, based on the lack of a clearly defined clinical syndrome and the unavailability of normative data on testosterone levels across the life span that can be used to define androgen deficiency. Based on the foregoing discussion, androgen replacement does not appear indicated for postmenopausal women with decreased libido.

Dehydroepiandrosterone Supplementation for Older Adults

Studies in rodents have reported a variety of beneficial effects of DHEA administration, including enhancement of immune function and prevention of a variety of disorders including cancer, obesity, and diabetes mellitus. However, these data have limited applicability to humans, because rodents have negligible production of adrenal androgens such as DHEA, and many of these studies used grossly supraphysiological doses of DHEA. In humans, some epidemiological studies have reported associations between DHEA levels and overall health. For example, DHEA levels are decreased in people with active rheumatoid arthritis, acquired immunodeficiency syndrome (AIDS), cancer, and cardiovascular disease, and DHEA levels are positively correlated with vigor and longevity. Additionally, high-functioning older adults have higher DHEAS levels than low-functioning individuals. Based on these findings and the marked decline in DHEA levels with aging, there has been considerable interest in the potential therapeutic effects of DHEA supplementation in older people.

Randomized controlled trials of DHEA in older adults have not revealed clear evidence of meaningful benefits. A 2-year trial of DHEA in people older than 60 years of age (75 mg daily in men and 50 mg daily in women, achieving circulating DHEA levels in the high-normal range for young adults) found no notable effects on body composition, physical performance, or insulin sensitivity. Earlier studies of DHEA supplementation at physiological to supraphysiological doses for up to 1 year reported inconsistent effects on body composition, glucose tolerance, and muscle strength. Several studies have reported small and inconsistent increases in bone mineral density that was deemed minimal in comparison to the effects of established osteoporosis treatments. A study of DHEA supplementation in 280 healthy older people 60 to 79 years of age reported an increase in libido in female subjects. However, androgen supplementation in older women remains controversial as noted above. Several randomized, placebo-controlled studies have failed to show improvements in well-being, mood, and cognition in healthy older adults receiving DHEA. No consistent effects of DHEA supplementation have been reported in vivo on immune function in older humans, for example, in studies of antibody responses to influenza vaccination or tetanus toxoid. It is possible that subgroups of older patients such as depressed or cognitively impaired people may benefit from DHEA supplementation, but these subgroups have not yet been defined.

To date, there have been no reports of significant adverse effects of DHEA supplementation in older people. DHEA is metabolized to sex steroids within prostate and breast tissue, but deleterious changes such as elevations in PSA and prostate volume have not been reported. Nevertheless, large and long-term studies on the scale of the Women's Health Initiative would be required to address these potential concerns definitively.

Adrenal Neoplasms

Benign adrenal neoplasms are common, with autopsy studies identifying these masses in approximately 6% of cases. Adrenocortical nodularity increases with aging, and the probability of identifying an adrenal "incidentaloma" on computerized tomography of the abdomen increases from 0.2% in people between 20 and 29 years of age to 6.9% in people older than 70 years of age. Most of these are adrenocortical adenomas, but adrenal carcinomas and pheochromocytomas also occur. One large survey reported that 4.2% of adrenal incidentalomas are pheochromocytomas. The goals of assessment are to determine whether the incidentaloma is functional (hormone-secreting) and to characterize it as benign or malignant.

Patients with adrenal incidentalomas should be queried for a history or episodes of hypertension, palpitations, headaches, and diaphoresis, suggestive of pheochromocytoma. Examination findings of proximal muscle wasting and weakness, purple striae, osteoporosis (height loss), hirsutism, and central obesity, suggestive of Cushing's syndrome, should be noted. Appropriate screening tests to determine whether the tumor is functional include a 24-hour urine collection for total and fractionated metanephrines and catecholamines, or plasma-free metanephrines to rule out pheochromocytoma, and in hypertensive patients, a morning plasma aldosterone concentration to plasma renin activity ratio. Androgen-secreting tumors are rare, and endocrine screening for androgen overproduction is not indicated in the absence of clinical signs and symptoms of hormone excess. Screening for corticosteroid hyperfunction is controversial. Many adrenal cortical adenomas have a degree of functional autonomy. In 57 patients (mean age 59 years) with adrenal incidentalomas screened with a 2-day low-dose DST, 12% had serum cortisol levels of 5 to 7.8 μg/dL, 67% had values of 1 to 5 μg/dL, and cortisol was undetectable in only 21%, whereas all control subjects suppressed cortisol to undetectable levels. Furthermore, higher cortisol levels after the DST were associated with larger adrenal incidentaloma size, higher midnight cortisol levels, and lower basal ACTH levels. Moreover, hypertension and obesity are significantly more prevalent in people with adrenal incidentalomas than in the general population. Indeed, most middle-aged patients with incidentalomas and cortisol nonsuppression after low-dose DST experienced improvement in hypertension, obesity, and diabetes control after adrenalectomy.

These data suggest that subtle autonomous glucocorticoid secretion is common in adrenal cortical adenomas, and that this secretory activity may be clinically significant. Some experts advocate screening individuals with adrenal incidentalomas for "subclinical" Cushing's syndrome using the overnight low-dose DST, with confirmatory tests in people with a positive result (24-hour urinary free cortisol, midnight salivary cortisol, and/or 2-day high-dose DST; and subsequent plasma ACTH) to rule out false-positives. However, tests of glucocorticoid function, such as the low-dose DST, have a high sensitivity but a relatively low specificity, therefore screening all older people with adrenal incidentalomas for subclinical Cushing's syndrome would result in a large proportion of false-positive results and additional evaluation in these cases. Furthermore, many of the tests proposed for confirmation of the diagnosis of subclinical Cushing's syndrome (e.g., 24-hour urinary free cortisol) lack sufficient sensitivity to identify mild hypercortisolemia, and there is no consensus on the appropriate laboratory criteria for this diagnosis. Of note, patients followed longitudinally for up to 7 years showed spontaneous normalization of hormonal hypersecretion in many cases, whereas a few others with apparently nonfunctioning adenomas developed subclinical hormonal hypersecretion. Finally, the long-term outcomes of adrenalectomy versus medical management of hypertension, diabetes, and obesity in older patients with adrenal cortical adenomas are unknown. Therefore, it may be prudent to restrict screening for corticosteroid hyperfunction to younger patients and those with a symptom complex including weight gain, muscle weakness, osteoporosis, hypertension, diabetes mellitus. and skin atrophy. suggesting Cushing's syndrome. However, screening is indicated in patients with adrenal incidentalomas who are scheduled for major surgery, because postoperative adrenal crisis may occur in patients with unrecognized subclinical Cushing's syndrome. For older patients undergoing surgery, laparoscopic adrenalectomy offers a less-invasive approach, but it is unknown whether adrenalectomy will prove superior to careful observation and management of the metabolic syndrome in these patients.

The other major issue in the evaluation of adrenal incidentalomas is assessment of malignancy risk. The size of the mass is a useful indicator of risk, with benign adenomas usually ranging in size from 1 to 6 cm, and adrenal carcinomas usually greater than 6 cm in diameter. In a survey of 1004 patients with adrenal incidentalomas, a size cutoff of 4 cm yielded optimal sensitivity but low specificity for malignant adrenal lesions. However, patients with carcinoma were significantly younger than were patients with adenoma. Imaging characteristics other than size may also be helpful in assessing malignant potential, including image attenuation on noncontrast CT, enhancement with contrast media, and magnetic resonance signal intensity on T2-weighted images. Although an increase in mass size has been considered suggestive of malignancy, excision of enlarging masses has generally identified benign underlying pathology. Indeed, studies of the natural history of adrenal incidentalomas indicate that with long-term follow-up, most of these lesions remain clinically insignificant and morphologically unchanged. Subclinical hormone hypersecretion develops in some individuals, but the risk of progression to overt hypersecretion is minimal. Furthermore, aggressive evaluation and management of adrenal incidentalomas in all older adults would be cost-prohibitive.

Based on the foregoing discussion, a conservative approach is warranted in the management of most older people with apparently nonfunctioning adrenal incidentalomas. In surgical candidates, tumors associated with overt hormonal hypersecretion and lesions larger than 6 cm should generally be removed. Masses less than 3 cm in size probably do not need further evaluation or follow-up. Lesions between 3 and 6 cm without other imaging characteristics suggesting malignancy may be followed with serial imaging studies, although the benefits of serial imaging have been questioned.

SYMPATHOADRENAL SYSTEM

Physiology

The sympathetic nervous system (SNS) plays a key role in the regulation of physiological homeostasis, including cardiovascular and metabolic functions. For example, postganglionic sympathetic neurons projecting to the heart and blood vessels regulate cardiac output and arterial blood pressure. The SNS stimulates release of epinephrine from the adrenal medulla, which in turn plays an important role in the regulation of both cardiovascular function and energy metabolism. SNS dysfunction has been implicated in the pathogenesis of a variety of age-associated disorders, including hypertension, obesity, congestive heart failure, type 2 diabetes mellitus, and sudden cardiac death.

NE is the primary neurotransmitter released by sympathetic postganglionic neurons. After release, most of the NE is taken up again into the presynaptic and postsynaptic axon terminals, whereas only a small fraction diffuses into the circulation. The adrenal medulla contains specialized postganglionic sympathetic neurons that enzymatically convert NE into epinephrine, the major secretory product of these cells.

There is a general consensus that SNS activity is increased with aging in humans. Basal plasma NE levels are increased in older people because of an increase in NE secretion and, to a lesser extent, a decrease in clearance. Furthermore, plasma NE responses to various stimuli such as upright posture, cold pressor tests, exercise, and hand grip are also increased with aging. By comparison, adrenal medullary function is relatively unchanged until 75 to 80 years of age. Clearance of epinephrine is increased with aging. However, in subjects younger than age 75 years, increased clearance appears to be balanced by a proportionate increase in epinephrine secretion, with no change in circulating epinephrine levels. However, in people older than age 80 years, levels of epinephrine are increased both at baseline and after cold-pressor testing, suggesting important effects of advanced age on both the sympathoneural and the sympathoadrenomedullary components of the SNS.

Although SNS tone is increased with aging, physiologic responses to adrenergic receptor-mediated stimulation generally decrease with aging. For example, the increased NE levels in older subjects do not increase basal heart rate, and stimulation of β-receptors by isoproterenol produces less of an increase in heart rate and contractility in aging, as compared to young individuals. Furthermore, aging subjects exhibit decreased β-receptor–mediated chronotropic responses to stimuli such as hypoxia, and decreased arterial vasoconstrictor responses to α-adrenergic stimulation. This decreased responsiveness to catecholamines appears to be a result of changes at both the receptor and the postreceptor level, including reduction in receptor number, decreased receptor affinity, and receptor–effector uncoupling.

Clinical

Hypertension

Clinical consequences of this age-related hyperadrenergic state may include the development of hypertension. Several studies report unchanged α-mediated arterial vasoconstriction with normal aging. Based on these studies, together with observations that β-adrenergic-mediated vascular smooth muscle relaxation is decreased with aging, it has been hypothesized that older people are predisposed to develop hypertension as a result of relatively unopposed α-adrenergic tone. However, this hypothesis was cast into doubt by studies that found a decrease in arterial α-adrenergic responsiveness to NE in normal older people, implying an appropriate compensatory response to elevated SNS tone with aging. When compared with older normotensive people, older hypertensive subjects exhibit an increase in vascular α-adrenergic receptor responsiveness despite equal or greater SNS activity. Therefore, a combination of an increase in systemic SNS tone and enhanced α-adrenergic receptor responsiveness may contribute to essential hypertension in older adults. In clinical practice, antihypertensive drugs that block CNS sympathetic outflow or SNS-mediated peripheral vasoconstriction may cause orthostatic hypotension in older adults, especially postprandially when gastrointestinal vasodilation occurs.

Metabolic Syndrome

Several lines of evidence suggest an important role of the SNS in the pathogenesis of the metabolic syndrome. First, various components of the metabolic syndrome such as obesity and hypertension are associated with an increase in SNS activity. For example, individuals with insulin resistance, hypertension, and obesity exhibit resting tachycardia, elevated plasma NE levels, increased secretion of NE from sympathetic nerves, and adrenoreceptor down-regulation. Second, increased sympathetic tone is associated with a decrease in insulin sensitivity. For example, experimental maneuvers in healthy subjects that decrease venous return cause an increase in NE release and peripheral vasoconstriction, together with an acute reduction in insulin sensitivity. Finally, adrenergic overactivity is associated with end-organ damage associated with the metabolic syndrome. Distensibility of medium and large arteries is decreased by sympathetic tone, which over time may promote atherogenesis.

Based on the foregoing discussion, inhibition of sympathetic overactivity is a potential therapeutic goal in people with the metabolic syndrome. This can be achieved either by adhering to an energy-restricted diet or by physical training. Of note, although moderate dietary sodium restriction is commonly recommended for people with hypertension, even a moderate restriction of sodium intake in people with the metabolic syndrome may precipitate SNS activation and potentially worsen insulin resistance. Angiotensin-converting enzyme inhibitors and angiotensin II receptor antagonists have sympathoinhibitory effects, and are useful antihypertensive agents in people with the metabolic syndrome.

Autonomic Insufficiency

Autonomic insufficiency may result from primary peripheral nervous system failure, coexisting diseases such as diabetes mellitus or multiple system atrophy, or drugs that interfere with SNS function. The most common clinical manifestation of these conditions is orthostatic hypotension, defined as a decrease in systolic blood pressure of at least 20 mm Hg, or a fall in diastolic blood pressure of at least 10 mm Hg within 3 minutes after arising from a supine to a sitting or standing position. In addition, the pulse rate may fail to increase despite a significant fall in blood pressure in more advanced cases. Other manifestations of autonomic insufficiency may include erectile dysfunction, urinary incontinence, urinary retention, constipation, gastroparesis, and anhidrosis. Aside from these clinical observations, and the identification of underlying disorders such as diabetes mellitus, routine laboratory testing of SNS function is not indicated. Management options for orthostatic hypotension associated with autonomic insufficiency are summarized in Table 107-6 Multiple interventions are usually employed simultaneously. Midodrine, an α_1-adrenergic receptor agonist with few cardiac or CNS side effects, is often better tolerated by older adults than fludrocortisone. For management of other clinical manifestations of autonomic insufficiency, see Chapter 49 (Sexual Dysfunction), Chapter 59 (Incontinence), and Chapter 93 (Constipation).

Pheochromocytoma

Pheochromocytoma is a rare tumor, with an incidence of less than 1% in patients with hypertension. Most cases are thought to occur in young and middle-aged adults, but epidemiologic and autopsy data indicate a progressive age-specific increase in the incidence rate. It is unclear whether some pheochromocytomas diagnosed at autopsy are nonfunctioning and of no clinical significance, or whether the disease is underdiagnosed in older patients. However, based on the

TABLE 107-6

Management Approaches For Orthostatic Hypotension Caused by Autonomic Insufficiency

Nonpharmacological
- Eliminate or reduce medications associated with postural hypotension
- Dangle legs for several minutes prior to arising from bed
- Dorsiflex ankles several times before arising from bed or chair
- Avoid rapid changes in position when arising from bed or chair
- Avoid dehydration
- Wear elastic support stockings to maximize venous return
- Liberalize dietary sodium intake
- Eat frequent, small meals to minimize postprandial hypotension
- Elevate head of bed up to 20 degrees
- For patients with a history of prolonged bedrest, increase amount of time spent sitting up each day

Pharmacological
- Fludrocortisone (mineralocorticoid, volume expander)
- Midodrine (α_1-adrenergic receptor agonist)
- When antihypertensive therapy is required, ACE-I, ARB, and β-blockers with intrinsic sympathomimetic activity are less likely to worsen OH

ACE-I, angiotensin converting enzyme inhibitors; ARB, angiotensin-receptor blockers; OH, orthostatic hypotension.

foregoing discussion, the age-related decrease in responsiveness to catecholamines may result in a muting or an absence of symptoms of excessive adrenergic stimulation such as diaphoresis and palpitations. Furthermore, pheochromocytomas present with protean symptoms and signs that may mislead the clinician, earning it the title of the "Great Masquerader." The diagnosis may be especially challenging in older adults with signs and symptoms of comorbid illnesses that further confound the diagnosis. Therefore, a high index of suspicion is necessary to make this diagnosis in older patients. A symptom complex of headaches, palpitations, and diaphoresis; refractory or severe hypertension of unknown cause; or a paradoxical blood pressure response to beta-blocking medications may suggest the diagnosis.

The diagnosis depends on the documentation of elevated 24-hour urinary total and fractionated catecholamines and metanephrines, or plasma metanephrines in a patient who is hypertensive or symptomatic at the time of specimen collection. Although some groups have advocated for the use of plasma free metanephrines as a sensitive and specific diagnostic test, debate remains regarding the relative merits of the various tests. Diagnostic accuracy may be improved by using a combination of tests. Of note, medications such as tricyclic antidepressants, alpha$_1$- and beta-adrenergic blocking agents, and calcium channel-blockers may cause false-positive results for one or more biochemical tests for pheochromocytoma. Imaging studies are useful for preoperative localization of tumor but generally not for diagnosis.

Surgical intervention is indicated in older patients with resectable pheochromocytomas, in view of the potential for surgical cure and the poor prognosis with medical management. Preoperative localization of tumor should be undertaken using abdominal CT or MRI scanning, with localization of extraadrenal foci using [123]I- or ^{131}I-metaiodobenzylguanidine (MIBG) scintigraphy. An additional benefit of MIBG scintigraphy is that the compound is taken up by adrenergic cells, confirming that the mass is adrenergic in cases where biochemical studies are indeterminate. 6-[^{18}F]fluorodopamine positron emission tomography scanning may be valuable in cases where conventional imaging modalities fail to locate the tumor despite compelling biochemical and clinical evidence of pheochromocytoma.

A careful cardiologic evaluation is warranted preoperatively in all patients with pheochromocytoma; the presence of coronary artery disease or cardiomyopathy may influence preoperative medical management. α-Receptor blockade is usually initiated preoperatively for blood pressure control even in normotensive patients, often in combination with β-blockers. However, β-receptor-blocking agents should not be given until after α-blockade is achieved, to avoid an increase in blood pressure induced by unopposed α activity. In addition, patients with pheochromocytoma have a contracted plasma volume and saline infusion is indicated for moderate volume expansion.

Occasionally, a pheochromocytoma will present as an adrenal incidentaloma with normal urinary metanephrines and catecholamines, and negative MIBG scintigraphy, but during surgery. its intraoperative behavior and subsequent histological findings indicate pheochromocytoma. It is important to take prophylactic measures during surgery for this possibility, including placement of an arterial line and arrangement for immediate access to intravenous nitroprusside.

RENIN–ANGIOTENSIN–ALDOSTERONE SYSTEM

Aldosterone secretion decreases with aging. Despite a concomitant decline in clearance rate, basal plasma aldosterone levels are 30% lower in healthy octogenarians compared to younger adults (Table 107-7). Aldosterone secretion is also reduced after stimuli such as sodium depletion or upright posture. However, these changes do not appear to be secondary to adrenal dysfunction because aldosterone responsiveness to ACTH is intact with aging. The primary defect responsible for these changes in aldosterone secretion is thought to be a reduction in plasma renin activity, which is decreased by 50% in older persons, as compared to younger adults. This decline

TABLE 107-7

Effects of Aging on Hormonal Regulation of Fluid and Sodium Balance

Antidiuretic hormone (ADH)	
Basal ADH levels	↑
ADH release after osmoreceptor stimulation	↑
ADH release after baroreceptor stimulation	↓
Renal responsiveness to ADH	↓
Aldosterone	
Basal aldosterone levels	↓
Aldosterone release after sodium depletion	↓
Aldosterone release after postural challenge	↓
Aldosterone release after ACTH stimulation	↔
Renin	
Plasma renin activity	↓
Atrial natriuretic hormone (ANH)	
Basal ANH levels	↑
ANH responses to stimuli	↑

↓, decreased; ↔, unchanged; ↑, increased.

TABLE 107-8

Risk Factors for Hyperkalemia in Older People

Diabetes mellitus*
Renal insufficiency or failure
Intravascular volume depletion
Adrenocortical insufficiency
Acidosis
Medications
   Aldosterone antagonists (spironolactone, eplerenone)
   Sodium channel antagonists ("potassium-sparing" diuretics: triamterene, amiloride)
   Trimethoprim-sulfamethoxazole
   Angiotensin-converting enzyme inhibitors
   Angiotensin antagonists
   Beta-adrenergic blocking agents
   Nonsteroidal anti-inflammatory agents
Potassium-containing salt substitutes
Tissue injury with rapid release of potassium from cells
   Crush injury
   Tumor lysis syndrome
   Hemolysis

*Multiple contributors, including insulin deficiency, renal insufficiency, hyporeninemic hypoaldosteronism, type IV renal tubular acidosis, and use of angiotensin-converting enzyme inhibitors.

in active renin concentration is thought to be a result of diminished conversion of inactive to active renin. In addition, age-related increases in atrial natriuretic hormone secretion contribute to the suppression of aldosterone secretion with aging, both directly and by inhibiting renal renin secretion, plasma renin activity, and angiotensin II levels. See Chapter 88 for additional information on effects of aging on salt and water regulation.

The clinical consequences of decreasing aldosterone levels with aging include a predisposition to renal sodium wasting, which, in combination with reduced thirst and decreased renal ADH responsiveness, further increases the potential for volume depletion and dehydration in geriatric patients. Furthermore, this state of relative hyporeninemic hypoaldosteronism places older adults at increased risk of hyperkalemia, especially patients with diabetes mellitus and renal insufficiency (Table 107-8). The addition of aldosterone antagonists, β-blocking agents, nonsteroidal antiinflammatory drugs, or heparin may lead to potentially life-threatening hyperkalemia in such patients.

GROWTH HORMONE AXIS

Physiology

Secretion of GH from the pituitary is regulated by the hypothalamic peptides GH-releasing hormone (GHRH) and somatostatin. These two peptides exert an opposing effect on GH secretion, with GHRH stimulating and somatostatin inhibiting GH secretion by the pituitary somatotropes. In humans, GH secretion appears to be controlled primarily by pulsatile GHRH secretion. In turn, insulin-like growth factor-1 (IGF-1 or somatomedin C), which is secreted by the liver and other peripheral tissues in response to GH, mediates most of the actions of GH. Furthermore, IGF-1 exerts a negative feedback effect on GH secretion through a direct effect at the pituitary level and indirectly by increasing somatostatin production. Most IGF-1 circulates in protein complexes with IGF binding protein-3 (IGFBP-3) or IGFBP-5. IGFBPs act in concert to regulate circulating levels of free IGF-1. In addition, IGFBPs appear to inhibit as well as stimulate IGF-1-mediated bioactivity, and in some cases, they may exert effects independent of IGF-1. Secretion of GH is pulsatile in response to pulsatile GHRH secretion, generally with very low circulating levels except for several pulses occurring during the first few hours of sleep, after meals or exercise, or without apparent cause. In young adult men, most of the GH is secreted within the first 4 hours after sleep onset, with large amplitude pulses occurring during slow-wave sleep, with IGF-1 levels remaining fairly constant over a 24-hour period. In contrast, young women have multiple episodes of GH secretion and a high basal output of GH during the daytime, with relatively low GH release during the night.

GH release is affected by numerous other factors, including other neurotransmitters and neuropeptides, medications, hormonal influences, blood glucose levels, degree of obesity, and physiologic states such as sleep and exercise. For example, the neurotransmitter dopamine and CNS-active dopaminergic agonists such as bromocriptine exert a stimulatory effect on GH release by promoting hypothalamic GHRH release. NE and α-adrenergic agonists also increase GHRH and GH release, whereas β-adrenergic agonists and dopamine- or α-receptor-blocking agents inhibit GH secretion. Furthermore, the GH-releasing effects of other stimuli such as exercise, stress, hypoglycemia, and arginine are thought to be mediated via α-adrenergic stimulation. Estrogens stimulate GH release, and premenopausal women have higher peak GH levels with exercise, arginine, and insulin-induced hypoglycemia than age-matched men. In contrast, GH secretion is inhibited in those treated chronically with glucocorticoids. Hyperglycemia is associated with decreased GH levels and GH responses to GHRH. Similarly, obese subjects exhibit decreased spontaneous GH secretion and reduced GH responsiveness to pharmacological stimulation compared to nonobese subjects, although IGF-1 levels are typically within normal limits. GH levels are acutely elevated during exercise, and there is indirect evidence that regular exercise may enhance GH secretion over the long term.

Age Effects

GH secretion reaches maximum levels at puberty, followed by a gradual but progressive decline with age. In adult men, GH secretion declines by approximately 14% per decade, such that by age 70 to 80 years, about half of all individuals have no significant GH secretion during a 24-hour period. Plasma IGF-1 levels exhibit a corresponding decline of 7% to 13% per decade, and by age 70 to 80 years, approximately 40% have plasma IGF-1 levels in the range found in GH-deficient children. In addition, serum levels of IGFBP-3 decline with aging in healthy adults, but it is unclear whether this affects the metabolic activity of IGF-1 with aging.

Collectively, these decreases in pituitary secretion of GH and circulating IGF-1 levels are often referred to as the somatopause. The age-related decrease in GH production appears to be primarily caused by a decrease in hypothalamic GHRH secretion and an increase in hypothalamic somatostatin release, rather than attenuation in pituitary responsiveness to GHRH. Accordingly, GH secretion and IGF-1 levels can be normalized with exogenous GHRH ad-

ministration. The age-related decrease in GH secretion is partially reversed by fasting in older people without an associated alteration in sleep quality, suggesting that lifestyle modification may augment endogenous GH secretion in older adults.

Growth Hormone Deficiency in Adults with Hypothalamic–Pituitary Disease

GH deficiency in adults with established hypothalamic–pituitary disease is associated with reduced lean body mass, muscle strength, and exercise capacity; diminished psychological well-being; insulin resistance; increased total body adiposity; higher waist-to-hip ratio of fat distribution; reduced bone density; adverse effects on lipid metabolism; and increased risk of death from cardiovascular disease, despite adequate replacement of other hormones including thyroxine, cortisol, and sex steroids. Many of these effects can be improved or corrected with daily subcutaneous administration of one of a number of recombinant human GH formulations, and GH supplementation is approved in the United States for adults with hypopituitarism and GH deficiency. Improvements in cardiac function, muscle strength, body composition, bone mass, metabolic indices, and health-related quality of life have been sustained in small trials lasting up to 10 years, and treatment has generally been well tolerated. The most commonly reported adverse effects of GH treatment in adults with hypopituitarism are fluid retention/edema, arthralgias, myalgias, and carpal/tarsal tunnel syndrome. These symptoms are most likely to occur in people who are older or obese, and are more common in those with the greatest increase in IGF-1 levels during treatment. However, these symptoms often resolve spontaneously during treatment and disappear with treatment cessation. Insulin sensitivity is further reduced in the short term with GH treatment, but later returns to baseline with prolonged treatment in studies of up to 7 years' duration. To date, there is no evidence that GH replacement increases the risk of diabetes mellitus in adults. Moreover, glycosylated hemoglobin and serum triglyceride levels tend to decline in patients treated with GH for more than 3 years. Retrospective studies have reported an increased rate of neoplasia as well as cancer-related mortality in patients with pituitary adenomas although it is unclear whether these findings reflect inherent risk, increased surveillance, or the effects of treatments received.

The diagnosis of GH deficiency in adults is suggested clinically by the presence of multiple pituitary hormone deficiencies and should be suspected in any patient with a history of hypothalamic–pituitary disease. However, laboratory criteria for distinguishing older adults with organic GH deficiency from those with normal age-related reductions in GH secretion have not yet been clearly defined. Furthermore, assessment of GH function is complicated by the need for GH stimulation tests, the lack of adequate normative data for many laboratories, assay variability, and the unavailability of appropriate age-adjusted normal values for diagnostic tests. Static GH levels are unsuitable for diagnosis, because GH is secreted episodically. IGF-1 levels decline during normal aging and are not a reliable indicator of GH deficiency secondary to pituitary disease in people older than 40 years of age, although IGF-1 levels below the age-adjusted normal range may suggest the diagnosis. Normal IGF-1 levels do not exclude the diagnosis of GH deficiency at any age. The insulin tolerance test is considered the most definitive test for GH deficiency in adults, but this test may be dangerous in older patients with ischemic heart disease. Arginine-induced GH secretion remains intact with normal aging, and the arginine/GHRH stimulation test has been proposed as a safer yet reliable alternative to distinguish GH deficiency secondary to hypopituitarism from normal age-related reductions in GH secretion. In patients with hypothalamic causes of suspected GH deficiency, arginine should be used without GHRH to avoid falsely normal results, because GHRH directly stimulates the pituitary. In adults with milder hypopituitarism, for example, two or fewer pituitary hormone deficiencies, it is advisable to use two independent stimulation tests to confirm GH deficiency.

As with younger adults, older people with GH deficiency related to hypopituitarism also appear to benefit from GH replacement. People with more severe biochemical and clinical manifestation of GH deficiency are more likely to derive benefit from GH replacement. In prospective cohort studies, GH-deficient adults older than age 65 years receiving GH replacement therapy for at least 12 months experienced significant improvements in knee flexion/extension and handgrip strength, total and low-density lipoprotein cholesterol levels, waist/hip ratio, and quality-of-life measures without significant deterioration in glucose homeostasis. The GH replacement dose in older GH-deficient adults is lower than that required by younger adults. In one study, a dose of 0.5 mg of GH per day resulted in elevated serum IGF-1 levels in half of older subjects, and 25% developed side effects on this dose. Most older subjects maintained IGF-1 levels within the normal range on 0.17 to 0.33 mg per day. By contrast, younger adults may require doses up to 1 mg per day. Treatment should begin at a low dose (e.g., 0.1–0.2 mg per day) with slow upward titration at no more than monthly or bimonthly intervals based on clinical and biochemical responses. Serum IGF-1 levels should be maintained within the normal adult range to optimize the beneficial effects of GH replacement while minimizing the potential for side effects such as carpal tunnel syndrome, arthralgias, fluid retention, and gynecomastia. Patients with an active malignancy should not receive GH supplementation. It should be noted that GH therapy is costly, which along with the need for daily sc injections may limit its use in an older population with limited resources. Longer-acting GHRH analogs and GH secretagogues are being developed for the treatment of adult GH deficiency, which will eventually increase the range of therapeutic options for older people with this disorder.

Growth Hormone Supplementation for Older People Without Hypothalamic–Pituitary Disease

Normal aging is associated with alterations in body composition similar to those in GH-deficient younger patients, including decreased muscle mass and strength, reduced bone mass, and increased adiposity. In turn, declining strength and bone mass are associated with increasing risk for falls and fractures in older people. These observations suggest that the reduction in GH secretion associated with aging (the somatopause) may contribute to alterations in body composition and increased frailty in older adults, and that GH supplementation, GHRH, or GH secretagogue treatment might be clinically useful in preventing or reversing these age-related changes.

Since the initial publication of a study by Rudman and colleagues that reported potentially beneficial changes in body composition with short-term GH supplementation in older men, interest in GH as an "antiaging" hormone has increased dramatically. It is estimated that 20,000 to 30,000 individuals in United States used GH for this purpose in 2004, and that up to one-third of the prescrip-

tions for GH worldwide are for "off-label" use. However, its use to prevent aging-related changes has remained controversial and it is illegal in the United States to distribute GH for use as an antiaging remedy.

A systematic review in 2007 of randomized, controlled trials of GH supplementation for up to 1 year in healthy older people found modest decreases in fat mass and increases in lean body mass in subjects receiving GH compared to placebo-treated subjects. These potentially beneficial effects on body composition were largely confined to men, possibly reflecting the observation that women require larger doses of GH over a longer period of time than men to achieve physiological replacement of GH. Although body composition improved (increase in lean mass and decrease in fat mass) in men treated with physiological amounts of GH for 6 months, muscle strength, endurance and functional status did not improve. Total serum cholesterol levels tended to decrease, but no significant changes occurred in bone mineral density or other serum lipid levels with GH supplementation. Older subjects receiving GH were more likely to develop peripheral edema, carpal tunnel syndrome, arthralgias, and gynecomastia. GH-treated subjects tended to have a higher incidence of impaired fasting glucose and type 2 diabetes mellitus, but this was not significant. Because of the limited study duration and small size of the study groups, no effect of GH treatment was reported on cancer risk or death. Overall, there is little evidence that GH supplementation improves other relevant outcomes in healthy older people, including strength, function, or quality of life. Based on the observations of minimal clinical benefit and a high rate of adverse effects, GH supplementation is not recommended as an antiaging treatment in healthy older adults.

THE HYPOTHALAMIC–PITUITARY–TESTICULAR AXIS

Age Effects

Significant age-related changes occur in male reproductive function with aging, including a decrease in sexual activity, libido, and fertility rates. However, in contrast to the relatively rapid and complete loss of gonadal function in women at the time of menopause, changes in testicular function in aging men occur gradually, vary considerably between individuals, and often do not result in severe hypogonadism. Many healthy older men exhibit a degree of primary testicular failure, with decreases in total and free or bioavailable testosterone levels, testosterone responses to exogenous gonadotropin administration, and daily sperm production, together with increased serum gonadotropin levels (Figure 107-4). Occasionally, community-dwelling older men present with overt testicular failure with total testosterone levels well below normal and symptoms of androgen deprivation including hot flashes, decreased libido, and gynecomastia. However, it is more common to see older patients with mildly decreased testosterone levels and relatively nonspecific symptoms such as impotence, loss of libido, osteopenia, and muscle weakness. In contrast, more marked testosterone deficiency is common in frail older men. For example, in male nursing home residents, it has been reported that 45% exhibit testosterone levels within the hypogonadal range.

Several factors contribute to this decrease in testosterone levels with aging (Table 107-9). First, testicular testosterone production

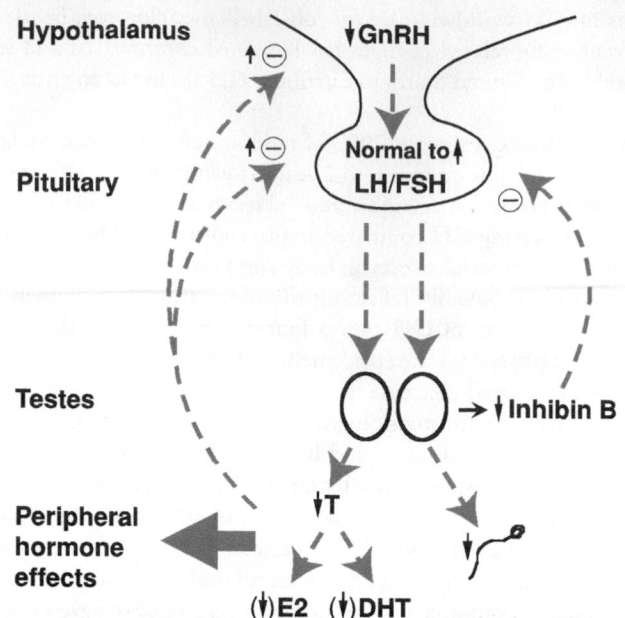

FIGURE 107-4. Age-related changes in male hypothalamic–pituitary–gonadal axis function. GnRH, gonadotropin-releasing hormone; LH, luteinizing hormone; FSH, follicle-stimulating hormone; E2, estradiol; DHT, dihydrotestosterone. Small solid arrows denote direction of change with aging.

is markedly reduced with aging, which is reflected in the decreased number and volume of Leydig cells in the aging testis. This reduction in testosterone production capacity may manifest as a more severe and prolonged depression of testosterone levels during intercurrent illness or other stresses in older men. Second, both production rates

TABLE 107-9

Age-Related Changes in Hypothalamic–Pituitary–Testicular Axis Function

Circulating levels of hormones and binding globulins
• Total T	↓
• Free/bioavailable T	↓↓
• SHBG	↑ (usually within normal range)
• Total E$_2$	→
• Free E$_2$	→/↓
• Total DHT	→/↑
• Free DHT	→/↓
• Inhibin B	↓
• LH	→/↑ (usually within normal range)
• FSH	→/↑ (may remain within normal range)

Other parameters of male reproductive function
• Testicular T production in response to LH	↓
• Daily sperm production	↓
• Sperm fertilizing capacity	→
• Bioactive/immunoreactive LH	↓
• Bioactive/immunoreactive FSH	↓
• Gonadotropin responsiveness to GnRH	→
• LH pulse frequency	↓

T, testosterone; SHBG, sex hormone binding globulin; E$_2$, estradiol; DHT, dihydrotestosterone; LH, luteinizing hormone; FSH, follicle-stimulating hormone; GnRH, gonadotropin-releasing hormone.

and metabolic clearance of testosterone are reduced in aging men, but in contrast to adrenal cortisol secretion and metabolism, the decrease in testosterone production is not completely offset by a decrease in clearance. Third, the normal circadian variation in testosterone levels observed in young men, with highest levels in the morning, is blunted with aging, resulting in reduced serum testosterone concentrations. Fourth, the concentration of the major testosterone binding protein, sex hormone-binding globulin (SHBG), increases with aging, Therefore, serum free or non-SHBG-bound (bioavailable) testosterone concentrations decline to a greater extent with aging than total testosterone. Finally, impairment of testicular function is associated with medical illnesses, medications, and malnutrition, which are commonly present in aging men. However, hypogonadism does not occur in all aging men; many healthy men older than age 80 years maintain serum testosterone levels within the normal young adult range.

In addition to these deficits in testicular function, hypothalamic/pituitary control of testicular function is also impaired with aging. Although gonadotropin levels increase with aging, they usually remain within normal limits, and the hormonal profile of a low testosterone and normal gonadotropin levels is consistent with aging-related secondary hypogonadism. Even in men with elevated levels of LH and FSH, the increases in gonadotropins are sometimes inappropriately low in comparison to younger men with similar reductions in testosterone levels, and FSH levels are more commonly elevated than LH levels. Furthermore, the ratio of bioactive to immunoreactive LH and FSH is decreased in older men, indicating that gonadotropin levels measured by radioimmunoassay may underestimate the extent of gonadotropin deficiency. Finally, healthy older men exhibit intact LH and FSH responsiveness to prolonged exogenous pulsatile GnRH administration but an inappropriately normal or decreased LH pulse frequency (an indicator of hypothalamic GnRH pulse-generator activity), as compared to young men. Based on the above evidence, it appears that age-related hypogonadism is a consequence of combined testicular and hypothalamic dysfunction.

The physiologic significance of the decrease in testicular androgen production associated with aging (often referred to as "late-onset hypogonadism," "partial androgen deficiency of the aging male," or "andropause") is uncertain. However, as testosterone levels decline with aging, various functional changes occur in androgen-dependent body tissues. In the testes, there are significant age-related decreases in the number of Sertoli cells, volume of seminiferous tubules, daily sperm production, and to some extent testicular volume. Serum levels of inhibin B, which is secreted by Sertoli cells and mediates feedback inhibition of pituitary FSH secretion, also decrease with aging. In studies controlled for the increased length of time between ejaculations in older men, sperm concentrations were unchanged with age, but older men exhibited lower ejaculated volume, decreased sperm motility, and a higher percentage of abnormal spermatozoa. However, these parameters remained within normal limits in most of the older subjects. Sperm fertilizing capacity by in vitro testing remains intact in healthy older men. Male fertility is thought to decrease with aging, mostly as a result of reduced sexual activity and sexual dysfunction. The causes of declining libido and sexual activity with aging are multifactorial, including the presence of chronic illnesses such as diabetes mellitus, vascular or neuropathic disease of the penis, medications, and depression (see Chapter 49).

Testosterone and other androgens are also important in the maintenance of normal body composition in men, including bone mass, muscle mass, strength, and adiposity. Bone mass declines progressively with age in men, and hypogonadism in men is associated with premature osteoporosis and an increased risk of fractures. Additionally, younger hypogonadal men exhibit excessive visceral adiposity and reduced lean body mass that are reversible with testosterone replacement, and supraphysiologic doses of testosterone increase muscle strength and lean body mass in healthy young men. Testosterone supplementation has been proposed not only to treat older men with frank hypogonadism caused by pathological disease in the hypothalamic–pituitary–testicular axis, but also to ameliorate age-associated changes in body composition, sexual functioning, and overall well-being in older men with low testosterone levels related to aging per se. The role of androgens in the evaluation and management of erectile dysfunction in older men and the potential benefits and risks of testosterone supplementation in older men are discussed in Chapter 49.

Laboratory Diagnosis of Hypogonadism

The signs and symptoms of hypogonadism in older men may include diminished energy, vitality, and libido; depressed mood; erectile dysfunction; increased total and abdominal obesity, and decreased lean body and muscle mass, strength, and bone mineral density; objective impairment of cognitive function (e.g., spatial ability, visual and verbal memory); mild anemia; and impaired subjective well-being. However, these manifestations are nonspecific and common in eugonadal older men, and may be attributable to other common age-associated comorbidities. Therefore, laboratory evidence as well as signs and symptoms are required to make the diagnosis of hypogonadism. Questionnaires have been developed as potential screening tools to diagnose androgen deficiency in older men, but they lack sufficient specificity to identify men requiring laboratory evaluation.

Currently, there are no clinically useful biomarkers of androgen action available, and the laboratory diagnosis of testosterone deficiency depends upon measurement of low circulating testosterone concentrations. As discussed previously, because SHBG levels increase with aging, total testosterone measurements may not fully reflect age-related reductions in biologically active testosterone. Therefore, older men with symptoms or signs consistent with androgen deficiency should be evaluated with a free or bioavailable (non-SHBG-bound) testosterone level using an accurate and reliable assay, e.g., free testosterone by equilibrium dialysis or calculated from measurements of total testosterone and SHBG. Free testosterone assays using the direct analog radioimmunoassay method do not accurately or reliably measure free testosterone and therefore are not recommended. Because testosterone levels exhibit considerable biological and assay variability, low values should be confirmed on repeat testing. Serum testosterone should be measured only after reversible causes of low testosterone such as acute illness and malnutrition are treated, or medications such as glucocorticoids or opiates are discontinued, if possible.

The laboratory evaluation of men with suspected hypogonadism should include serum LH and FSH levels to differentiate between primary (testicular) and secondary (hypothalamic/pituitary) hypogonadism, as well as a prolactin level if gonadotropins are inappropriately low-normal or low in the presence of reduced testosterone levels. Hyperprolactinemia inhibits hypothalamic GnRH secretion, resulting in a decrease in LH and FSH secretion, and could indicate the presence of a pituitary adenoma or a hypothalamic disorder. In patients with secondary hypogonadism suspected on the basis of low serum testosterone associated with low or inappropriately normal gonadotropins, additional studies may be warranted, including magnetic resonance imaging of the pituitary fossa, measurements of other pituitary hormones such as GH and thyroid hormone levels, and an ACTH stimulation test. Furthermore, bone densitometry measurement is indicated in hypogonadal men to evaluate for asymptomatic osteoporosis.

FURTHER READING

Arlt W. Androgen therapy in women. *Eur J Endocrinol.* 2006;154:1.

Bhasin S, Cunningham GR, Hayes FJ, et al. Testosterone therapy in adult men with androgen deficiency syndromes: an Endocrine Society Clinical Practice Guideline. *J Clin Endocrinol Metab.* 2006;91:1995.

Brzezinski A, Vangel MG, Wurtman RJ, et al. Effects of exogenous melatonin on sleep: a meta-analysis. *Sleep Med Rev.* 2005;9:41.

Craft S. Insulin resistance and Alzheimer's disease pathogenesis: potential mechanisms and implications for treatment. *Curr Alzheimer Res.* 2007;4:147.

Dorin, RI, Qualls CR, Crapo LM. Diagnosis of adrenal insufficiency. *Ann Intern Med.* 2003;139:194.

Hodak SP, Verbalis JG. Abnormalities of water homeostasis in aging. *Endocrinol Metab Clin N Am.* 2005;34:1031.

Kaufman JM, Vermeulen A. The decline of androgen levels in elderly men and its clinical and therapeutic implications. *Endocr Rev.* 2005;26:833.

Klee GG, Heser DW. Techniques to measure testosterone in the elderly. *Mayo Clin Proc.* 2000;75:S19.

Kudva YC, Sawka AM, Young WF, Jr. The laboratory diagnosis of adrenal pheochromocytoma: the Mayo Clinic experience. *J Clin Endocrinol Metab.* 2003;88:4533.

Liu H, Bravata DM, Olkin I, et al. Systematic review: the safety and efficacy of growth hormone in the healthy elderly. *Ann Intern Med.* 2007;146:104.

Mannelli M. Management and treatment of pheochromocytomas and paragangliomas. *Ann N Y Acad Sci.* 2006;1073:405.

Mazziotti G, Angeli A, Bilezikian JP, et al. Glucocorticoid-induced osteoporosis: an update. *Trends Endocrinol Metab.* 2006;17:144.

Miller M. Nocturnal polyuria in older people: pathophysiology and clinical implications. *J Am Geriatr Soc.* 2000;48:1321.

Minniti G, Esposito V, Piccirilli M, et al. Diagnosis and management of pituitary tumours: a review based on personal experience and evidence of literature. *Eur J Endocrinol.* 2005;153:723.

Molitch ME, Clemmons DR, Malozowski S, et al. Evaluation and treatment of adult growth hormone deficiency: an Endocrine Society clinical practice guideline. *J Clin Endocrinol Metab.* 2006;91:1621.

Supiano MA, Hogikyan RV, Sidani MA, et al. Sympathetic nervous system activity and alpha-adrenergic responsiveness in older hypertensive humans. *Am J Physiol.* 1999;276:E519.

Young WF, Jr. Clinical practice. The incidentally discovered adrenal mass. *N Engl J Med.* 2007;356:601.

Thyroid Diseases

Jerome M. Hershman ■ *Sima Hassani* ■ *Mary H. Samuels*

Thyroid disorders in the elderly population are common, often challenging diagnostically, and frequently overlooked. The clinical presentations of thyroid diseases maybe subtle, with nonspecific signs and symptoms that are attributed to other illnesses or to a normal aging process. Thyroid function tests can be misleading in the presence of concurrent acute or chronic diseases and may be affected by some medications. This chapter describes the most common thyroid disorders encountered in the elderly population.

THE AGING HUMAN THYROID

Anatomy

The thyroid gland is the largest endocrine organ in the human body, and weighs approximately 12 to 20 g in adults. The structural and functional changes of the thyroid gland that occur with aging are controversial. Some investigators report that there were no size or weight changes, others found increases to twice normal size after age 70 years, whereas other reports indicated that the thyroid gland undergoes atrophy, fibrosis, and decrease in weight. The thyroid gland is also more nodular with advancing age, and there is an increase in fibrosis and lymphocytic infiltration. Despite these changes, normal thyroid function is maintained by the vast majority of the elderly population. Estimation of the thyroid size and its palpation may be difficult in elderly patients because of cervical kyphosis, obesity, or chronic pulmonary disease.

Physiology

Iodine, an essential substrate for synthesis of thyroid hormone, is absorbed from the diet and enters the circulation as inorganic iodide that is distributed in extracellular fluids as well as in salivary, breast, and gastric secretions. The average daily iodine intake is about 250 μg/day in the United States. A 24-hour urinary iodine measurement is an index of dietary iodine intake.

Iodide is actively concentrated by the thyroid gland or cleared from the plasma by the kidney. The thyroid gland, compared with the kidneys, is the active participant in the competition for plasma iodide and adjusts the rate of entry of iodide into the thyroid tissue based on the changes in thyroid hormone synthesis rather than renal avidity for iodide ion. The active transport of iodide from plasma to follicular cell is carried out by the sodium iodide symporter, a transport protein on the follicular cell plasma membrane. The extracellular fluid iodide concentration is usually very low because of the rapid clearance of iodide from extracellular fluid by the thyroidal uptake and renal clearance.

Table 108-1 summarizes the aging effects on thyroid function. The renal and thyroidal iodide clearance rate diminishes with advancing age. Thyroid iodide clearance, estimated by a 24-hour radioactive iodine uptake by the thyroid gland, decreases in euthyroid subjects after age 60 years. Urinary iodine excretion also was found to be significantly reduced in subjects older than 80 years of age.

In the thyroid cell, the iodide is oxidized by the peroxidase enzyme and incorporated into tyrosines in thyroglobulin to form the thyroid hormone precursors monoiodotyrosine (MIT) and diiodotyrosine (DIT). The MIT and DIT within the large thyroglobulin molecule couple to form thyroxine (T_4) and triiodothyronine (T_3). In the plasma, the main binding protein is thyroid-binding globulin (TBG), which binds about 70% of serum T_4 and T_3. The other binding proteins are transthyretin and albumin. Only 0.02% of T_4 and 0.3% of T_3 are free and metabolically active because only the free hormone is rapidly transported into cells. Total serum T_4 and T_3 are readily measured. Free T_4 (FT_4) and free T_3 (FT_3) concentrations also can be measured to evaluate thyroid function.

The daily production rate of T_4 is about 85 μg/day and that of T_3 is about 30 μg/day in normal adults. About 85% of T_3 production is derived from T_4-to-T_3 conversion by 5′-deiodinase, a selenoprotein (Figure 108-1), in extrathyroidal tissues such as the

TABLE 108-1

Age-Related Changes in Thyroid Physiology

Renal iodide clearance ↓
Thyroid iodide clearance ↓
Total T_4 production ↓
T_4 degradation ↓
Serum T_4 concentration ↔
Serum TBG concentration ↔
T_3 concentration ↓
Reverse T_3 concentration ↑
TSH response to TRH ↑↔↓
Diurnal variation of TSH ↓↓

↓, Decreased; ↑, increased; ↔, unchanged. T_3, triiodothyronine; T_4, thyroxine; TBG, thyroid-binding globulin; TRH, thyrotropin-releasing hormone; TSH, thyroid-stimulating hormone.

liver, muscles, and kidneys. The other 15% of T_3 production is that secreted directly by the thyroid gland. Selenium deficiency results in reduced 5-deiodinase activity and serum T_3 concentration. Reverse T_3 (rT_3), inactive biologically, differs from T_3 because it is missing an iodine from the inner or tyrosyl ring of T_4 rather than from the outer ring or phenolic ring. T_4 is converted to rT_3 by 5-deiodinase in peripheral tissue. Total T_4 production and degradation decline with aging, but T_4 concentration and TBG concentration remain unchanged in healthy individuals throughout adult life. In contrast, the concentration of T_3 was reported to decrease by 10% to 20% with advancing age and the concentration of rT3 increases. These findings suggest that 5'-deiodinase activity decreases with increasing age.

Thyroid hormone regulation is through a negative feedback loop involving the hypothalamus, the anterior pituitary, and the thyroid gland (Figure 108-2). Thyrotropin-releasing hormone (TRH), synthesized and stored within the hypothalamus, stimulates the release of thyroid-stimulating hormone (TSH) from the anterior pituitary gland. TSH binds to the TSH receptor located on the outer side of the thyroid cell plasma membrane and increases thyroid hormone synthesis and secretion. In turn, T_4 and T_3 from the serum feedback on the pituitary and the hypothalamus to inhibit TSH and TRH production and secretion.

The secretory response of TSH to TRH stimulation in aging men has been reported to be decreased to 38% of the values in young men. This maybe an adaptive mechanism to the reduced need for thyroid hormone in old age. However, other reports of TRH-stimulated TSH secretion with aging have shown an unchanged or even increased response.

The serum TSH concentration has been either unchanged, lowered, or increased with aging in various reports. The heterogeneity of the populations studied may explain some of these discrepancies. Studies employing sensitive TSH assays have raised the question of whether the abnormal TSH reflects the prevalence of thyroid disorders or physiologic changes related to aging. In a random selection of the community-based population followed in the Framingham Heart Study, euthyroid older persons were found to have the same level of TSH as younger persons, although older euthyroid women had a slightly lower serum TSH level than middle-aged women. In a study of healthy centenarians (age range, 100–110 years), the median serum TSH level was lower than that of older individuals (age range, 65–80 years). The data of this study are consistent with TSH being well preserved until the eighth decade of life in healthy elderly subjects, whereas a decline in TSH may occur in those older

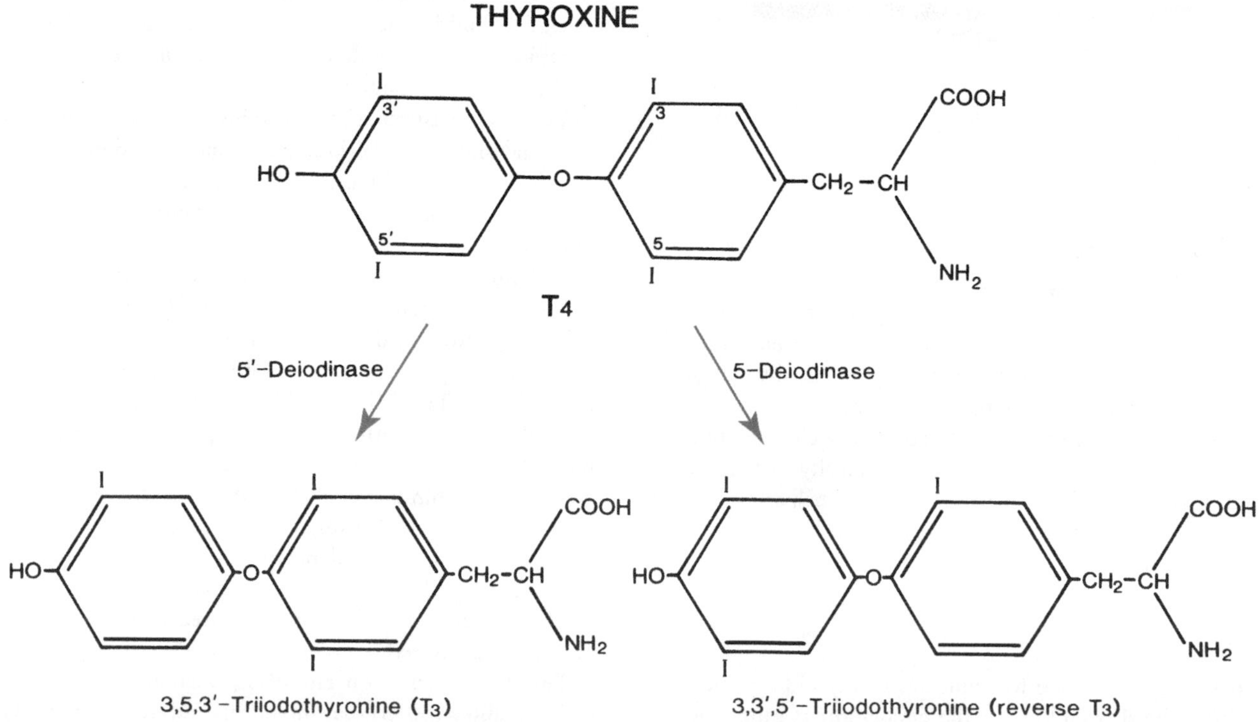

FIGURE 108-1. Structures of T_4 and the enzymatic pathways for deiodination of T_4 to its major active metabolite, T_3, and to reverse T_3 in peripheral tissues.

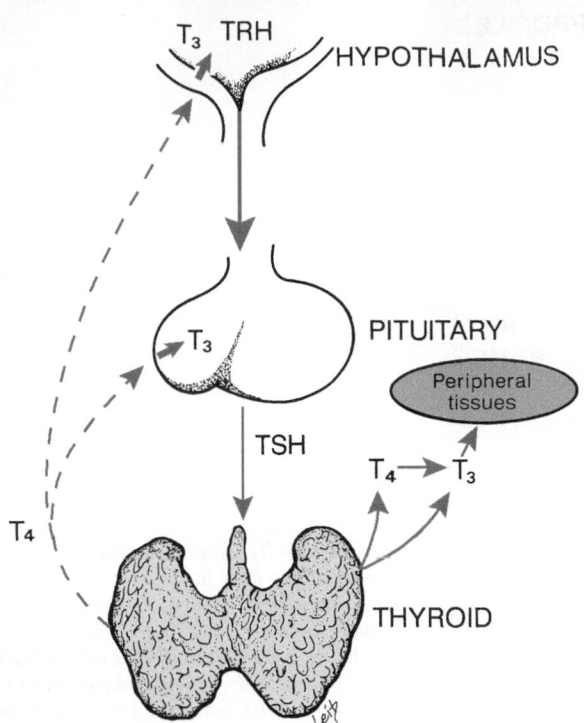

FIGURE 108-2. Feedback regulation for control of thyroid function that involves the hypothalamus–pituitary–thyroid axis. Arrows represent positive feedback; dashed lines denote the inhibitory feedback of T_4 and T_3 on pituitary thyroid-stimulating hormone (TSH) and hypothalamic thyrotropin-releasing hormone (TRH) secretion.

than 100 years of age. TSH levels rise about 50% in the late evening before the onset of sleep. Sleep attenuates this nocturnal peak of TSH secretion, and sleep deprivation exaggerates nocturnal TSH secretion. The diurnal variation of TSH levels has been reported to be absent in the elderly. The data from the healthy centenarians and individuals older than age 65 years also showed an age-related blunting of the nocturnal TSH peak. An increased prevalence of thyroid autoantibodies is also associated with human aging.

SCREENING FOR THYROID DISEASE

Both functional and anatomic abnormalities of the thyroid gland occur with increasing prevalence as patients age, and may present with nonspecific clinical findings. Therefore, the clinician should maintain a low threshold for testing if a patient presents with symptoms or signs that suggest the presence of thyroid disease or with atypical clinical findings (e.g., unexplained weight loss caused by apathetic hyperthyroidism). Testing should also be carried out in patients with a prior history of thyroid disease, other autoimmune disease, unexplained depression, cognitive dysfunction, or hypercholesterolemia.

Whether truly asymptomatic older subjects should be screened for thyroid disease is more controversial. The American Thyroid Association recommends screening all adults older than age 35 years for thyroid dysfunction and every 5 years thereafter. However, the American College of Physicians does not recommend routine screening of asymptomatic patients because of presumed lack of demonstrated efficacy or proven benefit in treatment of subclinical thyroid disease. In our opinion, the high prevalence of hypothyroidism and often subtle or nonspecific symptoms in patients older than 65 years of age justifies periodic screening for hypothyroidism.

In most ambulatory patients, the measurement of a serum TSH level is sufficient to screen for thyroid dysfunction. Modern TSH assays are sufficiently sensitive to distinguish normal from low or high values. TSH levels become abnormal before serum T4 or T3 levels because of the exquisite sensitivity of the pituitary gland to small increments in thyroid hormone feedback. However, there are certain patient populations where TSH levels alone may not provide accurate information about thyroid function. Patients with pituitary or hypothalamic disorders may have altered thyroid function with misleading TSH levels, and a full panel of thyroid tests is required to characterize their thyroid function. More commonly, patients with serious acute or chronic illnesses or receiving certain drugs may have altered thyroid hormone and TSH levels that do not accurately reflect their thyroid function. These common scenarios are described in the sections below on nonthyroidal illness and drug effects on thyroid function.

NONTHYROIDAL ILLNESS

The terms *sick euthyroid syndrome* or *nonthyroidal illness* (NTI) refer to altered serum thyroid hormone concentrations secondary to the physiologic stress of severe illness. By definition, patients with NTI have no apparent intrinsic thyroid disease. The types of illnesses responsible for thyroid function abnormalities include sepsis, surgery, trauma, burns, infections, malignancy, and chronic metabolic diseases such as malnutrition, starvation, and poorly controlled diabetes mellitus. An understanding of the effect of NTI on thyroid function tests is important, especially in the elderly patient who has multiple other underlying medical problems.

The effects of NTI on thyroid function have been described as the low T_3 and low T_4 states. The low T_3 state is associated with a decrease in extrathyroidal T_3 production, resulting in a low serum total T_3 level and usually low free T_3 level with a normal serum TSH concentration. With more severe illness, the serum T_4 level decreases. In severe NTI, the decreases in T_4 and T_3 maybe an adaptation to spare the patient from the catabolic effect of thyroid hormone during the periods of extreme stress. A reduction in serum T_3 concentration is the most common change of thyroid function tests in NTI with a frequency of 25% to 50%. The severity of the underlying illness correlates with the degree of the fall in serum T_3 concentration. The mechanisms responsible for low T_3 concentration are (1) a decrease in the peripheral conversion of T_4 to T_3 either because of inhibition of the 5′-deiodinase that is responsible for this conversion or because of a deficiency of a cofactor, such as glutathione, which is necessary for the activity of 5′-deiodinase; (2) a decrease in T_3 secretion from the thyroid gland; and (3) a decrease in tissue uptake of T_4 that limits the conversion of T_4 to T_3 in the extrathyroidal tissues. The serum rT_3 is increased in NTI because of the impaired rT_3 clearance as a consequence of the decreased activity of 5′-deiodinase with illness. The central question is how does the body maintain a euthyroid state when serum T_3 is reduced? The basis for an apparent euthyroid status in NTI is still unclear. There are several possible explanations: (1) T_3 concentrations may remain normal in the

CONTINUUM OF THYROID HORMONE AND THYROTROPIN PROFILES IN NONTHYROIDAL ILLNESS AND RECOVERY

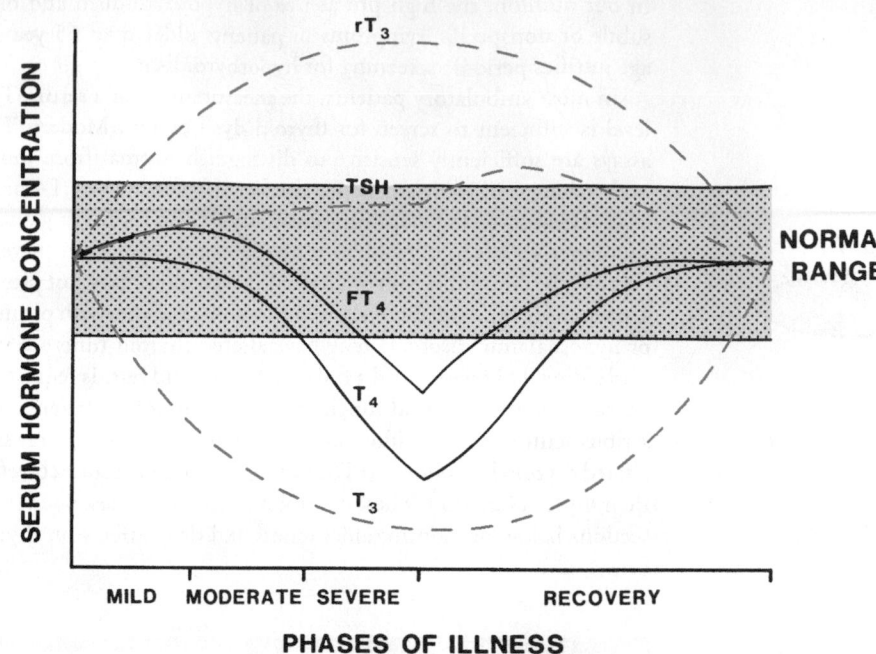

FIGURE 108-3. The relative changes in serum thyrotropin and thyroid hormone concentrations with increasing severity of nonthyroidal illness and with recovery. Serum T_4 and free T_4 falls with more severe illness, whereas serum T_3 is subnormal in mild illness. The recovery is generally a reverse of the illness pattern with a slight elevation of serum TSH in many instances.

intracellular compartment even though serum T_3 level is decreased; (2) T_3 maybe converted to triiodothyroacetic acid (Triac), which is metabolically active; and (3) studies of patients with various acute illnesses showed an increase in T_3-receptor messenger ribonucleic acids (mRNAs) and T_3-receptor protein that results in an increase in production of proteins that express the action of thyroid hormone, hence maintaining a euthyroid state in NTI.

The patients with the low T_4 state, also known as a low T_3/T_4 state, exhibit a low serum thyroxine level as well as low T_3 with a normal serum TSH concentration. Low serum total T_4 correlates with a poor prognosis. The mortality of critically ill patients with NTI is inversely related to serum T_4 concentration and has been reported to be as high as 84% in patients with serum T_4 concentration less than 3 μg/dL. There is no clear mechanism to fully explain the low T_4 state; however, possibilities include (1) reduced TBG concentration as a consequence of reduced hepatic protein synthesis; (2) inhibition of serum T_4 binding to TBG, probably by a substance released by injured tissue, or an acquired structural alteration of TBG that reduces its affinity for T_4; (3) alterations in hepatic uptake and metabolism of T_4; and (4) reduced secretion of T_4 caused by alteration in the structure of TSH, resulting in decreased biologic activity. Proinflammatory cytokines produced by the mononuclear cells (macrophages, lymphocytes, and monocytes) of the immune system in patients with NTI are probably responsible for the changes in thyroid function tests. Administration of proinflammatory cytokines such as tumor necrosis factor (TNF)-α and interleukin (IL)-1 to experimental animals made the animals sick and reduced serum T_4, T_3, and TSH concentrations. These cytokines inhibit thyroid iodide uptake by reducing the activity and transcription of the sodium iodide symporter, and they inhibit T_3 production by reducing the activity and transcription of 5′-deiodinase.

Recovery from the underlying illness results in improvement of the low T_3 and T_4 states. Serum T_4 level returns to normal faster than

serum T_3 level. Serum TSH concentration usually remains normal except in those patients receiving pharmacologic doses of dopamine or glucocorticoids, which reduce serum TSH levels. During the recovery stage, serum TSH usually remains in the normal range, but it may transiently increase above the normal range. Figure 108-3. diagrams the changes in thyroid hormone and serum TSH levels in NTI.

The effects of thyroid hormone replacement in NTI have been studied. Treatment of the low T_3 state with replacement doses of T_3 was found to be detrimental in a fasting model of NTI, resulting in an increase in protein catabolism and possibly muscle breakdown. T_3 given intravenously to cardiac patients undergoing open-heart surgery improved cardiac performance, but this was not confirmed in randomized trials. T_4 therapy in severe NTI had no beneficial effects and did not improve survival.

DRUGS AND THYROID FUNCTION

Altered sensitivity to drugs is particularly relevant in elderly patients with thyroid diseases. The metabolism and secretion of many drugs are attenuated in hypothyroidism and accelerated in thyrotoxicosis. Hypothyroidism results in increases in the plasma half-life of digoxin, insulin, glucocorticoids and morphine; consequently, sensitivity to the toxic effects of these drugs increases and doses should be decreased until the patient is euthyroid. Opposite metabolic changes in hyperthyroidism result in increased maintenance doses of these drugs while the patient is hyperthyroid. Resistance to the anticoagulant effect of warfarin in hypothyroidism is a result of slower-than-normal clearance of vitamin K-dependent coagulation factors; an augmented response is seen in hyperthyroidism.

Medications can affect many aspects of thyroid hormone secretion, absorption, transport, or metabolism, as listed in Table 108-2.

TABLE 108-2

Drugs That Affect Thyroid Function

Decrease TSH secretion
  Dopamine
  Glucocorticoids
  Octreotide
  Bexarotene

Increase thyroid hormone secretion
  Iodine and iodine-containing compounds
  Amiodarone
  Lithium
  Interferon alpha and IL-2

Decrease thyroid hormone secretion
  Thionamides (proplythiouracil, methimazole)
  Lithium
  Iodine and iodine containing compounds
  Amiodarone
  Aminoglutethimide
  Interferon alpha and interleukin 2
  Sunitinib

Decrease T_4 absorption
  Calcium
  Proton pump inhibitors
  Cholestyramine, Colestipol
  Aluminum hydroxide, sevelamer
  Ferrous sulfate
  Sucralfate
  Raloxifene (?)

Increase serum TBG
  Estrogen
  Tamoxifen and raloxifene
  Clofibrate
  Fluorouracil and capecitabine
  Mitotane
  Heroin
  Methadone

Decrease serum TBG
  Androgen
  Anabolic steroids (danazol)
  Glucocorticoid

Inhibit thyroid hormone binding to transport proteins
  Phenytoin and carbamazepine
  Furosemide
  Salicylates and salsalate
  Fenclofenac and meclofenamate
  Heparin
  Sulfonylureas

Decrease T4 5'-deiodinase activity
  Propylthiouracil
  Amiodarone
  Glucocorticoids

Increase hepatic T_4 and T_3 metabolism
  Phenobarbital
  Rifampin
  Phenytoin
  Carbamazepine
  Sertraline

A few drugs have been shown to suppress TSH secretion, most commonly seen in patients with critical illnesses receiving glucocorticoids and/or dopamine who can have low or undetectable TSH levels as a result. Low TSH levels are also seen during octreotide therapy for acromegaly or other rare endocrine diseases, and during administration of the retinoid X receptor ligand bexarotene for malignancies. Some of these patients develop central hypothyroidism and require thyroxine therapy.

A second major category of drugs that affect thyroid function include agents that directly increase thyroid hormone secretion. This may occur as a result of stimulation of a thyroid gland with underlying autonomous function, such as latent Graves' disease or a multinodular goiter. Iodine, iodine-containing radiocontrast agents, and amiodarone all act in this way to increase thyroid hormone synthesis and precipitate hyperthyroidism. A second mechanism is induction of destructive thyroiditis, leading to release of preformed thyroid hormone and transient thyrotoxicosis, as can occur with amiodarone, lithium, or the cytokines interferon alpha and IL-2.

Another class of drugs decreases thyroid hormone secretion. The thionamides proplythiouracil and methimazole are potent inhibitors of thyroid hormone synthesis and are used to treat hyperthyroidism. This class also includes iodine and iodine-containing agents, which can suppress thyroid hormone secretion in patients with underlying defective thyroid glands (e.g., Hashimoto's disease). It also includes some of the same drugs that cause thyroiditis, including amiodarone, lithium, and interferon alpha and IL-2. During drug-induced thyroiditis, the initial thyrotoxic phase is followed by a phase of reduced thyroid hormone secretion until the injured gland can recover synthetic function. The tyrosine kinase inhibitor, sunitinib, used to treat renal cancer and gastrointestinal stromal tumor, and aminoglutethamide, used to treat adrenal cancer, have also been reported to decrease thyroid hormone secretion.

A number of agents decrease thyroid hormone absorption from the gastrointestinal tract, including drugs commonly prescribed for elderly patients like calcium, ferrous sulfate, and proton pump inhibitors. These drugs do not affect thyroid hormone levels in euthyroid subjects, but they can lead to thyroxine malabsorption in patients taking exogenous thyroxine. Thyroxine should be given separately from these drugs, and the dose may have to be increased as well.

Drugs that cause increased serum TBG levels lead to increases in serum total T4 and total T3. Free T4, free T3, and TSH levels remain normal, attesting to the patient's euthyroid state. The most common cause of increased serum TBG and T_4 concentrations in postmenopausal women is estrogen replacement therapy. The serum TBG concentration is increased by 30% to 50% in women receiving 0.625 mg of conjugated estrogen daily. Less common are drugs that lower serum TBG (and therefore total T4 and total T3) levels.

Other drugs inhibit thyroid hormone binding to TBG and other transport proteins. Like agents that decrease TBG levels, this inhibition causes low total T4 levels, with normal free T4 and TSH levels, with the patient remaining euthyroid. The most frequently prescribed drugs in this category include high-dose aspirin or salsalate, high-dose furosemide, and heparin.

Drugs that inhibit 5' deiodinase activity include propylthiouracil, amiodarone, propronolol, and glucocorticoids. These agents block T4 to T3 conversion, but do not lead to clinical thyroid disease in euthyroid subjects.

The activity of the hepatic microsomal enzymes that metabolize T_4 and T_3 is increased by phenobarbital, rifampin, phenytoin, and carbamazepine. Hypothyroid patients treated with levothyroxine may become hypothyroid again when these agents are administered, and some patients require substantial increases of thyroxine dose.

HYPOTHYROIDISM

Definition

Hypothyroidism is a general term that refers to a state of decreased thyroid hormone availability to peripheral tissues. *Overt hypothyroidism* occurs when serum FT4 levels are below the normal range and usually is associated with some symptoms of hypothyroidism. Mild thyroid failure with an elevated serum TSH level and normal FT_4 concentration is referred to as *subclinical (biochemical) hypothyroidism.* Subclinical hypothyroidism is discussed in depth at the end of this section.

Prevalence

The prevalence of hypothyroidism varies based on the population under study (i.e., geriatric inpatient vs. primary care setting), age range, ethnicity, iodine content of the diet, and prevalence of antithyroid antibodies. In patients older than 60 years of age in the general population, the incidence of overt hypothyroidism is 2.3% to 10.3%. As dietary iodine intake increases, these rates also increase as a result of iodine effects to suppress the thyroid gland. In a comparative study of healthy elderly female patients, the prevalence of hypothyroidism in Regio Emilia, Italy, where there is low dietary iodine intake, was 0.9%, whereas a prevalence of 14% was found in Worcester, Massachusetts, where the dietary iodine is much higher.

Etiology and Pathogenesis

Table 108-3 lists the main causes of hypothyroidism. Primary hypothyroidism accounts for the vast majority of cases of thyroid failure. Less than 1% of cases are caused by central hypothyroidism.

In the areas of adequate iodine intake, chronic autoimmune (Hashimoto's) thyroiditis is the most common cause of primary hypothyroidism in elderly people, and is more common in women. Chronic autoimmune thyroiditis is characterized pathologically by a focal or diffuse lymphocytic infiltration of thyroid parenchyma and damaged or atrophic follicles. The thyroid maybe enlarged or atrophic. Thyroid atrophy has been attributed to blocking antibodies that bind to the TSH receptor and inhibit the action of TSH.

Autopsy reports from the United Kingdom and the United States reveal the presence of focal thyroiditis in 40% to 50% of women and in 20% of men with no prior history of thyroid diseases. The incidence of chronic autoimmune thyroiditis was significantly higher in Caucasians than in African-Americans in the same study. Antithyroid peroxidase (antimicrosomal) or antithyroglobulin antibodies are present in the serum of greater than 90% of patients with chronic autoimmune thyroiditis. The prevalence of positive thyroid antibodies increases with age, with frequencies as high as 33% in women

TABLE 108-3
Causes of Hypothyroidism in the Elderly Population

Primary hypothyroidism
    Chronic autoimmune thyroiditis (Hashimoto's thyroiditis)
    Radiation
        ^{131}I therapy for hyperthyroidism
        Radiation therapy for head and neck cancer
    Surgical thyroidectomy
    Drugs
        Iodine-containing drugs: amiodarone, radiocontrast agents
            containing iodine
        Antithyroid drugs (propythiouracil, methimazole)
        Other drugs that decrease TSH or thyroid hormone secretion
          (see Table 108-2)

Central hypothyroidism
    Hypothalamic tumors or infiltrative lesions
    Pituitary tumors or infiltrative lesions
    Pituitary surgery
    Radiation

older than 70 years of age. The presence of antithyroid antibodies increases the risk of developing subclinical or overt hypothyroidism, and also increases the risk of progression from subclinical to overt hypothyroidism.

The second most common cause of hypothyroidism is iatrogenic, caused by radiation treatment to the thyroid gland or thyroid surgery. Radiation-induced hypothyroidism is caused by either radioactive iodine treatment of hyperthyroidism or by external radiation therapy of head and neck cancers. Hypothyroidism has been reported in 76% of hyperthyroid patients treated with radioiodine and 20% to 47% of patients receiving radiotherapy for treatment of various malignancies of the head and neck region. This may take many years to develop, so patients having received radiation treatment at a young or middle age may develop hypothyroidism in old age.

Hypothyroidism in the elderly person maybe precipitated by certain drugs listed in Table 108-2. Patients with underlying autoimmune thyroid disease are more susceptible to developing iodine-induced hypothyroidism. This effect is a result of iodine-induced inhibition of thyroid hormone synthesis. Exposure of an elderly patient to iodine can occur as a result of administration of iodine-containing radiocontrast agents used during computed tomography (CT) scanning. Another source of exposure is the use of amiodarone, an iodine-containing drug used for treatment of arrhythmias. The incidence of amiodarone-induced hypothyroidism varies with the environmental iodine intake, with frequency of 10% to 30% in the United States. Overtreatment of hyperthyroidism with thionamide drugs (propythiouracil, methimazole) can lead to hypothyroidism. A number of other drugs that suppress TSH or T4 secretion (listed in Table 108-2) can precipitate hypothyroidism in elderly patients. Finally, there are drugs that interfere with exogenous thyroid hormone absorption, also listed in Table 108-2. These drugs do not cause hypothyroidism in euthyroid subjects, but they can lead to inadequate thyroid hormone dosing and hypothyroidism in thyroxine-treated patients who previously had normal TSH levels. Common culprits include calcium, ferrous sulfate, and proton pump inhibitors, all frequently prescribed in the elderly population.

Central hypothyroidism, resulting from an anatomic or functional disorder of the pituitary gland or the hypothalamus or both, is relatively rare. Thyroid hormone secretion is reduced secondary to deficient stimulation of the normal thyroid gland by TSH. The impairment of TSH secretion is caused by either primary or metastatic pituitary tumors, infiltrative lesions, external radiotherapy, or surgery.

Clinical Manifestations

The classic signs and symptoms of hypothyroidism include fatigue, weight gain, cold intolerance, dry skin, and constipation. Many elderly hypothyroid patients exhibit these classic findings, but they are often attributed to other comorbid conditions or to the aging process itself. This is because they are nonspecific and because hypothyroidism usually has an insidious onset and slow progression over months to years. Hypothyroidism may also present in a less typical fashion in elderly patients. Table 108-4 lists the common clinical features of symptomatic hypothyroidism in older patients, including findings that tend to occur at all ages, as well as neurologic, psychiatric, and cardiac features that particularly affect older patients. Table 108-5 compares signs and symptoms of overt hypothyroidism between elderly and younger patients. In the study summarized in this table, the mean serum TSH and FT$_4$ levels and duration of disease were similar between the two groups of patients. This study showed that the classic signs of overt hypothyroidism such as cold intolerance, paresthesias, weight gain, and muscle cramps were less frequent in older patients. The remainder of this section

TABLE 108-5

Comparison of Clinical Features of Overt Hypothyroidism in Elderly versus Young Patients

Symptoms and Signs	Elderly, ≥70 Years (%)	Young, ≤55 Years (%)
Bradycardia	12	19
Fatigue	68	83
Weight gain	24	59
Cold intolerance	35	65
Depression	28	52
Disorientation	9	0
Hypoactive reflexes	24	31
Weakness	53	67
Paresthesia	18	61
Dry skin	35	45
Hair loss	12	28
Reduced hearing	32	25
Muscle cramps	20	55
Snoring	18	22
Constipation	33	41

From Hassani S, Hershman JM. Thyroid diseases. In: Hazzard WR et al., eds. Principles of Geriatric Medicine & Gerontology. 5th ed. New York, New York: McGraw-Hill; 2003:843.

reviews some of the clinical aspects of hypothyroidism that are most relevant to the elderly population.

The neuropsychiatric features of hypothyroidism in the elderly population are initially nonspecific. Patients may report slowing of thought processes. As the patient becomes less motivated and responsive to others, disoriented, and less interested in usual activities, the diagnosis maybe confused with that of depressive mood disorder. Older people who present with deterioration in personality, retardation of thought or action, apathy, or global loss of intellectual function should be evaluated for hypothyroidism. As hypothyroidism becomes more severe, paranoia, delusions, hallucinations, and psychosis may develop. Because of these symptoms, hypothyroidism can be a cause of "pseudodementia" in some elderly people. However, hypothyroidism as a major contributing cause of dementia is rare; in one study of patients with dementia, the incidence of hypothyroidism was the same as in the general population. In another study of demented patients, 2.3% were found to have hypothyroidism, of whom only 25% improved with treatment.

Abnormalities in plasma lipids are among the most important metabolic changes that occur in hypothyroidism. Both hypercholesterolemia and hypertriglyceridemia can occur, and may exacerbate primary hyperlipidemia in older patients. In the majority of overt hypothyroid patients, hypercholesterolemia (plasma cholesterol level >250 mg/dL) is present. A reduction in cholesterol uptake because of reduced number of low-density lipoprotein (LDL) receptors results in an increase in low-density cholesterol-carrying apolipoprotein concentration. The synthesis rate of free fatty acids and triglycerides is normal in hypothyroidism; the hypertriglyceridemia is caused by a decreased fractional removal rate of triglycerides.

Thyroid hormone deficiency causes several cardiac abnormalities. Cardiomegaly is secondary to hypothyroid-induced pericardial effusion, bradycardia, diastolic hypertension, and/or atherosclerosis.

TABLE 108-4

Clinical Features of Hypothyroidism in Elderly Patients

Dry skin
Hair loss
Edema of face and eyelids
Cold intolerance
Neurologic
  Paresthesia (carpal tunnel syndrome)
  Ataxia
  Dementia
Psychiatric and behavioral
  Depression
  Apathy or withdrawal
  Psychosis
  Cognitive dysfunction
Metabolism
  Weight gain
  Hypercholesterolemia
  Hypertriglyceridemia
  Peripheral edema
Musculoskeletal
  Myopathy
  Arthritis/arthralgia
Cardiovascular
  Bradycardia
  Pericardial effusion
  Congestive heart failure

Pericardial effusion is found in approximately 30% to 50% of patients with overt hypothyroidism. The volume of the effusion correlates with the severity of the disease. The electrocardiogram may show ST and T wave changes, QT prolongation, and more often low-amplitude QRS complexes or a low voltage that is a result of pericardial effusion rather than a myocardial conduction defect. Cardiac tamponade and hemodynamic compromise are very rare. Bradycardia results from the effects of thyroid hormone deficiency on the cardiac conducting system. The slowing of the heart rate is moderate and its role in the development of fatigue in hypothyroid patients is unclear. Hypothyroidism may mask typical symptoms of coronary artery disease by causing depressed myocardial contractility and bradycardia, resulting in reduced myocardial oxygen consumption.

Exertional dyspnea and reduced exercise tolerance are present in 50% of elderly patients with overt hypothyroidism and maybe related to skeletal muscle dysfunction rather than impaired cardiac function. Anginal chest pain was reported in 25% of patients with overt hypothyroidism, suggesting an increased prevalence of coronary heart disease in these patients. Patients with a long-standing history of hypothyroidism are especially at risk of developing atherosclerotic vascular disease that may have been induced by diastolic hypertension and hypercholesterolemia. Hypothyroidism predisposes to diastolic hypertension by impairment of the diastolic relaxation phase. Approximately 1% of patients with diastolic hypertension may have hypothyroidism as the cause. Blood pressure normalizes with thyroid hormone replacement therapy in such patients.

Given the prevalence of hypothyroidism in the elderly population and the comorbidities listed above, it is not uncommon to be faced with an untreated elderly hypothyroid patient who requires surgery. A few small, retrospective studies suggest that surgery is relatively safe in hypothyroid subjects, and urgent surgery does not need to be postponed while therapy is started. However, particular attention must be given to anesthetic and drug administration since hypothyroid patients clear medications more slowly than euthyroid patients.

Diagnosis

The diagnosis of primary hypothyroidism is relatively straightforward since all cases are associated with elevated serum TSH levels. The serum-free T4 level will be low in overt hypothyroidism and will be normal in subclinical hypothyroidism. Serum T_3 concentrations are not helpful in diagnosing hypothyroidism since they are normal in about one-third of overtly hypothyroid patients and since they do not decrease below normal until the free T4 is already low. Therefore, TSH and free T4 levels are sufficient diagnostic tests for hypothyroidism.

There is some controversy regarding what TSH level indicates hypothyroidism. Most laboratories currently report upper limits of the TSH normal range to be approximately 4.5 to 5.0 mU/L. However, the upper normal range is lowered to 3.5 to 4.0 mU/L if subjects with antithyroid peroxidase antibodies are excluded, suggesting that the reported normal range includes subjects with incipient thyroid disease. This has led some experts to recommend a narrower TSH normal range, with TSH levels above 3.5 mU/L consistent with mild thyroid disease. If adopted, this would reclassify millions of patients as being hypothyroid or undertreated with thyroid hormone. There is almost no information on putative clinical effects in patients with

TSH levels of 3.5 to 5.0 mU/L, and therefore at this time it is premature to adopt this recommendation.

There are a few other caveats to the biochemical diagnosis of hypothyroidism. An elevated serum TSH level also may be seen during the recovery period from NTI or after withdrawal of certain drugs that suppress TSH levels. Therefore, the serum TSH measurement must be interpreted in the context of the clinical situation. Central hypothyroidism results in low serum T_4 and T_3 levels with a low or normal serum TSH concentration, rather than an elevated TSH level.

Treatment

The purpose of treatment of hypothyroidism, regardless of its cause, is to achieve a euthyroid state that is reflected by normal thyroid function tests. Synthetic levothyroxine is the preferred preparation for treatment of hypothyroidism because of its long half-life (approximately 7 days), reliable absorption, and relatively constant serum T_4 concentration after single daily doses. The replacement therapy dose of levothyroxine depends on the weight and age of the patient. Thyroxine requirements are decreased in the elderly because of a decline in the degradation of thyroid hormone. The average requirement of T_4 in elderly patients is 25% less than in young adults.

In elderly patients with coexisting cardiovascular disease, starting treatment with full replacement doses can result in exacerbation of angina and worsening of the underlying heart disease. Therefore, it is crucial that the starting dose of thyroxine should be small, such as 12.5 to 25 μg/day. The replacement dose titration needs to be done cautiously with close monitoring of the patient's symptoms and thyroid function tests. The dose should be adjusted at 6-week intervals by an increment of 12.5 to 25 μg until the patient is euthyroid and the serum TSH is in the mid-normal range. Once the serum TSH level is within the normal range, its measurement may be done every 6 to 12 months to monitor the dose and compliance. Patients with primary hypothyroidism can be monitored with a TSH alone, while patients with central hypothyroidism should be monitored by free T_4 measurement.

Levothyroxine absorption is decreased by food, a high-fiber diet, conditions associated with impaired gastric acid production, and a number of medications (see Table 108-2). Drugs that block its absorption include calcium carbonate, ferrous sulfate, proton pump inhibitors, cholestyramine, colestipol, sucralfate, and aluminum hydroxide. This malabsorption of thyroxine can be avoided to a large extent by instructing the patient to allow a time interval of at least 4 hours between the ingestion of the two drugs, but in some cases, an increase in thyroxine dose maybe required (such as during proton pump inhibitor therapy). Other medications accelerate thyroxine clearance, including rifampin, carbamazepine, phenytoin, and sertraline. Therefore, a higher levothyroxine replacement dose is required. Finally, estrogen therapy increases TBG levels, leading to a greater amount of administered thyroxine being bound to TBG and an increased thyroxine dose requirement.

Subclinical Hypothyroidism

Subclinical hypothyroidism is the term applied to the state in which serum TSH concentration is raised while free T_4 and T_3 concentrations are normal in a patient with no clinical features of hypothyroidism. Serum TSH concentrations bear a logarithmic relation to free T$_4$ levels; small decrements in free T$_4$ concentration (even within the population normal range) result in large increases in serum TSH concentration.

The prevalence of subclinical hypothyrodism is age dependent. The classic Whickham survey in Great Britain reported increasing prevalence of elevated TSH levels with age, up to 18% in women older than 74 years of age. The more recent Colorado Health Fair study reported a prevalence of elevated TSH levels of 9.5% in the entire study population, rising to 19% in those older than 74 years of age. Finally, the most recent National Health and Nutrition Examination Survey in the United States found that 12% to 14% of the population older than age 70 years had high serum TSH, as compared with approximately 2% of the population younger than age 40 years.

Most studies show that older women are at greatest risk for subclinical hypothyroidism. In the Whickham survey, the prevalence of subclinical hypothyroidism was more than threefold increased in older women compared to older men. In a survey in the United States, the prevalence of serum TSH elevation was 8.5% in women and 4.4% in men older than age 55 years. However, rates of subclinical hypothyroidism among older men in the Colorado Health Fair study approached those of older women.

The common causes of subclinical hypothyroidism are the same as the causes of overt hypothyroidism (see Table 108-3). The majority of patients have chronic autoimmune thyroiditis with positive antithyroid peroxidase antibodies. Those patients with high titers of antithyroid antibodies and more than twice the upper limit of serum TSH are most likely to develop overt hypothyroidism. In the 20-year follow-up study of patients with subclinical hypothyroidism in the Whickham Survey, the annual rate of thyroid failure was 4.3% in those with positive thyroid antibodies, as compared to 0.3% in thyroid-antibody-negative patients.

The clinical manifestations of subclinical hypothyroidism are debated; some studies have suggested adverse effects on serum lipids, cardiac function, or neuropsychiatric function. Cardiac and lipid effects have received particular attention since a large-scale survey of elderly women in Rotterdam showed that subclinical hypothyroidism increased the risk for myocardial infarction two- to threefold. Lipid abnormalities associated with subclinical hypothyroidism have primarily included cholesterol or LDL levels slightly higher than euthyroid control groups. Cardiovascular abnormalities associated with mild thyroid failure include left ventricular diastolic and endothelial dysfunction. The cardiac structure and function remain normal at rest, but ventricular function and cardiovascular and respiratory adaptation are impaired during exercise. Left ventricular ejection fraction is similar to the euthyroid state at rest, but reduced with exercise. In terms of neuropsychiatric function, previous cross-sectional studies have suggested increased rates of anxiety, depression, or cognitive impairment in subclinical hypothyroidism. However, a recent large cross-sectional study failed to find any association between subclinical hypothyroidism and numerous measures of mood and cognition.

Further studies have assessed the effects of thyroxine treatment on serum lipid concentrations, cardiac function, cognitive function, and psychiatric status in subclinical hypothyroidism. Results have been mixed, with some studies showing decreased cholesterol and LDL levels, improved cardiac function, or improved cognitive and affective symptoms. However, not all studies have demonstrated these effects, which are often of small magnitude and unclear clinical relevance. An expert consensus panel reviewed the efficacy of treating subclinical hypothyroidism. The panel concluded that treatment was reasonable in patients with TSH levels greater than 10 mU/L, those with symptoms, or those with elevated cholesterol levels. If implemented, the goal of therapy is to normalize the serum TSH concentration. In older people, 12.5 to 25 μg levothyroxine is recommended as the initial dose. With minimal TSH elevations and absence of clinical features, treatment is not necessary, but patients should be followed at intervals of 6 months.

Myxedema Coma

Myxedema coma is a rare syndrome that represents the result of severe untreated hypothyroidism. Most patients are older than 60 years of age. It is characterized by lethargy, progressive weakness, stupor, hypothermia, hyponatremia, cardiovascular shock, and coma. The mortality rate is very high in older patients, approximately 80% in untreated cases. Myxedema coma maybe precipitated by exposure to cold weather; drugs such as narcotics, sedatives, analgesics, anesthetics, or tranquilizers; pulmonary or urinary tract infections; and other coexisting medical conditions such as cerebrovascular accidents or congestive heart failure.

The patient may have a history of a previous thyroid disease, radioiodine therapy, or thyroidectomy. The medical history is of gradual onset of progressive weakness and impaired cognitive function, depression, and stupor. Physical findings include marked hypothermia, bradycardia, hoarseness, delayed reflexes, dry skin, and periorbital edema. Laboratory evaluation may indicate hyponatremia, elevated creatine phosphokinase level, neutropenia with a left shift, elevated serum cholesterol level, increased cerebrospinal fluid protein, carbon dioxide retention, and hypoxia. Serum tests reveal a low FT$_4$ level and a markedly elevated TSH concentration, except in central hypothyroidism, in which case an increased serum TSH is not found.

Myxedema coma is an acute medical emergency and treatment should be initiated immediately; 500-μg levothyroxine should be given by intravenous bolus because such patients absorb drugs poorly through the gastrointestinal tract. This is followed by daily administration of 50-μg thyroxine intravenously. Because the possibility of concomitant adrenal insufficiency (because of autoimmune adrenal or pituitary insufficiency) may exist, hydrocortisone hemisuccinate 100 mg intravenously should be administered followed by 50 mg every 6 hours. A serum cortisol level should be obtained prior to hydrocortisone infusion. If the serum cortisol level is greater than 20 μg/dL, then the corticosteroid can be discontinued. The patient's renal function, fluid status, and cardiopulmonary status must be monitored closely.

HYPERTHYROIDISM

Definition

Hyperthyroidism refers to a state of excessive thyroid hormone availability to peripheral tissues. *Overt hyperthyroidism* occurs when serum FT4 and/or T3 levels are above the normal range and usually is associated with symptoms of hyperthyroidism. Mild thyroid overactivity with a suppressed serum TSH level and normal FT$_4$ and

T3 concentrations is referred to as *subclinical (biochemical) hyper-thyroidism*. Subclinical hyperthyroidism is discussed in depth at the end of this section.

Prevalence

There is a considerable variation reported in the prevalence of hyperthyroidism in older subjects. Based on different ethnic and geographic regions and the criteria used for diagnosis, the prevalence varies from 0.5% to 2.3% in the elderly population. Approximately 10% to 17% of all hyperthyroid patients are older than age 60 years.

Etiology and Pathogenesis

By far the most common cause of hyperthyroidism in the general population is Graves' disease, or diffuse toxic goiter. In older patients, Graves' disease remains a common cause of hyperthyroidism, but other etiologies become more frequent. Graves' disease is an autoimmune disorder that results from the action of a thyroid-stimulating antibody on TSH receptors. TSH receptor antibodies are detectable in the serum of approximately 80% to 100% of untreated patients with Graves' disease. The cause of the extrathyroidal manifestations of Graves' disease, such as ophthalmopathy and dermopathy, is unknown. The proposed mechanism for the ophthalmopathy is the development of retrobulbar autoimmune inflammation caused by the release of cytokines, thickening of extraocular muscles, and swelling of orbital contents.

Toxic multinodular goiter is more common in the elderly population and has been reported in about one half of older patients with hyperthyroidism, especially in regions of relative iodine deficiency. It occurs most often in patients with a long-standing history of multinodular goiter. In most cases, the etiologic factor causing the transition from nontoxic to toxic multinodular goiter is unclear. However, there is generation of new follicles within the gland with functional autonomy independent from TSH stimulation. Autonomously functioning thyroid nodules synthesize and secrete thyroid hormones despite suppression of TSH secretion. Thyrotoxicosis can be precipitated in patients with nontoxic multinodular goiter by administration of a large iodine load such as radiocontrast agent or amiodarone.

Thyroiditis, either acute or subacute, occurs with less frequency in the aged as compared with younger patients with hyperthyroidism. Thyrotoxicosis results from extensive destruction of follicular cells by either an inflammatory or infectious process and release of T_4 and T_3 into the circulation. Certain drugs, including amiodarone, lithium, and cytokines such as interferon alpha and IL-2, may cause destructive thyroiditis and thyrotoxicosis.

Amiodarone-induced hyperthyroidism is particularly complex and difficult since the drug is prescribed to elderly patients with underlying cardiac disease or arrhythmias, which increases the risks of the superimposed hyperthyroidism. Amiodarone-induced thyrotoxicosis (AIT) in association with iodine excess is termed type 1 AIT, while destructive thyroiditis is called type 2 AIT. A combination of type 1 and type 2 AIT can also occur. Treatment can be difficult, and recommendations vary depending on whether the patient has type 1 or type 2 AIT. Unfortunately, distinguishing between the two types of AIT is sometimes impossible, especially in the acute situation, and patients are often treated simultaneously for both.

Hyperthyroidism resulting from a TSH-secreting pituitary adenoma or pituitary resistance to thyroid hormone is very rare. Clinical manifestations are similar to those of Graves' disease except that the patient does not have a suppressed TSH level.

Clinical Manifestations

The classic signs and symptoms of hyperthyroidism include weight loss with increased appetite, heat intolerance, excessive sweating, diarrhea or loose stools, tremor, tachycardia, and palpitations. Although they can be present, these classic findings are less common in older patients with hyperthyroidism. Absence of the typical manifestations of hyperthyroidism in the elderly patient was first described in 1931 by Lahey as "apathetic hyperthyroidism," in which there was only slight evidence of hypermetabolism. Instead, the dominant clinical findings maybe weight loss or cardiac or gastrointestinal manifestations, and the diagnosis of hyperthyroidism maybe overlooked. Table 108-6 lists the signs and symptoms of hyperthyroidism in the elderly patient. Recognition of these important clues will facilitate detection of the disease at an earlier stage.

Table 108-7 compares clinical findings of hyperthyroidism in elderly and young patients independent of etiology. In this study, thyroid hormone levels were similar in both groups, and there was no correlation between serum TSH and FT_4 levels and the prevalence of signs and symptoms of hyperthyroidism. The results of this study confirm that the presentation of hyperthyroidism in older patients is associated with fewer classic signs or symptoms and increased frequency of anorexia, atrial fibrillation, and a lack of goiter. Interestingly, palpable goiter is absent in approximately 50% of the older patients with hyperthyroidism, whereas 80% of the younger patients have thyroid enlargement on physical examination.

The cardiovascular manifestations of thyrotoxicosis may predominate in elderly patients, especially atrial fibrillation or supraventricular tachycardia. Occult hyperthyroidism should be ruled out in any elderly patient with a new onset of tachyarrhythmias. Elderly hyperthyroid patients with atrial fibrillation are at risk for systemic embolization and stroke, especially those with coexisting cardiac disease.

TABLE 108-6

Clinical Features of Hyperthyroidism in Elderly Patients

Cardiovascular
  Palpitations
  Chronic or intermittent atrial fibrillation
  Congestive heart failure
Psychiatric and behavioral
  Depression
  Apathy
  Lethargy
  Irritability
Gastrointestinal
  Decreased appetite
  Weight loss
  Nausea
  Constipation
Musculoskeletal
  Proximal muscle weakness
  Muscle atrophy

TABLE 108-7

Comparison of Clinical Features of Hyperthyroidism in Elderly versus Young Patients

Symptoms and Signs	Elderly, >70 Years (%)	Young, <50 Years (%)
Tachycardia	71	96
Fatigue	56	84
Weight loss	50	51
Tremor	44	84
Dyspnea	41	56
Apathy	41	25
Anorexia	32	4
Nervousness	31	84
Hyperactive reflexes	28	96
Weakness	27	61
Depression	24	22
Increased sweating	24	95
Diarrhea	18	43
Muscular atrophy	16	10
Confusion	16	0
Heat intolerance	15	92
Constipation	15	0

The excessive amounts of thyroid hormones in hyperthyroidism increase myocardial oxygen demand and may unmask coronary artery disease or exacerbate underlying cardiac conditions such as angina pectoris or congestive heart failure. Elderly patients with thyrotoxicosis and evidence of cardiac contractile dysfunction caused by hypertension, coronary artery disease, valvular heart disease, or atrial fibrillation are at higher risk of developing congestive heart failure.

Dyspnea on exertion and exercise intolerance are also common complaints of thyrotoxic patients. These symptoms can be caused by weakness of the skeletal and respiratory muscles rather than compromised cardiac function. Marked weakness and atrophy of muscles may have an insidious onset and slow progression in some elderly patients with thyrotoxicosis that has been long-standing as a result of delayed diagnosis because of its atypical presentation. Weakness involves mostly the proximal muscles, especially those of the shoulder girdle and the pelvis.

The classic gastrointestinal signs and symptoms of hyperthyroidism are increased appetite, rapid intestinal transit, resulting in more frequent defecation, and weight loss. However, some elderly patients with apathetic hyperthyroidism present with weight loss, anorexia, nausea, vomiting, and constipation. In a group of 880 patients with Graves' disease, weight loss became a major diagnostic finding in 80% of patients older than age 70 years. This weight loss is secondary to increased metabolic demands and reduced appetite. Thus, hyperthyroidism should be ruled out as a cause of weight loss in elderly patients before proceeding with an extensive evaluation for occult malignancy or gastrointestinal disease.

The neurobehavioral and psychiatric changes associated with hyperthyroidism in young adults include anxiety, emotional lability, insomnia, lack of concentration, restlessness, and tremulousness. In contrast to these features, apathy, lethargy, pseudodementia, and depressed mood frequently are present in older people with hyperthyroidism. Patients with an atypical depression (an increased prevalence of somatic complaints, anxiety, and fewer complaints of sadness or guilt) later in life should be evaluated for hyperthyroidism.

Diagnosis

The preferred approach to diagnosis of hyperthyroidism is the combination of free thyroxine or free thyroxine index level (either of which will be elevated) and a sensitive TSH assay (which will be suppressed). Although serum TSH level is suppressed in hyperthyroidism, there are other reasons for a suppressed TSH, so this test alone in a geriatric patient is not diagnostic of hyperthyroidism. In fact, most elderly subjects with low serum TSH levels are not hyperthyroid (see "Subclinical Hyperthyroidism" later in this chapter). Medications such as dopamine or glucocorticoids and conditions such as hypothalamic or pituitary disorders may cause suppression of the serum TSH level.

An elevation of serum T_3 level in addition to an elevated serum T_4 level is a strong confirmation of hyperthyroidism. However, the serum T_3 level is not increased in every elderly patient with hyperthyroidism and was found to be elevated in only 50% of such patients between 75 and 95 years of age. The relative absence of T_3 elevation may be a reflection of less conversion of T_4 to T_3 peripherally in the aged population.

Patients with a low serum TSH and normal FT_4 levels should have the T_3 level measured to identify T_3 thyrotoxicosis, a condition seen in 1% or 2% of hyperthyroid patients in the United States. T_3 thyrotoxicosis is more common in elderly patients with a solitary adenoma or with early toxic multinodular goiter. Its causes and treatment are the same as for hyperthyroidism in general.

Once hyperthyroidism is detected, a 24-hour radioactive iodine uptake should be done to exclude conditions causing thyrotoxicosis with low thyroid uptake: thyroiditis, exogenous intake of thyroid hormone, or iodine-containing drugs. If there is concern for a toxic nodule or toxic multinodular goiter, a 24-hour radioactive iodine scan can be added to the uptake measurement.

Treatment

The preferred mode of therapy for hyperthyroidism in the elderly is radioactive iodine-131. To avoid postradiation release of preformed thyroid hormone from glandular stores and subsequent exacerbation of hyperthyroidism, severely affected patients should be treated with antithyroid drugs for at least 3 months to achieve a normal or near-normal serum free T_4 level prior to use of [131]I. The usual doses are 5 to 15 mCi of radioactive ^{131}I for Graves' disease and 15 to 50 mCi for large multinodular glands. The antithyroid drugs should be discontinued 7 days before administration of the radioiodine dose and restarted 7 days after ^{131}I treatment. Beta-blockers are often used as an adjuvant, especially in cases of symptomatic tachycardia, and should be continued until the patient is euthyroid. The incidence of hypothyroidism in the first year after radioiodine treatment is dose-dependent, ranging up to 90%, and hypothyroidism continues to develop in subsequent years. Therefore, the patient should be monitored regularly for the development of hypothyroidism, and thyroxine therapy should be started promptly after the diagnosis of hypothyroidism is established.

Therapy with thionamide antithyroid drugs is also appropriate for otherwise healthy elderly patients with Graves' disease or toxic nodular goiters. Propylthiouracil and methimazole are the antithyroid drugs available in the United States. Methimazole is preferred over propylthiouracil since it can be given once a day and has a better side effect profile. When used for Graves' disease, thionamides are usually given for 12 to 18 months and then discontinued to see if a sustained remission has been achieved. Beta-blockers can be used temporarily until euthyroidism is achieved. Retrospective analysis of the therapeutic response to antithyroid drugs in patients with hyperthyroid Graves' disease has shown that euthyroidism was achieved in 2 to 3 months in patients older than age 60 years after treatment with methimazole. In long-term follow-up after thionamides are discontinued, recurrence rates are up to 50%. They were found to be the highest in patients younger than age 30 years and were significantly less with advanced age. If a relapse occurs after discontinuing a thionamide, the drug can be restarted, or radioactive iodine can be used. When used for toxic nodular goiters, thionamides have to be given indefinitely since these conditions do not remit.

Patients should be warned about the side effects of antithyroid drugs, which include rash, hepatic injury, and agranulocytosis. The latter two side effects are rare but potentially life-threatening. Routine monitoring of blood counts and liver function tests is not recommended, since these side effects can occur abruptly. If the patient develops sore throat, chills, fever, or signs of liver damage, the antithyroid drug should be stopped until the patient is assessed clinically. Fortunately, these side effects are reversible with supportive care.

Surgery for hyperthyroidism is only advised if there are obstructive symptoms from a large goiter or the presence of a nodule that is suspicious for malignancy. Preparation for thyroidectomy includes using a beta-adrenergic antagonist drug for several weeks before surgery in doses sufficient to lower the resting pulse rate to less than 90 beats per minute. If surgery must be done urgently, then sodium iopanoate has been reported to be safe and effective when given for 5 days together with a β-adrenergic antagonist. Although the mortality from subtotal thyroidectomy is very low, the complications of recurrent laryngeal nerve damage and hypoparathyroidism can result in lifelong disability. Because of the complications, surgery is rarely advisable in the elderly patient.

Atrial fibrillation in the context of hyperthyroidism is more common in elderly patients and is treated with standard agents while the hyperthyroidism is being treated. Atrial fibrillation may resolve once euthyroidism is achieved. Approximately 8% of hyperthyroid patients with atrial fibrillation may develop embolic stroke, with increasing rates in older patients with underlying structural heart disease; therefore, such patients should be given anticoagulation unless there is a contraindication. Anticoagulant doses must be carefully monitored, since hyperthyroidism affects clotting factor levels and drug metabolism.

Subclinical Hyperthyroidism

Subclinical hyperthyroidism is defined as a state of suppression of serum TSH with normal free thyroxine (FT_4) and triiodothyronine (T_3) levels in a patient who lacks clinical features of thyrotoxicosis. The most common cause of subclinical hyperthyroidism is iatrogenic because of the use of TSH-suppressive doses of thyroxine. This is done purposely in patients with thyroid cancer and inadvertently in patients with hypothyroidism. Other endogenous causes of subclinical hyperthyroidism are the same as for overt hyperthyroidism, including Graves' disease, toxic nodules or toxic multinodular goiters, and iodine or amiodarone administration.

In addition to subclinical hyperthyroidism, there are other reasons a patient might have a low or suppressed TSH. These include acute or chronic illness (the NTI syndrome described earlier in this chapter), drugs that suppress TSH levels, and transient thyroiditis. In fact, depending on the population, most patients with a low TSH level will have one of these other conditions, and not subclinical hyperthyroidism. For this reason, a thorough evaluation must be done before a patient receives a diagnosis of subclinical hyperthyroidism.

The prevalence of subclinical hyperthyroidism in older patients varies according to whether patients receiving exogenous thyroid hormone are included. If these patients are excluded, the prevalence is less than 2% of older subjects. The progression of subclinical hyperthyroidism to overt thyrotoxicosis is variable, with some patients eventually becoming hyperthyroid, while others remain stable or revert to a normal TSH level.

Most of the available data on pathophysiologic effects of TSH suppression have been derived from patients with either thyroid carcinoma or nontoxic nodular goiter on levothyroxine suppressive therapy. These effects have been studied in three main areas: symptoms and neuropsychiatric effects, bone loss, and cardiac effects. It should be noted that many of these studies included few if any older patients, so their generalizability to elderly people is unclear.

There are relatively few studies regarding symptoms and neuropsychiatric effects in patients with a suppressed TSH level, but some do suggest that these patients may have increased rates of hyperthyroid symptoms and decrements in mood or cognition. However, most of these studies suffer from bias, since patients were aware of their diagnoses and often treated with thyroxine. The largest and most recent cross-sectional study failed to find any associations between subclinical hyperthyroidism and a number of measures of mood and cognition.

Mild thyroid hormone excess is associated with increased bone turnover rate; the bone resorption rate exceeds the formation rate and bone loss results. However, there is extensive and conflicting information on whether this is clinically significant. Many studies in postmenopausal women with suppressed TSH have shown an accelerated bone loss in the hip, lumbar spine, and distal radius, whereas other studies have failed to demonstrate this. Two meta-analysis studies found a significant 10% loss of bone density in postmenopausal women with suppressed serum TSH. However, many women in these studies were treated with doses of thyroxine that would clearly be considered supraphysiologic today. The only large-scale study of fracture rates in women (the Study of Osteoporotic Fractures [SOF]), concluded that subclinical hyperthyroidism increased fracture rates at both the hip and the vertebrae. In sum, subclinical hyperthyroidism probably causes clinically relevant bone loss in postmenopausal women (not in men or premenopausal women), which can be attenuated with antiresorptive therapy.

Atrial fibrillation is probably the best documented and most serious consequence of subclinical hyperthyroidism. In the Framingham Heart Study of patients older than 60 years of age with subclinical hyperthyroidism, 28% of patients developed atrial fibrillation in a 10-year follow-up, as compared to 11% of the elderly population with normal TSH levels. This finding has since been replicated in other studies. In terms of cardiac structure and function, a number of studies have shown subtle but statistically significant increases in left ventricular mass and decreases in left ventricular diastolic function. Again, it should be noted that most of these subjects were young, and were receiving thyroxine in suppressive doses for thyroid cancer. Very little is known about cardiac structure and function in subclinical hyperthyroidism in elderly patients, but one could reasonably assume that the subtle decrements seen in young subjects may contribute to clinically relevant deterioration in cardiac function in older patients. In terms of mortality, one recent longitudinal study suggested an increase in cardiovascular mortality in older patients with subclinical hyperthyroidism, while a similar recent study failed to find such an association.

Therapy for subclinical hyperthyroidism should be considered in any patient with neuropsychiatric symptoms, osteoporosis, atrial fibrillation, or cardiac disease. A trial of antithyroid drugs to normalize the serum TSH level is warranted. In patients with more severe features, such as atrial fibrillation, ablation of the hyperfunctioning thyroid with radioactive ^{131}I can be considered.

THYROID NODULES

Prevalence

Thyroid nodules, either solitary or multiple, increase in frequency with advancing age. The lifetime risk of developing a palpable thyroid nodule was estimated to be 5% to 10% in the United States based on a prospective follow-up of more than 5000 patients in the Framingham, Massachusetts, population study. The prevalence of thyroid nodules was found to be higher in women than in men, approximately 5:1, in the same study. An ultrasound survey of 704 people in Sicily without a history of thyroid disease detected nodules in approximately 40% of those older than 60 years and 25% of those younger than 60 years. Three-fourths of the nodules were less than 10 mm in size, only 7% were 20 mm or larger, and the ratio of women to men with nodules was 1.4. Autopsy examination commonly has revealed thyroid nodules. A large autopsy series in the United States indicated that 50% of the population with no known history of thyroid disease had discrete nodules, 35% of whom had nodules greater than 2 cm in diameter.

Clinical Evaluation

In formulating an effective management of a patient with a thyroid nodule, a careful history and physical examination should be done to assess the risk of malignancy. The patient's age and gender are important risk factors for malignancy. Although thyroid nodules are found more frequently in women, the likelihood of a thyroid nodule being malignant is higher in men than in women. The cancer risk in a cold nodule was about sixfold higher in male patients older than 70 years according to a 10-year follow-up study of more than 5000 patients.

The history of radiation exposure during childhood is important because thyroid nodule or thyroid carcinoma can develop years later. Most patients received radiation therapy for treatment of benign conditions such as tonsillitis, acne, tinea capitis, impetigo, sinusitis, or an enlarged thymus. The earlier the age of exposure, the higher was the likelihood of cancer development. However, the latency period probably does not exceed 50 years, so the chance of radiation induction from childhood exposure is very low in the elderly person.

A family history of thyroid cancer suggests familial papillary thyroid cancer or familial medullary thyroid cancer as a component of multiple endocrine neoplasia (MEN) type 2. However, patients with MEN usually present in childhood or early adulthood rather than in the geriatric age group. Familial papillary thyroid cancer is much more common than familial medullary thyroid cancer. A history of goiter in the family maybe reassuring of a benign disorder.

Most thyroid nodules do not cause symptoms. Currently a large majority of nodules are found incidentally during a procedure such as carotid ultrasonography or CT scan or magnetic resonance imaging (MRI) of the neck in the elderly person, giving rise to the term *incidentaloma*. Pain may occur with a hemorrhage into a preexisting colloid nodule or a benign adenoma. Symptoms of rapid nodular growth over a period of weeks or months are suspicious of malignancy. Other symptoms that suggest malignancy are persistent hoarseness or change in voice consistent with recurrent laryngeal nerve dysfunction.

The physical examination of the patient with a thyroid nodule should include careful palpation of the neck with attention to the size and consistency of the nodule and the presence of adenopathy. The location of the nodule within the thyroid gland and the anatomy of the patient's neck maybe the limiting factors in palpatory examination of the neck. In general, most nodules larger than 3 cm in diameter are easily recognized on palpation. A hard and fixed nodule is more likely to be malignant, but many papillary carcinomas or follicular tumors are soft or cystic. Lymphadenopathy is strongly suggestive of malignancy in older patients; therefore, after finding a thyroid nodule, the neck should be examined carefully for the central and deep cervical lymph nodes.

A distinction between solitary and multiple nodules by neck examination maybe limited. In approximately 50% of patients with a clinically solitary nodule on palpation, the lesion subsequently was found to be a dominant nodule in a multinodular goiter on ultrasound or histologic examination. The relative risk of cancer in solitary versus multinodular thyroid glands is controversial. Older studies reported lower rates of thyroid carcinoma in palpable multinodular glands (5% to 13%) as compared with solitary nodules (9% to 25%), but recent studies have found similar incidences of cancer in multinodular and single nodule glands.

Diagnostic Tests

Laboratory and radiographic evaluation of thyroid function is useful to assist in determining whether a nodule is benign or malignant. Figure 108-4 illustrates a recommended approach to diagnostic evaluation. Nearly all patients with either thyroid carcinoma or a benign nodule are euthyroid. An abnormal thyroid function test in a patient with a thyroid nodule does not rule out thyroid cancer but may make thyroid carcinoma a less likely possibility. Low serum TSH concentration in the setting of a nodular goiter suggests the presence of either an autonomously functioning adenoma or a toxic multinodular goiter. Elevated antiperoxidase and antithyroglobulin antibody titers indicate lymphocytic thyroiditis, which may present as a nodule. The serum thyroglobulin level is not a useful test to distinguish benign from malignant nodules because it is increased with any goitrous process.

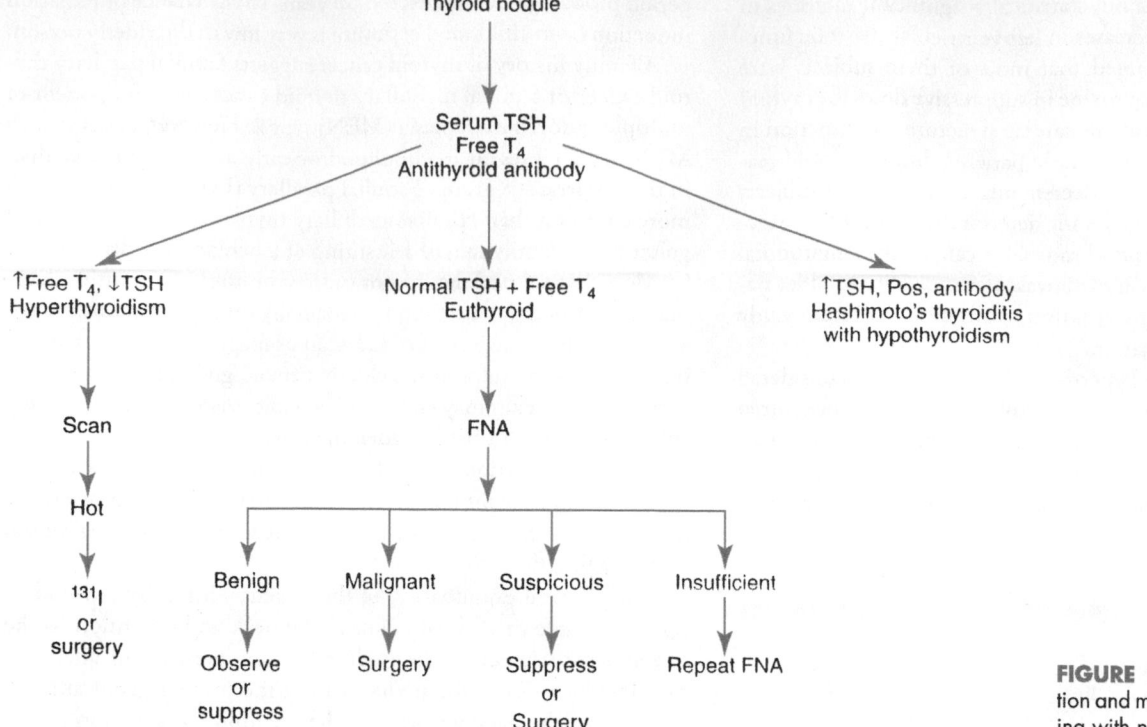

FIGURE 108-4. Algorithm for evaluation and management of patients presenting with nodular thyroid disease.

Thyroid ultrasound is a noninvasive test that discriminates cystic from solid lesions. It is useful for differentiating thyroid from nonthyroid neck masses and for localizing nodules deep within the gland. It is routinely used to guide fine-needle aspiration (FNA) biopsy. Thyroid ultrsonography is capable of identifying impalpable solid and cystic nodules as small as 0.2 mm in diameter. The clinical significance of nodules smaller than 8 mm detected by ultrasonography remains uncertain. The ultrasonographic features that suggest the diagnosis of malignancy are fine stippled calcifications and intranodular vascularity.

FNA biopsy is the most important diagnostic technique. It reliably identifies thyroid nodule cytology and is the most effective method to diagnose malignancy. In experienced hands, it is safe, with accuracy, sensitivity, and specificity of 98% to 99%. Use of FNA has been reported to result in reduction in thyroid nodule management costs by 25%, and the number of patients requiring surgery declined by more than 40%. FNA biopsy should be performed on solid nodules larger than 1.5 cm, on nodules with both a solid and cystic component larger than 2.0 cm, on the solid component of large cystic nodules, and on nodules with evidence of recent growth.

Results of FNA biopsies are divided into four basic categories: (1) benign, (2) suspicious (includes aspirates with some features of thyroid carcinoma but not conclusive), (3) malignant, and (4) insufficient. In a large series of patients with FNA biopsy of the thyroid, benign cytology was found in 69% (mainly colloid goiter), malignant cytology in 3.5%, and suspicious cytology in 10%. The suspicious category consists of variants of follicular neoplasm, but follicular adenomas are about 10-fold more common than follicular carcinomas. The presence of nuclear atypia in a follicular lesion gives a 44% prevalence of malignancy, and absence of nuclear atypia denotes a benign lesion. The insufficient or nondiagnostic cytology was reported as an average of 17% in the same report and has been attributed to lack of operator experience, nodular vascularity, or a small or posteriorly located nodule. Those patients with a nondiagnostic or "insufficient" cytologic diagnosis should have a repeat biopsy. An adequate specimen is obtained in a majority of repeat FNA of nodules.

By thyroid scans with radioiodine, nodules are classified into hyperfunctional or "hot" nodules, nonfunctional or "cold" nodules, or normal functioning or "warm" nodules. This classification is based on the extent of radioiodine incorporation into a nodule compared with the rest of the gland. In a study of more than 5000 patients with thyroid nodules undergoing preoperative scanning, approximately 85% of the nodules were cold, 10% were normal, and 5% were hot. These patients underwent thyroidectomy regardless of the scan result. Thyroid cancer was found in 16% of patients with cold nodules, in 9% with warm nodules, and in 4% with hot nodules. The last figure is higher than expected because most other studies show that a hot nodule is rarely malignant. The finding of a cold nodule has relatively low specificity because the majority of both benign and malignant solitary thyroid nodules appear hypofunctional relative to adjacent normal thyroid tissue. Because the thyroid scan generally is not useful for diagnosis of malignancy, it is not recommended in the initial evaluation of a thyroid nodule. In patients with nodules that are follicular lesions by FNA, radioiodine scan should be performed. Hot or functional nodules are rarely malignant.

Positron emission tomography (PET) has been used to localize recurrent thyroid cancers, but more quantitative studies of the uptake of the glucose analog [^{18}F]2-deoxy-2-fluoro-D-glucose are needed to determine its utility for diagnosis of a malignant thyroid nodule.

Management

The treatment of the thyroid nodule depends on the functional state of the nodule and cytologic diagnosis with FNA biopsy (see

Figure 108-4). The hyperfunctioning "hot" nodule is treated with radioiodine ablation or surgery. Older patients who refuse definitive therapy or who are poor candidates can be treated with thionamides, but these must be continued indefinitely, since hyperfunctioning nodules rarely remit. Patients treated with ^{131}I ablation become euthyroid in a few months, and hypothyroidism develops in only a small proportion of such patients.

The vast majority of thyroid nodules are benign and should be followed with observation alone or with thyroxine suppression therapy in selected patients. Spontaneous regression of thyroid nodules may occur. Thyroid hormone suppressive therapy is based on the assumption that growth of the nodule depends on TSH. The aim of therapy is to reduce serum TSH to the low-normal range. L-Thyroxine suppressive therapy is useful for nodules that do not decrease in size over several months of initial observation. Suppressive therapy in the treatment of benign thyroid nodules has been challenged in the past few years by failure of some studies to show a significant decrease in nodule size and concern about reducing mineral bone density or triggering atrial fibrillation, especially in the elderly. Several controlled studies showed greater than 50% reduction in nodular size in one fourth of patients with a single nodule. Generally, patients are followed by palpation at intervals of 4 months. Ultrasonographic examination can be performed to assess growth or shrinkage of a nodule if more objective documentation is required on an annual basis.

If the cytologic diagnosis indicates malignancy or is strongly suspicious for malignancy, the nodule should be removed surgically. In the 10% to 20% of "suspicious" cytologic findings for malignancy by FNA, approximately one-fourth of patients who undergo surgery are found to have a malignant lesion. Altogether, only approximately 5% to 10% of thyroid nodules are malignant.

THYROID CANCER

Thyroid cancer accounts for 2.2% of all new cancers in the United States. Mortality from thyroid cancer is 0.3% of all cancer deaths. Epidemiologic studies during the last two decades report an increased incidence of thyroid carcinoma in the United States because of improved diagnosis; however, the mortality has decreased because of earlier detection and improved treatment, in addition to a decline in incidence of anaplastic thyroid carcinoma.

Thyroid carcinoma is classified into five major types: papillary, follicular, medullary, anaplastic, and thyroid lymphoma. Most thyroid cancers are indolent and grow slowly over years, whereas a few grow aggressively and cause death in a year. Thyroid carcinomas tend to be more aggressive clinically and more poorly differentiated in elderly patients compared with younger individuals.

Papillary Thyroid Carcinoma

Papillary carcinoma, the most common type of thyroid cancer, accounts for more than 80% of all thyroid tumors. In autopsy studies, the prevalence of occult papillary carcinoma (<1 cm) was found to be 7% in patients older than 80 years of age. Papillary carcinoma arises from follicular thyroid cells and is often indolent and slow growing. The tumor tends to invade lymphatics and metastasize to the regional lymph nodes and the lungs. Hoarseness and vocal cord paralysis secondary to locally invasive thyroid cancer were found to

predict death from papillary carcinoma. Hematogenous spread also can occur to the bone and the central nervous system. The disease is more aggressive in the older patients. The prognosis of papillary thyroid carcinoma depends on the age of the patient at the time of initial diagnosis, the size of the primary lesion, local invasion, and the degree of metastases. Death rates are greater in adults older than 45 years of age. The 10-year survival was only 47% for patients older than 70 years of age.

In a 12-year follow-up of patients older than 47 years of age with papillary thyroid carcinoma, the death rate was 70% in patients with distant metastases versus 0.8% in patients with intrathyroidal disease. Thyroid tumors smaller than 1.5 cm in diameter rarely metastasize to distant sites, whereas larger tumors are associated with higher mortality rates. Extension of the tumor through the thyroid capsule and into the surrounding structures is associated with poorer prognosis. Cervical lymph node metastases occur in about 50% of patients and carry only a slightly higher rate of recurrence and mortality.

Surgery, either near-total or total thyroidectomy, is the initial treatment of choice for patients with papillary carcinoma. Near-total thyroidectomy is performed for extensive unilateral tumors with local metastases. Total thyroidectomy is performed for patients with extensive multifocal disease with metastases to the cervical lymph nodes, contiguous neck structures, or distant sites. The main disadvantage of total thyroidectomy is the higher incidence of hypoparathyroidism.

The prophylactic use of radioactive iodine-131 after surgery reduces the mortality rate and increases survival by destroying any residual thyroid tumor. It is used in nearly all older patients because of their worse prognosis based on age alone. Radioiodine therapy is also used to treat patients with residual or recurrent papillary cancer in the neck.

In order to scan and treat patients with ^{131}I, thyroxine therapy must be withheld for 4 to 6 weeks to allow serum TSH levels to rise. Alternatively, patients can be placed on 25-μg triiodothyronine (liothyronine) twice daily for 1 month instead of thyroxine; then the triiodothyronine is stopped for 2 weeks before administration of ^{131}I. This alternative procedure shortens the period of symptomatic hypothyroidism. Thyroid hormone in a suppressive dose is given after thyroidectomy to reduce thyroid cancer recurrence rates. TSH stimulates thyroid tumors that contain TSH receptors. The dose of thyroxine should be adjusted to keep the TSH suppressed without causing clinical thyrotoxicosis. The degree of suppression should be based on the staging of the patient. In patients with a good prognosis, TSH should be suppressed to the slightly subnormal range. In patients with worse prognosis, which includes many elderly patients, TSH should be suppressed to less than 0.1 mU/L without causing clinical thyrotoxicosis, if this can be done safely.

Recombinant human TSH (rhTSH) may be used to stimulate radioiodide uptake in scanning patients with well-differentiated thyroid cancer while they continue to take levothyroxine. This avoids the symptoms of hypothyroidism that occur after withdrawal of levothyroxine. rhTSH stimulates radioiodine uptake and thyroglobulin secretion in normal and abnormal thyroid tissue. A clinical trial comparing 48-hour ^{131}I whole-body scan results showed 89% concordance in patients receiving rhTSH, as compared to the withdrawal of levothyroxine therapy. Of the discordant results, 8% of scans were superior after levothyroxine withdrawal, while 3% were superior after stimulation with rhTSH (no significant difference).

Because stimulated serum thyroglobulin is a more sensitive assessment of recurrence, this has replaced radioiodine scans for follow-up of patients with differentiated thyroid cancer. The use of recently developed very sensitive assays of thyroglobulin may replace the need for stimulating thyroglobulin with rhTSH or thyroid hormone withdrawal because an undetectable sensitve serum thyroglobulin correlates well with a negative (low) stimulated serum thyroglobulin measurement.

Ultrasonography of the neck is also used for following patients after surgery because most recurrences are in the central neck region or in cervical lymph nodes.

Follicular Thyroid Carcinoma

Follicular thyroid carcinoma accounts for about 10% of all thyroid cancers in the United States and is relatively more common in regions of iodine deficiency. It occurs more frequently in elderly people. Approximately 80% of follicular cell neoplasms are benign. Larger follicular cell neoplasms are more likely to be malignant, especially in men and patients older than age 50 years. Follicular thyroid carcinoma is slightly more aggressive than papillary carcinoma. Cervical lymph node involvement is less common compared to papillary thyroid cancer, but distant metastasis is more frequent.

With minimally invasive follicular carcinoma, there is usually invasion of small vessels, whereas with more invasive tumors there is vascular and capsular invasion and penetration into the surrounding tissue, causing a poorer prognosis. Hürthle cell carcinoma is considered a variant of follicular thyroid carcinoma and carries an even worse prognosis. Follicular carcinoma also metastasizes to the lung, bone, central nervous system, and other soft tissues with higher frequency than papillary carcinoma. Tumor recurrence in distant sites is seen more frequently with follicular than with papillary carcinoma and occurs with higher prevalence in highly invasive tumors.

Treatment includes total thyroidectomy and ^{131}I therapy to ablate residual tumor. Radioiodine is the principal treatment of metastatic tumors. If the tumor does not concentrate the isotope, external radiation maybe effective. As with papillary carcinoma, thyroxine therapy should be given to suppress serum TSH levels to the subnormal range.

Medullary Thyroid Carcinoma

Medullary carcinoma accounts for 2% to 4% of thyroid cancers and is derived from the calcitonin-secreting cells or parafollicular cells. Elevated serum calcitonin levels establish the diagnosis and correlate with tumor mass. Approximately 20% are familial tumors and are associated with other endocrine neoplasias (MEN type 2A or 2B). The recognition of point mutations in the *ret* protooncogene on chromosome 10 has enhanced the ability to detect these neoplasms at an early and potentially curable stage in suspected family members. Approximately 80% of medullary carcinoma is sporadic and diagnosed later in life, mostly after age 50 years. Three fourths of patients with sporadic medullary carcinoma present with a thyroid mass and 15% have local symptoms of dysphagia, dyspnea, or hoarseness.

Immunohistochemical studies demonstrate the presence of calcitonin in the tumor that is also able to synthesize calcitonin gene-related peptide, ACTH, serotonin, prostaglandin, histamine, and carcinoembryonic antigen. Diarrhea occurs in 30% of patients with advanced disease and correlates directly with the tumor mass. Recurrence rate increases in frequency with age. About two thirds of patients older than age 70 years have persistent disease or a higher recurrence rate after surgery.

Anaplastic Thyroid Carcinoma

Anaplastic carcinoma of the thyroid, the most aggressive and lethal neoplasm, accounts for 2% of all thyroid carcinomas. It is often derived from a well-differentiated thyroid carcinoma. The peak occurrence of this tumor is in the seventh decade of life; three quarters of patients are 60 years of age or older and it is more common in women. Examination of the neck usually reveals a fixed, large, firm mass that often makes it difficult to detect neck nodes clinically. Hemorrhage and necrosis within the tumor may result in soft, fluctuant masses. Large axillary nodes are sometimes seen.

Treatment includes surgery, followed by external radiation and chemotherapy, which may result in disease-free intervals of 1 to 5 years. The mortality exceeds 80% at 12 months. Long-term survivors usually have only a small focus of anaplastic cells.

Thyroid Lymphoma

Thyroid lymphoma accounts for about 1% of thyroid malignancies. It is often engrafted on a background of chronic lymphocytic thyroiditis. At the time of presentation with lymphoma, the patient is usually older than 60 years of age. There is a female preponderance. This tumor arises from B-cell lymphocytes. It usually invades the walls of blood vessels and extends outside the thyroid gland. The usual clinical presentation is a rapidly enlarging thyroid mass in a patient with long history of a goiter or diagnosis of Hashimoto's thyroiditis that was treated with thyroid hormone. The patient may complain of neck pressure, local swelling of the thyroid gland, hoarseness, and dysphagia. FNA may suggest the diagnosis, but definitive diagnosis usually requires an open biopsy. Surgical removal of the lymphoma by total thyroidectomy is unwise. Treatment with external radiation and four to six courses of chemotherapy usually produces a permanent remission.

FURTHER READING

Bagchi N, et al. Thyroid dysfunction in adults over age 55 years. *Arch Intern Med.* 1990;150:785.

Bartolotta TV, et al. Incidentally discovered thyroid nodules: incidence, and greyscale and colour Doppler pattern in an adult population screened by real-time compound spatial sonography. *Radiol Med (Torino).* 2006;111:989.

Belfiore A, et al. Cancer risk in patients with cold thyroid nodules: relevance of iodine intake, sex, age, and multinodularity. *Am J Med.* 1992;363:363.

Cappola AR, Fried LP, Arnold AM, et al. Thyroid status, cardiovascular risk, and mortality in older adults. *JAMA.* 2006;295:1033.

Cooper DS. Subclinical hypothyroidism. *N Engl J Med.* 2001;345:260.

Cooper DS, et al. Management guidelines for patients with thyroid nodules and differentiated thyroid cancer. *Thyroid.* 2006;16:109.

Frates MC, et al. Management of thyroid nodules detected at US: Society of Radiologists in Ultrasound consensus conference statement. *Radiology.* 2005;237:794.

Frates MC, et al. Prevalence and distribution of carcinoma in patients with solitary and multiple thyroid nodules on sonography. *J Clin Endocrinol Metab.* 2006;91:3411.

Gussekloo J, van Exel E, De Craen AJ, Meinders AE, Frolich M, Westendorp RG. Thyroid status, disability and cognitive function, and survival in old age. *JAMA.* 2004;292:2591.

Hershman JM, et al. Serum thyrotropin and thyroid hormone levels in elderly and middle-aged euthyroid persons. *J Am Geriatr Soc.* 1993;41:823.

Kahaly GJ. Cardiovascular and atherogenic aspects of subclinical hypothyroidism. *Thyroid.* 2000;10:665.

Ladenson PW, et al. American thyroid association guidelines for detection of thyroid dysfunction. *Arch Intern Med.* 2000;160:1573.

Langton JE, Brent GA. Non-thyroidal illness syndrome: Evaluation of thyroid function in sick patients. *Endocrinol Metab Clin North Am.* 2002;31:159.

Lin JD, et al. Characteristics of thyroid carcinomas in aging patients. *Eur J Clin Invest.* 2000;30:147.

Mariotti S, et al. Complex alteration of thyroid function in healthy centenarians. *J Clin Endocrinol Metab.* 1993;77:1130.

Robbins RJ, Robbins AK. Clinical review 156: recombinant human thyrotropin and thyroid cancer management. *J Clin Endocrinol Metab.* 2003;88:1933.

Roberts LM, Pattison H, Roalfe A, et al. Is subclinical thyroid dysfunction in the elderly associated with depression or cognitive dysfunction? *Ann Intern Med.* 2006;145:573.

Toft AD. Subclinical hyperthyroidism. *N Engl J Med.* 2001;345:512.

Trivalle C, et al. Differences in the signs and symptoms of hyperthyroidism in older and younger patients. *J Am Geriatr Soc.* 1996;44:50.

Yamada T, et al. Age-related therapeutic response to antithyroid drugs in patients with hyperthyroid Graves' disease. *J Am Geriatr Soc.* 1994;42:513.

Diabetes Mellitus

Annette M. Chang ■ *Jeffrey B. Halter*

Diabetes mellitus is a common metabolic disorder affecting elderly people. Although it is recognized by its effects on carbohydrate metabolism to cause hyperglycemia, diabetes mellitus usually also affects lipid and protein metabolism. With time, effects of diabetes on the cardiovascular system, the kidneys, the retina, and the peripheral nervous system, often referred to as long-term complications of diabetes, substantially increase mortality and morbidity in older adults. Furthermore, diabetes may accelerate the risk and contribute to worse outcomes for other common age-related disorders. In general, diabetes mellitus in older adults is underdiagnosed and undertreated. A growing body of evidence assessing outcomes of interventions and an increasing number of therapeutic options for diabetes management has increased the importance of making a diagnosis and offering appropriate intervention strategies to elderly patients who have this potentially devastating disorder. There is also growing evidence of the ability to prevent the development of diabetes, including in older people. Management of diabetes is often considered to be synonymous with treatment of hyperglycemia. However, it is now recognized that appropriate diabetes management of an older patient must be much broader, addressing many factors that contribute to long-term complications.

DEFINITION AND CLASSIFICATION

Diabetes mellitus is a heterogeneous set of disorders affecting multiple body systems; however, diagnostic criteria are based on documentation of elevated circulating blood glucose levels. Because glucose levels vary during the course of the day, and even in the fasting state form a continuous variable in populations, the definition of a single cut point that separates normal from abnormal is somewhat arbitrary. The challenge of establishing appropriate diagnostic criteria for elderly subjects is made more difficult by well-described effects of aging on glucose metabolism (summarized later in this chapter in the section on "Effects of Aging"). Similar to criteria for hypercholesterolemia and hypertension, the diagnostic criteria for

diabetes mellitus are based on values that predict poor outcomes in population studies.

Table 109-1 summarizes the currently accepted diagnostic criteria, which were established by an expert panel convened by the American Diabetes Association (ADA) and published in 1997 with a follow-up report in 2003.

Type 1 Diabetes

Type 1 diabetes is a condition characterized by destruction of the insulin-producing beta cells of the endocrine pancreas, resulting in absolute deficiency of insulin. While evidence of cell-mediated autoimmunity is a hallmark of type 1 diabetes, some patients develop a type 1 diabetes phenotype with evidence of severe insulin deficiency and episodes of diabetic ketoacidosis (DKA) with no detectable autoimmunity. Such individuals have idiopathic type 1 diabetes. Although the incidence of new-onset type 1 diabetes in older adults is very low, effective treatment of type 1 diabetes may prevent or delay the development of long-term complications and increased mortality. Thus, people who develop type 1 diabetes earlier in life may live to old age and therefore become a part of the spectrum of diabetes mellitus in an older adult population.

Type 2 Diabetes

Approximately 90% of older adults with diabetes have type 2 diabetes mellitus. Hyperglycemia, often asymptomatic, is the hallmark and DKA is not part of the clinical syndrome. Obesity is often present, and resistance to insulin's metabolic effects is a characteristic feature. Impaired insulin secretion is also part of the picture, but severe absolute insulin deficiency is not. While there is a strong genetic predisposition to development of type 2 diabetes, its etiology remains unknown and is likely to be both highly heterogeneous and multifactorial. The interaction between genetics, lifestyle factors, and aging in the development of type 2 diabetes is discussed later in this chapter in the section on "Pathophysiology of Diabetes."

TABLE 109-1

1997 and 2003 American Diabetes Association Diagnostic Criteria for Diabetes Mellitus, Impaired Glucose Tolerance, and Impaired Fasting Glucose

Diabetes mellitus
  Classic diabetes symptoms plus a random glucose level ≥200 mg/dL (11.1 mmol/L)
  Fasting* glucose level ≥126 mg/dL (7.0 mmol/L)[†]
  Glucose level ≥200 mg/dL (11.1 mmol/L) at 2 hours during a standard OGTT[†]

Impaired glucose tolerance (IGT)
  Glucose level ≥140 mg/dL (7.8 mmol/L) and <200 mg/dL (11.1 mmol/L) at 2 hours during a standard OGTT

Impaired fasting glucose (IFG)
  Fasting glucose level ≥100 mg/dL (5.6 mmol/L) and <126 mg/dL (7.0 mmol/L)

OGTT, oral glucose tolerance test.
*No caloric intake for at least 8 hours.
[†]Either of these criteria should be confirmed on a separate day to establish a diagnosis of diabetes.

TABLE 109-2

Drugs That May Increase Glucose Levels

Diuretics
α-Adrenergic agonists
β-Adrenergic blockers
Alcohol
Ca^{2+} channel-blockers
Caffeine
Clozapine
Glucocorticoids
Growth hormone
Nicotine
Nicotinic acid
Nonsteroidal anti-inflammatory drugs
Female sex steroids (estrogen/progesterone)
Pentamidine
Phenytoin

Other Specific Types of Diabetes

The 1997 ADA classification for diabetes mellitus identifies a number of specific conditions that lead to development of diabetes mellitus, each of which is relatively uncommon. One group of disorders includes genetic defects of the pancreatic beta cell. The clinical phenotype for these genetic disorders is maturity-onset diabetes of youth (MODY). These genetic disorders have autosomal-dominant inheritance with first presentation of asymptomatic hyperglycemia early in life. Patients with MODY can live to old age, however, and therefore can be a part of the spectrum of diabetes in an elderly population. The metabolic disorder in some affected individuals maybe mild, whereas others may develop symptomatic hyperglycemia and long-term complications of diabetes mellitus similar to patients with typical type 2 diabetes. Another type of genetic defect has been identified in a few families in which insulin processing prior to secretion is impaired, which can predispose to development of hyperglycemia.

Other families have genetic defects affecting insulin action. Severe insulin resistance results, and when it is not adequately compensated for by increased insulin secretion, hyperglycemia occurs. Diseases of the exocrine pancreas can lead to damage to pancreatic beta cells, diminished insulin secretion, and hyperglycemia. Hyperglycemia also can occur in patients with excessive secretion of hormones that adversely affect carbohydrate metabolism, such as in acromegaly, Cushing's syndrome, glucagonoma, and pheochromocytoma. Similarly, tumors making aldosterone can cause hyperglycemia as a result of hypokalemia-induced inhibition of insulin secretion. A number of drugs or toxins can impair insulin secretion or insulin action and lead to the development of hyperglycemia. Table 109-2 lists such drugs. Several genetic neuromuscular disorders are associated with diabetes mellitus, but they are rare in the older adult population.

Gestational Diabetes Mellitus

Gestational diabetes mellitus (GDM) is a separate category in the 1997 ADA classification and refers to the first identification of an alteration in glucose metabolism during pregnancy. While GDM per se is not part of the spectrum of diabetes in older adults, a history of GDM maybe part of the background of an older woman presenting with type 2 diabetes. As GDM has been aggressively screened for and treated, increasing numbers of women reaching the geriatric age group will have this history, as GDM affects approximately 4% of all pregnancies in the United States. After pregnancy, 5% to 10% of women with gestational diabetes are found to have type 2 diabetes. Women who have had gestational diabetes have a 20% to 50% chance of developing diabetes in the next 5 to 10 years.

Diagnostic Criteria

The rationale for the circulating glucose level criteria shown in Table 109-1 is based on prediction of risk for diabetes-related complications. Thus, a 2-hour value during the oral glucose tolerance test (OGTT) greater or equal to 200 mg/dL is a strong predictor of diabetes complications, even when the fasting glucose level is less than 126 mg/dL. The term "isolated postchallenge hyperglycemia" (IPH) is sometimes used for individuals who meet the 2-hour OGTT criterion for diabetes, but who do not meet the fasting glucose criterion.

There is no age adjustment in the recommended criteria for the diagnosis of diabetes mellitus because the same glucose level cut points that predict complications appear to apply regardless of age. There is no current criterion for diagnosis of diabetes mellitus based on measurement of hemoglobin A1c, as no level of hemoglobin A1c accurately identifies people who meet glucose level diagnostic criteria.

The 1997 and 2003 ADA criteria shown in Table 109-1 also identify intermediate categories of altered glucose metabolism that identify an earlier stage (prediabetes) in the development of diabetes mellitus. Impaired glucose tolerance (IGT) is based on results of an OGTT and the category of impaired fasting glucose (IFG) is defined from fasting glucose levels. Because OGTTs are not routinely performed in clinical practice, the IFG category allows easy identification of some, but not nearly all, of the individuals who would meet criteria for IGT if an OGTT were performed. People with IGT and IFG are at increased risk for cardiovascular disease, as well as for subsequent development of overt diabetes mellitus. There is no recommended age adjustment for the criteria for either IGT or IFG, as these criteria predict risk for subsequent diabetes and cardiovascular disease similarly in older people.

Diagnostic Testing for Older Adults

One advantage of the 1997 and 2003 ADA recommendations is that a simple fasting glucose level can be used to classify patients and establish a diagnosis of diabetes mellitus, or even the intermediate stage of IFG. Unfortunately, many older individuals who meet diabetes criteria by OGTT will be missed by this method (see "Epidemiology of Diabetes and its Complications" later in this chapter). The ADA recommends that screening to detect prediabetes or diabetes with either fasting glucose level or 2-hour OGTT be considered in all individuals older than age 45 years at 3-year intervals, particularly in those with a body mass index (BMI) ≥ 25 kg/m^2. The rationale for such screening includes the high rate of undetected diabetes mellitus in population studies (discussed further subsequently in the section on "Epidemiology of Diabetes") and the substantial current evidence that early intervention delays the development of diabetes in people with prediabetes, including those older than 60 years of age. Yearly follow-up and retesting of people at higher risk should be considered. Such high-risk individuals include those who are overweight (BMI ≥ 25 kg/m^2; see Chapter 39), those with a strong family history of diabetes that includes a first-degree relative, those with a history of prior GDM, people with hypertension or dyslipidemia (particularly elevated triglyceride and/or low high-density lipoprotein [HDL] cholesterol levels), and those who have had IFG or IGT on previous testing. In addition, members of ethnic groups with higher risks of diabetes should be considered for more frequent testing. Such populations include African-Americans, Hispanics, Pacific Islanders, Asian Americans, and Native Americans.

What about testing to classify the type of diabetes mellitus? The ADA reports do not define criteria for classifying types of diabetes mellitus. In theory, it is possible to measure insulin levels and various pancreatic islet antibodies to identify most individuals with type 1 diabetes. At this time, however, the differentiation between types of diabetes is primarily based on clinical history. While clinical history is imprecise, it is sufficient under most circumstances to guide treatment interventions. Insulin therapy should be a key part of the approach to patients with type 1 diabetes and interventions targeted at enhancing endogenous insulin secretion are unlikely to be useful for such individuals, even in the early stages of their disease. Insulin can also be used in patients with other types of diabetes depending on the clinical situation (as described in more detail subsequently in the section on "Insulin"). Accurate classification maybe more important in the future. For example, if interventions are identified to prevent progression of autoimmune diabetes, it would be important to establish a specific diagnosis early so that such interventions could be used appropriately.

EPIDEMIOLOGY OF DIABETES AND ITS COMPLICATIONS

Diabetes Mellitus and Prediabetes

More than 50% of people in the United States with diabetes are older than 60 years of age. Figure 109-1 illustrates the dramatic age-related

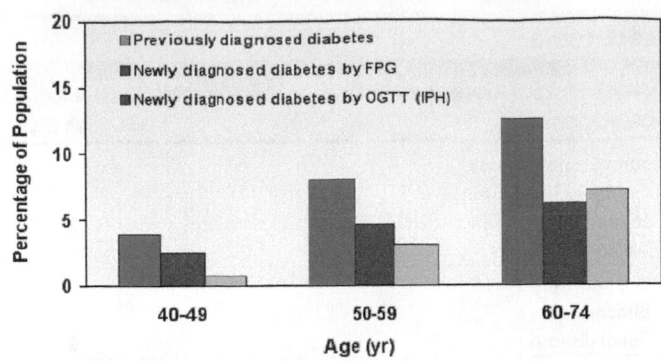

FIGURE 109-1. Prevalence of type 2 diabetes among elderly people according to age and ADA diagnostic criteria (National Health and Nutrition Examination Survey [NHANES] III). IPH, isolated postchallenge hyperglycemia. *(Data from Harris MI, et al. Prevalence of diabetes, impaired fasting glucose and impaired glucose tolerance in US adults. Diabetes Care. 1998;21:518, and Resnick HE, et al. American Diabetes Association diabetes diagnostic criteria, advancing age, and cardiovascular disease risk profiles: Results from the Third National Health and Nutrition Examination Survey. Diabetes Care. 2000;23:176.)*

increase in the prevalence rate of diabetes mellitus in men and women in the United States. This analysis from the Third National Health and Nutrition Examination Survey (NHANES III) was carried out from 1988 to 1994 by the National Center for Health Statistics of the Centers for Disease Control on a nationally representative sample of the U.S. noninstitutionalized population. Based on the 1997 ADA criteria, approximately 25% of people older than age 60 years have diabetes mellitus. The high prevalence rate was confirmed in the population-based Cardiovascular Health Study and extended to people older than age 75 years. Approximately half of these older affected persons had a physician diagnosis of diabetes mellitus, but the other half were previously undiagnosed. Among the 12% to 13% of previously undiagnosed older people, approximately half were detected by an elevated fasting glucose. However, the other half had IPH, requiring an OGTT to detect the presence of diabetes.

Comparison with similar data collected in the late 1970s during NHANES II indicates that the prevalence of diabetes increased by 30% to 40% during the interval between studies. Diabetes prevalence varies by ethnic group, with the lowest rates in non-Hispanic whites, higher rates in non-Hispanic blacks, and the highest rates in Mexican Americans. Even higher rates are observed in some Native American populations. These ethnic group differences appear to persist throughout the age range.

The prevalence, or percent of the population with diabetes mellitus at any given age, includes both incident or new cases plus all of those with diabetes who were diagnosed at an earlier age. Part of the dramatic age-related increase in prevalence of diabetes is a result of survival of people initially diagnosed at middle age. However, other studies of the incidence of diabetes indicate an age-related increase and the prevalence of undiagnosed diabetes in NHANES III and other studies also increases with age.

After excluding people who meet criteria for diabetes mellitus, the prevalence rate for IGT and IFG also both increase with age. In NHANES III, approximately 14% of the U.S. population older than 60 years of age had IFG and approximately 20% met criteria for IGT, rates substantially higher than for younger individuals. When prevalence rates for both diabetes and IGT are combined, the rate in

TABLE 109-3

Long-Term Complications of Diabetes in Elderly People

COMPLICATION	RELATIVE RISK*
Macrovascular disease	
Coronary heart disease	2
Stroke	2
Amputation	10
Microvascular disease	
Blindness	1.4
Renal disease	2
Neuropathy	Uncertain

*Risk compared to people of the same age who do not have diabetes.

elderly people in the United States exceeds 40%. It could be argued that a finding prevalent in nearly half of the population should not be considered "abnormal" and that the criteria for these conditions should thus be age-adjusted. However, these criteria identify older people at risk for progression to overt hyperglycemia and at increased risk for the complications of diabetes.

Diabetes Complications

Older adults with diabetes mellitus are susceptible to all the usual complications of diabetes. Although clinical outcomes of many of the diabetes complications including end-stage renal disease, loss of vision, myocardial infarction, stroke, peripheral vascular disease, and peripheral neuropathy all increase with age in the absence of diabetes, their incidence and cooccurrence are all exaggerated by the presence of diabetes, as summarized in Table 109-3. Diabetes-specific pathologic findings exist for some of these complications, but pathological information is generally not available for epidemiologic studies that depend on the more gross clinical outcomes. It is more difficult to be certain of the specific role of diabetes, and especially of hyperglycemia per se, in contributing to an outcome such as visual loss or end-stage renal disease in an older patient, as compared with a younger patient with diabetes, who would not otherwise be expected to have one of these problems.

In an older adult population, the presence of hyperglycemia and diabetes mellitus should be viewed as a risk factor for such complications, analogous to hypertension or hypercholesterolemia. Using this approach, there is substantial evidence that the presence of diabetes in an older adult increases risk for adverse outcomes, as summarized in Table 109-3. Overall, it is estimated that a diagnosis of diabetes is associated on average with a 10-year reduction in life expectancy. However, this figure becomes progressively reduced at advanced old age when risks of competing causes of mortality rise exponentially. Nonetheless, diabetes is associated with a higher mortality rate at any age, approaching twice the rate in older people of comparable age without diabetes in some studies. Similarly, the rates of myocardial infarction, stroke, and end-stage renal disease are increased approximately twofold, and the risk of visual loss is increased approximately 40% in older people with diabetes. This level of increased relative risk may appear modest on an individual level. However, since the elderly population has by far the highest rates of these conditions, the increase in absolute risk is more substantial. Thus a twofold relative risk increase represents a very large number of added ad-

verse outcomes. The risk for lower-extremity amputation is dramatically increased in older people with diabetes mellitus, approximately 10-fold greater than that for older people without diabetes.

PATHOPHYSIOLOGY OF DIABETES AND ITS COMPLICATIONS

Although the rate of new onset of type 1 diabetes is relatively low in older people, the mechanism for type 1 diabetes does not appear to be different in this population. Usually, patients with type 1 diabetes have markers of immune destruction of pancreatic beta cells such as islet cell antibodies, antibodies to insulin, or other pancreatic beta cell-specific antibodies. There are also strong human leukocyte antigen (HLA) associations.

Type 2 diabetes is by far the most prevalent form in older adults. Autoimmune destruction of pancreatic beta cells is not observed. Limited pathologic investigation suggests that total beta cell mass maybe moderately reduced, but severe loss of beta cell mass is uncommon. The pathophysiology of type 2 diabetes is unknown, but it appears to occur as a result of a complex interaction among genetic, lifestyle, and aging influences, as illustrated in Figure 109-2. The heterogeneity of type 2 diabetes likely reflects the varying contributions of each of multiple factors to the development of hyperglycemia in a given individual or family.

Effects of Aging

Many studies have demonstrated age-related glucose intolerance in humans, as illustrated in Figure 109-3. In normal people who do not meet criteria for either diabetes mellitus or IGT, there is a slight age-related increase in fasting glucose levels and a more dramatic slowing of return to normal of glucose levels following an oral glucose challenge.

Insulin Resistance

There is a decline in sensitivity to the metabolic effects of insulin with age. An age-related impairment of intracellular insulin signaling reduces insulin-mediated mobilization of glucose transporters, which are critical to glucose uptake and metabolism in insulin-dependent tissues such as muscle and fat. There is currently little evidence for an age-related impairment of insulin effects on protein or fat metabolism.

An absolute or relative increase of body adiposity, particularly central body adiposity, has been well-documented with advancing age and appears to account in large part for the age-related increase in insulin resistance. Decreased physical activity is associated with insulin resistance and exercise training can improve insulin sensitivity. Thus, diminished physical activity in an older individual can also contribute to decreased insulin sensitivity. Both in animal studies and in humans, it has been difficult to demonstrate a residual effect of aging on insulin action when the changes in body composition and physical activity are controlled for.

Impaired Insulin Secretion

The progression from normal glucose tolerance to IGT and type 2 diabetes in aging is characterized by progressive defects in pancreatic

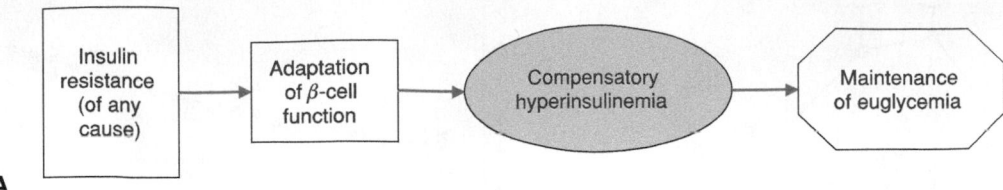

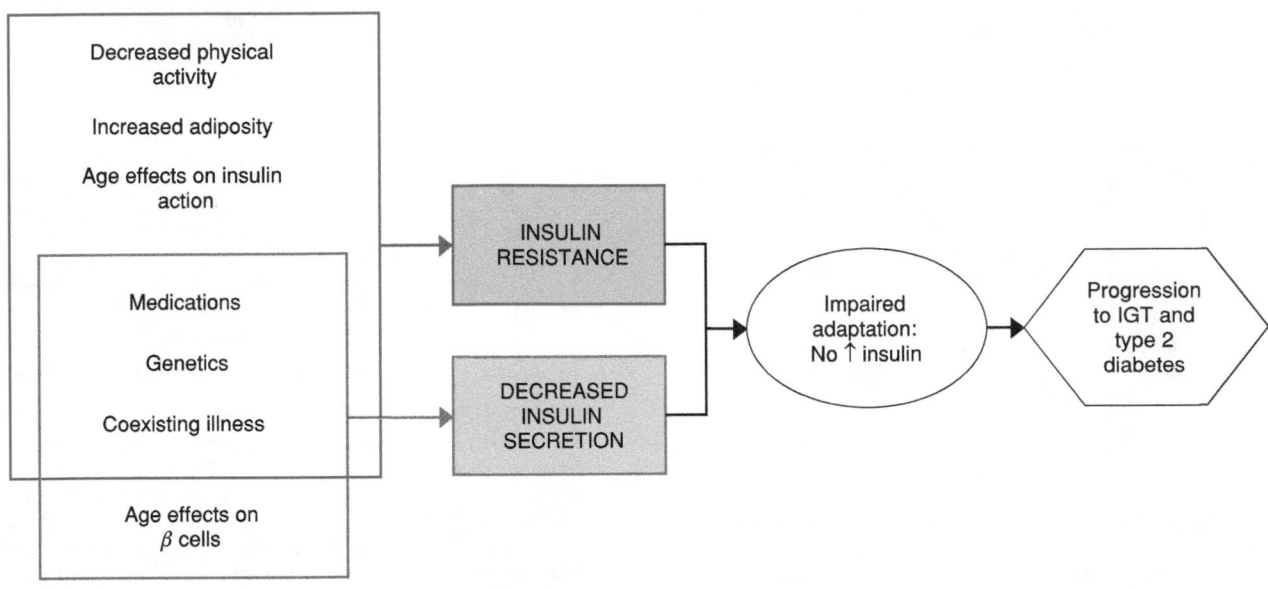

FIGURE 109-2. Model for age-related hyperglycemia. (A) Normal adaptation to insulin resistance. In normal individuals, pancreatic beta cell function compensates for insulin resistance with an adaptive response resulting in hyperinsulinemia, but maintenance of normal glucose levels (euglycemia). (B) Multiple risk factors for type 2 diabetes associated with aging predispose older adults to develop hyperglycemia. Some of these factors contribute to increased insulin resistance and some to decreased insulin secretion. As older individuals with impaired pancreatic beta cell function are unable to adapt adequately to insulin resistance, impaired glucose tolerance (IGT) and progression to type 2 diabetes can occur. A vicious cycle may ensue as hyperglycemia develops and leads to further deterioration of beta cell function and more severe insulin resistance. *(Adapted from Chang AM, Halter JB. Aging and insulin secretion. Am J Physiol Endocrinol Metab. 2003;284:E7.)*

beta cell function. Animal studies have demonstrated an age-related decline in beta cell function. However, there has been great variability in previous studies examining insulin secretion in older people. These human studies, however, may have failed to address adequately the importance of the normal adaptive response to insulin resistance. As most older individuals demonstrate insulin resistance, as already described, a compensatory increase of insulin secretion, leading to increased circulating insulin levels would be expected. As illustrated in Figure 109-2A, this is the normal adaptive response to insulin resistance that is observed in younger people who have obesity or other causes of insulin resistance. Such individuals have elevated fasting insulin levels and an increased insulin response to a glucose challenge. However, both basal and stimulated insulin levels in older adults are similar to those of insulin-sensitive young people, as illustrated in Figure 109-3, despite the coexistence of insulin resistance in the elderly subjects. Furthermore, when older and younger people are carefully matched for degree of insulin sensitivity, absolute impairments in betacell function with normal human aging have been demonstrated. Such defects are greater in older people with IGT, as

shown in Figure 109-4. Impaired pancreatic beta cell adaptation to insulin resistance is an important contributing factor to age-related glucose intolerance and risk for diabetes.

Interaction Between Impaired Insulin Secretion And Insulin Resistance

As summarized in Figure 109-2, in the setting of impaired beta cell function, there is a maladaptive response leading to impaired insulin secretion and progression to IGT and type 2 diabetes. Hyperglycemia, in turn, is known to contribute directly to insulin resistance and to impair pancreatic beta cell function, thereby setting up a vicious cycle of maladaptive mechanisms.

Coexisting illness is another factor affecting both insulin sensitivity and insulin secretion in an older person. Both hypertension and hyperlipidemia are common in older people and have been associated with diminished insulin sensitivity. In fact, a metabolic syndrome has been described that includes coexisting hypertension, hyperlipidemia, central obesity, and glucose intolerance. Some have

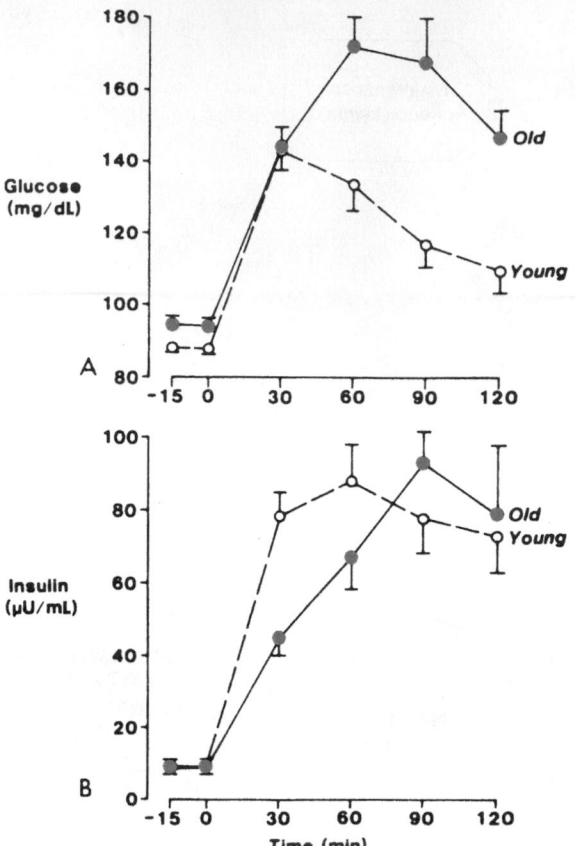

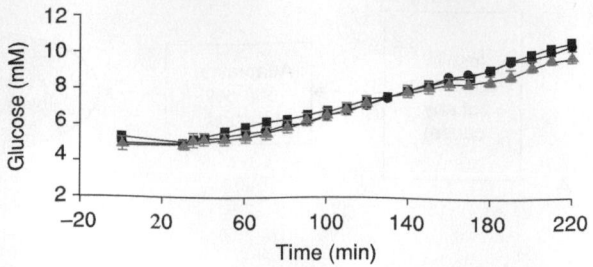

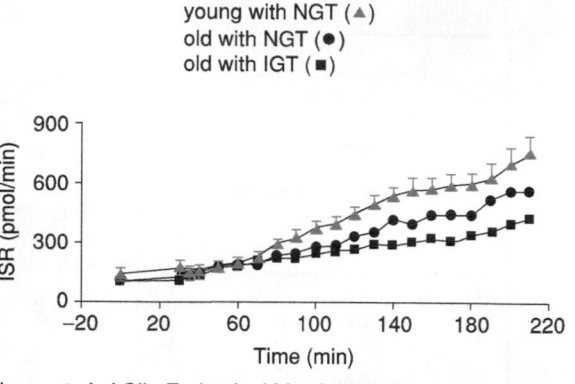

young with NGT (▲)
old with NGT (●)
old with IGT (■)

Chang et al, J Clin Endocrinol Metab 91: 3303–3309, 2006

FIGURE 109-3. Plasma glucose (*upper*) and insulin (*lower*) levels before and following oral ingestion of 100 g of glucose in healthy old (*n* = 18) and young (*n* =18) subjects matched for relative body weight and socioeconomic group. Subjects were eating an ad libitum diet. Note the slight elevation of fasting glucose levels in the old group and the delay in recovery of glucose levels following oral glucose. Also note the overall similarity of insulin levels between old and young subjects. *(Reprinted with permission from Chen M, et al. The role of dietary carbohydrate in the decrease glucose tolerance of the elderly. J Am Geriatr Soc. 1987;35:417.)*

FIGURE 109-4. Effect of age on insulin secretion rate (ISR) in humans with normal glucose tolerance (NGT) or impaired glucose tolerance (IGT) by American Diabetes Association criteria. Plasma glucose concentrations and ISR are shown over time during intravenous glucose infusions, comparing young with NGT (*n* =15, mean age = 26 yrs), old with NGT (*n* =16, mean age = 70 yrs), and old with IGT (*n* =14, mean age = 70 yrs). Glucose levels during variable rate glucose infusion begun at time 0 were well-matched in the three study groups, and degree of insulin resistance was also similar in the three study groups. ISR was significantly and progressively decreased in the two older groups, with the greatest impairment in old IGT (*P* = 0.0002, old IGT vs. young and old IGT vs. old NGT; and old NGT vs. young NGT). Data are means ± SE. *(Adapted from Chang AM, et al. Impaired β-cell function in human aging: response to nicotinic acid-induced insulin resistance. J Clin Endocrinol Metab. 2006;91:3303.)*

proposed that insulin resistance is a unifying feature linking the components of this metabolic syndrome; however, there is uncertainty about whether the insulin resistance in these circumstances is primary or a secondary result of these other conditions. Furthermore, any acute illness can precipitate hyperglycemia because of effects of stress hormones to cause insulin resistance combined with the α-adrenergic effects of catecholamines released during stressful illness to inhibit insulin secretion. Drugs that may be used by older people may also contribute to hyperglycemia by causing insulin resistance (see Table 109-2).

Finally, a pathogenetic sequence common to many syndromes in old age can be readily illustrated by diabetes in an elderly patient: Hyperglycemia becomes frank diabetes, leading to acute complications and such syndromes as hyperosmotic nonketotic coma or, with time, to microvascular or macrovascular complications such as renal disease, stroke, or myocardial infarction, with superimposed drug-induced aggravation of impaired glucose regulation and decreased physical activity, progressive disability, and functional decline; that is, a downward spiral of mutually reinforcing conditions perhaps triggered by an event such as influenza or a fall that would be readily withstood by a younger person, especially a younger person without diabetes.

Genetics

There is a strong genetic predisposition to type 2 diabetes mellitus. For example, the concordance rate for type 2 diabetes in identical twins approaches 100%. However, the genetic predisposition is complex and likely a key part of the heterogeneity of this disorder. As described previously, there are a few simple genetic abnormalities that cause a diabetes syndrome such as MODY. However, even within this narrow subtype of diabetes mellitus, there is considerable heterogeneity, as different families have now been described with defects in at least six different genes, all resulting in a similar phenotype. Furthermore, there is heterogeneity within each gene defect, as various alterations of the gene have been described in different families.

The situation in typical type 2 diabetes is likely to be much more complex, with multiple genes involved in different individuals in different families. Ultimately, there may be hundreds of different subtypes of type 2 diabetes identified as different combinations of genetic alterations are identified in different families. As these genes are identified and their functions determined, new therapeutic approaches to treatment may develop, enabling targeting of therapeutic interventions to the specific genetically determined defects present. Genome-wide scanning of large populations has now identified at least 10 genetic markers associated with type 2 diabetes. However, these markers in aggregate account for only a small percentage of type 2 diabetes risk.

In summary, the high rate of diabetes in older adults likely represents the interaction of genetic background with the linked age and lifestyle-related changes in insulin secretion and insulin action described here.

Mechanisms for Diabetes Complications

Chronic exposure to hyperglycemia may contribute directly to the development of diabetes complications in a number of ways. One mechanism may be the interaction of glucose with proteins to cause protein glycosylation and subsequent formation of advanced glycosylation end ("AGE") products. The AGE products can accumulate in proteins of slow turnover such as collagen, potentially leading to tissue damage and injury. Tissue exposure to high concentrations of glucose can also lead to accumulation of metabolic products of the aldose reductase system including nonmetabolized molecules such as sorbitol. Such accumulation can potentially affect cellular energy metabolism and contribute to cell injury and death. Given the complexity of the genetic background contributing to type 2 diabetes, the possibility also exists that some of the genetic background of an individual may directly contribute to the risk for one or more long-term complications of diabetes (e.g., end-stage renal failure) independently of the effects of hyperglycemia. However, such a possibility remains speculative. Interactions between diabetes and other comorbidities may contribute to the manifestation and severity of diabetes-related complications. Diabetic patients who also have hypertension are at greater risk for renal disease and for macrovascular disease than diabetic patients without hypertension. Similarly, neuropathy is more likely in a diabetic patient who is exposed to a neurotoxic agent.

PREVENTION

Type 2 diabetes is a gradually progressive disorder of carbohydrate metabolism that develops over a long period of time. It has been estimated that abnormalities of glucose regulation can be detected 8 to 10 years before the clinical diagnosis of type 2 diabetes is made. The importance of lifestyle factors in the pathophysiology of type 2 diabetes and the epidemiological associations of healthy lifestyles with reduced risk for diabetes suggest that lifestyle interventions might prevent the development of diabetes. Given the progressive nature of impairments of glucose regulation, there is great interest in trying to identify people early in this course who are at high risk and therefore candidates for intervention to prevent progression. There is now substantial evidence that high-risk individuals can be identified and that progression to type 2 diabetes can be delayed. People with IGT and obesity appear to benefit from such interventions. Individuals from high-risk ethnic groups or who have a history of GDM also appear to benefit.

In the largest of these studies, the multicenter Diabetes Prevention Program (DPP) in the United States, an effort was made to recruit older adults with IGT. A lifestyle intervention program including both caloric restriction and exercise was shown to be remarkably effective in reducing the rate of progression to type 2 diabetes, even though only 5% to 7% weight reduction was achieved. In the DPP, the lifestyle intervention program was even more effective in people older than age 60 years than in younger people at risk, reducing progression to diabetes by more than 70% as compared to a control group. Drug interventions have also been tested. Metformin was used in the DPP and was effective in slowing progression in younger adults, but had surprisingly much less effect in people older than age 60 years.

As more is learned about the genetics of type 2 diabetes, it may be possible to identify high-risk individuals early in life based on genotype and to effectively target interventions. The success of the initial intervention trials to prevent progression has raised the question, not yet resolved, about whether and how screening should be carried out to identify high-risk individuals for more widespread clinical interventions.

PRESENTATION

The finding of an elevated glucose level on routine laboratory testing is the most common presentation for type 2 diabetes in an elderly person. The classical clinical hallmarks of diabetes are symptoms associated with marked hyperglycemia, including polydipsia, polyuria, polyphagia, and weight loss. Older patients with type 2 diabetes may present with such symptoms, although it is relatively uncommon for them to do so. Some of these patients may have sufficient hyperglycemia to cause mild classical symptoms, while others may have had gradual unexplained weight loss. Other older patients may present with atypical symptoms from hyperglycemia such as falls, urinary incontinence, fatigue, or confusion. Because type 2 diabetes may go undetected for years, some older adults first present with symptoms or findings related to diabetes complications, such as visual loss with classic retinopathy on examination, proteinuria, or symptomatic peripheral neuropathy.

With the profound insulin deficiency of type 1 diabetes, mobilization of fatty acids occurs leading to accelerated production of ketoacids, potentially resulting in life-threatening DKA. Although type 1 diabetes usually occurs in early life, it can occur at any age, including first presentation in an elderly patient. Development of DKA is the classic form of presentation for a patient with type 1 diabetes, but it is now recognized that people with type 1 diabetes may have long periods of abnormal circulating glucose levels before the development of DKA. Furthermore, with early detection of such hyperglycemia and appropriate diabetes management, an episode of DKA might never occur. An older person with type 1 diabetes may be particularly more likely to present with an indolent course.

EVALUATION

Diabetes mellitus is a complex disorder that can have effects on many body systems, and its treatment may require a complex program including medication plus lifestyle changes. The choice of intervention strategies and the patient's capability to adhere to a diabetes treatment program may be limited by the presence of other health problems, as well as by the patient's living situation, economic status, availability of caregiver support, and the like. A comprehensive geriatric assessment (Chapter 11) is highly appropriate to provide the basis for developing a treatment plan for an older person with diabetes mellitus.

Medical Evaluation

Once a diagnosis of diabetes is established, a thorough medical evaluation is needed. Because the risk for developing diabetes complications is related to the duration of hyperglycemia, effort should be made to pinpoint the time of onset. Unless patients at risk have been followed up carefully with yearly measurement of a fasting glucose level, as currently recommended by the ADA, it may be difficult to establish a time of onset for type 2 diabetes mellitus in a given patient. Because of the usual uncertainty about time of onset, a careful search for existing diabetes complications is warranted even when a new diagnosis is made in an older adult. Such an evaluation is even more justified in a patient with a multiyear history of diabetes mellitus who is establishing a new relationship with a health care system or primary care provider. The evaluation for eye complications of diabetes should be carried out by an ophthalmologist with a detailed retinal examination, as early signs of diabetic retinopathy can easily be missed.

Evaluation of diabetic nephropathy should include a screening serum creatinine level. An elevated serum creatinine is a poor prognostic sign, suggesting that substantial kidney damage has already occurred and that an irreversible course of progressive renal insufficiency has already started. Depending on the patient's overall situation, referral to a nephrologist may be warranted to assess other potential causes of renal insufficiency. Urine screening for proteinuria should be carried out to detect earlier stages of diabetic nephropathy that are amenable to intervention. A positive qualitative urine for protein (dipstick method) indicates gross proteinuria. If confirmed on repeat testing, this finding in itself is an indication for treatment intervention. However, a negative qualitative urine protein test does not rule out early diabetic nephropathy. If the qualitative dipstick test is negative, a spot urine sample should be sent for quantitative measurement of urine protein and creatinine. A value greater than 30 mg/g, often referred to as microalbuminuria, suggests early diabetic nephropathy. Such a test should be repeated twice in subsequent months for confirmation. If two of three tests are positive, intervention is warranted.

A careful neurologic examination should be carried out for signs of diabetic neuropathy. This examination should include monofilament testing. This is a qualitative test with a 10-g nylon monofilament carried out at different points along the foot with simple yes or no responses by the patient about feeling the pressure of the monofilament. Vibration sense should also be tested with a tuning fork. This neuropathy evaluation should be carried out in conjunction with a careful foot examination to identify possible structural abnormalities that might contribute to risk for skin breakdown and damage.

The medical evaluation of an older patient with diabetes should also include information about other coexisting risk factors including hypertension, hyperlipidemia, and use of cigarettes. These conditions interact with diabetes to increase risk of adverse cardiovascular events and therefore need to be addressed in an overall patient management program. Blood pressure should be assessed both in the supine position and with upright posture, as an orthostatic drop in blood pressure may be another marker of diabetic neuropathy and is often associated with supine hypertension. The genitourinary system should also be assessed, as patients with diabetes may be prone to bladder dysfunction associated with autonomic neuropathy, thereby increasing the risk for urinary tract infection and kidney damage. Sexual dysfunction has been reported in a high percentage of older men with diabetes, suggesting an interaction between aging, neuropathy, and vascular disease in this population.

A thorough evaluation of the cardiovascular system also should be carried out, given the high rate of vascular disease in older people with diabetes mellitus. The history and physical examination should carefully assess evidence for cerebrovascular disease, coronary heart disease, and peripheral vascular disease. Suggestive history or physical findings should be documented with more in-depth testing including Doppler evaluation for carotid artery stenosis or extremity blood flow, or cardiovascular stress testing if there is any suggestion of coronary artery disease. Silent ischemia and myocardial infarction appear to be more common in people with diabetes mellitus. Thus, the threshold for stress testing should be rather low.

The drug history of an older patient with diabetes is important both to identify drug therapy that may be contributing to the patient's hyperglycemia (see Table 109-2), as well as to identify potential drug interactions that may affect diabetes management. The initial assessment should also include a diet history, a review of potential nutritional problems, and an oral health assessment, as dietary intervention is a key component of a treatment program for virtually all patients with diabetes. The assistance of a nutritionist who has a particular interest in diabetes is often very helpful for this part of the evaluation. Particular attention should be paid to dietary habits, ethnic food preferences, and meal patterns.

Other Evaluation Components

Diabetes Knowledge

Because of the complexity of diabetes management, usually requiring both lifestyle and medication interventions, the patient or caregivers must be actively involved in their own care and take responsibility for its many aspects. It is particularly important to review the patient's knowledge base regarding diabetes and its complications. Standardized diabetes knowledge tests are available, or an interview with a diabetes educator or suitably trained nurse can establish the status of the patient's knowledge base. The diabetes education program that becomes part of the treatment plan can then provide this base for new patients or fill in needed gaps for existing patients.

Functional Status

A review of activities of daily living and instrumental activities of daily living should be a part of comprehensive assessment of an elderly patient with diabetes mellitus. Diabetes puts the patient at increased risk for functional deficits. Such functional limitations must also be considered in developing a diabetes treatment program. In addition to general assessment of functional status, the ability of the patient and caregiver to carry out diabetes-specific functional tasks needs to be evaluated. For example, the ability to carry out home glucose monitoring or self-injection of insulin requires certain functional abilities.

Cognitive and Psychosocial Status

Given the complexity of diabetes management programs, an assessment of a patient's cognitive status is essential to developing an appropriate treatment plan. A screening cognitive test should be carried out, with more detailed testing as indicated by the screening test or a history of cognitive decline. Cognitive function may be affected directly by diabetes as a result of cerebrovascular disease, postulated direct effects of hyperglycemia to cause subtle impairments of cognition, as well as by diabetes treatment, which can result in hypoglycemia. Complex cognitive skills are required for a number of aspects of diabetes treatment. Similarly, the presence of other psychiatric disorders such as depression or bipolar disorder could have a major impact on the decision about diabetes treatment interventions. Both cognitive disorders and clinical depression are more common in older people with diabetes than in those without diabetes.

The patient's socioeconomic and living situation can also have an important impact on the diabetes treatment plan. The availability of caregivers in the home or nearby can compensate for some limitations in the patient's self-care abilities and influence lifestyle factors that can affect diabetes management. Economic issues may affect the patient's ability to adhere to a costly medical regimen, and cultural influences may need to be considered as a treatment plan is developed. The availability of a social worker or suitably trained nurse to assist in this aspect of the patient evaluation can be extremely helpful.

Overall Health Status

The presence of other medical problems needs to be documented, as decisions about the extent of intervention for diabetes need to be put in the context of the patient's overall health situation, disease burden, and prognosis in terms of functional status and estimated longevity. The presence of a coexisting illness such as congestive heart failure or uncontrolled cancer, which would substantially limit a patient's future life expectancy, will influence the decision about intensity of diabetes management.

DIABETES MANAGEMENT

General Approach

The first key step in developing a diabetes management program for an elderly patient is to establish the treatment goals. The overall treatment goal of a basic diabetes care plan is to prevent metabolic decompensation and to control other risk factors that may contribute to long-term complications in any patient with diabetes. Control of hyperglycemia as a means to reduce what some have termed glucose toxicity as a contributing factor to long-term diabetes complications is one part of an overall strategy of risk reduction. Such a strategy must include intensive effort at identifying and controlling hypertension, lipid disorders, and cigarette smoking. Thus, a complex, multifaceted treatment program is important for many older patients with diabetes. As other chapters cover the management of hypertension (Chapter 81) and lipid disorders (Chapter 110), these will be referred to only briefly in this chapter, which will focus on management of

TABLE 109-4

Factors to Consider in Setting a Diabetes Treatment Goal for Elderly Patients
Patient's estimated remaining life expectancy
Patient's preference and commitment
Beliefs of the primary care provider (e.g., whether glycemic control can prevent complications)
Availability of social support and services
Economic issues
Coexisting health problems
Major psychiatric disorder
Major cognitive disorder
Diabetes complications
Major limitation of diabetes functional status
Complexity of medical regimen
Risk of severe hypoglycemia

hyperglycemia. However, control of the traditional cardiovascular risk factors is absolutely critical to successful diabetes management. Unfortunately, many studies have documented the overall lack of success of standard clinical practice in achieving these goals.

It may be neither feasible nor appropriate to attempt to achieve a complex diabetes management program for some patients. Table 109-4 lists some of the factors to consider when deciding whether to strive for a treatment goal designed to minimize risk for diabetes complications. It is true that a limited remaining life expectancy shortens the time for long-term complications to develop and progress. Given the increasing life expectancy of older adults, only the very oldest segment of the population or those with coexisting illness that markedly shortens remaining life expectancy should be excluded from consideration for an aggressive treatment program. For example, it would be hard to justify abandoning risk reduction goals in an otherwise healthy 75-year-old woman with a recent diagnosis of diabetes, as such a person's remaining life expectancy may be 15 years or more. Given the potential complexity of treatment programs designed to minimize diabetes risks, the commitment on the part of an adequately informed patient is clearly critical. Availability of a supportive environment including a strong diabetes treatment team and adequate economic support for an intensive treatment program are also important. Such a treatment goal is also difficult to achieve without commitment of the health care team, which must believe that achievement of the treatment goal will really make a difference in the patient's long-term health.

Any decision about an intensive treatment program must take into account coexisting conditions and the overall complexity of the patient's medical regimen. For example, the existence of advanced diabetes complications in an elderly patient may provide a rationale for less strict control of hyperglycemia or dyslipidemia. A significant psychiatric or cognitive disorder may also preclude an intensive management program. The target for hyperglycemia control would need to be higher for a patient at risk for severe hypoglycemia (see the section on "Hypoglycemia" later in this chapter). On the other hand, some older adults are able to devote a substantial amount of time to their own health care and are able to manage complex multidrug interventions for multiple health problems. Based on the initial comprehensive patient assessment as described here, many older adults with diabetes may fit in a category for which an intensive treatment goal is appropriate.

Management of Cardiovascular Risk Factors

Management of hypertension and abnormal lipid metabolism is discussed in Chapters 81 and 110, respectively. Because of the high risk status of patients with diabetes, the Seventh Report of the Joint National Committee on Detection, Evaluation and Treatment of High Blood Pressure and the ADA recommend a blood pressure goal of less than 130/80. As described in Chapter 110, many diabetic patients have a dyslipidemia, requiring that attention be paid to triglycerides as well as cholesterol levels. Diabetes is considered a cardiac disease equivalent. Thus, an aggressive target for intervention (low-density lipoprotein [LDL] cholesterol <100 mg/dL) is recommended by the ADA and the National Cholesterol Education Program (NCEP), even in the absence of a known cardiac history. For people older than 40 years with diabetes, statin drug therapy to achieve an LDL reduction of 30% to 40% regardless of baseline LDL levels is recommended. In diabetic individuals with overt cardiovascular disease, the ADA also suggests an LDL cholesterol goal of <70 mg/dL as an option and recommends goals of triglyceride levels <150 mg/dL and HDL >40 mg/dL.

Use of aspirin reduces cardiovascular risk in patients with diabetes. Thus, older patients with diabetes should be treated with one aspirin per day unless there is a contraindication. Alternative approaches may be developed to reduce systemic glucose toxicity other than simply lowering circulating glucose levels. There have been efforts to develop drugs that inhibit formation of AGE products, although none are yet available clinically. In addition, aldose reductase inhibitors have been tested and continue to be under investigation.

Prevention of Microvascular Complications

Angiotensin-converting enzyme (ACE) inhibitors and angiotensin receptor blockers reduce the rate of progression from microalbuminuria to overt proteinuria and diabetic nephropathy. An ACE inhibitor or angiotensin receptor blocker should be added to a treatment program for any patient who has evidence of nephropathy. Also, rigorous blood pressure control is particularly important for such individuals.

Laser therapy reduces the rate of visual loss in patients with diabetic retinopathy. Thus, early detection is critical. Despite clear evidence of efficacy of retinopathy screening by ophthalmological examination and appropriate intervention, only 50% or fewer of diabetes patients receive recommended annual screening for retinopathy.

Other Diabetes Complications

Prevention of amputation in older people with diabetes requires careful attention to peripheral vascular disease, neuropathy, and foot care. While microvascular disease and peripheral neuropathy may contribute to skin damage and impaired healing, it is clear that patients with diabetes can benefit from treatment of large vessel disease, which is the primary factor responsible for lower-extremity ischemia in people with diabetes mellitus. As the development of neuropathy is insidious, patients should be instructed to examine their feet carefully on a daily basis, and a foot examination should be a routine part of a diabetes clinic visit. Although there is no

current therapeutic approach to reduce the rate of development of neuropathy other than reducing glucose levels toward normal, a number of drugs are under development that target neuropathy.

Painful neuropathy is a common complication of diabetes. The first step in the management of patients with neuropathy should be to aim for stable and optimal glycemic control. Many patients will require pharmacological treatment for painful symptoms. Many agents have efficacy for the management of painful diabetic neuropathy. Pain management can start with acetaminophen. Opioid analgesics may be necessary at times. Nonsteroidal anti-inflammatory drugs should be avoided in elderly patients, especially those with nephropathy. Two drugs have been approved by the Food and Drug Administration (FDA) for treatment of painful diabetic neuropathy: the norepinephrine and serotonin reuptake inhibitor, duloxetine, and the inhibitor of excitatory neurotransmitter release, pregabalin. Other drugs that have been used include tricyclic antidepressants, alpha-lipoic acid, gabapentin, carbamazepine, and locally administered capsaicin cream.

Management of Hyperglycemia

A major challenge in diabetes management is to set an appropriate treatment goal for hyperglycemia. The ADA recommends preprandial glucose levels of 90 to 130 mg/dL and a hemoglobin A_{1C} ≤7%, with hemoglobin A_{1C} as the primary target for glycemic control. However, the ADA also indicates that goals should be individualized and that certain populations (including elderly people) require special considerations. Similarly the California Healthcare Foundation/ American Geriatrics Society (CHF/AGS) Panel on Improving Care for Elders with Diabetes recommended in 2003 that the hemoglobin A_{1C} target should be individualized and that a target of ≤7% is reasonable for relatively healthy older adults who have good functional status. A more stringent glycemic goal (i.e., a normal hemoglobin A_{1C} <6%) may further reduce complications at the cost of increased risk of hypoglycemia. Thus, such a goal is not currently recommended, pending the results of ongoing intensive treatment trials. The CHF/AGS Panel also recommended a less stringent hemoglobin A_{1C} target such as 8% for frail elderly patients, for persons with a life expectancy less than 5 years, and for those in whom the risks of more intensive treatment appear clinically to outweigh the benefits.

Because of the difficulty in measuring the rates of diabetes complications and the long time it takes for them to develop, a detailed picture of the relationship between the degree of hyperglycemia and rate of development of complication has not yet been completed. A growing body of evidence from studies such as the National Institutes of Health's Diabetes Control and Complications Trial in people with type 1 diabetes and the United Kingdom Prospective Diabetes Study in people with type 2 diabetes has established that intensive diabetes management designed to achieve near normal glucose levels can reduce the rate of development of the microvascular complications of diabetes. At this point, there is also no evidence that the fundamental mechanisms contributing to diabetes complications differ between type 1 and type 2 diabetes. Until further information becomes available, the recommendations of the ADA and the CHF/AGS Panel seem reasonable for many elderly patients. Unfortunately, as in other patient groups, only a minority of older people with diabetes achieve these goals for hyperglycemia treatment, as illustrated in Figure 109-5.

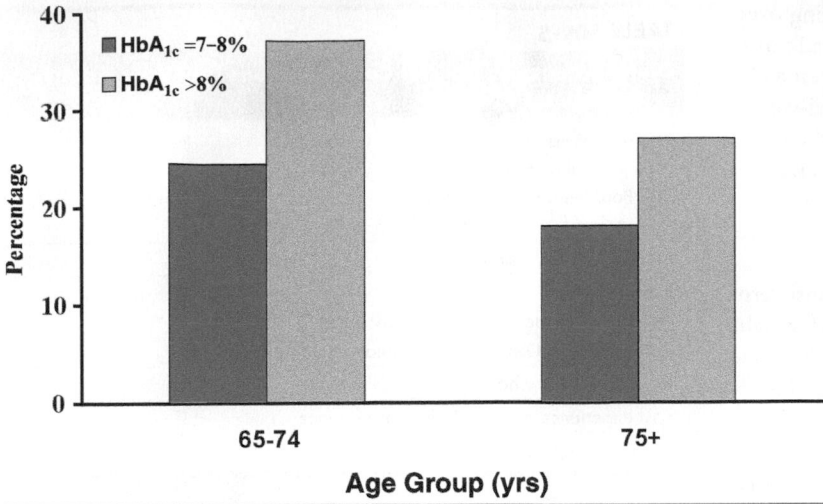

FIGURE 109-5. Percentage of elderly diabetes patients in NHANES III who did not achieve the level of hemoglobin A_{1C} (HbA$_{1C}$) recommended by the American Diabetes Association (HbA$_{1C}$ >7%). Patients were analyzed by age group and according to whether their HbA$_{1C}$ was in the range at which the ADA recommends therapeutic action (>8%) or not (7% to 8%). (Data from Shorr RI, et al. Glycemic control of older adults with type 2 diabetes: Findings from the Third National Health and Nutrition Examination Survey, 1988–1994. J Am Geriatr Soc. 2000;48:264.)

Regardless of whether a decision is made to try to prevent diabetes complications with intensive hyperglycemia management, a basic set of objectives should be part of the treatment plan for virtually all patients with diabetes. Metabolic decompensation with weight loss, muscle wasting, and a catabolic state is unlikely to occur if the average circulating glucose level is in the range of 200 mg/dL. This seems like a reasonable minimum target goal for basic diabetes care. Such a goal translates to a fasting glucose level in the range of 160 mg/dL and a hemoglobin A_{1C} value of 8% to 9%.

Basic Care

All patients with diabetes should receive a basic diabetes education about what diabetes is, what the long-term complications are, and the importance of periodic evaluation for them as well as basic lifestyle modifications that can improve risk and assist with diabetes management, including basic principles of diet and exercise. Basic diabetes care should include yearly follow-up and reevaluation for the development of diabetes complications, and intervention for those complications as appropriate. Recognition and treatment of hypoglycemia should also be part of the basic diabetes education program for any patient treated with insulin or a sulfonylurea drug.

Aggressive Care

Individuals who are selected for an aggressive treatment program should also receive all aspects of basic diabetes care. While the ADA and the CHF/AGS Panel recommended treatment goal of achieving a hemoglobin A_{1C} of 7% may require considerable effort and attention, it is important not to forget about aggressive detection and treatment of hypertension, dyslipidemia, and cigarette smoking. Regular monitoring for diabetes complications and institution of complication-specific interventions should also be carried out. In addition to basic diabetes education, the patient participating in an aggressive treatment program should be trained to carry out home blood glucose monitoring on a regular basis and should become familiar with various treatment approaches for hyperglycemia including diet, exercise, and medications. Such patients should participate in a formal diabetes education program to cover this material thoroughly. Access to a multidisciplinary diabetes care team should be part of an aggressive treatment program.

Specific Interventions for Hyperglycemia

A decision about setting a goal for either basic diabetes care or an aggressive treatment program should be made for each older person with diabetes. Once this decision has been made, a growing range of therapeutic options enables the treatment program to be individualized according to the specific situation of the individual patient, as determined in part by the initial comprehensive assessment carried out.

Diet

Dietary intervention has long been a cornerstone of hyperglycemia management. The ADA currently recommends that medical nutrition therapy be included in any diabetes care program, but that it should be individualized for each patient. Fundamental to any dietary recommendation is ensuring that essential dietary needs are met with adequate provision of vitamins and minerals. Over the years, dietary supplements have been proposed to assist in diabetes treatment such as vitamins C, E, or B complex, or minerals such as zinc or chromium to replace possible diabetes-related losses, thereby improving the metabolic state and possibly reducing the rate of various complications. There is, however, no convincing evidence that any of these dietary supplements improves hyperglycemia control or influences diabetes complications. Two aspects of diet need to be addressed in any dietary program: the total caloric intake, which is a key to maintenance of body weight or weight reduction; and dietary composition, or the distribution of fat, carbohydrate, and protein calories.

Caloric Intake Caloric restriction is usually part of the initial approach to management of overweight patients with diabetes mellitus. Because it is generally desirable to maintain muscle and bone mass, the target of caloric restriction is reduction in adiposity, particularly the central adiposity that seems to be critical in mediating obesity-related insulin resistance. One criterion for obesity is a BMI of 30 kg/m². A serious effort at weight reduction should be considered for any patient with a BMI in excess of 30 kg/m². A BMI greater than 25 kg/m² is used as a marker of overweight and may also be an indication for caloric restriction. As reviewed in Chapter 39, because of an age-related decline in lean body mass, older individuals may have increased adiposity and central adiposity without being overweight by usual BMI criteria. Documentation of central adiposity by waist measurement or computed tomography may suggest a role for caloric restriction in such individuals. Relatively normal-weight people with central adiposity likely already have diminished lean body mass, which will be further threatened by caloric restriction. For individuals who are not overweight and who do not have central adiposity, there is no role for caloric restriction as part of the hyperglycemia treatment program.

Although many types of diets are successful in the short-term in achieving weight reduction, long-term maintenance of weight reduction continues to be a major challenge. Some individuals are able to lose a significant amount of weight and maintain it. Therefore patients should be offered assistance with caloric restriction and supported for a weight loss program. In general, behavioral modification to change dietary habits is the most successful approach long-term. Relatively modest weight reduction can have a significant impact on the degree of insulin resistance and on control of glucose levels. Part of the approach should be to set a realistic goal of no more than 5% to 10% reduction of body weight, even if that will not achieve a normal BMI of less than 25 kg/m^2. The role for medications to assist weight loss in an older person with diabetes mellitus is uncertain. With the current explosion of knowledge about regulation of food intake in relation to obesity, it is likely that new medications will appear in the market to assist in weight reduction. These should be integrated into diet treatment if justified by results of clear studies of efficacy and risks in an older adult population, evidence lacking to date for any pharmacological weight loss agent.

Diet Composition

The average American diet includes approximately 45% of calories as carbohydrate, 40% as fat, and 15% as protein. While varying changes of overall dietary composition have been recommended in the past, there is currently no such recommendation. Current recommendations by the ADA are consistent with those of the American Heart Association and other groups, all of which recommend a diet relatively low in saturated fat (less than 7% of total calories), minimizing intake of trans fat, and limiting cholesterol intake to less than 200 mg per day. This recommendation for patients with diabetes especially makes sense given the very high rate of atherosclerosis-related complications in this patient population. These recommendations are not in conflict with the diet prescription if there is coexisting dyslipidemia that needs management.

Consistency of dietary intake in terms of meal composition, carbohydrate intake, and timing is particularly an issue in patients treated with insulin. The ADA's diet exchange program is one means of providing guidance to such patients to maintain consistency of dietary intake. Nutritional counseling can be particularly helpful in assisting patients to adhere to a dietary program.

Dietary Issues in Older People

As summarized in Table 109-5, there are a number of special issues to consider in dietary management of older adults with diabetes. Older adults with a significant mobility limitation may be relatively inactive and have low caloric utilization. Thus, caloric intake may need to be limited to rather low levels to achieve significant weight reduction. The potential benefit of caloric restriction and weight reduction under such circumstances needs to be balanced against the potential risk for complications related to undernutrition. Such patients also may have difficulty with access to food both in terms of food preparation and shopping to

TABLE 109-5

Dietary Therapy: Special Considerations for Older Adults with Diabetes Mellitus

Access to food
Functional disability
Poor meal preparation skills
Lack of formal or informal support to obtain food
Limited financial resources
Food intake
Decline in taste and smell appreciation
Poor dentition and/or xerostomia
Ingrained dietary habits
Past experience and ethnic food preference
Impaired cognitive function

bring food in. Furthermore, dietary habits established for a lifetime and often with a cultural background may be particularly difficult to modify. Older persons, especially men living alone, may have limited food preparation skills. The presence of impaired cognitive function may make following a dietary prescription particularly difficult. Any of these issues can be modified if there is sufficient caregiver support and/or social services that can assist with providing meals in the home setting.

Problems with taste and oral health, which are common in older people, may further limit adaptation to a prescribed diet. Oral health problems can be exacerbated by diabetes, which may increase the rate of periodontal disease. This may be a growing issue as more older adults are keeping their teeth for longer periods. Xerostomia is also more common in older people owing to decreased salivary gland flow, sometimes exacerbated by coexisting medication use.

Exercise

An exercise program may be an important adjunct to hyperglycemia management. By increasing caloric expenditure, an exercise program can facilitate the effectiveness of a weight reduction program for overweight people with diabetes mellitus. It may also help prevent reaccumulation of weight following caloric-restriction-facilitated weight loss. Simple increases of physical activity, such as with stretching exercises or walking, while potentially useful to improve overall functional capability, will have only a very modest effect on total caloric expenditure. There is, however, a growing body of evidence that exercise training can also enhance sensitivity to insulin by improving insulin-mediated glucose uptake. Thus, exercise training may have a beneficial affect beyond simply enhancing the effectiveness of a weight reduction program. Furthermore, patients with diabetes may benefit from the effects of exercise training to enhance cardiovascular function, lower blood pressure, and improve the lipid profile. A more detailed discussion of the effects of exercise training in older individuals is provided in Chapter 114.

Exercise training alone has not had consistent effects to improve circulating glucose levels in patients with diabetes mellitus. For all the reasons just indicated, exercise may be a useful adjunct to drug therapy and may well contribute to enhanced effectiveness of glucose-lowering agents. Given the high prevalence of coronary artery disease in older patients with diabetes mellitus, which may be asymptomatic or atypical in symptoms, it is important for such patients to have medically supervised stress testing before entering any challenging exercise training program. An additional issue to consider in an older person is the potential for foot and joint injury with upright exercise such as jogging. Particular attention should be given to the foot examination in an older person prior to and during the course of exercise training. Finally, because of its effects to enhance glucose uptake by muscle, exercise training may contribute to risk for hypoglycemia in patients treated with hypoglycemic agents. Issues related to hypoglycemia in older patients with diabetes are discussed in more detail later in the section on "Hypoglycemia".

Noninsulin Agents

A growing number of medications other than insulin are available for hyperglycemia management of older adults with diabetes mellitus. Table 109-6 lists the available drugs and summarizes some of the dosage and mechanism of action information. As the different classes of drugs have different mechanisms of action, there is increasing opportunity to individualize therapy as more is learned about the heterogeneity of type 2 diabetes. All of these agents are effective in lowering glucose levels in clinical trials of patients with type 2 diabetes mellitus. Some of them may also assist in lowering glucose levels as an adjunct to insulin therapy in patients with type 1 diabetes. The effectiveness of these agents must be considered in relation to the treatment goal set for the patient. For example, these agents are frequently successful in achieving the basic goal of hyperglycemia management; that is, to achieve an average glucose level in the range

of 200 mg/dL and avoid the catabolic effects associated with very poor diabetes control. These drugs have been much less successful in achieving the goals of aggressive hyperglycemia therapy, that is, a Hgb A_{1C} ≤7% and a fasting glucose level close to the normal range. In fact, even in carefully conducted clinical trials of relatively short duration, only a minority of patients with type 2 diabetes are able to achieve such rigorous goals for hyperglycemia management with one of these agents alone or even in combination. Thus, a therapeutic trial of one or more of these agents for older patients who have not achieved their goal for hyperglycemia management with lifestyle modifications in diet and exercise is warranted. Such therapeutic trials should be instituted over a limited time frame without losing sight of the overall therapeutic goal. For the substantial number of patients for whom such a trial does not successfully achieve or maintain the treatment goal, both the patient and health provider team should be prepared to move forward to a more aggressive regimen including treatment with insulin.

Sulfonylurea Drugs Sulfonylurea drugs have been on the market for many years and have been historically the predominant oral agents used in the elderly diabetes population. As first-generation sulfonylureas are rarely used, Table 109-6 only includes second-generation agents. Because of their long history, there is a substantial body of knowledge about the mechanism of action and side-effect profile of sulfonylureas. Their primary mechanism of action is to enhance insulin secretion by the beta cells of the endocrine pancreas. Indeed, there is a sulfonylurea receptor on pancreatic beta cells that is closely

TABLE 109-6

Drugs (Other Than Insulin) for the Management of Hyperglycemia			
GENERIC NAME	**BRAND NAME**	**USUAL DAILY DOSE**	**MECHANISM OF ACTION**
Sulfonylureas (Second Generation)			Enhance insulin secretion
Glimepiride	Amaryl	1–8 mg once	
Glipizide	Glucotrol	10–20 mg once or divided	
Glipizide, sustained release	Glucotrol XL	5–20 mg once or divided	
Glyburide	Diabeta, Micronase	2.5–20 mg once or divided	
Glyburide, micronized	Glynase	1.5–12 mg once or divided	
α-Glucosidase inhibitors			Decrease glucose absorption
Acarbose	Precose	25–100 mg tid	
Miglitol	Glyset	25–100 mg tid	
Biguanide			Decrease hepatic glucose production
Metformin	Glucophage	1500–2550 mg divided	
Thiazolidinediones			Enhance insulin sensitivity
Pioglitazone	Actos	15–45 mg once	
Rosiglitazone	Avandia	2–8 mg once or divided	
Meglitinide			Enhance insulin secretion
Repaglinide	Prandin	0.5–2 mg tid (before meals)	
D-Phenylalanine Derivative			Enhance insulin secretion
Nateglinide	Starlix	60–120 mg tid (before meals)	
DPP-4 inhibitor			Inhibitor of DPP-4, which degrades native GLP-1
Sitagliptin	Januvia	100 mg once orally	
GLP-1 Analog			Enhance glucose-dependent insulin secretion
Exenatide	Byetta	5 mcg-10 mcg sq bid (before meals)	Decrease glucagon secretion
			Slow gastric emptying
Amylin Analog			Reduces postprandial glucose in conjunction with mealtime insulin
Pramlintide acetate	Symlin	Adjunct to mealtime insulin sq tid (before meals)	

DPP-4 = Dipeptidyl peptidase-4; GLP-1 = Glucagon like Paptide-1.

linked to the signaling mechanism for glucose-induced insulin secretion. There is also some evidence that sulfonylurea drug treatment can enhance sensitivity to insulin in peripheral tissues. While enhancement of insulin action may be a direct effect of sulfonylureas on peripheral tissues, it is more likely that improved sensitivity to insulin is secondary to lowering of glucose levels, as hyperglycemia per se appears to contribute to insulin resistance in patients with diabetes mellitus.

Sulfonylurea drugs have established a long record of safety, with hypoglycemia being the main side effect about which to be concerned. Conservative dosing is recommended for older people. Glyburide has been associated with hypoglycemia in older people; however, it is also the sulfonylurea most frequently prescribed and is somewhat more potent than the other agents. These drugs should not be used in patients with renal insufficiency or with significant liver disease, as they depend on the liver for metabolism and the kidney for excretion. Hyponatremia has also been observed as a complication in some patients. Because of similar risk with use of thiazide diuretics, the combination of thiazide and sulfonylurea drugs should be avoided if hyponatremia is a concern.

α-Glucosidase Inhibitors

These agents work by inhibiting the key gastrointestinal (GI) enzyme responsible for breakdown of carbohydrates prior to absorption. They are particularly helpful to reduce postprandial increases of glucose levels and may be a useful adjunct to therapy with other agents. The major side effects are local to the GI tract (flatulence, diarrhea, abdominal pain) because these drugs are not absorbed to any significant degree. These agents may be useful and relatively safe in older people with fairly well-controlled diabetes. One can expect an approximate 0.5% decrease in hemoglobin A1c.

Biguanide

Metformin appears to work primarily by suppressing hepatic glucose production. Increased basal hepatic glucose production is an important contributing factor to fasting hyperglycemia in patients with diabetes mellitus. The precise mechanism by which metformin affects the liver is unknown, and there is somewhat inconsistent evidence for a small effect of metformin to enhance peripheral sensitivity to insulin as well. The most common side effect of metformin is some GI discomfort, which in some patients can be associated with decreased appetite and modest weight loss. While some have viewed this as a potential benefit for a patient on a weight-reduction program, this effect needs to be balanced against the degree of symptoms and the appropriateness of decreased caloric intake and weight loss in a given individual. The biguanide class of drugs is also known to be associated with development of life-threatening lactic acidosis under some circumstances. Although this complication appears to be rare in patients using metformin, this drug should be avoided in situations that may put people at risk for development of lactic acidosis. The drug should not be used in patients with chronic congestive heart failure, and it should be withheld during acute hospitalization for any major illness that could result in decreased tissue perfusion as a precipitating factor for lactic acidosis. Metformin also should be avoided in patients with significant liver disease or renal insufficiency (a creatinine level ≥ 1.5 mg/dL in men and ≥ 1.4 mg/dL in women). Creatinine clearance should be measured in people 80 years of age and older if metformin treatment is considered.

Thiazolidinediones

This class of drugs appears to work primarily by enhancing peripheral and hepatic sensitivity to insulin. This mechanism of action complements that of the other drug classes available. As peripheral resistance to insulin is a key part of the metabolic syndrome that predisposes to development of diabetes, use of a drug that targets this abnormality is attractive. These drugs have been shown to have similar efficacy and adverse events in older adults. One disadvantage is economic, as this is one of the more expensive class of drugs available and widely used for treatment of diabetes. These drugs may cause fluid retention and so should not be used in patients with heart failure. Overall analyses of the effectiveness of the thiazolidinedione rosiglitazone to reduce cardiovascular events or mortality have been disappointing, with some analyses showing increased, rather than decreased rates. Thus, the role of these agents in improving outcomes remains controversial.

Meglitinide

Repaglinide enhances insulin secretion, but by a mechanism that differs from the sulfonylureas. Repaglinide acts rapidly to enhance insulin secretion, and is designed to be used immediately before meals. It predominantly improved postprandial glucose levels, but also lowers fasting glucose. It is of moderate potency. Although there are no age differences in the pharmacokinetics of repaglinide, there is limited experience in older people. Repaglinide and glyburide achieved similar A1c lowering in one study of older people with type 2 diabetes, but less hypoglycemia with repaglinide. This agent should not be combined with gemfibrozil because of increased repaglinide levels.

D-Phenylalanine Derivative

Nateglinide acts directly on pancreatic beta cells to rapidly stimulate insulin secretion. Because of the rapid onset and short duration of action, it was developed to address mealtime needs for insulin secretion. It is to be taken shortly before a meal at a standard dose of 120 mg, although a 60 mg dose is also available. No dose adjustments are necessary in older people. Because of the glucose level dependency of its effect on insulin secretion and its short duration of action, its use has been associated with a low rate of hypoglycemia when used alone or in combination with other agents such as metformin. There are currently no known drug interactions, and nateglinide can be used in patients with renal insufficiency.

Dipeptidyl Peptidase-4 (DPP-4) Inhibition

The incretin hormones are intestinal hormones that are released as glucose levels increase with meals and cause glucose-dependent insulin secretion. Native incretin hormones (such as glucagon-like peptide-1 [GLP-1] and gastric inhibitory polypeptide [GIP]) have very short half-lives as they are degraded by the enzyme, dipeptidyl peptidase-4, and thus cannot be used for therapeutic treatment. Sitagliptin, which became available in 2006, inhibits DPP-4 and thus increases and prolongs the action of the incretin hormones. Sitagliptin is indicated for monotherapy or in combination with metformin or a thiazolidinedione. The recommended dosing is 100 mg by mouth daily, although 25 and 50 mg tablets are also available. This agent does not cause weight loss, but has few nonspecific side effects including nasopharyngitis and headache. No overall differences were noted in initial safety and efficacy studies including older people.

Glucagon-like Peptide-1 (GLP-1) Analog

Exenatide, a GLP-1 analog, became available in 2005. Similar to native GLP-1, but used in pharmacologic amounts, exenatide causes enhanced glucose-dependent insulin secretion, suppresses glucagon secretion, slows gastric emptying, and reduces food intake and body weight.

Exenatide is initiated at 5 mcg per subcutaneous injection via dosing pen twice daily at any time within the 60-minute period before the morning and evening meals. The dose can be increased to 10 mcg twice daily after 1 month of therapy. Exenatide primarily improves postprandial hyperglycemia, but also causes modest decreases in fasting glucose. Exenatide is approved for adjunctive therapy in patients treated with sulfonylurea and/or metformin and/or thiazolidinedione who have not achieved adequate glycemic control. There is limited experience in older people. Initial studies included people in late middle age and early sixties. Side effects include nausea/vomiting and hypoglycemia (with sulfonylurea treatment). Precautions include severe renal impairment and GI disease.

Combination Therapy Combinations of these oral agents or a combination of one or more of these oral/injectable agents with insulin are theoretically attractive because of the different modes of action of the various classes of drugs. Thus, combination therapy addresses various aspects of the pathophysiology of hyperglycemia in diabetes, offering the possibility of synergism in therapeutic efficacy without synergism in toxicity. Overall, the effects of such combinations are additive.

For elderly patients, the logic of combination therapy must be balanced against incremental costs and incremental risks of side effects with each additional drug. Furthermore, the potential for polypharmacy for multiple coexisting conditions such as hypertension, hyperlipidemia, osteoarthritis, and coronary artery disease needs to be considered. The overall treatment goal for the patient must also be kept in mind. Adding a second or third oral or injectable agent without achieving the target goal of near normoglycemia can be an indication to proceed to use of insulin.

Insulin Therapy

Use of insulin is required in patients with type 1 diabetes mellitus. Insulin is also often used in patients with type 2 diabetes either as a primary hypoglycemic agent or to maintain reasonable glucose control in the hospital setting during acute stressful illness or in the perioperative period when oral agents may be less acceptable or useful.

Advantages of Insulin There are now more than 75 years of clinical experience with use of insulin since its discovery in 1922 and the dramatic demonstration of its effectiveness to save lives of patients with type 1 diabetes in DKA. Many formulations of insulin with varying duration of action allow individualization of treatment plans. Insulin is the natural hormone that is deficient in relative or absolute terms in diabetes, so its use fits with the overall concept of hormone replacement for endocrine deficiency syndromes. Virtually all forms of insulin currently in use are identical to human insulin or with only slight molecular modifications, so the incidence of allergic reactions is very small. There are virtually no known drug interactions, at least from a pharmacokinetic point of view, and virtually no absolute contraindications to insulin use.

With appropriate dosage modification and monitoring of glucose levels, insulin can be used safely for patients with renal or hepatic insufficiency, patients unable to eat, and during major illness. Insulin itself is relatively inexpensive, although the overall program of insulin treatment, including frequent glucose monitoring, may become expensive. While appropriate insulin use can be a complex challenge, it encourages active self-care by the patient and/or care-

givers. Finally, and perhaps most important from the point of view of achieving treatment objectives, insulin can effectively lower glucose levels in virtually any patient and in sufficient dosage has at least the potential to normalize circulating glucose levels if the regimen intensity is sufficient.

Disadvantages of Insulin One disadvantage of insulin is that it requires injection to be effective. (Inhaled insulin became available in 2006, although it is not currently being marketed because of concerns about long-term pulmonary toxicity.) Injection may represent an insurmountable psychological barrier for a small number of patients. For others, insulin injections may not be feasible owing to functional limitations or insufficient caregiver support. Many older adults can, however, be trained to use insulin appropriately. Insulin is a potent agent and the dose must be carefully measured to minimize risk of hypoglycemia. Accidental overdosage is a risk. The most common issue to address with insulin management is risk for hypoglycemia, which is discussed in more detail later in the chapter in the section on "Hypoglycemia."

Insulin Regimens A range of therapeutic options is available for insulin, which can make a treatment program complex. If, however, a basic hyperglycemia treatment program is the goal for the patient, this can often be achieved with a single injection a day of a long-acting insulin analog, or two injections of intermediate-acting insulin in a patient with type 2 diabetes. Patients with type 1 diabetes may need three or four injections a day with mixtures of intermediate-acting and short-acting insulins to achieve even a basic treatment goal. Some patients with type 2 diabetes can also achieve an aggressive management goal with one or two injections of intermediate-acting insulin per day as long as a sufficient overall dose is provided. Mixtures of short- and intermediate-acting insulin, as well as increased frequency of insulin dosing, may be needed to meet an aggressive treatment goal in some patients with type 2 diabetes.

Newer, modified insulin preparations may help to target therapy. Insulin glargine (Lantus) is modified to slow degradation. It has a stable time course of action over 24 hours, so can be given once daily for basal insulin replacement. Insulin glargine is a clear solution with no need to re-suspend, which is a major cause of variability in absorption of long-/intermediate-acting insulins. Clinical trial and pharmacokinetic data suggest that insulin glargine can improve management of diabetic patients with a low incidence of nocturnal hypoglycemia, no pronounced peak, a long duration of action, and little interpatient absorption variability. Insulin glargine can be dosed as 0.2 units/kg/day subcutaneously once daily or initiated at 10 units once daily and adjusted as needed. Insulin glargine cannot be mixed with any other insulin. Insulin detemir (Levemir) is now also available. Insulin determir is highly bound to albumin, which delays its absorption from the subcutaneous space. Dosing can be initiated at 0.2 to 0.5 unit/kg/day (0.1 to 0.2 unit/kg/day for insulin naïve patients) with one injection daily in the evening or at bedtime. However, the lower dosage requires twice daily injection separated by 12 hours.

Insulin aspart (NovoLog) and insulin lispro (Humalog) were developed as agents with a very rapid onset of action and short duration. These insulins are used for injection just prior to meals and are less likely to result in postmeal hypoglycemia than longer-acting regular insulin. Insulin glulisin (Apidra) is a newer rapid-acting insulin, which can be given within 15 minutes before or within 20 minutes after starting a meal. Thus a combination of once-daily insulin glargine plus premeal injections of short-acting insulin may be used for intensive insulin therapy, with potentially similar results as with use of a subcutaneous insulin pump system delivering a continuous basal insulin infusion plus bolus injections with meals. Indeed, intensive insulin therapy of elderly people with type 2 diabetes using either of these two regimens achieved an average hemoglobin A$_{1C}$ of 7% over a period of 1 year with minimal adverse effects.

Amylin Analog: Adjunct to Mealtime Insulin Therapy

Amylin is cosecreted with insulin and is absent in type 1 diabetes and deficient in type 2 diabetes. Pramlintide acetate (Symlin) is an analog of amylin that overcomes the tendency of human amylin to aggregate and form insoluble particles. It reduces postprandial glucose in conjunction with mealtime insulin. It is used as an adjunct treatment in patients who use mealtime insulin therapy and have failed to achieve desired glucose control despite optimal insulin therapy with or without a concurrent sulfonylurea agent and/or metformin. Pramlinitide is administered as a subcutaneous injection via an insulin syringe before each major meal, but cannot be mixed with insulin. Pramlintide and insulin should always be given as separate injections and at separate sites at least 2 inches apart. Mealtime insulin is reduced by 50% with initiation of pramlintide with tailored dose escalation for type 1 and type 2 diabetes based on side effect of nausea and glucose levels.

Initiation of Insulin Therapy

In developing an insulin treatment regimen for an older adult, it is useful to keep in mind a target total dose range per 24 hours, even though the initial starting dose may be substantially lower. An estimate of 0.5 to 1.0 units per kilogram for a thin patient with type 1 diabetes and 1.0 to 2.0 units per kilogram for a typical type 2 diabetes patient with insulin resistance represent reasonable targets. Of course, there will be substantial variation among individuals in total dose needed, depending on the target treatment goal, patient adherence to lifestyle modification recommendations, degree of insulin resistance, and individual variation of insulin dose pharmacokinetic patterns. Thus, a low starting dose of a single injection of long-acting insulin 10 to 20 units daily, depending on the degree of obesity, is reasonable. Initiation of insulin treatment is usually done as an outpatient and in conjunction with a diabetes education program for the patient and family members.

Frequent follow-up should be provided initially to ensure that the treatment program is progressing smoothly and that hypoglycemia does not occur early on. Given the metabolic stability of most older patients with type 2 diabetes, there is no need to escalate the insulin dose rapidly. Doses can be adjusted in 2- to 5-unit increments every 3 to 5 days (or every 7 days for insulin glargine) while glucose levels are being monitored. Patients should be prepared from the outset to progress to at least two injections per day, although some patients may achieve the treatment goal with a single dose.

As insulin doses continue to be gradually adjusted upward, an obese patient with type 2 diabetes may need a total well in excess of 100 units per day to achieve an aggressive treatment goal. Also, as doses are increased, it makes sense to include a combination of short-acting insulin with intermediate-acting insulin to help cover meal-related increases of glucose levels.

As glucose levels are reduced, insulin sensitivity will likely improve owing to amelioration of organ direct effects of hyperglycemia. Thus, an overweight older patient who appears relatively unresponsive to a moderate dose of insulin initially may begin to respond dramatically to modest further increases of insulin dose. In fact, the patient may progress to having episodes of hypoglycemia even with reduction to a total insulin dose that previously was not very effective. It is apparent that close follow-up with the diabetes care team, careful attention to glucose monitoring, and coaching about symptoms of hypoglycemia are all critical to a successful treatment program. A suitably trained diabetes nurse educator can play a particularly critical role during this phase of treatment.

Combination of Insulin and Oral Agents

Combination therapy of insulin with one or more oral agents has also been considered, although there are little data available specifically in older adults. One regimen is use of an evening or bedtime injection of a long-acting insulin such as glargine (Lantus) to target control of the fasting glucose level plus oral agents for daytime use. A comparison of several insulin regimens added to oral therapy of people with type 2 diabetes with mean age of 62 years found that less than 25% of patients achieved a stringent hemoglobin A$_{1C}$ target of 6.5%. The average hemoglobin A$_{1C}$ was a little lower with multiple injections of short-acting insulin than with a single injection of detemir insulin, but the rate of hypoglycemia was higher with multiple injections.

There are theoretical advantages to combining insulin with an agent that enhances insulin sensitivity in a patient with insulin resistance or with an agent that reduces meal-related glucose excursions. However, insulin regimens alone with dose adjustments can achieve remarkably similar control of hyperglycemia as combinations of lower doses of insulin with an oral agent. Given the minimal incremental cost of additional insulin to a patient already on insulin and the potential for adverse drug reaction with any addition of a therapeutic agent, the practical gain of such combination therapy remains unclear.

Another theoretical advantage of combination therapy is that lower doses of insulin can be used to achieve similar glycemic control. It has been argued that high doses of insulin may have adverse cardiovascular effects. Such concerns are based in part on epidemiologic studies demonstrating that (in people without diabetes) higher circulating insulin levels are associated with coronary artery disease. There is also some evidence for direct effects of insulin on the cardiovascular system, some of which might be detrimental. There are, however, no convincing data linking dose of insulin in patients with diabetes to adverse cardiovascular effects.

Another concern about using a high dose of insulin is the potential for weight gain with an intensive insulin treatment program. For patients for whom the indication for insulin is a period of substantial weight loss caused by decompensated diabetes, insulin therapy should be expected to cause weight gain back toward baseline with accompanying restoration of lean body mass. For other patients, it may be necessary to balance the potential risk of weight gain versus the benefit of substantial lowering of circulating glucose levels. In general, weight gain with insulin therapy is modest (in the range of a few kilograms) except for those individuals who have lost substantial weight prior to insulin therapy. By emphasizing and reinforcing lifestyle modifications as insulin therapy is instituted, substantial weight gain can generally be avoided.

Follow-up Care

Diabetes mellitus is a chronic disease that requires long-term follow-up. Frequency and intensity of follow-up depend on the treatment goal for the patient and the type of treatment program that the patient is on. At a minimum, a patient should annually have a dilated retinal examination by an ophthalmologist, screening for early nephropathy, a foot examination and testing for neuropathy, measurement of circulating lipids, reassessment of blood pressure and smoking status, and review of key aspects of diabetes self-management and education. Measurement of hemoglobin A1c is a very useful way of assessing overall diabetes control and should be performed every 3 to 4 months for most patients. At regular follow-up visits, which can vary from monthly to every 3 months depending on the patient's situation, body weight and blood pressure should be assessed, a review of lifestyle components of the treatment program should be carried out, home glucose monitoring data should be evaluated, interim health problems and psychosocial problems should be reviewed, and appropriate adjustments in the overall treatment plan should be made. For patients with type 1 diabetes or type 2 diabetes with an aggressive treatment goal or with multiple diabetes complications, participation by a specialized diabetes care team in the overall management program should be carefully considered.

SPECIAL ISSUES

Hypoglycemia

Hypoglycemia is the primary short-term risk of a hyperglycemia treatment program, particularly one that is targeted at achieving near-normal control of glucose levels. Multiple mechanisms exist to maintain adequate circulating glucose levels because glucose is a fuel particularly targeted to meet the needs of the brain and other tissues that are not dependent on insulin for glucose uptake. The major peripheral tissues, muscle and fat, have a glucose transport system that primarily depends on insulin for activation. Brain cells, however, have a different type of glucose transporter molecule that is continually expressed on the cell surface and does not depend on insulin for activation. Thus, when insulin levels are low, as after an overnight fast, the brain does not have to compete with other major tissues for access to glucose. This is in contrast to fat-related fuel such as free fatty acids and ketones, which have ready access to muscle and fat tissue and therefore are less available to the brain. Because of the brain's dependency on glucose as a fuel, it is particularly vulnerable to injury from hypoglycemia, a fact that must be carefully considered as the overall benefits and risks of a diabetes treatment program are reviewed. An older diabetic adult on a hypoglycemic agent must be counseled to carry glucose tablets or food at all times. An older adult on insulin therapy and their family or caregiver should be given a glucagon emergency kit and teaching on its use.

Hypoglycemia Counterregulation

Table 109-7 lists factors that are important in recovery from hypoglycemia. The major source of endogenous glucose is the liver. The liver contributes to recovery from hypoglycemia by increasing glucose production under the influence of counterregulatory hormones. As the insulin effect fades during insulin-induced hypoglycemia, there is a decline in peripheral glucose uptake, preserving more circulating glucose for recovery. The degree of fall of glucose levels determines the magnitude of counterregulatory responses and

TABLE 109-7

Factors Affecting Recovery from Hypoglycemia
Hepatic glucose production
Glucose uptake by tissues
Degree of hypoglycemia
Wearing off of drug effect
Counterregulatory hormone responses
Behavioral responses

the speed with which normal glucose levels can be restored. Normally, there is a hierarchy of responses to hypoglycemia with release of counterregulatory hormones such as epinephrine and glucagon occurring before a patient becomes symptomatic and aware of hypoglycemia. The initial symptoms are caused by autonomic nervous system activation with tachycardia, nervousness, and a sweating response, all of which can alert the patient to the need to seek exogenous sources of glucose to facilitate recovery. Hunger is often a part of this behavioral response. However, as glucose levels fall lower and brain cell function becomes compromised, confusion, lethargy, and progression to coma can occur. Fortunately, the response to glucose administration is quick, and dramatic recovery normally occurs.

It is now recognized that the history of the glucose level that the brain is exposed to influences the counterregulatory response mechanisms, perhaps by affecting the brain glucose transport system. For example, there appears to be adaptation to chronic hyperglycemia in patients with diabetes, with resulting elevation of the glucose level at which counterregulatory responses begin to occur. Thus, a patient with diabetes may begin to develop symptoms of hypoglycemia at a glucose level in the range of 80 to 100 mg/dL, well above the symptomatic threshold in nondiabetic individuals of 50 to 60 mg/dL. Conversely, the brain appears to adapt to low glucose levels as well, with a shift downward of the glucose threshold for activation of counterregulatory responses. Prior exposure to hypoglycemia leads to diminished counterregulatory hormone responses. This can set up a vicious cycle by which patients are less able to counterregulate hypoglycemia and have more recurrent episodes. A key issue seems to be that as the glucose threshold for counterregulation drops, it becomes perilously close to glucose levels that can adversely affect brain function. Thus a patient may have a very narrow margin for error, proceeding from relatively normal function without symptoms to profound hypoglycemia and loss of consciousness. This so-called hypoglycemia unawareness syndrome is in part iatrogenic in origin and generally responds to strict avoidance of hypoglycemia.

Hypoglycemia in Elderly Patients

Table 109-8 summarizes a number of risk factors for hypoglycemia in an older patient with diabetes. As counterregulatory hormone responses are important for both symptom recognition and hypoglycemia counterregulation, impairment of autonomic nervous system reflexes can contribute to risk for hypoglycemia. In addition to risk of the hypoglycemia unawareness syndrome, some older patients may have autonomic neuropathy because of longstanding diabetes or other causes, and many older patients are treated with antiadrenergic agents for cardiovascular diseases. For example, β-adrenergic blocking drugs can potentially interfere with counterregulation of

TABLE 109-8

Risk Factors for Hypoglycemia in Older Diabetic Patients

Impaired autonomic nervous system function
Diminished glucagon secretion
Poor or irregular nutrition
Cognitive disorder
Use of alcohol or other sedating agent
Polypharmacy
Kidney or liver failure

hypoglycemia. Given the substantial benefit of β-adrenergic blockade to patients with cardiovascular disease, a combination with hypoglycemic drug therapy should not be viewed as an absolute contraindication, but only as a concern to keep in mind and share with the patient.

Fortunately, the counterregulatory system is redundant. Glucose counterregulation can be maintained quite well as long as there is an adequate glucagon response even when the adrenergic nervous system is blocked. However, some patients may have impaired glucagon secretion as well, particularly patients with longstanding type 1 diabetes or those with diabetes caused by inflammatory disease of the exocrine pancreas. Patients who have relatively poor nutrition and an irregular meal pattern are at increased risk of hypoglycemia, in part because of inadequate maintenance of muscle and liver glycogen stores. Use of alcohol or a sedating agent should be avoided in patients receiving hypoglycemic agents, particularly if an aggressive treatment program is being pursued. Clearly, a cognitive disorder will interfere with recognition of hypoglycemia and possibly affect decisions about responding to hypoglycemia. Patients with underlying renal or hepatic insufficiency may have problems eliminating hypoglycemic agents, particularly an issue for sulfonylurea drugs. Insulin is partly cleared by the kidney, and the insulin dose must often be reduced substantially in patients with renal insufficiency. A patient with severe hepatic insufficiency may have difficulty mobilizing a counterregulatory increase of glucose production. Finally, any complex drug regimen may include agents that influence the pharmacokinetics of hypoglycemic agents, or counterregulatory or behavioral responses to hypoglycemia, and therefore should be an issue when considering risk for hypoglycemia.

Despite all of these issues and concerns, many older patients with diabetes can be treated aggressively with low risk for hypoglycemia. By providing a strong educational program focused on hypoglycemia recognition and treatment and considering the risk factors outlined in Table 109-8, severe hypoglycemia can generally be avoided. Only subtle alterations of hypoglycemia counterregulatory mechanisms have been identified in healthy older adults, and patients who are hyperglycemic actually have elevated thresholds for counterregulation. Patients with type 2 diabetes are at less risk for severe hypoglycemia than are intensively treated patients with type 1 diabetes.

Hyperosmolar Coma and Diabetic Ketoacidosis

DKA and hyperosmolar coma are the extreme examples of impaired metabolism in patients with diabetes mellitus. DKA is relatively uncommon in older people, but it can occur in an older patient with type 1 diabetes mellitus. As in younger people, the hallmarks of DKA are substantial hyperglycemia, hyperosmolarity, and volume depletion, and the presence of systemic acidosis caused by marked elevation of ketoacids. Ketoacids result from metabolism of elevated free fatty acids released by lipolysis as a result of severe insulin deficiency. DKA can occur in a patient with type 1 diabetes when insulin is inappropriately discontinued, but in an older adult, this may be a result of a major underlying illness that interferes with the patient's self-care capability. In the setting of severe coexisting major illness in an older individual and decreased tissue perfusion, lactic acidosis may occur in the setting of hyperglycemia. It is important to document the presence of significant ketonemia to ensure that DKA is contributing to the systemic acidosis observed. Treatment of DKA should focus on immediate insulin replacement to inhibit lipolysis and reverse the ketoacidosis, vigorous replacement of fluids and salt to replace losses, and a thorough evaluation to identify underlying illness. Careful monitoring is required to ensure response and particularly to monitor the cardiovascular system for signs of failure.

Hyperosmolar coma, which occurs primarily in older people, is characterized by marked hyperglycemia, hyperosmolality, severe volume depletion, and associated renal insufficiency. The mortality rate is high because there is often a severe underlying illness such as pneumonia or a cardiovascular accident. Metabolic acidosis is notably absent, or, if present, it is caused by lactic acid rather than ketoacids. The reason for failure to mobilize fatty acids despite severe insulin deficiency in these patients is unclear. While insulin should be provided as part of the initial therapy, the focus should be on volume and sodium replacement and on identification and intervention for major underlying illness. In fact, as volume status is corrected, in the presence of recovering renal function, glucose levels can fall precipitously. Therefore attention must be paid to avoidance of hypoglycemia.

Diabetes in Long-Term Care

Diabetes mellitus is very common among nursing home residents. Because of the overall disease burden, degree of disability, and limited life expectancy of these patients, basic diabetes care should usually be the goal. As undernutrition may be a much more important health problem than obesity in this situation, diet therapy should focus on matching caloric intake to meet nutritional needs rather than restriction of calories. Furthermore, for a nursing home patient with limited remaining life expectancy, the priority should be to stimulate the patient's appetite and take advantage of opportunities for the patient to enjoy this aspect of life, rather than introduction of unnecessary dietary restrictions. Consistency of caloric intake is important for a patient treated with insulin and may be a particular challenge in a disabled nursing home resident.

Careful attention to skin and foot care is clearly important to avoid problems with healing and infection. Similarly, intensive exercise may not be appropriate for a nursing home resident. Efforts should focus on constructive leisure time activity. Given the staff support available, reliable insulin treatment should be available for a nursing home patient, and nursing home staff can also carry out glucose monitoring as needed. Staff needs to be trained to recognize symptoms of hypoglycemia, carry out testing as appropriate, and provide rapid intervention when hypoglycemia is present. In nursing home patients already at high risk for developing urinary tract infection, diabetes may increase this risk because of bladder dysfunction secondary to autonomic neuropathy. Particular attention should be paid to keeping the bladder free of infection and carrying out intermittent catheterization as needed.

FURTHER READING

American Diabetes Association. Standards of medical care in diabetes—2008. *Diabetes Care.* 2008;31:512.

Booth GL, et al. Relation between age and cardiovascular disease in men and women with diabetes compared with non-diabetic people: A population-based retrospective cohort study. *Lancet.* 2006;368:29.

Caruso LB, et al. What can we do to improve physical function in older persons with type 2 diabetes? *J Gerontol A Biol Sci Med Sci.* 2000;55A:M372.

Chang AM, Halter JB. Aging and insulin secretion. *Am J Physiol Endocrinol Metab.* 2003;284:E7.

Chang AM, et al. Impaired *β-cell function* in human aging: Response to nicotinic acid-induced insulin resistance. *J Clin Endocrinol Metab.* 2006;91:3303.

Gaede P, et al. Effect of a multifactorial intervention on mortality in type 2 diabetes. *N Engl J Med.* 2008;358:580.

Harris MI, et al. Prevalence of diabetes, impaired fasting glucose and impaired glucose tolerance in US adults. *Diabetes Care.* 1998;21:518.

Herman WH, et al. A clinical trial of continuous subcutaneous insulin infusion versus multiple daily injections in older adults with type 2 diabetes. *Diabetes Care.* 2005;28:1568.

Holman RR, et al. Addition of biphasic, prandial, or basal insulin to oral therapy in type 2 diabetes. *N Engl J Med.* 2007;357:1716.

Lindstrom J, et al. Sustained reduction in the incidence of type 2 diabetes by lifestyle intervention: follow-up of the Finnish Diabetes Prevention Study. *Lancet.* 2006;368:1673.

Maty SC, et al. Patterns of disability related to diabetes mellitus in older women. *J Gerontol Med Sci.* 2004;59A:148.

Nissen SE, Wolski K. Effect of rosiglitazone on the risk of myocardial infarction and death from cardiovascular causes. *N Engl J Med.* 2007;356:2457.

Resnick HE, et al. American Diabetes Association diabetes diagnostic criteria, advancing age, and cardiovascular disease risk profiles: results from the Third National Health and Nutrition Examination Survey. *Diabetes Care.* 2000;23:176.

Resnick HE, et al. Achievement of American Diabetes Association clinical practice recommendations among U.S. adults with diabetes, 1999–2002: The National Health and Nutrition Examination Survey. *Diabetes Care.* 2006;29:531.

Resnick HE, et al. Diabetes in U.S. nursing homes, 2004. *Diabetes Care.* 2008;31:287.

Shorr RI, et al. Glycemic control of older adults with type 2 diabetes: Findings from the Third National Health and Nutrition Examination Survey, 1988–1994. *J Am Geriatr Soc.* 2000;48:264.

Shorr RI, et al. Incidence and risk factors for serious hypoglycemia in older persons using insulin or sulfonylureas. *Arch Intern Med.* 1997;157:1681.

The Diabetes Control and Complications Trial (DCCT) Research Group: Effect of intensive diabetes management on macrovascular events and risk factors in the diabetes control and complications trial. *Am J Cardiol.* 1995;75:894.

The Diabetes Prevention Program Research Group: reduction in the incidence of type 2 diabetes with lifestyle intervention or metformin. *N Engl J Med.* 2002;346:393.

Tuomilehto J, et al. Prevention of type 2 diabetes mellitus by changes in lifestyle among subjects with impaired glucose tolerance. *N Engl J Med.* 2001;344:1343.

UK Prospective Diabetes Study Group. Intensive blood-glucose control with sulphonylureas or insulin compared with conventional treatment and risk of complications in patients with type 2 diabetes (UKPDS 33). *Lancet.* 1998;352:837.

Vijan S, et al. Screening, prevention, counseling and treatment for the complications of type 2 diabetes mellitus. *J Gen Intern Med.* 1997;12:567.

Wray LA, et al. The effect of diabetes on disability in middle-aged and older adults. *J Gerontol Med Sci.* 2005;60A:1206.

Dyslipoproteinemia

Leslie I. Katzel ■ *Jacob Blumenthal* ■ *John D. Sorkin* ■ *Andrew P. Goldberg*

DEFINITION

Dyslipoproteinemia, also referred to as dyslipidemia, encompasses a range of disorders of lipoprotein lipid metabolism that include both abnormally high and low lipoprotein concentrations, as well as abnormalities in the composition of these lipoprotein particles. Dyslipoproteinemias are clinically important because of their role in the pathogenesis of cardiovascular disease (CVD), which includes coronary artery disease (CAD), cerebrovascular disease, peripheral vascular disease, and renal disease. Thus the term dyslipoproteinemia is broader than the term hyperlipidemia, which focuses solely on the concentrations of the lipoproteins.

There is considerable evidence that dyslipoproteinemia is a risk factor for CVD in adults aged 60 to 80 years, with an expanding body of literature demonstrating dyslipoproteinemia as a risk factor for people older than 80 years of age. The consensus guidelines for the management of dyslipidemia are continually being reevaluated. Over the past several years, National Cholesterol Education Program (NCEP) Adult Treatment Panel (ATP) consensus guidelines have made the target lipoprotein concentrations more stringent for individuals with CVD. These guidelines have in turn led to more stringent recommendations for patients with CVD equivalents such as diabetes mellitus and renal disease, and for individuals with multiple CVD risk factors who are at increased risk for CVD events. Epidemiologic and clinical trial data suggest that the optimal concentration for low-density lipoprotein cholesterol (LDL-C) maybe <100 mg/dL, or even as low as 70 mg/dL for some high-risk patients. Similarly, the optimal concentration for high-density lipoprotein cholesterol (HDL-C) maybe >60 mg/dL. As discussed below, triglyceride, cholesterol, and LDL-C levels tend to rise with increasing age, before falling late in the sixth decade. HDL-C decreases at puberty and then is relatively constant across the age-span until the age of 70 years when it may increase (Figure 110-1). As a result, a majority of older individuals could be classified as having undesirable lipoprotein lipid concentrations and are candidates for lifestyle intervention and potentially for pharmacological therapy if their concentrations exceed treatment cut points. The changes in the treatment guidelines are reflected in secular changes in prescribing patterns of drugs to treat hyperlipidemia, as the number of older adults on cholesterol-lowering medications has quadrupled over the past 15 years. In 2002, more than 30% of Medicare patients between the ages of 65 and 84 years were prescribed a statin for cholesterol reduction.

Many older individuals have metabolic abnormalities that promote atherosclerosis, but are not routinely measured. These risk factors include elevated lipoprotein (a) [Lp (a)], elevated apolipoprotein (apo) B, small dense LDL particles (the atherogenic LDL pattern B phenotype), oxidized LDL, apo E4 genotype, insulin, high-sensitivity C-reactive protein (hsCRP), homocysteine, and other markers of inflammation. These biomarkers provide incremental benefit in predicting CVD risk beyond the routine measures that are included in the Framingham Risk score. The role of genetic analyses in the assessment of CVD risk is an evolving field of research. It is also becoming increasing clear that the measurement of structural markers of arterial vulnerability (carotid intimal-medial thickness, assessment of coronary artery calcium among others) and functional markers of arterial vulnerability (brachial artery reactivity assessment of endothelial function, arterial stiffness, and ankle-brachial blood pressure index [ABI]), similarly provide incremental benefit in predicting CVD risk in elderly people and help identify older individuals who might benefit from risk factor intervention.

Given the high prevalence of physical inactivity, hypertension and type 2 diabetes (T2DM) in the elderly, the geriatrician must have a firm understanding of the pathogenesis and treatment of disorders of lipoprotein metabolism in the geriatric population. This chapter reviews the epidemiology and mechanisms underlying age-associated changes in lipoprotein lipid concentrations, evidence that hyperlipidemia is a risk factor for coronary heart

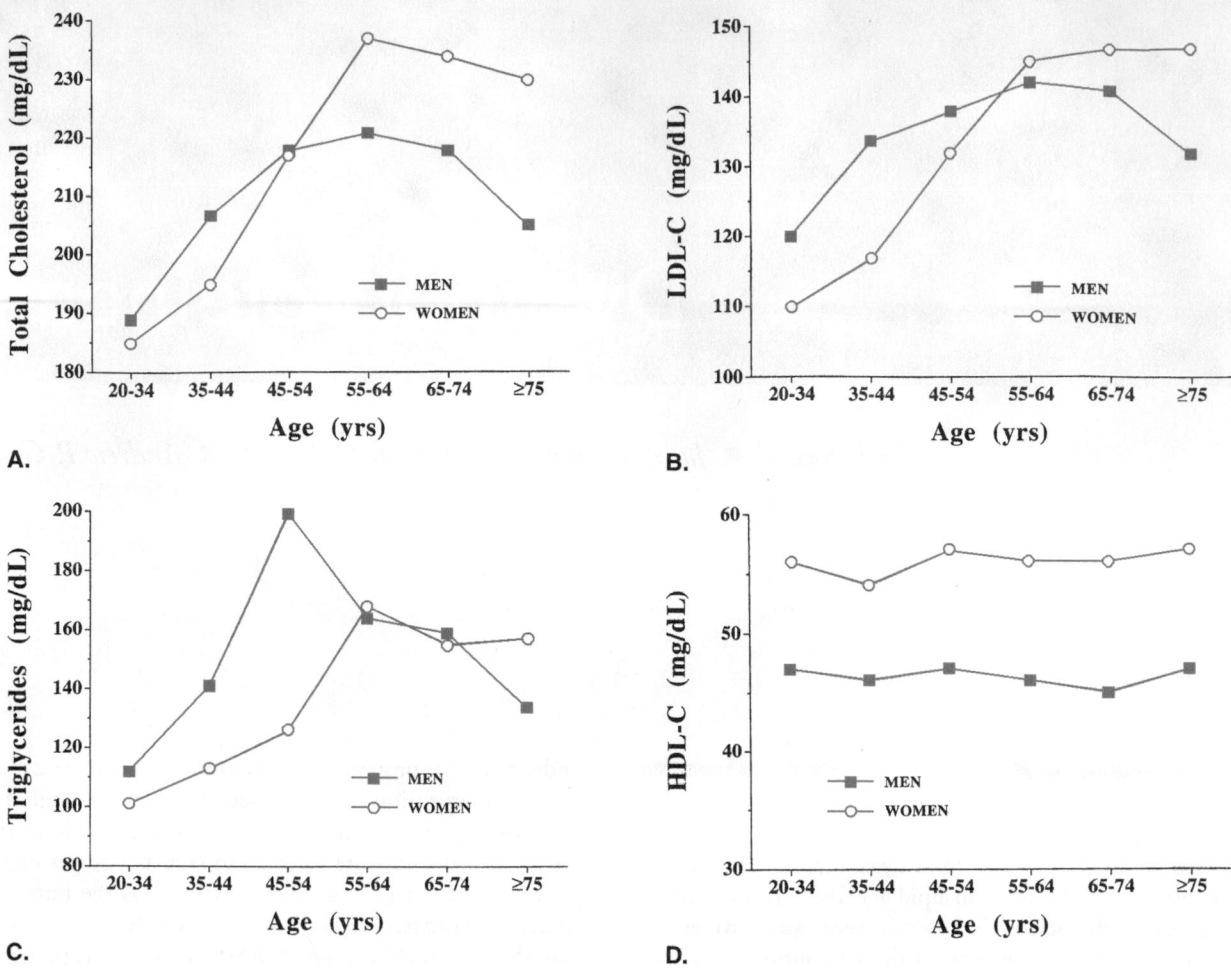

FIGURE 110-1. Time-series analyses of lipid concentrations in U.S. adults aged 20–75+ yr. Data are from the NHANES surveys of 1976–1980, 1988–1994, and 1999–2002 (http://www.cdc.gov/nchs/nhanes.htm). NHANES data are a representative sample of the civilian, noninstitutionalized population. Age groups are indicated on the abscissa, lipid concentrations in mg/dL on the ordinate. Each age group contains mean lipid concentrations obtained at three time points. Over 26 yr of follow-up, LDL cholesterol concentrations have dropped in men and women. There is more variability in the patterns of change for HDL (data not shown) and triglycerides; however overall over the last 26 yr, triglyceride concentrations have generally increased. Data represent values for all races combined. Concentrations are expressed as arithmetic means for LDL cholesterol and geometric means for triglycerides. (Data adapted from Carroll MD, Lacher DA, Sorlie PD, et al. Trends in serum lipids and lipoproteins of adults, 1960–2002. JAMA. 2005;294:1773–1781.)

disease (CHD) in the elderly population, and controversies regarding the screening and treatment of hyperlipidemia in elderly patients.

PATHOPHYSIOLOGY

Overview of Lipoprotein Subclasses and Lipoprotein Metabolism

Triglycerides (TG) and cholesterol of exogenous (dietary) and endogenous origin are transported in the blood stream as part of lipoprotein particles. These lipoprotein particles contain TG, cholesterol, cholesterol esters, phospholipids, and apolipoproteins (apo). Historically, the lipoprotein particles in the plasma have been classified on the basis of their density or by their electrophoretic mobility. Using ultracentrifugation, five major classes of plasma lipoproteins can be identified in ascending order of density: chylomicrons, very low-density lipoproteins (VLDL), intermediate density lipoproteins

(IDL), low-density lipoproteins (LDL), and high-density lipoproteins (HDL). The major classes of lipoproteins comprise subpopulations of lipoproteins that differ in composition, metabolic function, and atherogenic potential.

Lipoprotein metabolism involves the absorption of exogenous dietary fat from the GI tract, and the endogenous synthesis and secretion of triglyceride-rich lipoproteins by the liver. The physiological regulation of this process provides an understanding of the pathogenesis of atherosclerosis as the metabolic mechanisms by which therapies can target key regulatory sites to reduce CHD risk. In summarizing this process, we highlight a few key regulatory sites of normal and abnormal metabolic regulation and their consequences (Figure 110-2).

The major inherited forms of dyslipoproteinemia, and strategies for drug and dietary treatments for hyperlipidemia should be directed at these key regulatory sites of lipoprotein metabolism. Increased knowledge of the metabolic regulation of the lipoprotein subclasses by enzymes, cofactors, and transfer proteins, and various receptors has provided a framework for the understanding of pathogenesis of disorders of lipoprotein metabolism and their treatment.

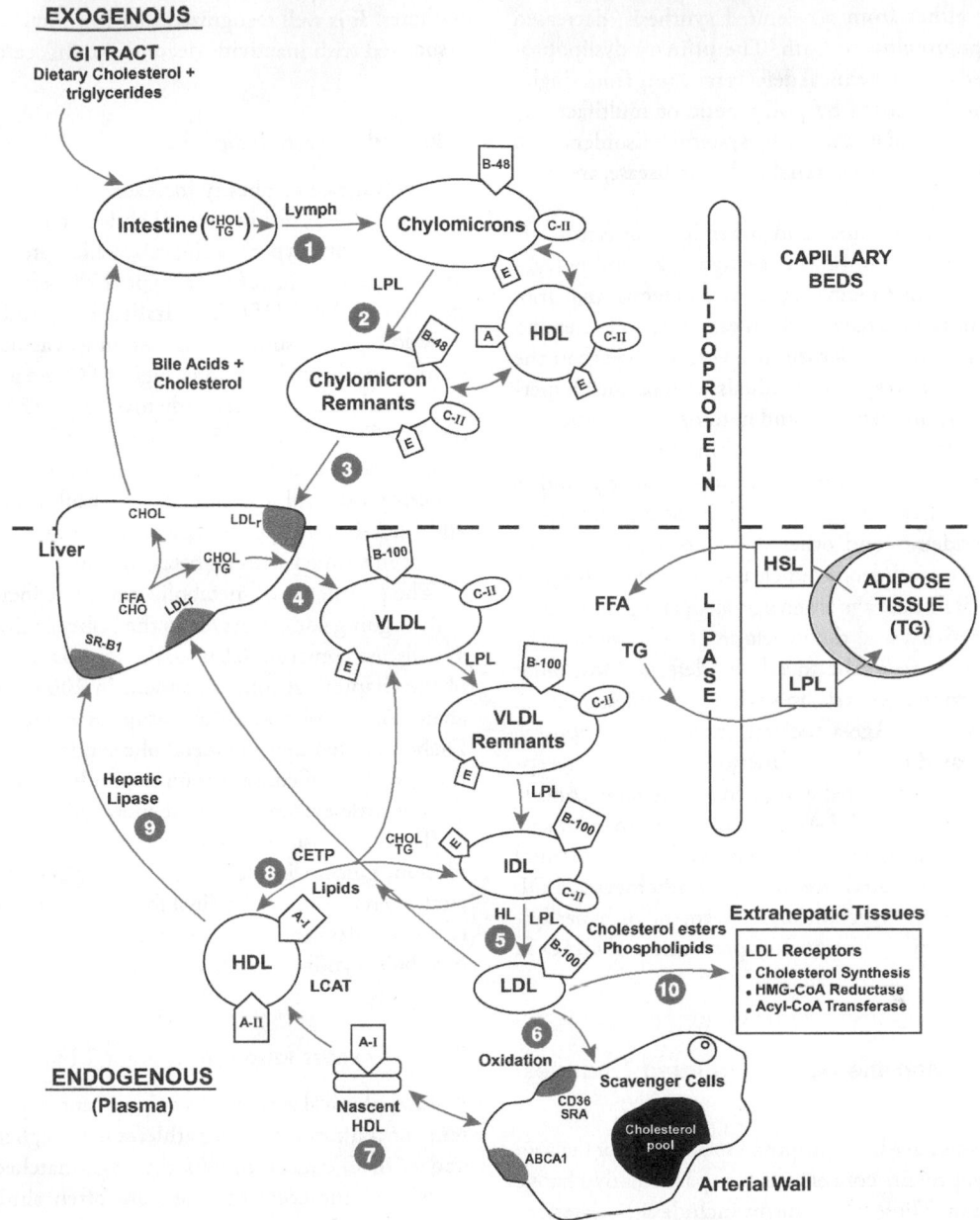

FIGURE 110-2. Schematic overview of the Apo B containing lipoproteins. Lipids in the diet are hydrolyzed in the small intestine, and the resultant fatty acids and monoglycerides are repackaged with apo B-48 into TG-enriched chylomicron particles by the intestinal enterocytes and secreted into the lymphatics (1). Dietary chylomicrons bypass the liver and enter the plasma via the thoracic duct. They acquire apo E and C-II from HDL, and are hydrolyzed by lipoprotein lipase (LPL) to smaller TG-depleted, cholesterol-rich chylomicron remnants (2). These remnants are taken up by the liver primarily by the LDL receptor-related protein receptor (LDL-R) and degraded, affecting endogenous TG synthesis and secretion (3). Endogenous TG is synthesized in the liver from carbohydrate and free fatty acid (FFA, derived from adipocyte hydrolysis by hormone-sensitive lipase) precursors assembled in the Golgi with apo B-100, E, C-II, C-III, and secreted as triglyceride-rich very low-density lipoproteins (VLDL-TG) (4). VLDL-TG are hydrolyzed by LPL to VLDL remnants and IDL, which are taken up by scavenger cells or apo E-specific hepatic receptors and degraded in the liver. VLDL remnants are removed irreversibly or hydrolyzed further by LPL and hepatic lipase to cholesterol-rich LDL particles (5). LDL has its cholesterol removed from plasma by the LDL receptor or oxidized and taken up by CD36 scavenger receptors on macrophages to generate an intracellular cholesterol pool. The hydrolysis of TG from VLDL-TG by LPL also generates free cholesterol, and phospholipids (PL), substrates for lecithin cholesterol acyl transferase (LCAT). Nascent HDL interacts with the ATP-binding cassette transporter-1 (ABCA1) on peripheral lymphoctes to remove excess cholesterol from cells and then binds with apo A-I, the principal activator of LCAT, to esterify cholesterol forming large, spherical cholesterol-ester-rich HDL2 particles (6). [Thus apo A-I and the ABCA1 transporter play critical roles in the formation of HDL and reverse cholesterol transport.] Cholesterol is transported back to the liver directly by HDL or via transfer to apo CII containing VLDL or IDL by the cholesterol ester transfer protein (CETP). Hepatic lipase stimulates HDL-C uptake by the hepatic scavenger class B type 1 receptor (SR-B1) (7). [Cholesterol is also synthesized endogenously from acetate precursors, regulated by the enzyme HMG-CoA reductase. The accumulation of intracellular free cholesterol suppresses endogenous cholesterol synthesis by inhibiting HMG-CoA reductase, the rate-limiting enzyme in cholesterol synthesis, stimulates cholesterol reesterification by acyl-CoA: cholesterol transferase, and downregulates LDL receptor synthesis (8).] However, if there is excess VLDL-TG production or dietary fat intake, CETP exchanges cholesterol from HDL with TG from VLDL, raising the TG and lowering the cholesterol composition of HDL (9). Hepatic lipase hydrolyzes HDL TG and phospholipid, converting HDL₂ back to smaller HDL₃ particles, reducing the efficient clearance of cholesterol from cells. Cholesterol can then be resecreted from the liver on VLDL, increasing endogenous LDL synthesis, excreted directly into the bile, or converted to bile acids for reabsorption (enterohepatic circulation) or excretion in stool and bile (10).

These disorders arise either from accelerated synthesis, decreased degradation of the lipoproteins, or both. The primary dyslipoproteinemias can be caused by biochemical defects resulting from single-gene mutations or can be caused by polygenetic or multifactorial causes. Secondary dyslipidemias, caused by systemic disorders such as obesity, diabetes, hypothyroidism, renal and liver disease, are more common in the elderly population.

Age, environmental factors, diet, and other lifestyle factors affect the phenotypic expression of both the single-gene and polygenetic disorders. The prevailing dogma is that dyslipidemias that arise from the single-gene mutations have both an earlier age of onset and clinical manifestations of atherosclerosis at a younger age than the polygenetic disorders. For example, individuals with familial hypercholesterolemia, both the homozygous and heterozygote genotypes, can be identified in childhood. Familial combined hyperlipidemia might not be phenotypically manifest until after puberty, and is usually clinically and biochemically diagnosed in the fourth decade. Familial hypertriglyceridemia and other disorders associated with increased TG production and decreased clearance may not become clinically apparent until middle age when age-associated increases in adiposity, physical inactivity, and the development of insulin resistance enhance the expression of the metabolic defects. Most older individuals presenting to the geriatrician with hypercholesterolemia have multifactorial disorders. Age-associated increases in adiposity, decreased fitness, decreased number or function of the LDL receptor, and hormonal changes associated with menopause act in concert with polygenetic factors to raise LDL-C concentrations in older age. Similarly, the interaction of genetic, lifestyle, and environmental factors increase the age-associated prevalence of atherogenic LDL pattern B phenotype. Early detection and treatment of hyperlipidemia is critical for primary and secondary prevention of CHD in the elderly.

Mechanisms Underlying the Age-Associated Changes in Lipids

A number of mechanisms have been proposed to account for the age-related changes in lipoprotein concentrations, particularly change in LDL-C concentration. These mechanisms include age-related increases in dietary fat content and adiposity, declines in physical activity and physical fitness, and decreases in the number and function of the hepatic LDL receptor.

Changes in Diet

Age-associated changes in dietary content are reviewed in Chapter 38. In men in the Baltimore Longitudinal Study of Aging (BLSA), total caloric intake, cholesterol intake, the percent of calories obtained from fat, and the percent of calories obtained from saturated fat declined with age. Such age-associated changes in dietary content would be expected to result in lower levels of total and LDL-C, a result that is opposite to the commonly observed age-associated increase in these parameters. Others have reported changes in the distribution of energy consumed in older adults with a larger relative contribution of calories consumed at breakfast and snacks, with fewer calories consumed at lunch and dinner. The increased snacking may result in a greater portion of calories from sweets and carbohydrates. It is well recognized that low total energy consumption is associated with inactivity, deconditioning, sarcopenia, and frailty.

Total and Visceral Adiposity

The prevalence of obesity increases with aging, with a preferential accumulation of fat in visceral abdominal sites. These changes are associated with hyperinsulinemia, which predisposes older adults to develop glucose intolerance, type 2 diabetes, and other metabolic risk factors for CHD. The Italian Longitudinal Study on Aging showed higher insulin concentration was associated with low HDL-C and apo AI concentrations, higher TG and glucose concentrations, hypertension, and higher body mass index (BMI), but not high total or LDL-C in a cohort of 5632 people aged 65 to 84 years. Among the subjects with diabetes, TG concentration was higher but HDL-C concentration did not differ across insulin quartiles; however, total and LDL-C concentrations were lower and white blood cell count higher in women with diabetes with high insulin concentrations.

The prevalence of metabolic syndrome increases with age. There is an ongoing controversy as to the utility of the metabolic syndrome as a disease construct (also see the "Special Issues" section at the end of the chapter). A joint statement in 2005 from the American Diabetes Association and the European Association for the Study of Diabetes noted that the metabolic syndrome is imprecisely defined, there is a lack of consensus on the underlying pathophysiology, and there is little evidence that the metabolic syndrome denotes greater CVD risk per se than the sum of its parts (low HDL-C, hypertension, glucose intolerance, hypertriglyceridemia, increased waist circumference). Longitudinal follow-up and the assessment of mortality will determine the relationship of hyperinsulinemia and the metabolic syndrome to CHD risk.

Physical Fitness (also see Chapter 114)

Regular physical activity has a significant impact on plasma lipoprotein concentrations. Older athletes have higher HDL-C, lower TG, and LDL-C concentrations than age-matched sedentary counterparts, and the concentrations are often similar to those seen in younger adults. The interpretation of these cross-sectional comparisons is confounded by differences in body composition, as the trained subjects are significantly leaner than the sedentary population. The differences in obesity contribute the most to the difference in TG and HDL-C concentrations between older athletes and their sedentary counterparts, while the differences in maximal aerobic capacity (VO_2 max) account for a small percentage of the variance in these lipoproteins. Current physical activity guidelines from the Centers for Disease Control and American College of Sports Medicine recommend that older adults participate in moderate-intensity aerobic activities 3 to 5 days a week for at least 30 minutes each session, daily stretching for flexibility, and strength-building activities 2 to 3 days per week (see Chapter 114). These guidelines are based on experimental and epidemiologic data that energy expenditure and metabolic responses to exercise training reduce lipoprotein lipid, insulin-glucose, and blood pressure associated CVD risk, and directly affect CVD mortality. Vigorous exercise improves cardiovascular fitness indexed as VO_2 max, reduces visceral adiposity, and has salutary effects on lipid profiles, insulin sensitivity, glucose metabolism, and blood pressure, thereby reducing major components and risk associated with the metabolic syndrome.

Lipoprotein Synthetic and Catabolic Rates

A number of studies have examined the metabolism of LDL in young and older subjects. Miller pooled data on the fractional catabolic rate of LDL apo B from four groups of subjects; normal men, normal women, individuals with heterozygous familial hypercholesterolemia, and in individuals with hypercholesterolemia. In these four groups the LDL apo B fractional catabolic rate decreased with age, whereas the LDL production rate did not change with age. The age-related rise in LDL was attributed to an acquired defect in the LDL receptor function. Similar findings subsequently were reported by Ericson, who suggested that there might be an age-associated reduction in hepatic LDL receptor expression. Kinetic studies with isotopes suggest that the age-associated increase in VLDL apo B-100 is caused by an increased rate of production, whereas the age-associated increase in LDL apo-B 100 is caused by increased residency time. Matthan and colleagues determined that decreased clearance of TG-rich lipoprotein and of LDL contributed to the increase in TG and LDL in postmenopausal women, rather than increased production of these particles. These studies did not control for differences in body composition and physical activity among age groups, factors which may elevate plasma-free fatty acid concentrations, glucose, and insulin concentrations in the older subjects and result in a raise in hepatic production of TG. We would contend that many of the purported age-related changes in lipoprotein concentrations reflect interactions between primary age-related changes in LDL metabolism and the effects of obesity, physical inactivity, diet, and other lifestyle habits, or secondary aging.

EPIDEMIOLOGY

Coronary Heart Disease

CHD remains the leading cause of death in older men and women. Despite secular declines in mortality rates from CHD, since 1950, as a result of the aging of the population since 1950, the number of CHD deaths in the United States has actually increased in people 65 to 74 years of age, and has more than doubled in those older than age 75 years. It is estimated that almost 16 million adults in the United States have prevalent CHD and 5.6 million have had a stroke. Based on National Health and Nutrition Examination Survey (NHANES) data, 23% of men and 15% of women aged 60 to 79 years have prevalent CHD. For those aged 80 years and older, 33% of men and 22% of women have prevalent CHD. However, these numbers severely understate the burden of CHD in the older adult population because much of the disease is clinically silent. Electron beam tomography, a noninvasive technique to detect subclinical coronary artery calcification, as indicator of atherosclerotic plaque burden and CHD, showed that two-thirds of the people older than 65 years of age in the Cardiovascular Health Study had either subclinical atherosclerotic disease or clinically apparent CHD. According to American Heart Association statistics, in 2004, 83% of the deaths from CHD and 88% of deaths from stroke occur in people older than 65 years of age. Furthermore, the projected growth of the population older than 80 years of age by 2030 suggests there will be a huge increase in the burden of disease from CHD and CVD. Many of these deaths and some of this burden maybe preventable (see "Prevention" later in the chapter).

Age-Associated Changes in Lipids

Many cross-sectional studies have examined age-associated changes in lipoprotein concentrations in both men and women. Unfortunately cross-sectional studies alone cannot distinguish changes caused by biological aging from those caused by lifestyle and those caused by disease. To do this longitudinal studies are needed. Knowledge of longitudinal changes in lipoproteins is limited because of the inherent difficulties in following cohorts of individuals over extended periods of time, and methodologies that limited widespread measurement of HDL-C and apolipoproteins prior to the mid-1970s. The window of opportunity to perform longitudinal studies of the natural history of lipoprotein changes with aging has closed, as treatment of clinically apparent dyslipidemia is standard clinical practice. In general, the cross-sectional studies demonstrate that total cholesterol, LDL-C, and TG concentrations increase in both men and women from the third to seventh or eighth decades of life, with a more pronounced increase in LDL-C concentration in women and important changes in women around the menopause. These increases in total cholesterol, LDL-C, and TG in general parallel changes in body composition seen with aging.

Typically, there is a decline in LDL-C and total cholesterol concentration in oldest age cohorts. For example, in NHANES III of 1988–1991, total cholesterol concentrations were on average 189 mg/dL in men aged 20 to 34 years and 221 mg/dL for men aged 55 to 64 years, but down to 205 mg/dL for men older than the age of 75 years. In the Honolulu Heart Study, total cholesterol levels were 8% lower in men older than age 85 years, as compared to men aged 71 to 74 years. This decline in cholesterol levels in the population older than age 75 years could reflect selective mortality, or be caused by changes in body composition, coexistent comorbid diseases, and poor nutrition. Indeed, longitudinal change in body weight over an 8-year period of time was an independent predictor of changes in total cholesterol, LDL-C, and HDL-C in older men and women in Rancho Bernardo, California.

The overall pattern of change in total cholesterol profiles across the age span in women is similar to that for men, but on average is 20 to 30 mg/dL above men from age 55 to 75 years. In NHANES III, 39% of women and 22% of men aged 65 to 74 years had a total cholesterol concentration above 240 mg/dL. However, the implications of "elevated" cholesterol in elderly people are not as straightforward as in younger age groups. In a subgroup of men aged 71 to 93 years from the Honolulu Heart Study, the age-adjusted incidence rates of coronary heart disease exhibited a significant U-shaped relationship with both total cholesterol and LDL.

In addition to the changes in the concentration of LDL, there are age-related changes in the LDL subclass population distribution that affect the atherogenicity and susceptibility of LDL to oxidation. The prevalence of individuals with a predominance of small, dense apo B-enriched LDL particles increases with age. In women, there are marked changes in lipoprotein concentrations and composition associated with menopause. In the Framingham Offspring Study, postmenopausal women had 16% higher values of total cholesterol, 62% higher TG, 23% higher LDL-C, and smaller LDL particles than premenopausal women. These changes in LDL composition adversely impact CAD risk, and are not detected by routine methods for measurement of lipoproteins.

There are also changes in HDL-C concentrations across the age span in both men and women. In men at puberty, there is a drop in HDL concentrations. The HDL-C concentration then remains fairly constant until the sixth or seventh decade of life, at which point there maybe an increase in the HDL-C concentration. This increase in HDL-C concentrations at older age noted in the cross-sectional studies also maybe the result of selective morbidity and mortality, as opposed to true age-associated changes in HDL metabolism. However, some studies have found lower HDL-C concentrations in postmenopausal women. Analogous to LDL, there are also compositional changes in the HDL subfractions associated with menopause that may increase CHD risk.

Based on ATP III guidelines, the marked age-associated increase in the prevalence of hypercholesterolemia (60% of men and 77% of women older than 65 years of age with total cholesterol > 200 mg/dL) make millions of older adults candidates for lifestyle intervention. Millions of older individuals with prevalent CHD, CHD equivalents (diabetes, stroke, peripheral vascular disease, chronic kidney disease), or with multiple risk factors for CHD events also are candidates for cholesterol lowering-drugs. Controversies on whom to treat and the target criteria are discussed in greater detail later in the chapter. As discussed in the next section, an increasingly informed and proactive older population, and changes in professional opinion toward ever more aggressive therapy for hyperlipidemia are reflected in the large number of elderly people prescribed HMG-CoA reductase inhibitors (statins).

SECULAR CHANGES IN LIPOPROTEIN LIPID CONCENTRATIONS AND PRESCRIBING PATTERNS

Secular Changes in Lipoprotein Lipid Concentrations

There have been substantial changes in lipoprotein lipid concentrations in the U.S. population over the past four decades (Figure 110-1). NHANES data demonstrates that from 1960 to 2002, secular changes in diet, increased use of lipid-lowering medications, and other factors resulted in lower mean total cholesterol concentration across the age span in both men and women. The greatest declines have occurred in the older populations. There was no change in mean HDL-C and a trend for an increase in TG. The increase in the proportion of adults using lipid-lowering medication, particularly in older age groups, likely contributed to the decreases in total and LDL-C concentration, while the heightened prevalence of obesity in the U.S. population probably contributed to the increase in plasma TG levels.

The secular decline in cholesterol concentration maybe accelerating. A retrospective analysis of data from nearly 80 million LDL-C tests performed at Quest laboratories across the United States from 2001 through 2004 for adult patients aged 20 years and older demonstrated that the average serum LDL-C concentration declined from 124 mg/dL at the beginning of 2001 to 112 mg/dL at the end of 2004. The decline in average LDL-C concentration was ob-

served across all age groups, but was most pronounced for tests performed on older patients. The decrease was greatest (approximately 13%) for people aged 70 years and older and least pronounced (approximately 7%) for the 20-to-39-year age range. These analyses were not adjusted for medication usage or disease, and patients referred for assessment of their lipoprotein lipids may not be representative of the general population.

This decline in cholesterol concentration could have a significant impact on CVD morbidity and mortality. Conversely, secular changes resulting in an increased prevalence of obesity may worsen the manifestations of the metabolic syndrome, i.e., raise TG concentration, lower HDL-C concentration, and shift the distribution of HDL and LDL lipoprotein particle distribution toward smaller, denser, more atherogenic particles, worsen insulin resistance, and raise blood pressure. Therefore, LDL-C concentration alone maybe misleading as in these older people there will be more LDL particles for any cholesterol concentration if the LDL particles are small and dense. Such changes may require a change in the approach to the identification and treatment of dyslipoproteinemia toward therapies that modify both the concentration and composition of HDL and LDL, and reduce the high number of apo B and dense LDL particles, as well as treat other components of the metabolic syndrome. Combination therapy of LDL-lowering drugs such as HMG-CoA reductase inhibitors with niacin, cholesterol absorption inhibitors (ezetimibe), or fibrates in combination with insulin sensitizers to reduce insulin resistance, glucose, and plasma triglyceride maybe required to achieve lipid-lowering targets (see "Management" later in the chapter.).

Secular Changes in HMG-CoA Reductase Inhibitor (Statin) Prescription Patterns

In 1997, fewer than 12% of the 38 million Medicare beneficiaries (4.4 million persons) used at least one statin. By 2002, roughly 27% of the 41 million Medicare beneficiaries (11 million individuals) used the drugs. The 2005 U.S. Agency for Healthcare Research and Quality (AHRQ) statistics (http://www.meps.ahrq.gov/mepsweb) indicates that statin use doubled between 1997 and 2002 in the Medicare recipients older than 65 years of age. The statistics from AHRQ's Medical Expenditure Panel Survey do not include Medicare patients in nursing homes or other institutional settings. When examined by age category, about 31% of those 65 to 74 years of age and 30% aged 75 to 84 years used a statin in 2002, but only 12% the of beneficiaries were older than 85 years.

Despite the large increase in number of prescriptions, many feel that statin therapy is underutilized. A study by Ko of elderly residents in Ontario demonstrated that paradoxically, older individuals with the highest cardiovascular risk and risk for death were the least likely to be prescribed statins. This was because of a largely sharp age-related decline in the prescribing of statins. This problem of underuse of statins is further compounded by patient noncompliance. Concerns about adverse side effects may also deter health care providers from prescribing these medications to the elderly. However, concerns about side effects are not supported by the available data, as a meta-analysis of 35 randomized controlled trials and examination of Medicare data bases demonstrate that statins as a class are safe with a risk of transaminase elevation in about 4/1000 patients and a risk of fatal rhabdomyolysis of about 0.15 per 1 million statin prescriptions (the risk was 12-fold higher in the now withdrawn cerivastatin). Contrary to some clinical observations, the rate of myalgias (5%) and creatine kinase elevations (1%) in the meta-analysis was similar to placebo. Concerns about statins causing an increased risk of cancer are probably unfounded, as epidemiological data suggest that statins may actually reduce the rates of several cancers. Of note, the protective effects of statin therapy may go beyond simple lipoprotein reduction to include possible anti-inflammatory, antioxidant, and antithrombotic effects, as well as effects on nitric oxide metabolism. Several studies are currently underway addressing the benefits of statins with a variety of comorbid medical conditions including congestive heart failure, cerebrovascular disease, type 2 diabetes, and aortic stenosis.

LIPOPROTEINS AS RISK FACTORS FOR CORONARY HEART DISEASE

Many case–control and prospective studies examining lipoprotein risk factors for atherosclerosis have focused on the impact of the traditional lipoprotein risk factors, that is, total cholesterol, LDL-C, and HDL-C. There is also substantial evidence that many older individuals have abnormalities in lipoprotein metabolism that are not detected by routine lipid profiles. These dyslipidemic syndromes include the apoE4 genotype, elevated levels of Lp(a), and the atherogenic LDL pattern B phenotype. These disorders of lipoprotein metabolism are more common than familial heterozygous hypercholesterolemia and familial multiple lipoprotein hyperlipidemia in both the general population and CHD patients, and may play major roles in the pathogenesis of CHD in older individuals. In this section, the evidence that dyslipidemia is a risk factor for CHD in the elderly population is reviewed.

Elevated Total and LDL-C Concentrations

There is convincing evidence that elevated levels of total cholesterol and of LDL-C increase the risk for CHD in middle-aged men. The evidence supporting elevated levels of LDL-C as a risk factor for CHD in the elderly population, particularly elderly women, is mixed. In pooled data presented at a National Heart, Lung, and Blood Institute (NHLBI) conference, in 21 of 24 studies of men aged 65 years and older, the relative risk was >1.00 for total cholesterol concentrations >240 mg/dL, as compared to cholesterol levels <200 mg/dL. The pooled relative risk was 1.32. By comparison, for women aged 65 years and older, in 10 of 16 studies, the relative risk was >1.00 for cholesterol >240 mg/dL, as compared to cholesterol levels <200 mg/dL. The pooled relative risk was 1.12. Although statistically significant, the relative risk for CHD in older individuals with hypercholesterolemia is lower than the relative risk observed in studies of men younger than 65 years of age.

There are many factors that may account for the disparities between the studies that have examined the relationship between cholesterol levels and CHD in the elderly. One explanation maybe a nonlinear relationship between cholesterol levels, CHD events, and total mortality, that is, a J- or U-shaped curve. In this situation, individuals with the highest or lowest cholesterol levels are at increased risk for CHD, as compared to those with intermediate levels. Another confounder in the association between cholesterol levels and CHD outcomes in the elderly person is that cholesterol levels measured at a given time may not accurately reflect the lifelong average exposure to plasma cholesterol, leading to spurious conclusions. For example, at age 70 years, the measured total cholesterol level maybe 220 mg/dL, whereas the average cholesterol level over the adult life span could have been 180 or 250 mg/dL. As a result, longitudinal studies that examine both the baseline cholesterol level and its change over time are needed to provide insight into the predictive values of cholesterol levels for subsequent CHD and all-cause mortality in the elderly population. For example, in a Finnish 30-year longitudinal study, there was a U-shaped relationship between the change in cholesterol level and coronary and all-cause mortality. The authors concluded that this U-shaped relationship may confound the association of cholesterol with CHD risk in the elderly. A potential way out of this conundrum is to focus on LDL cholesterol as advocated by the ATP III guidelines. Not only is this more closely linked to CVD, but increasing clinical trial data tie improvements in LDL-C to those in CHD clinical endpoints (see below).

The majority of studies report data on the relative risk of hypercholesterolemia for CHD morbidity and mortality. However, some investigators suggest that the attributable risk is a more useful parameter for making clinical decisions regarding treatment of hypercholesterolemia in the elderly. In this context, attributable risk is the difference in the CHD mortality rate in subjects with a high lipid concentration and the CHD mortality rate in subjects with a lower or desirable lipid concentration. Attributable risk provides an estimate of the degree to which cause-specific mortality (in this case CHD mortality) would be lowered if the putative risk factor were lowered to a normal level. Unlike relative risk, attributable risk is very sensitive to the underlying mortality rate in "normals", that is, the mortality rate in subjects with normal or desirable cholesterol levels. The MRFIT data permits an analysis of how the relative and attributable risks of hypercholesterolemia for CHD mortality vary with age. In MRFIT, the relative risk for CHD mortality for a man in the upper quintile of the population declined from over 7 in men aged 35 to 39 years to 2 for men aged 55 to 59 years (Figure 110-3). However, as a result of age-associated increases in the CHD death rate in men with "normal" cholesterol, the attributable risk for CHD in the upper versus lowest quintile increased progressively with age, from 0.7% for men aged 35 to 39 years compared to 1.9% for men aged 55 to 59 years. As a result of the age-related increase in the attributable risk for hypercholesterolemia, there maybe substantial public health benefit, i.e., the ability to prevent a large numbers of deaths by treating hypercholesterolemia in the elderly. Furthermore, as discussed in the Management section of this chapter, the number of subjects who have to be treated to prevent one death or the inverse of the attributable risk is substantially lower in older than in younger adults. Thus, pharmacologic interventions to decrease morbidity and mortality from CHD maybe more cost-effective in older compared to younger people.

Reduced Concentrations of HDL-C

A preponderance of studies demonstrate that measurement of HDL-C provides additional information on risk for CHD and stroke in the elderly. In the Framingham Study, 4- and 12-year follow-up data demonstrate inverse relationships between HDL-C concentrations and CHD incidence. In Framingham men 50 to 79 years of age, the relative risk for all-cause mortality in men with an HDL-C < 35 mg/dL compared to those whose HDL-C >54 mg/dL was 1.9 and risk of CHD mortality was 4.1. In women, the relative

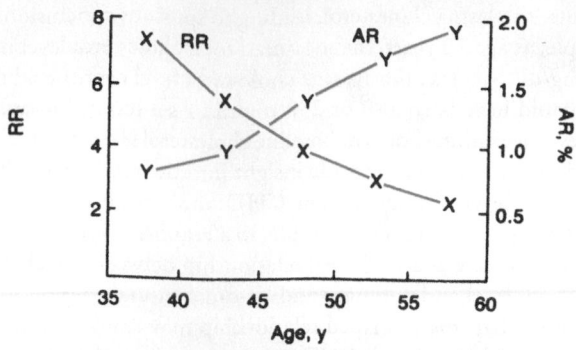

FIGURE 110-3. The effect of age on the relative and attributable risk of hypercholesterolemia for CHD death in patients of the Multiple Risk Factor Intervention Trial (MRFIT). Although the relative risk (RR) for CHD death for individuals with hypercholesterolemia declines with aging, because of age-associated increases in the absolute death rate from CHD, the attributable risk (AR) for CHD in the upper versus lowest quintile increased progressively with age. *(From Malenka DJ, Baron JA. Cholesterol and Coronary Heart Disease. The importance of patient-specific attributable risk. Arch Intern Med. 1988;148:2247–2252.)*

risk for all-cause mortality was 1.5 and the risk for CHD mortality was 3.1 (HDL-C < 45 mg/dL vs. > 69 mg/dL). In data from three Established Population for the Epidemiologic Study of the Elderly (EPESE) sites, subjects aged 71 to 80 years in the lowest HDL-C category (<35 mg/dL) were four times more likely to die from CHD than those with HDL-C above 60 mg/dL. A 10-year prospective study of lipid risk factors for CHD in 989 older subjects in Marshfield, Winconsin, showed that survival among men was associated with higher HDL-C and a lower total cholesterol/HDL ratio. However, there was no relationship between any of the lipid concentrations and all-cause mortality in women older than 65 years of age. There was a 1.24-fold increased risk of having peripheral arterial disease and a 1.36 risk of having a stroke for a 10 mg/dL decrement of HDL-C in older men and women, after controlling for other risk factors. Therapy with gemfibrozil increased HDL-C and reduced the risk of stroke in older men with prevalent CHD. These findings support the use of measurement of HDL-C along with total cholesterol to predict CHD risk in older individuals.

Measurement of apo A-I concentration, the main apolipoprotein constituent of HDL, or of apo B 100 (see next section), the primary apolipoprotein of LDL, or a combination of the two might provide superior discriminatory power than measurement of HDL-C and LDL-C in predicting CVD morbidity and mortality in older adults. In Swedish men aged 77 years who participated in the Uppsala Longitudinal Study of adult men, men in the first, second, and third quartiles of apo A-I values had a relative risk of subsequent death of 10.2, 5.0, and 3.0 compared to the quartile with the highest apo A-1 concentration. In older (>70 years) patients with diabetes, apo B concentration and the ratio of apo B to apo A-I predicted CHD events independent of LDL-C.

The association between low HDL concentration and CHD has accelerated the development of pharmacological treatments to raise HDL-C. Inhibition of cholesteryl ester transfer protein (CETP) is one strategy to raise HDL-C concentration, and initial studies with torcetrapib, a potent inhibitor of CETP, showed 60% increases in HDL accompanied by reductions in LDL-C beyond that that seen with atorvastatin. Unfortunately, a large-scale randomized clinical trial of torcetrapib was stopped prematurely because the torcetrapib

plus atorvastatin group had a substantially higher mortality rate than the group that received only atorvastatin. Increased rates of heart failure, angina, hypertension, and coronary revascularization were also seen in the torcetapib group. It is unclear whether these adverse results are restricted to this particular CETP inhibitor or to the entire class of CETP inhibitors.

Atherogenic LDL Pattern B Phenotype

LDL comprise a spectrum of heterogeneous particles that differ in size, chemical composition, and density. The LDL subpopulations differ in their metabolism and in their propensity for promoting atherosclerosis. There are two general phenotypic patterns of LDL particles distribution: individuals who have a predominance of large, buoyant LDL particles have the LDL pattern A phenotype, and those with a predominance of small, dense LDL particles have the LDL pattern B phenotype. Individuals with the LDL pattern B typically have other lipoprotein abnormalities, including mildly elevated TG and reduced HDL-C concentration, as well as hypertension, leading some to believe that the LDL B phenotype is a biochemical marker for the metabolic syndrome. Each of the metabolic components of the LDL pattern B phenotype promotes atherosclerosis, thus the term atherogenic LDL pattern B phenotype. Direct assessment of LDL size and LDL subclass distribution requires use of techniques such as gradient gel electrophoresis, density gradient ultracentrifugation, ultracentrifugation, and nuclear magnetic resonance, not routinely employed in clinical practice. Apo B concentration can be measured by most laboratories and provides an estimate of the total number of circulating LDL particles. Apo B levels tend to be higher in LDL pattern B and the ratio of LDL-C to apo B provides an indirect estimate of LDL particle size and number.

Most, but not all studies, demonstrate an association between LDL pattern B and increased risk for prevalent CHD and subclincal manifestations of atherosclerosis detected by assessment of carotid intima media thickness. In the Physicians' Health Survey, LDL pattern B was prospectively associated with a threefold increased risk of CHD, independent of total cholesterol, HDL, and body mass index. The prevalence of the atherogenic LDL pattern B phenotype increases markedly with age. Studies by Austin et al. demonstrated that the prevalence increases from 10% to 15% in young men to 30% to 35% in middle-aged men, and from 5% to 10% in young women to 15% to 25% in postmenopausal women. Several investigators propose that the atherogenic LDL pattern B phenotype maybe the most common abnormality in lipoprotein metabolism that predisposes to CHD. The NCEP III guidelines recognize small, dense LDL as a CVD risk factor.

The etiology of LDL pattern B is multifactorial. Family studies suggest that LDL pattern B is inherited as a Mendelian-dominant or polygenetic trait that interacts with other genes to increase apo B production. The phenotypic expression of the pattern is affected by age, visceral obesity, diet, sedentary lifestyle, and the presence of type 2 diabetes. Several studies link LDL pattern B to a number of genetic loci but there is no consensus on which of these, if any, is responsible for the syndrome.

If a preponderance of small LDL particles is harmful, one can hypothesize that individuals with larger, more buoyant LDL particles (LDL pattern A) would be less likely to have CVD and have greater longevity. In case–control studies, individuals with exceptional longevity (mean age 98 years) and their offspring have significantly larger HDL and LDL particle sizes than control families. The phenotype of larger LDL particles was associated with a lower prevalence of hypertension, CVD, metabolic syndrome, and increased homozygosity for the I405V variant in the CETP gene. These findings suggest that lipoprotein particle size is associated with longevity.

There is substantial evidence that individuals with the LDL pattern B have a different metabolic response to drug and dietary interventions than those with the "normal" LDL pattern A phenotype. Subjects with LDL patterns B and A had differential lipoprotein lipid responses to dietary interventions, exercise, weight loss, and therapy with statins, nicotinic acid, bile acid-binding resins, and fibrates. Certain classes of drugs appear more effective at lowering the concentration of the small, dense LDL particles than other drugs, and reductions in the concentration of these particles is associated with decreased CAD progression or regression in several studies that measured plaque size using angiography. In the St. Thomas' Atherosclerosis Regression Study (STARS) comparing usual care, intervention with lipid-lowering diet and lipid lowering diet + cholestyramine, small dense LDL was significantly reduced in the groups showing regression, and dense LDL concentration during the trial was the best predictor of arteriographic outcome with those with the lowest treated levels of dense LDL having the greatest regression. Similarly, in the Helsinki Heart Study (HHS), the subset of subjects having an elevated TG concentration and low HDL-C, that is, patients who presumably had LDL pattern B, received substantial clinical benefit from gemfibrozil. These findings have important implications for clinical practice.

Because statins lower the concentration of all LDL subclasses, their net effect on LDL subclass distribution or mean size of the LDL particles maybe only moderate. However, different statins have differential effect on the LDL subclass distribution. Pravastatin and simvastatin have a limited ability to modifying particle size and their subclasses while fluvastatin and atorvastatin seem to be much more effective. Rosuvastatin seems to be the most potent in altering particle size toward a less atherogenic profile. The clinician must realize that lipid-lowering drugs have differential effects on the lipoprotein subclasses that are not detected by routine measurements of TG, LDL-C, and HDL-C and could affect plaque regression. Advances in technology may make measurement of the lipoprotein subfractions and apolipoproteins part of the routine lipoprotein profile. Until that time, measurement of apo B concentrations and the LDL-C to apo B ratio can be used as surrogate markers for LDL particle size. This ratio can then be used to select drugs that target the patient's underlying metabolic abnormalities. However, until large-scale clinical trials comparing the effect of the different statins on morbidity and mortality in older individuals with different LDL subclass distributions and apolipoprotein profiles are performed, we will not know if the theoretical advantages of those medications particularly effective in decreasing dense LDL subfraction concentration result in improved clinical outcomes.

Apolipoprotein ε4 Allele

Apolipoprotein E is a constituent of chylomicrons, VLDL, and HDL, and modulates the metabolism of the apo B-containing lipoproteins. The gene that codes for apo E is polymorphic, with single amino acid substitutions that result in three common alleles designated ε2, ε3, and ε4. These alleles encode 3 common isoforms, E2, E3, E4, that determine the six common apo E genotypes ε2/2, ε2/3, ε2/4, ε3/3, ε4/3, and ε4/4. The relative frequencies of the ε2, ε3, and ε4 alleles in adult populations are approximately 8%, 78%, and 14% respectively. There are a number of studies that demonstrate that LDL-C concentrations are in part determined by the apo E gene locus. Individuals with the apo E2/3 genotype on average have LDL concentrations 20% lower than the common apo E3/3 genotype, whereas subjects with apo E4/3 have LDL-C concentrations 10% higher than apo E3/3. In addition, some individuals with apo E2/2 genotype have defective clearance of lipid remnants (dysbetalipoproteinemia, type III hyperlipidemia). The apo E genotype may also influence HDL concentrations, but the effect appears to be modified by gene–gene interactions with other loci (CETP, cholesterol 7-alpha-hydroxylase [CYP7A1], and others), as well as exercise and dietary factors.

A number of studies show that the apo ε4 allele is a risk factor for CHD. In the Framingham Offspring Study, apo E4 was a determinant of CHD risk independent of age, sex, hypertension, cigarette use, obesity, diabetes, or the concentrations of LDL-C and HDL-C. The odds ratio for CHD in men heterozygotic for apo E4 compared to men without any copy of the ε4 allele was 1.53, while in women it was 1.99. The ε4 allele also is associated with increased mortality and decreased survival into older age; thus, the frequency of the ε4 allele is lower in older compared to younger populations. In one cross-sectional study, the ε4 allele declined progressively across the age span: 0.198 in young adults to 0.116 in nonagenarian. Similarly, in another study, the frequency of the ε4 allele was lower in older women (0.098) compared to younger women (0.122), whereas the allele frequency of ε2 was higher and associated with lower total and LDL-C concentrations in the older cohort.

These cross-sectional studies are supported by results of longitudinal studies. In older Finnish men (mean age at entry 72 years), the death rate from CHD over 5 years of follow-up of men with the ε4 allele was double that of men with the other apo E genotypes. In the BLSA, in multivariate analyses, apo E4 was an independent predictor of coronary events (relative risk of 2.9) in middle-aged and older men over 20 years of longitudinal follow-up. These studies strongly support selective mortality as the cause for the progressive decrease in the prevalence of apo E4 in older populations. Conversely, a number of studies indicate that the ε2 allele promotes longevity, possibly through an association with lower concentration of apo B-containing lipoproteins. The apo E genotype may also affect the metabolic response to statin therapy. It is not known whether lifestyle or pharmacologic interventions specifically targeted at older individuals with the ε4 allele would reduce death from CHD and all-cause mortality.

Given its prevalence, the ε4 allele maybe the most common genetic lipid abnormality associated with CHD. The mechanism underlying the increased CHD in individuals carrying the ε4 allele is not known with certainty, but is in part caused by changes in LDL and TG-rich remnant metabolism. Patients with the ε4 allele tend to have lower HDL-C and higher TG concentrations than individuals with the common apo E3/3 genotype. In addition to being a genetic risk factor for CHD, there is an association between the ε4 allele and Alzheimer's disease, stroke, and Parkinson's disease. Understanding the mechanisms by which apo E polymorphisms modulate risk for atherosclerosis, mortality, and morbidity, and the affects of apo E on the brain and lipoprotein metabolism may shed light on the role of environmental change, lifestyle, and genetics on longevity. Ethical issues related to genetic screening, employment, and health insurance will need to be addressed prior to widespread measurement and treatment based on the apo E genotype in clinical practice.

Elevated Lipoprotein (a)

Lipoprotein (a) is a cholesterol-rich lipoprotein particle similar to LDL in which apolipoprotein (a) is covalently bonded to apo B. The genetic locus for apolipoprotein (a) is polymorphic and there are a large number of genetically determined isoforms of Lp(a). Genetic studies indicate that Lp(a) concentration is highly heritable, and one study estimated that 98% of the variance in Lp(a) concentration could be explained by the Apolipoprotein (a) locus. As a result, Lp(a) concentration is essentially constant across the life span. The pathogenicity of Lp(a) is attributed in part to the strong homology of apolipoprotein (a) and plasminogen, thereby providing a link between atherosclerosis and thrombosis. The Atherosclerosis Risk in Communities (ARIC) study showed that over a 10-year period, Lp (a) along with LDL-C, HDL-C, HDL_3-C, and TG concentrations were independent predictors of CHD events in middle-aged subjects, whereas apo B, apo A-I, and HDL_2-C were not. Lp(a) concentration was higher in subjects who developed CHD, but added only a small predictive value to that provided by LDL-C, HDL-C, and TG, and was not a predictor in black men. In a cohort of 5732 subjects aged 70 to 82 years enrolled in the prospective study of pravastatin in the elderly at risk PROSPER study, Lp(a) concentration was associated with a small increased risk of vascular disease over a period of 3 years. Niacin lowers the Lp(a) concentration, but other lipid-lowering drugs, such as resins and fibrates, have minimal effects. There are contradictory reports of the effects of statins and estrogen replacement therapy on Lp(a) concentrations.

Knowledge of a patient's Lp(a) concentration might provide the clinician with additional insight into the patient's risk for CHD, complementing the information provided by the standard lipoprotein profile. Unfortunately, there is no universally accepted standardization program for Lp(a) assays, thus limiting its utility because of the lack of reproducibility and reliability of measurement.

Summary

Despite impressive advances in our understanding of the pathogenesis of atherosclerosis, there are several ongoing questions to be resolved concerning the lipoprotein risk factors for CHD in the elderly population: (1) Do lipoprotein subfractions (Lp (a), LDL, HDL) predict CHD morbidity and mortality, as well as total mortality? (2) Should the interpretation of a given lipoprotein concentration take into account the age of the patient? (3) Does longitudinal measurement of lipoprotein concentrations improve prediction of CHD? (4) Would genetic screening for high CHD risk-associated polymorphisms identify individuals for whom early therapy might reduce CHD risk and prolong survival? and (5) What role should the noninvasive measurements of atherosclerotic plaque or calcium score have in the assessment of cardiovascular risk and treatment?

INTERVENTION TRIALS

Multiple clinical trials have assessed the effect of lowering LDL-C concentration on CHD and total mortality, and are summarized in Table 110-1. These studies demonstrate that treatment of hyper-

cholesterolemia in high-risk older adults aged 65 to 80 years with statins reduces CHD death rates. Collectively, these intervention studies support the use of statins in older individuals below the age of 80 years, particularly in those with prevalent CHD or CHD equivalents. Definitive evidence supporting treatment for those 80 years old and older is limited, and the ATP III recommends using good clinical judgment.

PRESENTATION

Dyslipoproteinemia is often diagnosed in asymptomatic individuals as part of a routine health maintenance evaluation for individuals with other risk factors for CVD. The primary clinical manifestations of dyslipoproteinemia are those related to symptomatic CVD. Physical findings directly related to dyslipidemia are relatively infrequent in elderly patients and include the development of yellowish nodules of fat, xanthomas or xanthelasmas, in the skin beneath eyes (xanthelamas palpebrarum), or overlying elbows, knees, and tendons.

Moderate elevations of TG may lead to fatty liver and pancreatitis and higher levels are linked to eruptive xanthomas over the trunk, back, elbows, buttocks, knees, hands, and feet. Severe hypertriglyceridemia (>2000 mg/dL) can give retinal arteries and veins a creamy white appearance (lipemia retinalis). Some forms of hyperlipidemia can lead to an enlarged liver and spleen, manifesting in discomfort or tenderness in the upper abdomen, and patients with the rare dysbetalipoproteinemia can have palmar and tuberous xanthomas.

EVALUATION

The NCEP recommends that all patients older than 20 years of age undergo lipid testing at least every 5 years. There is no defined upper age limit for this testing. The ATP III guidelines recommend a more comprehensive assessment, including measurements of fasting total cholesterol, LDL-C, HDL-C, and TG. If any of these concentrations are abnormal, the physician should evaluate the patient for causes of secondary dyslipidemia. These secondary causes include obesity, diabetes mellitus, hypothyroidism, obstructive liver disease (primary biliary cirrhosis, etc), nephrotic syndrome, chronic renal failure, the use of certain drugs (see "Special Issues" section at the end of the chapter), alcohol consumption, and smoking. The measurement of thyroid function is of particular importance in older subjects, as clinically silent hypothyroidism may occur with associated secondary dyslipidemia. In patients referred to a lipid clinic for hyperlipidemia, 3% had overt hypothyroidism and 4% had subclinical hypothyroidism.

The screening of older individuals, particularly those without overt CVD for dyslipoproteinemia, and the treatment of hyperlipidemia in older individuals remain controversial because of the paucity of data in older patients >80 years and in ethnic minority populations. The arguments for and against the treatment of hyperlipidemia in elderly patients are summarized in Table 110-2. The reader is referred to the May 2005 issue of the *Journal of Gerontology* for further discussion of the pros and cons of pharmacological therapy and interpretation of the NCEP III guidelines in the elderly population.

The foregoing arguments need to be viewed in the context of several secular changes. First, all the published screening guidelines

TABLE 110-1

Summary of Randomized Clinical Trials of Treatment of Dyslipidemia

TRIAL	POPULATION		INTERVENTION	OUTCOME	
	Characteristics	n		LDL	Comments
Scandinavian Simvastatin Survival Study (4S)	h/o Angina/MI TC 5.5–8mmol/L TG < 2.5 mmol/L	4444 ♂/♀ aged 50–75 yr	Dietary counseling ± Simvastatin (20 mg titrated to TC response)	25% reduction	Significantly reduced major coronary events and mortality—similarly in those younger than and 65 yr or older in age; 43% reduction in CHD mortality for those aged 65 yr or older
Pravastatin Limitations of Atherosclerosis in the Coronary Arteries (PLAC I)	h/o CAD and 130 ≤ LDL < 190 despite an AHA step I diet	408 ♂/♀ aged 50–75 yr	40 mg Pravastatin versus Placebo	28% reduction	Significantly reduced progression of atherosclerosis as well as incidence of coronary events—similarly in those younger than and 65 yr or older in age
Pravastatin, Lipids, and Atherosclerosis in the Carotid Arteries (PLAC II)	h/o CAD + diet-resistant elevated LDL	151 ♂/♀ aged 50–75 yr	Pravastatin (20 mg titrated to LDL response) versus Placebo	28% reduction	
Cholesterol and Recurrent Events (CARE)	h/o MI and baseline TC < 240, 115 < LDL < 175, TG < 350 mg/dL	4159 ♂/♀ aged 21–75 yr	40 mg Pravastatin versus Placebo	32% reduction	Reduced major coronary events and stroke in those 65–75 yr
West of Scotland Coronary Prevention Study (WOSCOPS)	LDL ≥154 despite dietary therapy, no h/o MI	6595 ♂ aged 45–64 yr	40 mg Pravastatin versus Placebo	26% reduction	Reduced cardiac endpoints to a greater extent, 31%, than would be predicted by its reduction of LDL-C
Medical Research Council/British Heart Foundation Heart Protection Study (HPS)	h/o DM, PVD, or CHD	20,536 ♂/♀ aged 40–80 yr	40 mg Simvastatin versus Placebo	44% reduction	Significant benefit on major vascular events irrespective of initial cholesterol levels and proportional across the age span
Prospective Study of Pravastatin in the Elderly at Risk (PROSPER)	h/o vascular disease or at high risk for CHD caused by HTN, smoking, or DM	5804 ♂/♀ aged 70–82 yr	40 mg Pravastatin versus Placebo	34% reduction	Significant reductions in major coronary events by 15%; no effect on stroke
The Reversal of Atherosclerosis with Aggressive Lipid Lowering (REVERSAL)	CAD and 125 < LDL < 210 after washout period	651 ♂/♀ aged 30–75 yr	40 mg of Pravastatin versus 80 mg of Atorvastatin	Pravastatin → 27% reduction Atorvastatin → 47% reduction	Both decreased atheroma volume. Greater benefit from Atorvastatin seen only among older individuals
Treating to New Targets (TNT)	Clinically evident CHD	10001 ♂/♀ aged 35–75 yr	Atorvastatin 10 mg versus 80 mg/day	35% reduction with 10 mg; additional 20% with 80 mg	Significantly greater reductions in the composite end point of death from CHD, nonfatal MI, resuscitation after cardiac arrest and stroke
Long-Term Intervention with Pravastatin in Ischemic Disease (LIPID)	h/o MI or hospitalization for USA and 155 < TC < 271	9014 ♂/♀ aged 31–75 yr	Dietary counseling ± 40 mg Pravastatin	18% reduction	Significantly reduced mortality by 21% as well as cardiovascular outcomes (MI death from CHD, stroke, coronary revascularization) with similar relative effects in older and younger patients
Pravastatin or Atorvastatin Evaluation and Infection Therapy (PROVE IT-TIMI22)	Recently hospitalized for ACS, TC ≤ 240	4162 ♂/♀ mean age 58 ± 11 yr	400 mg Gatifloxacin + 40 mg Pravastatin or 80 mg Atorvastatin	Pravastatin→ 10% Atorvastatin→42% reduction	Lower risk of recurrent MI or vascular death
Study Assessing Goals in the Elderly (SAGE)	Patients with CHD with evidence of ischemia on ambulatory monitoring	893 ♂/♀ aged 65–85 yr	80 mg Atorvastatin versus 40 mg Pravastatin	Pravastatin→ 32% Atorvastatin→56% reduction	Substantial reduction in ischemic burden on ambulatory monitoring in both groups, lower all cause mortality in Atorvastatin versus Simvastatin

TABLE 110-2

Considerations of Factors For and Against Treatment of Hyperlipidemia in the Elderly Patient

Factors favoring treatment of hyperlipidemia

CHD is the most common cause of death in old age

Attributable risk increases with age

Atherosclerosis is pathologically indistinguishable in elderly and middle-aged persons

Hypolipidemic drugs appear to be as efficacious in elderly persons as in middle-aged persons

Numerous clinical trials of lipid-lowering therapy found substantial reductions in cardiac morbidity and mortality in people age 65–80 yr

Factors against treatment of hyperlipidemia

Lack of evidence that primary or secondary prevention decreases CHD morbidity and mortality in individuals older than age 80 yr.

Drug side effects maybe greater

There maybe a lag time (2 yr) between the initiation of therapy and the reduction of morbidity and mortality from CHD

Cost for elderly persons on fixed incomes with limited insurance

The presence of other multiple comorbid diseases might limit life span or the quality of life

Polypharmacy and risk of drug side effects

---

assume that the clinician is faced with a de novo decision of whether the elderly patient should be screened for hyperlipidemia, when most of these individuals have had prior evaluations in middle-age or earlier. Indeed, cholesterol profiles are routinely obtained as part of the automated battery of laboratory tests in patients admitted to the hospital, and widespread cholesterol screening has occurred over the past 25 years. Thus most older individuals, particularly those at risk or with CVD, have already had multiple measurements of their lipid concentrations. Therefore, whether or not to screen de novo is often a moot point.

Second, given secular increases in the use of hypolipidemic drugs for both the primary and secondary prevention of CHD in middle-aged and older individuals, an increasing number of older patients presenting to the geriatrician will already be on lipid-lowering medications. For these patients, the geriatrician will have to decide on the appropriateness of continuing therapy. It will be difficult to discontinue medications in older patients with overt CVD and in those with multiple risk factors for CVD, unless there are compelling reasons.

Third, there is growing emphasis on maintaining or increasing functional independence and quality of life in the elderly. The prevention of coronary or vascular events that contribute to disability in the elderly must be factored into any decision related to the screening and treatment of hypercholesterolemia in the elderly. Some of the pharmacologic agents appear to have beneficial effects independent of their lipid-lowering effects. For example, statins may have antioxidant properties and have been associated with improvement in endothelial function, improved nitric oxide metabolism, and reduced inflammation. Some cross-sectional and epidemiological studies suggest that statin users have a lower prevalence of Alzheimer's disease than nonstatin users. Two completed studies demonstrate that the decline in cognitive function in older adults is significantly slower in patients treated with statins than in control groups. However, more recent randomized clinical trials do not demonstrate that statins cause a reduction in the incidence of Alzheimer's disease. Thus, some clinicians will place older patients on statins hoping for the secondary (pleiotropic) benefits despite a lack of convincing evidence that the therapy will be efficacious.

Fourth, the results of the PROSPER, HPS, and other studies (see Table 110-1) support the use of pharmacological interventions for the secondary prevention of CVD in older individuals up to the age of 80 years. We know of no definitive data demonstrating a lack of effectiveness among older individuals (>80 years). Delaying evidence-based preventive therapy while awaiting definitive studies maybe untenable in those living independently despite the cost.

Finally, the question of when and in which patients to pharmacologically intervene will be influenced by the development of new pharmacologic agents that target the underlying mechanisms of CVD. A multitude of new agents are currently in development and are undergoing clinical trials. New agents, including inhibitors of microsomal triglyceride transfer protein (MTP) that decrease the secretion of apo B containing proteins by the liver, may play a role, either alone or in combination, in the treatment of dyslipoproteinemia.

MANAGEMENT

Risk-Stratified Approach to Lipid Treatment

The approach to the management of hyperlipidemia in older persons (men ≥ 65 years; women ≥ 75 years) was extensively modified in the NCEP ATP III Report in 2001, and updated again in 2004. This report recommends the calculation of the Framingham Risk Score (http://hp2010.nhlbihin.net/atpiii/riskcalc.htm) as the primary means of identifying older persons at increased risk for coronary events. Based on the overall Framingham Risk Score, people are stratified into four main risk categories: high-risk, moderately high-risk, moderate risk, and low risk, with a portion of the high-risk patients being designated as very high risk. There are different treatment recommendations and therapeutic goals for the different risk categories with the most aggressive therapy directed at patients with the highest risk. Table 110-3 summarizes the ATP III updated risk categories.

Older people who have no risk factors other than their age with an absolute 10-year risk <10% are considered at low-risk. There is considerable controversy concerning the management of hyperlipidemia in older individuals who have no risk factors other than their age. For individuals in this risk category, the LDL-C goal is <160 mg/dL. According to the update, the absolute benefits for people at the lower levels of risk are less clear-cut and the recent clinical trials do not suggest a modification of treatment goals and cut points. The ATP III update emphasizes that therapeutic lifestyle changes, that is, diets low in saturated and *trans* fat, increased physical activity, and weight control are advocated for lowering cholesterol concentrations. The ATP III guidelines for pharmacological treatment in people at low risk have not changed the LDL concentration at which drug therapy should be considered, i.e., ≥160 mg/dL. However, many clinicians have taken a more aggressive therapeutic approach in older individuals in this category and have begun lipid-lowering therapy with statins to reduce LDL-C below 100 mg/dL.

TABLE 110-3

ATP III LDL-C Goals and Cut Points for TLC and Drug Therapy in Different Risk Categories and Proposed Modifications Based on Clinical Trial Evidence

RISK CATEGORY	LDL-C GOAL	INITIATE TLC	CONSIDER DRUG THERAPY*
High risk: CHD[†] or CHD risk equivalents[‡] (10-yr risk >20%)	<100 mg/dL (optional goal: <70 mg/dL)[§]	≥100 mg/dL[¶]	≥100 mg/dL** (<100 mg/dL: consider drug options)*
Moderately high risk: 2+ risk factors[‡] (10-yr risk 10–20%)[††]	<130 mg/dL[‡‡]	≥130 mg/dL[§]	≥130 mg/dL (100–129 mg/dL; consider drug options)[§§]
Moderate risk: 2+ risk factors[¶¶] (10-yr risk <10%)[††]	<130 mg/dL	≥130 mg/dL	≥160 mg/dL
Lower risk: 0–1 risk factor***	<160 mg/dL	≥160 mg/dL	≥190 mg/dL (160–189 mg/dL: LDL-lowering drug optional)

*When LDL-lowering drug therapy is employed, it is advised that intensity of therapy be sufficient to achieve at least a 30% to 40% reduction in LDL-C concentrations.

[†]CHD includes history of myocardial infarction, unstable angina, stable angina, coronary artery procedures (angioplasty or bypass surgery), or evidence of clinically significant myocardial ischemia.

[‡]CHD risk equivalents include clinical manifestations of noncoronary forms of atherosclerotic disease (peripheral arterial disease, abdominal aortic aneurysm, and carotid artery disease [transient ischemic attacks or stroke of carotid origin or >50% obstruction of a carotid artery]), diabetes, and 2+ risk factors with 10-yr risk for hard CHD >20%.

[§]Very high risk favors the optional LDL-C goal of <70 mg/dL, and in patients with high triglycerides, non-HDL-C <100 mg/dL.

[¶]Any person at high risk or moderately high risk who has lifestyle-related risk factors (e.g., obesity, physical inactivity, elevated triglyceride, low HDL-C, or metabolic syndrome) is a candidate for therapeutic lifestyle changes to modify these risk factors regardless of LDL-C concentration.

**If baseline LDL-C is <100 mg/dL, institution of an LDL-lowering drug is a therapeutic option on the basis of available clinical trial results. If a high-risk person has high triglycerides or low HDL-C, combining a fibrate or nicotinic acid with an LDL-lowering drug can be considered.

[††] Electronic 10-yr risk calculators are available at www.nhlbi.nih.gov/guidelines/cholesterol.

[‡‡]Optional LDL-C goal <100 mg/dL.

[§§]For moderately high-risk persons, when LDL-C concentration is 100 to 129 mg/dL, at baseline or on lifestyle therapy, initiation of an LDL-lowering drug to achieve an LDL-C concentration <100 mg/dL is a therapeutic option on the basis of available clinical trial results.

[¶¶]Risk factors include cigarette smoking, hypertension (BP ≥140/90 mm Hg or on antihypertensive medication), low HDL-C (<40 mg/dL), family history of premature CHD (CHD in male first-degree relative <55 yr of age; CHD in female first-degree relative <65 yr of age), and age (men ≥45 yr; women ≥55 yr).

***Almost all people with zero or 1 risk factor have a 10-yr risk <10%, and 10-yr risk assessment in people with zero or 1 risk factor is thus not necessary.

From Grundy SM, Cleeman JI, Merz CN, et al.; Coordinating Committee of the National Cholesterol Education Program. Implications of recent clinical trials for the National Cholesterol Education Program Adult Treatment Panel III guidelines. Arterioscler Thromb Vasc Biol.2004;24(8):e149–e161.

It is important to recognize that the relative risk of hyperlipidemia for CHD is lower in the elderly than in younger people because of competing causes of mortality and cumulative effects of comorbid diseases. However, because of both the high absolute risk in the elderly and the high attributable risk for CHD events, a given therapeutic treatment such as statin therapy will prevent a greater number of events in older than in younger people. Based on CARE (Cholesterol and Recurrent Events) data, Lewis and colleagues estimated that 225 cardiac events would be prevented for every 1000 older (>65 years) CHD patients with baseline cholesterol concentration <240 mg/dL treated with statin therapy for 5 years compared to 121 events prevented in younger patients. Twenty-seven fatal CHD events would be prevented per 1000 patients older than 65 years of age treated for 5 years with a statin. By contrast, only 11 fatal CHD events would be prevented in a comparable number of younger people with CHD treated for the same period of time. ATP III estimates that the number needed to treat (NNT) with statin therapy at age 65 years with the aim of preventing CHD events at age 80 years is only 10 for a 65-year-old person with a 10-year risk for hard CHD endpoint of 10%. The NNT for 65-year-old patient with a 20% 10-year risk for hard CHD endpoint is 5. Thus, the elderly with CHD and those with multiple risk factors would be expected to particularly benefit from pharmacologic therapy because of their high absolute and attributable risk.

There are a number of limitations to applying the Framingham Risk Score to older adults. Factors that increase the short-term risk for CHD are well known. However, the effect of risk factors on long-term risk are less clear, particularly at older ages because of the competing risks for non-CHD death. The usefulness of blood-based biomarkers beyond a standard lipid panel (e.g., LDL particle size, insulin, high sensitivity CRP, homocysteine, apolipoproteins,

etc.) and structural markers of subclinical diseases (such as extent of coronary atherosclerosis using the surrogate marker of coronary artery calcium assessed by computed tomography (CT) scan, increased carotid artery intimae medial thickness) to guide therapy needs further evaluation in the elderly population.

Therapeutic Lifestyle Intervention

Diets reduced in saturated fat and cholesterol and increased in fiber and complex carbohydrate content, weight loss, and regular aerobic exercise (Therapeutic Lifestyle Changes) are widely advocated for the initial treatment of hyperlipidemia. To reduce LDL-C, the American Heart Association and the American Diabetes Association recommend the following dietary composition: saturated fats should be <7% of energy intake; dietary cholesterol should be <200 mg/day; intake of trans-unsaturated fatty acids should be <1% of energy intake; total energy intake should be adjusted to achieve body-weight goals; total dietary fat should be moderated (25–35% of total calories) and should consist mainly of monounsaturated or polyunsaturated fat; dietary fiber should be >14 g per calories consumed; salt intake should be 1200 to 2300 mg/day; and alcohol intake should be moderate (limited to 1 drink per day in women and 2 drinks in men).

In obese individuals, moderate weight loss in combination with aerobic exercise will decrease total cholesterol and LDL-C concentrations by 10% to 15%, increase HDL-C by 15%, improve glucose tolerance, and lower blood pressure. Moreover, the lipid lowering response to lifestyle interventions is related to the initial lipoprotein profiles and probably selected gene polymorphisms. Individuals with the highest baseline cholesterol concentrations show the greatest improvements with weight loss and AHA diet interventions. However, the beneficial effects of low fat diets in reducing total and LDL-C concentrations maybe tempered by reductions in HDL-C. Without concomitant weight loss, the ratio of LDL-C to HDL-C may actually increase, not decrease when individuals are placed on diets low in saturated fat and cholesterol. This suggests that high carbohydrate diets might not be optimal for older women in whom HDL-C concentrations are a major determinant of CHD risk, but the beneficial effects of reduced atherogenic LDL-C concentrations may outweigh any putative harmful effects of reductions in HDL-C. The addition of monounsaturated fats to the diet may prevent declines in HDL-C.

Increased physical activity is often advocated as a means to reduce CVD risk factors. However, the majority of this benefit is likely because of the accompanying weight loss. Weight loss and aerobic exercise results in improved lipoprotein concentrations (as well as glucose tolerance and blood pressure) in middle-aged and older women and men, whereas aerobic training without weight loss yields substantially less beneficial effects. Nonetheless, a complete lifestyle intervention of achieving and maintaining optimal weight in conjunction with aerobic activity is likely to lead to the greatest improvements in CVD risk factors as well as maximize the long-term maintenance of these improvements. We advocate lifestyle interventions consisting of the AHA Step I diet, moderate weight loss, and daily moderate intensity exercise for 30 min/d in older individuals with overt manifestations of atherosclerosis, or in higher risk asymptomatic individuals with multiple CHD risk factors.

Pharmacological Therapy

In many older patients with hyperlipidemia at risk for CHD, therapeutic lifestyle intervention does not effectively lower LDL-C to within the target range. Several classes of drugs are available to treat hyperlipidemia. The commonly used lipid-lowering agents, their anticipated therapeutic effects, and side effects are summarized in Table 110-4. We briefly review their mechanism of action below.

The clinician should consult package inserts and other pharmacologic resources to obtain the most up-to-date information before prescribing these medications. A large number of nutraceuticals and dietary supplements are also employed to improve lipoprotein profiles. Their use is beyond the scope of this chapter. For many older adults, monotherapy with a statin can safely achieve LDL-C target goals.

HMG-CoA Reductase Inhibitors (Statins)

Statins inhibit hepatic HMG-CoA reductase, the enzyme catalyzing the rate-limiting step in hepatic cholesterol synthesis, thereby reducing cholesterol production. This has several effects: upregulation of LDL receptors by hepatocytes and consequent increased removal of apo E- and B-containing lipoproteins from the circulation and a reduction in the synthesis and secretion of lipoproteins from the liver. Statins lower LDL-C and increase the removal and reduce the secretion of remnant particles, that is, VLDL and IDL (non-HDL-C). Therefore statins are effective in treating patients who have an elevation of both LDL-C and TG.

Fibrates

The fibrates decrease the production of VLDL and increase the clearance of triglyceride-rich lipoproteins. The latter is mediated by the peroxisome proliferator activated receptor (PPAR)-α and by an increase in lipoprotein lipase, a key enzyme in the clearance of TG-enriched particles. Fibrates also increase HDL-C and apo A-I. Fibrates are indicated in the treatment of patients with high TG and low HDL-C.

Bile Acid Sequestrants

Bile acid resins are generally considered second-line agents for the treatment of hypercholesterolemia. The bile acid sequestrants bind bile acids in the intestine, which reduces the enterohepatic recirculation of bile acids. This promotes the upregulation of the enzyme 7-α hydroxylase and the conversion of more cholesterol in the hepatocyte into bile acids. This decreases the cholesterol content in the hepatocyte, which enhances LDL-receptor expression. This leads to increased clearance of LDL and VLDL remnants from the circulation. However, this also results in an increased synthesis of cholesterol by the liver, thereby partially negating the LDL-C-lowering effects of the sequestrants. Caution is indicated in the use of the resins in patients with elevated TG as the resins may increase hepatic VLDL production, thereby raising TG levels.

Nicotinic Acid (niacin)

Nicotinic acid inhibits lipoprotein synthesis and decreases the production of VLDL particles by the liver. It inhibits the peripheral mobilization of free fatty acids, thus reducing hepatic synthesis of TG and the secretion of VLDL, reducing the number of LDL particles. Nicotinic acid increases the production of apo A-I, thereby raising HDL-C.

Ezetimibe

Ezetimibe is an inhibitor of intestinal cholesterol absorption. It reduces the amount of biliary and dietary cholesterol delivered to the liver and reduces the cholesterol content of atherogenic particles remnant particles, VLDL, and LDL. The reduced delivery of intestinal cholesterol to the liver increases hepatic LDL receptor activity and increases clearance of circulating LDL. Current clinical trials question the added CHD preventive value of adding ezetimibe to statin therapy.

PREVENTION

The risk-based algorithms of ATP-III and Framingham Risk Score focus on 10-year risk. Age has a substantial effect on predicting absolute risk, and many elderly patients exceed thresholds for treatment solely based on their age. Estimation of lifetime risk may provide a more useful conceptual framework for the primary prevention of CVD. In the Framingham Heart Study, among men free of prevalent CHD at age 50 years, the lifetime risk of developing CHD was 52%, with an estimated 39% lifetime risk in women. Factors associated with survival to age 85 years included female gender, lower total cholesterol, lower systolic blood pressure, better glucose tolerance, not smoking, and higher education levels. At the age 50 years, the lifetime risk for men with optimal CHD risk profile for developing CHD was 5% versus 69% of men with two or more risk factors. In women, those with optimal CHD risk profile had an 8% risk versus 50% risk in women with two or more risk factors. Median survival

TABLE 110-4

Pharmacological Therapy for Hyperlipidemia

Drug Class	Dose	Anticipated Effect	Comment
Statins (HMG CoA reductase inhibitors)			
Lovastatin	20–80 mg/day, take with evening meal, take bid if >20 mg/day	40 mg reduces LDL by 31%	Statins remain the drugs of first choice for lowering LDL. For the statins, for every doubling above the standard dose one can expect ~6% decrease in LDL Changes in HDL-C are usually modest, in the 5–10% range, and not consistently dose-related; increases in HDL-C are greater in patients with low HDL-C and elevated triglycerides.
Pravastatin	10–80 mg/day, take at bedtime	40 mg reduces LDL by 34%	Statins are very safe: 95% of patients can tolerate them; 5% cannot. Common side effects include headache, upset stomach, fatigue, flu-like symptoms, and myalgia
Simvastatin	5–80 mg/day	20–40 mg reduces LDL 35–41%	One or both liver transaminases maybe elevated to more than three times the upper limit of normal in 0.5% (with starting doses) to as high as 2.5% (with high doses) in a dose-dependent manner. Myopathy defined as muscle symptoms (muscle weakness, aches, or soreness) plus CK >10 times the upper limit of normal is seen in 2–4 patients per 1000.
Fluvastatin	20–80 mg/day, 80 mg SR, take bid if >40 mg/day	40–80 mg reduces LDL 25–35%	
Atorvastatin	10–80 mg/day	10 mg reduces LDL by 31%	
Rosuvastatin	5–40 mg/day	5–10 mg reduces LDL by 39–45%	Statins have moderate TG-lowering in the range of 10–35%; reduction is dependent on the baseline TG concentration (the higher the baseline concentration, the greater the reduction) and the dose of the statin; the reduction in TG is greatest with the more potent statins.
Cholesterol absorption inhibitors			
Ezetimibe	10 mg/day	When used in monotherapy reduces LDL by 15–20%, additive effect when used with statin	Avoid use with cyclosporine, gemfibrozil; increased transaminases when used in combination with statin. Current clinical trials question the added CHD preventive value of adding ezetimibe to statin therapy.
Bile acid sequestrants			
Cholestyramine	2–8 g bid with max of 24 g/d	LDL-C reduced in dose dependent manner, range of 15–30%. Resins may raise TG although this side effect appears to be less with colesevelam	Mix with water, take before meals. Serious side effects for these sequestrants include fecal impaction and a variety of GI symptoms; medications may also lead to a deficiency of fat-soluble vitamins and loss of calcium in the urine. Extensive drug–drug interactions (consult pharmacist).
Colestipol	5–30 g/d divided qd to qid		Take other drugs >1 h before or 4 h after colestipol.
Colesevelam	625 mg tabs, take 6–7 tabs PO qd		May reduce dose and take BID if combined with a HMG Co-A reductase inhibitor; take with meals.
Nicotinic acid			
Niacin (immediate, sustained, and extended release)	Regular release form 1.5–3 g/d divided bid or tid, extended release 1–2 g PO QHS	Reduces LDL by 15–25%. Niacin is the most effective drug available for raising HDL-C. 1 gm/d can raise HDL by 25%	Unfortunately there are substantial prostaglandin-mediated side effects including cutaneous flushing, headache, warm sensation, and pruritus; other side effects include hyperpigmentation, acanthosis nigricans, dry skin, nausea, vomiting, diarrhea, and myositis. ASA 325 mg taken before dose may decrease flushing; need to monitor liver function, glucose and uric acid; extended release also sold in combination with lovastatin.
Fibrates			
Gemfibrozil	600 mg bid 30 min before morning and evening meal	Reduce TG by 25–50%, raise HDL by 15–25% with variable effect on LDL, range –5% to –20%. Can raise LDL in some patients	Drug class of choice for high TG, low HDL. Side effects include myositis, stomach upset, sun sensitivity, gallstones, irregular heartbeat, and liver damage. Contraindicated with ezetimbe/simvastatin; multiple other drug interactions (consult pharmacist).
Fenofibrate	Start 48 mg PO qd with max of 145 mg PO qd		Consider decreasing dose if lipids fall well below target; monitor CBC and LFTs periodically.
Clofibrate	1000 mg bid	Lowers LDL and HDL, rarely used	Clinical trials in 1970s and 1980s showed an increase in all-cause mortality, death from heart disease stroke and cancer in patients with clofibrate; Use is reserved for patients who fail other therapies; used for type III, IV, and V hyperlipidemia.

Data from multiple sources including Grundy SM, Cleeman JI, Merz CN, et al.; Coordinating Committee of the National Cholesterol Education Program. Implications of recent clinical trials for the National Cholesterol Education Program Adult Treatment Panel III guidelines. Arterioscler Thromb Vasc Biol.2004;24(8):e149–e161; McKenney JM. Selecting successful lipid-lowering treatments. http://www.lipidsonline.org/slides/slides.

was >11 years longer and 8 years longer, respectively, in men and women with optimal CHD risk factors. This suggests that there are impressive long-term benefits from optimal control of CVD risk factors.

The use of pharmacologic therapy to prevent CVD in older adults without prevalent CHD (true primary prevention of CVD) remains controversial (see review by Abramson). There is little clinical trial data to support statin therapy in older adults without prevalent CHD. Our position is that lifestyle intervention, particularly exercise training combined with weight loss, is beneficial to improve quality of life and function in older adults and should be universally recommended. Weight loss and medical nutrition therapy is particularly beneficial in individuals with the metabolic syndrome. The restriction of saturated fats, *trans*-unsaturated fats, and the inclusion of increased dietary fiber are recommended to improve lipids. Some would also advocate increasing monounsaturated and polyunsaturated fat in the diet and increased intake of omega three oils. For primary prevention of CVD in older adults, the horse is already out of the barn; about three quarters of older adults on statins are taking them for primary prevention. We advocate the noninvasive assessment of structural markers of arterial vulnerability (carotid intimal-medial thickness, assessment of coronary artery calcium) and functional markers of arterial vulnerability to identify older adults with evidence of subclinical disease who may particularly benefit from aggressive pharmacologic intervention. We recognize that a lack of standardization of these measures, paucity of clinical trial data supporting their use in primary prevention in older adults, and costs associated with these tests and subsequent evaluations for abnormal findings and incidental findings may limit their clinical utility.

SPECIAL ISSUES

Secondary Dyslipidemias Caused By Medications

A number of medications commonly used in older adults can adversely affect lipid profiles. Although diuretics and beta-blockers can adversely affect serum lipids, the beneficial effects of these medications on blood pressure outweigh their adverse effects. The effect of steroid hormones on lipoprotein lipids varies with the drug, dose, and route of administration. In general, anabolic steroids lower HDL-C and have a variable effect on LDL-C. The effects of progestins vary greatly depending on their androgenicity, and estrogens can cause hypertriglyceridemia. Glucocorticoids raise HDL-C, TG, and LDL-C. Retinoids increase TG and LDL-C and also reduce HDL-C. Interferons can cause hypertriglyceridemia. Medications used to prevent rejection following organ transplantation such as cyclosporine and CellCept (mycophenolate mofetil) can also cause dyslipidemia that may result in accelerated atherosclerosis. Antiretroviral therapy for human immunodeficiency virus (HIV), particularly protease inhibitors, can cause dyslipidemia characterized by elevated TG and LDL-C and other metabolic abnormalities (lipodystrophy syndrome) that increase risk for atherosclerosis.

Diabetic Dyslipoproteinemia and Metabolic Syndrome

Type 2 diabetes mellitus is a common condition in older adults and is a substantial risk for CVD (see Chapter 109). Diabetes is now considered a CAD equivalent for setting treatment goals because of the high long-term risk for the development of CAD, as well as increased risk for CVD events and subsequent morbidity and complications. Thus, older diabetes patients should have lipid, blood pressure and other CAD risk factors aggressively treated to target levels prescribed for patients with documented CAD. Furthermore, glucose toxicity affects coronary risk in older people with diabetes, and hyperglycemia is associated with a heightened incidence of silent ischemia during exercise stress testing.

Type 2 diabetes is commonly associated with dyslipidemia, characterized by hypertriglyceridemia, reduced HDL-C, a predominance of small-dense LDL particles, increased concentrations of apo B, and the accumulation of cholesterol-rich remnant particles, especially postprandially. The treatment of hyperlipidemia in T2DM is effective in reducing cardiovascular endpoints. Studies using statins (e.g., Heart Protection Study, 4S Study, Collaborative Atorvastatin Diabetes Study) all showed substantial 25% to 30% reductions in coronary events. However, most patients with T2DM have elevated TG and low HDL-C, lipoprotein lipids that are only modestly affected by statins. The results of the HHS, Veterans Affairs High Density Lipoprotein Intervention Trial (VA-HIT), the Bezafibrate Infarction Prevention Study (BIP), and the Fenofibrate Intervention and Event Lowering in Diabetes (FIELD) studies were inconsistent. Several additional large-scale clinical trials are underway to further examine the effects of lipid-lowering therapy on CVD events in diabetes. Pending their outcomes, we recommend statins to reduce total and LDL-C and raise HDL-C; however, when lifestyle changes and statins do not increase HDL-C to goal, we suggest the addition of niacin. Fenofibrate effectively lowers triglyceride and raises HDL-C in persons with hypertriglyceridemia, but we do not recommend combined therapy with statins because of the increased risk for myopathy in elderly patients.

There is a strong association between T2DM and manifestations of the metabolic syndrome, a constellation of risk factors associated with central obesity that cluster and promote accelerated arthrosclerosis and vascular complications. Described originally in 1988 by Reaven to include insulin resistance, glucose intolerance, hyperinsulinemia, increased TG, decreased HDL-C, and hypertension, many now consider inflammation, microalbuminuria, small dense LDL particles, dysfibrinolysis and coagulopathy, nonalcoholic fatty liver disease, and central adiposity to components of the syndrome. However, the NCEP, World Health Organization, and International Diabetes Federation criteria define multiple phenotypes based on cutoffs for blood pressure, glucose, waist circumference, HDL, and TG levels. Three of the components, hyperglycemia, high TG, and large waist, have variable associations with vascular events and are more closely predictive of T2DM. Furthermore, the metabolic syndrome criteria do not include LDL-C, cigarette smoking, or age, three important risk factors for vascular events. In addition, no underlying metabolic cause seems pathogenic for this syndrome, as there are many subjects with the syndrome who are not insulin-resistant. The notion that cut points for various risk factors are predictors of vascular events does not align itself with the dogma that risk factors have a linear and progressive association with CVD. Until there is greater uniformity and agreement on the components and cut points for the metabolic syndrome that define CVD risk, there is no clear rationale to cluster the vascular risk factors when prescribing treatment. As obesity approaches epidemic proportions in western society, the prevalence of T2DM will likely increase proportionately. We advocate aggressive risk factor modification that includes therapeutic lifestyle changes and physical activity to modify obesity, as well as pharmacological interventions for each component of the metabolic syndrome as indicated. Future advances in pharmacogenetics and therapeutics are likely to produce novel therapies for T2DM and the metabolic syndrome.

Hypocholesterolemia

The prevalence of hypocholesterolemia (typically defined as total cholesterol concentrations <160 mg/dL, sixth percentile Multiple Risk Factor Intervention Trial (MRFIT)], increases with age. A "J"-shaped relationship between cholesterol and mortality is reported in some studies, suggesting that hypocholesterolemic individuals are at increased risk of death. Any examination of the association between low cholesterol and morbidity or mortality can be confounded by the presence of active or subclinical/occult disease, such as chronic infection and inflammation, cancer, chronic involuntary weight loss, diabetes, and chronic obstructive pulmonary disorder (COPD). These diseases may either suppress hepatic cholesterol synthesis or accelerate cholesterol catabolism. This bias potentially can be eliminated by the longitudinal analysis of cohort data after excluding individuals with early deaths (who may have had an undiagnosed disease). Such studies, in a variety of populations, have revealed correlations of low cholesterol with nutritional and functional status, as well as mini-mental examination scores.

Data from the Framingham cohort reveals a relationship between total cholesterol and both coronary heart disease and all-cause mortality that is positive until around the seventh decade of life, when the relationships start to become negative. Biologically plausible mechanisms linking low total cholesterol to death include alterations in cell membrane structure and function, abnormalities in steroid hormone metabolism, and fat-soluble vitamin deficiencies. In data pooled from 19 cohort studies, men and women with cholesterol concentrations <160 mg/dL were at a 40% to 50% higher risk for noncardiovascular deaths that occurred more than 5 years after baseline measurement than individuals with cholesterol concentrations of 200–239 mg/dL.

Low normal cholesterol concentrations and declining cholesterol concentrations maybe markers for increased morbidity and mortality, even in apparently healthy community-dwelling older people. In the Honolulu Heart Study, persistence of low cholesterol concentrations over 20 years was associated with increased risk of death. In that study, the earlier in life that the patients exhibited hypocholesterolemia, the greater the risk of death. In an attempt to clarify whether low cholesterol was a consequence of disease, or a result of some genetic or lifestyle factor, Iribarren et al. studied the relationship between the 6-year trend in total cholesterol and subsequent 16-year mortality, and found that declining total cholesterol levels were associated with an increased rate of both disease-specific and all-cause mortality: 30% higher among those with a decline from the middle to the lowest tertile. These findings raise questions about whether it is advisable to lower cholesterol concentrations below 180 mg/dL (4.65 mmol/L) in elderly people.

In evaluating an older patient with hypocholesterolemia, the geriatrician must consider both the pattern of change of cholesterol concentrations over time and their relationship with other diseases and events. Hypocholesterolemia maybe a marker for occult malignancy and other diseases that result in increased morbidity and mortality.

Unfortunately, there are no firm guidelines for the evaluation of patients with hypocholesterolemia. Some advocate the performance of routine cancer evaluations in otherwise healthy community-dwelling individuals with hypocholesterolemia, while others favor either more or less aggressive evaluation. Randomized clinical trials are needed to determine the efficacy of aggressive nutritional intervention in older patients with hypocholesterolemia.

Management of Dyslipidemia in the Nursing Home Setting

The management of dyslipidemia in extended care facilities remains controversial. There is limited data on the value of treating elevated cholesterol in this situation. In a retrospective cohort study utilizing the Health Care Financing Administration's Minimum Data Set, nursing home residents with an active clinical diagnosis of CVD on statins were 31% less likely to have died at 1 year after adjusting for a broad variety of potential confounders than similar nonusers. In that study, there was no significant effect of treatment on declining physical function. A low-cholesterol diet had no effect on cardiovascular or overall mortality among a broad group of institutionalized individuals. On the other hand, precipitously declining cholesterol is linked to a greater than sixfold adjusted relative odds for death compared to nursing home residents with stable or increasing cholesterol. Therefore, based on the limited available data, we do not advocate the routine treatment of hypercholesterolemia in debilitated nursing home patients, but rather suggest good clinical judgment in identifying patients in whom the potential benefit outweighs the risks of drug toxicity and treatment costs.

FURTHER READING

Abramson J, Wright JM. Are lipid-lowering guidelines evidence-based? *Lancet.* 2007;369(9557):168–169.

American Heart Association Nutrition Committee; Lichtenstein AH, Appel LJ, Brands M, et al. Diet and lifestyle recommendations revision 2006: a scientific statement from the American Heart Association Nutrition Committee. *Circulation.* 2006;4(114):82–96.

Aronow WS. Should the NCEP III guidelines be changed in elderly and younger persons at high risk for cardiovascular events? *J Gerontol Med Sci.* 2005;60A:591–592.

Aronow WS. Managing hyperlipidemia in the elderly. Special considerations for a population at high risk. *Drugs Aging.* 2006;23:181–189.

Carroll MD, Lacher DA, Sorlie PD, et al. Trends in serum lipids and lipoproteins of adults, 1960–2002. *JAMA.* 2005;294:1773–1781.

Expert Panel on Detection, Evaluation, and Treatment of High Blood Cholesterol in Adults. Executive Summary of The Third Report of The National Cholesterol Education Program (NCEP) Expert Panel on Detection, Evaluation, And Treatment of High Blood Cholesterol In Adults (Adult Treatment Panel III). *JAMA.* 2001;285(19):2486–2497.

Grundy SM, Cleeman JI, Merz CN, et al.; Coordinating Committee of the National Cholesterol Education Program. Implications of recent clinical trials for the National Cholesterol Education Program adult Treatment Panel III guidelines. *Arterioscler Thromb Vasc Biol.* 2004;24(8):e149–e161.

Heart Disease and Stroke Statistics—2007 Update. A report from the American Heart Association Statistics Committee and Stroke Statistics subcommittee. *Circulation.* 2007;115:

Heart Protection Collaborative Group. MRC/BHF Heart Protection Study of cholesterol lowering with simvastatin in 20536 high-risk individuals; a randomized placebo-controlled trial. *Lancet.* 2002;360:7–22.

Heiss G, Tamin I, Davis CE, et al. Lipoprotein–cholesterol distributions in selected North American Populations: The Lipid Research Clinics Program Prevalence Study. *Circulation.* 1980;61:302–315.

Kolovou GD, Anagnostopoulou KK. Apolipoprotein E polymorphism, age and coronary heart disease. *Ageing Res Rev.* 2007;6:94–106.

Lloyd-Jones DM, Leip EP, Larson MG, et al. Prediction of lifetime risk of cardiovascular disease by risk factor burden age 50 years of age. *Circulation.* 2006;113:791–798.

Malenka DJ, Baron JA. Cholesterol and Coronary Heart Disease. The importance of patient-specific attributable risk. *Arch Intern Med.* 1988;148:2247–2252.

McKenney JM. Selecting successful lipid-lowering treatments. http://www.lipidson line.org/slides/slide01.cfm?tk=23. August 26, 2008.

Miller NE. Why does plasma low density lipoprotein concentration in adults increase with age? *Lancet.* 1984;263–266.

Packard CJ, Ford I, Robertson M, et al.; PROSPER Study Group. Plasma lipoproteins and apolipoproteins as predictors of cardiovascular risk and treatment benefit in the PROspective Study of Pravastain in the Elderly at Risk (PROSPER). *Circulation.* 2005;112:3058–3065.

Rizzo M, Berneis K. The clinical relevance of low-density-lipoproteins size modulations by statins. *Cardiovasc Drug Ther.* 2006;20:205–217.

Sacks FM, Tonkin AM, Shepherd J, et al. Effect of pravastatin on coronary disease events in subgroups defined by coronary risk factors: the Prospective Pravastatin Pooling Project. *Circulation.* 2000;102:1893–1900.

Vasan RS. Biomarkers of cardiovascular disease. Molecular basis and practical considerations. *Circulation.* 2006;113:2335–2362.

Wilson PWF, D'Agostino RB, Levy D, Belanger AM, Silbershatz H, Kannel WB. Prediction of coronary heart disease using risk factor categories. *Circulation.* 1998;97:1837–1847.

Hyperparathyroidism and Paget's Disease of Bone

Kenneth W. Lyles

HYPERPARATHYROIDISM

Background and Epidemiology

Hyperparathyroidism is a common disorder of calcium, phosphorus, and bone metabolism caused by increased circulating levels of parathyroid hormone (PTH). This disease is important to geriatricians because it occurs with increasing frequency in older patients. Widespread use of multiphasic biochemical screening tests led to an increase in the incidence of cases of primary hyperparathyroidism. In the population in Olmstead County, Minnesota, which is served by the Mayo Clinic, the annual incidence rose from 16 per 100,000 people before 1978 to a peak of 112 per 100,000 people 7 years later, then the rate declined. Now such screening tests are used less frequently and the incidence has fallen to 4 per 100,000 people. It is not clear why the incidence of hyperparathyroidism is decreasing, but it is postulated that there is a decreased exposure to ionizing radiation, or better supplementation with vitamin D.

Primary hyperparathyroidism may occur at any age but is found most commonly between the ages of 40 and 65 years. The incidence is approximately 1 per 1000. The disease affects women more than men by almost 2:1, and in women, this usually occurs in the first decade after menopause. In the United States, approximately 80% of patients with primary hyperparathyroidism have no signs or symptoms that are referable to their disease. With the development of sophisticated and specific technologies during the past 15 years, it has become feasible to evaluate patients with asymptomatic primary hyperparathyroidism in ways that have helped to establish prudent guidelines for surgical or medical management.

In hyperparathyroidism, PTH is inappropriately secreted by single or multiple glands in the presence of increased serum calcium levels. The disease is considered primary when autonomous hypersecretion of PTH is caused by a single adenoma, diffuse hyperplasia, multiple adenomas, or, rarely, a parathyroid carcinoma. Secondary hyperparathyroidism occurs when there is a prolonged hypocalcemic stimulus, as in cases of vitamin D deficiency or chronic renal failure. Tertiary hyperparathyroidism occurs in patients with chronic secondary hyperparathyroidism who develop autonomous hypersecretion of PTH and hypercalcemia, e.g., patients who undergo successful kidney transplants. This chapter focuses on primary hyperparathyroidism only.

Etiology and Pathology

The etiology of primary hyperparathyroidism is unknown. When calcium is infused into hypercalcemic hyperparathyroid patients, there is a failure to suppress the PTH levels. Furthermore, when cells from hyperparathyroid glands are incubated in vitro, higher levels of ionized calcium in the medium are required to suppress PTH release than are required to suppress PTH release from cells from normal glands. These data suggest that, in part, the abnormality occurring in the parathyroid gland is an elevation of the set point at which ionized calcium levels suppress PTH release. The receptor that is responsible for calcium-sensing in parathyroid glands has been cloned; it is a guanosine triphosphate (GTP)-binding protein that has a seven-amino-acid transmembrane domain. Mutations in this receptor are rare in primary hyperparathyroidism.

In most cases of hyperparathyroidism, no etiologic agent can be identified; these represent sporadic cases. Previous neck exposure to ionizing radiation is associated with an increased incidence of hyperparathyroidism. Lithium, when used for therapy of bipolar disorders, is associated with hypercalcemia and increased PTH levels in up to 10% of patients. Thiazide diuretics can cause hypercalcemia, but the persistence of hypercalcemia 6 weeks after stopping a thiazide usually means the agent has unmasked primary hyperparathyroidism. A few causes of hyperparathyroidism, usually parathyroid hyperplasia, are familial disorders that have an autosomal dominant mode of transmission, such as (1) familial hyperparathyroidism, (2) multiple endocrine neoplasia type I (Werner's syndrome: hyperparathyroidism, islet cell tumors, and pituitary tumors), and (3) multiple endocrine neoplasia type II (Sipple's syndrome: medullary carcinoma of the thyroid, pheochromocytoma, and hyperparathyroidism). Only rarely does hyperparathyroidism occur in multiple endocrine neoplasia type IIB or III (medullary carcinoma of the thyroid, pheochromocytoma, mucosal neuromas, and marfanoid body habitus).

The pathologic abnormality in the parathyroid gland(s) maybe an adenoma, four-gland hyperplasia, multiple adenomas, or carcinoma. Single adenomas cause 80% of the cases of hyperparathyroidism. Hyperplasia of all four glands is found in 15% of cases; parathyroid carcinomas and multiple adenomas comprise the remainder. Determining whether a single gland is an adenoma or chief cell hyperplasia is often difficult to ascertain by histologic features alone, so the gross pathology seen at operation is necessary to classify the disease. An adenoma is diagnosed when only one abnormal gland is found (all other glands are normal). Chief cell hyperplasia is diagnosed when more than one abnormal gland is found. Controversy currently exists regarding whether it is possible to have multiple adenomas. In several studies, enlargement of only two glands was documented, with the remaining two being normal. A rarer form of parathyroid hyperplasia is called "water-clear cell" hyperplasia, in which large, membrane-lined vesicles fill the cytoplasm. Finally, parathyroid carcinoma is diagnosed by finding mitotic figures in the gland or finding capsular or vascular invasion in pathological specimens obtained during surgery.

Signs and Symptoms

Patients with primary hyperparathyroidism can present with a varying spectrum of signs and symptoms ranging from a total lack of symptoms to acute hypercalcemic crisis. The diagnosis is most frequently made by routine calcium measurements with multichannel screening chemistries in a patient with either no symptoms or only weakness or easy fatigability. Acute hypercalcemic crisis is now a rare form of presentation.

Osteitis fibrosa cystica, with radiographic features of osteopenia, subperiosteal bone resorption, brown tumors, bone cysts, and "salt and pepper" skull, is rare. Patients with hyperparathyroidism show evidence of increased bone remodeling on bone biopsy, with increased amounts of osteoid surface and eroded surface when compared to normal subjects. However, dynamic parameters of bone remodeling show that the mineral apposition rate is unchanged. Although radiographic evidence of hyperparathyroid bone disease in hand films—with subperiosteal resorption and loss of the distal tuft of the phalanges—is rare in cases of primary hyperparathyroidism now, it is found in patients with secondary hyperparathyroidism from chronic renal failure.

Because osteoporosis is such a major health problem in older patients, attention has been directed at determining PTH's effect upon bone mass. With improved techniques to measure bone mass, it is possible to assess changes in both trabecular and cortical bone envelopes. Several early cross-sectional studies suggested that hyperparathyroid subjects have decreased amounts of trabecular bone in the vertebrae. More recent work shows that cortical bone as measured in the forearm or femur is reduced in the affected patients. Thus, elevated levels of PTH seem to have different effects upon cortical

bone. Four studies suggest that patients with hyperparathyroidism have an increase in vertebral compression fractures, but one study found no evidence of an increased incidence of vertebral fractures. A study in Sweden of more than 1800 patients reported no increase in hip fractures in women with hyperparathyroidism, but there was an increase in hip fractures in men.

Nephrolithiasis occurs in 20% of hyperparathyroid patients. Of patients with kidney stones, approximately 5% have hyperparathyroidism. PTH causes a proximal renal tubular acidosis, increasing bicarbonate loss and decreasing hydrogen ion excretion, as well as lowering the phosphate reabsorption threshold. These changes cause a hyperchloremic metabolic acidosis, and 30% of patients will be hypophosphatemic. Hyperparathyroidism can cause nephrocalcinosis and a subsequent decline in the glomerular filtration rate. Hypercalcemia can lead to nephrogenic diabetes insipidus because the renal tubule becomes unresponsive to the action of antidiuretic hormone. Asymptomatic patients with primary hyperparathyroidism have defects in their ability to concentrate urine.

Most other signs and symptoms of hyperparathyroidism can be attributed to the resultant hypercalcemia or, more specifically, the elevated ionized calcium level. *Gastrointestinal* (GI) disorders include anorexia, nausea, vomiting, and constipation. Peptic ulcer disease occurs with increased frequency, and, rarely, it maybe the first clue to a multiple endocrine neoplasia type I syndrome (hyperparathyroidism, islet cell tumors, especially gastrinoma, and, finally, pituitary tumors). Pancreatitis can also occur or be exacerbated by the hypercalcemia. *Central nervous system* disorders include impaired cognition, recent memory loss, anosmia, depression, lethargy, and coma. Thus, hypercalcemia and hyperparathyroidism are rare but important considerations in the differential diagnosis of depression and dementia in the elderly. *Neuromuscular* disturbances include a proximal weakness, more prominent in lower than in upper extremities. Many patients complain of malaise and fatigue. Rarely, pruritus can be caused by metastatic calcification in the skin. *Articular* disturbances include pseudogout from calcium pyrophosphate crystal deposition in articular cartilage, calcific tendinitis, and chondrocalcinosis. The main *cardiovascular* disturbance is an increased frequency of hypertension. Stefenelli et al. report that patients with surgically confirmed primary hyperparathyroidism showed a high incidence of left ventricular hypertrophy (82%) and aortic and/or mitral valve calcifications (46% and 39%, respectively). At 41 months after successful parathyroidectomy, there was regression of the left ventricular hypertrophy. Further studies are needed to confirm and expand upon these observations.

Physical signs are unusual in hyperparathyroidism. Soft-tissue calcification can cause pseudogout or cutaneous calcification. When present in the eye, deposits of calcium phosphate crystals can cause conjunctivitis. In the cornea, band keratopathy (a vertical line of calcium phosphate deposition parallel to and within the ocular limbus) is best appreciated with a slit lamp examination. Enlarged parathyroid glands are difficult to palpate in the neck; generally, when a nodule is found in the neck of a suspected hyperparathyroid patient, it represents thyroid rather than parathyroid tissue.

Diagnosis

Primary hyperparathyroidism is diagnosed by elevated serum calcium levels and, frequently, associated hypophosphatemia, without any other apparent disease or drug causing the abnormalities. The serum calcium should be measured fasting on several occasions with minimal or no venous stasis. Techniques for measuring PTH have improved significantly, making it possible to diagnose hyperparathyroidism directly rather than by exclusion as had been done previously. Thus, to prove hyperparathyroidism, serum PTH levels should be measured directly. Early assays measured the carboxy terminal portion of PTH. Because this fragment is cleared by the kidney, the diagnosis of hypercalcemia in patients with renal insufficiency was confounded. With improvement in assay techniques for the intact PTH molecule, using immunoradiometric (IRMA) and immuno-chemiluminescent (ICMA) assays, it is possible to show PTH elevations in 90% of patients.

Most clinical PTH assays have been validated so that the laboratory provides a range reflecting previous experience with the assay and showing where the patient's PTH and serum calcium levels fall in relation to the laboratory's other cases of hyperparathyroidism. In most nonparathyroid causes of hypercalcemia, PTH levels are suppressed, except in the unusual case of a malignant neoplasm that produces PTH. As is discussed in the section on "Differential Diagnosis," malignancy-associated hypercalcemia is always a concern in the differential diagnosis of hypercalcemia, but neoplasms that are actually proved to produce active PTH are unusual, most such cases being renal, pancreatic, ovarian, or hepatic carcinomas. In such instances, the PTH-related peptide secreted by the tumor does not usually cross-react with PTH of parathyroid origin in the immunoassays employed in most laboratories.

Serum phosphate levels maybe low in hyperparathyroidism, but they can be normal, especially if there is renal impairment. Although PTH does cause phosphaturia, other factors such as dietary intake and time of day may affect renal phosphate handling. Furthermore, patients with malignancy-associated hypercalcemia can have a decrease in the renal phosphate reabsorption threshold from hypercalcemia per se or from the tumor-derived peptides, which produce the hypercalcemia. Other serum electrolyte abnormalities, such as elevated chloride, low bicarbonate, and low magnesium levels, are not specific enough to be of diagnostic value. Both an elevated serum alkaline phosphatase level and increased urinary hydroxyproline level suggest significant skeletal involvement from hyperparathyroidism.

Patients who are being evaluated for hyperparathyroidism should have a 24-hour urine calcium and creatinine excretion measured. Patients with a calcium:creatinine ratio of 0.1 may have familial hypercalcemic hypocalciuria, a hereditary disorder with normal PTH levels that does not require surgery. It is caused by an inactivating mutation of the calcium-sensing receptor.

Routine use of preoperative localization of abnormal parathyroid tissue in hyperparathyroidism should not be part of the diagnostic evaluation because noninvasive imaging techniques require further development before being valid for such application. Some centers are evaluating the use of technetium-99m sestamibi scans or ultrasonography, but they should not be used routinely in evaluating patients for parathyroidectomy. Arteriography and selective venous catheterization looking for "stepped-up" levels is a technically difficult procedure and should be performed by experienced hands only when hyperparathyroidism persists after a failed neck exploration.

Differential Diagnosis

The differential diagnosis of hyperparathyroidism is that of hypercalcemia, which can be caused by a diverse group of diseases and drugs

TABLE 111-1

Differential Diagnosis of Hypercalcemia

Primary hyperparathyroidism
  Solitary adenoma
  Hyperplasia
  Multiple endocrine neoplasia

Malignancy-associated hypercalcemia
  Local osteolytic hypercalcemia
  Humoral hypercalcemia of malignancy
  $1,25(OH)_2D$-mediated hypercalcemia

Granulomatous disorders
  Sarcoidosis
  Berylliosis
  Tuberculosis
  Histoplasmosis
  Coccidiomycosis
  Candidiasis
  Eosinophilic granuloma
  Silicone implants

Medications
  Vitamin D and A intoxication
  Lithium
  Thiazide diuretics
  Estrogens/antiestrogens
  Theophylline

Immobilization plus
  Juvenile skeleton
  Malignancy
  Paget's disease of bone
  Primary hyperparathyroidism
  Renal failure

Milk alkali syndrome

Parenteral nutrition

Familial hypocalciuric hypercalcemia

Hypophosphatemia

Renal failure

Idiopathic hypercalcemia of infancy

Hyperthyroidism

Addison's disease

Hyperproteinemia

(Table 111-1). A major concern when hypercalcemia is encountered is whether it is caused by a neoplasm. The clinical setting must be considered. Most patients with malignancy-associated hypercalcemia have obvious neoplastic disease on thorough examination and routine diagnostic workup. Thus, a chest x-ray a mammogram, and a serum and urine protein electrophoresis should be ordered when evaluating hypercalcemia. Since primary hyperparathyroidism is a common disease in older women, an elderly female with hypercalcemia without obvious evidence of malignant disease will be more likely to have primary hyperparathyroidism than occult malignancy.

Familial hypocalciuria hypercalcemia (FHH) should be considered in an evaluation of hypercalcemia. Although uncommon, FHH can present with hypercalcemia, but there is usually a family history, reflecting an autosomal dominant mode of inheritance, and 24-hour urinary calcium:creatinine excretion ratio of 0.1 is highly suggestive.

At present, no adverse effects of the hypercalcemia have been reported from affected kindreds under supervision, and parathyroidectomy does not alter the hypercalcemia.

Drugs that cause hypercalcemia, such as thiazide diuretics and calcium supplements, can be excluded by withdrawing them for 4 weeks and making sure that serum calcium levels return to normal. Hypercalcemia caused by vitamin D intoxication can be diagnosed by measuring 25-hydroxyvitamin D levels and finding a level above 120 ng/mL. Hypercalcemia can be found in sarcoidosis, tuberculosis, and chronic fungal infections. The mechanism in all these diseases is believed to be increased production of 1,25-dihydroxyvitamin D by the granulomatous tissue, which causes increased calcium absorption from the GI tract. Other diseases causing hypercalcemia, such as hyperthyroidism, adrenal insufficiency, and vitamin D intoxication, should be diagnosed by their historical or clinical features.

Therapy

Treatment of hyperparathyroidism depends upon the way in which the patient presents to the physician. Because most cases are asymptomatic at presentation, no immediate therapy is usually necessary and a thorough diagnostic evaluation can be undertaken. When the patient presents with a hypercalcemic crisis (e.g., obtunded with serum calcium levels of greater than 12 mg/dL), management of the hypercalcemia must take precedence over diagnostic studies. Most hypercalcemic patients are dehydrated and may require several liters of parenteral fluids to lower the serum calcium into the 11.0 mg/dL range. Once hydration has been reestablished and the patient is stable, further decisions about therapy can be made.

At this time, there is no effective medical therapy for primary hyperparathyroidism. Beta-blockers, estrogen therapy in postmenopausal women, phosphate supplementation with potassium phosphate (Neutra-Phos-K), etidronate disodium (Didronel), or oral cellulose phosphate with dietary calcium restriction may lower serum calcium levels, while other aspects of the disease may progress. The second-generation bisphosphonates, alendronate, and risedronate can lower serum calcium levels, but long-term studies are needed to document their effect on the disease and whether they alter fracture rates. A new class of drug, calcimimetic agents, is under study. Calcimimetics activate the calcium sensing receptor in the parathyroid gland and inhibit PTH secretion. A long active calcimimetic agent, cinacolcet, is now approved by the Food and Drug Administration (FDA) for the treatment of secondary hyperparathyroidism with renal failure and for hypercalcemia from parathyroid cancer. This agent is not approved for the treatment of primary hyperparathyroidism, but early results suggest it may help control serum calcium levels. Therefore, long-term management of hyperparathyroidism must involve a decision about whether to intervene surgically or to follow the patient until there is an indication for surgery.

Because many cases of hyperparathyroidism are asymptomatic and without any potential complications of the disease at diagnosis, immediate surgery is not necessary, and some patients may never need an operation. A National Institutes of Health (NIH) consensus conference points out that because surgery is the only effective therapy for this disorder, the patient and the physician must realize that meticulous, long-term follow-up is necessary. Understanding of long-term complications is incomplete, and no study has randomized asymptomatic patients to surgery or medical follow-up.

There are indications for surgery in asymptomatic patients with primary hyperparathyroidism: (1) markedly elevated serum calcium (above 12.0 mg/dL); (2) history of life-threatening hypercalcemia; (3) reduced creatinine clearance (below 30% for age-matched normals); (4) nephrolithiasis; (5) markedly elevated 24-hour urinary calcium excretion (above 400 mg); and (6) reduced bone mass as measured by direct measurement (more than 2 standard deviations below age-matched normals). Surgery should be considered strongly in the following circumstances: (1) the patient desires surgery; (2) meticulous, long-term follow-ups are unlikely; (3) coexistent illness complicates management; and (4) the patient is young (younger than age 50 years). After successful surgery, recovery is rapid. Serum calcium levels normalize within hours to several days. There is a 90% reduction in recurrent renal stones in patients with nephrolithiasis. Bone mass also improves after surgery; patient can gain 12% to 20% of their femoral or lumbar density respectively in 4 years.

Patients with serum calcium levels below 11.0 mg/dL and no other evidence of disease maybe safely followed. There is agreement that malaise and fatigue are associated with hyperparathyroidism, but no prospective studies are available to show that these complaints improve with surgery. This is also true for neuropsychiatric disturbances in patients with serum calcium levels below 11.0 mg/dL. At present, no markers are available in lieu of direct measurements to suggest who will lose bone, develop nephrolithiasis, or have a decline in glomerular filtration rate. Therefore, patients with asymptomatic hyperparathyroidism require close follow-up; in addition, they should be educated about the signs and symptoms of hypercalcemia. Vitamin D deficiency can cause secondary hyperparathyroidism and patients with primary hyperparathyroidism may also be vitamin D-deficient. When vitamin D deficiency is found, patients should be given 400 IU of vitamin D daily. These patients should have yearly serum measurements of calcium and creatinine, determination of creatinine clearance, and yearly kidney–ureter–bladder radiography searching for nephrolithiasis. Most experts believe that bone mass measurements (spine, hip, and possibly radius) should be followed annually for 2 to 3 years until stable. Thus, if physician and patient decide not to operate for hyperparathyroidism, education and long-term follow-up are necessary.

For patients who require surgery, the most important aspect is referral to a surgeon who is experienced in neck dissections and identification of parathyroid glands. With an experienced surgeon, parathyroidectomy is usually not a major procedure unless the sternum must be split to find a substernal gland. All four glands should be identified and biopsied for histologic confirmation. Because 80% of the cases of hyperparathyroidism are caused by a single adenoma, removal of the offending gland is curative. When hyperplasia is identified, most surgeons remove 3.5 glands, marking the remaining portion of gland so it can be identified if necessary in the future. Transplantation of parathyroid tissue into the forearm after removal of all of the glands from the neck is used by some surgeons, especially when they anticipate removing more tissue should hyperplasia become a problem at a later time (e.g., with chronic renal failure).

Postoperatively, patients should be watched closely for 72 hours for signs of hypocalcemia. Nervousness, tingling, and a positive Chvostek or Trousseau sign may indicate hypocalcemia, which should be confirmed by total or ionized serum calcium levels. Many patients have transient hypocalcemia, and additional calcium should be given only if the level is below 8 mg/dL. Intravenous calcium as the chloride or gluconate salt maybe given for several days, but persistent hypocalcemia requires oral calcium in a dose of 1000 to 1200 mg daily. If hypocalcemia is severe, 1, 25-dihydroxyvitamin D (calcitriol) can be added at 0.5 to 1 μg/day in doses divided every 12 hours. Because calcitriol can cause hypercalcemia and hypercalciuria, serum and urine levels must be monitored. Patients who have developed hypocalcemia from skeletal uptake of calcium and phosphorus with healing of osteitis fibrosa cystica ("hungry bones") have normal or low serum phosphorus levels. This complication is currently rare because of early detection of the disease; treatment with calcium supplements and calcitriol can be necessary for up to 3 months. Permanent hypoparathyroidism is a rare complication of parathyroidectomy (when performed by experienced surgeons), but it can occur. Hypocalcemia with persistent hyperphosphatemia postoperatively suggests hypoparathyroidism. This can occur transiently from bruising of the glands as they are identified and biopsied at surgery, so follow-up is required to determine whether parathyroid function returns over time. Finally, hyperparathyroid patients can have low serum magnesium levels, another cause of hypocalcemia. Thus, the serum magnesium level should be checked if hypocalcemia develops postoperatively. Because serum magnesium levels may not reflect tissue stores, patients should receive parenteral magnesium if a low normal level is found.

PAGET'S DISEASE OF BONE

Epidemiology

Paget's disease of bone is a focal disorder of accelerated skeletal remodeling, first described by Sir James Paget in 1877. In his original description, Paget described six patients with enlarged skulls, hearing loss, bowed extremities, and kyphotic spines. He called the disease osteitis deformans and proposed an inflammatory basis to the lesion, which he said led to the progressive deformity of the affected bones over the lifetime of an individual.

Paget's disease is a disease of older people. In the United States, the disease occurs in 1.8% of people older than 60 years of age. Its prevalence increases to 10% to 15% by the ninth decade of life. Paget's disease affects men and women equally. The disorder is rarely recognized before age 40 years of age. The incidence and severity of Paget's disease of bone appears to be declining in New Zealand, Great Britain, Spain, and the United States. At this time, there is no explanation for this decline in prevalence and severity.

A cohort of subjects from Rotterdam was evaluated with serum alkaline phosphatase levels and radiographs. Of the subjects who had an elevated serum alkaline phosphatase level with normal measures of other liver enzymes activities, 20% were diagnosed with Paget's disease. Of the patients with normal serum alkaline phosphatase levels, Paget's disease was found using radiographs in 2.3%. The population prevalence in Paget's disease in the Netherlands is 3.6%. Importantly, 84% of subjects with Paget's disease in this country have a normal serum alkaline phosphatase level.

There are clear geographic distributions of Paget's disease. The disorder is most prevalent in England, western Europe, the United States, Australia, and New Zealand, but is uncommon in Scandinavia, China, Japan, and India.

Etiology

Although the etiology of Paget's disease of bone is unknown, there are two hypotheses currently promulgated that are not mutually exclusive: one, a viral etiology, and the other, a genetic susceptibility. Since the early 1970s, studies have suggested that paramyxoviruses may have a role in this disorder. Studies also document familial clusters of Paget's disease, suggesting a genetic component to this disorder.

Several paramyxoviruses (measles virus, respiratory syncytial virus, and canine distemper virus) are postulated to play a role in the etiology of Paget's disease. This hypothesis was based on finding nucleocapsid-like structures and antigens in osteoclast nuclei and cytoplasm. In addition, measles virus messenger RNA was found in osteoclasts and mononuclear cell progenitors. However, no virus has been cultured from pagetic cells, and despite use of sensitive techniques, no direct evidence of any type of paramyxovirus RNA or of virus infection has been found. In three other skeletal disorders—osteopetrosis, pyknodysostosis, and osteoclastoma—nuclear inclusions bodies have been identified. Transgenic mice with measles virus nucleocapsid protein introduced into osteoclasts develop skeletal lesions similar to those found in patients with Paget's disease.

Increased interleukin-6 (IL-6) levels have been reported in bone marrow plasma and the peripheral blood of pagetic patients, and IL-6 increases osteoclast formation when added to normal marrow cells. Cytokines in the marrow microenvironment are postulated to influence the development of osteoclast precursors and thus limit the lesions to local sites once the initial lesion occurs. What is still unknown is how the initial lesion begins.

The hypothesis that Paget's disease has a genetic etiology is supported by work showing that 15% to 30% of patients have a positive family history of the disorder. In one study from Spain, 40% of pagetic patients had an affected first-degree relative. Some of the more severely affected patients have disease involving the pelvis, the spine, the proximal femurs, and the skull, and the disease appears at an earlier age. Some such patients have a family history of the disorder. There are seven chromosomes where Paget's disease associated loci have been identified (PDB1-7). One of the PDB associated genes has been identified: the SQSTM1 gene, which is located in the PDB 3 region on chromosome 5p35. The SQSTM1/p62 protein is a scaffold protein in the RANK signaling cascade, but the pathogenic mechanism regarding Paget's disease is unclear presently.

A current hypothesis is that patients in middle to late life who have a genetic predisposition to Paget's disease of bone develop a viral infection, which causes the disease to become manifest. Still unknown is why it involves particular areas of the skeleton and why the disease generally becomes manifest after the age of 60 years.

Pathophysiology

Because Paget's disease of bone is a localized disorder of accelerated bone remodeling, it is useful to briefly review the normal bone remodeling process (also see Chapter 117). All areas of the skeleton must be remodeled throughout life to repair acquired microfractures and to strengthen parts of the skeleton placed under new or increased mechanical loads. The process begins when osteoclasts from bone marrow colony-forming units of the macrophage lineage come to a surface that needs remodeling. They excavate a cavity 50 μm in depth over a 2- to 4-week period and then undergo apoptosis. A new series of cells, osteoblasts, derived from bone marrow colony-forming units of fibroblast lineage, appear in the resorption cavity and fill it with layers of osteoid tissue known as *lamellae*. The cavity is filled with osteoid tissue and the osteoblast also form hydroxyapatite crystals on the collage, which provides strength to the matrix. The process of bone remodeling is tightly coupled so that increases or decreases in rates of bone resorption are followed for an increase or decrease in bone formation. Through this coupling process, it is possible for most people to maintain their skeleton as a serviceable, lightweight frame throughout life. We now know that the coupling process is mediated by cytokines and growth factors released by osteoblasts and osteoclasts, which serve to control the remodeling process. The final common pathway for control of osteoclast differentiation and function is the receptor activation of NF-κB (RANK) receptor activator of NF-κB ligand (RANKL) and osteoprotogerin (OPG). The pathway with IL-6 and macrophage colony stimulating factor are major regulators of osteoclast differentiation and function.

In pagetic lesions, the primary abnormality is in the osteoclast. A major histologic feature is the increased number and size of the osteoclasts and their nuclei. Normal osteoclasts have 10 nuclei while osteoclasts from areas of the skeleton with Paget's disease have up to 100 nuclei. There is a compensatory increase in the number and size of the osteoblasts in the areas of increased remodeling activity, which leads to large amounts of new bone formation. The increased rate of bone turnover disrupts the normal lamellar pattern of the osteoid tissue and results in immature woven or mosaic bone. This bone has increased amounts of fibrosis and vascularity as well as enlarged haversian canals. Thus, although the bone appears denser radiographically, it is more subject to fracture, can bow with weight bearing, and, especially in the skull, can enlarge as long as the remodeling activity is increased.

Clinical Manifestations

Patients with Paget's disease of bone present with a wide array of symptoms. Depending upon the clinical setting, 70% to 90% of patients with Paget's disease will have no symptoms. In a tertiary referral practice, 20% to 30% of patients will have symptoms. In contrast, in a primary care practice, only 10% of patients with the disease may have related symptoms. Many patients have the diagnosis made incidentally when an elevated serum alkaline phosphatase level is found on a multiphasic chemistry screening panel or radiography is performed that shows an asymptomatic bone lesion. The disease may affect any bone and can be monostotic or polyostotic. Symptoms depend on the bone(s) and the part of the bone involved as well as the activity of the bone remodeling. Many patients with radiographic evidence of Paget's disease have no symptoms.

The most commonly affected bones are the pelvis, lumbar spine, the skull, and proximal femurs. All areas of the skeleton can be affected by the disease. In patients with symptomatic Paget's disease, bone pain can be mild to severe. The pain is usually not related to physical activity. The pain can be variously described as dull aching, burning, or boring in nature. Acute pain may develop as a consequence of a pathologic fracture in an affected bone. Bone pain may also arise from increased vascularity or from stretching of the periosteum caused by the increased amount of new bone from the

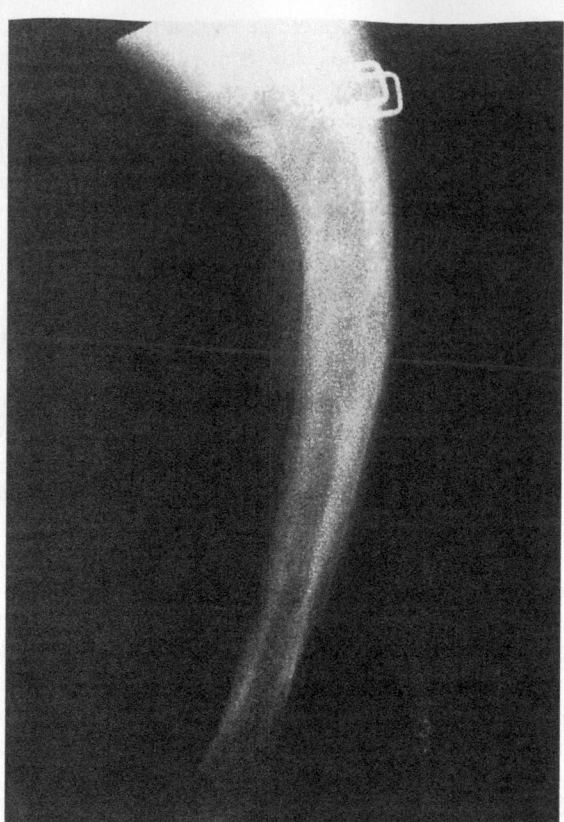

FIGURE 111-1. Left anteroposterior tibia and fibula radiograph from a 78-yr-old woman with Paget's disease of bone involving the tibia. At the proximal portion of the tibia are staples from a failed osteotomy 25 yr before. Note the lateral bowing of the tibia. There is the characteristic increase in cortical bone size from the abnormal remodeling process. In the distal portion of the tibia is seen the advancing lytic disease front, sometimes called a blade-of-grass lesion.

disorganized bone remodeling. Periarticular pain maybe the presenting symptom in 50% of cases and is an important diagnostic problem because Paget's disease commonly affects bone around major joints such as the hip and knee, as well as those of the spine, with narrowing of the joint spaces and formation of osteophytes.

Bowing of weight-bearing bone is another common feature, occurring most commonly in the femur, tibia, humerus, and ulna (Figure 111-1). The bowing seen in the femur and tibia is often associated with stress fractures on the convex surface of the bowed bone (Figure 111-2). Bone deformity alters force transmission through the adjacent joint causing premature loss of articular cartilage and secondary osteoarthritis especially in the hip and knee. In addition to deformities, the affected bone can enlarge. Degenerative arthritis in joints contiguous to pagetic lesions causes juxta-articular enlargement and altered subchondral bone support. Patients also develop osteoarthritis in unaffected knees as a result of favoring the nonpagetic knee. Protrusio acetabuli occurs in some patients with disease involving the ilium (Figure 111-3).

Neurologic complications reflect the predilection of the disease to affect the axial skeleton. Disease in the skull can cause nonspecific headaches, possibly from increased blood flow. Patients with skull involvement can develop deafness. Pagetic involvement of the temporal bone can cause conductive hearing loss. Involvement of the cochlea results in mixed sensory and conductive deafness.

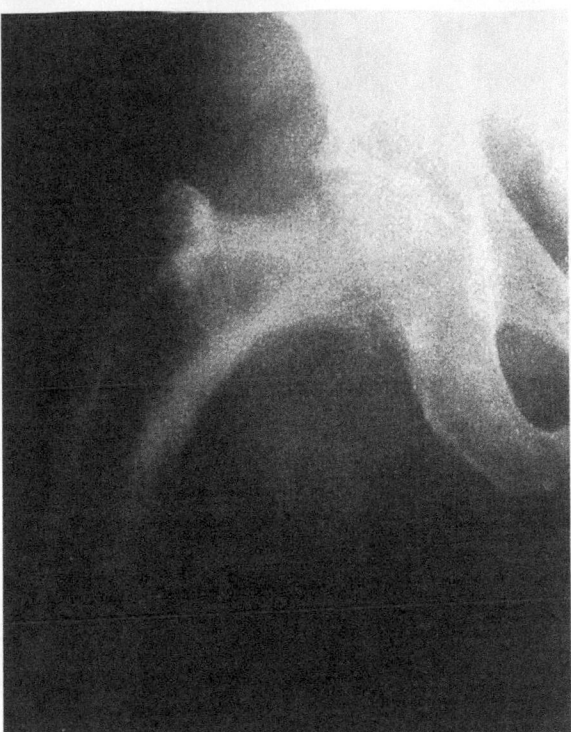

FIGURE 111-2. Right proximal femur and pelvis radiograph of a 68-yr-old man with Paget's disease of bone involving both the femur and ilium. The angle of the femoral neck and femur are decreased as the bone is less strong, a coxae vera deformity. Also note the lateral bowing of the femur with the stress fractures on the convex side of the femur.

Occasionally, the optic or trigeminal nerves maybe involved, resulting in visual loss or tic douloureux. Skull deformity may result in enlargement of the vault, with a characteristic appearance particularly of the forehead (frontal bossing) or of the maxilla (leontiasis osseum). Basilar invagination of the skull can cause symptoms from internal hydrocephalus or long tract signs from brainstem compression. Bone enlargement of vertebrae can cause spinal stenosis, resulting in spinal radiculopathy or cauda equina syndrome. Increased blood flow to the highly vascular pagetic bone has been postulated to provoke a

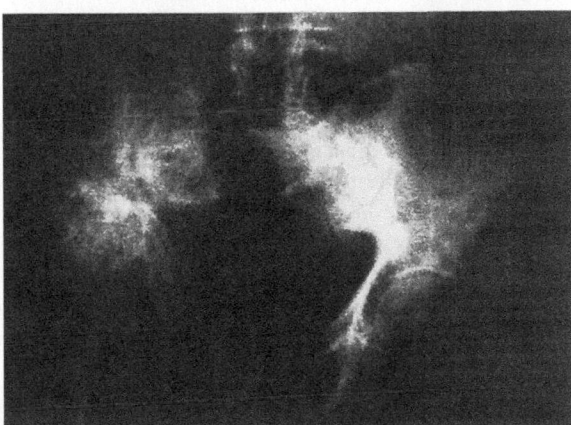

FIGURE 111-3. Anteroposterior pelvis radiograph from a 72-yr-old man with Paget's disease of bone involving the entire pelvis. Femurs are not involved with Paget's disease, but the right side of the pelvis has marked protrusio acetabuli.

"steal syndrome." In this situation, blood is shunted away from the neural elements, exacerbating the neurologic symptoms and signs accompanying the stenosis.

Pagetic bone fractures more easily because it is formed more rapidly than normal bone. In addition to incomplete fissure fractures on convex surfaces of bowed long bones, complete transverse fracture can occur with minimal trauma (Figure 111-4). These fractures are called chalk stick fractures because the bone breaks evenly as a piece of chalk would, rather than with jagged fragments as normal bone does. Such fractures also have a higher rate of nonunion, between 10% and 40%, occurring most commonly in the femur.

A serious but rare complication of Paget's disease (less than 0.1% of affected patients) is the development of malignant neoplasms. Osteosarcomas, chondrosarcomas, fibrosarcomas, and tumors of mixed histologic characteristics may develop, almost always in a preexisting pagetic lesion. Primary giant cell tumors and secondary spread of other cancers to existing pagetic lesions also occurs. When malignant neoplasms occur, they are very aggressive and unless the neoplasm can be removed totally (usually limb amputation), the disease is rapidly fatal. At present, there are no data showing that treatment of Paget's disease of bone reduces the occurrence of malignant neoplasms.

With high rates of bone remodeling, some patients with Paget's disease can develop nephrolithiasis. Occasionally, when patients with active polyostotic disease must be put in bed, for example, after a fracture, they can develop hypercalcemia and hypercalciuria. When this occurs, antiresorptive agents must be initiated on an emergent basis to reduce calcium release from bone resorption. Hyperuricemia and gout are reported to occur in patients with Paget's disease of bone. It is unclear whether abnormal purine metabolism is caused by the elevated bone remodeling or whether gout and Paget's disease are just two common diseases occurring in the same patient.

High-output cardiac failure has been reported to occur in patients with Paget's disease. Generally, patients have more than one third of their skeleton involved with bone turnover lesions; however, documented occurrences are rare.

A series of fibrosing or inflammatory disorders are reported to occur with Paget's disease: Dupuytren's contractures, Peyronie's disease, and Hashimoto's thyroiditis. Whether these inflammatory/fibrotic disorders are only associated with Paget's disease or in some fashion caused by the release of cytokines from the areas of increased turnover awaits further study. Angioid streaks and peripapillary chorioretinal atrophy are associated with Paget's disease of the bone but are more frequently seen with pseudoxanthoma elasticum, another connective tissue disease.

Diagnosis

All patients with Paget's disease of bone should receive a thorough history and physical examination. Because 30% to 70% of patients have the diagnosis made serendipitously, it maybe necessary to reevaluate the patient, seeking symptoms and signs of the disease. All patients with Paget's disease should have a total-body bone scan using a technetium-labeled bisphosphonate. Areas of rapidly remodeling bone will appear as hot spots and this technique is the most sensitive method for localizing pagetic areas. Areas that are hot on bone scan should then have radiographs to confirm the presence of abnormal remodeling. Radiographs of painful or deformed bones are usually diagnostic, showing the characteristic mixed appearance of

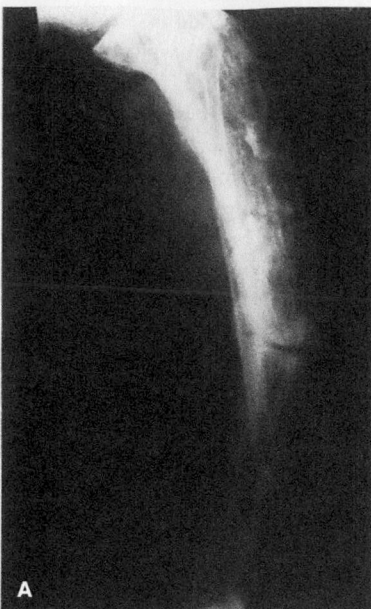
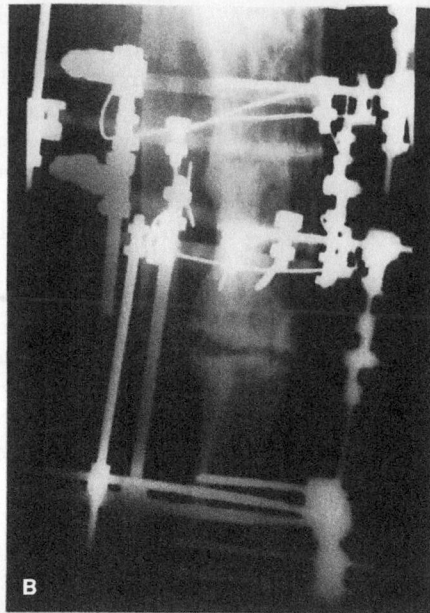
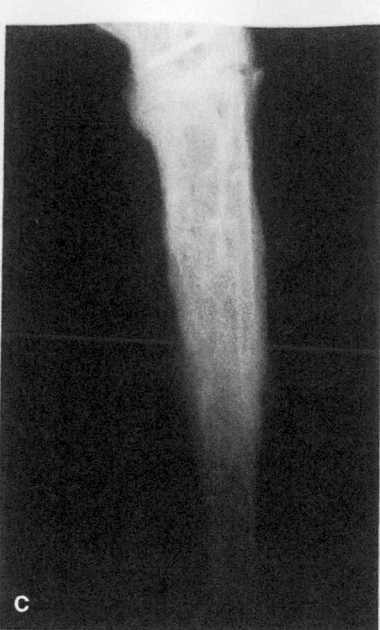

FIGURE 111-4. A series of left anteroposterior tibial radiographs from a 74-yr-old man with Paget's disease of bone in the left tibia. (A) The patient's tenth fracture; note chalk stick nature. The fracture did not heal with casting over 6 months. (B) The patient underwent tibial straightening with two osteotomies. He also wore an Ilizarov external fixation device for 1 yr and received 6 months of alendronate 40 mg daily. (C) The left tibia is much straighter. The patient now walks with a clamshell leg brace.

areas of lysis from increased osteoclastic resorption with sclerotic areas from excessive osteoblastic bone formation as well as cortical thickening. In the early stages of the disease, the changes maybe predominantly lytic with flame-shaped resorption fronts in long bones or osteoporosis circumscripta in the skull. A characteristic appearance that distinguishes Paget's disease from other conditions radiographically is the increased size and diameter of affected bones, particularly those of the spine or shafts of long bones. If spinal stenosis, hydrocephalus, or brainstem compression from basilar skull invagination is suspected, computed tomography (CT) or magnetic resonance imaging (MRI) scans may be necessary to confirm these diagnoses.

Measurement of a serum alkaline phosphatase level is the most useful biochemical test for Paget's disease. This enzyme is located in the plasma membrane of osteoblasts, and levels are elevated above the normal range in 90% of affected patients. Alkaline phosphatase activity reflects the number and functional state of osteoblasts in patients with the disease. The serum level of alkaline phosphatase correlates roughly with the extent of skeletal involvement as established by radionucleotide bone scans. Serial determinations of alkaline phosphatase provide useful, simple, and inexpensive biochemical indices of skeletal activity. Serum alkaline phosphatase levels do vary from day to day, so that for a change in levels to represent a change in disease activity or a response to therapy, the level should increase or decrease by 25% to be clinically significant. Because 10% of patients with Paget's disease have normal serum alkaline phosphatase levels, it can be helpful to measure bone specific alkaline phosphatase. This isoenzyme of alkaline phosphatase can be elevated when total alkaline phosphatase levels are normal and can also be useful in patients with coexisting liver disease. Measurement of serum osteocalcin level, a vitamin K-dependent protein made by osteoblasts, has not been useful in diagnosing or following patients with Paget's disease.

Increased bone resorption is the initial abnormality in Paget's disease. Bone resorptive activity can be assessed by measuring serum levels of collagen breakdown products, C-telopeptide or N-telopeptide. These collagen fragments can also be measured in urine specimens and creatinine should be assessed concomitantly. Markers of bone resorption change within 1 day to 1 week after the initiation of therapy for Paget's disease while it may take 1 to 2 months before serum alkaline phosphatase levels show a response to therapy. Once a diagnosis of Paget's disease has been made and the extent of the bone involvement quantitated, only serum alkaline phosphatase levels need to be followed. In some patients, bone pain can reoccur after successful suppression or disease activity with therapy. When this occurs, and serum alkaline phosphatase levels are normal, measurement of urinary levels of pyridinoline cross-links or n-telopeptide levels can show an increase in bone resorption activity.

Table 111-2 lists the diseases that should enter into the differential diagnosis of Paget's disease. These diseases can be categorized as either causing an elevated serum alkaline phosphatase level or causing a radiographic lesion similar to Paget's disease.

In most cases, the diagnosis of Paget's disease is not difficult. An asymptomatic or symptomatic bone lesion with an elevated serum alkaline phosphatase level can be easily resolved with the clinician and a radiologist. Occasionally, the author has seen an isolated skeletal lesion in the ilium or in a vertebral body that may not have the classical radiographic appearance of Paget's disease and the markers of bone turnover; serum alkaline phosphatase, urinary pyridinoline cross-links, or n-telopeptide levels are all normal. In these cases, a closed or open bone biopsy is necessary to rule out a neoplasm. Rarely, a patient with Paget's disease of bone may develop a metastasis from another cancer that is in a preexisting pagetic lesion. The author saw a man whose first recurrence of an adenocarcinoma from his lung primary appeared 2 years after resection of the primary lesion as a bone metastasis to an area of Paget's disease in his ilium.

TABLE 111-2

Differential Diagnosis of Paget's Disease of Bone

Causes of elevated serum bone alkaline phosphatase level
  Metastatic neoplasm to the skeleton
  Osteomalacia
  Hyperparathyroidism with osteitis fibrosa cystica
  Idiopathic hyperphosphatasia
Causes of skeletal lesions with similar radiographic appearance
  Metastatic neoplasm to the skeleton
  Vertebral hemangioma
  Fibrous dysplasia
  Chronic osteomyelitis
  Metaphyseal dysplasia (Engelmann's disease)
  Familial expansile osteolysis
  Sternocostal clavicular hyperostosis

Data from Crisp AJ. Paget's disease of bone. In: Maddison PJ et al., eds. Oxford Textbook of Rheumatology. Oxford: Oxford University Press; 1993:1025.

Finally, fibrous dysplasia can cause diagnostic confusion with Paget's disease because the lesion appears hot on bone scan. An experienced skeletal radiologist or a bone biopsy maybe required to clarify this diagnosis.

Therapy

As with any chronic disease, patient education about Paget's disease is the first and most important aspect of disease management is education of the patient about their illness. The Paget Foundation for Paget's Disease of Bone and Related Disorders, 120 Wall Street, New York, NY 10007, is helpful in providing information to patients and health care professionals, the Web site is http://www.paget.org/.

With current knowledge, not all patients with Paget's disease require treatment. In some cases, the symptoms that cause the patient to seek medical care are caused by an associated disorder. Thus, careful consideration of the symptoms and the physical and radiographic findings are necessary to determine whether treatment of the Paget's disease is indicated.

Patients with bone pain from associated osteoarthritis should be treated with aspirin, acetaminophen, or nonsteroid anti-inflammatory agents (NSAIDs). Because many patients are elderly, care should be taken to avoid renal and GI toxicity from NSAIDs. Some patients with severe joint destruction from Paget's disease who are not candidates for joint replacement may require narcotics to control their pain.

Patients who develop deformities or gait disturbances from their Paget's disease should be evaluated to correct or improve these impairments. A cane can be a very important therapeutic device for patients with disease in the pelvis or lower extremities. If the patient has a leg-length deformity, our group tries to correct the deformity with a shoe lift to 50% of the leg length discrepancy over 3 to 4 months. When this has been accomplished, the patients find they ambulate better. Patients with hearing impairments should be referred to an audiologist. When patients have maxillary or mandibular disease, they should be evaluated by a dentist.

Patients should be followed, once they are stable, semiannually or annually. An alkaline phosphatase should be checked annually, and radiographs performed when symptoms indicate a change in the disease.

TABLE 111-3

Indications for Treatment of Paget's Disease of Bone

- Symptoms caused by metabolically active Paget's disease
- In a patient planning to undergo elective surgery on a pagetic site
- Hypercalcemia with prolonged immobilization
- To decrease local progression and reduce the risk of future complications evening asymptomatic patient

Data from Siris ES, et al. Indications for treatment and review of current therapies medical management of Paget's disease of bones. J Bone Miner Res. 2006;21(2): P94–P98.

The ultimate goal of therapy for Paget's disease is to restore bone remodeling to normal levels so that all new bone formed is normal. At present, all available therapies only control the abnormal remodeling rates and do not cure the disease.

Two classes of drugs—bisphosphonates and calcitonin—are available to treat Paget's disease. Although both of these types of drugs control the increased bone remodeling by inhibiting bone resorption, bisphosphonates are more effective in controlling the increased remodeling rates. Now, calcitonin therapy is used when patients are allergic to bisphosphonates. A number of randomized controlled clinical trials have shown that bisphosphonates can improve the pain associated with Paget's disease of bone. Table 111-3 lists current recommendations for the types of patients who should receive therapy. Although no controlled clinical trials have been performed to support the second, third, and fourth points of the guidelines, such trials may never be performed. The recommendations are generally accepted by experts who treat large numbers of patients.

The development of potent "second and third generations" bisphosphonates has made these agents the drugs of choice for the treatment of Paget's disease. Bisphosphonates are analogs of inorganic pyrophosphate. Pyrophosphate binds avidly to the surface of the calcium phosphate mineral phase of bone and modulates the rate and extent of mineralization. Bisphosphonates have a carbon atom substituted for the oxygen atom in pyrophosphate. Bisphosphonates bind to bone mineral but are resistant to hydrolysis. Different side chains on the central carbon atom confer different activities to bisphosphonates. Bisphosphonates bind to bone mineral and are potent inhibitors of osteoclasts. The earliest bisphosphonate etidronate inhibited osteoclast activity, but it also impaired bone mineralization. Prolonged use of etidronate was associated with the development of osteomalacia.

There are now six bisphosphonates approved for the treatment of Paget's disease in the United States: alendronate, risedronate, tiludronate, pamidronate, etidronate, and zoledronic acid. Alendronate is given in doses of 40 mg daily for 6 months. More than 60% of patients who receive this drug normalize their serum alkaline phosphatase levels. Orally administered alendronate cause GI disturbances in 17% of patients; in some, esophagitis can be severe enough to cause discontinuation of the drug. Risedronate is given at a dose of 30 mg orally for 60 days. At this dose, 70% of patients experience normalization of their alkaline phosphatase levels. Although esophagitis can occur with risedronate, it is believed to occur less frequently than with alendronate.

A clinical trial of patients with Paget's disease of bone compared the effects of risedronate, 30 mg daily for 60 days versus intravenous zoledronic acid 5 mg in a single dose. The alkaline phosphatase levels were maintained within the normal range in the vast majority of patients treated with zoledronic acid, whereas patients treated with risedronate had an increase in their mean alkaline phosphatase level over a 2-year period. Thus, the advantage of the most potent bisphosphonate in normalizing and maintaining serum alkaline phosphatase levels over a 2-year period is apparent from this work.

Tiludronate is more potent than etidronate, but less potent than alendronate or pamidronate. It is given 400 mg orally for 3 months. This regimen is well-tolerated and will normalize alkaline phosphatase levels in 40% of patients. Pamidronate is another second-generation bisphosphonate that has been used in Europe for 15 years, but is approved in the United States only as an intravenous preparation. The approved regimen is 30 mg intravenously over 4 hours on 3 consecutive days. A second course of pamidronate maybe administered as needed. The advantage of pamidronate is that it can be given intravenously and thus GI toxicity is avoided.

There are several caveats when using nitrogen containing bisphosphonates. These agents are potent and require the person not be hypocalcemic or have a vitamin D deficiency. Rarely these drugs can cause an iritis and if they have, they should be avoided and the nonnitrogen containing bisphosphonates, etidronate or tiludronate, should be used. Patients receiving this class of drugs, especially intravenous pamidronate and zoledronic acid, should be instructed that they may experience an acute phase response within 96 hours after their dose of drug. This acute phase response can be managed with acetaminophen, aspirin, or ibuprofen taken for 72–96 hours post-dose. Finally, patients should be made aware of the risk, although it is small, associated with bisphosphonate-associated osteonecrosis of the jaw. It has been described in three patients treated with bisphosphonate for their Paget's disease of bone. However, in the three reported cases, the patients received more than the recommended dose to treat their disease.

Calcitonin is a safe treatment for Paget's disease. Salmon calcitonin must be administered subcutaneously, usually daily at first, and after 1 to 2 months, it is given three times a week. Calcitonin can normalize bone turnover indices in mild cases of Paget's disease, but it is clearly not as potent an antiresorptive agent as the bisphosphonates are. Usually, the biochemical response is partial, with about a two thirds reduction in serum alkaline phosphatase levels. In approximately 20% of patients, resistance to chronic salmon calcitonin develops after a successful initial treatment period. Neutralizing antibodies develop to calcitonin, but it is not clear whether these antibodies are responsible for the resistance. Side effects occur in approximately 20% of patients treated with either salmon calcitonin. These include nausea, facial flushing, and polyuria. Nasal salmon calcitonin is approved by the FDA for treatment of postmenopausal osteoporosis. It is not recommended for use in Paget's disease because only 40% of the drug is absorbed from the nasal mucosa, and, thus, does not provide a high enough dose of medication. If calcitonin is discontinued, exacerbation of biochemical abnormalities and symptoms usually occurs in 1 year.

Resistance to bisphosphonate is described but is poorly understood. Patients who receive salmon calcitonin, etidronate, and pamidronate have all been reported to have less reduction in their serum alkaline phosphatase levels or a more rapid return to an elevated alkaline phosphatase level after subsequent doses of bisphosphonate. The exact mechanism for this is not known. What is known is however that it is possible to switch the patients to a more potent bisphosphonate and with such therapy have reduction or normalization of alkaline phosphatase levels.

Plicamycin and gallium nitrate are two other drugs that have been used to treat Paget's disease. Both are approved for use in the treatment of hypercalcemia of malignancy and are effective antiresorptive agents. They are not approved by the FDA for use in Paget's disease and have been supplanted by the more effective second-generation bisphosphonates.

Patients with Paget's disease may need emergency or elective orthopedic surgical procedures because of complications of their Paget's disease. Fractures may require open reduction and internal fixation. Before any operative orthopedic procedure, it is desirable to reduce the remodeling activity to reduce excessive blood loss. Such a reduction in remodeling activity can be obtained with intravenous pamidronate or calcitonin if the surgery is emergent. Oral bisphosphonates maybe used if the procedure is elective. A goal of this form of therapy is to reduce alkaline phosphatase levels to normal. Surgery for spinal stenosis can be effective in relieving symptoms, but most experts suggest a course of bisphosphonates or calcitonin to try to improve symptoms before undertaking a decompression procedure. Total joint replacement especially for the hip is a highly effective way to control pain and improve mobility in patients with advanced Paget's disease and degenerative arthritis of the femur or ilium. Tibial osteotomy is effective in relieving knee pain in patients who have severe tibial bowing if the associated osteoarthritis is not too severe. An external fixation device (Ilizarov) has been used in patients with tibial Paget's disease, which allows an osteotomy to be performed and then gradual changes in external pressure to be used to straighten the bowed tibia or to allow a nonunion fracture to heal (see Figure 111-4). When any orthopedic procedure is performed, it is important to maintain the patient on antiresorptive medication after surgery so that prostheses will not loosen with accelerated remodeling or straightened limbs will not rebow.

ACKNOWLEDGMENTS

The author appreciates the help of Monica L. Harris in preparation of this chapter. Support for this work came from the VA Medical Research Service, AG11268 from NIA, and RR-30 from the Division of Research Resources, General Clinical Research Centers Program, NIH.

FURTHER READING

Beyens C, et al. Identification of sex-specific associations between polymorphisms of the osteoprotegerin gene, TNFRSF11B, and Paget's disease of bone. *J Bone Miner Res.* 2007;22:1062–1071.

Consensus Development Panel. Diagnosis and management of asymptomatic primary hyperparathyroidism: Consensus Development Conference statement. *Ann Intern Med.* 1991;114:593.

Cooper C, et al. The epidemiology of Paget's in Britain: Is the prevalence decreasing? *J Bone Miner Res.* 1999;14:192.

Crisp AJ. Paget's disease of bone. In: Maddison PJ, et al., eds. *Oxford Textbook of Rheumatology.* Oxford: Oxford University Press; 1993:1025.

Delmas BD, Meunier PJ. The management of Paget's disease of bone. *N Engl J Med.* 1997;336:558.

Helfrich MH, et al. A negative search for a paramyxoviral etiology of Paget's disease: Molecular molecular immunological and ultrastructural studies in UK patients. *J Bone Miner Res.* 2000;15:2315.

Hocking L, et al. Familial Paget's disease of bone: Patterns of inheritance and frequency of linkage to chromosome 18q. *Bone.* 2000;26:577.

Holick MF. Vitamin D deficiency. *N Engl J Med.* 2007;357:266.

Kenny AM, et al. Fracture incidence in postmenopausal women with hyperparathyroidism. *Surgery.* 1995;118:109.

Khosla S, et al. Primary hyperparathyroidism and the risk of fracture: A a population-based study. *J Bone Miner Res.* 1999;14:1200.

Larsson K, et al. The risk of hip fractures in patients with primary hyperparathyroidism: A a population-based cohort. *J Intern Med.* 1993;234:585.

Lyles KW, et al. A clinical approach to the diagnosis and management of bone. *J Bone Miner Res.* 2001;16:1379.

Lyles KW, et al. Peyronie's disease is associated with Paget's disease of bone. *J Bone Miner Res.* 1997;12:929.

Miller PD, et al. A randomized, double-blind comparison of risedronate and etidronate in the treatment of Paget's disease of bone. *Am J Med.* 1999;106:513.

Mirra JM, et al. Paget's disease of bone review with emphasis on radiologic features. Part I and Part II. *Skeletal Radiol.* 1995;24:163, 173.

Peacock M, et al. Cinacalcet hydrochloride maintains long-term normocalcemia in patients with primary hyperparathyroidism. *J Clin Endocrinol Metab.* 2005;90:135.

Rao DS, et al. Effect of vitamin D nutrition on parathyroid adenoma weight: Pathogenic and clinical implications. *J Clin Endocrinol Metab.* 2000;85:1054.

Reddy SV, et al. Bone marrow mononuclear cells from patients with Paget's disease contain measles virus nucleocapsid messenger ribonucleic acid that has mutations in a specific region of the sequence. *J Clin Endocrinol Metab.* 1995;80:2108.

Reid IR, et al. Comparison of a single infusion of zoledronic acid with risedronate for Paget's Disease. *N Engl J Med.* 2055;353:898–908.

Silverberg S, Bilezikian JP. Primary hyperparathyroidism: still evolving? *J Bone Miner Res.* 1997;12:856.

Siris ES, et al. Current recommendations for the medical management of Paget's disease of bone: US perspective. *J Bone Miner Res.* 2006;21(2):P94-P98.

Stefenelli T, et al. Cardiac abnormalities in patients with primary hyperparathyroidism: Iimplications for follow-up. *J Clin Endocrinol Metab.* 1997;82:106.

van Staa TP, et al. Incidence and natural history of Paget's disease of bone. *J Bone Miner Res.* 2002;17:465.

Aging of the Muscles and Joints

Richard F. Loeser, Jr. ■ *Osvaldo Delbono*

Aging-related changes present in the tissues that make up the musculoskeletal system contribute to a number of common chronic conditions seen in older adults. In fact, musculoskeletal disease is the most common cause of chronic disability in people older than age 65 years. This is attributable both to the prevalence of diseases affecting the musculoskeletal system and the central role of the musculoskeletal system in physical function. Despite the prevalence of musculoskeletal disease, however, there is still much to learn about the pathogenesis of these diseases, including the role of aging in their development.

A number of diverse tissues, including muscle, tendon, ligament, cartilage, and bone comprise the musculoskeletal system; aging-related changes, as well as changes secondary to disuse, have been noted to occur in all of these. As in other systems, it is often difficult to separate aging from disuse from disease. Because the musculoskeletal tissues must function in concert for normal joint motion and thereby appropriate movement to occur, it is easy to see why physical function so commonly declines with age. However, it is also clear that regular submaximal stress to the musculoskeletal system through exercise can prevent or slow the age-related decline in physical function as well as improve function of diseased tissues.

There are a number of age-related changes common to tissues of the musculoskeletal system, which have also been noted in other tissues within the body (Table 112-1). Because of the relatively slow turnover rate of cells and matrix components in musculoskeletal tissues, aging-related changes such as the accumulation of advanced glycation end-products (AGEs) in matrix proteins and oxidative damage to cell and matrix components can have particularly profound effects on the aging musculoskeletal system. This chapter reviews aging in each of the major components of the musculoskeletal system including cartilage, muscle, ligaments and tendons, and intervertebral disks. Although bone is a key player in the musculoskeletal system, aging changes in this tissue are discussed in more detail in Chapter 117.

ARTICULAR CARTILAGE

Normal Structure and Function

Articular cartilage is the tissue present on the ends of bones that comprise diarthrodial joints (Figure 112-1). This cartilage serves to provide a smooth surface with a very low coefficient of friction necessary for rapid, painless, and smooth joint motion. During joint motion, the opposing cartilage surfaces, separated by a thin layer of viscous and slippery synovial fluid, easily glide over each other. In addition to providing a form of lubrication for the joint surface, the synovial fluid also provides a large portion of the nutrition for the articular cartilage, which is an avascular and aneural tissue.

When a load is placed across the joint surface, such as occurs in the knee joint during ambulation, the thin gel-like cartilage is compressed. Compression of the cartilage helps to distribute the load evenly to the underlying bone, where force can be absorbed. Cartilage is too thin to absorb any substantial amount of force itself. Rather, the force of joint loading is absorbed by the muscle and bone associated with the loaded joint. This concept is relevant to the pathogenesis of diseases occurring in weight-bearing joints. If changes occur in muscle or bone that limit their ability to absorb mechanical loads, then the articular cartilage may experience abnormal stresses, which could adversely affect the tissue. Loading of the articular cartilage in the knee is also modulated by the presence of the medial and lateral menisci, which absorb approximately 50% of the load placed on the tibiofemoral regions. Damage to a meniscus can therefore significantly increase the load placed on the cartilage.

Complete compression of cartilage during joint motion is resisted by forces within the tissue generated primarily by the highly negatively charged proteoglycans. Proteoglycans are composed of a core protein to which are attached chains of glycosaminoglycans containing negatively charged sulfate groups. In articular cartilage,

Genral Mechanisms of Musculoskeletal Tissue Aging

Accumulation of modified and degraded extracellular matrix components

Increased collagen cross-linking by advanced glycation endproducts

Decreased numbers of mesenchymal stem cells to replace lost cells

Decreased mitogenic response to injury

Decreased synthetic capacity in response to growth factor stimulation

a large proteoglycan called aggrecan is present. Aggrecan is bound at its amino-terminus to a long strand of hyaluronic acid. Many aggrecan molecules are bound to a single strand of hyaluronic acid to form a large complex that is quite hydrophilic. Cartilage is approximately 70% to 75% water, and much of this water is bound to the negatively charged groups on proteoglycans, forming a gel-like substance. Water is partially extruded from the cartilage matrix during compression, resulting in exposure of negative charges that, as they are brought closer together, resist further compression. As the force is released, the proteoglycans reexpand, and water is drawn back into the cartilage bringing along nutrients from the synovial fluid. The role of joint motion in providing cartilage nutrition may be very relevant to changes occurring in cartilage with disuse.

In addition to proteoglycans, a number of other matrix proteins are responsible for the physical properties of cartilage, including several types of collagen (predominantly types II, VI, IX, and XI) and glycoproteins (including fibronectin and cartilage oligomeric protein). Collagen is quite abundant in cartilage, comprising about

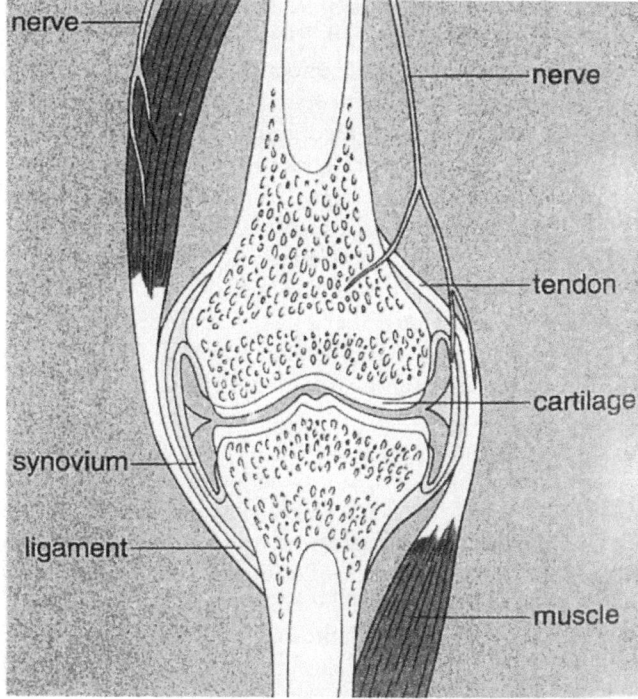

FIGURE 112-1. Components of the musculoskeletal system that comprise the joint include bone, cartilage, muscle, tendon, ligament, synovium, and meniscus (not shown). Note that the nerve supply to the joint does not include cartilage, and, therefore, age- or disease-related changes in cartilage are not directly responsible for joint pain. *(Reproduced with permission from Bullough PG. Atlas of Orthopedic Pathology, 4th ed. New York, New York: Gower Medical Publishing; 2004:9.4.)*

half of the dry weight of the tissue. The majority of the collagen in cartilage is type II collagen. Type II collagen forms long fibrils that provide the tensile strength of the tissue, while the proteoglycans provide the resiliency. The collagen fibers appear to hold aggrecan complexes in place and prevent the proteoglycan gel from complete expansion, which results in the generation of swelling or osmotic pressure within the tissue. Thus, in normal cartilage, the osmotic pressure generated by proteoglycans is balanced by the tensile force provided by the collagen fibrils. The nonfibrillar collagens and the other matrix proteins in cartilage are thought to be involved in the organization and maintenance of the collagen fibrillar network, in structural interactions between collagen and proteoglycans, and in mediating interactions between the chondrocytes and the extracellular matrix (ECM).

Regulation of Cartilage Matrix Turnover

Chondrocytes, the only cells present in cartilage, control the composition and organization of the cartilaginous matrix through the synthesis and degradation of selected ECM components. Together, the processes of synthesis and degradation result in ECM repair and remodeling. From studies performed in a number of tissues, including cartilage, it is becoming clear that ECM proteins can bind to cell surface receptors such as the integrin family of receptors, which, along with growth factors and cytokines, send signals to the cell to regulate matrix synthesis and degradation.

Several different types of enzymes capable of degrading cartilage ECM proteins are produced by chondrocytes, including the metalloproteinases, serine proteases such as elastase, and the cathepsins. The matrix metalloproteinases (MMPs) are prominent players in mediating cartilage catabolism. These include collagenases (MMP-1, MMP-8, and MMP-13), which cleave fibrillar collagens, the gelatinases (MMP-2 and MMP-9), which degrade denatured collagen, and stromelysin (MMP-3), which degrades proteoglycans. Other important MMPs in cartilage are the membrane-type (MT-MMPs), the ADAMs (a disintegrin and a metalloproteinase) and the ADAMTSs (a disintegrin and a metalloproteinase with a thrombospondin motif). The MT-MMPs are bound to the chondrocyte surface through transmembrane domains and can serve to activate other MMPs at the cell surface. An ADAM found in cartilage is ADAM-17, also known as tumor necrosis factor-α-converting enzyme (TACE), which functions to cleave tumor necrosis factor (TNF)-α to an active form. The ADAMTSs use the thrombospondin motif to interact with proteoglycans that can serve as substrates for these enzymes. ADAMTS-4 and ADAMTS-5 are aggrecanases that cleave the large proteoglycan aggrecan. The activity of the MMPs in cartilage is controlled in part by proteins called tissue inhibitors of metalloproteinase (TIMP). There is evidence for a reduction in the levels of TIMPs relative to the increased levels of MMPs in osteoarthritic (OA) cartilage.

A number of growth factors and cytokines are present in cartilage. These serve to regulate anabolic and catabolic processes involved in repair and remodeling (Table 112-2). In general, growth factors stimulate matrix synthesis, whereas the inflammatory cytokines inhibit synthesis and stimulate degradation. Insulin-like growth factor-1 (IGF-1), transforming growth factor-β (TGF-β), and osteogenic protein-1 (OP-1) appear to play a prominent role in regulating adult articular cartilage metabolism. They are expressed in cartilage and act in a paracrine and autocrine fashion to stimulate cartilage matrix

TABLE 112-2

Major Growth Factors and Cytokines Active in Cartilage

GROWTH FACTORS/CYTOKINES	ACTIVE
IGF-I	Promotes cell survival, stimulates matrix synthesis
OP-1 (BMP-7)	Stimulates matrix synthesis, inhibits some catabolic pathways
TGF-β	Mitogenic, stimulates matrix synthesis, stimulates chondro-osteophyte production
bFGF	Mitogenic, stimulates matrix synthesis, potentiates IL-1-induced protease release, may be more important in fetal and growth plate cartilage than adult
IL-1β	Inhibits matrix synthesis and stimulates matrix degradation
TNF-α	Similar to IL-1β
LIF	Stimulates matrix degradation
IL-6	Inhibits proteoglycan synthesis
IL-8	Neutrophil chemoattractant
MCP-1	Monocyte chemoattractant; stimulates MMP production

bFGF, basic fitbroblast growth factor; BMP-7, bone morphogenic protein-7; IGF-1, insulin-link growth factor-1; IL-1β, interleukin-1β; IL-6, interleukin-6; IL-8, interleukin-8; LIF, leukemia inhibitory factor; MCP-1, monocyte chemotactic protein-1; MMP, matrix metalloproteinase; OP-1, osteogenic protein-1; TNF-α, tumor necrosis factor-α; TGF-β, transforming growth factor β.

synthesis as well as inhibit cytokine-stimulated matrix degradation. IGF-1 also appears to promote chondrocyte survival in conjunction with signals from the matrix. As discussed later in this chapter, there is growing evidence that chondrocytes from older individuals are less responsive to growth factor stimulation than those from younger persons. This could contribute to aging-related changes in the tissue, as well as to disease progression with age.

The mitogenic properties of growth factors noted in cell culture studies may not be relevant to normal adult cartilage homeostasis in vivo. In the normal tissue, adult articular chondrocytes do not appear to proliferate or do so at such low rates that proliferating cells are not detected. Chondrocytes, however, are not postmitotic cells. When removed from cartilage by enzymatic digestion of the tissue and placed in cell culture, human chondrocytes can proliferate. Proliferation of chondrocytes in situ occurs during the development of OA, when the presence of clusters or "clones" of chondrocytes is a common pathologic finding. These clusters of cells are thought to represent an attempt at repair of damaged and lost tissue (Figure 112-2).

Normal articular cartilage in the adult contains fully differentiated cells and does not appear to contain its own source of undifferentiated mesenchymal cells available to repair or replace damaged or lost tissue. However, mesenchymal stem cells capable of differentiating into chondrocytes are present in the bone marrow, synovium, adipose tissue and periosteum. Current research is trying to use these cells for repair of cartilaginous lesions because endogenous repair responses in cartilage are inadequate to replace significant amounts of lost matrix, particularly after damage to the collagen network has occurred. The potential role of aging in the failed repair response in cartilage is discussed in the following sections.

AGE-RELATED CHANGES IN CARTILAGE

Changes in Cartilage Structure and Matrix Composition

A number of studies have examined age-related changes in articular cartilage by using tissue collected from various animal species or

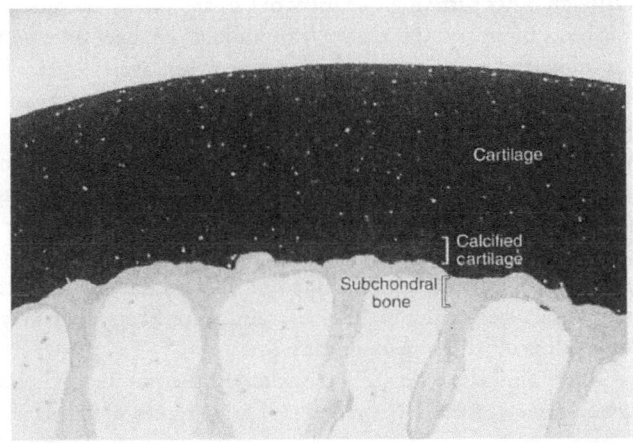

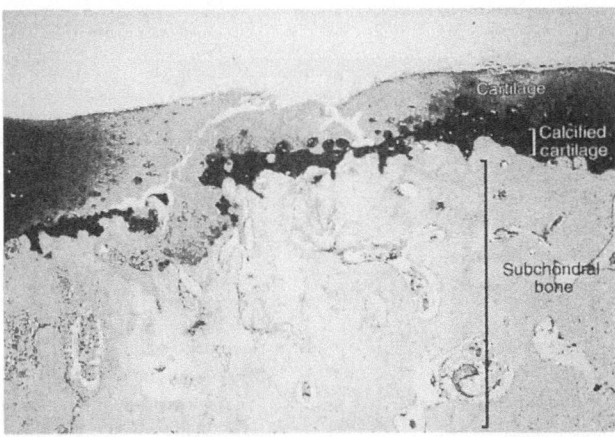

FIGURE 112-2. Normal (A) and osteoarthritic (B) cartilage. These sections from monkey knee joints are stained with toluidine blue, which binds to the negatively charged proteoglycans that are abundant in cartilage. In the osteoarthritic tissue, there is a loss of cartilage matrix staining, resulting from loss of proteoglycans. Other changes include fibrillation and cleft formation, presence of chondrocyte clusters, and a marked thickening of the subchondral bone. (Photographs are courtesy of Dr. Cathy S. Carlson.)

human tissues obtained either at autopsy or from surgical specimens. When surgical specimens are studied, they usually are obtained from subjects undergoing hip or knee replacement surgery for arthritis, in which case the tissue is taken from grossly normal appearing areas but may not be truly normal. Tissues have also been obtained during hip replacement surgery after femoral neck fracture, which is usually associated with osteoporosis. In these cases, the cartilage is felt more likely to be normal because osteoporosis and OA tend to occur in different patient populations, although this is not always true.

Problems in interpreting the results of cartilage aging studies include translating the biology from lower species of animals to humans and separating disease effects from aging effects. In addition, a number of changes have been reported to occur in cartilage when comparing immature versus middle-aged animals. These changes are probably best considered to be developmentally related rather than aging-related. With the above caveats in mind, there do appear to be a number of changes occurring in cartilage that can be related to aging and, importantly, many of the aging-related changes can be contrasted to changes seen in disease (Table 112-3).

Structurally, fibrillation of the articular cartilage surface becomes more prevalent with age, particularly in the knee joint on the vertical ridge of the patella and in the tibiofemoral areas not covered by the menisci. These changes could represent the presence of early OA, although other pathologic changes of OA are not always present and it is most often asymptomatic. Morphologic changes become more common and more extensive with advancing age (Figure 112-3). Similar to the articular cartilage, age-related changes in the menisci have also been noted. Recent studies that have examined the knee joints of older adults using magnetic resonance imaging have noted that damage to the meniscus is strongly associated with damage to the articular cartilage in the same area and meniscal damage predicts further cartilage loss. This work highlights the importance of the meniscus to the normal function of the knee joint. Since the peripheral areas of the menisci contain nerve fibers, they may also be a source of pain in people with OA.

There appears to be a slight decline in the number of chondrocytes present in cartilage with age. Early studies of cartilage from

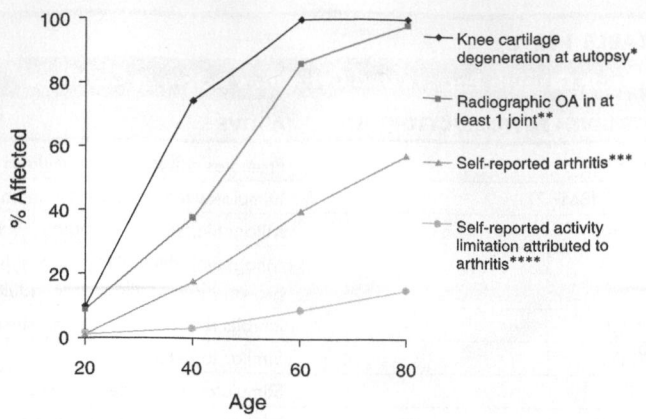

FIGURE 112-3. Effect of age on the prevalence of arthritis. *Knee cartilage degeneration at autopsy is the prevalence of significant histological changes of degeneration. **Radiographic evidence of OA (Kellgren and Lawrence Grade 2 or greater) present in at least one joint site (hands, feet, spine, knees, and hips) in a population survey in northern England. ***Self-reported arthritis and ****activity limitation attributable to arthritis derived from the National Health Interview Survey—US, 1989–1991. *(Reproduced with permission from Loeser RF. Aging and the etiopathogenesis and treatment of osteoarthritis. Rheum Dis Clin North Am. 2000;26:547.)*

the femoral head noted a 30% fall in cell density between the ages of 30 and 100 years. But more recent studies of knee joints have noted much lower cell loss with normal aging in the range of 1% to 2%. Cartilage from older individuals has also been noted to have microcracks in the calcified layer. The significance of these cracks is not clear, but if they extend to the underlying subchondral bone, they could provide a mechanism for the exchange of cytokines and growth factors between the two tissues; and if vascular invasion occurs, they could mediate remodeling of subchondral bone, which is a characteristic feature of OA.

A consistent biochemical finding in cartilage is an age-related decrease in hydration. A decrease in hydration could explain evidence obtained from magnetic resonance imaging of knee joints showing that some thinning of knee cartilage occurs with age, particularly at the femoral surface, which is more evident in women than men. The decrease in cartilage hydration is likely related to changes with age in the proteoglycans that bind the majority of the water in cartilage. The total proteoglycan content does not appear to change significantly, instead changes in proteoglycan structure have been reported that could affect its biophysical properties. Aggrecan molecules become smaller with age and are structurally altered as the result of proteolytic modification in the core protein as well as changes in the length and abundance of the attached glycosaminoglycan chains. Hyaluronic acid, to which the aggrecan molecules bind to form large aggregates, is also decreased in size with age. In addition, proteolysis of the aggrecan core protein between the G1 and G2 domains results in increased levels of molecules bound to hyaluronic acid that contain only the G1 region and therefore lack the remainder of the aggrecan molecule necessary for normal function. The half-life for the free binding region is calculated to be as long as 25 years, consistent with its accumulation in cartilage with aging. By occupying and competing for space on the hyaluronic acid strands, the bound G1 domains may reduce the number of newly synthesized aggrecan molecules bound to hyaluronic acid.

As with proteoglycans, there does not appear to be a significant reduction in the total amount of collagen present in cartilage with

TABLE 112-3

Contrasting Differences Between Aging and Osteoarthritis

AGING	OSTEOARTHRITIS
Decreased cartilage hydration	Increased cartilage hydration
Proteoglycans	Proteoglycans
Normal quantity	Decreased quantity
Smaller size	Smaller size
Ratio of CS 4/6* decreased	Ratio of CS 4/6* increased
Collagen	Collagen
Normal quantity	Decreased quantity
Increased stiffness	Decreased stiffness
Increased cross-linking	Cross-links lost during degradation
Chondrocytes	Chondrocytes
No or reduced proliferation	Increased proliferation
Reduced metabolic activity	Increased metabolic activity
No change in subchondral bone	Increased subchondral bone thickness

*Ratio of CS 4/6 is the ratio of chondroitin sulfate containing sulfate groups on either the fourth or sixth carbon.

Source: Data from Hamerman D: The biology of osteoarthritis. N Engl J Med 1989;320:1322.

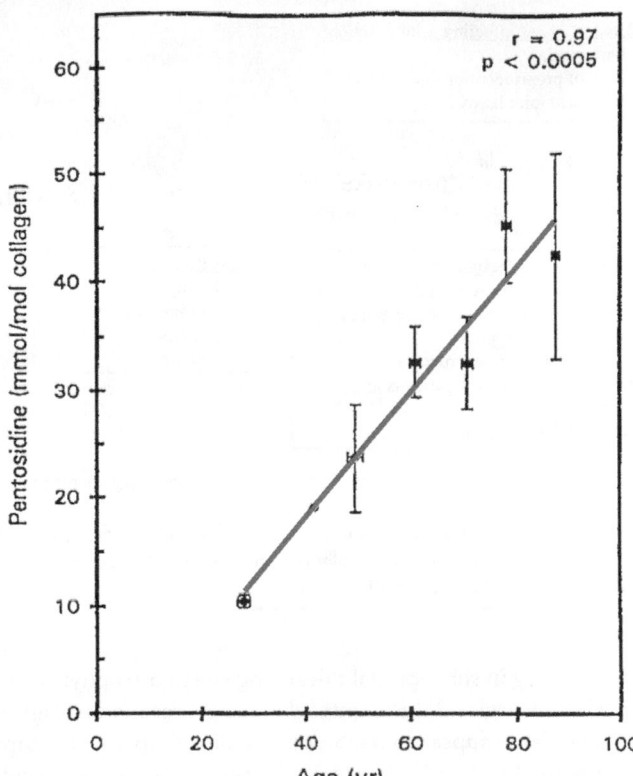

FIGURE 112-4. Age-related accumulation of advanced glycation end-products in cartilage. Pentosidine levels were measured in cartilage samples from 36 donors clustered into 10-year age intervals. Results shown are mean ± SEM (standard error of mean). *(Reproduced with permission from DeGroot et al. Age-related decrease in proteoglycan synthesis of human articular chondrocytes: The role of nonenzymatic glycation. Arthritis Rheum. 1999;42:1003.)*

age. However, important changes in collagen structure and function have been noted. The collagen network appears to become stiffer with age. The increased collagen stiffness is thought to be a result of increased collagen cross-linking. There is evidence for nonenzymatic glycosylation in cartilage from older adults that result in the formation of pentosidine residues that can cross-link collagen molecules. An age-related accumulation of AGEs has been noted in cartilage (Figure 112-4). Pentosidine and other AGEs have been found in collagen, as well as in aggrecan. The accumulation of pentosidine is reported to be greater in collagen than aggrecan because of the exceptionally long half-life of collagen in cartilage, which is calculated to be approximately 117 years.

In addition to increased cross-linking from the accumulation of advanced glycation end products, collagen fibril diameter tends to increase with age, and this may also contribute to changes in collagen stiffness. Increased collagen network stiffness could contribute to the decrease in hydration, as stiffer collagen would tend to cause greater proteoglycan compression and thereby push out more water from the matrix. Biomechanical studies suggest that the stiffer network is more prone to fatigue failure. With age there is a decrease in the tensile strength of cartilage as well as a decrease in overall tensile stiffness. Therefore, age-related changes in the overall composition of the cartilage matrix result in a tissue that is less capable of handling mechanical stress.

In addition to changes in type II collagen and aggrecan, age-related changes in several of the other less-abundant cartilage matrix proteins have been reported. These include a decrease in type IX collagen, a protein that may be important in holding together adjacent collagen fibers and an increase in link protein, the protein that helps bind aggrecan molecules to hyaluronic acid. While link protein is increased with age, it also appears to undergo proteolytic modification with age that could affect its function.

Aging and Chondrocyte Function

Changes in the proliferative and synthetic capacity of chondrocytes with age have been noted. There is evidence for an age-related decreased mitogenic response to serum and growth factor stimulation. There is also evidence for telomere shortening in chondrocytes isolated from older adults but it is not clear if telomere dysfunction is the cause of the reduced mitogenic response. In addition, a reduction in proteoglycan and protein synthesis in response to growth factor stimulation has been in seen in cartilage from older animals, including nonhuman primates. Likewise, decreased proteoglycan synthesis in response to serum stimulation has been noted in human cartilage from older adults. In the human samples, the decreased serum response correlated with the presence of advanced glycation end-products. Other studies also suggest that a decline in cell signaling in response to growth factors is responsible for the decreased mitogenic and synthetic responses.

A reduction in response to growth factor stimulation with age, disease, or both, could be significant in the development of OA, where catabolic processes are greater than anabolic. In addition, there appears to be an age-related increase in the ability of catabolic factors, including the cytokine interleukin-1β (IL-1β) and a fibronectin matrix fragment, to stimulate MMP production by chondrocytes. These age-related changes could contribute to the anabolic–catabolic imbalance that has been observed in OA.

An age-related finding in cartilage, which is also observed in many other soft tissues, is an increased prevalence of crystals and calcification. It is difficult to determine the relative effects of age and disease on cartilage calcification. Calcification or crystal formation within cartilage is a common feature of OA, particularly in advanced disease and, like OA, age is the strongest risk factor for the development of crystal-associated arthritis. Cartilage from older individuals often contains crystals composed of calcium pyrophosphate dihydrate or hydroxyapatite. Studies with animal tissues show that the increase in the formation of calcium pyrophosphate crystals may be caused by an age-related increase in the activity of transglutaminase, an enzyme that is involved in the biomineralization process. Also chondrocytes from older individuals produce more inorganic pyrophosphate in response to TGF-β stimulation, despite a decreased proliferative response to this and other growth factors.

Potential Role of Oxidative Stress in Cartilage Aging

The free radical theory of aging dates back to the 1950s and there is now a large body of evidence that oxidative damage can occur with aging in multiple tissues including musculoskeletal tissues. Oxidative damage in aging cartilage has been detected using antibodies to nitrotyrosine, which recognize a modification occurring after the reaction of protein tyrosine residues with the free-radical peroxynitrite generated from nitric oxide reacting with superoxide. In addition, age-related oxidative stress in human articular chondrocytes has been detected by measuring the ratio of intracellular oxidized to reduced glutathione. A reduction in levels of antioxidant enzymes with aging may contribute to an increase in oxidative stress and damage. As discussed further below, an increased level of reactive oxygen species (ROS) in aging chondrocytes could be important to the age-related increase in OA.

AGING AND THE DEVELOPMENT OF OSTEOARTHRITIS

Aging as a Risk Factor for OA

OA is a disease process that usually develops slowly over a long period and becomes manifest in the later years of life. OA is not seen clinically in children or adolescents and is rare in young adults, but becomes increasingly common in those older than age 55 years. In the Framingham cohort of subjects, radiographic knee OA was present in 27% of those aged 63 to 70 years and in 44% of those ages 80 years or older. A population survey in northern England that included x-rays of the hands, feet, spine, knees, and hips found evidence for radiographic OA in at least one joint in about 80% of the population by age 60 years (see Figure 112-3). Even so, not everyone develops OA with age; all joints are not equally affected by OA; and, perhaps most importantly, not every joint or every individual with radiographic or even pathologic evidence of the disease is symptomatic. In several studies, it has been found that only about 50% of people with radiographic OA are symptomatic.

Osteoarthritis appears to remain asymptomatic until sufficient damage occurs to structures capable of producing pain or results in changes in joint function. The percentage of people with symptoms increases with more severe radiographic disease and in particular people with bone marrow lesions noted on magnetic resonance imaging. These lesions appear in regions neighboring areas with the greatest cartilage loss and are associated with alignment abnormalities. An additional level of complexity is added by the physical, psychological, and sociological factors that contribute to the development of symptoms such as pain. The end result is a multifactorial, heterogeneous group of diseases in which symptoms do not always correlate with pathologic changes as visualized using methods such as plain radiographs.

Most likely the process leading to OA is initiated earlier in life under the influence of factors specific to each individual such as obesity, joint injury, abnormal joint anatomy, and genetically abnormal cartilage matrix proteins. These factors act by either directly altering the structure or metabolism of cartilage or bone or indirectly affecting the tissues by altering joint biomechanics. The changes noted in joint function and musculoskeletal tissues with age appear to increase the risk of developing OA and may contribute to progression of the disease. Abnormal effects on joint structure and function from one or more of the "OA factors" likely works in concert with aging to result in the development of the disease and to the expression of symptoms and disability (Figure 112-5).

As is the case with all diseases that are common in old age, osteoarthritis is really a group of diseases of various etiologies, resulting in common pathologic changes within diarthrodial joints. Pathologically, OA is characterized by changes in both cartilage and bone (see Figure 112-2). Fibrillation and loss of articular cartilage by degradation are accompanied by hypertrophic changes in the subchondral

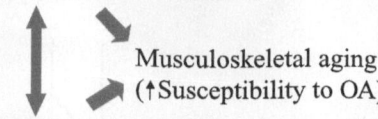
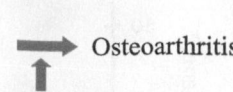

FIGURE 112-5. Relationship between musculoskeletal aging and the development of osteoarthritis. Changes that affect joint structure and function with aging increase the susceptibility to developing osteoarthritis but additional factors (OA factors) are usually also present which lead to the development of symptomatic osteoarthritis.

bone, resulting in subchondral thickening and in osteophyte formation at joint margins. Like many of the changes seen in cartilage, the changes in bone appear to be in opposite directions when comparing aging and OA (see Table 112-3). Thickening of the subchondral bone is a consistent finding in OA, whereas decreasing bone mass is commonly seen with age, at least in cortical and particularly in trabecular bone.

However, studies of aging in bone have not specifically assessed the region of the subchondral bone. The subchondral bone can remodel in response to mechanical loading, and this bony remodeling may play an important role in the OA disease process. It has been hypothesized that thicker and stiffer subchondral bone would place additional stress on the overlying cartilage during joint loading, resulting in mechanical failure of the cartilage. There is much debate about whether OA actually starts with changes in the subchondral bone rather than in cartilage. The answer as to which comes first may depend on the circumstances by which OA has developed. The importance of the subchondral bone to the OA disease process has been emphasized by studies that show increased activity in this region, detected by technetium bone scans, can predict disease progression in OA. Likewise, the presence of bone marrow lesions on magnetic resonance imaging (MRI) is also a risk factor for progression.

There is evidence for some degree of synovial inflammation in most patients with symptomatic OA, although the amount of synovial inflammation varies. A study that examined synovial tissue removed at the time of knee replacement found that about one third of patients had mild synovitis, one third moderate, and one third severe, suggesting that synovitis may play a role in disease progression in a subset of patients.

Contribution of Aging to the Anabolic and Catabolic Imbalance in OA

OA is often described as a "wear and tear" degenerative disease because the cartilage changes are most severe in the areas that receive the greatest mechanical stress. But the pathobiology of OA is much more complicated than either simple joint aging or wear and tear from repetitive use. Unlike an automobile part that can simply wear out with time, the tissues that comprise the joint contain living and metabolically active cells. The cells themselves are responsible for the destruction of the cartilage, likely under the influence of biomechanical forces, as well as for dynamic processes involved in continual regeneration, repair, and remodeling.

The cartilage changes found in OA appear to be caused by an imbalance between anabolic and catabolic activity. In OA, the chondrocytes are synthetically active, producing increased amounts of a number of matrix proteins, most likely as an attempt at repairing the damaged matrix. However, OA chondrocytes also produce increased amounts of degradative enzymes that overwhelm the repair response. Increased levels of several of the MMPs, including MMP-1, 2, 3, 9, and 13, as well as the aggrecanases (ADAMTS-4 and -5), have been noted in OA cartilage and appear to play a key role in matrix degradation. Matrix fragments, including hyaluronic acid fragments, collagen fragments, and fibronectin fragments, are produced as a result of the increased proteolytic activity and these fragments can in turn act on the cell to stimulate further matrix destruction. Cytokines, including IL-1, TNF-α, and others, are also increased in OA cartilage and contribute to the increased production of MMPs. Other factors associated with inflammation such as prostaglandins, nitric oxide, and ROS are also increased in OA cartilage. The increased local production of cytokines and inflammatory mediators in OA cartilage indicates that OA is really a process that involves cartilage inflammation.

Another characteristic of OA cartilage is the appearance of clusters of chondrocytes resulting from cell proliferation, thought to be part of the attempt at matrix repair. But areas practically devoid of cells can be seen adjacent to areas containing cell clusters. The overall number of cells in OA cartilage appears to decline, especially in the advanced stages of the disease. This decline is associated with the appearance of apoptotic chondrocytes, indicating that cell death is occurring, although significant cell death has not been confirmed at earlier stages of the disease. Therefore, it is not clear whether an imbalance between cell proliferation and death plays an important role

in the development of OA. If it does, then aging changes that reduce the proliferative capacity of the cells and changes which make the cells more susceptible to dying would contribute to the development of OA in older adults.

Similar to findings suggestive of a reduced response to growth factor stimulation with age in normal cartilage, studies indicate that chondrocytes from OA cartilage are also less responsive to growth factor stimulation. Lack of an anabolic response to IGF-I has been noted in several studies of OA chondrocytes. The decrease in response to IGF-I in OA may be related to increased levels of IGF-binding proteins, also noted in OA cartilage, which could decrease the amount of free IGF-1 available to bind to cell receptors. Although serum levels of IGF-1 decrease with age, there is no evidence that local levels in cartilage decrease. In fact, in OA cartilage levels of IGF-1 appear to be increased. If the cells maintain responsiveness to cytokines such as IL-1 while losing responsiveness to growth factors such as IGF-1, this could sway the balance of cartilage synthesis and degradation toward the catabolic side. This would be an important link between aging and the development of OA since an age-related resistance to growth factors such as IGF-I would allow degradative pathways to stay on, which would normally be shut down by growth factors released from matrix stores (Figure 112-6).

The basic cellular mechanisms that explain how aging contributes to the development of OA are just beginning to be understood. One hypothesis being tested is that production of ROS leading to oxidative stress alters the normal signaling pathways in the cartilage such that catabolic signaling is favored over anabolic. ROS are produced by chondrocytes in response to stimuli by cytokines as well as matrix fragments and are required as secondary messengers in cell signaling. ROS may also be produced in response to matrix damage from mechanical stimulation. Excessive levels of ROS could interfere with anabolic signaling pathways such as the IGF-I pathway and in this way tip the balance of anabolic and catabolic signaling (see Figure112-6). Restoring this balance represents an important goal for future OA therapies.

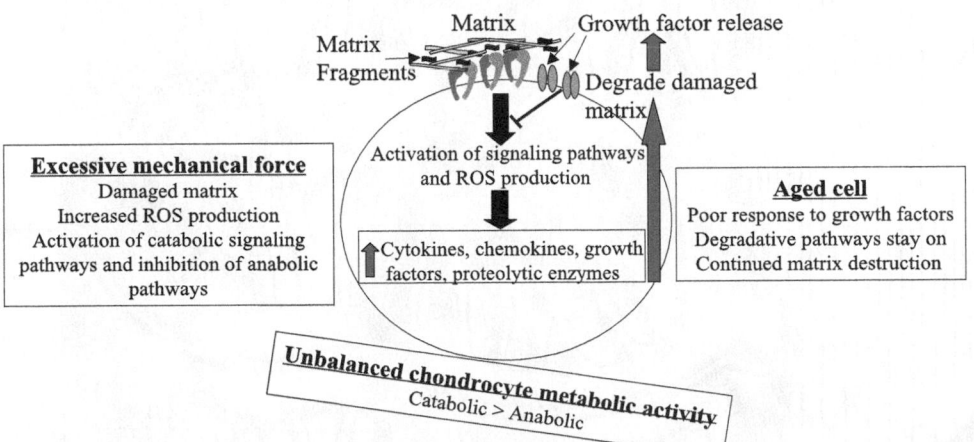

FIGURE 112-6. Theoretical model for pathways involved in cartilage destruction during the development of osteoarthritis. Excessive mechanical forces stimulate the chondrocyte directly or indirectly through signals generated by matrix damage including generation of matrix fragments. The resultant activation of signaling pathways, including ROS generation, results in increased production of cytokines, chemokines, and proteolytic enzymes. This catabolic response to injury serves to degrade the damaged matrix. Matrix degradation results in release of growth factors stored in the matrix, which would normally feedback on the cell and shut down the catabolic pathways. But aged chondrocytes have an insufficient response to growth factor stimulation resulting in continued matrix destruction from unbalanced catabolic and anabolic activity. *(Reproduced with permission from Loeser RF. Molecular mechanisms of cartilage destruction: mechanics, inflammatory mediators and aging collide. Arthritis Rheum. 2006;54:1357.)*

SKELETAL MUSCLE

Skeletal Muscle Structure and Function

All skeletal muscle is enclosed by a sheath of connective tissue called epimysium. Bundles of muscle fibers and individual contracting units of muscle fibers are surrounded by partitions of the connective tissue constituting the perimysium and the endomysium, respectively. Blood vessels, lymphatics, and nerves reach all the muscle compartments by way of these fibrous partitions. The connective tissue merges into stronger structures such as tendons, aponeuroses, raphes, the reticular layer of dermis, or the periosteum that provide support for muscle insertion and contraction.

Matured single muscle fibers are long multinucleated and cylindric units separated from other cells and surrounded by a membrane, the sarcolemma. Muscle fibers contain myofibrils made up of the contractile proteins myosin, actin, tropomyosin, and troponin and the structural supportive proteins actinin and titin. The particular spatial arrangement of the thick and thin contractile proteins is responsible for the characteristic cross-striations in skeletal muscle. Differences in the refractive index of the muscle fiber determine the alternation of light I band and dark A band (Figure 112-7). Z lines in the middle of the I bands are the limits of a sarcomere. The thick

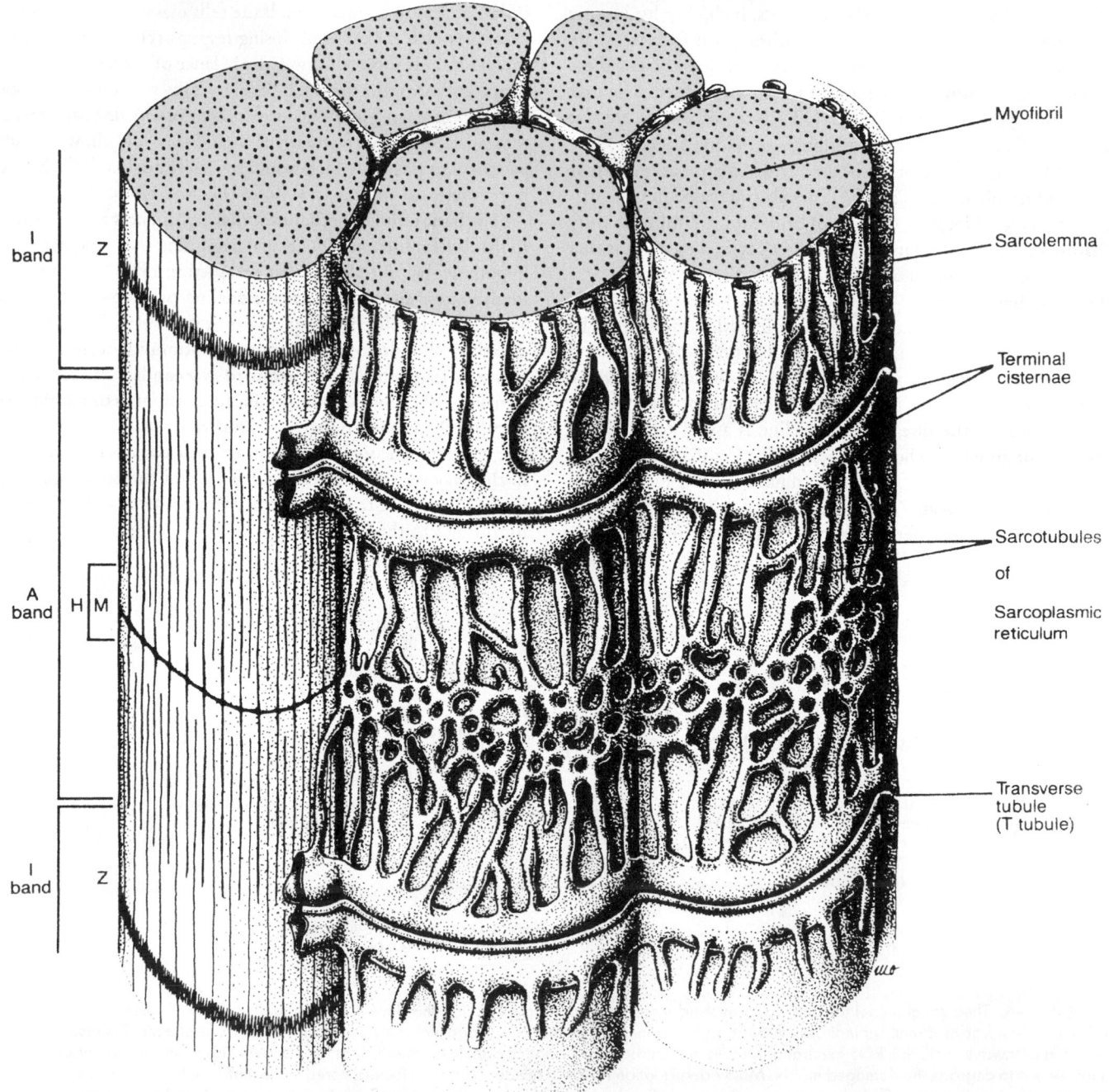

FIGURE 112-7. Diagram of a skeletal muscle fiber illustrating the spatial arrangement of contractile proteins and surrounding membrane system. *(Reproduced with permission from Cormack DH. Ham's Histology. 9th ed. Philadelphia: Lippincott, William and Wilkins; 1987:402.)*

filaments are made up of myosin, whereas the thin filaments are made up of actin, tropomyosin, and troponin.

Myosin is an actin-binding protein provided with a catalytic site that hydrolyzes adenosine triphosphate (ATP), the source of energy for muscle contraction. Actin molecules polymerize in long, thin double-helix filaments, forming a groove where tropomyosin molecules are located. Troponin molecules are located at regular intervals along the tropomyosin molecules. Troponin has three components: troponin T binds the other components to tropomyosin, troponin I inhibits the interaction of myosin with actin, and troponin C contains the binding sites for calcium that initiate muscle contraction.

Motor Unit

Lower spinal cord motor neurons provide a common pathway for transmitting neural impulses from upper motor levels of the central nervous system to the skeletal muscle. This information is directed to skeletal muscles via the ventral roots, peripheral nerves, and cranial nerves. Each motor neuron innervates muscle fibers within a single muscle and the motor neurons innervating a single muscle are grouped in the spinal cord, forming the motor neuron pool for that muscle. During development, polyinnervated muscles become innervated by a single motor neuron. Axonal branches establish synapses with multiple muscle fibers of a single muscle. The activation of a motor neuron brings all the muscle fibers to the mechanical threshold; therefore, a single motor neuron and its associated muscle fibers constitute the motor unit that is the smallest that can be activated to induce movement. On the basis of the speed of contraction, three types of motor units can be distinguished: fast-fatigable motor units, fatigue-resistant motor units, and slow-motor units that are in between the first two subtypes in terms of time to fatigue initiation. These differences in motor unit performance are based on physiologic and biochemical characteristics of their constituent muscle fibers.

Events in Muscle Contraction and Relaxation: Skeletal Muscle Excitation–Contraction Coupling

Skeletal muscle contraction is initiated by generation and conduction of action potentials by the motor neuron, release of acetylcholine at the motor end-plate, and binding to nicotinic acetylcholine receptors, and an increase in sodium and potassium conductance in the end-plate membrane. End-plate potentials at the muscle membrane lead to generation of action potentials and their conduction to the sarcolemmal infoldings (T-tubules).

The transduction of changes in sarcolemmal potential into elevations in intracellular calcium concentration is a key event that precedes muscle contraction. The muscle electromechanical transduction requires the participation of a protein located at the sarcolemmal T tubule, the dihydropyridine receptor (DHPR), in the early steps of this signal-transduction mechanism. The DHPR is a voltage-gated L-type Ca^{2+} channel (dihydropyridine-sensitive), and its activation evokes Ca^{2+} release from an intracellular store, the sarcoplasmic reticulum (SR) through ryanodine-sensitive calcium channels (RyR1) into the myoplasm. Figure 112-8 illustrates the typical arrangement of DHPR and RyR at the skeletal muscle triadic junction. The functional consequence of alterations in the number, function, or interaction of these receptors is a reduction in the amount of intracellular calcium mobilization and in the development of force. Calcium is bound to troponin C, leading to formation

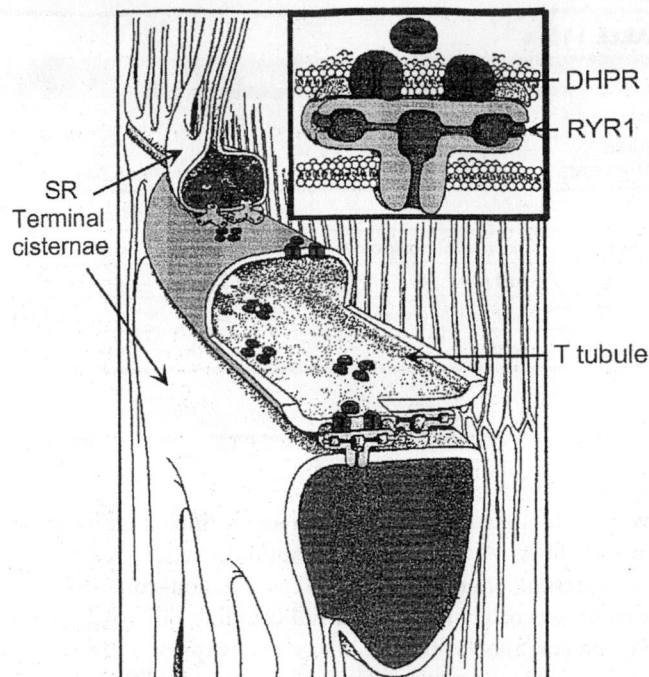

FIGURE 112-8. Schematic of the interaction between the dihydropyridine receptor (DHPR) and ryanodine receptor (RyR1) and their location at the sarcolemmal tubular system and sarcoplasmic reticulum terminal cisternae, respectively. *(Redrawn from Block BA, Imagawa T, Campbell KP, Franzini-Armstrong C. Structural evidence for direct interaction between the molecular components of the transverse tubule/sarcoplasmic raticulum junction in skeletal musicle. J Cell Biol. 1988 Dec;107(6 Pt 2):2587–2600; Brandt NR, Caswell AH, Wen SR, Talvenheimo JA. Molecular interactions of the junctional foot protein and dihydropyridine receptor in skeletal muscle triads. J Membr Biol. 1990 Feb;113(3):237–251; Wagenknecht T, Grassucci R, Frank J, Saito A, Inui M, Fleischer S. Three-dimensional architecture of the calcium channel/foot structure of sarcoplasmic reticulum. Nature. 1989 Mar 9;338(6211):167–170.)*

of cross-linkages between actin and myosin and sliding of thin on thick filaments, which produces shortening. Muscle relaxes as a result of calcium pumping back to the SR, release of calcium from troponin, and cessation of interaction between actin and myosin filaments.

Muscle Fiber Subtypes and Types of Contraction

Muscle fiber types can be determined using immunostaining or the adenosine triphosphatase (ATPase) stain based on the pH dependence of myosin ATPase activity, which relates closely to antigenic differences in myosin between fast- and slow-twitch muscles. Muscle fibers are classified by histochemical identification into type I and type II (A, B, and C) (Table 112-4), and into fast- and slow-twitch based on their contractile properties in response to brief stimulation (action potential). Fast-twitch fibers (type II, glycolytic, white) contract for less than 10 ms and are primarily concerned with fine, precise, and rapid movements. Slow-twitch fibers (type I, oxidative, red) exhibit twitch durations up to 100 ms and are involved in strong, gross, and sustained movements. Muscle fibers are integrated into motor units and are classified into fast-fatigable, fast-fatigue-resistant, and slow motor units according to their speed of contraction, maximum tension generated, and degree of fatigue.

TABLE 112-4

Histochemical Classification of Muscle Fibers

MUSCLE FIBER SUBTYPES	FUNCTIONAL AND HISTOCHEMICAL CHARACTERISTICS	ATPASE SATAIN		
		PH 9.4	pH 4.6	pH 4.2
Type I	Slow twitch, oxidative	Light	Dark	Dark
Type IIA	Fast twitch, oxidativeglycolytic	Dark	Light	Light
Type IIB	Fast twitch, glycolytic	Dark	Dark	Dark
Type IIC	Fetal	Dark	Dark	Dark

NEURAL CONTROL OF MUSCLE CONTRACTION

Several factors regulate muscle contraction, including innervation of muscle fibers. Alterations in innervation state leads to changes in gene expression of proteins involved in excitation–contraction (EC) coupling, ultimately resulting in EC coupling differences. During development, muscle fibers are innervated by spinal cord motor neurons. Fiber type is determined by interaction with different subpopulations of these motor neurons that activate contraction at different rates, ranging from 10 Hz (slow-twitch) to 100 Hz (fast-twitch fatigue-resistant) or 150 Hz (fast-twitch fatigue-sensitive). Interaction with motor neurons and induction of activity determines more than just fiber type. Depolarization of myotubes in culture triggers the appearance of dihydropyridine binding sites, suggesting that the induction of muscle activity during innervation induces DHPR expression.

Experimental denervation in fast-twitch muscle fibers, such as extensor digitorum longus (EDL), results in alterations in EC coupling. Denervated EDL fibers exhibit alterations indicative of reduced number or reduced functional DHPRs. Additionally, denervation affects DHPR function in other ways, slowing both DHPR activation and inactivation. Denervation also affects RyR1 function and expression. Morphological evidence from denervated EDL muscles shows a reduction in the number of "indentations" in SR terminal cisternae membranes. These indentations are the RyR1 feet at triad junctions. Accordingly, following denervation, RyR1 mRNA transcript levels have been shown to decrease.

DHPR in skeletal muscle is dependent upon the presence of RyR1 to function properly. Dyspedic myotubes, which do not express RyR1s as a result of a mutation, display drastically reduced DHPR function compared to normal myotubes. When dyspedic myotubes are transfected to express RyR1, DHPR function returns to normal levels. This evidence may indicate that denervation-induced reduction of DHPR expression may result from loss of innervation-driven gene expression, RyR1-driven DHPR gene expression, or a combination of both.

Although denervation removes nerve electrical influence from muscle, evidence indicates that electrical activity of a nerve is not the only controlling factor in muscle gene expression. Chronic blockade of nerve action potentials by infusion of tetrodotoxin, a specific sodium channel-blocker, without compromising axonal transport and nerve–muscle contact, increases expression of DHPR and RyR mRNA expression 4.5- and 2.5-fold, respectively. Accordingly, expression of both proteins was increased by 50% after 10 days of treatment with these agents. Muscle contraction analysis after elim-

inating axonal transport with a colchicine-containing cuff on the sciatic nerve in animal models indicate that alterations in EC coupling mechanisms may explain the decline in specific force.

While decreases in motor neuron electrical activation of and axonal delivery to skeletal muscle effect changes in gene expression, increases in nerve activity also causes changes in adult muscle gene expression. These changes are generally characterized by a fast-to-slow switch in myosin and Ca^{2+} ATPase isoforms. A 12-week endurance training program in rats, an activity that can lead to fast-to-slow transformations in muscle, was shown to increase DHPR expression as much as 60% in EDL muscles. Another method of increasing muscle activity, surgical ablation of synergistic muscles to induce hypertrophy of the plantaris muscle in rats, causes no change in DHPR or RyR1 expression in this predominately fast-twitch skeletal muscle. The possibility exists that the "protocol" used to increase activity plays an important role in regulating gene expression: endurance exercise training allows for long quiescent recovery periods between bouts of increased activity, while chronic low-frequency stimulation does not; and mechanical loading of muscle that induces hypertrophy apparently differs from these two protocols altogether.

In a rodent model, decreases in muscle activity without compromise of nerve–muscle interaction can be induced by mechanical unloading of muscle through the use of hindlimb unweighting. Hindlimb unloading is generally characterized by a slow-to-fast transition in fiber type, as evidenced by the increase in fast Ca^{2+} ATPase and myosin isoforms, as well as the speed of the unloaded muscle fiber shortening. This leads to marked atrophy of slow-twitch soleus muscles, but increases in DHPR mRNA and DHPR and RyR protein expression in the same soleus muscles. These results, taken together, indicate that electrical activity of the nerve, the pattern of nerve activation, axonal delivery of trophic factors to the muscle, muscle fiber type, fiber type transition direction (i.e., fast-to-slow or slow-to-fast), and type of muscle activity (i.e., endurance vs. strength training) are all variables that exist in tenuous balance to regulate muscle gene expression.

MECHANISMS UNDERLYING SKELETAL MUSCLE WEAKNESS IN OLD AGE

Age-related decreases in skeletal muscle mass and quality contribute to physical disability and loss of independence in the elderly population. In addition to decreased muscle mass, aging muscle is characterized by decreases in contractile force or weakness that have been reported to occur with age in several mammalian species including humans. Age-related weakness may be associated with fatigue, weakness discerned as an absolute decrease in muscle force, and fatigue as a progressive decline in force with prolonged physical activity. Muscle weakness is associated with limitations in activities of daily living, such as climbing stairs or rising from a chair, that lead to loss of independence. Muscle weakness is a risk factor for falling and also increases the risk for fractures resulting from a fall. Reduced heat and cold tolerance, impaired glucose homeostasis, and obesity have been also related to aging skeletal muscle. Decline in muscle performance with aging has been quantified in both untrained and highly trained individuals. These studies showed that although the individuals with higher levels of physical activity were stronger, the rate of decrease in the level of muscle performance in both groups was similar. These results suggest that age-related deficits are largely

TABLE 112-5

Suggested Pathogenesis of Skeletal Muscle Impairment with Aging

I. Neuronal alterations
  A. Spinal cord motor neurons
    1. Reduction in number
    2. Reduction in size
  B. Alterations in axonal flow
  C. Neuromuscular transmission alterations
    1. Decrease in nerve terminal numbers
    2. Reduced neurotransmitter release
    3. Decrease in acetylcholine receptor numbers
II. Primary muscle alterations
  A. Contraction-induced injury
  B. Alterations in muscle signal transduction (trophic factor/hormone resistance)
III. Combined neurogenic-muscular mechanism
  A. Muscle unloading
  B. Excitation–contraction uncoupling
IV. General mechanisms that involve skeletal muscle
  A. Oxidative stress
  B. Mitochondrial deoxyribonucleic acid mutations
  C. Age-related vasculopathy

inevitable and decreases in physical activity further contribute to this process.

Despite the importance of muscle strength in preventing disability, the biological mechanisms responsible for these phenomena are poorly understood. Cellular and molecular aspects have been explored both in human and more extensively in animal models of aging. The conclusions included in this section arise from investigations in human and nonhuman aging skeletal muscle. Factors that determine skeletal muscle impairment with aging can be divided into four groups: (1) neurogenic, (2) myogenic, (3) a combination of neural and muscular alterations, and (4) general mechanisms that involve skeletal muscle (Table 112-5).

Neurogenic Mechanisms of Skeletal Muscle Impairment with Aging

Neurogenic mechanisms of decline in muscle function with age include reduction in the number and/or size of spinal cord motor neurons, alterations in axonal flow, and the neuromuscular junction. Each of these factors, individually or in combination, leads to chronic muscle denervation and motor unit remodeling. Some older persons present electromyographic evidence of muscle denervation suggestive of motor neuron alterations. These patients never develop classical amyotrophic diseases (e.g., amyotrophic lateral sclerosis). Muscle denervation is associated with reinnervation, as demonstrated by the presence of muscle fiber grouping in histologic sections. Cycles of muscle denervation associated with reinnervation lead to motor unit remodeling.

The functional significance of motor unit remodeling still needs to be determined. The relative histologic areas corresponding to fast- and slow-twitch muscle fibers change with age, becoming predominantly slow muscle fibers. Age-related remodeling of motor units appears to involve denervation of fast muscle fibers with reinnervation by axonal sprouting from slow fibers. Therefore, motor unit remodeling leads to changes in fiber-type distribution in mixed fiber-type muscles.

Reinnervation of muscle fibers tends to compensate for denervation; however, a net loss of fibers across age has been detected. This obviously occurs when the rate of muscle fiber denervation surpasses the rate of axonal sprouting and reinnervation. Indirect studies show a decrease in the total number of fast-motor units and enlargement of the remaining motor units with age. Direct neuronal counting shows a reduction in the number and/or size of ventral spinal motor neurons at the cervical or lumbar regions with aging. Whether alterations in motor neuron, nerve terminal, or axonal transport account for muscle denervation is not clear.

Studies on conduction velocity in peripheral nerves do not show significant changes with aging. This would suggest that alterations in myelin or severe reductions in nerve axonal composition do not occur with age. Although denervation has been suggested as a contributing factor to aging skeletal muscle, the extension of denervation in individual muscles and its effect on human muscles remain to be determined. In addition, it is becoming apparent that denervation does not explain a significant deficit in specific maximum isometric tetanic force (muscle force normalized to cross-sectional area) recorded in aged skeletal muscles. Also, decreases in the number of spinal cord motor neurons occur after the eighth decade, when the loss in muscle mass and strength is already well established.

Myogenic Mechanisms of Skeletal Muscle Impairment with Aging

Primary muscular or myogenic factors refer to a group of alterations including contraction-induced injury and alterations in muscle signal transduction (trophic factor/ hormone resistance). The phenomenon of contraction-induced injury is related to increased mechanical frailty and decline in muscle restorative capacity with age. Muscles from older individuals or animals become injured when undergoing lengthening contractions. Also, older muscles recover more slowly and do not exhibit complete recovery when compared with those in younger controls. Eccentric contraction injury has also been demonstrated in older individuals. Insulin and IGF-1 resistance in aging skeletal muscle have been reported. The influence of weight and physical activity on trophic factor/hormone resistance are currently under investigation.

Combined Neurogenic–Muscular Mechanism

Combined mechanisms include muscle unloading and EC uncoupling. Muscle unloading associated with sedentary lifestyle is a major determinant of muscle atrophy in the elderly population. The decrease in physical activity is a combined process in which the lower the nerve activation, the lower the muscle contraction. This process leads subsequently to muscle atrophy. However, not all the motor units within a muscle seem to be affected to the same extent. Predominant atrophy of type II fibers has been reported in aging muscles from rodents; however, the clinical significance of this finding is uncertain because there are very few type IIB fibers in human muscles.

Alterations with age in muscle fiber signal transduction such as sarcolemmal excitation–SR calcium release uncoupling and impaired IGF-1-dependent modulation of muscle calcium channels have been demonstrated. Studies in muscle fibers deprived of sarcolemma (skinned muscle fibers) demonstrated that the force generated per unit cross-sectional area does not differ in adult and old mice during isometric contractions. These results suggest that muscle atrophy does not explain entirely the age-related decline in muscle strength. A deficit in specific contractile force (force normalized to muscle cross-sectional area) in aging skeletal muscle has been described in the literature. However, the significance of this finding in terms of the etiology and therapeutics of the age-related decline in muscle force has not been sufficiently investigated.

The deficit in specific force is a widespread phenomenon involving fast- and slow-twitch fibers in different muscles. Several mechanisms have been postulated to explain the skeletal muscle weakness associated with aging. However, it is not known whether the loss of specific and absolute force share common mechanisms. It appears that the age-related impairment in muscle force is only partially explained by the loss in muscle mass. Therefore, both the loss in specific and absolute forces contributes to the muscle weakness measured in the elderly and in animal models of aging.

Successful interventions aimed at counteracting age-associated functional deficits will require better insight into the mechanisms underlying the decline in muscle-specific force. Alterations in several mechanisms of signal transduction operate in aging skeletal muscles. Two of these mechanisms in particular are directly involved in development of muscle force: excitation-induced elevations in intracellular calcium and energy conversion from ATP into a mechanical response. It seems that changes in phosphorus metabolites involved in energy transduction (phosphocreatine, adenosine diphosphate [ADP], and ATP) and myosin isoforms do not change with aging. However, alterations in EC coupling have been demonstrated in human quadriceps.

Physiologic activation of the muscle membrane elicits elevations in intracellular Ca^{2+} that, in turn, induce muscle contraction by interaction with contractile proteins. Impairments in the mechanism of transduction of muscle activation into intracellular Ca^{2+} mobilization lead to decreases in muscle tension, clinically manifested as muscle weakness. The basic mechanism underlying EC uncoupling with aging is a molecular unlinkage between the two calcium channels, one that functions at the external membrane (sarcolemma) as a voltage-sensor, the other mediates calcium release from intracellular stores (SR). Alterations in EC coupling result from significant changes in either the number or regulation of these molecules, or both.

General Mechanisms of Aging that Involve Skeletal Muscle

General mechanisms that may adversely affect skeletal muscle directly or indirectly are oxidative DNA damage, mitochondrial DNA (mtDNA) mutations, and age-related vasculopathy. Superoxide radical and hydrogen peroxide that are continuously produced in aerobic cells undergo metal ion-catalyzed conversion into hydroxyl radicals. These hydroxyl radicals can cause oxidative damage, which, in turn, may be related to the development of mutations in mtDNA. Mitochondrial DNA mutations are associated with ischemic heart disease, late-onset diabetes, Parkinson's disease, Alzheimer's disease, and aging. The accumulation of damage to mtDNA by oxidation may be the basis for defects in oxidative phosphorylation capacity with age. A decline in oxidative phosphorylation capacity would be-

come symptomatic when tissue energetics fall below the threshold required for optimal organ function.

A group of factors that deserve attention are subclinical inflammation, vascular pathology, and muscle perfusion. Subclinical inflammation has been suggested as a mechanism for loss in muscle mass and weakness in the elderly, often called sarcopenia. Such inflammation-related loss may be mediated by tissue increases in TNF-α, IL-6, IL-1α, and/or IL-1β. Some evidence suggests that subclinical inflammation may contribute to the debilitating muscle atrophy associated with congestive heart failure, renal failure, or rheumatoid arthritis. In the extreme, this may lead to cachexia, generalized loss of muscle as well as fat mass, aggravated by the anorexia associated with starvation, acquired immunodeficiency syndrome, or advanced cancer. Thus, the involuntary decline in muscle mass characteristic of old age may represent a continuation in degree and rate of development with inflammation, subclinical or clinical, as an important mediating mechanism. The existence of an altered capillary bed in aging skeletal muscle is controversial at the present time. Reduced or increased numbers of capillaries have been reported in the literature, but less is known about muscle perfusion in physiologic conditions.

CLINICAL AND EXPERIMENTAL INTERVENTIONS AIMED AT DELAYING OR PREVENTING AGE-ASSOCIATED CHANGES IN SKELETAL MUSCLE COMPOSITION AND FUNCTION

We are just beginning to identify the specific changes in muscle with age. Withdrawal of anabolic stimuli to skeletal muscle, including decline in estrogen/androgen, growth hormone, insulin, or IGF-1 may lead to both loss in muscle mass and impairment in the intrinsic capacity of the muscle fiber to generate force. A key question to be addressed at this time in studies of both muscle and cartilage is: does a cell-signaling impairment with aging result from tissue resistance to trophic factors? Increasing evidence supports this concept. However, understanding this process requires further insight into a more general phenomenon, the role of trophic factors in mature tissue maintenance and restoration.

In healthy individuals, deficiency with aging in spontaneous and stimulated growth hormone secretion, as well as circulating IGF-1 and IGF-binding protein-3 levels, is associated with decreased lean body mass, decreased protein synthesis, and increased percent body fat. Administration of recombinant human growth hormone or growth hormone secretagogues improves nitrogen balance, increases lean body mass, and decreases body fat in older people with low IGF-1 levels. However, the effects on muscle strength do not seem to be proportional to the improvement in muscle mass with such replacements.

IGF-1 is a peptide structurally related to proinsulin, which has a primary role in promoting skeletal muscle differentiation and growth. In skeletal muscle, IGF-1 potentiates calcium current through L-type calcium channels in adult fibers but not in muscles from aging mammals, probably because of IGF-1 resistance. Using a transgenic mouse model overexpressing IGF-1 in skeletal muscle, increases in the number of DHPR have been reported. IGF-1 also has an effect on muscle mass, inducing hypertrophy in transgenic models or preventing atrophy in aging rodents. Virally mediated overexpression of IGF-1 in muscle prevents the age-related loss in type IIB fibers and contractile force in rodents. In summary, IGF-1 prevents EC uncoupling, changes in fiber type composition, and loss in absolute and specific force. One of the main stumbling blocks for IGF-1 application to human therapeutics is the need to design a strategy for safe delivery of IGF-1 in a sustained fashion.

Caloric restriction has beneficial effects on skeletal muscle structure and function. Transcriptional patterns of tissues from calorie-restricted animals, analyzed by DNA microarrays, suggest that calorie restriction retards the aging process by reducing endogenous damage and by inducing metabolic shifts associated with specific transcriptional profiles. Caloric restriction delayed the decline of gastrocnemius muscle mass and reduced the age-related loss of hindlimb skeletal muscle mass in rodents. Caloric reduction has been found to reduce the rate of age-related skeletal muscle mass loss in soleus, anterior tibialis, EDL, and hindlimb muscle of rats. The secondary or delayed onset injury induced by the free radicals in EDL muscle was alleviated by treatment with a free radical scavenger, polyethylene glycol–superoxide dismutase. Furthermore, 50% caloric restriction initiated at 17 months of age preserved the fiber number and fiber type composition in the vastus lateralis muscle of the aged rat. Our laboratory has demonstrated that calorie restriction prevents significantly age-dependent decrease in rat EDL and soleus muscles and the expression of proteins that play a crucial role in EC coupling. Whether this effect is recorded exclusively on muscle, motor neuron, or both was uncertain until recently when it was demonstrated that food restriction decreases motor neuronal loss with advancing age in the rat. Only sparse information about effects of calorie restriction on humans is available. Calorie restriction increases muscle mitochondrial biogenesis in healthy humans and reduces plasma endothelin-1 concentration, improving consequently obesity-induced endothelial dysfunction. The effect of calorie restriction on human skeletal muscle is currently unknown. Results from a human clinical trial (Comprehensive Assessment of Long-Term Effects of Reducing Intake of Energy [CALERIE]) sponsored by the National Institute on Aging will provide some clues on the effectiveness of this intervention on age-related diseases, and perhaps muscle changes with age.

Exercise is clearly one of the most effective interventions in reducing muscle impairment in the elderly. Exercise interventions such as resistance training are being used in an attempt to restore muscle force in the elderly. Strength training in sedentary young and sedentary older individuals improves muscle force, improves metabolic capacities, increases glycogen storage, and enhances oxidative enzyme activity. Aerobic training involving high-repetition, low-intensity muscle contractions leads to minimal strength gain when compared to the low-repetition, high-intensity stimulus of resistance training in which both strengthening as well as endurance activities are included. Further studies on the use of trophic factors and on the use of specific exercise interventions are needed to determine the best means of preventing or reversing the decline in muscle function with age.

TENDONS AND LIGAMENTS

Tendons and ligaments are composed of dense connective tissue that has a high content of fibrillar collagen to provide tensile strength. Tendons attach muscle to bone, while ligaments attach bone to bone. The integrity of these attachments is important for normal joint function. Ligaments serve to stabilize the joints, and tendons transmit the forces of muscle contraction to bone. There appears to be a general decline in joint range of motion with age that may be related, at least in part, to changes in tendons and ligaments.

The percent reduction in range of motion varies with the joint studied and is greatly influenced by both disuse and disease. In general, declines in the range of 20% to 25% have been reported. In addition to effects on joint motion, aging-related changes in tendons and ligaments may contribute to the development of injuries to these structures, resulting in conditions ranging from tendonitis to tendon and ligament tears or rupture. Although these injuries certainly occur in younger individuals, the amount of trauma required to produce them is reduced with age. In addition, ligamentous ruptures from injuries in younger individuals can predispose the affected joint to the development of OA later in life as a result from joint instability, altering joint biomechanics.

Biomechanical studies reveal that the strength of tendons and ligaments and their insertions to bone are reduced with age. In one study, it took approximately one third less loading to cause failure of the anterior cruciate ligament attachment in cadaver knees from individuals aged 60 to 97 years, as compared with a younger group individuals aged 22 to 35 years. A twofold decrease in the strength of the anterior longitudinal ligament of the spine has also been noted in subjects between the ages of 21 and 79 years in cadaver studies.

Shoulder problems are quite common in older adults and may be related to aging changes in the rotator cuff tendons. Changes with age including calcification, microtears, and fibrovascular proliferation have been reported in the region where the tendons attach to bone. These changes would result in a weakening in the attachment, predisposing the tissue to injury after minor trauma.

Biochemical studies of aging in tendons and ligaments have been limited but have shown changes with age, some of which are similar to changes noted in cartilage. Like cartilage, the tensile strength of these tissues depends on the collagen fibers, although the primary fibrillar collagen is type I rather than the type II found in cartilage. There is no clear evidence that collagen content in ligaments or tendons changes with age, but changes in cross-linking have been reported with the appearance of nonreducible cross-links with age, including cross-links formed by nonenzymatic glycation. Increased cross-linking may cause increased stiffness of the collagen and make it more prone to fatigue failure. Like cartilage, there appears to be a decrease in the water content of tendons and ligaments with age, but there is little information on changes in proteoglycans that, if altered, could explain the reduced water content as discussed earlier with respect to cartilage proteoglycans.

INTERVERTEBRAL DISKS

Imaging studies of normal subjects without recent back pain, as well as morphologic studies of autopsy material, show that disk degeneration increases directly with age, with at least some degree of degeneration universally present by the sixth decade of life. Because the presence of disk degeneration does not correlate well with symptoms of pain, it is often difficult to determine the clinical significance of these findings. Magnetic resonance imaging evidence of disk bulging and herniation increases with age but is often asymptomatic. On the other hand, disk herniation associated with extrusion of disk material is more likely to be associated with symptoms, particularly if the disk material extends beyond the posterior longitudinal ligament. It is also generally agreed that degenerative changes in the intervertebral disks likely contribute to a variety of conditions seen in older adults, including osteoarthritis, spondylosis, and spinal stenosis.

The intervertebral disks consist of an outer fibrous ring of dense connective tissue referred to as the annulus fibrosus and an inner gel-like material called the nucleus pulposus. The annulus fibrosus is composed of approximately 70% collagen by dry weight, whereas the nucleus pulposus is approximately 20% collagen and 50% proteoglycan. The superior and inferior boundaries of the disks are formed by end-plates consisting of a thin layer of cortical bone covered by hyaline cartilage that directly connects with the vertebral bodies. Aging changes occur within all these regions but are probably most pronounced in the nucleus pulposus.

The most common age-related change in the disk is dehydration. There is a marked decrease in water content, particularly in the nucleus pulposus, which becomes fibrotic, and, starting in young adults, contains fissures and cracks. Tears also become common in the outer annulus in young adults. These can lead to disk herniation, which has a peak incidence at about 40 to 50 years of age. With advancing age, the nucleus pulposus becomes more dehydrated and less likely to herniate. The decrease in water content is likely related to a decrease in proteoglycans in the nucleus pulposus as well as an increase in collagen cross-linking which, by making the collagen network stiffer, allows for less expansion of the proteoglycans. Similar to articular cartilage, there is evidence that increased collagen cross-linking with age is caused by the accumulation of advanced glycation end-products.

Many of the age-related changes noted in intervertebral disks are thought to be attributable to a decline in the diffusion of nutrients to the disc cells. Cells in the nucleus pulposus derive their nutrition by diffusion from vessels in the outside layers of the annulus and from the vertebral end plates. There appears to be a decline in the number of vessels in these regions with age, a disease which can be made worse by conditions including atherosclerotic vascular diseases and diabetes. There is a dramatic decline in the number of viable cells in the nucleus pulposus with age. This is associated with evidence of apoptotic cell death, likely because of the lack of nutrients.

Apoptotic cell death has also been noted in the end-plates. These structures become increasingly calcified with age. This contributes to the development of sclerosis. Because the facet joints of the spine are intimately linked with the end-plates and the disks, the age-related changes in these structures contribute significantly to the development of osteoarthritic changes in the spine. Degenerative disk disease accompanied by vertebral osteophytosis results in spondylosis, which, when severe, can cause spinal stenosis.

There is still much that is not known about aging in the intervertebral disks as well as in cartilage, muscle, ligaments, and tendons. It is necessary to continue to try to separate normal aging from changes in these tissues that lead to disease so that appropriate interventions can be designed to prevent and treat musculoskeletal disease in older adults.

FURTHER READING

Carrington JL. Aging bone and cartilage: cross-cutting issues. *Biochem Biophys Res Commun.* 2005;328:700.

Ding C, Cicuttini F, Blizzard L, Scott F, Jones G. A longitudinal study of the effect of sex and age on rate of change in knee cartilage volume in adults. *Rheumatology (Oxford)* 2007;46:273.

Freemont AJ, Hoyland JA. Morphology, mechanisms and pathology of musculoskeletal ageing. *J Pathol.* 2007;211:252.

Jarvik JG, Deyo RA. Imaging of lumbar intervertebral disk degeneration and aging, excluding disk herniations. *Radiol Clin North Am.* 2000;38:1255.

Loeser RF, Shakoor N. Aging or osteoarthritis: which is the problem? *Rheum Dis Clin North Am.* 2003;29:653.

Pelletier J-P, et al. Osteoarthritis, an inflammatory disease: potential implication for the selection of new therapeutic targets. *Arthritis Rheum.* 2001;44:1237.

Renganathan M, et al. Overexpression of IGF-1 exclusively in skeletal muscle prevents age-related decline in the number of dihydropyridine receptors. *J Biol Chem.* 1998;273:28845.

Roubenoff R, Hughes VA. Sarcopenia: current concepts. *J Gerontol.* 2000;55A:M716.

Verzijl N, et al. Effect of collagen turnover on the accumulation of advanced glycation end products. *J Biol Chem.* 2000;275:39027.

Wang Z-M, et al. Extension and magnitude of denervation in skeletal muscle from ageing mice. *J Physiol.* 2005;565(Pt 3):757.

Weindruch R. Interventions based on the possibility that oxidative stress contributes to sarcopenia. *J Gerontol A Biol Sci Med Sci.* 1995;50:157.

Zheng Z, et al. Insulin-like growth factor-1 increases skeletal muscle dihydropyridine receptor alpha 1S transcriptional activity by acting on the cAMP-response element-binding protein element of the promoter region. *J Biol Chem.* 2002;277:50535.

Biomechanics of Mobility

James A. Ashton-Miller ■ *Neil B. Alexander*

PREVALENCE OF MOBILITY PROBLEMS AMONG OLDER ADULTS

Problems with mobility in older adults are common. In the United States, among noninstitutionalized persons 65 years and older, approximately 13% have difficulty in performing activities of daily living. Approximately 9% have difficulty with bathing, 8% have difficulty with walking, and 6% have difficulty with bed or chair transfers. The rate at which these problems occur increases progressively after the age of 65 years and climbs sharply after the age of 80 years, so that, for example, more than 34% of noninstitutionalized persons who are 85 years or older have mobility problems.

AGE AND GENDER DIFFERENCES IN FALLS AND FALL-RELATED INJURY RATES

Perhaps the most serious problem of mobility impairment is the tendency of older adults to fall and to be injured by falls. Death rates from falls per 100,000 persons in 1999 were 9.1 for those between 65 and 74 years, 31.7 for those between 75 and 84 years, and 109.7 for those 85 years or older. For comparison, in those aged 75 years and older, the death rate from falls (67.9 per 100,000) is more than double that from motor vehicle accidents (29.8 per 100,000). Falls and fall injuries are of substantial concern because of their frequency and because of their physical, psychological, and social consequences. Even a fall that does not result in injury can have a substantially adverse effect on an older person's self-confidence, mobility, and independence. Indeed, fear of falling, which can accompany decreased mobility, can lead to decreased physical activity outside and avoidance of social activities because of the possibility of embarrassment as well as injury in connection with a fall.

Older females are substantially more prone to fall and to be injured in a fall than are older males. Three studies of rates of falls, involving more than 4500 adults ages 65 years or older, found those rates to range from 137 to 690 falls per 1000 persons per year, with older females falling from 1.3 to 2.2 times more often than older males. Three studies of rates of fall injuries requiring medical attention, involving more than 38,000 adults, found that fall injuries leading to hospital admission or death occurred in males and females at rates per 1000 persons per year of 1.88 and 0.83, respectively, for those aged 20 to 29 years and increased steadily with age to 6.97 and 15.58, respectively, for those aged 70 to 79 years. Correspondingly, female-to-male ratios of these serious fall injury rates increased with age from 0.44 to 2.24.

In 1996, there were 340,000 hip fractures requiring hospital admission. The direct medical and other costs for the injury have been estimated as being at least $16,300 in the first year following the injury. With current trends, approximately 500,000 hip fractures are expected to occur in the year 2040, with an associated total annual cost of $240 billion. Most hip fractures occur in old adults, and more than 95% of those hip fractures result from a fall; the remainder fracture spontaneously during a physically stressful activity or prior to the fall.

Hip fractures can be devastating, particularly in older women. In 1998, there were 863 hip fractures per 100,000 adults older than 65 years (1056 and 593 per 100,000 in women and men, respectively), with the highest rate in white women 85 years and older (2690 hip fractures per 100,000). Approximately 20% of women who fracture their hip do not survive the first year after fracture, and another 20% do not regain the ability to walk unassisted. The incidence of hip fractures rises much faster with age than that of falls. This increase in hip fractures with age is not fully accounted for by increases in the number of falls or decreases in bone mass of the hip with age. Therefore, other factors must increase susceptibility to hip fractures. The biomechanics of the fall arrest responses are likely to be among these factors. More than 85% of wrist fractures involve falls. The incidence of wrist fractures rises from the age of 50 to 65 years and then reaches a plateau after the age of 65 years, but why this occurs is not yet known.

Most falls (78.3%) in those 65 years and older occur in or within the immediate vicinity of the home. Much is known about the epidemiology of falls, but little is known about the mechanisms responsible for the remarkable increase with aging in falls and fall-related injury rates. Diagnosis of specific diseases does not discriminate elderly fallers from elderly nonfallers. Individual risk factors for falls may be grouped into intrinsic and extrinsic factors. Intrinsic factors include decreased level of physical activity, cognitive impairment, depression, visual deficits, sensory and strength deficits in the lower limbs, previous stroke, dizziness, medications, abnormal balance and gait, use of assistive devices, and age more than 80 years. Extrinsic factors include environmental factors including stairs and obstacles in the gait path that can cause trips or slips. The presence of multiple risk factors substantially increases the risk of a fall. Little is known about the changes with age in impending fall response biomechanics that must, in part, be responsible for the rate changes. For example, tripping is commonly self-reported by older persons as a cause of falls: In a 1-year study of 1042 persons greater than 65 years of age, tripping was reported to be the cause of the fall in 53% of the 356 falls that were documented. Whatever the underlying neurological and physiological mechanisms, responses to trips are ultimately expressed in terms of biomechanical factors.

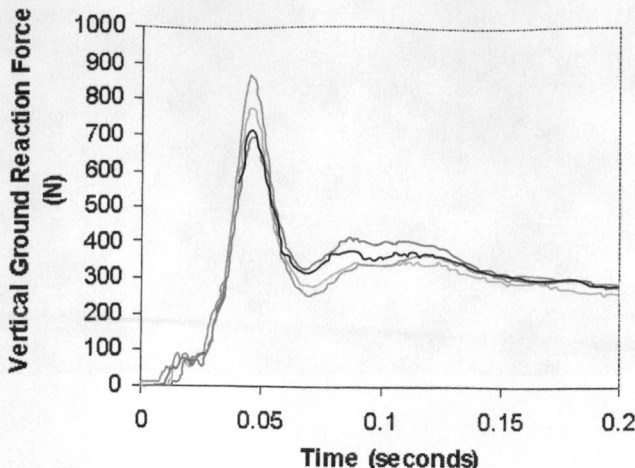

FIGURE 113-1. Example of the measured wrist impact force plotted versus time for one hand in four consecutive forward falls onto both arms for a young subject weighing 620 N. The subject fell onto a lightly padded surface from a shoulder height of 1 m. Note that (1) the time-to-peak force is less than any upper extremity neuromuscular reflex, rendering reflexes unable to protect the wrist, and (2) the magnitude of the peak impact force on one hand exceeds as much as one body weight for a brief time in two of the four trials, mainly as a result of the ground arresting the downward momentum of the upper extremity over a relatively short distance. *(Data from DeGoede KM, Ashton-Miller JA: Fall arrest strategy affects peak hand impact force in a forward fall. J Biomech. 2002;35:843.)*

Fall-Related Injury Biomechanics

There probably are a number of factors that determine whether a fall will result in an injury: the initial conditions under which the fall begins, the biomechanics of the response during the fall, the passive and active mechanisms for dissipating energy on impact with the ground or other surfaces, and the proneness to injury of the hard and soft tissues that are impacted. However, the biomechanics of fall arrests and of fall-related injuries have received little attention. Clear need exists to examine them, in order to improve assessments of risk and programs for both intervention and prevention.

The Biomechanics of Hip Fractures

The risk of bony fracture has been defined by Hayes and colleagues as the ratio of the magnitude of the force applied to the bone divided by the force necessary to cause fracture. A fall from standing height directly onto the greater trochanter carries a 21-fold higher risk for hip fracture than landing on another body part. This is because the loss in potential energy associated with such a fall is an order of magnitude greater than the average energy required to fracture the proximal femur in elderly cadaver specimens. Hence, falls in a lateral direction, which carry a higher risk for landing on the hip than other directions, must be avoided if possible. This is particularly true in an individual with reduced bone mineral density and reduced body mass index. Reductions in the latter are associated with less soft tissue over the hip to dissipate the impact energy. Hip pad protectors can be effective in reducing the risk of hip fracture in frail ambulatory elderly. By diverting the impact energy to adjacent tissues, the impact force on the hip may be more than halved. However, patient compliance has been problematic because the pads are uncomfortable to sleep with and the garment in which they are located can impede dressing and undressing.

The Biomechanics of Wrist Fracture

Once a fall is initiated, fall arrests have two post initiation phases: a preimpact phase and an impact phase. In a fall from standing height, the preimpact phase lasts approximately 0.7 seconds as the body falls to the ground. The impact phase lasts only tens of milliseconds for structures near the impact site (Figure 113-1) to a few tenths of a second at more proximal body sites further from impact. Thus, for structures near the impact site, like the hands and elbows in a forward fall, short- and long-loop neuromuscular reflexes are simply too long to be able to alter the fall arrest strategy during the impact phase.

The hands and arms are commonly used to protect the head and torso during a fall. The factors that determine the risk of Colles fracture, the most common upper extremity fall-related injury, are the height of the fall and the compliance of the surface. Moreover, at impact, the relative velocity of the hand as it strikes the surface, the elbow flexion angle, the angle of the lower arm with respect to the ground, and, of course, forearm bone mineral density status play a role. There is almost always time for older women or men to deploy their upper extremities in the event of a fall. But our research shows that a fall by an older woman from 25 cm or more onto a stiff surface, when landing with a straight arm, will almost certainly break the wrist. However, falling onto a slightly flexed arm will reduce this risk, although triceps and shoulder muscle strength is required to prevent the elbow from buckling. If the elbow buckles then the head, face, and cervical spine are placed at risk of injury. This justifies encouraging elderly people to maintain extensor muscle strength in the upper extremities so that they can better protect themselves in a fall.

AGE CHANGES IN COMPONENTS OF BIOMECHANICAL CAPABILITY

The biomechanical factors that underlie mobility impairments among older adults in general, and falling and fall injuries in particular, are not well understood. To come to that understanding, examination of the changes in biomechanical capabilities that occur with natural aging and with disease is merited. This section discusses the changes that occur in myoelectric latencies, reaction times, proprioception, joint ranges of motion (ROM), and muscular strengths and the rapid development of those strengths.

Myoelectric Latencies

The myoelectric latency or premotor time is the delay from a test stimulus cue to the onset of the first measurable change in myoelectric activity in a muscle. Myoelectric activity refers to the electrical signals sent through the nerves to initiate or modify the muscle contraction process. At the latency time, the muscle will not have yet developed any significant contractile force or, if already contracted, changed that force. Myoelectric latencies typically range from 30 to 50 milliseconds for myotatic reflexes involving the muscle spindles, 50 to 80 milliseconds when cerebellar or cortex neural pathways are involved, 80 to 120 milliseconds when afferent receptors and higher motor centers are involved, and 120 to 180 milliseconds for volitional actions.

Reaction Times

The term "reaction time" refers to the delay from a stimulus signaling a needed reaction to making a movement or developing a force. Reaction time is longer than myoelectric latency because it includes both the myoelectric latency and the finite time required for a muscle to develop or change its force magnitude after myoelectric activity begins. This additional time interval is called the motor time.

Researchers define reaction time in different ways. For example, in studies of postural control, reaction time is often defined as the delay between stimulus onset and the first measurable change in the forces exerted by the feet on the floor support. This reaction force is usually measured with an instrumented force plate. This force development reaction time incorporates the myoelectric latency and the motor time required for the muscles to contract in order to alter the body configuration enough to change the support force. This happens with little discernible foot movement or limb-segment acceleration. Reaction time has also been defined to be the delay from stimulus onset until the first detectable acceleration of a body segment. This might be termed segment acceleration reaction time. Reaction time has also been defined as the delay from stimulus onset until a limb has been moved to a target. This movement-to-target reaction time incorporates myoelectric latencies, body-segment acceleration reaction times, and body-segment movement times. Movement reaction times depend on how far body segments have to be moved. Reaction times also depend on how many choices a subject has in responding to a cue. Simple reaction times are those exhibited when no choices are given to the subject. Choice reaction times are those exhibited when the subject must decide between two or more courses of action, depending on which of two or more cues is presented. Choice reac-

tion time increases in proportion to the logarithm of the number of choices to be made. Choice reaction times are, therefore, considerably longer than simple reaction times. A speed-accuracy tradeoff is also found in reaction time measurements. As the accuracy requirement of the task is increased, reaction time increases. These differing definitions of reaction time and differing circumstances in which it is measured make it difficult to compare results from different studies of reaction times. Meaningful data on group differences in reaction times seem best obtained by comparing those times among different groups performing the same task, with the reaction time measure defined in the same way among the different groups.

Age and Gender Group Differences in Latencies and Reaction Times

Many studies report statistically significant age differences, but not gender differences, among healthy adults in myoelectric latencies. Myoelectric latencies are typically 10 to 20 milliseconds longer in healthy old than in young adults.

Age systematically increases force development reaction times. Older, compared with younger, adults require perhaps 10 to 30 milliseconds longer to volitionally develop from rest modest levels of ankle torque or to begin to take a step upon loss of balance. Systematic age differences in movement-to-target reaction times are often found. These increase on the order of 2 milliseconds per age decade between the second and 10th decades. Age differences increase when subjects are not warned several seconds in advance of the cue that it is imminent. Much larger increases with age occur in choice reaction times than in simple reaction times. For example, in 10-choice button pushing tasks, where choices were identified by letter or color or both, choice reaction times increased 27% to 86% more in subjects aged 65 to 72 years compared with those aged 18 to 33 years. No notable gender differences in reaction times have been reported.

Biomechanical Effects of Age Differences in Latencies and Reaction Times Are Minor

Despite these statistically significant age differences, of 10 to 20 milliseconds in latencies and of 15 to 30 milliseconds in some reaction times, these seem seldom critical to mobility function. Even rapid responses in time-critical situations take place during perhaps 200 to 500 milliseconds, so these latency and reaction time differences compared with the task execution times are not large. For example, among healthy older adults, the time required to fully contract a muscle is on the order of 400 milliseconds. The time to lift a foot in order to take a quick step is on the order of 200 to 400 milliseconds. Adults need warning times on the order of 400 to 500 milliseconds to be able to stop before reaching or to turn away from obstacles that come suddenly to attention.

Reaction times, which include muscle latencies, are task and strategy dependent. These are modifiable by central command. Reaction times of older adults are not always slower than those of young. Moreover, reaction times do not necessarily predict performance on complex mobility tasks. For example, one of our studies found that simple reaction times in lifting a foot immediately upon a visual cue did not predict how well the same young or older subjects could avoid stepping on a suddenly appearing obstacle during level gait. In fact, age-group differences in simple reaction times were substantially larger than age-group differences in the response times needed to avoid the obstacles successfully.

Proprioception

Proprioception describes awareness of body-segment positions and orientations. Relatively few studies have examined changes with aging in proprioception. One study found joint position sense in the knee to deteriorate with age. Joint angles could be reproduced to within 2 degrees by 20-year-olds, but only to within 6 degrees by 80-year-olds. Twenty-year-olds could detect passive joint motions of 4 degrees, but 80-year-olds could detect only motions larger than 7 degrees. Other studies have found no major decline with age in motion perception in finger and toe joints but have found declines with aging in sensing vibration. Proprioceptive acuity at a joint is significantly better when muscles at the joint are active than when these are passive. Proprioceptive thresholds during weight bearing are at least an order of magnitude lower than those typically reported during non-weight-bearing tests. Recent studies exploring the effect of age on thresholds for sensing ankle rotations show that healthy adults can sense quite small rotations in the sagittal and frontal planes under the weight-bearing conditions of upright stance. The probability of successful detection of rotation increases with increasing magnitude and speed of imposed foot rotation. A 10-fold reduction in the angular threshold was observed on increasing the speed of rotation from 0.1 to 2.5 degrees per second, but thresholds did not further reduce at higher speeds. In healthy adults between the third and eighth decades, age, rotation angle, and rotation speed also significantly affected the threshold for sensing the direction of foot rotation. Threshold angles were three to four times larger in older females than in younger females.

Individuals with central or peripheral proprioceptive impairments can exhibit articular pathology. Examples include Charcot changes occurring in the upper or lower extremities owing to central nervous system damage by syringeomyelia over several levels of the spinal cord and changes in the foot or ankle owing to lower extremity peripheral neuropathy often associated with diabetes. Indeed it is prudent to warn older diabetic patients planning an exercise program about the risk of developing Charcot feet if they try to return to activities requiring the feet to impact the ground in order to abruptly change direction (i.e., racquet sports or running), since they simply may not feel compression fractures of the bones comprising the arches of the feet. These can lead to skin breakdown, thereby increasing the risk for serious infection and even amputation.

Peripheral neuropathy increases the proprioceptive threshold at the ankle nearly fivefold compared with age-matched healthy controls. This increased threshold adversely affects postural stability and raises the risk of obstacle contact during gait, suggesting one mechanism that might underlie the 20-fold increase in fall risk and the 6-fold increase in fall-induced fractures that these patients have.

Joint ROM

Body joint ROM have generally been found to diminish with age, but not all findings are consistent. For example, studies have reported approximately a 20% decline between ages 45 and 70 years in hip rotation and 10% declines in wrist and shoulder ROM. Compar-

isons of the ROM of lower extremity joints for young and middle-aged adults with those for older adults showed declines ranging from negligible to 57%. At the age of 79 years, one-fifth of a large group of subjects had restricted knee joint motion and two-thirds had restricted hip joint motion. Among more than 3000 blue-collar workers with ages ranging from 20 to 60 years, a 25% decline with age was found in ability to bend to the side and a 45% decline in shoulder motion. Declines of 25% to 50% have been found in various ROM of the lumbar spine between ages of 20 to 80 years. However, a comparison between two groups with mean ages of approximately 65 and 80 years found no significant differences in 28 different joint ROM. At least one study suggests that passive or active stretching exercises can increase hip extension ROM in young adults by 8 to 17 degrees, and another study suggested that exercises with a focus on stretching improve spine flexibility in older adults.

The effects of decreased ROM on abilities to perform activities of daily living are not well understood in young or old adults. One study of adults with arthritis found that the ability to move around in one's environment correlated well with ROM in knee flexion, the ability to bend down correlated with hip flexion ROM, and the abilities in activities requiring use of hands and arms correlated well with ROM of the upper extremities. Another study found that restricted knee motion in 79-year-olds correlated with disability in entering public transport vehicles but that ROM impairment did not generally associate with commitment to institutional care. A third study found the majority of a group of 134 people aged 79 years to have enough spinal mobility to perform common activities of daily living.

Muscle Strength and Power

The loss of strength with age, even in healthy and physically active older adults (Table 113-1), has long been recognized. Isometric strengths peak at approximately the age of 25 years and then decline. The loss is approximately one-third by the age of 65 years. Isometric strength is more reliably measured, and considerably greater values are recorded, when the patient exerts force on a fixed force transducer, rather than one held by an examiner. To express the strength developed about the joint in units of torque, the force (in Newtons) developed by the limb segment against a force-measuring transducer is multiplied by its lever arm (in meters) about the joint being tested. Muscle strength about a joint is, therefore, expressed in torque units (i.e., Nm), and these torque units can be normalized by body size (i.e., body height * body weight) to facilitate gender or age comparisons. Dominant limb strengths are typically approximately 10% greater than nondominant strengths. It has long been recognized that mean strengths of female adults of any age are on the order of one-third lower than those of male adults (see Table 113-1). However, when those strengths are normalized by body size, then the difference may no longer be significant. Reports of strength values vary widely because these depend on many factors, for example substantially on whether subjects have impairments or experience pain or discomfort during testing, at which joint angles, whether under isometric or constant velocity conditions, and, at constant velocity, whether muscle shortening or lengthening is occurring. As an example, maximum knee extensor torque in healthy individuals decreases by 14%, 23%, 41%, and 53% of isometric values at joint rotation speeds of 30, 60, 90, and 180 degrees/s, respectively. Isokinetic

TABLE 113-1

Literature Values for Joint Torque Strengths (Unless Otherwise Noted, Mean Values in Nm)				
	HEALTHY YOUNG ADULTS*		**HEALTHY OLDER ADULTS†**	
DATA SOURCE	**Females**	**Males**	**Females**	**Males**
Toe flexors	14	24	11	16
Ankle dorsiflexors				
Sepic et al.	44	78	46	74
Thelen et al.	28	43	22	37
Ankle plantarflexors				
Sepic et al.	100	129	82	131
Thelen et al.	130	181	88	137
Knee flexors				
Borges	100	155	65	109
Knee extensors				
Borges	183	289	128	188
Hip flexors				
Cahalan et al.	66	108	51	89
Hip extensors				
Cahalan et al.	126	204	110	203
Hip abductors				
Cahalan et al.	90	108	55	72
Shoulder flexors‡				
Hughes et al.	32	58	16	38
Shoulder extensors‡				
Hughes et al.	40	72	22	40
Cervical spine extensors				
Jordan et al.	33	65	37	45
Grip strength‡ (N)				
Mathiowetz et al.	272	466	185	289

Most values quoted are for isometric strengths, but a few are for low-rate isokinetic strengths.

*Mean ages approximately 25–30 yr.

†Mean ages approximately 60–80 yr.

‡Nondominant limb.

Modified from Schultz AB. Mobility impairment in the elderly: challenges for biomechanics research. J Biomech. 1992;25:519.

dynamometers do not measure maximum torque or power accurately at speeds above 180 degrees/s because of substantial measurement artifacts.

The strength capacity needed at the very start of a recovery movement can best be measured by isometric strength. For the hip flexor muscles, which are needed to recover balance after tripping by swinging a leg forward rapidly and placing the foot on the ground ahead of the center of gravity, maximum hip flexor torque decreases linearly with increasing hip flexion angle, as a result of muscle shortening, and additionally with increasing hip flexion speed. So, given the typical bell-shaped hip flexion angular velocity versus time curve for a recovery step, it is the maximum power developed about the relevant joint that best predicts the fastest velocity that can be achieved mid-swing and, therefore, length of the recovery step. Since power is defined as the product of torque times angular velocity, high hip flexion power values would be attained by being able to develop a large torque about the joint at a high rotational velocity. Maximum power usually occurs in a shortening muscle at approximately one-third of the maximum movement velocity.

A prevalent casual belief is that many of the mobility impairments that arise in the elderly are caused by declines in muscular strength. This belief warrants careful consideration. Studies described subsequently suggest that the joint torques needed to maintain postural balance and even to rise from a chair are often well below the joint torque strengths that healthy older adults have available.

The decline with aging in the ability of muscles to produce power is perhaps well illustrated by records of elite athletic performances. In short-distance races, male elite runners more than 70 years old run approximately one-third slower than do elite young adult male athletes. In long-distance races, male elite runners more than 70 years old run approximately half as fast as elite young adult male athletes. By that age the maximum extensor muscle power that can be developed about the knee, for example, has declined by approximately 40%.

Age-related changes in muscle morphology and physiology help to explain these changes. Older adults are particularly prone to loss of isometric strength as well as torque at high velocities because of the irreversible loss of the largest (and fastest) motor units with age. Fast/slow muscle fiber innervation ratios also seem to change with age. By contrast, the maximum speed of unloaded shortening for specific muscle fiber types does not decrease significantly with aging. The reduction in muscle power reduction with age may also be caused by systemic factors, such as declines in cardiopulmonary function. It is thus likely that, in order to maintain muscle function in older adults, the focus should be on the assessment and training of both muscle power and strength.

Plantarflexion

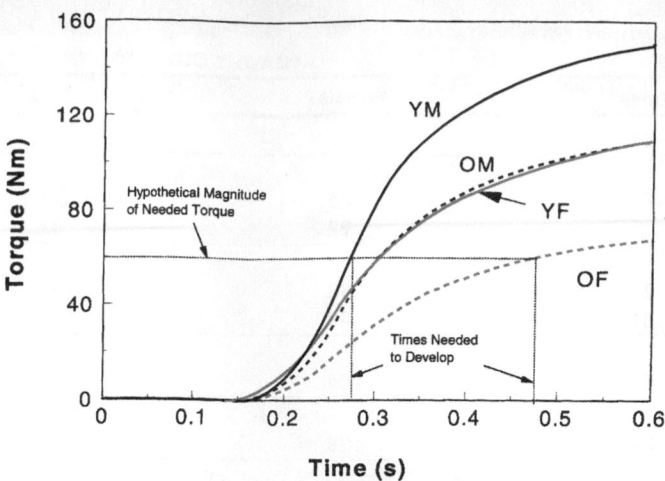

FIGURE 113-2. Age and gender differences in rapid development of ankle plantarflexor torque. The subjects tested were healthy young and older (Y, O) females and males (F, M). Time is measured from a light flash cue signaling the subjects to push against a pedal as hard and as fast as possible. The four subject groups exhibited nearly the same mean reaction times, approximately 160 milliseconds. However, the mean time needed to develop a given magnitude of torque varied substantially among the four age/gender groups. For example, were a plantarflexion torque of 60 Nm required to regain balance upon the initiation of a fall, YM would need approximately 275 milliseconds to develop that torque, and OF would need approximately 475 milliseconds. *(Data from Thelen DG et al: Effects of age on rapid ankle torque development. J Gerontol Med Sci. 1996;51A:M226.)*

Rapid Development of Joint Torque Strengths

Upon a substantial perturbation of standing balance, as already noted, fewer than 500 milliseconds are often available for the critical initial phase of balance restoration, yet 300 to 400 milliseconds can be required to develop maximum joint torques. Even older adults who are healthy and physically active have diminished abilities to develop large joint torques rapidly, compared with young adults. Moreover, older females have lower torque development rates than do older males. For example, in one study, the mean total time required to develop 60 Nm of ankle plantarflexion torque, when subjects were asked to develop maximum torque as fast as possible, was 311 milliseconds in young adult females and 472 milliseconds, or 161 milliseconds (52%) longer in older females. Corresponding times for males were 270 and 313 milliseconds (16% longer), respectively (Figure 113-2). Maximum rate of torque development tends to correlate highly with maximum voluntary torque strength, with correlation coefficients on the order of 0.8. Owing to slowing in peak rate of joint torque development abilities, capacities of even healthy old adults to recover balance or to carry out other time-critical actions that require moderate-to-substantial strengths, such as those required to avoid obstacles that come suddenly to attention, may be considerably reduced.

Source of Age Differences in Rapid Strength Development

Measurements of myoelectric signals in ankle dorsiflexor and plantarflexor muscles during rapid isometric and isokinetic exertions have been used to explore the extent to which this age-related slowing in rapid torque development might be attributed to neural factors, that is, those processes that precede the initiation of muscle contraction. In one study, latency times, muscle activation rates, and myoelectric activity levels of agonistic and antagonistic muscles were quantified. There were few marked age differences in the latencies or in the onset rates or magnitudes of agonistic or antagonistic muscles activities during maximum isometric and during isokinetic exertions. Myoelectric latency times were statistically associated with age, but, in the mean, these were only approximately 10 to 25 milliseconds longer in the old. Given the outcomes of this study, the differences observed in rapid torque development abilities in healthy elderly compared with healthy young adults seem largely because of differences in muscle contraction mechanisms once contraction is initiated, rather than to differences in the speeds of stimulus sensing or central processing of motor commands or to differences in the muscle recruitment decisions that precede contraction initiation.

AGE DIFFERENCES IN PERFORMANCE OF SIMPLE MOBILITY TASKS

To reach a better understanding of the biomechanical mechanisms that underlie mobility impairments in general, and falling and fall injuries in particular, attention to how the changes in biomechanical capabilities that occur with natural aging and with disease affect the performance of individual mobility tasks is merited. This section discusses age differences in performance of common mobility tasks, such as walking; turning, rising from chairs, beds, and floors; and regaining standing balance when it is disturbed.

Age-related declines in mobility task performances are seen in tasks that are physically and/or cognitively very challenging long before any declines are seen in tasks easily performed. Physical and cognitive capacities can decrease substantially without leading to any impairment if task performance demands are modest because these do not tax the functional reserve. Once capacity falls to a point at which task demand begins to equal capacity, performance ability begins to decline substantially. In healthy adults, the consequences of a decrement in capacity are unlikely to be seen in performances of easy tasks but are likely to be seen in performances of demanding tasks, accompanied, perhaps, by compensatory changes in performance strategies.

Assessment of Mobility Function

Mobility does associate with decrements in biomechanical variables. For example, in a recent study of community-dwelling older adults, self-reported difficulty with chair rise, ascending and descending stairs, and fast walking was found to be associated with a reduction of isometric knee extensor strength capacity below 3 Nm per kg body weight. A number of performance-based test batteries have been developed to globally assess a patient's mobility function, including that in changing positions, controlling upright posture, and walking. These batteries are designed to detect clinically significant changes that might, for example, place an individual at risk of falls or of developing mobility disability. Not all of these batteries are sensitive to the subtle age-related changes in performance found among healthy adults. Some do not include tasks that are sufficiently demanding. Others use rating systems that are not quantitative enough. Such batteries serve well for assessing more impaired older adults, but healthy older adults can often perform without difficulty all of the tasks the batteries include. Batteries are available that can elicit subtle age-related effects. These rate performance sensitively enough and include tasks with sufficient demand; for example, in one test patients are asked if health problems or physical impairments have resulted in adaptation in the way daily tasks are performed, to test the ability to balance on one leg for 10 seconds, and to measure average gait speed relative to a 0.5 m/s standard. For example, if patients have altered the way they perform daily tasks, cannot balance for 10 seconds on one foot, and walk at less than 0.5 m/s, then their risk of developing mobility disability in the next 18 months is more than 55%. A recent review of fall risk assessment measures showed that certain measures showed good sensitivity and specificity in acute care settings (e.g., "STRATIFY" and "Fall Risk Assessment Tool"), others performed well in extended care settings (e.g., "Morse Fall Scale" and "Timed Up and Go Test"), while yet others performed best in outpatient settings (e.g., "Elderly Fall Screening Test" and Timed Up and Go Test).

Ascribing Functional Decline Fully to Insufficient Motivation, Activity, or Training is Questionable

Performance records of elite older athletes suggest that physical inactivity, lack of motivation, and lack of training cannot fully explain functional decline in healthy older adults. Declines with age in physical performance abilities can be seen among even highly trained and highly motivated athletes. As already noted, top running speeds of short- and long-distance older elite runners are notably lower than those of young adult elite runners.

Gait

Hippocrates once said that walking is man's best medicine. We now know that gait speed is a powerful predictor of outcomes, including disease activity, mobility and activity of daily living (ADL) disabilities, institutionalization, and mortality. In older adults free of overt neurological, musculoskeletal, cardiorespiratory, or cognitive problems, comfortable gait speed declines minimally until approximately the age of 60 years and then declines by 1% to 2% per year through the age of 80 years; however, there is substantial variability among studies of age changes in comfortable gait speed (Figure 113-3). Speeds of less than 1.0 m/s, and 0.6 m/s in particular, have been suggested by Studenski and coworkers as identifying those at high risk of hospitalization and functional decline.

The causes of gait slowing with age are a subject of controversy. These may be multifactorial, including subtle age-related changes in joint stiffness, leg strength, and energy conservation strategies. Independently of age, comfortable walking speed associates nonlinearly with muscle strength (Figure 113-4) and maximum aerobic power. Much of the decline in speed has been attributed to reductions in step length. The earliest studies of gait in older adults found that men in their sixties demonstrated significantly shorter step and stride lengths and decreased ankle extension and pelvic rotation compared with younger males.

More recent studies have confirmed those findings, but not without exception. One found no significant age-group differences in step and stride lengths, velocity, or movements of the ankles, pelvis,

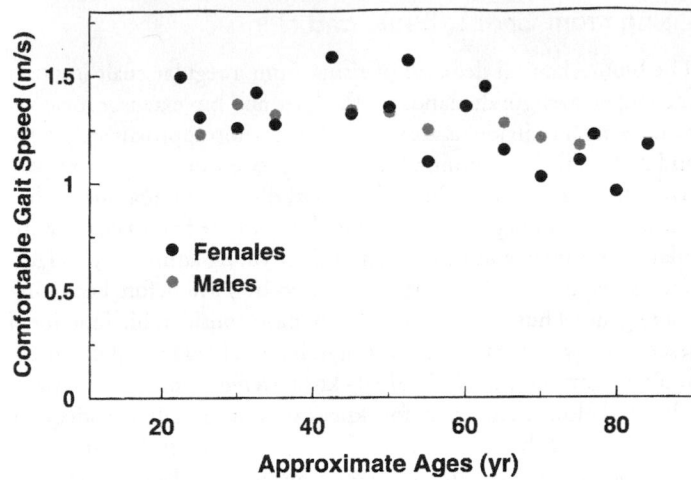

FIGURE 113-3. Age and gender differences in self-selected comfortable gait speeds. These data are graphed using those abstracted by Bohannon et al. (1996) from seven earlier literature reports. The mean speeds reported vary substantially. Nonetheless, the general trend is for comfortable gait speed to decline minimally until approximately the age of 60 yr and then to decline by 1% to 2% per yr through the age of 80 yr.

and total body mass center. Another concluded that increased variability in gait should not be regarded as a normal concomitant of old age. Still another found that among older adults, more than 40% of the variance in normal walking speed can be accounted for by differences in height, calf muscle strength, and the presence of health problems such as leg pain. A recent prospective study in older women showed that those with the poorest knee strength and balance scores were five times more likely to develop severe walking disability than those with normal function.

There is little evidence of an association between age-related reductions in stride length and gait speed and a tendency to fall. On the other hand, increased stride time variability is associated with a fivefold increase in the risk of falling.

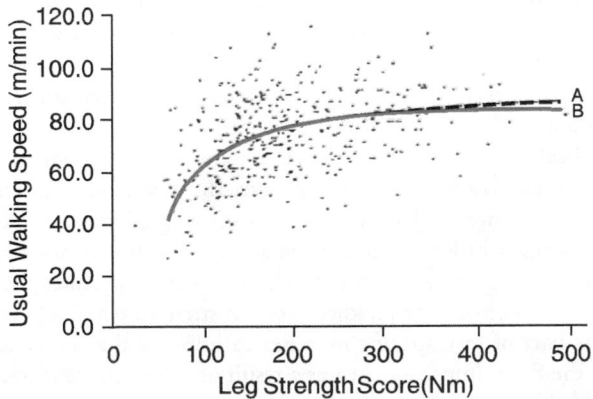

FIGURE 113-4. Comfortable gait speed is nonlinearly related to leg muscle strength score in a population-based sample of over 400 adults between the age of 60 and 96 yr. The strength score was formed from the summed isokinetic right knee and ankle flexor and extensor muscle strengths. The regression curve represents the fit for an average age of 76 yr. (Data from Buchner DM et al: Evidence for a non-linear relationship between Leg Strength and Gait Speed. Age and Ageing. 1996;25:390.)

Rising From Chairs, Beds, and Floors

The biomechanical demand of rising from a regular chair imposes the largest strength demands on the knee and hip extensor muscles: healthy older individuals are required to develop approximately 30% and 25% of their maximum knee and hip extensor strengths, respectively. It is instructive to think about how disease or impairments that affect muscle strength can affect the ability to rise from a chair. With bilateral symmetry in function and their young adult body weight, knee strength would have to be reduced by 70% before becoming inadequate. Thus, the healthy elderly have considerable functional reserve. However, if their body weight has doubled from their young adult weight, the older individual's knee strength would only have to fall 35% below age norms before knee extensor strength is inadequate to rise from a chair without arms. Likewise, a complete unilateral loss in knee extensor strength would mean that a healthy older individual could only tolerate a 35% loss in remaining knee strength before it becomes inadequate. In general, healthy older adults do rise more slowly than young adults, but the time differences for bed and chair rises are 2 seconds or less. When rising from the floor, age differences are larger, with older adults tending to take twice as long as young. Characteristic age-related changes in trunk, arm, and leg motions used to rise may account for these differences.

When rising from a chair, particularly without the use of hands for assistance, healthy old flex their necks, trunks, and legs and extend their thighs more than the young, resulting in a more anterior placement of their floor reaction force than young adults demonstrate. In one study of graded difficulty chair rise tasks, healthy young and older adults did not differ in the leg joint torques that they used to perform the series of tasks. Both young and older adults had enough strength to perform even the most challenging task. However, the old generally used a greater percentage of their available knee strength to rise from a chair, using near-maximum levels in challenging situations. Some of the older adults failed to rise when their postural control was challenged by a lowered seat and by a narrow foot support base. So, there are situations where older adults have adequate strength to rise from a chair but are limited by other factors, such as difficulty with postural control.

While rising from a bed, older adults, compared with young adults, tend to lengthen the time of contact of their arm with the bed surface. They are more likely to rotate and laterally flex their trunks, bear weight on their hip/gluteal area, and use their elbow to help pivot while rising. Declining trunk strength may account for some of these findings.

Many healthy older adults are unable to sit up in bed without the use of their hands. When rising from the floor, older adults tend to use key intermediate positions, such as getting to an all-fours position, in order to reduce the strength requirements and to enhance postural stability. In general, intermediate postures that reduce physical demands (e.g., knee extensor strength required) can be used as part of task-specific exercises to improve the ability to rise from the floor. Improvements as a result of these interventions, quantifiable biomechanically (such as increased momentum during the rise) and clinically (such as in time), are modest.

Turning in a Confined Space

In bathrooms and kitchens it is often necessary to use the feet to turn through angles as much as 180 degrees as one moves from one point to another. Falling while walking and turning has been shown to be 7.9 times more likely to result in hip fracture than falling while walking straight. In an effort to understand why turning is linked to such a high rate of injury, we have studied how age affects the kinematics of foot placement during turning by healthy young and older women. We found that subjects generally have a preferred direction of turning and that, in older women, the minimum foot separation distance during the turn was less when turning in the nonpreferred direction than in the preferred direction, raising the probability of foot–foot collisions, and hence a trip. The minimum foot separation distance during the turns was generally 55% more variable in the healthy older women than in young controls, despite the fact that they turned 20% more slowly.

Walking on Irregular Surfaces

There is often a need to cross irregular or uneven surfaces outside. Walking on an uneven or bumpy surface can pose a considerable challenge to an elderly person, as is evidenced by the fact that it is one of the two most frequent causes of falls in community-dwelling individuals. One of the first studies of gait on uneven surfaces compared subjects with age-related maculopathy against controls while walking across level, compliant, and uneven surfaces. Richardson and coworkers have shown that an irregular surface increases step width variability in healthy young and old controls and step time in peripheral neuropathic subjects who had to slow significantly on such surfaces. The irregular surface discriminated age and disease group differences in stepping pattern, as well as faller versus non-faller group differences better than did similar tests on a level surface. Application of bilateral ankle braces improved the step width variability in neuropathics patient walking on uneven surfaces.

Restoration of Standing Posture after Modest Disturbance

There is evidence of deterioration in many of the sensorimotor systems underlying postural control, even in elderly populations without obvious signs of disease. However, aging alone does not account for the heterogeneity of postural control problems in the elderly. Moreover, responses to postural perturbations are task and perturbation specific, so that a single assessment technique may not serve as a true indicator of the overall integrity of the balance control system.

Reports of age effects on sway while standing generally show sway to increase with age during adulthood, but not without exception. Age-related changes in postural control in healthy adults are minimal through the age of 70 years under situations of low task demand. Examples of low-demand tasks are standing on two feet with eyes open, or maintaining stance when it is perturbed by modest movements of the support surface or by gentle backward pushes. When task demand increases, age-group differences in postural control abilities become more apparent. For example, when a sway response no longer suffices to recover balance in the face of a perturbation, young adults tend to resort to a single step, whereas older adults tend to employ multiple steps in order to recover their balance. Task demand can be increased by decreasing visual input or by making the support surface more compliant. The most striking age-related differences often occur when several different demands are increased simultaneously. Studies have found that when both the support surface and the visual surround were rotated in phase

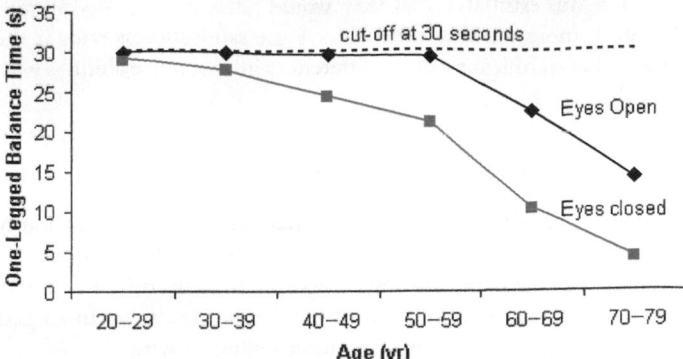

FIGURE 113-5. Age differences in ability to stand on one leg. Healthy adults were asked to balance on one leg for up to 30 seconds, with eyes open and then with eyes closed. The y-axis shows the time until balance was lost. Difficulty in performing the eyes open task did not arise until after the age of 50 yr, but when the eyes were closed, even the younger subjects had some difficulty. The older subjects had substantial difficulty with both tasks. (Data from Bohannon RW et al: Decrease in timed balance scores with aging. Phys Ther. 1984;64:1067.)

with body sway, 50% of older adults lost their balance on their first attempt to maintain stance, compared with 9% of younger controls. There is evidence that the age-group differences may increase after the age of 70 years. The mean time for standing on one leg with eyes open before losing balance for 20- to 29-year-olds was at least twice as long as that for 70- to 79-year-olds and nearly seven times longer with eyes closed. In contrast, mean stance time for 60- to 69-year-olds compared with 20- to 29-year-olds was only 20% less with eyes open and only three times less with eyes closed (Figure 113-5).

It is not known why these changes with age occur in postural control abilities. One-leg stance time differences might result from reduced ankle joint lateral muscle strength or endurance, increased muscle latency times, decreased cutaneous or joint proprioception, or decreased willingness to allow the center of the floor reaction to deviate from the center of the foot support area. Only a few studies to date have analyzed whole-body response biomechanics or even the body-segment motions that are used or the joint torques developed in response to postural disturbances. Those that have report that the required motions and torques are generally modest compared with the literature-reported capacities of healthy old adults.

Cognitive and Other Psychological Factors

Cognitive demand relative to cognitive capacity substantially influences physical task performance. As mobility task complexity increases, so do the cognitive demands placed on the individual. The need to perform two tasks simultaneously or to divide attention degrades performances of healthy elderly significantly more than for healthy young. For example, in a study of abilities to step over suddenly appearing obstacles while walking, the attention of groups of healthy young and older adults was divided by having them simultaneously respond in two reaction time tasks. Both young and old adults had a significantly increased risk of obstacle contact while negotiating obstacles when their attention was divided, but attention division diminished obstacle avoidance abilities of the old significantly more than it did in the young. These results suggest that

diminished abilities to respond to physical hazards present in the environment when attention is directed elsewhere may partially account for high rates of falls among the elderly. As an example, relative to controls, fallers tend to prematurely transfer their gaze from an obstacle that they are about to cross.

In our studies of relationships between neuropsychological status and physical performance, relatively minimal associations have been found in performance of simple tasks, such as in assessments of proprioception, joint ROM, and strengths. With tasks of increasing complexity, such as in chair rise, ambulation, and postural maintenance, visual attention abilities and psychomotor speed were found to be good predictors of performance. In performance of mobility tasks of substantial complexity, such as avoiding obstacles when attention is divided or stepping accurately under adverse conditions, measures of problem-solving ability and mental flexibility, along with psychomotor speed and attention, become performance predictors. These capacities include elements of executive control, an area of cognitive function increasingly recognized as critical to control of gait and fall avoidance. We have found that when embedding aspects of executive control into a walking task, such as the trails tests of visuomotor processing, older adults, particularly those with executive function impairment, perform more poorly.

Difficulties in walking seem to relate to cognitive impairment. Demented older adults have significantly shorter step lengths, lower frequencies of stepping, more step-to-step variability, and lower gait speed. Gait abnormalities in nondemented older adults can predict future occurrence of dementia, particularly vascular dementia. Difficulties in concurrent performance of cognitive and mobility tasks, such as a verbal task while walking, have been proposed as risk factors for falls. An extreme example, when the individual stops walking while talking, appears relevant only in those with significantly impaired gait or cognition. These findings reflect the inherent underlying cognitive demand in walking, particularly in those with already impaired gait. A geriatric rehabilitation program led to greater gains in walking speed in subjects with normal cognition than in those with impaired cognition. Moreover, walking speed appeared to be closely related to the ability to rise from a chair and to be a powerful predictor of patient placement upon discharge from the rehabilitation program. Of 116 older adults studied, none were able to live alone or even in a rest home if they were discharged with a walking speed of less than 0.15 m/s. Many frail elderly are aware of the difficulty of dividing one's attention while walking, as demonstrated by the ability of the simple but effective "Stops Walking When Talking Test" to predict impending falls in these patients.

AGE DIFFERENCES IN PERFORMANCE OF TIME-CRITICAL MOBILITY TASKS

Times Needed for Quick Responses to Maintain or Recover Balance

As already noted, the time available in which to recover from a substantial disturbance of upright balance or to safely arrest a fall is often less than 1 second. For example, when walking forward at a speed of 1.3 m/s, the comfortable walking speed typically self-selected by healthy young and old adults, only 200 to 300 milliseconds may be available in which to make initial responses appropriate for balance

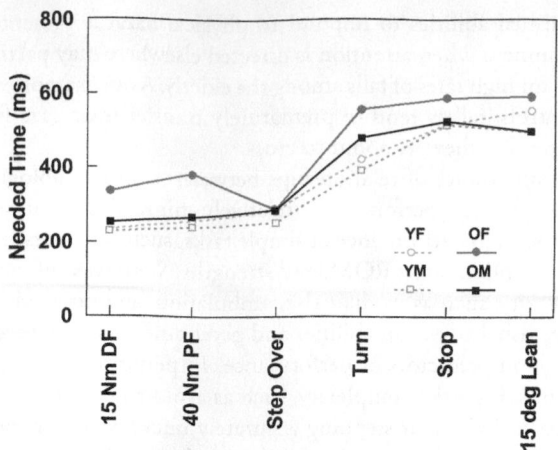

FIGURE 113-6. Summary of age and gender differences in times needed for various quick responses. Mean values across groups of healthy older females (OF), older males (OM), young females (YF), and young males (YM) of the times required for six different responses are shown. The responses are indicated by the horizontal axis labels. Each of the situations being responded to is further described in the text of this chapter. From left to right, the responses are the development of, respectively, (1) 15 Nm of ankle dorsiflexor flexor torque or (2) 40 Nm of ankle plantarflexor torque, as fast as possible; the achievement of a 50% rate of success in avoiding suddenly-appearing obstacles by, respectively, (3) stepping over the obstacle, (4) turning away before reaching the obstacle, or (5) stopping before reaching the obstacle; and (6) the replacement of the stepped foot on the ground when recovering balance by taking a single step up on sudden release from a 15-degree whole-body forward lean. The data points are connected by lines only to help distinguish the four subject groups.

recovery when tripping over an obstacle. If a large obstacle in the gait path, such as a moving vehicle, suddenly comes to attention 1 m ahead while walking at this speed, then a turnaway from the obstacle or a stop before reaching it would have to be accomplished within approximately 750 milliseconds. The term "time critical" is used here to refer to such situations. Differences in abilities to respond appropriately in at least some time-critical situations (Figure 113-6) may help explain age and gender differences in rates of falls and fall-related injuries.

Studies of Time-Critical Obstacle Avoidance Tasks

Avoiding Obstacles by Stepping over Them

The abilities of healthy and physically active young and older adults, who were walking forward at a speed of approximately 1.3 m/s, to step over an obstacle that suddenly appeared at seemingly random times and locations in front of them have been examined. The appearance of this obstacle was arranged to give the subjects available response times that varied from 200 to 450 milliseconds before they would have stepped on it. This task is a time-critical one, but because avoidance requires relatively minor changes in stepping pattern and relatively minor redistributions among segments of kinetic energies and forward momenta, the strength requirements of the task likely are modest. Few young or old could avoid obstacles if only 200 milliseconds were available. Most young and old reliably avoided obstacles that appeared so as to give 450 milliseconds warning time. Over all available response times used, the old had statistically significantly lower avoidance success rates than the young, but, in biomechanical

terms, it was estimated that they would have needed only 30 milliseconds more warning time to have the same success rates as the young. No significant gender differences in avoidance abilities were found.

Avoiding Obstacles by Turning Away Before Reaching Them

In a study of abilities to make sudden turns to avoid previously unseen obstacles, healthy old adults were substantially less successful than young when available response times were short. For example, for an available response time of 450 milliseconds, mean success rates in completing the turn without colliding with the obstacle were 68% in young and 27% in older adults. Moreover, males had substantially better success rates for given available response times than did females in corresponding age groups. This task is a time-critical one. Avoidance requires complete arrest of forward momenta and quick development of lateral momentum, but relatively minor redistributions among segments of kinetic energies. Therefore, the strength requirements of the task likely are moderate.

Avoiding Obstacles by Stopping Before Reaching Them

In a similar study of abilities to make sudden stops to avoid previously unseen obstacles, healthy old adults again were substantially less successful than young when available response times were short. For example, for an available response time of 525 milliseconds, mean success rates in stopping before passing forward of the obstacle were 58% for young females and male adults and 51% for older males, but only 23% for older females. This task is also a time-critical one. Avoidance requires complete arrest of forward momenta and total dissipation of body kinetic energy. Thus, the strength requirements of the task likely are substantial.

Studies of Time-Critical Balance Recovery Tasks

Once a fall begins as a result of a trip, quick recovery of balance may be needed to avoid injury. In one set of studies by Grabiner and coworkers, forward falls were induced in healthy older adults by an unexpected trip or backward movement of the support surface. Factors associated with a failure to recover balance were one or more of the following: too short a recovery step, slower response time, greater trunk flexion angle at toe-off, greater trunk flexion velocity at recovery foot contact with the ground, and buckling of the recovery limb. In the case of an unexpected trip, Grabiner and colleagues have shown that there are two basic recovery strategies: a so-called "elevating" strategy and a "lowering" strategy. In the elevating strategy, the swing foot that is obstructed by the obstacle is directly lifted up and over the obstacle and then swung forward as quickly as possible as a (slightly delayed) recovery step. If it should prove difficult to disentangle the foot from the obstacle (thereby obviating use of the elevating strategy), then the subject can switch to a lowering strategy: the swing foot that is impeded by the obstacle is immediately placed onto the ground behind the obstacle to become the stance limb, as the contralateral foot is lifted up and over the obstacle and used for the recovery step. Using a computer simulation of a simple inverted pendulum model to represent the forward fall of the body following the trip, this team found that the recovery foot placement must occur before the inclination of the center of mass exceeds a critical angle of from 23 to 26 degrees from the vertical. In modeling studies, a faster response time has been predicted to be more useful than a slower walking speed.

There is now evidence for two distinct phases of recovery from a trip in healthy adults: an early response and a later response. In the early response, a powerful stance limb plantarflexion moment and knee extensor and hip extensor moment are used to slow the forward angular momentum (and rotation) of the whole body around the point of obstacle contact, as well as torso flexion about the hip joint. The powerful plantarflexion moment helps to achieve this by orienting the ground reaction force in front of the whole-body center of mass. The resultant slowing of forward angular momentum allows more time for the necessary second part of the response: the powerful hip and knee flexor moment required to swing the recovery limb forward fast enough and far enough to land its foot in front of the onward traveling whole-body center of mass. Finally, as the recovery limb impacts the ground, sufficient resistance must be generated by its knee and hip extensor muscles to resist flexion buckling of the knee as the residual forward angular momentum of the body is attenuated. This resistance to buckling of the knee must come from the resistance of the knee extensor muscles to being forcibly lengthened. In other words, the knee extensor muscles must first be adequately activated, and then there must be sufficient knee extensor muscle mass to generate adequate elastic and viscous resistance to the sudden stretch of the knee extensor muscles. Inadequate activation or inadequate knee extensor muscle mass will mean that the task demands will exceed the capacity of the knee muscles to handle the challenge, the knee will then buckle and its owner will fall as the limb buckles under his/her weight.

Pijnappels and coworkers have shown that despite initial reactions not meaningfully slower, age adversely affects the ability of healthy individuals to generate an adequate stance limb ankle plantarflexor recovery response. This caused an age-related increase in failure to recover from a trip.

We have also studied the effect of age on the ability to recover from a forward fall by rapid step taking. Subjects were released from a forward-leaning position and instructed to regain standing balance by taking a single step forward. Lean angle was successively increased until a subject failed to regain balance as instructed. This task is a time-critical one, likely requiring the use of maximum strengths. The mean maximum lean angle from which older males could recover balance as instructed, 23.9 degrees, was significantly smaller than that for the young males, 32.5 degrees. Corresponding angles for the females were 16.2 and 30.7 degrees, but those numbers do not include five of the 10 older females who could not recover balance from even the smallest lean angle at which they were tested, approximately 13 degrees. Maximum lean angles were well correlated with the average forward step velocity and inversely correlated with the time required to unload the stepping foot, but were unrelated to myoelectric response latencies of ~70 milliseconds in both young and elderly. A gender difference has been found in torques used for recovery of balance. None of the males needed to use their maximum ankle, knee, or hip torque capacities; but the young females used maximal hip flexion torques, and the older females used maximum plantarflexor, knee flexion, hip flexion, and extension torques.

The results suggest that reduced abilities of healthy older adults to recover from forward falls result from an inability to generate adequate stance limb extensor torques and sufficiently rapid body-segment movements, rather than from delayed initiation of response.

This means that future interventions should target muscle training designed to increase hip, knee, and ankle muscle strengths and powers in order for the subject to maintain agility by making sufficiently rapid recovery movements.

Recovery from a Slip

An unexpected slip can be particularly challenging to recover from during gait. Healthy young subjects walking onto a level slippery floor attempt to correct an ongoing slip between 25% and 45% of stance phase (190–350 milliseconds after heel contact). In healthy young adults, the initial response to an unexpected slip is an early flexor synergy (starting at 146 milliseconds) in the muscles of the perturbed limb, presumably serving to limit how far the slipping foot slips; bilateral shoulder muscle activation (143 milliseconds) serving to produce bilateral arm elevation after approximately 288 milliseconds; and rapid protraction of the trailing swing foot onto the ground in order to rapidly enlarge the base of support rearward so as to be able to prevent a backward fall. This slows the acceleration of the whole-body center of mass by employing a flexor synergy in the trailing leg and decelerating the center of mass by using an extensor synergy of the leading leg. The trailing leg is rapidly placed back on the ground in order to provide a larger rearward base of support to decelerate the descending center of mass. Arm elevation movements help to dissipate forward momentum. After the first slip, healthy subjects exposed to successive slipping trials showed very rapid adaptation, with much less arm movement and more muscle cocontraction, often adopting a proactive "surfing" response whereby they slid forward on both feet.

The physical characteristics determining the potential for a slip as well as the required coefficient of friction (ratio of the shear to the normal foot forces) on slippery surfaces have been the subject of recent reviews. Redfern and coworkers have demonstrated on level floors and descending ramps that healthy subjects make significant proactive changes in gait (shorter stance phase duration, shorter normalized step lengths, and slower foot strike velocities) when anticipating the possibility for a slip. Properly corrected vision and good lighting can help foster such proactive strategies by elderly people.

Mechanisms Underlying Age and Gender Differences in Performance of Time-Critical Tasks with High Strength Demands

Some of the studies discussed here suggest that the source of both age and gender differences in performance of tasks that both are time critical and have high strength requirements lies primarily in strengths and speeds of muscle contraction, rather than in sensory processing or motor planning abilities. As pointed out earlier in this chapter, studies of myoelectric latencies for rapid ankle torque development have found no significant gender group differences. These have found statistically significant age-group differences, but the differences in the mean latencies were only approximately 10 to 20 milliseconds, whereas the total times needed to develop near-maximum torques were on the order of 400 to 600 milliseconds. They showed that age-group differences in the use of cocontraction were not responsible for the age-group differences in torque development rates. Studies of mean reaction times have also found statistically significant age-group differences in those times. However, those differences were only approximately 10 to 20 milliseconds, whereas the total response times ranged approximately from 400 to 800 milliseconds. No substantial gender differences were found in those reaction times. This suggests that, among healthy older compared with young adults and among females compared with males, differences in rapid torque development abilities, noted earlier in this chapter, and differences in performance of tasks that are both time critical and have high strength requirements seem largely because of differences in strengths and speeds of muscle contraction once contraction is initiated, rather than because of delays in initiating contraction.

The outcomes of the studies described, and those from other studies reported in the literature, suggest that healthy older compared with young adults, and healthy older females compared with older males, are more at risk of injury in tasks that both are time critical and have high strength requirements. Time-critical obstacle avoidance tasks involve rapid visual processing, rapid triggering of preplanned strategies, and rapid execution of movements, during which whole-body balance must be maintained. Among healthy adults, the times needed for the visual processing and response triggering phases are a few hundredths of a second longer for old than for young. In contrast, the times needed for movement execution are a few tenths of a second longer for old than for young. Almost exclusively because of these longer movement execution times, the warning times that older compared with younger adults need to perform successfully time-critical tasks with high strength requirements are a few tenths of a second longer. Although differences of a few tenths of a second in abilities to respond are not usually important, circumstances leading to needs for time-critical, high-strength responses probably combine at random. Sometimes, the consequence of needing a few tenths of a second longer to execute avoidance or recovery maneuvers may not be small, and that need, when circumstances combine unfavorably, may substantially lower the probability of regaining balance or avoiding a fall-related injury. The ability to perform these avoidance and recovery maneuvers usually involves stepping, and well-established clinical tests of these time-critical stepping responses do not yet exist. Tests of voluntary maximal distance and high-speed stepping are being evaluated.

CONCLUSIONS

Research findings to date regarding the biomechanics of mobility among healthy older adults suggest the following:

1. In activities such as ambulation, chair and bed rise, and postural responses to small perturbations, performances of healthy older adults are often remarkably similar to those of the young. Age-group differences among healthy adults that seem biomechanically significant have been found in only certain kinds of tasks.

2. Age differences in performances of many tasks apparently seldom arise from limitations in joint ROM. Only a few physical tasks present substantial joint ROM requirements.

3. Similarly, those differences apparently arise only in some circumstances from limitations in joint torque strengths. The strength requirements of many daily tasks, excluding time-critical tasks requiring high strengths and certain kinds of transferring tasks, are modest compared with the available strengths of healthy old adults.

4. There are substantial age and gender differences in abilities to develop joint torques rapidly, but these differences generally seem to be of importance chiefly in performing time-critical tasks requiring high strengths and/or powers.

5. When significant age differences in responses have been found, those differences appeared seldom to depend in major ways on age differences in latencies or reaction times. Under many circumstances, the age differences that do exist in sensing and neural processing times are small compared with total response times.

6. In performing time-critical tasks requiring high strengths, for which major age differences arise, these presumably arise because of age differences in the muscle contraction physiology underlying the biomechanical response execution.

7. Cognitive and other psychological factors, such as risk-taking preferences, have a substantial role in mobility task performance.

8. Age-related declines in mobility function appear during performances of tasks that are physically and/or cognitively very challenging at much younger ages than these appear in tasks that are easily performed.

9. Gait tests performed on an irregular surface appear to discriminate age and disease effects better than gait tests conducted on a flat surface.

FURTHER READING

Alexander NB, et al. Muscle strength and rising from a chair in older adults. *Muscle Nerve Suppl.* 1997;5:S56.

Alexander NB, et al. Task-specific resistance training to improve the ability of ADL-impaired older adults to rise from a bed and from a chair. *J Am Geriatr Soc.* 2001;49:1418.

Bohannon RW, et al. Decrease in timed balance scores with aging. *Phys Ther.* 1984;64:1067.

Bohannon RW, et al. Walking speed: reference values and correlates for older adults. *JOSTP.* 1996;24:86.

Chen HC, et al. Stepping over obstacles: dividing attention impairs performance of old more than young adults. *J Gerontol Med Sci.* 1996;51A:M116.

Cho BL, et al. Tests of stepping as indicators of mobility, balance, and fall risk in balance-impaired older adults. *J Am Geriatr Soc.* 2004;52:1168.

Cummings SR, Nevitt MC. A hypothesis: the causes of hip fractures. *J Gerontol Med Sci.* 1989;44:M107.

DeGoede KM, et al. Fall-related upper body injuries in the older adult: a review of the biomechanical issues. *J Biomech.* 2003;36:1043.

Faulkner JA, et al. Skeletal muscle weakness in old age: underlying mechanisms. *Ann Rev Gerontol Geriatr.* 1990;10:147.

Fitzpatrick R, McCloskey DI. Proprioceptive, visual and vestibular thresholds for the perception of sway during standing in humans. *J Physiol.* 1994;478:173.

Giordani B, Persad C. Neuropsychological influences on gait in the elderly. In: Hausdorff J, Alexander NB, eds. *Evaluation and Management of Gait Disorders.* Boca Raton: Taylor and Francis; 2005.

Greenspan SL, et al. Fall direction, bone mineral density, and function: risk factors for hip fracture in frail nursing home elderly. *Am J Med.* 1998;104:539.

Horak FB. Postural orientation and equilibrium: what do we need to know about neural control of balance to prevent falls? *Age Ageing.* 2006;35:7.

Leon J, Lair T. *Functional Status of the Noninstitutionalized Elderly: Estimates of ADL and IADL Difficulties.* National Medical Expenditure Survey Research Findings 4. Rockville, MD: Agency for Health Care Policy and Research; 1990. DHHS Publication No. PHS 90–3462.

Malmivaara A, et al. Risk factors for injurious falls leading to hospitalization or death in a cohort of 19,500 adults. *Am J Epidemiol.* 1993;138:384.

Richardson JK, Ashton-Miller JA. Peripheral nerve dysfunction and falls in the elderly. *Postgrad Med.* 1996;99:161.

Schultz AB, et al. What leads to age and gender differences in balance maintenance and recovery? *Muscle Nerve Suppl.* 1997;5:S60.

The American Geriatrics Society Panel of Falls in Older Persons. Guideline for prevention of falls in older persons. *J Am Geriatr Soc.* 2001;49:664.

Thelen DG, et al. Effects of age on rapid ankle torque development. *J Gerontol Med Sci.* 1996;51A:M226.

Tideiksaar R. *Falling in Old Age: Prevention and Management.* 2nd ed. New York, New York: Springer; 1997.

Exercise: Physiological and Functional Effects

Robert S. Schwartz ■ *Wendy M. Kohrt*

AGING, DISUSE, AND DISEASE

A common belief among the lay public, as well as among many health-care professionals, is that much of the disease and loss of function that commonly accompanies aging is inevitable and a result of the "aging process" itself. However, it has become clear that much of the physical decline and reduced physiological reserve previously blamed on aging is, in fact, caused by the complex interactions of true genetically determined aging, disease (often subtle or subclinical), disuse, and environmental exposure.

The myriad of possible interrelationships among these factors makes it difficult to ascribe specific causality for the loss of physical vigor or function. Thus, for example, preconceived societal notions about aging may predispose to greatly reduced expectations with regard to physical as well as mental performance. Such preconceptions may promote inactivity and disuse in women at an even earlier age than in men. With years of ensuing inactivity, disuse not only exaggerates and enhances any true age-related loss of endurance, strength, and flexibility, leading to further inactivity and disuse, but may also exacerbate previously subtle or subclinical diseases such as intra-abdominal obesity, glucose intolerance, osteopenia, hypertension, dyslipidemia, and coronary artery disease. These physiological disorders, the drugs used in their treatments, and the associated functional impairments and disability can, in turn, further limit activity and continue the vicious downhill spiral.

Physical activity level (and measured fitness) appears to be inversely related to the risk of mortality and is associated with a greater average life span (approximately 2 years in human studies). An inverse dose–response relationship has also been noted between physical activity and the risk of developing many important diseases (cardiovascular disease [CVD], stroke, hypertension, type 2 diabetes, osteoporosis, obesity, colon and breast cancer, anxiety, and depression). Many of these reports included older adults. Despite the clear advantages to physical activity, less than 40% of persons 65 years and older meet the CDC recommendations for activity, and this percentage falls significantly further in older age groups.

This chapter reviews the physiological effects of aging and exercise training on the most common measures of physical fitness: (1) endurance or maximal aerobic exercise capacity, (2) skeletal muscle strength and power, and (3) body composition. Next, it investigates the theoretical relationship between fitness and functional status, reviewing the available, albeit somewhat limited, data on the effects of increased activity on functional performance. The chapter then reviews the effects of aging and activity on disorders commonly observed in geriatric patients. Last, the risks associated with exercising are discussed and some suggestions are made with respect to prescribing an exercise program for older individuals.

While we and others commonly discuss health benefits of "exercise training," it is now abundantly clear that many benefits can be accrued simply through a more active (nonsedentary) lifestyle in the absence of formal "exercise training." This concept may be especially helpful in trying to encourage older individuals who feel unable or unwilling to engage in formal exercise training but can and will increase their physical activity.

AGING AND EXERCISE

Endurance (Aerobic) Exercise Capacity

Aging-Associated Changes in Endurance Exercise Capacity

The best physiological measure of endurance work capacity is the amount of oxygen consumed at maximal exercise (maximal aerobic power or Vo_{2max}). Cross-sectional studies have repeatedly demonstrated a significant age-related decrement in Vo_{2max} in both women and men. Together, these cross-sectional data suggest that exercise

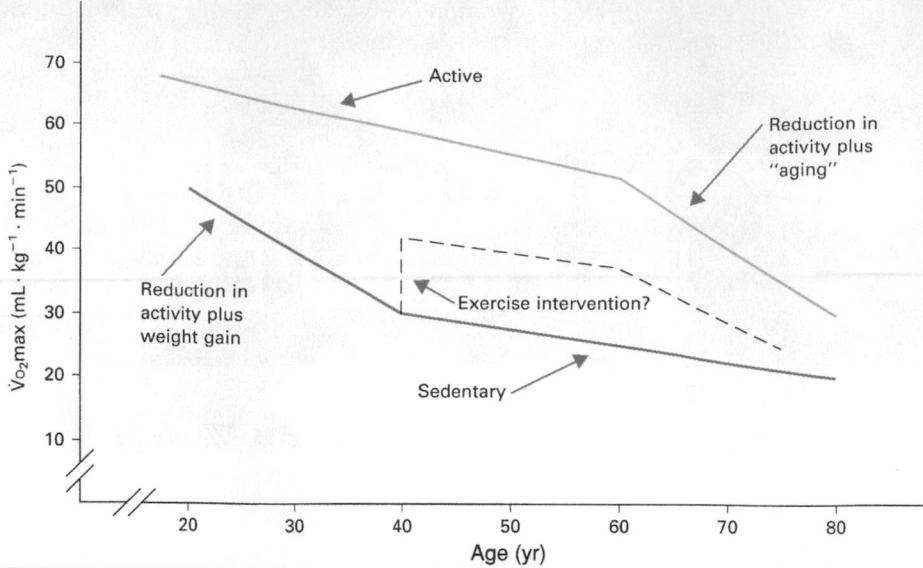

FIGURE 114-1. Possible interindividual differences in the age-related decline in Vo_{2max}. The possible effects of regular physical activity (or lack thereof) and the inevitable decline at advanced age are depicted. *(Reproduced with permission from Buskirk ER, Hodgson JL, Fed Proc. 1987;46:1824.)*

capacity declines by approximately 1% per year, when Vo_{2max} is expressed as milliliters of oxygen consumed per minute per kilogram of body weight (e.g., mL/min/kg). Longitudinal data in this area are somewhat more confusing, probably owing to (1) variation in the initial level of fitness of the subject populations, (2) spontaneous modifications in activity level between test periods, (3) alterations in body weight and composition, and (4) intervening illness. It is possible that the data are further influenced by a nonlinear decline over time (Figure 114-1), with a more rapid decline in Vo_{2max} in early adulthood in sedentary individuals followed by a less steep decline later in life. Longitudinal studies in both men and women demonstrate approximately a 0.5 mL/min/kg decline per year after a 4-year follow-up period. Almost half of this decrement could be accounted for by independent changes in adiposity and self-reported physical activity.

Both cross-sectional and longitudinal approaches have been used to determine whether habitual endurance training slows the age-related decline in Vo_{2max}. Cross-sectional comparisons of younger and older endurance athletes and normally active controls indicate that the slope of the regression line for age-related decline in Vo_{2max} is not as steep in athletes as in their more sedentary counterparts. In fact, these comparisons suggest that habitual exercise may attenuate the rate of decline in Vo_{2max} with aging by up to 50% (0.5% vs. 1.0% per year). Longitudinal studies of older endurance-trained men, followed for more than 10 to 22 years, indicate that the slower decline in Vo_{2max} occurs only in men who continue to train vigorously for competition. One study followed both sedentary and trained men, and the average rate of decline in Vo_{2max} was higher in the athletes than in the nonathletes (–2.9% vs.–1.5% per year). When athletes were characterized by the level of exercise training they maintained, the rate of decline was –0.3% per year in those who trained vigorously, –2.6% per year in those who trained moderately, and –4.6% per year in the low-training group. However, even in the low-training group, Vo_{2max} remained higher at follow-up (33.8 mL/min/kg; age 74 years) than in the sedentary controls (25.8 mL/min/kg; age 70 years). Thus, the higher fitness levels of active individuals may afford them protection later in life, by allowing them to remain above the threshold of exercise capacity necessary to remain functionally active.

The Peripheral Components of Endurance Capacity

Vo_{2max} is equal to the product of maximal cardiac output (Q_{max}) and the maximal ability of muscle to extract oxygen from the blood (a-Vo_2 difference) and, thus, is determined by both central (cardiovascular) and peripheral (primarily muscle) components. Studies have uniformly detected important changes in body composition associated with aging (see the following section on body composition), including increases in fat mass and decreases in fat-free mass (FFM) or lean body mass (LBM). Furthermore, with aging, muscle mass comprises a lesser percentage of what is usually measured as FFM. Several studies of carefully screened older subjects confirm that differences in FFM can explain some of the age-related differences in Vo_{2max}. In a cross-sectional study of very healthy men and women, muscle mass, as reflected by 24-hour creatinine excretion, was found to decline 23% between ages 30 and 70 years. When normalized for this decrease in muscle mass, the slope of the decline in Vo_{2max} with age flattened significantly, and the predicted age-related decline in Vo_{2max} between the ages of 30 and 70 years was reduced in both men (39% vs. 18%) and women (30% vs. 14%). Approximately half of the original age-related decline in Vo_{2max} could be explained by the age-associated loss of muscle mass. Other peripheral mechanisms might also account for some of the age-related decrement in Vo_{2max} by attenuating the a-Vo_2 difference, including a reduced ability to direct blood flow to the working muscles or a diminished ability of muscle cells in older (inactive) individuals to use oxygen.

The Central (Cardiovascular) Component of Endurance Capacity (See Chapter 74)

Declines in the central (cardiovascular) component of endurance capacity contribute substantially to the age-related reduction in Vo_{2max}. In the absence of hypertension or coronary artery disease (clinical or asymptomatic), resting cardiac output, heart rate, and heart size are normal in older individuals. However, as illustrated in Figure 114-2, a number of age-related changes in resting cardiac function have been defined. These cardiovascular changes detected at rest in the elderly person are quite similar to those observed with hypertension. Indeed, it has been hypothesized that mild vascular

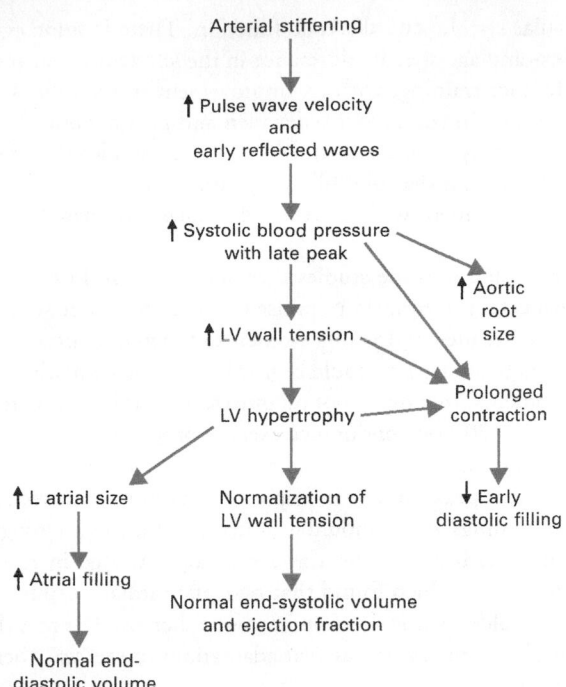

FIGURE 114-2. The interplay of vascular changes and adaptive cardiac changes that occur to varying degrees with aging in otherwise healthy individuals. *(Reproduced with permission from Lakatta EG, Eur Heart J. 1990;11(suppl C):22.)*

stiffness and ensuing subclinical hypertension may initiate this group of compensatory responses noted at rest.

As with most age-related abnormalities, alterations in cardiovascular physiology are most apparent and most clinically relevant during stress, such as physical exercise. In the setting of maximal exercise, striking differences between young and older individuals are apparent. By far the most salient and consistent is a marked decline in maximal heart rate with age. However, beyond this one finding, there is little agreement. While some studies suggest that most of the age-related decrement in Vo_{2max} is explained by a decline in cardiac output, others detect little decrease in maximal cardiac output with age. In fact, the majority of studies now support the concept that diminished central responses to maximal exercise substantially contribute to the reduced Vo_{2max} with aging. The degree to which this defect can be explained by a lower maximal heart rate or a reduced stroke volume response to exercise remains unclear.

The Physiological Effects of Endurance Exercise Training

Effects on Vo_{2max}

Certain individuals (e.g., master athletes) can maintain a reasonably high endurance exercise capacity well into old age. It is now clear that the fitness response to an endurance training program in previously sedentary, healthy older individuals is comparable to that in younger subjects. Depending on the type and duration of exercise employed, the improvement in Vo_{2max} typically varies between 10% and 30%, with similar responses in both men and women. Furthermore, when young and older subjects are trained in the same program at the same relative intensity, the relative increments in Vo_{2max} are similar.

Healthy older individuals can tolerate carefully supervised endurance training at relatively intense levels (e.g., 85% of heart rate reserve; HRR = 0.85 [(HR max − HR rest) + HR rest]) with acceptable attrition rates and few, if any, significant injuries. Indeed, it appears that speed is a more important determinant of injury than the actual overall intensity of the exercise. However, few older individuals choose to maintain this rigorous training intensity on their own, and a clinically more salient question is whether qualitatively similar adaptive responses can occur with lower-intensity training. Although not all studies agree, it appears that cardiovascular improvement can be obtained with moderate-intensity programs, where subjects train at approximately 50% of heart rate reserve. In addition, metabolic improvements can occur with low- to moderate-intensity exercise that is maintained over a sufficient period of time (see below). New recommendations suggest that multiple short (10 min) bouts of exercise may be comparable to a single larger training session.

Effects on Body Composition

As noted above, with aging there is a significant loss of FFM or LBM, mostly accounted for by a reduction in skeletal muscle mass. This decline has been estimated to be approximately 6% per decade between ages 30 and 80 years, although recent studies have suggested slower rates of decline. It is possible that the increasing prevalence of obesity has a "preserving" effect on LBM. Despite the loss of LBM with aging, body weight is sustained or increased as a result of the accumulation of adipose tissue. In fact, excess body fat is a stronger determinant of impaired physical function of older adults than is inadequate LBM. More importantly, with aging, fat is preferentially accumulated in a central distribution. This centralization of body fat seems to occur continuously with age (after puberty) in adult men, but, in women, a significant increase in central adiposity first occurs following menopause. This central distribution of adipose tissue mass is a major risk factor for many obesity- and age-related metabolic abnormalities and, in many studies, is independent of relative weight or other measures of obesity.

In cross-sectional studies comparing highly physically active older individuals with more sedentary controls, overall adiposity in the active group is consistently lower and, in fact, similar to younger individuals. This is true for both women and men, with the physically active groups having approximately 10% less body fat than sedentary controls. Furthermore, there is an inverse correlation between Vo_{2max} and central adiposity, as defined by waist-to-hip ratio, within a population of healthy older men. However, relatively little difference in FFM or LBM has been observed in active, as compared to sedentary, healthy elderly persons. Therefore, even highly endurance-trained older individuals have significantly less LBM than do younger individuals.

Longitudinal endurance training studies in previously sedentary individuals support these cross-sectional findings. Endurance training has consistently produced small but significant decrements in percent body fat and overall fat mass in older men and women. In two studies, a loss of 2.5% body fat (1.5–3 kg of fat mass) followed a 6- to 12-month intensive endurance-training program in older subjects. Associated with this modest decrement in overall adiposity was a preferential decrease in the central distribution of fat. In fact, following endurance training in older men, there was a small fall in waist-to-hip ratio, but a 20% decline in intra-abdominal fat as measured by computed tomography. In contrast to the modest but consistent decrements in adiposity, little or no change in overall FFM has been detected following endurance training in the elderly population, even when it is quite vigorous. The lack of improvement in overall FFM may be countered by significant changes in specific muscle groups. For example, cross-sectional mid-thigh muscle mass, measured by computed tomography, was found to increase by 10% in older men, despite no change in overall FFM. This finding suggests a redistribution of FFM with intensive endurance training in older men. The lack of accretion of FFM with endurance exercise in older individuals may reflect a reduced anabolic hormonal milieu, with lower levels of sex steroids, growth hormone, and insulin-like growth factor I.

Although highly trained athletes are leaner than less-active controls, the loss of weight or fat with endurance training is small when compared to dieting with caloric restriction. However, as noted above, the effects of exercise may be magnified by the preferential loss of central, and specifically intra-abdominal, fat with endurance training. Endurance training can increase the usually low resting metabolic rate in the elderly person by approximately 10%, even when corrected for any observed change in FFM. It should be noted that vigorous exercise in older subjects might be associated with a compensatory decrement in activity during nonexercising periods and, thus, no increment in overall energy expenditure. Concomitant exercise training was found to be associated with a lower rate of long-term recidivism in subjects participating in a dietary weight reduction program. Exercise may mitigate the drop in resting metabolic rate, lipolysis, and fat oxidation that usually accompany dietary caloric restriction, which would otherwise lead to rapid regain of lost weight. While there are fewer data available, it appears that strength training has many of the same effects of endurance training on adiposity.

A preliminary report of 10 days of continuous bed rest in healthy older subjects dramatizes the importance of activity and the tremendous costs of being sedentary. After even such a short period of time, healthy older subjects experienced a 30% reduction in muscle protein synthesis, a 1.5 kg loss of lean mass (most from the lower extremities), and a 16% decrement in lower extremity strength.

Effects on Cardiac Function

Although cross-sectional studies suggest a significant age-related decline in cardiac output (see previous discussion), training status appears to positively affect this end point, with a greater maximal cardiac output found in well-trained older men and women when compared to matched sedentary controls. Most of the higher Vo_{2max} in trained older individuals can be explained by their higher maximal cardiac output. In turn, a larger stroke volume explains the higher cardiac output, whereas no difference in maximal heart rate is detected between trained and untrained individuals. The relation between Vo_{2max} and left ventricular performance seems to be linear over a wide range of fitness levels, suggesting that similar improvements could be expected with training, no matter what the initial fitness level.

Longitudinal studies of endurance training in previously sedentary older subjects have provided conflicting results on cardiac function. Initially, some found no improvement in estimated cardiac output following either low- or high-intensity endurance training. However, studies using more sensitive methods and more vigorous exercise training interventions provided evidence of enhanced left

ventricular systolic and diastolic function. There is some evidence for a sex- and age-specific difference in the left ventricular response to endurance training, with an improvement in diastolic function demonstrated in young and older men and possibly only in young women. Others have been unable to show significant differences in left ventricular diastolic filling dynamics between older trained and sedentary men, with both being reduced compared to young controls.

The finding in some studies that older women do not increase maximal cardiac output in response to endurance exercise training, but that older men and young women and men do, raises the question of whether estrogens could be involved in this adaptation. When older women, either on or not on estrogen-based hormone therapy, underwent a 20-week endurance exercise program of stationary cycling, both groups of women had similar increases in estimated cardiac output at peak exercise in response to training. This contradicts previous findings, but it should be noted that the methodology used to evaluate cardiac function was not as sophisticated in this study as in the others, which found that maximal cardiac output did not increase in older women not on hormone therapy. The role that estrogens play in the cardiovascular adaptations to exercise, therefore, remains uncertain.

Effects on Endothelial Function

Vascular aging, including a decrease in large elastic artery compliance (increased stiffness) and vascular endothelial dysfunction, is a major independent risk factor for age-associated CVD in both women and men. In sedentary adults, arterial compliance and endothelial function decreases with advancing age even in the absence of clinical CVD. Cross-sectional studies demonstrate that the age-related loss of arterial compliance is attenuated in middle-aged and older endurance-trained men. Endurance training also mitigates the negative effects of estrogen deficiency on arterial compliance in postmenopausal women. Additionally, vascular endothelial function is preserved in endurance-trained men. Longitudinal studies demonstrate that short-term aerobic exercise programs (e.g., walking) can restore some of the age-associated loss of arterial compliance and completely restore endothelial function in previously sedentary middle-aged and older men. In previously sedentary postmenopausal women who chronically take hormone therapy, short-term aerobic exercise can restore arterial compliance to premenopausal levels.

SKELETAL MUSCLE STRENGTH AND POWER

Strength can be defined as the maximum force exerted by a muscle, and power is the rate of force development. Strength and power are not determined by muscle mass alone but also by intact neurological function. Consequently, as discussed in more detail below, strength and power can be increased by improving muscular function (e.g., muscle cell hypertrophy) or by improving neurological function (e.g., learning).

Strength assessment depends on the conditions of measurement, specifically the speed of muscular contraction, whether the muscle is shortening (concentric) or lengthening (eccentric) during the contraction, and the conditions of mechanical leverage. Muscle strength can be measured during isometric, isotonic, or isokinetic contractile activity. Isometric strength is the force generated against a fixed object, and isotonic strength is the force generated against a moving object (i.e., free weights and most resistance-exercise machines). Isokinetic strength also involves the generating force against a moving object, but, in this case, the speed of movement is controlled and constant. Muscle power can be determined simultaneously with the assessment of either isotonic or isokinetic strength by measuring the speed of movement.

Aging-Associated Changes in Muscle Strength and Power

For more than 100 years, cross-sectional studies have demonstrated that strength declines with age. After peak strength is reached sometime around the age of 40 years, cross-sectional studies show approximately a 30% to 40% reduction in strength by the age of 80 years. Longitudinal studies suggest that the true rate of decline may be underestimated by the cross-sectional data. For example, a longitudinal study estimated a 60% loss of handgrip strength between ages 30 and 80 years, while a cross-sectional analysis of the same data estimated loss at only 40%. Strength loss appears even more rapid at greater ages. Longitudinal studies have found approximately a 10% to 25% loss in quadriceps strength within only 5 to 7 years in 70-year-old adults. In the majority of these studies, muscle power was not measured. However, there is growing evidence that the rate of decline in muscle power is even greater than the decline in strength. Measurements of muscle strength and power for more than 10 years in the Baltimore Longitudinal Study on Aging indicated that the decline in muscle power was approximately 10% greater than the decline in strength.

It is now clear that the decline in muscle power is a stronger determinant than muscle strength of physical functional status in old age. This is not surprising if the decline in power is, indeed, more pronounced than the decline in strength. Leg muscle power was reduced in older women prone to falling, as compared with nonfallers, and was a stronger predictor than strength of self-reported functional status in elderly women. These findings suggest that intervention strategies should be aimed not only at preserving muscle mass and strength with aging, but also muscle power.

Muscle Mass

A close relationship exists between the size of a muscle, measured as cross-sectional area, and its ability to generate force. One would predict, then, that a 40% decline in muscle strength should be accompanied by a decline in muscle mass of a roughly equal amount—approximately 30% to 40%. This is the case, and, just as strength loss is more rapid at greater ages, loss of muscle mass is also reported as becoming more rapid with age. In laboratory animals, there is also an age-related decrease in muscle-specific force, which is the peak force per cross-sectional area. Single muscle fiber characteristics of tissue obtained from younger and older men and older women also indicate that the reduction in the capacity to generate force with aging is not solely a result of the reduction in fiber size or muscle mass and raise questions about how muscle fiber function and composition change with aging.

Muscle Fibers

Skeletal muscle is comprised of groups of individual muscle fibers. These fibers contain myofibrils, which are, in turn, composed of a number of myofilaments. The myofilaments contain the proteins actin and myosin and are arranged to form sarcomeres—the contractile units of muscle.

There are two major types of muscle fibers: slow twitch and fast twitch. Furthermore, there are at least three subtypes of fast-twitch fibers: a, b, and c. The fast-twitch fibers are variously referred to either as FTa, FTb, and FTc or as type 2a, type 2b, and type 2c. The slow-twitch fibers are referred to as ST or type 1 fibers. Type 1 fibers can sustain tension for long periods, are slow to fatigue, and have high oxidative (aerobic) capacity. Type 2 fibers can rapidly develop high tension, but only for short periods of time, and have high glycolytic (anaerobic) capacity. Types 2a, 2b, and 2c fibers all differ in their relative oxidative capacity.

The evidence that muscle mass decreases with aging is unequivocal. There is less certainty regarding the extent to which this is caused by a loss of muscle fibers versus a decrease in fiber size. There is a loss in the number of muscle fibers with age, but whether some fiber types are lost more rapidly with age remains controversial. Some evidence suggests that type 2 fibers are lost more rapidly than type 1 fibers. Opposing evidence suggests a more rapid reduction in type 2 fiber size with age but not a more rapid reduction in the total number of type 2 fibers. One factor that may contribute to the variation in these findings is the tremendous plasticity of skeletal muscle. Fiber cross-sectional area, and even the relative proportion of fiber types, may reflect the response to existing or recent physical activity patterns. That is, type 2 fiber loss and/or atrophy could be caused by an age-related change in activity patterns. As older adults perform fewer activities requiring rapid development of muscular force, they may have selective reduction in the type 2 fibers that are required for such activities.

Motor Units

Muscle function depends on the coordinated activity of groups of muscle fibers and the motor neuron that innervates them, i.e., the motor unit. The motor neuron appears to control the size, contraction time, resistance to fatigue, and enzyme activity of the muscle fibers it innervates. Hence, neuronal mechanisms could account for many age-related changes in muscle fibers. There is growing evidence that the number of motor units decreases with age. This conclusion is supported by electromyographic studies that suggest a loss of functional motor neurons with age. Indeed, the loss of motor units may even exceed the loss of neurons.

Muscle Quality

The concept that the quality as well as the quantity of muscle declines with aging has emerged in recent years, although there is no consensus regarding the factors that determine muscle quality or how it should be measured. It has been suggested that muscle quality encompasses many factors (e.g., structural composition, innervation, contractility, capillary density, fatigability, intramuscular fat content, protein metabolism, mitochondrial function, oxidative damage, and glucose metabolism). In general, there is an age-related deterioration in most factors that are thought to influence muscle quality. However, whether these are inevitable consequences of aging seems unlikely, as almost all respond favorably to increased physical activity.

Disuse versus Aging

There is some epidemiological evidence that regular physical activity may prevent some of the age-related loss in strength. However, when activities are classified as to their expected effects on muscle strength, epidemiological studies have probably focused on a relatively narrow range of activity near the middle of the continuum. At one end of the continuum is bed rest. Bed rest is associated with a dramatic loss of strength—estimated as high as 1% to 5% per day. At the other end of the continuum is vigorous strengthening exercise (discussed below), which produces substantial gains in strength in older adults.

It is this perspective, integrating findings from studies of bed rest, epidemiology, and experimental interventions, that most clearly suggests that age-related losses in strength are mainly a result of age-related changes in physical activity. As a corollary, epidemiologic studies of adults with similar activity at all ages should show little or no loss in strength. Indeed, a cross-sectional study of workers at a machine shop showed no decline in grip strength between the ages of 20 and 60 years. But aging per se appears to have some role in loss of strength, as, at some point during life, strength will begin to decline despite continued activity patterns.

The Physiological Effects of Strength Training

Strength training (resistance exercise) can be done in several ways. Unfortunately, at present there is no standard training program and little agreement on a preferred training method. In general, resistance exercise regimens typically involve either a high number of repetitions at a moderate level of resistance or a few repetitions at a high level of intensity. The former is aimed more at improving muscle endurance, while the latter is aimed more at increasing muscle strength. Analogous to the way in which strength can be measured, strength training can involve isometric, isotonic, or isokinetic exercises. The majority of equipment used for resistance training (i.e., free weights and machines) involves isotonic contractions. The relative level of intensity is usually based on the maximal weight that the subject can lift one time (the one-repetition maximum or 1RM).

Most resistance-training programs involve performing a prescribed number of sets (usually one to three) of each exercise, with a specific number of repetitions in each set, at a prescribed percentage of the 1RM. The number of repetitions that are performed depends on the relative intensity of each repetition. For example, at an intensity of 70% of the 1RM, people can typically perform 10 to 12 repetitions of an exercise, but at 80% of the 1RM usually only six to eight repetitions can be completed. When multiple sets of each exercise are performed, the relative intensity may be fixed for each set (e.g., 80%), increase with each set (70%, 80%, and 90%), or decrease with each set (90%, 80%, and 70%); whether one method is more effective is not certain. Once a subject can complete the proscribed number of repetitions in each set, a fresh prescription is written, based on a newly determined (higher) 1RM. New recommendations from the American College of Sports Medicine and the American Heart Association suggest one set of 10 to 15 repetitions for eight to 10 separate exercises on two nonconsecutive days should be undertaken by older adults.

In marked contrast to the effects of endurance exercise on vascular function and structure, the effects of chronic resistance training are less well studied and may be potentially detrimental. The age-related decrease in arterial compliance appears to be greater in resistance-trained compared with age-matched sedentary men, and resistance training is associated with a lower rather than a higher arterial compliance in middle-aged men. Additionally, large elastic artery compliance decreased following a 4-month resistance-training program in young healthy men. The reasons for these observations are unclear. One likely explanation is that acute intermittent elevations in arterial blood pressure that occur during resistance training may produce increases in the smooth muscle content of the arterial wall and enhance the load-bearing properties of collagen and elastin. A second possibility is that the higher baseline sympathetic nervous system activity in resistance-trained individuals may reduce arterial compliance via greater sympathetic adrenergic vasoconstrictor tone. It is possible that the nature of the adaptive process of the arterial wall may be even greater in older adults because their arteries have already undergone some untoward changes owing to the aging process. When combined with an endurance training program, the potentially detrimental effects of resistance training on arterial compliance appear to be mitigated. The effects of resistance-training on age-associated changes in vascular endothelial function are presently unknown.

Effect on Muscular Strength and Power

Historically, the majority of exercise intervention studies in older adults involved endurance exercise. More recently, there has been a dramatic increase in the number of resistance training studies. These have been primarily isotonic, fixed-resistance exercise programs lasting 2 to 6 months. Although almost all studies report that resistance training increases the strength of older adults, there is tremendous variability in the magnitude of the reported strength gains (from a few percent to almost 200%). A number of factors likely contribute to the variability, including the method of measuring strength, the duration of training, the exercise intensity, and baseline characteristics of the sample. Not surprisingly, the largest relative improvements in strength have been reported in frail elderly people in whom a small absolute increase in strength represents a large relative improvement because of their low starting strength levels. Progressive resistance training in older adults produces consistent enhancement in muscle strength, and some studies find functional improvements in areas such as gait speed, stair climb, and chair stand. However, there are few data of effects on disability measures.

A meta-analysis suggests that intensity of training is the most important factor affecting study results. Some studies used low- and moderate-intensity resistance training and reported only modest increases (10–25%) in strength. Other studies of healthy adults, physically unfit adults, and even frail adults have used more vigorous strength training, with resistance typically set at 80% of the 1RM. These studies report substantially larger strength gains (50–200%). Expressed in terms of the cross-sectional distribution of strength in the study samples, subjects improve from 1.0 to 3.5 standard deviations in strength over just a few months with these vigorous training protocols.

Duration of training also affects strength gain. Studies report weekly measurements of 1RMs, and strength continues to increase throughout the training interval, at least up to 6 months. Most studies of strengthening exercise fail to comment on the fact that their results show substantial variability in how older adults respond to strength training. The observed variability occurs despite the use of standard training protocols administered in supervised research settings. The causes of this observed variability remain to be explained.

Resistance training programs aimed at increasing muscular power feature fast concentric ("lift as fast as possible") and slow eccentric movements (lower for 2–4 seconds), as opposed to equally paced concentric and eccentric movements (2 seconds for each phase) that are typical of strength training. High-velocity or high-power training increases muscular power and improves physical function in older adults beyond that of traditional strength training. However, the optimum training loads have yet to be elucidated and depend, in part, on the desired outcome. For example, greater improvements in standing balance were found with light (20% 1RM), compared to heavier (50–80% 1RM), load high-velocity training, whereas training with the heavier loads was associated with greater improvements in muscular endurance and strength. Longer duration (2 years), high-velocity training may also impart greater benefits to bone. Importantly, in a *supervised* setting and with careful pre-exercise medical screening, adverse event rates have been comparable to that of traditional strength training regimes.

Physiological Mechanisms Explaining Gains in Strength with Exercise

Resistance exercise causes muscular hypertrophy in older adults, and muscle biopsies show hypertrophy of both type 1 and type 2 fibers. However, modest (10–20%) increases in fiber size or whole-muscle cross-sectional area have been reported to be accompanied by much larger (50–200%) increases in strength. This situation apparently violates the "rule" that muscle cross-sectional area is highly correlated with muscle strength. Actually, it is true in both older and younger adults that, after short-term strength training, there is a discrepancy between the increases in strength and muscle cross-sectional area. Some attribute the increase in strength that cannot be accounted for by hypertrophy as being caused by increased neural recruitment and discharge. In younger adults, the discrepancy appears to be transient, as highly trained individuals show the predicted ratio of strength to cross-sectional area. In older adults, it is unclear how the ratio of strength to cross-sectional area changes over the course of prolonged strength training. However, even very old individuals maintain the capability of increasing the synthesis rate of muscle contractile proteins in response to resistance exercise, suggesting that strength gains in elderly people are mediated both by neural mechanisms and by muscle hypertrophy.

Exercise, Physical Activity, and Functional Limitations

The question "Can regular physical activity prevent and/or reverse functional limitations and disability in older adults?" is of great public health importance. In discussing this question, we adopt the terminology and framework of the Nagi model of disablement. In the model, etiologic factors (risk factors) include genetic, behavioral, and environmental factors. The effects of these factors on the disabling process can be measured at four distinct levels:

1. Measurements of disease or pathology are made at the cell and tissue level.

2. Measurements of physiological impairment (e.g., muscle strength and Vo_{2max}) are made at the organ and organ system level.

3. Measurements of functional limitations are made at the behavioral, whole-organism level. Measures of functional limitations range from assessing simple movements (e.g., pushing with the foot) to more complicated movements (e.g., ability to walk as measured by gait speed) and to sequences of movement (e.g., ability to stand, walk, turn, and sit down).

4. Measurements of disability are made at the level of the interaction of the whole organism with the physical and social environment. For example, a person using a wheelchair has disabilities if stairs are the only means of getting inside and does not have disabilities if there is a ramp.

In this framework, risk factors cause disease, which causes physiological impairment, which causes functional limitations, which causes disability. (The model also includes the possibility of feedback loops and more complicated causal pathways.)

The discussion also makes a distinction between physical activity and exercise. Physical activity can be defined as any movement of the body produced by skeletal muscles that causes energy expenditure. Exercise is a subset of physical activity and can be defined as planned, structured, and repetitive body movement done specifically to improve fitness.

Evidence That Exercise Improves Functional Limitations

It is intuitive that adults who remain physically active are less likely to experience problems in performing activities of daily life, such as climbing stairs, walking, gardening, and housework. In the framework of the Nagi model, physical inactivity (risk factor) causes muscle weakness and low Vo_{2max} and other physiological impairments, which then cause functional limitations.

This intuition regarding the importance of physical activity in helping to maintain activities of daily life is supported by a number of important epidemiological studies. For example, in the Established Populations for Epidemiologic Studies of the Elderly, older adults who were physically active at the baseline examination were significantly less likely to experience mobility impairments during several years of follow-up. But the crucial issue is whether increasing physical activity levels in normally inactive older adults achieves the same health benefits found in naturally active older adults. A growing number of randomized trials address this issue. The emerging consensus is that exercise improves functional limitations in older adults. However, not all well-designed randomized trials show a beneficial effect of exercise. To illustrate how results vary among studies, consider the following randomized trials. A study of adults aged 75+ years, which compared resistance training and balance training, found that balance training, but not strength training, improved functional balance tasks. A study that compared strength training, aerobic training, and combined training found no effects of exercise on functional limitations. In a study of adults aged 68 to 85 years, walking exercise improved gait speed and SF-36 (Kidney Disease and Quality of Life Short Form 36 Health Survey) role physical scores, while aerobic movement and cycling exercises did not. In a study of older adults with knee osteoarthritis, aerobic exercise, and strengthening exercise caused similar, modest improvements in functional limitations for more than 18 months. Also, few studies have assessed whether regular physical activity (as opposed to exercise) affects functional limitations. This is important, as most adults who are sufficiently active according to public health guidelines do not also participate in regular, structured exercise programs.

The situation may be explained by the plausible argument that the effects of exercise on functional limitations should differ according to (1) type, frequency, duration, and intensity of exercise;

(2) the functional limitations of interest; (3) the method of measuring limitations; and (4) the target population. In particular, the effects of exercise on functional limitations should differ by target population because of a complicated, nonlinear relationship between physiological impairment and functional limitation. As noted above, high velocity training (power training) results in greater functional improvements than low velocity strength training in older adults. End points have included comprehensive performance-based functional assessment tests as well as tests of functional fitness. Power training also improves balance and slows contraction velocity at baseline, leading to balance improvement following the intervention.

Nonlinear Relationship Between Physiological Impairment and Functional Limitation

Note that nonlinear relationships and thresholds are implicit in the Nagi model. Healthy humans have excess physiological capacity not tapped during most daily activities, so humans can lose a fair amount of physiological reserve before functional limitations occur. Recent epidemiological studies confirm a nonlinear relationship, for example, between leg strength and walking speed. This nonlinear relationship is actually intuitive. After all, if strength was linearly related to walking speed, highly trained weight lifters would walk ridiculously fast (16–30 km/h) because they are several times as strong as normal adults, who walk at around 5 to 8 km/h. That is, above a certain threshold level of adequate physiological reserve, function is normal; below the threshold, function is impaired (Figure 114-3). The exact shape of the curve depends on the task and the physiological capacity of interest. The figure may oversimplify the situation, because most tasks have multiple physiological determinants that may interact to affect behavioral ability.

To illustrate the concepts of thresholds, consider that in steady-state measures of oxygen consumption, walking on a level grade at 5 km/h requires 3.2 METs (1 MET = 3.5 mL O_2/kg/min). With illness or inactivity, aerobic capacity falls below the level required for daily tasks. Because exercise can increase aerobic capacity, it should improve functional status when aerobic capacity is below the threshold needed for normal daily function. However, aerobic exercise would not affect ability to walk at 5 km/h in adults whose aerobic capacity already greatly exceeded 3.2 METs.

The implication of this model is that the effect of exercise on functional limitations depends on the target group. In frail adults with little or no physiological reserve, exercise theoretically produces a large improvement in function. In general, well-designed studies of exercise in frail adults report improvements in functional limitations with exercise. A randomized trial of 3 months of weight lifting in frail, very old nursing home residents found improvements in gait velocity and stair climbing. Even a 3-month supervised low-intensity exercise program produced a small improvement in physical performance in a group of frail older adults when compared to home-based flexibility training. Similarly, a 3-month task-specific resistance training program improved both the ability and the speed of bed and chair rises in a group of older patients living in a congregate care setting. In contrast, in healthy older adults, exercise would be expected to have much smaller effects on functional limitations, at least in basic activities of daily life. In general, the well-designed studies that do not report an effect of exercise training on functional limitations have enrolled relatively healthy older adults.

It follows that, if exercise has effects on functional limitations in healthy adults, effects will mainly occur with more difficult tasks, and a sensitive measurement tool may be required to ascertain the effects. One randomized trial of general exercise in healthy older adults suggests that this conclusion is true. The measurement used, the Continuous-Scale Physical Functional Performance, is sensitive to changes in functional limitations in the range of difficult tasks. In this study, there was a significant improvement in function noted in generally healthy older individuals following mixed endurance and strength exercise training.

EXERCISE AND COMMON GERIATRIC DISORDERS

Insulin Resistance and Glucose Intolerance

Aging is frequently associated with inactivity, increased adiposity, and a central distribution of fat. Because each of these potentially interrelated parameters can be associated with insulin resistance and glucose intolerance, the importance of aging alone has been unclear (see Chapter 109). Indeed, when secondary factors such as relative weight (e.g., body mass index [BMI]), central adiposity, and

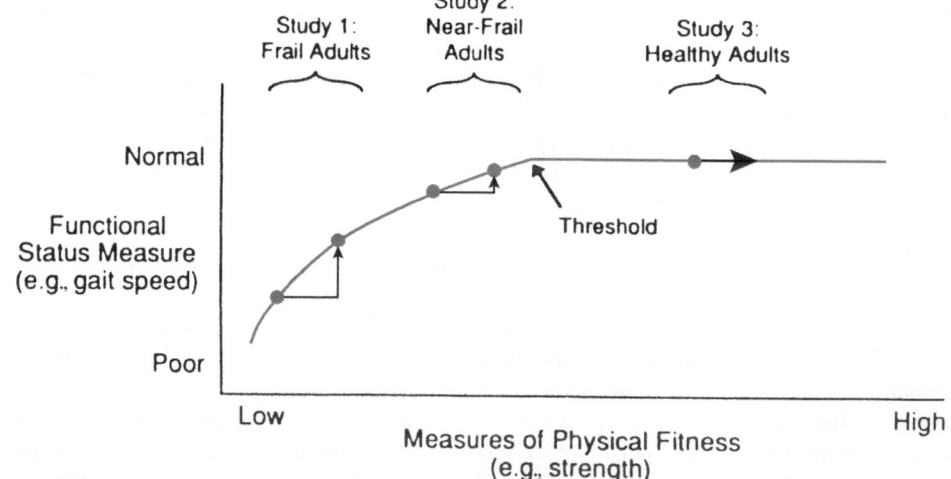

FIGURE 114-3. Theoretical relationship between physical fitness and functional status. The curvilinear relationship shows a threshold effect: above the threshold level of fitness, functional status is normal; below it, function is impaired. A curvilinear relationship implies that the benefit from exercise depends on the target group. Three hypothetical exercise studies are shown. Each study produces the same absolute improvement in fitness. In the frail adults of study 1, exercise produces a large improvement in functional status. In the healthy adults of study 3, no benefit is seen. Study 2 shows intermediate benefits. (Data from Buchner DM, et al. Evidence for a non-linear relationship between leg strength and gait speed. Age Ageing. 1996;25:386.)

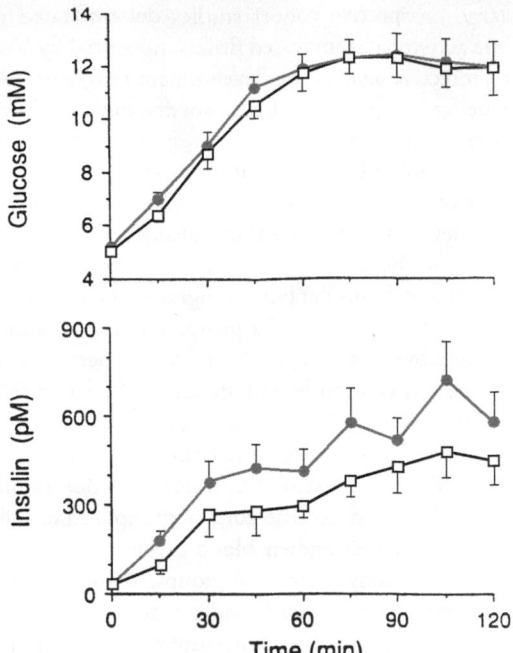

FIGURE 114-4. Glucose and insulin responses after a 100-g oral glucose load in 13 older subjects before and after 6-month exercise training. Data points, means ± standard error. *(Reproduced with permission from Kahn SE, et al. AM J Physiol. 1990;258:E937.)*

hypertension were statistically accounted for, age itself was not a significant independent determinant of the insulin resistance and/or glucose intolerance associated with "aging."

Immobilization or inactivity is known to be associated with a decline in insulin sensitivity and glucose tolerance. An important effect of physical activity on glucose and insulin metabolism with age is supported by findings of normal or near-normal insulin sensitivity and glucose tolerance in physically well-trained older individuals. Prospective studies have investigated the effects of endurance exercise training on glucose and insulin metabolism in older individuals. For example, following a 6-month intensive endurance training program, no change in fasting glucose or the oral glucose response curve was observed (Figure 114-4). However, both fasting insulin and insulin response to the oral glucose challenge declined, suggesting improved insulin sensitivity. Although quantitative measurement demonstrated a 36% improvement in insulin sensitivity, the sensitivity of the older men remained 30% to 60% lower than that of normal young controls. Because the improvement in insulin sensitivity was balanced by a reciprocal change in insulin secretion, overall glucose tolerance was unchanged. While both endurance exercise and weight loss may reduce insulin resistance in nondiabetic obese men, only weight loss appears to improve oral glucose tolerance. Strength training in older subjects may similarly enhance insulin action.

There are limited data on the effect of endurance exercise training in older patients with type 2 diabetes mellitus. In one study of patients aged 55 to 75 years old, no improvement in either glycosylated hemoglobin or insulin sensitivity was found after 26 weeks of endurance training. It is now generally agreed that most of the metabolic effects of exercise training are transitory and that the observed changes are related more to the effects of repeated acute bouts of exercise rather than a more sustained training effect. A modest

(7%) decline in glycosylated hemoglobin was detected in patients with type 2 diabetes following a 3-month strength-training intervention.

One potentially important role for exercise is in the prevention of type 2 diabetes mellitus in at-risk subjects, such as those with a strong family history of type 2 diabetes, personal history of gestational diabetes, central obesity, impaired glucose tolerance, hyperinsulinemia, hypertension, metabolic syndrome, or a sedentary lifestyle. Large, long-term prospective studies have detected significant reductions in the transition to type 2 diabetes in subjects with impaired glucose treated with a lifestyle intervention (diet and exercise). The Diabetes Prevention Program followed more than 3000 nondiabetic individuals with impaired glucose tolerance randomized to placebo, metformin, or lifestyle treatment for an average of approximately 3 years. The incidence of developing type 2 diabetes was 11.0, 7.8, and 4.8 cases per 100 person-years in the placebo, metformin, and lifestyle groups, respectively. While both the metformin and the lifestyle groups reduced the incidence of type 2 diabetes compared to placebo, the incidence rate with lifestyle intervention was 39% lower than with the metformin intervention group. These impressive reductions in the incidence in type 2 diabetes with the lifestyle intervention occurred with an average of only 6 kg of weight loss and an increase in leisure-time activity of only 6 MET-hr/week. While this study was not specific to older individuals, approximately 16% of the subjects were older than 60 years. It is noteworthy that the lifestyle intervention was even more effective in the older subjects than in younger age groups.

A post hoc analysis of the Diabetes Prevention Program showed a similar effect of interventions on the incidence of new metabolic syndrome (ATP III criteria) with the biggest effect in the lifestyle group. Approximately 50% of the Diabetes Prevention Program subjects met criteria for metabolic syndrome at baseline. Of these, after 3 years of intervention, metabolic syndrome resolved in 38% of the lifestyle, 23% of metformin, and 18% of the placebo group. In a small study of obese (BMI ≥30) older (age ≥65 years) subjects randomized to a similar lifestyle or control intervention or a control group for 26 weeks, metabolic syndrome resolved in 66% of the lifestyle group compared to none in the control group.

Thus, it appears that endurance training in older individuals produces a response similar to that noted in younger subjects. Insulin sensitivity is improved, as reflected by a decline in plasma insulin levels. Glucose tolerance improves modestly in type 2 diabetic patients but little or not at all in older subjects with normal or impaired glucose tolerance. Although there are fewer data for strength training; the qualitative and quantitative responses appear to be similar. It is as yet unclear whether these changes are related indirectly to alterations in body fat, fat distribution, and/or FFM, or whether these are directly related to the training itself through changes in muscle capillary density or blood flow, fiber type, enzymes, or glucose transporters. Despite relatively unimpressive effects of exercise on overall adiposity or glucose tolerance, exercise-induced changes could be important in the long term, given the accumulating data linking insulin resistance and hyperinsulinemia to diabetes mellitus, hypertension, dyslipidemia, and atherosclerosis. Exercise may play a major role in the prevention or delay in the onset of type 2 diabetes in subjects who are at high risk of its development. The role of exercise in the treatment and prevention of type 2 diabetes is described in a position paper by the American College of Sports Medicine.

Dyslipidemia

Dyslipidemia is common in the elderly population (see Chapter 110). Higher levels of physical activity are associated with less atherogenic lipoprotein profiles in cross-sectional studies in young and middle-aged individuals. Reduced plasma triglyceride (TG), very-low-density lipoprotein triglyceride concentrations, and higher high-density lipoprotein (HDL)-C, HDL2-C, and apolipoprotein A-I levels are consistently observed in trained subjects, when compared to sedentary controls. Of interest is the apparent lack of effect of physical activity on total and low-density lipoprotein cholesterol levels in many studies. However, in one prospective study in older adults (50–75 years), 6 months of endurance exercise positively affected low-density lipoprotein concentration and particle size, an effect that was independent of change in body fat. Neither cross-sectional nor intervention studies show a consistent effect of strength or strength training on lipoproteins.

In young and middle-aged individuals, there is a dose–response relationship between HDL-C and exercise for subjects running more than 10 miles/week but no effect for lower mileage. However, the duration and frequency of the training regimen may affect the relationship between exercise intensity and HDL-C. One study found no increase in HDL-C in older men and women who exercised vigorously or moderately for 1 year. After 2 years of participation, small but significant increments in HDL-C were noted at both exercise intensities. In fact, the increases were somewhat greater in the group that exercised more frequently (five vs. three times per week) at a lower intensity. Weight loss (or fat loss) may be necessary to attain an increase in HDL-C with exercise training, but intra-abdominal fat may be of particular importance in the increase in HDL-C with exercise. This small but metabolically important fat depot may be preferentially affected by exercise with little or no measurable loss of overall weight or adiposity.

There appears to be a difference in the effect of training on plasma lipoproteins between men and women, with women often demonstrating little or no improvement, especially with regard to HDL levels. The reason for this gender-related difference in response is not entirely clear but may relate to more favorable baseline lipoprotein concentrations in premenopausal women, or to differences in training effects on body composition or intra-abdominal fat depots between men and women.

Hypertension

Drug treatment of hypertension in the elderly population produces long-term benefits, with reductions in stroke, atherosclerotic CVD, or both (see Chapter 81). Despite the known benefits of antihypertensive therapy, the side-effect profile of many drug therapies, especially in elderly people, has led to a resurgence of interest in non-pharmacological treatments (e.g., weight loss, low-sodium diet, and endurance exercise), especially in patients with mild-to-moderate hypertension. The majority of cross-sectional and cohort studies find modestly lower systolic and diastolic blood pressures (approximately 5–10 mm Hg) in active subjects, but the magnitude of the difference is dependent on the type and intensity of exercise, as well as the position in which the blood pressure was measured (with greater differences when the subject is supine). As a whole, studies suggest a greater exercise effect in older subjects and those with mild-to-moderate hypertension.

Two large prospective cohort studies demonstrated that both leisure-time activity and increased fitness, measured by Vo_{2max} testing, were protective against the development of hypertension, with the effect being independent of age, obesity, and family history. In these studies, there tends to be a dose–response effect with the lowest risk of developing hypertension in the most active groups. In a cohort study of nearly 3000 middle-aged men and women, the relative risk of developing hypertension during the 10-year follow-up period was 1.7 in the least, as compared to the most, active group of men. A quantitatively similar but nonsignificant trend was noted for women. A 25-year follow-up of a prospective cohort study of men born in Malmo, Sweden, in 1914, found that hypertensive men who regularly exercised vigorously had an adjusted relative risk of 0.43 for total mortality and 0.33 for cardiovascular mortality.

Exercise intervention studies have frequently demonstrated small decrements in blood pressure after chronic endurance training. However, some of these had no true control group and are difficult to interpret given the well-known blood-pressure-lowering effect of participating in a study in control groups. A meta-analysis of 54 randomized controlled studies found a 3 to 4 mm Hg decline in both systolic and diastolic blood pressure with standard endurance training programs. While the number of studies comparing different intensities of exercise is small, it appears that the blood-pressure-lowering response to low- to moderate-intensity exercise is at least as good, if not superior, as that of more vigorous exercise. Indeed, even light T'ai Chi exercise can reduce blood pressure in sedentary older hypertensive patients. While older subjects with orthostatic hypotension must be careful of the hypotensive effect of an acute bout of strenuous exercise, chronic endurance exercise training may be useful in the treatment of patients predisposed to orthostatic dizziness and presyncope.

The blood-pressure-lowering effects of exercise are also found when ambulatory blood pressure monitoring is measured in older hypertensive patients, although it appears that most of the effect occurs during the daytime hours. Using ambulatory blood pressure monitoring, it appears that there is a positive relationship between blood pressure lowering (amount and duration) and the intensity of an acute bout of exercise.

There is, at present, no agreement on the possible etiology of any of the exercise-related effects on blood pressure in older individuals, although changes in body composition, fat distribution, sympathetic nervous system activity, and insulinemia have all been postulated. Both salt restriction and exercise have effects on arterial stiffness measures, with a threefold greater effect from salt restriction as compared to exercise. Weight loss alone or combined with exercise provides greater blood pressure lowering than exercise alone. Exercise also appears to restore the age-associated decline in cardiovagal baroreflex sensitivity in sedentary older subjects.

The available data on the effect of strength training on blood pressure are more limited, and at present there is no consensus. Excessive blood pressure elevations can be seen during high-intensity resistance training, especially if associated with Valsalva. However, with low- to moderate-intensity strength training and proper breathing techniques this is not a concern. Meta-analyses of randomized controlled trials of progressive-resistance-training effects on resting blood pressure revealed a 3 mm Hg drop in both systolic and diastolic blood pressure. Although less than found with endurance exercise, this degree of BP reduction has been associated with significant cardiovascular improvement. Despite the decline in resting BP with strength training, several studies have detected worsening of arterial compliance. The clinical significance of such findings remains to be determined. As noted above, the positive effects of endurance exercise on vascular resistance and endothelial function may not also be associated with resistance training.

Atherosclerotic CVD and Overall Mortality

An important effect of increased activity in reducing the risk of atherosclerotic CVD is supported by (1) population studies demonstrating a low prevalence of ischemic heart disease in extremely active societies, (2) retrospective studies comparing rates of heart disease in workers with active versus sedentary jobs, and (3) studies where activity mitigated the deleterious effects of a diet high in saturated fat and cholesterol in monkeys. Several large prospective cohort studies in humans also support this hypothesis. Paffenbarger's classic study of Harvard alumni found a greater than 50% reduction in the risk for heart attack in subjects expending more than 2000 kcal per week in leisure-time physical activity. Furthermore, it was present, not college, activity level that was inversely related to risk. Published multi-year follow-up studies of men who were middle aged at baseline confirm the importance of activity in protecting against CVD and reducing all-cause mortality. The 16-year follow-up of the Multiple Risk Factor Intervention study found excess CVD and all-cause mortality (29% and 22%, respectively) when comparing the least active (5 min of leisure-time physical activity per day) with those with light-to-moderate activity levels (23 min/d) and found no additional protection from more vigorous activity schedules. This study strongly supports the excess risks inherent with a sedentary lifestyle and suggests that even low-to-moderate activity can ameliorate much of this risk. The 20-year follow-up of the Goteborg Primary Prevention study evaluated both leisure- and workplace-related activity in men aged 47 to 55 years at baseline. They detected higher all-cause mortality in men with the greatest work-related activity, which was accounted for by smoking, alcohol, and occupational hazards. Leisure-time activity was associated with a relative risk of approximately 0.7 for both CVD and overall mortality when comparing the most and the least active groups. This protective effect of leisure-time activity was independent of other major risk factors. A 12-year follow-up of the Honolulu Heart study in 707 nonsmoking Japanese men living in Hawaii (ages 45–68 years at baseline) also noted a 50% increase in overall mortality in subjects who walked <1 mile/d, as compared to those who walked >1 mile/d. The cumulative all-cause mortality at 12 years in the group walking >2 miles/d (approximately 20%) was reached by the most sedentary group by 7 years of follow-up. At 12 years, the cumulative mortality in the sedentary group was twice that in the most active group (43/100 vs. 21/100).

Most of the older studies assessing the protection of activity against CVD and overall mortality were completed in male populations. Similar data have now been published in a 7-year follow-up of more than 40 000 postmenopausal women (ages 55–69 years at baseline). Those reporting regular physical activity had a relative risk of death of 0.77, as compared to those who reported none. While a dose–response effect was noted for increasing frequency of moderate activity, moderate activity as seldom as once a week was protective.

A study of nearly 16 000 healthy Finnish twins (ages 25–64 years at baseline) evaluated the effect of physical activity on mortality while controlling for possible hereditary influences. When subjects were classified as "conditioning" (six bouts of leisure-time exercise per month equivalent to 30 min of brisk walking), "sedentary" (no reported leisure-time activity), or "occasional exercisers" (the remainder), there was a significant trend for a reduced mortality risk with more vigorous exercise. In addition, when the total volume of exercise was estimated, there was also a trend toward a protective effect of increasing volumes of exercise. A 5% reduction in the hazard ratio was found for each quintile of increasing exercise volume. In twin pairs who were discordant for death during the follow-up period, the odds ratio for dying was 0.44 in the conditioning group and 0.66 in the occasional exercising group, when compared to the sedentary controls. When adjusted for smoking, occupation, and alcohol, these odds ratios did not quite reach significance, but the trend between the three activity categories remained significant.

While there is little argument about the positive effects of exercise on CVD and all-cause mortality, there remains some discrepancy about whether or not there is a threshold below which little protective effect is noted. It appears that the continuous inverse relationship between activity level and mortality is more easily detected when fitness level (Vo_{2max}) is used, rather that just a physical activity questionnaire. While activity questionnaires are clearly important in large population-based studies, these are more valid for either high-intensity activity or sedentary lifestyle and are less reliable for low or moderate levels of activity. In addition, it is possible that older studies that have used leisure-time physical activity questionnaires have consistently underestimated low-to-moderate levels of activity in women by failing to ascertain the activity involved in housework. Studies in older adults using quantitative methods to measure physical activity energy expenditure demonstrate an adjusted risk of all-cause mortality of 0.31 when the most active and least active tertiles are compared.

When fitness is used, not only is a continuous gradient of effect noted on mortality, but also the relative risk for mortality in the least-fit group (1.5 for men and 2.1 for women) is quite similar to the effect of smoking. Furthermore, when fitness level was measured at a mean interval of 5 years, an improvement in fitness (in a previously sedentary group) was associated with reduced mortality. For every minute increment in maximal treadmill time, there was an 8% decline in mortality risk. It should be noted that all of the above studies involved endurance exercise, and we are aware of no published studies assessing the relationship between CVD or all-cause mortality and strength training. The relationship between low cardiorespiratory fitness and CVD death was confirmed in an 11-year prospective follow-up of a cohort of nearly 1300 middle-aged Finnish men. Men in the low-fitness group (Vo_{2max} <27.6 mL/kg or <8 METs) were threefold more likely to have a CVD-related death than the high-fitness group (Vo_{2max} >37.1 mL/kg or >10.5 METs), when adjusted for age, smoking, and alcohol. This excess CVD death in the low-fitness group remained significant even when adjusted for lipids, diabetes, blood pressure, fasting insulin, and plasma fibrinogen. While there appeared to be a continuous effect of fitness on overall mortality, the major benefit seemed to occur for fitness levels above 9 METs. Low fitness was also found to be an important risk factor for non-CVD death, with a relative risk of 2.6, as compared to the high-fitness group. In this study, fitness was at least as good a predictor of both overall and CVD-related death as blood pressure, obesity, smoking, or diabetes.

In a study of fitness, obesity, and mortality, existing baseline CVD was the greatest predictor of overall mortality in the entire population, but low fitness conferred similar risk in the obese men.

Arthritis

Arthritis is an important cause of functional impairment in older adults. A description of age-related changes in joint function and the impact of arthritis on function in older adults is given in Chapter 112. Despite concerns that exercise could be harmful to arthritis patients, several randomized controlled trials have demonstrated that exercise, even vigorous exercise, is beneficial in arthritis. These studies have enrolled both young and older adults and have included functional status outcomes. Exercise has included endurance training, such as riding a stationary bicycle, and strength training by using weights.

The exercise trials in arthritis patients report a 10% to 25% improvement in functional status outcomes. Improvements include faster gait, improved physical function performance, lower depression scores, less subjective pain, and less frequent use of pain medications. Improvements have persisted as long as 9 months after discharge from supervised exercise classes. As a group, these studies provide strong evidence of a beneficial effect of exercise on functional status in patients with mild-to-moderate arthritis (both rheumatoid and osteoarthritis). In one study, endurance and strength training were directly compared, and similar positive effects were found. In a recent study using this same population, both resistance (RR = 0.6) and endurance (RR = 0.53) exercise reduced the loss of activities of daily living.

Osteoporosis

The decline in bone mineral density with age is well recognized (see Chapter 117), and there is an epidemic of osteoporotic fractures that affects women more than men and that primarily involves hip, vertebral, and wrist fractures. The extent to which the decline in bone mineral density with aging is a result of reduced physical activity is unknown.

The concept that mechanical loads are important to the integrity of the skeleton is more than 100 years old. Animal studies confirm the importance of mechanical strain to bone modeling and remodeling and have also identified the characteristics of loading forces that produce the greatest increase in bone mass. These studies demonstrated that (1) the osteogenic response to mechanical loading is optimized with relatively few repetitions of high-magnitude forces; (2) the application of force must be in a dynamic, rather than static, fashion; and (3) fast strain rates are more osteogenic than slow strain rates. Furthermore, the osteogenic response to mechanical loading is mediated locally in skeletal regions subjected to the strain, rather than systemically highlighting the need for exercises to specifically target regions of the skeleton at risk of fracture. Studies of laboratory animals suggest that bone cells lose sensitivity to mechanical loading after relatively few loading cycles. For example, four sets of 90 load applications per day was more osteogenic than one set of 360 loading cycles, and interposing an 8-hour recovery period between loading sessions resulted in a greater osteogenic response than when the recovery period was 0.5 hour. These concepts remain to be evaluated in humans. However, animal studies suggest that multiple short bouts of exercise per day may be more effective in preserving bone

health than a single, longer daily session. The concept of allowing bone to "rest" between loading cycles may also have implications for resistance training. For example, if the intent is to perform three sets of eight repetitions of several exercises, it might be of greater benefit to bone to perform one set of each exercise and then cycle back through for the second and third sets, rather than doing three consecutive sets of each exercise.

There are numerous cross-sectional studies of the effects of exercise on bone mass, comparing athletes who participate in different sports or physically active versus sedentary people. Interpretation of many of these studies is limited, because the area of bone density measurement frequently did not correspond to the bones that would be expected to receive the bulk of the mechanical stress from the given exercise. However, one well-conceived study found that the humerus in the dominant arm of tennis players had approximately 30% greater cortical bone thickness when compared to the nondominant arm. Other work suggests that the primary benefit of physical activity in adults may be to preserve, rather than increase, bone mass. Trabecular bone density was found to be roughly 5% to 10% higher in eumenorrheic runners when compared with eumenorrheic control women. Athletes who participate in muscle-building activities (e.g., weight lifting and body building) and in activities that involve jumping or vaulting (e.g., volleyball and gymnastics) also tend to have elevated bone mineral density. These data suggest that exercise in younger individuals may increase peak bone mass—an important negative risk factor for osteopenia later in life.

In postmenopausal women, exercise may increase bone mineral density by up to 5%, as compared to no-exercise controls, but average increases generally are only 1% to 3%. Although there are theoretical reasons why strength training may be a preferable intervention to increase bone mass, the magnitude of increase in bone mineral density in response to either resistance exercise or weight-bearing endurance exercise appears to be similar.

With the growing prevalence of obesity in the United States and other countries, it might be expected that the rate of osteoporosis will decline in the future. However, there are reasons why this may not occur. First, it is important to note that while low body weight is a risk factor for osteoporosis, increased body weight is not necessarily protective. In studies of overweight and mildly obese postmenopausal women, approximately one-third were osteopenic or osteoporotic. Second, the increased prevalence of overweight and obesity is likely to be accompanied by an increased prevalence of weight cycling (i.e., multiple cycles of weight loss and gain). Observational studies have found that women with a history of weight cycling have lower bone mineral density levels than noncyclers. Intervention studies have also found significant decreases in bone mineral density in response to modest weight loss (e.g., 5%) in postmenopausal women, even when calcium supplementation was provided and even when the weight loss was mediated by moderate-intensity exercise. It may be possible to prevent, or at least attenuate, bone loss during weight loss through the use of antiresorptive drugs.

There have been no randomized controlled intervention trials to evaluate the effectiveness of exercise to prevent fractures. However, results from prospective cohort studies, such as the Nurses' Health Study and the Study of Osteoporotic Fractures, suggest that the risk for hip fracture is reduced by ~50% in the most physically active quintile of the population. In evaluating just the potential benefit of walking activity, the Nurses' Health Study found a dose–response benefit for both duration and speed of walking, such that more hours per week spent walking and fast walking speed conferred reduced fracture risk. Even hours per week spent standing was inversely related to hip fracture incidence. Perhaps most importantly, changes in physical activity for several years were related to hip fracture incidence in the expected manner: decreases in physical activity were associated increased risk and vise versa. Such findings suggest that any type of ambulatory physical activity may confer skeletal benefits and that increased physical activity should be advocated at any age as a strategy to reduce fracture risk.

Exercise may help to prevent fractures both by preserving bone mass and strength and by reducing the incidence of injurious falls. Of course, many factors contribute to risk for falling, including some that would be expected to improve in response to exercise (e.g., poor muscle strength) and some that would not (e.g., poor vision). Exercise interventions involving balance, leg strength, flexibility, and endurance training can reduce fall risk in community-dwelling older women and men. Such interventions have not proven effective in nursing home residents, but that may relate to the diverse causes of falls in that population.

Cancer

Studies describing higher rates of cancer deaths in sedentary workers date back at least to the early 1960s, but these findings may have been skewed by greater alcohol and tobacco use in the higher-paid office workers. A more recent study demonstrated a dose–response relationship between fitness level and overall cancer death. In the 12-year follow-up of the Honolulu Heart Study, nearly one-third of the 208 deaths were from cancer. There was an inverse relationship between the daily distance walked and the risk of death from any cancer. The relative risk of cancer death was 2.4-fold greater in the sedentary group (<1 mile walked per day) when compared to the group walking >2 miles per day. At present, the most compelling data involve the relationship between activity and breast or colon cancer.

Both cohort and case–control studies in both men and women in a number of different ethnic populations have found a reduced relative risk of colon cancer when comparing the most to the least active groups, but the risk varies (range of relative risk, 0.4–0.9). In general, controlling for other cancer risks including tobacco, alcohol, age, obesity, and diet does not diminish the relationships. Evidence for a relationship between activity and rectal cancer appears to be substantially weaker. A negative result was reported from the Physicians Health study, where no level of reported physical activity was associated with a protection from colon cancer.

The risk for breast cancer has been linked to inactivity in 17 of 22 studies, with relative risks ranging from 0.20 to 0.89 when comparing the most active to the least active groups. These associations remain even after adjusting for potential confounding factors such as age, BMI, reproductive history, tobacco, and diet. The association holds for both pre- and postmenopausal women, although the risk factors for breast cancer in these two populations are felt to be different.

Mood and Cognition

Subjects who exercise regularly consistently report an improved sense of well-being and reduced tension and anxiety. Indeed, similar responses occur acutely and persist for several hours after a single bout of exercise. Exercise can also ameliorate some of the symptoms of depression and anxiety. Cohort studies of endurance exercise have found a dose–response relationship between exercise at baseline and the development of depression at a later time point. One randomized controlled trial found that resistance training was also of benefit in a group of older depressed patients. In this study, the intensity of training was independently related to the decline in the Beck depression score.

Several studies have now documented a positive effect of exercise on cognition. A report of 19 000 subjects aged 70 to 81 years in the Nurses Health study found better cognitive test scores in subjects with higher levels of overall long-term physical activity or walking. Regular physical activity was also associated with less age-related cognitive decline. In another study of 1740 older adults, a hazard ratio of 0.62 was found for incident dementia after 6 years of follow-up in subjects who exercised at least three times per week compared to less active individuals. Intervention trials show a mixed pattern of effect of activity on cognition. A meta-analysis of 18 exercise intervention trials on nondemented subjects found a moderate positive effect, with the greatest effect found for executive control processes. Of interest, the effect was stronger with mixed training paradigms and in women. A meta-analysis of 12 exercise training studies in demented subjects showed a similar moderate positive effect. MRI studies have also demonstrated better frontal and parietal activation and greater frontal and superior temporal lobe volume after endurance exercise training.

The bases for the exercise-associated improvements in cognition are presently under considerable investigation in animal models, which suggest that elevations in brain-derived neurotrophic factor may underlie an increase in neurogenesis in exercised animals. Other work is investigating the potential role that obesity and insulin resistance may play in the development of cognitive decline in patients with type 2 diabetes mellitus and metabolic syndrome.

Other Chronic Medical Disorders

While exercise rehabilitation has long been used in the treatment of patients with coronary artery disease, more recently, trials have begun to assess the effectiveness of exercise rehabilitation for the treatment of other common cardiovascular disorders. Exercise has also been found to provide improved functional outcomes in patients with peripheral arterial disease and claudication. In a randomized control trial, 6 months of endurance exercise improved distance walked until the onset of claudication (134%), distance to maximal claudication (77%), and walking economy (12%). More importantly, the daily physical activity in the trained group increased by almost 40%. While the most effective training appears to be walking, strength training may also provide some benefits.

Similarly, exercise rehabilitation has been shown effective in the treatment of some patients with congestive heart failure. Not only have increments in exercise duration and peak Vo_{2max} been found in these patients, but there may also be some improvements in the skeletal muscle myopathy, which have been described in congestive heart failure patients. Patients with chronic obstructive lung disease have been shown to benefit from exercise training with the ability to do more absolute work, and also to sustain a constant submaximal workload for a longer duration and with a lower minute ventilation.

RISKS ASSOCIATED WITH EXERCISE

Despite the recognition of exercise as a major public health objective for our entire population, there has been little systematic assessment of the health risks of exercise. This lack of information may be a result of the complex interplay of factors that may or may not predispose to injury: (1) host factors such as age, sex, fitness level, gait, balance, health status, and body weight; (2) exercise factors such as frequency, intensity, speed, duration, competition, and proper use of warm-up/cool-down periods; and (3) environmental factors such as surface, location, temperature, weather conditions, and use of proper supportive and protective equipment.

By far, the majority of injuries are caused by "overuse" and involve soft tissues. Approximately 10% of individuals (ages 16–65 years) participating in active sports or recreation reported having an injury within the last 4 weeks, with half of the incidents causing limitations in activity and 15% causing a hospital visit. Although the number of injuries might be expected to be reduced with less intensive and noncompetitive activity, it is also likely to be greater with increasing age. As noted previously, the speed of an activity may be a greater risk for injury than the intensity of the activity. Thus, fewer injuries would be expected from walking uphill as compared to jogging on a flat surface. Evidence also suggests that eccentric exercise (e.g., lowering a weight that has been lifted) may predispose to excess muscle injury. Patients with osteoporosis are at increased risk of fracture if they fall while exercising. Appropriate warm-up and cool-down periods, as well as emphasis on stretching and flexibility, are likely to be especially important in reducing soft-tissue injury in an older population.

A rigorous review of the potential exercise risks in an older population is outside the scope of this chapter, but two specific areas require comment. There is a significant transient increase in the risk of sudden death occurring during a bout of vigorous exercise, especially in previously sedentary individuals. However, the reduction in risk during the nonexercising period of the day more than makes up for the transient increase during exercise, producing an overall risk of sudden death in active men, which is 30% of that in sedentary men. These findings are supported by studies describing lower cardiovascular-related and overall mortality in active individuals. It should be emphasized that the relationship between the type, intensity, and duration of exercise and the reduction in cardiac risk remains unclear. The possible detrimental effects of resistance training on vascular function described above require additional investigation.

Exercise in older patients with diabetes mellitus also deserves additional comments. Careful attention to the possibility of both immediate and delayed episodes of exercise-induced hypoglycemia is critical, because of the sustained improvement in insulin sensitivity (24–48 hours) associated with vigorous exercise. Transient worsening of orthostatic hypotension can also occur following vigorous exercise, especially in hot weather. Meticulous foot care and supportive, well-fitted shoes are particularly critical for the exercising diabetic patient. Patients with proliferative retinopathy should avoid anaerobic (specifically isometric) exercise, such as power lifting, because of the increased ocular and systemic pressure occurring with the Valsalva maneuver. Diabetes is an important risk factor for ischemic heart disease, and its presence also puts the diabetic patient in a higher-risk category with respect to exercise-associated cardiovascular events.

RECOMMENDATIONS

There is now ample evidence strongly supporting the beneficial effects of exercise in older individuals on several important health-related end points. It is also clear, however, that we still do not yet know enough about different types of exercise regimens to accurately prescribe a specific program that can be aimed at a specific disorder. Several large prospective cohort studies as well as smaller clinical trials have demonstrated a dose–response relationship between the intensity of exercise and the improvement in most outcome measures (blood pressure being one possible exception). This gradient of effect seems even clearer when fitness is substituted for physical activity. However, significant cardiovascular and metabolic improvements can be obtained when less-intense exercise is maintained over sufficiently long periods of time and that less-intense exercise regimens are generally more acceptable (especially to older individuals) and appear to make long-term compliance more likely. Low-intensity programs may be necessary in frail populations, such as those with stroke, congestive heart failure, and chronic lung disease, in which more intensive exercise is not tolerated. While multiple short bouts of exercise (at least 10 min each) may be effective in improving certain outcome measures, longer sessions remain preferable if these can be tolerated. A potential disadvantage of vigorous exercise in older individuals is that it may have little effect on total daily energy expenditure if overall activity during nonexercising periods is reduced.

After a thorough review of the types and amounts of exercise required for promotion of health and prevention of disease, a distinguished panel, representing the American College of Sports Medicine and the American Heart Association, published consensus recommendations for physical activity for adults and a separate report for older adults in 2007 (Table 114-1). While the reports are similar, the differences in the recommendations for older adults

---

TABLE 114-1

Summary of Physical Activity Recommendations for Older Adults

1. Maintain a physically active lifestyle
2. Perform (a) moderate-intensity endurance activities a minimum of 30 min/d, 5 d/wk, (b) vigorous-intensity endurance activities a minimum of 20 min/d, 3 d/wk, or (c) a combination of moderate and vigorous activities
3. Perform 8–10 muscle strengthening activities that target all major muscle groups and require moderate to high effort (i.e., 10–15 repetitions) at least 2 d/wk
4. Perform activities that maintain or increase flexibility a minimum of 10 min/d, 2 d/wk
5. Perform activities that maintain or improve balance
6. Older adults with medical conditions for which physical activity is therapeutic should perform activities in a manner that is safe and effective for the conditions
7. Older adults who are not active at the recommended levels should increase physical activity level gradually. Many months of activity at less than recommended levels may be appropriate for some adults (e.g., those with low fitness) as they increase activity levels

Data from Nelson ME, et al. Physical activity and public health in older adults: recommendations from the American College of Sports Medicine and the American Heart Association. Circulation. 2007;116:1094–1105.

include (1) use of a relative scale of intensity, perceived effort, in place of an absolute measure of intensity in METs; (2) strength training exercise at a resistance that allows one set of 10 to 15 repetitions of eight to 10 different exercises; 3) inclusion of flexibility exercise; (4) balance exercise for those with a fall risk; and (5) use of a specific activity plan developed in consultation with a health-care provider, which can be tailored to specific chronic conditions and limitations, minimizes risk, and includes behavioral strategies to enhance adherence. The importance of reducing sedentary behavior and a gradual (stepwise) approach to increasing activity is stressed for all older adults.

For reasons of safety, in the past most experts recommended a pre-exercise assessment, including a complete history and physical examination, as well as an exercise stress test before vigorous exercise for all people older than 60 years. However, there are little data substantiating such a recommendation, and the significant cost of such an evaluation could greatly affect the practicality of using exercise as a public health measure and limit the participation of many older individuals in an exercise program. Furthermore, many older individuals have safely participated in community-based exercise programs for years with no such prior evaluation. New recommendations suggest that asymptomatic individuals who plan to exercise at moderate intensity do not need health-care provider screening before initiating an activity program. It is appropriate for patients to notify their physicians of their intent to begin an exercise program, because adjustments in medications or dosages may be necessary. The geriatric medicine axiom of "start low and go slow" should always be applied to beginning an activity program.

As discussed earlier, there are compelling reasons why an activity plan for older adults should also include activities that maintain and/or increase muscle strength. The Surgeon General's report on physical activity affirmed the accumulating evidence of the health benefits of strength-developing exercises.

Changes in lifestyle are difficult to maintain at any age, and recidivism rates for exercise programs are high. This problem may be reduced by (1) careful attention to warm-up periods and slow progression in an effort to reduce early injuries, (2) enthusiastic leadership, (3) regular assessment of improvement with personalized feedback and praise, (4) spousal and family support for participation, (5) flexible goals (time rather than distance) set by the participant, and (6) use of distraction techniques such as music. Because it is inevitable that a participant will, at some time, have a setback, it is important to provide strategies for coping with this stress at the beginning of any exercise program.

FURTHER READING

Albright A, et al. Exercise and type 2 diabetes. *Med Sci Sports Exerc.* 2000;32:1345.

Blair SN, et al. Influences of cardiorespiratory fitness and other precursors on cardiovascular disease and all-cause mortality in men and women. *JAMA.* 1996;276:205.

Bottaro M, et al. Effect of high versus low-velocity resistance training on muscular fitness and functional performance in older men. *Eur J Appl Physiol.* 2007;99:257–264.

Buchner DM, et al. Evidence for a non-linear relationship between leg strength and gait speed. *Age Ageing.* 1996;25:386.

Cress ME, et al. Exercise effects on physical functional performance in independent older adults. *J Gerontol.* 1999;54A:M242.

Diabetes Prevention Program Group. Reduction in the incidence of type 2 diabetes with lifestyle intervention or metformin. *N Engl J Med.* 2002;346:393.

Feskanich D, et al. Walking and leisure-time activity and risk of hip fracture in postmenopausal women. *JAMA.* 2002;288:2300.

Haskell WL, et al. Physical activity and public health: updated recommendation for adults from the American College of Sports Medicine and the American Heart Association. *Med Sci Sports Exerc.* 2007;39:1423–1434.

Kesaniemi YA, et al. Dose-response issues concerning physical activity and health: and evidence-based symposium. *Med Sci Sports Exerc.* 2001;33:S351–S358.

Kohrt WM, et al. American College of Sports Medicine Position Stand: physical activity and bone health. *Med Sci Sports Exerc.* 2005;36:1985.

Kramer AF, et al. Exercise, cognition, and the aging brain. *J Appl Physiol.* 2006;101:1237–1242.

Kujala UM, et al. Relationship of leisure-time physical activity and mortality. *JAMA.* 1998;279:440.

Latham NK, et al. Systematic review of progressive resistance strength training in older adults. *J Gerontol Med Sci.* 2004;59A:48–61.

Manini TM, et al. Daily activity energy expenditure and mortality in older adults. *JAMA.* 2006;296:171–179.

Nelson ME, et al. Physical activity and public health in older adults: recommendations from the American College of Sports Medicine and the American Heart Association. *Med Sci Sports Exerc.* 2007;39:1435–1445.

Orchard TJ, et al. The effect of metformin and intensive lifestyle intervention on metabolic syndrome: the Diabetes Prevention Program randomized trial. *Ann Intern Med.* 2005;142:611–619.

Von Stengel S, et al. Differential effects of strength versus power training on bone mineral density in postmenopausal women: a two year longitudinal study. *Br J Sports Med.* 2007;41:649–655.

Williams MA, et al. Resistance exercise in individuals with and without cardiovascular disease: 2007 update. *Circulation.* 2007;116:572–584.

Zoico E, et al. Physical disability and muscular strength in relation to obesity and different body composition indexes in a sample of healthy elderly women. *Int J Obesity.* 2004;28:234–241.

Mobility

Jennifer Brach ■ *Caterina Rosano* ■ *Stephanie Studenski*

INTRODUCTION

Mobility problems are pervasive in older adults. Mobility limitations affect personal independence, need for human help, and quality of life. Limited mobility predicts future health, function, and survival. Like other geriatric syndromes, mobility disorders are caused by diseases and impairments across many organ systems, so evaluation and management require multiple perspectives and disciplines. Healthcare providers should be able to assess and treat mobility problems. They should be able to measure and interpret clinical indicators of mobility such as gait speed, the short physical performance battery, and the performance-oriented mobility assessment. They should know the physiological and biomechanical mechanisms underlying normal and abnormal mobility, the differential diagnosis of the causes of mobility disorders, and the approaches to management of mobility problems.

DEFINITIONS AND METHODS OF CLASSIFICATION

Defining Mobility

Mobility is the ability to move one's own body through space. Mobility requires force production and feedback control systems to navigate the mass of the body through a three-dimensional environment. Walking is the fundamental mobility task for human life. Mobility also includes a wide range of other important activities that require moving one's body, from turning over in bed to climbing stairs. Mobility tasks have an inherent hierarchical order based on the biomechanical and physiological demands made on the body. This orderedness is apparent in the developmental tasks of infancy and childhood, when mobility independence is first achieved. The simplest and first mobility task is turning over in bed, followed by

sitting upright, transfers from lying to sitting and from sitting to standing, locomotion with an increased base of support (like crawling or using a walker), to independent two legged walking, then more challenging tasks like ascending and descending stairs, running, climbing ladders, and sports.

Mobility disability is best defined within a conceptual framework such as that of disablement (Table 115-1). Disability is caused by pathologic processes that lead to organ system impairments and functional limitations. Disability causes handicap by limiting life roles such as work or caregiving. Disability in mobility occurs at the level of the whole person and is manifested by the inability to carry out normal mobility activities like bathing or shopping. Mobility disability is caused by functional limitations in walking, transferring, or climbing stairs, which are, in turn, caused by problems with strength, endurance, coordination, balance, and range of motion. These functional limitations can be caused by numerous pathological processes. Disablement can be modified by psychological, social, and environmental factors. Mobility disability can precipitate a cycle of negative consequences because it often leads to decreased activity, which in turn worsens functional limitations and causes organ system deconditioning, including muscle weakness, loss of joint range of motion, and poor cardiovascular endurance.

Classification Methods for Mobility

Mobility classification is often driven by a tacit assumption of orderedness. No single current instrument assesses the full range of mobility from the lowest levels of rolling over in bed to the highest levels of endurance and coordination required for athletics or dance. Mobility assessment tools for older adults generally address one or more of the following three mobility levels: nonambulatory, ambulatory, and vigorous, corresponding broadly to Tinetti's levels of frail, transitional, and vigorous mobility status. Mobility levels are surprisingly stable. While day-to-day variability does occur, people in general tend to remain in one level or decline very gradually

TABLE 115-1

Mobility Disability and the Disablement Process

COMPONENT OF THE DISABLEMENT PROCESS	EXAMPLES RELATED TO MOBILITY DISABILITY
Pathological processes	Cardiopulmonary, neurological, and musculoskeletal conditions
Organ system impairments	Losses of strength, endurance, coordination, balance, and range of motion
Functional limitations	Problems with transfers, walking, and climbing stairs
Mobility disability	Dependence or difficulty with activities of daily living such as bathing or shopping
Handicap	Limitations in work, care giving

unless a major event has occurred. Within the nonambulatory level, there are important mobility skills that affect independence in personal care activities, care needs, and demand for human help; these activities include bed mobility, self transfer skills, and wheelchair mobility. Within the vigorous mobility level, the degree of fitness, as represented by the ability to perform demanding or challenging mobility activities, may be a useful indicator of the extent of "successful aging" and "physiological reserve." As an indicator of the extent of physiological reserve, vigorous mobility status may be a marker of ability to tolerate physiologic stressors such as acute illness, surgery, or periods of reduced activity.

Mobility can be assessed by self-report, professional observation, or direct measurement. Instruments to assess mobility from all three perspectives have been developed (Table 115-2). Each has advantages and disadvantages. These tools have been used to estimate the population incidence and prevalence of mobility disorders, predict

TABLE 115-2

Instruments Used to Screen and Classify Mobility

INSTRUMENT TYPE	INSTRUMENT NAME, REFERENCES	ITEMS	RANGE	COMMENTS
Self-report	Rosow-Breslau	Walk ½ or ¼ mile and climb stairs	Ambulatory to vigorous	Used as single items
	SF-36 physical function	10 items, many directly related to mobility, from walk across a room to walk 1 mile	Ambulatory to vigorous	Score 0–100 U.S. adult mean 84.2 Older adult mean 52.0 Insensitive at lower levels of mobility
	Long-term care survey	Walking inside and bed/chair transfers	Nonambulatory to ambulatory	Used as single items
	Mobility modifications	Self-report of changing the way one walks one-half mile of climbs stairs	Ambulatory	Used as single items
	Avlund mobility	Fatigue and need for help in six mobility activities from transfer to stairs and walking outside	Nonambulatory, ambulatory, and vigorous	Scores 0–6
Professional assessment	Barthel mobility items	Walking (or wheeling), transfers, and stairs	Nonambulatory, ambulatory, and vigorous	Mobility items integrated into total score
	Functional independence measure (FIM)	Transfers and locomotion (walk, wheelchair, and stairs)	Nonambulatory, ambulatory, and vigorous	Seven-level scoring of need for assistance with mobility items. Mobility items are integrated into total score
	Minimum Data Set (MDS)	Bed mobility, transfers, locomotion (includes wheelchair mobility), and walking	Nonambulatory to ambulatory	Used as single items
Performance	Short physical performance battery (SPPB)	Timed walk, chair rises, and tandem stands	Ambulatory	Score 0–12 Scores of 10–12, 7–9, and 4–6 associated with increasing risk of poor outcomes
	Gait speed	Timed walk, varying distances, instructions, and procedures	Ambulatory	Healthy older adult >1.0 m/s Slow <0.6 m/s Very slow < 0.4 m/s
	Timed up and go	Time to rise from chair, walk 10 feet, turn, walk back, and sit down	Ambulatory	<10 s—normal <20 s—able to move in community >30 s—needs assistance for mobility
	6-min walk	Distance covered in 6 min	Ambulatory to vigorous	Healthy older adult mean >500 m Older adults in assisted living <300 m
	Health ABC	Walking endurance: 400 m walk time, distance in 2 min Expanded SPPB: longer tandem stands, one foot stand, and narrow walk time	Ambulatory to vigorous	Supplements SPPB by increasing discrimination among healthy older adults. Useful for persons with scores of 10–12 on SPPB score range 0–4

the consequences of mobility problems, screen patient populations, determine care needs, and reimburse services in rehabilitation settings. More detailed instruments have been developed specifically for sorting out causes and mechanisms. Detailed instruments will be discussed separately in the section on causes of mobility limitations. Mobility measures have varying strengths and limitations, depending on characteristics such as reliability and validity, respondent burden, feasibility and convenience of use, and assessor skill required. Self-report measures are the easiest type of measure to obtain when gathering data from large populations. Self-report measures have high face validity in that they reflect the opinion of the person themselves. Since self-report measures usually ask about a period of time, such as recent weeks or months, these are capable of reflecting fluctuating ability over time. Self-report measures can be limited by problems with reliability, accuracy, and nonresponse. Because these are usually ordinal scales, they lack ability to discriminate small but important differences. Professional report measures reflect the opinion of an experienced assessor, can integrate over time, and may be more feasible when an individual is considered an unreliable informant or is unable to cooperate with testing. Professional report is limited by the need for assessor experience and training and can be vulnerable to problems with interassessor reliability unless extensive efforts to standardize assessment are made. Since professional reports are usually based on ordinal scales, ability to discriminate small but important differences might be limited. Mobility testing by measuring actual performance is somewhat more independent of opinion. Performance testing can produce very quantitative results, which discriminate small but important or subclinical differences. Performance measures are limited in that they require direct observation, subject cooperation, and standardization of instructions and procedures. These measure capability rather than actual daily mobility activities. The need for subject cooperation can lead to problems with nonresponse. Performance measures do not account well for short-term fluctuations over hours to weeks. Despite these limitations, performance testing may have direct applications in clinical settings because it can provide useful information and is brief and quantitative.

Psychological aspects of fear, mobility confidence, and activity avoidance can have great effect on mobility disability, separately or in combination with observable mobility limitations. Several instruments to assess psychological factors related to mobility disability have been developed (Table 115-3). Items from these scales might have use in the clinical setting.

EPIDEMIOLOGY

Prevalence

The epidemiology of mobility can be considered from the perspective of basic or higher-level mobility. Examples of basic mobility problems are getting around inside the house and transfers from bed or chair. Examples of higher-level mobility problems are getting around outside the house, ability to walk one-quarter or one-half mile, and ability to climb stairs. Basic mobility problems are uncommon in community-dwelling older persons but are very frequent in institutionalized older people. Among community-dwelling persons aged 65 years and older, approximately 5% are dependent in getting in and out of a chair or bed and 7.5% are dependent in getting around inside. Among institutionalized persons older than 65 years, approximately 80% are dependent in getting in and out of a chair or bed and getting around inside. Mobility disability increases dramatically with age; dependence in getting around inside increases from 5% of persons aged 65 to 74 years to 30% of persons aged 85+ years. Women tend to have higher rates of mobility disability than men and nonwhites than whites.

Approximately 13% of Americans older than 60 years report higher-level mobility problems in that they have difficulty going outside the home alone. There is a marked increase with age. There is also geographic variation; self-reported difficulty going outside the home alone is more common among older adults in the Southern United States. Higher-level mobility problems, defined as difficulty walking a quarter mile or climbing stairs, increase with age, are more common in women than in men, and appear to be decreasing during recent decades.

Risk of Adverse Consequences Associated with Mobility Status

Mobility problems have serious consequences. Mobility status predicts mortality. Older people with difficulty walking 2 km (a little more than a mile) or climbing one flight of stairs are twice as likely to die during the next 8 years compared to those with no difficulty. Mortality risk is even higher among those who both have mobility difficulty and are physically inactive. Poor mobility performance, even in the absence of self-reported mobility limitations,

TABLE 115-3

Instruments to Assess Psychological Factors Related to Mobility			
CONSTRUCT	**INSTRUMENT/QUESTION**	**# ITEMS**	**POPULATION**
Fear	Survey of Activities and Fear of Falling in the Elderly (SAFFE)	33	Community dwelling
	Fear	11	
	Activity	11	
	Activity restriction	11	
	Are you afraid of falling? (yes/no)	1	Community and LTC
	How would you rate your fear of falling? (five-point numerical rating 0–4)	1	
Self-efficacy/confidence	Falls Efficacy Scale (FES)*	10	Community dwelling, inpatients, and LTC
	Activities-specific Balance and Confidence Scale (ABC)	16	Community dwelling and patients
Avoidance	Has fear of falling made you avoid activities? (yes/no)	1	Community dwelling and LTC
	Modified SAFFE (mSAFFE)	17	Community dwelling

*Several modified versions exist (revised FES, adapted FES, modified FES, and FES United Kingdom).

is an independent predictor of death and nursing home placement. In community-dwelling older adults, baseline physical performance score was associated with a twofold increase of death. Among persons who report no mobility problems, gait speed less than 1.0 m/s has been associated with an increased risk of death compared to a gait speed of more than 1.0 m/s. In another community-based population, 9-year mortality for older persons with gait speeds less than 0.6 m/s was 78% compared to 48% in persons with gait speed between 0.6 and 1.0 m/s and was 26% in persons with gait speeds more than 1.0 m/s. A change in gait speed of approximately 0.1 m/s (equivalent to approximately 0.2 miles per hour) or a change of one point in the SPPB or 20 m in a 6-minute walk test appears to be clinically important. Older persons who have a 0.1 m/s decline in gait speed over 1 year have a doubled risk of dying during the subsequent 5 years. Older persons who have a 0.1 m/s improvement in gait speed over 1 year have a 40% decreased risk of dying in the following 8 years.

Poor mobility performance is an independent predictor of future self-care difficulty and mobility disability. Among community-dwelling persons older than 70 years with no baseline self-care disability and no higher-level self-reported difficulty in ability to walk one-half mile and climb stairs, baseline physical performance score was a powerful predictor of incident disability in both activities of daily living and in higher-level mobility disability. Mobility self-report and performance have been shown to predict disability and mortality in older populations from numerous countries and cultures, including Mexican American, British, Italian, French, Dutch, Spanish, Scandinavian, Australian, Japanese, and Chinese.

Poor mobility performance is also an independent predictor of hospitalization and nursing home placement. In a population-based study of older adults who reported no disability at baseline, poor baseline physical performance score was associated with a twofold increased risk of hospitalization and more days in the hospital over the following four years. The increased hospitalization risk was independent of baseline health status. The increased risk was mostly associated with hospitalization for geriatric conditions, such as dementia, pressure ulcer, hip fractures, other fracture, pneumonia, and dehydration.

Mobility may be part of an underlying constellation of core factors that link multiple outcomes associated with aging. Poor mobility as measured by timed chair stands is one of four factors proposed to be common risk factors for geriatric syndromes, including incontinence, falls, and functional decline. Conversely, good mobility, along with good cognition and nutritional status, is an independent predictor of recovery of independence after a period of disability. Abnormalities of gait and slow gait speed have been found to precede the onset of cognitive decline and dementia. Slow and abnormal gait is a risk factor especially for vascular dementia. Among older adults, simultaneous abnormalities of mobility, cognition, and mood are more common than would be expected by chance, perhaps implying potential common underlying causes.

Severe mobility disability, sometimes called immobility, has widespread and devastating consequences. It accelerates impairments in multiple organ systems, including bone, muscle, heart, circulation, lung, skin, blood, bowel, kidney, nutrition, and metabolism. Loss of organ system function can be rapid and severe; muscle strength can decline by 1% to 5% per day of enforced bed rest. Skin breakdown and pressure ulcer start to occur after only hours of persistent and unrelieved pressure. Major consequences of clinical significance include decreased plasma volume, orthostatic hypotension, accelerated loss of bone density, muscle weakness, decreased pulmonary ventilation, and constipation leading to fecal impaction. When even temporary bed rest is combined with the increased vulnerability of aging and acute illness, there is a marked increased risk of death, disability, and institutionalization.

PATHOPHYSIOLOGY

The causes of mobility problems are complex. Unique and complementary etiologic perspectives can all contribute to a better understanding of mobility. Three perspectives are described here: epidemiological, biomechanical, and biomedical. Each has advantages and disadvantages for the clinician and the researcher.

Epidemiological Perspective: Risk Factors

Epidemiological risk factors for the onset of higher-level mobility disability include demographics, health behaviors, psychological factors, and diseases. Demographic factors associated with increased risk include advancing age, lower income, and lower educational level. Behavior-related risk factors include current smoking, alcohol abstention, low physical activity, high body mass index, and high waist circumference. Physical activity, a health behavior that is a key to mobility, is influenced by multiple psychological, social, and environmental factors. Common reasons given by older adults for limiting or avoiding physical activity include lack of an exercise companion, lack of interest, fatigue, fear of falling, weather, and safety. Self-reported conditions identified as major barriers to physical activity by older adults include arthritis and past injury. Psychological factors that influence mobility include negative attitudes toward aging, fear of falling, and poor emotional vitality. Self-reported conditions associated with increased risk of new higher-level mobility disability include baseline and incident heart attack and stroke, baseline hypertension, diabetes, angina, dyspnea, exertional leg pain and incident cancer, and hip fracture.

Biomechanical Perspective: Direct Assessment of the Body in Motion

Age affects the biomechanics of walking. Normal gait can be defined in terms of the gait cycle with two main phases: stance and swing (Figure 115-1). A normal cycle begins with a push off from the forefoot, then a swing through and heel strike, timed tightly to be followed by the push off of the other leg. Normal gait has highly characteristic patterns of foot, ankle, knee, hip, pelvis, trunk, and arm motion. Gait biomechanics can also be viewed from the perspective of the pattern of steps (footprints) (Figure 115-2). Step length is the forward distance between two foot falls. Stride length is the distance covered by one foot until it falls again. Stride length is, therefore, twice the step length, assuming the step lengths are the same on both sides. Step width is the lateral distance between two foot falls. With age, gait speed slows, step length decreases, and the proportion of the gait cycle when both feet are in contact with the ground (double support time) increases. During gait, older people compared to young adults tend to have more thoracic kyphosis, more anterior pelvic tilt, increased hip flexion, and greater external rotation of the foot. Older people tend to generate less power about the ankle

Right Lower Extremity (LE)	Heel strike	Stance	Toe off	Swing
Ankle Joint:	Neutral position (90°)	Neutral position (90°)	Plantar flexion for push off	Dorsiflexion for foot clearance
Muscles:	Ankle dorsiflexors active to support position of ankle	Plantar flexor torque drives foot into floor, ankle dorsiflexors eccentrically active to slow foot	Plantar flexors active	Dorsiflexors active
		Weight rolls from heel to toe		
Knee Joint:	Extended to prepare for weight bearing	Slight knee flexion (shock absorbing) progressing to full extension for stable weight bearing	Extension progressing to passive knee flexion to prepare for swing	Knee flexion for foot clearance progressing to passive extension for limb advancement
Muscles:	Initially, knee extensors (quadriceps) active then both quadriceps and hamstrings active for knee stabilization.	Quadriceps eccentrically active to decelerate knee flexion		Hamstrings and gastrocnemius active for knee flexion, relax for knee extension.
Hip Joint:	Hip flexed ~30°	Progressive hip extension	Hyperextension of the hip progressing to hip flexion	Hip flexing to advance limb
Muscles:	Hip extensors active for stability.	Hip extensors active initially. Hip abductors active to keep pelvis neutral.	Hip flexion initiated by hip adductors and hip flexors.	Hip adductors and flexors active for swing, hamstrings active to terminate swing.
Left LE*	Toe off	Swing	Heel strike	Stance
SUPPORT	Double support	Single support (right)	Double support	Single support (left)

*Note: When the right LE is at heel strike, the left LE is approaching toe off and vice versa. When the right LE is in stance the left LE is in swing and vice versa.

FIGURE 115-1. Human walking.

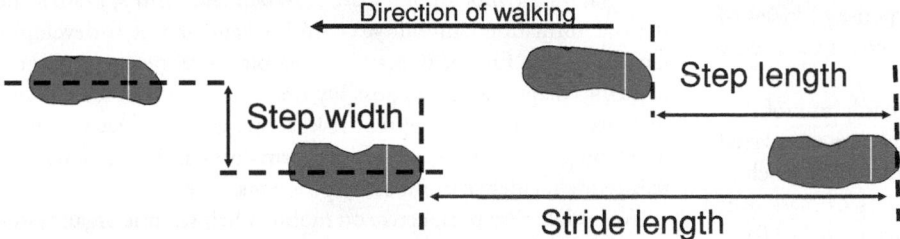

Step length = the distance between two consecutive footprints on opposite sides of the body.
Stride length = the distance between two consecutive footprints on the same side of the body.
Step width = the distance between the outer most borders of two consecutive footprints.

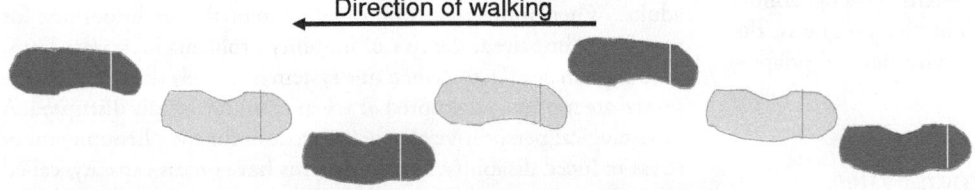

Dark (black) footprints represent foot placement during walking.
Quick clinical inspection for approximation of normal gait:
Step length = 1 step length between right and left steps (grey-dotted footprint).
Step width = 1 foot width (grey-dotted footprint) between right and left steps

FIGURE 115-2. Step patterns in human walking.

A. Usual gait: right and left step lengths approximately equal.

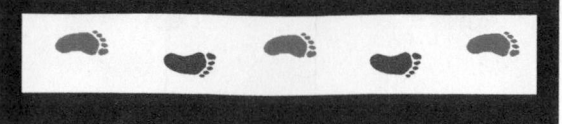

B. Asymmetric gait (limp): right step length consistently shorter than left step length. All left step lengths approximately equal and all right step length approximately equal.

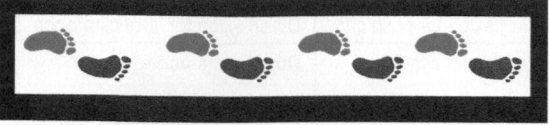

C. Variable gait: inconsistent right and left step lengths.

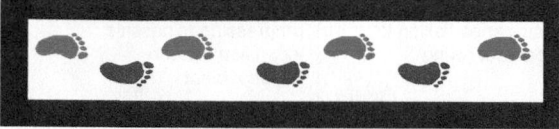

Red = left foot prints, Green = right foot prints

FIGURE 115-3. Gait patterns.

and use hip flexion to compensate more than young adults. Normal gait has a very regular spatial and temporal pattern. An irregular gait can be either regularly irregular, like a limp, or irregularly irregular, with no pattern at all (Figure 115-3). Irregularly irregular gait, often called gait variability, predicts falls and mobility disability.

Normal walking maximizes energy efficiency. When walking changes owing to biomechanical alterations caused by disease or aging, walking becomes more energy demanding. Normal walking also requires excellent control of balance and timing. When problems develop with balance and timing, the priority for safe walking may be to increase stability and support at the expense of losses of energy efficiency. Thus, many changes with aging increase the energy cost of walking and decrease gait efficiency.

A biomechanical perspective can be applied broadly to mobility and balance, based on the increasing biomechanical demand placed on the body in motion. Typically, tasks are considered more challenging as the base of support narrows and transfers of mass over the base become more demanding. Thus, difficulty increases from sitting to standing to walking, to climbing stairs, walking a line, or running. A biomechanical approach to postural alterations and body-segment movement abnormalities can be useful for identifying causes of, and solutions to, mobility problems. Specific abnormalities can be addressed by targeting rehabilitative programs, the type of assistive devices, or the design of environmental adaptations.

Physiological Perspective: Using Organ System Impairment to Link Function and Disease

The causes of mobility limitation can be assessed from a physiological perspective. There are three main physiological components of mobility. These components include balance control (neurological

system), force production (cardiopulmonary and muscular systems), and structural support (skeletal system—bone and joints). Ferrucci has created a framework that identifies six main physiological subsystems of the ability to walk: central nervous system, perceptual system, peripheral nervous system, muscles, bones and joints, and energy production. Another way of organizing the systems that affect walking is to consider inputs and outputs. In this approach, the physiological elements of mobility can be assigned to three main components based on a sequence of information from sensory inputs to central processing to effector factors that carry out instructions from the brain. Sensory inputs include vision, vestibular function, and peripheral sensation. Central processing includes level of consciousness, integration of sensory inputs, coordinated timing of multiple segmental body motions, and postural reflexes. Effector-related factors include endurance, pain, speed of reaction, and flexibility.

There are several important emerging areas of knowledge related to our understanding of the physiological contributors to walking. Brain abnormalities found on magnetic resonance imaging (MRI) are associated with alterations in central processing and abnormal gait. Small vessel cerebrovascular disease in the absence of stroke and MRI findings of "white matter disease" or focal grey matter atrophy are associated with slower gait speed, even among high-functioning older adults. These MRI findings predict the onset of mobility disability. Such brain abnormalities have been found to concurrently affect mobility, cognition, and mood and may suggest a shared underlying cerebrovascular process. Another emerging area of knowledge is related to subclinical losses of dopaminergic transmission in the brain in the aged. These losses of dopaminergic function also contribute to altered mobility and may present clinically in patterns that differ from traditional Parkinson disease. Dopamine deficiency in the aged may be related to cerebrovascular disease. Loss of oxygen-carrying capacity because of anemia has been recognized as a potential contributor to mobility limitations, especially in Caucasians, perhaps owing to decreased endurance but also possibly because of chronic subclinical ischemic effects on the brain. Research on the link among cardiovascular risk factors, brain structural abnormalities, mobility, cognition, and mood is developing rapidly. In the future, it may be possible to refine these observations into diagnosable and possibly treatable disorders. It is possible that attention to cardiovascular risk factors might reduce the risk of developing some of these brain abnormalities and thus potentially reduce the incidence of mobility problems.

A physiological perspective on mobility helps define organ system impairments, which can be linked to treatable diseases, conditions, and pathological processes, as described by the disablement process in Table 115-1. A physiological perspective is also helpful when accounting for the multiple interacting health problems of many older adults. When more than one organ system that is important for mobility is impaired, the risk of mobility problems increases. Thus, mobility can be affected when one system is severely disrupted, when several are modestly disrupted or when many are mildly disrupted. A physiological perspective also helps account for the phenomenon of stress-induced disability. Organ systems have excess capacity, called physiological reserve. Losses of organ system function can be clinically unapparent because these are losses of unused reserve or because one system is compensating for another. Many subclinical physiological losses may not be recognized until stress is placed on the system by further physiological decline or by an unexpected high demand on the system. When sufficient reserve is lost or a compensating organ system fails, mobility disability becomes overt. For example, when persons with many subclinical physiologic losses face an unexpected mobility demand, such as walking on ice at night, they may face a demand that is greater than their mobility capacity. Mobility reserve can now be assessed using recently developed tests. One way to challenge reserve is to perform simultaneous physical and cognitive tasks. Described as "dual tasks," older individuals may deteriorate significantly when asked to walk and talk or walk and perform a mental calculation. Mobility tests that incorporate obstacles also assess reserve. Tests of gait variability may be another way to detect subclinical change in mobility.

A physiological perspective can help define interventions, based on the disablement structure described in Table 115-1. Treatments could be aimed at managing the underlying pathological conditions that are causing the impairment (e.g., improving cardiac ejection fraction through treatment of congestive heart failure), treating the impairments themselves (e.g., strength training), or creating compensations and adaptations at the level of functional limitations (such as using a cane). A physiological approach offers a constructive way to connect biomechanical and clinical mobility assessment to a biomedical model of diagnosis and treatment.

Gait Speed as an Integrator of Multiple Approaches

Walking is the foundation of mobility, is influenced by biomechanical and physiological processes, and is a major driver of disability. Walking speed could be considered a "vital sign" in older adults. While there are several influences on measures of gait speed such as leg length, gender, or periods of acceleration and deceleration, in general gait speed can be interpreted clinically. Normal usual walking speed in the older adult should be at least 1 m/s. When measuring a fixed walk distance, this means that the time should be less than the distance in meters. For example, a 4-m walk speed should be less than 4 seconds. When measuring a fixed time, this means that the distance should be more than the time in seconds. For example, the distance walked in a 6-minute walk (360 seconds) should be more than 360 m. In a normal step frequency of walking (called the cadence), there are a little more than two steps per second or somewhat more than 120 steps per minute. With approximately two steps per second at a normal pace of 1 m/s, there is approximately m or 20 inches in a step. Clinically, this translates into approximately two shoes lengths per step, or an imaginary "shoe" in between each step (Figure 115-2).

As a general rule, there are links among walking speed, energy expenditure, and disability. Energy expenditure can be measured in metabolic equivalents (METs). One MET is the energy requirement for lying in bed. Two METs is twice the energy requirement for lying in bed and is approximately the energy requirement for self-care activities. The usual energy cost in METs of walking at various speeds has been reported in miles per hour, and walking speed can be translated directly between meters per second and miles per hour. Therefore, the energy requirements in METS and the expected activity level can be associated with gait speed, as described in Table 115-4. This conversion table allows clinicians and researchers to approximate the functional status of individuals or populations based on any measure of gait speed. Using METS as a basis for function, one might be able to define a sequence of mobility capacities, as described in Table 115-5.

TABLE 115-4

Translating Walking Speed: Walking Speed, METS, and Function

WALKING SPEED				
m/s	mph	6-min Walk Distance (m)	METS	FUNCTION
0.67	1.5	240	<2	Self-care
0.89	2.0	320	2.5	Household activities
1.0	2.2	360	2.7	
1.11	2.5	400	3.0	Carry groceries and light yard work
1.33	3.0	480	3.5	Climb several flights of stairs

EVALUATION

Strategy for the Clinical Encounter

There are no established standards for the overall evaluation and treatment of mobility problems in older adults. Currently, the best approach is similar to the ones used for other geriatric syndromes. These approaches are all based on a biopsychosocial model that incorporates biomedical, rehabilitative, and psychosocial elements and a multidisciplinary team. The initial goal of assessment is to classify the mobility problem into one of three large groups: nonambulatory, ambulatory, or vigorous. For the person who presents in a wheelchair or bed, one can screen for ability to stand or walk with assistance. For ambulatory individuals, a quick sorting strategy is to observe gait. Since most gait parameters are highly interrelated, abnormal gait can be grossly distinguished from normal by a few simple characteristics like use of a gait aid, gait speed less than 1 m/s (or step length less than twice foot length), or step asymmetry. Persons with

TABLE 115-5

Example of a Seven-Level Classification of Mobility Based on Energy Expenditure

Level 1	Able to perform sustained physical activity for at least 30 min at a vigorous pace like running, jogging, and tennis. Greater than 4 METs, sustained activity
Level 2	Able to perform sustained physical activity for at least 60 min at a usual pace like walking one or more miles. 3.5–4 METs, sustained activity
Level 3	Able to perform physical activity at a usual pace for at least 15 min like walking one-half mile. 2.5–3.5 METs, limited duration of activity
Level 4	Physical activity limited. Able to walk one block. May have slowed gait speed. May use an assistive device like a cane to walk. 2.0–2.5 METs
Level 5	Physical activity limited. May have difficulty walking one block but able to walk across a room. May use assistive device like a cane or a walker. <2 METs
Level 6	Mobility severely limited. Requires wheelchair for indoor mobility. Transfers independently. 1.5 METs
Level 7	Mobility profoundly limited; requires assistance with transfers from chair or bed. 1 MET

normal gait can be assessed for higher level fitness by use of one or more screening tests for higher level abilities such as single foot stand for 30 seconds, ability to tandem walk or ability to walk more than 450 to 500 m in 6 minutes. Persons with normal walking but inability to perform higher level tasks might be good candidates for exercise programs for well elders or for further evaluation if the mobility change is recent or causing problems. Further assessment of the non ambulatory or for those with abnormal gait depends in part on the treatment goals. The team can select a basic strategy; either to try to improve mobility or to compensate for irreversible mobility loss (Figure 115-4). This decision is based on the time course of the mobility loss, the potential to reverse impairments, the ability of the patient to participate in treatment, and preferences of the patient. For example, a person with severe cognitive deficits or severe irreversible motor paralysis might be considered more appropriate for compensation than for interventions to improve mobility. Planning for compensation might target mobility care needs and resources. For the person considered to have potential for improving mobility, the major decisions are the timing and value of interventions directly on mobility (usually through exercise and rehabilitation) and on underlying impairments (usually through medical team care). In some cases, it is clear that a person requires medical intervention first. For

example, in a person with poorly controlled congestive heart failure, medical treatment for symptom control probably needs to occur prior to rehabilitation. In other cases, it can be difficult to predict if intervention on multiple impairments should occur before or during rehabilitation efforts. For example in a person with depression, low vision and peripheral neuropathy, one could intervene with rehabilitation and exercise simultaneously with vision correction and antidepressants or one could try to correct the impairments first. This decision is based in part on whether the impairments are felt to create significant barriers to the success of rehabilitation. One could argue that in the absence of obvious barriers, a "trial" of rehabilitation should be started. Treatment can be initiated for impairments that cause barriers along the way. Alternatively, one could argue that it is more efficient to eliminate barriers prior to starting therapy. Since the time and effort of comprehensive mobility assessment and rehabilitation are both substantial, it is a challenge to determine where to apply efficiencies. Older adults with mobility problems often have numerous impairments identified as part of comprehensive assessment (see Chapter 11), some of which may be barriers and some may not. The process is likely to be inefficient, and like comprehensive geriatric assessment, hard to use in routine clinical practice. To the extent that there are "high payoff" areas based on prevalence

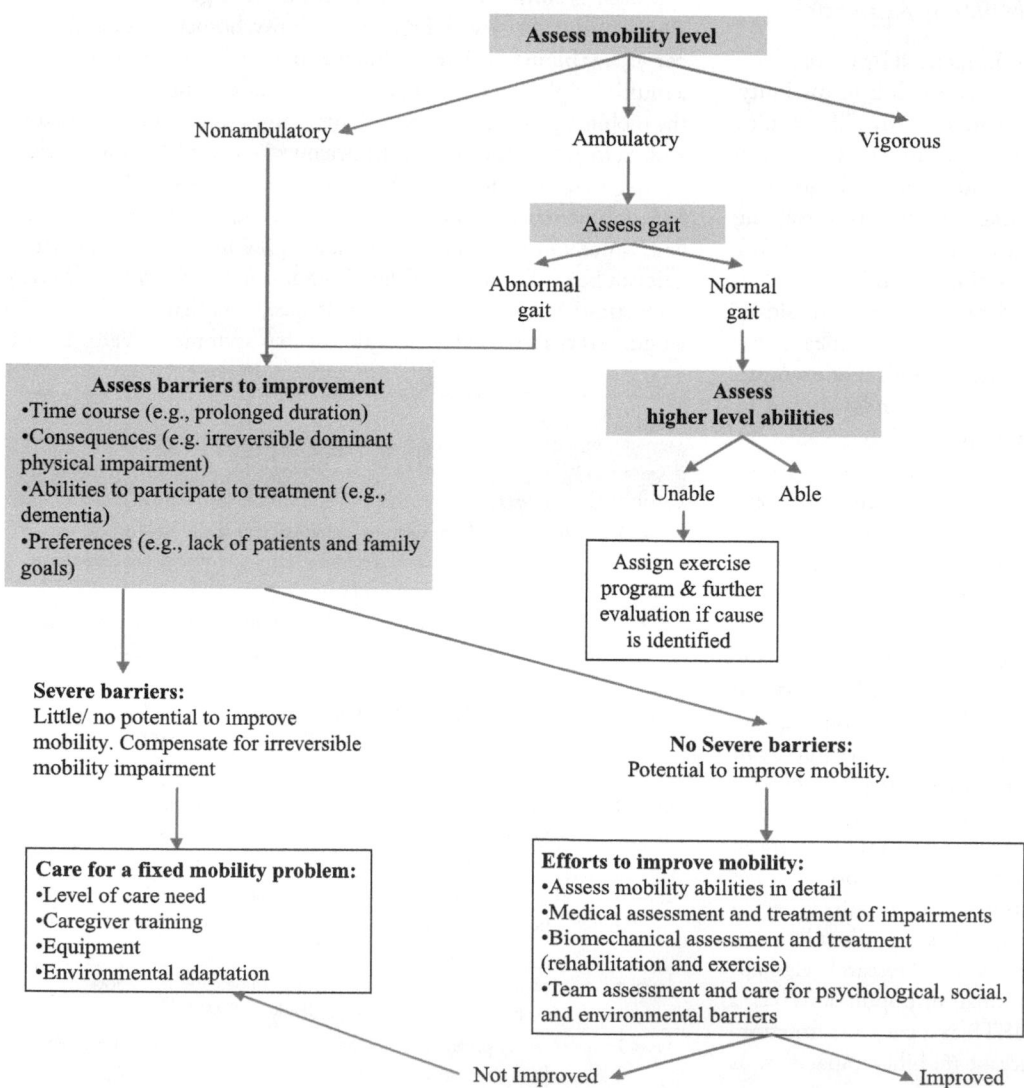

FIGURE 115-4. A clinical strategy for assessment and management of mobility problems.

TABLE 115-6

Brief Evaluation of Mobility Problems for Use in Primary Care

SYSTEM	SYMPTOMS LIMITING WALKING	CLINICAL FINDINGS
Cardiopulmonary (lung, heart, and blood)	Dyspnea and fatigue	FEV1, O_2 saturation with activity, hemoglobin, and ejection fraction
Neurological (frontal, motor, extrapyramidal, and peripheral)	Unsteady and hesitant	Tone, timed tapping, executive cognitive function, and peripheral sensation
Musculoskeletal (bones and joints, muscles)	Pain and stiffness	Knee, hip, low back range of motion, and pain. Manual muscle tests and chair rise

osteoarthritis, or dyspnea caused by congestive heart failure. When the cause of the mobility problem is less obvious, a referral to multidisciplinary team for comprehensive mobility assessment can be considered. Since the potential causes range across many organ systems, this strategy might be more efficient than referral to several organ system based specialists. Since research into mobility problems is an active and high priority area in aging, in the future, efficient clinical practice and referral may be better informed by evidence.

The comprehensive approach to the clinical assessment of treatable causes of mobility is currently a specialized referral function that is resource intensive. Evaluation starts with the clinical assessment of the severity, course and consequences of mobility limitation, and the determination of potential to improve mobility. Mobility performance is assessed in more detail, including biomechanical aspects of functional limitations during movement. Potential contributing factors are identified based on physiological impairments, and evidence is sought for psychosocial and environmental influences.

or responsiveness to intervention, it may be possible to prioritize and streamline the process. In primary care, the provider can offer a screening and triage function by recognizing mobility disorders and assessing potential for intervention. Table 115-6 gives examples of a quick system of assessment for symptoms and clinical findings based on the three main involved organ systems. The primary provider can identify and treat overt clinical impairments that can be detected quickly in the clinic, like weight-bearing pain caused by

Clinical Assessment of Mobility Performance

In ambulatory patients, simple assessment of gait speed is a useful place to start. The gait speed can be used to estimate function as described above. Gait can be assessed in more detail from a biomechanical perspective (Table 115-7). Gait can be examined for general characteristics like path deviations, irregular or variable stepping, or a widened base of support and for altered motion of the component parts: trunk, arms, hip, knee, ankle, and foot. Mobility tasks can be examined for performance difficulty or altered movement patterns

TABLE 115-7

Examples of a Biomechanical Assessment of Common Gait Abnormalities and Possible Causes

GAIT ELEMENT	GAIT ABNORMALITY	POSSIBLE CAUSES
Body segments		
Ankle and foot	Forefoot strikes floor simultaneously with initial heel contact (foot slap)	Weak ankle dorsiflexors and decreased proprioception
	Initial contact is by forefoot	Leg length discrepancy, plantar flexion contracture, and painful heel
	Heel and toe leave floor together during push off	Fixed ankle, weak plantar flexors, and painful forefoot
	Forefoot drags during swing (foot drop)	Weak ankle dorsiflexors
	Tendency to roll from plantar to medial surface of the foot while walking	Weak lateral ankle stabilizers and varus knee deformity
Knee	Knee flexed at initial contact	Painful knee, weak knee extensors, leg length discrepancy, and knee flexion contracture
	Decreased knee extension during swing	Knee pain or decreased range
	Hyperextension of the knee in stance	Weak knee extensors
Hip	Decreased hip flexion at initial contact	Weak hip flexors and decreased range of motion
	Increased hip flexion during swing (steppage gait)	Compensation for foot drop
	Decreased hip extension during late stance	Hip flexion contracture
	Hip circumduction with lateral movement of entire limb	Weak hip flexors and inability to flex leg
	Pelvis drops on one side, lateral instability when walking	Contralateral hip abductor or gluteus weakness
	Excessive elevation of the ipsilateral side of the pelvis during swing (hip/pelvic hiking)	Inadequate hip or knee flexion or excessive plantar flexion
Gait pattern		
Gait initiation	Hesitation	Parkinson disease, frontal lobe disorders, and normal pressure hydrocephalus
Stance width	Increased	Cerebellar disorders and peripheral neuropathy
Path	Weaving	Vestibular disorders
	Scissoring (steps cross over laterally)	CNS disorders
	Increased variability	CNS disorders (e.g., white matter hyperdensities and lacunar infarcts)

as task demands increase. Sometimes, the finding of an abnormal body-segment movement or gait characteristic suggests a specific impairment or disease. More often, the abnormality is nonspecific but is amenable to direct intervention in rehabilitation.

Clinical gait assessment tools that include many of these biomechanical elements include the Performance Oriented Mobility Assessment and the Gait Abnormality Rating Scale. A tool for analyzing the elements of bed mobility from the perspective of body segments has been proposed. Mobility and balance assessments can be based on a hierarchy of task difficulty. The Berg balance scale assesses 14 tasks of progressive difficulty from sitting balance to one leg standing and rising onto a step. Some scales have been designed to discriminate mobility capacity among the nonambulatory. The Hierarchical Assessment of Balance and Mobility assesses mobility, transfers, and balance and detects multiple levels within the bed and chair fast. The Physical Disability Index has eight mobility tasks including six items for nonambulatory persons. Mobility task scales usually have a functional rather than a biomedical perspective and are not designed to detect specific impairments. These scales can be used to identify areas for task practice or adaptation in rehabilitation and to assess the effects of treatment.

Differential Diagnosis Based on a Physiological Perspective

A clinical schema for the comprehensive evaluation of mobility that is derived from Ferrucci, Tinetti, and the author's own work is proposed in Table 115-8. Many impairments are detectable through the usual geriatric clinical history and physical examination. Some sensory systems are amenable to clinical evaluation. Vision can be assessed for acuity by Snellen chart, and fields by confrontation, dark adaptation by history, and depth perception can be assessed with a low-cost portable device resembling a shoe box with two pointers attached to cords. Peripheral sensation can be assessed by proprioception, vibratory threshold, and filaments. Vestibular function is difficult to test clinically, and many people with vestibular disease do not demonstrate vertigo or nystagmus. Tests of visual stabilization during head motion are in development and may become clinically useful. Some central systems can be assessed clinically. Perfusion can be assessed by history of orthostatic symptoms or presyncope and by direct assessment of orthostatic blood pressure change. Reaction time can be assessed by timed finger and foot tapping or grossly by observation of rapid alternating movements. Frontal lobe function can be assessed using the trail making B test or a dual task like walking and saying the days of the week in reverse order. Postural responses can be assessed by a test of the righting reflex. This test can be performed as a sternal nudge or rapid pull on the pelvic rim, with the goal to displace the center of mass sufficiently to require a displacement of the base of support, which generates a need to take a step. A normal response is a single brisk step backward. A grossly abnormal response is the "timber reaction" in which no lower extremity movement occurs. An equivocal response is several small steps. Since older adults can unexpectedly lack righting reflexes, it is essential to be positioned to catch the individual during this test. Absent righting reflexes are often found in Parkinson disease. Absent or decreased righting reflexes can also be found in other poorly defined central nervous system conditions. Poor trunk control, dysmetria, and a wide base of support in standing are seen in cerebellar disorders. Musculoskeletal and neurologic effector factors that can be assessed in the clinic include simple assessments of strength by manual muscle testing and by maneuvers that require the individual to move their own body mass, like chair rise, standing on the toes (with hands on examination table for stability), and squatting. Focal or asymmetric weakness may be caused by central, spinal cord, or peripheral nerve disorders. Flexibility can be assessed by range of motion. Flexibility in the neck and spine, as well as in the lower extremities, affects mobility. Weight-bearing pain and pain in the chest, back, or legs during motion or exertion can be assessed by history and maneuvers that reproduce the symptoms. Endurance can be assessed, in part, by history and examination of the heart, peripheral circulation, and lungs. A 6-minute walk test in the clinic might be feasible during comprehensive assessment.

Some impairments are hard to detect in the clinic and require further testing. Vestibular testing may be helpful when there is unsteadiness that is not well explained by other impairments or when specific vestibular symptoms are present. Electrodiagnostic testing of nerve conduction velocity or abnormal muscle activity may be indicated when neurological findings are suspicious. Exertional chest pain or dyspnea requires appropriate cardiac and pulmonary testing and a screen for anemia. Leg pain on exertion suggests testing for peripheral vascular disease or lumbar stenosis.

Psychosocial and Environmental Assessment

Mobility limitations are influenced by psychological, social, and environmental factors (Table 115-9). Depression can have a powerful effect on the desire to be mobile. Fear of falling, lack of confidence, and low self-efficacy can also adversely influence a person's mobility. Screens for these conditions can include a single question or multiple questions (Table 115-3) and should be part of a comprehensive mobility assessment. Apathy and lack of motivation are a common concern in geriatric rehabilitation. Formal and informal social support resources can be critical for the person with mobility limitations. Cultural and financial factors can influence attitudes toward disability and resources for addressing the problem. The safety and accessibility of the living environment can be a barrier or facilitator for persons with mobility problems. A home visit for assessment can offer many opportunities for creative problem solving.

MANAGEMENT

Intervening Directly on Mobility

Interventions directed at functional limitations are often rehabilitative in nature and involve exercise, adaptive equipment, and environmental modifications. Mobility limitations can be addressed through mobility task practice and exercise to improve specific impairments in strength, balance, endurance, and/or flexibility. Since deconditioning is almost always present as a direct consequence of reduced mobility and inactivity, and deconditioning has been found to be treatable in many older adults who are sick or frail, general conditioning programs of exercise are frequently indicated. Assistive and orthotic devices can improve stability and reduce weight-bearing pain. The evidence for the effectiveness of rehabilitation and exercise interventions is growing and has been examined in older adults with varying levels of mobility limitations. Chapter 29 on rehabilitation and Chapter 114 on exercise present these interventions in more detail.

TABLE 115-8

Assessment and Treatment of Organ or System Impairments That Cause Mobility Problems

Functional Domain	Organ System	Impairment	Assessment	Related Causes	Treatment
Sensory	Eye	Acuity	Near and far by Snellen chart	Presbyopia and cataracts	Lenses and surgery
	Eye	Peripheral vision	Confrontation	Glaucoma and stroke	Prisms
	Eye	Depth	Depth testing	Monocular	Lighting, contrast, and avoid multifocal lens while walking
	Eye	Dark adaptation	Self-report	Miotic agents for glaucoma	Change medications and lighting
	Vestibular	Otoliths	Ability to perceive vertical	Benign positional vertigo	Eppley maneuver and vestibular rehabilitation
	Vestibular	Semicircular canals	Ability to perceive rotation and acceleration	Meniere's disease	Medications and vestibular rehabilitation
	Peripheral nerve	Neuropathy	Filaments and vibratory sense	Diabetes and peripheral vascular disease	Haptic enhancement (see text) and footwear
Central	Circulation	Decreased brain perfusion	Hypotension and orthostasis	Medications, arrythmias, postprandial hypotension, and dehydration	Change medications, antiarrythmics, or pacemaker; increase fluid intake
	Brain	Motor processing	Level of consciousness, digit symbol substitution test, and trail making B test	Medications and CNS disorders (white matter hyperdensities, focal atrophy, and brain infarcts)	Change medication and blood pressure control
	Brain	Postural reflexes	Righting reflexes	Parkinson disease and other CNS disorders diseases	Trial of anti-Parkinson medications
Effector	Muscle	Strength	Manual muscle tests and strength-based motions (chair rise and squat)	Multiple neurological conditions and inactivity	Exercise, bracing, and medication adjustment
	Musculoskeletal	Flexibility	Contractures and range of motion (ROM)	Injury, arthritis, and inactivity	Active and passive ROM and orthotics
	Heart endurance	Cardiomyopathy	Dyspnea at rest or on exertion, fluid retention, and echocardiogram	Systolic or diastolic dysfunction	Standard care for systolic and diastolic dysfunction
	Lung endurance	Hypoxia or reduced air flow	Dyspnea rest or on exertion, hypoxia, and decreased peak flow	COPD, asthma, and other lung	Standard pulmonary care and oxygen
	Circulation endurance	Peripheral vasculature	Leg pain on exertion, decreased pulses, and bruits	Arteriosclerosis and venous insufficiency	Medical and surgical, and exercise
	Hematologic endurance	Anemia	Dyspnea or fatigue on exertion	Multiple causes	Treat based on cause and transfusion for severe
	Muscle endurance	Sarcopenia	Leg fatigue on exertion	Inactivity	Exercise and possibly trophic agents in the future
	Musculoskeletal pain	Bone and joint deficits	Weight-bearing pain	Osteoarthritis, osteoporotic fractures, periarticular conditions, and foot problems	Pain medications, injections, assistive devices, and orthoses
	Neurological pain	Spinal cord, roots, and nerves	Leg and back pain with activity	Spinal stenosis, radiculopathies, peripheral neuropathies, and CNS disorders	Injections, surgery, and medications

TABLE 115-9

Psychosocial and Environmental Assessment and Management of Mobility

Area	Type	Assessment	Management
Psychological	Depression	Standard screen (see Chapter 70)	Antidepressants and counseling
	Self-efficacy	Interview	Counseling
	Apathy	Interview and observation	Stimulants and social therapies
Social	Emotional and instrumental supports	Interview	Community programs and family engagement
	Culture	Interview	Cultural consultation
	Finances	Interview	Community resources
Environment	Physical barriers	Home visit	Environmental adaptations
	Access	Interview and home visit	Community programs

Treating Impairments

Some impairments can be linked to diseases and pathological processes that are amenable to treatment, and some impairments can be improved directly regardless of pathological cause (Table 115-8). Visual function for mobility can be modified by optimizing visual acuity with prescription glasses, by use of special prisms in the glasses (lenses that expand the visual field), and by making the best use of environmental lighting. Some vestibular disorders are amenable to rehabilitation through special head and eye exercises. Peripheral sensory disorders are often not correctable, but compensation can be achieved through the use of lighting to improve visual information and use of a cane to enhance haptic perception. Haptic perception is demonstrated by the remarkable decrease in sway with eyes closed, seen in persons with peripheral sensory or vestibular disorders, when they are allowed even minimal, nonsupporting contact with a stable surface such as a table or wall. Haptic sensation implies that another sensory input source can be used by the brain to provide information about body position when information from the feet is lost. When a cane is used to promote haptic sensation, it is providing information to the hand about body position and is not used as a weight-bearing device. Shoe inserts that increase sensory feedback are in development. Interventions for orthostatic hypotension include medication adjustment, compression stockings, and, in some cases, salt loading or medication such as fludorcortisone or midrinone. Treatment of arrhythmias, especially significant tachy- and bradyarrhythmias, when selected judiciously, might reduce dizziness and improve mobility. Delayed movement speed can be reduced if medications that exacerbate the problem are removed. The slowed gait of Parkinson disease can be responsive to medication although the balance disorder is not. Parkinson patients may move faster and thus increase their risk of fall injury when medications are initiated. Cardiac, pulmonary, and anemia-related symptoms that limit endurance may be managed medically. Strength and endurance are amenable to exercise training. Pain may be managed using medications, injections, orthotics, exercise, and sometime surgery.

Attention to Factors that Modify Behavior and Environment

The modifiable psychosocial factors that influence physical activity may offer opportunities to intervene (Table 115-9). Depression can be managed medically or with psychotherapy. In post acute care settings, methylphenidate has been used short term to treat apathy. Social support and encouragement can be promoted through group activities. Physical environmental adaptations in the home include ramps and railings, bathroom modifications, proper lighting, and strategic placement of stable furniture items. Further modifications are often indicated in institutional settings.

Care for the Immobile Person

Interventions to reduce the consequences of immobility include determining the level of care need and living setting, training others to properly position and move the patient, implementing a mobilization plan, use of pressure-reducing devices to prevent pressure ulcer, and, sometimes, using equipment to aid in transfers (see Chapter 58). Persons who are responsible for carrying out transfers of immobile patients, including health aides and family caregivers, need training in proper techniques that reduce injury to the patient and the assistant. Absolute bed rest is almost never indicated and should be discouraged in all settings. Mobilization, including walking, has been shown to be feasible even in the intensive care setting. An exception to routine mobilization might be for humanitarian reasons when an individual is actively dying, where routine mobilization might cause suffering without associated benefit. Mobilization rather than bed rest during hospitalization for acute illness has been one of the most consistent interventions in Acute Care of the Elderly units.

SUMMARY

Mobility disorders are widespread in older adults. Mobility limitations constrain many functions required for independent living and are powerful indicators of future problems. Mobility can be classified using simple screen. Evaluation starts with a triage function or simple measures like gait speed. Many common contributors to mobility limitations can be managed in the primary-care setting. A comprehensive mobility evaluation is resource intensive and requires a multidisciplinary team. Evaluation and management include a biomechanical approach to function, a biomedical approach to the physiological components of mobility, and a psychosocial and environmental approach to modifying factors.

FURTHER READING

Cesari M, Kritchevsky SB, Penninx BW, et al. Prognostic value of usual gait speed in well-functioning older people–results from the Health, Aging and Body Composition Study. *J Am Geriatr Soc.* 2005;53:1675.

Cham R, Perera S, Studenski SA, et al. Striatal dopamine denervation and sensory integration for balance in middle-aged and older adults. *Gait Posture.* 2007 Oct;26(4):516–525.

Creditor MC. Hazards of hospitalization of the elderly. *Ann Intern Med.* 1993;118:219.

Ferrucci L, Bandinelli S, Benvenuti E, et al. Subsystems contributing to the decline in ability to walk: bridging the gap between epidemiology and geriatric practice in the InCHIANTI study. *J Am Geriatr Soc.* 2000;48:1618.

Fried LP, Bandeen-Roche K, Chaves PHM, et al. Preclinical mobility disability predicts incident mobility disability in older women. *J Gerontol Med Sci.* 2000;55A:M43.

Gerety M, Mulrow C, Tuley MR. Development and validation of a physical performance instrument for the functionally impaired elderly: the physical disability index (PDI). *J Gerontol Med Sci.* 1993;48:M33.

Gill TM, Williams CS, Tinetti ME. Assessing risk for the onset of functional dependence among older adults: the role of physical performance. *J Am Geriatr Soc.* 1995;43:603.

Guallar-Castillon P, Sagardui-Villamor J, Banegas JR, et al. Waist circumference as a predictor of disability among older adults. *Obesity.* 2007;15:233.

Guralnik JM, Ferrucci L, Simonsick EM, et al. Lower-extremity function in persons over the age of 70 years as a predictor of subsequent disability. *N Engl J Med.* 1995;332:556.

Hausdorff JM. Gait variability: methods, modeling and meaning. *J Neuroeng Rehabil.* 2005;2:19.

Hoenig H, Ganesh SP, Taylor DH, et al. Lower extremity physical performance and use of compensatory strategies for mobility. *J Am Geriatr Soc.* 2006;54:262.

Jorstad EC, Hauer K, Becker C, et al.; on behalf of the ProFaNE Group. Measuring the psychological outcomes of falling: a systematic review. *J Am Geriatr Soc.* 2005;53:501.

Milbrandt EB. One small step for man. *Crit Care Med.* 2007;35:311.

Patel KV, Harris TB, Faulhaber M, et al. Racial variation in the relationship of anemia with mortality and mobility disability among older adults. *Blood.* 2007 Jun 1;109(11):4663–4670.

Penninx BWJH, Ferrucci L, Leveille SG, et al. Lower extremity performance in nondisabled older persons as a predictor of subsequent hospitalization. *J Gerontol Med Sci.* 2000;55:M691.

Penninx BWJH, Guralnik JM, Bandeen-Roche K, et al. The protective effect of emotional vitality on adverse health outcomes in disabled older women. *J Am Geriatr Soc.* 2000;48:1359.

Perera S, Mody SH, Woodman RC, et al. Meaningful change and responsiveness in common physical performance measures in older adults. *J Am Geriatr Soc.* 2006;54:743.

Podsiadlo D, Richardson S. The timed "up and go": a test of basic functional mobility for frail older persons. *J Am Geriatr Soc.* 1991;39:142.

Priplata AA, Niemi JB, Harry JD, et al. Vibrating insoles and balance control in elderly people. *Lancet.* 2003;362:1123.

Rantanen T, Guralnik JM, Ferrucci L, et al. Co impairments as predictors of severe walking disability in older women. *J Am Geriatr Soc.* 2001;49:21.

Rosano C, Brach J, Longstreth WT Jr, et al. Quantitative measures of gait characteristics indicate prevalence of underlying subclinical structural brain abnormalities in high-functioning older adults. *Neuroepidemiology.* 2006;26:52.

Satariano WA, Haight TJ, Tager IB. Reasons given by older people for limitations or avoidance of leisure time physical activity. *J Am Geriatr Soc.* 2000;48:503.

Simonsick EM, Newman AB, Nevitt MC, et al. Measuring higher level physical function in well-functioning older adults: expanding familiar approaches in the health ABC study. *J Gerontol Med Sci.* 2001;56A:M644.

Tinetti ME. Performance-oriented assessment of mobility problems in elderly patients. *J Am Geriatr Soc.* 1986;34:119.

Tinetti ME, Inouye SK, Gill TM, et al. Shared risk factors for falls, incontinence and functional dependence. *JAMA.* 1995;273:1348.

Verghese J, Wang C, Holtzer R, et al. Quantitative gait dysfunction and risk of cognitive decline and dementia. *J Neurol Neurosurg Psychiatry.* 2007 Sep;78(9):929–935.

West SK, Munoz B, Rubin GS, et al. Compensatory strategy use identifies risk of incident disability for the visually impaired. *Arch Ophthalmol.* 2005;123:1242.

Wolfson L, Whipple R, Amerman P, et al. Gait assessment in the elderly: a gait abnormality rating scale and its relation to falls. *J Gerontol Med Sci.* 1990;45:M12.

Woollacott M, Shumway-Cook A. Attention and the control of posture and gait: a review of an emerging area of research. *Gait Posture.* 2002;16:1.

Osteoarthritis

Shari M. Ling ■ *Yvette L. Ju*

INTRODUCTION

Osteoarthritis (OA) is defined as boney inflammation of a joint or joints. OA is the most common form of arthritis in the United States and Europe. Given the prolonged life expectancy in the United States and the aging of the "baby boomer" cohort, the prevalence of OA is expected to increase further. Although the precise cause of OA is unknown, it is likely that multiple causes and many factors influence disease expression.

EPIDEMIOLOGY, CAUSES, AND PREDISPOSING FACTORS

Epidemiological and observational studies provide important clues to the mechanisms by which OA develops and progresses and, thus, identify risk factors that might comprise intervention targets for OA prevention and management.

Age and Gender

Advanced age is the strongest risk factor for the development of OA across all anatomical sites. Prevalence rates for both radiographic OA and, to a lesser extent, symptomatic OA (moderate or severe) increase with age, with a steep rise after the age of 50 years in men and age of 40 years in women. Radiographic OA of the hand is the most prevalent form, followed by knee, then hip. It is not unusual to find incidental radiographic OA in an otherwise asymptomatic older patient. Symptomatic OA of the knee and hip OA are the most prevalent in both sexes, with symptomatic involvement of the hands increasing in women beginning at menopause.

Changes in the hormonal milieu are thought to contribute to OA pathogenesis and are supported by reports of reduced risk of incident hip OA in women receiving hormonal therapy. However, estrogen/progestin replacement has not been proven to reduce the chance of developing knee pain or disability in women with knee symptoms. Whether estrogen or hormonal therapy is beneficial with regard to OA thus remains controversial and further emphasizes that OA symptom and disease pathogenesis likely develop through different mechanisms.

Joint Trauma and Nontraumatic Biomechanical Factors

Joint trauma of a severity that causes swelling and discomfort lasting several days or longer has been shown to increase risk of knee OA. Prior surgical removal of a meniscus in the knee is also a predisposing factor to OA of the knee. Meniscectomy is associated with a sixfold increase in risk for development of radiographic OA, even if limited rather than total meniscal resection is employed. Obesity, female sex, and preexisting early-stage OA of the knee and concurrent hand OA compound the risks incurred following meniscectomy. Occupation- and sports-related *repetitive injury* and physical trauma contribute to the development of OA of specific joints (e.g., knees in soccer players, elbows of baseball pitchers, and upper limbs of air hammer operators) and account for occurrence at sites not usually affected by OA. Although the prevalence of knee OA is greater in adults who have engaged in occupations that require repetitive bending and strenuous activities, an association with intense exercise or recreational physical activity such as jogging has not been proven. *Joint malalignment* and *varus–valgus laxity* increase the risk of developing OA. Malalignment of the knee appears to explain some of the risk of knee OA progression attributable to obesity. Altered alignment, as in the case of acetabular dysplasia, may also increase risk of hip OA. Although laxity and malalignment may coexist, laxity independently increases risk of OA.

Obesity

Obesity and excess weight comprise an important risk factor for the development and progression of knee, hip, and even hand OA. It is estimated that persons in the highest quintile of body weight have up to 10 times the risk of knee OA than those in the lowest quintile.

Although mechanical factors are assumed to explain the increased risk of knee and hip OA associated with excess weight and obesity, the association with hand OA with weight raises the possibility of alternative mechanisms.

Muscle Strength

Weakness of the knee extensor muscles appears to be both a consequence and a risk factor for the development of knee and hand OA. However, muscle strengthening has not been proven to protect individuals from progression of OA. In fact, higher strength has been associated with greater risk of progression in malaligned knees, and also of proximal interphalangeal and carpal–metacarpal joint OA in men and metacarpophalangeal joint OA in men and women.

CLASSIFICATION AND PATHOPHYSIOLOGY

Classification

The term "primary OA" is used to denote idiopathic OA in contrast to "secondary OA" that results from damage induced by another process (gout, rheumatoid arthritis, and bacterial). Although OA can involve any joint, it is most prevalent in the fingers and thumb base of the hands, knees, hips, and also spine. The classification system developed by the American College of Rheumatology (Table 116-1) integrates patient age, radiographic features, clinical symptoms, and physical abnormalities of the hands, knees, and/or hips. Such classification systems define phenotypes of clinical presentation that may lend clarity to the development of specific treatment modalities in the future. OA that is radiographically apparent but not associated with clinical features specified in the ACR criteria is referred to as "radiographic OA."

Pathophysiology

Cartilage degeneration is the hallmark of this disease, with fibrillation and ulceration that begins superficially and eventually extends into deeper layers. In addition, subchondral bone abnormalities and focal synovial inflammation can also be observed. These pathological characteristics are thought to arise owing to disruption of the balance between degradative and repair processes necessary to maintain joint health. Inflammatory cytokines, matrix degrading metallopro-

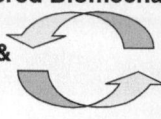

FIGURE 116-1. The process by which aging is theorized to increase risk of OA is depicted. Some of the mechanisms and mediators demonstrated in cellular and system aging are relevant to cartilage and periarticular structures. These changes may predispose the aging individual to altered biomechanics that increase risk of joint injury to which repair is attempted but eventually fails.

teinase enzymes, and chondrocyte apoptosis are likely contributors to this process. Osteophytes develop later and are thought to represent attempted repair. The process by which aging is theorized to increase risk of OA is depicted in Figure 116-1.

PRESENTATION

Symptoms

The most common initial symptom of OA is stiffness, which is most noticeable on awakening in the morning and after periods of inactivity. These symptoms are usually temporary and rarely persist for more than 30 minutes. As the disease progresses, patients experience pain with activity, which resolves on resting the joint. With further progression, patients report pain at rest and that awakens them from sleep. Validated questionnaires assessing the severity of painful symptoms referent to specific activities such as walking, stair climbing, and grasping are available and may prove useful in clinical settings, although these are primarily used in research studies of OA. Similarly, measures assessing the intensity and duration of stiffness may also prove useful—particularly in monitoring treatment

TABLE 116-1

Criteria for the Diagnosis of Osteoarthritis of the Hand, Knee, and Hip		
HAND	**KNEE**	**HIP**
Hand pain, aching, or stiffness	Knee pain	Hip pain
and	and	and
Hard tissue enlargement of two or more joints	Radiographic osteophytes	Two or more of the following:
and	and	*ESR <10 mm/h
Fewer than three swollen MCP joints	One or more of the following:	Radiographic femoral or acetabular osteophytes
and	Age ≥50 yr	Radiographic joint space narrowing
Two or more DIP joints with hard tissue enlargement	Morning stiffness <30 min	
or	Crepitus on motion	
Deformity in two or more select joints[†]		

*ESR, erythrocyte sedimentation rate.
[†]Select joints = DIP, PIP, and first CMC.

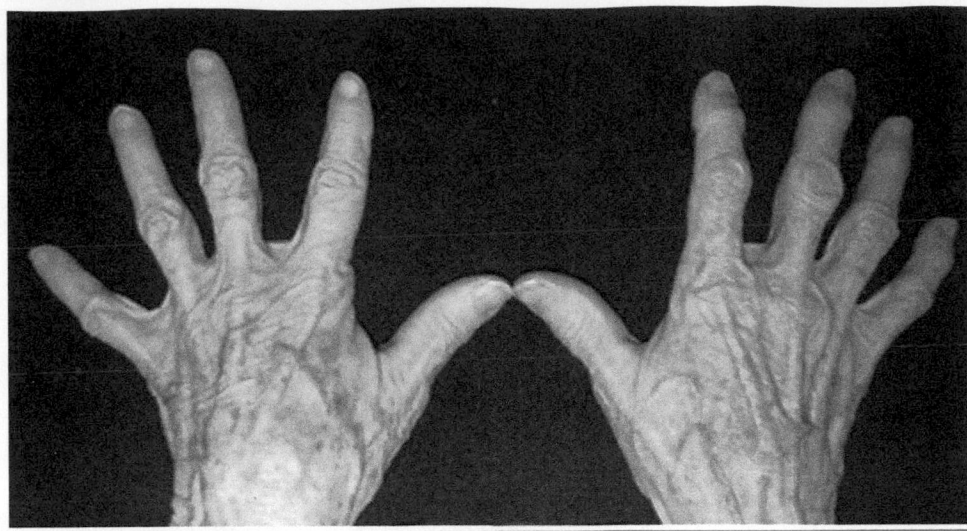

FIGURE 116-2. The features of bony prominence and deformity typical of hand OA are depicted here with Heberden's nodes of the distal and Bouchard's of the proximal interphalangeal joints of the fingers.

response. A history of systemic symptoms such as unintentional weight loss, excessive fatigue, and prolonged morning stiffness that extends beyond an hour suggests an "inflammatory" condition such as polymyalgia rheumatica or rheumatoid arthritis, rather than OA.

Physical Abnormalities

Physical examination of a joint with early OA may be completely normal. Subtle prominence of the finger joints and effusion of the knee may be present early. Joint tenderness, warmth, and painful motion may be present. Crepitus may be appreciated by palpating the joint during movement. Bony prominence develop later and are exemplified by Heberden's nodes of the distal and Bouchard's of the proximal interphalangeal joints of the fingers (Figure 116-2) (Color Plate 24). These are firm and bony on palpation, in distinction from more inflammatory etiologies that are boggy to palpation. As joint destruction ensues, crepitus and bony prominence become appreciable. Joint laxity or unexpected mobility may be observed on passive joint movement and may suggest incompetence of the supporting ligaments. As the disease progresses, joints may become malaligned and deformed. An example of this is knee deformity that is either

varus (knees pointing outward beyond the femoral–tibial line) or valgus (knees pointing inward). Joint motion becomes limited as the disease progresses. Disease severity may be manifested as OA involvement of multiple joints as well as the spine. In these cases, careful examination of each joint is required to ascertain the source of painful symptoms. For example, "hip pain" may arise from OA of the hip, but also may be pain referred from the knee or spine. Similarly, OA of the neck may manifest as shoulder pain. Accurate localization of the source of painful symptoms is required for effective management.

EVALUATION

Diagnostic Imaging

Conventional radiography remains the imaging modality of clinical choice to confirm a diagnosis of OA by the presence of osteophytes, as shown in Figure 116-3. Additional information obtainable from X-ray images includes joint space width and alignment, calcification of cartilage or periarticular structures, and soft-tissue swelling, bony

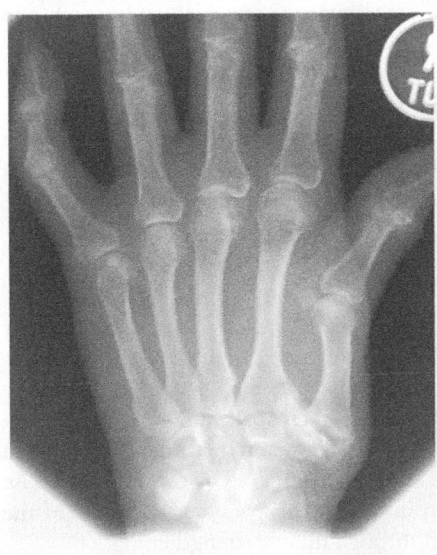

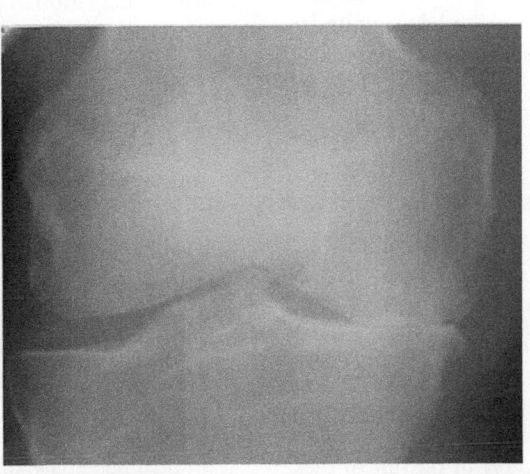

FIGURE 116-3. The radiographic characteristics of osteoarthritis shown in this knee X-ray include osteophytes at the joint margin, asymmetric joint space narrowing, subchondral sclerosis, and cysts. These features can be observed most commonly in the hands (A), knees (B), or hips.

A   **B**

defects (osteomas), and osteopenia and fracture. Scoring schema have been developed and used to assess disease severity as well as confirm disease presence. However, conventional radiographs have limited resolution and are, therefore, not capable of detecting early disease. Additionally, certain views are required to allow measurement of change in specific features (e.g., joint space width and osteophyte size) over time. Although X-rays can be useful in excluding conditions such as fracture and tumor, these can also be misleading because of the high prevalence of incidental radiographic abnormalities in older adults, as discussed further below. Therefore, X-ray abnormalities should be interpreted in the context of clinical history and physical findings or risk, mistakenly attributing symptoms from other illnesses (infection, aneurysm, etc.) to OA.

Magnetic Resonance Imaging

Magnetic resonance imaging (MRI) offers promise for earlier detection of OA, since focal defects in cartilage can be identified in painful knees that are still radiographically normal. Furthermore, MRI has contributed to our understanding that OA involves a variety of characteristics (e.g., osteophytes, cartilage defects, and bony abnormalities), which often occur together in one or several regions within a joint in a manner that is highly correlated with persistent painful symptoms, and has led the field to appreciate that OA is not a disease that is limited to cartilage. Moreover, changes in cartilage, bone, and synovium often occur together. MRI also allows visualization of structures important to functional stability of the joint (e.g., ligament and meniscus) and should be obtained to evaluate mechanical symptoms of locking or giveway weakness in knees, instability of the hip, and impingement symptoms of the shoulder. However, clinical discretion is required in determining whether visible structural defects require surgical correction. Additionally, MRI may be useful in distinguishing other intensely inflammatory conditions from OA.

Laboratory Studies

Laboratory studies are generally more helpful to exclude alternative diagnoses such as infectious arthritis, Lyme, or crystalline diseases (gout and CPPD) than to diagnose OA. Several reports of elevated concentrations of C-reactive protein in association with OA support our reconsideration of OA as a mildly inflammatory disease, but it is neither sensitive nor specific enough for diagnostic utility. Additional products of cartilage and bone turnover have been integrated into clinical OA studies but are not applicable to OA management. Collectively, these biologic indicators have contributed to our understanding of the OA process, but, at present, serum, urine, or synovial markers with acceptable test characteristics are not available for diagnostic or prognostic use.

MANAGEMENT

The objectives of OA management are to lessen painful symptoms and improve function and quality of life. The scope of OA management has appropriately broadened beyond medicinal agents to include physical and rehabilitative and other interventions. Primary-care practitioners can set in motion numerous services (e.g., rheumatology, physiatry, physical or occupational therapy, psychology, nutrition, social work, and orthopedic surgery) in pursuit of these

TABLE 116-2

Management of Osteoarthritis

Patient education
    OA education—cause and treatment
    Weight management
    Exercise

Nonmedicinal and rehabilitative
    Exercise
    Electrical stimulation
    Ultrasound
    Cryotherapy and thermotherapy
    Acupuncture
    Modalities
    Braces, orthotics, and assistive devices

Symptom-directed medicinal agents
    Topical agents
    Simple analgesics
    Nutriceuticals
    Nonsteroidal anti-inflammatory agents and cyclooxygenase-2 inhibitors
    Narcotic analgesics
    Intra-articular agents
    Potential structure-modifying agents

Surgical interventions
    Arthroscopy
    Osteotomy
    Arthroplasty
    Restorative surgery

objectives. Currently used management options are summarized in Table 116-2.

Patient Education

The effectiveness of OA management is highly dependent on patient compliance. Therefore, patient education should be considered the initial required element in OA management. Educational groups or classes provide an efficient and social vehicle to convey general information pertaining to OA and management strategies. Topics might include warning signs of medication toxicity, exercise, weight management, stress management, sleep hygiene, and general healthy living. Participants in self-management groups report less pain and reliance on nonsteroidal anti-inflammatory agents. Additional benefits of participation in these programs include boosting self-efficacy, increased physical activity, and lessening the frequency of arthritis-related physician visits. However, program participation does not obviate the need for individualized patient education in matters of medication compliance and drug toxicity monitoring.

Nonmedicinal Interventions

Weight loss in obese individuals with OA of the knee can reduce painful symptoms as well as slow disease progression and is, therefore, recommended for all patients who are overweight. In many cases, a structured weight management program with counseling may be required. Although a 10% reduction in weight is considered a reasonable objective, this should be achieved by combined exercise with dietary modification in older adult patients as a result of the additional benefits gained through muscle strengthening.

Type of exercise-isometric, isotonic, erc
Frequency number of repetitions and how often
Intensity ≤70% one MVC (Maximum Voluntary Contraction)
Precautions, e.g., avoid exertion postmeals

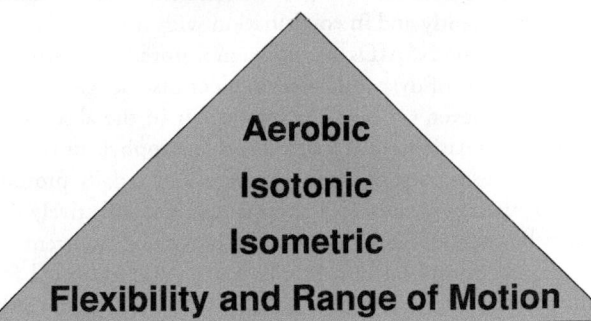

FIGURE 116-4. Prescribed exercise begins with selecting the form of exercise most appropriate to the patient's current functional and health status and finally to provide the details of intensity, duration, and frequency. Exercise precautions should be reviewed.

Exercise

Several studies have provided convincing evidence that resistive and aerobic exercise training is an effective means of reducing pain severity and disability in older adults with knee OA. General steps for composing an exercise prescription begin with reviewing absolute and relative contraindications and setting realistic objectives. Additional specifics are depicted in Figure 116-4 and include selecting the form of exercise most appropriate to the patient's current functional and health status, and finally to provide the details of intensity, duration, and frequency. Patients should be advised to watch for signs of excessive joint strain, including pain during activity, pain lasting more than 1 to 2 hours after exercise, swelling, fatigue, and weakness.

Mobilization exercises (i.e., stretching and flexibility training) are typically the first steps in restoring function and focus on relieving stiffness and increase joint mobility by increasing length and elasticity in muscles and periarticular tissues. *Isometric* exercises should be introduced early, given benefits of restoring muscle strength and joint stabilization without increasing pain. Straight leg raises, wall sits, and isometric leg presses are some examples of isometric quadriceps-strengthening exercises. Strengthening the quadriceps may realign and stabilize joints. *Isotonic exercises* can be introduced later to strengthen muscles as joints move. Squats, wall slides, and leg presses are some examples of isotonic exercise that strengthen both quadriceps and hamstring muscles concurrently. *Aquatic* exercise provides resistance exercise training while also unloading up to 50% to 60% of body weight. Finally, *aerobic* exercise improves fitness, exercise tolerance, and endurance. Walking and low-impact and aquatic aerobic programs improve overall general fitness and coordination. Patients with weight-bearing OA (knee and hip) should engage in strenuous activities cautiously. Some weight-bearing exercises such as stair climbing and heavy lifting (i.e., loads greater than 10% of body weight) may significantly increase loading on weight-bearing joints, as do speed walking and running.

Electrical Stimulation

Neuromuscular electrical stimulation delivers low-voltage electrical impulses through surface electrodes placed over motor points of the targeted muscle. Electrical stimulation induces muscle contraction. Neuromuscular electrical stimulation has been used to increase quadriceps muscle strength and lessen pain in older adults with disabilities with knee OA and may be an acceptable alternative for patients who are unable to participate in exercise owing to severe pain or contraindications.

Ultrasound

Therapeutic ultrasound is one of the most widely prescribed modalities for pain and loss of function caused by OA. Ultrasound uses high-frequency (0.8–1.0 MHz) sound waves to reduce painful symptoms by pulsed delivery for acute pain and inflammation or by continuous delivery for patients with chronic symptoms that have resulted in joint limitations.

Cryotherapy and Thermotherapy

Cold and heat are useful adjuncts for the treatment of OA and may decrease both pain and muscle spasms. Cold reduces the inflammation of arthritis, minimizes muscle spasm, and decreases the sensation of pain. Patients should limit use of ice or cold packs to 20 minutes or when the area becomes numb. Cautious use of heat can reduce pain and muscle spasm but should be limited to 20-minute intervals. Contrast therapy, which alternates between hot and cold treatment modalities, provides additional therapeutic benefits compared to either alone.

Acupuncture

Acupuncture has been included as a potentially useful adjunctive therapy in a comprehensive disease management program for OA. Transcutaneous electrical nerve stimulation delivers acupuncture-like stimulation in random order and is one of the modern changes to classical acupuncture.

Massage

Rubbing a painful joint is almost a reflex action for some clients. Massage is theorized to reduce pain by enhancing endorphin release. Massage relaxes muscle groups and may be a useful adjunct for patients with anxiety and depression.

Orthoses

Specific orthoses designed to reduce medial knee pain by unloading the medial compartment of the knee include a valgus unloader brace and a lateral wedge insole. Lateral wedge insoles of 5 and 10 degrees lateral significantly reduced knee varus torque during ambulation by 6% and 8%, respectively. A simpler change to a well-designed running shoe may also lessen pain and damage by decreasing the impact transmitted during ambulation.

Braces and Splints

Individuals with knee OA may experience knee instability, which can be described as buckling, shifting, or giving way of the knee. Neoprene braces are often requested by patients but unlikely to provide the required structural support, since multiple factors such as lower muscle strength and neuromuscular control and capsuloligamentous laxity likely contribute. However, neoprene braces may alleviate patellofemoral symptoms by improving patellar tracking and provide a greater sense of joint stability by improving joint proprioception.

Assistive Devices

A cane that is properly fitted to the level of the greater trochanter of the hip and held in the hand opposite to the affected knee or hip can reduce joint loading and symptoms significantly. Patients with advanced hand OA may require task modification or use of meal preparation devices, and hip OA may require additional devices to dress independently.

Symptom-Directed Medicinal Therapy

Alleviation of painful symptoms constitutes the primary focus of prescribed and over-the-counter medicinal management of OA. In general, treatments should use the least toxic and least expensive medications first. Furthermore, since there is no single best medication for any given patient, selection of specific agents should be based on each patient's symptom severity and weighed against potential adverse events. Finally, it is important to recognize the complexity of treating painful symptoms in older adult patients who are more likely to endure comorbid medical conditions and multiple medications.

Topical Agents

Topical agents have a role in the treatment of OA. Capsaicin, derived from capsicum, the common pepper plant, is known to be effective in management of OA of the hands when applied two to four times daily. Care should be taken to avoid the inadvertent application of capsaicin in the eyes and other mucous membranes. Topical nonsteroidal anti-inflammatory drugs (NSAIDs) may provide short-term relief of painful symptoms of knee OA. Although generally well tolerated, use of other topical analgesic agents (e.g., nonprescription formulations of menthol- and salicylate-based preparations) has not been proven more effective than placebo.

Simple Analgesics

Acetaminophen remains the first-line drug of choice for OA management. Acetaminophen should be used at a dose not to exceed 1 g four-times daily (maximum U.S. daily dose of 4 g) and is well tolerated. Despite some evidence of exacerbated renal insufficiency, it is a safer drug than are NSAIDs for patients with renal impairment. Acetaminophen should be used cautiously in patients with impaired liver function and should not be taken with alcohol.

Tramadol is an effective analgesic in management of OA symptoms. A starting dose of 25 mg daily for 3 days can be escalated slowly to a maximum dose thereafter to achieve the desired analgesia. Tramadol also has NSAID-sparing effects. Potential adverse effects include nausea and drowsiness. Seizures and allergic reactions have also been reported at higher doses. Although tramadol is not a controlled substance, it can be abused by patients with opioid dependence.

Non-steroidal anti-inflammatory Drugs

NSAIDs are the most commonly prescribed agents for treatment of both pain and inflammation in OA and appear to be more effective in relieving moderate-to-severe pain than acetaminophen. Although all NSAIDS inhibit cyclooxygenase enzymes, patient responses to specific agents may vary considerably. Patients vary in their benefit and adverse reactions to various NSAIDs. Difference in half-lives of the NSAIDs may influence patient adherence and dosing. Despite

their efficacy, NSAIDs should be prescribed with caution. Analgesia can often be achieved at low doses. Thus, treatment should begin with the lowest dose and increased incrementally to identify the lowest effective dose for each patient. Additionally, NSAIDs can be used intermittently and in combination with other analgesics.

Patients using NSAIDs should be monitored for gastrointestinal (GI) symptoms of dyspepsia, peptic ulcer disease, gastritis, and GI bleeding; however, GI bleeding may occur in the absence of prior symptoms. In patients at risk of GI events, prophylaxis is highly recommended using one of three strategies. Once-daily proton pump inhibitor therapy decreases dyspepsia and also effectively decreases the development of NSAID-associated ulcers and recurrent NSAID-related ulcer complications. Prophylaxis is also indicated for older adult patients taking low-dose aspirin who are at higher risk of GI toxicity. A second strategy to reduce GI events is cotreatment with misoprostol. Although misoprostol also decreases NSAID-induced ulcers and GI complications, its effectiveness depends on frequent dosing that in itself can cause diarrhea and dyspepsia. A third option for patients at high risk is to add a proton pump inhibitor. Cotreatment with H2 blockers and sucralfate may reduce GI symptoms but does not reduce the risk of ulcers or serious GI complications.

Cyclooxygenase-2 Inhibitors

Cyclooxygenase (COX)-2 inhibitors represent the third strategy for reducing NSAID-related GI complications. COX-2 inhibitors (celecoxib, rofecoxib, valdecoxib, etc.) can effectively relieve painful OA symptoms, with less risk of GI symptoms and serious GI adverse events when compared to nonselective NSAIDs. However, the potential benefits of COX-2 use should be weighed against the potential risks. First, data showing an increased risk of acute cardiovascular events in association with the use of selective COX-2 inhibitors have resulted in the removal of two of the three FDA-approved agents from the market (rofecoxib and valdecoxib) and a considerably more cautious approach to the use of the remaining agent (celecoxib). Although cotreatment with aspirin may be considered, concurrent use of low-dose aspirin may compromise the protective advantage of COX-2 selectivity in patients who have already experienced a GI bleed. Therefore, addition of a proton pump inhibitor may be required in patients at high risk. Finally, COX-2 selective agents are as likely as nonselective NSAIDS to reduce kidney function, particularly in older adults with renal compromise. Finally, coagulation parameters should be carefully monitored in patients who add any medication to their anticoagulants because of potential drug interactions. Thus, the risks and benefits of COX-2 selective antagonists must be carefully considered in each patient.

Nutriceuticals

Numerous nutriceutical products are advertised to reduce painful symptoms and to "promote joint health" with limited well-controlled studies to validate their efficacy. Oral glucosamine and chondroitin sulfate are popular nutritional supplements thought to relieve pain and limit OA progression. Two randomized placebo-controlled trials showed that glucosamine treatment slows rate of joint space narrowing for more than 3 years and chondroitin sulfate treatment for more than 2 years. Interestingly, some studies demonstrating structure modification do not have concomitant symptom improvement, with no consistent improvement in OA symptoms observed with glucosamine or chondroitin treatment across studies. Fortunately, glucosamine and chondroitin sulfate are relatively well tolerated. Earlier concerns of hyperglycemia, exacerbated diabetes, and possible effects of chondroitin effects on coagulation parameters have not been seen in recent studies. Thus, at present, a 3-month trial is likely safe but should be discontinued if symptoms do not abate. Other products such as S-adenosylmethionine or methylsulfonyl-methane, shark cartilage, and others remain commercially available and successfully marketed despite the absence of scientific support for their use in the treatment of painful OA.

Diacerein (50 mg twice daily) is an interesting compound that exerts anti-inflammatory effects by inhibiting interleukin-1 and collagenase production, with additional effects on neutrophil chemotaxis macrophage migration and phagocytosis. Diacerein does not alter renal or platelet cyclooxygenase activity and may, therefore, be tolerated by patients with prostaglandin-dependent renal function.

Narcotic Analgesics

Narcotic analgesics can be effectively prescribed in management of OA pain. Long-acting preparations of oxycodone can be considered for patients with persistent moderate-to-severe pain. For patients with persistent symptoms despite simple analgesics, codeine or propoxyphene can be prescribed. Short-term studies support the use of slow-release formulations of narcotics administered in low doses, such as oxycodone SR 10 mg, for patients with moderate-to-severe OA of the knee in whom pain is inadequately controlled by acetaminophen or NSAIDs alone. Improvements in pain and quality of sleep were comparable for short- versus long-acting narcotic preparations, with comparatively fewer GI side effects. These agents may be particularly useful for chronic management of patients with severe knee or hip OA in patients who are not surgical candidates owing to comorbid cardiac or pulmonary illness.

Structure-Modifying Medicinal Agents

Although definitive structure and disease-modifying therapies are not yet available for OA, several promising studies have been conducted, which provide hope that such therapy is within reach. Diacerhein has been proposed as a slow-acting, symptom-modifying, and perhaps disease-structure-modifying drug for OA. Doxycycline is of interest for its metalloproteinase-inhibiting activity and ability to limit joint space narrowing in obese women, but it does not appear to prevent disease development or improve symptomatic outcomes. Risedronate, a bisphosphonate indicated for treatment of osteoporosis, has recently been shown to reduce markers of cartilage degradation and bone resorption. Other agents of interest as potential OA structure modifiers include antagonists of interleukin-1 and inhibitors of matrix metalloproteinases, inducible nitric oxide synthetase, intracellular signaling pathways such as P38, MEK-1/2, peroxisome-proliferator-activated receptors, and vitamin D. Molecular strategies to inhibit destructive inflammatory cytokines and matrix metalloproteinases and promote to chondrocyte survival and synthesis of cartilage matrix components such as type II collagen and proteoglycans are additional areas of scientific development.

Intra-articular Therapies

Intra-articular therapies should be considered for patients with peripheral OA with symptoms despite maximal analgesics but may also be a viable therapeutic alternative for patients in whom NSAID or COX-2 inhibitor use is contraindicated or risky.

Intra-articular Glucocorticoid Agents

Intra-articular depot corticosteroids may be considered in management of accessible peripheral joints and are proven to achieve short-term relief from painful symptoms. When proper technique is employed, the risks of bleeding and septic arthritis are comparable to phlebotomy. Although recurrent administration is generally well tolerated and has not been observed to result in joint damage, more definitive surgical intervention should be considered.

Hyaluronic Acid Derivatives

The intra-articular delivery of synthetic and naturally occurring hyaluronan derivatives have gained popularity in management of mild-to-moderate OA of the knee and hip. Several injections are required for the different compounds, and some patients may experience a flare of symptoms after injection. In general, these agents are tolerated as well as corticosteroid injections. Thus far, long-term administration of these agents also appears to be safe.

Surgical Interventions

Surgical intervention should be considered in patients with OA who have persistent, function-limiting symptoms despite maximal medical management and who are healthy enough to withstand surgery. Several surgical options exist, each with specific indications.

Arthroscopy with Debridement

Arthroscopy allows direct visualization to assess structural integrity of the joint and is most appropriate for patients with mechanical symptoms (locking and giveway weakness) because of meniscal defects that are either repaired or removed. Arthroscopic lavage for OA of the knee and other joints is controversial but has been used in combination with viscosupplementation as a temporizing measure pending more definitive surgery.

Osteotomy

Osteotomy follows the principle of transferring load to the unaffected compartment of the knee. High tibial osteotomy is appropriate for OA, involving a single compartment in a varus malaligned knee. High tibial osteotomy achieves effective pain relief and restoration of mobility function in up to 90% of patients at 5 years, and 65% at 10 years. Postoperative alignment is the primary determinant of successful pain relief and may delay the need for joint replacement for up to 10 years. Therefore, young patients with varus malalignment who desire a fully active lifestyle that includes recreational sports are ideal candidates for osteotomy. When appropriately performed, osteotomy should not compromise later arthroplasty if it becomes necessary.

Arthroplasty

Arthroplasty, prosthetic joint replacement surgery, should be considered for patients who have function-limiting symptoms that have persisted despite receiving maximal medical and nonmedicinal treatment. Arthroplasty can replace either a single compartment (unicompartment) or the total joint.

Unicompartment Arthroplasty

It may be considered for patients who are nonobese with discrete pain and disease that is localized to the medial compartment of the knee and who have less than 10% varus malalignment, at least 90 degrees of motion without a flexion contracture, and who do not intend to return to high impact activities. Unicompartmental knee replacement can be achieved through a smaller surgical incision and shorter postoperative and rehabilitative course than total joint arthroplasty. Approximately 95% of unicompartment prostheses survive to 10 years.

Patellofemoral Arthroplasty

Isolated disease of the patellofemoral joint of the knee occurs in up to 10% of patients with OA of the knee. Several types of patellofemoral arthroplasties are available, but the results have been variable, highlighting the need for careful selection of patients. The most common complications following surgery are patella maltracking, excessive wear of the polyethylene implant, and disease progression in the other compartments of the knee joint.

Total Joint Arthroplasty

In contrast to patients with discrete symptoms, total joint arthroplasty is more appropriate for patients with diffuse OA of the knee or hip. Total knee replacement achieves rapid and long-term symptom relief in and functional recovery for 85% of patients with severe and diffuse disease of the knee or hip. With advances in design, prosthesis survival has improved to 90% at 15 years. However, arthroplasty revision is occasionally required for persistent and severe symptoms or prosthesis loosening. Flexion contracture and obesity are not contraindications for total joint arthroplasty but may complicate functional recovery.

Bilateral Knee Arthroplasty

For patients with severe bilateral knee OA, one might entertain bilateral simultaneous arthroplasty—that is replacement of both knees during a single operative session. Existing literature suggests that, in carefully selected patients, bilateral arthroplasty can be performed simultaneously and can achieve good outcomes without increasing perioperative risk.

Hand Surgery

Several different surgical procedures are available (trapeziectomy, trapeziectomy with ligament reconstruction, trapeziectomy with ligament reconstruction and tendon interposition, and joint replacement) and can lessen pain and improve function in patients with advanced OA of the thumb base. The specific type of procedure recommended will depend on durability and stability requirements of the patient's occupation and recreational activities.

Restorative Tissue Interventions

Transplantation of autologous chondrocytes has been used successfully to repair discrete defects in articular cartilage. Osteochondral transplantation is also promising. However, because the area of cartilage loss in OA in older adults is usually more extensive and because older chondrocytes are less metabolically active than young chondrocytes, transplantation to repair or replace diffusely degenerating cartilage is currently impractical.

PREVENTION

Since OA is likely a heterogeneous disease, it is not possible to identify one single factor that, if modified, would reduce risk of all forms of OA. Obesity has been implicated in the development and progression of knee and perhaps also hip and hand OA. Weight loss of this magnitude can alleviate painful symptoms, while also reducing the knee-joint load in overweight and obese older adults with knee OA. For every pound of weight lost, there is a fourfold reduction in the load exerted on the knee per step during daily activities. If this is accumulated for more than thousands of steps per day, the weight lost will be clinically meaningful. Additionally, although severe joint injuries increase risk of OA development, the role of repetitive, relatively minor, trauma in development of OA is not clear. Despite this, interventions to reduce joint injury in recreational sports and adaptations to improve mechanical efficiency for occupations requiring repetitive movements, or bending and lifting are prudent.

SPECIAL ISSUES

Pain and Incidental OA

Painful symptoms may be mistakenly attributed to OA as a result of the high prevalence of radiographic abnormalities in older adult patients. Conditions other than OA should be considered in patients who exhibit diffuse pain despite maximal medical and adjunctive therapy. Some of these alternative diagnoses are summarized in Table 116-3. Persistent pain with diffuse tenderness of periarticular regions warrant evaluation for metabolic disturbances that

TABLE 116-3

Differential Diagnosis of Osteoarthritis
Inflammatory joint disease
Rheumatoid arthritis
Crystalline diseases (gout, calcium pyrophosphate deposition disease, and hydroxyappetite)
Seronegative spondyloarthropathy (psoriatic arthritis and Reiter's)
Polymyalgia rheumatica
Bone disease
Osteomalacia and hypovitaminosis D
Paget's disease
Malignancy: myeloma and metastatic
Infectious diseases
Infectious arthritis
Osteomyelitis
Sepsis syndrome
Periarticular soft-tissue abnormalities
Tendonitis
Bursitis
Neuromuscular diseases
Neuropathy
Systemic diseases
Diabetes
Malignancy
Autoimmune (lupus and vasculitis)

affect bone, such as vitamin D deficiency or hyperparathyroidism. Fibromyalgia, characterized by pain, fatigue, nonrestorative sleep and soft-tissue tenderness, becomes more prevalent in late life and is also poorly responsive to conventional OA management.

Conditions Superimposed with OA

Pain caused by OA should be localized to that joint and reproduced on either palpation or movement of that joint. Occasionally, OA is accompanied by periarticular inflammation of the tendons (tendonitis) or bursae (bursitis), which are both elicited on active, but not passive, range of motion. Evaluation for other etiologies of pain is warranted by a few clinical "red flags." OA is not accompanied by constitutional symptoms of fever, unintentional weight loss, or severe fatigue. Presence of exquisite tenderness, erythema, and a tense effusion also cannot be explained by OA and warrant prompt evaluation for other causes (e.g., crystalline and infectious), particularly when abrupt in onset.

Functional Limitations

OA contributes to late-life functional limitations. Recent studies suggest that limitations develop early during the natural history of OA and can span mobility and hand function, including self-care tasks. Furthermore, gait patterns also change with weight-bearing OA to include slower walking speed, shorter stride length, reduced peak vertical ground reaction forces, and longer stance phase. Pain and muscle weakness appear to increase risk of functional limitations and disability and, therefore, comprise key targets of intervention. In addition, being overweight or obese not only increases risk of progressive knee OA but also contributes substantially to mobility limitations. Fortunately, pain relief achieved with weight reduction also improves walking speed in obese adults.

Falls

Patients with OA of weight-bearing joints (i.e., knee) are at increased risk of injurious falls and fracture. As discussed above, patients with advanced OA of the knee may have proprioceptive deficits. This deficit, usually bilateral, may contribute to the increased risk of falls observed in patients with weight-bearing OA. Recent studies suggest that pain may increase the propensity to trip on an obstacle and that relief of painful symptoms can decrease the propensity to trip and fall over an obstacle. This evidence underscores the importance of treating pain and enhancing muscle training in patients with OA.

Comorbidities

It is accepted that late-life physical disability is an important consequence of OA and other chronic age-associated diseases. However, beyond the limitations attributable to the cumulative effect of the number of chronic illnesses, specific comorbid disease pairs are of clinical importance and scientific interest. Comorbid OA and heart disease is one such disease pair that presents a significant clinical challenge. Patients with OA may engage in less strenuous activities, thereby having less opportunity to declare classic anginal symptoms. As discussed above, NSAIDs and COX-2 inhibitors that are commonly prescribed in management of OA symptoms must be used cautiously in patients with underlying heart disease. Finally, patients with significant heart disease would be ill-advised to undergo surgical procedures despite the severe symptoms and disability.

CONCLUSIONS

OA remains the most prevalent articular disease of older adults. Recommended treatments include safe and adequate pain relief by implementing combined medicinal with rehabilitative and behavioral interventions. Biological markers that will detect early disease and enable interventions capable of modifying or mitigating disease progression are being intensely pursued.

FURTHER READING

Altman RD. Status of hyaluronan supplementation therapy in osteoarthritis. *Curr Rheumatol Rep*. 2003;5(1):7–14.

Altman RD. Structure-/disease-modifying agents for osteoarthritis. *Semin Arthritis Rheum*. 2005;34(6 Suppl 2):3–5.

Altman RD, Gold GE. Atlas of individual radiographic features in osteoarthritis, revised. *Osteoarthritis Cartilage*. 2007;15(Suppl A):A1–A56.

Bennell K, Hinman R. Exercise as a treatment for osteoarthritis. *Curr Opin Rheumatol*. 2005;17(5):634–640.

Berman B. A 60-year-old woman considering acupuncture for knee pain. *JAMA*. 2007;297(15):1697–1707.

Brandt KD, Mazzuca SA. Lessons learned from nine clinical trials of disease-modifying osteoarthritis drugs. *Arthritis Rheum*. 2005;52(11):3349–3359.

Chan FK, Wong VW, Suen BY, et al. Combination of a cyclo-oxygenase-2 inhibitor and a proton-pump inhibitor for prevention of recurrent ulcer bleeding in patients at very high risk: a double-blind, randomised trial. *Lancet*. 2007;369(9573):1621–1626.

Clegg DO, Reda DJ, Harris CL, et al. Glucosamine, chondroitin sulfate, and the two in combination for painful knee osteoarthritis. *N Engl J Med*. 2006;354(8):795–808.

Ettinger WH Jr, Burns R, Messier SP, et al. A randomized trial comparing aerobic exercise and resistance exercise with a health education program in older adults with knee osteoarthritis. The Fitness Arthritis and Seniors Trial (FAST). *JAMA*. 1997;277(1):25–31.

Felson DT. Clinical practice. Osteoarthritis of the knee. *N Engl J Med*. 2006;354(8):841–848.

Felson DT, Goggins J, Niu J, Zhang Y, Hunter DJ. The effect of body weight on progression of knee osteoarthritis is dependent on alignment. *Arthritis Rheum*. 2004;50(12):3904–3909.

Fitzgerald GK, Piva SR, Irrgang JJ. Reports of joint instability in knee osteoarthritis: its prevalence and relationship to physical function. *Arthritis Rheum*. 2004;51(6):941–946.

Gossec L, Hawker G, Davis AM, et al. OMERACT/OARSI initiative to define states of severity and indication for joint replacement in hip and knee osteoarthritis. *J Rheumatol*. 2007;34(6):1432–1435.

Hawkey CJ, Fortun PJ. Cyclooxygenase-2 inhibitors. *Curr Opin Gastroenterol*. 2005;21(6):660–664.

Hochberg MC. Nutritional supplements for knee osteoarthritis–still no resolution. *N Engl J Med*. 2006;354(8):858–860.

Hunter DJ, Felson DT. Osteoarthritis. *BMJ*. 2006;332(7542):639–642.

Kraus VB. Biomarkers in osteoarthritis. *Curr Opin Rheumatol*. 2005;17(5):641–646.

Lewek MD, Ramsey DK, Snyder-Mackler L, Rudolph KS. Knee stabilization in patients with medial compartment knee osteoarthritis. *Arthritis Rheum*. 2005;52(9):2845–2853.

Ling SM, Xue QL, Simonsick EM, et al. Transitions to mobility difficulty associated with lower extremity osteoarthritis in high functioning older women: longitudinal data from the Women's Health and Aging Study II. *Arthritis Rheum*. 2006;55(2):256–263.

Loeser RF. Molecular mechanisms of cartilage destruction: mechanics, inflammatory mediators and aging collide. *Arthritis Rheum*. 2006;54(5):1357–1360.

McAlindon T, Formica M, LaValley M, Lehmer M, Kabbara K. Effectiveness of glucosamine for symptoms of knee osteoarthritis: results from an internet-based randomized double-blind controlled trial. *Am J Med*. 2004;117(9):643–649.

Messier SP, Royer TD, Craven TE, O'Toole ML, Burns R, Ettinger WH Jr. Long-term exercise and its effect on balance in older, osteoarthritic adults: results from the Fitness, Arthritis, and Seniors Trial (FAST). *J Am Geriatr Soc*. 2000;48(2):131–138.

Messier SP, Loeser RF, Miller GD, et al. Exercise and dietary weight loss in overweight and obese older adults with knee osteoarthritis: the Arthritis, Diet, and Activity Promotion Trial. *Arthritis Rheum*. 2004;50(5):1501–1510.

Mikesky AE, Mazzuca SA, Brandt KD, Perkins SM, Damush T, Lane KA. Effects of strength training on the incidence and progression of knee osteoarthritis. *Arthritis Rheum.* 2006;55(5):690–699.

Pelletier JP, Martel-Pelletier J. New trends in the treatment of osteoarthritis. *Semin Arthritis Rheum.* 2005;34(6 Suppl 2):13–14.

Raynauld JP, Buckland-Wright C, Ward R, et al. Safety and efficacy of long-term intraarticular steroid injections in osteoarthritis of the knee: a randomized, double-blind, placebo-controlled trial. *Arthritis Rheum.* 2003;48(2):370–377.

Rintelen B, Neumann K, Leeb BF. A meta-analysis of controlled clinical studies with diacerein in the treatment of osteoarthritis. *Arch Intern Med.* 2006;166(17):1899–1906.

Schnitzer TJ. Update on guidelines for the treatment of chronic musculoskeletal pain. *Clin Rheumatol.* 2006;25(Suppl 1):S22–S29.

Sharma L, Chang A. Overweight: advancing our understanding of its impact on the knee and the hip. *Ann Rheum Dis.* 2007;66(2):141–142.

Sharma L, Kapoor D, Issa S. Epidemiology of osteoarthritis: an update. *Curr Opin Rheumatol.* 2006;18(2):147–156.

Stitik TP, Altschuler E, Foye PM. Pharmacotherapy of osteoarthritis. *Am J Phys Med Rehabil.* 2006;85(11 Suppl):S15–S28.

Talbot LA, Gaines JM, Ling SM, Metter EJ. A home-based protocol of electrical muscle stimulation for quadriceps muscle strength in older adults with osteoarthritis of the knee. *J Rheumatol.* 2003;30(7):1571–1578.

Osteoporosis

Gustavo Duque ■ *Bruce R. Troen*

DEFINITION OF OSTEOPOROSIS

The term *osteoporosis* was first introduced in the nineteenth century based on histological diagnosis ("porous bone"). Osteoporosis is a "disease characterized by low bone mass and microarchitectural deterioration of bone tissue leading to enhanced bone fragility and a consequent increase in fracture incidence." Osteoporosis can be defined either by the presence of a fragility fracture or by bone mineral density (BMD) measurement. In defining BMD criteria for osteoporosis, the World Health Organization (WHO) used as the standard the BMD of young adult women who are at the age of peak bone mass. For each standard deviation below peak bone mass (or 1 unit decrease in T-score), a woman's risk of fracture approximately doubles. As seen in Table 117-1, a T-score <−2.5 defines osteoporosis; osteopenia (low bone mass) and normal bone mass are also defined. A BMD measurement allows early diagnosis of osteoporosis and intervention prior to fracture in older adults. In addition, women with osteopenia can be followed carefully for further bone loss. Although the original standards for definitions of osteoporosis were determined in white women, recent data indicate that the standards for men and Hispanic women are probably similar to those of white women. In addition, standards are now being developed for African-American women. However, defining osteoporosis solely by T-score does *not* effectively capture all patients at risk of a fracture. Greater than 50% of all hip fractures occur in those with T-scores that are better than −2.5. Failure to evaluate and treat such patients adds to the individual and societal cost and consequences of osteoporosis. Therefore, we are still faced with the challenge of improving the identification of the individual patient at risk of fracture and subsequently optimizing both prevention and treatment for the elderly.

Primary or idiopathic osteoporosis has been historically classified as postmenopausal or senile osteoporosis. Postmenopausal osteoporosis, formerly known as type I, occurs in women between 51 and 75 years of age and is related to estrogen deficiency seen with the menopausal transition. In contrast, senile osteoporosis typically occurs in persons older than 60 years of age. It affects both men and women and has a different pathophysiology, which involves reduced levels of bone turnover owing to a reduction in the numbers of bone-forming cells. Increasing evidence points to a progressive age-related alteration in stem cell physiology that favors adipogenesis and thereby reduces osteoblastogenesis and bone formation. Nevertheless, estrogen probably plays a role in the pathophysiology of senile osteoporosis as well. Secondary osteoporosis is the result of an underlying disease or medications that adversely affect bone. In this chapter, we will focus on the typical characteristics of senile osteoporosis from its pathophysiology to therapeutic approaches.

EPIDEMIOLOGY

In the United States, women have more than 250,000 and 500,000 hip and spine fractures per year, respectively. Men account for an additional 250,000 fractures per year; 75,000 are hip fractures. By using BMD, osteopenia is estimated to be present in 8 to 13 million men (28–47%) and in 13 to 17 million women (37–50%); osteoporosis is estimated to be present in 1 to 2 million men (3–6%) and in 4 to 6 million women (13–18%). On reaching the age of 90 years, one-third of women and one-sixth of men will suffer a hip fracture. Both women and men have a similar lifetime vertebral fracture risk of 12%.

The consequences of osteoporotic fracture include diminished quality of life, decreased functional independence, and increased morbidity and mortality. Pain and kyphosis, height loss, and other changes in body habitus resulting from vertebral compression fractures diminish quality of life in women and men. These changes lead to declines in functional status such as the inability to bathe, to dress, or to ambulate independently and may result in decrease pulmonary and gastrointestinal function. Approximately 50% of women do not fully recover prior function after hip fracture; older adults have a 20% to 25% mortality in the year following hip fracture. Men are at a

TABLE 117-1

World Health Organization Criteria for Osteoporosis	
WHO CLASSIFICATION	**BMD T-SCORE**
Normal	>-1
Osteopenia	≤ 1 but >-2.5
Osteoporosis	≤ -2.5
Severe osteoporosis	≤ -2.5 + fragility fracture

BMD, bone mineral density.

higher risk of dying after a hip fracture than women. Finally, the estimated annual cost of osteoporotic fractures in the United States is more than $14 billion, which is higher than the money spent treating cardiovascular disease. Therefore, prevention and early diagnosis and treatment of osteoporosis are vital to improving the health of older adults.

PATHOPHYSIOLOGY

New advances in the understanding of bone physiology have elucidated an active interaction among bone cells, growth factors, and hormones responsible for the maintenance of calcium levels, skeletal structure, and resistance to trauma. Bone is not simply a mineralized structure but a complex system of cell–cell, cell–matrix, and cell–hormone interactions influenced by genetic background, lifestyle, and diet.

Bone is composed of inorganic (calcium phosphate crystals) and organic compounds (90% collagen and 10% noncollagenous proteins). Noncollagenous proteins include albumin, osteopontin, osteocalcin, α_2-HS-glycoprotein, and growth factors, constituting the so-called bone matrix. The bone matrix is produced by osteoblasts and is the environment in which bone and external factors interact in a well-coordinated manner. There are two types of bone: cortical and trabecular. Cortical bone predominates in the long bones of the extremities, while trabecular bone predominates in the vertebrae and pelvis and makes up 80% of skeletal mass. While both types of bone have an active remodeling process, trabecular bone is metabolically more active than cortical bone and more acutely responsive to alterations in sex-steroid hormone status.

During childhood and adolescence, skeletal growth takes place at growth plates, areas in which cartilage proliferates and gradually undergoes calcification, resulting in new bone formation. However, bone remodeling is a lifelong process that maintains bone in order to harbor bone marrow, support the body, and protect vital organs and to provide a source of minerals. The process of remodeling replaces older, frailer bone with newer, more resistant bone in an organized manner. The end product of remodeling is the maintenance of skeletal homeostasis and the preservation of anatomical integrity. With aging or with menopausal transition, the once-coordinated mechanism of bone remodeling becomes uncoupled, leading to bone loss and increased risk of fracture.

Bone Cells

The cells involved in bone turnover are osteoclasts, osteoblasts, and osteocytes. Osteoclasts are macrophage-like cells that secrete proteolytic enzymes and hydrogen ions that are required for removal of the deposited bone matrix. The remodeling cycle begins when osteoclast precursors interact with other marrow cells and are activated, becoming multinucleated osteoclasts, which initiates resorption (Figure 117-1) (Color Plate 25). Bone resorption occurs within the resorption lacuna, a tightly sealed zone beneath the ruffled border of the osteoclast where it has attached to the bone surface. Resorption depends on acidification of this extracellular compartment leading to demineralization, and, subsequently, the organic matrix is degraded by cysteine proteases, chief of which is cathepsin K. Osteoclasts consequently create a functional extracellular lysosome, containing both an acidic environment and typical lysosomal enzymes.

In cortical bone, the resorption period lasts approximately 30 days; the final result is a resorption tunnel that will later be filled in by osteoblasts in a haversian manner. The apposition of these haversian channels takes the shape of a "cut onion," which gives the cortical bone its typical morphology. In trabecular bone, the erosion period lasts approximately 43 days, resulting in a trench between the trabeculae. The life span of osteoclasts is approximately 2 weeks; once these complete the role as bone-resorbing cells, these undergo apoptosis or programmed cell death.

Bone homeostasis depends the intimate coupling of bone formation and bone resorption. After bone is resorbed by osteoclasts, preosteoblasts differentiate into osteoblasts and migrate to the area of excavated bone and begin to deposit osteoid, which is eventually mineralized into new bone. Osteoblasts are fibroblast-like cells derived from pluripotent mesenchymal cells and localized on periosteal surfaces. Such pluripotent stromal cells can be induced to differentiate along the osteoblastic, adipocytic, fibroblastic, or chondrocytic lineages when required. When bone integrity has to be conserved, mesenchymal stromal cells are committed toward the osteoblastic lineage. Many factors are involved in the process of osteoblastogenesis, including the bone morphogenic protein family—bone morphogenic proteins 2, 4, and 7 are potent inducers of osteoblast differentiation (Table 117-2). A transcription factor called Runx2/Cbfa1 plays a key role in osteoblast differentiation; mice lacking Runx2/Cbfa1 do not form bone. A mature osteoblast is a cuboidal cell with a large nucleus and enlarged Golgi highly enriched in alkaline phosphatase. It produces type I collagen and specialized bone-matrix proteins as osteoid, the basic protein for further bone formation and mineralization. Osteoblasts produce alkaline phosphatase, the specific function of which has yet to be determined. Nevertheless, it is used as a marker of osteoblast differentiation and activity, and indirectly as a marker of subsequent osteoclast resorption. Mice lacking functional alkaline phosphatase suffer from hypophosphatasia characterized by impaired mineralization of cartilage and bone matrix. After osteoblasts complete their bone-forming function, they face one of three fates: (1) they become embedded in the newly formed matrix, becoming osteocytes; (2) they remain on the surface of the newly formed bone and become lining cells; or (3) they undergo apoptosis (see Figure 117-1). The ultimate fate of the osteoblast is determined by hormonal changes, the presence or absence of growth factors, and the aging process in bone.

Osteoclasts and osteoblasts belong to a temporary structure known as basic multicellular unit (see Figure 117-1). The coordinated process of bone resorption and formation by the basic multicellular unit lasts 6 to 9 months and results in newly mineralized bone. Osteoblasts are not only active as bone-forming cells, but these also play an important role in the regulation of osteoclast activity. The interaction between osteoblasts and osteoclasts requires a complex

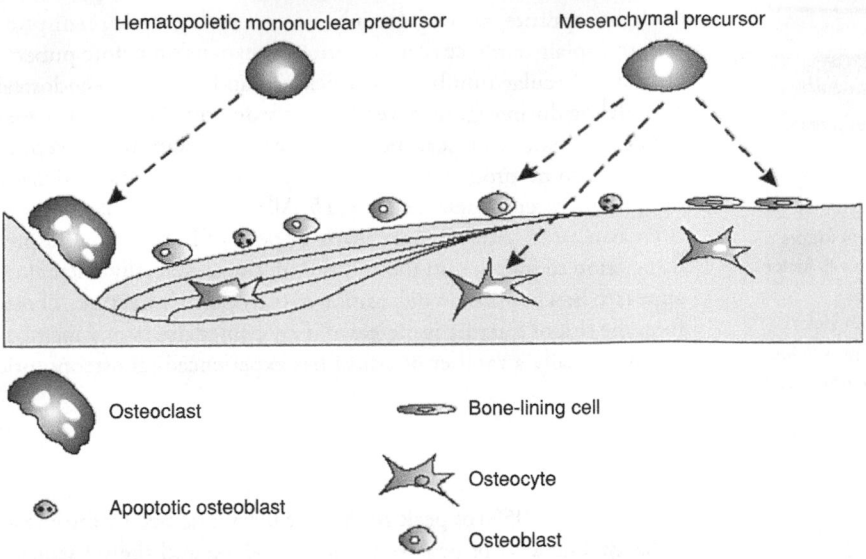

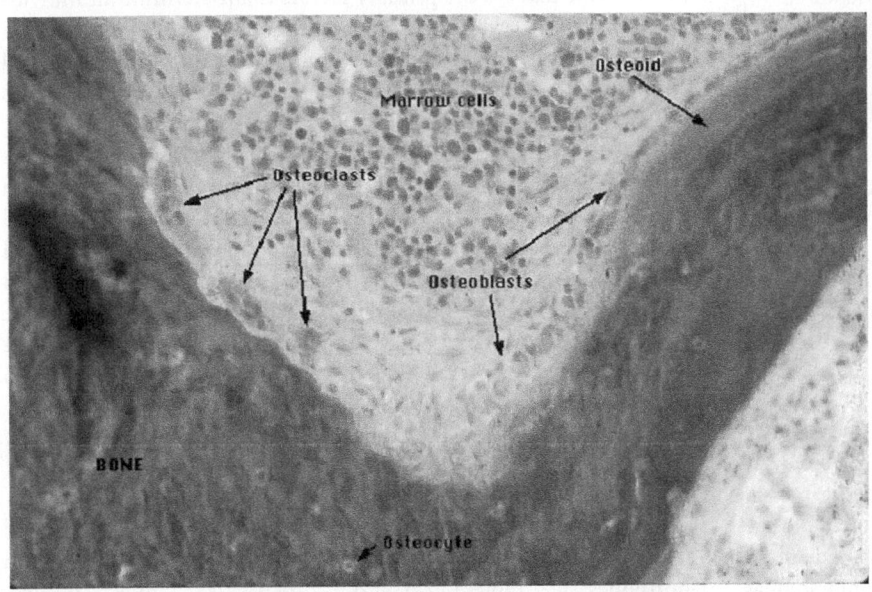

FIGURE 117-1. The cellular components of bone turnover. (A) Bone cell formation: After the expression of specific transcription factors, mesenchymal precursors differentiate into osteoblasts. In contrast, osteoclasts differentiate from mononuclear precursors and will act as bone-resorbing cells in the bone multicellular unit (BMU). After the completion of bone resorption, osteoclasts die by apoptosis and are replaced by active osteoblasts, which are responsible for the formation of new bone. Finally, osteoblasts end as either lining cells or as osteocytes embedded into the osteoid, or die by apoptosis. (B) Basic multicellular unit (BMU—also known as bone metabolic unit): Large multinucleated osteoclasts resorb bone on the left. Osteoblasts cascade into the resorption pit, laying down osteoid (unmineralized bone). The turquoise stain reflects mineralized bone. *(From Chan GK, Duque G. Age-related bone loss: old bone, new facts. Gerontology. 2002;48:62–71 [Figure 117-1A]; and Dr. Susan M. Ott http://courses.washington.edu/bonephys [Figure 117-1B].)*

system of factors and is facilitated by integrins and cadherins. Briefly, the major osteoclast/osteoblast interaction depends on the expression by osteoclast precursors and mature osteoclasts of a membrane receptor known as receptor activator of nuclear factor-κB (RANK), which belongs to the family of tumor necrosis factor (TNF) receptors. Osteoclast differentiation, maturation, and survival depend on the activation of RANK by its cognate ligand (RANK ligand—RANKL), which is produced by osteoblasts and osteoblast precursors after exposure to different stimuli such as hormones and cytokines (Figure 117-2) (Color Plate 26). Multiple other factors also act to either enhance or suppress osteoclast formation and activation and subsequent bone resorption (see Table 117-2).

RANKL is mainly a cytoplasmic membrane-bound molecule; to a lesser extent it is secreted. Mature osteoblasts also produce a decoy receptor for RANKL called osteoprotegerin (OPG). OPG binds to RANKL in a competitive manner and prevents the interaction between RANK and RANKL, thus decreasing osteoclastogenesis and osteoclastic bone resorption and increasing osteoclast apoptosis. Recently, a new group of molecules, known as ephrins, has been identified as key players in the regulation of osteoblast/osteoclast in-

teraction. This cellular communication is bidirectional and involves a transmembrane ligand known as ephrinB2, which is expressed by osteoclasts, and its receptor EphB4 expressed by osteoblasts (see Figure 117-2). This signaling seems to limit osteoclast activity while enhancing osteoblast differentiation. Consequently, osteoblastogenesis and osteoclastogenesis, along with corresponding bone formation and resorption, are tightly and ineluctably coupled. The differentiation and activation of both osteoblasts and osteoclasts depend critically on each other.

Osteocytes, the third group of bone cells, are the most abundant cell type in bone. Osteocytes are the focus of intense research; several functions recently described include the synthesis of matrix molecules like osteocalcin and an important role in direct communication with surface osteoblasts through molecules known as connexins. Connexins are believed to play a role in the activation and regulation of bone after physiological and mechanical stimuli. These modulate the response of bone during functional adaptation of the skeleton to mechanical forces and the need for repair of microdamage. More recently, sclerostins have been found to be secreted by osteocytes. Sclerostins inhibit osteoblast differentiation and

TABLE 117-2

Local Factors Regulating Bone Cell Interaction and Activity

Stimulators of bone resorption	Stimulators of bone formation
RANK ligand	Vitamin D
Interleukin-1, interleukin-6,	Estrogen
interleukin-8, interleukin-11	Androgen
Macrophage colony-stimulating factor	Insulin-like growth factors
Vitamin D	Transforming growth factor
Glucocorticoids	Mechanical force
Parathyroid hormone	Fibroblast growth factors
Tumor necrosis factor	Platelet-derived growth factor
Reduced mechanical force/low gravity	Bone morphogenetic proteins
Epidermal growth factor	
Platelet-derived growth factor	
Fibroblast growth factors	
Leukemia inhibitory factor	
Prostaglandins	
Thyroid hormone	

Inhibitors of bone resorption	Inhibitors of bone formation
Estrogen	Sclerostin
Androgen	Dickkopf
Osteoprotegerin	
Interferon-γ	
Interleukin-4	
Calcitonin	

activation, thereby regulating bone turnover and formation. The final fate of the osteocyte is unknown, but high numbers of apoptotic cells have been found in empty lacunae.

Genetics

Genetics plays a role in determination of peak bone mass. Racial differences in the incidence of osteoporosis have been reported, including a lower relative risk of fractures and higher peak bone mass in African-American women as compared with white women. No one gene, gene product, or polymorphism has yet been credibly identified to account for the variance seen in BMD in specific geographic areas. Several environmental factors, such as diet, topography, and yearly sunlight exposure, almost certainly interact with genetic predisposition to explain variance seen in periosteal expansion before puberty and in trabecular number and thickness and periosteal–endosteal remodeling during aging. Several recently described candidate genes for determination of peak bone mass are the vitamin D receptor, the peroxisome proliferator activator gamma, and the low-density lipoprotein receptor-related protein 5. All these polymorphisms have been associated with different levels of peak of bone mass and predisposition to fractures in the adulthood. More generally, there does appear to be a familial predisposition to osteoporotic fracture. Therefore, the risk of fracture is increased if an immediate family member (most typically a mother or sister) has experienced an osteoporotic fracture.

Mechanical Factors

Approximately 95% of peak adult bone mass is gained by the end of puberty. The level of peak bone mass attained and the subsequent rate of bone loss are the primary factors that determine an individual's bone mass in early and late adulthood. Initial bone formation does not require a mechanical stimulus, but further appositional and endochondral growth is dependent on the mechanical forces generated by the muscles. The magnitude of this loading is directly related to body mass and physical activity. There is some evidence that after mechanical load, microfractures may occur in bone, with subsequent activation of interleukins (ILs) and growth factors and stimulation of bone turnover. Osteocytes appear to be the critical mechanosensors in bone and, therefore, play an important role in this process. The decreased physical activity and immobility that are commonly seen in the elderly result in diminished mechanical forces upon the skeleton, which explains, in part, the age-related loss in mineral density.

Local Factors

Local factors are important in the regulation of bone turnover and in the interaction between bone matrix and systemic factors and hormones (see Table 117-2 and Figure 117-2) (Color Plate 26). The skeleton responds to mechanical forces by several regulatory

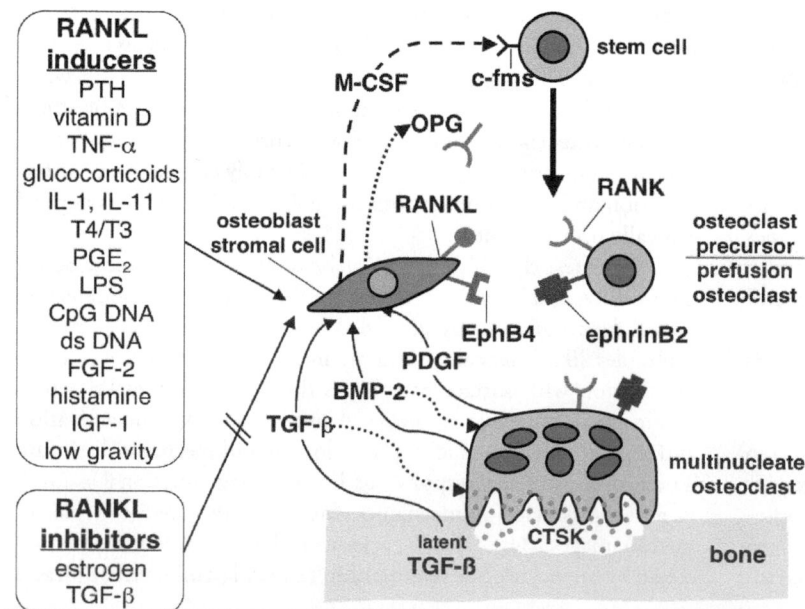

FIGURE 117-2. Osteoblast–osteoclast coupling and the regulation of RANK ligand expression. Osteoblast production of M-CSF and RANKL play critical roles in the differentiation and activation of osteoclasts. M-CSF acts to maintain monocytic stem cell survival, and subsequently RANKL acts to commit the cell toward osteoclast differentiation, fusion, polarization, and activation. EphB4 and ephrinB2 interact both to limit osteoclast activity and stimulate osteoblast differentiation. TGF-β acts only upon release from the extracellular matrix after osteoclastic resorption, which is mediated in large part by the excretion of CTSK. M-CSF, macrophage colony stimulating factor; RANKL, RANK ligand; TGF-β, transforming growth factor-β; BMP-2, bone morphogenetic protein-2; PDGF, platelet-derived growth factor; CTSK, cathepsin K. (Adapted from Duque G, Troen BR. Understanding the Mechanisms of Senile Osteoporosis: New Facts for a Major Geriatric Syndrome. J Am Geriatr Soc. 2008;56:935–941).

mechanisms including release of cytokines, such as macrophage colony-stimulating factor (M-CSF) and granulocyte colony-stimulating factor, which regulate cell differentiation. Mediators and regulators of cell–cell interaction include insulin-like growth factor (IGF)-1 and IGF-2, parathyroid hormone (PTH)-related peptide, IL-1 and IL-6, and TNF-α. The response to sex-steroid hormones is largely mediated by TNF-α, IL-6, IL-1, and prostaglandins. Although high levels of these factors are necessary for osteoblast–osteoclast regulation and pathogenesis of osteoporosis, their usually stable systemic levels suggest that alterations in local secretion and concentration are critical to bone physiology. These local factors largely determine the activation or inhibition of bone cells, cell recruitment and cell differentiation, and life span.

Systemic Hormones

A number of systemic hormones affect bone metabolism, including vitamin D, PTH, calcitonin, and sex-steroid hormones (estrogens and androgens) (see Table 117-2). The major effect of vitamin D is to maintain calcium homeostasis by increasing the efficiency of the small intestine in absorbing dietary calcium. Vitamin D also plays a role in both bone resorption by inducing RANKL expression by osteoblasts, thereby inducing osteoclast differentiation and activation, and bone formation by stimulating osteoblastogenesis and inhibiting apoptosis of mature osteoblasts. Hypovitaminosis D, which is widespread in the elderly, is associated with lower BMD, greater falls, and more osteoporotic fractures.

PTH is secreted by the parathyroid glands through a calcium sensor mechanism. When calcium levels decrease, PTH is released and exerts its function in two major target tissues: kidney and bone. In the kidney, PTH acts on the proximal tubule to reduce PO_4 resorption and to increase the activity of 1-α-hydroxylase, the enzyme that converts 25(OH) vitamin D to $1,25(OH)_2D_3$, the active form of vitamin D. In bone, PTH increases osteoclast-induced bone resorption by inducing RANKL expression and subsequent signaling via RANK. Hypovitaminosis D is often, but not always, accompanied by elevated PTH—secondary hyperparathyroidism. Acute and cyclical exposure to PTH in bone has an antiapoptotic as well as anabolic effect on osteoblasts. This is the basis for using PTH to treat severe osteoporosis (see below). Calcitonin is a hormone secreted by thyroidal C cells in mammals. Its main biologic effect is the inhibition of osteoclastic bone resorption. In vitro and in vivo studies in animals demonstrate that calcitonin causes the osteoclast to shrink and retract from the bone surface, which decreases its bone-resorbing activity and enhances bone formation by osteoblasts.

Sex-steroid hormones play a variety of roles in bone turnover. Although some aspects of its effects remain unclear, estrogen increases the level of OPG, inhibiting osteoclastogenesis. Estrogen also induces osteoclast apoptosis and regulates the action of IL-1, interleukin-1 receptor antagonist (IL-1Ra), IL-6, and TNF-α, and their binding proteins and receptors. Declining estrogen levels lead to increased expression of IL-1, IL-6, and TNF-α, all of which enhance bone resorption. In response to diminished estrogen, osteoblasts produce more RANKL and less OPG, which induces RANKL–RANK interaction and signaling, further stimulating osteoclast differentiation and activation. Since estrogen increases osteoblast differentiation and decreases osteoblast apoptosis, bone formation declines at the time of menopause. Overall, there is a high turnover state with predominant bone resorption, which results in bone loss and susceptibility to fractures. Androgens play an important role in the

formation of adolescent bone by regulating cytokines in the bone matrix. The effect of progesterone on bone seems to be indirect and limited, through its regulation of calcitonin secretion and thus bone resorption.

Women are at higher risk of osteoporosis because women have lower peak bone mass than men and experience accelerated bone loss during menopause, as described above. Histomorphometric data on the skeletal changes associated with postmenopausal bone loss show an increase in bone turnover in both cancellous and cortical bones. Biochemical markers also support high bone resorption after menopause. These markers return to normal with estrogen replacement. Trabecular bone is affected earlier in menopause than cortical bone because it is more metabolically active. Thus, rapid bone loss is seen primarily in the spine (3% per year) for approximately 5 years after menopause. Subsequently, there is a slower rate of bone loss that is more generalized (approximately 0.5% per year at many sites). A consistent finding in untreated postmenopausal women is a reduction in wall width of bone, indicating reduction in osteoblast activity. Although this could be related to the loss of the antiapoptotic effect of estrogen on osteoblasts, studies are inconclusive.

Age-Related Bone Loss

Age-related bone loss is a complex phenomenon, with many factors involved in its pathogenesis (Figures 117-3 and 117-4) (Color Plates 27 and 28). As an individual ages, distinct changes take place in trabecular bone, cortical bone, and bone marrow. The onset and triggers of age-related bone loss are not well defined, but densitometric studies show a slow and progressive decline in BMD after the third decade of approximately 0.5% per year, even though serum levels of estrogens are still within the normal range. With aging, osteoblastogenesis decreases, resulting in lower numbers of osteoblast precursors and increasing bone marrow adiposity (see Figure 117-3). The bone marrow of a young individual is virtually devoid of adipocytes. In older adults, however, adipose deposits may occupy up to 90% of the bone marrow cavity.

Although factors that are involved in osteoblast–adipocyte differentiation remain unclear, it is known that adipocytes can transdifferentiate into osteoblasts and osteoblasts can be induced to transdifferentiate into adipocytes (see Figure 117-4). It has been postulated that pluripotent mesenchymal cells within the bone marrow stroma are, by default, programmed to differentiate into adipocytes, but the presence of specific osteogenic factors in the bone marrow induces osteoblastic differentiation. If this hypothesis is proven true, then it could offer the potential for novel therapeutic approaches to osteoporosis in older adults. In addition, osteoblast apoptosis increases with aging. Histomorphometric data demonstrate that 50% to 70% of the osteoblasts present at the remodeling site cannot be accounted for after enumeration of lining cells and osteocytes. The discrepancy in osteoblast numbers is believed to be a consequence of osteoblast apoptosis. This phenomenon may account for the significant reduction in bone formation that is associated with aging. In men and women, the early changes associated with age-related bone loss are similar, as described above. However, women also experience accelerated bone loss of approximately 3% to 5% per year during menopause. In men, the decline in bone mass is gradual until very late in life, when the risk for fractures increases rapidly. Concomitant with the changes in osteoblast and adipocyte formation, multiple factors enhance osteoclastogenesis and bone resorption (see Figure 117-4). In particular, the interactions between osteoblast and

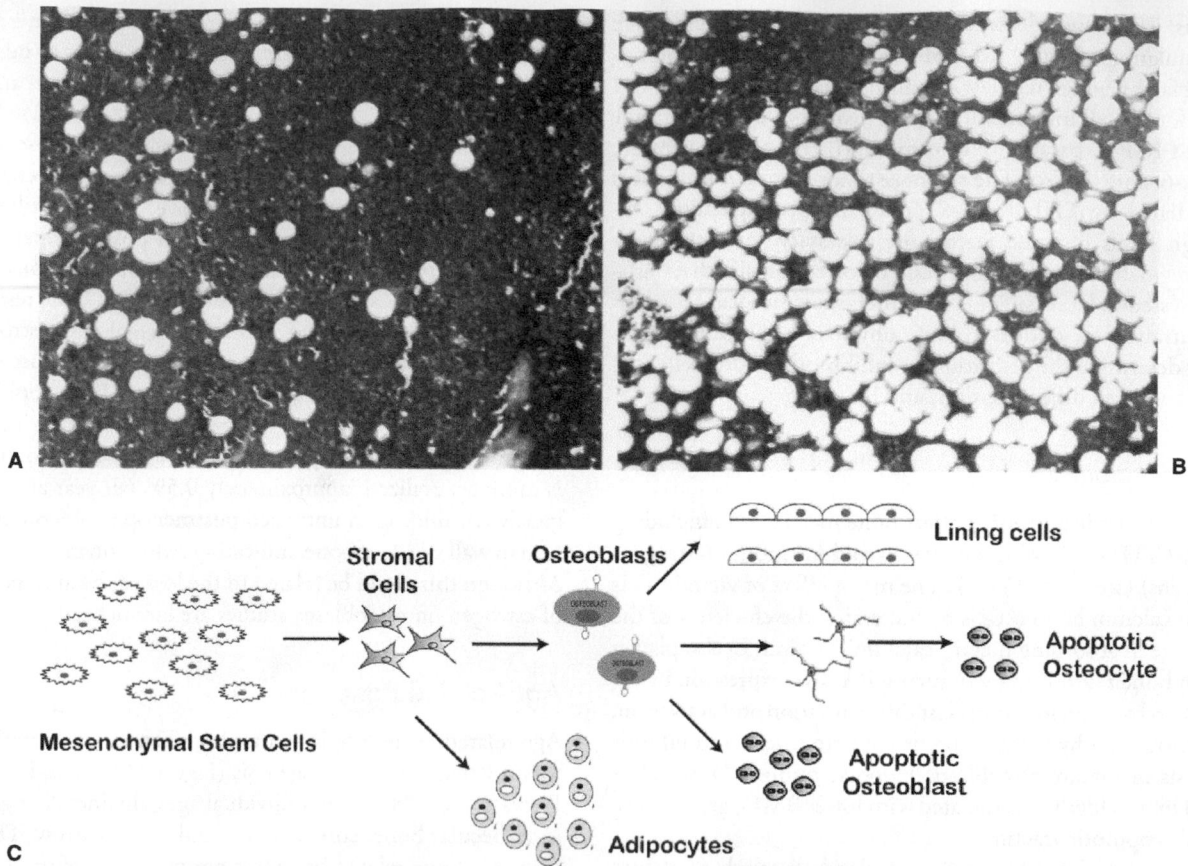

FIGURE 117-3. Cellular changes in senile osteoporosis. The panel on the right shows the much higher levels of bone marrow fat in the iliac crest of an 85-yr-old subject (A) compared with a 38-yr-old one in the panel on the left (B). There is also a marked reduction in the amount of hematopoietic tissue. (C) Changes in the confluence of mesenchymal stem cells (MSC) accompanied by a reduction in osteoblastogenesis result in the formation of fewer active osteoblasts in the bone multicellular unit. In addition, increasing levels of adipogenic differentiation leads to smaller numbers of differentiated osteoblasts. Finally, increasing osteoblast apoptosis reduces the number of active osteoblasts in the bone multicellular units.

osteoclasts, which are crucial to the dynamic equilibrium that maintains healthy bone, are altered. Consequently, the combination of decreased bone formation and increased bone resorption leads to diminished BMD, poorer bone structure and quality, and, ultimately, enhanced fragility and fractures.

In addition to cellular changes, there are two major changes in calciotropic hormones that have an impact on aging bone. Vitamin D levels decrease with age and reduce calcium absorption. Changes in the aging skin reduce the amount of 7-dehydrocholesterol, the precursor of cholecalciferol (vitamin D₃), as well as its rate of

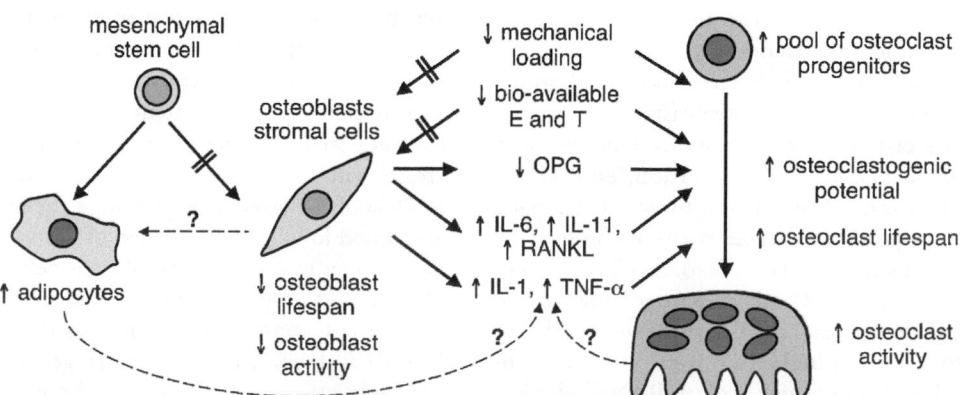

FIGURE 117-4. Changes in osteoblast–osteoclast interactions with aging. Aging predisposes to more adipogenesis and less osteoblastogenesis. In addition, transdifferentiation from osteoblasts to adipocytes may occur. Reduced physical activity/mechanical loading and decreased levels of bioavailable estradiol and testosterone exert diminished effects on osteoblasts (depicted by the arrows with the hatches), resulting in decreased osteoblast secretion of osteoprotegerin (OPG) and increased expression and secretion of RANKL, IL-1, IL-6, IL-11, and TNF-α. In turn, these compounds directly stimulate greater osteoclast formation and activity. The reduced OPG also permits greater binding of RANKL to RANK, which further facilitates increased osteoclastogenesis and resorption. (Adapted from Troen BR. Molecular mechanisms underlying osteoclast formation and activation. Exp Gerontol. 2003;38(6):605–614.)

conversion. Furthermore, declining renal function leads to reduction in the production and activity of 1-α-hydroxylase, the enzyme responsible for the activation of vitamin D_3. Consequently, a negative calcium balance ensues, which activates the calcium sensor receptor in parathyroid glands. PTH is secreted as a physiologic response, stimulating osteoclast activity, which maintains normal serum calcium levels at the expense of bone mineralization. This theory of secondary hyperparathyroidism was once the classic explanation for age-related bone loss. However, not all individuals with hypovitaminosis D exhibit secondary hyperparathyroidism. Therefore, it is just one of the elements of a syndrome that results in osteoporosis in older adults. However, this mechanism has been recently associated with additional important risk factors for fractures, which are sarcopenia and falls. Vitamin D and PTH appear to modulate neuromuscular function, particularly in the frail elderly. Serum levels of 25(OH) vitamin D lower than 35 nmol/L increase the risk of falls by 30%, which highly predisposes to fractures. Recent evidence has shown that patients with serum levels between 35 and 80 mmol/L, which were considered normal in the past, are still at risk of falls, suggesting that the therapeutic goal should be to obtain serum levels higher than 80 nmol/L.

In summary, age-related bone loss results from changes at the cellular level, including decreased osteoblastogenesis, shortened osteoblast life span, and increased adipogenesis, as well as from hormonal changes, including decreased levels and activity of sex-steroid hormones and vitamin D and increased levels and activity of PTH. These mechanisms have been demonstrated both in vitro and in vivo, mostly in murine models. New histomorphometric data in humans support these findings, although more studies are required to completely explain the pathophysiology and to offer specific therapeutic approaches.

Osteoporosis in Men

Although the pathophysiology of osteoporosis in men has been a subject of active research in recent years, the relative contribution of hormones and aging, per se, remains to be elucidated. It is well established that androgen levels decrease with aging. Testosterone levels decrease by approximately 1.2% per year and the binding protein levels increase with aging, resulting in lower bioavailable testosterone. There is evidence that androgens exert their effect on bone through the action of IGF-1. IGF-1 levels are increased during puberty and are closely related to sex-steroid levels. With aging, lower levels of sex-steroid hormones result in decreased levels of IGF-1, with a reduction in bone formation and bone mass. Dehydroepiandrosterone, another androgen, declines slightly at the sixth decade without major changes thereafter. Contradictory evidence is available about the importance of this decline in dehydroepiandrosterone and of its administration in the treatment of male osteoporosis. Thus, osteoporosis in men appears to result from cellular and hormonal changes, which include lower levels of testosterone, dehydroepiandrosterone, and IGF-1 with subsequent lower osteoblast activity and higher osteoblast apoptosis. However, further study is necessary to delineate the specific roles of these factors in the decline of BMD and high rate of fractures in men after the seventh decade of life. Case reports of low bone mass and increased bone turnover in men with estrogen deficiency—either from an estrogen receptor abnormality or from an absence of aromatase, the enzyme responsible for the conversion of testosterone to estrogen—suggest that estrogen is required for normal bone homeostasis in men. Serum estrogen levels better predict BMD in men than do serum testosterone levels. In older men in whom both gonadotropin secretion and aromatase conversion are suppressed, estrogen acts as the principal sex-steroid-regulating bone resorption. Blocking the conversion of testosterone to estrogen with the use of an aromatase inhibitor has been shown to increase bone resorption in a short-term study conducted in healthy older men, further supporting a role for estrogen in bone metabolism. Some of the effects of testosterone on bone may be mediated through aromatization of testosterone to estrogen, a possibility that warrants further study. Ongoing studies will provide further information on the role of estrogen in the pathogenesis of osteoporosis in older men.

PRESENTATION

Osteoporosis is frequently underdiagnosed and undertreated by medical professionals. Osteoporosis is a silent disease, and symptoms may not appear until an incident fracture. Men and women can have osteoporosis prior to a fracture, which is why it is so important to consider clinical risk factors (see below) and possible BMD measurement in those at risk of osteoporosis. Osteoporosis may be detected on plain x-rays (usually a chest x-ray) either by the presence of vertebral fractures or by "osteopenia" in the x-ray report. As many as a third or more of those with "osteopenia" on an x-ray may have T-scores worse than -2.5, and as many as half will have T-scores in the -2.5 to -1.0 range. Therefore, persons who are diagnosed with "osteopenia" by plain x-ray should have BMD measurement. Osteoporosis may also present as an acute fracture. Most fractures that occur in old age are caused, at least in part, by osteoporosis, and it is important to initiate a therapeutic regimen in these adults. Even after a fracture, the diagnosis is often not considered. Three-quarters of postmenopausal women with a distal radius fracture were either undiagnosed or not treated in one study. As many as 50% of women with a hip fracture leave the hospital without treatment. The overall risk of repeat fracture within the first year is 20%. Fractures that are likely related to osteoporosis and thus should trigger treatment with an approved agent include wrist, vertebral, and hip fractures. Those with such fractures do *not* require BMD testing. Frequently, these fractures are classified as fragility fractures, because there is often little or no trauma associated with the event.

Secondary Causes of Osteoporosis

The diagnosis of idiopathic or primary osteoporosis is made by bone density measurement prior to fracture or by incident fracture. Secondary osteoporosis is the consequence of diseases or drugs that affect bone either directly (involving changes in bone cells or bone matrix composition) or indirectly (by increasing endogenous or ectopic hormonal production). It is important to exclude diseases that may present as fracture or with low bone mass in the evaluation of women and men with osteoporosis. Table 117-3 lists the major secondary causes of osteoporosis along with laboratory tests used to exclude each disease. These laboratory tests should be considered in persons who present with acute compression fracture or who present with a diagnosis of osteoporosis by BMD measurement. Men are more likely to have a secondary cause of osteoporosis than are women. The most commonly reported secondary causes of osteoporosis in men include hypogonadism and malabsorption syndromes. Secondary osteoporosis can be either prevented or treated if suspected by the

TABLE 117-3

Recommendations for Evaluation of Secondary Causes of Osteoporosis

DISEASE	EVALUATION
Endocrine abnormalities	
Primary hyperparathyroidism	Ionized calcium, PTH
Paget's disease	Alkaline phosphatase
Osteomalacia	Serum + urine Ca, PO_4, alkaline phosphatase, and 25(OH)D
Hyperthyroidism	T_4 and thyroid-stimulating hormone
Hypogonadism (men only)	Bioavailable testosterone and prolactin
Cushing's syndrome	Urinary free cortisol
Neoplastic conditions	
Multiple myeloma	Complete blood count and serum and urine protein electrophoresis
Bone metastases	Serum calcium and bone scan
Other conditions	
Alcoholism	Medical history
Malabsorption syndromes	Medical history, antigliadin, and antiendomysial antibodies
Medications	
Glucocorticoids	Medical history
Anticonvulsants	25(OH)D and alkaline phosphatase
Heparin (long term)	Medical history
Excess thyroid hormone replacement	Thyroid-stimulating hormone

clinician. Immobilization predisposes to bone mineral loss; thus, a program of early mobilization of hospitalized elderly patients is important. Mild-to-moderate vitamin D deficiency may give rise to osteoporosis rather than to osteomalacia; oral replacement may prevent its occurrence. An additional secondary cause of osteoporosis in men relates to the use of luteinizing hormone-releasing hormone agonists in prostate cancer. Luteinizing hormone-releasing hormone agonists suppress the pituitary gland, decrease testosterone and estrogen to castrate levels, and render men. Several retrospective studies have found increased fracture rates in this population of men. A number of studies demonstrate rates of bone loss that are up to three- to fourfold higher in men treated with luteinizing hormone-releasing hormone agonists, as compared with annual rates of bone loss in normal aging men.

Other medications also may have a detrimental effect on bone. Consideration should be given to dose adjustment, discontinuation of the medications, or preventive treatment. Medications that adversely affect BMD include glucocorticoids, excess thyroid supplementation, anticonvulsants, methotrexate, cyclosporine, and heparin. In older adults, glucocorticoids and thyroid hormone are used quite commonly; accordingly, clinicians should consider the effects these medications may have on the already increased risk of fracture, when prescribing these to older adults.

The prevalence of osteoporosis in adults taking glucocorticoids is approximately 30%. Bone loss typically occurs in the first 6 months of therapy and increases with increasing glucocorticoid dose. Glucocorticoids both suppress bone formation through direct effects on osteoblasts and increase resorption through indirect effects on osteoclasts. Glucocorticoid-induced osteoporosis is preventable if treatment is considered when treatment with corticosteroids is initiated. Replacement of gonadal hormones and treatment with bisphospho-

nates or intermittent PTH has been shown to prevent bone loss in patients taking glucocorticoids. Other measures for prevention of bone loss are calcium and vitamin D supplementation and reduction of glucocorticoid dose to the lowest effective dose for the underlying disease. High doses of high-potency inhaled glucocorticoids may also result in bone loss, and the initiation of preventive measures is important.

EVALUATION

Bone Density Measurement

BMD, or bone mass measurement, is the best single predictor of fracture, although previous fracture, maternal history of hip fracture, and age are important additional independent predictors of fracture. BMD of the hip, spine, wrist, or calcaneus may be measured by a variety of techniques. The preferred method of BMD measurement is dual-energy x-ray absorptiometry. BMD of the hip, anteroposterior spine, lateral spine, calcaneus, and wrist can be measured using this technology. Quantitative computerized tomography is also used to measure BMD of the spine. Specific software can adapt computerized tomography scanners for BMD measurement. The advantages of dual-energy x-ray absorptiometry over quantitative computerized tomography include lower cost, lower radiation exposure, and better reproducibility over time. Peripheral dual-energy x-ray absorptiometry (measures wrist BMD) or ultrasonography of the calcaneus may be useful for general osteoporosis screening, and these have the advantage of reduced cost and portability. Peripheral bone densitometry (performed at the heel, finger, or forearm) is highly predictive of hip, spine, wrist, rib, and forearm fractures for the subsequent 12 months. Assessment of BMD should be considered for (1) postmenopausal women younger than 65 years with one or more additional risk factors (other than menopause); (2) all women older than 65 years, regardless of additional risk factors; and (3) women considering therapy for osteoporosis, if BMD testing would facilitate the decision. A study of more than 200 000 postmenopausal women from more than 4000 primary-care practices in 34 states reported that approximately 50% of this population had low BMD that was previously undetected, including 7% of women with osteoporosis. An additional study found that screening postmenopausal women with BMD reduced the incidence of hip fracture by 36%. These studies suggest that efforts should be made to increase BMD measurements in postmenopausal women. However, further investigation is required to determine if BMD screening is truly cost effective and to assess the usefulness of various clinical decision rules in medical practice. Postmenopausal women who present with a fracture do *not* require BMD to confirm a diagnosis of osteoporosis or to determine severity. In addition, postmenopausal women with a significant kyphosis and clinical risk factors also do *not* require BMD testing. Instead, both of these subsets of patients deserve treatment for osteoporosis. It is important to recognize that age is a much more important factor than BMD in determining fracture risk. The 10-year probability of a fracture in an 80-year-old is more than twice as great as the probability of fracture in a 50-year-old with the same BMD T-score (Figure 117-5).

BMD may also be used to establish the diagnosis and severity of osteoporosis in men and should be considered in men with

Age (years)	T-score 0	T-score -0.5	T-score -1.0	T-score -1.5	T-score -2.0	T-score -2.5	T-score -3.0
50	3.8	4.7	5.9	7.4	9.2	11.3	14.1
55	4.1	5.3	6.7	8.5	10.7	13.4	16.8
60	5.1	6.5	8.2	10.4	13.0	16.2	20.2
65	6.3	8.0	10.0	12.6	15.6	19.3	23.9
70	7.1	9.0	11.5	14.6	18.3	22.8	28.4
75	7.0	9.1	11.8	15.2	19.4	24.5	30.8
80	7.7	9.9	12.7	16.2	20.5	25.6	31.8

FIGURE 117-5. Ten-year probability of fracture in women by age and T-score. *(Data from Kanis et al. Osteoporos Int. 2001;12:989–995.)*

TABLE 117-4

Risk Factors for Osteoporotic Fracture

POTENTIALLY MODIFIABLE	NONMODIFIABLE
Current cigarette smoking	Personal history of fracture
Low body weight (<127 lb)	History of fracture in first degree relative
Estrogen deficiency	Advanced age
Early menopause (<45 yr of age)	
Prolonged premenopausal amenorrhea (>1 yr)	Female sex
	White or Asian race
Low calcium intake (lifelong)	Dementia
Alcoholism	
Taking sedative medication	History of corticosteroid medication
Impaired eyesight	Taking seizure medication
Recurrent falls	
Inadequate physical activity	Poor health/frailty
Arms usually required to stand	
Poor health/frailty	

low-trauma fracture, radiographic changes consistent with low bone mass, or diseases known to place an individual at risk of osteoporosis. Data relating BMD to fracture risk were originally derived from studies completed in women, but recent data suggest that similar associations may be valid in men as well. Assessment of BMD should also be strongly considered in both perimenopausal women and elderly men who are about to undergo long-term treatment with corticosteroids. Bone densitometry less frequently can be used to assess response to therapy. However, usually 2 years between tests are necessary to obtain accurate and useful information. Biochemical markers of bone turnover yield much quicker information about compliance and success of therapy (see below).

Clinical Risk Factors

While recent approaches to the patient with osteoporosis have based treatment on T-scores, assessment of clinical risk factors can improve identification of individual patients who are more likely to suffer from vertebral and nonvertebral fractures. This is particularly important, since the majority of fractures occur in postmenopausal women with T-scores that are better than −2.5. The age of the patient is the single most important contributor to fracture risk. Additional important factors include a previous fracture history as an adult, history of fracture risk in a first-degree relative, body weight less than 127 lb, current history of smoking, and corticosteroid use for more than 3 months (Table 117-4). Impaired vision, early estrogen deficiency, dementia, frailty, recent falls, low calcium and vitamin D intake, low physical activity, and alcohol consumption of more than two drinks per day are additional clinical risk factors. Prior recent fracture is a very strong predictor of future fracture. The increased risk is similar in both men and women and is the same as the risk of a first fracture in a woman who is 10 years older. Half of patients will re-fracture within 10 years, and half of those will occur within 2 years of the first fracture. Therefore, most elderly patients with a prior fracture are candidates for treatment. If additional clinical risk factors are present in such patients, BMD testing is not needed before initiating therapy. Conversely, in those patients without a history of fracture, clinical risk factors are useful in identifying women who should have BMD testing (Figure 117-6).

Since many osteoporotic fractures result from falls, it is essential to assess patients for fall risk and to institute preventive measures where appropriate. The causes of falls are often multifactorial and include medications, poor vision, impaired cognition, maladaptive devices, alcohol, orthostatic hypotension, impaired balance and gait, environmental hazards, and lower extremity weakness. Recent studies suggest that specific performance measures can help to identify those at greater risk of falling. Individuals who are unable to maintain a semitandem stand for 10 seconds with their eyes open are at increased risk. A normal gait velocity of less than 0.7 m/s also predicts a greater propensity to fall. Additional office-based screening tests that identify potential fallers include the inability to complete

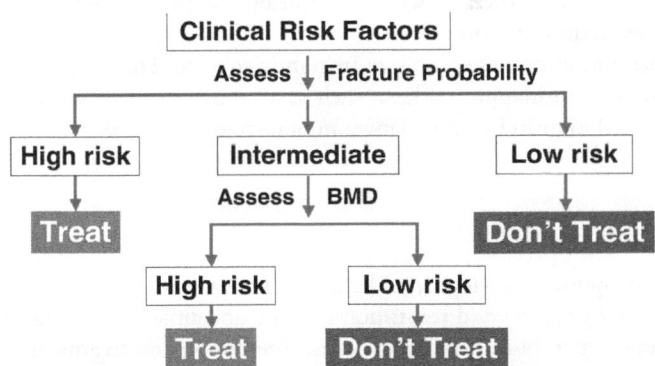

FIGURE 117-6. Approach to the osteoporosis patient. Clinical factors such as described in the text and in Table 117–4 help to assess contributions to fracture risk. The absence of these factors in younger women places them at low risk, and they do not require treatment. The presence of several factors in patients ≥70 yrs, particularly prior history of fracture and a fall history, suggests that treatment should be initiated without the need for densitometry. The greatest challenge lies in those patients who may have one or two clinical factors such as postmenopausal with poor calcium intake and low physical activity. Assessment of BMD can help stratify fracture risk and guide the decision to treat. The combination of clinical factors plus the BMD can be used in fracture risk calculators (for example, see http://courses.washington.edu/bonephys/FxRiskCalculator.html) to determine the cost effectiveness of treatment. *(From Kanis J. Annual meeting of the ASBMR, Philadelphia, PA; 2006.)*

the timed up and go test in 14 seconds, the inability to maintain a one leg stand for at least 5 seconds, and a score of less than 19 on the performance-oriented mobility assessment.

Biochemical Markers of Bone Turnover

Serum and urine biochemical markers that reflect collagen breakdown (or bone resorption) and bone formation are useful to monitor treatment of osteoporosis. Higher levels of resorption markers have been associated with increased hip fracture risk, decreased bone density, and increased bone loss in older adults in some studies. However, biochemical markers in many patients with osteoporosis will lie within the normal range. In addition, there is often substantial overlap of marker values in women with high and low bone density or rate of bone loss. Therefore, at this time, markers are not recommended for screening or diagnosis of osteoporosis. In addition, few studies have compared the response of a particular marker (or combination of markers) and bone density to therapy in order to determine the magnitude of decrease of a biochemical marker necessary to prevent bone loss or, more importantly, fracture. Markers are most useful in assessing the response of an individual patient to treatment. Markers of bone resorption and formation decrease in response to antiresorptive treatment and increase in response to PTH, a treatment with anabolic properties. The advantage of the serum versus urinary markers is that the intrapatient variability tends to be lower with serum markers, thus reducing error. It is important to assess a marker before initiating treatment. Many of the osteoclast-specific markers can then be rechecked as early as 6 weeks after beginning therapy. Bone markers yield quicker information, cost less, and incur no radiation when compared to repeating bone densitometry to assess response to therapy. The total alkaline phosphatase that is commonly obtained in routine serum chemistries, while not specific, is also useful to determine response to antiresorptives. However, it should be rechecked 12 weeks after beginning therapy. Successful antiresorptive therapy, which also means compliance, will result in a reduction of serum levels of markers of both resorption and formation, since these processes are tightly coupled. However, changes in bone formation markers, such as alkaline phosphatase, will lag several months behind changes in bone resoption markers.

MANAGEMENT

Osteoporosis develops in older adults when the normal processes of bone formation and resorption become uncoupled or unbalanced, resulting in bone loss. Osteoporosis prevention and treatment programs, then, should focus on strategies that minimize bone resorption and maximize bone formation, as well as strategies that reduce falls. A number of nonpharmacological and pharmacological options are available to health-care providers (see Tables 117-5 and 117-6). Modification of risk factors (see Table 117-4) is an important first step in preventing osteoporotic fractures in older adults.

Nonpharmacological

Exercise

Exercise is an important component of osteoporosis treatment and prevention programs. Data in older men and women suggest a posi-

TABLE 117-5

Treatment of Osteoporosis in Older Adults

Exercise	Walking and weight-bearing three times a week
Physical therapy	Postural exercises, gait and/or balance training, and muscle strengthening
Calcium (carbonate or citrate)	1200–1500 mg qd
Vitamin D (cholecalciferol)	Minimum 800 IU qd, may need 2000–5000 IU qd
Bisphosphonate	
• Alendronate	70 mg po once a week
• Risedronate	35 mg po once a week
• Ibandronate	150 mg po once a month, 3 mg IV push once every 3 months
• Zoledronate	5 mg IV infusion (15 min) once a year
Teraparatide	20 μg SC qd
Strontium ranelate	2 g po QHS

tive association between current exercise and hip BMD. Among regular exercisers, those who reported strenuous or moderate exercise had higher BMD at the hip than did those who reported mild or less-than-mild exercise. Similar associations were seen for lifelong regular exercisers and hip BMD. In a randomized study of women at least 10 years past menopause, the group receiving calcium supplementation plus exercise had less bone loss at the hip than did those assigned to calcium alone. Furthermore, high-intensity strength training effectively maintains femoral neck BMD as well as improves muscle mass, strength, and balance in postmenopausal women compared to nonexercising controls, suggesting that resistance training would be useful to help maintain BMD and to reduce the risk of falls in older adults.

Marked decrease in physical activity or immobilization results in a decline in bone mass; accordingly, it is important to encourage older adults to be as active as possible. Weight-bearing exercise, such as walking, can be recommended for older adults who should be encouraged to start slowly and gradually increase both the number of days and the time walked each day. Physical therapy is an important part of osteoporosis treatment programs, especially after acute vertebral compression fracture. The physical therapist can provide postural exercises, alternative modalities for pain reduction, and can suggest changes in body mechanics that may help prevent future falls and fracture. Gait training or balance training along with muscle strengthening can help to prevent falls, even for relatively frail elders. A meta-analysis of randomized clinical trial interventions to reduce falls concluded that all types of exercises achieved similar benefits in balance, endurance, flexibility, and strength. The key message is to prescribe a program for those patients who are mobile and functional enough, in addition to cognitively capable, to participate.

Nutrition

Calcium and vitamin D are required for bone health at all ages. Elemental calcium, 1200 to 1500 mg/day, for postmenopausal women and men older than 65 years is needed to maintain a positive calcium balance. The amount of vitamin D required is at least 800 IU/d, although recent evidence suggests that as much as 2000 IU of cholecalciferol per day and more are required to obtain appropriate

TABLE 117-6

Pharmacological Effect of Osteoporosis Medications on Bone Cellularity

COMPOUND	OSTEOBLAST	ADIPOCYTE	OSTEOCLAST
Bisphosphonates	↑ differentiation ↑ activity ↓ apoptosis		↓ differentiation ↓ activity ↑ apoptosis ↓ activity
Calcitonin			↑ apoptosis
PTH	↑ activity ↑ survival ↑ differentiation	↓ differentiation	↑ activity
SERMs			↓ differentiation ↓ activity
Strontium Ranelate	↑ activity ↑ differentiation ↑ activity	↓ differentiation	↓ activity ↓ survival ↑ activity
Vitamin D	↑ differentiation ↓ apoptosis	↑ transdifferentiation to osteoblasts	

PTH, parathyroid hormone; SERMs, selective estrogen receptor modulators; ↑, increase; ↓, decrease.
Duque G, Troen BR. Understanding the Mechanisms of Senile Osteoporosis: New Facts for a Major Geriatric Syndrome. J Am Geriatr Soc. 2008;56:935–941.

serum levels (25(OH) vitamin D ≥80 nmol/L) effective for fall and fracture prevention. Calcium plus vitamin D can increase or maintain bone density in pre- and postmenopausal women and prevent hip and other nonvertebral fractures in older adults. Serum levels of 25(OH) vitamin D up to 120 nmol/L are associated with greater BMD. Furthermore, women with acute hip fracture have lower 25(OH) vitamin D levels and higher PTH levels than do women admitted for elective hip replacement with or without osteoporosis by BMD, supporting a role for vitamin D deficiency and secondary hyperparathyroidism in hip fracture. In a recent meta-analysis, 800 IU/d of vitamin D reduced fracture risk and fall risk, whereas 400 IU/d did not. Thus, adequate calcium and vitamin D should be recommended to all older adults, regardless of BMD, in order to maximize bone health. Furthermore, supplementation with vitamin D enhances the BMD response to bisphosphonates.

Two recent prospective studies examined the effect of additional nutritional factors on bone loss and fracture risk in older adults. The Framingham Osteoporosis study found that higher baseline magnesium, potassium, and fruit and vegetable intakes were associated with higher baseline BMD. In men, increased potassium and magnesium intakes were associated with lower bone loss at the femoral neck. Additionally, this study showed a correlation of hip fractures with higher serum levels of homocysteine. Although homocysteine levels are associated with vitamin B-12, serum levels of this vitamin have not been associated with lower BMD, suggesting that the role homocysteine plays in bone biology remains to be elucidated. However, other studies have not found a clear association of homocysteine levels and fracture. Lower baseline protein intake or percent of total energy from animal protein, however, has been associated with greater bone loss at the femoral neck and lumbar spine. In another prospective cohort study, the Study of Osteoporotic Fractures, BMD was not associated with the ratio of animal to vegetable protein intake, but a higher ratio of animal/vegetable protein intake was associated with greater femoral neck bone loss and increased risk of hip fracture. These studies suggest that nutritional factors other than calcium and vitamin D are important for bone health in older adults. Prospective randomized studies are indicated to further elucidate the role of nutrition in prevention and treatment of osteoporosis in older adults.

Pharmacological

Estrogen Replacement Therapy

Multiple studies demonstrate that postmenopausal estrogen use will prevent bone loss at the hip and spine when initiated within 10 years of menopause, and other studies suggest that older women with low initial bone mass gain more bone than younger women. However, there have been few prospective studies of ERT (estrogen replacement therapy) and fracture prevention. One was a small study that demonstrated a reduction in vertebral fractures in postmenopausal women with transdermal estradiol, compared to placebo. The Women's Health Initiative study demonstrated a 24% reduction in all fractures and a 33% reduction in hip fractures in women taking estrogen plus progestin. However, the Women's Health Initiative study also concluded that the overall risks of estrogen plus progestin outweighed the benefits, including those associated with reduction of fractures.

Few studies have evaluated the use of estrogen in women in older than 70 years. Observational data, however, from the Study of Osteoporotic Fractures support a protective effect of current estrogen use against hip fracture, even in the oldest women. Furthermore, small short-term studies suggest that older women are responsive to estrogen treatment, and a recent study demonstrated that ERT increased BMD of the spine and hip in frail older women with just 9 months of treatment. Other studies suggest that low-dose estrogen, in combination with calcium and vitamin D, has an additive effect on bone turnover in women older than 70 years of age. Lower doses of estrogen are also effective in reducing bone resorption and bone loss in older women; the lower doses also result in fewer side effects than the usual replacement doses typically used by clinicians. In a randomized placebo-controlled study, 0.25 mg/day was as effective as 0.5 and 1.0 mg/day of 17β-estradiol in reducing biochemical markers of bone turnover in 75-year-old women, compared to placebo. In this study, the side-effect profile of 0.25 mg/day was similar to placebo and significantly different from the two higher doses. In a longer-term study, 0.3 mg/day conjugated equine estrogen plus 2.5 mg/day medroxyprogesterone acetate increased bone density of the hip and spine in older women who were vitamin D replete. While a recent report from the Women's Health Initiative study demonstrates cardiovascular benefit in women aged 50 to 59 years who took estrogen, at this time, better alternatives to treatment of osteoporosis in older patients exist. Therefore, in elderly patients, particularly those at least 5 to 10 years postmenopausal, estrogen is not recommended.

Bisphosphonates

Bisphophonates have gained wide acceptance as the primary antiresorptive treatment for osteoporosis. In postmenopausal women, both alendronate and risedronate reduce vertebral, nonvertebral, and hip fracture risk. Ibandronate has been shown to reduce vertebral fracture incidence. Although bisphosphonates have demonstrated their effectiveness in fracture prevention and gain in bone mass, their effectiveness in the very old (75 years and older) remains unclear because of the limited number of subjects included in the major trials. One of the major advantages of bisphosphonates is the dosing, since these can be given at different intervals from weekly to annually, depending on the medication used. Bisphosphonates act on the osteoclast, inhibiting differentiation and activity and inducing apoptosis. Additionally, there is recent evidence showing that bisphosphonates can enhance bone formation through the inhibition of bone marrow adipogenesis and induction of osteoblastogenesis. The only study using alendronate in older adults (>75 years) is a subpopulation of the Fracture Intervention trials. Alendronate reduced the risk for vertebral fracture, which was not affected by the subject's age. In addition, the absolute risk reductions for hip fractures in women aged 75 to 85 years with low BMD increased with age, supporting an increase in the cost effectiveness of bisphosphonate treatment in older patients. Currently, the recommended dose of alendronate is 70 mg weekly, together with calcium and vitamin D. Patients with low levels of 25(OH) vitamin D exhibit poorer response to bisphosphonate therapy. Conversely, supplementation with vitamin D enhances the BMD response to alendronate.

In the Hip Intervention Programme trial of risedronate, women aged 70 to 79 years with osteoporosis and women aged 80 years and older with at least one nonskeletal risk factor for hip fracture or a low BMD were assessed. This study did not show a reduction in nonvertebral fractures in women older than 80 years; however, it is possible that a proportion of them were not osteoporotic, as a result of the subject selection process. Indeed, even pooled data analysis from the Hip Intervention Programme, Vertebral Efficacy with Risedronate Therapy—Multinational (VERT-MN), and VERT North America (VERT NA) trials in patients older than 80 years with documented osteoporosis did not reveal a reduction in nonvertebral fracture risk (such as wrist, rib, and pelvis).

The efficacy of risedronate in women older than 80 years in reducing vertebral fracture risk was demonstrated using a post hoc pooling of data from three randomized, double-blind, controlled, 3-year fracture end point trials (Hip Intervention Programme, VERT-MN, and VERT NA). In individuals treated with risedronate ($n = 704$; 2.5 or 5 mg/day), the risk of new vertebral fractures was 81%

lower than for those treated with placebo ($n = 688$, $p < 0.001$) after 1 year. Additionally, the magnitude of the risk reduction associated with risedronate was larger in the first year of treatment of patients 80 years and older, but the efficacy was still apparent after 3 years of treatment. The recommended dose of risedronate is 35 mg weekly in combination with calcium and vitamin D.

The MOBILE (Monthly Oral iBandronate In LadiEs) study has shown efficacy for monthly ibandronate administration up on BMD, similar to that observed for the weekly administration of either alendronate or risedronate. In addition, it has also been approved for intravenous administration every 3 months to treat postmenopausal osteoporosis. However, its effectiveness in very old populations has not been studied. Recently, intravenous zoledronate, at a dose of 5 mg/IV yearly, has been assessed for its efficacy on fracture prevention in a population of 3889 patients (mean age 73 years) who were treated for 3 years. In this randomized control trial, intravenous zoledronate markedly lowered the risk of hip fracture by 41% and reduced nonverterbral fractures, clinical fractures, and clinical vertebral fractures by 25%, 33%, and 77%, respectively. The FDA has recently approved zoledronate for the treatment of osteoporosis. The zoledronate-treated subjects exhibited a small but statistically significant greater incidence of atrial fibrillation, which generally resolved within a month. A more recent study has demonstrated that treatment of hip fracture patients with zoledronate reduced subsequent vertebral and non-hip-non-vertebral fractures and also reduced overall mortality. In addition, no difference in the incidence of atrial fibrillation in the zoledronate-treated patients was found. Although these results suggest that zoledronate could become the treatment of choice for osteoporosis, with the advantage that compliance would be assured, the possibility of side effects suggests that more studies are required in the frail elderly population.

Bisphosphonates are generally safe, but administration can cause a rash or transient hypercalcemia. In addition, oral bisphosphonates can cause esophageal irritation and ulceration. Hence, patients need to take oral bisphosphonates with 8 oz of water and remain upright for at least 30 minutes. Intravenous bisphosphonates can acutely cause fever, myalgia, transient leukopenia, acute-phase reaction, arthralgia, headache, bone pain, and atrial fibrillation. However, the flu-like symptoms can be successfully ameliorated with acetaminophen. In addition, the symptoms are less prevalent with subsequent administration.

Longer-term administration has been associated with osteonecrosis of the jaw. It is important to stress that the great majority of cases of osteonecrosis of the jaw occur in patients with underlying neoplastic disease who have received high doses of intravenous pamidronate or zolendronate. The risk of osteonecrosis of the jaw in patients with postmenopausal osteoporosis taking oral bisphosphonates is exceedingly low. In fact, it has been estimated that the risk of osteonecrosis of the jaw is only 0.7/100 000 people per year, which is comparable to the risk of dying from lightning in New Mexico and much less than dying by anaphylaxis from a shot of penicillin (32/100 000 people per year).

Calcitonin

Calcitonin is a peptide hormone that is used to treat osteoporosis. It is available as a subcutaneous injection and a nasal spray. The advantages of a nasal spray over injectable calcitonin are fewer reported side effects and greater patient acceptance. Calcitonin has been shown to increase bone density in the spine and to reduce vertebral fractures.

In epidemiologic studies, calcitonin reduces hip fractures, although in clinical trials hip bone density does not increase. A recent 5-year study demonstrated a decrease in vertebral fracture in women on nasal spray calcitonin (200 IU/d), as compared to those women on placebo; in this study, 400 and 100 IU did not have any significant effect on vertebral fracture rate. Bone density at any site and markers of bone turnover did not change, compared to placebo. Nasal spray calcitonin does not appear to be as effective in preventing fractures as other approved agents; therefore, its use should be limited to those women who are unable to tolerate other treatments. The only current indication for the use of calcitonin is for analgesic treatment in acute compression fractures, in Paget's disease of bone and in bone pain because of metastatic disease.

Selective Estrogen Receptor Agonists

The selective estrogen receptor modulators are agents that act as estrogen agonists in bone and heart but act as estrogen antagonists in breast and uterine tissue. These medications have the potential to prevent osteoporosis or heart disease without the increased risk of breast or uterine cancer. Tamoxifen, an agent used in breast cancer treatment, has been shown to have beneficial effects on bone in several studies but has stimulatory effects on the uterus; it is not approved for treatment or prevention of osteoporosis. Raloxifene, a nonsteroidal benzothiophene, is a newer selective estrogen receptor modulator that has been approved for prevention and treatment of osteoporosis in postmenopausal women. In one study of postmenopausal osteoporotic women, raloxifene resulted in decreased bone turnover and increased BMD of the hip, spine, and total body bone density, as compared to placebo. Furthermore, raloxifene did not increase endometrial thickness for more than 2 years and had positive effects on the lipid profile. A later study examined the effect of 60 or 120 mg/day raloxifene on fractures. Raloxifene decreased the risk of new vertebral fractures (relative risk [RR] 0.5 [0.4–0.8] to 0.7 [0.6–0.9]). There was no difference in nonvertebral fracture incidence in the raloxifene-treated groups, as compared to placebo. BMD of the lumbar spine and femoral neck increased in both raloxifene-treated groups compared to placebo. Interestingly, the BMD increases with raloxifene were modest in this study, yet the reduction in vertebral fracture risk was clinically significant, suggesting that antiresorptive agents have effects on bone that are not reflected in BMD measurement. The major serious adverse effect of raloxifene was an increase in venous thromboembolic events, including deep vein thrombophlebitis and pulmonary embolism events (RR 3.1 [1.5–6.2]). However, raloxifene-treated women in this study had a reduced risk of breast cancer incidence (RR 0.3 [0.2–0.6]). In a 6-month study, raloxifene had effects on bone histomorphometry and bone turnover that were similar in direction to conjugated equine estrogen but were lower in magnitude.

Parathyroid Hormone

PTH, when administered daily subcutaneously, markedly increases bone mass and BMD. Multiple studies demonstrate significant reductions in vertebral and nonvertebral fracture risk. Administration of PTH increases osteocalcin, a marker of bone formation, more rapidly than deoxypyridinoline cross-links, a marker of bone resorption, suggesting early uncoupling of the bone remodeling cycle and providing a potential mechanism for the anabolic effect on bone. The PTH analog teraparatide effectively increases spinal BMD in osteoporotic men and women and reduces both vertebral and nonvertebral fractures in postmenopausal women. PTH also enhances BMD in glucocorticoid-dependent osteoporosis. The recommended dose is 20 μg SQ/d. Indications for PTH include a T-score worse than −3.5 or prevalent fractures in the setting of a T-score worse than −2.5. In addition, patients who continue to fracture or lose BMD after 2 years of bisphosphonate treatment are also candidates for PTH. The side effects that occurred more frequently in the PTH-treated groups were headache, nausea, dizziness, and hypercalcemia. The major limitations to the use of PTH in the elderly are its significant cost and the mode of administration, since subcutaneous dosages require an appropriate cognitive status, a high degree of motivation, and a significant level of functional independence. At present, studies suggest that PTH should *not* be combined with bisphosphonate therapy, since concurrent bisphosphonate treatment appears to blunt the BMD response to PTH. PTH therapy should continue no longer than 2 years. It is very important, however, to treat with an antiresorptive after discontinuation of PTH, in order to maintain gains in BMD.

Other Agents

Strontium Ranelate This agent appears to acts as both an anabolic and an antiresorptive medication for osteoporosis. Treatment with strontium ranelate reduces vertebral fractures by 40% in postmenopausal women with osteoporosis. The Treatment of Peripheral Osteoporosis study in postmenopausal women showed a reduction in the relative risk for all nonvertebral fractures of 16% and a decline of 19% for all major fragility fractures (hip, wrist, pelvis, sacrum, ribs, sternum, clavicle, and humerus) after 3 years of treatment at a dose of 2 g/d. In a subgroup analysis of high-risk women (age >74 years, femoral neck BMD T-score less than −3.0), the strontium reduced hip fractures by 36%. The fact that this agent is given as a soluble powder favors its acceptance and tolerance except for mild gastrointestinal adverse effects (nausea and diarrhea), which usually resolved by 3 months of treatment.

Denosumab Denosumab is a fully humanized monoclonal antibody directed against RANKL. It binds with high affinity and, therefore, blocks RANKL-stimulated osteoclast formation and activation. Although denosumab is still undergoing experimental trials, a phase 2 dose-ranging study in postmenopausal women with low BMD demonstrated that subcutaneous administration once every 6 months produced increases in lumbar spine and hip BMD at 12 months comparable to that seen with alendronate, both of which were significantly better than placebo. Adverse events were not significantly different from placebo- or alendronate-treated patients. More recently, a phase 3 trial (FREEDOM study) demonstrated that denosumab administered to post-menopausal woman once every six months for three years reduced vertebral, non-vertebral, and hip fractures by 68%, 20%, and 40%, respectively. These benefits were accompanied by increases in bone mineral density at both lumbar spine and total hip of 9.2% and 6.0%, respectively. There were no significant differences in adverse events between placebo and denosumab treatment.

Osteoporosis in Nursing Homes

There is increasing concern about the underdiagnosis and undertreatment of patients with osteoporosis in special settings, such as long-term care institutions. Institutionalized patients, whether mobile or immobile, are at high risk of osteoporosis. All institutionalized patients should be treated with a combination of vitamin D (minimal dose of 800 IU/d) plus calcium (1500 mg/day). Because the frail elderly may be markedly insufficient for vitamin D or exhibit an unpredictable response to supplementation, the serum level of 25(OH) vitamin D should be obtained before beginning supplementation. Preliminary reports suggest that between 1500 and 5000 IU/d may be needed. If the 25(OH) vitamin D level is ≤50 nmol/L, patients should be started on 2000 IU/d of cholecalciferol. For those who are frankly deficient (25(OH) vitamin D less than 20 nmol/L), 50,000 units of ergocalciferol weekly for 4 weeks should be administered, followed by 2000 IU of cholecalciferol per day. The serum level of 25(OH) vitamin D should again be assessed 8 to 12 weeks later. Additionally, the presence of risk factors and/or previous fractures strongly supports the use of pharmacological treatment with either antiresorptives or anabolics. The clinician should consider the patient level of functionality, quality of life, and life expectancy before starting pharmacological treatment for osteoporosis in a long-term care setting. However, since hip fractures lead to a decline in the quality of life and life expectancy, and fracture risk reduction can be achieved as quickly as 6 months of treatment, pharmacological approaches are justified in institutionalized patients who are at risk.

FURTHER READING

Adler RA. Epidemiology and pathophysiology of osteoporosis in men. *Curr Osteoporos Rep.* 2006;4:110–115.

Bischoff-Ferrari HA, Willett WC, Wong JB, et al. Fracture prevention with vitamin D supplementation: a meta-analysis of randomized controlled trials. *JAMA.* 2005;293:2257–2264.

Boonen S, Marin F, Mellstrom D, et al. Safety and efficacy of teriparatide in elderly women with established osteoporosis: bone anabolic therapy from a geriatric perspective. *J Am Geriatr Soc.* 2006;54:782–789.

Boonen S. Bisphosphonate efficacy and clinical trials for postmenopausal osteoporosis: similarities and differences. *Bone.* 2007;40:S26–S31.

Brown LB, Streeten EA, Shapiro JR, et al. Genetic and environmental influences on bone mineral density in pre- and post-menopausal women. *Osteoporos Int.* 2005;16:1849–1856.

Chan GK, Duque G. Age-related bone loss: old bone, new facts. *Gerontology.* 2002;48:62–71.

Chang JT, et al. Interventions for the prevention of falls in older adults: systematic review and meta-analysis of randomised clinical trials. *BMJ.* 2004;328:680.

Chapurlat RD, Delmas PD. Drug insight: bisphosphonates for postmenopausal osteoporosis. *Nat Clin Pract Endocrinol Metab.* 2006;2:211–219.

Chen P, Miller PD, Delmas PD, et al. Change in lumbar spine BMD and vertebral fracture risk reduction in teriparatide-treated postmenopausal women with osteoporosis. *J Bone Miner Res.* 2006;21:1785–1790.

Cherniack EP, Troen BR. Calciotropic hormones. In: Duque G., Kiel D., eds. *Senile Osteoporosis: Advances in Pathophysiology and Therapeutic Approach.* Springer-Verlag London Limited, pp. 34–46, 2008.

Colon-Emeric CS, Saag KG. Osteoporotic fractures in older adults. *Best Pract Res Clin Rheumatol.* 2006;20:695–706.

Dempster DW. Bone microarchitecture and strength. *Osteoporos Int.* 2003;14(Suppl 5):54.

Duque G. As a matter of fat: new perspectives on the understanding of age-related bone loss. *BoneKEy-Osteovision.* 2007;4:129–140.

Duque G, Troen BR. Skeletal aging. In: Chernoff, ed. *Geriatric Nutrition: The Health Professional's Handbook.* 3rd ed. Boston, MA: Jones and Bartlett; 2006:325–344.

Duque G, Troen BR. Understanding the Mechanisms of Senile Osteoporosis: New Facts for a Major Geriatric Syndrome. *J Am Geriatr Soc.* 2008;56:935–941.

Ganz DA, et al. Will my patient fall? *JAMA.* 2007;297(1):77.

Gimble JM, Zvonic S, Floyd ZE, et al. Playing with bone and fat. *J Cell Biochem.* 2006;98:251–266.

Hamann KL, Lane NE. Parathyroid hormone update. *Rheum Dis Clin North Am.* 2006;32:703–719.

Hampton T. Diabetes drugs tied to fractures in women. *JAMA.* 2007;297:1645.

Kanis JA, Oden A, Johnell O, et al. The use of clinical risk factors enhances the performance of BMD in the prediction of hip and osteoporotic fractures in men and women. *Osteoporos Int.* 2007;18(8):1033–1046.

Khosla S, Melton LJ. Osteopenia. *N Engl J Med.* 2007;356(22):2293–2300.

Lin JT, Lane JM. Rehabilitation of the older adult with an osteoporosis-related fracture. *Clin Geriatr Med.* 2006;22:435–447.

Lips P. Vitamin D status and nutrition in Europe and Asia. *J Steroid Biochem Mol Biol.* 2007;103:620–625.

Manuele S, Sorbello L, Puglisi N, et al. The teriparatide in the treatment of severe senile osteoporosis. *Arch Gerontol Geriatr.* 2007;44(Suppl 1):249–258.

Marie PJ. Strontium ranelate: new insights into its dual mode of action. *Bone.* 2007;40(Suppl 1):S5–S8.

Mundy GR, Elefteriou F. Boning up on ephrin signaling. *Cell.* 2006;126:441–443.

Roodman GD. Regulation of osteoclast differentiation. *Ann N Y Acad Sci.* 2006;1068:100–109.

Rosen CJ, Bouxsein ML. Mechanisms of disease: is osteoporosis the obesity of bone? *Nat Clin Pract Rheumatol.* 2006;2:35–43.

Roux C. Antifracture efficacy of strontium ranelate in postmenopausal osteoporosis. *Bone.* 2007;40:S9–S11.

Rubin J, Rubin C, Jacobs CR. Molecular pathways mediating mechanical signaling in bone. *Gene.* 2006;367:1–16.

Saquib N, von Muhlen D, Garland CF. Serum 25-hydroxyvitamin D, parathyroid hormone, and bone mineral density in men: the Rancho Bernardo study. *Osteoporos Int.* 2006;17:1734–1741.

Shoback D. Update in osteoporosis and metabolic bone disorders. *J Clin Endocrinol Metab.* 2007;92(3):747–753.

Suda T, Ueno Y, Fujii K, et al. Vitamin D and bone. *J Cell Biochem.* 2003;88:259–256.

Tanaka S, Nakamura K, Takahasi N, et al. Role of RANKL in physiological and pathological bone resorption and therapeutics targeting the RANKL-RANK signaling system. *Immunol Rev.* 2005;208:30–49.

Troen BR. Molecular mechanisms underlying osteoclast formation and activation. *Exp Gerontol.* 2003;38:605–614.

Troen BR. The regulation of cathepsin K gene expression. *Ann N Y Acad Sci.* 2006;1068:165–172.

Hip Fractures

Ram R. Miller ■ *Colleen Christmas* ■ *Jay Magaziner*

INTRODUCTION

Hip fracture is a major public health problem with significant consequences for the older patients, their families, and the health-care system. In 2003, there were 310,000 hospital admissions for hip fracture in the United States alone. Recent worldwide estimates are in the order of 1.6 million hip fractures annually. By the middle of this century, the number is expected to more than double. As seen in Figure 118-1, hip fracture incidence increases exponentially in both men and women with advancing age. The average age of a patient with hip fracture is 82 years. Although hip fractures are thought to be a condition faced primarily by older white women, approximately 20% of hip fractures occur in men, and, in the United States, 8% occur in nonwhites. Prominent risk factors for hip fracture are osteoporosis and propensity to fall. Underlying these essential conditions for having a hip fracture are the reduced bone strength and quality that are characteristic of osteoporosis and the multiplicity of medical, psychosocial, and environmental factors that lead to falls.

The direct medical and indirect nonreimbursed costs (e.g., unpaid caregiving services and lost wages of patients and caregivers) of hip fracture have been estimated at more than $15 billion annually in the United States. Of those who have a hip fracture, approximately 18% of women and 36% of men are expected to die within the first year of their fracture, with the most dramatic increases in mortality seen within the first few months of a fracture among those who are in the poorest health. Comparison of survival in women with hip fracture to similarly impaired women without fractures indicates that the fracture itself is responsible for nine extra deaths per 100 patients during the first 4 years following the fracture. There also is suggestion from epidemiological data on women that even in those with the fewest medical comorbidities and best functioning at the time of fracture, the mortality attributable to hip fracture continues to increase well beyond the first year post fracture. Causes of death in women and men are similar and approximately four times

greater than their nonfracture counterparts for heart disease, three times greater for cerebrovascular disease, and three times greater for chronic obstructive pulmonary disease. Interestingly, one recent study showed that men are far more likely than their nonfracture counterparts to die from infectious causes such as septicemia and pneumonia, in the first 2 years following hip fracture.

The intent of this chapter is to provide information about the medical and psychosocial status of the older patient who presents with a hip fracture and to discuss strategies for care and the role of the geriatrician in providing that care during the hospital stay and for the subsequent year or more of follow-up care.

WHAT TO EXPECT WHEN SEEING PATIENTS IN HOSPITAL

The cumulative effect of environmental exposures, lifestyle, and genetic influences results in a remarkably heterogeneous geriatric population. Aging impacts most organ systems, although the degree to which organs are impaired from aging varies from individual to individual. In addition, several chronic medical conditions may also exist in a given individual. Medical care of the patient with hip fracture must, therefore, be adapted to the individual patient's needs. This requirement for a tailored approach to care is both the challenge and the pleasure of geriatric medicine.

The changes that occur with aging physiology result in decreased resilience to stress, or the so-called "homeostenosis" in most organs. For example, older individuals have stiffening of their rib cages and decreased mucociliary clearance of their lungs, resulting in an increased propensity toward postoperative atelectasis and pneumonia and poorer tolerance of these complications when these do occur. By mechanisms that are yet to be understood, older individuals can more easily become delirious during the pre- and postoperative period. This complication not only increases the patient's risk of dying

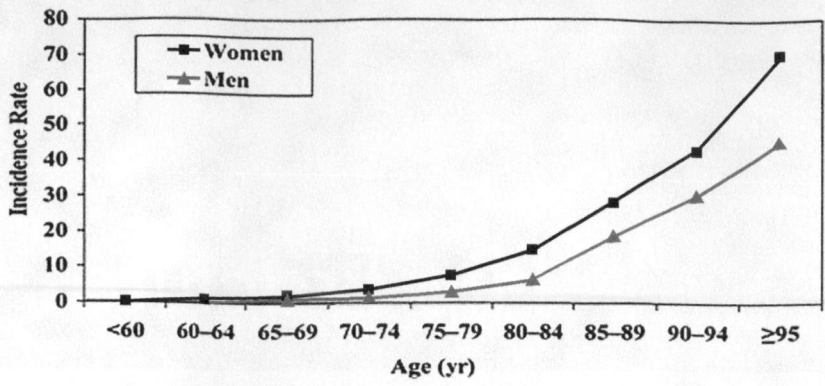

FIGURE 118-1. Age-specific incidence rates of hip fracture (per 1000 person-years): the Framingham study. *(Samelson et al. Am J Public Health. 2002;92(5):858–862.)*

in the coming year, but also can impact an individual's ability to participate in rehabilitation and significantly limit the patient's ability to recover after a fracture. Because of this decreased physiological reserve, older individuals are at particular risk of a wider range of iatrogenic complications and do not recover as well when complications and adverse events do occur. Thus, all interventions must be monitored very closely to quickly determine their impact on the patient.

Medical Presentation and Fracture Characteristics

Classically, a patient with hip fracture presents with a painful, shortened, and externally rotated lower extremity after a fall and landing on the affected hip. Usually, but not always, patients are unable to bear weight on the extremity. There are many exceptions to this description, however. While a small percentage of hip fractures occur without trauma preceding the fracture event, nearly a third do not recall or cannot give a clear history of the precipitating fall. In nondisplaced femoral neck fractures, the extremity may be neither shortened nor externally rotated, and patients with stable impacted

fractures or nondisplaced "hairline" fractures may be able to bear weight and ambulate. Occasionally, patients like this are sent home without fracture management but soon return for care, owing to continued pain and discomfort when ambulating. Thus, a better guiding principle is that all elderly patients with hip pain after trauma should be considered to have a hip fracture until proven otherwise. Similarly, patients having pain with gentle rolling of the lower extremity must be ruled out for hip fracture, irrespective of recollection of trauma.

Approximately half of all hip fractures occur in the area of the femoral neck (or "intracapsular fractures"), and the other half occur in the area between the greater and lesser trochanters ("intertrochanteric fractures" or "extracapsular fractures"). Far less common are fractures that occur within 5 cm below the lesser trochanter; these are called "subtrochanteric fractures." Patients with intertrochanteric fractures tend to be older than those with femoral neck fractures and are more likely to have multiple medical comorbidities pre-fracture. A schematic of the hip anatomy is shown in Figure 118-2, which also indicates the anatomy of the vascular supply

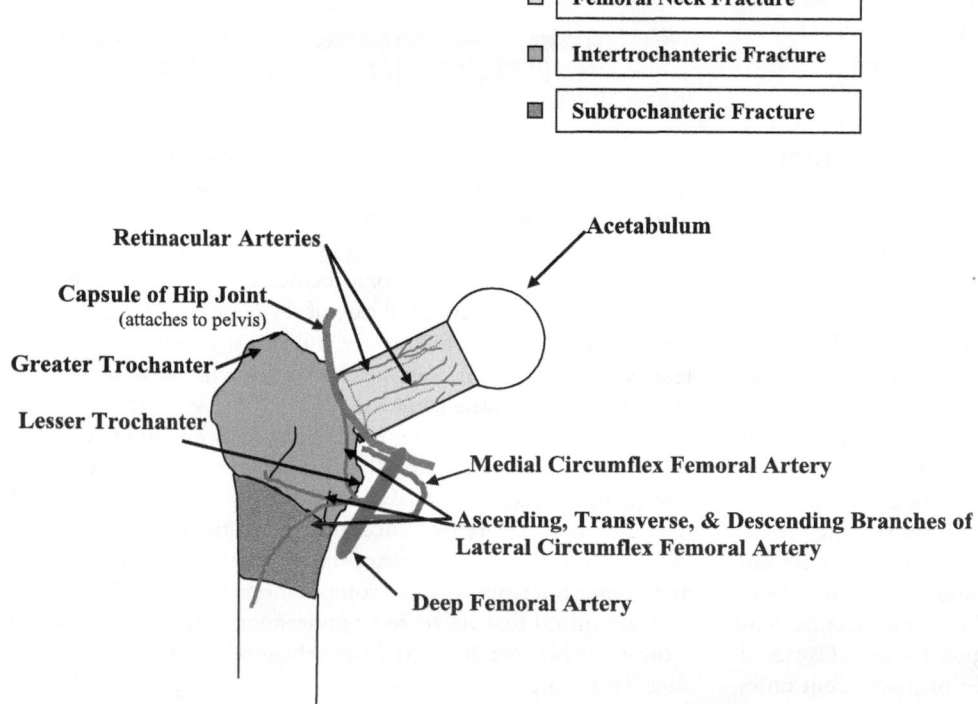

FIGURE 118-2. A schematic diagram of the anatomy of the hip.

to the hip region. This schematic is useful to understand the various surgical approaches to hip fracture care and the potential for blood loss at each site. As demonstrated in the schematic, the regions of the femoral neck and the femoral head derive their main blood supply from fine retinacular arteries that stem from the medial circumflex femoral artery. These delicate vessels are closely apposed to the femoral neck in this region. Therefore, a fracture in this region of the hip, particularly if any displacement occurs, is more likely to disrupt the vascular supply to the femoral neck and head, which can result in longer-term nonunion and osteonecrosis. Thus, fractures in the femoral neck region, particularly displaced fractures, are usually replaced rather than internally fixed. In contrast, the blood supply to the intertrochanteric area is plentiful and redundant, such that nonunion and osteonecrosis are less common in this region, and often fractures in this area heal well if internally reduced with screws, nails, or pins.

Cognitive Status

Dementia is a prominent risk factor for falls and fractures, so, not surprisingly, a significant number of patients with hip fracture have underlying cognitive impairment. Delirium is also a very common occurrence both at time of presentation to the emergency department and especially postoperatively, where up to 60% may develop confusion after hip fracture repair, with underlying dementia again being a powerful risk factor for the development of delirium. The presence of delirium and cognitive impairment very significantly portends a worse functional recovery for patients with hip fracture. Identification of underlying dementia and especially identification of risk factors for delirium are important both prognostically and so that some of the modifiable risk factors may be eliminated in hopes of reducing the occurrence of delirium. Given the high risk of delirium in this patient population, it is particularly important to prepare the patient and family emotionally for this potential complication, especially in those with identified risk factors for delirium, as the manifestations of delirium can be quite frightening to unprepared family members.

Risk factors for delirium in hospitalized patients have been well described by many sources. Some of the most consistently reported risk factors include advanced age, sensory impairment, male sex, presence of comorbid psychiatric disease, the use of psychoactive drugs, infection, polypharmacy, use of restraints, sleep deprivation, and undertreatment of pain. Allowing people to sleep at night and remain active during the day, minimizing sensory impairment, promptly removing unneeded tethers such as Foley catheters and IVs, providing daily orientation, and careful attention to pain and medications may be useful in reducing the incidence of delirium in patients with hip fracture, as has been demonstrated in geriatric general medical in-patients. Undertreatment of pain, particularly in cognitively intact individuals with fracture, appears to be a more powerful predictor of the development of delirium than use of narcotics. In one study, proactive geriatric consultation with recommendations on oxygen delivery, fluid balance, analgesia, elimination of unnecessary medications, regulation of bowel and bladder function, nutritional intake, mobilization, prevention of postoperative complications, assessment of environmental stimuli, and treatment of agitated delirium reduced the incidence of delirium overall by a third and the incidence of severe delirium by half.

The Geriatrician's Role in Caring for Patients with Hip Fracture on Entry into Acute Care and Recommendations Regarding Surgical Intervention

The geriatrician can serve a central role in caring for patients on entry into the acute hospital not only by evaluating the medical pre- and perioperative issues, and ensuring maximal medical stabilization prior to surgery, but also by providing vigilance and early detection of postoperative medical complications, by facilitating a smooth transition to rehabilitation or subacute care and by preparing the patient for long range preventive strategies to reduce future fractures.

Several studies demonstrate that services that use a multidisciplinary approach to acute care of the patients with hip fracture reduce medical complications and may shorten hospitalization, and the more involved the geriatrician is in providing or overseeing patient care, the greater the clinical benefits of the service. For example, a coattending model, in which both the geriatrics and the surgical services are responsible for the patient's care, is more effective than daily consultation, and daily consultation is more effective than twice-a-week consultation in most studies.

The geriatrician can first help by providing a "big picture" view of whether or not the patient will benefit from pursuing surgery to repair the hip or not. Although for most patients with hip fracture, surgical approaches will typically offer more benefits than nonsurgical approaches, surgical repair is usually presented as the only option, despite the fact that nonsurgical approaches may be equally or more appropriate for some selected patients. The clearest benefit of surgery over the usual nonsurgical approach of bed rest, pain management, bowel regimen, and prophylaxis against pressure ulcers and deep venous thrombosis is that surgery results in better anatomic alignment and better likelihood of ambulation. There is currently no evidence that surgery provides better pain control over bed rest. Thus, in patients who are unable to ambulate prior to the fracture and who are not likely to ambulate later, or for those in whom surgical risks are very high or life expectancy is very short, nonsurgical approaches may be considered. Geriatricians, like other providers, need to be careful not to prematurely judge the patient's likelihood of dying, since it may be difficult to base a prognosis on the presentation at the time of fracture and the determination of what might be most appropriate for a patient requires an understanding of that patient's prior status, goals, and priorities as well as the patient's medical conditions and psychosocial milieu to determine how the patient can best achieve those goals.

The majority of patients with a hip fracture will undergo surgical repair. The types of surgical approach and anesthesia employed are largely the purview of the surgeon and the anesthesiologist and often depend on local trends and the training of these physicians. Although, historically, regional anesthesia has been advocated over general anesthesia in frail elderly patients, observational studies suggest that there is little difference in short- and long-term outcomes with these two approaches.

In preparing a patient for hip fracture surgery, as with any surgery, one would determine the risks of cardiovascular, pulmonary, and other complications and strive to reduce those risks. (Refer to Chapter 35 for more details on the use of preoperative testing for risk stratification, preoperative pulmonary treatments, and the use of beta-blockers and other medications to reduce the risk of perioperative adverse cardiac events in high risk patients.) The geriatrician also is in a good position to step the patient and family through the many hospital and postacute care procedures and transitions that they can expect to encounter, thereby reducing uncertainty and alleviating anxiety at this unanticipated and challenging time.

Finally, while soliciting the preoperative history, the geriatrician is in a good position to use this opportunity to determine the patient's risk for subsequent falls and fractures. A thorough falls history should be obtained, including a complete description of the fall that led to the fracture as well as any previous falls, with particular attention to remediable risk factors to be altered prior to discharge back to home (see Chapter 54). Similarly, the geriatrician may begin to prepare the patient, family, and other providers about the need to evaluate for and treat osteoporosis to reduce the risk of subsequent fractures after discharge back to home (see Chapter 117).

POSTOPERATIVE CARE IN HOSPITAL

The Geriatrician's Role in Postoperative Care

Usually a patient will remain in the acute hospital for 2 to 5 days after surgery for hip fracture, although this may be longer in some health-care settings. Depending on the surgical approach used and the adequacy of the anatomic repair, most patients will resume a normal diet, have bladder catheters removed, and begin getting out of bed with physical therapy on postoperative day number 1. Early mobilization has been shown to be safe and is effective in minimizing deconditioning, reducing the risk of delirium, constipation, pneumonia, thromboembolism, and pressure ulcer formation. Adequate treatment of postoperative pain is useful in maximizing participation in physical therapy and increasing mobility.

The geriatrician must monitor the patient very closely for development of postoperative complications and is in a key position to detect subtle delirium that could be a harbinger of an ominous underlying complication, such as pulmonary embolus or pneumonia. Postoperative pulmonary complications are among the most lethal complications in this population, so the geriatrician should be particularly wary of these and enforce the use of deep breathing exercises with or without an incentive spirometer, early mobility, and use of physical and/or pharmacological approaches to reduce

the risk of deep venous thrombosis. Other important postoperative medical considerations the geriatrician may be particularly adept at managing are reducing polypharmacy, maximizing sensory input, explaining the treatments and progression of care to patients and family, and communicating across the transitions to reduce errors during this vulnerable time.

POSTFRACTURE CHANGES IN PHYSICAL AND PSYCHOSOCIAL FUNCTION AND IMPLICATIONS FOR CARE

Physical Function

Hip fractures have significant effects on functioning and body composition. Figure 118-3 shows the proportion of patients with hip fracture who were able to perform routine tasks involving lower extremities prior to their fracture and who are not able to perform them a year later. Twenty percent of those who could put their own pants on without assistance prior to their fracture will require assistance to do so a year later. More striking is the proportion of patients who will need assistance of another person or equipment to walk across a small room (40%), use the toilet (66%), or climb five stairs (90%). Instrumental tasks also are affected, with 62%, 53%, and 42% who could do their own housecleaning, get places out of walking distance independently, and shop without assistance, respectively, prior to their fracture, requiring assistance to perform these tasks a year later. Other functional consequences of hip fracture include increases in cognitive impairment and depressive symptoms, as well as increases in problems with gait and balance.

Psychological Status

The diagnosis of hip fracture conveys to patients and families a significant degree of psychological stress. Most lay persons are quite aware of the poor recovery of function for many individuals, the high rate of nursing home use and even long-term placement, and, for those who do return to the home, the high rates of dependency on others for care, at least transiently. Many patients and families

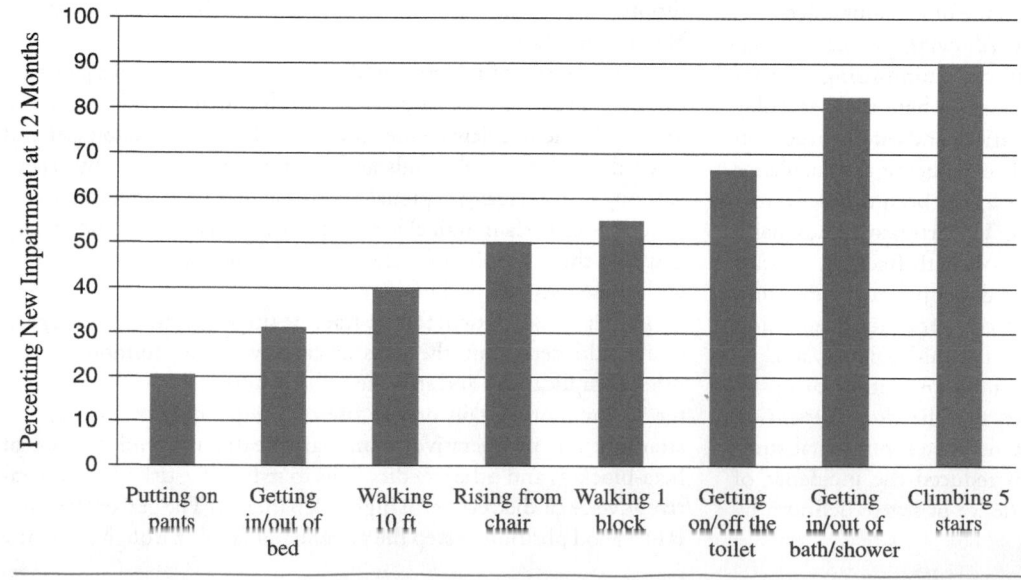

FIGURE 118-3. Lower extremity activities of daily living—percentage of those unimpaired pre-fracture with impairment at 12 months post fracture. (Magaziner et al. J Gerontol Med Sci 2000;55A(9):M498–M507.)

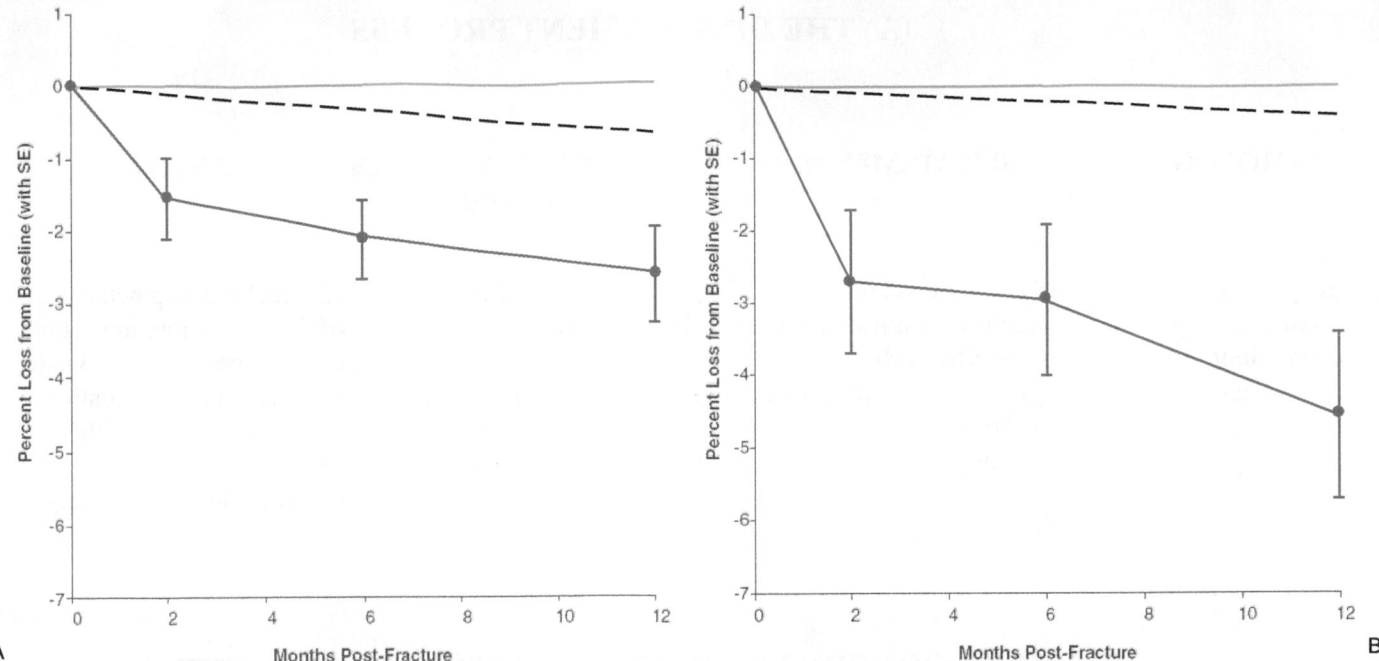

FIGURE 118-4. Expected and observed change in total hip bone mineral density (A) and femoral neck bone mineral density (B) during the 12 months following fracture. Legend for both panels: ● with solid line, hip fracture (observed mean and standard error); broken line, Study of Osteoporotic Fractures (SOF; expected mean based on interpolated data obtained for a 42.3-month period). *(Magaziner et al. Osteoporos Int. 2006;17:971–977.)*

believe that having a hip fracture signifies the "beginning of the end." It is likely that these facts, in addition to other physiological changes that happen with hip fracture or hip fracture repair, contribute to the high rates of postoperative depression that have been described. Patients may endorse depressive symptoms during their hospital stay and for up to 6 months after fracture; those who report symptoms of depression even transiently tend to recover less well than those who do not endorse depressive symptoms at all.

Physiologic Changes Post Hip Fracture

Changes in body composition also are notable after a hip fracture. The average woman who fractures a hip can expect to lose 3% to 6% of her muscle mass within 2 months of the hip fracture and to have an increase in fat mass of 3% to 4% during the postfracture year, under circumstances of usual care. Losses of bone mineral density also are profound in this already osteoporotic group of older women. In fact, older women lose nearly 3% of their total hip bone mineral density and more than 4.5% of their bone mineral density in the contralateral femoral neck during the year following a hip fracture. This is 12.5 times more than the loss of 0.5% that would have been expected in a group of women of the same age, comorbid disease status, and starting level of bone mineral density (Figure 118-4).

FUNCTIONAL RECOVERY POST HIP FRACTURE

Recovery in function following a hip fracture can be anticipated in many patients, despite the large numbers who fail to achieve prefracture levels, and this recovery appears to follow a sequence that may be instructive in deciding on the most appropriate intervention to recommend and/or provide during the postfracture year. After examining the patterns of recovery in several functional domains that are affected by hip fracture, it was noted that depression, upper

extremity activities of daily living, and cognitive function reach their peak recovery by approximately 4 months post fracture, while tasks associated with physical impairments such as balance and gait reach their natural plateau at approximately 9 months post fracture. Interestingly, the more complex tasks that are indicative of disability, such as performing lower extremity and instrumental tasks, recover by approximately a year if these are going to recover (Figure 118-5). This pattern of recovery seems to parallel the pattern by which disability develops according to the disablement process model proposed by Verbrugge and Jette (Figure 118-6).

When considering this pattern and the fact that different tasks recover at different postfracture times, it would seem worthwhile to consider delivery of targeted interventions in a way that addresses the specific deficits observed and takes full advantage of what we know

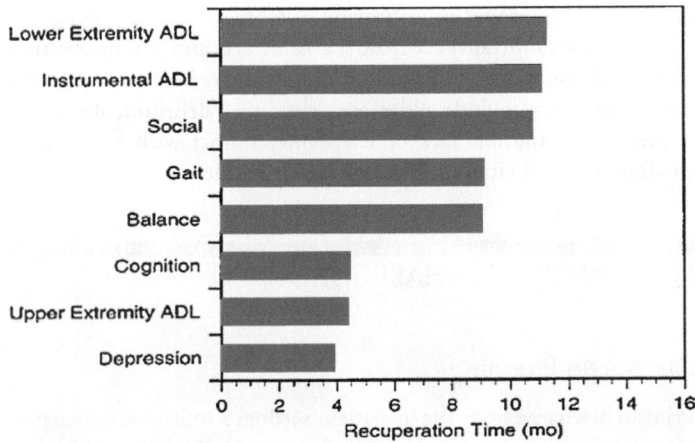

FIGURE 118-5. Time to recuperation following hip fracture in eight areas of function. *(Magaziner et al. J Gerontol Med Sci. 2000;55A(9):M498–M507.)*

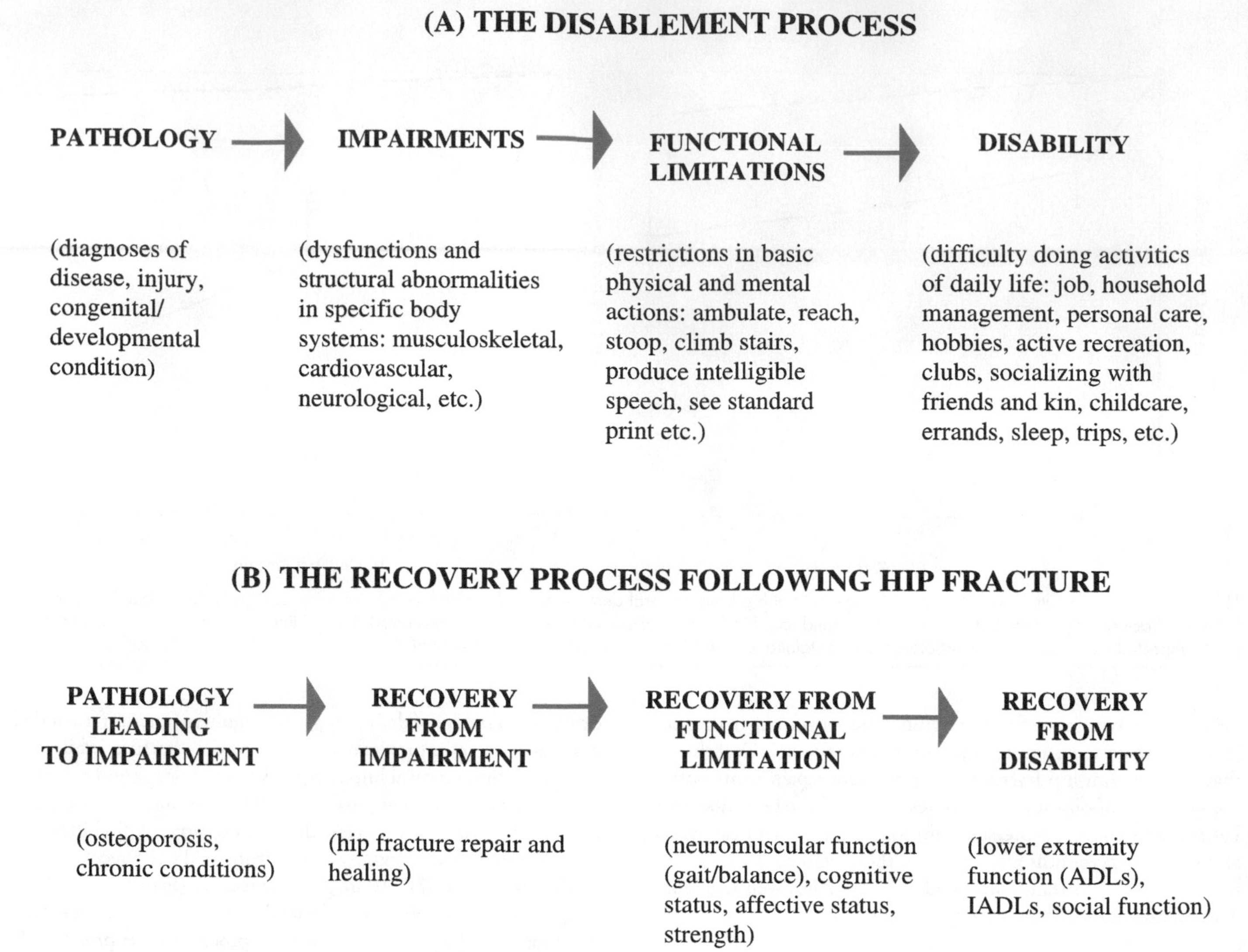

(A) THE DISABLEMENT PROCESS

PATHOLOGY → IMPAIRMENTS → FUNCTIONAL LIMITATIONS → DISABILITY

(diagnoses of disease, injury, congenital/ developmental condition)	(dysfunctions and structural abnormalities in specific body systems: musculoskeletal, cardiovascular, neurological, etc.)	(restrictions in basic physical and mental actions: ambulate, reach, stoop, climb stairs, produce intelligible speech, see standard print etc.)	(difficulty doing activities of daily life: job, household management, personal care, hobbies, active recreation, clubs, socializing with friends and kin, childcare, errands, sleep, trips, etc.)

(B) THE RECOVERY PROCESS FOLLOWING HIP FRACTURE

PATHOLOGY LEADING TO IMPAIRMENT → RECOVERY FROM IMPAIRMENT → RECOVERY FROM FUNCTIONAL LIMITATION → RECOVERY FROM DISABILITY

(osteoporosis, chronic conditions)	(hip fracture repair and healing)	(neuromuscular function (gait/balance), cognitive status, affective status, strength)	(lower extremity function (ADLs), IADLs, social function)

FIGURE 118-6. The disablement (A) and recovery (B) processes following hip fracture. (Verbrugge, Jette. Soc Sci Med. 1994;38:1–14 [Figure 118-6A]; Magaziner et al. J Gerontol Med Sci. 2000;55A(9):M498–M507. [Figure 118-6B])

about the recovery sequence. A sequence that might be appropriate is shown in Figure 118-7. It is also worthwhile to consider the risk factors for mortality and failure to recover with the ultimate goal of reducing risk as a way of improving outcomes. Among the known risk factors for mortality are male sex, older age, and having multiple comorbid conditions. Those factors known to be associated with poorer recovery include older age, male sex, delirium, dementia, depressive symptoms, lack of telephone contact with family after the fracture, and vitamin D deficiency at the time of fracture.

POSTFRACTURE REHABILITATION

Discharge Planning

Prior to discharge from the in-patient setting, a multidisciplinary assessment involving the geriatrician, the orthopedic surgeon, nursing, social work, physical therapy, and occupational therapy must be performed. The goal of this assessment is to decide on discharge plans and rehabilitation needs and goals. The following considerations should be taken into account: the patient's current level of function, the patient's postoperative medical and skilled nursing needs, the home environment, family and resources available, self-care skills, and requirements for activities of daily living. The geriatrician plays a key role in the coordination of the patient's care and communication with patients and families as patients transition through the health-care system, with regard to their medical needs, functional status, and living requirements. One critical role for the geriatrician is to ensure continuity of care. Recent studies have shown that, with each transition to a different site of care, there is the potential for an adverse effect on the care of patients with hip fracture, and physicians must, therefore, be vigilant to ensure adequate communication and good continuity of care to minimize this risk.

While the medical diagnoses and baseline functional status are important considerations of the ability of a patient to maximally recover function, return to a high quality of life may be even more dependent on the patient's support network and environment than the patient's medical illnesses. These factors will often dictate how long a patient needs to stay in in-patient rehabilitation before it is

Recovery Process	Possible Treatments
Treat Pathology	
Osteoporosis	Bone strengthening medications
Chronic conditions	Stabilize exacerbations, control complications
Treat Impairment	
Hip fracture	Surgical management to repair bone
Reduce Functional Limitations	
Neuromuscular training	Gait training, balance training, strength
Cognitive	Medical stabilization, orientation therapy
Affective	Medication, psychological therapy
Minimize Disability	
ADLs	Physical therapy
IADLs	Occupational therapy
Social activity	Social engagement therapies

FIGURE 118-7. Hip fracture treatments suggested by recovery sequence.

safe to discharge that patient back to home. For example, if a patient had been previously living independently in a three-story home where the bathroom and bedroom are on the second floor and the kitchen on the first, one could surmise that that individual would need one of three things to occur before the individual could be discharged home: (1) the patient would need to be able to negotiate a full flight of stairs independently and safely, (2) the patient would need to rearrange the home to live on the ground floor (e.g., move a hospital bed into the dining area and use a commode chair that someone emptied regularly) and be able to transfer and ambulate short distances on a level surface independently, or (3) the patient would need a responsible caregiver to assist with daily tasks. Obviously, to achieve option 1 would require more work for the patient and likely more time in the rehabilitation facility than option 3, and the more time a caregiver were available to assist the patient, the lower the target functional achievement needed for a safe discharge to home. Not all patients have access to assistance in their homes, but some families or friends are able to make significant adjustments to be able to provide this support, usually un-reimbursed, which can be a major stressor when the caregiver has taken a prolonged period away from work to do so. The geriatrician or internist may help the potential caregivers anticipate and prepare for the patients' upcoming needs by assessing the home environment and discussing these issues early in the course of the hip fracture treatment.

Rehabilitation Services

The majority of patients with hip fracture will undergo a period of rehabilitation therapy after the fracture. Rehabilitation services are provided to the patient with hip fracture only if both of the following requirements are fulfilled: (1) the patient has a functional loss and (2) the individual is able to participate in rehabilitation efforts. Based on these principles, individuals with severe cognitive impairment, or those with unresolved delirium and who may be unable to participate in standard rehabilitation and will require special attention, those with severe pre-fracture disability (e.g., bed-bound pre-fracture), and those with terminal illness may not qualify for rehabilitation services.

This rehabilitation typically takes place in one or more of the following settings: an inpatient rehabilitation setting, which can be either acute or subacute, or on an outpatient basis, either at home or in a clinic. In the United States, rehabilitation is typically limited by Medicare reimbursement and rarely goes beyond 30 days. In one study, approximately half of all patients were discharged to a skilled nursing facility for rehabilitation, 20% received rehabilitation in an acute rehabilitation facility, 15% were discharged to home, and 14% were discharged directly to long-term care.

Inpatient acute rehabilitation units are usually located in specialized units of an acute care hospital, in dedicated rehabilitation hospitals, or in skilled nursing facilities with specialized acute rehabilitation units. Patients with complex medical or rehabilitation needs and with good endurance may receive their rehabilitation in the acute setting. The requirements for acute rehabilitation are that the individual must be able to participate in therapy for at least 3 h/d and that they require at least two therapies (example physical therapy and occupational therapy).

Patients with less complex medical or rehabilitation needs, who may not be able to participate in 3 h/d of rehabilitation but who otherwise have a functional decline that would benefit from rehabilitation and are unable to be discharged to home, typically receive rehabilitation in the subacute setting. Subacute inpatient rehabilitation is usually delivered in skilled nursing facilities. These patients typically receive interventions from a licensed professional 5 days a week, however, on a less intense basis than in the acute rehabilitation setting.

Patients with more mild impairments or with good support at home may receive their rehabilitation on an outpatient basis, either at home or at an outpatient facility. In order to qualify for home rehabilitation, patients must have a functional decline that would benefit from rehabilitation, have good home supports that enable them to be discharged to home, and be homebound and therefore unable to attend rehabilitation at an outpatient clinic. Since rehabilitation will be delivered by home-care professionals in the patient's home, heavy equipment must not be required.

For individuals with less complex rehabilitation needs, services may be delivered in an outpatient clinic. Outpatient rehabilitation may follow rehabilitation in the acute, subacute, and home-care settings and may continue until the individuals attain their rehabilitation goals.

The Role of the Geriatrician in the Rehabilitation Setting

The geriatrician may also play a key role in the medical management in these rehabilitation settings, especially for the majority of patients with hip fracture who undergo rehabilitation in skilled nursing facilities. Regardless of the setting of rehabilitation, medical care depends on the following principles: continued postoperative hip fracture care, treatment of chronic medical conditions, prevention of complications from the functional decline and immobility following hip fracture, and prevention of future falls and fractures.

Despite ongoing therapy by rehabilitation professionals, increased risk for complications related to immobility, such as DVT, pressure ulcers, and constipation, persist into the rehabilitation setting. Thus, continued vigilance to their prevention and detection must be exercised. Based on current recommendations, DVT prophylaxis should be continued for 28 to 35 days after hip fracture surgery. Pressure ulcers are common after hip fracture surgery, with reports of an incidence rate of stage II or greater ulcers within 21 days of fracture of approximately 35%. Given the decreased mobility and frequency of use of narcotic analgesics for postoperative pain, constipation is a common occurrence and efforts should be made to prevent this with an adequate bowel regimen.

Many patients with hip fracture in the acute and subacute rehabilitation settings receive their medical care from a physician who was not their primary-care provider pre-fracture and who is not familiar with the patients' history or support system. Care for these patients represents a challenge for the attending physician, as these patients are typically older and with significant and complicated comorbid disease. More than 75% of patients with hip fracture have at least four comorbid medical conditions prior to their fracture. In addition to supervising the care of the hip fracture and any sequelae, the attending physician in inpatient rehabilitation setting must ensure that these chronic medical conditions continue to be addressed while the patient is being cared for in these settings.

What to Tell the Patient and Family to Expect in Terms of Function

Because hip fracture may result in persistent functional limitations and disability, patients with hip fracture may anticipate significant changes in their lifestyle. The geriatrician needs to provide support and encouragement during the initial recovery period following hip fracture surgery when pain and disability are greatest. Patients and their families can be reassured that patients are likely to experience significant improvements in their lower extremity function during the first few months postfracture, while at the same time cautioned that lower extremity limitations can be prolonged. Up to 50% of elders who had previously been independent may be dependent on mobility aids, such as a cane or a walker, for ambulation at 1 year post fracture. These limitations and fear of recurrent falls may result in limitation in their activities.

These declines in function may result in loss of independence in the older patient, and, as a result, the older patient with hip fracture may be facing the prospect of moving from their independent residence to a higher level of care for the first time. Individuals who have an injury, such as a hip fracture, as a result of a fall are 10 times more likely to be admitted to a skilled nursing facility. This may be one of the most frightening aspects of the postfracture recovery facing the patient with hip fracture, and helping them to understand that this is an expected reaction to having a hip fracture may help them to overcome this fear and resume their activities more quickly.

Older patients and those with other health problems may need to be told that their recovery may be slower than for others. Compared to younger patients, those who are older than 85 years have been found to require longer rehabilitation stays, have worse recovery of lower extremity function, are more likely to be discharged to long-term care, and are more likely to have persistent pain, which may be accompanied by Activities of Daily Living (ADL) limitations and reduced quality of life. Depression and cognitive limitations should also be discussed with patients and families. It is important for them to understand that depressive symptoms and cognitive limitations are common after a hip fracture. They should also be informed that these changes are not always persistent, as depressive symptoms and cognitive limitations will frequently resolve with limited intervention for the next 2 months, and that treatment for mild depression is often useful to avoid any lingering anxiety or depression that accompanies the hip fracture.

THE GERIATRICIAN'S ROLE IN CARING FOR PATIENTS WITH HIP FRACTURE FOLLOWING REHABILITATION

After the patient has returned home, the focus in follow-up care is on monitoring to be sure that the patient is making expected gains in recovery, on evaluation for contributing causes if expected gains are not achieved, and on preventing subsequent falls and injury. Most people will have recovered most of the function they will recover in the first 6 months after fracture, but the occurrence of complications may alter that course and many will continue to realize gains with longer amounts of time. A home safety evaluation is often high yield, done either by direct observation or by providing the patient or an involved care member a check list, as is determination of gait and balance with consideration for the use of an appropriate assistive device.

Problems with gait and balance remain a problem for older adults after hip fracture, and these individuals remain at high risk of recurrent falls. Community-based multidisciplinary fall risk assessment (example: home environment assessment, medication review, vision testing, postural blood pressure measurement, gait and balance testing, and targeted neurological, musculoskeletal, and cardiac examinations) followed by interventions directed at these risks has been shown to reduce fall risk and to be cost effective in older adults at risk of recurrent falls. Gait and balance training interventions in the clinical setting have also been shown to reduce recurrent falls rates.

Despite the fact that almost all older adults who have a hip fracture have preexisting osteoporosis, only a minority receives treatment for osteoporosis prior to the fracture and only this same minority typically receives these treatments after the fracture. The occurrence of a minimal trauma fracture, such as hip fracture, should provide an opportunity to address bone health in an older adult. A hip fracture is associated with an increased risk of subsequent fracture, including a second hip fracture. Although there is only one published randomized study on the secondary prevention of fractures in elders post

TABLE 118-1

Focus of the Geriatrician at Various Stages of Care for Patients with Hip Fracture

SETTING OF CARE	WHAT THE GERIATRICIAN IS FOCUSED ON
Acute hospital—preoperative	1. Do surgery or nonoperative approaches best meet this patient's goals? 2. What are the preoperative cardiac, pulmonary, cognitive, and other risks for this patient and what can be done to reduce these? 3. What must be done to prevent postoperative complications, especially pressure ulcers, delirium, anemia, and pneumonia? 4. Why did this person fall and how can this information be used to ensure that medical status is optimized for surgery or nonoperative management?
Acute hospital—postoperative	1. What can be done to prevent postoperative complications, such as pressure ulcers, delirium, anemia, and pneumonia? 2. Is pain adequately treated? 3. Is there delirium and how can it be addressed? 4. What is the next appropriate level of care and when is the patient ready to go there? 5. Who will next provide medical care and how can continuity of care be ensured?
Subacute setting—rehab	1. Is pain adequately treated? 2. Are there any complications requiring treatment, such as constipation, delirium, pneumonia, venous thrombosis, deconditioning, and pressure ulcers? 3. Are there signs of active depression limiting participation in rehabilitation and what can be done to address this during rehabilitation and after discharge? 4. Why did this person fall and what can be done to reduce the chances of future fractures? 5. Is this person on appropriate osteoporosis therapy? 6. What does this person need to do to be able to go home safely? 7. Who will next provide medical care and how can continuity of care be ensured?
Outpatient setting—primary care	1. Is this person receiving appropriate interventions to prevent falls and fractures and increase activity level and reengagement into community life? 2. Is this person safe in the current living arrangement? 3. Is recovery occurring in the expected sequence and in the expected time frame? 4. Is pain resolved?

hip fracture that demonstrated a benefit of a bisphosphonate therapy (i.e., zoledronic acid), interventions such as vitamin D and calcium supplementation, weight-bearing exercise, and pharmacological treatment with other antiresorptive agents such as bisphosphonates or the anabolic agent teriparatide, are also believed to be of benefit and should be considered.

Although hip protectors have recently received significant attention for their potential to reduce hip fractures, many older adults and their care providers may prefer their use to taking additional medication. The evidence for the efficacy of hip protectors in prevention of hip fracture is conflicting. Meta-analyses suggest that these offer little or no benefit for patients in randomized studies. As a result, these devices should not be considered as alternatives to the other fall reduction and bone-strengthening interventions listed above.

CONCLUSIONS

Care for the older patients with hip fracture represents one of the greatest challenges for the geriatrician because of the multiplicity of medical and psychosocial factors involved in their postfracture care. A summary of some of the key issues a geriatrician should focus on at various stages of hip fracture care appears in Table 118-1. Answering these questions requires vigilant attention preoperatively, postoperatively, in the rehabilitation setting, and after rehabilitation efforts have terminated. Although a hip fracture event has significant consequences for patients and their families, through this attention and communication with patients, families, and the other clinicians involved in the care of the patients as they transition through the various sites of care, it is the goal of the geriatrician to minimize long-term adverse effects and to ensure that the overall well-being of the patient is maximized.

ACKNOWLEDGMENTS

The overview of hip fractures presented in this chapter is derived, in part, from research supported by the National Institute on Aging Grant R37 AG09901 (Baltimore Hip Studies Project) and National Institute on Aging Grant P60 AG12583 (Claude D. Pepper Older Americans Independence Center Junior Faculty Award to Dr. Ram R. Miller). The authors also wish to express their appreciation for the research assistance provided by Christopher D'Adamo, Doctoral Candidate, Epidemiology, University of Maryland, Baltimore.

FURTHER READING

Boockvar KS, Litke A, Penrod J, et al. Patient relocation in the six months after hip fracture: risk factors for fragmented care. *J Am Geriatr Soc.* 2004;52(11):1826–1831.

Fox KM, Magaziner J, Hebel JR, Kenzora JE, Kashner TM. Intertrochanteric versus femoral neck hip fractures: differential characteristics, treatment, and sequelae. *J Gerontol Med Sci.* 1999;54(12):M635–M640.

Fox KM, Magaziner J, Hawkes WG, et al. Loss of bone density and lean body mass after hip fracture. *Osteoporos Int.* 2000;11(1):31–35.

Gilbert TB, Hawkes WG, Hebel JR, et al. Spinal anesthesia versus general anesthesia for hip fracture repair: a longitudinal observation of 741 elderly patients during 2-year follow-up. *Am J Orthop.* 2000;29(1):25–35.

Inouye SK, Bogardus ST Jr, Charpentier PA, et al. A multicomponent intervention to prevent delirium in hospitalized older patients. *N Engl J Med.* 1999;340(9):669–676.

Lyles KW, Colon-Emeric CS, Magaziner JS, et al. The HORIZON Recurrent Fracture Trial. Zoledronic acid and clinical fractures and mortality after hip fracture. *N Engl J Med.* 2007;357(18):1799–1809. [PMID:17878149]

Magaziner J, Hawkes W, Hebel JR, et al. Recovery from hip fracture in eight areas of function. *J Gerontol Med Sci.* 2000;55A(9):M498–M507.

Magaziner J, Simonsick EM, Kashner TM, et al. Predictors of functional recovery one year following hospital discharge for hip fracture: a prospective study. *J Gerontol Med Sci.* 1990;45(3):M101–M107.

Magaziner J, Wehren L, Hawkes WG, et al. Women with hip fracture have a greater rate of decline in bone mineral density than expected: another significant consequence of a common geriatric problem. *Osteoporos Int.* 2006;17:971–977.

Marcantonio ER, Flacker JM, Wright RJ, Resnick NM. Reducing delirium after hip fracture: a randomized trial. *J Am Geriatr Soc.* 2001;49(5):516–522.

Morrison RS, Magaziner J, McLaughlin MA, et al. The impact of post-operative pain on outcomes following hip fracture. *Pain.* 2003;103(3):303–311.

Samelson EJ, Zhang Y, Kiel DP, et al. Effect of birth cohort on risk of hip fracture: age-specific incidence rates in the Framingham study. *Am J Public Health.* 2002;92(5):858–862.

Siu AL, Boockvar KS, Penrod JD, et al. Effect of inpatient quality of care on functional outcomes in patients with hip fracture. *Med Care.* 2006;44(9):862–869.

Verbrugge LM, Jette AM. The disablement process. *Soc Sci Med.* 1994;38:1–14.

Wehren LE, Hawkes W, Orwig D, et al. Gender differences in mortality after hip fracture: the role of infection. *J Bone Mineral Res.* 2003;18(12):2231–2237.

Myopathy, Polymyalgia Rheumatica, and Temporal Arteritis

Yuri R. Nakasato ■ *Bruce A. Carnes*

SKELETAL MUSCLE, AGING, AND DISEASE

Skeletal muscle is a large and important organ system in the human body. Disorders and diseases of muscle are common in late life and have a major impact on function and quality of life. Many diseases affect muscle and are considered forms of myopathy. Myopathies are generally considered to be inflammatory or noninflammatory and will be addressed below. Loss of skeletal muscle mass owing to any disease or condition is called sarcopenia. Sarcopenia derives from the Greek and translates as "poverty of flesh." As a medical term, sarcopenia is nonspecific and can be caused by aging, disuse, wasting illness, or starvation or can be a secondary consequence of ischemia or neuropathy. Table 119-1 describes the characteristics of each of these forms of sarcopenia and highlights implications for care of the older adult. Sarcopenia can also develop in the course of some myopathies. Sarcopenia caused by aging itself is difficult to characterize since aging is often accompanied by the other contributors to loss of muscle described in Table 119-1.

Sarcopenia is now definable based on formal assessment of body composition using dual-energy x-ray absorptiometry. Similar to the use of relative bone mass to make the diagnosis of osteoporosis, dual-energy x-ray absorptiometry can yield estimates of lean body mass, which can be reported as absolute values or as scores relative to normal gender-specific values and skeletal size. In order to adjust for differences in skeletal size, the "relative skeletal muscle index" (RSMI) is defined as the predicted or measured (dual-energy x-ray absorptiometry) muscle mass (kg) divided by stature in square meters (RSMI = kg/m^2). On this scale, sarcopenia is defined by index values less than 2 standard deviations below the gender-specific mean for RSMI in a healthy, younger population. Thus, cutoff values for sarcopenia would be less than 7.26 kg/m^2 for males and 5.45 kg/m^2 for females. Since aging tends to alter body composition, with reduced muscle and bone and increased extracellular fluid volumes, the prevalence of sarcopenia increases with age. Sarcopenia

defined as RSMI less than 2 standard deviations below normal occurs in approximately 15% of people aged 60 to 69 years and approximately 40% of people older than 80 years.

MYOPATHIES

Idiopathic Inflammatory Myopathies (IIM)

Several of the most important diseases that primarily affect muscle are inflammatory in nature, are together termed idiopathic inflammatory myopathies, and carry labels using the term "myositis." The most common forms include polymyositis (PM), dermatomyositis (DM), and inclusion body myositis (IBM). Each will be described in the sections below. Since all three are often treated with glucocorticoids, a separate section discusses steroid treatment.

Polymyositis

PM is an IIM that affects all ages, with approximately one-third of cases in persons older than 65 years. Females are affected more than males. While the exact pathophysiology is not known, muscle biopsy shows inflammation that is mediated by T cells, mostly CD8+ T cells and macrophages causing perimysial and perivascular infiltrations. The inflammatory cells surround and invade non-necrotic muscle fibers, leading to necrosis at various stages alternating with regeneration and replacement by fibrous connective tissue and fat.

PM usually presents in an insidious fashion, and the course may be subacute or chronic with either no or mild pain. Common systemic features include fatigue, weight loss, arthralgias, and fever. Skin sensation and reflexes are typically normal. Symmetrical proximal weakness manifests in the neck flexors and extensors, as well as the shoulders and hips; dysphagia may occur in 25% of cases.

TABLE 119-1

Conditions That Contribute to Sarcopenia

	INTRINSIC MUSCLE AGING	DECONDITIONING/DISUSE	WASTING OWING TO CANCER, HIV, INFLAMMATORY CONDITIONS, OR CHRONIC DISEASES	STARVATION (PROTEIN MALNUTRITION) OR INCREASED METABOLIC DEMANDS	ISOLATED MUSCLE LOSS OWING TO LOCALIZED NERVOUS SYSTEM DISEASE OR CARDIOVASCULAR DISEASE
Myopathy	Not a myopathy, considered normal	Yes, considered abnormal	Yes, considered abnormal	Yes, considered abnormal	Yes, considered abnormal
Etiology	Normal intrinsic aging process	Loss of stimulation to muscle protein synthesis and maintenance of neuromuscular junctions. Similar to effects of low-gravity environment.	Increased inflammatory markers	Lack of sufficient protein reserves to counteract for muscle catabolism. Fasting results in decreased synthesis and increased breakdown of both myofibrillar and soluble muscle proteins and creates alternative sources of energy.	Peripheral vascular disease with consequent ischemia of an extremity, severance of a specific peripheral nerve with paralysis, cardiovascular accidents with paresias or paralysis, and loss of neuromuscular junctions because of similar conditions.
Creatinine kinase (CK)	Normal	Normal	Normal	Normal	Normal, unless there is an infarct of the region.
Potential implications for aging	Isolated effects of aging are hard to define, since most older adults also have other conditions that contribute to sarcopenia. The muscular system is integrated with other organ systems and is affected by disorders in other systems.	Levels of activity tend to decrease with aging. Many diseases reduce activity and cause secondary deconditioning.	Many wasting diseases increase in prevalence with age.	Calorie and protein intake can decrease with age and many conditions. Gastrointestinal absorption of nutrients may also decrease owing to several conditions that occur in older adults.	Cardiovascular and neurological conditions are common in older adults.
Usual presentation	Very chronic across decades of later life	Acute, subacute, or chronic	Acute, subacute, or chronic	Rarely acute. Usually subacute and chronic	Acute or subacute onset, eventually chronic
Caloric ingestion	Normal	Normal	Normal	Abnormal	Normal
Usual age of presentation	Starts around fourth decade of life	Any age	Any age	Any age	Any age
Approximate rate of loss	~1% per year	~1% per day	~1% per day	~1% per day	~1% per day
Usual outcome	Irreversible	Reversible	Potentially reversible	Reversible	Irreversible, partially reversible, or potentially reversible in rare cases
Histology	Muscle atrophy with no evidence of necrosis: loss of muscle cells, decrease in the size of existing muscle cells. Affecting type 2B cells more at the beginning, then affecting all types.	Muscle atrophy with no evidence of necrosis: decrease in size of muscle cells (fiber).	Muscle atrophy with no evidence of necrosis: decrease in the size of existing muscle cells. There could be loss of muscle cells.	Muscle atrophy with no evidence of necrosis: decrease in the size of existing muscle cells.	Muscle atrophy unless there is an infarction where muscle necrosis ensues.
Treatment	No cure. However, exercise can hypertrophy existing muscle cells and improve muscle function to compensate for the decrease in muscle cells and minimize the clinical impact of the muscle loss over time.	Aerobic and anaerobic exercise. Encourage physical therapy and occupational therapy.	Correction of the underlying cause and aerobic and anaerobic exercises	Nutritional correction and aerobic and anaerobic exercises	Rehabilitation exercise for recovery of remaining upper motor neurons for plasticity as in the case of stroke. Stent placement or angioplasty or surgery in the case of peripheral vascular disease. Aerobic and anaerobic exercise.

Creatinine kinase (CK) is elevated in 90% of cases, but myoglobinuria is usually not present. Anti-Jo-1 or anti-Mi2 antibodies may be present. Patients usually present with anemia and positive inflammatory markers. PM may be associated with inflammation in other organ systems such as pulmonary interstitial fibrosis or myocarditis and is sometimes a component of other connective tissue disorders. The electromyogram is abnormal in 90% of cases and shows motor unit action potentials (MUAPs) that are of short duration, of small amplitude, or polyphasic with early recruitment. Fibrillations and positive waves indicate active inflammation.

PM is treated mainly with steroids and cytotoxic agents. More detail about treatment is presented in the section below. With or without treatment, the disease may progress to dysphagia and respiratory failure. Prognosis for recovery is poorer in older adults, in part because of the effect of age on susceptibility to the complications of immunosuppressive drugs.

Dermatomyositis

DM is an IIM that affects all ages, with approximately one-quarter of cases developing in older adults. It has a female preponderance. While the pathophysiology is not fully understood, muscle biopsy shows endomysial inflammation with a more humoral component (CD4+ T cells and B cells). Perifascicular atrophy (atrophic fibers at the edges of the fascicles) may be caused by hypoperfusion, since capillary density is significantly reduced. Vessels are positive for complement membrane attack complex.

Presentation is insidious and the course is subacute with systemic features such as fatigue, weight loss, arthralgias, and fever. Pain is absent or mild. Sensation and reflexes are preserved. Photosensitivity rashes are common. Typical skin changes include heliotrope rash, Gottron's papules, V sign, Shawl's sign, and mechanic's hands. Heliotrope rash is a violet or purplish discoloration seen around the eyes and on the extremities. Gottron's papules are erythematous, raised areas at the bony prominences in the hands, elbows, and knees. V sign is a macular erythema on the chest in a V shape. Shawl sign is a macular erythema over the posterior thorax. Mechanic's hands are rough, cracked regions of skin on the palms and radial aspects of the fingers. Dysphagia occurs in approximately 25% of DM cases. Symmetrical proximal weakness appears in the neck flexors and extensors, as well as shoulders and hips. CK is elevated in 90% of cases, and myoglobinuria is usually not present. Jo-1 antibodies are associated with pulmonary interstitial fibrosis, and anti-Mi2 antibodies are associated with classic DM. Patients usually present with anemia and positive inflammatory markers. DM is sometimes associated with myocarditis and other connective tissue disorders. Electromyograms for DM and PM are indistinguishable.

Treatment involves steroids and cytotoxic agents. The disease sometimes progresses to dysphagia and respiratory failure. Prognosis, even with treatment, is worse for older than younger adults. Routine cancer screening is required, since 25% of cases with DM develop some type of associated cancer (mostly colon).

Inclusion Body Myositis

IBM is an IIM with a male preponderance and is the most common IIM in older adults. While the pathophysiology is not known, muscle biopsy shows endomysial infiltrates with CD8+ T cells, macrophages invading non-necrotic muscle fibers, as well as rimmed vacuoles and amyloid deposits in the muscle fibers.

The onset of IBM is more insidious than PM and DM, and its course is either subacute or chronic. Pain is absent or mild. Reflexes are either diminished or absent as a result of associated peripheral neuropathy. As opposed to the proximal muscle weakness that predominates in PM and DM, in IBM the proximal and distal muscles are equally involved. IBM might typically present with weakness of bilateral wrists, finger flexors, quadriceps, and foot dorsiflexors. IBM can present with atrophy of the quadriceps muscles. CK elevation in IBM is less than that for PM and DM. Skin involvement and myoglobinuria are usually not present.

The electromyogram shows a chronic myopathy with an active component (fibrillation). Fibrillations and positive waves indicate active inflammation. Nerve conduction studies reveal mild neurogenic features.

IBM is typically unresponsive to steroids. Up to one-third of cases will stabilize or improve with or without treatment. IBM medications, when used, are similar to those for PM and DM.

Treatment of Idiopathic Inflammatory Myopathies

Glucocorticoids are the first-line treatment for inflammatory myopathies. Initial dosage can be reduced for older compared to young adults, because overall muscle mass is expected to be lower with age. While prednisone dosing in young adults is calculated at 1.5 mg/kg (up to 100 mg/day), the dose in older adults is calculated at 1.0 mg/kg (up to 60 mg/day). The initial dose should be maintained until there is evidence of clinical response, especially a clinically detectable improvement in muscle strength. If there is no clinical response in 3 or 4 months, the patient should be considered steroid unresponsive and another immunosuppressive agent should be considered. Tapering begins with clinical response. Dosing can switch immediately to an alternate-day pattern (e.g., 60 mg every other day) or can be gradually converted to an alternate-day pattern (e.g., reduce the alternate or "off-day" dose by 10 mg per week). Continue the alternate-day regimen until either the patient's strength is normalized or improvement reaches a plateau (usually 4–6 months). Next, reduce the dosage by 5 mg every 2 to 3 weeks until the lowest dose capable of controlling symptoms and maintaining muscle strength is achieved. A maintenance dose of 10 to 25 mg every other day may be needed to achieve stability. This approach to tapering steroids can also apply to other inflammatory conditions such as polymyalgia rheumatica (PMR) and temporal arteritis.

Glucocorticoids are the only agents approved by the U.S. Food and Drug Administration (FDA) for treatment of inflammatory myopathies. The efficacy of other immunosuppressive agents in inflammatory myositis is unproven, and a recent systematic review found insufficient high-quality randomized controlled trials to make evidence-based conclusions. However, second-line use of other immunosuppressive agents might be considered in several circumstances. First, second-line agents might be helpful when a steroid-sparing effect is needed to avoid complications associated with steroid therapy. Second, such agents might be used when a relapse occurs repeatedly after attempts to taper steroids. Third, second-line agents might be attempted when first-line therapy with steroid has failed to show a clinical response after at least 3 months. Fourth, second-line agents might be added to steroids when the disease is progressing rapidly, with life-threatening manifestations such as severe weakness and/or respiratory failure. Table 119-2 summarizes the available agents. Some of these agents are very expensive,

TABLE 119-2

Disease-modifying Antirheumatic Drugs (DMARDs) That Can Be Considered as Second-Line Agents for Treatment of Idiopathic Inflammatory Myopathy*

Drug	Usual Dose	Main Side Effects
Methotrexate	7.5–20 mg oral or injection dose weekly	Diarrhea, mucosal ulcers, bone marrow toxicity, liver toxicity, and interstitial pneumonitis. Avoid methotrexate if patient has Jo-1 antibodies. Increased risk of opportunistic infections.
Azathioprine	50–150 mg oral dose daily	Bone marrow toxicity and liver toxicity. Increased risk of opportunistic infections.
Mycophenolate mofetil	2–3 g oral dose daily	Diarrhea and bone marrow toxicity. Increased risk of opportunistic infections.
Cyclophosphamide	50–150 mg oral dose daily	Nausea, vomiting, alopecia, bone marrow toxicity, and hemorrhagic cystitis. Increased risk of opportunistic infections.
Intravenous immunoglobulin (IVIg)	2 g/kg monthly (×3 months)	Patient deficient in serum IgA may be predisposed to anaphylactic reactions.
Cyclosporine A	100–400 mg oral dose daily	Bone marrow toxicity, hypertension, renal toxicity, liver toxicity, and increased risk of opportunistic infections.

*No DMARDs are FDA approved for treatment of inflammatory myopathy but are used as second-line agents under specific conditions. See text for further discussion.

and cost versus likelihood of benefit and harm should be carefully considered. It is good practice to involve the patient, and the family if the patient desires, in discussions about treatment options.

Complications of steroid use are a serious problem whenever they are prescribed and are a special problem in older people who are even more vulnerable to serious adverse events due to these agents. Table 119-3 lists the main complications of steroid use. Every effort should be made to minimize steroid exposure, to anticipate and prevent complications, and to educate the patient and family about what to expect.

OTHER MYOPATHIES

Steroid-Induced Myopathy

Steroid-induced myopathy is associated with either intrinsic or extrinsic excess of glucocorticoids. It can occur at any age and is more prevalent in women. Intrinsic corticosteroid excess may be secondary to diseases such as adrenal hyperplasia, neoplasia, and adrenocorticotropic hormone overproduction by pituitary or other neuroendocrine tumors. Extrinsic steroid use for less than 4 weeks is unlikely to cause myopathy.

The histopathological appearance of involved skeletal muscle is similar, whatever the source of the excess steroids. Excess glucocorticoids alter muscle lipid, carbohydrate, and protein metabolism. While muscle biopsy may show no inflammation, there is often evidence of type 2 muscle fiber atrophy with increased muscle glycogen. The prominent subsarcolemmal lipid deposits found in some biopsies indicate altered muscle lipid metabolism. Electron microscopy reveals mitochondrial aggregation, swelling, vacuolization, and myofibrillar degeneration.

The onset of steroid-induced myopathy is usually insidious and the course is either subacute or chronic, depending on the magnitude or duration of elevated steroid levels. Proximal weakness tends to involve legs more than arms, the strength of the neck flexors is unaffected, and the cranial nerve-innervated muscles and sphincters

TABLE 119-3

Adverse Effects of Glucocorticosteroids

SYSTEM	CONSEQUENCE	PREVENTION
Cardiovascular	Hypertension and hyperlipidemia	Manage cardiovascular risk factors; adjust cardiovascular medications upward or downward.
Muscle	Steroid-induced myopathy	Exercise (aerobic or anaerobic) to minimize impact of muscle atrophy.
Bone	Glucocorticoid-induced osteoporosis usually occurs during the first 6 months of therapy. Chronic use leads to increased risk of fracture and aseptic necrosis of femoral and humoral heads.	Get a baseline bone mineral density and start calcium 1500 mg a day plus vitamin D 800 IU. If therapy is prolonged, a bisphosphonate should be added.
Gastrointestinal	Peptic ulcer disease and upper gastrointestinal bleeding	Consider histamine-2 blockers or proton pump inhibitors.
Endocrine	Cushingoid habitus, glucose intolerance, and exacerbation of diabetes mellitus	Adjust diabetes medications during induction and tapering phase
Ophthalmic	Cataracts and glaucoma	Follow up with ophthalmology.
Immune	Immunosuppression and subsequent infections	Atypical presentation of infections occurs in the elderly. Acute abdomen may present differently. If possible, obtain a tuberculosis test (PPD) and give pneumococcal vaccination before starting treatment. Sepsis is more common.
Neurological	Psychosis with delirium	Taper the dose of steroids as soon as possible.
Skin	Thinning with capillary fragility; striae.	Minimize nonsteroidal anti-inflammatory drugs and aspirin if possible. Taper steroids as soon as possible.

are spared. The clinical examination is likely to reveal other signs of excess steroids, such as classic Cushingoid facies, central obesity, thin skin, and capillary fragility. CK is usually normal. The electromyogram typically shows no fibrillations. MUAPs are of low amplitude and short duration. Sharp waves or fibrillation potentials may also be present.

Treatment of steroid-induced myopathy is focused on reducing exposure to steroids, either by managing the underlying source of excess intrinsic steroids or by exploring options for tapering extrinsic steroids. Exercise may be helpful in preventing or ameliorating steroid-induced myopathy. Inactivity appears to increase glucocorticoid receptors in muscle while activity reduces these receptors and thus can help prevent atrophy. Since fluorinated steroids (triamcinolone, betamethasone, and dexamethasone) are more likely to cause muscle weakness, nonfluorinated steroids are preferred when chronic steroid treatment is planned. Consider the use of a steroid-sparing agent whenever long-term steroids are required to control inflammation. The course of recovery from steroid-induced myopathy after the source of excess steroids has been withdrawn is weeks to months.

Hypothyroidism-Related Myopathy

Hypothyroidism-related myopathy occurs when serum levels of thyroid hormone are low. Hypothyroidism reduces the basal metabolic rate and the number of adrenergic receptors on muscle cells, resulting in diminished glycogenolysis that, in turn, may contribute to muscle cramps and fatigability. Both protein synthesis and degradation are reduced with net protein catabolism. Hypothyroidism is more prevalent in older women than in men. The histopathological findings on muscle biopsy are nonspecific and include fiber size variation, type 2 fiber atrophy, internalization of nuclei, sporadic necrosis and regeneration, disrupted mitochondria, myofibrillar disorganization, and glycogen accumulation.

The onset is insidious and the course is chronic. Symptoms include nonspecific muscle soreness, weakness or stiffness, or cramping without actual weakness. Proximal muscle wasting and weakness are associated with weight gain. Myoedema (local contracture produced by tapping or pinching the muscle) and muscle enlargement may occur. Sensation is typically normal, but ankle reflexes are slow in the relaxation phase of the muscle and pseudomyotonia (a delay in relaxation with handgrip) can occur. Other clinical signs of hypothyroidism may be present (see Chapter 108 on thyroid disease). CK is elevated, but myoglobinuria usually is not present unless there is also rhabdomyalysis.

The electromyogram can be normal or may show low-amplitude polyphasic MUAPs, increased insertional activity, and occasional positive waves. Fibrillations or fasciculations indicating coincidental neuropathy may occur. Myoedema is electrically silent.

Treatment involves restoration of euthyroidism. Recovery takes weeks to months, and weakness may improve more slowly than the chemical and electromyographic abnormalities. Although most patients have recovered normal strength by 6 months, one-quarter of cases still have neuromuscular symptoms and 10% have weakness on physical examination 1 year after treatment.

Hyperthyroidism-Related Myopathy

Hyperthyroidism-related myopathy is associated with increased serum levels of thyroid hormone. It develops insidiously and progresses slowly. The mean age of onset is in the late forties. Hyperthyroidism in late life is more common in women than in men.

The muscle complications of hyperthyroidism are related to excess thyroid hormone effects, such as increased basal metabolic rate and heat production with increased consumption of mitochondrial oxygen, pyruvate, and malate, together resulting in skeletal muscle catabolism. Muscle biopsy is usually normal or may show mild abnormalities, including varying degrees of fatty infiltration, fiber atrophy, and nerve terminal damage. The clinical presentation includes myalgia, fatigue, and exercise intolerance. Although severe muscle wasting can occur, the muscle weakness is out of proportion to the amount of muscle wasting in up to half of cases. Distal muscle weakness develops later in the disease progression and is less severe than proximal weakness. Sphincters are spared and tendon reflexes are usually normal with 25% having shortened relaxation times. CK is usually normal but may be elevated in thyroid storms. Myoglobinuria is usually not present even during thyroid storm unless rhabdomyalysis is present.

The electromyogram is characterized by short-duration MUAPs and increased polyphasic potentials in proximal muscles. The EMG may be abnormal in up to one-third of cases with apparently normal muscle strength. The EMG is abnormal in distal muscles in only approximately 20% of cases. Spontaneous electrical activity is rare, and nerve conduction velocity is normal.

This myopathy is reversible if patients are returned to the euthyroid state. Adrenergic blocking agents may improve muscle strength acutely as may glucocorticoids that block the peripheral conversion of T3 to T4. See Chapter 111 for further discussion of hyperthyroid disease.

Statin-Induced Myopathy

Statin-induced myopathy is associated with use of statin-based cholesterol-lowering agents. It can present in a variety of fashions including myalgias, isolated CK elevation, weakness, or rhabdomyalysis. The risk of developing statin-induced myopathy is increased with higher dose of the statin, low body size, renal insufficiency, hepatic disease, hypothyroidism, age, diabetes, and drugs that use P-450 (CYP) 3A4 pathway (e.g., niacin, erythromycin, diltiazem, and cyclosporine). Muscle biopsy shows scattered muscle fiber necrosis with phagocytosis and small regenerating fibers. Electron microscopy demonstrates the subsarcolemmal accumulation of autophagic lysosomes. CK is often elevated, and myoglobinuria could present in cases of rhabdomyalysis.

The electromyogram is usually normal except when a generalized necrotizing myopathy has developed. In that case, there is increased insertional and spontaneous activity and small-amplitude, short-duration, polyphasic, or "myopathic" MUAPs. Fibrillation potentials or positive sharp waves can also occur.

Statin-induced myopathy is reversible with discontinuation of the offending agent. Since the severity of the condition varies widely, there may be situations where a mildly elevated CK without clinical consequences could be monitored and the drug continued, especially if there is a compelling need for the use of the statin. This option should be clearly discussed with the patient, who should be involved in the weighing of risks. See Chapter 75 for further discussion of statin use.

Other Myopathies

Mixed Connective Tissue Disorder (MCTD) has elements of systemic lupus erythematosus, scleroderma, and myositis and can present as a myopathy. Muscle biopsy in patients with MCTD is similar to those with DM/PM. Myalgias are common in MCTD, and half of MCTD cases have an inflammatory myositis. There is generalized weakness but little, if any, wasting. Patients may have normal or proximal weakness. The pelvic girdle is affected more than the shoulder girdle. Focal myositis may also occur. More severe cases can present with dysphagia and diaphragmatic dysfunction. CK is elevated and myoglobinuria is uncommon. Autoantibodies to ribonucleoprotein (anti-U1-snRNP) are a feature of MCTD but are not specific. The electromyogram is similar to DM/PM and has inflammatory features when myositis is present. Glucocorticoids are the main treatment and are prescribed as in PM and DM. See Chapter 120 for further discussion of autoimmune disease, including MCTD.

Osteomalacia is a metabolic bone disease characterized by unmineralized matrix because of lack of vitamin D. The disease can be associated with a myopathy. The risk of vitamin D deficiency is increased among older adults (see Chapters 116 and 117 on osteomalacia and on deficiency of vitamin D). This myopathy can present with proximal weakness, waddling gait, nonspecific bone pain, and tenderness with or without fractures. CK is typically normal. The electromyogram shows a myopathic process, and MUAPs are of low amplitude and short duration. Muscle biopsy shows minimal inflammatory infiltrates. This myopathy is reversible with administration of vitamin D.

Mitochondrial myopathies are associated with mitochondrial dysfunction. The clinical presentation of mitochondrial myopathy can be slow and progressive. Muscle biopsy shows ragged red fibers (Gomori trichrome stain). Patients usually present with droopy eyelids and double vision owing to ophthalmoplegia. CK is mildly elevated, and there is usually no myoglobinuria. The electromyogram is normal. There is no specific treatment other than physical therapy and vitamin supplementation to assure adequate nutrition.

Amyloid myopathy is associated with amyloidosis. The muscle biopsy shows extracellular amyloid deposits around the muscle fibers and blood vessel walls within the muscle. Sometimes there are inflammatory changes. Although rare, amyloid myopathy can occur in older people who have multiple myeloma. CK is usually elevated with no myoglobinuria. The electromyogram may reflect the inflammatory changes, but it is not specific. Treatment is aimed at the underlying cause (i.e., treatment of multiple myeloma, tuberculosis, etc.). See Chapter · · · for a more detailed discussion of multiple myeloma.

Alcohol-induced myopathy is related to chronic alcohol use. Since alcohol overuse is an important and often overlooked problem for older adults, alcohol-induced myopathy should be considered in older people presenting with a myopathic picture. The clinical presentation can be chronic, subacute, or acute and can be accompanied by weakness and myalgias. Muscle biopsy shows inflammation and necrosis in the acute and subacute form. Atrophy of type 2 fibers can be seen in the chronic presentation. CK is elevated, and myoglobinuria may be present with rhabdomyalysis. The electromyogram may show inflammatory changes in the acute or subacute presentation but may have noninflammatory myopathic changes in the chronic presentation. The myopathy can improve with alcohol abstinence. See Chapter 51 on alcohol and aging.

Late-onset muscular dystrophies are degenerative myopathies characterized by loss of muscle fibers, variation in fiber size, muscle fiber necrosis, and other nonspecific changes. Although these myopathies usually affect the young, these can develop de novo or worsen later in life. The dystrophies are characterized by the muscle groups that are affected and form three main patterns: (1) facioscapulohumeral

dystrophy, (2) oculopharyngeal dystrophy, and (3) limb girdle dystrophy. CK is usually elevated or normal with no evidence of myoglobinuria. The electromyogram shows a nonspecific myopathic pattern. There is no treatment or cure. Management is conservative with major goals to prevent aspiration and avoid deconditioning.

POLYMYALGIA RHEUMATICA

Polymyalgia rheumatica is a clinical syndrome characterized by aching and stiffness in the proximal portion of the extremities and torso. The annual incidence of PMR in the United States oscillates around 58.7/100 000 and its prevalence around 300/100 000. The incidence is higher in females, and it is most commonly found among persons of Northern European origin. PMR primarily affects the elderly and is rare in patients younger than 50 years old.

The etiology of PMR is unknown, but the systemic inflammation involved resembles that found in giant cell arteritis (GCA). In fact, 6% to 33% of patients with PMR will develop GCA. In addition to the vasculitis typical of the condition, synovitis (inflammation of the synovial lining of joints) can also be present. This form of synovitis is called "benign synovitis" because it does not progress to joint erosions.

The onset of PMR is often insidious, and its course is subacute or chronic. Fever, anorexia, weight loss, malaise, night sweats, and depression are common manifestations of the systemic inflammation associated with PMR. There is stiffness and pain around the muscles of the neck, shoulders, and pelvic girdle but no weakness. Glenohumeral joint synovitis and long-head biceps tenosynovitis can coexist in approximately 60% to 80% of patients. However, the passive range of motion of large joints is maintained. Laboratory findings usually include elevated erythrocyte sedimentation rate (ESR), elevated C-reactive protein, thrombocytosis, and normocytic normochromic anemia.

The diagnosis of PMR is made on clinical grounds. The differential diagnosis includes elderly-onset rheumatoid arthritis, seronegative rheumatoid arthritis, shoulder bursitis, trochanteric bursitis, and fibromyalgia, among others. Magnetic resonance imaging and ultrasound studies both show similar inflammatory shoulder lesions (synovitis). Bilateral subacromial/subdeltoid bursitis represents the imaging hallmark in PMR even in patients with normal erythrocyte sedimentation rate.

Corticosteroids are the main therapy. Initial treatment is usually prednisone up to 20 mg/day for 7 days. If there is no response, the dose can be increased to 30 mg/day for another week. Seek an alternative etiology if no response is observed. If the patient responds to the initial dose, then monitor for signs of GCA and start tapering the dose after muscle pain and stiffness have improved. A response to small doses of glucocorticoids is considered typical of PMR and can be used to affirm diagnosis, although symptoms, as a result of other conditions, may also respond transiently to steroids. Prednisone tapering must be pursued slowly in order to prevent recurrence of symptoms and can take up to 1 to 2 years.

TEMPORAL ARTERITIS (CLASSIC CRANIAL GCA)

GCA is a systemic vasculitis that mainly affects large vessels. It is a panarteritis. Temporal arteritis, also called cranial GCA, is a type of GCA that involves carotid artery branches, both external (mostly superficial temporal arteries and occipital arteries) and internal branches (ophthalmic arteries and posterior ciliary arteries).

There are several major subtypes of GCA and not all of them involve the cranial arteries. A form of large-vessel GCA, often called Takayasu's arteritis, produces a distinct spectrum of clinical manifestations and often occurs without involvement of the cranial arteries. It is characterized by upper extremity vascular insufficiency and it mainly affects young females. Large-artery GCA could also present as an aortic arch syndrome, with the arteritis spreading from medium-sized vessels to the subclavian and axillary vessels. The type of GCA that is most common in older adults is the cranial form.

The annual incidence of cranial GCA is around 7–27/100 000 and the prevalence around 200/100 000 in the United States. As was the case with PMR, it primarily affects females of Northern European origin who are older than 50 years of age.

The etiology of GCA is unknown. A plausible theory is that an antigen in the arterial wall activates T cells and macrophages that produce granulomatous reactions. This T-cell triggering occurs in the adventitia (where the vasa vasorum provides a port of entrance for inflammatory cells). The T cells secrete interferon-γ, a cytokine that regulates effector functions of macrophages recruited to the lesions. The recruited macrophages then differentiate into distinct subsets of tissue-injurious effector cells and produce a matrix of metalloproteinases and reactive oxygen intermediates. Macrophages and multinucleated giant cells also provide growth factors and angiogenic factors that support the response-to-injury program of the artery, which leads to the formation of lumen-occlusive intimal hyperplasia.

GCA can present either abruptly or insidiously. Its course can be subacute or chronic. While the sedimentation rate and C-reactive protein are usually elevated, these can be normal at initial presentation in a minority of patients. Thrombocytosis and normocytic normochromic anemia are common. Systemic manifestations include fever, anorexia, weight loss, malaise, night sweats, depression, and PMR. PMR occurs in approximately 41% of patients and may develop before, during, or after the diagnosis of GCA. Peripheral musculoskeletal manifestations occur in approximately one-quarter of patients and include peripheral arthritis of knees, wrists, and metacarpophalangeal joints. This arthritis pattern may satisfy the American College of Rheumatology criteria for rheumatoid arthritis. Other associated manifestations include distal extremity swelling with pitting edema, distal extremity swelling without edema, distal tenosynovitis, and carpal tunnel syndrome.

Headache with no particular anatomical pattern, accompanied by severe and sometimes throbbing pain, is a common manifestation of GCA. The pain often manifests as scalp tenderness or may localize to the temporal area and be elicited by touching, grooming, or wearing glasses. One or both temporal arteries can be swollen, thickened, tender, or nodular and have decreased pulses. Jaw claudication can be elicited by prolonged talking or chewing. As a type of claudication, pain comes on with activity and is relieved by rest. This symptom is attributed to reduced blood flow to the masseter and temporalis muscles. Jaw pain that stops when talking or chewing stops is a strong indicator of GCA with high specificity. Ocular symptoms are less common and are related to stenosis of the ophthalmic artery. Symptoms include transient or persistent partial or complete visual loss, or transient or persistent oculomotor deficits like diplopia. Unilateral or bilateral blindness is the most feared complication of GCA and may be permanent. It is attributed to occlusion of the posterior ciliary branches of the ophthalmic artery causing an-

terior ischemic optic neuropathy. Visual loss can also be secondary to central retinal artery occlusion, retrobulbar optic neuritis, or cortical blindness because of vertebral–basilar stroke. Other manifestations include odynophagia (painful swallowing), nonproductive cough, limb claudication elicited by the use of arms and paresthesias. More rare manifestations include ischemia of the tongue, face, or neck and facial swelling.

Imaging by angiogram may show beading and constrictions consistent with vasculitis. Biopsy of involved arteries shows discontinuous vascular inflammation, so arterial specimens should be at least 2 to 3 cm in length. In order to make the most of the opportunity to make the diagnosis by biopsy, frozen sections from the first temporal artery should be inspected, and if inflammatory infiltrates are absent, then the contralateral side should be biopsied.

The proper sequence for biopsy and steroid treatment is controversial. Immediate treatment with steroids may reduce pathologic findings of inflammation and produce false-negative biopsy results but may be indicated in the face of a high risk of vision loss if treatment is delayed. A temporal biopsy positive for GCA shows panarteritis, with lymphocytes and macrophages concentrated in the media at the media–intima junction. Multinucleated giant cells occur in approximately 50% of cases and tend to be grouped along the fragmented internal elastica lamina. Inflammatory infiltrates can sometimes be limited to the adventitia, indicating that panarteritis is not full-blown.

GCA increases the risk of cranial ischemic complications (CICs), which present as types of stroke. Stroke can develop even before GCA is diagnosed, or within the first month after starting prednisone therapy. Risk of CICs is increased when there is also thrombocytosis, a paucity of constitutional symptoms, jaw claudication, previous episodes of transient visual loss, and CICs at presentation. Some patients with GCA are particularly predisposed to ischemic complications; this predisposition is associated with a poor inflammatory response. GCA-induced strokes can involve a range of vascular territories including vertebral–basilar, temporal–occipital, cerebellar–occipital, temporal–occipital, and brain stem. Clinical consequences are protean and follow the pattern of the ischemic brain lesion. According to some authorities, posterior circulation strokes may be more common in GCA than in atherosclerosis.

Visual loss can occur in up to one-fifth of patients with GCA and may not be preceded by any systemic symptoms. It is sudden and painless; one or both eyes may be affected. Warning symptoms include amaurosis fugax, posture-related visual blurring, and diplopia. Funduscopic examination may reveal a pale edematous disc, or splinter hemorrhages at the disc margin or cotton wool spots in the peripapillary region. The risk of permanent visual loss is increased in patients with transient visual loss and/or jaw claudication and decreased in those with elevated liver enzyme levels and/or constitutional syndrome suggestive of systemic inflammation. Treatment markedly reduces the risk of vision loss to approximately 1% overall, but treatment is somewhat less effective if visual loss is present at diagnosis, in which case the subsequent risk of vision loss is halved to approximately 13%.

GCA is treated with oral glucocorticoids as described in the section above, which summarizes steroid treatment. Steroids provide dramatic relief of clinical symptoms and help prevent ischemic events. The central goal of GCA treatment is to prevent blindness and strokes. Low-dose aspirin may also help prevent CIC complications of GCA. Patients on low-dose aspirin are less likely to experience ischemic complications, especially if they are also receiving prednisone. Steroids are not always effective. CIC affecting the eye, face, and central nervous system can develop in 25% to 33% of patients even after receiving corticosteroids. If visual loss has occurred, partial therapeutic success is more likely if treatment is started within the first day of visual loss.

Steroid induction means starting with large parenteral loading doses of glucocorticoids. The goal of induction is to gain rapid control of symptoms, reduce the cumulative maintenance dose, and, perhaps, reduce glucocorticoid-related side effects. A typical induction would involve intravenous methylprednisolone at 15 mg/kg of ideal body weight/d (approximately 1000 mg/day for an average 70-kg patient) for 3 days. Patients simultaneously receive oral prednisone 40 mg/day. Induction doses sometimes vary in amount and duration of treatment. Further tapering is performed as described in the section on steroid use. In the absence of visual or cranial symptoms, prednisone can be initiated at 40 to 60 mg daily and tapered as described above. Since it can be difficult to completely wean patients with GCA and PMR from all steroids, slow tapering of low-dose steroids for months can be necessary. Typically when the daily dose is below 10 mg, dose is reduced by 1 mg/day every 2 weeks.

Relapse is defined as return of signs and symptoms and/or an increase in either erythrocyte sedimentation rate or C-reactive protein level while still on prednisone treatment. The prednisone dose should be increased, for example, by 10 mg daily if the patient is taking ≥25 mg/day. Once administered, maintain the new dosage for at least 2 weeks before tapering again according to a scheduled protocol. Recurrence is defined as a return of signs and/or symptoms and/or changes in laboratory parameters after all steroid therapies have been stopped for at least 1 month and may require reexposure to prednisone in varying doses.

Since it is often difficult to stop steroids in GCA and PMR, their use often becomes chronic, can last for years, and increases the probability of steroid complications. Steroid complications and their prevention are described in Table 119-3. Thus, there is a great need for steroid-sparing agents. While potentially helpful, clinical trials have not shown that use of methotrexate helps reduce steroid side effects. Given this lack of evidence, the use of methotrexate in GCA and PMR remains controversial. Other potentially steroid-sparing agents, including statins and tumor necrosis alpha inhibitors, are currently under study.

FURTHER READING

Alshekhlee A, Kaminski HJ, Ruff RL. Neuromuscular manifestations of endocrine disorders. *Neurol Clin.* 2002;20:35.

Baumgartner RN. Body composition in healthy aging. *Ann New York Acad Sci.* 2000;904:437.

Brack A, Martinez-Taboada V, Stanson A, Goronzy JJ, Weyand CM. Disease pattern in cranial and large-vessel giant cell arteritis. *Arthritis Rheum.* 1999;42:311.

Cantini F, Salvarani C, Olivieri I, et al. Inflamed shoulder structures in polymyalgia rheumatica with normal erythrocyte sedimentation rate. *Arthritis Rheum.* 2001;44:1155.

Choy EHS, Hoogendijk JE, Lecky B, Winer JB. Immunosuppressant and immunomodulary treatment of dermatomyositis and polymyositis. *Cochrane Neuromuscular Disease Group.* Cochrane Review November 02, 2005.

Cid MC, Font C, Oristrell J, et al. Associations between strong inflammatory response and low risk of developing visual loss and other cranial ischemic complications in giant cell (temporal) arteritis. *Arthritis Rheum.* 1998;41:26.

Di Martino SJ, Kagen LJ. Newer therapeutic approaches: inflammatory muscle disorders. *Rheum Dis Clin North Am.* 2006;32:121.

Flanigan KM, Lauria G, Griffin JW, Kunci RW. The neurology of aging. *Neurol Clin North Am* 1998;16:659.

Gonzales-Gay MA, Blanco R, Rodriguez-Valverde V, et al. Permanent visual loss and cerebrovascular accidents in giant cell arteritis. *Arthritis Rheum.* 1998;41:1497.

Gonzales-Gay, Garcia-Porrua C, Amor-Dorado JC, Llorca J. Giant cell arteritis without clinically evident vascular involvement in a defined population. *Arthritis Rheum (Arthritis Care Res).* 2004;51:274.

Marie I, Hatron PY, Levesque H, et al. Influence of age on characteristics of polymyositis and dermatomyositis in adults. *Arthritis Rheum.* 1999;78:139.

Mazlumzadeh M, Hunder GG, Easley KA, et al. Treatment of giant cell arteritis using induction therapy with high-dose glucocorticoids. *Arthritis Rheum.* 2006;54:3310.

Nesher G, Berkun Y, Mates M, Baras M, Rubinow A, Sonnenblick M. Low-dose aspirin and prevention of cranial ischemic complications in giant cell arteritis. *Arthritis Rheum.* 2004;50:1332.

Oddis CV, Rider LG, Reed AM, et al. ; for the International Myositis Assessment and Clinical Studies Group. International consensus guidelines for trials of therapies in the idiopathic inflammatory myopathies. *Arthritis Rheum.* 2005;52:2607.

O'Rourke K. Myopathies in the elderly. *Rheum Dis Clin North Am.* 2000;26:647.

Roubenoff R. Sarcopenia: effects on body composition and function. *J Gerontol Med Sci.* 2003;58A:M1012.

Ruegg DG, Kakebeeke TH, Gabriel JP, Bennefeld M. Conduction velocity of nerve and muscle fiber action potentials after a space mission or a bed rest. *Clin Neurophysiol.* 2003;114:86.

Salvarani C, Hunder GG. Musculoskeletal manifestations in a population-based cohort of patients with giant cell arteritis. *Arthritis Rheum.* 1999;42:1259.

Weyand CM, Goronzy JJ. Giant-cell arteritis and polymyalgia rheumatica. *Ann Intern Med.* 2003;139:505.

Rheumatoid Arthritis and Other Autoimmune Diseases

Raymond Yung

Our understanding of the pathogenesis and approach to treatment of autoimmune diseases continue to evolve. However, key questions concerning the epidemiology, pathogenesis and optimal treatment of these diseases in the elderly population remain unanswered. Despite the many exciting new therapeutic advances, immunosuppression in elderly patients with autoimmune diseases continues to pose a dilemma. Changing population demographics and the advent of biologics, coupled with the lack of the availability of a rheumatologist in many smaller communities, will significantly impact the geriatrician's role in the care of older adults with autoimmune diseases in the coming years. This chapter summarizes key recent advances, with specific references to the geriatric population.

RHEUMATOID ARTHRITIS

Definition

Rheumatoid arthritis (RA) is a chronic systemic inflammatory disease that preferentially affects diarthrodial joints. The current and most widely used classification criteria for RA were developed in 1987 by the American College of Rheumatology (ACR), based on the study of predominantly middle-aged patients attending hospital outpatient clinics (Table 120-1). While the criteria set is useful for diagnosing established and active disease in younger patients, its usefulness in detecting early disease and elderly-onset (>60 years old) rheumatoid arthritis (EORA) has not been established. This is important because the disease presentation in EORA may be distinct from that of young-onset RA (YORA).

One important advance that may lead to the eventual modification of the ACR classification criteria for RA is the discovery that the majority (70–90%, depending on the assay) of patients with RA has in their blood circulating anticyclic citrullinated peptide (anti-CCP) antibodies. Citrullination is a posttranslational modifi-

cation of protein-bound arginine into the nonstandard amino acid citrulline, and many citrullinated proteins have been found to be expressed in inflamed joints. Anti-CCP antibodies are as sensitive as, and more specific than, IgM rheumatoid factor (RF) in early and fully established disease. Furthermore, the presence of these antibodies is a marker for erosive disease and may predict the eventual development of RA in patients presenting with undifferentiated arthritis. These antibodies may also be detected in healthy individuals years before the onset of clinical RA. Unlike classical RF, the incidence of anti-CCP antibodies does not appear to increase with normal aging, making it a particularly useful marker for this disease in the elderly population.

In addition to classification criteria for the diagnosis of RA, the ACR has established criteria for functional status and for determining clinical remission in RA. The usefulness of these classification systems in older patients who often suffer functional disability from concomitant osteoarthritis, soft-tissue rheumatism, and cardiovascular or neurological diseases is unclear.

Epidemiology

Although the overall incidence of RA may be declining, the disease still affects approximately 1% of the population in the United States and in many western developed countries. Lower prevalence rates of 0.2% to 0.3% have been observed in China, Japan, some regions in Greece, and Africa. Southern Europeans may have a milder disease, with less extra-articular complications and less evidence of radiographic damage. Conversely, a much higher prevalence rate (up to 7%) and a more aggressive clinical course have been reported in several American-Indian and Alaska native populations. Gender and age are important factors in RA. Overall, women are affected by the disease two to three times more than men. However, this gender parity disappears in old age. The prevalence of RA increases with age and is commonest in the most elderly group studied (often 65 years and older or 70 years and older). Approximately 5% of

TABLE 120-1

Classification Criteria for Rheumatoid Arthritis* (R₃A₄)

Rheumatoid factor	Using a method with positive results in <5% of normal controls
Rheumatoid nodules	Subcutaneous nodules over bony prominences, extensor surfaces, or in juxta-articular regions
Radiographic changes	Typical changes of RA on hand and wrist radiographs, including erosions or unequivocal bony decalcification localized in or adjacent to the involved joints
Arthritis of the hand joints	Swelling of wrist, metacarpal phalangeal (MCP), or proximal phalangeal (PIP) joints for at least 6 weeks
Arthritis in three or more joints	Soft-tissue swelling or fluid present simultaneously for at least 6 weeks. Possible areas include PIP, MCP, wrist, elbow, knee, ankle, and metatarsal phalangeal joints
Arthritis that is symmetrical	Simultaneous involvement of the same joint areas on both sides of the body for at least 6 weeks
AM (morning) stiffness	Morning stiffness in and around the joints, lasting at least 1 h before maximal improvement at anytime in the disease course

*Requires at least four criteria for the classification of rheumatoid arthritis.
Modified with permission from Arnett FC et al. The American Rheumatism Association 1987 revised criteria for the classification of rheumatoid arthritis. Arthritis Rheum. 1987;31:315.

women older than the age of 55 years are affected by the disease. The incidence of RA also increases with age, with the peak incidence occurring in the sixth to eighth decades (Figure 120-1). The reason for the age-associated increase in disease susceptibility is currently unknown.

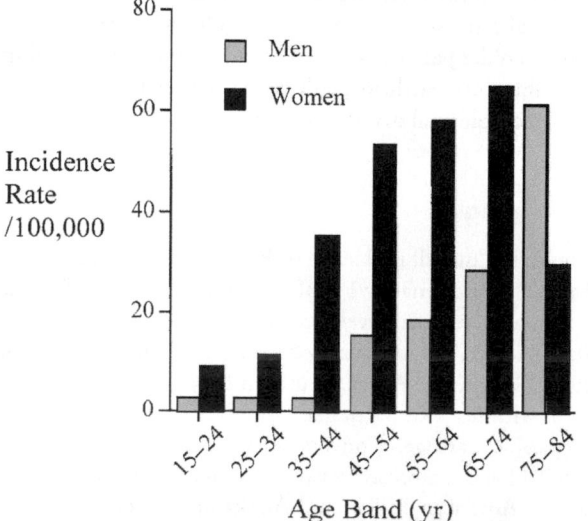

FIGURE 120-1. Age-related incidence of rheumatoid arthritis. *(Adapted from Symmons DPM, et al. The incidence of rheumatoid arthritis in the United Kingdom: results from the Norfolk Arthritis register. Br J Rheumatol. 1994;33:735.)*

Pathophysiology

RA begins as a disease of the synovium. Earlier on in the disease the normally one- or two-cell-layer-thick synovium becomes markedly hyperplastic and edematous, accompanied by prominent new blood vessel proliferation. Left unchecked, this is followed by the activation and recruitment of T cells into the RA joint, which set into motion a complex cascade of inflammatory responses (Figure 120-2). This results in further accumulation of inflammatory cells, panus formation, localized osteoporosis, bony erosions, and destruction of peri-articular structures, which are characteristic of this disease. Rheumatoid synovitis is accompanied by the accumulation of inflammatory joint fluid with white cell count typically in the range of 2000 to 20 000 cells per milliliter. Soluble proteins that have been implicated in the inflammatory process include a number of proinflammatory cytokines (interleukin [IL]-1, IL-6, IL-13, IL-15, and tumor necrosis factor [TNF]), metalloproteinases (stromelysin, collagenases, and gelatinases), transforming growth factor-β, granulocyte colony-stimulating factor, and activated complement components.

There appears to be a genetic susceptibility component to RA. The concordance rate for monozygotic twins is between 12% and 15%, approximately three times that of dizygotic pairs and much higher than the 1% background prevalence rate of the general population. The fact that most monozygotic twins are discordant for RA also highlights the importance of environmental factors. The association between RA and human leukocyte antigen (HLA) has been refined to alleles coding for a "shared" epitope (the sequences QRRAA or QKRAA) on the HLA-DRB1 genes. The presence of the DRB1*04 (DR4) allele (especially if both alleles are present) is a marker for increased susceptibility and severe disease. Population differences in the prevalence of the "shared epitope" may help to explain in part the geographic variation in the prevalence of RA.

An infectious etiology for RA has been postulated for more than half a century. The onset of RA can be heralded by polyarthralgias, fever, and malaise that are indistinguishable from an acute infection. The joints are known targets for diverse microorganisms from gonococci to *Borrelia burgdorferi* and *Mycobacterium tuberculosis*. Acute and chronic "reactive" arthritis can follow specific gastrointestinal (GI) or genital urinary infection. A transient RA-like illness can be seen in viral infections including parvovirus B19, Epstein–Barr virus, and human T-lymphotropic virus type 1.

Tantalizing evidence of a potential pathogenic role for microorganisms in RA includes the following: (1) Retroviral-like particles have been observed in RA synovial fluid. (2) Viral or bacterial superantigen can reawaken a latent or subclinical disease in animal models of inflammatory arthritis. (3) Heat shock proteins (viral and cellular) can act as autoantigens. Interestingly, both the dnaJ class of bacterial heat shock protein and the gp110 capsid protein of Epstein–Barr virus have the QKRAA "shared epitope" amino acid sequence.

Despite these observations, a direct role for infection in the pathogenesis in RA has not been proven. It is possible that transient exposure of the joints to microorganism protein with homology to normal antigen could attract lymphocytes to the synovium. This, in turn, may set up an autoimmune response through a molecular mimicry mechanism without requiring the presence of the inciting organism (the "hit and run" theory). Some investigators have shown that RA synovial cells may have defective apoptosis and a transformed phenotype. This opens up the possibility that environmental agents, including viruses, may transform synovial or lymphoid cells to cause

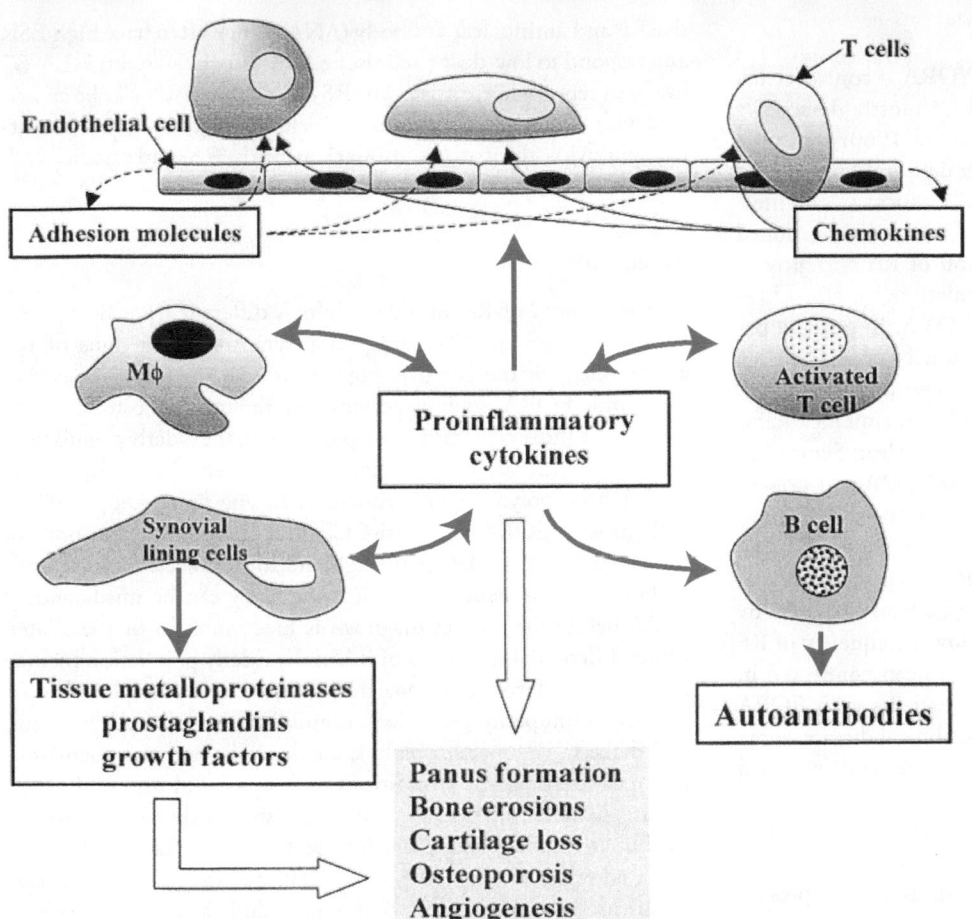

FIGURE 120-2. The inflammatory cascade in rheumatoid arthritis.

inflammation and tissue destruction without requiring the presence of the inciting agent.

Gender differences in reproductive hormones may explain the high female prevalence in RA. However, since the peak incidence of RA in women is in their fifties, high levels of female sex hormones may play a modifying, but not necessary, role in the pathogenesis of this disease.

The linkage of RA to specific major histocompatibility complex alleles, the abundance of specific T-cell subsets in synovial tissue and fluid, and other evidence from animal models of inflammatory arthritis all point to a central role of T lymphocytes in the immunopathogenesis of this disease. RA is considered to be a Th (T helper) 1-mediated disease based on the cytokine and more recently the chemokine receptor profile of T cells in synovial joints. Although it is tempting to postulate that RA-associated DRB1 epitope triggers disease by presenting an arthrogenic peptide to T cells, extensive search of unique peptides that are displayed selectively by RA-associated HLA molecules has so far been unsuccessful. Costimulatory molecules, including CD28 and CD60, may play a role in activating T cells in RA joints. However, their precise role in human disease is unclear. Signal transduction through the T-cell receptor is defective in RA, suggesting that non-T-cell-receptor-activating pathways may be important in T-cell activation in this disease.

Aging Effects

The reason for the age-associated increase in RA susceptibility is unclear. The traditional view that aging is associated with a "decline" in immune response does not explain the high incidence and severe onset of this autoimmune disease that is commonly seen in older adults. Decline in sex hormone production in postmenopausal years also cannot account for the high incidence of RA in elderly females. Unlike their younger counterparts, EORA occurs with equal frequency in males and females. Again, the rising incidence of RA in postmenopausal women suggests that while reproductive hormones may influence the disease manifestation, they are unlikely to play a major pathogenic role in the elderly population.

Animal studies suggest that aging is accompanied by a shift from a Th1 to a predominantly Th2 cytokine profile. However, such changes cannot explain the high incidence of RA, a predominantly Th1-mediated disease, in the elderly population either. Studies on the effect of age on the adenovirus vectors model of inflammatory arthritis have yielded conflicting results, with some strains showing more chronic and destructive arthritis in older female animals. The enhanced production of proinflammatory cytokines, including TNF-α and IL-1, in aging, may contribute to the clinical features of EORA. The recruitment and retention of T cells in the RA synovial joint are complex processes determined by the interaction of leukocyte adhesion molecules and chemokine receptors interacting with their respective ligands expressed by synovial and vascular endothelial cells. T cells from aged animals may express high levels of selective chemokine receptors that are important in the recruitment of T cells to RA joints. These lines of research may eventually provide the explanation for the increased susceptibility and severity of RA in elderly people.

Presentation

Whether EORA is a different disease from YORA is controversial. The clinical studies that address the issue were mostly descriptive or cross-sectional studies done in the 1950s and 1960s that have significant methodologic problems. The older definition of RA used in these studies also allowed terms such as "classical," "definite," and "probable" RA, which are no longer used today. As mentioned before, the most widely accepted classification of RA currently in use has not been validated in the elderly population.

Table 120-2 summarizes the features of EORA. In general, patients with EORA have a more equal gender distribution. The large joints, including the shoulder joint, are more often involved at presentation in EORA. Whether this is a result of concomitant rotator cuff disease that is prevalent in this age group is unclear. Symptoms in the proximal girdles have led to the belief that EORA may present with a polymyalgia rheumatica-like illness. Erythrocyte sedimentation rate (ESR) normally increases with age, especially in females. Elevated ESR is also more common in EORA. The prevalence of RF similarly increases after the age of 60 years, reaching 30% by the age of 90 years. Earlier reports suggest a lower frequency of RF in EORA than YORA. However, this has not been confirmed in more recent studies. As in younger patients, patients with EORA who are seropositive for RF have more severe clinical disease, more bony erosions on x-ray, worse functional outcome, and increased mortality. Whether patients with EORA who are seropositive have worse prognosis than do their younger counterparts is unclear. It is possible that the poor prognosis of EORA reported in some studies reflects the greater number of comorbid conditions that are present in older patients.

"Benign polyarthritis of the elderly" person occurs in up to a third of patients with EORA. They have a more explosive disease onset associated with systemic features such as fever and night sweats. The clinical features have led some to describe the disease as "infectious like." The disease is called benign because its general prognosis is good, with most people going into remission within 1 year with or without treatment. Within this group can be included a peculiar syndrome unique to the elderly population called the RS$_3$PE (remitting, seronegative, and symmetric synovitis with pitting edema) syndrome. This typically affects elderly men (2–3:1, male:female ratio) and is characterized by acute onset of symmetric polyarthritis/tenosynovitis with pitting edema involving both upper and lower extremities. As the name implies, these patients generally have nega-

tive RF and antinuclear antibody (ANA). They often have high ESR and respond to low-dose prednisone. The association with HLA-B7 has been reported inconsistently. RS$_3$PE may occasionally be associated with other rheumatic diseases, including polymyalgia rheumatica, spondyloarthropathies, psoriatic arthritis, RA, and sarcoid, and, rarely, malignancies.

Evaluation

The assessment of RA in older adults is different from that of the younger age group. The nonspecific symptoms and signs of RA are prevalent in the geriatric population. Rheumatic diseases that can mimic EORA, such as polymyalgia rheumatica, osteoarthritis, and crystal-induced arthritis, are prevalent in the elderly population. Anti-CCP antibody measurement may be useful in distinguishing EORA from polymyalgia rheumatica. In one small study, 65% of patients with EORA were anti-CCP antibody positive, but none of the patients with PMR or the aged healthy subjects had the antibodies. Arthritis associated with malignancy can be misdiagnosed as RA before the correct diagnosis is made months or years later. Other differential diagnoses of RA in the elderly population include inflammatory (erosive) osteoarthritis, late-onset spondyloarthropathy, endocrinopathy (e.g., hypothyroidism, hyperparathyroidism, and diabetic cheiroarthropathy), amyloidosis, and the edematous phase of scleroderma. Conditions such as sarcoidosis, adult Still's disease, hemochromatosis, and glycogen storage diseases can mimic RA but are unlikely to present for the first time so late in life.

In addition to the above considerations, the initial evaluation of an elderly patient with RA should include a careful assessment of the patient's living condition, social support, and cognitive and functional status. Many elderly patients have the misconception that there is no effective treatment for arthritis, and they should accept their physical suffering as part of normal aging. Older adults are often embarrassed about their arthritis pain. They may minimize their symptoms by using terms such as "aching" and "stiff" instead of pain. Unfortunately, many clinicians also do not take their symptoms seriously, resulting in the patients frequently feeling that their care resembles "a lick and a promise." Because pain is, by far, the commonest presenting symptom of RA, pain assessment should be an integral part of the patient's evaluation at presentation and in subsequent office visits. This can be difficult in the elderly patient who has significant cognitive or verbal impairment. Information from caregivers, nonverbal pain behavior, physical evidence of active joint inflammation, and decline in functions are important clues that more aggressive therapy may be necessary.

The ACR classification system for assessing the functional status of patients with RA is shown in Table 120-3. However, use of this classification for an elderly patient may be difficult because of functional disability from other coexisting diseases. This quick assessment tool is useful for describing the global functional status and allows patients to be grouped for studies. Patients with RA with the worst (class IV) functional status were reported to have extremely poor prognosis, with survival similar to patients with multiple vessel coronary artery disease and stage IV Hodgkin's lymphoma. Many clinicians now feel that the prognosis for RA has improved with the advent of better therapeutic regimens for RA in the past two decades. Whether this translates into prolonged survival remains to be determined. Concomitant medical conditions affecting the patient's hearing, eyesight, continence, and balance need to be

---

TABLE 120-2

Clinical Features of Elderly Onset Rheumatoid Arthritis

Age of onset >60 yr

Male:female ~1:1

Acute presentation

Oligoarticular (two to six joints) disease

Involvement of large and proximal joints

Systemic complaints, e.g., weight loss

Absence of rheumatoid nodules

Sicca symptoms common

Laboratory: high erythrocyte sedimentation rate; often negative rheumatoid factor

TABLE 120-3

American College of Rheumatology 1991 Revised Criteria for the Classification of Global Functional Status in Rheumatoid Arthritis

Class I	Completely able to perform usual activities of daily living (self-care, vocational, and avocational)
Class II	Able to perform usual self-care and vocational activities but limited in avocational activities
Class III	Able to perform usual self-care activities but limited in vocational and avocational activities
Class IV	Limited in ability to perform usual self-care, vocational, and avocational activities

Adapted with permission from Hochberg MC, Cahne RW, Dwosh I, Lindsey S, Pincus T, Wolfe F. The American College of Rheumatology 1991 revised criteria for the classification of global functional status in rheumatoid arthritis. Arthritis Rheum. 1992;25:498–502.

addressed to optimize functional ability and to prevent falls. Current and past medical histories are important elements of the initial evaluation. This information is important in determining the selection of specific treatment (see "Management" section). In contrast, family history is not as helpful in assessing elderly patients with RA.

In addition to excluding diseases mentioned above, a new patient suspected of having RA should be tested for the presence of anemia, cytopenia, liver or renal dysfunction, RF, and elevated ESR. The presence of extremely high RF should prompt the clinician to consider the possible diagnosis of cryoglobulinemia. Some patients have negative RF but positive ANA. These patients tend to have more severe disease, similar to the patients with positive RF. A workup for secondary Sjögren's syndrome should be done in patients with concurrent sicca symptoms (dry eye and dry mouth). In general, ESR is a better indicator of disease activity than changes in the titer of RF. For some patients C-reactive protein level may more closely parallel their clinical course than ESR.

Radiographic joint examination is an integral part of the evaluation of patients with RA. Elderly patients with RA for more than 10 years are at particular risk of cervical spine disease and atlantoaxial

joint instability. This is an important consideration before a patient is submitted to a surgical procedure, as overextension of the cervical spine during intubation may compromise the brainstem or spinal cord. Early x-ray changes include soft-tissue swelling and regional osteoporosis around the joint. Typical erosions in hands and feet involve the juxta-articular "bare areas" of bone not covered with cartilage (Figure 120-3). Isolated erosions in the first and second metacarpophalangeal joints may prompt the clinician to search for occult calcium pyrophosphate depositive disease, hyperparathyroidism, or hemochromatosis. Erosions are less common in the knee and hip joints. At these sites, RA typically causes cartilage loss and joint-space narrowing. Joint-space narrowing occurring predominantly in the lateral compartment of the knee and diffusely in the hip without bony proliferation is helpful features for distinguishing RA from osteoarthritis. To assess for joint-space narrowing of the knees, clinicians should request semiflexed weight-bearing films.

Because of the limitation of clinical examination in detecting subtle signs of inflammation, ultrasound and magnetic resonance imaging have been used for detecting synovitis. It is clear that these modalities are extremely sensitive for detecting active inflammation. One study found that the majority of patients with treated disease and considered by their physicians to be in remission continued to have magnetic resonance imaging evidence of active synovitis. The unanswered question is whether more aggressive treatments of patient with clinically inactive disease but imaging evidence of ongoing synovitis affect patient outcomes such as long-term disability. Elderly patients with RA have additional facets that need to be taken into consideration, such as a more limited lifespan and greater infection risk with immunosuppression. At this point, the utility of these sensitive imaging modalities in clinical practice is undefined.

There is no evidence that patients with EORA are more likely to develop extra-articular disease, as compared to those with YORA. However, the elderly population may be disproportionately affected because extra-articular manifestations are more common in chronic RA. High titer of RF is a risk factor for extra-articular RA, especially in male patients. Rheumatoid nodules are the most characteristic extra-articular manifestation of RA and are present in up to 40% of seropositive white patients. These are most commonly found in

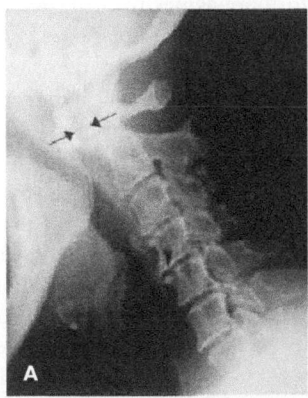
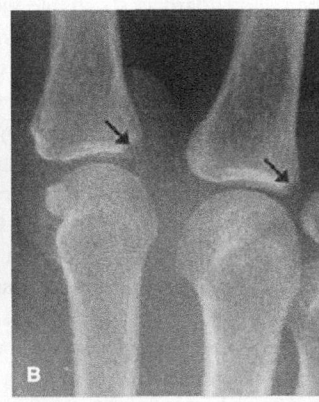
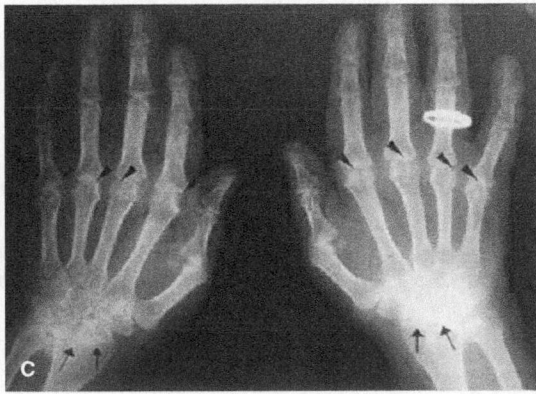

FIGURE 120-3. Radiographic changes of rheumatoid arthritis. (A) x-ray of the cervical spine in the flexed position showing severe atlantoaxial joint subluxation in a patient with chronic rheumatoid arthritis, with *arrows* highlighting the abnormal distance between the posterior surface of the anterior arch of the atlas and the anterior surface of the odontoid process. *Arrowhead* points to the erosion on the surface of C5. (B) Early erosive changes in the metacarpal phalangeal joints affecting the "bare area" of the bone not protected by cartilage. (C) Bilateral hand x-ray with advanced rheumatoid arthritis. Some of the features include juxta-articular osteoporosis, collapse of the carpal bones, radial deviation of the radiocarpal joint of the wrist (*arrows*), and erosion and destruction of metacarpal phalangeal joints (*arrowheads*). Note also the symmetric nature of the disease. *(Courtesy of Curtis Hayes, MD, University of Michigan.)*

areas of pressure such as the elbows, heels, and sacrum. Their presence does not correlate with disease activity and may increase in number during methotrexate therapy when synovitis is improving. Rheumatoid vasculitis affects vessels of all sizes. This complication may present as cutaneous vasculitis, mononeuritis multiplex, nail fold infarcts, or deep "punched-out" ulcers at atypical sites that fail to respond to conventional therapy. Pleuritis and pericarditis are found in 20% to 30% of patients with RA and do not usually cause any symptom. Other respiratory complications of RA include pulmonary granuloma (often in the upper lobes), Caplan's syndrome, fibrosing alveolitis, and bronchiolitis obliterans. Felty's syndrome (RA with splenomegaly and neutropenia) typically occurs in white patients with long-standing, chronic erosive RA. These patients are at increased risk of developing lymphoproliferative malignancies. Thrombocytopenia may occur, in part, because of splenic sequestration. Mild-to-moderate normochromic, normocytic anemia is extremely common in patients with chronic RA. Iatrogenic causes (e.g., nonsteroidal anti-inflammatory drugs [NSAIDs] and methotrexate) of anemia need to be excluded in all patients with RA who have anemia.

Management

Nonpharmacological Therapies

Successful management of RA involves patient participation in his/her care. In addition, family, social, and psychological supports are particularly critical in maintaining the older RA patients' independence. Older patients diagnosed with the disease may be particularly fearful of what it means to their independence or may become depressed. Establishing a good rapport, gaining the trust of the patient and the family, providing information about the nature of the disease, and setting realistic goals are all important elements of the initial management of RA. Many patients and their relatives also find it helpful to seek out support groups in their local area. Increasingly, elderly patients and their families are turning to the Internet, health magazines, and other nontraditional sources for information about treatment options, including over-the-counter complementary therapies. It is important that health-care professionals be aware of the pros and cons of these options. In this regard, resources such as The Arthritis Foundation's Guide to Alternative Therapies can be helpful. Unfortunately, the unexpected side effects of over-the-counter medications are increasingly being recognized. The latest information is often not available in traditional textbooks. Directing the patients to reputable websites such as that offered by the National Institute on Aging can be useful for more up-to-date information.

Nonpharmacologic therapies are crucial components of the total care of the patient with RA, which should be emphasized throughout the treatment course. In addition to their inherent usefulness, participation in these treatment modalities often provides the patients and their families with a sense of control over their chronic illness. The team approach that typifies geriatric medicine is eminently suitable for treating elderly patients with chronic arthritis. Physical and occupational therapy should be offered to every patient with RA, including those with mild and early disease. Education about rest/activity, use of cold/heat, massage, adaptive devices (to improve function and to prevent/correct joint deformity) are important. Performing exercises to strengthen muscles and ligaments for joint protection, gait training, and fall prevention can make a big

difference in the life of patients with RA. Community-based exercise programs such as PACE (Patients with Arthritis Can Exercise, the Arthritis Foundation) are a good resource for those who are able to participate. Psychological counseling and support groups are often helpful, especially to those who are socially isolated because of their arthritis. Depression is increasingly recognized as a common problem in the elderly and in those with chronic illness. Adequate treatment will help break the vicious cycle of pain, depression, and disability. Although nonpharmacologic therapies have not been shown to affect the course of RA, these can improve the patient's quality of life and help to reduce the requirement for pain medications that have significant potential for side effects in this vulnerable population.

Pharmacological Therapies

Recent years have seen an exciting explosion of new drugs available for the treatment of RA. Pharmaceutical companies have increasingly included the geriatric population in pre- and postmarketing clinical trials. Although this provides some reassurance to clinicians, knowing that these agents may be efficacious in the elderly population, it is important to remember that subjects participating in these studies rarely mirror the patients geriatricians see in their clinic who have multiple comorbidities and who already suffer from polypharmacy. The costs of these new agents may be out of reach for patients who do not have prescription coverage. Because of the complexity of modern treatment regimens, coupled with the need to monitor many potentially serious side effects, drug therapy for RA should ideally be instituted in consultation with a rheumatologist. Involvement of physicians experienced in the use of immunosuppressive therapies (e.g., hematologists and oncologists, or a gastroenterologist in the case of infliximab) will be helpful in patients living in isolated communities where there may not be a local rheumatologist.

The gradualism of the "pyramid approach" to RA treatment in the 1980s has been replaced with the widespread belief that rheumatoid inflammation should be suppressed as completely and as soon as possible once the diagnosis is confirmed. This change in philosophy is, in part, a result of the recognition that joint damage occurs much sooner than was previously believed. Results of well-designed clinical trials in the past decade have persuaded many that this new standard is attainable with more aggressive drug regimens. In the ACR updated *2002 Guidelines for the Management of Rheumatoid Arthritis*, it is suggested that the majority of patients with newly diagnosed RA should be started on disease-modifying antirheumatic drug (DMARD) therapy within 3 months of diagnosis.

Although NSAIDs are useful adjunct therapies for RA, many geriatricians are reluctant to prescribe this class of medication because of concern that elderly persons are vulnerable to the potential serious toxicity that can occur in almost every major organ system in the body. Meta-analysis of epidemiologic studies published in the 1990s found that NSAID use is associated with a 5- and 3.5-fold increased risk of serious upper GI tract disease in women and men, respectively. Age alone is a risk factor for upper GI bleeding (relative risk of 4.5 in 70–80 years age group, and 9.2 in those older than age 80 years). Because of the high background rate of upper GI events in the elderly population, the relative risk for GI bleeding only increases modestly in elderly patients on NSAID. Not surprisingly, elderly patients with history of GI bleeding are at the greatest risk of serious GI complications when they are placed on an NSAID. The concurrent use of glucocorticoids further increases the risk of GI bleeding.

The use of selective cyclooxygenase-2 (COX-2) inhibitors has decreased substantially in recent years when it was discovered that some of these agents are associated with an increased incidence of cardiac events in large population studies. In addition, COX-2 inhibitors shares similar renal toxicity, including hypertension, peripheral edema, and rising serum creatinine as traditional NSAIDs. Chronic use of these agents should, therefore, be avoided when possible. NSAID-induced renal complications are more likely to occur in patients who are on concurrent diuretics or angiotensin-converting enzyme inhibitors. One study showed that prolonged dosing of ibuprofen blocked the platelet inhibition effects of aspirin. Although other NSAIDs tested so far do not appear to have the same problem, this raises the concern that the aspirin/ibuprofen combination may not be ideal for patients having RA with cardiovascular risk factors. Concurrent use of low-dose ($\leq$325 mg/day) aspirin increases the already high risk for GI events in elderly patients taking traditional NSAIDs and may negate most of the GI-sparing effect of COX-2 inhibitors. At present, it appears that most at-risk elderly patients with RA requiring a traditional NSAID or a COX-2 selective agent plus aspirin should receive GI cytoprotection.

Low-dose glucocorticoid is effective for short-term symptom control in patients with active RA. There are also intriguing data showing that prednisone in early disease may be "disease modifying." Unfortunately, elderly patients commonly develop significant side effects but become functionally dependent on the drug. The lowest dose, and, if possible, alternate-day dosing should be prescribed. Assessment, prophylaxis, and treatment of osteoporosis, cardiovascular risk factors, diabetes, and GI complications are important. Judicious use of intra-articular steroid injections may provide local (and systemic) symptom relief and may be safer than oral glucocorticoids in elderly patients with poorly controlled diabetes, severe osteoporosis, and congestive heart failure.

Antimalarials including hydroxychloroquine and chloroquine are useful in mild cases of RA and are most often prescribed as part of a combination regimen. Hydroxychloroquine is often preferred over chloroquine because it has a lower incidence of ocular complications. Approximately 50% of hydroxychloroquine is protein bound in the plasma, a property that is important in elderly patients with low serum albumen and who are taking other highly protein-bound drugs. The mechanism of drug action is uncertain but is postulated to include changes in intracellular pH, which, in turn, affect antigen presentation by immune cells. An added benefit in patients with RA who are at increased risk of coronary heart disease is the drug's favorable effect on serum cholesterol level. There are also intriguing new data suggesting that patients with RA on hydroxychloroquine have up to 77% less risk of developing diabetes. The major side effect of hydroxychloroquine and chloroquine is retinal (macular) toxicity with the classical "bull's-eye" lesion. The patients most susceptible to this complication are those older than 70 years who are on >6.5 mg/kg daily dose or who have a cumulative dose of >800 g of the drug. Elderly patients with macular degeneration or inoperable dense cataract are not candidates for this drug.

Sulfasalazine is only occasionally used as monotherapy in the United States, although there are data showing that the drug may slow the progression of radiographic damage in RA. Its mechanism of immunosuppression is unclear but may include reducing immunoglobulin (Ig) levels, suppressed T- and B-cell proliferative response, and cytokine inhibition. Cytopenias (particularly leukopenia), GI symptoms (nausea and vomiting, and dyspepsia), and skin rashes are the commonest side effects. In addition to monitoring for hematologic toxicity, some experts recommend that liver enzyme levels should be tested regularly as well.

Methotrexate, an analog of folic acid, is the most commonly prescribed DMARD for RA in the United States. More than 50% of patients on methotrexate continue the drug beyond 3 years, longer than any other DMARD. The drug and its metabolites are potent inhibitors of dihydrofolic acid reductase and other distal enzymes in the folic acid metabolic pathway. The immunosuppressive effects may be partly a result of folate-dependent inhibition of lymphocyte proliferation. Methotrexate has also been reported to reduce the production of leukotriene B$_4$ and to directly alter phospholipase A$_2$ activity. Common side effects include cytopenias (particularly anemia), liver toxicity (fibrosis and cirrhosis), hypersensitivity pneumonitis, infections, mucosal ulceration, and alopecia. The elderly population is particularly susceptible to these side effects because methotrexate is excreted primarily by the kidneys and renal impairment is common in this group. Great caution and dose adjustment are, therefore, needed when using the drug to treat elderly patients with RA and those with a history of hepatitis. In addition, folic acid (1–3 mg/day) or folinic acid (leucovorin, 2.5–5 mg given 24 hours after methotrexate) supplementation reduces the incidence of many of methotrexate side effects and should be used routinely.

A number of other DMARDs are occasionally used as monotherapy for RA. Clinicians are often reluctant to use them because of their limited efficacy, high dropout rate, and potential serious side effects, especially in the elderly population. These include cyclosporin, azathioprine, gold, and penicillamine. Staphylococcal protein A immunoabsorption column may be useful in a small subset of patients with RA who have refractory disease. However, difficulty in administering treatment and high cost has prevented the treatment from being used widely.

Most combination therapies involve adding one or more DMARD to methotrexate. The triple therapy of methotrexate, hydroxychloroquine, and sulfasalazine is more efficacious than methotrexate alone. Similarly, patients treated with methotrexate and leflunomide experienced better outcomes than methotrexate alone. Interestingly, although methotrexate plus hydroxychloroquine is the commonest combination used in this country, its efficacy, as compared to methotrexate, has not been examined systematically. The main advantage of using combination therapy over the anticytokine treatments is cost. The argument that biologics may be cost effective because these reduce work disability may not apply to elderly, retired patients. However, whether the elderly tolerate combination therapies as well as monotherapy is uncertain. As high as 60% of patients receiving both methotrexate and leflunomide develop elevated liver enzyme levels. Combining methotrexate with a nephrotoxic drug such as cyclosporin has been used successfully in the treatment of RA but is potentially hazardous in the elderly patient who may already have underlying renal insufficiency and hypertension.

Biological Response Modifiers

The number of biological response modifiers available to clinicians has expanded considerably in the past few years, with many more in the late stages of clinical development. The success of these agents, which target soluble inflammatory proteins, T cells, and B cells, suggests that targeting the downstream mediators may be sufficient to modulate the disease. A critical issue is to determine which patient will best benefit from which class of biologic agent. While it is unlikely that primary-care providers will prescribe biologics for their patients with RA, understanding their use and potential side effects will be helpful in the day-to-day care of these patients. This portion of the chapter includes a general description of the currently available drugs and will emphasize the safety issues associated with these drugs, as these issues have great relevance to geriatrics health-care providers.

An important advantage of these agents is rapid onset of action, with many patients experiencing improvement within a few weeks of treatment. These agents appear to be effective in patients with both seropositive and seronegative rheumatoid. The decision as to which biological modifier to use will depend on individual patient characteristics such as comorbidity, patient preferences such as administration schedule, physician experience, and insurance coverage owing to the high cost of these drugs.

Leflunomide is an inhibitor of pyrimidine synthesis and has been available for the treatment of RA in the United States since 1998. The oral medication is rapidly metabolized to an active metabolite that is partially excreted in the bile and reabsorbed by the enterohepatic circulation. The plasma half-life of leflunomide is approximately 14 days. However, the excretion can be accelerated by oral cholestyramine. In clinical studies, leflunomide has been shown to be equal to methotrexate in efficacy. It is also the first drug to receive an FDA-approved label indication to retard structural damage in RA as evidenced by x-ray erosions and joint-space narrowing. The commonest side effects include diarrhea (20%), reversible alopecia (10%), and elevated liver function enzymes.

There are currently three TNF antagonists in clinical use. *Etanercept* is a recombinant soluble p75 TNF receptor fused to the Fc portion of human Ig G_1. The drug is usually given by subcutaneous injection once or twice a week, with or without concomitant methotrexate. *Infliximab* is a chimeric (mouse–human) anti-TNF monoclonal antibody that is given to patients intravenously every 4 to 8 weeks, usually in combination with methotrexate. *Adalimumab*, a fully human anti-TNF antibody, is given subcutaneously every 2 weeks, usually with methotrexate. Accumulating evidence suggests that patients who have "failed" one anti-TNF agent may still benefit from a trial of a different anti-TNF drug.

Anakinra is a recombinant human form of IL-1 receptor antagonist (IL-1ra) that blocks the binding of IL-1α and β to the IL-1 receptor. The drug is administered daily by subcutaneous injection with or without methotrexate. Anakinra has not been as popular as the anti-TNF agents among rheumatologists in part because of the high incidence of local skin injection site reactions and the requirement of daily injection. Furthermore, many have found the drug to be less efficacious as the anti-TNF agents, although there is no randomized comparison trial to date. Because the plasma clearance of the drug is reduced by 16%, 50%, and 70% to 75% in patients with mild (creatinine clearance 50–80 mL/min), moderate (creatinine clearance 30–49 mL/min), and severe (creatinine clearance <30 mL/min) renal insufficiencies, respectively, it is usually necessary to adjust the dose when used in older adults because of the frequency of reduced renal function in this population.

Rituximab is a chimeric anti-CD20 antibody, originally used for the treatment of a subset of patients with non-Hodgkin's lymphoma. The drug works by depleting B cells with CD20 on their surface. The drug is approved in the United States for the treatment of patients with RA with an inadequate response to anti-TNF agents. Since rituximab has nonhuman protein sequences, it should be used in conjunction with another immunosuppressive agent such as methotrexate. Patients are usually given one course of two infusions 2 weeks apart. It is possible to repeat the treatment 6 months later.

Abetacept is a recombinant fusion protein combining the extracellular domain of human CTLA-4 and an Fc domain of human IgG1 that has been modified to avoid complement fixation. The drug competitively binds to the costimulatory molecules CD80/CD86 to prevent these molecules from engaging CD28 on T cells and thereby prevents full T-cell activation. This, in turn, suppresses T-cell proliferation and inhibits the production of TNF-α, interferon (IFN)-γ, and IL-2. Abetacept is dosed according to the patient's body weight. Since most of the published data have examined the efficacy of a combination regimen using concomitant methotrexate, most patients should be on both drugs rather than abetacept monotherapy.

Safety and Other Issues with Biologics

While there is little doubt about the potential efficacy of the biologics in RA, there remains significant concern about their side effects, especially in vulnerable populations such as elderly patients with RA having multiple comorbidities. In addition, the significant cost associated with these drugs is prohibitive to many elderly patients without prescription drug coverage. One useful acronym for the safe use of biologics is SAFETY, outlined in Table 120-4. TNF is involved in host defense against foreign pathogens and in tumor surveillance. The most important risk associated with anticytokine therapy for elderly patients with RA is the increased incidence of fungal infections, tuberculosis, and atypical mycobacterial infections. As tuberculosis is usually caused by reactivation of latent infection, tuberculosis skin testing and a chest x-ray should be done prior to starting these agents. Whether yearly skin test and chest x-ray to detect new exposure are necessary in countries with a low incidence of tuberculosis is unclear. Yearly screening is recommended for selected patients who are at risk, such as those who travel regularly to TB endemic areas and nursing home residents.

TABLE 120-4

SAFETY of Novel Immunomodulatory Therapies: Optimizing Treatment

Stratify: Identify the patient's risk of adverse effects based on various factors, such as comorbidities (e.g., chronic obstructive pulmonary disease and diabetes mellitus), age, concomitant medication use, and a history of similar events (e.g., opportunistic infection).

Assess: Evaluate the patient for important risks (e.g., exposure to tuberculosis or hepatitis B or C virus infection, vaccination status, and status of comorbid conditions).

Fend off: Optimize the patient's health before treatment (e.g., wherever possible, vaccinate against infections and treat and/or control the patient's comorbidities).

Evaluate: Quickly evaluate adverse events, remembering that both typical and atypical presentations may be seen.

Treat: Aggressively manage adverse events to help minimize their severity.

Yearly: Reevaluate the patient on a regular basis.

Adapted with permission from Hennigan S, Kavanaugh A. Optimizing the use of TNF-α inhibitors. *J Musculoskel Med.* 2007;24:293–298.

Rituximab dramatically lowers the peripheral blood B-cell count for months after the infusion, and these patients also have lower IgG and IgM levels. The use of rituximab has been associated with the reactivation of JC polyoma virus infection, resulting in the disease progressive multifocal leukoencephalopathy. This complication, although very rare, highlights the potential for the development of all B-cell-dependent viral diseases in patients receiving the drug. Interestingly, progressive multifocal leukoencephalopathy has also been reported in patients with multiple sclerosis receiving natalizumab, a chimeric anti-α4 integrin antibody.

Rare cases of demyelinating disorders, aplastic anemia, lupus-like illnesses, and depression have also been associated with anti-TNF therapies. The long-term consequences of anticytokine suppression are unknown. One meta-analysis reported a fourfold higher rate of malignancies in patients treated with TNF inhibitors.

In addition to the concern about infection risk, abetacept can be potentially problematic in older adults with multiple comorbidities. Patients with chronic obstructive pulmonary disease have a higher incidence of adverse drug reaction and respiratory complaints such as chronic obstructive pulmonary disease exacerbation, cough, and dyspnea. Diabetic patients should be alerted to the fact that the abetacept formulation contains maltose and can give falsely elevated glucose readings in some glucose monitors on the day of the infusion.

Are biologics "cost effective" in the treatment of older adults with rheumatic diseases? Cost effectiveness for young patients with RA has been shown based on remaining in the work force, but there are no such data for the geriatrics cohort of retirees, and it is hard to define the economic value of improved functional status or quality of life. However, given the potential serious side effects that may more likely affect frail older adults, the author's approach is to start with traditional DMARDs such as methotrexate and hydroxychloroquine for such patients and move on to biologics only after these have failed or if the patients experience unacceptable side effects from the DMARDs.

As in other populations, cardiovascular disease is the single largest cause of death in patients with autoimmune inflammatory disorders. However, after accounting for the known traditional risk factors for heart diseases, patients with RA and lupus are at greater risk of developing coronary artery disease and stroke than those without these conditions. The reason for the increased incidence of cardiovascular disease in patients with these disorders of autoimmunity is not clear. Furthermore, a patient with rheumatoid arthritis who has a myocardial infarction has a similar prognosis as that of a diabetic patient with a similar event. Some findings suggest that conventional therapies, such as the use of lipid-lowering agents, may not reverse the cardiovascular risk associated with these inflammatory conditions. While not proven, it is hoped that use of more aggressive immunosuppressive regimens will help reduce the cardiovascular morbidity and mortality in these patients. However, the use of anti-TNF agents has been linked to an increased rate of congestive heart failure and cardiac mortality when these were used in heart failure clinical trials. Aging per se has been described by some as a state of chronic low-grade inflammation that has been termed "inflamm-aging," which may play a role in frailty and sarcopenia in both normal aging and chronic inflammatory conditions such as RA (see Chapter 4 for further details).

A disease-associated inflammatory state, chronic use of steroids, and the lack of exercise owing to arthritis-associated disability may all contribute to the high incidence of osteoporosis in older patients with rheumatic diseases. Since these are chronic conditions, aggressive treatment with antiresorptive agents, adequate calcium intake, and vitamin D to prevent and treat osteoporosis and fracture is critical.

Many RA therapies involve significant immunosuppression that may affect the patient's ability to mount an antibody response to immunization, worsening the already-impaired immune reaction as a result of immune senescence in older patients. It is, therefore, important that these patients are given their age-appropriate immunizations such as pneumococcal and flu vaccines preferably prior to receiving therapy with biologics. Patients already on biologics should avoid receiving any live vaccines.

Surgical Interventions

Surgeries can be useful to restore function and in many cases reduce pain in end-stage RA joints. These procedures include small-joint arthroplasty, joint fusion, and resection of metatarsal heads. Improvements in surgical techniques, prosthetic materials, perioperative care, and rehabilitation in the past two decades have resulted in much better outcomes in patients undergoing surgical treatments. However, it should be noted that there are very little long-term data examining the outcome of small joint arthroplasty. A number of ongoing National Institute of Health-sponsored studies will provide much needed data in the near future. Synovectomy and tendon repairs are important surgical procedures to prevent and treat tendon rupture that can have disastrous functional consequences in patients with RA. Careful planning and timing of various joint procedures in patients with RA are important. For example, it may be wise to first correct upper extremity deformities before lower-extremity surgery is performed to allow the use of the upper extremities to assist in transfer, rising from a chair, and stair climbing during rehabilitation.

Prevention

A major problem in attempting to prevent the disease is identifying those who are at risk of developing the disease in the first place. Although genetic studies provide some clues as to which segment of the population may be at risk, the available information is not precise enough to be of practical use. There is some evidence that oral contraceptive pill and hormone replacement therapy may reduce the risk of developing RA. Conversely, epidemiologic data suggest that smoking is associated with a slightly increased risk for the disease. During the past decade, there has been considerable interest in developing T-cell receptor peptide vaccines for RA. This approach has shown some promising results in an animal model of chronic inflammatory arthritis. Whether this will eventually lead to useful human vaccine is unclear. One study suggests that the use of aggressive drug therapy in patients with inflammatory arthritis but who do not yet fulfill the criteria for full-blown RA may reduce the number developing the disease. Whether this applies to EORA is unknown.

Special Issues

Patient Preference and Comorbidity

The choice of therapy should be made in conjunction with the patient and the caregivers. Although exercises are important to maintain joint and muscle functions in patients with RA, some elderly patients are unable to perform regular exercises because of their other medical conditions, or if they have lived an inactive lifestyle for many years and are reluctant to adopt any change. In these situations, emphasizing the positive aspects of exercise (physical, psychological, and social), setting realistic goals, and recommending exercise programs specially tailored for the elderly population are helpful. In this regard, finding a physical and occupational therapist accustomed to working with older adults is important. Too often the author has seen patients who refuse to return to their therapist because of unrealistic short-term exercise goals.

The importance of assessing a patient's risk of developing GI, renal, cardiac complication, and osteoporosis prior to starting NSAIDs and corticosteroids has already been emphasized. Patient preference is important when deciding on a specific DMARD. Elderly patients with poor eyesight are often reluctant to begin antimalarials out of fear of potential ocular complications, however small the risk may be. These drugs are contraindicated in elderly patients who cannot be monitored for retinal toxicity, including individuals with macular degeneration or untreated cataract. Older adults who do not want to give up drinking alcohol may choose not to take methotrexate. Some older women have refused to take methotrexate because the drug was part of their breast cancer chemotherapy in the distant past. Intramuscular methotrexate can be used in elderly patients who experience dyspepsia or who have difficulty swallowing. Methotrexate and biological response modifiers must be used with extreme caution or not at all in patients with chronic or active infection. Elderly patients with RA should have received all the appropriate immunizations prior to receiving DMARDs. Whether elderly patients with chronic lung disease taking DMARDs should receive *Pneumocystis carinii* prophylaxis is unclear. Assessment of the patient's tuberculosis status should be done prior to beginning anticytokine therapy. The appropriate use of biologics has already been discussed extensively.

Care Settings

The physician's choice of therapy has to take into account the patient's overall state of health and mobility, and the care setting. In most cases, home laboratory monitoring for DMARD toxicity can be arranged for patients with significant mobility problems. Instead of DMARDs, the use of corticosteroids (oral, intra-articular, or parenteral; low- or high-dose "pulse" treatment) may be a good option in patients with RA with active disease in the end stages of their lives. Therapeutic goals may also be different in a patient near the end of life, when either long-term treatment outcome or side effects may not be important considerations. An example will be a patient with RA who has end-stage dementia when judicious use of corticosteroid rather than high-dose immunosuppression for active disease may be more appropriate.

SYSTEMIC LUPUS ERYTHEMATOSUS

Systemic lupus erythematosus (SLE) is a prototypic autoimmune disease that predominantly affects the female population. The incidence of lupus has been increasing in the past few decades, with an estimated a quarter of a million patients now with the disease in this country. Late-onset lupus (LOL) is defined as symptoms beginning after the age of 55 years, representing approximately 10% of all cases of lupus. However, the United Kingdom General Practice Research Database (a population database covering 5% of the United Kingdom) has surprising data that the peak incidence of lupus in females occurs at age 50 to 54 years and for males it is 70 to 74 years (Figure 120-4). Comparable data are not available for the United States, since previous lupus surveillance studies have been confined to relatively small geographic areas. It is anticipated that an ongoing Centers for Disease Control and Prevention-sponsored study in southeastern Michigan will eventually provide a better estimate of the true age-specific incidence of this disease in the United States. Finally, improved therapies and greater appreciation of the importance of treating comorbid conditions such as coronary artery disease have resulted in more patients with lupus surviving into old age.

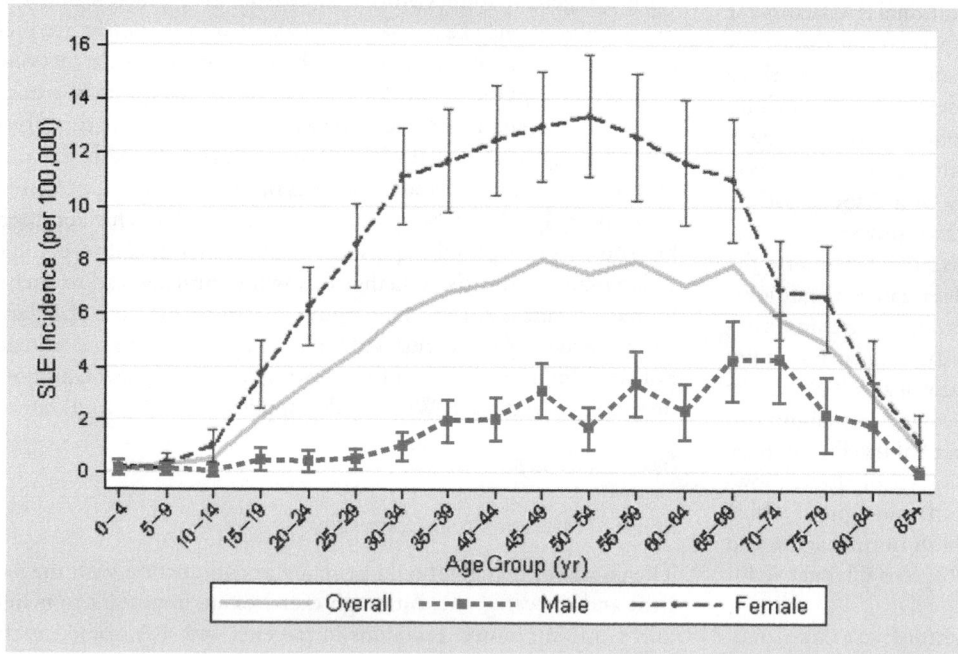

FIGURE 120-4. Incidence of systemic lupus erythematosus in the United Kingdom, 1990–1999. *(Reproduced with permission from Somers EC, et al. Arthritis Rheum. 2007; 57(4):612.)*

TABLE 120-5

Revised Classification Criteria for SLE

Serositis	Pleuritis, pericarditis, or peritonitis
Oral or nasal ulceration	Oral ulcers are often painless and occur in unusual parts of the oral cavity
Arthritis	Nonerosive polyarthritis involving the small joints
Photosensitivity	Skin rash when exposed to sunlight
Blood dyscrasia	Hemolytic anemia, leukopenia/lymphopenia, or thrombocytopenia
Renal disease	Proteinuria (>0.5 g/d), cellular casts, unexplained hematuria
ANA	≥1:160 titer in the absence of lupus-inducing drug
Immunological abnormalities	Anti-dsDNA, anti-Sm, or antiphospholipid antibody
Neuropsychiatric illness	Seizures or psychosis
Malar rash	Tends to spare the nasolabial folds
Discoid rash	Often scarring

ANA, antinuclear antibody; dsDNA, double-stranded deoxyribonucleic acid; Sm, Smith (antigen).
Data from Berney SM. Systemic lupus erythematosus. Hospital Physician. 1998; 1(3):2–12Berney SM (1998).

Diagnosis

The diagnosis of SLE is based on the presence of signs, symptoms, and laboratory features of autoimmunity. The 1982 ACR Classification Criteria for SLE was recently revised to include the presence of antiphospholipid antibodies (Table 120-5). It is important to recognize that these criteria were designed for research purposes and have not been validated in LOL. Low-titer ANA may be present in up to one-third of the elderly. Positive ANAs (titer ≥1:160) have high sensitivity but poor specificity for SLE when measured by indirect immunofluorescence using the standard Hep-2 substrate. In contrast, the presence of anti-dsDNA (double-stranded deoxyribonucleic acid) or anti-Sm (Smith) antibodies is highly specific for SLE. However, these antibodies are only detected in 31% to 86% and 0% to 24% of patients with LOL, respectively.

Pathogenesis

The cause of SLE is unknown. The concordance rate of SLE in monozygotic twins is between 25% and 50%, suggesting that genetic and environmental factors are both important. Human SLE is a polygenic disease. Genetic studies have identified at least 50 susceptibility or resistance loci in human and murine lupus (e.g., *sle*1, 2, 3). A defect or deficiency in gene product(s) regulating immune complex clearance, such as in some cases of inherited complement (C1, C4, and C2) deficiencies, is associated with a high likelihood of the development of SLE. Variability in the Fcγ receptor alleles is believed to play a role in determining the susceptibility to SLE in some racial and ethnic populations. Defective apoptosis as a consequence of mutations of the Fas or Fas-ligand gene is the central mechanism responsible for the lupus-like disease seen in the MRL/*lpr* and MRL/*gld* mice. However, such defects are exceedingly rare in humans, and, when present, these cause a much more limited autoimmune disease (the Canale–Smith syndrome).

Hormonal factors are important in the pathogenesis of SLE. The disease often affects females of childbearing age. The decline in fe-

male sex hormones in postmenopausal years was believed to be an important reason for a lower incidence of SLE in this age group, but the United Kingdom General Practice Research Database study raises questions about the validity of this association. There are also data showing that exogenous estrogens (hormone replacement therapy and oral contraceptive pill) may impose a small risk for developing lupus. The SELENA (Safety of Estrogens in Lupus Erythematosus National Assessment) trial showed that postmenopausal women receiving hormone replacement therapy have a slight increase in the number of mild-to-moderate lupus flares, but there was no increase in the number of severe flares. Similar to other autoimmune diseases, an inciting role for microbial organisms has been postulated but not proven.

An unanswered question is whether LOL is a different disease than the one that occurs at a younger age. It is well accepted that many older adults have a low level of circulating autoantibodies. Additionally, measures of various markers of immunosenescence suggest that patients with autoimmune diseases have accelerated aging of the immune system. Given the apparent high incidence of lupus in middle-aged and late life, a better understanding of how immune senescence can affect the normally tightly regulated process that prevents the development of autoimmunity is needed. One hypothesis is that defective T-cell activation in aging may result in suboptimal immune response to foreign antigen, which, in turn, may allow these cells to cross-react with self-antigens. Secondly, thymic involution and the accumulation of memory T cells in aging may "force" the proliferation of naïve T cells with high affinity for self-antigen. Thirdly, epigenetics, which refers to the regulation of gene expression through cellular processes including DNA methylation, histone modification, and RNA interference, has been shown to be affected by aging. Both DNA methylation and histone acetylation are important mechanisms for the development of lupus and potentially other autoimmune diseases. Whether the age-dependent epigenetic changes also affect genes that are important in the development of autoimmunity in aging is unknown. Finally, it has been postulated that age-related DNA methylation changes may "reawaken" X-chromosome genes that have previously been inactivated in females. This, in turn, may help to explain the gender differences in a disease such as lupus in the elderly population.

Presentation

Because of the lack of awareness of this disease in older people, the average time it takes from the onset of symptoms to the diagnosis of LOL is long, averaging between 2 and 3 years. The female:male ratio of LOL is approximately 4:1, much lower than the 9:1 ratio seen in the younger age group. It has been reported that the high prevalence of SLE in African-Americans is not so apparent in LOL. However, whether this merely reflects the demographics of the study locations is unclear.

The clinical features of patients with LOL are quite different from those who develop their lupus at a younger age (Table 120-6). The patients with LOL tend to have a milder disease and are less likely to develop alopecia, malar rash, photosensitivity, oral/nasal ulceration, glomerulonephritis, and lymphadenopathy. Patients with LOL may be more prone to develop cytopenias, serositis, and interstitial pneumonitis. Interestingly, the incidence of cancer, with the exception of non-Hodgkin's lymphoma, may be lower in LOL

TABLE 120-6

The Frequency of Symptoms and Signs of SLE in the Older Adults

SYMPTOMS/SIGNS	FREQUENCY (%)
Arthritis/arthralgia	60
Rash	47
Cytopenias	45
Interstitial pneumonitis	41
Serositis	32
Raynaud's phenomenon	28
Neuropsychiatric	25
Peripheral neuropathy	25
Glomerulonephritis	24

Adapted with permission from Kammer GM, Mishra N. Systemic lupus erythematosus in the elderly. Rheum Dis Clin North Am. 2000;266:475.

than in younger patients with lupus. The cause of death in patients with LOL is usually related to complications of treatment such as infections, cardiovascular disease, and stroke.

Management

The choice of therapy is largely dictated by the specific disease manifestations. Antimalarials (see above) are useful for many lupus symptoms including arthritis, serositis, mucositis, and skin disease. Available evidence strongly supports the long-term use of antimalarials in patients with lupus. Quinacrine, available from many compounding pharmacists, does not cause retinal damage and may be used in elderly patients who cannot take potentially retinotoxic drugs. NSAIDs are used by the majority of patients with lupus for symptomatic relief of arthralgias, myalgias, serositis, fever, and headaches. Their use in elderly patients must be weighed against their potential side effects. This class of drugs is best avoided in patients with lupus having renal involvement.

Local corticosteroid treatments such as (short-term) topical or intradermal injections can be helpful in cutaneous lupus. Systemic steroids are often reserved for more severe disease such as lupus pneumonitis, carditis, hemolytic anemia, or new-onset renal disease. Intravenous "pulse" methylprednisolone in doses of 1 g/d for up to 3 consecutive days can be lifesaving in rapidly progressive or fulminant disease.

The use of cytotoxic drugs such as cyclophosphamide has significantly reduced the morbidity and mortality associated with lupus nephritis. Monthly intravenous pulse cyclophosphamide is generally well tolerated and has fewer side effects than daily oral administration of the drug. Azathioprine, chlorambucil, or nitrogen mustard may be used in lupus patients with renal disease who are unable to tolerate high-dose corticosteroids or cyclophosphamide. Mycophenolate mofetil has gained significant acceptance in the treatment of many lupus manifestations and may be better tolerated than azathioprine. Cytotoxics should not be withheld from elderly patients with lupus with major organ involvement. The use of alkylating agents is associated with an increased risk of future cancer development. However, this may be a more important consideration in younger patients with a longer life expectancy. Gonad toxicity is not a very important issue in the elderly population.

SJÖGREN'S SYNDROME

Definition

Sjögren's syndrome is a chronic inflammatory autoimmune disease characterized by progressive lymphocytic and plasma cell infiltration of the exocrine glands, leading to dry mouth (xerostomia) and dry eye (keratoconjunctivitis sicca). The syndrome can occur in isolation (primary) or in association with other autoimmune diseases (secondary) such as RA, SLE, or polymyositis. In addition to the sicca symptoms (dry eyes and dry mouth) serologic evidence of autoimmunity and objective assessment of oral and ocular involvement need to be documented before the diagnosis of Sjögren's syndrome is made. The Schirmer test, in which a strip of Whatman No. 41 filter paper is placed in the lower conjunctival sac, is considered positive if less than 5 mm of the paper is wet after 5 minutes. Ocular involvement can also be documented by staining the conjunctiva with 1% Rose Bengal stain and slit-lamp eye examination. Minor salivary gland biopsy is the most commonly performed test used in diagnosing salivary gland involvement in Sjögren's syndrome. The test is considered positive when there is more than one focus (aggregate of ≥ 50 lymphocytes) per 4 mm^2 of biopsy specimen. Biopsy of the parotid, rather than of a minor salivary gland, should be done in patients complaining of parotid gland swelling. Saliva production is measured after overnight fasting without oral stimulation (brushing of teeth, smoking, etc.). A normal person should produce at least 1.5 mL of saliva in 15 minutes. Parotid sialography and salivary gland scintigraphy are alternate procedures for documenting salivary gland involvement.

Epidemiology

Depending on the definition and the age of the population studied, the prevalence of Sjögren's syndrome has been estimated to be between 0.04% and 4.8%, making it the second commonest autoimmune disease after RA. The disease is likely underdiagnosed as patients often fail to discuss their symptoms with their physicians or believe that the symptoms are part of the inevitable consequence of aging. One study on a geriatric population suggests that subclinical disease may occur in up to 3% of the nursing home population. Although the prevalence of sicca symptoms increases with age, the peak incidence of primary Sjögren's syndrome occurs in the fourth and fifth decades of life, with a 9:1 female:male ratio.

Pathogenesis

Most cases of Sjögren's syndrome occur sporadically, although there are examples of familial aggregation. An association with HLA antigens has been reported, including HLA-DR3, HLA-DR2, and HLA-DRw52 in white populations. In addition, HLA-DR3 and HLA-DQw2.1 are linked to the development of anti-Ro antibodies. Like most other autoimmune diseases, an environmental or viral trigger has been proposed for Sjögren's syndrome. One theory suggests that autoimmune lymphocytes are "homed" to salivary and lacrimal glands. This is followed by clonal expansion of the autoreactive cells in the glands, upregulation of major histocompatibility complex and adhesion molecules by epithelial cells, and secretion of proinflammatory cytokines by lymphocytes and epithelial cells. Defective apoptosis causing the failure to delete autoreactive cells has been proposed as a central mechanism explaining the lymphoid aggregates seen in the exocrine glands. α-Fodrin, a cytoskeletal protein, was recently identified as a candidate autoantigen in Sjögren's syndrome. Interestingly, neonatal immunization with this antigen can prevent the development of the disease in an animal model of Sjögren's syndrome.

Presentation and Clinical Features

Most patients with Sjögren's syndrome have a slowly progressive and benign course. The onset of the disease is insidious, and it may take up to 10 years for the full-blown disease to develop. Older patients with Sjögren's syndrome usually present with sicca symptoms. They may complain of difficulty chewing and swallowing dry foods, the frequent need to drink liquid especially at night, difficulty wearing dentures, abnormal taste, sore/burning sensation in the mouth, and intolerance to spicy foods. Xerostomia also predisposes these patients to dental decay and the development of oral candidiasis. Instead of the classical white candida plaque, patients with Sjögren's syndrome may have erythematous oral candidiasis. In addition to the feeling of dryness in the eyes, patients with ocular involvement may complain of an itching or burning sensation, the feeling that there is a foreign body in the eye, and photosensitivity. Unilateral or bilateral parotid gland swelling occurs in one-third of all patients with primary Sjögren's syndrome and is more commonly seen in the younger age group. The differential diagnosis of unilateral or bilateral parotid gland swelling includes viral (including HIV-1) and bacterial infections, sarcoidosis, salivary gland ductal obstruction, and neoplasm.

Approximately 60% of patients with Sjögren's syndrome develop extraglandular disease (Table 120-7). Nonerosive arthritis/arthralgia is the commonest extraglandular manifestation and may precede sicca symptoms. Any part of the pulmonary tree from the trachea to the pleural lining may be involved, causing cough, hoarseness, and shortness of breath. Pseudolymphoma and lymphoma should be suspected when an unexplained pulmonary nodule or lymphadenopathy is seen on chest radiograph. Patients with Sjögren's syndrome may experience dysphagia because of dryness of the oral pharynx or abnormal esophageal motility. Chronic atrophic gastritis, gastric lymphoma, vitamin B-12 deficiency, and antibodies to parietal cells have all been described in this disease. Autoimmune thyroid disease is present in 13% to 45% of patients with Sjögren's syndrome. Patients with Sjögren's syndrome often have elevated liver enzyme profile, especially if antimitochondrial antibodies are present. Interestingly, sicca symptoms are present in 50% of patients with primary biliary cirrhosis. Renal disease occurs in approximately 10% of patients with Sjögren's syndrome. Lymphocytic infiltration and immune complex deposition, proximal tubular acidosis with Fanconi syndrome, renal stones, electrolyte imbalance, and cryoglobulinemia have all been reported.

The association of RA and Sjögren's syndrome was first described by Henrik Sjögren in 1933. Although it is believed that RA is the commonest cause of secondary Sjögren's syndrome, its true prevalence in RA is unknown. Patients with secondary Sjögren's syndrome have milder disease with primarily sicca symptoms (dry eyes and dry mouth). Systemic complications such as salivary gland swelling, central nervous system disease, renal disease (interstitial nephritis or glomerulonephritis), and lymphoproliferative disease are uncommon.

Patients with Sjögren's syndrome often have polyclonal hypergammaglobulinemia, as well as selective increased production of specific autoantibodies. ANA and RFs are present in more than 75% and 66% of patients with Sjögren's syndrome, respectively. Anti-Ro and anti-La antibodies are detected in 70% and 40% of the affected patients. Interestingly, anti-La antibodies are less common in the secondary form of the disease.

Management

Simple lifestyle changes such as air humidification and avoidance of cigarette smoke are helpful. Nasal dryness can be treated with saline drops or gel. Vaginal dryness can be reduced using water-soluble lubricants and estrogen cream. Dry skin can be improved by using moisturizers and bath oil. Lipstick and lip balm can be used to reduce lip dryness. Meticulous oral hygiene and frequent dental visits are important to prevent complications such as dental decay and oral candidiasis. Frequent fluid replacement, topical fluoride treatment, the use of non-alcohol-based mouthwash, and sugarfree chewing gum can all be helpful. Unfortunately, artificial saliva substitutes that are currently available are not very helpful. Oral candidiasis can be treated with a prolonged course (1–4 months) of a noncariogenic antifungal drug (e.g., nystatin vaginal tablets 100,000 units two to three times a day), with separate treatment of dentures.

The mainstay of treatment for dry eye remains artificial tears. Preparations now available can penetrate into the epithelial cell layer, extending duration of action. However, these may occasionally cause blurring and leave residue on eye lashes. Because patients with Sjögren's syndrome generally require long-term tear replenishment, preservative-free artificial tears should be used. Topical low-dose cyclosporine can be used for Sjögren's eye disease. Tear drainage can also be reduced by the placement of occlusive elements (e.g., silicon implants) in the puncta or permanently by laser or thermal cautery. Soft contact lenses may be used to protect the cornea, especially

TABLE 120-7

Extraglandular Manifestations of Sjögren's Syndrome	
Cutaneous	Xerosis (including dryness of nasal passage, skin, and vagina), Raynaud's phenomenon, and cutaneous vasculitis
Pulmonary	Desiccation of the tracheobronchial tree, lymphocytic infiltration (alveolitis, interstitial pneumonitis, pseudolymphoma, and lymphoma), pleuritis/pleural effusion, vasculitis, and pulmonary hypertension
Gastrointestinal	Dysphagia, atrophic gastritis, malabsorption, pancreatic dysfunction and pancreatitis, hepatomegaly and hepatitis, and primary biliary cirrhosis
Renal	Interstitial nephritis, glomerulonephritis, distal renal tubular acidosis, and kidney stones
Hematological	Anemia and cryoglobulinemia
Neuromuscular	Sensory and trigeminal neuralgia, vasculitis; mononeuritis multiplex, neuropsychiatric disorders, seizures, encephalopathy, myelitis, aseptic meningitis, dementia, myopathy, and myositis
Endocrine	Autoimmune thyroid disease

in the presence of keratitis filamentosa. Because the contact lenses require wetting, the patient needs to be careful not to introduce infection to the eyes. Plastic wrap or swimming goggles can be used at night to reduce tear evaporation.

Whenever possible, drugs with significant cholinergic side effects should be discontinued. Muscarinic agonists (pilocarpine and cevimeline) may be helpful in alleviating dry mouth symptoms in patients with Sjögren's syndrome. Systemic corticosteroid and immunosuppressive drugs (e.g., cyclophosphamide) are sometimes used for severe extraglandular diseases such as interstitial pneumonitis, interstitial nephritis, and vasculitis. Musculoskeletal symptoms are often alleviated by the judicious use of NSAIDs, hydroxychloroquine, or sulfasalazine. IFN-α may improve salivary flow in a subset of patients with Sjögren's syndrome. Unfortunately, while treatments are helpful for symptomatic relief, the destruction of exocrine gland continues despite best current effort.

DRUG-INDUCED RHEUMATIC SYNDROMES

Polypharmacy and iatrogenic diseases are important geriatric issues. Medications are also increasingly recognized as common causes of rheumatic syndromes. These can be broadly categorized into drug-induced lupus (DIL), drug-induced myopathy/myositis, and drug-induced vasculitis.

Drug-Induced Lupus

More than 100 drugs have now been implicated in DIL (Table 120-8). However, specific criteria for the diagnosis of DIL have not been established. Compared to the idiopathic disease, patients with "classical" DIL have a milder illness and a more restricted autoantibody profile. Antihistone antibodies are present in high frequencies in DIL associated with drugs such as procainamide or hydralazine but are not as frequently seen in patients with drugs such as minocycline or anti-TNF agents. The incidence of DIL has been estimated to be approximately 15,000 to 20,000 per year, with between 30,000 and 50,000 patients currently affected in the United States.

Procainamide (procainamide-induced lupus, PIL) and hydralazine (hydralazine-induced lupus, HIL) are drugs historically associated with DIL and are well-defined DIL models. Patients with DIL are usually older and more likely to be men, reflecting the age and sex of the population receiving these drugs. One-third of patients receiving procainamide for more than a year will develop symptoms, and almost all will become ANA positive after 2 years. In contrast, fewer than 20% of hydralazine-treated patients will develop DIL. The risk for developing HIL is dose dependent and is highest in patients taking more than 200 mg/day and in those who have taken more than 100 g cumulative dose. Compared to patients with idiopathic lupus, patients with PIL and HIL have fewer renal, neuropsychiatric, and skin manifestations. Pleuropulmonary complaints are particularly common in PIL, while immune cytopenias are uncommon in DIL in general. By definition, all patients with DIL are ANA positive (mostly homogenous pattern). More than 90% of patients with PIL and HIL have antihistone antibodies, and 20% to 40% are RF positive.

Up to 19% of patients treated with IFN-α develop some form of autoimmunity. Approximately 12% of patients receiving this drug develop positive ANA, and between 0.15% and 0.7% will develop a

TABLE 120-8
Drugs Implicated in Drug-Induced Lupus

Acebutolol	Infliximab	Phenylbutazone
Aminoglutethimide	Interferon (α, γ)	Phenylethyla-cetylurea
Amiodarone	Interleukin-2	*Phenytoin*
Amoproxan	*Isoniazid*	Practolol
Anthiomaline	Labetalol	Prazosin
Atenolol	Lamotrigine	Primidone
Benoxaprofen	Leuprolide acetate	Prinolol
Canavanine (L-)	Levodopa	*Procainamide*
Captopril	Levomeprazone	Promethazine
Carbamazepine	Lithium carbonate	Prophythiouracil
Chlorpromazine	Lovastatin	Psoralen
Chlorprothixene	Mephenytoin	Pyrathiazine
Cimetidine	Mesalazine	Pyrithoxine
Cinnarazine	Methimazole	*Quinidine*
Clonidine	*Methyldopa*	Quinine
Clozapine	Methylsergide	Rifamycin
COL-3	Methylthiouracil	*Sulfasalazine*
Danazol	Metrizamide	(5-amino) salicylic acid
Diclofenac	*Minocycline*	Simvastatin
1,2-Dimethyl-3-hydroxypyride-4-1 (L)	Minoxidil	Spironolactone
	Nalidixic acid	Streptomycin
Disopyramide	Nitrofurantoin	Sulindac
Estrogens	Nomifensin	Sulfadimethoxine
Etanercept	Oral contraceptives	Sulfamethoxypyridazine
Ethosuximide	Olsalazine	Terbinafine
Flutamide	Oxyphenisatin	Tetracycline
Fluvastatin	Para-aminosalicylic acid	Tetrazine
Gold salts	*Penicillamine*	Thionamide
Griseofulvin	Penicillin	Thioridazide
Guanoxan	Perazine	Timolol eye drops
Hydralazine	Perphenazine	Tolazamide
Hydrazine	Phenelzine	Tolmetin
Ibuprofen	Phenopyrazone	Trimethadione
		Zafirlukast

Drugs with the strongest associations are in italic.
Adapted with permission from Yung RL, Richardson BC. Drug-induced rheumatic syndromes. Bull Rheum Dis. 2002;51(4):1.

lupus-like illness. Anti-dsDNA antibodies occur in 8%, and almost all the patients with IFN-α-induced lupus have elevated anti-dsDNA antibodies. The development of autoimmunity appears to be dependent on the dose and duration of treatment. Other rheumatic syndromes associated with IFN-α include RA, polymyositis, psoriatic arthritis, Reiter's syndrome, and sarcoidosis. Autoimmune thyroid diseases are common following IFN-α treatment. It is important to differentiate this from idiopathic hypothyroidism that is prevalent in the elderly population.

Patients receiving TNF antagonists often develop serologic evidence of autoimmunity. In one study, new ANA and anti-dsDNA antibodies were found in 33% and 9% of infliximab recipients, respectively. However, there is clear discordance between the development of autoantibodies and clinical autoimmunity, with only a handful of symptomatic patients reported, mostly with skin diseases. Approximately 13% of patients exposed to infliximab develop infliximab-specific antibodies. Patients receiving concurrent immunosuppressants such as methotrexate or azathioprine are less likely to develop these antibodies. The presence of antibodies to infliximab increases the likelihood of an infusion reaction but does not predict the development of autoantibodies or DIL.

Drug-Induced Myopathy/Myositis

Drug-induced muscle diseases include myopathy/myositis and rhabdomyolysis. In addition, drugs that impair consciousness (e.g., sedatives and hypnotics) and those that cause seizures (e.g., theophylline), hyperthermia (e.g., halothane and cocaine), malignant neuroleptic syndrome (e.g., haloperidol and phenothiazines), and dystonia (e.g., butyrophenones) can also result in muscle necrosis and elevated creatine phosphokinase (CPK).

Hydroxymethylglutaryl coenzyme A (HMG-CoA) reductase inhibitors (the "statins") are well known to cause different muscle complications varying from myalgias without elevated CPK, elevated CPK without any clinical symptom, to myopathy and rhabdomyolysis. The incidence of statin-induced myopathy (defined as a greater than 10-fold increased in CPK and muscle pain or weakness) is approximately 1 in 1000 patients taking the drug. The risk is greater when these drugs are used in conjunction with gemfibrozil, cyclosporin, niacin, erythromycin, itraconazole, and diltiazem. Other risk factors include renal insufficiency, hypothyroidism, advanced age, and serious infection. The mechanism of statin-induced myopathy is unclear. These agents may interfere with mitochondrial metabolic pathways. Myopathy associated with one statin does not predict the development of a similar problem with a different statin. However, there are rare reports of statin-induced rhabdomyolysis in patients with a previous history of statin-induced myopathy.

A number of drugs rheumatologists prescribe can cause significant muscle disease. Neuromyopathy occasionally develops in patients receiving colchicine. Older patients and those with renal impairment may develop this complication even if they are taking conventional doses of the drug. Patients receiving either chloroquine or hydroxychloroquine are at risk of developing a proximal myopathy and rarely cardiomyopathy. Steroid myopathy usually occurs when greater than 20 mg of prednisone is prescribed. The onset can be acute or insidious, involving the proximal muscle groups (especially the thighs and hip girdle). Serum creatinine kinase level is usually normal, but urine creatine may be elevated. Biopsy of the affected muscle classically shows type 2b fiber atrophy. Corticosteroid use is also associated with rhabdomyolysis when it is administered in the intensive care unit, often in the setting of concurrent paralytics or sedatives ("critical care myopathy"). Penicillamine used in the treatment of RA and Wilson's disease may cause polymyositis, myasthenia gravis, and other autoimmune disorders, including lupus, pemphigus, and Sjögren's syndrome.

Interest in over-the-counter "complementary" medicine has exploded in recent years. Several of these oral supplements have now been linked to the development of musculoskeletal syndromes. The best example is the eosinophilia–myalgia syndrome, believed to be caused by one or more contaminant(s) (the identity of which is still unclear) introduced during the manufacturing process of L-tryptophan by a single manufacturer from Japan. Patients who consumed the product developed peripheral eosinophilia, incapacitating myalgias, and tight skin and/or fasciitis. DL-Carnitine is sold in health food stores and is being promoted as a supplement to increase muscle strength. Although L-carnitine may improve fatigue and muscle strength in some individuals, the DL-carnitine preparation may rarely cause muscle weakness and a myasthenia-like syndrome.

Drug-Induced Vasculitis

Ingestion of a number of drugs is associated with the development of antineutrophil cytoplasmic antibody (ANCA)-positive vasculitis, including hydralazine, propylthiouracil, methimazole, penicillamine, and minocycline. Renal involvement is surprisingly common. The ANCAs often lack specificity and may have activity against myeloperoxidase, elastase, or antiproteinase 3 (PR-3). Discontinuation of the offending drug results in resolution of the clinical disease and a fall in the ANCA titer. Drug-induced vasculitis should be differentiated from drug-induced ANCA production, which is much more common.

Administration of hematopoietic growth factors, including granulocyte colony-stimulating factor and granulocyte-macrophage colony-stimulating factor, has been associated with the development of cutaneous and rarely systemic vasculitis. Interestingly, there is a particularly high prevalence of vasculitis among patients with chronic benign neutropenia receiving these growth factors. The risk of vasculitis increases when the absolute neutrophil count rises above $800/mm^3$, and the problem almost always subsides with decreasing absolute neutrophil count. A number of vasculitis mimics may also develop in association with hematopoietic growth factors, including Sweet's syndrome and pyoderma gangrenosum. Finally, the use of colony-stimulating factors in the settings of Felty's syndrome and malignancies is associated with a flare of preexisting RA.

There are numerous reports of postvaccination vasculitic syndromes (Table 120-9). Symptom onset usually occurs within days or weeks. Most cases resolve spontaneously or with steroid therapy. Some of these cases may be related to an infectious agent or coincidental primary/idiopathic disease. It is also possible that vaccination may trigger the onset of an underlying autoimmune process. The overall incidence of vaccination-induced vasculitis appears to be low. Clinicians should not withhold the appropriate vaccination from patients with preexisting autoimmune diseases or vasculitis based on these reports.

There are a number of reports linking the development of Churg–Strauss syndrome with the use of leukotriene inhibitors (particularly Zafirlukast) in patients with asthma. Onset of Churg–Strauss syndrome is often associated with exposure to the offending drug during a steroid taper. Many pulmonologists now believe that these cases represent unmasking of undiagnosed Churg–Strauss syndrome with tapering of the steroids, rather than a drug-induced disease.

TABLE 120-9

Vaccines Associated with Vasculitis	
Hepatitis B	Takayasu's, polyarteritis nodosa, cutaneous leukocytoclastic vasculitis, Churg–Strauss, cryoglobulinemia, and GCA
Influenza	PMR, GCA, HSP, cryoglobulinemia, microscopic polyangiitis, and cutaneous leukocytoclastic vasculitis
Pneumococcus	Cutaneous leukocytoclastic vasculitis
Varicella	Hypersensitivity vasculitis
Measles	HSP
BCG	PMR, GCA, urticarial vasculitis, and Kawasaki's disease
Tetanus	GCA
Meningococcal C	HSP

GCA, giant cell arteritis; HSP, Henoch–Schoenlein purpura; PMR, polymyalgia rheumatica.

Nevertheless, in the absence of further information, it remains possible that some cases of Churg–Strauss syndrome represent an idiosyncratic eosinophil-based response to leukotriene inhibitors.

RHEUMATIC SYNDROMES AND CANCER

Clinicians are often concerned that a patient's rheumatic complaints may represent the early systemic presentation of an occult tumor. Patients with autoimmune diseases are also at higher risk of developing cancers. Finally, immunosuppressive therapies used for treating autoimmune diseases may predispose the patients to malignancies as well.

Musculoskeletal Symptoms Associated with Cancer

An extensive search for an occult malignancy is not recommended in patients with most rheumatic syndromes unless there are specific symptoms or findings suggesting the possible presence of a tumor. Nevertheless, the possibility of metastatic disease should be considered in an elderly patient presenting with severe pain in or around a joint. Metastatic joint disease caused by lung or breast cancer is usually monoarticular or oligoarticular (two to five joints). Pain and synovitis are caused by synovial inflammation in response to tumor cells in and around the joint. Large joints (e.g., knee and hip) are most commonly affected. However, asymmetric polyarthritis can occur at the late stages of cancer. The vertebral column is a common place for metastatic disease. A malignancy workup should be done if an elderly patient presents with intractable or nocturnal back pain that is increasing in severity and if the patient has constitutional symptoms such as fever or weight loss. Multiple myeloma frequently causes lytic lesions and pathologic fractures. Light-chain amyloidosis occurs in 15% of these patients and is associated with a symmetric small-joint arthropathy. In addition, amyloid infiltration in the shoulder joint produces the classical "shoulder pad sign." Hyperuricemia and gout may develop in patients with large tumor bulk, especially during chemotherapy.

Hypertrophic osteoarthropathy is the most common rheumatic syndrome associated with malignancy and is almost always caused by metastatic lung cancer in the western world. Ankles, wrists, knees, and fingers are the sites most frequently affected. The cause is unknown, but a neurally mediated mechanism is suggested by improvement with vagotomy and atropine. Carcinomatous polyarthritis can precede or follow the diagnosis of the underlying cancer, most commonly breast in women and lung in men. The classical description is an acute-onset asymmetric seronegative polyarthritis in an elderly patient that resembles EORA. The arthritis often improves with cancer therapy and may relapse with tumor recurrence. A polymyalgia rheumatica-like disease has been linked to metastatic cancer. This is suggested by a younger age of onset, prominent constitutional symptoms, asymmetric involvement of proximal muscle groups, a relatively low sedimentation rate, and an incomplete response to prednisone. The Lambert–Eaton syndrome is characterized by an antibody-mediated defect in acetylcholine release at the neuromuscular junction. It is most commonly associated with small cell carcinoma of the lung. Ptosis, distal muscle involvement, and characteristic electromyogram findings distinguish the disease from common inflammatory myopathies. The combination of palmar fasciitis and polyarthritis is associated with gynecologic tumors, in particular, ovarian carcinoma. This is usually associated with late metastatic disease and carries a poor prognosis. Panniculitis with synovitis and serositis is a well-known accompaniment of pancreatic cancer. Finally, there are sporadic reports of steroid-resistant eosinophilic fasciitis associated with hematologic malignancies.

Rheumatic Diseases and Cancer

Patients with autoimmune diseases are at an increased risk of the development of a variety of malignancies. This tendency may be exacerbated by the use of specific immunosuppressive drugs. Patients with RA have a two- to fivefold increased risk of developing hematologic malignancies, including Hodgkin's and non-Hodgkin's lymphomas. The risk is even higher if secondary Sjögren's syndrome or a serum paraprotein is present. An increased risk for oral–pharyngeal cancers has been described in geographic locations where these tumors are prevalent. Interestingly, there are epidemiologic data showing that patients with RA may be at a lower risk of developing colorectal cancer. Whether this is related to the regular use of NSAIDs in this population is unknown. Patients with Sjögren's syndrome are 44 times more likely to develop lymphoma than are age-, sex-, and race-matched normal subjects. The risk may be higher if the patient is anti-Ro or anti-La positive. In some of these patients, there appears to be a progression from benign exocrinopathy to pseudolymphoma to lymphoma. These tumors are almost exclusively B-cell lymphomas with a high frequency of a t(14;18) chromosomal translocation. The malignant transformation is likely the result of chronic B-cell stimulation. The presence of a monoclonal IgM spike on serum protein electrophoresis may herald the transformation to malignant lymphoma. Hypogammaglobulinemia and loss of autoantibodies may eventually occur when the lymphoma cells replace the normal antibody-producing plasma cells.

Patients with polymyositis have a twofold increased risk of developing cancer, particularly in the 1 to 5 years following the diagnosis of the muscle disease. The risk of cancer in patients with dermatomyositis is much higher (four to five times), and the cancer may be discovered years before or after the muscle disease is diagnosed. Older age, the presence of digital vasculitis, and normal serum creatinine kinase level have been cited as possible risk factors for cancer development in patients with inflammatory myositis. Patients with overlap syndromes and those with myositis-specific antibodies do not appear to have a higher incidence of cancer than other patients with polymyositis or dermatomyositis. The cancers associated with inflammatory myositis are those that are commonly seen, including breast, lung, gynecologic, and GI malignancies. Interestingly, nasopharyngeal carcinomas are the dominant cancers associated with myositis in countries that have a high prevalence of these malignancies.

It is controversial whether patients with other autoimmune diseases are more likely to develop cancer. Some reports have described an increased risk of lymphoma (particularly non-Hodgkin's lymphoma) and possibly lung, breast, and cervical cancers in patients with SLE. Patients with scleroderma may be predisposed to skin cancer, and patients with systemic sclerosis who have pulmonary fibrosis are at risk of developing lung cancer.

Risk of Cancer with Immunosuppression

Epidemiologic studies have reported that patients with RA treated with methotrexate may be at increased risk of developing cancer and lymphoma. This is unclear, however, because most studies only examined the relative risk compared to that of the general population. Nevertheless, there are a large number of case reports or case series linking the occurrence of lymphoma (mostly diffuse large-cell non-Hodgkin's lymphomas) in patients with RA receiving low-dose weekly methotrexate. In most cases, cessation of therapy is associated with complete regression of the lymphoid cancer, suggesting a causative relationship. DNA analysis shows that approximately 50% of these lymphomas harbored the Epstein–Barr virus genome. It is, therefore, possible that the drug regimen may promote the malignant transformation of normal lymphoid tissue by the oncogenic virus. Patients with RA on azathioprine and cyclosporin A have a twofold increased risk of lymphoma relative to control patients with RA. A real association between the use of immunosuppressive therapy and the development of lymphoproliferative disorders is also supported by studies of patients with organ transplantation. The incidence of non-Hodgkin's lymphoma is 50-fold greater in patients with renal transplant, especially if they receive cyclosporin A as part of their immunosuppressive regimen.

The issue of cancer risk in patients on anti-TNF agents has already been discussed. Cyclophosphamide is commonly used to treat severe lupus manifestations, including nephritis and cerebritis. Patients with lupus on cyclophosphamide are more likely to develop bladder cancer, lymphoma (primarily non-Hodgkin's lymphoma), and possibly skin cancer. A small increased cancer risk has also been reported in patients with RA treated with the drug.

FURTHER READING

American College of Rheumatology Subcommittee on Rheumatoid Arthritis Guidelines. Guidelines for the management of rheumatoid arthritis: 2002 update. *Arthritis Rheum.* 2002;46:328.

Berney SM. Systemic lupus erythematosus. *Hospital Physician.* 1998;1(3):2–12.

Bongartz T, et al. Anti-TNF antibody therapy in rheumatoid arthritis and the risk of serious malignancies. *JAMA.* 2006;295:2275.

Hennigan S, Kavanaugh A. Optimizing the use of TNF-α inhibitors. *J Musculoskel Med.* 2007;24:293–298.

Hochberg MC, Cahne RW, Dwosh I, Lindsey S, Pincus T, Wolfe F. The American College of Rheumatology 1991 revised criteria for the classification of global functional status in rheumatoid arthritis. *Arthritis Rheum.* 1992;25:498–502.

Kammer GM, Mishra N. Systemic lupus erythematosus in the elderly. *Rheum Dis Clin North Am.* 2000;266:475.

Kremer LM. Rational use of new and existing disease-modifying agents in rheumatoid arthritis. *Ann Intern Med.* 2001;134:695.

Somers EC, et al. Incidence of systemic lupus erythematosus in the United Kingdom, 1990–1999. *Arthritis Rheum.* 2007;57(4):612.

Symmons DPM, et al. The incidence of rheumatoid arthritis in the United Kingdom: results from the Norfolk Arthritis register. *Br J Rheumatol.* 1994;33:735.

Wasko MCM, et al. Hydroxychloroquine and risk of diabetes in patients with rheumatoid arthritis. *JAMA.* 2007;298(2):187.

Yung RL, Richardson BC. Drug-induced rheumatic syndromes. *Bull Rheum Dis.* 2002;51(4):1.

Back Pain and Spinal Stenosis

Leo M. Cooney, Jr.

EPIDEMIOLOGY

Low back pain is a common problem in older individuals, but its etiology, natural history, and therapy are not well defined. Epidemiologic studies have reported the prevalence of back pain in older individuals from 6% to 47%. A recent Israeli study found that 44% of 70-year-olds and 58% of 77-year-olds reported back pain.

In the United States, back pain is the third most frequent symptom in those aged 75 years and older visiting their physicians. This pain is associated with depression, dependence in daily living activities, female gender, and poor self-reported health. The association of back pain and physical function has been quantified; the number of months with restricting back pain is associated with such markers of frailty as worsening rapid gait, chair stands, and foot tap performance. In the study of Medicare beneficiaries 65 years and older, back pain was second only to shortness of breath while climbing stairs in its association with impaired general physical health status.

Back pain is also becoming a substantial drain on health-care resources for older adults. While there was a 42% increase in total Medicare patients from 1991 to 2002, there was 131.7% increase in patients diagnosed with low back pain, and a 387% increase in low back pain charges.

It is clear that low back pain is a common problem for older individuals, is associated with poor outcome, and consumes a significant percentage of health-care resources. Our knowledge of the natural history and outcomes of this problem is limited. The studies during the past two decades that have helped to outline the natural history and outcome of back pain have been conducted exclusively in individuals younger than 60 years of age.

ETIOLOGY OF BACK PAIN

There is very little information in the literature on the natural history, associated features, and the etiology of older patients with back pain.

The clinician must first determine whether the problem is in the hip or back. It can be difficult to distinguish these conditions, as both can give buttock and low back pain. Pain that occurs when going from the supine to sitting position is more apt to be from the back, while groin pain, worsened with weight bearing, favors the hip. A complete examination of the passive range of motion of the hip, done with the patient in the supine position, should reveal 40 degrees of hip abduction, more than 100 degrees of flexion, 50 to 60 degrees of external rotation, and 20 degrees of internal rotation. In addition, a manual muscle examination of the lower extremities, which demonstrates mild weakness of the L4, L5 (hip abductor and great toe extensor) and L5, S1 (hip extensors) innervated muscles of the lower extremities, favors the back as the cause of pain. One recent study demonstrated that the presence of groin pain, a limp, and limited internal rotation of the hip all favored the hip as the cause of pain.

A number of discrete conditions may cause back pain in older individuals. These conditions include tumors, infections, vertebral compression fractures, osteoporotic sacral fractures sciatica, lumbar spinal stenosis, and mechanical causes. One approach to the assessment of back pain in older individuals is to evaluate those patients for the historical, physical, and diagnostic imaging features of these discrete conditions and then to appraise the patient with nonspecific low back pain without one of these conditions.

Tumor

The clinician must always be alert to nonmechanical, either referred or systemic, causes of low back pain. Visceral causes of back pain, such as abdominal aortic aneurysms or pancreatic cancer, are usually nonpositional, progressive, and associated with a normal examination of the lumbar spine and hip.

Tumors usually present with a gradual onset and progressive course, with persistent worsening of the pain over weeks and months. This insidious onset of pain, which is initially mild but progressive in severity, is quite distinct from the abrupt onset and positional characteristics of mechanical low back pain. Tumor pain is often nonpositional, lasts longer than 4 weeks, and is associated with systemic symptoms. One study found that an abnormal CBC and ESR are the best screening tests for tumor as a cause of back pain.

Infection

Although a rare cause of back pain, vertebral and disc infections can be difficult to distinguish from a mechanical cause of back pain; disc infections can cause the same abrupt onset, positional changes, and L4, L5 and L5, S1 neurologic abnormalities seen in mechanical disc disease.

Back pain is the most common musculoskeletal complaint seen in endocarditis. Because the disc is often involved in this condition, the signs and symptoms can mimic mechanical disc disease. Fever can be absent in older patients with infection. The clinician must be alert to a possible infectious cause of back pain for patients with a high risk of endovascular infection (artificial heart valves, indwelling venous catheters, intravenous drug abuse, etc.) and in patients with systemic symptoms and signs of inflammation.

Vertebral Compression Fractures

The abrupt onset of severe back pain, especially in a patient with risk factors for osteoporosis, should always call for a spinal x-ray to rule out a vertebral compression fracture (Table 121-1). At times, the initial x-ray is normal and the changes of vertebral collapse appear several days to weeks after the onset of pain. As there is no dislocation with osteoporotic vertebral fractures, neurological signs and symptoms are quite rare. Pain may be referred, however, into the chest, abdomen, or leg. Any movement, even rolling in bed, usually exacerbates the pain for the first several days. Pain then gradually improves over the next several weeks and resolves in 6 weeks.

Only approximately 30% to 40% of vertebral compression fractures are symptomatic. Most symptomatic fractures are in the lower thoracic and lumbar spine. Most mid and upper thoracic fractures are asymptomatic.

The presence of a vertebral fracture does increase the risk of a subsequent fracture. In a multicenter study of osteoporosis, the presence of a fracture increased the risk of subsequent fractures in the next year from 6.6% to 19.2%.

The role of osteoporosis and vertebral fracture in chronic back pain and disability is not clear. The finding that fractures are associated with increased mortality from pulmonary disease and cancer indicate that these fractures may be markers of frailty. While some studies have shown increased disability in patients with vertebral fractures, a British population-based study found no correlation between minor vertebral deformities and back pain. A study of women

TABLE 121-1

Characteristics of Vertebral Compression Fracture

Severe pain with lower thoracic and lumbar fracture

High and mid-thoracic fracture often asymptomatic

Pain resolves in 4–6 weeks

Increased risk for subsequent fracture

in Hawaii showed a correlation between recent fractures and back pain, but the prevalence of back pain among women with prevalent fractures was not significantly higher than those without these fractures. Finally, the Study of Osteoporotic Fractures found an increase in back pain and disability only if vertebral deformities were greater than 4 standard deviations from the mean.

Osteoporotic Sacral Fractures

There have been a number of reports of "sacral insufficiency fractures" as a cause of back pain. Older patients, usually women, complain of dull low back pain. This pain is also felt in the buttock area. The application of pressure to the sacrum is very painful. Associated neurologic defects have not been reported. The pain usually resolves spontaneously in 4 to 6 weeks. Approximately 50% of these patients had a preceding fall, and the majority of patients have old pelvic and vertebral compression fractures on x-ray.

Plain x-rays of the sacrum are normal, but technetium bone scans demonstrate the fractures. CT scans of the sacrum usually show displacement of the anterior border of the sacrum. A sacral insufficiency fracture should be considered if a woman with osteoporosis develops sudden pain in the low back and buttock with sacral tenderness.

Sciatica

Sciatica is usually defined as pain radiating to one leg below the gluteal fold. It is often felt in the buttock area, radiating into the posterior aspect of the leg down to the ankle. It may, however, be incomplete, as in the calf pain seen in the "pseudoclaudication" syndrome with lumbar spinal stenosis. The natural history of this condition is well defined in younger adults. Fifty percent of these patients have full resolution of symptoms within 6 weeks. While there are no studies of the natural history of sciatica in older patients, many clinicians do find that sciatica, which develops abruptly and occurs in all positions, usually has a good natural history, similar to that seen in younger individuals. Patients who develop sciatica as part of the lumbar spinal stenosis syndrome, with gradual progression of pain with shorter and shorter periods of standing and walking, have a more prolonged and persistent natural history.

Lumbar Spinal Stenosis

Narrowing of the lateral recess of the vertebral canal, as well as the anterior–posterior diameter of the canal, is frequently seen on diagnostic imaging tests of the lumbar spine in older individuals. These abnormalities have clinical significance only if the typical history of lumbar spinal stenosis is present (Table 121-2).

Changes in spinal dynamics with movement explain some of the clinical features of lumbar spinal stenosis. Flexion of the lumbar spine decreases the intraspinal protrusion of the disc, decreases the bulge of the yellow ligaments within the canal, and stretches and decreases the cross-sectional area of nerve roots, resulting in an increase in spinal canal volume in relation to nerve root bulk. Extension of the lumbar spine causes bulging of the disc into the canal, enfolding and protrusion of the yellow ligaments into the spinal canal, and a relaxation and increase of the cross-sectional diameter of nerve roots. Extension of the canal thus produces a decreased volume of the spinal canal in relation to nerve root bulk.

TABLE 121-2

Characteristics of Lumbar Spinal Stenosis

Pain with extended spine
  Prolonged standing
  Walking
  Walking down hill

Pain relieved on flexing spine
  Sitting
  Leaning on walker or grocery cart

Sciatic pain on walking

Incomplete sciatica—"pseudoclaudication"

These changes in dynamics explain the clinical picture of lumbar spinal stenosis. Positions that extend the spine (standing, walking down hill, prone lying, and extending the back) worsen symptoms, while positions that flex the spine (sitting, bending forward, placing weight on a walker or cart, and lying in a flex position) relieve the symptoms.

Patients with lumbar spinal stenosis present with pain, either in the lower back or legs, which comes on with prolonged standing and walking and is relieved with sitting. Individuals with this condition will often bend their spine more as they walk and find that they can walk further in a grocery store, supported by a cart. The leg pain can present with a classic picture of sciatica (pain radiating from the posterior aspect of the buttock down to the foot) or an incomplete "pseudoclaudication" syndrome, in which the patient feels pain only in the calf while standing and walking.

Lumbar spinal stenosis should not produce pain when going from lying to sitting and should not produce severe pain with bending, stooping, or lifting objects. In a masked study comparing radiologic and electrodiagnostic diagnoses to clinical impression, MRI findings and their interpretation did not relate in any important way to the clinical diagnosis of lumbar spinal stenosis.

Mechanical Low Back Pain

The majority of older people with low back pain do not have tumors, infections, lumbar spinal stenosis, or vertebral compression fractures (Table 121-3). They are best described as patients with mechanical back pain of uncertain etiology. Because the nucleus pulposus loses water content with aging, herniation of this structure is unusual beyond the age of 55 years.

A good deal of back pain in younger individuals is probably caused by displacement of the outer annulus fibrosis or inner nucleus pulposus of the intervertebral disc. The disc does not contain pain fibers: the perivertebral structures with the most sensitive pain fibers are the posterior longitudinal ligament and the dura mater, which lie

TABLE 121-3

Characteristics of Mechanical Low Back Pain

Intermittent sharp back pain

Pain comes on and subsides rapidly

Pain going from lying to sitting and with bending

Asymmetric loss of motion of lumbar spine

Weakness of L4, L5, L5, and S1 innervated muscles

---

posterior to the vertebrae and discs. The sinuvertebral nerve innervates these structures. Irritation of this nerve causes reflex spasms of the paravertebral muscles of the lumbar spine. It is, thus, logical to assume that soft-tissue displacement in this area will cause pain and limitation of some, but not all, of the planes of movement of the lumbar spine, spasm of the paravertebral muscles, and subtle weakness of the muscles innervated by the appropriate nerves roots (L4, L5, and S1—in most cases).

In a young lumbar spine, the central nucleus pulposus often herniates outside the annulus fibrosis and indents the pain-sensitive posterior longitudinal ligament and dura mater, producing pain that often lasts for several weeks and occasionally causing sciatica owing to nerve root irritation. Because of decreased water content, the nucleus pulposus becomes less gel-like as one ages and rarely herniates after the age of 55 years.

Older patients often have a syndrome of sharp pain in the lumbar area, worsened with bending movements, which comes on and subsides rapidly but recurs frequently. On physical examination, these patients often have asymmetric loss of range of motion in the lumbar spine, paravertebral muscle spasm, weakness of the L4-, L5-, and S1-innervated muscles, and pain going from the flexed to the erect position. Clinicians often use the term "unstable lumbar spine" to describe this syndrome, although the evidence for specific mechanical instability is lacking. Patients with this condition often have one intervertebral disc space narrowed and sclerotic out of proportion to other disc spaces, and anterior displacement of one vertebra on another (spondylolithesis). Maneuvers such as going from lying to sitting and bending forward often produce pain. Before considering major interventions, it is important to distinguish this condition, in which pain results from movement of the lumbar spine (e.g., lying to sitting), from lumbar spinal stenosis, in which pain results from prolonged extension of the spine (standing and walking).

Diffuse Idiopathic Skeletal Hyperostosis

Diffuse idiopathic skeletal hyperostosis (DISH) is a condition characterized by calcification of prevertebral and peripheral ligaments. Ossification of spinal ligaments is often confused with osteophytes, and the condition is frequently mislabeled as disc degeneration or osteoarthritis. Spinal involvement is characterized by the following: (1) the presence of flowing calcification and ossification along the anterolateral aspect of at least four contiguous vertebral bodies, (2) relative preservation of intervertebral disc height in the involved area, and (3) the absence of apophyseal joint bony ankylosis or other features of ankylosing spondylitis.

Most studies have not found any association with DISH and back pain, while other studies have noted an increase in ligamentous tenderness, stiffness, and immobility of the cervical, thoracic, and lumbar spine in individuals with this condition. The condition should be distinguished from disc disease with vertebral osteophytes and is a cause of significant spinal immobility in older individuals.

EVALUATION

The evaluation of the older patient with back pain must depend heavily on the history, physical examination, and observation of the patient. The history and physical examination remain the most helpful tools in the assessment of back pain in older persons, particularly because of the very high false-positive rate of spinal diagnostic imaging

TABLE 121-4
History Items That Help Differentiate Causes of Back Pain

Abrupt onset of pain
  Vertebral compression fractures
  Mechanical low back pain

Insidious onset, progressive course, nonpositional pain
  Tumor
  Infection
  Nonspinal visceral pain

Positional pain
  Pain when lying to sitting or bending
    Mechanical low back pain
  Pain when standing and walking, relieved with sitting
    Lumbar spinal stenosis
  Nonpositional
    Tumor
    Infection

TABLE 121-5
Physical Examination Findings That Help Differentiate Causes of Back Pain

Paravertebral muscle spasm
  Mechanical low back pain
  Vertebral compression fracture

Asymmetric loss of range of motion of lumbar spine
  Mechanical low back pain

Weakness of great toe extensor and hip abductor (L4, L5) and hip extensors (L5, S1)
  Mechanical low back pain
  Lumbar spinal stenosis

tests in this age group. Laboratory tests and diagnostic imaging studies have a secondary role in the assessment of these patients. The clinician must make sure that the clinical presentation of the patient fits the results of the diagnostic imaging tests before proceeding with interventions.

The role of the clinician in assessing and managing back pain in older individuals must thus focus on (1) identifying those conditions that require immediate attention (e.g., infections and tumors), (2) recognizing the usual patterns of pain for defined causes of back pain, (3) assisting the patient with therapy for these specific conditions, and (4) advising the patient on the natural history, precipitating events, and therapeutic approaches to nonspecific mechanical low back pain.

History

Patients with a mechanical cause for pain usually have intermittent, positional pain, often with the peak intensity of pain at the beginning of the syndrome (Table 121-4). Pain that is worse on going from lying to sitting and with bending, that occurs when one suddenly changes position, and that resolves quickly but recurs frequently, suggests mechanical disease of the lumbar spine as a result of soft-tissue displacement. Severe pain in any position, which comes on abruptly and is aggravated by even rolling over in bed, suggests a vertebral compression fracture. A woman with sacral and buttock pain, sacral tenderness, and osteoporosis should be evaluated for a sacral insufficiency fracture. Gradually worsening progressive pain, lasting more than a month, which is nonpositional and associated with systemic symptoms and signs, should suggest tumor. Hip disease can often mimic back problems. Pain that is worse when going from sitting to standing and that causes a limp indicates possible hip disease.

Physical Examination

Several findings on physical examination can be useful in determining discrete causes of back pain (Table 121-5). The physical examination of the lumbar spine is an essential component of the assessment of a patient with back pain (Figure 121-1). This is best done in the erect position. The examiner observes the patient for kyphosis or scoliosis and then palpates for paravertebral muscle spasm. The patient is then brought through the four ranges of motion of the lumbar spine, side flexion to the right, side flexion to the left, forward flexion, and extension, observing for asymmetric limitation of motion or reproduction of the patient's pain by these maneuvers (Figure 121-1). In the supine position, straight leg raise tests can indicate nerve root irritation if positive, but a negative test does not exclude any condition. The hips should be examined by testing the passive range of motion. The examiner should be able to abduct the leg to 40 degrees before the pelvis tilts. There should be 60 degrees of external rotation (heel toward the midline) and 20 degrees of internal rotation (heel away from the midline) of each hip (Figure 121-2).

Manual muscle testing of the lower extremity gives much useful information, as subtle L4, L5 and L5, S1 weakness is common in patients with mechanical back pain. L4, L5 is tested by resisting the patient's abducted leg at the lateral upper thigh (gluteus medius muscle) (Figure 121-2), by resisting the patient's ability to dorsiflex the foot (tibialis anterior muscle), and by resisting the great toe extensor (extensor hallucis longus) (Figure 121-3). L5, S1 (gluteus maximus muscle) is tested by trying to overcome hip extension (trying to pull the leg off the examining table, when the patient has been instructed to hold the leg firmly on the table). One can also test L5, S1 by resisting the patient's ability to evert the foot (peroneus longus and peroneus brevis).

Most patients with lumbar disc disease or lumbar spinal stenosis will have some abnormalities of the examination of the lumbar spine or of the muscles innervated by L4, L5 or L5, S1. Patient with vertebral compression fractures may have a good deal of tenderness in the lumbar spine but should have no neurologic abnormalities. Patients with osteoporotic sacral fractures will have sacral tenderness, but a normal lumbar spine examination and no lower extremity muscle weakness. Patients with sciatica almost always have L4, L5 and L5, S1 weakness. A patient with persistent, severe back pain, but with a normal examination of the lumbar spine, sacrum, and hips and no evidence of L4, L5 or L5, S1 muscle weakness, should be evaluated thoroughly for a possible neoplasm or infection.

Laboratory Tests and Imaging

The interpretation of diagnostic tests in older patients with back pain is a challenge, given the high rate of abnormal tests in asymptomatic individuals in this age group. As noted above, a CBC and an ESR

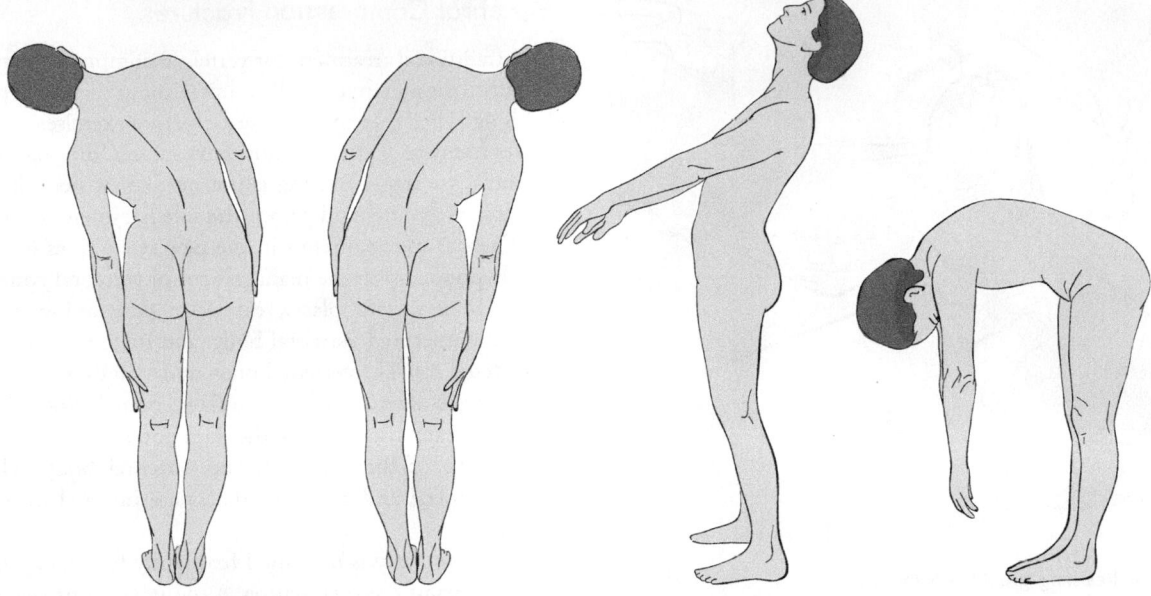

FIGURE 121-1. Range of motion of lumbar spine.

are reasonable screening tests if the patient's history and physical examination suggests a tumor or infection. A plain roentgenogram of the lumbar spine is more helpful in the evaluation of older patients than younger ones, as it may demonstrate a vertebral compression fracture, DISH, or spondylolithesis.

The clinician must be aware that changes in the lumbar spine are ubiquitous in older individuals and not well correlated with back pain. Kellgren and Lawrence's classic epidemiological study

in Leigh, England, found that 89% of the males and 57% of the females between the ages of 55 to 64 years had disc degeneration of the lumbar spine. A 1984 study of lumbar sacral spine x-rays found no association between back pain and Schmorl's nodes, the disc vacuum sign, traction spurs, and disc space narrowing between the third and fourth lumbar vertebrae, or between the fifth lumbar and first sacral vertebrae. There was an association between acute low back pain and disc space narrowing, and traction spurs between

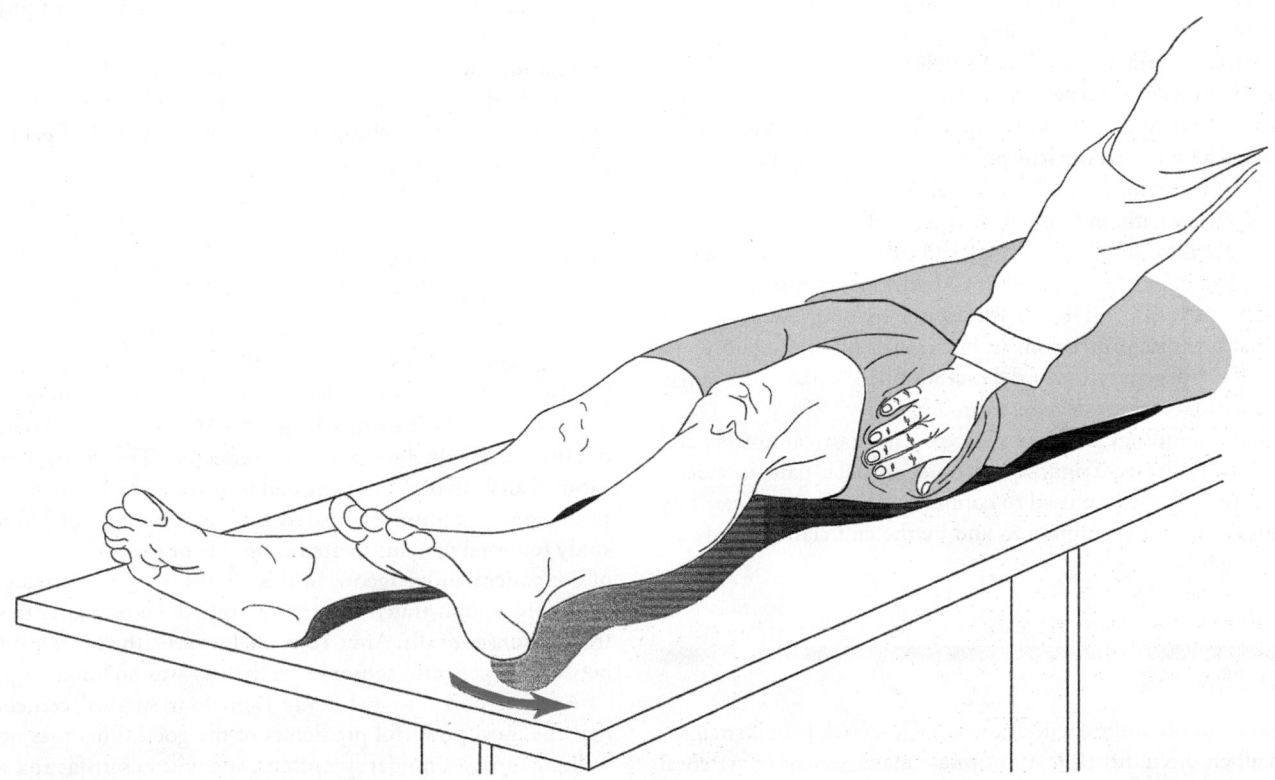

FIGURE 121-2. Resisting abduction of the leg.

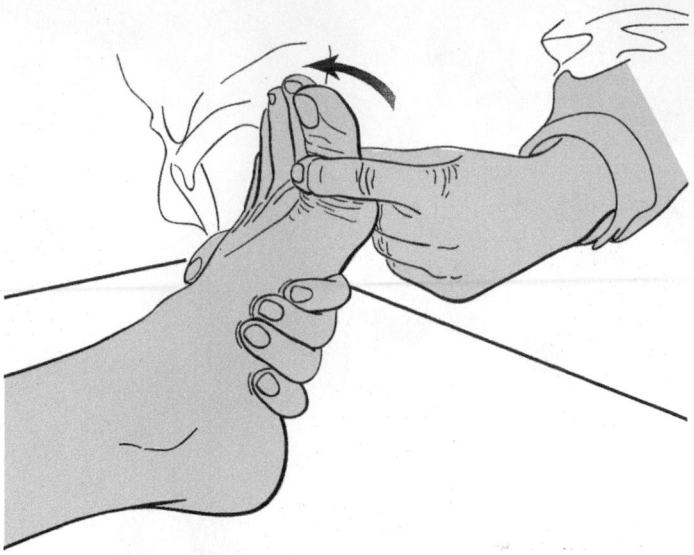

FIGURE 121-3. Resisting great toe extensor.

the fourth and fifth lumbar vertebra. A Lahey Clinic study found no correlation between vertebral osteophytes and low back pain but did find increased back pain in individuals with spondylolithesis (pars interarticularis defect and frontal slippage of one vertebra on an adjacent vertebra).

In a 1967 study, myelograms were performed on the lumbar spine in individuals who were undergoing these studies in the posterior fossa to evaluate acoustic neuromas. Thirty-seven percent of patients with no back pain had abnormal myelograms of the lumbar spine.

MRIs of the lumbar spine often demonstrate anatomic abnormalities in asymptomatic individuals, especially in the elderly. In a 1994 study of MRIs of the lumbar spine in patients without back pain, only 36% had a normal examination; 52% of these individuals had a disc bulge in at least one level, and 27% had disc protrusions. In another study of asymptomatic individuals, 36% of subjects older than 60 years had a herniated nucleus pulposus, 21% had spinal stenosis, and 93% had degenerative disc disease. A 1998 study found that 56% of asymptomatic individuals had tears of the annulus fibrosis of the lumbar disc. In a VA study of 198 subjects who had had no back pain for at least 4 months, 83% had moderate-to-severe degeneration of the disc, 64% had at least one bulging disc, and 32% had at least one disc protrusion. In individuals older than 65 years, 100% had disc degeneration and desiccation, 83% had a disc bulge, and 38% had facet joint degeneration.

The above findings indicate that the clinician cannot depend on imaging studies to diagnose the cause of back pain in elderly persons. These studies are used to confirm a diagnosis, indicated by the history, physical examination, and by the clinician's knowledge of applied anatomy.

MANAGEMENT

Therapy of tumors and infectious causes of low back pain is straightforward albeit often difficult. Appropriate management of vertebral compression fractures, lumbar spinal stenosis, and mechanical low back pain is less clear.

Vertebral Compression Fractures

The traditional treatment for vertebral compression fractures is bed rest until the patient can roll and sit without too much pain, avoiding prolonged bed rest; analgesia; and extensor exercises when the patient can participate. Calcitonin does have some additional analgesic effect in the acute stage. Bracing is not needed, as neurological sequelae are extremely rare, and pain is the sole parameter of recovery.

There is much interest in the new techniques of vertebroplasty and kyphoplasty in the management of vertebral compression fractures. In a vertebroplasty, extension positioning opens the cleft within a fractured vertebral body, and methylmethacrylate cement is injected into the vertebral body and stabilizes the fracture in this position. In a kyphoplasty, an inflated bone balloon displaces vertebral trabelate and elevates the superior end plate, allowing some restoration of the height of the vertebral body. The balloon is then removed and methylmethacrylate injected into the vertebral space.

Vertebroplasty is now used frequently for management of acute vertebral compression fractures. Although uncontrolled studies show encouraging relief of pain, the good natural history of the pain from compression fractures, and the potential complications and expense of this procedure, should lend caution to its use. Randomized controlled trials of this procedure are lacking. In a nonrandomized trial, the control patients were those who elected not to have the procedure. The pain score was significantly decreased in the vertebroplasty group as compared to the conservative therapy group in the first few days, but there were no significant differences in clinical outcomes at 6 weeks or 6 to 12 months. In a study of patients who had pain for greater than 1 year associated with compression fractures, kyphoplasty was performed on 40 patients, with 20 control patients who elected not to have the procedure. At 1 year, the patients with kyphoplasty had fewer new fractures, fewer back pain-related physicians' visits, and greater improvement in pain scores. Again, neither of these studies were randomized controlled trials. Most experts in this field suggest analgesics, calcitonin, and exercise in the acute phase, and moving on to vertebroplasty or kyphoplasty only if patients have persistent severe pain.

Lumbar Spinal Stenosis

The decision to proceed with extensive back surgery on an older patient is always a difficult one. A recent Cochrane review of surgery for degenerative lumbar spondylosis found that "there is still insufficient evidence of the effectiveness of surgery to draw any firm conclusions." On the other hand, the Maine Lumbar Spinal study did show that spinal surgery can be effective. This study is an observational analysis of patients treated by orthopedic surgeons and neurosurgeons in community-based practices throughout Maine. This study followed patients treated surgically or medically, at the choice of the patient and surgeon. In this cohort, patients initially treated surgically demonstrated better outcomes in all measures than those treated nonsurgically. After 10 years, however, the relative difference between surgery and conservative therapy was no longer significant.

Another observational study from four surgical centers found that the most powerful predictors of the good outcomes of greater walking capacity, milder symptoms, and greater satisfaction were the patient's report of good or excellent health before surgery, as well as low cardiovascular comorbidity.

The choice of nonsurgical treatment is difficult, as there are few randomized controlled trials of these therapies. Epidural steroid injections have been used for more than 50 years for sciatica. While there are a number of uncontrolled studies suggesting a good outcome with these injections for lumbar spinal stenosis, randomized controlled trials have had inconsistent results.

Physical therapy is advocated for this condition, but there are few controlled trials to validate this approach, and little evidence to justify advocating one treatment regimen over another. In a recent study of a relatively small number of patients (58), a program, which included thrust and nonthrust manipulation of the spine and lower extremities, manual strengthening, muscle strengthening exercises, and a body-weight-supported treadmill ambulation program, had better short- and long-term results than a regimen of lumbar flexion exercises, performance of a progressive treadmill walking program, and subtherapeutic ultrasound.

A recent randomized controlled multicenter trial of an intraspinous process decompression system did find that patients who underwent this procedure had a statistically significant improvement in neurogenic intermittent claudication versus controls.

In summary, it does seem reasonable to treat patients with lumbar spinal stenosis with a conservative approach including epidural steroid injections, physical therapy, and perhaps manipulative therapy. If this approach does not give relief in a reasonable period of time, then a surgical approach, decompressing the stenotic canal space, should be strongly considered. Those patients with high self-reported health and low cardiovascular morbidity seem to achieve the best surgical results. The role of the locally implanted intraspinous process decompression system is yet to be determined.

Mechanical Low Back Pain

The management of back pain in the older persons requires a logical, if not yet evidence based, approach to the patient, based on both an anatomical understanding of the most likely cause and precipitants of the patient's pain. For pain that is exacerbated by spinal movement (lying to sitting, bending, etc.), spinal instability is the most likely explanation, and thus attempts to stabilize the spine make the most sense. Stabilization may be achieved by isometric abdominal strengthening exercises, lumbar sacral corsets with metal stays, and back protection maneuvers (lifting with one's knees with the back straight, etc.). Spinal fusion is reserved for intractable cases of severe low back pain.

There is no therapy needed or indicated for DISH. The pain from sacral insufficiency fractures resolves in 4 to 6 weeks, and analgesics should suffice. Antiresorptive therapy for osteoporosis should be initiated to prevent future fractures.

Spontaneous sciatica improves without therapy in most older individuals. Epidural steroids may be helpful in the management of sciatica. Surgery should be considered only if the pain persists after 3 months of nonsurgical therapy.

Prolonged bed rest should be avoided in older persons, given the complications of this intervention in this age group. Patients should, however, avoid those activities that appear to precipitate their pain. Firm corsets should be considered to allow patients to stay mobile and active.

Analgesics should not be spared in the management of pain, but these must be used with care. There is little evidence that anti-inflammatory drugs are any better than simple analgesics, and these are associated with a high incidence of complications in this age group. Pain that occurs only with movement often does not respond well to analgesics. While narcotics may be very helpful with severe pain, the patient should be watched closely for confusion and constipation. Adjunctive pain therapy, with such agents as tricyclic antidepressants with limited anticholinergic side effects (nortriptyline and disimpramine) and gabapentin, may be helpful. The use of multiple analgesic classes may be effective at reducing pain while keeping side effects to a minimum.

FURTHER READING

Atlas S, Delitto A. Spinal stenosis. *Clin Orthop Relat Res.* 2006;443:198–207.

Bressler HB, Keyes WJ, Rochon PA, et al. The prevalence of low back pin in the elderly. *Spine.* 1999;24(17):1813–1819.

Brown MD, Gomez-Marin O, Brookfoeld KFW, et al. Differential diagnosis of hip disease versus spine disease. *Clin Orthop.* 2004;419:280–284.

Chang Y, Singer DE, Wu YA, et al. The effect of surgical and nonsurgical treatment on longitudinal outcomes of lumber spinal stenosis over 10 years. *JAGS.* 2005;53:785–792.

Cooper JK, Kohlmann T. Factors associated with health status of older Americans. *Age and Ageing* 2001;30:495–501.

Ettinger B, Black DM, Nevitt MC, et al. Contribution of vertebral deformities to chronic back pain and disability. *J Bone Miner Res.* 1992;7(4):449–456.

Gibson JN, Waddell G. Surgery for degenerative lumbar spondylosis: updated Cochrane review. *Spine.* 2005;30(20):2312–2320.

Haig AJ, Tong HC, et al. Spinal stenosis, back pain, or no symptoms at all? A masked study comparing radiological and electrodiagnostic diagnoses to the clinical impression. *Arch Phys Med Rehabil.* 2006;87:897–903.

Jacobs JM, Hemmerman-Rozenberg R, et al. Chronic back pain among the elderly: prevalence, associations, and predictors. *Spine.* 2006;31(7):E203–E207.

Jarvik JJ, Hollingworth W, Heagerty P, et al. The Longitudinal Assessment of Imaging and Disability of the Back (LAIDBack) study: baseline data. *Spine.* 2001;26(10):1158–1166.

Jensen MC, Brant-Zawadzki MN, Obuchowski N, et al. Magnetic resonance imaging of the lumbar spine in people without back pain. *NEJM.* 1994;331(2):69–73.

Joines JD, McNutt RA, Carey TS, et al. Finding cancer in primary care outpatients with low back pain. A comparison of diagnostic strategies. *J Gen Intern Med.* 2001;16:14–23.

Katz JN, Stucki G, Lipson SJ, et al. Predictors of surgical outcome in degenerative lumbar spinal stenosis. *Spine.* 1999;24(21):2229–2233.

Lindsey R, Silverman SL, Cooper C, et al. Risk of new vertebral fracture in the year following a fracture. *JAMA.* 2001;285(3):320–323.

Rao RD, Singrakhia MD. Painful osteoporotic vertebral fracture. *J Bone Joint Surg.* 2003;85-A(10):2010–2022.

Reid MC, Williams CS, Gill TM. Back pain and decline in extremity physical function among community-dwelling older persons. *J Gerontol Med Sci.* 2005;60A(6):793–797.

Weber M, Hasler P, Gerber H. Insufficiency fracture of the sacrum. *Spine.* 1993; 18(16):2507–2512.

Weiner DK, Kim YS, Bonino P, et al. Low back pain in older adults: are we utilizing healthcare resources wisely? *Pain Med.* 2006;7(2):143–150.

Whiteman JM, Flynn TW, Childs JD, et al. A comparison between two physical therapy treatment programs for patients with lumbar spinal stenosis. *Spine.* 2006;31(22):2541–2549.

Zucherman JF, Hsu KY, Hartjen CA, et al. A multicenter, prospective, randomized trial evaluating the X STOP interspinous process decompression system for the treatment of neurogenic intermittent claudication. *Spine.* 2005;30(12):1351–1358.

Primary Considerations in Managing the Older Patient with Foot Problems

Arthur E. Helfand

INTRODUCTION

Diseases and disorders of foot and their related structures in the older patient represent a significant health concern. The immobility that results from local foot conditions and the focal complications of systemic diseases have a significant impact on individuals' ability to maintain their independence, retain a quality of life, and become financial concerns for society in general. Two important factors involved in the older patient's ability to remain as a vital part of society are a keen mind and the ability to retain their mobility through ambulation.

The human foot is both a static and a mobile organ of function. It provides support for the body at rest and during propulsion and ambulation. It supports our ability to walk upright, which is a specific characteristic of modern humans. The ability to remain mobile and functional in society is a key activity of daily living and may well be the primary catalyst to independence for the older population. The loss of the ability to walk owing to some foot problem or change not only produces physical limitations but also has a significant impact on the patient's mental, social, and economic status. On average, 90% of the adult population older than 65 years will demonstrate some evidence of foot pain that alters independent activity. Foot and related complications also represent a significant factor for many hospital admissions, especially related to complications associated with diabetic and vascular ulceration and infection.

The goal of this chapter is to provide the geriatric health-care provider with a foundation of knowledge about the aging foot in health and disease. There is an extensive and unique comprehensive podiatric assessment and a medical vocabulary associated with the field of podiatry. An example of a comprehensive assessment and a list of podiatric terms are provided as appendices available in the online version of this text.

ETIOLOGICAL AND EPIDEMIOLOGICAL FACTORS

There are multiple factors that contribute to the etiology of foot problems in older patients. The primary factors include the aging process itself, years of use and abuse, repetitive stress, neglect, foot deformity, and the presence of multiple chronic diseases. Other significant factors include the degree of ambulation, limitation of activity, prior institutionalization, as well as prior and improper self-care. Foot problems are also affected by impaired vision, obesity, the inability to bend, and peripheral sensory loss. Local foot factors include altered biomechanics and pathomechanics, soft-tissue atrophy and plantar fat pad displacement, limited joint mobility, and contractures. Discomfort, pain (podalgia), ambulatory dysfunction, and pain when walking (pododynia dysbasia) become distressing and disabling.

In addition to factors of the host, agent factors that contribute to the development of foot conditions include hard flat surfaces for ambulation, trauma, foot-covering material and fabrication, foreign bodies, and foot-to-shoe-last incompatibilities. Environmental factors that affect the foot include customs and shoe styles; low income; adequate care and referral; nutrition; poor foot health education; cultural barriers; physical changes such as climate, flooring materials, and covering; the health-care system and insurance limitations; and the lack of school foot health programs.

ANATOMY OF THE FOOT AND CHANGES RELATED TO AGE

Figure 122-1 illustrates the major anatomic components of the foot. The human foot is an organ that is static and mobile. It provides support for the body at rest and during propulsion and ambulation.

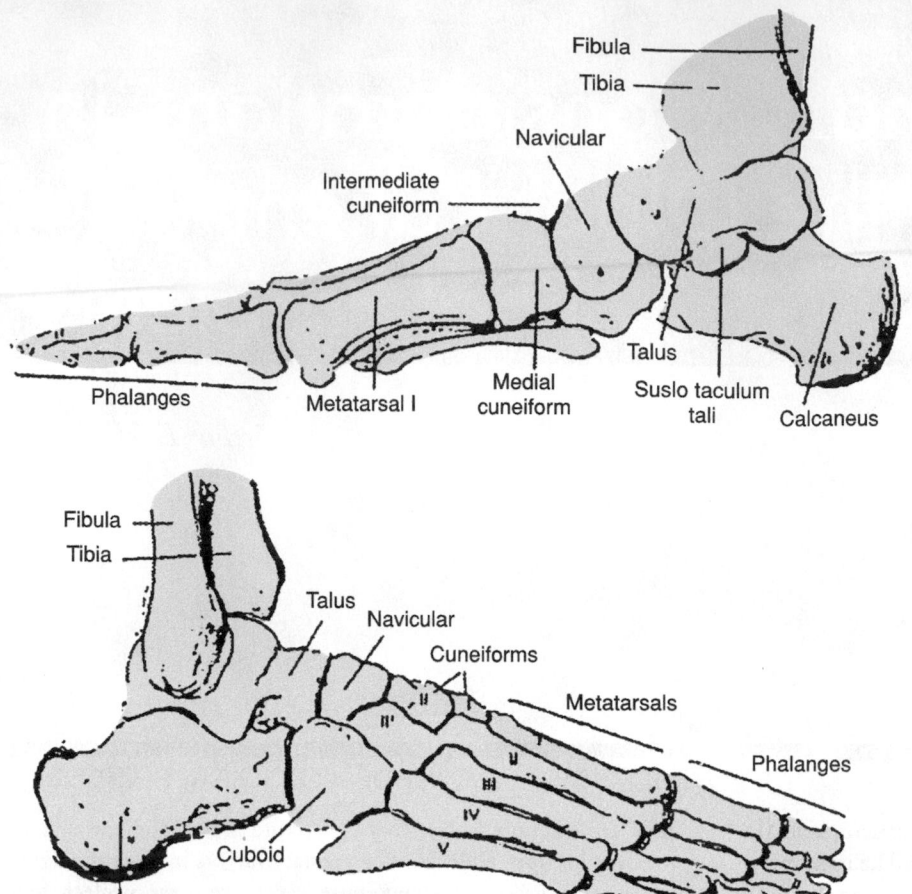

Fibula
Tibia
Navicular
Intermediate
cuneiform
Talus
Phalanges
Metatarsal I
Medial
cuneiform
Suslo taculum
tali
Calcaneus

Fibula
Tibia
Talus
Navicular
Cuneiforms
Metatarsals
Phalanges
Cuboid
Calcaneus

LATERAL. ASPECT OF RIGHT FOOT

FIGURE 122-1. Anatomy of the foot. (Adapted with permission from Pedorthic Footwear Association. Pedorthic Reference Guide. Columbia, MD; 1992, 1999, 2006.)

The human foot from a morphological standpoint is basically a modified rectangle that is also three dimensional.

The human foot is complex. Each foot has 26 bones (together constituting one-fourth of the body's total), ossicles, ligaments, muscles, tendons, arteries, veins, nerves, and its covering of skin. The foot normally bears weight on a triangular base, with the long sides being the inner and outer longitudinal arches and the metatarsal arch consisting of the bias along the five metatarsal heads. Weight is transferred from the calcaneus to the fifth and first metatarsal heads initially.

The talus, with the tibia and fibula, comprises the ankle joint. The talus has no muscular attachments and thus with the tendons and muscles, which parallel it, controls activity. The talus articulates with the calcaneus. The Achilles tendon attaches to the superior-posterior segment and is a significant structure to foot function. The cuboid is anterior to the calcaneus and is rectangular in shape, which adds to the structural support to the foot. The navicular is anterior to the talus and is coin shaped, which also provides muscular attachments to aid in function and stabilization. Anterior to the navicular and lateral to the cuboid are three wedge-shaped bones called the first, second, and third (medial, middle, and lateral) cuneiforms. These help provide stability to the foot. These bones comprise the "rear foot." The arches do not fall. The foot does rotate, pronate, supinate, invert, evert, and elongate and changes structurally in relation to Wolff's law (bone is deposited and resorbed in accordance with the stresses placed upon it) and Davis's law (soft tissue mod-

els itself along its imposed demands). The mid-foot consists of the remaining five tarsal bones, that is, the navicular, cuboid, and three cunieforms.

Anterior to the cuneiforms and cuboid bones are the five metatarsals. Each metatarsal consists of a base, a shaft, and a head. These are anatomically classed as long bones. Anterior to the metatarsals are the phalanges. Each of the lesser toes contains three phalanges. The first or great toe comprises two phalanges. The metatarsals and phalanges represent the forefoot.

Each osseous structure attaches by ligaments to another to form the joints of the foot. Their functional role is to maintain proximity by keeping the segments of bone articulating with each other. Their properties are strength and rigidity with limited elasticity, which permit the joints to maintain some degree of motion or movement. The basic change that occurs in aging bone is a loss of calcium (osteopenia and/or osteoporosis) and, in foot ligaments, the transition from elasticity to rigidity. The lateral longitudinal arch is formed by the calcaneus, cuboid, fourth, and fifth metatarsals. It is the lower structural arch. The medial longitudinal arch is formed by the calcaneus, talus, navicular, three cuneiforms, and the first, second, and third metatarsals. It is higher with its summit at the head of the talus and navicular. The pitch of the calcaneus (the angle formed by the plantar surface of the calcaneus and plane of support) determines, to a great degree, the height of that segment. The transverse arches of the foot include the posterior metatarsal arch, formed by the bases of the metatarsals and is reasonably firm, and the anterior metatarsal arch, formed by the five metatarsal heads, is flexible, and flattens during gait phases, with weight bearing, pronation, and supination.

The most predominant and significant membranous covering of the foot is known as the plantar fascia. It attaches to the plantar posterior segment of the calcaneus or tuberosity and fans out anteriorly to the metatarsal area. The plantar fascia covers all of the foot muscles, all of the ligaments, and all of the bones on the plantar aspect of the foot. It acts as a spring to aid in function as well as offers protection to plantar structures. It is a very elastic or flexible mass in youth, which becomes wasted and rigid with age. The dorsum of the foot does not have a strong fascial attachment. Most of the structures are subcutaneous.

The muscles that control the major functions of the foot have their origin in the leg. The posterior muscles include the tibialis posterior, flexor digitorum longus, flexor hallucis longus, plantaris, and calcaneal or Achilles tendon (formed by the gastrocnemius and soleus muscles). The lateral muscles include the peroneus longus and peroneus brevis. The anterior muscles include the tibialis anterior, extensor hallucis longus, and extensor digitorum longus. As individuals age and chronic disease becomes evident, there is a decrease in muscle strength that can result in ambulatory dysfunction, imbalance, foot drop, and a higher risk for falls.

The muscle on the dorsum of the foot is the extensor digitorum brevis. The muscles on the plantar surface of the foot are covered by the plantar fascia and are organized in four layers from superficial to deep. The muscles of the deepest fourth layer include the dorsal interossei (four), plantar interossei (four), and the tendons of the peroneus longus and tibialis posterior muscles. It is the atrophy of the interossei muscles that is a major factor in the development of hammertoes in the aging patient.

The nerves that control the foot include the lateral sural cutaneous, superficial and deep fibular (peroneal), medial dorsal cutaneous, dorsal digital, tibial, lateral calcaneal, medial plantar, lateral plantar, and saphenous nerves.

The arterial supply to the foot follows the femoral artery, to the popliteal artery, and divides to become the anterior and posterior tibial arteries. The anterior tibial artery becomes the dorsalis pedis artery on the dorsum of the foot, whose terminal branches are the dorsal metatarsal and dorsal digital arteries. The posterior tibial artery becomes the medial and lateral plantar arteries in the foot. The lateral calcaneal artery supplies the lateral segment of the calcaneal area of the foot. The venous return includes the dorsal venous arch, plantar cutaneous venous plexus, medial and lateral plantar veins, and the greater and lesser saphenous veins.

The skin of the foot is made up of fitted, flexible, elastic inner dermis, covered by a much less sensitive outer epidermis. The skin varies in thickness from one-half a millimeter (as in the eyelid) to 4 or 5 mm, in the sole of the foot. The skin of the foot undergoes many changes during the aging process. It becomes thinner, even parchment like; loses its elasticity, usually atrophies; and loses hair. It loses its hydration or water content because there is generally less perspiration and lubrication. The skin loses its suppleness, becomes brittle and dry, and injures easily. This condition, accompanied by a diminished blood supply, can be quite serious.

The normal toenail includes the nail matrix, nail bed, nail plate, lunula, eponychium, cuticle, and nail folds. The nail plate is a sheet of keratin and is important in clinical medicine, as it reflects the health events of the previous months. The nail plate grows slowly forward until it breaks free of the nail bed at the free edge. The tissue below the free edge is termed the hyponychium. The matrix is the area under the proximal nail fold, cuticle, and lunula. The arterial supply to the nail bed stems from small arterial branches from the dorsal and plantar anastomoses. Nail growth is affected by age, trauma, chemicals, environment, and disease.

Foot Changes with Age and Disease

The skin is one of the first structures to demonstrate change. There is a loss of hair below the knee and on the dorsum of the foot and toes. Atrophy follows with the skin appearing parchment like and xerotic. Brownish pigmentations are common and related to the deposition of hemosiderin. Hyperkeratotic lesions are associated with keratin dysfunction (hypertrophy and hyperplasia), with a residual to repetitive pressure, with atrophy of the subcutaneous soft tissue, and/or as space replacement as the body attempts to adjust to the changing stress placed on the foot.

Toenails undergo degenerative trophic changes (onychopathy), thickening (onychauxis and onychogryphosis), and/or longitudinal ridging (onychorrhexis) related to repeated microtrauma, disease, and nutritional impairment. Deformities of the toenails become more pronounced and complicated by xerotic changes in the periungual nail folds as onychophosis (hyperkeratosis) and tinea unguium (onychomycosis). These conditions are usually longstanding, chronic, and very common in the elderly and, in the case of onychomycosis, present a constant focus of infection.

Progressive loss of muscle mass and atrophy of soft tissue decreases function and a lack of activity that increases the susceptibility of the foot to injury, so that even minor trauma can result in a fracture and a marked limitation of activity. Atrophy of the interossei is a precipitating factor in the development of digital contractures (hammer toes), metatarsal prolapse, atrophy, and displacement of the plantar fat pad.

Peripheral vascular disease and arterial insufficiency produce trophic changes, rest pain, intermittent claudication, coldness, and color variations, such as rubor and cyanosis. There may be a loss of sensation and other changes related to neuropathy. The presence of hemorrhage subungually or in subhyperkeratotic tissue indicates marked vascular disease.

CLINICAL ASSESSMENT AND MEDICARE CONSIDERATIONS

The podiatrist provides clinical management based on important principles of podogeriatric assessment; recognizing primary changes in the aging foot; identifying complications related to systemic diseases and, in particular, diabetes mellitus and peripheral arterial occlusive disease; risk stratification; understanding Medicare reimbursement policies, serving as the patient's advocate; and being knowledgeable about primary management procedures. Given the many risk factors for foot diseases and conditions in older adults, specialized foot care is often required. Reasons to refer to a podiatrist for specialized foot care are listed in Table 122-1.

The Pennsylvania Department of Health's Diabetes Prevention and Control Program working with Temple University's School of Podiatric Medicine's Department of Community Health, Aging, and Health Policy and the Pennsylvania Diabetes Academy developed

TABLE 122-1

Reasons to Refer to a Podiatrist

- Signs suggesting generalized disease that include neuropathy, vascular disease infection, etc., and focal neoplastic disease
- In those cases where concomitant therapy is indicated
- Where initial management is not effective
- In the presence of skin, toenail, postural and structural deformities of the feet, and related structures
- In the presence of diabetes mellitus, neurosensory, peripheral vascular, and other risk diseases
- In the presence of foot problems combined with walking problems and/or a history of falls
- Where orthotics are indicated
- It the patient is unable to obtain and/or provide foot care
- If the patient complains of foot problems or has specific questions about care including information on footwear

TABLE 122-2

Conditions That Medicare Considers Qualifying for Routine Foot Care

Amyotrophic lateral sclerosis (ALS)
Arteriosclerosis obliterans (A.S.O., arteriosclerosis of the extremities, and occlusive peripheral arteriosclerosis)
Arteritis of the feet
Buerger's disease (thromboangiitis obliterans)
Chronic indurated cellulitis
Chronic thrombophlebitis*
Chronic venous insufficiency
Diabetes mellitus*
Intractable edema—secondary to a specific disease (e.g., congestive heart failure, kidney disease, and hypothyroidism)
Lymphedema—secondary to a specific disease (e.g., Milroy's disease and malignancy)
Peripheral neuropathies involving the feet
Associated with malnutrition and vitamin deficiency*
Malnutrition (general and pellagra)
Alcoholism
Malabsorption (celiac disease and tropical sprue)
Pernicious anemia
Associated with carcinoma*
Associated with diabetes mellitus*
Associated with drugs and toxins*
Associated with multiple sclerosis*
Associated with uremia (chronic renal disease)*
Associated with traumatic injury
Associated with leprosy or neurosyphilis
Associated with hereditary disorders
Hereditary sensory radicular neuropathy
Angiokeratoma corporis diffusum (Fabry's)
Amyloid neuropathy
Peripheral vascular disease
Raynaud's disease

*These conditions also must have been seen by their medical physician for management within 6 months prior to their foot care management.

a Comprehensive Clinical Podogeriatric and Chronic Diseases Assessment Protocol (Helfand Index—see online appendix). The format provides a methodology to assess foot problems associated with aging and chronic diseases, stratify those patients most at risk to develop complications, maintain a surveillance instrument related to patient care, and provide a means to evaluate data for outcome measurement, which would be valid, accurate, consistent, and relevant. The protocol instrument served as an adjunct to develop prevention and management programs for individual patients and their communities and as a component for comprehensive geriatric assessment. The protocol's application includes elements of primary, secondary, and tertiary prevention and stresses a need for patient and professional education as well as the need for appropriate multidisciplinary patient management.

As a part of the current Medicare regulations for coverage, there are a number of diseases and disorders that have been categorized as special risk conditions that qualify for coverage for "routine foot care." In Medicare terms, primary foot care refers to the débridement of hyperkeratotic lesions (heloma and tyloma) and hypertrophic onychodystrophy. Those patients who demonstrate neurosensory and vascular deficits and who present with clinical findings represent an exemption to the exclusion and become eligible for coverage, within utilization guidelines. Medicare has indicated that although not intended as a comprehensive list, the following metabolic, neurological, and peripheral vascular diseases commonly represent the underlying conditions that might justify coverage for "routine foot care." Table 122-2 lists the primary diseases and disorders that meet current Medicare requirements for routine foot care. This list is not comprehensive but illustrates major conditions.

The podiatrist obtains a history of present illness and past medical history and screens for risk conditions. The foot examination includes a dermatological, an orthopedic, a vascular, and a neurological examination. A full assessment is described in the online appendix and is summarized briefly here.

The basic dermatologic evaluation of the foot includes, but is not limited to, the following: focal hyperkeratatotic lesions, onychauxis, bacterial infection, ulceration, onychomycosis, onychodystrophy, onychocryptosis, cyanosis, xerosis, tinea pedis, verruca, hematoma, rubor, discoloration, and preulcerative changes.

Coverage for the débridement of onychomycosis also includes documentation of mycosis/dystrophy causing secondary infection

and/or pain, which results or would result in marked limitation of ambulation. The specific clinical findings include discoloration, hypertrophy, subungual debris, onycholysis, secondary infection, limitation of ambulation, and pain. In addition, evidence of dystrophy, onychodysplasia, onychauxis, and onychogryphosis are also frequently noted.

The initial foot orthopedic assessment includes an evaluation of the primary deformities related to biomechanical and pathomechanical changes that commonly cause pain and contribute to ambulatory dysfunction. Specific conditions are listed in online appendix. The foot type, muscle strength, and ranges of motion should be noted.

There should be some identification of gait and movement changes, including the use of mobility aids and if the patient is able to reach and see their feet. An evaluation of footwear is also performed. (See section "Footwear and Orthoses.")

As part of the assessment, the patient is evaluated for biomechanical risk for foot ulcers. Factors that increase pressure and stress should be considered. Those factors include body mass, gait (particularly antalgic), ambulatory speed, evidence of repetitive micro tissue trauma, change in weight diffusion, and weight dispersion.

Imbalance is the force on the foot that produces abnormal stresses. These factors include force (alteration in physical condition, either shape or position), compression stress (one force moves toward another), tensile stress (a pulling away of one part against another), shearing stress (a sliding or gliding of one part on the other), friction (the force needed to overcome resistance and usually associated with a sheering stress), elasticity (weight diffusion and weight dispersion), and fluid pressure (soft-tissue adaptation and conformity to stress).

The primary peripheral vascular assessment evaluation should include coldness, trophic changes, and palpation of the dorsalis pedis and posterior tibial pulses. If pulses are not present, the popliteal and femoral pulses should be identified. A history of night cramps, intermittent claudication and deep venous thrombosis, edema, atrophy, varicosities, and atrophy should be noted. Any amputation or partial amputation should be noted and the etiology identified, particularly related to diabetes mellitus, arterial occlusion, and/or infection.

The primary neurological assessment should include the following: Achilles, patellar, and superficial plantar reflexes; vibratory sense (pallesthesia); response to a loss of protective sensation using a 5.07 (10 g) nylon monofilament at bilateral and multiple sites; sharp, dull, and light touch reaction; joint position; burning; two-point discrimination; and related findings. The response to heat, cold, pain, and two-point discrimination are also important considerations. A Tip Therm can measure temperature sensation.

For Medicare purposes, the assessment for the evaluation and management of a diabetic patient with diabetic sensory neuropathy, resulting in a loss of protective sensation must include the criteria listed in Table 122-3.

The final segment of the assessment process is providing an initial impression and/or diagnosis and indicated referrals for management to include podiatric referral, medical specialty referral, patient education, special footwear, orthotics, vascular studies, clinical laboratory referrals, radiographic and other imaging studies, prescriptions as indicated for the management of diseases, and disorders of the foot and its related structures.

All of the assessment components including the focal diseases and disorders of the foot, its related structures, and the pedal manifestations and complications of acute and chronic diseases represent the multiple covariants involved in managing and treating older patients with foot conditions. One mandatory legal key to management includes the requirement for licensure by the individual providing and prescribing indicated medical and surgical care components.

TABLE 122-3

Medicare Coverage for Evaluation of the Patient with Loss of Protective Sensation (LOPS)

1. A diagnosis of LOPS
2. A patient history of diabetes mellitus
3. A physical examination consisting of findings regarding at least the following elements:
   a. Visual inspection of the forefoot, hindfoot, and toe web spaces
   b. Evaluation of protective sensation
   c. Evaluation of foot structure and biomechanics
   d. Evaluation of vascular status
   e. Evaluation of skin integrity
   f. Evaluation and recommendation of footwear
4. Patient education

PRIMARY MANAGEMENT—GUIDELINES AND PRINCIPLES

The management of foot problems in the older patient requires a review of their etiology, symptoms, signs, and clinical manifestations, including related diagnostic studies. The covariant complications, sequelae, relevant treatment, prognosis, and the overall management of the geriatric patient should reflect a reasonable approach that will reduce pain, improve the functional capacity of the patient, maintain that restored function, and provide for the comfort of the patient in activities of daily living and permit the individual to live life to the end of life. Management strategies include radiographs and other imaging studies, nonsteroidal anti-inflammatory drugs, local steroid injections, the use of physical modalities, exercise, and shoe modifications.

SKIN

A concern for older patients is dryness of the skin and/or xerosis. The etiology is as a result of a lack of hydration and lubrication and, to some degree, is a part of the normal aging and degenerative process. Keratin dysfunction can be associated with xerosis. Fissures develop as a result of stress and repetitive microtrauma and, when present, usually on the heel, present a potential hazard for the development of ulceration. Initial management includes the use of an emollient following hydration of the skin. Twenty percent urea is helpful to aid as a mild keratolytic. Creams and ointments containing lanolin can be used as long as the patient does not have an allergy to wool. A plastic or Styrofoam heel cup can be of assistance in minimizing trauma to the heel, reducing the potential for complications. Pruritus is common in the older adult patient and is usually more severe in the colder weather. It is related to dryness, scaliness, decreased skin secretions, keratin dysfunction, environmental changes, and defatting of the skin, which is usually precipitated by the constant use of hot foot soaks. The patient will scratch with excoriations noted on examination. Chronic tinea and allergic, neurogenic, and/or emotional dermatoses should be considered as part of the differential diagnosis and treated accordingly. Management consists of hydration, lubrication, protection, topical steroids if indicated, and judicious use of antihistamines in minimal doses to minimize the itching, which is usually the primary complaint. Particular care should be taken in the male patient with a history of prostatic hypertrophy. If excoriations are infected, proper antibiotic therapy should be instituted.

Hyperhidrosis and/or bromidrosis when present should be managed based on the etiology. If local, measures should be undertaken to control the excessive perspiration and odor. Hydrogen peroxide, isopropyl alcohol, and astringents may be used topically. Neomycin powder will help control the odor by reducing the bacterial decomposition of perspiration. Recommendations on footwear and stocking modifications should be considered. Particular care should be provided on colder climates, as dampness can predispose a patient to the vasospastic effects of cold.

Contact dermatitis may be the result of reactions to chemicals used in shoe construction, footwear fabrics, and/or stockings. Tannic acid, nickel, and synthetic fabrics are the common primary irritants. The skin lesions are usually well demarcated, self-limiting and usually bilateral in distributions. Skin testing can be employed to identify the primary irritant. The general principles of management include removing the cause, mild wet dressings, and the use of topical steroids.

Stasis dermatitis is the residual of venous insufficiency and chronic ulceration. It is more common in patients with dependent edema. Hemosiderin deposition may also be noted with discoloration and induration. Management locally consists of elevation, mild wet dressings, topical steroids, antibiotics as indicated, and supportive measures needed in the management of venous disease. Pyodermias and superficial bacterial infections should be managed locally in a similar manner and, when present with tinea, treatment directed toward both etiologies.

Tinea pedis in the older patient may be an extension of onychomycosis that serves as a focus of infection. It is more common in warmer climate and related to hyperhidrosis. Chronic keratotic tinea (dry squamous type) is more prevalent in older patients, with scales forming a moccasin pattern on the foot. Interdigital infection demonstrates pruritus, scaling, and fissuring and may macerate with excessive perspiration. The acute vesicular form demonstrates bullous lesions that can rupture and produce raw sensitive skin, which makes the patient more prone to secondary bacterial infection. Poor foot hygiene and the inability to bend or see their feet may delay the patients from seeking care until the condition becomes clinically significant and cellulitis is present. In a patient with diabetes or peripheral arterial disease, this complication can be limb threatening. There are a variety of topical medications, such as terbinafine, clotrimazole, butenafine, miconazole, ketoconazole, ciclopirox, naftifine, econazole, sertaconazole, etc., that can usually control this fungal infection. Solutions, powders, and/or creams (water washable or miscible) are best when the patient is unable to easily remove an ointment base. Other common dermatological manifestations that can be demonstrated in the older patient include atopic dermatitis, nummular eczema, neurodermatitis, lichen planus, and psoriasis.

Solitary and/or hemorrhagic bullae are related to shoe trauma and friction or are related to systemic diseases such as diabetes mellitus. Management is directed toward eliminating pressure, protection, and drainage when appropriate. Supportive dressings and shoe modifications should be used as indicated. Gait changes in the older patient magnify many of the foot-to-shoe-last incompatibilities that can result in local foot lesions. Hemorrhagic bullae related to diabetes mellitus are usually indicators of pending ulceration.

Hyperkeratotic lesions, such as tyloma (callous) and heloma (corn), and their varieties, such as hard (durum), soft (molle), vascular (vasculare), neurofibrous (neurofibrosum), seed (miliare), and subungual, are usually painful and secondary to repetitive stress, bony abnormality, deformity, keratin dysfunction, and a lack of hydration and lubrication to the skin. Intractable keratoma, eccrine poroma, porokeratosis, and verruca must be differentiated from these keratotic lesions, although each may present initially as a hyperkeratotic area. The biomechanical and pathomechanical factors that help create these problems are those associated with stress, i.e., compressive, tensile, and/or shearing. The loss of soft tissue as part of the aging process and atrophy of the plantar fat pad increase pain and limit ambulation. Contractures, gait changes, deformities, and the residuals of arthritis are all additional factors that need to be considered in management. The incompatibility of the foot type (inflare, straight, or outflare) to the shoe last is another factor to be considered. It is important to recognize that there is usually not one factor,

but a multiplicity of conditions including skin tone and elasticity, which results in the development of painful keratotic lesions in the elderly. Their management is not routine, and the term management signifies a period of continuing care, as with any other chronic condition in the elderly, to provide for ambulation and comfort.

The common sites for the development of hyperkeratotic lesions include dorsal or distal digital, plantar metatarsal heads, marginal calcaneal, and with deformities such as hammertoes, digital rotations, contractures, hallux valgus, bunion, and/or tailor's bunion (bunionette). These deformities are precipitating factors to foot-to-shoe-last incompatibilities that produce excessive pressure on segments of the foot. Management and treatment should be directed toward the functional needs of the patients and daily living activities. Considerations include débridement, padding, emollients, shoe modifications, last changes, orthoses, and surgical revision as indicated. Materials to provide soft-tissue replacement, such as Plastazote, Professional Protective Technology (PPT), foam, and silicone, produce weight dispersion diffusion as indicated. It is also important to recognize that keratotic lesions of long standing represent a hyperplastic and hypertrophic pathology. Even when weight bearing is removed, these tend to persist for some time. In a sense, hyperkeratotic lesions are a form of body protection to pressure and are symptoms of an abnormal condition. If permitted to remain untreated, enlarge, and condense, these become primary irritants. With pressure such as weight bearing and ambulation, these produce local avascularity, which can precipitate ulceration and their resultant sequelae. Ulcers in the foot usually begin with subkeratotic hemorrhage. Once débrided and managed properly, these usually heal but may be repetitive, unless adequate measures are instituted to reduce the pressure to the localized areas of stress and ulceration. The application of a topical emollient is also an important home or self-care measure. Even with all measures, the problem may persist because of residual deformity and systemic diseases, such as diabetes mellitus. Thus, management and monitoring are similar to any other chronic condition in the older adult and can have a significant impact on the social elements of society, for, without mobility and/or ambulation, the older patient is clearly institutionalized in some form.

TOENAILS

The onychial changes that occur with aging are the result of dystrophic changes, systemic complications, infection, long-term disorders, injury, and/or functional modification. Onychia is an inflammation involving the posterior nail wall and nail bed. It is usually precipitated by local trauma or pressure and a complication of systemic diseases, such as diabetes mellitus, and is the primary clinical sign of impending of infection. Mild erythema, swelling, and pain are the most prevalent findings. Treatment should be directed to removing all pressure from the area and the use of tepid saline compresses. Topical antibiotics can be used as a dressing. Lambs wool, tube foam, or shoe modification should be considered to reduce pressure to the toe and nail. If the onychia is not treated early, paronychia may develop with significant infection and abscess of the posterior nail wall. The infection progresses proximally and deeper structures become involved. The potential for osteomyelitis is greater in the presence of diabetes mellitus and vascular insufficiency. Necrosis, gangrene, and the potential for amputation become reality.

Management includes establishing drainage, culture and sensitivity, radiographs and scans as appropriate, saline compresses, and appropriate systemic antibiotics. Follow-up is essential to prevent cellulitis.

Deformities of the toenails are the result of repeated microtrauma, degenerative changes, and/or disease. The continued friction of the toenails over the years, against the inferior toe box of the shoe, is sufficient trauma to produce dystrophic change. The initial thickening is termed onychauxis. Onychorrhexis with accentuation of normal ridging, trophic changes, and longitudinal striations are onychopathic when related to disease and/or nutritional etiology. When débridement is not completed on a periodic basis, the nail structure elongates, continues to thicken, and becomes deformed with shoe pressure. Onychogryphosis or "ram's horn nail" is usually complicated by fungal infection. The resultant disability can prevent the elderly from wearing shoes. Pain is usually associated with shoe pressure and the deformity. Traumatic avulsion of the nail is a complication. The exaggerated curvature (onychodysplasia pincer toenails) may even penetrate the skin, with resultant infection and ulceration. Management should be directed toward periodic débridement of the onychial structures, both in length and in thickness, with as little trauma as possible. The degree of onycholysis (freeing of the nail from the anterior edge) and onychoschizia (splitting) helps determine the level of débridement. With the excess pressure of deformity, the nail grooves tend to become onychophosed (keratotic). Débridement and the use of mild keratolytics and emollients, such as ammonium lactate and 10% to 20% urea preparations provide some measure of home care for the patient. With onycholysis, subungual debris and keratosis develop, which increases discomfort and may generate pain. However, the patient may not present complaints of pain and discomfort caused by a loss of protective sensation.

Patients with neurosensory and vascular deficits usually demonstrate some form of onychodystrophy, such as onychorrhexis, onychophosis, deformity, hypertrophy, incurvation or involution, subungual hemorrhage (nontraumatic), onycholysis (freeing from the distal segment), onychomadesis (freeing from the proximal segment), autoavulsion, and onychomycosis. These individuals are at greater risk of infection, necrosis, gangrene, and possible amputation.

The most common nonbacterial infection of the toenails is onychomycosis. It is defined as a chronic, communicable disease. Culture, KOH microscopic examination, and the clinical presentation are of diagnostic importance. The clinical forms include distal–lateral subungual, white superficial, proximal subungual, total dystrophic, and candida onychomycosis. The superficial white form presents with fungal growth on the superior surface of the nail plate. Left untreated, invasion of the nail bed occurs with trophic changes. With the distal–lateral, proximal, and total dystrophic forms, the nail bed is primarily infected, with the possibility of paronychia and subsequent dystrophy. Onycholysis (freeing of the nail from the distal edge) and subungual keratosis occur owing to the long-standing chronic nature of this condition in older patients. The posterior nail wall and eponychium demonstrate xerotic changes and hypertrophy, as does the nail plate. Candida is most common in patients with some form of chronic mucocutaneous manifestation.

The older patient usually presents with a chronic infection, involving one or more of the nail plates. The entire thickness of the nail plates is usually involved with resultant hypertrophy and deformity because of the delay in management. Pain may be present with paronychia or deformity or diminished because of sensory deficits.

Mycotic onychia; paronychia; autoavulsion; subungual hemorrhage; a foul, musty odor; and degeneration of the nail plate are common findings. The options for treatment include oral antifungals such as terbinafine, itraconazole, and fluconazole and topical medications such as ciclopirox. A 50% urea–lactic acid combination in gel form will assist to chemically débride the infected nail structures. As a result of the chronicity of onychomycosis, matrix involvement enhances hypertrophy and deformity. Multiple prescriptions, diabetes mellitus, and vascular impairment may limit systemic management. Periodic débridement, topical urea, and topical fungicides are usually indicated for continuing management. Surgical excision may be indicated with excessive pain, as indicated. Onychomycosis must be viewed as a chronic infectious disease, deserving management as any other chronic condition, such as hypertension and/or diabetes mellitus.

Ingrown toenails (onychocryptosis) in the older patient are associated with deformity, trauma, and inappropriate self-care. When the nail penetrates the skin, an abscess and an infection result. If not managed early, periungual ulcerative granulation tissue may form, which increases the risk of serious complications. Deformity and involution (onychodysplasia) also increase the potential for penetration. In the early stage, a segment of the nail can easily be removed using an English nail splitter and an onychotome, drainage established, saline compresses employed, and antibiotics used as indicated. Measures should be taken to prevent the problem in the future. When ulcerative granulation tissue is present, excision, fulguration, desiccation, or the use of caustics is employed to reduce the granulation tissue. In all cases, removal of the penetrating nail is primary. Partial excision of the nail plate and matrix can be completed using regional anesthesia, followed by chemical cautery of the matrix area with CP Phenol. With this procedure, postoperative management includes isopropyl alcohol Zcompresses and topical steroid solutions. With aging, changes in the nail plate may occur, which, when viewed distally, appear "C" shaped (onychodysplasia). This abnormal curvature is incurvation or involution. When present, the pressure of the nail plate on the nail bed and folds produces onychophosis (hyperkeratosis in the nail folds) and discomfort, with complaints similar to an ingrown toenail. The condition may precipitate pressure ulcerations and infection. When this condition is severe, early and total removal of the nail plate and matrix should be considered to avoid complications as the patient ages.

Subungual heloma, when present, is usually associated with a subungual exostosis, spur or hypertrophy of the tufted end of the distal phalanx. Initial treatment consists of débridement and protection of the toe involved, as well as the use of a shoe with a high toe box. Surgical excision of the osseous deformity may be indicated if the condition cannot be managed in a conservative manner. A primary differential diagnosis is subungual melanoma that requires biopsy and prompt management. In all cases of suspected bone pathology, radiographs properly positioned to isolate the area of pathology will provide an appropriate diagnostic approach.

There are multiple onychopathies that occur in the older adult, which are associated with cutaneous and systemic disease. The most common ones include, but are not limited to, psoriasis, mucocutaneous lichen planus, anemia, diabetes mellitus, chronic obstructive pulmonary disease, myocardial infarction, Raynaud's disease, hyperthyroidism, hypothyroidism, vasospastic states, endocarditis, cardiac disease, hypertension, malignancy, rheumatoid arthritis, cirrhosis, alcoholism, peripheral arterial diseases, systemic medications, and local contact agents.

PATHOMECHANICS AND BIOMECHANICS

The human foot is primarily a rigid structure that supports heavy physical workloads that are static and dynamic. The foot itself is shaped like a modified rectangle and bears static forces in a triangular pattern. The transmission of weight and force starts at heel strike, proceeds anteriorly along the lateral segment of the foot, medially across the metatarsal heads, to the first metatarsal segment for the push-off phase of the gait cycle. The social activities of life, occupation, and disease produce morphological variations in both the structure and the function of the foot, in keeping with Wolff's and Davis' law, as the body adapts to the stress placed on it. The environment itself, that is, flat and hard surfaces, force the foot to absorb shock, creating prolonged periods of micro and repeated trauma.

As individuals age the problems magnify, by changing stance, gait, and the ambulatory status of the elderly. The primary considerations include balance; a shuffling gait; broadening the base of gait and stance; reduced toe clearance; changes related to hip, knee flexion, degenerative joint disease, and obesity; as well as specific gait change including circumduction, festinating, steppage, cerebellar, and sensory ataxic gait. Pain, slow speed, short step length, and a narrow stride and width are also important factors. The stress created on the foot and the inability of the patient to adapt to stress produces inflammatory changes in bone and soft tissue, such as osteitis, periostitis, synovitis, capsulitis, fasciitis, myositis, fibrositis, neuritis, and arthritis. Structural modifications of an external nature need to be considered along with the use of physical modalities and appropriate medication as indicated.

Foot problems of a pathomechanical or biomechanical nature usually arise from the interaction between normal morphological variations, the capacity to adapt to stress, and the stressors acting on the foot itself. Morphologic variations may be intrinsic, i.e., within the foot itself, or extrinsic, such as changes in the physiologic relationship of the legs, knees, thigh, hip, and back of the human foot. These changes may be bone and/or soft tissue. The common intrinsic changes include elements such as a hypermobile segment, pes cavus, atrophy of the interossei muscles producing digiti flexus or hammer toes, and the development of hallux valgus, or the so-called "bunion deformity."

The management of pathomechanical and/or biomechanical disorders should be directed toward eliminating the cause and redistributing weight to nonpainful areas of the foot, through weight diffusion and weight dispersion. In addition, the variations in an individual's capacity to adapt to change, particularly when surgical revision is considered, are significant. The primary treatment goals are to relieve pain, to restore maximum function, and to maintain that restored function once achieved. Bilateral weight- and non-weight-bearing radiographic and imaging studies are indicated as, patient management needs are considered from both a static and a dynamic phase.

The ability to adapt to stress is dependent on two major systems, the neuromuscular and vascular, which may be significantly comprised as part of the aging process and disease. The mechanical stressors are two in nature. The first is macrotrauma, which results from sudden injury, such as a fall, resulting in a fracture. The second might be termed microtrauma, which accounts for the hundreds of thousands of repetitive injuries to the foot from occupational activities, obesity, poor stance, modified gait, and foot-to-shoe-last incompatibilities. The systemic stressors are those factors affecting the foot as complications of diseases such as diabetes mellitus, all forms of arthritis, arteriosclerosis, etc. It is also obvious that the foot cannot be divorced or segmented from the body, nor can the foot itself be segmented. It is thus evident that the foot must be considered as a total "end" organ of locomotion and that the resultant mechanical, rotational, and/or positional changes comprise parts of a syndrome or a chain of events of a chronic and progressive process. Once a link in the chain breaks, every effort must be made to prevent further damage and minimize the associated complications of chronic disease. As such, chronic foot problems take years to develop and become significant when these create pain and affect ambulation, the activities of daily living, and the quality of life.

FOOT ORTHOPEDICS

There are a variety of residual foot deformities that can be present in multiple combinations in the older adult. These include, but are not limited to, hallux valgus, hallux varus, splay foot, hallux flexus, digiti flexus (hammertoe), digiti quinti varus, overlapping toes, underriding toes, prolapsed metatarsals, pes cavus, pes planus, pronation, hallux limitus, and hallux rigidus. Many of these changes are the result of and are related to degenerative joint disease (osteoarthritis), rheumatoid, and gouty arthritic changes.

Conservative modalities include shoe last changes, shoe modifications, orthoses, digital braces, physical medicine, exercises, and mild analgesics for pain. Surgical revision, arthroplasty, and joint replacement are also treatment options that should be considered with chronic pain, limitation of the quality of life, and as indicted. Age itself should not be the singular indication of contraindication for surgical consideration. Other factors must also be given to the patient's overall health, medical condition, mental status, and the ability to adapt to change in relation to ambulation, for to have an anatomically corrected joint and a patient who cannot ambulate without pain defeats the treatment needs of the elderly. Foot conditions need to be managed medically, physically, mechanically, and surgically, to keep the patient ambulatory and pain free.

Fractures of the foot and toes may be the result of direct trauma and/or stress, related to bone loss. Most uncomplicated and closed fractures that are in good position should be appropriately immobilized as indicated. Open fractures need surgical management. Digital fractures can usually be managed with silicone mold and surgical shoes and supportive dressings, as long as the joints distally and proximally are immobilized.

FOOTWEAR AND ORTHOSES

See Figure 122-2 for an overview of the anatomy of the shoe. Shoe selection should be based on the functional needs of the patient, a shoe last that conforms to the foot, the complications of other diseases and disorders, shoe size that is based on internal and external measurements, and fabrication of materials that will provide protection and support and permit maximum foot function. For example,

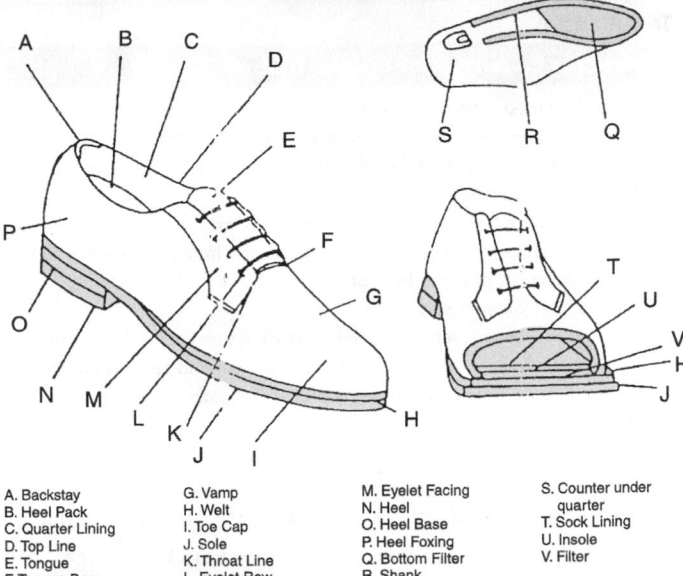

A. Backstay
B. Heel Pack
C. Quarter Lining
D. Top Line
E. Tongue
F. Tongue Bar
G. Vamp
H. Welt
I. Toe Cap
J. Sole
K. Throat Line
L. Eyelet Row
M. Eyelet Facing
N. Heel
O. Heel Base
P. Heel Foxing
Q. Bottom Filter
R. Shank
S. Counter under quarter
T. Sock Lining
U. Insole
V. Filter

FIGURE 122-2. Components of a shoe. (Adapted with permission from Pedorthic Footwear Association. Pedorthic Reference Guide. Columbia, MD; 1992, 1999, 2006.)

the stylish dress shoe has different social needs than a shoe for daily use and for walking and exercise.

For the most part, a shoe that provides some flexibility to allow for free mobility usually feels most comfortable unless there are deformities or other special conditions that require rigidity. The foot is basically a modified rectangle; thus, a quadrangular shoe would be the best last, to conform to the shape of the foot. With deformity, special lasts may be indicated. The shoe should have an acceptable heel height to avoid forcing the toes into the end of the shoe. The material of construction should be porous to allow for the evaporation of moisture. There should be some degree of moderate sole friction to avoid slippery and adhesive sole material. This consideration also needs to be evaluated in comparison to flooring surfaces and, in particular, high pile carpets. The shoe should be lightweight to reduce energy expenditure on the part of the patient. The wearing of shoes should be socially acceptable in appearance to the patient. Cost is a factor, and a reasonable price for the particular patient becomes essential given the limited incomes of older patients. For long-term care patients, these suggestions may well change for the incontinent nursing home patient; a soft washable foot covering may be the most practical solution.

Shoes are constructed over a last or model of the foot. The last may be inflare, straight, or outflare. It is essential that the flare of the foot match the flare of the shoe to avoid a foot-to-shoe-last incompatibility and permit abnormal pressure to develop. Shoe generally consist of an outsole, heel, rand, counter, quarter, vamp, back stay, quarter, filler, lining, upper, tip, toe cap, foxing, welting, insole, sock lining, tongue, eyelet, and laces or other closure.

Some of the basic shoe types include standard lasts, basic orthopedic shoe with its long counter and Thomas Heel, rigid shank shoes, high top lasts, extra-depth shoes, shoes with moldable interiors, custom-molded and fabricated footwear, and athletic footwear.

The basic shoe modifications that may be used for rthe older patient include medial (for valgus deformity) and lateral (for varus) heel seat wedges. Sole wedges are for alignment and support and to

help maintain a better gait pattern. Calcaneal wedges limit motion and alter gait. Metatarsal bars are used to shift or transfer weight from the metatarsal heads to the shaft. In addition, the bar produces a moderate heel rise to push off without additional metatarsal head weight bearing. Examples include the Denver, Hauser, Comma bar, etc. The Thomas Heel and long counter provide improved balance, increase calcaneal support, and increase the stability of the shank area. Long shoe counters are used to increase mid-foot support and control foot direction. Heel flares increase ankle stability either medially or laterally. The heel may be reversed to provide lateral stability.

A shank filler provides for a total contact shank area, increases stability, and enhances the weight-bearing surface. They can also be used for excessive valgus and varus. The spring extension can be used to increase push-off. The steel splint or plate is used to limit motion, usually at the first metatarsal–phalangeal joint, in relation to hallux limitus or rigidus. The rocker bottom, which is an extension of the metatarsal bar, is designed to prevent flexion and extension of the shoe. Shoe elevations can compensate for limb length discrepancies. The solid ankle cushion heel improves extension (planter flexion) or ankle motion. The solid ankle cushion heel can also be used with a metatarsal bar, rocker bar, springs, or double sole, which then limits some motion. The KEEL heel is used to eliminate lateral forces. Steel springs, cork, or wooden buildups may also be employed as indicated.

Internal shoe modifications include medial longitudinal pads or cookies, metatarsal pads, balance pads, calcaneal bars, heel pads and lifts, Barton and Thomas wedges, and tongue or bite pads, heel elevations, cushions, and wedges. Excavations and stretching or relasting are also important. Shoe selection and last determination as well as fit are essential for the older patient, particularly when orthoses are to be used.

Orthoses are used to protect, restore, and/or improve function that support, align, prevent, or modify deformities. Foot orthotics may or may not include a shoe and/or any modification to make an orthotic functional and effective. Orthoses are prescribed by healthcare professionals and are fabricated to meet the specific needs of the patient.

The primary prescription objectives include modifying foot function, compensate for existing deformities, weight dispersion, weight diffusion, soft-tissue supplementation, shock absorption, support, realignment, improved performance, restriction of motion, enhancement of motion, prevention of injury, reduction of weight load, stabilization, and the relief of pain.

The available orthoses include rigid, semirigid, and flexible forms, using a variety of materials. In addition, replaceable pads, insoles, heel orthoses, functional orthoses, latex shield, silicone molds, and digital orthoses are also used as indicated. The foot orthosis is a form of durable medical equipment that does provide support and compensate for malalignment, which may be present in the older patient. The orthosis is used to improve function and provide support. It may be used to evenly redistribute weight, as is the case of the total contact orthoses. It may accommodate painful areas and provide for filler in the postamputation period. For the older patient, correction is many times modified to become compensation and may limit motion, compensate for abnormal foot position, help equalize limb length discrepancy, and control position and motion.

Orthoses may be over-the-counter, custom-made, or customized and modified prefabricated components. They may be full length, to sulcus, to metatarsal head area, or may have extensions to compensate for metatarsal length discrepancies. Rigid orthoses are usually fabricated from metal or thermoplastics. With thermoplastics, the degree of rigidity and flexibility can be modified by the thickness and material selection, the weight and functional needs of the patient, and the use of soft material as a part of a top cover. Semirigid orthoses are usually fabricated from leather, rubber, cork, polypropylene, and celastic and may include steel springs in the shank area. Soft orthoses usually consist of materials that provide weight diffusion and weight dispersion or is multidensity to encompass both concepts. Silicone also is used both for plantar orthoses and as digital orthoses in the form of silicone molds. These custom-designed digital braces have a significant role to play in the management of the older patient, as these provide a great deal of flexibility, are cost effective, can easily be modified and/or changed, and can be custom designed to meet individual patient needs and diagnostic indications.

The general types include calcaneal orthoses such as heel stabilizer/cups, heel protectors, and shock-absorbing calcaneal seats. The full-length orthoses are usually soft and may have some degree of semirigid characteristics for stability. Multidensity and total contact orthoses usually fit this category. Schaffer, Whitman, and Mayer designs are still used, based on the indications and ability of the patient to adapt to this form of shell design. Metatarsal extensions and modifications are incorporated into these primary classifications and include, but are not limited to, the following examples: heel pad, heel spur pad, cutouts for weight dispersion, scaphoid pad, longitudinal arch reinforcement, wedges, Morton's extension, rear foot post, forefoot post, metatarsal pad, and heel lifts.

For the geriatric patient, the usual prescription includes some degree of flexibility to provide a functional accommodative orthotic. Some of the newer rigid materials, used in a thinner plate, do provide some flexibility and do permit a myotatic reflex to function. Geriatric orthoses usually provide some form of cushioning material that is both weight diffusive and weight dispersive. Keys are also strength, semiflexibility, and resiliency that compensate for change in the multiple systems involved in gait and the changes related to aging and chronic diseases.

The final determination of appropriate form and material depends on the weight of the patient, findings at examination, general functional needs, activities of daily living, and the physiological adaptability of the patient. Clinical needs and appropriate indications are essential considerations for relief of pain, restoration of a maximum degree of function, and maintaining that level of function, once achieved.

It is important to remember that footwear, as protection and foot covering, needs to be compatible with the foot and the patient's functional requirements. Shoe modifications enhance these requirements. The foot orthosis adds another link in the chain needed to keep the patient pain free and ambulatory. The foot, shoe, and orthoses must function as a unit and as a part of the patient's ambulatory system.

Therapeutic Shoes for Diabetics

The importance of footwear and appropriate orthoses for the older population has been clearly delineated in relation to the "at-risk" diabetic under Medicare. The "therapeutic shoe" provisions as currently projected demonstrate, in this singular disease, the important relationship between shoes and orthoses in the diabetic patients. It is important to note that this is just one example of need. See

---

TABLE 122-4

Criteria for Coverage for Special Diabetic Shoes

1. The patient must have diabetes mellitus
2. The patient has one or more of the following conditions:
   a. previous amputation of the other foot or part of either foot, or
   b. history of previous ulceration of either foot, or
   c. preulcerative callus formation of either foot, or
   d. peripheral neuropathy with a history of callus formation of either foot, or
   e. foot deformity of either foot, or
   f. poor circulation in either foot
3. The physician who is managing the patient's systemic diabetes condition has documented that indications 1 and 2 are met and certifies that the patient is being treated under a comprehensive plan of care for the diabetes and that the patient needs special shoes

---

Table 122-4 for criteria for coverage for diabetic shoes. Following the above, a podiatrist or other qualified physician knowledgeable in the fitting of therapeutic shoes and inserts may write the prescription. The footwear must be fitted and furnished by a podiatrist or other qualified individual such as a pedorthist, an orthotist, or a prosthetist.

ULCERATIONS

The management of ulcerations in the older patient depends on the etiology and the related complications associated with tissue loss. General principles include supportive measures to reduce trauma and pressure to the ulcerated area, such as dressings, orthoses, shoe modifications, and special shoes. The prevention and control of infection and maintaining a clean, healthy base to permit healing are essential. Issues that need to be considered include perfusion, size, depth of tissue loss, infection, and neuropathy including a loss of protective sensation. The débridement of keratosis when indicated is essential to prevent roofing of the ulcer. The use of physical modalities and measures such as low-voltage therapy (contractile currents) and exercises can assist in improving the local vascular supply to the ulcer and in helping to establish a clean base. Pressure ulcers of local origin are usually associated with a bony prominence, biomechanical abnormality, and external trauma as the result of stress associated with gait change. Atrophy of soft tissue and the residuals of arthritis provide a focus for the development of ulcerations. Tissue loss associated with systemic diseases is usually related to sensory loss, neuropathic joint change, and vascular insufficiency, as with diabetes mellitus and peripheral arterial disease. Management focuses on identifying the underlying diagnosis, local supportive measures, adequate treatment of the related systemic diseases, and efforts to minimize the potential for osteomyelitis and amputation risk, and maintaining the ambulatory status of the patient for as long as possible.

Methods to remove pressure from weight-bearing areas can be attained by the use of orthoses and/or shoe last changes; the use of pads, bars, wedges, and other modifications; increasing the sole thickness and using shock-absorbing material; and surgical shoes, total contact orthosis, special foot and ankle walkers, and ortho or heel wedge surgical shoes. Older patients who avoid the use of footwear at home, owing to their inability to bend, expose themselves to the potential of foreign bodies and foot injury.

DIABETIC AND PERIPHERAL ARTERIAL CONSIDERATIONS

Foot complications relating to diabetes have a significant impact on the quality of diabetic patients. The older diabetic presents with a covariant set of syndromes including dermopathy, onychopathy, vasculopathy, neuropathy, and myopathy. The symptoms are similar to those of aging in general but appear at an earlier age. Foot complications are also a major cause of hospitalization, and 50% to 75% of these amputations can be presented when the diagnosis is made early and interventions made that can affect outcomes. Emphasis is placed on preventing lower extremity amputations that can produce major life style changes and have a significant economic impact on the patient, their families, the health care system, and society in general. Programs such as "LEAP" (lower extremity amputation prevention, Department of Health and Human Services) and "PACT" (Prevention, Amputation, Care, and Treatment, Department of Veterans Affairs) are examples of these efforts. The older diabetic patients present the greatest risk for ulceration, infection, hospitalization, and amputation because of the multiple systems involved in the disease. Similar changes can be demonstrated with peripheral arterial disease, hemophilia, cardiac disease, chronic renal failure (dialysis), obesity, post stroke, and chronic obstructive pulmonary disease. Tissue loss in the elderly and amputation can terminate the patient's independent life of usefulness to themselves and society.

The pathogenesis of a diabetic foot ulceration in the older patient includes diabetes mellitus itself; trauma (direct and/or repetitive microtrauma); neuropathy—motor (weakness, atrophy, deformity, abnormal stress, high plantar pressure, and hyperkeratosis), sensory (loss of protective sensation), and autonomic (anhidrosis, xerosis, fissures, and decreased sympathetic tone); peripheral arterial disease—macrovascular (atherosclerosis and ischemia) and microvascular (structural and/or functional); osteoarthropathy (Charcot's joints); impaired response to infection; and reduced nutrient capillary blood flow, with subsequent ulceration and potential amputation. The risk increases with sensory deficits, altered biomechanics and neuropathy, increased tissue pressure (erythema and subkeratotic hematoma), bony deformity, decreased or absent pedal pulses, prior ulcerative history, and toenail pathology.

Hyperkeratotic lesions form as space replacements and provide a focus for ulceration caused by increased pressure on the soft tissues with an associated localized avascularity from direct pressure and counterpressure. Tendon contractures and hammertoes increase pressure. A warm foot with pulsations in an older diabetic with neuropathy is not uncommon. When ulceration is present, the base is usually covered by keratosis, which retards and many times prevents healing. Necrosis and gangrene are related to infection with eventual occlusion and gangrene. Foot drop and a loss of position sense are usually present. Pretibial lesions are indicative of this change as well as microvascular infarction. Arthropathy gives rise to deformity, altered gait patterns, and a higher risk for ulceration and limb loss.

In addition to the relationship of vascular and neuropathic changes, ulcerations must be related to trauma and, in particular, the effects of repeated microtrauma. Hyperkeratosis related to keratin dysfunction, space replacement, bony abnormality, and/or pathomechanics would react to pressure and trauma, which may be mechanical, thermal, and/or chemical in nature. Subhyperkeratotic hemorrhage is usually an early clinical sign of tissue breakdown. Regardless of the cause, the general principles of management include a decrease of local trauma by the use of orthotics, shoe modifications, specialized footwear, and efforts to maximize weight diffusion and weight dispersion techniques. Physical modalities, medication, and exercise can be employed to improve the vascular supply to the part, following adequate evaluation by Doppler and other techniques. Appropriate invasive techniques and bypass surgical procedures should be considered. Local débridement of the ulcerative site and adequate home wound care, appropriate antibiotics, topical enzymes, and tissue stimulants should be considered. Radiographs and bone scans should be ordered early on in the management process to deal with infection at its first signs. Culture and sensitivity, appropriate antibiotic therapy, and hospitalization should be considered to prevent, where possible, amputation. Wound care includes medical débridement, special dressings, autologous and epidermal grafts, and recognizing limb-threatening infection (deep ulceration, bone and/or joint involvement, systemic toxicity, ischemia, gangrene, and gas gangrene). Negative pressure wound therapy, hyperbaric oxygen, and transcutaneous oxygen measurement is additional considerations.

Asymptomatic diabetic older patients should be evaluated at least twice a year to identify problems at their earliest development. Patients with foot conditions requiring primary management should be followed every 30 to 60 days, depending on the degree of complications. A multidisciplinary care approach, which includes patients and their families, is an essential element in managing the elderly diabetic patients with foot problems.

CONCLUSION

The ability to retain ambulation is directly related to foot health as individuals age. Regardless of the care setting, that is, home, ambulatory facilities, long-term care programs, mental health facilities, assisted living, or other models, all practitioners must think comprehensively and recognize that team care must be an essential part of the management of the older individual. Foot health education, such as programs developed by the Pennsylvania Department of Health (Feet First and If the Shoe Fits), is available to both patients and professionals and should be employed as a part of all geriatric patient education programs. With the high prevalence and incidence of foot problems in the older patient, the ability to live life to the end of life will depend, to a great deal, on the ability to remain alert and mobile and to retain the qualities that make individuals want to live.

FURTHER READING

American College of Foot & Ankle Surgeons. Diabetic foot disorders – a clinical practice guideline. *Suppl J Foot Ankle Surg.* 2006;45(5):S1–S66.

Armstrong DG, Lavery LA. *Clinical Care of the Diabetic Foot.* Alexandria, VA: American Diabetes Association; 2005.

Baran RD, RPR, Tosti A, Haneke E. *A Text Atlas of Nail Disorders, Diagnosis and Treatment.* St. Louis: Mosby; 1996.

Birrer RB, Dellacorte MP, Grisafi PJ. *Common Foot Problems in Primary Care.* 2nd ed. Philadelphia: Henley & Belfus, Inc; 1998.

Bowker JH, Pfeifer MA. *Levin's & Oneal's the Diabetic Foot.* 6th ed. St. Louis, MO: Mosby; 2001.

Cavanagh PR, Boone EY, Plummer DL. *The Foot in Diabetes, a Bibliography.* Pennsylvania: Pennsylvania State University, State College; 2000.

Dauber R, Bristow I, Turner W. *Text Atlas of Podiatric Dermatology.* London: Martin Dunitz; 2001.

Edmonds ME, Foster AVM, Sanders LJ. *A Practical Manual of Diabetic Footcare.* Malden, MA: Blackwell Publishing; 2004.

Evans JG, Williams FT, Beattie BL, Michel JP, Wilcock GK. *Oxford Textbook of Geriatric Medicine*. 2nd ed. England: Oxford University Press; 2000.

Gabel LL, Haines DJ, Papp KK. *The Aging Foot, an Interdisciplinary Perspective*. Columbus, OH: The Ohio State University, College of Medicine and Public Health, Department of Family Medicine; 2004.

Helfand AE, ed. *Clinical Podogeriatrics*. Baltimore, MD: Williams and Wilkins; 1981.

Helfand AE, ed. *The Geriatric Patient and Considerations of Aging, Clinics in Podiatric Medicine and Surgery*. Vols. I and II. Philadelphia, PA: WB Saunders; 1993.

Helfand AE. A conceptual model for a geriatric syllabus for podiatric medicine. *J Am Podiatr Med Assoc*. 2000;90(5):258–267.

Helfand AE. *Assessing the Older Diabetic Patient*. CD. Harrisburg, PA: Pennsylvania Diabetes Academy, Pennsylvania Department of Health, Temple University, School of Medicine, Office for Continuing Medical Education, Temple University, School of Podiatric Medicine; December 2001.

Helfand AE. Foot problems. In: Mezzy MD, ed. *The Encyclopedia of Elder Care*. New York, New York: Springer; 2001:267–272.

Helfand AE. Podiatric medicine. In: Mezzy MD, ed. *The Encyclopedia of Elder Care*. New York, New York: Springer; 2001:512–514.

Helfand AE. Clinical podogeriatrics: assessment, education, and prevention. *Clin Podiatr Med and Surg*. 2003;20(3).

Helfand AE. Foot problems in older patients, a focused podogeriatric assessment study in ambulatory care. *J Am Podiatr Med Assoc*. 2004;94(3):293–304.

Helfand AE. Disorders and diseases of the foot, geriatric review syllabus. In: Cobbs EL, Duthie ED, Murphy JB, eds. *A Core Curriculum in Geriatric Medicine*. 6th ed. Malden, MA: Blackwell; 2006.

Helfand AE, ed. *Public Health and Podiatric Medicine – Principles and Practice*. 2nd ed. Washington, DC: APHA Pressn; 2006.

Helfand AE. In: Ham RJ, Sloane PD, Warshaw GA, Bernard MA, Flaherty R, eds. *Foot Problems, Primary Care Geriatrics – A Case Based Approach*. 5th ed. Philadelphia, PA: Mosby/Elsevier; 2007:523–532.

Helfand AE, ed. *Foot Health Training Guide for Long-Term Care Personnel*. Baltimore, MD: Health Professions Press; 2007.

Helfand AE, Bruno J, eds. *Rehabilitation of the Foot, Clinics in Podiatry*. Vol. 1, No. 2. Philadelphia, PA: W B Saunders Co.; 1984.

Helfand AE, Jessett DF. In: Pathy MSJ, Sinclair AS, Morley JR, eds. *Foot Problems, Principles and Practice of Geriatric Medicine*. 4th ed. Chichester: John Wiley; 2006.

International Diabetes Federation. *International Consensus on the Diabetic Foot*. Amsterdam, Netherlands: Text & CD; 2003.

Levy LA, Hetherington VJ. *Principles and Practice of Geriatric Medicine*. 2nd ed. Brooklandville, MD: Data Trace Publishing; 2006.

Lorimer D, French G, O'Donnell M, Burrow JG. *Neale's Disorders of the Foot, Diagnosis and Management*. 6th ed. New York, New York: Churchill Livingstone; 2002.

Merriman LM, Turner W. *Assessment of the Lower Limb*. 2nd ed. New York, New York: Churchill Livingstone, Elsevier; 2002.

Robbins JM. *Primary Podiatric Medicine*. Philadelphia, PA: WB Saunders; 1994.

Sanders LJ. *Diabetic Foot Ulcers and Amputations*. Alexandria, VA: American Diabetes Association; 2001.

Turner WA, Merriman LM. *Clinical Skills in Treating the Foot*. Edinburgh: Elsevier, Churchill, Livingstone; 2005.

Fibromyalgia and Myofascial Pain Syndromes

Cheryl D. Bernstein ■ *Debra K. Weiner*

Fibromyalgia and myofascial pain (MP) are among the most common musculoskeletal disorders from which older adults suffer. These disorders represent opposite ends of the pain spectrum with the discrete character of MP at one extreme and the widespread symptoms of fibromyalgia at the other. MP may be acute or chronic, and is associated with taut muscle bands and hypersensitive areas called trigger points. Fibromyalgia syndrome includes symptoms of sleep disruption, fatigue, and psychological distress in addition to widespread pain. Both fibromyalgia and MP syndromes may result in significant functional impairment and cause suffering and disability comparable to that of rheumatoid arthritis and osteoarthritis. Diagnosis of these disorders is grounded in appropriately targeted history and physical examination; these are the tools required to avoid unnecessary ordering of "diagnostic" tests and foster implementation of appropriate management strategies.

FIBROMYALGIA SYNDROME

Definition and Epidemiology

While a number of fibromyalgia classification criteria have been proposed, the criteria developed by the American College of Rheumatology are used most commonly. These criteria, which are 81% sensitive and 88% specific, allow fibromyalgia patients to be distinguished from patients with widespread pain caused by other rheumatological disorders (e.g., systemic lupus erythematosus, rheumatoid arthritis). They include a history of generalized body pain (i.e., pain in at least three of four body quadrants) for at least 3 months duration and at least 11 out of 18 specific tender points on physical examination. Although initially developed for classification of fibromyalgia, practitioners tend to regard them as required for diagnosis, although this is not accurate. Older adults who present with widespread pain and other supportive clinical features (see below) should be considered

to have fibromyalgia even if they do not precisely fulfill the ACR criteria. These criteria are best used as a general guide and to allow for study enrollment, not for strict use in the office setting.

The incidence of fibromyalgia syndrome (the proportion of new cases or first ever episodes) is difficult to measure in part because symptoms seem to ebb and flow over time. According to five large population studies, approximately 10% of the population has widespread pain. Of those with widespread body pain, approximately 2% meet ACR diagnostic criteria for fibromyalgia. Women are four to seven times as likely to have fibromyalgia compared to men, with the greatest prevalence in those 60 to 79 years of age. Patients with fibromyalgia also have been estimated to have a two- to sevenfold greater risk of suffering from depression, anxiety, headache, irritable bowel syndrome, chronic fatigue syndrome, systemic lupus erythematosus, and rheumatoid arthritis compared to healthy individuals.

Pathogenesis

While recent studies have added to our understanding of the pathogenesis of fibromyalgia, the exact cause is still unknown. Most studies suggest that abnormal central nervous system pain processing, known as central sensitization, plays a key role in fibromyalgia pathogenesis. Abnormal peripheral pain processing, peripheral sensitization, also contributes to fibromyalgia pathogenesis. The cause of sensitization is not known, but a variety of neuroendocrine and biochemical abnormalities are believed to be involved.

Peripheral Tissue Abnormalities

Early studies of fibromyalgia patients failed to consistently show abnormalities in the peripheral tissues. However, reexamination of this issue has uncovered differences between muscle samples from fibromyalgia subjects and healthy controls. One difference is higher levels of nitric oxide in muscles of fibromyalgia patients that may result in increased cell death. Other abnormalities that have been identified in muscles of fibromyalgia patients as compared with healthy individuals include lower phosphorylation potential and oxidative capacity as evidenced by lower levels of muscle phosphocreatine and ATP, as well as increased substance P, DNA fragmentation, interleukin-1, and perfusion deficits (see Staud reference). While the exact meaning of these abnormalities is unclear, the findings suggest an underlying difference in muscle metabolism of fibromyalgia patients as compared to people without fibromyalgia. Further study is needed to establish a relationship between these findings and the pain and fatigue fibromyalgia patients report.

Central and Peripheral Sensitization and Pain Amplification

Abnormalities of peripheral and central pain processing are well established in fibromyalgia. In the periphery, tissue sensitization results from changes in primary nociceptive afferents, increased neuronal excitability, and enlarged neuronal receptive fields. Central sensitization involves neuroplasticity in the brain and spinal cord. "Windup," a normal finding of increased pain sensations after repeated exposures to a painful stimulus, is an example of central sensitization. In studies of fibromyalgia patients, the "windup" response is exaggerated compared to controls. Staud and colleagues studied fibromyalgia patients and healthy controls after repeated exposure to heat stimuli. While both groups had higher pain ratings after repeated exposures to heat, the degree of windup and temporal summation was significantly greater in fibromyalgia subjects. In addition, the fibromyalgia subjects had more prolonged after sensations compared with control subjects. Peripheral and central sensitizations contribute to the exaggerated pain response of fibromyalgia patients.

Neuroendocrine Abnormalities

Altered activity of the hypothalamic–pituitary–adrenal axis (HPA), and abnormal levels of adrenocortical trophic hormone (ACTH) and urinary cortisol have been demonstrated in patients with fibromyalgia. Evidence suggests that the HPA axis may be less resilient than normal in fibromyalgia patients and that this and other HPA axis abnormalities may underlie the impaired response to stress that many of these patients exhibit. The review by Crofford provides an expanded discussion of the neuroendocrine abnormalities in fibromyalgia syndrome.

Biochemical Abnormalities

While there are no serologic tests to assist practitioners with making a diagnosis of fibromyalgia, a number of biochemical abnormalities have been identified in the context of research studies. Russell and colleagues have identified lower levels of serum serotonin and norepinephrine in patients with fibromyalgia compared to controls. Low platelet serotonin levels have also been identified. While cerebrospinal fluid (CSF) serotonin has not been measured in patients with fibromyalgia, its precursor and metabolic products have been demonstrated to exist at significantly lower levels in the CSF of fibromyalgia patients compared to controls. Norepinephrine's metabolite, methoxyhydroxyphenylglycol, and dopamine's metabolite, homovanillic acid, are also reduced in fibromyalgia patients.

Further discussion of the biochemical abnormalities found in fibromyalgia patients is found in the review by Mease.

Abnormal levels of nociceptive neurochemicals have also been found in patients with fibromyalgia. Several studies have shown that substance P, a neuropeptide involved in pain transmission, exists in significantly higher levels in the CSF of fibromyalgia patients compared to those without fibromyalgia (see the Russell reference). Nerve growth factor (NGF), which promotes production of substance P, also is elevated in the CSF of fibromyalgia patients.

Functional Imaging of Pain

Researchers have used functional magnetic resonance imaging (fMRI) to help understand fibromyalgia pathogenesis. Functional MRI measures regional blood flow in the central nervous system in response to various environmental stimuli and fMRI studies have demonstrated increased central nervous system activity that corresponds to fibromyalgia patients' subjective pain reports. In response to stimuli, which do not cause pain in controls, fibromyalgia patients report high pain scores and have augmented regional cerebral blood flow on fMRI.

Genetics

Mounting evidence points to fibromyalgia as a heritable disorder. This evidence includes familial aggregation of fibromyalgia as well as a reduced pain threshold in the first-degree female relatives of fibromyalgia patients, even in those without overt clinical symptoms. Gene polymorphisms in the serotonergic and dopaminergic systems and a higher prevalence of polymorphisms in the promoter region of the serotonin transporter gene (5HTT) in fibromyalgia patients as compared to healthy controls also have been identified.

Clinical Presentation

Patient History

Fibromyalgia patients often report that they feel pain "all over." Pain diagrams, on which patients are asked to shade painful areas of a human figure, are helpful in making a diagnosis. For fibromyalgia patients, these diagrams show diffuse shading on the right and left sides of the body as well as above and below the waist. We observe that some fibromyalgia patients shade, circle, or put an X through the entire figure. Patients generally rate their pain as moderate to severe in intensity. Over time, pain will fluctuate in severity but typically does not resolve completely. The quality of the pain may be variably described as deep aching, mild tenderness, or sharp sensations. Symptoms are generally constant throughout the day but often are worse in the morning and the evening. Triggers, including stress, cold weather, illness, and unaccustomed exertion, will likely increase pain. In addition to pain, 75% of patients report stiffness and over 50% report a sensation of swelling. Low back pain and chronic whiplash are relatively common, affecting 20% to 30% of the patients with fibromyalgia.

Fibromyalgia patients are likely to report a wide variety of nonmusculoskeletal symptoms, most commonly fatigue and difficulty sleeping. Sixty percent of patients report psychological and neuropsychological symptoms including anxiety, mental distress, and cognitive dysfunction. Thirty percent of patients report current

TABLE 123-1

Fibromyalgia Associated Symptoms and Syndromes

Musculoskeletal
Stiffness
Sensation of joint swelling

Nonmusculoskeletal
Fatigue
Difficulty sleeping
Dysesthesias
Paresthesias
Depression
Anxiety
Stress
Dyspnea
Palpitations
Difficulty concentrating
Tinnitus
Dizziness
Vertigo

Associated Syndromes
Headache
   Tension Type
   Cervicogenic
   Migraine
Irritable bowel syndrome
Pelvic pain
Restless leg syndrome
Interstitial cystitis
Myofascial pain syndromes

Associated Rheumatological Disorders
Systemic lupus erythematosus
Rheumatoid arthritis
Sjogren's syndrome

depression with over 50% of patients reporting a history of depression. Headaches are also common. Uncommon symptoms (<20% prevalence) include tinnitus, dizziness, vertigo, and Raynaud's phenomenon. Fibromyalgia may also coexist in 20% of rheumatoid arthritis patients, 30% of patients with systemic lupus erythematosus, and 50% of those with Sjögren's syndrome. Table 123-1 lists the symptoms and syndromes commonly associated with fibromyalgia.

Up to 80% of fibromyalgia patients report debilitating fatigue. This complaint encompasses mental fatigue and impaired concentration commonly referred to as "fibro fog," physical fatigue after exertion, and general sleepiness. In fibromyalgia patients, these symptoms most often occur in the absence of other medical illnesses. Poor sleep quality seen in fibromyalgia patients is known as nonrestorative sleep. Patients awaken feeling unrefreshed even after a full night's sleep. Other complaints include light sleep, frequent awakenings, and insomnia. As with other aspects of fibromyalgia, the cause of poor sleep and chronic fatigue is not fully known. Studies of sleep architecture in fibromyalgia patients have revealed abnormalities, which may account for daytime fatigue. One such finding is alpha wave intrusion into stage four sleep. In fibromyalgia patients, alpha waves, typically seen in stage one light sleep, are found in stage four slow wave deep sleep. In addition, fibromyalgia patients have a relative rapid eye movement (REM) sleep deficiency com-

pared to healthy controls. These abnormalities, while not specific to fibromyalgia, may cause significant fatigue.

Physical Examination

When evaluating the older adult with widespread chronic pain, the practitioner should be cognizant of multiple rheumatological disorders in addition to fibromyalgia syndrome such as generalized osteoarthritis, pseudogout, gout, rheumatoid arthritis, systemic lupus erythematosus, and polymyalgia rheumatica, as summarized in Table 123-2. A careful history and thorough physical examination for synovial and extrasynovial findings can help differentiate these conditions from fibromyalgia. Table 123-2 lists a number of key features on history and physical examination that may aid in the diagnosis. Other diagnostic considerations include hypothyroidism, vitamin D deficiency, demyelinating polyneuropathies, and paraneoplastic syndromes. A targeted laboratory panel may be helpful in teasing out these differential diagnostic considerations.

The characteristic physical examination finding in patients with fibromyalgia is the presence of tender points at the specific locations outlined in Table 123-3. A tender point is defined as a spot on the body that is painful with 4 kg of pressure (the amount of pressure required to blanch the examiner's thumbnail when palpating the palm of her own hand). Palpation of the tender points with 4 kg of pressure is needed, as below this level, most subjects will not report pain. Those who report pain when tested with 4 kg of pressure demonstrate a lower than normal pain threshold. Patients reporting pain in fewer than the 11 of 18 tender points included in the American College of Rheumatology classification criteria may still be diagnosed with fibromyalgia if they have otherwise supportive clinical features (e.g., sleep disturbance, fatigue, morning stiffness). Tender points exist in a number of conditions other than fibromyalgia, including cervical and lumbosacral facet arthrosis syndrome, sacroiliac joint syndrome, and chronic whiplash and therefore a careful history and examination are key diagnostic elements.

Treatment

A variety of pharmacologic and nonpharmacological interventions are available for the treatment of fibromyalgia. While many of these treatments are beneficial anecdotally, controlled research is limited and the optimal treatment remains unknown. Available research is limited by small sample size, short duration, and lack of blinding and randomization. Nonetheless, we have successfully employed a number of management approaches in our older adult patients with fibromyalgia. Medications, particularly antidepressants and some antiseizure medications, may be beneficial, particularly if therapy is aimed at addressing associated symptoms such as disrupted sleep, depression, and/or anxiety (Table 123-4). For improving overall function and well being, most experts agree that nonpharmacologic therapies have greater success and should be considered as essential to any well-formulated treatment plan.

Medications

Antidepressants

Antidepressants are among the most widely studied medications for the treatment of fibromyalgia. The analgesic effect of antidepressants

TABLE 123-2

Differentiation of Osteoarthritis from other Common Rheumatological Disorders: History, Physical Examination, and Other Diagnostic Features

| DISORDER | HISTORY | | PHYSICAL EXAMINATION | | OTHER DIAGNOSTIC FEATURES/COMMENTS |
	AM Stiffness	Location of Pain	Synovitis	Extrasynovial Disease	
Osteoarthritis	Generally short-lived, e.g., < 30 min	Weight-bearing appendicular joints, cervical and lumbar spine, DIPs, PIPs and first CMC. MCP and wrist involvement go against OA	Absent or mild	None related to arthritis itself.	Since OA is ubiquitous in older adults, x-rays should be used to rule out other disorders, not to diagnose OA.
Pseudogout	Pseudorheumatoid pattern may be associated with prolonged AM stiffness	Knee and wrist are most common locations; disease is often symmetrical	Acute flares are intensely inflammatory	Chondrocalcinosis on x-rays; eye deposits, bursitis, tendonitis, carpal and cubital tunnel syndromes may occur. Tophaceous soft tissue deposits uncommon.	Chondrocalcinosis may be asymptomatic. Identification of intracellular CPPD crystals offers a definitive diagnosis in acute flares. Acute and chronic forms occur.
Gout	Pseudo-rheumatoid pattern may be associated with prolonged AM stiffness	Joints of the lower extremities are most often involved, especially first MTP; disease is typically asymmetrical	Acute flares are intensely inflammatory	Tophi may deposit in soft tissues.	Hyperuricemia may be asymptomatic. Serum uric acid cannot diagnose gout. Identification of intracellular monosodium urate monohydrate crystals offers a definitive diagnosis in acute flares.
Rheumatoid arthritis	Prolonged, e.g., > 30 min. Duration of stiffness is used as one parameter of disease activity	Any synovial joint. The lumbar spine is typically spared.	Present	Not uncommon; rheumatoid nodules can develop in soft tissues. Many other possible manifestations including anemia, vasculitis (skin lesions, peripheral neuropathy, pericarditis, visceral arteritis, palpable purpura), pulmonary disease, etc.	Patients may be seronegative. If disease is suspected, patient should promptly be referred to a rheumatologist to retard disease progression.

Condition					
Systemic lupus erythematosus	Not a prominent feature	Depends upon tissues involved—may or may not be limited to joints. Comorbid fibromyalgia is not uncommon.	Generally absent; arthralgias are more common than arthritis	Common—e.g., anemia, skin rash, pleuritis, peritonitis, pericarditis, nephritis, meningitis, etc.	Anyone with suspected SLE should promptly be referred to a rheumatologist.
Fibromyalgia syndrome	Generally short-lived, e.g., < 30 min	Typically diffuse. Worst symptoms often involve the axial skeleton.	Absent. Joints themselves are not involved, although patients experience pain in joints and soft tissues	Many other disorders may coexist (see Table 123-4).	Fibromyalgia syndrome is not a diagnosis of exclusion, but one based upon careful history and physical examination (see text).
Polymyalgia rheumatica	Maybe prolonged, lasting several hours	Typically proximal—e.g., shoulder girdle, hip girdle, neck. If headaches, jaw claudication, and/or prominent systemic symptoms (e.g., fever), consider temporal arteritis.	May occur, especially in small joints of hands	Occurs if comorbid temporal arteritis and relates to involvement of arteries (e.g., Raynaud's phenomenon, bruits, claudication).	Because the erythrocyte sedimentation is very nonspecific, this test should be used to assist with confirmation of a suspected diagnosis. Note that cases of PMR and TA with a normal ESR have been reported.
Vitamin D deficiency	Absent	Typically described as diffuse, deep pain. Bony pain is often present.	Absent	Fatigue is a common feature with proximal muscular weakness (pelvic-girdle myopathy). Tenderness with palpation of bony structures.	Fatigue and difficulty climbing stairs are common complaints. Gait imbalance and falls may be seen. In severe cases, the profound weakness results in need for a wheelchair. Radiologic findings include fractures and Looser-Milkman pseudofractures (osteomalacia giving a striped appearance to bones). Direct measurement of serum 25(OH)D is the best marker for vitamin D deficiency.
Hypothyroidism	Absent	Diffuse myalgias and arthralgias.	Joint swelling may be present with noninflammatory joint effusions. Hand, knee, and wrist involvement. Avascular necrosis, gout and or pseudogout may co-exist	Myalgias, generalized weakness, and carpal tunnel may exist.	Fatigue, mental slowing, and depression often seen. Associated symptoms include hair loss, edema, cold intolerance, dry skin, constipation and weight gain.

CMC, carpometacarpal joint; CPPD, calcium pyrophosphate dehydrate; DIP, distal interphalangeal joint; ESR, erythrocyte sedimentation rate; MCP, metacarpophalangeal joint; MTP, metatarsophalangeal; OA, osteoarthritis; PIP, proximal interphalangeal joint; PMR, polymyalgia rheumatica; SLE, systemic lupus erythematosus; TA, temporal arteritis.

Reprinted from: Weiner DK. Office management of chronic pain in the elderly. American Journal of Medicine. 2007;120:306–315, with permission from Elsevier.

TABLE 123-3

Physical Examination in Older Adults with Low Back and Leg Pain: Detection of Soft Tissue and Biomechanical Abnormalities

FINDING	OPERATIONAL DEFINITION	EXAMINATION TECHNIQUE
Fibromyalgia tender points	Presence of pain when approximately 4 kg of force (i.e., enough force to blanch examiner's thumbnail bed) is applied to defined tender points	Have patient sit comfortably on examination table, arms resting in lap. Tell patient that you are going to apply pressure at several points on the body, and that you want to know if pressure on any point causes pain. Examine the following points bilaterally, using enough pressure to blanch thumb nail: (1) Occiput at suboccipital muscle insertions (2) Low cervical at the anterior aspects of the intertransverse spaces at C5-C7 (3) Trapezius, midpoint of upper border (4) Supraspinatus at origins, above the scapular spine near the medial border (5) 2nd rib at the 2nd costochondral junction, just lateral to the junction on the upper surfaces (6) Lateral epicondyle 2 cm distal to the epicondyle (7) Medial fat pad of the knee, proximal to joint line (8) Greater trochanter, just posterior to the trochanteric prominence (9) Gluteal at upper outer quadrant of buttocks in anterior fold of muscle
Functional leg length discrepancy	Pelvic asymmetry	Have patient stand with both feet on floor, shoes removed. Ask him to stand with feet together, and as erect as possible. Kneel behind patient. With palms parallel to floor, and fingers extended, place lateral surface of index finger of both hands atop pelvic brim bilaterally. Level of eyes doing the examination should be level with hands. Determine if right and left hands are at different heights.
Scoliosis (lateral/ rotational)	Lateral/rotational curvature along thoracolumbar spine	Have patient stand on floor with shoes removed. Stand behind patient. Run index finger along spinous processes (do not lift hand between vertebrae) a series of 3 times. If you do not detect scoliosis, then: Ask patient to bend forward. Determine if there is asymmetry in height of paraspinal musculature.
Sacroiliac joint pain	Pain with direct palpation of sacroiliac joint or with Patrick's test	*Direct palpation:* Have patient stand on floor with shoes removed. Stand behind patient. Exert firm pressure over sacroiliac joint, first on one side, then the other. Palpate right joint with right thumb, standing to left side of patient; palpate left joint with left thumb, standing to right of patient. *Patrick's (Fabere) test*—Have the patient lie supine on the examining table and place the foot of involved side on opposite knee Then slowly lower the test leg in abduction toward the examining table If patient reports pain in back (*not* groin, buttocks or leg), then test is positive
Myofascial pain, piriformis	Presence of pain on deep palpation of piriformis	Have patient lay supine on examination table Have patient flex right hip and knee, keeping sole of foot on table Cross bent leg over opposite leg; again place sole on table and exert mild medially directed pressure on lateral aspect of knee to put piriformis in stretch Exert firm pressure (4 kg) over middle extent of piriformis Repeat examination on opposite side
Myofascial pain, TFL ± iliotibial (IT) band pain	Presence of pain on deep palpation of tensor fascia lata and/or IT band	Have patient lying supine on examination table. Using thumbs of both hands, exert firm pressure (4 kg) over full extent of TFL and IT band. Repeat examination on opposite side.
Kyphosis	Deformity of thoracic spine creating forward flexed posture	Have patient stand on floor with shoes removed. Ask him to stand fully erect. Inspect posture from the side.
Myofascial pain of paralumbar musculature	Presence of pain on deep palpation of paralumbar musculature	Have patient stand on floor with shoes removed. Stand behind and to left of patient and brace him in front with left arm and palpate full extent of right paravertebral musculature with right thumb. Exert approximately 4 kg force. Repeat, palpating the left paravertebral musculature.
Vertebral body pain	Presence of pain on firm palpation of lumbar spinous processes	Position yourself behind patient, as for examination of paravertebral musculature above. Using dominant thumb, firmly palpate spinous processes L1–L5.
Hip disease	Pain and restricted motion of hip	*Hip internal rotation*—have patient lie supine on examining table with hip and knee bent to 90 degrees. Put the hip into maximum internal rotation and ask patient if he experiences pain. *Patrick's test*—As above.

Reprinted from: Weiner DK, Sakamoto S, Perera S, Breuer P. Chronic low back pain in older adults: prevalence, reliability, and validity of physical examination findings. J Am Geriatr Soc. 2006;54:11–20, with permission from Blackwell Publishing.

may result from increased central nervous system serotonin and norepinephrine, which act to block pain signals from the periphery. In addition to reducing pain, antidepressants may improve sleep and emotional well-being. Those used most commonly are the tricyclic antidepressants (TCAs), selective serotonin reuptake inhibitors (SSRIs), and serotonin norepinephrine reuptake inhibitors (SNRIs).

Among these classes of antidepressants, tricyclics are the oldest and have the strongest evidence for efficacy in fibromyalgia. Two

TABLE 123-4

Medications Used in Fibromyalgia Treatment

DRUG	RECOMMENDED DOSE	COMMENTS
Antiepileptic medications		Titrate slowly
Gabapentin	100–600 mg daily	May cause sedation or dizziness
	max dose 1800 mg daily	Dose adjustment for renal failure
Pregabalin	150–300 mg daily	
	max dose of 450 mg	
Tricyclic antidepressants (TCA)		Sedation and confusion
Nortriptyline	10–50 mg nightly	Avoid in narrow angle glaucoma
		Recommend baseline EKG to evaluate Q-T prolongation
		If present, avoid use
Serotonin reuptake inhibitors (SSRI)		SSRIs have superior tolerability compared to TCAs
Fluoxetine	20–80 mg daily	
Citalopram	20–40 mg daily	
Serotonin norepinephrine reuptake inhibitors (SNRI)		Avoid in those with uncontrolled hypertension
Venlafaxine	75–100 mg daily	Avoid in patients with liver disease
Duloxetine	30–60 mg daily	Avoid in those with narrow angle glaucoma
Analgesics		May cause sedation and confusion
Tramadol	50–100 mg every 6 h as needed	Avoid in patients with seizures
		May cause serotonin syndrome in combination with SSRIs or other antidepressants
		Dose adjustment for renal failure
Muscle Relaxants		Likely to cause sedation
Cyclobenzaprine	5–10 mg nightly	Similar side effects to tricyclic antidepressants

of the earliest placebo-controlled clinical trials demonstrated modest effectiveness of amitriptyline at doses of 25 to 50 mg nightly. Cyclobenzaprine, a muscle relaxant with structural similarity to the tricyclics, has shown efficacy in several short-term clinical trials. A recent meta-analysis of the literature on cyclobenzaprine has shown effectiveness in treating some symptoms and providing overall improvement but did not show reduction of fatigue or tender points (see Goldenberg reference).

While tricyclic medications may benefit patients with fibromyalgia, side effects may limit their use, even in low doses. The anticholinergic effects of this class are responsible for most of the adverse effects including sedation, confusion, constipation, and palpitations. As demonstrated by Dr. Weiner and colleagues, impaired mobility and falls have also been described in older adults. TCAs may also prolong the QT interval, which in the worst-case scenario results in torsade de pointes and death. Prior to their initiation, therefore, an EKG should be obtained and if there is evidence of QT prolongation, these medications should be avoided. Secondary tricyclic amines, desipramine, and nortriptyline have fewer side effects but are not as well studied.

The SSRIs and SNRIs may have fewer adverse effects than the TCAs, but there is only modest evidence for their efficacy. The SSRIs increase serotonin levels at lower doses and both serotonin and norepinephrine levels at higher doses. The first double-blind, randomized, placebo-controlled trial of fluoxetine failed to show any benefit compared to placebo. A crossover study found improvement in pain, function, and overall well-being after treatment with fluoxetine 20 mg daily or amitriptyline 25 mg daily compared to placebo, and a combination of both drugs produced a superior result compared to either drug alone. Two studies have evaluated citalopram. While one study failed to shown benefit of citalopram, Anderberg and col-

leagues demonstrated improvement in depression and overall well-being in fibromyalgia patients treated with citalopram (20–40 mg) compared to those in the placebo group.

Studies have also examined the dual serotonin and norephinephrine reuptake inhibitors (SNRIs) for the treatment of fibromyalgia. While benefits of venlafaxine were found in open-labeled studies, a randomized placebo-controlled trial showed no benefits of low-dose venlefaxine (75 mg daily) over placebo. The new SNRI duloxetine has been recently FDA approved for the treatment of FMS at 60 mg daily. Milnacipran, a new SNRI and a mild *N*-methyl-D-aspartate (NMDA) inhibitor, has demonstrated efficacy in the context of a large multicenter trial. It is available in Europe and Asia but not in the United States.

Antiepileptics

Aside from the antidepressants, very few drug classes have evidence for efficacy in the treatment of fibromyalgia. There is some support for the use of antiepileptic drugs. While the mechanisms of action of antiepileptic drugs are largely unknown, especially for the newest agents, it is believed that they reduce neuronal excitability, decrease ectopic neuronal discharge, and modulate the levels of a variety of neurotransmitters. A large study of pregabalin, an antiepileptic drug that binds to the alpha(2)-delta subunit of the voltage-gated calcium channel, found that fibromyalgia patients treated with pregabalin experienced significant improvement in pain, fatigue, social functioning, vitality, and general health perception compared to controls (see Crofford reference). Pregabalin is the first medication approved for fibromyalgia syndrome at a dose range of 300–450 mg daily. While the efficacy of gabapentin to treat fibromyalgia has not been rigorously examined, our clinical experience suggests that low-dose gabapentin (e.g., 100 to 600 mg/day) may be beneficial for reducing pain and improving sleep.

Analgesics

With the exception of tramadol, there are no data that demonstrate efficacy of analgesics for the treatment of fibromyalgia. Tramadol, a weak mu receptor agonist with dual serotonin and norepinephrine reuptake inhibition, is unique in its mechanism and has been shown to be effective in three randomized controlled trials. As with other opioids, prolonged use of tramadol may be linked to abuse and dependence and should be considered judiciously. Because of the sometimes refractory nature of pain in fibromyalgia, these patients not infrequently are treated with more potent opioids, which may result in a number of adverse effects including dysmobility and falls, delirium, increased depression, sedation, nausea, and vomiting. If opioids are being considered, a pain specialist's evaluation is often helpful.

Hormonal Supplements and Other Agents

Studies of hormonal supplements for patients with fibromyalgia have had mixed results. One study of 9 months of subcutaneous growth hormone showed benefit in fibromyalgia patients who had low insulin-like growth factor levels. Because this medication is quite costly ($1500 per month) and because the study results cannot be broadly generalized (i.e., most patients with fibromyalgia do not have low levels of insulin-like growth factor), it cannot be recommended for routine use. A number of other hormonal supplements have been tried anecdotally including thyroid hormone, dehydroepiandrosterone, and calcitonin but the absence of randomized controlled trials precludes recommending these agents for the treatment of fibromyalgia. Similarly, nutritional supplements, herbal medications, and vitamin therapy are not accompanied by rigorous data to support their use. While some studies and anecdotal reports suggest benefit from guafenesin, a 12-month randomized controlled trial of this medication showed no benefit for pain or symptom reduction.

Improving sleep and treating fatigue is often difficult. Sleep hygiene education, which includes keeping regular schedules, elimination of daytime naps, establishment of a restful sleep environment and exclusion of caffeine, is helpful for many patients. Benzodiazepines are typically not recommended for long-term use as they have addictive qualities when used long term and may disrupt the normal sleep cycle. Sedative antidepressants and muscle relaxants including cyclobenzaprine or tizanidine are useful in promoting sleep and well as improving other fibromyalgia symptoms.

Nonpharmacological Therapies

Nonpharmacological therapies for fibromyalgia include cognitive-behavioral techniques, exercise, acupuncture, balneotherapy (i.e., bathing), and massage. Exercise programs, particularly those that include an aerobic component, have been shown to reduce pain and improve function and well-being. Most therapists recommend individualizing programs based on patient abilities and symptoms. During pain flares, which may occur after physical exertion, programs should be modified but not ceased. Water aerobics may also be beneficial. Finally, strength training is beneficial to fibromyalgia patients who are typically deconditioned and may be up to 30% weaker than control subjects.

Data support the benefits of coupling exercise programs with educational sessions and cognitive-behavioral techniques. Cognitive-behavioral therapy (CBT) is useful for fibromyalgia patients who tend to catastrophize their painful symptoms. Patients can alter pain perception and manage pain flares through the use of coping skills and relaxation techniques. CBT is most useful as part of an interdisciplinary program that includes education and exercise. Both inpatient and outpatient interdisciplinary programs have been found beneficial.

The benefits of local therapies and complementary techniques for the treatment of fibromyalgia have also been evaluated. Several randomized controlled trials of acupuncture have shown effectiveness for relieving fibromyalgia symptoms although none have been performed exclusively in older adults. These data are encouraging, however, given the overall safety of this treatment modality. Weak evidence supports chiropractic treatment, massage therapy, interferential current and ultrasound for the treatment of fibromyalgia syndrome. Further studies are needed to determine the potential impact of all these modalities, and to identify potential long-term treatment benefits.

Assessing Response to Treatment

A number of standardized questionnaires are available to assess response to treatment. One of the most efficient and useful is the 20-question Fibromyalgia Impact Questionnaire (FIQ), which takes only a few minutes to complete and quantifies physical function, painful symptoms, and emotional well-being specifically in fibromyalgia patients (Figure 123-1, see Burckhardt reference).

MYOFASCIAL PAIN SYNDROMES

Background and Epidemiology

Myofascial Pain (MP) syndromes, that is, pain originating in physiologically abnormal muscles, affect a majority of older adults with chronic pain and can be the sole cause of pain or one of several contributors. MP may be localized or generalized and is characterized by motor and sensory abnormalities, with the hallmark features being taut bands and trigger points. Since the muscular system is the largest and most extensive organ system in the body, MP can occur in virtually any location. These disorders were originally described by Drs. Janet Travell and David Simons, the authors of the most authoritative text on this subject.

Pathogenesis

MP can be the result of direct or indirect muscular trauma, or aberrant neuronal input. Direct muscle trauma can take multiple forms, including disruption of normal muscular anatomy by surgery, for example, chronic chest wall pain following thoracotomy or chronic abdominal pain following abdominal surgery. Indirect trauma commonly results from abnormal body mechanics that place inordinate stress on certain muscles. Examples include tensor fascia lata (TFL) MP related to quadriceps weakness in patients with knee osteoarthritis. That is, when the quadriceps is weak, the TFL is relied upon more heavily to stabilize the leg when a person stands. Tensor fascia lata MP can also result from scoliosis or leg length discrepancy. This can be seen following total knee or hip replacement. Another

Name: _____   Date: / /

Directions: For questions 1 through 11, please circle the number that best describes how you did overall for the *past week*. If you don't normally do something that is asked, cross the question out.

	Always	Most	Occasionally	Never
Were you able to:				
Do shopping?	0	1	2	3
Do laundry with a washer and dryer?	0	1	2	3
Prepare meals?	0	1	2	3
Wash dishes/cooking utensils by hand?.....	0	1	2	3
Vacuum a rug?......................................	0	1	2	3
Make beds?	0	1	2	3
Walk several blocks?	0	1	2	3
Visit friends or relatives?	0	1	2	3
Do yard work?......................................	0	1	2	3
Drive a car?	0	1	2	3
Climb stairs?	0	1	2	3

12. Of the 7 days in the past week, how many days did you feel good?

     0   1   2   3   4   5   6   7

13. How many days last week did you miss work, including housework, because of fibromyalgia?

     0   1   2   3   4   5   6   7

Directions: For the remaining items, mark the point on the line that best indicates how you felt overall for the past week.

14. When you worked, how much did pain or other symptoms of your fibromyalgia interfere with your ability to do your work, including housework?

No problem with work ——————————————— Great difficulty with work

15. How bad has your pain been?

No pain ——————————————— Very severe pain

16. How tired have you been?

No tiredness ——————————————— Very tired

17. How have you felt when you get up in the morning?

Awoke well rested ——————————————— Awoke very tired

18. How bad has your stiffness been?

No stiffness ——————————————— Very stiff

19. How nervous or anxious have you felt?

Not anxious ——————————————— Very anxious

20. How depressed or blue have you felt?

Not depressed ——————————————— Very depressed

FIGURE 123-1. Fibromyalgia Impact Questionnaire (FIQ).

example of abnormal body mechanics causing MP is trapezius MP related to shoulder dysfunction (e.g., adhesive capsulitis or shoulder arthritis).

A number of explanations have been offered to clarify the pathogenesis of MP. Proposed etiologies for the apparent sustained muscular contraction that occurs with MP include neuronal sensitization in the spinal dorsal horn after tissue injury, primary muscle spindle dysfunction, and inflammatory changes in the muscle following injury. Electromyography has demonstrated "end-plate noise," or spontaneous electrical activity, within the taut bands of trigger points. More recently Gerwin and colleagues have hypothesized that facilitation of acetylcholine (ACh) release, inhibition of ACh breakdown, and removal from ACh receptors combined with upregulation of ACh receptors may underlie the persistent contraction of muscle fibers that plays a central role in myofascial pathology.

Central nervous system mechanisms also play a role in the pathogenesis of MP. These mechanisms are thought to explain the phenomenon of pain radiation in patients with myofascial dysfunction. As summarized in a recent review by Borg-Stein, "it is known from experimental data that under pathologic conditions, convergent connections from deep afferent nociceptors to dorsal horn neurons are facilitated and amplified in the spinal cord. Referral to adjacent myotomes occurs owing to spreading of central sensitization to adjacent spinal segments. This pattern results in referred pain and expansion of the region of pain beyond the initial nociceptive region." The process of central sensitization, as described in the section on fibromyalgia syndrome above, is also thought to play a role in MP syndromes.

Aberrant neuronal input in older adults can also result from axial spondylosis that injures spinal nerves, disrupts generation of neurotrophic factors, and results in muscle shortening and pain. This condition, formally described by Chan Gunn, is referred to as neuropathic MP. Axial spondylosis is ubiquitous in older adults, thus it is not surprising that MP commonly occurs in older adults with axial arthritis, even in the absence of frank radiculopathy (e.g., MP of the sternocleidomastoid and trapezius in patients with cervical spondylosis).

Clinical Presentation and Evaluation

MP may occur in virtually any body location and the pain may be relatively discrete or cover a large area. Patients may describe MP as dull, aching, or burning. Symptoms may mimic radiculopathy and other neuropathic pain syndromes. A number of features of the patient's history may point toward a diagnosis of MP. These include characteristic exacerbating and relieving factors. Patients with MP often report that the following factors exacerbate their pain: (1) excessive physical activity, (2) firm pressure over the painful muscle, (3) cold exposure, (4) psychological stress, (5) acute illness (e.g., viral infection). Patients report that the following factors tend to alleviate their pain: (1) mild activity, (2) gentle stretching, (3) gentle pressure (e.g., massage), (4) moist heat, (5) a brief rest period following activity. In addition to pain, patients with myofascial dysfunction typically experience restricted range of motion in involved areas. Myofascial pathology also may be associated with autonomic phenomena (e.g., piloerection, sweating, temperature changes), weakness, and depression. Myofascial taut bands (see below) also can entrap nerves that cause neuropathic symptoms such as paresthesias and numbness. Appetite and sleep disturbance and decrements in cognitive func-

tion can be part of any chronic pain disorder from which older adults suffer, including MP.

Physical examination is required to elicit the pathognomonic features of MP syndromes, that is, *taut bands* and *trigger points*. A taut band is a group of taut muscle fibers extending from a trigger point to the muscle attachments and a trigger point is defined as a hyperirritable spot in skeletal muscle that is associated with a hypersensitive palpable nodule in a taut band. Triggers points may be latent or active. A *latent trigger point* is one that is painful when compressed, but it is not associated with spontaneous pain (i.e., the patient does not report pain in this region when the practitioner is taking a history). Latent trigger points exist not uncommonly in contralateral muscle groups, perhaps because of compensatory muscle activity (e.g., pain in one leg related to myofascial pathology of the tensor fascia lata may cause a relatively antalgic gait with compensatory overuse of the contralateral tensor fascia lata). *Active myofascial trigger points* are those that are responsible for clinical symptoms. These points are always tender and prevent full muscle lengthening. When these points are compressed, typically a radiating pain pattern is elicited that corresponds to the pain that the patient reports in the context of the history of present illness. Sometimes a "jump sign" is elicited on physical examination, that is, a general pain behavior response demonstrated by the patient that may include verbal as well as nonverbal expression (e.g., crying out, grimacing, withdrawing). The examiner may also appreciate a "local twitch response," that is, a transient contraction of a taut band that traverses a trigger point and that occurs in response to stimulation of the trigger point (e.g., with needling or snapping palpation).

Accurate diagnosis of MP syndromes requires the use of precise physical examination technique, summarized in Table 123-5. Because effective treatment of MP involves recognition and treatment of the underlying cause (e.g., axial and appendicular arthritis, kyphosis, scoliosis, leg length discrepancy, Parkinson's disease) before examining the painful muscles, a general physical examination including comprehensive musculoskeletal, neurological, and mobility examinations must be performed. These examinations must be carried out with an eye toward identifying abnormalities that create muscular dysfunction. Examples in the neurological examination include abnormalities of resting muscle tone such as Parkinson's disease and poststroke changes. Examples in the musculoskeletal examination include decreased range of motion of the hips, knees, cervical spine, and shoulders; scoliosis; kyphosis; and functional leg length discrepancy (i.e., discrepancy in the height of the iliac crests, observed when standing behind the patient with the hands on top of the crests). Techniques used to comprehensively examine the lower back are described in Table 123-3. Examination of the patient's gait, allows an integrated assessment of body mechanics. Examination for underlying visceral pathology should also be performed, particularly in the presence of MP of the pelvic or abdominal musculature.

The most important aspect of preparing for the muscular examination is ensuring that the examiner and the patient are in a comfortable and relaxed position. When palpating the musculature of the upper body (e.g., trapezius, sternocleidomastoid), generally the patient should be sitting, with hands folded in the lap and the examiner should be standing squarely in front of him. When palpating the musculature of the lower back, the patient should be standing and the examiner should be standing to his side, bracing the front of the body with one arm and palpating the muscles with the other

TABLE 123-5

Physical Examination Technique for Examining the Patient with Myofascial Pain

1. Perform a general musculoskeletal examination looking for contributors to myofascial pain (e.g., spinal malalignment, leg length discrepancy, arthritis).
2. Place the patient in a comfortable and relaxed position.
   a. When examining the upper body, the patient should be sitting with forearms resting in lap.
   b. When examining the lower back, the patient may be standing, sitting, or side-lying.
   c. When examining the lower extremities, the patient should be lying in the supine position.
3. Place yourself in a comfortable and relaxed position.
   a. When examining the upper body, the examiner should be standing squarely in front of the patient.
   b. When examining the lower back, the examiner should be standing to the side of the patient, allowing for the use of one arm to brace the patient from the front and the other hand to palpate. If the patient is lying or sitting, stand to the side of the exam table and behind the patient.
   c. When examining the lower extremities, the examiner should be standing at the bedside.
4. When there is unilateral pain, always palpate the nonpainful side first.
5. Assess the movement of the skin over the subcutaneous tissue before palpating the muscles.
6. When palpating taut bands, sweep the examining hand firmly across the involved muscle, in a direction that is perpendicular to the orientation of the muscle fibers and in the same plane as the fibers.
7. When palpating trigger points, palpate firmly over the muscle in a direction that is perpendicular to the orientation of the muscle fibers and in a plane that is perpendicular to the fibers.
8. Physical examination targeting potential visceral pathology of the abdomen and/or pelvis should be performed if myofascial pain of these regions is diagnosed.

hand. If the patient is unable to stand, the paraspinal muscles can be palpated by having the patient in a side-lying position or sitting on the examining table with the examiner standing behind the patient. When palpating the musculature of the lower extremities, the patient should be in the supine position, with the examiner standing to the side of the patient.

Prior to palpating the musculature, the examiner should assess the movement of the skin over the subcutaneous tissues using very light palpation and simply gliding the skin in a direction of movement that is perpendicular to the orientation of the involved muscle fibers. Patients with chronic MP commonly have reduced movement of the skin over the involved region. After palpating the skin, the muscles should be examined. The nonpainful side of the body should be palpated prior to palpating the painful area. This strategy serves two purposes. First, it helps the patient to relax. Second, it allows comparison of normal with abnormal. Palpation of taut bands requires proper orientation of the examiner's hand in relation to the orientation of the muscle fibers. The hand should be placed perpendicular to the orientation of the fibers and the fingers swept firmly across the fibers. This motion allows for the tautness of the fibers to be appreciated. To elicit the radiating pain that is a pathognomonic feature of trigger points, the examiner should palpate the area firmly.

While a sweeping hand motion is needed to appreciate taut bands, this is not required to appreciate trigger points. Often, but not always, trigger points are associated with a "nodule." Depending on the location of the pain, the palpation technique may need to be modified. Travell and Simons offer two other techniques: (1) "pincer palpation," that is, palpation accomplished by grasping and rolling the muscle between the thumb and one or more fingers and (2) "deep palpation," that is, palpation accomplished by deep palpation through intervening tissue and application of pressure primarily in a direction that is perpendicular to the tissue plane. Following successful treatment of trigger points, taut bands and trigger points typically resolve, thus baseline examination is critical not only to arrive at a proper diagnosis, but to assess response to treatment.

Some examples of common MP syndromes include cervicogenic headaches, piriformis syndrome, trapezius MP (sometimes associated with "tension neckache"), pseudotrochanteric bursitis, upper and lower back pain, and postherpetic pain. These syndromes are discussed below.

Cervicogenic Headaches

Cervicogenic headaches are characterized by neck and pericranial pain and are often associated with structural abnormalities of the cervical spine including osteoarthritis and facet arthrosis. Typically, cervicogenic headaches are unilateral in location and range from moderate to severe in intensity. While cervicogenic headaches lack the pulsating quality of migraine headaches, they may have migraine-associated features such as photophobia, phonophobia, nausea, vomiting, and dizziness. Triggers of cervicogenic headache include a variety of neck postures and movements as well as pressure applied to the cervical paraspinal muscles, the suboccipital muscles, and the trapezius. Palpation of these muscles produces pain, which radiates over the head and may extend to the ipsilateral shoulder and arm.

Making the diagnosis of cervicogenic headache may be difficult especially if structural lesions of the cervical spine are not present. A careful history and examination that clearly implicate the cervical spine and its musculature as the source of the pain are essential for diagnosis. Some studies suggest that diagnostic blockade of cervical structures may be useful in patient evaluation; however, this is not typically needed.

Piriformis Syndrome

The piriformis muscle originates from the pelvic surface of the sacrum, passes through the greater sciatic foramen, and inserts into the medial side of the upper end of the greater trochanter. The fibers of the sciatic nerve course through the piriformis. Piriformis syndrome describes the occurrence of sciatica in association with piriformis MP that results from nerve entrapment by the myofascial taut bands in the piriformis. Patients with piriformis MP also may describe intense buttocks discomfort without sciatica. Because the piriformis acts to externally rotate the thigh at the hip joint, patients with piriformis MP sometimes demonstrate external rotation of the leg when standing or lying supine. Palpation of the piriformis can be performed with the patient standing or lying supine. The technique recommended for examining the patient in the supine position is described in Table 123-3. MP of the piriformis may involve the low back, buttock, and posterior thigh. Typically this MP is increased by sitting, standing, and walking.

Trapezius MP

The trapezius is a very large muscle and, therefore, associated MP can have a number of presentations. The fibers originate from the occiput, the ligamentum nuchae, and the vertebral spinous processes of the seventh cervical vertebra and all of the 12 thoracic vertebrae and they insert onto the distal third of the clavicle, the acromion, and the length of the spine of the scapula. The upper fibers elevate the scapula, the middle fibers pull the scapula medially, and the lower fibers pull the medial border of the scapula downward. The upper and lower fibers also assist the serratus anterior muscle in rotating the scapula when the arm is raised above the head.

Patients with MP of the trapezius typically do not complain of limitations in movement, but full rotation of the head and neck to the opposite side is often painful, and opposite side bending may be somewhat restricted. Radiating pain patterns vary according to which of the trapezius fibers contain trigger points (i.e., upper, middle, or lower). Trigger points that occur in the upper trapezius may cause pain that radiates up the posterolateral part of the neck to the mastoid process, causing so-called "tension neckache." Sometimes this pain may radiate to the angle of the jaw and/or the temple and back of the orbit. Dizziness also can occur. Trigger points of the middle fibers of the trapezius may be associated with a superficial burning pain very close to the spinous processes of the seventh cervical and the third thoracic vertebrae or with aching on the top of the shoulder or acromion process. Trigger points of the lower fibers of the trapezius, typically located along the lower border of the muscle, may refer pain to the high paracervical spinal musculature, the mastoid and the acromion, as well as aching and tenderness of the suprascapular region. Perpetuating factors include anything that causes abnormal biomechanics of the upper body such as a whiplash injury or prolonged computer work in an ergonomically unfriendly workspace.

Upper and Lower Back Pain

These syndromes may be caused by MP of the thoracolumbar paraspinal musculature. Numerous muscles constitute the paraspinal group, including both superficial and deep muscles. The superficial group is collectively referred to as the erector spinae and is the largest muscular mass of the back. It originates from the sacrum, the iliac crest, and the spinous processes of most of the lumbar and the last two thoracic vertebrae and insert into the ribs, the transverse processes of the cervical vertebrae, the thoracic vertebrae, and the mastoid process. The deep group comprises the semispinalis, multifidus, and rotatores. The primary function of the paraspinal musculature is spinal extension. Patients with parathoracic MP may experience pain that radiates to the region of the scapula or more medially, and sometimes to the anterior lower chest; patients with paralumbar MP may experience pain that radiates to the buttocks or the lower abdomen. Precipitation of MP may be caused by sudden muscular overload, for example when lifting objects using poor body mechanics, or associated with a vertebral compression fracture. Multiple vertebral compression fractures may also accumulate to cause hyperkyphosis and associated muscular strain. Physical examination typically reveals diminished spinal range of motion. Treatment of postural abnormalities is an important component of treating paraspinal MP. Physical therapy geared toward strengthening of paraspinal muscles is a key component of treatment, not only for the pain itself,

but also for reducing the risk of future vertebral compression fractures.

Pseudotrochanteric Bursitis

This syndrome is caused by MP that involves the tensor fasciae latae (TFL) muscle. The TFL originates from the outer edge of the iliac crest between the anterior superior iliac spine and the iliac tubercle and inserts into the iliotibial tract. It assists the gluteus maximus in maintaining the knee in extension when a person stands. It also flexes the hip. Patients with TFL MP experience pain in the region of the hip and thigh, sometimes extending to the knee. The pattern of pain radiation is not uncommonly confused with trochanteric bursitis and is thus sometimes referred to as pseudotrochanteric bursitis. Patients may also complain of poor sitting tolerance, difficulty walking rapidly, and lying on the involved side. They may also have difficulty lying on the opposite side unless a pillow is placed between the knees because of the tight iliotibial band. Physical examination may reveal restricted hip extension and adduction and TFL trigger points. When standing, patients with TFL MP tend to maintain the hip in slight flexion. Other disorders that should be considered in the differential diagnosis include L4 radiculopathy and meralgia paresthetica.

Postherpetic Pain

While postherpetic neuralgia is commonly thought of as a purely sensory phenomenon, MP has recently been described as a possible component of this disorder. The explanation for this association may be several-fold. The varicella zoster virus (VZV) can directly infect the ventral ventral horn of the spinal cord, but this mechanism is thought to be extremely uncommon. A more likely explanation for MP in the setting of postherpetic neuralgia lies in axial spondylosis (i.e., neuropathic MP, described above) or in guarding behavior.

We hypothesize that a spinal nerve already vulnerable from spondylosis that has caused muscle shortening may be particularly prone to the generation of MP following an acute insult such as VZV. The myofascial pathology that results may then further exacerbate neuropathic pain by entrapping the spinal nerves as they course through the taut bands of the muscles afflicted by myofascial dysfunction. This results in a feedback loop, as shown in Figure 123-2.

Myofascial pathology may also develop in the setting of postherpetic neuralgia as a result of guarding behavior. That is, the pain associated with reactivation of VZV can be excruciating, causing the patient to move their body in ways to protect the painful area. When

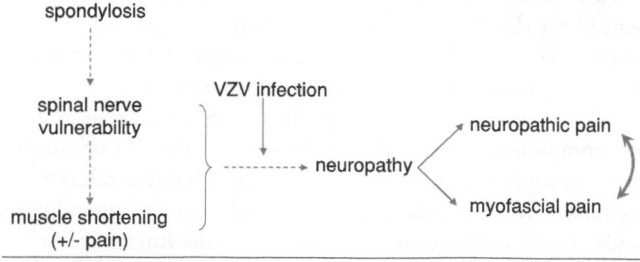

FIGURE 123-2. Theoretical relationship between reactivation of varicella zoster virus (VZV), neuropathic pain, and myofascial pain.

this type of behavior occurs over a prolonged period of time, muscles may develop contractions knots that are characteristic of MP. Whatever the mechanism by which postherpetic neuralgia may be complicated by the development of myofascial pathology, treatment of both the myofascial pathology and the neuropathy may be needed to afford optimal pain relief.

Other MP and Dysfunction Syndromes

Since muscles cover virtually the entire body, any body region may be affected by MP. Thus, MP should always be included in the practitioner's list of differential diagnoses for regional pain syndromes. Just as importantly, the practitioner must be aware that MP syndromes may occur in response to visceral disease; when myofascial dysfunction is identified in the abdomen and pelvis, the possibility of underlying visceral pathology must be kept in mind. Sometimes after the visceral pathology has been eradicated, MP may persist, which further complicates evaluation and treatment.

Some less common causes of MP syndromes include pelvic floor myofascial dysfunction causing chronic pelvic pain in both men and women, pelvic myofascial dysfunction causing urologic pain (e.g., interstitial cystitis and the urgency-frequency syndrome), masticatory myofascial dysfunction causing toothache, abdominal wall myofascial dysfunction causing chronic abdominal pain (e.g., following abdominal surgery or a gastrointestinal illness), and intercostal myofascial dysfunction causing postthoracotomy pain. As noted earlier in this chapter, myofascial dysfunction is not always associated with complaints of pain (i.e., in the case of latent trigger points). For example, masticatory myofascial dysfunction has been associated with tinnitus and myofascial dysfunction of the trapezius with dizziness. Cervical myofascial dysfunction may also be associated with dizziness, a sense of imbalance and tinnitus, and treatment (as outlined below) may alleviate these symptoms. Thus the practitioner must keep MP on his list of key differential diagnoses for the older adult who presents with a chief complaint of dizziness. For a more extensive discussion of these and other MP and dysfunction syndromes, the reader is referred to the authoritative two-volume text by Janet Travell and David Simons, *Myofascial Pain and Dysfunction—The Trigger Point Manual.* Another less detailed but very useful introductory text that practitioners may want to consider is *Trigger Point Therapy for Myofascial Pain—The Practice of Informed Touch,* 2005, edited by Finando and Finando; www.InnerTraditions.com

Management

The most important aspect of treating MP is attending to factors that perpetuate muscle dysfunction. Treatment of these factors and treatment of the trigger points themselves should occur in parallel. Ultimately a strengthening program to enhance muscular resilience should be implemented, and an aerobic program may also be beneficial to prevent recurrence. A summary of the overall approach to treating MP is provided in Table 123-6 and detailed discussion is provided below.

Treatment of Perpetuating Factors

A distinction must be made between *perpetuating factors* and *precipitating factors*. The factors that *perpetuate* MP in older adults typically are multiple and develop over a long period of time, creating an ac-

TABLE 123-6
Approach to Treating Myofascial Pain Syndromes

1. Identify and treat perpetuating factors. e.g., correct leg length discrepancy after total joint replacement, inject rotator cuff and provide physical therapy for rotator cuff tendonitis, treat knee osteoarthritis, begin or optimize medications for Parkinson's disease, prescribe rolling walker for those with kyphosis.
2. Refer to a physical therapist who is experienced in treating patients with chronic pain for *gentle* stretching and strengthening, treatment of perpetuating factors, and for education regarding activity pacing and flare self-management techniques.
3. Perform trigger point injections or dry needling to achieve a local twitch response.
4. If psychological stressors are identified as a perpetuating factor, refer for cognitive-behavioral therapy.
5. Prescribe systemic analgesics only as adjunctive therapy, not as the primary mode of treatment.
6. Refer patients who do not respond to these treatments for interdisciplinary management in a pain clinic.
7. Prescribe aerobic exercise for cardiovascular fitness and prevention of pain flares.

cumulation of factors that must be addressed as comprehensively as possible to afford an optimal therapeutic response. In the older adult with low back pain, for example, a combination of lumbar spondylosis, degenerative scoliosis, and hip arthritis may contribute to the injury pool. The physical factors that *precipitate* MP may be overt such as a fall with direct trauma to the piriformis that causes piriformis syndrome or they may be more subtle such as a flare of knee osteoarthritis that alters gait and precipitates tensor fasciae latae pain. Psychological stressors may also precipitate flares of MP or they may act as perpetuating factors.

As part of the search for perpetuating factors, the practitioner should specifically identify any repetitive movements that contribute to muscular dysfunction such as those that occur in wheelchair users and computer operators. Proper body mechanics during sitting, standing, walking, and sleeping should be taught by an occupational or physical therapist and efforts to modify repetitive movements and/or other mechanical stressors should be instituted. Direct or indirect acute trauma also should be identified. For example, if a patient has a sudden leg length discrepancy, such as that which may occur following total hip or knee replacement, prescription of a shoe lift by a physical therapist may be helpful. For patients with long-standing leg length discrepancy, a shoe lift may disrupt the patient's established compensatory strategies and lead to mobility dysfunction and falls. In these patients, the muscle dysfunction of the pelvis and lower extremities should be first addressed by a physical therapist before considering an orthotic device. Abnormal posture also should be corrected. This can be particularly helpful for the patient with cervicogenic headaches. In the older adult with severe kyphosis related to multiple vertebral compression fractures, restoration of normal posture may not be possible, and prescription of a walker to alleviate strain on the lower back musculature should be considered strongly.

To the extent that psychological stressors are playing a role in perpetuating MP, CBT may be useful. Vitamin D deficiency also should be identified and treated given its association with musculoskeletal pain (see Plotnikoff reference) although randomized controlled clinical trials evaluating its efficacy in patients with MP have not been performed. Patients who do not respond to these approaches in combination with trigger point treatment should be referred to an interdisciplinary pain clinic.

Trigger Point Treatment

Treatment of trigger points utilizes noninvasive and minimally invasive techniques. The goal of both forms of treatment is deactivation or release of the trigger points. Noninvasive treatment typically consists of gentle, sustained stretching of involved muscles perhaps with application of a vapocoolant spray. Stretching and correction of perpetuating factors are the mainstays of therapy. Trigger points also can be deactivated with injection of a local anesthetic (and sometimes a corticosteroid, although rigorous data attesting to the efficacy of this approach are lacking) or "dry needling" using a hypodermic or acupuncture needle. While trigger point injection has never been shown to be more effective than dry needling, injections may be associated with less pain during the procedure and less postneedling soreness. Regardless of which technique is utilized, achieving a local twitch response, as discussed above, is thought to be the essential therapeutic element of the procedure. It should be emphasized that the duration of pain relief following trigger point injection is largely dependent upon patient compliance, that is, the patient's willingness to maintain a stretching program and to eliminate perpetuating factors. An essential element of any physical therapy program for the treatment of MP, therefore, is instruction in a home exercise program that includes a daily stretching routine, identification and elimination of movements that may perpetuate myofascial dysfunction, and techniques to manage pain flares.

For the past decade, trigger point injections with botulinum toxin have been used to treat a variety of myofasical pain disorders. The effectiveness of botulinum toxin is often attributed to its paralytic effects. Antinociceptive effects of botulinum toxin, independent of chemical denervation, also have been suggested. Some studies have shown benefit of botulinum toxin injections in the treatment numerous MP syndromes including temporomandibular joint dysfunction, as well as myofascial neck and low back pain. The doses of botulinum toxin range from 25 to 100 units depending on the size of the muscle. Some research suggests that trigger point injections with botulinum toxin may provide a longer duration of relief than those with lidocaine and methylprednisolone. Use of botulinum is not FDA approved for the treatment of MP syndromes, and this off-label use should be explained to patients as part of obtaining informed consent.

Systemic analgesics should be regarded as adjunctive for the management of MP. Clonazepam is the only medication that has been found to help relieve pain in the context of a randomized controlled trial. Amitriptyline may benefit patients with tension-type headaches associated with MP. Both of these medications, however, are fraught with a number of serious adverse drug events such as delirium and falls. We have had some success with low-dose gabapentin (e.g., 300 mg twice a day) for the treatment of neuropathic MP, for example in patients with cervical spondylosis and MP of the paracervical musculature. Judicious use of cyclobenzaprine (e.g., 5–10 mg at bedtime) may be helpful for the patient with cervicogenic headaches.

A number of other treatments have been tried for MP, including topical medications such as capsaicin, lidocaine, and EMLA cream; repetitive magnetic stimulation; transcutaneous electrical nerve stimulation; biofeedback; massage; ultrasound; laser therapy; traditional Chinese acupuncture and Japanese acupuncture; nerve blocks; and cervical spine dorsal root rhizotomy for the treatment of cervicogenic headaches. The quality of evidence at the present time cannot recommend for or against prescription of any of these treatments.

CONCLUSION

Our understanding of the pathogenesis, diagnosis, and treatment of fibromyalgia and MP syndromes has grown significantly. We now understand fibromyalgia as a central sensitivity syndrome with patients demonstrating increased sensitivity to a variety of stimuli, especially pain. While the pathogenesis of fibromyalgia needs further study, there seems to be a genetic predisposition and a clear familial aggregation. Lower levels of central neurotransmitters and nociceptive chemicals are believed to be involved with fibromyalgia pathogenesis. Keys to the pathogenesis of MP syndromes lie in identifying perpetuating biomechanical factors.

For both fibromyalgia and MP syndromes, individualized approaches to treatment are recommended. Medications alone do not typically improve function, but may improve mood, sleep, and pain. Stretching and local modalities as well as identification and treatment of perpetuating factors should be considered first line for MP and aerobic exercise is a key component of the approach to treating fibromyalgia. While multidisciplinary treatment programs that include education, CBT, and exercise may be very effective for both fibromyalgia and MP syndromes, they are not widely offered and may be costly. Further studies are needed to advance the treatment of patients with these disorders, reduce the associated risk of functional compromise, and improve overall quality of life.

FURTHER READING

Anderberg UM, Marteinsdottir I, von Knorring L. Citalopram in patients with fibromyalgia—a randomized, double-blind, placebo-controlled study. *Eur J Pain.* 2000;4:27–35.

Borg-Stein J. Treatment of fibromyalgia, myofascial pain, and related disorders. *Phys Med Rehabil Clin North Am.* 2006;17:491–510.

Burckhardt CS, Clark SR, Bennett RM. The fibromyalgia impact questionnaire (FIQ): development and validation. *J Rheumatol.* 1991;18:728–733.

Crofford LJ, Rowbotham MC, Mease PJ et al. Pregabalin for the treatment of fibromyalgia syndrome: results of a randomized, double-blind, placebo-controlled trial. *Arthritis Rheumatism.* 2005;52(4):1264–1273.

Crofford, LJ. Neuroendocrine abnormalities in fibromyalgia and related disorders. *Am J Med Sci.* 1998;315(6)359–366.

Cummings TM, White AR. Needling therapies in the management of myofascial trigger point pain: a systematic review. *Arch Phys Med Rehabil.* 2001;82:986–992.

Fishman LM, Dombi G, Michaelsen C, et al. Piriformis syndrome: diagnosis, treatment, and outcome - a 10-year study. *Arch Phys Med Rehabil.* 2002;83:295–301.

Gerwin RD, Dommerholt J, Shah JP. An expansion of Simons' integrated hypothesis of trigger point formation. *Curr Pain Headache Rep.* 2004;8:468–475.

Goldenberg DL, Burckhardt C, Crofford L. Management of fibromyalgia syndrome. *JAMA.* 2004;292:2388–2395.

Gunn CC. Neuropathic myofascial pain syndromes. In: Loeser JD, Butler SH, Chapman CR, Turk DCe, eds. *Bonica's Management of Pain.* Philadelphia: Lippincott Williams & Wilkins; 2001.

Hong CZ. Lidocaine injection versus dry needling to myofascial trigger point: the importance of the local twitch response. *Am J Phys Med Rehabil.* 1994;73:256–263.

Mease P. Fibromyalgia syndrome: review of clinical presentation, pathogenesis, outcome measures, and treatment. *J Rheumatol.* 2005;32(suppl75):6–21.

Plotnikoff GA, Quigley JM. Prevalence of severe hypovitaminosis D in patients with persistent, nonspecific musculoskeletal pain. *Mayo Clinic Proc.* 2003;78:1463–1470.

Porta M. A comparative trial of botulinum toxin type A and methylprednisolone for the treatment of myofascial pain syndrome and pain from chronic muscle spasm. *Pain.* 2000;85:101–105.

Russell IJ, Orr MD, Littman B, et al. Elevated cerebrospinal fluid levels of substance P in patients with the fibromyalgia syndrome. *Arthritis Rheumatism.* 1994;11:1593–1601.

Simons DG, Travell JG, Simons LS. In: Simons DG, Travell JG, Simons LSe, eds. *Travell & Simons' Myofascial Pain and Dysfunction—The Trigger Point Manual, Volume I. Upper Half of Body, Volume II. Lower Half of Body.* Baltimore: Williams & Wilkins; 1999.

Staud, R. Biology and therapy of fibromyalgia: pain in fibromyalgia syndrome. *Arthritis Res Ther.* 2006;8:208.

Weiner DK, Hanlon JT, Studenski SA. Effects of central nervous system polypharmacy on falls liability in community-dwelling elderly. *Gerontology.* 1998;44(4):217–221.

Weiner DK, Schmader KE. Postherpetic pain: more than sensory neuralgia? *Pain Med.* 2006;7:243–249.

Wolfe F, Smythe H, Yunus MB, et al. The American College of Rheumatology 1990 criteria for the classification of fibromyalgia. *Arthritis Rheumatism.* 1990;33(2):160–172.

Infection in the Elderly

Kevin P. High

PREDISPOSITION OF THE ELDERLY TO INFECTION

There are a number of factors that increase the risk of infection in older adults when compared to young adults. The relationships between these risk factors, whether they are comorbidities, waning immunity, or age itself, may be very complex. For example, many older individuals have latent infection with *Mycobacterium tuberculosis* (i.e., asymptomatic infection) and do not manifest clinical illness despite an aging immune system and the presence of various comorbid conditions. However, superimposing malnutrition, perhaps caused by an intervening stress, may be the last insult necessary to tip the scales toward illness, resulting in clinical manifestations. This complex interplay of risk factors makes it difficult to determine the attributable risk of any one characteristic, and any risk factor in isolation cannot be considered "the cause" of infectious risk in the elderly. However, several well-recognized features associated with advanced age clearly do increase risk for clinical infection; these are reviewed in this chapter.

Comorbidities

In the elderly individual, the increased incidence of infection and mortality for many infectious diseases (Figure 124-1) is likely a direct result of the comorbid conditions (e.g., diabetes, renal failure, chronic pulmonary disease, edema, immobility) that accompany advanced age. Comorbidity most often results in reduced innate immunity, defined as those responses that are not specific to a given organism or antigen. These include nonspecific barriers such as skin integrity, cough, and mucociliary clearance, and those immune responses triggered by recognition of patterns of microbial products (e.g., endotoxin, lipoteichoic acid) without the need for prior exposure such as complement, tissue phagocytes, and toll-like receptors (TLRs). Perhaps the best clinical example in which comorbidity contributes heavily to infection risk is chronic obstructive pulmonary disease (COPD). This disease, most often caused by prolonged exposure to tobacco smoke, has a high prevalence in older adults. The impaired mucociliary clearance, alveolar macrophage dysfunction, and suppressed cough mechanism that accompany COPD substantially increase the risk for lower respiratory tract infection in the elderly. Comorbid diseases in elderly individuals with infection can also be more important predictors for worse outcomes. For example, community-acquired pneumonia (CAP) is typically treated on an outpatient basis and rarely causes mortality in patients younger than 50 years of age. However, multiple comorbid conditions and advanced age greatly increase the risk of mortality associated with CAP. In fact, while age itself dominates many CAP prognostic indices, advanced age alone is not a predictor of mortality in those persons older than 75 years of age where comorbidity dominates. Furthermore, cognitive decline and other barriers that reduce adherence to medical regimens often necessitate hospitalization of older adults in circumstances where their younger counterparts are often treated as outpatients, further increasing costs and enhancing the rate of complications.

Waning Immunity

While comorbidities substantially predispose older adults to infection, there are also age-related fundamental changes in the immune response that may predispose the elderly to infection (see Chapter 3), so called immune senescence. Immune senescence is not merely a global state of reduced immunity, but a dysregulation of immune responses at multiple levels. Some aspects of immunity are upregulated, including the inflammatory response, which demonstrates constitutive activation in older adults, as evidenced by elevated C-reactive protein and interleukin (IL)-6 blood levels, and cellular activation of nuclear factor-kappa B (NF-κB). However, other innate immune responses (e.g., natural killer [NK] cell activity) are frequently reduced in older adults, and though originally thought to be normal, more recent data suggest polymorphonuclear neutrophil (PMN) function may also be impaired with reduced microbial phagocytosis and killing.

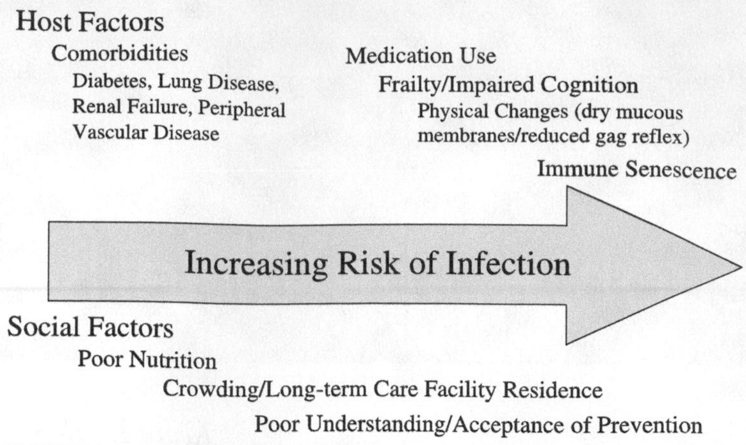

Host Factors
      Comorbidities   Medication Use
           Diabetes, Lung Disease,   Frailty/Impaired Cognition
           Renal Failure, Peripheral   Physical Changes (dry mucous
           Vascular Disease   membranes/reduced gag reflex)
                                       Immune Senescence

Increasing Risk of Infection

Social Factors
      Poor Nutrition
           Crowding/Long-term Care Facility Residence
                 Poor Understanding/Acceptance of Prevention

FIGURE 124-1. Multiple determinants model of infection risk in older adults. The relative contribution of host versus social factors varies by individual and it is the accumulation of multiple risk factors that results in higher infection risk.

The most consistent immune deficit identified in advance age is a reduction in adaptive immune responses. There are decreases in naïve T-cell subsets, marked depression of cytokine production (particularly IL-2) and important cellular surface receptors (IL-2 receptor and CD28), and suppression of T-cell responses by inflammatory cytokines that inhibit T cell immunity such as IL-10 and prostaglandin E_2.

Although there is little doubt that immune senescence exists, the clinical role of this phenomenon in the predisposition of the elderly person to infection remains uncertain. Many flaws plague the published observational studies, despite herculean efforts to minimize confounding using very strict criteria for entry (in most cases via use of the SENIEUR criteria). Ironically, less than 15% of the aged population meets SENIEUR criteria, and the generalizability and clinical relevance of the accumulated data remain in doubt. Is immune senescence irrelevant in patients with overwhelming comorbidity? Or is it the key factor that shifts the balance toward infection when young adults with comorbidity remain relatively well? A recent superb review highlights the confusing and often contrary results of human studies (see Castle, 2000).

Nutrition

Nutritional status is a major confounder in studies of immunity in the elderly population. Protein–energy malnutrition (PEM) is present in 30% to 60% of patients older than 65 years of age who are admitted to the hospital, and is linked to delayed wound healing, pressure ulcer formation, CAP, increased risk of nosocomial infection, extended lengths of stay, and increased mortality. In community-dwelling older adults, PEM frequently goes unrecognized, but even older adults with mild PEM (i.e., those with a serum albumin of 3–3.5 g/dL) demonstrate poor vaccine responses and diminished cytokine responses to immune stimuli. Despite the strong epidemiologic evidence linking PEM to infection in the elderly, the role of nutritional supplements for preventing infection remains controversial. Some studies of residents who live in long-term care facilities suggest use of supplements may increase caloric intake, but other reports indicate meal-time calorie consumption may reciprocally decrease, leading to no net change in protein or calories. Despite this controversy, there is widespread agreement that adequate nutrition should be encouraged and provided to debilitated elderly individuals, and that adequate nutrition is essential for proper wound healing, and may speed functional recovery from serious infectious diseases (i.e., pneumonia).

Specific micronutrient deficiencies are also common in older adults, and several have been linked to poor immune function (e.g., vitamin B-12 deficiency and inadequate pneumococcal vaccine responses). Several micronutrient supplementation trials have been performed that highlight the potential importance of adequate nutrition even in apparently healthy elderly. Vitamin E supplementation ($\geq$200 mg/day) in healthy elderly individuals enhances delayed-type hypersensitivity (DTH) and vaccine responses for a primary T-cell–dependent antigen (hepatitis B), but has no effect on T-cell-independent vaccine responses (pneumococcal vaccine) or the booster response to tetanus. A word of caution, however: a recent meta-analysis of vitamin E supplementation suggested increased mortality in those taking $\geq$400 mg/day, highlighting the dangers of megadose therapy with some vitamins (vitamins A, D, E, K). Multivitamin/mineral supplements have been examined in healthy, free-living elderly persons and consistently demonstrate improved serum vitamin levels, but results are inconsistent with regard to preventing clinical infection or boosting vaccine responses. Other studies in elderly residents of long-term care facilities suggest zinc (20 mg/day) plus selenium (100 μg/d), or specific commercial formulas may reduce the risk of infection, but more work is required to define the role of vitamin or mineral supplementation for augmenting immune response in the elderly population, and to determine whether there are specific subpopulations that could help identify target groups for therapy.

Social and Environmental Factors

There is an increasing recognition that the health of seniors is not only a function of biomedical variables but also socioeconomic status, biophysical environment, and delivery of health care services. This "determinants of health" perspective combines biomedical, behavioral, social, and environmental explanations of illness and health (Figure 124-1). Probably the best example of this with respect to infectious diseases in the elderly individual is that of respiratory tract infections. Population-based studies reveal that lower income is associated with higher rates of CAP and invasive pneumococcal infections among elderly individuals. Lower socioeconomic status may predispose to infection either because of increased exposure to infectious agents (e.g., crowding) or because of increased susceptibility. Although the evidence is limited, this might be a result of worse nutritional status, more frequent exposure to air pollution or tobacco smoke, or inadequate vaccination.

Long-term care residents highlight the concept of "multiple determinants of health," and the physical environment plays a particularly important role in infections in older adults who reside in long-term care facilities. This subset of the aging population has a particularly high incidence of respiratory and other infections (mainly urinary and skin infections). The close contact residents have with other residents plays a key role in the spread of respiratory infections such as influenza or with bacterial infections such as group A streptococcus (i.e., *Streptococcus pyogenes*). This combination of frail older individuals in a confined setting can lead to severe outbreaks with high mortality rates. The close proximity of residents, poor adherence to basic infection control measures, and the intense use of antibiotics are factors that lead to the spread of antibiotic-resistant bacteria such as methicillin-resistant *Staphylococcus aureus* (MRSA), vancomycin-resistant enterococci (VRE), and multiresistant gram-negative rods. Although the actual infectious threat many of these organisms pose to individual residents is uncertain, the potential reservoir creates a problem when such residents are transferred to acute care hospitals where these organisms can spread to other susceptible hosts.

DIAGNOSIS AND MANAGEMENT OF INFECTIONS IN THE ELDERLY PATIENT

Presentation of Illness

Infectious diseases frequently present with atypical features in older adults. Serious infections may be heralded by nonspecific declines in functional or mental status, or anorexia with decreased oral intake. Underlying illness (e.g., congestive heart failure [CHF] or diabetes) may be exacerbated, leading the elderly patient to seek medical attention. The most common sign that triggers the clinician to look for infection, fever, is often absent in the elderly patient. Several studies show that frail elderly individuals have lower mean baseline body temperatures than the currently accepted normal of 98.6°F (37°C). Animal models of aging demonstrate that temperature elevations in response to endogenous pyrogens (IL-1, IL-6, tumor necrosis factor [TNF]-α) are diminished with advanced age. The decline in basal temperature and blunted response to inflammatory stimuli make it less likely that a frail, older adult will achieve a body temperature commonly recognized as fever. It has been suggested that fever in frail older adults should be defined as (1) persistent elevation of body temperature of at least 2°F (1.1°C) over baseline values, or (2) oral temperatures of 99°F (37.2°C) or greater on repeated measures, or (3) rectal temperatures of 99.5°F (37.5°C) or greater on repeated measures. The sensitivity of detecting fever and infection in the nursing home setting has been improved using this definition, and reasonable specificity maintained. The importance of a "normal" or reduced temperature in the face of significant infection cannot be overemphasized. A blunted febrile response often leads to delayed diagnosis, and is an indicator of a poor prognosis.

Cognitive impairment also heavily contributes to the difficulty in diagnosing infection in the elderly. Subjects are often unable to communicate symptoms and clinicians should have a lower threshold to pursue objective assessments (e.g., laboratory and radiologic evaluations) in cognitively impaired elderly with changes in functional status.

Finally, age- and comorbidity-related changes in anatomy and physiology may confound interpretation of diagnostic evaluations.

Perhaps the best example of this is the diminished sensitivity for trans-thoracic echocardiography (TTE) for detecting vegetations on the heart valve in endocarditis. Studies suggest the additional echoes present as a result of age-related calcium deposition reduces sensitivity of TTE from 85% to 90% in adults aged 55 years and younger, to <50% for those older than 70 years of age.

Antibiotic Management

The profound physiologic changes associated with aging and comorbidities alter drug distribution, metabolism, excretion, and interactions (see Chapter 8) Antibiotic dose reductions are occasionally required in the elderly adult because of changes in renal function or predisposition of the elderly adult to important side effects such as changes in mental status (e.g., flouroquinolones). In addition, antibiotic interactions are more frequent because most elderly persons are taking multiple medications. Digoxin, warfarin, oral hypoglycemic agents, theophylline, antacids, and proton pump inhibitors all have significant interactions with commonly prescribed antibiotics. Drug concentrations can increase (e.g., enhanced digoxin toxicity associated with macrolides, tetracyclines, and trimethoprim) or decrease (e.g., reduced quinolone absorption with concomitant administration of antacids) with concomitant drug administration. These changes and the increased incidence of side effects in the elderly often lead clinicians to the dictum of "start low, go slow" when administering new medications in older adults. However, for antibiotics, this is not an appropriate strategy. Altered gastric motility, decreased absorption, increased adipose tissue, and coadministration of other drugs can decrease blood levels of antimicrobials in the elderly patient, and since systemic antibiotics reach tissues via blood flow, poor vascular perfusion to the site of infection, particularly in skin and soft-tissue infections of the lower extremities, may reduce efficacy. Adherence may be limited by poor cognitive function, inadequate understanding of the drug regimen, impaired hearing or vision, and polypharmacy, and studies suggest that any regimen requiring greater than twice daily dosing is associated with very poor adherence rates. Finally, there are data that suggest higher antibiotic levels are particularly important for efficacy in older adults. This is true for antibiotics that are "concentration-dependent" (i.e., the higher the concentration in relation to the minimal inhibitory concentration (MIC), the better the antibiotic kills). The activity of fluoroquinolones is concentration-dependent and the relationship between bacterial clearance and the serum/MIC ratio for levofloxacin suggests drug concentrations must be nearly twice as high in older adults than in young adults to clear infection. The reason for this is unclear, but may be caused by impaired defense mechanisms described above that aid clearance of bacteria.

Many ethical dilemmas surround antibiotic use in frail elderly persons and terminally ill patients. The 1998 American Medical Association (AMA) Council of Ethical and Judicial Affairs included antibiotics, along with mechanical ventilation, as "life-sustaining" treatment. Others argue that antibiotics are part of ordinary care, even those who are designated to be receiving "comfort measures only." While every clinical situation is unique, and no blanket recommendation can be made for the use or nonuse of antibiotics in the terminally ill, it seems prudent to include antibiotic administration in the discussion of advanced directives as a potentially life-sustaining maneuver and to treat it no differently than any other medical intervention such as surgery or mechanical ventilation.

Finally, although older adults are at the greatest risk for illnesses that are indications for outpatient parenteral antibiotic therapy (OPAT) (e.g., for treatment of endocarditis or osteomyelitis), OPAT was infrequently used in older adults primarily because of the fact that Medicare did not cover the cost of OPAT and older adults frequently had to be admitted to nursing homes or stay in acute care hospitals to obtain appropriate therapy. With the institution of Medicare Part D in 2006, OPAT is now covered, although navigating the system to obtain reimbursement for both the antibiotic and the necessary supplies for administration takes considerable skill. A recent study and accompanying editorial outline the safety, efficacy, and patient selection criteria for OPAT in older adults, and provides Web links to sites that assist with reimbursement issues (see Malani, 2008).

CLINICAL SYNDROMES IN THE ELDERLY

Infective Endocarditis

Although infective endocarditis (IE) was primarily a disease of young and middle-aged adults and associated with postrheumatic fever and congenital valvular lesions, it has become a disease of the elderly population, associated with degenerative valvular disorders and prosthetic valves (prosthetic valve endocarditis [PVE]). Furthermore, temporary and permanent pacemakers, pulmonary artery catheters, and other invasive devices are more frequently used in older adults and predispose subjects to IE.

Native valve IE in young adults is typically caused by viridans streptococci, *S. aureus,* and occasionally by HACEK organisms (*Haemophilus, Actinobacillus, Cardiobacterium, Eikenella, Kingella*). These same organisms predominate in the elderly patient, but comorbidities and prosthetic devices change the profile of causative agents; gastrointestinal (GI) and genitourinary (GU) organisms such as enterococci and gram-negative rods become more common in native valve IE. Coagulase negative staphylococci are a frequent cause of PVE, both from contamination at the time of surgery and from occult or documented bacteremia during the hospital stay. Other nosocomial bacteremias, often with more resistant organisms (e.g., *Enterobacter* spp.), can also result in PVE.

Endocarditis is difficult to diagnose in the elderly patient. Fever and leukocytosis are less common (55% and 25%, respectively, for elderly patients vs. 80% and 60%, respectively, for younger patients). As stated above, the prominence of degenerative, calcific valvular lesions and prosthetic valves lowers the sensitivity of TTE. Transesophageal echocardiography (TEE) may be more sensitive, and in at least one study, TEE improved the diagnostic yield by 45% over that of TTE. Age alone is not a major risk for mortality, with a 2-year survival of 75% for IE in all age groups unless major comorbidities exist.

Antibiotic treatment of IE is directed at identified pathogens or the most likely causes if blood cultures are negative (Table 124-1). Therapy is administered intravenously for 2 to 6 weeks. Combination regimens with aminoglycosides are particularly problematic in the elderly patient because of toxicity (both renal and ototoxicity), but is occasionally unavoidable in certain circumstances (e.g., enterococcal IE). Surgical therapy is required only when specific criteria are met, primarily recurrent embolic events or worsening heart failure.

Antibiotic prophylaxis is available for bacterial endocarditis for all "at-risk" patients and should be provided for dental, upper respiratory tract, GI, or GU procedures. Although the evidence supporting this practice is relatively weak, it has become the standard of care. Current recommendations for IE prophylaxis are available in sources listed in the references.

Bacteremia and Sepsis

Bacteremia rates are much higher in elderly patients than in younger patients, comprising up to 14% of all admissions in some geriatric units. Older patients with bacteremia are less likely than younger patients to have systemic signs such as fever, chills, or diaphoresis. Bacteremia in the elderly patient is more likely to arise from a GI or GU source than in young adults. Thus, the causative agent is more likely to be a gram-negative rod.

Despite a similar initial cytokine response to that of young adults with sepsis, the prognosis of sepsis in the elderly is worse. The 28-day mortality for sepsis in young adults is 26% to 33% versus 35% to 42% in adults older than age 65 years. Nosocomial gram-negative bacteremia carries a mortality rate of 5% to 35% in young adults, but 37% to 50% in older adults. A major contributing factor is reduced physiologic reserve because of age and comorbidities that reduce the ability of older adults to recover from a septic episode.

Antibiotic management of bacteremia and sepsis in the elderly patient is similar to that of younger adults, and the importance of initially broad coverage must be emphasized. Mortality is greatly reduced if an antibiotic that covers the eventually isolated organism is included in the initial regimen, whereas waiting to identify the organism and switching the antibiotic at that time has little to no effect on overall survival. Thus, it is imperative to include coverage for MRSA, resistant gram-negative rods, enterococci, and other resistant organisms when there is a high clinical suspicion for resistant organisms and the elderly, particularly nursing home residents, represent a high risk population. Immunomodulatory/adjunctive therapy for sepsis, activated protein C, has been approved and should be considered for those patients with sepsis and evidence of dysfunction in at least two organ systems. A subset analysis of the trial that led to FDA approval for activated protein C, demonstrated that elderly persons have a statistically greater chance of clinically important bleeding as an adverse event yet the benefit for in-hospital and long-term survival was even greater in older adults than in young persons.

Prosthetic Device Infections

As the prevalence of the U.S. population older than age 65 years has increased, permanent implantable prosthetic devices have become common. Prosthetic joints, cardiac pacemakers, artificial heart valves, intraocular lens implants, vascular grafts, penile prostheses, and a variety of other devices are primarily placed in the elderly. Foreign bodies interact with bacterial and host immune factors, often leading to infection. While it is impossible to review all prosthetic device infections in this chapter, several general concepts are presented. Prosthetic device infections are usually categorized by causative agents that typically present early (<60 days from implantation) or late (>60 days). Early infections are primarily caused by contamination at the time of surgery or events associated with the implantation hospitalization (e.g., bacteremia caused by IV or urinary catheters). Thus, the causative organisms for early prosthetic device infections are primarily skin and nosocomial flora. Coagulase-negative

TABLE 124-1

Suggested Empiric Antimicrobial Therapy for Common Infections in Older Adults

INFECTION	THERAPY	COMMENTS
Community-acquired		
Outpatient Therapy		
Acute sinusitis	Amoxicillin	Amox/clav or new macrolide (clarithromycin or azithromycin) if refractory; new macrolide if penicillin allergic
Chronic bronchitis	Amoxicillin-clavulanate	Infectious exacerbations only; new macrolide if penicillin allergic
Pneumonia	[Azithromycin or Clarithromycin + 2nd gen Ceph or Amox/clav] or Resp-FQ	Smoker/COPD most common
Cellulitis	Amox/clav or Cephalexin	Community-acquired MRSA much more common since 2005; include TMP-SMX or Minocycline if suspected (e.g., recurrent boils, very aggressive or abscess-forming skin/soft-tissue infection)
Infected neuropathic ulcer	Amox/clav	Initial outpatient treatment of diabetic foot infection
Symptomatic UTI	FQ, TMP-SMX	Uncomplicated cystitis or pyelonephritis
Infectious diarrhea	FQ	Oral rehydration is key
C. difficile diarrhea	Metronidazole (Vancomycin for serious disease)	Elevated white blood cell count common
Inpatient Therapy		
Pneumonia	[Ceftriaxone + Azithromycin or Clarithromycin] or Resp-FQ alone	Seriously ill (intensive care unit) combination therapy 3rd gen ceph + Resp-FQ consider Pseudomonas if severe COPD or structural lung disease
Pyelonephritis (no catheter)	3rd gen Cephalosporin or FQ	
Urosepsis (with catheter)	3rd gen Cephalosporin + ampicillin or vancomycin	Catheter-related urosepsis often polymicrobic; have to consider enterococcal species, in addition to gram-negative bacilli
Acute bacterial meningitis	Ceftriaxone + Vancomycin + ampicillin	Vancomycin needed because of small % of ceftriaxone-resistant S. pneumoniae; give dexamethasone with or prior to antibiotics if gram stain of CSF reveals bacteria
Intra-abdominal infection	[Ampicillin/sulbactam + Gentamicin] or Ampicillin + Gentamicin + Metronidazole] or Pip/tazo or carbepenem	Surgery often indicated for appendicitis, cholecystitis, ischemic colitis, abscess drainage, but rarely required for diverticulitis; tigecycline for patients with significant beta-lacatam allergy
Native valve endocarditis	Penicillin + Nafcillin	Vancomycin for penicillin-allergic patient
Infected diabetic foot ulcer	Ticar/clav or Pip/tazo	3rd gen Ceph and clinda for penicillin allergy; tigecycline for significant beta-lactam allergy
Cellulitis	Ampicillin/sulbactam	Add clinda if high suspicion for GAS; vancomycin if MRSA suspected; vancomycin + FQ for β-lactam allergy
Septic shock syndrome; with no obvious focus	Carbepenem; add clindamycin if GAS suspected	Aggressive supportive care; consider activated protein C if two or more end-organs with dysfunction; consider intravenous immunoglobulin if streptococcal toxic shock syndrome
Nursing home-acquired		
Infected pressure ulcer	FQ + clindamycin (po); ticar/clav or Pip/tazo (IV)	Pressure-relieving devices, nutrition, débridement essential; culture/x-ray to identify osteomyelitis or MRSA; NEVER do swab culture of surface to identify organism(s) – only surgical cultures of value
Pneumonia	Resp-FQ or (Ceftriaxone + Azithromycin)	Consider tuberculosis (primary or re-activation)
Urosepsis	Ciprofloxcin (po) Ceftriaxone (IM/IV)	Add enterococcal coverage if catheter
C. difficile colitis	Metronidazole (Vancomycin for serious disease)	Close attention to infection control as nosocomial spread documented; spores not killed by alcohol-based antiseptics, must wash hands with soap/water
Nosocomial/hospital		
Pneumonia	Cefepime or carbepenem or pip/tazo	Decision influenced by numerous factors: underlying medical conditions, mental status, respiratory support, prior antibiotic exposure, aspiration, risk of MRSA (add vancomycin)
Catheter-associated urosepsis	Vancomycin plus 3rd gen ceph or FQ	Culture to guide subsequent therapy
Intravenous catheter-associated infection (cellulitis, phlebitis, abscess, bacteremia)	Vancomycin	If immunocompromised, add cefepime or ceftazidime; surgery required for septic thrombophlebitis
C. difficile-related diarrhea	Metronidazole (Vancomycin for serious disease)	Discontinue the implicated antimicrobials if possible; attention to infection control and hand washing as noted above
Postoperative wound infection; incision/deep with cellulitis, abscess, or bacteremia	Cefazolin (mild infection) Vancomycin + 3rd gen ceph (severe infection)	Reopen and explore wound; definitive therapy guided by smears/cultures

2nd gen, second generation; 3rd gen, third generation; Amox/clav, amoxicillin-clavulanate; Carbepenem, imipenem-cilastatin or meropenem; ceph, cephalosporin; clinda, clindamycin; COPD, chronic obstructive pulmonary disease; FQ, Fluoroquinolone; GAS, group A streptococci (S. pyogenes); MRSA, methicillin-resistant S. aureus; Pip/tazo, Piperacillin-tazobactam; Resp-FQ, respiratory fluoroquinolone (gatifloxacin, levofloxacin, moxifloxacin); Ticar/clav, ticarcillin-clauvulanate; TMP-SMX, trimethoprim-sulfamethoxazole; vanco, vancomycin.

staphylococci predominate; *S. aureus* and diphtheroids are common as well. Gram-negative bacilli, fungi, or polymicrobial infection are rare causes of early infection except when the material itself or associated products such as dressing material are contaminated. Late infections tend to be caused by the same organisms that cause community-acquired bacteremia in the elderly population, and bacteremic seeding of the device is likely the mode of infection in these cases. Staphylococci, including coagulase-negative staphylococci, are the exception to this rule, playing a major role in prosthetic device infections in both the early and late periods. Thus, empiric anti-staphylococcal therapy is imperative in either early or late prosthetic device infection.

It is difficult to cure prosthetic device infections (i.e., eradicate the organism) with the device in place. However, in some instances, early antibiotic intervention combined with aggressive surgical débridement may result in cure without removing the device. Because prosthetic device infections often include biofilms and occur in the setting of other factors that limit antibiotic efficacy (e.g., poor circulation), it is preferable to use bactericidal antibiotics, and combinations with a second agent that penetrate these areas well (e.g., rifampin) may be most effective. If early, aggressive therapy is ineffective in controlling the infection, it is imperative that the device be removed. In prosthetic joint infection (the clinical entity of device-related infection most well-studied) two-stage procedures, where the device is removed and antibiotics given for an extended period (usually ≥6 weeks) with delayed reimplantation have the highest success rate. However, for life-saving devices, such as mechanical valves or implantable defibrillators, this is not an option.

A recent analysis of surgical débridement and long-term suppressive antibiotics versus two-stage removal/reimplantation for prosthetic hip infection used functional assessment, not just cure rate, as an important indicator outcome. Using Markov modeling, the two-stage procedure was preferred if the relapse rate in the débridement strategy was assumed to be >60% or the age of the patient with the infected arthroplasty was <79 years. However, débridement and suppressive antibiotics strategy were favored when these conditions were not met. Relapse rates of the débridement/retention with long-term antibiotic strategy are approximately 30% overall, but depend on the organism, duration of symptoms, which joint is infected, the susceptibility of the organism, and many other factors known and unknown. This model gives some guidance, but allows clinicians freedom to adjust strategy based on baseline functional status and infecting agent.

Prevention of prosthetic device infection is facilitated by the use of clean air systems and/or personal isolator systems in the operating room. Although there are limited data for efficacy, typical antimicrobial prophylaxis for clean surgery seems appropriate; prophylaxis other than at the time of surgery remain contentious. Perioperative antimicrobial prophylaxis for dental procedures is clearly indicated for prosthetic valves and is frequently employed for vascular grafts, particularly within the first few months after placement. There is no evidence to demonstrate benefit for prophylaxis in patients with prosthetic joints, intraocular lens implants, intracoronary artery stents, cerebrospinal fluid shunts, breast implants, or other less-commonly used prostheses. The American Dental Association (ADA) recommends "considering" antibiotic prophylaxis for patients with prosthetic joint at "high risk," which the ADA defines as joints within 2 years of placement, immunosuppressed patients (including immune compromise as a result of diabetes mel-

litus, rheumatoid arthritis, and malnourishment), or those with a previous joint infection.

Tuberculosis

Tuberculosis rates are again increasing in the United States after several years of decline, in large measure, caused by disease present in immigrants and the aging population. It has long been established that advanced age is a major risk factor for developing tuberculosis, and even with the increasing populations of young adults at risk as a result of the HIV epidemic and increasing immigrant populations, older adults still comprise approximately one quarter of all tuberculosis cases reported in the United States. Tuberculosis often presents differently in older adults than in young adults. Several studies have demonstrated that, when compared to young adults, older adults are less likely to present with fever, night sweats, cough, or hemoptysis, and more likely to present with nonspecific symptoms of dizziness, nonspecific pain or mental "dullness," a prior history of tuberculosis, and a concomitant diagnosis of underlying cancer. Radiographic and laboratory differences also occur with older adults being more likely to have widespread pulmonary parenchymal infiltrates whereas young adults are more likely to have isolated upper lobe infiltrates, and older adults are more likely to have evidence of malnutrition (i.e., reduced serum albumin).

Probably the most important issue in older adults remains the imperfections of diagnostic testing for tuberculosis. Using the tuberculin skin test (TST) in classic studies, William Stead and colleagues at the University of Arkansas defined the prevalence of TST positivity in older adult residents of long-term care facilities, the risk for reactivation of *M. tuberculosis* with and without prophylactic therapy, and the survival of older adults in each of these situations. Overall conclusions from these studies suggest that the sensitivity of the TST to detect latent infection declines with age, that tuberculosis is rare (<0.2%) in older residents in whom the TST is never positive, that TST-positive individuals develop clinical disease 2% to 5% of the time (much higher if the TST represents a recent conversion—7% to 12% incidence of clinical disease), and that isoniazid (INH) prophylaxis (usually provided as 300 mg daily for 12 months in the studies by Stead and colleagues) in TST-positive subjects reduces the risk of clinical disease to ≤0.3% for most subjects (the exception being those who are TST-positive and previously had active tuberculosis—in those cases, isonaizid therapy reduced the risk from 2–5% to 1.5–2%). The benefits of isoniazid prophylaxis are long-lasting with improved survival in TST-positive treated subjects (vs. untreated TST-positive subjects) apparent at 1.5 years and persisting up to at least 8 years.

From these data, it is clear that identifying TST-positive older adults is important for preventing active tuberculosis through INH prophylactic treatment. The confounding issues, however, surround interpretation of the TST. In the most recent guidelines from the American Lung Association, a TST is considered positive if >5 mm induration in HIV-positive persons, recent TB contacts, those with fibrotic changes on chest radiograph consistent with prior TB, and immunosuppressed patients (including those on ≥15 mg/day of prednisone for at least one month); >10 mm is considered positive for recent immigrants, injection drug users, residents and employees of healthcare facilities (including nursing homes), and persons with high-risk conditions (silicosis, diabetes mellitus, chronic renal failure, leukemia/lymphoma, head and neck or lung cancer, weight loss

≥10% of ideal body weight, s/p gastrectomy); for all other persons a TST >15 mm is considered positive.

New diagnostic tests for tuberculosis have been developed and include quantitation of interferon-γ release from whole blood or Elispot assays both measured after ex-vivo *M. tuberuculosis* antigen stimulation. Unfortunately, these newer assays have only demonstrated modestly improved sensitivity or specificity. The pooled sensitivity from multiple studies appears to be 71% for TST, 76% for interferon-γ release assays, and 88% for the Elispot assays. The specificity for the three tests is 66%, 97%, and 92%, respectively. None of the tests appears to be useful for following response to therapy.

The treatment of tuberculosis in older adults does not differ from that of young adults, but older adults are more susceptible to adverse effects and drug–drug interactions. Latent disease (TST-positive only without clinical signs and symptoms), if not previously treated, should be treated with 9 to 12 months of INH, whereas patients with clinical illness should initially receive four drugs (usually INH, rifampin, pyrizinamide, and ethambutol) pending culture and susceptibility testing. The duration of therapy is dependent on many factors including the site of infection, susceptibility test results, and clinical response.

Fever of Unknown Origin

Fever of unknown origin (FUO), classically defined as temperature >101°F (38.3°C) for at least 3 weeks and undiagnosed after 1 week of medical evaluation, has different causes in elderly adults and in young adults (Table 124-2) that should influence the diagnostic workup. The cause of FUO can be determined in virtually all cases and approximately one third of cases will have treatable infections (e.g., intraabdominal abscess, bacterial endocarditis, tuberculosis, or occult osteomyelitis). In contrast to young adults, connective-tissue disease (CTD) is a more frequent cause of FUO in adults older than age 60 years. A compilation of several recently published series suggests that 25% of all FUOs in the elderly patient are caused by CTDs. However, the CTD most likely to cause FUO in young adults is systemic lupus erythematosus (SLE), whereas SLE was absent in series of elderly patients and replaced by temporal arteritis

(TA) and polyarteritis nodosa (PAN). Neoplastic disease accounts for another 20%, most often a result of hematopoietic malignancies (e.g., lymphoma and leukemia). Importantly, however, multiple myeloma, a disease much more likely in older adults than in young adults, is almost never a cause of FUO. Drug fever is a common cause of FUO in the elderly, and Wegener's granulomatosis, deep venous thrombosis with or without recurrent pulmonary emboli, and hyperthyroidism occasionally cause FUO in older adults.

A reasonable approach to FUO in the elderly can be inferred from the most likely causative entities. A thorough history and physical examination; basic laboratory evaluations of complete blood counts with differential, serum chemistries and hepatic enzymes, thyroid function studies, erythrocyte sedimentation rate (ESR), placement of a purified protein derivative (PPD) skin test, a chest x-ray, and initial blood and urine cultures should begin the search. If the diagnosis continues to be elusive and the ESR is elevated, temporal artery biopsy even in the absence of typical history or objective physical findings should be strongly considered. If the source remains obscure, or if there is a low suspicion for TA, abdominal imaging with computed tomography (CT) or magnetic resonance imaging (MRI) should be performed. Further invasive diagnostic procedures, such as bone marrow and liver biopsy, or laparoscopy, should be considered in specific cases, but are low yield unless there are significant clues for involvement (e.g., cytopenias or hepatomegaly).

IMMUNIZATION OF THE ELDERLY

Immunization recommendations for older adults are constantly being updated. The latest consensus recommendations can be found online at the Centers for Disease Control (CDC) Web site at: http://www.cdc.gov/vaccines/recs/schedules/adult-schedule.htm

Pneumococcal Vaccine

Many reviews and meta-analyses have been performed to help assess the benefit of pneumococcal immunization in older adults. Although many have failed to reach statistical significance indicating benefit, the confidence intervals of negative studies have not ruled out benefit, particularly when only invasive disease end points (i.e., bacteremia and meningitis) were the outcomes selected. Some of the lack of clear benefit may be a result of waning of efficacy at the extremes of old age (>85 years), unrecognized immune compromise in many older adults, and the fact that the pneumococcal vaccine is really 23 different vaccines (i.e., 23 serotypes) and failure of any one serotype is considered a failure of the vaccine. Despite these ongoing scientific discourses, pneumococcal immunization for persons age 65 years and older has become standard practice, as well as for many patients younger than age 65 years with comorbid conditions. If more than 5 years has elapsed since the first dose and the patient was vaccinated prior to the age of 65 years, repeat vaccination is recommended and safe (Figure 124-2). The 23-valent polysaccharide vaccine, when given to adults older than age 65 years, is similar in cost-effectiveness to many procedures commonly employed in older adults (e.g., multiple screening procedures, angioplasty and coronary artery bypass grafting), even when one limits consideration of efficacy to only invasive disease (i.e., blood-borne infection), making no assumption for any benefit with regard to pneumonia. Pneumococcal

TABLE 124-2

Fever of Unknown Origin (FUO) in the Elderly Patient	
MAJOR CAUSES	**% OF CASES***
Infections	35
Intra-abdominal abscess	12
Tuberculosis	6
Infective endocarditis	10
Other	7
Collagen vascular disorders	28
Temporal arteritis/polymyalgia rheumatica	19
Polyarteritis nodosa	6
Other	3
Malignancy	19
Lymphoma/other hematological	10
Solid tumors	9
Other (pulmonary emboli, drug fever)	10
No diagnosis	8

*Percentages represent pooled data from three studies of FUO in the elderly patient.

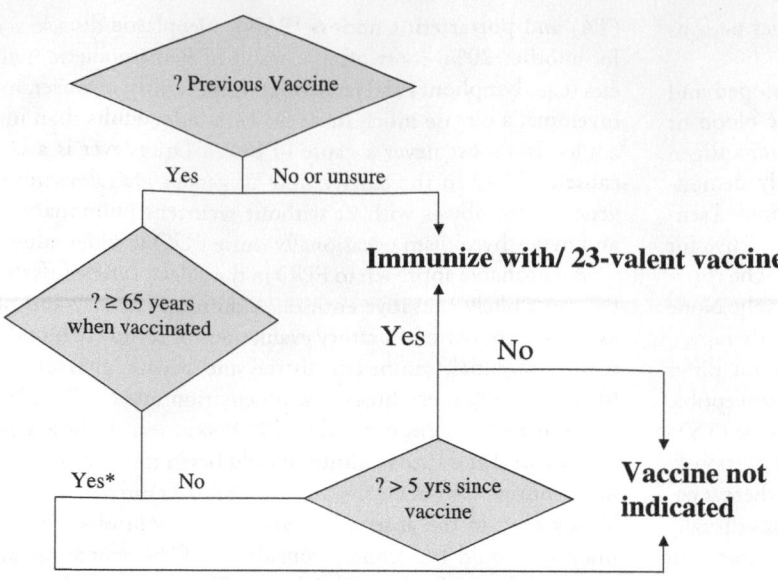

*re-vaccination not indicated for persons vaccinated at age ≥ 65 yrs.

FIGURE 124-2. Decision analysis for pneumococcal vaccine per current Advisory Committee on Immunization Practices recommendations.

vaccine can be given concurrently with other vaccines at a different anatomic site.

Implementing current pneumococcal vaccine recommendations remains the greatest obstacle to prevention of fatal *S. pneumoniae* disease in the elderly. According to CDC estimates, only 40% to 50% of eligible elderly persons receive pneumococcal vaccine. Many unvaccinated elderly patients diagnosed with invasive pneumococcal disease saw a medical practitioner within the prior 6 to 12 months. The CDC and its Advisory Committee on Immunization Practices (ACIP) have outlined several strategies for improving vaccine administration including (1) age-based: review immunizations in all persons at age 50 years, vaccinating those with qualifying comorbid conditions; (2) organizational (e.g., standing orders): routine administration in elderly and at-risk patients in office, nursing home, and hospital settings by a blanket order for all patients (this is the single-most effective strategy); (3) community-based: public health promotions focusing on underserved, often inner-city populations and community outreach programs (senior centers, civic organizations, etc.); and (4) provider-based: physician-reminder systems (chart checklists, computer "flags," prehospital discharge, etc.).

Protein–polysaccharide conjugate pneumococcal vaccines may be more effective and are approved for use in children. Conjugate vaccines reduce nasopharyngeal carriage of pneumococcus, thus reducing the incidence of both mucosal (i.e., otitis media) and invasive disease in children. Importantly, the conjugated pneumococcal vaccine reduces nasal carriage of pneumococci and has led to sharp declines in disease in older adults since many infections in older adults are acquired from children (Figure 124-3). This concept of "herd immunity," reducing the risk of disease in the most vulnerable older adults by immunizing children may have important implications for public health strategies to reduce the risk of infection in older adults who coincidentally are the most likely to experience poor responses to the currently available vaccines (see High, 2007).

Influenza

The current influenza vaccine is a killed virus that is modestly immunogenic with estimated efficacy rates of 60% for illness and 50% to 60% for mortality. Annual influenza immunization reduces rates

of respiratory illness, hospitalization, and mortality in the elderly population, and current ACIP recommendations are for all patients older than the age of 50 years or with underlying medical illnesses to be immunized just prior to influenza season each year. Medical personnel and caregivers for high-risk patients should also be immunized to reduce transmission to those at increased risk for complications. A live, attenuated influenza vaccine has been under development for years and appears to be more effective, but has not yet been approved for widespread use nor adequately studied in older adults (see Chapter 130 for additional details).

Zoster

Zoster is much more common, and the devastating effects of postherpetic neuralgia much more frequent in older adults than in young

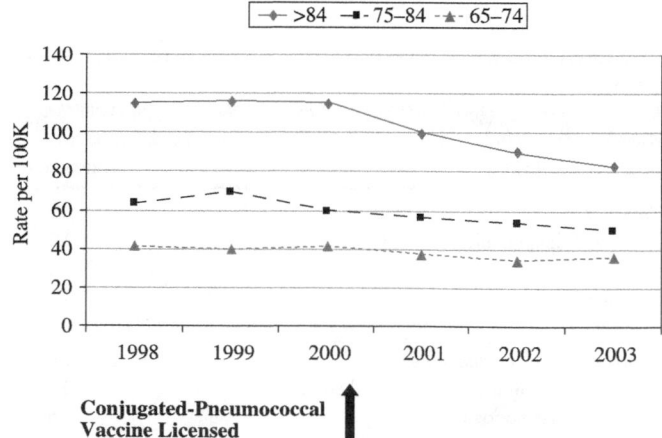

FIGURE 124-3. Reduction in the incidence of invasive pneumococcal disease in older adults after introduction of the conjugated pneumococcal vaccine in children. Presumably, the reduction in circulating pneumococcus in the community induced by protective immunity in children by the conjugated vaccine reduced exposure in older adults and consequently serious pneumococcal disease. All declines from 1998–1999 to 2003 are significant (–28%, –35%, –29% in the >84-, 75–84-, and 65–74-yr age groups, respectively). (Data from *JAMA.* 2005;294:2043.)

adults. In 2006, the FDA approved a vaccine that reduces the risk of zoster by about 50% and the risk of clinically significant postherpetic neuralgia by about 60%. The FDA approved the vaccine for use in those aged 60 years and older without a prior history of zoster. The ACIP however recommends the vaccine for all adults aged 60 years and older regardless of prior zoster history citing the safety of the vaccine and the unreliability of a zoster history (see Chapter 129 for additional details).

Other Vaccines

The elderly population is the group most at risk for tetanus in the United States, with older women being particularly susceptible because of a lower likelihood of receiving boosters associated with minor/moderate trauma. Subprotective levels of tetanus antibody (<0.01 U/mL) have been found in 43% to 61% of men and in 48% to 71% of women older than age 50 years. A complete vaccine series is indicated for persons with an uncertain history of tetanus immunization and for those who have received fewer than three doses. Boosters should be given at 10-year intervals, or more frequently with high-risk injuries such as burns, puncture wounds, or extensive soft-tissue injury.

Hepatitis vaccines may also be considered for the elderly patient under certain circumstances. Hepatitis B vaccine is indicated for all persons at risk for percutaneous or mucosal exposure to infected blood or body secretions. Older adults may have comorbidities (e.g., renal failure) that place them at risk, but they also commonly volunteer at health care facilities and should be considered at risk if they engage in any patient contact. Hepatitis A vaccine is indicated in more limited circumstances such as chronic hepatitis C, travel, and for men who have sex with men. Unfortunately, the efficacy of hepatitis A and B vaccines in older adults is unknown, but may be much lower than in young adults. Age-related declines in antibody titers to levels below those considered protective begin as early as age 35 years and by age 70 years, less than half of adults administered the hepatitis B vaccine, and only two thirds of those given the hepatitis A vaccine will produce serum antibodies to levels considered protective.

TRAVEL RECOMMENDATIONS FOR THE ELDERLY PERSON

Elderly persons are among the most widely traveled members of our society. The Centers for Disease Control and Prevention Web site (http://wwwn.cdc.gov/travel/contentVaccinations.aspx) has information on recommended vaccines. Many countries require cholera and yellow fever vaccines prior to entry, but a specific note of caution must be sounded for elderly adults. The yellow fever vaccine is a live-virus vaccine and recent data suggest that older adults are six times more likely than young adults to experience a serious adverse event. Furthermore, although still quite rare, reactions requiring hospitalization or resulting in death are 3.5- and 9-fold higher in adults aged 65 to 74 years and older than 75 years, respectively, when compared to young adults. Because the incidence of yellow fever in travelers is very low, particularly when travel is limited to urban centers, a compelling case to administer the vaccine should be elicited prior to administering yellow fever vaccine in older adults. Often the most compelling reason is that countries may deny access to those who

cannot prove recent immunization, but a physician's letter of exemption is often acceptable.

Other recommended immunizations include hepatitis A vaccine, which has replaced intramuscular immunoglobulin as the preferred method of prevention for hepatitis A. Hepatitis A immunization is strongly encouraged for individuals anticipating prolonged travel (usually longer than 3 weeks) in areas where water and sanitary conditions are uncertain. Similarly, typhoid vaccine may be indicated for travel for extended periods of time to rural areas with poor sanitation. Other considerations include rabies (particularly when traveling to rural areas of Southeast Asia where stray dogs are commonly encountered), hepatitis B, Japanese encephalitis, and meningococcal vaccines (particularly for travel to sub-Saharan Africa).

Malaria chemoprophylaxis can be difficult in the elderly. Side effects are more common for many agents (e.g., mefloquine may produce dizziness, change in mental status, and bradycardia or prolonged QT intervals), and coadministration may be difficult in those taking cardiac medications or with significant heart disease. There are multiple alternative regimens for malaria prophylaxis but recognition of current resistance patterns is critical. Clinicians are directed to the CDC Web site (www.cdc.gov/travel) for the most up-to-date information.

Diarrhea occurs in 25% to 50% of travelers to developing countries. Primary treatment consists of fluid and electrolyte replacement, but antimicrobial therapy with a quinolone is indicated when diarrhea is accompanied by fever, bloody stools, or is prolonged. Antimotility agents are safe when coadministered with antibiotics.

FURTHER READING

Bentley DW, Bradley S, High KP, et al. Practice guideline for evaluation of fever and infection in long-term care facilities. *Clin Infect Dis.* 2000;31:640.

Bradley S. Issues in the management of resistant bacteria in long-term care facilities. *Infect Control Hosp Epidemiol.* 1999;20:362.

Castle SC. Clinical relevance of age-related immune dysfunction. *Clin Infect Dis.* 2000;31:578.

Chintanadilok J, Bender BS. Sepsis. In: Yoshikawa TT, Norman DC, eds. *Infectious Disease in the Aging: A Clinical Handbook.* Totowa, NJ: Humana Press; 2001:33.

Fisman DN, Reilly DT, Korchmer AW, et al. Clinical effectiveness and cost-effectiveness of 2 management strategies for infected total hip arthroplasty in the elderly. *Clin Infect Dis.* 2001;32:419.

Herring A, Williamson J. Principles of antimicrobial use in older adults. *Clin Geriatr Med.* 2007;23:481–97.

High KP. Nutritional strategies to boost immunity and prevent infection in elderly individuals. *Clin Infect Dis.* 2001;33:1892.

High KP. Immunizations in older adults. *Clin Geriatr Med.* 2007;23:669–85.

Juthani-Mehta M, Quagliarello V. Prognostic scoring systems for infectious diseases: their applicability to the care of older adults. *Clin Infect Dis.* 2004;38:692.

Leder K, Weller PF, Wilson ME, et al. Travel vaccines and elderly persons: review of vaccines available in the United States. *Clin Infect Dis.* 2001;33:1553.

Loeb MB. Use of a broader determinants of health model for community-acquired pneumonia in seniors. *Clin Infect Dis.* 2004;38:1293.

Cox AM, Malani P, Wiseman SW, et al. Home intravenous antimicrobial infusion therapy: a viable option in older adults. *J Am Geriatr Soc.* 2007;55:645–650.

Marcus EL, Clarfield AM, Moses AE. Ethical issues relating to the use of antimicrobial therapy in older adults. *Clin Infect Dis.* 2001;33:1697.

Miller ER 3rd, Pastor-Barriuso R, Dalal P, et al. Meta-analysis: high-dosage vitamin E supplementation may increase all-cause mortality. *Ann Intern Med.* 2005;142:37.

Norman DC, Yoshikawa TT. Fever in the elderly. *Infect Dis Clin North Am.* 1996;10(1):93.

Tal S, Guller V, Gurevich A. Fever of unknown origin in the elderly. *Clin Geriatr Med.* 2007;23:649–668.

Van den Brande P. Revised Guidelines for the Diagnosis and Control of Tuberculosis: Impact on Management in the Elderly. *Drugs Aging.* 2005;22:663.

Werner GS, Schulz R, Fuchs JB, et al. Infective endocarditis in the elderly in the era of transesophageal echocardiography: Clinical features and prognosis compared with younger patients. *Am J Med.* 1996;100:90.

Wilson W, Taubert KA, Gewitz M, et al. *J Am Dent Assoc.* 2008;139(s):3s–24s.

Zevallos M, Justman JE. Tuberculosis in the elderly. *Clin Geriatr Med.* 2003;19:121.

General Principles of Antimicrobial Selection

Maureen Bolon ■ Stephen G. Weber

INTRODUCTION

When treating infection in older patients, selection of an antimicrobial regimen often precedes the identification of the causative pathogen and may sometimes be necessary even before the specific site of infection has been established. In these cases, the choice of therapy is typically based on the clinician's estimation of the most likely causative organism as well as properties of the available antimicrobial agents. This method of antimicrobial selection is described as "empiric," as opposed to "pathogen-directed," in which the causative organism has already been determined by the results of clinical cultures and antimicrobial susceptibility testing. This chapter addresses the unique challenges of selecting optimal empiric antimicrobial therapy for older patients with known or suspected infection.

To provide both a framework for discussion as well as a practical tool to be applied at the bedside, the process of selecting empiric antimicrobial therapy for older patients may be considered in three steps. First, to determine the potential causative pathogen as well as the appropriateness of initiating antimicrobial therapy, clinical and epidemiological clues are examined in order to establish the most likely site of infection. Next, estimation of the likelihood of antimicrobial resistance, together with consideration of the seriousness of the patient's infection and overall clinical status are used to determine the most appropriate breadth of antimicrobial coverage. Finally, pharmacological issues, including the pharmacokinetics of the available agents, potential toxicities and drug interactions are considered in order to facilitate the final selection of the most appropriate antimicrobial agent or agents. Once empiric therapy is initiated, the patient's clinical progress is closely followed and the antimicrobial regimen is broadened or narrowed according to the results of testing in the clinical microbiology laboratory. This process of choosing empiric therapy is summarized in Table 125-1.

In the section that follows, this systematic approach to the management of older patients with known or suspected infection is re-viewed in greater detail. Thereafter, the strategy is applied to the discussion of specific recommendations for antimicrobial therapy for a variety of infectious syndromes.

Identifying the Causative Pathogen

Clinical Features

When evaluating any patient with possible infection, determination of the most likely site of infection is a critical first step for the clinician who wishes to establish the causative pathogen in order to select the most appropriate antimicrobial regimen. The unique and often enigmatic manifestations of infection in older patients serve to complicate this endeavor. An understanding of the physiological factors that influence the clinical presentation of infection in older patients provides clinicians caring for this group with the necessary tools and increased sensitivity to detect evidence of infection in these vulnerable patients and lower the threshold to initiate empiric therapy even when only subtle signs or symptoms of infection are present.

The factors that increase vulnerability to infection and those that result in atypical or blunted manifestation of infection are often the very same in the elderly patient. These issues are addressed in greater detail in Chapter 124.

Epidemiological Context

Once clinical clues have raised the suspicion of infection and the decision has been made to initiate empiric antimicrobial therapy, epidemiological factors may offer additional information as to the most likely etiological agent. For example, a history of recent hospitalization or long-term care facility residence should increase concern for a wider diversity of infecting strains. For patients with this history, the relatively innocuous gram-positive flora that typically resides on

---

TABLE 125-1

Rational Stepwise Approach to the Selection of Antimicrobial Therapy for Older Patients

I. Estimate the most likely causative pathogen if not known
- Review clinical and epidemiological clues
- Identify the most likely site of infection

II. Determine the appropriate breadth of initial antimicrobial therapy
- Estimate the likelihood of antimicrobial resistance
- Consider the severity of patient's condition and comorbid diseases

III. Integrate pharmacological data to select the empiric choice of therapy
- Evaluate pharmacokinetic and pharmacodynamic data
- Consider the risk of drug toxicity and interactions

IV. Monitor clinical course and laboratory data to refine and narrow antimicrobial regimen
- Direct efforts at confirmation of microbiological diagnosis

---

the skin may be replaced by more aggressive gram-negative species that are more likely to infect surgical wounds, intravascular catheters and the urinary tract.

When considering epidemiological clues, knowledge of local outbreaks of infection should inform the diagnostic evaluation of a new case of illness in an individual patient. Seasonal factors should also be considered. For example, influenza may be an exceptionally common cause of respiratory infection from October to March, whereas other causes are more likely at other times of the year. The known geographic distribution of certain pathogens and infectious syndromes is also important for the clinician to keep in mind. The pathogen responsible for fever in a traveler returning from the Amazon Basin (malaria) is apt to be different than the organism causing the same presentation in an elderly resident of the desert Southwest (coccidiomycosis) or Martha's Vineyard (babesiosis).

Determining Breadth of Coverage

Severity of Infection

Following the identification of the site of infection and determination of the most likely causative organism, the next step in the management of the infected older patient is an evaluation of the severity of infection. While an accurate assessment of the severity of infection will inform a clinician's decision as to whether or not to start empiric therapy, the same information should influence the breadth of antimicrobial coverage once therapy is initiated. In general, the most appropriate response to evidence of a severe infection in an older patient on the part of the treating clinician should be rapid administration of one or more potent antimicrobial agents with efficacy against the most likely causative pathogen. There is evidence that rapid delivery of the first dose of therapy is particularly critical for the treatment of serious infections in older patients, such as sepsis, meningitis and pneumonia.

The severity of infection not only influences the choice of antimicrobial regimen, but may also influence antimicrobial dosing and the route of delivery selected. In all cases of severe infection, the goal is to ensure delivery of an adequate level of the antimicrobial agent to the site of infection in a sufficient concentration that will result in the killing of the pathogen. In general, parenteral administration of antimicrobial agents must be employed for serious

infections. Parenteral therapy may not be necessary for the entire duration of treatment, but should at least be used until the patient has demonstrated some response to therapy, such as resolution of fever or normalization of leukocytosis.

In general, use of an agent with a broad antimicrobial spectrum may be most appropriate in the early stages of treating a serious infection in an older patient. This should ensure that the agent is active against the pathogen, the identity of which is usually unknown at the time that therapy is initiated. Once the causative pathogen is identified, an agent with a narrower spectrum of activity can be used to more specifically target the pathogen without the attendant consequences of broad-spectrum therapy, such as disruption of the normal bacterial flora and selection of pathogens with antimicrobial resistance.

Antimicrobial Resistance

In addition to considering the severity of infection, the clinician pursuing a rational approach to antimicrobial selection for an older patient will incorporate the likelihood of antimicrobial resistance into their thinking. This is particularly an issue for patients in long-term care facilities or acute care hospitals where transmission of pathogens between patients is a particular concern. The high rates of antimicrobial use in long-term care and acute care facilities also leads to the selection of antimicrobial-resistant organisms. Inappropriate prescription of antimicrobials, reported to approach fifty percent of prescriptions in these settings, is a major contributor to the continued escalation of this problem.

In all cases of known or suspected infection with antimicrobial-resistant pathogens, knowledge of local susceptibility profiles for common pathogens should inform all decisions about antimicrobial choice. Institutions and laboratories should be encouraged to provide data on local susceptibilities to clinicians. Consideration should be given to an antimicrobial regimen with a broader spectrum of coverage until the causative pathogen is identified.

When infection with an antimicrobial-resistant pathogen is anticipated, it may be appropriate to consider the use of combination therapy—the concurrent use of two or more agents from different antibacterial classes. The rationale for the use of combination therapy is to increase the likelihood that the administered antibacterials are effective against the known or suspected pathogen, whether the increase in antimicrobial activity of the combination is additive or synergistic. The decision to initiate combination therapy must be weighed against the possibility of increased toxicity, additional expense, and further selection of resistant organisms. In general, while combination therapy may be appropriate for empiric therapy for a seriously ill older patient, the regimen can generally be narrowed to a single effective agent once a pathogen is isolated, identified and susceptibility results are available.

Pharmacological Considerations

Having established the need for empiric antimicrobial therapy and the most likely causative pathogen through careful examination of clinical and epidemiological clues and after considering the patient's severity of illness and the likelihood of antimicrobial resistance to determine the appropriate breadth of coverage, the clinician treating the infected older patient may still have a number of therapeutic options from which to choose. In making a final decision regarding the optimal antimicrobial regimen, he/she will need to draw

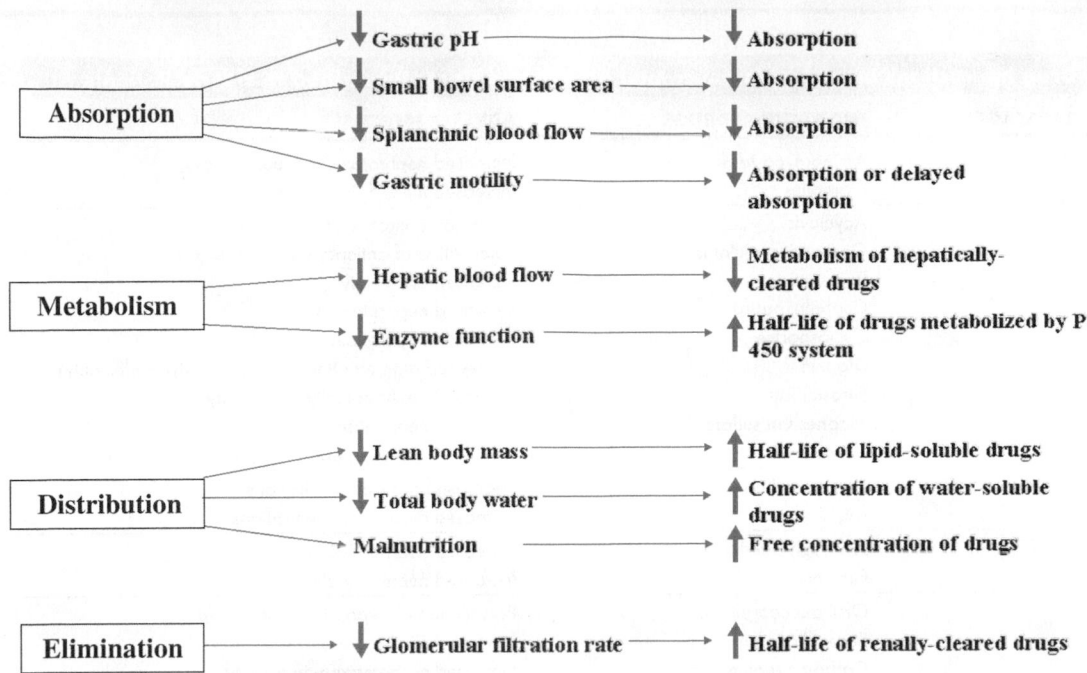

FIGURE 125-1. Pharmacokinetic issues to consider when prescribing antimicrobials to elderly patients.

upon an up to date knowledge of pharmacological principles, especially as they apply to this vulnerable population. While the recommended antimicrobial agent and dosing schedule for a particular infection should apply to most populations, there are unique pharmacological issues that affect the choice of therapy for older patients (Figure 125-1).

Pharmacokinetics

Theoretically, oral drug absorption may be reduced by physiological changes common in elderly populations, such as elevated gastric pH or reduced splanchnic blood flow. It is more likely, however, that coadministered medications are the primary culprits that interfere with the absorption of certain antimicrobial agents in this population. It may be appropriate to review timing of administration of medications such as antacids when a new antimicrobial agent is prescribed. While administration of parenteral therapy should avoid potential problems with oral absorption, the increased risk of intravascular catheter infection in this population must be weighed against the benefits of this approach.

Once absorbed, drug metabolism may be affected in the older adults. Age-related changes in hepatic function, such as reduced hepatic blood flow, smaller hepatic mass, and reduced enzyme function may lead to inefficient drug metabolism, which, in general, slows drug clearance. Patients prescribed other medications that interfere with antimicrobial metabolism may experience either higher or lower levels of antimicrobial than anticipated.

In many older patients, the volume of distribution of medications is altered. This can be because of the reduction in lean body mass, increase in proportion of adipose tissue, or reduction in total body water. Changes in protein-binding caused by malnourishment can also affect volume of distribution. These changes can lead to unpredictability in medication levels and are particularly important to keep in mind when choosing loading doses of antimicrobial agents.

Toxicity and Polypharmacy

Geriatric patients may be more prone to certain medication toxicities because of the vulnerability of the end organ. For example, exacerbation of hearing loss or impairment of the vestibular system is more likely to occur in geriatric patients treated with aminoglycosides. Renal impairment is of particular concern following aminoglycoside therapy, especially in older patients with pre-existing renal dysfunction. A list of frequently encountered adverse effects associated with specific antimicrobial agents is provided in Table 125-2.

The problem of polypharmacy in the geriatric population is thoroughly reviewed in Chapter 72. It is appropriate here, however, to consider the contribution of antimicrobial agents to this problem. In some respects, the individuals most susceptible to polypharmacy are also those at greatest risk for infection—frail older adults with multiple comorbid conditions. Drug–drug interactions are of primary concern when adding a new prescription for an antimicrobial to an already long medication list. A comprehensive list of potential interactions is presented in Table 125-3.

Final Considerations: Narrowing and Withholding Therapy

Ideally, microbiological cultures will have been obtained at the time infection is initially suspected in an older patient and the identity of the causative organism will be confirmed after 2 to 3 days of empiric therapy. With this information, the clinician will have the opportunity to narrow the breadth of coverage based on knowledge of antimicrobial susceptibility data. Optimally, the more focused regimen that is chosen demonstrates excellent penetration into affected tissue, is highly active against the causative pathogen, exhibits limited activity against commensal bacteria that are not implicated in the infection, and limits exposure of the patient to drug toxicity. In other words, therapeutic benefit is maximized with respect to

TABLE 125-2

Common Drug–Drug Interactions Involving Antimicrobial Agents and Drugs Prescribed to Elderly Patients

ANTIMICROBIAL CLASS/AGENT	INTERACTING DRUGS	ADVERSE EFFECT(S)
Acyclovir	Aminoglycosides	Increased nephrotoxicity/neurotoxicity
	Narcotics	Increased meperidine effect
Aminoglycosides	Acyclovir	Inreased nephrotoxicity/neurotoxicity
	Oral anticoagulants	Potentiation of anticoagulation effects
	Bumetanide	Increased ototoxicity
	Cephalosporins	Increased nephrotoxicity
	Cyclosporine	Increased nephrotoxicity
	Digoxin	Decreased digoxin effect (oral aminoglycosides only)
	Furosemide	Increased nephrotoxicity/ototoxicity
	Magnesium sulfate	Increased neuromuscular blockade
	Vancomycin	Possible increased nephrotoxicity and ototoxicity
Azithromycin	Aluminum/magnesium antacids	Decreased peak concentrations
	Digoxin	Increased digoxin concentrations
Cephalosporins	Aminoglycosides	Increased nephrotoxicity
	Furosemide	Increased nephrotoxicity
Clarithromycin	Oral anticoagulants	Potentiation of hypoprothrombinemia
	Benzodiazepines	Increased CNS toxicity
	Carbamazepine	Increased carbamazepine toxicity
	Corticosteroids	Increased effect and possible toxicity of methylprednisone
	Cyclosporine	Increased cyclosporine toxicity
	Digoxin	Increased digoxin concentrations
	Phenytoin	Possible increased or decreased effect
	Rifampin	Decreased clarithromycin concentrations
Erythromycin	Oral anticoagulants	Potentiation of hypoprothrombinemia
	Benzodiazepines	Increased CNS toxicity
	Carbamazepine	Increased carbamazepine toxicity
	Corticosteroids	Increased effect and possible toxicity of methylprednisone
	Cyclosporine	Increased cyclosporine toxicity
	Digoxin	Increased digoxin concentrations
	HMG-CoA reductase inhibitors	Increased risk of rhabdomyolysis
	Loratadine	Increased loratadine toxicity
	Phenytoin	Possible increased or decreased effect
	Valproic acid	Increased valproic acid toxicity
Fluconazole	Benzodiazepines	Increased CNS toxicity
	Coumarin anticoagulants	Increased prothrombin times
	Cyclosporine	Increased cyclosporine concentrations
	HMG-CoA reductase inhibitors	Increased risk of rhabdomyolysis
	Phenytoin	Increased phenytoin concentrations
	Rifampin	Increased fluconazole concentrations
	Sulfonylureas	Increased plasma concentrations and decreased metabolism of sulfonylureas
	Thiazides	Increased fluconazole concentrations
Fluoroquinolones	Antacids	Decreased fluoroquinolone effect
	Oral anticoagulants	Prolonged prothrombin times
	Cyclosporine	Increased risk of nephrotoxicity; increased serum cyclosporine concentrations
	Iron	Decreased serum fluoroquinolone concentrations
	NSAIDs	Possible increased risk of CNS stimulation
	Sucralfate	Decreased serum fluoroquinolone concentrations
Linezolid	SSRIs	Increased risk of serotonin syndrome
Metronidazole	Oral anticoagulants	Increased anticoagulant effect
Nitrofurantoin	Antacids	Possible decreased nitrofurantoin effect
	Fluoroquinolones	In vitro antagonism of quinolone activity
Rifampin (and other rifamycins)	Analgesics	Possible decreased concentrations and activity
	Oral anticoagulants	Possible decreased concentrations and activity
	Anticonvulsants	Possible decreased concentrations and activity
	Beta-blockers	Possible decreased concentrations and activity
	Clarithromycin	Decreased clarithromycin concentrations/increased rifamycin toxicity
	Corticosteroids	Possible decreased concentrations and activity

(continued)

TABLE 125-2

Common Drug–Drug Interactions Involving Antimicrobial Agents and Drugs Prescribed to Elderly Patients *(Continued)*

ANTIMICROBIAL CLASS/AGENT	INTERACTING DRUGS	ADVERSE EFFECT(S)
	Diazepam	Possible decreased concentrations and activity
	Digoxin	Decreased digoxin effect
	Fluconazole	Decreased fluconazole effect
	HMG-CoA reductase inhibitors	Decreased HMG effect
	Isoniazid	Possible increased hepatotoxicity
	Narcotics	Possible decreased concentrations and activity
	Verapamil	Possible decreased concentrations and activity
Sulfonamides	Oral anticoagulants	Increased anticoagulant e ffect
	Hypoglycemics	Increased hypoglycemic effect
Tetracyclines	Antacids	Decreased oral tetracycline effects
	Oral anticoagulants	Increased anticoagulant e ffect
	Bismuth subsalicylate	Decreased oral tetracycline effects
	Carbamazepine	Decreased doxycycline effect
	Digoxin	Increased digoxin effect
	Lithium	Increased lithium toxicity
	Phenytoin	Decreased doxycycline effect
	Rifampin	Possible4 decreased doxycycline effect
Vancomycin	Aminoglycosides	Possible increased nephrotoxicity and ototoxicity

NSAIDs, nonsteroidal anti-inflammatory drugs; SSRIs, selective serotonin reuptake inhbitors; CNS, central nervous system; HMG, hydroxy-3-methyl-glutaryl.

infection while the risk of toxicity and subsequent resistance is minimized. As an added benefit, narrow therapy is often less expensive than the broad-spectrum agents typically used for empiric coverage.

There are a number of scenarios in which it is appropriate to consider not initiating antimicrobial therapy. First and foremost, antibiotics may be specifically named in advanced directives and withheld when indicated in such documents. Withholding antibacterial agents is often justified for upper respiratory infections, as these are typically caused by viral pathogens. This is also true of many diarrheal illnesses. Some entities, such as asymptomatic bacteriuria, are not felt to represent true infection and, as such, affected patients do not benefit from therapy. There are a number of other instances in which a culture may demonstrate growth of bacteria in the absence of a clinical infection. Single blood cultures positive for skin flora, such as coagulase negative staphylococci, are generally felt to have been contaminated during the process of obtaining the culture and need not prompt initiation of treatment. Clinicians also must recognize that some positive culture results represent microbial colonization rather than invasive infection, such as bacteria that may grow from a culture swab of a skin ulcer without associated purulence, inflammation or cellulitis. Finally, for a clinically stable patient with a fever, it may be appropriate to follow closely while monitoring for signs and symptoms that clarify the source of the fever rather than initiating therapy. The caveat to this advice is that it is always appropriate to initiate empiric therapy in a patient with poor physiological reserve and/or evidence of sepsis with end organ dysfunction if there is a suspicion of infection.

SPECIFIC INFECTIOUS SYNDROMES

Pneumonia and Other Respiratory Infections

The physiology, microbiology, and management of pneumonia in older patients are discussed at greater length in Chapter 126. A lim-

ited discussion of the specific factors that influence the selection of antimicrobial therapy for older patients with respiratory infection is offered here in order to demonstrate the application of the paradigm for antimicrobial selection outlined in Table 125-1.

Anticipation of the causative pathogen is central to the appropriate selection of empiric antimicrobial therapy for older patients with respiratory infection. To this end, a number of clinical features have been associated with specific causative pathogens. However, these associations generally do not stand up to more rigorous scrutiny, especially in older patients. Of greater utility in predicting the causative pathogen in community-acquired pneumonia are the epidemiological features that distinguish one patient from the next, including nursing home residence and recent hospitalization.

In the absence of unique clinical or epidemiological features to suggest chronic respiratory infection (such as that cause by *M. tuberculosis*) or viral pneumonia, clinicians caring for older patients must make every effort to optimize their management of community-acquired pneumonia. For older patients, as for younger patients with pneumonia, there are a number of suitable therapeutic options to address the suspected pathogens (Table 125-4). These regimens are generally well tolerated, although clinicians must be alert to common toxicities, such as gastrointestinal distress caused by macrolides or mental status changes caused by fluoroquinolones.

The most appropriate duration of therapy for community-acquired pneumonia in the older patient has not been rigorously assessed. Conventionally, most patients will receive between 10 and 14 days of treatment.

Skin and Soft Tissue Infections

The skin of older patients is especially vulnerable to infection with a wide range of microorganisms as a result of the physiologic and physical changes to the integument that accompany aging. As is true for younger patients, the majority of skin and soft tissue infections in the older adults are caused by the gram-positive bacteria that normally colonize the skin. Streptococcal and staphylococcal species

TABLE 125-3

Adverse Effects of Antimicrobials Commonly Used in the Elderly Population

ANTIMICROBIAL CLASS/AGENT	COMMON ADVERSE EFFECTS
Acyclovir	Nephrotoxicity, CNS toxicity
Amantadine/rimantadine	CNS toxicity
Aminoglycosides	Nephrotoxicity, ototoxicity, vestibular toxicity
Azithromycin	GI toxicity (diarrhea, nausea, vomitting, abdominal pain), candidiasis/vaginitis
Beta-lactam agents	Rash, hypersensitivity reactions, bone marrow toxicity, CNS toxicity (seizure), interstitial nephritis, antibiotic-associated diarrhea, *C. difficile*-associated diarrhea
Clarithromycin	GI toxicity (diarrhea, nausea, vomitting, abdominal pain), CNS toxicity
Clindamycin	GI toxicity (esophagitis, gastritis, nausea, vomitting, abdominal pain), antibiotic-associated diarrhea, *C. difficile*-associated diarrhea
Erythromycin	GI toxicity (diarrhea), hepatotoxicity, QT prolongation, torsade de pointes, ototoxicity
Fluconazole	Hepatotoxicity
Fluoroquinolones	QT prolongation, torsade de pointes, CNS toxicity, peripheral neuropathy, tendone rupture, *C. difficile*-associated diarrhea
Isoniazid	Hepatotoxicity, peripheral neuropathy
Linezolid	Bone marrow suppression (thrombocytopenia), GI toxicity (nausea, vomitting, diarrhea), headache, peripheral neuropathy
Metronidazole	Dysgeusia, anorexia, GI toxicity (nausea, vomitting), CNS toxicity (dizziness, lightheadedness, headache), peripheral neuropathy, disulfram-like effects when alcohol is ingested
Nitrofurantoin	Pulmonary infiltrates, peripheral neuropathy
Rifampin	Rash, hypersensitivity reactions, nephrotoxicity, reddish-orange discoloration of the urine, tears, perspiration, saliva, hepatotoxicity
Sulfonamides	Rash, hypersensitivity, Stevens-Johnson syndrome, GI toxicity (nausea, vomitting), hyperkalemia, bone marrow suppression
Tetracyclines	Photosensitivity, GI toxicity (nausea, vomitting, diarrhea), hepatotoxicity, CNS toxicity (ataxia, dizziness, vertigo)
Vancomycin	Infusion-related histamine release (Red neck syndrome), ototoxicity, vestibular toxicity, nephrotoxicity (primarily when used in combination with other nephrotoxins), bone marrow toxicity (neutropenia)

predominate. However, it is important to recognize the potential for disruption of the native skin flora as a result of certain comorbidities, such as diabetes mellitus, organ recent antimicrobial therapy which may lead to a greater proportion of cutaneous infections caused by other less common pathogens. In such patients, cellulitis, furunculosis, or

folliculitis may be caused by gram-negative bacteria, including *Escherichia coli* and *Klebsiella* spp. Less commonly, *Pseudomonas aeruginosa* may be isolated as the cause of skin infection in an older patient.

The increased breadth of pathogens associated with skin and soft tissue infections among older patients is further complicated by the challenge of obtaining definitive microbiological diagnosis in such cases. Cultures of blood, skin swabs, and even skin biopsies are likely to be of low yield in establishing the causative pathogen of nonsuppurative infections like cellulitis. As a result, empiric therapy is the rule for treating patients with skin infection. When there is abscess material to be sampled, it is critical that specimens be collected as quickly as possible, preferably prior to the institution of antimicrobial therapy. Providing further rationale for incision and drainage of a furuncle is the fact that antimicrobial therapy may be unnecessary in the setting of adequate drainage. However, the decision to withhold antimicrobial therapy for furunculosis should only be contemplated in a stable patient with good baseline health without extensive soft tissue inflammation.

Once empiric therapy is started, the older patient with skin and soft tissue infection should be monitored closely for signs of improvement, as delayed recovery may be indicative of clinical failure as a result of inadequate antimicrobial coverage. Clinicians should monitor the patient for improvement in systemic signs of infection within the first 24 to 48 hours of antibiotic therapy and consideration should be given to modifying therapy for patients who appear to be failing.

Older patients, whether because of the phenomenon of immunosenescence, comorbid conditions, or immunosuppressive drug therapy, may be at increased risk for rapidly-progressive skin and soft tissue infection, including necrotizing fasciitis. In general, an older patient evaluated in the acute care setting for skin and soft tissue infection should be followed closely for early evidence of rapid spread of infection. Skin infection that measurably expands within the first hours of evaluation represents a potentially life-threatening emergency. In addition to broadening antimicrobial coverage, urgent surgical consultation is warranted.

The management of skin and soft tissue infections among all patients has been complicated in recent years by the emergence of strains of *Staphylococcus aureus*-resistant to methicillin in individuals without prior contact with the healthcare system or exposure to antibacterial agents. So-called community-associated methicillin-resistant *S. aureus* (MRSA) appears to be associated with particularly severe and recurrent skin infections. While the extent to which this emerging pathogen specifically affects older patients is not yet known, clinicians must be aware of this new epidemiological trend and adjust the choice of empiric therapy accordingly.

Despite concerns for gram-negative or antimicrobial-resistant pathogens, initial antimicrobial therapy active against streptococci and staphylococci remains appropriate for older patients with skin and soft tissue infection. Commonly-selected regimens include antistaphylococcal penicillin such as dicloxacillin (oral) or oxacillin (parenteral), or a first-generation cephalosporin such as cephalexin (oral) or cefazolin (parenteral). The rationale for choosing parenteral rather than oral therapy is based on the assessment of severity of illness. While penicillin offers adequate coverage for streptococcal infection, the typical absence of a confirmed microbiological diagnosis precludes this approach given the lack of activity of penicillin against nearly all staphylococci. For patients with allergy to β-lactam agents, clinicians may elect to treat with clindamycin, a macrolide or

TABLE 125-4

Common Pathogens and Optimal Treatments for Older Patients with Community-Associated Pneumonia

CLINICAL SETTING	COMMON PATHOGENS	RECOMMENDED EMPIRICAL REGIMEN
Community-acquired, not hospitalized	S. pneumoniae, atypical bacteria (M. pneumoniae, C. pneumoniae), viral pathogens	Respiratory fluoroquinolone, or azithromyc in plus high-dose amoxicillin
Community-acquired, hospitalized	S. pneumoniae, atypical bacteria (M. pneumoniae, C. pneumoniae)	Ceftriaxone plus azithromycin, or respiratory fluoroquinolone
Community-acquired, hospitalized in ICU	S. pneumoniae, Legionella spp.	3rd generation cephalosporin plus respiratory fluoroquinolone
Community-acquired, LTCF resident	S. pneumoniae, influeza, enterobactereciae, P. aeruginosa	3rd generation cephalosporin plus respiratory fluoroquinolone plus vancomycin (if S. aureus or MRSA suspected)
Hospital-acquired	P. aeruginosa, enterobactericiae	imipenem or piperacillin/tazobactam plus respiratory fluoroquinolone plus vancomycin (if S. aureus or MRSA suspected)

a tetracycline derivative (such as doxycycline). Antimicrobial agents active against MRSA are discussed in greater detail in the section on healthcare-associated infection.

Possible regimens for skin and soft tissue infection are generally well tolerated in older patients. There are limited drug interactions between these antibiotics and the pharmaceutical agents commonly prescribed to older adults. The duration of therapy should be approximately 2 weeks; however, there are limited data available comparing the effectiveness of different durations of therapy. In all cases, incision and drainage of any purulent collection offers not only the opportunity for microbiological diagnosis, but also improved likelihood of clinical resolution.

Gastrointestinal Infections

Infectious Diarrhea

As in other age groups, infectious diarrhea may represent nothing more than a harmless nuisance to the older patient. However, by some estimates 50–85% of the mortality associated with diarrheal illness in developed nations occurs in geriatric populations.

Certain epidemiologic factors may increase an elderly patient's risk for gastrointestinal infection with certain pathogens—such residence in a nursing home, known to be loci of norovirus outbreaks, or recent hospitalization or antimicrobial use, which should bring consideration of *Clostridium difficile* to mind. Clinical and epidemiological clues as to the causative pathogen may also be gained by inquiring about: how the illness began; stool characteristics (frequency and quantity); symptoms or signs of hypovolemia; travel history; whether the patient has ingested raw or undercooked meat, raw seafood, or raw milk; whether the patient's contacts are ill; the patient's sexual contacts, medications, and other medical conditions if any.

An older patient presenting with fever, tenesmus, and bloody stools should be evaluated for inflammatory or invasive diarrhea caused by *Salmonella, Shigella, Campylobacter, Yersinia,* or *C. difficile.* For this group, antimicrobial therapy may be appropriate. While clinicians may choose to treat empirically and not perform stool cultures, the utility of confirmatory testing for a microbiological diagnosis may be especially high in an institutional setting in which a number of individuals appear to have similar complaints. In ad-

dition, stool cultures can be beneficial to the care of the individual patient by identifying etiologic agents that do not require antimicrobial therapy (such as viral pathogens), thus avoiding unnecessary antibiotic use. Lastly, antimicrobial resistance has been observed in a number of enteric pathogens, including fluoroquinolone resistance in *Campylobacter* and multidrug resistance in *Salmonella.* As a general rule, it is probably wise to obtain stool testing from patients with diarrhea that has lasted longer than 1 day, is accompanied by fever, hematochezia, systemic illness, or dehydration, or in individuals who have recently been hospitalized or have received recent antimicrobials.

Having identified inflammatory diarrhea in an older individual and developed a suspicion about the likely pathogen based on epidemiologic clues, the next step is to determine whether or not to initiate antimicrobial therapy at all. Individuals with diarrhea caused by the *E. coli* O157:H7 strain may be more likely to develop hemolytic uremic syndrome after therapy with certain antimicrobials. Treatment of diarrhea caused by *Salmonella* spp. with fluoroquinolone agents can lead to a prolonged carrier state or relapse of symptoms. The decision to initiate antimicrobial therapy should be guided by an assessment of the patient's severity of illness as well as their comorbid medical conditions. Empiric recommendations are detailed in Table 125-5. Duration of therapy may range from 3 to 14 days depending upon the enteric pathogen, as outlined in Table 125-5. Anticipated toxicities may include exacerbation of intestinal distress by doxycycline or rash secondary to trimethoprim-sulfamethoxazole.

C. difficile-Associated Diarrhea

Advanced age is a well-established risk factor for *C. difficile*-associated diarrhea (CDAD). The vulnerability to CDAD in the geriatric age group is felt to be explained by age-related changes in the fecal flora, immunosenescense, and the presence of other comorid medical conditions.

Symptoms of CDAD can range from several loose stools a day without fever or clinical instability to a debilitating watery diarrhea associated with abdominal cramping, fever, leukocytosis with consequent dehydration and electrolyte losses. In advanced disease, a dangerous ileus may develop and the most severely ill patients may require colectomy. The range of manifestations highlights the need

TABLE 125-5

Antimicrobial Recommendations for Enteric Pathogens

ORGANISM	OPTIONS FOR THERAPY	SPECIAL CONSIDERATIONS
Aeromonas/Plesiomonas	Trimethoprim-sulfamethoxazole Fluoroquinolone	
Campylobacter spp.	Erythromycin	
C. difficile	Metronidazole Oral vancomycin	Discontinue antimicrobial therapy, if possible Recurrences can be managed with repeat courses of metronidazole
E. coli spp.		
Enterohemorrhagic (STEC)		Role of antimicrobials unclear, avoid administration. Avoid antimotility agents
Enteroinvasive	Trimethoprim- sulfamethoxazole Fluoroquinolone	
Enteropathogenic	Trimethoprim-sulfamethoxazole Fluoroquinolone	
Enterotoxigenic	Trimethoprim-sulfamethoxazole Fluoroquinolone	
Giardia lamblia	Metronidazole	
Salmonella, non-*typhi* spp.	Trimethoprim-sulfamethoxazole Fluoroquinolone Ceftriaxone	Be aware of possibility of trimethoprim-sulfamethoxazole and fluoroquinolone resistance
Shigella spp.	Trimethoprim-sulfamethoxazole Fluoroquinolone Ceftriaxone Azithromycin	

to remain vigilant for the possibility of *C. difficile* infection in patients recently treated with antimicrobials.

Contact with the healthcare system is a known risk for acquiring *C. difficile* colonization, which can then progress to infection following the administration of antibiotics. Nearly every antimicrobial agent has been implicated as a risk factor for CDAD and outbreaks have been seen both in acute care hospitals as well as long-term care facilities.

The initial approach to the management of CDAD includes discontinuing all precipitating antimicrobial agents (if possible), replacement of fluid and electrolyte losses, and avoidance of antimotility agents. Conservative management will not be sufficient for the majority of patients, and therapy with either metronidazole or vancomycin is needed. Although oral vancomycin is the only FDA-approved agent for treating CDAD, most guidelines recommend initiating therapy with oral metronidazole. This is because of the higher cost of vancomycin, the concern that use of vancomycin will lead to selection of vancomycin-resistant enterococci, and the fact that vancomycin was not been shown to be superior to metronidazole in head-to-head studies. Vancomycin may be considered for individuals who cannot tolerate oral metronidazole or for those patients who fail to improve with metronidazole therapy. Duration of therapy of 10 to 14 days is recommended.

It is estimated that recurrence of CDAD following the completion of therapy occurs in as many as half of cases. It is recommended that recurrence be managed with a repeated course of oral metronidazole of standard duration.

Probiotics such as *Sacharomyces boulardii* and *Lactobacillus rhamnosus* are microorganisms of low pathogenicity that may be used to re-populate the normal bowel flora that has been eliminated through the use of antimicrobial agents. Unfortunately, they have not been shown to be of great benefit. Use of probiotics should be avoided

in immunocompromised individuals because of the possibility of invasive infection caused by these organisms.

Bone and Joint Infections

Osteomyelitis

Bone infection presents both diagnostic and therapeutic challenges in all patient populations, but especially in older patients. Because manifestations of disease may be nonspecific, the first step in making the diagnosis of bone infection is the timely recognition of predisposing factors, such as loss of overlying skin and soft tissue integrity. The forms of osteomyelitis typically seen in older patients are vertebral osteomyelitis, generally secondary to bacteremic seeding, and contiguous osteomyelitis, which may or may not be associated with vascular insufficiency. In all forms of osteomyelitis in this population, identification of the causative pathogen greatly improves the likelihood of administering appropriate antimicrobial therapy. In most cases of spine infection as well as in cases of contiguous osteomyelitis, bone biopsy is almost always necessary to establish the pathological diagnosis and to identify the causative organisms so that appropriate therapy may be chosen. See Table 125-6 for anticipated pathogens and recommended regimens for treatment of osteomyelitis.

Vertebral osteomyelitis generally presents subacutely with fever and back pain; other constitutional symptoms such as night sweats or weight loss may also be present. The presentation in an elderly individual may be subtle or atypical and the presence of preexisting back pain may delay recognition of a new infectious process at this site. Knowledge of a primary site of infection from which the bone has been seeded is a clue to the pathogen, although frequently the primary site is unknown. Skin and soft tissue pathogens, particularly

TABLE 125-6

Subtypes of Bacterial Osteomyelitis Among Older Patients

	TYPICAL CLINICAL SETTING	COMMON PATHOGENS	RECOMMENDED EMPIRICAL REGIMEN
Spinal osteomyelitis	Bacteremic spread from other source of infection	S. aureus (including MRSA), streptococci	Vancomycin
Osteomyelitis from contiguous spread with vascular insufficiency	Diabetic foot ulcer	S. aureus, streptococci, enterococci, gram-negative pathogens, anaerobes	IV: ertapenem, ampicillin/sulbactam, vancomycin (if MRSA suspected) Orally: amoxicillin/clavulanate, fluoroquinolone plus clindamycin
Osteomyelitis from contiguous spread without vascular insufficiency	Pressure ulcer	S. aureus, streptococci, enterococci, gram-negative pathogens, anaerobes	imipenem, piperacillin/tazobactam, vancomycin (if MRSA suspected)

S. aureus, are most commonly involved, but genitourinary and respiratory infections, infected intravenous catheters, postoperative wounds, endocarditis, and dental sources are all considerations. In a patient with known or suspected exposure to tuberculosis, Pott's disease (tuberculosis of the spine) is a concern.

Because of the more chronic nature of the infection, empiric antimicrobial therapy may be safely withheld from the older patient with suspected vertebral osteomyelitis until cultures have been performed in order to increase the likelihood of identifying the infecting pathogen. A caveat to this is that patients experiencing neurological deficits, including new lower extremity sensory or motor deficits or bowel or bladder dysfunction, should receive prompt treatment with antimicrobials, as well as neurosurgical evaluation. While awaiting culture results once specimens have been collected, it may be reasonable to cover broadly for gram-positive skin and soft tissue organisms, particularly S. aureus, with a first-generation cephalosporin or an antistaphylococcal penicillin. In a patient with a history of MRSA or risk factors for MRSA, vancomycin is an appropriate addition. In a patient with known urinary tract infection or prostatitis, gram-negative coverage with a third-generation cephalosporin or a fluoroquinolone should be added. Once the infecting organism is identified, coverage can be narrowed and is generally continued for 4 to 6 weeks in intravenous or highly orally bioavailable form. Adverse effects associated with therapy for osteomyelitis include the complications of long-term intravenous access, such as line infection or thrombosis caused by the foreign body. Long-term β-lactam use may be associated with bone marrow suppression or hepatic toxicity. Prolonged vancomycin use may also result in bone marrow suppression or, infrequently, renal toxicity. Regular monitoring of blood counts and liver and kidney function is advised with prolonged use of any intravenous antimicrobial therapy, especially in older patients.

Osteomyelitis caused by contiguous spread of infection with vascular insufficiency generally refers to diabetic ulcers of the lower extremity, but may also occur in individuals with severe peripheral vascular disease. Patients typically present with a long-standing ulcer of the foot, possibly with concurrent cellulitis or purulent drainage. Polymicrobial infection is the rule; S. aureus, streptococci, enterococci, gram-negatives, and anaerobes are frequently seen. Bone biopsy for culture is valuable in identifying the causative organisms, as well as confirming the pathological changes of acute osteomyelitis, and is not associated with exacerbation of the infection. This infection may be slow to respond to antimicrobial therapy, particularly if

underlying issues of blood glucose control and vascular supply are not addressed. In many cases, the goal of therapy is to suppress infection and maintain functional status. Wound care and surgical management are equal partners to treatment with antimicrobial agents. Antimicrobial therapy is generally prolonged, but can often be administered orally, owing to the availability of oral agents with superior bone penetration, such as amoxicillin/clavulanate, trimethoprim-sulfamethoxazole, clindamycin, and ciprofloxacin.

Osteomyelitis caused by contiguous spread of infection without vascular insufficiency is most often associated with trauma, but pressure ulcers are a particular concern in bed-bound elderly individuals. These infections are generally polymicrobial in cause and may include staphylococci and streptococci. In the case of sacral pressure ulcers, Gram-negatives and anaerobes may be present given the proximity to the rectum and the likelihood of stool contamination of broken skin. Recommended empiric therapy should be broad, but can later be narrowed on the basis of cultures from deep tissue biopsy or debridement. Antimicrobial-resistant organisms are a concern, particularly in institutionalized patients, and culture-guided therapy may need to be administered for MRSA, VRE, or resistant gram-negatives. Surgical management is a critical component of therapy, the purposes of which include: drainage, debridement, obliteration of dead space, and wound protection. Proper wound care is also necessary, as is well described in Chapter 124.

Septic Arthritis

Septic arthritis is an infection with high morbidity and mortality. Elderly patients are particularly at risk, by virtue of pre-existing joint disease caused by rheumatoid arthritis, osteoarthritis, and gout, which are known risk factors for septic arthritis. Patients typically present with fever, pain, warmth, swelling, and decreased range of motion at the infected joint, although these may be absent in older patients. Gonococcal arthritis is common in young adults, but fairly infrequent in the elderly population, although it should be considered in the setting of appropriate risk factors. Gram-positive organisms are prominent, both because of the pathogenesis of bacteremic seeding from compromise of the skin and because of the proclivity of these organism to adhere to the connective tissue and extracellular matrix proteins of the joints. As such, S. aureus is the most commonly implicated organism and is associated with notably poor outcomes. Group B beta-hemolytic streptococcus (S. agalactiae) is seen in association with diabetes, cirrhosis, advanced age, and

TABLE 125-7

Common Pathogens and Optimal Treatments for Older Patients with Septic Arthritis

CAUSATIVE PATHOGEN	EPIDEMIOLOGICAL CLUES AND RISK FACTORS	OPTIMAL THERAPY
S. aureus	Usually bacteremic spread from other site of infection	Vancomycin if MRSA is suspected. Otherwise nafcillin or oxacillin
N. gonorrhea	Sexually active patient	3rd generation cephalosporin
S. pneumoniae	May follow pulmonary infection	3rd generation cephalosporin
Group B streptococcus	Diabetes, cirrhosis, neurological disease	Penicillin G or 3rd generation cephalosporin

neurologic disease. *S. pneumoniae* may occur following invasive pulmonary infection, but also occasionally in the absence of pneumonia. Gram-negative infections may occur following genitourinary infection, and are also associated with intravenous drug use, particularly *P. aeruginosa*. Coagulase negative staphylococci may be seen following joint arthroscopy.

Joint aspiration is necessary both to confirm the presence of septic arthritis and identify the causative organism. Gram stain of fluid is not particularly sensitive, so empiric therapy should be instituted before cultures results are available. Because the infection is rapidly destructive and has a high mortality, therapy should be initiated rapidly. If Gram stain is negative, an antimicrobial agent that covers staphylococci and streptococci as well as gram-negatives should be initiated, such as ceftriaxone. Many would also advise initial vancomycin therapy for the possibility of MRSA. Intravenous therapy is typically used for a 3-week duration. Surgical therapy is an important component of management, and joint drainage and irrigation should be performed to allow for decompression of the joint, improvement in blood flow, and removal of bacteria, toxins, and proteases. Open drainage should be considered in the case of a slow clinical response or inaccessible joint, such as the shoulder joint. See Table 125-7 for common pathogens and suggested empiric treatment for septic arthritis.

Prosthetic Joint Infection

This issue is covered in more detail in Chapter 116, but certain points will be highlighted here as they serve to illustrate key issues of antimicrobial management in the elderly population. One of the foremost of these is the well-established association between timing of infection relative to surgery and likely organisms isolated, an excellent example of how epidemiologic clues can help guide empiric antimicrobial therapy in older patients. The presentation of prosthetic joint infection is typically divided into 3 stages based on how soon after joint implantation the infection occurs (see Table 125-8).

TABLE 125-8

Bacteria Associated with Prosthetic Joint Infection by Time of Presentation

	TIMING	MOST COMMON PATHOGEN(S)
Early	0–3 months postoperative	S. aureus (including MRSA), gram-negative bacteria
Delayed	3–24 months postoperative	Coagulase-negative staphylococci, Proprionobacterium spp.
Late	>24 months postoperative	S. aureus (including MRSA), other pathogens from bacteremic spread

Early infections occur within the first 3 months following joint implantation and are typically caused by highly pathogenic organisms, such as *S. aureus* or Gram negatives that were inoculated during the original surgery. Delayed infections, occurring 3 to 24 months followings surgery, are also felt to have been inoculated during the original surgery, but involve less virulent pathogens, such as coagulase negative staphylococci and *Propionobacterium* that present in a subacute manner. Late infections, occurring more than 24 months after surgery, are felt to arise through hematogenous seeding of the prosthetic material, and, as such, involve virulent organisms typically associated with bacteremias, such as *S. aureus* from skin sources, and the appropriate organisms from respiratory, dental, and genitourinary sources.

Identification of the infecting organism may be facilitated by blood cultures, but often requires direct culture of joint fluid or tissue obtained from operative debridement or prosthetic removal. In the case of delayed infection, which is generally subacute, it is appropriate to withhold antimicrobial therapy until after cultures are obtained or if therapy has been initiated to stop therapy 2 to 4 weeks prior to obtaining operative cultures to improve the diagnostic yield of these cultures. Multiple tissue cultures are useful to confirm the pathogen status of organisms of low virulence like coagulase negative *Staphylococcus* or *Propionobacterium*. Empiric choice of antimicrobials should include coverage for resistant gram-positive organisms like MRSA or coagulase negative staphylococci—generally, vancomycin is used. Gram-negative coverage with a third-generation cephalosporin may be utilized if these less common culprits are suspected.

Once the causative organism is identified and directed therapy is chosen, it is necessary to consider addition of an agent like rifampin for its ability to penetrate biofilms. Bacteria growing on prosthetic material often form a biofilm—a community of bacteria growing within a polymeric matrix. Antimicrobials diffuse poorly through biofilms and bacteria within them assume a stationary growth phase that makes them less susceptible to antimicrobials with activity against dividing bacteria. Antimicrobial therapy for prosthetic infections must be prolonged in order to counter the resistance to therapy imparted by the biofilm. While intravenous agents such as antistaphylococcal penicillins, first-generation cephalosporins, or vancomycin are typically used along with rifampin, several older studies found that oral combinations of fluoroquinolones and rifampin also successfully treated prosthetic joint infections. Unfortunately, resistance to fluoroquinolones has become so prevalent in staphylococci that this is no longer a reliable combination. Rifampin should be used cautiously given its effect on hepatic metabolism and numerous consequent drug–drug interactions.

The most appropriate duration of therapy for prosthetic joint infection is typically prolonged and may range from several months to life-long therapy depending upon whether the infected prosthesis is removed.

Central Nervous System Infection

The manifestations of infection of the central nervous system (CNS) among both older and younger patients range from self-limited and benign to abrupt and lethal. Careful review of the patient's presenting complaints, history, examination and initial laboratory and radiographic data should permit a clear distinction between the infectious syndromes of the nervous system, including meningitis, encephalitis, and brain abscess. Figure 125-2 outlines the approach to managing an older patient with suspected CNS infection.

Meningitis

Signs and symptoms of bacterial infection of the CNS must be recognized in a timely manner in order to ensure the best possible clinical outcome. Unfortunately, the classical signs and symptoms of meningitis may be masked among older patients, contributing to a delay in diagnosis. Generally speaking, clinicians caring for older patients are well advised to have a low threshold to aggressively pursue the diagnosis of meningitis with early lumbar puncture and cerebrospinal fluid (analysis whenever confronted with a patient with the constellation of fever and headache or mental status change. While it is optimal to collect cerebrospinal fluid for Gram stain and culture prior to the administration of the first dose of antibiotic, therapy should not be delayed for an undue period while lumbar puncture is performed or radiological evaluation is completed.

In the setting of suspected meningitis in an elderly patient, empiric antimicrobial therapy should be selected that has sufficient coverage to address all clinically relevant pathogens. While meningococ-

cal meningitis occurs less frequently in elderly patients than in young adults and children, pneumoccocus remains a concern, and, in fact, is the most-commonly-isolated bacterial pathogen in this population. Older patients appear to be at increased risk for CNS infection with strains of pneumoccocus that are resistant to penicillin. While third-generation cephalosporins may be effective against penicillin-resistant *S. pneumoniae* infection at other sites, these agents may not be adequate for therapy of meningitis in this setting. As a result, supplemental therapy with vancomycin should be included in the initial empirical regimen to ensure coverage of resistant pneumococci.

Elderly patients are particularly susceptible to meningeal infection with *Listeria monocytogenes*. While a number of epidemiological clues can point to infection with *L. monocytogenes*, including exposure to specific contaminated food, such clinical risk factors need not be present to raise the concern for this infection. High dose ampicillin is the most appropriate choice for CNS infection with *L. monocytogenes*. Because the clinical signs and symptoms of CNS infection with *Listeria* overlap considerably with those attributable to infection with *S. pneumonia* and *N. meningitidis*, ampicillin should be included in the empiric regimen for all older patients even before microbiological identification and susceptibility testing has been completed.

Once the results of microbiological cultures and other laboratory studies are available, antimicrobial therapy for meningitis can be narrowed to focus on the causative pathogen while limiting toxicity and interactions with other pharmacological agents. The duration of therapy for pneumococcus should be approximately 2 weeks and for *Listeria* 3 weeks or longer depending upon clinical response.

If no causative bacterial pathogen is isolated despite the timely collection of CSF specimens and the clinical presentation (including

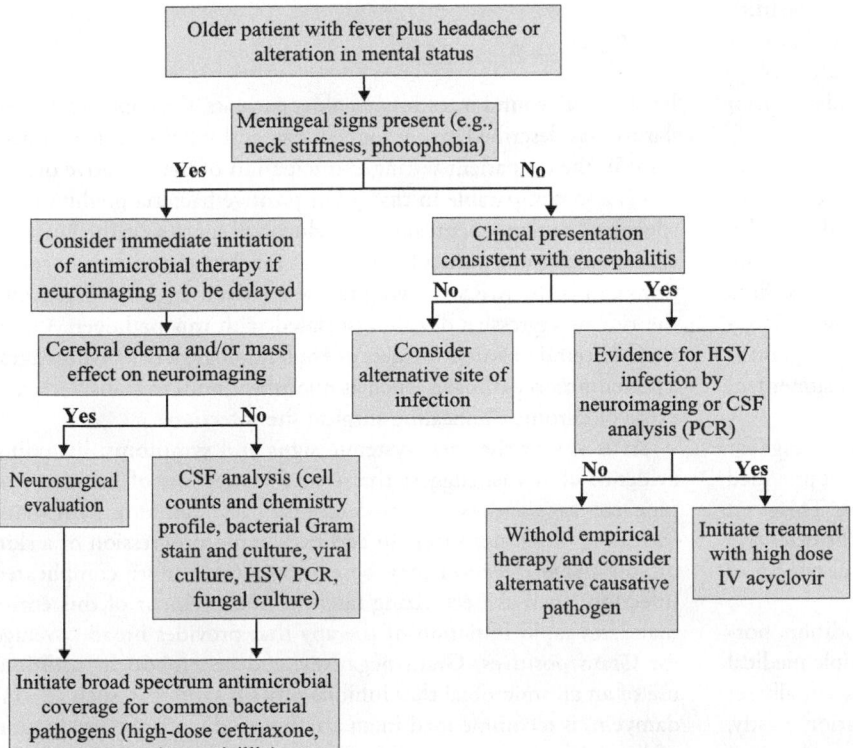

FIGURE 125-2. Approach to the older patient with suspected CNS infection.

clinical signs and symptoms as well as CSF cell counts, protein and glucose levels) is consistent with viral meningitis, antibacterial therapy should be discontinued so as to minimize the exposure to these potentially toxic drugs.

Encephalitis

In an older patient with fever and focal neurological signs and/or change in sensorium who lacks definitive clinical, physical examination or laboratory evidence for meningeal infection, the diagnosis of encephalitis must be considered swiftly. As was true for meningitis, prompt initiation of antimicrobial therapy may be critical to the recovery of affected individuals.

HSV encephalitis remains a prevalent cause of CNS infection among older patients. Clinicians should remain vigilant for the diagnosis, even in patients without other evidence of herpes virus infection or a known history of prior cutaneous involvement. Suspicion for this etiology is strengthened by characteristic in the temporal lobes visualized on MRI. Confirmatory diagnosis requires detection of HSV DNA by PCR of the spinal fluid. Because this testing may take several days in some centers, therapy should be initiated upon first suspicion of infection. The optimal therapy is parenteral acyclovir, which should be continued for 2 to 3 weeks.

Healthcare-Associated Infections

The approach to antimicrobial therapy for the older patient infected as a consequence of hospitalization or other contact with the healthcare system is sufficiently unique to warrant separate consideration. The same general themes that have been discussed regarding the management of other infections in the older adults apply to the special case of healthcare-associated infections. Clinical features of the patient's presentation and epidemiological clues should be integrated to deduce the most likely causative pathogen. Specimens should be collected expeditiously for microbiological testing prior to the initiation of antimicrobial therapy if possible. Finally, the overall severity of infection, along with understanding of the unique pharmacological challenges of treating older patients should be considered prior to the final decision regarding antimicrobial treatment.

The goal in all cases of suspected healthcare-associated infection is to determine the likely pathogen responsible for the patient's signs and symptoms. For hospitalized patients, the anticipated microbiology will be influenced not only by the actual site of infection, but by the geographical and temporal trends in antimicrobial flora and susceptibility within the institution itself. Integrating epidemiological and microbiological data from the hospital antibiogram is critical to the selection of empirical therapy for the treatment of healthcare-associated infections in the older adults.

In general, the breadth and intensity of antimicrobial coverage for hospitalized older patients will tend to be greater than that provided to even debilitated older patients in the outpatient setting. This need for broader, more potent therapy is a consequence of the extensive comorbid conditions and generally poorer physiological reserve of hospitalized older patients.

In addition to their generally weakened physical condition, hospitalized older patients are commonly exposed to multiple medical interventions. As a result, the risk of complicated and potentially severe drug interactions is greatly increased in this population. Lastly, because of comorbid conditions or other therapies, the volume of distribution, renal and hepatic clearance and other pharmacokinetic parameters may be significantly altered when older patients are hospitalized.

Healthcare-Associated Pneumonia

The microbiology of respiratory infection among hospitalized patients is fairly distinct when compared to that associated with community-acquired pneumonia. Specifically, commensal gram-positive and anaerobic bacteria are replaced by Enterobacteriaceae, including *E. coli* and *Klebsiella* spp, after an older patient is hospitalized for several days. Such changes in the oral flora coupled with the possibility of aspiration of oral contents into the lower respiratory tract should lead to the inclusion of therapy active against Enterobacteriaceae in an empirical regimen for healthcare-associated pneumonia. Agents with activity against *P. aeruginosa* are generally included as well because of the relatively high incidence and clinical severity of nosocomial infection caused by this organism. MRSA is also seen increasingly commonly in healthcare-associated pneumonia. Finally, while patients with witnessed or high-risk for aspiration generally are prescribed an antimicrobial agent with activity against oral anaerobes, the available literature and recent guidelines do not specifically support this intervention.

The specific choice and breadth of antimicrobial therapy will be strongly influenced by the severity of the patient's pneumonia. Common choices include combination β-lactam/β-lactamase inhibitors such as piperacillin/tazobactam, ceftazidime, and combinations of third-generation cephalosporins with fluoroquinolones. Vancomycin or linezolid should be included when there is concern for MRSA involvement. Recent guidelines have recommended a 7-day course of therapy for healthcare-associated pneumonia not caused by *P. aeruginosa*. Extending therapy to 10 to 14 days may be reasonable in individuals with poor baseline health or particularly severe manifestations of pneumonia.

Skin and Soft Tissue Infections

For surgical wound infections in older patients, the approach is similar to that described earlier for cellulitis and other soft tissue infections in the outpatient setting. Anticipation of the causative organism is also comparable in that gram-positive bacteria predominate, specifically streptococcal and staphylococcal species. In the hospital, clinicians must be particularly vigilant for skin and soft tissue infections caused by MRSA, owing to the relatively high incidence and the risk of aggressive disease associated with this pathogen. Occasionally certain clinical features or epidemiological clues will suggest a less common pathogen (such as nontuberculous mycobacteria as a cause of chronic nonhealing surgical site infection).

As is always the case, systemic signs and symptoms, including evidence of sepsis, suggest the need for selection of broader empiric coverage and even consideration of less common pathogens, including Gram negatives. In addition, rapid progression of a skin or soft tissue infection may be evidence for a more complicated infection, such as necrotizing fasciitis. Management of this entity mandates rapid initiation of therapy that provides broad coverage for Gram positives, Gram negatives, and anaerobes. In addition, use of an antimicrobial that inhibits protein synthesis, such as clindamycin, is recommended in an attempt to disrupt the production of bacterial toxins responsible for this potentially life-threatening infection.

TABLE 125-9

Antimicrobial Agents with Activity Against MRSA

	ROUTE OF ADMINISTRATION	NOTES
Trimethoprim/sulfamethoxazole, clindamycin, doxycycline	Orally or IV	Effective against many strains of community-associated MRSA. Ineffective against most hospital-acquired MRSA.
Vancomycin	Orally only (for systemic treatment)	Widely effective against nearly all MRSA strains isolated to date. Requires therapeutic monitoring to ensure efficacy and avoid toxicity
Daptomycin	IV only	Not effective for primary pulmonary infections
Linezolid	Orally or IV	Demonstrated effectiveness in skin and soft tissue infections. Associated with thrombocytopenia when administered for extended duration

While the optimal therapeutic regimen for patients with skin and soft tissue infection is subject to debate, a regimen with broad efficacy against gram-positive cocci and MRSA is requisite (see Table 125-9). Historically, the most common choice has been vancomycin. Familiar agents, such as clindamycin, trimethoprim-sulfamethoxazole, and minocycline, can be utilized for their activity against MRSA, but may have toxicities or limitations in coverage against streptococci, in the case of trimethoprim-sulfamethoxazole, that limit their use in all situations. The role to be played by newer agents such as linezolid and daptomycin remains to be seen. The toxicity and expense associated with these agents may preclude their use as the first choice of therapy. Additionally, it is recommended that linezolid not be used in combination with selective serotonin reuptake inhibitors (SSRIs) because of the concern for precipitating the serotonin syndrome. Duration of therapy typically mirrors that for nonhealthcare-associated skin and soft tissue infections—approximately 2 weeks—but in general, should be guided by the patient's response to treatment.

Urinary Tract Infection

Choosing antimicrobial therapy for healthcare-associated infections of the urinary tract presents several unique challenges. Standard culture methods enable detection of bacteria in the urine of hospitalized patients with a high sensitivity. In fact, the high sensitivity of culture results may even prove to be misleading. A large proportion of urine samples obtained from hospitalized older patients, particularly those with bladder catheters, may be found to be colonized with bacteria. In several studies, the prevalence of bacteriuria among catheterized patients has been found to approach 100% after 1 month with the catheter. As a result of these issues, in the setting of a sepsis-like syndrome occurring in an older hospitalized patient with bacterial growth in the urine as the sole evidence for the urinary tract as the primary site of infection, it is recommended that the search continue for a definitive source. Multiple cultures of the blood are essential to the informed management of such patients.

There are few unique clinical or epidemiological factors that influence appropriate selection of empiric antimicrobial therapy for older hospital patients with known or suspected urinary tract infection. For the most part, the antimicrobial regimen should include coverage for the Enterobacteriaceae that are most commonly associated with ascending urinary tract infections. Among the available agents, those that concentrate in the urine are particularly useful. Fluoroquinolones are frequently utilized in this capacity, although the rise of resistance to these agents mandates that therapy be guided by the bacterial susceptibility results obtained from urine cultures. A 3-day duration is appropriate for uncomplicated bladder infections.

However, in older hospitalized patients, the urinary tract infection will often be considered "complicated," necessitating a prolongation of therapy to 2 weeks.

Bacteremia

Bloodstream infection in hospitalized older patients can arise as a primary event affecting only the bloodstream or as a secondary manifestation of infection at a specific body site, such as bacteremic pneumococcal pneumonia. Among the former group, bloodstream infections complicating intravascular access devices remain most common. In all cases, the most common pathogens tend to be streptococci or staphylococci. However, when the endogenous flora that normally colonizes the skin and digestive tract of older patients are replaced by hospital-acquired pathogens, the diversity of pathogens causing bloodstream infection expands to include gram-negative bacteria and fungi.

Principal among the clinical and epidemiological factors that might influence the choice of empiric therapy is the detection of a primary site of infection in these patients. If infection of the lung, bladder, or a surgical wound is detected, therapy should be chosen to cover those pathogens most commonly associated with infection of that specific body site. Alternatively, clinical evidence of infection of a vascular access device, such as drainage or inflammation at a catheter insertion site, supports the diagnosis of a primary bloodstream infection. Most such cases, as has already been noted, will be caused by common gram-positive organisms.

Empiric coverage should generally be guided by the Gram stain or preliminary culture results. For gram positives, vancomycin should be used while awaiting identification and antimicrobial susceptibility testing, assuming that there is a high institutional prevalence of MRSA. For gram-negative pathogens, coverage should be informed by local antibacterial susceptibility trends as reported in an institutional antibiogram. The use of double coverage for gram-negative pathogens (and specifically for infection with *P. aeruginosa*) remains controversial. There is little direct evidence indicating a benefit of protracted coverage with more than one agent once final susceptibility results are available.

The optimal duration of therapy for bloodstream infection in the hospitalized older patient remains somewhat uncertain, but is influenced by whether or not the bacteremia is associated with a removable focus of infection. For patients with infected vascular access devices, best practice dictates the removal of the infected line. If this step is completed in a timely fashion, clinicians may opt to treat for as little as 7 to 14 days. However, this less intensive strategy would not be appropriate for patients with more complicated infection, including those with heart valve involvement or those with evidence of metastatic spread of infection, who may require several weeks of therapy.

FURTHER READING

Faulkner CM, Cox HL, Williamson JC. Unique aspects of antimicrobial use in older adults. *Clin Infect Dis.* 2005;40:997–1004.

Guerrant RL, Van Gilder T, Steiner TS, et al. Practice guidelines for the management of infectious diarrhea. *Clin Infect Dis.* 2001;32:331–350.

High K, Bradley S, Loeb M, Palmer R, Quagliarello V, Yoshikawa T. A new paradigm for clinical investigation of infectious syndromes in older adults: assessing functional status as a risk factor and outcome measure. *J Am Geriatr Soc.* 2005;53:528–535.

Kaye KS, Schmader KE, Sawyer R. Surgical site infection in the elderly population. *Clin Infect Dis.* 2004;39:1835–1841.

Khayr WF, CarMichael MJ, Dubanowich CS, Latif RH. Epidemiology of bacteremia in the geriatric population. *Am J Ther.* 2003;10:127–131.

Mader JT, Shirtliff ME, Bergquist S, Calhoun JH. Bone and joint infections in the elderly: practical treatment guidelines. *Drugs Aging.* 2000;16(1):67–80.

Mandell GL, Bennet JE, Dolin R, eds. *Principles and Practice of Infectious Diseases.* Philadelphia, PA: Churchill Livingstone, 2000.

Mandell LA, Wunderink RG, Anzueto A, et al., Infectious Diseases Society of America, American Thoracic Society. Infectious Diseases Society of America/American Thoracic Society consensus guidelines on the management of community-acquired pneumonia in adults. *Clin Infect Dis.* 2007;44(Suppl 2):S27–S72.

McCue JD. Antibiotic use in the elderly: issues and nonissues. *Clin Infect Dis.* 1999;28:750–752.

Mody L, Sun R, Bradley SF. Assessment of pneumonia in older adults: effect of functional status. *J Am Geriatr Soc.* 2006;54:1062–1067.

Nicolle LE, Bentley DW, Garibaldi R, Neuhaus EG, Smith PW. Antimicrobial use in long-term-care facilities. *Infect Control Hosp Epidemiol.* 2000;21:537–545.

Ross JJ. Septic arthritis. *Infect Dis Clin N Am.* 2005;19:799–817.

Ruhe JJ, Smith N, Bradsher RW, Menon A. Community-onset methicillin-resistant *Staphylococcus aureus* skin and soft-tissue infections: impact of antimicrobial therapy on outcome. *Clin Infect Dis.* 2007;44:777–784.

Simor AE, Bradley SF, Strausbaugh LJ, Crossley K, Nicolle LE, SHEA Long-Term-Care Committee. *Clostridium difficile* in long-term-care facilities for the elderly. *Infect Control Hosp Epidemiol.* 2002;23:696–703.

Weisfelt M, van de Beek D, Spanjaard L, Reitsma JB, de Gans J. Community-acquired bacterial meningitis in older people. *J Am Geriatr Soc.* 2006;54:1500–1507.

Whitley RJ. Herpes simplex encephalitis: adolescents and adults. *Antiviral Res.* 2006;71:141–148.

Yoshikawa TT. Antimicrobial resistance and aging: beginning of the end of the antibiotic era? *J Am Geriatr Soc.* 2002;50:S226–S229.

Yoshikawa TT. Epidemiology and unique aspects of aging and infectious diseases. *Clin Infect Dis.* 2000;30:931–933.

Zimmerli W, Trampuz A, Ochsner PE. Prosthetic-joint infections. *N Engl J Med.* 2004;351:1645–1654.

Pneumonia

Thomas J. Marrie

Pneumonia is a common, expensive (in 2002, the total cost was $8 billion to treat pneumonia in the United States), and often serious infection with considerable morbidity and mortality. The major burden of pneumonia in a community is borne by the elderly. Successful management of pneumonia, in any patient, but especially in the elderly requires considerable skills.

DEFINITIONS

From the viewpoint of the pathologist, pneumonia is an inflammatory response in the lung caused by an infectious agent that involves the alveoli and terminal bronchioles. It is manifested by increased weight of the lungs, replacement of the normal lung sponginess by consolidation and alveoli filled with white blood cells, red blood cells, and fibrin (Figures 126-1 and 126-2).

The clinician defines pneumonia as a combination of symptoms (fever, chills, cough, pleuritic chest pain, sputum), signs (hyper or hypothermia, increased respiratory rate, dullness to percussion, bronchial breathing, aegophony, crackles, wheezes, pleural friction rub), and an opacity (opacities) on a chest radiograph (Figure 126-3). In addition, laboratory findings; such as, increased white blood cell count and decreased level of oxygen saturation, may also be part of the definition.

The epidemiologist or clinical trialist defines pneumonia as two or more of the symptoms listed above, one or more of the physical findings listed above and a new opacity on chest radiograph that is not because of a condition other than pneumonia (such as, congestive heart failure, vasculitis, pulmonary infarction, atelectasis, or drug reaction).

Pneumonia may also be categorized according to the site of acquisition—community, hospital (nosocomial) or nursing home. Some authorities categorize nursing home acquired pneumonia as community-acquired, while others insist it more closely resembles nosocomial pneumonia and should be labeled institutionally ac-

quired pneumonia. However, nursing homes or long-term care facilities have residents who range from fully functional to those who are bedridden. We prefer to consider nursing home/long-term care facility acquired pneumonia as a separate category.

It is useful for the practicing clinician to remember definitions for the certainty with which an agent can be implicated as the cause of the pneumonia. An agent is said to be the definite cause of pneumonia if it is isolated from blood (although some blood isolates, such as coagulase negative staphylococci, are usually contaminants and not pulmonary pathogens), from pleural fluid or from pulmonary tissue; if it isolated from sputum and is a pathogen that does not colonize the upper airway (such as *Mycobacterium tuberculosis; Legionella* spp.; *Nocardia* spp.*)*; or if a microbial antigen is detected in urine (*Streptococcus pneumoniae; Legionella pneumophila*). Amplification of DNA or RNA of a microbial agent from pulmonary tissue or from nasopharyngeal secretions if that agent does not colonized the upper airway would allow categorization of the agent as the definite cause of the pneumonia. An agent is the presumptive or probable cause of pneumonia if it is isolated from a sputum sample which has >25 polymorphonuclear leucocytes per low power field and <10 squamous epithelial cells or if there is a fourfold or greater rise in antibody titer between acute and convalescent serum samples. Amplification of DNA or RNA of a viral agent from nasopharyngeal secretions would qualify that agent for status as a possible cause of the pneumonia.

EPIDEMIOLOGY

Data from the National Hospital Discharge Survey in the United States indicate that between 1990 and 2002 there were 21.4 million hospitalizations among those 65 years of age and older. Infectious diseases accounted for 48% of these hospitalizations and 46% of the infectious diseases hospitalizations were caused by the lower respiratory tract infections. Death resulting from these infections was

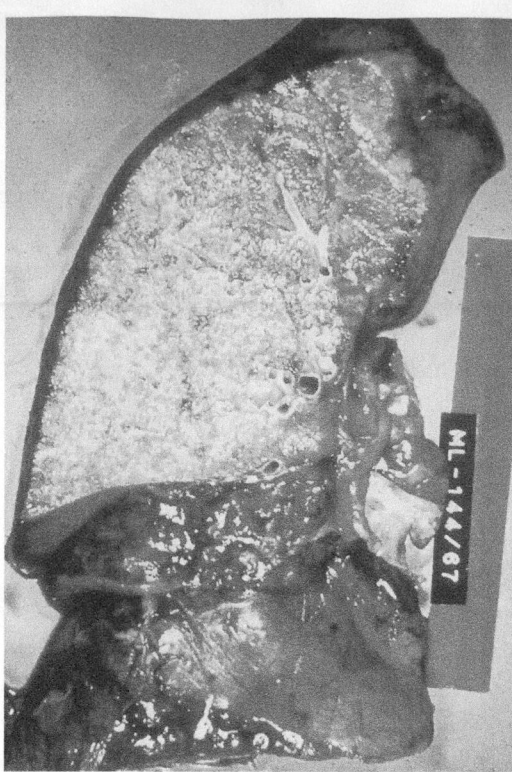

FIGURE 126-1. Photograph of a lung with pneumonia (white area) involving the entire upper lobe.

reported to be 48%. There has been a 20% increase in pneumonia as a first or any listed diagnosis in those 65 years of age and older from 1988 compared to 2002. The in-hospital mortality rate was 1.5 times higher for pneumonia compared with the other most common causes of hospitalization.

Pneumonia and influenza are listed as the 6th leading cause of death, and approximately 70% of hospitalized cases of pneumonia among adults occur in the elderly. Annual hospitalization rates for pneumonia and influenza were 23.1 per 1000 men aged 75 to 84 years of age and 13.3 per 1000 women in this age group. The cor-

responding numbers for men and women, respectively, in the 65 to 74 age group were 8.3 and 5.8 per 1000. Approximately 60% of the episodes of pneumonia among those 65 years of age and older are treated in the community. The admission rate for pneumonia is subject to considerable variation from region to region within a province or state and even from hospital to hospital within a single city. This variation cannot be explained solely on the basis of severity of illness and likely reflects variation in physician practice.

In a population-based study the following were identified as independent risk factors for community-acquired pneumonia: alcoholism, relative risk (RR) 9; asthma, RR 4.2; immunosuppression, RR 1.9; and age, RR 1.5 for those >70 years of age (vs. 60–69 years of age).

The overall mortality rate for patients with community acquired pneumonia (CAP) who require admission to hospital ranges from 6% to 15%. For those who require admission to an intensive care unit (ICU) for treatment of pneumonia, the mortality rate ranges from 45% to 57%. The annual per capita cost of pneumonia from an employer perspective is five times higher than the costs for typical beneficiaries. For elderly patients there is a burden of care for family members.

In an effort to determine the risk factors for pneumonia, investigators studied 101 patients aged ≥65 years old who were admitted with CAP, each patient with pneumonia was age and sex matched with a control subject who arrived at emergency within ± 2 days of the case and was subsequently admitted. By multivariate analysis, the following were identified as risk factors for pneumonia—suspected aspiration, low serum albumin, swallowing disorder, and poor quality of life. Significant predictors of a fatal outcome were bedridden state prior to onset of pneumonia; temperature ≤37°C; presence of a swallowing disorder; respiratory rate ≥30 breaths/minute; shock; creatinine greater than 1.4 mg/dL and ≥3 lobes involved on chest radiograph.

The attack rate for pneumonia in adults is highest among those residing in nursing homes with rates of 1.2 episodes of pneumonia per 1000 resident days. Pneumonia is the leading reason for transfer of nursing home patients to hospital. In many areas, nursing home/long-term care facility acquired pneumonia accounts for

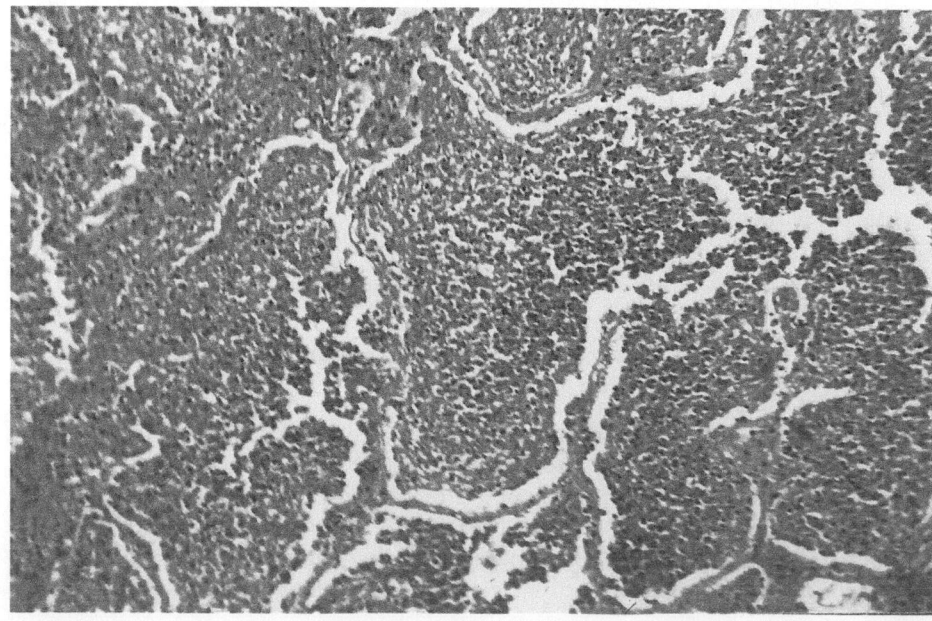

FIGURE 126-2. Photomicrograph of lung showing alveoli filled with inflammatory exudate. Magnification: 445x.

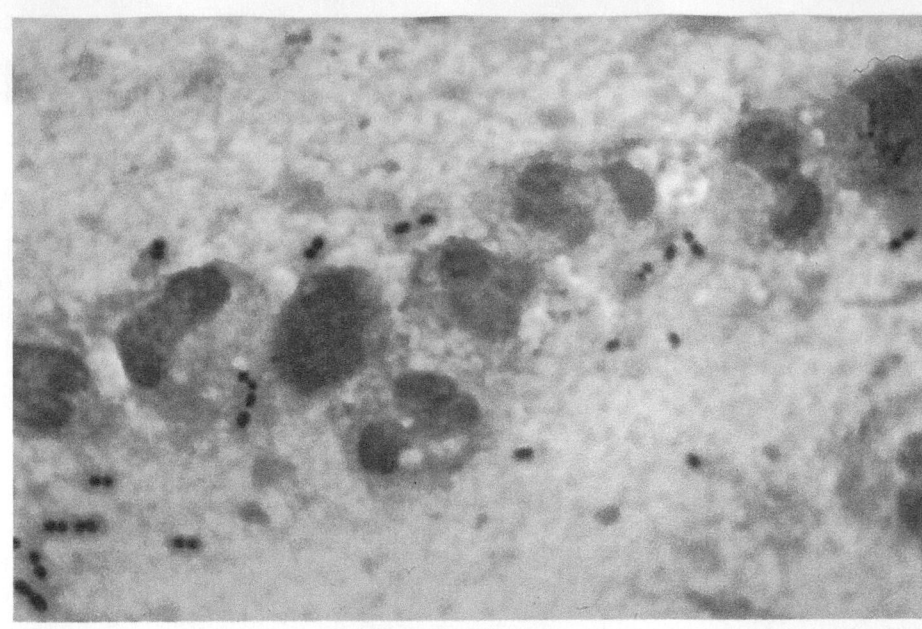

FIGURE 126-3. Gram stain sputum showing many polymorphonuclear leucocytes and gram-positive diplococci (*S. pneumoniae* was recovered on culture of this specimen). Magnification: 1000x.

10% to 18% of all pneumonia admissions. Lower respiratory tract infections are the fourth most common infection among residents of long term care facility (LTCFs) affecting 2.1% of the residents. In a nursing home population, old age, odds ratio (OR) 1.7; male sex OR 1.9; swallowing difficulty, OR 2; and inability to take oral medication were significant risk factors for pneumonia. In another study, profound disability (Karnofsky score of <10), bedfast state, urinary incontinence, presence of a feeding tube, or deteriorating health status were risk factors for pneumonia in this setting.

For specific etiologies of pneumonia, risk factors may differ from those for pneumonia as a whole. Thus, dementia, seizures, congestive heart failure, cerebrovascular disease, tobacco smoking, and chronic obstructive lung disease are risk factors for pneumococcal pneumonia. Fifty percent of patients with bacteremic pneumococcal pneumonia were homozygous for $Fc\gamma RIIa$-R31, which binds weakly to IgG_2, compared with 29% of uninfected controls suggesting that genetic factors may also be important risk factors for pneumococcal pneumonia.

Among HIV-infected patients the rate of pneumococcal pneumonia is up to 41.8 times higher than age matched patients who are not HIV-infected. Risk factors for Legionnaires' disease (LD) include male gender, tobacco smoking, diabetes, hematologic malignancy, cancer, end stage renal disease and HIV infection.

Both attack rates and mortality rates caused by pneumonia are highest in the winter months.

In a large study of 3474 adults hospitalized for the treatment of CAP, the mean length of stay (LOS) was 8.6 ± 6.3 days and the median LOS was 6.4 days. Patients were divided into those who stayed <7 days versus those who stayed >7 days and factors associated with these LOS were examined by multivariate analysis. Older age, ex-smoker status, home care prior to admission, reduced pre-morbid functional status and longer time to first dose of antibiotic were all associated with a longer stay. In contrast male gender, pathway use (refers to use of a critical pathway for treating CAP), residence at home without home care and shorter time to receipt of first dose of antibiotic were associated with a shorter stay. LOS was also independently associated with the hospital to which the patient was admitted. Thus, there are patient, institution, and physician factors that influence LOS in elderly patients with CAP.

ETIOLOGY

There are more than 100 microbial (bacteria, viruses, fungi, protozoa, and other parasites) causes of community-acquired pneumonia. *S. pneumoniae* is the most common cause of CAP accounting for approximately 50% of all cases. Advances in technology such as multiplex polymerase chain reaction are changing our knowledge of the etiology of pneumonia. It is apparent that viral pneumonia is more common in adults than was previously thought and in many instances a viral upper respiratory tract infection impairs ciliary clearance and pneumonia results from microaspiration of oropharyngeal microflora. Table 126-1 gives the most common causes of CAP. Table 126-2 identifies clues that might be obtained from the history to suggest a particular organism(s) as the cause of the pneumonia. It is important to remember that the relative frequency of each pathogen may vary geographically and seasonally. Many elderly persons travel

TABLE 126-1

Most Common Causes of Community-Acquired Pneumonia in the Older Adults

1. *S. pneumoniae*
2. *C. pneumoniae*
3. *Enterobacteriaceae*
4. *L. pneumophila* serogroups 1–6
5. *Haemophilus influenzae*
6. *Moraxella catarrhalis*
7. *S. aureus*
8. *Influenza A virus*
9. *Influenza B virus*
10. *Respiratory syncytial virus*
11. *Legionella* spp.
12. *M. tuberculosis*
13. HMPV
14. *Pneumocystis jiroveci*
15. Nontuberculous mycobacteria
16. *M. pneumoniae*
17. Hantavirus

TABLE 126-2

Clues to the Etiology of Pneumonia

FACTOR	POSSIBLE AGENT(S)
Travel	
Southeast Asia	*Burkholderia pseudomallei* (melioidosis); *M.tuberculosis*
Many countries	*M. tuberculosis*
Arizona, parts of California	*C. immitis*
Occupational History	
Health care workers	*M. tuberculosis*, acute HIV seroconversion with pneumonia (if recent needlestick injury from an HIV positive patient)
Veterinarian, farmer, abattoir worker	*C. burnetii*
Host Factor	
Diabetic ketoacidosis	*S. pneumoniae, S. aureus*
Alcoholism	*S. pneumoniae, Kelbsiella pneumoniae, S. aureus*, oral anaerobes; *Acinetobacter* spp.
Chronic obstructive lung disease	*S. pneumoniae, H. influenzae, Moraxella catarrhalis*
Solid organ transplant recipient	*S. pneumoniae, H. influenzae, Legionella* spp., *P. jiroveci*, (pneumonia occuring >3 mo *cytomegalovirus, Strongyloides stercoralis* after transplant)
Sickle cell disease	*S. pneumoniae*
HIV infection and CD4 cell count of <200/μL	*S. pneumoniae, P. jirovecii, H. influenzae, Cryptococcus neoformans, M. tuberculosis, Rhodococcus equi*
Dementia, stroke, altered level of consciousness	Aspiration pneumonitis
Structural lung disease (bronchiectasis)	*Pseudomonas aeruginosa*
Environmental Factors	
Exposure to: contaminated air conditioning, cooling towers, hot tub, recent travel stay in a hotel, exposure to grocery store mist machine, or visit to, or recent stay in a hospital with contaminated (by *Legionellaceae*) drinking water	*L. pneumophila* or other *Legionellaceae*
Exposure to: mouse droppings in an endemic area	Hantavirus
Pneumonia after windstorm in an area	*C. immitis* of endemicity
Outbreak of pneumonia in shelter for homeless men or jail	*S. pneumoniae, M. tuberculosis*
Outbreak of pneumonia occurs in military training camp	*S. pneumoniae, C. pneumoniae*, Adenovirus
Outbreak of pneumonia in a nursing home	*C. pneumoniae , S. pneumoniae*, Respiratory syncytial virus, Influenza A virus; *M. tuberculosis*
Pneumonia associated with mowing a lawn in an endemic area	*Francisella tularensis*
Exposure to bats, excavation or residence in an endemic area (Ohio and Mississippi river valleys)	*Histoplasma capsulatum*
Exposure to parturient cats in an endemic area	*C. burnetii*
Sleeping in a rose garden	*Sporothrix shenkii*
Camping, cutting down trees in an endemic area	*Blastomyces dermatiditis*

for pleasure, placing them at risk for a variety of pathogens (Table 126-2). Vacations in the sun to Arizona or parts of California can result in acquisition of the fungus *Coccidioides immitis* by inhalation. In most instances, the infection is asymptomatic. However, atypical pneumonia, hilar adenopathy or lung nodules may result. The latter are often misdiagnosed as carcinoma and the nodules excised. Elderly women who are receiving hormone replacement therapy may be at greater risk for the pulmonary nodule presentation of coccidioidomycosis. Legionellosis is also associated with travel.

S. pneumoniae

Worldwide *S. pneumoniae* continues to be the most common cause of CAP. It accounts for approximately 50% of all cases of pneumonia requiring admission to hospital for treatment and for 60% of all cases of bacteremic pneumonia. While there are more than 90 capsular polysaccharide types of *S. pneumoniae*, 80% of the strains that cause

invasive disease are present in the 23-valent-pneumococcal polysaccharide vaccine. These include serotypes 1, 2, 3, 4, 5, 6B, 7F, 9N, 9V, 10A, 11A, 12F, 14, 15B, 17F, 18C, 19A, 19F, 20, 22F, 23F, 33F. Vaccination of children with a 7-valent protein conjugate vaccine (contains serotypes 4, 6B, 9V, 14, 18C, 19F, 23F) has resulted in a decrease in invasive pneumococcal disease not only in children but also in elderly persons as well. Recently there has been emergence of outbreaks of invasive pneumococcal disease caused by serotype 5 among homeless adults.

One of the problems facing clinicians treating patients with CAP is drug-resistant *S. pneumoniae*. If an isolate is resistant to penicillin, it is likely also that it is resistant to three or more drug classes (multidrug resistant). Currently, 12% to 25% of *S. pneumoniae* isolates in North America are resistant to penicillin—approximately half demonstrate low-level resistance (minimal inhibitory concentration 0.1–1.0 mg/L) and half have high-level resistance (MIC ≥ 2 mg/L). In many communities, the levels of penicillin resistance are much higher than this. In the United States and Canada, approximately

20% of isolates of *S. pneumoniae* are resistant to erythromycin and the other macrolides. This resistance may be because of an efflux pump mechanism or to alteration of the target site of erythromycin action through a mutation in the *erm* gene. Approximately 70% of pneumococal erythromycin resistance in North America is as a result of an efflux pump mechanism and these isolates may respond to treatment with a macrolide. Isolates that are resistant as a result of the target site modification will not respond to treatment with a macrolide. Risk factors for penicillin-resistant *S. pneumoniae* (PRSP) include β-lactam antibiotic use within the previous 6 months; residence in a nursing home; residence in a day care center or being a parent of a resident in a day care center; and immunocompromised state. Age <5 years and nosocomial acquisition of the infection were independent predictions of macrolide resistance. Resistance among isolates of *S. pneumoniae* is also beginning to appear to fluoroquinolones, although at present it is uncommon with a 1% to 2% level of resistance. Risk factors for fluoroquinolone-resistant *S. pneumoniae* are presence of chronic obstructive pulmonary disease; nursing home residence; fluoroquinolone use within the last 12 months and nosocomial acquisition of the infection. More than 30% of *S.pneumoniae* isolates are resistant to trimethoprim-sulfamethoxazole and approximately 15% are resistant to tetracycline. In general, third-generation cephalosporins can be used to treat patients with drug-resistant *S. pneumoniae*. If central nervous system infection complicates the pneumonia, vancomycin should be added. Cefixime, cefibuten, cefaclor, and loracarbef have poor activity against *S. pneumoniae* and should not be used to treat pneumonia caused by this microorganism.

Early mortality (within the first 3 or 4 days) in patients with bacteremic pneumococcal pneumonia may not be influenced by antibiotic therapy. An APACHE II (the acute physiology and chronic health evaluation scoring system) score of ≥28 is associated with a mortality rate of 80% in patients with bacteremic pneumococcal pneumonia.

Staphylococcus aureus

Staphylococcus aureus is an uncommon cause of CAP, accounting for 1% to 5% of cases. However, it is approximately the third most frequent cause of bacteremic pneumonia and it is more common in patients with severe pneumonia who require treatment in an ICU. It is also more common as a cause of pneumonia among residents of long-term care facilities. *S. aureus* pneumonia has classically been described as a secondary bacterial pathogen in the setting of a primary influenza virus upper respiratory tract infection. In the setting of bacteremic *S. aureus* pneumonia one should always exclude endocarditis (often right sided), especially if there are multiple rounded opacities on the chest radiograph (septic emboli). Methicillin resistance (Methicillin-resistant *S. aureus* [MRSA]) among isolates of *S. aureus* was first reported in 1961 and is now common in both community and hospital acquired infections caused by this microorganism. Fortunately, vancomycin resistance, while it has been reported, is uncommon. More recently, community-acquired MRSA infections have been caused by strains producing the Panton-Valentine leukocidin (PVL). In 1932, Panton and Valentine described leukocidin as a virulence factor. Production of this leucocidin is now known to be associated with tissue necrosis. In one study, hemopytsis was found in 38% of 16 patients with severe pneumonia associated with *S. aureus* strains carrying PVL genes compared with 1 of 33 PVL negative patients. To date PVL *S. aureus* infections including pneumonia have been more common in young patients.

Chlamydophila pneumoniae

Chlamydophila pneumoniae is commonly implicated serologically as a cause of CAP. It is more frequent in those with chronic obstructive pulmonary disease. In the older adults, it usually manifests as reactivation of previous infection, while in younger adults it can be a primary infection. It is not necessary to include diagnostic studies for *C. pneumoniae* in working up a patient with CAP since in more than 50% of cases it is a copathogen and patients recover without specific treatment directed at *C. pneumoniae*. Outbreaks of pneumonia in nursing homes have been caused by this agent.

Mycoplasma pneumoniae

This microorganism is usually a cause of pneumonia in young adults; however, it can also cause pneumonia in older adults. It has rarely been responsible for outbreaks of pneumonia in nursing homes. *M. pneumoniae* has a number of extrapulmonary manifestations including—cold agglutinin induced hemolytic anemia; leukoerythrophagocytosis; encephalitis; cerebellar ataxia; stroke like syndromes; arthritis; erythema multiforme; and a maculopapular rash.

Legionnaires' Disease

The most common cause of LD is *L. pneumophila* serogroup 1, although just under half of the more than 40 recognized species in the Legionellaceae family can cause LD. *Legionella* spp. often cause a severe pneumonia with a high mortality rate. Epidemiologically, there is frequently a history of exposure to a contaminated water source. Outbreaks have been associated with exposure to a variety of aerosol-producing devices, including showers, a grocery store mist machine, cooling towers, whirlpool spas, decorative fountains, and evaporative condensers. It is also likely that aspiration of contaminated potable water by immunosuppressed patients is also a mechanism whereby *Legionella* is acquired. Outbreaks of pneumonia caused by *Legionella* spp. appear to be uncommon in nursing homes (but they have occurred) and are more likely to occur in a community or hospital setting. In the United States, rates of LD are higher in northern states and during the summer. From 1980 through 1998, there was a change in the methods of diagnosing LD in the US with a decline in the number of cases diagnosed by culture and direct fluorescent antibody test and serology and an increase in the number of cases diagnosed by the detection of antigen in the urine. These trends were associated with a decrease in the mortality rate from 26% to 10% for community-acquired cases and from 46% to 14% for nosocomial cases. Severe headache combined with hyponatremia are features that should raise a clinical suspicion of LD although the clinical features are usually not distinctive. *L. pneumophila* serogroup 1 accounts for most cases of LD in the United States. *Legionella longbeachae* accounts for 72% of the cases of LD in western Australia. In this area, cases have occurred in active gardeners and the organism has been isolated from potting soil. When patients with LD are compared with those with community-acquired pneumonia caused by other agents the patients with LD are more likely to have myalgias, headache, diarrhea, and a higher mean oral temperature at the time of presentation. They also present to hospital sooner after the onset of symptoms—4.7 days versus 7.7 days ($p = 0.02$). When patients with LD were compared with patients with bacteremic pneumococcal pneumonia the following features were associated with *L. pneumonia*—male sex, OR 4.6 95% confidence interval (CI) 1.48–14.5; heavy drinking 4.8 (1.39–16.42); previous β-lactam therapy 19.9 (3.47–114.2); axillary temperature >39 C 10.3 (2.71–38.84); myalgias 8.5 (2.35–30.74); gastrointestinal symptoms 3.5 (1.01–12.18). Negative associations included pleuritic chest pain, previous upper respiratory tract infection and purulent sputum.

In a study from Barcelona, 104 patients <65 years of age with LD were compared with the 54 patients who were older than 65 years of age. The older patients had more comorbidities and a greater likelihood of receiving corticosteroids while the younger patients were more likely to be male, smoke, have alcoholism and HIV. Fever, diarrhea and headache were less frequent in those older than 65 years of age. There was no difference in complications or requirement for mechanical ventilation. While the mortality rate was twice as high in the elderly, 11.2% versus 4.8%, the difference was not statistically significant.

Enterobacteriaceae

Enterobacteriaceae are commonly isolated from the sputum of elderly patients with CAP. The problem is distinguishing colonization from infection since these microorganisms commonly colonize the upper airway of elderly persons. Elderly patients who are bacteremic (usually secondary to pyelonephritis), with *Escherichia coli* in particular may have secondary seeding of the lungs.

M. tuberculosis

Nursing home residents account for 20% of cases of tuberculosis in older people. In the 1980s, approximately 12% of persons entering a nursing home were tuberculin positive, and active tuberculosis developed in 1% of isoniazid (INH) treated tuberculin positive patients compared with 2.4% of those who did not receive INH. The incidence of active tuberculosis among nursing home patients is 10 to 30 times greater than among community-dwelling elderly adults—thus, tuberculosis should always be considered in nursing home patients with pneumonia.

Viruses

There are a large number of viruses that affect the respiratory tract (predominately the upper respiratory tract). These include influenza A and B viruses; parainfluenza viruses 1,2,3,4; adenovirus; respiratory syncytial virus, human metapneumoviruses (HMPVs) A and B, severe acute respiratory syndrome (SARS) CoV, coronaviruses, hantaviruses and varicella. Viruses are estimated to be the cause of adult CAP in 10% to 31% of cases. In a prospective study of 338 nonimmunocompromised adults with a diagnosis of CAP in whom paired serology for respiratory viruses were obtained, 61 patients (18%) had a respiratory virus identified. Influenza virus was the most common (37 patients), followed by parainfluenza (11 patients), respiratory syncytial virus (5 patients), adenovirus (5 patients), and mixed viruses (3 patients). In most instances the virus infects the upper airway, impairs ciliary function so that bacteria which are microaspirated into the LRT are not cleared and bacterial pneumonia results.

Respiratory Syncytial Virus

In eight hospital-based studies of RSV-associated pneumonia in adults the rates of this infection ranged from 2% to 14% among the five studies that used complement fixation test to make the diagnosis and from 4% to 14% for the two studies that used an enzyme-linked immunoassay test. Direct fluorescent antibody testing of nasopharyngeal swabs for RSV should not be done in adults because of low sensitivity.

Human Metapneumovirus

HMPV was first described in 2001 in the Netherlands. HMPV can cause upper and lower respiratory tract infection in patients of all age groups, but symptomatic disease most often occurs in the young children or older adults. It is an emerging pathogen as a cause of CAP in adults in which it seems to behave like RSV.

Severe Acute Respiratory Syndrome

In November 2002, an outbreak of severe acute respiratory infection started in Guangdong Province in southern China and spread worldwide affecting more than 8000 persons. SARS was caused by a novel coronavirus that jumped the species barrier from civet cats to man. The case fatality rate of the 2003 Hong Kong outbreak was 11%, but higher mortality was seen in the elderly ($\geq$60 years of age) and pregnant women.

Other Coronaviruses

Human coronaviruses were first described in association with respiratory infections in 1935, but were largely ignored until the advent of SARS. HCoV-229E and HCoV-OC43 caused upper and lower respiratory tract infections prior to the SARS outbreaks. Since that time, human coronaviruses, HCoV-NL63 and CoV-HKU1 have been identified as additional etiologic agents in CAP.

Hantavirus

In May 1993, an outbreak of severe respiratory illness, caused by a previously unknown virus, Hantavirus, occurred in the southwestern United States. The illness was preceded by prodromal flu-like symptoms followed by noncardiogenic pulmonary edema. The virus accounting for the initial cases, Sin Nombre Virus, is spread to humans from infected mice. Subsequently other Hantaviruses have been found to cause Hantavirus pulmonary syndrome and the disease has been described in other parts of the United States, western Canada, and South America. It is important to recognize that Hantavirus does not cause pneumonia but instead causes an ARDS like picture, because of the host response to this virus.

Influenza A

Influenza continues to be a major cause of morbidity and mortality worldwide. Primary influenza pneumonia occurs when influenza virus infection directly involves the lung, typically producing a severe pneumonia. Influenza pneumonia occurs most frequently in certain groups of patients with underlying chronic illnesses who are classified as "high risk" for this infection. These high-risk groups include patients with heart or lung disease, diabetes mellitus, renal disease, hemoglobinopathy, or immunosuppression; residents of nursing homes or chronic care facilities; and otherwise healthy individuals older than 65 years of age.

The last major pandemic of influenza in 1918 caused the deaths of more than 20 million persons, and made almost 1 billion people ill. Epidemics of influenza typically occur during the winter months and are responsible for an average of 20,000 deaths per year in the United States.

There is increasing concern that we are on the verge of the next great pandemic. Health Canada predicts that 4.5–10.6 million Canadians will become clinically ill and 11,000 to 58,000 will die during the next pandemic. There is wide spread concern that the current strain of influenza A, H5N1 which has been circulating in South East Asia among birds with limited spread to humans will mutate and be the agent of the next pandemic. As of July 26, 2006, there had been 232 human cases and 134 deaths, a 57% mortality caused by this virus.

Aspiration Pneumonia

Aspiration pneumonia denotes two distinct clinical entities. (1) Aspiration pneumonitis: aspiration of gastric contents (usually sterile as long as there is gastric acid present) into the lungs with a resultant inflammatory response. (2) Pneumonia: aspiration of oropharyngeal flora into the lung with resultant bacterial infection.

In studies of medicare patients it was noted that the diagnosis of aspiration pneumonia increased 93.5% between 1991 and 1998. The mortality rate for patients with aspiration pneumonia was 23.1% compared with 7.6% for pneumococcal pneumonia. In elderly patients with CAP there is a high incidence of silent aspiration. Seventy-one percent of the elderly patients aspirated during sleep compared with 10% of control subjects. Just more than 28% of patients with Alzheimer's disease and 51% of those with a stroke aspirated when swallowing was tested using videofluoroscopy. Furthermore, feeding tube placement in patients shown to aspirate on videofluoroscopy was associated with increased rates of pneumonia and death over those who aspirated but did not receive such a tube. The manifestations of aspiration pneumonia vary according to the volume and the nature of the material aspirated. Gastric acid results in a chemical pneumonitis that can be very severe requiring assisted ventilation. There is an acute onset of dyspnea, tachypnea, bronchospasm, and cyanosis. The chest radiograph often shows diffuse opacities. Many elderly patients are achlorhydric, so this presentation may not occur in the elderly. Indeed clinically, aspiration pneumonitis is often indistinguishable from pneumonia in this population. A history or a witnessed account of an aspiration event (one or more of vomiting, coughing while eating, and displacement of a feeding tube, vomitus, or tube feeding on bed clothes or on the patient within 24 hours of the diagnosis of pneumonia) is present in only 40% of definite aspiration events among residents of a long-term care facility.

In the setting of aspiration of oropharyngeal contents if there is poor dental hygiene anaerobic bacteria may also be present and lung abscess is not uncommon. Particulate matter may be aspirated resulting in mechanical obstruction of the airway.

PATHOPHYSIOLOGY

There are three routes whereby pathogens gain access to the pulmonary parenchyma—hematogenous, airborne, and microaspiration. The latter is most common. Hematogenous spread may occur in the elderly patient bacteremic from a urinary tract source with secondary seeding of the lung. Most viruses and *Coxiella burnetii* cause infection via the airborne route. *Legionella* spp. may gain access to the lower respiratory tract via the airborne route or aspiration.

Once a pathogen is in an alveolus an inflammatory response is triggered. The pathogen serves as a chemoattractant for polymorphonuclear leucocytes. Pro-inflammatory mediators (tumor necrosis factor alpha, interleukins 1, 6) are liberated from the leucocytes amplifying the inflammatory response. Red blood cells, fibrin, and leucocytes fill the alveoli resulting in consolidation of the lung (see Figures 126-1 and 126-2). This inflammatory response results in fever, cough, purulent sputum, myalgia, and arthralgia, and if blood levels of the pro-inflammatory cytokines are high enough, septic shock ensues. In due course anti-inflammatory mediators, especially Il-10, are released leading to resolution of the inflammatory response.

Consolidation of the lung leads to dyspnea (as a result of decreased compliance) and hypoxemia. The latter is because of the ventilation-perfusion mismatch (consolidated lung is perfused but not ventilated).

PRESENTATION

Pneumonia may present with a sudden or insidious onset of symptoms. Table 126-3 gives the frequency of each symptom or sign of pneumonia at the time of presentation. Extrapulmonary symptoms such as nausea, vomiting, diarrhea, myalgia, and arthralgia are common. In one study, older patients with pneumonia complained of fewer symptoms than younger patients—patients aged 45 to 64, 65 to 74, and ≥ 75 years old had 1.4, 2.9 and 3.3 fewer symptoms than patients aged 18 to 44 years. Pneumonia can be one of the causes of insidious or nonspecific deterioration in general health and/or activities, for example, confusion or falls in the elderly; infection including pneumonia should be considered also as a cause of sudden deterioration of, or a slow recovery from, an existing primary disease in this group of patients. While these latter presentations are emphasized in teaching the care of the elderly, there is no data to indicate what percentage of elderly patients with pneumonia present in this fashion. A diagnosis of pneumonia based on physical examination has a sensitivity of 47% to 69% and a specificity of 58% to 75%; thus, a clinical diagnosis of pneumonia should be confirmed with a chest radiograph. Crackles, wheezes, and the signs of consolidation (dullness to percussion, bronchial breathing and aegophony) may be found. The most sensitive sign of pneumonia in an elderly adult is an increased respiratory rate (provided it is counted for 1 min) with a respiratory rate of >28 indicating severe pneumonia. The chest radiograph can be difficult to interpret in elderly patients, especially if it is a portable antero-posterior examination. There is at least a 25% inter-observer variation in the diagnosis of pneumonia in elderly patients on chest radiographs where one observer is a radiologist and the other is the attending physician. Computed tomography of the chest is very accurate for the diagnosis of pneumonia but obviously cannot be done on everyone in whom this entity is suspected.

TABLE 126-3

Frequency of Various Signs and Symptoms—Adults with Community-Acquired Pneumonia

SYMPTOMS AND SIGNS	%
Respiratory Symptoms	
Cough	85
Dyspnea	75
Sputum production	73
Pleuritic chest pain	57
Hemoptysis	20
Nonrespiratory Symptoms	
Fatigue	90
Fever	82
Anorexia	73
Chills	72
Sweats	70
Headache	50
Myalgia+	45
Nausea	40
Sore throat	29
Confusion	38
Vomiting	32
Diarrhea	30
Abdominal pain	29
Signs	
Altered mental status*	13
Respiratory rate ($\geq$30/min)	30
Heart rate ($\geq$125/min)	25
Temperature	
<35.0°C	0.7
$\geq$40.0°C	2.0
Systolic blood pressure, <90 mm Hg	5.9

*Altered mental status was defined as lethargy, stupor, coma or confusion representing an acute change from usual baseline state.

EVALUATION

Site of Care

The evaluation of a patient with pneumonia consists of an assessment of the severity of the pneumonia and use of this to guide the decision as to the optimal site of care—home, hospital (ICU or ward), or for those who are residents of a long-term care facility, whether to treat in the facility or transfer to hospital. A number of pneumonia specific severity of illness scoring systems have been developed (Tables 126-4 to 126-6). The pneumonia specific severity of illness scoring system

TABLE 126-4

British Thoracic Society Rule for Severity of Community-Acquired Pneumonia*

Respiratory rate >30 breaths/min
Diastolic BP <60 mm Hg
BUN >7 mM/L

*If 2 or more of the above are present, the pneumonia is severe and patient is likely to require admission to an ICU.

TABLE 126-5

CURB—65 Rule

Confusion
Urea >7 mM/L
Respiratory rate >30 breaths/min
Blood pressure: systolic <90 mm Hg or diastolic < 60 mm Hg
Age >65 yr
Assign one point for each when present
Mortality rate: 0–0.7%; 1–3.2%; 2–3%; 3–17%; 4–41.5%; 5–57%.

by Fine et al. predicts mortality. This system has been used to guide the admission decision—that is, all patients in classes I to III can be treated on an ambulatory basis while those who fall into classes IV and V should be admitted. However, subsequent experience has indicated that such an approach to the admission decision is flawed and the physician's judgment should be the most important element in the admission decision. The British Thoracic society rule (Table 126-4) is the simplest and accurately predicts pneumonia severity. It has been modified to become the CURB-65 rule (Table 126-5). More recently, Finnish investigators noted that acute aggravation of a coexisting illness (such as impairment of glucose control in diabetics or deterioration of congestive heart failure), a respiratory rate $\geq$25 breaths/minute, and a C-reactive protein level $\geq$100 were independently predictive of mortality. If none or 1 of these was present, the mortality rate was 2.2% while if all three were present it was 20%. It is noteworthy that a study designed to elucidate how physicians decided on the site of care for patients with pneumonia found the most common reason given for admitting a patient to hospital was that he or she looked sick. The problem with this approach is that there is a great deal of inter-observer variability in what constitutes "looks sick."

Transfer from a Nursing Home to Hospital

A number of studies have provided data to help us decide who should be transferred from a long-term care facility for the treatment of pneumonia. In one study the following were associated

TABLE 126-6

Severity of Nursing Home Pneumonia Scoring System

	SCORING POINTS
Respiratory rate >30	2
Pulse rate >125	1
Altered mental status	1
Dementia	1
Number of points	Mortality (%)
0	7.4
1	10.3
2	26.1
3	37.5
4	56.3
5	80

Data from Naughton BJ, Mylotte JM, Tayara A. Outcome of nursing home-acquired pneumonia: derivation and application of a practical model to predict 30-day mortality. J Am Geriatr Soc. 2000;48:1292.

TABLE 126-7

Criteria for Treatment of Pneumonia in a Nursing Home
Respiratory rate <30 breaths/min
Oxygen saturation ≥92% while breathing room air
Pulse rate <90 beats/min
Temperature 36.5°C to 38.1°C
Systolic and diastolic blood pressure within 10 mm Hg of usual readings
No feeding tube present
Conscious
Severity of pneumonia score 2 or less (see Table 126-6)
Availability of medical and nursing care
Wishes of patient and family

with failure of treatment of pneumonia in the nursing home: pulse rate >90 beats/minute; temperature >100.5° F; respiratory rate >30 breaths/minnute; feeding tube dependence and mechanically altered diets. If none of the above risk factors were present, the failure rate was 11%; while it was 23% for ≤2 and 59% when 3 or more of these risk factors were present. The model was not predictive of mortality. The authors of another study concluded that the following could be used as indicators of the need for hospitalization—very dependent for activities of daily living; low body temperature; decreased level of consciousness; and white blood cell count <5 or >20 × 10⁹/L. There was no significant difference in 30-day mortality rates between those initially treated in nursing homes (22%) and those initially treated in hospitals (31%); or between those treated with an oral regimen in the nursing home (21%) and those initially treated with an intramuscular antibiotic in nursing homes (25%). In a cluster randomized trial of 680 residents of 22 nursing homes with lower respiratory tract infections who were managed in the nursing home according to a clinical pathway or standard therapy, 10% of the 327 residents in the pathway were hospitalized compared with 22% in the standard therapy arm. There was no difference in mortality or health related quality of life between the two groups. However, there was a cost savings for just more than $1000 per resident treated.

Since nursing homes vary greatly in the facilities and nursing staff available to provide care to very ill patients, any decision that is made has to be done with the knowledge of available resources. The nursing home pneumonia severity of illness score in Table 126-6 and the criteria in Table 126-7 help in making the decision regarding who should be transferred from a long-term care facility to hospital for the treatment of pneumonia.

ICU Admission

Approximately 10% of patients admitted to hospital with pneumonia require intensive care. In this subgroup the mortality rate is approximately three times higher than the mortality rate for those patients with CAP who do not require intensive care. The decision to admit to an ICU is based on the severity of the pneumonia and often the need for mechanical ventilation (>50%); hemodynamic monitoring (30%); and shock (15%). Age alone should not be used to determine who is admitted to ICU. Elderly patients who require mechanical ventilation for the treatment of pneumonia can be weaned from the ventilator just as quickly as younger patients with pneumonia who require intubation, however, they require on

average 3 more days of ICU support and are more likely to require reintubation. ICU patients with pneumonia incur longer hospital stays (23 days vs. 9 days) and have a mortality rate that is approximately four times higher than patients with pneumonia who do not require ICU care.

Diagnostic and Therapeutic Evaluations

Diagnostic Evaluations

The specific evaluations that should be carried out for elderly patients with pneumonia are shown in Table 126-8. These are divided into three phases—those to be carried out in emergency department, in hospital and post discharge. The yield from blood cultures ranges from 6% to 15%. *S. pneumoniae* accounts for 60% of all cases of bacteremic CAP. *S. aureus* is the second most common cause of bacteremic CAP. The presence of *S. aureus* in the blood should prompt a search for endocarditis. MRSA is now quite common as a cause of community-acquired CAP. Aerobic gram-negative bacilli are the third most common cause of bacteremic CAP.

Sputum Gram stain and culture is perhaps the most controversial of all the diagnostic tests used in the evaluation of a patient with CAP for several reasons. Firstly, only approximately one-third of

TABLE 126-8

Evaluation of Elderly Patients with Pneumonia
I. In emergency department
Posterior-anterior and lateral chest radiographs
Blood cultures: two sets
Complete blood count (hemoglobin, white blood cell count, platelet count)
Electrolytes
Glucose
Creatinine
Blood urea nitrogen
Pulse oximetry: if the oxygen saturation is <92% (at sea level) or if patient has chronic obstructive pulmonary disease blood gas analysis should be done.
Sputum Gram stain and culture (do not withhold antibiotics waiting for patient to produce a sputum sample)
In selected patients: urine for legionella antigen and for pneumococcal antigen; sputum stain and culture for acid-fast bacilli; acute and convalescent serology; serum for testing for HIV infection; nasopharyngeal swab for direct detection of influenza A, B virus antigens; nasopharyngeal swab for detection of DNA of *Legionella* spp.; *M. pneumoniae*; *C. pneumoniae*.
II. In hospital
Daily assessment of pulse, temperature, respiratory rate, oxygenation status, and ability to eat and drink.
When the above parameters are stable asses functional and mental status.
Assess stability of comorbid illnesses.
Check for complications of pneumonia.
Check pneumococcal and influenza vaccination status and update if necessary.
If tobacco smoker offer access to smoking cessation programs.
III. Post discharge
Follow up chest radiograph to ensure that the pneumonia has cleared.
If pneumonia fails to clear radiographically, consider bronchoscopy.

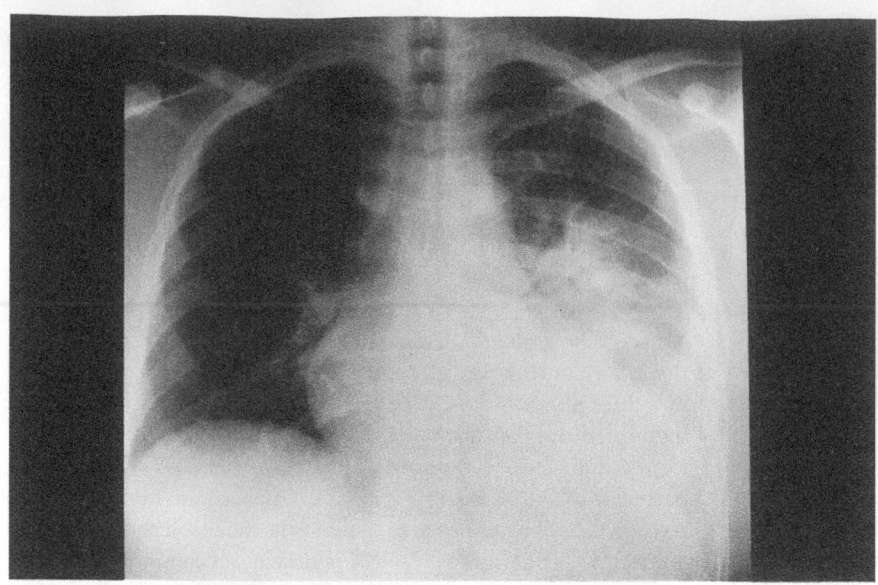

FIGURE 126-4. Chest radiograph showing left lower lobe opacity. This patient had Legionnaire's Disease.

elderly patients with pneumonia can provide an adequate sputum sample and one-third of these will yield a single pathogen; one-third yield multiple pathogens and one-third will be reported as negative or as showing oropharyngeal flora depending upon the reporting practice of the laboratory. The second problem is that the presence of a pathogen in sputum does not mean that it is in the lung and therefore the cause of the pneumonia. Nevertheless, sputum cultures should be done because a Gram stain on a good sputum specimen can give an immediate diagnosis (see Figure 126-3) and in some instances, a sputum stain and culture can be diagnostic such as with *M. tuberculosis* and in infection with *Nocardia* spp.

The chest radiograph is the gold standard for the diagnosis of pneumonia (Figures 126-4 to 26-8). Pneumonia on chest radiograph may be lobar, segmental or subsegmental and may be interstitial or alveolar. Remember that any disease that causes a pulmonary opacity can mimic pneumonia. Thus, pulmonary infarction, vasculitis, drug reactions, and pulmonary hemorrhage have been misdiagnosed

as pneumonia both clinically and radiographically. Suboptimal radiographs (portable single views) of elderly patients with suspected pneumonia are especially difficult to interpret. The inter- and intra-observer reliability of radiologists for the diagnosis of pneumonia is 80%.

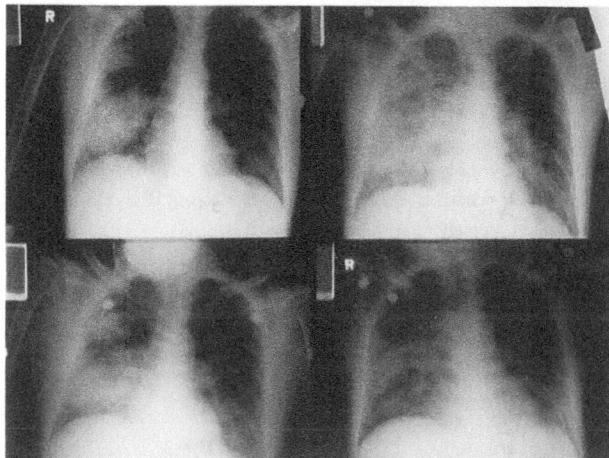

FIGURE 126-5. A series of chest radiographs of a patient with pneumococcal pneumonia. The upper-left radiograph shows right lower lobe opacity. The upper-right radiograph shows apparent progression of the pneumonia. At this time, the patient had an acute respiratory distress syndrome. Subsequent radiographs show resolution of the pneumonia.

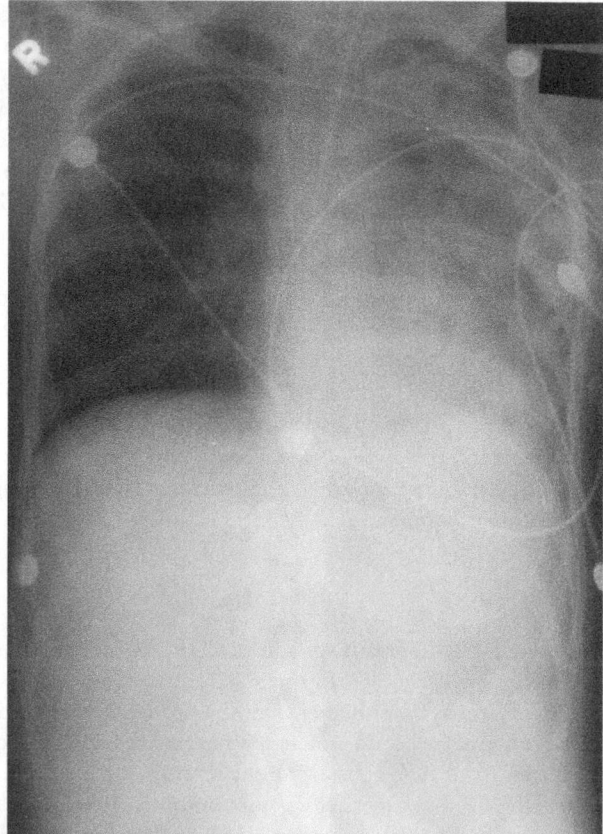

FIGURE 126-6. A chest radiograph showing diffuse opacification of the left lung. This patient, who had myotonic dystrophy, had a severe pneumonia caused by aspiration. Initially, this was a chemical pneumonitis but later nosocomial pneumonia developed.

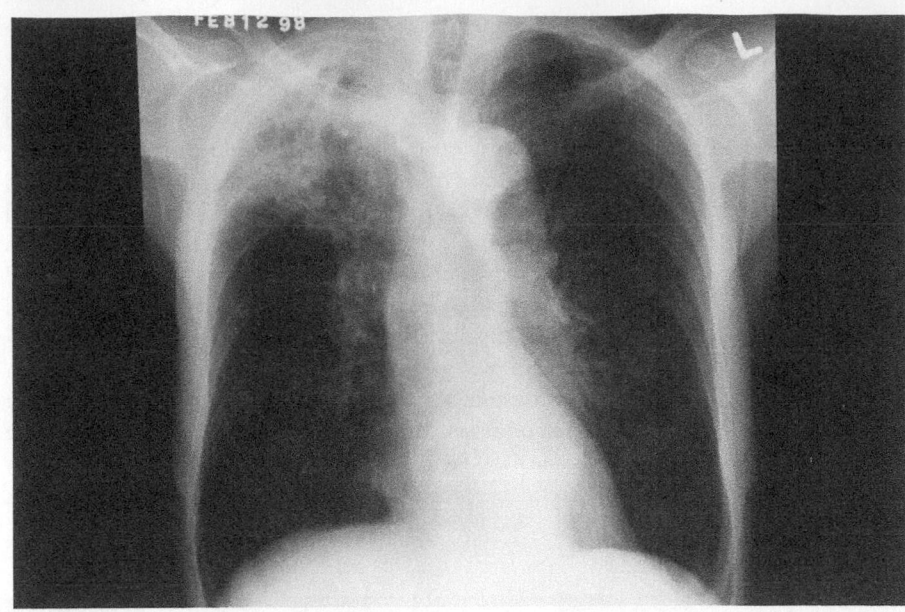

FIGURE 126-7. Chest radiograph showing patchy right upper lobe opacity. The clinical diagnosis was tuberculosis.

Legionella urinary antigen detects only *L. pneumophila* serogroup 1, for which it is 90% sensitive. However, it detects only approximately 60% of all cases of LD (since LD can be caused by *L. pneumophila* serogroups 2 to 6 and to many of the other species of Legionellaceae). Therefore, a negative test should not lead to a change in diagnosis or management if there is a strong clinical suspicion of LD.

An immunochromatic test is available to detect *S. pneumoniae* antigen in urine. This is done in a dipstick format with results available in 15 minutes. It is 80% sensitive when bacteremic pneumococcal pneumonia is used as the gold standard. The problem is defining the sensitivity and specificity of such tests in pneumonia where there is a presumptive diagnosis of pneumococcal pneumonia or in cases of pneumonia of unknown etiology. Currently, the test is best reserved for patients with severe pneumonia in whom blood cultures are negative and there is no sputum specimen available for culture.

Some authorities recommend drawing a blood sample for serology on all patients with pneumonia. A convalescent sample is drawn 2 to 6 weeks later. Serology remains the best way to diagnose pneumonia caused by Hantavirus, *C. burnetii* or *M. pneumoniae*.

Direct detection of influenza antigens in the upper airway is useful in making a rapid diagnosis of influenza and several commercial kits using direct immunofluoresence methodology (DFA) are available. It should be noted that a DFA assay on a nasopharyngeal swab is not useful for the detection of respiratory syncytial virus infection in adults. Amplification of DNA of respiratory pathogens from material collected via a nasopharyngeal swab using the polymerase chain reaction is useful for the diagnosis of LD. It can also be used to diagnose *Mycoplasma* or *Chlamydia* pneumonia. These latter two organisms may colonize the upper airway so detection of their DNA is only suggestive that they are the cause of the pneumonia. Multiplex nucleic acid amplification tests are now available so that a

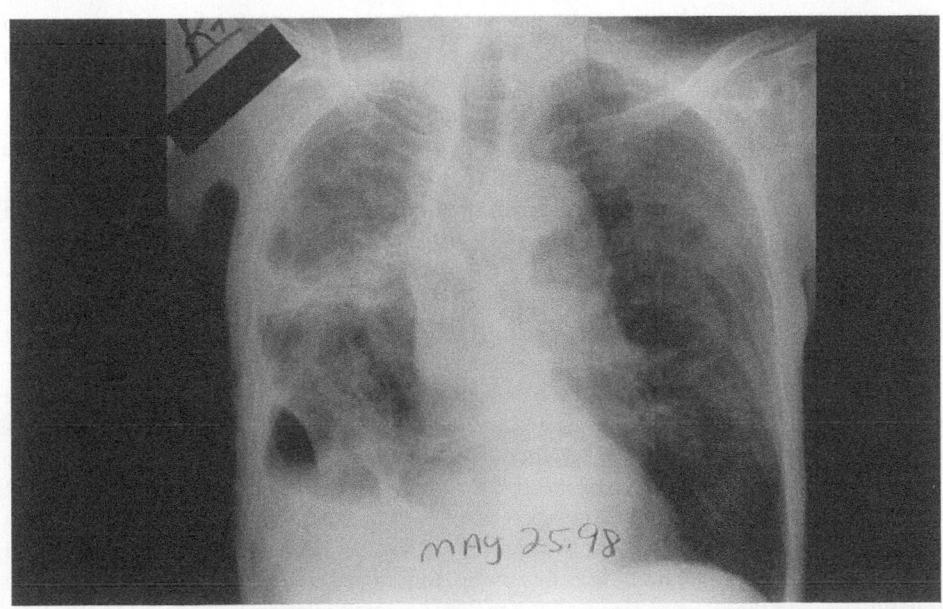

FIGURE 126-8. Chest radiograph of the same patient as in Figure 126-7 but approximately 3 months later. The patient did not respond to antituberculous therapy and was readmitted with weight loss, clubbing of the fingers and this radiograph was obtained. Note the diffuse patchy airspace disease and an air fluid collection at the right base. Aspiration of the pleural fluid revealed an empyema. *Fusobacterium necrophorum* was isolated. A bronchopleural fistula had developed and the patient had a prolonged recovery.

specimen (nasopharyngeal swab, pleural fluid, or lung tissue) can be tested for *Legionella* spp.; *M. pneumoniae*; *C. pneumoniae*; influenza viruses A and B, RSV, adenovirus; parainfluenza viruses; HMPVs and coronaviruses including SARS CoV.

Human immunodeficiency virus (HIV) does not respect age. Bacteremic pneumococcal pneumonia, *Pneumocystis carini* and *M. tuberculosis* are more common in HIV-infected patients. Thus, HIV serology may be part of the workup of the elderly patient with pneumonia.

C-reactive protein, serum procalcitonin and neopterin have been used in an attempt to distinguish viral from bacterial infection. An ultrasensitive assay for procalcitonin looks promising in that at a level of ≤ 0.25 μg/L, antibiotic therapy has been successfully discontinued in patients with pneumonia. The inference is that patients with this level of procalcitonin have viral pneumonia. Copeptin, which is cosynthesized with vasopressin is elevated in lower respiratory tract infections and the highest increase is in patients with pneumonia. However, since it is elevated in sepsis from any source it is not specific for pneumonia.

If a pleural effusion is present, a lateral decubitus film, with the affected side down, should be performed. If the effusion measures 1 cm or greater it should be aspirated and cultured for aerobes, anaerobes, fungi, and acid-fast bacilli. Cytology should always be performed on such specimens and the cell count, glucose, LDH, protein and pH determined. The specimen for pH should be collected in a blood gas syringe; the tip of the needle corked and submitted to the laboratory on ice.

Some patients will require invasive tests, such as bronchoscopy to make an etiological diagnosis. The decision to use such investigations depends upon the clinical setting.

Therapeutic Evaluations

The most frequently used therapeutic evaluation is repeated measurement of vital signs (including pulse oximetry) and repeated physical examination. In general, it is obvious when there is failure of therapy—see discussion on attainment of physiological stability under the discharge decision. In patients who are improving clinically there is a need for only one follow-up chest radiograph. The timing of when this is carried out is important. Chronic obstructive pulmonary disease is typically associated with delayed radiographic clearance of pneumonia. However, if the pneumonia has not resolved radiographically by 12 weeks, bronchoscopy should be done. In 2% of patients with CAP, the pneumonia is a manifestation of cancer of the lung (post obstructive pneumonia). In 50% of these patients, the diagnosis is suggested radiographically at the time of presentation. Hence, the importance of a follow-up chest radiograph to ensure that the pneumonia has cleared.

Computed tomography of the chest is useful in the assessment of a patient who is not improving. It can detect loculated pleural effusions (potentially empyema) and early cavitation before they are seen on conventional chest radiograph. The better detail and assessment of hilar and mediastinal adenopathy may also be helpful in suggesting alternative diagnoses.

Discharge Decision

This is often a complicated matter and involves not only the stability of the pneumonia but also the stability of comorbid illnesses and the functional and mental status of the patient. Once physiological stability is achieved (temperature <37.5°C; respiratory rate <22 [or a return to baseline for patients with chronic pulmonary compromise]; oxygen saturation of $\geq 92\%$ while breathing room air; stable blood pressure; and ability to eat and drink), clinical deterioration requiring admission to a critical care unit or telemetry monitoring occurred in less than 1% of patients. Indeed, in one study if discharge occurred once physiological stability has been reached, the length of hospital stay for pneumonia could be reduced by 1 day. There is no need to observe the patient in hospital once the switch from intravenous to oral antibiotic therapy has been made and the patient is physiologically stable. However, there are other factors to be considered in the discharge decision; such as the elderly person who can no longer care for himself or herself and requires placement in a long-term care facility or home care. A mini-mental status should be done prior to discharge and further assessment performed for those who score less than 25.

MANAGEMENT

Drugs

Antibiotics

Guidelines published by several different professional bodies for the empiric therapy of CAP suggest different antibiotics according to the severity of the pneumonia and certain epidemiological features, such as the likelihood that PRSP may be causing the infection. Unfortunately, most of these recommendations are not based on data from randomized clinical trials. Suggested treatment for ambulatory pneumonia is a macrolide or doxycycline. Telithromycin, a ketolide, is no longer used to treat ambulatory pneumonia because of hepatotoxicity. Tigecycline, a glycylcycline structurally derived from minocycline, is currently undergoing evaluation as an agent for the treatment of CAP. If PRSP is common in the community a "respiratory quinolone"; such as levofloxacin, moxifloxacin or gatifloxacin can be used. The Canadian guidelines for the treatment of CAP have added a new category to the treatment of pneumonia on an ambulatory basis; that is, "outpatient with modifying factors." This refers to patients with chronic obstructive lung disease who have received antibiotic therapy or oral corticosteroid treatment within the past 3 months. The antibiotic therapy of first choice in this setting is a respiratory quinolone; the second choice is amoxicillin-clavulinic acid with or without a macrolide; another possibility is a second-generation cephalosporin with or without a macrolide (Table 126-9). For patients requiring admission to a hospital ward, antibiotic therapy can be with a "respiratory quinolone" alone or with a macrolide plus a second or third-generation cephalosporin. For those who require admission to ICU, the recommended treatment is erythromycin or azithromycin or a fluoroquinolone with enhanced activity against *S. pneumoniae* plus cefotaxime, ceftriaxone, or a β-lactam/β-lactamase inhibitor (Table 126-9). Data from two studies (one a retrospective review of 12 945 Medicare inpatients with CAP, the other an observational study of 2963 patients with CAP) indicated that treatment with a second-generation cephalosporin plus a macrolide, or a nonpseudomonal third-generation cephalosporin plus a macrolide or a fluoroquinolone alone were associated with lower

TABLE 126-9

Antibiotic Therapy (First and Second Choices) of Community-Acquired Pneumonia When Etiology is Unknown

A. Patient to be treated on an ambulatory basis (previously healthy and no use of antimicrobials in the past 3 months)
  1. Macrolide (erythromycin 500 mg q 6h orally × 10 days, clarithromycin 500 mg twice daily orally × 10 days or azithromycin 500 mg orally once a day then 250 mg once a day orally × 4 days)
  2. Doxycycline 100 mg twice daily orally × 10 days. *If risk factors for PRSP or macrolide-resistant *S. pneumoniae* are present, consider a fluoroquinolone with enhanced activity against *S. pneumoniae*

  If chronic obstructive lung disease is present or antibiotics have been administered within the past 3 months.
  1. Fluoroquinolone with enhanced activity against *S. pneumoniae*; e.g., levofloxacin, moxifloxacin, gatifloxacin. Levofloxacin 750 mg once a day orally or IV. If creatinine clearance <50 mL/min reduce levofloxacin dose to 250 mg once a day. Moxifloxacin 400 mg once a day orally; Gatifloxacin 400 mg once a day orally or IV
  2. Combination therapy with a β-lactam antibiotic plus a macrolide

B. Patient to be treated in hospital ward
  1. Fluoroquinolone with enhanced activity against *S. pneumoniae*; e.g., levofloxacin, moxifloxacin, gatifloxacin. Levofloxacin 750 mg once a day IV or orally, If creatinine clearance <50 mL/min reduce levofloxacin dose to 250 mg once a day. Moxifloxacin 400 mg once a day orally; Gatifloxacin 400 mg once a day IV or orally
  2. Ceftriaxone 1 gm once a day IV or cefotaxime 2 g q 6 h IV plus azithromycin 500 mg once a day IV.

C. Patient to be treated in an ICU
  1. Azithromycin 1 gm IV then 500 mg IV once a day plus ceftriaxone 1 gm q12h. IV or cefotaxime 2 gm q6h IV (ceftazidime and an aminoglycoside if *Pseudomonas aeruginosa* infection is suspected; piperacillin/tazobactam; imipenem , meropenem, cefipime and ciprofloxacin also have activity against *P. aeruginosa*)
  2. Fluoroquinolone with enhanced activity against *S. pneumoniae* (not recommended as first choice because of lack of clinical trial data in the ICU setting)

  If MRSA infection is suspected in any of the above settings add Vancomycin 1 gm q12h IV or Linezolid 600 mg IV or orally q12h.

D. Patient to be treated in a nursing home
  1. Fluoroquinolone with enhanced activity against *S. pneumoniae* e.g., Levofloxacin 750 mg once a day orally or Moxifloxacin 400 mg once a day orally or Gatifloxacin 400 mg once a day orally
  2. Ceftriaxone 500–1000 mg IM once a day or cefotaxime 500 mg IM q12h plus a macrolide.

E. Aspiration pneumonitis/pneumonia
  1. Pneumonitis: history of, or witnessed aspiration of gastric contents and an opacity on chest X-ray
  Wait 24 hours—if still symptomatic antibiotic therapy as given below.
  2. Pneumonia:
    a. Poor dental hygiene and anaerobic infection suspected: metronidazole 500 mg q 12 h orally (clindamycin could be used but because of increased rate of *Clostridium difficile* with clindamycin use of metronidazole is preferred) plus one of the following: levofloxacin 500 mg once a day orally or moxifloxacin 400 mg once a day orally or gatifloxacin 400 mg once a day orally or ceftriaxone or cefotaxime.
    b. Anaerobic infection not suspected: as above but do not include anaerobic coverage.

*Risk factors for: PRSP—previous use (within 3 months) of β-lactam antibiotics, alcoholism, age <5 yr or >65 yr, in some areas residence in a nursing home; Macrolide-resistant *S. pneumoniae*—age <5 yr or nosocomial acquisition of infection.

30-day mortality rates. There is a suggestion that a β-lactam plus a macrolide therapy is associated with lower mortalty in patients with CAP independent of severity. There are also several observational studies that suggest that addition of a macrolide to a β-lactam is associated with lower mortality in patients with bacteremic pneumococcal pneumonia. There is also one prospective observational study which found that the mortality for critically ill patients with pneumococcal bacteremia was 23.4% for the group that received combination therapy versus 55.3% for the group with monotherapy. In the same prospective study, investigators examined the "impact of concordant antibiotic therapy (i.e., receipt of a single antibiotic with in vitro activity against *S. pneumoniae*) versus discordant therapy (inactive in vitro) on mortality was assessed at 14 days. Discordant therapy with penicillins, cefotaxime, and ceftriaxone did not result in a higher mortality rate." However, discordant therapy involving cefuroxime was associated with a significantly higher mortality rate. Prompt administration of antibiotics, within 4 to 8 hours of arrival at emergency department is associated with a lower mortality rate among elderly patients when compared with those who wait longer for antibiotic therapy.

The respiratory quinolones seem like ideal choices for the treatment of CAP since they are active against most of the microbial causes of pneumonia, including: penicillin-susceptible *S. pneumoniae* and PRSP, *H. influenzae*, *M. catarrhalis*, *S. aureus*, *M. pneumoniae*, *Legionella* spp., and *Chlamydia pneumoniae*. It is very important to remember that the respiratory quinolones (especially gatifloxacin [which was withdrawn from the market]) may cause dysglycemia. One study found that levofloxacin (and by inference other respiratory quinolones) was superior to ceftriaxone/cefuroxime for the treatment of mild to moderately severe CAP. New information indicates that levofloxacin 750 mg daily for 5 days is adequate for the treatment of CAP. There is concern that the widespread use of the respiratory fluoroquinolones will lead to the emergence of resistance among these respiratory pathogens. For this, reason the CDC working group on the management of CAP, in the era of pneumococcal resistance, recommended that macrolides or doxycycline should be first line therapy for the management of ambulatory pneumonia and that the new fluoroquinolones should be reserved for adults who have already failed one of the first line drugs; who are allergic to the first line drugs or who have documented infection with highly drug-resistant pneumococci. The CDC group recommends that first line treatment for moderately ill persons hospitalized with CAP should be with a parenteral β-lactam antibiotic; such as, cefuroxime, cefotaxime, ceftriaxone, or a combination of ampicillin sodium and sulbactam sodium and a macrolide; such as, erythromycin, azithromycin or clarithromycin.

In an International study of CAP it was found that 85% of patients in North America received treatment for both atypical and typical pathogens compared with 49% in Europe, 45% in Latin American, and 1% in Africa/Asia.

When to Switch from Intravenous to Oral Antibiotics in the Treatment of CAP

For patients who are treated with intravenous antibiotics, the question of when to switch to oral antibiotics arises. Studies have shown that the switch from intravenous to oral antibiotics can be safely done when the white blood cell count is returning toward normal, there are two normal temperature recordings 16 hours apart, and there is improvement in cough and shortness of breath. The respiratory quinolones are so well absorbed from the gastrointestinal tract, however, that intravenous therapy is only necessary in those who are hypotensive or who have nausea and/or vomiting.

Nonpharmacological Management

Because of fever and increased loss of water through the lungs caused by rapid breathing, dehydration is common in patients with pneumonia. Thus, rehydration with intravenous fluids is often necessary. Hypoxemia is common and supplemental oxygen is used to correct this. In the absence of bronchiectasis, chest physiotherapy is not useful. Patients with pleuritic chest pain may require analgesia. Intubation may be avoided in some patients with severe chronic obstructive pulmonary disease, who have pneumonia and impending respiratory failure, by use of positive pressure assisted ventilation via a tight fitting facial mask (BiPAP). Anti-pyretics should not be used unless the temperature is >39°C or unless the patient is quite uncomfortable from the fever. Twice daily measurements of temperature are useful for monitoring response of the pneumonia to treatment. Pneumonia in elderly patients frequently exacerbates baseline confusion or results in new onset of delirium. Indeed, all elderly patients with pneumonia should be assessed for the presence of delirium at the time of admission and daily for the first 4 to 5 days in hospital. Delirium requires both nonpharmacological and pharmacological management.

Ancillary Measures

Appropriate management of comorbid illnesses, some of which can be made worse by the pneumonia, is important.

In the PROWESS trial, drotrecogin alfa (activated protein C) resulted in a 28% relative reduction in mortality among patients with severe CAP. Currently, patients with CAP and an APACHE II score of >25 qualify for this drug, although the data suggest a beneficial effect beginning at an APACHE II score of 20.

Tissue factor pathway inhibitor may also have a beneficial effect in severe pneumonia, and currently trials of this compound are underway.

Low-dose corticosteroid therapy is beneficial to those seriously ill pneumonia patients who are relatively adrenal insufficient (<9 mcg/mL response in cortisol level to a dose of adrenocorticotrophic hormone). Hyperglycemia has been shown to be associated with higher mortality rates in patients who require hospitalization for community-acquired pneumonia, so it is likely that control of hyperglycemia will be beneficial for patients with pneumonia and elevated blood sugar.

PREVENTION

Pneumococcal Vaccine

Currently, there is a 23-valent capsular polysaccharide vaccine available for use in adults; with the most common capsular polysaccharide types of *S. pneumoniae* causing bacteremic pneumonia represented in the vaccine. Elderly subjects do not mount a good antibody response to this vaccine. However, the evidence indicates a beneficial effect from this vaccine. A booster dose is given 5 years after the first dose. A polysaccharide-protein conjugate vaccine is currently undergoing clinical trials, and promises to be more effective than the currently available capsular polysaccharide vaccine.

Influenza Vaccine

Yearly influenza vaccination of the elderly reduces the rate of admission to hospital for both pneumonia and congestive heart failure. Immunization of health care workers against influenza protects against nosocomial influenza.

Cessation of Tobacco Smoking

Tobacco smoking is associated with a twofold increase in risk for pneumococcal pneumonia. It is likely that cessation of tobacco smoking will reduce the rate of pneumonia, but there are no data from clinical trials to indicate this. Nevertheless, this recommendation is likely to have many benefits, including slowing the age related decline in lung function and reducing the risk of lung cancer.

Prevention of Aspiration Pneumonia

The "chin down" posture has been found to reduce the occurrence of aspiration both before and during the swallow. This posture results in a posterior shift of the anterior pharyngeal structures, narrowing the laryngeal entrance while widening the angle of the epiglottis to the anterior tracheal wall. The end result is protection of the airway. Cleaning of the teeth and gingival by caregivers after each meal reduced the latency time of the swallowing reflex and increased substance P in the saliva of patients with dysphagia caused by cerebrovascular disease. Substance P stimulates the neural pathways to improve the swallowing reflex.

SPECIAL ISSUES

Patient Preference

If there is a significant risk of mortality many prefer to be treated in hospital; otherwise they prefer to be treated at home. Sir William Osler termed pneumonia "Captain of the men of death." This is one condition where it is of utmost importance to know the wishes of your patient regarding ventilatory support and resuscitation. In one study 15% of patients with CAP, who required admission to hospital, had a do-not-resuscitate order (DNR) written within 24 hours of admission while an additional 7% had such an order written later. In multivariate analyses, the following were predictive of initial DNR: age, nursing home care, active cancer, dementia, neuromuscular disorders, altered mental status, low systolic blood pressure, tachypnea, abnormal hematocrit, abnormal blood urea nitrogen, and absence of alcohol or intravenous drug abuse. In similar analyses of DNR at any time, additional predictors included aspiration, low white blood count, chronic pulmonary disease, cerebrovascular disease, and congestive heart failure.

Patient Education

Patients (particularly those treated on an ambulatory basis) should be given written information on the expected course of the pneumonia, warning signs that indicate a need for reassessment, (such as increasing dyspnea, pleuritic chest pain, hemopytsis), and the requirement for a follow-up chest radiograph to ensure that the pneumonia has cleared.

Quality of Care Measures

The following have been adopted as quality of care measures for patients with CAP requiring admission to hospital: blood cultures prior to administration of antibiotics; measurement of oxygenation status; administration of antibiotics within 4 hours of presentation to emergency department; ascertainment of influenza; and pneumococcal vaccination status and administration of these vaccines as necessary. In addition, for those who smoke tobacco products, at the very least information re: cessation, and preferentially counseling regarding cessation of smoking. Two large studies have examined the quality of care in U.S. hospitals for a number of conditions including pneumonia. In one study, academic hospitals had higher performance scores for acute myocardial infarction than nonacademic hospitals and congestive heart failure but lower scores for pneumonia—69% versus 71%. Not-for-profit hospitals had significantly higher scores for all three conditions than did for profit hospitals. There were also regional differences with the Midwest and Northeast outperforming the West and the South. The number of beds was significantly associated only with pneumonia scores, with the smallest hospitals having the highest scores. Of 3484 hospitals most, approximately 98%, met the oxygenation assessment criteria; The pneumococcal vaccination criteria were very scattered—approximately 2% of the hospitals assessed immunization in 91% to 100% of cases; 18% did the assessment 0% to 10% of the time and approximately 60% of the hospitals assessed less than 50% of the patients. Only 3% of the hospitals gave antibiotics in the recommended time to 91% to 100% of the patients. In another study of U.S hospitals, the investigators examined hospital's performance on 18 standardized indications of quality of care for four conditions one of which was pneumonia. Data were collected more than a 2-year period in more than 3000 accredited hospitals. The measures assessed for CAP were—oxygenation assessment within 24 hours after admission; pneumococcal vaccination screening, blood cultures collected before initiation of antibiotic therapy; smoking-cessation counseling or advice; mean time from arrival to initial antibiotic administration. Over the course of the study the percentage of patients who had oxygenation assessment

done rose from 95% to 99%; pneumococcal vaccination from 28% to 50%; blood cultures from 82% to 83%; smoking cessation counseling from 34% to 67%; mean time to initiation of antibiotics 266 minutes to 227 minutes. With the exception of blood cultures all the rest were statistically significant

There are now a number of studies which have examined the effect of using guidelines on patient care, and while the design of these have differed, there is a strong suggestion that following guidelines has a "halo-effect" in improving patient care and results in decreased mortality and, in some instances, reduced LOS.

CONCLUSIONS

Management of pneumonia in the elderly is challenging yet very rewarding. Attention to vaccination status and advice regarding cessation of pneumonia can prevent many cases of pneumonia. Prompt treatment according to guidelines for empiric therapy and attention to the effect of pneumonia on comorbidities can optimize outcomes.

FURTHER READING

1. Medina-Walpole IS, Katz PR. Nursing home-acquired pneumonia. *J Am Geriatric Soc.* 1999;47:1005–1015.
2. Metlay JP, Schulz R, Li Y-H, et al. Influence of age on symptoms at presentation on patients with community-acquired pneumonia. *Arch Intern Med.* 1997;157:453–459.
3. Naughton BJ, Mylotte JM, Tayara A. Outcome of nursing home-acquired pneumonia: derivation and application of a practical model to predict 30-day mortality. *J Am Geriatr Soc.* 2000;48:1292.
4. Meehan TP, Fine MJ, Krumholz HM, et al. Quality of care, process and outcomes in elderly patients with pneumonia. *JAMA.* 1997;278:2080.
5. Gleason PP, Meehan TP, Fine JM, et al. Associations between initial antimicrobial therapy and medical outcomes for hospitalized elderly patients with pneumonia. *Arch Intern Med.* 1999;159:2562–2572.
6. Mandell LA, Marrie TJ, Grossman RF, et al. Canadian guidelines for the initial management of community-acquired pneumonia: an evidence-based update by the Canadian Infectious Diseases Society and the Canadian Thoracic Society. *Clin Infect Dis.* 2000;31:383–421.
7. Bartlett JG, Dowell SF, Mandell LA, et al. Practice guidelines for the management of community-acquired pneumonia in adults. *Clin Infect Dis.* 2000;31:347–382.
8. Gross PA, Hermogenes AW, Sacks HS, et al. The efficacy of influenza vaccine in elderly persons: a meta-analysis and review of the literature. *Ann Intern Med.* 1995;123:518–527.
9. Nichol KL, Margolis KL, Wuorenma J, et al. The efficacy and cost effectiveness of vaccination against influenza among elderly persons living in the community. *N Engl J Med.* 1994;31:778–784.
10. Riquelme R, Torres A, El-Ebiary M, et al. Community-acquired pneumonia in the elderly. A multivariate analysis of risk and prognositc factors. *Am J Respir Crit Care Med.* 1996;154:1450–1455.
11. Fine MJ, Auble TE, Yealy DM, et al. A prediction rule to identify low-risk patients with community-acquired pneumonia. *N Engl J Med.* 1997;336:243–250.
12. Williams SC, Schmaltz SP, Morton DJ, Koss RG, Loeb JM. Quality of care in US hospitals as reflected by standardized measures, 2002–2004. *NEJM.* 2005;353:255–264.
13. Capelastegui A, Espana PP, Quitana JM, Gorordo I, Ortega M, Idoiaga I, Bilbao A. Improvement of process-of-care and outcomes after implementing a guideline for the management of community-acquired pneumonia: a controlled before-and-after design study. *Clin Infect Dis.* 2004;39:955–963.
14. Marrie TJ, Wu L. Factors influencing in-hospital mortality in community-acquired pneumonia. *Chest.* 2005;127:1260–1270.
15. Sopena N, Pedro-Botet L, Mateu L, Tolschinsky G, Rey-Joly C, Sabria M. Community-acquired *Legionella* pneumonia in elderly patients: characteristics and outcome. *J Am Geriatrics Soc.* 2007;55:114–119.
16. Zhanel GG, Fontaine S, Adam H, et al. A review of new fluoroquinolones. Focus on their use in respiratory tract infections. *Treat Respir Med.* 2006;5:437–465.
17. Mandell LA, Wunderink RG, Anzueto A, et al. Infectious diseases society of America/American thoracic society consens guidelines on the management of community-acquired pneumonia in adults. *Clin Infect Dis.* 2007;44:S27–S72.

Urinary Tract Infections

Lindsay E. Nicolle

Urinary tract infection (UTI) is the most frequent bacterial infection in elderly populations. While urinary infection in the elderly person is usually asymptomatic, symptomatic infection occurs frequently with associated serious morbidity and, rarely, mortality. Optimal management of urinary infection in the elderly patient is challenging in the face of diagnostic uncertainty, concerns with excess antimicrobial use, and increasing antimicrobial resistance in both the community and nursing home. Current limitations in knowledge and optimal management strategies for this problem must be appreciated. In addition, the heterogeneity of the elderly populations means approaches may vary for different groups. The impact and management of urinary infection differs for women and men, and for the institutionalized and noninstitutionalized elderly person. There are also unique considerations for the subgroup of institutionalized elderly persons with chronic indwelling catheters. The discussion in this chapter is relevant to individuals without long-term indwelling catheters, unless otherwise stated.

PRESENTATIONS OF URINARY INFECTION

The bladder is normally sterile. While bacteriuria is always abnormal, it is not necessarily detrimental. "Bacteriuria", a positive urine culture without attributable signs or symptoms, is used interchangeably with "asymptomatic UTI" in this chapter. The majority of the elderly individuals with bacteriuria have evidence for a local host response. Some authors use the term "bladder colonization" in discussing asymptomatic bacteriuria. This term has not been shown to have clinical or biological relevance in elderly populations, and is not used in this discussion.

UTI encompasses a spectrum of presentations (Table 127-1). Acute uncomplicated urinary infection, also known as acute cystitis, is usually considered relevant only for premenopausal women. However, women who experience recurrent acute uncomplicated urinary infection prior to menopause often continue to experience these episodes after menopause. Complicated UTI occurs in either sex in the setting of a structurally or functionally abnormal urinary tract. A wide variety of genitourinary abnormalities are associated with infection, from prostatic hypertrophy and cystoceles to chronic renal failure and chronic indwelling catheters. A characteristic of complicated UTI is frequent and early post-therapy recurrence if the underlying genitourinary abnormality persists. These infections are also characterized by a wider variety of infecting organisms. The majority of functionally impaired older women and all men with urinary infection should be considered to have complicated infection.

Acute prostatitis is an infrequent, severe, febrile infection occurring primarily in young men. Chronic bacterial prostatitis occurs in older men. It is characterized by bacterial infection of the prostate with mild to moderate local symptoms, and is commonly associated with recurrent episodes of acute cystitis as organisms reinfect the urine from the prostate source. These symptoms respond to antimicrobial therapy. Presentations of chronic prostatitis/chronic pelvic pain syndrome in men without documentation of bacteria in the prostate are no longer thought to be attributable to infection, irrespective of the presence or absence of pyuria.

Recurrent urinary infection, either reinfection or relapse, is common for elderly persons. Reinfection is recurrent urinary infection with an organism isolated following antimicrobial therapy which differs from the pretherapy isolate. This is assumed to reflect entry of a new organism into the bladder during or following therapy. Superinfection is a new urinary infection (i.e., a reinfection) that occurs in the presence of existing bacteriuria, without an intervening episode of negative urine culture. Relapse is recurrent urinary infection when the organism-isolated post-therapy is similar to the pretherapy isolate. When relapse occurs, the organism has usually remained sequestered at some site in the urinary tract and was not eradicated with antimicrobial therapy.

TABLE 127-1

Potential Clinical Presentations of UTI

PRESENTATION	CHARACTERISTICS
Acute, uncomplicated urinary infection	Bladder infection in women with a normal genitourinary tract
Acute, nonobstructive pyelonephritis	Acute renal infection in women with a normal genitourinary tract
Complicated UTI	Bladder or renal infection in men and women with functional or structural genitourinary abnormalities
Asymptomatic bacteriuria (asymptomatic UTI)	Positive urine culture meeting standard quantitative criteria for significant bacteriuria with no signs or symptoms referable to the urinary tract, irrespective of the presence or absence of pyuria
Acute prostatitis	Febrile illness, usually with bacteremia and severe voiding symptoms associate with acute bacterial infection of the prostate
Chronic bacterial prostatitis	Symptomatic persistent relapsing documented bacterial infection of prostate, often manifested by recurrent acute cystitis

EPIDEMIOLOGY

Asymptomatic Infection

Elderly in the Community

There is a marked increase in the prevalence of asymptomatic bacteriuria with increasing age for women. The prevalence of bacteriuria is 2% to 3% in young women and increases to more than 10% for women older than age 65 years and 20% at 80 years or more (Table 127-2). Bacteriuria is uncommon in younger men but the prevalence of bacteriuria increases substantially with aging, particularly coincident with the development of prostatic hypertrophy. Approximately 5% of men older than age 70 years living in the community have bacteriuria. There are few studies describing the incidence of asymptomatic urinary infection in the elderly ambulatory populations. With yearly urine cultures obtained, it was reported to be 6.7/100 person years for diabetic and 3.0 for nondiabetic women aged 55 to 75 years. For 209 initially nonbacteriuric elderly ambulatory male outpatients of a veteran's hospital, 10% had at least one episode of bacteriuria during a mean of 2.8 years follow-up. Three-quarters of these episodes resolved spontaneously.

TABLE 127-2

Prevalence of Asymptomatic Bacteriuria in Elderly Populations

POPULATION	POSITIVE URINE CULTURE (%)	
	Women	Men
Community >70 yr of age	10–18	4–7
Long-term care	25–55	15–37

Institutionalized Older Adults

The prevalence of asymptomatic bacteriuria in institutionalized elderly populations is remarkably high (Table 127-2). This has been consistently observed in reports over several decades from many geographic areas of the world. It is somewhat higher in women, with 25% to 50% bacteriuric, compared to 15% to 40% of men. The variation in prevalence is primarily determined by characteristics of the institutionalized population. There may be an increased prevalence with increasing age of residents, although this is not consistent among studies. In fact, bacteriuria in the very elderly, those older than age 90 years, may be somewhat lower. The incidence of asymptomatic infection amongst these populations is also very high. In a group of previously bacteriuric women screened monthly, new infections occurred at a rate of 87 infections per 100 patient years. In elderly men resident in a veteran's hospital with urine cultures obtained every 2 weeks, an incidence of infection of 45 infections per 100 patient years was observed, with 10% of previously nonbacteriuric residents becoming bacteriuric in every 3-month period.

The remarkable occurrence of asymptomatic bacteriuria in elderly institutionalized populations has also been described in repeated prevalence surveys, with observations reported as both acquisition and loss of bacteriuria between surveys. Acquisition of bacteriuria at 1 month after initial negative screening was reported to be 11% for men and 12% for women. In another study, 8% of women acquired bacteriuria by 6 months, and 23% by 1 year. Reversion to negative urine cultures was observed in 22% of bacteriuric men at 1 year and, for women, 12% at 1 month, 31% at 6 months, and 27% at 1 year. Resolution of bacteriuria is often coincident with antimicrobial therapy.

Symptomatic Urinary Infection

Elderly in the Community

Clinically diagnosed urinary infection in an American community-living population older than 65 years of age was reported to be 13 per 100 person-years, 10.9 per 100 years in men and 14 per 100 years in women. The rate was 15 per 100 years in those aged 65 to 74 years, but 12 per 100 years in those older than age 75 years. In women 55 to 75 years enrolled in a group health plan in Washington State, symptomatic infection was 7/100 person years; 12/100 for women with diabetes and 6.7/100 for those without diabetes. Symptomatic infections were 0.17 per 1000 days in a cohort of 29 ambulatory elderly male veterans with bacteriuria. In initially bacteriuric residents of a geriatric apartment, the incidence of urinary symptoms was 0.9 per 1000 days during 6 months follow-up. Considering more severe presentations, hospitalization for acute pyelonephritis in persons older than 70 years was 10 to 15 per 10 000 population in one Canadian province, with hospitalization for women 1.3 times more frequent than men. An American study using 1997 administrative data reported pyelonephritis hospitalizations were 13.5/10 000 for women 60 to 79 years and 23.3/10 000 for women 80 years or older, and 6.3/10 000 and 12.9/10 000 for men, respectively.

Institutionalized Older Adults

The incidence of symptomatic urinary infection in long-term care facilities varies from 1.0 to 2.4 per 1000 resident days. Definitions to identify symptomatic urinary infection are, however, often imprecise and variable among studies. The reported incidence of symptomatic infection is only 0.27 to 0.4 per 1000 days for bacteriuric men or women when restrictive clinical definitions which require localizing genitourinary symptoms are used. An incidence of 0.6/1000 days was recently reported from a group of American facilities using standardized definitions, and 1.0/1000 resident days in a German nursing home. The incidence of fever from a urinary source in non-catheterized subjects in nursing homes was reported to be 0.5 to 1 per 1000 resident days using restrictive clinical or serologic criteria for identification of invasive urinary infection.

MORBIDITY AND MORTALITY

Asymptomatic Bacteriuria

Long-term adverse outcomes have not been attributed to asymptomatic bacteriuria for either ambulatory or institutionalized populations. Persistent asymptomatic urinary infection is not associated with an increased risk of development of renal failure or hypertension. In addition, despite a high prevalence of infection with urease-producing organisms such as *Proteus mirabilis,* complications from renal stone disease are not a common problem in institutionalized populations. Studies from Greece and Finland in the 1970s reported an association between asymptomatic bacteriuria and decreased survival for both elderly men and women. Subsequent studies in both community and institutionalized elderly populations in Finland, the United States, and Canada have not confirmed this observation. Thus, current evidence does not support an association between asymptomatic bacteriuria and decreased survival for elderly populations.

Symptomatic Urinary Infection

Symptomatic urinary infection is a common infection in the elderly population. Morbidity may occur along a continuum of limited voiding discomfort to disruption in daily activities or hospitalization for pyelonephritis or sepsis. An American study of 284 patients, older than 65 years of age, presenting to an emergency department reported 4.6% died during hospitalization; 9.5% required intensive care admission; 48.9% had greater than 2 days length of stay and 26.4% required more than 2 days intravenous antibiotics. Independent predictors of any of these adverse outcomes included mental status change, frequent past urinary infections, other non urinary infections, abnormal temperature, tachycardia, hypotension, elevated blood urea nitrogen, hyperglycemia, elevated white blood cell count and relative neutrophilia.

For the institutionalized population, deterioration in functional status may also contribute to morbidity, but this impact has not been rigorously evaluated. From 8% to 30% of transfers from long-term care to an acute care facility are necessitated by urinary infection. Urinary infection is the most common source of bacteremia in long-term care facility residents, although bacteremia is infrequent in residents without a chronic indwelling catheter. Antimicrobial pressure associated with treatment of UTIs, much of which may be asymptomatic, promotes emergence and persistence of resistant organisms in long-term care facilities. Antimicrobial therapy also contributes to morbidity through adverse effects. Urinary infection, however, is an infrequent cause of mortality, even with bacteremia from a urinary source.

PATHOGENESIS

Route and Site of Infection

Urinary infection occurs by the ascending route. The reservoir for infecting organisms is usually the gastrointestinal flora. Organisms colonize the periurethral area and ascend up the urethra into the bladder. Infecting organisms may subsequently reach the kidney. Renal infection is determined by virulence characteristics of the infecting organism or the presence of genitourinary abnormalities such as obstruction or reflux in the host. For men, ascending infection may also lead to prostate infection. Thus, urinary infection may be localized to the bladder, may involve the kidneys as well as the bladder and, for men, may also be localized in the prostate. Infection of the upper tract (kidney) is present in 50% of elderly women with asymptomatic infection. Renal localization is more frequent with increasing age, and in residents of nursing homes. The proportion of elderly men with a prostatic site of infection is unknown, but is likely substantial. In the institutionalized population, transfer of organisms which colonize the perineum or urinary drainage devices such as indwelling or external catheters may occur between patients. Rarely, infection may be hematogenous rather than ascending, with urinary infection secondary to bacteremia from a nonurinary source.

Microbiology

Infecting Organisms

The most frequent infecting organism isolated from urinary infection in either asymptomatic or symptomatic ambulatory elderly women is *Escherichia coli* (Table 127-3). For women with acute uncomplicated infection, the spectrum of virulence factors in urinary *E. coli* isolates is similar to younger women. Pyelonephritis strains are associated with *P. fimbriae,* and have an increased frequency of other virulence characteristics including capsule type, adhesins, and proteins such as iron binding proteins and hemolysins. *E. coli* isolated from persons with complicated urinary infection have a lower prevalence of virulence characteristics. In men, gram-positive organisms and other gram-negative organisms, particularly *P. mirabilis,* are more frequently isolated than *E. coli.*

E. coli remains the most frequent organism isolated from institutionalized women, although less common than in noninstitutionalized women. *P. mirabilis* is the most frequent in men (Table 127-3). *E. coli* may be more common in bacteremic infection than other gram-negative uropathogens. *E. coli* is also more likely to persist than other organisms in women with asymptomatic bacteriuria. Many other gram-negative organisms are isolated in the institutionalized population, including Enterobacteriaceae such as *Klebsiella pneumoniae, Serratia* spp., *Citrobacter* spp., *Enterobacter* spp., and *Morganella morganii,* as well as *Pseudomonas aeruginosa. Providencia stuartii* is an organism isolated virtually only from institutionalized subjects. When this organism is isolated, it is frequently the predominant organism in the ward or facility. Thus, it has a unique propensity for

TABLE 127-3

Distributions of Infecting Bacteria Isolated from Elderly Populations with Asymptomatic Urinary Infection and Without Indwelling Catheters

ORGANISM	POPULATION (% OF ISOLATES)			
	Community		Institutionalized	
	Women	Men	Women	Men
E. coli	68–72	19–50	47–77	11–27
P. mirabilis	0.8	0.6–4.7	2.3–27	30–36
K. pneumoniae	9–10	4.7–6.9	6.8–11	5.9–9.1
Citrobacter spp.	—	—	1.82.6	2.5–3.1
Enterobacter spp.	—	1.7–3.3	0.9–2	1.7–9.1
Providencia spp.	—	1.0	6.8	16
M. morganii	—	0.7	1.7	1.2–2.5
P. aeruginosa	—	4.7–9.4	5.1–9	13.2–19
Group B streptococci	10	—	0–13	0–1.7
Enterococcus spp.	4.8	18–25	4.5–8.0	5–23.7
Coagulase-negative staphylococci	5.6	8.9–39	0.9–4	1.7–4.5
Staphylococcus aureus	—	5.0	0–6	2.5–8.5

spread within the institutional setting. Gram-positive organisms include group B streptococci, which may be more common in persons with diabetes. *Enterococcus* spp. and coagulase-negative staphylococci are frequently isolated in men, but are seldom associated with symptomatic infection. Polymicrobial bacteriuria is common in both men and women resident in institutions, with more than one organism isolated in 10% to 25% of bacteriuric subjects.

Antimicrobial Resistance

Bacterial isolates from urinary infection in institutionalized populations are characterized by a higher frequency of antimicrobial resistance than organisms isolated in the community population. This is a consequence of intense exposure to antimicrobials together with facilitation of transmission of organisms in the institutional setting. The prevalence of resistant isolates varies widely among facilities. Resistant organisms of particular concern in urinary infection include vancomycin-resistant enterococci, extended spectrum beta lactamase producing *E. coli* and *K. pneumoniae*, and fluoroquinolone-resistant *P. aeruginosa*. For the elderly residents with urinary infection who present to emergency departments, prior antimicrobial use with either trimethoprim/sulfamethoxazole (TMP/SMX) or a fluoroquinolone is the most important risk factor for isolation of a resistant organism. Consistent associations for identification of resistant organisms in nursing home residents also include prior TMP/SMX exposure for TMP/SMX-resistant organisms, and prior fluoroquinolone exposure for fluoroquinolone-resistant organisms. The presence of an indwelling urethral catheter is also associated with isolation of fluoroquinolone-resistant *E. coli*.

Host Factors

Elderly in the Community

In the normal genitourinary tract, intermittent, complete voiding is the preeminent host defense against urinary infection. Most well-elderly women continue to empty their bladder completely. Sev-

eral host factors, however, contribute to the high frequency of urinary infection in elderly populations (Table 127-4). In ambulatory postmenopausal women associations with asymptomatic bacteriuria are urinary incontinence, increased postvoid residual urine, reduced mobility and estrogen treatment. For postmenopausal women who are diabetic, an additional risk factor is the duration of diabetes. A prospective study of risk factors for symptomatic UTI in women of age 55 to 75 years reported independent predictors were a prior history of urinary infection and diabetes. An initial case control study in the same women had reported sexual activity and incontinence to be associated with symptomatic infection, but these findings were not confirmed in the prospective study.

Any structural or functional abnormality which impairs voiding will increase the likelihood of urinary infection. Genitourinary abnormalities such as urethral or ureteric strictures, bladder

TABLE 127-4

Contributing Factors to the High Prevalence of Bacteriuria in Elderly Populations

Women	Genetic predisposition
	Loss of estrogen effect on genitourinary mucosa
	Changes in colonizing flora
	Cystoceles
	Increased residual volume
Men	Prostatic hypertrophy
	Bacterial prostatitis
	Prostatic calculi
	Urethral strictures
	External urine collecting devices
Both	Genitourinary abnormalities
	Bladder diverticulae
	Urinary catheters (intermittent, indwelling)
	Associated illnesses
	Neurologic disease with neurogenic bladder dysfunction
	Diabetes

diverticulae, and cystoceles occur with increased frequency in older populations, and contribute to bacteriuria. Studies in ambulatory women have tended to confirm an association of increased postvoid residual being associated with UTI. An association between urinary incontinence and UTI is consistently reported from both ambulatory and institutionalized women, but is unlikely to be causative. Women with incontinence have abnormal voiding, and voiding abnormalities are a major predisposing factor for development of bacteriuria or urinary infection. Thus, urologic abnormalities which lead to incontinence are also likely to promote bacteriuria. In multivariate analyses of associations with urinary incontinence, urinary infection frequently does not persist as an independent variable. Current evidence does not support a role for immunologic changes of aging being important contributors to the high frequency of urinary infection.

The association of estrogen decline in elderly women with urinary infection is complex, and observations sometimes conflicting. Loss of the estrogen effect on the genitourinary mucosa in postmenopausal women is associated with an increased colonization of the vagina with potential uropathogens. Postmenopausal women are less likely to have lactobacilli colonizing the vagina, and more likely to have *E. coli* and enterococci. These changes in vaginal flora, together with the higher pH in the absence of lactobacilli, are similar to changes observed in younger women with recurrent UTI, and have been suggested to facilitate urinary infection in older women. However, both case control studies and prospective, randomized trials, have consistently reported that systemic estrogen use in postmenopausal women is associated with an increased risk of symptomatic infection. It is suggested this is because women who use estrogen are more likely to be sexually active, but this hypothesis requires confirmation. Topical vaginal estrogen maintains a vaginal environment characterized by decreased pH and predominance of lactobacilli. Prospective, randomized clinical trials have reported that vaginal estrogen may decrease the frequency of infection. However, some case control studies report an association of topical vaginal estrogen with increased risk of urinary infection. Again, these studies may be biased by inclusion of women who are receiving topical estrogen because they are experiencing recurrent urinary infection.

Prostate hypertrophy is the most important factor promoting urinary infection in elderly men. This leads to obstruction and turbulent urethral urine flow which facilitates ascension of organisms into the bladder or prostate. Once bacteria are established in the prostate they are difficult to eradicate because of poor diffusion of antimicrobials into the prostate, and the increasing presence of prostate stones with age. These stones provide a nidus from which it may be impossible to eradicate bacteria. Frequent relapse of urinary infection from a prostate source is common, although months or even years may intervene between episodes.

Institutionalized Older Adults

The prevalence of asymptomatic bacteriuria in the institutionalized elderly population correlates with increasing functional impairment. The bacteriuric institutionalized elderly population are characterized by incontinence of bladder and bowel, immobility, and dementia. Impaired bladder emptying or ureteric reflux frequently accompany neurologic diseases which precipitate the requirement for institutional care, such as Alzheimer's disease, Parkinson's disease, and cerebrovascular disease. These voiding abnormalities promote the acquisition and persistence of urinary infection. No association of bacteriuria with other chronic diseases, including diabetes, or with specific medication use, has been reported. In contrast to observations in ambulatory women, bacteriuria has not been associated with elevated postvoid residual urine in women or men in the nursing home population. Oral estrogen and progesterone given to incontinent women resident in a nursing home was also not associated with a decreased prevalence of bacteriuria, despite vaginal pH and cytology showing a partial estrogen effect.

The use of external condom collecting devices for management of incontinence in men also promotes bacteriuria. Men who have incontinence managed with the use of these devices have a 2-fold-increased prevalence of bacteriuria when compared to men with incontinence in whom external catheters are not used. The initiation of condom catheter drainage is frequently temporally associated with onset of bacteriuria in a previously nonbacteriuric resident. With the external catheter, bacteria colonize the periurethral area in high concentrations and may ascend into the bladder, particularly if there is kinking or obstruction of the condom or drainage tube.

In long-term care facilities, host factors that predict symptomatic rather than asymptomatic infection have not been well characterized. Trauma to the genitourinary mucosa or obstruction of the genitourinary tract in the presence of asymptomatic urinary infection frequently precipitate fever, often with bacteremia from the urinary source. Identification of other host determinants of symptomatic infection requires further study.

Immune and Inflammatory Response

The elderly institutionalized individuals with asymptomatic bacteriuria usually have evidence for a local host response, and a substantial proportion also have evidence of a systemic response. More than 90% have pyuria. Approximately 30% of institutionalized subjects without bacteriuria, however, also have pyuria, presumably caused by other inflammatory processes of the genitourinary tract. Cytokines, such as interleukin (IL)-1α, IL-6, or IL-8, are measurable in the urine significantly more often in bacteriuric than nonbacteriuric subjects. Urine antibody levels against the infecting organism are elevated in most bacteriuric subjects, and markedly increased in more than one-third of subjects. Asymptomatic bacteriuria in hospitalized, functionally impaired elderly subjects is associated with circulating tumor necrosis factor receptors and a higher number of neutrophils in the blood, but not with increases in cytokines including tumor necrosis factor α, IL-6, or IL-1 receptor agonist, or with increased C-reactive protein. Approximately one-third of subjects with bacteriuria have markedly elevated serum antibody levels to their infecting uropathogens, and these elevated levels persist while bacteriuria persists. The clinical significance of the presence or degree of these abnormalities in asymptomatic subjects is unknown.

The response to symptomatic urinary infection in the elderly population is, generally, similar to that described for younger populations. There is evidence of local inflammation within the genitourinary tract with pyuria and elevated urinary cytokine and antibody levels. For systemic urinary infection, including fever and pyelonephritis, there is a systemic antibody response to the infecting organism, as well as elevated serum IL-6, C-reactive protein levels, and other inflammatory markers. These variables all decline together with resolution of systemic symptoms with appropriate treatment of the infection. Elderly individuals with systemic infection generally

TABLE 127-5

Clinical Presentations of Symptomatic UTI in Elderly Populations

Probable urinary infection
    Acute lower tract irritative symptoms (frequency, dysuria, urgency, increased incontinence)
    Acute pyelonephritis (fever, flank pain, and tenderness)
    Fever with urinary retention or obstruction of the urinary tract
    Fever with chronic indwelling urethral catheter
Unlikely caused by urinary infection
    Fever without localizing genitourinary signs or symptoms and no indwelling catheter
    Gross hematuria
    Nonspecific symptoms of clinical deterioration without localizing findings
Not caused by urinary infection
    Chronic incontinence
    Other chronic genitourinary symptoms

have a secondary antibody response, with antibody increases against antigens of the infecting organism in both urine and blood.

CLINICAL PRESENTATION

Symptomatic Urinary Infection

Clinical presentations of symptomatic infection may be similar to those in younger populations (Table 127-5). Acute lower tract infection (cystitis) presents with frequency, urgency, suprapubic discomfort, and dysuria. New or increased incontinence may also be a common presenting symptom in the elderly. Acute pyelonephritis presents with the classic triad of fever and costovertebral angle pain and tenderness, with or without associated lower urinary tract symptoms. The clinical diagnosis of symptomatic urinary infection is, however, frequently problematic, particularly in the highly functionally impaired elderly population. Difficulties in communication because of mental impairment or hearing loss and the presence of chronic symptoms associated with comorbid illnesses compromise the clinical assessment of changes in resident status.

Chronic genitourinary symptoms are common in elderly persons. These may include incontinence, frequency, urgency and dysuria. With the high prevalence of bacteriuria, especially amongst the institutionalized population, a positive urine culture frequently accompanies these chronic genitourinary symptoms. However, the chronic symptoms should not be attributed to bacteriuria, and are not improved by antimicrobial therapy. An unpleasant urinary odor may be associated with bacteriuria, likely attributable to polyamine production by infecting organisms in the urine. However, not all malodorous urine is bacterial infection, and infected urine is not universally malodorous. The appropriate approach to malodorous urine is through incontinence management and, perhaps, hydration, rather than considering this a symptom for which antimicrobial treatment is indicated.

Hematuria

Gross hematuria in institutionalized subjects occurs more frequently in men than in women. The majority of subjects with hematuria

are bacteriuric, approximately 75% in one study. However, urinary infection manifesting as hemorrhagic cystitis in this population is uncommon, and other diagnoses should always be sought. Bacterial hemorrhagic cystitis is reported to have an incidence of only 6.3 per 100,000 resident days. The most frequent causes of gross hematuria are bladder stones, tumors, or trauma associated with an indwelling catheter. Hematuria attributable to any genitourinary abnormality, however, in the presence of an infected urinary tract, is frequently complicated by secondary systemic urinary infection. As many as 30% of institutionalized subjects presenting with gross hematuria will subsequently become febrile. This is assumed to reflect organisms from the bacteriuric urinary tract entering the systemic circulation through whatever breach also produced the hematuria.

Clinical Deterioration Without Localizing Genitourinary Symptoms

It is sometimes suggested that urinary infection should be a consideration in any elderly person with "nonspecific" decline in clinical status. Such presentations may include acute delirium or confusion, lethargy, anorexia, or increased falls. The high prevalence of positive urine cultures in the institutionalized population means a positive urine culture is common with any clinical presentation. Thus, bacteriuria has a low predictive value for symptomatic urinary infection in the absence of localizing acute genitourinary symptoms. A diagnosis of urinary infection to explain general decline without localizing signs or symptoms should be entertained with skepticism. Further study defining clinical presentations of urinary infection in the functionally impaired elderly person is needed.

Fever without localizing signs or symptoms presents a diagnostic dilemma. As the expected prevalence of positive urine cultures in the noncatheterized institutionalized population is as high as 50%, attributing fever to urinary infection because of an associated positive urine culture is usually not a correct diagnosis. Only 10% to 15% of episodes of fever in bacteriuric institutionalized subjects without localizing genitourinary symptoms and without indwelling catheters are attributable to a urinary source. The positive predictive value of a positive urine culture for a urinary source of fever in the absence of genitourinary symptoms is less than 10%. Currently, however, clinical features that discriminate between a urinary and nonurinary origin, other than the presence of a chronic indwelling catheter, have not been identified.

LABORATORY EVALUATION

Microbiological Diagnosis

A definitive diagnosis of urinary infection requires isolation of appropriate quantitative counts of uropathogens from an optimally collected urine specimen (Table 127-6). When symptomatic urinary infection is a diagnostic consideration, a urine specimen for culture is essential to confirm the diagnosis and determine antimicrobial susceptibilities of the infecting organism to facilitate appropriate antimicrobial therapy. A urine specimen for culture should be obtained prior to antimicrobial therapy for all institutionalized residents, for all men, and for women with a clinical presentation consistent with pyelonephritis. Pretherapy urine culture may not be

TABLE 127-6

Quantitative Urinary Microbiology for Diagnosis of UTI

CLINICAL PRESENTATION*	QUANTITATIVE MICROBIOLOGY
Asymptomatic urinary infection	Same organism(s) $\geq 10^5$ CFU/mL on two consecutive cultures
Pyelonephritis or fever with localizing genitourinary symptoms	$\geq 10^4$ CFU/mL
Acute lower tract symptoms	$\geq 10^3$ CFU/mL of uropathogen
Specimen collected from:	
External collecting device (men only)	$\geq 10^5$ CFU/mL
Aspirated indwelling catheter	$\geq 10^3$ CFU/mL

*For both women and men unless otherwise stated.
CFU, colony-forming units.

indicated uniformly for well, ambulatory women presenting with symptoms consistent with cystitis and who have not recently received antimicrobial therapy. Pretherapy culture should be obtained from all women, however, in whom the diagnosis is uncertain, or who experience early symptomatic recurrence following antimicrobial therapy. While a positive urine culture cannot differentiate symptomatic from asymptomatic infection, a negative urine culture obtained prior to initiating antimicrobial therapy effectively excludes a diagnosis of UTI.

Urine Specimen Collection

A clean catch voided urine specimen collected to minimize contamination is preferred. Functionally impaired elderly subjects frequently cannot cooperate for optimal collection of a voided urine specimen. For incontinent women urine specimens may be contaminated with organisms which colonize the vagina and periurethral mucosa, compromising interpretation of the culture. The use of "pedibags" or bedpans has been proposed for urine specimen collection from such women, but these collection methods are subject to bacterial contamination, and not recommended. In-and-out catheterization should be used for urine specimen collection where a specimen is required from a woman who cannot provide a voided specimen. Catheterization should only be used where urine specimen collection is essential for clinical management as this procedure, itself, will precipitate bacteriuria in up to 5% of episodes.

Contamination with periurethral flora is less frequent in men than in women, and a clean-catch urine specimen can usually be obtained from men with voiding. Urine specimens from men who cannot cooperate for specimen collection may also be collected using external urine collecting devices. A standard approach for specimen collection which minimizes contamination should be followed. This includes cleaning of the glans, applying a clean condom and collecting bag, and immediate specimen collection after voiding.

Interpretation of Urine Culture

For asymptomatic urinary infection, two consecutive specimens with the same organism(s) isolated at $\geq 10^5$ colony-forming units (CFU)/mL are necessary (Table 127-6). With symptomatic infection, a single specimen with $\geq 10^5$ CFU/mL is sufficient. A bacterial quantitative count of $\geq 10^3$ CFU/mL is diagnostic for specimens obtained by in and out catheter. When urine specimens are collected

through external devices, a quantitative count of $\geq 10^5$ CFU/mL is necessary. Lower quantitative counts should be interpreted as contamination with colonizing periurethral organisms. In men with symptomatic infection, and for men or women with the clinical presentation of acute pyelonephritis, lower quantitative counts of $\geq 10^4$ CFU/mL of a single organism are generally considered sufficient for a microbiologic diagnosis of urinary infection. In the presence of renal failure, diuretic therapy, or with selected less common infecting organisms (e.g., *Candida albicans*) lower quantitative counts may also be consistent with infection. Rarely, with unusual pathogens (e.g., *Haemophilus influenzae* or *Ureaplasma urealyticum*), or with infection proximal to a complete obstruction, the urine culture may be negative. The urine culture, of course, may also be negative if the specimen for culture is obtained after antimicrobial therapy has been initiated. As infection with more than one organism may occur, especially in institutionalized subjects, cultures with multiple organisms isolated in appropriate quantitative counts should not be assumed to represent contamination.

Pyuria and Other Diagnostic Tests

Urinalysis or other screening tests for pyuria are not useful diagnostic tests for identification of urinary infection in elderly populations. Symptomatic urinary infection is consistently accompanied by pyuria, but pyuria also accompanies asymptomatic bacteriuria. More than 50% of bacteriuric elderly subjects living in the community have associated pyuria. In long-term care facilities, pyuria is almost a universal accompaniment of asymptomatic bacteriuria. Higher quantitative levels of pyuria are associated with renal rather than bladder infection. As many as 30% of long-term care facility residents without bacteriuria also have pyuria. The origins of pyuria in nonbacteriuric subjects have not been characterized, but are likely attributable to other inflammatory conditions within the urinary tract or, for women, contamination with vaginal secretions. Pyuria of any level with bacteriuria is not associated with poorer outcomes in elderly populations. Thus, the presence of pyuria does not identify "symptomatic" infection or indicate a need for therapy. While a finding of pyuria is not a useful diagnostic test, the absence of pyuria is helpful in excluding UTI.

Several rapid urine-screening tests have been proposed and evaluated for use in elderly populations as surrogate markers for identification of bacteriuria. The most widely used is the leukocyte esterase test, which screens for pyuria rather than bacteriuria. The nitrate-detection dipstick is also used. These tests have low sensitivity for bacteriuria and, when positive, cannot differentiate symptomatic from asymptomatic infection. None of these surrogate tests for bacteriuria have been demonstrated to have clinical utility in elderly populations, and they are not recommended for use in the management of urinary infection. A negative leukocyte esterase screen test, however, has high specificity and may be useful in excluding urinary infection.

MANAGEMENT

Asymptomatic Infection

As with other populations, ambulatory elderly women or men who experience recurrent episodes of symptomatic urinary infection also have a high prevalence of asymptomatic bacteriuria. There is no evidence that the asymptomatic bacteriuria causes symptomatic infection, and studies have consistently documented that treatment of asymptomatic bacteriuria is not effective in preventing symptomatic episodes. Clinical trials directly addressing treatment of asymptomatic bacteriuria in the elderly ambulatory men or women have not been reported. However, studies of management of asymptomatic bacteriuria in ambulatory women have often enrolled postmenopausal women. For instance, a study of diabetic women with asymptomatic bacteriuria and mean age more than 50 years reported that treatment of bacteriuria had no benefits, irrespective of age. Thus, treatment of asymptomatic infection in ambulatory populations is not recommended. It follows that routine screening for bacteriuria in asymptomatic elderly ambulatory populations is also not appropriate.

Antimicrobial treatment of asymptomatic bacteriuria in the institutionalized elderly is not beneficial. Clinical trials have consistently and repeatedly shown that therapy of asymptomatic urinary infection in either women or men in these settings does not decrease the occurrence of symptomatic urinary infection, improve chronic genitourinary symptoms, or improve survival. Chronic incontinence in bacteriuric subjects, in particular, is not improved with antimicrobial therapy. The prevalence of bacteriuria in a long-term care population is not decreased by efforts to eradicate bacteriuria in asymptomatic residents. Antimicrobial therapy for asymptomatic bacteriuria is, however, associated with negative outcomes, including an increased frequency of adverse drug effects, emergence of resistant organisms, and increased cost. Thus, for the institutionalized population, asymptomatic bacteriuria should not be treated with antimicrobial therapy. Similarly, the presence of pyuria in the absence of symptoms is not an indication for therapy. Routine screening for bacteriuria or pyuria in these populations is not recommended. The only exception would be if an invasive genitourinary procedure is planned. Antimicrobial therapy is indicated as prophylaxis to prevent bacteremia and sepsis following the procedure.

Symptomatic Urinary Infection

Choice of Antimicrobial

Antimicrobial selection for treatment of urinary infection is similar for elderly and younger populations. Consistent alterations in antimicrobial pharmacokinetics are observed in the elderly, including increased volume of distribution and decreased renal clearance. These changes are not, however, of sufficient consistency or magnitude that differences in selection or dosing of antimicrobials is recommended routinely on the basis of age alone. Therapy may be given either orally (Table 127-7) or, when oral administration cannot be tolerated or absorption is uncertain, parenterally (Table 127-8). The specific antimicrobial selected is determined by effectiveness of the agent for treatment of urinary infection, known or presumed susceptibilities of the infecting organism, whether oral or parenteral therapy is indicated, tolerance of the patient, and renal and hepatic function. Antimicrobial cost will also usually be a factor, especially for institutionalized populations. When the clinical presentation is not severe, therapy should be delayed until urine culture results with organism susceptibilities are available.

Oral Therapy The preferred oral therapy for susceptible gram-negative organisms would usually be nitrofurantoin or TMP/SMX,

TABLE 127-7

Oral Antimicrobial Regimens for Treatment of Acute UTI

AGENT	DOSE*
First line	
Nitrofurantoin	50–100 mg four times a day
TMP/SMX	160/800 mg, twice daily
TMP	100 mg twice daily
Amoxicillin[†]	500 mg three times daily
Other	
Amoxicillin/clavulanic acid	500 mg three times daily or 875 mg twice daily
Norfloxacin	400 mg twice daily
Ciprofloxacin	250–500 mg twice daily
Ofloxacin	200–400 mg twice daily
Levofloxacin	500 mg once a day
Cephalexin	500 mg four times a day
Cefaclor	500 mg
Cefadroxil	1 g once a day or twice daily
Cefixime	400 mg once a day
Cefuroxime axetil	250 mg twice daily
Cefpodoxime proxetil	100–400 mg twice daily

*Assumes normal renal function.
[†]For susceptible gram-positive organisms.

as these are relatively inexpensive agents with which there is extensive clinical experience. Nitrofurantoin should not be used for renal infection, *P. mirabilis*, *K. pneumoniae* or *P. aeruginosa* infection, or in patients with renal failure. Concerns about sulfa allergy have led some countries, including Sweden and Great Britain, to restrict the use of TMP/SMX. However, there is long experience with this antimicrobial and it remains a useful agent. Where sulfa allergy precludes use of the combination, TMP alone may be used.

TABLE 127-8

Parenteral Antimicrobial Regimens for the Treatment of UTI

AGENT	DOSE*
Preferred	
Gentamicin	1–1.5 mg/kg q8h or 4–5 mg/kg q24h
Tobramycin	1–1.5 mg/kg q8h or 4–5 mg/kg q24h
Ampicillin[†]	1 g q4–6h
Cefazolin	1–2 g q8h
Other	
TMP/SMX	160/800 mg q12h
Amikacin	5 mg/kg q8h or 15 mg/kg q24h
Piperacillin	3 g q4h
Piperacillin/tazobactam	4 g/500 mg q8h
Cefotaxime	1–2 g q8h
Ceftriaxone	1–2 g q24h
Cefepime	2 g q12h
Ceftazidime	0.5–2 g q8h
Aztreonam	1–2 g q6h
Imipenem/cilastatin	500 mg q6h
Vancomycin[†]	500 mg q6h or 1 g q12h
Ciprofloxacin	200–400 mg q12h
Levofloxacin	500 mg daily

*Assumes normal renal function.
[†]For gram-positive organisms.

There is, however, increasing TMP and TMP/SMX resistance in some populations, and local susceptibilities must be considered in choosing empiric therapy.

Fluoroquinolones have been widely used for treatment of UTI in both ambulatory and institutionalized elderly populations. A randomized, nonblinded study of oral suspensions of ciprofloxacin or TMP/SMX enrolled both ambulatory elderly and nursing home residents and reported 10 days of ciprofloxacin was superior to 10 days of TMP/SMX, and had fewer adverse effects. The difference was more marked in nursing home residents. Despite this, widespread use of fluoroquinolones as empiric first line therapy is of concern as this may promote resistance. The early fluoroquinolones, norfloxacin and ciprofloxacin, have had extensive use in elderly populations and are well tolerated. Levofloxacin may be associated with glucose abnormalities in diabetic patients. Moxifloxacin is not indicated for treatment of urinary infection because of limited urinary excretion. These agents are still most appropriately reserved for treatment of infections with organisms resistant to first-line agents, or in individuals who cannot tolerate alternate antimicrobials.

Amoxicillin is effective for treatment of infections with susceptible gram-positive organisms, such as group B streptococci or enterococci. It is not first-line therapy for gram-negative organisms because of the high prevalence of antimicrobial resistance. Amoxicillin/clavulanic acid and oral cephalosporins are also effective in the treatment of urinary infection, but are not recommended as first-line agents because of their broad-spectrum activity and cost.

Parenteral Therapy When parenteral therapy is indicated, aminoglycosides such as gentamicin or tobramycin remain the antibiotics of choice. These may be given either intravenously or intramuscularly. Ampicillin or vancomycin are added for empiric therapy if enterococcal infection is a concern. After assessment of the initial response to therapy, and when the pretherapy urine culture and susceptibility results are known, a decision should be made whether aminoglycoside therapy should be continued, changed to alternate parenteral therapy, or the therapeutic course completed with oral therapy. Ototoxicity and nephrotoxicity with aminoglycoside therapy are unlikely when therapy duration is limited to 48 to 72 hours. Aminoglycosides should not be used, however, in persons with renal failure. Many other parenteral antimicrobials are also effective (Table 127-8), but these are more costly and, again, there are concerns with promoting antimicrobial resistance with widespread use.

Resistant Organisms For vancomycin-resistant Enterococcus, nitrofurantoin usually remains effective therapy and is the treatment of choice for cystitis. Alternate therapies for renal or systemic infection would include linezolid or tigecycline, but there is little clinical experience with these agents for treatment of urinary infection at any age. Extended spectrum beta lactamase producing organisms are usually also resistant to TMP/SMX, fluoroquinolones, and aminoglycosides. Nitrofurantoin frequently remains effective and should be used for cystitis. Some of these strains are also susceptible to amoxicillin/clavulanic acid. If parenteral therapy is required, most strains remain susceptible to carbapenems, and ertapenem may be appropriate. Symptomatic candida infection is uncommon in noncatheterized individuals. The treatment of choice is fluconazole—the only azole with renal excretion. For fluconazole-resistant strains, such as *C. glabrata*, there is no clear consensus on optimal therapy. Amphotericin B bladder washout, or a single parenteral dose of am-

TABLE 127-9	
Recommended Duration of Antimicrobial Therapy for Treatment of Symptomatic UTI	
CLINICAL PRESENTATION	**DURATION**
Women	
Acute cystitis	3–7 days
Acute pyelonephritis	10–14 days
Men	
Acute cystitis	7–14 days
Acute pyelonephritis	14 days
Relapsing infection (likely prostatitis)	6–12 weeks

photericin B may be considered for bladder infection. For renal or systemic infection, amphotericin B deoxycholate or as lipid complex, voriconazole or caspofungin may be options, but no specific recommendations can be made.

Duration of Therapy (Table 127-9)

Treatment of symptomatic lower urinary infection in elderly women is less effective than for younger women. This is consistent for all durations of therapy, but shorter courses of therapy of a single dose or 3 days are likely proportionately less effective than 7-day courses in older women. Current guidelines and meta-analyses of clinical studies suggest that short course therapy should not be used for postmenopausal women with acute uncomplicated urinary infection. Despite this, the majority of postmenopausal women with acute cystitis will be cured by 3-day therapy. A recent randomized, double blind trial documented equivalent efficacy of 3 or 7 days ciprofloxacin for the treatment of acute cystitis in ambulatory elderly women older than 65 years of age. The mean age in this study was 79 years and women were carefully selected to exclude renal failure or complicated urinary infection. Thus, for well, ambulatory elderly women, 3 days fluoroquinolone therapy is an effective option.

Short course antimicrobial therapy is ineffective for treatment of asymptomatic bacteriuria in long-term care facility residents, but has not been evaluated for treatment of symptomatic infection. Longer antimicrobial courses are also associated with very high rates of recurrence, and the comparative efficacy of short or longer courses for symptomatic infection has not been evaluated. Seven days is currently recommended for women or men with bladder infection. Renal infection should be treated with 10 to 14 days of therapy. For men, retreatment with prolonged therapy of 6 or 12 weeks may achieve higher cure rates for prostate infection.

Prolonged suppressive antimicrobial therapy may be considered where there is persistent or recurrent morbidity attributable to urinary infection, and bacteria cannot be eradicated from the urinary tract. Such circumstances are uncommon, but might include recurrent invasive infection in the presence of an underlying genitourinary abnormality that cannot be corrected, persistent infected stones where suppressive therapy may prevent further stone enlargement, frequent symptomatic recurrences from a prostatic source, or with chronic renal failure. Antimicrobial selection for suppressive therapy is individualized, based on susceptibilities of the infecting organism and tolerance. For the elderly, it is usually continued indefinitely. It must be appreciated, however, that suppressive therapy is seldom indicated. When this approach is used, the therapy should be reevaluated regularly to ensure it remains appropriate and effective.

Outcome Following Therapy

Bacterial cure rates of 75% to 90% at 4 to 6 weeks post-therapy are anticipated for ambulatory elderly women treated for symptomatic infection. Recurrence may be symptomatic or asymptomatic. For ambulatory men with prostate infections, cure rates are only 40% to 50% at 4 to 6 weeks, even with more prolonged therapy. Prostatic infection may also be associated with very late relapses, occurring up to a year or more after therapy.

The outcomes following treatment of urinary infection for both men and women in the institutionalized population are similar to other populations with complicated urinary infection. Recurrent infection, either relapse or reinfection, occurs by 4 to 6 weeks for at least 50% of therapeutic courses. Thus, high microbiological recurrence rates are the norm. The goal of treatment is to ameliorate symptoms, not to sterilize the urine. Post-therapy urine cultures should be obtained only when symptoms persist or recur.

Controversies in UTI Management in Long-Term Care Facilities

UTI is one of the most frequent reasons for prescribing antimicrobial therapy in long-term care facilities. A substantial proportion of these antimicrobial courses are given for asymptomatic infection or presentations without localizing urinary symptoms. Symptomatic urinary infection is over-diagnosed and, in effect, asymptomatic bacteriuria is frequently treated on the basis of urinalysis findings or nonspecific changes in clinical status. While this problem has been appreciated for many years, limited progress toward a more rational antimicrobial approach in these facilities has been made.

Qualitative studies have characterized some variables which drive inappropriate antimicrobial use. When antimicrobial therapy is given, patients frequently are not assessed by physicians; nursing personnel are central to decision making and treatment. Ordering urine cultures and prescribing antibiotics are influenced by a wide range of nonspecific symptoms or signs in residents. The most commonly reported triggers for suspecting UTI in noncatheterized residents are changes in mental status, voiding patterns, or character of the urine. A strong odor to the urine or cloudy urine and fever are frequently assumed to be urinary infection. Dipstick analysis of the urine is often the initial testing procedure which, of course, frequently documents pyuria, and is interpreted as an indication for treatment despite the absence of acute localizing findings.

Guidelines and consensus statements recognize the problems with definitive diagnosis and have proposed management for potential urinary infection. The IDSA guidelines for evaluation of fever in long-term care facilities suggest diagnostic laboratory evaluation of suspected urinary infection in noncatheterized residents should be reserved for those with acute onset of symptoms and signs associated with urinary infection. These include fever, dysuria, gross hematuria, new or worsening urinary incontinence, and/or suspected bacteremia. A consensus conference proposed criteria for empiric antimicrobial treatment for non catheterized residents with suspected urinary infections which include presentations of either acute dysuria alone, or of fever (>37.9°C [100°F] or increase of 1.5°C [2.4°F] above baseline) and at least one of: new or worsening ur-

gency, frequency, suprapubic pain, gross hematuria, costovertebral angle tenderness, or urinary incontinence. These criteria assume that prior to institution of antimicrobial therapy a urine specimen for culture is obtained.

Intervention studies developed to improve antimicrobial use for urinary infection in long-term care facilities have also been reported. A Swiss study addressing the diagnosis and treatment of both urinary and respiratory infection assessed the impact of interventions which included a comprehensive, multidisciplinary educational program including distribution of guidelines followed by continuing lectures and feedback compared with usual practice. The intervention program was associated with a significantly increased adherence of antimicrobial therapy to the guidelines, together with an overall 54% reduction of antibiotic consumption for urinary infection and pneumonia combined. A comparative study in 24 Ontario and Idaho nursing homes evaluated a diagnostic and treatment algorithm based on the consensus recommendations for initiating antimicrobial therapy for UTI. The intervention included small group interactive sessions for nurses, videotapes, written material, outreach visits and one-on-one interviews with physicians. The intervention homes had a significant decrease in antimicrobial courses for suspected UTI, but total antimicrobial use was similar in intervention and usual care groups. This suggested that patients with nonspecific symptoms who were previously diagnosed as urinary infection were still receiving antimicrobial treatment, but given an alternate diagnosis. Approaches to improving antimicrobial use in long-term care facilities likely must be comprehensive, rather than focusing on a single infection.

PREVENTION

Asymptomatic Infection

The extraordinary frequency of urinary infection in the elderly populations is primarily attributable to aging changes and associated comorbidities. Prevention of urinary infection on a population basis would require modification of these contributing factors. Optimal management of comorbid illnesses is desirable, but the potential impact on bacteriuria is unknown. It is unlikely there are interventions which could substantially decrease the prevalence of bacteriuria.

Devices used for management of incontinence, including external urine collecting devices, intermittent catheterization and, of course, indwelling urethral catheters, contribute to bacteriuria. Avoidance or limitation of use of these devices will be effective in decreasing the frequency of bacteriuria. This may not, however, be an achievable goal in the individual elderly subject. In people with bladder emptying using intermittent catheterization, the frequency of urinary infection is similar with a sterile or clean technique, so in the long-term care setting a clean technique is appropriate, and less costly.

Symptomatic Infection

Some elderly women will experience recurrent episodes of acute cystitis, similar to younger women. Women who have recurrent symptomatic infections should be considered for referral to an urologist, as structural abnormalities in the lower urinary tract may predispose to recurrent infections. When these symptomatic episodes occur so

TABLE 127-10

Antimicrobial Regimens for Prophylaxis of Acute, Recurrent, Symptomatic Lower Tract Infection in Ambulatory Women

ANTIMICROBIAL	REGIMEN*
Preferred	
Nitrofurantoin	50–100 mg daily
TMP/SMX	80/400 mg daily or three times weekly
TMP	100 mg daily
Second line	
Cephalexin	125 mg daily
Norfloxacin	200 mg daily or three times weekly
Ciprofloxacin	125 mg daily

*Medication taken at bedtime. Topical estrogen use may prevent recurrent symptomatic infections in postmenopausal women. Patients with recurrent infections should be evaluated for a structural lesion (see text).

frequently that they are distressing to the patient or interfere with daily routine, and no correctable pathology has been identified, they may be prevented with long-term low-dose prophylactic antimicrobial therapy (Table 127-10). Prophylactic therapy is usually taken at bedtime, and initially continued for 6 months or 1 year. This approach is indicated for otherwise well women in the community with no genitourinary abnormalites. It would seldom be appropriate in women residents of long-term care facilities with neurological impairment of bladder emptying. Topical vaginal estrogen therapy may also decrease the frequency of acute symptomatic infection in selected women. However, studies of efficacy are conflicting and this intervention is not as effective as antimicrobial therapy. Currently, it does not seem appropriate to prescribe continuous topical vaginal estrogen solely to prevent recurrent UTI.

Ingesting large quantities of "natural" urinary antiseptics, particularly cranberry juice, has been proposed. Cranberry juice may be effective through interference with bacterial adherence. Female residents of a long-term care facility who drank large quantities of cranberry juice daily had a decreased prevalence of bacteriuria with pyuria, but not bacteriuria nor symptomatic episodes. A double blind, placebo controlled trial of cranberry juice in a geriatric assessment and rehabilitation ward found no significant decrease in symptomatic infection with cranberry juice, and no difference in antimicrobial use. While there seems no reason to discourage drinking cranberry juice, it is premature to endorse this as a means of preventing urinary infection or its complications in elderly populations.

There is an increased risk for systemic infection from a urinary source in the presence of obstruction of the genitourinary tract, such as the elderly man with prostatic hypertrophy. Continuing evaluation and early intervention if obstruction occurs should be effective in decreasing morbidity. Prophylactic antimicrobial therapy is indicated for bacteriuric subjects who will undergo an invasive genitourinary procedure likely to be associated with mucosal trauma. This includes cystoscopy in men and transurethral resection of the prostate, but not uncomplicated replacement of a long-term indwelling urethral catheter. Antimicrobial therapy must be initiated prior to the invasive procedure, preferably within 1 hour, and usually is not continued beyond the duration of the procedure. Studies suggest a single preprocedure dose of antimicrobial, selected based on the susceptibilities of the infecting bacteria, is adequate.

LONG-TERM INDWELLING CATHETERS

Epidemiology

From 5% to 10% of elderly residents of institutions have urine voiding managed with a chronic (long-term) indwelling catheter. A higher proportion of women have chronic indwelling catheters. The major indications for catheterization are retention, incontinence management, and to assist in healing pressure ulcers. Subjects with long-term indwelling catheters are always bacteriuric, usually with two to five organisms at any time. Morbidity from urinary infection is increased in the presence of a long-term indwelling catheter relative to bacteriuric residents without a catheter. Renal inflammation consistent with acute pyelonephritis is also identified at autopsy more frequently in elderly residents with an indwelling catheter. A chronic indwelling catheter is the single most important risk factor for bacteremia in the institutionalized elderly. Catheter obstruction is a frequent problem, but the incidence and time to obstruction varies among patients. Obstruction is caused by struvite formation by urease producing organisms such as *P. mirabilis* or *P. stuartii*. Mucosal trauma may occur with catheter change, and in the presence of infected urine may lead to fever. However, bacteriemia occurs infrequently, in less than 10% of catheter changes, and is usually asymptomatic. Residents with an indwelling urinary catheter also have an increased mortality compared to noncatheterized residents, but there is no evidence this is attributable to catheterization itself.

Biofilm Formation

Biofilm is uniformly present on the internal and external catheter surface. Initially, bacteria adhere to the conditioning protein film which coats the catheter immediately after it is placed. These bacteria excrete an extracellular polysaccharide material and organisms multiply and persist in colonies within this material. Urine constituents such as Tamm-Horsfall protein, magnesium, and calcium are also incorporated. Biofilm ascends the catheter surfaces within a few days of insertion of a new catheter.

The presence of the biofilm explains several clinically relevant observations. The microbiology of organisms present in the biofilm differs from that in the urine, with a greater number of organisms at higher quantitative counts isolated. Urine specimens obtained through a catheter *in situ* will sample the microbiology of the biofilm rather than urine. Biofilm formation is also responsible for catheter encrustation and obstruction through mineral deposition in the presence of an alkaline urine produced by urease producing organisms. This is the same process as struvite formation with urolithiasis. Finally, organisms grow in the biofilm in a relatively protected environment. Some antimicrobials are unable to diffuse into the biofilm. Antimicrobial therapy given to subjects with a chronic indwelling catheter encourages emergence of resistance in organisms resident in the biofilm. In addition, organisms may be relatively metabolically inactive and not susceptible to some antimicrobials. Host defenses, including neutrophils and immunoglobulins, also cannot diffuse into the biofilm and are ineffective in controlling growth of organisms in these colonies. Thus, the biofilm provides a protected environment where organisms persist despite antimicrobial therapy, and are a source of relapsing infection when therapy is discontinued.

Clinical Presentations

Presentations of urinary infection in patients with indwelling urethral catheters differ from those without a catheter. The most common presentation of symptomatic urinary infection is fever alone without localizing genitourinary signs or symptoms. Local findings such as obstruction or leaking of the catheter or evidence of trauma to the mucosa such as hematuria may occur. In the absence of localizing findings, the urinary tract is the likely source of fever in 30% to 40% of episodes. Local presentations of infection also occur. These include purulent urethritis, tunnel site infections in patients with suprapubic catheters, or periurethral abscesses. Men may develop a urethral fistula, epididymitis, orchitis, scrotal abscess, prostatitis or prostatic abscess. Urolithiasis with bladder or renal stones may also occur. A unique, uncommon, presentation is the "purple urine bag syndrome." This is thought to result when bacteria in the gut metabolize tryptophan to indole in the presence of decreased gut motility. The indole is absorbed and conjugated in the liver to indican, which is excreted into the urine and further metabolized to indoxyl by organisms present in the drainage bag. In an alkaline urine, indigo and indirubin are generated and dissolve in the plastic of the drainage bag, creating a purple color. While the presentation is dramatic, the condition is benign, and addressed by managing constipation and changing the drainage bag.

Management of Symptomatic Infection

Consensus recommendations for instituting empiric antimicrobial therapy for urinary infection in the presence of an indwelling urinary catheter suggest the presence of any one of fever (>37.9°C [100°F] or increase of 1.5°C [2.4°F] about baseline temperature), new costovertebral angle tenderness, rigors (shaking, chills) with or without identified cause, or new onset of delirium is sufficient. A urine specimen for culture should be obtained prior to antimicrobial therapy. The indwelling catheter should be changed and the specimen for culture obtained through the newly inserted catheter immediately prior to initiating antimicrobial treatment. This specimen is representative of urine rather than biofilm microbiology. Catheter replacement prior to antimicrobial therapy also leads to a more prompt resolution of fever, and a lower likelihood of symptomatic relapse post-therapy.

Considerations in choosing an antimicrobial are similar to those for subjects without indwelling catheters. When symptomatic urinary infection is diagnosed, antimicrobial therapy should be selected on the basis of the known or presumed infecting organisms and patient tolerance (Tables 127-7 and 127-8). The duration of antibiotic therapy is not well studied, but should be limited to prevent emergence of resistant organisms. Generally, only 5 to 7 days therapy is recommended if there is a prompt clinical response. There are no clinical studies, however, that define the optimal length of therapy, and clinical judgment is necessary.

Prevention

The most important intervention is to avoid catheter use or, when an indwelling catheter is indicated, to discontinue the catheter as soon as possible. This is not feasible for some long-term care facility residents, especially women. For men, incontinence management with an external condom collecting device is an option. A recent randomized trial in a VA hospital enrolling men with a mean age of 73 years, reported a significant decrease in adverse outcomes with condom drainage compared to an indwelling catheter. When possible, intermittent catheterization is preferred to a chronic indwelling catheter for retention, and may also be associated with fewer adverse effects. Use of a suprapubic catheter is sometimes suggested, but studies are inconsistent in documenting benefits with suprapubic catheter use. The surgical procedure for insertion may itself be associated with adverse effects. A suprapubic catheter, however, may have a role for selected individuals with difficulties with urethral catheter insertion or with discomfort with the urethral catheter.

Currently, there are no specific interventions which are documented to decrease the frequency of bacteriuria or complications of urinary infection in elderly patients who require chronic indwelling catheters. Maintenance of a closed drainage system for the catheter and tubing delays onset of bacteriuria in subjects with short-term indwelling catheters and is recommended for long-term indwelling catheters as well. The drainage bag should be maintained in a dependent position. The catheter should be secured in order to minimize urethral irritation, and to avoid contact with incontinent stool. Catheter care should minimize trauma, and facilitate prompt identification of obstruction. Routine catheter change, daily periurethral catheter care with antiseptics, or catheter irrigation with saline or antiseptics does not decrease the frequency of urinary infection, and these are not recommended practices.

Morbidity of UTI associated with chronic indwelling catheters is largely attributable to biofilm formation. Thus, development of catheter materials which limit biofilm formation would be an advance in preventing complications of catheter use. Use of a silicone rather than a latex catheter may delay onset of obstruction for selected patients. These catheters are more expensive, but should be considered for patients with repeated, early obstruction, as well as those with latex allergy. Some antimicrobial catheters may minimally delay onset of bacteriuria in short-term catheterization. To date, none of these have been shown to have a benefit for patients with chronic urinary catheters.

Summary

UTI is the most common infection which occurs in elderly populations. The management of UTI for elderly ambulatory individuals is similar to younger populations, and determined by the presentation as either acute uncomplicated urinary infection or complicated urinary infection. Treatment of symptomatic urinary infection requires optimal use of urine culture for diagnosis, appropriate antimicrobial selection, and appropriate duration of therapy. In the long-term care facility, the very high prevalence of asymptomatic bacteriuria interferes with ascertainment of symptomatic infection, especially in residents without localizing genitourinary symptoms. Bacteriuric elderly individuals who present with clinical decline without localizing findings should not be assumed to have a urinary source, despite a positive urine culture. A critical approach to diagnosis, investigation, and treatment is necessary. Further characterization of symptomatic presentations of urinary infection in the functionally disabled elderly, together with evaluation of management approaches such as non treatment with observation compared with empiric antimicrobial treatment, are needed. For residents with chronic indwelling catheters, optimal duration of antimicrobial therapy, management of complications, and evaluation of new catheter materials or alternatives to indwelling urethral catheters need to be addressed.

FURTHER READING

1. Bentley DW, Bradlry S, High K, et al. Practice guideline for evaluation of fever and infection in long term care facilities. *Clin Infect Dis.* 2000;31:640.

2. Jackson SL, Boylso EJ, Scliolrs D, et al. Predictors of urinary tract infection after menopause: a prospective study. *Am J Med.* 2004;117:903.

3. Loeb M, Bentley DW, Bradly S, et al. Development of minimum criteria for the initiation of antibiotics in residents of long term care facilities. *Infect Control Hosp Epidemiol.* 2001;22:316.

4. Loeb M, Brazil K, Lohfeld Letal, et al. Effect of a multifaceted intervention on number of antimicrobial prescriptions for suspected urinary tract infections in residents of nursing homes: cluster randomized controlled trial. *BMJ.* 2005;331:669.

5. Lutters M, Harbarln S, Jansscns JP, et al. Effect of a comprehensive, multidisciplinary, educational program on the use of antibiotics in a geriatric university hospital. *Jour Amer Ger Soc.* 2004;52:112.

6. McMurdo ME, Bissottl LY, Pricel RJ, et al. Does ingestion of cranberry juice reduce symptomatic urinary tract infections in older people in hospital? A double-blind, placebo controlled trial. 2005;34:256.

7. Nicolle LE, Frieson D, Haroting GK, et al. Hospitalization for acute pyelonephritis in Manitoba, Canada, during the period from 1989 to 1992. Impact of diabetes, pregnancy, and aboriginal origin. *Clin Infect Dis.* 1996;22:1051.

8. Nicolle LE, Strausbeugh LJ, Garibald RA, et al. Infections and antibiotic resistance in nursing homes. *Clin Microbiol Rev.* 1996;9:1.

9. Nicolle LE, Asymptomatic bacteriuria in the elderly. *Infect Dis Clin North Am.* 1997;11:647.

10. Nicolle LE. Urinary tract infection in long term care facility residents. *Clin Infect Dis.* 2000;31:757.

11. Nicolle LE. The chronic indwelling catheter and urinary infection in long-term care facility residents. *Infect Control Hosp Epidemiol.* 2001;22:316.

12. Nicolle LE. SHEA Long Term Care Committee: urinary tract infections in long-term care facilities. *Infect Control Hosp Epidemiol.* 2001;22:167.

13. Nicolle LE, Bradley S, Colgan R, et al: IDSA guidelines for the diagnosis and treatment of asymptomatic bacteriuria in adults. *Clin Infect Dis.* 2005;40:645.

14. Orr P, Nieolle LE, Duckworth H, et al. Febrile urinary infection in the institutionalized elderly. *Am J Med.* 1996;100:71.

15. Ouslander JG, Schapira M, Schnelle JF, et al. Does eradicating bacteriuria affect the severity of chronic urinary incontinence in nursing home residents? *Ann Intern Med.* 1995;12:749.

16. Raz R, Gennesin Y, Wasser J, et al. Recurrent urinary tract infection in postmenopausal women. *Clin Infect Dis.* 2000;30:152.

17. Raz R, Schiller D, Nicolle LE. Chronic indwelling catheter replacement prior to antimicrobial therapy for symptomatic urinary infection. *J Urol.* 2000;164:1254.

18. Rodhe N, Molstad S, England L, et al. Asymptomatic bacteriuria in a population of elderly residents living in a community setting: prevalence characteristics and associated factors. *Family Practice.* 2006;23:3003.

19. Schaeffer, AJ. Chronic prostatitis and the chronic pelvic pain syndrome. *N Engl J Med.* 2006;355:1690.

20. Vogel T, Verreault R, Gourdeau M, et al. Optimal duration of antibiotic therapy for uncomplicated urinary tract infection in older women: a double-blind randomized controlled trial. *Can Med Assoc Jour.* 2004;170:469.

Human Immunodeficiency Virus Infection

Amy C. Justice

Aging and human immunodeficiency virus (HIV) infection were once considered mutually exclusive conditions. Older people did not "get AIDS" (acquired immunodeficiency syndrome) and the younger people who did never had a chance to grow old. Now, thanks to the success of combination antiretroviral therapy (CART), people aged 50 years and older represent a growing proportion of all those living with HIV infection; from 2001 to 2004, the proportion grew from 17% to 23%. The U.S. Senate Subcommittee on Aging now predicts that by 2015, 50% of the U.S. population living with HIV infection will be 50 years of age or older.

As the prevalence of HIV infection grows in older population groups, the risk of new HIV infections is also likely to increase. This increased risk may be exacerbated by several factors. First, the use of sildenafil (Viagra) and related medications to effectively treat erectile dysfunction and enhance sexual performance may increase risky sexual behavior. Additionally, postmenopausal women may be less likely to request that condoms be used as they face no risk of pregnancy. Finally, age-associated erectile changes may make condom use difficult and age-associated declines in immunity may place older individuals at higher risk of transmission with each exposure.

Research in age, aging, and HIV has focused on comparing outcomes among persons aged 50 years and older to their younger counterparts. This cut point is supported in HIV for both sociological and medical reasons: people aged 50 years and older with HIV state they feel marginalized because of age and this group experiences a shortened survival and greater burden of comorbid disease. Additionally, some data suggests that chronic HIV infection causes an accelerated aging process; an HIV infected 50-year-old person may have more physiologically in common with an uninfected individual aged 60 or 70 years.

While few geriatricians are likely to choose to manage antiretroviral agents, geriatricians need to be aware of the new Centers for Disease Control and Prevention recommendations for HIV screening. Geriatricians will also be increasingly needed to comanage the effects of aging and cumulative frailty; comorbid medical and psychiatric conditions; and drug interactions and toxicities in people with HIV infection. Further, the study of HIV infection among aging individuals may provide a template for improving the management of complex chronic disease more generally especially among special populations of aging individuals—people of color, sexual minorities, those with few socioeconomic resources, and those aging with heavy substance use histories. These groups are often ignored or understudied when more common conditions of aging are addressed.

CLINICAL PRESENTATION

Little is known about the presentation of acute HIV infection in older patients. In younger patients, acute infection may be completely asymptomatic or present as a flu-like syndrome. Like older HIV-negative individuals, older people with HIV infection underreport symptoms as compared to younger individuals, and this underreporting may be especially pronounced in older black patients. In addition, the symptoms associated with HIV infection are also common among older patients without HIV infection.

Among those persons 50 years of age and older who are chronically infected with HIV and in care, the most common self-reported symptoms are fatigue, pain in hands or feet (peripheral neuropathy), problems sleeping, muscle or joint pain (myalgias or arthralgias), and problems with having sex. Prior to the start of antiretroviral therapy, people with HIV infection tended to have lower cholesterol values than demographically matched controls. Common laboratory abnormalities include leucopenia, anemia (predominantly normocytic), and transaminitis. Thus, unless the clinician has a high index of suspicion in the older patient, or routinely screens for HIV infection, it may be difficult to identify HIV-positive individuals. HIV-infected women enter menopause at a median age of 46 years compared to the median of 51 years among uninfected women. HIV-infected women also tend to experience more pronounced symptoms during menopause. Hypogonadism is also prevalent among men infected with HIV. Like the symptoms, signs, and laboratory abnormalities discussed above, most of the diagnoses made in older people with HIV are not unique to HIV infection.

DIAGNOSIS

Physicians and their older patients are likely to underestimate the risk of HIV infection. The patient may be misinformed or in denial. The physician may mistakenly believe that the patient is not having unprotected sex with multiple partners or using illicit drugs. Nationally, the median CD4 cell count at presentation for HIV care continues to indicate advanced HIV disease (counts below 200 per mm^3) and delayed treatment. This is especially true among older individuals.

Because untreated individuals are more likely to infect others, the benefit from treatment is less among those presenting with advanced disease and previous targeted screening policies have not improved the situation. The Centers for Disease Control and Prevention have revised their guidelines for HIV testing as of September of 2006 to encourage near universal screening. Specifically, current recommendations now call for HIV screening among:

- All patients aged 13 to 64 years in all health care settings
- All patients initiating treatment for tuberculosis
- All patients seeking treatment for sexually transmitted diseases
- All persons at high risk for HIV (at minimum on a yearly basis)

The Centers for Disease Control and Prevention goes further to say that opt-out screening (screening after notifying the patient that an HIV test will be performed unless the patient declines) is now recommended in all health care settings. Specific signed consent for HIV testing should not be required. General informed consent for medical care should be considered sufficient to encompass informed consent for HIV testing.

Regardless of age, any patient reporting any of the following: multiple sexual partners and unprotected sex; a prior diagnosis of a sexually transmitted disease (gonorrhea, syphilis, chlamydia, or trichomonas); or illicit drug use is at high risk for HIV infection and should be tested. Note that in some cases, an individual in a monogamous relationship may present with a sexually transmitted disease because their partner has more than one partner. These individuals are at risk for HIV as well and should be tested. While, intravenous drug use is a risk factor in itself; illicit drug use, IV or otherwise, is associated with risky sexual behavior. Hazardous alcohol use is also an important risk factor for unprotected sex with multiple partners. Because older patients may not spontaneously report these behaviors and conditions, physicians should routinely ask about them (Table 128-1).

HIV testing should be conducted as part of a diagnostic workup in any patient with unexplained anemia, peripheral neuropathy, oral candidiasis, widespread herpes zoster, recurrent bacterial pneumonia, or any of the more traditional AIDS-associated conditions (*Pneumocystis carnii* pneumonia, Kaposi's sarcoma, atypical mycobacterium, or tuberculosis). Finally, any patient for whom more common causes of debilitating fatigue or weight loss have been eliminated should be tested for HIV.

The blood test is simple, accurate (sensitivity and specificity >99.9%), and widely available. It involves two steps. The first step is a screening enzyme immunoabsorbent assay for HIV antibody. If this test is positive, a western blot is used to confirm the diagnosis.

TABLE 128-1

Short Sex and Drug History to Use with Older Adults

I now need to ask you some questions about some possible activities that may put you at risk for infectious diseases. Do you mind if we discuss your sexual health and other behaviors?

- Do you have sexual or intimate contact with another man or woman? If yes, with men, women, or both?
- Do you take disease precautions? If yes, explain your precautions? If no, why not?
- Do you take any recreational drugs that involve the use of needles? If yes, do you share needles? If yes, how do you clean them?
- Have you ever had a sexually transmitted disease? If yes, how was it treated?
- Do you drink alcohol before sex? Do you use any illicit drugs or other substances before sex?

Do you have any questions that you would like to ask me about your sexual health and practices?

Specifically, do you have any questions about AIDS or sexually transmitted diseases?

Adapted from Linsk NL. HIV among older adults: age-specific issues in prevention and treatment. AIDS Reader. 10(7):430, 2000.

If the first test is negative, the patient is considered uninfected. Even in low-risk populations such as blood donors, the false-positive rate of these combined tests is low (<0.001%). When an individual tests positive, it is important to inform them of these results with as much care as you would any other life-changing diagnoses like that of cancer or diabetes. It is particularly important that you facilitate their integration into a clinical practice with substantial experience in the treatment of HIV infection. Comanagement may be needed if the patient has a substantial burden of age-related comorbid conditions or frailty.

PROGNOSIS

Survival without treatment from the time of first AIDS-associated diagnosis is on the order of 1 to 2 years (median). Survival with current multiclass, combination antiretroviral treatment has not been fully characterized, but estimates suggest that current treatments confer between 10 and 25 additional years of survival. Of note, prognosis is poorer among those who present late for care or fail to adhere to their treatment regimen.

Throughout the epidemic, age at seroconversion has been strongly associated with survival. This is, in part, explained by delays in treatment. When treated, older people appear to adhere to multiclass, combination antiretroviral treatment better than their younger counterparts. However it remains unclear whether their immunologic response to treatment is as good as among younger individuals. Older individuals may also be more susceptible to short- or long-term adverse drug effects from antiretroviral therapy.

OVERLAPPING COMPLICATIONS, COMORBIDITIES, AND TOXICITY

Chronic HIV infection is a complex chronic disease in which it is often impossible to tell whether a new condition in an individual

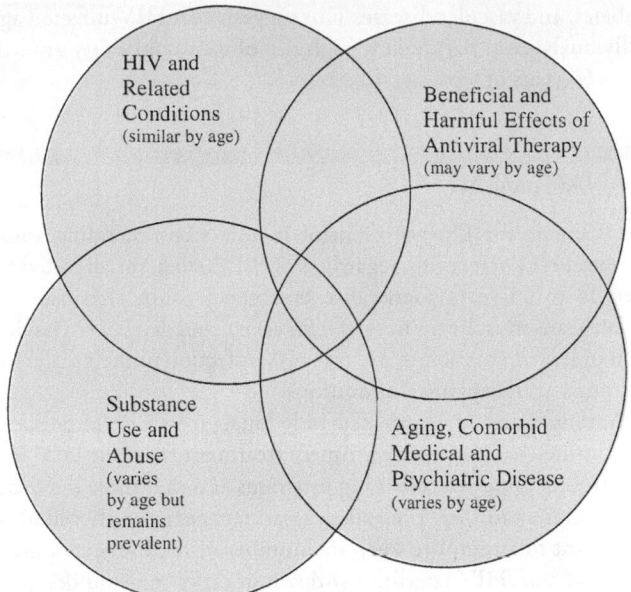

FIGURE 128-1. Outcomes among people aging with HIV infection.

TABLE 128-2

Comorbid and AIDS-Defining Medical Conditions by Age Among HIV-Infected Veterans (n = 876)

	OVERALL	<50 YEARS	50+ YEARS	P
Comorbid Condition (%)				
Hepatitis C	34	35	33	0.6
Hypertension	32	22	45	<0.0001
Diabetes	13	10	18	<0.0001
Obstructive lung disease	12	9	17	0.001
Non-AIDS cancers	7	3	13	<0.0001
Coronary artery disease	5	3	8	0.003
Congestive heart failure	5	4	6	0.3
Pancreatitis	4	5	4	0.7
Cerebral vascular disease	4	2	6	0.001
Peripheral vascular disease	2	1	3	0.1
Any Comorbid Medical Condition	**65**	**57**	**77**	**<0.0001**
AIDS-Defining Condition (%)				
Candidiasis	36	37	34	0.3
Bacterial pneumonia	27	27	28	0.9
Herpes simplex	21	21	20	0.9
Herpes zoster	18	19	16	0.3
Pnumocystis carinii pneumonia	16	19	12	0.004
Wasting	14	13	16	0.2
Tuberculosis	7	7	8	0.7
Fungi or parasites	5	6	4	0.2
Kaposi's sarcoma	3	3	5	0.1
Cytomegalovirus	2	3	2	0.3
Any AIDS-Defining Medical Condition	69	68	71	0.3

patient is the result of HIV disease progression, HIV treatment, or comoribidity (and/or its treatment) (Figure 128-1). In many cases, the likely answer is that there is no single etiology but rather the conditions results from a combination of some or all of these factors. Further, non-AIDS defining conditions among HIV-infected individuals tend to cluster into three main categories: medical conditions, substance use conditions, and psychiatric conditions. We are now challenged to develop diagnostic strategies and team management techniques to convert what was once a rapidly fatal disease to a well-tolerated (and well-managed) complex chronic disease.

HIV and Related Conditions

Most HIV-associated opportunistic infections and cancers do not vary significantly in prevalence when older patients are compared with their younger counterparts (Table 128-2). It is, however, important to note that the prevalence of these conditions has dropped significantly in the era of multiclass combination antiretroviral treatment. Furthermore, the conditions that are most prevalent are no longer *Pneumocystis carnii* pneumonia, Kaposi's sarcoma, or atypical mycobacterium infection. They are instead conditions that commonly occur in people without HIV infection such as esophageal candidiasis, bacterial pneumonia, tuberculosis, and herpes simplex and zoster. Further, HIV infection itself is also associated with anemia, renal insufficiency, hepatitis, wasting, and cognitive decline.

Benefits and Harms of Antiretroviral Treatment

As can be seen by the substantially improved survival seen with CART, individuals experience dramatic benefit from antiretroviral treatment. Some have suggested that this benefit may be muted among older individuals because of competing risk of death from comorbid conditions, to a possibly decreased immunological recovery on treatment, the likely increased risk of drug toxicity, and drug–drug interactions from cumulative organ system frailty.

Early reports from Phase I and II trials of antiretroviral therapies substantially underestimated the rates of toxicity likely as a result of the exclusion of individuals with prior organ injury from the trials. Longer term, postmarketing surveillance studies of populations receiving these drugs are beginning to describe the degree to which the earlier studies underestimated these effects. Common adverse antiretroviral drug effects include gastrointestinal intolerance (gas, bloating, nausea, and vomiting), diarrhea, chemical hepatitis, hyperlipidemia, hyperglycemia, peripheral neuropathy, bone marrow suppression (anemia, thrombocytopenia, neutropenia), fat redistribution, lactic acidosis, and bleeding diathesis. A subset of antiretrovirals are associated with nephrolithiasis, renal insufficiency, and failure. There is growing evidence that these adverse effects of treatment are more common among individuals with prior organ injury. Thus, aging individuals who are more likely to have prior hepatic injury, renal insufficiency, and preexisting hyperlipidemia or glucose intolerance may be at especially high risk for adverse effects of antiretroviral therapy. Longer term observation is required to determine whether HIV treatment incurs increased risk for cancer.

Substance Use and Abuse

As a group, patients infected with HIV who are aged 50 years or older are also more likely than their HIV-uninfected demographic counterparts to have consumed hazardous amounts of alcohol, used illicit drugs, and smoked cigarettes. As a result of these behaviors, these patients are also more likely than the general aging population to be coinfected with hepatitis C or B and to have liver, lung, and heart disease and to be at increased risk for a number of common cancers.

Among patients who continue to drink hazardously and or to use illicit drugs, ongoing organ injury and adherence to antiretroviral therapy are likely to be important issues. Patients should be asked directly about alcohol, cigarette, and illicit drug use, and encouraged to stop or curtail ongoing use. Any patient reporting current drug or alcohol use should be questioned closely regarding treatment adherence and monitored for alcoholic hepatitis. Current research suggests that even moderate levels of alcohol consumption may be hazardous among those aging with HIV infection.

Aging and Comorbid Medical and Psychiatric Disease

No one is immune from HIV infection. Nevertheless, HIV infection occurs more commonly among the homeless, members of inner-city minority or sexual minority populations, or those suffering from substance abuse and psychiatric illness as compared to the general population of people 50 years of age or older. General medical comorbidities such as hepatitis C, hypertension, diabetes, and obstructive lung disease are common in these populations. Depression and severe mental illnesses such as psychosis and posttraumatic stress disorder are also more common among older people with HIV infection than among the general population of people 50 years of age or older.

Risk for many forms of cancer may be elevated as well. Cancers that may be more common among those receiving treatment for HIV infection include liver cancer, lung cancer, and anal cancer. Finally, older people with HIV infection may have multiple reasons to have cognitive dysfunction, whether from cognitive diseases of aging (multi-infarct dementia or Alzheimer's disease) or from HIV (minor cognitive motor disorder or HIV-associated dementia). It should also be noted that older people in care for HIV infection may be on as many medications for their comorbid conditions as for HIV infection. The potential for drug–drug interactions and cumulative organ toxicity is substantial.

Thus, even before contracting HIV infection and receiving antiretroviral therapy, older people with HIV infection may be at greater risk of comorbid medical and psychiatric disease. Clearly, the prevalence of general medical comorbid conditions is high among older HIV-positive patients receiving antiretroviral treatment (see Table 128-2).

More recently, we have also come to recognize that long-term chronic HIV infection may be associated with a selective accelerated aging process. Evidence to support this theory includes the fact that, after adjustment for gender, race/ethnicity, and pack years of smoking, veterans with HIV infection have a greater risk of obstructive lung disease than uninfected veterans in every age category. Additional evidence comes from the observations that, even after adjustment for conventional risk factors for coronary artery disease, HIV-infected individuals appear to be experiencing cardiovascular events at an accelerated rate compared to uninfected control samples. Finally, a recent analysis comparing a national sample of HIV-infected veterans to 2:1 demographically matched uninfected veterans found significant positive interactions between age of 60 years or more years and HIV status for the risk of hypertension,

diabetes, and vascular disease. This suggests that HIV-infected aging individuals are at particularly high risk of multimorbidity once they reach 60 years of age.

MANAGEMENT

The Centers for Disease Control is now recommending routine universal HIV screening, regardless of risk factors, for all individuals aged 13 to 65 years. Generalist, emergency room physicians, and geriatricians must begin to screen for sexual and drug use behavior in their older patients and to include HIV infection in their differential diagnosis of unexplained conditions.

Among aging HIV-infected individuals it will be important to help insure that they receive timely treatment for their HIV infection through opt-out screening programs and that these individuals adhere closely to their prescribed treatment regimen. It will also be important to attempt to keep the number of total medications (for HIV and non-HIV conditions) down in order to avoid drug–drug interactions and cumulative toxicity and to screen regularly for evidence of liver, kidney, and bone marrow toxicity. Antiretroviral treatment timing and choice should be made balancing the individual's cumulative organ system frailty and their likely risk of adverse events against the substantial benefit of early and aggressive HIV treatment.

Recently published Infectious Disease Society of America Guidelines suggested that, "it is imperative that all persons in the United States be managed according to standard practices appropriate for the individual's age and sex regardless of HIV status." This statement ignores the fact that people receiving treatment for HIV infection do not enjoy a "normal" age-appropriate life expectancy. Whether or not a particular primary care practice is appropriate for an individual with HIV depends upon the frequency and impact of the condition, the degree to which outcomes associated with that condition can be modified by timely medical intervention, and the risk associated with the intervention. For example, colon cancer screening via colonoscopy has a slight risk of perforation at the time of screen and a substantial risk of discomfort for the patient. Patients probably need to live at least 5 to 7 years after their screening for the benefit of the screening in decreased risk of death from colon cancer to outweigh the risk of perforation and the pain and discomfort of the procedure. Conversely, more aggressive screening for anal cancer may be indicated because of the increased incidence of this condition among those with HIV infection. Thus, it would be unwise to apply all "age appropriate" primary care guidelines for those without to those with HIV infection without careful consideration for the individual's prognosis, preferences for care, and personal risk of these conditions.

Finally, because of the overlapping complications and comorbid medical and psychiatric disease experienced by most patients with HIV infection, comprehensive care requires a team approach. No one specialist or generalist can hope to stay on top of optimal care in all these domains. HIV specialists need to turn to generalists and geriatricians when determining the best way to manage overlapping comorbid medical disease and to psychologists, psychiatrists, and social workers when managing psychiatric diseases. The management of alcohol and drug abuse also requires the insights of generalists familiar with the medical complications of these behaviors and of psychiatrics, psychologists, and social workers familiar with methods of managing these behaviors. In turn, generalists and geriatricians will need careful guidance from HIV specialists in determining when to start antiretroviral treatment, choosing optimal drug combinations, and in determining when to stop or change therapy. For those who must manage patients far from specialty services, frequent telephone conferencing with specialists in HIV and with those experienced in the management of comorbid conditions is recommended.

FURTHER READING

Antiretroviral Therapy Cohort Collaboration (ART-CC). HIV treatment response and prognosis in Europe and North America in the first decade of highly active antiretroviral therapy. *Lancet.* 2006;368:451.

Braithwaite RS, Justice AC, Chang CC, et al. Estimating the proportion of patients infected with HIV who will die of comorbid diseases. *Am J Med.* 118:890, 2005.

Centers for Disease Control and Prevention. Revised Recommendations for HIV Testing of Adults, Adolescents, and Pregnant Women in Health Care Settings. *MMWR.* 2006;55(RR14):1.

Crothers K, Butt AA, Gibert CL, et al. Increased COPD among HIV-positive compared to HIV-negative veterans. *Chest.* 2006;130:1326.

Egger M, Junghans C, Friis-Moller N, Lundgren JD. Highly active antiretroviral therapy and coronary heart disease: the need for perspective *AIDS.* 2003;15:s193.

Engels EA. Human immunodeficiency virus infection, aging, and cancer. *J Clin Epidemiol.* 2001;54:S29.

Gebo KA. HIV and aging: implications for patient management *Drugs Aging.* 2006;23(11):897.

Goulet J, Fultz S, Rimland D, et al. Patterns of comorbidity among HIV-infected and matched HIV-uninfected veterans. *J Clin Infect Dis.* 2007;45(12):1593–601.

Justice AC. Prioritizing primary care in HIV: comorbidity, toxicity, and demography. *Top HIV Med.* 2006;14(5):159.

Linsk NL. HIV among older adults: age-specific issues in prevention and treatment. *AIDS Reader.* 2000;10(7):430.

Zingmond DS, Kilbourne AM, Justice AC, et al. Differences in symptom expression in older HIV-positive patients: The VACS and HCSUS experience. *J Acquir Immune Defic Syndr.* 2003;33(2):S84–92.

Herpes Zoster

Jack I. Twersky ■ *Kenneth Schmader*

DEFINITION

Herpes zoster is a neurocutaneous disease that is caused by the reactivation of varicella-zoster virus (VZV) from a latent infection of dorsal sensory or cranial nerve ganglia following varicella or primary infection with VZV earlier in life. Herpes zoster is characterized by unilateral, dermatomal pain and rash.

Postherpetic neuralgia (PHN) has been defined as any pain after rash healing or any pain from 1 to 6 months after rash onset. Pain experts currently define PHN as pain 90 to 120 days after rash onset to be consistent with established definitions of chronic pain and to eliminate neuropathic pain from acute inflammation. Some experts define the herpes zoster pain trajectory as an acute herpetic neuralgia that lasts for approximately 30 days after rash onset, a subacute herpetic neuralgia that lasts from 30 to 120 days after rash onset, and PHN as pain that persists 120 days and more after rash onset.

EPIDEMIOLOGY

Varicella-Zoster Virus Transmission

VZV is a double-stranded DNA that is transmitted from person to person via direct contact, airborne or droplet nuclei when a virus-naïve, VZV seronegative individual is exposed to the vesicular rash of varicella or herpes zoster. These exposed individuals may then develop varicella. Health care workers and staff in nursing homes and hospitals and children who have not received the varicella vaccine may not have had VZV primary infection and are potentially at risk for varicella. However, nearly all older adults are seropositive and latently infected with VZV. The exposure of a latently infected individual to herpes zoster does not cause herpes zoster or varicella.

Furthermore, there is no risk of VZV transmission when the herpes zoster rash is only maculopapular or crusted. All cases of herpes zoster are caused by the reactivation of endogenous VZV.

Herpes Zoster Incidence and Risk Factors

In general population studies from North America and Europe, the incidence of herpes zoster in persons of all ages is 1.2 to 4.8 cases per 1000 persons per year and in persons older than 60 years old, the incidence is 7.2 to 11.8 cases per 1000 per year. The lifetime incidence of herpes zoster is estimated to be about 20% in the general population and maybe as high as 50% among those surviving to 85 years or higher.

The cardinal epidemiological feature of herpes zoster is its increase in incidence with aging and with diseases and drugs that impair cellular immunity. The increase in the likelihood of herpes zoster with aging starts around 50 to 60 years of age and increases into late life in individuals older than 80 years of age (Figure 129-1). In the herpes zoster vaccine trial ("Shingles Prevention Study"), which was prospective, used active surveillance in a community-based population, and used polymerase chain reaction (PCR) for definitive diagnosis of herpes zoster cases, the incidence of herpes zoster in the placebo group ($n = 19\ 276$) was 11.8 cases per 1000 persons per year in adults 60 years of age and older. Immunocompromised patients at risk for herpes zoster include persons with human immunodeficiency virus (HIV) infection, Hodgkin's disease, non-Hodgkin's lymphomas, leukemia, bone marrow and other organ transplants, systemic lupus erythematosus, and those taking immunosuppressive medications. Other risk factors include white race, psychological stress, and physical trauma.

Current population figures and herpes zoster incidence data yield estimates of about 1 million new cases of herpes zoster each year in the United States, with more than half occurring in persons 60 years of age or older. The number of herpes zoster cases is expected to increase in the near future decades because of population

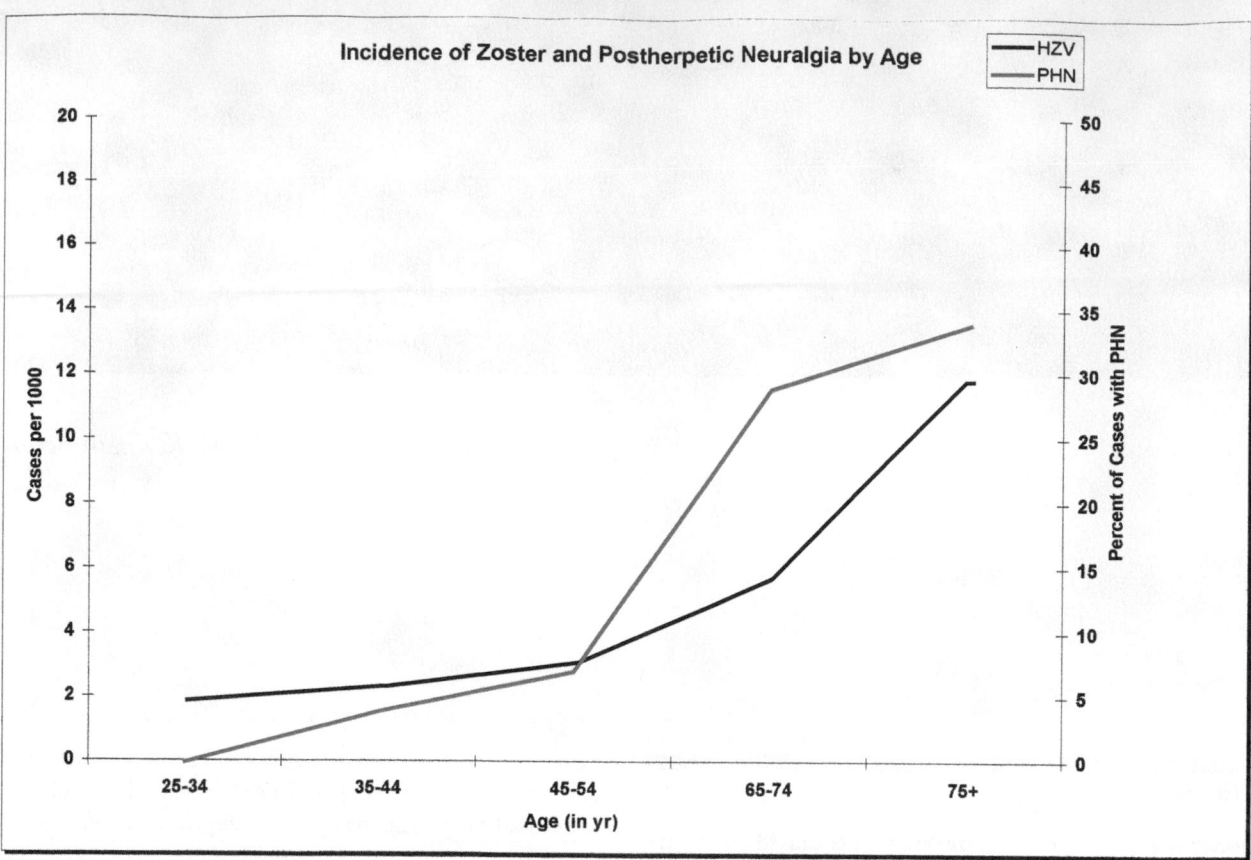

FIGURE 129-1. Incidence of zoster and postherpetic neuralgia by age. *(Data from Donahue JG, Choo PW, Manson JE, et al. The incidence of herpes zoster. Arch Intern Med.155:1605–1609, 1995; Choo PW, Galil K, Donahue JG, et al. Risk factors for postherpetic neuralgia. Arch Intern Med. 1997;157:1217–1224.)*

aging and the development of immunocompromising diseases (and their therapies) associated with aging. Whether varicella vaccination of children and the subsequent reduction in varicella incidence will contribute to an increase in the number of herpes zoster cases by reduced exogenous immune boosting in individuals latently infected with wild-type VZV is under investigation.

Postherpetic Neuralgia Incidence, Prevalence, and Risk Factors

Exact data on the incidence and prevalence of PHN are not available because of variable definitions and inadequate data in medical records and administrative databases. Useful figures for older patients who seek medical care come from a combined analysis of large trials of antiviral drugs for herpes zoster in outpatients aged 50 years and older. In this analysis, 49% to 54% of placebo recipients had pain 90 days after rash onset and 46% at 120 days after rash onset; 25% to 35% of antiviral recipients had pain 90 days after rash onset and 29% at 120 days after rash onset. In the placebo group of the Shingles Prevention Study, the incidence of PHN was 0.74 cases per 1000 person-years for subjects between 60 and 69 years and 2.14 for subjects older than 70 years (Figure 129-1). The figure illustrates that the rate of increase of PHN cases associated with aging is greater than the rate of increase of herpes zoster cases. Investigators have estimated that the prevalence of PHN ranges from 500 000 to 1 million in the United States.

Like herpes zoster, the most important epidemiological feature of PHN is its marked increase in incidence and severity with aging.

All epidemiological studies of PHN show that the risk of PHN is substantially increased in older adults. Other risk factors for PHN include the presence of prodromal pain, severe pain during the acute phase of herpes zoster, greater rash severity, more extensive sensory abnormalities in the affected dermatome and, possibly, ophthalmic nerve involvement. As the age of patient and severity of the episode of herpes zoster increases, the more likely the development of PHN.

CLINICAL FEATURES

Prodrome

VZV reactivates in the affected sensory ganglion and spreads in the peripheral sensory nerve, causing symptoms that frequently precede the rash by several days. These prodromal symptoms are located in the involved dermatome and range from a superficial itching, tingling, or burning to severe, deep, boring, or lancinating pain, paresthesia, or hyperesthesia. The pain can be constant or intermittent. The prodrome maybe mistaken for many other conditions in older adults, particularly in those patients with cognitive impairment. The prodrome may mimic pleurisy, a myocardial infarction, cholecystitis, appendicitis, renal colic, a collapsed intervertebral disk, glaucoma, trigeminal neuralgia, or unappreciated trauma. The prodromal symptoms usually last a few days, although it has been reported to last more than a week. Zoster sine herpete is a condition

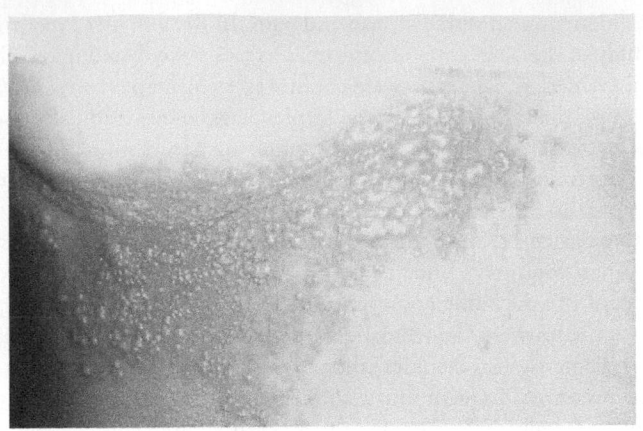

FIGURE 129-2. A patient with herpes zoster illustrates a range of lesions (e.g., large pustules, erythematous papules, and crusting).

when patients experience acute dermatomal neuralgia without ever developing a skin eruption.

Rash

When VZV reaches the dermis and epidermis, the initial cutaneous presentation of herpes zoster occurs as a unilateral, dermatomal, red, maculopapular eruption. Vesicles generally form within 24 hours and evolve into pustules, which dry and crust in 7 to 10 days. The rash usually heals over in 2 to 4 weeks. In normal individuals, new lesions may continue to appear for 1 to 4 days and occasionally for as long as 7 days. The T1 to L2 or V1 dermatomes are most commonly involved (Figure 129-2). Adjacent dermatomes can show satellite lesions but multiple lesions in contiguous dermatomes are not characteristic of herpes zoster. Atypical rashes may occur in older persons. The atypical rash maybe limited to a small patch located within a dermatome or may remain maculopapular without ever developing vesicles.

Acute Herpetic Neuralgia

Herses zoster-associated acute neuritis produces dermatomal neuralgic pain in many older adults. Some older patients never develop pain while others may experience the delayed onset of pain days or weeks after rash onset. The neuritis is described as burning, deep aching, tingling, itching, or stabbing. A subset of patients may develop severe pain, especially those with trigeminal nerve involvement. Acute herpetic neuralgia can have a profound adverse impact on functional status and quality of life in older adults. Acute herpes zoster pain can interfere with all activities of daily living but interference is greatest for instrumental activities of daily living, as well as sleep, general physical activity, and leisure activities. As overall pain burden increases, patients experience poorer physical, role, and emotional functioning.

Complications

Ophthalmic herpes zoster occurs in 10% to 15% of the cases. It is second in frequency to thoracic herpes zoster and is a result from VZV reactivation in the first division of the trigeminal nerve (cranial nerve V). Ophthalmic involvement may present with impaired vision as a result of local inflammation. In 30% to 40% of cases of ophthalmic

zoster, there is involvement of the nasociliary branch, which also innervates the side and tip of the nose. Symptoms and/or signs on the tip of the nose should immediately lead to a thorough search for involvement of the eye. VZV-induced damage to the cornea and uvea and other eye structures can cause corneal anesthesia and ulceration, glaucoma, optic neuritis, eyelid scarring and retraction, visual impairment, and blindness in patients who did not receive antiviral therapy. Secondary bacterial infections can cause panopthalmitis and enucleation. Ophthalmic herpes zoster is also associated with stroke occurring weeks to months after the onset of the rash. The cause of the stroke is a granulomatous arteritis of the carotid artery close to the involved first division of cranial nerve V. Arteriograms show segmental narrowing of cerebral arteries ipsilateral to the ophthalmic zoster. Herpes zoster-associated arteritis in the trigeminal distribution can also cause ipsilateral occlusion of the central retinal artery with resultant visual loss.

Herpes zoster can affect cranial nerves other than the first division of cranial nerve V in older adults. Involvement of the third division of cranial nerve V can produce lesions and pain in the mandibular area of the face and in the mouth. Cranial nerve VII and VIII involvement, or Ramsey Hunt syndrome, is characterized by facial palsy in combination with herpes zoster lesions of the ipsilateral external ear, ear canal, tympanic membrane, or hard palate. Symptoms include tinnitus, vertigo, deafness, problems with balance, and facial paresis. Involvement of cranial nerve IX, X may produce pharyngeal or laryngeal lesions and resulting pharyngitis or laryngitis. The patient may have multiple symptoms because more than one cranial nerve can be involved in an attack.

Motor paralysis is reported in 1% to 5% of patients with herpes zoster. Subclinical motor neuron involvement with herpes zoster probably occurs more frequently than reported because muscle weakness in the thoracic and lumbar dermatomes is difficult to appreciate. It results from VZV-induced destruction of motor neurons in the anterior spinal horn or motor radiculitis corresponding to the extension of VZV infection from the involved sensory ganglion. Paralysis involves muscle groups with innervation that is contiguous with that of the affected dermatome.

The most commonly observed affected muscles are those of the face with involvement of the cranial nerve VII and the extremities with herpes zoster of the accompanying dermatome. Painful Bell's palsy in an older adult strongly suggests herpes zoster. Motor deficits usually occur at the time of or within a few weeks after the onset of the rash. Full or partial recovery of motor function occurs in most patients within months of the onset of weakness but facial palsy has a much lower rate of recovery.

Herpes zoster myelitis, with detection of VZV in the spinal cord or cerebrospinal fluid, has been reported both as a complication of typical herpes zoster and of zoster sine herpete. The incidence of acute symptomatic myelitis and meningoencephalitis is low (0.2–0.5%), although lymphocytic pleocytosis, with or without an increase in the concentration of protein in the cerebrospinal fluid, is a regular feature of uncomplicated herpes zoster.

The most feared complication of herpes zoster among older adults is PHN. PHN patients describe the quality of their pain as burning, throbbing, stabbing, shooting, sharp, aching, gnawing, tiring, or tender. The pain maybe spontaneous and/or stimulus-evoked. Spontaneous pain maybe constant aching or burning and/or brief, intermittent shock-like sensations. Stimulus-evoked pain consists of allodynia or hyperpathia. Allodynia is pain elicited by an innocuous stimulus and is particularly problematic. A cold wind, clothes, or

Box 129.1 Clinical Pearls

There is no risk of VZV transmission when the herpes zoster rash is maculopapular or crusted i.e., there must be vesicles for VZV transmission

When Bell's palsy presents with pain think HZ. Corollary: If a patient presents with a painful facial paresis look in the ipsilateral ear for vesicles (Ramsey Hunt Syndrome).

A vesicle at the tip of the nose should raise suspicion for ophthalmological HZ

Acute and convalescent VZV IgG and IgM levels are needed to diagnose zoster sine herpete.

Increasing severity of pain and rash in herpes zoster increases the probability of developing PHN.

Patients who claim they have several episodes of shingles probably have HSV; definitive diagnosis requires microbiological testing (e.g., PCR, culture, IFA)

bed sheets against the allodynic skin may cause debilitating pain. Hyperpathia is an exaggerated pain after a mildly painful stimulus. A minor bump of the affected dermatome against an object can cause severe pain that lasts for hours. Patients may experience discomfort that is not described as pain such as numbness or itching. Postherpetic itch can be maddening and appears to be mediated by damage and dysfunction of peripheral and central itch-specific neurons.

PHN greatly interferes with the functional status and quality of life of older adults. Patients can suffer from a variety of constitutional symptoms including chronic fatigue, anorexia, weight loss, and insomnia. PHN is associated with depression and social isolation in older adults. Reduced quality of life and interference with activities of daily living (ADLs) increases significantly as pain severity increases. Instrumental and basic ADLs are all compromised by PHN. For example, the patient with allodynic skin may be forced to avoid bathing or clothing around the affected area. Instrumental ADLs commonly affected include traveling, shopping, cooking, and housework. Studies using standardized pain scales and measures of function and quality of life such as the SF-36, SF-12, EuroQol, and Nottingham Health Profile have shown that PHN significantly interferes with multiple ADLs, reduces health-related quality of life (HRQL), and impairs mental and physical health. Though most people eventually have relief of pain, some are refractory to all treatments and the pain can even get worse over time (see Box 129-1 on Clinical Pearls).

DIAGNOSIS

Differential Diagnosis

In patients who present with prodromal pain and no rash, herpes zoster is often confused with other causes of unilateral, localized pain in older adults, as noted above. One diagnostic clue to the presence of prodromal pain is localized cutaneous sensory abnormalities (e.g., hyperesthesia, dysesthesia) in the affected dermatome. Herpes zoster is easily diagnosed when an older adult patient presents with the typ-

ical dermatomal vesicular rash and pain. In the Shingles Prevention Study of the 1308 cases of suspected herpes zoster based upon clinical evaluation, 984 cases were confirmed to be herpes zoster (75%). During the rash phase, herpes simplex has the most similar presentation to herpes zoster. Evidence supporting herpes simplex includes a presentation in a younger population, multiple reoccurrences of lesions, and the absence of chronic pain. The lesions themselves are more difficult to distinguish, particularly when herpes zoster occurs in areas commonly affected by simplex (e.g., oral, genital, buttock lesions). In the Shingles Prevention Study, 3.4% of suspected herpes zoster cases were found to be herpes simplex virus. The differential diagnosis also includes contact dermatitis, burns, and vesicular lesions associated with fungal infections but the history and examination usually makes the distinction clear.

Laboratory Tests

The diagnosis of herpes zoster may need laboratory diagnostic testing when differentiating herpes zoster from HSV infection is necessary, for suspected organ involvement, and for atypical presentations, particularly in the immunocompromised host. The diagnostic tests include viral culture, immunofluorescent antigen (IFA) detection, PCR, and serology (Table 129-1). The best specimen is vesicle fluid, which contains abundant VZV. Lacking vesicle fluid, acceptable specimens include lesion scrapings, crusts, tissue biopsy, or cerebrospinal fluid. Crusts cannot be used for VZV culture. VZV isolation in culture of vesicular fluid is the "gold standard," but it is slower than other tests and not very sensitive as only 30% to 60% of vesicle culture specimens are positive. VZV antigen detection by IFA tests of vesicle scrapings or tissue biopsies takes hours to get results and is both specific and sensitive. These reasons make IFA the most useful test when specimens are available. Polymerase chain reaction is highly sensitive and so it can be used to test crust or other unusual samples. As the cost of PCR decreases over time, this will likely be the most commonly used test to confirm herpes zoster in the near future. Acute and convalescent VZV IgM and IgG levels maybe useful in making a retrospective diagnosis when there are no peripheral lesions or specimens are inadequate. Tzanck smears suggest herpes zoster when multinucleated giant cells and intranuclear inclusions are seen on slides but this does not differentiate herpes zoster from herpes simplex.

MANAGEMENT

Acute Herpes Zoster

Nonpharmacological Management

The principal goal of the treatment of herpes zoster in older adults is to decrease the length of the acute attack and to reduce or eliminate pain. Patients should be instructed to keep the rash clean and dry to decrease the chances of developing bacterial superinfection. Topical antibiotics should be discouraged. Cool compresses, calamine lotion, cornstarch, or baking soda may help to reduce local symptoms and speed the drying of the vesicles. When the vesicles have crusted over, a bland ointment or olive oil may help separate the adherent crusts. Occlusive ointments and topical steroids should be avoided.

TABLE 129-1

Laboratory Tests for Detecting Varicella-zoster Virus (VZV) and Diagnosing Herpes Zoster

TEST*	DETECTS	SENSITIVITY	SPECIFICITY	TURNAROUND	PROS	CONS
Culture	Whole VZV	Low (about 40%)	Very high (near 100%)	Days	Whole virus isolation is the standard for diagnosis. Only method that yields infectious VZV for further analysis. Readily available	Slow, insensitive, VZV difficult to grow on tissue culture
Immunoassays (IFA, EIA)	VZV antigen	High (90%)	High (90%)	Hours	Readily available. Good sensitivity and specificity.	Must be done in experienced laboratory, careful interpretation to avoid false positive and negatives
PCR	VZV DNA	Very high (near 100%)	Very specific (near 100%)	Hours	Superb sensitivity and specificity. Valuable for unusual specimens or when the clinician suspects. that IFA or culture has yielded false negative test results.	Expensive, not as readily available, must be done by experienced laboratory to avoid false positives
Serology (ELISA, FAMA, LA)	IgG, IgM antibody	High for antibody detection; unknown for HZ diagnosis	High for antibody detection; unknown for HZ diagnosis	Hours	Can be used to diagnose zoster sine herpete or HZ retrospectively using acute and convalescent VZV IgG titers.	Not clinically useful for diagnosing HZ at time of presentation; requires acute and convalescent (6 weeks later) samples

*IFA, immunofluorescence antigen; EIA, enzyme immunoassay; PCR, polymerase chain reaction; ELISA, enzyme-linked immunosorbent assay, FAMA, fluorescent antibody to membrane antigen; LA, latex agglutination.

Reassurance and education directly address concerns about contagiousness, for example, who is at risk for contracting VZV, zoster pain management, and potential disability. Social support, mental and physical activity, adequate nutrition, and a caring attitude are important interventions for coping with a herpes zoster attack.

Antiviral Therapy

The first line of drug therapy is aimed at inhibiting the replication of VZV. The guanosine analogs, acyclovir, famciclovir, and valaciclovir, are phosphorylated by viral thymidine kinase to a triphosphate form that inhibits VZV DNA polymerase and VZV replication. Valaciclovir and famciclovir are prodrugs, which have greater bioavailablity, resulting in higher blood levels and a less frequent dosing schedule. Randomized controlled trials indicate that oral acyclovir (800 mg five times a day for 7 days), famciclovir (500 mg q 8 hours for 7 days), and valaciclovir (1 gm three times a day for 7 days) reduce acute pain and the duration of chronic pain in older patients with herpes zoster who are treated within 72 hours of rash onset. The kidneys excrete these medications and the dose should be adjusted for renal insufficiency. They are safe and well-tolerated among older adults. The most common adverse effects are nausea, vomiting, diarrhea, and headache. The data from current clinical trials indicate that all three drugs are acceptable agents with factors other than efficacy determining the choice, such as cost and dosing schedule (Table 129-2). The effectiveness of antiviral agents has not been evaluated for treatment after 72 hours have elapsed since the onset of rash. An exception to the 72-hour threshold for treatment is made for patients who have ophthalmic zoster or patients that continue to have new vesicle formation. Topical antiviral therapy is not an effective treatment.

Analgesics

Acute herpes zoster pain requires the use of standardized pain measures (e.g., 0 to 10 rating scale), scheduled analgesia, and close monitoring to adjust dosing and detect adverse effects. Opioid and nonopioid analgesia are a standard of care for the acute pain syndrome. The choice of treatment will depend on the patient's pain intensity, comorbidities, and preferences. Patients with mild pain maybe managed with acetaminophen or nonsteroidal agents. Patients with moderate to severe pain usually require treatment with an opioid analgesic (e.g., oxycodone). There is a tendency among many clinicians to undertreat the pain and particularly to use opioid analgesia sparingly. Opioids have multiple adverse effects including nausea, constipation, and sedation, which maybe intolerable in some older adults. Among frailer patients, there is an increased risk for falls and confusion. Constipation should be anticipated and managed with

TABLE 129-2

Medications for the Management of Herpes Zoster

MEDICATION	DOSE (MG)	FREQUENCY	COST
Acyclovir	800	5 times/day	60 cents/pill
Famciclovir	500	3 times/day	$8.94 /pill
Valaciclovir	1000	3 times/day	$5.19 /pill

Data from http:// www.drugstore.com.

laxative therapy. Assessment of appropriate analgesia should include ability to sleep and manage routine activities as well as provide sufficient relief.

Corticosteroids

The anti-inflammatory effects of corticosteroids have been postulated to reduce herpes zoster symptoms but there remains controversy over their use. Randomized, controlled clinical trials demonstrated that corticosteroids do not prevent PHN when compared to placebo or acyclovir. These findings, the risk of VZV dissemination, and the adverse effects of corticosteroids in older adults argue against the routine use of these agents in herpes zoster. However, clinical trials have shown reductions in acute pain and one randomized controlled trial showed benefits in improvement in time to uninterrupted sleep, return to routine activities, and cessation of analgesic medications among patients with no relative contraindications to corticosteroids. In the trial, prednisone was administered orally at 60 mg/day for days 1 to 7, 30 mg/day for days 8 to 14, and 15 mg/day for days 15 to 21. Therefore, corticosteroids maybe useful in reducing moderate to severe acute pain unrelieved by antiviral agents and analgesics. Corticosteroids are used to treat VZV-induced facial paralysis and cranial polyneuritis to improve motor outcomes and provide pain relief. If prescribed, corticosteroids should always be used in conjunction with antiviral agents. The use of corticosteroids in older patients with hypertension, diabetes, gastritis, osteoporosis, psychosis, or cognitive impairment needs to be weighed carefully. The most common adverse effects of corticosteroids are dyspepsia, nausea, vomiting, edema, and granulocytosis. The doses and length of treatment would put the patient at risk for bone loss.

Adjuvant Agents

If moderate-to-severe herpes zoster pain is not inadequately relieved by antiviral agents in combination with oral analgesic medications and/or corticosteroids, then other therapies could be considered. Gabapentin or pregabalin, nortriptyline or desipramine, or neural blockade all have potential roles in the treatment of acute herpes zoster. There are no randomized controlled trials of gabapentin or pregabalin, or nortriptyline or desipramine, for acute herpes zoster pain nor are there trials showing these agents prevent PHN. The rationale for considering gabapentin or pregabalin is their known efficacy in relieving chronic neuropathic pain and a study using a single dose (900 mg) of gabapentin in acute herpes zoster pain showing pain reduction. The use of these anticonvulsant agents must be balanced against adverse effects of sedation, dizziness, ataxia, and peripheral edema. The rationale for considering nortriptyline or desipramine is their known efficacy in relieving chronic neuropathic pain and a trial using amitriptyline that showed treating acute herpes zoster resulted in a reduction in PHN at six months. This trial had major methodologic concerns including acyclovir use was unbalanced favoring the amitriptyline group and a question of whether the reduction in PHN was the result of treatment during acute herpes zoster or because the treatment with amitriptyline continued for 3 months after rash onset. The use of these tricyclic agents must be balanced against their adverse cardiac and anticholinergic effects. Neural blockade can reduce severe acute herpes zoster pain. A randomized controlled trial of antiviral therapy, oral analgesics, and a single epidural block with bupivacaine and methylprednisolone compared to antiviral therapy and oral analgesics alone showed that neural blockade reduces acute pain but does not prevent PHN. This modality requires referral to a pain specialist. Some patients have very severe pain refractory to usual outpatient treatments and require hospitalization for parenteral opioids and/or epidural analgesia.

Ophthalmic zoster requires ophthalmological consultation. Oral antiviral and analgesic therapy is the mainstay of treatment as it is for herpes zoster presenting on the rest of the body but other ocular therapies may be necessary. These treatments are best managed by an ophthalmologist and include antibiotic ophthalmic ointment to prevent bacterial infection of the ocular surface, topical steroids to reduce ocular inflammation, mydriatics as needed for iritis, and ocular pressure-lowering drugs as needed for glaucoma. Cool to lukewarm compresses may provide some comfort and oral corticosteroids maybe useful for patients with severe pain.

Postherpetic Neuralgia

Oral and Topical Pharmacotherapy

The treatment for PHN is problematic because the pain may last from months to a year or more and be associated with a decline in activities of daily living and quality of life. Based upon evidence of effectiveness from clinical trials and safety in older adult population, tricyclic antidepressants (TCAs), gabapentin, pregabalin, lidocaine patch, and opioids are considered first-line therapies because one or more high-quality randomized controlled trials demonstrated efficacy with these agents. Gabapentin, pregabalin, and the topical lidocaine patch 5% are approved by the FDA for the treatment of PHN.

Topical Treatments   The topical lidocaine patch 5% reduced PHN in randomized vehicle controlled trials. In one trial, which also included other neuropathic pain patients, the percentage of patients who obtained 50% reduction in pain was 31% with the lidocaine patch compared to 8% with placebo patch. The number needed to treat (NNT) for 50% pain reduction is 2.0. Up to three patches maybe applied over the affected area for 12 hours a day. It may take up to 2 weeks for these treatments to reach full effectiveness. Systemic lidocaine toxicity has not been reported from topical lidocaine. Capsaicin, a *trans*-8-methyl-*N*-vanillyl-6-nonenamide is known to deplete substance P, an endogenous neuropeptide that is involved in the transmission of nociceptive impulses from the sensory nerve endings to the central nervous system. This treatment has been shown to have a statistical benefit in studies but its clinical effect is small. It takes days to deplete substance P and many patients are unable to tolerate the burning it causes. Nonetheless, topical capsaicin maybe considered as a therapeutic option in PHN because it maybe effective in individual circumstances. Topical treatments should not be used in herpes zoster in the acute phase with open lesions.

Gabapentin and Pregabalin   Gabapentin is an anticonvulsant that has become a popular treatment partly because two randomized, placebo controlled studies showed a significant clinical benefit in pain relief with gabapentin and partly because of the favorable side effect profile. In those trials, 41% to 43% of patients on gabapentin reported moderate or better pain improvement compared to 12% to 23% of those on placebo. The NNT for 50% pain reduction was 4.6 (Table 129-3). Dosing is described in Table 129-3. Patients who

TABLE 129-3

Medication for Managing Postherpetic Neuralgia

MEDICATION	NUMBER NEEDED TO TREAT* (PERSONS)	SIDE EFFECTS OF MEDICATIONS	BEGINNING DOSE	TITRATION
Lidocaine patch	2.0	Dysesthesia vesicular rash, ulcerations, edema, or erythema at the application site.	Maximum of 3 patches daily for a maximum of 12 h	None needed
Gabapentin	4.4	Somnolence, dizziness, ataxia, peripheral edema and cognitive impairment.	100–300 mg at night	Increase by 100–300 mg a day every 1–7 days as tolerated in divided doses up to three times a day, maximum 3600 mg daily
Pregabalin	4.9	Somnolence, dizziness, ataxia, peripheral edema and cognitive impairment.	50–150 mg daily two to three times a day	Increase to 300 mg a day, given in 2 or 3 divided doses within 1 week; maximum dose generally 300 mg in older adults
Tricyclic antidepressant nortryptiline	2.6	Dry mouth, sedation, constipation and less risk for cognitive impairment and orthostatic hypotension.	10–25 mg qhs	Increase by 10–25 mg daily Every 3–7 days as tolerated; maximum dose 75–150 mg daily
Opioid oxycodone (dosage given for morphine equivalents)	2.7	Constipation, nausea sedation, impaired cognitive function, and falls.	2.5–15 mg every 4 h as needed	After 1–2 weeks, convert total daily dosage to long-acting opioid analgesic and continue short-acting medication as needed
Tramadol	4.7	Constipation, nausea sedation, impaired cognitive function, orthostasis, falls.	25 mg once daily	Increase by 25–50 mg daily in divided doses every 3–7 days as tolerated; maximum 300 mg daily in patients older than 75 yr of age

*NNT, number of patients needed to treat to achieve 50% reduction in pain.

Data from Hempenstall K, Nurmikko TJ, Johnson RJ, A'Hern RP, Rice ASC. Analgesic therapy in postherpetic neuralgia: a quantitative systematic review. PLOS Med. 2(e164): 0628–0644, 2005.

do not have at least partial relief at 1800 mg are unlikely to benefit from higher doses of gabapentin. Frail elderly patients often need smaller doses because of problems tolerating higher doses. Doses should be adjusted for creatinine clearance. Adverse effects include somnolence, dizziness, ataxia, and peripheral edema. Cognitive impairment may also occur in elderly patients.

Pregabalin is an anticonvulsant that is similar in structure and action to gabapentin. In placebo-controlled trials, the proportion of patients with greater than 50% decrease in mean pain scores was 50% in the pregabalin group compared to 20% in the placebo group. The NNT for 50% pain reduction is 4.9 (Table 129-3). The adverse effect profile of pregabalin is similar to gabapentin with dizziness, somnolence, peripheral edema, dry mouth, and gait disturbances as the most common adverse effects. The drug has few drug–drug interactions, can be given less frequently than gabapentin, and has a relatively rapid onset of action. Other anticonvulsants (e.g., phenytoin, levetiracetam, oxcarbazepine, tiagabine, topiramate, zonisamide, valproate) are possibly useful but cannot be considered first-line agents because of limited data for efficacy and/or significant adverse effects.

Tricyclic Antidepressants TCAs modulate nerve transmission. Multiple randomized controlled trials of TCAs demonstrated significant pain relief in patients with PHN with 44% to 67% of patients treated with TCAs reporting moderate to good pain relief compared to 5% to 19% of placebo of control drug recipients.

The NNT for 50% pain reduction is 2.8 (Table 129-3). In the only head-to-head comparison, nortriptyline demonstrated equivalent efficacy and was better tolerated when compared to amitriptyline in a PHN. Nortriptyline and desipramine are preferred over amitriptyline because they have less anticholinergic effects, resulting in less dry mouth, sedation, constipation, cognitive impairment, and orthostatic hypotension. Tricyclic antidepressants are associated with cardiac toxicity in patients with cardiovascular disease. They are contraindicated in patients with QT prolongation, familial histories of long-QT syndromes, atrioventricular block, bundle-branch block, or a recent acute myocardial infarction. An EKG looking for QT prolongation or heart block should be evaluated before initiating therapy and with each change in dose. Caution is necessary in the concomitant administration of TCAs and selective serotonin reuptake inhibitors (SSRIs). Tricyclic antidepressants are metabolized by the cytochrome P450 D26 enzyme system and SSRIs, especially fluoxetine, inhibit P450 D26 so toxic TCA plasma concentration could result. Dosing is described in Table 129-3.

Opioid and Opioid-Like Analgesics PHN pain responds to opioid treatment. In a randomized, crossover trial showing significant pain relief with oxycodone, 67% of patients expressed preference for oxycodone compared to 11% of the placebo recipients. The NNT for 50% pain reduction is 2.6. In another crossover study of PHN comparing opioid analgesics, TCAs, and placebo, controlled-release morphine and TCAs provided statistically significant benefits on pain relief. Patients preferred treatment with opioid analgesics compared to TCAs and placebo despite a greater incidence of side effects and more drop-outs during opioid treatment.

Although oxycodone has been shown to be an effective treatment, equianalgesic doses of other opiates are likely to be as effective. The most frequently reported adverse effects were constipation, nausea, and sedation. Impaired cognitive function, falls, and fractures are also more likely to occur in the older patients prescribed opioids. Starting at a low dose and slowly increasing the dose may reduce the probability of serious side effects. We start all patients receiving opioids on an aggressive bowel regimen. Dosing is described in Table 129-3. Tramadol is a mu opioid agonist and a norepinephrine and serotonin reuptake inhibitor. One randomized controlled trial in PHN found that 77% of subjects on tramadol versus 56% on placebo reported greater than 50% reduction. The adverse effects of tramadol include all the opioid adverse effects noted above as well as orthostatic hypotension, increased risk of seizures in patients with a history of seizures, and risk for serotonin syndrome in patients who use serotonergic medications, especially SSRIs and monoamine oxidase inhibitors. Dosing is described in Table 129-3.

Combination Pharmacotherapy

Combination Pharmacotherapy Many PHN patients do not respond to single drug therapy but there are relatively few data on optimal combinations of drugs. Combination therapy may augment a partial response to a single drug or produce better analgesia at lower doses of drug. However, combination therapy in older adults increases the risk of adverse effects and makes it difficult to determine which medication is responsible for adverse effects or benefits. In one study of combination therapy that included 22 patients with PHN, investigators studied the effects of morphine alone, gabapentin alone, or morphine–gabapentin combination in a randomized, double-blind, active placebo-controlled, four 5-week period crossover trial. The results showed that gabapentin and morphine combined achieved modestly better pain relief at lower doses of each drug than either as a single agent. However, the combination was associated with higher levels of sedation, dry mouth, and cognitive dysfunction than the maximal tolerated dose of each single agent. For patients with PHN who do not have an adequate response to any of the front-line medications, other drug and nondrug treatments deserve consideration. These patients should be referred to a pain specialist or pain center for consideration of more complex drug combinations, risky second-line medications, or invasive treatments.

Other Treatments

Noninvasive Treatments Transcutaneous electrical nerve stimulation (TENS), percutaneous electrical nerve stimulation (PENS), acupuncture, cold application, or psychological treatments maybe useful in some patients and have little risk, although their effectiveness in PHN has not been tested in controlled clinical trials. PHN patients who are good candidates for a trial of PENS or TENS are those that maybe experiencing associated myofascial pain in addition to neuropathic pain. The presence of myofascial pathology is indicated by taut muscle bands (i.e., a group of tense muscle fibers extending from a trigger point to the muscle attachments) and trigger point(s) (i.e., a hyperirritable spot in skeletal muscle that is painful on compression) in the affected dermatome.

Invasive Treatments Patients who remain in severe pain and have failed all other therapies can be considered for invasive interventions. which include neural blockade, spinal cord stimulation, and central nervous system drug delivery. Neural blockade techniques include sensory nerve, plexus, and sympathetic nerve blocks as well as epidural and intrathecal blockade with lidocaine-like drugs and/or corticosteroids. Spinal cord stimulation requires implantation of an electrode in the thoracic or lumbar epidural space and the placement of a percutaneous electrical stimulator. Central nervous system drug delivery systems place drug (e.g., morphine), as close as possible to central pain receptors in the spinal cord corresponding to the affected dermatome. In general, the risks of these interventions outweigh any potential benefits in older adults with PHN.

PREVENTION

Varicella Vaccine

The live, attenuated varicella vaccine is safe and effective in preventing varicella and is licensed for use in the United States. The Centers for Disease Control reported that varicella incidence declined by approximately 80% compared to prevaccination incidence rates in varicella surveillance areas in the year 2000. Vaccine uptake among children aged 19 to 35 months in the United States was 88% in 2004. These figures indicate that the varicella vaccine is having a dramatic impact on the epidemiology of varicella in the United States by markedly reducing the incidence of varicella. The effect of the varicella vaccine on older adults is a reduced likelihood of exposure to VZV and less chance of exogenous boosting of their cellular immunity against VZV. Whether this is clinically important is unknown but some experts speculate that latently infected individuals will be more likely to develop herpes zoster without this booster effect. The vaccine virus can establish a latent infection in children and reactivate at a later time. However, vaccine virus-associated herpes zoster will probably be less frequent and severe in vaccinated children as they become older adults because the vaccine virus is highly attenuated.

Zoster Vaccine

Regardless of the impact of the varicella vaccine, millions of latently infected older adults are at risk for herpes zoster for the foreseeable future. The zoster vaccine was developed to prevent or attenuate herpes zoster. It is similar to the varicella vaccine but it is formulated to yield much higher concentrations of live attenuated VZV and antigen than the varicella vaccine. The zoster vaccine, but not the varicella vaccine, significantly boosts VZV-specific cellular and humoral immunity in older adults. The increase in VZV-specific cellular immunity in older adults by the zoster vaccine forms the scientific rationale for testing the vaccine because cellular immunity to VZV declines with age.

The Shingles Prevention Study was a randomized, double-blind, placebo controlled trial to determine if the zoster vaccine would decrease the incidence and/or severity of herpes zoster and PHN among older adults. The study randomized 38 546 community-dwelling persons ≥60 years old to vaccine or placebo and followed them for herpes zoster and adverse events for a median of three years. There were 315 cases of herpes zoster among vaccine recipients compared to 642 cases among placebo recipients. There were 27 cases of PHN among vaccine recipients and 80 cases of PHN among placebo recipients. The vaccine reduced incidence of herpes zoster from 11.12 to 5.42 cases (51.3%) per 1000 person-years for an NNT of 59 over the 3.12 years of the study. The vaccine reduced the incidence PHN from 1.38 to 0.46 cases (66.5%) per 1000 person years for an NNT of 362 over the duration of the study. The zoster vaccine also reduced the pain burden of illness (a pain severity by duration measure) caused by herpes zoster by 61.1%. The efficacy of the zoster vaccine in reducing pain burden and PHN in the 60- to 70-year old group was mediated mostly by preventing herpes zoster, whereas efficacy in the greater than 70-year-old group was mediated mostly by attenuating herpes zoster since the vaccine was less effective in preventing HZ in that age group. Reactions at the injection site were more frequent among vaccine recipients but were generally mild. In 2006, the FDA licensed the zoster vaccine for the prevention of herpes zoster in immunocompetent adults 60 years of age and older and the Advisory Committee on Immunization Practices (ACIP) of the CDC unanimously recommended the vaccine for the prevention of HZ and PHN in immuncompetent adults 60 years of age and older.

Several key clinical questions are raised by the use of the zoster vaccine. What is the duration of the protective effect of the vaccine? The Shingles Prevention Study data indicate that vaccine efficacy persists for at least 4 years. Long-term follow-up studies are ongoing to determine the durability of the effectiveness of the zoster vaccine in a subset of study vaccine recipients. What is the effectiveness of the vaccine in very old and frail individuals? Neither the FDA nor the ACIP set an upper age limit on the use of the vaccine. These individuals are at highest risk for herpes zoster and PHN and reduction of herpes zoster pain severity and duration occurs in the "old–old" even when herpes zoster is not prevented. What is the efficacy of the zoster vaccine in individuals who have already had herpes zoster? Older adults with prior herpes zoster ask for the vaccine but the answer to this question is unknown because these individuals were excluded from the Shingles Prevention Study. Persons with recent episodes (within 3 to 5 years) of herpes zoster have a boost in immunity from reactivated wild-type VZV that is as strong or better than that obtained from the zoster vaccine so they may not benefit from the vaccine. However, other individuals with a more remote history of herpes zoster may benefit because herpes zoster can recur. The ACIP recommends the zoster vaccine for persons older than 60 years of age whether or not they report a prior episode of herpes zoster.

In summary, the incidence of herpes zoster and PHN increases greatly with aging so the majority of herpes zoster cases occur among older adults. Acute herpes zoster pain, other herpes zoster compli-

cations (e.g., ophthalmic zoster) and PHN interfere with functional status and lower quality of life in older people. Although not perfect, clinicians now have several tools to prevent and treat these conditions. Those tools include the zoster vaccine, early antiviral therapy, careful acute pain management, and a number of neuropathic pain treatments. The systematic application of these interventions will markedly reduce the suffering of older adults from herpes zoster and PHN.

FURTHER READING

Choo PW, Galil K, Donahue JG, et al. Risk factors for postherpetic neuralgia. *Arch Intern Med.* 1997;157:1217–1224.

Donahue JG, Choo PW, Manson JE, et al. The incidence of herpes zoster. *Arch Intern Med.* 1995;155:1605–1609.

Dubinsky RM, Kabbani H, El-Chami, Z, Boutwell C, et al. H. Practice parameter: treatment of post-herpetic neuralgia: An Evidence-Based Report of the Quality Standards Subcommittee of the American Academy of Neurology. *Neurology.* 2004;63:959–965.

Dworkin RH, Johnson RW, Breuer J, et al. Recommendations for the management of herpes zoster. *CID.* 2007:44 (Suppl 1):S1–S44.

Dworkin RH, Schmader KE. The epidemiology and natural history of herpes zoster and postherpetic neuralgia. In: Watson CPN, Gershon AA, eds. *Herpes Zoster and Postherpetic Neuralgia.* 2nd ed. Amsterdam: Elsevier; 2001:51.

Finnerup NB, Otto M, McQuay HJ, et al. Algorithm for neuropathic pain. *Pain.* 2005;118:289–305.

Gilron I, Bailey JM. Tu D, et al. Morphine, gabapentin, or their combination for neuropathic pain. *N Engl J Med.* 2005;352:1324–1334.

Hempenstall K, Nurmikko TJ, Johnson RJ, A'Hern RP, Rice ASC. Analgesic therapy in postherpetic neuralgia: a quantitative systematic review. *PLOS Med.* 2005;2(e164):0628–0644.

Hope-Simpson RE. The nature of herpes zoster: a long-term study and new hypothesis. *Proc Royal Soc Med (London).* 1965;58:9–20.

Jung BF, Johnson RW, Griffin DR, Dworkin RH. Risk factors for postherpetic neuralgia in patients with herpes zoster. *Neurology.* 2004;62:1545–1551.

Katz J, Cooper EM, Walther RR, Sweeney EW, Dworkin RH. Acute pain in herpes zoster and its impact on health-related quality of life. *Clin Infect Dis.* 2004;39:342–348.

Oxman MN, Levin MJ, Johnson GR, et al. A vaccine to prevent herpes zoster and postherpetic neuralgia in older adults. *N Engl J Med.* 2005;352:2271–2283.

Raja SN, Haythornthwaite JA, Pappagallo M, et al. Opioids versus antidepressants in postherpetic neuralgia: a randomized, placebo-controlled trial. *Neurology.* 2002;59:1015–1021.

Rowbotham M, Harden N, Stacey B, et al. Gabapentin for the treatment of postherpetic neuralgia: a randomized controlled trial. *JAMA.* 1998;280:1837–1842.

Seward JF, Watson BM, Peterson CL, et al. Varicella disease after introduction of varicella vaccine in the United States, 1995–2000. *JAMA.* 2002;287:606–611.

Van Wijck AJM, Opstelten W, Moons KG, et al. The PINE study of epidural steroids and local anaesthetics to prevent postherpetic neuralgia: a randomised controlled trial. *Lancet.* 2006;367:219–224.

Watson CPN, Babul N. Efficacy of oxycodone in neuropathic pain: a randomized trial in postherpetic neuralgia. *Neurology.* 1998;50:1837–1841.

Watson CPN, Vernich L, Chipman M, Reed K. Nortriptyline versus amitriptyline in postherpetic neuralgia: a randomized trial. *Neurology.* 1998;51:1166–1171.

Weiner DK, Schmader KE. Postherpetic pain: more than sensory neuralgia? *Pain Med.* 2006;7:243–249.

Whitley RJ, Weiss H, Gnann JW, et al. Acyclovir with and without prednisone for the treatment of herpes zoster: a randomized, placebo-controlled trial. *Ann Intern Med.* 1996;125:376–383.

Influenza and Respiratory Syncytial Virus

Mark B. Loeb

INFLUENZA

Influenza is an important threat to the health of older adults. Each year, it is estimated that 36,000 older adults in the United States die of influenza and pneumonia with the majority of these occurring in persons 65 years and older. Despite immunization, outbreaks of influenza occur regularly in nursing homes and other long-term care facilities. This section of the chapter will summarize the biological, epidemiological, and clinical features of influenza that are relevant to the elderly with a particular emphasis on prevention.

Clinically Relevant Biological Characteristics of Influenza Virus

To properly understand the impact of influenza in the elderly, it is important to be familiar with several key characteristics of the virus. The structure of influenza consists of an envelope with a central nucleic acid core comprised of single-stranded RNA. Key structural characteristics of the virus include the presence of hemagglutinin and neuraminidase proteins on the envelope. There are three types of influenza viruses A, B, and C. However only A and B are clinically relevant. Influenza A viruses are characterized by the structure of the hemagglutinin, a surface protein whose function is to bind to a glycoprotein on the surface of respiratory epithelial cells, allowing the virus to enter into the cell by forming an endosome and then using the protein making machinery of the cell to replicate itself. Annually new mutations are selected for resulting in small changes in the hemagglutinin ("antigenic drift") hence the reason why influenza vaccine needs to be given annually. The other surface projection, neuraminidase, cleaves terminal sialic acid residues from carbohydrate moieties on surfaces of infected cells, promoting the release of virions that go on to infect other cells. As discussed below, this is a key target for neuraminidase inhibitors, thus preventing the influenza virus from replicating.

An important feature of influenza is the segmented structure of the RNA at the core of the virus, with each of eight segments coding for a structural or enzymatic component of the virus. This gives the virus the potential to recombine with influenza viruses of animal origin, forming a virus with a novel genotype and hemaglutinnin to which there is no preexisting immunity. This is known as "antigenic shift" and was responsible for pandemics in 1957–1958 and 1968–1969. A recent concern is the changes in hemaglutinin from animal strains, such as avian influenza or H5N1, maybe able to attach to the human receptors, causing direct transmission from animals to humans. This is believed to have caused the 1918–1919 pandemic and is a current concern with avian influenza (H5N1). Of note is that the highest mortality rate occurring in the 1918–19 pandemic was not in the elderly, but in 18- to 25-year-olds. This may have been because of the fact that there were similar H1 viruses circulating in the early 1900s and individuals older than 50 years of age developed partial immunity with previous exposure. At present, there are only three hemaglutinins (H1, H2, H3) and two neuraminidases (N1, N2) that have developed a stable lineage in humans.

General Epidemiology of Influenza

Epidemics of influenza occur annually between November and April in the Northern hemisphere. A typical outbreak of influenza lasts for about 6 weeks, reaching a peak and slowly declining. However, in any given season, there maybe several strains circulating, with several peak periods of activity. It is for this reason that the annual influenza vaccine contains antigen from three influenza strains, two strains of influenza A, and one strain of influenza B.

Important Host Considerations in the Elderly

During the interpandemic period, older adults and particularly residents of long-term care facilities are among those at highest risk for complications of influenza. Rates of hospitalization for influenza in community dwelling elderly persons range from 125 to 228 hospitalizations per 100,000 persons. As with many other infectious diseases, the very old and the very young are at highest risk of complications. Children between the ages of 6 and 23 months similarly have high rates of hospitalization attributable to influenza, ranging from 144 to 187 hospitalizations per 1000 persons. The presence of chronic conditions, such as chronic lung disease, congestive heart failure, conditions that predispose to aspiration, and metabolic disease, increase the risk for complications following infection with influenza. Many of these conditions occur predominately in older age groups. Moreover, studies that have assessed complications have found that age older than 65 years alone is independently associated with increased risk for influenza complications.

Based on our current understanding, the cause of death as a result of influenza in the elderly in the interpandemic period is not viral pneumonia but typically a bacterial infection complicating the influenza infection. Infection with influenza virus therefore predisposes to *Streptococcus pneumoniae* or *Staphylococcus aureus* infection, resulting in bacterial pneumonia. Deficits in innate immunity (phagocytes natural killer cells) and acquired immunity (T-cell function, cytokine activity, antibody response) are all felt to play a role, as discussed in Chapter 3.

Clinical Presentation

Young, healthy individuals with influenza characteristically present with a sudden onset of fever, cough, myalgia, sore throat, and headache. Fever and cough have been shown in a systematic review to be the best predictors of influenza in the general population. In the elderly, the presentation usually is more subtle with cough and change in baseline temperature predominating. One of the most important factors in making the diagnosis of influenza, whether on clinical grounds or through diagnostic testing, is the local influenza activity. That is, if a community is experiencing an outbreak of influenza, particularly if the incidence of influenza is at its peak, fever and cough in an older person increase the likelihood of infection with influenza. However, it is important to bear in mind that the majority of studies that have assessed the diagnostic utility of clinical symptoms were done in samples with participants aged from 18 to 45 years, so less is known about the diagnostic utility of clinical signs and symptoms in the elderly.

In the nursing home setting, it is essential to obtain prompt diagnostic testing, because, as consistently demonstrated in longitudinal studies that have compared symptoms to etiologic agents, the clinical presentation is nonspecific. Even when there are peaks of influenza in the community, respiratory syncytial virus (RSV) or other respiratory viruses can circulate. It is essential to obtain testing, because it can lead to a change in management: an outbreak of influenza A in nursing home warrants chemoprophylaxis (see below) as well as immunization of nonimmunized residents in whom it is safe to do so.

Specific Diagnostic Tests

The traditional method to detect influenza has been viral culture. The main limitations of culture have been moderate diagnostic accuracy and delay in obtaining results, which may take 2 to 3 days. Rapid tests include direct fluorescent antigen (DFA), or direct immunofluoresence, where monoclonal antibodies labeled with fluorescent material are directed to influenza cell coat antigens. A result

can be reported within hours. Rapid enzyme-linked immunoassay (ELISA) tests are commercially available, however they are only available for influenza A and have a sensitivity of 60%. Nucleic acid amplification testing, such as polymerase chain reaction (PCR), is the most promising test since it is over 90% sensitive and specific and the turnaround time is rapid. The drawback however is that most laboratories do not have the resources to perform PCR on a routine basis.

Infection Control Aspects

The incubation period of influenza, the period of time from initial infection to development of symptoms, is typically 2 days, but can range from 1 to 4 days. An infected individual becomes contagious 1 day prior to the onset of symptoms. In adults, viral shedding at levels high enough to cause transmission occurs over 5 or 6 days. This is the rationale for keeping patients with influenza in isolation in hospital for 5 days after symptom onset. Although the extent to which influenza can be transmitted by airborne spread is controversial, the majority of spread of influenza is large droplet caused by coughing and sneezing. In terms of practical implications, use of "respiratory etiquette," coughing, and sneezing into tissues, for example, may help prevent spread to older adults who are susceptible to complications although supporting epidemiologic evidence is limited. In the hospital setting, the use of gloves, gowns, and a mask is recommended prior to entering a patient's room.

Immunization

In the United States, there are currently two types of influenza vaccine that are licensed, the inactivated trivalent vaccine, which is a split virus formulation with two strains of influenza A and one B, and a cold-attenuated live intranasal vaccine. Only the inactivated vaccine is licensed for persons older than of 65 years of age. A recent systematic review summarized randomized controlled trial and cohort study evidence for efficacy and effectiveness: 64 studies were included in assessment, resulting in 96 data sets. In nursing homes where there was a good vaccine match and high viral circulation the effectiveness of vaccines against influenza-like illness was 23% (6–36%) but it was not significant against influenza (relative risk [RR] 1.04: 95% CI 0.43–2.51). However, well-matched vaccines had a 46% (30–58%) efficacy for preventing pneumonia, 45% (16–64%) efficacy to prevent hospital, and 42% (17–59%) efficacy for preventing death from influenza or pneumonia.

In elderly individuals living in the community, the review showed that poorly matched vaccines were not significantly effective against influenza (RR 0.19; 95% CI 0.02–2.01), influenza-like illness (RR 1.05: 95% CI 0.58–1.89), or pneumonia (RR 0.88; 95% CI 0.64–1.20). Well-matched vaccines had a 26% (12–38%) efficacy for preventing hospital admission for influenza and pneumonia and a 42% (24–55%) efficacy for preventing all-cause mortality.

These data show that influenza immunization plays an important role in prevention. However, the data show only a modest effect of the influenza vaccine in community-dwelling elderly. One concern is the high effect size for preventing all cause mortality compared to the lack of significant effect for preventing influenza. A possible explanation is confounding by health status. That is, it maybe that "healthier" seniors are more likely to be immunized and as a result of their underlying health have higher survival rates than those who are not immunized. Empirical evidence of this relationship was demonstrated in a case–control study showing that when functional status is adjusted for, the efficacy of the influenza vaccine for preventing mortality is reduced.

Studies using seasonal regression modeling with both U.S. and Italian data show no reduction in mortality among the elderly with increased influenza vaccine coverage. These studies assessed trends in excess mortality after adjusting for age. One possible explanation of the results in these studies is that the influenza vaccine failed to protect the elderly against death because of immune senescence (see Chapter 3).

Influenza and Long-term Care

Residents of nursing homes and other long-term care facilities are at high risk for complications of influenza, including pneumonia, death, and hospitalization. This is likely because there is close contact between residents and staff in these facilities, increasing the exposure to and transmission of influenza, and because the majority of residents have comorbidities, including cognitive impairment, chronic lung diseases, and strokes. Outbreaks of influenza are well characterized in nursing homes, often described as "explosive" in that the onset is relatively abrupt. Such outbreaks are usually first detected by nursing home staff who notice a higher incidence of respiratory symptoms than usual on specific long-term units, although at least one surveillance study has shown that such outbreaks are commonly missed even when active surveillance by trained nurses is performed. Such outbreaks are best managed using a multifaceted approach that includes the following: cohorting residents, increasing adherence to hand hygiene, chemoprophylaxis with antiviral agents, and immunization of those not previously vaccinated. It should be noted that because of space limitations, it is usually not feasible to cohort ill residents together as a means of separating them from noninfected residents in long-term care facilities. Administering neuramindase inhibitors, such as oseltamivir or zanamavir, as chemoprophylaxis to noninfected residents helps to reduce further spread. In one randomized controlled trial where long-term units were randomized to zanamivir or to rimantidine, the risk of influenza was 3% in the zanamivir arm versus 8% in the rimantidine arm ($P = 0.038$). More recent data suggests that immunizing staff in nursing homes against influenza can benefit residents. There have been three cluster randomized controlled trials showing that immunizing healthcare workers against influenza reduces mortality in residents of long-term care facilities. Vaccinating nursing home staff against influenza may prevent deaths, use of health services, and influenza-like illness in nursing home residents.

Use of Antivirals to Prevent and Treat Influenza in Older Adults in the Community

There are four antivirals that are approved for treating influenza: amantadine, rimantadine, zanamivir, and oseltamivir. Amantadine and rimantadine are only active against influenza A while the neuraminidase inhibitors zanamivir and osteltamivir are active against influenza A and B. These agents are 70% to 90% effective for prophylaxis in preventing influenza and when used as treatment reduce clinical severity when given within 48 hours of symptom onset. Amantadine and rimantadine are not recommended when circulating strains with resistance have been detected, and in 2005, the Centers for Disease Control (CDC) noted that the majority of H3N2 influenza strains had become resistant to those agents. Also, the utility of amantadine is reduced in the elderly given the potential for central nervous system side effects. In contrast, zanamivir and oseltamivir are associated with few adverse effects. However, the feasibility of using these agents for treatment is reduced since the majority of patients in the community present over 48 hours following symptom onset.

Indirect Benefit of Immunization in Children to Protect Older Adults

There is good observational data to suggest that children play an important role in the spread of influenza in the community. For example, data from a 3-year longitudinal surveillance study of children and adults in New York State demonstrated that children were about twice as likely to acquire and shed influenza as compared to adults. In a longitudinal study conducted in Seattle from 1968 to 1974, elementary and junior high school students had the highest rates of influenza during epidemics, reaching 54%. In the Tecumseh, Michigan studies from 1976 to 1981, over one-third of children between the ages of 5 and 14 years had influenza virus isolated from specimens, the highest rate was among persons with febrile respiratory illness. Serological data revealed similar results, from 1977 to 1978, children in 5 to 9, 10 to 14, and 15 to 19 age groups had approximately a 30% infection rate with H3N2. This was over twice the rate seen in adults. There were similar infection rates with influenza B in children aged 5 to 14 years, rates 14-fold higher than those in adults older than 20 years of age.

Given that school-aged children appear to play an important role in introducing and transmitting influenza into households, and hence into the community, immunizing these children may interrupt spread to elderly persons who are at high risk for complications. In the Tecumseh studies, Monto and colleagues demonstrated that selectively immunizing 86% of children in this 7500-person community with inactivated influenza vaccine reduced influenza in adults by a third when compared to an adjacent community where children were not immunized. More evidence for the potential benefit of immunizing children with inactivated vaccine has been derived from an analysis of the effect of influenza vaccination in Japan. Japan began a program of immunizing school-aged children in 1962 and continued this policy until 1994. The effect of this policy was to dramatically reduce excess mortality rates to values similar to those in the United States. The fact that there was a rapid increase in excess deaths after 1994, the year in which mass immunization formally ended, supports the conclusion that the effects observed in earlier years were because of vaccine-induced herd immunity, although it is possible that social factors may have amplified the effects of this program. The authors explain their findings by hypothesizing that the high levels of vaccination in school children protected transmission of influenza to their grandparents. There have been several more recent observational studies where children have been immunized showing a reduced attack rate of influenza in adults. However, randomized clinical trial evidence of immunizing children to prevent influenza in older adults is limited.

RESPIRATORY SYNCYTIAL VIRUS

RSV has been long recognized as the major cause of bronchiolitis in children. Since the 1970s, there have been numerous reports about the burden of RSV in the elderly, particularly those residing in nursing homes. Although there is relatively less data about RSV in the elderly compared to influenza, it is now recognized as an important contributor to morbidity in both community-dwelling elderly as well as in residents of long-term care facilities. This section will describe the epidemiology of RSV in both settings including clinical, diagnostic, and management issues.

Characteristics of Respiratory Syncytial Virus

RSV is an enveloped RNA virus that can be classified into two major groups, A and B, based on antigenic and genetic properties. An import feature of RSV is that reinfections occur frequently throughout life and into older age. Because RSV infection does not produce robust immunity, developing a vaccine has been a major challenge.

General Epidemiology

Like influenza, RSV circulates during winter months in temperate climates. Epidemics last for roughly 4 to 5 months beginning in the August and lasting until early spring. Often clinical cases precede influenza epidemics. In contrast to influenza, the distribution of cases of RSV over time is fairly constant. The incubation period of RSV is 3 to 5 days. The majority of those who are infected show respiratory symptoms. In contrast to infants who shed higher titres (10^{5-6} plaque forming units/mL of secretion) for longer time periods (10–14 days), adults tend to shed lower titres of the virus 10^{2-3} plaque forming units/mL of secretion for 3 to 6 days. RSV is spread primarily by large droplets and fomites.

Community-Dwelling Elderly and Respiratory Syncytial Virus

The best data about RSV in elderly persons living in the community is derived from a cohort study conducted in Rochester, New York, from 1999 to 2003. This cohort was comprised of 608 healthy persons aged 65 years and older. Forty-six (8%) of the 608 participants developed RSV, compared to 56 (10%) of high risk elderly participants (defined as having congestive heart failure or chronic pulmonary disease). The impact of RSV infection was important in both the healthy elderly group and in the high risk group: 17% and 23%, respectively, in these groups made physician office visits. Morbidity was greater in the high-risk group, where 16% required hospitalization. The study was also useful because it allowed for a comparison to influenza: 42% of healthy elderly participants and 60% of high-risk participants required office visits for influenza, rates statistically significant higher than for RSV. A limitation of these comparisons is that other characteristics were not adjusted for.

Epidemiology of Respiratory Syncytial Virus in Long-term Care Facilities

Respiratory syncytial virus attack rates during nursing home outbreaks have been reported to be variable, ranging from 2% to 90%. However, most involved relatively small numbers of residents and included the use of diagnostic assays with varying levels of sensitivity. In one prospective study conducted in Rochester, where a sensitive enzyme immunoassay was used, the overall attack rate was 7% and the virus was identified as a cause of 27% of illness. One retrospective cohort study estimated the burden of illness in 81,000

nursing homes in Tennessee by linking cardiopulmonary hospitalization, medical utilization, and death to viral activity in the general community. According to these data, RSV accounted for 15 hospitalizations and 17 deaths per 1000 residents. However, these data are limited by the fact that the diagnosis of RSV was not confirmed at the individual level.

Clinical Features of Respiratory Syncytial Virus in the Elderly

It is important to note that the clinical features of RSV cannot be distinguished from those of other viruses, such as influenza, with the exception that fever is less pronounced than for influenza. The nonspecific nature of the clinical presentation indicates the need for diagnostic testing. Signs and symptoms include rhinorrhea, nasal congestion, sore throat, cough, and dyspnea.

Diagnosis

This can be done by viral culture, antigen detection in respiratory secretions, nucleic acid amplification, or serology. For diagnosis in real time, only the first three tests are appropriate. It is important to note that viral culture is only 50% sensitive. Similarly, detection of RSV antigens using immunofluorescence are insensitive in older adults. In contrast, reverse transcriptase-polymerase chain reaction (RT-PCR) is relatively sensitive and specific (73% and 90%. respectively).

Therapy

Care is mainly supportive in the older adult with RSV infection, including rehydration if required, oxygen, and antipyretics. The only licensed antiviral with activity versus RSV is ribavirin. Unfortunately, there is sparse data on which to base treatment recommendations in adults. A practical consideration is that the administration of this aerosolized drug to older adults using face masks maybe difficult.

Prevention

Transmission of RSV is believed to be caused by large droplet and fomites. Strategies such as increasing hand hygiene, particularly in nursing homes, may help to reduce spread. At the present time, there are no licensed RSV vaccines.

FURTHER READING

Elis SE, Coffey CS, Mitchel Jr EF, et al. Influenza and respiratory syncytial virus-associated morbidity and mortality in the nursing home population. *J Am Geriatr Soc.* 2003;51:761–767.

Falsey AR, Hennessey PA, Formica MA, Cox C, Walsh E. Respiratory syncytial virus infection in elderly and high-risk adults. *N Engl J Med.* 2005;352:1749–1759.

Falsey AR, Walsh EE, Betts RF, et al. Viral respiratory infections in the institutionalized elderly: clinical and epidemiological findings. *J Am Geriatr Soc.* 1992;40:115–119.

Falsey AR. Walsh EW. Respiratory syncytial virus infection in adults. *Clin Microbiol Rev.* 2000;371–384.

Fox JP, Hall CE, Cooney MK, Foy HM. Influenza virus infections in Seattle families, 1975–1979. Study design, methods and the occurrence of infections by time and age. *Am J Epidemiol.* 1982;116:212–227.

Glezen WP, Keitel WA, Taber LH, Piedra PA, Clover RD, Couch RB. Age distribution of patients with medically-attended illnesses caused by sequential variants of influenza A/H1N1: comparison to age-specific infection rates, 1978–1989. *Am J Epidemiol.* 1991;133:296–304.

Hall CB. Respiratory syncytial virus and parainfluenza virus. *N Engl J Med.* 2001;344:1917–1928.

Hayward AC, Harling R, Wetten S, et al. Effectiveness of an influenza vaccine programme for care home staff to prevent death, morbidity, and health service use among residents: cluster randomised controlled trial. *BMJ.* 2006;333:1241.

Jackson LA, Jackson ML, Nelson JC, Neuzil KM, Weiss NS. Evidence of bias in estimates of influenza vaccine effectiveness in seniors. *Int J Epidemiol.* 2006;35;337–344.

Long CE, Hall CB, Cunningham CK, et al. Influenza surveillance in community-dwelling elderly compared with children. *Arch Fam Med.* 1997;6:459–465.

Monto AS, Koopman JS, Longini IM, Jr. Tecumseh study of illness. XIII. Influenza infection and disease, 1976–1981. *Am J Epidemiol.* 1985;121:811–822.

Monto A, Davenport FM, Napier JA, Francis T. Modification of an outbreak of influenza in Tecumseh, Michigan by vaccination of schoolchildren. *J Infect Dis.* 1970;122:16–25.

Palese P. Influenza: old and new threats [review]. *Nat Med.* 2004;10 (12 Suppl):S82–S87.

Thomas RE, Jefferson T, Demicheli V, Rivetti D. Influenza vaccination for healthcare workers who work with the elderly. *Cochrane Database Syst Rev.* 2006 Jul 19, 3:CD005187.

Petric M, Comanor L, Petti CA. Role of the laboratory in diagnosis of influenza during seasonal epidemics and potential pandemics [review]. *J Infect Dis.* 2006;194 Suppl 2:S98–S110.

Reichert TA, Sugaya N, Fedson DS, et al. The Japanese experience with vaccinating school children against influenza. *N Engl J Med.* 2001;344:889–896.

Rivetti D, Jefferson T, Thomas R, et al. Vaccines for preventing influenza in the elderly. *Cochrane Database Syst Rev.* 2006;19;3:CD004876.

Index

Note: Page numbers followed by f indicate figures; page numbers followed by t indicate tables.